AF550857

The 5-Minute Clinical Consult 2027

35th EDITION

The 5-Minute Clinical Consult 2027

35th EDITION

Editor-in-Chief

Frank J. Domino, MD
Professor and Director of Predoctoral Education
Department of Family Medicine and Community Health
UMass Chan Medical School
Worcester, Massachusetts

Associate Editors

Robert A. Baldor, MD, FAAFP
Professor and Founding Chair
Department of Family Medicine
UMass Chan Medical School-Baystate
Springfield, Massachusetts
Designated Institutional Official
Baystate Franklin Medical Center
Greenfield, Massachusetts

Kathleen A. Barry, MD
Associate Professor
UMass Chan Medical School
Department of Family Medicine and Community Health
Hahnemann Family Health Center
Worcester, Massachusetts

Jeremy Golding, MD, FAAFP
Professor of Family Medicine and Obstetrics & Gynecology
UMass Chan Medical School
Department of Family Medicine and Community Health
University of Massachusetts Memorial Health Care
Hahnemann Family Health Center
Worcester, Massachusetts

Grace Shih, MD, MAS
Professor
Department of Family Medicine
University of Washington
Seattle, Washington

Mark B. Stephens, MD, MS, FAAFP
Associate Dean for Medical Education
Professor of Family and Community Medicine
Professor of Humanities
Penn State College of Medicine
University Park, Pennsylvania

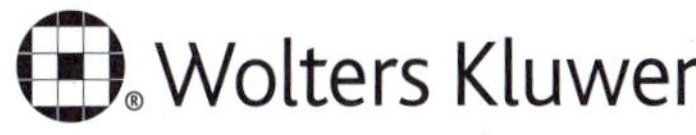

Philadelphia • Baltimore • New York • London
Buenos Aires • Hong Kong • Sydney • Tokyo

5MinuteConsult®

Acquisitions Editor: Joe Cho
Development Editor: Cindy Yoo
Editorial Assistant: Kristen Kardoley
Marketing Manager: Janet Feeney
Senior Production Specialist: Bridgett Dougherty
Manager, Graphic Arts & Design: Stephen Druding
Fulfillment Analyst: Lisa Bowling
Prepress Vendor: Absolute Service, Inc.

35th edition

9 8 7 6 5 4 3 2 1

Printed in Mexico

Library of Congress Cataloging-in-Publication Data available from the Publisher upon request.
ISBN-13: 978-1-9752-8572-2

shop.lww.com

QUADM0226

Retirement is near and thus my last dedication is for the pursuit of evidence-based knowledge and the art of healing, and to the patients who entrusted me with their care, my colleagues who inspired me, and the students who challenged me and reminded me why it all matters. I would be remiss if I did not recognize Dr. Frank Domino, as the Editor-in-Chief! Frank has mentored me, along with thousands of other clinicians on evidenced-based medicine and inspired us to utilize educated shared decision-making tools to enhance our patient's health.

After four decades as a practicing family physician, with the last two as an associate editor, I'm passing this work forward with gratitude and hope. This marks the end of my chapter in this work, but not its story. May it continue to evolve, enlighten, and empower those who seek to heal. I trust the next generation of writers to carry it further as they engage in an AI-assisted world. However, I urge all to reflect on the words of Dr. Bill Damon, a wise family physician mentor, who always counseled me on the value of listening and performing a physical exam in this high-tech world. "*Always touch the part that hurts and remember that oftentimes it's the heart.*"

My success is also due to my wonderful family, my devoted father John who motivated me to enjoy, not toil, with hard work and my loving mother Mary, who showed compassion and forgiveness to all. I've been blessed with children who continue to inspire me daily to be my best and make me proud to be a father. Anthony, Jocelyn, Daniel, John, Angelina, and Ella, you have endured my time away and tolerated my moods, while I have had the delight and joy of celebrating in your victories and achievements. Truly the best children one could wish for—*thank you*!

I must end but not before acknowledging the support of my precious wife, Carol. Although I'm "The Doctor" in the family, she has shown me the true nature of empathy, as the most caring person I know, and not a day goes by without my learning something new from her insights into the world around us. The next chapters in the book of my life will be exciting and rewarding because Carol will be at my side, providing love and care, despite my eccentricities and lack of patience with life's frustrations. I look forward to writing those chapters with her, our CAROB clan of nine brilliant children, and that group of rambunctious grandchildren!

Robert A. Baldor, MD, FAAFP

PREFACE

People do not seem to realize that their opinion of the world is also a confession of their character.

RALPH WALDO EMERSON

Opinion is such a luxury. Many societies prevent freedom of thought; and maybe even more manipulate and conflate opinion and fact. Luckily, we practice medicine. We dwell in the best evidence we can find and add our skill to give our patients the best care possible.

You are what you DO; people will judge you by your actions, not your intentions.

Be the example you want to see in the world.

Example is not the main thing influencing others; it is the only thing.

ALBERT SCHWEITZER

In the course of patient care, we strive to be neutral, objective, and patient centered. Yet, we must maintain scientific rigor. We need to act in a way that patients know we are supporting their best interests.

We need to make our example our confession of character.

Welcome to the 2027 edition of *The 5-Minute Clinical Consult*. Your clinical practice is full of challenges and unanswered questions. Your use of this amazing tool will provide you with the answers needed to help your patients live to their fullest.

The 5-Minute Clinical Consult is here to assist in fulfilling our role as health care providers. In each patient interaction, in addition to bringing your clinical expertise, remember how your patients view you—as their advocate, someone who prioritizes their well-being unlike anyone else.

Our editorial team has collaborated with hundreds of authors so that you may deliver your patients the best care. Each topic provides you with quick answers you can trust, where and when you need them most, either in print or online.

This highly organized content online provides you with the following:

- Differential diagnosis support from our expanded collection of algorithms
- Current evidence-based designations highlighted in each topic covering more than 500 commonly encountered diseases in print, with an additional 1,000 online adult and pediatric diseases and conditions topics
- FREE point-of-care CME and CE: 1/2-hour credit for every digital search
- More than 3,000 patient handouts in English and Spanish
- ICD-10 codes; additionally, SNOMED codes are available online.

Our Web site delivers clear answers to your clinical questions. It is an ideal resource for patient care. Integrating *The 5-Minute Clinical Consult* content into your workflow is easy and fast, and our patient education handouts can assist in helping you meet meaningful use compliance.

The site provides an easy-to-use interface, allowing smooth maneuverability between topics, algorithms, images, videos, and patient education materials as well as more than 400 online-only topics.

Evidence-based health care is the integration of the best medical information with the values of the patient and your skill as a clinician. We have updated our evidence-based medicine (EBM) content so you can focus on how to best apply it in your practice.

The algorithm section includes both diagnostic and treatment algorithms. This easy-to-use graphic method helps you evaluate an abnormal finding and prioritize treatment. They are also excellent teaching tools, so share them with the learners in your office.

This book and Web site are a source to solve problems and to help evaluate, diagnose, and treat patients' concerns. Use your knowledge, expressed through your words and actions, to address their anxiety.

The 35th edition means I have had the great fortune to help grow and support this content for half of its life. I am honored to play this role and hope to keep doing so for some years to come. I thank you, the reader, and the team at Wolters Kluwer for your support.

The 5-Minute Clinical Consult editorial team values your observations, so please share your thoughts, suggestions, and constructive criticism through our Web site's contact form.

FRANK J. DOMINO, MD

EVIDENCE-BASED MEDICINE

WHAT IS EVIDENCE-BASED MEDICINE?

We used to treat every otitis media with antibiotics. These recommendations came about because we applied logical reasoning to observational studies. If bacteria cause an acute otitis media, then antibiotics should help it resolve sooner, with less morbidity. Yet, when rigorously studied (via a systematic review), we found little benefit to this intervention.

The underlying premise of EBM is the evaluation of medical interventions and the literature that supports those interventions in a systematic fashion. EBM hopes to encourage treatments proven to be effective and safe. And when insufficient data exist, it hopes to inform you on how to safely proceed. EBM uses end points of real patient outcomes, morbidity, mortality, and risk. It focuses less on intermediate outcomes (bone density) and more on patient conditions (hip fractures).

Implementing EBM requires three components: the best medical evidence, the skill and experience of the provider, and the values of the patients. Should this patient be screened for prostate cancer? It depends on what is known about the test, on what you know of its benefits and harms, your ability to communicate that information, and that patient's informed choice. This book hopes to address the first EBM component, providing you access to the best information in a quick format. Although not every test or treatment has this level of detail, many of the included interventions here use systematic review literature support.

The language of medical statistics is useful in interpreting the concepts of EBM. Below is a list of these terms, with examples to help take the confusion and mystery out of their use.

Prevalence: proportion of people in a population who have a disease (in the United States, 0.3% [3 in 1,000] people >50 years old have colon cancer)

Incidence: how many new cases of a disease occur in a population during an interval of time; for example, "The estimated incidence of colon cancer in the United States is 104,000 in 2005."

Sensitivity: percentage of people with disease who test positive; for mammography, the sensitivity is 71–96%.

Specificity: percentage of people without disease who test negative; for mammography, the specificity is 94–97%.

Suppose you saw ML, a 53-year-old woman, for a health maintenance visit, ordered a screening mammogram, and the report demonstrates an irregular area of microcalcifications. She is waiting in your office to receive her test results; what can you tell her?

Sensitivity and specificity refer to people who are known to have disease (sensitivity) or those who are known not to have disease (specificity). But what you have is an abnormal test result. To better explain this result to ML, you need the positive predictive value.

Positive predictive value (PPV): percentage of positive test results that are truly positive; the PPV for a woman aged 50 to 59 years is approximately 22%. That is to say that only 22% of abnormal screening mammograms in this group truly identified cancer. The other 78% are false positives.

You can tell ML only 1 out of 5 abnormal mammograms correctly identifies cancer; the other four are false positives, but the only way to know which mammogram is correct is to do further testing.

The corollary of the PPV is the negative predictive value (NPV), which is the percentage of negative test results that are truly negative.

The PPV and NPV tests are population dependent, whereas the sensitivity and specificity are characteristics of the test and have little to do with the patient in front of you. So when you receive an abnormal lab result, especially a screening test such as mammography, understand their limits based on their PPV and NPV.

Treatment information is a little different. In discerning the statistics of randomized controlled trials of interventions, first consider an example. The Scandinavian Simvastatin Survival Study (4S) (*Lancet*. 1994;344[8934]:1383–1389) found using simvastatin in patients at high risk for heart disease for 5 years resulted in death for 8% of simvastatin patients versus 12% of those on placebo; this results in a relative risk of 0.70, a relative risk reduction of 33%, and a number needed to treat of 25.

There are two ways of considering the benefits of an intervention with respect to a given outcome. The absolute risk reduction is the difference in the percentage of people with the condition before and after the intervention. Thus, if the incidence of myocardial infarction (MI) was 12% for the placebo group and 8% for the simvastatin group, the absolute risk reduction is 4% (12% − 8% = 4%).

The relative risk reduction reflects the improvement in the outcome as a percentage of the original rate and is commonly used to exaggerate the benefit of an intervention. Thus, if the risk of MI were reduced by simvastatin from 12% to 8%, then the relative risk reduction would be 33% (4% / 12% = 33%); 33% sounds better than 4%, but the 4% is the absolute risk reduction and reflects the true outcome.

Absolute risk reduction is usually a better measure of clinical significance of an intervention. For instance, in one study, the treatment of mild hypertension has been shown to have relative risk reduction of 40% over 5 years (40% fewer strokes in the treated group). However, the absolute risk reduction was only 1.3%. Because mild hypertension is not strongly associated with strokes, aggressive treatment of mild hypertension yields only a small clinical benefit. Don't confuse relative risk reduction with relative risk.

Absolute (or attributable) risk (AR): the percentage of people in the placebo or intervention group who reach an end point; in the 4S, the absolute risk of death was 8%.

Relative risk (RR): the risk of disease of those treated or exposed to some intervention (i.e., simvastatin) divided by those in the placebo group or who were untreated

- If RR is <1.0, it reduces risk—the smaller the number, the greater the risk reduction.
- If RR is >1.0, it increases risk—the greater the number, the greater the risk increase.

Hazard ratio (HR): the probability of an event in a treatment group versus the probability of events in a control group at a given time (can be calculated at any time in the study; often applied to observational data); like RR, if HR is statistically <1.0, it reduces risk; if >1.0, it increases risk.

Relative risk reduction (RRR): the relative decrease in risk of an end point compared to the percentage of that end point in the placebo group

If you are still confused, just remember that the RRR is an overestimation of the actual effect.

Number needed to treat (NNT): This is the number of people who need to be treated by an intervention to prevent one adverse outcome. A "good" NNT can be a large number (100) if risk of serious outcome is great. If the risk of an outcome is not that dangerous, then lower (25) NNTs are preferred.

The NNT should be compared to a similar statistic, the number needed to harm (NNH). This is the number of people who have to be given treatment before one excess side effect or harm occurs. When the NNT is compared to the NNH, you and the patient can judge whether the benefit of the intervention is great enough to outweigh the risk of harm.

EVIDENCED-BASED GRADING

To help you interpret diagnostic and treatment recommendations within *The 5-Minute Clinical Consult*, we have graded the best information within the text and highlighted this content.

An "A" grade means the reference is from the highest quality resource, such as a systematic review. A systematic review is a summary of the medical literature on a given topic that uses strict, explicit methods to perform a thorough search of the literature and then provides a critical appraisal of individual studies, concluding in a recommendation. The most prestigious collection of systematic reviews is from the Cochrane Collaboration (www.cochrane.org).

A "B" grade means the data referenced comes from high-quality randomized controlled trials performed to minimize bias in their outcome. Bias is anything that interferes with the truth; in the medical literature, it is often unintentional, but it is much more common than we appreciate. In short, always assume some degree of bias exist in any research endeavor.

A "C" grade implies the reference used does not meet the A or B requirements; they are often treatments recommended by consensus groups (such as the American Cancer Society). In some cases, they may be the standards of care. But implicit in a group's recommendation is the bias of the author or the group that supports the reference.

BIAS

Bias is anything that interferes with the truth. There are many types of bias that should be considered by the publishers of medical information. Below describes a number of bias types that often affect our care without us knowing it is present.

Publication bias occurs when research is not published. The motivation to publish information that "didn't work" is low. It is estimated up to 40% of all medical research never gets published. When you read of an effective intervention, wonder if other studies did not show benefit and went unpublished.

Comparator bias occurs when research compares an intervention to not the standard of care. Knowing a new treatment is more effective than placebo for treating a condition is not helpful if you typically use a drug or procedure. Why not study comparing the new to the standard of care? Sometimes, the new treatment is no better than the current standard. And if a study was done to see if the new is better than the old and not published, you have an example of publication bias.

Selection bias involves choosing study populations that might be different than the average patient or just reporting a just subset of study participants from a study. Either will result in the data being skewed because it can only be applied to small subset of people.

Attrition bias and the concept of intention to treat. Attrition bias is when researchers address how a study deals with participants who do not adhere to the research protocol or drop out completely. Intention to treat analysis hopes to diminish attrition bias by statistically considering the nonadhering or dropped out patients as unsuccessfully benefiting from the intervention.

Commercial (funder) bias involves who paid for the research being done, and do they have a vested interest in the outcome. If the developer of a new drug does a large study, or a researcher has a personal financial interest in seeing a study succeed, they may consciously or unconsciously alter what is reported. The data may be accurate, but until this is studied by less vested interests, it is difficult to accept the conclusions.

A systematic review gathers all the literature on a topic, say using antibiotics to treat otitis media, and combines the data to determine if the sum of all the trials tells a different story than any single trial. The large number of participants in this type of research results in a much more statistically (and clinically) significant conclusion than any single paper.

A meta-analysis is a quantitative systematic review and demonstrates its outcomes in the form of a forest plot. The interpretation of a forest plot is to look for the diamond on the bottom. If it is totally to LEFT of the vertical line, it means risk of an outcome was reduced by the intervention. If it is fully to the RIGHT, then risk of that outcome was increased. And if the diamond touches the vertical line, it means there was no statistical influence of the intervention on the outcome.

We hope this brief introduction to EBM has been informative, clear, and helpful. If any of the information above seems unclear, or if you have a question, please contact us via the 5MinuteConsult Web site.

ACKNOWLEDGMENTS

This is the 35th edition of *The 5-Minute Clinical Consult*, a comprehensive point-of-care tool to assist in the care of patients. From beginning to end, one cannot find a more current and easy-to-use collection of clinically useful content.

Developing and maintaining a book and Web site of this magnitude requires an equally broad effort from its supporting team. I wish to thank the dedication and tireless efforts of many: Rebecca Schmidt, product lead, medical education and medical practice; Cindy Yoo, development editor; Joe Cho, acquisitions editor; and Lisa McAllister, vice president, medical practice. This 2027 edition is the direct result of the dedication and insights of our associate editors. I wish to thank Drs. Robert A. Baldor, Jeremy Golding, Mark B. Stephens, Kathleen A. Barry, and Grace Shih for their hard work and overwhelming commitment to *The 5-Minute Clinical Consult*.

I wish to especially thank my wife, Sylvia, and my daughter, Molly, who have given greatly for this book.

The challenge of completing a book covering this broad spectrum of medicine requires insights and skills far beyond my own. Many thanks to my mentors, Bob Baldor and Mark Quirk, who have been an enormous support—always there to encourage, reassure, and impart wisdom.

Many in the academic and health care worlds are due thanks for support, insight, and friendship: M. Diane McKee, Michele Pugnaire, Karen Rayla, Maryanne Adams, Erica White, Phil Fournier, Erik Garcia, Jeff Stovall, Jim Comes, Leah Honor, J. Herb Stevenson, Michael Kidd, Zainab Nawab, Sanjiv and Amita Chopra, Vasilios (Bill) Chrisostomidis, James (Jay) Broadhurst, Christina Kim, Madhavi Medipally, the staff of Shrewsbury Family Medicine, Ben Babbitt, Joyce Paquette, Priscila Velez, Brittany McLean, Michelle Leboeuf, Chad Ren, Joseph Frappier, my amazing colleagues Mark Powicki, Steve Messineo, Jill Terrien, Susan Feeney, Mariyan Montaque, Jillian Joseph, Jim Nairus, Kayla Chalmers, Danielle Ferreira, Rick Watson, and Sara Floros, and the faculty and students of the University of Massachusetts Medical School.

Medicine is a challenge I have fortunately not had to meet alone. Thanks to my parents, Frank and Angela (Jean); my brother, John, and his family, Marylou, Cate, and Jane; Frank, Mary Anne, Diane, and David Christian; the Diana and Hymie Lipschitz family; and the Bob and Ruth Pabreza family; they are responsible for who I am and my success in life.

I am blessed with the best of friends; without them, I would not be a physician. Thanks to Bob Bacic; Ron Jautz; Richard Onorato; John Horcher; Auguste Turnier; Bob Smith; Paul Saivetz; Bob and Nancy Gallinaro; Drew and Jill Grimes; Louay Toma; Laurie, Alan, Daniel, Jenny, and Matt Bugos; Alan Ehrlich; Andy Jennings; Bill Demianiuk; John and Kathleen Polanowicz; Phil and Carol Pettine; Mark and Linda Shelton; Steve Bennett; Vicki Triolo; and Bob and Laurie Jenal, Mike Rousse, Cliff Sterns, and Conor Wallace.

—Frank J. Domino, MD

CONTRIBUTING AUTHORS

Nawal Aamir, MD
Nephrology Fellow
Department of Medicine
UMass Chan Medical School/UMass Memorial Healthcare
Worcester, Massachusetts

Konstantin Abramov, MD, MHL
Associate Professor of Medicine
Department of Division of Renal Medicine
UMass Chan Medical School
Worcester, Massachusetts

Rashida Adenwala, MD
Family Medicine Attending Physician
Department of Family Medicine
Advocate Medical Group
Oak Lawn, Illinois

Adwoa A. Adu, MD
Family Medicine Physician
Department of Family Medicine
Prisma Health
Greenfield, South Carolina

Marium Palur Afzal, MD
Assistant Professor, MD
Department of Family Medicine
University of Texas Southwestern
Dallas, Texas

Francis Agama, MD, MS
Resident Physician
Department of Family Medicine
Baptist Memorial Hospital-DeSoto
Southaven, Mississippi

Arjola Agolli, MD, MBA
Family and Community Residency Program
Penn State Health
Reading, Pennsylvania

Yasir Ahmed, MD
Cornea, Cataract, and Refractive Surgeon
Eye Center of Texas
Houston, Texas

Rakan Al-Adwan, MD
Resident Physician
Department of Family Medicine
Advocate Christ Medical Center
Oak Lawn, Illinois

Daniel Albrecht, MD
Physician
Department of Family Medicine
Greenfield Family Medicine
Greenfield, Massachusetts

Fozia Akhtar Ali, MD, FAAFP
Professor/Clinical
Department of Family and Community Medicine
UT Health San Antonio
San Antonio, Texas

Rafia Ali, MD
Resident Physician
Department of Internal Medicine
Advocate Lutheran General Hospital
Park Ridge, Illinois

Saqeeb M. Ali, DO
PGY-3
Department of Internal Medicine
Ochsner Medical Center
Jefferson, Louisiana

Aya Allam, MD
Department of Family Medicine
Creighton University
Omaha, Nebraska

Mauro Amendola, MD, FAAFP
Associate Program Faculty
Department of Family Medicine Residency
Baptist Health
Southaven, Mississippi

Dhruval Amin, MD
Gastroenterology Fellow
Department of Gastroenterology
UMass Chan Medical School
Worcester, Massachusetts

Parth J. Amin, DO, MMS
Department of Population Health
Dell Medical School, The University of Texas at Austin
Austin, Texas

Ethan J. Anderson, DO
Resident
Department of Internal Medicine
Lutheran General Hospital
Park Ridge, Illinois

Matthew Anderson, MD
Resident Physician
Department of Internal Medicine
Stanford University School of Medicine
Palo Alto, California

Ann M. Aring, MD, FAAFP, FASAM
Associate Program
Director Family Medicine Residency
Ohio Health Riverside Methodist Hospital
Columbus, Ohio

Michael Arnold, MD[†]
Assistant Professor
Department of Family Medicine
Uniformed Services University of the Health Sciences
Bethesda, Maryland

Jason Assalita, DO
Residency Faculty
Department of Family Medicine
WellSpan Good Samaritan Hospital
Lebanon, Pennsylvania

Maximos Attia, MD, FAAFP
Associate Professor
Department of Family Medicine
Guthrie
Sayre, Pennsylvania

Frantz Aubry, MD
Clinical Fellow
Department of Psychiatry
One Brookdale Health
Brooklyn, New York

Camille D. Audette, DO
Fellow
Pediatric Emergency Department
UMass Memorial Children's Medical Center
Worcester, Massachusetts

Vicenda Augustin, MD
Resident Physician
Department of Family Medicine
Baptist Memorial DeSoto Hospital
Horn Lake, Mississippi

Sudeep K. Aulakh, MD, FACP, FRCPC
Director, Ambulatory Education
UMass Chan Medical School-Baystate
Springfield, Massachusetts

Ben Ayotte, MD
Clinical Assistant Professor, Division of Hospital Medicine
Department of Internal Medicine
Michigan Medicine, University of Michigan
Ann Arbor, Michigan

Melissa E. Badowski, PharmD, MPH
Clinical Associate Professor
Section of Infectious Diseases Pharmacotherapy, Department of Pharmacy Practice
University of Illinois at Chicago, College of Pharmacy
Chicago, Illinois

Nicole Baldera-Rodriguez, MD
Santo Domingo, Dominican Republic

Robert A. Baldor, MD, FAAFP
Professor and Founding Chair
Department of Family Medicine
UMass Chan Medical School-Baystate
Springfield, Massachusetts
Designated Institutional Official
Baystate Franklin Medical Center
Greenfield, Massachusetts

Katherine R. Baldwin, MD
Assistant Professor
Department of Pediatric Gastroenterology
Connecticut Children's Medical Center, University of Connecticut
Hartford, Connecticut

Kenneth A. Ballou, MD
Associate Professor of Clinical Medicine
Department of Family Medicine
University of California at Riverside School of Medicine
Riverside, California

Mrudula Bandaru, MD, BS
Resident
Department of Internal Medicine
George Washington University
Washington, District of Columbia

Tara Baney, MS, CRNP
Nurse Practitioner
Department of Family and Community Medicine
Penn State Health
State College, Pennsylvania

Kathleen A. Barry, MD
Associate Professor
UMass Chan Medical School
Department of Family Medicine and Community Health
Hahnemann Family Health Center
Worcester, Massachusetts

Faiz Bayo-Awoyemi, MD
Associate Program Director
Department of Family Medicine
Tufts University
Family Medicine Residency at Cambridge Health Alliance
Malden, Massachusetts

Frank B. Beacham, MD, MEHP
Physician
Department of Family Medicine
Prisma Health
Greenville, South Carolina

Christopher M. Beaumont, PA†
Assistant Professor
College of Allied Health Sciences, Uniformed Services University
Naval Undersea Medical Institute
Groton, Connecticut

Priscilla Becnel, MD, BS
Fellow and Associate Program Director, Internal Medicine Residency
Ochsner Medical Center
New Orleans, Louisiana

Trinity Simone Rosa Belgrave, BS, MS, MBBS
Resident
Department of Family Medicine Residency
Florida State University College of Medicine
Tallahassee, Florida

Markeeta Belmar, DO, MPH
Resident Physician
Department of Family Medicine
University of South Florida Morsani College of Medicine
Tampa, Florida

Brandis Belt, MD, MPH
Assistant Residency Director
Department of Family Medicine
Robert Wood Johnson—Somerset
Somerville, New Jersey

Brock A. Benedict, DO†
US Army
Family Physician
Womack Army Community Hospital
Fort Liberty, North Carolina

Brittney Bennett, MBBS
Department of Family Medicine Residency
Florida State University College of Medicine at Tallahassee Memorial HealthCare
Tallahassee, Florida

Ambreka Benons, MD
Psychiatry Resident
Brooklyn, New York

Christopher George Bentsen, MD
Resident Physician
Department of Internal Medicine
Advocate Lutheran General Hospital
Park Ridge, Illinois

Lukus A. Berber, MD
Resident Physician
Department of Internal Medicine
Advocate Lutheran General
Park Ridge, Illinois

Prarthna V. Bhardwaj, MD
Assistant Professor of Medicine
Department of Hematology Oncology
University of Massachusetts Medical School-Baystate
Springfield, Massachusetts

Sahil R. Bharwani, DO, MPH
Resident
Department of Hospital Medicine
Ochsner Clinic Foundation
New Orleans, Louisiana

Sonali Bhat, MD
Resident Physician
Department of Family and Community Medicine
Penn State Health Milton S. Hershey Medical Center
Hershey, Pennsylvania

Ghazaleh Bigdeli, MD, FCCP
Associate Professor
Department of Internal Medicine
Northeast Ohio Medical University
Rootstown, Ohio

Wendy S. Biggs, MD
Professor, Family Medicine
Central Michigan University College of Medicine
Saginaw, Michigan

Poorva Bindal, MD
Assistant Professor
Department of Internal Medicine/Hematology and Oncology
UMass Chan Medical School
Worcester, Massachusetts

Dmitry Bisk, MD
Associate Director
HonorHealth Scottsdale Osborn Family Medicine Residency Program
HonorHealth
Scottsdale, Arizona

Jennifer Cherry Bohannan, MD
Department of Family Medicine
Baylor Scott and White
Temple, Texas

Philip J. Bolduc, MD
Associate Professor
Department of Family Medicine and Community Health
UMass Chan Medical School
Worcester, Massachusetts

Frances J. Boly, DO
Department of Infectious Diseases
Advocate Christ Medical Center
Oak Lawn, Illinois

Kimberly A. Bombaci, MD
Assistant Professor
Department of Family Medicine
UMass Chan Medical School
Worcester, Massachusetts

Robert B. Bonanno, MD
Assistant Professor
Department of Family Medicine
Prisma Health
Greenville, South Carolina

Marie L. Borum, MD, EdD, MPH†
Professor of Medicine
Director of the Division of Gastroenterology and Liver Diseases
Department of Medicine
George Washington University School of Medicine and Health Care Sciences
Washington, District of Columbia

Deyanna M. Boston, MD
FMOB Program Director
Department of Family and Community Medicine
Assistant Professor
Creighton University School of Medicine
Omaha, Nebraska

William McCormick Bowen, MD
Program Director
UNM Santa Fe Family Medicine Residency
Santa Fe, New Mexico

Jennifer Bradford, MD, MPH
Assistant Professor
Family Medicine and Community Health
Director of Social Justice and Inclusion
Medical Director of Community HealthLink Detox Continuum
Worcester, Massachusetts

Alexandra Bray, MD
Assistant Professor
Department of Family Medicine
Oregon Health & Science University
Portland, Oregon

Anna Brickell, MD
Resident Physician
Department of Family Medicine
University of Arkansas for Medical Sciences
Jonesboro, Arkansas

Janae Zolna Brill, MD, MPH
Clinical Instructor
Department of Family Medicine of Southwest Washington
PeaceHealth
Vancouver, Washington

Bradley R. Brodie, MD
Resident Physician
Department of Family Medicine
Lakeland Regional Health
Lakeland, Florida

Katy (Ekaterina) Brodski-Quigley, MD, EdM
Physician, Urgent Care
Waltham, Massachusetts

Liana C. Brooks, MD
Resident Physician
UMass Chan Medical School
Worcester, Massachusetts

Phillip Charles Brown, MD
Department of Family Medicine
UCLA Santa Monica Medical Center
Santa Monica, California

Elizabeth L. Browning, DO
Core Faculty
Graduate Medical Education Family Medicine Baptist Memorial Hospital
Southaven, Mississippi

Laura Torrico Brusky, MD
Assistant Professor
Department of Family and Community Medicine
Medical College of Wisconsin
Milwaukee, Wisconsin

Laura Bujold, DO, MS
Assistant Professor of Family Medicine
Department of Family Medicine
University of Connecticut School of Medicine
Hartford, Connecticut

Carolina Isabel Burgos-Burgos, MD
Department of Family Medicine
University of Washington
Seattle, Washington

Liam P. Burke, MD
Assistant Professor
Department of Family Medicine and Community Health
UMass Chan Medical School
Worcester, Massachusetts

Patricia J. Burns, MD
Resident Physician
Department of Family and Community Medicine
University of Texas Health Science Center San Antonio
San Antonio, Texas

Harold J. Bursztajn, MD
Associate Professor of Psychiatry, Part-Time
Department of Psychiatry
Beth Israel Deaconess Medical Center
Harvard Medical School
Boston, Massachusetts

Jennifer Bustamante, DO
Assistant Professor
Family Medicine Residency
Nova Southeastern Dr. Kiran C. Patel College of Osteopathic Medicine—Evara Health Family Medicine Residency
Clearwater, Florida

Jennifer W. Caceres, MD
Associate Professor of Medicine
Department of Medicine
Schmidt College of Medicine at Florida Atlantic University
Boca Raton, Florida

David C. Cadena Jr., MD
Assistant Professor
Department of Family and Community Medicine
University of Texas Health Science Center San Antonio
San Antonio, Texas

Samantha Howard Caldwell, MD
Assistant Professor of Family Medicine
University of Tennessee Health Science Center
Memphis, Tennessee

Christine Ramos Camacho, MD, MS
Assistant Professor
Department of Family and Community Medicine
UT Health San Antonio
San Antonio, Texas

Justin Paul Canakis, DO
Resident Doctor
Department of Internal Medicine
George Washington University
Washington, District of Columbia

Brittany Lauren Carmack, MD
Assistant Professor
Department of Family Medicine
University of Arkansas for Medical Sciences
Arkansas, Jonesboro

Dana G. Carroll, PharmD, BCPS, CDCES, BCGP
Clinical Professor
Department of Pharmacy Practice
Auburn University Harrison School of Pharmacy
Tuscaloosa, Alabama

Matthew R. Carroll, DO
Resident
Department of Emergency Medicine
Rutgers Robert Wood Johnson Medical School
New Brunswick, New Jersey

Samantha Carroll, MD
Hospitalist
Department of Pediatrics
AdventHealth for Children
Orlando, Florida

Anthony Jay Carter, MD
Core Faculty
MS Delta Family Medicine Residency Program
Delta Health System
Greenville, Mississippi

Michael F. Cascio, MD, MHA
Resident Physician
Department of Family Medicine
Lakeside Medical Center
Belle Glade, Florida

Jennifer E. Cavin, MD
Assistant Professor
Department of Family Medicine
University of Texas Dell Medical School
Austin, Texas

William E. Cayley Jr., MD, Mdiv
Adjunct Clinical Professor
University of Wisconsin School of Medicine and Public Health
Prevea Family Medicine Residency
Eau Claire, Wisconsin

Jan Cerny, MD, PhD†
Associate Professor in Medicine
Department of Medicine, Division of Hematology/Oncology
UMass Chan Medical School
Worcester, Massachusetts

Ronald G. Chambers Jr., MD, FAAFP†
Medical Safe Haven Clinic Medical Director
Program Director
Department of Family Medicine
Dignity Health
Sacramento, California

Christine Chan, MD
Faculty
Hawai'i Island Family Medicine Residency
Hilo Benioff Medical Center
Hilo, Hawaii

Sangili Chandran, MD
Associate Professor
Department of Family Medicine
Roslyn Franklin University (Chicago Medical School)
Chicago, Illinois
Director, Primary Care Sports Medicine
Department of Family Medicine
Advocate Christ Hospital Medical Center
Oak Lawn, Illinois

Felix B. Chang, MD, DABMA, DABIHM, DABIM, FAAMA
Director, Inpatient Service
University of Massachusetts Fitchburg Family Medicine Residency Program
Hospitalist, Family Medicine
UMass Chan Medical School
Worcester, Massachusetts
Hospitalist
Department of Hospital Medicine
University of Massachusetts Memorial Medical Group
Leominster, Massachusetts

Jason Chao, MD, MS
Professor
Department of Family Medicine and Community Health
Case Western Reserve University and University Hospitals Cleveland Medical Center
Cleveland, Ohio

Parul Chaudhri, DO
Assistant Professor, Director of Osteopathic Education
Department of Family Medicine
University of Toledo
Toledo, Ohio

Janet Chen, DO
AdventHealth
Orlando, Florida

Jeffrey Chen, MD
Hospitalist
Department of Internal Medicine
University of Texas at Houston
Houston, Texas

John Cheng, MD
Associate Clinical Professor
Department of Family Medicine
Harbor-UCLA Family Medicine Residency Program
Torrance, California

Daniel Chilcote, DO
Primary Care Sports Medicine Fellow
Department of Community and Family Medicine
University Health
Kansas City, Missouri

Andrea Chin, MD, MSc
Resident Physician
Department of Family Medicine
UMass Chan Medical School
Worcester, Massachusetts

Cheyenne Chinea, OD, FAAO
Martinez, California

Grace H. Chiu, MD, FAAFP
Assistant Professor
Department of Clinical Medicine
UAMS, Northeast
Jonesboro, Arkansas

Ratnesh Chopra, MD
Assistant Professor
Department of Rheumatology
UMass Chan Medical School
Worcester, Massachusetts

Vasilios Chrisostomidis, DO
Associate Professor
Department of Family Medicine and Community Medicine
UMass Chan Medical School
Worcester, Massachusetts

Katherine Shoemaker Chu, MD
Penn State University College of Medicine
Hershey, Pennsylvania

Adrianna D. M. Clapp, MD, BSc
Assistant Professor
Department of Family Medicine
Mayo Clinic
Jacksonville, Florida

S. Lindsey Clarke, MD, FAAFP†
Medical University of South Carolina Area Health Education Consortium Professor (Greenwood/Family Medicine)
Director of Resident Education and Associate Program Director
Self Regional Healthcare
Greenwood, South Carolina

Karl T. Clebak, MD, MHA, FAAFP†
Associate Professor, Program Director
Department of Family and Community Medicine
Penn State Health Milton S. Hershey Medical Center
Hershey, Pennsylvania

Danielle N. Coderre, MD
Family Medicine Resident
Family Medicine and Community Health
UMass Chan Medical School
Worcester, Massachusetts

Erik Colegrove, MD
Department of Family Medicine
Central Michigan University
Mount Pleasant, Michigan

Irene Coletsos, MD, MS
Community Psychiatrist
Department of Behavioral Health
Vinfen, Department of Mental Health
Quincy, Massachusetts

Andrew Collyer, DO
Family Medicine Resident
Carl R. Darnall Army Medical Center
Fort Cavazos, Texas

Ellen Combs, MD
Resident
Department of Family Medicine
Prisma Health - Greenville School of Medicine
Greenville, South Carolina

Christina Conrad, DO
Department of Pediatric Emergency Medicine
Phoenix Children's Hospital
Phoenix, Arizona

Stephanie L. Conway-Allen, PharmD, RPh
Associate Professor
Department of Pharmacy Practice
Massachusetts College of Pharmacy and Health Sciences
Worcester, Massachusetts

Tonya M. Cook, PharmD
Faculty, Clinical Pharmacist
Department of Family Medicine Residency
St. Mary's Medical Center Family Medicine Residency
Grand Junction, Colorado

Valerie Coppenrath, PharmD
Associate Professor
Department of Pharmacy Practice
MCPHS University School of Pharmacy
Worcester, Massachusetts
Adjunct Faculty
UMass HealthAlliance Fitchburg Family Practice Medical Residency
Fitchburg, Massachusetts

Tatiana Cordova, MD
Associate Professor
Department of Family and Community Medicine
UT Health San Antonio
San Antonio, Texas

Jennifer M. Corliss, MD, FAAFP
Assistant Professor
Department of Family Medicine
University of Colorado
Denver, Colorado

Natalie Ann Correa, MD
Resident Physician
Department of Family Medicine and Community
UMass Chan Medical School
Worcester, Massachusetts

Jennifer Costa, MD
Assistant Professor
Department of Family Medicine
University of South Florida Morsani College of Medicine
Tampa, Florida

Corey J. Costanzo, DO, MPH, MS
Assistant Professor of Family Medicine
UMass Chan Medical School
Worcester, Massachusetts

Julie A. Creech, DO†
Family Medicine Physician, Sports Medicine Physician, Primary Care Sports Medicine Fellow United States Air Force
O'Fallen, Illinois

Laura Critchfield, PA-C
Assistant Professor
Department of Family and Community Medicine
Penn State Health Milton S. Hershey Medical Center
Hershey, Pennsylvania

Jason Cross, PharmD, BCPS, BCACP
Associate Professor of Pharmacy Practice
Massachusetts College of Pharmacy and Health Sciences University
Worcester, Massachusetts

Merly Cubelo, DO
Resident Physician
Department of Family Medicine
Lakeland Regional Health
Lakeland, Florida

Hongyi Cui, MD, PhD
Associate Professor of Surgery, Associate Director, Acute Care Surgery
Department of Surgery
UMass Memorial Medical Center
Worcester, Massachusetts

Shani H. Cunningham, DO, MEd, FAAP
Assistant Professor
Department of Pediatrics
Advent Health for Children
Orlando, Florida

Kirby W. Curtis, DO
Resident
Department of Family Medicine
UAMS Northeast
Jonesboro, Arkansas

Darnel Viray Dabu, MD, MPH, FAAFP, DipABLM
Faculty Physician
Department of Family Medicine
Lakeside Medical Center
Belle Glade, Florida

Jason I. Dailey, MD
Program Director
Psychiatry Residency
Carl R. Darnall Army Medical Center
Fort Cavazos, Texas

Cassandra Daisy, MD
Resident Physician
Department of Family Medicine and Community
UMass Chan Medical School
Worcester, Massachusetts

Puja Dalal, MD, FAAFP
Assistant Program Director
Director of POCUS
Novant Health Family Medicine Residency Program
Cornelius, North Carolina
Assistant Professor
Department of Family Medicine
University of North Carolina
Chapel Hill, North Carolina

Amanda d'Almeida, MD, MPH
Resident Physician
UCLA Family Medicine
University of California, Los Angeles
Santa Monica, California

Tina D'Amato, DO
Attending Family Physician
Charlotte Family Medicine
Charlotte, Vermont

Anthony Dambro, MD
Associate Professor
Department of Family and Community Medicine
Penn State College of Medicine
Hershey, Pennsylvania

Gena Damento, MD
Ophthalmologist
Department of Ophthalmology
Contra Costa Regional Medical Center
Martinez, California

Paul E. Daniel Jr., MD, MS
Hospitalist, Assistant Professor of Medicine
UMass Memorial Healthcare
Worcester, Massachusetts

Anne Darby, DO
Family Medicine Physician, Faculty
Penn State Health
Hershey, Pennsylvania

Akhil K. Das, MD, FACS
Professor
Department of Urology
Thomas Jefferson University
Philadelphia, Pennsylvania
Professor
Department of Urology
University of California Irvine
Orange, California

Amanda Kimberley Davis, MD, MBBS
Department of Family Medicine
Tallahassee Memorial Health Care FMRP
Tallahassee, Florida

Christopher R. Davis, MD, MPH
Pennsylvania State University
Hershey, Pennsylvania

Micheala Desere Davis, MD
Resident Physician
Department of Family Medicine
University of Tennessee
Memphis, Tennessee

Cailee A. Dean, DO
Resident Physician
Department of Family and Community Medicine
UMass Chan Medical School
Worcester, Massachusetts

Christian Dean, DO, MS, DiMM, FAWM
Jackson, Wyoming

Tyler M. Debbie, MD
Resident
Department of Emergency Medicine
Rutgers Robert Wood Johnson Medical School
New Brunswick, New Jersey

Tess A. Decater, MD, MPH
Chief Resident
Department of Internal Medicine
UMass Chan Medical School
Worcester, Massachusetts

Erin W. DeLaney, MD
Associate Professor
Department of Family and Community Medicine
University of Alabama at Birmingham
Birmingham, Alabama

Matthew DeLaney, MD
Professor
Department of Emergency Medicine
University of Alabama at Birmingham
Birmingham, Alabama

Leah N. Delfinado, MD
Residency Program Director
Designated Institutional Official
Department of Obstetrics and Gynecology
Advocate Healthcare
Chicago, Illinois

Konstantinos E. Deligiannidis, MD, MPH, FAAFP
Associate Professor
Department of Family Medicine
Donald and Barbara Zucker School of Medicine at Hofstra/Northwell
Medical Director
Northwell House Calls
Hempstead, New York

Henry Del Rosario, MD
Assistant Professor
Department of Family Medicine and Community Health
UMass Chan Medical School
Worcester, Massachusetts

Mario P. DeMarco, MD, MPH
Associate Professor of Clinical Family Medicine
Department of Family Medicine and Community Health
Perelman School of Medicine, University of Pennsylvania
Philadelphia, Pennsylvania

Jared Dendy, MD, FACP, ECNU
Department of Endocrinology
Ochsner Medical Center
Jefferson, Louisiana

Jaydip Desai, DO
Department of Emergency Medicine
Robert Wood Johnson
New Brunswick, New Jersey

Prit M. Dhagat, DO, MPH
Resident
Department of Family and Community Medicine
University of Texas Health Science Center San Antonio
San Antonio, Texas

Scott Michael Dickson, MD
Program Director
Regional Programs
University of Arkansas for Medical Sciences
Little Rock, Arkansas

Anastasia Dihel, MD
Resident Physician
Department of Family Medicine
Lakeside Medical Center
Belle Glade, Florida

Daniel D. Divilbiss, MD
Assistant Professor
Department of Family Medicine
AHEC/MUSC
Greenwood, South Carolina

Jill T. Wei Doherty, MD
Department of Family Medicine
Santa Monica Family Physicians
Santa Monica, California

Frank J. Domino, MD
Professor and Director of Predoctoral Education
Department of Family Medicine and Community Health
UMass Chan Medical School
Worcester, Massachusetts

Clare Donahue, DO
Assistant Professor
Department of Family Medicine
Western University of Health Sciences
Pomona, California

Meghana Doniparthi, MD
Physician
Department of Gastroenterology
Advocate Lutheran General Hospital
Park Ridge, Illinois

Andrea B. Dotson, MD, MSPH, IBCLC, NABBLM-C, FAAFP
Assistant Professor
Department of Family Medicine and Community Health
Durham, North Carolina

Joanna Drowos, DO, MPH, MBA
Associate Dean for Faculty Affairs
Associate Professor of Family Medicine
Charles E. Schmidt College of Medicine
Florida Atlantic University
Boca Raton, Florida

Michelle E. Duffelmeyer, MD
Director of Didactic Education
College of Health Science
Westfield State University
Westfield, Massachusetts

Ashten Duncan, MD, MPH, CPH
Resident Physician
Family and Community Medicine
University of New Mexico—Santa Fe Family Medicine Residency
Santa Fe, New Mexico

Nadir Ebrahim, MD, MBA
Resident
Department of Family Medicine
Baptist Memorial Hospital
Southaven, Mississippi

Mason Eghbali, MD
Resident Physician
Department of Internal Medicine
George Washington University
Washington, District of Columbia

Stephany Giraldo Eierle, DO, MPH
UMass Chan Medical School
Worcester, Massachusetts

Rebecca Feltman-Frank El Zoghbi, MD
Resident
Department of Psychiatry
Advocate Lutheran General Hospital
Park Ridge, Illinois

Ashraf Elamin, MD
Physician
Department of Nephrology
UMass Memorial Medical Center
Worcester, Massachusetts

Pamela Ellsworth, MD
Professor of Urology
University of Central Florida
Orlando, Florida

Meygan Lackey Elway, MD, MPH
Core Faculty
Department of Family Medicine
Boston University/Boston Medical Center
Boston, Massachusetts

Deborah R. Erlich, MD, MmedEd, FAAFP
Associate Professor
Department of Family Medicine
Family Medicine Clerkship Director
Tufts University School of Medicine
Boston, Massachusetts

Justin T. Ertle, MD
Assistant Professor
Department of Internal Medicine
Medical College of Georgia at Augusta University
Augusta, Georgia

Emily J. Eschleman, DO, MS, CAQSM
Attending Physician and Assistant Professor
Department of Family Medicine and Community
UMass Chan Medical School
Worcester, Massachusetts

Ricardo David Espinosa, MD
Department of Internal Medicine
Ochsner Medical Center
New Orleans, Louisiana

Tyler Evans, DO
Assistant Professor
Department of Family and Community Medicine
UT Southwestern Medical Center
Dallas, Texas

Vanessa Joyce M. Evardone, MD, BSMT
Fellow
Department of Geriatric Medicine
Florida Atlantic University (FAU) - West Palm Beach VA Medical Center
Boca Raton, Florida

Idil D. Ezhuthachan, MD, MS
Assistant Professor
Department of Pediatrics
Children's Healthcare of Atlanta
Assistant Professor
Department of Pediatrics
Emory University
Atlanta, Georgia

Michael Fahey, MD
Associate Professor of Pediatrics
Department of Pediatrics
UMass Memorial Medical Center
Worcester, Massachusetts

Peng Thim Fan, MD
Clinical Professor
Department of Medicine
David Geffen School of Medicine at UCLA
Los Angeles, California

Rhonda A. Faulkner, PhD[†]
Director of Behavioral Medicine
Department of Family Medicine
AMITA Health Saint Joseph Hospital Chicago
University of Illinois College of Medicine Master Affiliate
Chicago, Illinois

Dylan G. Fedor, DO, BSc
Resident Physician
Family Medicine Residency Program
University of Arkansas for Medical Sciences
Jonesboro, Arkansas

A. Susan Feeney, MS, DNP, FNP-BC
Assistant Professor
Director of Family and Adult Gerontology NP Programs
Tan Chingfen Graduate School of Nursing
UMass Chan Medical School
Worcester, Massachusetts

Neil J. Feldman, DPM
Podiatrist, Staff
UMass Medical Center
Worcester, Massachusetts

Allison H. Ferris, MD
Professor and Chair of Medicine
Department of Medicine
Florida Atlantic University Charles E. Schmidt College of Medicine
Boca Raton, Florida

Halle Elizabeth Field, MD
Assistant Professor
Department of Hospital Medicine
Ochsner Medical Center
New Orleans, Louisiana

Matthew J. Filippo, DO
Associate Professor, Teaching/Clinical Psychiatrist
Department of Psychiatry
Advocate Lutheran General Hospital
Park Ridge, Illinois

Alexa Finkelstein, BS
Medical Student
New York Institute of Technology College of Osteopathic Medicine
Old Westbury, New York

Theodore B. Flaum, DO
Associate Professor
Department of Osteopathic Manipulative Medicine
NYIT College of Osteopathic Medicine
Old Westbury, New York

Kyle J. Fletke, MD
Assistant Professor
Department of Family and Community Medicine
University of Maryland School of Medicine
Baltimore, Maryland

Suzanne Florczyk, PharmD
Clinical Pharmacist
Novant Health
Cornelius, North Carolina

Harry W. Flynn Jr., MD
The J. Donald M. Gass Distinguished Chair in Ophthalmology
Department of Ophthalmology
Bascom Palmer Eye Institute, UHealth-University of Miami Healthcare System
Miami, Florida

Jane Marie Forbes, MD
Assistant Professor
Department of Family Medicine
University of Virginia
Charlottesville, Virginia

Jennifer G. Foster, MD, MBA, FACP
Associate Professor of Medicine
Charles E. Schmidt College of Medicine
Florida Atlantic University
Boca Raton, Florida

Zoe J. Foster, MD, FAAFP
Program Director
Department of Family and Preventive Medicine
Prisma Health—University of South Carolina
Columbia, South Carolina

Maria Fowler, MD
Resident
Department of Family and Community Medicine
Penn State Health ilton S. Hershey Medical Center
Hershey, Pennsylvania

Nelson Franqui-Rios, MD
Resident Physician
Department of Internal Medicine–Pediatrics
University of South Florida Morsani College of Medicine
Tampa, Florida

Minjin Fromm, MD
UMass Chan Medical School
Worcester, Massachusetts

Moises Gallegos, MD, MPH, MEHP
Clinical Associate Professor
Department of Emergency Medicine
Stanford University School of Medicine
Stanford, California

Dennis Garcia-Rhodes, MD, MPH
Resident Physician
Department of Primary Care and Rural Medicine
Texas A&M University Health
Bryan, Texas

Taylor Gaudard, MD, IBCLC
Assistant Professor
Department of Family Medicine
Central Michigan University College of Medicine
Saginaw, Michigan

Hermione Gaw, MD
Resident Physician
Department of Family Medicine Residency
Dignity Health Sacramento
Sacramento, California

Kamini Geer, MD, MPH
Women's Health Fellowship Director
AdventHealth Winter Park
Winter Park, Florida

Scott Geiger, MD
Adjunct Faculty
Department of Urology
Penn State College of Medicine
Hershey, Pennsylvania

Michelle A. Georgia, DO
Resident Physician
Department of Pediatrics
University of Massachusetts
Worcester, Massachusetts
Fellow
Department of Pediatric Emergency Medicine
Children's Hospital of the King's Daughters
Norfolk, Virginia

Jenny T. Giang-Griesser, MD
Sea Mar Co-Site Director, Core Faculty
Swedish Cherry Hill Family Medicine Residency
Family Medicine Physician
Sea Mar Community Health Centers
Seattle, Washington

Corinne Gibbons, MD, MPH
Family Physician
Greater Lawrence Family Health Center
Lawrence, Massachusetts

Lawrence M. Gibbs, MD, MSEd, FAAFP
Program Director
Department of Family Medicine
HCA Healthcare Kansas City: Lee's Summit FMR
Lee's Summit, Missouri

Sonia Gilani, MD
Resident Physician
Department of Obstetrics and Gynecology
Advocate Illinois Masonic Medical Center
Chicago, Illinois

Jennifer L. Gilley, DO
Internal Medicine Resident
Department of Internal Medicine
Ochsner New Orleans
New Orleans, Louisiana

Daniel V. Girzadas Jr., MD
Department of Emergency Medicine
University of Illinois
Chicago, Illinois
Department of Emergency Medicine
Advocate Christ Medical Center
Oak Lawn, Illinois

Marni Klessman Gleiber, MD
Assistant Professor of Physical Medicine and Rehabilitation
Director of Ethics, Professionalism and Professional Identity Thread
Charles E. Schmidt College of Medicine Florida Atlantic University
Boca Raton, Florida

Joshua A. Go, DO
Assistant Professor
Department of Family Medicine
University of Washington
Seattle, Washington

Dori Goldberg, MD
Assistant Professor
Department of Dermatology
UMass Chan Medical School
Worcester, Massachusetts

Krystyna G. Golden, MD[†]
Resident Physician
Family Medicine Residency
Eglin Air Force Base Hospital
Eglin AFB, Florida
Sports Medicine Fellow
National Capital Consortium Sports Medicine Fellowship
Fort Belvoir, Virginia

Jeremy Golding, MD, FAAFP
Professor of Family Medicine and Obstetrics & Gynecology
UMass Chan Medical School
Department of Family Medicine and Community Health
UMass Memorial Health Care
Hahnemann Family Health Center
Worcester, Massachusetts

Tove Martine Goldson, MD, PhD
Assistant Professor
Department of Family and Community Medicine
Baylor College of Medicine
Temple, Texas

Anter Suarez Gonzales, MD
Assistant Professor
Department of Orthopedics
SUNY Downstate Health Sciences University
Brooklyn, New York

Juan C. Gonzalez, MD
Resident Physician
Department of Family Medicine
Advent Health
Winter Park, Florida

Tyler Gopee, DO
Resident
Department of Family Medicine
Garnet Health Medical Center
Middletown, New York

Robert S. Gordon III, DO, MS
Resident
Department of Internal Medicine
George Washington School of Medicine
Washington, District of Columbia

Emily Ann Gorman, DO
Assistant Program Director
Department of Family Medicine
OhioHealth Riverside Family Medicine
Columbus, Ohio

Kristina Gracey, MD, MPH
Assistant Professor
Department of Family Medicine and Community Health
University of Massachusetts
Worcester, Massachusetts

Corinne Grady, MD, MS
Resident Physician
Department of Family Medicine
Boston University School of Medicine
Boston Medical Center
Boston, Massachusetts

Kevin Gray, MD
Associate Professor
Department of Community and Family Medicine
University of Missouri—Kansas City School of Medicine
Kansas City, Missouri

Ramanpreet Grewal, MD
Family Medicine
Galesburg Cottage Hospital
Galesburg, Illinois

Simon B. Griesbach, MD[†]
Assistant Director
Department of Family Medicine
Waukesha Family Medicine Residency at ProHealth Care
Waukesha, Wisconsin
Clinical Adjunct Assistant Professor
Department of Family Medicine and Community Health
Madison, Wisconsin
Assistant Clinical Professor
Department of Family and Community Medicine
Medical College of Wisconsin
Milwaukee, Wisconsin

Andrew Grimes, MD
Physician Partner
USAD Central Texas
Austin, Texas

Sidhant Gugale, MD, MPH
Resident Physician
Department of Emergency Medicine
Rutgers Robert Wood Johnson Medical School
New Brunswick, New Jersey

Neena R. Gupta, MD[†]
Associate Professor
Department of Pediatrics
UMass Chan Medical School
Worcester, Massachusetts

Vikas Gupta, MD, MPH
Chair and Program Director
Department of Family Medicine
Montgomery Family Medicine Residency Program
Montgomery, Alabama

Claudia Liliana Gutierrez Cornejo, MD
Family Medicine Resident
UT Health San Antonio
San Antonio, Texas

Claudia Guzman, MD
Endocrinologist
Department of Endocrinology
Clínica Corominas
Santiago, Dominican Republic

Rebecca Gwaltney, MD, MPH
Assistant Professor
Department of Family Medicine and Community Health
University of Massachusetts
Worcester, Massachusetts

Emmeline Ha, MD[†]
Assistant Professor
Division of Family Medicine
The George Washington University
Washington, District of Columbia

Reem Hadi, MD
Board-Certified Family Physician
Forward Health
San Antonio, Texas

Katherine Haga, DO
Clinic Director
Novant Health Family Medicine Residency Program
Novant Health
Cornelius, North Carolina

Caitlyn Haines, MD
Assistant Professor
Department of Orthopedics and Rehabilitation
Department of Family and Community Medicine
Penn State College of Medicine
Hershey, Pennsylvania

Matthew A. Halfar, MD
Assistant Professor
Department of Family and Community Medicine
Creighton University
Omaha, Nebraska

Sigrun Hallmeyer, MD, FACCC
Advocate Health
Park Ridge, Illinois

Megan L. Hanna, MD
Adjunct Assistant Professor
Department of Family Medicine
University of South Carolina School of Medicine Greenville
Greenville, South Carolina
Faculty Member
Department of Family Medicine
Prisma Health Seneca Family Medicine Residency
Seneca, South Carolina

Thomas J. Hansen, MD[†]
System Vice President Chief Academic Officer
Department of Academic Affairs
Advocate Aurora Health
Downers Grove, Illinois

Maham Haq, MD
Department of Family Medicine
Advocate Christ Medical Center
Oak Lawn, Illinois

Allison Hargreaves, MD
Assistant Professor of Family Medicine and Community Health
UMass Chan Medical School
Worcester, Massachusetts

Chelsea Harris, MD
Faculty
Department of Family Medicine
Lawrence Family Medicine Residency
Lawrence, Massachusetts

Alyssa Jeanne Vest Hart, DO
Program Director
Department of Family Medicine
Ascension St. Joseph
Chicago, Illinois

Sydney Hartman-Munick, MD
Assistant Professor
Department of Pediatrics
UMass Memorial Medical Center/UMass Chan Medical School
Worcester, Massachusetts

Fern R. Hauck, MD, MS, FAAFP
Professor
Spencer P. Bass, MD, Twenty-First Century Professor of Family Medicine
Professor of Public Health Sciences
Director of Research and Faculty Development
University of Virginia School of Medicine
Charlottesville, Virginia

Madeline Hazle, MD
Resident
Department of Family and Community Medicine
UT Health San Antonio
San Antonio, Texas

Catherine Hendren, MD
Resident Physician
Department of Internal Medicine and Pediatrics
UMass Chan Medical School
Worcester, Massachusetts

Pablo I. Hernandez Itriago, MD, MHCM, FAAFP
Chief Medical Officer
Edward M. Kennedy Community Health Center
Assistant Professor
Department of Family Medicine
UMass Chan Medical School
Worcester, Massachusetts

Lisa Hertz, MD
Department of Gastroenterology
Long Beach Memorial Medical Center
Long Beach, California

Mark L. Higdon, DO, FAAFP
Clinical Associate Professor
University of North Carolina School of Medicine
Program Director
Novant Health Family Medicine Residency Novant Health
Cornelius, North Carolina

Ryunosuke Hisatomi, MD
Resident
Department of Family Medicine
LSU Health Shreveport
Shreveport, Louisiana

Joseph Daniel Hogue, MD, MBA
Program Director
Baptist Desoto Family Medicine Residency
Baptist Memorial Hospital-DeSoto
Southaven, Mississippi

Allison Holmes, DO
Assistant Professor for Family and Community Medicine
Department of Family and Community Medicine
Penn State Health
State College, Pennsylvania

Laura Horowitz, DO
Family Medicine Resident
Department of Family Medicine
ProHealth Care
Waukesha, Wisconsin

Steven A. House, MD, FAAFP, FAAHPM, HMDC
Professor, Program Director
Department of Family and Geriatric Medicine
University of Louisville/Glasgow
Glasgow, Kentucky

Sarah Hovland, MD, MPH
Assistant Professor
Department of Family Medicine
Baylor College of Medicine
Temple, Texas

Jordan Howard-Young, MD, MA-ID, DAAETS
Assistant Professor
Department of Family Medicine and Community Health, Department of Psychiatry
UMass Chan Medical School
Worcester, Massachusetts

Madeline Elaine Huff, MD, MS
Resident Physician
Department of Family Medicine
UT Dell Family Medicine Residency
Austin, Texas

Dennis E. Hughes, DO, FACEP
Attending Physician CoxHealth
Springfield, Missouri

Pamela R. Hughes, MD[†]
Military Program Director
Department of Family Medicine
St. Louis University Southwest Illinois Family Medicine Residency
O'Fallon, Illinois

Erik K. Hunsaker, MD
Resident
Department of Psychiatry
Carl R. Darnall Army Medical Center
Fort Cavazos, Texas

Adedapo Iluyomade, MD, MBA
Clinical Assistant Professor of Medicine
Department of Medicine
Herbert Wertheim College of Medicine, Florida International University
Preventive Cardiologist
Department of Cardiology
Miami Cardiac and Vascular Institute
Miami, Florida

Tamika Isaac, DO
Resident Physician
Department of Family Medicine and Community
UMass Chan Medical School
Worcester, Massachusetts

Allison Isabelli, DO
Resident Physician
Department of Internal Medicine
Advocate Christ Medical Center
Oak Lawn, Illinois

Bashyam Iyengar, MD, MPH
Faculty, Family Medicine
Ascension St. Vincent
Jacksonville, Florida

Duncan L. Jackson, MD
Department of Family Medicine Residency Program
Tallahassee Memorial Healthcare
Tallahassee, Florida

Vasudha Jain, MD
Core Faculty
Department of Family Medicine
Tidelands Health
Myrtle Beach, South Carolina

Lakshmi Gopinath Jaisankar, MD
Department of Family Medicine
Creighton University Graduate Medical Education
Omaha, Nebraska

Christian Javier, DO[†]
Resident
Department of Family Medicine
Dignity Health
Gilbert, Arizona

Kassandra M. Jean-Marie, MD
Resident Physician
Department of Family Medicine
Greenfield Family Medicine
Greenfield, Massachusetts

Oluwole Jegede, MD, MPH, FAPA
Assistant Professor
Department of Psychiatry
Yale University School of Medicine
New Haven, Connecticut

Tanner J. Jennings, DO
Physician
Department of Family Medicine
Texas A&M Family Medicine Residency
Bryan, Texas

Zaiba Jetpuri, DO, MBA, FAAFP
Associate Professor
Department of Family and Community Medicine
UT Southwestern Medical Center
Dallas, Texas

Can Angela Jiang, MD
Clinical Associate Professor
Department of Medicine
Stanford University School of Medicine
Palo Alto, California

Dongsheng Jiang, MD, MSc
Associate Professor
Department of Family and Community Medicine
Pennsylvania State University, College of Medicine
State College, Pennsylvania

Joanna Jiang, MD
Medical Resident
Ohio State University
Columbus, Ohio

Nasheena Jiwa, MD
Physician/Fellow
Department of Pulmonary and Critical Care
University of Connecticut Health Center
Farmington, Connecticut

Katherine G. W. Johnson, MD
Assistant Professor
Department of Family Medicine
Self Regional Healthcare
Greenwood, South Carolina

Shana-Kay Lambert-Johnson, MD
Resident Physician
Department of Family Medicine Residency Program
Medical City Fort Worth
Fort Worth, Texas

Julie Johnston, MD, FAAFP
Faculty Physician
Lawrence Family Medicine Residency
Lawrence, Massachusetts

William Johnston, MD
Department of Community and Family Medicine
University of Texas Southwestern
Dallas, Texas

Brandon D. Jones, MD
Core Faculty
Family Medicine Residency
Dignity Health East Valley Family Medicine Residency
Gilbert, Arizona

Myers Jones, MD
Resident
Department of Family Medicine
Prisma Health/University of South Carolina
School of Medicine Greenville (Seneca) Family Medicine Residency
Seneca, South Carolina

Melody A. Jordahl-Iafrato, MD, MPH, FAAFP
Associate Program Director
Community Hospital East Family Medicine Residency
Department of Family Medicine
Community Hospital East
Indianapolis, Indiana

Jillian K. Joseph, MPAS, PA-C
Instructor
Department of Family Medicine and Community Health
UMass Memorial Health
Worcester, Massachusetts

Kripalini Ephraim Joseph, MD
Department of Family Medicine
Prisma Health
Seneca, South Carolina

Nisarg Joshi, MD, BS
Junior Attending, Vitreoretinal Surgery Fellow
Department of Ophthalmology
University of South Florida
Tampa, Florida

July Jost, MD
Resident Physician
Department of Family Medicine
Texas A&M Family Medicine Residency Program
Bryan, Texas

Patrick Wakefield Joyner, MD, MS†
Assistant Professor
Department of Orthopedic Surgery
OrthoCollier
Naples, Florida

Khadija Kabani, DO, FAAFP
Associate Program Director
Department of Family Medicine
Methodist Health System
Dallas, Texas

Afsha Rais Kaisani, MD, FAAFP
Associate Program Director
Department of Family Medicine
HCA/Medical City Arlington Family Medicine Residency Program
North Richland Hills, Texas

Rasha Kakati, MD
Resident
Department of Family Medicine
University of Texas Southwestern
Dallas, Texas

Sukhjeet K. Kamboj, MD
Department of Family Medicine
WellSpan Good Samaritan Family Medicine Residency Program
Lebanon, Pennsylvania

Donna Marie Kaminski, DO, MPH, FAAFP
Assistant Director
Robert Wood Johnson Somerset Family Practice
Family Medicine Residency Program
Robert Wood Johnson University Hospital Somerset
Somerville, New Jersey

Rahul Kapur, MD
Assistant Professor
Family Medicine and Sports Medicine
Department of Family Medicine and Community Health
University of Minnesota Sports Medicine
University of Minnesota
Minneapolis, Minnesota

Beminet Kassaye, MD
Department of Internal Medicine
George Washington
Washington, District of Columbia

Naomi Kasturiarachi, DO
Resident
Department of Family Medicine
OhioHealth Riverside Methodist Hospital
Columbus, Ohio

Neelima Katukuri, MD, FACC, FSCAI
Advanced Structural Fellow
Division of Cardiology
UMass Memorial Medical Center
Worcester, Massachusetts

Shivam Kaushik, DO
Resident
Department of Emergency Medicine
Robert Wood Johnson Medical School
New Brunswick, New Jersey

Devin Patrick Kearns, DO
Resident Physician
Department of Family Medicine
St. Louis University Southwest Illinois Family Medicine Residency
O'Fallon, Illinois

Clara M. Keegan, MD
Associate Professor
Department of Family Medicine
The Robert Larner, M.D. College of Medicine at The University of Vermont
Burlington, Vermont

Caroline Kelley, DO
Resident
Department of Family Medicine
Methodist Health Systems
Dallas, Texas

Kaitlyn Kennedy, MD
Resident Physician
Department of Internal Medicine
UMass Chan Medical School
Worcester, Massachusetts

Matthew J. Kenney, DO†
Chief Resident, Family Medicine
Carl R. Darnall Army Medical Center
Fort Cavazos, Texas

Anila Khaliq, MD, FAAFP
Faculty
Department of Family Medicine
Touro College of Osteopathic Medicine
Middletown, New York

Muneeza Khan, MD, FAAFP
Associate Professor Chair
Department of Family Medicine
University of Tennessee Health Science Center
Memphis, Tennessee

Rohail Khan, MD
Resident
Department of Emergency Medicine
Rutgers Robert Wood Johnson Medical School
New Brunswick, New Jersey

Zehra Khan, MD
Resident Physician
Department of Family Medicine
Ascension Saint Joseph Hospital
Chicago, Illinois

Narmina Khanmammadova, MD
Fellow
Department of Urology
University of California Irvine
Orange, California

Myra Khawar, DO, MBS
Physician
Department of Family Medicine and Community
UMass Chan Medical School
Worcester, Massachusetts

Raphael Khella, DO
Resident
Department of Internal Medicine
Florida Atlantic University
Boca Raton, Florida

Catherine Peony Khoo, MD, FAAFP
Adjunct Clinical Assistant Professor of Family Medicine (Voluntary) at the Keck School of Medicine
Family Medicine Residency Program
California Hospital Medical Center
Los Angeles, California

Sally Khoury, MD
Department of Family Medicine
Baylor College of Family Medicine
Houston, Texas

Nicholas Kidd, MD
Assistant Professor
Department of Family Medicine
University of Virginia
Charlottesville, Virginia

Barbara M. Kiersz Mueller, DO, CFMDL1, AIT, IEC
Physician
Department of Developmental Pediatrics
THINK Neurology
Austin, Texas

Caleb Weiss Kiesow, MD, BS
Resident
Department of Family Medicine
SLU/SWIL USAF Family Medicine Residency
O'Fallon, Illinois

Jane J. Kim, MD
Resident
Department of Family Medicine
Penn State Hersey Medical Center
Hersey, Pennsylvania

Walter M. Kim, MD, PhD
Lecturer
Department of Medicine
Harvard Medical School
Associate Physician
Division of Gastroenterology, Hepatology and Endoscopy
Brigham and Women's Hospital Chief
Department of Gastroenterology
Lemuel Shattuck Hospital
Boston, Massachusetts

Brian J. Kimbrell, MD, FACS
Department of Trauma
Trauma Surgery/Surgical Critical Care
Sarasota, Florida

Shane R. Kinard, MD
Assistant Professor
Department of Medicine
Penn State Milton S. Hershey Medical Center
Hershey, Pennsylvania

Alex Kipp, MD, MALS
Core Faculty
Department of Family Medicine
Valley Family Medicine
Renton, Washington

Teri T. Kleinberg, MD, MSc
Instructor
Department of Family Medicine
UMass Chan Medical School
Worcester, Massachusetts

Laura K. Klug, PharmD
Associate Professor
Department of Pharmacy Practice and Family and Community Medicine
Creighton University
Omaha, Nebraska

Kelly Klump, MD
Resident Physician
Department of Family Medicine
Grand Stand Medical Center
Myrtle Beach, South Carolina

Anne M. Knierim, MD[†]
Resident Physician
Carl R. Darnall Army Medical Center
Fort Cavazos, Texas

Sharon Koehler, DO, FACS[†]
St John's Episcopal Hospital
Far Rockaway, New York

Sumira A. Koirala, MD, FAAFP
Faculty, Associate Professor of Family and Community Medicine
St. Elizabeth Boardman Family Medicine Residency
Bon Secours Mercy Health
Boardman, Ohio

Veerauo Vera Konkankit, MD, MSc
Family and Community Medicine Residency Core Faculty
Graduate Medical Education
Primary Care Physician
Department of Family Medicine
Yuma Regional Medical Center
Yuma, Arizona

Scott E. Kopec, MD
Associate Professor
Department of Medicine, Division of Pulmonary and Critical Care
UMass Chan Medical School
Worcester, Massachusetts

Peter Koppenheffer, MD
Assistant Professor of Family Medicine
Baystate Greenfield Family Medicine
Greenfield, Massachusetts

Matthew J. Kor, MD
Family Physician
Department of Family Medicine
Mark Twain Medical Center
San Andreas, California

Sharmilee Korets, MD
Associate Professor
Department of Gynecologic Oncology
UMass Chan School of Medicine
Worcester, Massachusetts

Electra Korn, MD
Fellow
Department of Urogynecology
UMass Memorial
Worcester, Massachusetts

Nora Elizabeth Kratz, MD
Resident Physician
Department of Family Medicine and Community Medicine
University of New Mexico
Albuquerque, New Mexico

Briana D. Krewson, DO, MPH
Department of Family Medicine
University of Wisconsin-Madison
Madison, Wisconsin

Anna Krzywiec, DO
Resident
Department of Emergency Medicine
Advocate Christ Medical Center
Oak Lawn, Illinois

Pankaj Ksheersagar, MD, FAAP
Assistant Professor
Family Medicine and Community Health
University of Massachusetts
Worcester, Massachusetts

Jameson Kuang, MD
Assistant Professor
Department of Internal Medicine–Pediatrics
University of South Florida Morsani College of Medicine
Tampa, Florida

Daniel B. Kurtz, PhD, BS[†]
Professor Emeritus
Department of Biology
Utica College
Utica, New York

Melinda Kwan, DO, MPH
Urgent Care Physician
Urgent Care Department
Southwest Medical Associates
Las Vegas, Nevada

Makayla B. Lagerman, MD
Resident Physician
Department of Family and Community Medicine
Penn State Milton S. Hershey Medical Center
Hershey, Pennsylvania

Shane L. Larson, MD[†]
Assistant Professor of Family Medicine
Uniformed Services University of the Health Sciences
Womack Army Medical Center
Fort Bragg, North Carolina

Kelley V. Lawrence, MD, NABBLM-C
Associate Program Director
Department of Family Medicine Residency
Novant Health
Cornelius, North Carolina
Assistant Dean
UNC School of Medicine Novant Health Charlotte Campus
Novant Health
Charlotte, North Carolina
Associate Professor
Department of Family Medicine
UNC School of Medicine
Chapel Hill, North Carolina

Cindy Le, MD
Physician Resident
Department of Internal Medicine
UMass Chan Medical School
Worcester, Massachusetts

Chanel M. Lear, DO, MBS
Resident
Department of Family Medicine
Evara Health
Clearwater, Florida

Daniel T. Lee, MD, MA
Clinical Professor
Department of Family Medicine
David Geffen School of Medicine at UCLA
Associate Program Director
Department of Family Medicine
UCLA Family Medicine Residency Program
Santa Monica, California

Hobart Lee, MD, FAAFP
Vice Chair
Department of Family Medicine
Loma Linda University School of Medicine
Loma Linda, California

Madeline E. Lee, MD
Department of Family and Community Medicine
Penn State Health Milton S. Hershey Medical Center
Hershey, Pennsylvania

Frederic Stuart Leeds, MD, MS, FAAFP
Associate Professor
Department of Family Medicine
Wright State University Boonshoft School of Medicine
Dayton, Ohio

Wodwentzky Lefranc, MD
Resident
Department of Family Medicine
Lakeside Medical Center
Belle Glade, Florida

Angelia Leipelt, BA, IBCLC, IBD, ICCE
Lactation Consultant
Maternity Department
Lucile Packard Children's Hospital Stanford
Palo Alto, California
Lactation Coordinator
Family Birth Center
Common Spirit Health - Methodist Hospital of Sacramento
Sacramento, California

Frances Leung, MD, MPH[†]
Sports Medicine Fellow
Harbor UCLA
Los Angeles, California

Gary I. Levine, MD
Associate Professor
Department of Family Medicine
Brody School of Medicine
East Carolina University
Greenville, North Carolina

Briana Lindberg, MD, CAQSM
Associate Program Director
Department of Family Medicine
Womack Army Medical Center Family Medicine Residency Program
Fort Bragg, North Carolina

Stephen W. Line, DO, CAQSM
Clinical Assistant Professor
Department of Primary Care and Rural Health
Texas A&M University
College Station, Texas

Timothy S. Lishnak, MD
Assistant Professor
Department of Family Medicine
University of Connecticut School of Medicine
Farmington, Connecticut

Sahoko Hirano Little, MD, PhD
Clinical Associate Professor
Department of Family Medicine
University of Michigan

Elizabeth A. Lorick, MD
Assistant Professor
Department of Family Medicine
University of Connecticut Health
Farmington, Connecticut

Kiran A. Lorick, MD
Assistant Professor
Department of Family Medicine
University of Connecticut Health
Farmington, Connecticut

Kevin Loughry, DO
Associate Program Director
Department of Internal Medicine
Advocate Christ Medical Center
Oak Lawn, Illinois

Jacquelynn Parks Luker, MD
Assistant Professor
Department of Family, Internal, and Rural Medicine
The University of Alabama
Tuscaloosa, Alabama

Andrew Lutzkanin, MD
Associate Professor
Department of Family and Community Medicine
Penn State College of Medicine
Hershey, Pennsylvania

Ann M. Lynch, BSP, PharmD
Adjunct Faculty
Department of Pharmacy Practice
Massachusetts College of Pharmacy and Health Sciences
Worcester, Massachusetts

Jonathan Edward MacClements, MD, FAAFP
Professor
Department of Medical Education and Population Health
Dell Medical School, The University of Texas at Austin
Austin, Texas

Nathan J. Macedo, MD, MPH
Assistant Professor
Department of Family Medicine
UMass Chan Medical School-Baystate
Springfield, Massachusetts

James Mack, DO
Robert Wood Johnson University Hospital
New Brunswick, New Jersey

Theodore E. Macnow, MD
Associate Professor of Pediatrics
Department of Pediatric Emergency
UMass Memorial Children's Medical Center/ UMass Chan Medical School
Worcester, Massachusetts

Maxwell Shayan Madani, MD
Washington, District of Columbia

Michael J. Maddaleni, MD, CAQSM
Department of Family Medicine/Sports Medicine
UMass Chan Medical School
Worcester, Massachusetts

Manju Mahajan, MD, FAAFP
Faculty
Department of Family Medicine and Community Health
Hahnemann Family Health Center
UMass Chan Medical School
Worcester, Massachusetts

Justin Maher, MD
Resident Physician
Baystate Medical Center
Greenfield, Massachusetts

Deepali Maheshwari, DO, MPH†
Fellow
Department of Obstetrics and Gynecology
UMass Chan Medical School
Worcester, Massachusetts

Janki Majithia, DO
Department of Family Medicine
Advocate Christ Family Medicine Residency
Oak Lawn, Illinois

Shivani Malhotra, MD, FAAFP
Associate Professor and Regional Chair
Department of Family Medicine
UAB Family Medicine Program
Huntsville, Alabama

Laura Mallinger, DO
Resident Physician
Department of Internal Medicine
Advocate Christ Medical Center
Oak Lawn, Illinois

Lee A. Mancini, MD, CAQSM, CSCS*D, CSN
Associate Professor
Department of Family Medicine and Community Health
Chief, Division of Sports and Exercise Medicine
Director, Primary Care Sports and Exercise Medicine Fellowship
University of Massachusetts
Worcester, Massachusetts

Ramandeep Mangat, MD
Resident
Department of Family Medicine
United Health Services
Johnson City, New York

Eric J. Mao, MD
Associate Professor
Department of Medicine, Division of Gastroenterology and Hepatology
University of California, Davis
Sacramento, California

Jill W. Marsh, MD
Assistant Professor
Department of Family and Community Medicine
UAB Heersink School of Medicine
Birmingham, Alabama

Laura Marsh, MD, CAQSM
Program Director
Sports Medicine Fellowship
Clinical Assistant Professor
Department of Primary Care and Rural Medicine
Texas A&M University
College Station, Texas

Bethany Marshall, PharmD
Clinical Pharmacy Specialist
Prisma Health
Sumter, South Carolina

William Edwin Martin, MD, MBA, MPH
Medical Director
Mediprise
Houston, Texas

Lisa C. Martinez, MD
Associate Professor
Department of Medicine
Florida Atlantic University
Boca Raton, Florida

Donnah Mathews, MD, FACP
Assistant Professor
Department of Internal Medicine
Alpert School of Medicine at Brown University
Providence, Rhode Island

Sean T. Matsuwaka, MD
Assistant Professor
Department of Rehabilitation Medicine
University of Washington
Seattle, Washington

Daniel R. Matta, MD, DFPHM, FAAFP
Family Medicine Residency Faculty
Department of Family Medicine
Tallahassee Memorial Hospital Family Medicine Residency Program
Tallahassee, Florida

Geoffrey Matthes, MD, MSc
Resident Physician
Internal Medicine
UMass Chan Medical School
Worcester, Massachusetts

Anysha K. Mattu, MD
Resident
Department of Family Medicine
Creighton University
Omaha, Nebraska

Douglas M. Maurer, DO, MPH, FAAFP†
Director, Medical Education
Department of Family Medicine
Madigan Army Medical Center
Tacoma, Washington

George Maxted, MD
Associate Clinical Professor
Department of Family Medicine
Tufts University School of Medicine
Adjunct Associate Clinical Professor
Department of Family Medicine
Boston University School of Medicine
Boston, Massachusetts

Beth K. Mazyck, MD
Associate Professor
Family Medicine and Community Health
UMass Chan Medical School
Worcester, Massachusetts

Andrew McBride, MD, CAQSM
Senior Instructor
Department of Family Medicine
University of Colorado School of Medicine
Aurora, Colorado

Adam McConnell, MD
Medical Director
SSM Family Medicine Residency
SSM Health St. Anthony
Oklahoma City, Oklahoma

Rachel KM McCool, MD
Resident Physician
Department of Family Medicine
David Grant Medical Center
Fairfield, California

Stephen McCormick, MD, MPH
Associate Professor
Donald and Barbara Zucker School of Medicine at Hofstra/Northwell
Hempstead, New York

Christopher McDaniel, MD
Associate Program Director
Baptist Memorial Medical Education
Southaven, Mississippi

Susan McDiarmid, EdD, MS, PA-C
Assistant Program Director
Physician Assistant Program
Westfield State University
Westfield, Massachusetts

Michelle Moran McDonough, MD
Co-Chief Resident
Department of Family Medicine Residency Program
Mayo Clinic-Mankato
Mankato, Minnesota

Marc McKenna, MD, CAQSM
Program Director
Chestnut Hill Family Medicine Residency
Philadelphia, Pennsylvania

Michael R. McNeely, MD†
Family Medicine Physician
Family Health Clinic
United States Air Force
JBER, Alaska

Emily M. Meara, MD
Department of Dermatology
UMass Chan Medical School
Worcester, Massachusetts

Madhavi Medipally, MD, FAAFP
Assistant Professor
University of Massachusetts
Worcester, Massachusetts

William B. Meier, MD
Resident
Department of Family Medicine
Creighton University School of Medicine
Omaha, Nebraska

Randi Cheree Melton, DO
Assistant Professor
Department of Family Medicine/Obstetrics
Tuscaloosa Family Medicine Residency Program
Tuscaloosa, Alabama

Donna I. Meltzer, MD
Clinical Associate Professor
Department of Family, Population and Preventive Medicine
Associate Vice Chair of Healthcare Quality, Patient Safety and Compliance
Department of Family Medicine
Renaissance School of Medicine at Stony Brook University
Stony Brook, New York

Taras Memko, MD
Resident
Department of Family Medicine
Lakeside Medical Center
Belle Glade, Florida

Adam Mendonca, MD[†]
Resident Physician
Department of Family and Community Medicine
Baylor College of Medicine
Houston, Texas

Chelsea Mendonca, MD[†]
Assistant Professor
Department of Family and Community Medicine
Baylor College of Medicine
Houston, Texas

Joseph L. Mercen, DO
Resident Physician
Department of Family Medicine
Mike O'Callaghan Medical Center
Las Vegas, Nevada

Marcelle Meseeha, MD, FACP
Assistant Professor
Department of Internal Medicine
Guthrie
Sayre, Pennsylvania

Daniel Michniuk, DO, MS
Core Faculty
Department of Internal Medicine
Advocate Lutheran General Hospital
Park Ridge, Illinois

Jan Estes Miller, MD
Associate Program Director
Family Medicine Residency
SSM Health St. Anthony
Oklahoma City, Oklahoma

Megan Mendez Miller, DO
Department of Family and Community Medicine
Penn State Health Milton S. Hershey Medical Center
Harrisburg, Pennsylvania

Erica Minor, DO
Resident Physician
Department of Psychiatry
Advocate Lutheran General Hospital
Park Ridge, Illinois

Tasaduq Hussain Mir, MD, FAAFP
Faculty
Department of Family Medicine
Medical City Arlington
Arlington, Texas

Farukh Ali Mirza, MD
Resident Physician
Department of Family Medicine
Baptist Memorial Hospital-DeSoto
Southaven, Mississippi

Mohammed Mirza, MD
Advocate Christ Hospital
Oak Lawn, Illinois

Naisargi Modi, MD
Resident Physician
Department of Internal Medicine
John H. Stroger, Jr. Hospital of Cook County
Chicago, Illinois

Cliff C. Moeckelmann, MD
Department of Family Medicine Residency
Community Health Care Family Medicine Residency
Tacoma, Washington

Hammad Mohsin, MD
Assistant Professor
Department of Psychiatry
Mather at Northwell Health
Port Jefferson, New York

Saadia Mohsin, MD
Physician Capital Health
Pennington, New Jersey

Nahid N. Molaie, MD
Associate Professor
Family Medicine Department Harbor-UCLA Medical Center
Torrance, California

Tamara Kailoa Montacute, MD, MPH
Clinical Associate Professor
Department of Medicine
Stanford University School of Medicine
Palo Alto, California

Nicholas Moore, MD, FAAFP, CAQSM
Medical Director
Motor City Orthopedics and Sports Medicine
Associate Director
Providence Sports Medicine Fellowship Program
Assistant Professor
Michigan State University College of Human Medicine
Novi, Michigan

Jared Morphew, MD
Assistant Professor
Department of Family and Community Medicine
UT Southwestern Medical Center
Dallas, Texas

Laquita Morris, MD
Assistant Professor
Department of Family Medicine
UMass Chan Medical School
Worcester, Massachusetts

Daniel Scott Morrison, MD
Associate Professor
Department of Emergency Medicine
Rutgers Robert Wood Johnson Medical School
New Brunswick, New Jersey

Christopher Morrow, PA-C[†]
United States Army

Matthew Morrow, DO
Resident Physician
Department of Family Medicine
UMass Memorial Hospital
Worcester, Massachusetts

Maydolis Mosquera Garcia, MD
Omaha, Nebraska

Christopher Moyer, MD
Creighton University
Omaha, Nebraska

Sahil Mullick, MD, FAAFP
Associate Program Director, Assistant Clinical Professor
Hospitalist, Director of Inpatient Service
Department of Family and Community Medicine
CHI Health Creighton University Medical Center - Bergan Mercy Hospital
Omaha, Nebraska

Mark T. Nadeau, MD[†]
Professor
Department of Family and Community Medicine
UT Health San Antonio
San Antonio, Texas

Sabari Nair, DO
Resident Physician
Department of Family Medicine
Lakeside Medical Center
Belle Glade, Florida

Munima Nasir, MD, FAAFP
Associate Professor
Department of Family and Community Medicine
Penn State Health Milton S. Hershey Medical Center
Hershey, Pennsylvania

Michelle Nelson, MD, FAAFP
Clinical Assistant Professor
Department of Family Medicine
Michigan State University College of Human Medicine
East Lansing, Michigan

Vicki R. Nelson, MD, PhD
Associate Professor
Department of Family Medicine
Prisma Health-Upstate
University of South Carolina School of Medicine Greenville
Greenville, South Carolina

Sandra N. New, DNP
Retired
Knoxville, Tennessee

Zakary S. Newberry, MD
Resident
Department of Family and Community Medicine
Penn State Health Milton S. Hershey Medical Center
Hershey, Pennsylvania

Jacob Thomas Newman, DO
Resident Physician
Department of Internal Medicine
The George Washington University Hospital
Washington, District of Columbia

Roland W. Newman II, DO
Assistant Professor
Associate Program Director—Family and Community Medicine Residency Program
Department of Family and Community Medicine
Penn State Health Milton S. Hershey Medical Center
Hershey, Pennsylvania

Andrew Timothy Ng, MBBS
Resident Physician
Department of Internal Medicine
Baystate Medical Center
Springfield, Massachusetts

Jeremy Ng, MD, CAQSM
Assistant Professor
Department of Primary Care Sports Medicine
Boston University School of Medicine
Boston Medical Center
Boston, Massachusetts

Melinda W. Ng, MD
Resident Physician
Department of Family Medicine
David Grant Medical Center
Fairfield, California

An-Thu N. Nguyen, DO
Resident Physician
Department of Family Medicine
HonorHealth
Scottsdale, Arizona

Elizabeth T. Nguyen, MD, CAQSM, FAAP
Department of Texas A&M Athletics
Department of Primary Care and Rural Medicine
Texas A&M University
College Station, Texas

Hieu Nguyen, DO
Assistant Professor
Department of Family Medicine
Western University of Health Sciences
Pomona, California

Nancy V. Nguyen, DO
Core Faculty, Methodist Hospital Family Medicine Residency Programs
Chair Family Medicine
Dignity Health Methodist Hospital of Sacramento
Sacramento, California

Tam T. Nguyen, MD
Washington Township Medical Group
Union City, California

Tu Dan Nguyen, MD, CAQSM
Director of Sports Medicine
Department of Family Medicine
Memorial Family Medicine Residency Program
Sugar Land, Texas

Jacqueline O. Nicholas, MD, BA
Department of Emergency Medicine
Robert Wood Johnson University Hospital
New Brunswick, New Jersey

Myles Stanley Nickolich, MD
Associate Professor of Medicine
Department of Medicine, Penn State Cancer Institute
Penn State College of Medicine
Hershey, Pennsylvania

Sarah E. Nickolich, MD
Assistant Professor
Department of Family and Community Medicine
Penn State Health Milton S. Hershey Medical Center
Hershey, Pennsylvania

Frederick W. Nielson, MD†
MAJ, USAF, MC
Department of Family Medicine
US Air Force
Eielson Air Force Base, Alaska

Matthew A. Niemi, MD
Associate Professor
Department of Medicine
UMass Medical School
Worcester, Massachusetts

Livia Yumi Maruoka Nishi, MD
Faculty
Department of Family Medicine with Obstetrics
FSU Tallahassee Memorial Hospital
Tallahassee, Florida

Jaret Nishikawa, MD
Resident Physician
Department of Family Medicine Residency and Sports Medicine
University of Washington
Seattle, Washington

Stanley Nkemjika, MD, MPH
Addiction Psychiatry Fellow
Department of Psychiatry and Human Behavior
Thomas Jefferson University
Philadelphia, Pennsylvania

Stephanie Núñez-González, MD, MPH
Resident Physician
Department of Family Medicine
University of South Florida Morsani College of Medicine
Tampa General Hospital
Tampa, Florida

Victoria Allon Nutting, DO, MS
Resident Physician
Department of Family Medicine Residency
Texas A&M University
College Station, Texas

Ogechukwu Nwanegwo, MD
Family Medicine Resident
Saint Louis University Southwest Illinois Family Medicine Program
O'Fallon, Illinois

Gabryel A. Obedoza, MD
Resident Physician
Department of Family Medicine
Cambridge Health Alliance
Malden, Massachusetts

Mateusz Ogledzinski, MD
Resident
Department of Family Medicine
Creighton University
Omaha, Nebraska

Smriti Ohri, MD
Associate Professor
Department of Family Medicine
Oregon Health and Science University
Portland, Oregon

Alicia Leandra Olowu, DO
Core Faculty
Department of Family Medicine
Garnet Health Medical Center
Middletown, New York

Toluwanimi V. Oludiran-Ayoade, MD, BSc
Department of Internal Medicine
Advocate Christ Medical Center
Oak Lawn, Illinois

Opeoluwa Olukorede, MD, MS
Family Medicine Resident
Department of Family Medicine
UMass Chan Medical School
Worcester, Massachusetts

Adedamola Ayo Omole, MD
Attending Physician
Department of Family Medicine
Adventist Health Hanford
Hanford, California

Janet A. Omole, MD
Resident Physician
Department of Internal Medicine
Advocate Christ Medical Center
Oak Lawn, Illinois

Keyona Oni, MD, IBCLC
Assistant Professor
Department of Family Medicine
Novant Health
Charlotte, North Carolina

Zoe Onion, MD
Resident
Department of Family Medicine
University of Massachusetts
Worcester, Massachusetts

Eugene Orientale Jr., MD
Professor Emeritus
Department of Family Medicine
University of Connecticut School of Medicine
Farmington, Connecticut

Jessica A. Orner, MD
Assistant Professor
Department of Family and Community Medicine
Penn State Health Milton S. Hershey Medical Center
Hershey, Pennsylvania

Bhreagh Orrell, MD
Department of Family Medicine
United Health Services Hospitals, Inc.
Johnson City, New York

Anthony Lloyd Overfield, MD
Resident Physician
Department of 96 HCOS
Eglin Family Medicine Residency
Eglin AFB, Florida

Saleha Ozair, MD
Resident Physician
Department of Internal Medicine
Larkin Community Hospital
Miami, Florida

Seniha Ozudogru, MD
Assistant Professor
Department of Neurology
University of Pennsylvania
Philadelphia, Pennsylvania

Kelly Pagidas, MD
Professor
Texas Christian University
Fort Worth, Texas

Amar Pandit, MD
Assistant Professor
Department of Medicine, Renal Division
UMass Chan Medical School
Worcester, Massachusetts

Christopher C. Paredes, MD
Regional Director
Northwell Health
New York, New York

Jon S. Parham, DO, MPH, FAAFP
Associate Professor
Department of Family Medicine
University of Tennessee Graduate School of Medicine
Knoxville, Tennessee

Susie J. Park, MD
Resident
Department of Internal Medicine
George Washington University Medical Center
Washington, District of Columbia

Naomi Parrella, MD, Dipl. ABOM, FOMA, FAAFP
Associate Professor and Medical Director
Department of Family Medicine
Department of Surgery
Rush University Medical Center
Chicago, Illinois

Michael T. Partin, MD
Assistant Professor
Department of Family and Community Medicine
Penn State Health Milton S. Hershey Medical Center
Hershey, Pennsylvania

Bindusri Paruchuri, MD
Advanced Women's Health Care Fellow
Department of Family Medicine
University of Tennessee
Memphis, Tennessee

Avignat S. Patel, MD
Senior Physician
Department of Pulmonary Critical Care Medicine
Lahey Hospital and Medical Center
Burlington, Massachusetts
Assistant Professor
Department of Medicine
Tufts University School of Medicine
Boston, Massachusetts

Avinash Patel, MD
Department of Family Medicine
Baptist Memorial Hospital-DeSoto
Southaven, Mississippi

Bhavin Bharat Patel, DO
Assistant Professor
Department of Hospital Medicine
UMass Chan Medical School
Worcester, Massachusetts

Bhumika Patel, DO
Resident Physician
Department of Family Medicine
University of Connecticut School of Medicine
Farmington, Connecticut

Birju B. Patel, MD, FACP, AGSF†
Adjunct Assistant Professor of Medicine
Emory University School of Medicine
Atlanta, Georgia

Jay Patel, DO
Resident
Department of Family Medicine
Dell Medical School, The University of Texas at Austin
Austin, Texas

Mahesh C. Patel, MD
Professor
Department of Internal Medicine-Infectious Diseases
University of Illinois at Chicago
Chicago, Illinois

Nihal K. Patel, MD
Assistant Clinical Professor
Department of Medicine
University of Connecticut School of Medicine
Harford, Connecticut

Ronak S. Patel, DO
Resident Physician
Department of Internal Medicine
Advocate Lutheran General Hospital
Park Ridge, Illinois

Sneha K. Patel, MD, MS
Resident Physician
Department of Family Medicine
Creighton University
Omaha, Nebraska

Amrutha Pavle, MD
Assistant Professor
Department of Family and Community Medicine
UT Southwestern Medical Center
Dallas, Texas

Amena Payami, DO
Family Medicine Resident Physician
AdventHealth East Orlando
Orlando, Florida

Elizabeth M. Payment, MD
Core Faculty
Department of Family Medicine
Advocate Christ
Oak Lawn, Illinois

Sean Pazurchek, DO, MPH
Resident
Department of Family Medicine
Baystate Health
Greenfield, Massachusetts

Rade N. Pejic, MD
Associate Professor
Department of Family Medicine
Tulane University School of Medicine
New Orleans, Louisiana

Bernadette Pendergraph, MD
Program Director
Department of Sports Medicine
Harbor-UCLA Medical Center
Harbor City, California

Austin Peppers, MD
Department of Family Medicine
Greenfield Family Medicine Residency
Greenfield, Massachusetts

Daniel Perez, MD
Faculty
Department of Family Medicine
Lakeside Medical Center
Belle Glades, Florida

Juan Perez, DO
Assistant Professor
Department of Family Medicine
Penn State University
Reading, Pennsylvania

Mayra A. Perez, DO
Clinical Assistant Professor
Department of Family and Community Medicine
UT Health San Antonio
San Antonio, Texas

Elimarys Pérez-Colón, MD
Associate Professor and Associate Program Director
Department of Internal Medicine–Pediatrics
University of South Florida Morsani College of Medicine
Tampa, Florida

Zoey Perham, MD
Resident
Department of Internal Medicine
Charles E. Schmidt College of Medicine
Florida Atlantic University
Boca Raton, Florida

Christine S. Persaud, MD, MBA
Assistant Professor, Program Director—Sports Medicine Fellowship
Department of Orthopaedic Surgery and Rehabilitation Medicine
SUNY Downstate Health Sciences University
Brooklyn, New York

Parvathi Perumareddi, DO
Associate Professor
Charles E. Schmidt College of Medicine
Florida Atlantic University
Boca Raton, Florida

Kelsey E. Phelps, MD†
Assistant Professor of Family Medicine
Louisiana State University Rural Family Medicine Residency
Bogalusa Louisiana State University
Bogalusa, Louisiana

D. Melessa Phillips, MD, MPH
Faculty
Mississippi Delta Family Medicine Residency
Delta Health System
Greenville, Mississippi

Sarah A. Pierotti, DO, FAAP, CAQSM
Program Director
Department of Sports Medicine
Advocate Lutheran General
Park Ridge, Illinois
Associate Clinical Professor
Department of Orthopedics
Rosalind Franklin University Medical School
North Chicago, Illinois

Grant Pierre, MD, CAQSM
Faculty UMass Sports Medicine Fellowship
Department of Family Medicine
University of Massachusetts
Worcester, Massachusetts

Anush Pillai, DO, FAAFP
Residency Program Director
Department of Family Medicine
Houston Methodist
Houston, Texas

Sreelakshmi Surendran Pillai, MD
Resident
Department of Family Medicine
Creighton University Medical Center
Omaha, Nebraska

Karly Pippitt, MD
Assistant Dean, Community Faculty
Department of Family and Preventive Medicine
University of Utah School of Medicine
Salt Lake City, Utah

William Andrew Pleasant, MD
Assistant Professor
Department of Emergency Medicine
Rutgers Robert Wood Johnson Medical School
New Brunswick, New Jersey

Alexander Pomerantz, MD, MPP
Fellow
Department of Primary Care Sports Medicine
Boston University School of Medicine
Boston Medical Center
Boston, Massachusetts

Yevgeniy Popov, DO, MPH
Assistant Professor
Department of Rheumatology
University of Massachusetts
Worcester, Massachusetts

Stacy E. Potts, MD, Med
Professor
Executive Vice Chair of Education
Department of Family Medicine and Community Health
UMass Chan Medical School
Worcester, Massachusetts

Anne C. Powell, MD
Chief, Division of Adolescent Medicine
Assistant Professor
UMass Chan Medical School
UMass Memorial Medical Center
Worcester, Massachusetts

James E. Powers, DO
Associate Dean for Clinical Integration; Professor of Emergency Medicine
Campbell University School of Osteopathic Medicine
Lillington, North Carolina

Priya Prasher, MBBS
Pediatric Emergency Medicine Fellow
Department of Emergency Medicine
Phoenix Children's Hospital
Phoenix, Arizona

Bethany Price, DO
Residency Faculty
Department of Family Medicine
Saint Mary's Family Medicine Residency
Grand Junction, Colorado

Bliss Puthenpurayil, MD
Department of Family Medicine
University of Texas Southwestern
Dallas, Texas

Natasha J. Pyzocha, DO, FAWM, FAAFP
Medical Director
98point6
Seattle, Washington

Juan Qiu, MD, PhD
Professor
Department of Family and Community Medicine
Pennsylvania State University College of Medicine
State College, Pennsylvania

Alexandria Quinere, MBS, DO
Resident Physician
Department of Family Medicine
Garnet Health Medical Center
Middletown, New York

Jeffrey D. Quinlan, MD, FAAFP[†]
Professor, Chair, and DEO
Department of Family Medicine
Roy J. and Lucille A. Carver College of Medicine, University of Iowa
Iowa City, Iowa

Nicholas Radigan, MD
Resident
Department of Family Medicine
Baystate Health
Greenfield, Massachusetts

Kalyanakrishnan Ramakrishnan, MD, FRCS
Professor
Department of Family and Preventive Medicine
University of Oklahoma Health Sciences Center
Oklahoma City, Oklahoma

Srinath Ramakrishnan, MD
Internal Medicine Resident
Department of Medicine
UMass Chan Medical School
Worcester, Massachusetts

Melinda M. Rathkopf, MD, MBA
Associate Professor
Department of Pediatric Allergy and Immunology
Emory University School of Medicine
Atlanta, Georgia

Tharani Ravi, MD
Associate Professor
Department of Family and Community Medicine
UT Health San Antonio
San Antonio, Texas

Raye Reeder, MD, MPH
Assistant Professor
Department of Family and Community Medicine
OU School of Community Medicine
Tulsa, Oklahoma

Robyn Lee Reese, DO
Fellow
Department of Gerontology
Harvard Multicampus Geriatric Medicine Fellowship Program
Boston, Massachusetts

Abdelrhman Refaey, MD
Resident Physician
Department of Internal Medicine
Holy Name Medical Center
Teaneck, New Jersey
Research Fellow
Department of Gastroenterology & Liver Diseases
The George Washington University School of Medicine and Health Sciences
Washington, District of Columbia

Tomas P.J. Reilly, MD
Department of Family Medicine
Baystate Health
Greenfield, Massachusetts

Caitlyn M. Rerucha, MD, MSEd, FAAFP, CAQSM
Assistant Professor, Family Medicine
Department of Family and Community Medicine
Uniformed Services University School of Medicine
Assistant Program Director, Family Medicine Residency Program
Carl R. Darnall Army Medical Center
Fort Cavazos, Texas

George Edsel Reusser, MD
Primary Care Physician
Associate Clinical Director
Family and Community Medicine Residency Core Faculty
Department of Family Medicine
Graduate Medical Education
Yuma Regional Medical Center
Yuma, Arizona

Mehak Riaz, MBBS, MSc
Medical Intern
Lemuel Shattuck Hospital
Boston, Massachusetts

Kristen Richard, MD
Pediatric Pulmonologist
Assistant Professor
Department of Pediatrics
UMass Memorial Medical Children's Center
UMass Chan Medical School
Worcester, Massachusetts

Jon Richards, MD, PhD
Department of Hematology/Oncology
Advocate Lutheran General Hospital
Park Ridge, Illinois

Michael Richardson, MD
Clinical Assistant Professor
Family Medicine
Tufts University School of Medicine
Boston, Massachusetts

Jacob Ringenberg, MD, CAQSM, MUSC, AHEC
Assistant Professor
Self Regional Healthcare
Greenwood, South Carolina

Candace Ripperda, MD
Clinical Assistant Professor
Department of Family Medicine
Baylor College of Medicine
Temple, Texas

Michele Roberts, MD, PhD
Paxton, Massachusetts

Cecile T. Robes, DO
Associate Professor
Department of Family Medicine
Novant Health Family Medicine Residency
Cornelius, North Carolina

Sean C. Robinson, MD, CAQSM
Assistant Professor
Department of Family Medicine and Sports Medicine
Oregon Health & Science University
Portland, Oregon

Sylvia M. Robinson, MD
Physician
Department of Pediatrics
Ann and Robert H. Lurie Children's Hospital of Chicago
Chicago, Illinois

Rashmi Rode, MD, FAAFP
Associate Professor
Department of Family Medicine
Baylor College of Medicine
Houston, Texas

Angela Rodgers, MD, FAAFP
Assistant Clinical Professor
Department of Family and Community Medicine
University of California, San Francisco
San Francisco, California
Core Faculty
Department of Emergency Medicine
Contra Costa Family Medicine Residency Program
Martinez, California

Rachel S. Rodriguez, MD, FAAFP
Assistant Professor
Department of Family Medicine
University of Colorado School of Medicine
Aurora, Colorado

Paloma Rodriguez, MD
Endocrinology and Metabolism Institute
Cleveland Clinic
Cleveland, Ohio

Kara Ann Romanowski, MD
Resident Physician
Department of Family and Community Medicine
Penn State Milton S. Hershey Medical Center
Hershey, Pennsylvania

Crystal L. Romero, MD, MPH
Clinical Assistant Professor
Department of Family Medicine
University of Florida
Gainesville, Florida

Leigh Romero, MD, CAQSM
Assistant Professor
Department of Population Health
Dell Medical School, The University of Texas at Austin
Austin, Texas

Jennifer M. Romeu, MD, FAAFP, MSM
Associate Program Director
Family Medicine Residency Program
Central Michigan University College of Medicine
Saginaw, Michigan

Scott Rosen, MD
Assistant Professor
Department of Internal Medicine
Baptist Memorial Medical Education
Southaven, Mississippi

Chad M. Ross, MD
Resident Physician
Department of Family Medicine/Graduate Medical Education
Baptist Memorial Hospital
Southaven, Mississippi

Laura Ross, MD
Hospitalist
Novant Health Huntersville Medical Center
Huntersville, North Carolina

Daniela Diaz Rubayo, MD
Resident Physician
Department of Urology
UMass Chan Medical School
Worcester, Massachusetts

Stacy P. Rubin, MD
Assistant Professor
Department of Internal Medicine
Charles E. Schmidt College of Medicine
Florida Atlantic University
Boca Raton, Florida

Abbas Rupawala, MD
Director
Inflammatory Bowel Diseases Center
Department of Medicine, Division of Gastroenterology
UMass Memorial Medical Center
Worcester, Massachusetts

Veronica Sabate, MD
Resident Physician
Department of Family and Community Medicine
University of Texas Health Science Center San Antonio
San Antonio, Texas

Anup Sabharwal, MD, MBA, FACC, FACE, FASPC, FNLA, FEAA
Professor
Department of Endocrinology, Diabetes, and Metabolism
Florida International University
Miami Beach, Florida

Richard A. Sacra, MD
Assistant Professor
Department of Family Medicine and Community Health
UMass Chan Medical School
Worcester, Massachusetts

Kristen EB Said, MD, MPH
Assistant Professor
Department of Family Medicine and Community Health
Duke University
Durham, North Carolina

Nida Ali Sajan, DO
Baylor Scott and White
Waco, Texas

Kyle M. Samyn, DO, MS
Sports Medicine Fellow
Department of Sports Medicine
Ascension Providence Hospital
Novi, Michigan

Jasmine Kaur Sandhu, MD
Family Medicine Resident
WellSpan Good Samaritan Hospital Family Medicine Residency Program
Lebanon, Pennsylvania

Vicente T. San Martin, MD
Medical Director
Department of Endocrinology
Macromedica
Santo Domingo, Dominican Republic

Sagar Saoji, MD
Resident Physician
Department of Family Medicine
Lakeside Medical Center
Belle Glade, Florida

Arindam Sarkar, MD, FAAFP
Assistant Professor
Department of Family and Community Medicine
Baylor College of Medicine
Houston, Texas

Brianna K. Sarowa, MD
Resident
Department of Family Medicine
SUNY Downstate Health Sciences University
Brooklyn, New York

Luay Sarsam, MD
Department of Cardiovascular Disease
Arnot Ogden Medical Center
Elmira, New York

Francesco Satriale, MD
Resident Physician
Department of Family and Community Medicine
Penn State Health Milton S. Hershey Medical Center
Hershey, Pennsylvania

Sarah A. Satriale, PA-C
Physician Assistant
Department of Family Medicine
Penn State Health
Hershey, Pennsylvania

Durr-e-Shahwaar Sayed, DO
Attending Physician
Department of Family Medicine
Inspira Medical Group
Woodbury, New Jersey

Payam Sazegar, MD†
Kaiser Permanente San Diego Family Medicine Residency
San Diego, California

Catherine Schaefer, MD, MS, BS
Program Director
Prisma Health Sumter
Family Medicine Residency
Department of Family Medicine
Prisma Health
Sumter, South Carolina

Kendal Schaetzle, DO
Christiana Care Family Medicine Residency
Wilmington, Delaware

Laura J. Schoerning, DO
Assistant Professor
Department of Family Medicine
UMass Memorial Medical Center
Worcester, Massachusetts

Jennifer Schwartz, MD†
Newton Wellesley Hospital
Newton, Massachusetts

Ingrid U. Scott, MD, MPH†
Jack and Nancy Turner Professor
Department of Ophthalmology
Professor of Public Health Sciences
Penn State College of Medicine
Hershey, Pennsylvania

Jarrett Keller Sell, MD, FAAFP, AAHIVS
Associate Professor
Department of Family and Community Medicine
Penn State Health Milton S. Hershey Medical Center
Hershey, Pennsylvania

Kristofer Lee Setterstrom, MD, BSc
Resident
Department of Family Medicine
St Johns Family Medicine Residency
St Paul, Minnesota

Haley Severin, DO, MS
Resident
Department of Family Medicine
University of Tennessee Health Sciences Center
Memphis, Tennessee

Anthony Shadiack, DO, CAQSM
Associate Program Director, Family Medicine
HCA Healthcare/Mercer University School of Medicine
Grand Strand Medical Center
Myrtle Beach, South Carolina

Blake R. Shaffer, MD†
Flight Surgeon/SOFME
AFSOC
Hurlburt AFB
Hurlburt Field, Florida

Aarsh Shah, DO
Resident Physician
Department of Emergency Medicine
Rutgers Robert Wood Johnson Medical School
New Brunswick, New Jersey

Chirag N. Shah, MD
Associate Professor
Department of Emergency Medicine
Rutgers Robert Wood Johnson Medical School
New Brunswick, New Jersey

Nehal R. Shah, MD†
Associate Professor of Medicine
Department of Internal Medicine/Rheumatology
Virginia Commonwealth University
Richmond, Virginia

Samir A. Shah, MD, AGAF, FACG, FASGE
Clinical Professor of Medicine
Department of Medicine/Gastroenterology
Alpert Medical School of Brown University
Chief of Gastroenterology
Department of Gastroenterology
The Miriam Hospital
Providence, Rhode Island

Ammar Shahid, MD†
Department of Sports Medicine
Tower Health and Drexel University
Philadelphia, Pennsylvania

Yara Shams, DO
Internal Medicine Faculty Attending
Advocate Christ Medical Center
Oak Lawn, Illinois

Raksha Sharma, MD
Department of Internal Medicine
Florida Atlantic University
Boca Raton, Florida

Jessalyn G. Shaw, MD
Assistant Professor
Department of Pediatrics
UMass Memorial Children's Medical Center
Worcester, Massachusetts

Vincent Shaw, MD
Program Director
Family Residency Program
Baton Rouge General Medical Center
Baton Rouge, Louisiana

Monika Shenouda, MD
Faculty Physician
Department of Graduate Medical Education-Family Medicine
California Hospital Medical Center
Los Angeles, California

Victoria Shepard, MD
Associate Program Director
Department of Population Health
Dell Medical School, The University of Texas at Austin
Austin, Texas

Grace Shih, MD, MAS
Professor
Department of Family Medicine
University of Washington
Seattle, Washington

Jeffrey Shih, MD
Associate Professor of Medicine
Medical Director, Ventricular Assist Device Program
Director, Advanced Heart Failure Program
Department of Medicine
University of Massachusetts
Worcester, Massachusetts

Humza Feroz Siddiqi, MD
Assistant Professor
Department of Family and Community Medicine
University of Texas Southwestern
Dallas, Texas

Irfan H. Siddiqui, MD
Attending Physician, Faculty
Department of Internal Medicine
Advocate Christ Medical Center
Oak Lawn, Illinois

Karlynn Sievers, MD
Associate Program Director
Department of Family Medicine
St. Mary's Family Medicine Residency Program
Grand Junction, Colorado

Matthew A. Silva, PharmD, RPh, BCPS
Professor
Pharmacy Practice
Massachusetts College of Pharmacy and Health Sciences - Worcester
Worcester, Massachusetts

Charanjot Singh, MD
Resident
Department of Family Medicine
WellSpan Good Samaritan Hospital
Lebanon, Pennsylvania

Madhavi Singh, MD†
Assistant Professor
Department of Family and Community Medicine
Penn State College of Medicine
Hershey, Pennsylvania

Navpreet K. Singh, MD
Department of Family Medicine and Sleep Medicine
Temple University
Philadelphia, Pennsylvania

Brian G. Skotko, MD, MPP
Emma Campbell Endowed Chair on Down Syndrome
Department of Pediatrics
Massachusetts General Hospital
Associate Professor
Department of Pediatrics
Harvard Medical School
Boston, Massachusetts

Karah A. Snider, DO
Chief Resident
Family Medicine Residency Program
Baptist Memorial Hospital-DeSoto
Southaven, Mississippi

Anastasia Sokhan, MD
Core Faculty
Department of Family Medicine
Lakeland Regional Health
Lakeland, Florida

Daniel J. Larez Solano, MD, MHA
Department of Family Medicine
Baptist Memorial Hospital-DeSoto
Southaven, Mississippi

D'Ann Wilson Somerall, FAANP, FNP-BC, DNP, CRNP, MAEd
Nurse Practitioner
Adjunct Assistant Professor
University of Alabama at Birmingham School of Nursing
Birmingham, Alabama

William E. Somerall Jr., MD, MAEd
Associate Professor
Department of School of Nursing
University of Alabama at Birmingham
Birmingham, Alabama

Kento Sonoda, MD
Assistant Professor
Department of Family and Community Medicine
Saint Louis University
St. Louis, Missouri

Alvin Soto Soto, MD
Resident Physician
Family Medicine Residency Program
Penn State Health St. Joseph Medical Center
Reading, Pennsylvania

Andrea Soto Abarca, MD
Resident
Department of Family Medicine
UT Health San Antonio
San Antonio, Texas

Mikayla L. Spangler, PharmD
Associate Professor
Department of Pharmacy Practice and Family Medicine
Creighton University
Omaha, Nebraska

Sawyer J. Sparks, DO
Chief Resident
Department of Family and Preventative Medicine
UAMS Northeast Family and Preventative Medicine
Jonesboro, Arkansas

Dana Sprute, MD, MPH, FAAFP
Associate Professor, Division of Family Medicine
Department of Population Health
Dell Medical School, The University of Texas at Austin
Austin, Texas

Akanksha Srivastava, MD
Resident Physician Department of OB/GYN
UMass Chan Medical School
Worcester, Massachusetts

Valerie Sarah Stark, MD, MPH
Resident Physician
School of Medicine & Health Sciences
George Washington University
Washington, District of Columbia

Mark B. Stephens, MD, MS, FAAFP
Associate Dean for Medical Education
Professor of Family and Community Medicine
Professor of Humanities
Penn State College of Medicine
University Park, Pennsylvania

Samuel Douglas Stringfellow, DO, BSc
Assistant Professor
UAMS Northeast Family Medicine Residency
University of Arkansas for Medical Sciences
Jonesboro, Arkansas

Adam Strosberg, DNP, ARNP-BC
Visiting Professor
Chamberlain University
Fort Lauderdale, Florida

Joshua T. Sutherland, MD, MS
Chief Resident
Department of Internal Medicine
Lutheran General Hospital
Park Ridge, Illinois

Jennifer E. Svarverud, DO†
Family Medicine Resident
Nellis Family Medicine Residency
Nellis Air Force Base, Nevada

Sasha S. Svendsen, MD
Assistant Professor
Department of Pediatrics
UMass Chan Medical School
Worcester, Massachusetts

Ryan Svoboda, MD, MS
Assistant Professor
Department of Dermatology
UMass Chan School of Medicine
Worcester, Massachusetts

Kayla Sweeten, MD
Department of Family Medicine
Baptist Memorial Hospital-DeSoto
Southaven, Mississippi

Valencia L. Swims, MD
Department of Family Medicine
Baptist Memorial
Southaven, Mississippi

Zubair A. Syed, MD
Associate Professor
Department of Family Medicine
UT Southwestern Medical Center
Dallas, Texas

Niloufar Akhavan Tabib, DO
Resident Physician
Department of Family Medicine
University of Massachusetts
Worcester, Massachusetts

Sandhya Tagaram, MD
Assistant Professor
Hospital Medicine
UMass Memorial Medical Center
Worcester, Massachusetts

Nergess T. Taheri, DO, MSBI
Assistant Program Director
Department of Family Medicine/Graduate Medical Education
Lakeside Medical Center
Belle Glade, Florida

Shelby Takeshita, MD†
Family Medicine Residency
David Grant Medical Center
Travis Air Force Base, California

Yuki Takeuchi, MD
Resident, Family Medicine
University of Rochester Medical Center
Rochester, New York

Irene J. Tan, MD, FACR†
Clinical Professor of Medicine
Department of Medicine
Sidney Kimmel School of Medicine, Thomas Jefferson University
Department of Medicine, Division of Rheumatology
Einstein Medical Center Philadelphia, Jefferson Health Systems
Philadelphia, Pennsylvania

Neil Tandon, MD
Resident Physician
Department of Family Medicine
University of Connecticut School of Medicine
Farmington, Connecticut

Madeline Taskier, MD
Research Instructor—Health Policy Fellow
Department of Family Medicine
George Washington University School of Medicine and Health Sciences
Washington, District of Columbia

Morris K. Taylor, MD
Resident
Department of Family and Community Medicine
Penn State Health Milton S. Hershey Medical Center
Hershey, Pennsylvania

Jason Teng, MD†
Attending Physician
Emergency Department
Virginia Hospital Center
Arlington, Virginia

Yuriko Terada, MD
Resident
Department of Family Medicine
University of Pittsburgh Medical Center Shadyside
Pittsburgh, Pennsylvania

Jayshree S. Thomas, DO
Fellow
Department of Population Health
The University of Texas at Austin Dell Medical School
Austin, Texas

Sarah M. Tiggelaar, MD, CLC
Assistant Professor
Department of Family Medicine
University of Rochester Medical Center
Rochester, New York

Edith Torres, DO
Resident
Department of Family and Community Health
UT Health San Antonio
San Antonio, Texas

Anna Marie Tran, DO
Resident Physician
Department of Family Medicine
Ascension St. Vincent's Hospital
Jacksonville, Florida

Thomas Triantafillou, MD
Assistant Professor
Department of Medicine
Advocate Christ Medical Center
Oak Lawn, Illinois

Alec L. Tributino, DO
Resident
Department of Family Medicine
University of Massachusetts
Worcester, Massachusetts

Anhthu Trinh, MD
Resident Physician
Department of Internal Medicine–Pediatrics
University of South Florida Morsani College of Medicine
Tampa, Florida

Zoltan Trizna, MD, PhD
Director
Department of Dermatology and Dermatological Surgery
Austin, Texas

Erin L. Trolley, MD
Department of Family Medicine
UMass Chan Medical School-Baystate Greenfield Family Medicine Residency Program
Greenfield, Massachusetts

Elizabeth Joyce Trout, MD, FAAFP, MLS (ASCP)
Resident
Department of Novant Health Family Medicine Residency
Novant Health
Cornelius, North Carolina

Jonathan C. Tsui, MD
Fellow Physician
Scheie Eye Institute, Department of Ophthalmology
University of Pennsylvania
Philadelphia, Pennsylvania

Mable Tsui, DO
Physician
Department of Family Medicine
Bayhealth
Dover, Delaware

Terrence Tsui, DO
Primary Care Sports Medicine Fellow
Department of Orthopedics
Bayhealth Medical Center
Dover, Delaware

Oswald Ramos Tuarez, MD
Sports Medicine Fellow
Department of Sports Medicine
Advocate Lutheran General
Park Ridge, Illinois

Sarah Tucker, MD
Fellow
Department of Pediatric Cardiology
Texas Children's Hospital
Houston, Texas

Alethea Y. Turner, DO, FAAFP
Associate Director
Family Medicine Residency Program HonorHealth
Scottsdale, Arizona

Rod J. Turner Jr., MD, CAQSM, MS
Assistant Professor
Department of Family Medicine
UTHealth Houston
Houston, Texas

Aneesh Tyle, MD
Physician
Department of Family Medicine
Ascension
Chicago, Illinois

Victoria Udezi, MD, MPH, FAAFP†
Assistant Professor
Department of Family Medicine
UT Southwestern Medical Center
Dallas, Texas

Idorenyin Emmanuel Udoeyop, MD
Department of Family Medicine
Creighton University
Omaha, Nebraska

George C. Umeh, MD
Physician
Bayhealth
Dover, Delaware

Ulunma Natalie Umesi, MD, MBA
Resident Physician
Brooklyn, New York
Child and Adolescent Psychiatry Fellow
Yale Child Study Center
New Haven, Connecticut

Santiago O. Valdes, MD, FAAP
Associate Professor
Department of Pediatric Cardiology
Baylor College of Medicine/Texas Children's Hospital
Houston, Texas

Virginia J. Van Duyne, MD
Associate Professor
Department of Family Medicine and Community Health
UMass Chan Medical School
Worcester, Massachusetts

Juan I. Vasquez Fuster, MD
Interventional Cardiology Fellow
Interventional Cardiology
UMass Memorial Medical Center
Worcester, Massachusetts

Stephanie Vaux Voyles, MD
Faculty Physician
Family Medicine Residency
St. Mary's Medical Center
Grand Junction, Colorado

Benjamin J. Velky, MD
Faculty Physician
Department of Family Medicine
Montgomery Center for Family Medicine
Assistant Professor of Family Medicine
Area Health Education Consortium
Medical University of South Carolina
Greenwood, South Carolina

Pavan S. Vemulakonda, MD
Resident
Department of Internal Medicine
George Washington University
Washington, District of Columbia

Brian Vickery, MD
Marcus Professor of Pediatric Immunology
Department of Pediatrics
Emory University and Children's Healthcare of Atlanta
Atlanta, Georgia

Maria del Pilar Montanez Villacampa, MD, FAAFP
Associate Professor
Department of Family and Community Medicine
UT Health San Antonio
San Antonio, Texas

Astrud San Antonio Villareal, MD, FAAFP†
Assistant Professor
Department of Family and Community Medicine
UT Southwestern Medical Center
Dallas, Texas

Ravjot Kaur Virdi, DO, MPH
Resident Physician
Department of Internal Medicine
Advocate Lutheran General Hospital
Park Ridge, Illinois

Francisco Vizcaino, MD
Family Medicine Resident
Department of Family and Community Medicine
Penn State Health St. Joseph Medical Center
Reading, Pennsylvania

Yongkasem Vorasettakarnkij, MD, MSc†
Assistant Professor
Department of Medicine
Chulalongkorn University
Cardiac Center
King Chulalongkorn Memorial Hospital, Thai Red Cross Society
Bangkok, Thailand

Aneeta Wadhawan, MD
Resident Physician
Department of Family Medicine
Creighton University
Omaha, Nebraska

Harmeet Wadhawan, MD
Omaha, Nebraska

Abdul Waheed, MD, MS, CPE, FAAFP
Professor, Tenured Track
Academic Chairman
Department of Family Medicine
Dignity Health Medical Group, AZ/Creighton University School of Medicine
Phoenix, Arizona

Anne Walsh, MMSc, PA-C, DFAAPA
Clinical Associate Professor
Department of Physician Assistant Studies
Chapman University
Irvine, California

Kellie Wang, PharmD
Pharmacist
Department of Pharmacy
Sarasota Memorial Hospital
Sarasota, Florida

Samuel C. Wang, MD
Faculty
Memorial Family Medicine Residency Program
Sugar Land, Texas

Kaleb R. Ward, DO
Resident Physician
Family Medicine Residency
HonorHealth
Scottsdale, Arizona

Daniel L. Warden, MD
Primary Care Sports Medicine Fellow
Department of Sports Medicine
Ascension Providence
Novi, Michigan

Muhammad Talha Waseem, MBBS
Department of Family Medicine
WellSpan Good Samaritan Hospital
Lebanon, Pennsylvania

Waiz Wasey, MD, FAAFP
Assistant Professor
Family Medicine, Sleep Medicine
Department of Family Medicine
Southern Illinois University
Springfield, Illinois

Leigh Weatherly, DO
Family Medicine
UMass Chan Medical School
Worcester, Massachusetts

Grant Wei, MD, FACEP
Associate Professor and Program Director
Department of Emergency Medicine
Robert Wood Johnson Medical School
New Brunswick, New Jersey

Lisa Weiss, MD, Med, FAAFP
Associate Professor
Bon Secours Mercy Health
Boardman, Ohio

Alexandre J. Wenk-Bodenmiller, MD
Assistant Professor
Department of Family Medicine and Community
UMass Chan Medical School
Worcester, Massachusetts

Maggie C. Wertz, MD
Faculty Physician
Eglin Family Medicine Residency
Eglin Air Force Base, Florida

Vernon L. Wheeler, MD
Family Medicine Obstetrics Faculty
Department of Family and Community Medicine
Carl R. Darnall Army Medical Center
Fort Cavazos, Texas

Beth A. Wichowski, DO
Department of Family Medicine
Baystate Franklin
Greenfield, Massachusetts

Joseph P. Wiedemer, MD
Associate Professor
Department of Family and Community Medicine
Penn State Health
State College, Pennsylvania

Melissa J. Wilcox, MD
Associate Program Director
Department of Family Medicine
Lost Coast Family Medicine Residency
Eureka, California

Susanne Wild, MD
Clinical Associate Professor
Department of Family Medicine
University of Arizona College of Medicine Phoenix Family Medicine Residency
Phoenix, Arizona

Amethyst Wilder, MD
Assistant Professor of Family Medicine
Department of Clinical Education
Mercer University School of Medicine
Savannah, Georgia

Eric L. Wilkerson II, MD
Core Faculty
Department of Family Medicine
Mississippi Delta Family Medicine Residency Program
Greenville, Mississippi

Brooks J. Willar, MD
Electrophysiology Fellow
Department of Cardiovascular Medicine
UMass Chan Medical School
Worcester, Massachusetts

Faren H. Williams, MD, MS†
Clinical Professor
Department of Orthopedics and Physical Rehabilitation
UMass Chan Medical School
Worcester, Massachusetts

Norton Winer, MD[†]
Assistant Clinical Professor of Neurology
Department of Neurology
University Hospitals Cleveland
Cleveland, Ohio

Fawn J. Winkelman, DO
Department of Osteopathic Family Medicine
Nova Southeastern University College of Osteopathic
Owner/Physician
Elite Medicine and Aesthetic Institute
Fort Lauderdale, Florida

Kathleen Wirshup, MD
Resident Physician
Department of Family Medicine
Boston University School of Medicine
Boston Medical Center
Boston, Massachusetts

Christopher M. Wise, MD
Professor of Internal Medicine
Department of Internal Medicine/Rheumatology, Allergy, and Immunology
Virginia Commonwealth University Health System
Richmond, Virginia

Jeffrey Wisinski, DO
Assistant Professor
Department of Family Medicine/Sports Medicine
Prisma Health
Columbia, South Carolina

William W. Wong, DO
Assistant Professor of Medicine
Department of Pulmonary and Critical Care Medicine
UMass Chan Medical School
Worcester, Massachusetts

Emma Wood, DO
Family Medicine
Baystate-Greenfield Family Medicine
Greenfield, Massachusetts

Sarah J. Wu, MD
Department of Internal Medicine
UMass Chan Medical School
Worcester, Massachusetts

Velyn Wu, MD, MACM
Assistant Clinical Professor
Department of Community Health and Family Medicine
University of Florida College of Medicine
Gainesville, Florida

Elliana Kae V. Yap, MD, BS
Medical Resident
Department of Family Medicine
UT Health Science Center San Antonio
San Antonio, Texas

Dinesh Yogaratnam, PharmD, BCPS, BCCCP
Associate Professor
Massachusetts College of Pharmacy and Health Sciences University
Worcester, Massachusetts

Jocelyn C. Young, DO, MSc
Clinical Assistant Professor
Department of Family Medicine
SUNY Upstate Medical University
Assistant Clinical Professor
Department of Family Medicine
United Health Services/Wilson Family Medicine Residency Program
Faculty Physician
Department of Family Medicine
United Health Services Hospitals
Johnson City, New York

Tiffany Yu, MD
Resident Physician
Department of Family Medicine
Adventist Health Hanford
Hanford, California

Betty Brenda Yue, MPA
Assistant Teaching Professor
Department of Family Medicine, MEDEX PA Program
University of Washington School of Medicine
Tacoma, Washington

Theresa Yurkonis, DO, MHSA
Assistant Professor
Department of Family and Community Medicine
Penn State Health Milton S. Hershey Medical Center/St. Joseph's Medical Center
Hershey, Pennsylvania

Alexandra Renee Zaballa, MD
Faculty
Department of Family Medicine
Swedish Cherry Family Medicine Residency
Seattle, Washington

Nida Zahra, MD, FAAFP
Associate Professor
Department of Family and Community Medicine
UT Southwestern Medical Center
Dallas, Texas

Touqir Zahra, MD, FACP
Assistant Professor
Department of Internal Medicine
Florida Atlantic University
Boca Raton, Florida

Syed Murtaza Haider Zaidi, MD, MBBS
Resident Physician
Department of Family and Community Medicine
Creighton University School of Medicine
Omaha, Nebraska

Batoul C. Zalkout, DO
Resident Physician
Department of Family Medicine
Advocate Aurora Health
Chicago, Illinois

Yuan Zhang, MD
Resident Physician
Department of Medicine
Stanford University School of Medicine
Palo Alto, California

Yuying Zhang, BS
Department of Dermatology
UMass Chan Medical School
Worcester, Massachusetts

Molly Zhao, MD
Resident Physician
Department of Family Medicine
University of Massachusetts
Worcester, Massachusetts

Anna K. Zheng, MD
Obstetrics Lead
Department of Family Medicine
Edward M. Kennedy Community Health Center Assistant Professor
Department of Family Medicine and Community Health
UMass Memorial Medical Center
Worcester, Massachusetts

Allen Zhou, MD
Internal Medicine Resident
Department of Hospital Medicine
Ochsner Medical Center
New Orleans, Louisiana

Mohammad Sameer Ahmed Zidan, MBBS
Resident Physician
Creighton University Family Medicine
Creighton University
Omaha, Nebraska

Erika Zimmons, DO, MS
Assistant Professor
Department of Family Medicine and Community Health
UMass Chan Medical School
Worcester, Massachusetts

Kira Zwygart, MD
Professor
Department of Family Medicine
University of South Florida Morsani College of Medicine
Tampa, Florida

[†]The views expressed are those of the authors and do not reflect the official policy of the Department of the Army, Department of the Navy, Department of the Air Force, the Department of Defense, or the United States Government.

CONTENTS

Topics

Diagnosis and Treatment: An Algorithmic Approach

This section contains flowcharts (or algorithms) to help the reader in the diagnosis of clinical signs and symptoms and treatment of a variety of clinical problems. They are organized by the presenting sign, symptom, or diagnosis.

These algorithms were designed to be used as a quick reference and adjunct to the reader's clinical knowledge and impression. They are not an exhaustive review of the management of a problem, nor are they meant to be a complete list of diseases.

ABDOMINAL PAIN, CHRONIC

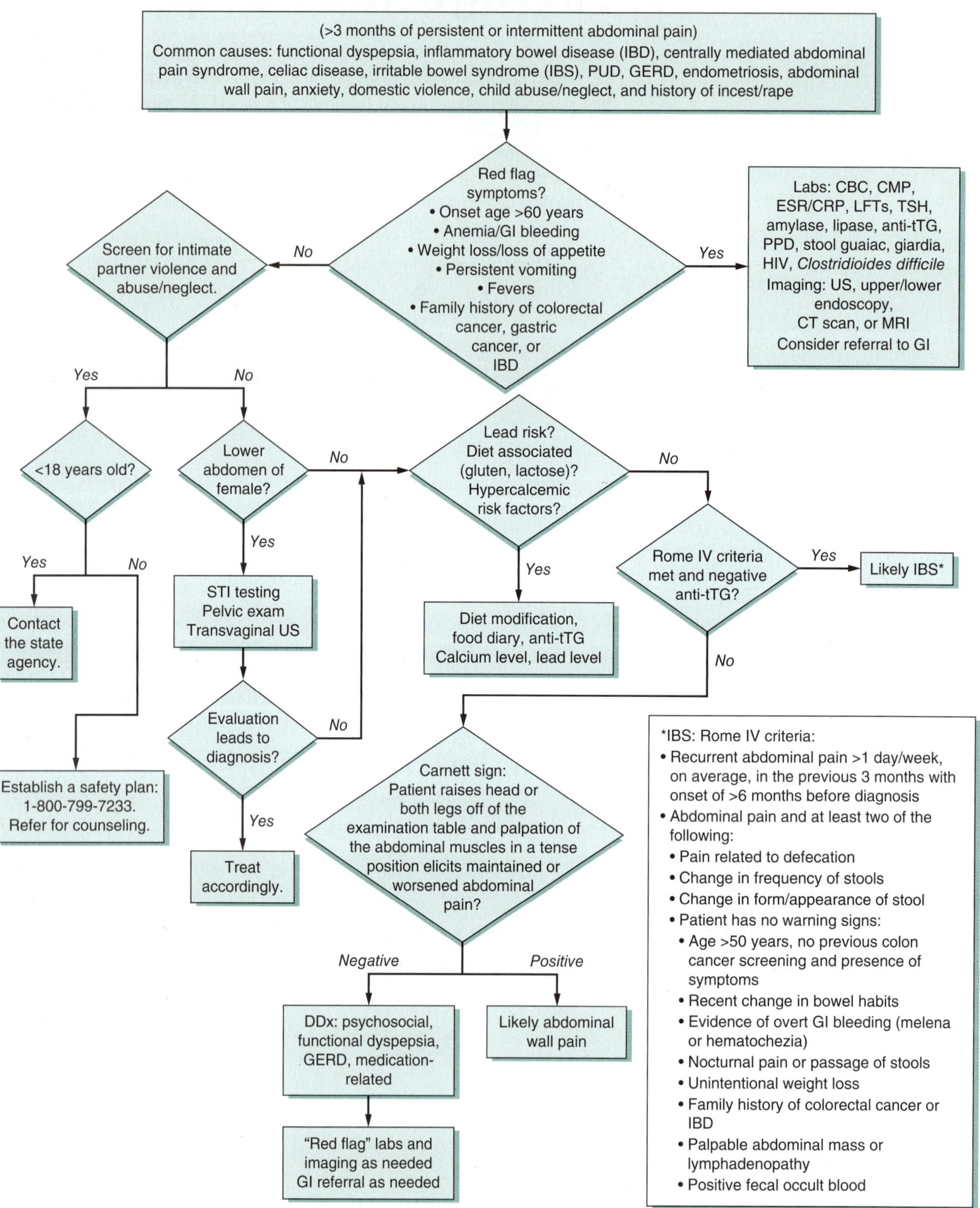

Kamini Geer, MD, MPH and Juan C. Gonzalez, MD

Sabo CM, Grad S, Dumitrascu DL. Chronic abdominal pain in general practice. *Dig Dis*. 2021;39(6):606–614.

ABDOMINAL PAIN, LOWER

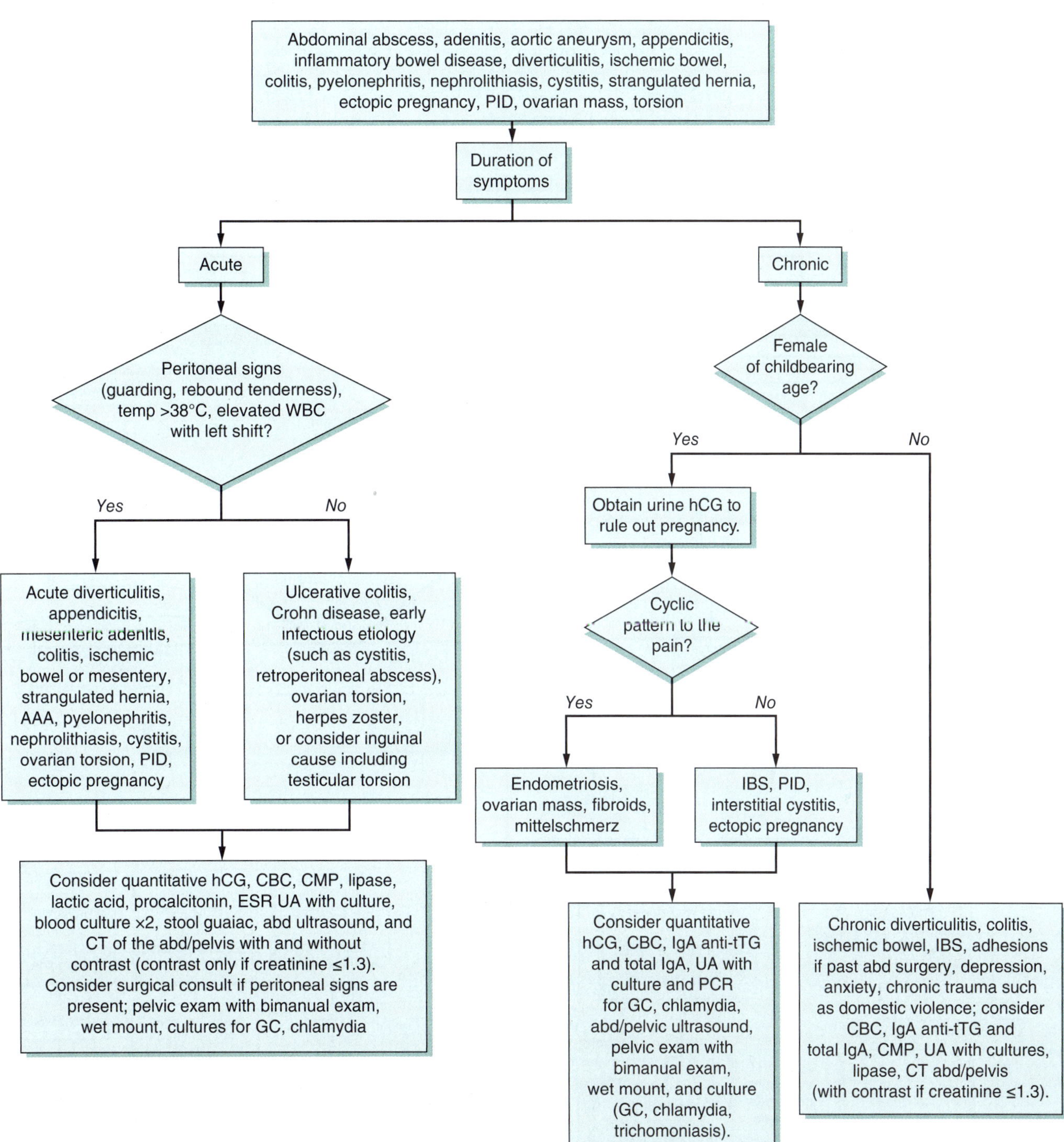

Kenneth A. Ballou, MD

Cullison KM, Franck N. Clinical decision rules in the evaluation and management of adult gastrointestinal emergencies. *Emerg Med Clin North Am*. 2021;39(4):719–732.

ABDOMINAL PAIN, UPPER

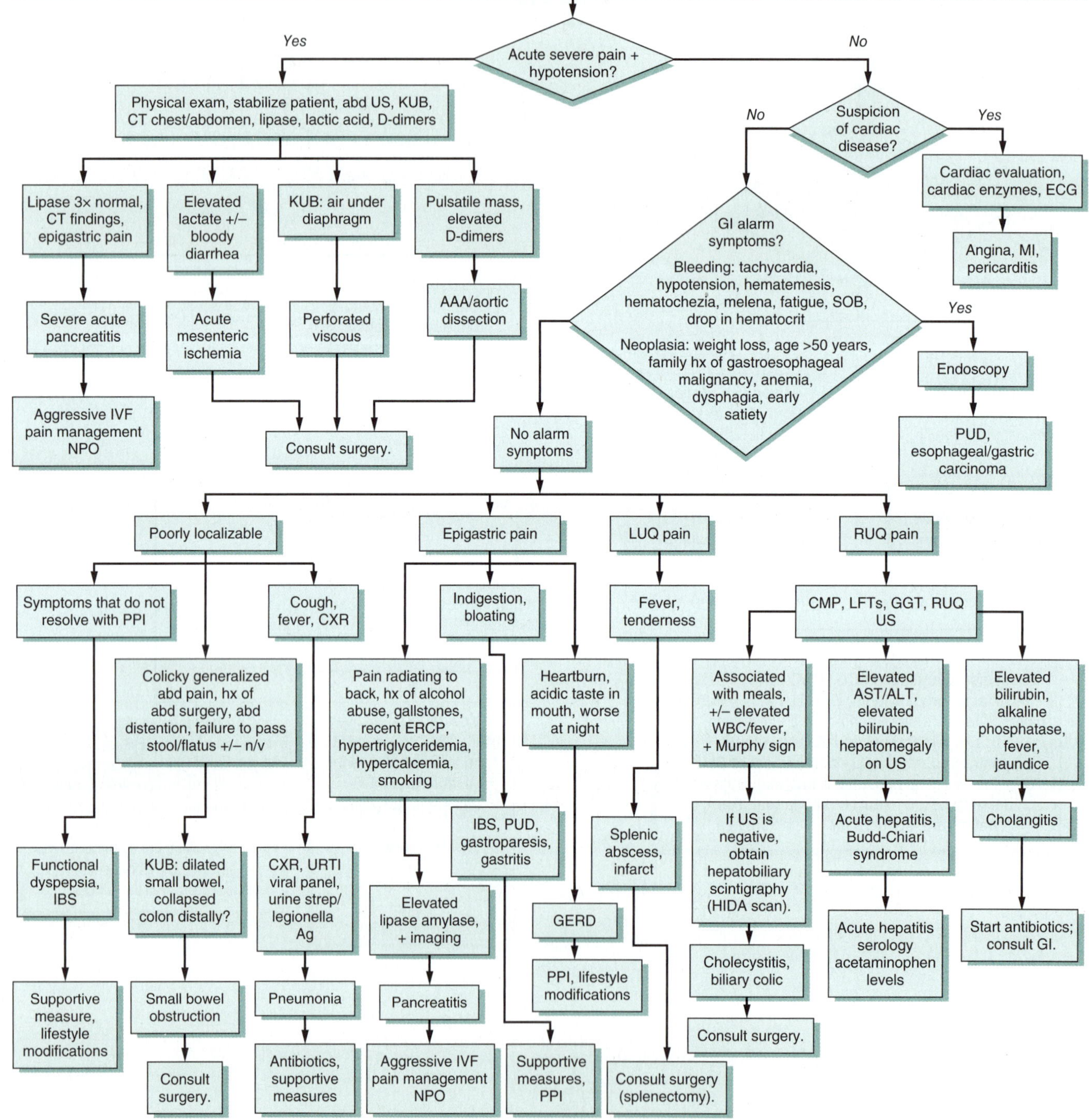

Tamika Isaac, DO and Rebecca Gwaltney, MD, MPH

Yew KS, George MK, Allred HB. Acute abdominal pain in adults: evaluation and diagnosis. *Am Fam Physician*. 2023;107(6):585–596.

ACETAMINOPHEN POISONING, TREATMENT

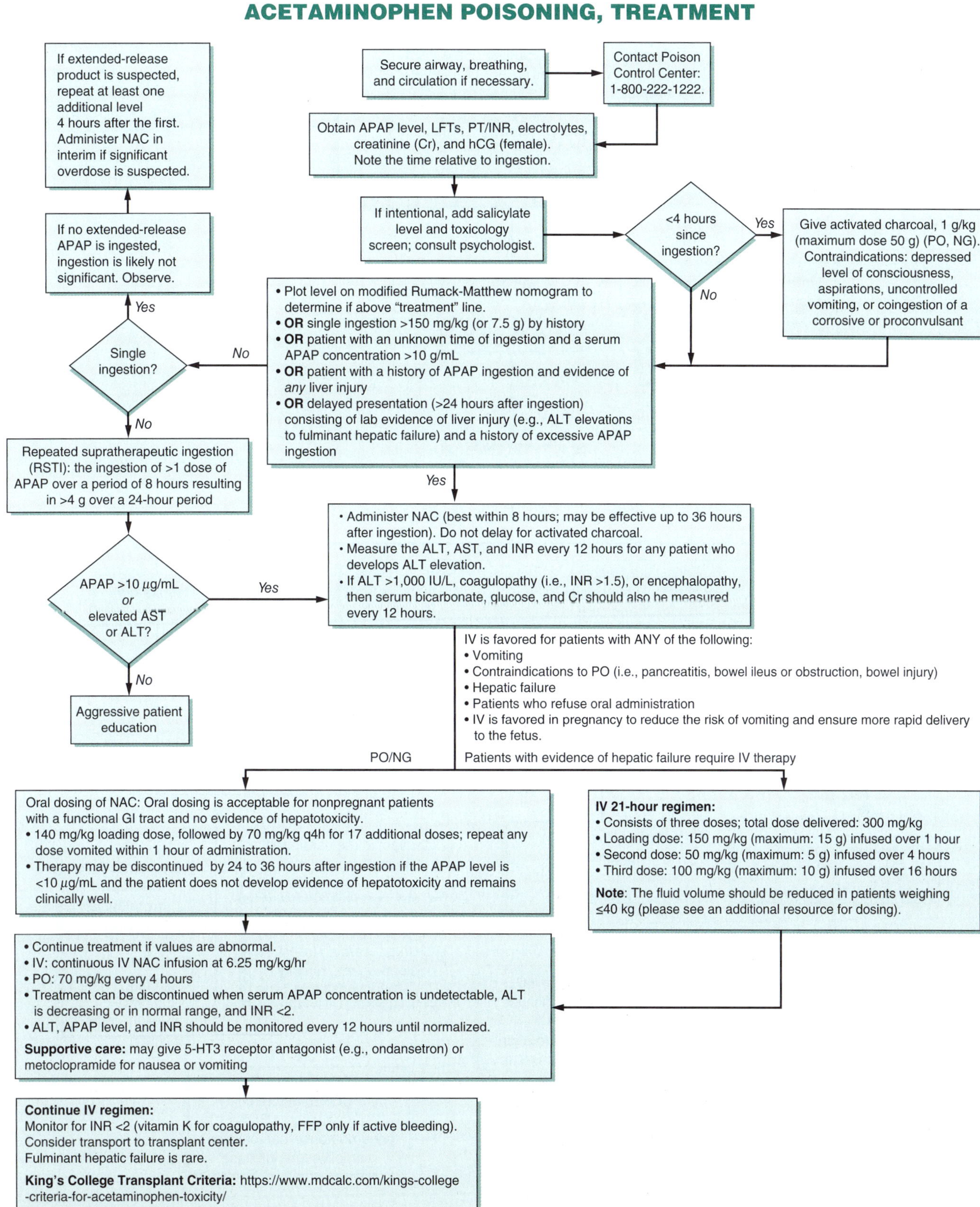

APAP, acetaminophen; NAC, *N*-acetylcysteine.

Pankaj Ksheersagar, MD, FAAP

Dart RC, Mullins ME, Matoushek T, et al. Management of acetaminophen poisoning in the US and Canada: a consensus statement. *JAMA Netw Open*. 2023;6(8):e2327739. doi:10.1001/jamanetworkopen.2023.27739.

ACIDOSIS

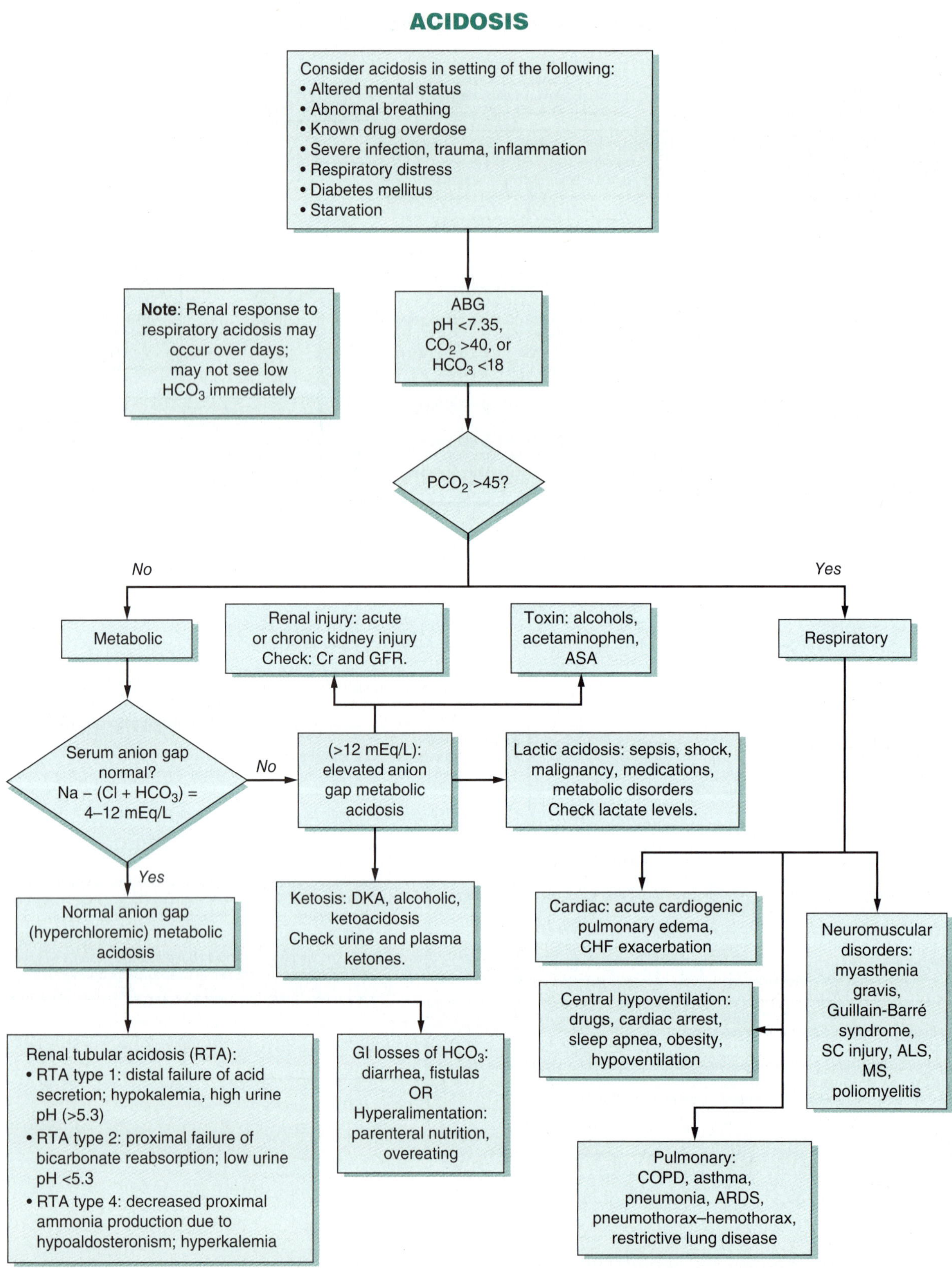

Shivani Malhotra, MD, FAAFP

Kraut JA, Madias NE. Serum anion gap: its uses and limitations in clinical medicine. *Clin J Am Soc Nephrol*. 2007;2(1):162–174.

ACNE

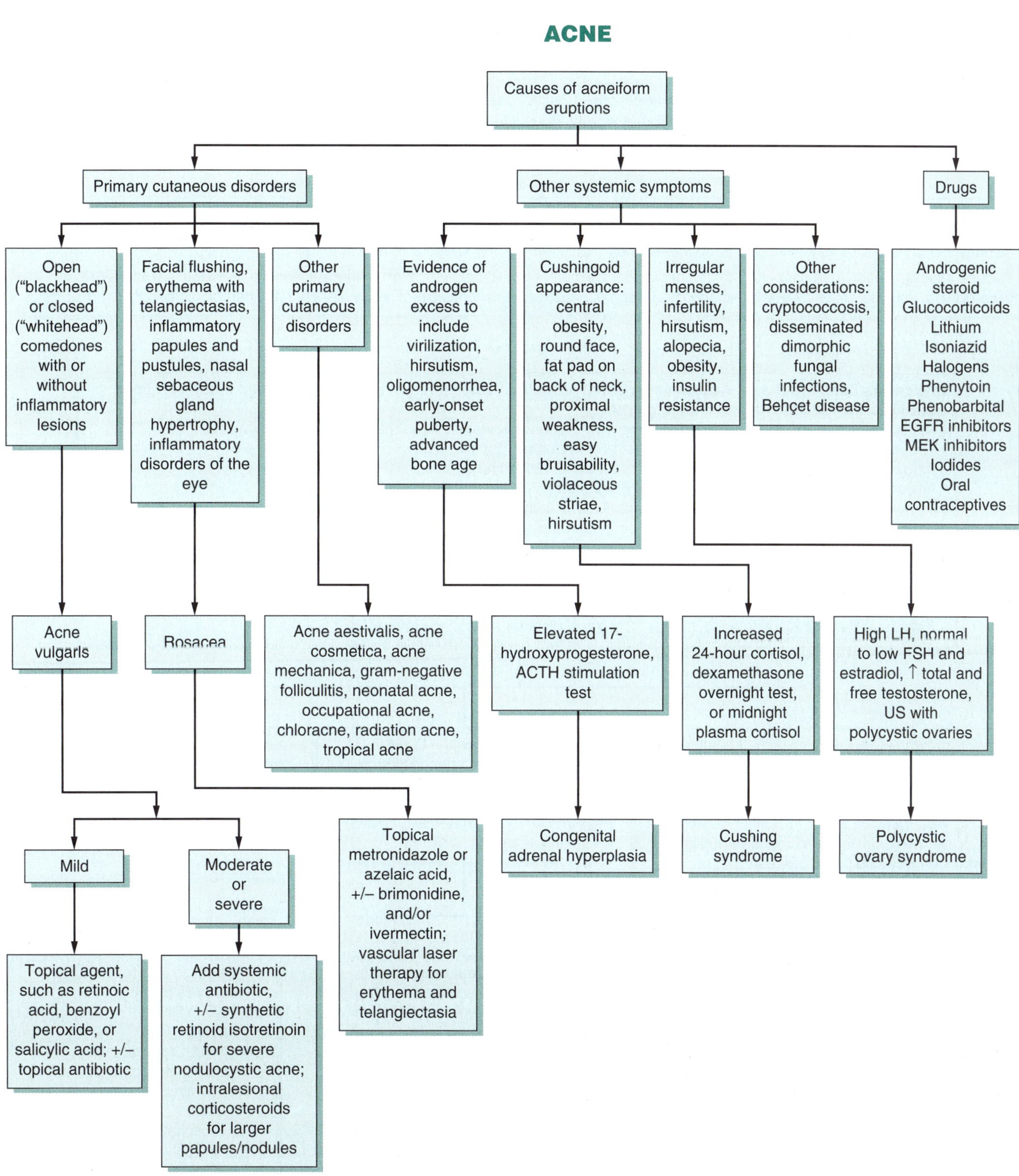

Justin Maher, MD and Nathan J. Macedo, MD, MPH

Reynolds RV, Yeung H, Cheng CE, et al. Guidelines of care for the management of acne vulgaris. *J Am Acad Dermatol*. 2024;90(5):1006.e1–1006.e30.

ALCOHOL WITHDRAWAL, TREATMENT

History: duration and quantity of alcohol intake for 2 weeks prior to presentation, time since last drink, previous episodes of alcohol withdrawal, concurrent substance use, currents medications (prescriptions and supplements), preexisting medical and psychiatric conditions, prior detoxification admissions, prior seizure activity, living situation, social supports, stressors, triggers

↓

Physical: Use *DSM-5* Criteria for Diagnosis of Alcohol Withdrawal, VS (fever, tachycardia, tachypnea, hypertension), **CIWA** (see below), MSE (arousal, orientation, hallucinations), HEENT (diaphoresis, scleral icterus), CV (arrhythmias), evaluate s/sx of liver failure (ascites, varices, caput medusae, asterixis, palmar erythema), neuro (nystagmus, tremor, seizure activity)

Include assessment of conditions likely to *complicate*, *exacerbate*, or *precipitate* alcohol withdrawal: anxiety, arrhythmias, CHF, CAD, dehydration, depression, GI bleeding, history of traumatic experience, infections, liver disease, pancreatitis, neurologic deficits.

↓

Clinical Institute Withdrawal Assessment (CIWA) of Alcohol Scale (For patients in the ICU who cannot respond to questions, the MINDS protocol should be used.)

- Nausea and vomiting 0–7 (0, none; 4, intermittent; 7, constant nausea; frequent dry heaves/vomiting)
- Tremor 0–7 (0, none; 4, moderate; 7, severe; even with arms not extended)
- Paroxysmal sweats 0–7 (0, none; 4, beads of sweat; 7, drenching sweats)
- Anxiety 0–7 (0, none; 4, moderate; 7, acute panic state)
- Agitation 0–7 (0, none; 4, moderately restless; 7, constantly thrashing about or pacing)
- Tactile disturbances 0–7 (0, none; 1–3, for pruritus or paresthesias; 4–7, for hallucinations)
- Auditory disturbances 0–7 (0, none; 1–3, for increased sensitivity; 4–7, for hallucinations)
- Visual disturbances 0–7 (0, none; 1–3, for increased sensitivity; 4–7, for hallucinations)
- Headache 0–7 (0, no headache; 4, moderate; 7, extremely severe)
- Orientation 0–4 (0, fully oriented; 1, cannot do serial additions or is uncertain about date; 2, disoriented to date but within 2 calendar days; 3, disoriented to date by >2 days; 4, disoriented to place or person)

↓

Mild withdrawal—CIWA 0–7 onset 5–8 hours after cessation or significant decrease in consumption: anxiety, restlessness, agitation, mild nausea, decreased appetite, sleep disturbance, facial sweating, mild tremulousness, fluctuating tachycardia and hypertension, possible mild cognitive impairment, no tremors or very mild tremulousness

→ **Good candidate for outpatient therapy:**

- Not pregnant
- No comorbid illnesses requiring hospitalization
- No history of seizures
- Not a suicide risk
- Low risk of delirium tremens
- No history of unsuccessful outpatient detoxification
- Good access to follow-up medical care
- Tolerating oral medication
- Adequate social support available

→ **Outpatient therapy contraindicated**: pregnant, history of seizures or withdrawal seizures, chronic or acute comorbid illness requiring inpatient observation, lack of ability to follow-up

High risk of delirium tremens:

- Age >30 years
- Heavy drinking >8 years
- Drinking >100 g ethanol per day (>8 drinks per day)
- Random BAC >200 mg/dL
- Elevated MCV
- Cirrhosis

(→ Admit to inpatient detoxification program)

Moderate withdrawal—CIWA 8–14 onset 24–48 hours after cessation: marked restlessness and agitation, moderate tremulousness with constant eye movement, diaphoresis, nausea, vomiting, anorexia, diarrhea

→ **Admit to inpatient detoxification program:**

- Replete thiamine IV as below before giving glucose and/or fluids containing dextrose to prevent Wernicke encephalopathy.
- VS q4h
- CIWA q4h
- Institute seizure precautions.
- IV fluids

Severe withdrawal/delirium tremens—CIWA 15–30 onset 48–96 hours after alcohol cessation: marked tremulousness, fever, drenching sweats, severe hypertension and tachycardia, delirium, seizures may also be present

→ **Admit to ICU for inpatient detoxification:**

- VS q15min
- CIWA q1h
- NPO, IV fluids
- Lateral decubitus position, restrain if necessary
- Glucose, sodium, potassium, phosphate, and magnesium replacement as needed

Treat as outpatient:
- Thiamine 100 mg once daily for 5 days
- Folic acid 1 g once daily for 5 days
- Evaluate daily until symptoms decrease.
- Assess blood pressure, heart rate, and CIWA-Ar score at each follow-up visit.
- Encourage referral to addiction specialist or inpatient treatment facility.
- Facilitate entry into a long-term outpatient therapy program (Alcoholics Anonymous).
- **If patient misses an appointment or resumes drinking, refer to addiction specialist or inpatient treatment facility.**
- Evaluate daily until symptoms decrease—usually for about 5 days. Face to face is preferred but can alternate with telemedicine visits if necessary.
- Discuss any additional postwithdrawal treatment options through primary care or a specialized alcohol treatment program.

Labs:
- Toxicology screen/EtOH level to assess need for and timing of withdrawal regimen
- CBC, electrolytes, phosphate, magnesium, vitamin B_{12}, folate.
- Amylase/lipase if suspected pancreatitis
- PT, PTT if suspected liver failure
- LFTs, GGT, PT, PTT, INR, Bilirubin
- UPT if premenopausal

Imaging:
- Head CT if history of trauma, mental status changes greater than expected, or focal neurologic changes
- Consider addition of EEG if focal neurologic signs or prolonged postictal state seizure.
- Consider addition of ECG if there is a history of cardiac problems.

Medications:
- Diazepam 5–20 mg IV q10min until calm and then q1h to maintain light somnolence for duration of delirium

If severe liver disease, severe asthma or respiratory failure, elderly, debilitated, or low serum albumin:
- Lorazepam 1–4 mg IV q10min until calm and then q1h to maintain light somnolence for duration of delirium

Example outpatient regimen:
Fixed diazepam schedule
Day 1: 10 mg q6h
Day 2: 10 mg q8h
Day 3: 10 mg q12h
Day 4/5: 10 mg at bedtime

Symptom-triggered diazepam schedule:
Give dose if CIWA >8.
Day 1: 10 mg q4h PRN
Day 2: 10 mg q6h PRN
Day 3: 10 mg q6h PRN
Days 4/5: 10 mg twice a day PRN
Pt with transaminitis, LFT >3 times normal *use* lorazepam (Ativan) in tapering doses over 5 days; may start with 2 mg q4h PRN

Fixed chlordiazepoxide (Librium) schedule:
Day 1: 50 mg PO q6h
Day 2: 25 mg q6h
Day 3: 25 mg q6h
Avoid in renal disease, liver disease, or elderly.

If benzodiazepines are contraindicated or if preference is to start with non-benzodiazepine agent, gabapentin is an alternative.

Immediate release: oral: initial: 300 mg/q6h on day 1, then 300 mg/q8h on day 2, then 300 mg/q12h on day 3, then 300 mg at night on day 4. In addition to scheduled doses, provide one additional PRN 300 mg dose per day for breakthrough withdrawal symptoms.

Carbamazepin can also be considered as monotherapy in mild alcohol withdrawal syndrome.

Discharge planning:
- CIWA scores <8–10 for 24 hours
- Begin 1:1 or group therapy.
- Discharge to treatment center, day program, home.
- Facilitate entry into Alcoholics Anonymous.
- Evaluate for outpatient treatment with benzodiazepine.
- Nutrition/social work consultation
- Close follow-up with primary care physician
- Discharge to treatment center or home (with or without plans for day program).

Medications:
Nutritional replacement
- Thiamine 100 mg IV/IM or PO once daily for 5 days
- Folic acid 1 g PO once daily for 5 days

Sympatholytic adjunctive therapy (no effect on prevention of withdrawal seizure and should be used with benzodiazepine therapy)
- Atenolol 50–100 mg once daily
- Clonidine 0.2 mg 3 times daily

For hallucinations associated with withdrawal:
- Haloperidol 2–5 mg IM/PO q1–4h max 5 mg/day
- Use only in conjunction with benzodiazepines and with extreme caution because haloperidol may lower seizure threshold.
- Frequent reassurance, re-orientation to time and place, and nursing care are recommended nonpharmacologic interventions.

Supportive care
- Frequent reorientation to time and place may be needed for patient.
- Decrease stimulation.
- Encourage PO fluid intake of noncaffeinated beverages.

Medications:
Long-acting benzodiazepines (diazepam or chlordiazepoxide) provide lower chance of recurrent withdrawal or seizures. Symptom-triggered regimen is preferred over fixed dose regimen. If patient is at greater risk of complications, can consider front-loading approach (CIWA-Ar score of ≥19)

Symptom triggered (Assess using CIWA q1h. Once moderate symptoms are controlled, can reduce assessment to q4–6h)
- Diazepam 10–20 mg (until CIWA-Ar <10)

  or
- Chlordiazepoxide 50–100 (until CIWA-Ar <10)

Front loading
- Diazepam 10 mg PO q1h until CIWA-Ar <10

Fixed schedule
- Diazepam 20 mg PO q2–3h for three doses

  or
- Chlordiazepoxide, 50 mg q6h for 4 doses, then 25 mg q6h for 8 doses

Short-acting benzodiazepines (lorazepam) may have lower risk when there is concern about prolonged sedation, for example, h/o liver disease, LFT >3 times normal limit, elderly patients, or those with severe hepatic insufficiency.
- Lorazepam 1–2 mg PO q2–4h until CIWA <8

Astrud San Antonio Villareal, MD, FAAFP and Victoria Udezi, MD, MPH, FAAFP

The ASAM clinical practice guideline on alcohol withdrawal management. *J Addict Med*. 2020;14(3S Suppl 1):1–72. *Erratum in: J Addict Med*. 2020;14(5):e280.

ALKALINE PHOSPHATASE ELEVATION

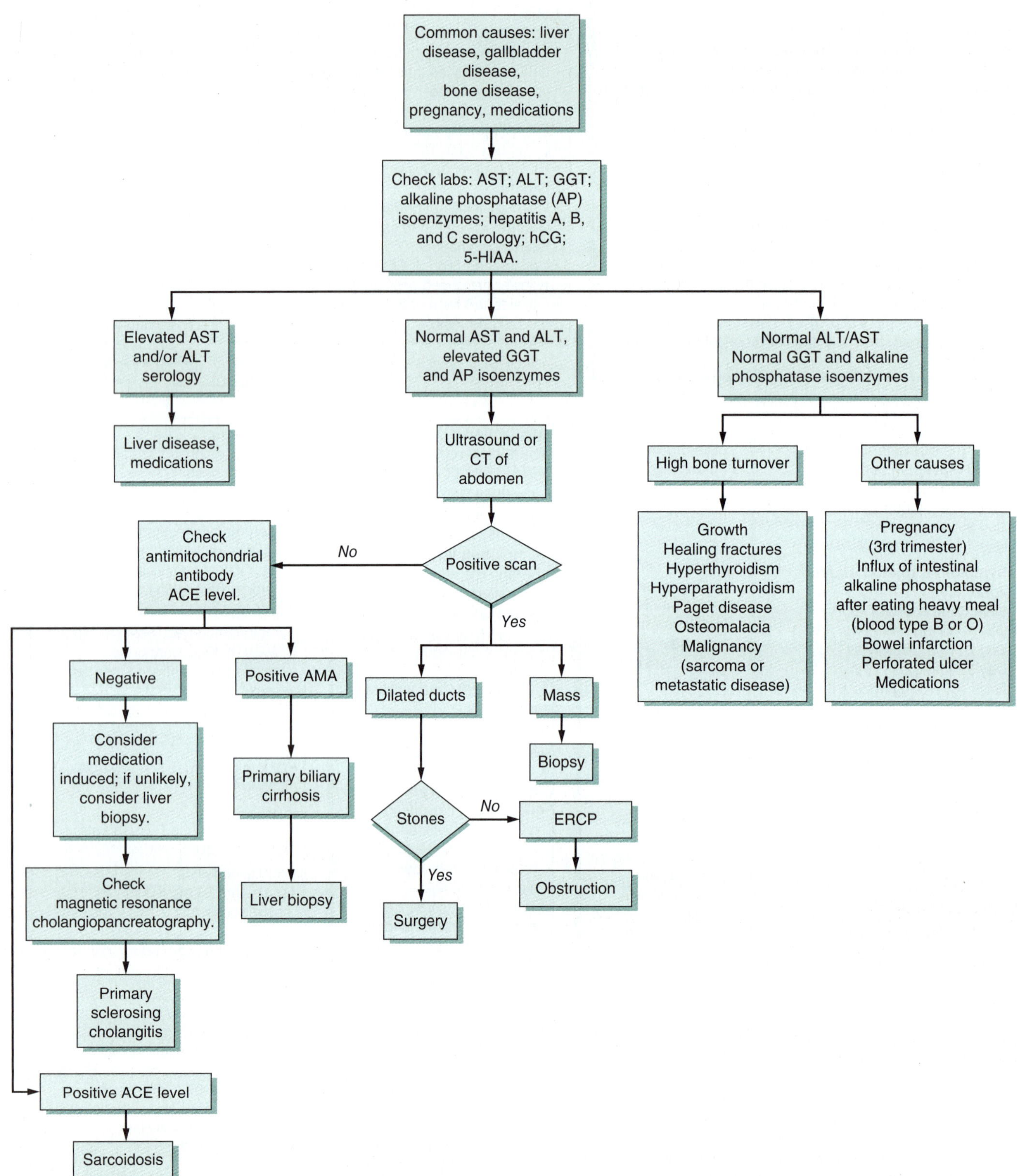

Reem Hadi, MD and Fozia Akhtar Ali, MD, FAAFP

Siddique A, Kowdley KV. Approach to a patient with elevated serum alkaline phosphatase. *Clin Liver Dis.* 2012;16(2):199–229.

AMENORRHEA, SECONDARY

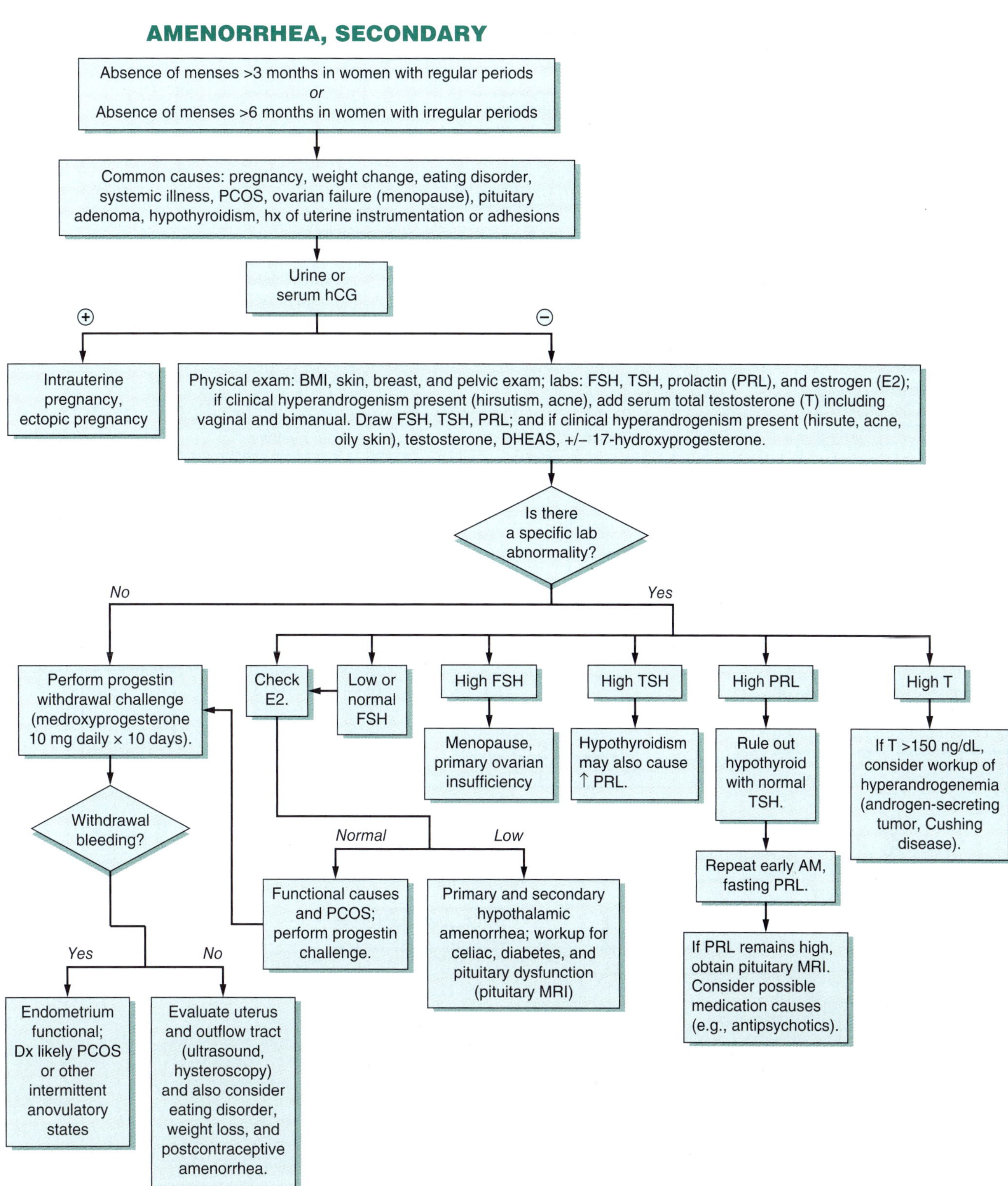

Rebecca Gwaltney, MD, MPH

Klein DA, Paradise SL, Reeder RM. Amenorrhea: a systematic approach to diagnosis and management. *Am Fam Physician*. 2019;100(1):39–48.

ANEMIA

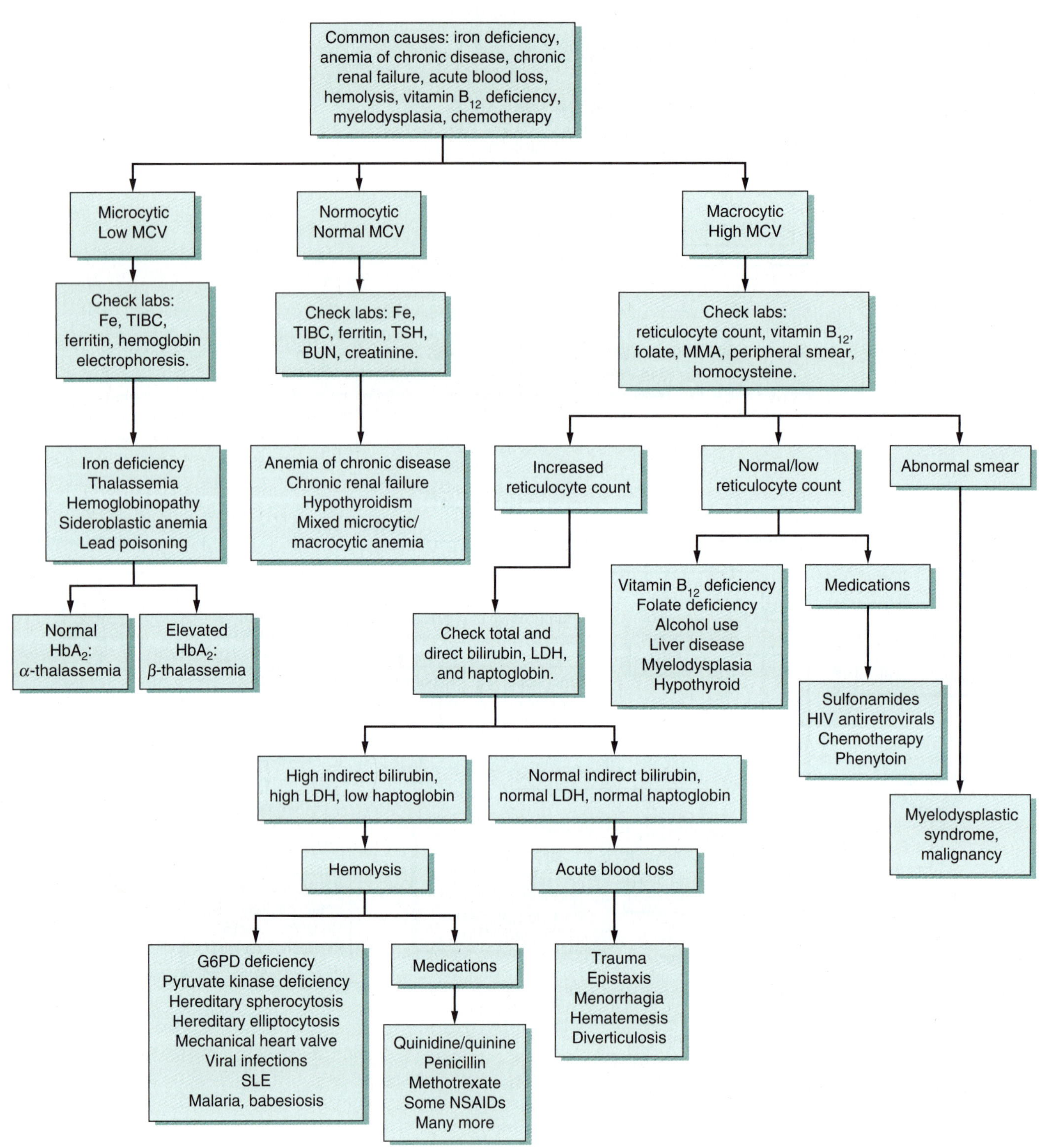

Kassandra M. Jean-Marie, MD

Lanier JB, Park JJ, Callahan RC. Anemia in older adults. *Am Fam Physician*. 2018;98(7):437–442.

AST ELEVATION

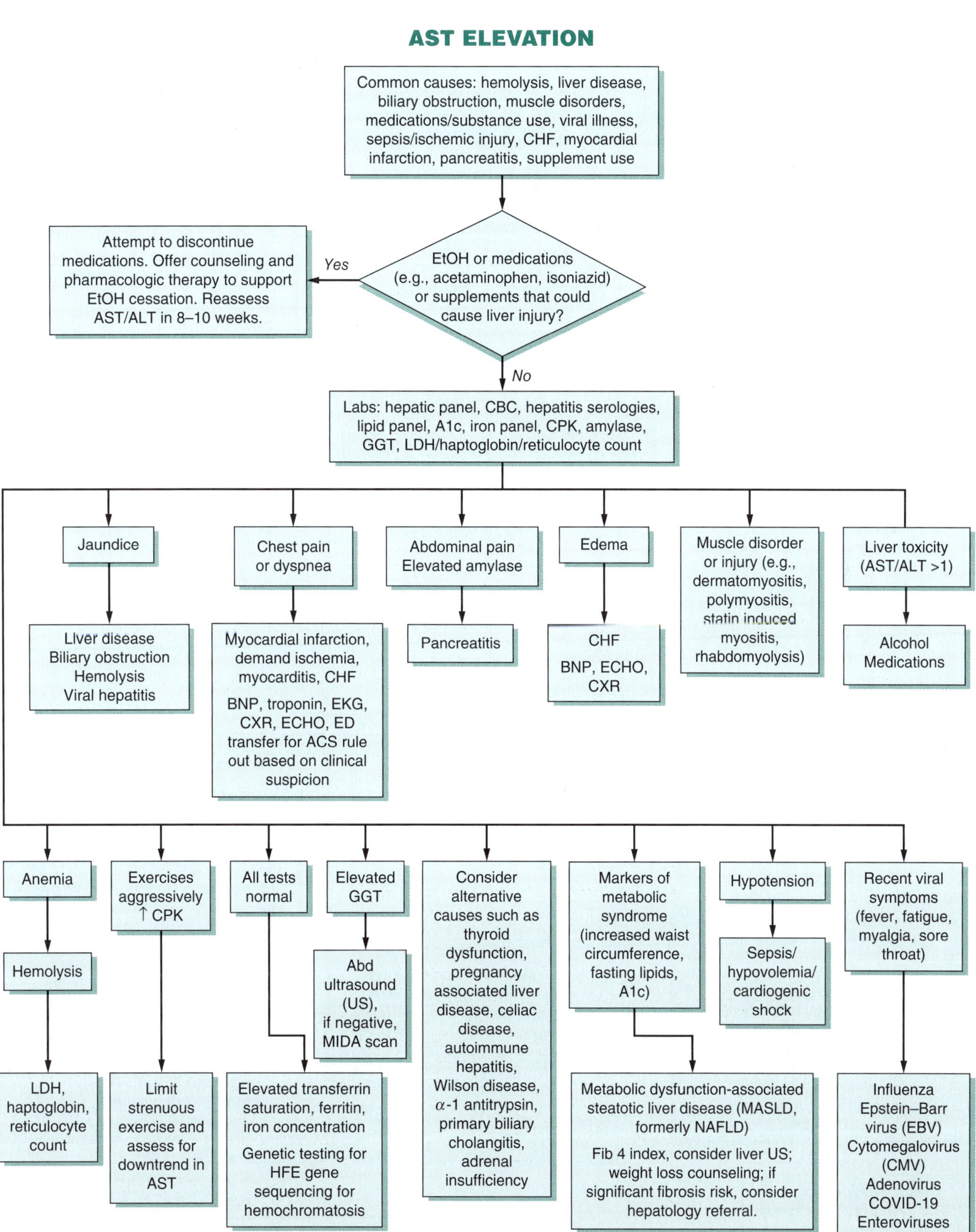

Natalie Ann Correa, MD and Myra Khawar, DO, MBS

Langan RC, Hines-Smith KA. Mildly elevated liver transaminase levels: causes and evaluation. *Am Fam Physician*. 2024;110(6):585–591. https://www.aafp.org/pubs/afp/issues/2024/1200/elevated-liver-transaminase-levels.html. Accessed November 19, 2025.

ASTHMA EXACERBATION, PEDIATRIC ACUTE

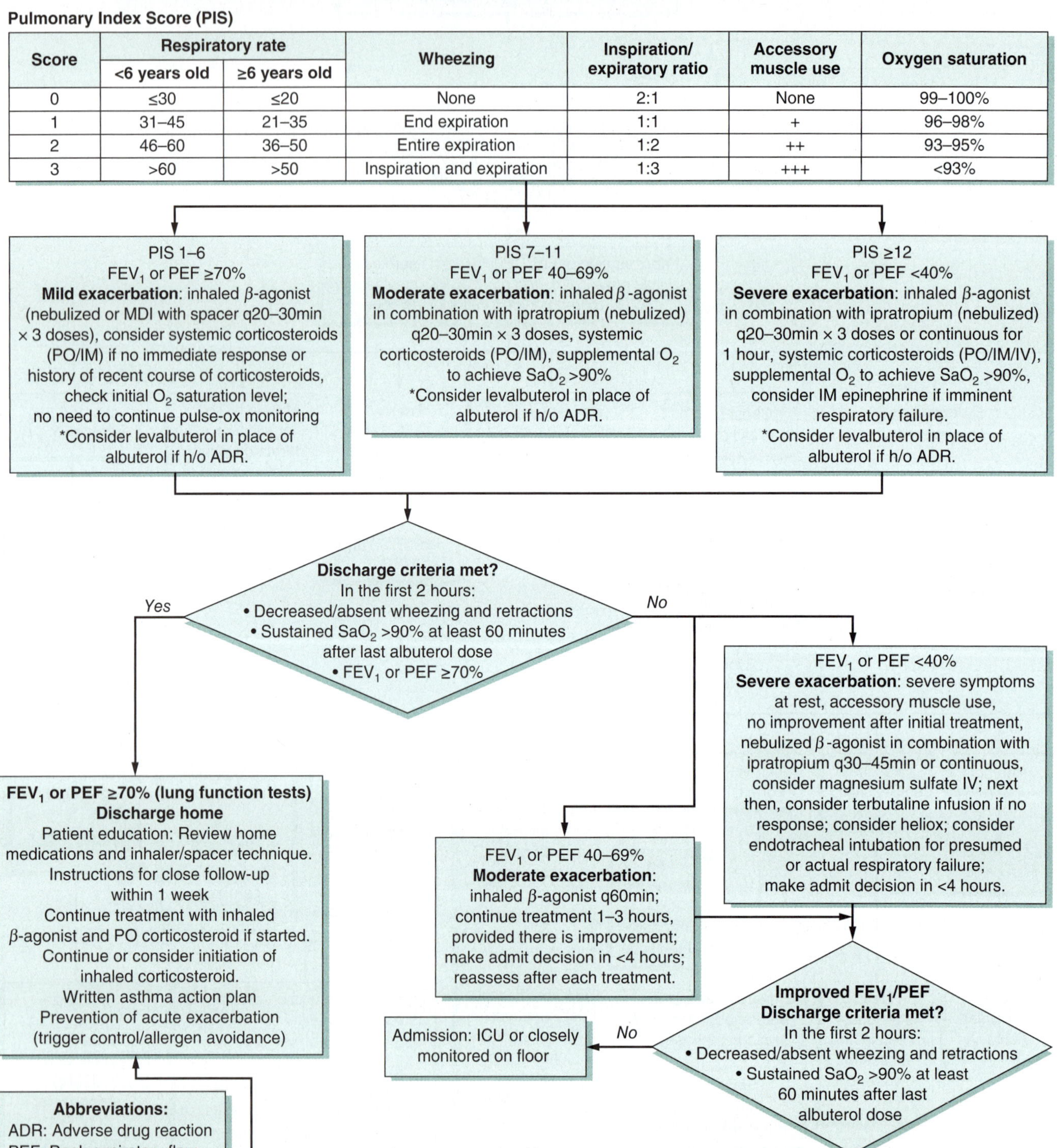

Pulmonary Index Score (PIS)

Score	Respiratory rate		Wheezing	Inspiration/ expiratory ratio	Accessory muscle use	Oxygen saturation
	<6 years old	≥6 years old				
0	≤30	≤20	None	2:1	None	99–100%
1	31–45	21–35	End expiration	1:1	+	96–98%
2	46–60	36–50	Entire expiration	1:2	++	93–95%
3	>60	>50	Inspiration and expiration	1:3	+++	<93%

Jan Estes Miller, MD and Adam McConnell, MD

Cloutier MM, Baptist AP, Blake KV, et al; for Expert Panel Working Group of the National Heart, Lung, and Blood Institute (NHLBI); National Asthma Education and Prevention Program Coordinating Committee (NAEPPCC). 2020 Focused updates to the asthma management guidelines: a report from the National Asthma Education and Prevention Program Coordinating Committee Expert Panel Working Group. *J Allergy Clin Immunol*. 2020;146(6):1217–1270.

ASTHMA TREATMENT AND MAINTENANCE, ADULTS AND ADOLESCENTS ≥12 YEARS

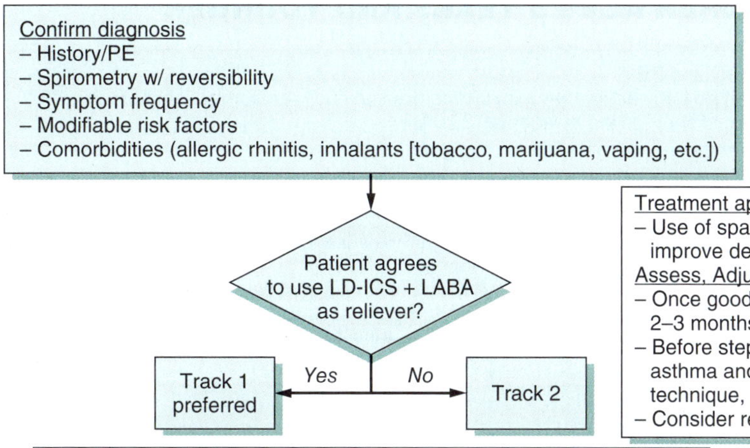

Confirm diagnosis
- History/PE
- Spirometry w/ reversibility
- Symptom frequency
- Modifiable risk factors
- Comorbidities (allergic rhinitis, inhalants [tobacco, marijuana, vaping, etc.])

Patient agrees to use LD-ICS + LABA as reliever?

Yes → Track 1 preferred

No → Track 2

Treatment approach
- Use of spacer for all MDIs (β-agonist, ICS) to improve delivery, decrease side effects

Assess, Adjust, Review
- Once good asthma control has been achieved for 2–3 months, consider stepping down therapy.
- Before stepping up, confirm symptoms are due to asthma and review/address common issues (inhaler technique, adherence, allergen exposure, etc.)
- Consider repeat lung function testing.

Track 1: Patient agrees to use LD-ICS + LABA as reliever (preferred).
Track 2: Patient prefers to use SABA as reliever and ICS as controller.

Symptoms	Step 1 Sx <2 times a month	Step 2 >2 times a month/ <4–5 times a week	Step 3 Daily symptoms/ waking ≥1/week	Step 4 Uncontrolled/ acute exacerbation	Step 5 Persistent symptoms/ exacerbations despite optimized step 4 treatments
Track 1	Preferred: As needed LD-ICS + formoterol	Preferred: As needed LD-ICS + formoterol	Preferred: LD-ICS + formoterol (MART)	Preferred: MD-ICS + formoterol (MART)	Preferred: Add on LAMA, HD-ICS, phenotype assessment Consider: Anti-IgE therapy (omalizumab) Anti-IL-5 therapy Anti-IL-4 antibody (dupilumab) Anti-TSLP (tezepelumab)
Track 2	Alternative: LD-ICS when SABA is used	Alternative: Daily LD-ICS and as needed SABA	Alternative: Daily LD-ICS + LABA	Alternative: Daily MD-ICS + LABA or HD-ICS + LABA	Alternative: Add on LAMA, HD-ICS, phenotype assessment; Consider: Anti-IgE therapy (omalizumab) Anti-IL-5 therapy Anti-IL-4 antibody (dupilumab) Anti-TSLP (tezepelumab)
		Other options: Daily LTRA	Other options: MD-ICS or HDM SLIT HDM SLIT	Other options: Add LAMA or Daily LTRA or HD-ICS	Other options: Add azithromycin or LD-OCS.

Adults and adolescents Inhaled corticosteroid	**Total daily ICS dose (μg) Low**	**Medium**	**High**
BDP (pMDI, HFA)	200–500	>500–1,000	>1,000
BDP (DPI or pMDI, extrafine particle, HFA)	100–200	>200–400	>400
Budesonide (DPI or pMDI, HFA)	200–400	>400–800	>800
Ciclesonide (pMDI, extrafine particle, HFA)	80–160	>160–320	>320
Fluticasone furoate (DPI)	100		200
Fluticasone propionate (DPI)	100–250	>250–500	>500
Fluticasone propionate (pMDI, HFA)	100–250	>250–500	>500
Mometasone furoate (DPI)	Depends on DPI device		
Mometasone furoate (pMDI, HFA)	200–400		400

BDP: beclomethasone dipropionate
pMDI: pressurized MDI
HFA: hydrofluoroalkane
DPI: dry powder inhaler
LD: low dose
MD: medium dose
HD: high dose
LD-OCS: low-dose oral corticosteroids
ICS: inhaled corticosteroids
SABA: short-acting β-agonist
LABA: long-acting β-agonist
MART: maintenance and reliever therapy
LAMA: long-acting muscarinic antagonist
LTRA: leukotriene receptor antagonist
HDM SLIT: house dust mite sublingual immunotherapy

Leigh Weatherly, DO

Global Initiative for Asthma. Global strategy for asthma management and prevention, 2022. https://www.ginasthma.org. Accessed December 23, 2024.

ASTHMA TREATMENT AND MAINTENANCE, CHILDREN AGES 5 YEARS AND YOUNGER

Diagnosis based on history and PE if:
(i) recurrent wheezing, (ii) no likely alternative explanation (foreign body, anatomical abnormality, CF), (iii) symptoms responsive to short-acting β_2-agonist (SABA)

↓

Treatment Approach:
- Recommend a pressurized metered-dose inhaler with spacer/holding chamber (with face mask for children aged <3 years and mouthpiece for children aged 3–5 years)
- Provide a written personalized asthma action plan, including seeking urgent care if child is acutely distressed or worsening despite SABA or same-day care if ≥4 puffs of SABA are needed within <4 hours.

↓

Management:
Step 1
- Use inhaled SABA as reliever via spacer/holding chamber.
- Address inhaler technique/spacer use and environmental factors (pet dander, tobacco, or heating fumes).

↓

Step 2
- If asthma symptoms occur more than twice a week or ≥1 severe exacerbations within a year, start daily inhaled corticosteroids (ICS); if good response to ICS for 2–3 months, consider a dose reduction.
- Alternative: daily leukotriene receptor antagonist (LTRA) or intermittent high-dose ICS

↓

Assess, Adjust, Review:
Stable/improved: Once good asthma control has been achieved for 2–3 months, consider stepping down therapy.
Not controlled: Before stepping up, confirm symptoms are due to asthma and review/address common issues (inhaler technique, adherence, allergen exposure, etc.).

↓

Step 3
- Double the low-dose ICS or add LTRA and continue SABA prn or refer to specialist for next steps.
- Review proper inhaler technique and treatment adherence, environmental factors, etc.

↓

Step 4
- Continue controller therapy and refer for specialist assessment; consider adding LTRA and/or LAMA.

↓

Acute Exacerbation: Initial home treatment:
- Inhaled SABA: 2 puffs of albuterol via age-appropriate spacer; repeat 2 more times at 20-minute intervals prn.
- Seek urgent medical care if child is acutely distressed, lethargic, fails to respond to initial bronchodilator therapy, or is worsening or if ≥4 puffs/day of inhaled SABA are required for symptom relief.

↓

Office Management:
- Assess severity using validated scoring tools (i.e., Pediatric Respiratory Assessment Measure [PRAM])
- Initiate SABA 2–6 puffs every 20 minutes for the first hour via pMDI/spacer or nebulized salbutamol (0.03 mL/kg of 0.5% solution, maximum 1 mL).
- Oxygen: to maintain saturation 94–98% or >94%
  - Systemic corticosteroids: oral prednisone or prednisolone 1–2.0 mg/kg (maximum 40 mg) for 3–5 days
  - *Or* dexamethasone 0.3–0.6 mg/kg (maximum 12 mg/day) for 1–2 days max (if relapses, use prednisolone at 1–2 mg/kg for 3–5 days)
- Immediate transfer to hospital if is no response to inhaled SABA within 1–2 hours, child is unable to speak or drink, respiratory rate is >40/min, cyanosis, unstable home, or oxygen saturation is <92% on room air.

Frank J. Domino, MD

Global Initiative for Asthma. Global strategy for asthma management and prevention, 2025. http://www.ginasthma.org. Updated November 15, 2025. Accessed December 22, 2025.

ASTHMA TREATMENT AND MAINTENANCE, CHILDREN AGES 6–11

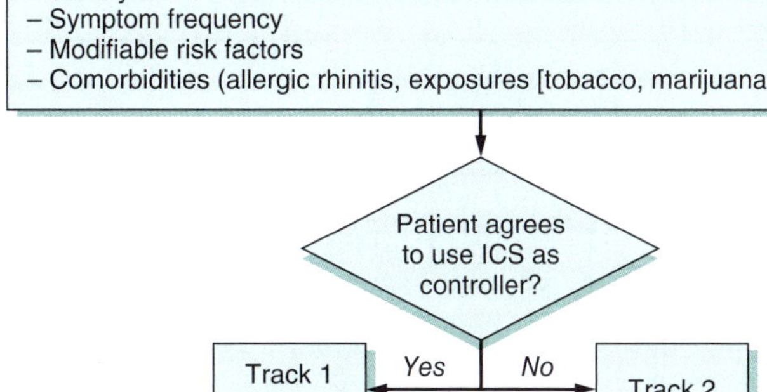

Treatment approach
- Use of spacer for all MDIs (β-agonist, ICS) to improve delivery, decrease side effects

Assess, Adjust, Review
- Once good asthma control has been achieved for 2–3 months, consider stepping down therapy.
- Before stepping up, confirm symptoms are due to asthma and review/address common issues (inhaler technique, adherence, allergen exposure, etc.).

Track 1: Patient agrees to use ICS as controller (preferred).

Track 2: Patient prefers to use SABA as reliever and ICS as controller.

Symptoms	Step 1 Sx <2 days a week	Step 2 Sx 2–5 days a week	Step 3 Sx most days or waking ≥1 time per week	Step 4 Symptoms most days Waking ≥1 week Low lung function	Step 5 Persistent symptoms/ exacerbations despite optimized step 4 treatments
Track 1	Preferred: LD-ICS when SABA is used	Preferred: LD-ICS + prn SABA	Preferred: LD-ICS-LABA + prn SABA MD-ICS + prn SABA or very LD-ICS + formoterol (MART)	Preferred: MD-ICS-LABA + prn SABA or LD-ICS + formoterol (MART) Refer to pediatric pulmonary	Preferred: HD-ICS-LABA + prn SABA *or* add on therapy: LAMA (tiotroprium), anti-IgE omalizumab Anti-interleukin-5/5Rα mepolizumab Anti-interleukin-4RA dupilumab
Track 2 (lacks efficacy evidence)	Alternative: no alternative for step 1 in track 2	Alternative: Daily LTRA or LD-ICS when SABA is used	Alternative: Daily LD-ICS + LTRA; + prn SABA	Alternative: Add tiotropium or LTRA; SABA or LD-ICS + formoterol as reliever	Alternative: As last resort, add on LD-OCS but consider side effects. SABA or LD-ICS + formoterol as reliever

Children 6–11 years Inhaled corticosteroid	Total daily ICS dose (μg) Low	 Medium	 High
BDP (pMDI, HFA)	100–200	>200–400	>400
BDP (pMDI, extrafine particle, HFA)	50–100	>100–200	>200
Budesonide (DPI, pMDI, standard particle, HFA)	100–200	>200–400	>400
Budesonide (nebules)	250–500	>500–1,000	>1,000
Ciclesonide (pMDI, extrafine particle, HFA)	80	>80–160	>160
Fluticasone furoate (DPI)	50		–
Fluticasone propionate (DPI)	50–100	>100–200	>200
Fluticasone propionate (pMDI, HFA, standard particle)	50–100	>100–200	>200
Mometasone furoate (pMDI, HFA)	100		200

BDP: beclomethasone dipropionate
pMDI: pressurized MDI
HFA: hydrofluoroalkane
DPI: dry powder inhaler
LD: low dose
MD: medium dose
HD: high dose
LD-OCS: low-dose oral corticosteroids
ICS: inhaled corticosteroids
SABA: short-acting β-agonist
MART: maintenance and reliever therapy
LTRA: leukotriene receptor antagonist
LABA: long-acting β-agonist
LAMA: long-acting muscarinic agonist

Catherine Hendren, MD, Kristen Richard, MD, and Michael Fahey, MD

Global Initiative for Asthma. Global strategy for asthma management and prevention, 2025. https://www.ginasthma.org. Accessed December 9, 2025.

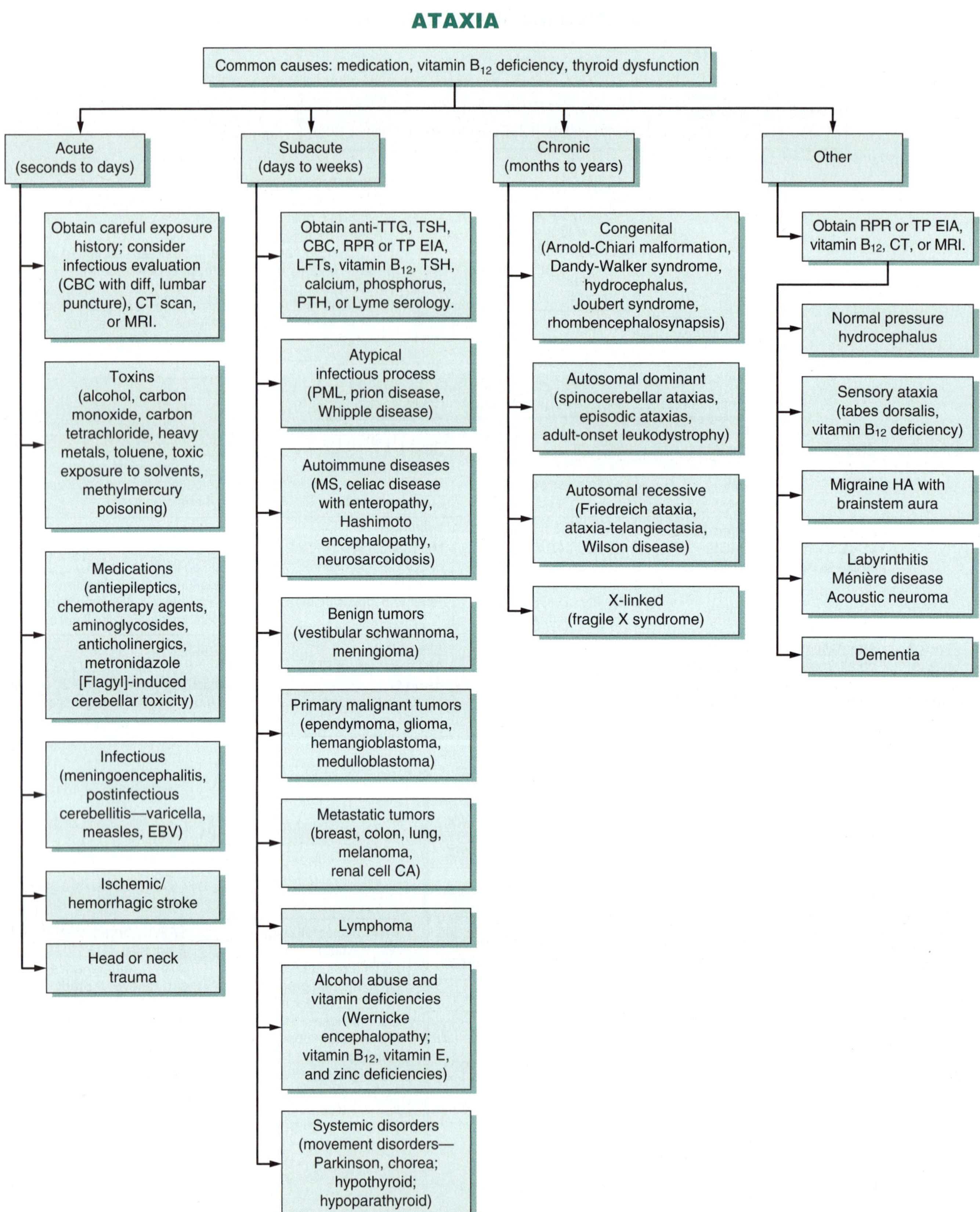

Fozia Akhtar Ali, MD, FAAFP and Claudia Liliana Gutierrez Cornejo, MD

Brunberg JA; for Expert Panel on Neurologic Imaging. Ataxia. *AJNR Am J Neuroradiol*. 2008;29(7):1420–1422.

AZOTEMIA AND UREMIA

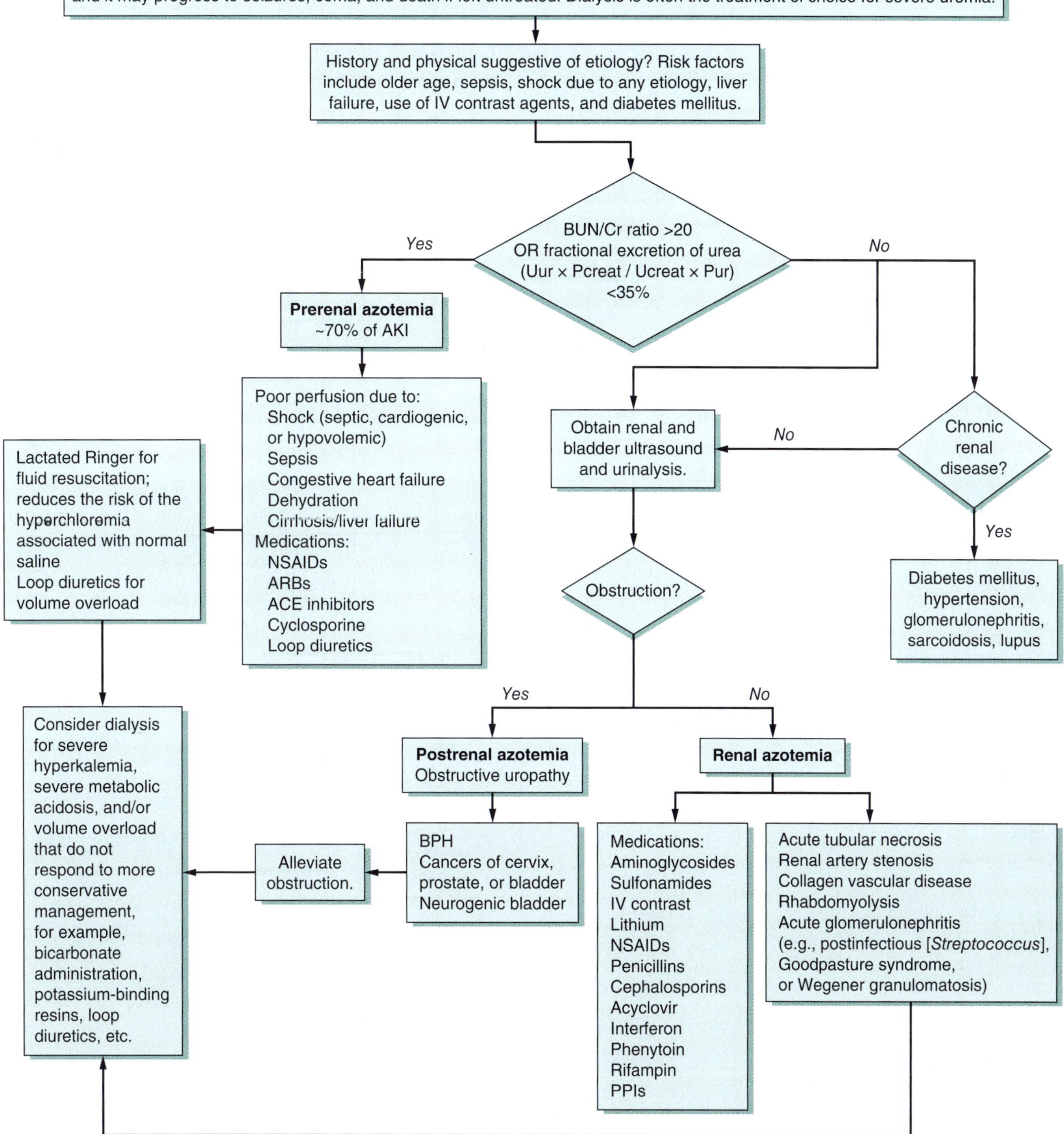

Steven A. House, MD, FAAFP, FAAHPM, HMDC

Mercado MG, Smith DK, Guard EL. Acute kidney injury: diagnosis and management. *Am Fam Physician*. 2019;100(11):687–694.

CARDIAC ARRHYTHMIAS

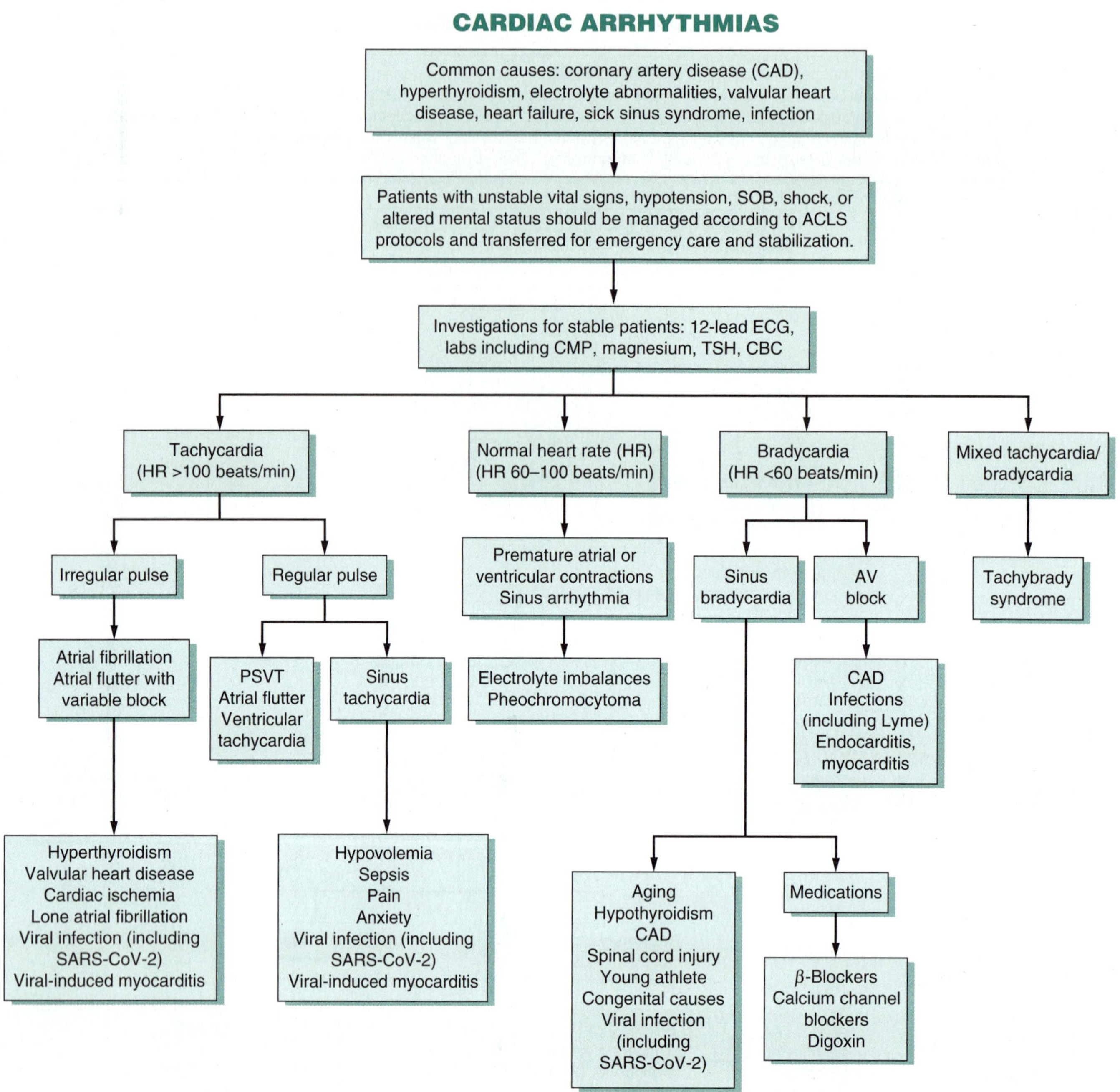

Anhthu Trinh, MD and Jameson Kuang, MD

Byrnes TJ, Costantini O. Tachyarrhythmias and bradyarrhythmias: differential diagnosis and initial management in the primary care office. *Med Clin North Am*. 2017;101(3):495–506.

CERVICAL CANCER SCREENING (PAP): NORMAL AND ABNORMAL IN NONPREGNANT WOMEN AGES 25–29 YEARS AND OLDER

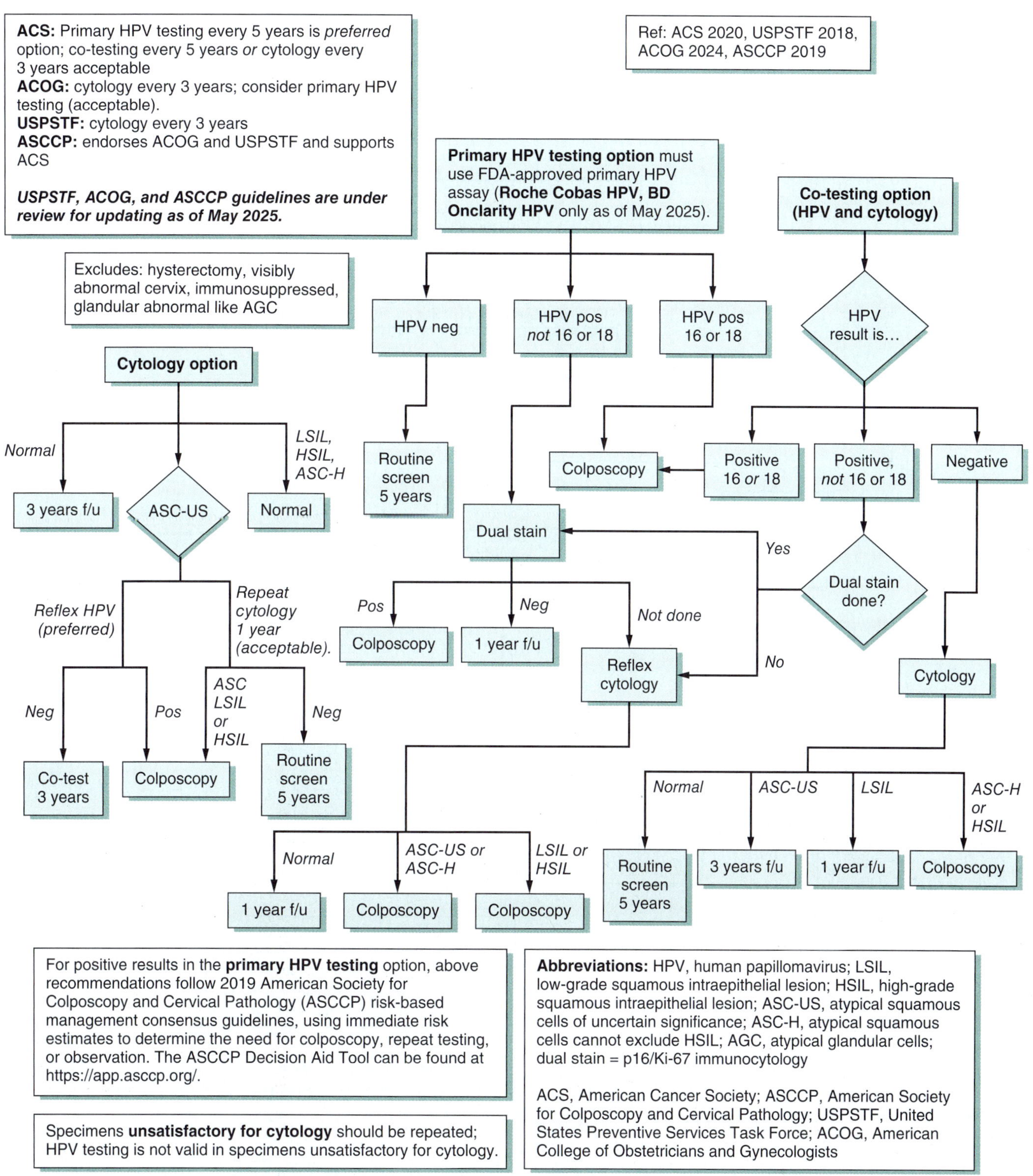

For positive results in the **primary HPV testing** option, above recommendations follow 2019 American Society for Colposcopy and Cervical Pathology (ASCCP) risk-based management consensus guidelines, using immediate risk estimates to determine the need for colposcopy, repeat testing, or observation. The ASCCP Decision Aid Tool can be found at https://app.asccp.org/.

Specimens **unsatisfactory for cytology** should be repeated; HPV testing is not valid in specimens unsatisfactory for cytology.

Abbreviations: HPV, human papillomavirus; LSIL, low-grade squamous intraepithelial lesion; HSIL, high-grade squamous intraepithelial lesion; ASC-US, atypical squamous cells of uncertain significance; ASC-H, atypical squamous cells cannot exclude HSIL; AGC, atypical glandular cells; dual stain = p16/Ki-67 immunocytology

ACS, American Cancer Society; ASCCP, American Society for Colposcopy and Cervical Pathology; USPSTF, United States Preventive Services Task Force; ACOG, American College of Obstetricians and Gynecologists

Manju Mahajan, MD, FAAFP and Jeremy Golding, MD, FAAFP

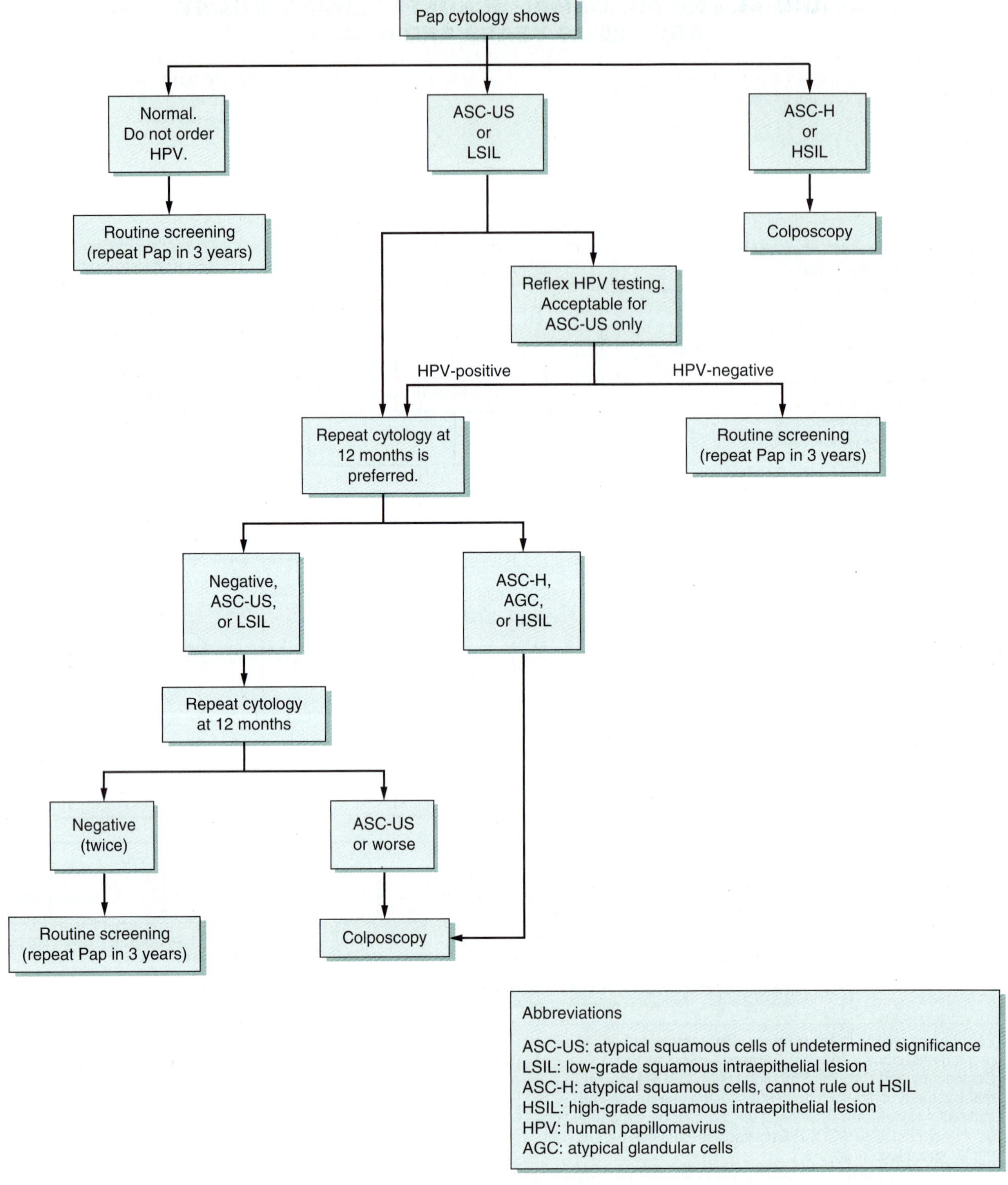

Abbreviations

ASC-US: atypical squamous cells of undetermined significance
LSIL: low-grade squamous intraepithelial lesion
ASC-H: atypical squamous cells, cannot rule out HSIL
HSIL: high-grade squamous intraepithelial lesion
HPV: human papillomavirus
AGC: atypical glandular cells

Manju Mahajan, MD, FAAFP and Jeremy Golding, MD, FAAFP

Perkins RB, Guido RS, Castle PE, et al; for 2019 ASCCP Risk-Based Management Consensus Guidelines Committee. 2019 ASCCP risk-based management consensus guidelines for abnormal cervical cancer screening tests and cancer precursors. *J Low Genit Tract Dis.* 2020;24(2):102–131.

CERVICAL CANCER SCREENING (PAP): NORMAL AND ABNORMAL IN AVERAGE-RISK, NONPREGNANT WOMEN AGES 30–65 YEARS

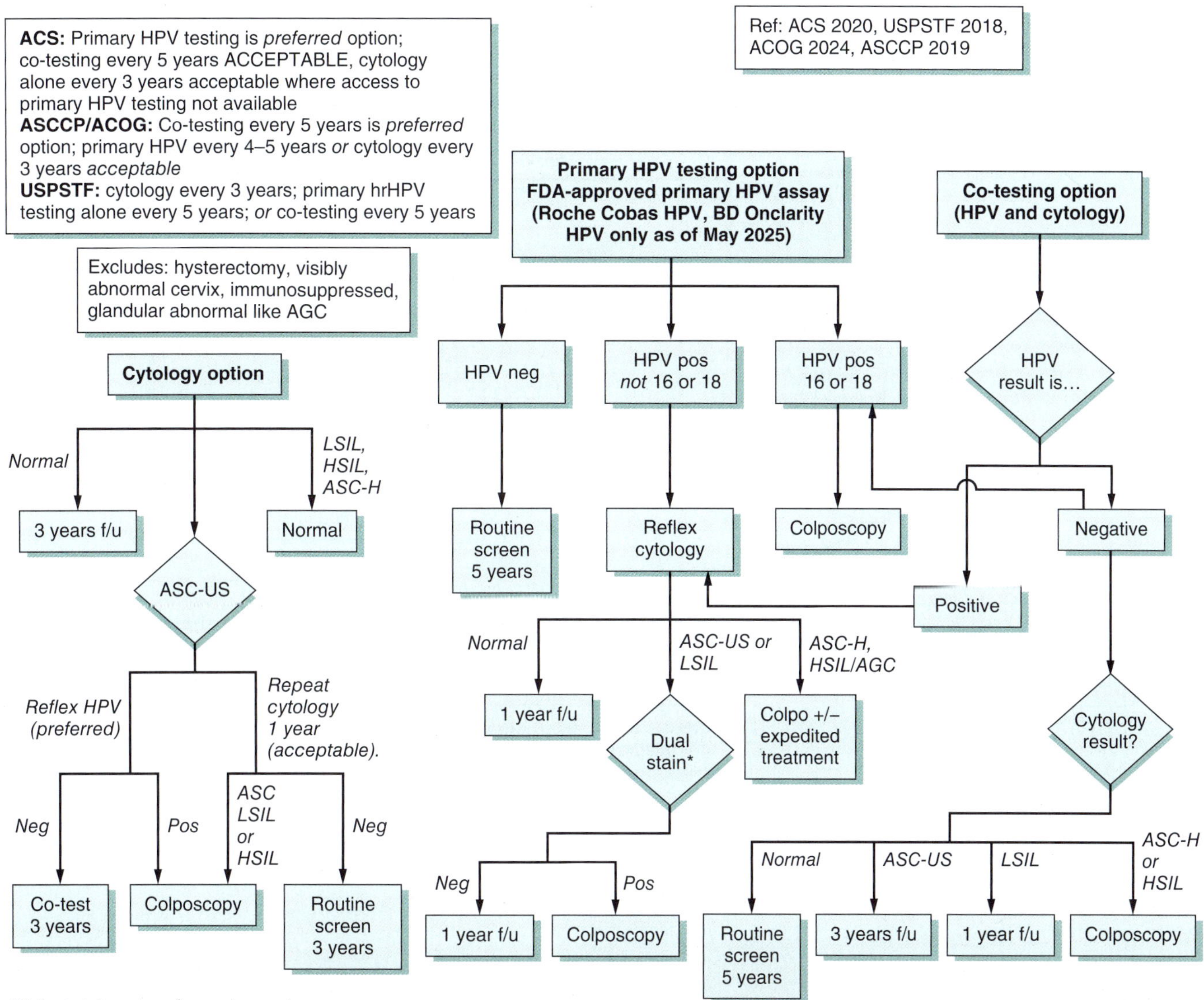

*If dual stain not performed, → colposcopy

For positive results in the **primary HPV testing** option, above recommendations follow 2019 American Society for Colposcopy and Cervical Pathology (ASCCP) risk-based management consensus guidelines, using immediate risk estimates to determine the need for colposcopy, repeat testing, or observation. The ASCCP Decision Aid Tool can be found at https://app.asccp.org/.

USPSTF, ACOG, and ASCCP guidelines are under review for updating as of May 2025.

Abbreviations: HPV, human papilloma virus; LSIL, low-grade squamous intraepithelial lesion; HSIL, high-grade squamous intraepithelial lesion; ASC-US, atypical squamous cells of uncertain significance; ASC-H, atypical squamous cells cannot exclude HSIL; AGC, atypical glandular cells; dual stain = p16/Ki-67 immunocytology

ACS, American Cancer Society; ASCCP, American Society for Colposcopy and Cervical Pathology; USPSTF, United States Preventive Services Task Force; ACOG, American College of Obstetricians and Gynecologists

Manju Mahajan, MD, FAAFP and Jeremy Golding, MD, FAAFP

CERVICAL HYPEREXTENSION INJURY

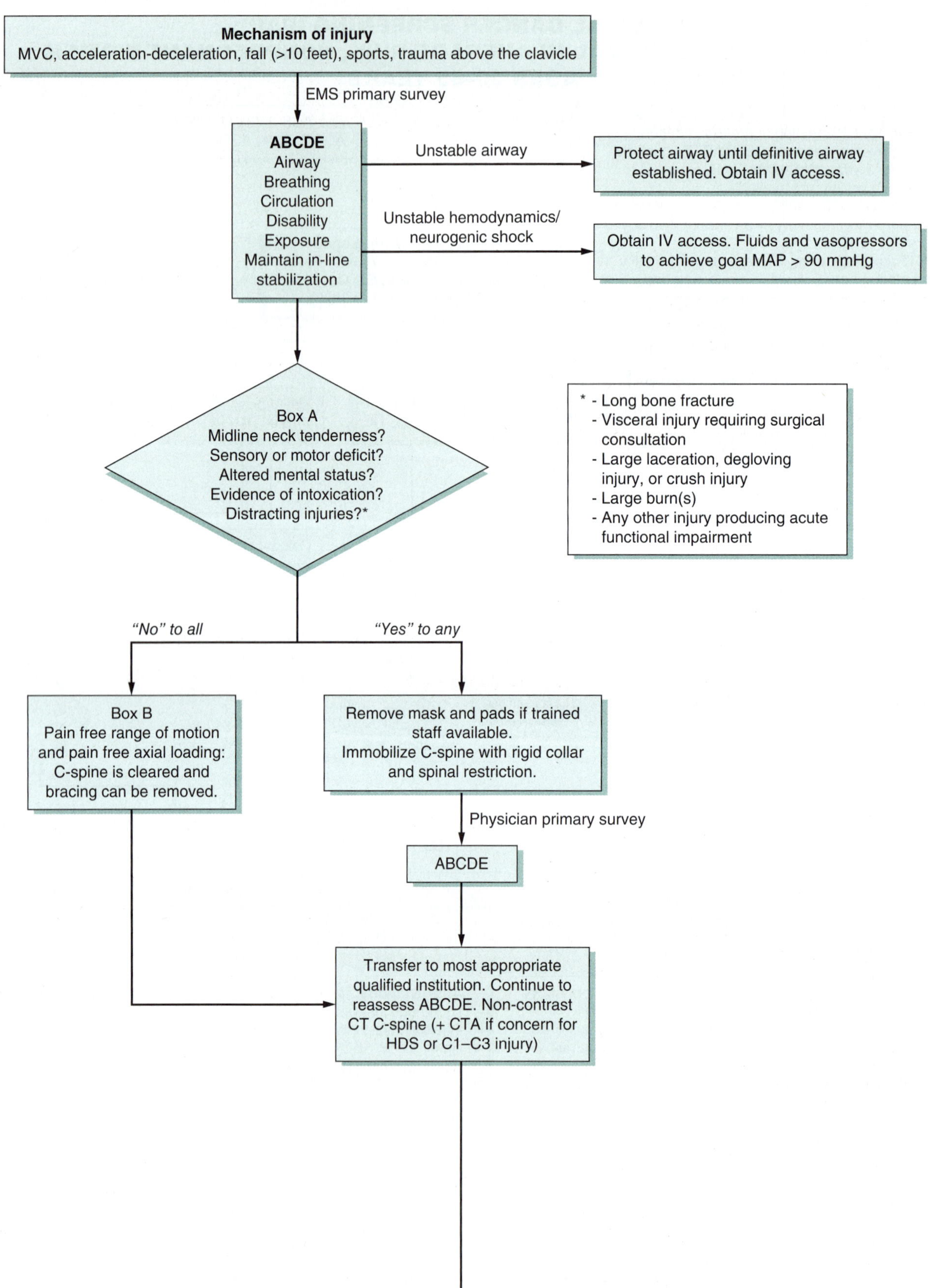

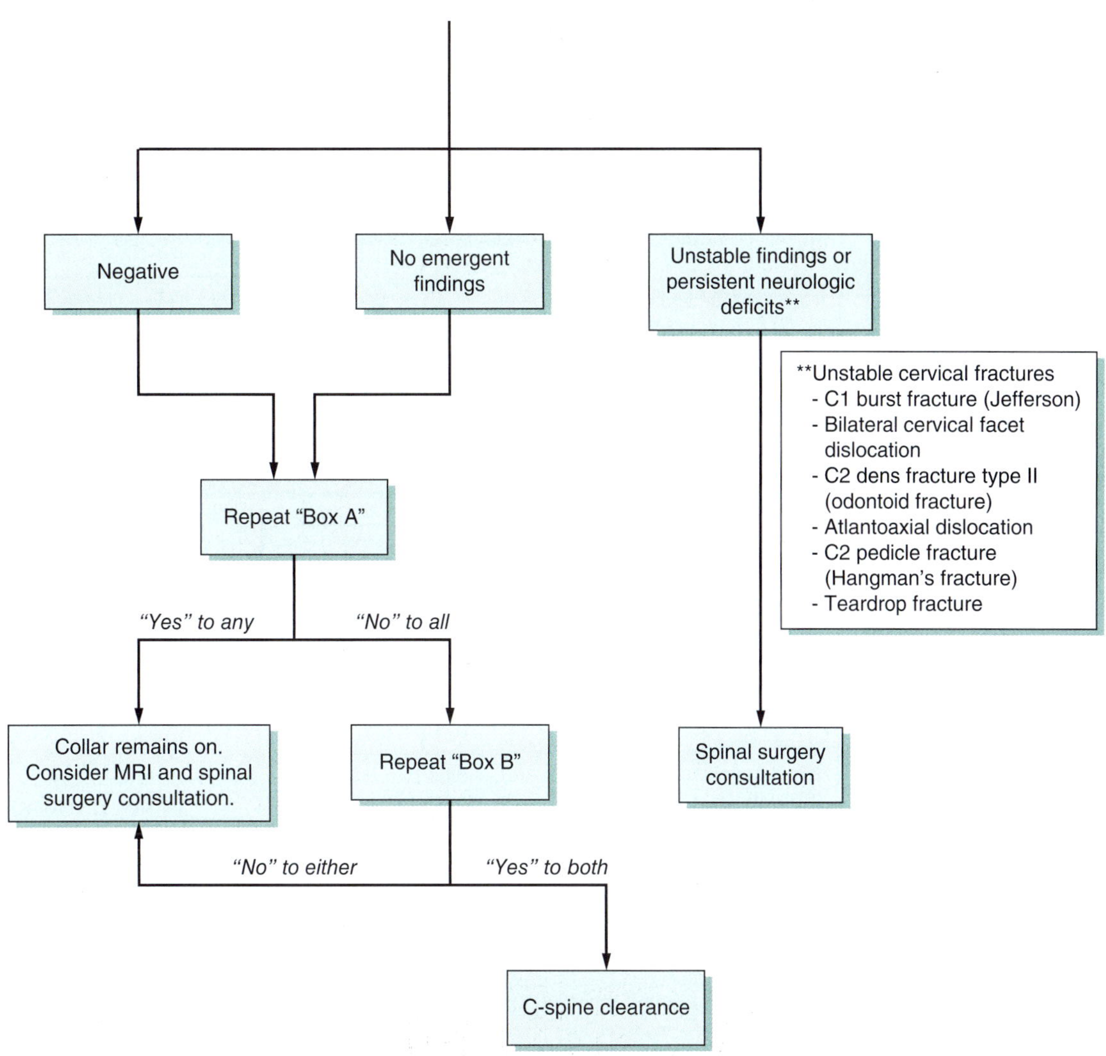

Alexander Pomerantz, MD, MPP and Jeremy Ng, MD, CAQSM

Okereke I, Mmerem K, Balasubramanian D. The management of cervical spine injuries—A literature review. *Orthop Res Rev*. 2021;13:151–162. doi:10.2147/ORR.S324622.

CHEST PAIN/ACUTE CORONARY SYNDROME

STEMI criteria
Any of the following
- 1 mm ST elevation in any two contiguous leads except V_2 and V_3
  – In women: 1.5 mm elevation in V_2 or V_3
  – In men aged <40 years: 2.5 mm elevation in V_2 or V_3
  – In men aged ≥40 years: 2 mm in V_2 or V_3

STEMI equivalents
- de Winter T waves
- ST depression in V_2 and V_3 and concerning posterior ECG
- LBBB or paced rhythm with Sgarbossa criteria*
- Hyperacute T waves

*Sgarbossa Criteria:
- Concordant ST elevation of ≥1 mm = 5 points
- Concordant ST-depression of ≥1 mm in V_1–V_3 = 3 points
- Discordant ST elevation of >5 mm = 2 points

Score of ≥3 has a 90% specificity for myocardial infarction; not sensitive

Chest pain

Consider noncardiac cause of chest pain: PE, aortic dissection, PTX, pericarditis, myocarditis, Boerhaave syndrome, costochondritis, GI related, trauma related, anxiety

ECG

STEMI criteria or STEMI equivalent

Alert cardiology.

162–325 mg ASA
O_2 if SpO_2 <90%
SL NTG q5min × 3 PRN for pain
(avoid in inferior STEMI)
Load with dual antiplatelet agent
- Clopidogrel 300 mg
~OR~
- Ticagrelor 180 mg
~OR~
- Prasugrel 60 mg

Heparin bolus
Avoid morphine if possible
(may interfere with antiplatelet agent).
Troponin, CXR

PCI available within 120 minutes?

Yes

PCI

Successful treatment?

No

Consider CABG.

Yes

Medical therapy

No

Administer thrombolytic within 30 minutes if unable to PCI within 120 minutes.

Medical therapy
- ASA 81 mg
- Clopidogrel 75 mg/day
- High-intensity statin
- β-Blocker unless CHF or shock
- Cardiac rehabilitation
- ACE inhibitor for patients with reduced EF
- Consider aldosterone antagonist if EF <40%.

No STEMI criteria or STEMI equivalent

ASA 162–325 mg, serial troponin, serial ECG if continuing chest pain, CXR

Serial ECG showing STEMI

Serial troponin positive?

Yes

- Admit.
- Heparin bolus
- ASA daily
- Consider nitrates, clopidogrel, β-blocker, ACEi, and statin.

Cardiology evaluation for consideration of cardiac catheterization

No

Risk stratify for CAD

High risk

Medium risk

Stress test

Positive

Negative

Review DDx: anxiety, GERD, PE, biliary dysfunction, MSK pain, domestic violence.

Low risk

Discharge home with PCP follow-up.

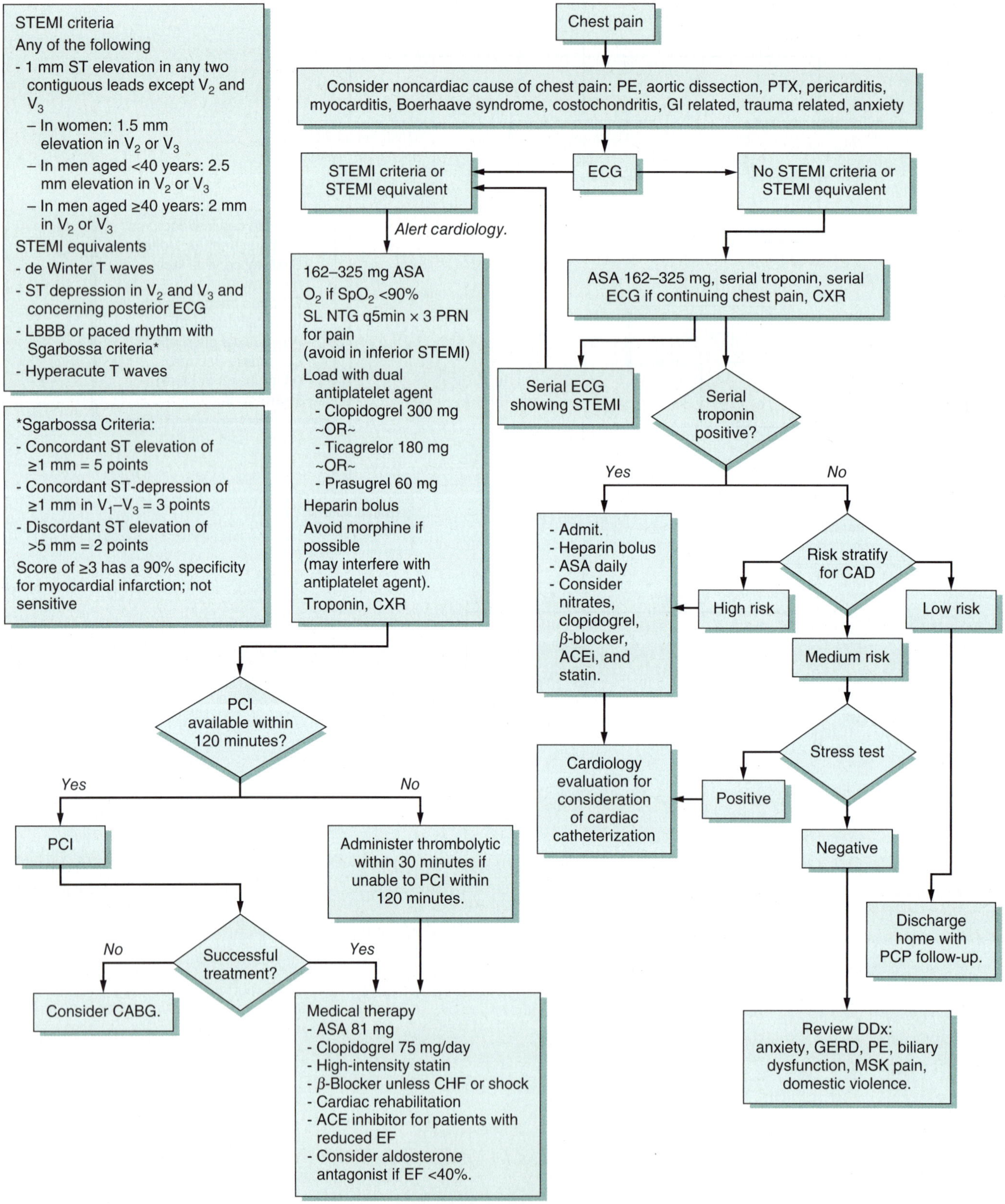

Jason Teng, MD and Moises Gallegos, MD, MPH, MEHP

Rao SV, O'Donoghue ML, Ruel M, et al. 2025 ACC/AHA/ACEP/NAEMSP/SCAI guideline for the management of patients with acute coronary syndromes: a report of the American College of Cardiology/American Heart Association Joint Committee on Clinical Practice Guidelines. *J Am Coll Cardiol*. 2025;85(22):2135–2237.

CHILD ABUSE: NONACCIDENTAL TRAUMA

When should you consider NAT in young children?

Skin Injury	**Age <6 months** • Any bruise or oral injury **Age 6 months–4 years** • Unexplained bruises in noncruising children • Bruises on the trunk, ear, neck, jaw line, cheek • Patterned bruising • Subconjunctival hemorrhage • Frenular tears
Burns	**Any age** • Unexplained burns • Burns in the shape of a heated object • Immersion burns • Burns on both the perineum and lower extremities
Fractures	**Age <6 months** • Any fracture **Age 6–11 months** • Linear parietal skull fractures without history • Any nonlinear parietal skull fracture • Any fracture of the ribs, femur, or humerus • Nonskull fractures in nonambulatory children • Any other fracture without history **Age 12–23 months** • Any rib or femur fracture • Nonsupracondylar humerus fracture • Any other fracture without history **Age 24 months–4 years** • Any rib fracture • Any other fracture without history
Intracranial	**Age <12 months** • Any subdural hemorrhage or hygroma **Age 12 months–4 years** • Acute subdural hematoma without history of high energy trauma (e.g., MVC, long-distance fall)
Visceral	**Age <12 months** • Any visceral injury **Age 12 months–4 years** • Unexplained traumatic visceral injury • Trauma to pancreas • Proximal hollow viscus injury

When should you consider NAT in older children?

- When a child makes a disclosure
- When there is no or inconsistent history to explain an injury
- When a prepubertal child displays sexualized behaviors
- When a prepubertal child has genital injury or infection
- Any pregnancy in a child <16 years old

Medical History

- If possible, interview the child separate from their guardian.
- Ask open-ended questions that do not introduce concepts of intentional injury or inappropriate behavior.
- When a child makes a disclosure, listen attentively, believe them, and thank them for telling you.

1. Obtain a focused injury history, especially a clear timeline.
2. PMH, that is, prior traumas, injuries, surgeries, hospitalizations
3. Family bleeding, bruising, bone, metabolic, or genetic history
4. Developmental and behavioral history
5. Social history, including living situation, other children in household, substance use, psychosocial stressors

Physical Examination

1. General assessment (alertness, demeanor, growth, evidence of neglect like severe caries, neglected wound care, etc.)
2. Skin exam, noting bruises, lacerations, burns, bites, etc.
3. Complete neurologic exam.
4. Consider secure photographs or sketches of physical signs.
5. If suspecting sexual violence, a specialized provider like a SANE nurse should perform the genital exam, if available.

Diagnostic Testing for Suspected NAT

1. Skeletal survey for those <24 months old
2. Head CT or MRI if <6 months old or concerned for head trauma
3. Consider basic lab evaluation: AST/ALT, urine toxicology
4. If bruising: CBC, PT, aPTT, von Willebrand factor VIII + IX
5. If fractures: Ca, Mg, phos, alk phos, PTH, vitamin D
6. If focal neuro findings or IC bleeding: Consult ophthalmology.

Management of Suspected NAT

1. Consult social work and child protection team.
2. Refer to child protection agencies when appropriate.
3. Document as objectively as possible.
4. Refer for mental health support early.

Cultural and Social Considerations

- Take the time to look into practices that differ from your own with a sense of curiosity and cultural humility, recognizing that parenting practices differ between cultures.
- NAT should never be the only thing on your differential.

- In many states, medical providers are mandated reporters when NAT is suspected, but we also have a responsibility to obtain a complete and accurate history to inform our degree of suspicion.
- The professional opinion of a medical provider is taken very seriously by child protective agencies and can have significant impact on the agencies' determinations.
- Although the investigation of cases of suspected NAT is intended to protect children, many forms of agency involvement, particularly family separation are inherently trauma inducing.

- Recognize that structural racism and other forms of oppression drive disparities in which families are suspected, referred, investigated, surveilled, and separated.
- Despite NAT being less likely to occur in families of color when controlling for other risk factors, children of color and Latinx children are overrepresented in child protective agencies, whereas cases of NAT among white, non-Latinx children are potentially missed.
- These structures of oppression, and the long history of medicine's involvement in their creation and perpetuation, create an understandable level of mistrust in some families.
- This mistrust can result in guarded responses, declining to volunteer information, or skepticism of medical recommendations, all of which may be misinterpreted by medical providers as suspicious.

Jordan Howard-Young, MD, MA-ID, DAAETS

Child Welfare Information Gateway. *Child Welfare Practice to Address Racial Disproportionality and Disparity.* Washington, DC: Children's Bureau; 2021. https://www.childwelfare.gov/pubPDFs/racial_disproportionality.pdf. Accessed November 30, 2024.

CHRONIC JOINT PAIN AND STIFFNESS

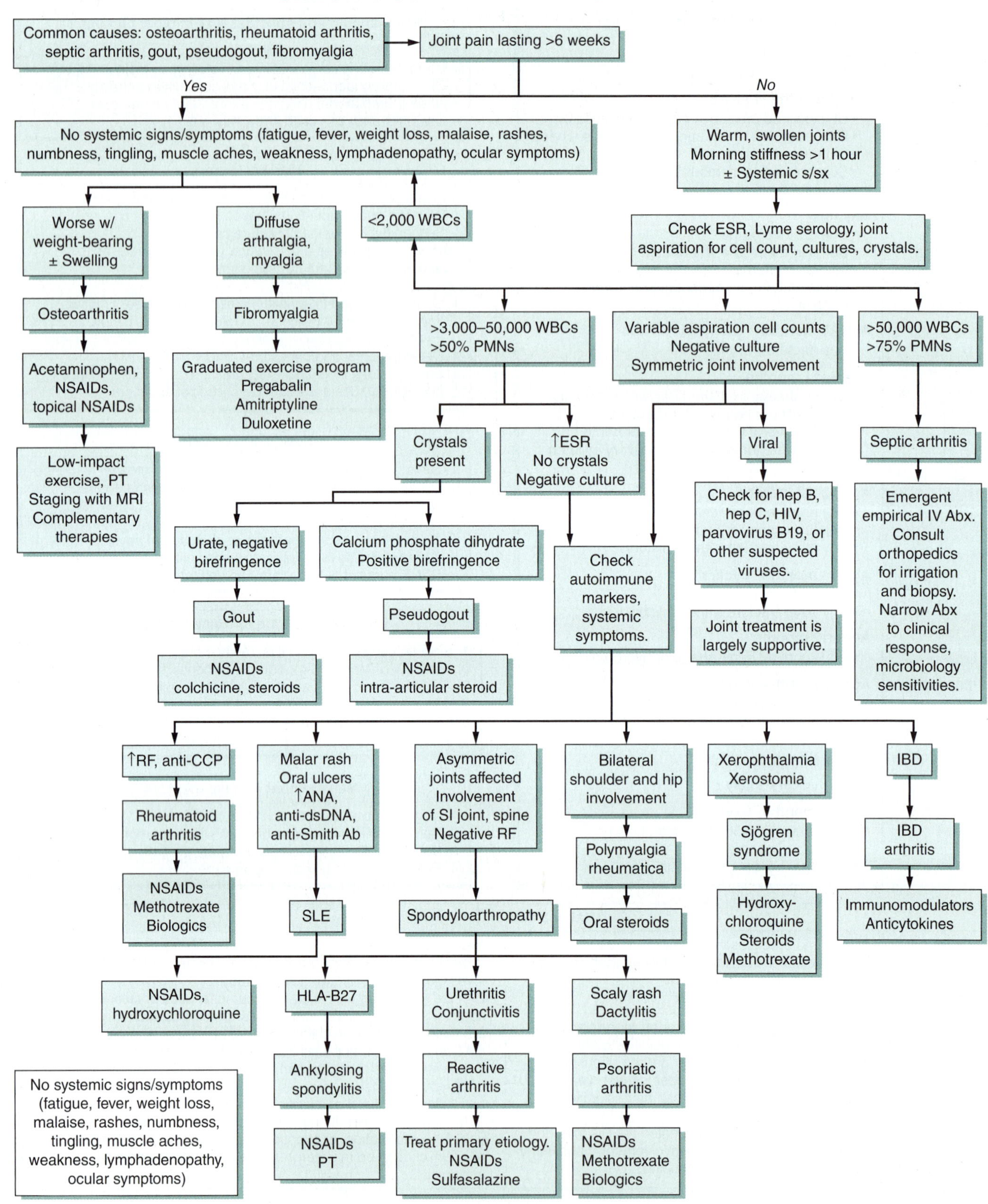

Bhumika Patel, DO and Laura Bujold, DO, MS

Foster ZJ, Day AL, Miller J. Polyarticular joint pain in adults: evaluation and differential diagnosis. *Am Fam Physician*. 2023;107(1):42–51.

CHRONIC OBSTRUCTIVE PULMONARY DISEASE (COPD), DIAGNOSIS AND TREATMENT

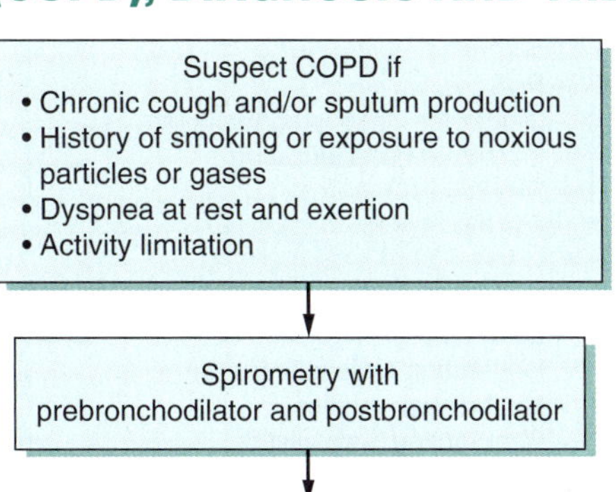

Suspect COPD if
- Chronic cough and/or sputum production
- History of smoking or exposure to noxious particles or gases
- Dyspnea at rest and exertion
- Activity limitation

↓

Spirometry with prebronchodilator and postbronchodilator

↓

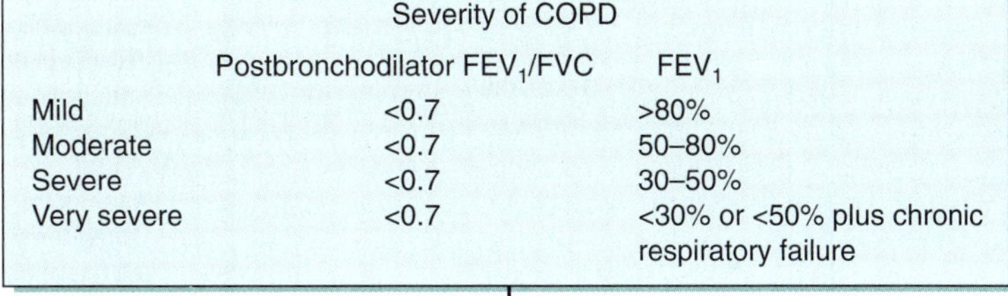

Severity of COPD

	Postbronchodilator FEV_1/FVC	FEV_1
Mild	<0.7	>80%
Moderate	<0.7	50–80%
Severe	<0.7	30–50%
Very severe	<0.7	<30% or <50% plus chronic respiratory failure

↓

Functional Dyspnea Scale

0	Not troubled with breathlessness except with strenuous exercise
1	Troubled by shortness of breath when hurrying or walking up a slight hill
2	Walks slower than people of same age due to breathlessness or has to stop for breath when walking at own pace on the level
3	Stops for breath after walking ~100 m or after a few minutes on the level
4	Too breathless to leave the house or breathless when dressing or undressing

↓

Diagnosis confirmed; initiate preventative measures:
- For >65 years of age and/or with chronic heart or lung disease, 1 dose of respiratory syncytial virus (RSV)
- Zoster vaccine for >50 years of age with COPD
- Influenza vaccine (yearly)
- Tdap
- COVID-19
- After age 18 years, 1 dose of 20-valent pneumococcal conjugate vaccine (PCV20) or 1 dose of PCV15 followed by PPSV23 or 1 dose PCV21. Patients who previously received PPSV23 only can receive either PCV20 or PCV15 1 year after the PPSV23.

↓

If actively smoking, aggressive smoking cessation counseling and offer approved pharmacotherapy.

↓

Lung cancer screening for ages 50–80 years old, 20-pack year history, and smoking within the last 15 years

↓

Group **A**/mild COPD	Group **B**/moderate COPD	Group **E**/severe COPD
– FDS = 0 or 1 – 0–1 exacerbations annually (not leading to hospitalization) Treatment: – Short-acting β-agonist or anticholinergic PRN	– FDS ≥2 – 0–1 exacerbations annually (not leading to hospitalization) Treatment: – Long-acting β-agonist plus long-acting anticholinergic combination inhaler – Short-acting β-agonist or anticholinergic PRN	– FDS ≥2 – 0–1 exacerbations annually (not leading to hospitalization) – ≥2 exacerbations annually or ≥1 exacerbation leading to hospitalization Treatment: – Long-acting β-agonist plus long-acting anticholinergic combination inhaler or inhaled corticosteroids plus long-acting β-agonist plus long-acting anticholinergic combination inhaler, if eosinophils are ≥100 – Short-acting β-agonist or anticholinergic PRN – Pulmonary rehabilitation: in person or virtual – Assess for supplemental oxygen. – Consider surgical options and/or add a phosphodiesterase-4 inhibitor. – Consider azithromycin 3 times a week to daily in patients with frequent exacerbations. – Consider dupilumab or ensifentrine.

William W. Wong, DO and Scott E. Kopec, MD

Global Initiative for Chronic Obstructive Lung Disease. 2024 Global strategy for prevention, diagnosis and management of COPD. https://goldcopd.org/2024-gold-report/. Accessed September 20, 2024.

CIRRHOSIS

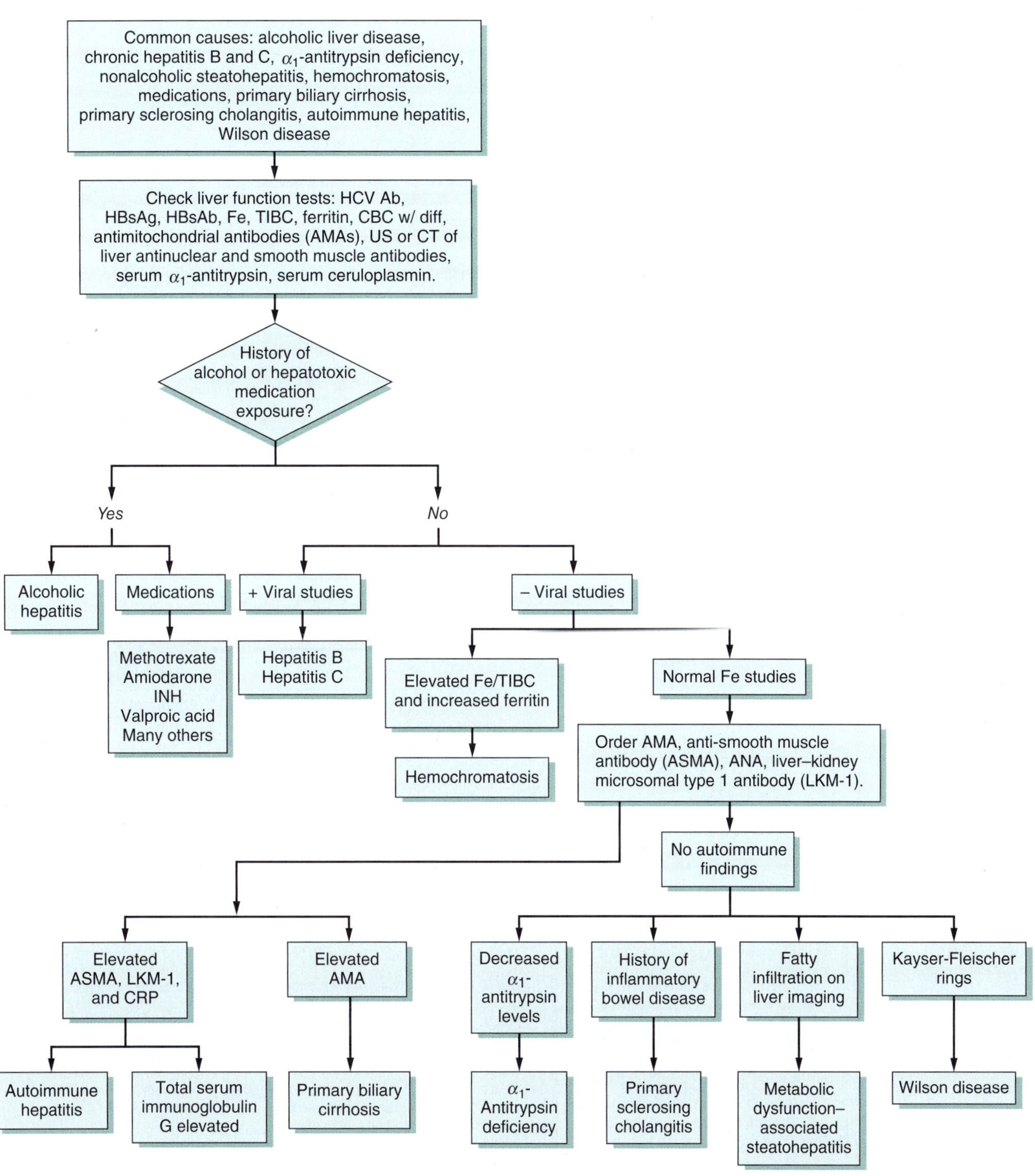

Chelsea Mendonca, MD and Adam Mendonca, MD

Smith A, Baumgartner K, Bositis C. Cirrhosis: diagnosis and management. *Am Fam Physician*. 2019;100(12):759–770.

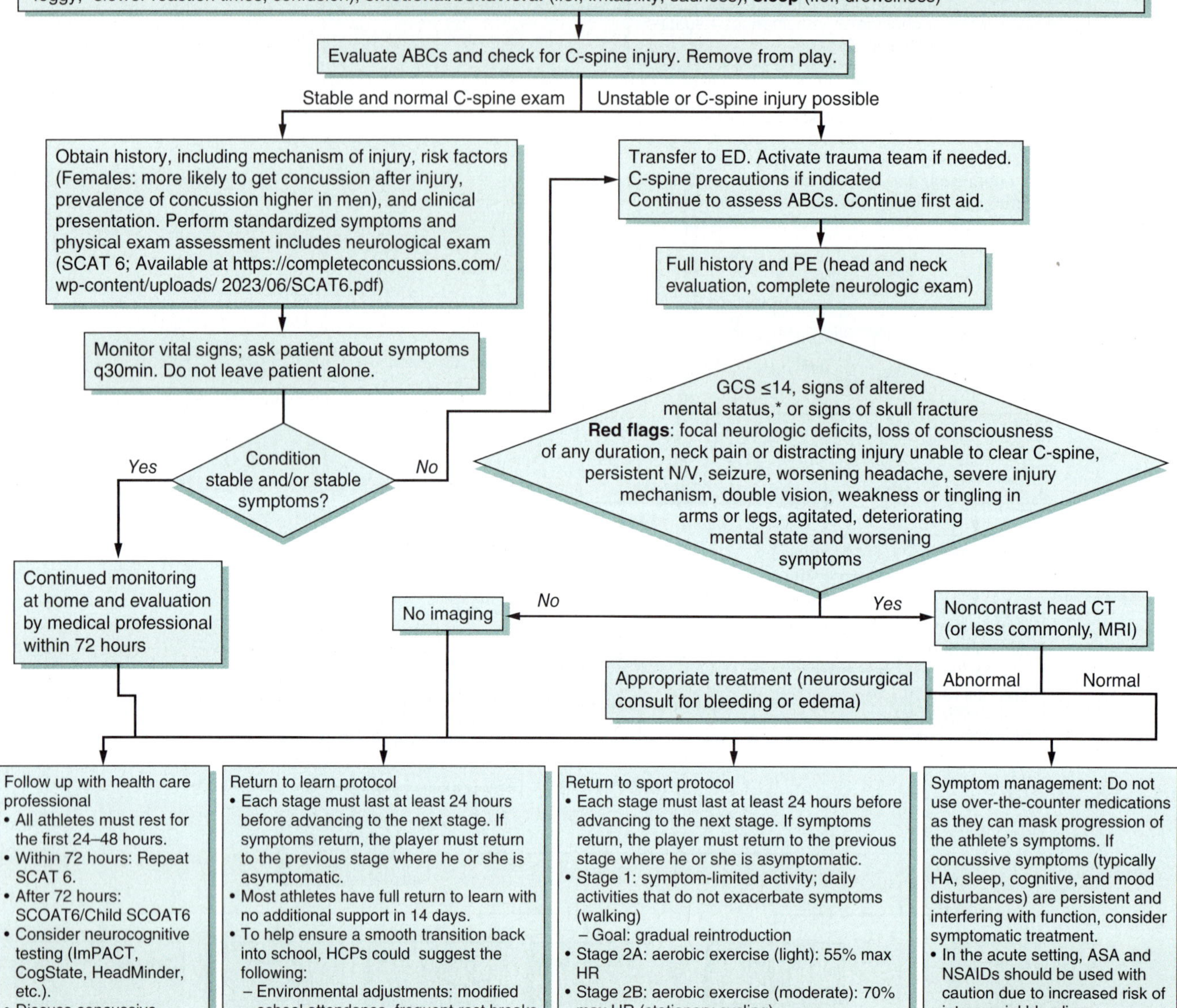

Follow up with health care professional
- All athletes must rest for the first 24–48 hours.
- Within 72 hours: Repeat SCAT 6.
- After 72 hours: SCOAT6/Child SCOAT6
- Consider neurocognitive testing (ImPACT, CogState, HeadMinder, etc.).
- Discuss concussive prevention tip: proper fitting mouth guards, limiting contact in practices, implementing protocols supporting optimal concussion management
- If at neurologic baseline, review and initiate return-to-play/ return-to-learn protocol.
- If not at neurologic baseline, consider ED evaluation, neuroimaging, specialist referral, and close follow-up.

Return to learn protocol
- Each stage must last at least 24 hours before advancing to the next stage. If symptoms return, the player must return to the previous stage where he or she is asymptomatic.
- Most athletes have full return to learn with no additional support in 14 days.
- To help ensure a smooth transition back into school, HCPs could suggest the following:
  - Environmental adjustments: modified school attendance, frequent rest breaks
  - Physical adjustments: avoid any activities that risk contact/collisions/falls
  - Curriculum adjustments: allow extra time for assignments, testing, projects
- Step 1: typical daily activities (i.e., reading)
  - Goal: return to typical activities
- Step 2: school activities (i.e., homework) outside of the classroom
  - Goal: increase tolerance to cognitive work
- Step 3: return to school part-time
  - Goal: increase academic activities
- Step 4: return to school full time
  - Goal: full academic activities and catch up on late/missed work

Return to sport protocol
- Each stage must last at least 24 hours before advancing to the next stage. If symptoms return, the player must return to the previous stage where he or she is asymptomatic.
- Stage 1: symptom-limited activity; daily activities that do not exacerbate symptoms (walking)
  - Goal: gradual reintroduction
- Stage 2A: aerobic exercise (light): 55% max HR
- Stage 2B: aerobic exercise (moderate): 70% max HR (stationary cycling)
  - Goal: increase HR
- Stage 3: individual sport-specific exercise
  - Goal: additional movement, change of direction
- Stages 4–6 should begin after the resolution of any symptoms, abnormalities, and cognitive function and any other clinical findings related to the current caution.
  - Stage 4: noncontact training drills
    - Goal: resume usual intensity of exercise, coordination, and increased thinking
  - Stage 5: full contact practice
    - Goal: restore confidence and assess functional skills
  - Stage 6: return to sport
    - Goal: normal game play

Symptom management: Do not use over-the-counter medications as they can mask progression of the athlete's symptoms. If concussive symptoms (typically HA, sleep, cognitive, and mood disturbances) are persistent and interfering with function, consider symptomatic treatment.
- In the acute setting, ASA and NSAIDs should be used with caution due to increased risk of intracranial bleeding. Acetaminophen and physical modalities are OK.
- If HA persists for a few days, consider typical abortive treatment. There is no established role for pharmacotherapy in the acute treatment of concussion-induced sleep, cognitive, or mood disturbances.
- If symptoms persist beyond 4 weeks, consider referral to specialist (neurology, sports medicine, etc.). Multidisciplinary approach is often needed.

**Signs of altered mental status: agitation, somnolence, repetitive questioning, or slow response to verbal communication.*

Anthony Shadiack, DO, CAQSM and Kelly Klump, MD

Putukian M, Purcell L, Schneider KJ, et al. Clinical recovery from concussion-return to school and sport: a systematic review and meta-analysis. *Br J Sports Med*. 2023;57(12):798–809.

CONGESTIVE HEART FAILURE: DIFFERENTIAL DIAGNOSIS

Common causes: CAD, MI, valvular disease, arrhythmia, idiopathic cardiomyopathy, pulmonary HTN, renal disease, medication nonadherence

↓

Diagnosis made clinically

↓

History: exercise intolerance, dyspnea on exertion or at rest, cough, orthopnea, paroxysmal nocturnal dyspnea, chest discomfort, fatigue, weight gain

↓

Exam: elevated jugular venous pressure, rales, S_3/S_4 gallop, hepatojugular reflux, increased abdominal distention, pallor, lower extremity edema

↓

Testing: chest x-ray, ECG, troponin, echo, BNP, BMP, LFTs, TSH, UA, uric acid

↓

Diagnosis of (C)HF: Framingham Diagnostic Criteria
Requires 2 major criteria or 1 major and 2 minor criteria

Major criteria
- Acute pulmonary edema
- Cardiomegaly
- Hepatojugular reflux
- Elevated jugular venous pressure
- Paroxysmal nocturnal dyspnea
- Rales
- S_3

Minor criteria
- Ankle edema
- Dyspnea on exertion
- Hepatomegaly
- Nocturnal cough
- Pleural effusion
- Tachycardia to >120 beats/min

97% and 89% sensitive for systolic and diastolic heart failure (HF), respectively

↓

- BNP <80 → (C)HF essentially ruled out
- BNP 80–500 → Indeterminate. Consider (C)HF AND alternative diagnoses:
  - COPD
  - Asthma
  - Lung disease
  - Pulmonary embolus
- BNP >500 → Likely (C)HF → LVEF <40% (HFrEF, systolic HF); EF 40–50% (HFmrEF); LVEF >50% (HFpEF, diastolic HF)

↓

Evaluate for causes of (C)HF.
- Ischemic: CAD/MI
- Nonischemic: HTN, idiopathic CM, valvular disease, HOCM, arrhythmia, myocarditis/pericarditis, collagen vascular disease
- Due to volume: medication noncompliance, renal failure

→ **Ischemic**
- History of CAD/MI
- Positive stress test
- CAD on cardiac catheterization
- Troponin elevation

↓

Cardiac catheterization unless contraindicated

→ **Nonischemic cardiomyopathy**

- Idiopathic cardiomyopathy
- Others: HTN, thyrotoxicosis, alcoholism, chemotherapy induced, cocaine, autoimmune, collagen vascular disease, infiltrative (amyloid, hemochromatosis), obstructive sleep apnea
- Tachycardia mediated (atrial fibrillation/flutter, SVT, frequent PVCs)
- Valvular disease cardiomyopathy
- Viral mediated (coxsackievirus, adenovirus, HIV, EBV)

Abbreviations:
HFpEF, heart failure with preserved ejection fraction; HFmrEF, heart failure with midrange ejection fraction; HFrEF, heart failure with reduced ejection fraction

Jeremy Golding, MD, FAAFP

King M, Kingery J, Casey B. Diagnosis and evaluation of heart failure. *Am Fam Physician.* 2012;85(12):1161–1168.

CONSTIPATION, DIAGNOSIS AND TREATMENT (ADULT)

Functional constipation
(Rome IV criteria)
- Two of the following for 12 weeks in past 6 months:
  - <3 stools per week
  - For 25% of time, any of the following:
    - Hard stools
    - Straining
    - Manual assist
    - Sense of incomplete evacuation
    - Sense of anorectal blockade
- Rare loose stools without laxative use
- Does NOT meet the criteria for IBS

Common causes: primary—functional, slow transit, pelvic floor dysfunction; secondary—IBS, diabetes mellitus, hypothyroidism, hypercalcemia, pregnancy, obstruction, medication side effect, pain, CKD

↓

History and physical: Diet, fluid intake, exercise, Rome IV criteria, digital rectal exam, abdominal exam, neurologic exam, stool quality (Bristol chart)

↓

Red flags: Unintentional weight loss, hematochezia, family Hx IBD or colon cancer, positive fecal occult, anemia, new onset in age >50 years, change in stool size, neurologic findings?
- *Yes* → Colonoscopy
- *No* → Medication Hx: anticholinergics, opiates, calcium channel blockers, antidepressants, antacids
  - *Yes* → Consider medication effect: Adjust and/or begin with empiric treatment. → Empiric treatment
  - *No* → Diagnostic testing: CBC, glucose, creatinine, calcium, TSH
    - Positive → Anemia (→ Colonoscopy), Hypothyroidism, Hypercalcemia, Diabetes mellitus
    - Negative → Empiric treatment

Empiric treatment: Lifestyle changes: gradually increase total fiber to 23–35 grams of fiber/day, (inulin up to 6 g/day or psyllium up to 35 g/day); pelvic floor therapy if appropriate. All patients should be given bowel retraining (https://www.med.unc.edu/ibs/wp-content/uploads/sites/450/2017/10/BowelRetrain.pdf).

↓

Symptoms improved?
- *Yes* → Continue therapy.
- *No* → Add polyethylene glycol and/or stimulant laxative. → Symptoms improved?
  - *Yes* → Continue therapy.
  - Partial → Add adjunctive agents such as lubiprostone and linaclotide.
  - *No* → Treatment failure → Anorectal manometry with balloon expulsion test
    - Normal ARM → Consider colonic transit time. → Add adjunctive agents such as lubiprostone and linaclotide.
    - Abnormal ARM → Pelvic floor dysfunction → Biofeedback; Consider MRI/defecography and surgical referral.

Bhumika Patel, DO and Laura Bujold, DO, MS

Sadler K, Arnold F, Dean S. Chronic constipation in adults. *Am Fam Physician*. 2022;106(3):299–306.

CONSTIPATION, TREATMENT (PEDIATRIC)

***Red flags:**
No meconium passed >48 hours in a term newborn
Constipation <1 month of age
Family history of Hirschsprung disease
Ribbon stools
Blood in the stools in the absence of anal fissures
Failure to thrive
Fever
Bilious vomiting
Severe abdominal distension
Abnormal thyroid gland
Abnormal position of the anus
Perianal fistula
Absent anal or cremasteric reflex
Decreased lower extremity strength/tone/reflex
Sacral dimple
Tuft of hair on spine
Gluteal cleft deviation
Anal scars
Extreme fear during anal inspection

Rome Criteria
Rome IV infants and children aged <4 years
- ≥1 month with two or more of following:
  - ≤2 bowel movements (BMs) per week
  - History of excessive stool retention
  - History of painful or hard BMs
  - History of large-diameter stools
  - Presence of large fecal mass in rectum
- If child is toilet trained, **criteria** include the following:
  - ≥1 episode per week of incontinence
  - History of large stools that may block toilet
- Potential accompanying symptoms
  - Irritability, decreased appetite, early satiety which resolve immediately after passing of a large stool

Rome IV diagnostic children and adolescents aged 4–18 years (developmental age ≥4 years)
- ≥1 month with two or more of following, at least once a week:
  - ≤2 BMs per week
  - ≥1 episode per week of incontinence after toilet training
  - History of retentive behavior or excessive volitional stool retention
  - History of painful or hard BMs
  - Presence of large fecal mass in rectum
  - History of large stools that may block toilet
- After appropriate evaluation, symptoms cannot be attributed to another medical condition.

Careful history and physical exam; digital rectal exam is not required for diagnosis.

Are red flags present?

Yes

Obtain based on symptoms: CBC, TSH, calcium, glucose, creatinine, tissue transglutaminase (tTG), and endomysium antibody (EMA).

Differential diagnosis:
Celiac disease
Hypothyroidism
Hypercalcemia
Hypokalemia
Diabetes mellitus
Drugs/toxins—opiates, anticholinergics, antidepressants, chemotherapy, heavy metals
Vitamin D intoxication
Botulism
Cystic fibrosis
Hirschsprung disease
Anal achalasia
Colonic inertia
Anal malformations
Pelvic mass
Spinal cord abnormalities
Abnormal abdominal musculature
Pseudoobstruction
Multiple endocrine neoplasia type 2B

Refer for specialty evaluation.

No

Functional constipation

Fecal impaction?

Yes

First line: polyethylene glycol (PEG) 3350 1.0–1.5 g/kg/day PO (as effective as enemas)

Second line: enemas daily for 3–6 days

No

Initial therapy: PEG 0.4 g/kg/day PO
Maintenance therapy: PEG 0.2–0.8 g/kg/day PO titrated to response; continue for 2 months until symptoms resolved for 1 month and then D/C gradually.

PEG is superior to lactulose.

Education: recognition of withholding behaviors; use of behavioral interventions: regular toileting routines, diaries, reward systems
Dietary/lifestyle recommendations:
– Normal fiber, fluid intake, physical activity
– No defined role for prebiotic or probiotic

A. Susan Feeney, MS, DNP, FNP-BC

Tabbers MM, DiLorenzo C, Berger MY, et al; for European Society for Pediatric Gastroenterology, Hepatology, and Nutrition, North American Society for Pediatric Gastroenterology. Evaluation and treatment of functional constipation in infants and children: evidence-based recommendations from ESPGHAN and NASPGHAN. *J Pediatr Gastroenterol Nutr.* 2014;58(2):258–274.

CONTRACEPTION

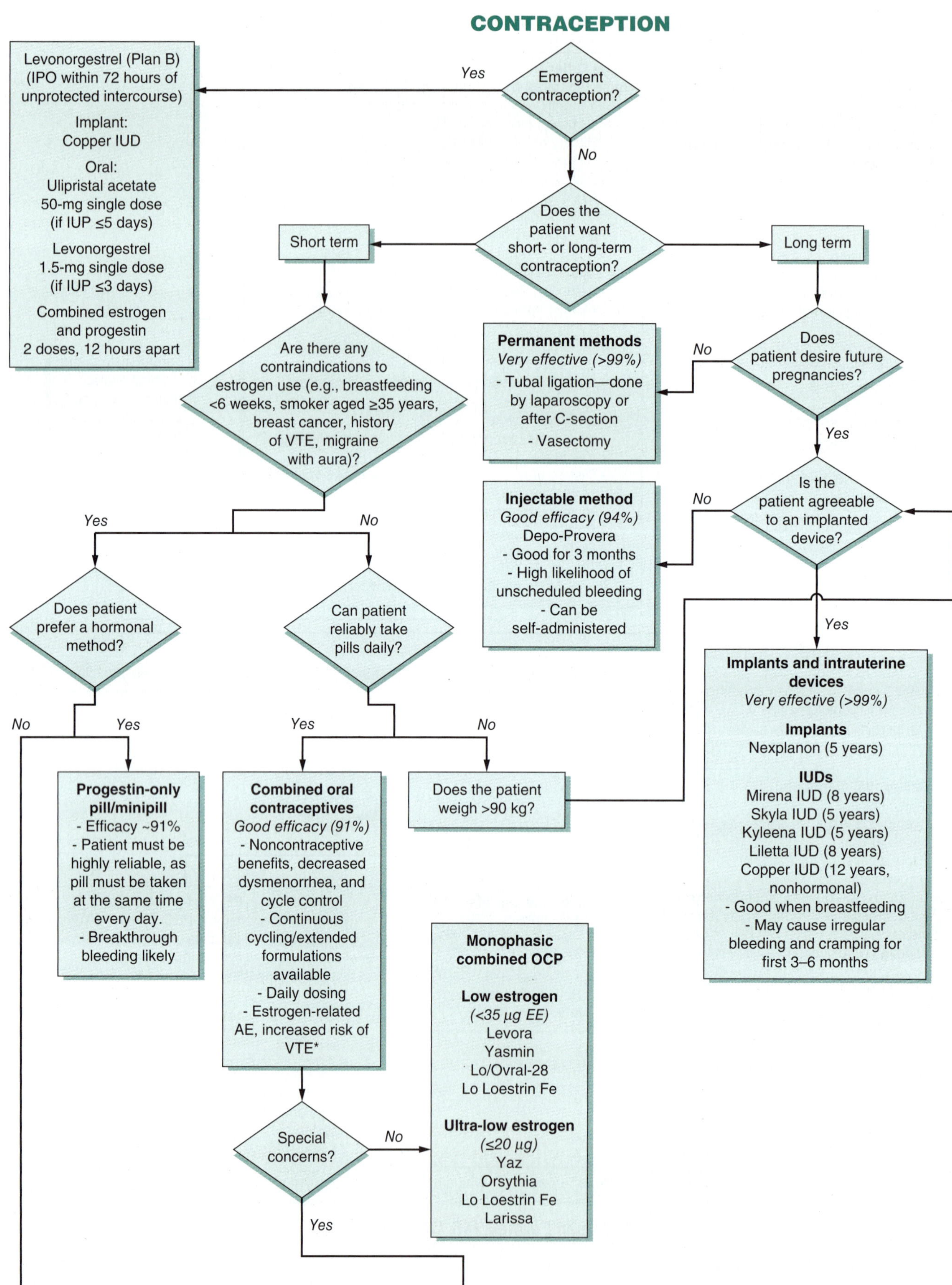

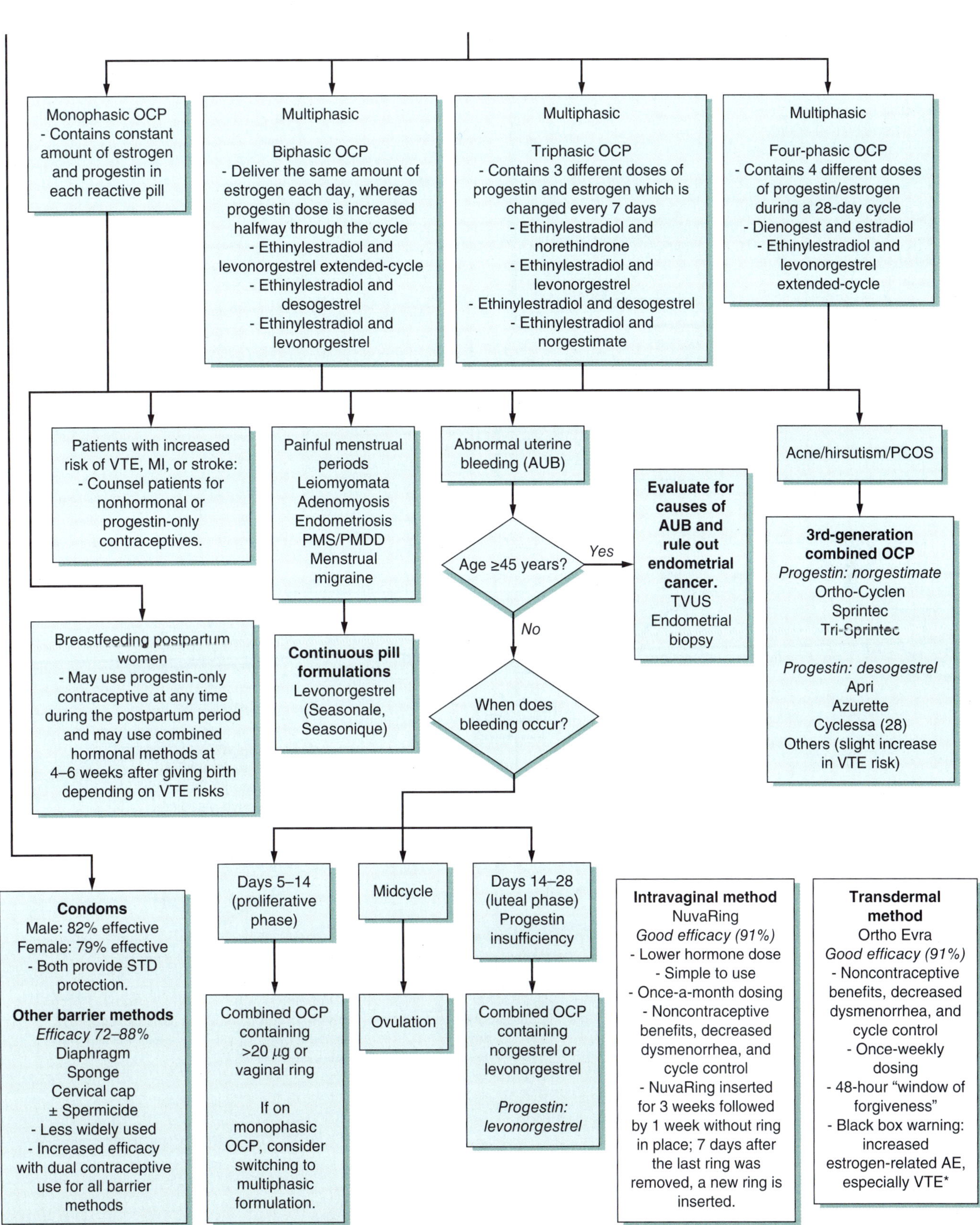

*Consult CDC MEC guidelines for contraindications to use.

Nicholas Radigan, MD and Peter Koppenheffer, MD

Madden T, Secura GM, Nease RF, et al. The role of contraceptive attributes in women's contraceptive decision making. *Am J Obstet Gynecol.* 2015;213(1):46.e1–46.e6.

DEEP VENOUS THROMBOSIS, DIAGNOSIS AND TREATMENT

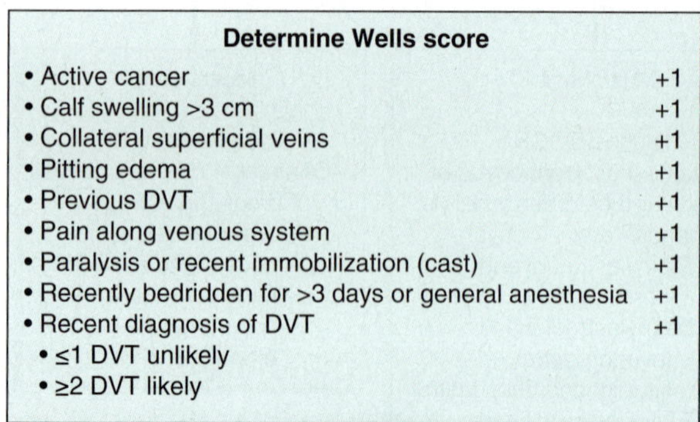

Determine Wells score

• Active cancer	+1
• Calf swelling >3 cm	+1
• Collateral superficial veins	+1
• Pitting edema	+1
• Previous DVT	+1
• Pain along venous system	+1
• Paralysis or recent immobilization (cast)	+1
• Recently bedridden for >3 days or general anesthesia	+1
• Recent diagnosis of DVT	+1

- ≤1 DVT unlikely
- ≥2 DVT likely

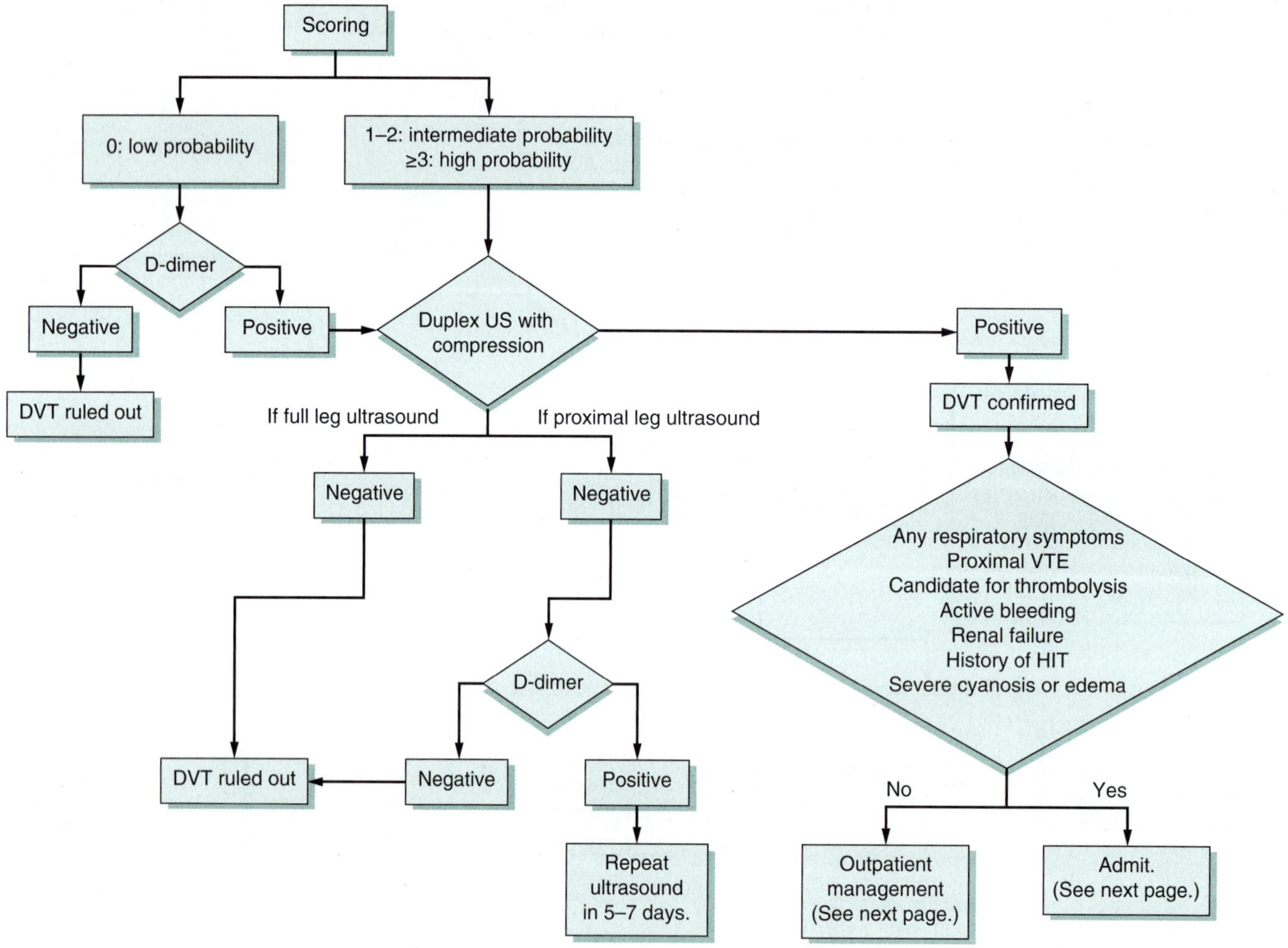

Scoring
- 0: low probability → D-dimer
  - Negative → DVT ruled out
  - Positive → Duplex US with compression
- 1–2: intermediate probability / ≥3: high probability → Duplex US with compression

Duplex US with compression
- If full leg ultrasound: Negative → DVT ruled out
- If proximal leg ultrasound: Negative → D-dimer
  - Negative → DVT ruled out
  - Positive → Repeat ultrasound in 5–7 days.
- Positive → DVT confirmed → Any respiratory symptoms / Proximal VTE / Candidate for thrombolysis / Active bleeding / Renal failure / History of HIT / Severe cyanosis or edema
  - No → Outpatient management (See next page.)
  - Yes → Admit. (See next page.)

Treatment

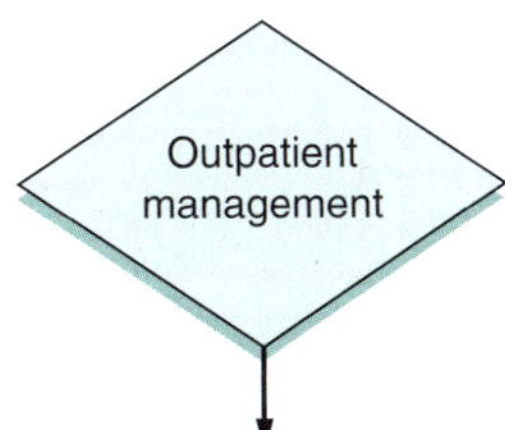

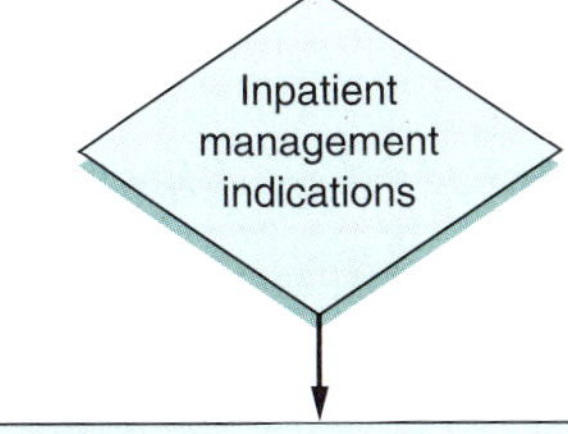

Therapy options:

Direct oral anticoagulants (rivaroxaban or apixaban) does not need bridge.

- Rivaroxaban
  - 15 mg BID with food for 21 days followed by 20 mg daily for at least 3 months
  - Avoid in patients with CrCl <30 mL/min.
- Apixaban
  - 10 mg BID for 7 days followed by 5 mg BID for at least 3 months

Low-molecular-weight heparin (LMWH), unfractionated heparin (UF), or fondaparinux with warfarin bridging

- Treatment with LMWH, UFH, or fondaparinux is recommended for at least 5 days *and* until INR ≥2 for 2 consecutive days.
  - Enoxaparin 1 mg/kg SC BID or
  - UFH preferred in patients with renal impairment
- Start warfarin on same days as LMWH, UFH, and fondaparinux.
  - Goal INR 2–3
  - Continue for 3–6 months after first DVT.
  - Warfarin is contraindicated in pregnancy.

LMWH, UF, or fondaparinux followed by dabigatran

- Dabigatran 150 mg BID after 7–10 days of LMWH and continue for at least 6 months
- Adjust dose for CrCl <50 mL/min.
- Do not use in CrCl <15 mL/min.

Inpatient management indications:

- Massive DVT
- Symptomatic PE
- High-risk bleeding with anticoagulation therapy
- Comorbid condition
- Phlegmasia cerulea dolens
- History of HIT

→

- IV UFH : 80 U/kg bolus or to a max 5,000 U → continuous infusion with initial dose 18 U/kg/hr → titrate to goal PTT 60–85 seconds *or*
- UFH 250 U/kg SC BID *or*
- Enoxaparin 1.5 kg/mg SC daily *or*
- Fondaparinux 5–10 mg SC daily depending on weight
- Consider catheter-directed thrombolysis or mechanical thrombectomy for extensive DVT.

Jason Teng, MD and Moises Gallegos, MD, MPH, MEHP

Ortel TL, Neumann I, Ageno W, et al. American Society of Hematology 2020 guidelines for management of venous thromboembolism: treatment of deep vein thrombosis and pulmonary embolism. *Blood Adv.* 2020;4(19):4693–4738.

DEHYDRATION, PEDIATRIC

Causes of dehydration in pediatric patients include gastrointestinal losses (vomiting, diarrhea), losses from skin (sweat, fever, burns), and urinary loses (glycosuria, diuretics).

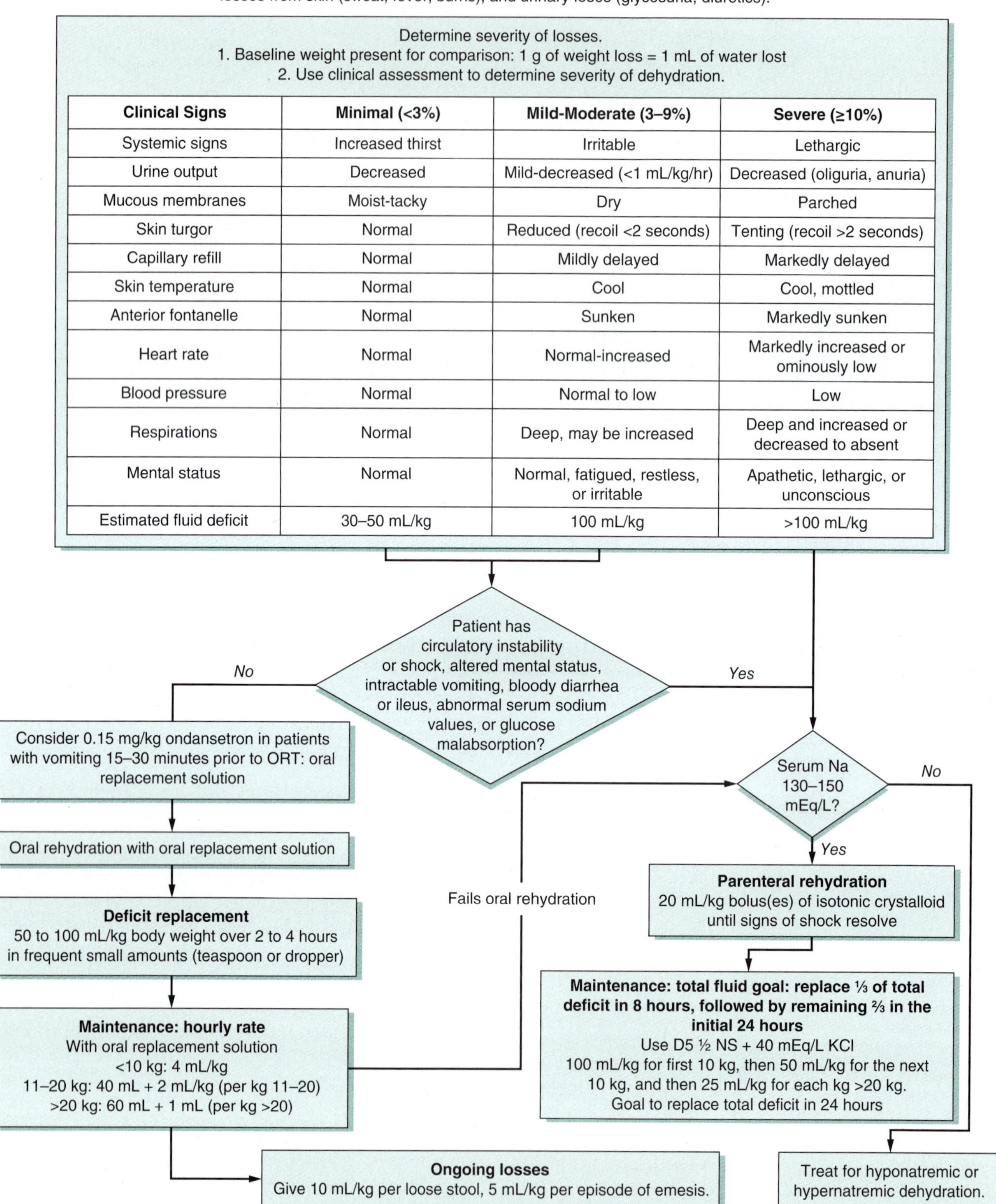

Determine severity of losses.
1. Baseline weight present for comparison: 1 g of weight loss = 1 mL of water lost
2. Use clinical assessment to determine severity of dehydration.

Clinical Signs	Minimal (<3%)	Mild-Moderate (3–9%)	Severe (≥10%)
Systemic signs	Increased thirst	Irritable	Lethargic
Urine output	Decreased	Mild-decreased (<1 mL/kg/hr)	Decreased (oliguria, anuria)
Mucous membranes	Moist-tacky	Dry	Parched
Skin turgor	Normal	Reduced (recoil <2 seconds)	Tenting (recoil >2 seconds)
Capillary refill	Normal	Mildly delayed	Markedly delayed
Skin temperature	Normal	Cool	Cool, mottled
Anterior fontanelle	Normal	Sunken	Markedly sunken
Heart rate	Normal	Normal-increased	Markedly increased or ominously low
Blood pressure	Normal	Normal to low	Low
Respirations	Normal	Deep, may be increased	Deep and increased or decreased to absent
Mental status	Normal	Normal, fatigued, restless, or irritable	Apathetic, lethargic, or unconscious
Estimated fluid deficit	30–50 mL/kg	100 mL/kg	>100 mL/kg

Bindusri Paruchuri, MD and Sarah M. Tiggelaar, MD, CLC

Santillanes G, Rose E. Evaluation and management of dehydration in children. *Emerg Med Clin North Am*. 2018;36(2):259–273. doi:10.1016/j.emc.2017.12.004.

DELIRIUM

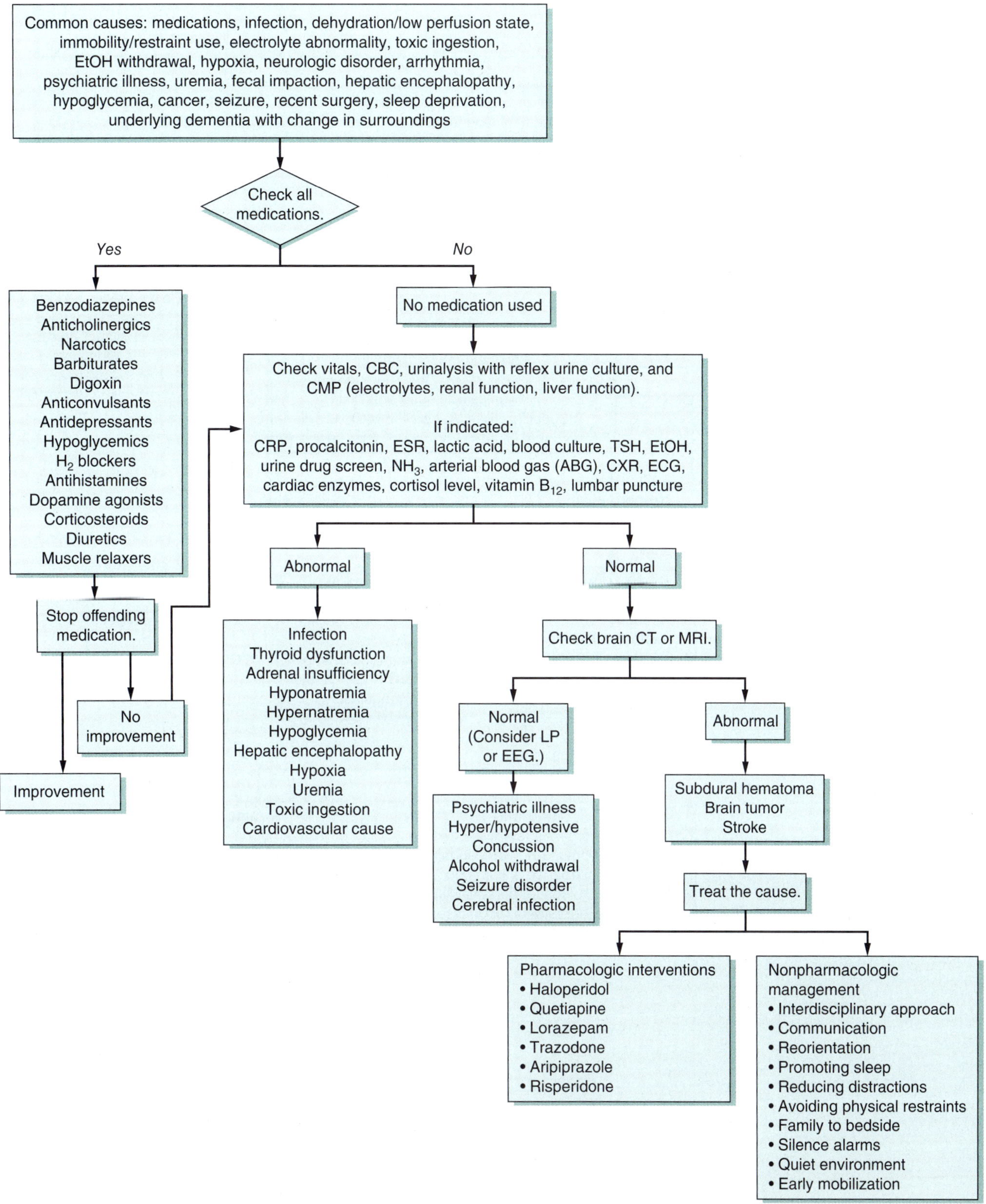

Frank J. Domino, MD

Thom RP, Levy-Carrick NC, Bui M, et al. Delirium. *Am J Psychiatry.* 2019;176(10):785–793.

DEMENTIA

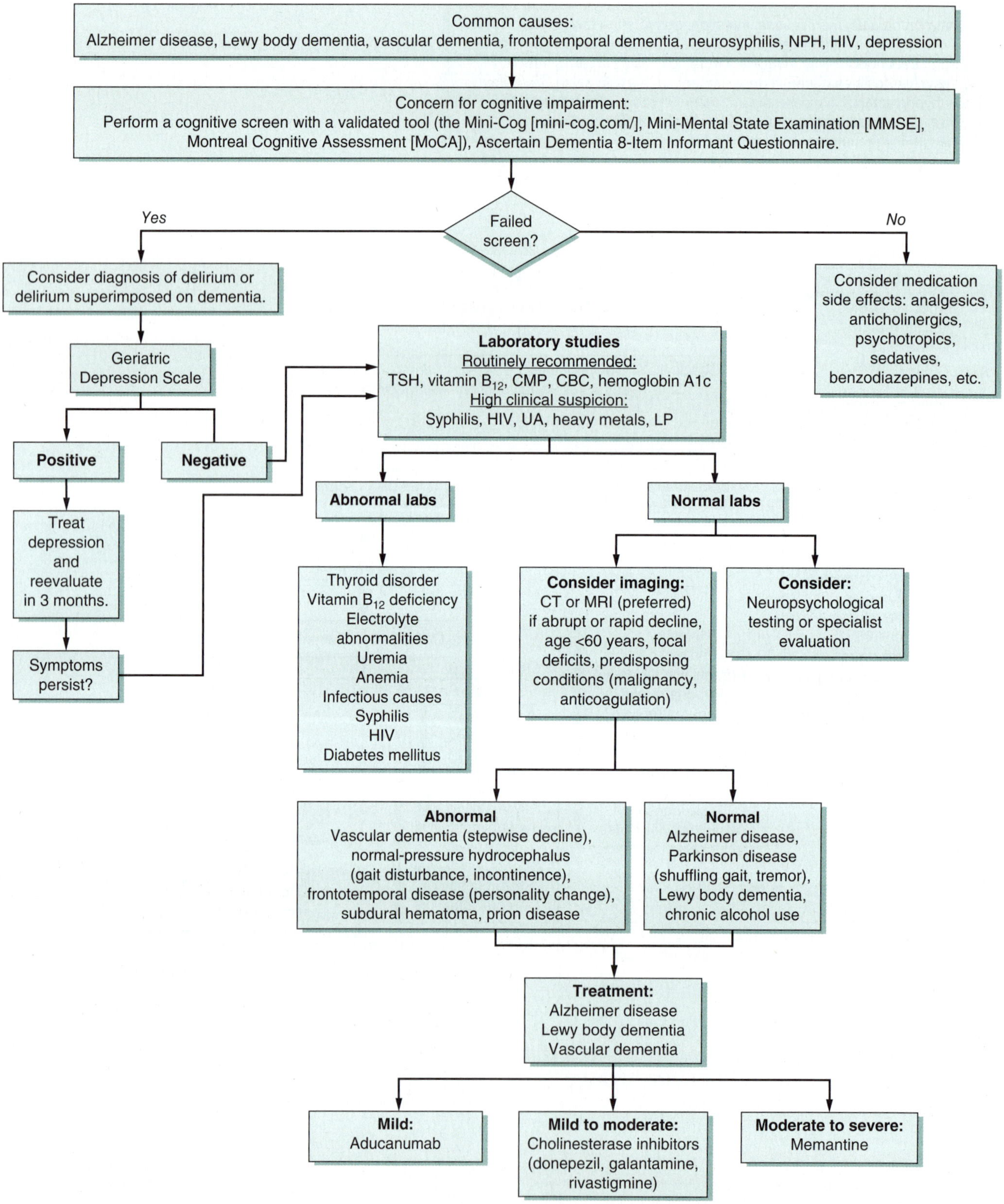

Common causes:
Alzheimer disease, Lewy body dementia, vascular dementia, frontotemporal dementia, neurosyphilis, NPH, HIV, depression

Concern for cognitive impairment:
Perform a cognitive screen with a validated tool (the Mini-Cog [mini-cog.com/], Mini-Mental State Examination [MMSE], Montreal Cognitive Assessment [MoCA]), Ascertain Dementia 8-Item Informant Questionnaire.

Failed screen?

Yes

Consider diagnosis of delirium or delirium superimposed on dementia.

Geriatric Depression Scale

Positive

Treat depression and reevaluate in 3 months.

Symptoms persist?

Negative

Laboratory studies
Routinely recommended:
TSH, vitamin B_{12}, CMP, CBC, hemoglobin A1c
High clinical suspicion:
Syphilis, HIV, UA, heavy metals, LP

Abnormal labs

Thyroid disorder
Vitamin B_{12} deficiency
Electrolyte abnormalities
Uremia
Anemia
Infectious causes
Syphilis
HIV
Diabetes mellitus

Normal labs

Consider imaging:
CT or MRI (preferred) if abrupt or rapid decline, age <60 years, focal deficits, predisposing conditions (malignancy, anticoagulation)

Consider:
Neuropsychological testing or specialist evaluation

Abnormal
Vascular dementia (stepwise decline), normal-pressure hydrocephalus (gait disturbance, incontinence), frontotemporal disease (personality change), subdural hematoma, prion disease

Normal
Alzheimer disease, Parkinson disease (shuffling gait, tremor), Lewy body dementia, chronic alcohol use

Treatment:
Alzheimer disease
Lewy body dementia
Vascular dementia

Mild:
Aducanumab

Mild to moderate:
Cholinesterase inhibitors (donepezil, galantamine, rivastigmine)

Moderate to severe:
Memantine

No

Consider medication side effects: analgesics, anticholinergics, psychotropics, sedatives, benzodiazepines, etc.

Adam Mendonca, MD and Chelsea Mendonca, MD

Falk N, Cole A, Meredith TJ. Evaluation of suspected dementia. *Am Fam Physician*. 2018;97(6):398–405.

DEPRESSIVE EPISODE, MAJOR

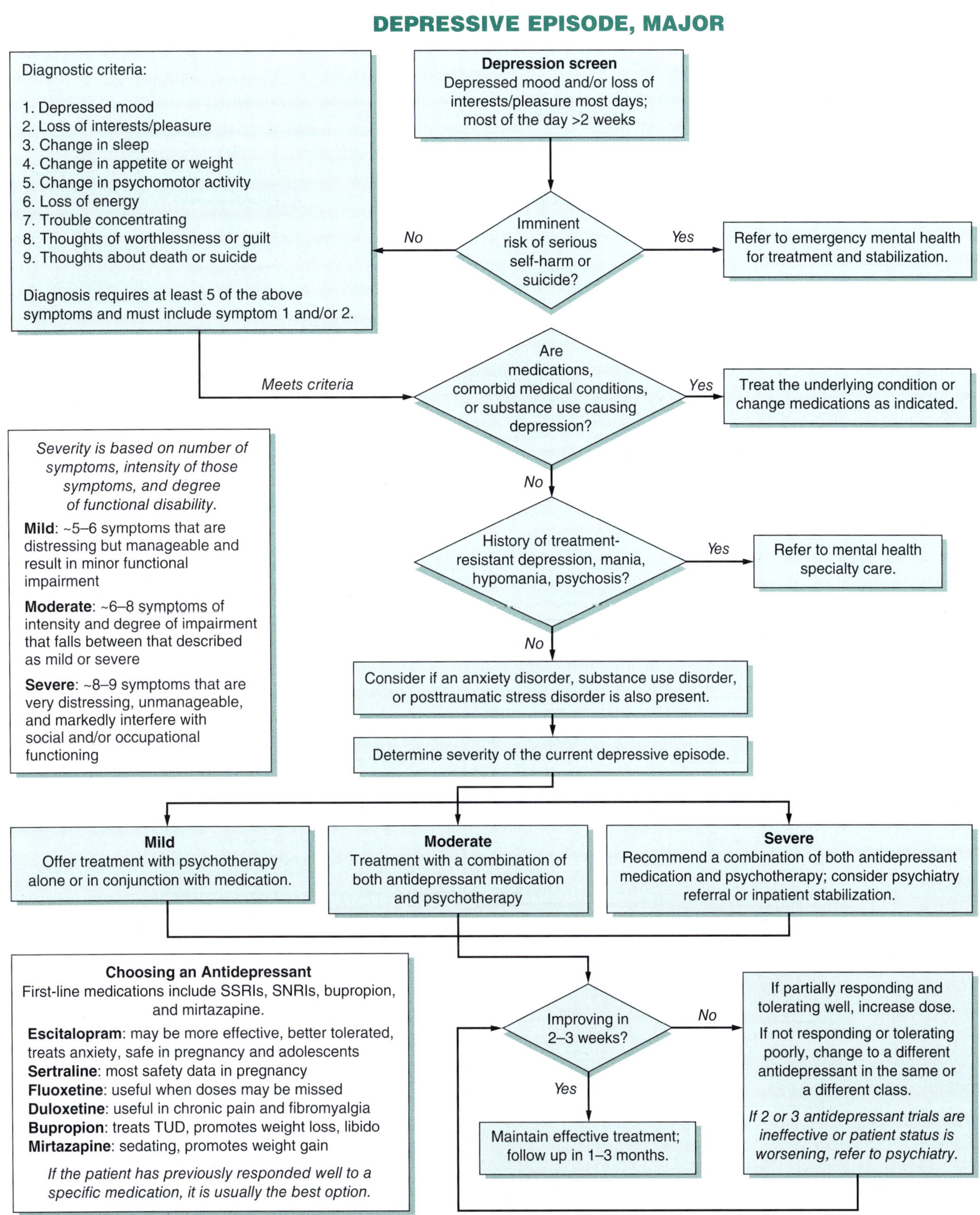

Jordan Howard-Young, MD, MA-ID, DAAETS and Stephany Giraldo Eierle, DO, MPH

U.S. Department of Veterans Affairs, U.S. Department of Defense. *VA/DoD Clinical Practice Guideline for Management of Major Depressive Disorder.* Washington, DC: U.S. Department of Veterans Affairs, U.S. Department of Defense; 2016.

DIABETIC KETOACIDOSIS (DKA), TREATMENT

DKA diagnostic criteria: serum glucose >250 mg/dL, arterial pH <7.3, serum bicarbonate <18 mEq/L, and elevated serum ketone level, SGLT2 inhibitors may precipitate euglycemic DKA
Complete initial evaluation. Check capillary glucose and serum/urine ketones to confirm hyperglycemia and ketonemia/ketonuria.

IV fluids

- Start 1.0 L of 0.9% NaCl/hr.
  - Severe/shock → Administer 9% NaCl at 1.0–1.5 L over the 1st hour and then, if serum-corrected Na is high or normal, give 0.45% NaCl at 250–500 mL/hr depending on hydration state. Hemodynamic monitoring and pressors
  - Mild dehydration → Evaluate corrected serum sodium (Na). Corrected Na = Measured Na + [0.016 × (Measured glucose − 100)]
    - Corrected serum Na ≥135 mEq/L → 0.45% NaCl (250–500 mL/hr)
    - Corrected serum Na <135 mEq/L → 0.9% NaCl (250–500 mL/hr)
    - → **Serum glucose <200 mg/dL** →
      - 5% dextrose with 0.45% NaCl at 150–250 mL/hr
      - Decrease insulin to 0.05–0.10 U/kg/hr IV.
      - If using SC insulin instead of IV, decrease rapid-acting SC bolus to 0.1 U/kg SC q2h.
    - → Keep serum glucose between 150 and 200 mg/dL until resolution of DKA. → Resolution of DKA*

Insulin

- Complicated:
  - pH <7
  - Stupor/coma
  - Bicarb <10 mEq/L
  - Anion gap >12 mEq/L
  - → Regular insulin 0.1 U/kg IV bolus 1–2 hours after starting IV fluids → Then 0.1 units/kg/hr continuous insulin infusion
- Uncomplicated DKA → Initiate rapid-acting insulin bolus 0.3 U/kg SC and then 0.2 U/kg SC 1 hour later. → Continue rapid-acting insulin 0.2 U/kg SC q2h.
- → If serum glucose does not fall by 50–70 mg/dL in the 1st hour, double IV dose or double SC bolus dose.

Potassium

- Urine output >50 mL/hr
  - K⁺ <3.5 mEq/L → Hold insulin until K⁺ >3.5 mEq/L. Give 20–40 mEq K⁺/hr. → K⁺ ≥3.5 and <5.0 mEq/L
  - K⁺ ≥3.5 and <5.0 mEq/L → Add 20–30 mEq K⁺ to each liter of IV fluid. Goal is K⁺ between 4 and 5 mEq/L. → Resolution of DKA*
  - K⁺ ≥5.0 mEq/L → Recheck every 2 hours.

Assess the need for bicarbonate.

- pH <6.9 → Give 100 mEq of $NaHCO_3$ in 400 mL sterile water. Give at rate of 200 mL/hr. Give with 20 mEq K⁺ if <5.0 mEq/L. → Repeat IV $NaHCO_3$ dose q2h until pH ≥6.9 and check serum K⁺. → Resolution of DKA*

Laboratory evaluation

- **Initial**: CBC, CMP, ABG, serum ketones, Mg, phosphate, UA, ECG, HbA1c; if indicated, CXR, BCx, UCx, amylase, lipase
- **Serial**: In addition to clinical monitoring and urine output, monitor glucose, BMP, phos, venous pH and β-hydroxybutyrate (BOHB).
- **Calculated**: effective osmolality, anion gap, corrected Na⁺, urine output
- **Frequency**: q1h initially and then q2–4h once stable until DKA resolution → Resolution of DKA*

Resolution of DKA* → Feed and change from IV to SC insulin (basal-bolus) regimen (0.5–0.8 U/kg/day for insulin-naive patients). Keep IV insulin running for 2–4 hours after initial SC dose. Look for causes of DKA. Reassess outpatient medication regimen and discontinue SGLT2 inhibitors if hx of DKA.

*Resolution of DKA criteria:
- Glucose level <200 mg/dL
- pH >7.3
- Serum bicarbonate level is ≥18 mEq/L.

Astrud San Antonio Villareal, MD, FAAFP, William Johnston, MD, and Tyler Evans, DO

American Diabetes Association Professional Practice Committee. 3. Prevention or delay of diabetes and associated comorbidities: standards of care in diabetes—2025. *Diabetes Care*. 2025;48(Suppl 1):S50–S58. doi:10.2337/dc25-S003.

DIARRHEA, CHRONIC

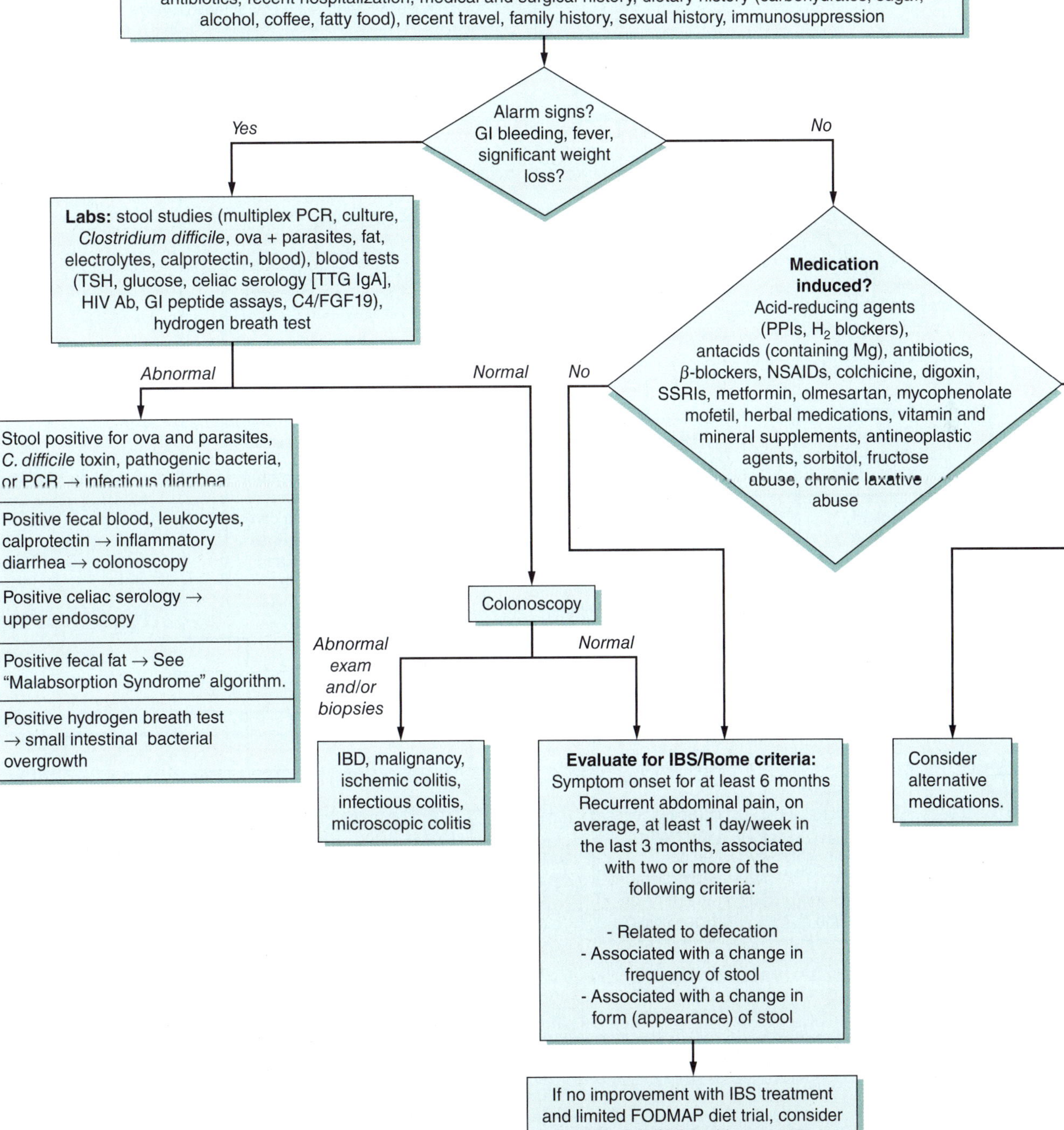

Jennifer M. Romeu, MD, FAAFP, MSM

Schiller LR. Evaluation of chronic diarrhea and irritable bowel syndrome with diarrhea in adults in the era of precision medicine. *Am J Gastroenterol.* 2018;113(5):660–669.

DIZZINESS

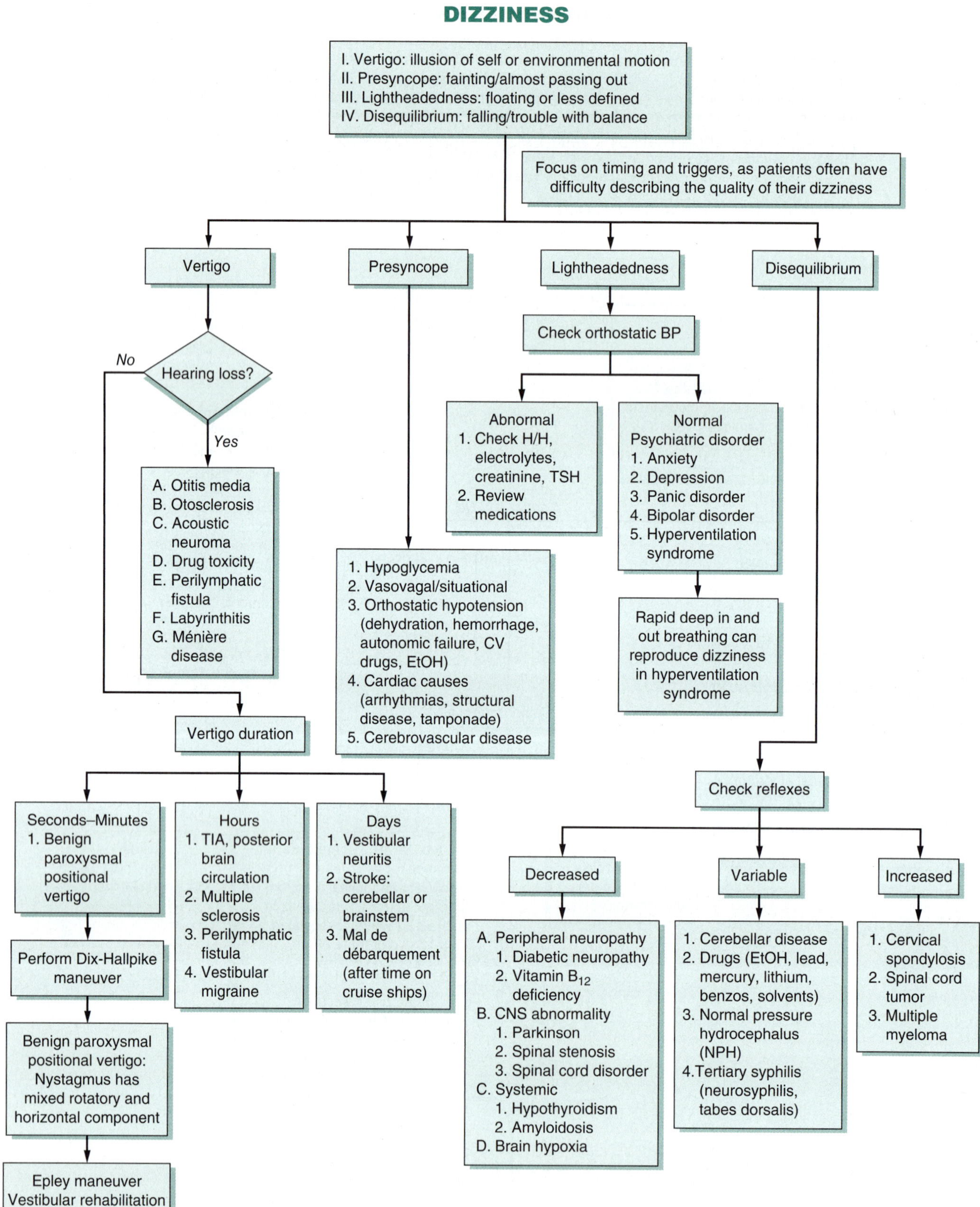

Jennifer G. Foster, MD, MBA, FACP

Stern SC, Cifu AS, Altkorn D, eds. *Symptom to Diagnosis: An Evidence-Based Guide.* 3rd ed. New York, NY: McGraw-Hill; 2014.

DYSPEPSIA

Dyspepsia: predominant symptom of epigastric pain for at least 1 month, associated with other symptoms, such as nausea, vomiting, or heartburn; common causes: GERD, peptic ulcer (<10%), gastroesophageal cancer (<1%), gastroparesis, functional dyspepsia (>70%)

Functional dyspepsia: dyspepsia with normal endoscopy. Main forms of functional dyspepsia: epigastric pain syndrome (intermittent pain/burning in epigastrium at least weekly) and postprandial distress syndrome (at least several episodes weekly of bothersome fullness after meals or early satiety). The two syndromes may both be present in the same patient.

Alarm features of dyspepsia: areas where gastric cancer is common (e.g., Southeast Asia), overt GI bleeding, progressive dysphagia and odynophagia, persistent vomiting, unintentional weight loss, family history upper GI cancer, palpable abdominal mass or lymphadenopathy, unexplained iron deficiency anemia

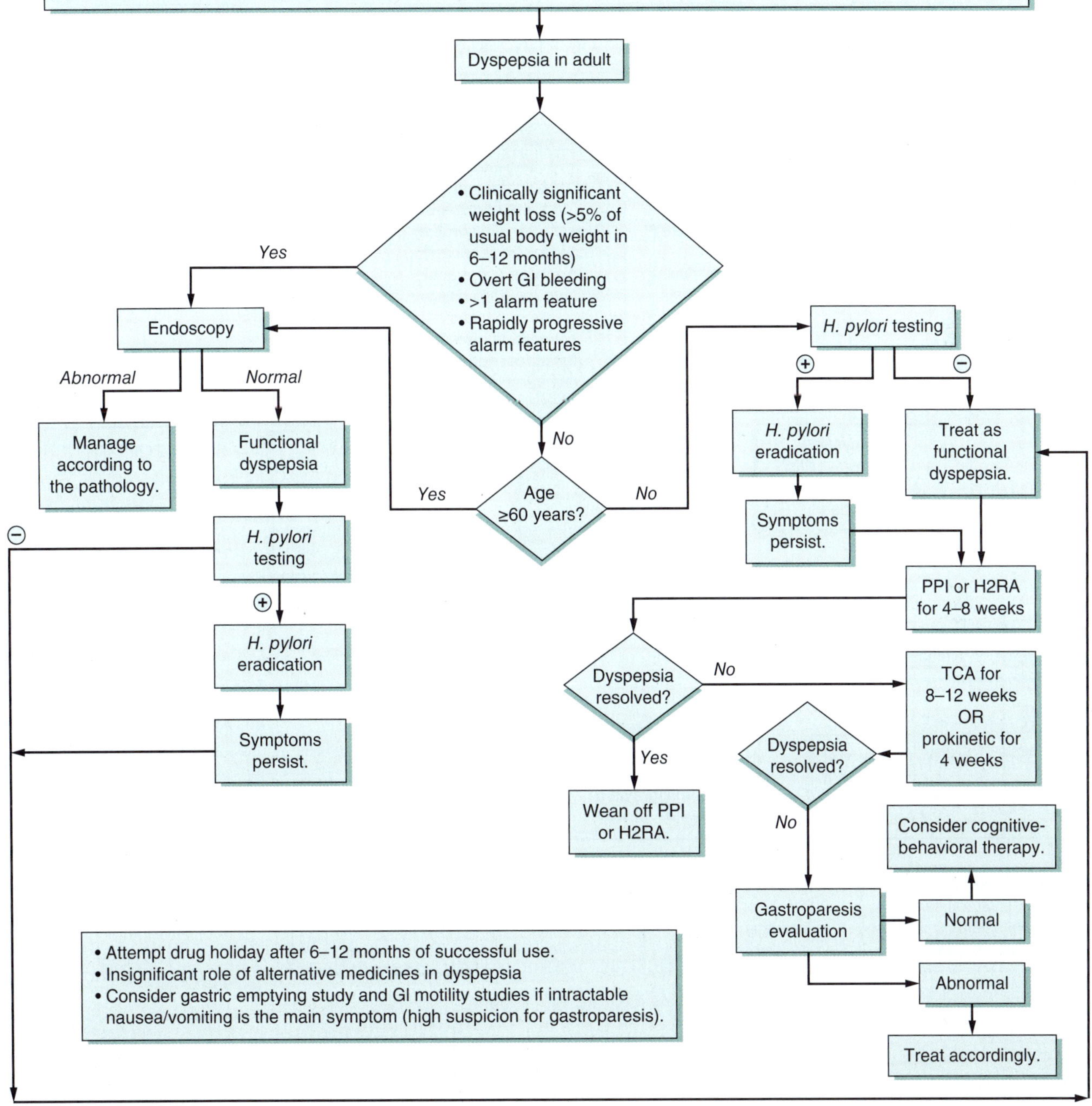

Adwoa A. Adu, MD

Moayyedi P, Lacy BE, Andrews CN, et al. ACG and CAG clinical guideline: management of dyspepsia. *Am J Gastroenterol*. 2017;112(7):988–1013.

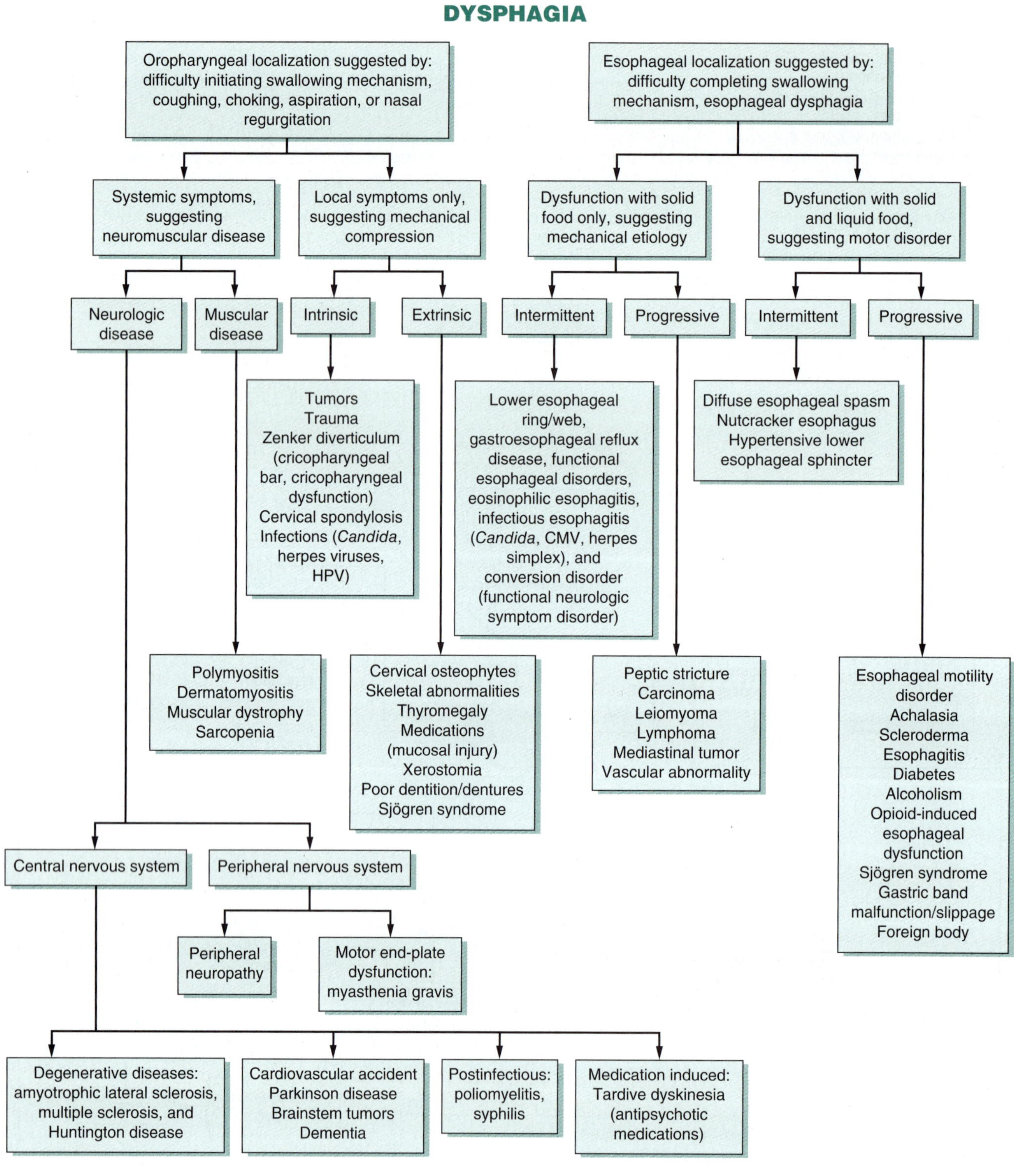

Joanna Drowos, DO, MPH, MBA

Wilkinson JM, Codipilly DC, Wilfahrt RP. Dysphagia: evaluation and collaborative management. *Am Fam Physician*. 2021;103(2):97–106.

ERYTHROCYTOSIS

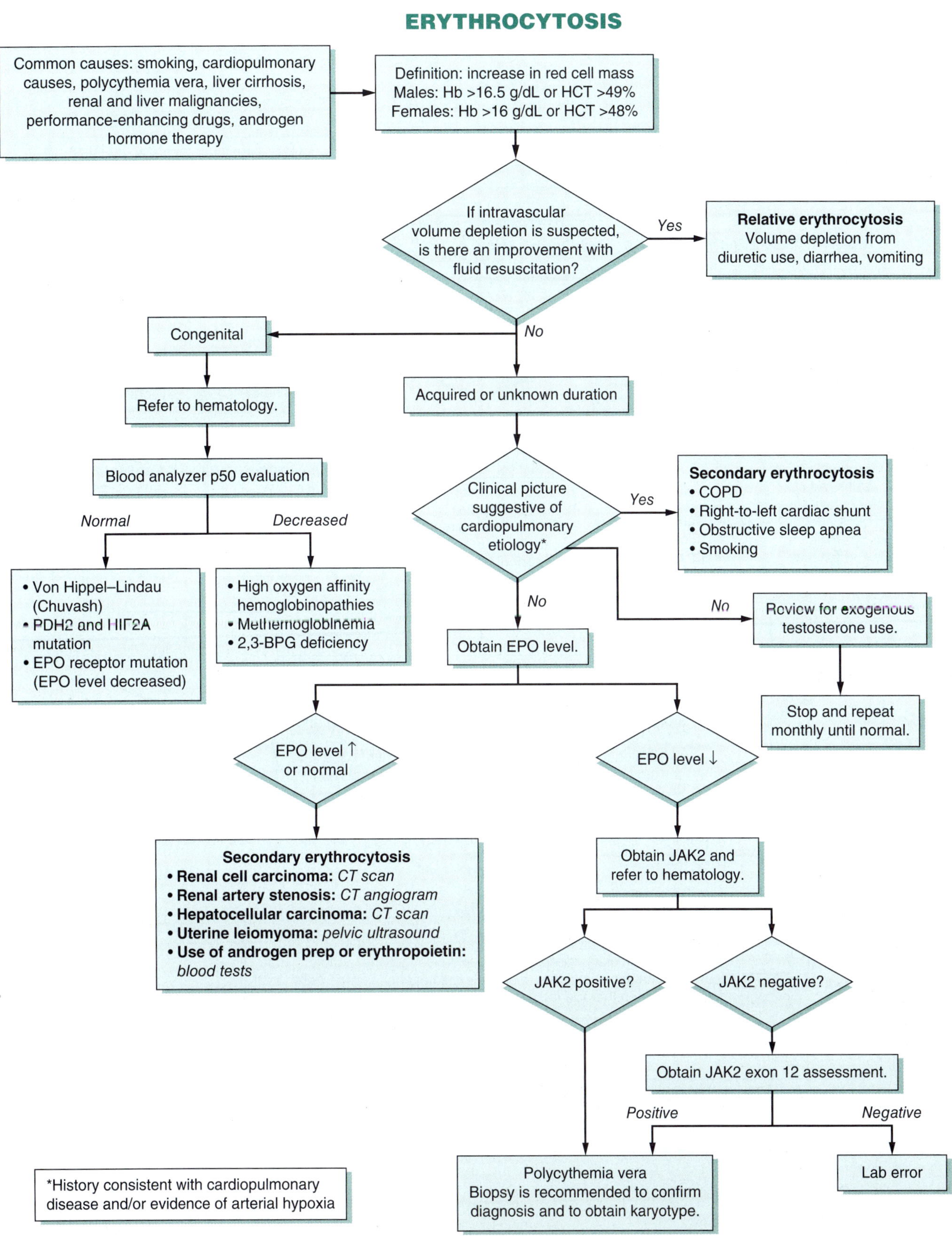

Frank J. Domino, MD

Tefferi A, Barbui T. Polycythemia vera and essential thrombocythemia: 2021 update on diagnosis, risk-stratification and management. *Am J Hematol*. 2020;95(12):1599–1613.

FATIGUE

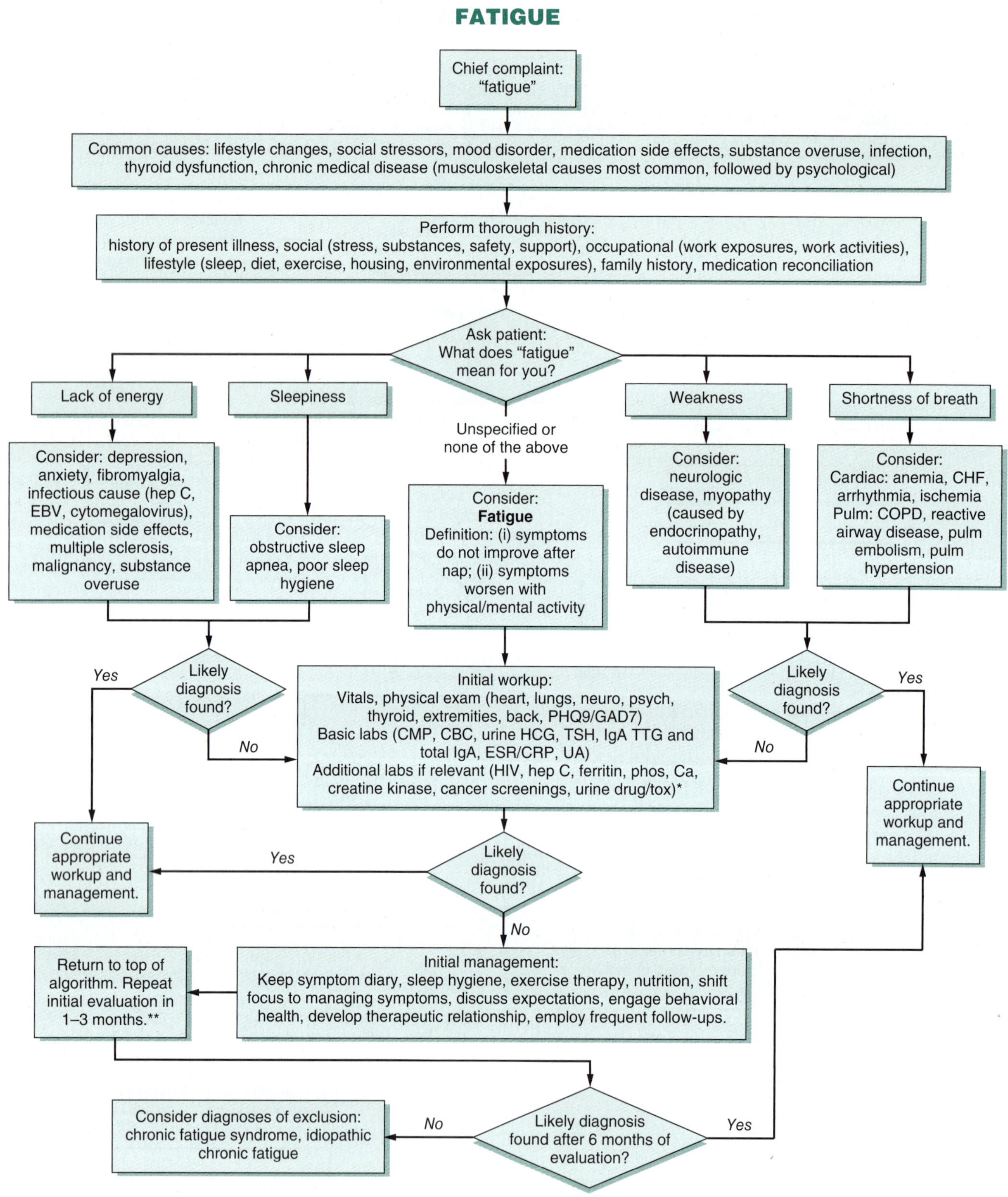

Stacy E. Potts, MD, Med

Wright J, O'Connor KM. Fatigue. *Med Clin North Am*. 2014;98(3):597–608.

FEVER IN FIRST 60 DAYS OF LIFE

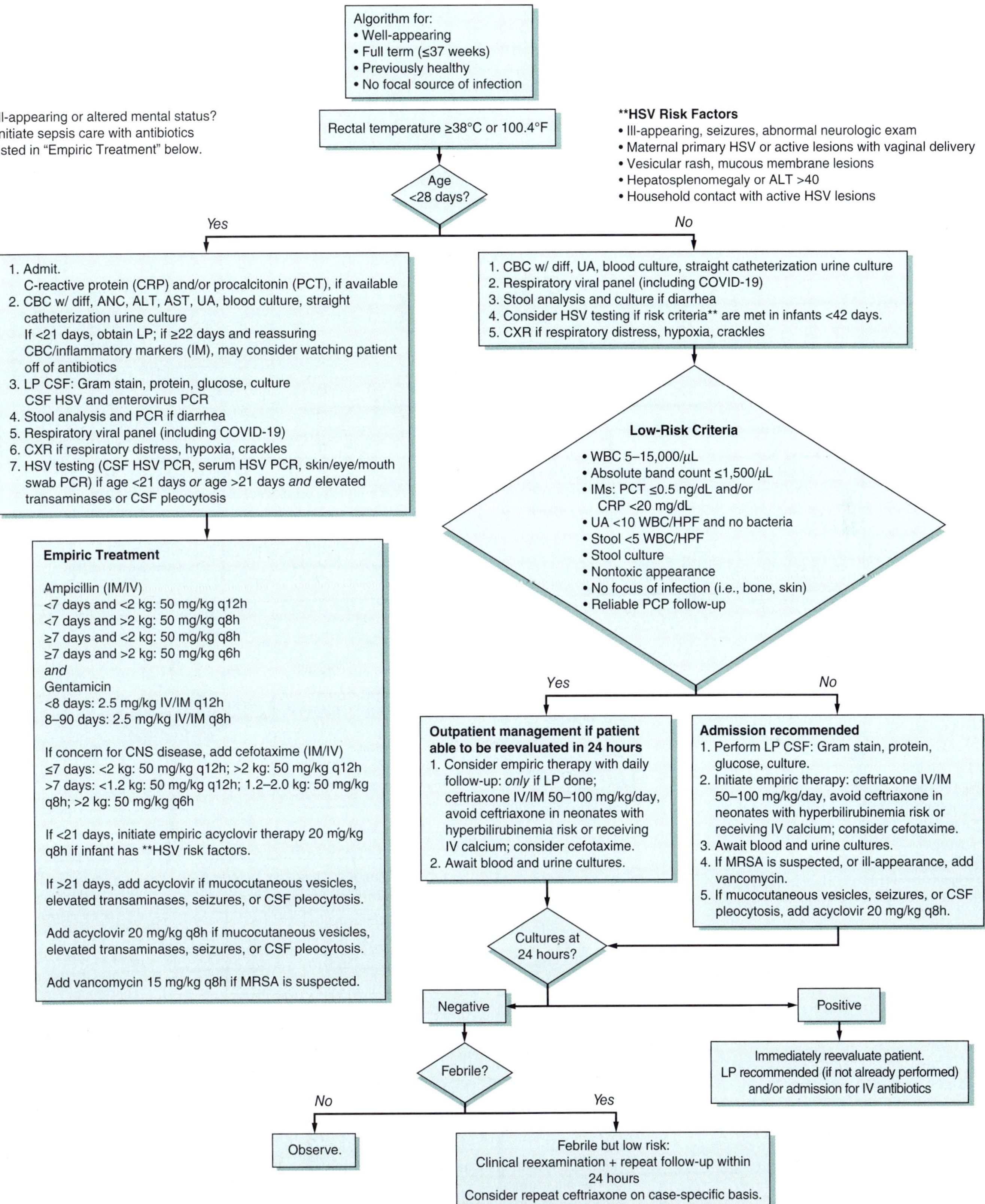

Markeeta Belmar, DO, MPH and Jennifer Costa, MD

Hile GB, Musick KL, Dugan AJ, et al. Occurrence of hyperbilirubinemia in neonates given a short-term course of ceftriaxone versus cefotaxime for sepsis. *J Pediatr Pharmacol Ther*. 2021;26(1):99–103. doi:10.5863/1551-6776-26.1.99.

FEVER OF UNKNOWN ORIGIN

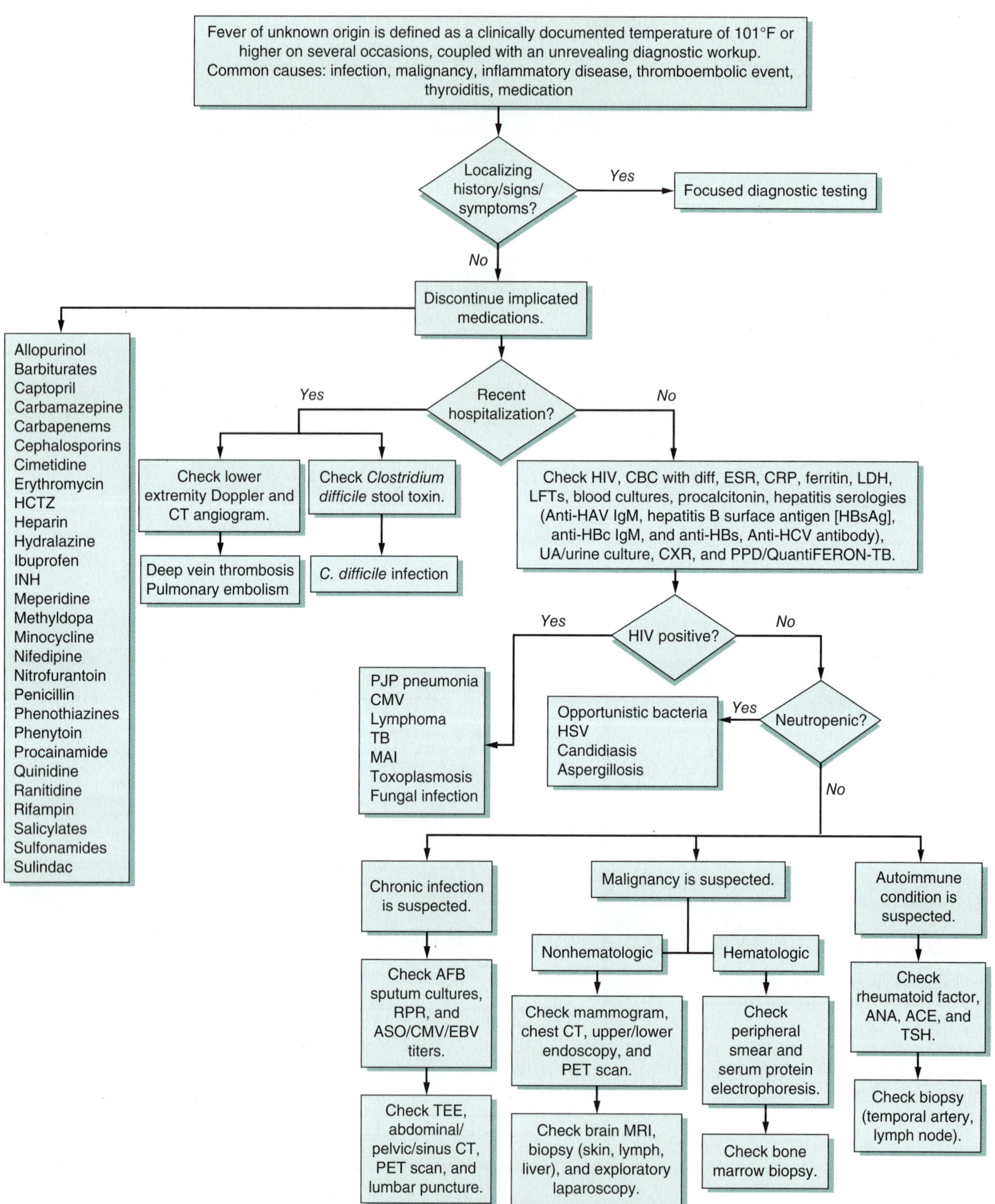

Meygan Lackey Elway, MD, MPH and Kathleen Wirshup, MD

David A, Quinlan JD. Fever of unknown origin in adults. *Am Fam Physician*. 2022;105(2):137–143.

GAIT DISTURBANCE

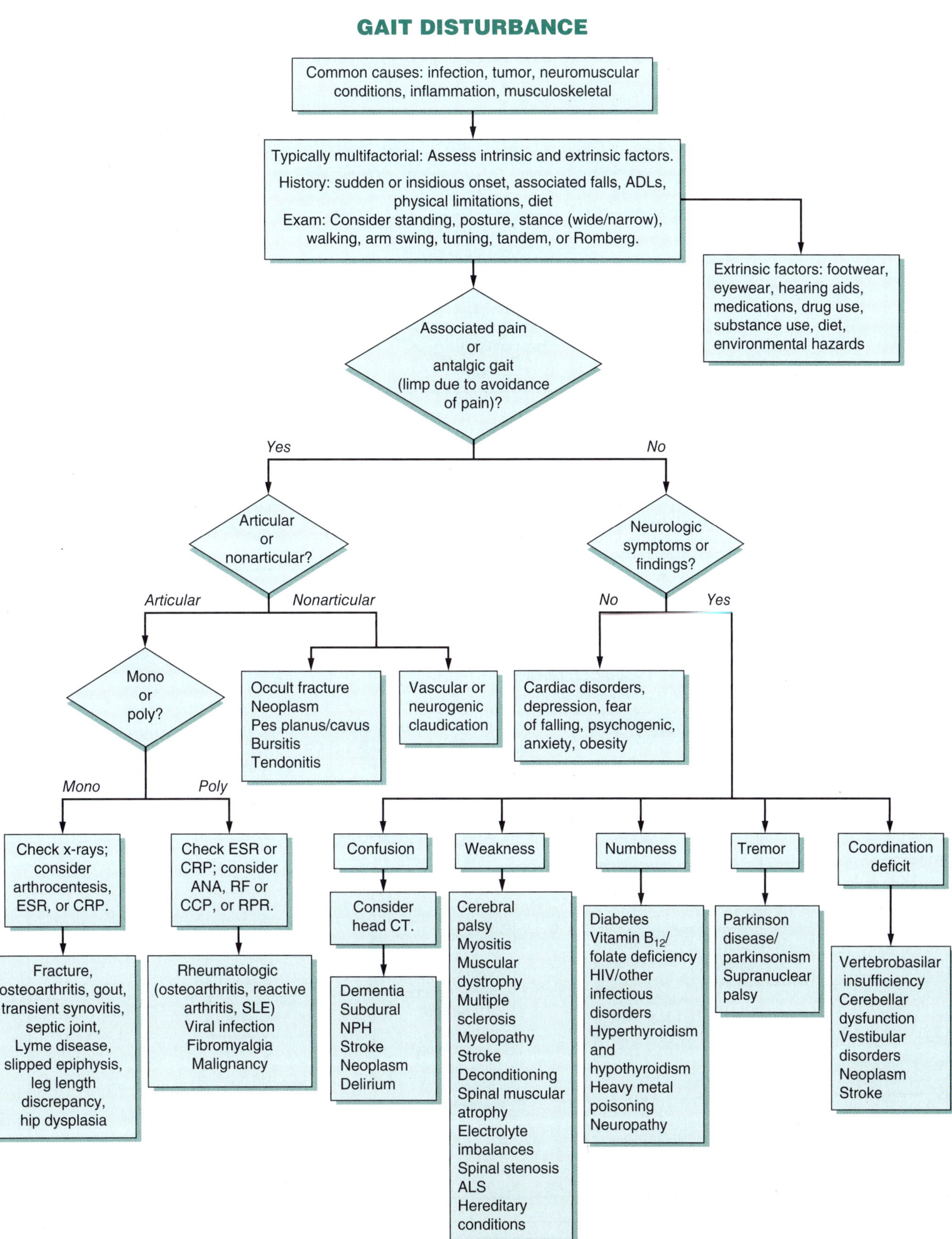

Can Angela Jiang, MD and Yuan Zhang, MD

Attaullah AHM, De Jesus O. *Gait Disturbances*. StatPearls; 2024. https://www.ncbi.nlm.nih.gov/books/NBK560610/. Accessed October 14, 2025.

GASTROESOPHAGEAL REFLUX DISEASE (GERD), DIAGNOSIS AND TREATMENT

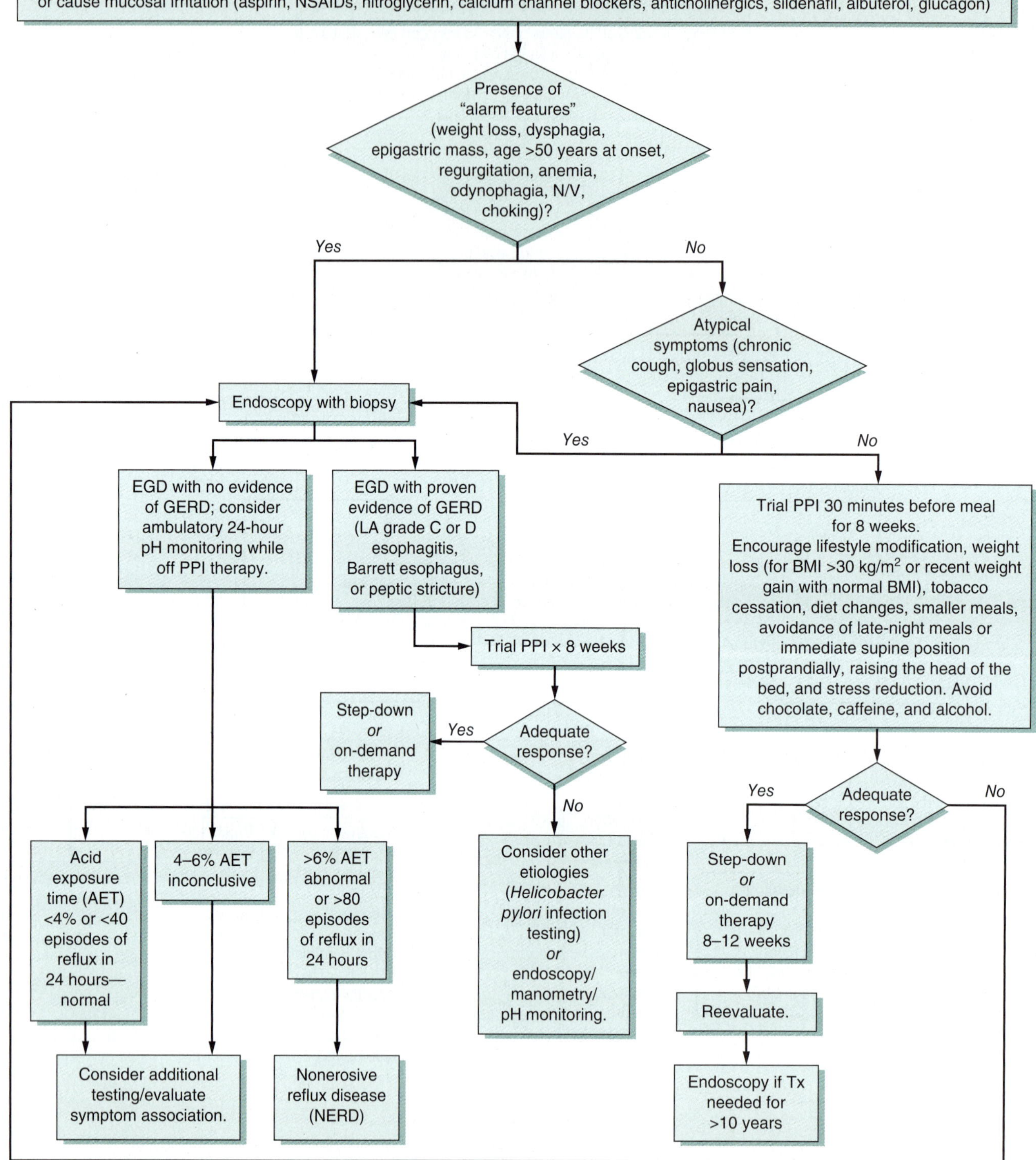

Nathan J. Macedo, MD, MPH

Fass R. Gastroesophageal reflux disease. *N Engl J Med*. 2022;387(13):1207–1216. doi:10.1056/NEJMcp2114026.

GENITAL ULCERS

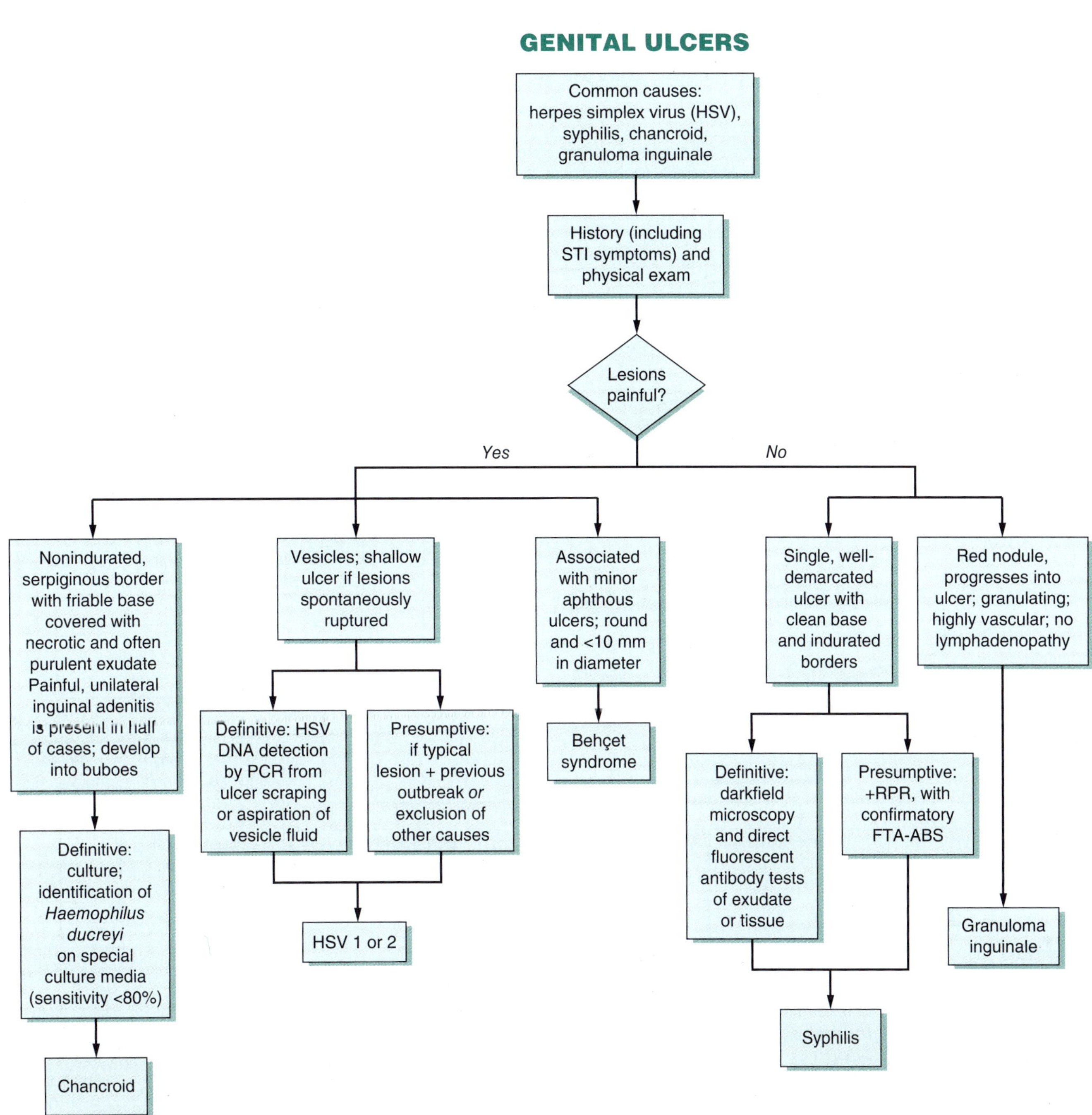

Arjola Agolli, MD, MBA

Roett MA. Genital ulcers: differential diagnosis and management. *Am Fam Physician*. 2020;101(6):355–361.

GRANULOCYTOSIS (LEUKOCYTOSIS)

WBC >11.0 × 10^9/L[1]

Common causes: infection, inflammation, drugs (steroid/lithium/β-agonists, G-CSF, GM-CSF, etc.), stress, smoking, asplenia/hyposplenism, pregnancy, myeloproliferative disorder, leukemia/lymphoma

Repeat CBC.
Order manual smear.

Leukocytosis confirmed?

- *No* → No further workup necessary.
- *Yes* → Leukocytosis explained by additional pertinent history and/or physical examination?
  - *Yes* → No further workup necessary.
  - *No* → Patient presents with weight loss, fatigue, fevers, night sweats, splenomegaly, lymphadenopathy, bruising? Abnormal red blood cell (RBC) and platelet count? Risk or history of prior malignancy?
    - *Yes* → Consider malignancy. Review peripheral blood smear. Hematology/oncology consultation Bone marrow biopsy and flow cytometry, cytogenetics, or molecular testing on bone marrow or peripheral blood
    - *No* → Determine affected cell line.

Lymphocytosis (≥3,500/mm³ [3.5 × 10^9/L])

- PLEOMORPHIC (REACTIVE) → Look for: Infections (viral, pertussis) Hypersensitivity Consider: Immunization Contact history Chest x-ray Viral panels
- MONOMORPHIC Suspect lymphoproliferative disorder. → Hematology/oncology consult

Monocytosis (≥1,000/mm³ [≥1.0 × 10^9/L])
Look for:
Chronic infection (EBV, fungal, protozoal, rickettsial)
Autoimmune
Splenectomy
Myelodysplastic syndrome
Consider:
Contact, travel, medical history, monospot test, PPD, ESR, CRP, ANA
→ If persistent >3 months → Hematology/oncology consult

INCREASED BLASTS → Hematology/oncology consult

Basophilia (≥300/mm³ [≥0.3 × 10^9/L])
Rare: Suspect myeloproliferative neoplasm (MPN) or CML.
Consider:
Karyotyping
BCR-ABL1
JAK2 V617F
→ Hematology/oncology consult

EOSINOPHILIA (>500/mm³ [0.5 × 10^9])
Look for reactive etiology:
Allergic conditions
Eosinophilic esophagitis
Drug reaction
Dermatologic conditions
Parasitic infections
Consider:
Drug, travel history
Full skin exam and biopsy if indicated
Allergy/immunology testing
Stool for ova and parasites
Upper GI endoscopy
→ If negative, rule out MPN, Hodgkin lymphoma. Consider: FISH/PCR for PDGFRA mutation → Hematology/oncology consult

Neutrophilia ≥7,700/mm³ (7.7 × 10^9/L)

- WBC >50,000 + blood smear findings (left shift, basophilia, dysplasia, blast): consistent with malignancy: CML/acute leukemia → Hematology/oncology consult
- WBC <50,000: leukemoid reaction → Look for: Infection Autoimmune/inflammatory disease Medications (including GM-CSF) Splenectomy Reactive (stressors, exercise, seizure, surgery, VTE, etc.) Consider: Medical, surgical drug, contact, social history ESR, CRP, ANA Blood smear review for nucleated RBCs Blood culture, lumbar puncture Additional system-specific studies, evaluation for MPNs

Hematology/oncology consult
Bone marrow biopsy
Flow cytometry, cytogenetics, and molecular analysis of bone marrow or peripheral blood

[1]for nonpregnant adults

Nelson Franqui-Rios, MD and Elimarys Pérez-Colón, MD

Gbenjo JTC, McCrary GLM, Wilson SE. Leukemia: what primary care physicians need to know. *Am Fam Physician*. 2023;107(4):397–405.

HEADACHE

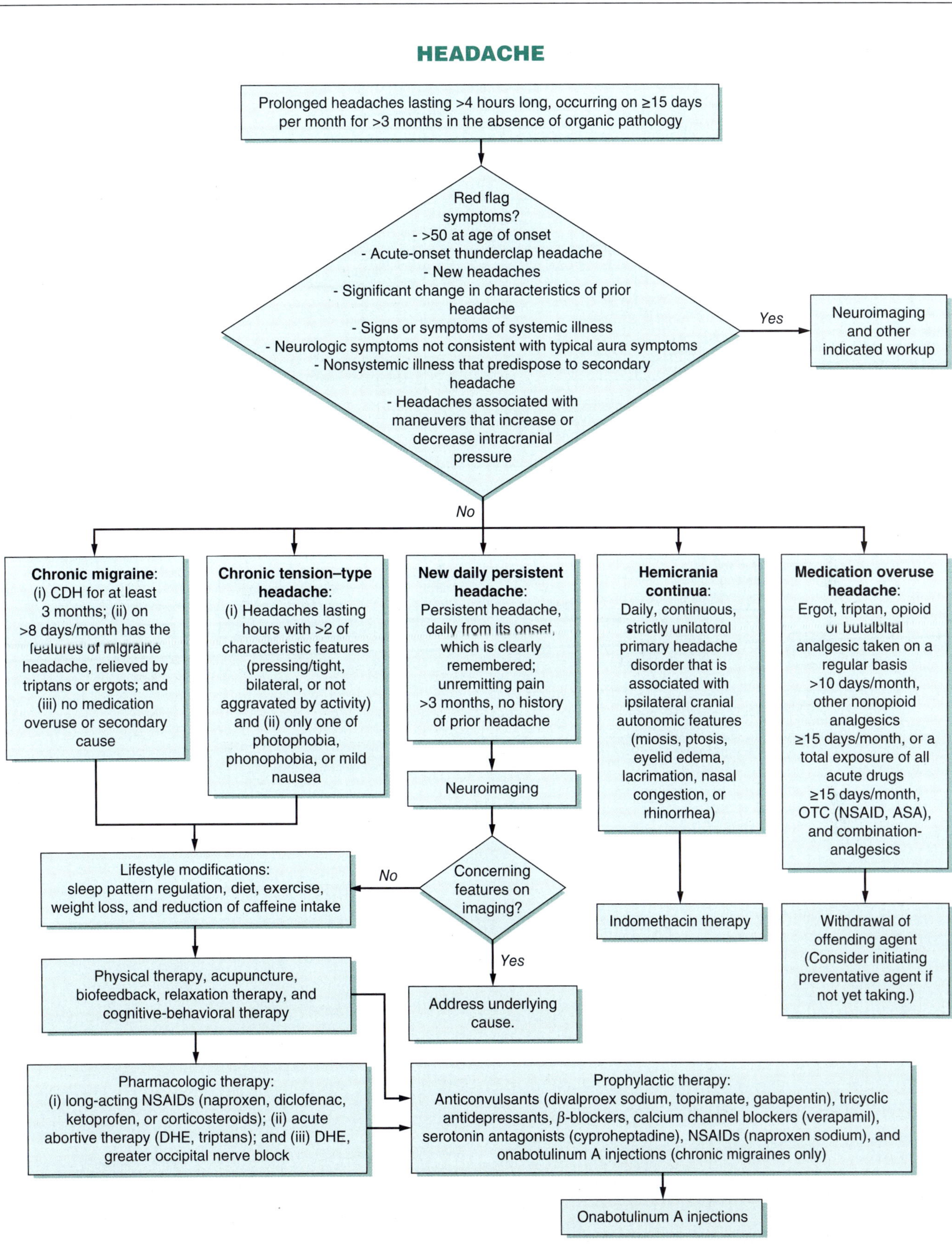

Karly Pippitt, MD

Dodick D, Dilli E. *Chronic Daily Headache*. Mt. Royal, NJ: American Headache Society; 2018. https://americanheadachesociety.org/wp-content/uploads/2018/05/David_Dodick_and_Esma_Dilli_-_Chronic_Daily_Headache.pdf. Accessed December 12, 2022.

HEART MURMUR

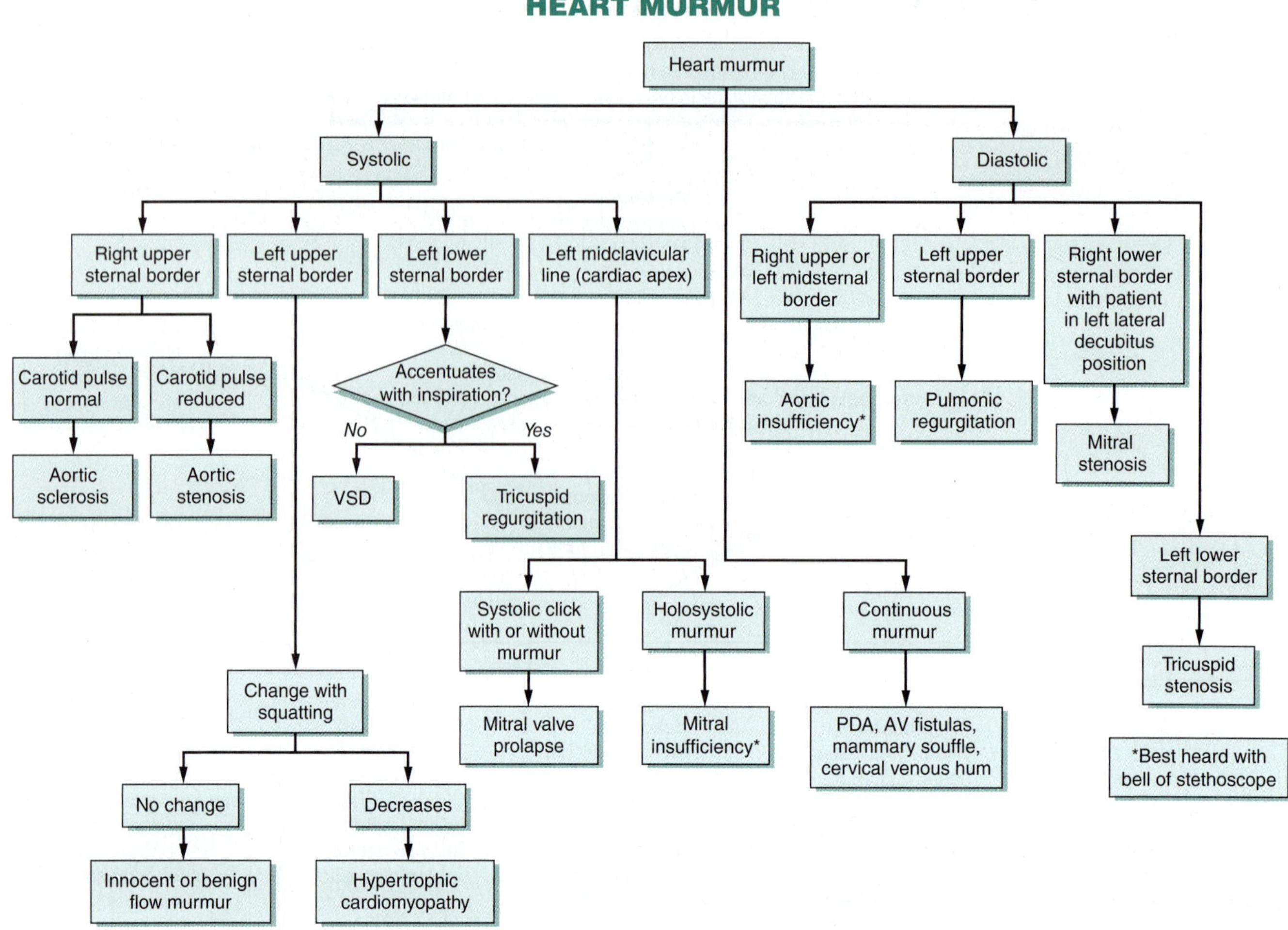

Navpreet K. Singh, MD

Bonow RO, Carabello BA, Chatterjee K, et al; for 2006 Writing Committee Members and American College of Cardiology/American Heart Association Task Force. 2008 Focused update incorporated into the ACC/AHA 2006 guidelines for the management of patients with valvular heart disease: a report of the American College of Cardiology/American Heart Association Task Force on Practice Guidelines (writing committee to revise the 1998 guidelines for the management of patients with valvular heart disease): endorsed by the Society of Cardiovascular Anesthesiologists, Society for Cardiovascular Angiography and Interventions, and Society of Thoracic Surgeons. *Circulation*. 2008;118(15):e523–e661.

HEMATEMESIS (BLEEDING, UPPER GASTROINTESTINAL)

Common causes:
PUD, Mallory-Weiss tear, esophagitis, gastritis, varices, epistaxis

Maintain two large-bore cannulas.
Transfuse pRBC to maintain Hb >7 mg/dL.

CBC, PT/INR, type and screen

Stable?

No → ABC steps
Fluid resuscitation
Make patient NPO.
Consult gastroenterology.

Start IV proton pump inhibitor.

Suspect variceal hemorrhage.

Start IV octreotide drip (3–5 days) and broad-spectrum antibiotics (5–7 days).

Perform upper endoscopy with variceal ligation banding within 6–24 hours.

Has the bleeding stopped?

Yes → Start prophylactic nonselective β-blocker after octreotide is completed. → Repeat endoscopy in 1–2 weeks and reband as needed.

No → Sengstaken-Blakemore tube → Consider emergent transjugular intrahepatic portosystemic shunt or surgery depending on local expertise.

Suspect nonvariceal hemorrhage.

Yes → Recent nosebleed?

Yes → Epistaxis

No → Perform upper endoscopy.

- No source identified → Consider repeat endoscopy and push enteroscopy.
- Arteriovenous malformation, Dieulafoy lesion → Endoscopic therapy with epinephrine, thermocoagulation, or clipping
- Erosive esophagitis → Continue proton pump inhibitor therapy.
- Peptic ulcer bleeding → Endoscopic therapy with epinephrine, thermocoagulation, and/or clipping → Has the bleeding stopped?
  - Yes → Continue proton pump inhibitor therapy; eradicate *Helicobacter pylori* infection if present and consider discontinuing NSAIDs/blood thinners if possible.
  - No → Reattempt upper endoscopy; otherwise, consider arteriography with embolization or surgery.
- Mallory-Weiss tear → Antiemetic and proton pump inhibitor; endoscopic treatment only if active bleeding

Manju Mahajan, MD, FAAFP and Cassandra Daisy, MD

Kamboj AK, Hoversten P, Leggett CL. Upper gastrointestinal bleeding: etiologies and management. *Mayo Clin Proc*. 2019;94(4):697–703.

HEMATURIA

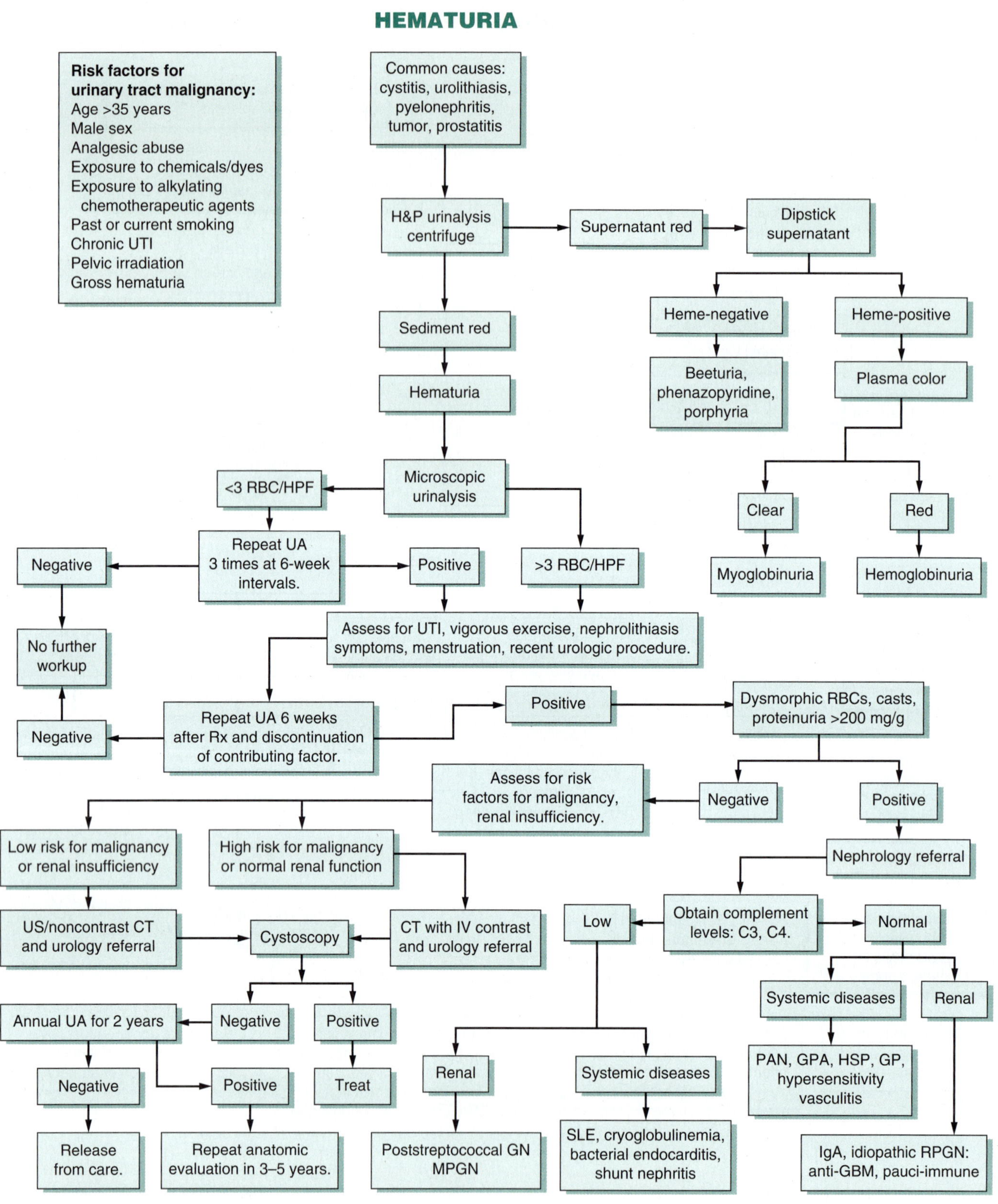

Michael T. Partin, MD and Karl T. Clebak, MD, MHA, FAAFP

Ingelfinger JR. Hematuria in adults. *N Engl J Med*. 2021;385(2):153–163.

HEPATOMEGALY

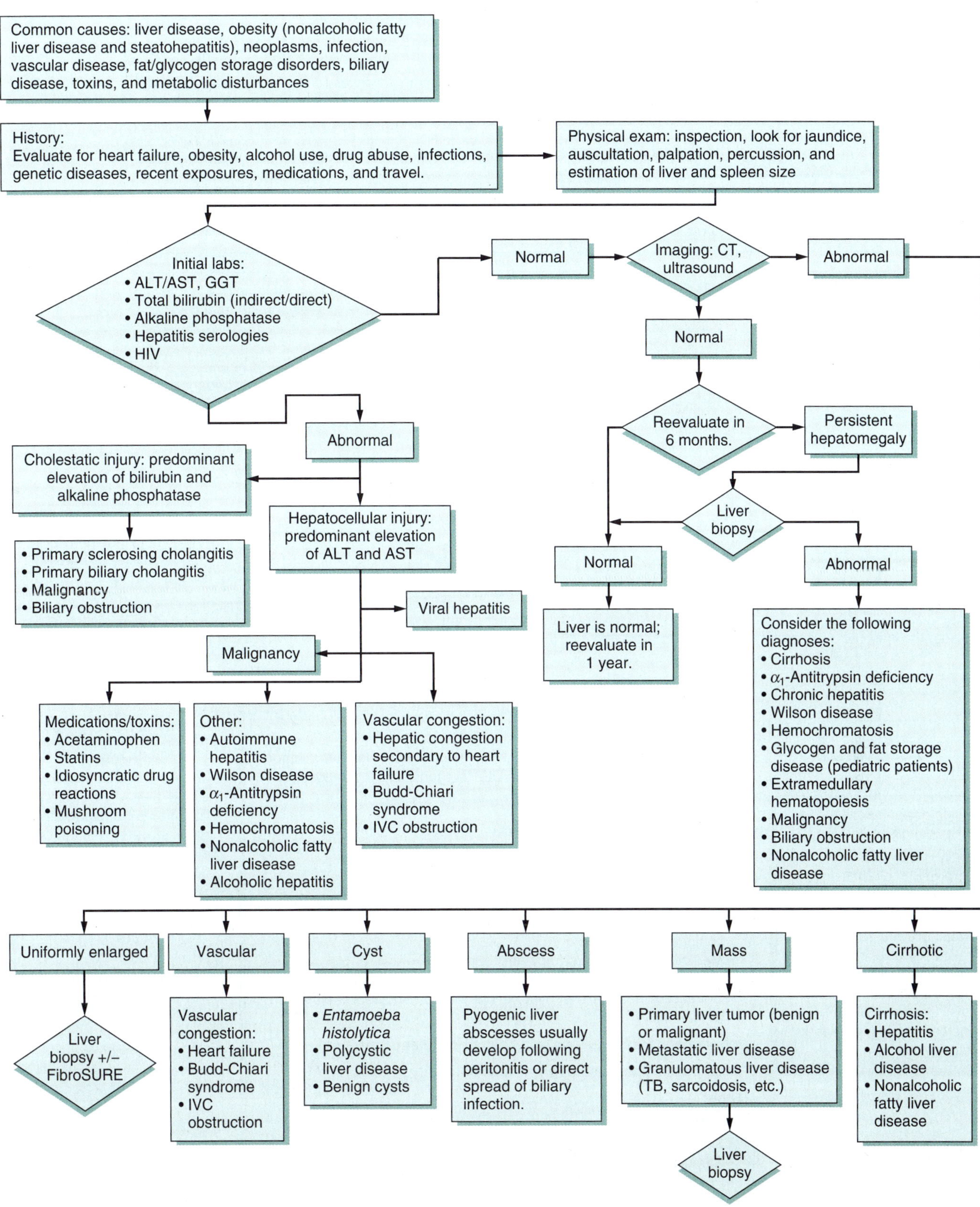

Manju Mahajan, MD, FAAFP

Kwo PY, Cohen SM, Lim JK. ACG clinical guideline: evaluation of abnormal liver chemistries. *Am J Gastroenterol.* 2017;112(1):18–35.

HYPERBILIRUBINEMIA AND JAUNDICE

Jaundice: a yellow discoloration of the skin, sclera and mucous membranes by bilirubin, a bile pigment formed by the breakdown of heme ring; detected when the serum bilirubin level >3 mg/dL

Bilirubin: a product of hemoglobin breakdown in the spleen; heme is converted to unconjugated bilirubin, bound to albumin, and transported to the liver where it is then conjugated.

Common causes of hyperbilirubinemia: Gilbert syndrome, hemolysis, hepatitis, and choledocholithiasis

History and physical: alcohol and drug use, fever, prodromal viral symptoms, weight loss, asterixis, mental status, bruising, spider angiomas, palmar erythema, gynecomastia, hepatomegaly, splenomegaly, right upper quadrant tenderness, ascites

Evaluation: CBC w/ diff; LFTs: AST, ALT, serum alkaline phosphatase (ALP), albumin, protein, total bilirubin (TB), and direct bilirubin (DB); prothrombin and/or international normalized ratio (INR), gamma-glutamyltransferase; US, CT, or MRCP

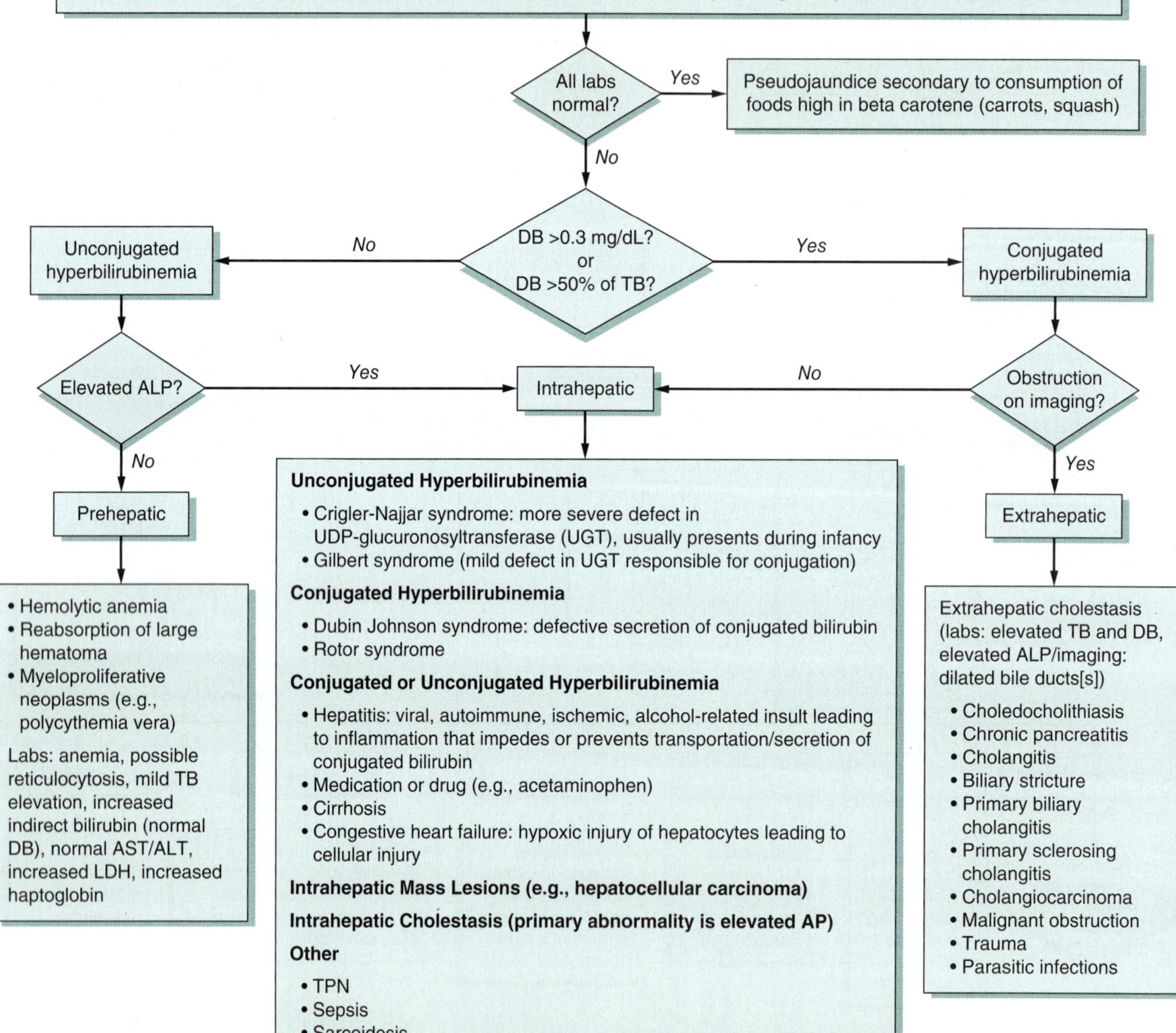

Catherine Peony Khoo, MD, FAAFP and Monika Shenouda, MD

Nelson M, Mulani SR, Saguil A. Evaluation of jaundice in adults. *Am Fam Physician*. 2025;111(1):25–30.

HYPERCALCEMIA

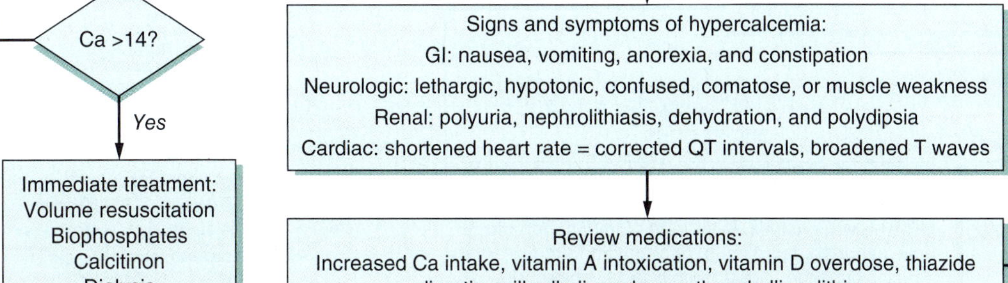

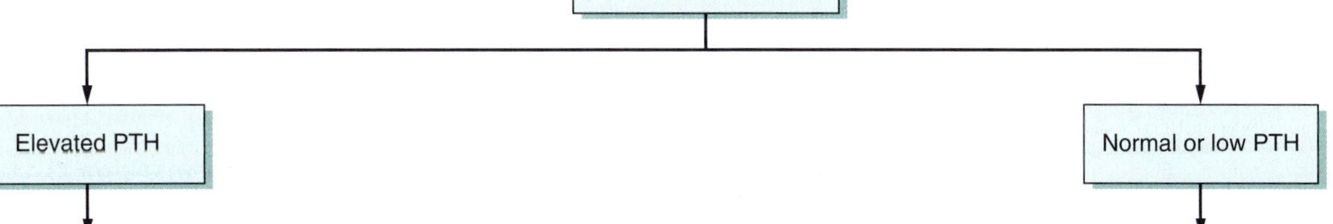

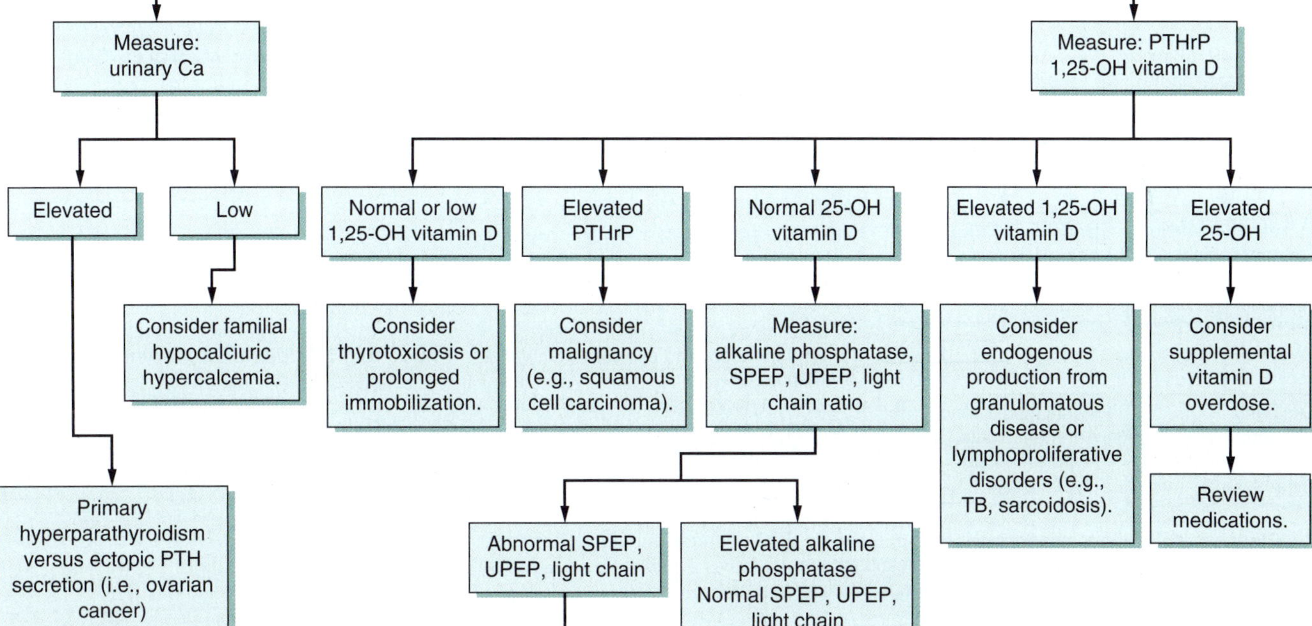

Vasudha Jain, MD

Renaghan AD, Rosner MH. Hypercalcemia: etiology and management. *Nephrol Dial Transplant*. 2018;33(4):549–551.

HYPERKALEMIA

K >5.5 mEq/L

Common causes: renal failure, hyperglycemia, specimen delay and hemolysis, renal insufficiency, acidosis, rhabdomyolysis, insulin deficiency, adrenal insufficiency, medications, massive blood transfusions, tumor lysis, ischemic bowel, CHF, DMII, MI, burns, excessive exercise, anemia, RAASi usage

Symptoms present?
- Weakness, nausea, paresthesias, palpitations, ileus, flaccid paralysis, fasciculation

ECG changes present?
- Peaked T waves, ↑ PR interval, ↑ QRS width, sine wave pattern, PEA
- K >6.5 mEq/L

No → Repeat test—by serum, not POC test.

Normal → Assess for pseudohyperkalemia: ICV with K, hemolysed sample (specimen delay, prolonged tourniquet), mechanical trauma, clotting, leukocytosis, thrombocytosis, fist clench >1 minute

Abnormal → Check medications: ACEI, ARBs, β-blockers, NSAIDs, penicillin K, TMP-SMX, digitalis, K-sparing diuretics, heparin, cyclosporine, tacrolimus, pentamidine, succinylcholine, direct renin agents, octreotide, mannitol

Check herbal and natural product use: Fruits, alfalfa, amino acids, dandelion, dried toad skin, hawthorn berry, horsetail, lily of the valley, mildewed, nettle, noni, juice, Siberian ginseng, OTC K salts, OTC K supplement

Suspicious medications or herbs/supplements found?

Yes → Discontinue use or modify under a physician's guidance.

No → Check: ABG, BMP, digoxin level (if applicable), CPK, urine K, BP, ECG, O_2 saturation

Urine K >30 mEq/L or spot urine K/Cr >200 mEq/g: transcellular shift → Acidosis, Rhabdomyolysis, Hyperglycemia, Burns

Urine K <30 mEq/L or spot urine K/Cr <20 mEq/g: impaired renal excretion → Renal insufficiency, Adrenal insufficiency, Hyporeninemic Hypoaldosteronism

Yes → Treat as acute hyperkalemia. Send to ED if not already admitted.

Acute hyperkalemia management: if ECG changes, moderate/severe symptoms, or K >6.5 mEq/L

Membrane stabilizers
- Calcium chloride (CaCl)—higher bioavailability (3 times higher than calcium gluconate): 10 mL of 10% CaCl over 2–5 minutes IV; may repeat in 5–10 minutes
- Calcium gluconate—less tissue toxicity: 30 mL of 10% Ca gluconate IV over 2–5 minutes; may repeat in 5–10 minutes
- Careful in potential dig toxicity as hypercalcemia can increase toxic effect of the drug
- Ca salts don't lower K.
- Action limited to 30–60 minutes

ICF shift
- Short-acting insulin: 10 units IV with glucose 50 g; works in 30–60 minutes
- β-Agonist: albuterol nebulizer; action in 30–60 minutes

K elimination
- K-binding agents
  - Sodium polystyrene sulfonate: works in several hours; 15–60 mg in 20% sorbitol (60–240 mL) orally or rectal = 0.5–1.0 mEq/g reduction
  - Patiromer sorbitex calcium: works in 7 hours; 4.2–16.8 g QD–BID; lowers K by 0.75 mEq/L
  - Sodium zirconium cyclosilicate: works in 1 hour; 10 g TID; lowers K by 0.7 mEq/L per 10-g dose
- Diuretics: loop diuretic in hypervolemic patients: furosemide 40 mg; works in 0.5–2.0 hours
- Dialysis: takes 1–8 hours; lowers K by 25–50 mEq/hr; peritoneal dialysis works in 1–4 hours and lowers K by 50–70 mEq/24 hr.
- $NaHCO_3$: only use in patient with metabolic acidosis; unsure of efficacy

Chronic hyperkalemia management: if K <6.5 and no ECG changes and no moderate/severe symptoms
- Dietary potassium counseling: Avoid salt substitutes.
- Manage RAASi therapy: Reduce or change medication if possible.
- Diuretic therapy
- Oral $NaHCO_3$ (if appropriate)
- Fludrocortisone: can increase fluid retention, HTN, vascular injury
- Consider potassium binders—see acute management (elimination section).
- Monitor potassium 2 times per year.
- Review medications, herbs, and supplements.
- Multidisciplinary approach: patient education, physician education, dietitian, pharmacist

Manju Mahajan, MD, FAAFP and Michael Richardson, MD

Palmer BF, Carrero JJ, Clegg DJ, et al. Clinical management of hyperkalemia. *Mayo Clin Proc*. 2021;96(3):744–762.

HYPERLIPIDEMIA

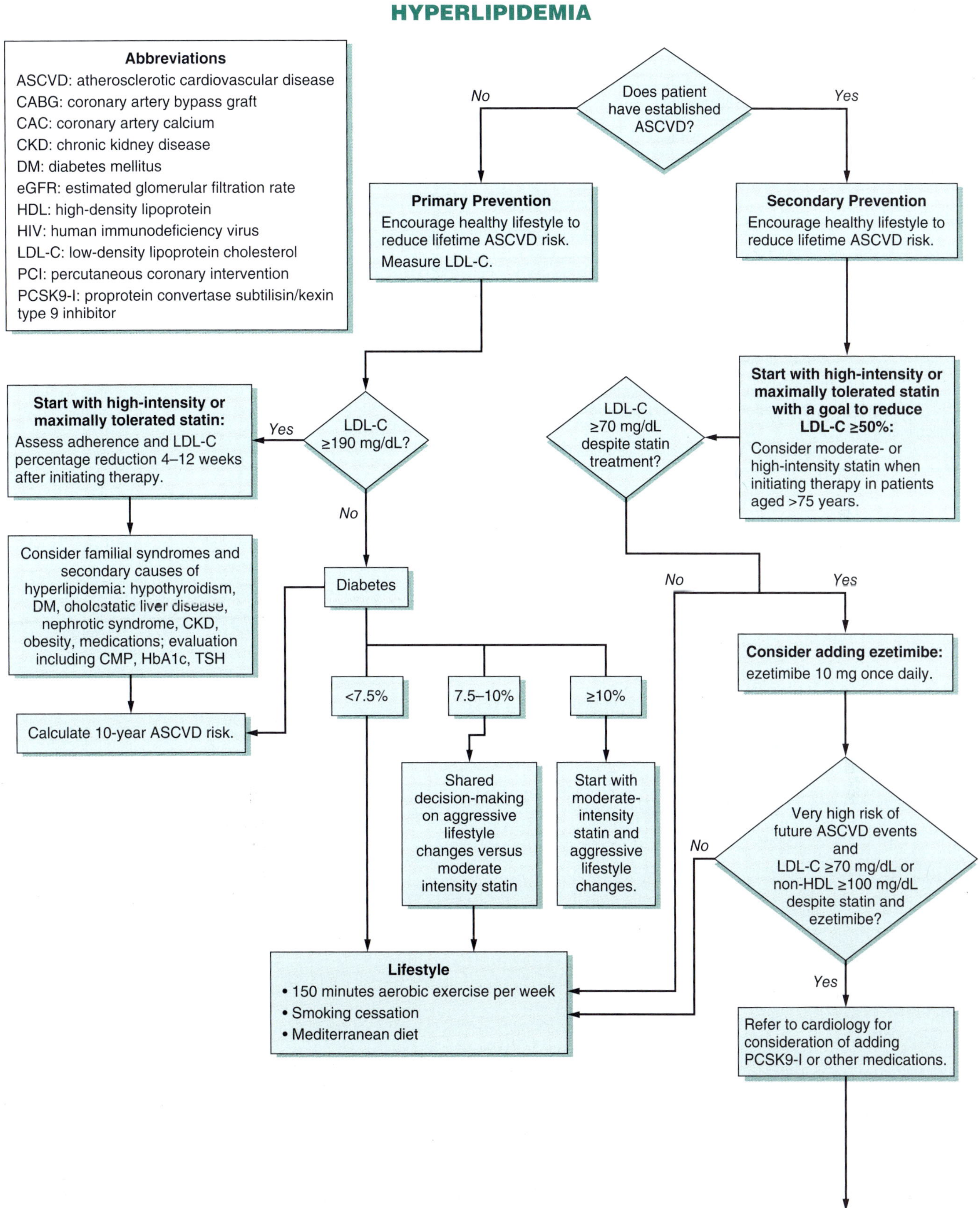

LDL-C reduction	≥50%	30–49%
Atorvastatin	40–80 mg/day	10–20 mg/day
Rosuvastatin	20–40 mg/day	5–10 mg/day
Simvastatin		20–40 mg/day
Pravastatin		40–80 mg/day
Lovastatin		40–80 mg/day
Fluvastatin		40 mg BID
Fluvastatin XL		80 mg/day
Pitavastatin		1–4 mg/day

Reassess 4–12 weeks after the start of treatment or after a change in medication dose:

Assess for medication and lifestyle adherence.

Measure LDL-C and determine percent reduction from baseline.

Reassess every 12 months.

Cardiovascular Risk Assessment
(10-year, Revised Pooled Cohort Equations 2018)

Available at
https://www.merckmanuals.com/medical-calculators/cvriskrevised2018-en.htm

Jason Cross, PharmD, BCPS, BCACP, Dinesh Yogaratnam, PharmD, BCPS, BCCCP, and Sudeep K. Aulakh, MD, FACP, FRCPC

Grundy SM, Stone NJ, Bailey AL, et al. 2018 AHA/ACC/AACVPR/AAPA/ABC/ACPM/ADA/AGS/APhA/ASPC/NLA/PCNA guideline on the management of blood cholesterol: executive summary: a report of the American College of Cardiology/American Heart Association Task Force on Clinical Practice Guidelines. *J Am Coll Cardiol*. 2019;73(24):3168–3209.

HYPERNATREMIA

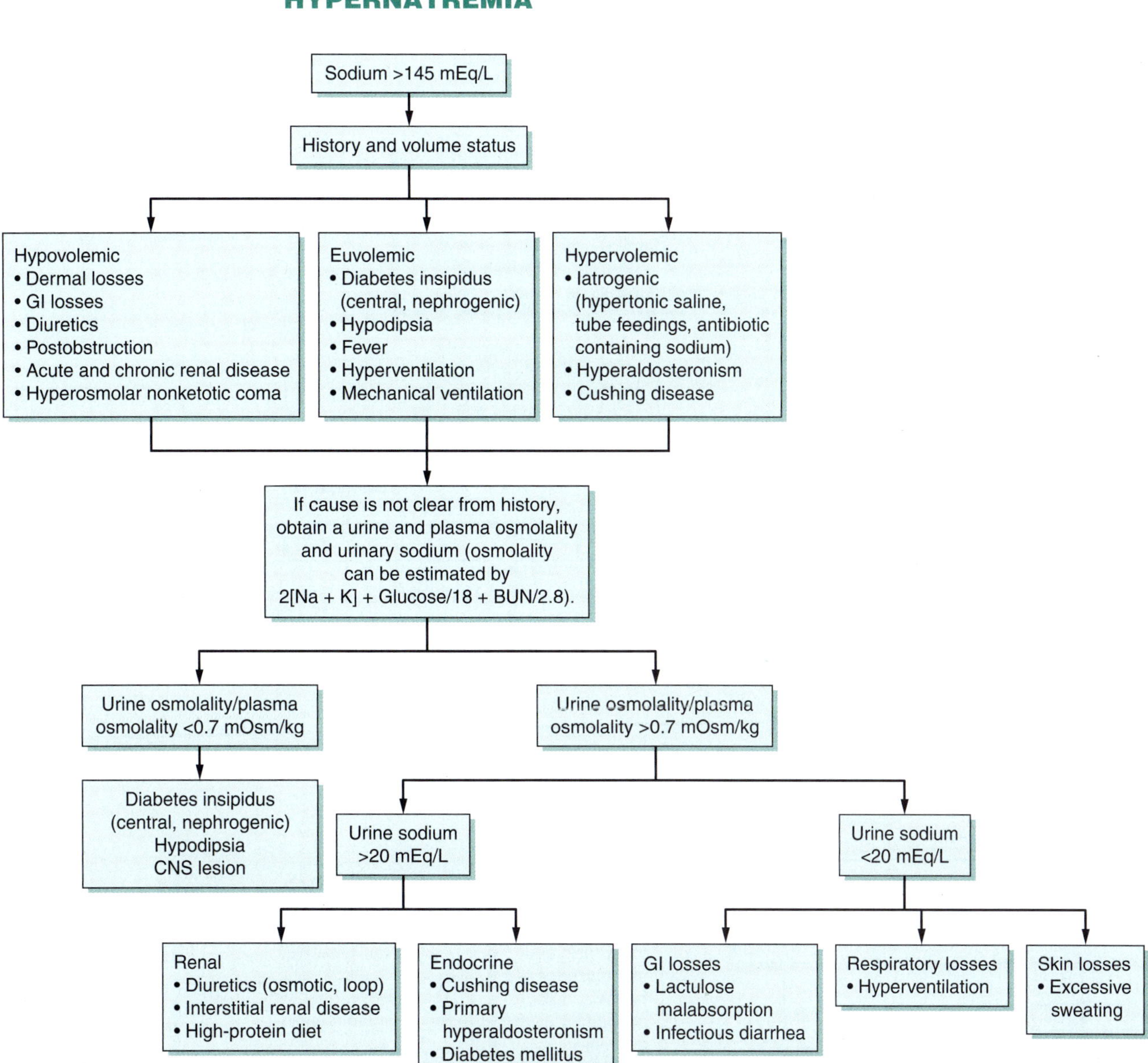

Neil Tandon, MD and Eugene Orientale Jr., MD

Braun MM, Barstow CH, Pyzocha NJ. Diagnosis and management of sodium disorders: hyponatremia and hypernatremia. *Am Fam Physician*. 2015;91(5):299–307.

HYPERTRIGLYCERIDEMIA

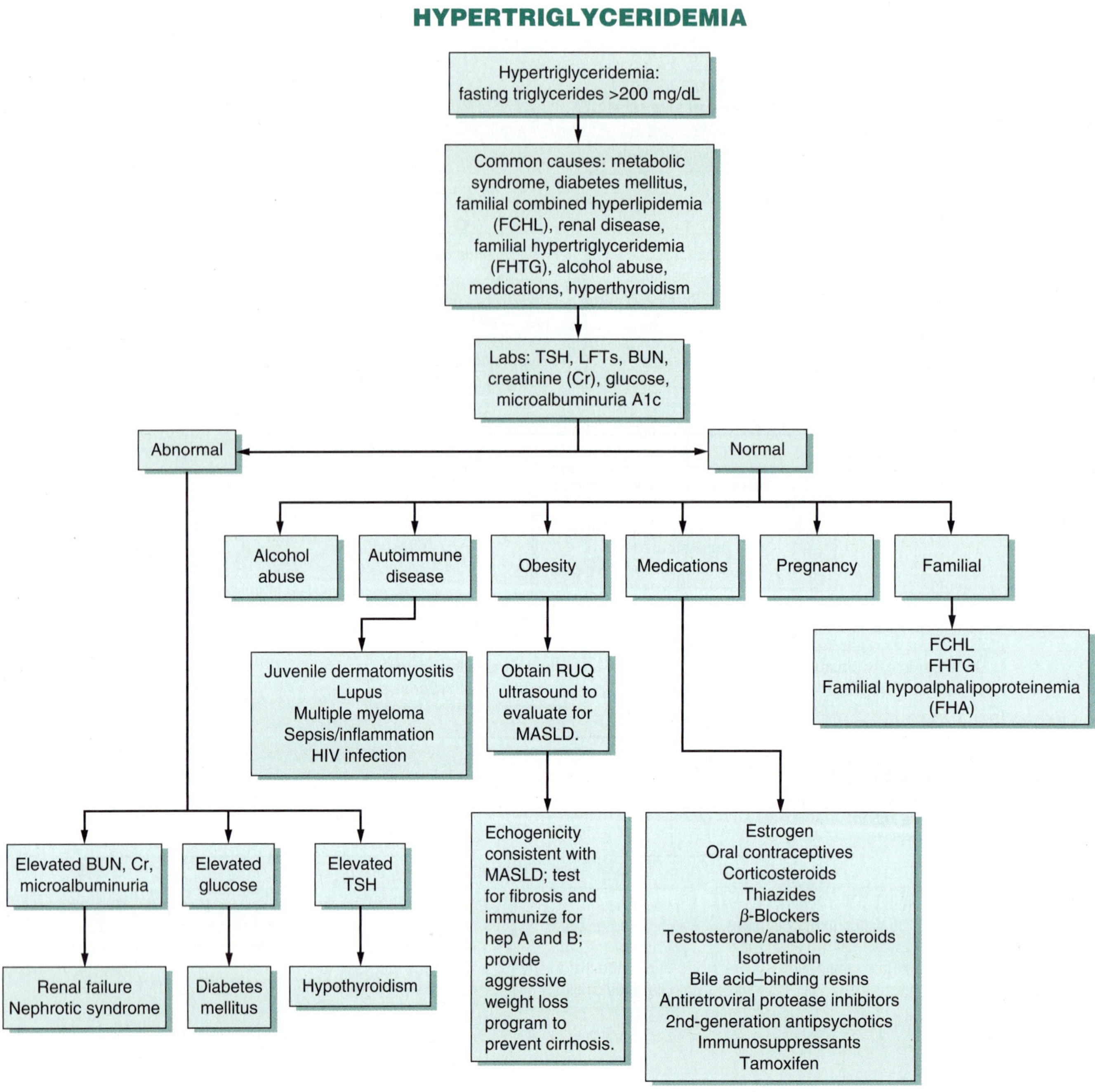

Frank J. Domino, MD

Berglund L, Brunzell JD, Goldberg AC, et al; for Endocrine Society. Evaluation and treatment of hypertriglyceridemia: an Endocrine Society clinical practice guideline. *J Clin Endocrinol Metab*. 2012;97(9):2969–2989.

HYPOALBUMINEMIA

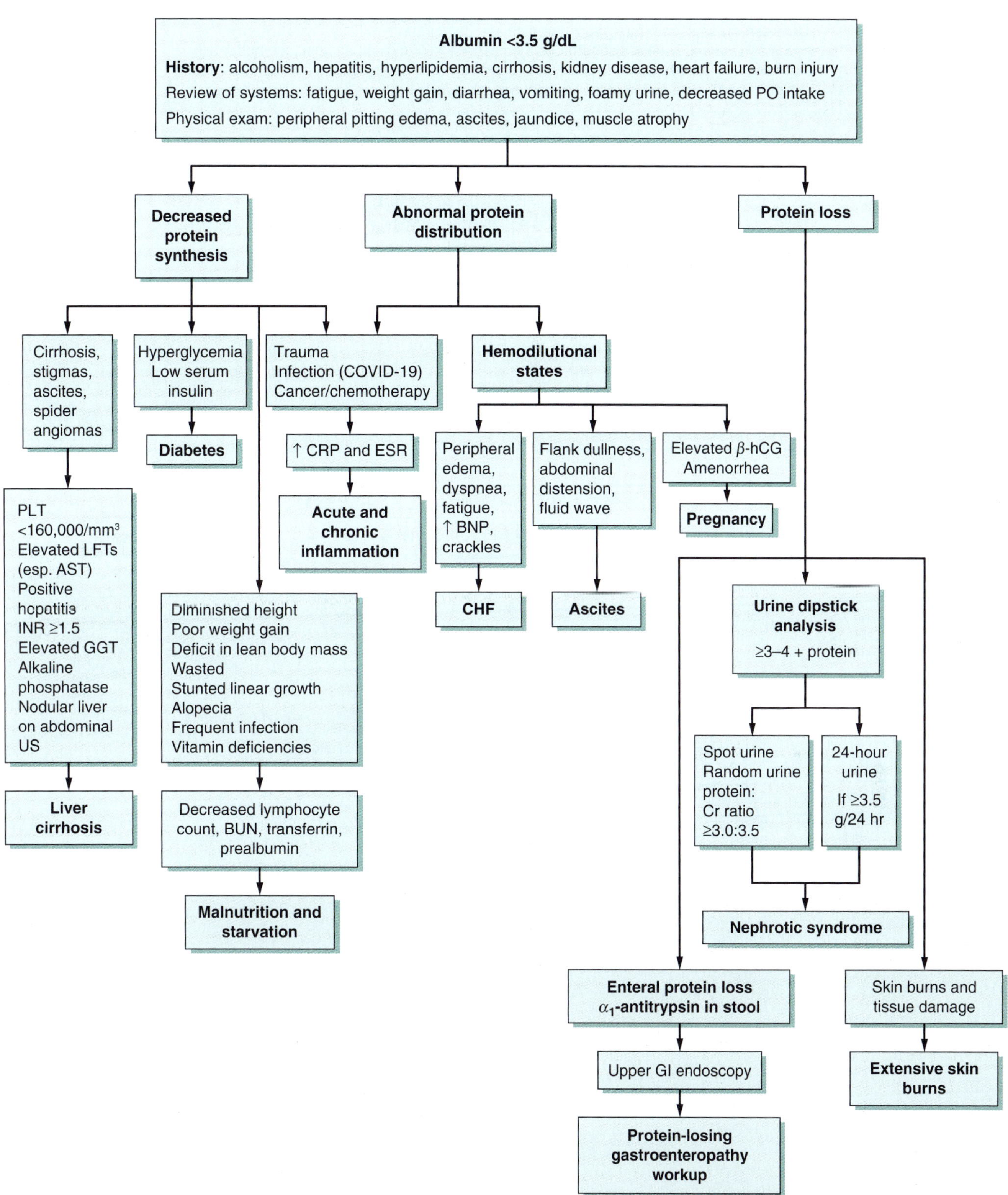

Anna Marie Tran, DO and Bashyam Iyengar, MD, MPH

Soeters PB, Wolfe RR, Shenkin A. Hypoalbuminemia: pathogenesis and clinical significance. *JPEN J Parenter Enteral Nutr*. 2019;43(2):181–193. doi:10.1002/jpen.1451.

HYPOCALCEMIA

Common causes: lab error, chronic renal failure, hypoparathyroidism, hypoalbuminemia, hypomagnesemia, hyperphosphatemia, medications (diuretics, phenytoin, chemotherapy, bone resorption inhibitors), PTH deficiency or resistance, vitamin D deficiency or resistance, blood transfusion, pancreatitis, rhabdomyolysis, tumor lysis syndrome, critical illness

↓

Check labs: Repeat serum calcium, ionized calcium, potassium, sodium, BUN, creatinine, magnesium, phosphorus, albumin, LFTs, PTH, alk phos, CK, lipase, ECG (for QTc), 25-hydroxyvitamin D.

↓

- Serum calcium <8.5 mg/dL, ionized or corrected calcium low, albumin normal or slightly low; if ionized calcium not available, correct serum calcium for albumin; calcium concentration falls by 0.8 mg/dL for every 1 g/dL fall in albumin.
  - Cr high → CKD, rhabdomyolysis, tumor lysis syndrome
  - Mg low → Hypomagnesemia
  - Mg and Cr Normal
    - High PTH
      - Low phos → Vitamin D deficiencies, rickets
      - High phos → Pseudohypoparathyroidism, calcium complexing (blood transfusion, pancreatitis), rhabdomyolysis, tumor lysis syndrome
    - Low PTH → Hypoparathyroidism (postsurgical, autoimmune, congenital, radiation, infiltrative)
- Serum calcium <8.5 mg/dL, ionized or corrected calcium normal, albumin low; if ionized calcium not available, correct serum calcium for albumin; calcium concentration falls by 0.8 mg/dL for every 1 g/dL fall in albumin.
  - Hypoalbuminemia → Cirrhosis, nephrotic syndrome, malnutrition, burns, chronic illness, sepsis

Timothy S. Lishnak, MD

Pepe J, Colangelo L, Biamonte F, et al. Diagnosis and management of hypocalcemia. *Endocrine*. 2020;69(3):485–495.

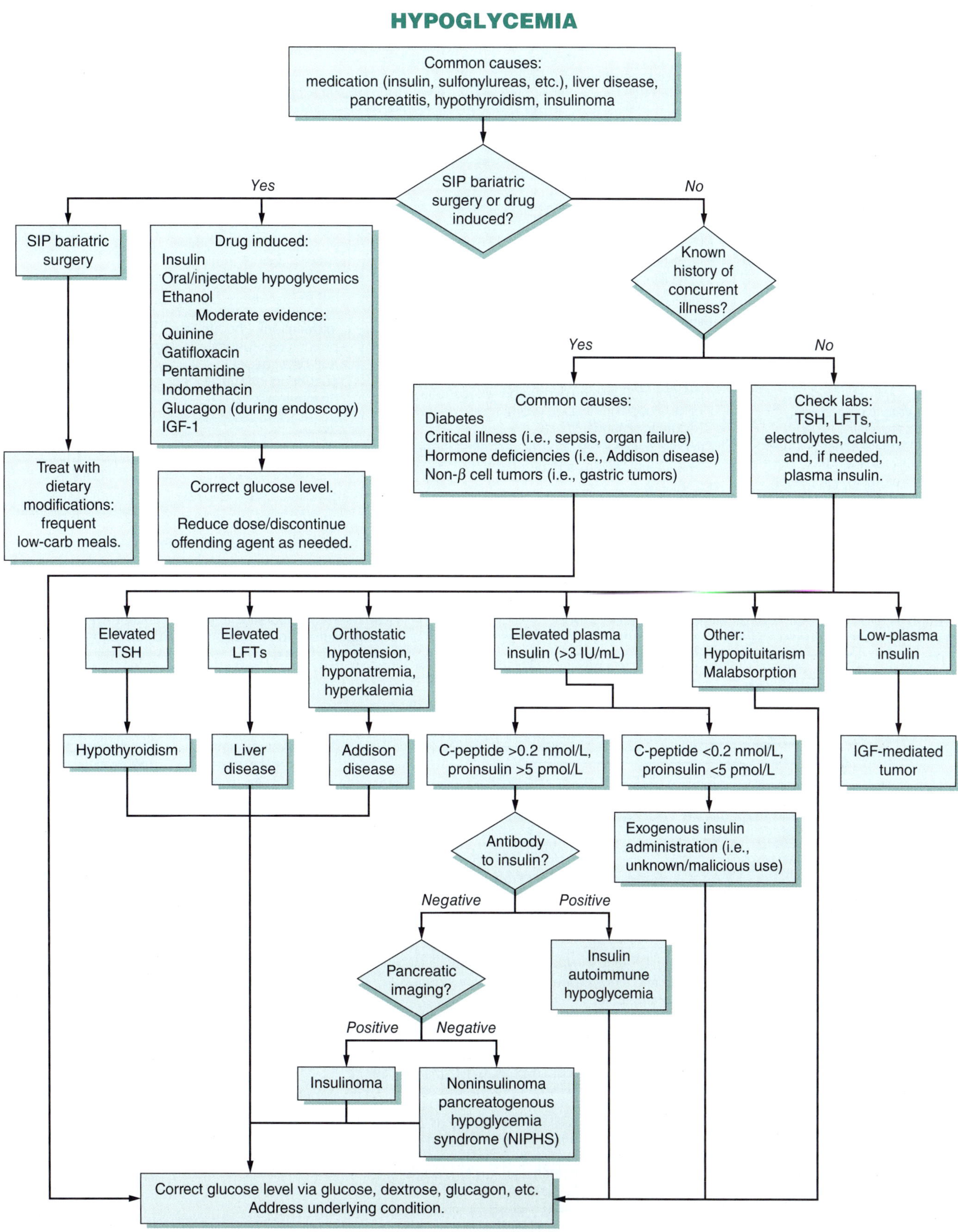

Frank J. Domino, MD

Kandaswamy L, Raghavan R, Pappachan JM. Spontaneous hypoglycemia: diagnostic evaluation and management. *Endocrine*. 2016;53(1):47–57.

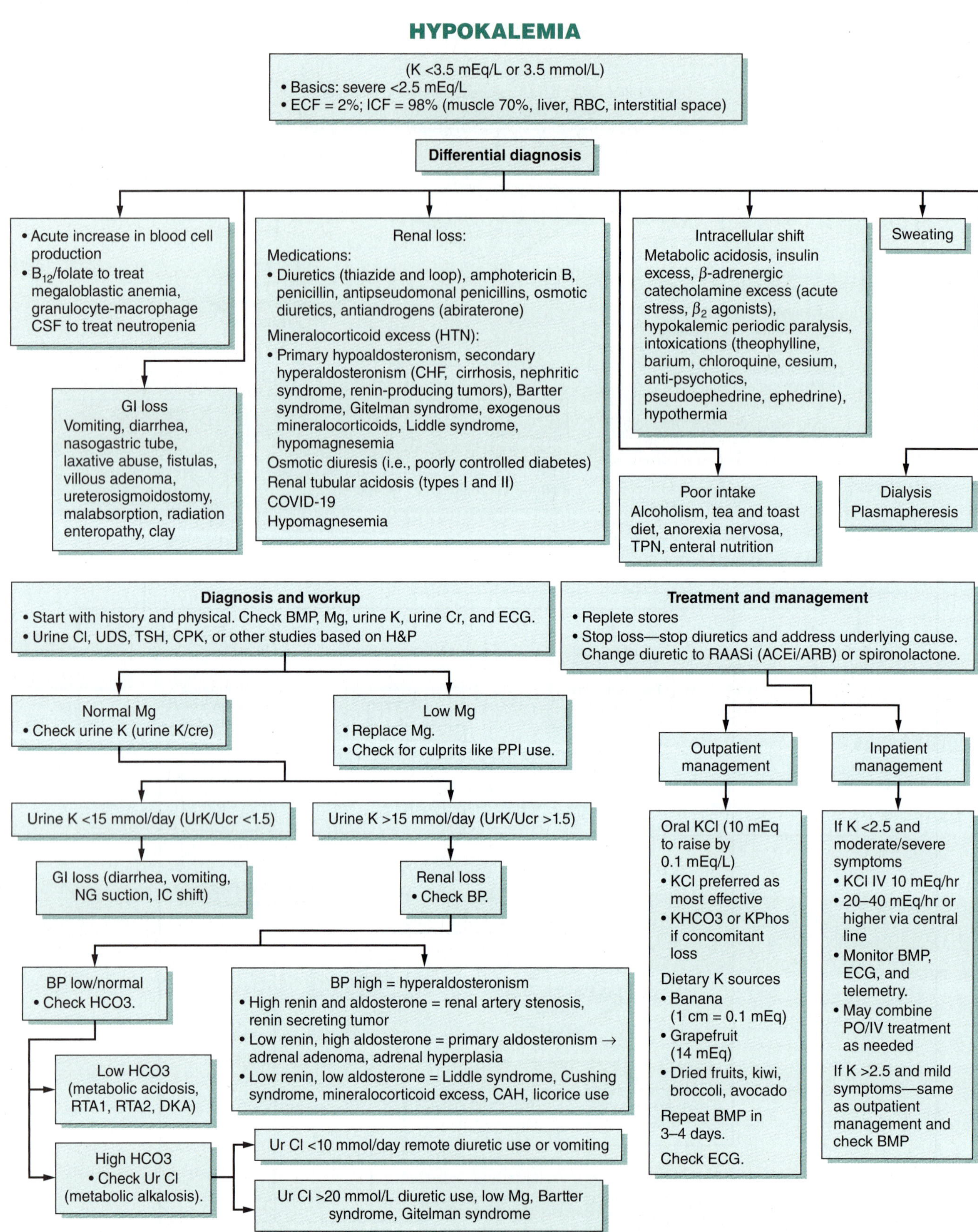

Lisa Weiss, MD, Med, FAAFP and Sumira A. Koirala, MD, FAAFP

Kardalas E, Paschou SA, Anagnostis P, et al. Hypokalemia: a clinical update. *Endocr Connect*. 2018;7(4):R135–R146.

HYPONATREMIA

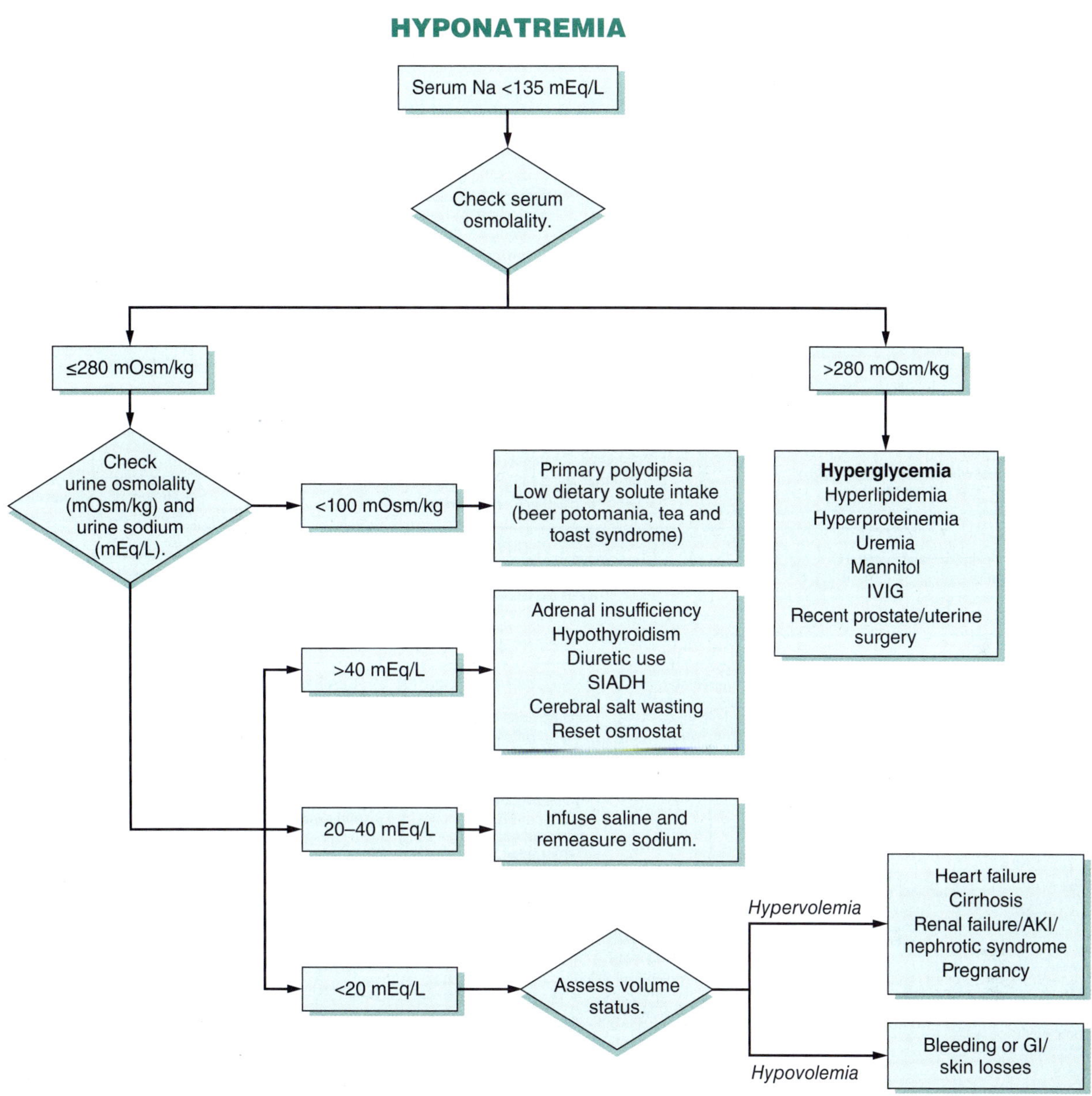

Chelsea Harris, MD and Corinne Gibbons, MD, MPH

Verbalis JG, Goldsmith SR, Greenberg A, et al. Diagnosis, evaluation, and treatment of hyponatremia: expert panel recommendations. *Am J Med*. 2013;126(10 Suppl 1):S1–S42.

HYPOTENSION

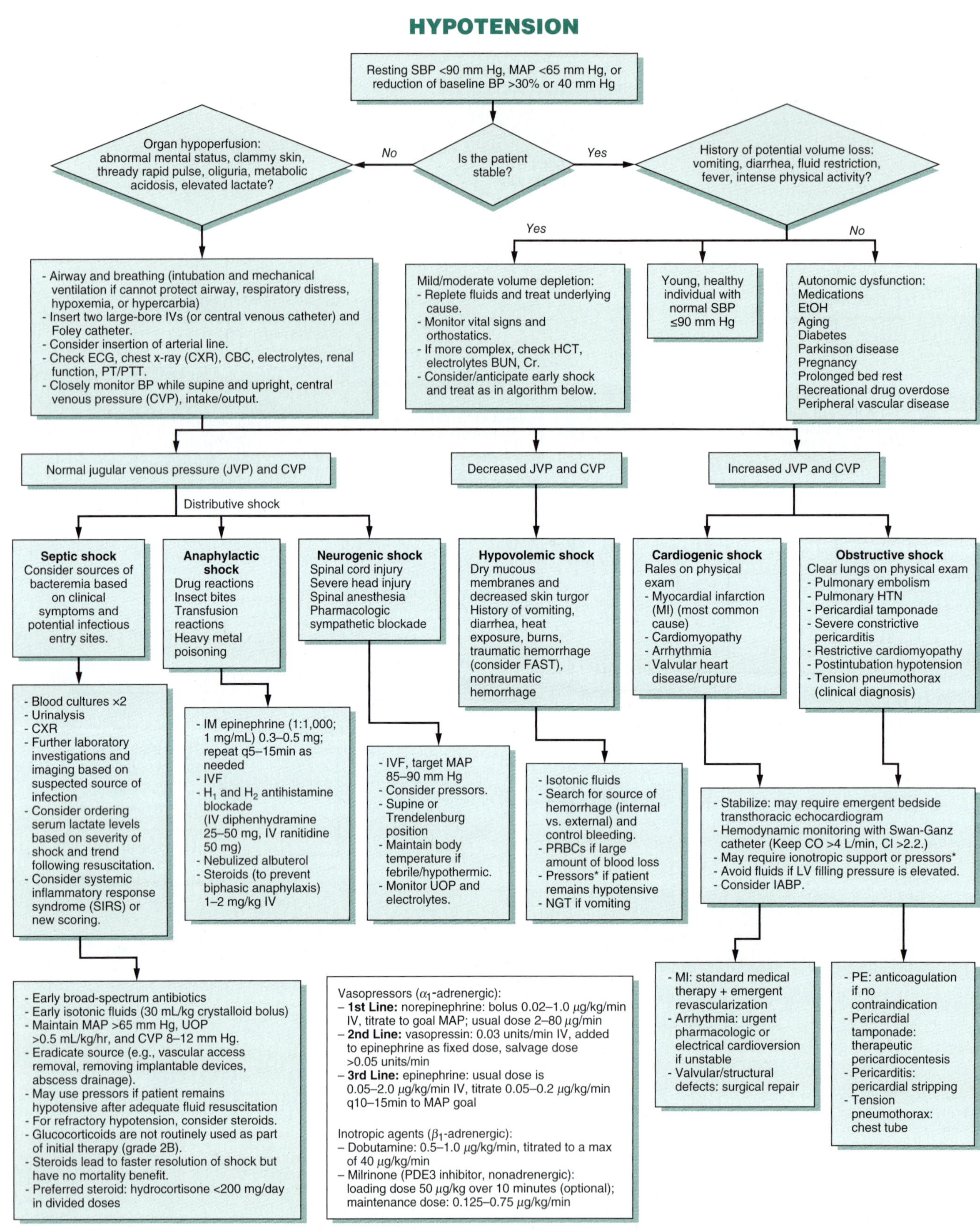

Tamara Kailoa Montacute, MD, MPH

Thompson K, Venkatesh B, Finfer S. Sepsis and septic shock: current approaches to management. *Intern Med J.* 2019;49(2):160–170.

INFERTILITY

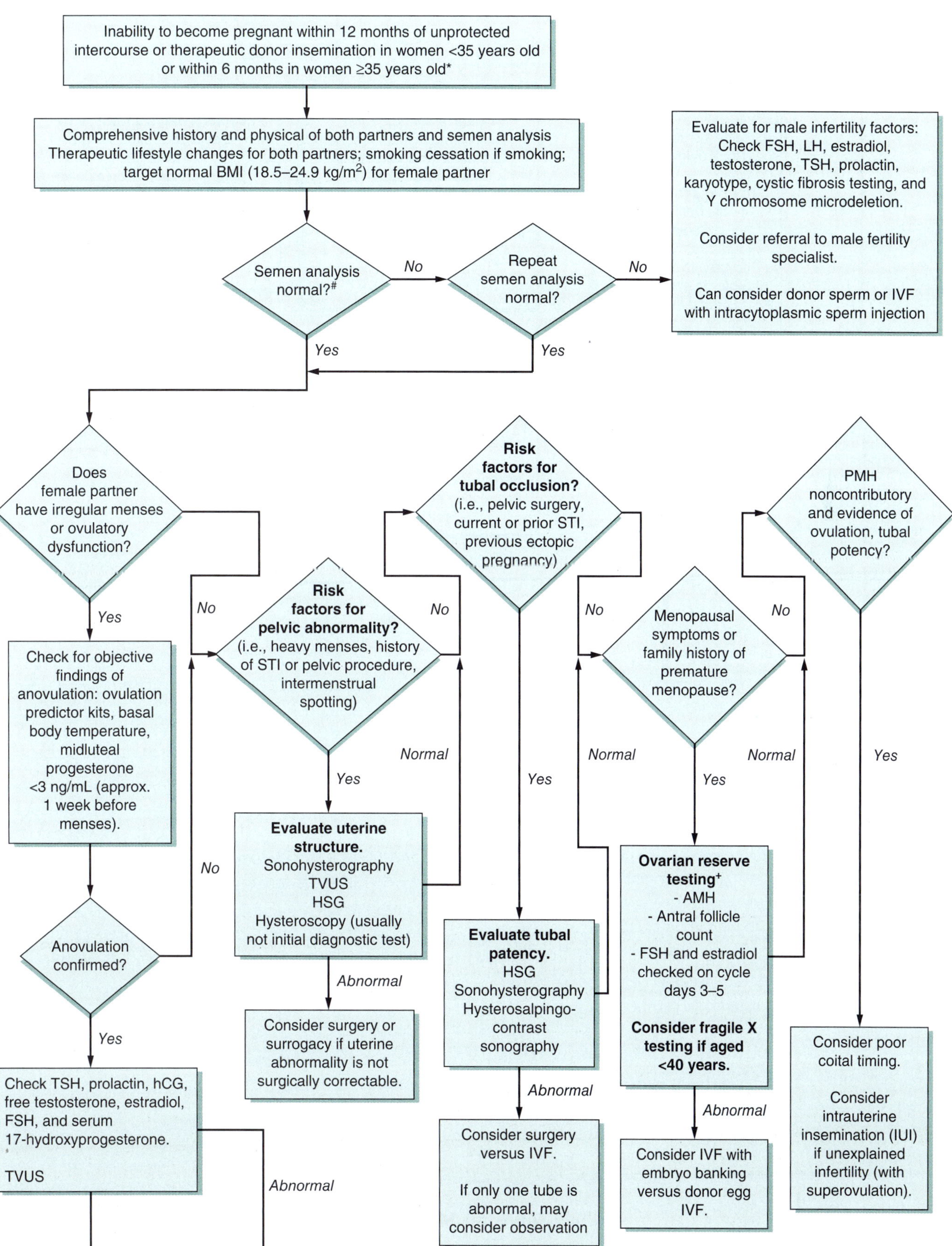

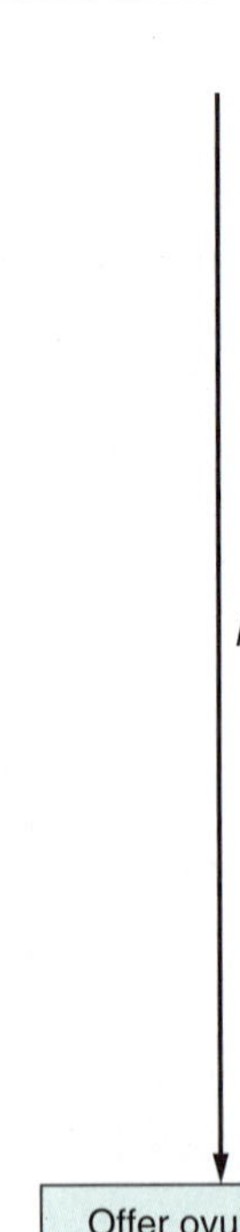

Offer ovulation induction meds (with preference for letrozole over clomiphene).

PCOS
Testosterone level may be increased.
Rotterdam criteria

Thyroid dysfunction
If abnormal thyroid studies

Pituitary abnormality
If prolactin abnormal or FSH and estradiol abnormal, consider brain MRI to evaluate for pituitary abnormality.

Nonclassical CAH
Consider if increased 17-hydroxyprogesterone.

***Common causes of infertility**
- Male factor (40–50%)
- Diminished ovarian reserve (premature menopause or advanced age)
- Tubal or uterine abnormality
- Ovulatory dysfunction (PCOS, thyroid abnormality, obesity/low BMI, eating disorder, hyperprolactinemia)
- Unknown (30%)

+Lab values consistent with reduced ovarian reserve
AMH <1 ng/mL
Antral follicle count <5–7
FSH >10 IU/L
Elevated estradiol (normal is <60–80 pg/mL)
History of poor response to IVF stimulation (<4 oocytes at egg retrieval)

#Lower limit cutoffs for normal semen analysis from WHO
Ejaculate volume 1.5 mL
pH ≥7.2.
Sperm concentration at least 15×10^6/mL
Minimum total sperm 39×10^6/ejaculate
Total motility 40%
No sperm agglutination

TVUS: transvaginal ultrasound
HSG: hysterosalpingogram
AMH: Anti-müllerian hormone
CAH: congenital adrenal hyperplasia

Julie Johnston, MD, FAAFP

Practice Committee of the American Society for Reproductive Medicine. Fertility evaluation of infertile women: a committee opinion. *Fertil Steril.* 2021;116(5):1255–1265.

KNEE PAIN

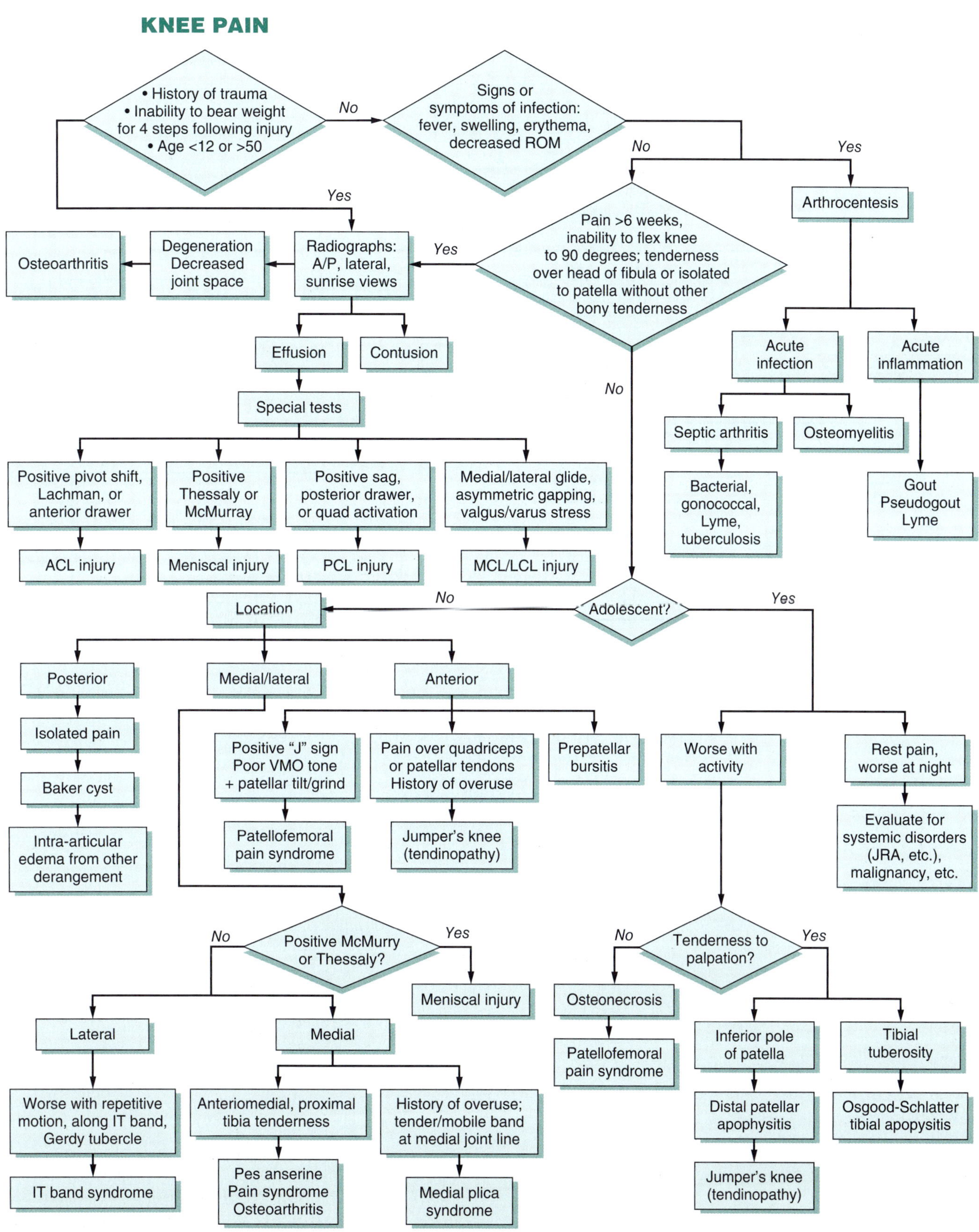

Tu Dan Nguyen, MD, CAQSM and Rod J. Turner Jr., MD, CAQSM, MS

Bunt CW, Jonas CE, Chang JG. Knee pain in adults and adolescents: the initial evaluation. *Am Fam Physician*. 2018;98(9):576–585.

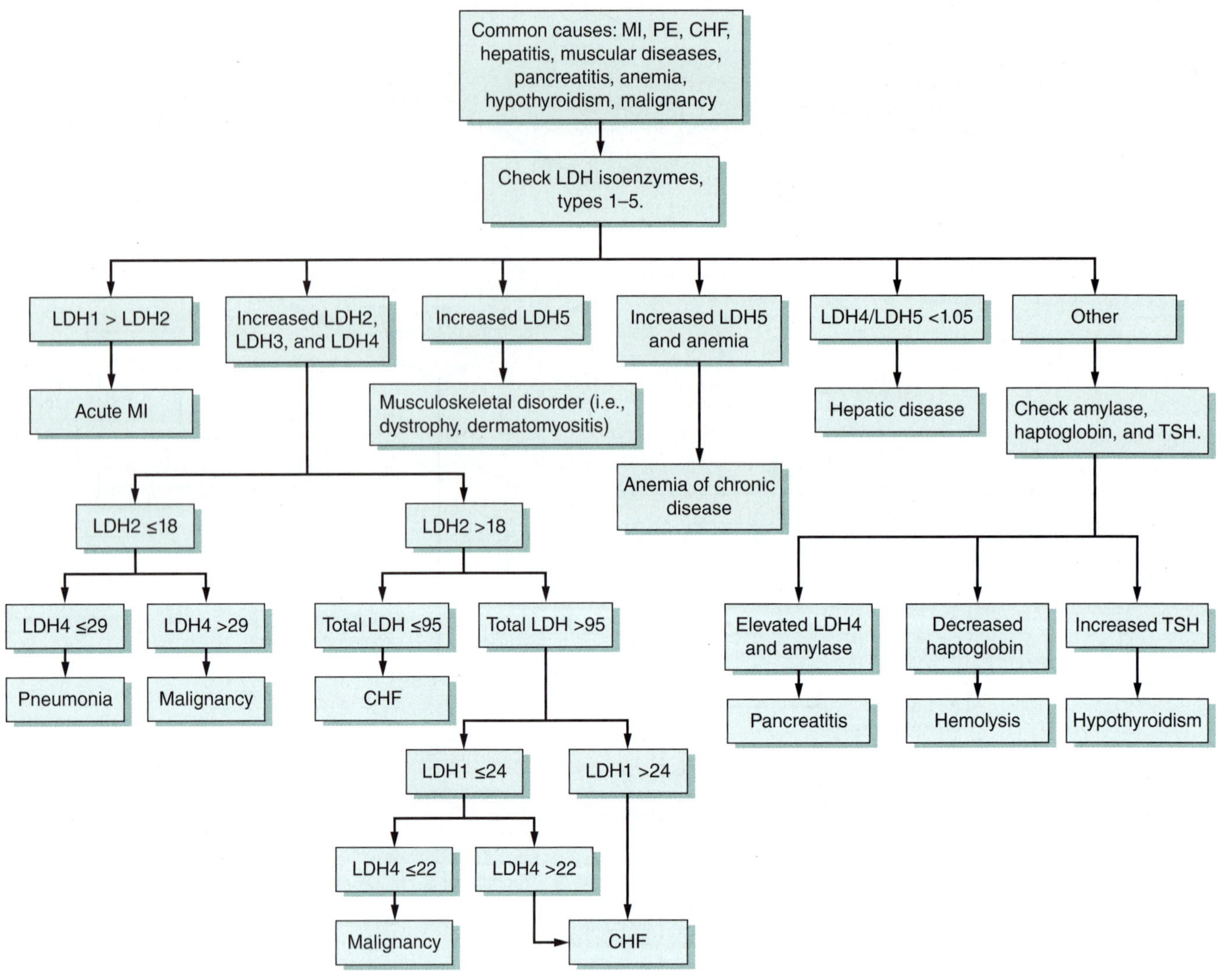

Meygan Lackey Elway, MD, MPH and Corinne Grady, MD, MS

Lossos IS, Breuer R, Intrator O, et al. Differential diagnosis of pleural effusion by lactate dehydrogenase isoenzyme analysis. *Chest.* 1997;111(3):648–651.

LOW BACK PAIN, CHRONIC

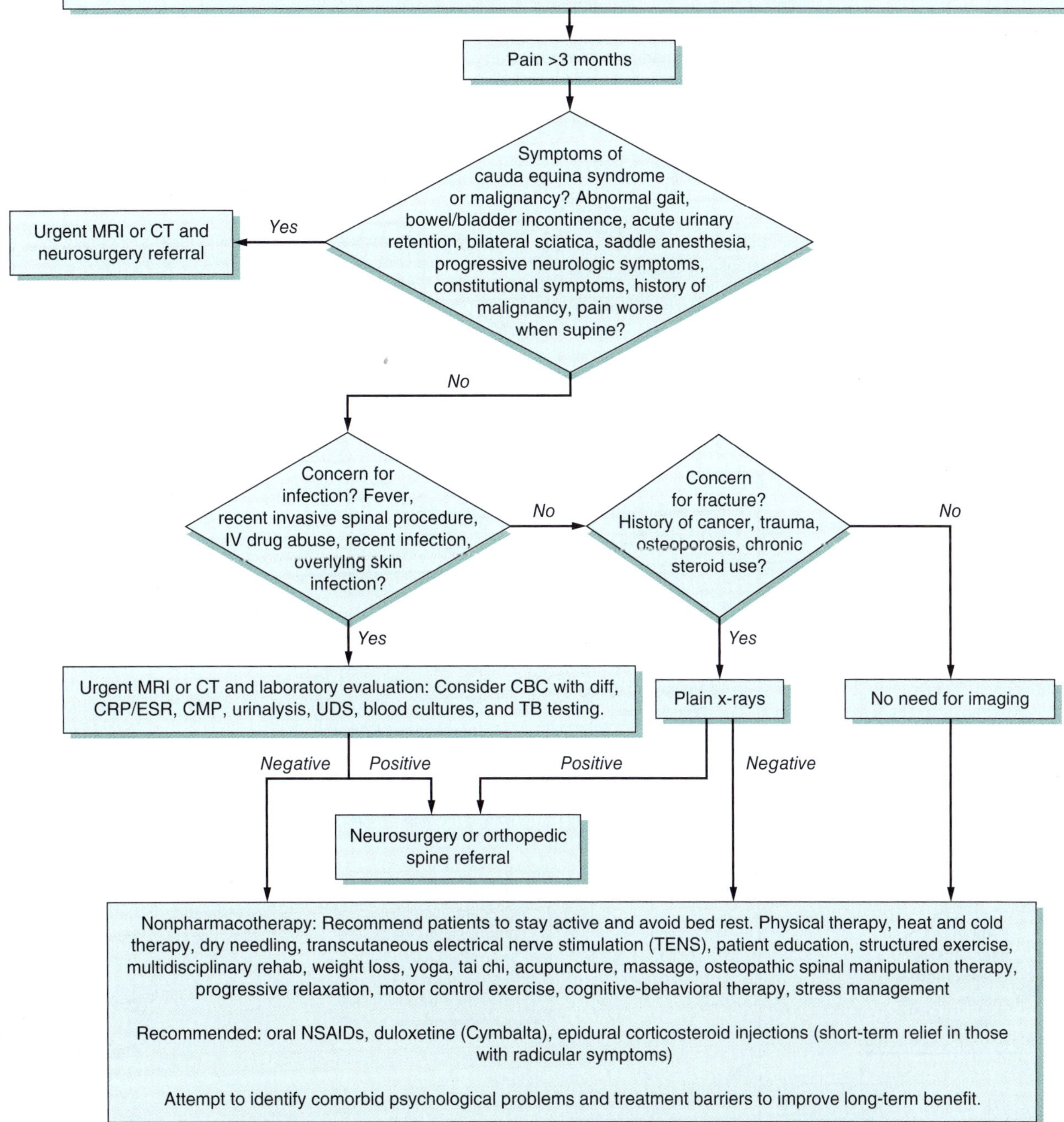

Danielle N. Coderre, MD and Emily J. Eschleman, DO, MS, CAQSM

Maharty DC, Hines SC, Brown RB. Chronic low back pain in adults: evaluation and management. *Am Fam Physician*. 2024;109(3):233–244.

LYMPHADENOPATHY

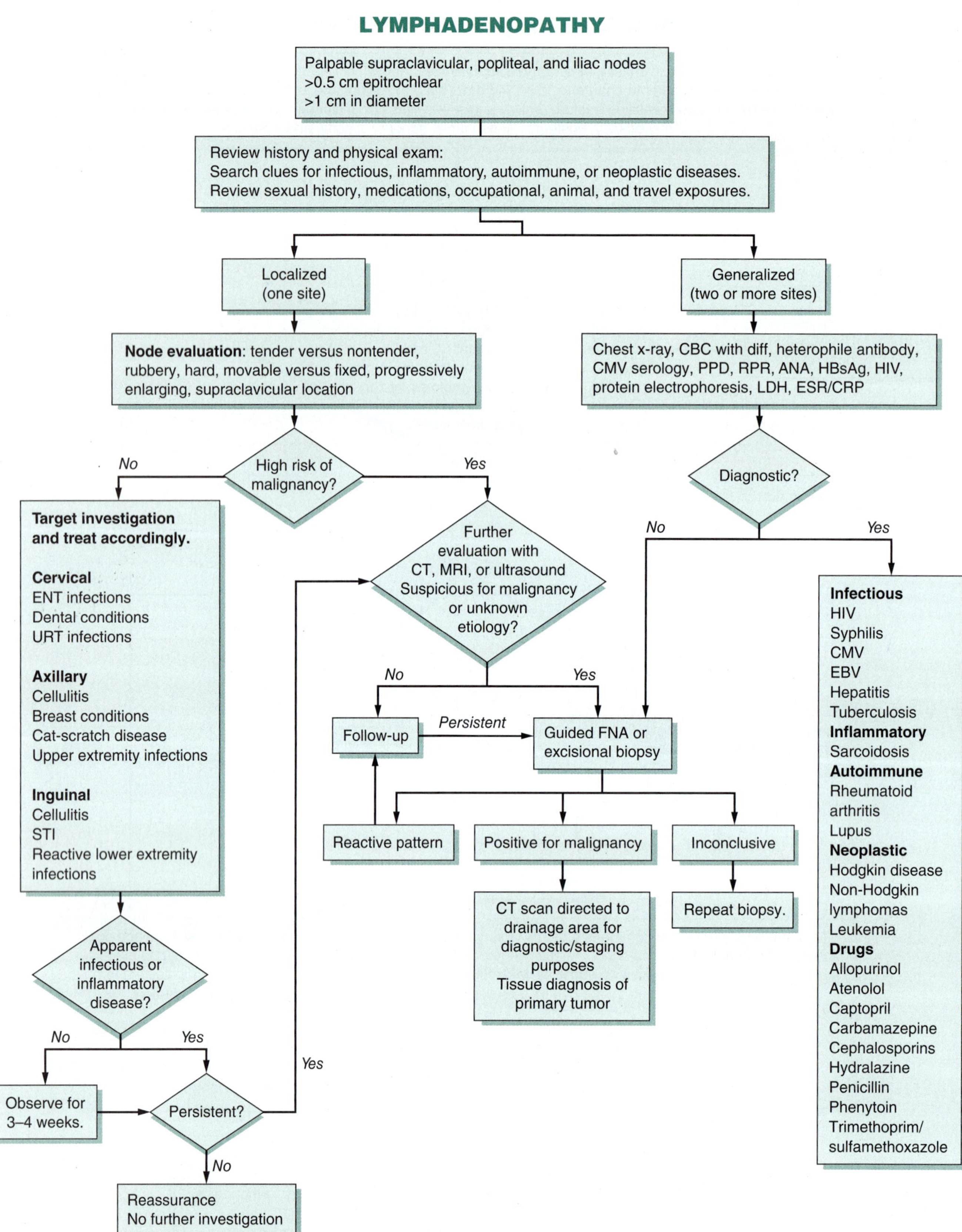

Katy (Ekaterina) Brodski-Quigley, MD, EdM

Gaddey HL, Riegel AM. Unexplained lymphadenopathy: evaluation and differential diagnosis. *Am Fam Physician*. 2016;94(11):896–903.

LYMPHOPENIA OR LYMPHOCYTOPENIA

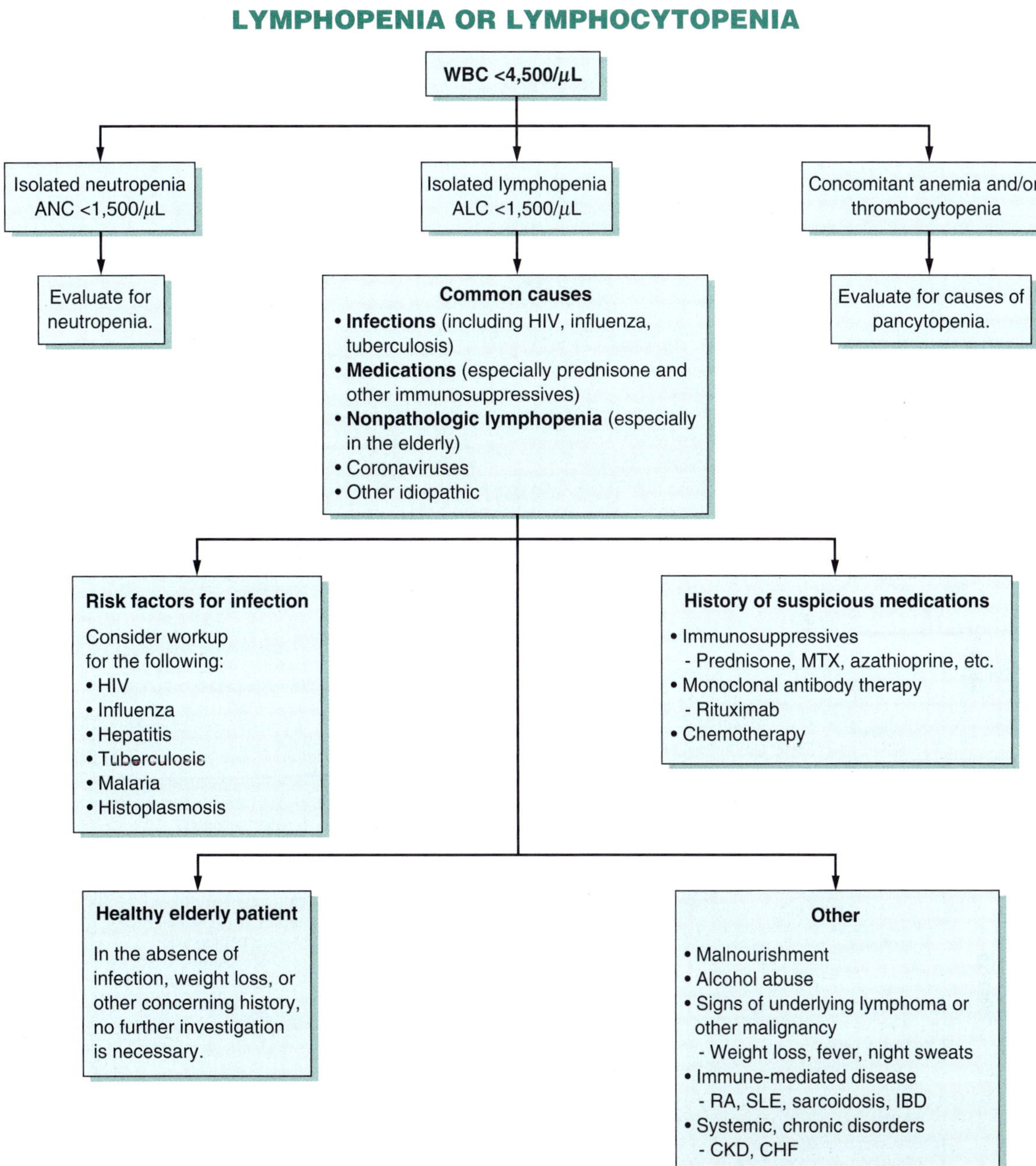

Jillian K. Joseph, MPAS, PA-C

Warny M, Helby J, Nordestgaard BG, et al. Incidental lymphopenia and mortality: a prospective cohort study. *CMAJ.* 2020;192(2):E25-E33. doi: 10.1503/cmaj.191024.

MENOPAUSE, EVALUATION AND MANAGEMENT PART I

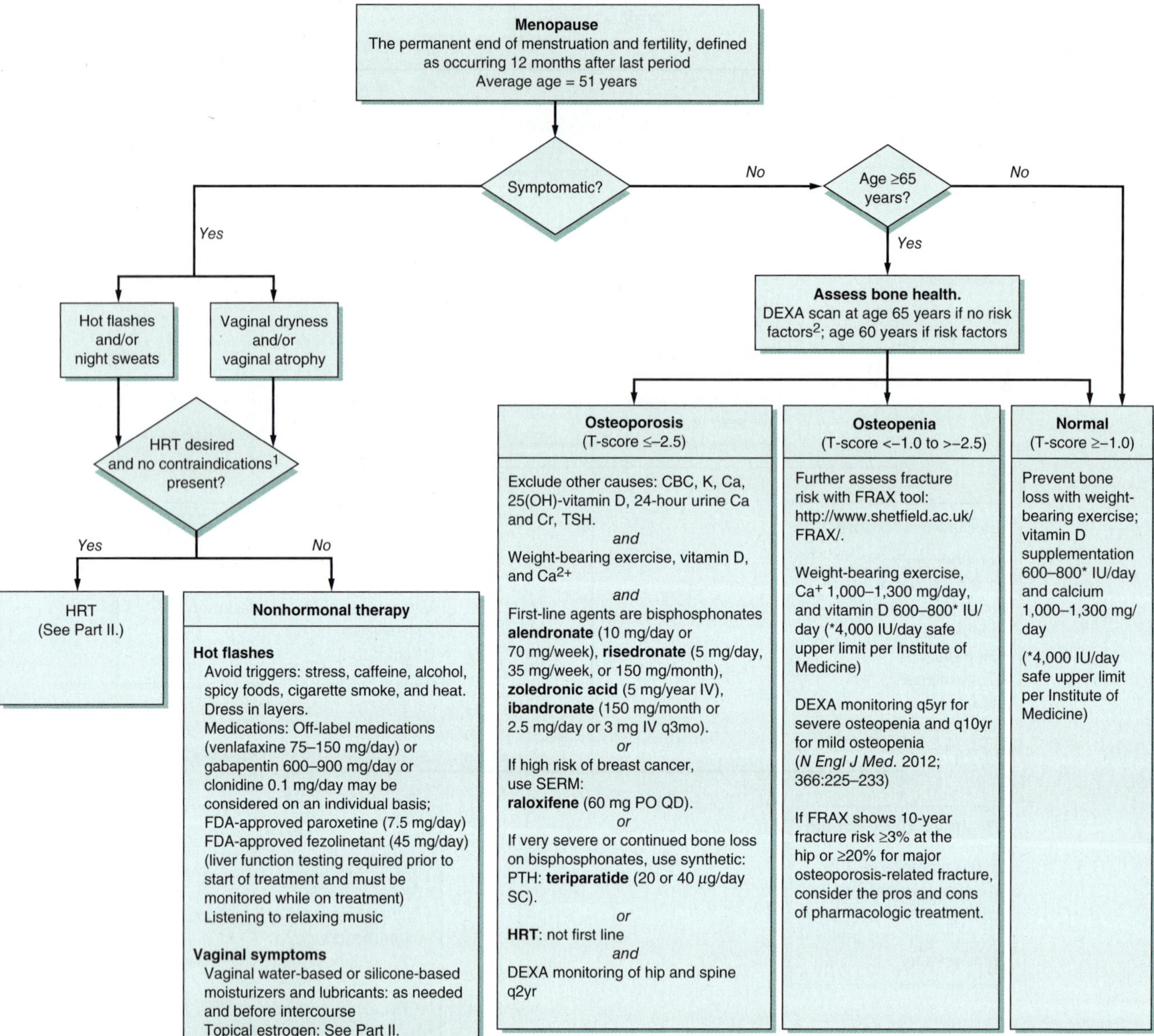

PART II

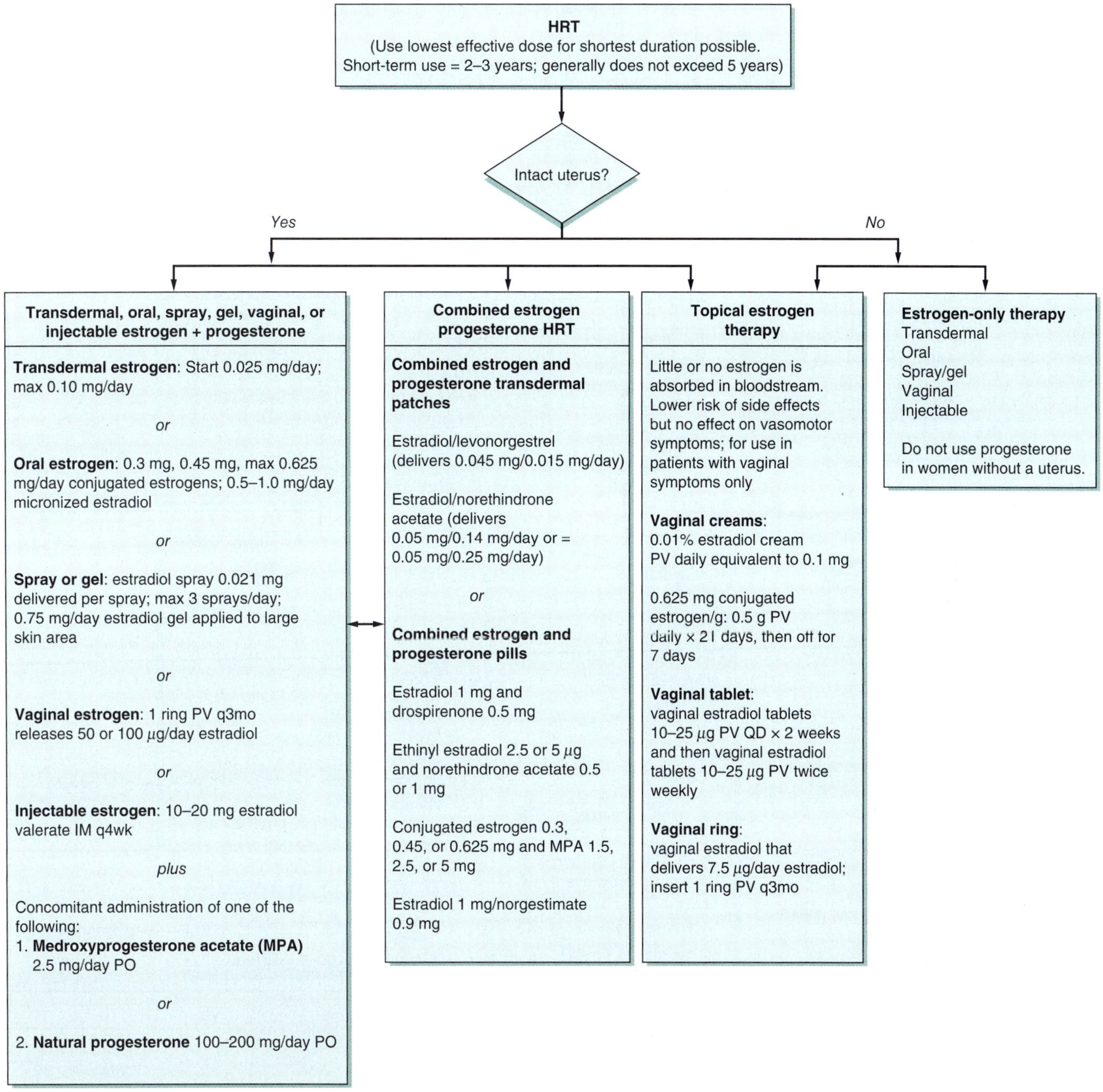

HRT
(Use lowest effective dose for shortest duration possible. Short-term use = 2–3 years; generally does not exceed 5 years)

Intact uterus?

Yes

Transdermal, oral, spray, gel, vaginal, or injectable estrogen + progesterone

Transdermal estrogen: Start 0.025 mg/day; max 0.10 mg/day

or

Oral estrogen: 0.3 mg, 0.45 mg, max 0.625 mg/day conjugated estrogens; 0.5–1.0 mg/day micronized estradiol

or

Spray or gel: estradiol spray 0.021 mg delivered per spray; max 3 sprays/day; 0.75 mg/day estradiol gel applied to large skin area

or

Vaginal estrogen: 1 ring PV q3mo releases 50 or 100 μg/day estradiol

or

Injectable estrogen: 10–20 mg estradiol valerate IM q4wk

plus

Concomitant administration of one of the following:
1. **Medroxyprogesterone acetate (MPA)** 2.5 mg/day PO

or

2. **Natural progesterone** 100–200 mg/day PO

Combined estrogen progesterone HRT

Combined estrogen and progesterone transdermal patches

Estradiol/levonorgestrel (delivers 0.045 mg/0.015 mg/day)

Estradiol/norethindrone acetate (delivers 0.05 mg/0.14 mg/day or = 0.05 mg/0.25 mg/day)

or

Combined estrogen and progesterone pills

Estradiol 1 mg and drospirenone 0.5 mg

Ethinyl estradiol 2.5 or 5 μg and norethindrone acetate 0.5 or 1 mg

Conjugated estrogen 0.3, 0.45, or 0.625 mg and MPA 1.5, 2.5, or 5 mg

Estradiol 1 mg/norgestimate 0.9 mg

Topical estrogen therapy

Little or no estrogen is absorbed in bloodstream. Lower risk of side effects but no effect on vasomotor symptoms; for use in patients with vaginal symptoms only

Vaginal creams:
0.01% estradiol cream PV daily equivalent to 0.1 mg

0.625 mg conjugated estrogen/g: 0.5 g PV daily × 21 days, then off for 7 days

Vaginal tablet:
vaginal estradiol tablets 10–25 μg PV QD × 2 weeks and then vaginal estradiol tablets 10–25 μg PV twice weekly

Vaginal ring:
vaginal estradiol that delivers 7.5 μg/day estradiol; insert 1 ring PV q3mo

No

Estrogen-only therapy
Transdermal
Oral
Spray/gel
Vaginal
Injectable

Do not use progesterone in women without a uterus.

Kelly Pagidas, MD

ACOG Practice Bulletin No. 141: management of menopausal symptoms. *Obstet Gynecol*. 2014;123(1):202–216.

MIGRAINE, TREATMENT

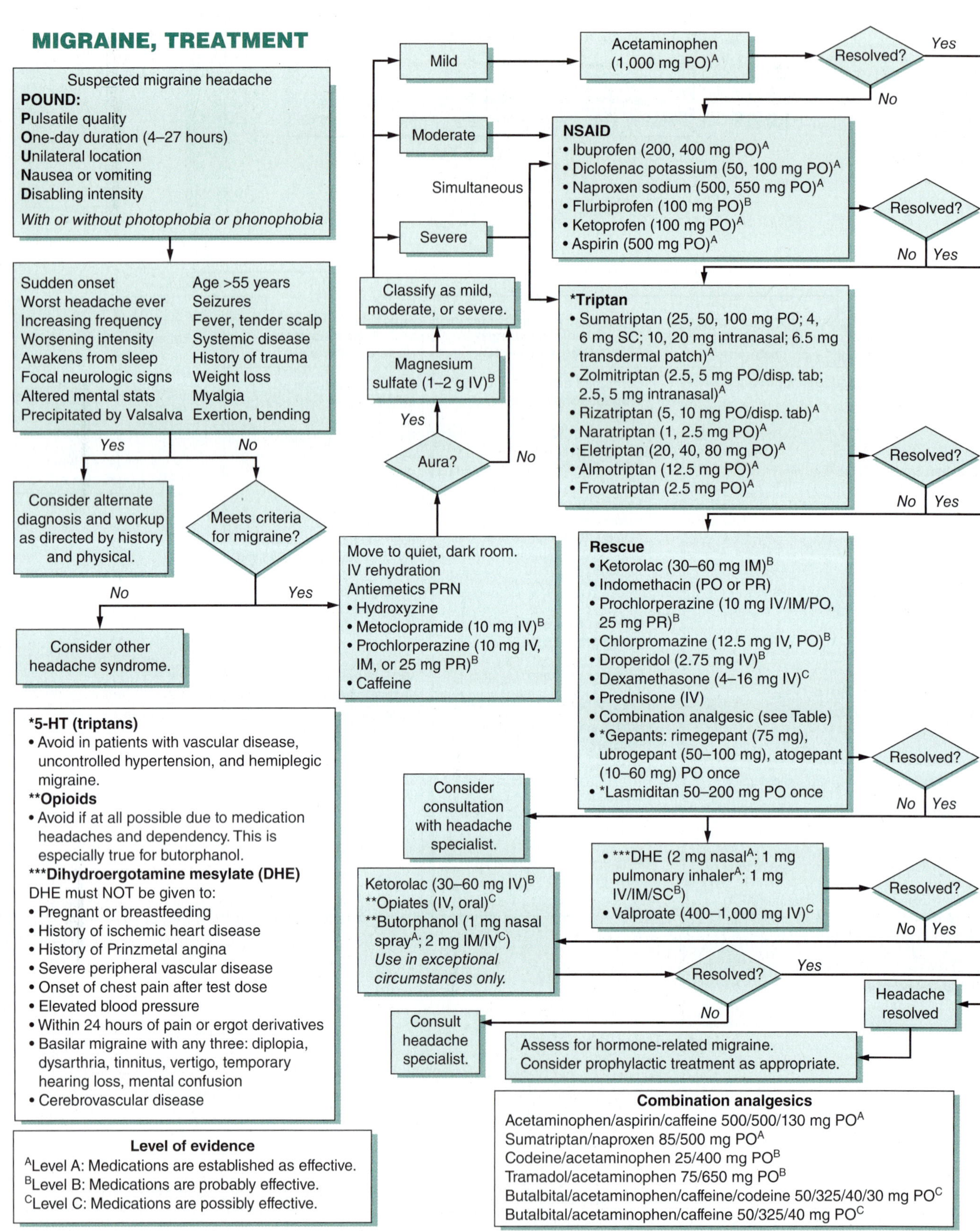

Katy (Ekaterina) Brodski-Quigley, MD, EdM

VanderPluym JH, Halker Singh RB, Urtecho M, et al. Acute treatments for episodic migraine in adults: a systematic review and meta-analysis. *JAMA*. 2021;325(23):2357–2369. doi:10.1001/jama.2021.7939.

NAIL ABNORMALITIES

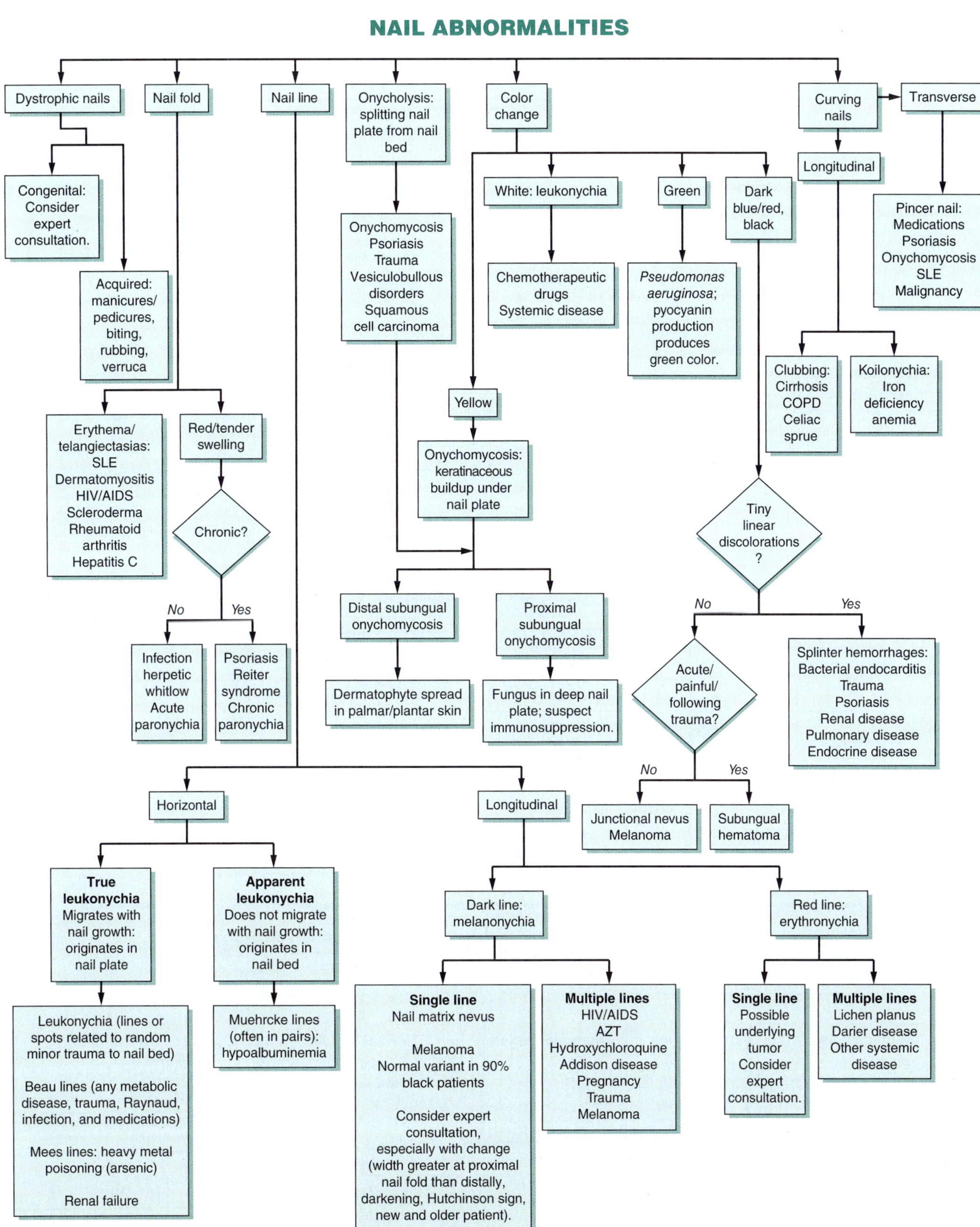

Natasha J. Pyzocha, DO, FAWM, FAAFP and Douglas M. Maurer, DO, MPH, FAAFP

Tully AS, Trayes KP, Studdiford JS. Evaluation of nail abnormalities. *Am Fam Physician*. 2012;85(8):779–787.

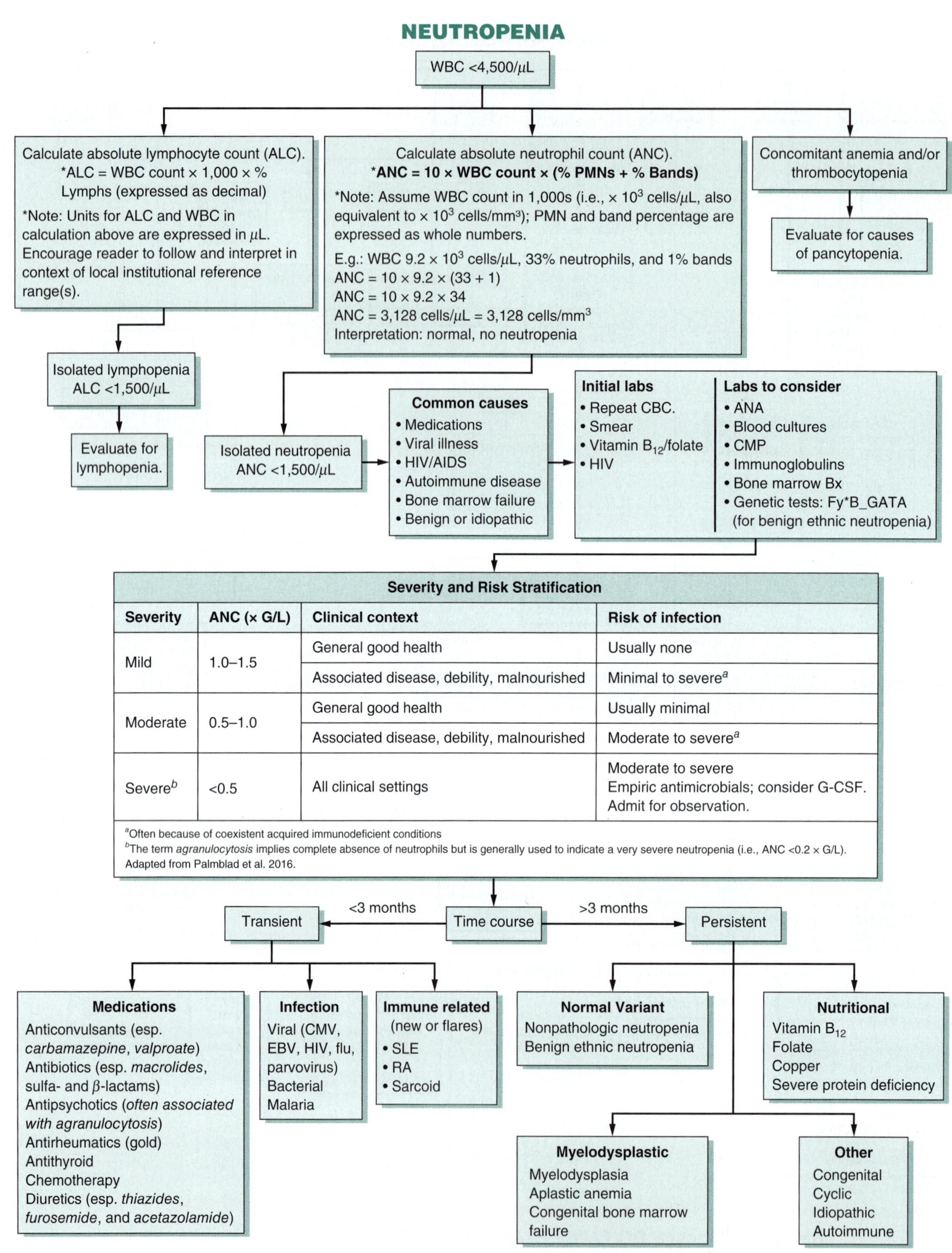

Severity and Risk Stratification

Severity	ANC (× G/L)	Clinical context	Risk of infection
Mild	1.0–1.5	General good health	Usually none
		Associated disease, debility, malnourished	Minimal to severe[a]
Moderate	0.5–1.0	General good health	Usually minimal
		Associated disease, debility, malnourished	Moderate to severe[a]
Severe[b]	<0.5	All clinical settings	Moderate to severe Empiric antimicrobials; consider G-CSF. Admit for observation.

[a]Often because of coexistent acquired immunodeficient conditions
[b]The term *agranulocytosis* implies complete absence of neutrophils but is generally used to indicate a very severe neutropenia (i.e., ANC <0.2 × G/L).
Adapted from Palmblad et al. 2016.

Ben Ayotte, MD and Matthew Anderson, MD

Frater JL. How I investigate neutropenia. *Int J Lab Hematol*. 2020;42(Suppl 1):121–132. doi:10.1111/ijlh.13210.

PAIN, CHRONIC, DIAGNOSIS

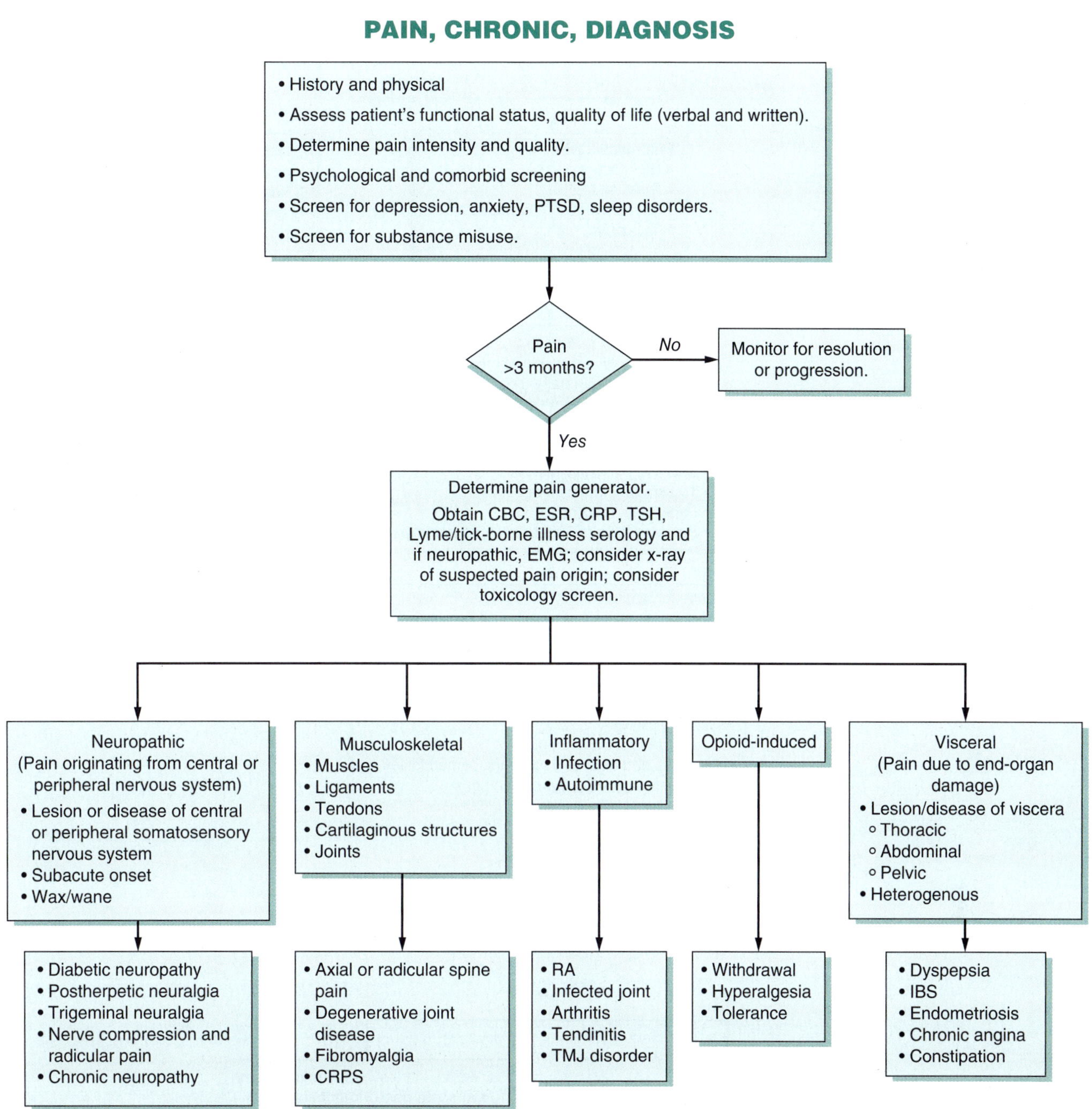

Jennifer Bradford, MD, MPH

Hooten M, Thorson D, Bianco J, et al. *Pain: Assessment, Non-Opioid Treatment Approaches and Opioid Management*. Bloomington, MN: Institute for Clinical Systems Improvement; 2017.

PAIN, CHRONIC, TREATMENT

Level I management (conservative and standard approach)

↓

Pharmacology
- NSAIDs*
- SSRI and SNRI**
- Anticonvulsant or antiepileptic**
- Topical agents*
- Muscle relaxers*
- Anxiolytics

*Nociceptive: acetaminophen, NSAIDs, topical agents, muscle relaxers
**Neuropathic

↓

Consider referral to both:
- Cognitive-behavioral therapy
- Physical therapy

↓

Interventional
- Sacroiliac joint injection
- Transforaminal epidural injection
- Facet joint injection
- Percutaneous radiofrequency neurotomy

↓

Complementary
- Acupuncture
- Herbal products (devil's claw, willow bark)
- Glucosamine/chondroitin

↓

Psychological
- Cognitive-behavioral therapy
- Diagnose and treat all psychiatric comorbidities (depression, anxiety, substance abuse).

↓

Goals met?
- Functional
- Barriers identified and addressed
- Reduced pain

Yes →

Outcomes assessment
- Document response to treatment.
- Reevaluate on scheduled basis.
- Recommend patient self-management (exercise, counseling, etc.).

No →

DIRE tool: https://www.mdcalc.com/dire-score-opioid-treatment

↓

Score ≥14?

Yes → May be chronic opioid candidate → Assess PEG score (https://www.mdcalc.com/calc/10405/pain-enjoyment-life-general-activity-peg-scale). → Assess opioid risk score (https://www.mdcalc.com/calc/10035/dire-score-opioid-treatment).

No → Level II management
- Biopsychosocial assessment
- Refer to multidisciplinary team.

Jennifer Bradford, MD, MPH

Mu A, Weinberg E, Moulin DE, et al. Pharmacologic management of chronic neuropathic pain: review of the Canadian Pain Society consensus statement. *Can Fam Physician*. 2017;63(11):844–852.

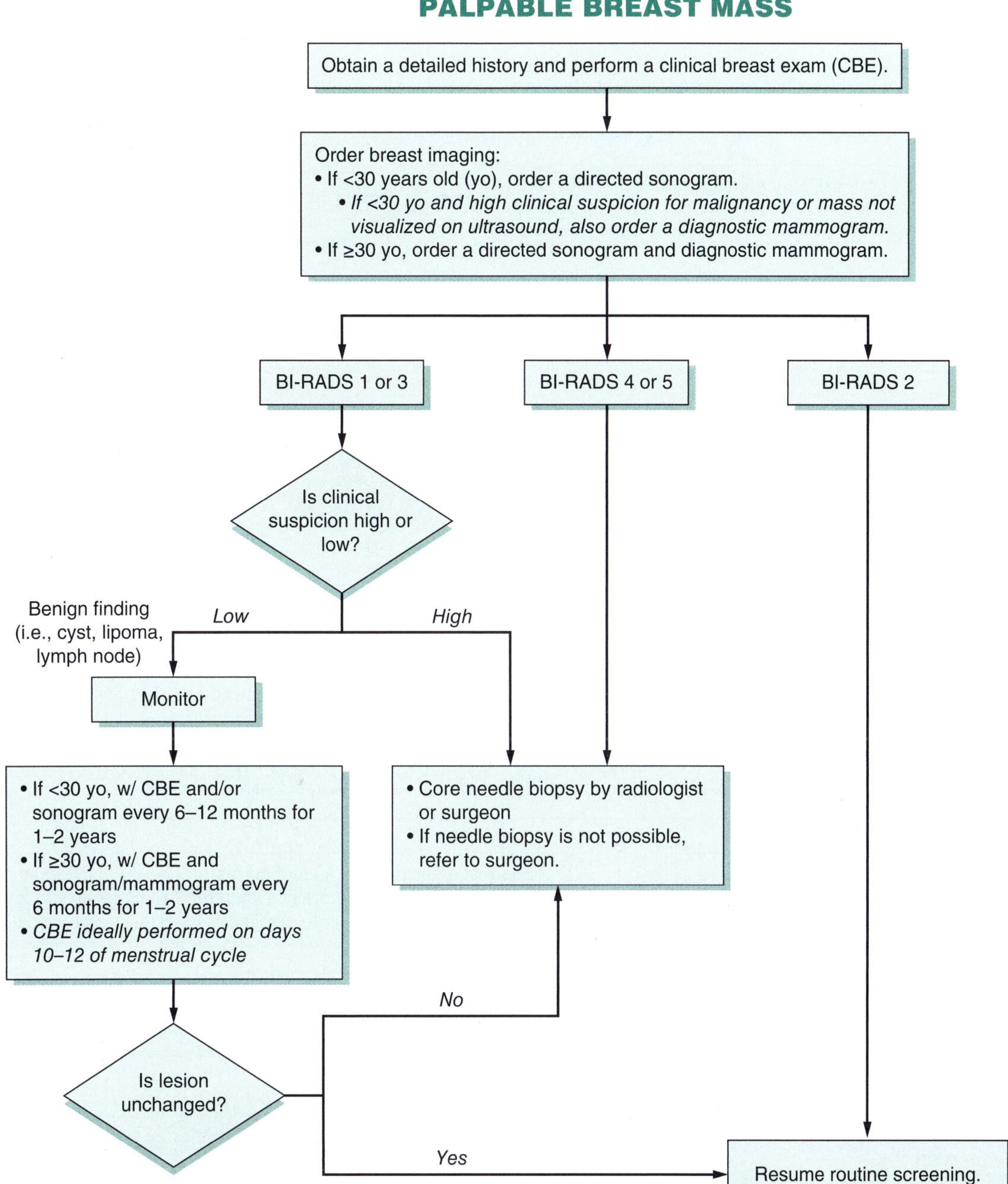

Stephanie Núñez-González, MD, MPH and Kira Zwygart, MD

Salzman B, Collins E, Hersh L. Common breast problems. *Am Fam Physician*. 2019;99(8):505–514.

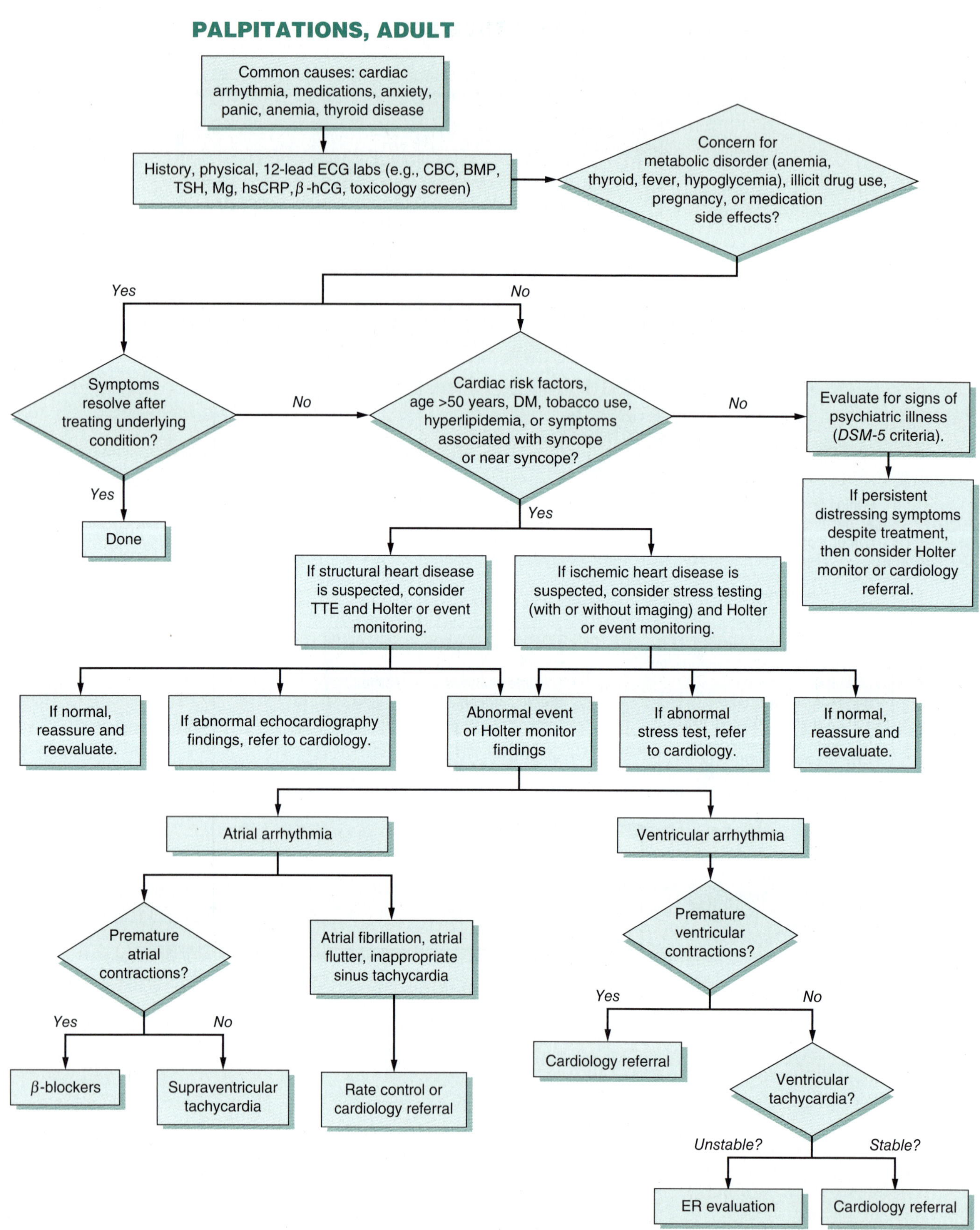

Elizabeth A. Lorick, MD

Gauer RL, Thomas MF, McNutt RA. Palpitations: evaluation, management, and wearable smart devices. *Am Fam Physician*. 2024;110(3):259–269.

PARKINSON DISEASE, TREATMENT

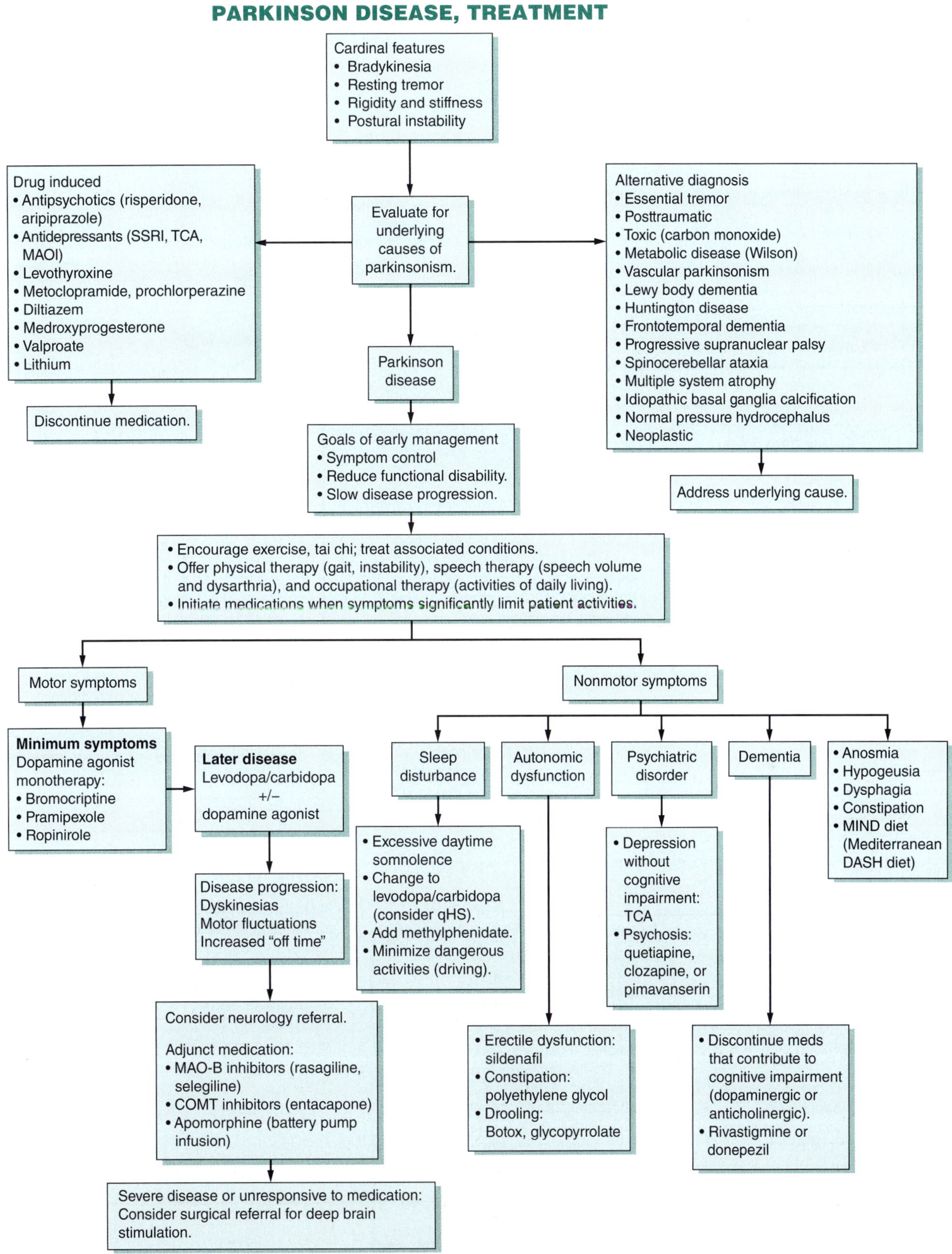

Saadia Mohsin, MD

Connolly BS, Lang AE. Pharmacological treatment of Parkinson disease: a review. *JAMA*. 2014;311(16):1670–1683.

PEDIATRIC EXANTHEMS, DIAGNOSTIC

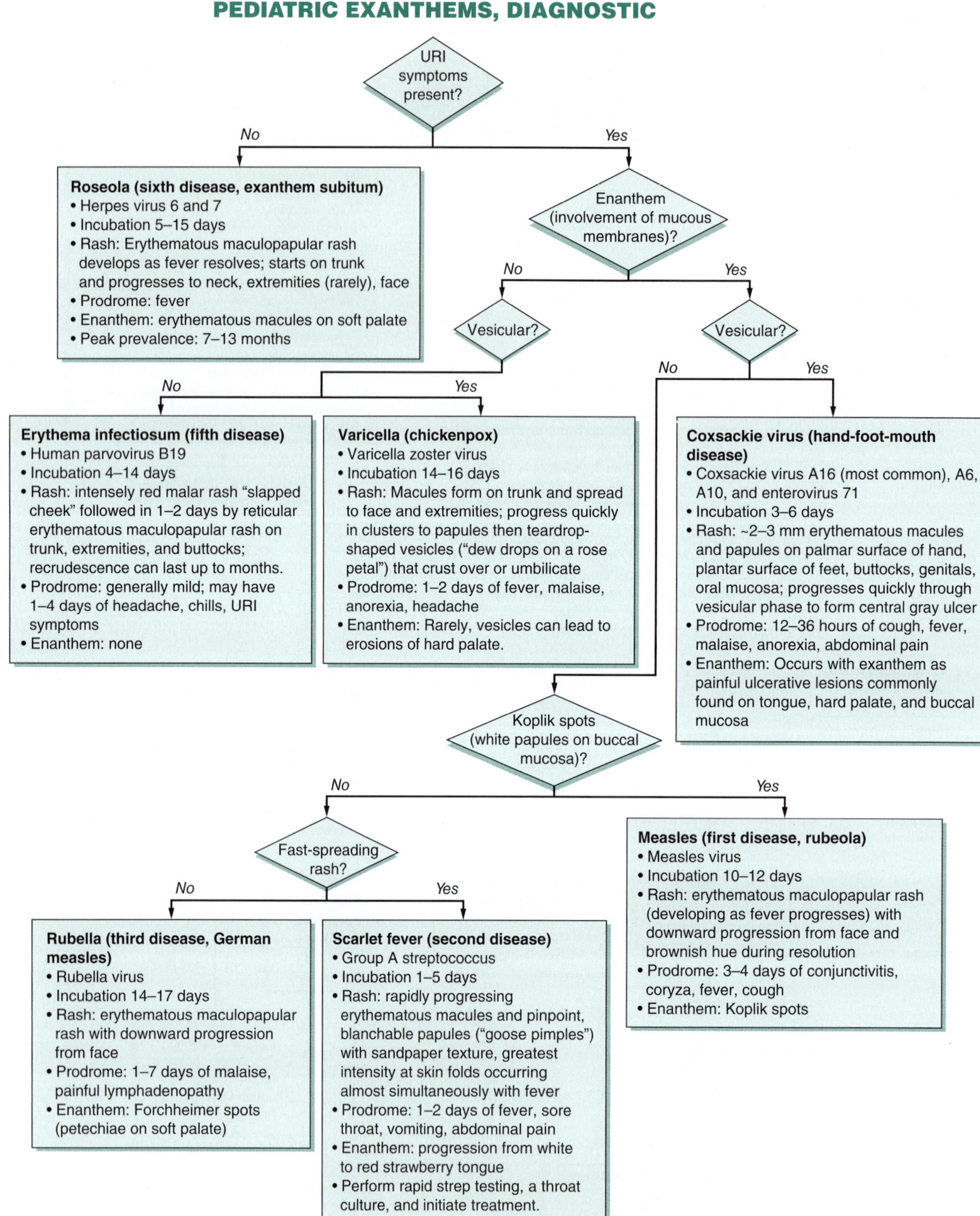

Jane Marie Forbes, MD and Fern R. Hauck, MD, MS, FAAFP

Dyer JA. Childhood viral exanthems. *Pediatr Ann*. 2007;36(1):21–29.

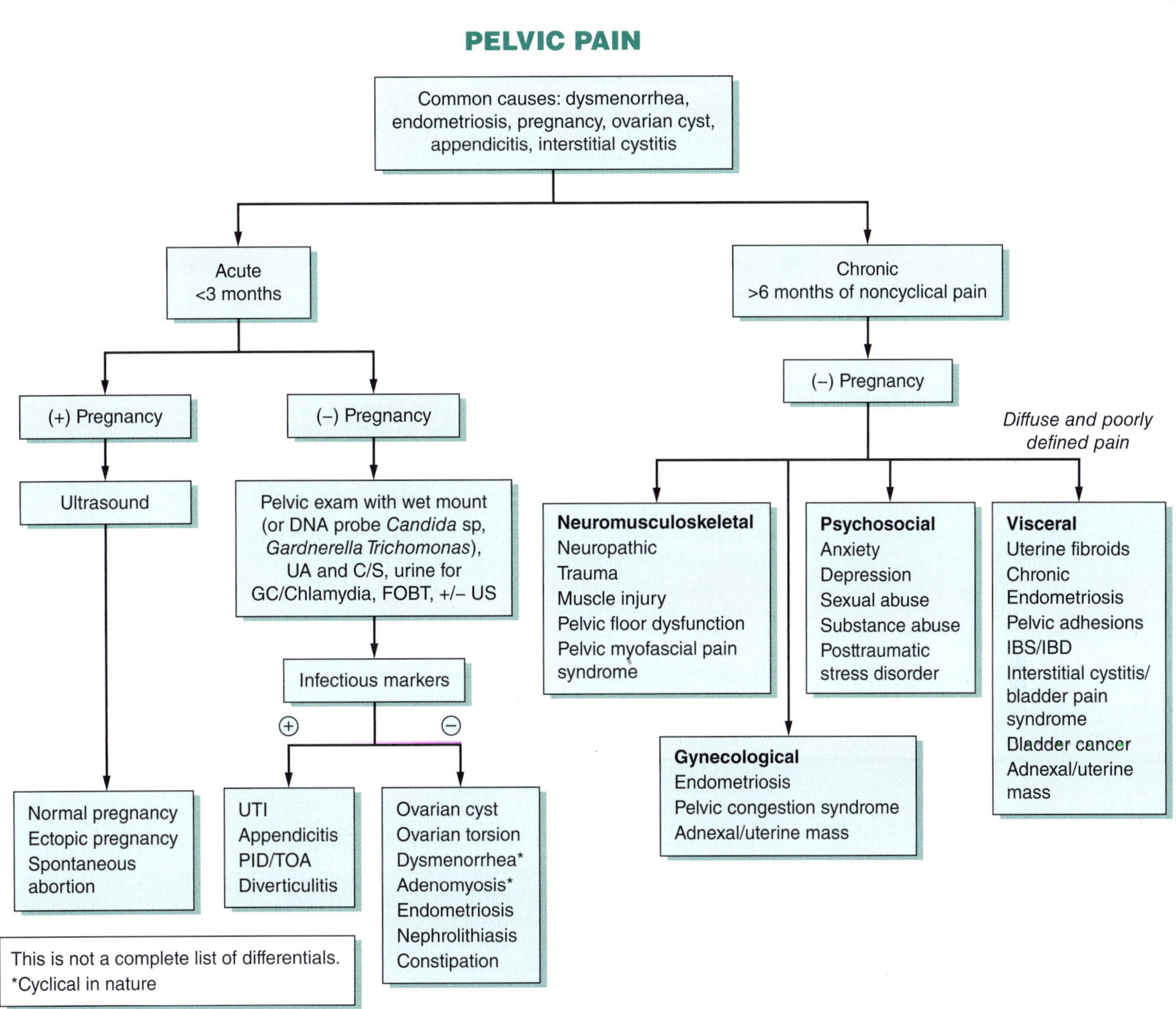

Wendy S. Biggs, MD and Taylor Gaudard, MD, IBCLC

Learman LA, McHugh KW; for American College of Obstetricians and Gynecologists' Committee on Practice Bulletins—Gynecology. ACOG Practice Bulletin Number 218: chronic pelvic pain. *Obstet Gynecol*. 2020;135(3):e98–e109.

POISON EXPOSURE AND TREATMENT

POISON EXPOSURE

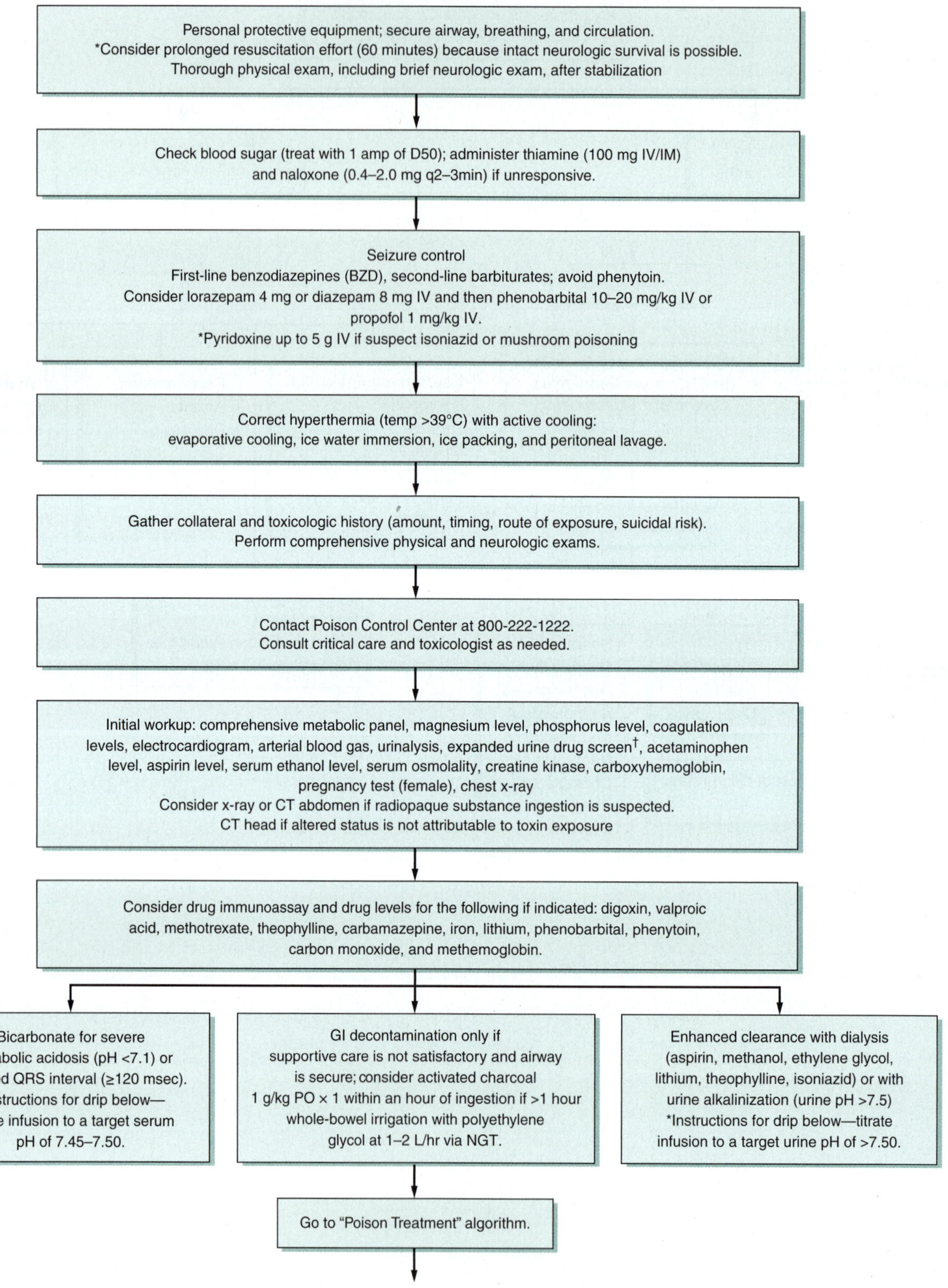

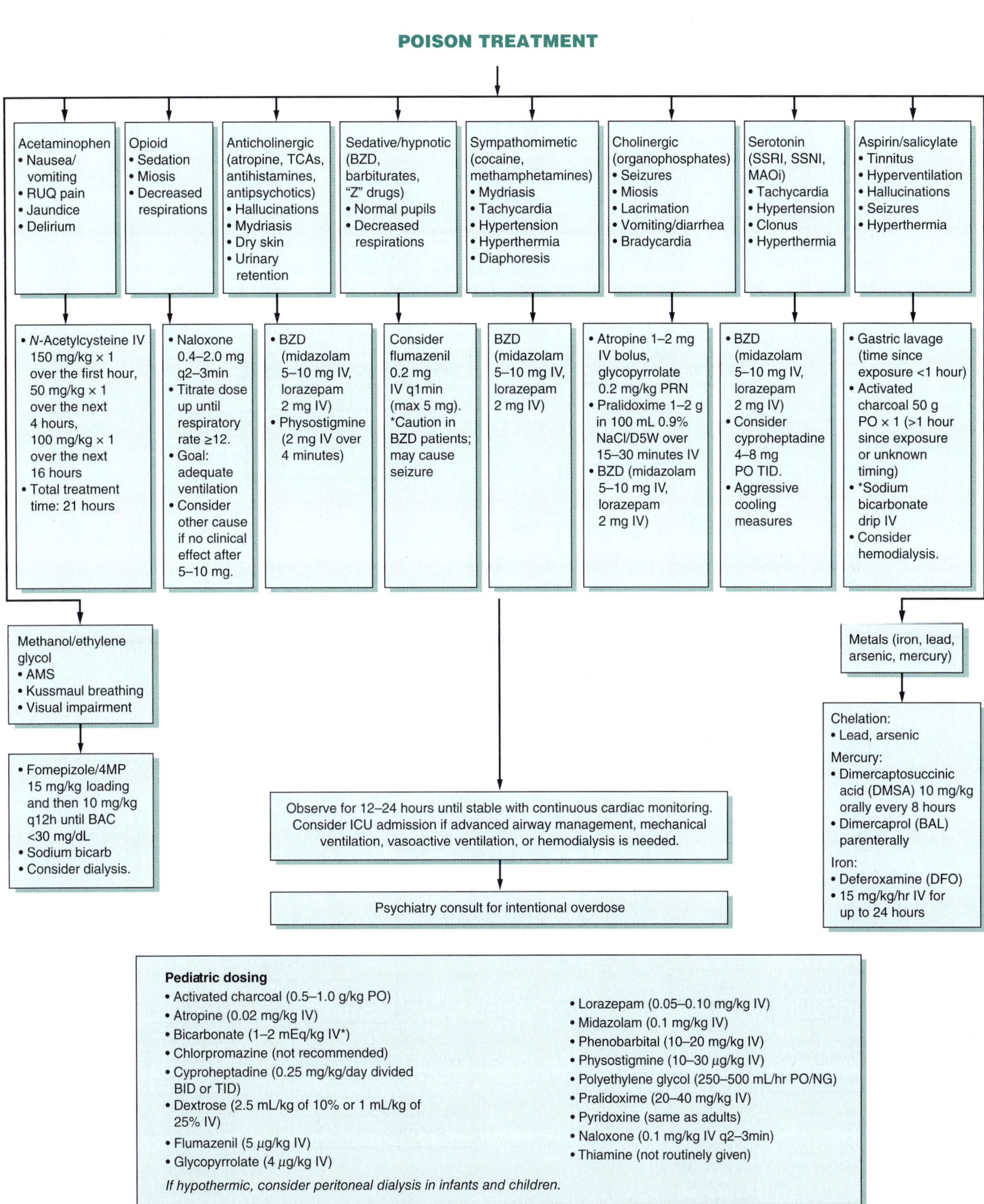

*To mix a bicarbonate drip: 150 mEq (3 amps) $NaHCO_3$ in 1 L of D5W and then start at a rate of 150–200 mL/hr.

†Urine drug screens should be interpreted cautiously because sensitivity and specificity are low, and they can have an unreliable clinical correlation with patient presentation.

Sean Pazurchek, DO, MPH and Emma Wood, DO

Vega IL, Griswold MK, Laskey D. Acute medication poisoning. *Am Fam Physician*. 2024;109(2):143–153.

PRECOCIOUS PUBERTY

- Signs of secondary sexual development in boys <9 years and girls <8 years
  - Common causes: medication, pituitary tumor, congenital adrenal hyperplasia, adrenal tumor, ovarian tumor, pseudoprecocious puberty
    - X-ray to determine bone age
      - Bone age > chronologic age
        - Basal LH levels
          - >5 mIU/mL
            - GnRH stimulation test, LH, FSH
              - LH, FSH increased
                - Gonadotropin-dependent (central) precocious puberty
                  - Estradiol, testosterone, TSH, MRI of brain
                    - CNS lesion
                    - Abnormal TSH
                      - Chronic primary hypothyroidism
                    - Negative
                      - Idiopathic precocious puberty
              - Absent LH response → Gonadotropin-independent (peripheral) precocious puberty
          - <5 mIU/mL
            - Gonadotropin-independent (peripheral) precocious puberty
              - Testosterone, estradiol, LH, FSH, cortisol, DHEA, DHEA-S, 17-hydroxyprogesterone, hCG (males), abdominal and pelvic US
                - In ♀, US + for ovarian cyst(s) or tumor
                - Elevated hCG in ♂
                  - Germ cell tumor
                - Very high levels of testosterone in ♂
                  - Leydig cell tumor
                - Elevated 17-hydroxyprogesterone
                  - Congenital adrenal hyperplasia
                - Pubertal values of testosterone in ♂ and estradiol in ♀, with bone and skin findings
                  - McCune-Albright syndrome
                - Elevated DHEA, DHEA-S, findings on imaging
                  - Adrenal tumor or cancer
                - Elevated testosterone in ♂ and estradiol in ♀
                  - Exogenous sex steroids
      - Bone age = chronologic age
        - Incomplete precocious puberty (premature adrenarche or thelarche)

Frank J. Domino, MD

Berberoğlu M. Precocious puberty and normal variant puberty: definition, etiology, diagnosis and current management. *J Clin Res Pediatr Endocrinol.* 2009;1(4):164–174.

PREOPERATIVE EVALUATION OF NONCARDIAC SURGICAL PATIENT

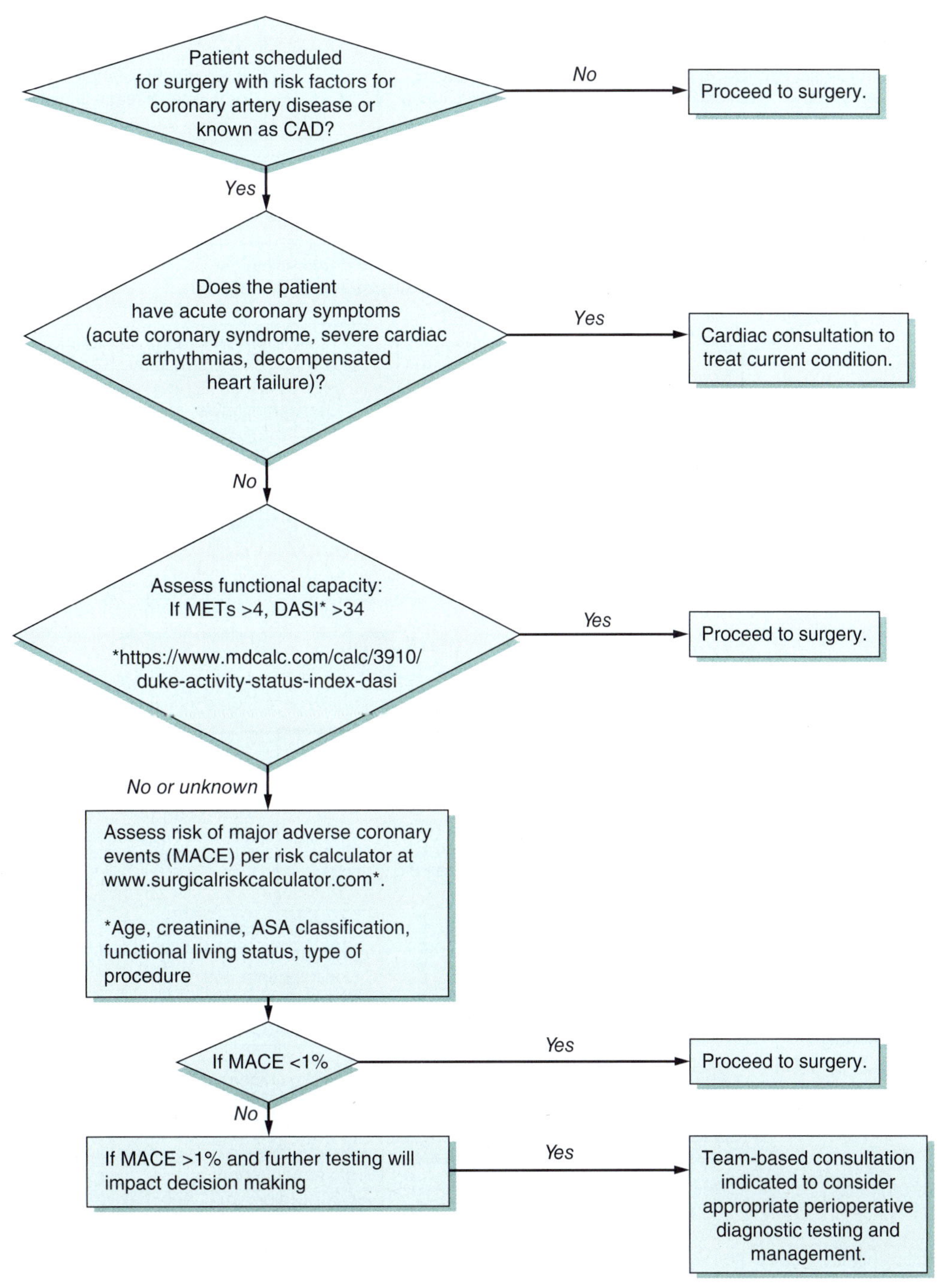

Andrew Grimes, MD

Thompson A, Fleischmann KE, Smilowitz NR, et al. 2024 AHA/ACC/ACS/ASNC/HRS/SCA/SCCT/SCMR/SVM guideline for perioperative cardiovascular management for noncardiac surgery: a report of the American College of Cardiology/American Heart Association Joint Committee on clinical practice guidelines. *Circulation*. 2024;150(19):e351-e442.

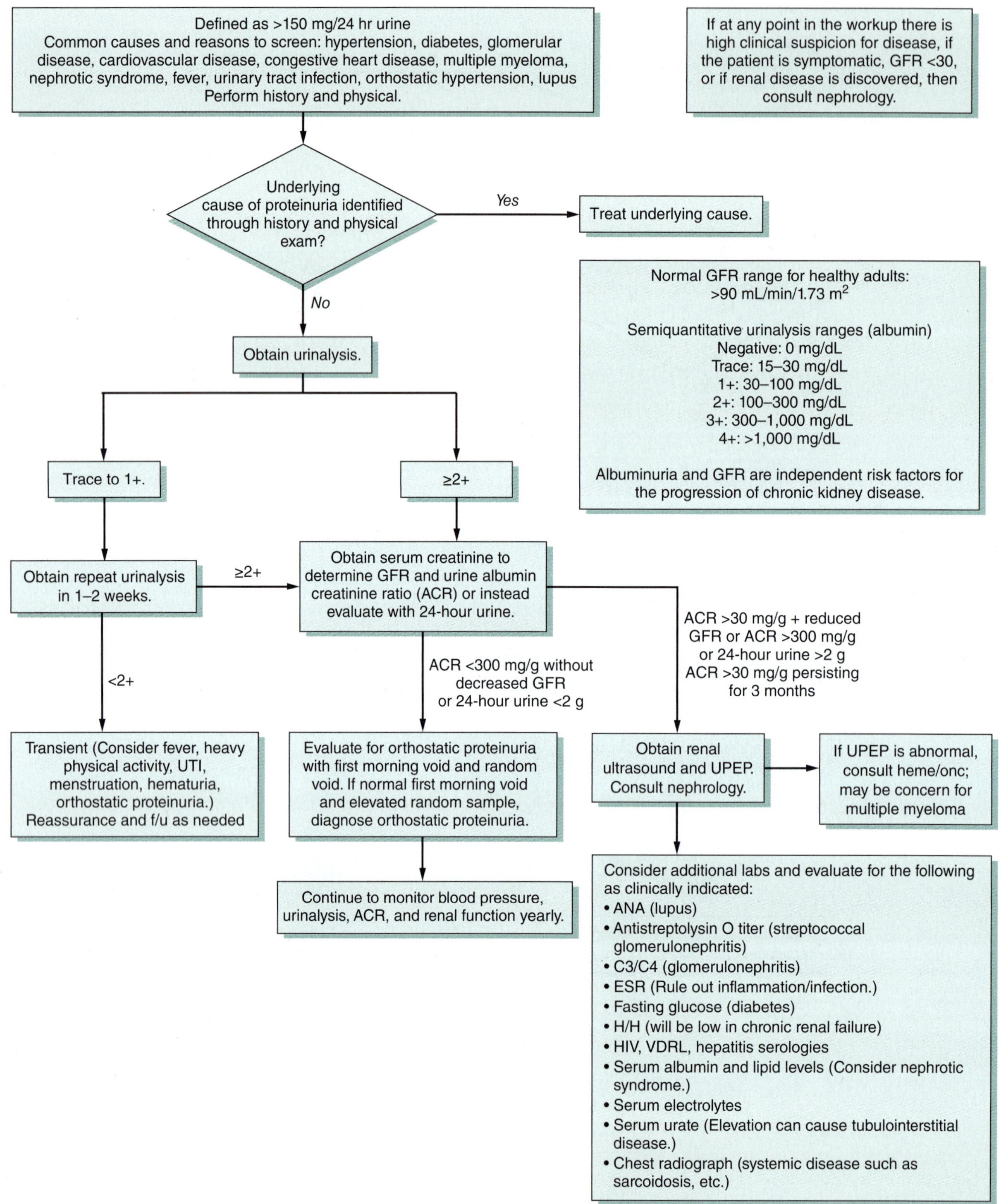

Pamela R. Hughes, MD and Joseph L. Mercen, DO

Kidney Disease: Improving Global Outcomes (KDIGO) CKD Work Group. KDIGO 2024 clinical practice guideline for the evaluation and management of chronic kidney disease. *Kidney Int*. 2024;105(4S):S117–S314.

PULMONARY EMBOLISM, DIAGNOSIS

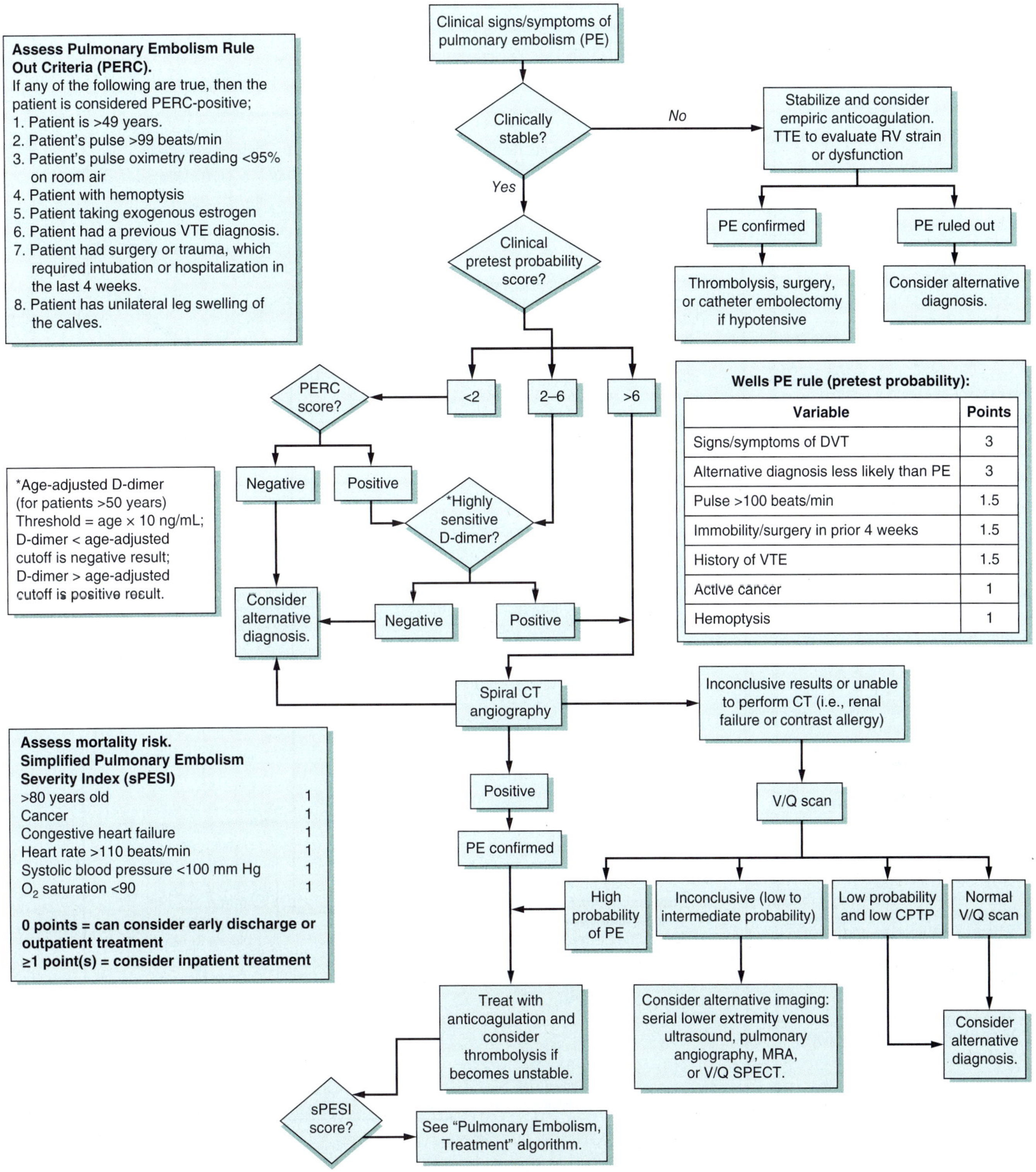

Assess Pulmonary Embolism Rule Out Criteria (PERC).
If any of the following are true, then the patient is considered PERC-positive;

1. Patient is >49 years.
2. Patient's pulse >99 beats/min
3. Patient's pulse oximetry reading <95% on room air
4. Patient with hemoptysis
5. Patient taking exogenous estrogen
6. Patient had a previous VTE diagnosis.
7. Patient had surgery or trauma, which required intubation or hospitalization in the last 4 weeks.
8. Patient has unilateral leg swelling of the calves.

Clinical signs/symptoms of pulmonary embolism (PE)

Clinically stable?

No → Stabilize and consider empiric anticoagulation. TTE to evaluate RV strain or dysfunction

- PE confirmed → Thrombolysis, surgery, or catheter embolectomy if hypotensive
- PE ruled out → Consider alternative diagnosis.

Yes → Clinical pretest probability score?

- <2 → PERC score?
  - Negative → Consider alternative diagnosis.
  - Positive → *Highly sensitive D-dimer?
- 2–6 → *Highly sensitive D-dimer?
  - Negative → Consider alternative diagnosis.
  - Positive → Spiral CT angiography
- >6 → Spiral CT angiography

*Age-adjusted D-dimer (for patients >50 years)
Threshold = age × 10 ng/mL;
D-dimer < age-adjusted cutoff is negative result;
D-dimer > age-adjusted cutoff is positive result.

Wells PE rule (pretest probability):

Variable	Points
Signs/symptoms of DVT	3
Alternative diagnosis less likely than PE	3
Pulse >100 beats/min	1.5
Immobility/surgery in prior 4 weeks	1.5
History of VTE	1.5
Active cancer	1
Hemoptysis	1

Spiral CT angiography

- → Consider alternative diagnosis.
- → Positive → PE confirmed → Treat with anticoagulation and consider thrombolysis if becomes unstable.
- → Inconclusive results or unable to perform CT (i.e., renal failure or contrast allergy) → V/Q scan
  - High probability of PE → Treat with anticoagulation and consider thrombolysis if becomes unstable.
  - Inconclusive (low to intermediate probability) → Consider alternative imaging: serial lower extremity venous ultrasound, pulmonary angiography, MRA, or V/Q SPECT.
  - Low probability and low CPTP → Consider alternative diagnosis.
  - Normal V/Q scan → Consider alternative diagnosis.

Treat with anticoagulation and consider thrombolysis if becomes unstable. → sPESI score? → See "Pulmonary Embolism, Treatment" algorithm.

Assess mortality risk.
Simplified Pulmonary Embolism Severity Index (sPESI)

>80 years old	1
Cancer	1
Congestive heart failure	1
Heart rate >110 beats/min	1
Systolic blood pressure <100 mm Hg	1
O_2 saturation <90	1

0 points = can consider early discharge or outpatient treatment
≥1 point(s) = consider inpatient treatment

Lawrence M. Gibbs, MD, MSEd, FAAFP

Teissandier D, Roussel M, Bannelier H, et al. Contemporary approaches to pulmonary embolism diagnosis: a clinical review. *Clin Exp Emerg Med*. 2024;11(2):127–135.

PULMONARY EMBOLISM, TREATMENT

Probability of pulmonary embolism above treatment threshold

Anticoagulation contraindicated?

Yes → IVC filter

No →

For all patients, assess for treatment at home versus in hospital through risk stratification. For example, Pulmonary Embolism Severity Index (PESI):
- If very low or low risk: Consider outpatient management.
- If intermediate, high, or very high risk: Consider inpatient management.

Massive pulmonary embolism?
- SBP <90 mm Hg for 15 minutes
- Fall in SBP >40 mm Hg for 15 minutes
- Requiring vasopressors
- Persistent bradycardia
- Cardiac arrest
- Evidence of end-organ ischemia

Yes → Thrombolysis contraindicated?

No → Benefits of thrombolysis may outweigh risks IF: hemodynamic instability, worsening oxygenation, severe RV dysfunction, or major myocardial necrosis. Thrombolysis indicated?

Yes → Thrombolysis contraindicated?

No → History of heparin-induced thrombocytopenia?

Thrombolysis contraindicated?
- Prior intracranial bleed
- Ischemic stroke <3 months
- Suspected aortic dissection
- Active bleeding diathesis
- Recent brain or spinal surgery
- Closed head or facial trauma

Yes →
- Interventional radiology or surgical embolectomy, per local expertise
- ECMO

No → Thrombolysis using tPA (can be given systemically or catheter directed based on bleeding risk)

Clinical improvement?

Yes → History of heparin-induced thrombocytopenia?

No → Interventional radiology or surgical embolectomy, per local expertise / ECMO

History of heparin-induced thrombocytopenia?

Yes →
- Consider oral anticoagulant. Apixaban or rivaroxaban do not need parenteral bridging, whereas dabigatran and edoxaban require 5–10 days of parental therapy.
- Alternatively, consider fondaparinux or argatroban (caution use of argatroban in liver disease) and vitamin K antagonist (warfarin) with at least 5 days of concomitant therapy. When used in combination, goal INR prior to discontinuation of the parenteral product is as follows: INR >2 (fondaparinux) or >4 (argatroban) × 24 hours. Of note, argatroban falsely elevates the INR, which can be misleading when given in combination with vitamin K antagonist. Once the INR is >4, discontinue the argatroban and recheck the INR in 4–6 hours with a goal INR 2–3.
- Prior to using vitamin K antagonist (warfarin) for new-onset heparin-induced thrombocytopenia, be sure platelets are >150,000.

No →

Begin:
- Oral anticoagulant therapy: Apixaban or rivaroxaban do not need parenteral bridging, whereas dabigatran and edoxaban require 5–10 days of parenteral therapy.

or

- Therapeutic dose low-molecular-weight heparin (LMWH)

or

- Heparin infusion to therapeutic aPTT or therapeutic LMWH and warfarin, discontinuing LMWH when INR >2 for at least 24 hours and minimum 5 days of concomitant therapy; goal INR 2–3

Emmeline Ha, MD and Jason Teng, MD

Ortel TL, Neumann I, Ageno W, et al. American Society of Hematology 2020 guidelines for management of venous thromboembolism: treatment of deep vein thrombosis and pulmonary embolism. *Blood Adv*. 2020;4(19):4693–4738.

RASH

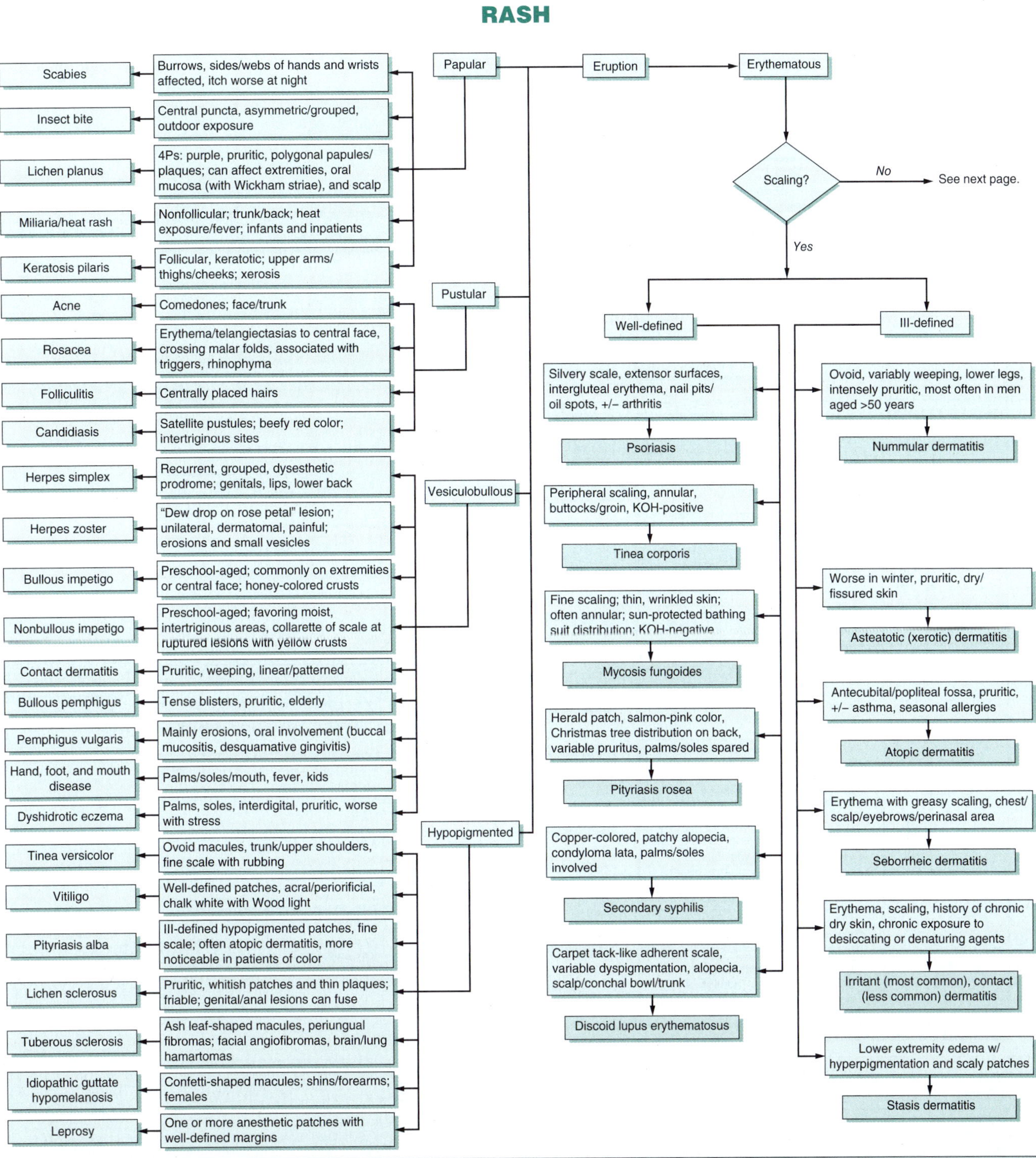

7 classes of topical steroids based on ability to constrict capillaries. Class I, strongest; class VII, weakest.

Class I	Class II	Class III	Class IV	Class V	Class VI	Class VII
Clobetasol propionate ointment, cream, 0.05% (Temovate)	Fluocinonide ointment, cream, gel, 0.05% (Lidex)	Triamcinolone acetonide ointment, 0.1% (Aristocort A)	Triamcinolone acetonide cream, 0.1% (Kenalog)	Fluocinolone acetonide cream, 0.025% (Synalar)	Desonide cream, 0.05% (DesOwen)	
Betamethasone dipropionate ointment, cream, 0.05% (Diprolene, Diprosone)	Amcinonide ointment, 0.1% (Cyclocort)	Betamethasone valerate ointment, 0.01% (Valisone)	Mometasone furoate cream, 0.1% (Elocon)	Fluticasone propionate cream, 0.05% (Cutivate)	Prednicarbate 0.1% cream (Dermatop)	Hydrocortisone, 0.5%, 1%, 2.5% (Hytone)
Halobetasol propionate ointment, cream, 0.05% (Ultravate)	Desoximetasone ointment, cream, 0.25%; gel, 0.05% (Topicort)	Fluticasone propionate ointment, 0.05% (Cutivate)	Hydrocortisone valerate ointment, 0.2% (Westcort)	Hydrocortisone valerate cream, 0.2% (Westcort)	Alclometasone dipropionate ointment, cream, 0.05% (Aclovate)	

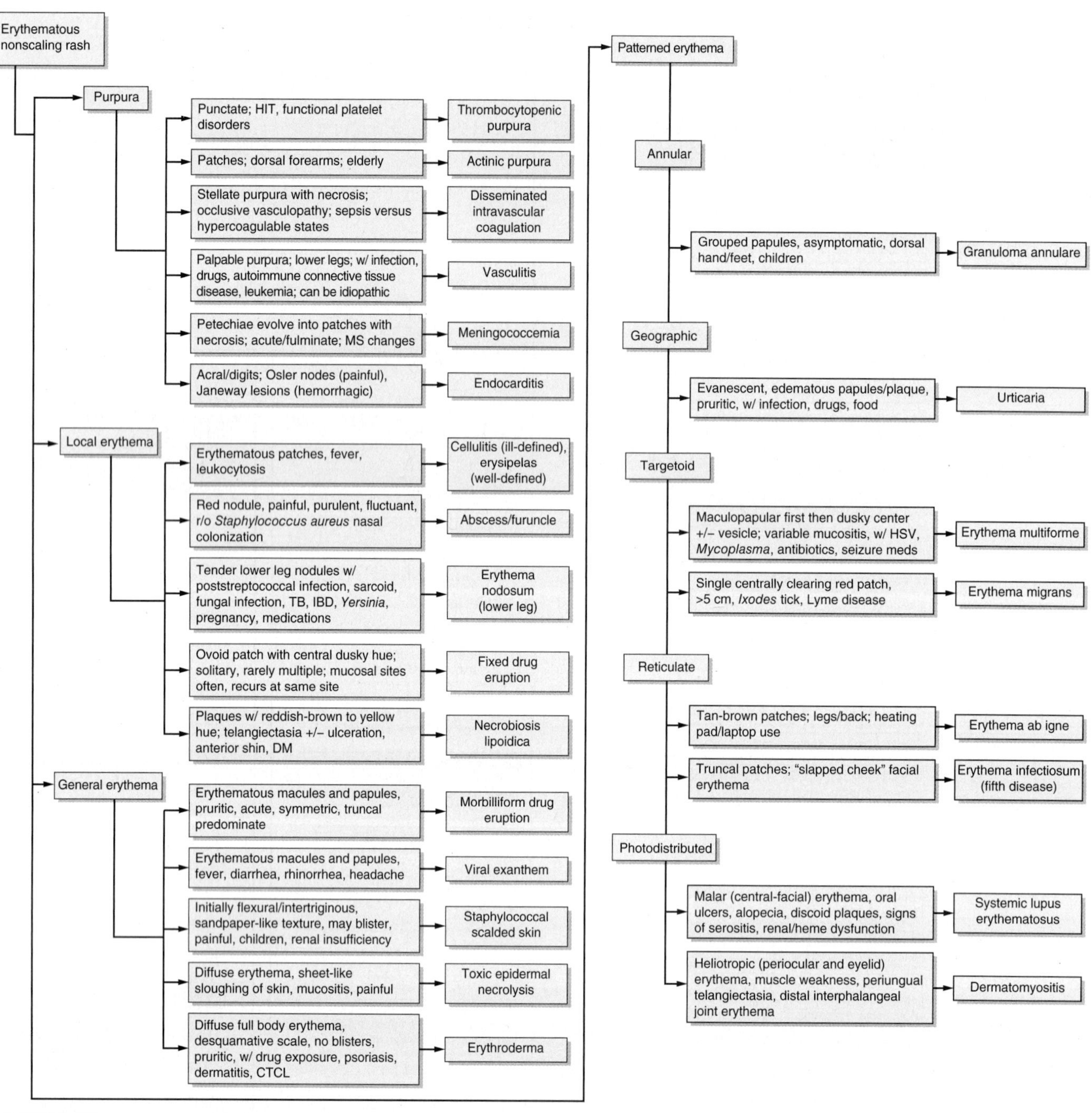

7 classes of topical steroids based on ability to constrict capillaries. Class I, strongest; class VII, weakest.

Class I	Class II	Class III	Class IV	Class V	Class VI	Class VII
Clobetasol propionate ointment, cream, 0.05% (Temovate)	Fluocinonide ointment, cream, gel 0.05% (Lidex)	Triamcinolone acetonide ointment, 0.1% (Aristocort A)	Triamcinolone acetonide cream, 0.1% (Kenalog)	Fluocinolone acetonide cream, 0.025% (Synalar)	Desonide cream, 0.05% (DesOwen)	
Betamethasone dipropionate ointment, cream, 0.05% (Diprolene, Diprosone)	Amcinonide ointment, 0.1% (Cyclocort)	Betamethasone valerate ointment, 0.01% (Valisone)	Mometasone furoate cream, 0.1% (Elocon)	Fluticasone propionate cream, 0.05% (Cutivate)	Prednicarbate 0.1% cream (Dermatop)	Hydrocortisone, 0.5%, 1%, 2.5% (Hytone)
Halobetasol propionate ointment, cream, 0.05% (Ultravate)	Desoximetasone ointment, cream, 0.25%; gel, 0.05% (Topicort)	Fluticasone propionate ointment, 0.05% (Cutivate)	Hydrocortisone valerate ointment, 0.2% (Westcort)	Hydrocortisone valerate cream, 0.2% (Westcort)	Alclometasone dipropionate ointment, cream, 0.05% (Aclovate)	

Jennifer G. Foster, MD, MBA, FACP, Lisa C. Martinez, MD, and Allison H. Ferris, MD

Ely JW, Stone MS. The generalized rash: part I. Differential diagnosis. *Am Fam Physician*. 2010;81(6):726–734;
Ely JW, Stone MS. The generalized rash: part II. Diagnostic approach. *Am Fam Physician*. 2010;81(6):735–739.

RECTAL BLEEDING AND HEMATOCHEZIA

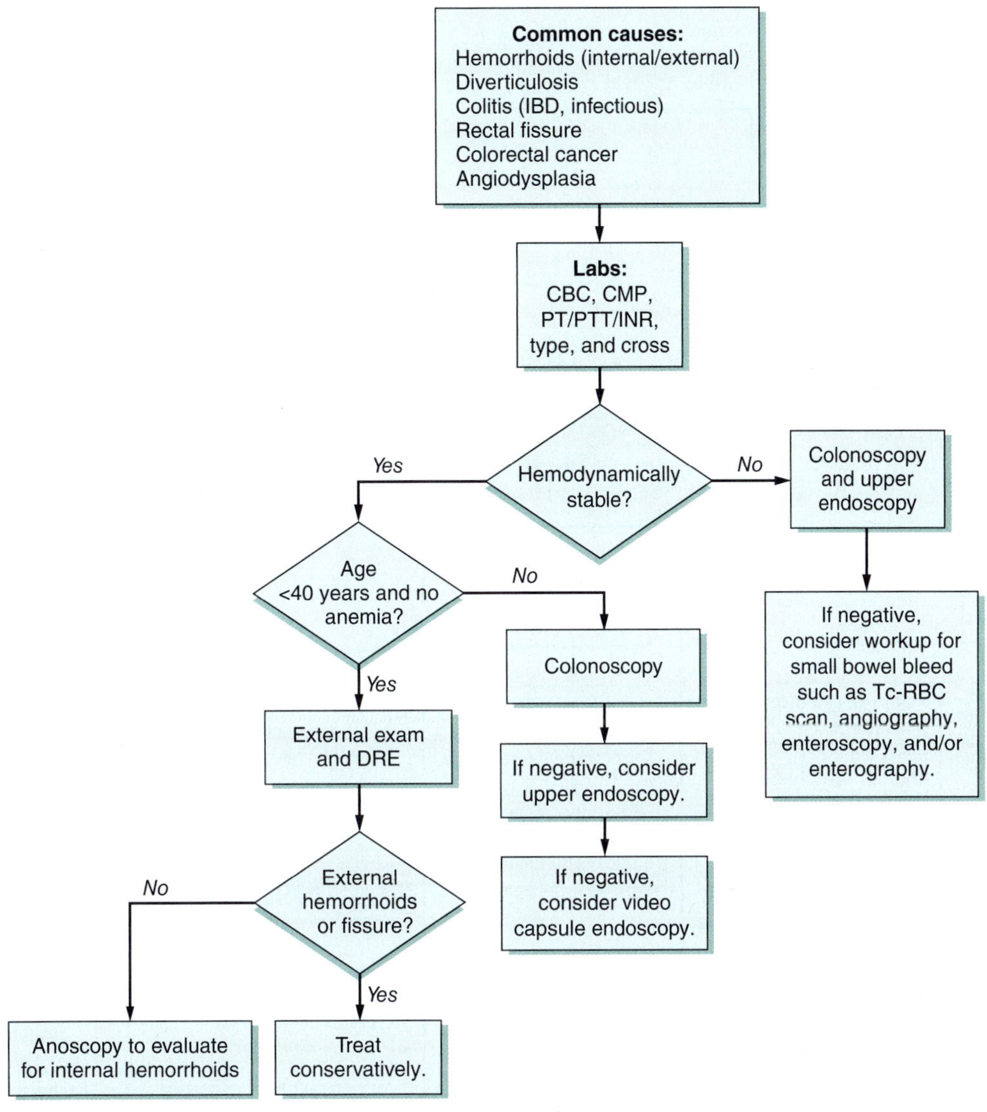

Tamika Isaac, DO and Rebecca Gwaltney, MD, MPH

Almadi MA, Barkun AN. Patient presentation, risk stratification, and initial management in acute lower gastrointestinal bleeding. *Gastrointest Endosc Clin N Am*. 2018;28(3):363–377.

RED EYE

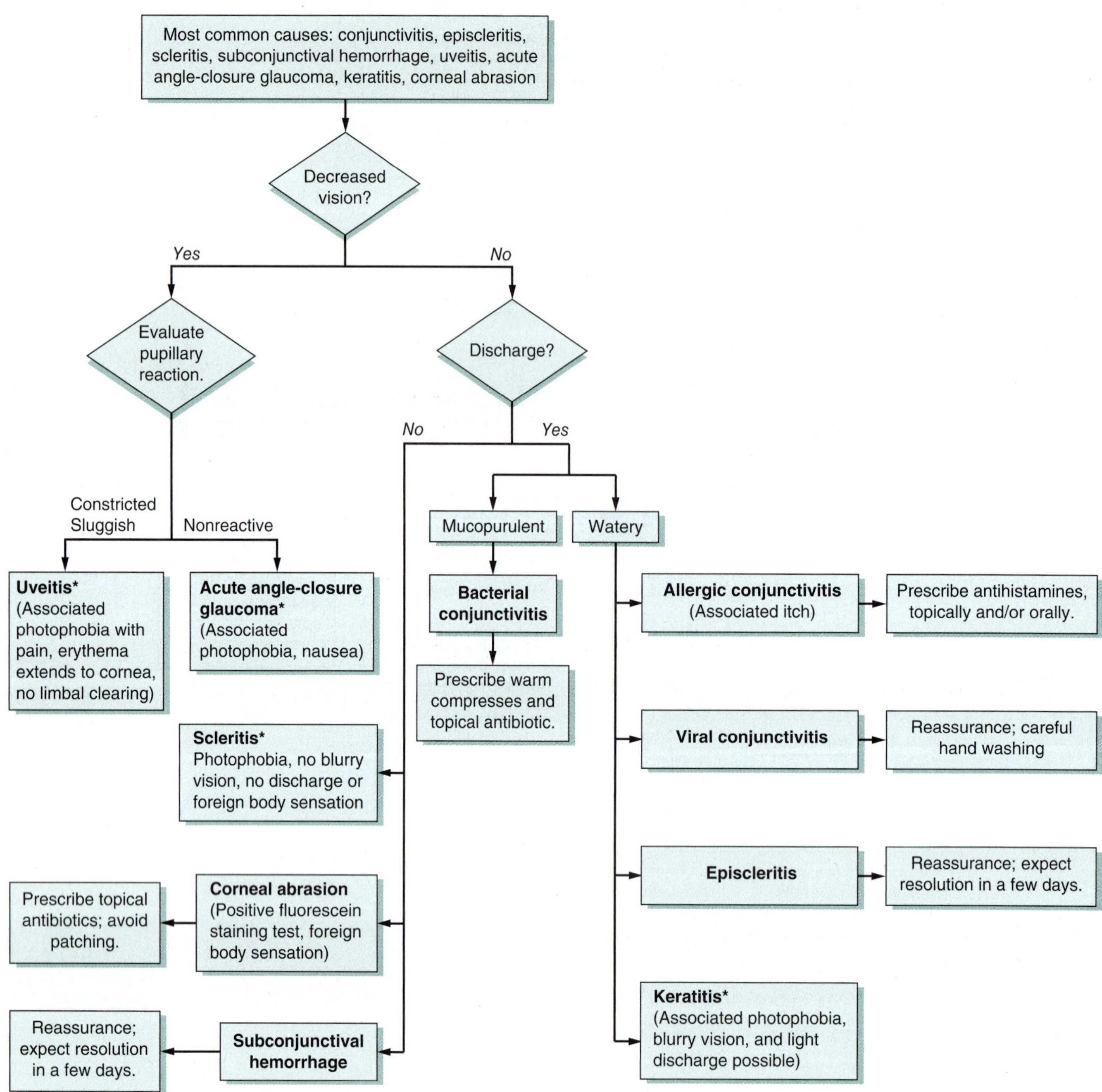

***Urgent ophthalmology consultation.**

Robert A. Baldor, MD, FAAFP

Cronau H, Kankanala RR, Mauger T. Diagnosis and management of red eye in primary care. *Am Fam Physician*. 2010;81(2):137–144.

SALICYLATE POISONING, ACUTE, TREATMENT

Assess airway, breathing, and circulation (ABC).
Provide appropriate ABC management. Avoid intubation unless patient is unable to protect airway. Intubation may increase acidosis and result in cardiovascular collapse.

Early toxicity: tachypnea, hyperpnea, nausea, vomiting, tinnitus, vertigo
Late toxicity: hyperthermia, hypotension, altered mental status

Does the patient exhibit signs of severe toxicity (altered mental status/coma, seizure, pulmonary edema, or need for endotracheal intubation and mechanical ventilation)?

Yes →

Initiate emergent hemodialysis.
Begin volume resuscitation and alkalinization using 150 mEq (3 amps) $NaHCO_3$ + 40 mEq KCl in 1 L D5W unless prohibited by cerebral/pulmonary edema. Administer 25 g (1 amp) D50 for altered mental status. Do not delay treatment for diagnostic studies.

No →

History and physical
Obtain careful history of ingestion (time, reported ingestion, coingestants, etc.) and perform thorough physical exam for hemodynamic instability, alterations in respiratory pattern, and changes in mental status.

Is the patient asymptomatic, stable, and known to have ingested <150 mg/kg?

Yes →

Evaluation/observation
Obtain first salicylate level, noting time since ingestion occurred.

ASA detectable?

No → Recheck if within 2 hours of presentation. Discharge after 6 hours observation if patient remains asymptomatic and levels are nondetectable.

Yes → Recheck levels q2h until persistently within therapeutic range, trending down, or nondetectable. Routinely reassess for changes in clinical status and initiate treatment if indicated.

Note: Volume resuscitation and alkalinization are the mainstays of therapy and should be given to all symptomatic patients unless pulmonary or cerebral edema is present. Respiratory alkalosis (pH >7.5) is *not* a contraindication to therapy. Do not delay for charcoal or diagnostic studies.

No →

Initial treatment
1. Early volume resuscitation with isotonic saline or LR at rate of 10–20 mL/kg body wt for first 2 hours then adjust to maintain urine output (UOP) of 1.0–1.5 mL/kg/hr.
2. Urinary alkalinization using 150 mEq (3 amps) $NaHCO_3$ + 40 mEq KCl mixed in 1 L D5W, infused at 2–3 mL/kg/hr
3. Administer first-dose activated charcoal at 1 g/kg (max 50 g) *only* if patient is alert, cooperative, has bowel sounds on exam, and can tolerate. Consider additional doses of 50 g q4h for 2 more doses if patient continues to meet the aforementioned criteria.

Obtain diagnostic studies.
Labs: salicylate level (note time since ingestion), ABG/VBG, basic electrolytes, BUN, creatinine, LFTs, coags, lactate, UA. Obtain tox screen if polysubstance overdose suspected.
Imaging: chest radiograph (to evaluate for pulmonary edema). Consider head CT for altered mental status to evaluate for cerebral edema or alternative causes of mental status changes.

Presence of salicylate level >90 mg/dL, arterial pH <7.3, pulmonary or cerebral edema, renal failure, or has patient deteriorated?

Yes → Initiate hemodialysis.

No →

Maintenance therapy and evaluation
1. Continue bicarbonate infusion to maintain UOP of 1–2 mL/kg/hr.
2. Measure urine pH hourly and titrate infusion to goal pH of 7.5–8.0.
3. Measure serum K hourly and replete if <4.5 mEq/L.
4. Measure ABG or VBG hourly and decrease rate of bicarbonate drip if serum pH exceeds 7.6.
5. Measure serum salicylate level q2h until salicylate level begins to decline and acid–base status is normal.

Disposition
Treatment should be continued with frequent clinical assessment for improvement. Treatment and testing may be stopped *only* when patient is asymptomatic, acid–base status is stable, *and* salicylate level has fallen into therapeutic range (10–30 mg/dL).

Kiran A. Lorick, MD

Vega IL, Griswold MK, Laskey D. Acute medication poisoning. *Am Fam Physician*. 2024;109(2):143–153.

SEIZURE, NEW ONSET

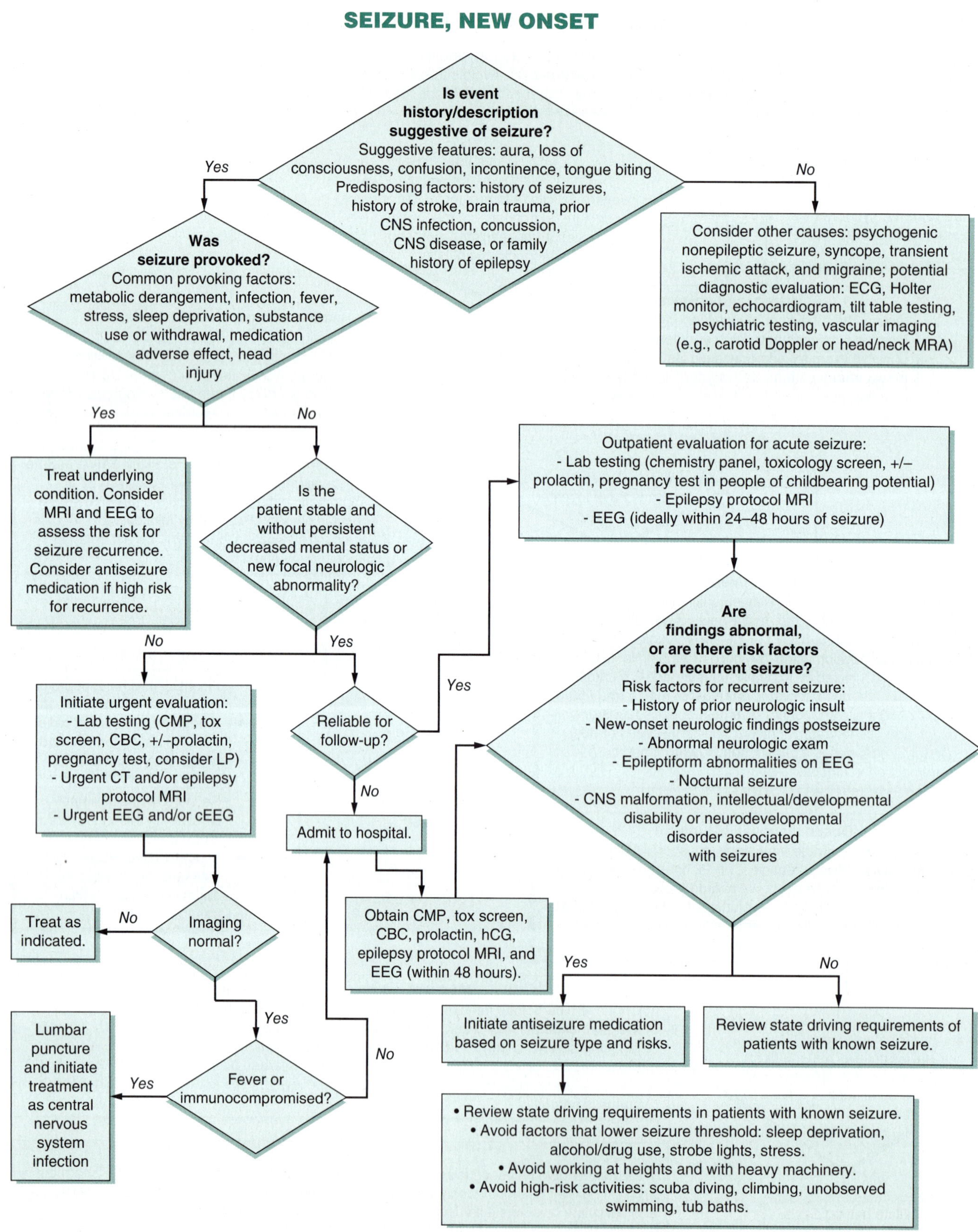

Yuki Takeuchi, MD and Kento Sonoda, MD

Gavvala JR, Schuele SU. New-onset seizure in adults and adolescents: a review. *JAMA*. 2016;316(24):2657–2668.

SHOULDER PAIN, TREATMENT

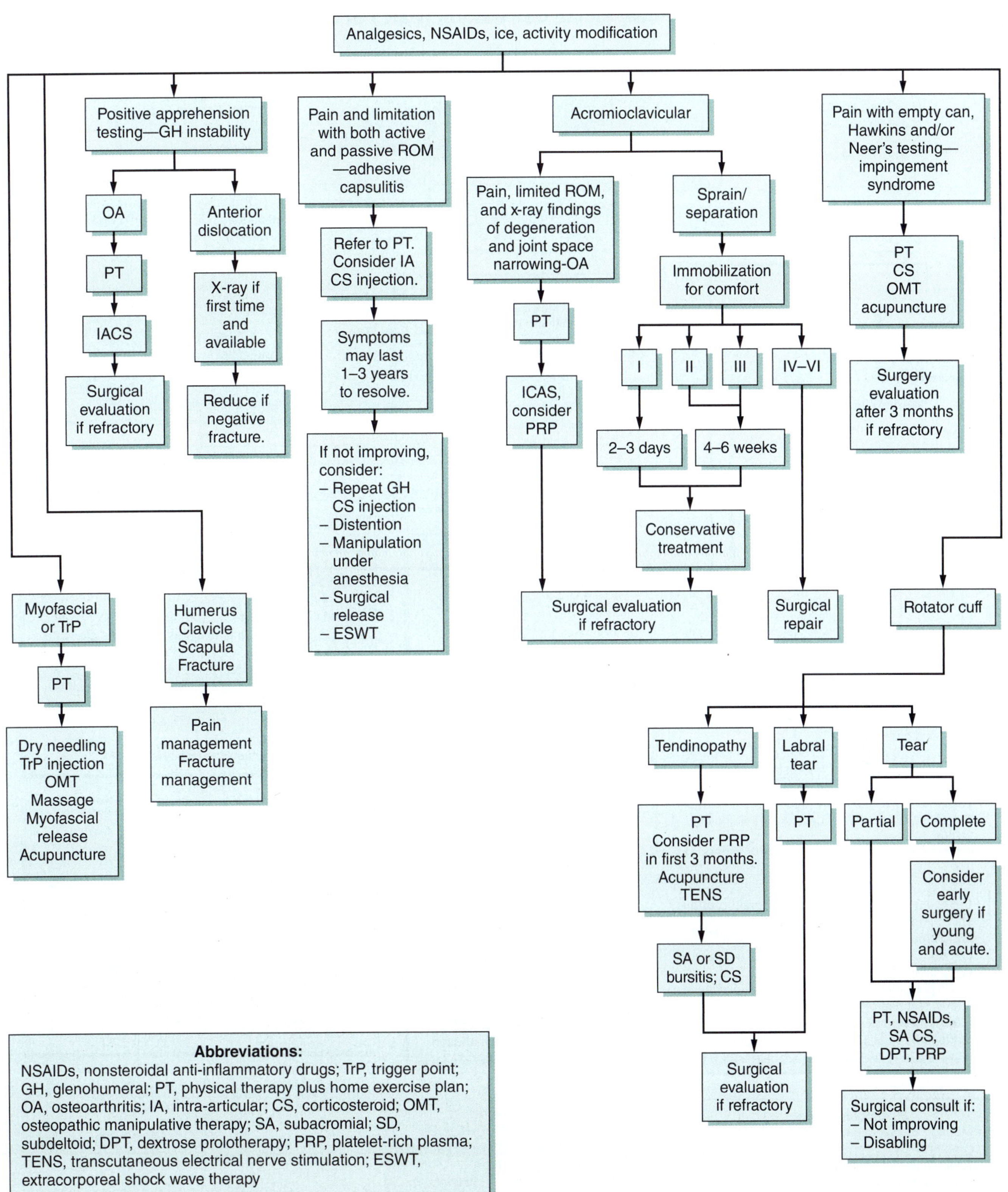

Abbreviations:
NSAIDs, nonsteroidal anti-inflammatory drugs; TrP, trigger point; GH, glenohumeral; PT, physical therapy plus home exercise plan; OA, osteoarthritis; IA, intra-articular; CS, corticosteroid; OMT, osteopathic manipulative therapy; SA, subacromial; SD, subdeltoid; DPT, dextrose prolotherapy; PRP, platelet-rich plasma; TENS, transcutaneous electrical nerve stimulation; ESWT, extracorporeal shock wave therapy

Vicki R. Nelson, MD, PhD

Greenberg DL. Evaluation and treatment of shoulder pain. *Med Clin North Am*. 2014;98(3):487–504.

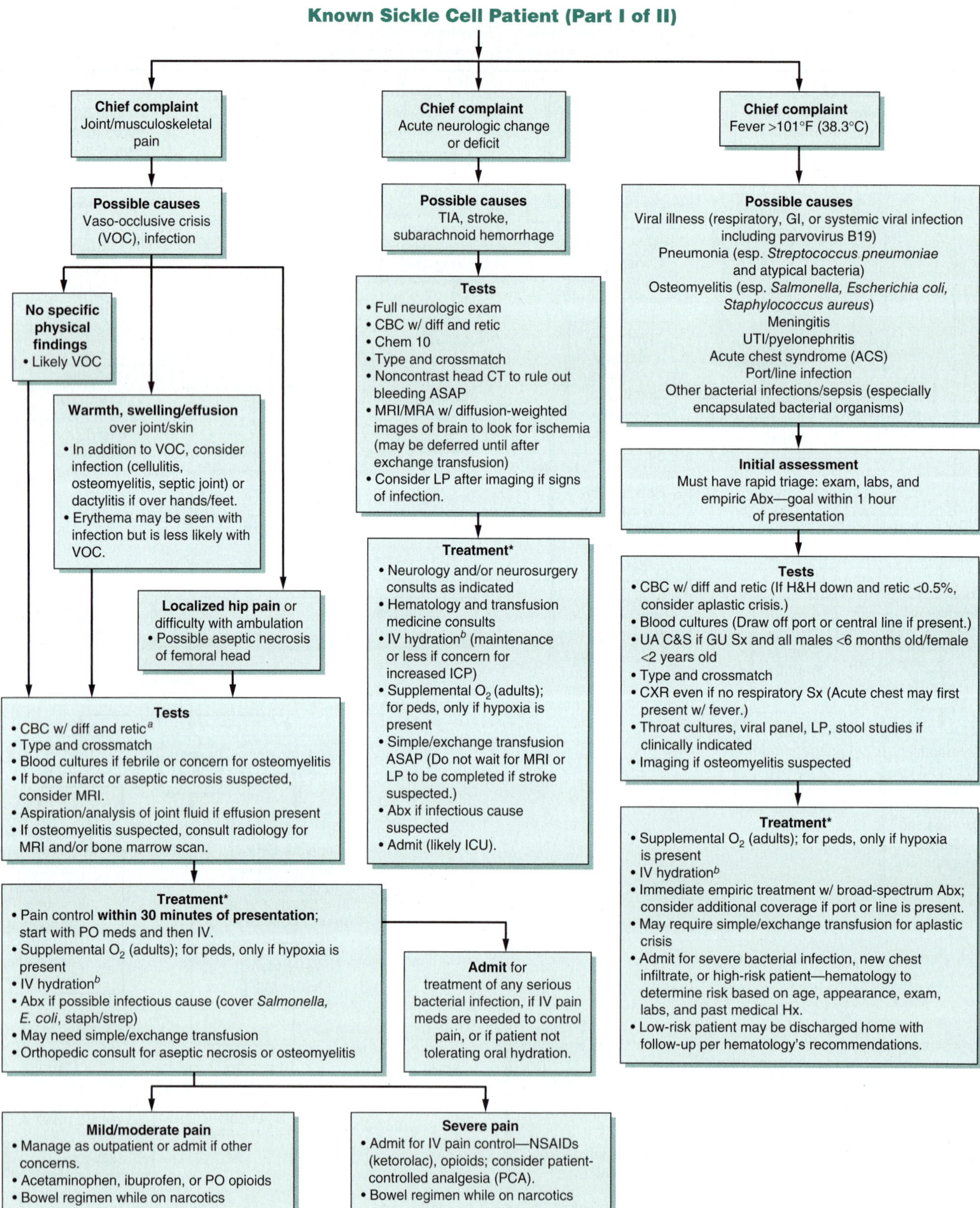

SICKLE CELL ANEMIA, ACUTE, EVALUATION AND MANAGEMENT
Known Sickle Cell Patient (Part I of II)
Chief complaint
Joint/musculoskeletal pain
Possible causes
Vaso-occlusive crisis (VOC), infection
No specific physical findings
• Likely VOC
Warmth, swelling/effusion over joint/skin
• In addition to VOC, consider infection (cellulitis, osteomyelitis, septic joint) or dactylitis if over hands/feet.
• Erythema may be seen with infection but is less likely with VOC.
Localized hip pain or difficulty with ambulation
• Possible aseptic necrosis of femoral head
Tests
• CBC w/ diff and retic[a]
• Type and crossmatch
• Blood cultures if febrile or concern for osteomyelitis
• If bone infarct or aseptic necrosis suspected, consider MRI.
• Aspiration/analysis of joint fluid if effusion present
• If osteomyelitis suspected, consult radiology for MRI and/or bone marrow scan.
Treatment*
• Pain control within 30 minutes of presentation; start with PO meds and then IV.
• Supplemental O2 (adults); for peds, only if hypoxia is present
• IV hydration[b]
• Abx if possible infectious cause (cover Salmonella, E. coli, staph/strep)
• May need simple/exchange transfusion
• Orthopedic consult for aseptic necrosis or osteomyelitis
Admit for treatment of any serious bacterial infection, if IV pain meds are needed to control pain, or if patient not tolerating oral hydration.
Mild/moderate pain
• Manage as outpatient or admit if other concerns.
• Acetaminophen, ibuprofen, or PO opioids
• Bowel regimen while on narcotics
Severe pain
• Admit for IV pain control—NSAIDs (ketorolac), opioids; consider patient-controlled analgesia (PCA).
• Bowel regimen while on narcotics
Chief complaint
Acute neurologic change or deficit
Possible causes
TIA, stroke, subarachnoid hemorrhage
Tests
• Full neurologic exam
• CBC w/ diff and retic
• Chem 10
• Type and crossmatch
• Noncontrast head CT to rule out bleeding ASAP
• MRI/MRA w/ diffusion-weighted images of brain to look for ischemia (may be deferred until after exchange transfusion)
• Consider LP after imaging if signs of infection.
Treatment*
• Neurology and/or neurosurgery consults as indicated
• Hematology and transfusion medicine consults
• IV hydration[b] (maintenance or less if concern for increased ICP)
• Supplemental O2 (adults); for peds, only if hypoxia is present
• Simple/exchange transfusion ASAP (Do not wait for MRI or LP to be completed if stroke suspected.)
• Abx if infectious cause suspected
• Admit (likely ICU).
Chief complaint
Fever >101°F (38.3°C)
Possible causes
Viral illness (respiratory, GI, or systemic viral infection including parvovirus B19)
Pneumonia (esp. Streptococcus pneumoniae and atypical bacteria)
Osteomyelitis (esp. Salmonella, Escherichia coli, Staphylococcus aureus)
Meningitis
UTI/pyelonephritis
Acute chest syndrome (ACS)
Port/line infection
Other bacterial infections/sepsis (especially encapsulated bacterial organisms)
Initial assessment
Must have rapid triage: exam, labs, and empiric Abx—goal within 1 hour of presentation
Tests
• CBC w/ diff and retic (If H&H down and retic <0.5%, consider aplastic crisis.)
• Blood cultures (Draw off port or central line if present.)
• UA C&S if GU Sx and all males <6 months old/female <2 years old
• Type and crossmatch
• CXR even if no respiratory Sx (Acute chest may first present w/ fever.)
• Throat cultures, viral panel, LP, stool studies if clinically indicated
• Imaging if osteomyelitis suspected
Treatment*
• Supplemental O2 (adults); for peds, only if hypoxia is present
• IV hydration[b]
• Immediate empiric treatment w/ broad-spectrum Abx; consider additional coverage if port or line is present.
• May require simple/exchange transfusion for aplastic crisis
• Admit for severe bacterial infection, new chest infiltrate, or high-risk patient—hematology to determine risk based on age, appearance, exam, labs, and past medical Hx.
• Low-risk patient may be discharged home with follow-up per hematology's recommendations.

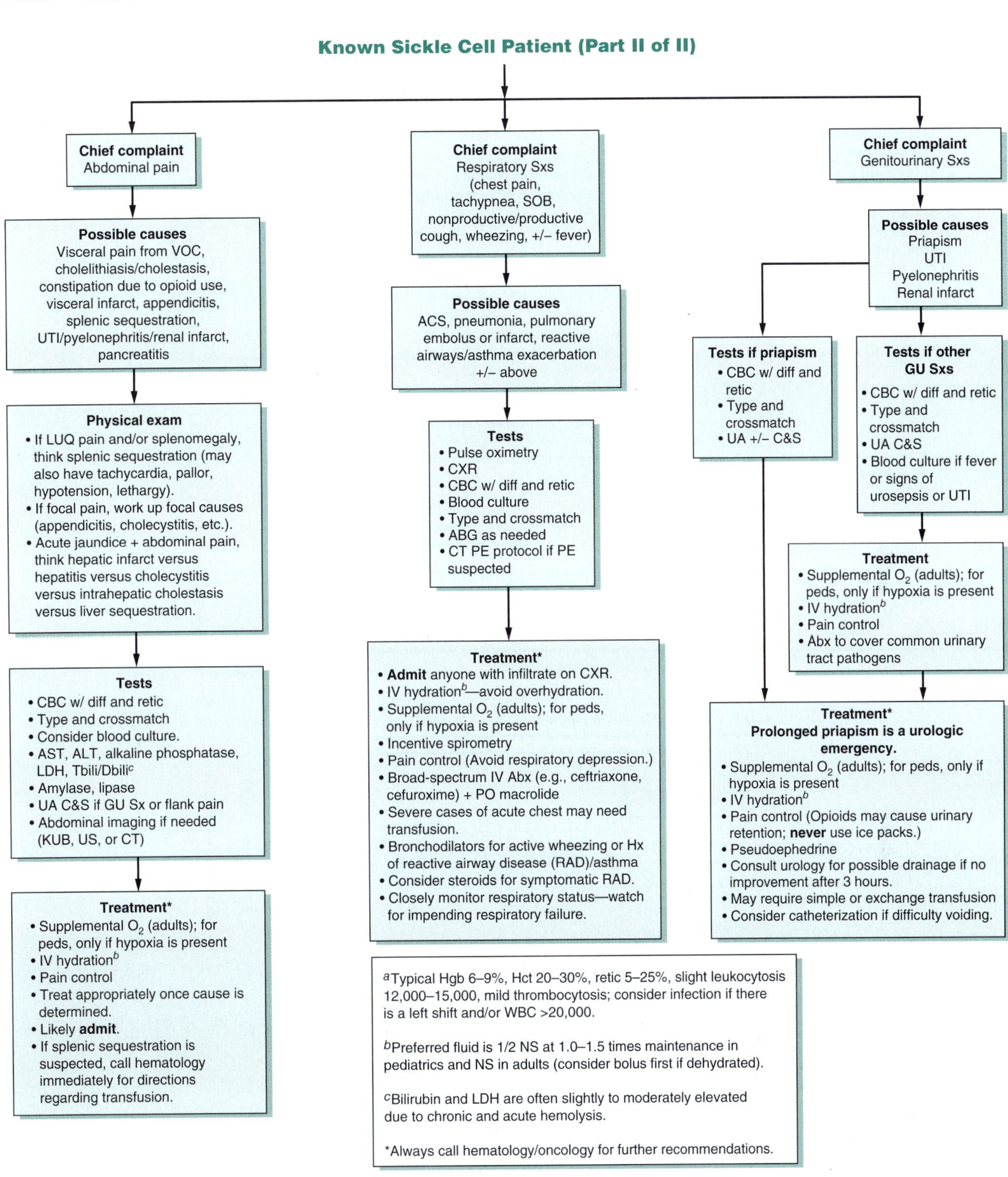

[a]Typical Hgb 6–9%, Hct 20–30%, retic 5–25%, slight leukocytosis 12,000–15,000, mild thrombocytosis; consider infection if there is a left shift and/or WBC >20,000.

[b]Preferred fluid is 1/2 NS at 1.0–1.5 times maintenance in pediatrics and NS in adults (consider bolus first if dehydrated).

[c]Bilirubin and LDH are often slightly to moderately elevated due to chronic and acute hemolysis.

*Always call hematology/oncology for further recommendations.

Paul E. Daniel Jr., MD, MS

National Heart, Lung, and Blood Institute. Evidence-based management of sickle cell disease: expert panel report, 2014. https://www.nhlbi.nih.gov/health-topics/evidence-based-management-sickle-cell-disease. Published September 2014. Accessed October 16, 2024.

This algorithm is meant to assist clinicians in the workup and management of common complications of sickle cell disease. It should not replace a physician's clinical judgment or be considered a standardized protocol for all patients.

SUICIDE, EVALUATING RISK FOR

Screen all depressed and anxious patients annually; if the patient has a loss or an anticipated loss, screen within 3 months of those events. Additional testing if the patient
1) Is known to be depressed
2) Has recently lost access to long-term opiate or benzodiazepine use
3) Is being bullied, threatened on social media (Inquire especially in young adults, who are less likely to show "classic" signs of depression and may be initially unwilling to reveal online harassment.)
4) Has been affected by the COVID-19 virus
5) Has a new medical or mental health diagnosis that they find distressing
6) Is a member of a sexual or gender minority
The pandemic itself has impacted individuals' emotional and economic well-being.

Over the past 2 weeks, how often have you been bothered by:
1) Little interest or pleasure in doing things?
2) Feeling down, depressed, or hopeless?

↓

Score each of the two questions on a scale of 0–3 (0 ["not at all"] to 3 ["nearly every day"]).

↓

- Score <3 — Negative depression screen
- Score ≥3 — Positive depression screen

↓ (Score ≥3)

Ask about suicidal ideation (if +, ask about a plan):
"Have you ever felt that life isn't worth living?"
"Did you ever wish you could go to sleep and not wake up?"
"Are you having thoughts about hurting yourself or others?"

↓

If any + (or if negative and you suspect patient is not being honest or is incompetent), get further expert advice.

↓

Higher risk

Question for:
- Mood instability (worsening anxiety or depression; sustained/self-righteous anger or vengeance)
- Losses or worry about potential losses
- Destabilizing events or worry that may occur (illness, injury, use of substances or relapse, job loss, lost professional opportunities, increased isolation)
- Personal or family history of suicide attempts
- Neurologic/psychiatric comorbidities (head injury, dementia, hallucinations, delusions)

↓

Preoccupation with suicide is a medical emergency, and measures should be taken *immediately* to keep the patient safe. This includes putting the patient under constant 1:1 supervision and inpatient admission and consultation.

Lower risk

↓

Close clinical follow-up

↓ (both branches)

Offer 24/7 resources to all patients (on a card or magnet):
In the United States: the National Suicide Prevention Lifeline:
English: 800-273-TALK (8255)
Spanish: 888-628-9454
Chat: https://suicidepreventionlifeline.org/chat

Irene Coletsos, MD, MS and Harold J. Bursztajn, MD

Posner K, Oquendo MA, Gould M, et al. Columbia Classification Algorithm of Suicide Assessment (C-CASA): classification of suicidal events in the FDA's pediatric suicidal risk analysis of antidepressants. *Am J Psychiatry*. 2007;164(7):1035–1043.

SYNCOPE

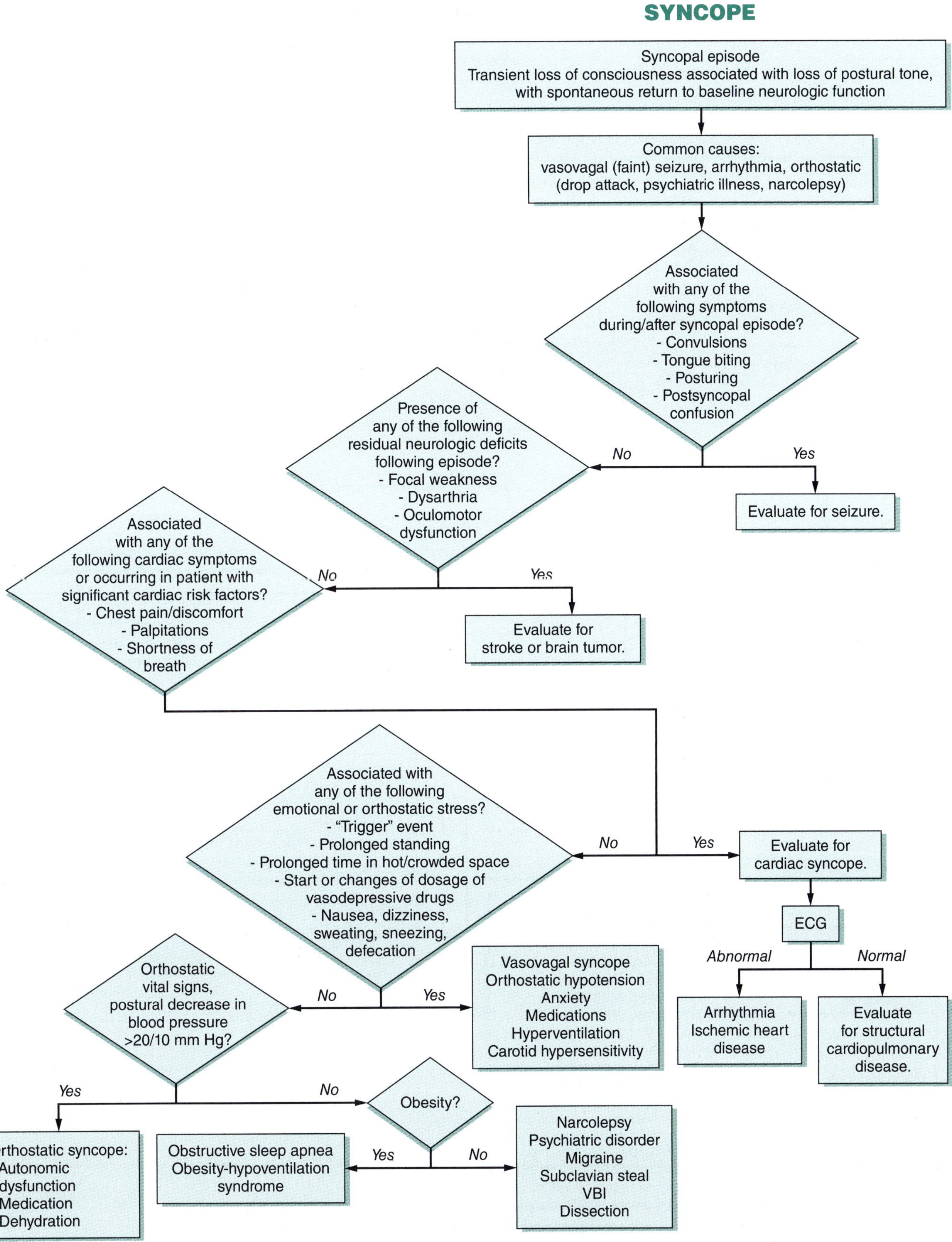

William E. Cayley Jr., MD, Mdiv

Runser LA, Gauer RL, Houser A. Syncope: evaluation and differential diagnosis. *Am Fam Physician*. 2017;95(5):303–312.

THROMBOCYTOPENIA

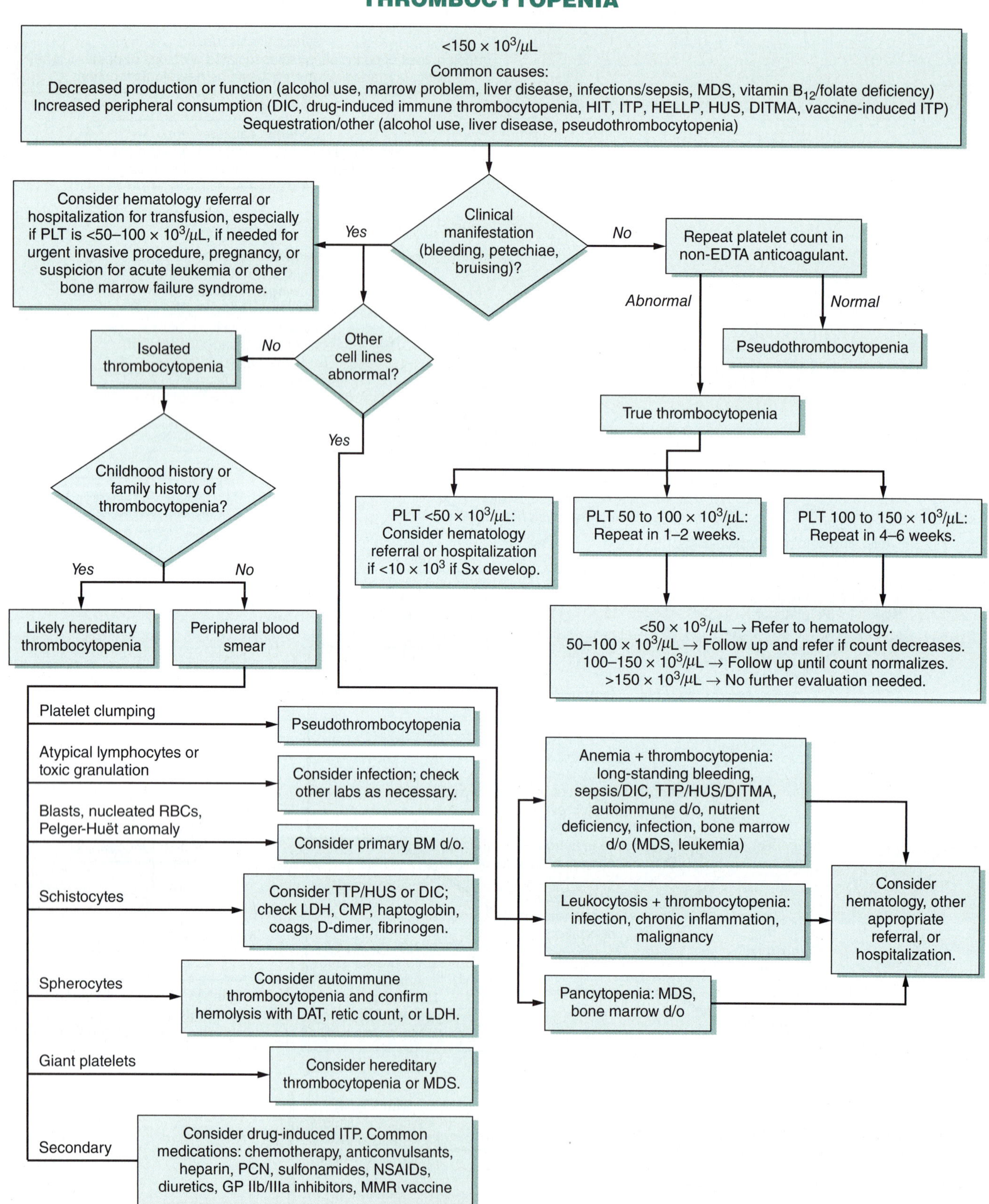

Jillian K. Joseph, MPAS, PA-C and Allison Hargreaves, MD

Gauer RL, Whitaker DJ. Thrombocytopenia: evaluation and management. *Am Fam Physician*. 2022;106(3):288–298.

TINNITUS

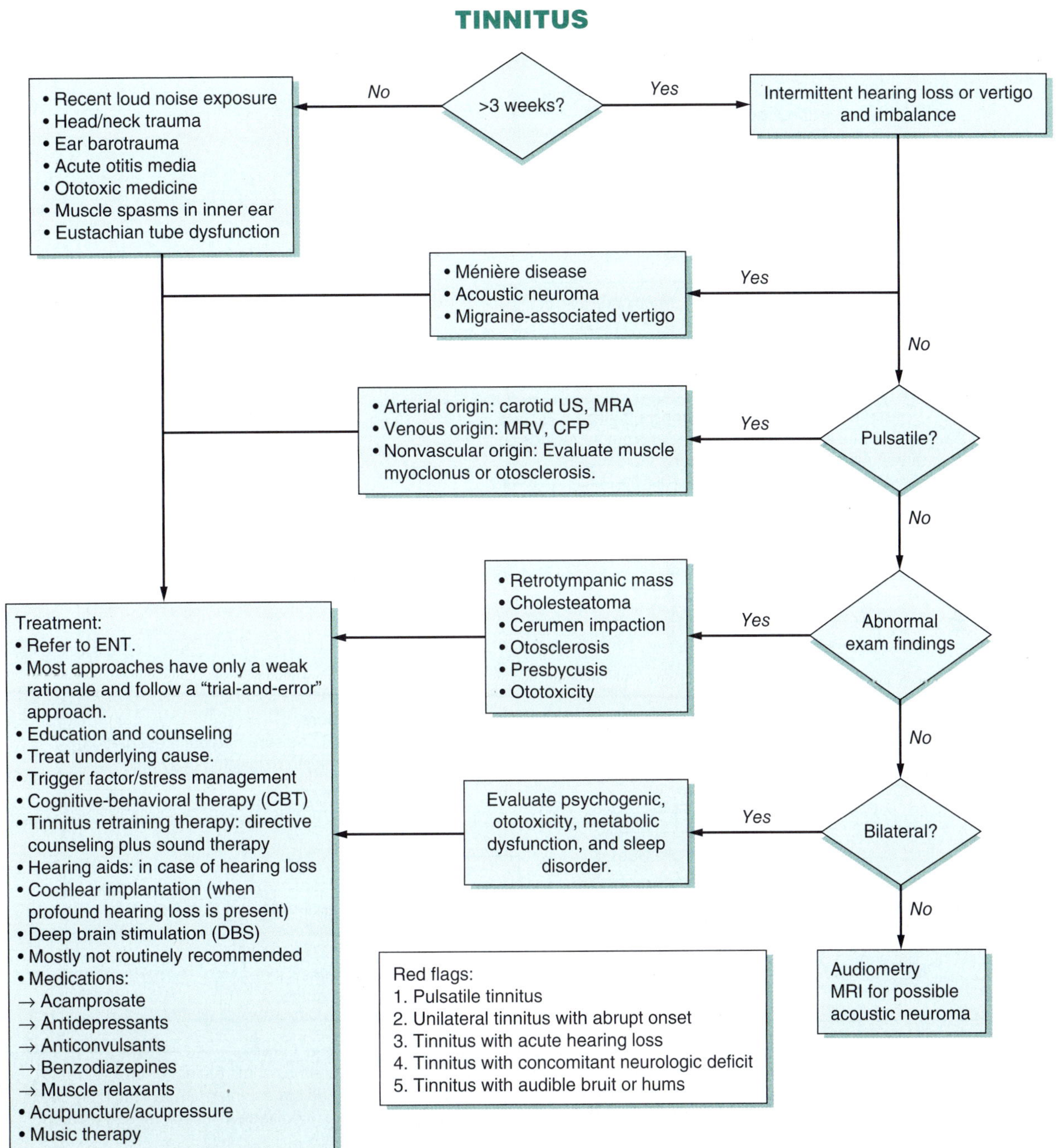

Dongsheng Jiang, MD, MSc

Kleinjung T, Peter N, Schecklmann M, et al. The current state of tinnitus diagnosis and treatment: a multidisciplinary expert perspective. *J Assoc Res Otolaryngol*. 2024;25(5):413–425. doi:10.1007/s10162-024-00960-3.

TRANSIENT ISCHEMIC ATTACK

TIA is defined as a transient episode of neurologic dysfunction caused by focal cerebral, spinal cord, or retinal ischemia without acute infarction.

↓

Common causes: migraine (+/– aura), carotid artery disease, stroke, seizure, syncope, subarachnoid hemorrhage, multiple sclerosis, ALS

↓

Clinical suspicion of a TIA should occur for an episode of sudden onset neurologic deficit, such as limb weakness, paresthesias, aphasia, dysarthria, dizziness, or gait instability.

↓

Risk factors: hypertension, dyslipidemia, diabetes mellitus, atrial fibrillation, cigarette smoking, obesity; less common, include family history of coagulation disorder, or history of COVID-19

↓

Initial assessment:
History
ECG
Blood glucose
Head CT no contrast

↓

Symptoms resolved?

- *No* → **Stroke protocol**
- *Yes* → CT or MRI evidence of stroke? (if CT is negative, MRI is necessary to rule out stroke)
  - *Yes* → **Stroke protocol**
  - *No* → **Differential diagnosis of TIA**: Most common include seizure, migraine, and syncope; others include peripheral vertigo, demyelinating disease, CNS infection, trauma, brain tumor, and other toxic/metabolic/infectious insults

↓

Workup:
MRI brain and vascular imaging (MRA or CTA or carotid duplex), ECG, echo, labs (LDL, A1c, fasting glucose, TSH, CBC, CMP, PT/INR, PTT); calculate ABCD^2 score.

→

ABCD^2 score
(age, blood pressure, clinical presentation, diabetes mellitus, duration of symptoms)

Age >60 years	1 pt.
SBP >140 mm Hg *or* DBP >90 mm Hg	1 pt.
Unilateral weakness	2 pts.
Speech impairment	1 pt.
Diabetes mellitus	1 pt.
Duration of TIA	
>60 minutes	2 pts.
10–59 minutes	1 pt.

↓

- ABCD^2 score of <3, either admit patient or provide rapid outpatient follow-up. Initiate aspirin (ASA) 81 mg daily within 24 hours and address modifiable risk factors (see below).

If ABCD^2 score is >3, admit patient, start ASA 81 mg daily, and administer clopidogrel 300 to 600 mg as loading dose followed by 75 mg daily for 21 days (90 days if intracranial stenosis identified on angiography).

Modifiable risk factors:
- Treat LDL to target LDL <70 mg/dL.
- Treat hemoglobin A1c to target <7.0%.
- Treat blood pressure to achieve normotension long-term.
- Tobacco cessation

Additional management/intervention may be based on suspected TIA etiology (small vessel, large vessel, embolic, cryptogenic).

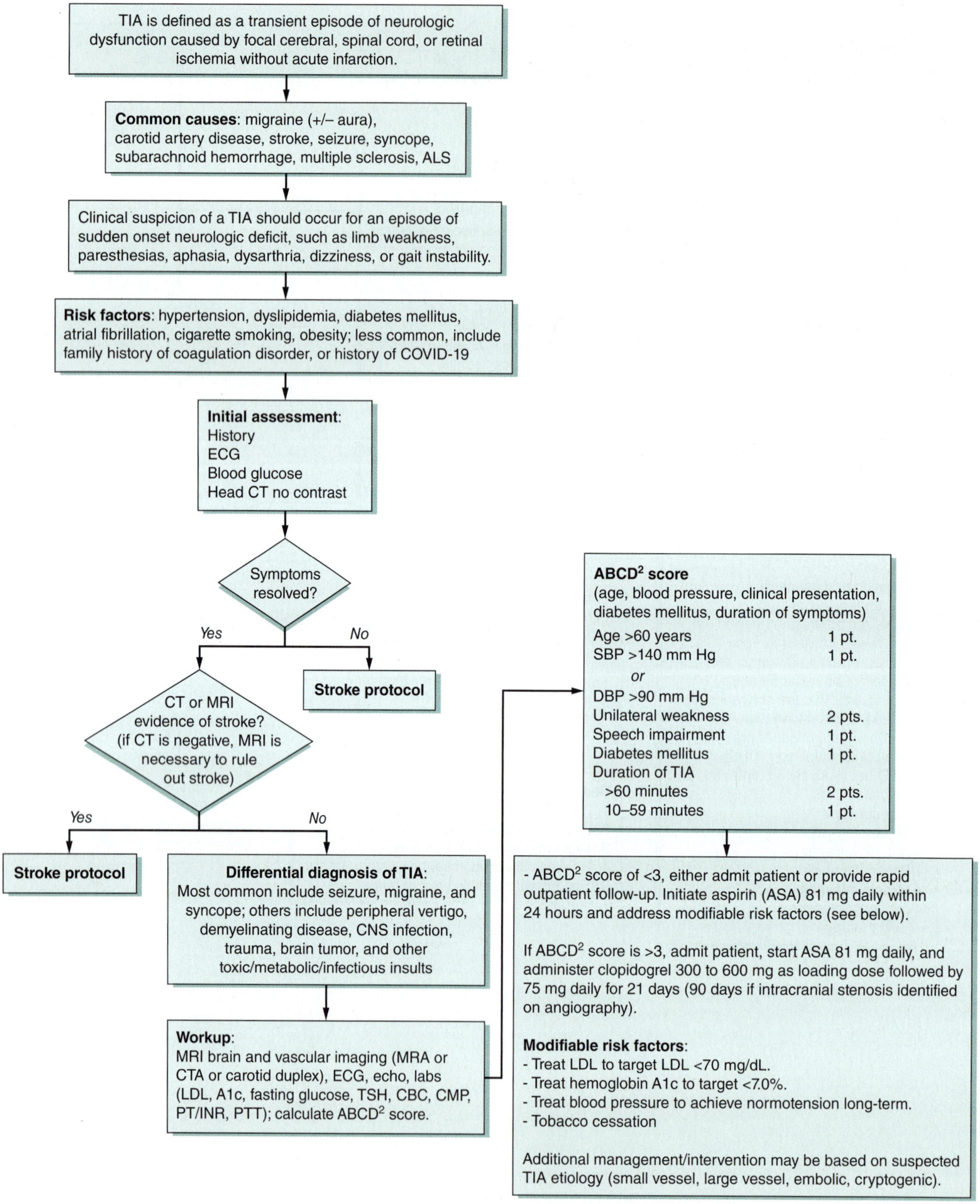

Shane R. Kinard, MD and Anne Darby, DO

Mendelson SJ, Prabhakaran S. Diagnosis and management of transient ischemic attack and acute ischemic stroke: a review. *JAMA*. 2021;325(11):1088–1098.

TREMOR

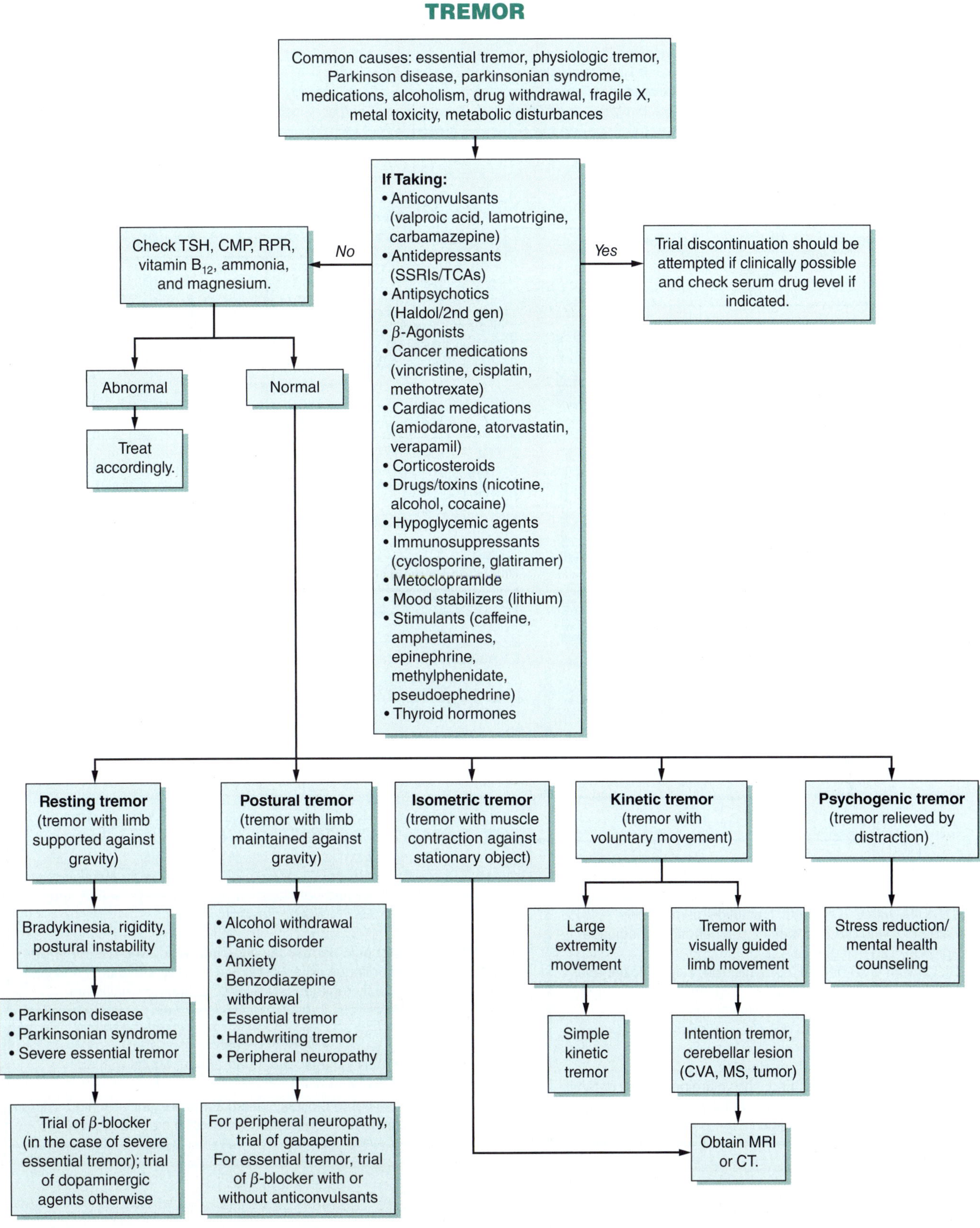

Marni Klessman Gleiber, MD

van de Wardt J, van der Stouwe AMM, Dirkx M, et al. Systematic clinical approach for diagnosing upper limb tremor. *J Neurol Neurosurg Psychiatry*. 2020;91(8):822–830.

TYPE 2 DIABETES, TREATMENT

First-line therapy: comprehensive lifestyle changes (including weight management and physical activity)
If HbA1c remains above goal, proceed below.
If initial HbA1c ≥8.5% or 1.5% above HbA1c target, can consider initiation of dual therapy (metformin + second agent)
If initial HbA1c ≥10%, BG >300 mg/dL, or symptoms of hyperglycemia, can consider basal insulin therapy

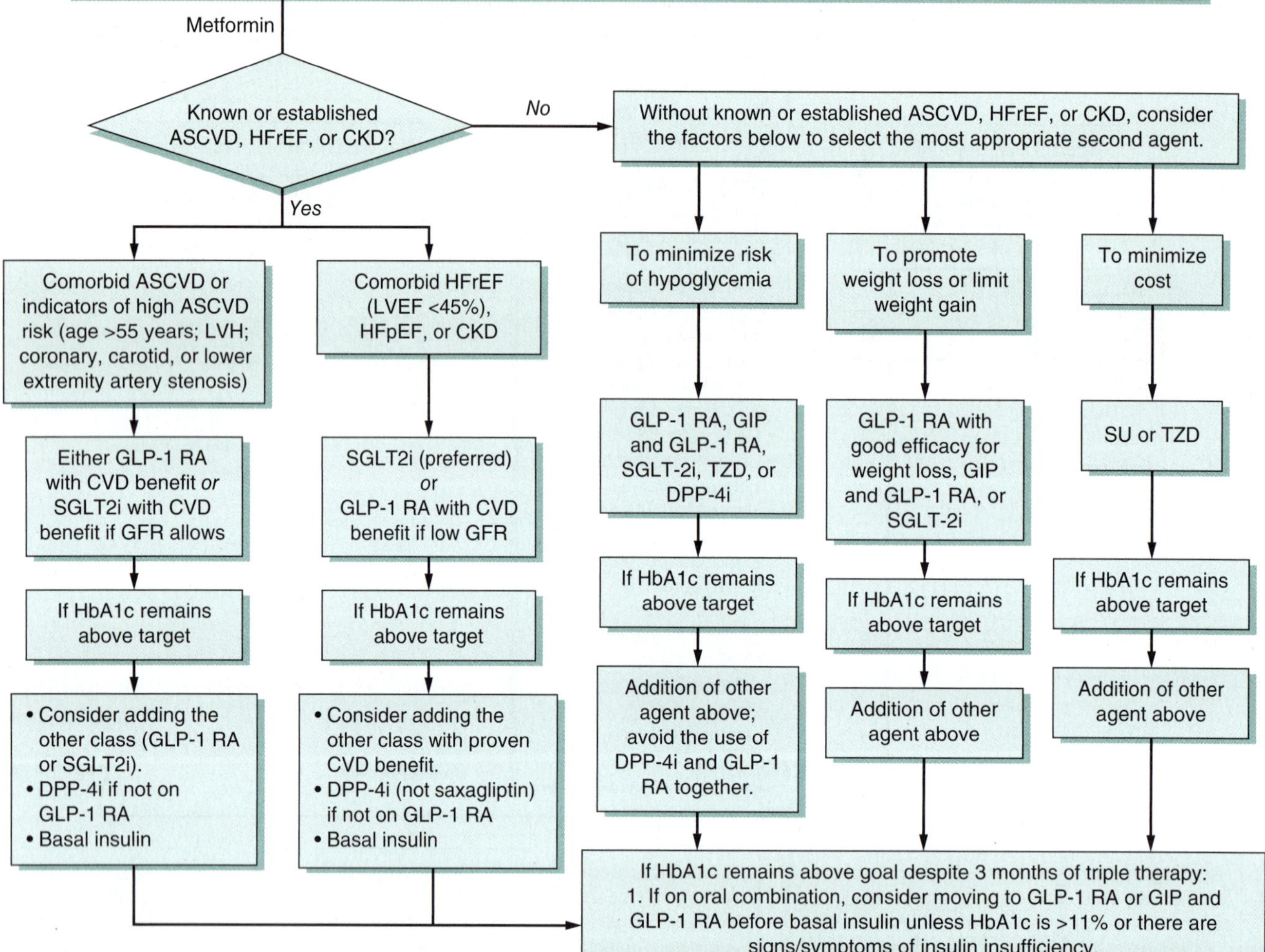

If HbA1c remains above goal despite 3 months of triple therapy:
1. If on oral combination, consider moving to GLP-1 RA or GIP and GLP-1 RA before basal insulin unless HbA1c is >11% or there are signs/symptoms of insulin insufficiency.
2. If on GLP-1 RA or GIP and GLP-1 RA, add basal insulin.
3. If on optimally titrated basal insulin, add GLP-1 RA or GIP and GLP-1 RA or mealtime insulin.

Metformin therapy should be maintained, if indicated, whereas other oral agents may be discontinued on an individual basis to avoid unnecessarily complex or costly regimens, side effects, and hypoglycemia.

GLP-1 RA with CVD benefit: liraglutide, semaglutide, dulaglutide; with greatest weight loss benefit: semaglutide, liraglutide, and dulaglutide
SGLT2i with CVD benefit: empagliflozin, canagliflozin, and dapagliflozin; requires renal dose adjustment
DPP-4i: linagliptin, saxagliptin, or sitagliptin; saxagliptin associated with increased risk of heart failure admissions
TZD: pioglitazone
SU: glimepiride, glyburide, or glipizide
Basal (long-acting) insulin: insulin glargine, insulin detemir, and insulin degludec; start at 10 U or 0.1–0.2 U/kg/day SQ.
GIP and GLP-1 RA: tirzepatide

Glycemic Goals
- An HbA1c goal for newly diagnosed, nonpregnant adults with no comorbidities is <7%.
- If older age, multiple comorbidities, limited life expectancy, or high risk for hypoglycemia, higher HbA1c goals (such as <8%) may be appropriate.

Christine Chan, MD

Vaughan EM, Santiago-Delgado ZM. Management of type 2 diabetes mellitus with noninsulin pharmacotherapy. *Am Fam Physician*. 2024;109(4):333–342.

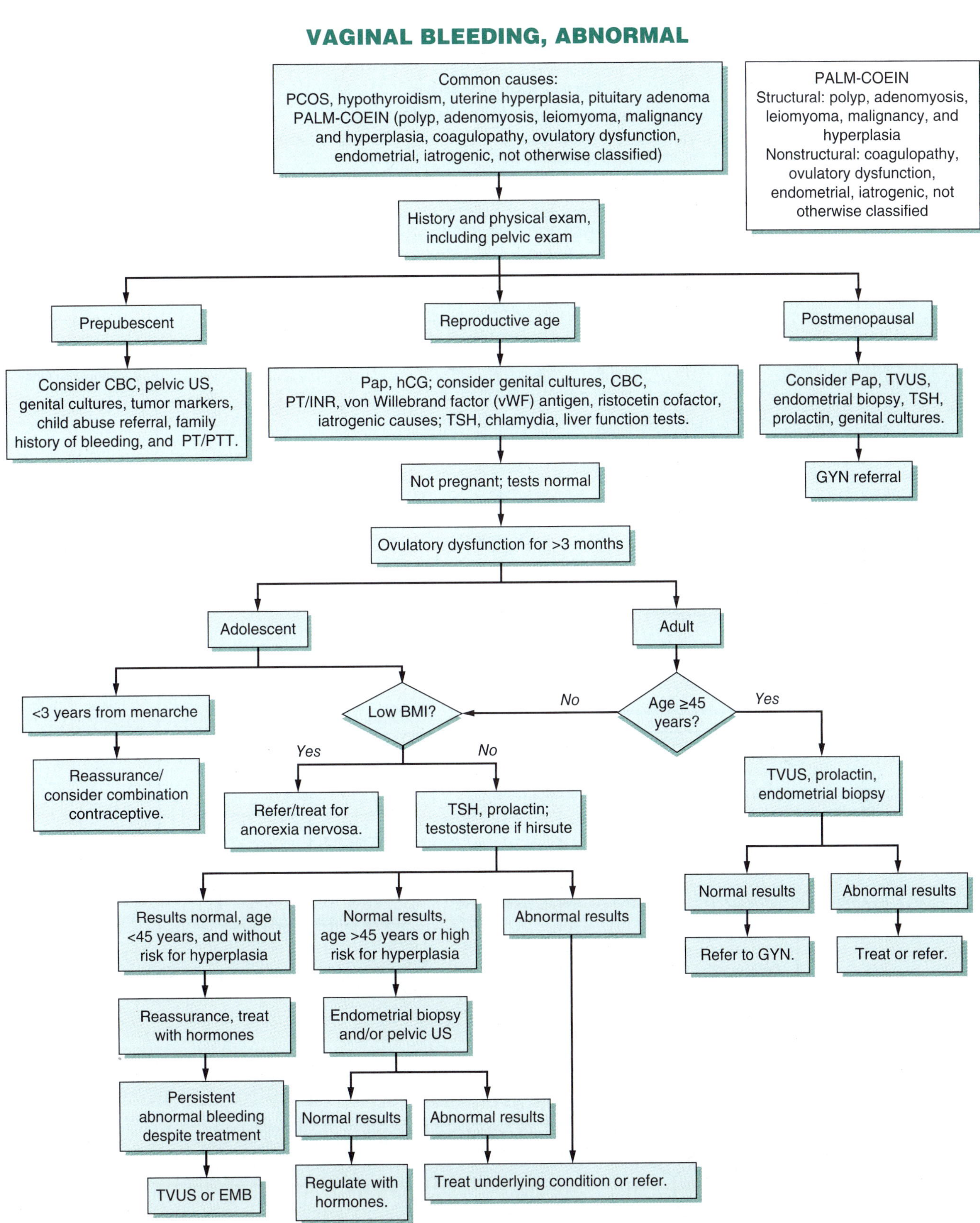

Andrea Chin, MD, MSc and Kimberly A. Bombaci, MD

Wouk N, Helton M. Abnormal uterine bleeding in premenopausal women. *Am Fam Physician*. 2019;99(7):435–443.

VITAMIN D DEFICIENCY

Risk factors/common causes:

- Age >65 years
- Insufficient sunlight exposure (homebound, veiled)
- Renal disease
- Liver disease
- Depression
- Dark skin
- Insufficient dietary intake
- Obesity (BMI >30 kg/m^2)
- Immigrants to colder climates
- Chronic use of glucocorticoids
- Periosteal bone pain (e.g., sternum, tibia)
- GI malabsorption (celiac, cystic fibrosis, inflammatory bowel disease, exocrine pancreatic insufficiency, short bowel syndrome)
- Pregnancy
- Medications: anticonvulsants, antiretroviral, and glucocorticoids
- Gastrectomy or extensive bowel surgery
- Wearing clothing that covers a large portion of the body

Significant risk factors?

No → Low suspicion for vitamin D deficiency → Supplement with 600–2,000 IU of vitamin D per day.

Yes → Age <18 years?

Yes →

Requirements:
<1 year old: 400 IU/day
>1 year old: 600 IU/day
To reach levels >30 ng/mL, may require 1,000 IU/day
Obese children: 2–3 times more vitamin D for their age group
Maintenance dose:
0–6 months old: 1,000–2,000 IU/day
6 months–1 year old: 1,500–2,000 IU/day
1–3 years old: 2,500–3,000 IU/day
4–8 years old: 3,000 IU/day
>8 years old: 2,000 IU/day
Vitamin D deficiency:
0–1 year old: 2,000 IU/day for 6 weeks or 50,000 IU weekly for 6 weeks followed by maintenance 400–1,000 IU/day
1–18 years old: 2,000 IU/day for 6 weeks or 50,000 IU weekly for 6 weeks followed by maintenance 600–1,000 IU/day

No → **Lab:** serum 25-hydroxyvitamin D concentration

- Level <20 ng/mL (vitamin D deficiency) → Treatment → Start 50,000 IU vitamin D_2 once a week for 8–12 weeks and then begin 2,000–3,000 IU vitamin D per day.
- Level 20–29 ng/mL (vitamin D insufficiency) → Treatment → 2,000–4,000 IU vitamin D per day
- Level ≥30 ng/mL normal → Maintenance → Supplement with 600–2,000 IU of vitamin D per day.

After 6 months, consider repeating serum 25-hydroxyvitamin D level.

Recheck serum 25-hydroxyvitamin D concentration.

Level <20 ng/mL?

No → Supplement with 600–2,000 IU of vitamin D per day.

Yes → Consult endocrinology if no malabsorptive disease.

Parvathi Perumareddi, DO

Holick MF, Binkley NC, Bischoff-Ferrari HA, et al; for Endocrine Society. Evaluation, treatment, and prevention of vitamin D deficiency: an Endocrine Society clinical practice guideline. *J Clin Endocrinol Metab*. 2011;96(7):1911–1930.

WEIGHT LOSS, UNINTENTIONAL

Unintentional weight loss of >5% over 6–12 months?
- *No* → If >12 months, consider age-related physiologic changes.
- *Yes* → **Decreased PO intake?**

- Most patients with unintentional weight loss do *not* have undiagnosed cancer.
- Psychogenic causes such as depression, anorexia, or substance abuse disorders account for 15–25% of cases.
- 25% of cases of unintentional weight loss will have no identifiable cause; this generally confers a favorable prognosis.

Decreased PO intake?
- *No* → **Suspicion of metabolic factors or a catabolic state?**
  - *Yes* →
    - Age-appropriate or history-relevant malignancy screening: CBC, CMP, LDH, UA, TSH, CRP, ESR, CXR and FOBT/colonoscopy, HIV
    - Endocrine: hyperthyroidism, severe diabetes, hypercalcemia, or adrenal insufficiency
    - Infectious causes: HIV, HCV, TB, or hepatitis C
    - Chronic conditions: severe CHF or COPD
  - *No* → **Suspicion of malabsorption?**
    - *Yes* →
      - Check tTG-IgA, stool studies, and endoscopy.
      - Gastric: *Helicobacter pylori*, peptic ulcer disease, gastroparesis or early satiety
      - Intestinal: diarrhea, gluten enteropathy, inflammatory bowel disease, ileal resection
      - Pancreatic: steatorrhea or pancreatic insufficiency
- *Yes* →
  - **Psychogenic cause** → Screen for depression, dementia, paranoia, grief, eating disorder, and substance or alcohol use.
  - **Unable to secure preferred foods** → Consider food insecurity, financial difficulty, and elder abuse/neglect.
  - **Loss of appetite** →
    - Medication contributors: anticonvulsants, SGLT2 inhibitors, bupropion, digoxin, excess thyroxine replacement, or recent discontinuation of steroids, metformin, and GLP-1 agonists
    - Substances: nicotine, caffeine, cocaine, PCP, amphetamines, herbal supplements (hoodia, ephedra, or guarana)
  - **Dysphagia** →
    - Oropharyngeal: GERD, globus pharyngeus, hiatal hernia, stroke, MS, ALS, Sjögren syndrome or poor dentition
    - Esophageal: eosinophilic esophagitis, pill esophagitis (e.g., ferrous sulfate, bisphosphonate, NSAIDs) or achalasia
  - **Nausea** → Medication contributors: digoxin, dopamine agonists, SSRIs, antibiotics, antiretrovirals, NSAIDs, opiates, iron, or metformin
  - **Dry mouth** → Medication contributors: clonidine, loop diuretics, anticholinergics, or chemotherapy agents
  - **Altered taste** →
    - Medication contributors: GLP-1 agonists, spironolactone, topiramate, allopurinol, methimazole
    - Other conditions: long COVID-19, cirrhosis, zinc deficiency, or thrush

Arindam Sarkar, MD, FAAFP and Chelsea Mendonca, MD

Gaddey HL, Holder KK. Unintentional weight loss in older adults. *Am Fam Physician*. 2021;104(1):34–40.

ABNORMAL (DYSFUNCTIONAL) UTERINE BLEEDING

Alexandra Renee Zaballa, MD • Jenny T. Giang-Griesser, MD

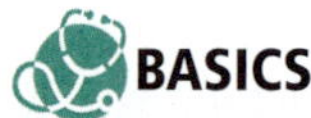

BASICS

DESCRIPTION
- Abnormal uterine bleeding (AUB) is uterine bleeding that is abnormal in terms of menstrual regularity, frequency, duration, or volume (1).
- May be acute or chronic (occurring >6 months)
- The International Federation of Gynecology and Obstetrics (FIGO) now uses AUB rather than dysfunctional uterine bleeding (DUB).

EPIDEMIOLOGY
Adolescent and perimenopausal women are affected most often.

Incidence
5% of reproductive-aged women will see a doctor in any given year for AUB.

Prevalence
10–30% of reproductive-aged women have AUB (1).

ETIOLOGY AND PATHOPHYSIOLOGY
- The breakdown of etiologies for AUB varies by population and age. Anovulation accounts for 90% of AUB among adolescents related to an immature hypothalamic pituitary ovarian (HPO) axis.
- The mnemonic PALM-COEIN was developed to describe AUB in reproductive-aged women.
- PALM (structural causes): Polyp, Adenomyosis, Leiomyoma, and Malignancy and/or hyperplasia
- COEIN (nonstructural causes): Coagulopathy, Ovulatory disorders, Endometrial, Iatrogenic, and Not yet classified
- Coagulopathy
  - Approximately 20% of patients with heavy menstrual bleeding have a bleeding disorder.
  - von Willebrand disease and platelet dysfunction are the most common coagulopathies associated with AUB.
- Diseases causing ovulatory dysfunction: hyperprolactinemia, immature hypothalamic-pituitary-adrenal axis (adolescence), intense exercise/stress, polycystic ovary syndrome (PCOS), starvation (including eating disorders), thyroid disorders
- Medications (iatrogenic causes): anticoagulants, antipsychotic medications (mostly first generation), copper intrauterine device, hormonal contraception or other hormone therapy, tamoxifen (estrogen receptor antagonists),
- Other causes of AUB not defined in PALM-COEIN: ectopic pregnancy, threatened or incomplete abortion or hydatidiform mole, upper genital tract infections, advanced or fulminant liver disease, chronic renal disease, nutritional deficiencies, inflammatory bowel disease, excessive weight gain, increased exercise

Genetics
Inherited bleeding disorders such as von Willebrand disease and rare inherited clotting factor deficiencies and platelet function defects

RISK FACTORS
- Bleeding disorders are a major risk factor.
- Among adolescents, conditions including PCOS, thyroid disease, stress, and eating disorders increase the risk of an immature HPO axis.

GENERAL PREVENTION
There is no known direct preventive measure for AUB.

Menstrual Cycle Terms	Descriptive Terms	Definition
Frequency (interval between the start of each menstrual cycle)	Infrequent	>38 days
	Normal	≥24 and ≤38 days
	Frequent	<24 days
Regularity (variation of menstrual cycle length, measured over 12 months)	Regular	Regular: shortest to longest cycle variation ≤7 to 9 days
	Irregular	Irregular: shortest to longest cycle variation ≥10 rays
Duration of menstruation	Shortened	<4.5 days
	Normal	≤8 days
	Prolonged	>8 days
Volume (total blood loss each menstrual cycle)	Light	Patient considers light
	Normal	Patient considers normal
	Heavy	Patient considers heavy

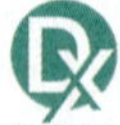

DIAGNOSIS

Definitions of normal and AUB; the FIGO recommendations on terminologies and definitions for normal and AUB

HISTORY
- Menstrual history: onset, frequency, regularity and volume; volume should be quantified by pad/tampon use, presence and size of clots; passing blood clots or changing pads/tampons at least hourly suggest heavy menstrual bleeding (1).
- A history of postcoital bleeding may indicate cervicitis, ectropion, or rarely cervical cancer.
- Associated abdominopelvic pain may suggest infection, structural lesions, or endometriosis.
- Gynecologic history: gravidity and parity, STI history, previous Pap smear results
- Family history of abnormal bleeding or personal history of heavy menstrual bleeding since menarche, or symptoms such as frequent bruising, bleeding gums, epistaxis, postpartum hemorrhage, or bleeding with surgical and dental procedures.
- Review of systems (Exclude symptoms of pregnancy, bleeding disorders, stress, exercise, recent weight change, visual changes, headaches, galactorrhea)

ALERT
Postmenopausal bleeding is any bleeding that occurs >1 year after the last menstrual period; cancer must always be ruled out (1).

PHYSICAL EXAM
Evaluate for:
- Signs of PCOS (i.e., hirsutism and acne)
- Signs of thyroid disease (i.e., thyroid nodules)
- Signs of insulin resistance (i.e., acanthosis nigricans)
- Signs of pituitary lesions (i.e., visual field defects, galactorrhea)
- Findings suggestive of bleeding disorder include petechiae, ecchymosis, skin pallor, or swollen joints (although absence does not exclude the possibility of underlying bleeding condition) (2).
- Pelvic exam: Examine all potential bleeding sites, including the urethra, perineum, and anus.
- Perform cervical cancer screening if not up-to-date.

Pediatric Considerations
- Premenarchal children with vaginal bleeding should be evaluated for foreign bodies, physical/sexual abuse, possible infections, and signs of precocious puberty.
- Pelvic examination can be deferred in adolescents if the patient is not sexually active, neither trauma nor infection is suspected, and the response to initial treatment is adequate (1).

DIFFERENTIAL DIAGNOSIS
See "Etiology and Pathophysiology."

DIAGNOSTIC TESTS & INTERPRETATION

Initial Tests (lab, imaging)
- All patients: pregnancy test and complete blood count
- If coagulopathy is suspected: prothrombin time (PT), activated partial thromboplastin time (aPTT), and fibrinogen level; note that these results may be normal in women with von Willebrand or other bleeding disorders.
- Consider other tests based on differential diagnosis and risk factors:
  - Suspected hormonal abnormalities: TSH, prolactin level
  - Age ≥45 years or elevated risk of endometrial carcinoma: endometrial biopsy (EMB)
  - Concern for infection: STI screening (GC/CT, trichomonas), KOH prep, vaginitis panel
  - Suspected congenital adrenal hyperplasia: 17-hydroxyprogesterone
  - Suspected PCOS: Consider testosterone and/or dehydroepiandrosterone sulfate (DHEA-S).
- Imaging
  - Indications for pelvic imaging include abnormalities palpated on bimanual exam or symptoms that persist despite initial treatment.
  - Transvaginal ultrasound is the first-line approach for most patients.
- Procedures: endometrial sampling/biopsy for certain patients (see "Diagnostic Procedures/Others")

Follow-Up Tests & Special Considerations

- Depending on results of initial tests, or if a patient's medical history is suggestive of underlying bleeding condition, specific tests for von Willebrand disease or other coagulopathies may be indicated, including von Willebrand-ristocetin cofactor activity, von Willebrand factor antigen, and factor VIII (2).
- If transvaginal ultrasound imaging is not adequate or further evaluation of cavity is necessary, then sonohysterography (also known as saline infusion sonohysterography) or hysteroscopy is recommended.
- It is appropriate to initiate medical therapy in females <35 years of age if low risk of uterine anatomic/histologic abnormality or adenomyosis prior to performing an EMB.
- American College of Obstetricians and Gynecologists (ACOG) recommends endometrial sampling for postmenopausal women with AUB, but states that a thin, homogeneous endometrial thickness (ET) <4 mm does not require endometrial sampling unless bleeding is persistent or recurrent, whereas ET >4 mm should prompt further evaluation (based on ACOG 2018 guidance). Sampling of thin endometrium is often unsatisfactory for histologic evaluation.
- Incidentally found endometrial measurement >4 mm without associated bleeding in postmenopausal women should not trigger evaluation; however, assessment based on individual risk factors is appropriate.

Diagnostic Procedures/Other

- EMB
  - Women age >45 years with AUB to rule out cancer or premalignancy
  - Postmenopausal women with ET ≥4 mm
  - Women aged 18 to 45 years with AUB, a history of unopposed estrogen and failed medical management
  - Women of any age without risk factors if they have abnormal findings following imaging
  - Perform on or after day 18 of cycle, if known; secretory endometrium confirms ovulation occurred.
- Hysteroscopy with targeted biopsy if suspected intrauterine lesion with negative EMB; NPV for endometrial cancer with negative hysteroscopy at any age is 99.5%.

Test Interpretation

Pap smear could reveal carcinoma or inflammation indicative of cervicitis. Most EMBs show proliferative or dyssynchronous endometrium (suggesting anovulation) but can show simple or complex hyperplasia without atypia, hyperplasia with atypia, or endometrial adenocarcinoma.

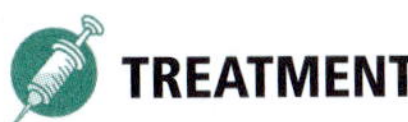

TREATMENT

MEDICATION

First Line

- Management should be directed at the suspected cause of the AUB. For those with known structural, infectious, or endocrine etiologies, appropriate medical or surgical therapies should be selected. Those with unknown etiologies can be triaged into acute or chronic bleeding.
- Acute bleeding
  - Conjugated equine estrogen
    - Hemodynamically unstable: 25 mg IV q4–6h for 24 hours); shown to stop bleeding in 72% of participants within 8 hours of administration compared with 38% of participants treated with placebo (3)
    - Hemodynamically stable: 2.5 mg conjugated equine estrogen (Premarin) PO q6h for 21 days should control bleeding in 12 to 24 hours (2)[A].
  - Oral contraceptive pills (OCPs): 1 monophasic pill containing 35 μg of ethinyl estradiol PO 3 times daily for 7 days (3)
  - Tranexamic acid (TXA) 10 mg/kg IV (max 600 mg/dose) q8h or 20 to 25 mg/kg PO q8h (3)
  - Intrauterine tamponade by filling 26F Foley bulb with 30 mL saline
  - Dilation and curettage (D&C) if no response after 2 to 4 doses of Premarin or sooner if bleeding >1 pad per hour
- Chronic bleeding:
  - The 20-μg-per-day formulation of levonorgestrel-releasing intrauterine system (Mirena) is the most effective for decreasing heavy menstrual bleeding (71–95% reduction in blood loss) and performs similarly to hysterectomy with quality-adjusted life years considered (1).
  - Progestins: medroxyprogesterone acetate (Provera) 10 mg/day for 5 to 10 days each month; daily progesterone for 21 days per cycle results in significantly less blood loss; medroxyprogesterone acetate (Depo-Provera) 150 mg q12w.
  - OCPs: 1 monophasic pill containing 35 μg daily estrogen plus progesterone
  - TXA (Lysteda) 1.0 to 1.5 g by mouth 3 times a day.
  - NSAIDs (naproxen sodium 500 mg BID, ibuprofen 600 to 1,200 mg/day) decrease amount of blood loss and pain compared with placebo.
- Additional considerations:
  - Do not use estrogen if contraindications exist including breast cancer, suspicion for endometrial hyperplasia or carcinoma, history of DVT, liver disease, migraine with aura, or smoking in women >35 years of age (relative contraindication).
  - Do not use TXA in patients at increased risk of thrombosis.
  - Both TXA and NSAIDs are effective, well-tolerated, non-hormonal choices that are taken only when patient is bleeding. TXA is safe to use while patient is attempting to conceive.
  - The need for surgical treatment depends on clinical stability of patient, severity of bleeding, contraindications to medical management, and response to medical management (3).

ISSUES FOR REFERRAL

If an obvious cause for vaginal bleeding is not found in a pediatric patient, refer to a pediatric endocrinologist or pediatric/adolescent gynecologist.

ADDITIONAL THERAPIES

- Antiemetics if treating with high-dose estrogen or progesterone
- Iron supplementation if anemia (usually iron deficiency) is identified.

SURGERY/OTHER PROCEDURES

Surgical options include D&C, endometrial ablation, uterine artery embolization, and hysterectomy (3).

ADMISSION, INPATIENT, AND NURSING CONSIDERATIONS

- Admission for inpatient care recommended if there is significant hemorrhage causing acute anemia with signs of hemodynamic instability; with acute bleeding, replace volume with crystalloid and blood, as necessary.
- Discharge criteria: hemodynamic stability and control of vaginal bleeding

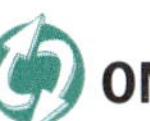

ONGOING CARE

FOLLOW-UP RECOMMENDATIONS

Once stable from acute management, recommend follow-up evaluation in 2 to 4 months for further evaluation.

Patient Monitoring

Women should keep a menstrual diary to document bleeding patterns and their response to therapy.

DIET

No dietary restrictions, although a 5% reduction in weight can induce ovulation in anovulation caused by PCOS

PATIENT EDUCATION

https://www.acog.org/womens-health/faqs/abnormal-uterine-bleeding

PROGNOSIS

- Varies with pathophysiologic process
- Most anovulatory cycles can be treated with medical therapy and do not require surgical intervention.

COMPLICATIONS

Iron deficiency anemia, impaired quality of life, hemodynamic instability

REFERENCES

1. Wouk N, Helton M. Abnormal uterine bleeding in premenopausal women. *Am Fam Physician*. 2019;99(7):435–443.
2. Committee on Practice Bulletins—Gynecology. Practice bulletin no. 128: diagnosis of abnormal uterine bleeding in reproductive-aged women. *Obstet Gynecol*. 2012;120(1):197–206. doi:10.1097/AOG.0b013e318262e320.
3. ACOG committee opinion no. 557: management of acute abnormal uterine bleeding in nonpregnant reproductive-aged women. *Obstet Gynecol*. 2013;121(4):891–896. doi:10.1097/01.AOG.0000428646.67925.9a.

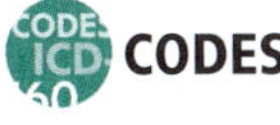

CODES

ICD10

- N93.9 Abnormal uterine and vaginal bleeding, unspecified
- N93.8 Other specified abnormal uterine and vaginal bleeding

CLINICAL PEARLS

- AUB is a clinical diagnosis defined by deviations in normal menstrual parameters cause by many etiologies. PALM-COEIN is a commonly used diagnostic algorithm for AUB.
- Approximately 20% of AUB is caused by bleeding disorders. Anovulation accounts for 90% of AUB in adolescents.
- EMB should be performed in:
  - Women age >45 years with AUB
  - Women aged 18 to 45 years with AUB and a history of unopposed estrogen and failed medical management

ABNORMAL MENSTRUAL BLEEDING (AUB) IN REPRODUCTIVE-AGE WOMEN

Nergess T. Taheri, DO, MSBI • Anastasia Dihel, MD

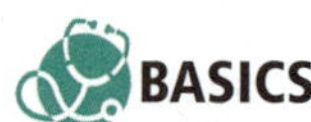

BASICS

This article focuses on heavy menstrual bleeding (HMB) in nonpregnant reproductive-age women.

DESCRIPTION

- HMB is a form of abnormal uterine bleeding (AUB) and is defined as a volume of menstrual blood loss that interferes with the patient's physical, social, emotional, and/or material quality of life.
- Based on current terminology, menorrhagia is regular bleeding that is heavy or prolonged with cyclic (ovulatory) menses.
- It is based on the patient's perspective as increased volume of menstrual flow, regardless of the duration, frequency, or regularity.
- This volume as defined by clinical trials is >80 mL of blood lost per cycle (one third of the patients documented); however, self-assessment can be inaccurate. Indirect assessment has been developed for better measurement.
- There is consensus to abandon the use of the term *menorrhagia* as it is found to be confusing and/or poorly defined.

EPIDEMIOLOGY

- In the United States, AUB accounts for 20–30% of all gynecologic visits and results in more than half of hysterectomies performed annually for benign uterine disorders.
- The prevalence varies with age, most commonly occurring at menarche and perimenopause.
- HMB is linked to decreased quality of life and increased health care costs, with significant morbidity due to anemia.

Incidence

HMB can present as an acute or chronic condition.

Prevalence

- Ranges from 9% to 14% in studies based on objective assessment, measuring the volume
- Much higher 20–52% in studies based on subjective assessment
- Multiple aspects contribute to the underreporting of the symptom HMB prevalence.
- Lack of awareness, social, cultural, or religious practices
- Normalization of HMB by society, families, HCPs

ETIOLOGY AND PATHOPHYSIOLOGY

- Any derangement in the structure of the uterus, in the clotting pathways, or disruption of the hypothalamic-pituitary-ovarian axis can cause HMB.
- The pathophysiology of HMB is outlined with reference to the International Federation of Gynecology and Obstetrics (FIGO) PALM-COEIN classification system of AUB (1). More research needs to be done to elaborate the many causes of this condition.
- HMB can be caused by structural issues such as (PALM acronym):
  - Polyp (AUB-P)
  - Adenomyosis (AUB-A)
  - Leiomyoma (AUB-L)
  - Malignancy/hyperplasia (AUB-M)
- Excessive estrogen stimulation likely causes polyps, which are abnormal outgrowths of hypertrophied endometrial tissue. It does not demonstrate the normal cyclical changes of normal endometrium causing irregular and intermenstrual HMB.
- Adenomyosis may cause HMB by affecting normal myometrial contraction, but the exact cause is unknown.
- Leiomyomas are common benign myometrial neoplasms thought to form as a result of chromosomal abnormalities and grow in response to estrogen and progesterone. The exact cause for HMB lacks sufficient evidence to support the many proposed theories.
- Excess estrogen can promote endometrial hyperplasia and insufficient reduction in progesterone to promote shedding may underlay heavy bleeding.
- It can also be caused by nonstructural causes which include (COEIN acronym):
  - Coagulopathy (AUB-C)
  - Ovulatory (AUB-O)
  - Endometrial (AUB-E)
  - Iatrogenic (AUB-I)
  - Not yet classified (AUB-N)
- Ovulatory dysfunction is associated with a thick stratum functionalis caused by excessive estrogen stimulation of the endometrium. Endometrial shedding tends to be noncyclical with irregular bleeding noted.
- HMB can also be classified as ovulatory or anovulatory bleeding.
- Conditions in not otherwise classified category include pelvic inflammatory disease (PID), chronic liver disease, and cervicitis
- Rare etiologies include arteriovenous malformations, myometrial hyperplasia, and endometritis

Pediatric Considerations

Due to immaturity of the hypothalamic-pituitary-ovarian axis, adolescents are at risk for irregular and HMB. Of note, adolescents with heavy bleeding should be evaluated for possible bleeding disorders, especially von Willebrand disease and qualitative platelet dysfunction.

RISK FACTORS

Obesity

GENERAL PREVENTION

- Combined oral contraceptives may prevent HMB particularly when progesterone is dominant. Lower estrogen doses result in less menstrual bleeding.
- Progesterone-only contraceptives may reduce overall blood loss but often result in irregular bleeding.

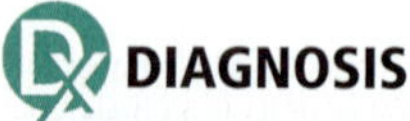

DIAGNOSIS

The first part of diagnosis involves a thorough history and physical exam (PE).

HISTORY

- It is important to obtain a proper understanding of the patient's bleeding episode and to ask questions focused on PALM-COEIN etiologies to determine the patient's cause of abnormal bleeding.
- Recent or current pregnancy
- Menstrual history and bleeding patterns: menarche, LMP, menses frequency, regularity, duration, the volume flow, intermenstrual and postcoital bleeding. To determine the quantity of blood loss, pads changed every 2 to 3 hours represents at least 80 mL of blood loss.
- Sexual history: Evaluate for PID, STI, pain, fever, discharge.
- History of obstetric or gynecologic surgery, contraceptive use, IUD, medication use, chronic medical conditions
- Initial screening for underlying disorder of hemostasis:
  - HMB since menarche; two or more of family history of bleeding symptoms, frequent gum bleeding, epistaxis 1 to 2 times per month, or bruising 1 to 2 times per month; one of the following: bleeding associated with dental work, surgery-related bleeding, or postpartum hemorrhage
  - Positive screen comprises any of the above categories and warrants further testing and hematology referral.
  - Anovulatory bleeding is noted to be irregular, unpredictable, and the patient lacks typical ovulatory symptoms such as midcycle pain or premenstrual symptoms.

PHYSICAL EXAM

- Assess hemodynamic stability, and if unstable (tachycardia, hypotension, positive orthostatic), need to be stabilized in the emergency department before proceeding with additional evaluation
- The goal of PE is to look for signs of systemic illness, such as fever, ecchymoses, an enlarged thyroid gland, or evidence of hyperandrogenism such as hirsutism or acne. Acanthosis nigricans may be seen in polycystic ovary syndrome (PCOS), galactorrhea can suggest hyperprolactinemia.
- A complete pelvic examination should be performed, inspecting the vulva, urethra, vagina, anus, and perineum. Note signs of trauma like lacerations. It is also prudent to note any hemorrhoids as a possible source of bleeding.
- Bimanual exam is done to feel for uterine or cervical abnormalities or enlargement. Pelvic and adnexal masses would also be palpated during this exam.
- Cervical cancer screening

DIFFERENTIAL DIAGNOSIS

- Normal menses
- Complication of pregnancy
- Other sources of bleeding (e.g., cervical, vaginal, gastrointestinal)

DIAGNOSTIC TESTS & INTERPRETATION

Initial Tests (lab, imaging)

- Initial testing on all patients should include pregnancy test and CBC.
- If the patient is acutely bleeding heavily, type and crossmatch should be ordered.
- Laboratory evaluation for disorder of hemostasis: PTT, PT/INR, fibrinogen
- Initial testing for von Willebrand disease: von Willebrand factor antigen, ristocetin cofactor assay, factor VIII
- Other tests may include TSH with reflex T4, CMP, iron studies, and STI panel.
- For ovulatory dysfunction: thyroid function testing, human chorionic gonadotropin, prolactin, and follicle-stimulating hormone
- Transvaginal ultrasound; additional imaging at clinicians discretion

Follow-Up Tests & Special Considerations

- Saline infusion sonohysterography, diagnostic hysterography, and hysterosalpingography can be performed to diagnose endometrial polyps and submucosal leiomyoma (2).
- MRI can be performed to better visualize the changes of adenomyosis and determine if uterine sparing treatment is an option in patients with leiomyoma (2). MRI can also detect leiomyosarcoma.

Diagnostic Procedures/Other

If a patient is >45 years of age or <45 years of age with risk factors, endometrial biopsy with or without hysteroscopy is performed for possible endometrial hyperplasia or carcinoma.

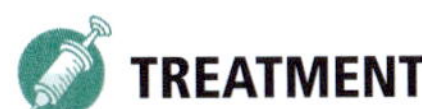

TREATMENT

MEDICATION

First Line

- Acute bleeding
  - Conjugated equine estrogen 25 mg IV every 4 to 6 hours for 24 hours with IV antiemetic agents
  - Monophasic combined OCP containing 35-μg ethinyl estradiol TID for 7 days and then 1 daily
  - Medroxyprogesterone 20 mg or norethindrone 20 mg TID for 7 days
  - Tranexamic acid 10 mg/kg IV (maximum 600 mg per dose) or 1.5 g PO every 8 hours for 5 days
  - Desmopressin in patients with von Willebrand disease: intranasal inhalation, IV, SC
  - Other factor-specific deficiencies
- Chronic bleeding
  - Ibuprofen 600 mg every 6 hours or 800 mg every 8 hours; naproxen 500 mg initially and repeat 3 to 5 hours later and then 250 to 500 mg BID; mefenamic acid 500 mg TID (with food)
  - Monophasic 30- to 35-μg estrogen-containing OCP daily with or without inert pills
  - Medroxyprogesterone 5 to 10 mg or norethindrone 5 to 10 mg daily
  - Tranexamic acid 1.3 g PO every 8 hours up to 5 days
  - Depot medroxyprogesterone 150 mg SC every 3 months. Levonorgestrel 19.5- to 52.0-mg intrauterine devices (IUDs) (3)[A] (19.5-mg levonorgestrel-releasing intrauterine system [LNG IUS] is a slightly smaller device); etonogestrel subdermal implant

Second Line

- Danazol, GnRH agonists, aromatase inhibitors, selective estrogen receptor modulators (SERMs), and selective progesterone receptor modulators (SPRMs) are used as second-line agents in management of bleeding caused by leiomyoma and adenomyosis.
- Of note, SPRMs are not currently available in the United States.

ISSUES FOR REFERRAL

Refer to gynecology if a primary care physician is uncomfortable placing an IUD, performing endometrial sampling, if there is persistent bleeding despite treatment, or malignancy is suspected. Depending on etiology, refer to hematology, oncology, or interventional radiology.

ADDITIONAL THERAPIES

- Iron replacement therapy PO (preferred) or IV (if unable to tolerate oral) for anemia
- MRI-guided focused ultrasound (MgFUS) had been approved by the FDA for the treatment of uterine fibroids and has been used with success in decreasing bleeding in patients with adenomyosis.

SURGERY/OTHER PROCEDURES

- Intrauterine tamponade, uterine artery embolization, endometrial ablation, dilation and curettage can be considered in the setting of acute severe bleeding.
- Surgical procedures are directed to the specific identified pathology.
  - Endometrial and cervical polyps—polypectomy
  - Adenomyosis—hysterectomy
  - Leiomyoma—for women who do not desire fertility laparoscopic radiofrequency ablation, uterine artery embolization or hysterectomy can be performed. For women who desire fertility, myomectomy is preferred.
  - Malignancy—hysterectomy with or without adjuvant chemotherapy and radiotherapy
- Conservative surgery (i.e., myomectomy, endometrial ablation, or uterine artery embolization) is more effective for controlling bleeding symptoms at 1 and 2 years than oral medications or the levonorgestrel-releasing IUD, but by 5 years, there is no difference in long-term results or patient satisfaction.
- Hysterectomy, the definitive treatment, may be necessary for failure of medical management or presence of another indication such as malignancy.

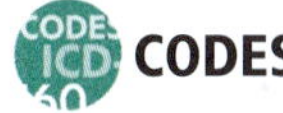

ONGOING CARE

PATIENT EDUCATION

Worldwide, many women do not report AUB to their health care providers. It is important to have an open discussion on menstruation, and patient should be educated on any pertinent lifestyle changes, treatment options, and when to seek emergency care.

PROGNOSIS

Favorable but vastly dependent on etiology. The main goal is to rule out malignancy and improve patient's quality of life.

COMPLICATIONS

Anemia, infertility, endometrial cancer

REFERENCES

1. Muncro MG, Critchley HOD, Fraser IS, et al. The two FIGO systems for normal and abnormal uterine bleeding symptoms and classification of causes of abnormal uterine bleeding in reproductive years: 2018 revisions. *Int J Gynaecol Obstet*. 2018;143(3):393–408.
2. Marnach ML, Laughlin-Tommaso SK. Evaluation and management of abnormal uterine bleeding. *Mayo Clin Proc*. 2019;94(2):326–335.
3. Sangkomkamhang US, Lumbiganon P, Pattanittum P. Progestogens or progestogen—releasing intrauterine systems for uterine fibroids (other than preoperative medical therapy). *Cochrane Database Syst Rev*. 2020;11(11):CD008994. doi:10.1002/14651858.CD008994.pub3.

ADDITIONAL READING

- Centers for Disease Control and Prevention. About bleeding disorders in women. https://www.cdc.gov/female-blood-disorders/about/index.html. Accessed September 8, 2025.
- Centers for Disease Control and Prevention. Materials about signs and symptoms. https://www.cdc.gov/female-blood-disorders/communication-resources/signs-and-symptoms.html. Accessed September 8, 2025.
- Cheong Y, Cameron IT, Critchley HOD. Abnormal uterine bleeding. *Br Med Bull*. 2019;131(1):119.
- Committee on Practice Bulletins—Gynecology. Practice bulletin no. 128: diagnosis of abnormal uterine bleeding in reproductive-aged women. *Obstet Gynecol*. 2012;120(1):197–206.
- Hill S, Shetty MK. Abnormal uterine bleeding in reproductive age women: role of imaging in the diagnosis and management. *Semin Ultrasound CT MR*. 2023;44(6):511–518.

CODES

ICD10

- N92.0 Excessive and frequent menstruation with regular cycle
- N92.3 Ovulation bleeding
- N92.2 Excessive menstruation at puberty

CLINICAL PEARLS

- HMB is often associated with a structural uterine disorder.
- A thorough history and PE is a key part of determining the cause of AUB.
- Additional tests and imaging may be warranted depending on the suspected etiology.
- Treatment is based on etiology, desire for fertility, and medical comorbidities.
- The goal of initial therapy is to stop bleeding, treat anemia, and restore quality of life.
- Women >45 years of age or <45 years of age with risk factors for malignancy require endometrial sampling.
- Up to 20% of women with HMB may have underlying coagulation disorder.
- Progestin-only contraception may be considered to suppress menstruation.
- Patients with Hx of SARS and/or COVID-19 may also report changes in their menstrual cycle.

ABNORMAL PAP AND CERVICAL DYSPLASIA

Anna K. Zheng, MD • Leigh Weatherly, DO • Jeremy Golding, MD, FAAFP

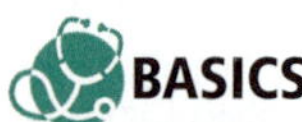

BASICS

DESCRIPTION

- Cervical dysplasia: precancerous epithelial changes in the transformation zone of the uterine cervix and endocervical canal associated with persistent infection of high-risk human papillomavirus (HPV) types; potential precursor to invasive disease
- Cervical intraepithelial neoplasia or CIN encompasses a range of histologic findings. Biopsy material is typically obtained from colposcopy after an abnormal Pap smear result.
  - CIN I: mild dysplasia; low-grade lesion; cellular changes are limited to the lower 1/3 of the squamous epithelium.
  - CIN II: moderate dysplasia; high-grade lesion; cellular changes are limited to the lower 2/3 of the squamous epithelium.
  - CIN III or carcinoma in situ: severe dysplasia; high-grade lesion; cellular changes involve the full thickness of the squamous epithelium.
- System(s) affected: reproductive

Pediatric Considerations

Fewer than 0.1% of cervical cancers occur before age 21 years. Screening any asymptomatic individual with a cervix age <21 years is not recommended (1),(2).

Geriatric Considerations

- Screening any immunocompetent individual with a cervix and age >65 years who has had adequate prior screening and no history of CIN II+ in the last 25 years is not recommended (3).
- Screening should continue beyond age 65 years per 2019 ASCCP Risk-Based Management Consensus Guidelines if there is risk for invasive disease (3),(4).

Pregnancy Considerations

- CIN diagnosed during pregnancy is most often stable or regresses postpartum, with regression rates reported between 39% and 69% in various cohorts (5).
- Colposcopy without endocervical sampling is recommended to exclude the presence of invasive cancer in high-risk individuals.
- Management is conservative, with treatment deferred until postpartum unless there is suspicion of invasive disease (6).

EPIDEMIOLOGY

Incidence of CIN III peaks between ages 25 and 29 years; invasive disease peaks 15 years later. Cervical cancer most commonly occurs in those aged 35 to 44 years. >15% of cervical cancer cases occur in those >65 years of age (occurs in those who did not get regular screening). Each year in the United States 14,000 new cases of cervical cancer are diagnosed, approximately 100,000 people are treated for cervical dysplasia, and 4,000 die of cervical cancer (3),(6).

Incidence

The age-adjusted incidence rate in the United States is approximately 11.5 per 100,000 women aged 15 to 75 years (1),(3),(6).

Prevalence

In the United States, the prevalence of cervical cancer is much lower due to widespread screening and HPV vaccination, per drop in incidence rate. Globally, cervical cancer remains the fourth most common cancer in women, and the leading cause of cancer-related death in women in several regions of sub-Saharan Africa (6).

ETIOLOGY AND PATHOPHYSIOLOGY

Transient HPV infection among sexually active individuals is very common.

- High-risk HPV types: 16, 18, 45, 31, 33, 35, 39, 51, 52, 56, 58, 59, and 68 together account for >95% of cervical cancer cases, although 16 and 18 account for 70% of cases (3) types for cervical cancer.
- Most HPV infections are transient, becoming undetectable within 1 to 2 years. Persistent infections are what place women at significant risk for developing precancerous lesions. Compared to younger women, women age >30 years are less likely to clear a new HPV infection.
- Low-risk types: HPV viral types 6, 11, 42, 43, and 44 are considered common low-risk types and may cause genital warts. HPV 6 and 11 (cause 90% of benign anogenital warts) can lead to low-grade squamous intraepithelial lesion (LSIL) and CIN I.

RISK FACTORS

- HIV infection and other immunosuppressive conditions
- In utero exposure to diethylstilbestrol
- Multiple sexual partners and partners with multiple partners
- Early age at first intercourse
- Lack of access to screening
- History of abnormal Pap smears, HPV infection, CIN, STI or a combination of these
- Increased risk associated with low socioeconomic status, tobacco use, high parity, oral contraceptive use (6)

GENERAL PREVENTION

Immunization: Immunization decreases high-risk HPV infections, CIN II/III cervical pathology, and invasive cervical cancer. Per the Advisory Committee on Immunization Practices (ACIP), offer HPV vaccine to adolescents 11 to 12 years of age and can start vaccination as early as 9 years old. Gardasil 9: The U.S. Food and Drug Administration (FDA) approved in October 2018 for use in females and males ages 9 to 26 years and via shared clinical decision for ages 27 to 45 years; 88% effective preventing dysplasia due to HPV types 16 and 18 (75% of cervical cancer), types 6 and 11 (anogenital warts), and protection against five additional HPV types, which cause approximately 25% of CIN II+ lesions. Current studies show maximum benefit from vaccination when administered before 14 years of age, prior to first sexual intercourse, and shared decision-making is recommended for vaccination of individuals ages 27 to 45 years because vaccination in this age group is not expected to be effective nor cost-effective of cancer prevention on a population level (3).

- Vaccine schedule: Only 2 doses are required when the first dose is given before 15 years of age, 6 to 12 months apart. 3 doses are recommended at interval of 0, 2, and 6 months when the first dose is given at ≥15 years of age.
- Immunocompromising conditions: 3 doses needed
- Safe sex practices: condom use; advise smoking cessation.
- Screening
  - Pap smear has been the main screening test for cervical cellular pathology, with or without cotesting for HPV.
  - Screening recommendations by age and source with follow-up for abnormal results: See algorithms "Cervical Cancer Screening (Pap): Normal and Abnormal in Women Ages 21–24 Years," "Cervical Cancer Screening (Pap): Normal and Abnormal in Nonpregnant Women Ages 25–29 Years and Older," "Cervical Cancer Screening (Pap): Normal and Abnormal in Average-risk, Nonpregnant Women Ages 30–65 Years" (1),(3) (USPSTF/ASCCP/ACOG).
  - Frequency of screening recommendation for average risk: USPSTF/ASCCP/ACOG generally agree by age and screen, but several guidelines are under revision in 2025. In general:
    - <21 years: Do not screen.
    - 21 to 29 years: Screen with cytology alone every 3 years American Cancer Society (ACS) primary HPV testing every 5 years starting at age 25 is preferred.
    - 30 to 65 years: "primary" HPV testing alone (with an FDA-approved assay for this purpose), HPV testing with cytology (cotesting) every 5 years or cytology alone every 3 years (3),(6)
    - >65 years who have had adequate prior screening, immunocompetent and average risk: Do not screen (1),(3).
  - 2020 ACS guidelines: recommends beginning screening at the age of 25 years and prefers primary HPV testing alone (2) if available; ages 21 to 24 years: no screening (3)
- Special circumstances: patients after hysterectomy with removal of the cervix and with no history of CIN II+ in past 25 years: Do not screen (1),(3).
- HIV-positive patients: Centers for Disease Control and Prevention (CDC) recommends to initiate screening with a Pap test within 1 year of sexual debut but no later than age 21, or at the time of HIV diagnosis if not previously screened; ages 21 to 29 years: screen annually until three consecutive negative test results, then every 3 years; age ≥30 years for life: annual Pap testing with HPV cotesting (preferred); if both cytology and HPV are negative, screening can be every 3 years.

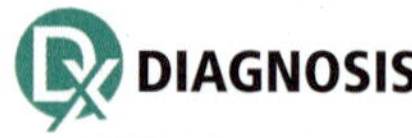

DIAGNOSIS

HISTORY

Usually asymptomatic until there is invasive disease

PHYSICAL EXAM

Exam with or with speculum occasionally may reveal external HPV lesions. Examine for exophytic or ulcerative cervical lesions, with or without bleeding.

DIFFERENTIAL DIAGNOSIS

Acute or chronic cervicitis secondary to infectious or noninfectious causes (e.g., peri- or postmenopause); cervical glandular hyperplasia; uterine malignancy

DIAGNOSTIC TESTS & INTERPRETATION

- ThinPrep is a liquid-based cytology method favored over conventional collection by reducing obscuring factors such as blood, inflammation, and poor fixation.
- Sample both the ectocervix and endocervix with cytobrush and spatula.
- Cervicovaginal primary HPV testing alone is >95% sensitive for detecting precancer, although sensitivity of cytology alone is 50–70%. In 2025, the only HPV tests approved by the FDA for primary HPV testing in cervical cancer screening are the Cobas HPV test (Roche Molecular Diagnostics) and the Onclarity HPV test (Becton Dickinson). These tests have a sensitivity for high-grade cervical abnormalities of 95–99%. The sensitivity and specificity of assays approved for HPV cotesting (HPV and cytology testing together) demonstrate a similar or slightly lower sensitivity, but specificity for high-grade lesions is lower than with primary HPV assays, resulting in somewhat more false positives.
- Cytology: Bethesda 2014 system (cytologic grading) of epithelial cell abnormalities: Report specimen *Adequacy* and *general categorization*; adequacy (amount of cellular material), presence or absence of endocervical cells, and specimen type (conventional or liquid based); categorization negative for intraepithelial lesion or malignancy (NILM) versus epithelial cell abnormality:
  - Squamous cell abnormalities:
    - Atypical squamous cells (ASCs) (of undetermined significance [ASC US]; ASCs cannot exclude high-grade squamous intraepithelial lesion or HSIL [ASC-H])
    - Low-grade squamous intraepithelial lesion (LSIL): encompasses HPV/mild dysplasia/CIN I
- HSIL: encompasses moderate/severe dysplasia, carcinoma in situ, CIN II and CIN III
- Glandular cell abnormalities:
  - Atypical glandular cells (AGCs): favor neoplasia, or not otherwise specified
  - AGCs: AIS adenocarcinoma in situ (AIS), adenocarcinoma

Diagnostic Procedures/Other

- Clinical action depends on immediate risk of CIN III+ for cases age ≥25 years (4). See "https://www.asccp.org/management-guidelines or ASCCP smartphone app" and "https://www.asccp.org/mobile-app" The 2019 ASCCP guideline differentiates between those aged 21 to 24, 25 to 29, and 30 years and older.
- The following algorithms are based upon ASCCP risk estimates:
  - Cervical Cancer Screening (Pap): Normal and Abnormal in Women Ages 21–24 Years
  - Cervical Cancer Screening (Pap): Normal and Abnormal in Nonpregnant Women Ages 25–29 Years and Older
  - Cervical Cancer Screening (Pap): Normal and Abnormal in Average-risk, Nonpregnant Women Ages 30–65 Years

Test Interpretation

Atypical squamous or columnar cells, coarse nuclear material, increased nuclear diameter, koilocytosis (HPV hallmark)

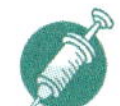

TREATMENT

ASCCP smart-phone application includes 2019 guidelines: Evidence-based management phone application includes algorithms to guide Pap smear and post-colposcopic diagnostics and therapeutics are available online at https://www.asccp.org/mobile-app and https://www.asccp.org/management-guidelines (4).

GENERAL MEASURES

Office evaluation and observation; promote smoking cessation; promote safe sex ectocervix practices; promote immunization.

MEDICATION

Infective/reactive Pap smear: Treat organism/condition found on Pap smear results. Condyloma acuminatum treatment options: See chapter "Condylomata Acuminata."

SURGERY/OTHER PROCEDURES

- Expedited treatment that bypasses colposcopy biopsy is recommended for nonpregnant patients ≥25 years of age with immediate CIN III+ risk of >60% and is acceptable for immediate CIN III+ risk between 25% and 60%, although stressing the importance of shared decision-making (4).
- Observation is preferred to treatment for CIN I (4). Colposcopy can be deferred for certain patients and repeat HPV testing or cotesting in 1 year is recommended if immediate CIN III+ risk is low (<4%).
- Excisional treatment (e.g., loop electroexcision, LEEP) is preferred to ablative treatment for histologic HSIL (CIN 2 or CIN 3). For AIS, excision is recommended (4).
- If cervical malignancy, see "Cervical Malignancy."

ONGOING CARE

FOLLOW-UP RECOMMENDATIONS

After successful treatment (excision or ablation) and initial posttreatment management, individuals should reenter screening with HPV testing or cotesting at 3-year intervals for at least 25 years (4).

PATIENT EDUCATION

HPV vaccination, smoking cessation, protected intercourse, regular screening with Pap smear per guidelines

PROGNOSIS

- Progression of CIN to invasive cervical cancer is slow, and the likelihood of regression is high: Up to 43% of CIN II and 32% of CIN III lesions may regress. CIN III has a 30% probability of becoming invasive cancer over a 30-year period, although only about 1% if treated. Lesions discovered early are amenable to treatment with excellent results and few recurrences.
- The 5-year survival rate for cervical cancer patients is 66.3%. The 5-year relative survival rate for patients diagnosed with localized disease is 91.9%.

COMPLICATIONS

Aggressive cervical surgery may be associated with cervical stenosis, cervical incompetence (leading to preterm labor), and scarring affecting cervical dilatation in labor.

REFERENCES

1. Curry SJ, Krist AH, Owens DK, et al. Screening for cervical cancer: U.S. Preventive Services Task Force recommendation statement. *JAMA*. 2018;320(7):674–686.
2. Fontham ETH, Wolf AMD, Church TR, et al. Cervical cancer screening for individuals at average risk: 2020 guideline update from the American Cancer Society. *CA Cancer J Clin*. 2020;70(5):321–346.
3. Perkins RB, Wentzensen N, Guido RS, et al. Cervical cancer screening: a review. *JAMA*. 2023;330(6):547–558.
4. Perkins RB, Guido RS, Castle PE, et al. 2019 ASCCP risk-based management consensus guidelines for abnormal cervical cancer screening tests and cancer precursors. *J Low Genit Tract Dis*. 2020;24(2):102–131.
5. Larish A, Long ME. Diagnosis and management of cervical squamous intraepithelial lesions in pregnancy and postpartum. *Obstet Gynecol*. 2024;144(3):328–338.
6. Tewari KS. Cervical cancer. *N Engl J Med*. 2025;392(1):56–71.

ADDITIONAL READING

American Society for Colposcopy and Cervical Pathology. ASCCP diagnostic and management guidelines. https://www.asccp.org/management-guidelines. Accessed September 8, 2025.

SEE ALSO

- Cervical Malignancy; Condylomata Acuminata; Trichomoniasis; Vulvovaginitis, Prepubescent
- Algorithms: Cervical Cancer Screening (Pap): Normal and Abnormal in Nonpregnant Women Ages 25–29 Years and Older; Cervical Cancer Screening (Pap): Normal and Abnormal in Women Ages 21–24 Years; Cervical Cancer Screening (Pap): Normal and Abnormal in Average-risk, Nonpregnant Women Ages 30–65 Years

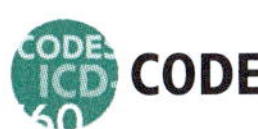

CODES

ICD10

- R87.619 Unspecified abnormal cytological findings in specimens from cervix uteri
- N87.9 Dysplasia of cervix uteri, unspecified
- N87.1 Moderate cervical dysplasia

CLINICAL PEARLS

- Vaccine should be offered prior to onset of sexual activity for maximum effectiveness.
- Know and adhere to recognized screening guidelines to avoid the harms of over screening.
- Optimal screening strategy is in evolution. HPV-only screening using an approved assay is now preferred to cytology or cotesting strategies, but the approved assays are not yet widely available in 2025.

ACETAMINOPHEN POISONING

Janet Chen, DO

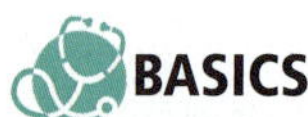

BASICS

DESCRIPTION

- A disorder characterized by hepatic necrosis following large acetaminophen ingestions. Clinical manifestations of acetaminophen toxicity vary with time of ingestion and are generally classified into four stages.
- Single, large ingestions of acetaminophen account for a majority of poisonings. Toxicity can also occur with ingestions of lesser amounts in individuals who regularly abuse alcohol, are chronically malnourished, or take medications impacting hepatic metabolism. Ingestions >12 g in adults and >250 mg/kg in children are likely to cause toxicity.

EPIDEMIOLOGY

- Two-thirds of hospitalizations due to acetaminophen toxicity are due to intentional ingestion. Most (80%) are adults, and 70% are women. 50% of poison control calls related to acetaminophen are related to unintentional ingestions in children <5 years old.
- The second leading factor associated with liver transplantation worldwide
- >50,000 emergency department visits, >2,500 hospitalizations, and nearly 500 deaths annually in the United States are associated with acetaminophen ingestion.

Prevalence

In 2021, >80,000 calls to US poison control centers reinvolved acetaminophen products.

ETIOLOGY AND PATHOPHYSIOLOGY

- Pharmacokinetics
  - With oral therapeutic ingestion, acetaminophen is entirely absorbed from the duodenum and reaches peak serum concentrations of 10 to 20 μg/mL after up to 2 hours. This peak may be delayed with toxic ingestions.
  - Therapeutic adult doses of acetaminophen are 325 to 1,000 mg q4–6h to a maximum dose of 4 g/day. Therapeutic pediatric doses are 10 to 15 mg/kg q4–6h, not to exceed 5 doses in 24 hours or 75 g/kg/day.
  - The elimination half-life of acetaminophen ranges from 2 to 4 hours but may be delayed in extended-release formulation.
- Pathophysiology
  - Ingestion of supratherapeutic doses of acetaminophen or subtherapeutic ingestions in individuals with compromised liver function can cause acetaminophen poisoning and result in hepatocellular damage. The liver metabolizes 96% of ingested acetaminophen and 2–4% is excreted in urine. Therapeutic doses break down into 90–95% benign metabolites and 5–10% of the toxic metabolite, N-acetyl-p-benzoquinone imine (NAPQI). NAPQI is rapidly conjugated with hepatic stores of glutathione to form a nontoxic metabolite to be excreted in the urine. Toxic ingestions of acetaminophen saturate the glucuronidation and sulfation pathways, depleting glutathione stores and result in accumulations of NAPQI that cause hepatocellular damage.

RISK FACTORS

Concurrent poisoning with other hepatotoxic substances; psychiatric illness or history of suicide attempts; ingestion of large amounts of alcohol; chronic malnutrition and risk related to previous weight loss surgery

GENERAL PREVENTION

- Poison Control: 800-222-1222 for consultations and management guidance
- U.S. Food and Drug Administration labeling guidance: https://www.fda.gov/Drugs/GuidanceCompliance-RegulatoryInformation/Guidances/default.htm

Geriatric Considerations

There is an increased risk of hepatic damage in elderly patients due to decreased hepatic metabolism and co-ingestion of other hepatotoxic medications. Recommendation is to limit acetaminophen to ≤3,000 mg/day in seniors and in patients with liver disease and/or alcohol abuse disorders.

Pediatric Considerations

Hepatic damage after ingestion of toxic acetaminophen doses can be less severe in young children, potentially because they have more stores of glutathione.

Pregnancy Considerations

There is an increased incidence of spontaneous abortion in pregnant patients with acetaminophen poisoning. Abortion incidence and possible fetal death is increased if *N*-acetylcysteine (NAC) treatment is delayed. IV NAC is generally preferred in pregnancy due to greater bioavailability.

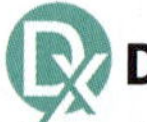

DIAGNOSIS

Signs and symptoms of poisoning develop over the first 24 hours following large ingestions. Presentation of symptoms varies, and it is divided into four stages:

- Stage 1—first 24 hours after ingestion
  - Patient may be asymptomatic in first 8 hours following ingestion. Symptoms may include nausea, emesis, anorexia, and diaphoresis. Laboratory results are usually unremarkable at this time.
- Stage 2—days 2 to 3 following ingestion
  - Typically less nausea, vomiting, diaphoresis, and malaise than in stage 1. Right upper quadrant pain and hepatomegaly may become evident. Elevated aminotransferases are usually seen.
- Stage 3—days 3 to 4 following ingestion
  - Stage 1 symptoms reappear. Severe poisonings may result in jaundice, confusion, somnolence, and coma. Marked liver enzyme elevations, peak at this point; prolonged prothrombin time (PT)/international normalized ratio (INR); typically negative acetaminophen levels. Multiorgan failure and death most commonly occur in this stage.
- Stage 4—days 5+ after ingestion
  - Possible recovery stage in patients with resolving stage 3 symptoms. Recovery may be prolonged, but is typically without long-term sequelae. Laboratory abnormalities typically resolve. Fulminant hepatic failure occurs in <1% of adults and is rare in children <6 years of age.

HISTORY

Focus on specific ingestion (extended release, hydrocodone-acetaminophen, coingestants, etc.), how much, what time, other medical history?

PHYSICAL EXAM

In general, a full physical examination is warranted.

- Assess individual's appearance for somnolence, fatigue, pallor, diaphoresis, and signs of dehydration.
- Signs of hepatotoxicity: hepatomegaly and right upper quadrant pain

DIFFERENTIAL DIAGNOSIS

- Consider coingestants: alcohol, opiates, and/or aspirin.
- Other ingested toxins that produce severe acute hepatic injury, includes the mushroom *Amanita phalloides* and products containing yellow phosphorus or carbon tetrachloride; other causes of hepatitis: alcoholic, viral, ischemic

DIAGNOSTIC TESTS & INTERPRETATION

Initial Tests (lab, imaging)

- Draw plasma acetaminophen levels on all patients ≥4 hours after ingestion (levels peak at 4 hours). Draw labs at 6 and 8 hours if extended-release form was ingested. Poison Control may help guide the frequency of exams and vitals and provide other recommendations.
  - If a sustained-released product has been ingested, obtain two serum acetaminophen levels 4 to 6 hours apart. Treat if either level is above the possible toxicity line.
  - For chronic toxicity or patients who present 24 hours post ingestion, treat based on clinical effects, LFTs, and the acetaminophen level.
- Liver function tests: alanine transaminase (ALT), aspartate transaminase (AST), PT/INR, bilirubin, lactate dehydrogenase (LDH)
  - With severe poisonings, PT/INR rise in parallel with LFT changes. With toxic ingestions, AST, ALT, and bilirubin levels begin to rise in stage 2 and peak in stage 3. Improvement in ALT with therapy is an encouraging clinical sign.
- Additional labs: electrolytes, glucose, BUN, creatinine, urinalysis, urine drug screen (UDS), serum alcohol and salicylate.
  - Screen for coingestants with the above labs and consider searching for other medications/substances depending upon the clinical history. Obtain a pregnancy screen (urine or serum) as it can influence management.
  - Consider an arterial blood gas (ABG): anion gap metabolic acidosis due to accumulation of 5-oxoproline may rarely be seen.

Follow-Up Tests & Special Considerations

During recovery, liver tests should normalize and complete restoration of liver function without long-term sequelae is expected.

Diagnostic Procedures/Other

Advanced imaging of the liver and/or kidney with ultrasound or CT should be considered when acute hepatitis or kidney injury is present to rule out alternative causes. Otherwise, imaging is not required and any abnormal findings, if present, may be nonspecific.

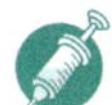

TREATMENT

- Immediately contact a local Poison Control center for recommendations. Call (800) 222-1222 in the United States.
- NAC is a benign prodrug that provides cysteine as a substrate to detoxify acetaminophen metabolites and replenish glutathione stores in the liver. NAC administration may reduce mortality from 5% to 0.7%.
- The Rumack-Matthew nomogram:
  - A plot used to determine if acetaminophen levels are high enough to warrant treatment with NAC during acute toxic ingestions. The nomogram is not intended for sustained-release products or chronic ingestions.
  - Give NAC when acetaminophen plasma levels measured ≥4 hours after ingestion are at the "treatment line" or higher on the Rumack-Matthew nomogram.
  - Treatment line acetaminophen plasma levels on the nomogram correspond to >150 μg/mL (993 μmol/L), >75 μg/mL (497 μmol/L), and >37 μg/mL (244 μmol/L) at 4, 8, and 12 hours after ingestion, respectively.
- Initiate NAC (Mucomyst) within 8 hours of ingestion whenever possible; single-dose activated charcoal (1 g/kg PO) may be effective if given within 1 to 4 hours of ingestion. *Never* delay oral NAC for activated charcoal.
- Ipecac and gastric lavage are no longer recommended for routine use at home or in health care facilities (1).

MEDICATION

First Line

- Empirically start NAC within 8 hours prior to lab results. It may be effective up to ≥36 hours after ingestion.
  - NAC may be given PO or IV, depending on situation and availability. IV NAC has been shown to decrease the length of hospitalization compared to PO NAC (1).
  - A two-bag regimen should be used to administer a total of 300 mg/kg IV NAC (Acetadote, Cetylev) over a 20-hour period to reduce adverse effects of NAC administration. Begin with a 200 mg/kg IV dose over 4 hours followed by a 100 mg/kg IV dose over 16 hours.
  - Use an oral loading dose of 140 mg/kg and then 70 mg/kg q4h for 17 additional doses (72-hour regimen).
- NAC precautions:
  - PO NAC may cause significant nausea and vomiting due to its sulfur content and is often poorly tolerated; consider a nasogastric tube.
  - IV NAC (Acetadote) may cause anaphylactoid reactions, (3–6%) including rash, bronchospasm, pruritus, angioedema, tachycardia, or hypotension (higher rates seen in asthmatics and those with atopy). Reactions usually occur with the loading dose. To prevent this, slow or temporarily stop the infusion; may concurrently treat with antihistamines.
  - Nausea can be treated with metoclopramide, 1 to 2 mg/kg IV, or ondansetron, 0.15 mg/kg IV.
  - NAC failure rates range from 3–7% (1).
- Give single-dose activated charcoal within 1 to 4 hours of ingestion (especially in cases of coingestants). Do not delay NAC administration for use of activated charcoal.

Second Line

In massive ingestions (levels >1,000 mg/L, severe acidosis, coma/hypotension) or when severe renal failure is present, hemodialysis may improve survival (1).

ISSUES FOR REFERRAL

- Behavioral health evaluation for intentional ingestions
- Child abuse reporting if neglect led to overdose

ADMISSION, INPATIENT, AND NURSING CONSIDERATIONS

- Consider hospitalization for toxic ingestions with vital instability and/or laboratory abnormalities. Consider transfer to a psychiatric facility for intentional ingestions when medically stable.
- IV fluids are generally provided for hydration purposes.

ONGOING CARE

FOLLOW-UP RECOMMENDATIONS

- Evaluate all patients at an accredited health care facility. Evaluate patients with evidence of organ failure, increased LFTs, or coagulopathy for emergency liver transplant (ELT) at a transplant center.
- Restrict activity if hepatic damage is significant. Outpatient management is adequate for nontoxic accidental ingestions.

DIET

No special diet, except with severe hepatic damage

PATIENT EDUCATION

Counsel patients to avoid acetaminophen (Tylenol, others) or other forms of acetaminophen, particularly if using combination product(s) containing acetaminophen. Educate parents/caregivers during well-child visits regarding appropriate OTC dosing and medication storage. Educate patients on long-term acetaminophen therapy.

PROGNOSIS

- Complete recovery with early therapy is possible.
- 10% of adult patients with severe liver complications develop necrosis, hepatic encephalopathy, or require transplant.
- Hepatic failure is rare in children <6 years of age.

COMPLICATIONS

Recovery after acute poisoning is complete and sequelae are rare.

REFERENCES

1. Chiew AL, Gluud C, Brok J, et al. Interventions for paracetamol (acetaminophen) overdose. *Cochrane Database Syst Rev*. 2018;2(2):CD003328.

ADDITIONAL READING

Dart RC, Mullins ME, Matoushek T, et al. Management of acetaminophen poisoning in the US and Canada: a consensus statement. *JAMA Netw Open*. 2023;6(8):e2327739. doi:10.1001/jamanetworkopen.2023.27739.

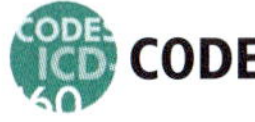

CODES

ICD10

- T39.1X4A Poisoning by 4-Aminophenol derivatives, undetermined, init
- K71.10 Toxic liver disease with hepatic necrosis, without coma
- T39.1X1A Poisoning by 4-Aminophenol derivatives, accidental, init

CLINICAL PEARLS

- Immediately call local Poison Control Center for management recommendations (800) 222-1222 United States.
- Give NAC when plasma acetaminophen concentrations (measured ≥4 hours after ingestion) are in the possible risk or higher levels. This corresponds to acetaminophen levels >150 μg/mL (993 μmol/L), >75 μg/mL (497 μmol/L), and >37 μg/mL (265 μmol/L) at 4, 8, and 12 hours after ingestion, respectively.
- Start NAC within 8 hours of ingestion for best chance of hepatic protection. Empirically give NAC in patients presenting near 8 hours. A two-bag IV dosing regimen over 20 hours is preferred.
- All patients with acetaminophen liver injury (even after 8 hours) should receive NAC.
- If using oral NAC, dilute with a palatable beverage. Serve in a cup with lid and straw.
- For extended-release acetaminophen, follow plasma levels at 4, 6, and 8 hours after ingestion. Start NAC if any level is elevated.

ACNE ROSACEA

Jennifer M. Romeu, MD, FAAFP, MSM

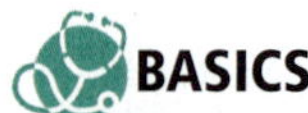

BASICS

DESCRIPTION

- Rosacea is a chronic condition characterized by recurrent and sometimes fixed episodes of facial flushing, erythema (due to dilatation of small blood vessels in the face), papules, pustules, and telangiectasia (due to increased reactivity of capillaries) in a symmetric, central facial distribution; sometimes associated with ocular symptoms (ocular rosacea)
- Four subtypes:
  - Erythematotelangiectatic rosacea (ETR)
  - Papulopustular rosacea (PPR)
  - Phymatous rosacea
  - Ocular rosacea
- System(s) affected: skin/exocrine
- Synonym(s): rosacea

Geriatric Considerations

- Chronic inflammatory dermatosis with middle-age onset
- Effects of aging might increase the side effects associated with oral used for treatment (at present, data are insufficient due to lack of clinical studies in elderly patients aged ≥65 years).

EPIDEMIOLOGY

Prevalence

- Predominant age of onset: 30 to 50 years
- Predominant sex: female > male. However, males are at greater risk for progression to later stages.
- More common in Fitzpatrick skin types I and II, however, it may be underreported in other skin types due to background pigmentation. This may lead to a delay in diagnosis for patients with darker skin types (1).

ETIOLOGY AND PATHOPHYSIOLOGY

- No proven cause
- Possibilities include the following:
  - Thyroid and sex hormone disturbance
  - Immune system and neurocutaneous dysregulation (2)
  - Alcohol, coffee, tea, spiced food overindulgence (unproven)
  - Demodex follicular parasite (suspected)
  - Exposure to cold, heat
  - Emotional stress
  - Dysfunction of the GI tract (possible association with *Helicobacter pylori*)

Genetics

- People of Northern European and Celtic background commonly afflicted
- Associated with three human leukocyte antigen (HLA) alleles: HLA-DRB1, HLA-DQB1, and HLA-DQA1 (MHC class II)

RISK FACTORS

- Exposure to spicy foods, hot drinks
- Environmental factors: sun, wind, cold, heat

GENERAL PREVENTION

No preventive measures known however avoidance of patient specific triggers can minimize severity of flare ups (3).

COMMONLY ASSOCIATED CONDITIONS

- Seborrheic dermatitis of scalp and eyelids
- Keratitis with photophobia, lacrimation, visual disturbance
- Corneal lesions
- Blepharitis
- Uveitis

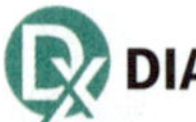

DIAGNOSIS

HISTORY

- Usually have a history of episodic flushing with increases in skin temperature in response to heat stimulus in mouth (hot liquids), spicy foods, alcohol, sun exposure
- Acne may have preceded onset of rosacea by years; nevertheless, rosacea usually arises de novo without preceding history of acne or seborrhea.
- Excessive facial warmth and redness are the predominant presenting complaints. Itching is generally absent.

PHYSICAL EXAM

- Rosacea has four subtypes:
  - The rosacea diathesis: episodic erythema, "flushing and blushing"
  - ETR: persistent erythema with telangiectases
  - PPR: persistent erythema, telangiectases, papules, pustules
  - Phymatous: persistent deep erythema, dense telangiectases, papules, pustules, nodules; rarely persistent "solid" edema of the central part of the face (phymatous)
- Progression from one subtype to another is hypothetical.
- Facial erythema, particularly on cheeks, nose, and chin; at times, entire face may be involved.
- Inflammatory papules are prominent; pustules and telangiectasia may be present.
- Comedones are absent (unlike acne vulgaris).
- Women usually have lesions on the chin and cheeks, whereas the nose is commonly involved in men.
- Ocular findings (mild dryness and irritation with blepharitis, conjunctival injection, burning, stinging, tearing, eyelid inflammation, swelling, and redness) are present in 50% of patients.

DIFFERENTIAL DIAGNOSIS

- Drug eruptions (iodides and bromides)
- Granulomas of the skin
- Cutaneous lupus erythematosus
- Carcinoid syndrome
- Acne vulgaris
- Seborrheic dermatitis
- Steroid rosacea (abuse)
- Systemic lupus erythematosus
- Lupus pernio (sarcoidosis)

DIAGNOSTIC TESTS & INTERPRETATION

- Diagnosis is based on physical exam findings.
- A recent change in classification has been proposed based on the phenotype that reflects the clinical presentation and to better focus treatment options, which are targeted to address the main clinical presentation.

Test Interpretation

Histology of affected skin may reveal:

- Inflammation around hypertrophied sebaceous glands, producing papules, pustules, and cysts
- Absence of comedones and blocked ducts
- Vascular dilatation and dermal lymphocytic infiltrate
- Granulomatous inflammation

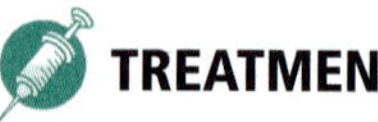

TREATMENT

GENERAL MEASURES

- Proper skin care and photoprotection are important components of management plan. Use of mild, nondrying soap is recommended; local skin irritants should be avoided.
- Avoidance of triggers
- Reassurance that rosacea is completely unrelated to poor hygiene
- Treat psychological stress if present.
- Topical steroids should not be used because they may aggravate rosacea.
- Establishing a skin care routine (4)
  - Avoid oil-based cosmetics. Others are acceptable and may help women tolerate symptoms.
- Electrodesiccation or chemical sclerosis of permanently dilated blood vessels
- Possible evolving laser therapy
- Support physical fitness.

MEDICATION

First Line

- Topical metronidazole preparations
  - Once (1% formulation) or twice (0.75% formulations) daily for 7 to 12 weeks was significantly more effective than placebo in patients with moderate to severe rosacea. A rosacea treatment system (cleanser, metronidazole 0.75% gel, hydrating complexion corrector, and sunscreen SPF 30) may offer superior efficacy and tolerability to metronidazole (5).
- Topical azelaic acid (Finacea) 15% gel
  - Very effective as initial therapy for PPR subtype; topical alone is effective for maintenance.
- Topical ivermectin 1% cream
  - Recently found to be more effective than metronidazole for treatment of PPR
  - Upregulates anti-inflammatory cytokine IL-10 and has anti-parasitic activity against *Demodex folliculorum*
- Topical brimonidine tartrate 0.5% gel
  - Effective in reducing erythema associated with ETR subtype
  - α_2-Adrenergic receptor agonist; potent vasoconstrictor
- Topical oxymetazoline 1% cream
  - α_{1A}-Adrenergic receptor agonist recently approved for the treatment of persistent erythema associated with rosacea in adults
- Oral doxycycline 40 mg dose
  - As effective as 100-mg dose and has a correspondingly lower risk of adverse effects but is much more expensive
  - Precautions: Tetracyclines may cause photosensitivity; sunscreen is recommended.
  - Significant possible interactions:
    - Tetracyclines: Avoid concurrent administration with antacids, dairy products, or iron.
    - Broad-spectrum antibiotics: may reduce the effectiveness of oral contraceptives; however, this finding has only been confirmed with rifampin; consider adding barrier method.

Second Line

- Topical erythromycin
- Topical timolol maleate 0.5%
- Topical clindamycin (lotion preferred)
  - Can be used in combination with benzoyl peroxide; commercial topical combinations are available.
- Possible use of calcineurin inhibitors (tacrolimus 0.1%; pimecrolimus 1%).
  - Pimecrolimus 1% is effective to treat mild to moderate inflammatory rosacea.
- Topical permethrin 5% cream
  - Similar efficacy compared to metronidazole for severe cases
- Oral isotretinoin at 0.3 mg/kg for a minimum of 3 months
  - Can be used to treat ETR/PPR recalcitrant to other treatments

Pediatric Considerations

Tetracyclines: not for use in children <8 years of age

Pregnancy Considerations

- Tetracyclines: not for use during pregnancy
- Isotretinoin: teratogenic; not for use during pregnancy or in women of reproductive age who are not using reliable contraception; requires registration with iPLEDGE program

ADDITIONAL THERAPIES

Cyclosporine 0.05% ophthalmic emulsion may be more effective than artificial tears for ocular rosacea.

SURGERY/OTHER PROCEDURES

Laser treatment is an option for progressive telangiectasias or rhinophyma.

- Pulsed dye laser (585 nm or 595 nm) is effective in treating telangiectases and erythema.
- CO_2 fractional ablative laser can be used to treat rhinophyma.
- Potassium titanyl phosphate (KTP) laser is effective for treating telangiectases.

ONGOING CARE

FOLLOW-UP RECOMMENDATIONS

Outpatient treatment

Patient Monitoring

- Occasional and as needed
- Close follow-up and laboratory assessment for patients using isotretinoin per prescribing instructions and iPLEDGE program guidance
- Consider ophthalmology evaluation in patients with ocular symptoms.

DIET

Avoid alcohol and hot drinks of any type.

PROGNOSIS

- Slowly progressive
- Subsides spontaneously (sometimes)

COMPLICATIONS

- Rhinophyma (dilated follicles and thickened bulbous skin on nose), especially in men
- Conjunctivitis
- Blepharitis
- Keratitis
- Visual deterioration

REFERENCES

1. Maruthappu T, Taylor M. Acne and rosacea in skin of colour. *Clin Exp Dermatol*. 2022;47(2):259–263. doi:10.1111/ced.14994.
2. van Zuuren EJ, Arents BWM, van der Linden MMD, et al. Rosacea: new concepts in classification and treatment. *Am J Clin Dermatol*. 2021;22(4):457–465. doi:10.1007/s40257-021-00595-7.
3. Goh CL, Wu Y, Welsh B, et al. Expert consensus on holistic skin care routine: focus on acne, rosacea, atopic dermatitis, and sensitive skin syndrome. *J Cosmet Dermatol*. 2023;22(1):45–54. doi:10.1111/jocd.15519.
4. Sharma A, Kroumpouzos G, Kassir M, et al. Rosacea management: a comprehensive review. *J Cosmet Dermatol*. 2022;21(5):1895–1904. doi:10.1111/jocd.14816.
5. Leydon JJ. Efficacy of a novel rosacea treatment system: an investigator-blind, randomized, parallel-group study. *J Drugs Dermatol*. 2011;10(10):1179–1185.

ADDITIONAL READING

Al Mokadem SM, Ibrahim AM, El Sayed AM. Efficacy of topical timolol 0.5% in the treatment of acne and rosacea: a multicentric study. *J Clin Aesthet Dermatol*. 2020;13(3):22–27.

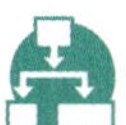

SEE ALSO

- Acne Vulgaris; Blepharitis; Dermatitis, Seborrheic; Lupus Erythematosus, Discoid; Uveitis
- Algorithm: Acne

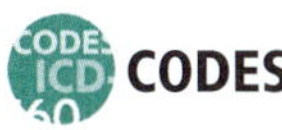

CODES

ICD10

- L71.9 Rosacea, unspecified
- L71.8 Other rosacea

CLINICAL PEARLS

- Rosacea usually arises de novo without any preceding history of acne or seborrhea.
- Rosacea may cause chronic eye symptoms, including blepharitis.
- Avoid alcohol, sun exposure, and hot drinks.
- Medication treatment resembles that of acne vulgaris, with oral and topical antibiotics.

ACNE VULGARIS

Gary I. Levine, MD

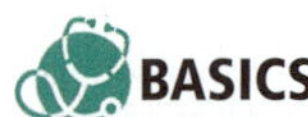

BASICS

DESCRIPTION

Acne vulgaris is a disorder of the pilosebaceous units, and a chronic inflammatory dermatosis notable for open/closed comedones, papules, pustules, nodules.

Geriatric Considerations

Favre-Racouchot syndrome: comedones on face/head due to sun exposure

Pregnancy Considerations

- May result in a flare or remission of acne; typically, improves in 1st, may worsen in 3rd trimester
- Can use topical benzoyl peroxide (BP), azelaic acid, erythromycin or clindamycin; salicylic acid, oral erythromycin, azithromycin, cephalexin, or amoxicillin
- Avoid topical tretinoin, trifarotene and adapalene—may cause retinoid embryopathy; class C
- Contraindicated: isotretinoin (Category X), tazarotene, tetracycline, doxycycline, minocycline, sarecycline, spironolactone

Pediatric Considerations

- Neonatal acne (neonatal cephalic pustulosis)—newborn to 8 weeks; lesions limited to face; usually self-limited, Rx topical ketoconazole 2% cream
- Infantile acne—6 weeks to 1 year; lesions on face, neck, back, chest; topical/systemic Rx
- Early to middle childhood acne—1 to 7 years; rare; consider hyperandrogenism.
- Preadolescent acne—7 to 12 years; common, 47% of children, usually due to adrenal awakening, comedonal lesions
- Do not use tetracyclines in those <8 years old; other therapies similar to adolescent

EPIDEMIOLOGY

- Predominant age: early to late puberty, may persist in 20–40% into 4th decade
- Male > female (teen), female > male (adult)

Prevalence

- 80–95% of adolescents affected; 8% of adults aged 25 to 34 years; 3% at 35 to 44 years
- African Americans 37%, Hispanic 32%, White 24%
- 9.4% globally, 8th most common disease worldwide

ETIOLOGY AND PATHOPHYSIOLOGY

- Androgens (testosterone and dehydroepiandrosterone sulfate [DHEA-S]) stimulate sebum production/qualitative sebum changes, proliferation of keratinocytes in follicles. Keratin plug obstructs follicle os, causing sebum accumulation or follicular distention.
- *Cutibacterium acnes* phylotype IA1 a gram-positive anaerobe, colonizes/proliferates within a biofilm in the plugged follicle. *C. acnes* promotes proinflammatory mediators/cytokines (IL-1), causing inflammation of follicle/dermis.

Genetics

Familial association in 50%

RISK FACTORS

- Increased endogenous androgenic effect
- Oily cosmetics, cocoa butter, polyvinyl chloride, chlorinated hydrocarbons, cutting oil
- Occluding skin surface (e.g., sports equipment such as helmets and shoulder pads), cell phones, hands against skin, pandemic masks ("maskne"—subset of acne mechanica)
- Numerous drugs, including androgenic steroids (e.g., steroid abuse, some birth control pills), lithium, phenytoin
- Endocrine disorders: PCOS, Cushing syndrome, congenital adrenal hyperplasia, androgen-secreting tumors, acromegaly
- Psychological stress
- High-glycemic load, possibly high-dairy diets (skim milk), and whey protein supplements may exacerbate acne.
- Severe acne may worsen with smoking.

GENERAL PREVENTION

Avoidance of risk factors

COMMONLY ASSOCIATED CONDITIONS

Rarely: acne conglobata, hidradenitis suppurativa

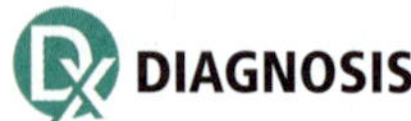

DIAGNOSIS

HISTORY

Ask about duration, relation to menses, medications, cleansing products, stress, smoking, exposures, diet, family history.

PHYSICAL EXAM

- Closed comedones (whiteheads), open comedones (blackheads)
- Nodules or papules, pustules, cysts
- Scars: ice pick, rolling, boxcar, atrophic macules, hypertrophic, depressed, sinus tracts
- Consistent grading is useful; no specific universal grading system is recommended.
- Grading system (American Academy of Dermatology, 1990)
  - Mild: few papules/pustules; no nodules
  - Moderate: some papules/pustules; few nodules
  - Severe: many papules/pustules/nodules
  - Very severe: acne conglobata, acne fulminans, acne inversa
- Most common areas affected are face, chest, back, and upper arms (greatest concentration of sebaceous glands).
- Adult female—facial lesion distribution not limited to mandibular and perioral lesion location

DIFFERENTIAL DIAGNOSIS

Folliculitis: gram-negative, gram-positive, and pityrosporum, acne (rosacea, cosmetica, steroid induced), perioral dermatitis, pseudofolliculitis barbae, drug eruption, keratosis pilaris, sarcoidosis, seborrheic dermatitis, lupus erythematosus

DIAGNOSTIC TESTS & INTERPRETATION

Initial Tests (lab, imaging)

Only indicated if additional signs of androgen excess; if so, test for free and total testosterone, DHEA-S and consider LH/FSH (PCOS).

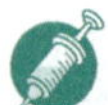

TREATMENT

- Comedonal (grade 1): keratinolytic agent
- Mild inflammatory acne (grade 2): BP +/− topical retinoid or BP +/− topical antibiotic +/− topical retinoid (1)[A]
- Moderate inflammatory acne (grade 3): Add time-limited systemic antibiotic to grade 2 regimen.
- Severe inflammatory acne (grade 4): as in grade 3, or isotretinoin
- Topical retinoid plus a topical antimicrobial agent (such as BP) is first-line treatment for more than mild disease (2)[A].
- Topical retinoid + antibiotic (topical or PO) is better than either alone for mild/moderate.
- Topical retinoids are first-line agents for maintenance therapy (2)[A]. Avoid long-term antibiotics for maintenance.
- Avoid oral or topical antibiotics as monotherapy. Use with topical BP +/− topical retinoid.
- Recommended vehicle type: dry or sensitive skin: cream, lotion, or ointment; oily skin, humid weather: gel, solution, wash; hair-bearing areas: lotion, hydrogel, or foam
- Apply topical agents to entire affected area, not just visible lesions.
- Mild soap daily to control oiliness; avoid abrasives.
- Avoid drying agents; use gentle cleanser/noncomedogenic moisturizer to decrease irritation with keratinolytic agents.

MEDICATION

ALERT

Most prescription, branded and many generic, topical medications are very expensive.

- Keratinolytic agents (α-hydroxy acids, salicylic acid, topical retinoids, azelaic acid) (Side effects include dryness, erythema, and scaling; start with lower strength or alternate day Rx, increase as tolerated.)
- Tretinoin (Retin-A, Retin-A Micro, Avita, Atralin, Altreno), 1st generation, varying strengths and formulations: Wash skin. Apply pea-sized dose at bedtime. Retin-A Micro, Atralin, and Avita are less irritating and stable with BP; may cause an initial flare; may be eased by every other day application for first 2 to 4 weeks
  - Avoid in pregnant and lactating women.
  - Cost varies based on formulation—$50 to $150 per tube for generic.
- Adapalene (Differin): 0.1%, apply topically HS, 3rd generation
  - Effective; less irritation than tretinoin or tazarotene (2)[A]
  - May be combined with BP (Epiduo)—0.1 or 0.3%/2.5%—very effective in skin of color
  - 0.1% gel is available as over-the-counter (OTC), *much less* expensive than other Rx retinoids ($10 to $15)
- Tazarotene (Tazorac): Apply at bedtime, 3rd generation. Most irritating; teratogenic, $400 per tube
- Trifarotene (Aklief): 0.005% cream, apply in PM, 4th generation retinoid, greater selectivity, truncal acne, safer, $600

- Azelaic acid (Azelex) 20% topical cream BID, Finevin 15% gel
  - Keratinolytic, antibacterial, anti-inflammatory reduces postinflammatory hyperpigmentation.
  - Side effects: erythema, dryness, scaling, hypopigmentation
  - Effective in postadolescent acne; safe in pregnancy Category B
  - 20% Rx >$400 per tube, OTC 10% and 15% formulations cost $10 to $40 per tube
- Salicylic acid: 0.5–2%, less effective/less irritating than tretinoin; α-Hydroxy acids, can use with BP, OTC
- Topical BP: generates free O_2 radicals, no resistance in *C. acnes*
  - 2.5% as effective as stronger preparations (5% and 10%), gel penetrates better into follicles.
  - When used with tretinoin, apply BP in morning and tretinoin at night (tretinoin is photolabile).
  - Microencapsulated BP 3% and tretinoin 0.1% (Twyneo) (expensive)
  - Side effects: concentration dependent irritation; may bleach clothes; photosensitivity
- Topical antibiotics (other than BP): Do not use as monotherapy due to antibiotic resistance.
  - Erythromycin 2%, clindamycin 1%, minocycline 4% foam (Amzeeq), metronidazole gel or cream: once daily
  - BP–erythromycin (Benzamycin): especially effective with azelaic acid
  - BP–clindamycin (BenzaClin, DUAC, Clindoxyl)
  - Tretinoin 0.025%–clindamycin 1.2% gel (Veltin), apply HS
  - BP–salicylic acid (Cleanse & Treat, Inova): similar in effectiveness to BP–clindamycin
  - Sodium sulfacetamide (Sulfacet-R, Novacet, Klaron): useful in acne with seborrheic dermatitis or rosacea
  - Dapsone (Aczone) 5% or 7.5% gel: useful in adult females with inflammatory acne; may cause yellow/orange skin discoloration when mixed with BP; very rare methemoglobinemia, OK in glucose-6-phosphate dehydrogenase (G6PD) deficiency (G6PD testing not required), expensive—$350 per tube
- Oral antibiotics: Use for shortest possible period, generally 6 to 12 weeks of therapy; limit to 3 months, max 6 months if necessary; use when acne is more severe, trunk involvement, unresponsive to topical agents, or at greater risk for scarring; do not use as monotherapy.
  - Tetracycline: 250 to 500 mg BID, less effective than doxycycline or minocycline, photosensitivity, esophagitis
  - Minocycline: 100 to 200 mg/day, divided daily—BID; side effects include photosensitivity, urticaria, gray-blue skin, vertigo, autoimmune hepatitis, lupus; extended-release preparation better tolerated
  - Doxycycline: 20 to 200 mg/day, divided daily—BID; photosensitivity
  - Sarecycline: 60 to 150 mg daily (1.5 mg/kg), narrow spectrum, less side effects, $1,000/month
  - Erythromycin: 500 to 1,000 mg/day; divided BID–QID; decreasing effectiveness due to *C. acnes* resistance
  - Trimethoprim-sulfamethoxazole (Bactrim DS, Septra DS): QD or BID
  - Azithromycin (Zithromax): 500 mg 3 days/week × 1 month and then 250 mg every other day × 2 months
  - Amoxicillin: 1,000 to 1,500 mg/day
- Oral retinoids
  - Isotretinoin: 0.5 to 1 mg/kg/day divided BID to maximum 2 mg/kg/day divided BID for very severe disease; 60–90% cure rate; usually given for 12 to 20 weeks; maximum cumulative dose = 120 to 150 mg/kg; 20% of patients relapse and require retreatment, 0.25 to 0.4 mg/kg/day in moderately severe acne
    - Side effects: teratogenic (spontaneous abortion 20%, embryopathy 18–28%), pancreatitis, excessive drying of skin, hypertriglyceridemia, hepatitis, blood dyscrasias, hyperostosis, premature epiphyseal closure, night blindness, erythema multiforme, Stevens-Johnson syndrome, possible suicidal ideation, psychosis
    - Avoid taking tetracyclines or vitamin A during isotretinoin use.
    - Monitor for pregnancy, psychiatric/mood changes, CBC, lipids, glucose, and LFTs at baseline and every month.
    - Patient and provider must register with iPLEDGE program (https://ipledgeprogram.com/), two forms of effective contraception required, monthly urine hCG
  - Isotretinoin micronized (Absorica LD): 0.4 to 0.8 mg/kg/day BID × 15 to 20 weeks, may have fewer side effects, $1,100/month
- Medications for women only
  - FDA-approved oral contraceptives (in order of possible effectiveness)
    - Drospirenone/ethinyl estradiol (Yaz), or drospirenone/ethinyl estradiol/levomefolate (Beyaz) > norgestimate/ethinyl estradiol > norethindrone acetate/ethinyl estradiol
    - Most combined contraceptives are also effective; may take 3 to 6 months
  - Spironolactone (Aldactone); 25 to 200 mg/day; antiandrogen; reduces sebum production, not FDA-approved for acne Rx
- Clascoterone topical (Winlevi): 1% cream, antiandrogen, can use in both sexes >12 years old, no systemic side effects, expensive, $500 to $675

ISSUES FOR REFERRAL

Diagnostic uncertainty, acne fulminans, acne conglobata, severe nodulocystic acne, poor response to treatment, management of acne scars, consideration of isotretinoin Rx

ADDITIONAL THERAPIES

- Acne hyperpigmented macules: topical hydroquinone (1.5–10%), azelaic acid (20%) topically, topical retinoids, corticosteroids: low dose, dapsone 5% gel (Aczone): sunscreen
- Light-based treatment—ultraviolet A/ultraviolet B (UVA/UVB), blue or blue/red light; pulse dye, infrared laser; photodynamic therapy with 5-aminolevulinic acid has best evidence.

SURGERY/OTHER PROCEDURES

- Comedo extraction after incising the layer of epithelium over closed comedo
- Inject large cystic lesions with 0.05 to 0.3 mL triamcinolone (Kenalog 2 to 5 mg/mL); 30-gauge needle, inject through pore, slightly distend cyst, can cause local atrophy.
- Acne scar treatment: retinoids, steroid injections, cryosurgery, electrodesiccation, microdermabrasion, chemical peels, laser resurfacing, pulsed dye laser, microneedling, fillers, punch elevation, thread lifting

COMPLEMENTARY & ALTERNATIVE MEDICINE

Evidence suggests tea tree oil (from *Melaleuca alternifolia*), some plant extracts, and green tea extract may be useful.

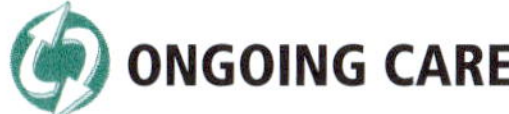

ONGOING CARE

FOLLOW-UP RECOMMENDATIONS

Limit use of oral antibiotics to 3 months; taper topical antibiotic as lesions resolve; consider adapalene + BP for maintenance.

DIET

High-glycemic index foods, milk chocolate, skim milk may worsen acne. Paleo diet and high omega-3 fatty acid foods are helpful.

PATIENT EDUCATION

Lesions may worsen initially; improvement typically seen after a minimum of 4 weeks of treatment.

PROGNOSIS

Gradual improvement over time (usually within 8 to 12 weeks after beginning therapy)

COMPLICATIONS

- Acne conglobata: severe confluent inflammatory acne with systemic symptoms; facial scarring, psychological distress, including anxiety, depression, and suicidal ideation
- Postinflammatory hyperpigmentation, keloids, scars—more common in skin of color

REFERENCES

1. Reynolds RV, Yeung H, Cheng CE, et al. Guidelines of care for the management of acne vulgaris. *J Am Acad Dermatol*. 2024;90(5):1006.e1–1006.e30.
2. Kolli SS, Pecone D, Pona A, et al. Topical retinoids in acne vulgaris: a systematic review. *Am J Clin Dermatol*. 2019;20(3):345–365.

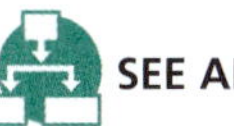

SEE ALSO

- Acne Rosacea
- Algorithm: Acne

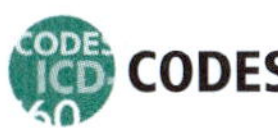

CODES

ICD10

L70.0 Acne vulgaris

CLINICAL PEARLS

Decrease topical frequency to every day or to every other day to lessen irritation.

ACUTE CORONARY SYNDROMES: NSTE-ACS (UNSTABLE ANGINA AND NSTEMI)

Jeremy Golding, MD, FAAFP • Alexandre J. Wenk-Bodenmiller, MD

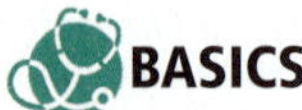

BASICS

DESCRIPTION

- Unstable angina (UA) and non–ST-segment elevation myocardial infarction (NSTEMI) are acute coronary syndromes without ST-segment elevation (NSTE-ACS) that are differentiated from one another based on the absence of cardiac damage in UA (no elevation in cardiac biomarkers) that is present in NSTEMI.
- UA and NSTEMI are difficult to distinguish initially because elevation in cardiac biomarkers levels may not be detectable until several hours after presentation. Initial management for both syndromes is similar.
- Patient history alone is not sufficient to make a diagnosis of ACS and the clinical dilemma of distinguishing between cardiac and noncardiac chest pain involves a combination of patient history, ECG, and cardiac biomarkers.

EPIDEMIOLOGY

Incidence

- The estimated annual incidence of new and recurrent myocardial infarction (MI) is 550,000 and 200,000, respectively.
- In the United States, the average age at first MI is 65.6 years for males and 72 years for females, and males outnumber females at a 3:2 ratio.

ETIOLOGY AND PATHOPHYSIOLOGY

- NSTE-ACS is due to a sudden decrease in myocardial blood flow, resulting in an imbalance between myocardial oxygen consumption and demand, sometimes with resultant tissue injury (NSTEMI). This can be due to acute plaque rupture or plaque erosion and leads to a partially occluding thrombus in the coronary artery, rather than a total or complete occlusion as seen in STEMI.
- Other mechanisms of NSTE-ACS include:
  - Prinzmetal angina or coronary vasospasm induced by tobacco use, hyperventilation, magnesium deficiency, cocaine, or methamphetamines.
  - Increased myocardial oxygen demand resulting in supply-demand mismatch (type 2 NSTEMI) due to underlying causes such as pulmonary embolism, sepsis, shock, arrhythmias/tachycardia
  - Coronary microvascular dysfunction or endothelial dysfunction without epicardial coronary obstruction (MI with no obstructive coronary artery [MINOCA])
  - Less commonly: coronary arterial aneurysm, spontaneous coronary artery dissection, and thromboembolism

Genetics

Genetic polymorphisms of MMP-3 5A/6A and ACE I/D along with conventional ischemic heart disease risk factors can increase the risk of occurrence of STEMI, while having no influence on the pathogenesis of NSTEMI or UA.

RISK FACTORS

- Traditional/classic: age, male sex, prior MI, hypertension (HTN), tobacco use, diabetes mellitus (DM), dyslipidemia, and family history of premature CAD (defined as age of onset prior to 55 years in males and 65 years in females)
- Novel/emerging risk factors: sedentary lifestyle, overweight/obesity (metabolic syndrome), inflammation (psoriasis, rheumatoid arthritis), cigarette or smoking, psychosocial factors (anxiety/depression/stress), chronic kidney disease (CKD), obstructive sleep apnea, environmental pollutants

GENERAL PREVENTION

Smoking cessation, normal body mass index, stress management, regular physical activity, glycemic control for patients with diabetes and blood pressure control in patients with HTN, risk-based lipid control, aspirin in those with documented CAD

DIAGNOSIS

HISTORY

- Chest heaviness/tightness lasting ≥10 minutes; at rest, typically retrosternal and can radiate to the neck, jaw, interscapular area, upper extremities, or epigastrium; pain is typically described as a pressure, tightness, heaviness, squeezing, or fullness.
- Associated symptoms of palpitations, dyspnea, nausea/vomiting, diaphoresis, light-headedness, syncope, or dysphoria can occur.
- Atypical symptoms: stabbing or pleuritic pain, epigastric/abdominal pain, indigestion, hiccups, or isolated dyspnea; more common in those aged >75 years, in women, or those with diabetes, renal insufficiency, and dementia; and may present without chest pain and with symptoms of dyspnea, diaphoresis, and extreme fatigue which represent "anginal equivalents"

PHYSICAL EXAM

- Tachycardia or bradycardia, HTN or hypotension, widened pulse pressure, tachypnea, fever, poor dental hygiene
- Dysrhythmia, jugular venous distention (JVD), new murmur (third and fourth heart sounds), rub or gallop, diminished peripheral pulses, carotid bruits
- Tachypnea, ↑ work of breathing, crackles
- Pain reproducible with movement or palpation is unlikely to be cardiac.
- Cool skin, pallor, diaphoresis, signs of dyslipidemia (xanthomas, xanthelasma)

DIFFERENTIAL DIAGNOSIS

- Cardiac: aortic dissection, myocarditis, pericarditis, pericardial effusion/cardiac tamponade, heart failure, hypertensive emergency, stress cardiomyopathy (takotsubo), dysrhythmia, and mitral valve disease
- Pulmonary: pulmonary embolism, pneumothorax, pneumonia, pleuritis, bronchitis, pneumonitis, and pleuritis
- Psychiatric: panic attacks, anxiety
- Musculoskeletal: costochondritis, rib fracture
- Gastroenterology: gastroesophageal reflux disease, esophageal spasm, esophagitis, esophageal rupture or perforation, hiatal hernia, penetrating or perforating peptic ulcer, biliary or pancreatic pain

DIAGNOSTIC TESTS & INTERPRETATION

Initial Tests (lab, imaging)

- 12-lead ECG: should be obtained within 10 minutes of presentation; applies to both UA and NSTEMI (1)[C]
- CBC, BMP (to evaluate for electrolyte abnormalities), and serum troponin biomarkers (negative by definition in UA) which can be elevated within the first 2 to 3 hours since the onset of chest pain (1)
- Chest x-ray, computed tomography with contrast (to exclude other etiologies if applicable), transthoracic echocardiography are recommended.

Follow-Up Tests & Special Considerations

Fasting lipid profile, preferably within 24 hours, activated partial thromboplastin time (aPTT), TSH, HbA1c, and urine drug screen (in selected patients)

Diagnostic Procedures/Other

- Routine invasive management for NSTEMI/UA reduces recurrent MI and rehospitalization but does not confer a survival benefit and increases bleeding risk. For low- to intermediate-risk patients with resolution of symptoms and nondiagnostic ECG with negative biomarkers, consider risk-stratifying using noninvasive cardiac testing (exercise treadmill test, exercise stress echocardiography, or myocardial perfusion imaging) (1)[C].
- Alternatively, coronary computed tomography angiography can be performed as well in the same population at low to intermediate risk (1)[C].
- In patients with NSTE-ACS who are at intermediate or high risk of ischemic events, an invasive approach with the intent to proceed with revascularization is recommended during hospitalization (1)[C].

Test Interpretation

- ECG results in the setting of NSTE-ACS:
  - New ST-segment depression ≥0.5 mm in ≥2 contiguous leads and/or T-wave inversions ≥1 mm in ≥2 contiguous leads
  - Caution: ST depression and/or tall R wave in V_1/V_2 with upright T waves may indicate transmural STEMI of posterior wall. ECG with posterior leads (V_7–V_9) should be performed.
  - If initial ECG is nondiagnostic but symptoms persist with suspicion for ACS, perform serial ECGs at 15- to 30-minute intervals to evaluate for dynamic changes.
- Troponin concentration rises 3 to 6 hours after the onset of ischemic symptoms but can be delayed 8 to 12 hours.
  - Numerous troponin assays exist with specific cutoffs for NSTEMI. A cardiac troponin >99th percentile of the upper reference limit or an increase specific to the troponin assay after 1 to 2 hours is suggestive of NSTEMI. In patients with symptoms suggestive of ACS, negative troponin at 6 hours effectively rules out infarct in most patients (1).
  - CK-MB has better specificity than troponin in post-PCI MI. Troponin elevation will resolve in 3 to 10 days, CK-MB will return to normal within 3 to 4 days (1).
  - Repeat biomarkers 8 to 12 hours from onset of symptoms to assess for peak. A rapid rise and fall of biomarkers is characteristic of an MI as compared with alternative causes of elevated troponin (1).

TREATMENT

GENERAL MEASURES

- Initial ABCDs, assess clinical stability (adequate oxygenation) and determine next step. Administer supplemental oxygen if O_2 saturation <90%, respiratory distress, or other high-risk features for hypoxemia.
- Risk stratify (TIMI or GRACE score) to select invasive approach (coronary angiography within 24 hours of admission) versus ischemia-guided therapy; urgent invasive management is required for very high-risk patients.
- TIMI risk score: age >65 years, ≥3 CAD risk factors, known CAD with >50% stenosis, aspirin use within the last 7 days, severe angina in the preceding 24 hours, elevated cardiac markers, and ST deviation >0.5 mm; a score of 0 to 2 is low, 3 to 4 is intermediate, 5 to 7 is high risk.
- GRACE risk score: age, heart rate, systolic BP, creatinine, Killip class CHF, cardiac arrest, ST-segment deviation, and elevated cardiac enzymes; useful to predict death and MI in the hospital and at 6 months
- Bed/chair rest with continuous ECG monitoring, maintaining O_2 saturation >90%, and tight BP control; discontinue NSAIDs. Support smoking cessation. Correct electrolyte abnormalities with potassium goal around 4 mEq/L and magnesium at 2 mg/dL.

MEDICATION

First Line

- Antiplatelet therapy: Dual antiplatelet therapy for all patients with NSTE-ACS, with an oral P2Y12 inhibitor is indicated for at least 12 months in patients with ACS who are not at high-bleeding risk (1)[C].
- Aspirin, nonenteric coated, initial dose of 162 to 325 mg chewed or crushed; maintenance dose of 75 to 100 mg/day indefinitely (1)[C]
- Antithrombotic therapy: Initiate anticoagulant (unfractionated heparin (1)[B], enoxaparin (1)[C], or fondaparinux (1)[C]) on presentation. Stop after PCI or after 48 hours for a conservative approach. Warfarin has not been shown to be beneficial and can increase the risk of major bleeding.
- P2Y12 inhibitors should be given at the time of diagnosis unless a surgical approach is planned in a high-bleeding risk patient (1)[C]. Ticagrelor or prasugrel is recommended over clopidogrel in pts undergoing PCI.
  - Ticagrelor, loading dose 180 mg PO, followed by 90 mg PO twice daily; avoid in patients with 2nd- and 3rd-degree heart block; can cause dyspnea in some patients; contraindicated in patients with severe liver dysfunction, *or*
  - Prasugrel 60 mg PO, followed by maintenance dose of 10 mg PO daily; often reserved for post-PCI patients treated with coronary stents; contraindicated in patients aged ≥75 years or those with history of CVA/TIA, *or*
  - Clopidogrel, loading dose 300 to 600 mg PO, followed by maintenance dose of 75 mg PO daily; use with caution with thrombocytopenia and CKD (adding clopidogrel to aspirin may reduce the combined outcome of mortality).
- Nitroglycerin sublingual 0.4 mg every 5 minutes for total of 3 doses and then assess need for IV nitroglycerin based on blood pressure and pain relief (1)[C]. Nitroglycerin-induced hypotension may be attenuated with right ventricular infarction.
- Morphine sulfate (initial dose of 2 to 4 mg), with increments of 2 to 8 mg, can be repeated at 5- to 15-minute intervals for relief of severe, persistent chest pain (1)[C].
- Oral β-blocker therapy (metoprolol succinate, carvedilol, and bisoprolol) should be initiated within 24 hours in patients without signs of heart failure, cardiogenic shock, or other contraindications to β-blockade (1)[C]
- Lipid-lowering therapy: Initiate or continue high-intensity statin therapy (preferred due to nonlipid benefit on vascular function) with atorvastatin 80 mg daily or rosuvastatin 20 to 40 mg daily regardless of the patient's baseline LDL level (1)[C]. Non-statin lipid-lowering is recommended for patients already on maximum statin with LDL-C >70 mg/dL.
- ACE inhibitor (ACEi) or angiotensin receptor blockers (ARBs) should be started and continued indefinitely in all patients with LVEF <40%, and in those with diabetes or HTN, (1)[C].
- Aldosterone antagonist (spironolactone or eplerenone) is recommended in NSTEMI for patients without significant renal dysfunction or hyperkalemia who are on a therapeutic dose of ACEi/ARB and β-blocker and have LVEF ≤40%, DM, or heart failure.

Second Line

Nondihydropyridine calcium channel blockers (CCB) (verapamil or diltiazem) are used to reduce myocardial oxygen demand when β-blockers are contraindicated if left ventricular ejection fraction (LVEF) is normal (1)[C].

ISSUES FOR REFERRAL

- Cardiology consultation is indicated for NSTE-ACS.
- Referral to exercise-based cardiac rehabilitation program prior to hospital discharge is associated with decreased morbidity and mortality.

ADDITIONAL THERAPIES

Influenza vaccine reduces mortality (2).

SURGERY/OTHER PROCEDURES

Some patients often undergo exercise stress testing a few weeks or more after hospital discharge as part of a cardiac rehabilitation program for activity counseling.

ONGOING CARE

FOLLOW-UP RECOMMENDATIONS

- Patients with low-risk suspected ACS who have normal serial ECGs and cardiac troponin levels may have a treadmill ECG, stress myocardial perfusion imaging, or stress echocardiography within 72 hours after discharge.
- With LVEF <40%, repeat LVEF 1 to 3 months postdischarge.

DIET

- One-third of deaths caused by cardiovascular disease (CVD) can be prevented through healthy lifestyle choices.
- The Mediterranean diet is associated with reduced CVD mortality while DASH diet is associated with reduced risk of CAD.
- There is an association with increased sodium intake and CVD risk, but reducing dietary sodium has not been shown to reduce CVD risk.

PATIENT EDUCATION

- May resume exercise, sexual activity within 2 weeks in asymptomatic patients after outpatient reevaluation
- Exercise recommendations for adults include at least 150 minutes of moderate-intensity aerobic activity per week and are associated with reduced CVD risk.

PROGNOSIS

- 50% of patients with UA progress to MI within 30 days if left untreated.
- Between 9% and 19% of those with ACS die in the first 6 months after initial diagnosis, with about one-half of these deaths occurring within the first 30 days.

REFERENCES

1. Rao SV, O'Donoghue ML, Ruel M, et al; for Peer Review Committee Members. 2025 ACC/AHA/ACEP/NAEMSP/SCAI guideline for the management of patients with acute coronary syndromes: a report of the American College of Cardiology/American Heart Association Joint Committee on clinical practice guidelines. *J Am Coll Cardiol*. 2025;85(22):2135–2237.
2. Nohria R, Viera AJ. Acute coronary syndrome: diagnosis and initial management. *Am Fam Physician*. 2024;109(1):34–42.

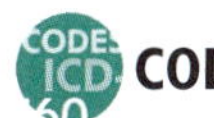

CODES

ICD10

- I24.9 Acute ischemic heart disease, unspecified
- I20.0 Unstable angina
- I21.4 Non-ST elevation (NSTEMI) myocardial infarction

CLINICAL PEARLS

NSTEMI is diagnosed in patients who present with symptoms consistent with ACS and elevated troponin levels, but without ECG changes suggestive of STEMI. UA presents similarly to NSTEMI, but without elevated troponin levels and is treated, initially, with medical management.

ACUTE CORONARY SYNDROMES: STEMI

Juan I. Vasquez Fuster, MD • Brooks J. Willar, MD

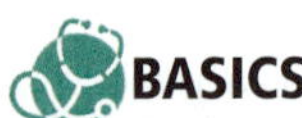

BASICS

DESCRIPTION

Acute myocardial infarction (AMI) is the rapid development of myocardial necrosis resulting from a sustained and complete absence of blood flow to a portion of the myocardium. ST-segment elevation myocardial infarction (STEMI) occurs when coronary blood flow ceases, usually following complete atherothrombotic occlusion of an epicardial coronary artery, resulting in transmural ischemia. This is accompanied by release of serum cardiac biomarkers and ST-segment elevation on an electrocardiogram (ECG).

EPIDEMIOLOGY

Incidence

There are >800,000 cases of AMI reported annually in the United States. Early revascularization and AMI management has improved mortality, with a 30-day survival of 95%.

Prevalence

Atherosclerotic heart disease is the leading cause of morbidity and mortality in the United States. ~7.5 million people in the United States are affected by AMI. Prevalence increases with age and is higher in men (5.5%) compared to women (2.9%). Coronary artery disease (CAD) accounts for ≥12% of total U.S. health expenditures.

ETIOLOGY AND PATHOPHYSIOLOGY

- Atherosclerotic CAD: Atherosclerotic lesions can be fibrotic, calcified, or lipid laden. Thin-capped atheromas are more likely to rupture, causing atherothrombotic occlusion.
- Nonatherosclerotic causes:
  - Embolism from either infective vegetations, or thrombi originating within the right atrium across the foramen ovale ("paradoxical"), from the left atrium or from within the left ventricle
  - Spontaneous coronary artery dissection: prevalent in fibromuscular dysplasia (FMD) and in young women
  - Mechanical or iatrogenic obstruction: chest trauma, dissection of the aorta and/or coronary arteries (e.g., from catheterization procedures)
  - Coronary artery spasm from increased vasomotor tone; anginal variant
  - Arteritis and other etiologies: hematologic causes (disseminated intravascular coagulation [DIC], severe anemia), aortic stenosis, cocaine, IV drug use, severe burns, prolonged hypotension

RISK FACTORS

Advancing age, hypertension, tobacco use, diabetes mellitus, dyslipidemia, family history of premature onset of CAD, sedentary lifestyle

GENERAL PREVENTION

Smoking cessation/abstinence; healthy diet; weight loss/control; regular physical activity and exercise; control of hypertension, hyperlipidemia, and diabetes mellitus

COMMONLY ASSOCIATED CONDITIONS

Abdominal aortic aneurysm, cerebrovascular disease, atherosclerotic peripheral vascular disease

DIAGNOSIS

HISTORY

- Symptoms:
  - Classically, sudden onset of chest heaviness/tightness, with or without exertion, lasting minutes to hours, often with pain/discomfort radiating to neck, jaw, interscapular area, upper extremities, and/or epigastrium
  - Patients with inferior MI may present primarily with abdominal discomfort.
- Previous history of myocardial ischemia (stable or unstable angina, AMI, coronary bypass surgery, or percutaneous coronary intervention [PCI])
- Assess risk factors for CAD, history of bleeding, noncardiac surgery, family history of premature CAD.
- Medications: Ask if recent use of phosphodiesterase type 5 inhibitors (if recent use, avoid concomitant nitrates).
- Tobacco, alcohol, and/or drug abuse (especially cocaine)

PHYSICAL EXAM

- General: restlessness, agitation, hypothermia, fever
- Neurologic: dizziness, syncope, fatigue, disorientation (especially in the elderly)
- Cardiovascular (CV): dysrhythmia, hypotension, widened pulse pressure, S3 and S4, jugular venous distention (JVD)
- Respiratory: dyspnea, tachypnea, crackles, rales
- GI: abdominal pain, nausea, vomiting, hiccups
- Skin: cool skin, pallor, diaphoresis

Geriatric and Gender Considerations

- Elderly patients may have an atypical presentation, including silent or unrecognized MI. They may often present with syncope, weakness, shortness of breath, unexplained nausea, epigastric pain, altered mental status, or delirium.
- Women or patients with diabetes mellitus may present with typical and/or "atypical" symptoms such as fatigue, dyspnea, and malaise.

DIFFERENTIAL DIAGNOSIS

Unstable angina, aortic dissection, pulmonary embolism (PE), perforating gastric ulcer, pericarditis (myocarditis), Takotsubo cardiomyopathy, dysrhythmias, gastroesophageal reflux disease (GERD), esophageal spasm, biliary/pancreatic pain, hyperventilation syndrome, anxiety/panic

DIAGNOSTIC TESTS & INTERPRETATION

Initial Tests (lab, imaging)

- 12-lead ECG:
  - ≥1 mm ST elevation in a regional pattern, involving at least two contiguous leads, with or without abnormal Q waves; in leads V_2/V_3, ST elevation of 2 mm for men and 1.5 mm for women are necessary.
  - STEMI of posterior wall: ST depression ± tall R waves in V_1–V_2
  - Absence of Q waves represents partial or transient occlusion or early infarction.
  - Consider right-sided and posterior chest leads if inferior MI pattern (examine V_3R, V_4R, V_7–V_9).
  - In the setting of ventricular pacing or a prior left bundle branch block (LBBB), the Sgarbossa criteria or BARCELONA algorithm may be helpful.
- 2-Dimensional transthoracic echocardiography is useful in evaluating regional wall motion in MI, left ventricular function, mechanical complications, and mural thrombus.
- Once diagnosis is suspected, emergent coronary angiography with PCI is preferred.

Follow-Up Tests & Special Considerations

Serum biomarkers

- Troponin I and T (cTnI, cTnT) rise 3 to 6 hours after onset of ischemic symptoms.
- Elevations in cTnI persist for 7 to 10 days, whereas cTnT elevations persist for 10 to 14 days after MI.
- High-sensitivity troponin is highly sensitive and provides faster recognition of AMI.
- Myoglobin fraction of creatine kinase-MB (CK-MB) adds little diagnostic value in assessment of possible AMI to troponin testing.

Pregnancy Considerations

Pregnant patients presenting with STEMI will need discussion of risks and benefits of invasive coronary angiography with radiation exposure to fetus. Management should otherwise be the same as in nonpregnant patients.

Diagnostic Procedures/Other

- Portable chest x-ray; transthoracic echocardiography; chest computed tomography angiography (CTA) scan may occasionally be of value acutely in equivocal presentations to evaluate for alternative diagnoses (aortic dissection, PE, ventricular aneurysm).
- Coronary angiography is the definitive test.

ALERT

Patients with chronic kidney disease need special attention to amount of contrast media used.

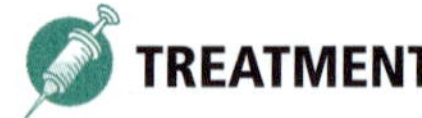

TREATMENT

GENERAL MEASURES

Following emergent revascularization, admit the patient to the coronary care unit (CCU) or a telemetry unit with continuous ECG monitoring, bed rest, and use:

- Antiarrhythmics as needed for unstable dysrhythmia
- Dual antiplatelet therapy (DAPT) with continuation of aspirin 81 mg/day with clopidogrel 75 mg/day or prasugrel 10 mg/day or ticagrelor 90 mg twice daily

MEDICATION

Medication recommendations are based on the 2013 American College of Cardiology (ACC)/American Heart Association (AHA) guideline (1)[C] and 2017 European Society of Cardiology (ESC) guideline (2)[C].

First Line

- Supplemental oxygen 2 to 4 L/min for patients with oxygen saturation <90% or respiratory distress
- Nitroglycerin (NTG) sublingual 0.4 mg q5min for a total of 3 doses, followed by NTG IV if ongoing pain and/or hypertension and/or management of pulmonary congestion if no contraindications exist such as systolic <90 mm Hg or >30 mm Hg below baseline, right ventricle (RV) infarct, use of phosphodiesterase type 5 (PDE-5) inhibitors such as sildenafil or vardenafil within 24 hours or within 48 hours of tadalafil

- Morphine sulfate 4 to 8 mg IV with 2 to 8 mg IV repeated at 5- to 15-minute intervals to relieve pain, anxiety, or pulmonary congestion
- Antiplatelet agents:
  - Aspirin (ASA), non–enteric-coated, initial dose 162 to 325 mg chewed
  - A loading dose of a P2Y12 inhibitor is recommended for patients with STEMI for whom PCI is planned. Prasugrel or ticagrelor is preferred.
    - Prasugrel 60 mg loading dose; prasugrel is contraindicated in patients with previous stroke/transient ischemic attack. Do not recommend in patients aged >75 years or in patients with lower body weight (<60 kg).
    - Ticagrelor 180 mg loading dose; ticagrelor may cause transient dyspnea.
    - Clopidogrel 600 mg loading dose should be given if neither prasugrel nor ticagrelor is available.
    - Cangrelor may be considered in patients not pretreated with oral P2Y12 receptor inhibitors at the time of PCI or in those who are unable to take oral agents.
    - Standard recommendation for duration of DAPT is 6 to 12 months after PCI, depending on bleeding and ischemia risks.
- Anticoagulation therapy:
  - Unfractionated heparin (UFH) 70- to 100-U/kg IV bolus *or*
  - Enoxaparin 0.5 mg/kg IV bolus *or*
  - Bivalirudin 0.75 mg/kg IV bolus and then 1.75 mg/kg/hr infusion for up to 4 hours after procedure
- PCI versus fibrinolysis: The goal is to keep total ischemic time within 120 minutes. Door-to-needle time should be within 30 minutes or door-to-balloon time within 90 minutes.
  - Coronary reperfusion therapy
    - Primary PCI (balloon angioplasty, coronary stents) in the following:
      - Symptom onset of ≤12 hours
      - Symptom onset of ≤12 hours and contraindication to fibrinolytic therapy irrespective of time delay
      - Cardiogenic shock or acute severe heart failure (HF) irrespective of time delay from onset of MI
      - Evidence of ongoing ischemia 12 to 24 hours after symptom onset
  - Procedural considerations: Radial access is recommended over femoral access. PCI of infarct-related artery (IRA) is indicated.
  - Fibrinolysis
    - If presenting to a hospital without PCI capability and cannot be transferred to a PCI-capable facility to undergo PCI within 120 minutes of first medical contact
    - If no contraindications, administer within 12 to 24 hours of symptom onset, if there is evidence of ongoing ischemia.
      - Alteplase (tPA): 15 mg IV bolus, followed by 0.75 mg/kg (up to 50 mg) IV over 30 minutes and then 0.5 mg/kg (up to 35 mg) over 60 minutes; maximum 100 mg over 90 minutes
      - Reteplase (rPA): 10 units IV bolus; give second bolus 30 minutes apart.
      - Tenecteplase (TNK-tPA) (preferred agent in United States due to ease of administration and its use in the more modern trials of efficacy and safety): 30 to 50 mg (based on weight) IV bolus; recommend reducing to half dose in patients ≥75 years of age.
    - Adjunctive antiplatelet therapy with fibrinolysis
      - Aspirin: 162 to 325 mg loading dose followed by 81 mg/day indefinitely
      - Clopidogrel (300 mg loading dose for patients <75 years of age, 75 mg dose for patients >75 years of age); clopidogrel 75 mg/day should be continued for at least 14 days and up to 1 year.
    - Adjunctive anticoagulation therapy with fibrinolysis: Use anticoagulants (UFH, enoxaparin, or fondaparinux) as ancillary therapy to reperfusion therapy for a minimum of 48 hours and preferably duration of admission (up to 8 days) or until revascularization, if performed.
- Glycoprotein IIb/IIIa receptor antagonists at the time of primary PCI in selected patients if there is no reflow or thrombotic complications (abciximab, eptifibatide, or tirofiban)
- ACE inhibitors should be initiated orally within 24 hours of STEMI in patients with anterior infarction, HF, diabetes, or ejection fraction (EF) ≤0.4 unless contraindicated.
- High-intensity statin therapy should be started as early as possible.
- Mineralocorticoid receptor antagonist (spironolactone, eplerenone) is recommended in patients with EF <40% and HF or diabetes, who are already receiving an ACE inhibitor and a β-blocker (BB), if there is no renal failure or hyperkalemia.

Second Line

Calcium channel blockers may have a limited role in specific circumstances in patients intolerant of BB and without left ventricular (LV) systolic dysfunction: treating coronary spasm, lowering blood pressure, reducing heart rate in atrial fibrillation. Immediate-release nifedipine is contraindicated in STEMI.

ISSUES FOR REFERRAL

Transfer high-risk patients who receive fibrinolytic therapy as primary reperfusion therapy at a non–PCI-capable facility to a PCI-capable facility as soon as possible.

SURGERY/OTHER PROCEDURES

Urgent coronary artery bypass graft (CABG) surgery is indicated in patients with STEMI and coronary anatomy not amenable to PCI who have ongoing or recurrent ischemia, cardiogenic shock, severe HF, or other high-risk features.

ADMISSION, INPATIENT, AND NURSING CONSIDERATIONS

All STEMI patients should be admitted to a CCU or an intensive cardiac care unit for evaluation and treatment.

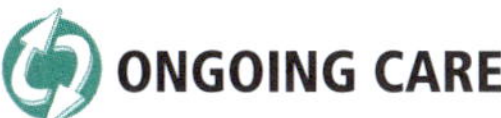

ONGOING CARE

FOLLOW-UP RECOMMENDATIONS

STEMI patients should follow up with a cardiologist 1 to 2 weeks postdischarge, every 3 months for the 1st year and then yearly. Emphasize medication adherence and encourage smoking cessation. Strongly consider referral to an exercise-based cardiac rehabilitation program.

DIET

Low-fat/healthy-fat diet: reduced intake of saturated fats (to <7% of total calories), eliminate *trans*-fatty acids (to <1% of total calories); Mediterranean diet is healthy.

PATIENT EDUCATION

May resume sexual activity ≥1 week after uncomplicated MI or 6 to 8 weeks after CABG; smoking cessation and low-fat diet

COMPLICATIONS

HF, myocardial wall rupture, left ventricular aneurysm, pericarditis, dysrhythmias, acute mitral regurgitation, and depression (common)

REFERENCES

1. O'Gara PT, Kushner FG, Ascheim DD, et al. 2013 ACCF/AHA guideline for the management of ST-elevation myocardial infarction: a report of the American College of Cardiology Foundation/American Heart Association Task Force on practice guidelines. *J Am Coll Cardiol*. 2013;61(4):e78–e140.
2. Ibanez B, James S, Agewall S, et al; for ESC Scientific Document Group. 2017 ESC guidelines for the management of acute myocardial infarction in patients presenting with ST-segment elevation: the task force for the management of acute myocardial infarction in patients presenting with ST-segment elevation of the European Society of Cardiology (ESC). *Eur Heart J*. 2018;39(2):119–177.

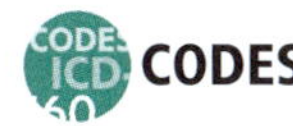

CODES

ICD10

- I24.9 Acute ischemic heart disease, unspecified
- I21.3 ST elevation (STEMI) myocardial infarction of unspecified site
- I25.10 Athscl heart disease of native coronary artery w/o ang pctrs

CLINICAL PEARLS

Early revascularization with PCI within 90 minutes of presentation at a PCI-capable hospital, or within 120 minutes if transfer to a PCI-capable hospital is required. Fibrinolytic therapy should be initiated within 30 minutes if presenting to a hospital without PCI capability and the patient cannot be transferred to a PCI-capable facility to undergo PCI within 120 minutes of first medical contact.

ACUTE KIDNEY INJURY

Sandhya Tagaram, MD

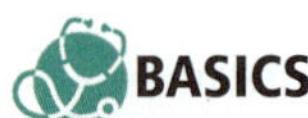

BASICS

DESCRIPTION

- An abrupt loss of kidney function, acute kidney injury (AKI) is defined as (1):
  - Increase in serum creatinine (SCr) of ≥0.3 mg/dL within 48 hours
  - ≥50% increase in baseline SCr within 7 days
  - Urine output of <0.5 mL/kg/hr for 6 hours
- Staging is based on SCr or urine output:

Stage	1	2	3
Increase in baseline creatinine	1.5 times	2.0–2.9 times	3.0 times
Increase in creatinine	≥0.3 mg/dL	N/A	≥4.0 mg/dL
Urine output	<0.5 mL/kg/hr for 6–12 hours	<0.5 mL/kg/hr for ≥12 hours	<0.3 mL/kg/hr for ≥24 hours

- The result is retention of nitrogenous waste, electrolyte, acid–base, and volume abnormalities (1).

EPIDEMIOLOGY

Incidence

- 5% of hospital and 30% of ICU admissions have AKI. 25% of patients develop AKI while hospitalized; 50% of these cases are iatrogenic.
- Developing AKI as an inpatient is associated with >4-fold increased risk of death (2).

ETIOLOGY AND PATHOPHYSIOLOGY

Three categories: prerenal, intrarenal, and postrenal

- Prerenal (reduced renal perfusion, typically reversible):
  - Decreased renal perfusion (often due to hypovolemia) leads to a decrease in glomerular filtration rate (GFR).
  - Caused by hypotension, volume depletion (GI losses, excessive sweating, diuretics, hemorrhage); renal artery stenosis/embolism; burns; heart/liver failure; if decreased perfusion is prolonged or severe, can progress to ischemic acute tubular necrosis (ATN)
- Intrarenal (intrinsic kidney injury, often from prolonged or severe renal hypoperfusion)
  - ATN—from prolonged prerenal azotemia, radiographic contrast material, aminoglycosides, nonsteroidal anti-inflammatory drugs (NSAIDs), or other nephrotoxic substances
  - Glomerulonephritis (GN)
  - Acute interstitial nephritis (AIN; drug induced), arteriolar insults, vasculitis, accelerated hypertension, cholesterol embolization (following an intra-arterial procedure), intrarenal deposition/sludging (uric acid nephropathy and multiple myeloma [Bence Jones proteins])
- Postrenal (obstruction of the collecting system)
  - Extrinsic compression (e.g., benign prostatic hypertrophy [BPH], carcinoma, pregnancy); intrinsic obstruction (e.g., calculus, tumor, clot, stricture, sloughed papillae); decreased function (e.g., neurogenic bladder), leading to obstruction of the urinary collection system

Genetics

No known genetic pattern

RISK FACTORS

- Chronic kidney disease (CKD); comorbid conditions (e.g., diabetes mellitus, hypertension, heart failure, liver failure); advanced age; radiocontrast material exposure (intravascular), female gender, African American.
- Medications that impair autoregulation of GFR (NSAIDs, angiotensin-converting enzyme inhibitors [ACEI], angiotensin II receptor blockers [ARB], cyclosporine/tacrolimus)
- Nephrotoxic medications (e.g., aminoglycoside antibiotics, platinum-based chemotherapy); hypovolemia (e.g., diuretics, hemorrhage, GI losses); sepsis, surgery, rhabdomyolysis, burns; solitary kidney (risk in nephrolithiasis); BPH; malignancy (e.g., multiple myeloma)

GENERAL PREVENTION

- Maintain adequate renal perfusion with isotonic fluids, vasopressor support if necessary.
- Avoid nephrotoxic agents.

COMMONLY ASSOCIATED CONDITIONS

Hyperkalemia, hyperphosphatemia, hypercalcemia, hyperuricemia, hydronephrosis, BPH, nephrolithiasis, congestive heart failure (CHF), uremic pericarditis, cirrhosis, CKD, malignant hypertension, vasculitis, drug reactions, sepsis, severe trauma, burns, transfusion reactions, recent chemotherapy, rhabdomyolysis, internal bleeding, dehydration

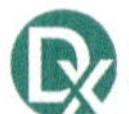

DIAGNOSIS

AKI is usually asymptomatic until the patient has experienced severe loss of function. Oliguria can be present, but it is neither specific nor sensitive.

HISTORY

- Thorough medication history; changes in oral intake, urine output, and body weight
- Prerenal: thirst, orthostatic symptoms, vomiting, diarrhea, bleeding
- Intrarenal: nephrotoxic medications, radiocontrast material, other toxins
- Postrenal: Colicky flank pain that radiates to the groin suggests ureteric obstruction such as a stone; nocturia, frequency, and hesitancy suggest prostatic disease; suprapubic and flank pain are usually secondary to distension of the bladder and collecting system; anticholinergic drugs inhibit bladder emptying.
- Uremic symptoms: lethargy, altered mental status, nausea, vomiting, anorexia, metallic taste

PHYSICAL EXAM

- Uremic signs: altered mental status, seizures, myoclonus, pericardial friction rub, peripheral neuropathies
- Prerenal signs: tachycardia, decreased jugular venous pressure (JVP), orthostatic hypotension, dry mucous membranes, decreased skin turgor; comorbid stigmata of sepsis, liver disease, or heart failure
- Intrinsic renal signs: pruritic rash, livedo reticularis, subcutaneous nodules, ischemic digits despite good pulses
- Postrenal signs: suprapubic distension, flank pain, enlarged prostate

DIAGNOSTIC TESTS & INTERPRETATION

Multiple emerging biomarkers (e.g., kidney injury molecule-1 [KIM-1]; neutrophil gelatinase-associated lipocalin [NGAL] and cystatin C) to assist in the prediction, diagnosis, and severity of AKI

Initial Tests (lab, imaging)

- Compare to baseline renal function (creatinine [Cr] and GFR) (1)[A]
- Urinalysis: dipstick for blood and protein; microscopy for cells, casts, and crystals (1)[A]
- Sterile pyuria (especially WBC casts) suggests AIN; triad of fever, rash, and eosinophilia present in 10% of cases
- Proteinuria, hematuria, and edema, often with nephritic urine sediment (RBCs and RBC casts), suggest GN or vasculitis.
- Casts: transparent hyaline casts—prerenal etiology; pigmented granular/muddy brown casts—ATN; WBC casts—AIN; RBC casts—GN
- Urine eosinophils: ≥1% eosinophils suggest AIN (poor sensitivity)
- Urine electrolytes in an oliguric state
  - FE_{Na} = [(urinary Na × SCr) / (serum Na × urinary Cr)]
  - FE_{Na} <1% suggests prerenal etiology and >2% indicates intrinsic cause
  - If on diuretics, use FE_{urea} instead of FE_{Na}. FE_{urea} (percent) = [(SCr × urine urea) / (serum urea × urinary Cr)] × 100; FE_{urea} <35% suggests prerenal etiology and >50% suggests intrinsic disease
- CBC, BUN, SCr, electrolytes (including Ca/Mg/P); consider arterial or venous blood gas (ABG/VBG).
- Common lab abnormalities in AKI
  - Increased: potassium, phosphate, magnesium, uric acid
  - Decreased: hemoglobin, calcium
- Calculate creatinine clearance (CrCl) to ensure appropriate medication dosing
- Imaging:
  - Renal ultrasound (US): first line; excludes postrenal causes; identifies kidney size, nephrolithiasis
  - Doppler-flow renal US: evaluates for renal artery stenosis/thrombosis
  - Abdominal x-ray (kidney, ureter, bladder [KUB]): identifies calcification, renal calculi, kidney size
- Novel biomarkers such as urinary IL-18, NGAL, KIM-1, plasma cystatin C, TIMP-2, and *IGFBP7* under investigation (3)

Follow-Up Tests & Special Considerations

- Consider CK (rhabdomyolysis) and immunologic testing (if GN or vasculitis suspected).
- Advanced imaging if initial tests unrevealing
  - Prerenal: US as effective as CT for obstruction; noncontrast helical CT: most sensitive test for nephrolithiasis
  - Radionuclide renal scan: evaluates renal perfusion, function (GFR), and presence of obstructive uropathy and extravasation. MRI: acute tubulointerstitial nephritis with increased T2-weighted signal.
  - Avoid gadolinium contrast in at-risk patients (those with diabetes mellitus and GFR <45 mL/min/1.73 m^2, or those without diabetes and GFR <30 mL/min/1.73 m^2). If necessary, use intravenous fluids before and after contrast administration.

Diagnostic Procedures/Other

Cystoscopy with retrograde pyelogram evaluates for bladder tumor, hydronephrosis, obstruction, and upper tract abnormalities without risk of contrast nephropathy.

Test Interpretation

Kidney biopsy: if patient does not respond to therapy or if diagnosis remains unclear; most useful to evaluate intrinsic AKI of unclear causes

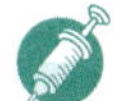

TREATMENT

Fluid resuscitation is the mainstay of treatment of AKI, both in prerenal and in some forms of intrinsic kidney injury. In severe cases of kidney injury, renal replacement therapy (RRT) may be required. The most important aspect of treating AKI is determining the underlying cause.

GENERAL MEASURES

- Identify and correct prerenal and postrenal causes; stop nephrotoxic drugs and renally dose others. Strictly monitor intake/output and daily weight; optimize cardiac output to maintain renal perfusion. Optimize nutrition and treat any infections. Remove obstruction by placing a Foley catheter, suprapubic catheter, or nephrostomy tube as clinically indicated.
- Indications for RRT: volume overload, severe hyperkalemia, or metabolic acidosis refractory to medical management; advanced uremic complications (pericarditis, encephalopathy, bleeding diathesis); pulmonary edema

MEDICATION

First Line

- Find and treat the underlying cause. Correct electrolyte imbalances—particularly hyperkalemia.
  - If patient is oliguric and not volume overloaded, a monitored fluid challenge may help.
- Furosemide can be used to manage volume overload and/or hyperkalemia. Furosemide stress test may predict the likelihood of progressive AKI, need for RRT, and mortality.
- Fenoldopam, a dopamine agonist, has been equivocal in decreasing risk of RRT and mortality in AKI; not currently recommended (1)[C]
- Hyperkalemia with ECG changes: Give IV calcium gluconate, isotonic sodium bicarbonate (only if acidemic, and avoid use of hypertonic "amps" of $NaHCO_3$), glucose with insulin, and/or high-dose nebulized albuterol (to drive K^+ into cells); Kayexalate and/or furosemide (to increase K^+ excretion); hemodialysis if severe/refractory.
- Fluid restriction may be required for oliguric patients to prevent worsening hyponatremia.
- Effective strategies for AKI prevention: isotonic IVF, once-daily dosing of aminoglycosides; use of lipid formulations of amphotericin B, use of iso-osmolar nonionic contrast media.
- Risk of contrast-induced AKI is reduced by avoidance of hypovolemia:
  - Inpatients: isotonic saline 1 mL/kg/hr 6 to 12 hours preprocedure, during the procedure, and 6 to 12 hours postprocedure
  - Outpatients: isotonic saline 3 mL/kg/hr × 1 hour preprocedure, 1.0 to 1.5 mL/kg/hr × 4 to 6 hours during and after the procedure for a total of 6 mL/kg

Second Line

- Tamsulosin or other selective α-blockers for bladder outlet obstruction secondary to BPH
- Dihydropyridine calcium channel blockers may have a protective effect in posttransplant ATN.

ISSUES FOR REFERRAL

- Consider nephrology consultation for potential initiation of RRT; persistent and prolonged anuria or oliguria and/or refractory elevation in BUN and/or Cr despite appropriate fluid and/or electrolyte replacement, and/or underlying structural or functional renal disease (e.g., glomerulonephropathies, SLE nephritis, cryoglobulinemia), and/or renal transplant patients.
- Consider urology consult for obstructive nephropathy.

SURGERY/OTHER PROCEDURES

- Relieve obstruction by retrograde ureteral catheters/percutaneous nephrostomy.
- Hemodialysis catheter placement

COMPLEMENTARY & ALTERNATIVE MEDICINE

Many herbal and dietary supplements are potentially nephrotoxic (aristolochic acid, ochratoxin A, Djenkol bean, impila [*Callilepis laureola*]), orellanine, cat's claw, Chinese yew (*Taxus celebica*), morning cypress (*cupressus funebris* [Endl]), St. John's wort.

ADMISSION, INPATIENT, AND NURSING CONSIDERATIONS

- Treat life-threatening complications: hyperkalemia, metabolic acidosis, volume overload, and advanced uremia.
- Monitor strict intake and output through fluid balance and daily weights.
- Consider urinary catheter placement to quantify urine output, weighing risks of catheter-associated urinary tract infection (CAUTI). Remove as soon as possible. Stabilize renal function and ensure treatment plan prior to discharge; dialysis if necessary.

ONGOING CARE

FOLLOW-UP RECOMMENDATIONS

Nephrology follow-up if persistent renal impairment and/or proteinuria

DIET

- Total caloric intake of 20 to 30 kcal/kg/day (1)
- Restrict Na^+ to 2 g/day (unless hypovolemic); consider K^+ restriction (2 to 3 g/day) if hyperkalemic. If hyperphosphatemic, consider use of phosphate binders, although no evidence of benefit in AKI. Avoid magnesium- and aluminum-containing compounds.

PATIENT EDUCATION

- Keep well hydrated. Avoid nephrotoxic drugs, such as NSAIDs and aminoglycosides.
- Acute Kidney Injury (AKI). National Kidney Foundation: https://www.kidney.org/atoz/content/AcuteKidneyInjury

PROGNOSIS

- In cases of prerenal and postrenal AKI, short duration of AKI correlates with good rates of recovery.
- Among patients who require RRT for AKI, recovery more likely with higher baseline GFR, AKI from ATN due to sepsis or surgery; recovery less likely with preexisting heart failure

COMPLICATIONS

Death, sepsis, infection, CKD, seizures, paralysis, peripheral edema, CHF, arrhythmias, uremic pericarditis, bleeding, hypotension, anemia, hyperkalemia, uremia

REFERENCES

1. Ostermann M, Lumlertgul N, Jeong R, et al. Acute kidney injury. *Lancet*. 2025;405(10474):241–256. doi:10.1016/S0140-6736(24)02385-7.
2. Gonsalez SR, Cortês AL, da Silva RC, et al. Acute kidney injury overview: from basic findings to new prevention and therapy strategies. *Pharmacol Ther*. 2019;200:1–12.
3. Gameriero J, Fonseca JA, Outerelo C, et al. Acute kidney injury: from diagnosis to prevention and treatment strategies. *J Clin Med*. 2020;9(6):1704.

ADDITIONAL READING

Tamargo C, Hanouneh M, Cervantes CE. Treatment of cute kidney injury: a review of current approaches and emerging innovations. *J Clin Med*. 2024;13(9):2455.

SEE ALSO

- Glomerulonephritis, Acute; Hepatorenal Syndrome; Hyperkalemia; Prostatic Hyperplasia, Benign (BPH); Chronic Kidney Disease; Reye Syndrome; Rhabdomyolysis; Sepsis; Renal Insufficiency
- Algorithm: Anuria or Oliguria

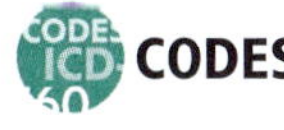

CODES

ICD10

- N17.0 Acute kidney failure with tubular necrosis
- N17.1 Acute kidney failure with acute cortical necrosis
- N17.8 Other acute kidney failure

CLINICAL PEARLS

- Three categories of AKI:
  - Prerenal: decreased renal perfusion (often from hypovolemia) leading to a decrease in GFR; reversible
  - Intrarenal: intrinsic kidney damage; ATN most common due to ischemic/nephrotoxic injury
  - Postrenal: extrinsic/intrinsic obstruction of the urinary collection system
- Indications for emergent hemodialysis: severe hyperkalemia, metabolic acidosis, or volume overload refractory to conservative therapy; uremic pericarditis, encephalopathy, or neuropathy; and selected alcohol and drug intoxications
- Management of ATN is supportive; no specific treatments are proven to effectively hasten recovery.
- Fluid management remains a mainstay of treatment in prerenal and intrinsic kidney injury.

ADHESIVE CAPSULITIS (FROZEN SHOULDER)

Erin L. Trolley, MD

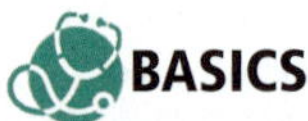

BASICS

DESCRIPTION

- Adhesive capsulitis (AC) or frozen shoulder:
  - Presents as progressive painful restriction in range of movement of the glenohumeral (GH) joint
  - Course usually involves diminishment of pain, but can have residual pain and limits of active and passive range of motion (ROM).
- Subtypes:
  - Primary AC:
    - Idiopathic
    - Usually associated with diabetes mellitus (DM)
    - Commonly resolves in 9 to 24 months
  - Secondary AC:
    - Commonly due to prolonged immobilization
    - Most commonly due to a complication of rotator cuff impingement syndrome (rotator cuff tendonitis) that remains incompletely treated
    - Sometimes called "shoulder-hand-syndrome"
      - A complex regional pain syndrome (CRPS) or reflex sympathetic dystrophy (RSD) characterized by shoulder pain, diffuse swelling, and decreased ROM
- Clinical course:
  - Phase 1 (2 to 9 months): painful phase
    - Pain is constant.
    - Diagnosis may be difficult if restricted movement is not present in early disease.
  - Phase 2 (4 to 12 months): stiffening or freezing phase
    - Movement becomes restricted, especially with external rotation.
  - Phase 3 (12 to 42 months): resolution or thawing phase
  - Gradual return to normal shoulder mobility

EPIDEMIOLOGY

Incidence

- 2.4/1,000 people per year
- Female:male ratio (1.4:1)

Prevalence

2–5% in the general population, 10–20% among diabetes (1)

ETIOLOGY AND PATHOPHYSIOLOGY

Underlying fundamental processes:

- Idiopathic
- Inflammation:
  - Mast cells, T cells, B cells, and macrophages have been identified histologically, suggesting an inflammatory process. Studies confirm presence of elevated inflammatory cytokines such as IL-1, IL-6, TNF-α, COX-1, and COX-2 (1).
  - Elevated markers for neoangiogenesis (CD34) and neoinnervation (GAP43, PGP9.5, NGFR p75) have been associated with AC, which helps explain the acute painful phase. Additionally, one study showed that over expression of TGF-β led to the development of AC in rats (1).
- Scarring:
  - Fibroblasts and myofibroblasts have been identified histologically.
  - Capsular contracture reduces the joint volume to 3 to 4 mL (normal 10 to 15 mL).
  - Intracellular adhesion molecule-1 (ICAM-1) facilitates leukocyte endothelial transmigration (elevated in both AC and DM).
  - This scarring primarily effects the rotator interval (coracohumeral ligament [CHL], biceps tendon, and GH capsule). A contracted CHL is an essential finding in AC (1).
- Contracture of the GH capsule from loss of synovial layer, capsular adhesions, and loss of capsular volume are seen in AC.

RISK FACTORS

- Shoulder immobilization; often due to impingement syndrome (most significant risk factor)
- Increasing age
- Female gender
- Diabetes
- Thyroid disease
- Atherosclerotic cardiovascular disease (ASCVD): cerebrovascular accident (CVA)/myocardial infarction (MI)/hyperlipidemia
- Antiretroviral medication use
- Parkinson disease
- Trauma/surgery
- Prior history of AC in contralateral shoulder

GENERAL PREVENTION

- Active lifestyle, while avoiding shoulder injury
- Optimization of diabetes, atherosclerotic disease, thyroid, and autoimmune conditions

COMMONLY ASSOCIATED CONDITIONS

DM, autoimmune disorders, Parkinson disease, highly active antiretroviral therapy (HAART) use, CVA/MI, cervical disc disease, thyroid disorders

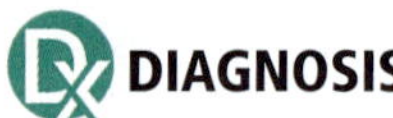

DIAGNOSIS

HISTORY

- Identify possible risk factors.
- Progressive and worsening stiffness of the GH joint
- Most patients will experience diffuse shoulder pain at disease onset, followed by progression to shoulder stiffness.
- Rule out other pain invoking conditions such as fractures, osteoarthritis (OA), subacromial pathologies such as bursitis and rotator cuff tendinopathy, cervical radiculopathy, and GH arthrosis (1).

PHYSICAL EXAM

- Limitation in both active and passive ROM due to true mechanical restriction
- Capsular pattern of ROM restriction is demonstrated.
  - External rotation most affected, followed by abduction and flexion, respectively
- Pain with rotator cuff impingement tests
- Inability to reach overhead or back pocket
- Scapular substitution frequently accompanies active shoulder movement
- Loss of arm swing with gait

DIFFERENTIAL DIAGNOSIS

- Rotator cuff strain/tear/impingement syndrome
- GH or acromioclavicular (AC) joint OA
- Cervical strain/radiculopathy/OA
- Subacromial bursitis
- Parsonage-Turner syndrome (brachial plexus inflammation secondary to a trigger such as an infection, trauma, or autoimmune condition)
- Myofascial pain syndrome
- Calcific tendonitis
- Fracture
- Shoulder subluxation/dislocation
- Bony neoplasm/metastasis

DIAGNOSTIC TESTS & INTERPRETATION

AC is a clinical diagnosis that can further be guided by labs and imaging if needed. No single lab or imaging alone can make the diagnosis.

Initial Tests (lab, imaging)

- No labs are required for diagnosis of idiopathic AC.
  - If risk factors for an associated condition are present, laboratory evaluation is indicated for further workup (diabetes, thyroid diseases, stroke, autoimmune disease, Parkinson disease) consider obtaining appropriate labs (thyroid-stimulating hormone (TSH), hemoglobin A1C (HbA1c), erythrocyte sedimentation rate (ESR), C-reactive protein (CRP).
- Imaging
  - Plain radiographs of the affected shoulder are the preferred initial test in order to rule out other pathologies such as GH, OA, fractures, dislocation, or tumors (posteroanterior, external rotation, axillary, and supraspinatus outlet views)
- Magnetic resonance imaging (MRI)
  - Not indicated unless there is a concomitant pathology in the shoulder or neurologic deficit
  - Thickening of the joint capsule and the CHL along with edema and increased joint fluid may be visualized
  - Rotator interval/axillary joint capsule enhancement and inferior GH and/or CHL hyperintensity are the most diagnostic signs with sensitivity and specificity >80% (2).
- Ultrasound (US)
  - Indicated if there is neurologic deficit on exam or concomitant pathology in shoulder, should be performed on case-by-case basis.
  - May reveal thickening of the CHL, thickening of soft tissues of the joint capsule, and increased joint fluid
  - Doppler may show increased vascularity surrounding the intra-articular (IA) portion of the biceps tendon and CHL.

Follow-Up Tests & Special Considerations

- Shared decision-making regarding treatment
- Pain referral for CRPS/RSD

Diagnostic Procedures/Other

Injection test can be helpful in differentiating AC from subacromial pathologies such as rotator cuff tendinopathy (which should improve with injection of local anesthetics, in contrast to AC). This should only be done if the diagnosis is still uncertain after a thorough history and physical.

TREATMENT

- Self-limited condition in most patients
- Physical therapy with exercises within the limits of pain
- Manage patient expectations; resolution often takes 18 months of medication and rehabilitation.
- Treat any underlying medical conditions associated with AC such as DM and thyroid disorders.

MEDICATION

- Medication can be used to provide symptomatic relief.
- Acetaminophen or nonsteroidal anti-inflammatory drugs (NSAIDs) are first line of treatment.
- Glucocorticoid injections:
  - Single IA corticosteroid injections and multi-site injections showed great statistical and clinical outcomes for pain when used in the beginning of the disease.
    - IA corticosteroid injections in patients with frozen shoulder for <1 year duration showed greater benefits compared to other interventions and such benefits were shown to last as long as 6 months.
  - A course of physical therapy after an injection, for 4 to 6 weeks, with or without IA corticosteroid appeared to be associated with short-term benefits of improving pain and ROM.
  - Injection may be diluted with a local anesthetic such as lidocaine.
    - Triamcinolone 20 to 40 mg or methylprednisolone 20 to 40 mg can be used.
  - Hydrodilation with normal saline combined with IA corticosteroid injection may expedite ROM recovery compared to corticosteroid injection alone (1).
- Although a short course of oral glucocorticoid can temporarily provide pain relief and improved mobility, the benefits were not greater than a few weeks. Studies have shown that IA corticosteroid injections are more effective than oral steroid treatment (1).

First Line

Conservative treatment

- Home exercises including "climbing the wall"
  - Climbing the wall: Face a wall and place the hand from the affected shoulder flat on the surface of the wall; use the fingers to "climb" the wall; pause 30 seconds every few inches. Repeat the exercise after turning the torso 90 degrees to wall (abduction).
- Patients may perform home exercises/physical therapy in conjunction with NSAIDs or glucocorticoid injections.
- Oral steroids are usually not recommended.

Second Line

If there is no improvement in 6 to 8 weeks of conservative treatment, more invasive treatment may be indicated.

- Hydrodilatation:
  - Injection of 10 to 20 mL of saline or 1% lidocaine along with glucocorticoid
- Continuation of physical therapy

ISSUES FOR REFERRAL

Surgical referral can be considered if symptoms have been present for >1 year and patients fail to make progress with appropriate management for 3 months.

ADDITIONAL THERAPIES

- Exercise and physical therapy:
  - Gentle ROM exercises should be offered to every patient.
    - Exercises should be performed daily and as tolerated. A structured plan should be given to the patient.
  - Physical therapy has been found to be beneficial especially in phases 2 and 3 of AC. Best data supports its use in conjunction with other treatment such as corticosteroid injections.
- Laser has been suggested as a possible treatment, particularly for pain relief; not enough evidence for support
- Suprascapular nerve block can provide temporary pain relief and may be a therapeutic option for AC refractory to IA corticosteroid injections; however, there is a lack of high-quality evidence for support (1).
- Other therapies that have been studied include whole-body cryotherapy and IA injection of botulinum toxin type A, both of which have demonstrated to improve pain and ROM but with limited evidence (1).

SURGERY/OTHER PROCEDURES

- Should be reserved for patients who do not respond to conservative measures for at least 1 year.
- Some of the most common procedures include manipulation under anesthesia (MUA), arthroscopic capsular release (ARC), distension arthrogram, among others. One study comparing ARC, MUA, and physiotherapy showed that while all three treatments led to substantial improvements in pain and function, none of the treatments were clinically superior to another.

ONGOING CARE

FOLLOW-UP RECOMMENDATIONS

- After establishing a diagnosis, assess the need for pain control and start the patient on NSAIDs, in combination with a gentle exercise program with guidance with physical therapy.
- Follow-up in 3 to 4 weeks: if no significant improvement, may consider IA corticosteroid injections
- Physical therapy should be concurrently used because it can hasten the rate of recovery and increase ROM.
- For secondary AC, consider evaluation and management of underlying condition.
- If no improvement, consider surgical intervention.

PATIENT EDUCATION

- Patient education is important; discuss prognosis and reinforce that patient will likely see improvement in symptoms with treatment compliance.
- Climbing the wall: Face a wall and place the hand from the affected shoulder flat on the surface of the wall; use the fingers to "climb" the wall; pause 30 seconds every few inches. Repeat the exercise after turning the torso 90 degrees to wall (abduction).
- In case of secondary AC, address the importance of treating underlying causes.

PROGNOSIS

- Recovery is dependent on onset of treatment, symptoms, and comorbidities in patient.
- Variable duration, lasting 1 to 3 years without intervention
- Patients with idiopathic frozen shoulder have a good rate of recovery.

REFERENCES

1. Le HV, Lee SJ, Nazarian A, et al. Adhesive capsulitis of the shoulder: review of pathophysiology and current clinical treatments. *Shoulder Elbow*. 2017;9(2):75–84.
2. Suh CH, Yun SJ, Jin W, et al. Systematic review and meta-analysis of magnetic resonance imaging features for diagnosis of adhesive capsulitis of the shoulder. *Eur Radiol*. 2019;29(2):566–577.

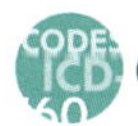

CODES

ICD10

- M75.00 Adhesive capsulitis of unspecified shoulder
- M75.01 Adhesive capsulitis of right shoulder
- M75.02 Adhesive capsulitis of left shoulder

CLINICAL PEARLS

- Frozen shoulder or AC is generally a self-limiting global restriction in ROM of the shoulder joint. Up to 15% will have long-term disability.
- Natural course consists of a painful phase, freezing phase, and thawing phase. It occurs mostly in older women; total prevalence is 2–5% of the general population and roughly 10–20% of the diabetic population.
- An active and passive ROM restriction will be present. Most commonly, patients will have is an inability to externally rotate the shoulder. Other signs include pain on provocation of subacromial space and inability to reach overhead or for back pocket.
- Plain x-rays are the preferred initial imaging modality. MRI and US are done only if there is concomitant pathology or neurologic deficit.
- Treatment includes pain control and physical therapy; can progress to glucocorticoid therapy with a consideration for surgery
- Resolution of symptoms may take up to 24 months.
- Given the prevalence in patients who are middle-aged, it is also referred to as the "50-year-old shoulder."

ADVANCE CARE PLANNING

Jessica A. Orner, MD

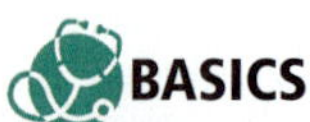

BASICS

DESCRIPTION

- Advance care planning (ACP) (1) is a process that allows patients to have a voice in current and future decisions about their care based on their individual values, wishes, and preferences. There is a recent shift from "planning" to "preparation" emphasizing the fluid and ongoing nature of these conversations.
- There are several methods of addressing a patient's priorities in their care:
  - Facilitated conversations with family and significant others
  - Advance directives, including living wills (LWs) and heath care durable powers of attorney, also known as a medical power of attorney (MPOA)
  - Physician/medical orders for life-sustaining treatment (POLST/MOLST) and directives to physicians
- ACP is an important aspect of patient-centered care as the population ages and individuals lose decision-making capacity, when new chronic medical conditions are diagnosed, or in the setting of severe acute illnesses.
- ACP helps to interpret patient wishes in the context of individual illness circumstances, negotiate conflicts in decisions, and allow patients to determine what is in their best interest based on personal values.
- Definitions
  - Advance directives (2): written instructions to guide decision-making in the event a patient is unable to provide informed consent
    - LWs and MPOAs usually only take effect if the patient has been determined to lack capacity to decide care for himself or herself; otherwise, patient preference takes precedence (even if contradictory to the LW).
    - If done appropriately, these help patients avoid languishing in poor quality of life states or receiving unwanted care which can be associated with complex ethical dilemmas.
  - LW: a patient's explicit written instructions of his or her wishes regarding medical care
    - Each state has specific legal requirements. Certain states do not recognize LWs but have other "medical directive" forms. LWs and medical directives can take effect immediately (e.g., when a patient is diagnosed with a terminal illness) or when a patient can no longer make decisions for himself or herself.
    - LWs have direct treatment instructions.
    - Challenges of LWs include lack of standardization, narrow scope, and limited updating on changes in disease trajectory.
    - LWs do not expire and they can be revised.
    - The LW is NOT a medical directive, so it cannot prevent life-sustaining treatment in an emergent situation (as a POLST/MOLST can [see next]).
  - MPOA: a written document designating a surrogate medical decision maker in the event a patient cannot speak for himself or herself
    - A health care proxy (HCP)/MPOA speaks on behalf of the patient to make decisions aligned as closely as possible to the patient's health care wishes. Ideally, this is someone the patient knows and trusts. It is also helpful if this individual has had discussions with the patient about his or her values and desires.
    - Different states have varying rules regarding precedence if there is a conflict between an LW provision and an HCP decision. When there is conflict, engage with palliative care, ethics, and legal.
    - If a patient has had goals of care discussions with friends or family but does not have a legally named HCP, those discussions can still help inform the decision-making process and elicit patient values.
  - POLST/MOLST: a medical directive which, unlike an LW, directs point-of-care decision-making by EMS/first responders
    - Designed to minimize confusion in emergent situations, these are adjunctive documents to LWs and MPOAs that provide clear instruction regarding resuscitation, intubation, and other life-sustaining treatments.
    - They are portable and follow a patient across different care settings. Given their simplicity, a POLST/MOLST is more likely to be followed than an LW, which can be difficult to locate.
    - Although EMS/first responders may be concerned about the legal implications of withholding life-sustaining treatment, POLST forms provide legal protection if patient wishes are followed.
- There are no authoritative guidelines for when to initiate discussions about ACP; age 65 years may be an appropriate time. Additionally, patient values and wishes should be discussed following a new diagnosis of a serious illness or a significant change in disease trajectory. Each conversation must be individualized.
- ACP should be completed while patients are able to make decisions about their future care. Every effort should be made to initiate discussions and complete required forms prior to incapacitating health changes.
- Nursing home residents and patients with dementia often do not have capacity to complete legal documents related to LW and MPOA.

Pediatric Considerations

For children with serious acute or terminal illness, it is a difficult (but important) part of treatment.

- Provider fears about increasing parental distress when discussing ACP are unfounded.
- ACP may unburden parents from difficult decisions and is associated with increased positive emotions, understanding of the patient's illness, and provider rapport.

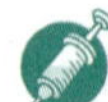

TREATMENT

- Suggested discussion points:
  - For all adult patients:
    - Assess willingness to engage in ACP. Do not force patients if they are not ready to have this potentially emotionally challenging conversation.
    - Discuss what values are most important to patients.
    - Ask patients to identify who they would like to make decisions for them if they were unable to do so.
    - Encourage patients to inform trusted family or friends about new diagnoses or changes in health.
    - Document decisions concisely and clearly.
  - For any patient with a chronic, serious, or terminal illness:
    - Ensure accurate understanding of the current medical situation and prognosis.
    - Discuss the natural course of disease progression, including time course, potential interventions (risks/benefits), and end-of-life expectations.
      - For example:
        - Chronic obstructive lung disease: exacerbations, decreased ability to perform activities of daily living, supplemental oxygen, mechanical ventilation
        - Malignancy: possibility of chronic pain, inability to swallow/poor appetite necessitating alternative feeding options, ascites and therapeutic procedures, treatment side effects
    - Discuss what matters most to the patient and other decision makers.
  - For older patients:
    - Consider routine discussions of ACP around age 65 years. It is crucial to speak with patients while they still have decision-making capacity. Discussions should be repeated regularly, especially if clinical course deteriorates, to ensure patient preferences have not changed.
    - Provide online resources for completing LWs.
    - Refer patients to legal or notary services for AD/MPOA, as applicable.
    - Complete POLST/MOLST forms in clinic, if applicable in your state.
  - For any change in clinical status (including frequent ER visits or hospitalizations):
    - Changes in functional status should prompt a discussion about prognosis and future wishes. Hospitalizations are important milestones to discuss recovery or decline.
    - Consider palliative care services.
    - Consider support services to prevent caregiver burnout.

- At the end of life, if it is the patient's desire, it is important to engage hospice services in a timely manner.
  - ACP discussions are often complicated by social, familial, cultural, spiritual, and medical factors. It is important to be sensitive to each patient's individual context.
  - Do not force the conversation if a patient is resistant or unprepared to discuss ACP.
    - Motivational interviewing can be used to gauge interest and readiness to discuss ACP.
    - Addressing implications for friends and family who may be burdened with decision-making may help promote ACP conversations.
  - The first time ACP is brought up often serves as an introduction to the topic and an opportunity for the patient to consider options. Subsequent visits can address specific scenarios and choices.
  - Avoid medical jargon (i.e., CPR, mechanical ventilation, parenteral nutrition, etc.) when addressing options. Patients may not understand the severity or implications of advanced life-saving interventions. It may be more effective to describe how a particular intervention may affect the patient and what the resulting quality of life may look like.

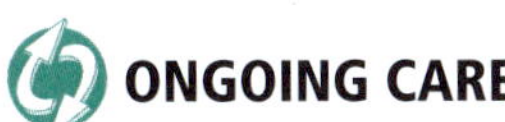

ONGOING CARE

Reimbursement: The Centers for Medicare & Medicaid Services reimburses physicians for ACP discussions.

- Current CPT codes are 99497 for the first 16 to 45 minutes of discussion and completion of forms, and 99498 as an add-on for a total of 46 to 75 minutes (3).
- There are no limits to the number of times ACP can be reported in a given period of time.
- An advance directive does not have to be completed in order to bill for services.
- No specific diagnosis is required for the ACP codes.

FOLLOW-UP RECOMMENDATIONS

Patient Monitoring

- There are no specific guidelines for how often an LW or durable powers of attorney (DPOA) discussion should be revisited after completion.
- When there is a new diagnosis or a significant change in clinical status, have the patient consider how it would affect his or her ACP decision-making.
- Have patients display POLST/MOLST forms prominently for ease of visibility to EMS, such as on their refrigerator.

PATIENT EDUCATION

- See "Additional Reading" for links: The National Hospice and Palliative Care Organization; National Institute on Aging; Aging with Dignity; National Healthcare Decisions Day; and the American Bar Association have resources to help patients.
- Online platforms such as Prepare for your Care and MyDirectives allow patients to specify their wishes electronically.
- DeathWise is a nonprofit organization with worksheets patients can use for the health, financial, care of body, and service components of ACP.

COMPLICATIONS

- Often LWs, MPOAs, and POLST/MOLSTs are completed, but physicians do not have access to them. Electronic health records are a convenient place to store documents, but they may be difficult to retrieve.
  - Any ACP form should be part of the medical record with open access (if possible) to facilitate appropriate decision-making.
- Emergency rooms are vulnerable to uncertainty about what interventions patients want if they cannot communicate for themselves and guiding documents are often not readily available. POLST forms can help avoid confusion.
- There is often misunderstanding on the part of both doctors and patients regarding do-not-resuscitate (DNR) and do-not-intubate (DNI) orders.
  - DNR/DNI orders can be reversed and should be readdressed as a patient's clinical status changes.
  - DNR/DNI in a person with a chronic progressive illness does not necessarily mean DNR/DNI for an acute reversible process.

REFERENCES

1. Sedini C, Biotto M, Crespi Bel'skij LM, et al. Advance care planning and advance directives: an overview of the main critical issues. *Aging Clin Exp Res*. 2022;34(2):325–330.
2. American Association of Retired Persons. Advance directive forms. http://www.aarp.org/caregiving/financial-legal/free-printable-advance-directives/. Accessed October 30, 2024.
3. Centers for Medicare & Medicaid Services. Medicare Learning Network: Advance Care Planning. https://www.cms.gov/Outreach-and-Education/Medicare-Learning-Network-MLN/MLNProducts/Downloads/AdvanceCarePlanning.pdf. Accessed November 12, 2024.

ADDITIONAL READING

- Aging with Dignity. Five wishes. https://www.agingwithdignity.org/. Accessed September 26, 2025.
- American Bar Association. Toolkit for health care advance planning. https://www.americanbar.org/groups/law_aging/resources/health_care_decision_making/consumer_s_toolkit_for_health_care_advance_planning.html. Accessed September 26, 2025.
- CaringInfo: http://www.caringinfo.org/
- DeathWise: https://www.deathwise.org/
- Heyland DK. Engaging seriously ill older patients in advance care planning. https://psnet.ahrq.gov/webmm/case/404/engaging-seriously-ill-older-patients-in-advance-care-planning. Accessed September 26, 2025.
- Malhotra C. Reimagining and rebranding advance care planning. *Age Ageing*. 2024;53(10):afae233.
- Moody SY, Bell CL, Lindenberger EC, et al. Adaptive care planning: a paradigm shift. *J Am Geriatr Soc*. 2024;72(2):337–345.
- My Directives: https://www.mydirectives.com/
- National Healthcare Decisions Day: https://theconversationproject.org/nhdd/
- National Hospice and Palliative Care Organization: https://allianceforcareathome.org/
- National Institute on Aging: https://www.nia.nih.gov/
- Prepare for your Care: https://prepareforyourcare.org/en/prepare/welcome

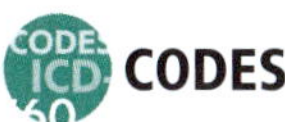

CODES

ICD10

- Z71.89 Other specified counseling
- Z51.5 Encounter for palliative care
- Z66 Do not resuscitate

CLINICAL PEARLS

- ACP is an important and underutilized element of compassionate and comprehensive patient-centered care.
- The primary barriers to discussing advanced directives from the patient perspective include lack of knowledge, fear of burdening family, and a desire for physicians to initiate the discussion.
- The primary barriers to discussing advanced directives from the physician perspective include discomfort with the topic and lack of time to fully address the topic.
- Fewer unwanted interventions occur in emergency room and inpatient settings when ACP is actively reviewed and patient wishes are documented and conveyed appropriately.

AIR TRAVEL EMERGENCIES

Theodore E. Macnow, MD • Michelle A. Georgia, DO • Camille D. Audette, DO

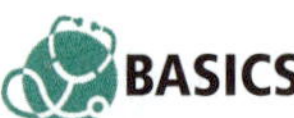

BASICS

DESCRIPTION

Physicians commonly help with in-flight medical events (IMEs). Many IMEs fall outside practitioner's normal scope of practice. The aircraft environment is cramped with limited medical resources. Despite these obstacles, health care workers should be prepared to render assistance when called upon in IME settings.

EPIDEMIOLOGY

Incidence

- ~3 million passengers travel daily worldwide. In the United States, 1.7 million individuals travel by plane every day.
- Airlines estimate an IME occurs on ~1 in 600 flights. Most (~90%) continue to their final destinations.
- The likelihood of encountering an IME is increasing because of larger aircraft, longer flights, and an aging population.
- The most common IMEs involve syncope/near syncope (32.7%), gastrointestinal (14.8%), respiratory (10.1%), and cardiovascular symptoms (7%) (1).

ETIOLOGY AND PATHOPHYSIOLOGY

Hypobaric hypoxia: Atmospheric pressure of oxygen drops from 160 mm Hg at sea level to 120 mm Hg at cruising altitude in a pressurized cabin. In healthy people, the drop in arterial oxygen tension is associated mean in-flight oxygen saturations of 93% (range: 85 to 98).

ALERT

Passengers with chronic obstructive pulmonary disease (COPD) or other pulmonary disorders have a lower baseline PaO_2, so any drop in oxygen tension may result in more significant hypoxemia. Passengers with unstable angina or heart failure may not be able to compensate for hypoxia. Alcohol consumption on airplanes by healthy individuals causes more significant and prolonged hypoxia and tachycardia during sleep.

- Gas expansion: Gases expand about 30% in flight. This can lead to a pneumothorax, sinus pressure, and tympanic membrane rupture in children with ear infections.
- Venous thromboembolism: There is an increased risk of deep vein thromboses (DVTs) on longer flights and in passengers with underlying medical conditions because of prolonged sitting, hypoxic conditions, and dehydration.
- Stress: Traveling is mentally and physically stressful, which may lead to psychiatric emergencies or acute coronary syndrome (ACS).
- Insomnia: Passengers have disrupted circadian rhythms, which may trigger seizures and contribute to medication nonadherence.
- Turbulence: Turbulence is increasing due to ongoing climate changes. Motion sickness is common and traumatic injury can result from falling luggage.
- Medication nonadherence: Missed medication administrations may occur due to travel time changes and medications in checked luggage.
- Decreased access to food and drink: Vasovagal syncope may result from dehydration. Diabetics may suffer hypoglycemia.
- Low air humidity: Cabin air is <20% relative humidity, which contributes to dehydration, epistaxis, and asthma or COPD exacerbations.
- Viral infections: Parainfluenza and influenza are the most common viruses communicated by proximity. The cabin air is filtered and not infectious.

ALERT

Transmission of SARS-CoV-2 virus can occur on air travel. Like other viruses, the risk is mostly from proximity to infected passengers rather than cabin air flow.

RISK FACTORS

- Recent surgery: Passengers are at risk for wound dehiscence, bowel perforation, and compartment syndrome from gas expansion.
- COPD, asthma, CHF, or coronary artery disease: Passengers may suffer from hypoxemia and not be able to compensate appropriately.
- Recent cast placement: Passengers are at risk for compartment syndrome due to tissue edema.
- Hypercoagulability: Passengers with inherited or acquired hypercoagulable conditions, pregnancy, certain medications, heart disease, or recent surgery are at increased risk for DVTs.
- Recent scuba diving: Passengers are at risk for decompression syndromes.
- Long flights: The effects of hypoxia are cumulative and time dependent.

GENERAL PREVENTION

General guidelines:

- Travelers should discuss medication timing with their doctor and bring necessary medications and equipment onboard with them in carry-on luggage.
- Supplemental in-flight oxygen is required for patients with a baseline PaO_2 <70 mm Hg or who are unable to walk a flight of stairs or 150 feet without becoming short of breath or experiencing angina (2)[C].

Pregnancy Considerations

Women are generally safe to fly if there are no other complications. Some airlines restrict travel after 36 weeks' gestation.

Pediatric Considerations

- Travelers with children should bring liquid formulations of medication in allowed quantities on the plane. Children with asthma should have a rescue inhaler with spacer and facemask.
- Specific guidelines:
  - Avoid flying 10 to 14 days after surgery (varies by type of surgery).
  - Casts may need to be bivalved if applied 24 to 48 hours before a flight.
  - Avoid scuba diving 24 hours before flying.
  - DVT prevention (2)[C]:
    - Adequately hydrate.
    - Stand, stretch, and exercise legs in flight.
    - Passengers with risk factors may need compression stockings, aspirin, or anticoagulation.

DIAGNOSIS

HISTORY

- Symptoms vary based on emergency; gather as much history as possible.
- Ask about past medical and surgical history, medications and compliance, and allergies.
- Inquire about illicit drug or alcohol use, and any recent activities (i.e., scuba diving).
- Document findings and recommendations and save a secure copy.

PHYSICAL EXAM

- Wear all available PPE. Protective gloves are available on board.
- May need to obtain blood pressure by palpitation due to noise
- Assess vital signs, general appearance, and mental status. Look for signs of dehydration including skin perfusion.
- If stethoscope available—auscultate as good as possible.

ALERT

Assess for tension pneumothorax by listening for decreased lung sounds and contralateral tracheal deviation. A tension pneumothorax requires needle decompression.

DIFFERENTIAL DIAGNOSIS

- **Syncope or near-syncope**: vasovagal syncope, dehydration, hypoglycemia, intoxication, medication reaction or toxicity, ACS, arrhythmia, cerebrovascular accident, pulmonary thrombosis/air embolism, and hypoxia
- **Chest pain**: ACS, pulmonary embolism, pneumothorax, bronchospasm, aortic dissection, gastroesophageal reflux, musculoskeletal etiology, and anxiety
- **Shortness of breath**: COPD or asthma exacerbation, pneumonia, pulmonary thrombosis/air embolism, toxic exposure
- **Stroke-like symptoms**: cerebrovascular accident, transient ischemic attack, hypoglycemia, seizure, syncope, intracranial mass, and complex migraine
- **Seizure**: seizure, syncope, hypoglycemia, eclampsia, cardiac arrest
- **Gastrointestinal illness**: motion sickness, food-borne illness, gastritis, enteritis, gastroesophageal reflux, pancreatitis, medication, or substance withdrawal
- **Obstetric emergency**: preterm labor, miscarriage, eclampsia, placenta previa
- **Allergic reaction**: urticaria, anaphylaxis, dermatitis
- **Cardiac arrest**: arrhythmia, pulmonary embolism, respiratory arrest, ACS, intoxication, syncope
- **Altered mental status**: Use or withdrawal from drugs or alcohol (consider gastrointestinal absorption from smuggling), hypoglycemia, panic attack, DKA, hypoxia, psychiatric emergency

DIAGNOSTIC TESTS & INTERPRETATION

The automated external defibrillator (AED) may be used as a cardiac monitor. Consider prescribed or personal wearable technology and smart devices to provide ongoing diagnostic information such as heart rate, pulse oximetry, limited ECG, or glucose monitoring (3).

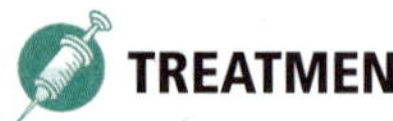

TREATMENT

GENERAL MEASURES

- **First aid and CPR**: If there is no pulse or not breathing, start CPR, BLS, ALS, and PALS as appropriate. Airline crew members are trained in first aid and CPR.
- **Ask for help**: Ask the flight crew and other passengers for equipment, medications, expertise, and lifting assistance.
- **Oxygen**: All flights have oxygen at 2 to 5 L/min by facemask. This oxygen delivery at cruising altitude mimics conditions at sea level. Oxygen should be applied in all cases of respiratory distress, chest pain, seizures, and altered mental status.

- **Ground-based physician support**: Many airlines contract with companies that offer in-flight medical advice, interpreter services, recommendations for diversion, and even telemedicine technology.
- **Request to fly at lower attitude**: Flying <22,500 feet with cabin pressurization mimics sea level oxygen pressure. Flying lower uses more fuel and is slower; so, it may not be optimal to reach a hospital quickly.
- **Request a diversion**: The pilot can request an expedited landing, medical services on arrival, or a closer destination. Medical emergencies that involve resuscitation, persistent abnormal vital signs, chest pain, stroke symptoms, respiratory distress, unconsciousness, obstetrics, or psychiatric emergencies should be considered for diversion.

MEDICATION

- All U.S. commercial aircraft have an emergency medical kit (EMK) as well as basic first aid kits on the aircraft. The contents vary among countries, airlines, and aircraft. Many airlines have adopted a more extensive EMK.
- The minimal contents in the EMK required by the Federal Aviation Administration are described in Table 1.

Table 1. FAA-Mandated Contents of Emergency Medical Kit

Equipment	Oropharyngeal airways (3 sizes)
	Cardiopulmonary resuscitation mask
	Manual resuscitation devices, 3 masks
	Adhesive tape, 1 inch
	Alcohol sponges
	IV administration set
	Needles
	Protective gloves
	Sphygmomanometer
	Stethoscope
	Tape scissors
	Tourniquet
	Instructions on kit use
Medications	Analgesic, nonnarcotic
	Antihistamine, 50 mg, injectable
	Antihistamine tablets, 25 mg
	Aspirin tablets, 325 mg
	Atropine, 0.5 mg, 5 mL
	Bronchodilator, inhaled (i.e., albuterol)
	Dextrose, 50%/50 mL, injectable
	Epinephrine 1:1,000, 1 mL, injectable
	Epinephrine 1:10,000, 2 mL, injectable
	Lidocaine, 5 mL, 20 mg/mL, injectable
	Nitroglycerine tablets
	Saline solution (minimum 500 cc)

- Depending on the airline, local policies, and country of operation, nurse practitioners and physician assistants may be able to open and use the EMK.
- All aircraft are equipped with an AED.

ALERT

Not usually found in the EMK are glucometers, intubation equipment, ACLS drugs, narcotics, insulin, or antibiotics. In a 2019 survey, only 35% of EMKs contain naloxone. Ask other passengers for needed medications or equipment.

Pediatric Considerations

The most common cause of airplane diversion in the pediatric population was secondary to seizures. Most EMKs do not contain anticonvulsant medications. EMKs do not include liquid or suppository medications. Consider crushing tablets or asking other passengers for medication or equipment. A toilet paper roll or cut soda bottle can be taped to an albuterol pump to make a spacer.

ADDITIONAL THERAPIES

- **Cardiac arrest**: CPR; early defibrillation; epinephrine 1:10,000 q3–5 minutes, (adults: 1 mg IV, pediatric: 0.01 mg/kg IV); lidocaine or atropine when indicated; recommend diversion.
- **ACS**: oxygen by facemask, aspirin 325 mg PO, nitroglycerin (0.4 mg sublingually q5 to 10 minutes if systolic blood pressure >100 mm Hg). Apply AED. Recommend diversion.
- **Asthma/COPD exacerbation**: oxygen, albuterol 2.5 mg inhaled (repeat as needed), steroid (if available), epinephrine 1:1,000, (autoinjector: adult: 0.3 mg, pediatric [<25 kg]: 0.15 mg IM; ampule: adult 0.3 mg, pediatric 0.01 mg/kg) if significant respiratory distress; consider diversion.
- **Allergic reaction**: diphenhydramine (PO or IV, adult: 25 to 50 mg, pediatric: 1 mg/kg); If anaphylaxis, epinephrine 1:1,000, (autoinjector: adult: 0.3 mg, pediatric [<25 kg]: 0.15 mg IM; ampule: adult 0.3 mg, pediatric 0.01 mg/kg); NS (IV, adults: 1L, pediatric: 20 cc/kg); steroid (if available); divert if anaphylaxis.
- **Vasovagal syncope**: Elevate legs. If alert and oriented, offer oral liquids. Consider IV fluid bolus. Consider hypoglycemia and offer oral glucose. Monitor blood pressure. Consider diversion if the patient remains symptomatic or has persistent abnormal vital signs.
- **Gastrointestinal**: Oral antiemetic and antacid may be available from the EMK or other passengers. If there is abdominal pain; consider diversion.
- **Tension pneumothorax**: Needle thoracostomy is preferred over 2nd intercostal space midclavicular line.
- **Psychiatric emergency**: Consider intoxication, hypoglycemia/hyperglycemia, and hypoxia. Attempt verbal de-escalation. The airline protocol should be used for physical restraint. Ask patient and other passengers if they have oral anxiolytics. Monitor the patient for signs of respiratory distress or ACS if restrained. Consider diversion.
- **Opioid ingestion**: Rescue breathing as needed; naloxone if available in EMK or from other passengers 0.4 to 0.8 mg IV or 2 mg intranasal or IM

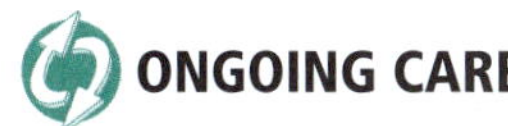

ONGOING CARE

PROGNOSIS

- The Aviation Medical Assistance Act of 1998 covers any person with a medical license qualified to provide medical care in the United States who act to the best they can within their training and do not demonstrate gross negligence or willful misconduct. No physician has been successfully sued in the United States for volunteering care in an IME.
- When overhead paged for assistance, health care workers responded 76% of the time, physicians in 48% of cases. 60% of IMEs improve with help from a health care provider.

REFERENCES

1. Martin-Gill C, Doyle TJ, Yealy DM. In-flight medical emergencies: a review. *JAMA*. 2018;320(24):2580–2590. doi:10.1001/jama.2018.19842.
2. Air Travel. CDC Yellow Book 2024. Centers for Disease Control and Prevention. https://wwwnc.cdc.gov/travel/yellowbook/2024/air-land-sea/air-travel. Accessed September 13, 2025.
3. Kim DS, Webster E, Rodriguez F, et al. High-flying precision medicine: leveraging wearable technology for in-flight emergencies. *PLOS Digit Health*. 2025;4(4):e0000834. doi:10.1371/journal.pdig.0000834.

CLINICAL PEARLS

- Medical emergencies on airplanes are common. Most are minor.
- Equipment and drugs on board airplanes vary widely.
- Flights are equipped with AEDs and oxygen.
- Many airlines partner with ground-based physician support.
- Use passengers as a resource for help, information, and supplies.

ALCOHOL USE DISORDER (AUD)

Jason Assalita, DO • Charanjot Singh, MD • Muhammad Talha Waseem, MBBS

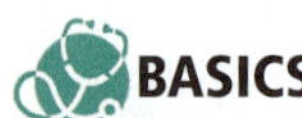

BASICS

DESCRIPTION

- Any pattern of alcohol use causing significant physical, mental, or social dysfunction; key features are tolerance, withdrawal, and persistent use despite problems.
- The severity of alcohol use disorder (AUD) exists on a spectrum but is classified as mild, moderate, or severe based on the number of clinical criteria that are met. Manifestation of 2 to 3 of the *DSM-5* criteria for substance use disorders is considered mild disease, 4 to 5 is classified as moderate, and ≥6 is severe AUD.
- *DSM-5* criteria for AUD
  - Impaired control
    - Alcohol cravings
    - Unable to cut down or quit using alcohol
    - A large amount of time is spent using or recovering from alcohol.
    - Drinking larger amounts or over longer time than intended
  - Social dysfunction/physical risk
    - Alcohol use during hazardous situations or continued alcohol use that leads to hazardous situation
    - Continued use of alcohol despite a negative impact on relationships
    - Failure to meet obligations at work or school
    - Social or occupational activities that were once important to the person are abandoned.
    - Continued alcohol use despite known physical or psychological consequences (i.e., hypertension, hyperlipidemia, cirrhosis, depression, anxiety)
    - Physiologic dependence
    - Tolerance or withdrawal
    - Loss of control over the amount of alcohol used
- National Institute on Alcohol Abuse and Alcoholism (NIAAA) criteria for low-risk alcohol use
  - Low-risk alcohol use: NIAAA criteria for low-risk drinking is no more than 14 drinks a week or no more than 4 drinks per occasion. For women, low-risk drinking involves no more than 7 drinks a week or 3 per occasion. Alcohol use that exceeds these levels does not always result in AUD but can still be problematic for an individual.
  - The safest level of use is considered no use as even low-level use is associated with reduction in gray matter and cognitive impairment.
  - Binge drinking: drinking that brings blood alcohol levels to 0.08 g/dL; this is usually 4 drinks for women and 5 drinks for men in 2 hours.
- Measuring alcohol use
  - A standard drink includes 14 g (0.6 fluid oz) of pure alcohol. This includes the following:
    - 12 oz of beer, that are 5% alcohol
    - 5 oz of wine, that are 12% alcohol
    - 1.5 oz of distilled spirits that are 40% alcohol

Geriatric Considerations

- Multiple drug interactions
- Signs and symptoms of AUD may be different or attributed to a chronic medical problem or dementia.
- Accelerated aging from frequent alcohol use together with increased consumption in middle-aged and older adults increases risk of cognitive decline and dementia.

Pediatric Considerations

- Children of alcoholics are at increased risk; 2.5% of adolescents have AUD; 13.4% of youth aged 12 to 20 years report binge drinking in the past month; negative effect on maturation and normal brain development
- Early-onset drinkers (those who start drinking before age 21 years) are 4 times more likely to develop a problem than those who begin after age 21 years.

EPIDEMIOLOGY

Predominant age 18 to 25 years, but all ages affected; male > female (3:1)

- Young drinkers through college age commonly engage in heavy to binge drinking (4 drinks for women and 5 drinks for men in 2 hours) to extreme binge-drinking (>15 drinks in one session) on weekends.
- New data reflects increased drinking in middle-aged to older adults and binge drinking, especially in women, increasing risk of cognitive decline and dementia. Drinking particularly increased during the COVID-19 pandemic.

Prevalence

- 23% of Americans aged ≥18 years reported binge drinking in the past month; 6% reported heavy alcohol use in the past month; 15 million adults (6%) aged >18 years has AUD.
- AUD affects ~11% of the US population and contributes to 140,000 deaths annually.
- In the United States, harmful alcohol use is the third leading cause of preventable death and has become a major public health crisis.
- <20% of individuals with AUD receive treatment.

ETIOLOGY AND PATHOPHYSIOLOGY

- Multifactorial: genetic, environment, psychosocial
- Alcohol is a CNS depressant, facilitating γ-aminobutyric acid (GABA) inhibition and blocking *N*-methyl-D-aspartate receptors.

Genetics

50–60% of risk is genetic.

RISK FACTORS

- Family history; depression; anxiety disorders; bipolar disorder; eating disorders
- Tobacco and/or other substance abuse
- Male gender; lower socioeconomic status; unemployment; poor self-esteem
- Posttraumatic stress disorder; antisocial personality disorder; criminal behavior

GENERAL PREVENTION

- Counsel patients with family history and risk factors.
- USPSTF recommends screening adults for alcohol use and providing brief counseling to those with risky drinking habits.
- Screening and brief intervention (SBI)

COMMONLY ASSOCIATED CONDITIONS

- Cardiomyopathy; atrial fibrillation; hypertension
- Peptic ulcer disease; cirrhosis; fatty liver; cholelithiasis; hepatitis; pancreatitis
- Diabetes mellitus; malnutrition; upper GI malignancies
- Peripheral neuropathy, seizures
- Abuse and violence
- Behavioral disorders (depression, bipolar, schizophrenia): >50% of patients have a comorbid substance abuse problem.

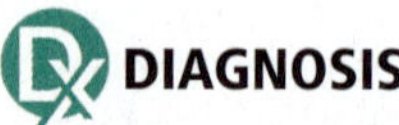

DIAGNOSIS

Use *DSM-5* criteria listed previously

HISTORY

- Thorough behavioral history
- Anxiety, depression, insomnia, psychological and social dysfunction, marital or relationship problems, domestic violence
- Complaints about alcohol-related behavior; frequent trauma, MVAs, ED visits

PHYSICAL EXAM

- General: fever, diaphoresis, agitation
- Cardiovascular: hypertension, dilated cardiomyopathy, tachycardia, arrhythmias
- Respiratory: aspiration pneumonia
- GI: stigmata of chronic liver disease, peptic ulcer disease, pancreatitis, esophageal malignancies, esophageal varices
- Musculoskeletal: poorly healed fractures, myopathy, osteopenia, osteoporosis, bone marrow suppression
- Neurologic: tremors, cognitive deficits (e.g., memory impairment), peripheral neuropathy, Wernicke-Korsakoff syndrome (from severe acute deficiency of thiamine: Korsakoff psychosis is a chronic neurologic sequela of Wernicke encephalopathy). Wernicke encephalopathy has the traditional triad of ophthalmoplegia, ataxia, and confusion.
- Dermatologic: burns (e.g., cigarettes), bruises, poor hygiene, palmar erythema, spider telangiectasias

DIFFERENTIAL DIAGNOSIS

- Other substance use disorders
- Depression, dementia; cerebellar ataxia; cerebrovascular accident (CVA); benign essential tremor; seizure disorder
- Hypoglycemia; diabetic ketoacidosis; viral hepatitis

DIAGNOSTIC TESTS & INTERPRETATION

Screening

- CAGE questionnaire: (Cut down, Annoyed, Guilty, and Eye opener): >2 "yes" answers is 74–89% sensitive, 79–95% specific for AUD; less sensitive for white women, college students, elderly; not an appropriate tool for less severe forms of alcohol abuse
- Single question for unhealthy use: "How many times in the last year have you had X or more drinks in 1 day?" (X = 5 for men, 4 for women); 81.8% sensitive, 79% specific for AUDs
- Alcohol Use Disorders Identification Test (AUDIT): 10 items, if score is >5: 70–92% sensitive, better in populations with low incidence of alcoholism: https://www.nams.sg/helpseekers/alcohol/self-assessment-tool/Pages/default.aspx
- AUDIT-C is a three-item screening tool. Scores over 4 for men and 3 for women are concerning for alcohol misuse.
  - Q#1: How often did you have a drink containing alcohol in the past year?
  - Q#2: How many drinks containing alcohol did you have on a typical day when you were drinking in the past year?
  - Q#3: How often did you have ≥6 drinks on one occasion in the past year?

Initial Tests (lab, imaging)

- CBC; liver function tests (LFTs); electrolytes; BUN/creatinine; lipid panel; INR, thiamine; folate; hepatitis A, B, and C serology
- Amylase, lipase (if GI symptoms present)
- Serum levels increased in chronic abuse:
  - AST/ALT ratio >2; γ-glutamyl transferase (GGT); carbohydrate-deficient transferrin; uric acid
  - Elevated mean corpuscular volume (MCV); ↑ prothrombin time; triglycerides and cholesterol (total)
- Often decreased: Serum protein, albumin; thiamine, folate
- CAT scan or MRI of brain: cortical atrophy, lesions in thalamic nucleus, and basal forebrain
- Abdominal ultrasound (US): ascites, periportal fibrosis, fatty infiltration, inflammation
- Calculate MELD score.

Follow-Up Tests & Special Considerations

Abdominal US every 6 months to screen for hepatocellular carcinoma (HCC) among individuals with cirrhosis

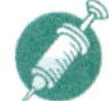

TREATMENT

For management of acute withdrawal, see "Alcohol Withdrawal."

GENERAL MEASURES

- Brief interventions and counseling by clinicians have proven effective for problem drinking.
- Treat comorbid problems (sleep, anxiety, etc.), but use extreme caution in prescribing medications with cross tolerance to alcohol (benzodiazepines).
- Group programs and/or 12-step programs help patients accept treatment and develop insight (i.e., Alcoholics Anonymous groups).

MEDICATION

First Line

- Long-term treatment of AUD is initiated after resolution of acute withdrawal:
  - FDA approved
    - Naltrexone: 50 mg/day PO or 380 mg IM once every 4 weeks; most evidence-based FDA-approved medication for AUD; opiate antagonist reduces craving and likelihood of relapse and decreases number of heavy drinking days among people with AUD (IM route may enhance compliance and efficacy); will precipitate withdrawal if patient is on opioids
    - Acamprosate: 666 mg (two 333-mg tablets) PO TID after withdrawal completed; consider if contraindication to naltrexone; reduces relapse risk; if helpful, use for 1 year; caution in stage 4 chronic kidney disease (CKD) (GFR <30)
    - Disulfiram: 500 mg PO for 1 to 2 weeks followed by 250 mg/day; FDA approved but not considered first line given unproven efficacy and severe risks; may provide psychological deterrent; most effective if used with close supervision; extreme caution with use given potential for severe emesis in population at risk for esophageal varices; severe reactions may involve myocardial infarction, upper GI bleed, seizure, and death; CYP2E1 inhibitor, causes increase in serum levels of phenytoin, warfarin, and isoniazid leading to toxicity (1).
- Supplements for all
  - Thiamine: 100 mg/day (first dose IV prior to glucose to avoid Wernicke encephalopathy)
  - Folic acid: 1 mg/day
  - Multivitamin: daily
- Contraindications
  - Naltrexone: caution during pregnancy, acute hepatitis, cirrhosis
  - Acamprosate: caution if GFR <30

ALERT

Treat acute symptoms if in alcohol withdrawal; give thiamine 100 mg/day with first dose prior to glucose.

Second Line

Non–FDA-approved medications for long-term treatment of AUD (initiate after resolution of acute withdrawal)

- Topiramate: 25 to 300 mg/day PO or divided BID; may enhance abstinence (off-label FDA use)
- Baclofen: initial dose 5 mg TID; initial dose may be titrated to 10 mg TID with max dose 60 mg/day in three divided doses; well tolerated in patients with cirrhosis; doses beyond 60 mg/day provide no identifiable benefit.
- Selective serotonin reuptake inhibitors may be beneficial if comorbid depression exists.
- Varenicline may provide benefit to patients with AUD who also smoke.

ISSUES FOR REFERRAL

Addiction specialist, 12-step or long term program, behavioral health professional

ADDITIONAL THERAPIES

Psychosocial interventions complement pharmacologic therapy and include cognitive behavioral therapy (CBT), motivational enhancement therapy (MET), and 12-step programs

ONGOING CARE

FOLLOW-UP RECOMMENDATIONS

Weekly follow-up at the outset is often ideal with progressive spacing to 4-week follow-up as condition stabilizes.

Patient Monitoring

- Outpatient detoxification: daily visits (not recommended for patients with heavy alcohol abuse)
- Early outpatient rehabilitation: weekly visits; detoxification alone is not sufficient.

DIET

- Calorie intake: Recommended calorie intake for men is 2,200 to 3,000 kcal/day and for women 1,800 to 2,400 kcal/day. An increase of 10–20% is recommended in people with malnutrition.
- Vitamin and minerals: rich in vitamins B_6, B_9, and B_1, zinc, vitamin A, vitamin D, and vitamin K as alcohol causes deficiency of these vitamins. Typical diet would include whole grains, nuts, legumes, cereals, seafood, green leafy vegetables, citrus fruits.
- Protein: Recommended intake in AUD without encephalopathy is 1.2 to 1.5 g/kg of body weight per day to prevent muscle wasting.
- For patient with encephalopathy, normal to high protein intake >1.2 g/kg/day.
- Carbohydrates: should provide 50–60% of total calories
- Fats: Typically, fats should contribute 25–30% of the total recommended calories.
- Salts: For patients with liver damage recommended is <2,000 mg/day. In severe cases of ascites, <1,500 mg/day is recommended.

PATIENT EDUCATION

- Center for Substance Abuse Treatment: https://www.samhsa.gov/about/offices-centers/csat
- Alcoholics Anonymous: https://www.aa.org/
- Secular Organizations for Sobriety: https://aaagnostica.org/secular-organization-for-sobriety-sos/

PROGNOSIS

- Chronic relapsing disease; mortality rate more than twice general population, death 10 to 15 years earlier
- Abstinence benefits: survival, mental health, family, employment
- 12-step programs, cognitive behavior, and motivational therapies are often effective during 1st year following treatment.

REFERENCES

1. Haber PS. Identification and treatment of alcohol use disorder. *N Engl J Med*. 2025;392(3):258–266. doi:10.1056/NEJMra2306511.

ADDITIONAL READING

- NIAAA. Rethinking drinking. https://www.rethinkingdrinking.niaaa.nih.gov. Accessed September 26, 2025.
- NIAAA: Helping patients who drink too much: a clinician's guide. https://www.niaaa.nih.gov/guide. Accessed September 26, 2025.

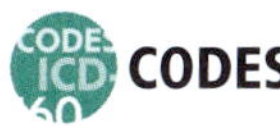

CODES

ICD10

- F10.10 Alcohol abuse, uncomplicated
- F10.20 Alcohol dependence, uncomplicated
- F10.239 Alcohol dependence with withdrawal, unspecified

CLINICAL PEARLS

- CAGE questionnaire: >2 "yes" answers is 74–89% sensitive, 79–95% specific for AUD; less sensitive for white women, college students, elderly; not an appropriate tool for less severe forms of alcohol abuse
- Single question for unhealthy use screening: "How many times in the last year have you had X or more drinks in 1 day?" (X = 5 for men, 4 for women); 81.8% sensitive, 79% specific for AUD
- NIAAA criteria for "at-risk" drinking: men >14 drinks a week or >4 per occasion; women: >7 drinks a week or >3 per occasion

ALCOHOL WITHDRAWAL

Ulunma Natalie Umesi, MD, MBA • Oluwole Jegede, MD, MPH, FAPA

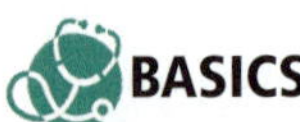

BASICS

DESCRIPTION

Alcohol withdrawal syndrome (AWS) is a spectrum of symptoms resulting from abrupt cessation or reduction in alcohol intake, after a period of prolonged use. Presentation ranges from minor symptoms such as tremors, and insomnia, to major complications such as seizures, and delirium tremens. Symptoms generally start within a few hours of the last drink and peak at 24 to 48 hours; life-threatening symptoms can begin several days after the last drink.

EPIDEMIOLOGY

Incidence

In the United States, about 10.2% of people ≥12 years old (~29 million individuals) have an alcohol use disorder (AUD) annually, based on the 2023 National Survey on Drug Use and Health (NSDUH).

ETIOLOGY AND PATHOPHYSIOLOGY

- Consumption of alcohol stimulates γ-aminobutyric acid (GABA), resulting in decreased excitability, with chronic ingestion, this repeated stimulation downregulates GABA inhibitory effects.
- Concurrently, alcohol ingestion inhibits glutamate on the central nervous system (CNS), with chronic alcohol use upregulation of excitatory *N*-methyl-D-aspartate glutamate receptors.
- When alcohol is abruptly stopped, the joint effect of a downregulated inhibitory system (GABA modulated) and upregulated excitatory system (glutamate modulated) results in brain hyperexcitability no longer suppressed by alcohol; clinically seen as AWS

Genetics

Several genes may increase an individual's susceptibility to AUD by affecting alcohol metabolism, brain chemistry, and reward systems. For example, the ADH1B gene which regulates the rate of liver metabolism of alcohol and the ALDH2 gene is involved with acetaldehyde metabolism, certain variants can cause a build-up of acetaldehyde, making drinking uncomfortable and potentially reducing the risk of AUD. Numerous other genes influence the brain's sensitivity to alcohol's effects (e.g., DRD2, OPRM1 genes).

RISK FACTORS

- Long duration of heavy alcohol consumption
- Recent binge-drinking behavior (NIAAA)
- Prior history of alcohol withdrawal episodes
- Elevated blood pressure on presentation, comorbid medical conditions, or surgical illness
- Physiologic dependence on benzodiazepines (BZDs) or barbiturates

Geriatric Considerations

Older adults with AUD are more susceptible to withdrawal.

Pregnancy Considerations

- Inpatient hospitalization for acute alcohol withdrawal recommended
- TWEAK—screening tool for alcohol use; helpful for use in pregnant people

GENERAL PREVENTION

The U.S. Preventive Services Task Force recommends screening all adults for AUD.

- Screening tools include CAGE, CAGE-AID, AUDIT, AUDIT-C to detect unhealthy alcohol use.

COMMONLY ASSOCIATED CONDITIONS

With chronic AUD:

- Electrolyte abnormalities
- Cirrhosis, esophageal varices, GI bleed, pancreatitis
- Macrocytic anemia
- Hypertension, atrial fibrillation
- Wernicke-Korsakoff syndrome

DIAGNOSIS

- *Diagnostic and Statistical Manual of Mental Disorders 5th Edition* diagnostic criteria for AWS:
  - Two (or more) of the following present within a few hours after the cessation or reduction of heavy and prolonged alcohol ingestion:
    - Autonomic hyperactivity
    - Hand tremor
    - Insomnia
    - Psychomotor agitation
    - Anxiety
    - Nausea or vomiting
    - Generalized seizures
    - Transient visual, auditory, or tactile hallucinations or illusions
- Clinical manifestations
  - Autonomic hyperactivity: onset a few hours of cessation and peak 24 to 48 hours
  - Neural excitation: Alcohol withdrawal–associated seizures are often brief, and typically occur 12 to 48 hours after last drink.
  - Alcohol withdrawal delirium: onset 48 to 72 hours after cessation

HISTORY

- Duration and quantity of alcohol intake, time since last drink
- Prior symptoms of alcohol withdrawal, or history of prior admissions for AUD
- Concurrent substance use
- Preexisting medical and psychiatric conditions, prior seizure activity
- Social history: living situation, social support, stressors, and triggers

PHYSICAL EXAM

Assess for conditions that are exacerbated by AWS.

- Cardiovascular: arrhythmias, heart failure, coronary artery disease
- GI: GI bleed, liver disease, pancreatitis
- Neuro: full neurologic workup, oculomotor dysfunction, gait ataxia, neuropathy
- Psych: orientation, memory (may be complicated by hepatic encephalopathy), perceptual disturbances
- General: hand tremor (6 to 8 cycles per second), infections
- The Clinical Institute Withdrawal Assessment for Alcohol-Revised (CIWA-Ar) scale

DIFFERENTIAL DIAGNOSIS

- Cocaine, amphetamines, anticholinergic drug intoxications
- Opioid, marijuana, and other sedating substances withdrawal
- Neuroleptic malignant syndrome
- Sepsis, CNS infection, or hemorrhage
- Mania, psychosis, anxiety, or panic disorder
- Thyroid crisis

DIAGNOSTIC TESTS & INTERPRETATION

Initial Tests (lab, imaging)

- Blood alcohol level, urine drug screen
- Complete blood count; comprehensive metabolic panel; lipase; amylase, GGT

Follow-Up Tests & Special Considerations

- For patients reporting abdominal pain, with elevated amylase or lipase, consider abdominal ultrasound or CT.
- Electrocardiogram for patients aged >50 years or with history of cardiac problems

Diagnostic Procedures/Other

Consider head CT, EEG and lumbar puncture depending on the clinical presentation

Test Interpretation

Rate of metabolism of alcohol varies but is generally 10 to 15 mg/dL/hr; patients with prolonged alcohol use metabolize at a faster rate of 20 to 30 mg/dL/hr. Using these calculations can approximate when withdrawal symptoms may increase.

- Blood alcohol concentration (BAC): <100 mg% loss of coordination and mood changes
- BAC: 100 to 199 neurologic impairment, slower reaction time, or ataxia
- BAC: 200 to 299 obvious intoxication is present, unless person has marked tolerance.
- BAC: >300 can be associated with slurred speech, amnesia, coma, and death.

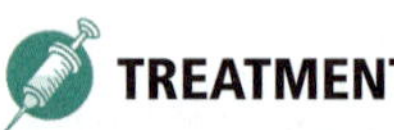

TREATMENT

GENERAL MEASURES

- Goals of therapy:
  - Provide a safe humane withdrawal, while protecting the individual's dignity.
  - Prepare for ongoing treatment of dependency.
- The Clinical Institute Withdrawal Assessment of Alcohol-Revised (CIWA-Ar) scale is useful for deciding medication dosing and frequency for AWS. Severity of symptoms are rated on a scale from 0 to 7, with 0 being without symptoms and 7 being the maximum score (except orientation and clouding of sensorium, scale 0 to 4) (1).
  - Nausea and vomiting
  - Tactile disturbances
  - Tremor
  - Auditory disturbances
  - Paroxysmal sweats
  - Visual disturbances
  - Anxiety
  - Headache or fullness in head
  - Agitation
  - Orientation and clouding of sensorium

- Mild withdrawal: score ≤8: likely resolve without medication
- Moderate withdrawal: 8 to 14: often require management with medication
- Severe withdrawal: ≥15 are associated with the highest risk of seizures and development of DTs.
- Frequent reevaluation with CIWA-Ar score is crucial.

MEDICATION

First Line

- BZD monotherapy has been the treatment of choice for CIWA-Ar scores >10, based on the following considerations (1):
  - Agents with rapid onset control agitation more quickly (e.g., IV diazepam).
  - Long-acting BZDs (diazepam, chlordiazepoxide) are more effective at preventing breakthrough seizures and contribute to reduction in rebound symptoms.
  - Short-acting BZDs (lorazepam, oxazepam) are preferable when prolonged sedation is a concern (e.g., elderly patients); oxazepam, lorazepam, and temazepam are preferable when there is hepatic impairment.
- Symptom-triggered regimens are associated with lower BZD amounts and reduce hospitalization length of stay.
- Fixed-schedule regimens are helpful if nursing staff do not have training for symptom triggered regimens, or if history of CAD, or past withdrawal seizures.
- Symptom-triggered regimen: Administer one of the following medications every 4 to 6 hours, with added doses PRN when CIWA-Ar ≥8. Assess need for further medications 1 hour after each dose.
  - Chlordiazepoxide: 50 to 100 mg PO
  - Diazepam: 10 to 20 mg PO
  - Oxazepam: 30 to 60 mg PO
  - Lorazepam: 2 to 4 mg PO
- Fixed-schedule regimen: Administer one of the following medications every 6 hours:
  - Chlordiazepoxide: 50 mg PO for 4 doses and then 25 mg PO for 8 doses
  - Diazepam: 10 mg PO for 4 doses and then 5 mg PO for 8 doses
  - Lorazepam: 2 mg PO for 4 doses and then 1 mg PO for 8 doses
  - Important to monitor closely and provide additional BZDs if CIWA-Ar ≥8
- Folic acid: 1 mg daily
- Thiamine: 50 to 100 mg daily; do not administer IV glucose before giving thiamine because this may precipitate Wernicke encephalopathy and Korsakoff psychosis.
- Phenobarbital is supplanting BZDs. This barbiturate targets GABA receptors and glutamate receptors in the CNS. It is used to treat alcohol withdrawal, as it can provide faster and more definitive therapy than BZDs, which are more commonly used. Phenobarbital can also treat alcohol withdrawal seizures, unlike phenytoin, which is ineffective (2).

Second Line

- Gabapentin: reduces alcohol consumption, cravings, and may be effective for mild withdrawal
- β-Blockers (e.g., atenolol or propranolol) and α_2-agonists (e.g., clonidine) help to control hypertension and tachycardia but do not prevent severe symptoms such as DT or seizures; not used as monotherapy
- Carbamazepine: associated with reduced seizures and effective at mild withdrawal; should not be used as a monotherapy
- An antipsychotic (haloperidol) can be used for significant agitation and alcoholic hallucinosis but requires close observation because of lower seizure threshold.

SURGERY/OTHER PROCEDURES

For individuals with AUD undergoing surgery, proactive steps should be taken to prevent AWS by conducting a thorough assessment of their alcohol use history prior to surgical procedure.

COMPLEMENTARY & ALTERNATIVE MEDICINE

Complementary and alternative medicine (CAM) can be a helpful for individuals recovering from AUD, as they address the emotional and mental aspects of recovery. Practices such as mindfulness meditation, acupuncture, herbal supplements, yoga, and nutritional support have been reported to reduce cravings, improving mental well-being, and managing stress.

ADMISSION, INPATIENT, AND NURSING CONSIDERATIONS

Criteria for admission:

- CIWA-Ar score >15 or severe withdrawal
- Presence of ataxia, nystagmus, confusion
- Severe nausea or vomiting that prevents ingestion of medications
- Pregnancy
- History of seizure disorder, withdrawal seizures, or DTs
- Concurrent psychiatric or medical illness that requires treatment

ONGOING CARE

FOLLOW-UP RECOMMENDATIONS

- Managing alcohol withdrawal is only first step toward treating patient's underlying AUD, discharge arrangements should include outpatient substance use counseling, peer support groups, and/or residential treatment facility (3).
- Prescribe medication for AUD (MAUD):
  - Acamprosate (666 mg PO TID): glutamate and GABA modulator indicated to reduce cravings
  - Naltrexone (50 mg/day PO; 380 mg IM every 28 days): opiate receptor antagonist, reduce craving; initiate therapy after patient is opioid free for at least 7 days.
  - Disulfiram (250 mg/day PO): creates adverse reaction to alcohol by interfering with aldehyde dehydrogenase, blocking alcohol metabolism, leading to an accumulation of acetaldehyde

Patient Monitoring

Follow-up to monitor for relapse

DIET

Ensure adequate vitamin B_{12}, folate, and thiamine supplementation.

PATIENT EDUCATION

- Alcoholics Anonymous: http://www.aa.org/
- Self-Management and Recovery Training (SMART Recovery): http://www.smartrecovery.org/ (not spiritually based)
- FamilyDoctor.org: Alcohol Withdrawal Syndrome
- Substance Abuse and Mental Health Services Administration (SAMHSA): https://www.samhsa.gov/substance-use/

PROGNOSIS

Mortality from severe withdrawal (DTs) is 1–5%. Mortality rate may be much higher without treatment.

REFERENCES

1. Rastegar DA, Fingerhood MI. *The American Society of Addiction Medicine Handbook of Addiction Medicine*. 2nd ed. New York, NY: Oxford University Press; 2020.
2. Celik M, Gold MS, Fuehrlein B. A narrative review of current and emerging trends in the treatment of alcohol use disorder. *Brain Sci*. 2024;14(3):294. doi:10.3390/brainsci14030294.
3. Tiglao SM, Meisenheimer ES, Oh RC. Alcohol withdrawal syndrome: outpatient management. *Am Fam Physician*. 2021;104(3):253–262.

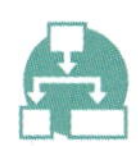

SEE ALSO

Substance Use Disorders

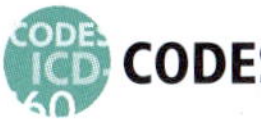

CODES

ICD10

- F10.239 Alcohol dependence with withdrawal, unspecified
- F10.230 Alcohol dependence with withdrawal, uncomplicated
- F10.231 Alcohol dependence with withdrawal delirium

CLINICAL PEARLS

- Any BZD dose should be patient specific, sufficient to achieve and maintain a "light somnolence" (e.g., sleeping but easily arousable), and should be tapered off carefully to prevent BZD withdrawal.
- Phenobarbital is slowly supplanting BZD as first-line treatment for withdrawal.
- Administer thiamine before patient receives glucose, so to not precipitate Wernicke encephalopathy.
- Avoid administering diazepam and lorazepam intramuscularly because of erratic absorption.
- Managing AWS is the first step toward treating AUD. Ensure patient has outpatient follow-up to continue treatment.

ALOPECIA

Melinda W. Ng, MD

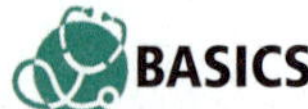

BASICS

Absence of hair from areas where it normally grows

DESCRIPTION

- Phases of the hair follicle cycle
  - Anagen phase (growth phase): 90% scalp hair follicles, lasts 2 to 6 years
  - Catagen phase (transition phase): regression of follicle, <1% follicles, lasts 3 weeks
  - Telogen phase (resting phase): club hair ready for shedding, lasts 2 to 3 months
- Scarring (cicatricial) alopecia
  - Inflammatory disorders leading to permanent follicle destruction and hair loss
  - Includes lymphocytic, neutrophilic, and mixed cicatricial alopecia
- Nonscarring (noncicatricial) alopecia
  - Mild or no inflammation, no destruction of follicle
  - Includes focal (alopecia areata [AA], traction alopecia), patterned (androgenic alopecia, female pattern hair loss), or diffuse hair loss (telogen effluvium, anagen effluvium)
- Structural hair disorders: brittle hair from abnormal hair formation or external insult

EPIDEMIOLOGY

Prevalence

- Androgenic alopecia:
  - In men, 30% White by age 30 years, 50% by age 50 years, and 80% by age 70 years
  - In women, 70% >65 years of age
- AA: 1/1,000 with lifetime risk 1–2%, men and women affected equally
- Scarring alopecia: rare, 3–7% of all hair disorder patients

ETIOLOGY AND PATHOPHYSIOLOGY

- Scarring (cicatricial) alopecia
  - Inflammatory disorders leading to permanent destruction of the follicle
  - Slick smooth scalp without follicles evident
  - Three subtypes based on inflammation: lymphocytic, neutrophilic, and mixed
  - Primary scarring includes discoid lupus, lichen planopilaris, frontal fibrosing alopecia, central centrifugal cicatricial alopecia, acne keloidalis nuchae, folliculitis decalvans, dissecting cellulitis of scalp, primary fibrosing, among others
  - Secondary scarring from infection, neoplasm, radiation, surgery, and other physical trauma, including tinea capitis
  - Central centrifugal cicatricial alopecia most common form of scarring hair loss in African American women; etiology unknown but possibly from hair care practices
- Nonscarring (noncicatricial) alopecia
  - Focal hair loss
    - AA: Patchy hair loss, usually autoimmune, T cell–mediated inflammation resulting in premature transition to catagen then telogen phases
      - May progress to alopecia totalis (entire scalp) or alopecia universalis (loss of all hair)
      - Nail disease frequently seen (10–20% of patients with AA)
      - High psychiatric comorbidity
    - Alopecia syphilitica: "moth-eaten" appearance, secondary syphilis
    - Pressure-induced alopecia: hair loss from long periods of pressure on one area of scalp
    - Temporal triangular alopecia: congenital patch of hair loss in temporal area
    - Traction alopecia: due to physical stressor of tight braids/ponytails/hair weaves
  - Patterned hair loss
    - Androgenic alopecia: hair transitions from terminal to vellus hairs
    - Male pattern hair loss: thinning in bitemporal or vertex areas (Norwood Hamilton classification, type I to VII); results from increased androgen receptors, and increased 5-α reductase leads to increased testosterone conversion in follicle to dihydrotestosterone (DHT); this leads to decreased follicle size and vellus hair.
    - Female pattern hair loss: thinning on frontal and vertex areas; unclear etiology, possible association with polycystic ovary syndrome, adrenal hyperplasia, and pituitary hyperplasia
  - Trichotillomania: intentional pulling of hair from scalp; presents various patterns
- Diffuse
  - Telogen effluvium: sudden shift of many follicles from anagen to telogen phase resulting in decreased hair density but not bald areas
    - May follow major stressors, including childbirth, injury, illness; occurs 2 to 3 months after event
    - Can be chronic with ongoing illness (SLE, renal failure, IBS, HIV, thyroid/pituitary dysfunction)
    - Adding or changing medications (oral contraceptives, anticoagulants, anticonvulsants, SSRIs, retinoids, β-blockers, ACE inhibitors, colchicine, cholesterol-lowering medications, etc.)
    - Malnutrition from malabsorption, eating disorders; poor diet can contribute.
  - Anagen effluvium
    - Interruption of the anagen phase without transition to telogen phase; days to weeks after inciting event
    - Chemotherapy is the most common trigger. Radiation, anticancer drugs, and severe protein-calorie malnutrition can also trigger.
- Inherited and acquired structural hair disorders
  - Multiple inherited hair disorders including Menkes disease, monilethrix, and so forth; these result in the formation of abnormal hairs that are weakened.
  - May also result from chemical or heat damaging from hair processing treatments

Genetics

Family history of early patterned hair loss is common in androgenic alopecia, also in AA.

RISK FACTORS

- Genetic predisposition
- Chronic illness including autoimmune disease, infections, cancer
- Physiologic stress including pregnancy and childbirth
- Poor nutrition
- Medication, chemotherapy, radiation
- Hair chemical treatments, braids, weaves/extensions

GENERAL PREVENTION

Minimize risk factors where possible.

COMMONLY ASSOCIATED CONDITIONS

- See "Etiology and Pathophysiology."
- Vitiligo: 4.1% patients with AA, may be the result of similar autoimmune pathways

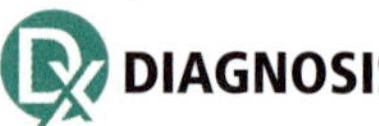

DIAGNOSIS

The diagnosis is clinical, made by history and examination.

HISTORY

- Description of hair loss problem: rate of loss, duration, distribution, degree of hair loss, hair care practices, and hair breakage versus hair shedding
- Associated symptoms: pruritus, pain, burning
- Hair care practices: use of prolonged heat, coloring, bleaching, chemical relaxers, and hairstyling (braids/ponytails)
- Medications
- Medical illness: recent illness/surgeries, pregnancy, thyroid disorder, iron deficiency, poisoning/exposures
- Psychological stress
- Dietary history and weight changes
- Family history of hair loss or autoimmune disorders

PHYSICAL EXAM

- Pattern of hair loss
  - Generalized, patterned, focal
  - Assess hair density, vellus versus terminal hairs, broken hair.
- Scalp scaling, inflammation, papules, pustules
- Presence of follicular ostia to determine class of alopecia
- Hair pull test
  - Pinch 25 to 50 hairs between thumb and forefinger and exert slow, gentle traction while sliding fingers up.
    - Normal: 1 to 2 dislodge
    - Abnormal: ≥6 hairs dislodged
    - Broken hairs (structural disorder)
    - Broken-off hair at the borders patch that are easily removable (in AA)
- Hair loss at other sites, nail disorders, skin changes
- Clinical signs of thyroid disease, lupus, or other diseases
- Clinical signs of virilization: acne, hirsutism, acanthosis nigricans, truncal obesity

DIFFERENTIAL DIAGNOSIS

Search for type of alopecia and then for reversible causes.

DIAGNOSTIC TESTS & INTERPRETATION

Initial Tests (lab, imaging)

- No testing may be indicated depending on clinical appearance.
- For diffuse nonscarring alopecia, consider TSH, serum iron and ferritin, CBC. Depending on clinical history and exam, consider LFT, BMP, zinc, RPR, ANA, prolactin.
- If suspected hyperandrogenic state in female patten hair loss, consider free and/or total testosterone level and dehydroepiandrosterone sulfate.

Follow-Up Tests & Special Considerations

Consider visualization under dermatoscope; will see exclamation point hairs for AA

Diagnostic Procedures/Other

- Light hair pull test: Pull on 25 to 50 hairs; ≥6 hairs dislodged is consistent with shedding (effluvium, AA).
- Direct microscopic exam of the hair shaft
  - Anagen hairs: elongated, distorted bulb with root sheath attached
  - Telogen hairs: rounded bulb, no root sheath
  - Exclamation point hairs: club-shaped root with thinner proximal shaft (AA)
  - Broken and distorted hairs may be associated with multiple hair dystrophies.
- Biopsy: scarring (cicatricial) alopecia or if diagnosis remains unknown
  - Recommend two 4 mm punch biopsies.
  - In scarring alopecia, take the biopsy at the edge of inflammation.
    - Lymphocytic inflammation with perifollicular fibrosis
  - In nonscarring alopecia, take the biopsy at an area with thinning hair but not complete hair loss.
    - Androgenic alopecia: ratio of terminal: vellus hair follicle <2:1, variable size of hair shafts, follicular miniaturization
    - Telogen effluvium: increased ratio of catagen: telogen, no change in number of hair follicles, no miniaturization of follicle
    - AA: increased ratio of catagen: telogen, no change in number of hair follicles, follicular miniaturization
- Ultraviolet light fluorescence and potassium hydroxide prep (to rule out tinea capitis)

TREATMENT

GENERAL MEASURES

- Consider potential harms and benefits to the patient prior to treatment. Many will gain an improved quality of life.
- Treat underlying medical causes (e.g., thyroid disorder, syphilis).
- Traction alopecia: change hair care practices, education
- Trichotillomania: often requires psychological intervention to induce behavior change

MEDICATION

- **AA**: Extent of hair loss and patient are the most important factors influencing the approach to treatment. Spontaneous remission rates range from 8% for extensive disease (>50% scalp involvement) to 68% (<25% scalp involvement) (1).
  - <10 years old: topical 0.1% mometasone cream +/− topical 5% minoxidil foam/solution BID (1)[C]
  - ≥10 years old:
    - <50% scalp involvement: topical corticosteroids +/− intralesional corticosteroids +/− topical 5% minoxidil (1)[C]
      - 0.05% clobetasol propionate foam
      - Triamcinolone acetonide 2.5 mg/mL
        - For scalp, inject 0.1 mL into deep dermal layer 1 cm apart with 0.5 inch 30-G needle, every 4 to 6 weeks; max 40 mg per session
        - Adverse effects: itching, burning, acne, skin atrophy
    - >50% scalp involvement; in addition to above:
      - Topical immunotherapy: diphenylcyclopropenone (DPCP) or 3% squaric acid dibutylester (SADBE) (1)[C]
        - 2% DPCP for initial sensitization and then 0.001% DPCP applied with increased concentration weekly until patient develops desired effect; must be applied by physician/nurse weekly. Instruct patient to wash off after 1 to 2 days.
        - Avoid topical immunotherapy in pregnant women due to teratogenic effects; other side effects: severe eczema and cervical and occipital lymphadenopathy, among others
      - JAK inhibitor +/− intralesional corticosteroid (2)[C]
        - Baricitinib 2 mg once daily. Increase to 4 mg once daily if the response is not adequate after 3 months of treatment. Reduce back to 2 mg once daily when adequate response is achieved. If no response in 6 months, discontinue drug.
        - Obtain baseline labs prior to initiation: CBC, LFTs, lipid panel, viral hepatitis panel, latent TB, renal insufficiency, pregnancy.
- **Androgenic alopecia**: Treatment must be continued indefinitely; can use in combination
  - Minoxidil (Rogaine) (3)[A]: topical 2% solution 1 mL BID or 5% foam daily for women; topical 5% 1 mL BID solution or foam for men; adverse effects: skin irritation, hypertrichosis of face/hands, tachycardia; Category C in pregnancy
  - Finasteride (Propecia) (3)[A]: 1 mg daily for men and women (off-label)
    - Adverse effects: loss of libido, gynecomastia, depression; caution in liver disease
    - Absolutely no use/contact during pregnancy, Category X, contraception required in female use
  - Spironolactone (Aldactone) (3)[A]: 100 to 200 mg/day (off-label); adverse effects: dose-dependent, hyperkalemia, menstrual irregularity, fatigue; Category D in pregnancy
  - Combination: Finasteride + minoxidil has superior efficacy to monotherapy.

SURGERY/OTHER PROCEDURES

- Wigs, hairpieces, extensions, scarfs, hats
- Surgical: graft transplantation, flap transplantation, or excision of the scarred area; used primarily in scarring alopecia
- Platelet-rich plasma: has been shown to restore dormant hair follicles and stimulate new hair growth

COMPLEMENTARY & ALTERNATIVE MEDICINE

- Many herbal medications are available; no clear evidence at this time
- Volumizing shampoos can help remaining hair look fuller.

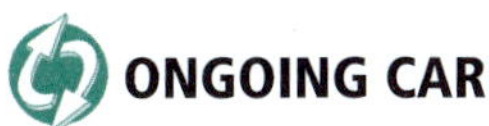

ONGOING CARE

DIET

If nutritional deficit noted, supplementation may be necessary.

PATIENT EDUCATION

National Alopecia Areata Foundation: https://www.naaf.org

PROGNOSIS

- *Cicatricial alopecia*: hair follicles permanently damaged; prognosis depends on type of alopecia and available treatments.
- *AA*: often regrows within 1 year even without treatment; recurrence is common. 10% have severe, chronic form; poor prognosis more likely with long duration, extensive hair loss, autoimmune disease, nail involvement, and young age
- *Traction alopecia*: excellent prognosis with behavior modification
- *Androgenic alopecia*: Prognosis depends on response to treatment.
- *Telogen effluvium*: maximum shedding 3 months after the inciting event and recovery following correction of the cause; usually subsides in 3 to 6 months but takes 12 to 18 months for cosmetically significant regrowth; rarely, permanent hair loss, usually with long-term illness

REFERENCES

1. Strazzulla LC, Wang EHC, Avila L, et al. Alopecia areata: an appraisal of new treatment approaches and overview of current therapies. *J Am Acad Dermatol*. 2018;78(1):15–24.
2. King B, Ohyama M, Kwon O, et al. Two phase 3 trials of baricitinib for alopecia areata. *N Engl J Med*. 2022;386(18):1687–1699. doi:10.1056/NEJMoa2110343.
3. Kanti V, Messenger A, Dobos G, et al. Evidence-based (S3) guideline for the treatment of androgenetic alopecia in women and in men—short version. *J Eur Acad Dermatol Venereol*. 2018;32(1):11–22.

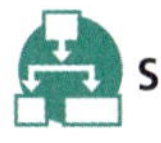

SEE ALSO

- Hyperthyroidism; Lichen Planus; Lupus Erythematosus, Systemic (SLE); Polycystic Ovarian Syndrome (PCOS); Syphilis; Tinea (Capitis, Corporis, Cruris)
- Algorithm: Alopecia

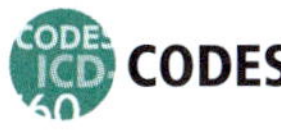

CODES

ICD10

- L65.9 Nonscarring hair loss, unspecified
- L64.9 Androgenic alopecia, unspecified
- L63.9 Alopecia areata, unspecified

CLINICAL PEARLS

- History and physical are necessary in determining type of alopecia for appropriate treatment.
- Treatment of underlying medical condition or removal of triggering medication will often resolve hair loss.
- Educating the patient about the nature of the condition and expectations is key to care.
- Alopecia can affect the psychological condition of the patient, and it may be necessary to address this in any type of hair loss.

ALTITUDE ILLNESS

Andrew McBride, MD, CAQSM • Christian Dean, DO, MS, DiMM, FAWM

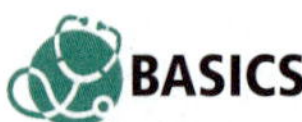

BASICS

DESCRIPTION

- A spectrum of cerebral and pulmonary syndromes ranging from mild discomfort to fatal illness that occur on ascent to higher altitudes as a direct result of inadequate acclimatization
- Categories of altitude: high, 1,500 to 3,500 m; very high, 3,500 to 5,500 m; and extreme, 5,500 to 8,850 m (1)
- Altitude illness can affect anyone, including experienced and fit individuals. For most, it is an unpleasant (self-limited) syndrome that does not require medical intervention (2).
- Acute mountain sickness (AMS): symptoms associated with a physiologic response to a hypobaric, hypoxic environment; onset usually occurs within 6 to 12 hours after ascending >2,500 m. Neurologic symptoms predominate, ranging from mild to moderate headache and malaise to severe impairment.
- High-altitude pulmonary edema (HAPE): noncardiogenic pulmonary edema; typically after ≥2 days at altitudes >3,000 m, rare between 2,500 and 3,000 m
- High-altitude cerebral edema (HACE): a potentially fatal neurologic syndrome considered to be the end stage of AMS; onset after at least 2 days at altitudes >4,000 m
- System(s) affected: nervous/pulmonary
- Synonym(s): mountain sickness

Geriatric Considerations

- Risk does not increase with age.
- Age alone should not preclude travel to high altitude; allow extra time to acclimate.
- Worsening of preexisting medical problems referred to as altitude-exacerbated conditions

Pediatric Considerations

- Altitude illness seems to have the same incidence in children as in adults; diagnosis may be delayed in younger children.
- Any child who experiences behavioral symptoms after recent ascent should be presumed to have an altitude-related illness.

Pregnancy Considerations

- The risk during pregnancy is unknown.
- No evidence suggests that exposure to high altitudes (1,500 to 3,500 m) poses a risk to a normal pregnancy.

EPIDEMIOLOGY

Most epidemiologic studies are limited to relatively homogeneous male populations.

Incidence

- Incidence and severity increase with altitude and rate of ascent.
- AMS: >25% of unacclimatized persons who ascend to 3,500 m; 40–50% in trekkers and climbers near 4,000 m; >50% at altitudes above 6,000 m (1)
- HACE: 0.01% of general population at around 2,500 m; however, increases to 1–2% in trekkers, climbers, and soldiers around 4,000 m (1)
- HAPE: 0.01–0.10% in the general pollution at 2,500 m; 2–6% in trekkers and mountaineers at 4,000 m (1)

ETIOLOGY AND PATHOPHYSIOLOGY

- Hypobaric hypoxia and hypoxemia are the pathophysiologic precursors to altitude illness.
- The conditions of AMS and HACE represent a pathophysiologic continuum (1).
- Symptoms of AMS may be the result of cerebral swelling, either through vasodilatation induced by hypoxia or through cerebral edema.
- Other mechanisms include impaired cerebral autoregulation, release of vasogenic mediators, and alteration of the blood–brain barrier.
- HAPE is a noncardiogenic pulmonary edema characterized by exaggerated pulmonary hypertension leading to vascular leakage through overperfusion, stress failure, or both.

Genetics

Protective polymorphisms in EPAS1, EGLN1, and NOS genes may reduce susceptibility to AMS and HAPE.

RISK FACTORS

- Individuals with a prior history of AMS, HACE, or HAPE
- Failure to properly acclimatize at a lower altitude
- Ascent rate (sleeping elevation) >500 m/day (2)
- No known evidence links menstrual cycle phases to increased AMS risk
- Trips to extreme altitude
- Increased duration at high altitude
- Higher altitude during sleep cycle
- Cardiac congenital abnormalities
- Younger age (<50 years) (1)
- Iron deficiency

GENERAL PREVENTION

- General guidelines
  - Pre-acclimatization (exposure of hypoxia prior to ascent) protects against altitude illness.
  - Slow increase in sleeping elevation (gradual ascent); no more than 500 m elevation gain/day above 2,500 to 3,000 m
  - Lower sleeping elevation: "Climb high and sleep low" for anyone going >3,500 m.
  - Avoid heavy exertion for the first 1 to 3 days at altitude.
  - Avoid respiratory depressants (alcohol and sedatives).
  - Pre-ascent physical conditioning is not preventive.
- Pharmacologic prophylaxis
  - Acetazolamide, dexamethasone, and ibuprofen (see "Treatment")
  - For prevention of HAPE only (if at risk): Consider nifedipine, dexamethasone, and tadalafil (see "Treatment").

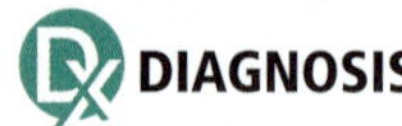

DIAGNOSIS

HISTORY

- AMS:
  - Symptoms include headache and at least one of anorexia, irritability, marked fatigue, nausea, vomiting, dizziness, light-headedness, dyspnea with exertion, or insomnia.
  - Often these symptoms resolve spontaneously after 18 to 36 hours, without requiring descent (1).
  - Severity has been studied using the Lake Louise questionnaire, which ranks four symptoms from 0 (none) to 3 (severe).
    - Headache, gastrointestinal symptoms, fatigue and/or weakness, and dizziness/light-headedness
    - AMS is considered diagnostic with a headache score of at least 1 point and a total score of at least 3 points.
    - Mild: 3 to 5 points, moderate: 6 to 9 points, severe: 10 to 12 points
    - Recommend calculating score after 6 hours at altitude (to exclude travel and acute hypoxia symptoms) (1).
- HAPE symptoms: hypoxia, reduced exercise tolerance, exertional dyspnea, cough followed by dyspnea at rest, cyanosis, and productive cough that may contain pink frothy sputum (2); begins within 1 to 3 days of reaching a new altitude, rarely occurring after 4 days
  - At least two of these symptoms: dyspnea, cough, asthenia, reduced physical performance, chest tightness, or congestion *plus*
  - At least two of these symptoms: crackles, rhonchi, tachypnea, or tachycardia
- HACE symptoms: altered mental status (irrational behavior, lethargy, obtundation, coma); ataxia: In <1% of cases, AMS can develop into HACE (1).

PHYSICAL EXAM

- HAPE
  - Labored breathing
  - Lung crackles, rhonchi, or wheezing
  - Tachycardia
  - Pink frothy sputum and central cyanosis in severe illness
- HACE
  - Abnormal mental status exam (behavioral change, lethargy, obtundation, coma)
  - Truncal ataxia
  - Papilledema, retinal hemorrhage, cranial nerve palsies
  - Focal neurologic deficits (rare)

DIFFERENTIAL DIAGNOSIS

- AMS/HACE
  - Dehydration
  - Hypoglycemia
  - Hyponatremia
  - Ingestion of toxins, drugs, or alcohol
  - Subarachnoid hemorrhage, CNS mass, cerebrovascular accident
  - Complicated migraine
  - Carbon monoxide exposure
  - CNS infection
  - Acute psychosis
- HAPE
  - Pneumonia, mucous plugging
  - Cardiogenic pulmonary edema
  - Spontaneous pneumothorax, pulmonary embolism
  - Asthma, bronchitis
  - Myocardial infarction
  - Hyperventilation syndrome
- Onset of symptoms >3 days at a given altitude, the absence of headache, or the lack of rapid response to oxygen or descent suggests an alternative diagnosis.

DIAGNOSTIC TESTS & INTERPRETATION

Initial Tests (lab, imaging)

- AMS: Laboratory studies are nonspecific and rarely required for diagnosis; increasing optic nerve sheath diameter on portable ultrasound (POCUS)
- HAPE: severe hypoxemia demonstrated with oximetry or blood gas analysis
  - B-lines with POCUS
  - Chest radiographs usually show patchy infiltrates.
- ECG may show sinus tachycardia or right-sided heart strain (2).

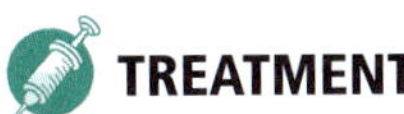

TREATMENT

GENERAL MEASURES

- Individuals without previous altitude exposure should adhere to acclimatization guidelines.
- Stop ascent, acclimatize at the same altitude, and/or descend if symptoms do not abate over 24 hours. Definitive treatment is to descend to a lower altitude. Dramatic improvement accompanies even modest reductions in altitude.
- Oxygen helps relieve symptoms. Give continuously by cannula or mask, and titrate to SaO_2 >90% (2).
- AMS and HACE
  - Acetazolamide reduces mild to moderate symptoms of AMS 250 mg PO BID
  - Dexamethasone may also be effective in treating moderate AMS 2 mg PO q6h
  - Immediate descent in severe cases of AMS (2)[A]
- HACE
  - Acetazolamide may be used as prophylaxis. 125 to 250 mg PO BID
  - Dexamethasone prophylaxis 2 mg PO q6h
  - Immediate descent (2)[A]
  - Supplemental oxygen (highest flow available; maintain SaO_2 >90%) (2)[A]
  - Portable hyperbaric therapy if available and unable to descend (2)[B]
- HAPE
  - Supplemental oxygen (highest flow available; maintain SaO_2 >90%) (2)[A]
  - Minimize exertion and keep patient warm.
  - Immediate descent or evacuation to a lower altitude (2)[A]
  - Portable hyperbaric therapy (2 to 15 psi using Gamow bag or Chamberlite) is an effective and practical alternative when descent is not possible (2)[C].
  - Nifedipine (see "Medication")

MEDICATION

First Line

- Oxygen: 2 to 15 L/min to maintain SaO_2 >90% until symptoms improve
- Acetazolamide: If patient has a history of problems at altitude and/or plans to ascend >500 m/day above 2,500 m, consider therapy for primary prevention. Avoid in patients with a history of anaphylaxis to sulfonamide or history of Stevens-Johnson syndrome (2).
  - Primary prevention of AMS: adult dosing 125 mg PO BID starting 24 hours before ascent and continued for 2 to 4 days at a stable altitude (2)[A]; pediatric dosing 2.5 mg/kg (maximum 125 mg) q12h (2)[C]
  - Treatment of AMS: 250 mg PO BID until symptoms resolve; pediatric dose: 2.5 mg/kg q12h (2)[C]
- Dexamethasone: may significantly reduce the incidence and severity of AMS; adverse side effects are rare.
  - Prevention of AMS: 2 mg PO q6h or 4 mg PO q12h, starting 1 day before ascent and discontinued cautiously after 2 days at maximum altitude; do not use for pediatric prevention (2)[A].
  - Prevention of HAPE: 8 mg PO q12h (2)[C]; reserved for those who cannot tolerate or do not have access to nifedipine or tadalafil.
  - Treatment of AMS: 4 mg PO/IV/IM q6h; pediatric dose: 0.15 mg/kg dose q6h (2)[C]
  - Treatment of HACE: 8 mg PO/IV/IM initially and then 4 mg q6h; pediatric dose: 0.15 mg/kg dose q6h (2)[C]
- Nifedipine (reduces pulmonary arterial pressure)
  - Prevention of HAPE: 30 mg extended-release PO BID starting 1 day prior to ascent and continued for 2 days at maximum altitude (2)[B]
  - Treatment of HAPE: 30 mg extended-release PO q12h (likely unnecessary if oxygen is available) (2)[C]
- Tadalafil: Consider for the prevention of HAPE when nifedipine is not tolerated or is unavailable (2).
  - Prevention HAPE: 10 mg PO BID 1 day prior to ascent in HAPE susceptible individual (2)[C]
  - Can be used for treatment of HAPE when descent is impossible or delayed, access to supplemental oxygen or portable hyperbaric therapy is impossible, and nifedipine is unavailable (2)[C]
- Adjunct therapy
  - Salmeterol:
    - Possible treatment of HAPE (not well studied): 125 μg inhaled BID starting 1 day before ascent and continued for 2 days at maximum altitude
    - Not recommended for HAPE prevention (2)[B]
  - NSAIDs:
    - Aspirin: 325 mg PO q4h for total 3 doses
    - Ibuprofen: 600 mg PO q8h 3 times daily for 1 to 2 days for prophylaxis (2)[B]; can also be used to treat headache at high altitude (2)[C]
  - Antiemetics
    - Prochlorperazine: 10 mg PO/IM q6–8h
    - Promethazine: 25 to 50 mg PO/IM/PR q6h
  - Acetaminophen: can be used in the treatment of headache at high altitude (2)[C]
- Other trialed therapies
  - *Ginkgo biloba*, inhaled budesonide, and acetaminophen should not be used for AMS prevention (2)[C]. Acetaminophen may be used to treat headache at high altitude.
  - Remote ischemic preconditioning (RIPC), as well as supplementation of antioxidants, dietary nitrites, leukotriene receptor blockers, phosphodiesterase inhibitors, salicylic acid, spironolactone, sumatriptan, or iron lack quality evidence supporting their use (2).
  - Coca-containing products have been used in the Andes but have not been well studied (2).
  - Furosemide: not recommended for prophylaxis; should not be used for treatment in HAPE (2)[C]

ADMISSION, INPATIENT, AND NURSING CONSIDERATIONS

Outpatient treatment for mild cases

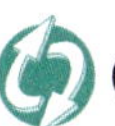

ONGOING CARE

FOLLOW-UP RECOMMENDATIONS

Patient Monitoring

- For mild cases, no follow-up is needed.
- For more severe cases, follow closely until symptoms subside.

PATIENT EDUCATION

Counsel patients about the risks of high-altitude travel and how to recognize symptoms of high-altitude illness.

PROGNOSIS

Most cases of mild to moderate AMS are self-limiting and often do not require medical intervention. Patients may resume ascent once the symptoms subside. If identified early, HAPE and HACE respond well to descent/evacuation, supplemental oxygenation, and pharmacologic treatment.

COMPLICATIONS

High-altitude retinal hemorrhages are usually painless but can cause visual changes.

REFERENCES

1. Savioli G, Ceresa IF, Gori G, et al. Pathophysiology and therapy of high-altitude sickness: practical approach in emergency and critical care. *J Clin Med*. 2022;11(14):3937.
2. Luks AM, Beidleman BA, Freer L, et al. Wilderness Medical Society Clinical practice guidelines for the prevention, diagnosis, and treatment of acute altitude illness: 2024 update. *Wilderness Environ Med*. 2024;35(Suppl 1):2S–19S.

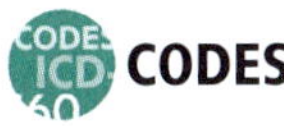

CODES

ICD10

- T70.20XA Unspecified effects of high altitude, initial encounter
- T70.20XD Unspecified effects of high altitude, subsequent encounter
- T70.20XS Unspecified effects of high altitude, sequela

CLINICAL PEARLS

- Slow ascent and timely descent are important to prevent and treat high-altitude illnesses.
- Lack of symptom resolution with appropriate descent suggests an alternative diagnosis.
- High-flow oxygen, followed by oxygen titrated to maintain SaO_2 >90%, is the first-line treatment for all patients with more than mild altitude illness.

ALZHEIMER DISEASE

Fozia Akhtar Ali, MD, FAAFP • Veronica Sabate, MD

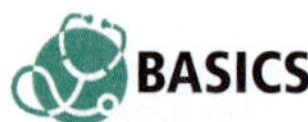

BASICS

DESCRIPTION

- Alzheimer disease (AD) is a neurodegenerative condition with insidious inset and progressive impairment of behavioral and cognitive functions.
- AD is the most common type of dementia: 2/3 of cases in >65 years old
- AD is the seventh leading cause of death in the United States.
- People ≥65 years with new AD live 4 to 8 years on average.
- AD is underdiagnosed (~50%), and >50% with AD unaware of diagnosis
- Economic burden in 2023: ~$245 billion, projected $1.1 trillion by 2050 (1)
- Dementia should be distinguished from:
  - Age-related cognitive decline: lifelong changes in mental ability and memory; part of normal aging
  - Mild cognitive impairment (MCI): decline in cognitive abilities (memory and thinking skills) that is greater than expected for a person's age but does not interfere significantly with activities of daily living (ADLs).
    - MCI: People are generally able to live independently, from a cognitive perspective.
    - MCI: affects 17–22% of those ≥65 years, with 32–38% developing dementia ≤5 years (1)
- AD diagnostic classification:
  - Preclinical AD: no cognitive symptoms, AD biomarkers present
  - MCI due to AD: very mild impairment
  - Dementia due to AD:
    - Mild: impairment in some activities
    - Moderate: impairment in many activities
    - Severe: impairment in most activities
- System(s) affected: nervous
- Synonym(s): presenile dementia; senile dementia of the Alzheimer type

EPIDEMIOLOGY

- Predominant age: >65 years
- Incidence: females = males
- Prevalence: females > males

Incidence

New cases of AD in the United States: 484,000/year

- 65 to 75 years: 4 new cases per 1,000 people
- 75 to 84 years: 32 new cases per 1,000 people
- ≥85 years: 76 new cases per 1,000 people

Prevalence

~6.9 million in United States; ~50 million worldwide (1)

- Projected to double in United States by 2050
- 1 in 9 (10.9%) of those aged ≥65 years have AD dementia.
- 33.3% of those aged ≥85 years have AD dementia.
- ~200,000 in United States with early-onset AD (age <65 years)

ETIOLOGY AND PATHOPHYSIOLOGY

- Progressive, irreversible disease, worsening cognitive impairment
- β-Amyloid plaques outside of neurons and τ protein tangles inside of neurons, resulting in loss of connections and neuron death
- Age, genetics, systemic diseases, lifestyle behaviors may influence AD progression.

Genetics

- Autosomal dominant: <5% of AD, usually early onset (age <65 years)
- Familial inheritance AD (non-autosomal dominant): 15–25% of AD

RISK FACTORS

- Nonmodifiable risk factors (1),(2):
  - Age: greatest risk factor, the percentage of people with AD increases dramatically with age
  - Family history
  - Genetic mutations: in 2022, researchers identified 31 new genes that appear to affect biologic process known to be at play in AD:
    - APOE-e4 gene variant: e4 heterozygous 2- to 3-fold risk; e4 homozygous 8-fold risk
    - Mutations
  - Racial and ethnic differences in AD exist.
- Modifiable risk factors:
  - Cardiovascular: hypertension; hyperlipidemia, diabetes, and smoking
  - Obesity and diet (Dietary Approaches to Stop Hypertension [DASH], Mediterranean, Mediterranean-DASH Intervention for Neurodegenerative Delay [MIND])
  - Lack of physical activity
  - Cerebrovascular (stroke) risks and injury
- Other potentially modifiable risk factors:
  - Fewer years of formal education (<8th grade)
  - Lack of continuous brain activity—learning
  - Traumatic brain injuries: repetitive mild and moderate/severe
  - Lack of social engagement
  - Late-life depression
  - Poor quality and inadequate sleep
  - Hearing and vision deficits
  - High alcohol consumption
  - Environmental factors (e.g., air pollution)

GENERAL PREVENTION

- HTN management, increased physical activity, varicella zoster vaccine and cognitive training may delay/prevent cognitive decline, MCI, and AD.
- NSAIDs, estrogen, and vitamin E do not delay AD onset; insufficient evidence for statins and proton pump inhibitors
- Healthy lifestyles may prevent or delay AD.
- Treat psychiatric conditions and avert delirium during hospitalizations.

COMMONLY ASSOCIATED CONDITIONS

- Down syndrome
- Depression

DIAGNOSIS

- "Welcome to Medicare" preventive visit and Medicare Annual Wellness Visit both require assessment of cognitive function.
- Diagnosis of dementia requires exclusion of delirium. Delineating specific dementia type requires a thorough H&P, cognitive, and other diagnostic tests.
  - 2000 *DSM-IV-TR* criteria: progressive impairment in two or more areas of memory, executive function, attention, language, or visuospatial skills and significant interference in ability to function in work, home, or social interactions
  - 2013 *DSM-5* uses term "neurocognitive disorder" instead of dementia; impairment in one or more cognitive areas sufficient to disrupt independent living: complex attention, executive function, learning and memory, language, perceptual motor, social cognition

HISTORY

- Include informant: family member, caregiver, or friend.
- Alzheimer's Association 10 signs:
  - Memory loss that disrupts daily life
  - Difficulty completing familiar tasks
  - Challenges in planning and problem-solving
  - New problems with words in speaking or writing
  - Trouble with visual images or spatial relationships
  - Changes in mood or personality
  - Misplacing things, losing ability to retrace steps
  - Decreased or poor judgment
  - Withdrawal from work or social activities
  - Confusion with time and place

PHYSICAL EXAM

- Exam to rule out other causes of dementia or delirium
- Noncognitive portions of physical exam often normal for age except in severe AD (2)
- Neuro: speech, language, vision, hearing, gait, balance, reflexes, muscle strength and tone, tremor, abnormal movements (akathisia, bradykinesia/dyskinesia)
- Late stage: skin lesions, nutrition-hydration status
- Brief cognitive testing, such as Mini-Cog, Montreal Cognitive Assessment (MoCA), Mini-Mental State Examination (MMSE)
- Assess depression: Patient Health Questionnaire-9, Geriatric Depression Scale (GDS)
- Functional assessment: instrumental activities of daily living (IADLs), Functional Activities Questionnaire (FAQ)

DIFFERENTIAL DIAGNOSIS

- Other dementias (most common):
  - Vascular (large and microvessel, mixed); mixed type (with AD)
  - Frontotemporal lobar degeneration; dementia with Lewy bodies
  - Parkinson disease; normal pressure hydrocephalus
  - Creutzfeldt-Jakob disease; Huntington disease; Wernicke-Korsakoff syndrome
- Metabolic: hyper-hypothyroid, vitamin-nutrient deficiency, uremia/renal, hepatic, hyponatremia
- Autoimmune: vasculitis, end-stage multiple sclerosis
- Infectious: HIV, syphilis, Lyme disease, varicella-zoster virus, prion
- Depression; brain tumor: primary or metastatic; subdural hematoma (usually acute presentation)
- Medications, drug-alcohol reactions/addiction

DIAGNOSTIC TESTS & INTERPRETATION

Neuropsychological testing for atypical symptoms, young age, unclear presentation, or need to determine independent decision-making

Initial Tests (lab, imaging)

- To help rule out other causes of dementia (1),(2)
  - Complete blood count with differential; homocysteine level
  - Chemistry panel; thyroid function, syphilis testing, lipid panel, vitamin B_{12}
  - Special considerations: ESR, HIV, folate, C-reactive protein, HbA1c

- Imaging (biomarkers): Different professional standards exist; may help determine cause of dementia
  - Consider MRI (preferred) or computed tomography (CT) scan if MRI contraindicated.
    - Initial AD evaluation; recent or rapid decline, age <65 years, history of stroke, atypical presentation, concern for cancer, high bleeding risk
  - Single photon emission CT (SPECT) and positron emission tomography (PET): rarely indicated; *insufficient evidence to use alone*

Follow-Up Tests & Special Considerations

- Consider genetic testing with concern for autosomal dominant and familial AD.
- Cerebrospinal fluid biomarker testing not currently indicated

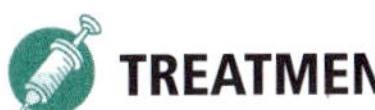

TREATMENT

GENERAL MEASURES

- Optimize treatment of risk factors and associated comorbid conditions (e.g., hearing, vision or balance issues).
- Advanced care planning (Living Will, health care proxy) early in illness before individual loses ability for independent decisions
- Assess caregiver support and burnout.

ALERT

American Geriatrics Society recommends "Don't prescribe cholinesterase inhibitors (ChEIs) for dementia without periodic assessment for perceived cognitive benefits and adverse gastrointestinal effects" in its Choosing Wisely statement.

MEDICATION

First Line

- Acetylcholinesterase inhibitors (ChEIs) (2)[A]
  - Best in mild to moderate disease; *may* be effective in Lewy body dementia
  - ChEIs equally effective; side effects: GI, bradycardia, syncope
  - When used for at least 6 months, may provide mild benefit in cognition and behavior
  - Try different ChEIs if no benefit.
  - Donepezil (Aricept): Start at 5 mg/day PO; may increase to 10 mg/day after 1 month, may increase to 23 mg/day after 3 months if needed
  - Orally disintegrating tablets; generic available
  - Caution with digoxin or β-blockers (Donepezil may prolong PR interval.)
  - Rivastigmine (Exelon): Start at 1.5 mg PO BID, increase by 1.5 mg BID every 2 weeks; goal of 3 to 6 mg/day total
  - Capsule, solution, or patch (reduced side effects)
  - Galantamine (Razadyne): Start at 4 mg BID for 4 weeks, increase by 4 mg BID every month: goal of 8 to 12 mg/day dose.
  - Tablets, solution, extended-release (ER) capsule, and transdermal formulations
- Vitamin E—2,000 IU/day, mixed data, side effects exist (2)[B]
- Memantine, an *N*-methyl-D-aspartate (NMDA) receptor antagonist for moderate to severe AD
  - Monotherapy or in combination with acetylcholinesterase inhibitors (2)[A]
  - Memantine immediate release: 5 mg/day; increased by 5 mg/day weekly; goal dose 10 mg BID
  - Memantine ER: 7 mg/day up to 28 mg/day, adding 7 mg/day qwk PRN
- Aducanumab (Aduhelm): monoclonal antibody therapy targeting β-amyloid; Biogen, the manufacturer, decided to discontinue development and commercialization of the drug in January 2024.
- Neuropsychiatric symptoms: assessment for delirium and reversible causes (sleep, hearing, environment; for moderate to severe symptoms—consider second-line care)

Second Line

- For moderate to severe depression: selective serotonin reuptake inhibitors (SSRIs) preferred
- Insomnia: Medications have little efficacy for sleep in AD (2)[A].
  - Avoid antihistamines in elderly.
  - Caution and use the lowest dose possible: trazodone
- Moderate agitation, anxiety/restlessness: may consider low-dose risperidone or SSRIs (citalopram) (2)[B].
- Cautious use of low-dose risperidone for severe psychosis
- Precautions
  - Avoid anticholinergic drugs when possible.
  - Benzodiazepines may produce paradoxical excitation or daytime drowsiness.
  - Triazolam (Halcion) can produce confusion, memory loss, and psychotic behavior.
  - Donepezil: caution with anticholinergics, sick sinus syndrome, and history of peptic ulcers

ISSUES FOR REFERRAL

Consider geriatric psychiatry and behavioral health referral for AD patients with behavioral symptoms requiring psychotropic medications.

ADDITIONAL THERAPIES

- Exercise to reduce restlessness; cognitive stimulation therapy
- Consider occupational, music, aroma, and pet therapy.

ONGOING CARE

FOLLOW-UP RECOMMENDATIONS

Patient Monitoring

- Medication reconciliation each visit, including OTCs
- Recommend: healthy lifestyle: exercise, nutrition, sleep, activities that promote positive social connections (bingo, arts and craft, etc.)
- Inform about unproven products advertised to improve brain health: some medications, nutritional supplements, and brain games.
- Frequently assess medication side effects and effectiveness (ChEIs/memantine).
- Late AD may require skilled care placement.
- Advanced care planning is Medicare reimbursable.
- National Highway Traffic Safety Administration's safe driving assessment: https://www.nhtsa.gov/older-drivers/driving-safely-while-aging-gracefully

DIET

A heart-healthy diet emphasizes fruits, vegetables, whole grains, fish, chicken, nuts, legumes and healthy fats such as olive oil while limiting saturated fats, red meat, and sugar.

PATIENT EDUCATION

- Alzheimer's Association: https://www.alz.org/
- Early advanced care planning, such as advanced directives, financial planning, caregiver support

PROGNOSIS

Average survival from diagnosis is 4 to 8 years; and initial diagnosis is often delayed.

COMPLICATIONS

- Hostility, agitation, wandering, falls, "sundowning," depression, suicide
- Infections, inadequate nutrition/hydration, drug toxicity

REFERENCES

1. Alzheimer's Association. 2023 Alzheimer's disease facts and figures. *Alzheimer's Dement*. 2023;19(4):1598–1695. doi:10.1002/alz.13016.
2. Atri A. The Alzheimer's disease clinical spectrum: diagnosis and management. *Med Clin North Am*. 2019;103(2):263–293.

ADDITIONAL READING

The Gerontological Society of America. The GSA KAER toolkit for primary care teams. The Gerontological Society of America; 2020. https://www.geron.org/publications/kaer-toolkit

SEE ALSO

Delirium; Depression; Hypothyroidism, Adult; Substance Use Disorders

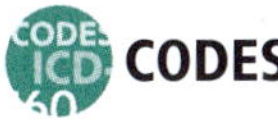

CODES

ICD10

- G30 Alzheimer's disease
- G30.1 Alzheimer's disease with late onset
- G30.9 Alzheimer's disease, unspecified

CLINICAL PEARLS

- AD is very common, >33.3% in those >85 years, and greatly underdiagnosed.
- Imaging not needed for diagnosis for typical AD.
- Consider advance care planning (e.g., advanced directives) and caregiver support as soon as diagnosis is made.
- Atypical antipsychotic medications increase mortality.

AMENORRHEA

Michelle E. Duffelmeyer, MD

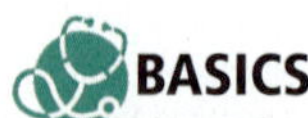

BASICS

DESCRIPTION

- Primary amenorrhea
  - No menses by age 13 years with absence of secondary sexual characteristics *or*
  - No menses by age 15 years with normal secondary characteristics
- Secondary amenorrhea: cessation of menses for 3 months if previously normal menstrual cycles or 6 months if a history of irregular cycles
- System(s) affected: endocrine/metabolic; reproductive

Pregnancy Considerations

Pregnancy is by far the most common cause of secondary amenorrhea.

EPIDEMIOLOGY

Prevalence

- Primary amenorrhea: <1% of female population
- Secondary amenorrhea: 3–4% of female population
- No evidence for race and ethnicity affecting prevalence

ETIOLOGY AND PATHOPHYSIOLOGY

Absence of menses that can be temporary, intermittent, or permanent due to dysfunction of the hypothalamus, pituitary, uterus, ovaries, or vagina

- Primary amenorrhea
  - Gonadal dysgenesis (e.g., Turner syndrome [45,X]) or failure (e.g., autoimmune, idiopathic)
  - Anatomic abnormalities (e.g., müllerian agenesis, imperforate hymen, transverse vaginal septum)
  - Hypothalamic-pituitary abnormalities
    - Functional hypothalamic amenorrhea (abnormal GnRH secretion, stress, exercise, anorexia nervosa)
    - Physiologic delay of puberty
    - Central lesions (tumors, hypophysitis, granulomas)
    - Pituitary dysfunction (hyperprolactinemia, abnormal follicle-stimulating hormone [FSH], luteinizing hormone [LH], or GnRH)
    - Thyroid dysfunction
  - Polycystic ovary syndrome (PCOS)
  - Androgen insensitivity syndrome
  - Congenital adrenal hyperplasia
- Secondary amenorrhea
  - Pregnancy
  - Hypothalamic dysfunction (reduced GnRH secretion)
    - Functional hypothalamic amenorrhea (stress, anorexia nervosa, and/or excessive exercise)
    - Hypothalamic tumors
    - Severe systemic illness (e.g., diabetes mellitus type 1 or celiac disease)
  - Pituitary disease (e.g., hyperprolactinemia, Sheehan syndrome, Cushing syndrome)
  - Thyroid disease
  - PCOS
  - Ovarian disorders (e.g., primary ovarian insufficiency [due to chemotherapy, radiation, fragile X syndrome] or ovarian tumors)
  - Anatomic abnormalities (e.g., intrauterine adhesions [Asherman syndrome])
- Pathophysiology varies, depending on etiology.

Genetics

May occur with Turner syndrome or testicular feminization

RISK FACTORS

- Obesity
- Excessive exercise (commonly associated "female athlete triad")
- Eating disorders
- Malnutrition
- Stress (emotional or illness-induced)
- Family history of amenorrhea or early menopause
- Treatment with antipsychotic medications

GENERAL PREVENTION

Maintenance of proper body mass index (BMI) and healthy lifestyle with respect to food and exercise

COMMONLY ASSOCIATED CONDITIONS

- Primary ovarian insufficiency may be associated with autoimmune abnormalities (autoimmune thyroiditis, type 1 diabetes).
- PCOS is associated with insulin resistance and obesity.
- Decreased exposure to estrogen may increase risk for osteopenia or osteoporosis.

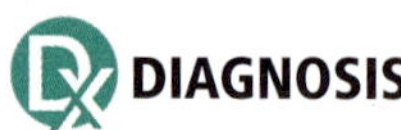

DIAGNOSIS

HISTORY

- Review of systems, including weight change, symptoms of pregnancy or menopause, virilizing changes, cyclic pelvic pain, galactorrhea, headaches, vision changes, fatigue, palpitations, polyuria/polydipsia
- Growth and pubertal development history, including age of breast development, pubertal growth spurt, and adrenarche (early sexual maturation)
- History of chronic illness, trauma, surgery, medications (including contraceptives), prior chemotherapy or radiation
- Obstetrical history
- Psychiatric history
- Social history, including diet and exercise history, drug abuse, sexual history, and stress
- Family history of delayed or absent puberty

PHYSICAL EXAM

- General appearance
- Vital signs, height, weight, growth percentile and BMI, hypotension, bradycardia, hypothermia (anorexia nervosa)
- HEENT exam: evidence of dental erosions, trauma to palate (bulimia), visual field defect, funduscopic changes, cranial nerve findings (prolactinoma), webbed neck (Turner syndrome), thyromegaly
- Skin exam: evidence of androgen excess (acne, hirsutism), acanthosis nigricans (PCOS), fine downy hair on body (anorexia nervosa), striae, vitiligo, easy bruisability
- Breast: state of development, evidence of galactorrhea (prolactinoma), shield chest (Turner syndrome)
- Pelvic exam: presence or absence of pubic hair (if sparse: androgen insensitivity or deficiency); clitoromegaly (androgen excess); distention or bulging of external vagina (imperforate hymen); thin, pale vaginal mucosa without rugae (estrogen deficiency and ovarian failure); presence of cervical mucus (evidence for estrogen production); blind vaginal pouch (müllerian agenesis, androgen insensitivity syndrome); ovarian enlargement (tumors, PCOS)

DIAGNOSTIC TESTS & INTERPRETATION

If normal-appearing vagina and uterus are not seen on physical exam, pelvic ultrasound is recommended to visualize anatomy of uterine and ovarian and evaluate for outflow obstruction.

Initial Tests (lab, imaging)

- Primary amenorrhea
  - Serum human chorionic gonadotropin (hCG), prolactin (PRL), thyroid-stimulating hormone (TSH), and FSH
  - If no or minor breast development:
    - Low FSH suggests primary hypothalamic-pituitary etiology or constitutional delay of puberty.
    - High FSH suggests gonadal failure, and karyotype analysis should be performed.
  - If normal breast development:
    - If low FSH, evaluate for anatomic abnormalities. If uterus is absent or abnormal, perform karyotype analysis, testosterone level, and dehydroepiandrosterone sulfate (DHEA-S).
- Secondary amenorrhea
  - Serum hCG, PRL, TSH, and FSH
    - PRL >50 ng/mL: Suggests empty sella syndrome or pituitary adenoma; however, levels can transiently increase with stress. Repeat level, and if elevated, perform MRI for evaluation.
    - PRL elevated, but <50 ng/mL: Repeat fasting in the morning and before exercise.
    - If FSH high: Consider primary ovarian insufficiency or natural menopause.
  - To determine endogenous estrogen production, perform a progestin challenge (see "Treatment"): if withdrawal bleed, likely chronic anovulation (most commonly PCOS). If no withdrawal bleed, perform estrogen and progestin challenge (see "Treatment"):
    - If no bleed: Consider outflow tract obstruction or hypoestrogenism.
    - If bleed occurs: Check FSH/LH: elevated in premature ovarian failure; decreased in pituitary tumors, eating disorders, chronic illness.
- If there is evidence for hyperandrogenism, measure total testosterone, DHEA-S, and 17-OH levels. Initiate evaluation for androgen-secreting tumor if testosterone >200 ng/dL.
- US may show ovarian cysts (PCOS), presence or absence of uterus, and endometrial thickness (consider MRI if unable to tolerate US probe).

Follow-Up Tests & Special Considerations

- Women <30 years with ovarian failure (see below) should have karyotype analysis and be investigated for premutations of *FMR1* gene (fragile X syndrome) and for adrenal antibodies.
- If absence of uterus or foreshortened vagina, karyotype analysis should also be performed.
- Laparoscopy: diagnosis of streak ovaries (Turner syndrome) or polycystic ovaries
- Hysterosalpingogram: Rule out Asherman syndrome and other etiologies of outflow obstruction.

Diagnostic Procedures/Other

- If constitutional delay is suspected, obtain bone age.
- If hypothalamic amenorrhea from functional suppression is suspected, consider dual energy x-ray absorptiometry (DEXA) scan to assess bone loss.

TREATMENT

GENERAL MEASURES

Identify and correct underlying pathology if possible.

MEDICATION

- Progestational challenge and replacement medroxyprogesterone (Provera): 10 mg/day for 10 days will result in withdrawal bleed within 7 days of last dose if hypothalamic–pituitary–gonadal axis is intact (i.e., amenorrhea is a consequence of anovulation and lack of progesterone), although the predictive value with regard to adequacy of estrogen effect on the endometrium is inconsistent (1),(2).
- Estrogen replacement: cycling with a combination oral contraceptive (containing 35 or 50 μg of estrogen) or conjugated estrogen (Premarin) 0.625 mg for 25 days with medroxyprogesterone added as above for the last 10 days will result in a withdrawal bleed if the uterus and lower genital tract are normal (response to challenge indicates hypothalamic-pituitary axis pathology).
- Use of hormonal therapies will not correct the underlying problem. Other drugs might be required to treat specific conditions (e.g., dopamine agonist cabergoline or for hyperprolactinemia).
- Use of hormonal replacement therapy is not recommended for long-term management of amenorrhea in older women but may be safe for symptom management in young women. Give to maintain secondary sex characteristics and to prevent osteoporosis in adolescents and young women.
- Combination estrogen/progesterone contraceptives (oral contraceptive pills [OCPs], patch, ring) replace estrogen and prevent pregnancy.
  - Have a positive effect on bone mineral density in oligomenorrheic/amenorrheic women but not in functional hypothalamic amenorrhea
  - Can decrease hirsutism in PCOS
- Calcium supplementation: 1,500 mg/day if cause is hypoestrogenism
- Because PCOS is related to insulin resistance, metformin is used to correct metabolic abnormalities, improve ovulation, and restore normal menstrual patterns. Of note, treatment with has shown an increase in clinical pregnancy rates but not in live birth rates.
- Contraindications to estrogen administration
  - Pregnancy, thromboembolic disease, previous myocardial infarction or cerebrovascular accident, estrogen-dependent malignancy, severe hepatic impairment or disease
- Precautions
  - Patients with amenorrhea who desire pregnancy should not be given hormone replacement therapy but should receive treatment for infertility based on the specific cause.

ISSUES FOR REFERRAL

Many causes of amenorrhea require referral to specialists in OB/GYN, endocrine, surgery, and/or psychiatry.

SURGERY/OTHER PROCEDURES

- Hymenectomy for primary amenorrhea if due to imperforate hymen
- Lysis of adhesions in Asherman syndrome is often effective in restoring regular menses and fertility.
- If karyotype is XY, gonads must be removed due to increased risk of tumors.
- Patients with congenital short vagina can undergo surgery to create a functioning vagina.
- Treatment of prolactinomas may include surgical resection.

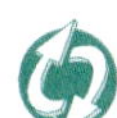

ONGOING CARE

FOLLOW-UP RECOMMENDATIONS

If excessive exercise is suspected, activity level should be reduced by 25–50%.

Patient Monitoring

- Depends on the cause and treatment chosen
- If hormonal replacement is used, discontinue after 6 months to assess spontaneous resumption of menses.

DIET

- Correct overweight or underweight by dietary management and behavior modification.
- If PCOS is the etiology, a weight loss diet will help restore ovulation.

PATIENT EDUCATION

- Educate on the circumstances and complications of her condition and its underlying etiology.
- Specific educational resources are helpful.
- Discuss the expected duration of amenorrhea (temporary or permanent), its effect on fertility, and the long-term sequelae of untreated amenorrhea (e.g., osteoporosis, vaginal dryness).
- Appropriate contraceptive advice should be given because fertility returns before menses.
- Additional support may be needed if amenorrhea is associated with a reduction in, or loss of, fertility.

PROGNOSIS

Reflects the underlying cause. In functional hypothalamic amenorrhea, one study demonstrated 83% reversal rate in the presence of an obvious contributing factor.

COMPLICATIONS

- Estrogen-deficiency symptoms (e.g., hot flashes, vaginal dryness) and osteoporosis in prolonged hypoestrogenic amenorrhea
- Increased risk of endometrial cancer in patients whose amenorrhea is secondary to anovulation with estrogen excess (obesity, PCOS)
- Premature ovarian failure may increase cardiovascular risk.

REFERENCES

1. American College of Obstetricians and Gynecologists. Amenorrhea: absence of periods. https://www.acog.org/womens-health/faqs/amenorrhea-absence-of-periods. Accessed July 3, 2025.
2. Klein DA, Paradise SL, Reeder RM. Amenorrhea: a systematic approach to diagnosis and management. *Am Fam Physician*. 2019;100(1):39–48.

SEE ALSO

- Hyperthyroidism; Hypothyroidism, Adult; Osteoporosis and Osteopenia
- Algorithms: Amenorrhea, Primary (Absence of Menarche by Age 16 Years); Amenorrhea, Secondary; Delayed Puberty

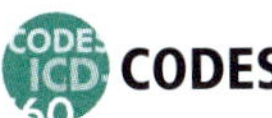

CODES

ICD10

- N91.1 Secondary amenorrhea
- N91.2 Amenorrhea, unspecified
- N91.0 Primary amenorrhea

CLINICAL PEARLS

- Evaluate whether amenorrhea is primary or secondary and exclude pregnancy. TSH and PRL are usual first blood tests.
- Progestin challenge may cause withdrawal bleed in women with intact hypothalamic–pituitary–gonadal axis.

ANAL FISSURE

Anne Walsh, MMSc, PA-C, DFAAPA • Lisa Hertz, MD

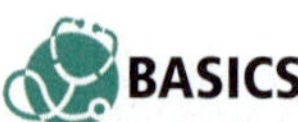

BASICS

DESCRIPTION

Anal fissure (fissure in ano): longitudinal tear in the lining of the anal canal distal to the dentate line, most commonly at the posterior midline; characterized by a knifelike tearing sensation on defecation, often associated with bright red blood per rectum; this common benign anorectal condition is often confused with hemorrhoids; may be acute or chronic (>4–8 weeks in duration) and may be associated with the presence of hypertrophic papilla and sentinel pile (skin tag)

EPIDEMIOLOGY

- Affects all ages; common in infants 6 to 24 months; not common in older children, suspect abuse or trauma; elderly less common due to lower resting pressure in the anal canal
- Sex: male = female; women more likely to get anterior midline fissures (25%) versus men (8%)

Incidence

Exact incidence is unknown (1), as patients often treat with home remedies and do not seek medical care. However, one cohort study found the average lifetime risk in the United States to be 7.8%, equal to that of appendectomy (2).

Prevalence

- 80% of infants, usually self-limited
- 10–20% of adults, most of whom do not seek medical advice

ALERT

Secondary fissures:

- Lateral fissure: Rule out infectious disease.
- Atypical fissure: Rule out Crohn disease.

ETIOLOGY AND PATHOPHYSIOLOGY

High resting pressure within the anal canal (usually as a result of constipation/straining) coupled with decreased perfusion of the posterior canal leads to ischemia of the anoderm, resulting in splitting of the anal mucosa that extends from the dentate line toward the anal verge during defecation and spasm of the exposed internal sphincter.

RISK FACTORS

- Constipation (25% of patients)
- Diarrhea (6% of patients)
- Passage of hard or large-caliber stool
- Low fiber diet
- High resting pressure of internal anal sphincter (prolonged sitting, obesity)
- Trauma (sexual activity or abuse, foreign body, childbirth, mountain biking)
- Prior anal surgery with scarring/stenosis
- Inflammatory bowel disease (Crohn disease)
- Infection (chlamydia, syphilis, herpes, tuberculosis)
- Hirschsprung disease (congenital absence of distal colonic ganglion cells causing chronic constipation)

GENERAL PREVENTION

All measures to prevent constipation; avoid straining and prolonged sitting on toilet.

COMMONLY ASSOCIATED CONDITIONS

Posterior midline location: constipation from any cause, including irritable bowel syndrome (IBS); other multiple locations: Crohn disease, tuberculosis, leukemia, and HIV

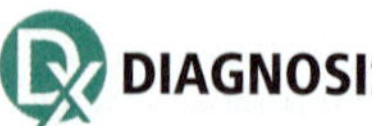

DIAGNOSIS

Physical exam (visual inspection of the anus) is required to confirm the clinical diagnosis.

HISTORY

- Severe, sharp rectal pain, often with and following defecation but can be continuous; bright red blood on the stool or on the paper when wiping
- Occasionally, anal pruritus or perianal irritation

PHYSICAL EXAM

- Gentle retraction of the buttocks with close inspection of the anal verge will reveal a tender, smooth-edged tear in the anodermal tissue, typically posterior midline, occasionally anterior midline, rarely eccentric to midline. Digital rectal exam and anoscopy are painful and can be deferred if inspection confirms the diagnosis.
- Minimal edema, erythema, or bleeding may be seen.
- Chronic fissures may demonstrate rolled edges, exposed muscle fibers, hypertrophic papillae at proximal end, and a sentinel pile (tag) at distal end.

DIFFERENTIAL DIAGNOSIS

- Thrombosed external hemorrhoid: tender, firm, blue-purple nodule at anal verge
- Perirectal abscess: tender, warm erythematous induration or fluctuant mass
- Perianal fistula (abnormal communication between rectum and perianal epithelium): a small opening with feculent or purulent drainage; possible erythema/edema of surrounding skin
- Pruritus ani: shallow perianal excoriations and erythema

DIAGNOSTIC TESTS & INTERPRETATION

Diagnostic Procedures/Other

- Avoid anoscopy/sigmoidoscopy initially unless necessary for differential diagnoses or chronic fissures.
- Due to pain, some patients may require exam under anesthesia in order to confirm the diagnosis.

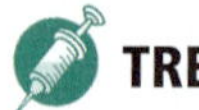

TREATMENT

The goal of treatment is to prevent repeated tearing of the anal mucosa and resultant spasm of the internal anal sphincters by decreasing the patient's high sphincter tone and addressing its underlying cause.

GENERAL MEASURES

- Wash area gently with warm water; consume a high-fiber diet, increase fluids, add daily fiber supplement and stool softener; avoid constipation and maintain healthy weight.
- Medical therapy for chronic fissures is usually initiated in a stepwise manner when needed: topical nitrates, topical calcium channel blockers, botulinum toxin injections.

MEDICATION

First Line

Acute fissures—50% will heal spontaneously with supportive measures (1)[C]. Over the counter therapies (3),(4) include the following:

- Stool softeners (docusate) orally 1 to 3 times daily to mitigate hard stools
- Osmotic laxatives (polyethylene glycol) orally 1 to 2 times daily as needed to treat constipation
- Fiber supplements (psyllium, methylcellulose, inulin) orally daily with 8 oz of fluid and increased overall fluid intake to prevent constipation
- Topical analgesics (2% lidocaine gel or 3% cream) application 2 to 3 times daily as needed for pain control
- Topical lubricants/emollients (Balneol lotion, glycerin ointment, petroleum jelly) for comfort during and postdefecation
- Topical hydrocortisone 1% cream 2 times daily short term for inflammation/pruritus
- Sitz baths (plain, warm-hot water soak of perineum for 10 to 20 minutes) 2 to 3 times daily after bowel movements

Second Line

Chronic fissures—will not heal without treatment, due to persistent internal sphincter spasm and ischemia.

- Chemical sphincterotomy—first-line treatment. Prescription therapies include the following:
  - Topical calcium channel blockers (nifedipine 0.2–0.3% gel, diltiazem 2% ointment) applied 2 to 4 times per day to relax the internal sphincter thereby reducing the resting anal pressure; no better than nitrates for healing but fewer side effects (1)[C]. Oral calcium channel blockers confer lower healing rates, more side effects, and equal rates of recurrence.
  - Botulinum toxin (Botox) 4 mL (20 units) injected into the internal sphincter muscle to inhibit the release of acetylcholine from nerve endings causing short-term paralysis. Lower doses similar to topical nitrates for healing with fewer side effects; higher doses (80 to 100 units) improve healing rates and patient satisfaction.

ISSUES FOR REFERRAL

- Persistent symptoms despite medical therapy, which is usually tried for 90 to 120 days prior to colorectal surgery referral. Select patients with chronic fissures may be referred directly for surgical therapy due to proven superior healing rates (1)[C].
- Late recurrence, which is common (50%) particularly if the underlying issue remains untreated (constipation, IBS)
- Secondary fissures (suspected infectious or inflammatory bowel disease [IBD])

ADDITIONAL THERAPIES

Anococcygeal support (modified toilet seat) may offer an advantage in chronic fissures to avoid surgery.

SURGERY/OTHER PROCEDURES

- Surgery is typically reserved for failure of medical therapy (chronic/recurrent anal fissures).
- Lateral internal sphincterotomy (LIS) involves division of the internal sphincter muscle and is the surgical procedure of choice (95% healing rate) (1)[C].
  - Risk for fecal or flatus incontinence: up to 47% short term, up to 15% long term
  - Open and closed techniques have similar results and are equally acceptable (1)[C].
  - May be repeated for recurrent fissures with similar outcomes (1)[C]
  - Not typically performed on women of childbearing potential due to increased risk of fecal incontinence with or without subsequent obstetrical injury (1)
- Anocutaneous flap safe alternative to LIS in patients without anal hypertonia; less incontinence but lower healing rates (1)[C]
- Botulinum toxin injections also first-line treatment; less effective (60–80% healing) than surgery but fewer complications
  - Risk for fecal or flatus incontinence: 18% short term, reversible
  - May be repeated as needed with same efficacy, which varies based on dose and injection site; higher doses and injection out of fissure conferred both higher healing rates and higher complication rates (namely, fecal and flatal incontinence)
  - Higher doses combined with fissurectomy may be as effective as surgical sphincterotomy.
- Controlled pneumatic balloon dilation may be used by gastroenterologists if surgical referral is not available; should not be used first line as benefits are not well documented. Uncontrolled manual dilation is no longer recommended.

COMPLEMENTARY & ALTERNATIVE MEDICINE

Alternative therapies (hibiscus and other herbal extracts, clove and coconut oil, essential oils, homeopathic and ayurvedic medications, anal self-massage) need further study before they can be recommended as first-line treatment.

ONGOING CARE

FOLLOW-UP RECOMMENDATIONS

Prevention of anal fissures is recommended by addressing patient-specific issues that predispose to constipation (diet, dehydration, medication side effects, sedentarism, etc.).

DIET

High fiber (>25 g/day; augment with daily fiber supplements); increase water/fluid intake, decrease caffeine and alcohol intake.

PATIENT EDUCATION

- Avoid prolonged sitting or straining during bowel movements; drink plenty of fluids; treat constipation with osmotic laxatives; increase physical activity; adopt a weight loss plan if obese.
- Avoid use of triple antibiotic ointment and long-term use of steroid creams to the anal area.
- Use a finger cot or glove when applying nitroglycerin ointment and apply the first dose before bedtime to minimize side effects.
- Topical medications should be applied directly to anal verge; no need to insert rectally

PROGNOSIS

Most acute fissures heal within 6 weeks with conservative medical therapy. Medical therapy is less likely to be successful for chronic anal fissures (40% failure rate) but should remain first-line treatment.

COMPLICATIONS

- Chronic fissure is a complication of nonhealing acute fissure.
- Recurrence is a common complication especially when the underlying cause (constipation/straining) is not addressed.
- Abscess and fistula formation are less common complications.
- Fecal and flatal incontinence is more commonly associated with surgery (5–47% postop), which may become permanent (up to 8% long term, primarily to flatus).

REFERENCES

1. Stewart DB Sr, Gaertner W, Glasgow S, et al. Clinical practice guideline for the management of anal fissures. *Dis Colon Rectum*. 2017;60(1):7–14 doi:10.1097/DCR.0000000000000735.
2. Salati SA. Anal fissure—an extensive update. *Pol Przegl Chir*. 2021;93(4):46–56. doi:10.5604/01.3001.0014.7879.
3. Oad S, Qadir MU, Alam F, et al. Efficacy of botulinum toxin in the treatment of chronic anal fissure: a comprehensive systematic review. *Ann Med Surg (Lond)*. 2025;87(8):5142–5152. doi:10.1097/MS9.0000000000003471.
4. Vitoopinyoparb K, Insin P, Thadanipon K, et al. Comparison of doses and injection sites of botulinum toxin for chronic anal fissure: a systematic review and network meta-analysis of randomized controlled trials. *Int J Surg*. 2022;104.106798. doi:10.1016/j.ijsu.2022.106798.

ADDITIONAL READING

American Neurogastroenterology and Motility Society. Anal fissure. https://motilitysociety.org/pdf/brochures/anal_fissure_handout.pdf.

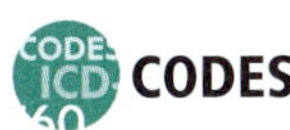

CODES

ICD10

- K60.2 Anal fissure, unspecified
- K60.0 Acute anal fissure
- K60.1 Chronic anal fissure

CLINICAL PEARLS

- Pain with defecation and minimal bleeding are typical symptoms.
- Most acute fissures health with conservative measures.
- Avoid anoscopy or sigmoidoscopy initially unless necessary for differential diagnoses (e.g., secondary fissures).
- Best chance to prevent recurrence is to treat the underlying cause (e.g., chronic constipation).

ANEMIA, CHRONIC DISEASE

Kassandra M. Jean-Marie, MD

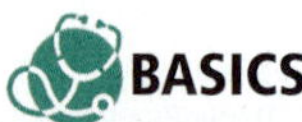

BASICS

DESCRIPTION

- Otherwise known as anemia of chronic inflammation
- During chronic systemic infection, inflammation, or malignancy, the production of proinflammatory mediators causes inhibition of erythropoiesis as well as the imbalance in iron homeostasis (1).
- A normocytic, normochromic, hypoproliferative anemia and classically has low serum iron levels, deceased total iron-binding capacity (TIBC), and elevated ferritin levels (1).
- Anemia is typically mild to moderate with hemoglobin (Hgb) rarely <8 g/dL.

EPIDEMIOLOGY

Prevalence

Anemia of chronic disease (ACD) is the second most common anemia after iron deficiency anemia (IDA). Worldwide, estimates suggest up to 40% of all anemias can be considered from ACD or with ACD as a contributing factor, affecting >1 billion individuals.

ETIOLOGY AND PATHOPHYSIOLOGY

- Production of red blood cells (RBCs) is decreased as a result of functional iron deficiency.
- Three major pathways are involved as a result of proinflammatory cytokines: iron restriction, inflammatory suppression of erythropoietin (EPO), and decreased erythrocyte survival (2).
- Iron overload and the proinflammatory cytokines IL-1, IL-6, and BMP6 increase the production of the iron-regulating hormone hepcidin (1).
  - Hepcidin binds to ferroportin causing internalization and degradation, preventing efflux of iron from stores in macrophages and hepatocytes.
  - Hepcidin decreases iron absorption by duodenal enterocytes.
  - Newer studies show hepcidin may directly block iron export and limit erythropoiesis (2).
- EPO production and the response to EPO by erythroid bone marrow is suppressed by proinflammatory cytokines such as IL-1, TNF-α, and IFN-γ (1).
- Inflammatory cytokines may also cause erythrophagocytosis and oxidative damage, reducing RBC survival.
- It is unclear if the severity of anemia corresponds to the severity of disease.

RISK FACTORS

Hepatic disease, renal disease, infections, malignancies, old age, autoimmune causes

GENERAL PREVENTION

Prevention of ACD involves timely identification and treatment of the underlying condition.

COMMONLY ASSOCIATED CONDITIONS

- Chronic inflammatory diseases: rheumatoid arthritis (RA), systemic lupus erythematosus (SLE), sarcoidosis, temporal arteritis, inflammatory bowel disease (IBD)
- Cancer and hematologic malignancies
- Hepatic disease or failure
- Congestive heart failure (CHF) or coronary artery disease
- Chronic kidney disease (CKD)
- Chronic obstructive lung disease
- Acute or chronic infections
  - Viral: HIV, HCV
  - Bacterial: abscess, subacute bacterial endocarditis, tuberculosis, osteomyelitis
  - Fungal
  - Parasitic
- Malignancies
- Cytokine dysregulation (anemia of aging)
- Hypometabolic states: protein malnutrition, thyroid disease, panhypopituitarism, diabetes mellitus, Addison disease

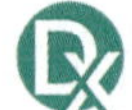

DIAGNOSIS

Diagnosis is typically made in conjunction with clinical picture and labs.

HISTORY

- ACD is often discovered incidentally on routine CBC with differential.
- ACD presents with the underlying causative infectious, inflammatory, or malignant process without any source of occult bleeding; often, patients will have mild and vague anemia symptoms, such as fatigue, light-headedness, and palpitations (1).
- Those with a cardiovascular condition may experience symptoms of angina, shortness of breath (SOB), and reduced exercise capacity with even a moderately low Hgb level (10 to 11 g/dL).

DIFFERENTIAL DIAGNOSIS

- IDA
- Anemia of CKD
- Drug-induced marrow suppression or hemolysis
- Endocrine disorders
- Thalassemia
- Sideroblastic anemia
- Dilutional anemia

DIAGNOSTIC TESTS & INTERPRETATION

Initial Tests (lab, imaging)

- CBC with differential, serum iron, transferrin saturation (TSAT), ferritin, TIBC, ESR/CRP, hepcidin
- Common findings include: normal MCV, low iron, increased, low TSAT, increased ferritin, TIBC can be low or normal, increased hepcidin.
- Hgb (1)
  - Typically, <13 g/dL in males or <12 g/dL in females
  - An Hgb of <8 g/dL suggests a concurrent secondary cause for the anemia and warrants additional workup.
- MCV
  - Usually normal (80 to 100 fL), but microcytosis (<80 fL) may be present with concurrent iron deficiency or long-standing disease
- RBC morphology
  - Normocytic and normochromic
- Serum ferritin
  - Nonspecific acute phase reactant
  - Normal or slightly elevated (usually >100 μg/L) (2)
  - Serum ferritin levels <30 μg/L suggest coexisting iron deficiency.
- Serum iron levels
  - Low due to increased retention and decreased release from stores (<50)
- TIBC
  - Low (<300)
- Absolute reticulocyte count
  - Inappropriately low (reticulocyte index, 20,000 to 25,000/mL) due to reduced erythropoiesis
- Serum B_{12} and folate
  - Diminished due to decreased absorption or lacking in diet

	IDA	ACD	IDA + ACD
Iron	Low	Low	Low
Reticulocyte count	Low	Low	Low
Transferrin, TIBC	High	Low	Normal/high
Transferrin saturation	Low	Normal	Low
Ferritin	Low	Normal/high	Normal
sTfR index	High	Low/normal	High
Hepcidin	Low	High	Normal
EPO	High	Normal/high	High
Inflammatory markers	Normal	High	High

Follow-Up Tests & Special Considerations

It is important to note that, although uncommon, ACD may be the first indication of a serious underlying condition. If a patient presents with signs and symptoms of ACD, it is essential to investigate and identify the underlying cause if it is not already known.

Diagnostic Procedures/Other

- Traditional gold standard: anemia, hypoferremia, and low TSAT combined with bone marrow biopsy with Prussian blue stainable iron (1)
  - Staining is qualitative and may not be accurate.
- Reticulocyte Hgb concentration <28 pg
- Measuring the hepcidin level via enzyme-linked immunosorbent assay can help differentiate IDA from ACD (3).
- Soluble transferrin receptor (sTfR) and the sTfR/log ferritin index
  - Ratio reflects erythropoiesis within bone marrow and differentiates among ACD, IDA, and ACD + IDA.
    - However, sTfR alone may have greater clinical value than the sTfR index because unlike ferritin, transferrin is not affected by chronic disease/inflammation.
      - Elevated sTfR indicates IDA whereas normal values are more consistent with ACD.
- Functional test: supplemental iron increase H/H in IDA and little effect on ACD
- Although a known cause of anemia may be present, iron, B_{12}, and folate deficiencies should be ruled out.

TREATMENT

GENERAL MEASURES

- Primary management should focus on the underlying cause of ACD (1).
  - Treatment of the primary disease will generally restore Hgb back to baseline.
- In cases where primary treatment is not possible (e.g., terminal cancer, end-stage renal disease), additional treatment can be considered.
  - The two main forms of treatment are EPO-stimulating agents (ESAs) and transfusions.
  - ACD is frequently responsive to ESAs (epoetin-α, darbepoetin) in pharmacologic doses.
  - Replete iron to maximize ESA effectiveness.
  - Transfusion should only be initiated in severe anemia or acute symptoms.
- Currently, no target Hgb exists, but treatment to Hgb >13 g/dL is associated with adverse outcomes (1).
- Coexisting B_{12} or folate deficiency should be considered and corrected in severe cases of anemia.
  - Reduced dietary intake of nutrients is common among patients who are chronically ill.
  - Patients who regularly undergo hemodialysis will often lose these during treatment.

MEDICATION

- ESAs
  - Specifically approved for CKD, but there is evidence that they may also have applications in RA, IBD, HIV, and certain cancers (do not use in breast, cervical, head and neck, lymphoid, and non–small cell lung cancers); do not administer to patients with active malignancy not receiving curative therapy.
  - Indication for ESA therapy is an Hgb <10 g/dL.
  - ESAs have not been shown to improve symptoms or outcomes in mild anemia of CHF.
- Epoetin-α (1)
  - Indications
    - Hgb <10 g/dL
    - Fatigue or exertional intolerance
    - CKD (eGFR <60 mL/min)
    - Anemia due to IBD, RA, hepatitis C
    - Chemotherapy in patients with specific malignancies (palliative therapy)
  - Dosing and schedule
    - Lowest effective dose to maintain an Hgb level generally between 10 g/dL and 12 g/dL (1)
    - CKD associated: Start 50 to 100 U/kg SC/IV 3 times per week.
  - Patients with cancer who are undergoing chemotherapy: 150 U/kg SQ 3 times per week or 40,000 U once a week
  - Adverse effects:
    - Increased risk of cardiovascular complications, mortality, and thromboembolism
    - Pure red cell aplasia (decrease in Hgb, low reticulocyte count, normal WBC and platelets)
    - Risk of tumor progression in certain cancer patients
- Darbepoetin-α
  - Long-acting, molecularly modified EPO preparation with a half-life 3 to 4 times longer than recombinant human EPO, reducing the frequency of injections to weekly or biweekly
  - Dosing and schedule
    - Administer SC/IV q1–2wk; hold if Hgb >12 g/dL; IV route is preferred in hemodialysis patients.
  - Adverse effects
    - Similar to EPO
- Epoetin-α or darbepoetin-α dose adjustments
  - Follow FDA-approved labeling.
  - Treatment beyond 6 to 8 weeks without appropriate rise of Hgb (>1 to 2 g/dL) is not recommended.

First Line

The best treatment for ACD is to address the underlying disease. Either epoetin-α or darbepoetin-α may be used as first-line treatment.

ADDITIONAL THERAPIES

- Iron supplementation (PO or IV)
  - Indicated in combined ACD and IDA
  - Forms
    - Oral: ferrous sulfate; poorly tolerated (GI side effects); incomplete absorption (due to hepcidin)
    - Intravenous: ferric gluconate, iron sucrose, iron dextran (potential allergic and anaphylactoid reactions), ferumoxytol
  - Adverse effects: may stimulate hepcidin production and exacerbate iron restriction
  - Benefits: relatively safe, inexpensive, may decrease ESA requirements (DRIVE study)
- Transfusions
  - 1 to 2 U packed RBCs (1)
    Indications
    - Life-threatening/severe anemia: A "restrictive threshold" of Hgb 7 to 8 g/dL to guide transfusion in asymptomatic patients should be used.
    - Patients with underlying cardiac or pulmonary disease, active ACS, elderly patients, or patients with acute bleeding or hemorrhagic shock may require transfusion at Hgb of higher threshold (>10 g/dL).
    - Symptomatic anemia (chest pain, SOB, reduced exercise capacity) and/or ECG changes
    - Lack of response to medical therapy
  - Possible adverse effects: infection (HIV, hepatitis), volume overload, transfusion reaction
  - Specific benefits: rapid correction of anemia
  - When an infection occurs during EPO therapy, it is best to cease EPO therapy and rely on transfusion therapy instead until the infection is properly treated.
- Future directions (1)
  - Hepcidin-antagonizing strategies
  - Anti-BMP, anti–IL-6 antibodies
  - Ferroportin stabilizers
  - Vitamin D (lowers hepcidin)
  - Heparin (impairs hepcidin transcription)

ONGOING CARE

FOLLOW-UP RECOMMENDATIONS

Patient Monitoring

- Hgb should not be increased >12 g/dL because normalization of Hgb has been associated with higher mortality.
- Baseline and periodic monitoring of TSAT and ferritin levels every 3 months may be of value.

DIET

Many chronic conditions associated with ACD are impacted by diet. A well-balanced diet rich in fruits, vegetables, and legumes, including iron rich foods, may be beneficial in treatment.

PATIENT EDUCATION

Patients receiving medical therapy should be advised about the following possible risks: mortality, cardiovascular complications, thromboembolism, progression of cancer

COMPLICATIONS

- Adverse effects of ACD: mortality; cardiovascular complications; symptoms affecting daily life
- Adverse effects of ESAs:
  - Heightened risk of mortality and/or cardiovascular complications in CKD patients
  - Heightened risk of mortality and/or tumor progression in cancer patients
  - Elevated risk of thromboembolism

REFERENCES

1. Gangat N, Wolanskyj AP. Anemia of chronic disease. *Semin Hematol*. 2013;50(3):232–238.
2. Weiss G, Ganz T, Goodnough L. Anemia of inflammation. *Blood*. 2019;133(1):40–50.
3. Karlsson T. Evaluation of a competitive hepcidin ELISA assay in the differential diagnosis of iron deficiency anaemia with concurrent inflammation and anaemia of inflammation in elderly patients. *J Inflamm (Lond)*. 2017;14:21

SEE ALSO

Anemia, Iron Deficiency

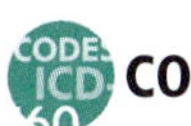

CODES

ICD10

- D63.1 Anemia in chronic kidney disease
- D63.8 Anemia in other chronic diseases classified elsewhere

CLINICAL PEARLS

- ACD is the second most common anemia seen clinically.
- One of the most common diagnostic problems is making the distinction between ACD, IDA, and combined ACD + IDA.
  - Common findings include normal MCV, low iron, increased, low TSAT, increased ferritin, TIBC can be low or normal, increased hepcidin.
- Hgb should be kept in low to normal range, do not replete beyond 12 g/dL.

ANEMIA, IRON DEFICIENCY

Deborah R. Erlich, MD, MMedEd, FAAFP

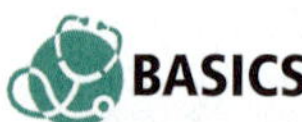

BASICS

DESCRIPTION

- Low serum iron associated with low hemoglobin (Hgb) or microcytic, hypochromic red blood cells (RBCs)
- Because normal Hgb varies with age and sex, anemia is defined as Hgb level 2 standard deviations below normal for age and sex (1).
- Onset acute (rapid blood loss) or chronic (slow blood loss, deficient iron intake, or poor absorption)
- Both low Hgb per RBC and fewer RBC in total lead to blood oxygen deficiency, which can have serious systemic consequences.
- System(s) affected: hematologic, lymphatic, immunologic, cardiac, and gastrointestinal (GI) systems

Geriatric Considerations

- Iron deficiency anemia (IDA) is associated with increased hospitalization, morbidity, and mortality in older adults.
- Older patients with suspected IDA should undergo endoscopy to evaluate for occult GI malignancy.

Pediatric Considerations

- Risks for IDA in children include low birth weight, history of prematurity, lead exposure, low income status, immigrant status, and drinking cow's milk before 12 months of age.
- The U.S. Preventive Services Task Force (USPSTF) did not find sufficient evidence for screening low-risk infants; the Centers for Disease Control and Prevention (CDC) recommends screening high-risk infants at 6 to 12 months, and the American Academy of Pediatrics (AAP) recommends universal screening at 12 months (1).
- Should screening be done, include both Hgb and ferritin.

Pregnancy Considerations

- The USPSTF did not find sufficient evidence for screening pregnant women for IDA; the CDC recommends screening women for anemia at the first prenatal visit and giving low-dose iron to all pregnant women, whereas the American College of Obstetricians and Gynecologists (ACOG) recommends screening all pregnant women for IDA and treating those who test positive for IDA.
- Iron supplements are recommended during pregnancy to improve maternal hematologic indexes, although significant clinical outcomes have not been proven (2)[A].

EPIDEMIOLOGY

- Iron deficiency is the most common nutritional deficiency in the world and IDA is the most common cause of anemia (50%).
- Predominant age: all ages but especially toddlers and menstruating and pregnant women
- Predominant sex: female
- Common in developing and developed countries

Incidence

- Adults: men 2%, women 15–20% annually
- Infants and toddlers: 3–5% annually
- Pregnant patients: may be as high as 20% (1)

Prevalence

2 billion people worldwide

- Infants and children aged 6 to 59 months: 40%
- Men: 2–5%
- Menstruating women: 30%

ETIOLOGY AND PATHOPHYSIOLOGY

Depletion of iron stores leads to decrease in both reticulocyte count and production of Hgb. Causes:

- Blood loss (menses, GI bleeding, trauma)
- Poor iron intake
- Poor iron absorption (e.g., atrophic gastritis, postgastrectomy, celiac disease)
- Increased demand for iron (e.g., infancy, adolescence, pregnancy, breastfeeding)

RISK FACTORS

- Premenopausal woman
- Frequent blood donor
- Pregnancy/lactation, young maternal age
- Strict vegan diet
- Use of NSAIDs
- Hospitalized with frequent blood draws
- Living in or visiting countries with endemic hookworm infection

GENERAL PREVENTION

- Consider screening asymptomatic pregnant women and high-risk children at 1 year of age (guidelines vary) (1)[C].
- Supplementation in asymptomatic children 6 to 12 months if at risk for IDA (e.g., malnutrition, abuse) (1),(2)
- Iron-rich and vitamin C–rich diet for menstruating women
- Iron 30 mg/day for asymptomatic pregnant women (2)

COMMONLY ASSOCIATED CONDITIONS

- Celiac disease, GI tract malignancy, peptic ulcer disease (PUD), *Helicobacter pylori* infection, irritable bowel disease
- Hookworm or other parasitic infestations
- Hyper metrorrhagia
- Pregnancy
- Obesity treated with gastric bypass surgery
- Malnutrition
- Medications such as NSAIDs or antacids

DIAGNOSIS

HISTORY

Asymptomatic in most cases; symptoms may occur in severe anemia:

- Weakness, fatigue, malaise, headaches, and/or inability to concentrate
- Exertional dyspnea
- Angina with coronary artery disease
- Melena
- Pica (chewing dirt, ice, or other non-food items)

PHYSICAL EXAM

- Pallor (skin, conjunctivae, sublingual)
- Tachycardia, tachypnea
- Cool extremities
- Brittle nails/hair
- Signs of heart failure

DIFFERENTIAL DIAGNOSIS

- GI bleeding (e.g., gastritis, PUD, carcinoma, varices, celiac disease)
- Chronic intravascular hemolysis (e.g., paroxysmal nocturnal hemoglobinuria, malfunctioning prosthetic valve)
- Defective iron usage (e.g., thalassemia trait, sideroblastosis, G6PD deficiency)
- Defective iron reutilization (e.g., infection, inflammation, cancer, hypothyroid, chronic diseases)
- Hypoproliferation (e.g., decreased erythropoietin from hypothyroidism, renal failure)
- Other anemias such as anemia of chronic disease, thalassemia, lead poisoning

DIAGNOSTIC TESTS & INTERPRETATION

Initial Tests (lab, imaging)

- Obtain: Hgb, HCT, ferritin, serum iron, total iron binding capacity (TIBC)
- Hgb (to define anemia):
  - $<$13 g in men and $<$12 g in women
  - Hgb 2 standard deviations below normal for age and sex (1)
  - Patients with comorbidities (e.g., chronic hypoxemia, smokers, high altitudes) may be anemic at higher Hgb levels.
- Mean corpuscular volume (MCV): $<$80 Fl
  - MCV may be low normal in mild anemia or hidden by large cells (reticulocytes, macrocytes).
- Ferritin is most sensitive and specific for diagnosing iron deficiency as cause of anemia:
  - $<$15 μg/L diagnoses IDA (1).
  - $<$45 μg/L recommended by American Gastroenterological Association (AGA) as cutoff to reduce false negatives (3).
  - $>$100 μg/L rules out iron deficiency.
- Iron studies:
  - Decreased: ferritin, serum iron, transferrin saturation (TF = [serum iron] × 100 / TIBC)
  - Increased: TIBC, transferrin
- Red cell distribution width (RDW) increases with a mixed population of cells (e.g., mixed IDA and vitamin B_{12} deficiency).
- CBC with differential, peripheral smear, reticulocyte count, and index
  - Peripheral smear usually shows hypochromia and microcytosis but may be normal, and reticulocyte production index is low (1).
- When comorbidity is suspected:
  - Consider testing for G6PD deficiency.
  - Evaluate for thalassemia.
    - Very low MCV $<$80, elevated Hgb A2 or Hgb F, family history, and especially high or high normal RBC count
    - Microcytosis with ovalocytosis and unresponsive to iron suggests the thalassemia trait.
- Celiac disease: IgA antiendomysial antibodies (IgA anti-EmA) and/or IgA antitissue transglutaminase (IgA anti-TTG)
- TSH for hypothyroidism
- An empiric trial of iron at 3 mg/kg/day may help diagnose decreased iron stores in children; reticulocytes become elevated in 7 to 10 days or Hgb increases $>$1 g/dL weekly, indicating iron deficiency.

- Drugs that may alter lab results:
  - Iron supplements or multivitamin–mineral preparations that contain iron
- Disorders that may alter lab results:
  - Elevated ferritin: acute inflammation, liver disease, Hodgkin disease, acute leukemia, solid tumors, fever, renal dialysis
  - Elevated Hgb: smoking, chronic hypoxemia, high altitude

Diagnostic Procedures/Other

- Stool guaiac (low sensitivity, so if negative, consider further evaluation)
- Stool for ova and parasites if at risk
- Colonoscopy and endoscopy to evaluate for bleeding sites and colorectal and gastric carcinoma for:
  - Premenopausal women with negative gynecologic workup and/or lack of response to iron
  - Men and postmenopausal women (1)[C]
- Bone marrow aspiration rarely performed

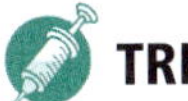

TREATMENT

GENERAL MEASURES

- Search for underlying cause and correct it.
- Avoid transfusions, except in rare cases.

MEDICATION

- Elemental iron 100 to 200 mg/day for adults (whether pregnant or not) (2)
- Elemental iron 3 to 6 mg/kg/day for children
- Ferrous sulfate 325 mg TID, ferrous gluconate 300 mg 1 to 3 tablets BID–TID or ferrous fumarate 324 mg 1 tablet BID on an empty stomach 1 hour before meals (1)[C]
- Common side effect is GI discomfort, especially constipation; consider a stool softener.
- Concomitant vitamin C enhances absorption.
- Medications that reduce gastric acid secretion, such as proton pump inhibitors and H_2 antagonists, reduce iron absorption (1).
- IV iron is indicated for patients who cannot tolerate oral replacement (e.g., pregnant people or patients with GI disorders); insufficiently respond to oral replacement; or who have Hgb <6 g/dL, bariatric surgery status, heavy uterine bleeding, malabsorption, inflammatory bowel disease, or ongoing/severe losses.
- IV iron is superior to oral iron in efficacy and toxicity and can be given in healthy adults in high-dose, low-frequency treatments. Although rare, allergic reactions should be monitored and prepared for. Premedication with antihistamines do not prevent infusion reactions.
- Six available IV iron formulations: ferric gluconate (FG), iron sucrose (IS), low molecular weight iron dextran (LMWID), ferric carboxymaltose (FCM), iron isomaltoside-1000 (ISM), and ferumoxytol (FXT)
- Liquid iron preparations (used for children) can also be used in adults when tablets are not absorbed or well tolerated.
- Formula to determine elemental iron needed: elemental iron (mg) = dose (mL) = 0.0442 (desired Hgb [g/dL] − current Hgb [g/dL]) × LBW (lean body weight in kg) + (0.26 × LBW)
  - For males: LBW = 50 kg + 2.3 kg for each inch of height >5 feet
  - For females: LBW = 45.5 kg + 2.3 kg for each inch of height >5 feet
  - Normal Hgb (males and females)
    - >15 kg (33 lb) . . . 14.8 g/dL
    - <15 kg (33 lb) . . . 12 g/dL
- Relative contraindications for oral iron: tetracycline, allopurinol, antacids, penicillamine, fluoroquinolones, vitamin E
- Precautions:
  - Iron overdose is toxic; absorption is limited to 1 to 2 mg daily; keep tablets and liquids out of reach of children.
- Blood transfusion is indicated for severe acute blood loss or severely symptomatic patients (e.g., demand ischemia due to anemia). Hgb threshold varies by risk factors and clinical scenario. Pregnant women with Hgb <6 g/dL should be transfused (1)[C].

ISSUES FOR REFERRAL

- Men and postmenopausal women with IDA (Test for colon cancer.)
- Pregnant women with Hgb level <9 g/dL
- Nonpregnant adults with Hgb <6 g/dL
- Failure to respond to a 4- to 6-week trial of oral iron

ONGOING CARE

FOLLOW-UP RECOMMENDATIONS

Patient Monitoring

- Monitor patients every 3 months after Hgb normalizes for a year and then yearly (1)[C].
- Hgb increases 1 g/dL every 3 to 4 weeks.
- Iron stores may take up to 4 to 8 weeks to correct after Hgb normalizes.

DIET

- Iron-rich foods include red meat, poultry, fish and eggs (all heme iron sources, best absorbed); and lentils, beans, dark green vegetables, raisins, tofu, and iron-fortified breads/cereals (non-heme iron sources, less well absorbed).
- Foods containing ascorbic acid (vitamin C), such as citrus, tomatoes, dark green leafy vegetables, and berries, enhance iron absorption
- Avoid milk or dairy products within 2 hours of iron tablet ingestion.
- Limit milk to 16 oz/day (adults).
- Limit tea, coffee, and caffeinated beverages.
- Increase fluid and dietary fiber to decrease likelihood of constipation.
- Limit foods with high levels of chemicals (phytates and polyphenols).

PATIENT EDUCATION

https://familydoctor.org/condition/anemia/

PROGNOSIS

- IDA can be resolved with iron therapy if the underlying cause is treated.
- Treat coexisting subclinical hypothyroidism. Failure to treat hypothyroidism results in poor response to iron therapy.

COMPLICATIONS

- Ischemic events or heart failure, especially in elderly
- Poor growth, failure to thrive, motor and cognitive developmental delay in children

REFERENCES

1. Short MW, Domagalski JE. Iron deficiency anemia: evaluation and management. *Am Fam Physician*. 2013;87(2):98–104.
2. McDonagh M, Cantor A, Bougatsos C, et al. *Routine Iron Supplementation and Screening for Iron Deficiency Anemia in Pregnant Women: A Systematic Review to Update the U.S. Preventive Services Task Force Recommendation.* Evidence Syntheses No. 123. Rockville, MD: Agency for Healthcare Research and Quality; 2015.
3. Ko CW, Siddique SM, Patel A, et al. AGA clinical practice guidelines on the gastrointestinal evaluation of iron deficiency anemia. *Gastroenterology*. 2020;159(3):1085–1094.

ADDITIONAL READING

National Institutes for Health Office for Dietary Supplements. Iron: fact sheet for health professionals. https://ods.od.nih.gov/factsheets/Iron-HealthProfessional/. Accessed June 29, 2025.

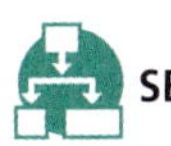

SEE ALSO

Algorithm: Anemia

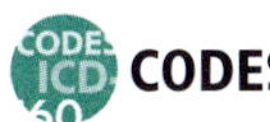

CODES

ICD10

- D50.9 Iron deficiency anemia, unspecified
- D50 Iron deficiency anemia
- O99.01 Anemia complicating pregnancy

CLINICAL PEARLS

- IDA due to poor dietary iron intake is the most common anemia.
- Blood loss and reduced iron stores due to poor utilization or malabsorption are risk factors for IDA.
- Children and premenopausal women are at the greatest risk for IDA.

ANEMIA, SICKLE CELL

Joseph P. Wiedemer, MD • Dongsheng Jiang, MD, MSc

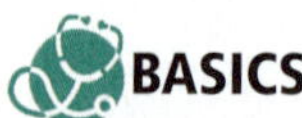

BASICS

DESCRIPTION

- Hereditary, hemoglobinopathy marked by chronic hemolytic anemia, acute episodes of painful crises, and increased susceptibility to infections
- The heterozygous condition (HbAS), sickle cell trait, is usually asymptomatic without anemia.
- Synonym(s): sickle cell disease (SCD); HbSS disease

EPIDEMIOLOGY

Prevalence

- ~100,000 Americans have sickle cell anemia (SCA), and ~3 million people in the United States have sickle cell trait.
- The condition affects mainly people of African descent. Hispanic, Middle Eastern, Asian Indian, and Mediterranean ancestry may also be affected.

ETIOLOGY AND PATHOPHYSIOLOGY

- Hemoglobin S (HbS) results from the substitution of the amino acid valine for glutamic acid at the sixth position of the β-globin chain.
- HbS polymerization occurs in the RBC with increased concentrations of HbS and in deoxygenated states, resulting in RBC sickling.
- Sickle RBCs exhibit increased adhesion, are inflexible and have decreased ability to maneuver through small vessels leading to increased blood viscosity, stasis, and vaso-occlusion of small arterioles and capillaries, resulting in ischemia.
- Sickle cell crises:
  - Vaso-occlusive crisis: tissue ischemia and necrosis; progressive organ failure/tissue damage from repeated episodes
  - Aplastic crisis: suppression of RBC production by severe infection (e.g., parvovirus and other viral infections)
  - Hyperhemolytic crisis: accelerated hemolysis with reticulocytosis; increased RBC fragility/shortened lifespan
  - Sequestration crisis: splenic sequestration of blood (only in young children as spleen is later lost to autoinfarction)
- Hand–foot syndrome: Vessel occlusion/ischemia affects small blood vessels in hands or feet.

Genetics

- Autosomal recessive; homozygous condition, HbSS; heterozygous condition, HbAS
- The heterozygous condition can also be combined with other hemoglobinopathies: Sickle cell hemoglobin C (HbSC) disease and Sβ + thalassemia are clinically similar to the heterozygous condition, whereas Sβ thalassemia is clinically similar to the homozygous condition.

RISK FACTORS

- Vaso-occlusive crisis: hypoxia, dehydration, high altitudes, stress, fever, infection, acidosis, cold, anesthesia, strenuous physical exercise, alcohol, smoking
- Aplastic crisis: severe infections, human parvovirus B19 infection, folic acid deficiency
- Hyperhemolytic crisis: acute bacterial infections, exposure to oxidant

GENERAL PREVENTION

- Prevention of crises
  - Avoid hypoxia, dehydration, cold, infection, fever, acidosis, and anesthesia.
  - Prompt management of fever, infections and pain.
  - Avoid alcohol and smoking. Avoid high-altitude areas.
- Minimizing trauma: Aseptic technique is imperative.

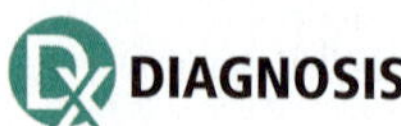

DIAGNOSIS

HISTORY

- Often asymptomatic in early months of life due to presence of fetal hemoglobin
- In those >6 months of age, the earliest symptoms: irritability and painful swelling of the hands and feet (hand–foot syndrome); pneumococcal sepsis or meningitis, severe anemia and acute splenic enlargement (splenic sequestration), acute chest syndrome, pallor, jaundice, or splenomegaly
- Manifestations in older children include anemia, severe or recurrent musculoskeletal or abdominal pain, aplastic crisis, acute chest syndrome, splenomegaly or splenic sequestration, and cholelithiasis.
- Painful crises in bones, joints, abdomen, back, and viscera account for 90% of all hospital admissions.
- Acute chest syndrome: tachycardia, fever, bilateral infiltrates caused by pulmonary infarctions

DIAGNOSTIC TESTS & INTERPRETATION

Initial Tests (lab, imaging)

- Screening test: Sickledex test/Hb electrophoresis (diagnostic test of choice); SCA (FS pattern)
  - 80–100% HbS, variable amounts of HbF, and no HbA1
  - Sickle cell trait (FS pattern): 30–45% HbS, 50–70% HbA1, minimal HbF.
- Hemoglobin ~5 to 10 g/dL; RBC indices: mean corpuscular volume (MCV) normal to increased; mean corpuscular hemoglobin concentration (MCHC) increased; reticulocytes 3–15%
- Leukocytosis; bands in absence of infection, platelets elevated; peripheral smear: sickled RBCs, nucleated RBCs, Howell-Jolly bodies
- Serum bilirubin mildly elevated (2 to 4 mg/dL); ferritin very elevated in patients with multiple previous transfusions; serum lactate dehydrogenase (LDH) elevated, fecal/urinary urobilinogen high
- Haptoglobin absent or very low
- Urine analysis: hemoglobinuria, hematuria (sickle cell trait may have painless hematuria), increased albuminuria (Monitor for progressive kidney disease.)
- Imaging depends on clinical circumstances.
  - Bone scan to rule out osteomyelitis
  - CT/MRI to rule out CVA; high index of suspicion required for any acute neurologic symptoms other than mild headache
  - Chest x-ray: may show enlarged heart; diffuse alveolar infiltrates in acute chest syndrome
  - Transcranial Doppler: Start at age 2 years; repeat yearly. Transcranial Doppler ultrasound identifies children age 2 to 16 years at higher risk of stroke; may be normal in clinically silent strokes
  - ECG to detect pulmonary hypertension and echocardiogram every other year from age 15 years and older

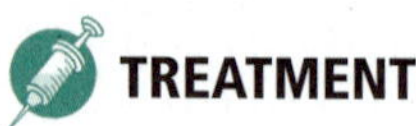

TREATMENT

GENERAL MEASURES

- Painful crises: hydration, analgesics; oxygen regardless of whether the patient is hypoxic
- Retinal evaluation starting at school age to detect proliferative sickle retinopathy
- Occupational therapy, cognitive and behavioral therapies, support groups
- All standard childhood vaccinations should be administered accordingly.
- Adults 19 to 64 years of age: Pneumococcal 20-valent conjugate vaccine (Prevnar 20) is recommended.
- Meningococcal vaccine:
  - 6 weeks old: Hib-MenCY at ages 2, 4, 6, and 12 months
  - 9 months old: 2 doses of MCV4 separated by 3 months
  - ≥2 years of age: 2 doses of MCV4-D-CRM separated by 2 months; boosters recommended every 5 years

MEDICATION

First Line

- Four FDA approved medications for SCD treatment (1),(2):
  - Hydroxyurea: decrease in painful events including acute chest syndrome; age ≥9 months; dose: initial: 20 mg/kg daily; maintenance: 20 to 35 mg/kg, maximum dose of, 2,500 mg daily
  - L-glutamine: reduction in vaso-occlusive episodes (VOE) and hospitalization; age ≥5 years; dose: weight <30 kg: 5 gm BID; 30 to 65 kg: 10 gm BID; >65 kg: 15 gm BID
  - Crizanlizumab: reduction in VEO; age ≥16 years; loading: 5 mg/kg IV every 2 weeks for 2 doses; maintenance: 5 mg/kg IV every 4 weeks
  - Voxelotor: increase Hb; age ≥4 years; dose: <40 kg: 600 to 900 mg once daily; ≥40 kg: 1,500 mg once daily

- Prophylactic penicillins indicated in infants and children starting at 2 months: A dose of 125 mg BID is recommended for children aged <3 years. A dose of 250 mg BID is recommended for children aged 3 to 5 years. Amoxicillin 20 mg/kg/day is an alternative to penicillin. Penicillin can be discontinued at age 5 years unless the patient has had a splenectomy or invasive pneumococcal infection.
- Supplemental oxygen
- Painful crises (mild, outpatient)—nonopioid analgesics (ibuprofen)
- Painful crises (severe, hospitalized)—parenteral opioids (e.g., morphine on fixed schedule); patient-controlled analgesia (PCA) pump may be useful. Patients given strong opioids in the acute care setting should be safely monitored.
- Acute chest syndrome: Patients may deteriorate quickly; monitor patients with vaso-occlusive crisis with incentive spirometry. Treat with aggressive management with oxygen, analgesics, antibiotics, and simple or exchange transfusion.
- Empiric antibiotics to cover *Mycoplasma pneumoniae* and *Chlamydia pneumoniae* (cephalosporins or azithromycin). If osteomyelitis, cover for *Staphylococcus aureus* and *Salmonella* (e.g., ciprofloxacin).
- Precautions: Avoid high-dose estrogen oral contraceptives; consider Depo-Provera. G-CSF use is contraindicated as it may lead to vaso-occlusive episodes and multiorgan failure.

Second Line

Folic acid: 0 to 6 months old: 0.1 mg/day; 6 to 12 months old: 0.25 mg/day; 1 to 2 years of age: 0.5 mg/day; >2 years of age: 1 mg/day

ADDITIONAL THERAPIES

- Transfusion: It increases oxygen-carrying capacity and improves blood flow in severe anemia.
  - It is the main treatment during an acute episode and is helpful in splenic sequestration, aplastic crisis, stroke, acute chest syndrome, multiple organ failure, priapism, etc.
  - Prophylactic transfusions for primary or secondary stroke prevention in children
  - Preoperative transfusions have been shown to reduce the risk of perioperative complications with goal Hgb >10g/dL.
- Chelation with oral deferasirox if the patient is multiply transfused (after age 2 years).
- Red cell exchange is indicated to minimize the level of HbS (<30%) as well as prevent iron overload.
- Hematopoietic cell transplantation (HCT) (3): up to 80–100% survival rate.
- Gene therapy (3): It uses autologous cell engineering to modify hematopoietic cells for transplant, so no donor is needed. Both lovotibeglogene autotemcel (lovo-cel) and exagamglogene autotemcel (exa-cel) are potentially curative treatments but long-term data on their efficacy and safety are still unknown.

SURGERY/OTHER PROCEDURES

- Hematopoietic stem cell transplant (HSCT): curative
- Endothelin-1 has therapeutic potential for prevention of renal and pulmonary complications of SCD.
- Oral therapy with L-glutamine
- Monoclonal antibodies that bind P-selectin

ADMISSION, INPATIENT, AND NURSING CONSIDERATIONS

Admission criteria/initial stabilization: severe pain, suspected infection or sepsis, evidence of acute chest syndrome

ONGOING CARE

FOLLOW-UP RECOMMENDATIONS

Patient Monitoring

- Treat infections early. Any temperature of ≥101°F (38.3°C) requires immediate medical attention.
- Monitor for hepatitis C and hemosiderosis in patients who receive chronic transfusions.
- Periodic eye evaluations: starting at age 10 years for proliferative sickle retinopathy; rescreen 1- to 2-year intervals.
- Biannual examination for hepatic, renal, and pulmonary dysfunction
- Neuroimaging screening for risk of stroke: transcranial Doppler beginning at age 2 years and continuing up to age 16 years
- Baseline pulmonary evaluation at each visit to assess for wheezing, shortness of breath, or cough (indicators of disease severity and pulmonary hypertension); echocardiography for symptomatic patients; right heart catheterization for diagnosis
- Screening for albuminuria should be performed annually starting at age 10 years, with introduction of ACE/ARB therapy for management of confirmed albuminuria.
- SCD may be considered a provoking factor for VTE, but decisions on anticoagulation duration and prophylaxis should be a shared decision-making process.

DIET

- Avoid alcohol (leads to dehydration); maintain hydration.
- Multivitamin without iron is recommended; vitamin D deficiency and decreased bone marrow density in SCD patients

PROGNOSIS

- Anemia occurs in infancy; sickle cell crises at 1 to 2 years of age; some children die in their 1st year.
- In adulthood, fewer crises but more complications; median age of death is 42 years for men and 48 years for women.

COMPLICATIONS

- Alloimmunization, bone infarct and osteomyelitis, aseptic necrosis of femoral head
- Cerebral strokes (peak age 6 to 7 years), impaired mental development, even without history of stroke
- Cholelithiasis/abnormal liver function
- Chronic leg ulcers, poor wound healing
- Impotence, priapism, hematuria/hyposthenuria, renal complications (proteinuria)
- Retinopathy, splenic infarction (by age 10 years)
- Acute chest syndrome (infection/infarction) leading to chronic pulmonary disease
- Infections (pneumonia, osteomyelitis, meningitis, pyelonephritis); sepsis (leading cause of morbidity and mortality)
- Hemosiderosis (secondary to multiple transfusions)
- Risk of opioid tolerance and substance abuse in chronic, uncontrolled patients

REFERENCES

1. Kavanagh PL, Fasipe TA, Wun T. Sickle cell disease: a review. *JAMA*. 2022;328(1):57–68. doi:10.1001/jama.2022.10233.
2. Brandow AM, Liem RI. Advances in the diagnosis and treatment of sickle cell disease. *J Hematol Oncol*. 2022;15(1):20. doi:10.1186/s13045-022-01237-z.
3. Walia R, Fertrin KY, Sabath DE. History, advances, and challenges of sickle cell disease treatment. *Clin Lab Med*. 2024;44(4):679–691. doi:10.1016/j.cll.2024.07.004.

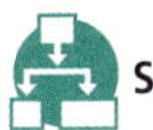

SEE ALSO

Algorithm: Anemia

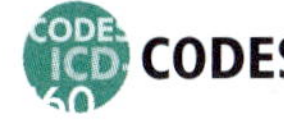

CODES

ICD10

- D57.212 Sickle-cell/Hb-C disease with splenic sequestration
- D57.211 Sickle-cell/Hb-C disease with acute chest syndrome
- D57.21 Sickle-cell/Hb-C disease with crisis

CLINICAL PEARLS

- Painful crises in bones, joints, abdomen, back, and viscera account for 90% of all hospital admissions. Management of pain should follow individualized pain plans or hospital protocol for SCD crises without discrimination.
- Four medications are FDA approved for SCA and hydroxyurea remains a cornerstone.
- HCT and gene therapies are potentially curative.

ANEURYSM OF THE ABDOMINAL AORTA

Jeffrey Chen, MD

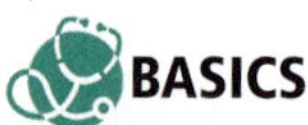

BASICS

DESCRIPTION

- There are two types of aneurysms: true and false. A true aneurysm involves all three vessel wall layers. False aneurysms or pseudoaneurysms occur when the intimal and medial layers are disrupted and the dilated segment is surrounded by the adventitia only. Ruptures are usually higher with false aneurysms due to poor support of the aneurysmal wall.
- Abdominal aortic aneurysm (AAA) is the most common true arterial aneurysm. False aneurysms of the abdominal aorta are usually due to trauma or infection.
- The average diameter of the infrarenal aorta is 2 cm; an aortic diameter of ≥3 cm is considered aneurysmal.
- In men, AAA diameters are predictive of clinical events. In women, aneurysms are still defined as >3 cm, but the aortic scaling index (ASI; diameter [cm] / body surface area [m^2]) is more predictive of clinical events.
- System(s) affected: cardiovascular; neurologic; heme/lymphatic/immunologic
- Synonym(s): aortic aneurysms; AAA

Geriatric Considerations

Incidence of AAA, risk of rupture, and operative morbidity and mortality all rise with age.

Pediatric Considerations

Rare in children; may be associated with umbilical artery catheters, connective tissue diseases, arteritides, or congenital abnormalities

EPIDEMIOLOGY

- Estimated prevalence of AAA in developed countries is 2–8%. Age-related increase is seen more with men than women.
- Ultrasound studies show that 4–8% of older men have an occult AAA.
- 90% of all AAA >4 cm are related to atherosclerotic disease, with the vast majority located infrarenally.
- Predominant gender: male > female

Incidence

- Roughly 15,000 deaths per year and the 15th leading cause of death in the United States.
- 0.4% to 0.67% in Western populations or 2.5 to 6.5 aneurysms per 1,000 patient-years
- If stratified into years, the incidence of AAA is increased in the older populations. For example, the incidence increases from 55 to 298 per 100,000 patient-years if comparing men aged 65 to 74 years versus men >85 years of age.

Prevalence

- The prevalence of AAA-associated mortality has decreased by 50% since the 1990s, likely due to the decline in cigarette smoking, increased screening for AAA detection, and early interventions.
- With the increasing life expectancy in developed countries, the prevalence of AAA is expected to increase, but the decreased prevalence of smoking will have the opposite effect.

ETIOLOGY AND PATHOPHYSIOLOGY

- AAAs are caused by degradations of abnormal production of elastin and collagen, the structural components of the aortic wall.
- There are many causes of aortic aneurysms: inflammation, degenerative disorders, vasculitis, infections, and trauma. However, the vast majority of AAA are caused by inflammation with atherosclerosis as the inciting factor.
- Although most aortic aneurysms are caused by inflammatory or degenerative destruction of elastin and collagen; infections, trauma, and connective tissues disorders can also degrade elastin and collagen, leading to similar presentations.
- The natural course of an AAA is progressive expansion, based on multiple factors, the most important being ongoing smoking.

Genetics

- Familial AAA have a variable polygenetic inheritance pattern.
- Monogenetic inheritance patterns such as: Marfan syndrome (fibrillin-1 defect), Ehlers-Danlos syndrome (type IV collagen defect), or Loeys-Dietz syndrome are more commonly associated with thoracoabdominal aortic aneurysms.

RISK FACTORS

Older age, male sex, Caucasian race, family history, smoking, hypertension (HTN), hyperlipidemia, atherosclerosis, peripheral aneurysms, obesity

GENERAL PREVENTION

- Address cardiovascular disease risk factors.
- Follow screening guidelines: U.S. screening for detection of AAA in male patients, aged 65 to 75 years, who have ever smoked.

COMMONLY ASSOCIATED CONDITIONS

- HTN, myocardial infarction (MI), heart failure, carotid artery atherosclerosis, lower extremity peripheral arterial disease, tobacco abuse
- Screening for thoracic aneurysm should also be considered.
- 20% of patients with AAA have concurrent thoracic aneurysm (1).

DIAGNOSIS

Asymptomatic AAA (majority)

- USPSTF recommends a one time screen for an AAA by abdominal ultrasonography for men aged 65 to 75 years with a smoking history (2)[A].
- Selective screening for AAAs in nonsmoker men aged 65 to 75 years can be offered based on personal or family history and patient's preferences (2)[A].
- Women with a first-degree relative with an AAA can be offered screening via abdominal ultrasonography (1)[C].

ALERT

- Symptomatic: The triad of shock, pulsatile mass, and abdominal pain always suggest rupture of AAA, and immediate surgical evaluation is recommended (1).
  - Hemodynamically stable patients (shock is absent as the rupture is contained) may undergo a CT abdomen with IV contrast for evaluation of an AAA.
  - Unstable patients (rupture is uncontained) undergo a focused bedside ultrasound and surgical repair if AAA is present.

- Unusual presentations:
  - Primary aortoenteric fistula: erosion/rupture of AAA into duodenum
  - Aortocaval fistula: erosion/rupture of AAA into vena cava or left renal vein: 3–6%

HISTORY

- Abdominal, back, or flank pain
- AAA risk factors, hypotension if presenting in an emergency situation
- Found on routine screening if presenting in an outpatient setting

PHYSICAL EXAM

- Pulsatile supraumbilical mass
- Encroachment by aneurysm
  - Vertebral body erosion, gastric outlet obstruction, ureteral obstruction
  - Lower extremity ischemia secondary to embolization of mural thrombus
- Rupture leads to tachycardia, hypotension, evidence of shock and anemia, and possible flank contusion (Grey Turner sign).

DIFFERENTIAL DIAGNOSIS

- Other abdominal masses
- Other causes of abdominal or back pain (e.g., peptic ulcer disease, renal colic, diverticulitis, appendicitis, incarcerated hernia, bowel obstruction, GI hemorrhage, arthritis, metastatic disease, MI)

DIAGNOSTIC TESTS & INTERPRETATION

Initial Tests (lab, imaging)

- If rupturing AAA is considered: complete blood chemistry (chemistries, PT/INR, PTT, type and cross), ECG
- Ultrasound: simplest and least expensive diagnostic procedure with a high sensitivity (94–100%) and specificity (98–100%); test of choice for an asymptomatic AAA (1)[C]
- Surveillance of asymptomatic aneurysm
  - 2.6 to 2.9 cm: Screen at 10-year intervals.
  - 3 to 3.9 cm: Screen at 3-year intervals.
  - 4 to 4.9 cm: Screen at 12-month intervals.
  - 5 to 5.4 cm: Screen every 6 months.
- CT scans are preferred preoperative study (caution with IV contrast in renal failure) if a symptomatic AAA is suspected.
- MRI/MRA can visualize AAA but is often not possible in emergent situations.
- Abdominal x-rays can be diagnostic if calcifications exist; not a diagnostic tool of choice

Follow-Up Tests & Special Considerations

- Evaluation for coronary artery disease is appropriate prior to elective AAA repair, including stress test, echocardiography, and ECG if appropriate.
- If AAA was discovered at any location, then full assessment of entire aorta, including thoracic aorta and aortic valve, is recommended (1)[C].

Diagnostic Procedures/Other

ALERT

Use clinical judgment: Patients with known AAA having abdominal or back pain symptoms may be rupturing despite a negative CT scan.

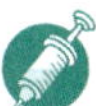

TREATMENT

GENERAL MEASURES

- Treat atherosclerotic risk factors: HTN, dyslipidemia, diabetes mellitus, and smoking (2)[A].
- Smoking was associated with a 0.35 mm/year AAA growth, twice as fast as AAA growth in nonsmokers, and is the most important AAA outcome predictor (1).
- Emergent treatment in unstable or symptomatic patients requires immediate vascular surgery consultation, adequate IV access and resuscitation, type and cross for multiple units, and rapid bedside ultrasound (1).
- Less acute prevention of AAA rupture is elective repair and risk factor modification.

MEDICATION

- β-Blockers, aspirin, and statins theoretically reduce the rate of growth of AAAs by decreasing shear wall stress, inflammation, and prevention of an intraluminal mural thrombus. However, there are conflicting RCT and meta-analysis trials. Because concomitant atherosclerosis is often a precipitating factor in AAAs, their use is recommended for reduced mortality in patients with coronary artery disease or its equivalents (3)[A].
- The use of ACE inhibitors has shown to be inconclusive with regard to growth of AAA; however, studies do indicate a decreased rate of AAA rupture (3)[A].
- Doxycycline and roxithromycin, theorized to decreased wall inflammation, have not been shown to have any effect on AAA (4).

SURGERY/OTHER PROCEDURES

Current recommendations are the following:

- Elective
  - 5.5-cm diameter is threshold for repair in "average" patient (1)[C].
  - Younger, low-risk patients with long-life expectancy may prefer early repair.
  - Saccular aneurysms should be considered for elective repair (1)[C].
  - Women or AAA with high risk of rupture: Consider elective repair at 4.5 to 5 cm.
    - Consider delayed repair in high-risk patients.
    - 5% perioperative mortality for open elective repair (1)
- High risk of rupture
  - Expansion >0.5 cm/year; poorly controlled HTN; smoking/severe COPD
- High-risk patients for elective repair
  - Risk factors for open repair include age >75 years, COPD, chronic kidney disease with Cr >1.75, and suprarenal clamp site.
  - The leading cause of early mortality after AAA repair is coronary artery disease, with open AAA repair being much higher risk than endovascular AAA repair (1)[C].
- The RCT IMPROVE trial showed a similar 30-day mortality for patients with ruptured AAA who underwent endovascular repair versus open repair (35.4% vs. 37.4%); 1-year follow-up all-cause mortality between the two groups (41.1% vs. 45.1%) (4)[A].
- Perioperative morbidity rates are lower for EVAR, suggesting that an EVAR is preferable in patients with a ruptured AAA with poor prognostic factors for an open repair, such as SBP <80 mm Hg, age >80 years, Cr >1.3 on admission, ischemic heart disease, female sex, and hemoglobin <9.0 on admission (2),(4)[A].
- Contraindications for AAA endovascular repair are an aortic neck length >32 mm and a ruptured AAA with aortic neck length <7 mm. In these patients, an open AAA repair is performed due to anatomical constrictions.

ADMISSION, INPATIENT, AND NURSING CONSIDERATIONS

Risk of abdominal compartment syndrome after repair, 4–12%; usually associated with large fluid resuscitation

ONGOING CARE

FOLLOW-UP RECOMMENDATIONS

Patient Monitoring

- May do a CT scan 5 years after an open repair for possible late aortic dilatation or pseudoaneurysm (2)[C]
- Follow-up imaging should be tailored to patient. Once renal function stabilizes postoperatively, a CT can be performed to evaluate the endograft (2)[C].
- Aggressive risk factor modification always recommended postoperatively (2)[A].

DIET

Low-fat, low-salt, and low-caffeine diet; optimize nutrition prior to elective repair.

PATIENT EDUCATION

Smoking cessation, aerobic exercise, and aggressive control of atherosclerotic risk factors such as HTN

PROGNOSIS

- Naturally progressive disorder, expands at an average rate of 0.3 to 0.4 cm/year; a fast expansion is considered >0.6 cm per year and should be evaluated for operative management.
- Possibility of rupture increases with an aneurysm diameter of >5.5 cm or a fast rate of expansion (>0.5 cm over a 6-month period), continued cigarette use, female sex, recent surgery, uncontrolled HTN, and aneurysm couture.

COMPLICATIONS

- Emergent AAA repair and elective AAA repair have similar complications, with a higher incidence in emergent AAA repair.
- Complications include MI, respiratory failure, and acute kidney injury in the early period.
- Late complications such as aortic graft infection, aortoenteric fistula, and graft occlusion have similar rates between emergent and elective repair.
- Ischemic bowel and abdominal compartment syndrome are complications usually after a ruptured open AAA repair given the massive blood loss, increased operative time, and magnitude of fluid resuscitation.

REFERENCES

1. Chaikof EL, Dalman RL, Eskandari MK, et al. The Society for Vascular Surgery practice guidelines on the care of patients with an abdominal aortic aneurysm. *J Vasc Surg*. 2018;67(1):2–77.e2.
2. LeFevre ML; for U.S. Preventive Services Task Force. Screening for abdominal aortic aneurysm: U.S. Preventive Services Task Force recommendation statement. *Ann Intern Med*. 2014;161(4):281–290.
3. Guessous I, Periard D, Lorenzetti D, et al. The efficacy of pharmacotherapy for decreasing the expansion rate of abdominal aortic aneurysms: a systematic review and meta-analysis. *PLoS One*. 2008;3(3):e1895.
4. Braithwaite B, Cheshire NJ, Greenhalgh RM, et al; for IMPROVE Trial Investigators. Endovascular strategy or open repair for ruptured abdominal aortic aneurysm: one-year outcomes from the IMPROVE randomized trial. *Eur Heart J*. 2015;36(31):2061–2069.

ADDITIONAL READING

Aggarwal S, Qamar A, Sharma V, et al. Abdominal aortic aneurysm: a comprehensive review. *Exp Clin Cardiol*. 2011;16(1):11–15.

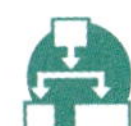

SEE ALSO

Aortic Dissection; Arteritis, Temporal; Ehlers-Danlos Syndrome; Marfan Syndrome; Polyarteritis Nodosa; Turner Syndrome

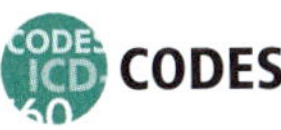

CODES

ICD10

- I71.4 Abdominal aortic aneurysm, without rupture
- I71.3 Abdominal aortic aneurysm, ruptured

CLINICAL PEARLS

- Men with a smoking history aged 65 to 75 years should undergo a one-time screening abdominal ultrasound to evaluate for an AAA. Men and women with a first degree relative with an AAA should be considered for a screening abdominal ultrasound.
- Larger AAAs should be screened more often, with elective repair with AAA >5.5 cm or an expansion of >0.5 cm every 6 months.
- Patients with a ruptured AAA present in shock, with abdominal pain and a pulsatile mass. A bedside ultrasound should be done quickly to evaluate for an AAA, or an emergent CT scan can be performed if the patient is hemodynamically stable.
- AAA are treated either open or endovascularly as an elective or emergent procedure. 30-day and 1-year mortality between the two methods remain the same; however, there is increased mortality with an emergent AAA repair.
- Patients require aggressive risk factor modification, especially smoking cessation.

ANGIOEDEMA

Tess A. Decater, MD, MPH • Scott Kopec, MD

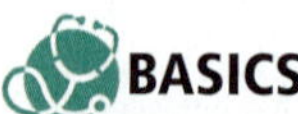

BASICS

Angioedema (AE) is a localized, self-limiting, noninflammatory edema of the deep dermis, subcutaneous, or submucosal tissues caused by vasodilation and increased vascular permeability (1).

DESCRIPTION

- AE can occur with urticaria, but when it presents without wheals, it should be diagnosed as a distinct disease (1).
- AE develops in minutes to hours and resolves in hours to days but can be life-threatening if the upper airway is involved.
- Two major classifications of AE exist, both with unique subtypes (1):
  - Acquired AE (AAE): involves all cases that are not considered to be hereditary AE (HAE)
    - Idiopathic histaminergic (IH-AAE): no cause identified, responds to antihistamine treatment
    - Idiopathic non-histaminergic (InH-AAE): no cause identified, no response to antihistamine treatment
    - Angiotensin-converting enzyme inhibitor (ACEI)-related AAE (ACEI-AAE)
    - C1-inhibitor (C1-INH) deficiency–related AAE (C1-INH-AAE)
  - HAE: mediated by changes in the genes that regulate complement cascades and result in excessive bradykinin production
    - HAE with C1-INH deficiency (C1-INH-HAE): caused by genetic mutations of the SERPING1 gene resulting in a C1-INH functional deficiency (1)
      - Type 1: reduced production of functionally normal C1-INH protein
      - Type 2: normal or elevated amount of functionally abnormal C1-INH protein
    - HAE with non-C1-INH mutation, including HAE-normal-complement (nC1-INH-HAE) and HAE of unknown cause (U-HAE): caused by specific non-SERPING1 gene mutations or unknown cause. Patients have a normal C1-INH level and/or function (1)
- Synonym(s): angioneurotic edema; Quincke edema

EPIDEMIOLOGY

- Predominant age of onset
  - AAE:
    - IH-AAE, InH-AAE, ACEI-AAE: any age
    - C1-INH-AAE: >40 years (2)
  - HAE:
    - Types 1 and 2: infancy to 2nd decade of life (3)
    - nC1-INH-HAE: mean age ~27 years (3)
- Predominant gender: male = female, except nC1-INH-HAE with an FXII mutation, which predominantly affects females

Prevalence

- AAE:
  - IH-AAE: most common form of AE
  - ACEI-AAE: In the United States, ACEI-AAE accounts for one-third of the patients who present to the emergency department for AE (2).
    - Risk factors: Black, female sex, >65 years old, concurrent use of NSAIDs. Note: Race is now recognized as a social, not biologic, construct, and decisions about initiation of ACEI should not be influenced by self-identified race.
  - C1-INH-AAE: 1:500,000
- HAE
  - C1-INH-HAE: 1:50,000 to 100,000
  - C1-INH-HAE type 1 accounts for 85% of cases of HAE (1).
  - C1-INH-HAE type 2 accounts for the remaining 15% (1).

ETIOLOGY AND PATHOPHYSIOLOGY

- AAE:
  - IH-AAE: due to release of vasoactive substances
  - ACEI-AAE: thought to be due to elevated plasma levels of bradykinin and other vasodilatory products, such as substance P (2)
  - C1-INH-AAE: overactivation of the classical complement pathway resulting in consumption of C1-INH either secondary to an underlying lymphoproliferative disorder or because of the formation of a C1-INH autoantibody that neutralizes C1-INH function (2)
    - The most commonly associated lymphoproliferative disorders include monoclonal gammopathy of uncertain significance and Hodgkin's lymphoma (2).
    - Less commonly it can also be associated with other malignancies and autoimmune diseases (e.g., systemic lupus erythematous) (2)
- HAE:
  - Attacks can be triggered by prolonged mechanical pressure, cold, heat, trauma, emotional stress, hormonal fluctuations, infections, and medical procedures.
  - C1-INH-HAE
    - Type 1: decreased production of C1-INH
    - Type 2: normal or high levels of C1-INH, however, is dysfunctional.
  - nC1-INH-HAE: Normal C1-INH levels and/or function with presence of mutations in key non-C1-INH components of the kinin-kallikrein system including factor XII (F12), angiopoietin-1 (ANGPT1), plasminogen (PLG), and kininogen 1 (KNG1) (1)
  - U-HAE: normal C1-INH levels and/or function with unknown cause

Genetics

- All subtypes of HAE have an autosomal dominant inheritance pattern
- C1-INH-HAE: 75% of cases have a reliable history of angioedema (usually first degree relative); 25% of cases occur because of spontaneous de novo mutations (1).

RISK FACTORS

- Consuming medications and foods that can cause allergic reactions
- Positive family history

GENERAL PREVENTION

- Avoid known triggers.
- Do not use ACEI in C1-INH-HAE type 1 or 2.

COMMONLY ASSOCIATED CONDITIONS

- Quincke disease (AE of the uvula)
- Urticaria

DIAGNOSIS

- AAE:
  - Lack of positive family history of AE
  - Assess for: Exposure to common allergens: foods, (shellfish, nuts, eggs, milk, wheat soy), latex, insect bites/stings, medication (antibiotics, aspirin, narcotics, NSAIDs, and oral contraceptives [OCPs])
    - Allergy can be confirmed with positive skin prick test.
    - Exposure to ACEI
    - Exposure to physical stimuli (cold or vibration)
  - If ACEI, allergy, or other causes have been ruled out, then deemed idiopathic (IH-AAE). If AE recurs despite prophylactic antihistamine use, then deemed InH-AAE.
- HAE:
  - Positive family history of AE in first-degree relative
  - C1-INH-HAE, nC1-INH-HAE, and U-HAE require laboratory confirmation.

HISTORY

- Acute, typically asymmetric, nonpitting edema with onset in minutes to hours
- In comparison with urticaria, AE presents without wheals, typically is nonpruritic but can cause a painful, burning sensation.
- Identify potential triggers as listed above.
- Family history of AE
- History of autoimmune disease or malignancy

PHYSICAL EXAM

- Vitals: Symptoms of hypotension, tachycardia, and tachypnea indicate systemic involvement and increased severity.
- Tense, nondependent, nonpitting, asymmetric skin swelling that is skin colored or slightly erythematous
- Commonly affects the mucus membranes of the face including periorbital, lips, tongue, or larynx but can involve any part of the body
- Evaluate for involvement of oropharynx or symptoms such as stridor.
- GI tract involvement is more common in forms of HAE and may manifest as intermittent, unexplained abdominal pain.
- In C1-INH-HAE, erythema marginatum, a serpentine, erythematous discoloration on the extremities and trunk, is the single recognized physical prodrome (3).

ALERT

- Increased risk for early intubation and tracheostomy with involvement of the anterior tongue, base of the tongue or larynx, stridor within 4 hours of onset of symptoms, and drooling
- Patients with HAE are at higher risk for intubation, tracheostomy, and death, although these complications can occur with any subtype.

DIFFERENTIAL DIAGNOSIS

Urticaria; anaphylaxis; contact dermatitis; food/drug allergy; erysipelas; connective tissue disease: systemic lupus erythematosus, dermatomyositis; lymphedema; insect bite reaction; diffuse subcutaneous infiltrative process

DIAGNOSTIC TESTS & INTERPRETATION

Initial Tests (lab, imaging)

- Initial diagnosis should be based on history and clinical assessment alone.
- Laboratory testing includes CBC, ESR, complement testing (C4, C1 INH, C1 INH function), allergy testing, and screening for paraproteinemia (SPEP, UPEP).
- Complement testing assists in distinguishing between various types of AE; this assessment should be done in collaboration with an allergy specialist:
  - Low serum C4 is a sensitive but nonspecific screening test for hereditary and acquired C1-INH deficiency.
  - If C4 is normal, determine C1-INH level and function and recheck C4 during an acute attack.
  - If C4 level and C1-INH level and function are still normal, consider other causes and/or requires genetic assessment (i.e., F12 gene)
  - If C4 level, C1-INH level, and C1-INH function are low, these indicate C1-INH-HAE type 1.
  - C1-INH-HAE type 2 is characterized by low C4 and low C1-INH function, but C1-INH level can be normal or elevated.
- For recurrent AE with urticaria, complement levels should be obtained in addition to allergy testing for potential triggers.
- Abdominal radiographs and CT scan can demonstrate GI AE or ileus.
- Acquired C1-INH deficiency may occur in association with an underlying lymphoproliferative disorder. In rare cases, AE can be a paraneoplastic disease. Imaging (CT scan, radiography, etc.) would be done as part of a neoplastic workup for patients with AAE.
  - Also note: Compared to other types of AE, in C1-INH-AAE, C1q is low 70–80% of the time and C1-INH antibody may be positive (2)

Follow-Up Tests & Special Considerations

If C4 and C1q antigen are low (as in AAE), neoplastic and autoimmune workup is warranted. CBC, a peripheral smear, protein electrophoresis, immunophenotyping of lymphocytes, and imaging studies are often undertaken to rule out hematologic malignancies or cancer.

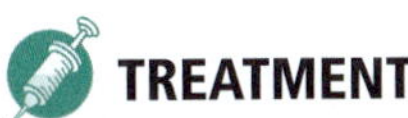

TREATMENT

GENERAL MEASURES

- Intubation if airway is threatened
- Eliminate suspected trigger.
- Volume replacement is essential for patients who are unstable or refractory to initial therapy.

MEDICATION

First Line

- If AE presenting with signs of anaphylaxis (hypotension, respiratory compromise): epinephrine 1:1,000; 0.1 mg/kg (maximum 0.3 mg for children, 0.5 mg for adults) intramuscularly q5–15min
- If cause of AE is unknown, use first-line therapy:
  - Epinephrine, if airway involvement
  - H_1 antagonist (IV diphenhydramine, adult: 25 to 50 mg, children: 1 mg/kg, maximum 50 mg). In older adults, side effects can include delirium, urinary retention, constipation, and increased ocular pressure.
  - H_2 antagonists (IV ranitidine, adult: 50 mg, children: 1 mg/kg, maximum 50 mg)
  - Corticosteroids (IV hydrocortisone, adult: 200 mg, children: maximum 100 mg; or IV methylprednisolone, adult: 50 to 100 mg, children: 1 mg/kg, maximum 50 mg)
- AAE
  - IH-AAE
    - Acute treatment: first-line therapy, as above
    - Prevention: second-generation antihistamines (cetirizine, fexofenadine, loratadine, etc.) administered daily; may need to escalate to higher than standard doses, up to four times labeled dosing, before considering treatment failure or alternative diagnosis, that is, InH-AAE (2)
  - InH-AAE
    - Acute treatment: Attempt first-line therapy as above, but these medications are generally not effective.
    - Prevention: specialty referral for immunosuppressive agents, can consider tranexamic acid (TXA) (2)
  - ACEI-AAE
    - Acute treatment:
      - Remove causative agent. Although despite discontinuation, recurrent AE can occur for several weeks to months (2).
      - May be ineffective: first-line therapy, as above
      - Off label: bradykinin receptor antagonist (icatibant), C1-INH replacement (Berinert, Ruconest), kallikrein inhibitor (ecallantide), TXA
    - Prevention: Remove causative agent; angiotensin receptor blockers (ARBs) are an appropriate substitute as they have a low incidence of cross-reactivity.
  - C1-INH-AAE
    - Acute treatment:
      - Off label: bradykinin receptor antagonist (icatibant), C1-INH replacement (Berinert, Ruconest), kallikrein inhibitor (ecallantide)
      - H1/H2 antagonists, corticosteroids, and epinephrine are ineffective and not recommended.
      - Associated improvement through treatment of underlying disease
    - Prevention: possible remission through treatment of underlying disease
- HAE
  - Patients no not improve with antihistamines or oral corticosteroids. Epinephrine only provides transient benefit but does not alter the fundamental course of the attack (2)
  - C1-INH-HAE
    - Berinert (human C1 esterase inhibitor) 20 IU/kg IV (2)
    - Ruconest (recombinant C1 esterase inhibitor) 50 to 100 IU/kg IV (2)
  - nC1-INH-HAE/U-HAE:
    - Treatment choice should be driven by allergy/immunology specialist and may include: C1-INH agents, icatibant, ecallantide, progesterone, danazol, and TXA (2)
  - Prevention: Avoid triggers such as ACEIs, estrogen-containing contraceptives, and estrogen hormone replacement (2).

Second Line

HAE acute treatment: FFP can be considered if first-line treatments unavailable, however, can potentially worsen attack, so caution is required.

ISSUES FOR REFERRAL

Patients presenting with first episode of AE with a positive family history or recurrent AE will benefit from management from allergy/immunology specialist.

ADMISSION, INPATIENT, AND NURSING CONSIDERATIONS

Need for admission is based on severity of airway involvement. Ishoo criteria can be used for risk stratification. All patients with respiratory distress or in need of airway support will benefit from treatment in an intensive care unit.

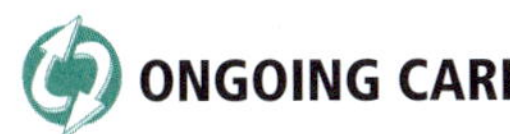

ONGOING CARE

PATIENT EDUCATION

Educate on avoidance of identified triggers, types of treatment, when to seek emergency care, and wearing medical alert bracelet.

PROGNOSIS

- AE symptoms often resolve in hours to 2 to 4 days. If airway is compromised, AE can be life-threatening.
- Patients with HAE have an average of 20 attacks per year; each may last 3 to 5 days. Prophylaxis can decrease the frequency of events and number of missed days of school or work.

REFERENCES

1. Proper SP, Lavery WJ, Bernstein JA. Definition and classification of hereditary angioedema. *Allergy Asthma Proc*. 2020;41(Suppl 1):S03–S07.
2. Kesh S, Bernstein JA. Isolated angioedema: a review of classification and update on management. *Ann Allergy Asthma Immunol*. 2022;129(6):692–702.
3. Azmy V, Brooks JP, Hsu FI. Clinical presentation of hereditary angioedema. *Allergy Asthma Proc*. 2020;41(Suppl 1):S18–S21.

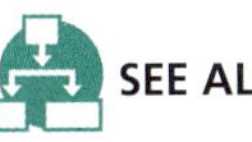

SEE ALSO

Anaphylaxis; Urticaria

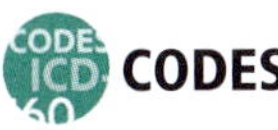

CODES

ICD10

- T78.3XXA Angioneurotic edema, initial encounter
- D84.1 Defects in the complement system

CLINICAL PEARLS

- AE is an acute, localized swelling of skin, mucosa, and submucosa caused by extravasation of fluid into the affected tissues.
- There are two major classifications of AE: AAE and HAE.
- Onset is in minutes to hours and often resolves in hours to days, but it can be life-threatening if the upper airway is involved.
- Any recurrent AE requires referral for specialist management
- ARBs are an appropriate substitute for patients with ACEI-AAE as they have a low incidence of cross-reactivity.

ANKLE FRACTURES

Joshua A. Go, DO • Jaret Nishikawa, MD • Sean T. Matsuwaka, MD

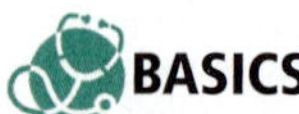

BASICS

- Ligaments: syndesmotic, lateral collateral, and medial collateral (deltoid) ligament
- Mortise joint: tibial plafond, fibula above (forming medial and lateral malleolus) and talus below
- Bones: tibia, fibula, calcaneus, talus, navicular

DESCRIPTION

- Danis-Weber classification: based on level of fibular fracture in relationship to tibiotalar joint
  - Type A (30%): below ankle joint; usually stable
  - Type B (63%): at the level of the ankle joint; may be stable or unstable
  - Type C (7%): above ankle joint; usually unstable
- Lauge-Hansen (LH) classification: based on foot position and direction of applied force relative to the tibia
  - Supination-adduction (SA)
  - Supination-external rotation (SER): most common (40–75% of fractures)
  - Pronation-abduction (PA)
  - Pronation-external rotation (PER)
- Stability-based classification
  - Stable
    - Isolated lateral malleolar fractures (Weber A/B) without talar shift and negative stress test
    - Isolated nondisplaced medial malleolar fractures
  - Unstable
    - Bimalleolar or trimalleolar fractures
    - High fibular fractures (Weber C) or lateral malleolar fracture with medial injury and positive stress test
    - Lateral malleolar fracture with talar shift/tilt (bimalleolar equivalent)
    - Displaced medial malleolar fractures
- Pilon fracture: tibial plafond fracture due to axial loading (unstable)
- Maisonneuve: fracture of proximal 1/3 fibula associated with ankle fracture or ligament disruption (unstable); high risk of peroneal nerve injury

Pediatric Considerations

- Ankle fractures more common than sprains in children because ligaments are stronger than physis.
- Talar dome fracture: suspect in child with nonhealing ankle "sprain" or recurrent effusions
- Tillaux fracture: isolated Salter-Harris III of distal tibia with growth plate involvement
- Triplane fracture: Salter-Harris IV with fracture lines oriented in multiple planes: 2-, 3-, and 4-part variants

EPIDEMIOLOGY

- Ankle fractures are responsible for 9% of all adult and 5% of all pediatric fractures.
- Peak incidence: females 45 to 64 years; males 8 to 15 years

Incidence

187 per 100,000 people per year

ETIOLOGY AND PATHOPHYSIOLOGY

- Most common: falls (38%), inversion injury (32%), sports-related (10%)
- Plantar flexion (joint less stable in this position)
- Axial loading: tibial plafond or pilon fracture

RISK FACTORS

- Age, fall, fracture history, polypharmacy, intoxication
- Obesity, sedentary lifestyle
- Sports, physical activity
- History of smoking or diabetes
- Alcohol or slippery surfaces

GENERAL PREVENTION

- Nonslip, flat, protective shoes
- Fall precautions in elderly

COMMONLY ASSOCIATED CONDITIONS

- Most ankle fractures are isolation injuries, but 5% have associated fractures.
- Sprains
- Tibiotalar or subtalar dislocation
- Other axial loading or shearing injuries (i.e., vertebral compression or pelvic fractures)

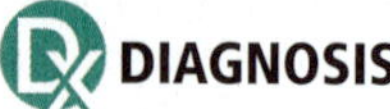

DIAGNOSIS

HISTORY

- Location of pain, timing, and mechanism
- Weight-bearing status after injury
- History of ankle injury or surgery
- Other injured areas (spine, hip, knee)
- Neurovascular symptoms
- Comorbidities (diabetes, smoking)
- Tetanus status
- Assess for safety and fall risk.

PHYSICAL EXAM

- Examine skin integrity (open vs. closed fracture).
- Assess point of maximal tenderness.
- Palpate joints above and below.
- Neurovascular status
- Weight-bearing
- Special tests: anterior drawer (ATFL [anterior talofibular ligament]), talar tilt (ligaments), squeeze test, and external rotation stress test for the tibiofibular syndesmosis
- An ankle fracture is stable if:
  - Isolated to lateral, medial, or posterior malleolus
  - Nondisplaced or at/below level of the mortise
  - Not associated with ligamentous injury
- An ankle fracture is unstable if two or more sites of significant injury are present.

DIFFERENTIAL DIAGNOSIS

- Ankle sprain, including syndesmotic ("high ankle") sprain
- Other fractures: talus, 5th metatarsal, calcaneus
- Achilles tendon injury
- Do not miss: Maisonneuve fracture, talar neck fracture (high risk of avascular necrosis), septic arthritis, pathologic fracture, compartment syndrome

DIAGNOSTIC TESTS & INTERPRETATION

- Plain radiographs: first line based on pretest probability (Ottawa Ankle Rules [OAR])
- OAR: Overall sensitivity of 98% in adults increases to 99.6% if applied within the first 48 hours after trauma (1)[A].
- OAR—x-ray in patients aged 18 to 55 years if:
  - Tenderness at posterior edge of distal 6 cm of tibia or tip of medial malleolus, or
  - Tenderness at posterior edge or distal 6 cm of fibula or tip of lateral malleolus, or
  - Inability to bear weight both immediately and in ED for 4 steps, or
  - Tenderness at navicular or 5th metatarsal (Ottawa Foot Rules)
- Three standard views
  - Anteroposterior (AP)
  - Lateral: Talar dome/distal tibia incongruity indicates instability.
  - Mortise (15- to 25-degree internal rotation view): symmetry of mortise; space between the medial malleolus and talus (i.e., medial clear space) should be ≤4 mm.
- If initial x-ray is normal, but severe symptoms persist past 48 to 72 hours, obtain repeat x-ray.
- To determine stability of lateral malleolar fractures, presence or absence of medial injury:
  - Medial clear space >4 mm on weight-bearing x-ray concerning for deltoid ligament injury and an unstable fracture
- In children aged >1 year, OAR sensitivity is 98.5%.
- OAR not valid for intoxicated patients, those with multiple injuries, or sensory deficits (neuropathy)

Pediatric Considerations

- Consider tenderness over distal fibula with normal films as Salter-Harris I.
- Stress views are unnecessary in children and may cause physeal damage.
- Salter-Harris V often missed and diagnosed with leg length discrepancy or angular deformity after Salter-Harris I; rare, 1% of fractures

Follow-Up Tests & Special Considerations

- CT recommended for operative planning in trimalleolar, Tillaux, triplane, pilon fractures, or fractures with intra-articular involvement
- CT may be considered for radiographically occult talus fracture if clinical suspicion warrants.
- MRI not routinely indicated; does not increase sensitivity for detecting complex ankle fractures
  - MRI useful for chronic instability, osteochondral lesions, occult fractures, and unexpected stiffness in children (1)[A]

Diagnostic Procedures/Other

- Ultrasound can be used for presence of medial (deltoid) injury, but weight-bearing x-ray must still be done to assess stability of lateral injury.
- Bone scan or MRI for stress fracture (1)[A]

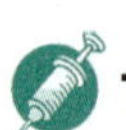

TREATMENT

GENERAL MEASURES

- Initial management: splinting, ice, elevation, analgesics, immobilize for non–weight-bearing
- Closed ankle fractures—must determine stability
  - Stable = nonoperative management
  - Unstable = surgery
  - Lateral shift of talus ≥2 mm or displacement of either malleolus by 2 to 3 mm = surgery
  - In adults with displaced fractures: Insufficient evidence whether surgery or nonoperative management produces superior long-term outcomes.
- Stable syndesmosis injury = nonoperative
- Fracture-dislocations: urgent reduction
  - Do not wait for imaging if neurovascular compromise, obvious deformity, or skin tenting.
  - Flex hip and knee 90 degrees for easier reduction.
  - Postreduction: neurovascular exam and x-rays

MEDICATION

First Line

- NSAIDs and/or acetaminophen for pain: short-term relief 3 to 7 days (1)[A]
- Initial IM pain injection (i.e., ketorolac)
- For suspected open fractures: tetanus booster, broad-spectrum cephalosporin, and aminoglycoside within 3 hours post-injury
- Intra-articular or hematoma block

Second Line

Cryotherapy can help reduce pain and swelling of soft tissue injuries when applied soon after the injury for 3 to 5 days (1)[A].

ISSUES FOR REFERRAL

- Indications for referral to orthopedic surgery:
  - Open fractures (immediate)
  - Neurologic or vascular deficits (immediate)
  - Fracture-dislocations require rapid reduction and referral.
  - Loss of joint congruency
  - Loss of joint stability
  - Unstable fracture should be referred within a 1 to 2 days of injury.
- All other fractures: Follow up in 1 week and remain non–weight-bearing. Consult orthopedics if uncomfortable with routine fracture management.

ADDITIONAL THERAPIES

- Nonoperative = cast immobilization
- No difference in type of immobilization (Air-Stirrup, cast, orthosis)
- Initially non–weight-bearing with crutches and then advance to 50% with crutches; full weight-bearing after 6 weeks postinjury
- If removable cast, gentle range-of-motion exercises at 4 weeks
- Open ankle fractures (2%)
  - Remove gross debris/contamination in ED.
  - Surgical emergency: best if repaired within 24 hours

SURGERY/OTHER PROCEDURES

- Surgical options
  - Open reduction and internal fixation (ORIF); preferred in athletes and unstable fractures
  - External fixation may be preferred in extreme tissue injury or comminuted fractures; may have more malunion compared to ORIF but no difference in wound complications
- Timing of surgery
  - Immediately if neurovascular compromise, open fracture, unsuccessful reduction, tissue necrosis
  - Otherwise, delay >5 days post-injury because inflammation can affect wound healing.
- Length of recovery is usually 6 to 8 weeks.
- Rehab after surgery
  - Early weight-bearing (within 3 weeks after surgery) can lead to improved ankle function, but the clinical significance is unclear (2)[A].
  - Effectiveness of physical therapy versus structured exercise program versus home exercises for improved ankle function is uncertain (2)[A].
  - Removable versus nonremovable ankle support for improved ankle function showed no clinically significant difference (2)[A].

Pediatric Considerations

- Salter-Harris I and II = nonoperative
  - Distal tibia: long leg cast for 4 to 6 weeks and then short leg cast for 2 to 3 weeks
  - Distal fibula: posterior splint or ankle brace 3 to 4 weeks, weight-bearing; if displaced, then short leg cast 4 to 6 weeks, non–weight-bearing
  - Limit reduction attempts because of potential injury to growth plate.
  - Reduction not recommended if presenting ≥1 week postinjury
  - Intra-articular displacement of ≥2 mm in child with >2 years growth remaining = ORIF
- Salter-Harris III and IV:
  - Distal tibia: if >2 mm displacement = ORIF
  - Distal fibula: rare, usually stable after tibial reduction
  - Tillaux and triplane: ORIF if displaced ≥2 mm

Geriatric Considerations

- Higher surgical risk due to age/comorbidities
- Osteoporosis increases risk of implant/fixation failure.
- Risks from surgery/anesthesia: wound healing problems, pulmonary embolism, mortality, amputation, reoperation

ADMISSION, INPATIENT, AND NURSING CONSIDERATIONS

- Admit if:
  - Emergency surgery required
  - Patient nonadherent, lacks social support, unable to maintain non–weight-bearing status, or has significant associated injuries
  - Concerning mechanism of injury (i.e., syncope, myocardial infarction, head injury)
  - Nursing: non–weight-bearing; maintain splint/cast; apply ice; keep leg elevated; pain control; assist ADLs
- Discharge criteria:
  - Ambulates with walker or crutches
  - Medical workup (if needed) completed
  - Orthopedic follow-up arranged

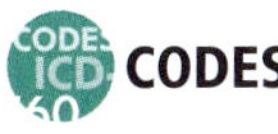

ONGOING CARE

FOLLOW-UP RECOMMENDATIONS

Patient Monitoring

- Orthopedic follow-up: serial x-rays
- In children, sclerotic lines on x-ray (Parker-Harris growth arrest lines) indicate growth disturbance.
- Immobilize for 4 to 6 weeks and then progressive activity, weight-bearing, with removable splint or boot.
- Physical therapy referral: no difference in outcomes between stretching, manual therapy, and exercise program (2)[A]

PATIENT EDUCATION

- Ice and elevate for 2 to 3 weeks; use crutches/cane as instructed; splint/cast care (avoid getting wet, etc.)
- Notify physician if swelling increases, paresthesias, pain, or change in color of extremity (infection, compartment syndrome from cast)

PROGNOSIS

- Good results can be achieved without surgery if fracture is stable.
- Most return to activity within 3 to 4 months
- Most athletes return to preinjury activity levels.
- Increasing age, not injury severity, associated with worsening mobility after fracture

COMPLICATIONS

- Delayed union, malunion, or nonunion (0.9–1.9%)
- Loss of fixation, further surgery, amputation
- Deep venous thrombosis
- Complex regional pain syndrome, extensor retinaculum syndrome in children
- Infection (osteomyelitis)
- Posttraumatic arthritis, degenerative joint disease, growth arrest in children

REFERENCES

1. Polzer H, Kanz KG, Prall WC, et al. Diagnosis and treatment of acute ankle injuries: development of an evidence-based algorithm. *Orthop Rev (Pavia)*. 2012;4(1):e5.
2. Lewis SR, Pritchard MW, Parker R, et al. Rehabilitation for ankle fractures in adults. *Cochrane Database Syst Rev*. 2024;9(9):CD005595.

CODES

ICD10

- S82.899A Oth fracture of unsp lower leg, init for clos fx
- S82.899B Oth fracture of unsp lower leg, init for opn fx type I/2
- S82.56XA Nondisp fx of medial malleolus of unsp tibia, init

CLINICAL PEARLS

- OAR are nearly 100% sensitive in determining the need for x-rays.
- Assess neurovascular status, ability to bear weight, and associated injuries.
- Assess joint above/below to avoid overlooking extent of injury (i.e., Maisonneuve fracture).
- Normal x-rays with point tenderness suggest Salter-Harris type I fractures in children.
- Assessment of fracture stability often dictates conservative versus operative management.

ANKYLOSING SPONDYLITIS

Elizabeth T. Nguyen, MD, CAQSM, FAAP • Dennis Garcia-Rhodes, MD, MPH

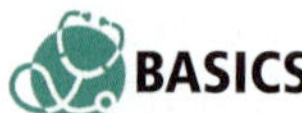

BASICS

DESCRIPTION

- Ankylosing spondylitis (AS) is an axial inflammatory spondyloarthropathy (axSpA) characterized by chronic low back pain (>3 months duration) and evidence of sacroiliitis (sclerosis, erosions, and changes in joint width) on plain radiography.
  - Assessment of Spondyloarthritis International Society (ASAS) published within an updated consensus that axial spondyloarthritis and AS are equivalent and can be used interchangeably, therefore referred to now as axSpA (1).
- Systems affected: musculoskeletal (MSK); ophthalmic; cardiovascular; neurologic; pulmonary; gastrointestinal (GI)
- Synonyms: Marie-Strümpell disease; "bamboo spine"; Bekhterev disease

EPIDEMIOLOGY

- Peak onset typically during 3rd decade of life; rarely occurs after age 45 years
- Male > female (approximately 2 to 3:1) for axSpA
  - Studies vary with effect of gender on axSpA.
  - Peripheral disease
    - Higher prevalence of anterior uveitis in men versus higher prevalence of peripheral arthritis and psoriasis in women

Incidence

- Approximately 7 per 100,000 affected
- Higher incidence in Europe and United States given presence of HLA-B27 gene; more studies are needed for this to assess incidence of axSpA in other areas.

Prevalence

Prevalence of axSpA among adults varies from 0.3 to 1.4% although highly influenced by presence of HLA-B27.

ETIOLOGY AND PATHOPHYSIOLOGY

- Autoinflammation at sites of bacterial exposure (e.g., intestines) or mechanical stress in genetically susceptible individuals
- Inflammation at the insertion of tendons, ligaments, and fasciae to bone (enthesopathy) causes erosion, remodeling, and new bone formation.

Genetics

- Majority of patients with axSpA are *HLA-B27* positive.
- Other genetic associations include endoplasmic reticulum aminopeptidase 1 (*ERAP1*), interleukin 23 receptor (*IL23R*).

RISK FACTORS

- Positive family history
  - Concordance rates of 63% for HLA-B27–positive monozygotic twins and 27% for dizygotic twins
- Gut microbiome theory
  - 57–70% of patients with AS had asymptomatic intestinal inflammation in terminal ileum.
- Current smoking (not history of smoking)

COMMONLY ASSOCIATED CONDITIONS

- Peripheral arthritis
- Enthesopathy: Achilles tendonitis, plantar fasciitis (prevalence 35–60%)
- Uveitis (prevalence 6–30%)
- Psoriasis (prevalence 10%)
- Dactylitis "sausage digit"
- Inflammatory bowel disease (IBD) (prevalence of 4–6%)

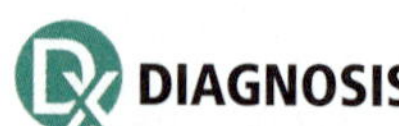

DIAGNOSIS

HISTORY

- Inflammatory back pain
  - Insidious onset typically at age <45 years; duration >3 months; insidious onset; nighttime awakenings secondary to back pain; pain and stiffness increase at rest and improve with activity.
- Alternating buttock/hip pain and constitutional symptoms (fatigue, poor sleep, weight loss, low-grade fever) are common and may appear before radiographic evidence of the disease.
- Other symptoms associated with enthesopathy (Achilles tendon pain, plantar fascia pain), dactylitis (sausage digits), iritis (unilateral pain, red eye, photophobia, vision changes/blurring)

PHYSICAL EXAM

- Sacroiliac (SI) joint tenderness, loss of lumbar lordosis, and cervical spine rotation
  - Low sensitivity and specificity for physical examination of sacroiliitis
- Diminished range of motion in the lumbar spine in all three planes of motion
- Peripheral oligoarthritis/dactylitis seen mostly with peripheral axSpA
- Extra-articular manifestations: uveitis, psoriasis, IBD

DIFFERENTIAL DIAGNOSIS

- Mechanical low back pain
- Other types of arthritis: reactive, infectious, inflammatory
- Osteoarthritis or erosive osteochondritis of the axial spine
- Infectious discitis, unilateral sacroiliitis
- Vertebral compression fracture
- Fibromyalgia—tender points can mimic enthesitis findings.

DIAGNOSTIC TESTS & INTERPRETATION

- ESR and C-reactive protein (CRP) may be mildly elevated or normal; if high, correlates with disease activity and prognosis
- HLA-B27 testing
- SI joints:
  - Can do a single, anteroposterior view; oblique view may also provide useful information but require slightly higher radiation levels.
  - Radiographic interpretation can vary in results for interpretation of sacroiliitis and can be challenging.
- If pelvic radiographic negative or equivocal, consider pelvic MRI to evaluate for active inflammation.
- Spine: lateral view preferred
  - Can help rule out other causes of back pain
- In adults with AS of unclear activity while on a biologic, conditionally recommendations are to obtain a spinal or pelvis MRI to assess activity; no recommendation to obtain spinal or pelvis MRI to confirm inactivity of adults with stable AS (2)

Initial Tests (lab, imaging)

Diagnosis is based off of the ASAS criteria

- Overall sensitivity of 82% and specificity of 89%
- 2009 ASAS classification:
  - If a patient has low back pain for at least 3 months, is <45 years old and there is concern for axSpA based off of history and physical, obtain an anterior-posterior x-ray of the SI joints.
    - If sacroiliitis suspected on imaging plus at least ≥1 axSpA feature *or*
    - HLA-B27–positive plus at least ≥2 axSpA features (as below):
      - axSpA features include arthritis, colitis, Crohn disease, dactylitis, elevated CRP, enthesitis, family history of axSpA, good response to nonsteroidal anti-inflammatory drugs (NSAIDs), positive HLA-B27, inflammatory back pain, psoriasis, or uveitis
- 1984 modified New York criteria for axSpA—must fulfill radiologic criteria and at least ≥1 clinical criteria.
  - Clinical criteria
    - Low back pain and stiffness >3 months that improves with exercises and not relieved by rest
    - Limitation of motion of lumbar spine in flexion and extension
    - Limitation of chest expansion relative to normal values correlated for age and sex
  - Radiologic criteria
    - Sacroiliitis at least grade 2 bilaterally or grade 3 to 4 unilaterally
  - If patients have negative radiographic imaging and negative HLA-B27 but two to three axSpA features, can consider MRI of SI joint

Follow-Up Tests & Special Considerations

- Routine monitoring of radiographic changes with serial spine radiographs is not recommended (2).
- If significant change in course of disease occurs, causes other than inflammation, such as spinal fracture, should be considered and appropriate evaluation should be performed.

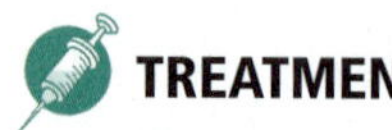

TREATMENT

GENERAL MEASURES

- Symptom control, maintaining spinal flexibility and normal posture, reducing functional limitations, maintaining work ability, and decreasing disease complications are primary treatment goals.
- Exercise, smoking cessation, and physical therapy are important components of nonpharmacologic management (1).

MEDICATION

First Line

- NSAIDs are first-line pharmacologic agent for pain and stiffness in AS.
  - Naproxen, up to 500 mg BID; celecoxib, up to 200 mg BID; ibuprofen, up to 800 mg TID
  - In adults with stable AS, when continuous use is not needed to control symptoms, conditionally recommend per American College of Rheumatology (ACR) on-demand treatment with NSAIDs.
    - The decision on continuous use of NSAIDs should be based more so on symptom control and not for control of structural disease progression (1).
- Precautions
  - Consider CVD, GI, and renal risks of NSAIDs. Use with caution in patients with a bleeding diathesis or on anticoagulants.
- Injection of intra-articular corticosteroids into SI joints can provide transient relief for patients with mainly peripheral symptoms (i.e., isolated sacroiliitis or enthesitis) with limited response to NSAIDs, but systemic corticosteroids are not recommended for patients with purely axial disease.

Second Line

- Recommended for active disease after lack of response to at least two different NSAIDs over 2 to 4 weeks and primarily axial disease (vs. mainly peripheral symptoms)
- Biologic agents: tumor necrosis factor inhibitors (TNFi), interleukin-17 inhibitors (IL-17i), and Janus kinase inhibitors (JAKi)
  - TNFi: infliximab, etanercept, adalimumab, certolizumab, golimumab
  - IL-17i—secukinumab, ixekizumab, bimekizumab
  - JAKi—tofacitinib
- In adults with active AS despite treatment with NSAIDs, recommend treatment with TNFi first and then treatment with secukinumab (IL-17i) or ixekizumab (IL-17i) over sulfasalazine, methotrexate, or tofacitinib (JAKi) (3).
  - If history of recurrent uveitis or active IBD: can use TNFi monoclonal antibody
  - If history of significant psoriasis: IL-17i preferred
- Precautions with TNFi
  - TNFi increase the risk of serious bacterial, mycobacterial, fungal, opportunistic, malignancies, and viral infections. Screen for tuberculosis and hepatitis B.
  - Immunizations (especially live vaccines) should be updated before initiating anti-TNFs; live vaccines are contraindicated once patients receive anti-TNFs.
- Disease-modifying antirheumatic drugs (DMARDs), such as methotrexate and sulfasalazine, are ineffective for axial disease; sulfasalazine may be effective for peripheral arthritis; this class may be considered in patients with contraindications to TNF agents (2).
- Recommendations for tapering if in remission or switching choices differ currently between ACR and ASAS-EULAR

ISSUES FOR REFERRAL

- Coordinate care with a rheumatologist for diagnosis, monitoring, and management (anti-TNF therapy).
- Management of extra-articular manifestations and other systemic conditions may require referral to appropriate specialty.

ADDITIONAL THERAPIES

Addressing psychological impact of axSpA via cognitive behavioral therapy may be beneficial in disease management.

SURGERY/OTHER PROCEDURES

- Evaluate for C-spine ankylosis/instability before intubation in patients with AS undergoing surgery.
- Consider total hip arthroplasty in patients with refractory pain or disability and radiographic evidence of structural damage, independent of age.
- Spinal corrective osteotomy can be considered in patients with severe disabling deformity although less evidence for this and recommendations differ (i.e., between ACR and ASAS-EULAR).

ONGOING CARE

FOLLOW-UP RECOMMENDATIONS

Patient Monitoring

- Monitor posture and range of motion with 6- to 12-month visits; increase frequency if higher disease activity.
- Bath Ankylosing Spondylitis Disease Activity Index (BASDAI) or Ankylosing Spondylitis Disease Activity Score (ASDAS) can be used to measure disease activity.
  - Some studies have considered the ASDAS to be a more appropriate scoring system for assessment of disease activity.
- Fall prevention/evaluation
- Regular-interval monitoring of CRP or ESR
- Screening for osteopenia/osteoporosis with dual energy x-ray absorptiometry scan

PATIENT EDUCATION

- Maintain physical activity and posture. Avoid trauma/contact sports.
- Swimming, water aerobics, tai chi, and walking are excellent activities.
- Arthritis Foundation: https://www.arthritis.org
- Spondylitis Association of America: https://www.spondylitis.org

PROGNOSIS

- Extent and rapidity of progression of condition are highly variable.
- Most patients will show a clinical response to treatment but sustained remission in only about 1/3 of the clinical practice. (3)

COMPLICATIONS

- MSK/spine: osteoporosis, spinal fusion causing kyphosis, C-spine fracture or subluxation, cauda equina syndrome (rare)
- Pulmonary: restrictive lung disease, upper lobe fibrosis (rare)
- Cardiac: conduction defects at atrioventricular (AV) node, aortic insufficiency, aortitis, pericarditis (extremely rare)
- Eye: uveitis, cataracts
- Renal: IgA nephropathy, amyloidosis (<1%)
- GI: microscopic, subclinical ileal, and colonic mucosal ulcerations in up to 50% of patients, mostly asymptomatic

REFERENCES

1. Ramiro S, Nikiphorou E, Sepriano A, et al. ASAS-EULAR recommendations for the management of axial spondyloarthritis: 2022 update. *Ann Rheum Dis*. 2023;82(1):19–34.
2. Ward MM, Deodhar A, Gensler LS, et al. 2019 Update of the American College of Rheumatology/Spondylitis Association of America/Spondyloarthritis Research and Treatment Network Recommendations for the treatment of ankylosing spondylitis and nonradiographic axial spondyloarthritis. *Arthritis Care Res (Hoboken)*. 2019;71(10):1285–1299. doi:10.1002/acr.24025.
3. Navarro-Compán V, Sepriano A, Capelusnik D, et al. Axial spondyloarthritis. *Lancet*. 2025;405(10473):159–172.

ADDITIONAL READING

- Mease PJ. Fibromyalgia, a missed comorbidity in spondyloarthritis: prevalence and impact on assessment and treatment. *Curr Opin Rheumatol*. 2017;29(4):304–310.
- Walsh JA, Magrey M. Clinical manifestations and diagnosis of axial spondyloarthritis. *J Clin Rheumatol*. 2021;27(8):e547–e560.

SEE ALSO

Arthritis, Psoriatic; Arthritis, Rheumatoid (RA); Reactive Arthritis (Reiter Syndrome)

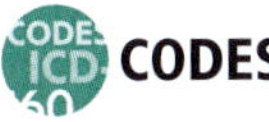

CODES

ICD10

- M45.0 Ankylosing spondylitis of multiple sites in spine
- M45.6 Ankylosing spondylitis lumbar region
- M45.7 Ankylosing spondylitis of lumbosacral region

CLINICAL PEARLS

- Diagnosis of AS is suggested by a history of inflammatory back pain, restricted spinal motion, radiographic evidence of sacroiliitis, and response to NSAIDs.
- HLA-B27 testing supports the diagnosis if clinical features are not definitive.
- MRI is more sensitive at detecting SI joint inflammation than plain radiography.
- Physical therapy is important in helping to maintain posture and mobility.
- NSAIDs and TNFi are the mainstays of pharmacologic treatment of AS.

ANOREXIA NERVOSA

Jennifer E. Cavin, MD

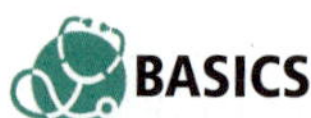

BASICS

DESCRIPTION

- An eating disorder characterized by the restriction of food intake leading to significantly low weight with intense fear of weight gain and distorted perception of body weight and shape
- *Diagnostic and Statistical Manual of Mental Disorders*, 5th edition (*DSM-5*) divides anorexia into two types:
  - Restricting type: characterized by restricting intake of calories or extreme amounts of exercise without binge-eating and purging behaviors within the last 3 months
  - Binge-eating/purging type: regular engagement in binge intake or purging behaviors (self-induced vomiting, misuse of laxatives, diuretics, or enemas) within the past 3 months
- System(s) affected: nervous, cardiovascular, endocrine, metabolic, pulmonary, gastrointestinal, reproductive, ophthalmic, taste, and dermatologic
- Severity of anorexia nervosa (AN) is based on BMI; severe is <16 kg/m^2.

EPIDEMIOLOGY

Prevalence

- Estimated lifetime prevalence among U.S. adults of 0.8%
- Median age of onset age: 17 years
- Predominant sex: female > male (10:1 to 20:1 female-to-male ratio)

ETIOLOGY AND PATHOPHYSIOLOGY

- Complex relationships among genetic, biologic, environmental, psychological, and social factors that result in the development of this disorder.
- Serotonin, norepinephrine, and dopamine neuronal systems are implicated.

Genetics

- Aggregates in families—11-fold risk amongst female relatives of a proband with the disorder
- Evidence of high concordance rates in monozygotic than in dizygotic twins
- GWAS study showing 8 loci exceeding genome wide significance on chromosomes 1, 3, 10, and 11.

RISK FACTORS

- Body dissatisfaction, negative self-evaluation
- Perfectionism, high parental demands, academic pressure, severe life stressors
- Personal history of other psychiatric disorders—including anxiety and obsessive compulsive disorder
- History of sexual or physical abuse or parental maltreatment
- Participation in sports or activities that emphasize leanness: ballet, figure skating, gymnastics, cheerleading
- Type 1 diabetes mellitus
- Family history of substance abuse, affective disorders, or eating disorders

GENERAL PREVENTION

Prevention programs for adolescents and young women ≥15 years of age can reduce risk factors and future onset of eating disorders.

- Encourage realistic and healthy weight management strategies and attitudes.
- Promote self-esteem; reduce focus on thin as ideal.
- Decrease co-occurring anxiety/depressive symptoms and improve stress management.

COMMONLY ASSOCIATED CONDITIONS

- Suicide, mood and anxiety disorders
- Substance use disorder
- Cluster C personality disorder

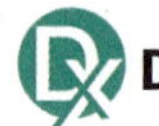

DIAGNOSIS

DSM-5 diagnosis of AN requires these three criteria:

- Restriction of energy intake that leads to a low body weight
- Intense fear of weight gain or becoming obese, or continuous behavior that prevents weight gain, despite being considered underweight
- Distorted perception of body weight, body shape, and undue influence of weight on self-worth, or denial of the medical seriousness of low body weight

HISTORY

- Onset may be insidious or stress related.
- Patient unlikely to self-identify problem
- Restriction of required energy intake, leading to significantly low body weight
- Fear of weight gain and/or distorted body image and preoccupation with body size (even of certain body parts and weight control)
- Elaborate food preparation and eating rituals.
- Other possible signs and symptoms:
  - Extensive exercise
  - Amenorrhea
  - Weakness, fatigue, cognitive impairment
  - Cold intolerance
  - Constipation, bloating, early satiety
  - Growth arrest, delayed puberty
  - Fractures
- Screening recommended by the USPSTF (SCOFF)
- Do you make yourself Sick because you feel uncomfortably full? (Yes is abnormal.)
- Do you worry you have lost Control over how much you eat? (Yes is abnormal.)
- Have you recently lost more than One stone (14 lb or 6.35 kg) in a 3-month period? (Yes is abnormal.)
- Do you believe yourself to be Fat when others say you are too thin? (Yes is abnormal.)
- Would you say that Food dominates your life? (Yes is abnormal.)

PHYSICAL EXAM

- May be normal
- Abnormal vital signs: hypothermia, bradycardia, orthostatic hypotension
- Body weight <85% of expected (may wear extra clothes or hide heavy objects to increase weight on scale)
- Cardiac: dysrhythmias, midsystolic click from mitral valve prolapse
- Skin/extremities: dry skin; lanugo hair on extremities, face, and trunk; hair loss; peripheral edema
- Neurologic and abdominal exams: to rule out other causes of weight loss and vomiting
- Gynecologic: amenorrhea

DIFFERENTIAL DIAGNOSIS

- Hyperthyroidism, adrenal insufficiency
- IBS, malabsorption
- Immunodeficiency, chronic infections
- Uncontrolled diabetes
- Bulimia, body dysmorphic disorder, restrictive eating disorder not otherwise specified
- Depressive, anxiety, or conversion disorders

DIAGNOSTIC TESTS & INTERPRETATION

Initial Tests (lab, imaging)

- Vitals: hypotension, bradycardia, hypothermia
- UA: low specific gravity, ketone, low urine creatinine excretion
- CBC: anemia, leukopenia, thrombocytopenia
- Low-serum LH, FSH; low-serum testosterone in men
- Thyroid function tests: low thyroid-stimulating hormone with normal T_3/T_4
- LFT: abnormal liver enzymes
- Chem 7: altered BUN, creatinine clearance; electrolyte disturbances including hyponatremia, hypokalemia
- Hypoglycemia, hypercholesterolemia, hypercortisolemia, hypophosphatemia, hypomagnesemia
- Low vitamin D and hypocalcemia
- 12-Lead EKG to assess for prolonged QT interval
- If underweight for >6 months: DEXA scan to assess for diminished bone density

Follow-Up Tests & Special Considerations

Weighting is an anxiety-provoking test but an important marker to assess progress. Ask staff to be nonjudgmental. Try to weight patients in a gown, as many intend to exaggerate their weight by hiding heavy objects or wearing baggy clothes.

Test Interpretation

- Osteoporosis/osteopenia, pathologic fractures
- Sick euthyroid syndrome, dehydration

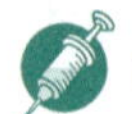

TREATMENT

GENERAL MEASURES

- OP treatment: for patients who are not medically unstable, are highly motivated, and able to control eating and exercising behaviors
  - Interdisciplinary team (primary care physician, mental health provider, dietitian)
  - Average weekly weight gain goal: 0.5 to 1.0 kg, with stepwise increase in calories
  - CBT, other forms of psychotherapy
  - Focus on health, not weight gain alone.
  - Build trust and a treatment alliance.
  - Involve the patient in establishing diet and exercise goals.
  - Help the patient to recognize feelings that lead to disordered eating.
  - In chronic cases, goal may be to achieve a safe weight rather than a healthy weight.

- Inpatient treatment if medically unstable, or with comorbid psychiatric issues, or unable to control eating and exercise behaviors
  - If possible, admit to a specialized eating disorders unit.
  - Monitor vital signs, electrolytes, cardiac function, edema, and weight.
  - Assess risk for refeeding syndrome—potentially fatal shift in fluid and electrolyte balance with restoration of nutrition characterized by hypophos phatemia, hypokalemia, seizures, CHF, rhabdomyolysis, peripheral edema
  - Initial supervised meals may be necessary.
  - Stepwise increase in activity
  - Tube feeding or TPN is used only as a last resort.
- CBT has demonstrated effectiveness as a means of improving treatment adherence and minimizing dropout among patients with AN.

MEDICATION

First Line

- No medications are available that effectively treat patients with AN, but pharmacotherapy may be used as an adjuvant to CBTs.
- If medications are used, start with low doses due to increased risk for adverse effects.
- SSRIs may:
  - Help to prevent relapse after weight gain.
  - Treat comorbid depression or OCD.
  - Use of atypical antipsychotics is being studied with generally positive findings to date. Specifically, olanzapine is potentially beneficial as an adjuvant treatment of underweight individuals in the inpatient settings.
- Attend to black box warnings.
- Bupropion should be avoided because it is associated with a higher incidence of seizures.

Second Line

- Management of osteopenia:
  - Primary treatment is weight gain.
  - Supplements—Elemental calcium 1,200 to 1,500 mg/day plus vitamin D 800 IU/day
  - No indication for bisphosphonates in AN
  - Weak evidence for use of hormone-replacement therapy
- Psyllium to prevent constipation

ISSUES FOR REFERRAL

Patients with AN benefit from an interdisciplinary team

ADMISSION, INPATIENT, AND NURSING CONSIDERATIONS

- Suggested physiologic values to admit: heart rate <40 beats/min, BP <90/60 mm Hg, symptomatic hypoglycemia, temperature <97°F (36.1°C), dehydration, other cardiovascular abnormalities, weight <75% of expected, rapid weight loss, lack of improvement while in OP therapy
- Suggested psychological indications: poor motivation/insight, lack of cooperation with OP treatment, inability to eat, need for nasogastric feeding, suicidal intent or plan, severe coexisting psychiatric disease, problematic family environment
- Suggested lab indications: potassium <3 mmol/L, prolonged QTC (>0.499 ms), urine specific gravity >1.03 or <1.01

Pediatric Considerations

- Children often present with nausea, abdominal pain, fullness, and inability to swallow.
- Additional indications for hospitalization: heart rate <50 beats/min, orthostatic BP, hypokalemia or hypophosphatemia, rapid weight loss even if weight not <75% below normal

Geriatric Considerations

- Late-onset AN (>50 years of age) may be a long-term disease or triggered by death of loved one, marital discord, divorce, or depression.
- Always consider other organic causes of weight loss.

ONGOING CARE

FOLLOW-UP RECOMMENDATIONS

- Family and individual therapy is extremely important for long-term outcomes.
- Emphasize importance of moderate activity for health.

Patient Monitoring

- Level of exercise activity
- Weigh weekly until stable, then monthly.
- Depression, suicidal ideation

DIET

Dietary consultation and nutritional education programs

PATIENT EDUCATION

- http://www.mayoclinic.org/diseases-conditions/anorexia/home/ovc-20179508
- National Alliance on Mental Illness: http://www.nami.org/Learn-More/Mental-Health-Conditions/Eating-Disorders

PROGNOSIS

- Prognosis: ~50% recover, 30% improve, 20% are chronically ill
- Mortality: 5–18% (annual mortality rate of 5 per 1,000 person-years)

ALERT

High risk of suicide (approximately 1 in 5 individuals with AN who died had committed suicide)

COMPLICATIONS

- Refeeding syndrome
- Cardiac arrhythmia, cardiac arrest, cardiomyopathy, congestive heart failure
- Delayed gastric emptying, necrotizing colitis
- Seizures, Wernicke encephalopathy, peripheral neuropathy, cognitive deficits
- Osteopenia, osteoporosis

Pregnancy Considerations

- Behaviors may persist, decrease, or recur during pregnancy and the postpartum interval.
- Increased risk for preterm labor, operative delivery, and infants with low birth weight; anemia, genitourinary infections, and labor induction should be managed as high risk.

ADDITIONAL READING

- Crone C, Fochtmann LJ, Attia E, et al. The American Psychiatric Association practice guideline for the treatment of patients with eating disorders. *Am J Psychiatry*. 2023;180(2):167–171. doi:10.1176/appi.ajp.23180001.
- Hoek HW, van Elburg AA. Feeding and eating disorders in the DSM-5 [in Dutch]. *Tijdschr Psychiatr*. 2014;56(3):187–191.
- Muratore AF, Attia E. Current therapeutic approaches to anorexia nervosa: state of the art. *Clin Ther*. 2021;43(1):85–94. doi:10.1016/j.clinthera.2020.11.006.
- Williams PM, Goodie J, Motsinger CD. Treating eating disorders in primary care. *Am Fam Physician*. 2008;77(2):187–195.

SEE ALSO

- Amenorrhea; Bulimia Nervosa; Osteoporosis and Osteopenia
- Algorithm: Weight Loss, Unintentional

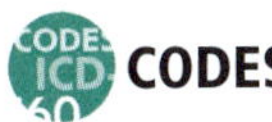

CODES

ICD10

- F50.01 Anorexia nervosa, restricting type
- F50.02 Anorexia nervosa, binge eating/purging type
- F50.00 Anorexia nervosa, unspecified

CLINICAL PEARLS

- "Are you satisfied with your eating patterns?" or "Do you worry that you have lost control over how you eat?" may help to screen those with an eating problem.
- Assess for suicide risk.
- To care for a patient with AN, an interdisciplinary team that includes a medical provider, a dietitian, and a behavioral health professional is the most accepted approach.

ANTIPHOSPHOLIPID ANTIBODY SYNDROME

Yara Shams, DO • Allison Isabelli, DO

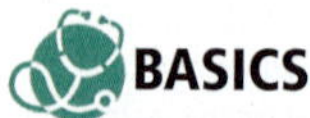

BASICS

DESCRIPTION

- Antiphospholipid syndrome (APS) is an autoimmune thrombophilic disorder characterized by recurrent arterial or venous thrombosis and/or recurrent fetal loss in the presence of antiphospholipid antibodies (APAs).
- The three most common antibodies include lupus anticoagulant (LAC), anticardiolipin antibodies (aCL), and/or anti–β_2 glycoprotein-I (GPI) antibody. The APAs enhance clot formation by binding phospholipid-binding plasma proteins. Thrombotic manifestations of the syndrome can cause morbidity and mortality.
- Classification of APS
  - Primary APS: primary autoimmune condition
  - Secondary APS: most commonly associated with autoimmune diseases, such as systemic lupus erythematosus (SLE), systemic sclerosis, Sjögren syndrome; transient APAs have been linked to certain infections, drugs, and malignancies.
- Classification based on clinical manifestations
  - Thrombotic APS
    - Characterized by recurrent venous (most common), arterial (e.g., cerebrovascular accidents [CVAs], myocardial infarction limb ischemia), or microvascular thromboembolism (e.g., pulmonary hemorrhage, livedoid vasculopathy, adrenal hemorrhage)
  - Obstetric APS
    - Complications include maternal venous thromboembolism (VTE), stroke, preeclampsia, and placental insufficiency. Fetal complications include fetal demise, fetal growth retardation, miscarriage, and preterm birth.
  - Catastrophic antiphospholipid syndrome (CAPS) a.k.a. Asherson syndrome (<1%)
    - Characterized by thrombotic microangiopathy resulting in multiorgan failure
    - High mortality if treatment is delayed

EPIDEMIOLOGY

Appears to be more common in females than males

Incidence

- Incidence of APS is around 1 to 2 individuals per 100,000 persons per year.
- In patients with positive APAs without prior risk of thrombosis, the annual incident risk of thrombosis is 0–3.8%. This risk is increased to 5.3% in those with triple positivity. 10–15% of recurrent first and second trimester fetal loss may be attributable to APS.

Prevalence

- Prevalence around 40 to 50 cases per 100,000 persons per year
- APAs are present in 1–5% of the general population and in ~40% of those with SLE. A higher prevalence of 10–15% is seen in those with VTE, fetal loss, and stroke.

ETIOLOGY AND PATHOPHYSIOLOGY

- Anti–β_2-GP1 antibodies play a central role in the pathogenesis of APS. The procoagulant effect is mediated by various possible mechanisms:
  - Endothelial effects: inhibition of prostacyclin production and disruption of annexin V (a protein with anticoagulant property)
  - Platelet activation resulting in adhesion and aggregation
  - Interference of innate anticoagulant pathways (such as inhibition of protein C)
  - Complement activation
- Pregnancy-related complications are also a result of autoantibody-mediated effects:
  - Interference with expression of trophoblastic adhesion molecules resulting in abnormal placentation and placental thrombosis
- Proposed mechanisms: excess production of natural antibodies, molecular mimicry due to infections, exposure of phospholipid antigens during platelet activation, cardiolipin peroxidation, and genetic predisposition
- A "second hit" by environmental factors is often required to manifest APS.

Genetics

Most cases of APS are acquired.

RISK FACTORS

- Cardiovascular risk factors: hypertension (HTN), hyperlipidemia, diabetes, obesity, smoking, combined oral contraceptive use
- Underlying autoimmune disease (SLE, rheumatoid arthritis, collagen vascular disease, Sjögren syndrome, idiopathic thrombocytopenic purpura, Behçet syndrome)
- APA positivity
- Surgery, immobilization, pregnancy

GENERAL PREVENTION

Risk factor modification:

- Control HTN and diabetes.
- Smoking cessation
- Avoidance of oral estrogen contraceptives in high-risk patients
- Start thromboprophylaxis in established cases
- Preconception assessment

COMMONLY ASSOCIATED CONDITIONS

- Autoimmune diseases: SLE (most common autoimmune condition associated with APS), scleroderma, Sjögren syndrome, dermatomyositis, and rheumatoid arthritis
- Malignancy
- Infections: viral (e.g., HIV, Hep C), bacterial, parasitic, and rickettsial
- Certain drugs associated with APA production without increased risk of thrombosis: phenothiazines, hydralazine, procainamide, and phenytoin
- Hemolysis, elevated liver enzymes, and low platelet count in association with pregnancy (HELLP) syndrome
- Sneddon syndrome (rare APS variant syndrome presenting with livedo reticularis and stroke)

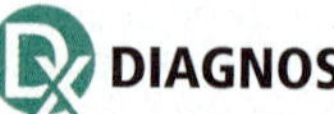

DIAGNOSIS

- Revised Sapporo criteria (Sydney criteria) was classically used.
  - At least one of the following clinical criteria:
    - Vascular thrombosis
      - ≥1 clinical episodes of arterial, venous, or small vessel thrombosis, confirmed by unequivocal imaging studies or histopathology without associated inflammation in the vessel wall
      - Superficial venous thrombosis does not meet the criteria for APS.
    - Complications of pregnancy (any one of the following):
      - ≥3 consecutive spontaneous abortions before the 10th week of pregnancy, unexplained by maternal/paternal chromosomal abnormalities or maternal anatomic/hormonal causes
      - ≥1 unexplained deaths of morphologically normal fetus (documented by ultrasonography or by direct examination) at ≥10th week of gestation
      - ≥1 premature births of morphologically normal newborn babies at ≤34th week of pregnancy due to severe preeclampsia, eclampsia, or placental insufficiency
  - *And* the presence of at least one of three laboratory findings (confirmed on ≥2 occasions at least 12 weeks apart):
    - LAC detected in blood
    - Anticardiolipin IgG and/or IgM antibodies present at moderate or high levels in the blood via a standardized ELISA
    - Anti–β_2-GP1 IgG and/or IgM antibodies in blood at a titer >99th percentile by standardized ELISA
- The new 2023 ACR/EULAR APS classification criteria—must fulfill entry criteria as well as 3 points from clinical criteria and >3 points from laboratory criteria
  - Entry criteria
    - At least one clinical criterion
    - Positive antiphospholipid antibody testing within 3 years of the clinical criterion
  - Six clinical criteria
    - Macrovascular VTE
    - Macrovascular arterial thromboembolism
    - Microvascular thrombosis
    - Obstetric complications
    - Cardiac valve: thickening or vegetation
    - Hematology: thrombocytopenia
  - Laboratory (aPL) criteria
    - LAC positivity
    - Anticardiolipin/Anti–β_2-GP1 positivity

HISTORY

- History of VTE or arterial thrombosis
- History of recurrent fetal loss or other obstetric complications
- Bleeding from thrombocytopenia if severe or acquired factor II deficiency
- Personal or family history of autoimmune disease
- Not all patients with APAs are symptomatic; these individuals are discovered incidentally, such as in cases of elevated PTT, autoimmune disease condition evaluation, or a false-positive rapid plasma reagin (RPR) test for syphilis.

PHYSICAL EXAM

- Signs of venous thrombosis
- Skin manifestations, including a vasculitic rash in the form of palpable purpura or livedo reticularis, superficial thrombophlebitis, or lower extremity ulcers
- Cardiac murmurs if valvular involvement
- Focal neurologic or cognitive deficits in setting of CVA/transient ischemic attack (TIA)

DIFFERENTIAL DIAGNOSIS

- Thrombophilic conditions
  - Inherited: deficiency of protein C, protein S, antithrombin III; mutation of factor V Leiden, prothrombin gene mutation
  - Acquired: neoplastic and myeloproliferative disorders, hyperviscosity syndromes, nephrotic syndrome
- Embolic disease secondary to atrial fibrillation, LV dysfunction, endocarditis, cholesterol emboli
- Disseminated intravascular coagulation
- Paroxysmal nocturnal hemoglobinuria
- Heparin-induced thrombocytopenia
- CAPS: hemolytic-uremic syndrome, TTP, or malignant HTN

DIAGNOSTIC TESTS & INTERPRETATION

- Diagnostic tests of choice—confirmed 12 weeks apart
  - LAC assay: combines at least two out of three screening tests (prolongation of aPTT, dilute Russell viper venom time [dRVVT], and kaolin clotting) with two confirmatory tests
  - IgG and IgM aCL by ELISA
  - Anti–β_2-GP1 IgG and IgM antibodies
- A weakly positive LAC result should be considered clinically important.
- Anti–β_2-GP1 antibodies are important in the pathogenesis of thrombosis. A positive LAC assay recognizes antibodies against β_2-GP1 and prothrombin.
- Tissue thromboplastin inhibition test
- Platelet neutralization procedure, mixing tests

Initial Tests (lab, imaging)

- CBC, PT/INR, aPTT, LAC, aCL, anti–β_2-GP1 antibodies
- Prevalence of APAs in SLE ranges from 11% to 87%; hence, it is important to screen for SLE.
- Imaging is based on clinical picture, suspected sites of thrombosis, and organ involvement.

Follow-Up Tests & Special Considerations

- The results of LAC are difficult to interpret in patients treated with warfarin. Unfractionated heparin or low-molecular-weight heparin (LMWH) and fondaparinux do not affect the LAC assay.
- Repeat testing at 12 weeks to assess for persistence of APAs.

Diagnostic Procedures/Other

Biopsy of the affected organ system may be necessary to distinguish from vasculitis.

Test Interpretation

Usual finding is thrombosis and minimal vascular or perivascular inflammation:

- Acute changes: capillary congestion and noninflammatory fibrin thrombi
- Chronic changes: ischemic hypoperfusion, atrophy, and fibrosis

TREATMENT

MEDICATION

First Line

- Primary thromboprophylaxis: controversial in patients with APS and no clinical symptoms. Low-dose aspirin or heparin can be considered in patients with a high risk of thrombosis.
- Secondary thromboprophylaxis: All symptomatic, nonpregnant patients with APS need indefinite anticoagulation. The target INR depends on the severity and type of thrombosis:
  - Venous thrombosis (first episode): warfarin with target INR of 2 to 3
  - Arterial thrombosis or recurrent venous thrombosis despite anticoagulation: consideration of warfarin with target INR 3 to 4 although there is a lack of consensus
  - LMWH and fondaparinux are alternatives.
- Direct oral anticoagulants (DOACs) have been approved for treatment of DVT/PE; however, studies in APS are lacking.
  - The 16th International Congress on Antiphospholipid Antibodies Task Force concluded that there is insufficient evidence to recommend DOACs in APS and recommend warfarin in most patients.
  - A 3-year, open-label, randomized noninferiority trial in 2019 did not show noninferiority of rivaroxaban to dose-adjusted VKAs for thrombotic APS and moreover showed a nonstatistically significant near doubling of the risk for recurrent thrombosis.
- Other therapies:
  - Danaparoid, fondaparinux, and argatroban can be considered in heparin-induced thrombocytopenia.
  - Statins can decrease proinflammatory and prothrombotic state in APS and may be considered as adjunctive therapy in refractory cases, although not recommended in those without hyperlipidemia or other indication for statins.
  - Recommended to replenish vitamin D in cases of vitamin D deficiency/insufficiency
  - Hydroxychloroquine can be added in recalcitrant APS.
  - Rituximab and eculizumab may have a role in refractory cases of APS.
- CAPS:
  - Anticoagulants and high-dose steroids may suffice in less severe cases. Aggressive treatment with either IVIG or plasma exchange is often required in severe cases. These measures have improved survival up to 66%. Rituximab or eculizumab may also have benefit in treatment of severe CAPS.
  - Treatment of precipitating factors is also crucial.
- Treatment in pregnancy:
  - Low-dose aspirin and LMWH or unfractionated heparin are the drugs of choice. There is no role for warfarin given potential teratogenicity.
    - Patients with APAs and no prior thrombotic events may be offered low-dose aspirin during pregnancy if deemed high risk; treatment decisions should be individualized though.
    - For women with no prior history of thrombosis and ≥3 early miscarriages, treat with either aspirin 81 mg alone or in combination with unfractionated subcutaneous heparin or LMWH (prophylactic dose).
    - In those with a previous late pregnancy loss (>10 weeks gestation) or preterm delivery (<34 weeks) due to severe preeclampsia, a combination of aspirin and heparin is recommended.
    - In those with a history of thrombosis, low-dose aspirin plus either therapeutic low-dose heparin or therapeutic LMWH is preferred.
    - Refractory cases: Up to 30% of patients have recurrent pregnancy loss despite the use of aspirin and heparin. Such cases are best managed in consultation with a maternal–fetal medicine specialist.
  - Prophylactic-dose heparin is recommended in the postpartum period (unless patient is on therapeutic anticoagulation) given high risk of thrombosis up to 6 weeks postpartum.
  - Preconception assessment and treatment with low-dose aspirin, vitamin D, and folate should be offered in selected patients.

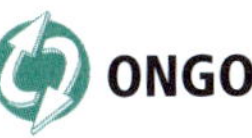

ONGOING CARE

DIET

Patients on warfarin should limit foods rich in vitamin K (kale, spinach, sprouts, greens).

PATIENT EDUCATION

- Compliance with warfarin therapy to keep INR at goal
- Awareness of drug and diet interactions with warfarin
- Avoid oral hormonal contraceptives.

PROGNOSIS

- Pulmonary HTN, neurologic involvement, myocardial ischemia, nephropathy, gangrene of extremities, and CAPS are associated with a worse prognosis.
- 30% risk of recurrent thrombosis in the absence of adequate anticoagulation

COMPLICATIONS

- Pregnancy complications and pulmonary HTN are associated with higher morbidity and mortality.
- Thrombotic complications are the most common cause of death.

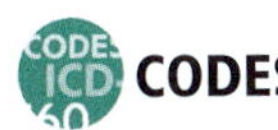

CODES

ICD10

- D68.61 Antiphospholipid syndrome
- D68.69 Other thrombophilia
- D68.62 Lupus anticoagulant syndrome

CLINICAL PEARLS

- APS is a multisystem autoimmune disorder with recurrent venous/arterial thrombosis and fetal loss and positive APAs.
- Both clinical and laboratory criteria are required for diagnosis. The latter must be confirmed on two separate occasions at least 12 weeks apart.
- APS requires lifelong anticoagulation.

ANXIETY (GENERALIZED ANXIETY DISORDER)

Rhonda A. Faulkner, PhD • Aneesh Tyle, MD

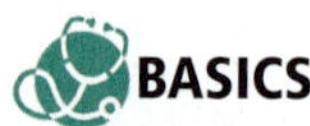

BASICS

DESCRIPTION

- Persistent, excessive, and difficult-to-control worry associated with significant symptoms of motor tension, autonomic hyperactivity, and/or disturbances of sleep or concentration
- System(s) affected: nervous (increased sympathetic tone and catecholamine release), cardiac (tachycardia), pulmonary (dyspnea), and GI (nausea, irregular bowels)

EPIDEMIOLOGY

Prevalence

- Lifetime prevalence in United States of America: 5.1–11.9%
- Onset at any age but typically during adulthood; median age of onset in the United States is 31 years.
- Female > male (2:1)

ETIOLOGY AND PATHOPHYSIOLOGY

- May be mediated by abnormalities of neurotransmitter systems (serotonin, norepinephrine, γ-aminobutyric acid [GABA])
- Associated with altered regional brain function (increased activity in the amygdala and prefrontal cortex)

Genetics

A serotonin transporter gene (*5HT1A*) may contribute to GAD.

RISK FACTORS

- Adverse life events (illness, poverty, etc)
- Family history
- Comorbid psychiatric disorders (1)

GENERAL PREVENTION

- Physical activity and cardiorespiratory fitness are associated with decreased generalized anxiety.
- Cognitive-behavioral therapy (CBT) and parental intervention in children with early anxiety may protect against GAD (1).

COMMONLY ASSOCIATED CONDITIONS

- Major depressive disorder (>60%), dysthymia, bipolar disorder, schizophrenia
- Alcohol/drug abuse; cigarette smoking
- Panic disorder, agoraphobia, phobia, social anxiety disorder, anorexia nervosa, PTSD, ADHD
- Somatoform and pain disorders

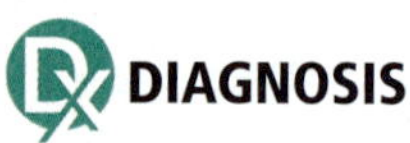

DIAGNOSIS

HISTORY

Diagnosis is primarily through history. Pathologic anxiety must be distinguished from normal anxiety reactions.

- *DSM-5* criteria are as follows:
  - Symptoms of excessive anxiety and worry occur more often than not for at least 6 months.
  - Difficult to control the worry
  - At least three additional criteria for diagnosis of GAD in adults; only one in children
    - Restlessness or feeling keyed up or on edge
    - Easily fatigued
    - Difficulty concentrating or mind going blank
    - Irritability
    - Muscle tension
    - Sleep disturbances (difficulty falling or staying asleep)
  - Persistent worry must cause significant distress or impairment in social, occupational, or other areas of functioning.
  - Focus of anxiety and worry is not consistent with or limited to the occurrence of other types of psychiatric disorders and is not directly related to PTSD.
  - Symptoms are not the result of a substance, another medical condition, or other *DSM-5* diagnosis.

PHYSICAL EXAM

No specific physical findings in GAD; patients may exhibit irritability, bitten nails, tremor, or clammy hands.

DIFFERENTIAL DIAGNOSIS

- Cardiovascular: ischemic heart disease, mitral valve prolapse, cardiomyopathies, arrhythmias, congestive heart failure
- Respiratory: asthma, chronic obstructive pulmonary disease, pulmonary embolism
- CNS: stroke, seizures, dementia, migraine, vestibular dysfunction, neoplasms
- Metabolic and hormonal: hyperthyroidism or hypothyroidism, pheochromocytoma, adrenal insufficiency, Cushing syndrome, hypokalemia, hypoglycemia, hyperparathyroidism
- Drug-induced anxiety: alcohol, sympathomimetics (cocaine, amphetamine, caffeine), corticosteroids, herbals (ginseng)
- Withdrawal: alcohol, sedative-hypnotics
- Psychiatric: panic disorder, OCD, PTSD, social phobia, adjustment disorder, and somatization disorder

DIAGNOSTIC TESTS & INTERPRETATION

Initial Tests (lab, imaging)

- Lab tests are normal. Initial tests may include TSH, CBC, BMP, urine drug screen, and ECG.
- GAD-2: two-question self-reporting scale (22% positive predictive value [PPV]/78% negative predictive value [NPV])
- PHQ-4 provides a very brief screen for both anxiety and depression (1).

Diagnostic Procedures/Other

Psychological testing

- GAD-7: provides more detailed information for treatment
- Hamilton Anxiety Scale (HAM-A), Anxiety Disorders Interview Schedule (ADIS-IV)
- Children: ADIS-IV Parent and Child Version, Multidimensional Anxiety Scale for Children (MASC), Screen for Child Anxiety Related Emotional Disorders (SCARED)

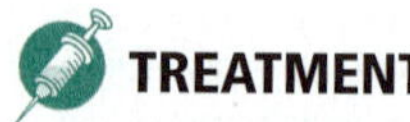

TREATMENT

GENERAL MEASURES

- Assess for suicidality.
- Identify and treat coexisting substance abuse and other psychiatric conditions.
- Delayed treatment may result in poorer outcomes compared with treatment within 1 year of symptom onset.
- Remission may not occur until 4 to 6 months of treatment. Treat for ≥12 months.
- Psychotherapeutic approaches
  - Psychological treatments are effective in treating GAD: number needed to treat (NNT) = 2 (2)[A].
  - CBT: most well-studied psychological treatment; may improve comorbid conditions; treatment of choice (1)[A]
  - Psychodynamic psychotherapy: patient discovering and verbalizing unconscious conflicts (1)[C]

MEDICATION

First Line

- SSRIs and SNRIs have demonstrated efficacy, are well-tolerated, do not cause abuse/dependence, and treat comorbid depression. Data to compare between agents are limited (3)[A].
- Medication selection based on side effect profile, drug–drug interactions, and/or patient treatment history/preference.
- For SSRIs/SNRIs, start at lowest available dose, uptitrate q2–4wk, use highest tolerated FDA-approved dose for at least 4 to 6 weeks before deeming ineffective or switching to a different SSRI/SNRI. Taper gradually to discontinue.
- Switching between medications without adequate dose or duration of therapy can lead to ineffective treatment.
- Common side effects of SSRIs: nausea, diarrhea, insomnia, agitation or sedation, drug interactions, weight gain, and sexual side effects (decreased libido, delayed orgasm)
- Common side effects of SNRIs: nausea, dizziness, insomnia, sedation, constipation, sweating, and blood pressure elevation
- SSRI: escitalopram (Lexapro): initially 10 mg/day; may titrate to a max of 20 mg/day (4)[A]
- SNRIs:
  - Duloxetine (Cymbalta): initially 30 mg/day; may titrate by 30 mg/day qwk to a max of 120 mg/day; doses >60 mg/day rarely more effective (4)[A]
  - Venlafaxine XR (Effexor XR): initially 37.5 to 75.0 mg; may titrate up by 75 mg q4d to a max of 225 mg/day (4)[A]
- Pregabalin (Lyrica): decreases anxiety scores and reduces relapse at 75 to 300 mg BID; less sexual dysfunction and sleep disruption than SSRIs; taper to discontinue; rapid onset of action (off-label) (4)[A]

Second Line

- Sertraline (Zoloft): initially 25 mg/day; may titrate by 25 to 50 mg/day qwk to a max of 200 mg/day (4)[B]
- Buspirone (BuSpar): less dependence risk; 15 mg/day divided BID–TID initially; max of 60 mg/day divided BID–TID (4)[B]
- Fluoxetine (Prozac): 10 to 20 mg/day; may titrate up to 60 mg/day (off-label) (4)[B]

- Mirtazapine (Remeron): 15 mg nightly; titrate in increments of 15 mg qwk; max dose 45 mg daily; use as monotherapy or adjunct to SSRI; most common side effect is drowsiness (off-label) (4)[B].
- Paroxetine (Paxil): initially 10 to 20 mg/day; may titrate by 10 mg/day qwk to a max of 50 mg/day (no added benefit >20 mg/day); efficacious but poorly tolerated (4)[A]
- Quetiapine (Seroquel): optimal dose 150 mg/day; efficacious but less well tolerated than SSRIs; consider as augmentation (4)[A].
- Citalopram (Celexa) likely has efficacy for GAD but does not have FDA indication.
- Fluvoxamine (Luvox): start at 50 mg/day, also treats OCD
- Gabapentin: Start 300 mg/daily; can titrate up to 2,400 mg/day (split TID); rapid onset; taper to discontinue; similar to pregabalin
- Benzodiazepines: efficacious in the short term, less effective long term, risk for dependence/abuse (3),(4)[A]
  - Clonazepam (Klonopin): 0.25 mg BID; may increase to 4 mg/day divided BID
  - Diazepam (Valium): 2 to 5 mg BID–QID; may increase to max of 40 mg/day
  - Lorazepam (Ativan): 0.5 mg BID–TID; may increase to 6 mg/day divided TID
  - Alprazolam (Xanax): 0.25 mg TID; may increase to 4 mg/day
- Hydroxyzine (Vistaril, Atarax): CNS depressant, antihistamine, anticholinergic; decreased risk of dependence: usual dose: 50 to 100 mg PO QID; limit use in the elderly (2)[B].
- Newer SRIs (SSRI + 5HT agonists): Vilazodone (Viibryd), Vortioxetine (Trintellix)—approved for MDD, studies ongoing for GAD; less sexual side effect than traditional SSRIs

Geriatric Considerations

- SSRIs/SNRIs still first line
- Avoid TCAs and long-acting benzodiazepines; monitor for dizziness, somnolence with pregabalin, gabapentin

Pediatric Considerations

- CBT is first-line treatment for mild to moderate GAD.
- CBT with SSRI is first-line treatment for severe GAD.
- Black box warning (SSRIs): Antidepressants increase the risk of suicidal thinking and behavior in children, adolescents, and young adults (5).
- SSRIs and SNRIs have all been shown to be effective, with SSRIs as the first-line choice (sertraline, escitalopram, fluoxetine)
- Anxiety and ADHD often co-occur. Treat the more debilitating first, and consider using nonstimulating medications.

Pregnancy Considerations

- Buspirone: Category B, secreted in breast milk; inadequate studies to assess risk
- Benzodiazepines: Category D, may cause lethargy and weight loss in nursing infants; avoid breastfeeding if the mother is taking chronically or in high doses. Use shortly before delivery is associated with floppy infant syndrome.
  - Prenatal exposure to diazepam increases absolute risk of oral cleft by 0.01% (6).
- SSRIs: If possible, taper and discontinue. After 20 weeks' gestation, there is increased risk of pulmonary hypertension; mild transient neonatal syndrome of CNS; and motor, respiratory, and GI signs. Studies regarding risk of autism show mixed results. Most are Category C, except for:
  - Paroxetine: Category D, conflicting evidence regarding risk of congenital cardiac defects and other congenital anomalies in 1st trimester, fetal echocardiography should be performed in mothers with 1st trimester exposure.
  - Hydroxyzine: Category C, case reports of neonatal withdrawal

ALERT

- Benzodiazepines: age >65 years, respiratory disease/sleep apnea, contraindicated with narrow-angle glaucoma, precaution with open-angle glaucoma; sudden discontinuation increases seizure risk. Long-term use has potential for tolerance and dependence; use with caution in patients with history of substance abuse.
- Buspirone: hepatic and/or renal dysfunction; monoamine oxidase inhibitor (MAOI) treatment
- SSRIs: Use caution in those with comorbid bipolar disorder; may increase risk of serotonin syndrome, especially in combination with other serotonergic drugs

COMPLEMENTARY & ALTERNATIVE MEDICINE

- Probable benefit but more study needed for acupuncture, yoga, massage, tai chi, and aromatherapy (7)[B]
- Mindfulness-based stress reduction is noninferior to escitalopram in treating anxiety (3).
- Kava: some evidence for benefit in mild to moderate anxiety, but concern regarding potential hepatotoxicity (7)[B]
- Strong evidence to support regular physical activity (7)[A]
- Possible benefit from repetitive transcranial magnetic stimulation for pharmacotherapy treatment refractory patients
- Cannabidiol may have beneficial role in the treatment of anxiety-related disorders and COVID-19 disease-related anxiety; more longitudinal studies are needed.
- Psilocybin with behavioral intervention may have a substantial additive benefit.

ONGOING CARE

FOLLOW-UP RECOMMENDATIONS

Patient Monitoring

- Follow up within 2 to 4 weeks from starting new medications.
- Medications should be continued past the initial period of response and recommend continued treatment for 12 months.
- Monitor all patients for suicidal ideation, especially those on SSRIs and SNRIs.
- Clinical follow-up with patient every q6mo is recommended.

DIET

Limit caffeine; avoid alcohol and nicotine.

PATIENT EDUCATION

- Regular exercise may be beneficial.
- Psychoeducation regarding normal versus pathologic anxiety and the physiology of anxiety can be helpful.

PROGNOSIS

Probability of recovery is 40–60%, but comorbid psychiatric disorders and poor relationships with family make relapse more likely.

REFERENCES

1. Patel G, Fancher TL. In the clinic. Generalized anxiety disorder. *Ann Intern Med*. 2013;159(11):ITC6-1–ITC6-12.
2. Cuijpers P, Sijbrandij M, Koole S, et al. Psychological treatment of generalized anxiety disorder: a meta-analysis. *Clin Psychol Rev*. 2014;34(2):130–140.
3. Huh J, Goebert D, Takeshita J, et al. Treatment of generalized anxiety disorder: a comprehensive review of the literature for psychopharmacologic alternatives to newer antidepressants and benzodiazepines. *Prim Care Companion CNS Disord*. 2011;13(2):PCC.08r00709.
4. Slee A, Nazareth I, Bondarpnek P, et al. Pharmacological treatments for generalised anxiety disorder: a systemic review and network meta-analysis. *Lancet*. 2019;393(10173):768–777.
5. O'Leary KB, Khan JS. Pharmacotherapy for anxiety disorders. *Psychiatr Clin North Am*. 2024;47(4):689–709. doi:10.1016/j.psc.2024.04.012.
6. Armstrong C. ACOG guidelines on psychiatric medication use during pregnancy and lactation. American Family Physician. https://www.aafp.org/pubs/afp/issues/2008/0915/p772.html. Accessed September 9, 2025.
7. Sarris J, Moylan S, Camfield DA, et al. Complementary medicine, exercise, meditation, diet, and lifestyle modification for anxiety disorders: a review of current evidence. *Evid Based Complement Alternat Med*. 2012;2012:809653.

SEE ALSO

Algorithms: Anxiety; Depressive Episode, Major

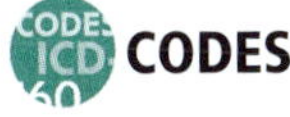

CODES

ICD10

F41.1 Generalized anxiety disorder

CLINICAL PEARLS

- Psychiatric comorbidities, especially depression, are common with GAD; patients are at increased risk for suicidality.
- CBT and SSRIs/SNRIs are the treatments of choice.
- Start medication at low doses, with careful titration to therapeutic dosing, to minimize side effects and maximize efficacy.
- Benzodiazepines may be used initially but should be tapered and withdrawn if possible.

AORTIC VALVULAR STENOSIS

Grant Wei, MD, FACEP • Chirag N. Shah, MD • Sidhant Gugale, MD, MPH

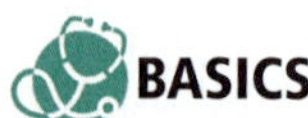

BASICS

DESCRIPTION

- Aortic stenosis (AS) is a narrowing of the aortic valve (AV) area from leaflet fibrosis or calcification, leading to obstruction of the left ventricular (LV) outflow tract.
- AS has a long asymptomatic latency period.
- Development of severe obstruction, syncope, angina, and symptoms of congestive heart failure (CHF) have high mortality without surgical intervention.

EPIDEMIOLOGY

- AS is the most common acquired valve disease leading to operative intervention in Europe and North America (1).
- Cause by age at presentation: <30 years, congenital; typically presents as bicuspid or unicuspid valve; 30 to 65 years, congenital or rheumatic fever (RF); >65 years, degenerative calcification of AV

Prevalence

- Affects 1% of population aged 65 to 74 years, 2% of aged 75 to 84 years, 4% of aged >84 years
- Bicuspid aortic valve present in 1–2% of population predisposes to AS at an earlier age.

ETIOLOGY AND PATHOPHYSIOLOGY

- An increase in LV systolic pressure is required to preserve cardiac output leading to concentric LV hypertrophy (LVH), preserving ejection fraction but adversely affecting heart function. LVH impairs coronary blood flow during diastole by compressing coronary arteries and reducing capillary ingrowth into hypertrophied muscle.
  - LVH results in diastolic dysfunction by reducing ventricular compliance. Diastolic dysfunction necessitates stronger left atrial (LA) contraction to augment preload and maintain stroke volume. Loss of LA contraction by atrial fibrillation can induce acute deterioration.
- Diastolic dysfunction may persist after AS interventions due to interstitial fibrosis.
- Degenerative calcific changes to the AV caused by endothelial dysfunction and lipid deposition, followed by an inflammatory response, fibrosis, and calcification.
- Congenital: unicuspid valve, bicuspid valve, tricuspid valve with fusion of commissures, hypoplastic annulus

Genetics

Bicuspid aortic valves display genetic variants leading to accelerated calcification in AS.

RISK FACTORS

- Congenital unicommissural valve or bicuspid valve
- RF—zost cases are associated with mitral valve disease.
- Degenerative calcific changes
  - Most common cause of acquired AS in the US. Risk factors include hypercholesteremia, hypertension, cigarette smoking, male gender, age, diabetes mellitus, and arterial hypertension.

GENERAL PREVENTION

Optimal management of hypertension, cardiac comorbid conditions, and smoking cessation; angiotensin-converting enzyme (ACE) and ARB inhibitors decrease LV fibrosis.

COMMONLY ASSOCIATED CONDITIONS

- Coronary artery disease (CAD) (50% of patients); hypertension (40% of patients)
- Aortic insufficiency (common in calcified bicuspid valves and rheumatic disease)
- Mitral valve disease: 95% of patients with AS from RF also have mitral valve disease.
- LV dysfunction and CHF
- Acquired von Willebrand disease: Impaired platelet function and decreased von Willebrand factor results in bleeding in 20% of AS patients. Severity of coagulopathy is directly related to severity of AS.
- Gastrointestinal arteriovenous malformations (AVMs)
- Cerebral or systemic embolic events due to calcium emboli.

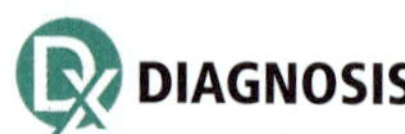

DIAGNOSIS

HISTORY

- Primary symptoms: angina (most common), syncope (often exertional), and heart failure.
- Palpitations
- Neurologic events (transient ischemic attack or cerebrovascular accident) secondary to embolization
- Geriatric patients may have subtle symptoms (fatigue and exertional dyspnea).
- Symptoms do not always correlate with valve area (severity of AS) but most commonly occur when AV area is <1 cm^2, jet velocity is >4 m/s, or the mean transvalvular gradient is ≥40 mm Hg.

PHYSICAL EXAM

Auscultation

- Harsh, systolic crescendo–decrescendo murmur is best heard at 2nd intercostal space on the right sternal border and radiates into the carotid arteries. Peak of murmur correlates with severity of stenosis; later peaking murmur suggests greater severity.
- High-pitched blowing diastolic murmur suggests associated aortic insufficiency.
- Paradoxically split S_2 or absent A_2. Normally split S_2 reliably excludes severe AS.
- S_4 due to stiffening of the left ventricle

DIFFERENTIAL DIAGNOSIS

- Mitral regurgitation: High-frequency, pansystolic murmur, best heard at the apex, often radiates to the axilla.
- Hypertrophic obstructive cardiomyopathy: also systolic crescendo–decrescendo murmur but best heard at left sternal border and may radiate into axilla. Murmur intensity increases by changing from squatting to standing and/or by Valsalva maneuver.
- Discrete fixed subaortic stenosis: 50–65% has associated cardiac deformity (patent ductus arteriosus [PDA], ventricular septal defect [VSD], aortic coarctation).
- Aortic supravalvular stenosis: Williams syndrome, homozygous familial hypercholesterolemia.

DIAGNOSTIC TESTS & INTERPRETATION

Initial Tests (lab, imaging)

- Chest X-ray (CXR)
  - May be normal in compensated, isolated valvular AS; boot-shaped heart reflective of concentric hypertrophy; poststenotic dilatation of ascending aorta, and/or calcification of aortic valve
- ECG: often normal, nondiagnostic ECG. May show LVH, LA enlargement, and nonspecific ST- and T-wave abnormalities.
- Echo indications
  - Initial workup
    - Transthoracic echocardiogram (TTE): primary test in the diagnosis and evaluation of AS (1)[C]; assesses valve anatomy, severity of disease; LV wall thickness, size, function; and pulmonary artery pressure
  - Based on AS severity, asymptomatic patients should have repeated TTE.
    - Mild: every 3 to 5 years, moderate: 1 to 2 years, and severe: 6 to 12 months
- Echo findings
  - Aortic valve thickening, calcification; decreased aortic valve excursion; reduced AV area; transvalvular gradient across aortic valve; LVH and diastolic dysfunction; LV ejection fraction altered; wall-motion abnormalities suggesting CAD; evaluate for concomitant aortic insufficiency or mitral valve disease.

Diagnostic Procedures/Other

- Exercise stress testing
  - Asymptomatic patients with severe AS: helpful to uncover subtle symptoms or changes, abnormal BP (increase <20 mm Hg), and ECG changes (ST depressions). 1/3 of patients develop symptoms with exercise testing; *stop* testing at this point.
  - Symptomatic patients: *do not* perform exercise stress testing as it may induce hypotension or ventricular tachycardia.
  - CHF patients: Dobutamine stress echocardiography is reasonable to evaluate patients with low-flow/low-gradient AS and LV dysfunction.
- Cardiac catheterization
  - Perform prior to aortic valve replacement (AVR) in patients with suspected CAD; determines need for coronary artery bypass graft (CABG)
- CT calcium scoring
  - Patient with low-flow, low-gradient AS with preserved EF
  - Calcium score >1,200 AU for women and >2,000 AU for men help predict severity AS and clinical outcomes.

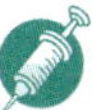

TREATMENT

MEDICATION

- No effective medical therapy for severe or symptomatic AS
- Currently, more research into the pro-inflammatory cytokines, clotting factors, and proteins involved in promoting calcification in AS are potential novel targets for medications
  - PCSK9 inhibitors, simvastatin/ezetimibe combination, and medications lowering lipoprotein A are promising therapeutics to prevent mild AS from worsening.
- Prevention: currently no recommended medical therapy; statins have been thought to slow progression if initiated during mild disease. However, this has not been supported by large, randomized controlled trials.
- Antibiotic prophylaxis against recurrent RF is indicated for patients with rheumatic AS (penicillin G 1,200,000 U IM q4wk; duration varies with age and history of carditis).
- Antibiotic prophylaxis is no longer indicated for prevention of infective endocarditis.
- Comorbidities: hypertension: ACE inhibitors. Be cautious of vasodilators, which may cause hypotension.

SURGERY/OTHER PROCEDURES

- AVR is recommended for most symptomatic patients with evidence of significant AS on echocardiography. If the AV area is >1.5 cm^2 and the gradient is <15 mm Hg, there is no benefit from AVR.
- Transcatheter aortic valve replacement (TAVR) versus surgical aortic valve replacement (SAVR) has shown no difference in all-cause mortality in 1 year in severe, asymptomatic aortic stenosis in ages ≥70 years with moderately increased operative risk. (2)[A]
- In patients ≥65 years with severe, symptomatic AVS, TAVR was noninferior to SAVR when looking at all-cause mortality or stroke in one year (2)[A]. TAVR is less likely to cause major or life-threatening bleeds than SAVR.
- Indications for AVR surgery
  - Symptomatic and severe high-gradient AS by history or exercise testing when surgical risk is low or intermediate
  - Asymptomatic, severe AS, and LVEF <50%
  - Severe AS when undergoing other cardiac surgery
- AVR surgery is reasonable in patients who are asymptomatic with severe AS with low surgical risk, decreased exercise tolerance, or have an exercise fall in blood pressure.
- TAVR offers a less invasive option for some patients (1)[C]
  - For those who are at high surgical risk and considered inoperable, TAVR has been shown to be superior to medical therapy.
  - For those who are at high surgical risk, TAVR has demonstrated noninferiority to surgical AVR.
  - For those who are at low or intermediate surgical risk, TAVR now a reasonable alternative to surgical AVR
  - Valve-in-valve TAVR can be considered in high-risk patients with failed surgically implanted bioprosthetic valves.
- Percutaneous balloon valvuloplasty may have role in palliation or as a bridge to valve replacement in hemodynamically unstable or high-risk patients but is not recommended as an alternative to valve replacement as the improvements in hemodynamics are transient.
- Many types of replacement valves exist:
  - Mechanical prosthetic valves experience minimal structural degeneration even after 25 years; however, they require anticoagulation with warfarin with INR of 2.0 to 3.0.
  - Stented biologic valves are made from bovine AVs or valves created from bovine pericardium mounted on a stent frame.
  - Stentless biologic valves improve on the hemodynamics of the stented biologics by removing the metal cages, but are more operatively challenging to implant.
  - Homografts are rarely used (except in cases of endocarditis) due to higher rates of structural valvular degeneration.
  - The Ross procedure functionally transfers the patient's pulmonic root to the aortic position.
  - TAVR procedures use balloon-expandable valves or self-expanding valves.

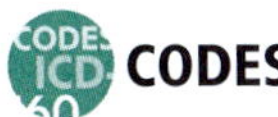

ONGOING CARE

FOLLOW-UP RECOMMENDATIONS

Report symptoms referable to AS (angina, syncope). Asymptomatic patients: yearly history and physical; serial ECHO: yearly for severe AS, every 1 to 2 years for moderate AS, every 3 to 5 years for mild AS

PATIENT EDUCATION

Physical activity limitations

- Asymptomatic mild AS: no restrictions; asymptomatic moderate to severe AS: Avoid strenuous exercise. Consider exercise stress test prior to starting exercise program.

PROGNOSIS

- Although survival in asymptomatic patients is comparable to that in age- and sex-matched control patients, it decreases rapidly after symptoms appear.
- 25% mortality per year in symptomatic patients who do not undergo valve replacement; average survival is 2 to 3 years without AVR surgery; median survival in symptomatic AS: heart failure: 2 years; syncope: 3 years; angina: 5 years
- Perisurgical mortality: AVR surgery has 4% mortality rate; AVR + CABG has 6.8% mortality rate; adverse postoperative prognostic factors: age, heart failure New York Heart Association (NYHA) class III/IV, cerebrovascular disease, renal dysfunction, CAD.

REFERENCES

1. Baumgartner H, Falk V, Bax JJ, et al; for ESC Scientific Document Group. 2017 ESC/EACTS guidelines for the management of valvular heart disease. *Eur Heart J*. 2017;38(36):2739–2791.
2. Blankenberg S, Seiffert M, Vonthein R, et al; for DEDICATE-DZHK6 Trial Investigators. Transcatheter or surgical treatment of aortic-valve stenosis. *N Engl J Med*. 2024;390(17):1572–1583.

CODES

ICD10

- I35.0 Nonrheumatic aortic (valve) stenosis
- I06.0 Rheumatic aortic stenosis
- Q23.0 Congenital stenosis of aortic valve

CLINICAL PEARLS

- AS is diagnosed on physical exam by a systolic crescendo–decrescendo murmur and delayed/diminished pulses.
- Symptomatic AS most commonly presents as angina, syncope, and heart failure.
- Symptomatic AS has a very poor prognosis unless treated with surgical intervention.

APPENDICITIS, ACUTE

Grant Wei, MD, FACEP • Rohail Khan, MD • Chirag N. Shah, MD

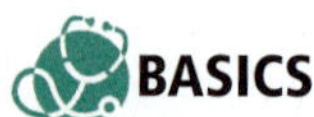

BASICS

DESCRIPTION

- Acute inflammation of the appendix
- Simple or uncomplicated appendicitis occurs when there is no clinical or radiologic sign of perforation. Complicated or perforated appendicitis is defined by a palpable mass and phlegmon, perforation, or abscess on imaging.
- Arising from the base of the cecum in right lower quadrant (RLQ), the appendix can be anterior, posterior, medial, or lateral to the cecum as well as in the pelvis. Vascular supply provided by appendicular artery, a branch of the ileocolic artery; nerve supply derived from the superior mesenteric plexus
- Most common cause of acute surgical abdomen worldwide

EPIDEMIOLOGY

- Predominant age: 10 to 30 years; rare in infancy; although uncommon, can be more challenging to diagnose in elderly
- Predominant sex: slight male predominance
  - Ages 10 to 30 years: male > female (3:2)
  - Peak incidence in 2nd and 3rd decade of life
  - Age >30 years: men = women

Incidence

- 1 case per 1,000 people per year
- Lifetime incidence 1 in every 15 people (7–8%)

Pregnancy Considerations

- Most common extrauterine surgical emergency
- Incidence similar in pregnancy
- Higher rate of perforation; more likely to present with peritonitis

ETIOLOGY AND PATHOPHYSIOLOGY

Obstruction of the appendiceal lumen is thought to lead to distention, ischemia, and bacterial overgrowth. Without intervention, appendicitis can lead to perforation and subsequent abscess formation or generalized peritonitis. Causes of obstruction:

- Fecaliths (most common)
- Lymphoid tissue hyperplasia (in children)
- Vegetables, fruit seeds, and other foreign bodies
- Intestinal worms (ascarids)
- Strictures, fibrosis, neoplasms

Genetics

First-degree relative with history of appendicitis increases risk; no direct genetic link found.

RISK FACTORS

Male adolescents, familial tendency, intra-abdominal tumors

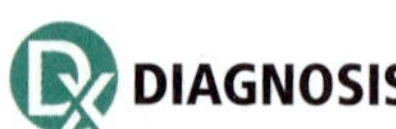

DIAGNOSIS

- Diagnosis relies on history and physical examination with supporting laboratory studies and imaging.
- Multiple scoring systems are available to quantify a clinician's gestalt for acute appendicitis. Traditionally, the modified Alvarado scoring system (sensitivity 89%, specificity 71%) has been used, but currently, the Raja Isteri Pengiran Anak Saleha Appendicitis (RIPASA) scoring system appears to be more effective (sensitivity 96%, specificity 86%) (1)[A].
- RIPASA scoring system
  - Patient demographics
    - Sex: men (1 point), women (0.5 point)
    - Age: <40 years (1 point), >40 years (0.5 point)
  - Symptoms
    - Right iliac fossa pain (0.5 point)
    - Migration of pain to RLQ (0.5 point)
    - Anorexia (1 point)
    - Nausea and vomiting (1 point)
    - Duration of symptoms: <48 hours (1 point), >48 hours (0.5 point)
  - Signs
    - Right iliac fossa tenderness (1 point)
    - Right iliac fossa guarding (2 points)
    - Rebound tenderness (1 point)
    - Rovsing sign (2 points)
    - Fever >37°C (2 points)
  - Investigations
    - Elevated WBCs (1 point)
    - Negative urinalysis (1 point)
  - Additional criterion: not a Singapore national (1 point)
    - Because it was developed in Singapore, which has many foreign nationals, the "foreign national registration identity card" was included in the score as it was found to have some predictive capacity. This is harder to apply to other populations.
- RIPASA score >7.5 is very accurate for the diagnosis of acute appendicitis.
- Pediatric appendicitis score—helps predict the likelihood of acute appendicitis (diagnosis is still clinical).

HISTORY

- Classic history is vague periumbilical pain, followed by anorexia, nausea, and vomiting. Over the next 4 to 48 hours, pain migrates to the RLQ.
- Only 50% of patients present with a classic history.
- Pain before vomiting (~100% sensitive), abdominal pain (~100%), pain migration (50%)
- Anorexia (~100%), nausea (90%), vomiting (75%), obstipation
- Atypical symptoms and pain suggest a retrocecal or pelvic appendix.

PHYSICAL EXAM

- Fever; temperature >100.4°F (may be absent); tachycardia
- RLQ tenderness; maximal tenderness at McBurney point (1/3 the distance from the anterior superior iliac spine to the umbilicus)
- Voluntary and involuntary guarding
- Rovsing sign: RLQ pain with palpation of left lower quadrant
- Psoas sign: pain with right thigh extension (retrocecal appendix)
- Obturator sign: pain with internal rotation of flexed right thigh (pelvic appendix); local and suprapubic pain on rectal exam (pelvic appendix)
- Pelvic and rectal exams are helpful to assess other causes of lower abdominal pain (e.g., pelvic inflammatory disease, prostatitis).
- Serial exams can be useful in indeterminate cases.

DIFFERENTIAL DIAGNOSIS

- GI
  - Gastroenteritis, inflammatory bowel disease
  - Diverticulitis, ileitis
  - Cholecystitis, pancreatitis
  - Intussusception, volvulus
- Gynecologic
  - Pelvic inflammatory disease, ectopic pregnancy
  - Ovarian cyst, ovarian torsion, tubo-ovarian abscess
  - Endometriosis
  - Ruptured graafian follicle
- Urologic
  - Testicular torsion, epididymitis
  - Kidney stones, prostatitis, cystitis, pyelonephritis
- Systemic: Diabetic ketoacidosis, Henoch-Schönlein purpura, sickle cell crisis, porphyria
- Other
  - Acute mesenteric lymphadenitis
  - No organic pathologic condition
  - Hernias
  - Psoas abscess
  - Rectus sheath hematoma
  - Epiploic appendagitis
  - Pneumonia (basilar)

Pediatric Considerations

- Decreased diagnostic accuracy of history and physical exam
- Higher fever; more vomiting and diarrhea

Pregnancy Considerations

- Appendicitis is more difficult to diagnose in pregnancy.
- Normal inflammatory response is suppressed.
- Appendix displaced out of pelvis by gravid uterus

Geriatric Considerations

Decreased diagnostic accuracy, more likely to be an atypical presentation

DIAGNOSTIC TESTS & INTERPRETATION

Initial Tests (lab, imaging)

- Leukocytosis: WBC >10,000/mm^3 (70%)
- Polymorphonuclear predominance—"left shift" (>90%)
- Urinalysis: hematuria, pyuria (30%)
- Human chorionic gonadotropin (hCG) (If positive, rule out ectopic pregnancy.)
- C-reactive protein: nonspecific inflammatory marker; when paired with an elevated WBC, increases predictive value for appendicitis
- Drugs may alter lab results: antibiotics, steroids
- Imaging if the diagnosis is not clear; helps to detect complications (abscess, perforation)
- Plain films: minimal utility, nonspecific findings, may visualize fecalith
- CT scan with contrast: sensitivity 91–98%; specificity 95–99%; imaging modality of choice; consider radiation dose, particularly in young patients.
- Ultrasound: alternative in pregnancy, children, and women with suspected gynecologic pathology; sensitivity and specificity vary with skill of the ultrasonographer. Increasing use in adult populations, with positive predictive value approaching 100% in some studies; can rule in appendicitis but cannot reliably exclude the diagnosis; an effective strategy is to start with ultrasound and, if negative, obtain a CT scan if suspicion warrants.

- MRI: increasing use in pregnant patients; may help in patients with contrast allergies and renal failure; limitations include cost, availability, and time required to complete study.
- Radioisotope-labeled WBC scans: may be used in patients with indeterminate CT scans and suspected appendicitis as an alternative to observation or surgery; limitations include availability and time required to complete the study.

Diagnostic Procedures/Other

- Exploratory laparotomy/laparoscopy
- Acceptable appendectomy rates vary based on age and gender and may be higher for females of childbearing age than males.

Test Interpretation

- Acute appendiceal inflammation, local vascular congestion, obstruction
- Gangrene, perforation with abscess (15–30%)
- Fecalith

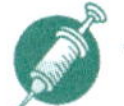

TREATMENT

GENERAL MEASURES

- Surgery (appendectomy) has been the standard of care for acute, uncomplicated appendicitis. Evidence suggests nonoperative management with antibiotics may be noninferior to appendectomy after 30 days, but carries a 29% rate of recurrence with need for appendectomy within 90 days. Surgical treatment of uncomplicated appendicitis has a higher complication-free success rate (82%) than that of antibiotic treatment alone (67%) in both adult and pediatric patients.
- Generally, surgery is indicated for complicated or perforated appendicitis with abscess formation. For larger drainable abscesses, percutaneous drainage, and antibiotics are recommended.
- Studies suggest that antibiotic treatment in adults with imaging confirmed acute appendicitis is a safe alternative to surgery and results in 2/3 of patients avoiding appendicectomy during the first year (2)[A].

MEDICATION

First Line

- Uncomplicated acute appendicitis: perioperative dose of antibiotic: single dose of cefoxitin or ampicillin/sulbactam (Unasyn) or cefazolin plus metronidazole
- Nonoperative antibiotic of choice: intravenous ertapenem for 2 days followed by 5 days PO levofloxacin and metronidazole (3)[B]
- Gangrenous or perforating appendicitis
  - Broadened antibiotic coverage for aerobic and anaerobic enteric pathogens
  - Piperacillin and tazobactam (Zosyn) or ticarcillin and clavulanate (Timentin) or a 3rd-generation cephalosporin plus metronidazole are initial options.
  - Adjust dosage and choice of antibiotic based on intraoperative cultures.
  - Continue antibiotics for at least 7 days postoperatively or until patient becomes afebrile with normal WBC count.

Second Line

- Uncomplicated acute appendicitis: clindamycin plus one of the following: ciprofloxacin, levofloxacin, gentamicin, or aztreonam
- In the case of acute appendicitis complicated by abscess formation or phlegmon in pediatric patients, some studies show initial conservative management with antibiotics alone to carry fewer risks and complications than emergent appendectomy.
- Gangrenous or perforated appendicitis: ciprofloxacin or levofloxacin plus metronidazole or monotherapy with a carbapenem (imipenem and cilastatin, meropenem, ertapenem)

ISSUES FOR REFERRAL

All cases of appendicitis require emergent surgical consultation.

ADDITIONAL THERAPIES

A newer option for the treatment of acute appendicitis is currently being studied—endoscopic retrograde appendicitis therapy (ERAT). Studies thus far indicate high technical and clinical success rates (>99%), with very low rates of complication (0.19%) and a much lower recurrence rate (6.01%) than treatment with antibiotics only.

SURGERY/OTHER PROCEDURES

- The American College of Surgeons, Society for Surgery of the Alimentary Tract, and others recommend surgery as the treatment of choice.
- Antibiotic treatment might be used as an alternative in specific patients or if surgery is contraindicated.
- Nonoperative management with antibiotics with up to a reported 39% recurrence rate at 5 years for uncomplicated acute appendicitis

ADMISSION, INPATIENT, AND NURSING CONSIDERATIONS

- Admit all patients with appendicitis.
- Fluid resuscitation with normal saline (NS) or lactated Ringer (LR) solution
- Correct fluid and electrolyte deficits.
- Discharge when tolerating oral intake, return of bowel function, afebrile, normal WBC

ONGOING CARE

FOLLOW-UP RECOMMENDATIONS

- Return to work in 1 to 2 weeks is typical following most cases of uncomplicated appendicitis.
- Restrict activity for 4 to 6 weeks after surgery: no heavy lifting (>10 lb) or strenuous physical activity.
- If managed nonoperatively and patient is >40 years, consider colonoscopy to rule out malignancy.

PATIENT EDUCATION

Postoperative warning signs:

- Anorexia, nausea, vomiting
- Abdominal pain, fever, chills
- Signs/symptoms of wound infection

PROGNOSIS

- Generally uncomplicated course in young adults with unruptured appendicitis
- Extremes of age and appendiceal rupture increase morbidity and mortality.
- Morbidity rates
  - Nonperforated appendicitis: 3%
  - Perforated appendicitis: 47%
- Mortality rates
  - Unruptured appendicitis: 0.1%
  - Ruptured appendicitis: 3%
  - Patients >60 years of age make up 50% of total deaths from appendicitis.
  - Older patients with ruptured appendix: 15%

Pediatric Considerations

- Rupture earlier
- Rupture rate: 15–60%

Pregnancy Considerations

- Rupture rate: 40%
- Fetal mortality rate: 2–8.5%

Geriatric Considerations

Rupture rate: 67–90%

COMPLICATIONS

- Intestinal fistulas
- Intestinal obstruction, paralytic ileus, incisional hernia
- Liver abscess (rare), pylephlebitis
- Stump appendicitis: recurrence of appendicitis at appendiceal stump after appendectomy

REFERENCES

1. Alvarez-Lozada LA, Fernandez-Reyes BA, Arrambide-Garza FJ, et al. Clinical scores for acute appendicitis in adults: a systematic review and meta-analysis of diagnostic accuracy studies. *Am J Surg*. 2025;240:116123.
2. Scheijmans JCG, Haijanen J, Flum DR, et al. Antibiotic treatment versus appendicectomy for acute appendicitis in adults: an individual patient data meta-analysis. *Lancet Gastroenterol Hepatol*. 2025;10(3):222–233.
3. Dahiya DS, Akram H, Goyal A, et al. Controversies and future directions in management of acute appendicitis: an updated comprehensive review. *J Clin Med*. 2024;13(11):3034.

SEE ALSO

Algorithm: Abdominal Rigidity

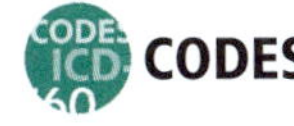

CODES

ICD10

- K35.80 Unspecified acute appendicitis
- K35.2 Acute appendicitis with generalized peritonitis
- K35.3 Acute appendicitis with localized peritonitis

CLINICAL PEARLS

- Anorexia with periumbilical pain localizing to RLQ is the classic history for acute appendicitis.
- Diagnosis is more challenging in children, pregnant patients, and the elderly due to varying symptoms and signs.
- In equivocal cases, CT scan is the diagnostic test of choice. Ultrasound and MRI are alternatives.
- Acute appendicitis is the most common surgical emergency during pregnancy.

APPROACH TO TRAVEL MEDICINE COUNSELING

Sukhjeet K. Kamboj, MD • Jasmine Kaur Sandhu, MD

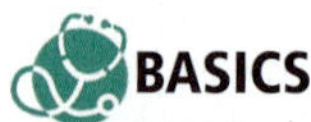

BASICS

DESCRIPTION

A pretravel consultation is recommended to assess health risks based on destination(s), duration of travel, planned activities, health status, medical history, and vaccination history.

EPIDEMIOLOGY

Incidence

In 2024, global travel rebounded to near prepandemic levels, with an estimated 1.4 billion international arrival. Travel-related incidents range from infectious diseases to injuries.

Prevalence

20–70% of travelers from the United States returning from international trips report some kind of illness during or after travel (1). Gastrointestinal illness is the most common, followed by dengue and malaria.

RISK FACTORS

Risks vary by destination, length of the trip, planned activities, age, and health status of the traveler.

- Traveler details
  - Past medical history (age, gender, medical conditions, allergies, current medications)
    - Flying is contraindicated within 2 weeks of an uncomplicated myocardial infarction and within 10 days of thoracic or abdominal surgery (2).
      - Flying is often discouraged after the 36th week of pregnancy, and most cruise lines restrict travel after 24th week of pregnancy.
  - Immunization history
- Trip details
  - Itinerary (countries/specific regions, rural or urban; side trips); timing (length, season, time until departure; reason for travel; special activities (disaster relief, medical care, high altitude or climbing, diving, cruise ship, rafting, cycling, extreme sports)
  - Counselling should include about limitations of treatment of the complications occurred due to procedures/surgeries or medications received during the overseas medical tourism trip.

GENERAL PREVENTION

- Routine vaccinations
  - *Haemophilus influenzae* type b
  - Hepatitis A
  - Hepatitis B
  - Influenza
  - Measles, mumps, rubella—more common in countries without routine childhood immunization
  - Meningococcal—or sub-Saharan Africa especially during the dry season (December through June); Saudi Arabia requires the quadrivalent vaccine for Hajj pilgrims (3).
  - Pneumococcal
  - Polio—wild poliovirus type 1 circulates currently in Afghanistan and Pakistan (3).
  - Rotavirus—recommended for children
  - TdaP
  - Varicella; zoster
  - Human papillomavirus (HPV)—sexual activity during travel may lead to HPV infection.
- Travel-specific vaccinations (destination dependent)
  - Japanese encephalitis—most of Asia and parts of Western Pacific; two-dose series; must be given at least 1 week prior to travel
  - Rabies—if immunoglobulin is difficult to obtain, consider vaccination to simplify postexposure prophylaxis.
  - Tick-borne encephalitis (not available in United States) is endemic in European and Asian countries.
  - Typhoid—highest risk in India, Pakistan, and Bangladesh. Avoid giving to pregnant women, immunocompromised patients, or if antibiotics taken in the previous 72 hours (3). Oral vaccine available for 6 years and older at least 1 week prior to travel. Injectable vaccine available for 2 years and older given at least 2 weeks prior to travel.
  - Yellow fever—highest risk in sub-Saharan Africa and the Amazon regions of South America (3). Approved for ages 9 months or older as a single dose 10 days before travel.
  - Cholera—recommended if traveling to areas of active transmission of cholera. Oral vaccine is available and approved for age 2 years onward as a single dose that can be administered 10 days prior to travel (3).
- Malaria prophylaxis
  - Based on destination, types of planned activities, and patient preferences; CDC has up-to-date recommendations.
  - Chloroquine-sensitive malaria (3),(4); most of these have to be given 1 to 2 weeks prior to travel and continue for 4 weeks after leaving the malaria endemic area.
    - Chloroquine—in the dose of 300-mg base (500-mg salt) orally once weekly for adults. Pediatric dose is 5 mg/kg base (8.3 mg/kg salt) orally once weekly (up to 300-mg base per dose).
    - Hydroxychloroquine—adult dose: 310-mg base (400-mg salt) orally once weekly; pediatric dose: 5 mg/kg base (6.5 mg/kg salt) orally once weekly (up to 310 mg base per dose)
  - Chloroquine-resistant malaria (3),(4)
- Atovaquone/proguanil (Malarone)—begin 1 to 2 days before travel and continue for 1 week after leaving malaria-endemic area.
  - Adult dose: 250 mg/100 mg atovaquone/proguanil PO daily; pediatric dose: tablets contain 62.5 mg/25 mg atovaquone/proguanil hydrochloride; 5 to 8 kg: 1/2 pediatric tablet daily; >8 to 10 kg: 3/4 pediatric tablet; >10 to 20 kg: 1 pediatric tablet daily; >20 to 30 kg: 2 pediatric tablets daily; >30 to 40 kg: 3 pediatric tablets daily; >40 kg: 1 adult tablet daily; contraindications: pregnant women, breastfeeding (child less than 5 kg) and individuals with severe renal impairment
- Doxycycline—begin 1 to 2 days before travel and continue for 4 weeks after leaving malaria-endemic area; adult dose: 100 mg orally daily; pediatric dose: ≥8 years old 2.2 mg/kg up to adult dose of 100 mg daily; contraindications: pregnant women and children <8 years old
- Mefloquine—begin 1 to 2 weeks before travel and continue for 4 weeks after leaving malaria-endemic area; not recommended for people with cardiac conduction abnormalities (especially ventricular arrhythmias), major psychiatric disorders, or seizures
  - Adult dose: 228-mg base (250-mg salt) orally once weekly; pediatric dose: ≤9 kg: 4.6 mg/kg base (5 mg/kg salt) orally once weekly; 10 to 19 kg: 1/4 tablet once weekly; 20 to 30 kg: 1/2 tablet once weekly; 31 to 45 kg: 3/4 tablet once weekly; >45 kg: 1 tablet once weekly
- Tafenoquine—begin 200 mg daily for 3 days prior to travel, weekly during travel, and continue for 1 week after leaving malaria-endemic area.
  - Contraindication: pregnant women, children, individuals with glucose-6-phosphate dehydrogenase (G6PD) deficiency or unknown status of G6PD deficiency, and with psychotic disorders
- Primaquine: Begin 1 to 2 days before travel and continue for 7 days after leaving malaria-endemic area.
  - Adult dose: 30-mg base (52.6-mg salt) daily; pediatric dose: 0.5 mg/kg base (0.8 mg/kg salt) up to adult dose daily
  - Contraindications: pregnant women and people with G6PD deficiency or unknown status of G6PD deficiency
- Protection against mosquitoes and ticks
  - Avoid peak exposure times dusk, dawn and daylight for different species.
  - Appropriate clothing; minimize exposed skin; check for ticks; Use bed netting
  - Insecticides and repellants—reapply regularly
- Zika virus
  - Transmitted via mosquito bite (Aedes species) or via sexual intercourse
  - Most infections are asymptomatic. Pregnant women should avoid travel to any area with risk of Zika virus transmission. If planning a pregnancy, consider waiting 2 to 3 months after travel to a Zika-endemic area before conceiving.
- SARS-coronavirus-2 (COVID-19)
  - COVID-19 primary series and boosters as recommended
- Mpox
  - Recent rise in Mpox cases; transmitted via contaminated fomites, skin lesions, or body fluids from an infected person; symptoms include flu-like symptoms followed by a rash (vesiculopustular) and may have umbilication; vaccine available; recommended for travelers to countries experiencing outbreaks (e.g., Burundi, Kenya, Rwanda, Tanzania, Uganda, and Zambia) at least 6 weeks prior to travel; postexposure prophylaxis (PEP) for those exposed to Mpox

- Traveler's diarrhea
  - Symptoms range from mild abdominal cramping, loose stools to severe abdominal pain, fever, vomiting, and bloody diarrhea. Nausea and vomiting may both be present, although usually resolve within 12 to 24 hours; approximately 75–90% bacterial, 10–25% viral, 10% protozoal (2)
  - High-risk areas include Asia, Middle East, Africa, Mexico, and Central and South America (3).
  - Intermediate-risk areas include countries in Eastern Europe, South Africa, and some Caribbean islands (3).
  - Strategies to minimize diarrhea (3)
    - Wash hands or use sanitizer containing >60% alcohol prior to eating. Avoid raw or undercooked meat, fish, or shellfish, salads, uncooked vegetables, unpasteurized fruit juices, or unpasteurized milk or milk products. Avoid unpeeled raw fruit. Only drink beverages that are sealed, boiled, chlorinated, or otherwise confirmed to be safe and purified.
    - Prophylaxis for high-risk patients
    - Bismuth subsalicylate reduces incidence of travelers' diarrhea by 50%; 2 oz of liquid or two chewable tablets QID (not recommended for children <3 years or pregnant women). Note the darkening of stool as a side effect (3).
  - Treatment based on severity of disease (3)
    - Mild—no medication necessary
    - Moderate—Antibiotics such as fluoroquinolones, azithromycin, or rifaximin. Loperamide can be used as a monotherapy.
    - Severe—incapacitating diarrhea. Azithromycin 1 g if symptoms not resolved in 24 hours and then continue daily dosing for 3 days. Alternate dosing is 500 mg daily for 3 days. Ciprofloxacin 750 mg single dose as alternative. If symptoms do not resolve, continue for 3 days.
  - Adjunct medications
    - Loperamide—4 mg initially followed by 2 mg after each loose stool (max 16 mg/day); not recommended for children <6 years old; 6 to 8 years—2 mg initial dose, followed by 1 mg after each loose stool (max 4 mg/day); 9 to 11 years—2 mg after initial dose, followed by 1 mg after each loose stool (max 6 mg/day)
    - Diphenoxylate: 5 mg (2 tablets) TID or QID until control achieved (max 20 mg/day); pediatric dose: not recommended for children <2 years; children over 2: 0.3 to 0.4 mg/kg/day in 4 divided doses
- Altitude illness
  - More likely at an altitude of 8,000 feet (2,500 m) or higher; elevation at destination, rate of ascent, and exertion impact risk (3)
  - Acute mountain sickness (AMS)—generally presents with headache 2 to 12 hours after arrival; other symptoms include fatigue, loss of appetite, nausea, and vomiting; usually resolves within 24 to 48 hours of acclimatization (3)
  - High-altitude cerebral edema (HACE)—lethargy, drowsiness, confusion, ataxia; requires immediate descent (3)
  - High-altitude pulmonary edema (HAPE)—symptoms include shortness of breath, weakness, and cough; requires supplemental oxygen and immediate descent
  - Preventive measures/medications:
    - Ascend gradually. Avoid alcohol.
    - Acetazolamide—AMS/HACE prevention dose: 125 mg BID (250 mg BID if >100 kg); pediatric dose: 2.5 mg/kg q12h. AMS treatment dose: 250 mg BID; pediatric dose: 2.5 mg/kg q12h; used as an adjunct to dexamethasone (3)
    - Dexamethasone—usually reserved for treatment; prevention dose: 2 mg q6h or 4 mg q12h; should not be used for prophylaxis in pediatric patients. AMS treatment dose: 4 mg q6h PO, IV, or IM. HACE treatment dose: 8 mg once and then 4 mg q6h PO, IV, or IM; pediatric dose: 0.15 mg/kg/dose q6h up to 4 mg
      - Nifedipine—for prevention and treatment of HAPE; dose: 30 mg SR q12h (3)
      - Tadalafil—for prevention of HAPE only; dose: 10 mg BID (3)
      - Sildenafil—for HAPE prevention; dose: 50 mg q8h (3)
- Jet lag
  - Before travel, adjust sleep cycle (and possibly meal times) 1 to 2 hours earlier or later (depending on direction of travel) for several days prior to departure. Drink plenty of water to remain hydrated. Avoid caffeine and alcohol. Short-term sedative hypnotics (nonbenzodiazepine), such as zolpidem, can help if not otherwise contraindicated and used sparingly. If using benzodiazepines, use short-acting agents, such as temazepam.
- Motion sickness
  - Prevention—avoid known triggers, strategic positioning (front of car, over wing of aircraft). Scopolamine patch can behind ear at least 4 hours prior to exposure and every 3 days as needed. Avoid use in children.
  - Dimenhydrinate 1.0 to 1.5 mg/kg 1 hour before travel and every 6 hours during the trip as needed for symptom management
- Environmental hazards
  - Avoid walking barefoot and swimming in freshwater where there is a risk for schistosomiasis or leptospirosis.
  - Use sunscreen.
- If scuba diving, avoid flying or altitude exposure >2,000 feet (3).
  - ≥12 hours after surfacing from nondecompression dive; ≥18 hours after repetitive dives or multiple days of diving; 24 to 28 hours after a dive that required decompression stops
- Other considerations
  - Consider travel insurance.

REFERENCES

1. Center for Disease Control and Prevention. *CDC Yellow Book 2026*. https://www.cdc.gov/yellow-book/hcp/contents/index.html. Accessed May 18, 2025.
2. Potin M, Carron PN, Genton B. Injuries and medical emergencies among international travelers. *J Travel Med*. 2024;31(1):taad088. doi:10.1093/jtm/taad088.
3. Center for Disease Control and Prevention (CDC). *CDC Yellow Book 2024: Health Information for International Travel*. Oxford University Press; 2023.
4. Rupert J, Groh T, Allen R. The pretravel consultation. *Am Fam Physician*. 2025;111(3):245–253.

ADDITIONAL READING

- Centers for Disease Control and Prevention. Travelers' health. https://www.cdc.gov/travel Accessed September 9, 2025.
- UN Tourism World Tourism Barometer. Global Tourism Statistics. https://www.unwto.org/un-tourism-world-tourism-barometer-data. Accessed September 9, 2025.

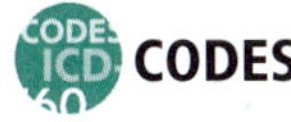

CODES

ICD10

- Z71.9 Counseling, unspecified
- Z71.89 Other specified counseling

CLINICAL PEARLS

- The CDC Travelers' Health website is useful for destination-specific travel advice (https://wwwnc.cdc.gov/travel/).
- Pre-Travel Provider Rapid Evaluation portal (Pre-Travel PREP) (https://gten.travel/prep/prep) and Heading Home Healthy (https://www.headinghomehealthy.org/) are other resources to help travelers stay healthy and safe.
- Patients should seek advice several weeks prior to anticipated travel.

ARTERITIS, TEMPORAL

Irfan H. Siddiqui, MD • Janet A. Omole, MD • Toluwanimi V. Oludiran-Ayoade, MD, BSc

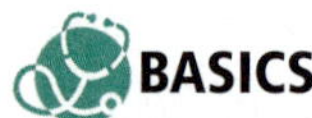

BASICS

DESCRIPTION

- Also known as giant cell arteritis (GCA), Horton disease, and cranial arteritis
- Temporal arteritis is a chronic inflammatory disease involving large- and medium-sized arteries, most commonly cranial arteries originating from aortic arch. Inflammation of the aorta is observed in 50% of cases.
- New headache is a common presenting symptom and occurs in more than 2/3 of patients. Other symptoms include jaw claudication, vision loss, fatigue, fever, weight loss, symptoms of polymyalgia rheumatica (PMR), and aortic arch syndrome (decreased or absent peripheral pulses, discrepancies of blood pressure, arterial bruits). Onset of symptoms is usually subacute; however, acute presentations can also occur.
- Considered medical emergency due to risk of irreversible vision loss if not treated due to arteritic anterior ischemic optic neuropathy, central or branch artery occlusion, posterior ischemic optic neuropathy, or rarely cerebral ischemia.

EPIDEMIOLOGY

- Most common form of systemic vasculitis affecting persons ≥50 years old
- 80% of cases occur ages 70 to 80 years.
- Women are affected approximately 3 times more than men in persons of Northern European descent.
- Most common vasculitis in individuals of Northern European descent

Incidence

- Incidence varies by ethnicity; in the United States, approximately 1% in women and 0.5% in men
- Prevalence in Northern Europeans is 2 per 1,000 persons.
- Peaks in patients 70 to 80 years old, >80% of patients

ETIOLOGY AND PATHOPHYSIOLOGY

- The exact etiology of GCA remains unknown, although current theory suggests that advanced age, ethnicity, and specific genetic predisposition lead to a maladaptive response to endothelial injury, intimal hyperplasia, and ultimately vascular stenosis.
- GCA is a chronic, systemic vasculitis primarily affecting the elastic lamina of medium- and large-sized arteries. Histopathology of affected arteries is marked by transmural inflammation of the intima, media, and adventitia, as well as patchy infiltration by lymphocytes, macrophages, and multinucleated giant cells. Mural hyperplasia can result in arterial luminal narrowing, resulting in subsequent distal ischemia.
- Current theory regarding the etiology of GCA is that a maladaptive response to endothelial injury leads to an inappropriate activation of T-cell–mediated immunity via immature antigen-presenting cells. The subsequent release of cytokines within the arterial vessel wall can attract macrophages and multinucleated giant cells, which form granulomatous infiltrates and give diseased vessels their characteristic histology. This also leads to an oligoclonal expansion of T-cells directed against antigens in or near the elastic lamina. Ultimately, this cascade results in vessel wall damage, intimal hyperplasia, and eventual stenotic occlusion.
- In recent years, GCA and PMR have increasingly been considered to be closely related conditions.
- Varicella zoster virus has been proposed as possible immune trigger for GCA; however, this has not been substantiated, and adjunctive treatment with antivirals remains controversial.

Genetics

The gene for *HLA-DRB1*04, HLA-DQA1,* and *HLA DQB1* have been identified as risk factors for GCA, and polymorphisms of *ICAM-1* and *PTPN-22* have also been implicated.

RISK FACTORS

- Increasing age (>70 years) is the greatest risk factor
- Females
- Genetic predisposition—occasional family clustering has been reported.
- Environmental factors influence susceptibility.
- History of smoking
- Early menopause (<43 years) and lower BMI at menopause in women 50 to 69 years old

COMMONLY ASSOCIATED CONDITIONS

Population studies have shown 40–60% of patients diagnosed with GCA also have PMR symptoms, and 16–21% of patients with PMR have GCA.

DIAGNOSIS

HISTORY

- Most common presenting symptom is headache (2/3 of patients).
- Constitutional symptoms (fever, fatigue, weight loss)
- Any visual disturbances (amaurosis fugax, diplopia)
- Vision loss (20% of patients); unilateral is most common, often proceeds to bilateral if untreated
- Jaw claudication (Presence of symptom significantly increases likelihood of a positive biopsy.)
- Scalp tenderness or sensitivity
- Claudication of upper extremities or tongue
- Symptoms of PMR (shoulder and hip girdle pain and stiffness)
- Distal extremity swelling/edema
- Upper respiratory symptoms

PHYSICAL EXAM

- Temporal artery abnormalities (beading, prominence, tenderness)
- Typically, appear "ill"
- Decreased peripheral pulses in the presence of large vessel diseases
- Funduscopic exam shows pale and edema of the optic disc, scattered cotton wool patches, and small hemorrhages.
- Unlike other forms of vasculitis, GCA rarely involves the skin, kidneys, and lungs.
- Supraclavicular, axillary, and supraorbital bruits

DIFFERENTIAL DIAGNOSIS

- Migraines
- Herpes zoster
- Other vasculitis (Takayasu arteritis, Wegner, PAN)
- Other rheumatologic condition (RA, PMR, MCTD)
- Primary angiitis of the central nervous system
- Idiopathic aortitis
- VEXAS syndrome
- Nonarteritic anterior ischemic optic neuropathy
- Infection (such as endocarditis, tertiary syphilis, HIV, herpes zoster, hepatitis B and C)

DIAGNOSTIC TESTS & INTERPRETATION

- American College of Rheumatology 1990 classification criteria are as follows:
  - Age >50 years
  - New localized headache
  - Temporal artery abnormality (tenderness to palpation, decreased or absent pulses)
  - ESR >50 mm/hr
  - Abnormal temporal artery biopsy showing vasculitis with predominance of mononuclear cell infiltration or granulomatous inflammation
- Three or more of the American College of Rheumatology criteria demonstrate a sensitivity of 94.5% and a specificity of 91.2%.

Initial Tests (lab, imaging)

- ESR >50 mm/hr (86% sensitivity), although nonspecific (27%); infrequently, may be normal
- C-reactive protein (CRP) >2.45 mg/dL is a more sensitive marker of inflammation (97% sensitivity) and is associated with increased odds of a positive biopsy result.
- Although a normal ESR and/or CRP renders the diagnosis of GCA unlikely; 4% of patients with GCA have both ESR and CRP in normal range.
- Acute-phase reactants (fibrinogen, interleukin-6) are frequently elevated but very nonspecific and reserved for diagnostically difficult cases.
- Mild anemia: very nonspecific but may be associated with a lower rate of ischemic complications
- Color Doppler US of the temporal artery may identify vascular occlusion, stenosis, or edema ("halo sign"); it is low cost and noninvasive but also very operator dependent and does not significantly improve on the clinical exam. It may aid in the diagnosis of larger vessel involvement.
- Atherosclerotic disease with carotid intima-media thickness >0.9 mm may mimic halo sign.
- MRI and MRA may be beneficial in diagnosis (78% sensitive, 90% specific) if performed within 5 days of steroids.
- Positron emission tomography (PET), like MRI/MRA and color Doppler, may be useful in diagnostically difficult cases to quantify the inflammatory burden and early in the course of disease, as the metabolic changes occur prior to structural vascular damage, but it also lacks studies to support its use.

Follow-Up Tests & Special Considerations

- Development of aortic aneurysms (late and potentially serious complication of GCA) can lead to aortic dissection.
- Due to the risk of irreversible vision loss, treatment with high-dose steroids should be started on strong clinical suspicion of GCA, prior to the temporal biopsy being done.

Diagnostic Procedures/Other

- Gold standard diagnostic study: histopathologic examination of the temporal artery biopsy specimen (Do not delay starting medication if suspicion as pathology remains up to 14 days after starting steroids.)
- The temporal artery is chosen because of its accessibility in the systemic disease; alternatively, facial artery or other cranial arteries may be used.
- Length of biopsy specimen should be at least 7 to 10 mm to avoid false-negative results because skip lesions may occur.
- Diagnostic yield of biopsy may be increased if procedure is coupled with imaging (high-resolution MRI or color Doppler US).
- Bilateral temporal artery biopsy should not be performed, unless the initial histopathology is negative and the suspicion for GCA remains high.
- May be negative in up to 42% of patients with GCA, especially in large vessel disease, and a negative biopsy alone should not dictate treatment
- Biopsy results are not affected by prior glucocorticoids; so treatment should not be delayed.

Test Interpretation

- Inflammation of the arterial wall, with fragmentation and disruption of the internal elastic lamina
- Multinucleated giant cells are found in <50% of cases and are not specific for the disease.
- GCA occurs in three histologic patterns: classic, atypical, and healed.

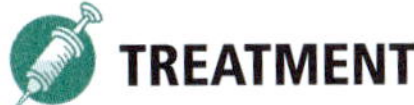

TREATMENT

MEDICATION

First Line

Glucocorticoids:

- The typical dose of prednisone is between 60 and 80 mg/day (or 1 mg/kg/day), and the dose may be titrated up to relieve symptoms. Steroids should not be in the form of alternate day therapy because this is more likely to lead to a relapse of vasculitis (1)[A].
- IV steroids indicated if vision loss has been noted, otherwise PO steroids are equally effective (1)[C]
- Given risk of irreversible vision loss, immediate steroid therapy should be initiated prior to confirmation by biopsy.
- The initial dose of steroids is continued for 2 to 4 weeks and slowly tapered over 9 to 12 months. Tapering may require ≥2 years (1)[A]. Assess for relapse during taper by monitoring symptoms, ESR, CRP.
- Tocilizumab (an IL-6 receptor antagonist) 162 mg SQ weekly or biweekly in addition to prednisone may be superior to prednisone alone, although it does carry a black box warning regarding increased risk of opportunistic infections.
- It has been suggested that low-dose aspirin might be effective for patients with GCA.

Second Line

- Methotrexate as an adjunct to glucocorticoid therapy may have a modest effect in decreasing the relapse rate of GCA.
- Cyclophosphamide have shown some benefit in patients who have not adequately responded to glucocorticoids.
- Azathioprine and abatacept can also be used as adjuncts to glucocorticoids.
- Therapies directed at TNF as adjunct to steroids have not shown significant benefit (1)[B].

ISSUES FOR REFERRAL

- Visual symptoms or threatened vision
- Uncertain diagnosis
- Refractory or relapsing disease
- Severe systemic involvement
- Steroid sparing therapy
- Atypical or large vessel involvement
- Complications of treatment

SURGERY/OTHER PROCEDURES

- Aortic aneurysm/dissection repair
- Carotid endarterectomy or stenting
- Endovascular stenting
- Cataracts/glaucoma surgery (for steroid-induced ocular complications)
- Osteoporotic fracture repair

ONGOING CARE

FOLLOW-UP RECOMMENDATIONS

Sun avoidance and protection of the head and the face from photodamage may eventually prove to be important preventive measures for GCA.

Patient Monitoring

- GCA is typically self limited and lasts several months or years.
- Overall, GCA does not seem to decrease longevity. Nevertheless, it may lead to serious complications such as visual loss, which occurs in about 15–20% of patients.
- Another complication of GCA is the development of aortic aneurysms, usually affecting the ascending aorta. Yearly chest x-rays may be useful to identify this problem.
- About 50% of the patients with GCA will eventually develop PMR (stiffness of shoulder and hip girdle).
- Low-dose aspirin should be given as indicated by atherosclerosis guidelines.

DIET

Calcium and vitamin D supplementation should be administered for osteoporosis prevention associated with prolonged corticosteroid therapy.

PATIENT EDUCATION

- Consequences of discontinuing steroids abruptly (adrenal insufficiency, disease relapse)
- Risks of long-term steroid use (infection, hyperglycemia, weight gain, impaired wound healing, osteoporosis, hypertension)
- Possibility of relapse and importance of reporting new headaches and vision changes to provider immediately

PROGNOSIS

- Variable duration of disease, from 1 year to chronic course
- Life expectancy is not affected by the disease unless severe aortitis is present.
- Once vision loss has occurred, it is unlikely to be recovered, but treatment resolves the other symptoms and prevents future vision loss and stroke.
- In most patients, glucocorticoid therapy can eventually be discontinued without complications. In patients with chronic disease, however, prednisone may need to be continued for years.
- Disease relapse is possible (40–70%).

COMPLICATIONS

- Vision loss with delayed diagnosis
- Glucocorticoid-related toxicity
- Ischemic strokes
- Aortic aneurysm/dissection
- Tissue necrosis of the jaw
- Chronic pain and disability

REFERENCES

1. Borchers AT, Gershwin ME. Giant cell arteritis: a review of classification, pathophysiology, geoepidemiology and treatment. *Autoimmun Rev*. 2012;11(6–7):A544–A554.

ADDITIONAL READING

De Miguel E, Beltran LM, Monjo I, et al. Atherosclerosis as a potential pitfall in the diagnosis of giant cell arteritis. *Rheumatology (Oxford)*. 2018;57(2):318–321.

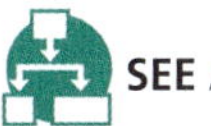

SEE ALSO

Depression; Fibromyalgia; Headache, Cluster; Headache, Tension; Polymyalgia Rheumatica; Polymyositis/Dermatomyositis

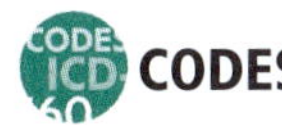

CODES

ICD10

- M31.6 Other giant cell arteritis
- M31.5 Giant cell arteritis with polymyalgia rheumatica

CLINICAL PEARLS

- Due to the risk of irreversible vision loss, treatment with high-dose steroids (prednisone 60 mg/day) should be started immediately in patients suspected of GCA.
- Temporal artery biopsy is the gold standard for diagnosis. Temporal artery biopsy is not likely to be affected by a few weeks of treatment.
- Treatment consists of a very slow steroid taper. Bone protection therapy and low-dose aspirin should be considered.
- Normal ESR level = value of age / 2 for men and age + 10 / 2 for women
- Patients on corticosteroids should be placed on therapy to minimize osteoporosis, unless there are contraindications.

ARTHRITIS, JUVENILE IDIOPATHIC

Zaiba Jetpuri, DO, MBA, FAAFP • Rasha Kakati, MD • Zubair A. Syed, MD

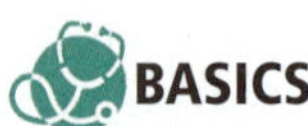

BASICS

DESCRIPTION

- Juvenile idiopathic arthritis (JIA) is the most common chronic pediatric rheumatologic disease.
- JIA is diagnosed before 16 years of age.
- JIA can be associated with significant disability and commonly involves ≥6 weeks of joint swelling, restricted range of motion, warmth, redness, and/or pain.
- Seven (International League of Associations for Rheumatology [ILAR]) subtypes determined by clinical characteristics in first 6 months of illness:
  - Systemic (sJIA): 10%; preceded by febrile onset of ≥2 weeks with rash, serositis, hepatosplenomegaly, or lymphadenopathy; arthritis may not be present initially; pathogenic role for IL-6 and IL-1
  - Polyarticular (PA): ≥5 joint involvement; large and small joints
    - PA with positive rheumatoid factor (RF): 2–7%; RF positive on two tests ≥3 months apart (1)[C]; uncommon in <9 years old
    - PA with negative RF: 15–20%; 50% of patients antinuclear antibodies (ANA) positive
  - Oligoarticular (OA): 30–60%; involvement of 1 to 4 joints; asymmetric large joints; risk for chronic uveitis in ANA positive females and axial skeletal involvement in older boys (1)[C]; types: (i) persistent (40%): knee, ankle, elbow; (ii) extended type (20%): >4 joints after first 6 months
  - Psoriatic arthritis: 5%; arthritis with psoriasis or arthritis with >2 of the following: dactylitis, nail changes (pitting), psoriasis in first-degree relative peaks age 2 to 4 years, and then again after age 10 years; HLA-B27 positive in 10–12%
  - Enthesitis-related arthritis: 1–11%; arthritis and/or enthesitis plus at least two of the following: sacroiliac or lumbosacral pain, Reiter syndrome or acute anterior uveitis in first-degree relative, acute symptomatic anterior uveitis, human leukocyte antigen HLA-B27 positive, history of ankylosing spondylitis, sacroiliitis with inflammatory bowel disease, onset of arthritis in male >6 years old
  - Undifferentiated arthritis (11–21%): presents with overlapping symptoms in ≥2 categories above or arthritis that does not fulfill above categories (1)[C]
- Systems affected: musculoskeletal, hematologic, lymphatic, immunologic, dermatologic, ophthalmologic, gastrointestinal
- Synonyms: juvenile chronic arthritis; juvenile arthritis; juvenile rheumatoid arthritis (JRA); Still disease (1)[C]

EPIDEMIOLOGY

54% of cases occur in children 0 to 5 years old.

Incidence

2 to 20/100,000 children <16 years old in developed nations

Prevalence

16 to 150/100,000 children <16 years old in developed nations

ETIOLOGY AND PATHOPHYSIOLOGY

- Humoral and cellular immunodysregulation due to immune response toward a self-antigen; T lymphocytes play a key role.
- Environmental triggers, possibly infections: Rubella or parvovirus B19; heat shock proteins
- Immunoglobulin or complement deficiency

Genetics

Strong genetic component; HLA and non-HLA-related genes (e.g., TNFα)

RISK FACTORS

Female sex 3:1

GENERAL PREVENTION

Maintain immunizations and infection prevention.

COMMONLY ASSOCIATED CONDITIONS

Other autoimmune disorders, chronic anterior uveitis, nutritional impairment, growth issues

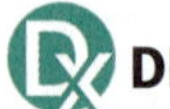

DIAGNOSIS

Clinical criteria: age of onset <16 years old and ≥6 weeks duration of objective arthritis (and no other form of childhood arthritis) in ≥1 joints

HISTORY

- Arthritis for ≥6 weeks
- Intermittent fevers, fatigue, malaise, myalgias, weight loss, morning stiffness, rash, lymphadenopathy

PHYSICAL EXAM

- Arthritis: swelling, effusion, loss of musculoskeletal landmarks, limited range of motion, tenderness, pain with motion, warmth, limp
- Rash: Salmon-pink, macular rash of differing sizes is characteristic, particularly around the axillae and waist but can be found anywhere. Rash is more prominent with fever, heat, touch, or minor trauma such as scratches.
- Rheumatoid nodules (uncommon), lymphadenopathy, hepato- or splenomegaly, enthesitis, dactylitis (mainly in psoriatic type)
- Uveitis is seen in all types of JIA but at different rates for subtypes (1)[C].

DIFFERENTIAL DIAGNOSIS

- Legg-Calvé-Perthes, toxic synovitis, growing pains, Perthes disease
- Septic arthritis, osteomyelitis, avascular necrosis, viral infection, mycoplasmal infection, Lyme disease/ Lyme arthritis
- Reactive arthritis: postinfectious, rheumatic fever, Reiter syndrome
- Inflammatory bowel disease
- Hemoglobinopathies, hemarthrosis, rickets, malaria
- Malignancy: leukemia (particularly acute lymphocytic leukemia), bone tumors (osteoid osteoma), lymphoma, neuroblastoma
- Vasculitis, immunoglobulin A vasculitis, Kawasaki disease
- Systemic lupus erythematosus, dermatomyositis, mixed connective tissue disease, sarcoidosis, systemic sclerosis, collagen disorders, juvenile fibromyalgia
- Farber disease
- Accidental or nonaccidental trauma

DIAGNOSTIC TESTS & INTERPRETATION

Initial Tests (lab, imaging)

- CBC: leukocyte count is normal or elevated; lymphopenia, reactive thrombocytosis, anemia
- Liver function test (LFT) elevation
- Renal function tests
- ESR and C-reactive protein (CRP) typically elevated especially in sJIA subtype; CRP often disproportionately high
- Myeloid-related proteins (MRP 8/14) associated with flares
- ANA positive: typically in OA (up to 70%) and PA subtypes. ANA-positive patients have increased risk of uveitis.
- RF positive: 2–10% (usually PA); poor prognosis
- Ferritin elevation: common in sJIA
- HLA-B27 positive: enthesitis-related arthritis
- Fever workup: blood and urine cultures, viral studies, chest radiograph, joint-fluid aspiration/analysis
- Ultrasound initially used to detect effusion and/or synovitis
- Radiograph of affected joint(s):
  - *Early* changes: soft tissue swelling, periosteal reaction, juxta-articular demineralization
  - *Later* changes: joint space loss, articular surface erosions, subchondral cyst formation, sclerosis, joint fusion
- CT is best for bony abnormalities.
- MRI can assess synovial hypertrophy and cartilage degeneration; MRI more sensitive to monitor disease activity and clinical responsiveness to treatment in peripheral joints.
- Radionuclide scans: to rule out infection/malignancy

Follow-Up Tests & Special Considerations

Use pediatric (not adult) controls when interpreting results of dual-energy x-ray absorptiometry.

Diagnostic Procedures/Other

Synovial biopsy: if synovial fluid cannot be aspirated or if infection is suspected despite negative synovial fluid culture

Test Interpretation

Synovial biopsy can show synovial cell hyperplasia, hyperemia, infiltration of small lymphocytes, and mononuclear cells.

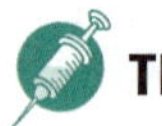

TREATMENT

GENERAL MEASURES

- Goal is to control active disease, minimize extra-articular manifestations, and achieve clinical remission
- Moist heat or electric blanket for morning stiffness.
- Aerobic exercise to improve functional capacity

MEDICATION

First Line

- ≤4 joints
  - NSAIDs: adequate in ~50%; symptoms often improve within days; full efficacy 2 to 3 months; may increase serum methotrexate (MTX) levels
  - Intra-articular long-acting corticosteroids: immediately effective; improve synovitis, joint damage, contractures, prevent leg length discrepancy; indicated in patients with oligoarthritis who fail a 2-month NSAID trial or with poor prognosis (1)[C]
- ≥5 joints: If high disease activity or a failed 1 to 2 months NSAID trial → MTX

Second Line

- 30–40% of patients require addition of disease-modifying antirheumatic drugs (DMARDs): synthetic (MTX, sulfasalazine, leflunomide), biologic (tumor necrosis factor [TNF] antagonists [etanercept, infliximab, adalimumab], rituximab, and newer biologic therapies, IL-1 and IL-6 receptor antagonists), and target-specific (e.g., janus kinase inhibitors).
  - MTX: 10 mg/m^2/week PO or SC
  - Sulfasalazine: OA and HLA-B27 spondylarthritis
  - TNF antagonists: excellent response among OA and PA; poor response in sJIA
    - Etanercept: 0.8 mg/kg (max of 50 mg/dose) given SC q1wk or 0.4 mg/kg SC twice a week (max of 25 mg/dose)
    - Infliximab: 5 mg/kg q6–8wk
    - Adalimumab: if weight 15 kg to <30 kg, 20 mg SC q2wk; if weight ≥30 kg, 40 mg SC q2wk
  - IL-6 inhibitors: excellent response in sJIA, OA, and PA
  - IL-1 inhibitors (e.g., Anakinra): excellent response in sJIA; poor response in OA and PA
- Refractory cases:
  - If biologic DMARD fails after 3 to 6 months, trial of a different biologic or a targeted synthetic DMARD (i.e., step-up therapy)
    - Rituximab: for RF-positive PA who have failed two TNF-α inhibitors
    - Tocilizumab: for RF-pJIA who have failed two TNF-α inhibitors
    - IL-17 inhibitors: for enthesitis-related disease refractory to TNF antagonists
    - Janus kinase inhibitors emerging for treatment of refractory cases
- Combination synthetic DMARD and biologic DMARD have shown better outcomes than step-up therapy at 3 years (STOP-JIA trial).

ISSUES FOR REFERRAL

- Patients with sJIA can be very ill initially although definitive diagnosis can only be made after ≥6 weeks of arthritis. Prompt pediatric rheumatology referral is favored upon suspicion.
- Orthopedics as needed for articular complication
- Ophthalmology to evaluate for uveitis/screening
- Behavioral health if difficulty coping with disease

ADDITIONAL THERAPIES

- Systemic glucocorticoids usually only if:
  - Bridging therapy during initiation of DMARD therapy in patients with severe disease
  - Severe sJIA
  - Macrophage activation syndrome (MAS)
- Physical and occupational therapy

SURGERY/OTHER PROCEDURES

- Total hip and/or knee replacement for severe disease
- Soft tissue release if splinting/traction unsuccessful
- Correct limb length or angular deformities
- Synovectomy is rarely performed.

COMPLEMENTARY & ALTERNATIVE MEDICINE

Some anti-inflammatory benefit to omega 3 and turmeric

ADMISSION, INPATIENT, AND NURSING CONSIDERATIONS

- Hospitalize if:
  - Unable to ambulate
  - Signs/symptoms of pericarditis
  - Persistent fever or diagnostic confusion to facilitate workup
  - Need for surgery
- Discharge when fever and serositis resolved.

ONGOING CARE

FOLLOW-UP RECOMMENDATIONS

Patient Monitoring

- Disease activity
  - Juvenile Arthritis Disease Activity Score (JADAS) questionnaire
  - Growth: height, weight, and BMI
  - Pain and quality of life
- Medication
  - NSAIDs: periodic CBC, urinalysis, LFTs, renal function tests
  - MTX: monthly LFTs, CBC, BUN, creatinine. MRP-8/14 can be helpful to predict relapse.
  - Biologic DMARD: CBC and LFT

DIET

Well-balanced, nutrient-dense diet

PATIENT EDUCATION

- Psychosocial needs; school issues; behavioral strategies for dealing with pain and noncompliance; available health care resources; support groups
- http://www.rheumatology.org/I-Am-A/Patient-Caregiver

PROGNOSIS

- 50–60% of patients will ultimately achieve remission
- Functional ability depends on adequacy of therapy (disease control, maintaining muscle and joint function)
- Poor prognosis: patients with active disease at 6 months; PA disease; extended pauciarticular disease course; female gender; RF positive; ANA positive; persistent morning stiffness; rapid appearance of erosions; hip involvement
- 30–100% of patients have flares after medication discontinuation; 50% of those patients cannot regain disease control

COMPLICATIONS

- Uveitis
  - Acute anterior uveitis: rapid-onset eye pain, conjunctival erythema and photophobia; common with HLA-B27 positive
  - Chronic anterior uveitis: initially asymptomatic and requires ophthalmologic screening every 3 to 6 months; can lead to blindness; commonly seen in OA, RF-negative PA and psoriatic subtypes; highest risk in ANA-positive females <6 years old
- Band keratopathy, glaucoma, growth failure, micrognathia (if temporomandibular joint involvement), debilitating joint disease, disseminated intravascular coagulation, hemolytic anemia
- MAS: severe, life-threatening; persistent fever, coagulopathy pancytopenia, elevated ferritin, liver injury, central nervous system dysfunction; associated with sJIA
- Serositis: pleural effusions, interstitial lung disease, pulmonary hypertension, pericarditis; lung disease prevalence is increasing with the use of IL-1 and IL-6 inhibitors and can lead to hypoxic respiratory failure
- Treatment-associated complications:
  - NSAIDs: peptic ulcer, GI hemorrhage, CNS reactions, renal disease, leukopenia
  - DMARDs: bone marrow suppression, hepatitis, renal disease, dermatitis, mouth ulcers, retinal toxicity
  - TNF antagonists: higher risk of infection
  - Osteoporosis, avascular necrosis
  - MTX: Folate supplementation decreases hepatic/GI symptoms; may reduce stomatitis

REFERENCES

1. Saad N, Onel K. Overview of juvenile idiopathic arthritis. *Open Orthopaed J*. 2020;14:101–109.

ADDITIONAL READING

Ringold S, Angeles-Han ST, Beukelman T, et al. 2019 American College of Rheumatology/Arthritis Foundation Guideline for the Treatment of Juvenile Idiopathic Arthritis: Therapeutic Approaches for Non-Systemic Polyarthritis, Sacroiliitis, and Enthesitis. *Arthritis Rheumatol (Hoboken, N.J.)*. 2019;71(6):846–863. doi:10.1002/art.40884.

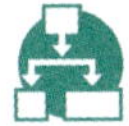

SEE ALSO

Arthritis, Rheumatoid (RA); Reactive Arthritis (Reiter Syndrome); Uveitis

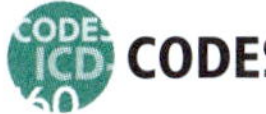

CODES

ICD10

- M08.90 Juvenile arthritis, unspecified, unspecified site
- M08.80 Other juvenile arthritis, unspecified site
- M08.00 Unsp juvenile rheumatoid arthritis of unspecified site

CLINICAL PEARLS

- JIA is the most common form of arthritis in children.
- Consider JIA in any child presenting with a limp.
- High-titer RF correlates with disease severity; prognosis worse if positive RF titers
- NSAIDs are typically first-line choice of medication.
- DMARDs improve JIA-associated symptoms.

ARTHRITIS, PSORIATIC

Kevin Loughry, DO

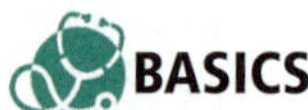

BASICS

A chronic, destructive, seronegative arthropathy in patients with long-standing psoriasis

DESCRIPTION

- Psoriatic arthritis (PsA) is a seronegative spondyloarthropathy characterized by inflammatory arthritis and enthesitis.
- Five patterns of arthritis in PsA:
  - Asymmetric oligoarthritis: <5 joints
  - Distal interphalangeal (DIP) joint predominant: osteoarthritis-like, associated with nail psoriasis
  - Symmetric polyarthritis: may be indistinguishable from rheumatoid arthritis (RA)—typically milder
  - Spondyloarthritis: asymmetric and discontinuous, unlike ankylosing spondylitis (AS)
  - Arthritis mutilans: destructive, resorptive arthritis; produces "opera-glass" or "telescoping" digit
- Psoriasis may be limited in extent.
  - Course of arthritis and extent of psoriasis do not correlate.
  - Other extra-articular features, such as iritis, are less common.
  - Damaging joint disease may occur in 40–60%. Characteristic radiologic changes include "pencil-in-cup" deformity and periostitis.
- Rheumatoid factor (RF) and anti–cyclic citrullinated peptide (anti-CCP) antibody are usually negative. HLA-B27 may be positive.

EPIDEMIOLOGY

- Peak onset age: 30 to 50 years
- Predominant gender: female = male
- Polyarthritis is more common in women.
- Spondylitis in up to 25%, more common in males
- Psoriasis precedes arthritis in most patients by an average of 12 years. Arthritis preceding psoriasis occurs in up to 15% of patients, usually children. Arthritis and psoriasis may present simultaneously.
- Psoriasis occurs in 2–3% of the U.S. population; 6–42% will develop PsA (1).

Prevalence

Prevalence: 1 to 2/1,000 population (1)

ETIOLOGY AND PATHOPHYSIOLOGY

- CD4+/CD8+ T cells; tumor necrosis factor-α (TNF-α); interleukins 1 (IL-1), 6, 8, 10, 17, and 23; and matrix metalloproteases present in synovial fluid
- Osteoclast precursor cell upregulation
- Unknown, probably multifactorial: immunologic, genetic, environmental factors

Genetics

- 30–40% concordance in identical twins
- HLA-B27 in 15–50% with PsA (spondylitis pattern) versus 90% in AS
- Other HLA associations in PsA: HLA-B7, HLA-B38, HLA-B39, HLA-Cw6

RISK FACTORS

- Psoriasis
- Family history of PsA
- Obesity

GENERAL PREVENTION

No known prevention strategies; unknown whether early treatment of psoriasis prevents onset of PsA

COMMONLY ASSOCIATED CONDITIONS

Psoriasis

DIAGNOSIS

- A history of inflammatory arthritis, dactylitis, or enthesitis in patients with existing psoriasis helps establish the diagnosis. It can be difficult to differentiate PsA from other inflammatory arthropathies.
- Use the CASPAR (Classification Criteria for Psoriatic Arthritis) system (91% sensitivity, 99% specificity) to screen patients for PsA. Inflammatory articular disease (joint, spine, or entheseal) with ≥3 points from the following five categories:
  - Evidence of current psoriasis, a personal or family history of psoriasis (2 points)
  - Typical psoriatic nail dystrophy, including onycholysis, pitting, and hyperkeratosis (1 point)
  - Negative RF (ELISA preferred) (1 point)
  - Current or prior history of dactylitis (1 point)
  - Radiologic evidence of new bone formation (excluding osteophyte formation) on plain radiographs of the hand or foot (1 point)

HISTORY

History and physical exam help establish the diagnosis of PsA.

- (Generally) long-standing history of psoriasis
- Morning stiffness of hands, feet, or low back for >30 minutes
- Pain of involved joints
- Swelling or redness of peripheral joints
- Low back or buttock pain
- Ankle or heel pain
- Dactylitis or uniform swelling of an entire digit

PHYSICAL EXAM

- Affected peripheral joints may have overlying erythema, warmth, and swelling.
  - Synovitis
  - Dactylitis
  - Swelling of tendons (e.g., Achilles tendon) and tenderness at insertion sites (e.g., calcaneus)
  - Limited range of motion of axial skeleton
  - Pain with stress of the sacroiliac joint
- Well-demarcated pink-to-red erythematous plaques with a white silvery scale; common locations include scalp, ears, trunk, periumbilical area, buttocks, gluteal cleft, elbows and forearms, knees and legs, and palms and soles.
- Nails may be dystrophic with pits, oil spots, crumbling, leukonychia, and red lunulae.

DIFFERENTIAL DIAGNOSIS

- Reactive arthritis
- Psoriasis and RA
- Psoriasis and osteoarthritis
- Psoriasis and polyarticular gout
- Psoriasis and AS

DIAGNOSTIC TESTS & INTERPRETATION

Initial Tests (lab, imaging)

- Serum RF (usually negative)
- Anti-CCP (usually negative)
- Antinuclear antibodies (usually negative)
- Acute-phase reactants (ESR and C-reactive protein) may be elevated.
- HLA-B27 is noted in 50–70% with axial disease and <15% with peripheral disease.
- Baseline radiographs of affected joints
- Plain radiographs may aid diagnosis, assess joint damage, disease progression, and response to therapy.
- Juxta-articular new bone formation (periostitis) and marginal joint erosions that progress centrally ("pencil-in-cup" erosions) are characteristic radiographic features.
- In patients with psoriasis, detection of enthesitis on ultrasound may be associated with higher risk of PsA.

Follow-Up Tests & Special Considerations

Follow-up radiographs; interval based on severity

Diagnostic Procedures/Other

Biopsy of skin or synovium is not usually required. Nail scrapings can exclude fungal causes of nail changes.

Test Interpretation

When anti-CCP antibody-positive, correlates with erosive disease.

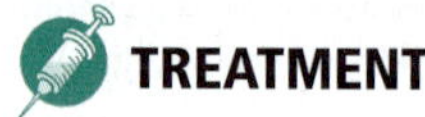

TREATMENT

GENERAL MEASURES

Physical therapy and/or occupational therapy benefit all stages of disease.

- Treatment algorithms for PsA are based on severity of joint symptoms, extent of structural damage, and severity of psoriasis. Patients with moderate to severe arthritis should be started on disease-modifying antirheumatic drugs (DMARDs) or biologic disease-modifying antirheumatic agents (bDMARDs) to reduce or prevent joint damage and preserve joint integrity and function.
- In addition to pharmacotherapy, patients should be educated on lifestyle modifications such as smoking cessation, diet, weight reduction, joint protection, physical activity, exercise, work participation, and stress coping mechanisms (2).

MEDICATION

First Line

- NSAIDs to control symptoms of mild disease; intermittent intra-articular glucocorticoid injections may help.
- There are no systematic trials of NSAIDs for PsA. Dose NSAIDs to suppress mild inflammation. NSAIDs selection is based on patient preference and dosing convenience. Sample NSAIDs include ibuprofen 400 to 800 mg PO TID–QID; naproxen 250 to 500 mg PO BID–TID; diclofenac 100 to 150 mg QD; and indomethacin 100 to 150 mg QD.

- Monotherapy is as effective as combination therapy (≥2 drugs from the following: analgesics, NSAIDs, opioids, opioid-like drugs, and neuromodulators [antidepressants, anticonvulsants, and muscle relaxants]).
- In patients with the polyarthritis phenotype, or monoarthritis/oligoarthritis and poor prognostic factors such as structural damage, elevated acute phase reactants, dactylitis, or nail involvement, rapid imitation of a conventional DMARDs are preferred.

Second Line

- Recommended DMARDs include methotrexate, sulfasalazine, and leflunomide. There is no evidence to support the use of combination DMARDs therapy. Methotrexate is the preferred conventional DMARDs in patients with clinical significant skin involvement.
- Initial dosing regimens for DMARDs: methotrexate (1 test dose of 2.5 to 5.0 mg PO to assess for significant bone marrow suppression and then 15 to 25 mg once weekly), sulfasalazine (2 to 3 g/day PO divided in BID dosing), leflunomide (loading dose of 100 mg/day PO for 3 days and then 20 mg/day PO)
- Oral glucocorticoids are not recommended.
- In patients with axial predominant disease or enthesitis, bDMARDs may be initiated even if they have not tried and failed conventional DMARDs if adequate control is not achieved with NSAIDs (3).
- Dosing regimens for anti–TNF-α agents (preferred bDMARDs in axial disease, monoclonal antibodies if concomitant inflammatory bowel disease).
  - Adalimumab 40 mg SC q2wk
  - Certolizumab pegol 200 mg q2wk; for maintenance dosing or 400 mg q4wk
  - Etanercept 50 mg SC weekly
  - Golimumab 50 mg SC monthly
  - Infliximab 5 mg/kg at 0, 2, and 6 weeks, q8wk afterward
- Anti–interleukin-17 agents include:
  - Ixekizumab 80 mg q4wk
  - Secukinumab 150 mg weekly from 0 to 4 weeks and then monthly
  - Brodalumab 210 mg SC × 1 weekly from 0 to 2 and then q2wk (4)
- Anti–interleukin-12/interleukin-23 agents include:
  - Ustekinumab is currently dosed at 45 or 90 mg (depending on weight) at 0, 4, and 12 weeks and then q12wk thereafter.
- IL-23 selective inhibitor include:
  - Risankizumab 150 mg SC × 1 on week 0, 4, then q12wk
  - Guselkumab 100 mg SC × 1 at 0 and 4 weeks and then q8wk
- PDE4 inhibitors include:
  - Apremilast 30 mg PO BID
- JAK 1, JAK 2, and JAK 3 inhibitors include (generally third line after failure of, or contraindication to, other bDMARDs):
  - Tofacitinib citrate dosed at 5 mg PO BID immediate release or 11 mg once daily extended release (1)
  - Upadacitinib dosed at 15 mg PO QD
- Selective T-cell costimulation blocker:
  - Abatacept dosed at 125 mg once weekly SC or according to body weight. Following the initial IV infusion (using the weight-based dosing), repeat IV infusion (using the same weight-based dosing) q2wk and q4wk after the initial infusion, and q4wk thereafter (1).
- Above medications are FDA-approved for PsA.
- Do not use anti-TNF agents in the setting of active infection (including TB and hepatitis B). Do not use anti-TNF agents with concurrent live vaccinations, with New York Heart Association classes III to IV congestive heart failure, with malignancy, or in patients with a history of demyelinating disease.
- Do not use biologic therapies in patients with active infection, with concurrent live vaccinations, or with history of malignancy.
- Do not use JAK inhibitors (JAKi) in patients with active infection or malignancy or those with risk factors for cardiovascular and thromboembolic disease.

Pregnancy Considerations

- Avoid teratogenic medications (e.g., methotrexate, leflunomide) during pregnancy.
- Adalimumab, etanercept, golimumab, infliximab, ustekinumab, and certolizumab pegol, secukinumab, are currently listed as Category B medications. Apremilast, abatacept, tofacitinib citrate, ixekizumab, and guselkumab are listed as pregnancy Category C medication. Upadacitinib is pregnancy Category D.

ISSUES FOR REFERRAL

- Rheumatology
- Dermatology

SURGERY/OTHER PROCEDURES

Joint fusion or replacement for advanced destruction

ONGOING CARE

FOLLOW-UP RECOMMENDATIONS

Epidemiologic data suggest a relationship between psoriasis, metabolic syndrome, type 2 diabetes, Crohn disease, myocardial infarction, and stroke. Control of weight, blood pressure, lipids, and glucose is recommended (2).

PATIENT EDUCATION

- National Psoriasis Foundation: https://www.psoriasis.org/about-psoriatic-arthritis/
- Arthritis Foundation: http://www.arthritis.org/about-arthritis/types/psoriatic-arthritis/
- American College of Rheumatology: https://www.rheumatology.org

PROGNOSIS

- Course is typically insidious with chronic joint disease and recurring/remitting skin disease.
- Prognosis is more favorable than for RA (except for patients who develop arthritis mutilans).

COMPLICATIONS

- Disability
- Psychosocial impact of PsA: anxiety and depression

REFERENCES

1. Ritchlin CT, Colbert RA, Gladman DD. Psoriatic arthritis. *N Engl J Med*. 2017;376(10):957–970.
2. Ruta S, Cespedes RJ, Cuellar L, et al. Psoriatic arthritis: differential features at the time of clinical presentation in a large cohort of patients with polyarthralgia. *Eur J Rheumatol*. 2023;10(1):12–17. doi:10.5152/eurjrheum.2022.22035.
3. Gossec L, Kerschbaumer A, Ferreira RJO, et al. EULAR recommendations for the management of psoriatic arthritis with pharmacological therapies: 2023 update. *Ann Rheum Dis*. 2024;83(6):706–719.
4. Singh JA, Guyatt G, Ogdie A, et al. Special article: 2018 American College of Rheumatology/National Psoriasis Foundation guideline for the treatment of psoriatic arthritis. *Arthritis Rheumatol*. 2019;71(1):5–32.

ADDITIONAL READING

- Norden A, Oulee A, Ivanic M, et al. The use of ultrasound to detect enthesitis as a potential guide for intervention in patients with psoriasis at risk of psoriatic arthritis: a systematic review. *Int J Dermatol*. 2023;62(8):973–979.
- Ruyssen-Witrand A, Perry R, Watkins C, et al. Efficacy and safety of biologics in psoriatic arthritis: a systematic literature review and network meta-analysis. *RMD Open*. 2020;6(1):e001117.

CODES

ICD10

- L40.50 Arthropathic psoriasis, unspecified
- L40.51 Distal interphalangeal psoriatic arthropathy
- L40.53 Psoriatic spondylitis

CLINICAL PEARLS

- One in four patients with psoriasis develops PsA.
- The severity of psoriasis correlates with the likelihood of developing arthritis, not the severity of arthritis.
- Commonly overlooked locations of psoriasis include scalp, ears, umbilicus, and gluteal cleft.
- Osteoarthritis and polyarticular gout may mimic or coexist with PsA.
- The polyarticular pattern of PsA mimics RA. The presence of both enthesitis and psoriasis helps differentiate PsA from RA.
- Therapies for PsA are rapidly expanding and include NSAIDS; DMARDs; immunosuppressants, biologics and JAKi.

ARTHRITIS, RHEUMATOID (RA)

Peng Thim Fan, MD

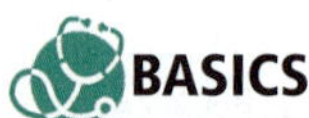

BASICS

DESCRIPTION

Rheumatoid arthritis (RA) is a symmetric, inflammatory disease primarily causing synovial inflammation and leading to the destruction of bone and cartilage (1).

EPIDEMIOLOGY

Incidence

Annual incidence: United States is approximately 40 per 100,000 persons.

Prevalence

- Prevalence: 0.5–1% of the general population worldwide. In the United States, the prevalence is the same as globally, between 0.5% and 1%.
- Female:male 3:1; onset is typically between 30 and 50 years, but it can occur at any age.
- The lifetime risk of developing RA: 3.6% in women and 1.7% in men

ETIOLOGY AND PATHOPHYSIOLOGY

RA is a chronic inflammatory disease caused by an unchecked synovial proliferation. A pannus forms and erodes into cartilage and bone causing loss of cartilage and bony destruction with progressive joint deformity leading to significant disability.

Genetics

RA has strong familial associations; a parent with RA increases the risk by 3-fold over standard incidence, a sibling by 4.6, and a parent and sibling with RA increases the risk by 9.3. HLA-DRB1 linked to a higher risk of RA.

RISK FACTORS

Disruption of the gut microbiome by infection (e.g., *Porphyromonas gingivalis*) may provoke autoreactive T cells contributing to inflammation and joint-specific immune responses. Cigarette smoking and gingivitis also exacerbate the inflammatory process.

GENERAL PREVENTION

Smoking cessation, a well-balanced diet, achieving a healthy weight, regular physical activity, regular dental checkups and good dental hygiene; diet rich in omega-3 fatty acids

COMMONLY ASSOCIATED CONDITIONS

Fatigue, sleep disturbances, depression, fibromyalgia, osteoporosis, atherosclerotic coronary artery disease, lung disease (pleuritis, pleural effusion, interstitial fibrosis and pulmonary nodules), episcleritis, scleritis, Sjögren disease.

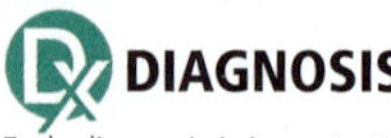

DIAGNOSIS

Early diagnosis is important. 50–70% of patients have radiographic joint damage within 2 years of disease onset.

HISTORY

- Joint pain is the primary symptom. It is insidious in onset, often symmetrically involving small (peripheral) synovial-lined joints. The axial skeleton is spared and RA is not associated with cervical, thoracic, or lumbar spine pain or limited movement.
- Morning stiffness (≥1 hour) is common.
- Improvement of pain and stiffness with activity, low-grade fever, and weight loss are other historical features.
- Joint deformity is a longer term sequela.

PHYSICAL EXAM

- Symmetric swelling, tenderness, and reduced range of motion of metacarpophalangeal (MCP), proximal interphalangeal (PIP), and metatarsophalangeal (MTP) joints. The distal interphalangeal (DIP) joints are spared. The shoulder, elbow, knee, and ankle joints may be involved.
- Ulnar deviation, boutonnière deformity, MCP joint subluxation, radial deviation at the wrist, hammertoe deformity, extensor tendon rupture are uncommon findings, described in the literature in long-standing poorly managed RA. With our current effective treatment of RA, they are preventable.
- Subcutaneous nodules
- Extra-articular manifestations: keratoconjunctivitis, episcleritis, scleritis, rales, crackles, pericardial friction, rubs, splinter hemorrhage, palpable purpura, skin ulceration, nail fold infarcts, sensory and/or motor deficit, osteoporosis
- Cervical spine instability occurs with atlantoaxial subluxation at C1–C2. These patients may present with long tract signs of spinal cord compression.

DIFFERENTIAL DIAGNOSIS

Psoriatic arthritis, systemic lupus erythematosus (SLE), inflammatory myopathies, mixed connective tissue disease, scleroderma, tophaceous gout, polymyalgia rheumatica; fibromyalgia, a disorder of pain perception, may mimic or complicate RA by causing widespread symmetrical joint pains and prolonged morning stiffness.

DIAGNOSTIC TESTS & INTERPRETATION

A definitive diagnosis of RA requires these criteria:

- Inflammatory arthritis affecting ≥3 joints
- Positive rheumatoid factor (RF) and/or anti-CCP antibody
- Elevated levels of erythrocyte sedimentation rate (ESR) or C-reactive protein (CRP)
- Exclusion of other diseases with similar features: psoriatic arthritis, viral arthritis, polyarticular gout, calcium pyrophosphate deposition disease, SLE, and other connective tissue diseases
- The duration of joint symptoms is >6 weeks. Most viral arthritis do not persist beyond 4 weeks except for parvovirus B19 and Chikungunya that may cause prolonged arthritis.

Initial Tests (lab, imaging)

- Recommended laboratory studies
  - Complete blood count (CBC), comprehensive metabolic panel, urinalysis, TSH (free T4)
  - ESR and CRP
  - RF and anti-CCP
  - ANA (if extra-articular features, related to SLE)
- Recommended imaging
  - X-rays of hands and feet to look for juxta-articular demineralization, joint space narrowing, and erosions
  - Doppler ultrasound of affected joints (may be more sensitive than x-rays)
  - MRI scan of hands, wrists, and feet if x-rays are negative and the clinical picture suggests RA.

Follow-Up Tests & Special Considerations

- Laboratory monitoring starting and monitoring methotrexate therapy: hepatitis B and C, CBC, liver and renal function before; CBC and liver function every 4 weeks during treatment for 6 months and then every 6 weeks thereafter
- For initiation of a biologic DMARD (bDMARD) or targeted synthetic DMARD (tsDMARD): Test for latent tuberculosis (Quantiferon-Gold, T-spot or PPD skin test.) If positive, then start prophylaxis against TB for a month before starting the DMARD and give a complete course of prophylaxis

Diagnostic Procedures/Other

- Joint aspiration to exclude crystal arthropathy and septic arthritis, especially when only a single joint is inflamed
- Synovial fluid analysis in RA: yellowish-white, turbid, white blood cell increased (3,500 to 50,000 cells/mm), protein: ~4.2 g/dL (42 g/L), serum-synovial glucose difference >30 mg/dL

Test Interpretation

- Anti-CCP antibodies are present in 60–70% of patients with RA but are 90–98% specific for RA. They are often present many years before clinical arthritis. It correlates with erosive disease.
- RF is positive in 50% of patients at the time of diagnosis and an additional 20–35% becomes positive in 6 months.
- Imaging: x-ray to follow the progression and identify the destruction of the disease; x-rays are repeated yearly until the disease is in full remission. MRI of hands and wrists (erosions, pannus, synovitis), and ultrasound can assess synovial thickening/erosions.

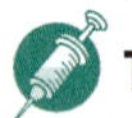

TREATMENT

A treat-to-target approach is strongly recommended over usual care for patients who have not been previously treated with DMARDS (both traditional and biologics).

GENERAL MEASURES

Smoking cessation, well-balanced diet, regular physical activity, good dental hygiene

MEDICATION

- NSAIDs as initial treatment are useful for relieving joint pain and swelling. Because they are not disease modifying, they should not be used alone, and they may be stopped once the disease is controlled.
- Conventional synthetic disease-modifying antirheumatic drugs (csDMARDs) are recommended as first line: HCQ, leflunomide, methotrexate (MTX), and sulfasalazine (SSZ) are the most common—MTX is the most used first-line RA drug worldwide and is generally preferred as the first-line DMARD. Start MTX at 7.5 mg for the first week and raise to 20 mg weekly. Folic acid 1 mg daily is given to reduce nausea, GI distress, oral ulcers, and possibly fatigue. Leucovorin may work for more sensitive patients. SQ MTX may work when oral is not adequately effective; the dosage can be raised to 25 mg SQ weekly. MTX is an effective drug able to achieve a remission of disease in 1/3 of patients with early RA.

- Leflunomide has roughly the same efficacy as MTX and the two in combination may confer better efficacy. SSZ is less effective but may be preferred in patients who are positive for hepatitis B or C. Hydroxychloroquine (HCQ) is the best tolerated but the least effective. It is best used in patients who are negative for both RF and anti-CCP because the "double negative" RA patients generally have milder joint inflammation. HCQ may cause retinal toxicity with long-term use; the dosage for prolonged use should not exceed 5 mg/kg/day and yearly eye examination with retina monitoring is recommended.
- Corticosteroids are not recommended in the 2021 ACR Guidelines but high-dose prednisone with rapid taper may be effective. Prednisone 5 mg daily may be helpful and potentially disease modifying; a slow taper may sustain improvement. Use of prednisone beyond 6 months is not recommended.
- An alternative to using a biologic agent when response to MTX alone is inadequate is to use "triple therapy"—combining MTX with SSZ and HCQ. Efficacy is comparable to using a tumor necrosis factor-alpha inhibitors (TNFi) like etanercept, but adherence is a problem because of the many pills needed daily.
- TNFis: etanercept, infliximab, adalimumab, certolizumab, and golimumab have the longest safety data and are the initial choice for of a bDMARD when the response to MTX is inadequate. Etanercept is an engineered biologic combination of the TNF-α receptor extracellular domain with IgG Fc. Infliximab, adalimumab, and golimumab are monoclonal antibodies to TNF. Certolizumab binds TNF via the Fab fragment. All are comparable in efficacy. Certolizumab does not cross the placenta and is the preferred agent in pregnant women.
- Other bDMARDs are used in TNFi failures: tocilizumab and sarilumab inhibit IL-6, abatacept reduces T-cell activation, rituximab depletes B cells, and anakinra (less effective) blocks IL-1.
- The tsDMARDs are oral agents that block the transmission of signal from the cell-surface receptor to the nucleus by disrupting the JAK-STAT pathway and thereby stopping gene expression. They are called Jakinibs. They work rapidly and show a beneficial response within 4 weeks if they are effective for that patient. Three drugs are available to date: tofacitinib, baricitinib, and upadacitinib. They are comparable in efficacy. They have a higher risk for reactivating herpes zoster. A long-term safety trial showed that tofacitinib had a higher risk of MACE events and of cancer compared to the TNFis. Therefore, they should be used in TNFi failures and not as initial treatment.
- All the biologic and targeted synthetic agents work better in combination with MTX even in those who previously had an inadequate response to MTX.

First Line

csDMARDs, especially MTX; a 3-month trial is needed to assess efficacy. A treat-to-target approach is best. An objective assessment of disease activity is performed every 3 months using a tool such as DAS-28, CDAI, or SDAI. A target of remission (minimal or no disease activity) is required for early disease (e.g., DAS-28 <2.6) or low disease activity for patients with long-standing disease (e.g., DAS-28 2.6 to 3.2). If this goal is not achieved, then change of treatment is mandatory until the target is reached.

Second Line

- bDMARD such as a TNFi, with or without MTX; alternatively, the other classes of biologic agents.
- An oral Jakinib may be used in patients who fail a TNFi or other bDMARD.
- A treat-to-target approach every 3 months; change biologic agent or Jakinib if target is not reached or side effects are not tolerated.

ISSUES FOR REFERRAL

- Primary care providers should familiarize and feel comfortable using MTX and other cDMARDs.
- Rheumatology for management of biologics and Jakinibs
- Pulmonology: interstitial lung disease
- Ophthalmology: scleritis, episcleritis, screening patients on HCQ (Plaquenil)

SURGERY/OTHER PROCEDURES

Synovectomy, tendon alignment, arthroplasty

COMPLEMENTARY & ALTERNATIVE MEDICINE

Psychosocial interventions, physical and occupational therapy

ADMISSION, INPATIENT, AND NURSING CONSIDERATIONS

For serious infection

ONGOING CARE

FOLLOW-UP RECOMMENDATIONS

Patient Monitoring

Drug toxicity monitoring regularly, monitoring for extra-articular manifestation.

DIET

Avoid fatty foods and eat lots of fruits and vegetables. Eating 3.5 oz fish rich in omega-3 fatty acid twice a week improves joint pain, swelling, and tenderness. A Mediterranean diet improves some activity measures.

PATIENT EDUCATION

Smoking cessation; good dental hygiene; avoid alcohol and pregnancy while on MTX.

PROGNOSIS

Excellent for early RA; remission is achievable in 80% of patients. Aggressive treatment is needed for patients positive for both RF and anti-CCP and for those with extra-articular disease. Aggressive suppression of inflammatory disease activity has also reduced risk for cardiovascular diseases: strokes and MI

COMPLICATIONS

Joint deformities, malignancies (lymphoma, lung cancer, skin cancer), pulmonary disease, infection, cardiovascular diseases

REFERENCES

1. Kim JW, Suh CH. Systemic manifestations and complications in patients with rheumatoid arthritis. *J Clin Med*. 2020;9(6):2008. doi:10.3390/jcm9062008.

ADDITIONAL READING

- Di Matteo A, Bathon JM, Emery P. Rheumatoid arthritis. *Lancet*. 2023;402(10416):2019–2033. doi:10.1016/S0140-6736(23)01525-8.
- He J, Maharaj AB. Highlights of advancement in rheumatoid arthritis research and clinical practice. *Best Pract Res Clin Rheumatol*. 2025;39(1):102040. doi:10.1016/j.berh.2025.102040.
- Peterson E, Gallagher MK, Wilbur J. Rheumatoid arthritis: diagnosis and management for the family physician. *Am Fam Physician*. 2024;110(5):515–526.

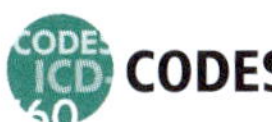

CODES

ICD10

- M06.9 Rheumatoid arthritis, unspecified
- M05.60 Rheu arthritis of unsp site w involv of organs and systems
- M05.30 Rheumatoid heart disease w rheumatoid arthritis of unsp site

CLINICAL PEARLS

- Early treatment with DMARDs is essential; treat-to-target approach
- MTX is the first-line treatment for active disease.
- Biologic agents continue to rapidly evolve and are a critical element of the ongoing treatment of RA. Selection of specific agents is dependent on individual patient characteristics and is best done with rheumatologic support.
- Ongoing monitoring is important to assess for infection risk, vaccine status, and cardiovascular morbidity.

ARTHRITIS, SEPTIC

Terrence Tsui, DO

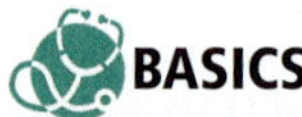

BASICS

DESCRIPTION

- Infection due to bacterial invasion of the joint space
- Septic arthritis is a medical emergency that leads to rapid irreversible damage to the joint.
- Synonyms: suppurative arthritis; infections arthritis; pyarthrosis; pyogenic arthritis; bacterial arthritis

EPIDEMIOLOGY

Incidence

- May occur at any age, bimodal incidence with peaks in childhood and age >55 years; knee most commonly affected in adults; hips in children
- 40 to 60 cases per 100,000 population/year overall
- Disseminated gonococcal infection is 3 cases per 100,000 population/year.

Prevalence

- 27% of patients presenting with monoarticular arthritis have nongonococcal septic arthritis.
- Given rising prevalence of prosthetic joints, infected hardware is now the most common form of septic arthritis (~2–10% of all joint recipients).

ETIOLOGY AND PATHOPHYSIOLOGY

- Nongonococcal: *Staphylococcus aureus* (most common in adults, accounts for >50% of cases [1])
  - MRSA risk increased in elderly, intravenous drug users (IVDU), postsurgical
  - *Streptococcus* spp. (second most common in adults)
  - Gram-negative rods (GNR): IVDU, trauma, extremes of age, immunosuppressed
- *Neisseria gonorrhoeae* (most common in young, sexually active adults)
- Polymicrobial infections typically occur after penetrating trauma such as bite wounds or organic foreign body penetration.
- Other: rickettsial (e.g., Lyme), fungal, mycobacterial
- Risk by specific age:
  - <1 month: *S. aureus*, group B *Streptococcus* (GBS), GNR
  - 1 month to 4 years: *Kingella Kingae, Staphylococcus* and *Streptococcus N. meningitidis*
  - 16 to 40 years: *N. meningitidis*, *S. aureus*
  - >40 years: *S. aureus*
- Patients with native joint infection are at increased risk for infection of prosthesis (of the same joint should it require replacement).
- Specific high-risk groups:
  - Rheumatoid arthritis (RA): *S. aureus*
  - IVDU: *S. aureus*, GNR, opportunistic pathogens
  - Neonates: GBS
  - Immunocompromised: Gram-negative bacilli, fungi
  - Trauma patients with open injuries: mixed flora
- Pathogenesis:
  - Hematogenous spread (most common)
  - Direct inoculation by microorganisms secondary to trauma or iatrogenic (e.g., joint surgery)
  - Adjacent spread (e.g., osteomyelitis)
- Pathophysiology:
  - Microorganisms initially enter through synovial membrane and spread to the synovial fluid.
  - Resulting inflammatory response releases cytokines and destructive proteases leading to systemic symptoms and joint damage.

RISK FACTORS

- Low socioeconomic status, alcoholism
- Cellulitis and skin ulcers
- Prior orthopedic surgery
- Intraarticular injection
- Trauma
- History of previous joint disease
  - Inflammatory arthritis (RA: 10-fold increased risk)
  - Osteoarthritis
  - Crystal arthritides
- Systemic illness: diabetes mellitus, liver disease, HIV, malignancy, end-stage renal disease/hemodialysis, immunosuppression, sickle cell anemia
- Risks for hematogenous spread: IVDU, severe sepsis/systemic infection

GENERAL PREVENTION

Prompt treatment of skin and soft tissue infections

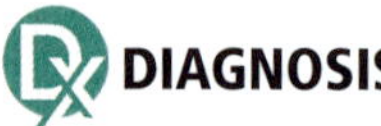

DIAGNOSIS

HISTORY

- Can present with a combination of fever, chills, joint pain, swelling, warmth, and decreased range of motion (ROM)
- Nongonococcal arthritis: mostly monoarticular (80%)
  - Typically large joints: knee (50%), hip (20%), shoulder (8%), ankle (7%)
  - Most patients report fever.
  - IV drug users may develop infection in axial joints (e.g., sternoclavicular joint).
  - Prosthetic joint infections present differently and may only have pain and decreased function without systemic signs of infection; may present with drainage from site of surgical incision
  - Patients on chronic immunosuppressive drugs and those receiving articular corticosteroid injections may have atypical presentations (absent fever or joint pain).
- Pediatric considerations:
  - Infants may avoid use of limb (often mistaken for neurologic problem).
  - Refusal to walk and/or a new limp
  - Hip pain may commonly refer to knee and/or thigh.
- Gonococcal arthritis
  - Bacteremic phase: Migratory polyarthritis, tenosynovitis, high fever, chills, pustules (dermatitis–arthritis syndrome)
  - Localized phase: less symptomatic—often monoarticular, low-grade fever
- Approximately 22% of all patients with culture-proven septic arthritis had no associated risk factors or underlying joint disease.

PHYSICAL EXAM

- Physical exam has poor sensitive and specificity for septic arthritis; however, common findings include:
  - Fever (60–80% of cases)
  - Limited ROM
  - Joint effusion and tenderness
  - Erythema and warmth over affected joint
  - Pain with passive ROM
- Infants with septic hip arthritis maintain the joint in flexion and external rotation as position of comfort.
- Purpura associated with disseminated gonococcal infection

DIFFERENTIAL DIAGNOSIS

- Crystal arthritis: gout, pseudogout
- Infectious arthritis: fungi, spirochetes, rheumatic fever, HIV, viral
- Inflammatory arthritis: RA, spondyloarthropathy, systemic lupus erythematosus, sarcoidosis, psoriatic arthritis
- Osteoarthritis
- Trauma: meniscal tear, fracture, hemarthrosis
- Other: bursitis, cellulitis, tendinitis

DIAGNOSTIC TESTS & INTERPRETATION

Initial Tests (lab, imaging)

- Need high index of suspicion as high-grade fever and serum leukocytosis may be absent in 1/3 of cases (2).
- Synovial fluid analysis is the gold standard of diagnosis.
  - Obtain prior to antibiotic therapy when possible.
  - Include Gram stain, culture, cell count/differential, and crystal analysis.
  - Use blood culture bottles to increase yield.
  - Gram stain (sensitivity 29–65%); culture (positive in 80%)
  - >50,000 WBCs/HPF with >90% polymorphonuclear leukocytes is suggestive.
    - *Synovial WBC* (sWBC) *count alone is insufficient to rule in or rule out septic arthritis.*
    - Likelihood of septic arthritis increases as sWBC rises >100,000/HPF.
  - Analysis of synovial fluid leukocyte esterase is associated with a high negative predictive value (NPV) (3).
  - Crystals (e.g., urate or calcium pyrophosphate) *do not exclude concurrent infectious arthritis*.
  - Prosthetic joint: WBC count is unreliable; a lower number of sWBCs may indicate infection.
- Serum tests:
  - ESR >15 mm/hr has sensitivity up to 94% but poor specificity.
  - CRP >20 mg/L has sensitivity of 92%.
  - Synovial lactate is a potential biomarker to rule out septic arthritis when <250 U/L; however, more study is needed.
  - Blood cultures positive in ~50% of adult cases (20% of pediatric cases) (4)
- Other tests:
  - Disseminated gonococcus: culture blood, cervix, urine, urethra, pharynx in addition to joint fluid
  - Suspect Lyme arthritis: PCR and serum titers for *Borrelia* IgM and IgG indicate exposure.

- Pediatrics: No single lab test distinguishes septic arthritis from transient synovitis.
  - The combination of fever, non–weight-bearing, and elevated ESR/CRP is suspicious; obtain synovial fluid for analysis when possible.
- Imaging:
  - Can help identify effusion but does not further differentiate causes of arthritis
  - Plain films
    - Nondiagnostic for septic arthritis; useful for trauma, soft tissue swelling, osteoarthritis, or osteopenia
    - May show nonspecific inflammatory arthritic changes (i.e., erosions, joint destruction, or joint space loss)
  - Ultrasound
    - Useful for guiding arthrocentesis
  - MRI:
    - Highly sensitive for effusion, may help differentiate between transient synovitis and septic arthritis in children
    - Other imaging
      - CT is not routinely indicated.
      - Bone scans are not performed unless there is concurrent suspicion for osteomyelitis.

Diagnostic Procedures/Other

Arthrocentesis in all suspected cases (prior to starting antibiotics): Avoid contaminated tissue (e.g., overlying cellulitis) when performing arthrocentesis.

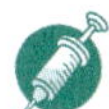

TREATMENT

GENERAL MEASURES

- Admit for parenteral antibiotics and monitoring
  - Begin antibiotics immediately after arthrocentesis.
  - In cases of sepsis or septic shock, empiric antibiotic therapy should *not* be delayed (5)[B].
- Drainage of purulent material in conjunction with antibiotics is mainstay of treatment (5)[C].
  - Pediatric: Surgical drainage and irrigation is recommended if hip involvement due to high risk of avascular necrosis.
  - Prosthetic joint: antibiotics and consult with orthopedics for consideration of revision arthroplasty, resection arthroplasty, or débridement
- Antibiotic therapy for a total of 4 weeks in most cases (5)
  - Each case should be evaluated individually and contextually, consulting infectious disease specialists when appropriate.

MEDICATION

First Line

- Initial antibiotic choice is guided by Gram stain or most likely organism based on age, clinical history, and risk factors.
- Nongonococcal
  - Gram-positive cocci: vancomycin 15 to 20 mg/kg 2 to 3 times daily or linezolid 600 mg twice daily
  - Gram-negative bacilli:
    - Cefepime 2 g twice daily or ceftriaxone 2 g daily or ceftazidime 2 g 3 times daily or cefotaxime 2 g 3 times daily
    - For cephalosporin allergy: Consider treatment with ciprofloxacin 400 mg 3 times daily.
  - Negative Gram stain: vancomycin 15 to 20 mg/kg 2 to 3 times daily plus 3rd-generation cephalosporin until cultures and susceptibilities return
  - Duration of therapy: typically 2 weeks of IV and additional 1 to 2 weeks PO while monitoring therapeutic response closely; if there is contiguous osteomyelitis, then 4 to 6 weeks for antibiotic therapy is needed (4),(5).
- Gonococcal:
  - Ceftriaxone 1 g IV/IM daily for 7 to 14 days
    - Continue at least 24 to 48 hours after symptom resolution.
    - May require concurrent drainage of affected joint
    - Concomitant treatment for *Chlamydia* (doxycycline 100 mg twice daily or azithromycin 1 g once)
- If patient shows improvement and CRP declines after 2 to 4 days of antibiotics, consider switch to PO/IM. Duration depends on clinical response (10 to 14 days up to 3 to 4 weeks) potential choices include:
  - Vancomycin: 15 mg/kg every 6 to 8 hours, adjusted based on renal function and serum levels
  - Ceftriaxone: 50 mg/kg IM once daily
  - Ceftazidime: 50 mg/kg every 8 hours
  - Clindamycin: 10 to 13 mg/kg every 6 to 8 hours
- Other considerations:
  - Narrow antibiotic therapy based on culture results.
  - Consider *Salmonella* in pediatric patients with history of sickle cell disease.
    - 3rd-generation cephalosporins
  - Lyme arthritis: doxycycline 100 mg PO twice daily or amoxicillin 500 mg PO 3 times daily for 28 days if no neurologic involvement, otherwise ceftriaxone dose 2 g IV daily

ISSUES FOR REFERRAL

- Infectious disease specialist consult for IVDU and immunosuppressed patients
- Orthopedic consultation for prosthetic joint infections and to assess drainage modality for all joint infections

ADMISSION, INPATIENT, AND NURSING CONSIDERATIONS

Mean duration of hospitalization is 12 days.

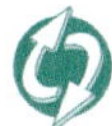

ONGOING CARE

Mobilization of the joint is recommended to start as soon as possible once infection is under control and after drains have been removed and surgical wounds closed (5).

FOLLOW-UP RECOMMENDATIONS

Patient Monitoring

- Can monitor synovial fluid to verify decreasing WBC and sterile fluid after initial treatment
- If no improvement in 24 hours, reevaluate and consider arthroscopy.
- Follow up at 1 week and 1 month after stopping antibiotics to exclude relapse.
- CRP can be used to monitor appropriate treatment response (5).

PROGNOSIS

- Early treatment improves functional outcome.
- Delayed recognition/treatment is associated with higher morbidity and mortality.

COMPLICATIONS

- Mortality rates between 3% and 25%
- Limited joint ROM, ankylosis, osteomyelitis, postinfectious synovitis
- Secondary osteoarthritis; flail, fused, or dislocated joint; sepsis, septic necrosis
- Osteomyelitis, postinfectious synovitis
- Limb length discrepancy (primarily in cases prior to skeletal maturity)

REFERENCES

1. Chan BY, Crawford AM, Kobes PH, et al. Septic arthritis: an evidence-based review of diagnosis and image-guided aspiration. *AJR Am J Roentgenol*. 2020;215(3):568–581.
2. Ross JJ. Septic arthritis of native joints. *Infect Dis Clin North Am*. 2017;31(2):203–218.
3. Dey M, Al-Attar M, Peruffo L, et al. Assessment and diagnosis of the acute hot joint: a systematic review and meta-analysis. *Rheumatology (Oxford)*. 2023;62(5):1740–1756.
4. Woods CR, Bradley JS, Chatterjee A, et al. Clinical practice guideline by the Pediatric Infectious Diseases Society (PIDS) and the Infectious Diseases Society of America (IDSA): 2023 guideline on diagnosis and management of acute bacterial arthritis in pediatrics. *J Pediatric Infect Dis Soc*. 2024;13(1):1–59.
5. Ravn C, Neyt J, Benito N, et al. Guideline for management of septic arthritis in native joints (SANJO). *J Bone Jt Infect*. 2023;8(1):29–37.

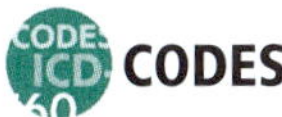

CODES

ICD10

- M00.079 Staphylococcal arthritis, unspecified ankle and foot
- M00.829 Arthritis due to other bacteria, unspecified elbow
- M00.011 Staphylococcal arthritis, right shoulder

CLINICAL PEARLS

- Arthrocentesis and synovial fluid analysis are mandatory in cases of suspected septic arthritis.
- Gram stain has variable sensitivity in septic arthritis. sWBC count is generally >50,000/HPV but is unreliable as a sole diagnostic feature and should be interpreted in context.
- Early IV antibiotics and appropriate drainage of infected joints are critical to successful management.
- Crystalline disease may coexist with septic arthritis.

ARTHROPOD BITES AND STINGS

James E. Powers, DO

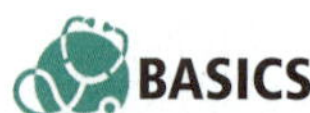

BASICS

DESCRIPTION

- Arthropods are the largest division of the animal kingdom. Two classes, insects and arachnids, have the greatest impact on human health. Arthropods affect humans by inoculating venom, microorganisms, or irritative substances through a bite or sting; by invading tissue, or by contact allergy to their skin, hairs, or secretions.
- Anaphylactic reactions and transmission of infectious microorganisms are the greatest concerns.
- Sequelae of bites, stings, or contact include:
  - Local redness with itch, pain, and swelling: common, usually immediate and transient; large local reactions that increase over 24 to 48 hours. Systemic reactions with anaphylaxis, neurotoxicity, organ damage, or other systemic toxin effects; tissue necrosis or secondary infection

EPIDEMIOLOGY

Incidence

Arthropod bites and stings account for up to 1 million emergency department visits annually in the United States.

Prevalence

Widespread, with regional and seasonal variations

ETIOLOGY AND PATHOPHYSIOLOGY

- Arthropods: four medically important classes
  - Insects: *Hymenoptera* (bees, wasps, hornets, fire ants), mosquitoes, bed bugs, flies, lice, fleas, beetles, caterpillars, and moths
  - Arachnids: spiders, scorpions, mites, and ticks
  - Chilopods: centipedes
  - Diplopods: millipedes
- Four general categories of pathophysiologic effects:
  - Toxic effects of venom: local (tissue inflammation or destruction) versus systemic (neurotoxic or organ damage)
  - Allergic: Antigens in saliva or venom may cause local inflammation, anaphylaxis, or serum sickness. α-Gal syndrome, an immunoglobulin E (IgE)-mediated hypersensitivity to mammalian red meat, is associated with bites from the lone star tick.
  - Trauma: Mechanical injury from biting or stinging causes pain, swelling, and portal of entry for bacteria and secondary infection. Retention of arthropod parts can cause a granulomatous reaction.
  - Infection: Arthropods transmit bacterial, viral, and protozoal diseases.

Genetics

Family history of atopy may increase risk of more severe allergic reactions.

RISK FACTORS

Previous sensitization; although most arthropod contact is inadvertent, certain activities, occupations, and travel exposures increase risk. Greater risk for adverse outcomes in young, elderly, immunocompromised, and those with cardiac or respiratory disease; increased risk of anaphylaxis in patients with mastocytosis

GENERAL PREVENTION

- Avoid common arthropod habitats.
- Insect repellents (effective for mosquitoes, ticks, and flies)
  - N,N-diethyl-meta-toluamide (DEET)
    - Broad spectrum of activity against biting arthropods (1)[A]
    - Concentrations of 20–35% offer approximately 5 hours of protection (1)[A]; safe for children >2 months of age, and pregnant and lactating women (1)[A]
  - Picaridin
    - 20% spray comparable to 20% DEET for mosquito and tick protection
  - p-Menthane-3,8-diol (PMD; lemon eucalyptus extract)
    - 30% concentrations give 4 to 5 hours of protection against mosquitoes and ticks; not for use on children <3 years old
  - Many other products but lack evidence regarding efficacy, duration of action, and safety
- Barrier methods:
  - Use of light-colored pants, long-sleeved shirts, and hats may reduce arthropod impact; permethrin: synthetic insecticide derived from chrysanthemum plant; permethrin-impregnated clothing provides protection against arthropods. Permethrin should not be applied directly to skin; mosquito nets: advised for travelers to disease-endemic areas; permethrin-treated nets may offer additional protection.
- Risk of tick-borne diseases decreased by removal of ticks within 24 hours of attachment.

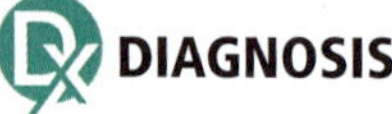

DIAGNOSIS

HISTORY

- Sudden onset of pain or itching with visualization of arthropod
- Many cases unknown to patient or asymptomatic initially; consider in patients presenting with localized erythema, urticaria, wheals, papules, or pruritus
- May identify arthropod by its habitat or by remnants brought by the patient; history of exposure useful but not always reliable; travel, occupational, social, and recreational history may identify risk factors for arthropod exposure.
- Patients with anaphylaxis-associated α-gal syndrome generally present 2 to 6 hours after eating red meat or being exposed to mammalian products.

PHYSICAL EXAM

- If stinger is present, remove by flicking or scraping away from skin.
- Anaphylaxis is a clinical diagnosis. Signs and symptoms include:
  - Erythema, flushing, urticaria, angioedema: Caution—skin involvement absent in up to 20% of cases; itching/edema of lips, tongue, uvula; drooling; respiratory distress, wheeze, repetitive cough, stridor, dysphonia
  - Hypotension, dysrhythmia, syncope, confusion, chest pain, vomiting
- If no evidence of anaphylaxis, the exam focuses on the sting or bite itself. Common findings include local erythema, swelling, wheals, urticaria, papules, or bullae; excoriations from scratching may be present.
- Thorough exam to look for arthropod infestation (lice, scabies) or attached ticks. Body lice usually found in seams of clothing; skin scraping or dermoscopy to identify scabies; signs of secondary bacterial infection after 24 to 48 hours: increasing erythema, pain, fever, lymphangitis, or abscess

DIFFERENTIAL DIAGNOSIS

- Urticaria and localized dermatologic reactions:
  - Contact dermatitis, drug eruption, mastocytosis, bullous diseases, dermatitis herpetiformis, tinea, eczema, vasculitis, pityriasis, erythema multiforme, viral exanthem, cellulitis, abscess, impetigo, folliculitis, erysipelas, necrotizing fasciitis
- Anaphylactic-type reactions
  - Cardiac, hemorrhagic, or septic shock; myocardial infarction; acute respiratory failure, asthma; angioedema, urticarial vasculitis; flushing syndromes (catecholamines, vasoactive peptides); syncope; scombroid

DIAGNOSTIC TESTS & INTERPRETATION

Initial Tests (lab, imaging)

Seldom needed; basic lab parameters usually normal; IgE immunoassays to galactose-α-1,3-galactose can be helpful in diagnosing α-gal syndrome.

Follow-Up Tests & Special Considerations

- Severe envenomations may affect organ function and require monitoring of corresponding lab values.
- Potential arthropod-borne diseases:
  - Ticks: Lyme disease, Rocky Mountain spotted fever, relapsing fever, anaplasmosis, babesiosis, tularemia; ehrlichiosis, Powassan disease; Heartland virus; Bourbon virus; noninfectious complications include tick paralysis and α-gal sensitization resulting in red meat allergy.
  - Flies: tularemia, leishmaniasis, African trypanosomiasis, bartonellosis, loiasis, anthrax
  - Fleas: plague, tularemia, murine typhus
  - Chigger mites: scrub typhus
  - Body lice: epidemic typhus, relapsing fever
  - Kissing bugs: Chagas disease
  - Mosquitoes: malaria, yellow fever, dengue fever, West Nile virus, chikungunya, Zika virus, lymphatic filariasis, Rift Valley fever virus; Japanese Eastern, equine, and St. Louis encephalitis
- Refer patients with anaphylaxis or significant systemic symptoms to an allergist for formal testing (1)[A].

Diagnostic Procedures/Other

Skin and immunologic tests help identify specific allergens. Baseline serum tryptase levels for follow-up of anaphylaxis.

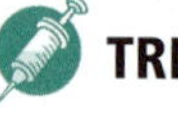

TREATMENT

Most treatments are based on consensus recommendations, clinical experience, or retrospective studies.

ALERT

- Anaphylaxis is potentially life-threatening. Most deaths occur within 30 to 60 minutes.
- Give epinephrine immediately if anaphylaxis suspected; delay associated with increased morbidity and mortality (2)[A]
- Antihistamines and steroids do not replace epinephrine and are never initial therapy in anaphylaxis (2)[A].

GENERAL MEASURES

Routine management of arthropod bites and stings is directed at relieving itching, pain, and swelling; includes local wound care, ice compress, topical corticosteroids, systemic antihistamines, and analgesics

MEDICATION

First Line

- For arthropod bites/stings with anaphylaxis (2)[C]
  - Epinephrine: most important: IM injection in midanterolateral thigh
    - IM dose: epinephrine 1:1,000 (1 mg/mL): 0.01 mg/kg to a maximum dose of 0.3 mg for children and 0.5 mg for adults; can repeat every 5 to 15 minutes
  - High flow oxygen up to 100%
  - Establish 1 to 2 large-bore IV lines; normal saline bolus 20 to 30 mL/kg/; repeat as needed
  - Antihistamines: H_1 and H_2 antagonists are poorly effective in treating cardiovascular and respiratory impacts of anaphylaxis; may have adjunctive role after treatment with epinephrine.
  - Short-acting β-2 agonists (albuterol) may be used if symptoms of bronchoconstriction but do not replace need for epinephrine.
  - *Corticosteroids: 2012 Cochrane review showed no benefit in acute anaphylaxis*; no clear benefit in reducing risk for biphasic reactions; use of steroids such as methylprednisolone is still common practice but their use should never delay or replace treatment with epinephrine.
- Arthropod bites/stings without anaphylaxis
  - Routine wound care; antibiotics only if an infection
  - Tetanus booster, as indicated
  - Oral antihistamines may be helpful in control of itching/hives. Commonly used H_1 and H_2 antagonists include diphenhydramine and cetirizine.
    - H_2 antagonists such as famotidine may be helpful in treating hives and itching but are not FDA approved for this purpose.
  - Oral steroids: Consider short course of prednisone or prednisolone for severe pruritus or local reactions.
  - Consider topical corticosteroids.
    - OTC 1% hydrocortisone; may consider higher potency such as triamcinolone 0.1%, fluocinolone 0.025%
  - Other specific therapies:
    - Scorpion stings: Treat excess catecholamine release (nitroprusside, prazosin, β-blockers); atropine for hypersalivation; consider antivenom if severe symptoms and in consultation with a toxicologist (1)[B].
    - Black widow bites: Treat muscle spasms with benzodiazepines and opioid analgesics; antivenom available for severe symptoms and in consultation with a toxicologist (1)[B]
    - Consult Poison Control for questions regarding envenomation management: 1-800-222-1222.
  - Fire ants: characteristically cause sterile pustules; leave intact—do not open or drain.
  - Brown recluse spider: local wound care, tetanus prophylaxis as indicated, pain control, supportive treatment; surgical consult if débridement needed (1)[C]
  - Ticks: early removal to reduce risk of disease transmission
  - Pediculosis: head, pubic, and body lice
    - First line: permethrin 1% topical lotion (3)[A]; alternatives: pyrethrins; ivermectin PO shown to be effective but not FDA-approved for pediculosis. Repeat treatment in 7 to 10 days.
    - Body lice usually treated successfully by bathing and laundering clothing and linens in hot water (3)[A].
  - *Sarcoptes scabiei*—scabies:
    - Permethrin 5% cream is generally considered first-line treatment: Apply to entire body. Wash off after 8 to 14 hours. Repeat in 1 week (3)[A].
    - Ivermectin: 200 μg/kg PO once; repeat in 2 weeks shown to be effective but not FDA-approved for scabies.

ISSUES FOR REFERRAL

Patients with anaphylaxis or significant systemic symptoms should be referred to an allergist for formal testing (1)[A].

SURGERY/OTHER PROCEDURES

Débridement and delayed skin grafting may be required for severe brown recluse spider bites.

COMPLEMENTARY & ALTERNATIVE MEDICINE

- Ice, cool compresses; calamine lotion commonly used but no clear benefit.
- A paste of 3 tsp of baking soda and 1 tsp water may help salve bites.

ADMISSION, INPATIENT, AND NURSING CONSIDERATIONS

Admission required for anaphylaxis, vascular instability, neuromuscular events, renal damage/failure, or severe pain, infection

ONGOING CARE

All patients experiencing an anaphylactic reaction must be prescribed one or more epinephrine autoinjectors and be educated on anaphylactic risks, recognition, and self-treatment. Epinephrine nasal spray, approved by the FDA for the treatment of anaphylactic reactions, is an alternative to epinephrine autoinjectors for patients with anaphylaxis.

FOLLOW-UP RECOMMENDATIONS

Venom immunotherapy is the cornerstone of treatment for *Hymenoptera* stings; 80–98% effective so patients with anaphylaxis should be referred to allergist for testing.

Patient Monitoring

Monitor for delayed effects, including infectious diseases from arthropod bites; serum sickness reactions, vasculitis (rare)

DIET

Patients with suspected or confirmed α-gal syndrome should avoid ingesting red meats, including beef, pork, venison, and lamb. Allergic reactions to mammalian dairy products are also possible.

PATIENT EDUCATION

Provide instruction on symptomatic care, arthropod avoidance, and infection and vector-borne disease surveillance. For patients with anaphylaxis, provide action plan and instructions on the use of epinephrine (2)[C].

PROGNOSIS

- Excellent for local reactions and mild systemic symptoms
- In anaphylaxis, immediate treatment with epinephrine significantly reduces morbidity and mortality.

COMPLICATIONS

- Anaphylaxis, including delayed reactions associated with α-gal syndrome
- Secondary bacterial infection; arthropod-associated infectious diseases
- Scarring
- Psychological effects, phobias

REFERENCES

1. Herness J, Snyder MJ, Newman RS. Arthropod bites and stings. *Am Fam Physician*. 2022;106(2):137–147.
2. Cardona V, Ansotegui IJ, Ebisawa M, et al. World Allergy Organization anaphylaxis guidance 2020. *World Allergy Organ J*. 2020;13(10):100472. doi:10.1016/j.waojou.2020.100472.
3. Finnikin SJ, Wilcock J, Edwards PJ. Presentation and management of insect bites in out-of-hours primary care: a descriptive study. *BMJ Open*. 2023;13(9):e070636. doi:10.1136/bmjopen-2022-070636.

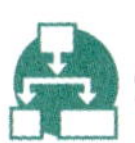

SEE ALSO

- Centers for Disease Control: Preventing Tick Bites
- Centers for Disease Control: Alpha-gal Syndrome

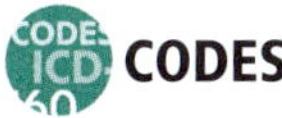

CODES

ICD10

- T63.481A Toxic effect of venom of arthropod, accidental, init
- T63.301A Toxic effect of unsp spider venom, accidental, init
- T63.484A Toxic effect of venom of oth arthropod, undetermined, init

CLINICAL PEARLS

- Urgent administration of epinephrine is the key to successful treatment of anaphylaxis.
- Local treatment and symptom management are sufficient in most arthropod bites and stings.
- Tick-borne illness is on the rise in the United States.

ASCITES

Tasaduq Hussain Mir, MD, FAAFP • Afsha Rais Kaisani, MD, FAAFP • Shana-Kay Lambert-Johnson, MD

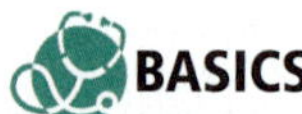

BASICS

DESCRIPTION

Ascites is the pathologic accumulation of fluid in the peritoneal cavity and the most common complication of cirrhosis (1). It may occur in conditions that cause generalized edema (e.g., nephrotic syndrome, heart failure, malignancy)

- Amount of fluid accumulation:
  - Grade 1: mild ascites—only detected by ultrasound; responsive ascites
  - Grade 2: moderate ascites—moderate symmetric distension of abdomen visible on exam; recurrent ascites
  - Grade 3: large or gross ascites—marked distension of the abdomen; refractory ascites (RA)
    - Ascitic fluid that recurs after paracentesis or cannot be prevented by treatment
- Men generally have no fluid in peritoneal cavity; women may have up to 20 mL depending on menstrual phase.

EPIDEMIOLOGY

- Children: most commonly associated with nephrotic syndrome, malignancy, portal hypertension and congenital heart disease with right-sided heart failure
- Adults: cirrhosis (81%), cancer (10%), heart failure (3%), tuberculosis (TB) 2%, other (6%)
- 50% of patients with decompensated cirrhosis develop ascites.

Incidence

Approximately 50–60% of cirrhotic patients develop ascites within 10 years (2). Presence of ascites in cirrhotic patients is a poor prognostic indicator with median survival of ~1 year after onset.

Prevalence

10% of patients with cirrhosis have ascites.

ETIOLOGY AND PATHOPHYSIOLOGY

- Portal hypertension versus nonportal hypertension
  - Cannot confirm etiology without paracentesis
  - Serum-ascites albumin gradient (SAAG): (serum albumin level: ascites albumin level) helps to differentiate
- High portal pressure (SAAG ≥1.1 g/dL)—reflects portal hypertension
  - Cirrhosis, hepatitis (alcoholic, viral, autoimmune, medications), acute liver failure, liver malignancy (primary or metastatic), heart failure or constrictive pericarditis, Budd-Chiari syndrome, and portal vein thrombosis
- Normal portal pressure (SAAG <1.1 g/dL)—excludes portal hypertension
  - Peritoneal carcinomatosis, TB, severe hypoalbuminemia (nephrotic syndrome; severe enteropathy with protein loss), Meigs syndrome (ovarian cancer), lymphatic leak (chylous ascites), pancreatitis, inflammatory (vasculitis, lupus serositis, sarcoidosis), other infections (parasitic, fungal), hemoperitoneum (trauma or ectopic pregnancy)
- Pathogenesis of ascites in the setting of portal hypertension (cirrhotic ascites): backward transmission of increased pressure to the visceral capillary bed with subsequent dilation and shift of fluid to the peritoneal cavity.
  - This decreases intravascular volume and leads to hypotension. Systemic hypovolemia triggers renin-angiotensin-aldosterone system.

Genetics

Genetic predisposition might play a role.

RISK FACTORS

- Cirrhosis—hepatitis B and C; alcohol abuse
- Metabolic dysfunction associated steatotic liver disease (MASLD)
- Congestive heart failure (CHF); advanced kidney disease; malignancy
- TB

GENERAL PREVENTION

Lifestyle—appropriate diet; physical activity; safe sexual practices; avoid alcohol misuse and hepatotoxic medications.

COMMONLY ASSOCIATED CONDITIONS

Nephrotic syndrome, liver cancer, heart failure

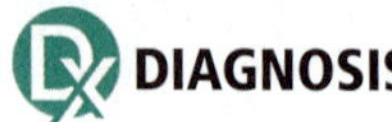

DIAGNOSIS

History, physical examination, and diagnostic abdominal paracentesis are key to diagnosis.

HISTORY

- Address risk factors (e.g., EtOH use, TB exposure, prior malignancies, sexual partners, transfusion history, metabolic syndrome, increased risk of nonalcoholic steatohepatitis progressing to cirrhosis, previous history of cardiac illness).
- Assess for symptoms of underlying disease (chest pain, dyspnea, orthopnea, peripheral edema, asterixis, weight loss, night sweats, chronic cough).
- Assess for complications (fever/abdominal pain might indicate spontaneous bacterial peritonitis [SBP], progressive dyspnea due to increased abdominal girth).
- Progressive abdominal distention may be painful.

PHYSICAL EXAM

- Abdominal distention with flank/shifting dullness is the most sensitive (83%) and specific (56%) exam finding; requires >1,500 mL of fluid to detect
- Signs of right-sided heart failure: peripheral edema (penile/scrotal, pedal), increased jugular venous pressure
- Stigmata of chronic liver cirrhosis (palmar erythema, spider angiomata, dilated abdominal wall collateral veins)
- Other signs of advanced liver disease: jaundice, muscle wasting, gynecomastia, leukonychia, asterixis
- Signs of underlying malignancy: cachexia; supraclavicular (Virchow) node suggests upper abdominal malignancy.

DIFFERENTIAL DIAGNOSIS

Obesity; large ovarian tumors; bowel obstruction; massive splenomegaly

DIAGNOSTIC TESTS & INTERPRETATION

Diagnostic abdominal paracentesis is the most cost-effective method.

Initial Tests (lab, imaging)

- Abdominal ultrasound (can detect small volumes of ascitic fluid ~100 mL)—highly sensitive, cost-effective, no radiation
- Diagnostic paracentesis to rule out infection with clinically new-onset ascites or new abdominal pain in patient with ascites
- Ascitic fluid should be sent for analysis for cell count, protein, gram stain, and culture (2)[C].
  - Cell count and differential: Polymorphonuclear (PMN) leukocytes ≥250 cells/mm^3 is diagnostic of SBP.
  - Albumin to calculate SAAG (obtained by subtracting ascitic fluid albumin from serum albumin obtained on the *same* day):
    - <1.1 g/dL indicates a low portal pressure exudative process (i.e., inflammatory, biliary/pancreatic, carcinomatosis, TB).
    - ≥1.1 g/dL indicates portal hypertensive/transudative process (cirrhosis, CHF, constrictive pericarditis, thrombosis).
    - Other tests (based on clinical scenario to rule out etiologies other than cirrhosis) (2)[C]
- Portal US Doppler can detect thrombosis or cirrhosis.
- CT scan for intra-abdominal pathology (malignancy)
- MRI preferred for evaluation of liver disease or confirmation of portal vein thrombosis

Follow-Up Tests & Special Considerations

- All patients with cirrhosis should be evaluated for hepatocellular carcinoma with ultrasound every 6 months.
- Complete metabolic panel (CMP), complete blood count (CBC), PT/INR should be checked every 6 months to calculate Child-Pugh and Model for End-Stage Liver Disease (MELD).

Diagnostic Procedures/Other

Laparoscopy: if imaging and paracentesis are nondiagnostic

- Allows for direct visualization and biopsy of peritoneum, liver, and intra-abdominal lymph nodes
- Preferred for evaluating suspected peritoneal TB or malignancies

Test Interpretation

Cytology may reveal malignant cells: adenocarcinoma (ovary, breast, GI tract) or primary peritoneal carcinoma (most commonly associated with ascites).

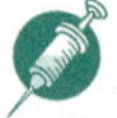

TREATMENT

For all patients, first-line treatment consists of:

- Daily weight
- Restrict dietary sodium to ≤2 g/day if the cause is due to portal hypertension (high SAAG).
- Water restriction (1 to 1.5 L/day) only necessary if evidence of hyponatremia (serum sodium <120 to 125 mEq/L)
- Avoid alcohol and ensure adequate nutrition if liver disease.
- Baclofen may be used to reduce alcohol craving/consumption in EtOH cirrhosis.

GENERAL MEASURES

Prophylactic antibiotics to prevent SBP should be started in patients who have a prior history of SBP, or in those with ascitic fluid protein <1.5 g/dL (15 g/L) and evidence of advanced liver disease (Child-Pugh score ≥9 or bilirubin ≥3 mg/dL), kidney disease (serum creatinine ≥1.2 mg/dL, BUN ≥25 mg/dL, or serum sodium ≤130 mmol/L), or acute GI bleeding.

MEDICATION

ALERT

- Aggressive diuresis can induce acute kidney injury (AKI), encephalopathy, and hyponatremia. Monitor creatinine and electrolytes. Serum creatinine >2 mg/dL or serum sodium <120 mmol/L warrants withdrawal of diuretics.

- Avoid nonsteroidal anti-inflammatory drugs (NSAIDs) (can exacerbate oliguria/azotemia).
- Angiotensin-converting enzyme (ACE) inhibitors and angiotensin receptor blockers (ARBs) may be harmful due to an increased risk of hypotension and renal failure. Avoid in RA.
- Consider discontinuing β-blockers in patients with RA, SBP, worsening hypotension (SBP <90 mm hg), AKI, hyponatremia <130 mEq/L, or azotemia.

First Line

- Sodium restriction and diuretics are the mainstay of treatment for patients with elevated portal pressures; other causes (e.g., carcinomatosis) are less likely to respond.
  - Spironolactone 100 to 400 mg daily PO; typical initial dose is 100 to 200 mg in AM.
  - Furosemide 40 to 160 mg daily PO; typical initial dose is 40 mg in AM.
  - Most common and preferred regimen is spironolactone and furosemide together (initial ratio of 100:40 mg/day)for maximum efficacy and potassium homeostasis.
- Diuretic-intractable/RA (10% of patients—50% mortality in 6 months) defined as:
  - Persistent or worsening ascites despite maximum doses of spironolactone (400 mg/day) and furosemide (160 mg/day) for at least 1 week
  - Recurrence of grade 2 or 3 ascites within 4 weeks of achieving minimal ascites.
  - Diuretic-induced complications like hepatic encephalopathy, hyponatremia to <125 mEq/L, renal impairment with creatinine rise of 100% to >2
- Additional management:
  - Discontinue diuretics if urinary sodium excretion with diuretics is less than 30 mmol/day.
  - Therapeutic paracentesis or serial large-volume paracentesis (LVP).
  - IV furosemide reduces eGFR dramatically in ascitic patients and is better avoided.

Second Line

- Midodrine 7.5 mg TID can be used for RA or hypotensive patients may improve survival (2)[B]. Titrate to blood pressure response.
- Alternatives to spironolactone: amiloride up to 40 mg/day; triamterene up to 200 mg/day in divided doses (2)[C]
- Alternatives to furosemide: torsemide up to 100 mg/day; bumetanide up to 4 mg/day (2)[C]
- Vaptans: FDA recommended avoiding use in chronic liver disease due to potential for inducing serious liver injury (3)[A].

ISSUES FOR REFERRAL

Liver transplant is the definitive treatment for portal hypertension. Consider referral for transplant in patients with decompensated liver disease, whether ascites is present/controlled (2)[B]. Patients with cirrhosis and MELD score of 15 or more should be referred for liver transplant.

SURGERY/OTHER PROCEDURES

- Therapeutic paracentesis
  - Initial therapy if tense ascites is present (2)[C]. Serial (generally every 2 weeks) paracenteses can be used in patients with elevated portal pressures. Continue diuretics at 50% of the previous dose if transitioning to serial paracentesis in patients failing diuretic monotherapy.
  - Replace albumin if removing >5 L of ascites; 6 to 8 g/L removed
- Transjugular intrahepatic portosystemic shunt (TIPS): effective for diuretic RA.
- Automated low flow ascites pump drains ascitic fluid from peritoneal cavity to urinary bladder for elimination; used in patients with contraindication to TIPS placement or liver transplant
- Peritoneovenous shunt (LeVeen or Denver shunt): drains ascites directly into the inferior vena cava and reserved for patients with RA not candidates for TIPS or liver transplant and unable to tolerate repeat paracentesis (2)[C]
- Indwelling catheters with external drainage: useful in malignant ascites as palliative measure

ADMISSION, INPATIENT, AND NURSING CONSIDERATIONS

Admit patient in hospital who have cirrhosis and present with new abdominal pain, fever, and hypotension.

ONGOING CARE

FOLLOW-UP RECOMMENDATIONS

Patient Monitoring

CMP, CBC, PT/INR should be checked every 6 months to calculate Child-Pugh and MELD.

DIET

Low sodium diet (<2 g/day)

PROGNOSIS

Prognosis varies depending on underlying cause. Ascites in itself is rarely life-threatening but can signify life-threatening underlying disease.

COMPLICATIONS

- SBP: ascitic fluid PMN leukocyte count $\geq$250 cells/mm^3 or positive culture
- Hepatorenal syndrome
  - Type 1—rapid acute worsening of renal function evolving in the setting of a known precipitating factor
  - Type 2—slowly progressive in the setting of RA
- Cellulitis: common in obese patients with brawny edema; treat with diuretics and antibiotics (2)[B].
- Hepatic hydrothorax: pleural effusion due to transdiaphragmatic movement of ascitic fluid
- RA unresponsive to the medical management requiring paracentesis and surgical procedures like TIPS

REFERENCES

1. Tapper EB, Parikh ND. Diagnosis and management of cirrhosis and its complications: a review. *JAMA*. 2023;329(18):1589–1602. doi:10.1001/jama.2023.5997.
2. Cornman-Homonoff J, Fortune BE, Kolli KP, et al. Management of ascites: AJR Expert Panel Narrative Review [published online ahead of print April 9, 2025]. *AJR Am J Roentgenol*. 2025. doi:10.2214/AJR.23.30768.
3. Rogal SS, Hansen L, Patel A, et al. AASLD practice guidance: palliative care and symptom-based management in decompensated cirrhosis. *Hepatology*. 2022;76(3):819–853. doi:10.1002/hep.32378.

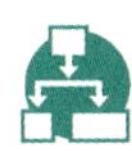

SEE ALSO

- Cirrhosis of the Liver; Hepatorenal Syndrome
- Algorithms: Congestive Heart Failure: Differential Diagnosis; Nephrotic Syndrome

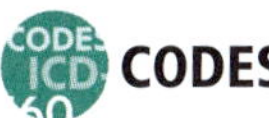

CODES

ICD10

- R18.8 Other ascites
- R18.0 Malignant ascites
- K70.31 Alcoholic cirrhosis of liver with ascites

CLINICAL PEARLS

- Ascites is most commonly caused by cirrhosis-related portal hypertension.
- Patient with new-onset ascites should undergo diagnostic paracentesis; SAAG is reliable diagnostic tool to differentiate cause.
- Management includes sodium restriction, diuretics, serial paracentesis and evaluation for transplant.
- Avoid NSAIDs, ACE inhibitors, ARBs, and nonselective β-blockers.
- Inability to adhere to dietary sodium restriction is the most common cause of "diuretic-intractable ascites."
- SBP is a critical complication requiring empiric treatment.

ASTHMA

Sarah J. Wu, MD • Scott Kopec, MD

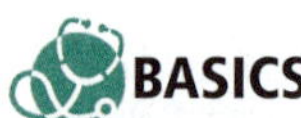

BASICS

DESCRIPTION

- A heterogeneous disease characterized as chronic inflammation of the airway
- Patient may experience symptoms-free periods alternating with sporadic flare-up (exacerbations) brought on by triggers (e.g., exercise, allergens, weather changes, viral respiratory infections).
- There are many different asthma phenotypes, with the most common including allergic asthma, nonallergic asthma, adult-onset, asthma with fixed airflow limitation, asthma of obesity, and cough variant asthma.
- Asthma severity is assessed retrospectively from treatment required to control symptoms.
  - Mild: well controlled with step 1 or 2 treatment (i.e., with as-needed ICS-formoterol alone or with low-intensity maintenance controller treatment)
  - Moderate: well controlled with step 3 or 4 treatment (i.e., low- or medium-dose inhaled corticosteroids [ICS] long-acting β-agonists [LABA])
  - Severe: remains "uncontrolled" with optimized treatment with high-dose ICS-LABA or that requires high-dose ICS-LABA to prevent it from becoming "uncontrolled"

EPIDEMIOLOGY

Incidence

The yearly incidence rate of asthma in United States ~3.8/1,000 at-risk adults and 12.5/1,000 at-risk children (1). Incidence varies by demographic group.

Prevalence

Asthma affects 262 million individuals worldwide.

- In 2021, 7.7% of the U.S. population had asthma (2).
- African Americans are three times more likely to die from asthma.
- Asthma affects about 10% of children ages 5 to 18 years in the United States.
- Obesity is associated with increased prevalence and incidence of asthma.
- Rate of asthma deaths is largest among those ages ≥65 years.

ETIOLOGY AND PATHOPHYSIOLOGY

Asthma is defined by airway hyperresponsiveness. Several theorized contributory mechanisms, including inflammatory cell infiltration and degranulation, subbasement fibrosis, mucus hypersecretion, epithelial injury, significant smooth muscle hypertrophy and hyperreactivity, and angiogenesis lead to reversible bronchospasm, which lead to intermittent airway obstruction.

Genetics

Broadly, there is a genetic association between asthma and genes that are involved in the production of inflammatory cytokines (e.g., interleukin [IL]-13 and IL-4) that lead to IgE production, recruitment of inflammatory cells (e.g., eosinophils, basophils, T cells) and the differentiation of T cells into Th2 cells. The subsequent inflammation leads to increased airway hyperresponsiveness. The immunotherapies lebrikizumab, tralokinumab, and dupilumab target these cytokine signaling pathways.

RISK FACTORS

- Genetic predisposition, sex, obesity, preterm or small for gestational age (SGA)
- Environmental: viral infections, animal and airborne allergens, tobacco smoke exposure, e-cigarette use, pollution, stress
- Aspirin or NSAIDs hypersensitivity

GENERAL PREVENTION

- Avoidance of environmental tobacco exposure during pregnancy and first year of life (1)
- Encourage vaginal delivery and breastfeeding (1).
- Avoid use of broad-spectrum antibiotics during first year of life (1).
- Avoid allergens and triggers in new-onset asthma.

COMMONLY ASSOCIATED CONDITIONS

- Atopy: eczema, allergic conjunctivitis, allergic rhinitis
- Obesity (associated with higher asthma rates)
- Gastroesophageal reflux disease (GERD)
- Obstructive sleep apnea (OSA)

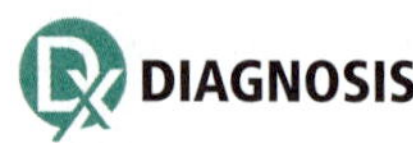

DIAGNOSIS

HISTORY

History of variable respiratory symptoms:

- More than one symptom such as wheeze, dyspnea, cough, chest tightness
- Symptoms that are worse at night, vary in time and intensity, and are worse with common triggers

PHYSICAL EXAM

- May be normal
- Focus on
  - Rhinitis, nasal polyps, swollen nasal turbinates
  - Expiratory wheezing, prolonged expiratory phase Note: Wheezing may be absent in severe exacerbation due to severely reduced airflow.
  - Skin: eczema

DIFFERENTIAL DIAGNOSIS

- In children: upper airway disease (allergic rhinitis or sinusitis), large airway obstruction (e.g., foreign body aspiration, vocal cord dysfunction, vascular ring or laryngeal web, laryngotracheomalacia, enlarged lymph nodes, tumor), small airway obstruction (e.g., viral bronchiolitis, cystic fibrosis, bronchopulmonary dysplasia, heart disease, primary ciliary dyskinesia, bronchiectasis)
- In adults: chronic obstructive pulmonary disease (COPD), bronchiectasis, heart failure, pulmonary embolism, tumor, pulmonary infiltration with eosinophilia, Churg-Strauss syndrome, medication-induced cough (ACE inhibitors), vocal cord dysfunction
- Chronic upper airway cough syndrome, aspiration, GERD

DIAGNOSTIC TESTS & INTERPRETATION

Initial Tests (lab, imaging)

- Blood tests are not required but may find eosinophilia or elevated serum IgE levels (allergic asthma).
- The gold standard of diagnosis is documented variable expiratory airflow limitation.
- Chest x-ray to exclude alternative diagnoses

Follow-Up Tests & Special Considerations

Assess asthma symptoms control with simple screening tools, such as consensus-based Global Initiative for Asthma (GINA) symptom control tool or Primary Care Asthma Control Screening tool (PACS). Use the review, assess, adjust method of ongoing management.

Diagnostic Procedures/Other

- Allergy skin testing is not useful for diagnosis of asthma but may be to evaluate atopic triggers.
- Measurement of fractional exhaled nitric oxide (FeNO) suggests eosinophilic airway inflammation.

Test Interpretation

Spirometry or peak expiratory flow (PEF) is used to diagnose asthma. Examples of positive tests include an increase in baseline in FEV1 ≥12% or FVC ≥200 mL on spirometry with methacholine challenge, excessive variability in diurnal PEF over 2 weeks (10% in adults, 13% in children), fall in FEV1 on bronchial challenge test (with positive result varying depending on method of testing), or significant increase in lung function after 4 weeks of daily ICS treatment (≥12% FEV1 in adults and children) (1).

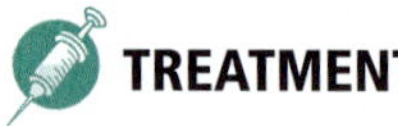

TREATMENT

GENERAL MEASURES

- Focus on symptom control and prevention of exacerbations.
- Smoking cessation
- Use of holding chambers ("spacers") with inhaled agents improves clinical outcomes.
- Encourage physical activity, weight loss, smoking cessation, avoidance of irritants, emotional stress.
- Avoidance of occupational exposure
- Annual influenza vaccine; consider pneumococcal vaccine.

ALERT

Treatment of asthma with short-acting β-agonists (SABAs) alone is no longer recommended by the GINA guidelines for adults and adolescents. ICS therapy is essential to reduce risk of death and severe exacerbations.

Pediatric Considerations

Treatment for children 6 to 11 years old:

- Step 1 for asthma symptoms 1 to 2 days/week or less: as needed low-dose ICS *plus* SABA
- Step 2 for asthma symptoms 2 to 5 days/week:
  - Maintenance low-dose ICS *plus* as-needed SABA
  - Or daily leukotriene receptor antagonist (LTRA)
- Step 3 for asthma symptoms 4 to 5 days/week or waking due to asthma ≥1 time/week:
  - Maintenance low-dose ICS-LABA *plus* as-needed SABA
  - Or maintenance medium-dose ICS *plus* as-needed SABA
  - Or very-low-dose ICS-formoterol maintenance and reliever therapy (MART)
  - Or daily low-dose ICS *plus* LTRA *plus* as-needed SABA
- Initial asthma presentation is during an acute exacerbation: Treat for exacerbation with short course of OCS and commence step 3 or step 4 of treatment

- Tiotropium is not indicated in children aged <12 years.
- Reliever for all management steps in children aged 6 to 11 years is as-needed SABA.

Pregnancy Considerations

- Do not use bronchial provocation test nor step down controller treatment until after delivery. Cessation of ICS during pregnancy is a significant risk factor for exacerbation.
- Poorly controlled asthma results in low birth weight, increased prematurity, and perinatal mortality.
- All short-acting agents (SABA) are pregnancy Category C as well as ICS.
- LTRAs montelukast and zafirlukast are Category B but are not studied extensively in pregnancy.

Geriatric Considerations

- Asthma is underdiagnosed in geriatric populations due to overlapping comorbidities, such as COPD, heart failure, and OSA.
- Elderly patients are at higher risk from side effects of high-dose ICS such as pneumonia, decreased bone mineral density, retinopathy, and cataracts. They are also vulnerable to side effects of long-acting muscarinic antagonists (LAMAs), such as urinary outlet obstruction and narrow-angle glaucoma (3).
- LTRAs may be beneficial in elderly asthmatics who prefer a pill and/or have difficulty adhering to inhalers.

MEDICATION

First Line

- Categories of medications (1)
  - SABA: e.g., levalbuterol, albuterol
  - ICS
  - LABA: formoterol, salmeterol, vilanterol, indacaterol
  - Controller medications: contain ICS; used to control symptoms and reduce exacerbations
  - Reliever medications: contain ICS-formoterol, ICS-SABA, and/or SABA; used for as-needed relief of breakthrough symptoms and short-term prevention of exercise-induced bronchoconstriction (EIB)
    - Combination ICS-LABA with non-formoterol LABA cannot be used as a reliever as the non-formoterol LABAs have a slower onset of action and should not be used more than once daily.
    - ICS-formoterol should not be used as the reliever for patients on maintenance ICS-LABA with a non-formoterol LABA.
  - MART: only ICS-formoterol inhalers; the most recent GINA guidelines recommend treatment based on 2 tracks for patients >12 years old (1).
- Track 1: Reliever is low-dose ICS-formoterol; preferred because it reduces the risk of severe exacerbations compared to SABA reliever
  - Steps 1 to 2 for asthma symptoms ≤1 to 5 days/week, with normal or mildly reduced lung function: symptom-driven treatment with as-needed low-dose ICS-formoterol
  - Step 3 for asthma symptoms ≥4 to 5 days/week, waking from asthma >1 time/week, or low lung function: low-dose ICS-formoterol as daily maintenance treatment and as-needed for breakthrough symptoms (MART therapy)
  - Step 4 for daily asthma symptoms, waking from asthma >1 time/week, with low lung function: maintenance medium-dose ICS-formoterol MART therapy
  - Initial asthma presentation is an acute exacerbation: Treat with short course of oral corticosteroids (OCS) and commence medium-dose MART.
- Track 2: Maintenance with regular daily low-dose ICS *plus* as-needed SABA. Less preferred as adherence with ICS can be poor and patients who take SABA alone are at risk of increased exacerbations.
  - Step 1 for asthma symptoms ≤1 to 5 days/week: symptom-driven treatment with as-needed SABA *plus* low-dose ICS
  - Step 2 for asthma symptoms ≤3 to 5 days/week, with normal or mildly reduced lung function: maintenance ICS inhaler *plus* as-needed SABA
  - Step 3 for asthma symptoms ≥4 to 5 days/week, waking from asthma >1 time/week, or low lung function: maintenance low-dose ICS-LABA *plus* as-needed SABA or maintenance medium-dose ICS *plus* as-needed SABA
  - Step 4 for daily asthma symptoms, waking from asthma >1 time/week, with low lung function: maintenance medium- or high-dose ICS-LABA *plus* as-needed SABA or as-needed ICS-SABA
  - Initial asthma presentation is an acute exacerbation: Treat with short course of OCS and commence medium- or high-dose ICS-LABA *plus* as-needed SABA.

Second Line

LTRAs and anti-IgE therapy are options for augmenting treatment in patients with uncontrolled symptoms.

ISSUES FOR REFERRAL

- Specialized testing (e.g., bronchoprovocation)
- Specialized treatments (e.g., immunotherapy)
- Poorly controlled asthma, frequent exacerbation, or multiple emergency department visits
- Occupational asthma due to legal implications

ADDITIONAL THERAPIES

- Allergen immunotherapy when there is a clear relationship between symptoms and exposure
- Management of acute exacerbation of asthma: mild symptoms: Patients who are speaking in full sentences, HR <120 beats/minute, oxygen saturation 90–95%, and peak flow >50% of predicted can be managed as outpatient with ICS-formoterol *or* SABA/ICS *plus* prednisone. Step up dose of ICS-containing treatment for 2 to 4 weeks.
- Severe symptoms: Patients who are not able to speak in full sentences, are using accessory muscles to breathe, are drowsy/confused, and/or have no lung sounds on auscultation ("silent chest"), HR >120 beats/minute, oxygen saturation <90%, PEF <60% predicted or personal best, or are not responding to treatment in 48 hours should be considered for inpatient treatment of asthma exacerbation with oral or IV corticosteroids and scheduled nebulizers.

SURGERY/OTHER PROCEDURES

Bronchial thermoplasty is a therapeutic option for adult patients with severe persistent asthma uncontrolled by ICS and LABA.

ADMISSION, INPATIENT, AND NURSING CONSIDERATIONS

Admitted patients should receive systemic corticosteroids and resume or commence, ICS-containing therapy upon discharge.

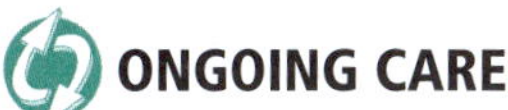

ONGOING CARE

FOLLOW-UP RECOMMENDATIONS

ICS-containing treatment should be stepped up for 2 to 4 weeks, and reliever medication reduced to as-needed use.

Patient Monitoring

- Patients should be seen in follow-up early, ideally before discontinuation of OCS.
- Consider stepping down treatment once symptoms are controlled for 3 months.

DIET

Maternal obesity during pregnancy poses an increased risk for asthma in the child (1).

PROGNOSIS

Prognosis is good with adherence to inhaler regimens.

COMPLICATIONS

- Atelectasis, pneumonia, medication-specific side effects/adverse effects/interactions
- Respiratory failure; death: ~50% of asthma deaths occur in the elderly (age >65 years)

REFERENCES

1. Global Initiative for Asthma. 2024 GINA strategy report: global strategy for asthma management and prevention. https://ginasthma.org/2025-gina-strategy-report/. Accessed November 11, 2025.
2. Pate CA, Zahran HS. The status of asthma in the United States. *Prev Chronic Dis*. 2024;21:E53. doi:10.5888/pcd21.240005.
3. Khosa JK, Louie S, Lobo Moreno P, et al. Asthma care in the elderly: practical guidance and challenges for clinical management—a framework of 5 "Ps." *J Asthma Allergy*. 2023;16:33–43. doi:10.2147/JAA.S293081.

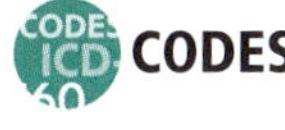

CODES

ICD10

- J45.20 Mild intermittent asthma, uncomplicated
- J45.52 Severe persistent asthma with status asthmaticus
- J45.51 Severe persistent asthma with (acute) exacerbation

CLINICAL PEARLS

- SABA *plus* ICS or formoterol/ICS is the most effective rescue therapy for acute asthma symptoms.
- Holding chambers should be used by all.
- ICSs are the preferred long-term control therapy for patients of all ages.

ATELECTASIS

Kaitlyn Kennedy, MD • Scott Kopec, MD

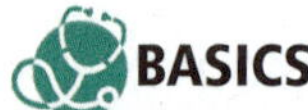

BASICS

DESCRIPTION

- Atelectasis is defined as the incomplete expansion of lung tissue due to collapse or closure of the airways.
- Broadly categorized as:
  - Obstructive: due to airway blockage
  - Nonobstructive: multiple etiologies including loss of contact between the parietal and visceral pleurae, replacement of lung tissue by scarring or infiltrative disease, surfactant dysfunction, and parenchymal compression
- Atelectasis can be further classified by:
  - The amount of lung involved (lobar, segmental, subsegmental)
  - Location within the lung
- Often asymptomatic; symptoms depend on the rate of collapse, the amount of lung involved, and whether the patient has underlying lung disease and/or comorbidities.
- Reduced respiratory gas exchange can cause hypoxemia.

EPIDEMIOLOGY

- Mean age is 60 years, but all ages are susceptible
- Male = female; no racial or socioeconomic predilection
- No significant pre-disposing risk factors related to underlying COPD, asthma, or age
- Frequently occurs in immobilized patients and patients on mechanical ventilation
- Increased risk in postoperative patients especially in patients undergoing cardiothoracic, thoracic, or upper abdominal procedures
- Patients with lung or chest wall injury (i.e., rib fractures)
- Obesity and pregnancy are associated with an increased risk.

Incidence

Postoperative atelectasis, especially after major cardiovascular or gastrointestinal (GI) procedures; can be seen in up to 90% of patients

Prevalence

Rounded atelectasis can be seen in up to 65–70% of patients with significant asbestos exposure

ETIOLOGY AND PATHOPHYSIOLOGY

Physiologically, atelectasis occurs when collapsing forces (positive pleural pressure, surface tension) overcome expanding forces (alveolar pressure, elastic recoil) of the lung. This then causes an impairment in oxygenation of the blood from the lung, and causes reduced lung compliance.

- Obstructive (resorptive) atelectasis is caused by intrinsic airway blockage and is the most common variety. It can be caused by luminal blockage (i.e., foreign body, mucus plug, asthma, cystic fibrosis, trauma, mass lesion) or airway wall abnormality (i.e., congenital malformation, emphysema).
  - Distal to the obstruction, alveolar air is rapidly reabsorbed into the deoxygenated venous system, causing complete collapse of the alveolar tissue.
  - The patency and function of the collateral ventilatory systems in each lobe (pores of Kohn, canals of Lambert, and fenestrations of Boren) depends on multiple patient factors including age, underlying lung disease, and FiO_2, as well as the amount of collateral ventilation systems.
  - In patients with emphysema, the fenestra of Boren become enlarged, which acts as a compensatory mechanism and can lead to a delay in atelectasis despite an obstructing lesion or mass.
- Nonobstructive atelectasis
  - Passive atelectasis (i.e., during a pleural effusion, pneumothorax, or large emphysematous bulla) occurs with the parietal and visceral pleura connection is disrupted coupled with the associated loss of normal negative pressure within the pleura space.
  - Compression atelectasis occurs with space-occupying lesions, cardiomegaly, abscess, or significant lymphadenopathy. The increased chest wall pressure compresses the alveoli.
  - Adhesive atelectasis occurs in the setting of acute respiratory distress syndrome (ARDS), radiation, smoke inhalation, posttraumatic lung contusion, or uremia. The underlying surfactant dysfunction causes increased surface tension and alveoli collapse.
  - Cicatrization atelectasis is common in granulomatous disease (i.e., sarcoidosis, TB), toxic or radiation exposure, and drug-induced fibrosis (i.e., amiodarone, cyclophosphamide). The scarring and fibrosis reduces lung expansion.
  - Replacement atelectasis: occurs when a tumor fills alveoli of a lobe causing complete lobar collapse
- Rounded atelectasis is a distinct form of atelectasis seen in patients with asbestos exposure.
- Muscular weakness due to neuromuscular blockers or in neuromuscular diseases with respiratory muscle involvement.

Pediatric Considerations

Children are at a higher risk of developing atelectasis due to their less developed collateral ventilation and compensatory mechanisms. Atelectasis is common in children with aspiration of foreign bodies.

RISK FACTORS

- Critical care, surgery, and prolonged immobilization
- General anesthesia (including long-acting muscle relaxants, postoperative epidural anesthesia)
- Positive fluid balance
- Massive blood transfusion (≥4 units)
- Nasogastric tube placement
- Hypothermia
- Mechanical ventilation with high tidal volume (Vt) (Vt >10 mL/kg) and plateau pressure (>30 cm H_2O)
- Patient risk factors for postoperative atelectasis:
  - Age >60 years and <6 years
  - Chronic obstructive pulmonary disease (COPD), obstructive sleep apnea, congestive heart failure (CHF), pulmonary hypertension
  - Alcohol abuse, smoking
  - Poor cough effort
  - Albumin <3.5 g/dL, hemoglobin <10 g/dL
  - BMI >27 kg/m^2 (weak evidence)
  - ASA class II+ functional dependence in activities of daily living (ADLs)

GENERAL PREVENTION

- Early mobilization, deep breathing exercises, coughing, and frequent changes in body position
- Preoperative physical therapy lowered rates of atelectasis, pneumonia, and length of stay (LOS) in patients undergoing elective cardiac surgery (1)[A]
- Mechanical ventilation settings with high Vt (Vt >10 mL/kg) and plateau pressures (>30 cm H_2O), and without positive end-expiratory pressure (PEEP) are associated with postoperative pulmonary complications (i.e., pneumonia, respiratory failure) (2):
  - Minimize ventilator-induced injury by employing low Vt and plateau pressures at sufficient PEEP (3)[C].
  - Ensure lower FiO_2 during anesthetic induction and intraoperatively to prevent nitrogen washout (2)[A].

COMMONLY ASSOCIATED CONDITIONS

- Obstructive lung diseases (COPD and asthma)
- Chest wall and lung trauma
- Infections of the lung such as respiratory syncytial virus (RSV), bronchiolitis, and bacterial pneumonia
- ARDS, neonatal RDS, pulmonary edema, pulmonary embolism, pneumonia, pleural effusion, pneumothorax
- Cystic fibrosis
- Bronchial stenosis, pulmonic valve disease, pulmonary embolism, and pulmonary hypertension
- Neuromuscular disorders (muscular dystrophy, spinal muscular atrophy, spinal cord injury, and Guillain-Barré syndrome)

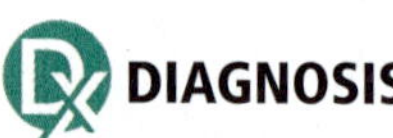

DIAGNOSIS

HISTORY

- Frequently asymptomatic
- Tachypnea and sudden-onset dyspnea
- Nonproductive cough
- Pleuritic pain on affected side
- History of recent intubations, smoking, COPD, pulmonary insufficiency, exposure to radiation, asbestos, or other air pollutants

PHYSICAL EXAM

- Signs of hypoxia or cyanosis
- Tracheal or precordial impulse displacement toward the affected side; dullness to percussion
- Bronchial breathing in patent airway
- Wheezing or absent breath sounds in occluded airway
- Diminished chest expansion

DIFFERENTIAL DIAGNOSIS

Generally, the differential for the collapse of lung tissue as seen with atelectasis is broad and can be considered by mechanism or by presentation:

- Airway obstruction: mucous plug, foreign body, neoplasm, postoperative complication
- External compression: pleural effusion, pneumothorax, lymphadenopathy
- Parenchymal disease: pneumonia, pulmonary edema, fibrosis, ARDS

DIAGNOSTIC TESTS & INTERPRETATION

Initial Tests (lab, imaging)

- CBC and respiratory Gram stain, culture, and viral panel if infection suspected
- ABG: Despite hypoxemia, $PaCO_2$ level is usually normal or low.
- Chest x-ray (CXR): PA and lateral

Follow-Up Tests & Special Considerations

- Chest CT with contrast or MRI may be indicated to visualize airway and mediastinal structures and identify cause of atelectasis in unclear cases.
- Chest ultrasound may differentiate atelectasis versus pleural effusion or consolidation.
- Pulmonary function tests (PFTs) can help identify obstructive or restrictive disease and decreased respiratory muscle pressures.
- Hypoalbuminemia (albumin <3.5 g/L) is a powerful marker of increased risk for postoperative pulmonary complications, including atelectasis.

Diagnostic Procedures/Other

Flexible fiber-optic bronchoscopy can be considered in unexplained or refractory cases.

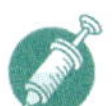

TREATMENT

GENERAL MEASURES

- Identify and treat the underlying etiology.
- Pain control to facilitate deeper breathing
- Lie on the unaffected side, encourage frequent coughing, deep breathing exercises, and early mobility.
- Nebulized albuterol or 3% hypertonic saline to increase mucociliary
- PEEP for prevention following surgery or general anesthesia (2)[A]
- Regular use of incentive spirometry (3)[A]
- Mechanical ventilation with PEEP in severe respiratory distress or hypoxemia
- Continuous positive airway pressure (CPAP) may be beneficial in patients with hypoxemia in the setting of few secretions (3)[A].
- Patients with postoperative atelectasis and significant secretions should be suctioned frequently and undergo chest physiotherapy.

MEDICATION

First Line

Pharmacotherapy should address underlying etiology:

- Effective analgesia to permit deep inspiration and coughing
- Antibiotics for infection
- Chemotherapy or radiation for malignancy
- Bronchodilators and corticosteroids for asthma
- Mucolytics can be considered to promote airway clearance.

Pediatric Considerations

- Dornase alfa may be effective clearing mucinous secretions in refractory mucous plugging in children (used in cystic fibrosis).
- Chest physiotherapy (i.e., percussion, drainage, deep insufflation, and saline lavage) is the most commonly used therapy in the inpatient setting.
- Other physically stimulating modalities (mechanical insufflation-exsufflation, intrapulmonary percussive ventilation, intermittent positive pressure breathing) may have utility in patients with neuromuscular disease and cystic fibrosis to enhance mucus clearance.
- Applying continuous distending pressure has shown some benefit in the treatment of preterm infants with RDS and has the potential to reduce lung damage particularly if used early.
- In obstructive atelectasis, bronchoscopy remains controversial. However, in the presence of a mucus plug or cast, bronchoscopy may be beneficial.

Second Line

Fiber-optic bronchoscopy to improve airway clearance has been efficacious in several studies; however, there is debate regarding its efficacy in the treatment of atelectasis. It may be beneficial in those with unsuccessful attempts or contraindications to chest physiotherapy (i.e., chest wall trauma).

SURGERY/OTHER PROCEDURES

Appropriate surgical resection for underlying disease (i.e., tumor, severe lymphadenopathy)

ALERT

The association between postoperative atelectasis and fever is likely coincidental rather than causal.

ADMISSION, INPATIENT, AND NURSING CONSIDERATIONS

Ensure adequate oxygenation (may start with 100% FiO_2 then taper) and humidification. Note: if obstructive atelectasis is suspected, then judiciously increase FiO_2 to prevent nitrogen washout, which can hasten atelectasis.

ONGOING CARE

FOLLOW-UP RECOMMENDATIONS

Patient Monitoring

- Frequency/adequacy of monitoring will vary by underlying cause and concurrent comorbidities.
- For uncomplicated cases of atelectasis, outpatient monitoring may be appropriate.

PATIENT EDUCATION

Maximize mobility as tolerated and encourage frequent coughing and deep breathing exercises. Seek further treatment or return to ED for worsening symptoms or shortness of breath.

PROGNOSIS

- Postoperative atelectasis usually spontaneous resolves within 24 hours but can persist for days.
- Resolution of lobar atelectasis due to endobronchial obstruction depends on treatment of underlying disease or malignancy.

COMPLICATIONS

- Pneumonia or other pulmonary infections
- Acute atelectasis: hypoxemia, respiratory failure, postobstructive drowning of the lung
- Chronic atelectasis: bronchiectasis, pleural effusion, empyema

REFERENCES

1. Hulzebos EH, Smit Y, Helders PP, et al. Preoperative physical therapy for elective cardiac surgery patients. *Cochrane Database Syst Rev*. 2012;11(11):CD010118.
2. Lagier D, Zeng C, Fernandez-Bustamante A, et al. Perioperative pulmonary atelectasis: part II. clinical implications. *Anesthesiology*. 2022;136:206–236. doi:10.1097/ALN.0000000000004009.
3. Marret E, Cinotti R, Berard L, et al; and the PPV study group. Protective ventilation during anaesthesia reduces major postoperative complications after lung cancer surgery: a double-blind randomised controlled trial. *Eur J Anaesthesiol*. 2018;35(10):727–735. doi:10.1097/EJA.0000000000000804.

ADDITIONAL READING

- Guimarães MM, El Dib R, Smith AF, et al. Incentive spirometry for prevention of postoperative pulmonary complications in upper abdominal surgery. *Cochrane Database Syst Rev*. 2009;(3):CD006058.
- Zeng C, Lagier D, Lee JW, et al. Perioperative pulmonary atelectasis: part I. biology and mechanisms. *Anesthesiology*. 2022;136(1):181–205. doi:10.1097/ALN.0000000000003943.

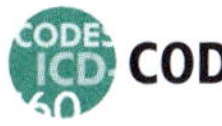

CODES

ICD10

- P28.10 Unspecified atelectasis of newborn
- J98.11 Atelectasis
- P28.19 Other atelectasis of newborn

CLINICAL PEARLS

- Low serum albumin (<3.5 g/L) is a strong predictor of postoperative pulmonary complications, including atelectasis.
- Anesthesia-induced atelectasis occurs in almost all anesthetized patients but can be reduced by employing PEEP intraoperatively or when reversing anesthesia.
- Early mobilization, coughing, deep breathing exercises, and treating the underlying cause are the mainstays of therapy.
- Bronchogenic carcinoma can present as atelectasis and must be excluded in all patients aged >35 years.
- No strong clinical evidence supports atelectasis as an early cause of postoperative fever.

ATRIAL FIBRILLATION AND ATRIAL FLUTTER

Brooks J. Willar, MD

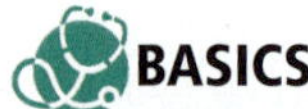

BASICS

This topic covers both atrial fibrillation (AFib) and atrial flutter (AFlut).

DESCRIPTION

- AFib: paroxysmal or continuous supraventricular tachyarrhythmia typically originating from the left atrium characterized by rapid, uncoordinated atrial electrical activity and an irregularly irregular ventricular response. The ventricular rate can become rapid because the atrioventricular (AV) node is bombarded with very frequent atrial electrical impulses (400 to 600 beats/min).
- AFlut: paroxysmal or continuous supraventricular tachyarrhythmia with rapid but organized atrial electrical activity. In typical AFlut, the atrial rate is between 250 and 350 beats/min and is often manifested as "saw-tooth" flutter (F) waves on the ECG, inverted in the inferior leads and upright in V_1. AFlut can have a regular ventricular response and commonly occurs with 2:1 or 3:1 AV block, but also can have an irregular ventricular rate when there is variable AV block.
- AFib and AFlut are related arrhythmias, sometimes seen in the same patient. Distinguishing the two is important because there may be implications for management.
- Clinical classifications:
  - Paroxysmal: self-terminating episodes, usually <7 days
  - Persistent: sustained >7 days, usually requiring pharmacologic or electrical cardioversion to restore sinus rhythm
  - Permanent: Long standing AFib where sinus rhythm cannot be restored/maintained.
  - Nonvalvular AFib: absence of moderate-to-severe mitral stenosis or a mechanical heart valve
- Lone AFib occurs in patients <60 years (with possible genetic predisposition) who have no clinical or echocardiographic evidence of cardiovascular disease, including hypertension (HTN).

EPIDEMIOLOGY

- Incidence/prevalence increases significantly with age.
- Young patients with AFib, particularly lone AFib, are most commonly males.

Incidence

- AFib: from <0.1%/year <40 years of age to >1.5%/year >80 years of age
- Lifetime risk: 25% for those ≥40 years of age
- AFlut is less common.

Prevalence

- Estimated at 0.4–1.0% in general population, with 8.6 million patients in North America
- Increases with age, up to 8% in those ≥80 years of age

ETIOLOGY AND PATHOPHYSIOLOGY

- Cardiac: HTN, acute coronary syndrome (ACS), congestive heart failure (CHF), valvular heart disease, cardiomyopathy, pericarditis, and infiltrative heart disease
- Pulmonary: pulmonary embolism (PE), chronic obstructive pulmonary disease (COPD), obstructive sleep apnea, pneumonia
- Ingestion: ethanol, caffeine, nicotine
- Endocrine: hyperthyroidism, diabetes mellitus (DM)
- Obesity and sleep apnea
- Idiopathic: lone AFib
- Postsurgical: cardiac and noncardiac surgery
- Patients with paroxysmal episodes are usually associated with premature atrial beats and/or bursts of tachycardia, originating in pulmonary veins.
- Many patients with AFib are thought to have some degree of atrial fibrosis or scarring.
- Autonomic (vagal and sympathetic) tone may play a role in triggering the arrhythmia.
- The presence of AFib is associated with electrical and structural remodeling processes that promote arrhythmia maintenance in the atria, termed "AFib begets AFib."

Genetics

Familial forms are rare but do exist. There are ongoing efforts to identify the genetic underpinnings of such cases.

RISK FACTORS

Age, HTN, obesity, sleep apnea, and type 2 DM are the most important risk factors for both AFib and AFlut.

GENERAL PREVENTION

AHA guidelines (1)[C], based on strong class 1 evidence recommend comprehensive lifestyle and risk factor modification, including weight loss, exercise, smoking cessation, alcohol reduction, and optimal blood pressure control as central to *both* primary and secondary prevention of AFib.

COMMONLY ASSOCIATED CONDITIONS

HTN, stroke and other cardiac diseases

DIAGNOSIS

HISTORY

Symptoms vary from none to mild (palpitations, lightheadedness, fatigue, poor exercise capacity) to severe (angina, dyspnea, syncope).

PHYSICAL EXAM

- AFib: irregularly irregular heart rate and pulse, pulse deficit
- AFlut: similar to AFib but may have regular pulse

DIFFERENTIAL DIAGNOSIS

- Multifocal atrial tachycardia
- Sinus tachycardia with frequent atrial premature beats
- Supraventricular tachycardia (Wolff-Parkinson-White [WPW], AV nodal reentry tachycardia [AVNRT]), atrial tachycardia (ATach)

DIAGNOSTIC TESTS & INTERPRETATION

- Screening with ECG to detect asymptomatic cases of AFib has not been shown to detect more cases than screening focused on pulse palpation (2)[A].
- AFib: The ECG is diagnostic, with findings of low-amplitude fibrillatory waves without discrete P waves and an irregularly irregular pattern of QRS complexes. There can be tachycardia in the absence of heart rate–controlling medications.
- AFlut: The ECG is diagnostic. Saw-tooth F waves are the classic sign, generally best seen in the inferior leads, although ventricular rate may need to be slowed to see the waves. QRS complexes may be regular or irregular; there can be tachycardia.
- Ambulatory rhythm monitoring (e.g., telemetry, Holter monitoring, event recorders) is helpful in confirming suspected paroxysmal AFib or AFlut and monitoring for recurrence. Many "smartwatches" can detect dysrhythmia consistent with AFib, but should be confirmed by a physician.

Initial Tests (lab, imaging)

Thyroid-stimulating hormone, electrolytes, complete blood count, complete metabolic panel, 2D transthoracic echocardiogram, prothrombin time/international normalized ratio (INR) (if anticoagulation is contemplated); digoxin level (if appropriate)

Follow-Up Tests & Special Considerations

- Occasional Holter monitoring and/or exercise stress testing to assess for adequacy of rate and/or rhythm control
- Chest x-ray (CXR) for cardiopulmonary disease
- ECG for signs of cardiac hypertrophy, ischemia, and/or other arrhythmias
- Transesophageal echocardiogram to detect left atrial appendage (LAA) thrombus if cardioversion is planned
- Sleep study may be useful if sleep apnea is suspected.

Test Interpretation

Evaluate for presence of atrial dilatation and fibrosis, atrial thrombus (especially in atrial appendage), valvular heart disease, cardiomyopathy.

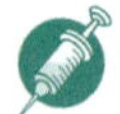

TREATMENT

- Two primary issues in the medical management of AFib and/or AFlut: decisions on heart rate control (control ventricular rate while allowing AFib to continue) or rhythm control (terminate AFib and restore normal sinus rhythm), and decision to anticoagulate or not. In general, newer guidelines emphasize careful risk stratification for anticoagulation, especially for those at intermediate annual stroke risk (1)[C]. This means incorporating stroke risk modifiers such as AFib burden, sex, blood pressure control, and other clinical factors to facilitate shared decision-making, rather than relying on CHA_2DS_2VASc score alone.
- Anticoagulation therapy to prevent thromboembolism (primarily stroke) reduces risk of stroke by about 2/3. If risk is sufficiently low, or risk of bleeding is high (HAS-BLED tool may assist in evaluation), no anticoagulation or LAA closure devices (see below) may be indicated. Clinical judgment and patient preference remain important.
- There is a new emphasis on early and continued rhythm control, including catheter-ablation as first-line therapy for selected patients with symptomatic paroxysmal AFib, based on emerging evidence that early rhythm control improves outcomes (1)[C].

MEDICATION

- American Heart Association/American College of Cardiology anticoagulation guidelines (the same for AFib and AFlut):
  - CHA_2DS_2VASc scoring (**C**HF [1 point], **H**TN [1 point], **A**ge ≥75 years [2 points], **D**M [1 point], prior **S**troke or transient ischemic attack [TIA] or thromboembolism [2 points], **V**ascular disease [1 point], **A**ge 65 to 74 years [1 point], female **S**ex **c**ategory [1 point]). CHA_2DS_2VASc is the recommended stroke risk assessment for patients with nonvalvular AFib.
    - In patients with nonvalvular AFib and a CHA_2DS_2VASc score of 0 in males or 1 in females, anticoagulant therapy may be omitted.
    - In patients with nonvalvular AFib and a CHA_2DS_2VASc score of 1 in males and 2 in females (with one nonsex related risk factor), oral anticoagulant therapy may be considered.
    - In patients with nonvalvular AFib with any high-risk factors for stroke (prior TIA/cerebrovascular accident [CVA]/thromboembolism) or a CHA_2DS_2VASc score ≥2 in men or ≥3 in women should receive oral anticoagulants unless contraindicated.
  - Direct-acting oral anticoagulant (DOAC)/non-vitamin K oral anticoagulant (NOAC) agents are recommended over warfarin for most patients with nonvalvular AFib who should receive anticoagulant therapy. Oral anticoagulants include warfarin with maintenance of an INR of 2 to 3, dabigatran (Pradaxa), rivaroxaban (Xarelto), apixaban (Eliquis), or edoxaban (Savaysa). Patients with valvular AFib should be treated with warfarin to maintain an INR of 2 to 3 or 2.5 to 3.5 dependent on the type and location of the prosthesis.
  - The selection of an anticoagulant should be individualized; consider the risks of each agent, cost, patient preference, and tolerability.

ALERT

Renal and hepatic functions should be evaluated prior to initiation of direct thrombin or factor Xa inhibitors. Limited information is available about safety in patients on renal dialysis. Apixaban should be dose reduced to 2.5 mg BID if patient meets any 2 of the following: ≥80 years, weight ≤60 kg, or Cr >1.5 mg/dL. Rivaroxaban should be taken with a meal and should be dose reduced to 15 mg daily if CrCl <50 mL/min. Specific reversal agents for life-threatening bleeding or urgent procedure are available:

- Idarucizumab (Praxbind) for dabigatran
- Coagulation factor Xa (recombinant), inactivated-zhzo (Andexxa) for apixaban and rivaroxaban
- In addition to anticoagulation, initial rate control must be achieved followed by a decision regarding long-term strategy: rate-control alone or rhythm control. Four classes of medications are available to achieve ventricular rate control: β-blockers (i.e., metoprolol), nondihydropyridine calcium channel blockers (i.e., verapamil, diltiazem), digoxin, and amiodarone. Optimal target for ventricular rate has not been firmly established, but there is evidence that aggressive control of the ventricular rate (<80 beats/min) offers no benefit beyond more modest rate control (i.e., resting heart rate <110 beats/min).
- Patients in whom rate control cannot be achieved or who continue to have persistent symptoms despite reasonable heart rate control may require attempts at restoration of sinus rhythm.
- Restoration of sinus rhythm using electrical or pharmacologic cardioversion may significantly reduce the symptom burden of AFib or AFlut in many patients and may also be useful for controlling ventricular rate.
- Early rhythm control is associated with a lower risk of adverse cardiovascular outcomes.

ISSUES FOR REFERRAL

AHA recommends a multidisciplinary care model which encourages collaboration between primary care and specialty teams to optimize risk factor management and patient education.

SURGERY/OTHER PROCEDURES

- Electrophysiologic study and ablation may be considered for patients with either AFib or AFlut. In the case of AFlut, ablation is a procedure viewed as a first-line therapy. Ablation of AFib may be first-line therapy in patients with paroxysmal AFib as well as symptomatic patients with heart failure with reduced ejection fraction (HFrEF) to lower mortality and reduce hospitalization. Ablation should also be considered in patients who have failed a trial of antiarrhythmic medications.
- Cardiac surgery (e.g., the maze procedure, occlusion of the LAA) may be considered in patients planning to undergo cardiac surgery for other reasons.
- Percutaneous LAA occlusion with the WATCHMAN device may be considered in those at increased risk of stroke and systemic embolism with contraindications to long-term anticoagulation and those undergoing AFib ablation.

COMPLEMENTARY & ALTERNATIVE MEDICINE

The use of herbal remedies, dietary supplements, and vitamins should be thoroughly assessed to avoid medication interactions.

ADMISSION, INPATIENT, AND NURSING CONSIDERATIONS

- Patients with significant symptoms, RVR, AFib/AFlut triggered by an acute process (e.g., ACS, CHF, PE), or in whom antiarrhythmic therapy is being started likely require admission to the hospital for a period of stabilization.
- Acute therapy for symptomatic patients with AFib or AFlut:
  - IV β-blockers or nondihydropyridine calcium channel blockers (e.g., diltiazem, verapamil) for control of ventricular rate in patients without preexcitation (caution if wide QRS complex); caution in the use of calcium channel blockers in patients in decompensated heart failure.
  - IV amiodarone or digoxin may be considered in patients with severe left ventricular dysfunction or hemodynamic instability.
- Urgent direct-current cardioversion is recommended in patients with hemodynamic instability or inadequate rate control.
- Consider the initiation of anticoagulation therapy.

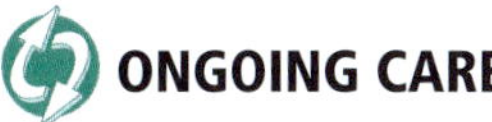

ONGOING CARE

FOLLOW-UP RECOMMENDATIONS

Patient Monitoring

- Adequate anticoagulation levels with warfarin should be determined weekly during initiation and at least monthly when stable.
- If NOACs are employed, hepatic and renal functions should be reevaluated at least annually.

DIET

Patients on warfarin should attempt to consume a stable amount of vitamin K.

PATIENT EDUCATION

Blood pressure control, weight management, reduction or elimination of alcohol, and management of other risk factors has demonstrated beneficial effects on controlling AFib.

PROGNOSIS

AFib and AFlut may increase morbidity and mortality, but the overall prognosis is a function of underlying heart disease and adherence with therapy.

COMPLICATIONS

- Embolic stroke
- Peripheral arterial embolization
- Bleeding with anticoagulation
- Tachycardia-induced cardiomyopathy with prolonged periods of inadequate rate control

REFERENCES

1. Joglar JA, Chung MK, Armbruster AL, et al. 2023 ACC/AHA/ACCP/HRS Guideline for the diagnosis and management of atrial fibrillation: a report of the American College of Cardiology/American Heart Association Joint Committee on Clinical Practice Guidelines. *Circulation*. 2024;149(1):e1–e156.
2. Jonas DE, Kahwati LC, Yun JDY, et al. Screening for atrial fibrillation with electrocardiography: evidence report and systematic review for the US Preventive Services Task Force. *JAMA*. 2018;320(5):485–498.

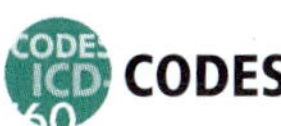

CODES

ICD10

- I48.91 Unspecified atrial fibrillation
- I48.92 Unspecified atrial flutter
- I48.0 Paroxysmal atrial fibrillation

CLINICAL PEARLS

Reevaluation of the need for and choice of anticoagulation therapy at periodic intervals is recommended to reassess stroke and bleeding risks.

ATRIAL SEPTAL DEFECT

Frank J. Domino, MD

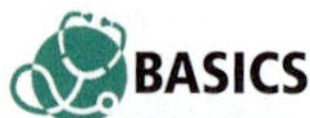

BASICS

DESCRIPTION

- Atrial septal defect (ASD) is a congenital defect of the interatrial septum characterized by absent or insufficient tissue. Patent foramen ovale (PFO) is not considered an ASD, because no septal tissue is missing.
- Types classified by location and abnormal embryogenesis (1)
  - 75%: ostium secundum defect, located in the midseptum
  - 15–20%: ostium primum defect, located in the inferior septum, associated with cleft mitral valve and failure of endocardial cushion development
  - 5–10%: sinus venosus defect, located in the superior-posterior septum near the orifice of the superior vena cava, associated with partial defect in right upper pulmonary venous return
  - <1%: coronary sinus defect, absence of the entire common wall between the coronary sinus and the left atrium
- Hemodynamic effects
  - Left-to-right shunting in late ventricular systole and early diastole
  - Degree depends on size of the defect and relative pressures of the two ventricles.
  - Causes excessive blood flow through the right-sided circulation, ultimately leading to reactive pulmonary hypertension and heart failure
- Systems affected: cardiovascular; pulmonary

Pediatric Considerations

- Most cases of ASD are detected and corrected in the pediatric population.
- The smaller the defect and the younger the child, the greater the chance of spontaneous closure.

EPIDEMIOLOGY

Incidence

- Predominant age: present from birth, may be diagnosed at any age
- Female to male ratio 2–4:1
- No race predilection
- 1/1,500 live births
- Ostium secundum alone accounts for >90% of all congenital heart lesions in the adult population (2).

Prevalence

ASDs account for 13% of congenital heart disorders.

ETIOLOGY AND PATHOPHYSIOLOGY

- The flow across ASD is usually left-to-right because of higher left-sided pressures:
  - Minimal right-to-left shunting in early ventricular systole, especially during inspiration
  - Increased right-sided pressure/pulmonary arterial hypertension can cause reversal of shunt flow (Eisenmenger syndrome) with resulting cyanosis and clubbing.
- Symptoms typically occur due to right ventricular and pulmonary vascular volume overload and right-sided heart failure.

Genetics

- Majority of cases are spontaneous, although rare familial cases exist.
- 25% prevalence in Down syndrome
- 5% with chromosomal abnormalities

RISK FACTORS

- Family history, other congenital heart defects
- Maternal age >35 years
- Gestational exposures: thalidomide, alcohol, tobacco, elevated blood glucose

COMMONLY ASSOCIATED CONDITIONS

- 70% ASDs are isolated but may occur as a component of other complex cardiac structural defects, including anomalous pulmonary venous return.
- May be associated with rare underlying genetic syndromes, including Holt-Oram (ASD present in 66%), Ellis-van Creveld, VACTERL syndrome, Down syndrome, or Noonan syndrome

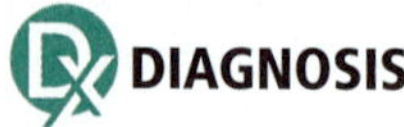

DIAGNOSIS

HISTORY

- Most ASDs are small, asymptomatic in throughout childhood, and only found as an incidental cardiac murmur on routine physical examination.
- Infants with large ASDs may present with right-sided heart failure (more advanced, only 10% at diagnosis), tachypnea, recurrent respiratory infections, or failure to thrive.
- Uncorrected defects usually become symptomatic by 40 years of age and may present with palpitations (most frequently), exercise intolerance, dyspnea, syncope, peripheral edema, cyanosis, or fatigue.
- Children and young adults are rarely symptomatic but may present with exercise intolerance or atrial arrhythmias.

PHYSICAL EXAM

- Children and young adults are mostly asymptomatic, although they can rarely exhibit cyanosis and hyperdynamic precordium.
- Signs vary according to extent of shunting.
- Cardiac palpation
  - Hyperdynamic precordium over the right ventricle
  - Palpable pulmonary artery pulse at the left upper sternal border
- Cardiac auscultation
  - *Fixed, widely split S_2 (key physical finding)*
  - May also have
    - Systolic ejection murmur (pulmonic flow murmur)
    - Low-pitched diastolic rumble (tricuspid flow murmur)
    - Diastolic murmur (pulmonic regurgitation)
    - Systolic murmur (mitral regurgitation)
    - Fourth heart sound in the setting of right-sided heart failure
- Signs of Eisenmenger syndrome:
  - Cyanosis and clubbing
  - Jugular venous distention and edema

DIFFERENTIAL DIAGNOSIS

- Other congenital heart disease
- Right bundle branch block (for widely split S_2)

DIAGNOSTIC TESTS & INTERPRETATION

Initial Tests (lab, imaging)

- Best initial test is transthoracic echocardiogram (TTE) with Doppler imaging of the entire atrial septum: sensitive for secundum (89%), primum (100%), and sinus venosus (44%) defects.
- If TTE is nondiagnostic or shows evidence of right ventricular overload, progression to transesophageal echocardiography (TEE) is warranted.
- Oximetry at rest and with activity: Cyanosis or SpO_2 <90% may suggest Eisenmenger syndrome (right-to-left shunting). In certain subsets of patients, these signs may only appear with activity (3).
- ECG is not typically diagnostic but may show various signs of right- or left-sided heart strain, inverted P wave in lead III (in sinus venosus), or leftward axis (ostium primum or sinus venosus).

Follow-Up Tests & Special Considerations

- Bubble contrast enhancement may be helpful.
- TEE may be required to define ASD morphology and to locate the pulmonary veins; often used prior to percutaneous closure. TEE has excellent sensitivity and specificity.

Diagnostic Procedures/Other

- Echocardiography is first line as noted above.
- Cardiac catheterization: used to characterize ASDs and concomitant heart disease and to assess presence of pulmonary vascular resistance or hypertension (particularly if considering surgery); this procedure is not indicated in young patients unless part of a planned closure, evaluating another disease simultaneously, or other visualization methods are insufficient (3).
- Cardiac magnetic resonance: noninvasive follow-up to echocardiography, used to evaluate sinus venosus defects/pulmonary veins, shunt fraction, and right ventricular function (3)
- Exercise testing: may be used to document change over time
- Chest x-ray: may be used to identify right ventricular or pulmonary artery enlargement
- Cardiac CT: may further define ASD but with significant radiation exposure

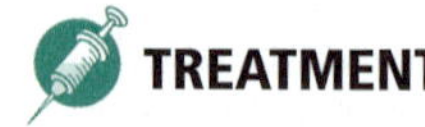

TREATMENT

GENERAL MEASURES

- 75% of small secundum ASDs (<8 mm) will close spontaneously by 18 months of age; however, close follow-up is warranted.
- Surgical closure is usually required for primum and sinus venosus defects.

MEDICATION

First Line

- Treatment of secondary cardiac or pulmonary vascular disease
  - Atrial fibrillation/supraventricular tachycardia (SVT) with anticoagulation and cardioversion/sinus rhythm or rate-control
  - Heart failure with diuretics, oxygen, digoxin, etc.
  - Remodeling therapy with prostaglandins, endothelin blockers, and PDE-5 inhibitors for patients with severe pulmonary arterial hypertension (3)
- Consider pulmonary vasodilator therapy for adults with progressive/severe pulmonary vascular disease.

Second Line

- Antibiotic prophylaxis is NOT recommended for unrepaired/isolated ASDs or as prophylaxis against infective endocarditis during dental procedures.
- To prevent thrombus formation after device deployment, aspirin alone or a combination of aspirin and clopidogrel 75 mg for at least 6 months is recommended.

SURGERY/OTHER PROCEDURES

- The majority of small secundum defects, <6 mm, close spontaneously by 2 years of age. Closure is generally indicated in children with defects >8 mm, defects of any size in children aged >5 years with related symptoms
- Closure for secundum defects is not recommended in asymptomatic patients before 2 years of age given the possibility of spontaneous closure. It is also contraindicated in patients with irreversible, severe pulmonary hypertension without continued shunting.
- In adults, secundum closure via percutaneous transcatheter device or surgery to reduce subsequent morbidity and mortality indicated in patients with right heart enlargement with or without symptoms, pulmonary systemic flow ratio of 2:1 (or >1.5:1 and <21 years old per the AHA), or symptoms including documented orthodeoxia/platypnea or paradoxical embolism. Treatment with a closure device does not significantly affect aortic/mitral valve function.
- Surgical repair is standard for a sinus venosus, coronary sinus, or primum ASD.
- Percutaneous closure with a closure device is considered the treatment of choice of secundum ASD in adults (3),(4). It is safe and effective with satisfactory long-term clinical follow-up. In addition, the use of closure device does not significantly affect aortic or mitral valve function (4).
- Maze procedure may be considered before or after closure for patients with intermittent or chronic atrial tachyarrhythmias.

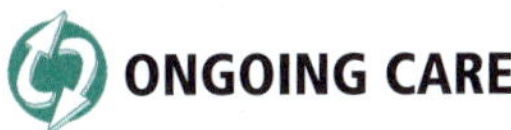

ONGOING CARE

FOLLOW-UP RECOMMENDATIONS

- Outpatient cardiologist visits: every 3 months to 5 years depending on physiologic stage of the defect (3)
- ECG: every 1 to 5 years depending on physiologic stage of the defect
- TTE: every 1 to 5 years depending on physiologic stage of the defect
- Exercise stress test: every 6 to 24 months for advanced disease

Patient Monitoring

- In otherwise asymptomatic healthy children, follow up until defect has closed or become negligible in size.
- ASDs repaired in adulthood may require periodic long-term follow-up.
- ASDs repaired in childhood generally do not have late complications.
- Pregnancy is well tolerated in cases with repaired/small unrepaired ASDs but is not recommended in cases of unrepaired ASD/Eisenmenger syndrome due to increased risk of maternal and fetal mortality.
- Recommend consultation in patients with unrepaired ASDs prior to scuba diving or high-altitude travel.

PATIENT EDUCATION

For patient education materials on this topic, consult the American Heart Association or Mayo Clinic ASD webpages.

PROGNOSIS

- ASD closure in asymptomatic, minimally symptomatic, and symptomatic adults reduces morbidity especially if performed before 25 years of age (2),(3).
- ASD repair deferred until after adolescence may not decrease long-term risk of future atrial arrhythmias.
- In one study, prognosis after ASD closure saw a >20% reduction in pulmonary resistance by pretreatment with PAH therapies and pulmonary remodeling treatments (3).
- Unoperated ASDs: up to 25% mortality by 27 years, up to 90% mortality by 60 years, increased rates of atrial arrhythmias, reduced functional capacity, greater degrees of pulmonary arterial hypertension (2),(3)

COMPLICATIONS

- Unrepaired: congestive heart failure, stroke, atrial arrhythmias, increased infection risk (pulmonary, cerebral abscess, infective endocarditis); rarer complications include pulmonary arterial hypertension/Eisenmenger syndrome, and paradoxical embolism (3).
- Surgically repaired: late-onset arrhythmias 10 to 20 years after surgery (5%), perioperative atrial tachyarrhythmias (10–13% of patients), increased risk of arrhythmia-associated embolic events (2)
- Device closure: device embolization (1%), cardiac perforation, thrombus formation, endocarditis, supraventricular arrhythmias, and device erosions

REFERENCES

1. Bradley EA, Zaidi AN. Atrial septal defect. *Cardiol Clin*. 2020;38(3):317–324.
2. Oster M, Bhatt AB, Zaragoza-Macias E, et al. Interventional therapy versus medical therapy for secundum atrial septal defect: a systematic review (Part 2) for the 2018 AHA/ACC Guideline for the Management of Adults With Congenital Heart Disease: a report of the American College of Cardiology/American Heart Association Task Force on Clinical Practice Guidelines. *J Am Coll Cardiol*. 2019;73(12):1579–1595.
3. Stout KK, Daniels CJ, Aboulhosn JA, et al. 2018 AHA/ACC guideline for the management of adults with congenital heart disease: executive summary: a report of the American College of Cardiology/American Heart Association Task Force on Clinical Practice Guidelines. *J Am Coll Cardiol*. 2019;73(12):1494–1563.
4. Scacciatella P, Marra S, Pullara A, et al. Percutaneous closure of atrial septal defect in adults: very long-term clinical outcome and effects on aortic and mitral valve function. *J Invasive Cardiol*. 2015;27(1):65–69.

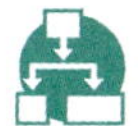

SEE ALSO

Aortic Valvular Stenosis; Coarctation of the Aorta; Patent Ductus Arteriosus; Pulmonary Valve Stenosis; Tetralogy of Fallot; Ventricular Septal Defect

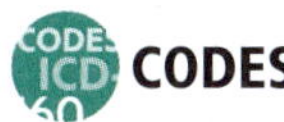

CODES

ICD10

- Q21.2 Atrioventricular septal defect
- Q21.1 Atrial septal defect
- I23.1 Atrial septal defect as current complication following acute myocardial infarction

CLINICAL PEARLS

- ASD is often missed due to subtle clinical presentation.
- Ideally, hemodynamically significant ASDs should be closed in early childhood, although some benefit from closure is present in older patients.
- Many ASDs can be treated by catheter-directed percutaneous closure rather than open-heart surgery.
- Routine endocarditis prophylaxis is not recommended for unrepaired ASDs.
- Generally, symptomatic and hemodynamically significant ASDs are repaired; optimal management of asymptomatic small ASDs is unclear.
- PFOs, unlike large ASDs, are very common and generally require no treatment in asymptomatic individuals.

ATTENTION DEFICIT/HYPERACTIVITY DISORDER, ADULT

Beth A. Wichowski, DO

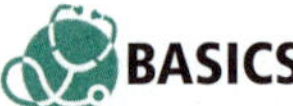

BASICS

- Adult attention deficit hyperactivity disorder (adult ADHD) is a pattern of behaviors that include inattention and/or hyperactivity or impulsivity. It is present in multiple settings that impair social, academic, or work performance.
- Complications of adult ADHD include employment, financial and interpersonal difficulties, as well as increased risk for driving accidents and suicide.
- Adult ADHD typically begins in childhood and 30–60% will continue to meet criteria as adults.

DESCRIPTION

- Symptoms include difficulty concentrating, impulsivity, and hyperactivity/overactivity. Impairment in executive functioning and emotional dysregulation are common features.
- The three main types of ADHD are:
  - Hyperactivity-impulsivity predominant
  - Inattentive predominant
  - Combined
    - The combined type is the most common, followed by the inattentive and hyperactive types.

EPIDEMIOLOGY

Prevalence

ADHD affects approximately 4.4–5.2% of adults between 18 and 44 years of age (1). ADHD is more common in men than women, who are less likely to be referred for assessment and more likely to be undiagnosed or misdiagnosed.

ETIOLOGY AND PATHOPHYSIOLOGY

Genetics

ADHD appears to have a genetic component, with heritability of approximately 0.8, suggesting that genetic factors would account for about 65% of phenotypic variance.

RISK FACTORS

- Risk is increased among offsprings of mothers who smoked or had obesity and diabetes during pregnancy. Risk is also increased with childhood lead exposure. Unknown whether these associations are causal.
- Premature birth; very low birth weight; and extreme neglect, abuse, or social deprivation; as do certain infections during pregnancy, at birth, and in early childhood
- Neurodevelopmental disorders (e.g., autism, learning disabilities)

COMMONLY ASSOCIATED CONDITIONS

- Substance use and substance abuse disorders
- Mood and anxiety disorders
- Obsessive-compulsive disorder (OCD)
- Tic disorders
- Delayed sleep-wake phase disorder

DIAGNOSIS

- Diagnosis is made from patient's history and detailing patient's current level of functioning in at least two different settings (e.g., work and home).
- It is important to gather history of patient's childhood and school performance.

HISTORY

- Commonly reported symptoms of ADHD include poor concentration, disorganization, failure to complete projects, poor performance at work, and difficulty controlling temper
- *DSM-5* criteria include (1):
  - At least five symptoms of inattention or hyperactivity/impulsivity
  - Several symptoms must be present before age 12 years (if not diagnosed in childhood, this is established by a historical assessment of childhood symptoms)
  - Symptoms must be present in two or more settings (home, work, etc.).
  - There must be clear evidence that symptoms interfere with or reduce quality of social, academic, or work functioning.
  - Symptoms must be present for >6 months.
- History of medication or substances that have side effects that impact attentiveness and mimic ADHD symptoms
- History of thyroid disorders, head injury or trauma, liver disease, seizure disorders
- Ask about cardiovascular disease, neurodevelopmental disorders including autism spectrum disorder, tic disorders, learning disabilities
- Ask about family history of ADHD and other psychiatric and neurologic problems.

PHYSICAL EXAM

- Physical exam is key to ruling out other medical conditions.
- Focus on thyroid and neurologic examinations for new onset of symptoms in adulthood
- Record BP and baseline weight; monitor if starting medical treatment.

DIFFERENTIAL DIAGNOSIS

Hearing impairment; hyperthyroid/hypothyroid; sleep deprivation; sleep apnea; phenylketonuria; OCD; lead toxicity; substance abuse (2)

DIAGNOSTIC TESTS & INTERPRETATION

- Adult ADHD screening tools:
  - Retrospective scales include the Childhood Symptom Scale and the Wender Utah Rating Scale
  - Current symptom scales include the Adult ADHD Rating Scale IV, Adult Self Report Scale Symptom Checklist, and the Connor Adult Rating Scale (1). These scales can take 5 to 20 minutes to complete.
- Provider/patient screening checklist
  - https://add.org/wp-content/uploads/2015/03/adhd-questionnaire-ASRS111.pdf
  - https://nyulangone.org/files/psych_adhd_screener_0.pdf

Initial Tests (lab, imaging)

- Thyroid-stimulating hormone (TSH)
- ECG with concerns for cardiac disease in patient or family history
- Urine toxicology screen to rule out concomitant substance abuse disorder

Follow-Up Tests & Special Considerations

- Liver function test monitoring
- Consider polysomnography in patients with sleep disorder symptoms to rule out sleep apnea.
- A history of childhood behaviors is helpful, but adult patients often don't accurately recall childhood symptomology.
- Inquire about family history of ADHD, family and personal substance abuse, and tic disorders to facilitate formulation of an accurate diagnosis and recognition of high-risk behaviors.
- Caution against stimulant use in pregnancy because of high risk of low fetal birth weight and preterm birth. Risks and benefits of treatment must be discussed in detail with patient and preferably with their spouse (3)[B].
- Caution against use of stimulants in adult patients with cardiac history.

ALERT

Mood disorders, generalized anxiety disorders, and substance abuse can also coexist with adult ADHD; treating both the ADHD and comorbid conditions will improve the patient's prognosis.

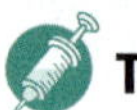

TREATMENT

- Most of the research and medication trials have been performed in children.
- There is increasing evidence that medications used in children are also effective in adults (2)[A].

ALERT

Because stimulant medication may induce dependency, substance abuse, and diversion, it is recommended to do pill counts, screen urine for drugs, monitor behavior, and query prescription databases. Misuse of amphetamines may cause sudden death and serious cardiovascular adverse events.

GENERAL MEASURES

When substance abuse is not present, stimulants are first-line treatment for ADHD and highly efficacious. Patients may require trials of different dosages, formulations, and medications before an optimal response in symptoms and functions is achieved. Non-stimulants are useful when there is abuse potential, comorbid conditions, or poor response to stimulants.

MEDICATION

- Titrate slowly to effective dose to avoid side effects.
- Stimulants are more effective than antidepressants or nonstimulants, but up to 30% discontinue medications because of side effects.
- Stimulants can be grouped into those related to methylphenidate and those related to amphetamine. Both groups include both short- and long-acting preparations. Recent evidence suggests that adherence and persistence rates improve in those using long-acting agents (1).
- Antidepressants studied for ADHD include bupropion, which has been shown to have a medium effect compared with stimulants (2)[A].

First Line

D and D-L stimulant classes:

- Stimulants: methylphenidate (Concerta, Ritalin), dexmethylphenidate (Focalin), dextroamphetamine /amphetamine (Adderall), dextroamphetamine (Dexedrine), lisdexamfetamine (Vyvanse)
  - Methylphenidate preparations are available in short-acting, intermediate acting, long acting, and patch formulations.
  - Methylphenidate hydrochloride extended-release (Ritalin LA) may be used for patients naive to stimulants. It can be started at 20 mg daily and dose titrated by 10 mg increments weekly to symptoms response; max 60 mg/day
  - Concerta ER is another option in adults up to 65 years of age; starting dose of 18 mg/day; adjust in increments of 18 mg weekly until symptoms improve; max 72 mg/day
  - Dextroamphetamine is commonly used (half-life of 4 to 6 hours) with an initial dose of 5 mg BID; titrate up by 5 mg weekly to max 20 mg BID.
  - Dextroamphetamine/amphetamine (Adderall) is a 75%/25% mix that also comes in an extended-release form. Initial dosing can be started at 5 mg BID for short-acting or 20 mg daily for long acting and increased by 5 mg/week for short-acting and 10 mg/week long acting to a max 60 mg total daily.
  - Lisdexamfetamine (Vyvanse) is an extended-release stimulant that is a prodrug requiring metabolization to active component, dextroamphetamine.
  - Common side effects of stimulants include hypertension (HTN), tachycardia, insomnia, weight loss, stomach upset, increased anxiety/irritability, or worsening of tics (2)[A].
- Nonstimulants:
  - Atomoxetine (Strattera) has been shown effective in adults with ADHD when compared to placebo (4)[B]. It may be given as a single dose or split dose and has low abuse potential. Onset of effect may take up to 4 weeks. Atomoxetine may be particularly useful when anxiety, mood or tics co-occur with ADHD. There are rare cases of liver damage associated with these medications. Monitor for increased suicidal thinking.
  - Antidepressants: best used for those at high risk or with history of substance abuse disorder. Bupropion (Wellbutrin) is effective in adults with ADHD symptoms, especially if comorbid depression (3)[A].
  - Tricyclic antidepressants (desipramine and nortriptyline) have also shown to be effective in ADHD (1).
  - α_2-Agonists (guanfacine, clonidine) have been found to be effective in children and adolescents; however, they have not been studied extensively in adults (5)[C]. These may be used with comorbid tics and/or disruptive behavior disorders.
  - Combining stimulants with a nonstimulant medication such as atomoxetine, guanfacine, or clonidine has shown positive effects among patients who are resistant to stimulants alone.

ADDITIONAL THERAPIES

- Cognitive-behavioral therapy (CBT) can be useful in conjunction with medication to help patient modify and cope with symptoms. CBT helps reduce impairments resulting from executive dysfunction (EDF) that is not optimally ameliorated with medication (1).
- Among adults with ADHD and EDFs, addition of memantine as an adjunct to extended-release methylphenidate was associated with improved executive functioning, supporting the need for further research.

COMPLEMENTARY & ALTERNATIVE MEDICINE

- Mixed evidence that fatty acid supplementation in addition to medication may be beneficial (6).
- Eliminating artificial food coloration only shows a mild benefit in decreasing symptoms (7).
- Behavioral therapy

ONGOING CARE

Transfer from pediatric to adult care must be closely coordinated to avoid hiatus in treatment.

FOLLOW-UP RECOMMENDATIONS

- Close follow-up of medication as dose is titrated to monitor for side effects.
- Reinforce behavioral change (e.g., self-initiated through CBT), which is essential goal of long-term management.
- Repeat screening checklists to quantify benefits; however, self-report of symptoms are limited in reliability, given that adults with ADHD have likely compensated for symptoms since childhood.

DIET

- Limit caffeine intake while prescribed stimulant medication.
- Limit intake of processed foods.

PATIENT EDUCATION

Support groups (e.g., https://chadd.org/ and https://add.org/)

COMPLICATIONS

Co-occurring psychiatric conditions such as MDD, anxiety disorders, OCD, and tic disorders.

REFERENCES

1. Young JL, Goodman DW. Adult attention-deficit/hyperactivity disorder diagnosis, management, and treatment in the DSM-5 era. *Prim Care Companion CNS Disord*. 2016;18(6). doi:10.4088/PCC.16r02000.
2. Castells X, Ramos-Quiroga JA, Bosch R, et al. Amphetamines for attention deficit hyperactivity disorder (ADHD) in adults. *Cochrane Database Syst Rev*. 2011;(6):CD007813.
3. Verbeeck W, Tuinier S, Bekkering GE. Antidepressants in the treatment of adult attention-deficit hyperactivity disorder: a systematic review. *Adv Ther*. 2009;26(2):170–184.
4. Asherson P, Bushe C, Saylor K, et al. Efficacy of atomoxetine in adults with attention deficit hyperactivity disorder: an integrated analysis of the complete database of multicenter placebo-controlled trials. *J Psychopharmacol*. 2014;28(9):837–846.
5. Hirota T, Schwartz S, Correll CU. Alpha-2 agonists for attention-deficit/hyperactivity disorder in youth: a systematic review and meta-analysis of monotherapy and add-on trials to stimulant therapy. *J Am Acad Child Adolesc Psychiatry*. 2014;53(2):153–173.
6. Millichap JG, Yee MM. The diet factor in attention–deficit/hyperactivity disorder. *Pediatrics*. 2012;129(2):330–337.
7. Sonuga-Barke EJS, Brandeis D, Cortese S, et al. Nonpharmacological interventions for ADHD: systematic review and meta-analyses of randomized controlled trials of dietary and psychological treatments. *Am J Psychiatry*. 2013;170(3):275–289.

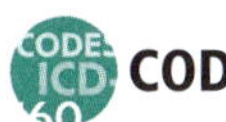

CODES

ICD10

- F90.9 Attention-deficit hyperactivity disorder, unspecified type
- F90.1 Attn-defct hyperactivity disorder, predom hyperactive type
- F90.0 Attn-defct hyperactivity disorder, predom inattentive type

CLINICAL PEARLS

- Adult ADHD typically results in disruptions in school, work, or relationship settings; symptoms include inattention, easy distractibility, hyperactivity, and impulsive behavior. It is associated with low self-esteem, problematic interpersonal relationships, and difficulty meeting academic and job expectations.
- Psychotropic medications with cognitive behavioral treatments are the cornerstone of management.
- Substance misuse is a common co-occurring condition, particularly in those who were not managed with stimulant medication in childhood for ADHD symptoms. Recommend use of nonstimulant medication in those at high risk of substance misuse.

ATTENTION DEFICIT/HYPERACTIVITY DISORDER, PEDIATRIC

Anne C. Powell, MD • Sydney Hartman-Munick, MD

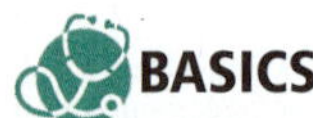

BASICS

DESCRIPTION

- Attention deficit/hyperactivity disorder (ADHD) is a neurodevelopmental disorder that manifests in early childhood characterized by distractibility, impulsivity, hyperactivity, and/or inattention.
- Three subsets: predominantly hyperactivity (ADHD-H), predominantly inattentive (ADHD-I), or combined (ADHD-C)
- System(s) affected: nervous

EPIDEMIOLOGY

- Predominant age: onset <12 years; lasts into adolescence and adulthood
- Predominant sex: assigned male at birth > assigned female at birth (2:1); ADHD-I is more common in patients assigned female at birth.

Prevalence

9–15% of children aged 4 to 17 years

ETIOLOGY AND PATHOPHYSIOLOGY

Not definitive—suggested pathogenesis includes imbalance of catecholamine metabolism and structural brain differences. Environmental influences are controversial.

Genetics

ADHD has a high heritability rate of up to 75%.

RISK FACTORS

- Family history (genetic component)
- Medical causes (affecting brain development)—including prenatal tobacco exposure and prematurity

COMMONLY ASSOCIATED CONDITIONS

- Mood disorders—depression, anxiety
- Behavior disorders—oppositional defiant disorder, conduct disorder
- Autism spectrum disorder
- Physiologic disorders—sleep disorders, tics
- Learning disabilities, developmental coordination syndrome, language disorder
- Substance use disorders

DIAGNOSIS

- American Academy of Pediatrics (AAP) guidelines recommend *DSM-5-TR* criteria to establish diagnosis.
- *DSM-5-TR* (1) criteria for children aged <17 years: ≥6 inattention criteria and/or ≥6 hyperactivity/impulsivity criteria; symptoms must occur often; can be present before age of 12 years, for >6 months; can be noticed in ≥2 settings (e.g., home, school); reduced quality of social or scholastic functioning; can be excessive for development level of child; and are not better explained by or occur with another mental disorder (e.g., depression, anxiety, or personality disorder).
- Inattention
  - Careless mistakes in tasks; difficulty sustaining attention or in organizing
  - Does not seem to listen
  - Does not follow through or finish tasks
  - Avoid tasks that require sustained mental effort
  - Loses things
  - Forgetful in daily activities
  - Distracted by external stimuli
  - Forgetful
- Hyperactivity/impulsivity
  - Fidgets
  - Difficulty remaining seated
  - Runs/climbs excessively or inappropriately; difficulty playing quietly
  - Acts as if "driven by a motor" or seeming to always be "on the go"
  - Talks excessively
  - Blurts out answers before question is complete
  - Has difficulty waiting turn
  - Interrupts others
- Children undergoing extreme stress (divorce, illness, homelessness, abuse) may demonstrate ADHD behaviors secondary to stress.
- If diagnostic behaviors are noted in only one setting, explore the stressors in that setting.
- The diagnostic behaviors are more noticeable in tasks that require concentration or boredom tolerance.

HISTORY

- Birth and development history
- Psychosocial evaluation of home environment
- School performance and school absences
- Psychiatric history or history of comorbid disorder(s)
- Cardiac history

PHYSICAL EXAM

- Baseline weight, heart rate, blood pressure for future monitoring
- Note any soft neurologic signs such as tics, clumsiness, mixed handedness.
- Assess hearing and vision.

DIFFERENTIAL DIAGNOSIS

- Activity level appropriate for age
- Dysfunctional family situation or abuse
- Learning disability (e.g., dyslexia)
- Hearing/vision/language disorder
- Autism spectrum disorders
- Oppositional/defiant disorder or conduct disorder
- Seizure disorder
- Neurodevelopmental syndromes (e.g., fragile X)
- Lead poisoning
- Sequelae of central nervous system infection/trauma
- Medication effect
- Any of the comorbid conditions above

DIAGNOSTIC TESTS & INTERPRETATION

- Behavior rating scales completed by parents, caregivers, and teachers prior to initiation of therapy and then repeated after therapy (Vanderbilt ADHD forms)
- National Institute for Children's Health Quality. Caring for Children with ADHD: a resource toolkit for clinicians; https://www.nichq.org/resource/caring-children-adhd-resource-toolkit-clinicians
- Testing for learning disability: request from school

Initial Tests (lab, imaging)

Rarely needed; consider lead.

Diagnostic Procedures/Other

ECG prior to stating stimulant medication if positive family history of premature CV disease

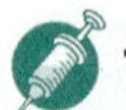

TREATMENT

GENERAL MEASURES

- Always develop a behavioral health plan with parents and school.
- Identify treatment goals based upon behaviors which are most harmful to the child's development.
- Coordinate school and home behavioral plan.
- Children aged 4 to 5 years should begin with behavioral interventions.
- Children aged 6 to 17 years should begin with behavioral interventions and consider medication if behavioral goals are not being met over time.
- Behavioral counseling can be beneficial for both parents and child, including parent training, academic training, and social training.
- Behavioral modifications should involve repeated positive reinforcement with limiting negative comments, reward systems, environmental changes at both home and school (time out, quiet time), etc.

MEDICATION

- Stimulant medications are often considered first line as they have the highest efficacy but also carry greater risks.
- Atomoxetine may be used first line, especially if there is risk of diversion in the home, growth concerns (poor weight gain, sleep issues, etc.), or if parents wish to try nonstimulant medication.
- Stimulant choice should be based on cost, formulary, convenience, and duration. A second type of stimulant should be tried if the first treatment fails.

First Line

Stimulant:

- Methylphenidate
  - Short acting
    - Ritalin, Methylin: onset within 30 minutes; duration 3 to 5 hours
  - Intermediate acting
    - Metadate ER: onset within 20 to 60 minutes and lasts for 8 hours
  - Long acting
    - Methylphenidate CD: combination of immediate release and delayed release for duration over 8 to 12 hours (bimodal)
      - Cotempla XR-ODT: combination of immediate release and extended release for duration up to 12 hours
      - Quillivant XR: combination of immediate release and extended release with duration up to 12 hours
      - Quillichew ER: continuous release over 6 to 8 hours with duration up to 13 hours
      - Ritalin LA: combination of immediate release and delayed release over 8 to 12 hours
      - Concerta/Relexxii: combination of immediate release and continuous release for duration over 10 to 12 hours
      - Aptensio XR: combination of immediate release and controlled release for duration of 12 hours
      - Adhansia XR: combination of immediate release and controlled release for duration of 16 hours

- Jornay PM: night-time dosing where <5% of drug available within the first 10 hours of administration with a peak concentration at 14 hours and steady decline after
- Daytrana transdermal patch: onset 2 hours after application with duration of 9 to 12 hours

- Dexmethylphenidate
  - Focalin: duration 5 to 6 hours
  - Focalin XR: combination of immediate release and delayed release over 10 to 12 hours
- Serdexmethylphenidate-dexmethylphenidate
  - Azstarys: 70% prodrug delayed and 30% immediate release drug; onset within 1 hour and duration of 13 hours
- Amphetamine
  - Immediate release
    - Evekeo/Evekeo ODT: onset within 20 to 60 minutes with duration 4 to 6 hours
  - Extended release
    - Dyanavel XR: combination of immediate and extended release for duration of 13 hours (liquid + tab)
    - Adzenys XR-ODT: combination of immediate release and extended release; duration over 10 to 12 hours
- Dextroamphetamine
  - Immediate release
    - Dexedrine, ProCentra: onset within 20 to 60 minutes for duration of 4 to 6 hours
  - Extended release
    - Dextroamphetamine SR: combination of immediate release and continuous release; duration over 8 to 12 hours
      - Xelstrym patch: onset 2 hours after application with duration of 9 to 12 hours
- Dextroamphetamine/amphetamine mixed salts
  - Short acting
    - Adderall: onset within 20 to 60 minutes with duration of 4 to 6 hours
  - Long acting
    - Adderall XR: combination of immediate and continuous release for duration of 10 to 12 hours
    - Mydayis: combination of immediate and 2 different delayed-release beads; duration up to 16 hours
- Lisdexamfetamine
  - Vyvanse: prodrug converted to dextroamphetamine with effect over 10 hours

ALERT

Precautions:

- If not responding, check compliance and consider another diagnosis.
- Some children experience withdrawal (tearfulness, agitation) after a missed dose or when medication wears off. A small, short-acting dose at 4 PM may help to prevent this.
- Stimulants can be used as drugs of abuse and should be monitored carefully.
- Drug holidays are not recommended but may be tried in weight loss or ADHD-I.

- Common adverse effects:
  - Anorexia, insomnia, growth delay, GI effects, CV effects, and headache
  - Rare priapism, psychosis, tics, suicidal thinking
- Significant possible interactions: may increase levels of anticonvulsants, SSRIs, tricyclics, and warfarin
- High-caffeine energy drinks, albuterol inhalers, and decongestants may increase side effects.
- The FDA reports permanent skin discoloration with Daytrana patches.

Second Line

Nonstimulant:

- Serotonin-norepinephrine reuptake inhibitor (SNRI)
  - Atomoxetine (Strattera): effects last at least 10 to 12 hours, but must be taken daily without drug holidays
  - Viloxazine (Qelbree): lasts throughout the day, must be taken daily without drug holidays
- α_2-Agonist
  - Modest efficacy, high side effects; consider consultation before use.
    - Clonidine XR (Kapvay): duration at least 10 to 12 hours
    - Guanfacine XR (Intuniv): duration at least 10 to 12 hours

ALERT

- SNRIs carry a "black box" warning regarding potential exacerbation of suicidality (similar to SSRIs). Close follow-up is recommended.
- Side effects similar to stimulants including CV/GI effects, and the rare side effects of tics and priapism.
- Associated with hepatic injury in a small number of cases; check liver enzymes if symptoms develop.

ISSUES FOR REFERRAL

Refer for children if there are additional mental health issues, developmental issues, or poor response to treatment.

COMPLEMENTARY & ALTERNATIVE MEDICINE

Parents of children with ADHD use herbals and complementary treatments frequently (20–60%) but very limited evidence to support any intervention including video game therapies and trigeminal nerve stimulation.

ONGOING CARE

FOLLOW-UP RECOMMENDATIONS

Patient Monitoring

- Office visits to monitor side effects and efficacy: End points are improved grades, rating scales, family interactions, and peer interactions
- Monitor growth (especially weight), HR, and BP.

PATIENT EDUCATION

- Excellent reference: http://www.parentsmedguide.org
- Teachers reference: ADDitude toolkit for parents and teachers

PROGNOSIS

- Relative deficits in academic and social functioning may persist into late adolescence/adulthood.
- Encourage career choices that allow autonomy and mobility.

COMPLICATIONS

Primarily from untreated ADHD

- Increased failing in school, parental abuse, social isolation, poor self-esteem, risk of substance abuse, automobile accidents, and injuries.

REFERENCES

1. American Psychiatric Association. *Diagnostic and Statistical Manual of Mental Disorders: DSM-5-TR*. 5th ed. Text rev. Washington, DC: American Psychiatric Association Publishing; 2022.

ADDITIONAL READING

Felt BT, Biermann B, Christner JG, et al. Diagnosis and management of ADHD in children. *Am Fam Physician*. 2014;90(7):456–464.

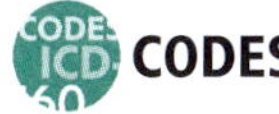

ICD10

- F90.2 Attention-deficit hyperactivity disorder, combined type
- F90.0 Attention-deficit hyperactivity disorder, predominantly inattentive type
- F90 Attention-deficit hyperactivity disorders

CLINICAL PEARLS

- Identify treatment goals before initiating any intervention and make treatment plan based on these goals.
- Behavioral therapy for child and parents, and coordination with teachers and behavioral specialists in schools.
- AAP recommends behavioral interventions for age 4 to 5 years and behavioral interventions plus stimulant medications as first-line treatment for age 6 to 17 years.
- Multiple medications—stimulants first line; titrate to patient response with close monitoring of response and side effects.

ATYPICAL MOLE (DYSPLASTIC NEVUS) SYNDROME

Sahil Mullick, MD, FAAFP • Lakshmi Gopinath Jaisankar, MD

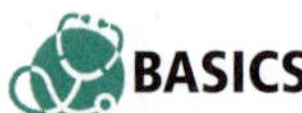

BASICS

Atypical mole syndrome (AMS), also known as dysplastic nevi syndrome (DNS), B-K mole syndrome, Clark nevi syndrome, or familial atypical multiple mole melanoma (FAMMM) syndrome, is a condition characterized by a large number of pigmented nevi with architectural disorder, which arise sporadically or by inheritance and are associated with an increased risk of melanoma.

DESCRIPTION

There is no consensus on criteria for AMS.

- Elevated total body nevi count, including clinically atypical nevi, is usually >50 and often >100.
  - Larger number in hereditary AMS versus sporadic atypical nevi (as few as <10)
- Increased risk of melanoma
  - Up to 90% occurrence by age 80 years in certain high-risk individuals
  - Earlier onset than in sporadic melanoma
  - More arise de novo than from an existing nevus (1)[A]
  - Higher risk for appearance at unusual sites (e.g., scalp, eyes, and sun-protected areas)
- Median age of diagnosis for melanoma in AMS is 10 to 20 years earlier than the general population, with documented cases of melanoma as early as in the 2nd and 3rd decades of life.

EPIDEMIOLOGY

Incidence

Uncertain due to phenotype variability, limited data

Prevalence

Affects between 2% and 8% of fair-skinned adults as well as those with high exposure to ultraviolet radiation

ETIOLOGY AND PATHOPHYSIOLOGY

- Cyclin-dependent kinase inhibitor 2A (*CDKN2A*) mutations have been observed in familial DNS and multiple melanomas. The *CDKN2A* gene on 9p21 encodes for the proteins p16 and p14. p16 binds to CDK4/6 and is a negative cell-cycle regulator via inhibition of the CDK-cyclin D interaction needed for cell cycle progression from G1 to S. p14 functions by stabilizing the tumor-suppressor protein p53 in the G1 phase of the cell cycle.
- Familial cases of germline *CDKN2A* mutations are transmitted in an autosomal dominant fashion.
- No clear somatic mutation patterns in sporadic cases

Genetics

CDKN2A gene mutation is observed in 25–40% of hereditary cases, with autosomal dominant inheritance but variable expressivity and incomplete penetrance.

RISK FACTORS

Family history of melanoma or multiple nevi, sun exposure, neonatal blue-light phototherapy, history of painful sunburns

GENERAL PREVENTION

- Primary prevention with sun avoidance, sun protection (may be especially important in presence of already-dysplastic nevi (2)
- Secondary prevention of melanoma with routine skin exams, biopsy of suspect lesions, and environmental risk mitigation as above

COMMONLY ASSOCIATED CONDITIONS

- Malignant melanoma, including ocular melanoma
- Ocular nevi
- Pancreatic cancer in *CDKN2A* mutation

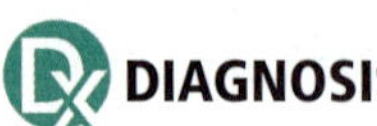

DIAGNOSIS

AMS is a clinical diagnosis with various classifications schemes proposed. Although not widely accepted, diagnostic criteria, as defined by the NIH, require the three features of (i) malignant melanoma in ≥1 first- or second-degree relatives; (ii) numerous melanocytic nevi (frequently >50), some of which are clinically atypical; and (iii) nevi that have certain histologic features (3).

HISTORY

- Changing lesions: bleeding, scaling, size, texture, nonhealing, hyper- or hypopigmentation
- Large number of nevi
- Congenital nevi
- Sun exposure
- Prior skin biopsies
- Prior melanoma
- Immunosuppression (e.g., AIDS, chemotherapy, pancreatic cancer)
- First- or second-degree relatives with:
  - AMS
  - Melanoma
  - Pancreatic cancer

PHYSICAL EXAM

- Full-body skin exams, with photography to track new and changing nevi
- Goal to distinguish melanoma from atypical mole (AM)
- ABCDE mnemonic for skin lesions concerning for melanoma: Asymmetry, Border irregularity, Color variegation, Diameter >6 mm, and Evolving lesion
  - AM is often defined as ≥5 mm and at least two other features.
  - Melanoma typically has several characteristics of ABCDEs, with increased specificity for melanoma if lesion diameter is >6 mm.
- "Ugly duckling sign" (4)[B]:
  - Melanoma screening strategy for increasing accuracy of diagnosis of melanoma by identifying malignant nevi straying from the predominant nevus pattern when numerous atypical nevi are present
- Most common features of AM on dermoscopy include (5):
  - Reticular pattern most common
  - Uniform pigmentation most common followed by multifocal hypo- or hyperpigmentation
  - Homogenous brown globules
  - Pigmentation with central heterogeneity and abrupt termination
- Dermatoscopic features more suggestive of melanoma include (6):
  - Depigmented areas
  - Whitish veil
  - Homogenous areas distributed irregularly, in multiple areas, or >25% of total lesion
  - ≥4 colors

DIFFERENTIAL DIAGNOSIS

- Common nevus: acquired or congenital
- Melanoma
- Seborrheic keratosis
- Dermatofibroma
- Lentigo
- Pigmented actinic keratosis
- Pigmented basal cell carcinoma
- Blue rubber bleb nevus syndrome

DIAGNOSTIC TESTS & INTERPRETATION

Diagnosis is first suspected with history and physical exam and then confirmed by biopsy and histopathology.

Initial Tests (lab, imaging)

- Dermoscopy can be used for a more detailed exam of nevus to aid in distinguishing between benign and malignant lesions as well as for further classification to any of the 11 subtypes; however, the degree of success is dependent on the skill of the examiner.
- Reflectance confocal microscopy (RCM) may provide more specificity than dermoscopy in distinguishing AM from melanoma.
- When the total nevus count is high and following each nevus is impractical, total body photography may aid in the evaluation of evolving nevi as well as in documenting new nevi.

Follow-Up Tests & Special Considerations

Genetic testing is available for *CDKN2A* mutations, but it is not recommended outside of research studies because results cannot be adequately used for management or surveillance.

Diagnostic Procedures/Other

- Biopsy is recommended for any lesion where melanoma cannot be excluded or in the presence of clinically concerning features (e.g., recent growth) (7)[B].

- Biopsy entails full-thickness biopsy of the entire lesion with a narrow 1- to 3-mm margin of normal skin down to fat for adequate depth assessment.
  - Excisional biopsy, elliptical or punch excision, provides the most accurate diagnosis and should be performed when possible.
  - Scoop shave biopsy can also be used, but care must be taken to not transect the lesion.
- Reexcision of mild to moderately dysplastic nevi with positive margins likely does not change pathologic diagnosis or outcomes (2),(8)[A], but for severely dysplastic nevi which shares features with melanoma, consider reexcision, with surgical margins of 2 to 5 mm (9)[C].
- Genetic testing can help diagnosis in ambiguous situations, but studies are limited.

Test Interpretation

"Dysplastic nevus" is a term more accurately reserved as a histologic diagnosis. Features may include melanocyte proliferation in the dermoepidermal junction extending through at least three rete ridges in a specific pattern, fusing of rete ridges, dermal fibrosis, neovascularization, and interstitial lymphocytic inflammation (9).

TREATMENT

MEDICATION

No medications have been shown to treat AMS (9)[C].

ISSUES FOR REFERRAL

- Routine skin exams and total-body photography for those patients at high risk for melanoma
- Ophthalmologic exams for ocular nevi/melanoma screening/papilledema
- Oncology or specialized genetics study group involvement if strong family predisposition to pancreatic cancer

ADDITIONAL THERAPIES

- Topical chemo- and immunotherapies have been unsuccessfully attempted to treat AMS (9)[C].
- Laser treatment should be avoided because it is both unsafe and ineffective for melanocytic nevi (9)[C].

SURGERY/OTHER PROCEDURES

Surgical excision of all atypical nevi is not recommended because most melanomas in AMS appear de novo on healthy skin and therefore has low clinical value and is not cost-effective. Excision of all atypical nevi also leads to both poor cosmetic outcomes and a false sense of security. Lesions suspicious for melanoma should be biopsied or removed surgically.

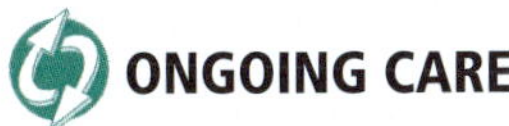

ONGOING CARE

FOLLOW-UP RECOMMENDATIONS

Close follow-up with a dermatologist or other physician experienced with assessment of atypical nevi:

- Total body skin exam (including nails, scalp, genital area, and oral mucosa) every 6 months initially, starting at puberty; may be reduced to annually once nevi are stable
- Total body photography at baseline and intervals to track new and changing nevi
- Dermoscopic evaluation of suspicious lesions
- Excision of suspicious lesions
- Ocular exam for those with familial AMS

Patient Monitoring

Monthly self-exams of skin

PATIENT EDUCATION

For young adults with fair skin, counsel to minimize exposure to ultraviolet radiation to reduce risk of skin cancer (USPSTF grade B).

- Fair skin: light eye, hair, or skin color, freckles
- Educate on sun avoidance, proper application of sunscreen, use of protective clothing (e.g., hats), avoidance of tanning booths and sunburns.
- Teach "ABCDE" mnemonic + "ugly duckling sign" to assess nevi and identify potential melanomas.
- Provide instruction on skin self-exam techniques.
- A sample listing of patient-centric review sources on this topic are as follows:
  - Verywell Health: https://www.verywellhealth.com/the-abcdes-of-skin-cancer-514388
  - Skin Cancer Foundation: https://www.skincancer.org/risk-factors/atypical-moles/
  - Melanoma Research Foundation: https://melanoma.org/melanoma-education/what-melanoma-looks-like/

PROGNOSIS

- Most AMs either regress or do not change.
- Multiple classification schemes have been developed over the years to delineate risk of melanoma in patients with AMS. Individuals with a family history of melanoma are at greatest risk. The Rigel classification system can be applied in the clinical setting. Points are assigned based on incidence of melanoma, with 1 point given for a personal history with melanoma and 2 points for each family member with melanoma (modified nuclear family consisting of first-degree relatives plus grandparents and uncles/aunts) and stratified as follows:
  - Score = 0, Rigel group 0, 6% 25-year accumulated risk for melanoma
  - Score = 1, Rigel group 1, 10% risk
  - Score = 2, Rigel group 2, 15% risk
  - Score ≥3, Rigel group 3, 50% risk
- The *CDKN2A* mutation has also been associated with a 60–90% risk of melanoma by age 80 years and a 17% risk for pancreatic cancer by age 75 years. In patients with melanoma, presence of the *CDKN2A* mutation may not worsen overall survival rates.

COMPLICATIONS

- Malignant melanoma
- Poor cosmetic outcomes from biopsy

REFERENCES

1. Dessinioti C, Befon A, Stratigos AJ. The association of nevus-associated melanoma with common or dysplastic melanocytic nevus: a systematic review and meta-analysis. *Cancers (Basel)*. 2023;15(3):856.
2. Spaccarelli N, Drozdowski R, Peters MS, et al. Dysplastic nevus part II: dysplastic nevi: molecular/genetic profiles and management. *J Am Acad Dermatol*. 2023 Jan;88(1):13–20.
3. Goldsmith LA, Askin FB, Chang AE, et al. Diagnosis and treatment of early melanoma: NIH consensus development panel on early melanoma. *JAMA*. 1992;268(10):1314–1319.
4. Gaudy-Marqueste C, Wazaefi Y, Bruneu Y, et al. Ugly duckling sign as a major factor of efficiency in melanoma detection. *JAMA Dermatol*. 2017;153(4):279–284.
5. Hofmann-Wellenhof R, Blum A, Wolf IH, et al. Dermoscopic classification of atypical melanocytic nevi (Clark nevi). *Arch Dermatol*. 2001;137(12):1575–1580.
6. Salopek TG, Kopf AW, Stefanato CM, et al. Differentiation of atypical moles (dysplastic nevi) from early melanomas by dermoscopy. *Dermatol Clin*. 2001;19(2):337–345.
7. Wiedemeyer K, Hartschuh W, Brenn T. Dysplastic nevi: morphology and molecular and the controversies in-between. *Surg Pathol Clin*. 2021;14(2):341–357.
8. Vuong KT, Walker J, Powell HB, et al. Surgical re-excision vs. observation for histologically dysplastic naevi: a systematic review of associated clinical outcomes. *Br J Dermatol*. 2018;179(3):590–598.
9. Duffy K, Grossman D. The dysplastic nevus: from historical perspective to management in the modern era: part I. historical, histologic, and clinical aspects. *J Am Acad Dermatol*. 2012;67(1):1.e1–1.e18.

ADDITIONAL READING

Perkins A, Duffy RL. Atypical moles: diagnosis and management. *Am Fam Physician*. 2015;91(11):762–767.

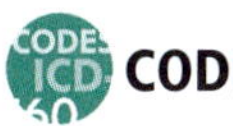

CODES

ICD10

- D22.9 Melanocytic nevi, unspecified
- D22.4 Melanocytic nevi of scalp and neck
- D22.30 Melanocytic nevi of unspecified part of face

CLINICAL PEARLS

- In describing nevi, "atypical" is a clinical term, whereas "dysplastic" is a histologic term.
- AMS is a risk factor for melanoma, although most atypical moles/dysplastic nevi are not precursors of melanoma. Melanoma in AMS tends to arise from healthy skin despite a large number of atypical nevi.
- ~20% of individuals with familial AMS will develop pancreatic cancer by age 75 years.
- Patients with AMS tend to produce neoplasms in unusual sites such as the scalp, eyes, and sun-protected areas (e.g., gluteal folds).

AUTISM SPECTRUM DISORDERS

Tasaduq Hussain Mir, MD, FAAFP • Afsha Rais Kaisani, MD, FAAFP

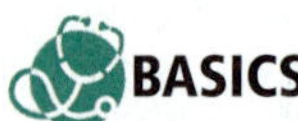

BASICS

DESCRIPTION

- Autism spectrum disorder (ASD) is a developmental disorder impacting roughly 1 in 59 children across the United States and other high-income countries. American Academy of Pediatrics (AAP), in contrast to the U.S. Preventive Services Task Force (USPSTF), recommends screening for ASD at 18 and 24 months of age. It is important to distinguish ASD from symptoms that could be better explained by other intellectual disability.
- Symptoms must cause functional impairment; severity levels:
  - Level 1: requiring support—noticeable impairment
  - Level 2: requiring substantial support—marked deficits
  - Level 3: requiring very substantial support—severe impairments interfering with functionality

EPIDEMIOLOGY

Onset in early childhood; predominant sex: male > female, approximately 4:1 ratio

Pediatric Considerations

Symptom onset can often be seen in children <3 years of age but may not become apparent until social demands exceed capacity.

Prevalence

- Estimated prevalence has increased from approximately 1.1% in 2008 to 2.3% in 2018 among children aged 8 years in the United States (1).
- Higher prevalence contributed to changes in diagnostic criteria, increased awareness, improved ascertainment, and access to care (1).
- Higher percentage of ASD observed in Black, Hispanic, and Asian and Pacific Islander children than in White children, which could reflect improvements in identification among these groups (1).

ETIOLOGY AND PATHOPHYSIOLOGY

- No single cause has been identified. Variety of genetic and environmental factors have been associated with ASD, but none with absolute specificity for ASD development (1).
- ASD has no association with immunization.

Genetics

- Genetic concordance: A 2009 Swedish population-based cohort study of 2 million subjects showed a cumulative risk of 59% for monozygotic twins.
- The American College of Medical Genetics and Genomics practice guidelines lists the risk of siblings of children diagnosed with ASD without an identifiable cause to be 7% if the affected child is female, 4% if the affected child is male, >30% if there are ≥2 affected children.

RISK FACTORS

- Male sex, advanced paternal age, family history, very low birth weight
- Perinatal insults including toxic exposures, teratogens, prenatal infections, use of selective serotonin reuptake inhibitors (SSRI) or valproate during pregnancy

GENERAL PREVENTION

- Screening for early intervention is associated with improved prognosis, yet median age of diagnosis in the United States is >4 years.
- Routine screening for ASD with a validated tool is recommended at 18- and 24-month well-child visits to assist with early detection.
- Screening is indicated after 24 months if parents or clinician have concerns about ASD as less severe presentations may pass earlier routine screening.
- Children with false positives for ASD frequently have some form of developmental disorder and benefit from early intervention.
- Screening difficult due to variability of signs and symptoms of ASD and lack of unanimous consensus of social developmental milestones, thus leading to delayed diagnosis

COMMONLY ASSOCIATED CONDITIONS

- Intellectual disability (seizure in severe cases)
- Attention deficit hyperactivity disorder (ADHD), anxiety, depression, or obsessive behavior
- Motor impairments including hypotonia, apraxia, toe walking, or gross motor delays
- Phenylketonuria (PKU), tuberous sclerosis, fragile X syndrome, Angelman syndrome, Rett syndrome, CHARGE syndrome, Joubert syndrome, Smith-Lemli-Opitz syndrome, Timothy syndrome, and fetal alcohol syndrome (rare)
- Sleep issues: insomnia, circadian rhythm sleep-wake disorder, sleep-related movement disorder
- Change in bowel habits, abdominal pain

DIAGNOSIS

Based on developmental history and behavior

HISTORY

Listen to parents' concerns and test early for suspicion of a neurodevelopmental disorder.

- Impairment in social-emotional reciprocity: failure of normal back-and-forth conversations
- Deficits in nonverbal communication: abnormal eye contact or body language; deficits in understanding and use of gestures; lack of facial expression and nonverbal communication
- Deficits in developing, maintaining, and understanding relationships:
  - Difficulties adjusting behavior to suit various social contexts; difficulties in sharing imaginative play or in making friends; absence of interest and developing peer relationships
- Repetitive and stereotyped behavior patterns
  - Stereotyped or repetitive motor movements, use of objects, or speech
  - Insistence patterns of behavior with intolerance to change
  - Fixated interests that are abnormal in intensity or focus
  - Hyperreactivity or hyporeactivity to sensory input or unusual interest in sensory aspects of the environment
- History of seizure disorder
- Family history of autism, genetic disorders, learning disabilities, psychiatric illness, or neurologic disorders

PHYSICAL EXAM

- Measurement of growth parameters: height, weight, head circumference (Macrocephaly is present in 25% of ASD.)
- Vision, hearing, speech/language, and communication assessments
- Developmental and sensorimotor testing
- Complete neurologic exam
- Examination for dysmorphic features consistent with genetic disorders
- Wood lamp skin exam to rule out skin manifestations of neurocutaneous disorders
- Red flags: early symptoms of ASD
  - By 9 months—does not respond to name or show facial expressions of emotions
  - By 12 months—no simple interactive games
  - By 18 months—no pointing

DIFFERENTIAL DIAGNOSIS

- Behavioral disorder: anxiety, obsessive-compulsive, reactive attachment
- Development disorders: elective mutism, Rett syndrome, language disorder, hearing impairment, intellectual disability/global developmental delay, social communication disorder, ADHD
- Others: fetal alcohol disorder, tic disorder, fragile X syndrome, acquired epileptic aphasia

DIAGNOSTIC TESTS & INTERPRETATION

- The AAP recommends developments and behavioral screening for all children during well-child visits at 9, 18, and 30 months.
- Recommendation for ASD screening at 18 and 24 months
- The Modified Checklist for Autism in Toddlers (M-CHAT): commonly used test to screen for ASD in children 12 to 30 months; additional information needed for children <12 months (M-CHAT) (2)[B]
- The Modified Checklist for Autism in Toddlers Revised, Follow-up (M-CHAT-R/F): improved PPV, lower false-positive rate in children aged 16 to 30 months, especially those with cultural barriers (M-CHAT-R/F) (2)[B]; children with M-CHAT-R total score >2 are considered at risk and require follow-up.
- Infant and toddler checklist (parent questionnaire): identifies language delay in low-risk patients between 6 and 24 months; useful in identifying infant siblings of children with ASD at increased risk for ASD (2)[B]
- Screening Tool for Autism in Toddlers and Young Children (STAT) shows promising evidence as level 2 screening to detect 2-year-olds with autism with other developmental disorders (2)[B].
- Autism Diagnostic Interview, Revised (ADI-R) is a semi-structured interview with the parent(s) and the Autism Diagnostic Observation Schedule, 2nd Edition (ADOS-2) is a semi-structured direct observation of a child's behavior with sensitivity of 80% and 91%, respectively, and specificity of 72% and 76%, respectively (1).
- ASD screening tools for older children: Autism Spectrum Quotient-Child and Childhood Autism Spectrum Test (ages 4 to 11 years), Autism Spectrum Screening Questionnaire (ages 7 to 16 years), the Developmental Behaviour Checklist (ages 4 to 18 years with intellectual disabilities), and Asperger Syndrome Diagnostic Scale (higher functioning children aged 5 to 18 years)

Initial Tests (lab, imaging)

- Chromosomal microarray (CMA), DNA analysis (fragile X), and whole exome sequencing
- Complete blood count, thyroid-stimulating hormone, creatine kinase, and PKU screening; consider lead testing.
- Complete metabolic panel if systemic signs or symptoms are present.
- TORCH (toxoplasmosis, others [syphilis, varicel-lazoster, parvovirus B_{19}], rubella, cytomegalovirus, HIV, and herpes) infection workup if microcephaly is present.
- MRI if focal neurologic symptoms

Follow-Up Tests & Special Considerations

- Children with ASD have the same general health care needs as other children and should receive the same preventative care.
- Follow-up appointments and testing recommended as indicated for comorbidities
- Consider additional hearing tests with audiometry and brainstem auditory evoked response (BAER) or consultation to audiology.
- Speech and language evaluation
- Evaluation by multidisciplinary team: psychiatrist, genetic counselor, neurologist, psychologist, other autism specialists
- Monitoring of intellectual level

Diagnostic Procedures/Other

Electroencephalogram if displaying signs or symptoms suggestive of epilepsy or specific developmental disorders associated with abnormal encephalographic findings (1)

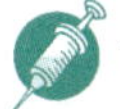

TREATMENT

Goal of therapy is to improve function and well-being (1).

GENERAL MEASURES

Two categories of evidence-based interventions exist: comprehensive treatment model (CTM) and focused interventions (1),(2)

- CTMs are replicable, intense, and specifically designed programs that address a broad range of symptoms and specific skill(s) or symptom(s). Some examples of CTMs include early intensive behavioral intervention with applied behavior analysis, focused on learning and reinforcing acceptable behaviors: Treatment and Education of Autistic and Related Communication-Handicapped Children (TEACCH) and the Early Start Denver Model (ESDM).
  - Treatment addresses social communication, language, play skills, and maladaptive behavior to improve cognitive, language, and adaptive skills.
- Focused intervention practices: designed to address social communication or learning a specific task and generally arranged to be delivered over a short period of time
  - Cognitive-behavioral therapy: shown to reduce anxiety in older children with ASD

MEDICATION

First Line

- FDA-approved psychotropic medications for irritability, aggression, and emotional dysregulation in individuals with ASD:
  - Risperidone: age >5 years—0.25 mg/day in <20 kg; 0.5 mg/day in >20 kg with effective dose ranges 0.5 to 3.0 mg/day PO divided doses
  - Aripiprazole: ages 6 to 17 years; PO; initial dose 2 mg daily for 2 days, increase up to 5 mg daily/week; max 15 mg/day
- Stimulants (such as methylphenidate, atomoxetine and guanfacine extended-release): efficacious in treating concomitant symptoms of ADHD
- SSRIs: limited evidence for ASD; initial choice for anxiety and depressive mood
- Melatonin used for patients with concomitant sleep disorders; shown mixed efficacy

ISSUES FOR REFERRAL

Refer early for evaluation of behavior and language, genetic counseling, and audiology. Refer to geneticist if ASD associated with genetic syndrome. Consider referrals to psychiatry, ophthalmology, otolaryngology, neurology, and nutrition. Refer family members to support groups.

COMPLEMENTARY & ALTERNATIVE MEDICINE

- Medications such as secretin, intravenous immunoglobulin, vitamins, and minerals have no benefit; may carry risks
- Music, massage, therapeutic horseback riding, and other pet therapies merit further review.

ONGOING CARE

Planning for transition to adulthood should begin around 12 to 14 years of age, with adaptation for developmental abilities.

FOLLOW-UP RECOMMENDATIONS

Patient Monitoring

- Constant monitoring by caregivers; evaluation every 6 to 12 months by physician for symptom and medical management
- Intellectual and language testing every 2 years in childhood
- Siblings of children with ASD should be monitored for symptoms of ASD.

DIET

Insufficient evidence for recommendations of any certain dietary modifications for ASD.

PROGNOSIS

- Prognosis influenced by IQ, early intervention, strength of early language skills, and psychiatric comorbidities
- General expected course is for a lifelong need for supervised structured care; some patients will develop gainful employment, independent living, and social relationships.

COMPLICATIONS

Increased risk for physical and sexual abuse; with pica, increased risk of lead poisoning; gastrointestinal issues

REFERENCES

1. Hirota T, King BH. Autism spectrum disorder: a review. *JAMA*. 2023;329(2):157–168. doi:10.1001/jama.2022.23661.
2. Hyman SL, Levy SE, Myers SM, et al. Identification, evaluation, and management of children with autism spectrum disorder. *Pediatrics*. 2020;145(1):e20193447.

ADDITIONAL READING

Sanchack KE, Thomas CA. Autism spectrum disorder: primary care principles. *Am Fam Physician*. 2016;94(12):972–979.

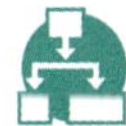

SEE ALSO

Algorithm: Intellectual Disability

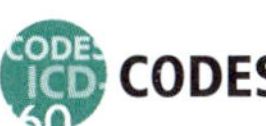

CODES

ICD10

- F84.5 Asperger's syndrome
- F84 Pervasive developmental disorders
- F84.2 Rett's syndrome

CLINICAL PEARLS

AAP ALARM mnemonic:

- **A**SD is prevalent (screen all children between 18 and 24 months).
- **L**isten to parents when they feel something is wrong.
- **A**ct early: Screen children with delayed language and social developmental milestones.
- **R**efer to multidisciplinary teams.
- **M**onitor support for patient and families.

BABESIOSIS

Frederick W. Nielson, MD

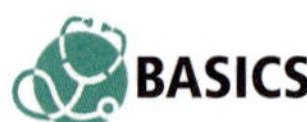

BASICS

DESCRIPTION

- Rare tick-borne hemolytic disease caused by intraerythrocytic protozoan parasites of the genus *Babesia microti* transmitted by *Ixodes scapularis*.
- Transmission primarily occurs in Northeast and upper Midwest. Asymptomatic infection is common in these areas. Disease is rarely found outside the United States although sporadic cases have been reported in Central America, Europe, and even China; all within the Northern Hemisphere.
- Incubation period varies from 5 to 33 days:
  - Most patients do not recall specific tick exposure.
  - After transfusion of infected blood, the incubation period can be up to 9 weeks.
- System(s) affected: cardiovascular, gastrointestinal, hemic/lymphatic/immunologic, musculoskeletal, nervous, pulmonary, renal/urologic

Pediatric Considerations

Transplacental and perinatal transmission is rare. Atovaquone has been used safely in children who weigh >5 kg.

Pregnancy Considerations

Safety data on use of atovaquone in pregnant women are limited. However, there are limited safety data available to suggest administration of quinine plus clindamycin during pregnancy may be safe. For this reason this drug combination, rather than atovaquone plus azithromycin is generally recommended for treatment of symptomatic babesiosis during pregnancy.

Geriatric Considerations

Morbidity and mortality are higher in elderly populations, especially with those who have comorbidities.

EPIDEMIOLOGY

- Babesiosis affects patients of all ages. Most patients present between ages 50 and 80 years.
- Coinfection with other tick-borne illness (anaplasmosis, ehrlichiosis, Lyme Disease) is common.

Incidence

- Cases reported to the CDC hover around 2,000 per year (data last reported in 2020): https://www.cdc.gov/parasites/babesiosis/data-statistics/index.html
- In patients at high risk for tick-borne diseases, seroconversion data show antibodies to *B. microti* in 7 of 671 individuals (1%).

Prevalence

Prevalence is difficult to estimate due to lack of surveillance and asymptomatic infections.

ETIOLOGY AND PATHOPHYSIOLOGY

- Of the 100 species known, only 6 species have been found to be pathogenic in humans. *B. microti* (most common in the United States) and *Babesia divergens* and *Babesia bovis* (in Europe) cause most human infections. *B. divergens* and a new strain *Babesia duncani* appear to be more virulent. Other species are identified in case reports. All share morphologic, antigenic, and genetic characteristics.
- Ixodid (hard-bodied) ticks are the primary vectors.
- The white-footed deer mouse is the primary reservoir.
- Infection is passed to humans through the saliva of a nymphal-stage tick during a blood meal. Sporozoites introduced at the time of the bite enter red blood cells and form merozoites through binary fission (classic morphology on blood smear). Humans are a dead-end host for *B. microti*.
- In the United States, transmission may occur via blood transfusion from donors who are asymptomatic at the time of blood donation.

RISK FACTORS

Those residing in endemic areas are at elevated risk for contracting babesiosis. Complications from the disease are highest in those with asplenia, who are immunocompromised or elderly.

GENERAL PREVENTION

- Avoid endemic regions during the peak transmission months of May to September.
- Appropriate insect repellent is advised during outdoor activities, especially in wooded or grassy areas.
  - 10–35% N,N-diethyl-meta-toluamide (DEET) provides adequate skin protection.
  - Acaricides, such as permethrin, provide impregnated clothing with even further protection.
- Daily skin checks to ensure early removal of ticks is essential.

COMMONLY ASSOCIATED CONDITIONS

Coinfection with *Borrelia burgdorferi* (Lyme disease), *Ehrlichia,* and *B. microti* in endemic areas is relatively common.

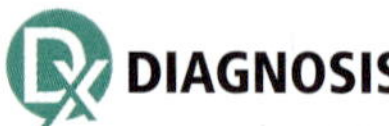

DIAGNOSIS

HISTORY

- Travel history to endemic regions as well as exposure history are helpful.
- The tick must remain attached for at least 24 hours before the transmission of *B. microti* occurs.
- Severe disease is more common in patients with comorbidities (immunosuppression, chronic disease), so maintaining a proper index of suspicion after exposure history may prompt workup and treatment.
- The disease presentation is similar to malaria (1): fever (68–89%), fatigue (78–79%), chills (39–68%), sweats (41–56%), headache (32–75%), myalgia (32–37%), anorexia (24–25%), cough (17–23%), arthralgias (17–32%), nausea (9–22%); other symptoms include abdominal pain, vomiting, and diarrhea.

PHYSICAL EXAM

- High fever (up to 104°F [40°C])
- Hemodynamic instability (shock in extremely ill)
- Hepatomegaly and splenomegaly (mild if noted)
- Rash (uncommon; if rash is present, consider concurrent Lyme disease.)
- CNS involvement includes headache, photophobia, neck and back stiffness, altered sensorium, and emotional lability.
- Jaundice and dark urine may develop later in course of illness.

DIFFERENTIAL DIAGNOSIS

- Bacterial sepsis
- Hepatitis
- Lyme disease, ehrlichiosis, babesiosis, Rocky Mountain spotted fever
- Leishmaniasis
- Malaria
- HIV, EBV
- HELLP syndrome (in pregnancy)

DIAGNOSTIC TESTS & INTERPRETATION

Initial Tests (lab, imaging)

- Diagnosis requires a high index of clinical suspicion. Nonspecific laboratory clues include evidence of mild to severe hemolytic anemia, normal to slightly depressed leukocyte count, thrombocytopenia, elevated LDH or transaminase level, elevated BUN and creatinine, proteinuria, and hemoglobinuria.
- Definitive diagnosis is made by blood smear.
  - Wright- or Giemsa-stained peripheral blood smear demonstrates intraerythrocytic parasites.
  - Dividing "cross-like" tetrads of merozoites (Maltese cross) are pathognomonic.
  - Serial blood smears may be required (low parasite load early in the illness).
  - Can be confused with *Plasmodium falciparum* on peripheral smear
- Detection of *B. microti* by polymerase chain reaction (PCR) is more sensitive and equally specific in acute cases. PCR can also be used to monitor disease progression. Newer real-time PCR tests have a sensitivity and specificity approaching 100%.

Follow-Up Tests & Special Considerations

Monitoring intraerythrocytic parasitemia helps guide treatment.

TREATMENT

GENERAL MEASURES

- In areas endemic for Lyme disease and ehrlichiosis, doxycycline 100 mg BID PO empirically treats coinfection until serologic testing is complete.
- Drug resistance has emerged in severely immunocompromised patients.
- Consider treating asymptomatic patients if parasitemia persists for >3 months; otherwise, do not treat in absence of symptoms.

MEDICATION

First Line

- Mild to moderate infection with *B. microti*:
  - 7 to 10 days of atovaquone 750 mg PO (with a fatty meal) BID *plus*
  - Azithromycin 250 to 500 mg/day PO QD
- Pediatrics: atovaquone 20 mg/kg (max 750 mg) BID and azithromycin 10 mg/kg (max 500 mg) on day 1 and then 5 mg/kg (max 250 mg) (2)[C]
- For severe *B. microti* infection oral quinine 650 mg TID or QID *plus* clindamycin 600 mg QID for 7 to 10 days
  - Pediatrics: clindamycin 7 to 10 mg/kg (max 600 mg) TID or QID and quinine 8 mg/kg (max 650 mg) TID
- Persistent or relapsing babesiosis: Treat for 6 weeks, including 2 weeks after Babesia is no longer detected on blood smear.

Second Line

- Combination of quinine sulfate 650 mg PO TID and clindamycin 600 mg PO TID or 1.2 g parenterally BID for 7 to 10 days is the most commonly used treatment. Pediatric: quinine 8 mg/kg (max 650 mg) q6–8h for 7 to 10 days and clindamycin 7 to 10 mg/kg (max 600 mg) PO q6–8h for 7 to 10 days; some experts prefer this regimen for severe infections (2)[C].
- Other drugs including tetracycline, primaquine, sulfadiazine (Microsulfon), and sulfadoxine/pyrimethamine (Fansidar) have been evaluated. Results vary. Pentamidine (Pentam) is moderately effective in diminishing symptoms and decreasing parasitemia.

ALERT

- Clindamycin can lead to *Clostridium difficile*–associated diarrhea.
- It is helpful to know G6PD status before using quinine therapy.

ISSUES FOR REFERRAL

Consultation with hematology and infectious disease for exchange transfusion may be considered in severe disease (blood parasitemia is >10%, there is massive hemolysis, and asplenia).

ADMISSION, INPATIENT, AND NURSING CONSIDERATIONS

Targeted organ damage due to disease by prompt inpatient management; select patients with severe babesiosis and organ compromise may be considered for exchange transfusion.

ONGOING CARE

FOLLOW-UP RECOMMENDATIONS

Patient Monitoring

- If left untreated, silent babesiosis may persist for months or years.
- Alkaline phosphatase levels >125 U/L, WBC counts >5 × 10^9/L, history of cardiac abnormality, history of splenectomy, presence of heart murmur, and parasitemia of ≥4% are associated with disease severity.
- The need for monitoring depends on disease severity. In cases of severe infection hematocrit and parasitemia levels can be followed until clinical improvement is evident and parasitemia is <5%. For mild to moderate disease anticipate clinical improvement within 48 hours and complete resolution within 3 months.
- Sporadic cases of persistent, relapsing low-grade parasitemia have been reported so frequent and flexible testing for patients who are treated may be considered.

COMPLICATIONS

- Many remain asymptomatic.
- Complications in hospitalized patients: CHF (12%), DIC (18%), ARDS (21%), renal failure (6%), coma/lethargy (9%), death (9%)
- Other reported complications include neutropenia and myocardial infarction.
- In asplenic patients, warm autoimmune hemolytic anemia has been reported.

REFERENCES

1. Waked R, Krause PJ. Human babesiosis. *Infect Dis Clin North Am*. 2022;36(3):655–670.
2. Krause PJ, Auwaerter PG, Bannuru RR, et al. Clinical practice guidelines by the Infectious Diseases Society of America (IDSA): 2020 guideline on the diagnosis and management of babesiosis. *Clin Infect Dis*. 2021;72(2):e49–e64. doi:10.1093/cid/ciaa1216.

ADDITIONAL READING

- Centers for Disease Control and Prevention. Parasites-Babesiosis. Resources for Health Professionals. https://cdc.gov/babesiosis/hcp/clinical-care/index.html. Accessed October 26, 2025.
- Vannier E, Hunfeld KP, Smith RP, et al. Management of human babesiosis—approaches and perspectives. *Expert Rev Anti Infect Ther*. 2025;23(9):739–752. doi:10.1080/14787210.2025.2526843.

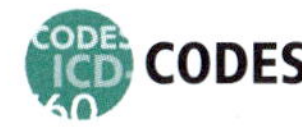

CODES

ICD10

B60.0 Babesiosis

CLINICAL PEARLS

- Ticks must remain in place for 24 hours to transmit infection. Encourage daily "tick checks" if people are exposed in high-risk areas.
- Most patients do not recall tick exposure, and incubation can last up to a month.
- Left untreated, silent babesiosis may persist for months or years and may not require treatment.
- First-line treatment for mild or moderate disease is atovaquone plus azithromycin.
- Patients with mild-to-moderate disease should show clinical improvement within 48 hours after starting therapy. Symptoms should fully resolve in 3 months.
- Coinfection with *B. burgdorferi* and *Ehrlichia* species is common in endemic areas, consider adding doxycycline until serologic testing is completed.

BACK PAIN, LOW

Vasilios Chrisostomidis, DO

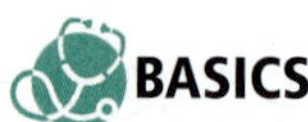

BASICS

DESCRIPTION
- Low back pain (LBP) is a common chief complaint presenting to primary care and acute care settings.
  - 2.5 million were diagnosed with LBP in the United States between 2008 and 2015 (1).
  - Annual expenditure in the United States on LBP care >$100 billion dollars (1)
- Defined as "a pain between the costal margins and the inferior gluteal folds..." (2)
- Suggested classification is by duration (2):
  - Acute: most cases resolve in 4 to 6 weeks
  - Recurrent: repetitive occurrence of symptoms in a year
  - Chronic: at least 3 months in duration
- LBP has significant implications on work-life balance.
  - LBP is the leading cause of loss of productivity worldwide (1).
  - LBP is the leading cause of years lived with disability across 126 countries (1).
- It is necessary to rule out "red" flag symptoms indicating the need for immediate intervention.
- System(s) affected: musculoskeletal, neurologic
- Synonym(s): lumbago, lumbar sprain/strain, low back syndrome

EPIDEMIOLOGY

Incidence
Annually, 7% in the United States (1)

Prevalence
Prevalence increases with age (2):
- 1–6% in children 7 to 10 years old
- 18% in adolescents
- 28–42% in adults 40 to 69 years old (peak prevalence by age)

ETIOLOGY AND PATHOPHYSIOLOGY
Recent subcategorization by primary type of pain (1):
- Mechanical, including facet arthropathy, myofascial pain, sacroiliac joint dysfunction
- Inflammatory, including spondyloarthropathies
- Neuropathic/radicular (16–55% of chronic LBP)—classical symptoms radiating down legs in dermatomes (1)
  - Herniated disk is a common cause.
  - Spinal stenosis results from age related degeneration.
  - Less common causes to consider: metastatic disease, herpes zoster
- Nociplastic—amplified pain from central nervous system (1)

RISK FACTORS
- Age
- High-risk activity (lifting, sudden twisting, bending)
- Obesity
- Sedentary lifestyle
- Physically strenuous work
- Psychosocial factors—anxiety, depression, stress
- Poor flexibility
- Smoking

GENERAL PREVENTION
There is no strong existing evidence for prevention; however, routine physical activity has been shown to be beneficial.

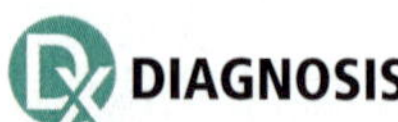

DIAGNOSIS

HISTORY
- Onset of pain (sudden or gradual)
- Inciting event, injury, or trauma
- Frequency of pain (episodic or constant with or without fluctuation)
- Characterization and location of pain:
  - Facet pain commonly radiates to sacroiliac joint/PSIS region.
  - Sacroiliac pain often refers to the thigh and can radiate below the knee.
  - Irritation, impingement, or compression of lumbar nerve roots often results in leg pain rather than back pain.
  - Pain from the L1–L3 nerve roots radiates to the hip and/or thigh; pain from the L4–S1 nerve roots radiates below the knee.
- Red flags (1)
  - Patient history: cancer, trauma, age (<16 years, >50 years), weight loss, immunodeficiency, osteoporosis
  - Medications: IV drug use, corticosteroid use
  - Symptoms: fever, pain at night/at rest, saddle anesthesia, bowel/bladder dysfunction, gait abnormality, night sweats

Pediatric Considerations
A patient <4 years old with LBP should raise suspicion of abuse or a nonmechanical cause; consider malignancy, inflammatory, and infectious processes.

PHYSICAL EXAM
- Follow the "IPASS" system: inspection, palpation, active/passive range of motion, strength, special tests
  - Observe posture, gait, positioning, muscle atrophy
  - Evaluate for point tenderness at midline spinous processes and paraspinal muscle
  - Lumbar spine range of motion evaluation—flexion, extension, rotation, sidebending
- Completely evaluate reflexes, strength, pulses, sensation
  - Slump test:
    - Have patient sit on table and slump shoulders forward.
    - Then have patient touch chin to chest and attempt to have them extend one leg at a time.
    - Symptom reproduction radiating down dermatomal distribution of lower extremities is consistent with lumbar radiculopathy, such as from a disk herniation.
  - Straight leg test:
    - With the patient supine, passively raise the patient's leg straight to at least 60 degrees keeping the knee straight and ankle dorsiflexed.
    - Pain, especially radiating down the leg, may also imply lumbar radiculopathy, such as from a disk herniation.
  - Stork test:
    - Have patient stand on one leg with opposite hip held in flexion.
    - Extend back.
    - Pain in lumbosacral area is a positive test—consider spondylolisthesis versus facet OA.
  - Evaluate for saddle anesthesia; anal wink reflex if concern for cauda equina syndrome exists
- Consider special testing of the hips for differentiation from sacroiliac-related back pain (e.g., FABER, FADIR).
- Evaluate mental and emotional well-being.

DIFFERENTIAL DIAGNOSIS
- Intrinsic spine: fracture, disk herniation, stenosis, muscle strain, spondylolysis/spondylolisthesis/spondylosis (3)
- Systemic: infectious, inflammatory, malignancy, connective tissue disorder (3)
- Referred: abdominal aortic aneurysm, herpes zoster, other pelvic and retroperitoneal diagnoses (3)

B

DIAGNOSTIC TESTS & INTERPRETATION

Initial Tests (lab, imaging)

- Initial diagnosis is typically made clinically via history and physical exam.
- Imaging is *not* recommended in initial presentation, unless red flag symptoms are present.

Follow-Up Tests & Special Considerations

- MRI is recommended for chronic LBP or if surgical/procedural intervention is considered (2).
- X-ray can be considered if concern for fracture, spondylolysis, or spondylolisthesis exists.
- Blood work can be considered if inflammatory, infectious, or rheumatologic conditions are a concern.

Diagnostic Procedures/Other

Emergent neurosurgical consult for acute neurologic deficits or suspected cauda equina syndrome

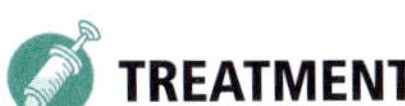

TREATMENT

GENERAL MEASURES

- The American College of Physicians recommends initial treatment with nonpharmacologic options: heat, massage, acupuncture, or spinal manipulation, as they are most effective for (4) improving pain and function with NSAIDs offering the best balance of medication benefit versus harm (5).
- First-line management:
  - Limit bed rest and support early return to routine duties.

MEDICATION

First Line

- NSAIDs (both traditional and COX-2 agents) are equally effective and should be used for acute LBP assuming contraindications do not exist (2).
- Non-benzodiazepine muscle relaxants: Systematic reviews find very low certainty evidence that non-benzodiazepine antispasmodics in the first weeks of treatment provide small reductions in pain intensity but cause an increased risk of adverse events (fatigue, dizziness, etc.).

Second Line

- Rarely needed for acute
- TCAs/SSRIs/SNRIs—assist with neuropathic symptoms and associated mental health concerns
- Gabapentinoids—assist with chronic neuropathic symptoms
- Opioids—rarely needed; use very low dose and shortest possible duration; educate on misuse.

ISSUES FOR REFERRAL

- With referred nerve pain (sciatica), early referral for physical therapy improves time resolution.
- If not responding to initial measures, can consider (2):
  - Osteopathic manipulative therapy, massage therapy TENS unit
- For subacute or chronic pain, referral to PM&R for epidural corticosteroid injection or radiofrequency denervation if long-term radicular symptoms persist
- Failure of conservative measures or presentation of alarm symptoms warrants further evaluation.

ADDITIONAL THERAPIES

There is no strong evidence to support bracing, therapeutic ultrasound, traction, insoles, or inversion table treatment (2).

COMPLEMENTARY & ALTERNATIVE MEDICINE

- Osteopathic manipulation has been found to be effective for nonspecific LBP and for chronic back pain.
- There is no strong evidence to support use of dry needling or meditation (2).

ONGOING CARE

FOLLOW-UP RECOMMENDATIONS

- Initial follow-up is recommended in 2 to 4 weeks for acute flare.
- Longer interval follow-up of 6 to 12 weeks may be beneficial for chronic LBP.

REFERENCES

1. Knezevic NN, Candido KD, Vlaeyen JWS, et al. Low back pain. *Lancet*. 2021;398(10294):78–92. doi:10.1016/S0140-6736(21)00733-9.
2. Bailly F, Trouvin AP, Bercier S, et al. Clinical guidelines and care pathway for management of low back pain with or without radicular pain. *Joint Bone Spine*. 2021;88(6):105227. doi:10.1016/j.jbspin.2021.105227.
3. Casazza BA. Diagnosis and treatment of acute low back pain. *Am Fam Physician*. 2012;85(4):343–350.
4. Qaseem A, Wilt TJ, McLean RM, et al. Noninvasive treatments for acute, subacute, and chronic low back pain: a clinical practice guideline from the American College of Physicians. *Ann Intern Med*. 2017;166(7):514–530. doi:10.7326/M16-2367.
5. Gianola S, Bargeri S, Del Castillo G, et al. Effectiveness of treatments for acute and subacute mechanical non-specific low back pain: a systematic review with network meta-analysis. *Br J Sports Med*. 2022;56(1):41–50. doi:10.1136/bjsports-2020-103596.

ADDITIONAL READING

- Andronis L, Kinghorn P, Qiao S, et al. Cost-effectiveness of non-invasive and non-pharmacological interventions for low back pain: a systematic literature review. *Appl Health Econ Health Policy*. 2017;15(2):173–201.
- Phillips SF, Butts JF, Silvis M. Low back pain in youth: recognizing red flags. *J Fam Pract*. 2020;69(8):E1–E8.

SEE ALSO

Algorithm: Low Back Pain, Acute

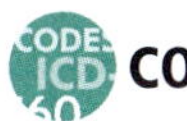

CODES

ICD10

- M54.5 Low back pain
- G89.29 Other chronic pain
- M53.3 Sacrococcygeal disorders, not elsewhere classified

CLINICAL PEARLS

- LBP is a common cause for health care expenditure, disability, and loss of productivity worldwide.
- If no alarm symptoms are present, imaging is not beneficial in initial workup.
- Initial management should include heat, massage, acupuncture, or spinal manipulation, physical therapy for sciatica, activity modification, and NSAIDs.
- Referral for surgical evaluation is necessary if alarm symptoms develop.

BACTERIURIA, ASYMPTOMATIC

Bindusri Paruchuri, MD

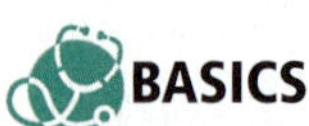

BASICS

DESCRIPTION

Asymptomatic bacteriuria (ASB) is specific bacterial growth of $\geq 10^5$ CFU/mL in one and two consecutive midstream urine samples for men and women, respectively >18 years old. This definition applies to individuals with no clinical symptoms.

EPIDEMIOLOGY

Incidence

- Premenopausal females: 1–6%
- Pregnancy: 2–10%
- Older females and males: 4–19%
  - ~22% of women >90 years old (1)
- Institutionalized older population: 15–50%

Prevalence

- Variable: increases with age, female gender, sexual activity, neurogenic bladder, and presence of genitourinary (GU) abnormalities
- Pregnancy: 2–10%
- Short- and long-term indwelling catheter 9–23% and 100%, respectively
- Long-term care residents in women 25–50% and men 15–40%

ETIOLOGY AND PATHOPHYSIOLOGY

- Pathophysiology: Most cases are secondary to the ascension of bacteria from the urethra to bladder.
- Microbiology is similar to that of other urinary tract infections (UTI), with bacteria originating from the periurethral area, vagina, or gut.
- Organisms are less virulent in ASB than those causing UTI.
- The most common organism is *Escherichia coli*. Other common organisms are *Klebsiella pneumoniae*, *Enterobacter*, *Proteus mirabilis*, *Staphylococcus aureus*, group B *Streptococcus* (GBS), and *Enterococcus*.

Genetics

Genetic variations that reduce toll-like receptor-4 function (*TLR4*) have been associated with ASB by lowering innate immune response and delaying bacterial clearance.

RISK FACTORS

- Pregnancy
- Older age
- Female gender
- Sexual activity, use of diaphragm with spermicide
- GU abnormalities: neurogenic bladder, urinary retention, urinary catheter use (indwelling, intermittent, or condom catheter), or pathologic urinary fistulas
- Institutionalized elderly population
- Diabetes mellitus
- Immunocompromised status
- Spinal cord injuries or functional impairment
- Hemodialysis

COMMONLY ASSOCIATED CONDITIONS

Depends on the risk factors

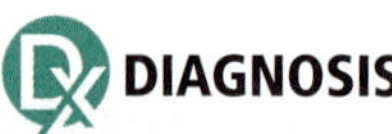

DIAGNOSIS

HISTORY

- Asymptomatic
- Lack of symptoms attributable to UTI such as fever, acute dysuria (<1 week), new or worsening urinary urgency/frequency/incontinence, or acute gross hematuria

PHYSICAL EXAM

- Afebrile
- No suprapubic and costovertebral angle tenderness

DIFFERENTIAL DIAGNOSIS

- UTI
- Uncomplicated cystitis
- Contaminated urine specimen

DIAGNOSTIC TESTS & INTERPRETATION

Initial Tests (lab, imaging)

- Urinalysis (UA):
  - The presence of pyuria, leukocyte esterase, and nitrite in ASB is common.
- Urine culture (clean catch)
- Screening urine culture in asymptomatic patients is indicated in only two conditions:
  - Pregnancy: screening between 12 and 16 weeks' gestation or at first prenatal visit if later
  - Prior to transurethral resection of prostate (TURP) or any urologic interventions when mucosal bleeding is anticipated
- Screening for ASB in men and nonpregnant women is not recommended.

Follow-Up Tests & Special Considerations

- Noncontaminated urine specimen should be used for urine culture.
- In pregnancy, periodic screening urine culture should be done after ASB treatment but not required in GBS bacteriuria (2).

Test Interpretation

- Patient with significant bacteriuria with or without pyuria and without symptoms referable to UTI should be diagnosed as ASB per Infectious Diseases Society of America.
  - Significant bacteriuria is defined based on type of urine specimen, sex, and the amount of bacteria.
  - By midstream, clean catch specimen
    - Male: >100,000 CFU/mL of single bacteria species
    - Female: the same criteria as male but needs two positive consecutive specimens
      - In pregnancy, if >10,000 CFU/mL of GBS, treatment is indicated (grade B)
    - By catheterized specimen male and female: >100 CFU/mL of one bacterial species; required one-time collection only
- The presence of pyuria or leukocyte esterase is common but not a marker of infection.
- Positive nitrite is an indicator of the presence of bacteriuria but cannot differentiate UTI from ASB or poor collection technique.

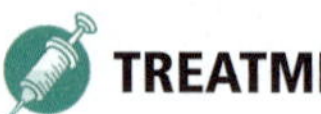

TREATMENT

GENERAL MEASURES

ALERT

- Antibiotic treatment of ASB is indicated in only two conditions:
  - Pregnancy
    - Rationale: Treatment prevents up to 70% of pregnant women from developing acute pyelonephritis, which reduces the risk of low birth weight and preterm delivery that are perinatal complications.
  - Prior to TURP
    - Rationale: Antibiotic treatment can effectively prevent postprocedure bacteremia and sepsis.
- Treatment of ASB in other conditions (nonpregnant women, diabetic women, indwelling catheter, patients with spinal cord injury, or the elderly living in the community) does not provide any known clinical benefit, does not reduce the risk of symptomatic infection nor improve morbidity or mortality. It increases health care cost, adverse drug side effects, development of resistant organisms, and reinfection rate.
- Recommendation against screening all nonrenal solid organ transplant or after 1 month following renal transplant. Inadequate evidence to guide management in nonurologic procedure (3)[A]

MEDICATION

- Pregnancy
  - Intrapartum antibiotic prophylaxis with IV penicillin or clindamycin (penicillin allergy) is recommended for women with GBS bacteriuria occurring at any stage of pregnancy and of any colony count to prevent GBS disease in the newborn.
  - No consensus on choice of antibiotics and duration of treatment in pregnancy; however, the cure rate is higher for the 4 to 7 days of treatment than 1-day treatment.
  - Choice of antibiotics should be guided by bacterial pathogen, local resistance rate, adverse effects, and comorbidities of patients.
  - Common oral antibiotics (FDA-B) that have been used
    - Nitrofurantoin 100 mg BID for 5 days (low level of resistance, may cause hemolysis in glucose-6-phosphate dehydrogenase deficiency)
    - Amoxicillin/clavulanate 500/125 mg BID for 5 to 7 days
    - Cefuroxime 250 mg BID for 5 days
    - Cephalexin 500 mg BID for 5 days
    - Fosfomycin 3 g for 1 single dose (not effective when glomerular filtration rate is <30 mL/minute, may be used in highly resistant bacteria such as methicillin-resistant *S. aureus* [MRSA], vancomycin-resistant enterococci [VRE], and extended-spectrum β-lactamase [ESBL]-producing organism bacteria)
  - Avoid trimethoprim in 1st trimester and near term. Avoid sulfa after 32 weeks' gestation. This is due to a theoretical risk of kernicterus. However, this may be used if other options are unavailable or contraindicated.
  - Contraindicated: fluoroquinolones (FDA-C), tetracyclines (FDA-D)
- Prior to invasive urologic interventions
  - Initiate antibiotic the night before or immediately before the procedure.
  - Antibiotic should be continued until the indwelling catheter is removed postprocedure.

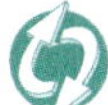

ONGOING CARE

FOLLOW-UP RECOMMENDATIONS

No consensus on rescreening frequency of ASB in pregnancy; per American College of Gynecology (ACOG) guidelines, follow-up urine culture, after treatment, is recommended. Although more data is needed to determine the effectiveness of this recommendation.

Patient Monitoring

Development of any signs/symptoms of UTI should warrant antibiotic treatment.

DIET

Daily cranberry juice or cranberry capsules twice daily may reduce the frequency of ASB during pregnancy, but it has not been confirmed in large study.

PATIENT EDUCATION

Patient should seek medical attention when UTI symptoms develop.

COMPLICATIONS

- Late pregnancy pyelonephritis occurs in 20–35% of women with untreated bacteriuria (20- to 30-fold higher than women with negative initial screening urine cultures or in whom bacteriuria was treated). Pyelonephritis is associated with premature delivery and worse fetal outcomes (infant with group B streptococcal infections, low-birth-weight infant). Antimicrobial treatment will decrease the risk of subsequent pyelonephritis from 20–35% to 1–4% and the risk of having a low-birth-weight baby from 15% to 5%.
- If bacteriuria remains untreated in patients who undergo traumatic urologic procedures, up to 60% develop bacteremia after the procedure and 5–10% progress to severe sepsis/septic shock.

REFERENCES

1. Owens DK, Davidson KW, Krist AH; for US Preventive Services Task Force. Screening for asymptomatic bacteriuria in adults: US Preventive Services Task Force recommendation statement. *JAMA*. 2019;322(12):1188–1194. doi:10.1001/jama.2019.13069.
2. Zolotor AJ, Carlough MC. Update on prenatal care. *Am Fam Physician*. 2014;89(3):199–208.
3. Nicolle LE, Gupta K, Bradley SF, et al. Clinical practice guideline for the management of asymptomatic bacteriuria: 2019 update by the Infectious Diseases Society of America. *Clin Infect Dis*. 2019;68(10):e83–e110. doi:10.1093/cid/ciy1121.

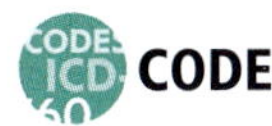

CODES

ICD10

- N39.0 Urinary tract infection, site not specified
- B96.20 Unsp Escherichia coli as the cause of diseases classd elswhr
- B96.1 Klebsiella pneumoniae as the cause of diseases classd elswhr

CLINICAL PEARLS

- ASB is a common and benign disorder for which treatment is not indicated in most patients.
- The presence of pyuria, leukocyte esterase, and nitrite is common in ASB and not an indication for antimicrobial treatment.
- Antibiotic treatment is indicated for ASB in pregnancy, patients who require TURP, or any urologic interventions with mucosal bleeding.
- Treatment of ASB in other conditions does not decrease the frequency of UTI or improve outcome.
- Overtreatment of ASB may result in negative consequences such as antimicrobial resistance, adverse drug reaction, and unnecessary cost.

BALANITIS, PHIMOSIS, AND PARAPHIMOSIS

Abdul Waheed, MD, MS, CPE, FAAFP • Christian Javier, DO • Brandon D. Jones, MD

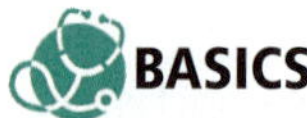

BASICS

DESCRIPTION

- Balanitis:
  - Balanitis is an inflammation of the glans penis.
  - Posthitis is an inflammation of the foreskin or prepuce.
  - Balanoposthitis is inflammation of both the glans penis and the foreskin.
  - Balanitis xerotica obliterans (BXO) is lichen sclerosus of the glans penis (uncommon).
- Phimosis and paraphimosis:
  - Phimosis: when the foreskin is too tight to retract back to expose glans penis; can be physiologic (normal) or pathologic
  - Paraphimosis: a urologic emergency where the foreskin is retracted over the glans penis and cannot return to normal position which can lead to strangulation, vascular compromise, and even necrosis
- System(s) affected: renal/urologic; reproductive; skin/exocrine; psychosocial

ALERT

- Recurrent infections and irritations (for example condom catheter) can lead to pathologic phimosis.
- Phimosis may lead to acute urinary retention.
- Paraphimosis is a urologic emergency; if left untreated, can lead to necrosis and autoamputation

EPIDEMIOLOGY

- Balanitis: occurs in all ages but most common in children <4 years old and uncircumcised elderly; lifetime incidence for uncircumcised males is 68% (1).
- Phimosis/paraphimosis: 8% of boys aged 6 years and 1% of men >16 years of age; predominant age involvement is infancy and adolescence; unusual in adults and middle age but risk returns in elderly
- In transgender or intersex individuals, a similar syndrome may present with clitoromegaly or post-vaginoplasty.

ETIOLOGY AND PATHOPHYSIOLOGY

- Balanitis:
  - Infectious etiologies include: fungal (*Candida albicans*—most common, dermatophytes); bacterial (streptococcal spp.—second most common); sexually transmitted (chlamydia, gonorrhea, trichomonas, HPV, syphilis); scabies, mpox, circinate erosive balanitis (often part of reactive arthritis syndrome—formerly Reiter syndrome)
  - Trauma: Damage to skin represents compromise of an important immune mechanism which can occur through direct skin injury such as zipper injuries or friction.
  - Fixed drug eruption: predictable and repeated onset after exposure to sulfa, tetracyclines, or other drugs
  - Various dermatoses can produce balanitis as a presenting symptom (see differential diagnosis below).
  - Smegma: an oily or waxy substance secreted under the foreskin and composed of desquamated epithelial cells as well as various fats and proteins; may be a direct skin irritant in some cases, as well as a nidus for infection by dermatophytes, candida, and bacteria
- Phimosis:
  - Physiologic: present at birth; resolves spontaneously during the first 2 to 3 years of life through nocturnal erections, which slowly dilate the phimotic ring
  - Acquired: recurrent inflammation, trauma, or infections of the foreskin; needs attention and treatment
- Paraphimosis:
  - often iatrogenically or inadvertently induced by the foreskin not being pulled back over the glans after voiding, cleaning, cystoscopy, or catheter insertion
  - may be post-circumcision especially infants, especially in cases where prepuce is not removed adequately or heals with adhesions and scarring at the corona

Geriatric Considerations

- Balanitis: Condom catheters, poor hygiene, and poorly controlled diabetes mellitus (DM) may predispose to balanitis.
- Phimosis & Paraphimosis: Incontinence or post-micturition dribbling can lead to constant moisture resulting in irritant contact inflammation, scarring, and adhesion formation; may lead to urologic emergency with acute urinary retention and incarceration and strangulation of the glans

Pediatric Considerations

Balanitis is more prevalent in children <4 years of age; oral antibiotics may predispose male infants to Candida balanitis; age is key when determining likely etiology, as children may be more or less prone to specific infections than adults (1). Phimosis/paraphimosis: Most phimosis referrals seen in pediatric urology clinics are normal physiologic, resolves on its own resulting in a fully retractable prepuce in 99% by the age of 16 years. Inappropriate care of physiologic phimosis can lead to acquired phimosis by repeated forced reduction of the foreskin. Uncircumcised penises require no special care and with normal hygiene, most foreskins will become retractile over time.

Genetics

Not a heritable condition in and of itself, though genetics may play a role in specific etiologies.

RISK FACTORS

- Balanitis: presence of foreskin, DM (uncontrolled BG, use of SGLT2 inhibitors may worsen risk of candida colonization), insufficient hygiene, chemical or physical irritants (diaper dermatitis, latex condoms, urine, smegma), morbid obesity, nursing home environment, condom catheters, hidradenitis suppurativa (lymphedema may predispose)
- Phimosis: irregular hygiene, DM or repeated balanitis in older patients, frequent diaper dermatitis in infants
- Paraphimosis: presence of foreskin, post-procedure complication (leaving foreskin retracted after catheter placement), inadequate return of the retracted foreskin over the glans after initial retraction, penile coital trauma, poor education about care of the foreskin

GENERAL PREVENTION

- Balanitis:
  - Regular hygiene and avoidance of allergens
  - Without regular cleaning under the foreskin, substances such as smegma, urine, or other irritants may accumulate under the foreskin, possibly also becoming a nidus for infection.
  - Regular hygiene should be performed daily by gently retracting the foreskin and using warm water and soap to cleanse the area. Allow it to dry fully before replacing the foreskin.
  - Overly aggressive hygiene (overexposure to soaps, cleansing agents, friction irritation) may increase the risk.
  - Circumcision reduces the risk of balanitis by 68% as compared to the uncircumcised.
  - Proper hygiene and avoidance of allergen
- Phimosis and paraphimosis:
  - Appropriate care of the foreskin is necessary.

COMMONLY ASSOCIATED CONDITIONS

- Balanitis: posthitis (inflammation of the foreskin), phimosis, paraphimosis, infections (see above under "Etiology and Pathophysiology" section), lichen sclerosus/BXO, worsening soft tissue infections, cellulitis, Fournier gangrene (rare), penile intraepithelial neoplasia (Bowen disease, erythroplasia of Queyrat, etc.); balanitis appears to increase risk of penile cancers (relative risk 3.8); consider sexual abuse, especially in children with the appropriate history.
- Phimosis/paraphimosis: uncircumcised, lower urinary tract symptoms from bladder outlet obstruction of different etiologies, urinary incontinence, and inflammatory dermatosis including Lichen sclerosus/BXO

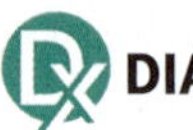

DIAGNOSIS

Primarily clinical based upon history and physical examination

HISTORY

- Balanitis: symptoms of inflammation including pain, drainage, dysuria, odor, ballooning of foreskin with voiding, redness
- Phimosis: painful erections, recurrent balanitis, foreskin balloons when voiding, inability to retract foreskin at appropriate age, acute urinary retention
- Paraphimosis: uncircumcised fully, pain, drainage, voiding difficulty, recent penile catheterization, cleaning, foreskin manipulation

PHYSICAL EXAM

- Balanitis: Inflammation of the foreskin or glans penis establishes the diagnosis with erythema, tenderness, edema, discharge, drainage, odor/foul smell, ulceration, and or scaling crusting with or without plaque formation.
  - Infectious signs: discharge, erythema, weeping, crusting, ulceration
  - Dermatopathologic signs: plaques, erythema, ulceration, lichenification, scaling, xerosis, gross deformity
  - Extragenital signs may be present with certain syndromes like different dermatosis or reactive arthritis.

- Phimosis: Foreskin that will not retract is the hallmark of diagnosis.
  - Painful erections
  - Foreskin ballooning while urinating
  - Acute urinary retention can sometimes be a presentation with abdominal and penile pain.
  - Preputial orifice has fine white fibrous ring of scar in pathologic phimosis.
- Paraphimosis: any combination of symptoms of phimosis above with edema, pain, swelling, change in color of the glans with foreskin stuck around the corona of the glans; may have recent history of catheterization or foreskin manipulation

DIFFERENTIAL DIAGNOSIS

- Balanitis: Focus attention on primary balanitis versus secondary balanitis where the manifestations are beyond the penis.
  - Balanoposthitis: similar to balanitis but in both glans penis and foreskin
  - Posthitis: similar to balanitis but involves only the foreskin
  - Contact dermatitis, psoriasis, eczema, lichens planus, lichens sclerosis, lichens sclerosus et atrophicus, BXO, erythroplasia of Queyrat, scabies
  - Reactive arthritis (formerly known as Reiter syndrome)
  - Zoon balanitis (2): characterized by intradermal infiltration of plasma cells (2)
    - Consider if single red-orange erythematous patch, typically among the elderly
    - May also have overlying smaller macules called cayenne pepper spots
  - Penile Intraepithelial Neoplasia (PIN)
- Phimosis/paraphimosis:
  - Penile lymphedema, which can be related to insect bites, trauma, or allergic reactions
  - Penile tourniquet syndrome: foreign body around penis, most commonly hair especially in pediatric population
  - Anasarca

DIAGNOSTIC TESTS & INTERPRETATION

Initial Tests (lab, imaging)

Consider pathogen specific testing if infectious etiology is suspected, for example KOH prep for fungal, gram stain and culture for bacterial, and/or other tests specific to sexually transmitted infections. Use specific tests for secondary balanitis, for example ESR and CRP. For reactive arthritis, consider HbA1c for candida.

Follow-Up Tests & Special Considerations

Depends upon specific etiology

Diagnostic Procedures/Other

Biopsy, if persistent

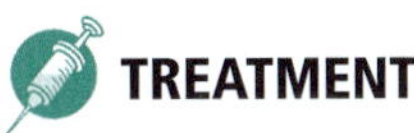

TREATMENT

GENERAL MEASURES

- Regular hygiene should be performed daily by gently retracting the foreskin and using warm water and soap to cleanse the area.
- Overly aggressive hygiene (overexposure to soaps, cleansing agents, friction irritation) may increase the risk.
- Consider circumcision for paraphimosis, phimosis, and recurrent balanitis.

MEDICATION

- Balanitis
  - General principles:
    - Specific treatments depend upon the specific etiology.
    - Set START and STOP criteria for steroid use: Limit the intensity and dose to smallest possible, consider limiting to 1 to 2 weeks. Consider using high potency weekend pulse dosing instead of using medium dose for daily use. Consider appropriate referral to dermatology (3).
  - Allergic/irritant: hydrocortisone 1% BID
  - Fungal infections: clotrimazole (Lotrimin) 1% BID for 1 to 2 weeks, nystatin (Mycostatin) BID–QID until the resolution; fluconazole: 150 mg PO single dose in severe cases
  - Bacterial infections: topical bacitracin QID
  - Full cellulitis: cephalosporin or sulfa drug PO or parenteral
  - Zoon balanitis: conservative treatment with regular hygiene, topical steroids QID, circumcision (2)
  - Suspected penile intraepithelial neoplasia with mass/deformity needs prompt referral for biopsy and treatment.
- Phimosis: 0.05% fluticasone propionate daily for 4 to 8 weeks with gradual traction placed on foreskin or 1% pimecrolimus BID for 4 to 6 weeks; not for use in children <2 years of age
- Paraphimosis:
  - Manual reduction under sedation; place the middle and index fingers of both hands on the engorged skin proximal to the glans. Place both thumbs on glans and, with gentle pressure, push on the glans and pull on the foreskin to attempt reduction. If unsuccessful, a dorsal slit will be necessary, with eventual circumcision after the edema resolves.
  - Osmotic agents: granulated sugar placed on edematous tissue for several hours to reduce edema
  - Puncture technique: Multiple punctures of foreskin with a 21-gauge needle will allow edematous fluid to escape and thus allow reduction.

ISSUES FOR REFERRAL

Recurrent infections; development of meatal stenosis; suspected malignancy

SURGERY/OTHER PROCEDURES

- Balanitis and phimosis: Consider circumcision as preventive and management measure.
- For paraphimosis: Prompt referral for surgical procedure is required; may consider applying hair removal cream if hair-torniquet is suspected cause

ADMISSION, INPATIENT, AND NURSING CONSIDERATIONS

- Admission criteria/initial stabilization: uncontrolled DM, necrotizing infection, sepsis
- Appropriate hygiene if condom catheters are used

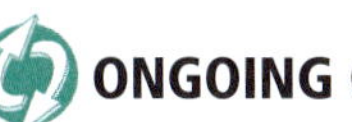

ONGOING CARE

FOLLOW-UP RECOMMENDATIONS

Patient Monitoring

Balanitis:

- Every 1 to 2 weeks until etiology has been established
- Persistent balanitis may require biopsy to rule out malignancy or BXO.
- Evaluation for resolution of phimosis

DIET

Weight reduction, if obese

PATIENT EDUCATION

- Need for appropriate hygiene
- Appropriate foreskin care
- Avoidance of known allergens such as soaps
- No sexual activity for 2 to 3 weeks after circumcision.

PROGNOSIS

Should resolve with appropriate treatment

COMPLICATIONS

- Meatal stenosis
- Premalignant changes from chronic irritation
- UTIs
- Acquired phimosis
- Unreducible paraphimosis can lead to gangrene.
- Posthitis (inflammation of the prepuce)

REFERENCES

1. Morris BJ, Krieger JN. Penile inflammatory skin disorders and the preventive role of circumcision. *Int J Prev Med*. 2017;8:32.
2. Lam K, Cook DK. Chronic balanitis: when should we be concerned? *Aust J Gen Pract*. 2020;49(12):839–841.
3. Teichman JMH, Mannas M, Elston DM. Noninfectious penile lesions. *Am Fam Physician*. 2018;97(2):102–110.

SEE ALSO

Reactive Arthritis (Reiter Syndrome)

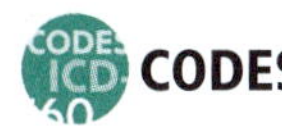

CODES

ICD10

- N48.1 Balanitis
- N47.1 Phimosis
- N48.0 Leukoplakia of penis

CLINICAL PEARLS

- Balanitis is an inflammation of the glans penis. Posthitis is an inflammation of the foreskin. BXO is lichen sclerosus of the glans penis.
- With recurrent infections and a plaque, a biopsy should be done to rule out BXO or malignancy.
- If there is a true phimosis that interferes with appropriate hygiene, treat the phimosis with steroids or circumcision.

BARRETT ESOPHAGUS

Dhruval Amin, MD

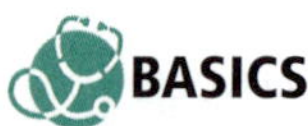

BASICS

DESCRIPTION
- Presence of intestinal metaplasia of ≥1 cm that replaces the native stratified squamous epithelium likely a consequence of chronic gastroesophageal reflux disease (GERD)
- Endoscopically recognized by its salmon-colored mucosa and histologically by intestinal metaplasia and goblet cells
- Only known precursor lesion for development of esophageal adenocarcinoma (EAC)

EPIDEMIOLOGY
- Predominant age >50 years, more common in men; estimated to be present in 1–2% of adult population
- Very rare in pediatric population

Incidence
- 5–12% of patients with chronic GERD symptoms will harbor Barrett esophagus (BE) (1).
- Incidence of EAC is rising in the United States (2) since 1970s; attributed to changes in smoking and obesity rather than reclassification or overdiagnosis
- Annual incidence of adenocarcinoma in all Barrett patients estimated at 0.5% per year

Prevalence
Potentially as many as 1.5 to 2 million U.S. adults

ETIOLOGY AND PATHOPHYSIOLOGY
- Chronic gastric reflux exposure damages the esophageal lining which promotes a more resilient intestinal cell type growth to better withstand the acidic conditions.
- Columnar cells in the esophagus have higher malignant potential than squamous cells. Activation of *CDX2* gene and overexpression of HER2/neu (ERBB2) oncogene promotes carcinogenesis.
- Elevated levels of COX-2 are associated with BE.
- Classic progression: normal epithelium → esophagitis/reflux exposure → metaplasia (BE) → dysplasia (low → high grade) → adenocarcinoma

Genetics
Familial predisposition to GERD and BE with multiple genetic markers have been identified.

RISK FACTORS
- Chronic reflux (>5 years)
- Male sex, age >50 years
- White race
- Smoking history, intra-abdominal obesity
- Family history—at least one first-degree relative with BE or EAC

GENERAL PREVENTION
Weight loss, smoking cessation, robust intake of fruits and vegetables, and moderate wine consumption may decrease risk of BE and lower progression to esophageal cancer.

COMMONLY ASSOCIATED CONDITIONS
GERD, obesity, hiatal hernia

DIAGNOSIS

Endoscopically with biopsies

HISTORY
- Assess underlying risk factors.
- Common GERD symptoms: heartburn, regurgitation
- Atypical symptoms include chest pain, odynophagia, chronic cough, water brash, globus sensation, laryngitis, or wheezing.
- Symptoms suggestive of complicated GERD or cancer include weight loss, anorexia, dysphagia, odynophagia, hematemesis, or melena.

ALERT
BE is not by itself symptomatic; up to 50% of EAC and BE patients do not report GERD.

PHYSICAL EXAM
- No physical exam findings are specific for BE.
- Findings generally similar to GERD

DIFFERENTIAL DIAGNOSIS
Erosive esophagitis; uncomplicated GERD; hiatal hernia

DIAGNOSTIC TESTS & INTERPRETATION
Endoscopy with multiple biopsies demonstrating intestinal metaplasia extending ≥1 cm proximal to the gastroesophageal junction (GEJ) is required to diagnose BE.
- Gastric cardia-type epithelium on pathology does not have clear malignant significance and may reflect sampling error.
- Specialized intestinal metaplasia at the GEJ: unclear significance; cancer risk is difficult to assess with varying definitions of GEJ landmarks.

ALERT
- Endoscopic screening is controversial. Consider one-time screening for patients with chronic GERD (>5 years) and/or frequent GERD symptoms with ≥3 risk factors: age >50 years, white ethnicity, central obesity, smoking history, family history of BE or EAC (ACG), or patients with multiple risk factors (3)[B].
- Screening for BE in the general population with GERD is *not* routinely recommended (3)[C].

Initial Tests (lab, imaging)
None
- *Helicobacter pylori* testing is *not* indicated.
- No current biomarkers are effective for diagnosis; some under investigation for risk stratification

Diagnostic Procedures/Other
- Endoscopy: Visualization of epithelial change with biopsy confirmation is standard.
- Classify disease extent: long segment (≥3 cm) versus short segment (<3 cm)
- Systematic endoscopic biopsies confirm diagnosis:
  - Seattle protocol: four-quadrant biopsies at regular intervals with biopsies of visible mucosal irregularities; more time-consuming but higher diagnostic yield than random biopsies
  - Chromoendoscopy (dye or virtual) should be used in addition to white light endoscopy.
- Nonendoscopic swallowable capsule sponge devices combined with biomarkers are an alternative to endoscopy for screening.

Test Interpretation
- Specialized intestinal metaplasia (also called specialized columnar epithelium) is diagnostic of BE.
- Diagnosis of dysplasia (and grade) should be confirmed by two gastrointestinal pathologists before treatment. Benign BE is established by a single pathologist report.
- Cardia-type columnar epithelium may predispose to malignancy (unclear risk).
- If screening endoscopy reveals erosive esophagitis, repeat after 8 to 12 weeks of proton pump inhibitor (PPI) therapy to exclude underlying BE; defer biopsies until healing occurs (3)[C].

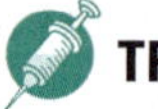

TREATMENT

Should be individualized according to patient's age, comorbidities, and availability of endoscopic and surgical treatments

MEDICATION
- The goal of medical therapy is to control GERD and reduce esophagitis.
- Neither suppression of gastric acid production via high-dose PPIs nor reduction in esophageal acid exposure via antireflux surgery induces regression of BE. These therapies may, however, decrease progression/cancer risk.

First Line
- Patients with BE should be treated with a daily PPI regardless of GERD symptoms. Refractory GERD may be managed with twice daily PPI if needed.
- Dose PPIs 30 to 60 minutes before a meal (ideally, the first meal of the day).

ALERT
Titrate PPI therapy to symptoms; routine pH monitoring is *not* recommended.

ISSUES FOR REFERRAL
- Most patients with low-grade dysplasia (except those who do not desire intervention) and all those with high-grade dysplasia or intramucosal carcinoma should be referred for endoscopic eradication of their BE.
- Refer patients considering esophagectomy (rare) to a high-volume institution.

ADDITIONAL THERAPIES

- Aspirin combined with high-dose twice-daily PPI may reduce progression to dysplasia (not yet routinely recommended).
  - COX-2 selective inhibitor celecoxib use not shown to affect progression of Barrett dysplasia to adenocarcinoma
  - Consider low-dose aspirin in patients with BE and risk factors for cardiovascular disease.
- Statins, alone or in combination with aspirin or NSAIDs, may be effective in chemoprevention.
- No dysplasia: No other therapy is generally indicated; continue regular surveillance every 3 to 5 years (4)[C].
- Treatment of dysplasia:
  - Low-grade dysplasia: Refer for endoscopic therapy (usually radiofrequency ablation or cryotherapy) (4)[C].
  - High-grade dysplasia: Refer for endoscopic mucosal resection and/or endoscopic therapy to prevent progression to adenocarcinoma (4)[C].
  - Intramucosal carcinoma: endoscopic resection if possible, followed by ablation of remaining BE, with surgery as a backup
  - More advanced carcinoma: Refer to oncology and surgery to discuss resection.
  - Indeterminate grade dysplasia should have a reevaluation with biopsies on increased PPI dosage.
  - Endoscopic eradication is successful in >90% of patients but often requires multiple sessions and can be associated with complications (4). Patients with prior ablation need ongoing surveillance for recurrence.

ALERT

Endoscopic eradication is not recommended for most BE without dysplasia.

SURGERY/OTHER PROCEDURES

ALERT

- Antireflux surgery does not appear to decrease risk of esophageal cancer.
- Esophagectomy is definitive but should only be considered after failure of minimally invasive endoscopic eradication therapy for high-grade dysplasia. Morbidity and mortality are higher than with endoscopic treatment.

COMPLEMENTARY & ALTERNATIVE MEDICINE

Multivitamin, vitamin C, or vitamin E once a day may reduce progression to EAC in patients with BE.

Geriatric Considerations

Surveillance or no treatment in patients who are poor operative candidates; discontinue surveillance in patients who are not candidates for treatment.

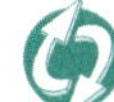

ONGOING CARE

FOLLOW-UP RECOMMENDATIONS

- Surveillance is recommended in high-risk patients with histologically confirmed BE.
- Patients diagnosed with BE on initial exam require surveillance based on presence and grade of dysplasia (3)[C].
- No dysplasia: Survey every 3 to 5 years.
  - Discontinue surveillance if life expectancy is ≤5 years.
- Low-grade dysplasia not planning for ablation: Survey every 6 to 12 months (3),(4)[C].
  - Routine surveillance if patients have confirmed absence of low-grade dysplasia after two consecutive endoscopies
- Low-grade dysplasia with eradication therapy: Survey at 1 year and then every 2 years.
- Indefinite for dysplasia: Repeat after 3 to 6 months of increased acid suppression, and if unchanged, survey every 12 months.
- High-grade dysplasia without eradication therapy: Survey every 3 months; with eradication therapy: survey at 3, 6, and 12 months and then annually.

ALERT

- Adherence to recommended surveillance protocols may improve rates of dysplasia and cancer detection.
- Continue surveillance even if the patient has had endoscopic ablation therapy, antireflux surgery, or esophagectomy.

DIET

Avoid foods that trigger reflux: caffeine, alcohol, chocolate, peppermint, carbonated drinks, garlic, onions, spicy foods, fatty foods, citrus, and tomato-based products.

PATIENT EDUCATION

- Lifestyle modifications: smoking cessation and weight loss; avoid supine position after meals; avoid tight-fitting clothes; elevate the head of bed.
- No evidence that treating GERD reverses BE or necessarily prevents esophageal cancer.

PROGNOSIS

Annual incidence of esophageal cancer in patients with BE is estimated 0.12–0.6% per year:

- Low-grade dysplasia: may be transient; cancer risk 0.7–0.8% per year (4)
- High-grade dysplasia: cancer risk 5–9% per year (3),(4)
- Promising areas for research include the use of biomarkers for risk stratification, chemoprevention of neoplastic progression, advanced imaging, capsule endoscopy for screening, and the use of vitamins and antioxidants for prevention and treatment.

COMPLICATIONS

Same as GERD: stricture, bleeding, ulceration

REFERENCES

1. Shaheen NJ, Falk GW, Iyer PG, et al. Diagnosis and management of Barrett's esophagus: an updated ACG guideline. *Am J Gastroenterol*. 2022;117(4):559–587. doi:10.14309/ajg.0000000000001680.
2. Muthusamy VR, Wani S, Gyawali CP, et al; for CGIT Barrett's Esophagus Consensus Conference Participants. AGA clinical practice update on new technology and innovation for surveillance and screening in Barrett's esophagus: expert review. *Clin Gastroenterol Hepatol*. 2022;20(12):2696–2706.e1. doi:10.1016/j.cgh.2022.06.003.
3. Bryce C, Bucaj M, Gazda R. Barrett esophagus: rapid evidence review. *Am Fam Physician*. 2022;106(4):383–387.
4. Qumseya B, Sultan S, Bain P, et al; for ASGE Standards of Practice Committee Chair. ASGE guideline on screening and surveillance of Barrett's esophagus. *Gastrointest Endosc*. 2019;90(3):335–359.e2.

ADDITIONAL READING

- Cotton CC, Eluri S, Shaheen NJ. Management of dysplastic Barrett's esophagus and early esophageal adenocarcinoma. *Gastroenterol Clin North Am*. 2022;51(3):485–500. doi:10.1016/j.gtc.2022.06.004.
- Sarem M, Martínez Cerezo FJ, Salvia Favieres ML, et al. Low-grade dysplasia in Barrett's esophagus: a problematic diagnosis. *Gastroenterol Hepatol*. 2023;46(8):637–644. doi:10.1016/j.gastrohep.2022.10.002.

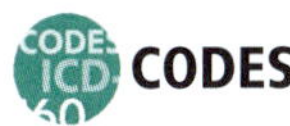

CODES

ICD10

- K22.70 Barrett's esophagus without dysplasia
- K22.719 Barrett's esophagus with dysplasia, unspecified
- K22.710 Barrett's esophagus with low grade dysplasia

CLINICAL PEARLS

- Patients with BE and no dysplasia can be managed with endoscopic surveillance. Patients with low-grade dysplasia may be managed with either endoscopic surveillance or endoscopic eradication. Patients with BE and high-grade dysplasia can be managed with endoscopic eradication.
- The highest incidence of BE is in White men >50 years of age.
- Esophagectomy is generally limited to patients with invasive carcinoma or those failing to respond to endoscopic therapy.

BASAL CELL CARCINOMA

Karl T. Clebak, MD, MHA, FAAFP • Kara Ann Romanowski, MD

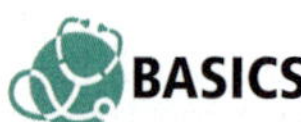

BASICS

DESCRIPTION

Basal cell carcinoma (BCC) is the most common type of skin cancer, originating from the basal cell layer of the epidermis and its appendages.

- Rarely metastasizes but is locally invasive and can cause local tissue destruction and disfigurement, especially in soft tissue, cartilage, and bone

EPIDEMIOLOGY

BCC is the most common cancer in the United States, Europe, and Australia (highest in Australia); similar rates are seen across North America, Europe, and Asia; the most common skin cancer worldwide

Incidence

- Annual incidence in the United States is estimated to be 4.3 million; 2 times more common than squamous cell carcinoma (SCC)
- Lifetime risk is ~30% in white populations and ~20% overall.
- Most common skin cancer in Asian and Hispanic individuals; second most common skin cancer in African American/Black individuals (1). Recent reports suggest an increasing incidence of BCC in Hispanic individuals.
- Predominant age: generally >60 years
- Predominant sex: men > women (1.5:1 ratio)

ETIOLOGY AND PATHOPHYSIOLOGY

UV radiation induces inflammation and cyclooxygenase activation in the skin.

Genetics

Several genetic conditions increase the risk of developing BCC:

- Albinism (recessive alleles)
- Xeroderma pigmentosum (autosomal recessive)
- Bazex-Dupre-Christol syndrome (rare, X-linked dominant)
- Nevoid BCC syndrome/Gorlin-Goltz syndrome (rare, autosomal dominant)
- Cytochrome P450 CYP2D6 and glutathione S-transferase detoxifying enzyme gene mutations (especially in truncal BCC, marked by clusters of BCCs and a younger age of onset)
- Mutations in the tumor suppressor gene patched, or activated mutations in smoothened, resulting in upregulation of hedgehog pathway signaling
- Epidermolysis bullosa simplex

RISK FACTORS

- Chronic sun exposure (UV radiation); increased susceptibility in the following phenotypes:
  - Light complexion: skin type I (burns, but does not tan) and skin type II (usually burns, sometimes tans)
  - Freckles
  - Red or blond hair
  - Blue or green eyes
- Tendency to sunburn
- Prolonged exposure to water, sand, or snow increases UV risk.
- Male sex; rising risk in women due to tanning beds
- History of nonmelanoma skin cancer
- Family history of skin cancer
- Immunosuppression (e.g., transplant, HIV, lymphoma)
- Exposure to carcinogenic substances (e.g., arsenic)
- Xeroderma pigmentosum
- Photosensitizing medications

GENERAL PREVENTION

- Use broad-spectrum sunscreens of at least SPF 30 daily at least 15 minutes before outdoor activity. Reapply every 2 hours or after swimming.
- Avoid sun overexposure and tanning beds. Use physical barriers methods such as protective clothing, hats, and sunglasses.
- The USPSTF concludes the current evidence is insufficient to assess the balance of benefits and harms of visual skin examination by a clinician to screen for skin cancer in adults. Consensus guidelines recommend a whole-body skin examination every 6 to 12 months for the first 2 years following BCC diagnosis and then at least annually for life.

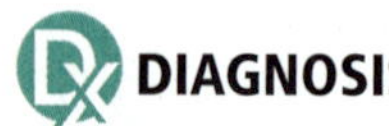

DIAGNOSIS

HISTORY

- Exposure to risk factors, family history of skin cancer
- History of a growing, ulcerating, or bleeding skin lesion often in a sun-exposed area

PHYSICAL EXAM

- 75–80% are found in the head/neck region.
- Nodular (60–80%): pink, pearly papule with rolled border, ulceration, telangiectasias
- Pigmented: translucent papule with dark pigment, mimics melanoma (2)
- Superficial: red, scaly plaque with central clearing; trunk/extremities
- Morpheaform: scar-like plaque, ill-defined, ulcerated; head/neck
- Infiltrative: firm plaques with crust, often cooccurs with nodular
- Fibroepithelial: rare, soft pedunculated papule; lower back

DIFFERENTIAL DIAGNOSIS

- SCC
- Sebaceous hyperplasia
- Epidermal inclusion cyst
- Intradermal nevi (pigmented and nonpigmented)
- Molluscum contagiosum
- Actinic keratosis
- Nummular dermatitis
- Psoriasis
- Melanoma (pigmented lesions)
- Atypical fibroxanthoma
- Fibroma
- Keratoacanthoma
- Papilloma
- Tinea

DIAGNOSTIC TESTS & INTERPRETATION

Initial Tests (lab, imaging)

- Biopsy is necessary to confirm the diagnosis.
- Dermoscopy may improve diagnostic accuracy of BCCs.

Diagnostic Procedures/Other

- Clinical diagnosis and histologic subtype are confirmed through skin biopsy and pathologic examination.
- Shave biopsy is typically sufficient and used for nodular lesions. For flat lesions, a 2- to 4-mm punch biopsy or a shave biopsy with a scoop technique allows for the assessment of depth of tumor and perineural invasion. Excisional biopsy rarely used.
- MRI is preferred for staging of advanced disease. CT and PET/CT are of value for further metastatic workup.

Test Interpretation

- Nodular BCC
  - Extending from the epidermis are nodular aggregates of basaloid cells.
  - Tumor cells are uniform; rarely have mitotic figures; large, oval, hyperchromatic nuclei with little cytoplasm, random central organization surrounded by a peripheral palisade
  - Increased mucin in dermal stroma
- Superficial BCC
  - Appear as buds of basaloid cells attached to undersurface of epidermis
  - Peripheral palisading
- Morpheaform BCC
  - Thin cords and strands of basaloid cells; embedded in dense, fibrous, scar-like stroma
  - Less peripheral palisading and retraction, greater subclinical involvement
- Infiltrating BCC
  - Like morpheaform BCC but no scar-like stroma and thicker, spiky, irregular strands
  - Less peripheral palisading and retraction, greater subclinical involvement
- Micronodular BCC
  - Small, nodular aggregates of tumor cells
  - Less retraction artifact and higher subclinical involvement than nodular BCC

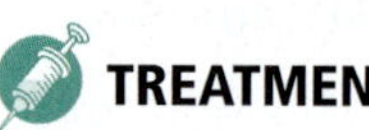

TREATMENT

GENERAL MEASURES

- Low-risk BCC: curettage and electrodesiccation (C&E), standard excision, radiation therapy
- High-risk BCC: standard excision, Mohs surgery, radiation therapy

MEDICATION

- For patients who cannot tolerate or refuse surgery, with low-risk superficial/nodular BCC
  - 5-Fluorouracil (5-FU) cream for superficial low-risk lesions; apply BID for 3 to 10 weeks.
  - Imiquimod (Aldara) cream approved for treatment of low-risk superficial BCC; daily dosing for 6 to 12 weeks; 80% clearance rate (3)[A]

- Emerging therapies:
  - Vismodegib and sonidegib, sonic hedgehog pathway inhibitors; for patients with advanced BCC failing other options as well as metastatic disease; also beneficial for multiple BCC and BCC nevus syndrome
  - Intralesional injection: Intralesional methotrexate, rituximab, 5-FU, interferons, IL-2, and bleomycin show variable success. Adverse effects are uncommon and are typically dose related including local effects at the treatment site and flu-like symptoms.
  - Laser therapy: used as monotherapy or adjunct for superficial BCC; one study using superpulsed CO_2 therapy for superficial/nodular BCC showed no recurrence at 3 years (3)[B].

First Line

Surgical excision is first line (see "Surgery/Other Procedures").

ADDITIONAL THERAPIES

- Radiation therapy
  - Useful for patients, typically older (>60 years), who cannot not undergo surgery and for unresectable tumors
  - Used after surgery as adjuvant therapy, if tumor margins were not cleared
  - Cure rate is ~90%.
  - Recurrence rates are 16%.
- Photodynamic therapy (PDT)
  - PDT uses photosensitizing agents (injected or topical) which becomes accumulated in the target cells with subsequent light irradiation.
  - Methyl aminolevulinate and 5-aminolevulinic acid, photosensitizers, are activated by specific wavelengths of light that destroy local tissue.
  - Currently approved in Canada, Europe, Australia, and New Zealand; off-label treatment for BCC in the United States; clearance rates are reported between 70% and 90%.

SURGERY/OTHER PROCEDURES

- Surgical excision is first-line treatment; treatment selection varies with extent and location of lesion as well as tumor border demarcation.
- High-risk areas
  - Inner canthus, nasolabial sulcus, philtrum, preauricular area, retroauricular sulcus, lip, temple, "mask areas" of the face
- C&E
  - If nodular lesion <1 cm, in low-risk area, not deeply invasive
  - Avoid in the hair-bearing areas due to risk of the tumor extending down follicular structures.
  - 5-year cure rate of 91–97%; recurrence as high as 19% for high-risk lesions (3)
  - Pathology sample sent at time of C&E to ensure absence of high-risk pathology
- Excision with postoperative margin assessment
  - Treatment of choice for low-risk lesions <2 cm in diameter
  - Goal is 4-mm margin in low-risk BCC. For high-risk cases, a minimum margin of 6 mm is recommended.
  - 5-year cure rate of 98%
- Cryosurgery
  - Cryosurgery may treat low-risk or selected high-risk BCCs alone or with curettage. Histology must be known beforehand, as margins can't be assessed post freeze/thaw cycles.
  - Reserved for nodular and superficial BCC, not indicated for tumors with depth exceeding 3 mm
  - Avoid in hair-bearing, lower extremities, and facial areas due to cosmesis (3).
  - Typically, used for tumors with low risk of recurrence; reported cure rates between 94% and 99%
  - Mean recurrence rates range from 0% to 39% across different studies.
- Mohs surgery
  - Surgical procedure where thin layers of the tumor are progressively removed and examined to determine tumor boarder, allowing only cancer-free tissue to remain
  - Preferred microsurgically controlled surgical treatment for lesions in high-risk areas, recurrent lesions, and lesions exhibiting an aggressive growth pattern
  - 5-year recurrence rates up to 10.1% in primary BCC, 17.4% in recurrent BCC
  - Requires referral to appropriately trained dermatologic surgeon

COMPLEMENTARY & ALTERNATIVE MEDICINE

Nicotinamide 500 mg BID lowers incidence of nonmelanoma skin cancers; β-carotene has not been shown effective.

ONGOING CARE

FOLLOW-UP RECOMMENDATIONS

- Consensus guidelines recommend a whole-body skin examination every 6 to 12 months for the first 2 years following BCC diagnosis and then at least annually for life.
- Sunscreen, shade, between 10 AM and 4 PM.
- Oral retinoids may prevent the development of new BCCs in patients with Gorlin-Goltz syndrome, renal transplant recipients, and patients with severe actinic damage.

Patient Monitoring

- Follow-up every 6 to 12 months for 2 to 5 years, then annually. Consider reducing frequency if no recurrence after 2 years.
- Increased risk of other skin cancers
- Recurrence:
  - Local: Follow consensus guidelines for primary treatment.
  - Regional: surgery and/or radiation therapy
  - Metastatic: multidisciplinary tumor board consultation

PATIENT EDUCATION

- Monthly skin self-exam
- Educate on adequate vitamin D intake. Use broad-spectrum UVA/UVB sunscreen SPF 15 or higher.
- Avoid sun exposure in infants; use sunscreen after 6 months.

PROGNOSIS

- Proper treatment yields 90–95% cure.
- Most recurrences occur within 5 years, especially in head/neck lesions.
- Development of new BCCs: Many patients (30–50%) will develop a new lesion within 5 years.
- Cure rates with 5-FU, imiquimod, PDT, or cryotherapy may be 10% lower than surgery.

COMPLICATIONS

- Recurrence rates > 5 years postoperatively are up to 56% in primary BCC, 14% in recurrent BCC; long-term follow-up in high-risk tumors is indicated.
- Usually, recurrences will appear within 5 years.
- Metastasis: rare (<0.1%) but metastatic disease usually fatal within 8 months
  - Head and neck location, depth, tumor diameter >4 cm are risk factors for metastasis and death.

REFERENCES

1. Hogue L, Harvey VM. Basal cell carcinoma, squamous cell carcinoma, and cutaneous melanoma in skin of color patients. *Dermatol Clin*. 2019;37(4):519–526.
2. Cameron MC, Lee E, Hibler BP, et al. Basal cell carcinoma: epidemiology; pathophysiology; clinical and histological subtypes; and disease associations. *J Am Acad Dermatol*. 2019;80(2):303–317.
3. Cameron MC, Lee E, Hibler BP, et al. Basal cell carcinoma: contemporary approaches to diagnosis, treatment, and prevention. *J Am Acad Dermatol*. 2019;80(2):321–339.

ADDITIONAL READING

Dzubow L, Goldberg LH, Lebwohl M, et al. *Basal Cell Carcinoma Prevention Guidelines*. New York, NY: The Skin Cancer Foundation; January 2021. http://www.skincancer.org/skin-cancer-information/basal-cell-carcinoma/bcc-prevention-guidelines. Accessed October 13, 2021.

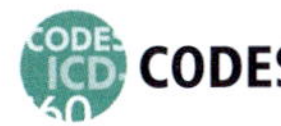

CODES

ICD10

- C44.711 Basal cell carcinoma of skin of unspecified lower limb, including hip
- C44.51 Basal cell carcinoma of skin of trunk
- C44.61 Basal cell carcinoma of skin of upper limb, including shoulder

CLINICAL PEARLS

- BCC is the most common cancer and skin malignancy, originating from the basal cell layer of the skin appendages.
- Chronic sun exposure and fair skin type increase risk with 80% on face and neck.
- Nodular type most common; telangiectasia seen at the borders

BED BUGS

Fawn J. Winkelman, DO • Adam Strosberg, DNP, ARNP-BC

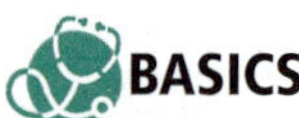

BASICS

DESCRIPTION

- Nocturnal obligate blood parasites residing in furniture and bedding
- 5 to 7 mm oval, reddish brown, flat, wingless morphology
- Microscopic evidence suggests a mature bed bug *Cimex lectularius* is approximately the size of an apple seed (1).

EPIDEMIOLOGY

Incidence

- Bed bug infestations are increasing in incidence and becoming more difficult to treat due to increased resistance to insecticides (particularly pyrethroids) (2).
- Increased travel, use of secondhand furniture, and high turnover rates of hotel guests have also contributed to rising incidence.

Prevalence

- Infestations have increased by 10–30% across the United States (1) in public places (schools, hospitals, hotels/motels, aircraft) over the past decade.
- The global population of bed bugs (*C. lectularius* and *C. hemipterus*, family Cimicidae) has undergone a significant resurgence since the late 1990s. The global bed bug population is increasing annually.
- There are over 75 species of Insecta: Hemiptera: Cimicidae ("bed bugs") with the two genera and species implicated in human infestations being *C. lectularius* and *C. hemipterus* (1).
- *C. lectularius* lives in urban environments and *C. hemipterus* lives in tropical climates.

ETIOLOGY AND PATHOPHYSIOLOGY

- Insect family Cimicidae
- Three species bite humans: *C. lectularius, C. hemipterus*, and *Leptocimex boueti*.
- Most prevalent species is *C. lectularius*.
- Found in tropical and temperate climates
- Hide in crevices of mattresses, box springs, headboards, and baseboards
- Infestations occur in hotels/motels, hospitals, cinemas, vehicles, aircraft, and homes.
- Unlike other infestations, bed bug infestations are not associated with alterations in personal hygiene.
- Reactions range from an absent or minimal response to the typical pruritic, erythematous maculopapular rash. Less commonly, there is an urticarial or anaphylactoid response.
- Skin reactions are due to host immunologic response to parasite salivary proteins.
- Urticarial reactions are mediated via immunoglobulin (Ig) G antibody response to salivary proteins.
- Bullous reactions caused by an IgE-mediated hypersensitivity to nitrophorin in bug saliva
- Bugs are attracted to body warmth and exhaled carbon dioxide.
- Bites do not transmit other known pathogens.

RISK FACTORS

- Immunocompromise
- High hotel turnover
- Secondhand furniture in home

GENERAL PREVENTION

- Integrated pest management (IPM) strategies entail a mixture of chemical and nonchemical controls to limit bed bug infestations.
- Traps typically use carbon dioxide and heat to attract and trap bugs but can be cost prohibitive.
- Vector control: Vacuum regularly; reduce clutter; seal cracks in walls; inspect luggage and clothing.
- Launder all bedding and clothing in >130°F (50°C) for 2 hours or place in 20°F (−5°C) or cooler environment for at least 5 days.
- If present in the home, eradicate using professional extermination services. Some pest control companies use canines to detect live bed bugs and eggs based on pheromones from the bed bugs.

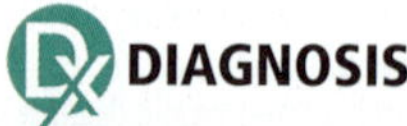

DIAGNOSIS

HISTORY

- Recent travel
- Bed bug sighting; blood specks on sheets
- New skin lesions in the morning
- Intense pruritus, pain, or burning

PHYSICAL EXAM

- Characteristic lesions are erythematous pruritic papules in an irregular linear pattern (1).
- Found on body surfaces exposed during sleeping such as face, neck, arms, legs, and shoulders
- May appear hours to days after being bitten
- Patients are usually asymptomatic but may present with papular urticaria, diffuse urticaria, bullous lesions, and/or anaphylactoid symptoms.

DIFFERENTIAL DIAGNOSIS

- Urticaria; insect or spider bite; scabies
- Dermatitis herpetiformis

DIAGNOSTIC TESTS & INTERPRETATION

Initial Tests (lab, imaging)

- Skin scraping with mineral oil preparation
- Skin biopsy

Test Interpretation

- Skin scraping is negative with mineral oil, which helps to exclude scabies.
- Skin biopsy shows nonspecific perivascular eosinophilic infiltrate consistent with arthropod bite reaction.

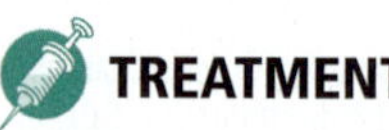

TREATMENT

GENERAL MEASURES

- Treatment should address three areas: treatment of the skin; eradication of the infestation; and assessment for potential behavioral health consequences (1).
- Most patients present for the treatment of skin irritation and lesions.
- Disease is self-limited and resolves within 1 to 2 weeks.
- Treat symptomatically.

MEDICATION

First Line

- Oral antihistamines (i.e., diphenhydramine, hydroxyzine)
- Topical antipruritics (i.e., pramoxine/calamine ointment or doxepin cream)
- Topical low-potency to mid-potency corticosteroids for 2 weeks (i.e., hydrocortisone, triamcinolone)
- Systemic corticosteroids (severe cases)

ADDITIONAL THERAPIES

- If secondarily infected, use topical or oral antibiotics against *Staphylococcus* and *Streptococcus* spp. (i.e., cephalexin, tetracycline, doxycycline, clindamycin, topical mupirocin).
- Epinephrine for anaphylaxis
- Professional extermination may be necessary.
- The CDC recommends a comprehensive IPM program—remove clutter, seal cracks, heat treatment, vacuum, and nonchemical pesticides.
- New approaches (more research necessary) include xenointoxication (oral arthropodicidal agent) toxic to the bed bugs.

COMPLEMENTARY & ALTERNATIVE MEDICINE

- Bed bugs may be eradicated with heat.
- Tropical bed bugs (*C. hemipterus*) require a higher average temperature to eradicate.

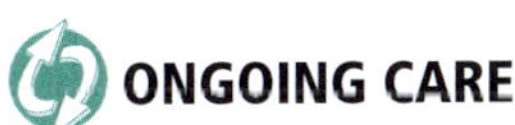

ONGOING CARE

FOLLOW-UP RECOMMENDATIONS

- Not necessary as disease is self-limited
- May need specific care in extreme cases or if anaphylactoid reactions
- Consider behavioral health consultation depending on the severity of the patient's emotional reaction to the infestation.

Patient Monitoring

Tips for travel:

- Inspect rooms by checking mattresses and luggage racks (best done with a flashlight).
- Reduce clutter.
- Keep luggage and bags off the bed and bedding.

PATIENT EDUCATION

- Avoid scratching to prevent superinfection.
- Inspect bedding, furniture, and luggage regularly.
- Centers for Disease Control and Prevention: https://www.cdc.gov/parasites/bedbugs/
- Environmental Protection Agency: https://www.epa.gov/bedbugs
- Myth 1: *Bed bugs are invisible*. They are nocturnal and hide during the daytime. Adult bugs are ~1/4-inch long, and eggs are the size of a pin head.
- Myth 2: *Bed bugs reproduce rapidly*. Their life cycle is 4 to 5 weeks, longer than the housefly.
- Myth 3: *Bed bugs can live without feeding*. Bugs can live 3 to 5 months without a blood meal.
- Tips to prevent and control bed bugs
  - Ensure infestation is bed bugs (not fleas, other insects, and/or ticks).
  - Regularly wash and heat dry your clothing and bedding, especially if it touches the floor.
  - EPA tips: https://www.epa.gov/bedbugs/top-ten-tips-prevent-or-control-bed-bugs
  - Bed Bug Information Clearinghouse: https://www.epa.gov/bedbugs/bed-bug-information-clearinghouse

COMPLICATIONS

- Bed bug dermatitis, allergic reactions, asthma exacerbations, anaphylaxis
- Significant psychological distress (insomnia, depression, anxiety, delusional parasitosis)
- Secondary bacterial infections
- Transmission of blood-borne diseases (rare)

REFERENCES

1. Leung AKC, Lam JM, Barankin B, et al. Bed bug infestation: an updated review. *Curr Pediatr Rev*. 2024;20(2):137–149. doi:10.2174/1573396320666230406084801.
2. Shipman KE, Weaving G, Shipman AR. Bedbugs: how to diagnose and manage cases of infestations. *Clin Exp Dermatol*. 2023;48(5):453–461. doi:10.1093/ced/llac140.

ADDITIONAL READING

National Pesticide Information Center: http://npic.orst.edu/

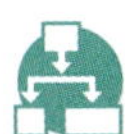

SEE ALSO

United States Environmental Protection Agency. Do-it-yourself bed bug control. https://www.epa.gov/bedbugs/do-it-yourself-bed-bug-control. Accessed August 5, 2023.

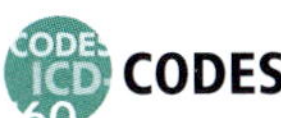

CODES

ICD10

- S00.96XA Insect bite (nonvenomous) of unspecified part of head, initial encounter
- S10.96XA Insect bite of unspecified part of neck, initial encounter
- S40.269A Insect bite (nonvenomous) of unspecified shoulder, initial encounter

CLINICAL PEARLS

- 90% of infestations occur within 3 feet of bedding.
- Wash bedding/clothing regularly in hot water and vacuum carpet daily or steam clean daily.
- Inspect furniture, bedding, and luggage regularly.
- Avoid use of "bug bombs" and chemical pesticides as bed bugs are largely resistant to over-the-counter (OTC) pesticide products (permethrin, cyfluthrin, bifenthrin, and deltamethrin or fluvalinate and esfenvalerate).

BEHAVIORAL PROBLEMS, PEDIATRIC

Sahil Mullick, MD, FAAFP • Christopher Moyer, MD

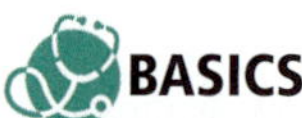

BASICS

DESCRIPTION

Behavior that disrupts ≥1 area of psychosocial functioning; common problems:

- Noncompliance: active or passive refusal to do as requested by parent/authority figure
- Temper tantrums: loss of internal control that causes crying, whining, breath holding, aggressive behavior
- Sleep problems: difficulty going to sleep or staying asleep, nightmares, night terrors
- Nocturnal enuresis: bed-wetting in children >5 years of age for ≥3 months with no medical problems
  - Primary: never dry for a minimum of 6 months (1)
  - Secondary: return of enuresis dry period of ≥6 months (1)
  - Monosymptomatic enuresis: bed-wetting only
  - Nonmonosymptomatic enuresis: bed-wetting plus daytime incontinence, urgency, voiding difficulties or voiding <4 or >7 times per day
- Functional encopresis: repeated involuntary fecal soiling; can be retentive in 80% (functional constipation) or nonretentive (20%)
- Problem eating: "picky eating," difficult mealtime behaviors
- Thumb-sucking: problematic if persists after primary teeth eruption

EPIDEMIOLOGY

- Noncompliance: more common in males; decreases with age
- Temper tantrums (2):
  - ≥12 months, up to 2 to 3 years old
  - 20% of 2-year-olds; 18% of 3-year-olds; 10% of 4-year-olds
- Sleep problems (3):
  - 10–30% of children, varies by age group
  - Bedtime resistance in 10–15% of toddlers
  - Nightmares in 10–50% of preschoolers; peak age 6 to 10 years
  - Night terrors in 1–6.5% early childhood; peak age 4 to 12 years
  - Sleepwalking in 3–5%; peak age 4 to 8 years
  - Nocturnal enuresis: 5–10% of 7-year-olds; 3% of teenagers wet the bed.
    - Monosymptomatic nocturnal enuresis is 2 × boys > girls.
    - Resolves spontaneously at a rate of approximately 15% per year
- Functional encopresis: rare in children aged <3 years, approximately 1–4% of 4-year-olds and 1–2% of children ≥7 years; more common in boys
- Problem eating: Prevalence peaks at 50% at 24 months; no relation to sex/ethnicity/income (4)
- Thumb-sucking: decreases with age; most children spontaneously stop between 2 and 4 years of age (4).

Prevalence

- Sleep problems in 25–50% of children ≥6 months; 20% in preschool/early school-ages; 20–40% in middle childhood, with girls > boys (5).
- Adolescents 16 to 18 years old, 12% seen in males compared to 23% in females
- Higher prevalence seen with ADHD, autism, and neurodevelopmental disorders (5).

ETIOLOGY AND PATHOPHYSIOLOGY

Genetics

Nocturnal enuresis: 45% risk if one parent has history, 75% if both parents have history after 5 years of age

RISK FACTORS

Adverse childhood experiences (ACEs) associated with behavioral problems in middle childhood (5)

COMMONLY ASSOCIATED CONDITIONS

- Noncompliance: Rule out depression, compulsive behaviors, adjustment disorder, inappropriate discipline.
- Temper tantrums: stress, normal development
- Sleep problems: inconsistent bedtime routine/schedule, stimulating bedtime environment; associated with hyperactive behavior, poor impulse control, poor attention in young children; acute/chronic anxiety is associated with insomnia. Long-acting stimulant medications may disturb sleep quality.
- Enuresis: associated with constipation, obstructive sleep apnea (OSA), neurodevelopmental conditions (ASD, ADHD)
- Functional encopresis: enuresis, ADHD, emotional stressors

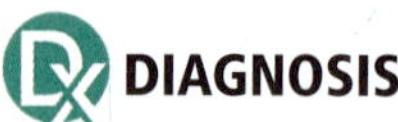

DIAGNOSIS

HISTORY

- Noncompliance: history from caregivers, teachers; direct child observation, child–caregiver interaction
  - Criteria: problematic for at least some adults, leading to difficult interactions for at least 6 months
  - Reduces child's ability to take part in structured activities
  - Creates stressful relationships with other children
  - Disrupts academic progress; places child at risk for physical injury
- Temper tantrums: stiffening limbs, arching back, dropping to floor, shouting, screaming, crying, pushing/pulling, stomping, hitting, kicking, throwing, or running away (2)[C]
- Sleep history: bedtime routine, excessive daytime sleepiness, nighttime wakings, regularity and duration of sleep, and snoring (BEARS) screen.
- Nocturnal enuresis: onset and duration; dry overnight previously; daytime wetting or any associated genitourinary symptoms; fluid intake and voiding patterns, family history of enuresis; medical, developmental and psychosocial history; constipation; sleep problems; child and caregiver's motivation for treatment; voiding diary (6)[C]
- Encopresis: fecal continence ever attained; triggering event; how often and where the child stools; pain or blood with defecation; how much stool passed accidentally; history of trauma or abuse; rectal prolapse; prior surgery
- Problem eating: review child's diet, growth curves, nutritional needs, caregiver's response to behavior (4)

PHYSICAL EXAM

- Nocturnal enuresis: generally normal; look for poor growth, tonsillar hypertrophy, constipation, or occult spinal dysraphism (6)[C].
- Functional encopresis: abdominal exam for masses or tenderness; rectal exam for tone, size of rectal vault, fecal impaction, masses, fissures, hemorrhoids; back for dimpling or hair tufts

DIFFERENTIAL DIAGNOSIS

- Temper tantrums: language deficits, autism, or disruptive mood dysregulation disorder (DMDD)—distinguishable because of baseline irritable mood between outbursts and older age (6 to 18 years)
- Nocturnal enuresis: bladder dysfunction, UTI, kidney disease or structural abnormality, OSA, diabetes insipidus, spinal dysraphism
- Functional encopresis: neurologic disorders, ectopic anus, Hirschsprung disease

DIAGNOSTIC TESTS & INTERPRETATION

Initial Tests (lab, imaging)

- Enuresis: urinalysis to rule out UTI, inability to concentrate urine, glycosuria (6)[C]
- Functional encopresis: TSH; rule out celiac disease if poor growth or family history.
- Imaging if evidence of spinal dysraphism or if both encopresis and daytime enuresis; barium enema if suspect Hirschsprung disease

Follow-Up Tests & Special Considerations

- Sleep disorders: sleep study if history of snoring and/or observed apnea (OSA); daytime ADHD-type symptoms may be present.
- Nocturnal enuresis: urodynamics (bladder dysfunction), renal ultrasound (kidney disease), MRI (spinal dysraphism)

Diagnostic Procedures/Other

- Pediatric Symptom Checklist: https://brightfutures.org/mentalhealth/pdf/professionals/ped_sympton_chklst.pdf
- National Initiative for Children's Healthcare Quality (NICHQ) Vanderbilt Assessment (ADHD screen): https://www.myadhd.com/vanderbiltparent6175.html
- Child Sexual Behavior Inventory: completed by female caregiver to assist with differentiation of normative versus abnormal behaviors particularly those related to sexual abuse: https://www.nctsn.org/measures/child-sexual-behavior-inventory

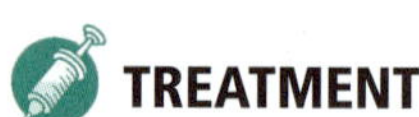

TREATMENT

GENERAL MEASURES

- Educate caregiver about specific behavioral problem.
- Parent training programs effective for many child behavior problems.
- Noncompliance: Consider parent training programs; normal screening for ADHD, obsessive-compulsive disorder (OCD), oppositional defiant disorder (ODD), or conduct disorder (CD)

- Temper tantrums: Remind caregiver this is a normal development.
  - Identify triggers: over tiredness, changing activities, and try to prevent tantrums
  - Other methods for dealing with a tantrum include one of the following:
    - Ignoring; hold/restrain child until calm; providing child with clear, firm, and consistent instructions and enough time to obey (2)[C].
- Sleep problems: Educate importance of bed routine and consistency.
  - Specific recommendations:
    - Graduated extinction: Ignore cries for specified period; check in at increasing intervals.
    - Fading: gradual decrease in direct contact; goal is for the child to fall asleep independently.
    - If fearful, special routines or aromatherapy sprays, so child feels more secure.
- Nocturnal enuresis
  - Emphasize that it is not caused by poor parenting skills or under the child's control.
  - Poor evidence for waking child to void or limiting fluids; void prior to bedtime.
  - Nonmonosymptomatic: aggressive treatment of constipation; generally treat daytime symptoms first; may require referral
  - Monosymptomatic: positive reinforcement for dry nights; enuresis alarm used nightly; discontinue after 6 weeks if no progress; if helpful, use until 14 consecutive dry nights achieved (6)[C].
- Functional encopresis
  - Disimpaction: manually, or with enemas
  - Maintenance therapy: No quick fix, results take months to achieve, and relapses are common.
    - Medical: increase fiber, fluids, polyethylene glycol, lactulose, sorbitol, magnesium citrate
    - Behavior modification: postmeal toileting 2 to 3 times a day, star charts, rewards
- Problem eating: Avoid punishment, prodding, or rewards. Offer a variety of healthy foods at every meal; limit milk to 24 oz per day and decrease juices.
- Normative sexual behavior: No treatment needed; caregivers should not punish; gently redirect behavior in public setting.
  - Sexual curiosity common in children 2 to 5 years old, including interest in looking at others, intruding on physical boundaries, and touching their mother's breasts.
- Thumb-sucking: Praise children when not sucking their thumb, offer soothing alternatives (e.g., stuffed toys), and use negative reinforcement such as a bandage around or bitters on the thumb (4).

MEDICATION

Most pediatric behavioral issues respond well to nonpharmacologic therapy:

- Sleep disorders: Cognitive-behavioral therapy and sleep hygiene are first-line treatment; no recommended pharmacotherapy
  - After behavioral methods are exhausted, melatonin 0.5 to 10.0 mg PO can be tried with behavior modification. However, this is not approved by the FDA for children.
- Encopresis: laxatives, rectal suppositories, enema for constipation
- Nocturnal enuresis:
  - First line: Desmopressin decreases urine production; response in 1/3 of patients; safe for long-term use and few side effects; chronic polydipsia can lead to hyponatremia and is a contraindication; dose: 0.2 to 0.4 mg 1 hour before bedtime, 1 to 2 weeks trial
  - Second line: tricyclic antidepressants (e.g., imipramine) used by specialists (6)[C]
  - Third line: anticholinergics (e.g., oxybutynin) at night; side effects: dry mouth, headache, constipation

ISSUES FOR REFERRAL

- Severe tantrums, >5 years old, self-injurious behaviors, slow recovery time from tantrums, more tantrums inside the home than outside, or more aggressive behaviors may require referral to psychologist or psychiatrist (2)[C].
- Chronic insomnia or anxiety: Refer to child psychologist or psychiatrist.
- Enuresis and OSA symptoms, refer for sleep study. Surgical correction of obstructive airway often improves enuresis and daytime wetting (6)[C].
- Developmentally inappropriate or sexual behaviors: If more frequent or earlier than expected, becomes a preoccupation, or recurs after corrective efforts. If abuse is not suspected, consider referral to a child psychologist. If abuse is suspected, must report to child protective services.
- If fecal disimpaction (either manual vs. medical) is unsuccessful, consult gastroenterology or surgery. If no improvement >6 months of therapy, refer to gastroenterology.
- Resistant thumb-sucking threatening permanent dentition and bite: Evaluate by a pediatric dentist for use of habit-breaking dental appliances (4)[C].

ONGOING CARE

DIET

Avoid foods with high-sugar and caffeine. Balanced meals decrease aggressive and noncompliant behaviors.

PATIENT EDUCATION

- See *Parent Training Programs: Insight for Practitioners* at: https://files.eric.ed.gov/fulltext/ED511666.pdf
- American Academy of Pediatrics. *Caring for Your Baby and Young Child: Birth to Age 5*. 8th ed. AAP Books; 2024.

REFERENCES

1. Guzman JA, Palmer LS. Nocturnal enuresis. *Pediatr Rev*. 2024;45(8):479–481. doi:10.1542/pir.2023-006166.
2. Prutipaisan W, Chunsuwan I, Hansakunachai T, et al. Characteristics of temper tantrums in 1–6-year-old children and impact on caregivers. *Clin Exp Pediatr*. 2025;68(2):170–177. doi:10.3345/cep.2024.00766.
3. Baddam SKR, Canapari CA, Van de Grift J, et al. Screening and evaluation of sleep disturbances and sleep disorders in children and adolescents. *Child Adolesc Psychiatr Clin N Am*. 2021;30(1):65–84.
4. Nasir A, Nasir L. Counseling on early childhood concerns: sleep issues, thumb-sucking, picky eating, school readiness, and oral health. *Am Fam Physician*. 2015;92(4):274–278.
5. Hunt TKA, Slack KS, Berger LM. Adverse childhood experiences and behavioral problems in middle childhood. *Child Abuse Negl*. 2017;67:391–402. doi:10.1016/j.chiabu.2016.11.005.
6. Nevéus T, Fonseca E, Franco I, et al. Management and treatment of nocturnal enuresis—an updated standardization document from the International Children's Continence Society. *J Pediatr Urol*. 2020;16(1):10–19.

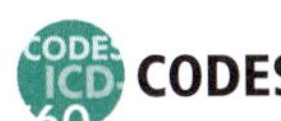

CODES

ICD10

- F91.9 Conduct disorder, unspecified
- F91.1 Conduct disorder, childhood-onset type
- F91.2 Conduct disorder, adolescent-onset type

CLINICAL PEARLS

- Well-child visits provide opportunities for screening for these common conditions.
- In extreme disobedience, screen children for ADHD, OCD, ODD, or CD.
- Parental education, including a review of age-appropriate discipline, is a key component of treatment.
- Temper tantrums in toddlers are common, often occurring at least one per day.

BELL PALSY

Megan L. Hanna, MD • Kripalini Ephraim Joseph, MD • Myers Jones, MD

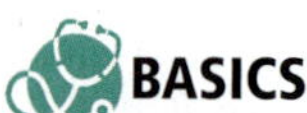

BASICS

DESCRIPTION

An acute, unilateral, self-limiting facial nerve (cranial nerve VII) palsy; Bell palsy is often idiopathic, resulting in the inability to voluntarily move the facial muscles of the affected side. It is associated with edema and compression of cranial nerve VII (CN VII).

EPIDEMIOLOGY

- No race, geographic or gender predominance
- Affects all ages, with the highest incidence being in patient ages 15 to 45 years
- Occurs with equal frequency on the left and right sides of the face

Incidence

- Global studies have demonstrated annual incidence of up to 53 per 100,000.
- Lifetime risk is 1 in 60.

ETIOLOGY AND PATHOPHYSIOLOGY

- The etiology of Bell palsy remains unclear.
- Inflammation of CN VII causes edema, subsequent compression, and possible degeneration of both the nerve and the associated vasculature.
- Activation of a latent herpes virus (herpes simplex type 1 [HSV-1] or herpes zoster) in cranial nerve ganglia is thought to account for many cases.

RISK FACTORS

- Pregnancy, with increased risk seen in patients with chronic hypertension, maternal obesity, and severe preeclampsia
- Immunosuppression
- Diabetes mellitus
- Viral upper respiratory infection
- Chronic hypertension
- Obesity
- Extremes of temperature

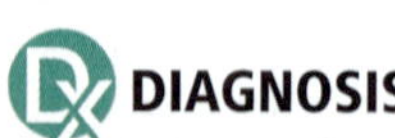

DIAGNOSIS

The diagnosis is clinical, based on a thorough history and examination (1).

HISTORY

- Onset: typically rapid (over 24 to 48 hours)
- Presentation: unilateral (very rarely bilateral) facial weakness involving both the upper and lower portion of the face (includes the forehead)
- Course: progressive, peaking at up to 3 weeks after onset. Symptoms may take up to several months to improve.
- Although strokes may present with facial weakness, facial nerve palsy is not usually the sole presenting symptom.
- Associated symptoms:
  - Mastoid or postauricular pain
  - Hyperacusis
  - Dysgeusia: alteration of taste on the ipsilateral anterior 2/3 of the tongue (chorda tympani branch of the facial nerve)
  - Numbness on the ipsilateral side of the face
  - Decreased lacrimation or salivation
- Thorough travel history (or if they live in a Lyme endemic area) or presence of skin rashes may help to elicit a more likely cause for the patient's facial nerve weakness (such as herpes zoster, Lyme disease, or sarcoidosis).

PHYSICAL EXAM

- Neurologic/HEENT
  - Flaccid paralysis of muscles on the affected side, including the forehead
    - Impaired ability to raise the eyebrow
    - Impaired closure of the eye
    - Smoothing of the brow
    - Impaired ability to smile, grin, or purse the lips
    - Flattening of the nasolabial fold
    - Bell phenomenon: upward diversion of the eye with attempted closure of the lid
- Central (upper motor neuron) versus peripheral (lower motor neuron) lesion:
  - In contrast to peripheral lesions, the forehead muscles are usually spared in central lesions.
  - Subtle deficits in other cranial nerves, especially trigeminal, glossopharyngeal, and hypoglossal, may be present, but if these signs are prominent, the diagnosis of Bell palsy is doubtful.
- Skin: Examine for erythema migrans (Lyme disease) and vesicular rash (herpes zoster virus).
- House-Brackmann scale is used to assess severity of Bell palsy (2).
  - Grade I: normal function
  - Grade II: (minimal) slight weakness on close inspection, slight synkinesis, complete eyelid closure with minimal effort
  - Grade III: (moderate) obvious but not disfiguring facial asymmetry, synkinesis is noticeable but not severe, complete eyelid closure with effort, mouth is slightly weak with maximal effort
  - Grade IV: (severe) disfiguring facial asymmetry or obvious facial weakness, forehead cannot move, incomplete eyelid closure, mouth is asymmetrical with maximal effort
  - Grave V: total paralysis

DIFFERENTIAL DIAGNOSIS

- Up to 50% of cases of peripheral facial nerve palsy may not be due to Bell palsy
- Consider other differentials if any of the following "red flags" exist:
  - Sparring of the forehead
  - Gradual onset over weeks to months
  - Concomitant vertigo, tinnitus, or hearing loss
  - Constitutional symptoms and/or cervical lymphadenopathy
  - Evidence of Lyme disease
  - Failure to improve within 3 months or worsening of weakness over several months
- CN VII palsy etiologies include:
  - Congenital causes: genetic syndromes, birth-related trauma, developmental hypoplasia of facial muscles
  - Acquired causes: infective (Ramsay Hunt syndrome, Lyme, TB, HIV), inflammatory (vasculitis, sarcoidosis, autoimmune), neoplastic (benign, malignant), cerebrovascular (stroke, aneurysm), iatrogenic (Botox), traumatic
- Clinical approach:
  - Recurrent, ipsilateral palsy: neoplasm of the nerve (schwannoma) or adjacent structures (parotid, temporal bone, or cerebellopontine angle)
  - Bilateral palsy: neurologic (Guillain-Barré syndrome, particularly if patient presents with ataxia and ophthalmoplegia) or associated with neoplasm (lymphoma, disseminated carcinomatosis, malignant pachymeningitis); rare: cryptococcal meningitis associated with HIV, autoimmune (MS, myasthenia gravis, Sjögren, sarcoidosis, or granulomatosis with polyangiitis)
  - Palsy at birth: segmental developmental palsy (associated with synkinesis, recovers spontaneously)
  - Facial palsy syndromes: Ramsay-Hunt (rash in the ear [zoster oticus] and/or mouth caused by VZV); Melkersson-Rosenthal (orofacial edema, recurrent facial palsy, and fissured tongue); Heerfordt-Waldenström (parotid enlargement, anterior uveitis, facial palsy, and fever)

DIAGNOSTIC TESTS & INTERPRETATION

Bell palsy is a clinical diagnosis. Routine lab testing or diagnostic imaging in new-onset Bell palsy is not necessary. However, further testing (MRI of head or orbits/face/neck with and without intravenous contrast) may be considered in:

- Atypical presentation of facial palsy
- Recurrent facial palsy or symptoms for more than 2 months
- Slowly progressive disease >3 weeks
- Lack of improvement after 4 months

Initial Tests (lab, imaging)

Depending on the clinical scenario, blood testing may include:

- CBC, CRP/ESR to rule out inflammatory process
- Rapid plasma reagin (RPR), Lyme serology and/or HIV test if indicated
- Titers for VZV, rubella, cytomegalovirus, hepatitis A, hepatitis B, and hepatitis C
- Polymerase chain reaction (PCR) for HSV-1 or herpes zoster virus

Follow-Up Tests & Special Considerations

- Facial radiographs: to evaluate for fractures
- Contrast-enhanced CT: to evaluate for stroke or temporal bone fracture
- MRI: to evaluate for brain or parotid neoplasms
- Invasive diagnostic procedures are not indicated because biopsy could further damage the nerve.

Diagnostic Procedures/Other

- Electrodiagnostic studies may be offered to patients with complete paralysis for prognostic purposes but does not change the management.
- Parotid gland biopsy: considered in cases of no recovery with negative imaging at 7 months

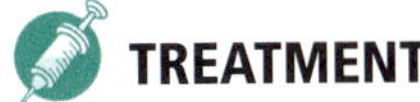

TREATMENT

GENERAL MEASURES

- Artificial tears should be used frequently to lubricate the cornea.
- The ipsilateral eye should be patched or taped shut at night to avoid drying and infection.

MEDICATION

- Recovery from Bell palsy is possible without treatment, particularly in patients who do not have a complete palsy.
- Patients should be prescribed oral corticosteroids, which decrease inflammation and limit nerve damage, increasing the number of patients who make full recovery and reducing disabling sequelae (NNT = 10) (2)[A].
  - Should be started within 72 hours of symptoms onset
  - A 10-day course of oral steroids is recommended. This may be either:
    - Prednisolone 50 mg PO daily for 10 days
    - Prednisone 60 mg daily for 5 days and then tapering dose (by 10 mg/day) the next 5 days
  - Precautions: Use with discretion in patients with peptic ulcer disease and diabetes.
  - Contraindications: documented hypersensitivity, preexisting infections (TB, systemic mycosis)
- Antiviral therapy alone has no benefit over placebo (3). The use of antivirals as a monotherapy in new-onset Bell palsy is not recommended.
- For patients with new-onset Bell palsy, antivirals, in addition to steroids, might be offered to reduce incidence of long-term sequelae (synkinesis) (NNT = 12) (3)[A]. Patients offered antivirals should be counseled that a benefit from antivirals has not been established, and if there is a benefit, it is likely to be modest at best (3)[B].
  - If antiviral is being used, consider valacyclovir 1,000 mg PO TID for 7 days or acyclovir 400 mg 5 times per day for 10 days.

Pediatric Considerations

In the pediatric population, early treatment with oral prednisolone does not appear to improve complete recovery. The vast majority of pediatric patients improve without treatment (4).

Pregnancy Considerations

Steroids should be used cautiously during pregnancy. Acyclovir and valacyclovir are considered category B drugs in pregnancy by the U.S. Food and Drug Administration.

ISSUES FOR REFERRAL

- Refer to ophthalmology for persistent weakness in eyelid closure.
- In the setting of bilateral, recurrent or prolonged symptoms, patients should be referred to speciality care (ENT or neurology) and may require neuroimaging to rule out neoplasms.
- In children, refer to neurology or neurosurgery if condition is associated with trauma, age <2 years and/or symptoms lasting >4 weeks.

ADDITIONAL THERAPIES

- In patients who make an incomplete recovery following the use of steroids with or without antiviral therapy, consider botulinum toxin to treat facial asymmetry, facial tightness, and synkinesis (5).
- Physical therapy remains an alternative treatment option when systemic disease or allergies render pharmacologic treatment intolerable.
- Physical therapy should be offered to patients with severe paralysis (House-Brackmann grade V or VI) or persistent paralysis (>3 months).

SURGERY/OTHER PROCEDURES

- There is insufficient evidence to decide whether surgical intervention is beneficial or harmful in the management of Bell palsy.
- Decompression surgery should not be performed >14 days after the onset of paralysis because severe degeneration of the facial nerve is likely irreversible after 2 to 3 weeks.

COMPLEMENTARY & ALTERNATIVE MEDICINE

Electrical stimulation, acupuncture, photobiomodulation, Kabat rehabilitation, and facial exercises offer unclear benefit. More high-quality trials are needed to confirm therapeutic value and optimize protocols.

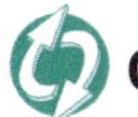

ONGOING CARE

FOLLOW-UP RECOMMENDATIONS

Patient Monitoring

- Start steroid treatment immediately.
- Patients who do not recover complete facial nerve function should be referred to ENT, neurology, or ophthalmology for further management.

PATIENT EDUCATION

Bell Palsy, American Academy of Family Physicians: https://familydoctor.org/condition/bells-palsy

PROGNOSIS

- Most patients achieve spontaneous recovery within 2 weeks. >80% recover within 3 months.
- Up to 90% of children and pregnant women completely recover.
- 85% of untreated patients will experience the first signs of recovery within 3 weeks of onset.
- Up to 30% of patients do not recover facial function completely.
- 7% may have recurrence, which may be on the affected or opposite side.
- 5% experience severe sequelae, and a few patients experience permanent facial weakness and dysfunction.
- Poor prognostic factors include the following:
  - Age >60 years
  - History of recurrence
  - Complete facial weakness
  - Diabetes mellitus; hypertension
  - House-Brackmann grade >II

COMPLICATIONS

- Corneal abrasion or ulceration
- Steroid-induced hyperglycemia, psychological disturbances, avascular necrosis of the hips, knees, and/or shoulders
- Chronic spasm of facial muscles (synkinesia) or blepharospasms due to aberrant regeneration of the facial nerve can affect up to 26% of patients 1 year after onset of Bell palsy.

REFERENCES

1. Gilden DH. Clinical practice: Bell's palsy. *N Engl J Med*. 2004;351(13):1323–1331.
2. Dalrymple SN, Row JH, Gazewood J. Bell palsy: rapid evidence review. *Am Fam Physician*. 2023;107(4):415–420.
3. Gagyor I, Madhok VB, Daly F, et al. Antiviral treatment for Bell's palsy (idiopathic facial paralysis). *Cochrane Database Syst Rev*. 2019;9(9):CD001869.
4. Babl FE, Herd D, Borland ML, et al. Efficacy of prednisolone for bell palsy in children: a randomized double-blind placebo-controlled, multicenter trial. *Neurology*. 2022;99(20):e2241–e2252.
5. Shinn JR, Nwabueze NN, Du L, et al. Treatment patterns and outcomes in botulinum therapy for patients with facial synkinesis. *JAMA Facial Plast Surg*. 2019;21(3):244–251.

ADDITIONAL READING

- Baugh RF, Basura GJ, Ishii LE, et al. Clinical practice guideline: Bell's palsy. *Otolaryngol Head Neck Surg*. 2013;149(Suppl 3):S1–S27.
- Peitersen E. The natural history of Bell's palsy. *Am J Otol*. 1982;4(2):107–111.

SEE ALSO

Herpes Simplex; Herpes Zoster (Shingles); Lyme Disease; Sarcoidosis; Ramsay-Hunt Syndrome

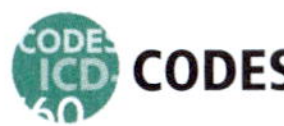

CODES

ICD10

G51.0 Bell's palsy

CLINICAL PEARLS

- Look closely at the voluntary movement on the upper part of the face on the affected side; in Bell palsy, all the muscles are involved (weak or paralyzed), whereas in a stroke, the upper muscles (forehead) are spared (because of bilateral innervation).
- No need to obtain routine labs or diagnostic imaging in a typical new-onset Bell palsy.
- Initiate steroids immediately following the onset of symptoms and consider addition of antiviral therapy (may reduce risk of long-term synkinesia).
- Protect the affected eye with lubrication and taping nightly.
- In areas with endemic Lyme disease, consider Lyme until proven otherwise.

BIPOLAR I DISORDER

Maria del Pilar Montanez Villacampa, MD, FAAFP

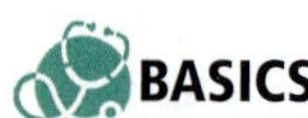

BASICS

DESCRIPTION

- A chronic disorder of at least one manic or mixed (mania and depression) episode that causes marked impairment, psychosis, and/or hospitalization
- Symptoms are not caused by a substance or general medical condition.

Geriatric Considerations

In new onset in older patients (>50 years of age), a workup for organic or chemically induced pathology is recommended.

Pediatric Considerations

Need for clarity of symptoms is critical to differentiate between attention deficit/hyperactivity disorder (ADHD), oppositional defiant disorder (ODD), disruptive mood dysregulation, and other diagnoses with overlapping symptoms that can occur in childhood.

Pregnancy Considerations

- Pregnancy does not reduce risk of mood episodes.
- Need to weigh risk of fetal and maternal exposure to mood episode to that of medication
- Avoid divalproex (Depakote) due to high teratogenicity risk.
- Postpartum carries high risk of severe acute episode with psychosis and/or infanticidal ideation.

EPIDEMIOLOGY

Onset usually between 15 and 30 years of age, average prior to age 25 years.

Incidence

1% of the world's population

Prevalence

- 0.5–1% lifetime prevalence
- Manic episodes more common in men; depressive episodes more common in women

ETIOLOGY AND PATHOPHYSIOLOGY

- Dysregulation of biogenic amines or neurotransmitters (particularly serotonin, norepinephrine, and dopamine)
- MRI findings suggest abnormalities in prefrontal cortical areas, striatum, and amygdala that predate illness onset.

Genetics

- Monozygotic twin concordance 40–70%; dizygotic 5–25%
- 50% have at least one parent with a mood disorder.

GENERAL PREVENTION

Treatment adherence and education help to prevent relapses.

COMMONLY ASSOCIATED CONDITIONS

Substance abuse (60%), ADHD, anxiety disorders (~50%), and eating disorders

DIAGNOSIS

The diagnosis of BP-I requires at least one manic or mixed episode (simultaneous mania and depression). Although a depressive episode is not necessary for the diagnosis, 80–90% of people with BP-I also experience depression. Refer to the *DSM-5* for additional information.

HISTORY

- Collateral information makes diagnostics more complete and is often necessary for a clear history.
- History: safety concerns (e.g., Suicidal/homicidal ideation? Safety plan? Psychosis present?), physical well-being (e.g., Number of hours of sleep? Weight change? Substance abuse?), personal history (e.g., Talkative? Risky driving? Excessive spending? Credit card debt? Promiscuity? Other risk-taking behavior? Legal trouble?), substance use (e.g., Did the mood change precede or occur during or after substance use?)

PHYSICAL EXAM

- Mental status exam in acute mania
  - General appearance: disorganized or discombobulated, psychomotor agitation
  - Speech: disorganized, pressured, difficult to interrupt
  - Mood/affect: euphoria, irritability, expansive, labile
  - Thought process: flight of ideas (streams of thought occur to patient at rapid rate), easily distracted
  - Thought content: grandiosity, paranoia, hyperreligiosity
  - Perceptual abnormalities: 3/4 of manic patients experience delusions, grandiose, or paranoia.
  - Suicidal/homicidal ideation: aggression toward self or others; suicidal ideation is common with mixed episode.
  - Insight/judgment: poor/impaired
- With mixed episodes, patients may exhibit a combination of manic and depressive mental states.

DIFFERENTIAL DIAGNOSIS

- Other psychiatric considerations: unipolar depression ± psychotic features, schizophrenia, schizoaffective disorder, personality disorders (particularly antisocial, borderline, histrionic, and narcissistic), ADD ± hyperactivity, substance-induced mood disorder
- Medical considerations: epilepsy (e.g., temporal lobe), brain tumor, infection (e.g., AIDS, syphilis), stroke, traumatic brain injuries, dementia, endocrine (e.g., thyroid) disease, electrolyte imbalances, multiple sclerosis, autoimmune disorders (e.g., SLE psychosis), toxins (e.g., drugs, alcohol), medications (e.g., steroids)
- In children, consider ADHD and ODD.

DIAGNOSTIC TESTS & INTERPRETATION

- The Mood Disorder Questionnaire is a self-assessment screen for history of mood elevation (thus presumed bipolar diagnosis) (sensitivity 73%, specificity 90%).
- Patient Health Questionnaire-9 helps to determine the presence and severity of a depressive episode.

Initial Tests (lab, imaging)

- TSH, CBC, BMP, B12, LFTs, RPR, HIV, ESR
- Drug/alcohol screen with each presentation
- Consider brain imaging (CT, MRI) with initial onset of mania to rule out organic cause (e.g., tumor, infection, or stroke), especially with onset in elderly and if psychosis is present.

Diagnostic Procedures/Other

Consider EEG if presentation suggests temporal lobe epilepsy (hyperreligiosity, hypergraphia).

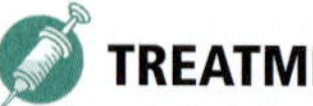

TREATMENT

GENERAL MEASURES

- Ensure safety; daily schedule especially sleep; clean from substances; avoid blue light (screens) in evening; exercise; a healthy diet
- Psychotherapy for depression (e.g., cognitive-behavioral therapy, social rhythm, interpersonal) in conjunction with medications

MEDICATION

- Acute mania (1),(2)[B]
  - First line
    - Lithium monotherapy (side effects concerns: renal toxicity, hypothyroidism, diabetes insipidus)
    - Atypical antipsychotic: quetiapine, risperidone/paliperidone, aripiprazole, asenapine, or cariprazine monotherapy
    - Divalproex
    - Lithium or divalproex plus atypical antipsychotic
  - Second line
    - Olanzapine; carbamazepine; lithium plus divalproex; lithium or divalproex plus olanzapine; ziprasidone; haloperidol, cariprazine
    - Electroconvulsive therapy (ECT)
- Acute bipolar I depression (2)
  - First line
    - Quetiapine
    - Lithium, lamotrigine, lurasidone, cariprazine
  - Second line
    - Divalproex, lumateperone
    - Bupropion adjunctive
    - Olanzapine + fluoxetine
      - Olanzapine side effects concerns: weight gain, metabolic syndrome, and extrapyramidal symptoms (EPS) warrant vigilance and monitoring by the clinician.
    - ECT
- Treatment mood stabilizer(s) or other psychotropic medications; when combining, use different classes (e.g., an atypical antipsychotic and/or an antiseizure medication and/or lithium).
  - Lithium: 600 to 1,200 mg/day divided BID–QID; start 600 to 900 mg/day divided BID–TID, titrate based on blood levels. *Warning*: caution in kidney and heart disease; use can lead to diabetes insipidus or thyroid disease over time. Pregnancy requires close monitoring and risks to fetus (Ebstein anomaly). *Monitor*: Check ECG for those aged >40 years, TSH, BUN, creatinine, electrolytes at baseline and every 6 months; check level 5 to 7 days after initiation or dose change, then every 2 weeks × 3, and then every 3 months (plasma range: 0.8 to 1.2 mmol/L).

- Anticonvulsants
  - Divalproex sodium, valproic acid: Start 250 to 500 mg BID–TID; maximum 60 mg/kg/day; black box warnings: hepatotoxicity, pancreatitis, thrombocytopenia, pregnancy Category D (high risk for multiple major malformations); recommendation: avoiding in reproductive age women; monitor CBC and LFTs at baseline and every 6 months. Check level 5 days after initiation and dose changes (plasma range: 50 to 125 μg/mL).
  - Carbamazepine: 800 to 1,200 mg/day PO divided BID–QID; start 100 to 200 mg PO BID and titrate up to lowest effective dose. *Warning*: Do not use with tricyclic antidepressant (TCA) or within 14 days of using MAOI; caution in kidney/heart disease; risk of aplastic anemia/agranulocytosis, enzyme inducer; pregnancy Category D; monitor CBC and LFTs at baseline and every 3 to 6 months; check level 4 to 5 days after initiation and dose changes (plasma range: 4 to 12 μg/mL).
  - Lamotrigine: 200 to 400 mg/day; start 25 mg/day for 2 weeks, then 50 mg/day for 2 weeks, then 100 mg/day for 1 week, and then 150 mg/day. *Warning*: Titrate slowly (risk of Stevens-Johnson syndrome); caution with kidney/liver/heart disease; pregnancy relative safety but needs close follow-up.
  - Oxcarbazepine: 300 mg PO QD; titrate to 1,800 to 2,400/day max.
- Atypical antipsychotics
  - Side effects: orthostatic hypotension, metabolic side effects (glucose and lipid dysregulation, weight gain), tardive dyskinesia, neuroleptic malignant syndrome (NMS), prolactinemia, increased risk of death in elderly with dementia-related psychosis, pregnancy growing data on relative safety; watch for metabolic AE above.
  - Monitor LFTs, lipids, glucose at baseline, 3 months and annually. Check for EPS with Abnormal Involuntary Movement Scale (AIMS) and assess weight (with abdominal circumference) at baseline; at 4, 8, and 12 weeks; and then every 3 to 6 months. Monitor for orthostatic hypotension 3 to 5 days after starting or changing dose.
  - Aripiprazole: 15 to 30 mg/day; IM preparation available; for mania and maintenance
  - Asenapine: 5 to 10 mg sublingual BID; for mania
  - Cariprazine: 1.5 to 3.0 mg/day for depression; 3 to 6 mg/day; for mania and depression
  - Lumateperone: 42 mg QD for depression
  - Lurasidone: 20 to 60 mg/day for depression
  - Olanzapine: 5 to 20 mg/day; most likely to cause metabolic side effects (weight gain, diabetes); for mania, depression, and maintenance
  - Paliperidone: 6 mg QAM; may cause agranulocytosis, cardiac arrhythmias; IM preparation available
  - Quetiapine: for mania, 200 to 400 mg BID; for bipolar depression, 50 to 300 mg QHS; XR dosing 50 to 400 mg QHS for mania, depression and maintenance; XR has less sedative effect.
  - Risperidone: 1 to 6 mg/day divided QD–QID; IM preparation available (every 2 weeks) for mania and maintenance
  - Ziprasidone: 40 to 80 mg BID; less likely to cause metabolic side effects; for mania and maintenance
- Avoid TCAs and serotonin-norepinephrine reuptake inhibitor (SNRI) that increase risk of mood cycling risk.

ISSUES FOR REFERRAL

Patients benefit from a multidisciplinary team, including a primary care physician, psychiatrist, therapist, and/or behavioral health consultant.

ADDITIONAL THERAPIES

- Modest evidence supports full spectrum 10,000 lux midmorning light, transcranial magnetic stimulation, ketamine infusion, armodafinil/modafinil, and levothyroxine bipolar depression.
- Blue-blocking glasses or dark therapy for mania
- A regular sleep and wake-up schedule is helpful.

ADMISSION, INPATIENT, AND NURSING CONSIDERATIONS

- To admit involuntarily, the patient must have a psychiatric diagnosis (e.g., BP-I) and present a danger to self or others, or the mental disease must be inhibiting the person from obtaining basic needs (e.g., food, clothing, shelter).
- Nursing: Alert staff to potentially dangerous or agitated patients. Acute suicidal threats need continuous observation.

ONGOING CARE

FOLLOW-UP RECOMMENDATIONS

- Regularly scheduled visits support adherence with treatment.
- Frequent communication among primary care doctor, psychiatrist, and therapist

Patient Monitoring

Mood charts are helpful to monitor symptoms.

DIET

Omega-3 fatty acids and probiotics; data limited

PATIENT EDUCATION

- National Alliance on Mental Illness (NAMI): http://www.nami.org/
- National Institute of Mental Health (NIMH): http://www.nimh.nih.gov/index.shtml
- International Bipolar Foundation (IBPF): https://ibpf.org/

PROGNOSIS

- Frequency and severity of episodes are related to medication adherence, consistency with therapy, quality of sleep, and support systems.
- 40–50% of patients experience another manic episode within 2 years of first episode.
- 25–50% attempt suicide, and 15% die by suicide.
- Substance abuse, unemployment, psychosis, depression, and male gender are associated with a worse prognosis.

REFERENCES

1. American Psychiatric Association. Diagnostic and Statistical Manual of Mental Disorders (DSM-5-TR). 5th ed. Text rev. Washington, DC: American Psychiatric Publishing; 2022.
2. Huang H, Nissen N, Lim CT, et al. Treating bipolar disorder in primary care: diagnosis, pharmacology, and management. *Int J Gen Med*. 2022;15:8299–8314.

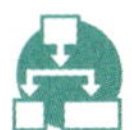

SEE ALSO

Algorithm: Depressive Episode, Major

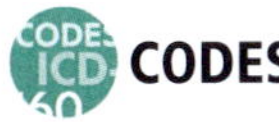

CODES

ICD10

- F31.9 Bipolar disorder, unspecified
- F31.10 Bipolar disorder, current episode manic without psychotic features, unspecified
- F31.30 Bipolar disord, crnt epsd depress, mild or mod severt, unsp

CLINICAL PEARLS

- BP-I is characterized by at least one manic or mixed episode that causes marked impairment; major depressive episodes usually occur but are not necessary.
- 25–50% of BP-I patients attempt suicide, and 15% die by suicide.
- There is no known way to prevent BP-I, but treatment adherence and education helps reduce further episodes.
- Goal of treatment is to decrease the intensity, length, and frequency of episodes as well as greater duration of euthymia (healthy mood) between episodes.

BIPOLAR II DISORDER

Maria del Pilar Montanez Villacampa, MD, FAAFP

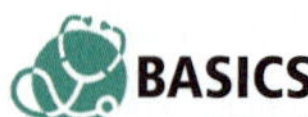

BASICS

DESCRIPTION

Chronic mental health condition characterized by at least one episode of major depression (with or without psychosis) and at least one episode of hypomania, a nonsevere mood elevation

Geriatric Considerations

In new onset in older patients (>50 years of age), a workup for organic or chemically induced pathology is strongly recommended.

Pediatric Considerations

Need for clarity of symptoms is critical to differentiate between attention deficit hyperactivity disorder (ADHD), oppositional defiant disorder (ODD), disruptive mood dysregulation, and other diagnoses with overlapping symptoms that are common in childhood.

Pregnancy Considerations

- Pregnancy does not protect against risk of mood episodes.
- Need to weigh risk of exposure to mood episode to that of medication
- Avoid divalproex (Depakote) due to high teratogenicity risk.
- Postpartum caries high risk of severe acute episode with psychosis and/or infanticidal ideation.

EPIDEMIOLOGY

Onset usually between 15 and 30 years of age

Prevalence

- 0.5–1% lifetime prevalence
- More common in women

ETIOLOGY AND PATHOPHYSIOLOGY

Dysregulation of biogenic amines or neurotransmitters (particularly serotonin, norepinephrine, and dopamine)

Genetics

Heritability estimate: >77%

RISK FACTORS

Genetics, major life stressors, or substance misuse

GENERAL PREVENTION

Treatment adherence and education can help to prevent further episodes.

COMMONLY ASSOCIATED CONDITIONS

Substance misuse, ADHD, anxiety disorders, and eating disorders

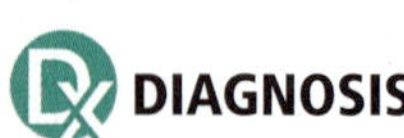

DIAGNOSIS

DSM-5 criteria: one hypomanic episode and at least one major depressive episode. Mood elevation symptoms cause unequivocal change in functioning noticed by others but not severe enough to cause marked impairment (1)[C].

- Hypomania is a distinct period of persistently elevated, expansive, or irritable mood, different from usual euthymic mood, including increase in activity or energy lasting at least 4 days:
  - The episode must include at least three of the "DIG FAST" symptoms *plus increased energy* below (four if the mood is only irritable):
    - Distractibility
    - Insomnia, decreased need for sleep
    - Grandiosity or inflated self-esteem
    - Flight of ideas or racing thoughts
    - Agitation or increase in goal-directed activity (socially, at work or school, or sexually)
    - Speech pressured/more talkative than usual
    - Taking risks: excessive involvement in pleasurable activities that have high potential for painful consequences (e.g., sexual or financial)
- Major depression: Depressed mood or diminished interest and four or more of the "SIG E CAPS" symptoms are present during the same 2-week period:
  - Sleep disturbance (e.g., trouble falling asleep, early-morning awakening)
  - Interest: loss or anhedonia
  - Guilt (or feelings of worthlessness)
  - Energy, loss of
  - Concentration, loss of
  - Appetite changes, increase or decrease
  - Psychomotor changes (retardation or agitation)
  - Suicidal/homicidal thoughts
  - Rapid cycling is ≥4 mood episodes in 12 months (major depression or hypomania).
  - Mixed specifier: when three or more symptoms of opposite mood pole are present during primary mood episode, for example, hypomania with mixed features (of depression)
- Note: If symptoms have *ever* met criteria for a full manic episode, for example, hospitalization was necessary secondary to manic/mixed symptoms or psychosis was present, then the diagnosis is BP-I.

HISTORY

- Collateral information makes diagnostics more complete and is often necessary for a clear history.
- History: safety concerns (e.g., Suicidal/homicidal ideation? Safety plan? Psychosis present?), physical well-being (e.g., Number of hours of sleep? Substance abuse?), personal history (e.g., Risky driving? Excessive spending? Credit card debt? Promiscuity? Other risk-taking behavior? Legal trouble?), substance use (e.g., Did the mood change precede, or occur subsequent to, substance use?)

PHYSICAL EXAM

- Mental status exam in hypomania
  - General appearance: usually appropriately dressed may be bright colors or eye-catching style, often with psychomotor agitation
  - Speech: may be pressured, talkative, difficult to interrupt
  - Mood/affect: euphoria, irritability, congruent, or expansive
  - Thought process: may be easily distracted, difficulty concentrating on one task
  - Thought content: usually positive, with "big" plans
  - Perceptual abnormalities: none
  - Suicidal/homicidal ideation: low incidence of homicidal or suicidal ideation
  - Insight/judgment: usually stable/may be impaired by distractibility or grandiosity
- Mental status exam in depression
  - General appearance: unkempt, psychomotor retardation, poor eye contact
  - Speech: low, soft, monotone
  - Mood/affect: sad, depressed/congruent, flat
  - Thought process: ruminating thoughts, generalized slowing
  - Thought content: preoccupied with negative or nihilistic ideas
  - Perceptual abnormalities: 15% of depressed patients experience hallucinations or delusions.
  - Suicidal/homicidal ideation: Suicidal ideation is very common.
  - Insight/judgment: often impaired

DIFFERENTIAL DIAGNOSIS

- Other psychiatric considerations: BP-I disorder, unipolar depression, personality disorders (particularly borderline, antisocial, and narcissistic), ADHD, substance-induced mood disorder
- Medical considerations: epilepsy (e.g., temporal lobe), brain tumor, infection (e.g., AIDS, syphilis), stroke, endocrine (e.g., thyroid disease), multiple sclerosis, autoimmune (e.g., SLE psychosis), medications (e.g., steroids)

DIAGNOSTIC TESTS & INTERPRETATION

- Mood Disorder Questionnaire, self-assessment screen for history of mood elevation (thus presumed bipolar diagnosis)
- Hypomania Checklist-32 distinguishes between BP-II and unipolar depression (sensitivity 80%, specificity 51%).
- Patient Health Questionnaire-9 helps to determine the presence and severity of depression.

Initial Tests (lab, imaging)

- Rule out organic causes of mood disorder during initial episode.
- Drug/alcohol screen is prudent with each presentation.
- With initial presentation: Consider CBC, chem 7, TSH, LFTs, ANA, vitamin B12, RPR, HIV, and ESR.
- Consider brain imaging (CT, MRI) with initial onset of hypomania to rule out organic cause, especially with onset in the elderly.

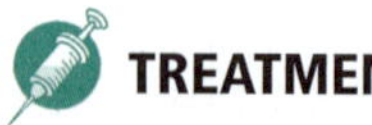

TREATMENT

GENERAL MEASURES

- Ensure safety.
- Psychotherapy for depression, stress reduction (e.g., CBT, social rhythm, interpersonal, family focused) in conjunction with medications
- Regular circadian rhythm/daily sleep and activity schedule, exercise, a healthy diet
- Sobriety, substance free

MEDICATION

- Acute mood elevation
  - First line
    - Quetiapine; lithium
    - Atypical, other: cariprazine, risperidone, aripiprazole, ziprasidone, asenapine,
    - Divalproex (avoid in reproductive age women)
  - Second line
    - Haloperidol; paliperidone, olanzapine, cariprazine
    - Lithium plus divalproex
    - Lithium or divalproex plus atypical

- Acute bipolar II depression
  - First line
    - Quetiapine, lurasidone
  - Second line
    - Lithium; lamotrigine; cariprazine
    - Bupropion adjunct
    - ECT
- When combining, use different classes (e.g., an atypical antipsychotic and/or an antiseizure medication and/or lithium).
  - Lithium: 600 to 1,200 mg/day divided BID–QID; start 600 to 900 mg/day divided BID–TID, titrate based on blood levels. *Warning*: caution in kidney and heart disease; use can lead to diabetes insipidus or thyroid disease. Pregnancy requires close monitoring. *Monitor*: Check ECG >40 years, TSH, BUN, creatine, electrolytes at baseline and every 6 months. Check level 5 to 7 days after initiation or dose change, then every 2 weeks × 3, and then every 3 months (goal: 0.6 to 1.2 mmol/L).
  - Anticonvulsants
    - Divalproex sodium, valproic acid: Start 250 to 500 mg BID–TID; maximum 60 mg/kg/day; black box warnings: hepatotoxicity, pancreatitis, thrombocytopenia, pregnancy Category D; monitor CBC and LFTs at baseline and every 6 months; check level 5 days after initiation and dose changes (goal: 50 to 125 μg/mL).
    - Lamotrigine: 200 to 400 mg/day; start 25 mg/day for 2 weeks, then 50 mg/day for 2 weeks, then 100 mg/day for 1 week, and then 150 mg/day. (Note: Use half dosing if adjunct to valproate.) *Warning*: Titrate slowly (risk of Stevens-Johnson syndrome); caution with kidney/liver/heart disease; depression prevention indication does not treat mood elevation.
  - Atypical antipsychotics
    - Side effects: orthostatic hypotension, metabolic side effects (glucose and lipid dysregulation, weight gain), tardive dyskinesia, neuroleptic malignant syndrome (NMS), akathisia, prolactinemia (except aripiprazole), sedation, increased risk of death in elderly with dementia-related psychosis
    - Monitor LFTs, lipids, glucose at baseline, 3 months and annually; check for EPS with Abnormal Involuntary Movement Scale (AIMS) and assess weight (with abdominal circumference) at baseline; at 4, 8, and 12 weeks; and then every 3 to 6 months; monitor for orthostatic hypotension 3 to 5 days after starting or changing dose.
    - Aripiprazole: 10 to 30 mg/day; less likely to cause metabolic side effects, IM dosing once a month to once every 6 months, for hypomania and maintenance
    - Asenapine: 5 to 10 mg sublingual BID
    - Cariprazine: 1.5 mg to 3.0 mg for depression, up to 6 mg for mood elevation
    - Lurasidone: 20 to 60 mg/day for depression
    - Paliperidone: 6 mg every morning; may cause agranulocytosis, cardiac arrhythmias, for hypomania and maintenance
    - Quetiapine: 200 to 400 mg BID for hypomania; 50 to 600 mg for bipolar depression QHS; XR dosing 50 to 400 mg QHS, high sedation and metabolic profile
    - Risperidone: 1 to 6 mg/day divided QD–QID; IM preparation available (q2wk); watch for hyperprolactinemia and abnormal involuntary muscle movements, for hypomania and maintenance.
    - Ziprasidone: 40 to 80 mg BID; less likely to cause metabolic side effects, for hypomania and maintenance
- Unipolar antidepressants
  - Bupropion (Wellbutrin): dosing: 150 to 300 mg PO QD; not FDA-approved; use only with antimanic agent.
  - Avoid TCAs and SNRIs—increases mood cycling risk

ISSUES FOR REFERRAL

Patients benefit from a multidisciplinary team, including a primary care physician, psychiatrist, therapist, and/or behavioral health consultant.

ADDITIONAL THERAPIES

- Modest evidence supports full spectrum bright light, transcranial magnetic stimulation, vagus nerve stimulation, ketamine infusion (2),(3), and hormone therapy (e.g., thyroid) in bipolar depression.
- Blue-blocking glasses or dark therapy for mood elevation, regular sleep wake cycle, awakening the same time every morning

ADMISSION, INPATIENT, AND NURSING CONSIDERATIONS

- To admit involuntarily, the patient must have a psychiatric diagnosis (e.g., BP-I) and present a danger to self or others, or the mental disease must be inhibiting the person from obtaining basic needs (e.g., food, clothing).
- Nursing: Alert staff to potentially dangerous or agitated patients. Acute suicidal threats need continuous observation.

ONGOING CARE

FOLLOW-UP RECOMMENDATIONS

Regularly scheduled visits support adherence with treatment.

Patient Monitoring

Mood charts are helpful to monitor symptoms.

DIET

May benefit from omega-3 fatty acids and probiotics; data limited

PATIENT EDUCATION

- National Alliance on Mental Illness (NAMI): http://www.nami.org/
- National Institute of Mental Health (NIMH): http://www.nimh.nih.gov/index.shtml
- International Bipolar Foundation (IBPF): https://ibpf.org

PROGNOSIS

- Frequency and severity of episodes are related to medication adherence, consistency with therapy, quality of sleep, and support systems.
- 25–50% attempt suicide and 15% die by suicide.
- Substance abuse, unemployment, psychosis, depression, and male gender are associated with a worse prognosis.

REFERENCES

1. American Psychiatric Association. *Diagnostic and Statistical Manual of Mental Disorders*. 5th ed. Arlington, VA: American Psychiatric Association; 2013.
2. Huang H, Nissen N, Lim CT, et al. Treating bipolar disorder in primary care: diagnosis, pharmacology, and management. *Int J Gen Med*. 2022;15:8299–8314. doi:10.2147/IJGM.S386875.
3. Marzani G, Price Neff A. Bipolar disorders: evaluation and treatment. *Am Fam Physician*. 2021;103(4):227–239.

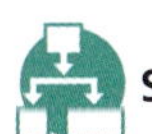

SEE ALSO

Algorithm: Bipolar Disorder I

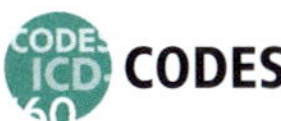

CODES

ICD10

F31.81 Bipolar II disorder

CLINICAL PEARLS

- BP-II is characterized by at least one episode of major depression and one episode of hypomania.
- Patients may not recognize symptoms and/or decline treatment during a hypomanic episode; they may enjoy the elevated mood and productivity.
- Patients with BP-II are at great risk for both attempting and completing suicide.

BITES, ANIMAL AND HUMAN

Kellie Wang, PharmD • Brian J. Kimbrell, MD, FACS

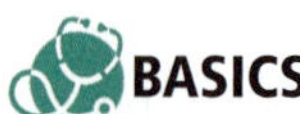

BASICS

DESCRIPTION

Animal bite rates vary by species: dogs (60–90%), cats (5–20%), rodents (2–3%), humans (2–3%), and (rarely) other animals, including snakes.

EPIDEMIOLOGY

All ages, but children > adults

Incidence

- 3 to 6 million animal bites per year in the United States; account for 1% of all injury-related ED visits
- 1–2% will require hospital admission, and 20 to 35 victims die from dog bite complications, annually.

ETIOLOGY AND PATHOPHYSIOLOGY

- Dog bites are more common than cat bites; most dog bites are from a known domestic pet; ~90% of cat bites are provoked. Dog bites are more common in children, cat bites in adults. Cat bites are more prone to serious infection (deep puncture wounds).
- Human bite wounds are typically incurred by striking another in the mouth with a clenched fist; human bites also occur incidentally (e.g., paronychia, thumb-sucking, or bites to the face, breasts, or genital areas).
- Animal bites can cause tears, punctures, scratches, avulsions, or crush injuries.
- Contamination by oral flora leads to infection.
- Dog and cat bites most commonly involve *Pasteurella* spp., *Capnocytophaga*, streptococci, staphylococci. Human bites most commonly involve *Eikenella* spp., *Staphylococcus*, *Streptococcus*, and anaerobes.

RISK FACTORS

- Clenched-fist human bites are frequently associated with the use of alcohol or drugs.
- Patients presenting >8 hours following the bite are at greater risk of infection.

GENERAL PREVENTION

- Instruct about animal hazards.
- Educate pet owners; appropriate pet vaccinations

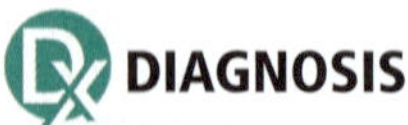

DIAGNOSIS

HISTORY

- Detailed history of the incident (provoked or unprovoked), type of animal, site of the bite, animal's vaccine status, whereabouts of animal, and geographic setting
- Underlying patient medical history—particularly comorbid diseases and immunosuppression
- Ascertain patient immunization history (tetanus and rabies, in particular)

PHYSICAL EXAM

- Dog bites: hands and face most common site of injury in adults and children, respectively; more likely to have associated crush injury
- Cat bites: predominantly involve the hands, followed by lower extremities, face, and trunk; more often puncture-type wound
- Human bites
  - Intentional bite: semicircular or oval area of erythema and bruising, with or without break in skin
  - Clenched-fist injury: wounds over the metacarpophalangeal joints from striking the fist against another's teeth
- Signs of wound infection include fever, erythema, swelling, tenderness, purulent drainage, and lymphangitis.
- Signs of tenosynovitis (hand or finger bites): finger held in flexion, fusiform swelling, pain along tendon sheath, pain with active or passive extension of the affected digit
- Document neurovascular status.

Pediatric Considerations

Human bite marks on a child with an intercanine distance >3 cm are likely from an adult and should raise concerns about child abuse.

DIFFERENTIAL DIAGNOSIS

Evaluate for other possible causes of trauma.

DIAGNOSTIC TESTS & INTERPRETATION

Initial Tests (lab, imaging)

- Gram stain and culture wound drainage; 85% of bite wounds will yield a positive culture; most are polymicrobial.
- Obtain aerobic and anaerobic blood cultures before starting antibiotics if bacteremia is suspected.
- Plain radiograph or CT scan for suspected foreign body or bone or joint injury (Baseline imaging is also helpful for later comparison if osteomyelitis is suspected, especially in clenched-fist injuries.)

ALERT

Cat bites are twice as likely to become infected as dog bites and have higher risks of osteomyelitis, tenosynovitis, and septic arthritis.

Follow-Up Tests & Special Considerations

- Plain radiograph and/or MRI for suspected osteomyelitis
- CT scan for severe skull bites
- Ultrasound can detect abscess formation.
- If wound fails to heal, culture for atypical pathogens (e.g., fungi, *Nocardia*, and mycobacteria); keep bacterial cultures for 7 to 10 days (some pathogens are slow-growing).

Diagnostic Procedures/Other

Surgical exploration may be needed to determine the extent of injuries or to drain deep infections (e.g., tendon sheath), especially in severe hand wounds.

Test Interpretation

Most common microorganisms include:

- Dog bites (1)
  - *Pasteurella* spp. present in 50% of bites
  - Streptococci spp., *S. aureus*, *S. intermedius*, *Neisseria* spp., *C. canimorsus*, *Bacteroides* spp., *Fusobacterium* spp.
- Cat bites
  - *Pasteurella* spp. in 75% of bites
  - *Streptococcus* spp. (including *Streptococcus pyogenes*), *Staphylococcus* spp. (including methicillin-resistant *S. aureus* [MRSA]), *Neisseria* spp., *Moraxella* spp., *Porphyromonas* spp., *Fusobacterium* spp., *Bacteroides* spp.
- Human bites
  - *Eikenella corrodens* (15–29%), *Streptococcus* spp., *S. aureus* (including MRSA), and various anaerobic bacteria (e.g., *Fusobacterium*, *Peptostreptococcus*, *Prevotella*, and *Porphyromonas* spp.)
  - Although rare, case reports suggest transmission of viruses (Hepatitis B/C, HIV, and herpes simplex).
- Aquatic bites
  - *S. aureus*, *Streptococcus* spp., *Vibrio* spp. (saltwater, brackish water), *Aeromonas* spp. (freshwater), *Mycobacterium* spp., *Pseudomonas* spp.
- Reptile bites
  - *Pseudomonas aeruginosa*, *Proteus* spp., *Salmonella*, *Bacteroides fragilis*, and *Clostridium* spp.
- Rodent bites
  - *Streptobacillus moniliformis* or *Spirillum minus*, which causes rat-bite fever
- Ungulate (hooved animal) bites
  - Pigs are the most likely to bite; commonly polymicrobial infections (*Staphylococcus* and *Streptococcus* spp., *Haemophilus influenzae*, *Pasteurella*, *Actinobacillus*, and *Flavobacterium* spp.)

ALERT

Asplenic patients and those with underlying hepatic disease are at risk for bacteremia and fatal sepsis after dog bites infected with *C. canimorsus*.

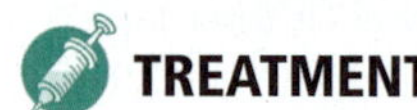

TREATMENT

GENERAL MEASURES

- Elevate the injured extremity to prevent swelling.
- Copious irrigation of the wound with normal saline via a catheter tip to reduce risk of infection
- Complete and submit bite report per local policy.
- Contact local health department to determine rabies prevalence in biting species: https://www.cdc.gov/rabies/resources/contacts.html

MEDICATION

- Prophylactic antibiotics are recommended only for human bites and high-risk wounds (deep puncture, crush injury, venous or lymphatic compromise, hands or near joint, face or genital area, immunocompromised hosts, requiring surgical repair, asplenic, advanced liver, edema).
- Duration of antibiotic therapy: preemptive, 3 to 5 days; treatment of cellulitis/skin abscess, 5 to 10 days
- Refer to most common microbial organisms to determine appropriate antibiotic coverage for unusual animals.
- Determine the need for antirabies therapy: rabies immunoglobulin and rabies vaccine for those bitten by wild animals (primary vector in the United States is bat or raccoon), rabid pets, unvaccinated pets depending on detail of the incident, or in situations where the animal cannot be quarantined for 10 days.
- Consider tetanus toxoid (Td) for previously immunized with >10 years since their last dose (2)[C]; tetanus, diphtheria, and pertussis (Tdap) formulation is generally preferred to Td (2)[C].

ALERT

- Anti-HBs negative patients bitten by HBsAg-positive individuals should receive both hepatitis B immunoglobulin (HBIG) and hepatitis B vaccine.
- HIV postexposure prophylaxis is generally not recommended for human bites unless there is significant blood exposure to broken skin.
- Snake bite: If venomous, transport for appropriate evaluation and antivenom; be sure patient is stable for transport.
- Monkey bite: All monkey bites can transmit rabies, bites of macaque monkeys may transmit herpes B virus which is potentially fatal. Contact CDC and consider an antiviral, such as valacyclovir, that is active against herpes B virus.

First Line

- For prophylactic and empiric antibiotic treatment, amoxicillin and clavulanate is first line (2)[B].
  - Adults: amoxicillin and clavulanate 875/125 mg PO BID
  - Children: amoxicillin and clavulanate (dose is based on amoxicillin component) 45 mg/kg/day divided q12h; maximum 875 mg per dose
- Patients with deep or severe wound infections, systemic infections requiring IV therapy, and the immunocompromised:
  - Adults: ampicillin and sulbactam 3 g IV q6h *or* piperacillin and tazobactam 3.375 g IV q6h (2)
  - Children: ampicillin and sulbactam (dose based on ampicillin component) 200 mg/kg/day IV divided q6h; maximum 3 g per dose

Second Line

- Alternative oral regimens
  - Adults: clindamycin (300 mg PO TID) plus either trimethoprim-sulfamethoxazole (TMP-SMX; 1 DS tablet PO BID) *or* ciprofloxacin (500 to 750 mg PO BID)
  - Children: clindamycin (25 to 30 mg/kg/day PO in 3 divided doses; maximum 400 mg per dose) plus TMP-SMX (8 to 10 mg/kg/day of trimethoprim PO in 2 divided doses; maximum 160 mg TMP per dose)
- Alternative IV regimens
  - Adults: ciprofloxacin 400 mg IV q12h *or* levofloxacin 750 mg IV daily, with metronidazole 500 mg IV q8h

ALERT

- Consider community-acquired MRSA as a possible pathogen (from human skin or colonized pet); if high suspicion, doxycycline or TMP-SMX provide good coverage
- Avoid 1st-generation cephalosporins (e.g., cephalexin), penicillinase-resistant penicillins (e.g., dicloxacillin), and clindamycin (when not administered with another agent) because they lack activity against *Pasteurella multocida* (dog and cat bites) and *E. corrodens* (human bites).

Pregnancy Considerations

For pregnant women who cannot take penicillins or cephalosporins due to severe allergy, consider azithromycin; observe closely due to increased risk of treatment failure.

ISSUES FOR REFERRAL

- Consider surgical consultation for deep, severe, or complex bite wounds.
- Deep wounds to the hand and face should be referred to a hand surgeon or plastic surgeon.
- Bites from primates or unusual species of animals should be referred to infectious disease specialist.

SURGERY/OTHER PROCEDURES

- Débride devitalized tissue; débridement of puncture wounds is not advised.
- Consider primary closure if the irrigated wound is clean, the bite is <12 hours old, and in bites to the face (cosmesis).
- Infected wounds and those at high risk for infection (cat bites, human bites, bites to the hand, crush injuries, presentation >12 hours from injury) should be left open.
- Delayed primary closure in 3 to 5 days is an option for infected wounds; large, gaping wounds should be reapproximated with widely spaced sutures or adhesive strips.

ADMISSION, INPATIENT, AND NURSING CONSIDERATIONS

Patients with deep or severe wound infections, systemic infections requiring IV therapy, and immunosuppression generally require inpatient admission.

ONGOING CARE

FOLLOW-UP RECOMMENDATIONS

Patient Monitoring

- Recheck for infection in 24 to 48 hours.
- Base revisions of antibiotic therapy on culture results and clinical response.

PATIENT EDUCATION

Educate patients about how to be safe around animals and avoid animal bites.

PROGNOSIS

Wounds should improve and close over 7 to 10 days.

COMPLICATIONS

- Tenosynovitis
- Endocarditis
- Extensive soft tissue injuries with scarring, gas gangrene
- Hemorrhage
- Meningitis, osteomyelitis
- Posttraumatic stress disorder
- Sepsis, septic arthritis

REFERENCES

1. Baxter M, Denny KJ, Keijzers G. Antibiotic prescribing in patients who presented to the emergency department with dog bites: a descriptive review of current practice. *Emerg Med Australas*. 2020;32(4):578–585.
2. Stevens DL, Bisno AL, Chambers HF, et al. Practice guidelines for the diagnosis and management of skin and soft tissue infections: 2014 update by the Infectious Disease Society of America. *Clin Infect Dis*. 2014;59(2):e10–e52.

ADDITIONAL READING

Elcock KL, Reid J, Moncayo-Nieto OL, et al. Biting the hand that feeds you: management of human and animal bites. *Injury*. 2022;53(2):227–236.

SEE ALSO

Bartonella Infections; Cellulitis; Rabies

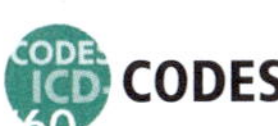

CODES

ICD10

- S61.459A Open bite of unspecified hand, initial encounter
- S01.85XA Open bite of other part of head, initial encounter
- S20.97XA Other superficial bite of unspecified parts of thorax, initial encounter

CLINICAL PEARLS

- Cleanse, débride, and culture animal and human bites.
- Antibiotic prophylaxis is recommended for human bites and high-risk wounds.
- Consider rabies and tetanus vaccination.
- Animal and human bites require close follow-up to assess for signs of infection or other complications.

BLADDER CANCER

Jon S. Parham, DO, MPH, FAAFP

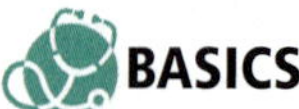

BASICS

A primary cancer tumor originating in cells lining the urinary bladder lumen

DESCRIPTION

- Bladder cancer (BC) cell types: urothelial carcinoma, 90% (formerly named transitional cell), and others (squamous cell and adenocarcinoma)
- The spectrum of BC relates to tumor penetration into muscularis propria layer or not:
  - Nonmuscle invasion (NMIBC); 70% occurrence
  - Muscle invasion (MIBC); 25%
  - Metastatic disease (MIBC plus spread beyond the bladder); 5%

EPIDEMIOLOGY

Primarily white men aged >55 years who smoke tobacco

Incidence

- Estimated 4.2% of all new cancer cases; 83,190 new cases; and 16,840 deaths in United States for 2024
- Median age at diagnosis is 73 years.
- Two times more common in whites
- Male > female (3 to 4:1); but in smokers, risk is 1:1.
  - Fourth most common solid cancer in men and the 10th most common cause of cancer death in United States
  - Women are diagnosed in more advanced stages than men (hematuria mimicking gynecologic illnesses).
- 17.4/100,000 new US cases age-adjusted rate for 2021

Prevalence

In 2022, there were 744,039 cases in the United States; far exceeding population of Wyoming or Vermont

ETIOLOGY AND PATHOPHYSIOLOGY

Related but distinct in genetic alterations related to risk factors

- NMIBC, frequent chromosome 9 deletion and activation of RAS-MAPK pathway
- MIBC, dysfunction of tumor suppressors

Genetics

- Same sex, monozygotic twins have 10% increased BC risk.
- Patient with Lynch syndrome has up to 20% lifetime BC risk due to altered DNA mismatch repair genes.

RISK FACTORS

- Male
- Advanced age, primary risk factor, due to chronic exposure to risky substances
- Tobacco smoking is the key modifiable risk factor; 50% attribution
- Smokeless tobacco, secondhand tobacco smoke exposure or e-cigarettes
- Other risk factors:
  - Occupational exposures to benzidine; magenta, auramine dyes; aluminum and rubber production; certain paints, plastics, carbon black dust (printing ink), petroleum, diesel exhaust, and chimney soot
  - Arsenic or pesticide exposure in drinking water
  - History of bladder radiation, pelvic irradiation, or certain chemotherapy drugs like cyclophosphamide or ifosfamide
  - Chronic lower UTI or chronic indwelling urinary catheter
  - Pioglitazone (diabetes), aristolochic acid (herbal supplement), cyclophosphamide, and chlornaphazine

ALERT

Microscopic (≥3 RBC/high-power field) or gross hematuria found in a smoker needs cystoscopy and axial upper tract imaging, regardless of anticoagulation or antiplatelet status, unless there is a documented UTI with urgency and frequency that responds to UTI treatment or if related to a gynecologic or other nonmalignant genitourinary cause.

GENERAL PREVENTION

- Avoid tobacco exposure.
- https://www.cdc.gov/tobacco/quit_smoking/index.htm or 800-QUIT NOW (800-784-7669)
- Counseling of avoidance if risky occupational exposure
- Prompt follow-up for individuals with any hematuria, regardless of anticoagulation or anti-platelet status

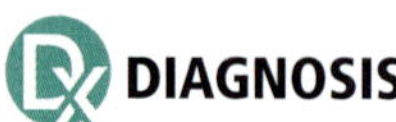

DIAGNOSIS

HISTORY

- Painless hematuria: most common symptom of BC
  - 4% BC risk with microhematuria; 16.5% BC risk with gross hematuria (1)[C]
- Urinary symptoms persisting (frequency, urgency, dysuria, decreased urine flow)
- Abdominal or pelvic pain in advanced BC

PHYSICAL EXAM

Normal in early cases; pelvic or abdominal mass in advanced disease; wasting in systemic disease

DIFFERENTIAL DIAGNOSIS

- UTI; nephrolithiasis
- Noninfectious hemorrhagic cystitis
- Urinary tract trauma; renal cell carcinoma
- Interstitial cystitis/nephritis
- Papillary urothelial hyperplasia
- Other urinary tract neoplasms

DIAGNOSTIC TESTS & INTERPRETATION

Core testing: urinalysis/microscopy, cystoscopy, upper tract imaging

Initial Tests (lab, imaging)

- Urinalysis with microscopy in patients with gross or microscopic hematuria or irritating urinary symptoms
- Cystoscopy and axial upper tract imaging in all hematuria, except in the presence of a benign cause or low-risk, asymptomatic, microhematuria patients with shared decision-making to repeat urinalysis with microscopy in 6 months
- Specific American Urology Association guideline (2020): work up even if microhematuria alone
- Endoscopic transurethral resection of bladder tumor (TURBT) is diagnostic for histologic grade, tumor depth, and possibly therapeutic. Repeat TURBT needed in 4 to 6 weeks if incomplete resection, in certain histologic stages, or if lamina propria and detrusor muscle are not sampled.
- Imaging:
  - Renal ultrasound may be used with low- and intermediate-risk microscopic hematuria patients.
  - Urogram (CT or MRI) if gross hematuria or high-risk microhematuria, or renal ultrasound or retrograde pyelogram (1)[C]
    - Because tumor invasion of detrusor muscle is poorly seen in regular CT urography, dual energy CT is recommended then.
  - T2-weighted and functional sequenced MRI views are most revealing if obtained before TURBT or at least 2 weeks after TURBT.
  - MRI without contrast can be used in special situations:
    - Severe renal dysfunction or severe contrast allergy
    - Detrusor muscle invasion seen poorly on CT, or if need to avoid radiation (2)[C]
- Urine cytology for gross hematuria or post-treatment follow-up is low in sensitivity (37%) but high in specificity (95%).
- Urine tumor markers are *not* accurate enough to replace cystoscopy.
- Enhanced cystoscopy, narrowband, or blue light types improve sensitivity and specificity in diagnosis and resection (1)[B].

Follow-Up Tests & Special Considerations

- Special case initial imaging: vesicle imaging-reporting and data system (VI-RADS) using multiparametric MRI
  - Sensitivity: 83–90%, specificity: 90–97% with level 3 as threshold likelihood of invasion of muscle wall
  - Diffusion-weighted and dynamic contrast-enhanced MRI and dual-energy spectral CT scan are options to diagnose end-stage bladder tumors (2)[C].
- Metastatic disease workup: chest x-ray or CT and abdomen/pelvis CT
  - If metastatic disease suspicion:
    - Liver function tests and alkaline phosphatase (AP) blood testing
    - Nuclear medicine bone scan if bone pain or if AP is elevated (1)[C].
    - Preferred imaging study for micrometastases in normal size lymph nodes: unknown (2)[C]
    - Immuno-oncologic biomarkers like programmed death-ligand 1 link may target specific treatment (2)[C].

Test Interpretation

- TURBT characterizes as superficial (NMIBC) or invasive (MIBC).
- Superficial cancer (70%)
  - Ta: noninvasive papillary carcinoma, low grade, tend to recur
  - Tis: carcinoma in situ (CIS); flat lesion, always high grade
  - T1: extends into submucosa, lamina propria; usually high grade

- Invasive cancer (30%), always high grade
  - T2: invasion into: muscle, superficial (pT2a); deep (pT2b)
  - T3: invasion into: perivesical fat, microscopic (pT3a); macroscopic (pT3b)
  - T4: invasion into adjacent organs
    - T4a: invades prostate, uterus, vagina, or bowel
    - T4b: invades abdominal wall, pelvic wall, or other organs
- N1–N3: invades lymph nodes
- M: metastasis to bone or soft tissue (1)[C]

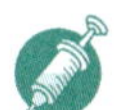

TREATMENT

- NMIBC, risk group:
  - Low:
    - Solitary Ta ≤3 cm diameter
      - Primary: TURBT: enhanced cystoscopy, in <24 hours single-dose chemotherapy (1)[B], reject adjuvant intravesical therapy, may fulgurate small lesions (1)[C]
  - Intermediate:
    - Recurrence <1 year, low-grade Ta, or solitary low-grade Ta >3 cm diameter, or multifocal low-grade Ta, or high-grade Ta ≤3 cm diameter, or low-grade T1
    - Primary: TURBT: enhanced cystoscopy; in T1, restage TURBT at 4 to 6 weeks, <24 hours single-dose chemotherapy, or consider induction intravesical therapy (chemotherapy or bacille Calmette-Guérin [BCG] (1)[B]), or do maintenance chemotherapy or BCG for 1 year in responders (1)[C]
    - Alternatives: If persistent or recurrent disease/cytology after intravesical therapy, do prostatic urethra and upper tract evaluation; or offer repeat induction course of BCG; or pembrolizumab in BCG-failure patients or offer clinical trial (1)[C].
  - High:
    - T1 high grade; or any high-grade recurrent Ta; or Ta >3 cm high-grade or multifocal; or any CIS; or any high-grade disease, BCG failure; or any variant histology;
      or any lymphovascular invasion (LVI); or any prostatic urethral involvement that is high grade
    - Primary: TURBT: enhanced cystoscopy (1)[B]; in high-grade Ta, restage TURBT at 4 to 6 weeks (1)[C], or in T1, restage TURBT at 4 to 6 weeks, or induction BCG, or in responders, maintenance BCG for 3 years (1)[B]
    - Alternatives: Consider radical cystectomy in high-grade T1 persistently or T1 with variant histology, LVI, or CIS; or recurrent or persistent disease after intravesical therapy do prostatic urethra evaluation; offer second BCG induction course; or if failed BCG, use pembrolizumab; or offer clinical trial (1)[C].
- MIBC, nonmetastatic: primary and alternative treatment
  - Cisplatin ineligible: initial radical cystectomy
  - Cisplatin eligible: neoadjuvant cisplatin-based chemotherapy (i.e., dose-dense methotrexate), vinblastine, doxorubicin, and cisplatin (ddMVAC) or gemcitabine plus cisplatin, then radical cystectomy or chemoradiation and concurrent maximal TURBT
  - If patient declines primary, alternative is partial cystectomy, or in ideal patients, maximal TURBT.
- MIBC, metastatic: primary and alternative treatment:
  - Cisplatin ineligible: If tumor expresses PD-L1 or patient is ineligible for any platin-based therapy, try atezolizumab/pembrolizumab; or if negative PD-L1, try combination carboplatin-based chemotherapy; or gemcitabine +/− paclitaxel; or ifosfamide, gemcitabine, doxorubicin
  - Cisplatin eligible: chemotherapy (gemcitabine + cisplatin vs. ddMVAC)
  - Alternative treatment:
    - Postplatinum failure: pembrolizumab (preferred); or atezolizumab versus nivolumab versus durvalumab versus avelumab; or erdafitinib
    - Postplatinum and checkpoint inhibitor immunotherapy failure: enfortumab vedotin (1)[C]

MEDICATION

See above listed treatment, by category

ISSUES FOR REFERRAL

Unexpected hematuria or delayed referral to urologist

ADDITIONAL THERAPIES

Radiosensitization in BCG-unresponsive NMIBC may help to preserve bladder (2)[C].

SURGERY/OTHER PROCEDURES

Surgery is definitive therapy:

- Superficial cancer: TURBT
- Invasive cancer: Radical cystectomy, full pelvic lymphadenectomy, and exenteration, plus urine diversion
- Meticulous lymph node dissection is prognostic, therapeutic, and essential in curative treatment (1)[B].

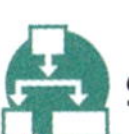

ONGOING CARE

FOLLOW-UP RECOMMENDATIONS

- NMIBC
  - Urine cytology alone has *not* been shown to be sufficient for follow-up.
  - Low risk: cystoscopy at 3 to 4 months, 6 to 9 months, and then yearly for 5 years; no upper tract imaging, no urinary biomarkers if normal cystoscopy
  - Intermediate/high risk: cystoscopy with cytology at 3 to 4 months, then each 3 to 6 or 4 months for 2 years, then each year or 6 months ongoing; upper tract imaging each 1 to 2 years; urinary biomarker use may indicate response to BCG or to resolve equivocal cytology.
- Follow-up for invasive cancers depends on the metastasis and approach to treatment but involves cystoscopy (if no cystectomy), urine cytology, advanced imaging urography or renal ultrasound in years 5 to 10, chest imaging (x-ray or CT), FDG PET/CT (if no metastasis), serum laboratory tests (1)[C].

Patient Monitoring

BCG patients require lifelong follow-up.

DIET

Continue adequate fluid intake.

PATIENT EDUCATION

- Smoking cessation, occupational exposures
- Cancer.NET: https://www.cancer.net/cancer-types/bladder-cancer

PROGNOSIS

- Death rates, 2016–2020, men 7.1, women 2 per 100,000 age adjusted to 2000 US standard population
- NMIBC
  - 5-year relapse-free survival at risk level: low, 43%; intermediate, 33%; high, 23%
  - 5-year progression-free survival at risk level: low, 93%; intermediate, 74%; high, 54%
  - BCG treatment decreases risk of recurrence and progression in high-risk superficial lesions (1)[B].
- MIBC and advanced BC
  - Nonmetastatic: 36–48% overall survival rate at 5 years
  - Metastatic disease: regional, 36%; distant, 5% relative survival rate at 5 years (1)[C]

COMPLICATIONS

Neobladder patients at risk for azotemia (absorption of ammonium chloride) and metabolic acidosis (bicarb loss) (1)[C]

REFERENCES

1. Lenis AT, Lec PM, Chamie K, et al. Bladder cancer: a review. *JAMA*. 2020;324(19):1980–1991.
2. Compérat E, Amin MB, Cathomas R, et al. Current best practice for bladder cancer: a narrative review of diagnostics and treatments. *Lancet*. 2022;400(10364):1712–1721.

ADDITIONAL READING

- Kumbham S, Rahman KMM, Foster BA, et al. A comprehensive review of current approaches in bladder cancer treatment. *ACS Pharmacol Transl Sci*. 2025;8:286–307.
- Lopez-Beltran A, Cookson MS, Guercio BJ, et al. Advances in diagnosis and treatment of bladder cancer. *BMJ*. 2024;384:e076743.

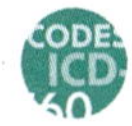

SEE ALSO

- Hematuria
- Algorithm: Hematuria

CODES

ICD10

- C67.8 Malignant neoplasm of overlapping sites of bladder
- C67 Malignant neoplasm of bladder
- C67.6 Malignant neoplasm of ureteric orifice

CLINICAL PEARLS

- Painless hematuria (when there is no benign explanation) must be evaluated with at least cystoscopy; regardless of anticoagulation or antiplatelet use.
- The U.S. Preventive Services Task Force does *not* recommend routine screening for BC.

BORDERLINE PERSONALITY DISORDER

Robert B. Bonanno, MD • Ellen Combs, MD

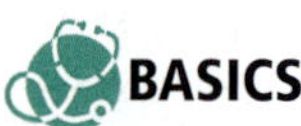

BASICS

DESCRIPTION

Borderline personality disorder (BPD) is a psychiatric disorder characterized by a consistent and pervasive pattern of emotional dysregulation including: distorted sense of self, rapidly labile mood, impulsive behaviors (including suicidality or self-injury), fear of abandonment, and volatile or chaotic interpersonal relationships. It is often manifested during adolescence but is typically diagnosed in early adulthood. It is considered a cluster B personality type.

EPIDEMIOLOGY

Onset during adolescence or early adulthood; however, may go undiagnosed for years

- More common among women in clinical settings (1)[C]
- Severity of symptoms often remits over time

Prevalence

- 0.7–2.7% lifetime prevalence in the United States (1)[C],(2)[C]
- 6% of primary care population
- 10–18% in outpatient psychiatric practices
- 9–25% of inpatient psychiatric milieu

ETIOLOGY AND PATHOPHYSIOLOGY

Undetermined but generally accepted that BPD is multifactorial in etiology including (1)[C]:

- Environmental factors (i.e., history of childhood sexual and/or physical abuse, history of childhood neglect, ongoing conflict in home, maladaptive parenting styles, socioeconomic status, parental substance use)
- Neuroimaging studies have shown hyperactivity of the amygdala, decreased prefrontal cortex activation, and decreased brain volumes/white matter connectivity in frontal and limbic structures.
- Dysregulation of various neurotransmitter systems, including serotonin, oxytocin, and endogenous opiates, may also play a role.

Genetics

Estimated heritability of BPD is 40%

RISK FACTORS

- Childhood trauma (e.g., sexual and/or physical abuse and neglect)
- Lack of secure parental attachment beginning in early childhood, family adversity, maternal psychopathology
- Low socioeconomic status or parental substance abuse

COMMONLY ASSOCIATED CONDITIONS

High rate of associated comorbid psychiatric disorders such as depression, anxiety, bipolar, chronic pain, obesity, and substance use disorders (SUDs) (1)[C]

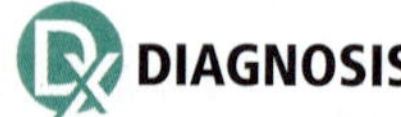

DIAGNOSIS

HISTORY

- Obtain collateral information (i.e., from family, partner) about patient behaviors
- History of interpersonal difficulties, affective instability, and impulsivity
- History of self-injurious behavior, possibly with suicidal threats or attempts
- History of substance use

PHYSICAL EXAM

- Perform a physical exam and consider laboratory workup as indicated.
- Consider laboratory evaluation if personality changes due to a physiologic etiology from a medical condition.
- Physical exam may show signs of self-mutilation such as cutting or burning.

DIFFERENTIAL DIAGNOSIS

- Mood disorders:
  - Screen for or differentiate between bipolar, anxiety, and depressive disorders as well as PTSD.
- Psychotic disorders:
  - Though auditory and visual hallucinations may be present (1)[C], they typically are in the context of situational crises and are not accompanied by disordered thoughts, bizarre delusions, flat affect, or other negative symptoms.
- Attention deficit hyperactivity disorder (ADHD)
- Other medical conditions (autoimmune, endocrine, traumatic/structural, infectious)
- SUD

DIAGNOSTIC TESTS & INTERPRETATION

- Diagnosis requires a comprehensive psychiatric evaluation including structured interviews within which the clinician may consider using specific assessment tools to aid in diagnosis, such as the Revised Diagnostic Interview of Borderlines or the Structured Clinical Interview for the DSM-5 Alternative Model for Personality Disorders (2)[C].
- The McLean Screening instrument for BPD may be used as a screening tool if BPD is suspected (2)[C].

Initial Tests (lab, imaging)

Individualized based on level of suspicion for other general medical conditions (autoimmune, endocrine, traumatic/structural, infectious)

Follow-Up Tests & Special Considerations

Referral for comprehensive psychological testing may be considered if diagnosis is uncertain or confounded by other conditions.

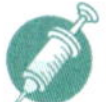

TREATMENT

- Dialectical behavioral therapy (DBT) psychotherapy for BPD appears to be the most established treatment, although other psychotherapy modalities have shown some benefit (2)[C]:
  - DBT combines cognitive behavioral techniques for emotional regulation and processes including distress tolerance, acceptance, and self-awareness.
- Other empirically supported treatments to consider include transference-focused (psychodynamic) psychotherapy, mentalization-based therapy, and schema-focused therapy.

GENERAL MEASURES

Focus on patient management rather than on "fixing" behaviors:

- Schedule consistent appointment follow-ups to alleviate patient anxiety.
- Use team-based communication to mitigate "splitting" behaviors by patient.
- Set appropriate boundaries for communication and expectations between the provider and patient: use motivational interviewing and problem-solving techniques.
- Medications may aid in symptom management if comorbid conditions are present.

MEDICATION

- No specific medications are approved by the FDA to treat BPD; limited evidence exists for symptom management with second-generation antipsychotics, mood stabilizers and omega-3 fatty acids (2)[C].
- Consider risk of self-harm and suicidal behavior when prescribing.

ADMISSION, INPATIENT, AND NURSING CONSIDERATIONS

- Hospitalizations should be limited and of short duration to adjust medications, implement psychotherapy for crisis intervention, and stabilize patients from psychosocial stressors.
- Inpatient hospitalization should be considered for the following reasons:
  - Persistent/severe suicidal ideation, self-harm or risk to others
  - Comorbid substance use and/or nonadherence to outpatient or partial hospitalization treatments
  - Severe comorbid disorders (i.e., eating disorders, mood disorders, psychosis)

ONGOING CARE

FOLLOW-UP RECOMMENDATIONS

- Schedule visits that are short, more frequent, and focused to relieve patients' anxiety about relationships with their physician/provider and to help reduce risk of provider burnout.
- Emphasize importance of healthy lifestyle modifications (i.e., exercise, rest, sleep, nutrition, stress management).

Patient Monitoring

Monitor for suicidal ideation/behaviors or other self-harm behaviors.

PATIENT EDUCATION

Include patients in the treatment plan so that they are aware of their behavior and its impact.

PROGNOSIS

Symptom severity often remits over time.

REFERENCES

1. American Psychiatric Association. *Diagnostic and Statistical Manual of Mental Disorders*. 5th ed., text rev. Arlington, VA: American Psychiatric Association; 2022.
2. Mendez-Miller M, Naccarato J, Radico JA. Borderline personality disorder. *Am Fam Physician*. 2022;105(2):156–161.

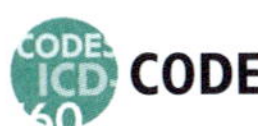

CODES

ICD10

F60.3 Borderline personality disorder

CLINICAL PEARLS

- BPD is a chronic condition with one of the characteristic features being mood dysregulation in which individuals react out of proportion to stressors, often stemming from a lack of self-identity and a feeling of emptiness.
- Clear boundaries should be established with the treatment team.
- Psychotherapy (such as DBT) is first-line treatment while pharmacotherapy has only limited evidence of benefit.

BRAIN INJURY, TRAUMATIC

Gabryel A. Obedoza, MD • Faiz Bayo-Awoyemi, MD

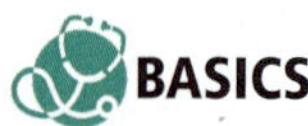

BASICS

DESCRIPTION

- Traumatic brain injury (TBI) is defined as an alteration in brain function caused by an external force.
- Mild TBI (mTBI) is defined by Glasgow Coma Scale (GCS) score 13 to 15 and short-lived neurologic symptoms (loss of consciousness [LOC], posttraumatic amnesia, altered mental status [AMS], or transient neurologic deficit).
- System(s) affected: neurologic; psychiatric; cardiovascular; endocrine/metabolic; gastrointestinal; pulmonary
- Synonym(s): head injury, concussion

EPIDEMIOLOGY

Incidence

- Majority (>70%) of TBIs are mild.
- 2.87 million ED visits with 288,000 hospitalizations per year in the United States
- 56,000 TBI-related deaths per year; ~43% of patients who survive will experience long-term disabilities.
- Young children (ages 0 to 4) and older adults (≥75 years old) have highest incidence (1).

ETIOLOGY AND PATHOPHYSIOLOGY

- Centers for Disease Control and Prevention (CDC) TBI data in 2017, mechanism of injury of hospitalized patients (male vs. female percentage)
  - Unintentional falls (35.6 vs. 23.9)
  - Motor vehicle crashes (22.5 vs. 10.8)
  - Unintentionally being struck by or against an object (2.3 vs. 0.9)
  - Intentional self-harm (0.8 vs. 0.3)
  - Assault (7.5 vs. 1.7)
  - Children 0 to 17 years
    - Falls (7.7)
    - Motor vehicle crashes (6.8)
- Contact sports account for 45% of TBI emergency room visits for children related to sports and recreation.
- Mechanical damage with actuation of complex cellular and molecular cascades that promote cerebral edema, ischemia, and apoptotic cell death

RISK FACTORS

Alcohol and drug use, prior/recurrent head injury, contact sports, seizure disorder

Geriatric Considerations

Subdural hematomas (SDHs) are common after a fall or blow in elderly; symptoms may be subtle and not present until days after trauma.

GENERAL PREVENTION

- Safety education and fall prevention
- Seat belts; bicycle and motorcycle helmets
- Banning certain types of contact in sports that carry increased risk of concussion

Geriatric Considerations

Learning about individual fall risk can help prevent injuries resulting in TBI for adults ≥75 years old.

Pediatric Considerations

- Incidence is high in children age 0 to 4 due to falls and developing motor skills. Risk also increases in adolescence due to sports and motor vehicle accidents.
- Child abuse: Consider if dropped or fell <4 feet (e.g., off bed, couch), suspicious history, significant injury present, injury inconsistent with developmental age (e.g., rolling off bed in an infant), or any retinal hemorrhages.

DIAGNOSIS

HISTORY

- LOC, headache, vomiting, amnesia, confusion, "brain fog," dizziness, sensitivity to light, mood disturbances, irritability, sleep disturbances (2)
- Epidural hemorrhage from blunt trauma: 30% with a "lucid interval" (initial LOC followed by recovery of consciousness and then LOC recurs and persists)

PHYSICAL EXAM

- Neurologic and cognitive testing is important.
- For mTBI: neurologic exam (cranial nerves, motor strength), balance testing, cognition/memory, vestibulo-ocular reflex (VOR) testing (3)
- For severe brain injury: Repeat neurologic exams every 30 minutes until 2 hours after GCS reaches 15, then hourly for 4 hours, and then every 2 hours.
- Evidence of increased intracranial pressure (ICP) (elevated BP, decreased pulse rate, or slow/irregular breathing [Cushing triad]—only 30% have all three)
- Signs of basilar skull fracture: raccoon eyes, Battle sign, hemotympanum, CSF rhinorrhea or otorrhea

DIFFERENTIAL DIAGNOSIS

Other causes of AMS (e.g., toxicologic, infectious, metabolic, vascular)

DIAGNOSTIC TESTS & INTERPRETATION

Initial Tests (lab, imaging)

- mTBI and concussions cognitive screening tests
- Evaluate for coagulopathy.
- Perform drug and alcohol screening.
- Noncontrasted head CT is the study of choice to review bone windows, tissue windows, and subdural space if indicated.

Pediatric Considerations

- Can use Pediatric Emergency Care Applied Research Network (PECARN) criteria to assess if mechanism of injury or symptoms are severe enough to warrant head CT.
- Skull radiographs are not indicated unless abuse is suspected, in which case they can detect fractures not seen under CT.

Follow-Up Tests & Special Considerations

For mTBI, reassess symptoms and repeat exam every 1 to 2 weeks until symptom-free and able to return to sport/activity without issue.

Pediatric Considerations

Stepwise return to activity after initial 24 to 48 hours of complete cognitive rest; return to school activities should precede return to sport/physical activity.

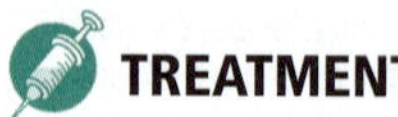

TREATMENT

GENERAL MEASURES

Acute management depends on injury severity. Most patients need no interventions.

- Immediate goal: Determine who needs further therapy, imaging studies (CT), and hospitalization to prevent further injury.
- For the mildly injured patient
  - Early education is beneficial for recovery.
  - Graduated return to cognitive and physical activity when there are no evident signs or symptoms (physical, cognitive, emotional, or behavioral) on neuropsychologic and clinical evaluation.
- For the moderate to severely injured patient
  - Avoid hypotension or hypoxia. Head injury causes increased ICP secondary to edema, and cerebral perfusion pressure (CPP) should be maintained between 60 and 70 mm Hg (4)[A].
  - 30-degree head elevation decreases ICP and improves CPP.
  - Hyperventilation (hypocapnia) for patients with impending herniation while preparing for definitive treatment or intraoperatively
  - Mild systematic hypothermia lowers ICP but leads to increased rates of pneumonia.
  - 3% hypertonic saline and mannitol effectively reduce ICP.
- Seizure prophylaxis with phenytoin or levetiracetam for 1 week postinjury or longer for patients with early seizures, dural-penetrating injuries, multiple contusions, and/or SDHs requiring evacuation

MEDICATION

First Line

- Individuals with severe brain injuries who can't communicate, may benefit from using the Nociception Coma Scale (NCS) to assess pain.
- Increased ICP
- Hypertonic saline: 2 mL/kg IV decreases ICP without adverse hemodynamic status; preferred agent
- Mannitol: 0.25 to 2.0 g/kg (0.25 to 1.0 g/kg in children) given over 30 to 60 minutes in patients with adequate renal function. Prophylactic use is associated with worse outcomes.
- Sedation
  - Propofol: preferred due to short duration of action; avoid high doses to prevent propofol infusion syndrome. When combined with morphine, it can also effectively decrease ICP and decrease use of other medications.
  - Midazolam: similar sedating effect to propofol but may cause hypotension

- Seizures
  - Phenytoin (Dilantin): 15 mg/kg IV (1 mg/kg/min IV, not to exceed 50 mg/min); stop infusion if QT interval increases by >50%.
- Headaches and sleep disturbance
  - Tricyclic antidepressants such as amitriptyline are often used with variable efficacy.
- Mood disturbances
  - Selective serotonin reuptake inhibitors (SSRIs) are commonly used for post-injury depression and mood symptoms.

ALERT
Avoid corticosteroid use because it increases mortality rates and risk of developing late seizures.

ISSUES FOR REFERRAL
- Consult neurology if symptoms are persistent for >4 weeks or if worsening symptoms.
- Consult neurosurgery for penetrating head trauma, abnormal head CT that meet brain injury guidelines (BIG)-3 criteria as below.

ADDITIONAL THERAPIES
Cognitive rehabilitation therapy and physical therapy

SURGERY/OTHER PROCEDURES
- Early evacuation of trauma-related intracranial hematoma decreases mortality especially with GCS <6 and CT evidence of hematoma, cerebral swelling, or herniation.
- CSF drainage reduces ICP but has not been demonstrated to have long-term benefit.
- CSF leakage often resolves in 24 hours with bed rest, but if not, may require surgical repair.

COMPLEMENTARY & ALTERNATIVE MEDICINE
Music therapy in conjunction with multimodal stimulation improves awareness in comatose TBI patients.

ADMISSION, INPATIENT, AND NURSING CONSIDERATIONS
TBI severity can be defined by the BIG as BIG-1, BIG-2, or BIG-3. Criteria and therapeutic plan listed below: (5)

- BIG-1:
  - Normal neurologic exam
  - Not intoxicated
  - Any of the following non-contrast head CT findings: SDH <4 mm, epidural hematoma (EDH) <4 mm, intraparenchymal hemorrhage (IPH) <4 mm in one location, traced subarachnoid hematoma (SAH), no intraventricular hemorrhage (IVH)
  - No skull fracture
  - Negative history of anticoagulation or antiplatelet use
  - Repeat neurologic physical exam check every 2 to 4 hours.
  - Observation for 6 hours, only repeat non-contrast head CT for neurologic changes, otherwise no need for repeat head CT.
  - Can be discharged if neurologic exam at baseline after 6 hour observation
  - Neurosurgical consultation not required.
- BIG-2:
  - Normal neurologic exam
  - Any of the following non-contrast head CT findings: SDH 5 to 7 mm, EDH 5 to 7 mm, IPH 3 to 7 mm in two locations, localized SAH, no IVH
  - Non-displaced skull fracture
  - Negative history of anticoagulation or antiplatelet use
  - Repeat neurologic exam every 2 hours.
  - Inpatient admission required.
  - Only repeat non-contrast head CT for neurologic changes, otherwise no need for repeat head CT.
  - Neurosurgical consultation not required.
- BIG-3:
  - Abnormal neurologic exam.
  - Any of the following non-contrast head CT findings: SDH >8 mm, EDH >8 mm, IPH >8 mm in multiple locations, scattered SAH, presence of IVH.
  - Displaced skull fracture
  - Positive history of anticoagulation or antiplatelet use
  - Repeat neurologic exam hourly.
  - Inpatient admission required, consider ICU admission.
  - Neurosurgery consult required.
- C-spine immobilization should be considered in all head trauma.
- Use normal saline for resuscitation fluid.

ONGOING CARE

FOLLOW-UP RECOMMENDATIONS
- Schedule regular follow-up within a week to determine return to activities.
- Rehabilitation indicated following a significant acute injury. Set realistic goals.
- For patients on anticoagulants, net benefit to restarting therapy after discharge despite increased bleeding risk.
- Screen for depression and PTSD after TBI as the prevalence of these conditions are higher in those with history of TBI.

PATIENT EDUCATION
Patient should be discharged to the care of a competent adult with clear instructions on signs and symptoms that warrant immediate evaluation (e.g., changing mental status, worsening headache, focal findings, or any signs of distress). Patients should be monitored but not awakened from sleep.

PROGNOSIS
- Gradual improvement may continue for years.
- Mortality rate for TBI is 30 per 100,000 annually in the United States.
- Poor prognostic factors: low GCS on admission, nonreactive pupils, old age, comorbidity, midline shift, nonambulatory
- 50% of patients with mTBI will return to work by 1 month after injury, and >80 by 6 months.
- Past history of mood disorders, ADHD, and/or learning disorder may increase risk of post-concussive symptoms or contribute to prolonged recovery in mTBI.

COMPLICATIONS
- Chronic SDH, which may follow even "mild" head injury, especially in the elderly; often presents with headache and decreased mentation
- Seizures: incidence of late seizures after TBI, >30 years is 2% for mild injuries, 4% for moderate injuries, and >15% for severe injuries.

REFERENCES

1. Haarbauer-Krupa J, Pugh MJ, Prager EM, et al. Epidemiology of chronic effects of traumatic brain injury. *J Neurotrauma*. 2021;38(23):3235–3247.
2. Patricios JS, Schneider KJ, Dvorak J, et al. Consensus statement on concussion in sport: the 6th International Conference on Concussion in Sport–Amsterdam, October 2022. *Br J Sports Med*. 2023;57:695–711.
3. Haider MN, Leddy JJ, Du W, et al. Practical management: brief physical examination for sport-related concussion in the outpatient setting. *Clin J Sport Med*. 2020;30(5):513–517.
4. Tsang KK, Whitfield PC. Traumatic brain injury: review of current management strategies. *Br J Oral Maxillofac Surg*. 2012;50(4):298–308.
5. Joseph B, Obaid O, Dultz L, et al; for AAST BIG Multi-institutional Study Group. Validating the brain injury guidelines: results of an American Association for the Surgery of Trauma prospective multi-institutional trial. *J Trauma Acute Care Surg*. 2022;93(2):157–165. doi:10.1097/TA.0000000000003554.

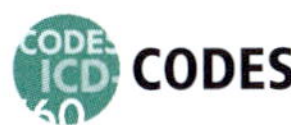

CODES

ICD10
- S06.9X0A Unsp intracranial injury w/o loss of consciousness, init
- S06.5X0A Traum subdr hem w/o loss of consciousness, init
- S06.6X0A Traum subrac hem w/o loss of consciousness, init

CLINICAL PEARLS

- TBI involves two distinct phases: the primary mechanical insult and secondary dysregulation of the cerebrovascular system with cerebral edema, ischemia, and cell-mediated death.
- Indications for imaging include evidence of skull fracture, altered consciousness, neurologic deficit, persistent vomiting, scalp hematoma, abnormal behavior, coagulopathy, age >65 years.
- Treatment should be tailored to individual's symptoms and severity and treatment often includes combining pharmacologic and nonpharmacologic regimens.

BREAST ABSCESS

Kelley V. Lawrence, MD, NABBLM-C • Puja Dalal, MD, FAAFP • Keyona Oni, MD, IBCLC

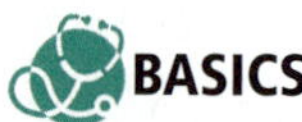

BASICS

DESCRIPTION

- Breast abscess: localized accumulation of infected fluid within the breast parenchyma
- Mastitis: breast inflammation with or without infection. This can be associated with lactation (puerperal) or nonlactational.
- Associated with lactation or fistulous tracts secondary to squamous epithelial neoplasm or duct occlusion
- System(s) affected: skin/exocrine, immune
- Synonym(s): mammary abscess; peripheral breast abscess; subareolar abscess; puerperal abscess

Pregnancy Considerations

Most commonly associated with postpartum lactation.

EPIDEMIOLOGY

- Most common benign breast problem during pregnancy and puerperal period
- Predominantly reproductive age and perimenopausal (between ages 18 and 50 years)
  - Puerperal abscess: lactational
  - Subareolar abscess: reproductive age through postmenopause:
    - 90% of nonlactational breast abscesses are subareolar.
- Predominant sex: female
- Higher incidence associated with diabetes, smoking, and obesity

Incidence

Ranges between 3% and 11% of women with mastitis

Prevalence

Transient condition usually as a complication of mastitis; mastitis prevalence ranges between 1% and 10% (1).

ETIOLOGY AND PATHOPHYSIOLOGY

- Puerperal abscesses:
  - Associated with hyperlactation and dysbiosis (disrupted milk microbiome); these can lead to ductal narrowing and inflammation and subsequently to reduced milk flow, obstruction, plugged lactiferous duct causing stasis, microbial growth, and infection.
  - Mammary dysbiosis is a consequence of multiple factors including genetic, breastfeeding related, medical, and microbial
    - Likely that bacteria (often from infants oral flora) gain entry through cracks/fissures in the nipple
    - Insufficient treatment of mastitis
    - Unattended postpartum engorgement and other situations leading to breast milk stasis
- Subareolar abscess:
  - Associated with squamous metaplasia of the lactiferous duct epithelium, keratin plugs, ductal ectasia, and fistula formation
- Microbiology
  - *Staphylococcus aureus* is the most common cause for lactational abscesses.
  - Methicillin-resistant *S. aureus* (MRSA) is a significant cause.
  - Other common causes include coagulase-negative *Staphylococcus* and Streptococcus species.
  - Less common causes:
    - *Escherichia coli*, Enterobacteriaceae, *Corynebacterium*, and *Pseudomonas*
    - Anaerobes
    - Polymicrobial

Genetics

Maternal genetics may play a role as protective and predisposing factors for mammary dysbiosis which is associated with the pathophysiology.

RISK FACTORS

- Smoking, maternal age >30
- Primiparous, pregnancy ≥41 weeks' gestation
- Diabetes
- Obesity
- Nipple piercing
- Milk stasis:
  - Infrequent or missed feeds
  - Poor latch, weak or uncoordinated suckling
  - Damage or irritation of the nipple, nipple inversion or retraction
  - Inefficient removal of milk (by baby or pump)
  - Oversupply of milk
  - Illness in mother or baby
  - Rapid weaning
  - Plugged duct(s)
  - Pressure on the breast (i.e., tight bra, car seatbelt)
- Medically related risk factors:
  - Steroids (oral or topical)
  - Breast implants
  - Lumpectomy with radiation
  - Inadequate antibiotics to treat mastitis
  - Topical antifungal medication used for nipple pain/infection

GENERAL PREVENTION

- Frequent movement of milk with on-demand feeding and/or pumping to prevent mastitis
- Early treatment of mastitis with movement of milk on a regular basis, reduction in inflammation (with use of ice and/or NSAIDs), pain control (with acetaminophen) and antibiotics (if indicated)
- Smoking cessation to minimize occurrence/recurrence

COMMONLY ASSOCIATED CONDITIONS

Lactation, mastitis, weaning

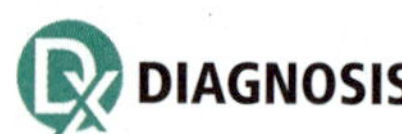

DIAGNOSIS

HISTORY

- Tender breast lump, usually unilateral
- Breastfeeding, weaning, or returning to work
- Recent or recurrent mastitis
- Systemic malaise (usually less than with mastitis)
- Localized erythema, warmth, edema, pain
- Fever, nausea, vomiting
- Prior breast infection
- Decreased breast milk supply on affected breast
- Spontaneous nipple drainage
- Diabetes
- Smoking
- Perimenopausal/postmenopausal

PHYSICAL EXAM

- Fever, tachycardia (not always present)
- Erythema or hyperpigmentation of overlying skin
- Palpable mass, sometimes fluctuant
- Tenderness on palpation
- Induration
- Local edema
- Draining pus or skin ulceration
- Nipple and/or skin retraction
- Regional lymphadenopathy
- Puerperal abscesses are generally peripheral; nonlactational abscesses are more commonly found in periareolar/subareolar region.

DIFFERENTIAL DIAGNOSIS

- Engorgement
- Plugged milk duct
- Mastitis
- Galactocele (sometimes referred to as a milk lake)
- Fibrocystic breasts
- Fat necrosis
- Tuberculosis (potentially associated with HIV infection)
- Sarcoid
- Granulomatous mastitis
- Syphilis
- Foreign body reactions (e.g., to silicone and paraffin)
- Mammary duct ectasia
- Carcinoma (inflammatory or primary squamous cell)

DIAGNOSTIC TESTS & INTERPRETATION

Initial Tests (lab, imaging)

- US helps distinguish abscess from mastitis.
- Elevated WBC, elevated ESR
- Culture of expressed breast milk or aspirate to identify pathogen
  - The presence of pathogenic bacteria or high bacteria count (e.g., $> 10^3$/mL) indicates mastitis; low predictive value, clinical context is needed.

Follow-Up Tests & Special Considerations

Mammogram to rule out malignancy; with US and biopsy ordered when indicated

Diagnostic Procedures/Other

- Aspiration (+/− US guided) for culture
  - Can be diagnostic and therapeutic
  - Does not exclude malignancy
  - Cytology (particularly in nonlactating patient)
- Mammography has limited value in the acute assessment of mastitis.
- Point-of-care ultrasound (POCUS) emerging as helpful for diagnosis and management of breast abscess in the outpatient setting

Test Interpretation

- Abscesses on US can be hypoechoic, well-circumscribed, and/or macrolobulated
  - If US is negative for pocket of fluid, consider alternative diagnoses.
  - If multiloculated on imaging, refer to breast surgical/interventional specialist.
- Use culture sensitivities to guide antibiotic therapy when possible.

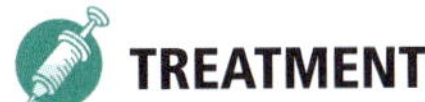

TREATMENT

GENERAL MEASURES

- Cold and/or warm compresses for pain control (2)[A]
- Continue to move milk (via direct feeding or pumping) to drain the affected breast (2)[A].
- US-guided needle aspiration to drain abscess; without drainage, antibiotics are ineffective (2)[A],(3)[A].
  - Acceptable to start antibiotics while working to get patient to drainage/aspiration

MEDICATION

First Line

- Continuation of movement of milk on a regular basis (2)[A]
- Drainage for source control and culture; adjust antibiotics if indicated based on culture and sensitivities (3)[A].
- First line for nonsevere and no MRSA risk factors (2)[A]:
  - Dicloxacillin or flucloxacillin 500 mg QID for 10 to 14 days
  - Cephalexin 500 mg QID for 10 to 14 days
- If risk factors for MRSA, including past MRSA infection, recent hospitalization (for something other than delivery) in the last 12 months, antibiotic use in the last 6 months, or severe β-lactam hypersensitivity (2)[A]:
  - Clindamycin 300 to 450 mg PO TID, 10 to 14 days
  - Trimethoprim-sulfamethoxazole (TMP-SMZ) 1 to 2 tabs PO BID, 10 to 14 days

Second Line

- Clindamycin 300 mg 4 times daily for 10 to 14 days (2)[A]
- TMP-SMZ DS BID for 10 to 14 (2)[A]
  - Not recommended for mothers of children with G6PD deficiency; use with caution in mothers with premature infants or infants with hyperbilirubinemia, especially <30 days old.
- Consult infectious disease specialist if inadequate response to antibiotic treatment plus drainage.

ISSUES FOR REFERRAL

If showing signs of hemodynamic instability, patient should be referred for inpatient stabilization and care (rare).

ADDITIONAL THERAPIES

- NSAIDs for analgesia, anti-inflammatory effect, and/or antipyresis (2)[A]
- Rest, adequate fluid intake, good nutrition (2)[A]
- Application of heat to the breast just prior to feeding/milk expression may help with adequate milk flow (2)[A].
- Cold packs applied after a feeding/milk expression can reduce pain and edema (2)[A].

SURGERY/OTHER PROCEDURES

- Current best practice recommendation suggests:
  - Aspiration (using 18- to 21-gauge needle) with or without US guidance for abscesses <3 cm (1)[A],(3)[A] (Serial aspirations may be necessary.)
    - US-guided aspiration of breast abscess is preferred to incision and drainage (I&D) in most cases due to better cosmesis and faster recovery.
  - Consider US-guided percutaneous catheter placement if abscess is >3 cm (3)[A].
  - Consider I&D using a no. 15 blade scalpel if abscess is >5 cm, recurrent, or chronic (3)[A].
- Biopsy nonpuerperal abscesses to rule out malignancy; remove all fistulous tracts in nonlactating patients as well (3)[A].

COMPLEMENTARY & ALTERNATIVE MEDICINE

- Lecithin supplementation (to support milk flow as an emulsifying agent)
- Probiotics (to support microbiome)
- Acupuncture (may help with breast engorgement and prevention of breast abscess)
- Breast lymphatic massage (may ease engorgement)
- Judicious use of cabbage leaves applied over affected area (to decrease inflammation and milk production)

ADMISSION, INPATIENT, AND NURSING CONSIDERATIONS

- Outpatient, unless systemically immunocompromised, septic, or requiring inpatient antibiotic treatment
- Hospital-grade breast pump should be made available to patient from time of admission.

ONGOING CARE

- If lactating, continue effective milk movement to prevent recurrence.
- If planning to wean from breastfeeding, avoid abrupt discontinuation of feeding.
- Recommend smoking cessation to decrease risk of nonlactational abscess recurrence.

FOLLOW-UP RECOMMENDATIONS

Patient Monitoring

- Ensure complete resolution to exclude malignancy.
- Close outpatient follow-up until resolution as abscesses may require serial aspirations or drainage

DIET

No dietary patterns have been associated with breast abscess formation; however, these can affect the microbiome (2)[A].

PATIENT EDUCATION

- Wound care, rest, breast milk movement
- Continue with breastfeeding or pumping to prevent engorgement.

PROGNOSIS

- Drained abscess heals from inside out (in 8 to 10 days)
- Subareolar abscesses frequently recur, even after I&D and antibiotics; may require surgical removal of ducts

COMPLICATIONS

- Fistula: mammary duct or milk fistula
- Poor cosmetic outcome
- Early cessation of breastfeeding

REFERENCES

1. Louis-Jacques AF, Berwick M, Mitchell KB. Risk factors, symptoms, and treatment of lactational mastitis. *JAMA*. 2023;329(7):588–589.
2. Mitchell KB, Johnson HM, Rodríguez JM, et al; and the Academy of Breastfeeding Medicine. Academy of Breastfeeding Medicine Clinical Protocol #36: the mastitis spectrum, revised 2022. *Breastfeed Med*. 2022;17(5):360–376.
3. Pileri P, Sartani A, Mazzocco MI, et al. Management of breast abscess during breastfeeding. *Int J Environ Res Public Health*. 2022;19(9):5762.

ADDITIONAL READING

Zhou F, Li Z, Liu L, et al. The effectiveness of needle aspiration versus traditional incision and drainage in the treatment of breast abscess: a meta-analysis. *Ann Med*. 2023;55(1):2224045. doi:10.1080/07853890.2023.2224045.

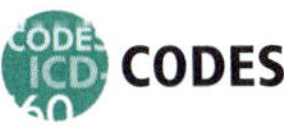

CODES

ICD10

- N61 Inflammatory disorders of breast
- O91.13 Abscess of breast associated with lactation
- O91.12 Abscess of breast associated with the puerperium

CLINICAL PEARLS

- Up to 11% of cases of puerperal mastitis progress to abscess formation (most often due to inadequate therapy).
- Risk factors for mastitis and breast abscess include a combination of genetic, microbial, breastfeeding, and medical factors.
- Treat abscesses not associated with lactation with antibiotics that cover anaerobic bacteria and work up for malignancy.
- The treatment of choice for most breast abscesses is the combination of antibiotics plus aspiration.
- US-guided aspiration of breast abscess is preferred to I&D in most cases due to better cosmesis and faster recovery.
- If abscess is <5 cm, surgical I&D is recommended.
- If lactating, continue to move milk (feeding on-demand and/or pumping at regular intervals).

BREAST CANCER

Ravjot Kaur Virdi, DO, MPH • Sigrun Hallmeyer, MD, FACCC

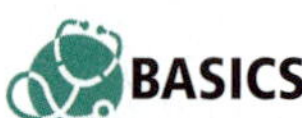

BASICS

DESCRIPTION

- Breast cancer is a malignant neoplasm of breast epithelial, glandular, or stromal cells.
- Histologic subtypes
  - Noninvasive
    - Ductal carcinoma in situ: confined to ducts; may show mammographic microcalcifications; high risk for ipsilateral invasive carcinoma
    - Lobular carcinoma in situ: confined to terminal ductal lobular units; low risk for ipsilateral/contralateral invasive carcinoma
  - Invasive
    - Invasive ductal carcinoma: 70–80% of cases; unilateral; cords/nests of cells
    - Invasive lobular carcinoma: 8% of cases; bilateral 20% of the time; single-file stromal infiltration
    - Inflammatory breast cancer: rare; dermal lymphatic invasion; peau d'orange
  - Paget disease: rare; nipple/areolar involvement; red/scaly rash, pruritus, ulceration, nipple retraction, discharge
- Molecular subtypes (receptor-defined)
  - Hormone receptor positive (HR+): estrogen receptor (ER) and/or progesterone receptor (PR)
  - Human epidermal growth factor receptor 2 (HER2) status is determined by immunohistochemistry (IHC) and confirmed by fluorescence in situ hybridization (FISH):
    - Negative (0): no HER2 expression (IHC 0, FISH−)
    - Ultralow: minimal expression (IHC ≤10% faint staining, FISH−)
    - Low: low expression (IHC 1+ or 2+, FISH−)
    - Positive: overexpression (IHC 3+ or 2+ with FISH+)
  - No ER, PR, HER2 expression (triple negative)

EPIDEMIOLOGY

Incidence

- 2018 to 2022: U.S. incidence was 130.8/100,000 women/year.
- Median age: 63 years
- Rates increased by 0.6%/year from 2013 to 2022
- Highest rates in North America, Australia/New Zealand, Western/Northern Europe

Prevalence

- Most diagnosed cancer worldwide
- Second most common malignancy in women after non-melanoma skin cancers
- ~4 million U.S. women lived with breast cancer in 2022.
- Lifetime risk for women (2018 to 2021) is ~13%.
- 15.5% of all new cancer cases in the United States

ETIOLOGY AND PATHOPHYSIOLOGY

- Etiology: increased hormone exposure, genetic mutations, lifestyle/environmental factors
- Arises from uncontrolled proliferation of mammary epithelial cells, starting as ductal/lobular carcinoma in situ, progressing to invasive carcinoma with stromal infiltration, and spreading via lymphatics/blood to distant sites

Genetics

- 5–10% of breast cancers are hereditary.
- Tumor suppressor genes:
  - BRCA1 and BRCA2: autosomal dominant DNA repair defects; seen in male breast cancer
  - Other: TP53, PTEN, CHEK2, PALB2
- Oncogenes: HER2 receptor expression, PIK3CA and ESR1 mutations

RISK FACTORS

- Characteristics: female sex, age >65 years, postmenopausal, dense breasts, obesity
- Genetic: BRCA or other mutations, first-degree relative with breast cancer
- Prolonged estrogen exposure: early menarche, late menopause, nulliparity, late first pregnancy, lack of breastfeeding, hormone replacement therapy, oral contraceptives
- Lifestyle/environmental: alcohol, smoking, high-fat diet, prior chest radiation

GENERAL PREVENTION

- Early detection in average-risk women: biennial mammogram from age 40 to 74 per U.S. Preventative Services Task Force (1)
- Family history: screening 10 years before earliest family diagnosis (but not before age 30 years)
- High-risk women (≥20% lifetime risk): annual MRI + mammogram starting age 30 years
- Transgender individuals
  - Trans men: no screening after bilateral mastectomy; otherwise, follow cisgender guidelines.
  - Trans women: if ≥5 years of hormone therapy, screen as cisgender women; if <5 years, screening based on risk factors
- Risk-reducing interventions for BRCA or other high risk gene carriers:
  - Prophylactic bilateral mastectomy ± salpingo-oophorectomy
  - Chemoprevention (5 year duration):
    - Premenopausal and age ≥35 years: selective ER modulator (tamoxifen)
    - Postmenopausal: selective ER modulators (tamoxifen, raloxifene) or aromatase inhibitors (anastrozole, letrozole, exemestane)

COMMONLY ASSOCIATED CONDITIONS

Breast, ovarian, prostate, and pancreatic cancer in BRCA+ patients

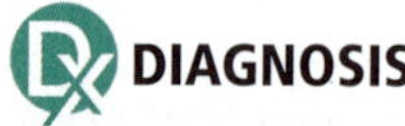

DIAGNOSIS

HISTORY

Personal/family cancer history, tobacco/alcohol use, hormonal/reproductive history, prior chest radiation, prior abnormal mammogram/need for biopsy, history of atypia, and breast symptoms

PHYSICAL EXAM

- Hard, palpable mass embedded in breast tissue
- Axillary/supraclavicular adenopathy
- Skin erythema, thickening, peau d'orange, nipple retraction
- Metastatic signs: bone pain, liver pain/jaundice, dyspnea, or cough weight loss

DIFFERENTIAL DIAGNOSIS

- Benign conditions: cellulitis, mastitis, abscess, fat necrosis, fibroadenoma, cysts, fibrocystic changes
- Other malignant conditions: breast lymphoma, metastasis to breast

DIAGNOSTIC TESTS & INTERPRETATION

Initial Tests (lab, imaging)

- Initial imaging (1):
  - Age <30 years: ultrasound (US) ± mammogram
  - Age ≥30 years: diagnostic mammogram + US
- Imaging reports use breast imaging reporting and data system (BI-RADS): 0 = incomplete imaging; 1 = negative; 2 = benign; 3 = likely benign (≤2% risk); 4 = consider biopsy; 5 = highly concerning (≥95% risk); 6 = biopsy-proved cancer

Follow-Up Tests & Special Considerations

Biopsy all suspicious lesions

- Preferred: image-guided core needle biopsy
- Alternatives: excisional or punch biopsy, fine-needle aspiration
- Indeterminate results → surgical excision

Diagnostic Procedures/Other

- Receptor testing: ER, PR, HER2
- Axillary staging: sentinel lymph node biopsy or axillary lymph node dissection
- Distant metastasis workup: labs (CBC, CMP, alkaline phosphatase); consider CT, MRI, PET-CT, and bone scan.

Test Interpretation

American Joint Committee for Cancer tumor-node-metastasis criteria for staging considers primary tumor size, lymph node involvement, and distant metastasis.

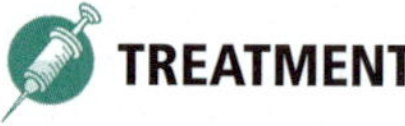

TREATMENT

GENERAL MEASURES

- Systemic therapy may impair fertility → refer to fertility specialists.
- Premenopausal patients need contraception counseling.

MEDICATION

Therapy guided by tumor characteristics

- HR+: endocrine therapy ± chemotherapy
- HER2+: targeted therapy + chemotherapy
- Triple negative: chemotherapy

First Line

- Chemotherapy (2):
  - Anthracyclines (doxorubicin, epirubicin):
    - Contraindications: cardiac disease, high cumulative dose
    - Adverse effects: cardiotoxicity, myelosuppression, alopecia
  - Taxanes (paclitaxel, docetaxel):
    - Contraindications: hypersensitivity
    - Adverse effects: neuropathy, neutropenia
  - Alkylating agents (cyclophosphamide, carboplatin):
    - Contraindications: severe bone marrow suppression, hypersensitivity
    - Adverse effects: cyclophosphamide (hemorrhagic cystitis, infertility, secondary malignancies); carboplatin (nephrotoxicity, ototoxicity)
- Endocrine therapy:
  - Premenopausal: tamoxifen *or* ovarian suppression (gonadotropin-releasing hormone [GnRH] agonist) + aromatase inhibitor
  - Postmenopausal: tamoxifen *or* aromatase inhibitor
    - Contraindications: tamoxifen (thromboembolism history, endometrial cancer); aromatase inhibitors (osteoporosis)
    - Adverse effects: tamoxifen (thromboembolism, endometrial cancer, hot flashes); aromatase inhibitors (bone loss)
- CKD4/6 inhibitors (palbociclib, ribociclib, abemaciclib): combined with endocrine therapy in HR+ advanced disease and approved for high-risk early disease and/or advanced/metastatic disease
  - Contraindications: severe infection, baseline cytopenias
  - Adverse effects: fatigue, diarrhea, alopecia, pancytopenia
- HER2-targeted therapy (trastuzumab, pertuzumab):
  - Contraindications: preexisting cardiomyopathy, reduced ejection fraction
  - Adverse effects: dilated cardiomyopathy, infusion reactions
- Poly ADP ribose polymerase (PARP) inhibitors (olaparib, talazoparib): used adjuvantly for high-risk, early-stage BRCA+ cancer and first line in BRCA+ metastatic disease
  - Contraindications: pregnancy, severe marrow suppression
  - Adverse effects: myelosuppression, diarrhea

Second Line

- Immunotherapy (pembrolizumab): used neoadjuvantly for triple negative cancer regardless of PD-L1 status (2)
- Antibody-drug conjugates:
  - Ado-trastuzumab, trastuzumab deruxtecan: for HER2+ refractory disease
  - Sacituzumab govitecan: for triple negative cancer refractory to two prior systemic therapies

ISSUES FOR REFERRAL

Multidisciplinary team: medical oncology, breast surgeon, radiation oncology, geneticist, plastic surgery, fertility specialist, physical/occupational therapy

ADDITIONAL THERAPIES

Radiation: adjuvant or palliative therapy

- Common sites: partial/whole breast, locoregional nodes, chest wall

SURGERY/OTHER PROCEDURES

Breast-conserving surgery, mastectomy, breast reconstruction

COMPLEMENTARY & ALTERNATIVE MEDICINE

- Integrative medicine: Meditation/yoga, acupuncture, massage, nutrition, and exercise improve quality of life, reduce stress, and help manage side effects.
- Psychosocial: support groups and counseling improve coping

ADMISSION, INPATIENT, AND NURSING CONSIDERATIONS

- Admission criteria:
  - Poor social support/hospice needs
  - Unstable vitals, uncontrolled pain
  - Severe lab/radiology abnormalities (cytopenias, hypercalcemia, liver failure, cord compression)
  - Severe treatment toxicities
- Inpatient care: stabilize; empiric antibiotics (sepsis), corticosteroids (cord/brain mets), denosumab (hypercalcemia), procedures (thoracentesis)
- Nursing: Monitor vitals/neurologic status; manage symptoms, medications, and adherence.
- Discharge: instructions on medications, red-flag symptoms, follow-ups

ONGOING CARE

FOLLOW-UP RECOMMENDATIONS

Patient Monitoring

- Exam every 3 to 6 months × 3 years, then every 6 to 12 months × 2 years, then annually
- Labs: not recommended in asymptomatic survivors
- Mammograms per screening guidelines
- Annual pelvic exam if receiving tamoxifen
- Bone density scans if taking aromatase inhibitor

DIET

- No breast cancer-specific guidelines
- Mediterranean diet linked to lower recurrence and mortality

PATIENT EDUCATION

- Self-monitoring: regular breast/chest wall exams
- Recurrence prevention: Adhere to endocrine therapy, maintain healthy lifestyle, and keep up with screenings.

PROGNOSIS

- Worse outcomes with advanced aged, black race.
- Poorer prognosis with HR−, HER2+, or triple negative tumors
- 2019 to 2023 death rate in the United States: 19.2/100,000 women/year
- 5-year relative survival: 91.7%
- Median age at death: 71 years

COMPLICATIONS

- Metastatic spread: bone, lung, liver, brain
- 40% of cases reoccur
- 7–11% of patient develop malignant pleural effusions
- Surgical: lymphedema; long thoracic nerve injury

REFERENCES

1. Cadet MJ, Ajay G, Drago CI, et al. Understanding recommendations from various breast cancer screening guidelines. *J Nurse Pract*. 2025;21(1):105238. doi:10.1016/j.nurpra.2024.105238.
2. Sukhun SA, Temin S, Barrios CH, et al. Systemic treatment of patients with metastatic breast cancer: ASCO resource—stratified guideline. *JCO Global Oncol*. 2024;10:e2300285. doi:10.1200/GO.23.00285.

ADDITIONAL READING

National Cancer Institute. Cancer Stat Facts: Female Breast Cancer. Surveillance, Epidemiology, and End Results Program. National Institute of Health. https://seer.cancer.gov/statfacts/html/breast.html. Accessed October 24, 2025.

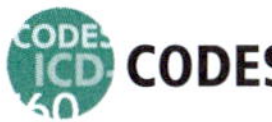

CODES

ICD10

- C50.52 Malignant neoplasm of lower-outer quadrant of breast, male
- C50.929 Malignant neoplasm of unspecified site of unspecified male breast
- C50.812 Malignant neoplasm of overlapping sites of left female breast

CLINICAL PEARLS

- Mammography is the cornerstone of early detection.
- Key risk factors include family history, BRCA mutations, estrogen exposure, and prior chest radiation.
- Clinical signs include palpable masses, nipple changes, and peau d'orange.
- HR+ tumors respond to endocrine therapy, HER2+ to targeted agents, while triple-negative cancers rely on chemotherapy/immunotherapy.
- Long-term follow-up includes regular exams, mammography of intact breasts, and lifestyle guidance. Optimal care requires coordination among a multidisciplinary team.

BREASTFEEDING

Angelia Leipelt, BA, IBCLC, IBD, ICCE • Ronald G. Chambers Jr., MD, FAAFP

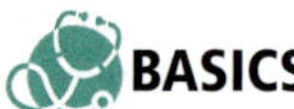

BASICS

- Breast/chest feeding is the natural process of feeding human milk directly from the breast.
- Breast milk is the preferred nutritional source and the normal and physiologic way to feed all newborns and infants.
- Breast milk contains over 200 active components which provide nutrition, fight pathogens, promote healthy gut microbiome, and aid in maturity of immune system.
- The American Academy of Pediatrics (AAP), the American Academy of Family Physicians (AAFP), and the American Congress of Obstetricians and Gynecologists (ACOG) recommend exclusive breastfeeding for 6 months, with continuation of breastfeeding for ≥2 year as desired by birth parent and infant (1).

DESCRIPTION

- Maternal benefits (as compared with those who do not breast/chest feed) include the following:
  - Rapid involution/decreased postpartum bleeding
  - Decreased risk of postpartum depression and increased bonding
  - Postpartum weight loss
  - Decreased risk of breast cancer and association of decreased risk of pre- and postmenopausal ovarian cancer (2), decreased risk of type 2 diabetes, hypertension, hyperlipidemia, rheumatoid arthritis, and cardiovascular disease
  - Decreased risk of prematurity
  - Increased bone density
- Infant benefits include the following:
  - Ideal food: easily digestible, nutrients well absorbed, less constipation
  - Lower rates of virtually all infections via maternal antibody protection
    - Fewer respiratory and GI infections
    - Decreased risk of ear infections, bacterial meningitis, pneumonia, and sepsis
    - Decreased incidence of otitis media and necrotizing enterocolitis
  - Decreased incidence of obesity and type 1 and 2 diabetes
  - Decreased incidence of allergies, clinical asthma, and atopic dermatitis in childhood
  - Decreased risk of developing celiac disease and inflammatory bowel disease
  - Decreased risk of childhood leukemia
  - Decreased risk of sudden infant death syndrome (SIDS)
  - Enhanced neurodevelopmental performance including intelligence (3)
  - Increased attachment between birth parent and baby

EPIDEMIOLOGY

Incidence

- According to CDC's Breastfeeding Scorecard, U.S. breastfeeding rates are on the rise in 2022: any breastfeeding: 83.2% (however, differs among different sociodemographic and culture)
- Breastfeeding at 6 months: 55.8%
- Breastfeeding at 12 months: 35.9%
- Exclusive breastfeeding at 3 months: 45.3%
- Exclusive breastfeeding at 6 months: 24.9%

ETIOLOGY AND PATHOPHYSIOLOGY

- The mechanism of milk production is based on several hormones: Prolactin triggers milk production and oxytocin releases milk based on supply and demand. Endocrine control system triggers making of colostrum at 5 months' gestation.
- Alveoli make milk in response to hormone prolactin. Sucking stimulates secretion of prolactin, which triggers milk production.
- Stimulation of areola causes secretion of oxytocin. Oxytocin is responsible for let-down reflex when myoepithelial cells contract and milk is ejected into milk ducts.
- Endocrine/metabolic: Cystic fibrosis, diabetes, galactosemia, phenylketonuria, and thyroid dysfunction may cause delayed lactation or decreased milk.

GENERAL PREVENTION

Most vaccinations can be given to breastfeeding mothers, including COVID-19 immunization. The CDC recommends that the diphtheria-tetanus-acellular pertussis, hepatitis B, inactivated influenza virus (as opposed to live attenuated), measles-mumps-rubella (MMR), and inactivated polio and varicella vaccines can be given. The CDC recommends avoiding the yellow fever or smallpox vaccine in breastfeeding mothers.

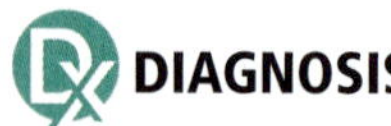

DIAGNOSIS

PHYSICAL EXAM

Breast/chest examination during pregnancy; assess for scars, lumps, or flat/inverted nipples. Confirm history of infertility, endocrine disorders, breast and hormonal pathology, overall health and psychosocial concerns, perinatal complications, and previous breastfeeding problems.

ALERT

A breast lump should be followed to complete resolution or worked up if present and not just attributed to changes from lactation.

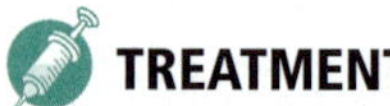

TREATMENT

GENERAL MEASURES

Breast/chest feeding initiation

- Initiate breast/chest feeding immediately after birth, ideally placing the infant naked on birth parent's chest uninterrupted skin-to-skin *in first hour.*
- As baby opens wide, bring baby close, tucking baby in "belly to belly." Line baby's nose to nipple, baby tilts its head back with wide open mouth, bring baby close as baby latches to ensure baby's gum takes in more of the areola.
- Baby's lips are flanged, rounded cheeks, no clicking or popping sounds, and absence of nipple pain when latched.
- Feed baby 2 to 8 times for the first 24 hours and 8 or more times per 24 hours, feeding 10 or more minutes.
- Observation of a nursing session by an International Board Certified Lactation Consultant (IBCLC), nurse, or experienced physician
- Avoid supplementation with infant formula or water and/or artificial nipples unless medically indicated.
- Contraindications to breastfeeding are few (WHO).
  - Maternal HIV (in industrialized world) or human T-cell leukemia virus (HTLV) infection
  - Active untreated tuberculosis
  - Active herpes simplex virus (HSV) lesions on the breast
  - Substances of abuse without evaluation and discontinuation of use
  - Review medications that will pass into human milk.
  - Infants with galactosemia or maple syrup urine disease should not be fed with breast milk. Infants with phenylketonuria may be fed breast milk under close observation.
  - Mothers who develop varicella 5 days before through 2 days after delivery
  - Suspected or confirmed Ebola virus disease
  - Maternal hepatitis is *not* a contraindication.

ISSUES FOR REFERRAL

- Refer to IBCLC, experienced nurser, or physician for inpatient and/or outpatient teaching.
- Frequent follow-up if having problems with latching, nipple/breast pain, breast infection, overactive let down, oversupply or inadequate milk production
- Appropriate screening/referral for postpartum depression as related to unresolved pain with breastfeeding.

COMPLEMENTARY & ALTERNATIVE MEDICINE

Galactagogues

- Metoclopramide, domperidone, fenugreek, goat's rue, and milk thistle have mixed results in improving milk production, but efficacy and safety data are lacking in literature.

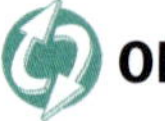

ONGOING CARE

FOLLOW-UP RECOMMENDATIONS

See mother and baby within 48 to 72 hours after hospital discharge, especially if first time breastfeeding.

- Risk factors for suboptimal initiation
  - Breast surgery or reduction surgery prior to pregnancy may disrupt breast milk production.
  - Severe postpartum hemorrhage may lead to Sheehan syndrome associated with difficulty breastfeeding due to poor milk production.
  - Other factors: delivery mode, duration of labor, gestational age, maternal infection, parity, culture, birth parent–infant separation, maternal anxiety, maternal depression, use of artificial nipple or use of non–breast milk fluids

Patient Monitoring

- Monitor maternal breast milk supply concerns.
- Monitor infant's weight, behavior, and output closely.
- Supplementation with pumped milk and/or infant formula if infant has lost ≥10% of birth weight.
- Supplementation without persistent breast stimulation, frequent feedings, or breast pump use will decrease milk production and decrease breastfeeding success.

B

DIET

- For chestfeeding/breastfeeding
  - Healthy choices from protein-rich foods, vegetables, fruits, and whole grains. Drink plenty of fluids to satisfy thirst and optimal hydration.
  - Breastfeeding/chestfeeding parent may require ~500 more calories per day.
  - Limit caffeine to <300 mg/day.
  - Alcohol should be avoided. Possible long-term effects of alcohol in maternal milk remain unknown.
- For infants:
  - In 2008, the AAP increased its recommended daily intake of vitamin D for infants from 200 to 400 IU. For exclusively breastfed babies, this will require taking a vitamin supplement, such as Poly-Vi-Sol or Vi-Daylin vitamin drops, 0.5 mL/day, beginning in the first few days of life.
  - In 2010, the AAP recommended adding supplementation for breastfed infants with oral iron 1 mg/kg/day beginning at age 4 months. Preterm infants fed by human milk should receive an iron supplement of 2 mg/kg/day by 1 month of age, and this should be continued until the infant is weaned to iron-fortified formula or begins eating complementary foods that supply the 2 mg/kg of iron.

PATIENT EDUCATION

- Support measures to normalize breast/chest feeding have been shown to be successful with respect to infant/child and maternal health outcomes.
  - Emphasize importance of exclusive breast/chest feeding for the first 6 weeks of life to allow adequate buildup of sufficient milk supply.
  - Regular promotion of the advantages of breast/chest feeding and risks of not breastfeeding
- Breast milk usually transitions to mature milk about 3 to 5 days postpartum.
- Signs of adequate nursing
  - Baby feeding on demand (8 to 12 feedings per 24 hours by day 2)
  - Baby should have 6 to 8 wet diapers per day and 3 to 4 bowel movements per day by day 6 to 8.
  - Proper latching and positioning
  - Baby satisfied; appropriate weight gain (average of 1 oz/day in first few months)
- Weaning
  - Solid food may be introduced at 4 months with continuation of breastfeeding.
  - Breast/chest-feeding parent returning to work/school should begin alternative feeding methods 1 to 2 weeks prior. Initiate breast pumping plan.
- Family planning
  - Options include lactational amenorrhea method (LAM), barrier methods, implants, medroxyprogesterone (Depo-Provera), oral contraception, and intrauterine devices (IUDs). ACOG recommends that progesterone-only pills be used 2 to 3 weeks postpartum and that medroxyprogesterone (Depo-Provera), IUDs, combined OCPs, and etonogestrel implant (Nexplanon) can used between 2 and 28 days postpartum can protect against pregnancy.
  - Monitor for changes in milk supply after starting a contraceptive.

COMPLICATIONS

- Breast milk jaundice should be considered if jaundice persists for >1 week in an otherwise healthy, well-hydrated newborn. It peaks at 10 to 14 days.
- Plugged duct
  - Mother is well except for sore lump in one or both breasts and is without fever. Use moist, cold compress or ice pack on lump prior to, and during, nursing; more frequent nursing on affected side. Avoid excessive pumping on affected breast.
- Mastitis (see "Mastitis")
  - Sore lump in one or both breasts plus maternal fever and/or redness on skin overlying lump
  - Use cold compress or ice pack on lump prior to nursing to reduce pain and inflammation.
  - Antibiotics covering for *Staphylococcus aureus* (most common organism)
  - Other possible sources of fever should be ruled out, that is, endometritis and pyelonephritis.
  - Mother should get increased rest; use acetaminophen (Tylenol) PRN.
  - Fever should resolve within 48 hours or consider changing antibiotics. Lump should resolve. If it continues, an abscess may be present, requiring surgical drainage.
- Milk supply inadequate
  - Review health concerns; breast changes; infant weight loss; signs of adequate supply; technique, feeding frequency, and duration of nursing; use of lactation aids during feeding or additional supplementation with non-breast milk fluids.
- Sore nipples
  - Check positioning techniques and improve latch-on.
  - Baby should be taken off the breast by breaking the suction with a finger in the mouth.
  - Check for signs of thrush in baby and on mother's nipple. If affected, treat both.
  - Check for evidence of ankyloglossia (tongue tie) in the infant. Correction of ankyloglossia may lead to decreased nipple soreness and improved breastfeeding.
  - Nipple bleb (a blister on the nipple that can be filled with serous fluid or another fluid) due to improper positioning; cold compress or ice pack and improve position/latch techniques.
- Flat or inverted nipples
  - When stimulated, inverted nipples will retract inward; flat nipples remain flat; check for this on initial prenatal physical. Assess latch if using nipple shield to aid in latching and review rationale for use with breastfeeding.
- Engorgement
  - Begins 3 to 5 days after birth and subsides within 12 to 48 hours
  - Signs are warm, hard, sore breasts.
    - Frequent nursing; breastfeed long enough to empty breasts.
    - Pump to relieve discomfort.
    - Explore reasons for ongoing problems.

REFERENCES

1. Johnston M, Landers S, Noble L, et al. Breastfeeding and the use of human milk. *Pediatrics*. Revised 2012;129(3): e827–e841.
2. World Health Organization. Breastfeeding. https://www.who.int/health-topics/breastfeeding. Accessed October 15, 2024.
3. U.S. Department of Health and Human Services. *The Surgeon general's Call to Action to Support Breastfeeding.* Washington, DC: U.S. Department of Health and Human Services, Office of the Surgeon General; 2011.

ADDITIONAL READING

- American Academy of Pediatrics, American College of Obstetricians and Gynecologists. *Breastfeeding Handbook for Physicians.* 3rd ed. Elk Grove Village, IL: American Academy of Pediatrics; 2023.
- Mitchell KB, Johnson HM, Rodríguez JM, et al; for Academy of Breastfeeding Medicine. Academy of Breastfeeding Medicine clinical protocol #36: the mastitis spectrum, revised 2022. *Breastfeed Med*. 2022;17(5):360–376.

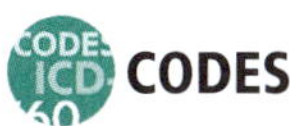

CODES

ICD10

Z39.1 Encounter for care and examination of lactating mother

CLINICAL PEARLS

- Support systems improve duration of breastfeeding.
- Almost all can breast/chest feed with accurate information, support from family, the health care system, and society at large.
- Breast milk is the optimal food for infants, with myriad health benefits for the chest/breastfeeder and for the child being fed.

BRONCHIECTASIS

Sarah J. Wu, MD • Scott Kopec, MD

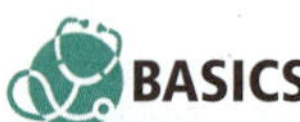

BASICS

DESCRIPTION

Bronchiectasis is an irreversible syndrome with symptoms of chronic productive cough, recurrent exacerbations, and characteristic findings on cross-sectional imaging of bronchial wall dilation and thickening.

EPIDEMIOLOGY

Incidence

Incidence of bronchiectasis is estimated to be 200 cases per 100,000 in the United States and is increasing.

Prevalence

Overall estimated prevalence of bronchiectasis in the United States is 701 per 100,000 (1).

ETIOLOGY AND PATHOPHYSIOLOGY

- Bronchiectasis often arises as a complication of inherited or acquired disease states but may arise as an isolated diagnosis.
- Vicious cycle hypothesis (1):
  - An initial pulmonary insult causes airway inflammation, dysfunction, and structural disease.
  - Dysfunctional airways are further impaired in their ability to clear infections.
  - A pattern of lung damage/inflammation and progressive airway dysfunction is established, leading to clinical decline.
- Neutrophil extracellular traps (NETs) levels and neutrophil elastase activity correlate with disease activity and may serve as potential therapeutic targets (1).

Genetics

There is no single genetic locus or condition that gives rise directly to bronchiectasis. It is, however, associated with multiple inheritable conditions, as detailed below. Bronchiectasis is commonly divided into cystic fibrosis (CF)-associated bronchiectasis and non-CF bronchiectasis.

RISK FACTORS

- Severe lower respiratory tract infection
- Tuberculosis (TB), non-TB mycobacterium, pertussis, and viruses, including adenovirus and measles
- Certain systemic diseases such as connective tissue diseases and inflammatory bowel disease

GENERAL PREVENTION

- Routine immunization against respiratory infections (pertussis, measles, *Haemophilus influenzae* type B, influenza, and *Streptococcus* pneumonia)
- Genetic counseling for patients with inheritable conditions which predispose to bronchiectasis who wish to conceive
- Encourage and support smoking cessation in all patients who smoke.

COMMONLY ASSOCIATED CONDITIONS

- Many cases are idiopathic, and bronchiectasis may be an isolated pulmonary diagnosis.
- Acquired conditions associated with bronchiectasis include recurrent lower respiratory tract infections (bacterial pneumonia, TB, allergic bronchopulmonary aspergillosis [ABPA]), GERD, conditions of airflow obstruction (asthma/chronic obstructive pulmonary disease [COPD], obstructing airway mass), connective tissue disorders, and chronic aspiration.
- Inherited conditions associated with bronchiectasis include CF, primary ciliary dyskinesia, congenital airway abnormalities (tracheobronchomalacia, tracheobronchomegaly, familial congenital bronchiectasis [Williams-Campbell syndrome]), α_1-antitrypsin deficiency, and primary immunodeficient conditions (X-linked agammaglobulinemia, common variable immune deficiency, hyper-IgE syndrome).

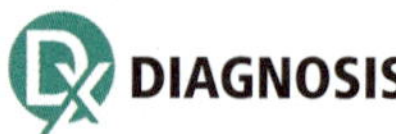

DIAGNOSIS

HISTORY

- Symptoms are commonly present for many years and include cough, sputum production, dyspnea, fatigue, rhinosinusitis, anorexia, and >1 lower respiratory tract infection a year requiring antibiotic therapy.
- Patients often report a history of recurrent exacerbations of symptoms, defined as a deterioration in ≥3 of the following symptoms for at least 48 hours *and* if a clinician determines that a change in treatment is needed (2): cough, sputum volume/consistency/purulence, breathlessness or exercise intolerance, fatigue or malaise for at least 48 hours, and/or hemoptysis.

PHYSICAL EXAM

Basal, coarse rales, and wheezing may be present.

DIFFERENTIAL DIAGNOSIS

Differential diagnosis primarily consists of other causes of chronic cough (e.g., COPD, asthma, chronic rhinosinusitis, lung cancer, GERD).

DIAGNOSTIC TESTS & INTERPRETATION

Initial Tests (lab, imaging)

For patients in which bronchiectasis is expected, consider ordering the following studies (2):

- Pulmonary function testing to detect chronic obstructive or restrictive lung disease
  - Normal or obstructive pattern on spirometry is most commonly seen in bronchiectasis.
- Chest x-ray is used primarily to evaluate for alternative or comorbid diagnoses: In moderate to severe disease, chest radiographs may show atelectasis, dilated airways, and/or peripheral opacifications.
- Computed tomography (CT) with slice thickness ≤1 mm is the test of choice to diagnosis bronchiectasis.
- Sputum sample for bacterial, mycobacterial, and fungal culture

Follow-Up Tests & Special Considerations

- In addition to sputum culture, current guidelines suggest that all patients with confirmed bronchiectasis should also undergo workup with CBC with differential, quantitative serum immunoglobulins, and ABPA testing (skin prick testing, Aspergillus-specific IgE antibodies) (2).
- Children with suspected bronchiectasis are recommended to also undergo testing for possible CF and primary ciliary dyskinesia (3).
- Consider testing for co-infectious such as TB and HIV.

Diagnostic Procedures/Other

Bronchoscopy and bronchioalveolar lavage may have a role in facilitating airway clearance and diagnosing underlying infectious organisms during an acute exacerbation but is not routinely used during diagnosis (4).

Test Interpretation

- CT chest findings suggesting bronchial dilation are required to diagnose bronchiectasis (≥1 of the following) (1):
  - Bronchoarterial ratio >1 (inner or outer airway diameter to adjacent pulmonary artery)
  - Lack of tapering of the airways
  - Radiographically visible airways in the perimeter within 1 cm of costal pleural surface or touching mediastinal pleura
- Other CT chest findings commonly associated with bronchiectasis may include mucus plugging, bronchial wall thickening, "tree in bud" nodularity, and mosaic perfusion.
- Location of disease may suggest but not prove etiology (1).
  - Predominantly upper lobe disease is seen in CF-associated bronchiectasis.
  - Centrally located disease is common in ABPA.
  - Right middle lobe disease is associated with nontuberculous mycobacterial (NTM) infection.

TREATMENT

- In adults, existing guidelines recommend stepwise treatment based on severity (2):
  - Step 1 (initial treatment):
    - Treat the underlying cause.
    - Educate on airway clearance techniques and consider referral for pulmonary rehabilitation.
    - Recommend pneumococcal polysaccharide vaccine and annual influenza vaccination.
    - Create a self-management plan with patients.
  - Step 2 (if ≥3 exacerbations per year despite adherence to step 1):
    - Evaluate adequacy of physiotherapy.
    - Consider trial of mucolytics in appropriate patients (notable difficulties with sputum expectoration).
    - Ensure patient is referred to a specialist team if not already followed.
  - Step 3 (if ≥3 exacerbations per year despite adherence to step 2):
    - Initiate long-term antibiotics (≥6 to 12 weeks) based on review of sputum cultures.
    - Initiate long-term (≥3 months) inhaled antibiotics if sputum culture is positive for *Pseudomonas aeruginosa*.
    - Combined therapy if lack of response *or* move on to step 4
  - Step 4 (if ≥3 exacerbations per year despite adherence to step 3):
    - Long-term macrolide therapy
    - If sputum is positive for non-TB mycobacteria, avoid macrolide monotherapy as this can give rise to macrolide-resistant mycobacteria.
  - Step 5 (if ≥3 exacerbations per year despite adherence to step 4): IV antibiotics every 2 to 3 months should be considered.

- At all stages, obtain sputum cultures and treat exacerbations with prompt administration of empiric antibiotics: Recommended duration of antibiotics is 14 days (2).
- Different guidelines exist for treatment of bronchiectasis in children/adolescents.
  - All patients should be seen by a pediatric chest physiotherapist for education on airway clearance techniques.
  - Exacerbations of bronchiectasis should be treated with a 14-day course of appropriate antibiotics.
  - Eradication therapy should be considered for children/adolescents with a new detection of *P. aeruginosa*.
  - Children/adolescents with ≥3 exacerbations per year should receive long-term macrolides.
  - Inhaled hypertonic saline should not be used routinely, only in selected patients with high daily symptoms and frequent exacerbations.

GENERAL MEASURES

- Examples of airway clearance techniques include forced expiration (Huff cough), chest physical therapy (postural drainage, hand or mechanical chest clapping), positive expiratory pressure (PEP) devices, oscillatory PEP devices, and high-frequency chest wall oscillation (HFCWO).
- Examples of mucolytics recommended for non-CF bronchiectasis include nebulized hypertonic saline. Inhaled mannitol and *N*-acetylcysteine have not been shown to have clinical benefit in non-CF bronchiectasis.

MEDICATION

First Line

- First-line antibiotics are selected based on sputum microbiology (2).
- Duration of antibiotics for treatment of exacerbations is 14 days (2).
- Eradication therapy should be considered for patients with new sputum isolation of *P. aeruginosa* (2). Eradication: oral fluoroquinolone for 2 weeks followed by inhaled antibiotics for a total duration of 3 months

Second Line

Long-acting bronchodilators, systemic steroids, and surgical interventions should not be standard treatment for all patients and should be offered on a case-by-case basis (2).

ISSUES FOR REFERRAL

Indications for specialty referral include the following (2):

- ≥3 exacerbations per year
- Positive sputum cultures for *P. aeruginosa*, MRSA, or NTM; or diagnosis or ABPA
- Patients on long-term antibiotics (≥3 months)
- Rapidly deteriorating condition (or other indication for lung transplantation)

ADDITIONAL THERAPIES

- Mucoactive medications, such as nebulizer hypertonic saline, can be considered in patients who have difficulty with sputum expectoration despite airway clearance techniques (2).
- Long-acting bronchodilators may benefit some patients with significant breathlessness.
- Pulmonary rehabilitation should be considered for patients with symptomatic breathlessness.
- Support/encourage optimization of nutrition, exercise, and psychological support.

SURGERY/OTHER PROCEDURES

- Patients with localized bronchiectasis and frequent exacerbations despite adequate treatment may benefit from surgery.
- Lung transplantation may be indicated in patients experiencing rapidly progressive deterioration.
- Patients with refractory issues with sputum expectoration may benefit from bronchial aspiration or bronchial wash.

COMPLEMENTARY & ALTERNATIVE MEDICINE

Yoga may have a positive effect on dyspnea and quality of life, and alternative Eastern methods such as acupuncture and herbal medicines have also been studied. However, these treatments currently do not have the strength of quality of evidence to be included in guidelines on the management of bronchiectasis.

ADMISSION, INPATIENT, AND NURSING CONSIDERATIONS

Factors which may prompt inpatient admission for treatment of bronchiectasis may include need for supplemental oxygen or other vital sign instability, need for IV medications, or outpatient treatment failure.

ONGOING CARE

FOLLOW-UP RECOMMENDATIONS

Children and adults with CF and non–CF-related bronchiectasis should be treated by comprehensive interdisciplinary chronic disease management programs.

Patient Monitoring

See patients in clinic at least every 3 to 6 months for the following:

- Assess adherence to respiratory physiotherapy/pulmonary rehabilitation regimen and consider re-referral if additional education is required.
- Routine monitoring of sputum cultures every 6 to 12 months
- Consideration of repeat testing (i.e., pulmonary function testing, CT imaging) based on individual clinical factors
- Consideration of adjunctive therapies (i.e., mucolytics, bronchodilators)

DIET

There is no diet specific to treating bronchiectasis. Dietary recommendations should also be tailored to any coexisting conditions, such as CF or inflammatory bowel disease.

PATIENT EDUCATION

Bronchiectasis, American Lung Association: https://www.lung.org/lung-health-diseases/lung-disease-lookup/bronchiectasis

PROGNOSIS

- Validated symptoms severity scores can be used to aid in determination of short- and long-term prognosis.
  - Bronchiectasis Severity Index: https://bronchiectasis.com.au/assessment/medical/bronchiectasis-severity-index
  - FACED Score: https://bronchiectasis.com.au/assessment/medical/faced-score
- *Pseudomonas* infection, low body mass index, and advanced age are associated with poorer prognosis.

COMPLICATIONS

Hemoptysis, pneumothorax, sepsis, lung abscesses, pulmonary hypertension, cor pulmonale

REFERENCES

1. O'Donnell AE. Bronchiectasis—a clinical review. *N Engl J Med*. 2022;387(6):533–545.
2. Polverino E, Goeminne PC, McDonnell MJ, et al. European Respiratory Society guidelines for the management of adult bronchiectasis. *Eur Respir J*. 2017;50(3):1700629. doi:10.1183/13993003.00629-2017.
3. Chang AB, Fortescue R, Grimwood K, et al. European Respiratory Society guidelines for the management of children and adolescents with bronchiectasis. *Eur Respir J*. 2021;58(2):2002990. doi:10.1183/13993003.02990-2020.
4. Liu Y, Lu HW, Gu SY, et al. Bronchoscopic airway clearance therapy for acute exacerbations of bronchiectasis. *EBioMedicine*. 2021;72:103587. doi:10.1016/j.ebiom.2021.103587.

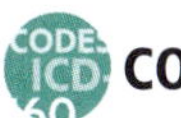

CODES

ICD10

- Q33.4 Congenital bronchiectasis
- A15.0 Tuberculosis of lung
- J47.0 Bronchiectasis with acute lower respiratory infection

CLINICAL PEARLS

- Symptoms of bronchiectasis include chronic productive cough, wheezing, and dyspnea often accompanied by repeated respiratory infections.
- A chest x-ray has poor sensitivity and specificity for the diagnosis; a noncontrast multidetector chest CT is the most important diagnostic tool.
- Current practice guidelines recommend treating acute exacerbations with a 14-day course of antibiotics. Frequent exacerbations may be treated with prolonged and aerosolized antibiotics.

BRONCHIOLITIS

Dennis E. Hughes, DO, FACEP

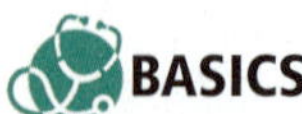

BASICS

DESCRIPTION

- Inflammation and obstruction of small airways and reactive airways generally affecting infants and young children; manifests as an upper respiratory infection (URI) prodrome followed by increased respiratory effort, crackles, and wheezing
- Usual course: insidious, acute, progressive with a variable duration; some experience persistent symptoms (primarily cough) for 14 to 21 days.
- Leading cause of hospitalizations in infants and children in most Western countries; it is the most common cause of lower respiratory tract infections (LRTI) in children <24 months of age.
- Predominant age: newborn to 2 years (peak age <6 months); neonates are not protected despite transfer of maternal antibody.
- Predominant sex: male > female

EPIDEMIOLOGY

Incidence

- Accounts for ~$1.7 billion in health care costs in the United States; incidence is estimated at 3.2/1,000. Almost 100% of children experience RSV infection by two seasons.
- Usually seasonal (October to May in the Northern Hemisphere) and often occurs in epidemics—in subtropical regions, RSV is endemic year-round.
- Responsible for 18.8% (90,000 annually) of all pediatric hospitalizations (excluding live births) in children aged <2 years
- Incidence is increasing since 1980 (with concomitant increase in relative rate of hospitalization from 2002 to 2007); of those <12 of age months with condition, the hospitalization rate is ~2–3%.

Prevalence

There is a 21–25% prevalence of bronchiolitis in children <12 months of age, decreasing to 13% from 12 to 24 months of age in the United States.

ETIOLOGY AND PATHOPHYSIOLOGY

RSV accounts for 70–85% of all cases (children <12 months of age), but rhinovirus, parainfluenza virus, metapneumovirus, adenovirus, influenza virus, *Mycoplasma pneumoniae*, and *Chlamydophila pneumoniae* have all been implicated:

- Infection results in necrosis and lysis of epithelial cells and subsequent release of inflammatory mediators.
- Edema and mucus secretion, which combined with accumulating necrotic debris and loss of cilia clearance, result in airflow obstruction.
- Ventilation-perfusion mismatching, which may result in hypoxia
- Air trapping is caused by dynamic airways narrowing during expiration, which increases work of breathing.
- Bronchospasm appears to play little or no role.

RISK FACTORS

- Secondhand cigarette smoke
- Low birth weight, premature birth (especially those infants born <35 weeks' gestation)
- Immunodeficiency—both congenital and acquired
- Formula-fed infants
- Contact with infected person (primary mode of spread)
- Children in daycare environment
- Congenital cardiopulmonary disease
- Comorbid neurologic disorder
- <12 weeks of age

GENERAL PREVENTION

- Handwashing or use of alcohol-based hand rubs (preferred)—this simple exercise has been estimated to have the largest impact on prevention of transmission.
- Contact isolation of infected babies
- Persons with colds should keep contact with infants to a minimum.
- Breastfeeding of infants for at least 6 months has been associated with reduced morbidity of disease.
- Palivizumab (Synagis), a monoclonal product, administered monthly, October to May, 15 mg/kg IM; used for RSV prevention *only* in high-risk patients (see American Academy of Pediatrics [AAP] recommendations)
- CDC recommends (August 2024) that pregnant women receive RSV vaccine (Pfizer Abrysvo—currently only option) between 32 and 36 weeks gestation (if gestational age corresponds to RSV season—September through January). Current data show significant (67%) reduction in hospitalization risk in infants.

Pediatric Considerations

Prior infection does not seem to confer subsequent immunity.

COMMONLY ASSOCIATED CONDITIONS

- Upper respiratory congestion
- Conjunctivitis
- Pharyngitis
- Otitis media
- Diarrhea

DIAGNOSIS

History and physical examination should be the basis for the diagnosis of bronchiolitis; ancillary testing is only indicated if clinical picture is unclear (no single group of tests confirmatory for bronchiolitis).

HISTORY

- Irritability
- Anorexia
- Fever
- Noisy breathing (due to rhinorrhea)
- Cough
- Grunting
- Cyanosis
- Apnea
- Vomiting

PHYSICAL EXAM

- Tachypnea
- Retractions (increased work of breathing)
- Rhinorrhea
- Wheezing
- Upper respiratory findings: pharyngitis, conjunctivitis, otitis

DIFFERENTIAL DIAGNOSIS

- Other pulmonary infections such as pertussis, croup, or bacterial pneumonia
- Aspiration
- Vascular ring
- Foreign body
- Asthma
- Heart failure
- Gastroesophageal reflux
- Cystic fibrosis

DIAGNOSTIC TESTS & INTERPRETATION

Laboratory and other ancillary testing (including chest x-ray) are not required if clinical diagnosis is bronchiolitis. Recent meta-analysis found no single history or physical factor that predicted air-space disease on chest radiograph.

Initial Tests (lab, imaging)

- Arterial oxygen saturation by pulse oximetry; results need to be interpreted in clinical context. Transient hypoxemia is a common phenomenon in healthy infants; capnography not found to aid in prediction of disease severity or need for hospitalization; AAP guidelines (2014/2019), 2013 Choosing Wisely campaign and 2020 BEEP suggest intermittent verses continuous pulse oximetry be considered.
- Rapid respiratory viral antigen testing is not necessary during RSV season because the disease is managed symptomatically but may be useful for epidemiologic, hospital cohorting, or in the very young to reduce unnecessary other workup; also indicated in infants admitted while receiving palivizumab prophylaxis (If positive, prophylaxis may be discontinued as recent data suggests no benefit in using palivizumab prophylaxis during active disease).
- The AAP does not recommend routine RSV testing in infants and children with bronchiolitis.
- Chest x-ray findings are variable and may include atelectasis, peribronchial cuffing, hyperinflation, and perihilar infiltrates (AAP, others do not recommend routine chest radiographs in clinical picture of acute bronchiolitis).

Diagnostic Procedures/Other

Point-of-care ultrasound (POCUS) is being used to assist with diagnosis of pneumonia in bronchiolitis with accuracy comparable to radiographs. Also, use of a POCUS-derived scoring system may prognosticate patients who need escalation of therapy.

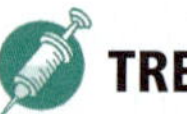

TREATMENT

- The cornerstone of therapy is supportive to include upper airway suctioning, prevention of significant and prolonged hypoxia, and dehydration.
- Positive-pressure ventilation (PPV) in the form of continuous positive airway pressure (CPAP) can be used in cases of respiratory failure. There is limited clinical evidence other than observational studies.

- Recent clinical practice guidelines do not support the routine use of corticosteroids, bronchodilators, or epinephrine. Despite these recommendations against such treatments, some estimated 50% of patients receive some combination of medication or other treatments during their course. Many experienced clinicians feel that trials of therapy (other than supportive care) are warranted based on clinical appearance (i.e., bronchodilators in wheezing patients).
- Parental education and support is vital.

GENERAL MEASURES

To prevent the transmission of RSV (most common infectious etiology of bronchiolitis), it is recommended that caregivers disinfect hands with alcohol-based skin cleaners both before and after contact with patients. Family should also be instructed on similar measures to reduce transmission.

MEDICATION

First Line

- Humidified oxygen for hypoxia of <90% (many feel that transient pulse oximetry in 85–90% range during sleeping in clinically well-appearing infant may be observed)
- Nebulized hypertonic saline (3%) can be effective in reducing LOS in hospitalized patients and a recent Cochrane review (2023) suggested use in the ED may reduce need for hospitalization (1)
- Antibiotics only if secondary bacterial infection present (rare); not indicated for routine use
- High-flow nasal cannula oxygen widely used in various settings to improve oxygen saturation with resultant reduction in end-tidal CO_2 ($ETCO_2$) and respiratory rate, but overall effectiveness remains unproven to date. Recent RCT (2023) found no benefit comparing HF to LF oxygen therapy in hospitalized infants (2).

Second Line

Consider NG or IV fluids in those infants or children unable to maintain intake and adequate hydration due to work of breathing.

ADDITIONAL THERAPIES

- Ribavirin and palivizumab for patients at high risk (for prophylaxis per CDC/AAP guidelines)
- Heliox therapy (70% helium and 30% oxygen) may be of benefit early in moderate to severe bronchiolitis to reduce degree of respiratory distress due to air flow restriction, but Cochrane Review found little evidence of sustained benefit at 24 hours.
- Although not routinely recommended, inhaled β-agonists (albuterol) can be effective in selected cases (particularly in patients with a history of bronchospasm). Many clinicians will attempt an empiric trial of bronchodilators in a primary presentation to judge the clinical response (some argue that this condition maybe asthma equivalent).

ADMISSION, INPATIENT, AND NURSING CONSIDERATIONS

- Bronchiolitis can be associated with apnea in children <6 weeks of age.
- Respiratory rate >45 breaths/min with respiratory distress or apnea
- Hypoxia is common, so clinical criteria are more helpful (sustained pulse oximetry <94% used by many as cutoff).
- Ill or toxic appearance
- Underlying heart condition, respiratory condition, or immune suppression
- High risk for apnea (aged <30 days, preterm birth [aged <37 weeks])
- Dehydrated or unable to feed (<50% of normal intake suggested as threshold for hospitalization consideration)
- Uncertain home care
- Use of respiratory distress assessment instrument may aid in determining admission. The five best predictors of admission are the following: age, respiratory rate, heart rate, oxygen saturation, and duration of symptoms were recently incorporated into a scoring instrument.
- Supplemental oxygen for pulse oximetry <94% on room air if clinically indicated (i.e., retractions, increased WOB, etc.); AAP recommends O_2 saturation >90% if infant is otherwise well.
- IV fluids indicated only if tachypnea precludes oral feeding; weight-based maintenance rate plus insensible losses
- Discharge criteria:
  - Normal respiratory rate and no oxygen requirement: Recent small studies suggest that after a period of observation, children can be safely discharged on home oxygen with home health follow-up. Despite reassuring appearance, the clinical course is unpredictable, so follow-up and parental education is important.

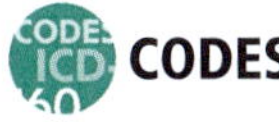

ONGOING CARE

FOLLOW-UP RECOMMENDATIONS

Patient Monitoring

- Hospitalization is usually required only if oxygen is a requirement or infant is unable to feed/drink (due to tachypnea).
- For a hospitalized patient, monitor as needed depending on the severity of the infection.
- If the patient is receiving home care, follow daily by telephone call for 2 to 4 days; the patient may need frequent office visits.

PATIENT EDUCATION

- American Academy of Pediatrics: http://www.aap.org
- American Academy of Family Physicians: http://www.familydoctor.org

PROGNOSIS

- Recovery time is variable. 40% can have symptoms at 14 days and 10% at 4 weeks.
- Mortality statistics differ but probably <1%.
- High-risk infants (bronchopulmonary dysplasia, congenital heart disease) may have a prolonged course.

COMPLICATIONS

- Bacterial superinfection
- Bronchiolitis obliterans
- Apnea
- Respiratory failure
- Death
- Increased incidence of development of reactive airway disease (asthma)

REFERENCES

1. Zhang L, Mendoza-Sassi RA, Wainwright CE, et al. Nebulised hypertonic saline solution for acute bronchiolitis in infants. *Cochrane Database Syst Rev*. 2023;4(4):CD006458. doi:10.1002/14651858.CD006458.pub5.
2. Kooiman L, Blankespoor F, Hofman R, et al. High-flow oxygen therapy in moderate to severe bronchiolitis: a randomised controlled trial. *Arch Dis Child*. 2023;108(6):455–460. doi:10.1136/archdischild-2022-324697.

ADDITIONAL READING

- Joseph MM, Edwards A. Acute bronchiolitis: assessment and management in the emergency department. *Pediatr Emerg Med Pract*. 2019;16(10):1–24.
- Oppenlander KE, Chung AA, Clabaugh D. Respiratory syncytial virus bronchiolitis: rapid evidence review. *Am Fam Physician*. 2023;108(1):52–57.

CODES

ICD10

- J21.9 Acute bronchiolitis, unspecified
- J21.0 Acute bronchiolitis due to respiratory syncytial virus
- J21.8 Acute bronchiolitis due to other specified organisms

CLINICAL PEARLS

- Bronchiolitis is the leading cause of hospitalizations in infants and children—especially <3 months of age.
- Diagnosis is a clinical one of children in the first 2 years of life, associated with rhinorrhea, cough, labored breathing, and irritability.
- RSV causes the majority of bronchiolitis. CXR is not indicated.
- Parental education and support is essential.
- Treatment: nasal and upper airway suctioning mainstay of treatment

BRONCHITIS, ACUTE

Ghazaleh Bigdeli, MD, FCCP

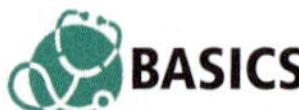

BASICS

- Acute bronchitis is defined as an acute, self-limited inflammation of the tracheobronchial tree, most commonly caused by viral infections. It presents with a cough (with or without sputum production) lasting <3 weeks in individuals without chronic pulmonary disease. Importantly, acute bronchitis occurs in the absence of pneumonia, as confirmed by lack of radiographic evidence, and should not be confused with exacerbations of chronic lung conditions like chronic obstructive pulmonary disease (COPD) or asthma.
- It is primarily a clinical diagnosis, and in the absence of pneumonia or other underlying lung disease, it does not require routine antibiotic therapy.

DESCRIPTION

- Acute bronchitis is a lower respiratory tract infection that causes reversible bronchial inflammation, involving the large airways, without evidence of pneumonia, that occurs in the absence of chronic obstructive lung disease.
- Cough, the predominant symptom, may last as long as 3 weeks.
- Generally self-limited, with complete healing and full return of function
- Most infections are viral if no underlying cardiopulmonary disease is present.
- Synonym(s): tracheobronchitis
- Geriatric patients:
  - More severe illness may occur in those with underlying heart or lung disease (e.g., congestive heart failure (CHF), COPD), especially if caused by influenza.
  - Monitor closely for secondary infections or decompensation.
- Pediatric patients:
  - Often associated with viral upper and lower respiratory infections
  - Recurrent episodes warrant evaluation for asthma, anatomic airway anomalies, or immunodeficiency.
  - Respiratory syncytial virus (RSV) may cause severe or fatal outcomes in infants, especially with prematurity or chronic lung disease.

EPIDEMIOLOGY

Incidence

- Acute bronchitis is one of the most common diagnoses in primary care settings, with approximately 5% of adults and 6–10% of children being affected annually (1),(2).
- The condition is most prevalent during the fall and winter months, corresponding with the peak season for viral respiratory infections like influenza, rhinovirus, and RSV.
- Age distribution:
  - Adults: Acute bronchitis is more common in younger adults and those with lower socioeconomic status or underlying respiratory conditions such as asthma or COPD.
  - Children: Acute bronchitis is frequent among preschool-aged children, who are more susceptible to viral respiratory infections. In children, the condition is often associated with other upper and lower respiratory infections, such as the common cold or RSV.

ETIOLOGY AND PATHOPHYSIOLOGY

- Primary causes:
  - Viral infections (90%+ of cases):
    - Common viruses include rhinovirus, influenza, parainfluenza, RSV, adenovirus, and coronavirus.
  - Bacterial infections (less common):
    - Includes *Mycoplasma pneumoniae*, *Chlamydia pneumoniae*, *Bordetella pertussis*, *Streptococcus pneumoniae*, and *Haemophilus influenzae*
    - Typically seen in secondary infections or specific populations (e.g., immunocompromised)
  - Environmental and underlying conditions: Tobacco exposure, air pollution, or preexisting lung diseases (COPD, asthma) increase susceptibility.
- Pathophysiology of acute bronchitis
  - Viral inflammation:
    - Infection leads to bronchial epithelial inflammation with edema and mucus hypersecretion.
    - Viral damage impairs ciliary function, reducing mucus clearance.
  - Immune response:
    - T lymphocytes, neutrophils, and macrophages are recruited to the airway to fight infection.
    - Pro-inflammatory cytokines (e.g., IL-6, TNF-α) contribute to symptoms (e.g., cough, wheezing).
  - Mucus hypersecretion: Goblet cells produce excessive mucus, leading to viscous sputum and contributing to productive cough; can cause bronchial obstruction and wheezing.
  - Bronchospasm and airway narrowing: In patients with reactive airway disease, infection may trigger bronchospasm, resulting in dyspnea and chest tightness.

Genetics

No known genetic pattern

RISK FACTORS

- Infants
- Elderly
- Air pollutants
- Smoking
- Secondhand smoke
- Environmental changes
- Chronic bronchopulmonary diseases
- Chronic sinusitis
- Tracheostomy or endobronchial intubation
- Bronchopulmonary allergy
- Hypertrophied tonsils and adenoids in children
- Immunosuppression
  - Immunoglobulin deficiency
  - HIV infection
  - Alcoholism
- Gastroesophageal reflux disease (GERD)

GENERAL PREVENTION

- Avoid smoking and secondhand smoke.
- Control underlying risk factors (i.e., asthma, sinusitis, and reflux).
- Avoid exposure, especially daycare.
- Pneumovax, influenza immunization

COMMONLY ASSOCIATED CONDITIONS

- COPD
- Asthma
- CHF
- Cystic fibrosis
- Diabetes
- GERD
- Immunocompromised states (e.g., HIV, organ transplant, chemotherapy)
- Recent upper respiratory infections (e.g., common cold, influenza)
- Sinusitis or rhinitis
- Allergic rhinitis

DIAGNOSIS

- Acute bronchitis should be suspected in patients with an acute onset but persistent cough (often lasting 1 to 3 weeks) who do not have clinical findings suggestive of pneumonia (e.g., fever, tachypnea, rales, signs of parenchymal consolidation) and do not have COPD.
- In most cases, the diagnosis can be made based on the history and physical examination.
- Testing is generally reserved for cases in which pneumonia is suspected, clinical diagnosis is uncertain, or when results would change management.

HISTORY

- Cough for >5 days and no evidence of pneumonia, asthma, exacerbation of COPD
- Cough is initially dry and nonproductive, later, mucopurulent sputum, which may indicate secondary infection.
- Dyspnea, wheeze, and fatigue may occur.
- Fever may suggest pneumonia or influenza infection.

PHYSICAL EXAM

- General appearance:
  - Typically well-appearing but may appear mildly distressed due to cough
- Vital signs:
  - Normal temperature or low-grade fever (rarely high fever)
  - Normal pulse and blood pressure
  - Possible tachypnea (rapid breathing)
- Respiratory examination:
  - Cough: Predominant symptom can be productive or nonproductive.
  - Wheezing: may be present, especially in patients with underlying asthma or reactive airway disease
  - Crackles: may be heard in early phase or due to mucous in airways
  - Normal or slightly decreased breath sounds
  - Tactile fremitus: may be normal or slightly decreased
  - Increased respiratory rate due to cough and irritation
- Cardiovascular exam:
  - Normal heart sounds, no murmurs or gallops
  - No signs of heart failure (e.g., jugular venous distention, peripheral edema)
- Other findings:
  - No signs of consolidation (e.g., dullness to percussion, egophony, fremitus increase)
  - Sinus tenderness may be present if there's a concurrent upper respiratory infection.

DIFFERENTIAL DIAGNOSIS

- Pneumonia
- COVID-19
- Postnasal drip syndrome
- Common cold
- Acute sinusitis
- Bronchopneumonia
- Influenza

- Bacterial tracheitis
- Bronchiectasis
- Asthma
- Reactive airway dysfunction syndrome (RADS)
- Allergy
- Eosinophilic pneumonitis
- Retained foreign body
- Heart failure
- GERD
- ACE inhibitors use

DIAGNOSTIC TESTS & INTERPRETATION

Initial Tests (lab, imaging)

- None normally needed; diagnosis is based on history and physical exam showing no postnasal drip or rales.
- For a complicated picture, consider the following:
  - CBC with differential
  - Influenza titers (if appropriate for time of year)
  - Viral panel/testing for SARS-CoV-2 (COVID-19) is recommended for all patients during the COVID-19 pandemic.
- No testing needed unless concerned about pneumonia
- Pulse oximetry if underlying pulmonary disease is present
- CXR are only indicated if:
  - Dyspnea, bloody sputum, or rusty sputum color
  - Pulse >100 beats/min
  - Respiratory rate >24 beats/min
  - Oral body temperature >100°F (37.8°C)
  - Focal consolidation, egophony, or fremitus on chest examination

Follow-Up Tests & Special Considerations

- Arterial blood gases: hypoxemia (rarely)
- Sputum culture in those patients intubated or with tracheostomy

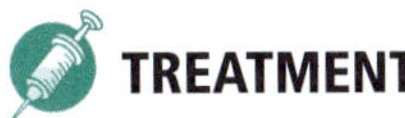

TREATMENT

GENERAL MEASURES

- Stop smoking and avoid secondhand smoke.
- Steam inhalations or vaporizers
- Adequate hydration
- Antitussives (honey 1 tbsp every 2 to 3 hours PRN)
- Antibiotics are not recommended.
- Treat associated illnesses (e.g., GERD).

MEDICATION

ALERT
Antibiotics are not recommended unless a treatable pathogen has been identified or significant comorbidities are present. This should be explained to patients who likely expect an antibiotic to be prescribed.

First Line

- Supportive; increased fluids (Cough results in increased fluid loss.)
- Antipyretic analgesic such as aspirin, acetaminophen, or ibuprofen
- Decongestants if accompanied by sinus symptoms or postnasal drip
- Cough suppressant for troublesome cough (not with COPD); nonpharmacologic therapy honey (1 tbsp every 1 to 4 hours as needed), throat lozenges, hot tea; smoking cessation and avoidance of secondhand smoke is a reasonable first step.
- Pharmacologic therapy: benzonatate (Tessalon)
- Guaifenesin with or without dextromethorphan and mucolytic agents have not been found to be beneficial and are not recommended.
- Inhaled β-agonist (e.g., albuterol) or in combination with high-dose inhaled corticosteroids for cough with bronchospasm in those with known airflow obstruction (1)[B]
- If influenza is highly suspected and symptom onset is <48 hours: oseltamivir (Tamiflu), zanamivir (Relenza), IV peramivir (Rapivab), or baloxavir marboxil (Xofluza)
- In case of positive COVID-19 infection, patients can be treated with antiviral medications or monoclonal antibodies based on National Institute of Health (NIH) COVID-19 treatments. Nirmatrelvir (Paxlovid) is the first choice treatment for mild to moderate COVID-19 in patients with a higher risk of severe illness.
- Antibiotics *only* if a treatable cause (i.e., pertussis) is identified.
  - Doxycycline: 100 mg/day × 10 days if *Moraxella*, *Chlamydia*, or *Mycoplasma* suspected
    - Quinolone for more serious infections or other antibiotic failure or in elderly or patients with multiple comorbidities
    - Clarithromycin (Biaxin): 500 mg q12h or azithromycin (Zithromax) for atypical or pertussis infection
- Contraindication(s): Doxycycline and quinolones should not be used during pregnancy or in children.
- Precautions:
  - Antibiotic use can be associated with *Clostridium difficile* infections.
  - Cough and cold preparations should not be used in children aged <6 years.

ISSUES FOR REFERRAL

- Comorbidities such as COPD
- Cough lasting >3 months

ADDITIONAL THERAPIES

- Antipyretic for fever (e.g., acetaminophen or ibuprofen)
- Inhaled β-agonist (e.g., albuterol) or in combination with high-dose inhaled corticosteroids for cough with bronchospasm
- Oral corticosteroids probably not indicated with exception in COVID-19 infection

ADMISSION, INPATIENT, AND NURSING CONSIDERATIONS

- Hypoxia—may require supplemental oxygen.
- Respiratory failure that may require CPAP/bilevel ventilation
- Severe bronchospasm
- Exacerbation of underlying disease
- Bronchodilators if patient is bronchospastic
- Discharge criteria: improvement in symptoms and comorbidities

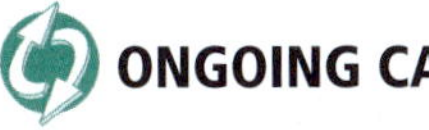

ONGOING CARE

FOLLOW-UP RECOMMENDATIONS

- Usually a self-limited disease not requiring follow-up
- Cough may linger for several weeks.
- In children, if recurrent, need to consider other diagnoses, such as asthma (2).

DIET

Increased fluids (3 to 4 L/day) while febrile

PATIENT EDUCATION

American Academy of Family Physicians: https://familydoctor.org

PROGNOSIS

- Cough may persist for several weeks after an initial improvement.
- Bronchiolitis obliterans and organizing pneumonia (rare)

COMPLICATIONS

- Superinfection such as bronchopneumonia
- Bronchiectasis
- Hemoptysis
- Acute respiratory failure
- Chronic cough

REFERENCES

1. Becker LA, Hom J, Villasis-Keever M, et al. Beta2-agonists for acute cough or a clinical diagnosis of acute bronchitis. *Cochrane Database Syst Rev*. 2015;(9):CD001726.
2. Gonzales R, Anderer T, McCulloch CE, et al. A cluster randomized trial of decision support strategies for reducing antibiotic use in acute bronchitis. *JAMA Intern Med*. 2013;173(4):267–273.

ADDITIONAL READING

Smith SM, Fahey T, Smucny J, et al. Antibiotics for acute bronchitis. *Cochrane Database Syst Rev*. 2017;6(6):CD000245. doi:10.1002/14651858.CD000245.pub4.

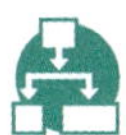

SEE ALSO

- Asthma; Chronic Obstructive Pulmonary Disease and Emphysema
- Algorithm: Cough, Chronic

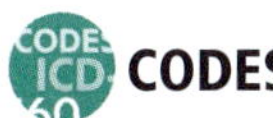

CODES

ICD10

- J20.9 Acute bronchitis, unspecified
- J68.0 Bronchitis and pneumonitis due to chemicals, gases, fumes and vapors
- B97.0 Adenovirus as the cause of diseases classified elsewhere

CLINICAL PEARLS

- Acute bronchitis is a common and generally self-limited disease.
- Treat cough with honey (1 tbsp every 2 to 4 hours as needed), benzonatate (Tessalon), guaifenesin with dextromethorphan.
- It does not require treatment with antibiotics. This needs to be explained to patients who expect antibiotics to be prescribed.
- Cough may linger for several weeks after the resolution of other symptoms.
- Recurrent or seasonal episodes may suggest another disease process, such as asthma.
- Fever is uncommon and should prompt investigation for pneumonia or influenza.

BULIMIA NERVOSA

Elizabeth M. Payment, MD

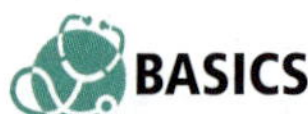

BASICS

DESCRIPTION

An eating disorder which includes binge eating and inappropriate compensatory behaviors; symptoms include the following:

- Episodes of binge eating (greater than one would typically eat in a similar situation over a 2-hour sitting), lack of self-control for eating at least once a week for 3 months
- Inappropriate compensations to prevent weight gain
  - For example, caloric restriction (most common), excessive exercise, self-induced vomiting, inappropriate laxative or diuretics use
- Alternating binge eating and compensations for prolonged time not during anorexia nervosa
- Distorted self-body image
- *DSM-5* classifies severity based on inappropriate compensatory behaviors per week:
  - Mild (1 to 3), moderate (4 to 7), severe (8 to 13), extreme (≥14)
- System(s) affected: oropharyngeal, endocrine/metabolic, gastrointestinal, dermatologic, cardiovascular, pulmonary, psychiatric

EPIDEMIOLOGY

- Mean age of onset: 18 to 21 years
- Predominant sex: female > male (13:1)

Prevalence

Approximately 0.5% of females and 0.08% males in the United States.

ETIOLOGY AND PATHOPHYSIOLOGY

Combination of biologic, psychological, environmental, and social factors.

Genetics

Heritability estimated to be up to 41%

RISK FACTORS

- Female gender
- History of obesity and dieting
- Body dissatisfaction; critical comments about weight, body shape, or eating; low self-esteem
- Depression, social anxiety, severe life stressor
- Poor impulse control, substance abuse
- Family history of substance abuse, affective disorders, eating disorder, or obesity
- Diabetes
- Childhood trauma (sexual or physical abuse, neglect)

GENERAL PREVENTION

- Realistic and healthy weight management strategies and attitudes
- Decrease body dissatisfaction and promote self-esteem.
- Reduce focus on thin as ideal.

COMMONLY ASSOCIATED CONDITIONS

- Major depression, dysthymia, anxiety, obsessive-compulsive, bipolar disorders
- Substance use disorder
- Personality disorders: borderline, schizotypal, antisocial (1)
- Nonsuicidal self-injury (33%) and suicidal attempts (21%) (2)

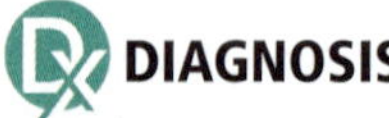

DIAGNOSIS

HISTORY

- Patients unlikely to self-identify binge eating or purging behaviors; corroborate with parent/relative.
- Unhappiness and/or preoccupation with weight and diet attempts
- Pattern of binge eating and compensatory behaviors
  - Binging
  - Vomiting (often with little effort)
  - Vigorous aerobic exercise
  - Distress/shame related to loss of control
  - Use of diuretics, laxatives without medical indication
- Depressed mood and self-depreciation following the binges
- Other possible signs and symptoms
  - Requesting weight loss help and mildly underweight to overweight
  - Diet pill, diuretic, laxative, ipecac, and thyroid medication use/abuse, frequent fluctuations in weight
  - Menstrual disturbances or amenorrhea
  - Fatigue and lethargy
  - Abdominal pain, bloating, constipation, diarrhea, rectal prolapse
  - Sore throat and thermal tooth sensitivity
  - Omission/underdosing insulin in diabetes patients

PHYSICAL EXAM

- Often with normal/fluctuating weight or overweight range
- Tachycardia
- Erosion of dental enamel (8.33%)
- Perimylolysis, cheilosis, gingivitis
- Sialadenosis (parotid gland swelling and/or asymptomatic, noninflammatory parotid gland enlargement)
- Epigastric tenderness to palpation
- Russell sign: scars, calluses, abrasions, bruising on hand, thumb
- Peripheral edema

DIFFERENTIAL DIAGNOSIS

- Anorexia, binge eating/purging type; distinguished by body mass index (BMI) <18.5 kg/m^2
- Binge eating disorder
- Major depressive disorder/borderline personality disorder
- Other metabolic disorders: Addison disease, celiac disease, diabetes mellitus, hyperthyroidism, hypothyroidism, hyperpituitarism
- Genetic syndromes: Kleine-Levin syndrome, Prader-Willi syndrome
- Pregnancy

DIAGNOSTIC TESTS & INTERPRETATION

- All lab results may be within normal limits and are unnecessary for diagnosis.
- Psychological self-report screening tests may be helpful but tend to increase false positives.
- SCOFF questionnaire is recommended by United States Preventative Task Force (sensitivity 0.86 and specificity of 0.83) (3)
- Eating disorder screen for primary care (ESP)
- Primary Care Evaluation of Mental Disorders Patient Health Questionnaire

Initial Tests (lab, imaging)

- CBC, CMP, and LFTs
  - Hypokalemia, hyponatremia, hypochloremia, hypocalcemia, hypomagnesemia, hypophosphatemia, hypoproteinemia, hypoglycemia
  - Serum amylase levels and pH derangements
  - Elevated BUN
- Urinalysis: increased urine specific gravity

Diagnostic Procedures/Other

- Pregnancy test
- Electrocardiogram: bradycardia or arrhythmias, conduction defects, depressed ST segment due to hypokalemia

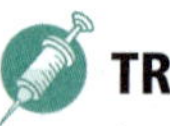

TREATMENT

Cognitive-behavioral therapy (CBT) and nutritional rehabilitation should be considered as first-line treatment (4),(5). Combination treatment with CBT and medications are more effective than psychotherapy alone, and psychotherapy alone is more effective than medication alone.

GENERAL MEASURES

- Multidisciplinary team (primary care clinician, behavioral health provider, nutritionist)
- CBT for bulimia nervosa (5)
- Family therapy for adolescents
- Nutritional education, relaxation techniques

MEDICATION

First Line

- Selective serotonin reuptake inhibitors (SSRIs) (6)[A], particularly fluoxetine titrated by 20 mg daily every week to 60 mg/day, is effective in reducing symptoms. Higher doses than standard doses for depression are often needed.
  - Maintain full therapeutic dose for at least 6 to 12 months after remission (7).
- If there is no adequate response to treatment, evaluate for medical nonadherence or adjust treatment every 4 to 8 weeks.

Second Line

- Select different SSRIs (sertraline, escitalopram, and fluvoxamine). Paroxetine is not often used for increased risk of weight gain.
- Third-line therapies include TCAs, MAOIs, and trazodone.
- The anticonvulsant topiramate may help to diminish binge-purge episodes.
- Ondansetron (Zofran) 4 to 8 mg TID between meals may decrease nausea and vomiting.
- Bupropion is contraindicated due to association with seizures with electrolyte abnormalities.

ISSUES FOR REFERRAL

A multidisciplinary approach should be used which include a primary care physician, behavioral health provider, and nutritionist.

COMPLEMENTARY & ALTERNATIVE MEDICINE

Bright light therapy is potentially effective at improving disordered eating and mood (8).

ADMISSION, INPATIENT, AND NURSING CONSIDERATIONS

- Admission to a specialized eating disorders unit for ≥1 of the following:
  - ≤75% ideal BMI for age and sex
  - Dehydration; electrolyte disturbance (hypokalemia, hyponatremia, hypophosphatemia)
  - ECG abnormalities (e.g., prolonged QTc or severe bradycardia)
  - Severe bradycardia (<50 beats/min daytime; <45 beats/min at night)
  - Hypotension (systolic <90 mm Hg)
  - Hypothermia (body temperature <96°F [35.6°C])
  - Orthostasis
  - Acute food refusal, uncontrollable bingeing and purging
  - Acute medical complications of malnutrition (e.g., syncope, seizures, cardiac failure, pancreatitis)
  - Comorbid psychiatric or medical condition that prohibits or limits appropriate outpatient treatment (e.g., severe depression, suicidal ideation, obsessive-compulsive disorder, type 1 diabetes mellitus) (9)
- During admission:
  - Supervised meals and bathroom privileges
  - Gradually shift control to patients as they demonstrate improvement.

ONGOING CARE

FOLLOW-UP RECOMMENDATIONS

Patient Monitoring

- Binge-purge activity, including antecedents and consequences, level of exercise activity
- Self-esteem, comfort with body and self, ruminations, and depressive symptoms
- Repeat any abnormal lab values weekly until stable.

DIET

- Balanced diet, normal eating pattern
- Nutritional rehabilitation aims to restore a structured and consistent meal pattern: three meals and two snacks per day

PATIENT EDUCATION

National Alliance on Mental Illness: https://www.nami.org/Learn-More/Mental-Health-Conditions/Eating-Disorders/Overview

PROGNOSIS

- An estimated 45–70% will have a full recovery or improvement of symptoms, and 20–30% may experience relapse (10).
- Positive prognostic factors: younger age at presentation, shorter duration of illness, less frequent symptoms, absence of laxative use, close social relationships, and a good therapeutic response within the first month of treatment
- Negative prognostic factors: overemphasis on body shape and weight, history of physical abuse, disturbed family relationships, poor motivation, self-injurious behaviors, and presence of a personality disorder (10)

COMPLICATIONS

- Substance use disorder
- Osteopenia/osteoporosis/stress fracture
- Gastric dilatation/Boerhaave syndrome/Mallory-Weiss tears
- Spontaneous pneumomediastinum
- Potassium depletion, cardiac arrhythmia, cardiac arrest
- Suicide

REFERENCES

1. Udo T, Grilo CM. Psychiatric and medical correlates of *DSM-5* eating disorders in a nationally representative sample of adults in the United States. *Int J Eat Disord*. 2019;52(1):42–50. doi:10.1002/eat.23004.
2. Mandelli L, Arminio A, Atti AR, et al. Suicide attempts in eating disorder subtypes: a meta-analysis of the literature employing *DSM-IV*, *DSM-5*, or *ICD-10* diagnostic criteria. *Psychol Med*. 2019;49(8):1237–1249. doi:10.1017/S0033291718003549.
3. Kutz AM, Marsh AG, Gunderson CG, et al. Eating disorder screening: a systematic review and meta-analysis of diagnostic test characteristics of the SCOFF. *J Gen Intern Med*. 2020;35(3):885–893. doi:10.1007/s11606-019-05478-6.
4. Linardon J, Wade TD, de la Piedad Garcia X, et al. The efficacy of cognitive-behavioral therapy for eating disorders: a systematic review and meta-analysis. *J Consult Clin Psychol*. 2017;85(11):1080–1094. doi:10.1037/ccp0000245.
5. Hay PP, Bacaltchuk J, Stefano S, et al. Psychological treatments for bulimia nervosa and binging. *Cochrane Database Syst Rev*. 2009;2009(4):CD000562.
6. Bacaltchuk J, Hay P, Trefiglio R. Antidepressants versus psychological treatments and their combination for bulimia nervosa. *Cochrane Database Syst Rev*. 2001;2001(4):CD003385.
7. Yager J, Devlin MJ, Halmi K, et al. Guideline watch: practice guideline for the treatment of patients with eating disorders. *FOCUS*. 2014;12(4):416–431. doi:10.1176/appi.focus.120404.
8. Beauchamp MT, Lundgren JD. A systematic review of bright light therapy for eating disorders. *Prim Care Companion CNS Disord*. 2016;18(5). doi:10.4088/PCC.16r02008.
9. Golden NH, Katzman DK, Sawyer SM, et al; for Society for Adolescent Health and Medicine. Position paper of the Society for Adolescent Health and Medicine: medical management of restrictive eating disorders in adolescents and young adults. *J Adolesc Health*. 2015;56(1):121–125. doi:10.1016/j.jadohealth.2014.10.259.
10. Castillo M, Weiselberg W. Bulimia nervosa/purging disorder. *Curr Probl Pediatr Adolesc Health Care*. 2017;47(4):85–94. doi:10.1016/j.cpped.2017.02.004.

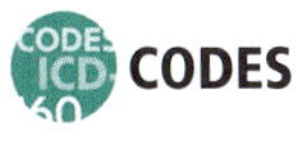

ICD10

F50.2 Bulimia nervosa

CLINICAL PEARLS

- Asking "Are you satisfied with your eating patterns?" and/or "Do you worry that you have lost control over how much you eat?" may help to screen for an eating problem.
- Screening with SCOFF or ESP is recommended for eating disorders.
- Use a multidisciplinary team approach when resources are available.
- SSRIs, particularly fluoxetine (60 mg daily), is a useful first-line medication and/or adjunctive treatment with CBT.
- Pharmacotherapy alone is reasonable if specialized nutritional rehabilitation and psychotherapy are not available.
- Combination therapy has the highest rates of improvement.

BUNION (HALLUX VALGUS)

Theresa Yurkonis, DO, MHSA

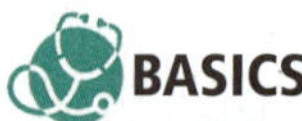

BASICS

DESCRIPTION

- Lateral deviation of the great toe ("Hallux abducto valgus" derives from the Latin for "big toe askew.")
- Associated medial deviation of the 1st metatarsal, leading to a medial prominence of the 1st metatarsophalangeal (MTP) joint
- Progressive subluxation of the 1st MTP joint in later stages

EPIDEMIOLOGY

- More common in adults; female:male 15:1
- More common in shoe-wearing populations especially constrictive footwear between the age of 20 and 39 years
- More commonly observed in those with connective tissue disorders including Marfan syndrome, Ehlers-Danlos and Down syndrome

Prevalence

- Adults (ages 18 to 65 years): estimated prevalence of 23%
- Elderly (>65 years): estimated prevalence of 36%
- Juvenile hallux valgus: estimated prevalence of 7.8

ETIOLOGY AND PATHOPHYSIOLOGY

Multifactorial and controversial; contributing factors may include underlying anatomy and repetitive external forces

- The 1st metatarsal, proximal phalanx, and distal phalanx form the anatomy of the hallux with two sesamoid bones (medial and lateral) contributing to the 1st MTP joint. The sesamoid bones are embedded in the flexor hallucis brevis tendon and articulation allows for force generation.
- The hallux valgus angle (HVA) is formed by the intersection of the longitudinal axes of the proximal phalanx and the 1st metatarsal. Normal is <15 degrees, ≥20 degrees is pathologic, and 45 to 50 degrees is classified as severe.
- Absence of muscles that directly stabilize the 1st MTP allows relatively unopposed forces to influence lateral deviation of the proximal phalanx and medial deviation of the 1st metatarsal head.
- Medial MTP joint capsule and medial collateral ligament are chronically stretched and may eventually rupture, decreasing stability and causing progressive subluxation of the 1st MTP joint.
- Lateral joint capsule and collateral ligaments also contract.
- Lateral and plantar migration of abductor hallucis muscle moves the great toe into plantar flexion and lateral pronation.
- Juvenile bunions are thought to be caused more in a deformity in the MTP joint with more severely elevated distal metatarsal articular angles (DMAAs) with MTP congruity being the main significant factor.

Genetics

- Cohort and twin studies suggest heritability possible following an autosomal dominant pattern with incomplete penetrance.
- Genome-wide association studies suggest sex-specific differences in genetic mechanisms.

RISK FACTORS

- Genetic predisposition
- Abnormal biomechanics (i.e., flexible flat feet)
- Foot deformities: joint laxity, hindfoot pronation, contracture of Achilles tendon, pes planus (fallen arches), metatarsus primus varus
- Amputation of 2nd toe
- Inflammatory joint disease
- Neuromuscular disorders (cerebral palsy, stroke)
- Improper footwear (high heels, narrow toe box, restrictive footwear)
- No association with obesity or occupation (except for ballet dancing)

GENERAL PREVENTION

Proper footwear may decrease the progression of the disease.

COMMONLY ASSOCIATED CONDITIONS

- Medial bursitis of the 1st MTP joint (most common)
- Hammertoe deformity of the 2nd phalanx
- Plantar callus
- Metatarsalgia
- Degeneration of cartilage covering the 1st metatarsal head and sesamoids
- Pronated feet; ankle equinus
- Onychocryptosis (ingrown toenail)
- Entrapment of the medial dorsal cutaneous nerve
- Synovitis of the MTP joint

DIAGNOSIS

- Based on clinical exam
- Radiographs are used for staging.

HISTORY

Focus on duration of symptoms, activity modification, type of footwear, and previous interventions.

- Painful MTP joint (most common symptom in adults)
- Abnormal position of great toe
- Enlargement of the MTP joint medially (patients complain of a "bump")
- Shoes do not fit properly.
- Plantar foot pain and pain with ambulation
- Skin irritation, blister, or callus at the 1st MTP

PHYSICAL EXAM

- Observe gait; may be antalgic due to pain
- Medial prominence at the MTP joint
- Skin changes: erythema, blistering, callus, or ulceration at the MTP joint
- Great toe overriding or underriding the second toe
- Examine the entire 1st metatarsal and toe for:
  - 1st MTP range of motion
  - 1st tarsometatarsal (TMT) mobility
  - Neurovascular integrity
  - Degenerative osteoarthritis
- Examine entire foot and ankle for other abnormalities.

DIFFERENTIAL DIAGNOSIS

- Trauma: turf toe, sesamoiditis, stress fracture
- Infection: osteomyelitis, septic arthritis
- Joint disorder: osteoarthritis, rheumatoid arthritis, pseudogout, gout
- Tendon disorder: tendinosis, tenosynovitis, tendon rupture
- Other: bursitis, ganglion cyst, foreign body granuloma

DIAGNOSTIC TESTS & INTERPRETATION

Initial Tests (lab, imaging)

- Weight-bearing AP and lateral radiographs (sesamoid view optional) to assess:
  - Joint congruency and degenerative changes
  - Lateral sesamoid bone displacement
  - Rounded 1st metatarsal head
  - Longer 1st metatarsal
- Radiographic parameters include but are not limited to:
  - HVA: Long axis of the 1st MT and proximal phalanx is normally <15 degrees.
  - Intermetatarsal angle (IMA): Between long axis of 1st and 2nd metatarsal is normally <9 degrees.
  - DMAA: Between 1st metatarsal long axis and line through base of distal articular cap is normally <8 degrees.
  - Hallux valgus interphalangeal angle (IPA): Between long axis of distal phalanx and proximal phalanx is normally <10 degrees.

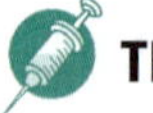

TREATMENT

- Primary indication for treatment is pain.
- There are conservative (nonoperative) and surgical approaches.
- Only surgical approaches can correct the hallux valgus deformity.
- Surgical treatment is generally more effective in improving pain but has risks.

GENERAL MEASURES

Nonoperative treatment options may improve pain and delay the progression of hallux valgus deformity, although high-quality evidence is limited (1)[B]:

- Proper fitting footwear: low-heeled, wide-toe shoes to decrease stress on MTP joint

- Orthotics in general to correct foot alignment (pes planus and overpronation) unfortunately have not been shown to prevent or slow progression of the angle but may improve pain (1),(2)[B], but custom orthotics for bunions specifically showed some improvement in both (1)[A].
- Splinting: in theory, stabilizes and balances soft tissue structures around the MTP but there is limited evidence showing improvement in degree of angulation or pain in mild hallux valgus (2)[C]
- Available over-the-counter nighttime splints unfortunately did not show improvement in short-term pain but possible long-term outcomes (2)[C],(3)[C].
- Foot mobilization and exercise, combined with a toe separator, may improve pain scores, strength and range of motion in moderate hallux valgus (4)[B].
- Botox injections have been shown to moderately improve pain and angulation (2)[B].
- Taping with manual therapy, multimodal physical therapy all showed some promise in reducing long-term pain (2)[B]

MEDICATION

- Topical NSAIDs or capsaicin cream and oral analgesic medications (NSAIDs, acetaminophen) can be used to relieve pain.
- Corticosteroid injections may improve pain (rarely used outside postoperative setting).

ISSUES FOR REFERRAL

Surgery is indicated for patients with severe pain, dysfunction, or persistent symptoms that do not abate with conservative therapy.

SURGERY/OTHER PROCEDURES

- >150 different surgical techniques exist to treat hallux valgus.
- No single technique is proven superior; no universally accepted standard exists for procedure selection.
- Minimally invasive techniques continue to evolve and may achieve better outcomes than open techniques.
- Choice of technique depends on disease severity, radiographic findings, and patient/surgeon-specific factors:
  - Arthrodesis: fusion of the 1st MTP joint; used for severe and/or recurrent hallux valgus; fusion of the 1st TMT joint (modified Lapidus) is considered for TMT joint hypermobility.
  - Arthroplasty: removing the joint or replacing it with a prosthesis; high revision rates
  - Exostectomy/bunionectomy: removing the medial bony prominence of the MTP joint (less common now)
  - Soft tissue realignment: alters the function of surrounding ligaments and tendons; used for minor deformities or as an adjunct to bony correction techniques
  - Osteotomy and realignment: common and includes wide variety of techniques:
    - Distal—used for mild to moderate deformity (e.g., distal chevron osteotomy)
    - Proximal—used more often to correct severe deformity
  - Mini TightRope procedure: use of a FiberWire to correct misalignment.
- Some patients may have little to no improvement in symptoms despite interventions; establish realistic expectations prior to surgery.
- In pediatric patients, surgery should generally be delayed until skeletal maturity.

COMPLEMENTARY & ALTERNATIVE MEDICINE

Marigold ointment may reduce pain and soft tissue swelling related to bunion.

ONGOING CARE

FOLLOW-UP RECOMMENDATIONS

- Postoperative treatment includes physical therapy, physiotherapy, supportive footwear, continuous passive motion, or manual manipulation.
- Time until full weight-bearing depends on the surgical procedure.

PROGNOSIS

- Patient outcome varies depending on biomechanical factors, severity of the deformity, and treatment modality used.
- Recurrence after surgery is common (25%) and increases with degree of preoperative HVA and IMA and postoperative HVA and sesamoid position.

COMPLICATIONS

- Risks associated with surgery include infection, persistent pain, and poor cosmetic result.
- Additional risks vary with the surgical procedure.
- Other complications may include:
  - Early swelling
  - Hallux varus
  - Recurrence of bunion
  - Metatarsal fracture
  - Decreased sensation over the 1st metatarsal or phalanx
  - Avascular necrosis

REFERENCES

1. Li G, Shen J, Smith E, et al. The evaluation of orthotics in reducing hallux valgus angle in patients with hallux valgus over a twelve-month treatment. *Int J Environ Res Public Health*. 2022;19(19):12531. doi:10.3390/ijerph191912531.
2. Hurn SE, Matthews BG, Munteanu SE, et al. Effectiveness of nonsurgical interventions for hallux valgus: a systematic review and meta-analysis. *Arthritis Care Res (Hoboken)*. 2022;74(10):1676–1688. doi:10.1002/acr.24603.
3. Chadchavalpanichaya N, Chueluecha C. Effectiveness of hallux valgus strap: a prospective, randomized single-blinded controlled trial. *Siriraj Med J*. 2017;63(2):42–46.
4. Abdalbary SA. Foot mobilization and exercise program combined with toe separator improves outcomes in women with moderate hallux valgus at 1-Year Follow-up: a randomized clinical trial. *J Am Podiatr Med Assoc*. 2018;108(6):478–486.

ADDITIONAL READING

- Arbeeva L, Yau M, Mitchell BD, et al. Genome-wide meta-analysis identified novel variant associated with hallux valgus in Caucasians. *J Foot Ankle Res*. 2020;13(1):11.
- Barnish MS, Barnish J. High-heeled shoes and musculoskeletal injuries: a narrative systematic review. *BMJ Open*. 2016;6(1):e010053.
- Kwan MY, Yick KL, Yip J, et al. Hallux valgus orthosis characteristics and effectiveness: a systematic review with meta-analysis. *BMJ Open*. 2021;11(8):e047273.

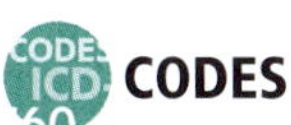

CODES

ICD10

- M20.10 Hallux valgus (acquired), unspecified foot
- M20.11 Hallux valgus (acquired), right foot
- M20.12 Hallux valgus (acquired), left foot

CLINICAL PEARLS

- Avoid footwear with high heels, pointed toe boxes, or inadequate toe space to reduce development or progression of bunions.
- Trial of night splints, physical therapy with or without taping, manual therapy, or BOTOX may be considered
- Surgery generally results in superior outcomes for pain relief in appropriately selected patients, but long-term efficacy has not been proven.
- No single surgical method has shown to be superior for long-term pain relief.
- Establish realistic expectations prior to surgery to improve patient satisfaction with surgical outcomes.

BURNS

Grant Wei, MD, FACEP • Chirag N. Shah, MD • Tyler M. Debbie, MD

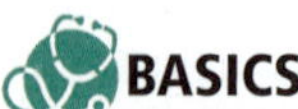

BASICS

DESCRIPTION

- Tissue injuries caused by application of heat, chemicals, electricity, or irradiation
- Extent of injury (depth of burn) results from the intensity and duration of exposure.
  - Superficial burn (formerly 1st degree) involves superficial layers of epidermis.
  - Partial-thickness burn (formerly 2nd degree) involves varying amounts of epidermis (with blister formation) and part of the dermis.
  - Full-thickness burn (formerly 3rd degree) involves destruction of all skin elements (full thickness) with coagulation of the subdermal plexus.
- System(s) affected: endocrine/metabolic, pulmonary, skin/exocrine

Geriatric Considerations

- Prognosis is worse for severe burns.
- Patients >60 years of age account for 11% of all burns.

Pediatric Considerations

Consider child abuse or neglect when dealing with hot water burns in children; abuse accounts for 15% of pediatric burns. Special concerns are sharply demarcated wounds, immersion injuries, and suspect stories. Involve child protective services early.

EPIDEMIOLOGY

- Fourth most common trauma worldwide
- Predominant age: 20 to 30 years; 13% are infants; 11% are >60 years of age
- Predominant gender: Males account for 70%.

Incidence

Per year in the United States

- 1.2 to 2 million burns; 700,000 emergency room visits; 45,000 to 50,000 hospitalizations; 3,900 deaths from burn-related complications
- In children: 250,000 burns; 15,000 hospitalizations; 1,100 deaths
- Estimated total cost of $2 billion annually for burn care.
- House fires cause 75% of deaths.
- Burn deaths decreasing nationally due to improved prevention and treatment.
- Increase in burns from the illegal production of methamphetamines. Patients can present with a combination of chemical burns, thermal burns, and explosion injuries.

ETIOLOGY AND PATHOPHYSIOLOGY

- Open flame and hot liquid are the most common causes of burns (heat usually ≥45°C): flame burns more common in adults; scald burns are more common in children.
- Caustic chemicals or acids (may show little signs or symptoms for the first few days)
- Electricity (may have significant injury with very little damage to overlying skin)
- Excess sun exposure (radiation)

RISK FACTORS

- Water heaters set too high.
- Workplace exposure to chemicals, electricity, or irradiation
- Young children and older adults with thin skin are more susceptible to injury.
- Carelessness with burning cigarettes: related to 18% of fatal fires in 2006
- Inadequate or faulty electrical wiring
- Lack of smoke detectors: Lacking or nonfunctioning smoke alarms are implicated in 63% of residential fires.
- Arson: cause of 12.4% of fires that resulted in fatalities in 2012
- Low socioeconomic status has been associated with an increased risk of unintentional injury and mortality.

GENERAL PREVENTION

Home safety education should be a key mechanism for injury prevention.

- Families educated on home safety were more likely to have safe hot water temperatures.
- Safety education results in more families having functioning smoke alarms and increased use of fireguards.

COMMONLY ASSOCIATED CONDITIONS

- Smoke inhalation syndrome
  - May involve thermal burn to respiratory mucosa (e.g., trachea, bronchi) as well as carbon monoxide inhalation
  - Occurs within 72 hours of burn
  - Should be suspected in all burns occurring in an enclosed space or exposure to explosions
- Cyanide toxicity: Consider smoke inhalation, especially from fires involving artificial items/fabrics.

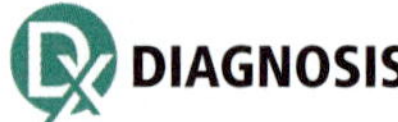

DIAGNOSIS

HISTORY

History of source of burn. In children or elderly: Check for consistency between the history and the burn's physical characteristics.

PHYSICAL EXAM

- Superficial: erythema of involved tissue, skin blanches with pressure; skin may be tender.
- Partial thickness: Skin is red and blistered; skin is very tender.
- Full thickness: Burned skin is tough and leathery; skin is nontender.
- Rule of 9s
  - Each upper extremity: adult and child 9%
  - Each lower extremity: adult 18%; child 14%
  - Anterior trunk: adult and child 18%
  - Posterior trunk: adult and child 18%
  - Head and neck: adult 10%; child 18%
- Quick estimate: The surface area of the patient's hand (palmar surface plus fingers) is 1% of the body surface area (BSA).
- Check for any signs suggestive of potential airway involvement, such as singed nasal hair, facial burns, carbonaceous sputum, progressive hoarseness, inflamed oropharynx, circumferential burns around the neck, or tachypnea.

DIAGNOSTIC TESTS & INTERPRETATION

- Children: glucose (hypoglycemia may occur in children because of limited glycogen storage)
- Smoke inhalation: arterial blood gas, carboxyhemoglobin
- Electrical burns: ECG, urine myoglobin, creatine kinase isoenzymes
- Electrolyte abnormalities may occur which can cause seizures or arrhythmias

Initial Tests (lab, imaging)

- Labs: hematocrit; type and screen; electrolytes, including BUN and creatinine; urinalysis
- Imaging: chest radiograph; xenon scan is useful in suspected smoke inhalation.

Diagnostic Procedures/Other

Bronchoscopy may be necessary for smoke inhalation to evaluate the lower respiratory tract.

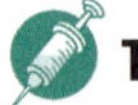

TREATMENT

- Prehospital care
  - Remove the patient from the source of the burn and extinguish and remove all burning clothing.
  - Room-temperature water may be poured onto the burn in the first 15 minutes following burn exposure.
  - Wrap the patient to prevent hypothermia.
  - All patients receive 100% oxygen via face mask
- Hospitalization for all severe burns
  - Partial-thickness burns >10% of BSA
  - Any full-thickness burn
  - Burns of hands, feet, face, or perineum
  - Electrical or lightning burns
  - Inhalation injury
  - Chemical burns
  - Circumferential burn
- Transfer to a burn center for
  - Partial- and full-thickness burns >10% of BSA in patients aged <10 years and >50 years of age
  - Partial-thickness burns >20% of BSA and full-thickness burns >5% BSA in any age range
  - Full-thickness burns in any age group
  - Burns of hands, feet, face, or perineum
  - Electrical or lightning burns
  - Inhalation injury
  - Chemical burns
  - Circumferential burn
  - Burns in patients with additional trauma (fractures, etc.) in which the burn is the more severe injury; otherwise, transfer to a trauma center for stabilization.
  - Burn injuries in patients with medical comorbidities that could affect management, mortality, or recovery (1)[A]

GENERAL MEASURES

- Based on depth of burns and accurate estimate of total BSA involved (rule of 9s)
- Tetanus prophylaxis (if not current)
- Remove all rings, watches, and other items from injured extremities to avoid tourniquet effect.
- Remove clothing and cover all burned areas with dry sheets.
- Flush area of chemical burn (for ~2 hours).
- For all major burns, use 100% oxygen administration; consider early intubation.
- Do not apply ice to burn site.
- Nasogastric tube (high risk of paralytic ileus)
- Foley catheter
- Analgesia
- ECG monitoring in the first 24 hours following electrical burn
- Daily or BID cleansing with dressing changes

- Burn fluid resuscitation
  - Calculate fluid resuscitation from the time of burn, not when treatment begins.
  - 2 to 4 mL of Ringer lactate × body weight (kg) × % total BSA burn (50% fluid given in first 8 hours, remaining 50% in the next 16 hours); in children, this is provided in addition to maintenance fluids and is adjusted according to urine output and vital signs. Protocol-based resuscitation leads to superior outcomes.
  - Colloid solutions are not recommended during the first 12 to 24 hours of resuscitation.
  - Other: Use of biologic membranes or skin substitutes may be indicated for burn coverage.
- Inhalation injury
  - Intubation and ventilation with positive end-expiratory pressure assistance. Employ lung protective ventilation strategies.
  - Hyperbaric oxygen treatment may be useful in patients with carbon monoxide levels >25% patients with coma, focal neurologic deficit or ischemic ECG changes, and pregnant patients.

MEDICATION

First Line

- IV morphine or hydromorphone for severe pain
- Oral analgesics, such as acetaminophen with codeine, acetaminophen with oxycodone, or acetaminophen with hydrocodone for moderate pain
- Neosporin or bacitracin ointment
- Use of silver sulfadiazine dressing has been shown to have poorer healing outcomes than alternative dressings (2)[A].
- Mupirocin: has potent inhibitory activity against methicillin-resistant *Staphylococcus aureus* (MRSA) (2)[A]
- Acticoat A.B. (a dressing consisting of two sheets of high-density polyethylene mesh coated with nanocrystalline silver) has a more controlled, prolonged release of silver, allowing less frequent dressing changes.
- Electrical burn with myoglobinuria will require alkalinization of urine and mannitol.
- Consider H_2 blockers (e.g., famotidine) or proton pump inhibitors (e.g., lansoprazole, pantoprazole) for stress ulcer prophylaxis in severely burned patients.
- Tetanus toxoid/tetanus immunoglobulin
- There is no clear indication for prophylactic systemic antibiotics.
- Use of negative pressure wound therapy may result in a low-protease environment with higher levels of angiogenic factor (vascular endothelial growth factor [VEGF]) during wound healing, leading to a more chaotic, hyperkeratinized, thickened epidermis when compared with a standard hydrocolloid dressing.
- Consider EMLA cream for small (<25 cm^2) burns in adults, as recent literature suggests it is safe and effective (3)[A].

Second Line

- Mafenide (Sulfamylon) for full-thickness burn, best against *Pseudomonas* (*caution*: metabolic acidosis, painful)
- Silver nitrate 0.5% (messy, leeches electrolytes from the burn, causes water toxicity)
- Povidone-iodine (Betadine) may result in iodine absorption from burn and "tan eschar," making débridement more difficult (2)[A].
- Travase (enzymatic débridement)

SURGERY/OTHER PROCEDURES

- Escharotomy may be necessary for constricting circumferential burns of extremities or chest due to compartment syndrome (1)[A].
- Tangential excision with split-thickness skin grafts: Early excision of burns results in a significant reduction in mortality (excluding patients with inhalational injury) and a significant decrease in hospital length of stay (1)[A].
- Various dressings (e.g., biosynthetic, biologic) are available to help reduce the number of dressing changes and promote healing (2)[A].

ONGOING CARE

FOLLOW-UP RECOMMENDATIONS

Early mobilization is the goal.

DIET

- High-protein, high-calorie diet when bowel function resumes
- Nasogastric tube feedings may be required in early postburn period.
- Total parenteral nutrition if NPO is expected for >5 days
- Early initiation of enteral nutrition in the first 24 hours of admission results in shorter intensive care unit (ICU) stays and lower wound infection rates.

PATIENT EDUCATION

- Use of sunscreen: Skin grafts or newly epithelialized skin are highly sensitive to sun exposure and thermal extremes.
- Isolate household chemicals.
- Household smoke detectors with particular emphasis on maintenance
- Family/household evacuation plan
- Proper storage and use of flammable substances

PROGNOSIS

- Superficial burn: complete resolution
- Partial-thickness burn: epithelialization in 10 to 14 days (deep partial-thickness burns probably will require skin graft)
- Full-thickness burn: no potential for reepithelialization; skin graft is required.
- Length of hospital stay and need for ICU care depends on extent of burn, smoke inhalation, comorbidities, and age.
- Burn size is correlated to complications; >60% total BSA burned in children and >40% in adults are at increased risk for mortality and morbidity.
- A 50% survival rate can be expected with a 62% burn rate in patients aged 0 to 14 years, 63% burn rate in patients aged 15 to 40 years, 38% burn rate in patients aged 40 to 65 years, and 25% burn rate in patients >65 years of age.
- 90% of survivors can be expected to return to an occupation comparable to their preburn employment.

COMPLICATIONS

- Gastroduodenal ulceration (Curling ulcer)
- Marjolin ulcer: malignant squamous cell carcinoma developing in old burn site
- Infection (discoloration, green fat, edema, eschar separation). Biopsy is the best to diagnose wound infection.
- Burn wound sepsis: most commonly *S. aureus* (including MRSA), vancomycin-resistant enterococci, and gram-negative organisms. Pneumonia.
- Decreased mobility with possibility of future flexion contractures. Hypertrophic scarring is common with burns.

REFERENCES

1. Miroshnychenko A, Kim K, Rochwerg B, et al. Comparison of early surgical intervention to delayed surgical intervention for treatment of thermal burns in adults: a systematic review and meta-analysis. *Burns Open*. 2021;5(2):67–77.
2. Jiang Q, Chen ZH, Wang SB, et al. Comparative effectiveness of different wound dressings for patients with partial-thickness burns: study protocol of a systematic review and a Bayesian framework network meta-analysis. *BMJ Open*. 2017;7(3):e013289.
3. Rangatchew F, Schoelzer L, Drzewiecki KT, et al. EMLA cream in burns: a systematic review of safety, analgesic efficacy, and effects on burn pathophysiology. *J Plast Reconstr Aesthet Surg*. 2024;95:386–401.

ADDITIONAL READING

- Jeschke MG, van Baar ME, Choudhry MA, et al. Burn injury. *Nat Rev Dis Primers*. 2020;6(1):11.
- Regan A, Hotwagner DT. *Burn Fluid Management*. National Library of Medicine. https://www.ncbi.nlm.nih.gov/books/NBK534227/. Accessed October 15, 2024.
- Roshangar L, Soleimani Rad J, Kheirjou R, et al. Skin burns: review of molecular mechanisms and therapeutic approaches. *Wounds*. 2019;31(12):308–315.

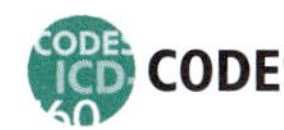

CODES

ICD10

- T23.029A Burn of unspecified degree of unspecified single finger (nail) except thumb, initial encounter
- T23.039A Burn of unspecified degree of unspecified multiple fingers (nail), not including thumb, initial encounter
- T23.079A Burn of unspecified degree of unspecified wrist, initial encounter

BURSITIS, PES ANSERINE (PES ANSERINE SYNDROME)

Jennifer Schwartz, MD

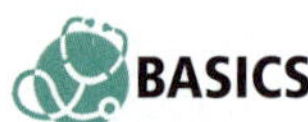

BASICS

DESCRIPTION

- The pes anserinus is the combined insertion of the sartorius, gracilis, and semitendinosus tendons on the anteromedial tibia. The sartorius, gracilis, and semitendinosus muscles help to flex the knee and protect against valgus and rotational stresses.
- The pes anserine bursa lies deep to the pes anserinus and the medial collateral ligament (MCL).
- *Pes anserine tendino-bursitis (PATB)* is due to irritation of the bursa and/or tendons in this area. Clinically, it is difficult to distinguish pes anserine tendonitis from pes anserine bursitis due to proximity of the structures.

ETIOLOGY AND PATHOPHYSIOLOGY

PATB is thought to occur due to the following:

- Excessive valgus and rotational stresses on the knee (due to overuse or underlying biomechanical factors)
- Degenerative changes
- Direct trauma

RISK FACTORS

- More common in middle age, overweight females
- Other risk factors include the following:
  - Pes planus; genu valgum
  - Long distance/hill running, cycling, swimming ("breaststroker's knee")
  - Sports with side-to-side/cutting activity (soccer, basketball, racquet sports)

GENERAL PREVENTION

- Avoid repetitive valgus/rotational stresses to the knee and treat underlying biomechanical risk factors
- Control weight
- Adequate hamstring stretching

COMMONLY ASSOCIATED CONDITIONS

- Osteoarthritis (OA)—always think about concurrent PATB in patients with OA.
  - Increased incidence of PATB in patients with symptomatic OA; PATB commonly contributes to knee pain in patients with OA.
  - Higher grades of OA are associated with a thicker pes anserine bursa and a larger area of bursitis.
- Medial meniscal tear
- Type II diabetes, rheumatoid arthritis, gout (chronic PATB)

DIAGNOSIS

Largely a clinical diagnosis (although sensitivity and specificity of clinical findings may be low and PATB can be confused with other medial sided knee pathologies) (1)[C]

HISTORY

- Medial knee pain at the pes anserine insertion
  - Pain is located 4 to 6 cm below the medial joint line on the anteromedial aspect of the tibia.
- Pain is exacerbated by knee flexion:
  - Going up or down the stairs
  - Getting up out of a chair or from a sitting position
  - Sitting cross-legged

PHYSICAL EXAM

- Tenderness to palpation or localized swelling at the pes anserine insertion
  - Caution: many patients without PATB will have tenderness to deep palpation in this area. Be sure to examine both sides and correlate physical exam with history before making a diagnosis.
- Pain worsens with flexion of the knee against resistance.
- Findings that suggest an alternative diagnosis: joint effusion, tenderness directly over the joint line, locking of the knee, systemic signs such as fever

DIFFERENTIAL DIAGNOSIS

- Medial compartment OA
- MCL injury
- Medial meniscal injury
- Medial plica syndrome
- Tibial stress fracture
- Septic arthritis

DIAGNOSTIC TESTS & INTERPRETATION

Initial Tests (lab, imaging)

- Primarily a clinical diagnosis
- Lab work not indicated; imaging is not routinely indicated unless there is a concern for underlying bony injury/fracture, ligamentous injury, or meniscal tear.

Follow-Up Tests & Special Considerations

- X-ray
  - Can demonstrate underlying OA.
- Ultrasound (US)
  - Can demonstrate focal edema within the pes anserine bursa but this may not correlate with clinical findings
  - Many patients with a clinical diagnosis of PATB have no morphologic changes of the pes anserine complex on US.
- MRI: T2-weighted axial images are preferred.
  - May see fluid in the pes bursa on MRI in a subset of asymptomatic patients
  - No large studies have evaluated the correlation between a clinical diagnosis of PATB and radiographic evidence of pes anserine pathology on MRI.

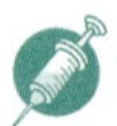

TREATMENT

- Pes anserine bursitis is often self-limited, but it can recur.
- Conservative therapy is preferred:
  - Relative rest and activity modification to avoid offending movements (especially knee flexion)
  - Ice to the affected area
  - NSAIDs for pain control
  - Physical therapy (PT) for knee strengthening and treatment of other underlying pathology
  - Kinesio taping
    - Kinesio taping can provide temporary relief of PATB pain.
    - One study found taping to be more effective than PT + Naprosyn to decrease pain from PATB.
  - Corticosteroid injection
    - Steroid injections and PT found to be equally effective for acute pain in PATB. Steroid injections may be preferred in some cases due to immediate results or risk of low PT compliance. However, symptom improvement from steroid injection alone may be less sustained than those from PT (2)[C].

- When considering intra-articular steroid injection for symptomatic OA, also consider steroid injection at the pes anserine bursa. In patients with OA, intra-articular injection alone may not be sufficient to control pain if there is also underlying PATB.
- Steroid injections may be superior to platelet-rich plasma (PRT)/extracorporeal shock wave therapy (ECSWT) in decreasing pain and improving function in PATB (and are often more accessible) and so are a better first-line procedural option (3)[C].

– ECSWT
  - ECSWT is also a safe and effective treatment for PATB. Data varies as to how ECSWT compares to other therapies for pain control. However, ECSWT may have a longer lasting effect and eventually lead to more consistent symptom improvement versus steroid injection

– PRP
  - May be an effective treatment for PATB.

– Weight loss to improve biomechanical forces at the knee.

MEDICATION

First Line

- NSAIDs: that is ibuprofen (800 mg PO TID) or naproxen (500 mg PO BID)
- Corticosteroid injection combined with local anesthetic:
  - Inject at the point of maximal tenderness using standard aseptic technique.
  - ~2 mL of anesthetic (i.e., 1% lidocaine) and 1 mL of steroid (i.e., 40 mg of methylprednisolone) are injected into the bursa using a small (e.g., 25-gauge, 1-inch) needle.
  - Insert needle perpendicular to the skin until bone is felt and then withdraw slightly before injecting.
  - Avoid injecting directly into the tendon.
- US-guided injection superior to blind injection

ADDITIONAL THERAPIES

- Hamstring and Achilles stretching
- Quadriceps and adductor strengthening

SURGERY/OTHER PROCEDURES

- No role for surgery in routine isolated cases
- Drainage or removal of bursa may be used in severe/refractory cases.

ONGOING CARE

Physical therapy with home exercise program focusing on flexibility and strengthening

DIET

Consider dietary changes as part of a comprehensive weight-loss program if obesity is a contributing factor.

PROGNOSIS

- Most cases of pes anserine syndrome respond to conservative therapy.
- Recurrence is common, and multiple treatments may be required.

REFERENCES

1. Atici A, Bahadir Ulger FE, Akpinar P, et al. Poor accuracy of clinical diagnosis in pes anserine tendinitis bursitis syndrome. *Indian J Orthop*. 2021;56(1):116–124.
2. Sarifakioglu B, Afsar SI, Yalbuzdag SA, et al. Comparison of the efficacy of physical therapy and corticosteroid injection in the treatment of pes anserine tendino-bursitis. *J Phys Ther Sci*. 2016;28(7):1993–1997.
3. Gouda W, Abbas AS, Abdel-Azis TM, et al. Comparing the efficacy of local corticosteroid, platelet-rich plasma, and extracorporeal shockwave therapy in the treatment of pes anserine bursitis: a prospective, randomized, comparative study. *Adv Orthop*. 2023;2023:5545520.

ADDITIONAL READING

- Alvarez-Nemegyei J. Risk factors for pes anserinus tendinitis/bursitis syndrome: a case control study. *J Clin Rheumatol*. 2007;13(2):63–65.
- Homayouni K, Foruzi S, Kalhori F. Effect of kinesio-taping versus non-steroidal anti-inflammatory drugs and physical therapy for treatment of pes anserinus tendino-bursitis: a randomized comparative clinical trial. *Phys Sportsmed*. 2016;44(3):252–256.
- Khosrawi S, Taneri P, Ketabi M. Investigating the effect of extracorporeal shock wave therapy on reducing chronic pain in patients with per anserine bursitis: a randomized, clinical-controlled trial. *Adv Biomed Res*. 2017;6:70.
- Luo WH, Li Y. Current evidence does support the use of KT to treat chronic knee pain in short term: a systematic review and meta-analysis. *Pain Res Manag*. 2021;2021:5516389.
- Majidi L, Saeb F, Alaei B, et al. Comparison of the effectiveness of local corticosteroid injection and extracorporeal shockwave therapy in patients with pes anserine bursitis: an open-label randomized clinical trial. *Med J Islam Repub Iran*. 2023;37:10.
- Rowicki K, Płomiński J, Bachta A. Evaluation of the effectiveness of platelet rich plasma in treatment of chronic pes anserinus pain syndrome. *Ortop Traumatol Rehabil*. 2014;16(3):307–318.

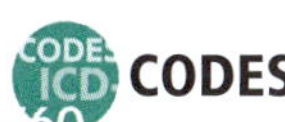

CODES

ICD10

M70.50 Other bursitis of knee, unspecified knee

CLINICAL PEARLS

- Consider pes anserine syndrome in patients presenting with medial knee pain, especially those with persistent symptoms associated with medial sided OA. Intra-articular injections for OA may not provide full relief if PATB is also present and contributing to symptomatology.
- Tenderness over the insertion of the pes anserine tendon on the medial aspect of the tibia 4 to 6 cm distal to the joint line is common in asymptomatic patients as well—correlation of the entire clinical picture is necessary for accurate diagnosis.
- Treatment is typically conservative and PT, NSAIDS, and/or kinesio taping can be helpful. A local steroid/anesthetic injection may also provide pain relief and enhance rehabilitation, but is often a more temporary option. Also consider ECSWT/PRP for refractory cases.

CANDIDIASIS, MUCOCUTANEOUS

Karlynn Sievers, MD • Tonya M. Cook, PharmD

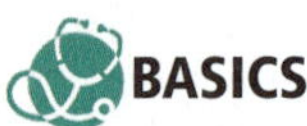

BASICS

DESCRIPTION

- Heterogeneous group of mucocutaneous infections with commensal *Candida* spp.
- Characterized by superficial infection of the skin, mucous membranes, and nails
- >20 *Candida* spp. cause infection in humans. *C. albicans* is responsible for 70% of fungal infections worldwide.
  - *C. auris* is an emerging global pathogen with a high propensity to develop drug resistance (1).
- Candidiasis affects:
  - Aerodigestive system
    - Oropharyngeal candidiasis (thrush): mouth, pharynx
    - Angular cheilitis: corner of the mouth
    - Esophageal candidiasis
    - Gastritis and/or ulcers, associated with thrush; alimental or perianal
  - Other systems
    - Candida vulvovaginitis: vaginal mucosa and/or vulvar skin
    - Candidal balanitis: glans of the penis
    - Candidal paronychia: nail bed or nail folds
    - Interdigital candidiasis: webs of the digits
    - Candidal diaper dermatitis and intertrigo (within skin folds)
- *Synonym(s): monilia; thrush; yeast; intertrigo*

ALERT
Vaginal antifungal creams and suppositories can weaken condoms and diaphragms.

Pregnancy Considerations

- Vaginal candidiasis is common during pregnancy—extend treatment (typically a full 7-day course).
- Vaginal yeast infection at birth increases the risk of newborn thrush but is of no overall harm to baby.

EPIDEMIOLOGY

- Common in the United States; particularly with immunodeficiency and/or uncontrolled diabetes
- Age considerations
  - Infants and seniors: thrush and cutaneous infections (infant diaper rash)
  - Women (prepubertal through postmenopausal): yeast vaginitis

Incidence

Unknown—mucocutaneous candidiasis is common in immunocompetent patients. Complication rates are low.

Prevalence

Candida spp. are normal flora of oral cavity, GI tract that are present in >70% of the U.S. population.

ETIOLOGY AND PATHOPHYSIOLOGY

C. albicans (responsible for 80–92% vulvovaginal and >80% of oral isolates); altered cell–mediated immunity against *Candida* spp. (either transient or chronic) increases susceptibility to infection.

Genetics

Chronic mucocutaneous candidiasis is a heterogeneous, genetic syndrome that typically presents in infancy.

RISK FACTORS

- Immune suppression (antineoplastic treatments, transplant patients, cellular immune defects, HIV/AIDS)
- Malignant diseases
- Corticosteroid use
- Smoking and alcoholism
- Hyposalivation (Sjögren disease, drug-induced xerostomia, radiotherapy)
- Broad-spectrum antibiotic therapy
- Douches, chemical irritants, birth control pills, intrauterine devices, and concurrent vaginitides
- Denture wear, poor oral hygiene
- Endocrine alterations (diabetes mellitus [DM], pregnancy, renal failure, hypothyroidism)
- Uncircumcised men at higher risk for balanitis

GENERAL PREVENTION

- Use antibiotics and steroids judiciously; rinse mouth after using inhaled steroids.
- Minimize perineal moisture (wear cotton underwear; frequent diaper changes; avoid douching).
- Clean dentures often; use well-fitting dentures and remove during sleep.
- Optimize glycemic control in diabetics.
- Preventive regimens during cancer treatments, especially in patients with hematologic malignancies
- Treat with HAART in HIV-infected patients; antifungal prophylaxis is not recommended unless HIV-infected adults have frequent or severe recurrences.

COMMONLY ASSOCIATED CONDITIONS

HIV, DM, cancer, and other immunosuppressive conditions

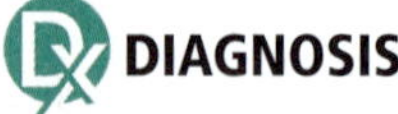

DIAGNOSIS

HISTORY

- Infants/children
  - Oral: adherent white patches on oral mucosae or on the tongue that do not wipe away easily
  - Perineal: erythematous rash with characteristic satellite lesions; painful if skin layer eroded
  - Angular cheilitis: painful fissures at mouth corners
- Adults
  - Vulvovaginal lesions; whitish "curd-like" discharge; pruritus; burning
  - Balanitis: erythema, erosions, scaling; dysuria
- Immunocompromised hosts
  - Oral: white, raised, painless, distinct patches; red, slightly raised patches/petechiae
  - Esophagitis: dysphagia, odynophagia, retrosternal pain; usually concomitant thrush
  - GI symptoms: abdominal pain
  - Folliculitis: follicular pustules

PHYSICAL EXAM

- Infants/children
  - Oral: white, raised, distinct patches within the mouth; when wiped off, reveals red base
  - Perineal: erythematous maculopapular rash with satellite pustules or papules
  - Angular cheilitis: tender fissures in mouth corners, often cracked and bleeding
- Adults
  - Vulvovaginal: thick, whitish, cottage cheese–like discharge; vagina or perineum erythema
  - Balanitis: erythema, linear erosions, scaling
  - Interdigital: redness, excoriation at base and web spaces of fingers and/or toes, possible maceration
- Immunocompromised hosts
  - Oral: white, raised, nontender, distinct patches; red, slightly raised patches; thick, dark-brownish coating; deep fissures
  - Esophagitis: Often, oral thrush is visible.
  - Folliculitis: follicular pustules

DIFFERENTIAL DIAGNOSIS

- For oral candidiasis, consider leukoplakia; lichen planus; geographic tongue; herpes simplex; erythema multiforme; pemphigus, burning mouth syndrome
- Baby formula or breast milk can mimic thrush—easier to remove than thrush.
- Hairy leukoplakia: does not rub off; dorsum and lateral margins of tongue
- Angular cheilitis from vitamin B or iron deficiency, staphylococcal infection, or edentulous overclosure
- Bacterial vaginosis and *Trichomonas vaginalis* tend to have more odor, itch, and a different discharge.

DIAGNOSTIC TESTS & INTERPRETATION

Initial Tests (lab, imaging)

- 10% KOH slide preparation: mycelia (hyphae) or pseudomycelia (pseudohyphae) yeast forms
- Associated with normal vaginal pH (<4.5)

Diagnostic Procedures/Other

- If first-line treatment fails, obtain samples for culture.
- Esophagitis or hyperplastic candidiasis may require endoscopy with biopsy (if suspicious for cancer).

Test Interpretation

Biopsy: epithelial parakeratosis with polymorphonuclear leukocytes in superficial layers; periodic acid–Schiff staining reveals candidal hyphae.

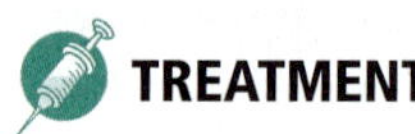

TREATMENT

GENERAL MEASURES

Screen for immunodeficiency (diabetes, HIV, autoimmune disease).

C

MEDICATION

First Line

- Vaginal (choose 1)
  - Miconazole (Monistat) 2% cream: one applicator or 200 mg (one suppository), intravaginally QHS for 7 days
  - Clotrimazole (Gyne-Lotrimin, Mycelex): intravaginal suppository (100 mg QHS for 7 days; 200 mg QHS for 3 days; 500 mg daily for 1 day) or 2% cream (one applicator QHS for 3 days)
  - Fluconazole 150 mg PO single dose
- Oropharyngeal
  - Mild disease
    - Clotrimazole (Mycelex): oral 10-mg troche; 20 minutes 5 times daily for 7 to 14 days
    - Nystatin suspension: 100,000 U/mL swish and swallow 400,000 to 600,000 U 4 times per day
    - Nystatin pastilles: 200,000 U each, QID daily for 7 to 14 days (1)
    - Denture wearers
      - Nystatin ointment: 100,000 U/g under denture and corners of mouth for 3 weeks
  - Moderate-to-severe disease
    - Fluconazole: 200 mg load and then 100 to 200 mg (>14 days of age: 6 mg/kg × 1 dose and then 3 mg/kg q24h × 7 to 14 days [max 100 mg/day])
- Esophagitis
  - Fluconazole: PO 400 mg load and then 200 to 400 mg/day for 14 to 21 days or IV 400 mg (6 mg/kg) daily
  - Alternative options are available if fluconazole is not tolerated; systemic antifungal therapy is always required (2).

Pregnancy Considerations

2% miconazole cream, intravaginally, for 7 days in uncomplicated candidiasis; systemic amphotericin B for invasive candidiasis

Second Line

- Vaginal
  - Topical antifungals, with no one preferred agent recommended (2)
  - Alternatively, fluconazole 150 mg in a single dose (2)
  - For recurrent cases (≥4 symptomatic episodes in 1 year): induction therapy with 10 to 14 days of topical or oral azole and then fluconazole 150 mg once per week for 6 months
    - In HIV patients: Concerns with this regimen include emergence of drug resistance.
- Oropharyngeal
  - Miconazole oral gel (20 mg/mL): QID, swish and swallow.
  - Itraconazole (Sporanox) suspension: 200 mg (20 mL) daily; swish and swallow for 7 to 14 days.
  - Posaconazole (Noxafil) oral suspension: 400 mg BID for 3 days and then 400 mg daily for up to 28 days
  - Amphotericin B (Fungizone) oral suspension (100 mg/mL): 1 mL QID daily, swish and swallow; use between meals.
- Esophagitis
  - Amphotericin B (variable dosing) IV dose of 0.3 to 0.7 mg/kg daily or an echinocandin should be used for patients who cannot tolerate oral therapy.
  - For refractory disease:
    - Could consider amphotericin B, itraconazole, posaconazole, voriconazole, isavuconazole (1)
  - Echinocandins (may be first choice in severe disease in patients with immunodeficiency) (1)
  - Several new agents are under investigation (1).
- Continue treatments for 2 days after infection gone:
  - Contraindications
    - Ketoconazole, itraconazole, or nystatin (if swallowed): severe hepatotoxicity
    - Amphotericin B: can cause nephrotoxicity
- Precautions
  - Miconazole: can potentiate the effect of warfarin but drug of choice in pregnancy
  - Fluconazole: renal excretion; rare, hepatotoxicity; resistance frequent
  - Posaconazole: can cause GI discomfort or QT prolongation (1)
  - Voriconazole: transient visual disturbances; clinical hepatitis, cholestasis, and fulminant liver failure (rare) (1)
- Possible interactions (rarely seen with topical treatment)
  - Fluconazole
    - Rifampin and tolbutamide: decreased fluconazole concentrations
    - Warfarin, phenytoin, cyclosporine: altered metabolism; check levels.
  - Itraconazole: potent CYP3A4 inhibitor; carefully assess all coadministered medications.

ISSUES FOR REFERRAL

- Evaluate patients with recurrent superficial candidal infections for immunodeficiency.
- GI candidiasis

ADDITIONAL THERAPIES

- For infants with thrush: Boil pacifiers and bottle nipples; assess mother's breasts/nipples for *Candida* infection.
- For denture-related candidiasis: Remove dentures at night. Disinfect dentures (using soak solution of white vinegar, 2% chlorhexidine gluconate solution, or 0.1% hypochlorite solution) and treat orally.

COMPLEMENTARY & ALTERNATIVE MEDICINE

Probiotics: *Lactobacillus* and *Bifidobacterium* may inhibit *Candida* spp.

ADMISSION, INPATIENT, AND NURSING CONSIDERATIONS

Proper oral hygiene; protocols for brushing, denture care, and oral cavity moistening reduce oral candidiasis.

ONGOING CARE

FOLLOW-UP RECOMMENDATIONS

Patient Monitoring

Immunocompromised persons benefit from regular evaluation and screening.

DIET

Active culture yogurt or other live lactobacillus may decrease colonization; indeterminate evidence

PATIENT EDUCATION

- Advise patients at risk for recurrence about potential for overgrowth with antibacterial therapy.
- Oral "azole" medications should be avoided in the 1st trimester. Thereafter, only give orally when benefits outweigh risks.

PROGNOSIS

Benign prognosis in immunocompetent patients; may have significant morbidity in immunosuppressed persons

COMPLICATIONS

In HIV patients, moderate immunosuppression (e.g., CD4 200 to 500 cells/mm^3) may be associated with chronic candidiasis. With more severe immunosuppression (e.g., CD4 <100 cells/mm^3), esophagitis or systemic fungal infections are possible.

REFERENCES

1. Cinicola BL, Uva A, Duse M, et al. Mucocutaneous candidiasis: insights into the diagnosis and treatment. *Pediatr Infect Dis J*. 2024;43(7):694–703. doi:10.1097/INF.0000000000004321.
2. Lu H, Hong T, Jiang Y, et al. Candidiasis: from cutaneous to systemic, new perspectives of potential targets and therapeutic strategies. *Adv Drug Deliv Rev*. 2023;199:114960. doi:10.1016/j.addr.2023.114960.

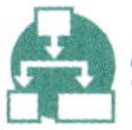

SEE ALSO

Candidiasis, Invasive; HIV/AIDS

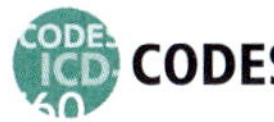

CODES

ICD10

- B37.9 Candidiasis, unspecified
- B37.2 Candidiasis of skin and nail
- B37.89 Other sites of candidiasis

CLINICAL PEARLS

- Candidiasis is typically a clinical diagnosis. KOH preparations are a simple confirmatory office test. Culture and biopsy are rarely needed.
- Person-to-person transmission is rare.
- Obtain a biopsy if there is concern for oral cancer.
- Oral antifungal medications are hepatically metabolized and may have serious side effects.

CANNABIS USE DISORDER

Ulunma Natalie Umesi, MD, MBA • Stanley Nkemjika, MD, MPH

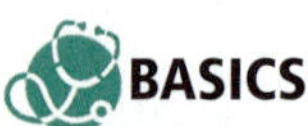

BASICS

DESCRIPTION

- Cannabis use leading to clinically significant impairment or distress, manifested by ≥2 of the following symptoms within a 12-month period:
  - Consumption of larger amounts over a longer period of time than intended
  - Persistent desire or inability to cut down or control amount used
  - Inordinate amount of time spent in activities is necessary to obtain, use, or recover from use.
  - Presence of craving for cannabis
  - Recurrent use resulting in failure to fulfill major role obligations at work, school, or home
  - Continued use despite having persistent or recurrent social or interpersonal problems due to cannabis use
  - Important social, occupational, or recreational activities are given up or reduced.
  - Recurrent use in physically hazardous situations
  - Continued use despite knowledge of a persistent physical or psychological problem caused or exacerbated by cannabis
  - Tolerance defined by using increased amounts of cannabis to achieve the desired effect or intoxication or diminished effect with continued use of the same amount
  - Withdrawal occurs following cessation of prolonged use, and has at least three behavioral symptoms such as anxiety, restlessness, depression, irritability, insomnia, odd dreams, or physical symptoms such as tremors and/or decreased appetite.
- According to *DSM-5-TR*, cannabis use disorder (CUD) is defined as being mild, moderate, or severe based on presenting symptoms; mild: 2 to 3; moderate: 4 to 5; severe: ≥6

EPIDEMIOLOGY

- The WHO ranks the United States first among 17 European and North American countries for prevalence of cannabis use.
- It is estimated that 4.5 to 7.0 million persons in the United States meet criteria for CUD.
- Chronic pain remains the most common reason for medical cannabis licensure. 10–30% of lifetime cannabis users meet criteria for CUD
- Cannabis-associated psychosis is associated with high-potency cannabis.
- >90% of Americans approve of cannabis for medical use.
- Carriers of the AKT1 gene is associated with developing psychosis with use of cannabis

Incidence

Around 17.7 million adults reported daily or near-daily cannabis use in 2022. (This surpasses the number of daily alcohol users (~14.7 million).

Prevalence

- Lifetime prevalence: As of 2019, approximately 46% of U.S. adults report having used cannabis at least once in their life
- Prevalence in North America (2015): Estimated 11.6% of the population were recent (past year) cannabis users, totaling about 36.7 million people

Gene	Function	Association with CUD
CHRNA2	Nicotinic receptor subunit	Genome-wide association study data support
CADM2	Risk behavior, synaptic function	Linked to impulsivity and cannabis use
FOXP2	Brain development, language	Inconsistent association with CUD
ANKK1/DRD2	Dopamine signaling	Involved in reward and addiction risk
CNR1	Cannabinoid receptor (CB1)	Direct link to THC effects
ARID1B	Neurodevelopmental processes	Rare variants linked to CUD

- Global prevalence (2013): 128 to 232 million people aged 15 to 65 years used cannabis—equating to 2.7–4.9% of the global population.
- Meta-analysis across 33 countries (2000 to 2024) demonstrated that in legalized countries, pooled cannabis-use prevalence ~12% (95% CI: 10–14.3%). In non-legalized countries, cannabis-use prevalence was lower, at ~5.4% (95% CI: 4.3–6.9%)

ETIOLOGY AND PATHOPHYSIOLOGY

- The two most known therapeutically active cannabinoids in cannabis are δ9-tetrahydrocannabinol (THC) and cannabidiol (CBD).
- THC is the psychoactive component responsible for cannabis' analgesic, antiemetic, and intoxicating properties. THC concentrations in cannabis have risen over the past 20 years from 4% to 20%. Additionally, high concentration oils and resins are used to increase THC potency.
- CBD is the nonpsychoactive component responsible for the perceived and experienced antianxiety, antidepressant, antipsychotic, antispastic, anticonvulsant, and antineoplastic properties of cannabis.
- Strains of cannabis vary, with varying THC/CBD ratios
- Smoking cannabis results in 25–50% absorption of THC, which rapidly passes into the circulation. The oral bioavailability of THC is much less (3–10%). Effects of smoked cannabis occur within minutes and last several hours; effects from cannabis consumed in foods or beverages appear more slowly, taking 30 minutes to 2 hours to have an effect.
- Only 5% of those with CUD seek treatment from a health care provider.

Genetics

Studies have identified specific genetic variants associated with an increased risk of developing CUD

RISK FACTORS

- Individuals 18- to 29-year-olds, are at more risk for severe CUD.
- Higher potency cannabis use increases risk of CUD and increases severity of symptoms.
- Frequency of use affects risk of CUD; monthly users are at 4-fold increased risk, weekly users at 8-fold and daily users at 17-fold increased risk
- Family history of chemical dependence, comorbid psychiatric disorders, other substance use (i.e., alcohol, tobacco). Lower educational achievement (rates of dependence are lowest among college graduates); low socioeconomic status and ease of acquisition of cannabis and synthetic versions of cannabis
- Among youths with mood disorders, CUD is a risk marker for nonfatal self-harm, all-cause mortality, and death by unintentional overdose and homicide.

COMMONLY ASSOCIATED CONDITIONS

- Mood disorders
- Anxiety disorders
- Cannabis hyperemesis syndrome (CHS)

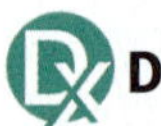

DIAGNOSIS

- Ask for frequency and amount used (e.g., "How often do you use cannabis? Daily? Weekly?"; "How long does a typical 'eighth' [1/8 oz] last?").
- Usage is quantified as: occasional = 1/8 oz/week, moderate = 1/4 oz/week, heavy = 1/2 oz/week. (1 oz = 28.5 g which is equivalent to about 50 to 60 cigarettes).
- Unexplained deterioration in school or work performance is an indicator of potential abuse, particularly in young people.
- Changes, problems, or dissolution of social relationships or engagement with previously enjoyed recreational activities (outside those related to cannabis use) may also indicate problematic use
- If possible, obtain collateral history from close contacts

HISTORY

- Clinical presentation of acute intoxication:
  - Euphoria, elation, laughter, heightened sensory perception, altered perception of time, increased appetite
  - Poor short-term memory, concentration
  - Fatigue, depression
  - Occasionally, distrust, fear, anxiety, panic
  - With large doses, acute psychosis: delusions, hallucinations, loss of sense of identity
- Withdrawal symptoms:
  - Irritability; anxiety, restlessness, nausea; weight loss; decreased appetite
  - Insomnia; depressed mood, tremors

PHYSICAL EXAM

- Evaluate for:
  - Conjunctival injection; xerostomia; nystagmus; increased heart rate
  - Decreased coordination; altered mental status
- Withdrawal findings (nonspecific-similar to other drugs of abuse) include:
  - Restlessness/agitation; irritability; tremor; diaphoresis
  - Increased body temperature

DIAGNOSTIC TESTS & INTERPRETATION

Cannabinoids can be detected in urine weeks to months after chronic cannabis use. Blood testing is preferred for interpreting acute effects and levels. In the United States, there is no consensus for acceptable legal limits for cannabis levels while driving. Hair testing can be unreliable and may reflect second-hand exposure. In general, testing identifies cannabis use (not necessarily CUD).

Initial Tests (lab, imaging)

- Standard urine toxicology (UTox) typically includes cannabis
  - Synthetic cannabis (i.e., k2) may need to be specially ordered.
- Chronic exposure to cannabis use (in adolescents) has shown a dose-dependent association with prefrontal cortex thinning.

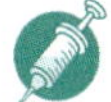

TREATMENT

- There are no FDA-approved medications for the treatment of CUD. There is insufficient evidence to recommend for or against pharmacotherapy for CUD. CBD is a promising candidate for CUD treatment (1).
- Behavioral interventions for initial treatment:
  - Cognitive-behavioral therapy (CBT) and motivational enhancement therapy (MET) are generally first-line, often augmented by contingency management planning.
  - Social network behavior therapy; 12-step approach; family-oriented therapy
  - Brief intervention; relapse prevention; community reinforcement approach
- Treating co-occurring behavioral health disorders may help reduce use.
- To help manage withdrawal:
  - Reduce amount used before quitting entirely. Delay first use of cannabis until later in the day.
  - Consider nicotine replacement therapy if concomitant tobacco use is present. Avoid cues and triggers associated with use.
- With marked irritability and restlessness, consider very low-dose diazepam for 3 to 4 days.
- Provide individual and immediate support network with information regarding problematic use, misuse, addiction, and withdrawal.
- Withdrawal symptoms peak on day 2 or 3; generally subside by day 7. Vivid dreams can continue for 2 to 3 weeks.

MEDICATION

- No effective medication is currently approved to specifically treat cannabis intoxication or cannabis misuse.
- A recent review of medication options for treatment of CUD concluded that
  - SSRI (low strength evidence—did not reduce cannabis use or assist with cravings); antipsychotics (insufficient evidence for benefit); anxiolytics (low-strength evidence that buspirone has no benefit over placebo); mood stabilizers (insufficient evidence for any benefit)
  - Gabapentin (insufficient evidence) was not helpful in management.
- Oral FDA-approved cannabinoids such as dronabinol or nabiximol may help abate cannabis withdrawal symptoms.
- Options to assist with cravings include naltrexone 50 mg PO daily or N-Acetylcysteine 1,200 mg PO TID.
- Treatment of withdrawal is targeted towards symptom management such as anxiety, insomnia, and nausea.

ISSUES FOR REFERRAL

There is potential for co-occurring substance use disorders with varying severity regarding withdrawal.

ADMISSION, INPATIENT, AND NURSING CONSIDERATIONS

THC use is not considered a significant cause of respiratory depression. However, cross-contamination with substances leading to respiratory depression should be considered during an admission/inpatient evaluation.

ONGOING CARE

FOLLOW-UP RECOMMENDATIONS

- Monitor cessation by testing urine over several weeks for the inactive cannabis metabolites (carboxy-THC).
- Drug screening of heavy smokers may remain positive for cannabis up to 6 weeks after last use.

PATIENT EDUCATION

- National Institute on Drug Abuse (NIDA): http://www.drugabuse.gov
- Substance Abuse and Mental Health Services Administration: https://www.samhsa.gov
- National Institutes of Health: https://www.ncbi.nlm.nih.gov

COMPLICATIONS

- Acute adverse effects:
  - Acute panic or paranoid reactions can occur, especially in drug-naive individuals or those with a history of psychosis or other behavioral health conditions.
  - Cannabis use is an independent risk factor for heart failure.
  - In states where cannabis has been legalized there has been an increase in ED visits for acute myocardial infarction.
  - Psychotic symptoms with high-doses/high-potency use have been observed.
  - Driving under the influence of cannabis increases the risk for motor vehicle accidents.
  - Adverse long-term effects on cognitive dysfunction and increased risk of stroke
- Chronic adverse effects:
  - Abnormal brain development; diminished lifetime achievement
  - Chronic bronchitis and impaired respiratory function in regular smokers
  - Cannabis use is associated with an increased risk of fibrosis in hepatitis C patients.
  - Cannabis may contribute to or result in pancreatitis.
  - CHS is characterized by episodes of cyclic nausea and vomiting in association with chronic cannabis use; symptoms may start at any point during cannabis use, even months/years after onset of use.

REFERENCES

1. Shah K, Farwa UE, Vanaparti A, et al. Global epidemiology of cannabis use disorders and its trend from 1990 to 2019: benchmarking analysis of the global burden of disease study. *J Family Med Prim Care*. 2024;13(3):881–889. doi:10.4103/jfmpc.jfmpc_824_23.

ADDITIONAL READING

Gorelick DA. Cannabis-related disorders and toxic effects. *N Engl J Med*. 2023;389(24):2267–2275. doi:10.1056/NEJMra2212152.

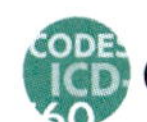

CODES

ICD10

- F12.10 Cannabis abuse, uncomplicated
- F12.20 Cannabis dependence, uncomplicated
- F12.288 Cannabis dependence with other cannabis-induced disorder

CLINICAL PEARLS

- It is estimated that 4.5 to 7 million persons in the United States meet criteria for CUD.
- Acute cannabis intoxication is manifested by conjunctival injection, increased heart rate, euphoria, heightened sensory perception, altered perception of time, increased appetite, poor short-term memory and concentration, and fatigue. Large doses/high-potency use may result in acute psychosis, panic or paranoid reactions, delusions, or hallucinations.
- Withdrawal symptoms include weight loss, decreased appetite, insomnia, and depressed mood. These symptoms peak on day 2 or 3 and resolve by day 7.
- Treatment of withdrawal is targeted towards symptom management
- CBT, motivational interviewing, MET, and contingency management are four behavioral interventions with the best evidence for efficacy in treating CUD.

CAPACITY (COMPETENCE) DETERMINATION AND INFORMED CONSENT

Jessica A. Orner, MD

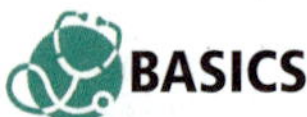

BASICS

- Personal autonomy in decision-making is a fundamental personal freedom.
- Capacity determination is an inherent element of the informed consent process.
- It is universally presumed that patients 18 years old and older (or an emancipated minor under individual state laws) have legal and clinical capacity to give informed consent for health care testing, interventions, and treatment or to refuse the same no matter the harm or benefit until proven otherwise.

DESCRIPTION

- Capacity:
  - Involves a clinical evaluation by a credentialed health care provider
  - Focuses on perceived ability of patient to participate and understand the process of informed consent
- Competence:
  - A legal determination of abilities, performed by a court judge
  - Refers executive functioning and ability to make decisions (i.e., finances, living wills)
    - Involves medical information but does not need to be limited to only medical issues
- *Capacity* is the currently preferred term to competence: legal capacity and medical capacity.
- A capacity determination is needed when arriving at a health care decision for testing, treatment, or an intervention involving risk of harm or no improvement.
  - Any treating health care provider can evaluate capacity, including the provider also obtaining informed consent (although a psychiatrist or neuropsychiatric consultant is often asked to weigh in, other health care providers can determine capacity).
- Medical capacity is determined by four elements:
  - Understanding risks and benefits of a procedure as well as alternatives
  - Appreciating those risks/benefits
  - Reasoning to make an informed decision
  - Communicating those informed decisions
    - Interviews with a guardian or designated health care power of attorney (POA) (if indicated)
- The four "Cs" of capacity are:
  - Context: comprehension of their health status
  - Choices: able to describe options
  - Consequences: able to explain possible outcomes
  - Consistency: continuity of choice selection
- Adequate cognition is a fundamental component but not the sole determinant of capacity (1).

EPIDEMIOLOGY

Most adults in the United States do not have an advanced directive—population studies show approximately 1/3 have completed an advanced directive (2).

Incidence

Need for capacity determination has been increased due to:

- Increasingly older population
- Prolonged chronic disease states
- Better patient rehabilitation opportunities
- Safer anesthetics and advanced postsurgery care

Prevalence

Prevalence varies based on the patient risk factors (pretest probability) and physician experience:

- ~3% of healthy outpatient seniors lack capacity.
- Highest rate of incapacity (68%) is in learning disabled patients.

ETIOLOGY AND PATHOPHYSIOLOGY

- Dementia is the most common reason individuals are found incapable of making health care decisions in the outpatient setting.
- Capacity is a dynamic state; reassessment is necessary with each significant health care decision and informed consent.

RISK FACTORS

- For incapacity:
  - Longevity, multiple comorbidities, hospitalized for medical reasons
  - Never married, never worked outside home
- Insufficient informed consent:
  - Patient factors:
    - Health illiteracy
    - Education level
    - Excessive information
  - Provider factors:
    - Inexperience with process (house staff for example)
    - Insufficient discussion time

GENERAL PREVENTION

Early assessment and periodic reassessment of capacity in:

- Dynamic patient conditions, like electrolyte imbalance, closed head injuries, delirium states
- After procedures with anesthesia or analgesics
- Enhancement and dissipation of mind-altering substances

COMMONLY ASSOCIATED CONDITIONS

- Dementia/Alzheimer disease, Parkinson disease, and traumatic brain injury
- Schizophrenia, depression, and substance abuse
- Acute illness, metabolic derangement

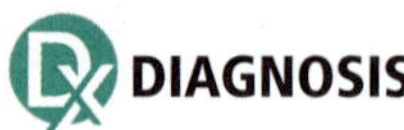

DIAGNOSIS

In patients without capacity, physicians are unable or unwilling to recognize the incapacity 42% of the cases (1)[C].

HISTORY

Family or frequent observers are resources regarding behavior patterns and reasoning displayed by patients.

- Engage in a deliberate approach, initially assessing for:
  - Communication barriers: physical impairments, lack of language fluency, medical jargon
  - Reversible causes of incapacity: metabolic derangements, medication side effects, serious illness, delirium
  - Health belief system; cultural differences; religious, political viewpoints, or adverse historical events

PHYSICAL EXAM

Verbal patient responses, facial expression, and body language can inform capacity assessment or suggest "warning signs" to obtain more formal evaluation.

DIAGNOSTIC TESTS & INTERPRETATION

Initial Tests (lab, imaging)

Screening for capacity occurs with:

- Informal patient conversations
- Discussions inherent to medical history taking
- Informed consent discussions

Follow-Up Tests & Special Considerations

- Four common tools for the formal evaluation of capacity
  - MacArthur Competence Assessment Tool-Treatment (MacCAT-T)—gold standard
    - Assesses: understanding, reasoning, appreciation, expression of choice
    - Semi-structured interview, 20 minutes
  - Aid to capacity evaluation (ACE)
    - Semi-structured interview, 7 questions
    - Found predictive for medical and psychiatric patients, except for schizophrenic patients (3)[A]
  - Assessment of Capacity for Everyday Decision-Making (ACED)
    - Semi-structured interview
    - Used with cognitively impaired seniors to measure capacity to perform independent activities of daily living
  - Capacity assessment tool (CAT)
    - Structured interview
    - Assesses capacity to discern between two intervention choices
- Special situation/considerations for assessment of capacity for informed consent
  - Communication impairments
    - Availability of translators of all languages, including for deaf/mute and blind combined with deafness
    - Health literacy level accommodation
  - Patient participation in research or experimental intervention protocols
  - Patient refusal to participate in informed consent
  - Child or adolescent as patient

Diagnostic Procedures/Other

Cognitive screening (e.g., Mini-Mental State Examination and Montreal Cognitive Assessment) can contribute to (but not substitute for) capacity determination.

Test Interpretation

Capacity definition is state specific, but all incorporate the four elements. Capacity determination in the informed consent process is determined by the treating provider (1)[C].

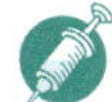

TREATMENT

GENERAL MEASURES

Steps to take if a patient fails to have capacity or fails to display ability to participate in informed consent:

- Determine the acuity of the need for decision making (e.g., decisions regarding emergency care—"loss of life or limb"—are made by treating provider).
- Correct any reversible causes of impaired capacity (e.g., electrolyte rebalance or language translation).
- Reframe questions that help determine capacity or simplify explanation in informed consent.
- Find and use the advanced directive or reach out to health care POA to help guide patient's medical decisions and wishes.
- Seek out next of kin to become a proxy decision maker with understanding of patient's values.
- Court-appointed guardian process is lengthy and usually is not necessary.

ISSUES FOR REFERRAL

Specialist consultation is not usually necessary to determine capacity for medical decision-making. As indicated, consider consulting with the following expert services: psychiatry, neuropsychiatry, medical ethics, health care attorney.

ADMISSION, INPATIENT, AND NURSING CONSIDERATIONS

~16% ICU patients do not have a medical POA or default surrogate decision maker.

- Court can appoint a fiduciary.

ONGOING CARE

The following, in rank order, have responsibility for medical decision-making/informed consent if patient lacks capacity:

- Spouse (unless legally separated)
- Adult child
- A parent
- An adult sibling
- An adult who has provided unique care and has a special knowledge of the patient values and is accessible

FOLLOW-UP RECOMMENDATIONS

- Reassessment of patient's capacity is a provider responsibility:
  - At each significant medical decision point
  - If the patient shows signs of change in capacity
- If capacity is uncertain, the final decision should favor the patient.

REFERENCES

1. Barstow C, Shahan B, Roberts M. Evaluating medical decision-making capacity in practice. *Am Fam Physician*. 2018;98(1):40–46.
2. Yadav KN, Gabler NB, Cooney E, et al. Approximately one in three US adults completes any type of advance directives for end-of-life care. *Health Aff (Millwood)*. 2017;36(7):1244–1251.
3. Downey VA, Zun L. Who has the ability to consent? *Prim Care Companion CNS Disord*. 2020;22(4):20m02619.

CLINICAL PEARLS

- Use a structured approach in assessing decision-making capacity, including an assessment of language barriers, identification and remediation of reversible causes of incapacity, and a comprehensive interview to assess the ability to consent. Include appropriate formal assessment tools.
- Capacity is dynamic. Reassess at new (or changing) significant health care decision/informed consent points.
- The order of succession for decision-making is spouse, adult child, parent, adult sibling, adult with close relationship.
- Integrate formal assessment with individual patient context to determine capacity.

CARBON MONOXIDE POISONING

Beth A. Wichowski, DO

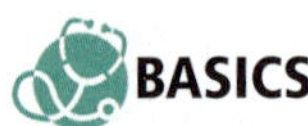

BASICS

DESCRIPTION

Carbon monoxide (CO) is an odorless, tasteless, colorless gas produced during the incomplete combustion of carbon-based compounds. If inhaled, CO may cause nonspecific symptoms and is potentially fatal (1).

- CO inhalation leads to displacement of oxygen (O_2) from binding sites on hemoglobin to form carboxyhemoglobin (COHb). The formation of COHb leads to tissue hypoxia from decreased O_2 carrying capacity and a left shift of the oxyhemoglobin dissociation curve (resulting in less O_2 delivery to a tissue at a given arterial O_2 pressure). CO binds to mitochondrial cytochrome oxidase, impairing adenosine triphosphate (ATP) production. It also binds to myoglobin, resulting in decreased contractility and vascular smooth muscle relaxation.

Pregnancy Considerations

Tissue hypoxia due to CO poisoning may cause significant fetal abnormalities because CO has a stronger affinity and a longer half-life when bound to fetal hemoglobin. The fetus is therefore susceptible to adverse outcomes even if the mother is unaffected.

EPIDEMIOLOGY

Incidence

- CO poisoning is the third leading cause of poisoning death in the United States. There are approximately 500 deaths annually from CO poisoning.
- Accounts for 50,000 ER visits annually (16 cases per 100,000 population); 1–3% are fatal
- Approximately 15,000 intentional poisoning occur per year, accounting for 2/3 reported deaths (10-fold higher than unintentional poisonings); results in approximately 1,200 to 1,600 deaths a year in the United States due to fire and non-fire related poisoning
- Vague symptoms may cause patients to not seek care, leading to underdiagnosis.
- May have concurrent co-exposures such as cyanide poisoning or intoxicants

Prevalence

- More prevalent during the winter months in areas with colder climate.
- Environmental CO exposure is usually <10 parts per million (ppm).
  - Tobacco users can increase exposure to 400 to 500 ppm while actively smoking.
  - After using a gas stove, indoor concentrations may reach 100 ppm.
  - Gas powered generators in an enclosed garage can reach 1,000 ppm in 15 minutes.
  - 4 hours of exposure to 70 ppm can result in a CO concentration of 10% and 350 ppm over 4 hours can result in a concentration of 40%.
- Occupational exposure to methylene chloride, found in industrial solvents such as paint remover, is metabolized to CO in the liver and can result in exposure and toxicity.

ETIOLOGY AND PATHOPHYSIOLOGY

- CO is rapidly absorbed through the lungs, binding hemoglobin with 210 to 240 times the affinity of O_2. This stabilizes hemoglobin in the relaxed high affinity state (R state), reducing O_2-carrying capacity and delivery, leading to left shift of the oxyhemoglobin dissociation curve. CO inactivates cytochrome oxidase. This leads to decreased ATP production, especially in tissues with high metabolic demands (brain, heart). The electron transport chain continues, generating superoxide radicals, leading to further damage.
- CO also causes direct cellular toxicity as well as generating reactive O_2 species and oxidative stress.
- Direct CO toxicity results from CO binding to myoglobin resulting in myocardial and skeletal muscle dysfunction as well as binding to guanylate cyclase that results in cerebral vasodilation and syncope.
- CO displaces nitric oxide (NO) from platelets, leading to platelet activation and aggregation. Oxidative stress, lipid peroxidation, and apoptosis are additional effects. NO also causes vasodilation and profound hypotension.
- Mitochondrial dysfunction and hypoxia lead to myocardial stunning and injury. Proteases released from neutrophil degranulation interact with xanthine hydrogenase forming xanthine oxidase. This inhibits endogenous defense against oxidative stress.
- CO also initiates an inflammatory cascade that can lead to oxidative degradation of nervous system lipids and delayed neurologic damage.

RISK FACTORS

- Intentional exposure (suicide gesture)
- Patients at extremes of age (particularly with underlying cardiovascular or neurologic disease)
- Patients with severe COPD regardless of current tobacco smoke exposure; closed or improperly ventilated spaces
- Fires and fire-related injuries; high-risk vocations: coal miners, auto mechanics, paint stripping, work in the solvent industry; exposure to exhaust from motor vehicles, faulty furnaces, stoves, generator use (power outages and storms), and other fuel burning devices

GENERAL PREVENTION

- Appropriate ventilation around fuel-burning cooking stoves; installation of in-home CO monitors or alarms
- Post-exposure determination of CO source to limit future exposures, eliminate source, and initiate treatment
- Public policy to ensure building code safety; limiting occupational exposures for those who work with automobiles, paint, solvents, or mines

COMMONLY ASSOCIATED CONDITIONS

- CO and cyanide poisoning often occur simultaneously after smoke inhalation and have synergistic effects.
- Intentional poisoning often occurs in the context of coingestion of other substances (~40%).
- Up to 50–75% of fire-related injuries have a component of CO poisoning.

DIAGNOSIS

- Clinical triad of (i) relevant symptoms, (ii) history of CO exposure, (iii) and elevated COHb levels (2)
- An elevated COHb level of >3% in a nonsmoker and >10% in smokers. People living in high pollution areas and heavy tobacco users may have higher levels at baseline (1).
- The COHb level does not correlate with the severity of the illness or long-term prognosis but is necessary for the diagnosis (2). Older pulse oximeters do not differentiate COHb from oxyhemoglobin, with normal oximeter readings in a hypoxic patient.

HISTORY

- The diagnosis of CO poisoning is dependent on duration and mechanism of exposure. No single symptom is sensitive or specific. A high index of suspicion is necessary.
- Common symptoms include
  - Headache (91% of patients), dizziness (77%) and weakness (53%) most common symptoms; confusions/impaired judgment (1)
  - Nausea/vomiting, fatigue, chest pain, and shortness of breath
- Patients may also present with visual disturbances, seizures, syncope, arrhythmias, rhabdomyolysis, and loss of consciousness.
- Some patients may present with cardiopulmonary symptoms such as chest pain, palpitations, or shortness of breath.
- Long-term (subacute) exposure is defined as >24 hours and occurs with repeated exposure to low concentrations of CO. Symptoms include chronic fatigue, emotional distress, memory deficits, difficulty working, sleep disturbances, vertigo, neuropathy, recurrent infections, polycythemia, paresthesia, abdominal pain, and diarrhea.
- Delayed neurologic symptoms can appear 2 to 40 days later and is a poorly defined syndrome with incidence of 1–47% after CO exposure and can be manifested with a wide variety of neurologic complications (3).
- Exclude pregnancy in all female patients.

PHYSICAL EXAM

- Pulse oximetry does not distinguish between oxygenated hemoglobin, deoxygenated hemoglobin, COHb, and methemoglobin. Therefore, patients exposed to CO must have COHb levels measured with a co-oximeter or blood gas analysis; respiratory depression or tachypnea, and cyanosis; tachycardia, hypotension, cardiac dysrhythmias (2)
- Patients often report confusion or have altered mental status.
- Classical "cherry red" skin coloring of lips and skin is rare (<1% of cases).
- Examine for signs of burns of the skin and oropharynx (enclosed space fires) or other secondary injuries.
- Confusion/CNS depression, ataxia, visual field defects, papilledema, and nystagmus

DIFFERENTIAL DIAGNOSIS

- Cyanide toxicity (co-existent); methylene chloride (dichloromethane) inhalation or ingestion
- Viral syndromes
- Behavioral and mental health disorders (major depressive disorder)
- Infections (meningitis or encephalitis); metabolic causes (hypoglycemia, electrolyte impairment)
- Alcohol intoxication, opiates, acetylsalicylic acid (ASA) overdose; trauma; CNS lesions; coingestion of other substance

DIAGNOSTIC TESTS & INTERPRETATION

Initial Tests (lab, imaging)

- Diagnosis requires a recent history of CO exposure, consistent symptoms, and demonstration of an elevated COHb level.
- Do not use noninvasive COHb measurement
- Arterial or venous blood gas:
  - COHb levels of >3% in nonsmokers, >10% in smokers; COHb may be low despite significant poisoning (e.g., treatment with O_2 or significant time elapses before the level is drawn)
  - Significant metabolic acidosis; anion gap >16; elevated lactate confers worse prognosis and should prompt consideration of cyanide toxicity; PaO_2 tends to be normal because O_2 dissolved in blood is not affected by CO.
- Serum chemistries, CBC, troponin, lactic acid, chest x-ray (CXR)
- ECG
- Cardiac enzymes in patients with moderate or severe poisoning
- Pregnancy test in all women of childbearing age
- Toxicology screen (particularly important in intentional poisoning); CK to evaluate for rhabdomyolysis
- Head CT/MRI scan can help to rule out other neurologic causes.

Follow-Up Tests & Special Considerations

- Consider CO poisoning in younger patients with chest pain or symptoms suggestive of ischemia.
- Consider the diagnosis in afebrile patients with vague or "flulike" symptoms. CO poisoning and the flu are both common during the winter time. Patients may present as a group (coworkers, family members, school children) with similar symptoms. Patients with intentional poisoning should undergo behavioral evaluation when stable.
- For diagnosis of delayed neurologic symptoms from CO exposure, consider MRI of brain and formal neuropsychiatric testing.

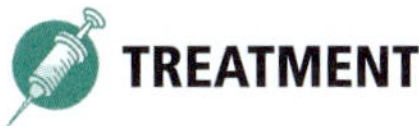

TREATMENT

GENERAL MEASURES

- Prompt removal from the CO source and initiation of O_2 therapy to displace CO.
- Supportive care as necessary; intubation and mechanical ventilation may be necessary for severe intoxication, particularly if the patient is unable to protect their airway or if there are signs of respiratory failure.
- Poison Control: 800-222-1222 (United States)

MEDICATION

First Line

100% O_2 via non-rebreathing reservoir facemask until COHb is normal (<3%) and patient is asymptomatic, regardless of O_2 saturation or PO_2

- CO has a half-life of 250 to 320 minutes in room air and this half-life is reduced to 90 minutes with O_2 therapy via a non-rebreather mask.
- Consider high-flow nasal cannula, especially in patients unable to tolerate non-rebreather facemask.
- Concurrent treatment of associated disorders such as cyanide poisoning, intentional overdose, etc.

Second Line

Hyperbaric oxygen (HBO_2) therapy (not always readily available); for severe poisoning (neurologic symptoms, high COHb) preferably within 6 hours

ADDITIONAL THERAPIES

- HBO_2 is associated with lower long- and short-term mortality rates and long-term neuropsychiatric symptoms, although criteria for starting therapy remains unclear.
- HBO_2 currently recommended for exposure >24 hours; CO levels >25% (>20% if pregnant); altered mental status; cardiovascular ischemia; severe acidosis; HBO_2 not as likely to be helpful if >24 hours since exposure; greatest benefit occurs if initiated as early as possible, goal is within 6 hours of exposure; however, American College of Medical Toxicology and American Academy of Clinical Toxicology have not published guidelines (1).
- Empirically treat patients for cyanide poisoning who present with CO poisoning from a house fire, if the pH is <7.2 or plasma lactate is >10 mmol/L (2).
- Expert consensus favors HBO_2 therapy for pregnant women.
- Locate a HBO_2 chamber in the United States through the Undersea and Hyperbaric Medical Society website (https://www.uhms.org) or via the Divers Alert Network Emergency Hotline (+1-919-684-9111).
- Estimated only 75 chambers available for high acuity emergency basis within the United States (3)

ADMISSION, INPATIENT, AND NURSING CONSIDERATIONS

- Patients whose symptoms do not improve after 4 to 5 hours of 100% O_2 should be transported to the nearest HBO_2 facility. Hospitalize patients with severe poisoning, ECG or laboratory evidence of end-organ damage, and those with concerning medical or social factors. Admit unconscious patients with CO poisoning to ICU following intubation.
- Patients with accidental poisoning and mild symptoms that resolve in the ED can be safely discharged.

ONGOING CARE

FOLLOW-UP RECOMMENDATIONS

- All patients treated for acute CO poisoning should follow up in 1 to 2 months after discharge (2).
- If there are behavioral or cognitive concerns, pursue neuropsychological evaluation, particularly following intentional CO poisoning. Long-term cognitive, psychiatric, speech, occupational, and physical rehab may be necessary.

Patient Monitoring

Repeat measurement of COHb levels with arterial blood gases.

PATIENT EDUCATION

- Professional installation and maintenance of combustion devices
- CO detector in bedrooms and by potential CO sources; consider proper ventilation in stoves that use natural gas in the household (4).
- Centers for Disease Control and Prevention: https://www.cdc.gov/carbon-monoxide/about/index.html

PROGNOSIS

Although most patients completely recover, chronic neuropsychiatric impairment is described in 12–68% of patients.

COMPLICATIONS

- High-activity metabolic tissues are at higher risk.
- Cardiac: myocardial ischemia/infarction; left ventricular dysfunction; dysrhythmia (prolonged QT)
- Pulmonary: inhalation injury; pulmonary edema; pneumonia; acute respiratory failure
- Neurologic: encephalopathy; vestibulomotor defects; hippocampal atrophy; cognitive dysfunction; Parkinsonism
- Behavioral: depression, anxiety, irritability, moodiness, violent behavior

Geriatric Considerations

Increased number of comorbid leading to possibility of complications and worse outcomes

REFERENCES

1. Chenoweth JA, Albertson TE, Greer MR. Carbon monoxide poisoning. *Crit Care Clin*. 2021:37(3):657–672.
2. Savioli G, Gri N, Ceresa IF, et al. Carbon monoxide poisoning: from occupational health to emergency medicine. *J Clin Med*. 2024;13(9):2466.
3. Nañagas KA, Penfound SJ, Kao LW. Carbon monoxide toxicity. *Emerg Med Clin North Am*. 2022:40(2):283–312.
4. Sun L, Héroux MÈ, Xu X, et al. Associations between residential fossil fuel combustion and indoor concentrations of nitrogen dioxide, carbon monoxide, and aldehydes in Canadian homes. *J Expo Sci Environ Epidemiol*. 2025;35(4):649–660.

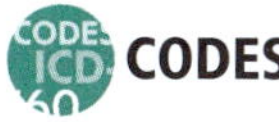

CODES

ICD10

- T58.0 Toxic effect of carbon monoxide from motor vehicle exhaust
- T58.2 Toxic effect of carbon monoxide from incomplete combustion of other domestic fuels
- T58.9 Toxic effect of carbon monoxide from unspecified source

CLINICAL PEARLS

- CO poisoning warrants a high index of suspicion. Consider in patients exposed to fire; during the winter months, in young patients with chest pain; and when patients present as a group.
- Noninvasive pulse oximeters are not reliable for the diagnosis of CO poisoning. COHb levels aid in diagnosis but do not reliably predict disease severity. Clinical assessment is imperative.
- If CO poisoning is suspected, remove individuals from the source and immediately administer 100% O_2.
- Although not required in all cases, consider HBO_2 for the treatment of CO poisoning if it is available.

CARDIOMYOPATHY

Neelima Katukuri, MD, FACC, FSCAI

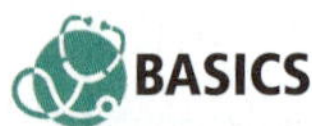

BASICS

DESCRIPTION

- Cardiomyopathies are myocardial diseases which result in structural and functional heart abnormalities in the absence of coronary artery disease, congenital heart disease, valvular disease, or hypertension which could sufficiently explain the clinical myocardial dysfunction.
- Results in 5–10% of cases of heart failure
- Classification of cardiomyopathies
  - Primary (mainly involves the heart)
    - Genetic
      - Hypertrophic cardiomyopathy (HCM)
      - Arrhythmogenic right ventricular cardiomyopathy/dysplasia (ARVC/D)
      - Left ventricular (LV) noncompaction (LVNC)
      - Glycogen storage (Danon type, PRKAG2)
      - Conduction defects
      - Mitochondrial myopathies
      - Ion channel disorders: long QT syndrome (LQTS), Brugada syndrome, short QT syndrome, and catecholaminergic polymorphic ventricular tachycardia (CPVT)
    - Mixed (genetic and nongenetic)
      - Dilated cardiomyopathy (DCM)
      - Restrictive (nonhypertrophied and nondilated)
    - Acquired
      - Myocarditis, stress cardiomyopathy, peripartum, tachycardia induced, infants of type 1 diabetic mothers
  - Secondary (multiorgan involvement; see list)
    - Specific: ischemic, valvular, hypertensive, and congenital heart disease

EPIDEMIOLOGY

Incidence

DCM: 5 to 8 new cases per 100,000 population annually

Prevalence

- DCM: roughly 1:2,500; most common reason for heart transplantation
- HCM: 1:500 of the adult population; 50% sporadic and rest are familial

ETIOLOGY AND PATHOPHYSIOLOGY

- HCM: hypertrophied (>15 mm), nondilated left and/or right ventricle which is disproportionate to hemodynamic stress on the heart
- ARVC/D: involves the right ventricle with progressive loss of myocytes and fatty/fibrofatty tissue replacement; can be associated with myocarditis (adenovirus or enterovirus)
- LVNC: congenital cardiomyopathies with "spongy" appearance of the LV myocardium
- LQTS: most common ion channelopathy with prolonged ventricular repolarization and QTc
- DCM: Ventricular chamber enlargement and systolic dysfunction with normal LV wall thickness result in progressive heart failure and further complications; strong genetic component with infectious and toxic etiologies
- RCM: normal/decreased ventricular volume with restrictive physiology, biatrial enlargement, and impaired ventricular filling
- Myocarditis: acute or chronic inflammation of the myocardium produced by toxins, drugs, or infectious causes
- Peripartum cardiomyopathy (PPCM): a form of DCM with LV systolic dysfunction and heart failure of unknown etiology
- Stress cardiomyopathies: triggered by profound psychological stress resulting in acute but rapidly reversible LV systolic dysfunction
- Endocrine: diabetes mellitus, hyperthyroidism, hypothyroidism, hyperparathyroidism, pheochromocytoma, acromegaly
- Nutritional deficiencies: beriberi, pellagra, scurvy, selenium, carnitine, kwashiorkor
- Autoimmune/collagen: systemic lupus erythematosus, dermatomyositis, rheumatoid arthritis, scleroderma, polyarteritis nodosa
- Infectious causes
  - Viral (e.g., HIV, coxsackievirus, adenovirus)
  - Bacterial and mycobacterial (e.g., diphtheria, rheumatic fever)
  - Parasitic (e.g., toxoplasmosis, *Trypanosoma cruzi*)
- Infiltrative (1): amyloidosis, Gaucher disease, Hurler disease, Hunter disease, Fabry disease
- Storage: hemochromatosis, glycogen storage disease (type II, Pompe), Niemann-Pick disease
- Neuromuscular/neurologic: Duchenne and Emery-Dreifuss muscular dystrophies, Friedreich ataxia, myotonic dystrophy, neurofibromatosis, tuberous sclerosis
- Toxic: alcohol, drugs, and chemotherapy (anthracyclines, cyclophosphamide, trastuzumab [Herceptin]), radiation, heavy metal, chemical agents
- Inflammatory (granulomatous): sarcoidosis
- Idiopathic
- Endomyocardial: endomyocardial fibrosis, hypereosinophilic syndrome (Loeffler endocarditis)

Genetics

- Genetic causes are well recognized in HCM; less common in DCM; careful ascertainment of family history, counseling patients with HCM about the potential for genetic transmission of HCM, and options for genetic testing are cornerstones of care (2).
- Most familial cardiomyopathies are inherited in autosomal dominant pattern (3). Prevalence would be expected to be equal among the sexes, but women are consistently less represented than men in clinical studies across different cardiomyopathies (30–40%) (3). Differences may be explained by various systematic biases in health care attendance and in diagnostic measurements and criteria.
- Involves mutations in sarcomere contractile proteins

RISK FACTORS

Same as etiology

GENERAL PREVENTION

Some cardiomyopathies which are not inherited can be prevented. Preventive measures include healthy eating habits and lifestyle. Regular moderate intensity exercise, avoidance of polysubstance abuse, management of stress, and maintenance of healthy body weight are recommended. Control of underlying comorbidities like blood pressure and diabetes are also beneficial.

COMMONLY ASSOCIATED CONDITIONS

Cardiomyopathy is commonly associated with coronary artery disease. Infections or noncardiac disease may cause cardiomyopathy, such as viral infections including COVID-19, connective tissue disorders like rheumatoid arthritis and lupus, endocrine disorders like multiple endocrine neoplasia syndromes, systemic infiltrative disorders (e.g., amyloidosis, sarcoidosis), and thyroid related conditions are few conditions associated with cardiomyopathy.

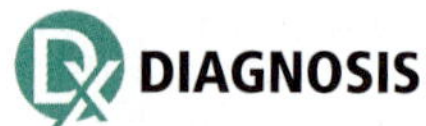

DIAGNOSIS

HISTORY

- Dyspnea at rest or with exertion, paroxysmal nocturnal dyspnea, orthopnea
- Right upper quadrant pain or bloating, edema
- Chest pain

PHYSICAL EXAM

- Tachypnea
- Cheyne-Stokes breathing
- Low pulse pressure
- Cool extremities
- Jugular venous distention
- Bibasilar rales
- Tachycardia
- Displaced point of maximal impulse (PMI)
- S_3 gallop
- Blowing systolic murmur
- Hepatosplenomegaly
- Ascites
- Edema

DIFFERENTIAL DIAGNOSIS

- Severe pulmonary disease
- Primary pulmonary hypertension
- Recurrent pulmonary embolism
- Constrictive pericarditis
- Some advanced forms of malignancy
- Anemia

DIAGNOSTIC TESTS & INTERPRETATION

Initial Tests (lab, imaging)

- ECG: LV hypertrophy, interventricular conduction delay, atrial fibrillation, evidence of prior Q-wave infarction
- Chest radiograph: cardiomegaly, increased vascular markings to the upper lobes, pleural effusions

- Initial diagnostic testing is via echocardiography. Depending on underlying risk factors further diagnostic work up can be considered. Ischemic cardiomyopathy (most common) is usually easily diagnosed and treated by cardiac catheterization; Holter monitor for patients where tachycardia induced cardiomyopathy when clinical suspicion for arrhythmias is high
  - In DCM: four-chamber enlargement and global hypokinesis; mural thrombi may be seen.
  - In HCM: Severe LV hypertrophy is present; systolic anterior motion of mitral valve, MR, dynamic flow obstruction
  - In RCM: low voltage, pseudoinfarction pattern (qw)
- Cardiac MRI
  - Useful to characterize certain nonischemic cardiomyopathies like myocarditis or infiltrative disease
  - In HCM: hypertrophy + patchy delayed enhancement
- Stress myocardial perfusion imaging (MPI): useful to rule out ischemia

Follow-Up Tests & Special Considerations

Genetic tests, genetic counselling

Diagnostic Procedures/Other

Cardiac catheterization: to rule out ischemia

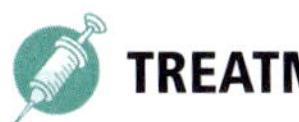

TREATMENT

MEDICATION

First Line

- Treat associated heart failure (3)[C]. See "Heart Failure, Chronic."
- If nonobstructive physiology: transplant evaluation
- If refractory: Options include surgical myectomy and alcohol septal ablation.
- Caution with use of diuretics (decrease in preload can worsen output) and digoxin (increased contractility can worsen obstruction).
- Negative ionotropes/chronotropes: β-blockers, CCB
- Implantable cardioverter-defibrillator (ICD): if VT/VF/SCD prevention; consider if family history of SCD.
- Counsel to prevent dehydration and extreme exertion
- If associated Afib: Anticoagulation, rate control with β-blocker
- Immunosuppression: in cases of DCM associated with myocarditis and collagen vascular disease
- Tafamidis (TTR binder): for restrictive cardiomyopathy associated with TTR amyloid

Second Line

Mavacamten was FDA approved in 2022 for treatment of symptomatic obstructive HCM in adults to improve functional capacity and symptoms. Treatment with this medication should be considered when response to first line of treatment fails, there is poor quality of life while on first line of treatment or more than two hospitalizations in six months. LV assist device (LVAD) is a treatment for cardiomyopathy as bridge to transplant (BTT), bridge to candidacy (BTC) when patient has temporary contraindications to transplant or as destination therapy (DT) when patient has permanent contraindication to heart transplant. Unlike donor hearts, LVADs have less wait time and are readily available.

ISSUES FOR REFERRAL

- Management by a heart failure team improves outcomes and facilitates early transplant referral (3).
- Refer for transplant evaluation if refractory to medical management.

ADDITIONAL THERAPIES

Alcohol septal ablation or septal myomectomy can be considered to treat HCM.

COMPLEMENTARY & ALTERNATIVE MEDICINE

Clinical evidence supporting use of complementary and alternative medicine (CAM) for cardiomyopathy is limited and controversial. Some CAM therapies can be beneficial when added to standard medical therapy as these therapies are often underreported to medical providers and so there is lack of evidence to support such therapies.

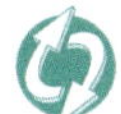

ONGOING CARE

FOLLOW-UP RECOMMENDATIONS

In addition to regular follow-up visits to health care provider, diet and weight monitoring, remote monitoring devices such as CardioMEMS can be considered in selected eligible patients.

Patient Monitoring

Multidisciplinary care team involving caregiver, social worker, and home health care in elderly patients can reduce recurrent hospital admissions associated with cardiomyopathy. Depression is common, so ongoing assessment is recommended.

DIET

Low fat, low salt, fluid restriction

PROGNOSIS

~20–40% of patients in NYHA FC IV die within 1 year. With a transplant, 1-year survival rate is as high as 94%.

COMPLICATIONS

Worsening congestive heart failure syncope, renal failure, arrhythmias, or sudden death

REFERENCES

1. Seward JB, Casaclang-Verzosa G. Infiltrative cardiovascular diseases: cardiomyopathies that look alike. *J Am Coll Cardiol*. 2010;55(17):1769–1779.
2. Ommen SR, Ho CY, Asif IM, et al. 2024 AHA/ACC/AMSSM/HRS/PACES/SCMR guideline for the management of hypertrophic cardiomyopathy: a report of the American Heart Association/American College of Cardiology joint committee on clinical practice guidelines. *Circulation*. 2024;149(23):e1239–e1311.
3. Arbelo E, Protonotarios A, Gimeno JR, et al; for ESC Scientific Document Group. 2023 ESC guidelines for the management of cardiomyopathies. *Eur Heart J*. 2023;44(37):3503–3626.

SEE ALSO

- Alcohol Use Disorder (AUD); Alcohol Withdrawal; Amyloidosis; Diabetes Mellitus, Type 1; Diabetes Mellitus, Type 2; Hypertension, Essential; Hypertrophic Cardiomyopathy; Hypothyroidism, Adult; Protein–Energy Malnutrition; Rheumatic Fever; Sarcoidosis
- Algorithm: Congestive Heart Failure: Differential Diagnosis

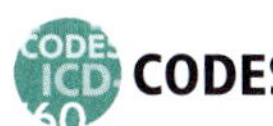

CODES

ICD10

- I42.9 Cardiomyopathy, unspecified
- I42.0 Dilated cardiomyopathy
- I42.5 Other restrictive cardiomyopathy

CLINICAL PEARLS

- Cardiomyopathy represents the end-stage of numerous disease processes involving the heart muscle.
- Ischemic, hypertensive, postviral, familial, alcoholic, and incessant tachycardia-induced are the most common cardiomyopathy varieties seen in the United States.
- Core therapy for heart failure involves salt restriction, diuretics, ACE inhibitors, β-blockers, aldosterone antagonists, digoxin, and electrical treatments, such as cardiac resynchronization and implantable defibrillators, as appropriate.

CAROTID SINUS HYPERSENSITIVITY

Bhreagh Orrell, MD • Ramandeep Mangat, MD

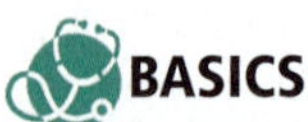

BASICS

Carotid sinus hypersensitivity (CSH) is an exaggerated response to stimulation or pressure applied to the carotid sinuses that results in bradycardia, vasodilation, and hypotension which presents clinically as syncope or presyncope.

DESCRIPTION

- The carotid sinuses play a central role in maintaining blood pressure (BP) homeostasis.
- The carotid sinuses are located near the bifurcation of the internal and external carotid arteries and contain baroreceptors that are responsive to changes in arterial pressure.
- An endogenous increase in BP or external pressure applied to a carotid sinus can cause an increase in the baroreceptor firing rate and activate vagal efferents and/or inhibit the sympathetic discharge to the heart and blood vessels which results in a slowing of the heart rate and drop in BP.
- In CSH, stimulation of one or both carotid sinuses (such as mechanical forces with turning the neck) causes an exaggerated baroreceptor response that can result in dizziness or syncope.
- There are three definitions for CSH (1):
  - Standard criteria: a pause in heart rate of ≥3 seconds in response to carotid sinus massage (CSM) and/or ≥50 mm Hg drop in systolic BP or both of the above
  - Krediet criteria: a pause in heart rate of ≥6 seconds in response to CSM and/or a fall in MAP to a value <60 mm Hg for ≥6 seconds
  - Kerr criteria: a pause in heart rate in response to CSM >95th percentile of the population response (7.3 seconds asystole), and/or vasodepression in response to CSM >95th percentile of the population response (>77 mm Hg fall in systolic BP), or both
- CSH is generally divided into three subtypes, based on response to CSM:
  - Cardioinhibitory (70–75%): asystole for at least 3 seconds
  - Vasodepressive (5–10%): fall in systolic BP of at least 50 mm Hg
  - Mixed (20–25%): combination of the first two subtypes
- Carotid sinus syndrome (CSS) typically (but not consistently) refers to CSH *with syncope and may be classified as*:
  - Spontaneous CSS: syncope after accidental mechanical manipulation (trigger) of the carotid sinuses (e.g., shaving, tight collars, or tumors)
  - Induced CSS: syncope diagnosed by CSM, although no mechanical trigger is found

EPIDEMIOLOGY

- Disease of elderly; most often occurs in male patients aged >65 years
- Associated with a history of coronary artery disease (CAD) and hypertension (HTN), with right CSH > left CSH

Prevalence

- In 2006, CSH was found in 39% of unselected adults >65 years of age using standard diagnostic criteria and found to be comparable with 2019 review of prevalence data (2).
- CSH may be a cause of the symptoms in 30% of elderly patients with unexplained syncope.

ETIOLOGY AND PATHOPHYSIOLOGY

- The exact site that causes the hypersensitivity response remains unknown. Changes in any part of the reflex arc or the target organs may give rise to this condition. It may be a part of a generalized autonomic disorder associated with autonomic dysregulation.
- Associated with resting sympathetic overactivity and increased baroreflex sensitivity
- Bradycardia and asystole seen in cardioinhibitory and mixed CSH subtypes appear to be mediated by vagal efferents, whereas vasodilatation and arterial hypotension in the vasodepressor and mixed subtypes are attributed to decrease sympathetic tone.
- Symptomatic CSH has been shown to be associated with impaired cerebral autoregulation, found to be normal in asymptomatic CSH.
- Atherosclerosis may diminish carotid sinus compliance, resulting in a reduction in afferent impulse traffic in the baroreflex pathway.
- CSH is often idiopathic but can be caused by:
  - Carotid body tumors
  - Inflammatory and malignant lymph nodes in the neck
  - Extensive scarring from prior neck surgery in the area of the carotid sinus
  - Metastatic cancer

RISK FACTORS

- Advanced age
- Male gender
- CAD
- HTN
- DM

COMMONLY ASSOCIATED CONDITIONS

- Carotid sinus syncope
- Sick sinus syndrome
- Atrioventricular block
- CAD
- HTN
- Orthostatic hypotension
- Vasovagal syncope
- Alzheimer disease
- Parkinson disease

DIAGNOSIS

HISTORY

- Recurrent syncope: usually sudden, unexplained, of short duration, seemingly spontaneous, and with complete recovery, although fractures and other injuries may occur
- Unexplained falls: Evidence of a causal relationship is suggested between falls and the cardioinhibitory subgroup.
- Dizziness: manifests as transient light-headedness or presyncope but not usually as true vertigo; associated more with vasodepressor and mixed subtypes
- Syncope may be associated with prodrome or retrograde amnesia.
- Causative or exacerbating factors
  - Any CSM-like maneuver such as shaving, wearing tight collars, or turning one's head sharply
  - Neck tumors, extensive neck scarring secondary to radical dissection or radiation fibrosis, and neck trauma
  - Certain medications can potentiate symptoms associated with CSH:
    - Digoxin or β-blockers (especially with cardioinhibitory subtype)
    - Physostigmine, morphine, methacholine increase vagal sensitivity and may predispose to cardioinhibitory subtype of CSH

PHYSICAL EXAM

Normal unless carotid baroreceptor is stimulated, then results in:

- Bradycardia
- Hypotension
- Pallor
- Diaphoresis

DIFFERENTIAL DIAGNOSIS

- Neurocardiogenic syncope
- Postural hypotension
- Situational syncope
- Postural tachycardia syndrome (POTS)
- Primary autonomic insufficiency
- Hypovolemia
- Dysrhythmias
- Sick sinus syndrome
- Cerebrovascular insufficiency
- Other causes of syncope (e.g., metabolic, psychogenic)

DIAGNOSTIC TESTS & INTERPRETATION

Initial Tests (lab, imaging)

- Orthostatic vital signs
- CBC, BMP, and fingerstick glucose
- ECG may demonstrate sinus pause(s) or atrial-ventricular block.
- Carotid duplex scan to rule out carotid stenosis in presence of a bruit

Diagnostic Procedures/Other

- CSM is considered in patients >40 years of age with syncope of unknown etiology after a negative initial evaluation.
- Commonly accepted technique for accurate diagnosis involves the following steps:
  - Patient in supine position for 5 minutes with continuous BP monitoring and ECG (on footplate-type tilt table for increased diagnostic accuracy); baseline BP and ECG are recorded.
  - For 5 to 10 seconds, apply firm longitudinal massage over the right carotid sinus (between the superior border of the thyroid and the angle of the mandible) at the site of maximal pulsation:
    - Note that light pressure over the carotid sinus will not reliably produce a hypersensitivity response.
    - Record symptoms, BP, and note ECG changes.
    - Discontinue if asystole ≥3 seconds.
  - If initial test nondiagnostic, apply pressure to the left carotid sinus while the patient remains supine; if still nondiagnostic, repeat in 70-degree head-up tilt (first on the right then, if necessary, the left), allowing time for hemodynamic adjustment to the head-up position.

- Evidence behind the testing strategy
  - Right side first: Up to 66% with CSH have positive response on the right; if a positive right response, no need to repeat test on the left side
  - 30% of CSM exams are found to be nondiagnostic in the supine position; positive predictive value increases from 77% to 96% with a specificity of 93% by performing CSM in the 70-degree position.
- Absolute contraindications for CSM testing
  - Carotid bruit present: must examine via carotid ultrasound with Doppler first:
    - No testing if >70% stenosis
    - Supine only testing if 50–70% stenosis
  - Myocardial infarction, transient ischemic attack, or stroke within the past 3 months
- Relative contraindications to CSM testing
  - History of ventricular tachycardia or ventricular fibrillation
  - False-positive results with CSM are relatively common in the elderly. Care should be taken to exclude other causes of syncope.
  - Neurologic and cardiovascular complications have been reported during CSM. Cardiovascular complications (primarily arrhythmia) are extremely rare. Transient neurologic symptoms and signs occur in up to 0.9% of patients. Persistent neurologic deficits are extremely rare following CSM. Correctly performed CSM should be considered a safe, low-risk procedure.

Test Interpretation

Standard positive response criteria (asystole ≥3 seconds and/or drop in systolic BP ≥50 mm Hg) are based on historical observations, although expert review of more recent data suggest these criteria may be too sensitive (3)[C].

- Specificity of the CSM technique increases if reproduction of a patient's syncope is demonstrated during a test (3)[B].

TREATMENT

GENERAL MEASURES

- No treatment is required for isolated CSH in asymptomatic individuals. Educate patients about CSH and monitoring and avoidance of triggers (tight collars, manipulation of the neck)
- High dietary salt intake and increased fluid intake may be helpful to maintain intravascular volume in patients with vasodepressor subtype and absence of other cardiovascular disease.
- Evaluation for driving restrictions

MEDICATION

First Line

No single agent has demonstrated long-term effectiveness for treatment of recurrent and symptomatic CSH.

Second Line

- Fludrocortisone or midodrine may be used to improve orthostatic symptoms in patients with vasodepressor subtype (not approved by FDA for this indication). However, fludrocortisone causes sodium and water retention and should be used with caution in elderly patients with heart disease. An adverse effect with midodrine is that it increases mean ambulatory BP.
- Atropine may be used in the acute setting in patients with cardioinhibitory subtype with bradycardia.
- Some evidence of benefit from sertraline and fluoxetine in patients unresponsive to pacemakers

ADDITIONAL THERAPIES

CSH and sick sinus syndrome coexist in 26% of cases. Pacemaker placement is beneficial for both.

SURGERY/OTHER PROCEDURES

- 2017 ACC/AHA/HRS Guideline for the Evaluation and Management of Patients With Syncope (4) notes that evidence is very limited and thus recommendation strength not high. Available evidence does not support the use of pacing for reflex-mediated syncope beyond patients with recurrent vasovagal syncope and asystole documented by implantable loop recorder.
- Permanent pacing may reduce the frequency of symptoms but may not completely eliminate them.
- Surgery for patients with CSH secondary to mass effect from tumor burden
- Carotid sinus denervation by surgery or radiation therapy is no longer recommended because of the high rate of complications.

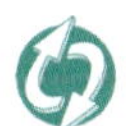

ONGOING CARE

DIET

High dietary salt intake and increased fluid intake may be helpful to maintain intravascular volume in patients with vasodepressor subtype and absence of other cardiovascular disease.

PATIENT EDUCATION

- Avoid precipitating maneuvers (as described above) that place pressure on the neck, such as tight collars and neck ties.
- With syncope, restrict driving or other potentially hazardous activities until the patient is cleared by the physician
- Avoid precipitating medications like vasodilators and those temporally related to symptoms.
- Teach patient to assume supine position if prodromal symptoms or presyncope occurs.
- Explain diagnosis, provide reassurance, and explain risk of recurrence.

PROGNOSIS

- The presence of CSH has not been demonstrated to confer an independent mortality risk however may result in falls and/or syncope related injuries which could be fatal in certain circumstances.
- Untreated CSS patients have a syncope recurrence rate as high as 62% within 4 years.
- Patients with cardioinhibitory CSH who received a pacemaker had a significant reduction in their mean number of falls, from 9.3 to 4.1 falls in a 1-year follow-up period.

COMPLICATIONS

CSH, according to Kerr criteria, is associated with increased mortality. Further evaluation is needed to predict future falls, syncope, and ability of criteria to identify patients who would benefit from pacing (1)[B].

REFERENCES

1. McDonald C, Pearce MS, Newton JL, et al. Modified criteria for carotid sinus hypersensitivity are associated with increased mortality in a population-based study. *Europace*. 2016;18(7):1101–1107.
2. Kadermuneer P, Sandeep R, Haridasan V, et al. Prevalence and one-year outcome of carotid sinus hypersensitivity in unexplained syncope: a prospective cohort study from South India. *Indian Heart J*. 2019;71(1):1–6.
3. Runser LA, Gauer RL, Houser A. Syncope: evaluation and differential diagnosis. *Am Fam Physician*. 2017;95(5):303–312.
4. Varosy PD, et al. Pacing as a treatment for reflex-mediated (vasovagal, situational, or carotid sinus hypersensitivity) syncope: a systematic review for the 2017 ACC/AHA/HRS guideline for the evaluation and management of patients with Syncope: a report of the American College of Cardiology/American Heart Association Task Force on Clinical Practice Guidelines and the Heart Rhythm Society. *Circulation*. 2017;136(5):e123–e135.

ADDITIONAL READING

Parry SW. Should we ever pace for carotid sinus syndrome? *Front Cardiovasc Med*. 2020;7:44.

SEE ALSO

- Syncope
- Algorithm: Sinus Node Dysfunction (Sick Sinus Syndrome)

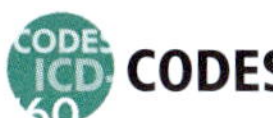

CODES

ICD10

G90.01 Carotid sinus syncope

CLINICAL PEARLS

- Consider CSH as a potential cause for syncope, dizziness, or unexplained falls, especially in the elderly.
- Diagnose CSH via CSM (using firm pressure for 5 to 10 seconds), producing asystole of at least 3 seconds and/or a drop in systolic BP of at least 50 mm Hg.
- Remember to auscultate for carotid artery bruit prior to considering CSM.
- Consider dual-chamber pacemaker in patients with recurrent syncope and cardioinhibitory or mixed CSH subtypes.
- The finding of CSH does not exclude other causes of syncope.

CAROTID STENOSIS

Rade N. Pejic, MD

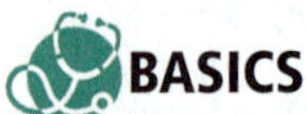

BASICS

Carotid stenosis may be caused by atherosclerosis, intimal fibroplasia, vasculitis, adventitial cysts, or vascular tumors. However, atherosclerosis is the most common etiology.

DESCRIPTION

- Narrowing of the carotid artery lumen is typically due to atherosclerotic changes in the vessel wall. Atherosclerotic plaques are responsible for 90% of extracranial carotid lesions and up to 30% of all ischemic strokes.
- A "hemodynamically significant" carotid stenosis produces an internal carotid artery peak systolic velocity (PSV) >125 cm/sec on carotid duplex imaging.
- Carotid lesions are classified by the following:
  - Symptom status
    - Asymptomatic: homogenous and stable
    - Symptomatic: heterogeneous and unstable; present with stroke or transient cerebral ischemic attack
  - Degree of stenosis
    - Total occlusion: no detectable patent lumen
    - Near occlusion: markedly narrow lumen on color Doppler ultrasound (US)
    - High grade: PSV >230 cm/sec; 70–99% stenosis
    - Moderate grade: PSV 125 to 230 cm/sec; 50–69% stenosis
    - Low grade: PSV <125 cm/sec with visible plaque or intimal thickening; <50% stenosis
    - Normal: PSV <125 cm/sec and no visible plaque or intimal thickening

EPIDEMIOLOGY

More common in men and with increasing age (see "Risk Factors")

Incidence

Unclear (Asymptomatic patients often go undiagnosed.)

Prevalence

- Moderate stenosis
  - Age <50 years: men 0.2%, women 0%
  - Age >80 years: men 7.5%, women 5%
- Severe stenosis
  - Age <50 years: men 0.1%, women 0%
  - Age >80 years: men 3.1%, women 0.9%

ETIOLOGY AND PATHOPHYSIOLOGY

- Atherosclerosis at the carotid bifurcation begins during adolescence. The carotid bulb has unique blood flow dynamics. Hemodynamic disturbances cause endothelial injury and dysfunction. Plaque formation in vessel wall results and stenosis then ensues.
- Initial cause is not well understood, but certain risk factors are frequently present (see "Risk Factors"). Tensile stress on the vessel wall, turbulence, and arterial wall shear stress seem to be involved.

Genetics

- Increased incidence among family members
- Genetically linked factors
  - Diabetes mellitus (DM), race, hypertension (HTN), family history, obesity, hyperlipidemia
  - In a recent single nucleotide polymorphism study, the following genes were strongly associated with worse carotid plaque: *TNFSF4*, *PPARA*, *TLR4*, *ITGA2*, and *HABP2*.

RISK FACTORS

- Nonmodifiable factors: advanced age (>65 years old), male sex, family history, coronary artery disease (CAD), peripheral artery disease, aortic aneurysmal disease, congenital arteriopathies
- Modifiable factors: smoking, diet, dyslipidemia, physical inactivity, obesity, HTN, DM
- Possible factors: *Chlamydia pneumoniae* and *Cytomegalovirus*

GENERAL PREVENTION

- Antihypertensive treatment to maintain blood pressure (BP) <140/90 mm Hg; see "Hypertension, Essential."
- Smoking cessation to reduce the risk of atherosclerosis progression and stroke
- Lipid control: plaque stabilization and regression of carotid atherosclerotic lesions seen with statin therapy

COMMONLY ASSOCIATED CONDITIONS

- Transient ischemic attack (TIA)/stroke
- CAD/myocardial infarction (MI)
- Peripheral vascular disease (PVD)

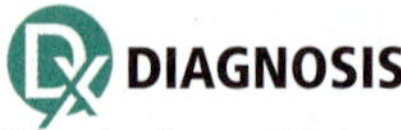

DIAGNOSIS

Screening for carotid stenosis is not recommended for asymptomatic low-risk patients; harms likely outweigh benefits (1). However, screening may be considered for certain asymptomatic high-risk patients and is strongly recommended in the setting of symptoms suggestive of stroke or TIA.

HISTORY

- Identification of modifiable and nonmodifiable comorbidities (See "Risk Factors.")
- History of cerebral ischemic event
- Stroke, TIA, amaurosis fugax (monocular blindness), aphasia
- CAD/MI
- Peripheral arterial disease
- Review of systems, with focus on risk factors for
  - Cardiovascular disease
  - Stroke (HTN and arrhythmias)

PHYSICAL EXAM

- Lateralizing neurologic deficits: contralateral motor and/or sensory deficit
- Amaurosis fugax: ipsilateral transient visual obscuration from retinal ischemia
- Visual field defect
- Dysarthria, aphasia (in the case of dominant hemisphere involvement, usually left)
- Carotid bruit (low sensitivity and specificity)

DIFFERENTIAL DIAGNOSIS

- Aortic valve stenosis
- Aortic arch atherosclerosis
- Arrhythmia with cardiogenic embolization
- Migraine
- Brain tumor
- Metabolic disturbances
- Functional/psychological deficit
- Seizure

DIAGNOSTIC TESTS & INTERPRETATION

Initial Tests (lab, imaging)

Workup for suspected TIA/stroke may include the following:

- CBC with differential
- Basic metabolic panel
- ESR (if temporal arteritis is a consideration)
- Glucose/hemoglobin A1c
- Fasting lipid profile
- Duplex ultrasonography is the recommended initial diagnostic test in patients with known or suspected carotid stenosis. Duplex US identifies ≥50% stenosis, with 98% sensitivity and 88% specificity.

Follow-Up Tests & Special Considerations

Other noninvasive imaging techniques can add detail to duplex results:

- CT angiography
  - 88% sensitivity and 100% specificity
  - Requires IV contrast with risk for subsequent renal morbidity
- MR angiography
  - 95% sensitivity and 90% specificity but tends to overestimate the degree of stenosis
  - Evaluates cerebral circulation (extracranial and intracranial) as well as aortic arch and common carotid artery
  - The presence of unstable plaque can be determined

Diagnostic Procedures/Other

Cerebral digital subtraction angiography is the gold standard for diagnosis:

- Delineates the anatomy pertaining to aortic arch and proximal vessels
- The procedure is invasive and has multiple risks:
  - Contrast-induced renal dysfunction (1–5% complication rate)
  - Thromboembolic-related complications (1–2.6% complication rate) and neurologic complications
  - Should be used only when other tests are not conclusive

Test Interpretation

- Stenosis consistently occurs at the carotid bifurcation with plaque formation most often at the level of the proximal internal carotid artery:
  - Plaque is thickest at the carotid bifurcation.
  - Plaque occupies the intima and inner media and avoids outer media and adventitia.
- Plaque histology
  - Homogenous (stable) plaques seldom hemorrhage or ulcerate:
    - Fatty streak and fibrous tissue deposition
    - Diffuse intimal thickening
  - Heterogenous (unstable) plaques may hemorrhage or ulcerate:
    - Presence of lipid-laden macrophages, necrotic debris, cholesterol crystals
    - Ulcerated plaques
  - Soft and gelatinous clots with platelets, fibrin, and red and white blood cells

TREATMENT

Therapeutic lifestyle modifications, smoking cessation, BP control, glycemic control, statins, and antiplatelet medications are the primary treatments for both asymptomatic and symptomatic carotid stenosis.

GENERAL MEASURES

- Therapeutic lifestyle modifications: heart-healthy diet, weight loss, and exercise of 30 min/day at least 5 days/week
- Patients should be advised to quit smoking and offered smoking cessation intervention.

MEDICATION

- Control of HTN with antihypertensive agents to maintain BP <140/90 mm Hg. In carefully selected individuals, tighter BP control might reduce cerebrovascular events but this remains uncertain.
- Antihypertensive treatment with an ACE-I or ARB reduces the stroke risk in individuals with diabetes.
- Glycemic control in diabetic patients using lifestyle modifications, metformin, SGLT-2 inhibitors, and GLP-1 agonists
- Statin therapy using the maximally tolerated statin dosage
- Aspirin: 75 to 325 mg/day
- If the patient has sustained a TIA or ischemic stroke, antiplatelet therapy with
  - Aspirin alone (75 to 325 mg/day) *or*
  - Clopidogrel alone (75 mg/day), *or*
  - Aspirin plus extended-release dipyridamole (25 and 200 mg BID, respectively)
  - A combination of clopidogrel plus aspirin is *not* recommended within 3 months post-TIA or CVA.

ISSUES FOR REFERRAL

- For acute symptomatic stroke, order imaging and consult neurology.
- For known carotid stenosis, some suggest duplex imaging every 6 months if stenosis is >50% and patient is a surgical candidate.

SURGERY/OTHER PROCEDURES

- Symptomatic carotid stenosis (history of ischemia ipsilateral to stenosis)
  - Carotid endarterectomy (CEA) is of some benefit in 50–69% symptomatic stenosis, highly beneficial for those with 70–99% stenosis without near occlusion, and has no benefit in people with carotid near-occlusion or total occlusion (2).
  - CEA is recommended for patients with a life expectancy of at least 5 years. The anticipated rate of perioperative stroke or mortality must be <6%.
  - Treatment with aspirin (81 to 325 mg/day) is recommended for all patients who are having CEA. Aspirin should be started prior to surgery and continued for at least 3 months postsurgery but may be continued indefinitely.
  - Carotid artery stenting (CAS) provides similar long-term outcomes as CEA.
    - CAS has an increased risk of adverse cerebrovascular events in the elderly compared to the young but similar mortality risk.
    - CAS is suggested in selected patients with neck anatomy unfavorable for arterial surgery and those with comorbid conditions that greatly increase the risk of anesthesia and surgery.
    - Dual antiplatelet therapy with aspirin (81 to 325 mg/day) plus clopidogrel (75 mg/day) is recommended for 30 days post-CAS.
  - Transcarotid revascularization (TCAR) appears to avoid the pitfalls of CAS with similar outcomes to CEA (3).
- Asymptomatic patients: As compared with CAS, CEA is the preferred option for the management of asymptomatic carotid stenosis if a surgical option is chosen although TCAR is now an alternative in select patients. CAS has the potential for increased risks of periprocedural stroke and periprocedural death (4)[A].

ADMISSION, INPATIENT, AND NURSING CONSIDERATIONS

- Any patient with a presentation of acute symptomatic carotid stenosis should be hospitalized for further diagnostic workup and appropriate therapy.
- Rapid evaluation for symptoms compatible with TIA should be obtained in the emergency department (ED) or inpatient setting.
- Discharge criteria: 24 to 48 hours post-CEA, if ambulating, taking adequate PO intake, and neurologically intact

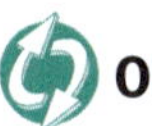

ONGOING CARE

FOLLOW-UP RECOMMENDATIONS

Patient Monitoring

- Duplex at 2 to 6 weeks postoperatively
- Duplex every 6 to 12 months
- Reoperative CEA or CAS is reasonable, if there is rapidly progressive restenosis.
- Patients with any of the following: renal failure, heart failure, diabetes, and age >80 years have a high readmission rate following CEA; thus, intensive medical therapy and rigorous follow-up is recommended.

DIET

Heart-healthy diet low in saturated fat and no trans fat

PATIENT EDUCATION

For patient education materials on this topic, consult the following: https://medlineplus.gov/carotidarterydisease.html

COMPLICATIONS

- Untreated: TIA/stroke (risk of ipsilateral stroke approximately 1.68% per year)
- Postoperative (status post CEA)
  - Perioperative (within 30 days)
    - Stroke/death, cranial nerve injury, hemorrhage, hemodynamic instability, MI
  - Late (>30 days postoperatively)
    - Recurrent stenosis, false aneurysm at the surgical site

REFERENCES

1. Krist AH, Davidson KW, Mangione CM, et al; for US Preventive Services Task Force. Screening for asymptomatic carotid artery stenosis: US Preventive Services Task Force recommendation statement. *JAMA*. 2021;325(5):476–481. doi:10.1001/jama.2020.26988.
2. AbuRahma AF, Avgerinos ED, Chang RW, et al. Society for Vascular Surgery clinical practice guidelines for management of extracranial cerebrovascular disease. *J Vasc Surg*. 2022;75(1S):4S–22S. doi:10.1016/j.jvs.2021.04.073.
3. Columbo JA, Martinez-Camblor P, Stone DH, et al. Procedural safety comparison between transcarotid artery revascularization, carotid endarterectomy, and carotid stenting: perioperative and 1-year rates of stroke or death. *J Am Heart Assoc*. 2022;11(19):e024964. doi:10.1161/JAHA.121.024964.
4. Moresoli P, Habib B, Reynier P, et al. Carotid stenting versus endarterectomy for asymptomatic carotid artery stenosis: a systematic review and meta-analysis. *Stroke*. 2017;48(8):2150–2157. doi:10.1161/STROKEAHA.117.016824.

SEE ALSO

Algorithms: Stroke; Transient Ischemic Attack

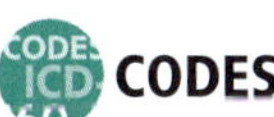

CODES

ICD10

- I65.29 Occlusion and stenosis of unspecified carotid artery
- I65.21 Occlusion and stenosis of right carotid artery
- I65.22 Occlusion and stenosis of left carotid artery

CLINICAL PEARLS

- Atherosclerosis is responsible for 90% of all cases of carotid artery stenosis.
- Duplex US is the best initial imaging modality.
- Antiplatelet therapy and aggressive treatment of vascular risk factors are the mainstays of medical therapy.
- Compared with CEA, CAS increases the risk of any stroke but decreases the risk of MI. For every 1,000 patients opting for stenting rather than endarterectomy, 19 more patients would have strokes and 10 fewer would have MIs.
- TCAR appears to avoid the pitfalls of CAS with similar outcomes to CEA.

CARPAL TUNNEL SYNDROME

Daniel R. Matta, MD, DFPHM, FAAFP • Duncan L. Jackson, MD

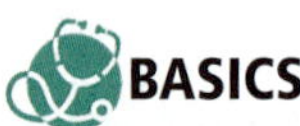

BASICS

DESCRIPTION

- Symptomatic compression neuropathy of the median nerve that runs in the carpal tunnel caused by increased pressure leading to motor sensory findings
- Most common nerve entrapment syndrome (90% of all neuropathy cases)
- The dorsal aspect of the carpal tunnel is composed of the carpal bones. The transverse carpal ligament defines the palmar boundary. The carpal tunnel contains nine flexor tendons and the median nerve.
- Symptoms most commonly affect the dominant hand; >50% of patients will experience bilateral symptoms.
- Most expensive upper extremity musculoskeletal disorder; >$2 billion per year
- Carpal tunnel release (CTR) is one of the most frequently performed hand/wrist procedures, with approximately 600,000 CTR procedures per year.
- Median time lost by U.S. workers with carpal tunnel syndrome (CTS) = 28 days
- System(s) affected: musculoskeletal, nervous

ALERT

Increased incidence during pregnancy (up to 20–45%) and chronic hemodialysis (2–31%)

EPIDEMIOLOGY

Predominant age: 40 to 60 years; predominant sex: female > male (3:1 to 10:1)

Incidence

- Two peaks: late 50s (female); late 70s (both genders)
- Incidence increases with age

Prevalence

- About 3% of the population (4% in women and 2% in men); 3.8 cases per 1,000 individuals per year in United States
- 14% in diabetics without neuropathy and 30% in patients with diabetic neuropathy

ETIOLOGY AND PATHOPHYSIOLOGY

- Combination of mechanical trauma, inflammation, increased pressure, and ischemic injury to the median nerve within the carpal tunnel
- Acute CTS caused by rapid and sustained pressure in carpal tunnel, usually secondary to trauma, may require urgent surgical decompression.
- Distal radius fractures and volar lunate dislocations increase risk.
- Chronic CTS divided into four categories:
  - Idiopathic: combination of edema and fibrous hypertrophy without inflammation
  - Anatomic: persistent median artery, ganglion cyst, infection, space-occupying lesion in carpal tunnel
  - Systemic: associated with conditions such as obesity, diabetes, hypothyroidism, rheumatoid arthritis, amyloidosis, scleroderma, renal failure, and drug toxicity
  - Exertional: repetitive use of hands and wrists, repeated palmar impact, use of vibratory tools

Genetics

- Unknown; however, a familial type has been reported.
- More likely to experience CTS if there is a first-degree relative with CTS

RISK FACTORS

- Prolonged postures in extremes of wrist flexion and extension including activities such as gardening, cycling, or tennis; repetitive exposure to vibration (motorcycle riding)
  - There is insufficient evidence to implicate computer use in the development of CTS.
  - Jobs most at risk for CTS: use of vibratory tools, food processing and packing, dairy and poultry workers, and assembly workers
- Alterations of fluid balance: pregnancy, rheumatoid arthritis, obesity, renal failure, hypothyroidism, congestive heart failure, hemodialysis
  - CTS is the most common neuropathy in patients with rheumatoid arthritis.
- Neuropathic factors: diabetes, alcoholism, vitamin deficiency, or exposure to toxins
- More common in patients with concomitant migraine headaches

GENERAL PREVENTION

There is no known prevention for CTS. It is recommended to take occasional (e.g., hourly) breaks when doing repetitive work involving hands or if prolonged occupational exposure to vibratory tools.

COMMONLY ASSOCIATED CONDITIONS

- Diabetes, obesity; pregnancy; hypothyroidism; amyloidosis
- Osteoarthritis of small joints of hand and wrist
- Hyperparathyroidism, hypocalcemia
- Hemodialysis

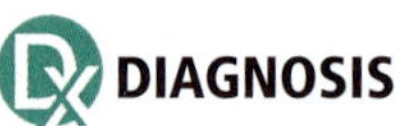

DIAGNOSIS

HISTORY

- Nocturnal pain, numbness, and tingling of the thumb, index, long, and radial portion of the ring fingers. Symptoms characteristically are relieved by shaking or rubbing the hands known as a positive Flick sign. This has a sensitivity of 93% and specificity of 96%.
- Hand weakness during tasks such as opening jars is often noted early in the disorder.
- Atypical presentation involves paresthesias in radial digits, with pain radiating proximally along median nerve to elbow and sometimes the shoulder
- During waking hours, symptoms occur when driving, talking on the phone, and occasionally when using the hands for repetitive maneuvers.

PHYSICAL EXAM

- Durkan compression test: Direct compression of median nerve at carpal tunnel for 30 seconds elicits symptoms (87% sensitivity; 90% specificity).
- Positive Phalen sign: Holding the wrist in fully flexed position for 60 seconds precipitates paresthesias, numbness, or pain (68% sensitivity; 73% specificity).
- Positive Tinel sign: Tapping over the palmar surface of the wrist proximal to the carpal tunnel may produce an electric sensation along the distribution of the median nerve (50% sensitivity; 77% specificity).
- Square-sign test: positive if measurement of wrist width/height ≥0.7 (53% sensitivity, 80% specificity)
- Hand elevation test: Hands held above head for 1 to 2 minutes, positive if symptoms are reproduced (85% sensitivity, 95% specificity)
- Loss of two-point discrimination
- Decreased sensation to pain
- Upper extremities and neck should be evaluated to exclude causes such as cervical radiculopathy.
- Wasting of thenar musculature is a late sign and should not be used to rule out CTS (16% sensitivity, 94% specificity).

DIFFERENTIAL DIAGNOSIS

- Cervical spondylosis (carpal tunnel may also occur with cervical spine disease; "double crush")
- Generalized peripheral neuropathy
- Brachial plexopathy, in particular upper trunk
- CNS disorders (multiple sclerosis, cerebral infarction)
- Thoracic outlet syndrome
- Pronator syndrome (median nerve compression at the elbow)
- Anterior interosseous syndrome
- Ulnar nerve compression
- Musculoskeletal disorders of the wrist:
  - Trauma or distal radius fracture
  - Degenerative joint disease
  - Rheumatoid arthritis
  - Ganglion cyst
  - De Quervain tenosynovitis
  - CMC arthritis
- Scleroderma
- Raynaud syndrome

DIAGNOSTIC TESTS & INTERPRETATION

- The most accurate screening forms are the CTS-6, Boston Carpal Tunnel Questionnaire (BCTQ), Kamath and Stothard questionnaire, and Katz and Stirrat hand symptom diagram.
- No laboratory test is diagnostic.
  - TSH, HbA1c, ESR, and serum chemistries help exclude secondary conditions associated with CTS.
- The most sensitive indicator is median sensory distal latency, which is prolonged in CTS.

Initial Tests (lab, imaging)

- X-rays of the wrist to evaluate for degenerative joint disease but are not necessary to diagnose CTS; magnetic resonance imaging is of limited benefit.
- Ultrasound—rapid, noninvasive, painless modality; sensitivity 87%; specificity 91%; hypoechoic median nerve cross-sectional area ≥11.5 mm^2

Diagnostic Procedures/Other

Electrodiagnostic studies

- Sensitivity 85%; specificity 95%
- Most useful with low pretest probability and suspicion of alternate peripheral neuropathy, radiculopathy, or "double-crush" phenomenon with compression at multiple locations
- Nerve conduction studies compare latency and amplitude of median nerve signals across the carpal tunnel.
- Positive result is useful for ruling in CTS, but a negative result does not exclude CTS (most notably in mild cases).
- Findings usually used to grade severity of CTS
- 15–25% of patients with clinically defined CTS may have normal electrodiagnostic studies.

Test Interpretation

Axon loss or muscle denervation signifies severe disease and should prompt referral for surgery.

TREATMENT

GENERAL MEASURES

- Strong evidence supports immobilization (brace/splint/orthosis) and the use of local steroid (methylprednisolone) injection in improving patient-reported outcomes (American Academy of Orthopaedic Surgeons strong recommendation).
- Corticosteroid injections may improve symptoms, short-term function and may reduce the likelihood of needing surgical intervention and the benefits may persist up to 1 year; treatment response 47% to 77% up to 1 month and 50 % at 1 year
- A trial of nonoperative management is generally recommended for patients with mild to moderate CTS symptoms.
- A half of patients with nonsevere symptoms spontaneously improve within 2 years.
- Use of the CTS clinical severity rating should guide treatment options.
- Consider surgical intervention if symptoms do not improve after 4 to 6 months of nonoperative management.

MEDICATION

First Line

Mainstay treatments for mild to moderate CTS include night splinting (12 weeks) and local corticosteroid injection or oral nonsteroidal anti-inflammatory agents.

- Over-the-counter analgesia such as NSAIDs and acetaminophen have not shown any benefit for CTS.
- Short courses of prednisone (<2 weeks) are effective for short-term relief but less effective than corticosteroid injection.
- Local corticosteroid injection is effective for treatment of mild and moderate CTS with benefits lasting up to 6 months and a reduced need for surgery up to 12 months (1).
- Splinting remains first line due to its simplicity, affordability, and tolerability; should be worn for 1 to 2 months. Symptoms usually improve in 2 weeks and may continue to improve up to 6 months with consistency.
- Nighttime splinting only is as effective as continuous wear splints and neutral splint may be more effective than an extension splint.
- No evidence supports multiple trials of injection; thus, surgery should be considered for those with refractory or recurrent symptoms.
- Those with moderate to severe disease benefit from early surgery.

ISSUES FOR REFERRAL

Preoperative electrodiagnostic studies are generally obtained prior to any surgical intervention.

SURGERY/OTHER PROCEDURES

- Surgical intervention for patient with moderate to severe CTS and findings of nerve injury or for patients unsuccessful with nonsurgical management; surgical decompression is an outpatient procedure.
- Completely dividing the transverse carpal ligament provides symptom relief in $>95\%$ of patients.
- Splinting after surgical intervention is not recommended as it does not appear to improve symptoms and may impede recovery.
- Incisional healing generally takes 2 weeks; an additional 2 weeks may be required before using the affected hand for tasks requiring strength.
- Complete resolution of numbness in 93.8% of patients with severe CTS by EMG at follow-up of 9.3 years.
- The approach should be based on surgeon and patient preference.
  - There is no difference in long-term outcomes between a mini-open CTR (i.e., a small longitudinal palmar incision not crossing the wrist crease) and an endoscopic CTR (2).
  - Patients undergoing endoscopic release are at greater risk for transient nerve injury (median neurapraxia).
  - Ultrasound-guided CTR shows promise but needs further investigation.

COMPLEMENTARY & ALTERNATIVE MEDICINE

- No evidence to support of vitamin B_6 in the prevention or treatment of CTS
- Acupuncture shown to be as effective as short-term oral prednisolone therapy and may be used as an alternative therapy or as an adjuvant.
- No data to support chiropractic therapy as a treatment for CTS.

ADMISSION, INPATIENT, AND NURSING CONSIDERATIONS

Outpatient

ONGOING CARE

FOLLOW-UP RECOMMENDATIONS

Patient Monitoring

- Patients treated nonoperatively (splinting, injections) require follow-up over 4 to 12 weeks to ensure adequate progress.
- There is only limited, low-quality evidence to suggest that rehabilitation exercises such as wrist immobilization, ice therapy, and multimodal hand rehabilitation are beneficial.
- 7–20% of patients treated surgically may experience recurrence.

PROGNOSIS

- One prospective cohort study found after 1 year approximately 30% of nonsevere cases improved, 40% remained stable and 20% worsened.
- Risk factor for progression includes old age and the duration of symptoms.
- Approximately 85% of patients that initially respond to conservative therapy will experience reemergence of symptoms within 4 years.
- A positive Phalen test and thenar wasting are factors that have been associated with poorer outcomes with conservative management.
- Patients with severe CTS may not recover completely after surgical release. Paresthesias and weakness may persist, but nighttime symptoms generally resolve.
- If untreated, more severe cases of CTS can lead to numbness and weakness in the hand, atrophy of the thenar muscles, and permanent loss of median nerve function.

COMPLICATIONS

- Injury to the median nerve or its recurrent (motor) branch
- Pillar pain (tenderness adjacent to the actual ligament release sites of the trapezial ridge and hook of hamate) in the months following CTR (prevalence of 6–36%)
- Complications post-op include wound infection, complex regional pain syndrome, vascular injuries of the superficial palmar arch, painful scar formation.

REFERENCES

1. Ashworth NL, Bland JDP, Chapman KM, et al. Local corticosteroid injection versus placebo for carpal tunnel syndrome. *Cochrane Database Syst Rev*. 2023;2(2):CD015148. doi:10.1002/14651858.CD015148.
2. American Academy of Orthopaedic Surgeons. Management of carpal tunnel syndrome evidence-based clinical practice guideline. aaos.org/cts2cpg. Published May 18, 2024. Accessed September 15, 2025.

ADDITIONAL READING

Wipperman J, Penny ML. Carpal tunnel syndrome: rapid evidence review. *Am Fam Physician*. 2024;110(1):52–57.

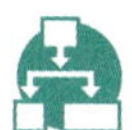

SEE ALSO

- Arthritis, Rheumatoid (RA); Hypoparathyroidism; Lupus Erythematosus, Systemic (SLE); Scleroderma
- Algorithms: Carpal Tunnel Syndrome, Pain In Upper Extremity

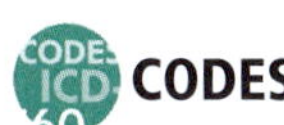

CODES

ICD10

- G56.0 Carpal tunnel syndrome
- G56.01 Carpal tunnel syndrome, right upper limb
- G56.02 Carpal tunnel syndrome, left upper limb

CLINICAL PEARLS

- Paresthesias associated with CTS are confined to the thumb, index, long, and radial 1/2 of the ring fingers of the affected hand.
- Thenar atrophy is a late finding, indicating nerve damage, and is associated with a higher likelihood of failure with conservative management.
- The Durkan (carpal compression) test is superior to Tinel sign (tapping on median nerve over carpal tunnel) and Phalen maneuver (holding wrists in flexion) for the clinical diagnosis of CTS. The Flick sign has the highest sensitivity and specificity.
- Steroid injection and night splinting are the mainstays of treatment for mild to moderate CTS.
- Surgical release of the carpal tunnel is $>90\%$ effective long term.

C

CATARACT

Ingrid U. Scott, MD, MPH • Yasir Ahmed, MD • Harry W. Flynn Jr., MD

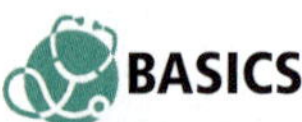

BASICS

DESCRIPTION

- A cataract is any opacity or discoloration of the lens, localized or generalized; the term is usually reserved for changes that affect visual acuity (1).
- Etymology: from Latin *cataracta*, for "waterfall"; named after foamy appearance of opacity
- Leading cause of blindness worldwide, estimated 20 million people (1)
- Types include the following:
  - Age related: approximately 90% of cases
  - Metabolic (diabetes via accelerated sorbitol pathway, hypocalcemia, Wilson disease)
  - Congenital (1/250 newborns; 10–38% of childhood blindness)
  - Systemic disease associated (myotonic dystrophy, atopic dermatitis [AD])
  - Secondary to associated eye disease, so-called complicated (e.g., uveitis associated with juvenile rheumatoid arthritis or sarcoid, tumor such as melanoma or retinoblastoma)
  - Traumatic (e.g., heat, electric shock, radiation, concussion, perforating eye injuries, intraocular foreign body)
  - Toxic/nutritional (e.g., corticosteroids)
- Morphologic classification:
  - Nuclear: exaggeration of normal aging changes of *central* lens nucleus, often associated with myopia due to increased refractive index of lens (Some elderly patients consequently may be able to read again *without spectacles*, so-called "second sight.")
  - Cortical: outer portion of lens; may involve anterior, posterior, or equatorial cortex; radial, spoke-like opacities
  - Subcapsular: Posterior subcapsular cataract has more profound effect on vision than nuclear or cortical cataract; patients particularly troubled under conditions of miosis; near vision frequently impaired more than distance vision
- System(s) affected: nervous

Geriatric Considerations

Some degree of cataract formation is expected in all people >70 years of age.

Pediatric Considerations

See congenital cataract; may present as leukocoria

Pregnancy Considerations

See congenital cataract (i.e., medications, metabolic dysfunction, intrauterine infection, and malnutrition)

EPIDEMIOLOGY

Incidence

- ~48% of the 37 million cases of blindness worldwide result from cataracts (1).
- Leading cause of treatable blindness and vision loss in developing countries (1)

Prevalence

An estimated 50% of people 65 to 74 years of age and 70% of people >75 years of age have age-related cataract.

ETIOLOGY AND PATHOPHYSIOLOGY

- Age-related cataract:
  - Continual addition of layers of lens fibers throughout life creates hard, dehydrated lens nucleus that impairs vision (nuclear cataract).
  - Aging alters biochemical and osmotic balance required for lens clarity; outer lens layers hydrate and become opaque, adversely affecting vision.
- Congenital:
  - Usually unknown etiology
  - Drugs (corticosteroids in 1st trimester, sulfonamides)
  - Metabolic (diabetes in mother, galactosemia in fetus)
  - Intrauterine infection during 1st trimester (e.g., rubella, herpes, mumps)
  - Maternal malnutrition
- Other cataract types:
  - Common feature is a biochemical/osmotic imbalance that disrupts lens clarity.
  - Local changes in lens protein distribution lead to light scattering (lens opacity).

Genetics

Congenital (e.g., chromosomal disorders [Down syndrome])

RISK FACTORS

- Aging
- Cigarette smoking
- Ultraviolet (UV) sunlight exposure
- Diabetes
- Prolonged high-dose steroids
- Positive family history
- Alcohol

GENERAL PREVENTION

- Use of UV protective glasses
- Avoidance of tobacco products
- Effective control of diabetes
- Care with high-dose, long-term steroid use (systemic therapy > inhaled treatment)
- Protective methods using pharmaceutical intervention (e.g., antioxidants, acetylsalicylic acid [ASA], hormone replacement therapy [HRT]) show no proven benefit to date.

COMMONLY ASSOCIATED CONDITIONS

- Diabetes (especially with poor glucose control)
- Myotonic dystrophy (90% of patients develop a visually innocuous change in 3rd decade; becomes disabling in 5th decade)
- AD (10% of patients with severe AD develop cataracts in 2nd to 4th decades; often bilateral)
- Neurofibromatosis type 2
- Associated ocular disease or "secondary cataract" (e.g., chronic anterior uveitis, acute [or repetitive] angle-closure glaucoma or high myopia)
- Drug induced (e.g., steroids, chlorpromazine)
- Trauma

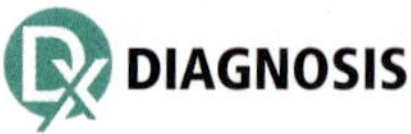

DIAGNOSIS

HISTORY

- Age-related cataract:
  - Decreased visual acuity, blurred vision, distortion, or "ghosting" of images (1)
  - Problems with visual acuity in any lighting condition
  - Falls or accidents; injuries (e.g., hip fracture)
- Congenital: often asymptomatic; leukocoria; parents notice child's visual inattention or strabismus.
- Other types of cataract:
  - May also present with decreased visual acuity
  - Appropriate clinical history or signs to help with diagnosis

PHYSICAL EXAM

- Visual acuity assessment for all cataracts
  - Glare testing allows further assessment of visual dysfunction.
- Age-related cataract: lens opacity on eye examination
- Congenital:
  - Lens opacity present at birth or within 3 months of birth
  - Leukocoria (white pupil), strabismus, nystagmus, signs of an associated syndrome (as with Down or rubella syndrome)
  - *Note*: must always rule out ocular tumor; early diagnosis and treatment of retinoblastoma may be lifesaving.
- Other types of cataract: may present with decreased visual acuity associated with characteristic physical findings (e.g., metabolic, trauma)

DIFFERENTIAL DIAGNOSIS

- An opaque-appearing eye may be due to opacities of the cornea (e.g., scarring, edema, calcification), lens opacities, tumor, or retinal detachment. Biomicroscopic examination (slit lamp) or careful ophthalmoscopic exam should provide a diagnosis.
- In the elderly, visual impairment is often due to multiple factors such as cataract and macular degeneration, both contributing to visual loss.
- Age-related cataract is significant if symptoms and ophthalmic exam support cataract as a major cause of vision impairment.
- Congenital lens opacity in the absence of other ocular pathology may cause severe amblyopia.
- *Note*: Cataract *does not* produce a relative afferent pupillary reaction defect. Abnormal pupillary reactions mandate further evaluation for other pathology.

DIAGNOSTIC TESTS & INTERPRETATION

- Visual quality assessment: Glare testing, contrast sensitivity is sometimes indicated.
- Retinal/macular function assessment: potential acuity meter testing
- Workup of the underlying process

Diagnostic Procedures/Other

- Optical biometry to measure the eye axial length and corneal keratometry for placement of intraocular lens
- Corneal topography to measure corneal curvature and power

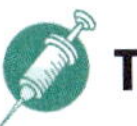

TREATMENT

- Outpatient (usually)
- ~1.64 million cataract extractions in the United States yearly (2)

GENERAL MEASURES

Eye protection from UV light

MEDICATION

There are currently no medications to prevent or slow the progression of cataracts.

ISSUES FOR REFERRAL

If the patient has cataracts and symptoms do not seem to support recommendation for surgery, a second opinion by another ophthalmologist may be indicated.

SURGERY/OTHER PROCEDURES

- Age-related cataract:
  - Surgical removal is indicated if visual impairment producing symptoms are distressing to the patient, interfering with lifestyle or occupation, or posing a risk for fall or injury (2)[A].
  - Because significant cataracts may develop gradually, the patient may not be aware of how it has changed their lifestyle. The physician may note a significant cataract, and the patient reports "no problems." Thus, evaluation requires an effective physician–patient relationship.
  - Preoperative evaluation: by the primary care physician:
    - Patients on anticoagulants may need to be temporarily discontinued 1 to 2 weeks before surgery if possible (but usually not necessary, thus need to discuss with ophthalmologist).
    - Patients who have ever taken an α-blocker such as tamsulosin (Flomax) should alert their ophthalmologist due to increased risk of intraoperative floppy iris syndrome [IFIS] even in patients who no longer use these drugs.
  - Anesthesia: usually topical with sedation and monitoring of vital signs, sometimes local injection as well
  - Surgical technique: cataract extraction via phacoemulsification through small incisions created by blade or laser, followed by implantation of a prosthetic intraocular lens; lenses have power calculated based on the size of the eye and curvature of the cornea usually to correct for distance vision; surgery performed on one (usually worse) eye, with contralateral surgery after recovery and if deemed necessary
    - Laser-assisted cataract surgery: Laser allows automated completion of certain steps of cataract surgery such as incisions, opening the lens capsule, and breaking up the cataract before surgical removal with phacoemulsification (3).
    - Light adjustable lens: allows refractive adjustments postoperatively which is especially valuable in patients with a history of prior corneal refractive surgery
  - Postoperative care: usually protective eye shield as directed, topical antibiotic, NSAIDs, and steroid ophthalmic medications; avoid lifting or bending for at least a week; keeping eye protected in general
- Congenital cataract:
  - Treatment is surgical removal of cataract. Newborns may require surgery within days to reduce the risk of severe amblyopia. The use of lens implants is controversial because the eyes are growing.
  - Postoperative care: long-term patching program for the good eye to combat amblyopia; refractive correction of operative eye, with multiple repeat examinations; challenging for physician and parents

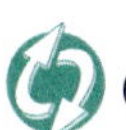

ONGOING CARE

FOLLOW-UP RECOMMENDATIONS

Patient Monitoring

- As the cataract progresses, the glasses or contact lens prescription may change to maintain vision. When this is no longer successful and interferes with patient's activities of daily living, surgery is indicated.
- Following surgery, spectacle correction may still be required to maximize near and/or far visual acuity. Refraction is usually prescribed several weeks after surgery.

PATIENT EDUCATION

Medline Plus on cataracts at: https://www.nlm.nih.gov/medlineplus/cataract.html

PROGNOSIS

- Ocular prognosis is good after cataract removal if no prior or coexisting ocular disease: 94.3% of otherwise healthy eyes achieve best-corrected visual acuity of 20/40 or better. Success rates are lower with comorbidities such as diabetes and glaucoma (4).
- Posterior capsular opacification can occur after cataract surgery and can cause a decrease in vision (14.7–42.7% of eyes, usually treated with Nd:YAG laser capsulotomy in the office with a rate of 4–25.3%).
- In congenital cataracts, prognosis is often poorer because of the high risk of amblyopia.

COMPLICATIONS

- Vary widely from delay in visual recovery or protracted visual discomfort to blindness and loss of the eye
- Complications are uncommon in general (<2% of eyes). Among the complications, a posterior capsular rupture is significant as it may require additional steps during surgery (5)[B].
- Poor preoperative visual acuity is related to surgical complications.

REFERENCES

1. Asbell PA, Dualan I, Mindel J, et al. Age-related cataract. *Lancet*. 2005;365(9459):599–609.
2. Riaz Y, Mehta JS, Wormald R, et al. Surgical interventions for age-related cataract. *Cochrane Database Syst Rev*. 2006(4):CD001323.
3. Kolb CM, Shajari M, Mathys L, et al. Comparison of femtosecond laser-assisted cataract surgery and conventional cataract surgery: a meta-analysis and systematic review. *J Cataract Refract Surg*. 2020;46(8):1075–1085.
4. Biber JM, Sandoval HP, Trivedi RH, et al. Comparison of the incidence and visual significance of posterior capsule opacification between multifocal spherical, monofocal spherical, and monofocal aspheric intraocular lenses. *J Cataract Refract Surg*. 2009;35(7):1234–1238.
5. Lundström M, Barry P, Henry Y, et al. Visual outcome of cataract surgery; study from the European Registry of Quality Outcomes for Cataract and Refractive Surgery. *J Cataract Refract Surg*. 2013;39(5):673–679.

SEE ALSO

- Floppy Iris Syndrome
- Algorithm: Cataracts

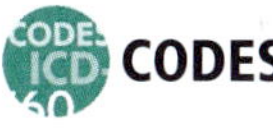

CODES

ICD10

- H26.049 Anterior subcapsular polar infantile and juvenile cataract, unspecified eye
- H26.069 Combined forms of infantile and juvenile cataract, unspecified eye
- H26.231 Glaucomatous flecks (subcapsular), right eye

CLINICAL PEARLS

- Cataracts are the leading cause of blindness worldwide; most cataracts are age-related.
- The primary indication for cataract surgery is visual impairment leading to significant lifestyle changes for the patient.
- For congenital cataracts, always consider ocular tumor because early diagnosis and treatment of retinoblastoma may be lifesaving.

CELIAC DISEASE

Michelle E. Duffelmeyer, MD

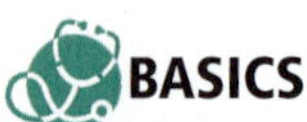

BASICS

DESCRIPTION

- A non–IgE-mediated immune enteropathic reaction to gliadin, a protein component of dietary gluten (found in wheat, barley, rye, and other grains) primarily affecting the small intestine in genetically predisposed individuals
- Presentations
  - Typical
    - Diarrheal illness characterized by villous atrophy with symptoms of malabsorption (steatorrhea, weight loss, vitamin deficiencies, anemia, dermatitis herpetiformis (DH) rash); resolves with a gluten-free diet (GFD)
    - <50% of adults present with gastrointestinal (GI) symptoms.
  - Atypical
    - Minor GI symptoms, with a myriad of extraintestinal manifestations (e.g., anemia, elevated LFTs, dental enamel defects, neurologic symptoms, infertility)
  - Asymptomatic (silent) disease
    - Found when screening first-degree relatives
    - Positive laboratory tests and genetics, without signs/symptoms; normal histology on biopsy
- System(s) affected: GI
- Synonym(s): celiac sprue; gluten-sensitive enteropathy; nontropical sprue

EPIDEMIOLOGY

Celiac disease (CD) is now recognized globally and incidence is increasing (1).

Incidence

Predominant sex: female > male (0.6%/0.4%) (2)

Prevalence

- 1% worldwide is estimated and is distributed in areas with susceptible human leukocyte antigen (HLA) genotype and gluten exposure.
- Exact worldwide prevalence of CD is unclear; recent meta-analysis showed 1.4% based on serology and 0.7% bases on biopsy (2).

ETIOLOGY AND PATHOPHYSIOLOGY

Sensitivity to gluten, specifically gliadin protein fraction; tissue transglutaminase (tTG) modification of the gliadin protein leads to immunologic cross-reactivity, inflammation, and tissue damage (villous atrophy) with subsequent GI symptoms and malabsorption.

Genetics

Homogenicity for HLA-DQ2/DQ8 increases risk of CD and enteropathy-associated T-cell lymphoma.

RISK FACTORS

First-degree relatives

Pediatric Considerations

No other risk factors (e.g., grain processing, genetically modified organisms, hygiene and illness during childhood, breastfeeding, time of introduction of solid foods, pollution, tobacco use, and medication) definitively explain why some susceptible individuals develop celiac, whereas others do not.

- If a first-degree relative has confirmed CD, then testing of the patient is warranted (3).
- Patients with type 1 diabetes should be tested for CD if there are any signs or symptoms (3).

COMMONLY ASSOCIATED CONDITIONS

- DH: 85% of patients with DH have CD. All patients with DH should follow a GFD.
- Secondary lactase deficiency
- Osteopenia and osteoporosis
- Infertility
- Thyroid disease: Hashimoto thyroiditis
- Type 1 diabetes
- Symptomatic iron deficiency: 10–15% have CD.
- Elevated AST and ALT (with no direct cause)
- Hyposplenism
- Oral aphthous ulcers
- Irritable bowel syndrome (IBS)
- Restless leg syndrome
- CD is associated with an increased risk for adenocarcinoma and lymphoma of the small bowel.
  - The risk of lymphoproliferative malignancies depends on small intestinal histopathology.
  - Little to no increased risk in latent CD (seropositive but normal biopsy)
- Associated autoimmune conditions (type 1 diabetes, autoimmune thyroiditis, primary biliary cirrhosis, autoimmune hepatitis, psoriasis, Sjögren disease)
- Associated genetic conditions (Down syndrome, IgA deficiency, Turner syndrome, Williams syndrome)

Pregnancy Considerations

- Prevalence of CD: 2.5 to 3.5 times higher in women with unexplained infertility
- Up to 19% of men with CD have androgen resistance. Semen quality and the likelihood of pregnancy increase with GFD.
- Higher rates of low birth weight, prematurity, spontaneous abortions, intrauterine growth restriction, and stillbirths

Pediatric Considerations

Children with type 1 diabetes, Down syndrome, Turner syndrome, Williams syndrome, IgA deficiency, and autoimmune thyroid disease are at risk for CD (3)[C].

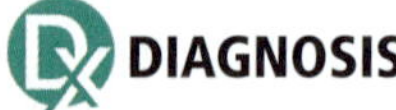

DIAGNOSIS

HISTORY

- Diarrhea and cramping are the most common GI symptoms.
- Other symptoms include steatorrhea (fatty stools); abdominal pain or distension; nausea, vomiting, flatulence; weight loss, weakness, fatigue; muscle cramps; bone and joint pain; paresthesias in hands and feet; constipation.
- Clinical signs include delayed puberty; iron deficiency anemia; recurrent aphthous stomatitis; dental enamel hyperplasia; anxiety, depression; migraines; anorexia; encopresis
- In children, malabsorption may manifest as failure to thrive, short stature, or chronic fatigue (3).

PHYSICAL EXAM

Physical examination is often normal. Findings can include:

- Cardiovascular: orthostatic hypotension, peripheral edema
- Oropharynx: aphthous stomatitis, glossitis, angular cheilitis
- Skin: DH (symmetric erythematous papules and blisters on elbows, knees, buttocks, and back), pallor
- Abdomen: distention

DIFFERENTIAL DIAGNOSIS

- Gluten allergy type II allergic reaction with signs of anaphylaxis
- Nonceliac gluten sensitivity—GI symptoms and/or systemic symptoms improved by GFD but without biomarkers characteristic of CD
- Short bowel syndrome, small intestinal bacterial overgrowth
- Lactose intolerance; gastroesophageal reflux disease (GERD)
- Pancreatic exocrine insufficiency, Crohn disease, Whipple disease
- Tropical sprue; intestinal lymphoma
- Microscopic colitis, autoimmune enteropathy
- HIV enteropathy
- Acute enteritis, radiation enteritis, eosinophilic gastroenteritis
- Giardiasis
- IBS, dyspepsia

DIAGNOSTIC TESTS & INTERPRETATION

Tissue biopsy is the gold standard for diagnosis.

Initial Tests (lab, imaging)

- Biopsy and histologic examination of duodenal bulb during routine upper endoscopy increase the diagnostic yield of CD. A sampling of the duodenal bulb and the distal duodenum is recommended to improve histologic confirmation of CD. Do not base diagnosis solely on serology in adults. Patients with symptoms highly suggestive of CD or those with positive serologies should undergo endoscopy for small bowel biopsy while on a gluten-containing diet.
- tTG-IgA is the preferred serologic test in patients aged >2 years.
- Total serum IgA to screen for IgA deficiency

ALERT

Positive tTG-IgA has high sensitivity and specificity (sensitivity, 95–98%; specificity, 95%) if on a normal (non–gluten-free) diet for at least 4 weeks. If positive, consider duodenal biopsy as next step.

- IgA-deficient patients have false-negative tTG-IgA antibodies.
- IgA deficiency is 10 to 15 times more prevalent in patients with CD.

Follow-Up Tests & Special Considerations

- If the patient is IgA deficient *or* if tTG-IgA is negative, follow up with anti-DGP IgA and IgG.
  - Sensitivity, 94%; specificity, 99% (~tTG-IgA)
- Do not use HLA DQ serotyping for initial diagnosis. Consider if discrepant serology-histology results in patients unable to test on GFD and children with Down syndrome.
- Consider bone mineral density testing at the time of diagnosis and after 1 year (if osteopenia/osteoporosis on initial testing) or 2 years (if normal initially and patient still symptomatic or nonadherent to diet).
- Younger age on diagnosis, less severe initial histologic damage, and male gender increase the likelihood of achieving mucosal recovery.
- Members of a family who have more than one individual with CD are at higher risk. Screen family members, including second-degree relatives.
- Vitamin B_{12}, folate, vitamin D, and iron studies

Pediatric Considerations

- Test symptomatic pediatric patients with IgA and IgA anti-tTG antibodies (Ab).
- Periodic monitoring with IgA anti-tTG Ab can assess dietary adherence.
- Negative serology cannot rule out CD.
- Consider HLA for high-risk children with negative serology.
- Limit IgA anti-endomysial antibodies to patients with illnesses that increase false-positive tTG Ab, such as type I diabetes or autoimmune liver disease.

Diagnostic Procedures/Other

- Endoscopy with a minimum of four biopsies of distal duodenum and two of duodenal bulb at the time of initial evaluation correctly diagnose 95% of children.
- Video capsule endoscopy is a promising alternative with a sensitivity and specificity of 80% and 95%, particularly helpful if antibody screening and clinical picture are consistent with CD despite nondiagnostic duodenal biopsies.

Test Interpretation

Small-bowel biopsy

- Villous atrophy, hyperplasia and lengthening of crypts, infiltration of plasma cells, and intraepithelial lymphocytosis in lamina propria
- Villous atrophy is also caused by Crohn disease, radiation enteritis, *Giardia*, and other food intolerances.

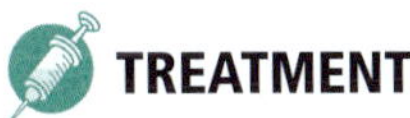

TREATMENT

GENERAL MEASURES

- GFD—avoid wheat, barley, rye, and other grains that contain gluten.
  - Rice, corn, and nut flour are safe and palatable substitutes.
  - Grains: uncontaminated oats, rice, corn, tapioca, quinoa, amaranth, sorghum
- Levels of IgA antigliadin normalize with gluten abstinence.
- Lifelong abstinence is required; immune response to gluten will recur with the resumption of gluten intake.

MEDICATION

First Line

Usually, no medications; GFD is the primary treatment.

Second Line

- In refractory disease, consult with GI to consider the choice, dosing, and duration of second-line treatment with steroids or immunomodulators.
- Depending on disease severity, patients may develop nutritional deficiencies that require appropriate supplementation.

ISSUES FOR REFERRAL

- Additional nutritional support with a qualified dietitian
- Refractory CD
- Child with positive celiac serology

COMPLEMENTARY & ALTERNATIVE MEDICINE

- Many alternative therapies are under development. Future treatment may include predigestion of gluten with peptidase, tight junction blockade, transglutaminase 2 or HLA DQ2/DQ8 blockers, and induction of immune tolerance.
- Patients with CD are at increased risk for pneumococcal infection. Pneumococcal vaccination should be considered, especially for those between the ages of 15 and 64 years who may not have received vaccination.

ONGOING CARE

FOLLOW-UP RECOMMENDATIONS

- Consultation with a registered dietitian
- Screen for osteoporosis and treat accordingly.
- Follow-up with GI at 3 to 6 months for serology and 12 months for repeat biopsy, if indicated

Patient Monitoring

- Repeat EGD if no clinical response to GFD or relapse in symptoms.
- Follow anti-tTG IgA or deaminated antigliadin antibodies to measure response/compliance with diet (vs. antigliadin IgA or IgG).

DIET

- Remove gluten: wheat, rye, barley, and products with gluten additives (processed food/meat, medications, hygiene products)
- Dietary change is challenging (especially identifying sources of "hidden" gluten) and should be coordinated with a skilled registered dietitian.

PATIENT EDUCATION

- Discuss how to recognize gluten in various products; highlight potential complications and outcomes of failing to follow a GFD; support groups and self-education
- Celiac Disease Foundation: https://www.celiac.org/; quick start GFD guide for celiac disease and non-celiac gluten sensitivity: http://celiac.org/wp-content/uploads/2013/12/quick-start-guide.pdf
- National Celiac Association: https://nationalceliac.org/; Beyond Celiac: https://www.beyondceliac.org/

PROGNOSIS

- Good prognosis if adherent to GFD
- Patients should see improvement within 7 days of dietary modification.
- Symptoms usually resolve in 4 to 6 weeks.

COMPLICATIONS

- Malignancy: Untreated and refractory patients have increased cancer risk, but successful treatment decreases risk to population baseline.
- Refractory disease (rare ~1–2% of all patients)
  - May respond to prednisone
  - May need total parenteral nutrition
- Osteoporosis, dehydration, electrolyte depletion, vitamin deficiencies

REFERENCES

1. Shiha MG, Chetcuti Zammit S, Elli L, et al. Updates in the diagnosis and management of celiac disease. *Best Pract Res Clin Gastroenterol*. 2023;64–65:101843. doi:10.1016/j.bpg.2023.101843.
2. Singh P, Arora A, Strand TA, et al. Global prevalence of celiac disease: systematic review and meta-analysis. *Clin Gastroenterol Hepatol*. 2018;16(6):823.e2–836.e2.
3. Rubio-Tapia A, Hill ID, Semrad C, et al. American College of Gastroenterology guidelines update: diagnosis and management of celiac disease. *Am J Gastroenterol*. 2023;118(1):59–76.

SEE ALSO

Algorithms: Diarrhea, Chronic; Malabsorption Syndrome

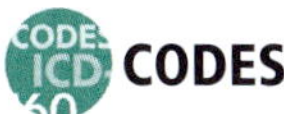

CODES

ICD10

K90.0 Celiac disease

CLINICAL PEARLS

- Screen for CD in patients with nonspecific GI symptoms, presumed IBS, DH, unexplained transaminitis, or unexplained iron deficiency anemia.
- Test total IgA levels along with tTG-IgA in patients >2 years of age. Positive serology should lead to consideration of duodenal biopsy for definitive diagnosis.
- Complete diagnostic testing while on a gluten-containing diet.
- Standard of treatment is a GFD. Patient symptoms should improve in 7 days if fully compliant.

CELLULITIS

Karl T. Clebak, MD, MHA, FAAFP • Madeline E. Lee, MD

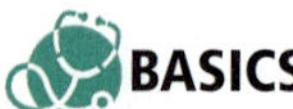

BASICS

Skin and soft tissue infections (SSTIs) cause >650,000 U.S. hospital admissions yearly; ~25% require inpatient care

DESCRIPTION

- An acute bacterial infection of the dermis and subcutaneous tissue
- Types and locations:
  - Periorbital: bacterial infection of the eyelid and surrounding tissues
  - Orbital: infection of the eye posterior to the septum; sinusitis is the most common risk factor.
  - Facial: often follows URI or otitis media
  - Buccal: infection of cheek in children associated with bacteremia (common before *Haemophilus influenzae* type B vaccine)
  - Peritonsillar: pediatric, with fever, sore throat, and muffled speech
  - Perianal: sharply demarcated, bright, perianal erythema
  - Necrotizing: gas-producing bacteria in the lower extremities; more common in diabetics

EPIDEMIOLOGY

- Predominant sex: male = female
- Seasonality increased hospitalizations for cellulitis in the summer with fewer in the winter months

Incidence

1.5 to 24.6 per 1,000 person-years with recurrent cellulitis with an incidence rate ranging from 16% to 53% within 3 years.

Prevalence

Visits to U.S. ambulatory practices for purulent SSTI range from 5.4 to 11.3 million visits annually.

ETIOLOGY AND PATHOPHYSIOLOGY

Cellulitis is caused by bacterial penetration through a compromise in the epidermis, the protective barrier of the skin, into the deep dermis and subcutaneous tissues.

- Microbiology
  - β-Hemolytic streptococci (groups A, B, C, G, and F), staphylococci (*Staphylococcus aureus*, including MRSA), and gram-negative aerobic bacilli are most common.
  - *S. aureus* seen in periorbital and orbital cellulitis and people who inject IV drugs
  - *Pseudomonas aeruginosa* seen in diabetics and other immunocompromised patients, or through nail/sharp metal puncture through soles of shoes
  - *H. influenza* causes buccal cellulitis.
  - Clostridia and non–spore-forming anaerobes: necrotizing cellulitis (crepitant/gangrenous)
  - *Streptococcus agalactiae*: cellulitis following lymph node dissection
  - *Pasteurella multocida* and *Capnocytophaga canimorsus*: cellulitis preceded by bites
  - *Streptococcus iniae*: immunocompromised hosts
  - Rare causes: *mycobacterium*, fungal (mucormycosis, aspergillosis)

Genetics

No genetic pattern

RISK FACTORS

- Skin barrier disruption (e.g., trauma, bites, intravenous drug user [IVDU], ulcers, fissures)
- Inflammation from excoriating skin disorders or radiation therapy
- Edema due to venous insufficiency; lymphatic obstruction due to surgery or congestive heart failure
- Advanced age, male gender, diabetes, hypertension, cancer, obesity
- Dermatomycosis, tinea pedis, onychomycosis, presence of *S. aureus* and/or streptococci in the toe webs
- Previous episode of cellulitis
- Recurrent cellulitis:
  - Cellulitis recurrence score (predicts recurrence of lower extremity cellulitis based on presence of lymphedema, chronic venous insufficiency, peripheral vascular disease, and deep venous thrombosis)
  - Seen in patients with immunosuppression, diabetes, vascular disease, chronic kidney disease, or drug use

GENERAL PREVENTION

- Good skin hygiene keeping skin well hydrated to avoid dryness and cracking
- Management of edema including elevation, compression stockings, pneumatic pressure pumps
- Maintain glycemic control and proper foot care in diabetic patients.

COMMONLY ASSOCIATED CONDITIONS

Abscess, lymphedema, venous insufficiency, stasis dermatitis, obesity

DIAGNOSIS

Clinical diagnosis presenting as an area of local inflammation consisting of pain, swelling, and/or erythema which may be associated with a systemic inflammatory response

HISTORY

- Disruptions of the skin barrier such as previous trauma, surgery/vein stripping, animal/human/insect bites, dermatitis, IVDU, and fungal infection are portals of entry.
- Pain, itching, and/or burning
- Fever, chills, and malaise

PHYSICAL EXAM

- Assess vital signs for hemodynamic stability.
- Painful erythema with induration and warmth; often poorly demarcated; may include signs of lymphangitis (streaking)
- Regional lymphadenopathy
- Purulent drainage
- Orbital cellulitis: proptosis, globe displacement, limitation of ocular movements, vision loss, diplopia
- Facial cellulitis: malaise, anorexia, vomiting, pruritus, burning, anterior neck swelling

DIFFERENTIAL DIAGNOSIS

Toxic shock syndrome, venous stasis dermatitis, deep vein thrombosis, thrombophlebitis, bursitis, dermatitis, herpes zoster, osteomyelitis, malignancy, drug reaction, sunburn, insect bites, erythema nodosum

DIAGNOSTIC TESTS & INTERPRETATION

Initial Tests (lab, imaging)

- If there are signs of systemic disease (fever, heart rate >100 bpm, or systolic blood pressure <90 mm Hg): CBC, blood cultures, CPK, CRP, ESR; consider serum lactate levels.
- Swab breaks in skin, ulcerations, blister fluid for culture. Microbiologic diagnosis is generally not needed.
- Plain radiographs, CT, and MRI are useful if osteomyelitis, fracture, necrotizing fasciitis, retained foreign body.
- MRI and ultrasound are most useful for evaluation of potential underlying abscesses.
- Procalcitonin is not useful in diagnosing early cellulitis.

Diagnostic Procedures/Other

Consider lumbar puncture in children with *H. influenzae* type B or if meningeal signs and facial cellulitis.

TREATMENT

GENERAL MEASURES

- Elevate limb to reduce swelling.
- Cool compresses or sterile saline dressings relieve pain.
- Edema: compression stockings, pneumatic pumps; diuretic therapy for CHF patients
- Mark the borders of erythema to monitor progression and response to therapy.
- Tetanus immunization if needed

MEDICATION

First Line

- Target treatment if known pathogen and/or with certain exposures (animal bites)
- Empiric antibiotic selection:
  - Nonpurulent cellulitis
    - With nonpurulent drainage, target treatment toward β-hemolytic streptococci and MSSA.
    - Outpatient: Treat for 5 days; extend if no improvement (1)[C].
      - Oral: for mild cellulitis
        - Cephalexin 500 mg PO q6h; children: 25 to 100 mg/kg/day in 3 to 4 doses (max 4,000 mg/day)
        - Dicloxacillin 500 mg PO q6h; children <40kg: mild-moderate disease: 12.5 mg/kg/day divided into 4 equal doses qh6; severe disease: 25 mg/kg/day divided into 4 equal doses q6h
        - Clindamycin 300 to 450 mg PO q6–8h; children: 20 to 30 mg/kg/day in 4 doses (max 1.8 g/day)

- IV: for rapidly progressing cellulitis
  - Cefazolin 1 to 2 g IV q8h; children: 100 mg/kg/day IV in 2 to 4 divided doses (max 6 g/day)
  - Oxacillin 2 g IV q4h; children: 150 to 200 mg/kg/day IV in 4 to 6 doses (max 12 g/day)
  - Nafcillin 2 g IV q4h; children: 150 to 200 mg/kg/day IV in 4 to 6 doses (max 12 g/day)
  - Clindamycin 600 to 900 mg IV q8h; children: 25 to 40 mg/kg/day IV in 3 to 4 doses (max 4.8 g/day)

– Purulent cellulitis (probable CA-MRSA)
  - Culture purulent wounds and follow-up in 48 hours.
  - Start trimethoprim-sulfamethoxazole (TMP-SMX), clindamycin, or doxycycline 3rd- or 4th-generation fluoroquinolone for patients with cellulitis likely caused by CA-MRSA (2)[A].
  - Incise and drain abscesses and start empiric antibiotic therapy; modify based on culture results; tailor duration based on clinical response:
    - Oral
      - Clindamycin 300 to 450 mg PO; children: 40 mg/kg/day in 3 to 4 doses, max 1.8 g/day
      - TMP-SMX 1 DS tab PO BID; children: dose based on TMP at 8 to 12 mg/kg/day divided in 2 doses
      - Doxycycline 100 mg PO BID; children >8 years old: ≤45 kg: 4 mg/kg/day divided in 2 doses; >45 kg: 100 mg PO BID
      - Minocycline 200 mg PO once and then 100 mg PO BID; children >8 years old: 4 mg/kg PO once and then 4 mg/kg PO BID, max 400 mg/day
      - Linezolid 600 mg PO BID; children <12 years old: 10 mg/kg/dose (max 600 mg/dose) PO TID; ≥12 years old: 600 mg PO BID, limit tyramine food content <100 mg/meal.
      - Tedizolid 200 mg PO once daily; children >12 years old: 200 mg PO daily; dosing is not established.
    - IV
      - Vancomycin 20 to 35 mg/kg one time loading dose then 15 to 20 mg/kg/dose IV q8–12h, adjusted based on blood levels
      - Daptomycin 4 mg/kg/dose IV once daily for moderate infection; if bacteremia is present or suspected: 8 to 10 mg/kg IV once daily
      - Linezolid 600 mg IV q12h
      - Tedizolid 200 mg IV q daily
      - Ceftaroline 600 mg IV q12h
      - Tigecycline 100 mg IV once, thereafter 50 mg IV q12h

- Necrotizing cellulitis: requires broad-spectrum coverage to cover aerobic and anaerobic species including MRSA: ampicillin-sulbactam 1.5 to 3.0 g q6–8h IV or piperacillin-tazobactam 3.37 g q6–8h IV plus ciprofloxacin 400 mg q12h IV plus clindamycin 600 to 900 mg q8h IV; consider intensive care and emergent surgical consultation.
- Freshwater exposure: penicillinase-resistant: penicillin plus gentamicin or fluoroquinolone; salt water exposure: doxycycline 200 mg IV in 2 divided doses
- Bites: The combination of amoxicillin and clavulanic acid is recommended for human and dog bites. Ticarcillin and clavulanic acid or the combination of a 3rd-generation cephalosporin (i.e., ceftriaxone) plus metronidazole provides adequate parenteral therapy for animal or human bites. If allergic to penicillin, use fluoroquinolone plus metronidazole.
- Facial cellulitis in adults: ceftriaxone IV
- Diabetic foot infection:
  – Mild to moderate: cephalexin or cephalexin plus doxycycline or TMP-SMX plus amoxicillin clavulanate
  – Severe: ampicillin-sulbactam or imipenem-cilastatin or meropenem; alternative: combinations of targeting anaerobes as well as gram-positive and gram-negative aerobes
- If severe infection, toxicity, immunocompromised patients, or worsening infection despite empirical therapy, admit for empiric antibiotic therapy covering MRSA.
- Recurrent streptococcal cellulitis: penicillin 250 mg BID, or if penicillin-allergic, use erythromycin 250 mg BID.
- Dalbavancin, a 2nd-generation lipoglycopeptide antibiotic with MRSA coverage, can be used to treat cellulitis and be administered rarely as once a week.

Pediatric Considerations

- Avoid doxycycline in children ≤8 years old and during pregnancy.
- The Melbourne ASSET tool is helpful in determining the need for IV antibiotics in pediatric populations (sensitivity 60%, specificity 93%).

SURGERY/OTHER PROCEDURES

- Débridement for gas and purulent matter
- Intubation or tracheotomy may be needed for cellulitis of the head or neck.

ADMISSION, INPATIENT, AND NURSING CONSIDERATIONS

- Severe infection, suspicion of deeper or rapidly spreading infection, tissue necrosis, or severe pain
- Marked systemic toxicity or worsening symptoms that do not resolve after 24 to 48 hours of therapy
- Patients with underlying risk factors or severe comorbidities

ONGOING CARE

FOLLOW-UP RECOMMENDATIONS

Patient Monitoring

- Repeat relevant labs if patient is toxic or not improving.
- Symptomatic improvement usually occurs in 24 to 48 hours, but visible improvement may take 72 hours.

DIET

Glucose control in diabetics

PATIENT EDUCATION

Good skin hygiene including moisturizing to prevent skin barrier breakdown

PROGNOSIS

Older age, BMI, and diabetes lower response to antibiotics.

COMPLICATIONS

- Local abscess
- Bacteremia, sepsis
- Superinfection with gram-negative organisms
- Lymphangitis
- Thrombophlebitis/thrombosis
- Bacterial meningitis
- Gangrene

REFERENCES

1. Stevens DL, Bisno AL, Chambers HF, et al. Practice guidelines for the diagnosis and management of skin and soft tissue infections: 2014 update by the Infectious Diseases Society of America. *Clin Infect Dis*. 2014;59(2):147–159.
2. Clebak KT, Reedy-Cooper A, Partin MT, et al. A guide to the Tx of cellulitis and other soft-tissue infections. *J Fam Pract*. 2021;70(5):214–219. doi:10.12788/jfp.0198.

ADDITIONAL READING

Rrapi R, Chand S, Kroshinsky D. Cellulitis: a review of pathogenesis, diagnosis, and management. *Med Clin North Am*. 2021;105(4):723–735. doi:10.1016/j.mcna.2021.04.009.

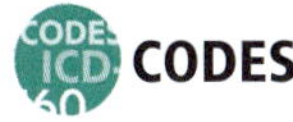

CODES

ICD10

- L03.032 Cellulitis of left toe
- L03.312 Cellulitis of back [any part except buttock]
- L03.211 Cellulitis of face

CLINICAL PEARLS

- *S. aureus* and group A *Streptococcus* are the most common organisms causing cellulitis.
- Consider MRSA if cellulitis does not respond to antibiotics within 48 hours or if purulence present.
- Rapid expansion of infected area with discoloration and severe pain may suggest necrotizing fasciitis, requiring urgent surgical evaluation.
- Venous stasis dermatitis often mimics cellulitis leading to improper use of antibiotics.

CELLULITIS, ORBITAL

Frances J. Boly, DO • Laura Mallinger, DO

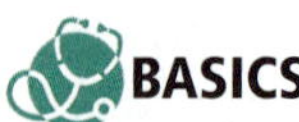

BASICS

DESCRIPTION
- Acute, severe, vision-threatening infection of orbital contents posterior to the orbital septum; preseptal (previously referred to as periorbital) cellulitis is anterior to the septum. Location determines the appropriate workup and treatment.
- Synonym(s): postseptal cellulitis

EPIDEMIOLOGY
- More common in children
- Orbital cellulitis is much less common than preseptal cellulitis (1).

Incidence
The incidence of orbital cellulitis has declined since introduction of routine *Haemophilus influenzae* type b (Hib) vaccination.

ETIOLOGY AND PATHOPHYSIOLOGY
- Sinusitis is classically associated with orbital cellulitis. Local skin conditions surrounding the eyelids and lashes are typically associated with preseptal cellulitis. The ethmoid sinus is separated from the orbit by the lamina papyracea ("layer of paper"), a thin bony separation, and is often the source of contiguous spread of infection to the orbit. The ethmoid sinus is present at birth. The orbital septum is a connective tissue barrier that extends from the skull into the lid and separates the preseptal from the orbital space.
- Cellulitis in the closed bony orbit causes proptosis, globe displacement, orbital apex syndrome (mass effect on the cranial nerves), optic nerve compression, and vision loss.
- Cultures of surgical specimens in adults often grow multiple organisms. In over 1/3 of cases, no pathogen is recovered. Blood cultures typically do not grow an organism.
- Most common organisms: *Staphylococcus aureus*, *Streptococcus pneumoniae*, *Streptococcus anginosus*
- Haemophilus is no longer the leading cause of orbital cellulitis. MRSA is increasingly a consideration.

Genetics
No known genetic predisposition

RISK FACTORS
- Sinusitis (present in 80–100% of cases). Pansinusitis is often observed in adults (1).
- Orbital trauma, retained orbital foreign body (FB), ophthalmic surgery, and/or history of sinus surgery (1)
- Dental, periorbital, skin, or intracranial infection; acute dacryocystitis (inflammation of the lacrimal sac) and acute dacryoadenitis (inflammation of the lacrimal gland)
- Immunosuppressed patients are at increased risk for adverse outcomes.

GENERAL PREVENTION
Routine Hib vaccination; appropriate treatment of bacterial sinusitis; proper wound care and perioperative monitoring of orbital surgery and trauma; avoid trauma to the sinus and orbital regions.

COMMONLY ASSOCIATED CONDITIONS
- Sinusitis, especially pansinusitis in adults; trauma and intraorbital FB; preseptal cellulitis
- Adverse outcomes include neutropic keratitis, secondary glaucoma, septic uveitis or retinitis, exudative retinal detachment, meningitis, cranial nerve palsies, panophthalmitis, inflammatory or infectious neuritis, retinal vein occlusion, central retinal artery occlusion, orbital abscess, subperiosteal abscess, orbital apex syndrome, subdural or brain abscess, and death.

DIAGNOSIS

HISTORY
- Complaints of acute onset red, swollen, tender eye or eyelid, and pain with eye movements
- History of surgery, trauma, sinus or upper respiratory infection, dental infection
- Malaise, fever, stiff neck, mental status changes
- Specific signs of orbital cellulitis include the following:
  - Proptosis, double vision, ophthalmoplegia, vision loss (or decreased field of vision), pain with eye movement, decreased color vision (differentiating green and red)

ALERT
- Differentiating orbital from preseptal cellulitis is the critical diagnostic step. Preseptal cellulitis can be identified by exam or following CT scan.
- Both preseptal and orbital cellulitis present with a red, swollen painful eye or eyelid.
- Diplopia, ophthalmoplegia, painful extraocular movements, proptosis, vision loss, and fever suggest orbital involvement.
- Contrast CT is the imaging method of choice and must be done for suspicion of orbital cellulitis (2).
- Treat with immediate intravenous (IV) antibiotics, hospital admission, and ophthalmology referral.
- Monitor frequently for vision loss, cavernous sinus thrombosis, abscess, and meningitis.

PHYSICAL EXAM
Vital signs
- Assess visual acuity (with glasses if required).
- Lid exam and palpation of the orbit; pupillary reflex for afferent pupillary defect
- Extraocular movements; assess for pain with eye movement—if present, then concerning for orbital cellulitis.
- Red desaturation: Patient views red object with one eye and compares to the other; reduced red color may indicate optic nerve involvement.
- Proptosis; pain with palpation; confrontation visual field testing
- Chemosis
- Ophthalmoplegia (restricted eye movements)

DIFFERENTIAL DIAGNOSIS
- Preseptal cellulitis
  - Eyelid erythema with or without conjunctival erythema, afebrile, no pain on eye movement, no diplopia, normal eye exam, vision intact
- Metastatic tumors and autoimmune inflammation may masquerade as orbital cellulitis in rare cases; usually present with painless slow onset of symptoms
- Idiopathic orbital inflammatory disease (orbital pseudotumor); orbital FB
- Arteriovenous fistula (carotid-cavernous fistula)
- Cavernous sinus thrombosis; acute thyroid orbitopathy; orbital tumor; trauma, insect bite, ruptured dermoid cyst
- Clinical signs help distinguish preseptal from orbital cellulitis. Preseptal infection causes erythema, induration, and tenderness of the eyelid and/or periorbital tissues, and patients rarely show signs of systemic illness. Local skin trauma, lacerations, or bug bites can be seen. Extraocular movements and visual acuity are intact.
- Orbital cellulitis also presents with red, swollen, painful eye or eyelid. More specific symptoms include proptosis, conjunctival edema, ophthalmoplegia, painful eye movements, and decreased visual acuity.

DIAGNOSTIC TESTS & INTERPRETATION
- CBC with differential, C-reactive protein (often >120 mg/L), ESR; inflammatory markers higher in orbital than preseptal cellulitis; an elevated neutrophil-to-lymphocyte ratio (NLR) suggests infection.
- Swab cultures of eye secretions or nasopharyngeal aspirates are often contaminated by normal flora but may identify causative organism(s).
- Blood cultures (usually negative) should be obtained prior to initiation of antibiotic therapy in ill-appearing or febrile patients.

Initial Tests (lab, imaging)
- CT scan of orbits and sinuses with axial and coronal views, with and without contrast, is imaging modality of choice. US and MRI are alternatives.
  - Thin section (2 mm) CT, coronal and axial views with bone windows to differentiate preseptal from orbital cellulitis, confirm extension into orbit, detect coexisting sinus disease, and identify orbital or subperiosteal abscesses that may require surgery; deviation of medial rectus indicates intraorbital involvement.
- MRI offers superior soft tissue resolution for identification of cavernous sinus thrombosis but is less effective for bone imaging.
- US is used to rule out orbital myositis, locate FBs or abscesses, and follow progression of drained abscess.

Follow-Up Tests & Special Considerations
- Frequent eye exam and vital signs (q4h)
- Identify associated conditions, such as meningitis or orbital abscess.

Diagnostic Procedures/Other

Consult ophthalmology for slit lamp and dilated funduscopic exam; to evaluate proptosis, color vision, automated visual field; and need for surgery.

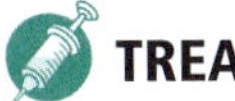

TREATMENT

Admit patients with orbital cellulitis for monitoring and treatment with broad-spectrum IV antibiotics.

MEDICATION

- Empiric antibiotic therapy to cover pathogens associated with acute sinusitis (*S. pneumoniae*, *H. influenzae*, *M. catarrhalis*, *Streptococcus pyogenes*) as well as for *S. aureus*, *S. anginosus*, and anaerobes
- Modify IV antibiotic treatment when culture and sensitivity results are available. Duration of IV therapy is usually a week. Additional PO therapy depends on response.
- PO antibiotic therapy for 2 to 3 weeks or longer (3 to 6 weeks) is recommended for patients with severe sinusitis and bony destruction.

First Line

IV therapy (preferred initially)

- Vancomycin
  - For MRSA coverage
    - Children: 40 to 60 mg/kg/day IV divided into 3 or 4 doses; maximum daily dose 4 g
    - Adults: 15 to 20 mg/kg/day IV every 8 to 12 hours; maximum 2 g for each dose
  - Plus one of the following:
    - Ceftriaxone
      - Children: 50 mg/kg per dose IV QD or BID; maximum daily dose 4 g/day
      - Adults: 2 g IV/day
    - Cefotaxime
      - Children: 150 to 200 mg/kg/day in 3 doses; maximum daily dose 12 g
      - Adults: 2 g IV every 4 hours
    - Ampicillin-sulbactam
      - Children: 300 mg/kg/day in 4 divided doses; maximum daily dose 8 g of ampicillin
      - Adults: 3 g IV every 6 hours
    - Piperacillin-tazobactam
      - Children: 240 mg/kg/day in 3 divided doses; maximum daily dose 16 g of piperacillin
      - Adults: 4.5 g IV every 6 hours
    - Metronidazole
      - For anaerobic
        - Adults: 500 mg IV or 500 mg PO q8h daily
  - If allergic to penicillin treat with a combination of vancomycin plus:
    - Ciprofloxacin
      - Adults: 400 mg IV BID or 500 to 750 mg orally BID
      - Children: 20 to 30 mg/kg/day divided every 12 hours; maximum dose of 1.5 g orally daily or 800 mg IV daily
    - Levofloxacin
      - Adults: 500 to 750 mg IV or orally QD
      - Children 5 years or older: 10 mg/kg per dose q24h; maximum 500 mg/day
      - Children 5 years or younger: 10 mg/kg per dose every 12 hours
- Oral therapy (if good response)
- Clindamycin (alone)
  - Adults: 300 mg q8h
  - Children: 30 to 40 mg/kg/day in 3 to 4 divided doses, max of 1.8 g/day
- Clindamycin or Trimethoprim-Sulfamethoxazole
  - Adults: 1 to 2 DS tablets every 12 hours
  - Children: 10 to 12 mg/kg per day of trimethoprim divided q12h
- Plus one of the following:
  - Amoxicillin
    - Adults: 875 mg orally q12h
    - Children: 45 mg/kg per day in divided doses every 12 hours or 80 to 100 mg/kg per day in divided doses every 8 hours; Maximum dose 500 mg per dose
  - Amoxicillin-clavulanic
    - Adults: 875 mg q12h
    - Children: 40 to 45 mg/kg per day in divided doses every 8 to 12 hours or 90 mg/kg per day divided every 12 hours (600 mg/5 mL suspension)
  - Cefpodoxime
    - Adults: 400 mg q12h
    - Children: 10 mg/kg/day divided every 12 hours, not to exceed 200 mg per dose
  - Cefdinir
    - Adults: 300 mg bid
    - Children: 7 mg/kg bid, not to exceed 600 mg/day

ALERT

In severe orbital cellulitis, in suspected or proven MRSA infection, vancomycin remains the parenteral drug of choice. Use in conjunction with agents to cover gram-negative bacteria.

- Vancomycin: 1 g IV q12h for adults; 40 mg/kg/day IV divided q8–12h; max daily dose 2 g for children

Second Line

Any number of antibiotic regimens have been reported as successful. There is no definitive consensus for best choice (1).

ISSUES FOR REFERRAL

Always admit to the hospital and consult with ophthalmology. Consider consultation with ID and ENT; neurology/neurosurgery if intracranial spread is suspected.

ADDITIONAL THERAPIES

- Steroid use is controversial. PO steroids as an adjunct to IV antibiotics for orbital cellulitis may speed resolution of inflammation.
- Nasal decongestants are often recommended.
- Topical erythromycin or nonmedicated ophthalmic ointment protects the cornea from exposure in cases with severe proptosis.
- Children may be treated with amoxicillin/clavulanate 20 to 40 mg/kg/day divided TID or in adults 250 to 500 mg TID.

SURGERY/OTHER PROCEDURES

- IV antibiotic therapy is the initial therapy. 80–90% of cases respond to medical therapy without surgery.
- Surgical intervention warranted for visual loss, complete ophthalmoplegia, well-defined large abscess (>10 mm) on presentation or no clinical improvement after 24 to 48 hours of antibiotic therapy

ADMISSION, INPATIENT, AND NURSING CONSIDERATIONS

Patients with orbital cellulitis should be admitted for IV antibiotics and serial eye exams to evaluate progression of infection or involvement of optic nerve.

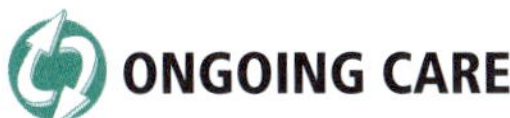

ONGOING CARE

FOLLOW-UP RECOMMENDATIONS

Patient Monitoring

Serial visual acuity testing and slit lamp exams

ALERT

Bedside exam q4h is indicated, as complications can develop rapidly.

PATIENT EDUCATION

Maintain proper handwashing and good skin hygiene. Avoid skin or lid trauma.

PROGNOSIS

Historically, blindness occurred in 20% and death in 17% of cases before antibiotics. Vision loss occurs in 3–11% of cases (1).

COMPLICATIONS

- Vision loss, CNS involvement, and death
- Permanent vision loss
- CNS complications: Intracranial abscess, meningitis, cavernous sinus thrombosis

REFERENCES

1. Pelletier J, Koyfman A, Long B. High risk and low prevalence diseases: orbital cellulitis. *Am J Emer Med*. 2023;68:1–9. doi:10.1016/j.ajem.2023.02.024.
2. Khan SA, Hussain A, Phelps PO. Current clinical diagnosis and management of orbital cellulitis. *Expert Review of Ophthalmology*. 2021;16(5):387–399.

ADDITIONAL READING

Miranda-Barrios J, Bravo-Queipo-de-Llano B, Baquero-Artigao F, et al. Preseptal versus orbital cellulitis in children: an observational study. *Pediatr Infect Dis J*. 2021;40(11):969–974. doi:10.1097/INF.0000000000003226.

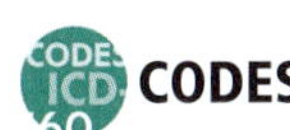

CODES

ICD10

- H05.019 Cellulitis of unspecified orbit
- H05.011 Cellulitis of right orbit
- H05.012 Cellulitis of left orbit

CLINICAL PEARLS

- Orbital cellulitis is a medical emergency—most cases arise from sinusitis.
- CT of orbits and sinuses with axial and coronal views with and without contrast is diagnostic modality of choice.
- Patients with orbital cellulitis must be admitted for visual monitoring and IV antibiotic therapy.
- Older age (>10 years) and diplopia predict need for surgical intervention in children.
- Ophthalmoplegia, mental status changes, contralateral cranial nerve palsy, or bilateral orbital cellulitis raise suspicion for intracranial involvement.

CELLULITIS, PERIORBITAL

Jennifer M. Romeu, MD, FAAFP, MSM

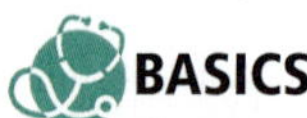

BASICS

DESCRIPTION

- An acute bacterial infection of the skin and subcutaneous tissue anterior to the orbital septum; does not involve the orbital structures (globe, fat, and ocular muscles)
- Synonym(s): preseptal cellulitis

ALERT

It is essential to distinguish periorbital cellulitis from orbital cellulitis. Orbital cellulitis is a potentially life-threatening condition. *Orbital cellulitis is posterior to the orbital septum; symptoms include restricted eye movement (ophthalmoplegia), pain with eye movement, proptosis, and vision changes.*

EPIDEMIOLOGY

- Occurs more commonly in children; mean age 21 months
- 3 times more common than orbital cellulitis

Incidence

Increased incidence in the winter months (due to increased cases of sinusitis)

ETIOLOGY AND PATHOPHYSIOLOGY

- The anatomy of the eyelid distinguishes periorbital (preseptal) from orbital cellulitis:
  - A connective tissue sheet (orbital septum) extends from the orbital bones to the margins of the upper and lower eyelids; it acts as a barrier to infection of deeper orbital structures.
  - Infection of tissues anterior to the orbital septum is periorbital (preseptal) cellulitis.
  - Infection deep to the orbital septum is orbital (postseptal) cellulitis.
- Periorbital cellulitis typically arises from a contiguous infection of soft tissues of the face.
  - Sinusitis (via lamina papyracea) extension
  - Local trauma; insect or animal bites
  - Foreign bodies
  - Dental abscess extension
  - Hematogenous seeding
- Common organisms
  - *Staphylococcus aureus*, typically MSSA (MRSA is increasing.)
  - *Staphylococcus epidermidis*
  - *Streptococcus pyogenes*
  - *Streptococcus pneumonia* (1)
- Atypical organisms
  - *Acinetobacter* spp.; *Nocardia brasiliensis*
  - *Bacillus anthracis; Pseudomonas aeruginosa*
  - *Neisseria gonorrhoeae; Proteus* spp.
  - *Pasteurella multocida; Mycobacterium tuberculosis; Trichophyton* sp. (ringworm)
- Since vaccine introduction, the incidence of *Haemophilus influenzae* disease has decreased (should still be suspected in unimmunized or partially immunized patients).

Genetics

No known genetic predisposition

RISK FACTORS

- Contiguous spread from upper respiratory infection
- Acute sinusitis
- Conjunctivitis
- Blepharitis
- Dental infection
- Local skin trauma/puncture wound
- Insect bite
- Bacteremia

GENERAL PREVENTION

- Avoid trauma around the eyes.
- Avoid swimming in fresh or salt water with facial skin abrasions.
- Routine vaccination: particularly *H. influenzae* type B and *Streptococcus pneumoniae*

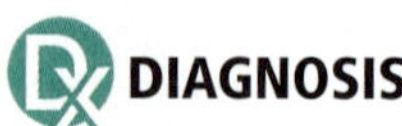

DIAGNOSIS

HISTORY

- Induration, erythema, warmth, and/or tenderness of periorbital soft tissue, usually with normal vision and normal eye movements
- Chemosis (conjunctival swelling), proptosis; pain with extraocular eye movements can occur in severe cases of periorbital cellulitis and are concerning for orbital cellulitis.
- Fever (not always present)
- History of recent upper respiratory illness, sinusitis, or insect bite/local trauma (2)

ALERT

Pain with eye movement, fever, and conjunctival swelling raise the suspicion for orbital cellulitis.

PHYSICAL EXAM

- Vital signs and general appearance (Patients with orbital cellulitis often appear systemically ill.)
- Inspect eyes and surrounding structures—eyelids, lashes, conjunctiva, and skin.
  - Erythema, swelling, and tenderness of lids without orbital congestion
  - Violaceous discoloration of eyelid is more commonly associated with *H. influenzae*.
- Evaluate for skin breakdown.
- Look for vesicles to rule out herpetic infection.
- Inspect nasal vaults and palpate sinuses for signs of acute sinusitis.
- Examine oral cavity for dental abscesses.
- Test ocular motility and visual acuity.

DIFFERENTIAL DIAGNOSIS

- Orbital cellulitis
  - Orbital cellulitis may have the same signs and symptoms as periorbital cellulitis, with fever, proptosis, chemosis, ophthalmoplegia, decreased visual acuity, pain with ocular movement.
- Abscess
- Dacryocystitis
- Hordeolum (stye)
- Angioedema (allergic inflammation) (2)
- Orbital or periorbital trauma
- Idiopathic inflammation from orbital pseudotumor
- Orbital myositis
- Rapidly progressive tumors
  - Rhabdomyosarcoma
  - Retinoblastoma
  - Lymphoma
- Leukemia

DIAGNOSTIC TESTS & INTERPRETATION

Initial Tests (lab, imaging)

- CBC with differential diagnosis
- Blood cultures (not performed routinely) (2)
- Wound culture of purulent drainage (if present)
- Imaging is indicated if there is suspicion for orbital cellulitis (marked eyelid swelling, fever, and leukocytosis or failure to improve on appropriate antibiotics within 24 to 48 hours).
  - CT to rule out orbital cellulitis if there is suspicion based on history and exam:
    - CT with contrast, thin sections (2 mm); coronal and axial views with bone windows
    - The classic sign of orbital cellulitis on CT scan is bulging of the medial rectus.
    - CT head can be considered to rule out intracranial involvement (when suspecting abscess) (2)

Follow-Up Tests & Special Considerations

- Children with periorbital or orbital cellulitis often have underlying sinusitis.
- If a child is febrile, <15 months old, and appears toxic, admit for blood cultures, antibiotic therapy, and consider lumbar puncture.

TREATMENT

MEDICATION

- Treat periorbital cellulitis with oral antibiotics and ensure close follow-up.
- Empiric antibiotic treatment should cover the most likely organisms (*Staphylococcus* and *Streptococcus*).
- Observe local prevalence of MRSA to determine need for coverage.
- No evidence that IV antibiotics are more effective than PO in reducing recovery time or preventing secondary complications in simple periorbital cellulitis
- Insufficient evidence for benefit of steroid use (3)

First Line

- Uncomplicated periorbital cellulitis
  - Usually due to skin flora, including *Staphylococcus* and *Streptococcus*
  - Amoxicillin-clavulanate 875 mg PO BID for 7 to 10 days
  - Clindamycin 300 mg PO TID
  - Trimethoprim-sulfamethoxazole (TMP-SMX) 1 to 2 DS tablets PO q12h if MRSA is suspected (often used in combination with cephalexin 500 mg PO TID or dicloxacillin 500 mg QID to cover streptococci concurrently)
  - If not immunized by *H. influenzae*, consider antibiotic with beta-lactam coverage (2)
  - 3rd-generation cephalosporin (e.g., cefdinir 300 mg PO BID)
- Dental abscess
  - Amoxicillin-clavulanate 875 mg PO BID or clindamycin 300 mg PO TID
- Bacteremic cellulitis
  - May be associated with meningitis
  - Ceftriaxone 1 g IV q24h plus vancomycin 15 mg/kg/dose IV q8–12h or clindamycin 600 to 900 mg IV q8h to cover MRSA
  - Duration of therapy: A 10- to 14-day course is usually sufficient. Follow patients treated with oral antibiotics for presumed periorbital cellulitis closely (daily follow-up until improvement occurs), for response to antibiotics, and possible progression to orbital cellulitis. If symptoms do not improve within 24 hours, reevaluate for IV antibiotic therapy.

ISSUES FOR REFERRAL

Consult ENT and ophthalmology if there is concern for orbital cellulitis or if patients do not respond quickly to first-line treatment.

SURGERY/OTHER PROCEDURES

- Usually not indicated in uncomplicated cases
- If there is an abscess or potential compromise of critical structures, orbital surgery is indicated.
- Diplopia is the strongest clinical predictor for surgery.

ADMISSION, INPATIENT, AND NURSING CONSIDERATIONS

- If the patient is stable and there are no systemic signs of toxicity, mild cases in adults and children >1 year of age can be safely managed on an outpatient basis.
- Consider hospitalization and IV antibiotics:
  - If patient appears systemically ill
  - Children <1 year of age
  - Patients not immunized against *S. pneumoniae* or *H. influenzae*
  - If patients do not improve or deteriorate within 24 hours of oral antibiotics
  - High suspicion for orbital cellulitis (eyelid swelling with reduced vision, diplopia, abnormal light reflexes, or proptosis)
- No strict guidelines indicate when to switch from parenteral to PO therapy. In general, a switch from IV to oral antibiotics is reasonable once eyelid edema and erythema have significantly improved.
- A 10- to 14-day course of antibiotics is indicated.

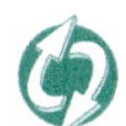

ONGOING CARE

FOLLOW-UP RECOMMENDATIONS

Patient Monitoring

Follow for signs of orbital involvement, including decreased visual acuity or painful/limited ocular motility.

PATIENT EDUCATION

- Maintain good skin hygiene.
- Avoid skin trauma.
- Report early skin changes (swelling, redness, and pain) if recurrent after a course of therapy.

PROGNOSIS

- With timely treatment, patients do well.
- Recurrent periorbital cellulitis occurs with ≥3 periorbital infections in 1 year with at least 1 month of in between episodes; must be differentiated from treatment failure due to antibiotic resistance

COMPLICATIONS

- Orbital cellulitis; orbital abscess formation
- Scarring
- Vision loss
- Cavernous sinus thrombosis
- Osteomyelitis

REFERENCES

1. Vanga S, Daniel AR, Gould MB, et al. A diagnostic challenge: periorbital or orbital cellulitis? *Cureus*. 2023;15(11):e48439. doi:10.7759/cureus.48439.
2. Bae C, Bourget D. *Periorbital Cellulitis*. Treasure Island, FL: StatPearls Publishing; 2024.
3. Kornelsen E, Mahant S, Parkin P, et al. Corticosteroids for periorbital and orbital cellulitis. *Cochrane Database Syst Rev*. 2021;4(4):CD013535. doi:10.1002/14651858.CD013535.pub2.

ADDITIONAL READING

Miranda-Barrios J, Bravo-Queipo-de-Llano B, Baquero-Artigao F, et al. Preseptal versus orbital cellulitis in children: an observational study. *Pediatr Infect Dis J*. 2021;40(11):969–974. doi:10.1097/INF.0000000000003226.

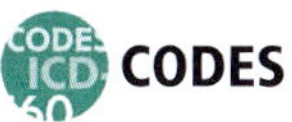

CODES

ICD10

L03.211 Cellulitis of face

CLINICAL PEARLS

- Periorbital (preseptal) and orbital (postseptal) cellulitis occur most commonly in children.
- CT scan of sinuses and orbits can differentiate periorbital cellulitis from orbital cellulitis.
- Orbital cellulitis typically presents with fever, pain with eye movement, ophthalmoplegia, diplopia, and/or proptosis.
- Prompt imaging and consultation is necessary if there is a concern for orbital cellulitis.

CEREBRAL PALSY

Zakary S. Newberry, MD • Anthony Dambro, MD

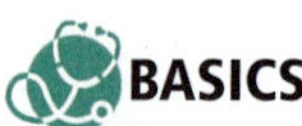

BASICS

DESCRIPTION

Cerebral palsy (CP) is a group of clinical syndromes characterized by motor and postural dysfunction due to permanent nonprogressive disruptions in the developing brain. Motor impairment resulting in activity limitation is necessary for this diagnosis. CP is classified by the nature of the movement disorder and its functional severity.

EPIDEMIOLOGY

Incidence

- Most common cause of childhood disability
- Overall, 1.5 to 2.5/1,000 live births

Prevalence

- Prevalence increases as gestational age (GA) at birth decreases:
  - 146/1,000 for GA of 22 to 27 weeks
  - 62/1,000 for GA of 28 to 31 weeks
  - 7/1,000 for GA of 32 to 36 weeks
  - 1/1,000 for GA of ≥37 weeks
- Prevalence increases as birth weight decreases (1).

ETIOLOGY AND PATHOPHYSIOLOGY

- Multifactorial; CP results from static injury or lesions in the developing brain, occurring prenatally, perinatally, or postnatally.
- Cytokines, free radicals, and inflammatory response are likely contributing factors.
- Spastic CP is most common, usually related to premature birth, with either periventricular leukomalacia or germinal matrix hemorrhage.

Genetics

There are reports of associations between CP and polymorphisms of certain genes: thrombophilic, cytokines, and apolipoprotein E.

RISK FACTORS

- Prenatal: congenital anomalies, multiple gestation, in utero stroke, intrauterine infection (cytomegalovirus [CMV], varicella), intrauterine growth retardation (IUGR), clinical and histologic chorioamnionitis, antepartum bleeding, maternal factors (cognitive impairment, seizure disorders, hyperthyroidism), abnormal fetal position (e.g., breech)
- Perinatal: preterm birth, low-birth weight, periventricular leukomalacia, perinatal hypoxia/asphyxia, intracranial hemorrhage/intraventricular hemorrhage, neonatal seizure or stroke, hyperbilirubinemia
- Postnatal: traumatic brain injury or stroke, sepsis, meningitis, encephalitis, asphyxia, and progressive hydrocephalus

GENERAL PREVENTION

- Prenatal: routine prenatal care; magnesium sulfate for preterm deliveries and preeclampsia; corticosteroids during preterm delivery
- Perinatal: delayed cord clamping, therapeutic hypothermia in the setting of hypoxic brain injury within 6 hours of delivery
- Postnatal: treatment of group B *streptococcus*, routine vaccinations, safety measures regarding car seating, swimming pools, and shaking of the baby (2)[A]

COMMONLY ASSOCIATED CONDITIONS

- Epilepsy
- Intellectual, speech, and language impairments
- Behavioral and sleep disorders
- Hearing and visual impairments
- Gait disorders
- Thyroid dysfunction (2)[A]
- Feeding impairment, swallowing dysfunction, and aspiration
- Poor dentition
- GI conditions: constipation, vomiting, gastroesophageal reflux
- Osteopenia
- Urologic conditions (incontinence, neurogenic bladder)
- Orthopedic disorders(contractures, hip subluxation/dislocation, foot deformities, scoliosis)

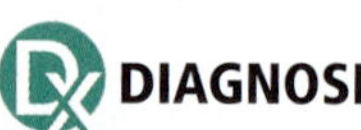

DIAGNOSIS

Diagnosis should be made as early as possible to optimize potential for neuroplasticity. Due to the complexity of the condition, diagnosis is multifaceted and relies on clinical features, physical assessment, and neuroimaging.

HISTORY

History should include prenatal, perinatal, and postnatal risk factors as well as discussion around:

- Neurobehavioral signs (poor feeding/frequent vomiting/irritability)
- Timing of motor milestones
- Abnormal spontaneous general movements
- Asymmetry of movements such as early hand preference

PHYSICAL EXAM

- Assessment should include the following:
  - Tone: may be increased in the setting of spasticity or decreased
  - Reflexes: may be hyperreflexic, asymmetric, or persistently primitive
  - Range of motion: may be decreased in the setting of contractures
  - Movement: may have ataxia, abnormal gait, or delayed motor milestones
- There is international consensus on clinical features to prompt referral for evaluation:
  - Hand preference before 12 months of age
  - Stiffness/tightness in legs between 6 and 12 months of age
  - Hands fisted beyond 4 months of age
  - Persistent head lag beyond 4 months of age
  - Not able to sit unsupported beyond 9 months of age
  - Consistent asymmetry of posture/movements beyond 4 months of age (3)[C]
- There is further consensus for warning signs to prompt monitoring:
  - Persistent Moro reflex beyond 6 months of age
  - Consistent toe walking or asymmetric walking after 12 months of age (3)[C]

DIFFERENTIAL DIAGNOSIS

Benign congenital hypotonia, brachial plexus injury, familial spastic paraplegia, dopa-responsive dystonia, transient toe-walking, muscular dystrophy, metabolic disorders (e.g., glutaric aciduria type 1), mitochondrial disorders, genetic disorders (e.g., Rett syndrome)

DIAGNOSTIC TESTS & INTERPRETATION

- Systematic review of current evidence support a combination of standardized tools and neuroimaging in diagnosis.
  - Prior to 5 months of corrected age, most predictive tools include the following:
    - MRI (86–89% sensitivity)
    - Prechtl qualitative assessment of general movements (98% sensitivity)
    - Hammersmith Infant Neurological Examination (HINE) (90% sensitivity)
  - After 5 months of corrected age, most predictive tools include:
    - MRI (86–89% sensitivity)
    - HINE (90% sensitivity)
    - Developmental Assessment of Young Children (83% C index) (4)[A]
- Laboratory testing is not needed to make diagnosis but it can help exclude other etiologies.
  - Testing for metabolic and genetic syndromes (5)[C]
    - Considered if no specific etiology is identified by neuroimaging or if there are atypical features in clinical presentation
    - Detection of certain brain malformations may warrant genetic or metabolic testing to identify syndromes.
  - Diagnostic testing for coagulopathies should be considered in children with hemiplegic CP with cerebral infarction identified on neuroimaging (5)[C].

Diagnostic Procedures/Other

- Screening for comorbid conditions: developmental delay/intellectual impairment, vision/hearing impairments, speech and language disorders, feeding/swallowing dysfunction, or seizures
- Electroencephalograms (EEGs) should only be obtained if there is a history of suspected seizures.

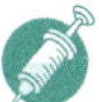

TREATMENT

CP cannot be cured. Treatment consists of an interdisciplinary approach regarding several therapeutic interventions to progress development, prevent secondary impairments, treat symptoms, and improve quality of life.

GENERAL MEASURES

- Early intervention for children 0 to 3 years of age (6)[A]
- Various therapies enhance the following function:
  - Traditional physiotherapy to improve posture stability and gait, motor strength and control, and prevent contractures
  - Physical and occupational therapy to increase functional activities of daily living (7)[A]
  - Speech therapy for verbal and nonverbal speech and to aid in feeding
- Equipment optimizes participation in activities:
  - Orthotic splinting (ankle–foot orthosis)
  - Spinal bracing (body jacket) may slow down scoliosis
  - Augmentative communication with pictures, switches, or computer systems for nonverbal individuals
  - Crutches, walkers, gait trainers, and wheelchairs for mobility and standers for weight-bearing

MEDICATION

Medications are used to provide symptom relief related caused by spasticity.

First Line

- Diazepam (8)[C]
  - A γ-aminobutyric acid-A ($GABA_A$) agonist that facilitates CNS inhibition at spinal and supraspinal levels to reduce spasticity
  - Used for short-term treatment for generalized spasticity; insufficient evidence on motor function
  - Adverse effects: ataxia and drowsiness
  - Adult dose: 2 to 12 mg/dose PO q6–12h
  - Pediatric dose ($<$12 years of age and $<$15 kg): $<$8.5 kg: 0.5 to 1.0 mg HS; 8.5 to 15.0 kg: 1 to 2 mg HS; children 5 to 16 years of age and $\geq$15 kg: 1.25 mg TID
- Baclofen (8)[C]
  - A $GABA_B$ agonist, facilitates presynaptic inhibition of monosynaptic and polysynaptic reflexes
  - Adverse effects: drowsiness and sedation
  - Abrupt withdrawal symptoms: spasticity, hallucinations, seizures, confusion, hyperthermia
  - Adults: Initial dose is 5 mg TID; increase dosage every 3 days to maintenance dose of 20 mg TID, 80 mg/day maximum.
  - Pediatric dose ($>$2 years of age): initial 10 to 15 mg/day; titrate to effective dose (maximum of 40 mg/day). $<$8 years of age: 60 mg/day maximum; $>$8 years of age: 60 mg/day maximum
- In a head-to-head study, neither diazepam nor baclofen have been found to be superior in efficacy or safety (9)[B].

Second Line

- Intrathecal baclofen (baclofen pump) (8)[C]
  - Continuous intrathecal route allows greater maximal response with smaller dosage to reduce spasticity.
  - May help ambulatory individuals with gait but no improvement seen in nonambulatory patients
  - Adverse effects: infection, catheter malfunction, CSF leakage
- Botulinum toxin type A (8)[C]
  - Acts at neuromuscular junction to inhibit the release of acetylcholine to reduce tone
  - Injected directly into muscles of interest for localized spasticity; insufficient evidence on motor function
  - Higher functional benefit when combined with occupational therapy
  - Lasts for 12 to 16 weeks following injection

ADDITIONAL THERAPIES

Multidisciplinary care teams including primary care, ophthalmology, neurology, orthopedics, and physiatry along with physical, occupational, and speech therapists (2)[A]

SURGERY/OTHER PROCEDURES

- Dorsal root rhizotomy selectively cuts dorsal rootlets from L1–S2; decreases spasticity in lower limbs when done in conjunction with physiotherapy but associated with adverse effects; evidence is lacking as to long-term outcomes.
- Surgical treatment of joint dislocations/subluxation, scoliosis management, tendon lengthening, gastrostomy

COMPLEMENTARY & ALTERNATIVE MEDICINE

- Therapeutic horse riding or hippotherapy improves postural control and balance (7)[A].
- Aquatherapy improves gross motor function in patients with various motor severities.

ONGOING CARE

PROGNOSIS

Reduced lifespan is strongly associated with level of functional impairment and intellectual disability.

REFERENCES

1. Sadowska M, Sarecka-Hujar B, Kopyta I. Cerebral Palsy: Current opinions on definition, epidemiology, risk factors, classification and treatment options. *Neuropsychiatr Dis Treat*. 2020;16:1505–1518.
2. Paul S, Nahar A, Bhagawati M, et al. A review on recent advances of cerebral palsy. *Oxid Med Cell Longev*. 2022;2022:2622310.
3. Boychuck Z, Andersen J, Bussières A, et al. International expert recommendations of clinical features to prompt referral for diagnostic assessment of cerebral palsy. *Dev Med Child Neurol*. 2020;62(1):89–96.
4. Novak I, Morgan C, Adde L, et al. Early, accurate diagnosis and early intervention in cerebral palsy: advances in diagnosis and treatment. *JAMA Pediatr*. 2017;171(9):897–907.
5. Ashwal S, Russman BS, Blasco PA, et al; for the Quality Standards Subcommittee of the American Academy of Neurology, Practice Committee of the Child Neurology Society. Practice parameter: diagnostic assessment of the child with cerebral palsy: report of the Quality Standards Subcommittee of the American Academy of Neurology and the Practice Committee of the Child Neurology Society. *Neurology*. 2004;62(6):851–863.
6. Spittle A, Orton J, Anderson PJ, et al. Early developmental intervention programmes post-hospital discharge to prevent motor and cognitive impairments in preterm infants. *Cochrane Database Syst Rev*. 2012;(12):CD005495.
7. Mahendra R, Upadhyay J, Amita R, et al. A systematic review on etiology, epidemiology, and treatment of cerebral palsy. *Int J Nutr Pharmacol Neurol Dis*. 2017;7:76–83.
8. Reilly M, Liuzzo K, Blackmer AB, et al. Pharmacological management of spasticity in children with cerebral palsy. *J Pediatr Health Care*. 2020;34(5):495–509.
9. Goyal V, Laisram N, Wadhwa RK, et al. Prospective randomized study of oral diazepam and baclofen on spasticity in cerebral palsy. *J Clin Diag Res*. 2016;10(6):RC01–5.

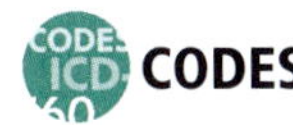

CODES

ICD10

- G80.9 Cerebral palsy, unspecified
- G80.1 Spastic diplegic cerebral palsy
- G80.2 Spastic hemiplegic cerebral palsy

CLINICAL PEARLS

- Management should focus on maximizing functioning and quality of life using multidisciplinary team approach.
- Regression of motor skills does not occur with CP.

CERVICAL HYPEREXTENSION INJURIES

Terrence Tsui, DO

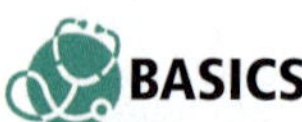

BASICS

DESCRIPTION

- Class of neck injuries typically seen in rapid, forceful extension of the cervical spine
- Flexion–extension injuries ("whiplash") are usually from motor vehicle accidents (MVAs), typically side-impact or rear-end collisions.
- Increasing incidence in elderly due to falls
- Diagnosed clinically, after acute injury using National Emergency X-Ray Utilization Study C-Spine (NEXUS) criteria and/or Canadian C-Spine Rule (CCR) to determine if CT is required to rule out significant cervical spine injury.
- May involve:
  - Injury to vertebral and paravertebral structures: fractures, dislocations, ligamentous tears, and disk disruption/subluxation
  - Spinal cord injury (SCI): traumatic central cord syndrome (CCS), SCI without radiologic abnormality (SCIWORA)
  - Blunt cerebrovascular injury (BCVI): vertebral artery or carotid artery dissection
  - Soft tissue injury: cervical strain/sprain (i.e., whiplash), cervical stingers (see "Brachial Plexopathy")

EPIDEMIOLOGY

- Predominant age: SCI average age of injury 43 years, CCS average age 53 years
- High-energy trauma (e.g., road accidents) and sports injuries are more common in young adults (average age 29 years), whereas low-energy trauma (e.g., falls) are usually implicated in the >65 years age group.
- Most (~80%) new SCI cases are male (1).

Incidence

In the United States

- CCS: 4/100,000 people/year
- BCVI: estimated 1/1,000 of hospitalized trauma patients; incidence increased with cervical spine or thoracic injury.
- Whiplash is the most common injury in MVAs and accounts for 28% of all ED visits for MVAs.
- Incidence of whiplash is 70 to 328/100,000 with rates highest in 20- to 24-year-old women.

ETIOLOGY AND PATHOPHYSIOLOGY

Blunt trauma due to MVAs, falls, sports injuries, and violence (primarily gunshot wounds)

RISK FACTORS

- Chronic pain and/or disability: litigation, previous neck pain or injury, female gender, report of headache/low back pain at onset, low education level
- Fractures: osteoporosis, conditions predisposing to spinal rigidity, such as ankylosing spondylitis or other spondyloarthropathies
- CCS: preexisting spinal stenosis present in >50%
  - Acquired: prior trauma, spondylosis
  - Congenital: Klippel-Feil syndrome (congenital fusion of any two cervical vertebrae)

GENERAL PREVENTION

Seat belts, higher neck rest, rule changes, proper technique, and proper use of protective equipment for sports activities can prevent or minimize injury.

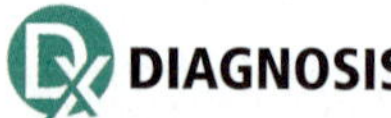

DIAGNOSIS

HISTORY

Usually acute presentation with mechanism of cervical hyperextension and complaints of neck pain, stiffness, or headaches ± neurologic symptoms

PHYSICAL EXAM

- External signs of trauma on the head and neck such as abrasions, lacerations, or contusions provide clues to mechanism and associated injuries.
- Presence, severity, and location of neck tenderness help localize involved structure(s):
  - Posterior, midline bony tenderness raises concern for underlying fracture.
  - Paraspinal or lateral soft tissue tenderness suggests muscular/ligamentous injury.
  - Anterior tenderness concerning for vascular injury
- Carotid bruit raises concern for carotid dissection.
- Trauma patients presenting with Glasgow Coma Scale (GCS) <15 warrant close attention and reassessment.
- Neurologic exam: paresthesias, weakness suggests SCI or stroke secondary to BCVI:
  - CCS often presents as
    - Distal > proximal symptom distribution, upper extremity > lower extremity
    - Extremity weakness/paralysis predominates
    - Variable sensory changes below level of lesion (including paresthesias and dysesthesia)
    - Bladder/bowel incontinence may occur.

DIFFERENTIAL DIAGNOSIS

- Acute or chronic disc pathology
- Osteoarthritis
- Cervical radiculopathy
- Bilateral brachial plexus injuries
- Carotid or vertebral artery dissection

DIAGNOSTIC TESTS & INTERPRETATION

Initial Tests (lab, imaging)

- Low-risk patients can be cleared clinically (without CT) using either the CCR or the NEXUS criteria (1):
  - CCR: Stable and alert (GCS >15) trauma patient with no history of cervical spine disease/surgery can be cleared if all the following conditions are met:
    - Able to actively rotate neck 45 degrees left and right
    - No dangerous mechanism or extremity paresthesias
    - Age <65 years
    - At least one "low-risk factor" (i.e., simple rear-end MVA, ambulatory at any time, no midline cervical tenderness, delayed onset of neck pain, or sitting position in the ED)
  - NEXUS C-spine rule: clinically cleared if all the following are met:
    - No midline tenderness
    - No evidence of intoxication
    - Normal level of alertness
    - No focal neurologic deficit
    - No distracting injury
  - Reported sensitivity/specificity: CCR (99.4%/45.1%), NEXUS (90.7%/36.8%)
- In patients with high-risk mechanism or concerning historical/physical exam, recommend imaging based on the suspected injury and level of clinical suspicion:
  - X-ray cervical spine: rarely indicated, in some patients who cannot be cleared clinically but are still in low-suspicion category: sensitivity for C-spine injury 31.6%
  - Axial CT from occiput to T1 with coronal and sagittal reconstructions has replaced plain radiography as the test of choice for cases with moderate to high clinical suspicion of C-spine injury, given high sensitivity (90–100%).

- MRI: test of choice in CCS with direct visualization of traumatic cord lesions (edema or hematomyelia), soft tissue compressing cord, and/or stenosis of canal; detects ligamentous injury and abnormalities of intervertebral disks and soft tissues; MRI is less helpful for fractures.
- CT angiography: visualization of cervical and cerebral vascular structures to detect BCVI, sensitivity approaches 100% when a $\geq$16-slice CT scanner is used. MR angiography is an alternative, although sensitivity of 47–50% limits utility.

Test Interpretation

- CCS: thought to be due to white matter axonal disruption of the lateral column, particularly the corticospinal tracts
- BCVI: intimal disruption, leading to thrombosis and embolization
- Acute cervical strain/sprain: Models suggest myofascial tearing, edema, and inflammation.

Geriatric Considerations

- Degenerative changes of the C-spine may be confused with acute traumatic change; osteopenia may limit fracture visualization on x-ray—CT is more accurate.
- Degenerative disease and osteopenia increase risk of upper cervical spine injuries (even with low-velocity trauma).

Pediatric Considerations

PECARN C-spine imaging rule: unique to pediatric population predicted to cut CT radiation exposure in half (2)

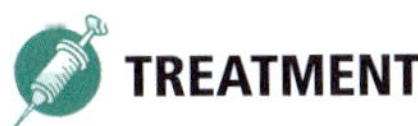

TREATMENT

GENERAL MEASURES

- Whiplash/WAD
  - Mainly supportive, offer reassurance
  - Limited or no benefit to cervical collar; if provided, use for $<$72 hours and encourage early mobilization (2)
  - Provide adequate nonopioid pain control.
  - Arrange primary care follow-up; neck pain can continue even 1 year after trauma.
- Fractures
  - Stability determined by imaging
  - Decompression and stabilization are indicated for:
    - Incomplete SCIs with spinal canal compromise
    - Clinical deterioration or failure to improve despite conservative management
  - Odontoid and hangman fracture: Treat according to type.
- CCS: neck immobilization with cervical collar, PT/occupational therapy (OT)

MEDICATION

- Cervical strain/sprain, whiplash: NSAIDs or acetaminophen. Muscle relaxants may help with muscle tightness and sleeping at night.
- Fractures: pain control with analgesics
- CCS: Within 8 hours of injury, consider methylprednisolone 30 mg/kg IV over 15 minutes and then continuous infusion 5.4 mg/kg/hr IV for 23 hours. Further improvement in motor function recovery may be seen if infusion is continued for 48 hours, especially if initial bolus administration is delayed after injury.
- BCVI: anticoagulation with IV heparin, followed by warfarin therapy for 3 to 6 months and then long-term antiplatelet therapy; antiplatelet agent as sole initial therapy in patients with contraindications to anticoagulation

ISSUES FOR REFERRAL

- If cervical spine injury is suspected, immobilize patient and send to ED for evaluation and clearance.
- Emergent consultation from a spine surgeon for any concern for unstable fracture or SCI

ADMISSION, INPATIENT, AND NURSING CONSIDERATIONS

Varies by injury; clinical judgment, imaging findings, concomitant injuries, and need for operative intervention

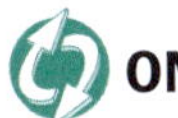

ONGOING CARE

PROGNOSIS

- Presenting neurologic status is the most important factor in determining prognosis.
- BCVI
  - Patients have fewer neurologic sequelae with early diagnosis and antithrombotic therapy. There is unequal efficacy of anticoagulation and antiplatelet agents in preventing stroke.
- CCS
  - Spontaneous recovery of motor function in $>$50% over several weeks. Younger patients are more likely to regain function.
  - Leg, bowel, and bladder functions return first, followed by upper extremities.
- WAD: Prognostic factors for development of late whiplash syndrome ($>$6 months of symptoms affecting normal activity) include increased initial pain intensity, pain-related disability, and cold hyperalgesia.

REFERENCES

1. Jara-Almonte G, Pawar C. Emergency department management of cervical spine injuries. *Emerg Med Pract*. 2021;23(10):1–28.
2. Leonard JC, Harding M, Cook LJ, et al. PECARN prediction rule for cervical spine imaging of children presenting to the emergency department with blunt trauma: a multicentre prospective observational study. *Lancet Child Adolesc Health*. 2024;8(7):482–490.

ADDITIONAL READING

- Carr MT, Harrop JS, Houten JK. Traumatic central cord syndrome. *Clin Spine Surg*. 2024;37(9):379–387.
- Futch BG, Seas A, Ononogbu-Uche F, et al. Shifting trends in the epidemiology of cervical spine injuries: an analysis of 11,822 patients from the National Electronic Injury Surveillance System over two decades. *J Neurotrauma*. 2024;41(17–18):2158–2167. doi:10.1089/neu.2024.0194.
- Martínez-Palacios K, Rubiano AM, Demetriades AK, et al. Traumatic central cord syndrome: an integrated neurosurgical and neurocritical care perspective. *Brain Spine*. 2025;5:104281.

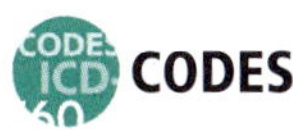

CODES

ICD10

- S13.4XXA Sprain of ligaments of cervical spine, initial encounter
- S13.101A Dislocation of unspecified cervical vertebrae, init encntr
- S14.109A Unsp injury at unsp level of cervical spinal cord, init

CLINICAL PEARLS

- Use NEXUS or CCR to determine need for CT in every patient with a potential neck injury.
- Always perform imaging if clinical judgment suggests the need to do so.
- Inquire about preexisting cervical spine conditions, especially in the elderly, because this may increase risk of injury or change radiographic interpretation.
- Consider BCVI when neurologic deficits are inconsistent with level of known injury or in the setting of a significant mechanism of injury.

CERVICAL MALIGNANCY

Jeremy Golding, MD, FAAFP

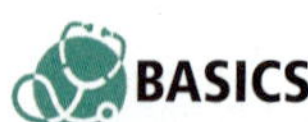

BASICS

DESCRIPTION

Cervical cancer is a malignant neoplasm arising from the cells of the uterine cervix. Most cervical cancers, almost 90%, are squamous cell carcinomas and begin in the squamocolumnar junction where the exocervix and endocervix meet, also known as the transformation zone. A small percentage of cervical cancers are adenocarcinomas and begin in the glandular cells of the endocervix.

EPIDEMIOLOGY

Incidence

- According to the American Cancer Society (ACS), the annual incidence of cervical cancer in the United States between 2015 and 2019 was 7.7 cases per 100,000 person-years.
- According to the World Health Organization (WHO), cervical cancer is the fourth most common cancer in women globally with around 660,000 new cases and around 350,000 deaths in 2022 (1).
- In the United States, cervical cancer is most frequently diagnosed in the 35 to 44 age group, with average age at diagnosis being 50 years. Women <20 years of age rarely get cervical cancer. However, over 20% of cervical cancer cases are in women >65 years of age.

Prevalence

In 2023, the ACS estimates 13,960 new cases of invasive cervical cancer and 4,310 deaths due to cervical cancer in the United States.

ETIOLOGY AND PATHOPHYSIOLOGY

- Human papillomavirus (HPV) infection with high-risk (HR) serotypes, especially HPV 16 and HPV 18, is the most important etiologic factor.
- HPV infection has high prevalence with most sexually active adults having it at one point in their lives.
- HR HPV accounts for 99% of all cervical cancer.

Genetics

There is a broad separation of HPV types and the HR types that can be tested for include HPV 16, 18, 31, 33, 35, 39, 45, 51, 52, 56, 58, 59, 66, and 68.

RISK FACTORS

- Persistent HPV infection is the primary risk factor for developing cervical cancer.
- Other risk factors include lack of or decreased access to health care and ability to obtain regular Pap tests; early coitarche especially before the age of 18; multiple sexual partners; unprotected sex; a history of sexually transmitted infections (STIs); low socioeconomic status; first birth prior to age of 2 years; high parity (≥3 full-term deliveries); cigarette smoking (doubles the risk); immunosuppression (HIV/AIDS, chemotherapy); diethylstilbestrol (DES) exposure in utero; oral contraceptive use of ≥5 years (risk back to baseline after ≥10 years of nonuse), family history of cervical cancer

GENERAL PREVENTION

- The cornerstone of prevention includes not only routine screening with a Pap test (or HPV test) but also vaccination against HR-HPV.
- The three FDA-approved vaccines are four-serotype Gardasil 4, nine-serotype Gardasil 9, and two-serotype (HPV 16 and 18) Cervarix, but only Gardasil 9 is currently distributed.
- Vaccination is recommended for:
  - Everyone through the age of 26
  - Girls and boys ages 11 or 12 years in 2 doses, 6 to 12 months apart. It can also be given as early as 9 years of age.
  - Children ≥15 years should receive 3 doses over the course of 6 months.
  - Immunocompromised patients ages 9 to 26 years, men who have sex with men, and the LGBTQ community
- Current guidelines from the US Preventive Services Task Force (USPSTF 2018), ASCCP (2021), and ACOG (2021) recommend screening as follows (2):
  - Women aged 21 to 29 years: cytology alone every 3 years
  - Women aged 30 to 65 years: cytology alone every 3 years, HR-HPV testing (using an assay specifically approved by the FDA for HPV-screening-only testing) alone every 5 years, or cytology plus HR-HPV cotesting every 5 years
- An alternative screening algorithm using a risk-based strategy and specific FDA-approved high-risk HPV tests followed by cytology for positive screens is a recommended alternative.
- Management of abnormal results obtained from screening should involve personalized risk assessment for the individual patient using ASCCP management guidelines (available via web-based and mobile applications) (2)

COMMONLY ASSOCIATED CONDITIONS

Condyloma acuminata, preinvasive/invasive lesions of the vulva, vagina, oral, anal, and oropharyngeal cancers

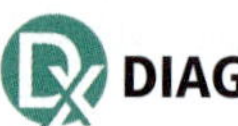

DIAGNOSIS

HISTORY

- Patients with HPV infection may be asymptomatic. Early stages can be discovered incidentally as a result of cervical cancer screening.
- The most common symptoms of cervical cancer are irregular or heavy bleeding, postcoital vaginal bleeding, unusual discharge, pain with sex, or pelvic pain.

PHYSICAL EXAM

- A thorough pelvic exam is essential. Many patients have a normal exam, especially with microinvasive disease. Lesions may be exophytic, endophytic, polypoid, papillary, ulcerative, or necrotic.
- In women with symptoms of cervical cancer, bimanual and rectovaginal examination should be performed to evaluate uterine size, vaginal wall, rectovaginal septum, and parametrial, uterosacral, and pelvic sidewall involvement.
- Enlarged supraclavicular or inguinal lymphadenopathy, lower extremity edema, ascites, or decreased breath sounds with lung auscultation may indicate metastases or advanced stage disease.

DIFFERENTIAL DIAGNOSIS

- Cervical condyloma, leiomyoma, or polyp
- Metastasis from endometrial carcinoma or gestational trophoblastic neoplasia.

DIAGNOSTIC TESTS & INTERPRETATION

Initial Tests (lab, imaging)

- Pap test
- Colposcopy with directed biopsies and/or biopsy of gross lesions are the definitive means of diagnosis.
- In advanced disease, may need to check CBC, UA, BUN, creatinine, and liver function tests (LFTs)
- Computed tomography (CT) scan of the chest, abdomen, and pelvis and/or a positron emission tomography (PET) scan for metastatic workup
- 2018 FIGO staging recommendations emphasize MRI of the pelvis to image extent of tumor and nodal involvement in patients who are surgical candidates or for planning radiation therapy.

Follow-Up Tests & Special Considerations

- Exam under anesthesia may be helpful in determining clinical stage, disease extent, and suitability for surgery.
- Endocervical curettage and cervical conization as indicated to determine depth of invasion and presence of lymphovascular involvement
- Cystoscopy to evaluate bladder invasion, proctoscopy for invasion into rectum

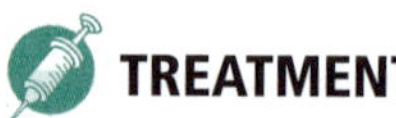

TREATMENT

GENERAL MEASURES

Improve nutritional state, correct anemia (Hb <12 g/dL), and treat pelvic infections. Lymph node evaluation is key to staging and treatment. Correction of urinary tract obstruction is important prior to beginning chemoradiation. Pretreatment evaluation should be done prior to chemotherapy for lymph nodes involvement using PET/CT scan.

MEDICATION

- Chemoradiation with a cisplatin-containing regimen is the preferred treatment for certain stages of cervical cancer
- Neoadjuvant chemotherapy may improve survival for early and locally advanced tumors. Adjuvant chemotherapy after chemoradiation may improve progression-free survival in patients who receive primary chemoradiation for stages IIB to IVA tumors.
- The addition of the antiangiogenesis drug bevacizumab to standard combination chemotherapy (cisplatin/topotecan or cisplatin/paclitaxel) for recurrent, persistent, or metastatic disease has been shown to improve overall survival.

First Line

- Chemoradiation is the primary treatment of choice for stages IB3 to IVA. The preferred regimen is weekly cisplatin or cisplatin with 5-fluorouracil along with radiation. If cisplatin is not a good option, then carboplatin can be used.
- The preferred first-line for recurrent or metastatic disease is a combination of cisplatin/carboplatin/paclitaxel/bevacizumab/topotecan.

Second Line

Other alternative medications include docetaxel (Taxotere), ifosfamide (Ifex), 5-fluorouracil (5-FU), irinotecan (Camptosar), gemcitabine (Gemzar), and mitomycin. Bevacizumab (Avastin) can also be added to chemo regimen.

ISSUES FOR REFERRAL

Multidisciplinary management of patients as needed and in a timely fashion

ADDITIONAL THERAPIES

- Chemoradiation (without surgery) is the first-line therapy for tumors stage IB3 and higher. Combination of external-beam pelvic radiation and brachytherapy is usually employed.
- If para-aortic lymph node metastases are suspected, extended-field radiation or lymph node dissection prior to radiation therapy may be performed.

SURGERY/OTHER PROCEDURES

- Removal of precursor lesions (cervical intraepithelial neoplasia [CIN]) by loop electrosurgical excision procedure (LEEP), cold knife conization, laser ablation, or cryotherapy
- Open hysterectomy is superior to laparoscopic hysterectomy for cervical cancer treatment for patients with stages IA1, IA1, and IB1.
- Stage IA2 (lesions with >3 mm but ≤5 mm depth): option of radical hysterectomy with lymph node dissection or radiation depending on clinical setting; robotic radical hysterectomy (RRH) has demonstrated to be superior to laparoscopic radical hysterectomy and open radical hysterectomy in intraoperative blood loss, length of hospital stay, and intraoperative and postoperative complications; RRH can be regarded as a safe and effective therapeutic procedure for the management of cervical cancer.
- Stages IA2 to IB1: Fertility-sparing radical trachelectomy may be considered in selected patients.
- Stages IB1 to IIA (gross lesions without obvious parametrial involvement): option of radical hysterectomy with lymph node sampling or primary chemoradiation with brachytherapy and teletherapy, depending on clinical setting (1); in stage IB, when comparing adjuvant radiotherapy with no adjuvant radiotherapy, there is no significant difference in survival at 5 years between women who received radiation and those who received no further treatment (risk ratio [RR] = 0.8, 95% confidence interval [CI] 0.3–2.4). However, women who received radiation had a significantly lower risk of disease progression at 5 years (RR 0.6, 95% CI 0.4–0.9).
- Stage IVA (lesions limited to central metastasis to the bladder and/or rectum): Primary pelvic exenteration may be feasible.
- Stage IVB (lesions spread to distant organs): Treatment goal is palliation; therefore, early referral to palliative care should be made.

Pregnancy Considerations

- Management is guided by consideration of stage of lesion, gestational age, and maternal assessment of risks and benefits from treatment. Abnormal cytology is best followed up by colposcopy with directed biopsies.
- In pregnant women with early stages (IA1, IA2, IB) diagnosed before 3 months' gestation, treatment may be delayed to allow for fetal maturity.
- In pregnant women diagnosed with stage 1 cervical cancer in 2nd or 3rd trimester, a cold knife conization or radical trachelectomy may be suggested with plan for early C-section delivery.
- In pregnant women with advanced disease (stage 2 or higher) diagnosed in 2nd or 3rd trimester, chemotherapy may be recommended. Cisplatin, carboplatin, and paclitaxel usually do not harm the fetus if given in the second or third trimester but could possibly cause early labor or low-birth weight.

ADMISSION, INPATIENT, AND NURSING CONSIDERATIONS

- Admission may be needed for active bleeding, dehydration, treatment complications, and ureteral blockage (with hydronephrosis or urosepsis).
- Active vaginal bleeding can be controlled with timely vaginal packing and radiation therapy.

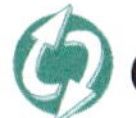

ONGOING CARE

FOLLOW-UP RECOMMENDATIONS

Patient Monitoring

- With completion of definitive therapy and based on individual risk factors, patients are evaluated with physical/pelvic examinations: every 3 to 6 months for 2 years, every 6 to 12 months until the 5th year, and yearly thereafter.
- Pap smears may be performed yearly but have a low sensitivity for detecting recurrence.
- CT and PET scan are useful in locating metastases when recurrence is suspected; preferably 3 to 4 months post-treatment
- Signs of recurrence include vaginal bleeding, unexplained weight loss, leg edema, and pelvic or thigh pain.

PATIENT EDUCATION

The Society of Gynecologic Oncology: https://www.sgo.org/; the Foundation for Women's Cancer: https://foundationforwomenscancer.org/

PROGNOSIS

- If detected early, invasive cervical cancer can be treated successfully. Survival rates were calculated based on women diagnosed with cervical cancer between the years of 2012 and 2018. Rates were calculated for each Surveillance, Epidemiology, and End Results (SEER) stage.
  - The 5-year survival rate for localized disease is estimated at 92%.
  - The 5-year survival rate for regional disease is estimated at 59%.
  - The 5-year survival rate for distant disease is estimated at 17%.
  - The 5-year survival rate for all SEER stages combined is estimated at 67%.
- An elevated squamous cell carcinoma antigen (SCC-Ag) serum levels estimated by ELISA technique can be used to predict the clinical response to neoadjuvant chemotherapy and residual disease. Persistently elevated SCC-Ag level at 2 to 3 months after RT had a significantly higher incidence of treatment failure. Serum SCC-Ag levels are also useful for monitoring treatment efficacy, disease progression, recurrence, and poor prognosis in SCCs. The combination of clinical pelvic examination and SCC-Ag levels provides useful information for the further need of treatment.

COMPLICATIONS

- Loss of ovarian function from radiotherapy or indication for bilateral oophorectomy
- Hemorrhage, pelvic infection, genitourinary fistula, bladder dysfunction, sexual dysfunction
- Ureteral obstruction with renal failure, bowel obstruction, pulmonary embolism, lower extremity lymphedema

REFERENCES

1. World Health Organization. Cervical cancer. https://www.who.int/news-room/fact-sheets/detail/cervical-cancer. Accessed November 24, 2024.
2. Gavinski K, DiNardo D. Cervical cancer screening. *Med Clin North Am*. 2023;107(2):259–269.

ADDITIONAL READING

Tewari KS, Monk BJ. Evidence-based treatment paradigms for management of invasive cervical carcinoma. *J Clin Oncol*. 2019;37(27):2472–2489.

SEE ALSO

Abnormal Pap and Cervical Dysplasia

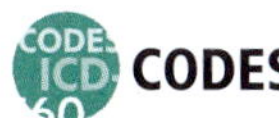

CODES

ICD10

- C53.9 Malignant neoplasm of cervix uteri, unspecified
- C53.0 Malignant neoplasm of endocervix
- C53.1 Malignant neoplasm of exocervix

CLINICAL PEARLS

Improving access to cervical cancer screening is likely to have the greatest impact in the reduction of the burden of disease. With HPV immunization and screening, the disease should be almost completely preventable.

CHILD ABUSE

Sasha S. Svendsen, MD • Jessalyn G. Shaw, MD

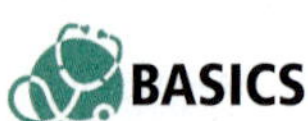

BASICS

DESCRIPTION

- Types of abuse: neglect (most common and highest mortality), physical abuse, emotional/psychological abuse, sexual abuse, and sexual exploitation
- Neglect includes physical (e.g., failure to provide necessary food or shelter or lack of appropriate supervision), medical (e.g., failure to provide necessary medical or mental health treatment), educational (e.g., failure to educate a child or attend to special education needs), and emotional (e.g., inattention to a child's emotional needs, failure to provide psychological care, or permitting the child to use alcohol or other drugs).
- System(s) affected: gastrointestinal (GI), endocrine/metabolic, musculoskeletal, nervous, renal, reproductive, skin/exocrine, pulmonary, cardiac, immune, and psychiatric
- Synonym(s): nonaccidental trauma; child maltreatment; inflicted injury

EPIDEMIOLOGY

Prevalence

Children's Bureau report for federal fiscal year (FFY) 2023 (1):

- Child protective services agencies received ~4.4 million referrals alleging maltreatment, with a national screened-in referral rate of 28.7 referrals per 1,000 children.
- Approximately 3 million children received either an investigation or alternative response. Of those investigated, 546,159 children (7.4 per 1,000) were found to be victims of abuse or neglect.
- Neglect is the most common type of reported maltreatment at 65%, followed by physical abuse at 11%, and sexual abuse at 8%. 11% of children experience multiple forms of maltreatment.
- The overall rate of child fatalities was 2.73 deaths per 100,000 children in the national population. The rate of child fatalities is slightly higher in boys compared to girls.
- The majority of perpetrators are the parents of their victims (76%).

RISK FACTORS

- American Indian or Alaska Native children had the highest rates of victimization.
- Children from birth to 1 year old had the highest rate of victimization 21 per 1,000 infants and highest rate of mortality.
- Females have a slightly higher rate of victimization versus males.
- Military families are at risk, especially with deployment.
- Child risk factors: chronic illness, physical/congenital disability, developmental delay, preterm, unintended pregnancy
- Caregiver risk factors: poverty, substance misuse, lower educational status, parental history of abuse, parental mental health issues, young and/or unmarried mother, poor support network, and domestic violence

GENERAL PREVENTION

- Screen for risk factors at prenatal, postnatal, and pediatric visits.
- Physicians can educate parents on a range of normal behaviors to expect in infants and children: for example anticipatory guidance on ways to handle crying infants; methods of discipline for toddlers

COMMONLY ASSOCIATED CONDITIONS

Failure to thrive, prematurity, developmental delays, poor school performance, poor social skills, low self-esteem, anxiety, or depression

DIAGNOSIS

- Relatively minor skin injuries, frenulum tears, or bruising in precruising infants may be the first indications of child physical abuse; these relatively minor, unexplained injuries have been termed "sentinel injuries."
- Of children <1 year old with injuries determined to be from abuse, 28% had a prior sentinel injury (80% a bruise) (2).
- Infants with injuries caused by child abuse often present with vague complaints.
- Documentation
  - Critical elements include:
    - Brief statement of child's disclosure or caregiver's explanation, including any alternate explanations offered (Use direct quotations when possible.)
    - Time the incident occurred and date/time of disclosure
    - Whether witnesses were present
    - Developmental abilities of child
    - Objective medical findings
    - Other at-risk children in the household (siblings)
- *Do not* use terms such as "rule out" and "alleged." Clearly state objective findings and medical provider's opinion.
- Obtain history from caregiver separately from the child.
- Any description of abuse given by the child should be documented word for word using quotation marks in the child's own language and attributed to the child whenever possible.
- The child should not be rewarded after a disclosure (e.g., "Tell me what happened, and you can go back to your mom. . .").
- Documentation should include disposition of patient and record any report made to child welfare.

HISTORY

- Use nonjudgmental, open-ended questions (ask: who, what, when, and where; *never* why).
- Document past medical history, developmental history, child's temperament, and thorough social history including objective documentation of family interactions.
- History of a sentinel injury should prompt consideration of abuse.
- The following historical elements may suggest abusive injury:
  - History that is inconsistent with the injury or with the child's developmental level
  - No explanation offered for the injury or injury blamed on sibling or another child
  - Important detail of explanation changes dramatically.
  - Different witnesses provide different history.
  - There is unreasonable delay in seeking treatment.
  - Denial of trauma in a child with injury
- Nonspecific symptoms of abuse:
  - Behavior changes; self-destructive behavior; anxiety and/or depression
  - Sleep disturbances, night terrors; school problems

PHYSICAL EXAM

- Examine child in a comfortable setting:
  - Explain what the exam will involve and why procedures are needed.
  - Allow child to choose who will be in the room.
  - Completely undress the child and have them wear a gown to perform a complete physical examination, including thorough skin exam.
- Complete a general assessment for signs of physical abuse, neglect, and self-injurious behaviors:
  - Measurements, photographs, and careful objective descriptions are critical for accurate diagnosis.
- A thorough physical exam includes:
  - Skin (completely undress, including diaper to visualize buttocks)
  - Head (including fontanels), eyes, ears, nose, and mouth (including all 3 frenula)
  - Chest/abdomen
  - Anogenital area (visualization of external genital structures with labial separation and traction—no speculum)
  - Extremities
  - Review growth charts
- Physical abuse findings
  - Skin markings (e.g., lacerations, burns, bruises, patterned injuries, bites)
  - Immersion injuries with clearly demarcated borders
  - Oral trauma (e.g., torn frenulum, loose teeth)
  - Ear bruising
  - Eye trauma (e.g., hyphema, subconjunctival hemorrhage)
  - Head/abdominal blunt trauma
  - Fractures
  - Patterns suggestive of abuse:
    - Bruises seen away from bony prominences (e.g., face, back, abdomen, arms, buttocks, ears, hands)
    - Multiple bruises in clusters or uniform shape
    - Patterned injuries (such as bite marks or the imprint of an object like a hand, belt, or cord) should be considered highly concerning for inflicted injury.
    - TEN-4-FACESp method to identify bruises suggestive of child abuse (3):
      - T: torso; E: ear; N: neck
      - 4: any bruise, anywhere on a child ≤4 months
      - F: frenulum; A: angle of jaw; C: cheeks; E: eyelids; S: subconjunctivae; p: patterned bruising

- Sexual abuse findings
  - Unexplained penile, vaginal, hymenal, perianal, or anal injuries/bleeding/discharge
  - Pregnancy or sexually transmitted infections (STIs)
- Neglect findings
  - Low-growth parameter trends, unclean, unkempt, rashes
  - Fearful or overly trusting
  - Abnormal development or growth parameters

DIFFERENTIAL DIAGNOSIS

- Physical trauma mimics
  - Accidental injury; toxic ingestion
  - Bleeding disorders (e.g., von Willebrand disease, hemophilia)
  - Metabolic or congenital conditions
  - Conditions with skin manifestations (e.g., congenital dermal melanocytosis, Henoch-Schönlein purpura, meningococcemia, erythema multiforme, hypersensitivity, staphylococcal scalded skin syndrome, varicella, impetigo)
  - Cultural practices (e.g., cupping, coining)
- Neglect mimics
  - Endocrinopathies (e.g., diabetes mellitus), constitutional growth delay
  - GI (clefts, malabsorption, irritable bowel), seizure disorder
- Skeletal trauma mimics
  - Obstetrical trauma, nutritional (scurvy, rickets)
  - Infection (congenital syphilis, osteomyelitis)
  - Osteogenesis imperfecta

DIAGNOSTIC TESTS & INTERPRETATION

Initial Tests (lab, imaging)

- Directed by history and physical exam findings:
  - Complete blood count, coagulation studies
  - Liver and pancreatic function tests (abdominal trauma)
  - Urinalysis and stool guaiac (abdominal trauma/flank/back/genital trauma)
- In cases of suspected neglect:
  - Stool exam, calorie count, purified protein derivative and anergy panel, sweat test, lead and zinc levels
- In cases of suspected sexual abuse:
  - STI testing:
    - Urine NAAT: gonorrhea, chlamydia, *Trichomonas*
    - Serum: HIV, hepatitis B and C serologies, syphilis
  - Urine/serum pregnancy test
- In cases of suspected physical abuse:
  - Skeletal survey: 22 radiographs surveying each bone of the body, examining for evidence of acute or healing fractures
    - Recommended for:
      - Infants aged <6 months with bruising, regardless of pattern
      - Children aged <2 years with bruising concerning for abuse or domestic violence (see TEN-4-FACESp)
      - All children aged <2 years with fractures and poorly explained injuries
      - All children aged <2 years who live with an abused child should be evaluated
      - May also consider for older child in which the patient has impaired mobility or communication skills
  - Noncontrast head CT:
    - Consider brain magnetic resonance imaging (MRI) of head/neck/spine for further evaluation of more subtle findings, brain parenchyma, intracerebral edema, or hemorrhage.
    - Recommended for:
      - All abused children with skull fracture found on skeletal survey
      - All infants aged <6 months (perhaps <1 year) when any physical abuse is suspected
      - All infants in whom nonaccidental head injury is suspected
  - CT scan of abdomen with IV contrast:
    - Children with clinical concern for abdominal injury (abdominal bruising, peritonitis, or a positive abdominal ultrasound) or history of blunt abdominal trauma and abdominal tenderness
  - Dilated fundoscopic exam: Presence of extensive retinal hemorrhages is highly concerning for abusive head trauma.
    - For any child with intracranial hemorrhage; within 24 to 72 hours of initial presentation
- High risk imaging findings:
  - Fractures in nonambulatory patients (Children who are not walking or cruising rarely have bruising or fractures from "short falls.")
  - Corner or bucket-handle fractures
  - Posterior rib fractures in infants
  - Injury to liver/spleen/pancreas in blunt abdominal trauma

Follow-Up Tests & Special Considerations

In cases of sexual abuse where there is concern for exposure to body fluids, forensic evidence kit collection may be indicated up to 120 hours post assault.

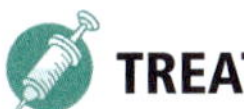

TREATMENT

MEDICATION

First Line

- Consider antibiotics for postexposure prophylaxis in postpubertal children as indicated for STIs. Of note, do not prophylactically treat prepubertal children with antibiotics for STIs.
- If exposure to body fluids is of concern, consider HIV postexposure prophylaxis.

ALERT
Emergency contraception reduces rate of pregnancy after sexual assault:

- Levonorgestrel (Plan B): single dose of 1.5 mg or two 0.75 mg doses taken together or 12 hours apart; effective up to 72 hours *or*
- Ulipristal (Ella): 30 mg single dose as soon as possible; effective up to 120 hours

ISSUES FOR REFERRAL

When responding to possible abuse, consider:

- The child's safety
  - Is the child at imminent risk for additional harm if sent back to the environment where the possible perpetrator has access to the child?
  - Are there other children in the home/environment who may also be at risk?
- Mental health referrals for the victim and other family members, including siblings
- Any follow-up with medical subspecialties, as needed
- Continue to support the caregivers through the process when possible.

ADMISSION, INPATIENT, AND NURSING CONSIDERATIONS

Admission if moderate/severe injuries, psychological trauma, inability to coordinate safe discharge plan

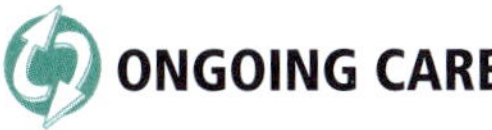

ONGOING CARE

PATIENT EDUCATION

- National Child Abuse hotline: 1.800.4.A.CHILD
- National Toll-Free Crisis Hotline Numbers: https://www.childwelfare.gov/pubs/reslist/tollfree/
- Trauma resources: National Child Traumatic Stress Network (NCTSN): https://www.NCTSN.org

PROGNOSIS

Without intervention, child abuse is often a chronic and escalating phenomenon.

COMPLICATIONS

Sexual, physical, and emotional abuse in childhood are risk factors for poorer adult mental and physical health.

REFERENCES

1. U.S. Department of Health & Human Services, Administration for Children and Families, Administration on Children, Youth and Families, Children's Bureau. (2024). Child Maltreatment 2022. https://www.acf.hhs.gov/cb/data-research/child-maltreatment. Accessed September 11, 2025.
2. Sheets LK, Leach ME, Koszewski IJ, et al. Sentinel injuries in infants evaluated for child physical abuse. *Pediatrics*. 2013;131(4):701–707.
3. Pierce MC, Kaczor K, Lorenz DJ, et al. Validation of a clinical decision rule to predict abuse in young children based on bruising characteristics. *JAMA Netw Open*. 2021;4(4):e215832.

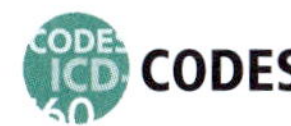

CODES

ICD10

- T74.12XA Child physical abuse, confirmed, initial encounter
- T74.32XA Child psychological abuse, confirmed, initial encounter
- T74.22XA Child sexual abuse, confirmed, initial encounter

CLINICAL PEARLS

- Mandated reporting is required for suspected child abuse and neglect; the medical provider does not have to prove abuse.
- Bruising in nonambulatory children should be considered as a potential sentinel injury for physical abuse if no plausible explanation is given.
- Neglect is the most common and lethal form of abuse.

CHLAMYDIA INFECTION (SEXUALLY TRANSMITTED)

Mark B. Stephens, MD, MS, FAAFP

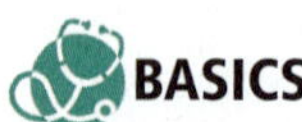

BASICS

DESCRIPTION

- *Chlamydia trachomatis* remains the most common bacterial sexually transmitted infection worldwide and in the United States.
- Transmitted through vaginal, anal, or oral sex; and vertically during vaginal delivery
- Most cases are asymptomatic. Untreated disease can lead to pelvic inflammatory disease (PID), ectopic pregnancy, and infertility.

Pregnancy Considerations

Perinatal acquisition may result in neonatal pneumonia and/or conjunctivitis.

EPIDEMIOLOGY

Incidence

- Mandatory reporting started in 1985
- 1.6 million cases reported in 2023

Prevalence

- ~500/100,000 people in the United States; highest prevalence in ages 20 to 24 years
- Females have twice the reported incidence and prevalence than males (higher screening rates in women). Use of highly sensitive nucleic acid amplification test (NAAT) urine screening may increase identification in males.
- Estimated ~2% of young sexually active individuals in the United States are affected.

ETIOLOGY AND PATHOPHYSIOLOGY

C. trachomatis serotypes D to K are associated with genital tract infections. Chlamydia is an obligate intracellular organism and has a biphasic life cycle. Chlamydia derives from the Greek word for "cloak." Its extracellular elementary body (EB) is metabolically inactive and infectious. Once taken up by host cell (columnar epithelium of the genital tract), the EB prevents lysosomal phagocytosis and transforms to reticulate body (RB) which uses energy from host cell to synthesize RNA, DNA, and proteins. EBs are released to infect neighboring cells or to infect other individuals through sexual contact.

RISK FACTORS

- Number of lifetime and concurrent sexual partners
- Lack of barrier contraception during intercourse
- Higher rates reported Black/Hispanic/Native American and Alaskan Native populations
- Men who have sex with men (MSM) may be at higher risk for rectal and pharyngeal chlamydia; consider testing with NAAT when appropriate (1).

GENERAL PREVENTION

- Screening recommended if with new or >1 sex partner in past 6 months. Screen if with rectal pain, discharge, tenesmus, or testicular pain; and test all individuals with urethral or cervical discharge.
- All sexually active women ≤25 years of age should be screened at least yearly. Repeat testing in ~3 months is recommended for those who screen positive because reinfection rate is high regardless of whether the sexual partner is treated or not (2)[A].
- Consider screening sexually active men ≤25 years of age particularly in high-risk populations.
- Screen high-risk MSM annually with genital and extragenital screening (3)[A].
- NAAT is the preferred screening test in all circumstances except child sexual abuse involving boys or rectal/oropharyngeal testing in prepubescent girls. For these situations, culture and susceptibility testing is preferred (3)[A].
- Acceptable to screen women for chlamydia on same day as intrauterine device (IUD) insertion—treat if positive (no need to remove IUD in this circumstance)
- Doxycycline post-exposure prophylaxis ("Doxy-PEP") is an emerging prevention strategy for chlamydia, syphilis, and possibly gonorrhea, currently best studied in MSM and transgender women with a history of bacterial STI within the past year.

COMMONLY ASSOCIATED CONDITIONS

- Individuals with female anatomy
  - PID: ~10% develop PID within 12 months if untreated.
  - Infertility, ectopic pregnancy
  - Chronic pelvic pain
  - Urethral syndrome (dysuria, frequency, and pyuria in the absence of infection)
- Individuals with male anatomy
  - Epididymitis and nongonococcal urethritis
  - Reiter syndrome (HLA-B27)
  - Proctitis
- Neonates
  - Inclusion conjunctivitis (occurs in ~40% of exposed neonates)
- Diseases caused by other chlamydial species
  - Lymphogranuloma venereum (LGV): *C. trachomatis* serotypes L1 to L3
  - Trachoma: *C. trachomatis* serotypes A to C

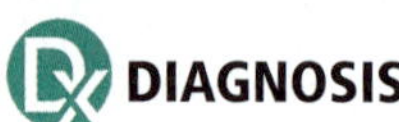

DIAGNOSIS

Many patients are asymptomatic.

Pregnancy Considerations

- Test all patients at first prenatal visit.
- Repeat testing 3 to 4 weeks after treatment for all pregnant patients with confirmed chlamydial infection. Test again after 3 months.
- Repeat screening in 3rd trimester for high-risk patients (2)[A].

HISTORY

- Thorough sexual history, including number of lifetime and recent sex partners, prior history of STIs, use of barrier protection, commercial sex work, oral or anal receptive intercourse, and partner fidelity
- Most common symptoms in females: mucopurulent vaginal discharge, dysuria (urethral syndrome), bartholinitis, abdominopelvic pain (endometritis, salpingitis/PID), right upper quadrant pain (Fitz-Hugh–Curtis syndrome)
- Most common symptoms in males: dysuria, urethral discharge (urethritis), scrotal pain (epididymitis), rectal pain or discharge (proctitis), acute arthritis (Reiter syndrome)

PHYSICAL EXAM

- All patients: external genitalia (rash, lesions), urethral discharge, inguinal lymphadenopathy, pharyngeal exudate, and perianal lesions
- People with female anatomy: cervix (discharge), bimanual examination for cervical motion tenderness, uterine, ovarian/adnexal tenderness, or mass
- LGV (*C. trachomatis* serovars L1, L2, or L3): Primary lesion is a small papule that may ulcerate at the site of transmission after an incubation period of 3 to 30 days. Unilateral tender lymphadenopathy. With rectal transmission, LGV causes an invasive proctocolitis.

DIFFERENTIAL DIAGNOSIS

- *Neisseria gonorrhoeae*: urethritis, proctitis, epididymitis, cervicitis, PID, Bartholin abscess
- *Mycoplasma* or *Ureaplasma urealyticum*: urethritis, epididymitis, Reiter disease, PID
- *C. trachomatis* (serotypes L1 to L3): LGV, proctitis
- Trichomoniasis

DIAGNOSTIC TESTS & INTERPRETATION

Initial Tests (lab, imaging)

- NAAT (vaginal, endocervical, rectal, pharyngeal, and urethral swabs, first-stream urine sample): sensitivity >95%; specificity >99%
- First-stream urine is as sensitive as cervical swab. Self-collected vaginal swabs are most sensitive (3)[A].
- Lab result may remain positive for 3 weeks after successful treatment.
- Test for concurrent STIs, including gonorrhea, HIV, and syphilis; perform cervical cancer (Pap smear) screening according to recommended guidelines.

Follow-Up Tests & Special Considerations

See "Patient Monitoring."

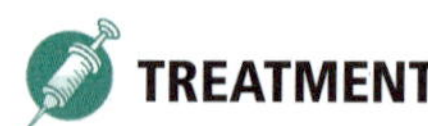

TREATMENT

GENERAL MEASURES

- Offer patients concurrent testing for gonorrhea, HIV (after counseling and consent), and syphilis. Ensure up to date with recommended cervical cancer screening.
- Consider treating gonorrhea empirically.
- Test and treat all partners (all partners within the past 60 days).

MEDICATION

First Line

- https://www.cdc.gov/std/treatment-guidelines/chlamydia.htm
- Treatment of chlamydial urethritis, cervicitis, proctitis, and pharyngitis
- Doxycycline 100 mg PO BID for 7 days (preferred)
  - Alternative regimens: azithromycin 1 gm PO × 1 (recommended in pregnancy) *or* levofloxacin 500 mg PO daily for 7 days
- First-line PID treatment (outpatient)
  - Ceftriaxone 250 mg IM × 1 *plus* doxycycline 100 mg PO for 14 days with or without metronidazole 500 mg PO BID for 14 days or (please note updated uncomplicated gonorrhea treatment guidelines published December 2020, which recommend 500 mg of ceftriaxone IM for patients <150 kg, and 1 gm for patients >150 kg.)
  - Cefoxitin 2 g IM × 1 with probenecid 1 g PO × 1 *plus* doxycycline 100 mg PO for 14 days with or without metronidazole 500 mg PO BID for 14 days
- Azithromycin and ceftriaxone may be given simultaneously in the office to treat both chlamydia and gonorrhea. This reduces nonadherence.
- Doxy-PEP (post-exposure prophylaxis) after unprotected sex for MSM and transgender women; 200 mg as soon as possible after sex (within 3 days)

ALERT

Use azithromycin with caution in patients with known QT prolongation, hypokalemia, hypomagnesemia, bradycardia, or who are currently treated with antiarrhythmics.

Pregnancy Considerations

- Tetracyclines (doxycycline) and quinolones (levofloxacin) are contraindicated in pregnancy.
- Approved treatments:
  - Azithromycin 1 g PO *or*
  - Amoxicillin 500 mg PO TID for 7 days *or*
  - Erythromycin base 500 mg PO QID for 7 days

ALERT

Tetracyclines and quinolones are contraindicated in young children:

- <45 kg: erythromycin base or ethinyl succinate 500 mg/kg/day PO QID for 14 days
- >45 kg but <8 years of age: azithromycin 1 g PO once
- >8 years of age: adult regimen
- Investigate possible sexual abuse in children with chlamydial infections.

Second Line

For chlamydial urethritis/cervicitis

- Erythromycin base 500 mg PO QID for 7 days *or* erythromycin ethylsuccinate 800 mg PO QID for 7 days
- Levofloxacin 500 mg PO daily for 7 days *or* ofloxacin 300 mg PO BID for 7 days

ADDITIONAL THERAPIES

Patient-delivered partner therapy (PDPT) or expedited partner therapy (EPT): Provide medications or prescriptions for sexual partners of persons infected with STIs without clinical assessment; only allowed in some states.

- EPT reduces recurrence more effectively than traditional partner referral.
- https://www.cdc.gov/std/ept/legal/

ADMISSION, INPATIENT, AND NURSING CONSIDERATIONS

- Inpatient treatment of PID: pregnancy, lack of response or intolerance to oral medicines, suspicion of poor compliance, severe clinical illness, pelvic abscess, and possible need for surgical intervention
- Otherwise, treat PID as outpatient unless moderately or severely ill.

ONGOING CARE

FOLLOW-UP RECOMMENDATIONS

Abstain from sexual contact for at least 7 days after treatment (single-dose treatment such as azithromycin) or until completion of the full course of other antibiotics (doxycycline, levofloxacin).

Patient Monitoring

- Test of cure is not routinely recommended except in pregnancy. Do not repeat NAAT <3 weeks after testing; may be falsely positive due to nonviable organisms
- Test of cure in 3 to 4 weeks in pregnancy as well as test for reinfection in 3 months
- Consider rescreening higher risk pregnant people in 3rd trimester even if initial screening negative.
- Test for reinfection (not cure) 3 months after treatment or, if not possible, then at next presentation to medical care if within 12 months.
- Sexual partners should be treated.

PATIENT EDUCATION

- Counsel regarding safe sexual practices, barrier protection, and abstinence.
- Complete antibiotic course (patient and partners).

PROGNOSIS

Prognosis is good following therapy.

COMPLICATIONS

- Chlamydial infection enhances transmission of and susceptibility to HIV.
- Individuals with female anatomy: tubal infertility (most common cause of acquired infertility), ectopic pregnancy, chronic pelvic pain
  - Annual screening of sexually active women would prevent 61% of chlamydia-related PID.
- People with male anatomy: transient oligospermia and postepididymitis urethral stricture (rare)

REFERENCES

1. Hocking JS, Geisler WM, Kong FYS. Update on epidemiology, screening and management of Chlamydia trachomatis infection. *Infect Dis Clin North Am*. 2023;37(2):267–288. doi:10.1016/j.idc.2023.02.007.
2. Sharma V, Khan MM. Current progress and future perspective of *Chlamydia trachomatis* infection: a rising threat to women's health. *Curr Microbiol*. 2025;82(7):314. doi:10.1007/s00284-025-04287-x.
3. Luetkemeyer AF, Donnell D, Dombrowski JC, et al; for the DoxyPEP Study Team. Post-exposure doxycycline to prevent bacterial sexually transmitted infections. *N Engl J Med*. 2023;388(14):1296–1306. doi:10.1056/NEJMoa2211934.

ADDITIONAL READING

Dutra K, Lazenby G. An update on gonorrhea and chlamydia. *Obstet Gynecol Clin North Am*. 2023;50(2):299–310.

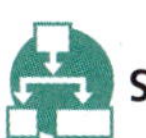

SEE ALSO

Cervicitis, Ectropion, and True Erosion; Epididymitis; Gonococcal Infections; HIV/AIDS; Pelvic Inflammatory Disease (PID); Syphilis; Urethritis

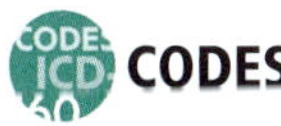

CODES

ICD10

- A56.8 Sexually transmitted chlamydial infection of other sites
- A56.01 Chlamydial cystitis and urethritis
- A56.02 Chlamydial vulvovaginitis

CLINICAL PEARLS

- *C. trachomatis* is common in young sexually active individuals. Annual screening is recommended in sexually active women 25 years of age and younger and in other individuals with known risk factors.
- To prevent recurrence, treat patients and their partners concurrently. Test for reinfection 3 months afterward.
- Doxycycline is the treatment of choice unless otherwise contraindicated.
- Test of cure is only recommended for pregnant patients 3 to 4 weeks after treatment for an identified chlamydia infection. Repeat screens in 3rd trimester for high-risk patients.
- Post-exposure prophylaxis with 200 mg of doxycycline (Doxy-PEP) in MSM has been shown to significantly reduce the incidence of gonorrhea, chlamydia, and syphilis.

CHOLELITHIASIS

Hongyi Cui, MD, PhD

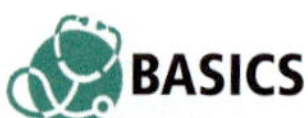

BASICS

DESCRIPTION

The presence of cholesterol, pigment, or mixed stones (calculi) within the gallbladder

Pediatric Considerations

Most gallstones in children are pigment stones associated with blood dyscrasias.

EPIDEMIOLOGY

Incidence

2% of the U.S. population develops gallstones annually.

Prevalence

- 8–10% of the U.S. population with gallstones; 20% >65 years of age
- Female > male (2 to 3:1)

ETIOLOGY AND PATHOPHYSIOLOGY

- Gallstone formation is a complex process mediated by genetic, metabolic, immune, and environmental factors. Gallbladder sludge (a mixture of cholesterol crystals, calcium bilirubinate granules, and mucin gel matrix) serves as the nidus for gallstone formation. Bile supersaturated with cholesterol (cholesterol stones) precipitates as microcrystals that aggregate and expand. Stone formation is enhanced by biliary stasis or impaired gallbladder motility.
- Decrease in bile phospholipid (lecithin) or decreased bile salt secretion
- Excess unconjugated bilirubin in patients with hemolytic diseases; passage of excess bile salt into the colon with subsequent absorption of excess unconjugated bilirubin in patients with inflammatory bowel disease (IBD) or after distal ileal resection (black or pigment stones)

RISK FACTORS

- Age peaks in patients 60 to 80 years of age; female gender, pregnancy, multiparity, obesity, and metabolic syndrome
- Caucasian, Hispanic, or Native American descent
- High-fat diet rich in cholesterol
- Cholestasis or impaired gallbladder motility in association with prolonged fasting, long-term total parenteral nutrition (TPN), following vagotomy, long-term somatostatin therapy, and rapid weight loss
- Hereditary (p.D19H variant for the hepatic canalicular cholesterol transporter ABCG5/ABG8).
- Medications (birth control pills, estrogen at high doses, long-term corticosteroids)
- Viral hepatitis, biliary tract infection, and stricture (promotes intraductal formation of pigment stones)

GENERAL PREVENTION

- Regular exercise and dietary modification may reduce the incidence of gallstone formation.
- Lipid-lowering drugs (statins) may prevent cholesterol stone formation by reducing bile cholesterol saturation.
- Ursodiol (Actigall) taken during rapid weight loss helps prevent gallstone formation.

COMMONLY ASSOCIATED CONDITIONS

90% of people with gallbladder carcinoma have gallstones and chronic cholecystitis.

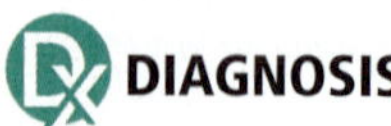

DIAGNOSIS

HISTORY

- Most patients are asymptomatic (80%): 2% become symptomatic each year. Over their lifetime, <50% of patients with gallstones develop symptoms.
- Episodic right upper quadrant or epigastric pain lasting >15 minutes and sometimes radiating to the back (biliary colic—due to transient cystic duct obstruction); pain is usually postprandial, particularly following a fatty meal but sometimes awakens patients from sleep (nocturnal); most patients develop recurrent symptoms after a first episode of biliary colic.
- Other symptoms include nausea, vomiting, indigestion or bloating sensation, and fatty food intolerance.
- Gallstone-related complications (such as gallstone pancreatitis [GP]) may be first manifestation of gallstone disease.

PHYSICAL EXAM

- Physical exam is *usually normal* in patients with cholelithiasis in the absence of an acute attack.
- Epigastric and/or right upper quadrant tenderness (Murphy sign) is a traditional physical finding associated with acute cholecystitis. Murphy sign has limited sensitivity and specificity.
- Charcot triad: fever, jaundice, right upper quadrant pain historically associated with cholangitis
- Reynolds pentad: fever, jaundice, right upper quadrant pain, hemodynamic instability, mental status changes; also classically associated with ascending cholangitis
- Flank and periumbilical ecchymoses (Cullen sign and Grey Turner sign) in patients with acute hemorrhagic pancreatitis
- Courvoisier sign: palpable mass in the right upper quadrant in patient with obstructive jaundice most commonly due to malignant tumors within the biliary tree or pancreas

DIFFERENTIAL DIAGNOSIS

- Peptic ulcer diseases and gastritis; hepatitis
- Pancreatitis; cholangitis; gallbladder cancer; gallbladder polyps
- Acalculous cholecystitis; biliary dyskinesia; choledocholithiasis

DIAGNOSTIC TESTS & INTERPRETATION

Ultrasound (US) is the preferred diagnostic modality for cholelithiasis (high sensitivity and specificity).

Initial Tests (lab, imaging)

- Leukocytosis and elevated C-reactive protein level are common in acute calculus cholecystitis.
- US is the preferred imaging modality. US detects gallstones in 97–98% of patients.
- Thickening of the gallbladder wall (≥5 mm), pericholecystic fluid, and direct tenderness when the probe is pushed against the gallbladder (sonographic Murphy sign) are associated with acute cholecystitis.
- CT scan has no advantage over US except for detecting distal common bile duct (CBD) stones.
- MR cholangiopancreatography (MRCP) is reserved for cases of suspected CBD stones. However, MRCP has no therapeutic value, and preoperative MRCP is not more cost-effective than initial cholecystectomy with cholangiography in the diagnosis of patients with suspected CBD stones and patients with mild to moderate GP.
- Endoscopic US is as sensitive as endoscopic retrograde cholangiopancreatography (ERCP) for detection of CBD stones in patients with GP.
- Hepatobiliary iminodiacetic acid (HIDA) scan is useful in diagnosing acute cholecystitis secondary to cystic duct obstruction. It is also useful in differentiating acalculous cholecystitis from other causes of abdominal pain. False-positive tests can result from a fasting state, insufficient resistance of the sphincter of Oddi, and gallbladder agenesis.
- Cholecystokinin (CCK)-HIDA is specifically used to diagnose gallbladder dysmotility (biliary dyskinesia).
- 10–30% of gallstones are radiopaque calcium or pigment-containing gallstones (visible on plain x-ray). A "porcelain gallbladder" is a calcified gallbladder (also visible by x-ray) associated with chronic cholecystitis and gallbladder cancer.

Test Interpretation

Pure cholesterol stones are white or slightly yellow. Pigment stones may be black or brown. Black stones contain polymerized calcium bilirubinate, most often secondary to cirrhosis or hemolysis; these almost always form within the gallbladder. Brown stones are associated with biliary tract infection, caused by bile stasis, and as such primarily form in the bile ducts.

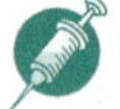

TREATMENT

GENERAL MEASURES

- Treat symptomatic cholelithiasis. For adult patients with uncomplicated symptomatic cholelithiasis, surgery is no more effective than conservative management in the short term (≤18 months).
- Conservative therapy is preferred during pregnancy; surgery in the 2nd trimester if necessary.
- Prophylactic cholecystectomy for patients with calcified (porcelain) gallbladder (risk for gallbladder cancer), patients with large stones (≥3 cm), patients with sickle cell disease, pediatric gallstones, patients planning an organ transplant, and patients with recurrent pancreatitis due to microlithiasis

Geriatric Considerations
Gallstones are more common in the elderly. Age alone should not alter the therapeutic plan.

MEDICATION
First Line
- Analgesics for pain relief
  - NSAIDs are the first-choice treatment for pain control which is equivalent to opioid therapy.
  - Opioids are an option for patients who cannot tolerate or fail to respond to NSAIDs.
- Antibiotics for patients with acute cholecystitis
- Prophylactic antibiotics in low-risk patients do not prevent infections during laparoscopic cholecystectomy (LC).

ISSUES FOR REFERRAL
Patients with retained or recurrent bile duct stones following cholecystectomy should be referred for ERCP.

SURGERY/OTHER PROCEDURES
- Surgery should be considered for patients who have symptomatic cholelithiasis or gallstone-related complications (e.g., cholecystitis) or in asymptomatic patients with immune suppression, porcelain gallbladder, giant gallstones (≥3 cm) or family history of gallbladder cancer.
- Open and LC have similar mortality and complication rates. LC is the current gold standard.
- In well-selected patients, robotic cholecystectomy (RC) is an alternative to LC. RC is associated with higher cost, and has not been shown to be superior to LC in terms of pain and risk of complication.
  - Conversion to open procedure is based on clinical judgment.
  - In 10–15% of patients with symptomatic cholelithiasis, CBD stones are detected by intraoperative cholangiogram (IOC). CBD stone(s) can be removed by laparoscopic CBD exploration or postoperative ERCP.
  - Indocyanine green (ICG) near-infrared florescence cholangiography has been shown to reduce bile duct injuries and conversions to open surgery during laparoscopic or robotic cholecystectomy for patients with acute and chronic cholecystitis.
- Early LC (<24 hours after diagnosis of biliary colic) decreases hospital stay and operating time. For patients with acute cholecystitis, early LC (<7 days of clinical presentation) is safe and may shorten the total hospital stay versus delayed LC (>6 weeks after index admission with acute cholecystitis) (1)[A].
- Percutaneous cholecystostomy (PC) is used for high-risk patients with cholecystitis or gallbladder empyema. Interval cholecystectomy is recommended.
- Symptomatic patients who are not candidates for surgery or those who have small gallstones (5 mm or smaller) in a functioning gallbladder with a patent cystic duct are candidates for oral dissolution therapy (ursodiol [Actigall]). The recurrence rate is >50% once medication is discontinued.
- Transpapillary cystic duct stenting via ERCP or EUS-guided transmural (cholecystogastrostomy or cholecystoduodenostomy) gallbladder drainage via deployment of a lumen-apposing metal stent (LAMS) are novel options for managing severe acute cholecystitis, gallbladder hydrops, or empyema in patients unfit for surgery. It can be used as a bridge to LC.

ADMISSION, INPATIENT, AND NURSING CONSIDERATIONS
For patients with symptomatic cholelithiasis, LC is typically an outpatient procedure. For patients with complications (i.e., cholecystitis, cholangitis, pancreatitis), inpatient care is necessary; acute phase: NPO, IV fluids, and antibiotics; adequate pain control with narcotics and/or NSAIDs

ONGOING CARE

FOLLOW-UP RECOMMENDATIONS
Patient Monitoring
- Follow for signs of symptomatic cholelithiasis.
- Follow patients on oral dissolution agents with serial liver enzymes, serum cholesterol, and imaging.

DIET
A low-fat diet may help.

PATIENT EDUCATION
- Change in lifestyle (e.g., regular exercise) and dietary modification (low-fat diet and reduction of total caloric intake) may reduce gallstone-related hospitalizations.
- Patients with asymptomatic gallstones should be educated about the typical symptoms of biliary colic and gallstone-related complications.

PROGNOSIS
- <50% of patients with gallstones become symptomatic.
- Cholecystectomy-related mortality is <0.5% in elective cases and 3–5% in emergency cases; morbidity is <10% in elective cases and 30–40% in emergency cases. ~10–15% of patients have associated choledocholithiasis. After cholecystectomy, stones may recur within the biliary tree in patients with associated risk factors.

COMPLICATIONS
- Acute cholecystitis (90–95% secondary to gallstones)
- GP; ERCP ± sphincterotomy offers no clear benefit in patients with mild GP but reduces complications in those with severe GP (2)[A].
- CBD stones with obstructive jaundice and acute cholangitis. In patients undergoing ERCP for CBD stones, early LC reduces the risk of recurrent biliary events (2)[B]; biliary-enteric fistula and gallstone ileus
- Gallbladder cancer; Mirizzi syndrome (extrinsic bile duct obstruction caused by gallstones lodged in gallbladder or cystic duct)

REFERENCES

1. Patel H, Jepsen J. Gallstone disease: common questions and answers. *Am Fam Physician*. 2024;109(6):518–524.
2. Garcia-Pagan JC, Francoz C, Montagnese S, et al. Management of the major complications of cirrhosis: beyond guidelines. *J Hepatol*. 2021;75(Suppl 1):S135–S146.

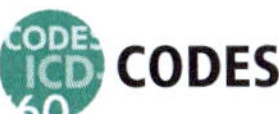
SEE ALSO

Cholangitis, Acute; Choledocholithiasis

CODES

ICD10
- K80.20 Calculus of gallbladder w/o cholecystitis w/o obstruction
- K80.21 Calculus of gallbladder w/o cholecystitis with obstruction
- K80.01 Calculus of gallbladder w acute cholecystitis w obstruction

CLINICAL PEARLS
- Most gallstones are asymptomatic.
- Transabdominal US is the imaging modality of choice for cholelithiasis (sensitivity, 97%; specificity, 95%).
- LC is the preferred surgical procedure for symptomatic cholelithiasis and gallstone-related complications.
- Acute acalculous cholecystitis is associated with bile stasis and gallbladder ischemia.
- Prophylactic cholecystectomy is not routinely indicated in patients with asymptomatic gallstones.

CHRONIC COUGH

Scott Kopec, MD

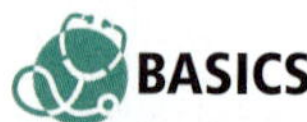

BASICS

DESCRIPTION

- Chronic cough is defined as a cough that persists for >8 weeks in adults.
- In children, chronic cough is often defined as a cough of >4 weeks in duration.
- Subacute cough describes a cough lasting 3 to 8 weeks.
- Patients present because of fear of the causative illness (e.g., cancer), annoyance, self-consciousness, and hoarseness.
- System(s) affected: gastrointestinal (GI), pulmonary

EPIDEMIOLOGY

- Predominant age: all age groups
- Predominant sex: male = female, with females more likely to seek out medical attention

Incidence

Persistent unexplained cough occurs in up to 10% of patients presenting with chronic cough and up to 46% referred to specialty cough clinics.

Prevalence

Chronic cough is one of the most common reasons for primary care visits.

ETIOLOGY AND PATHOPHYSIOLOGY

Varies with findings and disorders implicated

- Often multiple etiologies, but most are related to bronchial irritation. Frequent etiologies (account for >90% of cases) in nonsmokers include the following:
  - Upper airway cough syndrome (UACS) and other upper airway abnormalities, including allergic and vasomotor rhinitis syndromes
  - Chronic rhinitis with postnasal drip (allergic, nonallergic, chronic sinusitis, etc.)
  - Postviral cough
  - Asthma
  - Gastroesophageal reflux disease (GERD)
- Other causes:
  - ACE inhibitors
  - Chronic smoking or exposure to smoke or pollutants
  - Aspiration
  - Bronchiectasis
  - Infections (e.g., pertussis, tuberculosis)
  - Nonasthmatic eosinophilic bronchitis (NAEB)
  - Cystic fibrosis
  - Sleep apnea
  - Restrictive lung diseases
  - Neoplasms: bronchogenic or laryngeal
  - Psychogenic (habit cough)
- Cough hypersensitivity syndrome: a syndrome of cough with characteristic trigger symptoms not adequately explained by other medical conditions
- Etiologies of chronic cough in young children differ from those in older children and adults: Most common causes include asthma, protracted bacterial bronchitis, and UACS; somatic (psychogenic) and tic (habit) should only be considered if extensive testing has ruled out other causes (1).

RISK FACTORS

Most common causes: smoking and pulmonary diseases

COMMONLY ASSOCIATED CONDITIONS

Patients with UACS, asthma, and GERD may present with chronic cough as the only symptom and not the usual symptoms associated with the diagnoses.

DIAGNOSIS

HISTORY

- Patient's age, associated signs/symptoms, medical history, medication history (i.e., ACE inhibitors), environmental and occupational exposures, potential for aspiration, and smoking history may make some causes more likely.
- The character of cough or description of sputum quality is rarely helpful in predicting the underlying cause.
- Cough diaries have not correlated well with objective measures.
- Hemoptysis or signs of systemic illness preclude empiric therapy.

PHYSICAL EXAM

- Signs and symptoms are variable and related to the underlying cause; usually, a nonproductive cough with no other signs or symptoms
- Possible signs and symptoms of UACS, sinusitis, GERD, congestive heart failure, chronic stressors
- Absence of additional signs/symptoms of a particular condition not necessarily helpful

DIAGNOSTIC TESTS & INTERPRETATION

- Clinical trial of empiric therapy directed at likely underlying etiology and/or simple testing such as a chest x-ray (CXR)
- Extensive testing if indicated by the history and physical

Pediatric Considerations

Children with chronic cough not responsive to an inhaled β-agonist and without overt stressors should undergo spirometry (if age-appropriate) and foreign body evaluation (CXR).

Initial Tests (lab, imaging)

- Peak flow may be indicated.
- If considering neoplasm, heart failure, or infectious etiologies, CXR or B-type natriuretic peptide (BNP) may be indicated.
- In cases of failure to respond to initial trial of empiric therapy, CXR may also be beneficial.

Follow-Up Tests & Special Considerations

- If considering chronic obstructive pulmonary disease (COPD), asthma, or restrictive lung disease: spirometry
- If suspicious of cystic fibrosis: sweat chloride testing
- If suspicious of hypereosinophilic syndrome, tuberculosis, or malignancy: sputum for eosinophils and cytology
- If abnormal CXR or underlying pulmonary disorder: chest CT
- Consider pulmonary consultation and/or GI for endoscopy.

Diagnostic Procedures/Other

If diagnosis suggested and inadequate response to initial measures, other procedures can be considered:

- Pulmonary function testing
- Purified protein derivative (PPD) skin testing
- Allergen testing
- 24-Hour esophageal pH monitor
- Bronchoscopy, if history of hemoptysis or smoking with normal CXR
- Endoscopic or video fluoroscopic swallow evaluation or barium esophagram
- Sinus CT
- Ambulatory cough monitoring and cough challenge with citric acid, capsaicin, or other bronchodilator (at specialized cough clinic)
- Echocardiogram

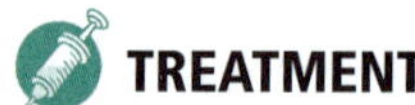

TREATMENT

GENERAL MEASURES

- With chronic cough, empiric treatment should be directed at the most common causes as clinically indicated (UACS, asthma, GERD) (1)[C].
- Empiric trial of nasal steroids and/or antihistamines should be considered if allergic symptoms or postnasal drip is present.

- With concomitant complaints of heartburn and regurgitation, GERD should be considered as a potential etiology (1).
- In patients with cough associated with the common cold, nonsedating antihistamines were not found to be effective in reducing cough (1).
- Many patients will have resolution of cough after smoking cessation.
- When indicated, ACE inhibitor therapy should be switched in patients in whom intolerable cough occurs. It may take several days or weeks for cough to resolve after stopping ACE inhibitor therapy.
- Empirically treat postnasal drip and GERD.
- Empiric proton pump inhibitor (PPI) are not recommended in children or adults in the absence of a GERD diagnosis (1).
- Multimodality speech pathology therapy had a positive benefit on cough severity in some adults.
- Attempt maximal therapy for single most likely cause for several weeks and then search for coexistent etiologies.

MEDICATION

- Treatments (nasal steroids, classic antihistamines, antacids, bronchodilators, inhaled corticosteroids, PPIs, antibiotics) should be directed at the specific cause of cough.
- If history and physical exam suggest GERD, may want to trial empiric PPI therapy prior to further diagnostic testing
- The FDA issued a public health advisory stating that OTC cough and cold medicines, including antitussives, expectorants, nasal decongestants, antihistamines, or combinations, should not be given to children <2 years. Subsequently, manufacturers have changed labeling to state "do not use" in children <4 years. In 2017, the FDA issued a contraindication to codeine for cough treatment in children <12 years.
- Routine empiric treatment of children with chronic cough with leukotriene receptor antagonists lacks evidence and cannot be recommended.

First Line

In adults: nasal steroids: fluticasone, budesonide, others, 1 spray BID for those with allergic rhinitis symptoms or postnasal drip or an empiric trial of PPI (omeprazole, others) once a day

Second Line

- A peripherally acting antitussive agent has been used: In patients >10 years, benzonatate (Tessalon Perles) 100 to 200 mg PO TID as needed (maximum 600 mg/day)
- Gabapentin was evaluated in a randomized, double-blind, placebo-controlled trial of patients with refractory chronic cough found improved cough-specific quality of life versus placebo. If likely etiologies fail, consider a therapeutic trial × 6 months.
- A comparative effectiveness review of 49 studies with common opioid and nonanesthetic antitussives found limited evidence and limited efficiency for treating cough in adults.
- Studies evaluating inhaled corticosteroid use in chronic cough for patients without additional indication such as asthma did not show consistent benefits.

ISSUES FOR REFERRAL

Patients with chronic cough may benefit from evaluation by pulmonary, gastroenterology, ear/nose/throat (ENT), and/or allergy specialists. Consider specialist cough clinic.

ONGOING CARE

FOLLOW-UP RECOMMENDATIONS

Consider stepwise withdrawal of medications after resolution of cough.

DIET

Dietary modification: Patients with GERD may benefit by avoiding ethanol, caffeine, nicotine, citrus, tomatoes, chocolate, and fatty foods.

PATIENT EDUCATION

- Reassure patient most cases of chronic cough are not life threatening and the condition can usually be managed effectively.
- Counsel that several weeks may be needed for significant reduction or elimination of cough.

PROGNOSIS

- >80% of patients can be effectively diagnosed and treated using a systematic approach.
- Cough from any cause may take weeks to months until resolution, and resolution depends greatly on efficacy of treatment directed at underlying etiology.

COMPLICATIONS

- Cardiovascular: arrhythmias, syncope
- Stress urinary incontinence
- Abdominal and intercostal muscle strain
- GI: emesis, hemorrhage, herniation
- Neurologic: dizziness, headache, seizures
- Respiratory: pneumothorax, laryngeal, or tracheobronchial trauma
- Skin: petechiae, purpura, disruption of surgical wounds
- Medication side effects
- Other: negative impact on quality of life

REFERENCES

1. Michaudet C, Malaty J. Chronic cough: evaluation and management. *Am Fam Physician*. 2017;96(9):575–580.

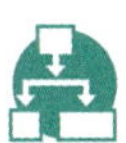

SEE ALSO

- Asthma; Bronchiectasis; Eosinophilic Pneumonias; Gastroesophageal Reflux Disease; Laryngeal Cancer; Lung, Primary Malignancies; Pertussis; Pulmonary Edema; Rhinitis, Allergic; Sinusitis; Tuberculosis
- Algorithm: Cough, Chronic

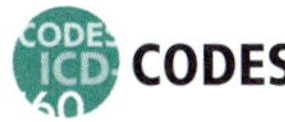

CODES

ICD10

- R05 Cough
- J44.9 Chronic obstructive pulmonary disease, unspecified
- J41.0 Simple chronic bronchitis

CLINICAL PEARLS

- Chronic cough is defined as a cough that persists for >8 weeks in adults.
- In patients with chronic cough, most frequent etiologies include a history of smoking, asthma, UACS, and GERD.
- The FDA issued a public health advisory stating that OTC cough and cold medicines should not be given to children <2 years. OTC cough expectorant and suppressant product labels state "do not use" in children <4 years. Codeine is contraindicated for cough treatment in children <12 years.

CHRONIC KIDNEY DISEASE

Cindy Le, MD • Konstantin Abramov, MD, MHL

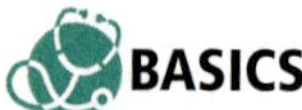

BASICS

Chronic kidney disease (CKD) is defined as structural or functional abnormalities of the kidney, as determined by either pathologic abnormalities or markers of damage (abnormalities in blood or urine tests, histology, imaging studies) or a glomerular filtration rate (GFR) <60 mL/min/1.73 m². Findings present for ≥3 months. CKD is classified based on the cause, GFR category (G1 to G5), and albuminuria category (A1 to A3).

DESCRIPTION

- Kidney Disease: Improving Global Outcomes (KDIGO) categories by GFR estimation (in mL/min/1.73 m²):
  - G1: kidney damage with normal or increased GFR ≥90
  - G2: mild ↓ GFR 60 to 89; G3a: mild to moderate ↓ GFR 45 to 59
  - G3b: moderate to severe ↓ GFR 30 to 44
  - G4: severe ↓ GFR 15 to 29
  - G5: kidney failure: GFR <15 or dialysis
- CKD per albumin-to-creatinine ratio (ACR) category:
  - A1: normal to mildly increased: <30 mg/g or <3 mg/mmol
  - A2: moderately increased: 30 to 300 mg/g or 3 to 30 mg/mmol
  - A3: severely increased: >300 mg/g or >30 mg/mm

EPIDEMIOLOGY

- African Americans are 3.6 times more likely to develop CKD than White people.
- Similar in both sexes; however, rate of end-stage renal disease (ESRD) is 1.6 times higher in males than females.

Incidence

Estimated annual incidence of 1,700/1 million population

ETIOLOGY AND PATHOPHYSIOLOGY

- Progressive destruction of kidney nephrons; GFR will drop gradually, and plasma creatinine (Cr) values will approximately double, with 50% reduction in GFR and 75% loss of functioning nephrons mass. Hyperkalemia usually develops when GFR falls to <20 to 25 mL/min/1.73m². Anemia develops from decreased renal synthesis of erythropoietin.
- Renal parenchymal/glomerular
  - Nephritic: hematuria, red blood cell (RBC) casts, hypertension (HTN), variable proteinuria
    - Focal proliferative: IgA nephropathy, systemic lupus erythematosus (SLE), Henoch-Schönlein purpura, Alport syndrome, proliferative glomerulonephritis, crescentic glomerulonephritis
    - Diffuse proliferative: membranoproliferative glomerulonephritis, SLE, cryoglobulinemia, rapidly progressive glomerulonephritis (RPGN), Goodpasture syndrome
  - Nephrotic: proteinuria (>3.5 g/day), hypoalbuminemia, hyperlipidemia, and edema
    - Minimal change disease, membranous nephropathy, focal segmental glomerulosclerosis
    - Amyloidosis, diabetic nephropathy
- Vascular: HTN, thrombotic microangiopathies, vasculitis (granulomatosis with polyangiitis [GPA]), scleroderma, crush injury
- Interstitial tubular: infections, obstruction, toxins, allergic interstitial nephritis, multiple myeloma, connective tissue disease, cystic disease, nephrolithiasis
- Postrenal: obstruction (benign prostatic hyperplasia [BPH]), neoplasm, neurogenic bladder

Genetics

- Alport syndrome, Fabry disease, sickle cell anemia, SLE/autoimmune disease, and autosomal dominant polycystic kidney disease can lead to CKD.
- Polymorphisms in gene that encodes for podocyte nonmuscle myosin IIA are more common in African Americans than Caucasians and appear to increase risk for nondiabetic ESRD.

RISK FACTORS

Type 1 or 2 diabetes mellitus (DM) (most common); age > 60 years; low socioeconomic status; obesity; smoking; drug use; chronic infection (hepatitis B/C, HIV); cardiovascular disease (HTN, renal artery stenosis, atherosclerosis); prior kidney transplant; BPH; autoimmune disease; vasculitis; connective tissue disease; nephrotoxic drugs (nonsteroidal anti-inflammatory drugs [NSAIDs], lithium, sulfonamide, aminoglycosides, vancomycin, PPIs, allopurinol, loop diuretics, chemotherapeutic agents); congenital anomalies; obstructive uropathy; renal aplasia/hypoplasia/dysplasia/reflux nephropathy

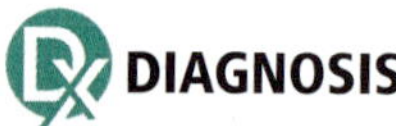

DIAGNOSIS

HISTORY

Patients with CKD stages 1 to 3 are usually asymptomatic; can present with oliguria, nocturia, polyuria, change in urinary frequency, bone disease, edema, HTN, dyspnea, fatigue, depression, weakness, pruritus, ecchymosis, anorexia, nausea, vomiting, hyperlipidemia, claudication, erectile dysfunction, decreased libido, amenorrhea

PHYSICAL EXAM

Check for volume status (pallor, BP/orthostatic; edema; jugular venous distention; weight); skin for sallow complexion or uremic frost; ammonia-like odor; murmurs; bruits; pericarditis; pleural effusions; enlarged prostate; CNS changes such as asterixis; confusion; seizures; coma; and peripheral neuropathy.

DIAGNOSTIC TESTS & INTERPRETATION

Initial Tests (lab, imaging)

- GFR can be estimated using the Modification of Diet in Renal Disease (MDRD) and Chronic Kidney Disease-Epidemiology Collaboration (CKD-EPI) equations
- Cr clearance using the Cockcroft-Gault formula to determine medication dosage
- UA to assess for evidence of damage (WBC casts in pyelonephritis, RBC casts in glomerulonephritis/vasculitis, sodium (Na), Cr, urea, albuminuria)
- US (initial imaging test of choice to assess for cysts, masses, hydronephrosis, kidney size)

Follow-Up Tests & Special Considerations

- Hematology: normochromic, normocytic anemia; increased bleeding time
- Chemistry: elevated BUN, Cr, hyperkalemia, metabolic acidosis, increased parathyroid hormone (PTH), hyperlipidemia, hyperphosphatemia, decreased 25-(OH) vitamin D, hypocalcemia, decreased albumin
- Serology: antinuclear antibody (ANA); double-stranded DNA, antineutrophil cytoplasmic antibody; complements (C3, C4, CH50); antiglomerular basement membrane (anti-GBM) antibodies; hepatitis B, C; and HIV screening
- Serum and urine immunoelectrophoresis

ALERT

Drugs that may alter lab result:

- Cimetidine: inhibits Cr tubular secretion
- Trimethoprim: inhibits Cr and K^+ secretion and may cause/worsen hyperkalemia
- Cefoxitin and flucytosine: increases serum Cr
- Diltiazem and verapamil (like angiotensin-converting enzyme inhibitors [ACE-Is]/angiotensin receptor blockers [ARBs]) have significant antiproteinuric effects in patients with CKD.

Diagnostic Procedures/Other

- Biopsy: hematuria, proteinuria, acute/progressive renal failure, nephritic or nephrotic syndrome
- ECG: assess for abnormal heart rhythms due to electrolyte imbalances

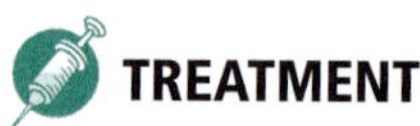

TREATMENT

MEDICATION

- HTN: Adults with elevated blood pressure and CKD G1 to G3 should be treated to a target systolic blood pressure of 120 mm Hg using standardized office measurements. Renal transplant patients should have a target blood pressure of <130/80 mm Hg (1)[C].
  - ACE-I or ARB recommended for diabetic and nondiabetic adults with albumin excretion >30 mg/24 hr based on evidence of benefits.
    - An ACE-I or ARB can still be considered in patients with no albuminuria. Those patients, however, are at less risk for CKD progression.
    - Avoid combining ACE-I, ARB, and DRI therapy in diabetic and nondiabetic patients with CKD.
    - Advise contraception in women who are receiving ACE-I or ARB therapy and discontinue in women who are considering pregnancy or have become pregnant (2)[C].
  - Calcium channel blockers (CCB) or ARB is first line in adult kidney transplant patients for prevention of allograft failure and minimization of possible drug-induced side effects.
  - In children with CKD, 24-hour mean arterial pressure by ABPM should be lowed to <50th percentile for age, sex, and height. In this population, an ACE-I or ARB is first line.
  - A combination between a low-Na diet plus the use of an ACE-I or ARB leads to significant reduction in proteinuria (3)[C].

- Secondary hyperparathyroidism
- For GFR <45 mL/min/1.73 m^2, monitor for hyperphosphatemia, hypocalcemia, and vitamin D deficiency if intact PTH is elevated.
- Calcimimetic agents (oral cinacalcet or IV etelcalcetide) are not FDA approved for use in patients with CKD not on dialysis. These should be reserved for ESRD patients (3)[C].
- Hyperphosphatemia: Maintain normal serum phosphate levels using the following:
  - Stages 3 to 5 CKD (not on dialysis): Restrict dietary phosphate to 800 to 1,000 mg/day.
  - Noncalcium phosphate binders (with meals): sevelamer, lanthanum
  - Calcium binders have not been associated with improvement in mortality or cardiovascular outcomes (3)[C].
  - Vitamin D: inactive vitamin D_2 (ergocalciferol) or vitamin D_3 (cholecalciferol), calcitriol (active vitamin D 1,25 [OH]): Vitamin D may increase absorption of phosphate by intestines and should not be started until serum phosphate concentration is controlled.
- Anemia: Treat with iron replacement therapy with or without erythropoietin-stimulating agents (ESAs). Consider ESA if Hb >9 g/dL and <10 g/dL. ESA initiation not recommended for Hb >10 g/dL. If using ESA, goal Hb range 10 to 11 g/dL, not to exceed 11.5 g/dL.
- Hyperlipidemia: statins with low-density lipoprotein (LDL) goal <70 mg/dL
- Glycemic control: Goal HbA1c range 6.5–8%. HbA1c may be falsely low in patients with decreased RBC; glucose logs may be more accurate reflection of glycemic control.
  - Metformin use should be reviewed for GFR between 30 and 44 mL/min/1.73 m^2 and discontinued if GFR <30 mL/min/1.73 m^2.
  - Use SGLT2 inhibitors along with metformin in patients with type 2 DM and GFR >30 mL/min/1.73 m^2 (2)[C].
  - SGLT2 inhibitors can be used for patients with and without DM to control disease progression.
  - Use of GLP-RA in addition to optimize glycemic control
- Metabolic acidosis: Start treatment with Na bicarb when bicarbonate <22 mEq/L with goal to maintain in normal range.

ISSUES FOR REFERRAL

- Nephrology consult:
  - GFR <15 mL/min/1.73 m^2: immediate, GFR 15 to 29 mL/min/1.73 m^2: urgent, GFR 30 to 59 mL/min/1.73 m^2: nonurgent referral, GFR 60 to 89 mL/min/1.73 m^2: not required unless with comorbidities
  - Rapid decline of eGFR (>5 mL/min/1.73 m^2 per year), nondiabetics with heavy proteinuria (24-hour urine protein >500 mg, urine PCR >0.5, urine ACR >300), diabetics with >3 g proteinuria or hematuria, management of complications (metabolic management, electrolyte abnormalities, acidosis, etc.)
- Urology consult for hematuria, renal masses, complex renal cysts, symptomatic nephrolithiasis, hydronephrosis
- Registered dietitian/psychology/social work/physical therapy/occupational therapy consultation to assist with dietary options, behavioral modification, access to food resources, and mobility
- Renal replacement: Prepare for dialysis or transplant when GFR <30 mL/min/1.73 m^2.

ADDITIONAL THERAPIES

- Aspirin for secondary prevention for patients with established cardiovascular disease
- For mild pain associated with CKD, acetaminophen is considered first-line therapy. Oral, parental, and even topical NSAIDs are generally not recommended.
- For moderate to severe pain, opioids may be indicated, but the risk of overdose or toxicity is increased because many are renally excreted. Oxycodone, fentanyl, and methadone are preferred, but dose adjustment is still recommended. Meperidine is contraindicated in CKD. Codeine and morphine should be used with caution.
- Chronic pain syndromes may be treated with anticonvulsants and gabapentinoids, which should be renally dosed.

COMPLEMENTARY & ALTERNATIVE MEDICINE

Caution with herbal supplements as these are generally not regulated and may contain excessive amounts of potassium and phosphorus. They may also interact with metabolism of prescription drugs.

ADMISSION, INPATIENT, AND NURSING CONSIDERATIONS

- For use of contrast in imaging, patients should have eGFR > 30 mL/min/1.73 m^2. Volume expansion with IV isotonic saline prior to and following iodinated contrast is recommended.
- Metformin should be held prior to iodinated contrast imaging and resumed after 48 hours.

ONGOING CARE

FOLLOW-UP RECOMMENDATIONS

Patient Monitoring

- Monitor for changes in blood pressure, serum Cr, and serum potassium within 2 to 4 weeks of initiation of ACE-I or ARB. If >30% increase in Cr, correct AKI, reassess medications, reduce/stop the current ACE-I or ARB dose. Discontinue therapy in the setting of symptomatic hypotension or uncontrolled hyperkalemia.
- For patients taking metformin, monitor eGFR annually and vitamin B_{12} levels after taking metformin >4 years.
- Monitor Cr levels in pregnant patients with CKD closely.
- Monitor Hgb annually for GFR 30 to 59 mL/min/1.73 m^2 and biannually for GFR <30 mL/min/1.73 m^2, calcidiol levels, HbA1c 2 to 4 times a year, volume status, electrolytes, kidney function (urine albumin, GFR, serum Cr).
- Calcium, phosphate, PTH, alkaline phosphatase beginning at CKD stage G3

DIET

<2 g Na per day; limit processed foods, refined carbohydrates, sweetened beverages. Restrict potassium and phosphorus if indicated. In CKD stage 3 to 5, restrict protein to 0.8 g/kg/day. Mediterranean diet is generally recommended. Restrict fluids depending on volume status; can consider iron and vitamin D supplementation (4)[C]

PROGNOSIS

Progression is defined as 25% decrease in GFR from baseline. Rapid progression is decrease in GFR by >5 mL/min/1.73 m^2/year. Patients with CKD gradually progress to ESRD.

COMPLICATIONS

HTN, anemia, secondary hyperparathyroidism, renal osteodystrophy, sleep disturbances, infections, malnutrition, electrolyte imbalances, platelet dysfunction/bleeding, pseudogout, gout, metabolic calcification, sexual dysfunction

REFERENCES

1. Kidney Disease: Improving Global Outcomes (KDIGO) CKD Work Group. KDIGO 2024 clinical practice guideline for evaluation and management of chronic kidney disease. *Kidney Int*. 2024;105(4S):S117–S314.
2. Kidney Disease: Improving Global Outcomes (KDIGO) Diabetes Work Group. KDIGO 2020 clinical practice guideline for diabetes management in chronic kidney disease. *Kidney Int*. 2020;98(4S):S1–S115.
3. U.S. Department of Veterans Affairs. VA/DoD Clinical Practice Guideline: Management of Chronic Kidney Disease. 2019. https://www.healthquality.va.gov/guidelines/CD/ckd/. Accessed September 27, 2025.
4. Ikizler TA, Burrowes JD, Byham-Gray LD, et al. KDOQI Clinical Practice Guideline for Nutrition in CKD: 2020 Update. *Am J Kidney Dis*. 2020;76(3)(Suppl 1):S1–S107.

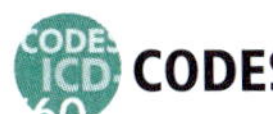

CODES

ICD10

- N18.9 Chronic kidney disease, unspecified
- Q63.9 Congenital malformation of kidney, unspecified
- N18.3 Chronic kidney disease, stage 3 (moderate)

CLINICAL PEARLS

- ACE-I and ARB are first line for HTN treatment in CKD with albuminuria.
- Consider nonurgent nephrologist referral for GFR ≤59 mL/min/1.73 m^2 and urgent nephrologist referral for GFR ≤29 mL/min/1.73 m^2.
- Restrict Na in diet (<2 g/day) and potassium, phosphorus, if indicated. In CKD stage 3 to 5, restrict protein to 0.8 g/kg/day if diabetic.
- CKD progression should be monitored closely and managed by a multidisciplinary team to ensure proper nutrition, pain control, mobility, and access to care.

CHRONIC OBSTRUCTIVE PULMONARY DISEASE AND EMPHYSEMA

Kaitlyn Kennedy, MD • Scott Kopec, MD

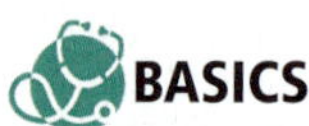

BASICS

DESCRIPTION

The 2025 Global Initiative for Chronic Obstructive Lung Disease (GOLD) defines chronic obstructive pulmonary disease (COPD) as follows:

- COPD is a heterogenous lung condition characterized by chronic respiratory symptoms (dyspnea, cough, sputum production, and/or exacerbations) due to abnormalities of the airways (bronchitis, bronchiolitis) and/or alveoli (emphysema) that cause persistent, often progressive, airflow obstruction.
- COPD was the third leading cause of death and 90% of these deaths occur in low- to medium-income countries.

EPIDEMIOLOGY

Incidence

The incidence of COPD is 8.9/1,000 person-years.

Prevalence

Global prevalence of COPD based on the Burden of Obstructive Lung Diseases (BOLD) program is 10.3% and is projected to rise.

ETIOLOGY AND PATHOPHYSIOLOGY

COPD is the end-result of lifetime environmental exposures including noxious gasses or particles leading to pathologic processes in the airways, lung parenchyma, and pulmonary vasculature.

- Impaired gas (carbon dioxide and oxygen) exchange, persistent airway obstruction, destruction of lung parenchyma

Genetics

α_1-Antitrypsin deficiency caused by SERPINA1 gene, an inherited disorder due to two autosomal codominant alleles, is rare, although it is the best documented genetic risk factor for COPD.

RISK FACTORS

- History of severe childhood respiratory infections and/or asthma and airway hyperreactivity
- Smoking tobacco or marijuana: including passive smoking and water pipe
- Lower level of education and lower socioeconomic status
- Indoor air pollution (especially indoor biomass cooking worldwide): wood, animal dung, crop residues, coal, open fires or poorly functioning stoves
- Occupational organic and inorganic dusts, chemical agents and fumes
- Outdoor air pollution (particulate matter, ozone, oxides of nitrogen and sulfur, heavy metals, greenhouse gasses)
- Aging: including healthy aging as well as the cumulative summation of lung exposure over time

GENERAL PREVENTION

- Smoking cessation and general avoidance of noxious material is the most important preventative measure.
- Reduction of exposure to dusts, fumes, and gases; air pollutants, efficient ventilation, nonpolluting cooking stoves; avoid potential irritants.

COMMONLY ASSOCIATED CONDITIONS

- Pulmonary: lung cancer, respiratory failure, obstructive sleep apnea, pulmonary hypertension (HTN), asthma, bronchiectasis
- Cardiovascular: HTN, cardiovascular disease (CVD), peripheral vascular disease (PVD) arrhythmia (especially low FEV_1), heart failure
- Ear/nose/throat (ENT): chronic sinusitis, laryngeal carcinoma
- Gastrointestinal (GI): gastroesophageal reflux disease (GERD); musculoskeletal
- (MSK): osteoporosis
- Heme: polycythemia, anemia
- Neuro-psych: depression, anxiety, insomnia, cognitive impairment

DIAGNOSIS

The diagnosis of COPD requires these features to meet diagnostic criteria:

- Dyspnea, chronic cough, sputum production, and/or wheezing with a history of recurrent lower respiratory tract infections, and/or a history of exposure to risk factors for the disease
- A postbronchodilator forced expiratory volume in 1 second (FEV_1)/forced vital capacity (FVC) ratio of <0.7, which confirms the presence of persistent airflow limitation

HISTORY

- Review risk factors: smoking and environmental exposures (household/outdoor)
- History, including smoke exposure, asthma, allergies, sinusitis, respiratory infections in childhood, HIV, tuberculosis (TB)
- Family history of COPD or other chronic respiratory disease
- Common symptoms:
  - Chronic, persistent, progressive dyspnea worse with exercise
  - Recurrent wheeze, chest tightness, chronic progressive cough, coughing spells with sputum production
  - Recurrent lower respiratory tract infections
  - Fatigue; weight loss, muscle wasting, anorexia in severe COPD; edema (cor pulmonale)

PHYSICAL EXAM

- Prolonged expiration, wheezing
- Barrel chest, diminished breath sounds, distant heart sounds
- Accessory muscle use, pursed lip breathing, cyanosis, exertional dyspnea
- Clubbing not typical for COPD, however, may indicate another process (e.g., lung cancer, bronchiectasis, or interstitial lung disease)
- Cyanosis

DIFFERENTIAL DIAGNOSIS

- Asthma (including occupational), reactive airways dysfunction syndrome (RADS)
- Respiratory infection (TB)
- Interstitial lung disease, bronchiectasis, primary alveolar hypoventilation, bronchiolitis obliterans
- Lung cancer
- Chronic pulmonary embolism
- Sleep apnea
- Congestive heart failure (CHF)
- GERD
- Cystic fibrosis
- Vasculitis (i.e., granulomatosis with polyangiitis)

DIAGNOSTIC TESTS & INTERPRETATION

Initial Tests (lab, imaging)

- The United States Preventative Service Task Force (USPSTF) recommended against screening for COPD in asymptomatic adults for the general population.
- Spirometry: lung volumes and carbon monoxide diffusing capacity of lungs (DLCO)
- CBC to evaluate eosinophilia or polycythemia
- BMP may reveal elevated CO_2 as an indicator of chronic CO_2 retention.
- Imaging (CXR, CT chest)

Follow-Up Tests & Special Considerations

- Pulse oximetry to assess need for oxygen, both at rest and with exertion
- α_1-Antitrypsin screening for those with COPD age <45 years, have a blood relative with this disease, or spirometry out of proportion to tobacco use
- Low dose CT (LDCT) is recommended by the USPSTF for those at an increased risk of lung cancer (e.g., ages 50 to 80 years with >20 pack-year smoking history).

Diagnostic Procedures/Other

Pulmonary function testing without/with bronchodilator

- Decreased postbronchodilator FEV_1:FVC ratio <0.7; this is the diagnostic criteria for airway obstruction; repeat spirometry recommended if between 0.6 and 0.8.
- Reduced FEV_1, normal or increased FVC with normal or increased total lung capacity and increased residual volume; diffusing capacity is normal or reduced.
- Typically, not bronchodilator responsive (change in FEV_1 or FVC of $\geq 12\%$)

Test Interpretation

- Staging: GOLD criteria staging in the presence of FEV_1/FVC <0.7
  - Grade 1: FEV_1 $\geq 80\%$ predicted
  - Grade 2: FEV_1 50–80% predicted
  - Grade 3: FEV_1 30–50% predicted
  - Grade 4: FEV_1 $<30\%$ predicted
- Symptom severity assessment: GOLD severity assessment based on symptom burden and risk of exacerbation
- The ABE assessment tool incorporates severity of patient's symptoms and exacerbation history.
  - Group A: low risk, less symptoms: 0 to 1 exacerbation per year and no prior hospitalization for exacerbation; and COPD assessment test (CAT Score) <10 or mMRC grade 0 to 1
  - Group B: low risk, more symptoms: 0 to 1 exacerbation per year and no prior hospitalization for exacerbation; and CAT score ≥ 10 or mMRC grade ≥ 2
  - Group E: high risk, more or less symptoms: ≥ 2 exacerbations per year or ≥ 1 hospitalization for exacerbation; and CAT score <10 or ≥ 10 or mMRC grade 0 to grade ≥ 2

TREATMENT

GENERAL MEASURES

- GOLD severity assessment based on symptom burden and risk of exacerbation in conjunction with:
  - CAT score
  - Modified Medical Research Council Dyspnea Scale (mMRCD)
- Treatment based upon GOLD severity assessment (see "First Line")
- Smoking cessation: This is the most important intervention to decrease risk of disease progression.
- Home oxygen: In patients with severe resting chronic hypoxemia ($PaO_2 \leq 55$ mm Hg or <60 mm Hg if there is cor pulmonale or secondary polycythemia), long-term oxygen therapy improves survival.
- All patients should receive COVID-19, pneumococcal, influenza, and pertussis vaccines and those aged >50 years should also receive the varicella zoster vaccine.
- Inhaler techniques need to be assessed regularly.
- Pulmonary rehabilitation
- Noninvasive positive pressure ventilation (NPPV) may decrease mortality and prevent rehospitalization.

MEDICATION

First Line

- GOLD group A: one or no moderate exacerbations requiring systemic steroids and/or antibiotics with no hospitalizations or ED visits for COPD exacerbations *and* dyspnea with exercise or walking uphill (CAT score <10 or mMRC grade 0 to 1): short or long-acting bronchodilator
  - Short-acting β-agonists: albuterol, levalbuterol
- GOLD group B: one or no moderate exacerbations requiring systemic steroids and/or antibiotics with no hospitalizations or ED visits for COPD exacerbations *and* dyspnea with simple walking, needing stop and catch breath (CAT score ≥ 10 or mMRC grade ≥ 2)
  - Combined long-acting β-agonists (LABA)–long-acting muscarinic antagonists (LAMA) rather than steroids
- LABA: formoterol, arformoterol, salmeterol
- LAMA: tiotropium, aclidinium, umeclidinium, glycopyrrolate
- GOLD group E (former groups C and D are now merged into group E): two or more moderate exacerbations requiring systemic steroids and/or antibiotics, or a hospitalization or ED visit for a COPD exacerbation
  - Combined LABA–LAMA rather than steroids
    - LABA: formoterol, arformoterol, salmeterol
    - LAMA: tiotropium, aclidinium, umeclidinium, glycopyrrolate
    - Add to LABA/LAMA an inhaled corticosteroid (ICS) if blood eosinophil count is ≥ 300 cells/uL.
  - If patients have concomitant asthma, they should be treated like patients with asthma, making the use of an ICS necessary.
  - For those on a LABA/LAMA and ICS who continue to have exacerbations, consider adding a macrolide (azithromycin) or roflumilast.
- Rescue short-acting bronchodilators SABA should be prescribed to all patients for immediate symptom relief.
- Once initial therapy is implemented, patients should be reassessed for attainment of treatment goals and identification of any barriers to treatment to make any treatment modifications.
- Acute COPD exacerbations: Mild-to-moderate exacerbations can be treated with short-acting bronchodilators and possibly short courses of steroids and/or antibiotics (5 to 7 days). Severe exacerbations require inpatient admission (see below).
- Mepolizumab and dupilumab: Reserved for patients with poorly controlled moderate to severe COPD and eosinophilia (>300 eosinophils/μL). Patients should be referred to specialists.

Second Line

ALERT

Precautions:

- β-Agonists: sinus tachycardia, arrhythmias in susceptible patients; can consider levalbuterol
- Anticholinergics: minimal systemic absorption in inhaled form; urinary retention possible
- ICS: increased risk of pneumonia; oral candidiasis
- Corticosteroids: weight gain, diabetes, adrenal suppression, osteoporosis, infection (pneumonia)
- Macrolides: Long-term use can possibly lead to bacterial resistance and hearing impairment (monitor QTC interval).
- Ensifentrine: A dual phosphodiesterase 3 (PDE3) + phosphodiesterase 4 (PDE4) inhibitor may play a role for recalcitrant COPD.

ISSUES FOR REFERRAL

Severe exacerbation, frequent hospitalizations, rapid progression, weight loss, or surgical evaluation

ADDITIONAL THERAPIES

Pulmonary rehabilitation program for patients with high symptom burden

SURGERY/OTHER PROCEDURES

Lung reduction surgery, bronchoscopic lung reduction, surgical bullectomy, lung transplantation

ADMISSION, INPATIENT, AND NURSING CONSIDERATIONS

- An exacerbation of COPD is defined as dyspnea and/or cough and sputum that has worsened over <14 days while ruling out other processes such as pneumonia and heart failure.
- Severe acute exacerbation: Maintain oxygenation, short-acting inhaled β-agonists/inhaled anticholinergic agents, and oral or IV corticosteroids prednisone (up to 1 mg/kg/day commonly 40 mg/day for 5 days). Antibiotics for moderate/severe exacerbations with increased sputum volume or sputum purulence; optimal antibiotic therapy has not been determined; NPPV
- Have patient delineate an advance directive.

C

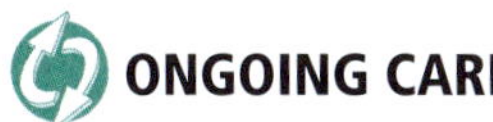

ONGOING CARE

FOLLOW-UP RECOMMENDATIONS

Pulmonary rehabilitation program for patients with high symptom burden and risk of exacerbations

PATIENT EDUCATION

American Lung Association: https://www.lung.org/lung-disease/copd/

PROGNOSIS

- Supplemental oxygen, when indicated, is shown to increase survival (may only require at night).
- Smoking cessation improves prognosis.
- NPPV may improve hospitalization-free survival in selected patients after recent hospitalization, especially in those with persistent hypercapnia in the daytime ($PaCo_2 >53$ mm Hg).
- Four-year mortality estimates range from 28% for mild-to-moderate COPD to 62% for moderate-to-severe COPD.

COMPLICATIONS

- Malnutrition, poor sleep quality, infections, secondary polycythemia
- Acute or chronic respiratory failure, bullous lung disease, pneumothorax
- Arrhythmias, cor pulmonale, pulmonary HTN

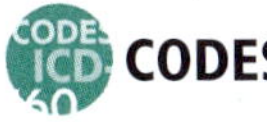

CODES

ICD10

- J44.9 Chronic obstructive pulmonary disease, unspecified
- J43.9 Emphysema, unspecified
- J42 Unspecified chronic bronchitis

CLINICAL PEARLS

- Smoking cessation
- Home oxygen evaluation is important because supplemental oxygen improves mortality.
- Influenza/pneumococcal vaccines should be current.
- Discuss advance directives before patient is seriously ill.

CHRONIC PAIN MANAGEMENT: AN EVIDENCE-BASED APPROACH

Mark B. Stephens, MD, MS, FAAFP

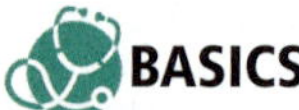

BASICS

- Chronic pain lasts longer than 3 months and involves sensory, emotional, and cognitive components. Chronic pain is classified in International Classification of Diseases, 11th revision (ICD-11) as a distinct diagnostic entity.
- An epidemic of undertreated pain coexists with an epidemic of prescription drug abuse in the United States.
- Racial disparities in pain treatment persist showing implicit bias that impacts analgesic prescribing. Structured decision support and standardized assessments are recommended to minimize this bias.
- Management should be multimodal. Nonpharmacologic and nonopioid treatments are recommended as first line for chronic primary pain.

EPIDEMIOLOGY

Incidence

- Chronic pain affects ~20% of U.S. adults. 8% experience severe chronic pain that limits major activities.
- The economic burden related to chronic pain is estimated to be over $600 billion annually taking into account both direct costs and lost productivity.

Prevalence

In the United States, an estimated 20% (50 million) of adults report some level of chronic pain on cross-sectional household surveys. The prevalence is higher among women and those with lower socioeconomic status (1).

ETIOLOGY AND PATHOPHYSIOLOGY

- Chronic pain involves peripheral sensitization, central sensitization, maladaptive neuroplasticity, and dysregulated descending inhibition.
- Neuroimaging studies show structural and connectivity changes in the insula, anterior cingulate cortex, amygdala, supporting chronic pain as a CNS disease.
- Chronic overlapping pain conditions (e.g., fibromyalgia, temporomandibular pain, and chronic headache) appear to have same neuromodulatory pain mechanisms.

Genetics

Genetic polymorphisms may affect individual's response to certain opioids (2).

RISK FACTORS

- Traumatic: motor vehicle accidents, repetitive motion injuries, falls
- Postsurgical: back surgeries, amputations, thoracotomies
- Psychiatric comorbidities include substance abuse, mood disorders, posttraumatic stress disorder (PTSD). Sedentary behavior is an independent and modifiable risk factor for chronic pain.
- Disordered sleeping is an independent amplifier of pain severity.
- Adverse childhood experiences (ACEs) increase lifetime risk of experiencing chronic pain.

GENERAL PREVENTION

- Prevent work-related injuries through ergonomic workplace design.
- Encourage regular physical activity.
- Varicella vaccine and rapid treatment of shingles to lower risk of postherpetic neuralgia
- Tight glycemic control for diabetic patients
- Address alcohol and substance use; encourage tobacco cessation.

COMMONLY ASSOCIATED CONDITIONS

Any chronic disease and/or its treatment can cause chronic pain.

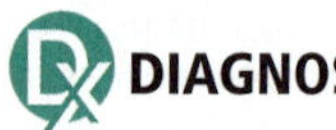

DIAGNOSIS

Chronic pain is the presence of unpleasant sensory and emotional experience lasting for >3 months. Two general categories of pain:

- Nociceptive pain (response to tissue damage):
  - *Somatic*: skin, bone, soft tissue disease; described as well localized, sharp, stabbing, aching
  - *Visceral*: visceral inflammation/injury; described as poorly localized, dull, aching; may refer to sites remote from lesion; can wax and wane
- Neuropathic pain: damaged peripheral or central nerves; described as burning, tingling, and/or numbness

HISTORY

- Pain history: location, onset, intensity, duration, quality, temporal pattern, exacerbating agents, alleviators, prior treatments.
- Assess how pain affects patient's functioning and quality of life.
- Screen for personal or family history of substance use disorders and dependence, mental health conditions, and/or sexual abuse.
- Screen for other chronic pain syndromes (fibromyalgia, etc.).
- Standardized tools: pain severity—Brief Pain Inventory (short form); mood—Patient Health Questionnaire-9 (PHQ-9)
- Stratify patients who would be at increased risk for developing an opioid use disorder if opioids were indicated; substance abuse—Screener and Opioid Assessment for Patients with Pain (SOAPP; https://www.mcstap.com/docs/SOAPP-5.pdf)
- PEG-3 score; over the past week:
  - Rate your average Pain (0 to 10 scale).
  - Rate how pain has interfered with your Enjoyment of life (0 to 10 scale).
  - Rate how pain has interfered with your General activity (0 to 10 scale).
  - Add three scores together and divide by 3; gives final score of 0 (no pain) to 10 (severe pain)
- Opioid Risk Tool (ORT) (https://nida.nih.gov/sites/default/files/opioidrisktool.pdf)

PHYSICAL EXAM

Exam is guided by history and includes neurologic functional and behavioral assessments.

DIFFERENTIAL DIAGNOSIS

- Complex regional pain syndrome is a disorder of a body region, which is characterized by pain, swelling, limited range of motion, vasomotor instability, skin changes, and bone demineralization. It frequently affects one body region and begins after a fracture, soft tissue injury, or surgery.
- Aberrant drug-taking behaviors could be related to inadequate analgesia, disease progression, opioid-resistant pain, opioid-induced hyperalgesia, opioid tolerance, substance use disorder, self-medication of nonpain symptoms, criminal intent (diversion), and poor health literacy.

DIAGNOSTIC TESTS & INTERPRETATION

Base testing on history, exam, and differential diagnosis.

Initial Tests (lab, imaging)

- Kidney and liver function should be evaluated prior to initiation of certain medications.
- Urine toxicology screening and testing for those prescribed controlled substances to assess adherence to prescribed medications and to detect the presence of illicit substances:
  - The array of qualitative and quantitative analyses will be dependent on lab availability.
  - Qualitative analysis is a screening test and quantitative analysis is for confirmation of individual drug levels.
  - If you have questions about your toxicology test, contact the toxicologist associated with your lab.

Follow-Up Tests & Special Considerations

Depending on prescribed medications, patients may need follow-up kidney and liver function as well as toxicology testing.

- Avoid routine imaging for chronic low back pain in the absence of red flag signs/symptoms.
- For methadone, baseline ECG and annual ECG if methadone daily dose >120 mg or lower doses if prescribed multiple QT-prolonging medications.

Diagnostic Procedures/Other

Consider interventional pain clinic for complex injections and nerve blocks.

Test Interpretation

- Be aware of false positive and negative results of your screening or toxicology testing for commonly prescribed medications like SSRIs, sleep agents, and over-the-counter medications like diphenhydramine.
- Confirmatory quantitative analysis should be performed if there is a positive qualitative result that may alter the treatment plan.

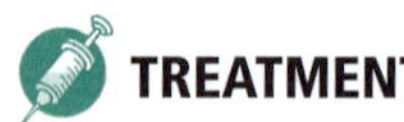

TREATMENT

GENERAL MEASURES

- Goals of treatment are to restore function and decrease pain.
- Treatment should be multimodal and include both pharmacologic and nonpharmacologic interventions.
- Address untreated sleep disorders or psychiatric conditions because they can make pain control more difficult.
- Focus on disease-modifying treatment options (e.g., allopurinol for gout).

MEDICATION

- Management depends on type of pain (neuropathic vs nociceptive).
- Use sequential time-limited trials of medications; start at low doses and gradually increase until effect or dose-limiting side effects are reached.
- Combination acetaminophen/NSAID products with opioids can lead to serious acetaminophen/NSAID toxicities if patients exceed recommended doses. Patient and family education is critical.
- Note: Be aware of implicit bias. People of color are at greatest risk for undertreatment regardless of pain type or type of analgesia.

First Line

- For nociceptive pain:
  - NSAIDs remain the cornerstone of therapy: Avoid in kidney disease and heart failure. Most common side effect is GI distress/gastritis.
    - Topical NSAIDs are recommended over oral NSAIDs for knee/hand osteoarthritis and older adults (aged >75 years).
  - Acetaminophen may have limited efficacy for some forms of chronic musculoskeletal pain (e.g., chronic back pain) and can be useful if NSAIDs are contraindicated: Up to 3 to 4 g/day in healthy adults. Limit to <2 g/day in patients with hepatic disease of significant comorbidities.
  - Topic agents
    - NSAIDs (diclofenac gel 1–3% BID)
    - Lidocaine (4% gel OTC is less effective but more affordable than 5% patch)
    - Capsaicin 0.075–0.1% QD–QID (up to 8% is used in some specialty settings)
- For neuropathic pain:
  - Gabapentin 100 to 300 mg qhs initially; can titrate to 1,800 to 3,600 mg/day in divided doses. Benefit generally plateaus ~1,800 mg/day. Sedation is primary dose-limiting effect.
  - Pregabalin 50 mg TID or 75 mg BID initially. Titrate to 150 to 300 mg/day. 600 mg/day is maximum.
  - Duloxetine 30 mg/day initially; titrate to 60 mg/day.
  - Tricyclic antidepressants (desipramine [25–100 mg QD but start with 10 mg QD in frail elderly] and nortriptyline [25–100 mg QD but start with 10 mg QD in frail elderly]); should use with caution in any elderly patients
  - Consider combining antidepressant or antiseizure medication with topical therapies like lidocaine or capsaicin.

Second Line

- Opioid prescribing: Use for moderate to severe chronic pain in accordance with approved guidelines. Prescribe the lowest possible effective dose. Start <50 MME/day. Reassess every 2 to 4 weeks initially. Use Prescription Drug Monitoring Program (PDMP) with single-source prescribing, controlled substance agreement (CSA), and urine toxicology screening to minimize misuse.
  - Buprenorphine (partial opioid agonist) preferred over full opioid agonists due to lower overdose potential
  - Morphine, oxycodone, hydromorphone, oxymorphone, fentanyl; check institutional opioid equianalgesic table.
    - Avoid morphine in patients with renal insufficiency.
    - Methadone should only be prescribed by experienced providers due to many drug interactions and risk of potentially fatal cardiac arrhythmias.
    - No evidence supports any of these opioids as superior to other or having improved side effect profile; however, genetic polymorphisms do exist as aforementioned.
  - Once stable dose of opioids is established, change to sustained-release formulations if pain is likely to be long term; short-acting formulations for breakthrough/episodic pain only
  - Common side effects: constipation, nausea, sedation, mental status changes, and pruritus; respiratory depression and opioid overdose are possible at any dose especially if combined with other centrally active agents.
  - Coprescribe nasal naloxone for patients on chronic opioids (see "Ongoing Care")
- Evidence on use of cannabis for chronic pain is low quality and controversial.

ADDITIONAL THERAPIES

- Cognitive-behavioral therapy (CBT), mindfulness-based stress reduction and regular exercise therapy have strongest evidence for effectiveness in different contexts of chronic pain.
- Acupuncture may be particularly helpful for chronic low back pain, chronic headaches, and chronic osteoarthritis.
- Spinal cord stimulation may help patients with refractory neuropathic pain.
- Interdisciplinary care teams are superior to single sources of care.

SURGERY/OTHER PROCEDURES

Consider interventional procedures, including joint injections, nerve blocks, spinal cord stimulation, and intrathecal medication among others, as needed.

COMPLEMENTARY & ALTERNATIVE MEDICINE

- Biofield therapies (e.g., Reiki, therapeutic touch) are less well studied but can be considered if the harm assessment is minimal for the individual patient.
- Yoga as effective as standard physical therapy for moderate to severe chronic low back pain.

ONGOING CARE

FOLLOW-UP RECOMMENDATIONS

Patient Monitoring

- Create a shared, written pain agreement outlining the frequency of follow-up visits and rate of toxicology testing and discuss patient expectations for chronic pain management.
- Patients should be reevaluated for safety and efficacy of the prescribed pain regimen.
- Assess and document benefits, risks, pain levels, functioning, and quality of life.
- *Universal precautions*:
  - Informed consent for opioid therapy; written agreement between patient and clinician
  - One prescriber and one pharmacy; no after-hours prescriptions or early refills
  - Mandatory police reporting for medication thefts; random urine drug tests, pill/patch counts
  - Continue with physical therapy, counseling, and psychiatric medications.
  - Participate in state's prescription drug monitoring program: http://www.cdc.gov/drugoverdose/pdmp/
  - Taper and discontinue medications if patient does not benefit or if side effects outweigh benefits. If medications are abused or diverted, more rapid taper may be appropriate.
  - If substance use disorder is suspected, always offer treatment for substance abuse.
  - Tapering opioids should involve shared decision-making between patient and clinician with an individualized taper plan to each patient based on risks and benefits (3)[C].
  - Patients on long-term opioid therapy may see improvement in pain, function, and quality of life with voluntary dose reductions.
- Nasal naloxone should be prescribed for all patients prescribed full agonist opioids. Naloxone kit: two prefilled intranasal mucosal atomization device; takes effect in 2 to 5 minutes, lasts 30 to 90 minutes

PATIENT EDUCATION

American Chronic Pain Association: https://theacpa.org

COMPLICATIONS

- Estimates of opioid use disorder (OUD) in patients on long-term opioid therapy vary widely (~3–19%), depending on setting, populations, and definitions of misuse.
- Definitions
  - Substance use disorder: chronic biopsychological disease characterized by impaired control over drug use, compulsive use, and continued use despite harm
  - Physical dependence: withdrawal syndrome produced by abrupt cessation or rapid dose reduction
  - Tolerance: state of adaptation when a drug induces changes that diminish its effects over time
  - Diversion: selling drugs or giving them to persons other than for whom they are prescribed

REFERENCES

1. Rikard SM, Strahan AE, Schmit KM, et al. Chronic pain among adults—United States, 2019–2021. *MMWR Morb Mortal Wkly Rep*. 2023;72(15):379–385.
2. Vieira CMP, Fragoso RM, Pereira D, et al. Pain polymorphisms and opioids: an evidence based review. *Mol Med Rep*. 2019;19(3):1423–1434.
3. Dowell D, Ragan KR, Jones CM, et al. CDC Clinical Practice Guideline for prescribing opioids for pain—United States, 2022. *MMWR Recomm Rep*. 2022;71(3):1–95.

ADDITIONAL READING

- Bril V, England J, Franklin GM, et al. Evidence-based guideline: treatment of painful neuropathy. *Neurology*. 2023;101(6):251–263. doi:10.1212/WNL.0000000000021329.
- Clauw DJ. Chronic overlapping pain conditions and the neurobiology of pain sensitization. *N Engl J Med*. 2023;389(2):115–126. doi:10.1056/NEJMra2212337.
- Häuser W, Petzke F, Sommer C. Evidence-based non-pharmacologic therapies for chronic pain. *Pain*. 2023;164(Suppl 1):S1–S15. doi:10.1097/j.pain.0000000000002790.

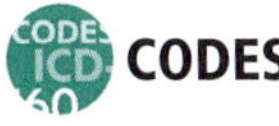

CODES

ICD10

- G89.29 Other chronic pain
- G89.21 Chronic pain due to trauma
- G89.28 Other chronic postprocedural pain

CLINICAL PEARLS

- Chronic pain is a complex neuroplastic CNS condition, not persistent tissue injury.
- Exercise is the most consistently effective therapy for chronic pain.
- If low-dose neuropathic medications fail at low doses, consider combination therapy which can be more effective than monotherapy at higher doses.
- Buprenorphine should be considered as a lower risk option when opioid therapy is required.
- Proper evaluation and treatment sleep disorders can reduce pain by up to 20–40%.
- Early referral for multidisciplinary care improves outcomes and reduces long-term opioid use.

CIRRHOSIS OF THE LIVER

Liam P. Burke, MD

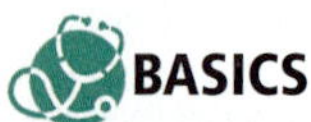

BASICS

DESCRIPTION

A chronic inflammatory disease with hepatocellular dysfunction, fibrosis, necrosis, and vascular remodeling possibly leading to liver failure and/or cancer

EPIDEMIOLOGY

- Diagnosis: typically at 40 to 60 years old; male > female
- Liver disease and cirrhosis are the 9th leading cause of death in the United States. Age-adjusted mortality is 22/100,000.
- Metabolic dysfunction-associated steatotic liver disease (MASLD) is now the most common cause of cirrhosis.

Incidence

>30,000 new cases of cirrhosis per year

Prevalence

- 2.2 million of Americans have cirrhosis.
- Highest in non-Hispanic Blacks, Mexican Americans, and those below the poverty level

ETIOLOGY AND PATHOPHYSIOLOGY

- Chronic hepatitis C virus (HCV) (24%); alcohol related (28%); MASLD (~26%); hepatitis B virus (HBV) (2%); other (~20%): hemochromatosis, autoimmune hepatitis, primary biliary cirrhosis (PBC), secondary biliary cirrhosis, biliary atresia, idiopathic biliary fibrosis, primary sclerosing cholangitis, Wilson disease, α_1-antitrypsin deficiency, granulomatous disease (e.g., sarcoidosis); drug-induced liver disease (e.g., methotrexate, α-methyldopa, amiodarone); venous outflow obstruction (e.g., Budd-Chiari syndrome, veno-occlusive disease)
- Hepatocellular injury leads to chronic inflammatory changes, extracellular matrix deposition, cellular hyperplasia (regenerating nodules), fibrous infiltration, and angiogenesis. Distortions in blood flow result in portal hypertension.

Genetics

Hereditary hemochromatosis, Wilson disease, and α_1-antitrypsin deficiency in adults increase cirrhosis risk.

RISK FACTORS

Alcohol abuse, intravenous drug abuse, obesity

GENERAL PREVENTION

- Mitigate risk factors (e.g., screen for and address hepatitis C and alcohol overuse); >80% of CLD is preventable.
- Advise weight loss in overweight or obese patients.

COMMONLY ASSOCIATED CONDITIONS

HCV, alcohol and drug abuse, diabetes, depression, obesity

DIAGNOSIS

HISTORY

- Review risk factors (alcohol use, viral hepatitis, and familial primary liver cancer, liver disease, or autoimmune disease).
- Symptoms
  - Fatigue, malaise, weakness, anorexia, weight loss (weight gain if ascites/edema)
  - Right upper abdominal pain; tea-colored urine, clay-colored stools
  - Edema, abdominal swelling/bloating, pruritus; bruising, bleeding, hematemesis, hematochezia, melena
  - Absent/irregular menses, chronic anovulation; diminished libido, erectile dysfunction

PHYSICAL EXAM

Physical exam may be normal until end-stage disease—many relate to manifestations of portal hypertension and/or hyperestrinism.

- Spider angiomas, palmar erythema, jaundice, scleral icterus, ecchymoses, caput medusa, hyperpigmentation, decreased body hair, facial telangiectasias
- Hepatomegaly, splenomegaly, abdominal fluid wave, shifting dullness
- Gynecomastia, Dupuytren contractures
- Pretibial/presacral pitting edema, and clubbing (mostly in hepatopulmonary syndrome [HPS])
- Asterixis, altered mental status (AMS) (hepatic encephalopathy [HE]), muscle wasting, fetor hepaticus

DIFFERENTIAL DIAGNOSIS

Steatohepatitis, other causes of portal hypertension (e.g., portal vein thrombosis, lymphoma); metastatic or multifocal cancer in the liver; vascular congestion (e.g., cardiac cirrhosis); acute alcoholic hepatitis

DIAGNOSTIC TESTS & INTERPRETATION

- Diagnosis is increasingly noninvasive.
- Fibrosis-4 (FIB-4) index (based on patient age; aspartate aminotransferase [AST]; alanine aminotransferase [ALT] and platelet count) followed by liver elastography when indicated (>15 kPa suggests cirrhosis)
- FIB-4 < 1.45 reliably rules out advanced hepatic fibrosis.
- FIB-4 1.45 to 3.25 intermediate risk of fibrosis
- FIB-4 >3.25 highly suggestive of advanced liver fibrosis

Initial Tests (lab, imaging)

- AST/ALT often mildly elevated, typically AST > ALT, and may normalize as cirrhosis progresses; elevated alkaline phosphatase (ALP), γ-glutamyl transpeptidase (GGT), and total/direct bilirubin; anemia from hemolysis, folate deficiency, or splenomegaly
- Thrombocytopenia (<110; 95% specific for cirrhosis); FIB-4 < 1.45 or AST-to-platelet ratio index <0.7 unlikely cirrhotic; FIB-4 >3.25 suggests cirrhosis.
- Hypoalbuminemia, low cholesterol, prolonged prothrombin time (PT) and partial thromboplastin time (PTT), elevated international normalized ratio (INR)
- Hyperammonemia, elevated BUN, hyperkalemia, and hyponatremia indicate progression
- Hepatorenal syndrome (HRS): creatinine clearance <40 mL/min (or serum creatinine >1.5) with urine volume <500 mL/day and urine sodium <10 mEq/L
- RUQ ultrasound to screen for hepatocellular carcinoma (HCC) and to assess parenchyma, and hepatic and portal veins. Elastography evaluates parenchymal scarring/fibrosis.

Follow-Up Tests & Special Considerations

Consider:

- Hepatitis serologies; ethanol and GGT if alcohol abuse suspected; antimitochondrial antibody check for PBC; anti-smooth muscle and antinuclear antibodies for autoimmune hepatitis
- Transferrin saturation (>50%) and elevated ferritin to screen for hemochromatosis; if abnormal, check hemochromatosis (HFE) genetics/mutation analysis; α_1-antitrypsin phenotype screen; ceruloplasmin to screen for Wilson disease; if low, check copper excretion (serum copper plus 24-hour urine copper); α-fetoprotein level to screen for HCC

Diagnostic Procedures/Other

- Liver biopsy: recommended if noninvasive markers incongruent with imaging; percutaneous if INR <1.5 and no ascites
- Endoscopy (EGD) in cirrhosis to screen for esophageal varices/portal hypertensive gastropathy
- Known liver nodularity or splenomegaly on MRI or CT indicate cirrhosis
- Magnetic resonance elastography: in obese or MASLD patients

Test Interpretation

Fibrous bands and regenerative nodules are histologic features of cirrhosis.

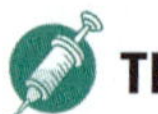

TREATMENT

Outpatient care for all acute and chronic HCV patients, except during major GI bleeding, AMS, sepsis/infection, rapid hepatic decompensation, or renal failure

GENERAL MEASURES

- Abstain from alcohol, drugs, hepatotoxic medicines, and herbs. PCV-20, hepatitis A/B, and influenza vaccinations; weight loss, exercise, and control of lipids/glucose
- Determine if uncompensated disease: ascites, spontaneous bacterial peritonitis (SBP), hepatic encephalopathy (HE), coagulopathy, variceal hemorrhage.

MEDICATION

First Line

Treat the underlying cause first (note prescribing precautions in decompensated cirrhosis) to delay progression of disease.

- HCV: Treatment with direct acting antivirals (DAAs) to eradicate viral RNA recommended if without cirrhosis (e.g., FIB-4 <3.25, FibroScan <12.5 kPa, normal biopsy, or platelet count >150,000) with glecaprevir-pibrentasvir for 8 weeks in genotypes 1 to 6, or sofosbuvir-velpatasvir for 12 weeks in genotypes 1, 2, 4, 5, and 6; if cirrhosis, past treatment failure, eGFR <30 mL/min/m^2, pregnancy, hepatitis B, HIV, suspected HCC, then specialty referral; monitor INR for those taking warfarin and for hypoglycemia in diabetes
- HBV: When no cirrhosis with PCR DNA >20,000 in HBeAg-positive and ALT >2 × ULN in HBeAg-negative disease, goal is to reduce HCC and decompensation risk. First line is entecavir 0.5 to 1.0 mg PO daily, then tenofovir 300 mg PO or telbivudine 600 mg PO daily; often prescribed indefinitely without return to HBeAg negative status.

- MASLD: weight loss of 5% of body weight reduces steatosis, and >10% loss with improved fitness up to >150 min/week of physical activity reduces MASH and fibrosis. Minimize saturated fats and refined carbohydrates. Consider glucagon-like peptide-1 receptor antagonists, SGLT2 inhibitors or pioglitazone in diabetes mellitus +/− MASH; resmetirom approved in MASLD with F2 or F3 without maintained weight loss
- Alcoholic hepatitis: Treat alcohol withdrawal; if Maddrey Discriminant Function score >32, patients may benefit from prednisolone 40 mg/day beginning on hospital day 3 for 28 days with 2 week taper to reduce short-term mortality; pentoxifylline for patients who cannot tolerate steroids
- Hereditary hemochromatosis: phlebotomy every 1 to 2 weeks until serum ferritin is 50 to 100 μg/L then 2 to 6 times per year as needed. Deferoxamine 40 mg/kg/day over 8 to 12 hours for 5 to 7 days in dyserythropoietic syndrome and chronic hemolytic anemia to reduce iron overload quickly.
- PBC: ursodeoxycholic acid (ursodiol) 13 to 15 mg/kg PO divided BID with food. For pruritus, if ursodiol is ineffective, then cholestyramine 4 to 8 g PO BID is next therapy, followed by antihistamines, rifampin 150 to 300 mg PO BID or naltrexone 50 mg/day. Evaluate for fat-soluble vitamin deficiencies, metabolic bone disease, hypercholesterolemia, hypothyroidism, and anemia.
- Wilson disease: initial treatment with penicillamine 1,000 to 1,500 mg/day PO BID–QID or trientine 750 to 1,500 mg/day PO BID–TID on empty stomach; trientine 750 to 1,500 mg/day PO BID–TID is better tolerated. After 1 year, zinc acetate 150 mg/day PO BID–TID for maintenance; zinc for presymptomatic, pregnant, and pediatric populations
- Autoimmune hepatitis: Treat if AST or ALT >10 times ULN, or if either >5 times ULN and γglobulins >2 times ULN with prednisone 30 mg/day for 1 week, then 20 mg/day for 1 week, then 10 mg/day for 2 weeks with maintenance of 5 mg/day. At outset test for TPMT activity, and if not low or negative, add azathioprine 50 to 100 mg/day throughout; treat to normal transaminases. At 24 months of remission trial, withdrawal of steroids with AZA maintenance for 3 months then trial AZA taper by 50 mg q3mo.
- Esophageal varices: variceal bleed prophylaxis with propranolol >40 mg, carvedilol 6.25 mg or nadolol 40 mg PO daily, to lower heart rate to 55 to 60 bpm; PPI indicated when varices require banding, and for portal hypertensive gastropathy
- Ascites/edema: low-sodium (<2 g/day) diet and spironolactone 100 to 400 mg/day with or without furosemide 40 to 160 mg/day PO; torsemide as substitute for furosemide. If serum sodium <120 mmol/L, then 1.0 to 1.5 L/day water restriction; if new onset, rule out SBP. If prior SBP, consider SBP prophylaxis with TMP-SMX DS or norfloxacin 400 mg PO daily.
- HE: lactulose 15 to 45 mL BID; titrate to induce 2 to 3 loose bowel movements daily to resolve AMS. Add rifaximin 550 mg PO BID if needed.
- Prophylactic antibiotics for invasive procedures, GI bleeding, or history of spontaneous bacterial peritonitis

Second Line

HBV: adefovir 10 mg PO daily second line; lamivudine not recommended as first-line agent due to resistance

ISSUES FOR REFERRAL

Evaluate for liver transplant at onset of ascites, variceal bleeding, HE, jaundice, liver lesion suggestive of HCC, or when evidence of hepatic dysfunction develops (Child-Turcotte-Pugh [CTP]) >7 and Model for End-Stage Liver Disease (MELD) >10.

SURGERY/OTHER PROCEDURES

Varices: endoscopic ligation, 4 to 6 treatments (if acute bleed, use pre-esophagogastroduodenoscopy [EGD] octreotide as vasoconstrictor); transjugular intrahepatic shunt (TIPS) second-line or salvage therapy for acute bleed; ascites: if tense, therapeutic paracentesis every 2 weeks PRN; caution if pedal edema is absent; fulminant hepatic failure: liver transplantation; HCC: curable if small with radiofrequency ablation or resection and transplant

COMPLEMENTARY & ALTERNATIVE MEDICINE

- Zinc sulfate 220 mg BID for dysgeusia and appetite; adjunct for HE
- Milk thistle may lower transaminases and improve symptoms.
- Vitamin E 800 IU daily in MASH with caution and monitoring for vitamin K–dependent antagonism diathesis

ADMISSION, INPATIENT, AND NURSING CONSIDERATIONS

Major GI bleeding, AMS, sepsis/infection, rapidly progressing hepatic decompensation, renal failure

ONGOING CARE

- Monitor liver enzymes, sodium, creatinine, platelets, and PT q6–12mo; calculate MELD score.
- Serial α-fetoprotein and liver ultrasound screening q6mo in patients with cirrhosis; MRI with contrast best follow-up test for HCC if α-fetoprotein elevated and/or liver mass found on ultrasound; EGD at cirrhosis diagnosis and every 3 years (compensated) and every 1 year (decompensated) to screen for varices

FOLLOW-UP RECOMMENDATIONS

Regular physical conditioning may help with fatigue.

Patient Monitoring

- Monitor for fatigue, weakness, reduced appetite, itchy skin at each visit.
- AMS, jaundice, or abdominal pain are major concerns.

DIET

Protein (1.2 to 1.5 g/kg body weight daily), high fiber, multivitamin (without iron), sodium restriction (<2 g/day), combined with fluid restriction, essential if ascites/edema

PATIENT EDUCATION

- Educate about when to seek emergency care (e.g., hematemesis, AMS).
- Drug, alcohol, and smoking cessation (no cannabis)
- Update required immunizations; HCV transmission precautions

PROGNOSIS

- 5 to 20 years of asymptomatic disease from time of initial diagnosis.
- After onset of complications, death typically within 5 years without transplant.
- 5% per year develop HCC. 50% develop ascites over 10 years; 50% 5-year survival after ascites develop. Acute variceal bleeding is the most common fatal complication; 30% mortality. Median survival after complications (ascites, variceal bleeding, HE) is 1.5 years. With transplant, 85% survive 1 year; after transplant, ~5% annual mortality; <25% of eligible patients receive a transplant due to organ shortage.

COMPLICATIONS

Ascites, edema, infections, HE, GI bleeding, esophageal varices, gastropathy, colopathy, HRS, HPS, HCC, hepatic failure

ADDITIONAL READING

Volk ML, Clarke C, Asrani SK, et al. Cirrhosis quality collaborative. *Clin Gastroenterol Hepatol*. 2022;20(5): 970–972. doi:10.1016/j.cgh.2022.01.043.

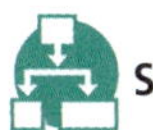

SEE ALSO

Algorithm: Cirrhosis

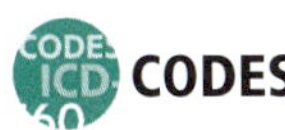

CODES

ICD10

- K74.60 Unspecified cirrhosis of liver
- K70.30 Alcoholic cirrhosis of liver without ascites
- K74.69 Other cirrhosis of liver

CLINICAL PEARLS

- 80% of CLD is preventable (primarily alcohol abuse, hepatitides).
- After diagnosis of cirrhosis, abdominal ultrasound q6–12mo for early detection of HCC.
- Update necessary immunizations and treat underlying cause (e.g., HCV, alcohol).
- Always rule out SBP in patients presenting with initial episode of ascites.

CLOSTRIDIUM DIFFICILE INFECTION

Fozia Akhtar Ali, MD, FAAFP • Patricia J. Burns, MD

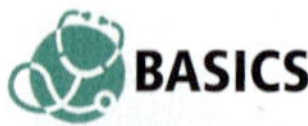

BASICS

DESCRIPTION

- *Clostridioides difficile* is a gram-positive, spore-forming, anaerobic bacillus that releases toxins to produce clinical disease.
- Associated with antibiotic use, recent hospitalization, residence at long-term care facilities, weakened immune system, and age >65 years
- Severity of infection ranges from asymptomatic carrier to diarrhea, colitis, sepsis, perforation, and death.
- Typically, person-to-person transmission of spores via the fecal-oral route but may also occur through exposure to contaminated surfaces or equipment
- System(s) affected: gastrointestinal

EPIDEMIOLOGY

Incidence

- Colonization with *C. difficile* found in:
  - 2–10% of community, 3–18% of inpatients, 4–20% of long-term residents (1)
- Estimated incidence of *C. difficile* infection 116.1/100,000/year, hospitalization rates are increasing (2).
- National incidence of health care–associated *C. difficile* infection 54/100,000 persons
- National incidence of community-acquired *C. difficile* infection 62.1/100,000 persons

Prevalence

- *C. difficile* accounted for 12% of health care–associated infections in 2010
- >2 million cases of C. difficile–associated disease in U.S. hospitals from 1993 to 2005

ETIOLOGY AND PATHOPHYSIOLOGY

- Anaerobic toxin-producing, gram-positive bacillus bacteria existing in vegetative and spore forms
- Has 1-week incubation period with spores that can survive for 5 months in harsh conditions and outside the body
- Spread by fecal-oral contact; acid-resistant spores pass through stomach to reside mostly in the colon.
- Colonic colonization causes disruptions in barrier functions of the normal microbiome.
- *C. difficile* is noninvasive. Toxins mediate disease: Toxins A (enterotoxin) and B (cytotoxin) attract neutrophils and monocytes, degrading colonic epithelial cells and causing clinical disease.
- The hypervirulent strain BI/NAP1/027 of *C. difficile* is associated with higher rates of colectomy and death.

Genetics

No known genetic factors

RISK FACTORS

- Host risk factors
  - Age >65 years; hospitalization or long-term health care facility
  - Comorbidities, including inflammatory bowel disease, immunosuppression, chronic liver disease, and end-stage renal disease
  - Enteral feeding; previous *C. difficile* infection
- Factors that disrupt normal colonic microbiota:
  - Exposure to antibiotics (including perioperative prophylaxis)
  - Commonly implicated antibiotics: ampicillin, amoxicillin, clindamycin (most common), cephalosporins, fluoroquinolones, and carbapenems
  - Chronic acid suppression
- Recurrence from prior infection: Recurrence rates are ~25%; recurrence more likely with each additional episode
- Risk increases with length of hospital stay, duration of antibiotics exposure, and number of antibiotics used (3)

Geriatric Considerations

C. difficile is the most common cause of acute diarrheal illness in long-term care facilities.

Pediatric Considerations

- Neonates have a higher rate of *C. difficile* colonization (25–80%) but are generally less symptomatic than adults.
- Frequently serve as carrier for infection in adults

GENERAL PREVENTION

- Antibiotic stewardship programs decrease the incidence of *C. difficile* infection
- Society for Healthcare Epidemiology of America (SHEA)/Infectious Diseases Society of America (IDSA) guidelines for prevention:
  - For health care workers, patients, and visitors
    - Contact precautions, including gloves and gowns, on entry to room; alcohol-based hand sanitizers are not effective. Handwashing with soap and water before and after patient interaction is recommended.
    - Accommodate patients with *C. difficile* infection in private rooms if possible.
  - Environmental cleaning and disinfection
    - Disinfect with hypochlorite or other spore-killing solution.
    - Identify and reduce environmental sources of *C. difficile*.
  - Antimicrobial restrictions: Minimize the frequency and duration of antibiotic therapy.

COMMONLY ASSOCIATED CONDITIONS

Pseudomembranous colitis, toxic megacolon, sepsis, colonic perforation

DIAGNOSIS

HISTORY

- Common presenting symptoms include diarrhea and abdominal cramping or pain.
- Age and underlying comorbidities
- Recent antibiotic (Risk of *C. difficile* infection may persist for 3 months after antibiotic is discontinued.); proton pump inhibitor or H_2-receptor blocker use
- Diarrhea (defined as >3 stools in 24 hours) that is watery, foul-smelling, and sometimes bloody (1)
- Fever (<10%), anorexia, nausea
- Recent hospitalization or stay at nursing facility

PHYSICAL EXAM

- Abdominal exam: Look for tenderness, increasing distension, diminished bowel sounds, peritoneal signs.
- Initial presentation can be fulminant and rapidly fatal; assessment of severity is key to management.
- Look for signs of systemic illness including fever, tachycardia, hypotension, dehydration.

DIFFERENTIAL DIAGNOSIS

- Infectious causes: *Salmonella*; *Shigella*; *Campylobacter*; Shiga toxin–producing *Escherichia coli* infection
- Noninfectious causes
  - Intestinal obstruction; ischemic bowel disease; inflammatory bowel disease: ulcerative colitis, Crohn disease
  - Gastrointestinal cancer; drug-associated diarrhea; foodborne illness
  - Other antibiotic associated diarrhea (75% of antibiotic diarrhea not associated with *C. difficile*)

DIAGNOSTIC TESTS & INTERPRETATION

Initial Tests (lab, imaging)

- Two-step testing
  - Glutamate dehydrogenase (GDH) assay (sensitivity, 85–95%; specificity, 89–99%) *or*
  - Nucleic acid amplification tests (NAATs) followed by:
  - Specific toxin assay
- Repeat testing during the same episode of diarrhea is not recommended. Stool carriage persists for 3 to 6 weeks after successful treatment and can remain positive in 60% of patients.
- Routine radiologic examination is not recommended in the absence of signs of systemic disease or clinical suspicion for complicated/severe disease.
  - Plain films may show thumbprinting and colonic distension.
  - CT may show mucosal thickening, colonic wall thickening, pericolonic inflammation, or signs of complicated infection in severe cases (i.e., extraluminal air).

Follow-Up Tests & Special Considerations

Two-step testing can help to differentiate colonization from infection. Initial screening with NAAT (detects gene coding for toxin) or GDH (enzyme produced by both toxigenic and nontoxigenic *C. difficile* strains) followed by confirmation with EIA (detects toxins produced by *C. difficile*) is helpful. If NAAT/GDH is negative and EIA is negative, infection is unlikely. If both are positive, infection is likely. If discordant, then colonization is possible. The clinical status of the patient helps to differentiate this as well.

Diagnostic Procedures/Other

Endoscopy can evaluate for presence of pseudomembranes and exclude other conditions.

- Although not all patients with *C. difficile* infection have pseudomembranes, their presence is pathognomonic.
- Flexible sigmoidoscopy may miss 15–20% of pseudomembranes (from the proximal colon).

C

Test Interpretation

SHEA/IDSA guidelines

- Mild or moderate disease: leukocytosis with white blood cell (WBC) count <15,000 cells/μL and a serum creatinine level <1.5 times the premorbid level
- Severe, uncomplicated disease: leukocytosis with WBC count >15,000 cells/μL or a serum creatinine level >1.5 times the premorbid level
- Severe, complicated disease: hypotension, sepsis, markedly elevated WBC count, lactic acidosis, hypoalbuminemia, and imaging findings of complicated disease

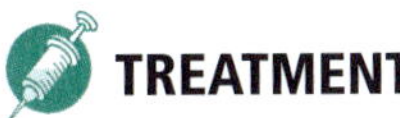

TREATMENT

GENERAL MEASURES

- Antimotility agents are contraindicated.
- Avoid indiscriminate use of antibiotics.
- Proton pump inhibitors are associated with recurrent infection but have not been shown to be causal.
- Discontinue offending antibiotic, whenever possible.

MEDICATION

First Line

- Initial episode (nonsevere or severe disease):
  - Fidaxomicin 200 mg PO BID ×10 days; preferred over vancomycin 125 mg PO QID × 10 days
  - If unable to PO, then IV metronidazole or intraluminal (PO) vancomycin
- First recurrence
  - Fidaxomicin: 200 mg PO BID × 10 days *or* 200 mg PO BID × 5 days, followed by once every other day × 20 days
  - Vancomycin: 125 mg PO TID × 10 to 14 days, then 125 mg PO BID × 7 days, then 125 mg PO once daily × 7 days, then 125 mg PO q2–3 for 2 to 8 weeks *or* 125 mg PO TID × 10 days
- Second recurrence
  - Fidaxomicin: 200 mg PO BID × 10 days *or* 200 mg PO BID ×5 days, followed by once every other day × 20 days
  - Vancomycin: 125 mg PO QID × 10 to 14 days, then 125 mg PO BID × 7 days, then 125 mg PO once daily × 7 days, then 125 mg PO q2–3 days × 2 to 8 weeks *or* 125 mg PO QID × 10 days, then rifaximin PO 400 mg TID × 20 days
- Fulminant infection (hypotension, shock, ileus, megacolon): Consider surgical and critical care consultation.
  - Vancomycin 500 mg PO QID (nasogastric tube, or rectally) + metronidazole 500 mg IV q8h

Pediatric Considerations

Metronidazole and vancomycin are preferred for initial and recurrent infections, fidaxomicin is not approved for patients <18 years old.

ALERT

- When using vancomycin to treat *C. difficile* infection, use oral or rectal formulations. IV formulations (not excreted into the colonic lumen) are ineffective.
- Monitor creatinine levels very closely.

Second Line

- Oral metronidazole 500 mg PO TID for 10 to 14 days
- Vancomycin: for patients who cannot tolerate or have failed metronidazole therapy and for pregnancy
- Fecal transplant: stool from healthy, screened donor; either rectal or oral; effective for recurrent infections in adult and pediatric populations (80–90% cure rate) after offending antibiotic stopped; recipient gut flora transformed in as few as 3 days.

SURGERY/OTHER PROCEDURES

- Severe abdominal pain or signs of hemodynamic instability should prompt further evaluation and consultation.
- Perforation of the colon (4)

ALERT

BI/NAP1/027 strain is associated with fulminant colitis.

COMPLEMENTARY & ALTERNATIVE MEDICINE

- Adjunctive IV immunoglobulin (IVIG) has shown promise; more data needed before routine use
- Probiotics *Lactobacillus acidophilus* and *Saccharomyces boulardii* have inhibitory effects on *C. difficile* and can help prevent *C. difficile* infection and should be prescribed when started on antibiotics.
- Other investigational treatments:
  - Newer antibiotics (rifalazil, tolevamer, and ramoplanin); monoclonal antibodies to modulate toxin effects
  - Vaccine form of *C. difficile* antitoxin antibody

ADMISSION, INPATIENT, AND NURSING CONSIDERATIONS

- Admission criteria/initial stabilization: hypovolemia; inability to keep up with enteric losses; hematochezia; electrolyte disturbances
- IV fluids to maintain volume status
- Discharge criteria: decreased diarrhea severity and frequency; tolerating oral diet and medications

ONGOING CARE

FOLLOW-UP RECOMMENDATIONS

Do not repeat testing for toxins because patients may shed for weeks following an acute infection.

Patient Monitoring

- Relapses of colitis occur in 15–30%.
- Relapses typically occur 2 to 10 days after discontinuing antibiotics.

DIET

- Regular diet
- NPO if severe colitis and surgical evaluation pending

PATIENT EDUCATION

Educate patients about *C. difficile* transmission, the importance of contact precautions when interacting with patients with *C. difficile*, the importance of handwashing with soap and water as alcohol-based sanitizers does not inactivate spores, and avoidance of unnecessary use of antibiotics.

PROGNOSIS

- Most patients improve with conservative management and oral antibiotics.
- 1–3% of patients develop severe/fulminant colitis requiring emergency colectomy.

REFERENCES

1. Cymbal M, Chatterjee A, Baggott B, et al. Management of *Clostridioides difficile* infection: diagnosis, treatment, and future perspectives. *Am J Med*. 2024;137(7):571–576. doi:10.1016/j.amjmed.2024.03.024.
2. Barbut F, Mostaghat I, Ehmig M, et al. Laboratory diagnosis of *Clostridioides difficile* infection: past, present and future. *Anaerobe*. 2025;93:102974. doi:10.1016/j.anaerobe.2025.102974.
3. Johnson S, Lavergne V, Skinner AM, et al. Clinical practice guideline by the Infectious Diseases Society of America (IDSA) and Society for Healthcare Epidemiology of America (SHEA): 2021 focused update guidelines on management of *Clostridioides difficile* infection in adults. *Clin Infect Dis*. 2021;73(5):e1029–e1044. doi:10.1093/cid/ciab549.
4. Giles J, Roberts A. Clostridioides difficile: current overview and future perspectives. *Adv Protein Chem Struct Biol*. 2022;129:215–245. doi:10.1016/bs.apcsb.2021.11.003.

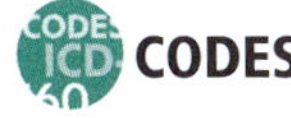

CODES

ICD10

- A04.7 Enterocolitis due to Clostridium difficile
- A04.71 Enterocolitis due to Clostridium difficile, recurrent
- A04.72 Enterocolitis due to Clostridium difficile, not specified as recurrent

CLINICAL PEARLS

- *C. difficile* is spread by fecal-oral contact.
- Alcohol-based hand sanitizers are ineffective against *C. difficile*. Wash hands thoroughly with soap and water.
- Testing and treatment of asymptomatic patients is not recommended.
- *C. difficile* and organismal by-products (e.g., toxin) are identifiable from stool samples.
- Patients may shed organism or toxin for weeks after treatment. Repeat toxin assays following treatment are not helpful.
- Vancomycin and fidaxomicin are first-line treatments.
- Consider probiotic use when prescribing antibiotics to potentially decrease risk of development of *C. difficile* infection.

COLIC, INFANTILE

Daniel T. Lee, MD, MA • Phillip Charles Brown, MD • Amanda d'Almeida, MD, MPH

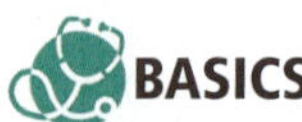

BASICS

DESCRIPTION

- Colic is defined as excessive crying in an otherwise healthy infant.
- A commonly used criteria is the Wessel criteria or the Rule of Three, when crying lasts for:
  - >3 hr/day
  - >3 days/week
  - Persists >3 weeks
- Many clinicians do not strictly adhere to the criterion of persistence for >3 weeks because few parents or clinicians will wait that long before evaluation or intervention.
- The Rome IV criteria refined the criteria for clinical purposes and for research purposes
- The Rome IV clinical diagnostic criteria must include all the following:
  - An infant who is <5 months when symptoms start and stop
  - Recurrent and prolonged periods of crying, fussing, or irritability without obvious cause and unable to console
  - No evidence of failure to thrive, fever, or illness
- Additional Rome IV criteria for clinical research purposes:
  - Caregiver reports crying/fussing for ≥3 hr/day during ≥3 days within a week.
  - Total daily crying is ≥3 hours when measured by at least one prospectively kept 24-hour diary.
- Colic usually peaks at 6 weeks of life.
- Some clinicians consider that colic represents the extreme end of the spectrum of normal crying, whereas most consider that colic a distinct clinical entity.

EPIDEMIOLOGY

Incidence

- Predominant age group is between 2 weeks and 4 months of age.
- Equal predominance among males and females, breast-fed versus formula fed, full term versus preterm, and first-born versus subsequent-born.
- Possibly more common in industrialized countries and in White infants

Prevalence

- Wide range from 10% to 40% of infants; however, more likely affects 10–25% of infants
- Causes 10–20% of pediatric visits during the early weeks of an infant's life

Pediatric Considerations

This is a problem during infancy.

ETIOLOGY AND PATHOPHYSIOLOGY

The cause is unknown. Factors that may play a role include the following:

- Infant gastroesophageal reflux disease
- Intolerance to cow's milk, soy milk, or breast milk protein
- Intolerance to lactose and functional lactose overload (i.e., breast milk with lower lipid content can have faster transit time in the intestine, leading to more lactose fermentation in the gut and hence gas and distension)
- Intolerance to other substances in the maternal diet such as cruciferous vegetables, cow's milk, chocolate, and onion have been suggested.
- Intestinal immaturity leading to incomplete absorption of carbohydrates in the small intestine, which result in excessive gas when the unabsorbed carbohydrate is fermented by colonic bacteria
- Alterations in intestinal or fecal microflora
- Swallowing air during the process of crying, feeding, or sucking
- Overfeeding or feeding too quickly; underfeeding has also been proposed.
- Inadequate burping after feeding
- Family tension and/or stress
- Parental anxiety, depression, and/or fatigue
- Parent–infant interaction mismatch
- Infant's inability to console himself or herself when dealing with stimuli
- Hypersensitivity after exposure to prolonged environmental stimuli
- Fruit juice intolerance
- Increases in the gut hormone motilin, causing hyperperistalsis
- Tobacco smoke and nicotine exposure
- Immature motor regulation
- Increased serotonin concentration
- Possible early manifestation of childhood migraine

RISK FACTORS

- Physiologic predispositions in an infant may play a role, but no definitive risk factors have been established.
- Maternal smoking or exposure to nicotine replacement therapy during pregnancy is associated with higher incidence of infantile colic.
- Infants with a maternal history of migraine headaches are twice as likely to have colic.

GENERAL PREVENTION

Colic is generally not preventable.

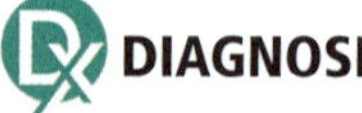

DIAGNOSIS

HISTORY

- Evaluation for Wessel criteria or Rome IV criteria
- Thorough history to rule out organic causes
- Episodes usually have a clear beginning and end and generally occur more often in the afternoon and evening.
- The crying is generally spontaneous, without preceding events triggering the episodes.
- The crying is typically different from normal crying. Colicky crying may be louder, more turbulent, variable in pitch, and appears more like screaming.
- Episodes of colic may be associated with hypertonia, which may include facial flushing, circumoral pallor, tense abdomen, arching of the back, tightening of the arms, clenching of the fingers, or drawing up of the legs.
- The infant may be difficult to soothe or console despite all the parents' efforts.
- The infant acts normally when not colicky.
- Assess the support system of caregivers and families, including coping skills.

PHYSICAL EXAM

- A comprehensive physical exam is normal.
- Because excessive crying may be a risk factor for abuse, be sure to examine the child carefully for signs of shaken baby syndrome or other types of child abuse.

DIFFERENTIAL DIAGNOSIS

Organic causes account for <5% of cases of inconsolable crying in infants. These may include:

- Infectious causes such as meningitis, sepsis, otitis media, diaper rash, thrush, or UTI
- Inadequate feeding or difficulty feeding due to causes such as tongue-tie
- Gastrointestinal causes such as gastroesophageal reflux disease, intussusception, lactose intolerance, constipation, anal fissure, testicular torsion, or strangulated hernia
- Trauma, which includes foreign body, corneal abrasion, occult fracture, digit or penile hair tourniquet, or child abuse

DIAGNOSTIC TESTS & INTERPRETATION

Initial Tests (lab, imaging)

Infantile colic is a clinical diagnosis. No lab or imaging testing is typically performed unless clinical symptoms imply other causes (UTI, weight loss or poor weight gain, abnormal physical exam, etc.).

Diagnostic Procedures/Other

A thorough history and physical exam should be performed to rule out other causes. Otherwise, no diagnostic procedures are indicated.

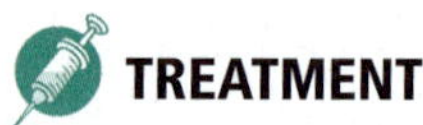

TREATMENT

GENERAL MEASURES

- Soothe by holding and rocking the baby (1)[B].
- Use a pacifier (1)[B].
- Use gentle rhythmic motions (e.g., strollers, infant swings, car rides) (1)[B].
- Use white noise (e.g., vacuum cleaner, clothes dryer, white noise machine) (1)[B].
- Crib vibrators or car ride simulators have not proven to be helpful
- Provide a warm bath (1)[B].
- Increased carrying or use of infant carriers has not been shown to improve colic (1)[B].
- Frequent burping does not significantly lower colic events (and may increase rate of regurgitation).
- Rubbing the infant's abdomen
- Employ the 5 Ss (need to be done concurrently):
  - Swaddling: tight wrapping with blanket (with arms snug and straight and hips loose); may be especially beneficial in infants <8 weeks old
  - Side/stomach: holding baby on side or stomach
  - Shushing: loud white noise
  - Swinging: rhythmic, jiggle motion while supporting baby's head and neck
  - Sucking: on a nipple, finger, or pacifier
  - "Stay Calm." The baby may not understand what is said but rather how it is said (e.g., "Everything will be fine; I am here now.").

MEDICATION

- No medication has been found to be universally beneficial in treating infantile colic.
- Probiotics are safe, and some studies have suggested their efficacy. Their use is discussed in the "Complementary & Alternative Medicine" section.
- Dicyclomine (Bentyl) may have some benefit, but the potential serious adverse effects, such as apnea, seizures, and syncope, have precluded its use. Furthermore, the manufacturer has made the medication contraindicated for infants <6 months (2)[B].
- Simethicone has not been shown to be beneficial (2)[B].
- Proton pump inhibitors and H_2 receptor antagonists have not been shown to be beneficial.

ISSUES FOR REFERRAL

Excessive vomiting, poor weight gain, recurrent respiratory diseases, or bloody stools should prompt referral to a specialist.

COMPLEMENTARY & ALTERNATIVE MEDICINE

- There is no clear evidence that probiotics are effective at preventing infantile colic.
- Limited studies on strains of *Lactobacillus reuteri* DSM 17938 and *Bifidobacterium* as probiotics suggest they may decrease daily crying times in breastfed infants (more studies need to be conducted in formula-fed infants) (3).
- Randomized control trials across multiple countries showed the strain *Lactobacillus reuteri* DSM 17938 decreased crying time in infants that are primarily breastfed, but this data may not be generalizable to all populations.
- There is anecdotal evidence that car rides, both real and simulated, can be effective. You can find a 10-hour recording of a simulated car ride at the following link: https://www.youtube.com/watch?v=8KAXmle-T_4.
- Providing "white noise," such as running a vacuum cleaner, clothes dryer, white noise generator, or infant sound machine, may also help. Avoid excessively loud and/or prolonged noise to minimize potential adverse effects on hearing or auditory development.
- Decrease environmental stimuli by turning off TVs, phones, and music and by turning down or off lights in the room.
- Herbal teas and supplements may help but are not recommended because of limited, inconclusive evidence.
  - Herbal teas containing mixtures of chamomile, vervain, licorice, and balm mint used up to TID may be beneficial. However, the study used high dosages, raising clinical concerns that this therapy may impair needed milk consumption in infants and be impractical to administer. In addition, preparations used in the study may not be commercially available in the United States.
  - There is evidence supporting the effectiveness of different preparations of fennel, such as oils, teas, and herbal compounds, in treating infantile colic.
  - Medications described as "soothing" that include activated charcoal are growing in popularity but are not recommended at this time and also have their own risks.
- A home-based intervention focusing on reducing infant stimulation and synchronizing infant sleep-wake cycles with the environment, as well as on parental support, has been shown to be effective.
- Use of music may help.
- Chiropractic treatment, craniosacral therapy, and acupuncture have not been shown to be effective.
- Infant massage has not been shown to be helpful.

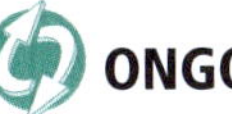

ONGOING CARE

FOLLOW-UP RECOMMENDATIONS

Frequent outpatient visits as needed for parental reassurance, education, and monitoring and to ensure the health of the infant and parents.

Patient Monitoring

Follow for proper feeding, growth, and development.

DIET

- If breastfeeding:
  - Continue breastfeeding; switching to formula unlikely to help.
  - Low likelihood of therapeutic benefit from eliminating milk products, eggs, wheat, nuts, soy, and/or fish from the diet of breastfeeding mothers, but this may be beneficial if the mother is atopic or if the infant has symptoms of cow's milk allergy (1)[B].
- If formula feeding:
  - Feeding the infant in a vertical position using a curved bottle or bottle with a collapsible bag may help to reduce air swallowing.
  - If no intervention or dietary change has been effective, consider a 1-week trial of hypoallergenic formulas such as whey hydrolysate (e.g., Good Start) or casein hydrolysate (e.g., Alimentum, Nutramigen, Pregestimil) (1)[B],(2)[C].
  - Adding fiber to formula also has not been shown to be helpful (1)[B].
- Supplementing with sucrose solution may be helpful, but the effect may be short-lived (<1 hour) (1),(2)[B].
- Switching to soy protein formula is unlikely to be helpful.
- Despite the proposed mechanism of functional lactose overload, use of lactase enzymes in formula or breast milk or given directly to the infant has no therapeutic benefit (1)[B].

PATIENT EDUCATION

- Caregiver support, in the form of reassurance and education, is critical.
- Reassure parents that colic is not the result of something they are doing or not doing.
- Reassure parents that colic is normal and that the infant is not sick.
- Advise parents about having proper rest breaks, adequate sleep, help in caring for the infant, and even a rescue plan in case parents become overwhelmed.
- Parents need to develop their own personal coping strategies to deal with colic episodes to avoid risk of harm to infant.
- Explain the spectrum of crying behavior.
- Avoid overfeeding or underfeeding.
- Instruct parents regarding beneficial feeding techniques such as improved bottles (low air, curved) and sufficient burping after feeding.
- Information for parents of colicky infants can be found at the following link from the American Academy of Family Physician: https://www.aafp.org/afp/2004/0815/p741.html.

PROGNOSIS

- Colic usually subsides by 3 to 5 months of age.
- Despite apparent abdominal pain, colicky infants eat well and gain weight normally.
- A few studies in toddlers up to 4 years old indicate temper tantrums may be more common among formerly colicky infants.
- Colic has no bearing on the baby's intelligence or future development.

COMPLICATIONS

- Colic is self-limiting, and there are no proven lasting effects to the infant.
- There may be associations with increased risk/incidence of postpartum depression among either or both parents, child abuse, caregiver burnout, and early cessation of breastfeeding.

REFERENCES

1. Johnson JD, Cocker K, Chang E. Infantile colic: recognition and treatment. *Am Fam Physician*. 2015;92(7):577–582.
2. Wade S, Kilgour T. Extracts from "clinical evidence": infantile colic. *BMJ*. 2001;323(7310):437–440.
3. Pereira AR, Rodrigues J, Albergaria M. Effectiveness of probiotics for the treatment of infantile colic. *Aust J Gen Pract*. 2022;51(8):573–576.

ADDITIONAL READING

- Anheyer D, Frawley J, Koch AK, et al. Herbal medicines for gastrointestinal disorders in children and adolescents: a systematic review. *Pediatrics*. 2017;139(6):e20170062.
- Gelfand AA, Thomas KC, Goadsby PJ. Before the headache: infant colic as an early life expression of migraine. *Neurology*. 2012;79(13):1392–1396.

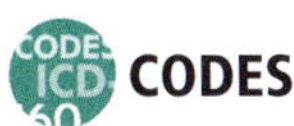

CODES

ICD10

R10.83 Colic

CLINICAL PEARLS

- Colic is defined as excessive crying in an otherwise healthy infant (3 hr/day, 3 days/week, persists >3 weeks).
- Colic usually subsides spontaneously by 3 to 5 months of age.
- Provide advice, support, and reassurance to parents.
- Prevent caregiver burnout by advising parents to get proper rest breaks, sleep, and help in caring for the infant.

C

COLITIS, ISCHEMIC

Marie L. Borum, MD, EdD, MPH • Abdelrhman Refaey, MD

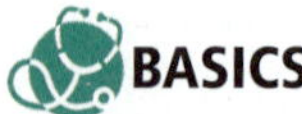

BASICS

Ischemic colitis (IC) results from decreased blood flow to the colon with resultant inflammation and tissue damage.

DESCRIPTION

- IC is self-limited and reversible in 80% of patients: 20% of patients progress to full-thickness necrosis requiring surgical intervention.
- Most commonly, ischemia is related to a nonocclusive reduction in blood flow.
- Presentation varies, but patients with acute IC typically present with localized abdominal pain and tenderness. Frequent loose, bloody stools may be seen within 12 to 24 hours of onset.
- Laboratory and radiographic findings are nonspecific and must be correlated with clinical presentation.
- Colonoscopy is the gold standard for diagnosis of IC.
- Most patients recover with supportive care (IV fluids, bowel rest, and clinical monitoring).

EPIDEMIOLOGY

- More common in the elderly; can affect patients of all ages
- More common in women (57–76%—particularly after age 69 years)
- Rare in patients <60 years old; average age at diagnosis is 70 years.

Incidence

Approximately 23 cases per 100,000 person-years (range 4.5 to 44) in the general population (may be underestimated due to nonspecific clinical manifestations)

Prevalence

Prevalence is not well established due to the acute and self-limited nature of most cases.

ETIOLOGY AND PATHOPHYSIOLOGY

- Local colonic hypoperfusion compromises the ability to meet metabolic demands. Reperfusion injury may also play a role.
- The colon is perfused by both the superior and inferior mesenteric arteries (SMAs and IMAs) and branches of the internal iliac arteries. Occlusion of larger branches of the SMA or IMA, rarely leads to ischemic consequences due to extensive collateral circulation.
- Watershed areas of the colon (splenic flexure and rectosigmoid junction) are supplied by narrow terminal branches of the SMA and IMA, respectively, and are most susceptible to ischemic damage.
- The left colon is more commonly affected than the right; isolated right-sided disease has the worst prognosis.
- The rectum is often spared because of additional blood supply from the internal iliac arteries.
- Type I: unidentified etiology (usually attributed to localized nonocclusive ischemia)
  - Likely small vessel disease; treat supportively.
- Type II: etiology identified
  - Treat the underlying cause.
    - Hypoperfusion from shock, trauma
    - Embolic occlusion of mesenteric vessels
    - Hypercoagulable states, vasculitis; sickle cell disease
    - Arterial thrombosis; venous thrombosis
    - Mechanical obstruction of the colon (e.g., tumor, adhesions, hernia, volvulus, prolapse, diverticulitis)
    - Surgical complications
    - Medications (intestinally active vasoconstrictive substances, medications that induce hypotension and thus, hypoperfusion); cocaine use disorder
    - Aortic dissection
    - Strenuous physical activity (e.g., long-distance running)
- Repeated episodes of ischemia and inflammation may result in chronic colonic ischemia, possible stricture formation, recurrent bacteremia, and sepsis. These patients may have unresolving areas of colitis and require segmental colonic resection.

Genetics

- Various coagulopathies have been related to IC including deficiencies of protein C, protein S, antithrombin III, and factor V Leiden mutation.
- Routine coagulation testing is not justified except in younger patients and patients with recurrent IC.

RISK FACTORS

- Age >60 years (90% of patients)
- Smoking (most common cause of recurrent IC)
- Hypertension, diabetes mellitus
- Rheumatologic disorders/vasculitis
- Cerebrovascular disease, ischemic heart disease
- Atherosclerotic disease
- Recent abdominal surgery (i.e., ileostomy)
- Constipation, constipation-inducing medications
- History of vascular surgery
- Chronic obstructive pulmonary disease
- Hypoalbuminemia; hemodialysis
- Hypercoagulability, oral contraceptive
- NSAID use
- Immunomodulators
- IBS
- Following colonoscopy
- Severe COVID-19 infection

GENERAL PREVENTION

Standard practices, counseling and treatment of risk factors as indicated

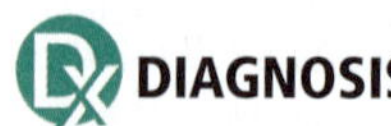

DIAGNOSIS

- Diagnosis is based on history, risk factors, and physical examination.
- Laboratory values and radiographic findings are usually nonspecific but may help predict severity.
- Colonoscopy is diagnostic.

HISTORY

- Abdominal pain is the most common symptom (1). Pain may be out of proportion to physical examination findings.
- Sudden-onset, mild to moderate abdominal pain with tenderness over the affected segment of bowel (2)
- Sudden urge to defecate followed by passage of either bright red or maroon stool typically within 12 to 24 hours of abdominal pain onset (2)
- Lower GI bleeding is rarely heavy.

PHYSICAL EXAM

- Individual signs and symptoms are poorly predictive of IC (3)[C].
- Vital signs: hypotension; tachycardia
- Tenderness over the involved segment of bowel (2)
- Abdominal distention with vomiting (due to possible associated ileus)
- In the uncommon setting of transmural ischemia, patients may develop peritoneal signs.

DIFFERENTIAL DIAGNOSIS

- Infectious colitis
- Inflammatory bowel disease (ulcerative colitis, Crohn disease)
- Colon cancer, diverticulitis
- Pseudomembranous colitis (3)[A]
- Radiation colitis

DIAGNOSTIC TESTS & INTERPRETATION

- Depends on clinical presentation, extent of colonic involvement, transmural involvement, acuity
- CT scan is the initial diagnostic test for patients with nonspecific abdominal pain (3)[A].
- Colonoscopy for definitive diagnosis
- Radiographic tests and laboratory values are otherwise nonspecific (3)[A].

Initial Tests (lab, imaging)

- The following lab markers of ischemia are not specific to IC but can help determine disease severity (3)[A]:
  - CBC (leukocytosis) (3)[A]
  - BMP, ABG (signs of metabolic acidosis) (3)[A]
  - Lactate, LDH, CPK, amylase (3)[A]
  - Alkaline phosphatase (3)[A]
  - Albumin (2)
- Abdominal plain film: rarely may see thumbprinting and mural thickening; may predict more severe disease
- Abdominal CT scan with contrast:
  - Thickening of the colonic wall and pericolonic fat stranding (2)
  - Other findings include hyperdense mucosa, submucosal edema, and mesenteric inflammation.
  - Pneumatosis, pneumoperitoneum, and free peritoneal fluid suggest advanced ischemia.
  - Double halo sign is highly suggestive of IC but is rarely present.
- Multiphasic CTA should be performed for suspected right-sided IC or if acute mesenteric ischemia cannot be excluded (2)[B].

Follow-Up Tests & Special Considerations

- Stool cultures, fecal leukocytes, stool ova, and parasites to rule out infection (3)[A]
- Patients undergoing aortic surgery may benefit from postoperative colonoscopy within 2 to 3 days to look for signs of IC (2).
- If indicated, cardiac workup including electrocardiogram, Holter monitoring, or transthoracic echocardiogram to exclude cardiogenic embolism (3)[A]
- Drug and toxicology screening (2)
- If colon cancer screening is indicated, perform several weeks following recovery from the ischemic insult.

Diagnostic Procedures/Other

- Colonoscopy with biopsy is gold standard; sigmoidoscopy used to evaluate postoperative left-sided ischemia.
- Cyanotic hemorrhagic tissue and edematous mucosa suggest ischemia (2).
  - Segmental distribution (watershed), hemorrhagic nodules, and rectal sparing (2)
  - "Colon single-stripe sign" is a single line of erythema, with a 75% histopathologic yield (2).
  - Routine biopsy is no longer advised, as results are typically nonspecific.
- In cases of isolated right IC, noninvasive vascular imaging studies are recommended to evaluate acute SMA occlusion (2).

Test Interpretation

Biopsied specimens reveal mucosal infarction and ghost cells, which show normal cellular outlines but lack intracellular contents.

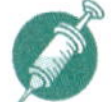

TREATMENT

- Treatment depends on disease severity.
- In the absence of colonic necrosis or perforation, most patients respond to supportive care:
  - Bowel rest (2)
  - IV fluids to maintain hemodynamic stability (2)
  - Avoid intestinally active vasoconstrictive medications (2)[A].
  - Avoid systemic corticosteroids—may worsen ischemia and increase risk of perforation.
- If ileus is present, place nasogastric tube.
- If radiographic abnormalities are present, serial abdominal x-rays help follow improvement (2)[A].
- If signs of clinical deterioration are present despite supportive care (increased abdominal pain, peritoneal signs, persistent diarrhea, bleeding, or sepsis), consider surgery.

MEDICATION

Specific medications have been associated with IC, including:

- Constipation-inducing medications (i.e., opioids)
- Immunomodulators (anti-TNFα inhibitors, type 1 interferon-α/β)
- Illicit drugs (cocaine, amphetamines)

First Line

Consider broad-spectrum antibiotics covering aerobic and anaerobic bacteria to avoid bacterial translocation secondary to colonic mucosal damage (2).

- Ciprofloxacin 400 mg IV BID or 500 mg PO BID
- Metronidazole 500 mg PO/IV TID

Second Line

A 3rd-generation cephalosporin may be used instead of a fluoroquinolone.

ISSUES FOR REFERRAL

- If cardiac workup reveals CHF or cardiac arrhythmias, initiate appropriate treatment (2).
- If signs of clinical deterioration are present despite supportive care (increased abdominal pain, peritoneal signs, persistent diarrhea, bleeding, or sepsis), consider surgery.

SURGERY/OTHER PROCEDURES

- 20% of patients require surgical intervention (1).
- Surgery may be indicated for:
  - Peritoneal signs, increased abdominal tenderness, new-onset shock, lactic acidosis, or acute renal failure
  - Pneumatosis intestinalis, portal vein air, or free peritoneal air
  - Diarrhea, lower GI bleeding, or exudative colitis persisting past 14 days
- Most common surgical intervention is colectomy with end ileostomy (3)[A].
  - Cholecystectomy may prevent resuscitation-related acute acalculous cholecystitis.

COMPLEMENTARY & ALTERNATIVE MEDICINE

- *Ginkgo* biloba extract has been studied as an adjunct to general treatment.
- Weight loss supplements/herbal supplements (ephedra, ma huang, bitter orange, white willow bark) have been implicated in cases of IC.

ADMISSION, INPATIENT, AND NURSING CONSIDERATIONS

- ICU patients represent a difficult population to diagnose IC given the concurrent comorbidities and clinical care (sedation/ventilation) that can mask the characteristic signs and symptoms.
- Consider bedside colonoscopy in critically ill patients.

ONGOING CARE

FOLLOW-UP RECOMMENDATIONS

Patient Monitoring

- Vital sign monitoring depending on initial presentation
- Observation for further episodes of bloody stool or melena
- Consideration of serial CBCs
- Serial abdominal exams

DIET

- Bowel rest until symptoms resolve
- Parenteral nutrition for patients needing prolonged bowel rest who have contraindications to surgery

PATIENT EDUCATION

Risks of IC with the use of weight loss medications/herbal supplements

PROGNOSIS

- In most patients, IC symptoms resolve in 24 to 48 hours.
- Radiographic or endoscopic resolution within 2 weeks
- Right-sided IC is the most significant predictor of outcome. Right-sided IC has a 2-fold increase in mortality and a 4-fold increase in morbidity (2).
- Secondary cardiovascular prevention minimizes recurrence.
- Male gender, low hemoglobin, low serum albumin, high BUN, and presence of metabolic acidosis are poor prognostic factors.
- Chronic kidney disease, chronic obstructive pulmonary disease (COPD), long-term care facilities increase mortality in IC.

COMPLICATIONS

About 20% of patients develop chronic IC with persistent diarrhea or stricture formation requiring surgery.

REFERENCES

1. Huber TS, Björck M, Chandra A, et al. Chronic mesenteric ischemia: clinical practice guidelines from the Society for Vascular Surgery. *J Vasc Surg*. 2021;73(1 Suppl):87S–115S.
2. Maimone A, De Ceglie A, Siersema PD, et al. Colon ischemia: a comprehensive review. *Clin Res Hepatol Gastroenterol*. 2021;45(6):101592. doi:10.1016/j.clinre.2020.101592.
3. Ahmed M. Ischemic bowel disease in 2021. *World J Gastroenterol*. 2021;27(29):4746–4762.

ADDITIONAL READING

Rizwan R, Feuerstadt P. Bad blood: ischemic conditions of the large bowel. *Current Opin Gastroenterol*. 2022;38(1):72–79. doi:10.1097/MOG.0000000000000797.

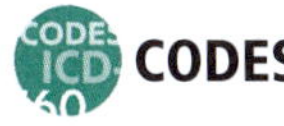

CODES

ICD10

- K55.9 Vascular disorder of intestine, unspecified
- K55.0 Acute vascular disorders of intestine
- K55.1 Chronic vascular disorders of intestine

CLINICAL PEARLS

- Suspect IC in patients with multiple risk factors who present with abdominal pain and loose bloody stools.
- Risk factors include advanced age, smoking, hypertension, diabetes mellitus, cardiovascular or rheumatologic disease, recent abdominal surgery, medications (such as constipation inducing, NSAIDs, and immunomodulators), IBS, hemodialysis, and COPD
- Colonoscopy with biopsy is the diagnostic gold standard.
- Most often, IC is self-limited and responds well to conservative management with IV fluids, bowel rest, and empiric broad-spectrum antibiotics.
- Peritoneal signs or lack of clinical improvement suggests more extensive ischemia and need for surgical intervention.

COLON CANCER

Kento Sonoda, MD • Yuriko Terada, MD

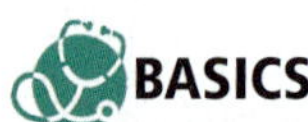

BASICS

DESCRIPTION

- Colon and rectal cancers (CRC) are often grouped together but are two distinct clinical entities that differ in their prognosis, presentation, staging, and management.
- CRC is the third leading cause of cancer-related deaths in men, the fourth leading cause in women, and the second leading cause when numbers for men and women are combined in the United States.

EPIDEMIOLOGY

Incidence

- Estimated that in 2025 in the United States, there are 107,320 new cases of colon cancer and 46,950 new cases of rectal cancer per the American Cancer Society.
- Colorectal cancer is expected to cause about 52,900 deaths in 2025.
- Internationally, CRC is the third most common cancer and the second leading cause of cancer death.

Prevalence

Lifetime risk for developing colorectal cancer in the United States is ~1 in 23 (4.3%) for men and 1 in 25 (4%) for women.

ETIOLOGY AND PATHOPHYSIOLOGY

- Progression from the first abnormal cells to colon cancer occurs over 10 to 15 years.
- High-risk polyps: multiple polyps, villous, sessile serrated, or dysplastic polyps and larger polyps; hyperplastic polyps are less likely to evolve into CRC.

Genetics

- About 5% of CRC cases are linked to an inherited gene. Patients with genetic causes should consider family members having early screening.
  - Many of these are inherited in an autosomal dominant fashion:
    - *APC*, a tumor suppressor gene, is altered in familial adenomatous polyposis (FAP).
    - Genes encoding DNA mismatch repair (MMR) enzymes are implicated in hereditary nonpolyposis colon cancer (HNPCC), formerly Lynch syndrome, including *hMLH1*, *hMSH2*, *hMSH6*, *hPMS2*, *EPCAM*, and others.
    - STK11, a tumor suppressor gene, is altered in Peutz-Jeghers syndrome.
  - A smaller portion of patients with familial CRC may have a recessive gene.
    - MUTYH defects lead to issues with the base excision repair gene. This MUTYH-associated polyposis (MAP) may present as a variant form of FAP.
- Sporadic cases of CRC have been linked to oncogenes: *KRAS*, *PIK3CA*, *APC*, *TP53*, *BRCA 1*, *BRCA 2*, *BRAF*.

RISK FACTORS

- Age: The incidence of colon cancer increases between 40 and 50 years old. ~87% of those with new CRC diagnosis will be >50 years old; younger patients are more likely to have advanced disease at the time of diagnosis.
- Personal history of colorectal polyps: The risk increases with multiple polyps, villous polyps, larger polyps (>1 cm), and presence of dysplasia.
- Personal history of cancer
  - 30% increase in risk of developing metachronous (new primary tumors unrelated to the patients' previous cancers) colon cancer
  - 2–4% incidence of local recurrence with colon cancer, 3–5% incidence of synchronous colon cancer
  - History of radiation therapy to the abdomen/pelvis
- Personal history of inflammatory bowel disease (IBD)
  - The risk of CRC begins ~8 years after the onset. Prevalence of CRC in ulcerative colitis and Crohn disease is ~3%, with a cumulative risk of CRC of 2% at 10 years, 8% at 20 years, and 18% at 30 years.
  - Ulcerative colitis with pancolitis up to 10-fold risk of CRC, 8 to 10 years after initial diagnosis
- Anal human papillomavirus
- Family history of CRC
  - Having a single first-degree relative with a history of CRC increases risk ~1.7-fold.
  - Risk is more than double for with a history of CRC or polyps in:
    - Any first-degree relative <50 years of age; ≥2 first-degree relatives, regardless of age; one first-degree and one second-degree relative
- Inherited syndromes
  - HNPCC
    - Often develops at younger age (~48 years)
    - With right-sided lesions
  - FAP: Affected individuals develop hundreds to thousands of polyps in colon and rectum, typically presenting during childhood with CRC present by age 40 years in untreated patients; most have prophylactic colectomies
  - Peutz-Jeghers syndrome
    - Individuals may have hyperpigmented mucocutaneous lesions (mouth, hands, feet) and large polyps in GI tract discovered as an adolescent.
    - 81–93% risk for cancers including CRC, cancers of pancreas, breast, cervix, testes, and lung
- Race and ethnicity: African Americans have the highest CRC incidence and mortality rates in the United States.
- Lifestyle factors: smoking, obesity, sedentary activity, insulin resistance, low intake of calcium, whole-grain, and/or fiber-rich foods, high consumption of red and processed meat, excessive alcohol

GENERAL PREVENTION

- Lifestyle factors and medications that may reduce risk:
  - Regular physical activity, diet high in fiber 30 g/day), and fruits and vegetables
  - There is conflicting evidence on folic acid, calcium, vitamin D, magnesium, NSAIDs, fish oil, and statins.

ALERT

The U.S. Preventive Services Task Force (USPSTF) states all adult ≥45 years should be offered screening regardless of the presence of the risk factors (recommendation for 45 to 49 years old with Grade B and 50 to 75 years old with Grade A) (1). For ages 76 to 85 years old, screening should be based on overall health status and life expectancy and should involve shared decision-making.

- Screening methods (2):
  - Visualization-based tests:
    - Colonoscopy every 10 years (primary screening modality)
    - Flexible sigmoidoscopy every 10 years with a high-sensitivity fecal immunochemical test (FIT) annually
    - Flexible sigmoidoscopy every 5 to 10 years
    - Capsule colonoscopy every 5 years (considered 3rd tier for those unwilling)
  - Stool-based tests
    - FIT
    - Multitarget stool DNA test (Cologuard) every 3 years
    - High-sensitivity guaiac fecal occult blood test (gFOBT) annually
  - Imaging-based tests:
    - CT colonography every 5 years
    - For patients who have a positive noncolonoscopy-based CRC test (stool-based, flexible sigmoidoscopy, CT colonography), a colonoscopy is recommended.
- Colonoscopy:
  - People who have a first-degree relative or two second-degree relatives with CRC or advanced polyps before age 60 years should begin colonoscopy at age 40 or ≤10 years than the youngest age of the affected relative, whichever is earlier. Repeat every 5 years.
  - Patients with IBD should start surveillance colonoscopies every 1 to 2 years and 8 to 10 years after diagnosis.
  - Genetic testing may be appropriate for individuals with a strong family history of CRC or polyps:
    - Family members of a person with HNPCC should start colonoscopy starting at age 20 to 25 years or 2 to 5 years prior to the youngest age of the affected relative at the time of cancer diagnosis, whichever occurs first and repeated every 1 to 2 years.
    - Individuals with suspected FAP should have colonoscopy every 1 to 3 years, beginning at age 10 to 14 years.

- Frequency of follow-up of polyps:
  - 2 to 6 months: following piecemeal (unable to remove with single loop) removal of a large polyp ≥20 mm
  - 1 year:
    - Known FAP or at risk based on family history
    - >10 adenomatous polyps
  - 1 to 2 years: IBD (Crohn disease or ulcerative colitis)
  - 3 years:
    - 5 to 10 tubular adenomas <10 mm
    - 5 to 10 sessile serrated polyps
    - Tubular adenoma ≥10 mm
    - Sessile serrated polyp ≥10 mm
    - Adenoma with villous or tubulovillous histology and/or high-grade dysplasia
    - Sessile serrated polyp with dysplasia
    - Traditional serrated adenoma
  - 3 to 5 years:
    - 3 to 4 sessile serrated polyp <10 mm without dysplasia
    - 3 to 4 adenomas <10 mm
    - Hyperplastic polyps ≥10 mm
    - History of colon cancer s/p surgery if initial 1-year follow-up is normal
  - 5 to 10 years: 1 to 2 sessile serrated polyp <10 mm without dysplasia
  - 7 to 10 years: 1 to 2 adenomas <10 mm
  - 10 years:
    - Normal screening colonoscopy with no polyps
    - ≤20 hyperplastic polyps <10 mm
- Some international organizations recommend screening for anal cancer via rectal swab at:
  - 35 years old for those with HIV especially men who have sex with men and transgender women
  - 45 years old for those without HIV especially men who have sex with men and transgender women.

COMMONLY ASSOCIATED CONDITIONS

- HNPCC, Gardner, Crail (Turcot), FAP, Peutz-Jeghers, juvenile polyposis syndromes, MAP, and cystic fibrosis (CF)
- IBDs including Crohn disease and particularly ulcerative colitis with pancolitis

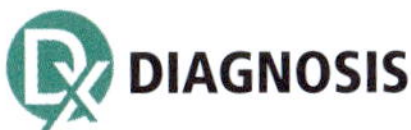

DIAGNOSIS

HISTORY

- Microcytic, iron-deficiency anemia in men of any age and postmenopausal women (diagnostic colonoscopy)
- Symptoms may indicate advanced disease.
  - Abdominal pain or cramping, change in bowel habits or caliber of stool (tenesmus, constipation, diarrhea)
  - Rectal bleeding, dark stools, or blood in stool
  - Weakness or fatigue, unintentional weight loss

PHYSICAL EXAM

- Signs of anemia (pallor, systolic flow murmurs, etc.), weight loss
- Palpable abdominal mass (late presentation), hepatomegaly, ascites, and lymphadenopathy

DIFFERENTIAL DIAGNOSIS

>95% of colon cancers are adenocarcinomas. Others include carcinoid tumors, lymphomas, gastrointestinal stromal tumors (GIST), and Kaposi sarcoma in HIV.

DIAGNOSTIC TESTS & INTERPRETATION

Initial Tests (lab, imaging)

Tumor marker CEA has low value for diagnosis of cancer due to its low sensitivity and specificity. However, CEA levels can be useful in predicting prognosis and monitoring patients with a confirmed diagnosis of CRC.

Follow-Up Tests & Special Considerations

- Contrast CT chest, abdomen, and pelvis to evaluate for metastatic disease
- Intraoperative ultrasound may be used to evaluate solid organs (e.g., the liver) after tumor resection.
- Positron emission tomography (PET) may be used to detect metastatic disease.
- Staging of colon cancer
  - The SEER staging
    - Localized: no signs with spread outside the colon or rectum
    - Regional: signs with spread outside the colon or rectum but only to nearby structures
    - Distant: signs with spread to distant sites of the body (i.e., the liver, lungs, or distant lymph nodes)

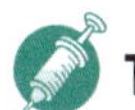

TREATMENT

ADDITIONAL THERAPIES

Adjuvant chemotherapy is most clearly beneficial for stage III (node-positive) disease, in which improvements of 30% can be achieved in both disease recurrence and overall survival, compared with controls. Chemotherapeutic regimens for metastatic disease may extend overall survival from a median of 6 months to 2 years. Often used therapies are FOLFOX (folinic acid, 5-fluorouracil, oxaliplatin), FOLFIRI (folinic acid, leucovorin, 5-fluorouracil, irinotecan), or CAPEOX (capecitabine, oxaliplatin). Neoadjuvant chemotherapy, immunotherapy, and targeted therapy (bevacizumab, ramucirumab, ziv-aflibercept, pembrolizumab, panitumumab, cetuximab, nivolumab, regorafenib, encorafenib) could also be used.

SURGERY/OTHER PROCEDURES

- Localized cancer
  - Surgery is the primary treatment with regional lymph node dissection.
  - Primary anastomosis can be possible for local cancers.
    - Obstructing lesions tend to require resections with diversion followed by colectomy with regional lymphadenectomy.
- Locally advanced cancers: multivisceral resection
- Metastatic cancer: It can be reasonable to aggressively resect metastatic lesions isolated to the liver/lungs in addition to the primary tumors.

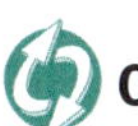

ONGOING CARE

FOLLOW-UP RECOMMENDATIONS

Patient Monitoring

Monitoring after completion of primary treatment for stage I, II, and III cancer without evidence of disease

- Stage I: colonoscopy in a year; if normal, repeat in 3 years and then every 5 years.
- High-risk stage I, stage II, and stage III: CEA and history and physical every 3 to 6 months for 2 years and then every 6 months for 5 years; chest, abdominal, and pelvic CT annually for 5 years or 2 times in 5 years; colonoscopy in a year, if normal repeat in 3 years and then every 5 years.

PATIENT EDUCATION

Centers for Disease Control and Prevention: https://www.cdc.gov/cancer/colorectal/basic_info/screening/tests.htm

PROGNOSIS

- Overall 5-year relative survival rate (colon cancer, rectal cancer): 63%, 67%
- 5-year relative survival rate (colon cancer, rectal cancer): localized: 91%, 90%; regional: 73%, 74%; distant: 13%, 18%

COMPLICATIONS

- Chemotherapy: hair loss, nausea, vomiting, diarrhea, easy bruising, fatigue, skin change, and increased risk for infections
- Radiation therapy: skin irritation, nausea, rectal pain, incontinence, bladder irritation, fatigue, sexual problems, scarring, fibrosis, and adhesion

REFERENCES

1. Davidson KW, Barry MJ, Mangione CM, et al; for US Preventive Services Task Force. Screening for colorectal cancer: US Preventive Services Task Force recommendation statement. *JAMA*. 2021;325(19):1965–1977.
2. Shaukat A, Kahi CJ, Burke CA, et al. ACG clinical guidelines: colorectal cancer screening 2021. *Am J Gastroenterol*. 2021;116(3):458–479.

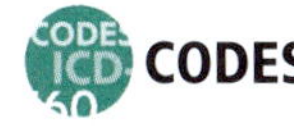

CODES

ICD10

- C18.9 Malignant neoplasm of colon, unspecified
- C18.2 Malignant neoplasm of ascending colon
- C18.8 Malignant neoplasm of overlapping sites of colon

CLINICAL PEARLS

Microcytic, iron deficiency anemia in men and postmenopausal women is CRC until proven otherwise and a colonoscopy should be performed.

COLONIC POLYPS

Maximos Attia, MD, FAAFP • Marcelle Meseeha, MD, FACP

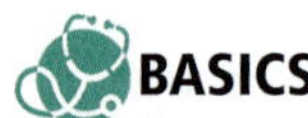

BASICS

DESCRIPTION

- Intraluminal colonic tissue growth; most commonly sporadic or part of polyposis syndromes
- Generally slow growing with low malignant potential; due to high prevalence in population; however, resection is generally recommended to eliminate risk.
- Size classification:
  - Diminutive ≤5 mm, small 6 to 9 mm, large ≥10 mm
- Morphologic classification:
  - Depressed, flat, sessile, or pedunculated
- Clinical significance:
  - >95% of colonic adenocarcinomas arise from polyps.

EPIDEMIOLOGY

Colorectal polyps are more common in non-Caucasian men in Western countries.

Incidence

Incidence increases with age.

Prevalence

- 15–20% of all adults
- 30% of U.S. population aged >50 years
- 6% of children
- 12% of children with lower GI bleed

ETIOLOGY AND PATHOPHYSIOLOGY

- Mucosal
  - Neoplastic
    - Adenomatous polyps (tubular >80%, villous 5–15%, tubulovillous 5–15%)
    - Serrated polyps
    - Sessile serrated polyps are common, more in proximal colon, with low malignant potential if no dysplasia and significant malignant potential if dysplastic.
    - Traditional serrated adenoma is uncommon, more often noted in distal colon, with significant malignant potential.
  - Nonneoplastic polyps (hyperplastic, juvenile polyps, hamartomas, inflammatory pseudopolyps)
    - Hyperplastic polyps are very common, more in distal colon, with very low malignant potential.
    - Juvenile polyps are common in childhood, benign hamartomas, more in rectosigmoid, and not premalignant.
- Submucosal (lipomas, lymphoid aggregates, carcinoids)

Genetics

- Inactivation of tumor suppressor genes as adenomatous polyposis coli (APC) or mismatch repair genes (*MLH1*) causes polyps to grow into cancer.
- Familial adenomatous polyposis (FAP) is autosomal dominant. By age 40 years, almost all patients develop colorectal cancer (CRC).
- MUTYH-associated polyposis (MAP) is autosomal recessive caused by biallelic mutations in MUTYH gene.
- Juvenile polyposis syndrome (JPS) is autosomal dominant. 50–60% of patients have a mutation in the SMAD4 or BMPR1A gene. By age 35 years, 20% of patients develop CRC.

RISK FACTORS

- Family history of intestinal polyposis, polyps, or CRC
- Advancing age; male
- High-fat, low-fiber diet; tobacco use
- Excessive alcohol intake: >8 drinks a week
- Inflammatory bowel disease is associated with a decreased prevalence of colon polyps (but with higher risk of colon cancer).

GENERAL PREVENTION

- Low-fat, high-fiber diet
- Avoid smoking.
- Decrease alcohol intake.
- Use of NSAIDs and calcium is associated with decreased incidence and recurrence of polyps.
- No lower rates of CRC with azathioprine, 6-mercaptopurine, folate, calcium, multivitamins, or statins

COMMONLY ASSOCIATED CONDITIONS

Hereditary polyposis syndromes:

- Adenomatous
  - FAP
    - Classic (CFAP), attenuated (AFAP)
  - MAP
  - FAP variants:
    - Gardner syndrome, Turcot syndrome
- Hamartomatous
  - Peutz-Jeghers syndrome (PJS), JPS, Cowden syndrome

ALERT

JPS imposes a higher risk of CRC, although juvenile polyps are not premalignant.

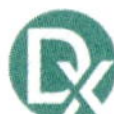

DIAGNOSIS

Screening for average-risk adults should begin at age 45 years, with colonoscopy every 10 years if no polyps are identified.

HISTORY

- Generally asymptomatic
- Painless rectal bleeding, bright or dark red, mixed with stools, dripping, or on wiping
- Diarrhea or mucous stool
- Abdominal pain
- Constipation
- Chronic bleeding, resulting in iron deficiency anemia
- McKittrick-Wheelock syndrome; large hypersecretory rectosigmoid villous adenoma, resulting in persistent severe diarrhea, electrolyte disorder, dehydration, and prerenal acute renal failure
- Social and family history

PHYSICAL EXAM

- Usually normal
- Rectal polyps noted as prolapsed or palpated on digital rectal examination (DRE)
- Fecal occult blood test (FOBT) by DRE is less effective than FOBT by stool passed spontaneously.

DIAGNOSTIC TESTS & INTERPRETATION

Initial Tests (lab, imaging)

- CBC; anemia with chronic bleeding
- Basic metabolic panel; electrolyte disorder with hypersecretory adenomas
- FOBT, insensitive screening test, because small polyps don't usually bleed:
  - Guaiac (gFOBT)—uses a chemical indicator with color change in presence of blood
  - Immunochemical FOBT (iFOBT or fecal immunochemical test [FIT])—uses antibodies against human hemoglobin
- Stool DNA test is more sensitive and less specific than FIT.

Diagnostic Procedures/Other

- Colonoscopy is the gold standard test for detection of polyps and allows for concurrent polypectomy; not a perfect screening test, with increased miss rate with right-sided colon polyps, smaller polyp size, low quality of colon prep, less endoscopist experience
- Computed tomographic colonography (CTC) is less sensitive with flat polyps and requires excellent bowel preparation.
- Double-contrast barium enema

- Colon capsule endoscopy
- Enhanced optical technologies can potentially differentiate between neoplastic and nonneoplastic colonic lesions (1)[A].
- Enhanced optical technologies include:
  - Narrowed spectrum endoscopy (narrow-band imaging [NBI])
  - Image-enhanced endoscopy (i-scan)
  - Fujinon intelligent chromoendoscopy (FICE)
  - Confocal laser endomicroscopy (CLE)
- Patients with >10 colorectal adenomas should undergo genetic testing for APC and MUTYH.

Test Interpretation

- Tubular adenoma
  - Gross: tends to be polypoid
  - Micro: dysplastic epithelium, tubular architecture
- Villous adenoma
  - Gross: tends to be sessile
  - Micro: dysplastic epithelium, fingerlike projections
- Tubulovillous adenomas have a combination of tubular and villous architecture.
- Hyperplastic polyps are composed of hyperplastic colonic mucosa.
- Hamartomatous polyps include muscularis mucosa.
- Juvenile polyp
  - Gross: pedunculated, smooth red mass, 1 to 3 cm

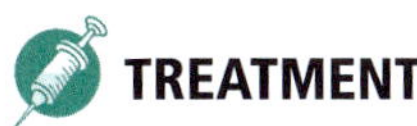

TREATMENT

SURGERY/OTHER PROCEDURES

- Colonic polypectomy; diagnostic, therapeutic:
  - Snare polypectomy with electrocautery for pedunculated polyps
  - Endoscopic mucosal resection for sessile polyps
  - Endoscopic submucosal dissection
- Colorectal surgery; prophylactic in FAP and MAP and when there are numerous polyps or persistent bleeding:
  - Total colectomy ileorectal anastomosis
  - Proctocolectomy ileal pouch anal anastomosis
- Chemoprevention: NSAIDs and calcium may reduce incidence and recurrence of polyps in patients with FAP and MAP (2).

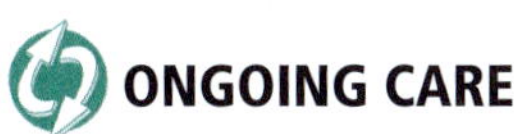

ONGOING CARE

FOLLOW-UP RECOMMENDATIONS

Follow-up colonoscopy in (3):

- 10 years if no polyps or distal small hyperplastic polyps (<10 mm) (3)[B]
- 3 to 5 years in hyperplastic polyps ≥10 mm (3)[C]
- 10 years if 1 to 2 small tubular adenomas (<10 mm) (3)[B]
- 3 to 4 years if 3 to 4 small tubular adenomas (<10 mm) (3)[C]
- 3 years if 5 to 10 small tubular adenomas (<10 mm); any adenoma >10 m or any high-grade/dysplastic features (3)[B]
- 1 year if >10 adenomas (3)[C]
- 6 months if adenoma ≥20 mm or sessile serrated polyp (SSP) ≥20 mm, with piecemeal resection (3)[B]
- 5 to 10 years if 1 to 2 small SSPs (<10 mm) (3)[C]
- 3 to 5 years if 3 to 4 small SSPs (<10 mm) (3)[C]
- 3 years if 5 to 10 small SSPs; any SSP ≥10 mm; any SSP with dysplasia or any traditional serrated adenoma (<10 mm) (3)[C]
- Different consideration is given for polyps that meet criteria for serrated polyposis syndrome (3)[B].

Patient Monitoring

- Colonoscopy for CRC screening starts at age 45 years (earlier for at-risk patients). The U.S. Preventive Services Task Force, American College of Gastroenterology (ACG), and the American Cancer Society (ACS) recommend that people at average risk of CRC start screening at age 45 years through age of 75 years, may extend to 85 years, based on life expectancy and overall health.
- Stop screening if life expectancy is <10 years.
- In CFAP and AFAP, screen for extracolonic manifestations: thyroid cancer, desmoid tumors, and gastroduodenal polyposis (every 6 months to 5 years).
- In families, lifetime screening for mutation carriers:
  - In CFAP: with sigmoidoscopy or colonoscopy, every 1 to 2 years starting at age of 10 to 11 years
  - In AFAP and MAP: with colonoscopy, every 1 to 2 years starting at age of 18 to 20 years
- After colorectal surgery, surveillance of the rectum (every 6 to 12 months) or pouch (every 6 months to 5 years) is indicated.
- First-degree relatives of patients with JPS require screening by colonoscopy and upper endoscopy after age 12 years.
- Genetic evaluation is recommended for any patient with >10 adenomas cumulatively over lifespan (3).

DIET

Low-fat, high-fiber diet (insufficient evidence)

PATIENT EDUCATION

Importance of colonoscopy as a screening tool

PROGNOSIS

- Regression or no change in size, more with small hyperplastic polyps and with patients on NSAIDs
- Recurrence: Juvenile polyps recur in 45% of children with multiple polyps and 17% with solitary polyps.
- Risk factors for colon cancer:
  - Polyp pathology
    - Adenomatous
    - Serrated
    - With high-grade dysplasia
    - With >25% villous histology
    - Polyp size >1 cm in diameter
    - Polyps located in proximal colon
    - >3 polyps
- Recurrence rates <10% postpolypectomy
- Ineffective endoscopic resection of precancerous lesions results in lingering cancer.

COMPLICATIONS

- Polyps: progression to cancer
- Polypectomy: bleeding 2–11%, perforation 0–1%, higher with endoscopic submucosal dissection
- Colonoscopy: complications related to anesthesia and procedure itself

REFERENCES

1. Shaukat A, Kahi CJ, Burke CA, et al. ACG clinical guidelines: colorectal cancer screening 2021. *Am J Gastroenterol*. 2021;116(3):458–479.
2. Kotula AE, Korde YV, Oyler HJ, et al. Colorectal polyps: pathophysiology, malignant potential, and advancements in therapeutic strategies. *Med Oncol*. 2025;42(8):287. doi:10.1007/s12032-025-02861-8.
3. Gupta S, Lieberman D, Anderson JC, et al. Recommendations for follow-up after colonoscopy and polypectomy: a consensus update by the US Multi-Society Task Force on Colorectal Cancer. *Gastrointest Endosc*. 2020;91(3):463–485.e5.

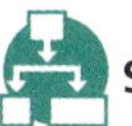

SEE ALSO

Colon Cancer; Rectal Cancer

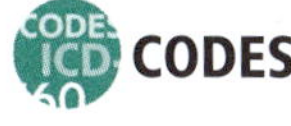

CODES

ICD10

- K63.5 Polyp of colon
- D12.6 Benign neoplasm of colon, unspecified
- K51.40 Inflammatory polyps of colon without complications

CLINICAL PEARLS

- Colonoscopy is the gold standard for diagnosing polyps. Colonoscopy should begin at age 45 years for average-risk individuals.
- Biopsy small hyperplastic polyps to differentiate adenomatous and serrated polyps.
- Use of NSAIDs and calcium is associated with decreased incidence and recurrence of polyps.
- The progression of disease from normal mucosa to polyp to carcinoma takes years.

COMMUNITY ACQUIRED METHICILLIN-RESISTANT *STAPHYLOCOCCUS AUREUS* (CA-MRSA) SKIN INFECTIONS

Morris K. Taylor, MD • Andrew Lutzkanin, MD

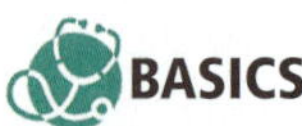

BASICS

DESCRIPTION

- Community-acquired methicillin-resistant *Staphylococcus aureus* (CA-MRSA) has unique properties that allow the organism to cause skin and soft tissue infections (SSTIs) in healthy hosts:
  - CA-MRSA has a different virulence and disease pattern than hospital-acquired MRSA (HA-MRSA).
- CA-MRSA infections generally impact patients who have not been recently (<1 year) hospitalized or had a medical procedure (e.g., dialysis, surgery, catheters).
- Incidence of CA-MRSA increased in the United States from 2000 until 2010 to 2013 when it plateaued for adults and decreased for children.
- CA-MRSA typically causes mild to moderate SSTIs (abscesses, furuncles, and carbuncles).
- Severe or invasive CA-MRSA disease is less frequent but can include:
  - Osteomyelitis
  - Sepsis
  - Septic thrombophlebitis
  - Necrotizing fasciitis
  - Necrotizing pneumonia with abscesses
- HA-MRSA can still cause SSTIs in the community.
- System(s) affected: skin, soft tissue

EPIDEMIOLOGY

- Predominant age: all ages, generally younger
- Predominant sex: women > men

Incidence

- SSTI incidence for adult ambulatory care peaked in 2010 at 35 per 1,000 population and has since plateaued.
- SSTI incidence for pediatric ambulatory care visits peaked in 2011 at 26 per 1,000 population, decreasing to 13 per 1,000 in 2015.
- The incidence of MRSA-related hospitalizations decreased from 2010 to 2014.
- Among people who inject drugs, the incidence of MRSA-related skin abscesses is increasing. Patients should receive substance misuse disorder care and be linked with syringe exchange programs.

Prevalence

- Local epidemiology patterns vary.
- 25–30% of U.S. population colonized with *S. aureus*; up to 7% are colonized with MRSA.
- CA-MRSA isolated in ~60% of SSTIs presenting to emergency departments (range 15–74%).
- CA-MRSA accounts for up to 75% of all community staphylococcal infections in children.

ETIOLOGY AND PATHOPHYSIOLOGY

- First noted in 1980; current epidemic began in 1999. The USA300 clone is predominant.
- CA-MRSA is distinguished from HA-MRSA by:
  - Lack of a multidrug-resistant phenotype
  - Presence of exotoxin virulence factors
  - Type IV staphylococcal cassette cartridge (contains the methicillin-resistant gene *mecA*)

Genetics

Staphylococcal cassette chromosome mec (SCCmec) IV element and Panton-Valentine leukocidin genes appear to relate to invasive disease/abscess formation.

RISK FACTORS

~50% of patients have no obvious risk factor. Recognized risk factors include:

- Antibiotic use in the past month, particularly cephalosporins and fluoroquinolones
- Abscess; reported "spider bite"
- Skin trauma
- Intravenous (IV) or intradermal drug use, HIV infection
- Hemodialysis catheter presence, history of MRSA infection
- Close contact with a similar infection; children, particularly in daycare centers
- Resident in long-term care facility, competitive athletes, incarceration

GENERAL PREVENTION

- Colonization (particularly of the anterior nares) is a risk factor for subsequent *S. aureus* infection. It is unclear whether this is similar for CA-MRSA. Oropharyngeal and inguinal colonization are equally prevalent.
- CA-MRSA is transmitted easily through environmental and household contact.
- CDC guidance for prevention of MRSA in athletes: https://www.cdc.gov/mrsa/prevention/athletes.html

COMMONLY ASSOCIATED CONDITIONS

Many patients are otherwise healthy.

DIAGNOSIS

HISTORY

- Review risk factors.
- "Spider bite" is commonly confused with MRSA—patients often report a history of spider bite.
- Prior CA-MRSA skin infection
- Risk factors alone cannot rule in or rule out a CA-MRSA infection.

PHYSICAL EXAM

- Abscess, sometimes with surrounding cellulitis. Nonsuppurative cellulitis is a much less common presentation of CA-MRSA.
- Erythema, warmth, tenderness, swelling, fluctuance; folliculitis, pustular lesions; tissue necrosis

DIFFERENTIAL DIAGNOSIS

SSTIs due to other organisms

DIAGNOSTIC TESTS & INTERPRETATION

Initial Tests (lab, imaging)

- Wound cultures establish definitive diagnosis. Culture a purulent lesion if there are systemic signs of illness or if the patient is immunocompromised (1)[B].
- Susceptibility testing; many labs use oxacillin instead of methicillin.
- "D-zone disk-diffusion test" evaluates for inducible clindamycin resistance if CA-MRSA is resistant to erythromycin.
- Ultrasound may help identify abscesses versus a non-drainable phlegmon; evidence suggests abscesses shallower than 0.4 cm may not need incision and drainage (I&D) (2).
- Look for fascial plane edema on CT or MRI if necrotizing fasciitis is suspected. *Do not delay* surgical intervention to obtain imaging in such cases.

Diagnostic Procedures/Other

(I&D) for purulent lesions; needle aspiration not recommended (1); an effective alternative to I&D is the loop drainage technique.

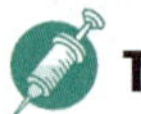

TREATMENT

- For purulent infections, surgical drainage for abscesses, wound culture, and narrow-spectrum antimicrobials
- Use antibiotics active against HA-MRSA for patients with abscesses if no response to initial antibiotic treatment, impaired host defenses, or systemic inflammatory response syndrome (SIRS) and hypotension (1).
- Packing may not improve outcomes. Moist heat may work for small abscesses.
- Extended antibiotic coverage for CA-MRSA is not warranted for nonsuppurative cellulitis.
- Consider decolonization (nasal mupirocin and chlorhexidine washes) in patients with recurrent infections.
- Most CA-MRSA infections are localized SSTIs and do not require hospitalization or vancomycin.
- Base initial antibiotic coverage on local CA-MRSA prevalence and individual risk factors.
- CDC guidance: https://www.cdc.gov/mrsa/media/pdfs/FlowChart-Poster-P.pdf

GENERAL MEASURES

- Modify therapy based on culture and susceptibility.
- Treat underlying conditions that may predispose susceptibility to bacterial infection (e.g., tinea pedis).
- Restrict contact (e.g., sports competition) if wound cannot be covered.
- Elevate affected area.

MEDICATION

ALERT

Studies have shown a role for narrow-spectrum antibiotics in addition to surgical drainage. Clindamycin or trimethoprim/sulfamethoxazole (TMP/SMX) for abscesses <5 cm results in improved cure rates at 7 to 14 days (number needed to treat is 7 to 14).

First Line

Antibiotics for CA-MRSA SSTIs: 7- to 14-day course (depends on severity and clinical response):

- TMP/SMX: DS (160 mg TMP and 800 mg of SMX) 1 to 2 tablet(s) PO q12h; children, 8 to 12 mg/kg/day PO of trimethoprim component in 2 divided doses
- Doxycycline or minocycline: 100 mg PO q12h; children, >8 years of age and <45 kg, 2 to 5 mg/kg/day PO in 1 to 2 divided doses, not to exceed 200 mg/day; >8 years of age and >45 kg, use adult dosing; taken with a full glass of water

- Clindamycin: 300 to 450 mg PO q6h; children, 30 to 40 mg/kg/day PO in 3 divided doses; taken with full glass of water; check D-zone test in erythromycin-resistant, clindamycin-susceptible *S. aureus* isolates (a positive test indicates induced resistance—choose a different antibiotic).
- CA-MRSA is resistant to β-lactams (including oral cephalosporins and antistaphylococcal penicillins) and often macrolides, azalides, and quinolones.
- Although most CA-MRSA isolates are susceptible to rifampin, this drug should *never* be used as a single agent because of concerns for resistance. The role of combination therapy with rifampin in CA-MRSA SSTIs is not clearly defined.
- There has been increasing resistance to clindamycin, both initial (~33%) and induced.
- Although CA-MRSA isolates are susceptible to vancomycin, oral vancomycin cannot be used for CA-MRSA SSTIs due to limited absorption.

Second Line

Treat severe CA-MRSA SSTIs requiring hospitalization and HA-MRSA SSTIs using:

- Vancomycin: generally, 1 g IV q12h (30 mg/kg/day IV in 2 divided doses); children: 40 mg/kg/day IV in 4 divided doses; vancomycin-like antibiotics that require only 1 or 2 doses are also available.
- Linezolid: 600 mg IV/PO q12h; children, uncomplicated: <5 years of age, 30 mg/kg/day IV/PO in 3 divided doses; 5 to 11 years of age, 20 mg/kg/day IV/PO in 2 divided doses; >11 years of age, use adult dosing; children, complicated: birth to 11 years of age, 30 mg/kg/day IV/PO in 3 divided doses; for older children, use adult dosing.
  - Linezolid seems to be more effective than vancomycin for treating people with SSTIs, but current studies have high risk of bias.
- Clindamycin: 600 mg IV q8h; children, 10 to 13 mg/kg/dose IV q6–8h up to 40 mg/kg/day
- Daptomycin: 4 mg/kg/day IV; children, 1 to <2 years of age, 10 mg/kg IV once daily; 2 to 6 years of age, 9 mg/kg IV once daily; 7 to 11 years of age, 7 mg/kg IV once daily; 12 to 17 years of age, 5 mg/kg IV once daily; ≥18 years of age, adult dosing
  - Do not use if pulmonary involvement.
- Ceftaroline: 600 mg IV q12h; children, 0 (gestational age ≥34 weeks and postnatal age ≥12 days) to <2 months, 6 mg/kg IV q8h; 2 months to <2 years of age, 8 mg/kg IV q8h; ≥2 years to <18 years of age and ≤33 kg, 12 mg/kg IV q8h; ≥2 years to <18 years of age and >33 kg, 400 mg IV q8h *or* 600 mg IV q12h; ≥18 years of age, adult dosing

Pediatric Considerations

- Tetracyclines are not recommended for patients age <8 years for CA-MRSA (in contrast with their position as treatment of choice in tickborne rickettsial diseases).
- TMP/SMX is not recommended for patients aged <2 months.
- Daptomycin is not recommended in pediatric patients <1 year of age (risk of neuromuscular, and/or nervous system side effects).
- Daptomycin dosage adjustment for pediatric patients with renal impairment has not been established.
- Ceftaroline dosage adjustment for pediatric patients with CrCl ≤50 mL/min/1.73 m^2 has not been established.

Pregnancy Considerations

- Tetracyclines are contraindicated.
- TMP/SMX not recommended in 1st or 3rd trimester

Geriatric Considerations

A recent review notes no prospective trials in this age group and recommends use of general adult guidelines.

ISSUES FOR REFERRAL

Consider consultation with infectious disease specialist if: Refractory CA-MRSA infection; plan to attempt decolonization.

SURGERY/OTHER PROCEDURES

Concern for serious SSTIs (including necrotizing fasciitis) mandates prompt surgical evaluation.

ADMISSION, INPATIENT, AND NURSING CONSIDERATIONS

- Consider admission if:
  - Systemically ill; extensive soft tissue involvement; comorbidities that may delay or complicate resolution of SSTI; immunocompromised status; failure to improve despite appropriate oral antibiotic therapy
  - Presence of SSTI complications (sepsis, necrotizing fasciitis) and comorbidities
- Alternatives to inpatient admission include observation units and outpatient parenteral antimicrobial therapy (OPAT) in carefully selected cases.
- Nursing: contact precautions
- If admitted for IV therapy, assess the following before discharge:
  - Afebrile for 24 hours; clinically improved; able to take oral medication
  - Has adequate social support and is available for outpatient follow-up

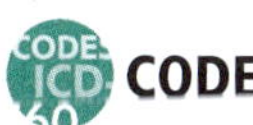

ONGOING CARE

Patients who present with IV drug use should be effectively connected to ongoing substance use disorder care.

FOLLOW-UP RECOMMENDATIONS

Patient Monitoring

For outpatients: promptly return for care with systemic symptoms, worsening local symptoms, or failure to improve within 48 hours; consider a follow-up within 48 hours of initial visit to assess response and review culture.

PATIENT EDUCATION

- Cover draining wounds with clean, dry bandages.
- Clean hands regularly with soap and water or alcohol-based gel; hot soapy shower daily
- Do not share items that may be contaminated (including razors or towels). Clean clothes, towels, and bed linens.
- CDC MRSA education: https://www.cdc.gov/mrsa/about/index.html

PROGNOSIS

In outpatients, improvement should occur within 48 hours.

COMPLICATIONS

- Necrotizing pneumonia or empyema (after an influenza-like illness); necrotizing fasciitis
- Sepsis syndrome; pyomyositis and osteomyelitis
- Disseminated septic emboli; endocarditis

REFERENCES

1. Stevens DL, Bisno AL, Chambers HF, et al; for Infectious Diseases Society of America. Practice guidelines for the diagnosis and management of skin and soft tissue infections: 2014 update by the Infectious Diseases Society of America. *Clin Infect Dis*. 2014;59(2):e10–e52.
2. Howarth K, Thoppil J, Salazar GA. Emergency department management of cellulitis and other skin and soft-tissue infections. *Emerg Med Pract*. 2022;24(5):1–24.

ADDITIONAL READING

- Hindy JR, Haddad SF, Kanj SS. New drugs for methicillin-resistant *Staphylococcus aureus* skin and soft tissue infections. *Curr Opin Infect Dis*. 2022;35(2):112–119. doi:10.1097/QCO.0000000000000800.
- Kao CM, Fritz SA. Infection prevention-how can we prevent transmission of community-onset methicillin-resistant *Staphylococcus aureus*? *Clin Microbiol Infect*. 2025;31(2):166–172. doi:10.1016/j.cmi.2024.01.004.

CODES

ICD10

- A49.02 Methicillin resis staph infection, unsp site
- A41.02 Sepsis due to Methicillin resistant Staphylococcus aureus
- J15.212 Pneumonia due to Methicillin resistant Staphylococcus aureus

CLINICAL PEARLS

- Incise and drain abscesses and send purulent material for culture and sensitivity.
- Local susceptibility patterns of CA-MRSA should guide empiric antibiotic treatment.
- Expect clinical improvement within 48 hours.
- TMP/SMX; doxycycline and clindamycin remain first-line oral agents for uncomplicated CA-MRSA infections.

COMPLEMENTARY AND ALTERNATIVE MEDICINE

Kelley V. Lawrence, MD, NABBLM-C • Mark L. Higdon, DO, FAAFP • Katherine Haga, DO

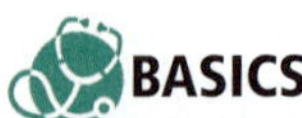

BASICS

DESCRIPTION

Complementary and alternative medicine (CAM) are systems, practices, and products that are not typically part of mainstream medical care. "Complementary" practices are used alongside standard treatments, while "alternative" therapies are used in place of conventional medicine. Integrative medicine is the coordinated combination of complementary medicine with conventional medicine. Functional medicine aims to create personalized interventions for patients based on consideration of each patient's genetics, environmental, and lifestyle influences. CAM modalities often emphasize lifestyle medicine/strategies (which focuses on prevention and treatment of chronic diseases through behavioral modifications) and take a complete biopsychosocial approach to care. Of note, most CAM modalities fall outside of the western medical paradigm and therefore the evidence for these treatments in a standard randomized controlled study format is limited.

- Common examples:
  - Meditation, mindfulness, relaxation
  - Yoga, qigong, tai chi
  - Specialized diets
  - Herbal and dietary supplements
  - Massage
  - Osteopathic manipulative therapy
  - Chiropractic therapy
  - Acupuncture (including needling, moxibustion, cupping), acupressure
  - Ayurvedic medicine, East Asian medicine, naturopathic medicine
  - Biofeedback (including heart rate variability, thermal, EEG, EMG)
- Common reasons patients choose CAM:
  - Additive therapy to address issues not covered by conventional medical treatment
  - Conventional medicine has been unsuccessful in fully addressing the ailment.
  - Preventative health care and/or a desire for a more holistic/natural/noninvasive approach to well-being
  - Concern about medication or treatment side effects
  - Cultural or familial belief systems

EPIDEMIOLOGY

- Approximately 36.7% of adults in the United States reported using at least one form of CAM in 2022, increased from 19.2% in 2002.
- CAM is more commonly used by women and those with higher education levels.
- CAM is most frequently used to treat musculoskeletal issues; 59–90% of patients claim that the use of alternative therapy helped their chronic pain.

Prevalence

An estimated 60–70% of North Americans have tried at least one form of CAM.

COMMONLY ASSOCIATED CONDITIONS

Acute/chronic pain, osteoarthritis, fibromyalgia, insomnia, fatigue, cancer-related symptoms and treatment side effects, headaches, irritable bowel syndrome, depression/anxiety, low libido, weight loss, asthma, eczema, tinnitus, autoimmune disease, PMS

DIAGNOSIS

HISTORY

- Patient's beliefs, goals, and expectations
- Patient's attitudes and experiences with conventional and alternative medical treatments
- Impact of medical condition on patient's life
- Nutritional habits, exercise regimen, sleep hygiene
- Social interactions, support system, mood, spirituality
- Environmental exposures, air, food, and water quality
- All drugs being taken, including prescription drugs, vitamins, herbals, supplements, and over-the-counter medications

PHYSICAL EXAM

- Focused physical exam based on patient presentation
- Skin, hair, and nails assessment may suggest nutritional or metabolic issues.
- Tongue analysis can indicate digestive and systemic health issues.
- Pulse diagnosis can provide insight to the body's internal state of balance.
- If indicated, osteopathic structural exam: Observe gait and posture; screen for somatic dysfunctions, focusing on tissue texture changes, asymmetry, motion restriction, and tenderness.

DIAGNOSTIC TESTS & INTERPRETATION

- Diagnostic testing often evaluates for imbalances and overall well-being rather than fully manifested pathologies.
- Functional lab markers like food sensitivity tests (IgG antibodies or ELISA), micronutrient assessment, genomic and nutrigenomic testing, detailed stool analyses, and salivary or urine hormone panels
- Bioelectrical impedance analysis to assess body composition
- Heart rate variability can provide insight into the body's ability to adapt to stress.
- Consider PHQ-9, and GAD-7 for behavioral health evaluation.
- Testing for inflammatory markers, vitamin deficiencies, endocrine and/or metabolic imbalances

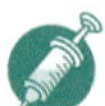

TREATMENT

Variable quality evidence supports the safety and efficacy of:

- Cancer-related fatigue (CRF)
- Back pain: chiropractic therapy, OMT, massage therapy
- Nausea, including that associated with chemotherapy: ginger
- Migraine prophylaxis: petasites (butterbur extract), riboflavin, CoQ10, magnesium
- Migraine treatment: OMT and acupuncture (1)[C]
- Anxiety, depression, and stress: music therapy, meditation, mindfulness-based stress reduction, yoga, massage therapy, relaxation techniques, acupuncture, exercise, light therapy (2)[C]
  - Combining acupuncture with antidepressants showed higher remission rates compared to antidepressant monotherapy (3)[C].
- Fatigue: qigong, acupuncture, ginseng (2)[C]
- PMS
- Lactation

ISSUES FOR REFERRAL

- Patient perception of medical professional stigma towards CAM
- Minimal provider education and training in CAM
- Confirm certification and training of CAM providers when referring or recommending CAM to a patient.

ADDITIONAL THERAPIES

- CRF: tai chi; qigong and cognitive behavioral therapy
- Anxiety:
  - Omega-3 fatty acids 1 to 2 g combined EPA and DHA
  - Ashwagandha (*Withania somnifera*) 300 mg PO bid
  - Passionflower (*Passiflora incarnata*) 500 mg dried extract
  - Lavender (*Lavandula angustifolia*) 80 mg Silexan capsule
  - Magnesium glycinate 200 to 400 mg
- Migraines:
  - Magnesium glycinate, citrate, oxide, or L-threonate 500 mg QHS
  - Riboflavin 200 mg PO BID with meals (can take 3 months for effect)
  - CoQ10 150 to 300 mg daily
- Cognitive impairment in patients with dementia: Gingko (*Ginkgo biloba*) 240 mg PO daily
- Depression:
  - St. John's wort (*Hypericum perforatum*) 300 mg PO up to TID
  - 5-HTP 150 to 300 mg PO daily
  - SAMe 200 mg PO BID
  - Omega-3 combined EPA and DHA 1 g PO daily

- Adjunctive therapies for depression:
  - Light therapy: 10,000 lux for 30 minutes in the early morning
  - Exercise: 30-minute moderate intensity 3 times/week
  - Yoga: 2 to 4 sessions weekly
- Insomnia:
  - Valerian root can improve sleep quality and reduce sleep latency.
  - Progressive muscle relaxation
  - Light therapy to regulate sleep-wake cycle
  - Melatonin (2 mg taken 1 to 2 hours before bedtime)
- Premenstrual syndrome:
  - Acupuncture, yoga, exercise, magnesium and calcium have been shown to be effective in reducing menstrual pain and PMS symptoms.
  - Chaste tree (Vitex) 250 to 500 mg powdered herb daily
- Lactation:
  - For increasing milk supply:
    - Fenugreek 1 to 6 g/day (capsule) or 1 to 2 g TID as a tea
    - Silymarin 420 mg/day in divided doses
  - For decreasing milk supply: peppermint, parsley, sage orally; cabbage leaves applied topically

Geriatric Considerations

- *Ginkgo biloba* can help improve cognition in patients with dementia.
- Incorporating integrative medicine into palliative care may be beneficial.
- Tai chi and yoga may reduce the risk/fear of falls and improve mobility in the elderly.
- Gentle chair yoga, as well as massage, acupuncture, and Reiki may be beneficial for fatigue in elderly cancer patients.

Pediatric Considerations

- Carob bean juice and preparations including *Matricaria chamomilla* and apple pectin were shown to significantly reduce the duration of diarrhea.
- Probiotics have shown efficacy in gastrointestinal disorders and eczema.
- Peppermint oil can decrease the duration, frequency, and severity of pain in children suffering from undifferentiated functional abdominal pain.
- Mindfulness and yoga can improve anxiety, stress, and reduce ADHD symptoms.
- Different fennel preparations were found to be useful in treating infantile colic.
- An RCT found saffron to be as effective as methylphenidate in the short-term treatment of ADHD in children.
- Iron is a leading cause of accidental poisoning in children <6 years of age.

ONGOING CARE

FOLLOW-UP RECOMMENDATIONS

Maintain contact and share records between primary care provider and CAM providers.

Patient Monitoring

When discussing current medication regimen, ask specifically for over-the-counter and herbal supplements.

PATIENT EDUCATION

- The National Center for Complementary and Integrative Health: https://nccih.nih.gov/
- The Cleveland Clinic: Complementary Medicine: What Is It, Types & Health Benefits (https://clevelandclinic.org)
- Osher Center for Integrative Health: patient educational resources (https://www.fammed.wisc.edu/integrative/resources/)
- Downloadable phone app: About Herbs from Memorial Sloan Kettering Cancer Center

COMPLICATIONS

- Patients may delay seeking medical care or consider replacement of curative conventional treatment.
- Ginkgo, goldenseal, and St. John's wort account for most reported herb–drug interactions.
- Herbs with possible adverse effects:
  - Black cohosh (*Actaea racemosa*) may reduce the effectiveness of statins.
  - Ginkgo (*Ginkgo biloba*) can increase bleeding time.
  - Goldenseal (*Hydrastis canadensis*) interferes with many prescription medications.
  - Licorice (*Glycyrrhiza* spp.) may deplete serum potassium with long term use.
  - Senna (Cassia senna) depletes serum potassium.
  - St. John's wort (*Hypericum perforatum*) induces CYP3A4 pathway, increasing drug metabolism including cyclosporine, tacrolimus, warfarin, protease inhibitors, theophylline, venlafaxine, digoxin, oral contraceptives.
  - Wormwood (*Artemisia absinthium*) can elevate serotonin level, raise blood pressure.
  - Yohimbe (*Pausinystalia yohimbe*) may elevate blood pressure.

REFERENCES

1. Florczyk S, Elliott T, Lawrence K, et al. Headache treatment options. *J Am Board Fam Med*. 2024;37(4):737–744. doi:10.3122/jabfm.2023.230450R1.
2. Berman S, Mischoulon D, Naidoo U. Complementary medicine and natural medications in psychiatry: a guide for the consultation-liaison psychiatrist. *Psychosomatics*. 2020;61(5):508–517.
3. Gartlehner G, Dobrescu A, Chapman A, et al. Nonpharmacologic and Pharmacologic treatments of adult patients with major depressive disorder; a systematic review and network meta-analysis for a clinical guideline by The American College of Physicians. *Ann Intern Med*. 2023;176(2):196–211.

ADDITIONAL READING

- American Osteopathic Association. Tenets of Osteopathic Medicine. https://osteopathic.org/about/leadership/aoa-governance-documents/tenets-of-osteopathic-medicine
- Rakel D. *Integrative Medicine*. 5th ed. Philadelphia, PA: Elsevier; 2022.
- Urits I, Schwartz RH, Orhurhu V, et al. A comprehensive review of alternative therapies for the management of chronic pain. *Eur J Pain Therapy*. 2021;10(2):415–431.

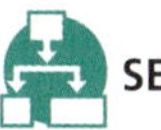

SEE ALSO

- Natural Medicines Database for herb–drug interactions (https://naturalmedicines.therapeuticresearch.com/)
- ConsumerLab.com (https://www.consumerlab.com/) and US Pharmacopeia (https://www.usp.org/) for dietary supplement quality and safety reviews
- Environmental Working Group (https://www.ewg.org/) for safety of supplements, water, and personal care products

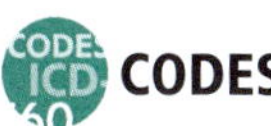

CODES

ICD10

Z76.89 Persons encountering health services in other specified circumstances

CLINICAL PEARLS

- CAM allows clinicians to take a holistic approach to health, by focusing on treating the patient, and not just the disease.
- Outcomes of CAM are best measured in terms of the patient's symptom relief, satisfaction, and functional status.
- OMT, chiropractic therapy, massage, tai chi, and acupuncture may help with chronic pain.
- Yoga, light therapy, and exercise are helpful for depression.
- Peppermint oil can help with abdominal pain associated with IBS.
- Ginkgo, goldenseal, and St. John's wort account for most herb–drug interactions.
- Tai chi can help with balance and reduce the risk of falls in the elderly. Tai chi is also an effective adjuvant therapy for fibromyalgia.

COMPLEX REGIONAL PAIN SYNDROME

Dennis E. Hughes, DO, FACEP

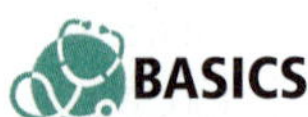

BASICS

DESCRIPTION

- Complex regional pain syndrome (CRPS) is a pain syndrome that can be chronic and debilitating. It is divided into two subtypes and can result in significant physical and psychosocial short- and long-term disability. Most cases are a result of a physical insult to an extremity such as trauma or surgery. The lack of a dermatomal distribution (i.e., the pain is regional) distinguishes CRPS from other pain syndromes.
  - Type I: no nerve injury (reflex sympathetic dystrophy [RSD])
  - Type II: associated with a demonstrable nerve injury (causalgia)
- Synonyms: traumatic erythromelalgia; Weir Mitchell causalgia; causalgia; RSD; posttraumatic neuralgia; sympathetically maintained pain

EPIDEMIOLOGY

- Peak age: 50 to 70 years
- Predominant gender: female > male (3:1, 60–81%), with postmenopausal women affected disproportionally.
- Rarely seen in pediatrics—cases in this age group predominantly involve lower extremities in females.
- Recent studies found 3.8% occurrence after wrist fracture and 7% occurrence after intra-articular ankle fracture—both independent strong risk for CRPS. Fractures and sprains are associated ~60% of cases, the remaining 40% have less precise or no recognized inciting event. Upper extremities are more commonly involved.
- CRPS is more prevalent in patients that report higher than commonly expected pain in early phases of trauma. Latency depends on normal injury recovery time—prolonged pain (>2 months) after injury hints at diagnosis.

Incidence

Incidence of 5.46 to 26.2/100,000 for type I and 0.82/100,000 for type II in the United States

ETIOLOGY AND PATHOPHYSIOLOGY

- Poorly understood activation of abnormal sympathetic reflex that lowers pain threshold. The process is multifactorial and involves both central and peripheral nervous systems. It can progress in a variable fashion over time.
  - Increased excitability of nociceptive neurons in the spinal cord; "central sensitization"
  - Exaggerated responses to normally nonpainful stimuli (hyperalgesia, allodynia)
  - The exaggerated inflammatory response results in afferent neurons releasing increased amounts of neuropeptides.
- Type II is associated with physical injury to nerve. This represents a minority of cases.
- Emerging information reveals CNS changes (functional, anatomic, biochemical) in addition to spinal level changes. Increased levels of immunomodulators suggest autoimmune component. The lack of a definitive pathophysiologic mechanism has led to suggest that CRPS is a "functional neurologic syndrome."

Genetics

No known genetic pattern

RISK FACTORS

- Minor or severe trauma (upper extremity fracture—particularly distal radius noted in a significant number of those with CRPS)
- Surgery (particularly carpal tunnel release)
- Lacerations, burns, frostbite
- Casting/immobilization after extremity injury
- Penetrating injury (case reports of CRPS developing after snakebites)
- Polymyalgia rheumatica
- Myocardial infarction, cerebral vascular accident
- Reports of CRPS development after "innocuous" events such as IV catheters and IM injections

GENERAL PREVENTION

- Early mobilization and avoiding prolonged immobilization has proven benefit in reducing incidence of CRPS.
- One study of wrist fractures found that addition of 500 mg/day of vitamin C lowered rates of CRPS.
- There is evidence that limiting use of tourniquets, liberal regional anesthetic use, and ensuring adequate perioperative analgesia can reduce the incidence of CRPS-I.

COMMONLY ASSOCIATED CONDITIONS

- Serious injury to bone and soft tissue
- Herpes zoster postherpetic neuralgia results from partial or complete damage to afferent nerve pathways that occurs in a dermatomal distribution.
- Signal exists for patients having comorbid painful conditions or psychiatric diagnosis at increased risk of developing CRPS.

DIAGNOSIS

Unprovoked pain is the hallmark of the condition, and the diagnosis of CRPS is excluded by the existence of conditions that would otherwise account for the degree of symptoms (1). Budapest clinical diagnostic criteria can aid in establishing diagnosis:

- Continuing pain which is disproportionate to any inciting event
- At least one symptom in three of the four following categories:
  - Sensory: hyperalgesia and/or allodynia
  - Vasomotor: skin, temperature, color asymmetry
  - Sudomotor/edema: edema, sweating changes, or sweating asymmetry
  - Motor/trophic: decreased range of motion or motor dysfunction and/or trophic changes (hair, nail, skin)
- Must display one sign at the time of the evaluation in two or more of the following:
  - Sensory: hyperalgesia (to pinprick) or allodynia (to light touch, pressure, or joint movement)
  - Vasomotor: evidence of temperature, skin, color asymmetry
  - Sudomotor/edema: evidence of edema or sweating changes or asymmetry
  - Motor/trophic: decreased range of motion; motor dysfunction; or trophic changes in hair, nails, skin
- There is no other diagnosis that explains the signs and symptoms.

HISTORY

The patient commonly complains of persistent burning pain, swelling, and poor function after extremity injury. The severity of the preceding injury may vary from fracture to relatively minor trauma.

PHYSICAL EXAM

- The affected extremity appears swollen with erythematous, shiny skin with brittle nails, and reduced hair.
- The patient usually exhibits limited range of motion—both active and passive in the affected extremity.

DIFFERENTIAL DIAGNOSIS

- Infection
- Hypertrophic scar
- Neuroma
- CNS tumor or syrinx
- Deep vein thrombosis or thrombophlebitis
- Thoracic outlet syndrome
- Connective tissue disorder
- Factitious

DIAGNOSTIC TESTS & INTERPRETATION

The diagnosis of CRPS does not require any specific testing—it is a clinical diagnosis. It is a symptom-based diagnosis of exclusion. Testing is performed to rule out other potential etiologies of clinical symptoms.

Initial Tests (lab, imaging)

- CBC, erythrocyte sedimentation rate (ESR)
- Plain radiographs may show patchy demineralization within 3 to 6 weeks of onset of CRPS that are more pronounced than would be seen from disuse alone.
- Three-phase bone scanning has varying sensitivity but is most accurate for support of the diagnosis when there is diffuse activity (especially on phase 3).
- Bone density

Diagnostic Procedures/Other

- Electromyelography (EMG) shows nerve injury with type II CRPS.
- Sudomotor function testing (resting sweat testing, resting skin temperature, quantitative sudomotor axon reflex testing; all related to increased autonomic activity of the affected limb)

Test Interpretation

- Partial or complete damage to afferent nerve pathways and probably reorganized central pain pathways
- Nerves most commonly involved are median and sciatic.
- Atrophy in affected muscles
- Incomplete nerve plexus lesion

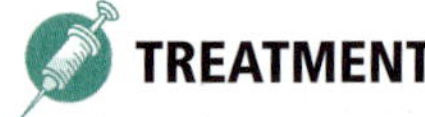

TREATMENT

GENERAL MEASURES

Discourage maladaptive behaviors (pain medication seeking, secondary gain). Principal of functional restoration is a stepwise and multidisciplinary approach. Early and aggressive mobilization seems to lessen the duration. Avoidance of opiates cannot be overemphasized (2).

MEDICATION

First Line

NSAIDs are recommended early in course but have mixed support in literature. The following have literature support of a suggestive benefit in treatment of CRPS-I:

- Corticosteroids (prednisone 30 mg/day × 2 to 12 weeks with taper) are the only class of drugs that have direct clinical trial support early in the course. A recent retrospective case review found that patients showed significant improvement with various measurable physical parameters after treatment with prednisolone (30 mg starting dose tapering by 5 mg every 3 days for a total of 3 weeks treatment). Prolonged use of corticosteroids has no proven benefit and may contribute to osteopenia.
- Gabapentin 600 to 1,800 mg/day for 8 weeks following diagnosis
- DMSO 50% cream applied to affected extremity up to 5 times daily
- *N*-Acetylcysteine 600 mg TID
- Bisphosphonates (alendronate) at 40 mg/day (however, optimal dose uncertain)
- Nifedipine 20 mg/day showed benefit early in the course of the condition.
- Tricyclic and heterocyclic antidepressants are commonly used because they have benefit in managing neuralgia as well the associated depression present in many patients with CRPS.

ISSUES FOR REFERRAL

- After 2 months of the illness, psychological evaluation generally is indicated to identify and treat any comorbid conditions. Depressive symptoms frequently develop.
- Physical therapy and occupational therapy early for guided motor and mirror therapy

ADDITIONAL THERAPIES

Type I

- Physical and occupational therapy (beneficial to the overall prognosis for recovery) and should be initiated early in the course of treatment
  - "Mirror therapy" has shown good results.
  - Case reports of patients responding favorably to passive ROM treatment under sedation followed by multiple physical therapy sessions
- Transcutaneous nerve stimulation
- Psychotherapy
- Use of sub-dissociative (0.2 to 0.5 mg/kg) infusions of ketamine has shown some promise, but effects seem to be time limited; systemic literature review failed to find and high-quality support for ketamine treatment.

SURGERY/OTHER PROCEDURES

- Type II responds more favorably to nerve-directed treatment.
  - Sympathetic blocks
  - Cervicothoracic or lumbar sympathectomies have little data to support their use and should be used judiciously and after all other therapies have failed.
- Anesthetic blockade (chemical or surgical) of sympathetic nerve function
  - Transient relief suggests that chemical or surgical sympathectomy will be helpful.
  - Little in the way of quality clinical trials exist to support local sympathetic blockage as the gold standard of therapy.
- IV regional sympathetic block with guanethidine or reserpine by pain specialist or anesthetist
- Transcutaneous electric nerve stimulation (controversial)
- Inject myofascial painful trigger points.
- Dorsal root ganglion (DRG) stimulation higher rate of success than spinal cord stimulation in recent comparative study; more specific target as DRG home of soma of sensory neurons
- Intrathecal analgesia
- Amputation as a last resort in severe cases, with patients reporting improved quality of life
- Single case study of topical 5% lidocaine revealed significant pain reduction and improved range of motion and function.
- Osteopathic manipulation (case report literature)

COMPLEMENTARY & ALTERNATIVE MEDICINE

- Vitamin C (500 mg/day) may help to prevent CRPS in those with wrist fracture.
- Cognitive behavioral therapy
- Acupuncture
- Hypnosis and guided imagery has been successful in improving pain scores.
- Relaxation training (alternate muscle relaxing and contracting)
- Biofeedback
- Whirlpool baths

ADMISSION, INPATIENT, AND NURSING CONSIDERATIONS

Only for proposed surgical therapy

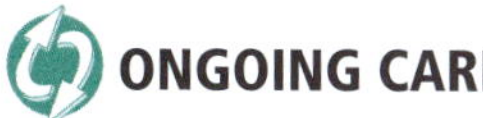

ONGOING CARE

FOLLOW-UP RECOMMENDATIONS

Weekly, to monitor progress and initiate additional modalities as needed

PATIENT EDUCATION

- Counsel to remain active physically.
- Reflex Sympathetic Dystrophy Syndrome Association: https://rsds.org/; 203-877-3790

PROGNOSIS

Most improve with early treatment, but symptoms may be lifelong if there is limited response to initial treatments.

COMPLICATIONS

- Depression
- Disability
- Opioid dependence

REFERENCES

1. Harden RN, McCabe CS, Goebel A, et al. Complex regional pain syndrome: practical diagnostic and treatment guidelines, 5th edition. *Pain Med*. 2022;23(Suppl 1):S1–S53. doi:10.1093/pm/pnac046.
2. Abd-Elsayed A, Stark CW, Topoluk N, et al. A brief review of complex regional pain syndrome and current management. *Ann Med*. 2024;56(1):2334398. doi:10.1080/07853890.2024.2334398.

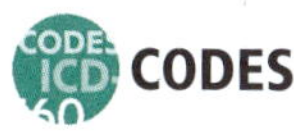

CODES

ICD10

- G90.52 Complex regional pain syndrome I of lower limb
- G90.523 Complex regional pain syndrome I of lower limb, bilateral
- G56.4 Causalgia of upper limb

CLINICAL PEARLS

- A pain syndrome disproportioned to injury
- Pain control and early mobility are the key to recovery.
- Avoid use of opiate analgesics.
- Use a multidisciplinary approach.

C

CONDYLOMATA ACUMINATA

Victoria Shepard, MD • Parth J. Amin, DO, MMS

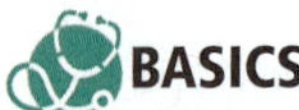

BASICS

- Condylomata acuminata are soft, skin-colored, fleshy lesions (commonly called genital warts) that are caused by human papillomavirus (HPV). The flat, papular, or pedunculated warts can appear singly or in groups (a single wart is a "condyloma"; multiple warts are "condylomas" or "condylomata"); typically appear on the anogenital skin (penis, scrotum, introitus, vulva, perianal area); and may occur in the anogenital tract (vagina, cervix, rectum, urethra, anus) or outside the genital tract (conjunctival, nasal, oral, and laryngeal warts).
- System(s) affected: skin/exocrine, reproductive, occasionally respiratory

DESCRIPTION

Pediatric Considerations

Consider sexual abuse if seen in children, although children can be infected by other means (e.g., transfer from wart on another child's hand or prolonged latency period). Consider screening for STDs.

Pregnancy Considerations

- Warts often grow larger, increase in number, and become more friable in pregnancy (1). They can regress spontaneously after delivery.
- Neonatal infection is thought to occur through vertical transmission. Incidence remains controversial.
- Few documented cases of infant laryngeal papillomas due to HPV transmission at the time of delivery; although rare, the condition is life-threatening. Cesarean section solely to prevent transmission of HPV to the newborn is not indicated (1).
- Cervical infections are a risk factor for preterm birth.
- HPV vaccination is contraindicated in pregnancy.
- Treatment during pregnancy is somewhat controversial because it can be incomplete, but accepted treatments are trichloroacetic acid (TCA), cryotherapy, electrocautery, or surgical excision.
- The safety of sinecatechins, podophyllin, and podofilox in pregnant women has not been established, and these agents are not recommended for use during pregnancy (1). Imiquimod appears to pose low risk but should be avoided until more data are available.

EPIDEMIOLOGY

- HPV types 6 and 11 are associated with 90% of condylomata acuminata. Types 16, 18, 31, 33, and 35 may be found in warts and may be associated with high-grade intraepithelial dysplasia in immunocompromised states such as HIV.
- Highly contagious; incubation period may be from 1 to 8 months. Initial infections may go unrecognized.
- Predominant age: 15 to 30 years
- Predominant sex: 1:1 male to female
- Most infections are transient and clear spontaneously within 2 years.

Incidence

After the introduction of the HPV vaccine, the incidence of condyloma acuminata decreased by more than 50% for females under 24 and similarly for males (1).

Prevalence

- Most common viral sexually transmitted infection (STI) in the United States. Most sexually active men and women will have acquired a genital HPV infection, usually asymptomatic, at some time.
- Estimated 6.2 million Americans become infected with genital HPV each year.
- Peak prevalence in ages 17 to 33 years
- 10–20% of sexually active women may be actively infected with HPV. Studies in men suggest a similar prevalence.
- Pregnancy and immunosuppression favor recurrence and increased growth of lesions.

ETIOLOGY AND PATHOPHYSIOLOGY

HPV is a circular, double-stranded DNA molecule. There are >120 HPV subtypes. HPV types 6 and 11 cause 90% of genital warts and do not cause anogenital cancers. Rarely oncogenic strains of HPV exist alongside HPV 6 and 11 (1).

RISK FACTORS

- High risk sexual activity
- History of STI
- Immunosuppression (particularly HIV)
- Cigarette smoking
- Use of oral contraceptives
- Radiation therapy

GENERAL PREVENTION

- HPV vaccination is for prevention of HPV infections and HPV-associated cancers.
- The Advisory Committee on Immunization Practices (ACIP) recommends routine vaccination at age 11 or 12 years for females (since 2006) and males. Vaccination can start at as early as 9 years old.
  - A 2-dose schedule (0, 6 to 12 months) will have efficacy equivalent to a 3-dose schedule (0, 1 to 2, 6 months) if the HPV vaccination series is initiated before the 15th birthday.
  - For any immunocompromised patient regardless of age, a 3-dose schedule (0, 1 to 2, and 6 months) is recommended (1).
  - The 9-valent HPV (9vHPV; Gardasil 9) vaccine protects against the two most common HPV serotypes (types 6 and 11, which cause most anogenital warts) and the two most cancer-promoting types (16 and 18) as well as 31, 33, 45, 52, and 58.
- Use of condoms is partially effective, although warts may be easily spread by lesions not covered by a condom (e.g., 40% of infected men have scrotal warts.)
- After treatment, encourage abstinence until treatment is completed.

COMMONLY ASSOCIATED CONDITIONS

- Cervical dysplasia; >90% of cervical cancer associated with HPV types 16, 18, 31, 33, and 35
- 60% of oropharyngeal and anogenital squamous cell carcinomas are associated with HPV.
- STIs (e.g., gonorrhea, syphilis, chlamydia), AIDS

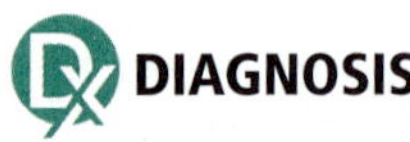

DIAGNOSIS

HISTORY

- Sexual history, condom use, and other lifestyle topics
- Most warts are asymptomatic, but symptoms include pruritus, burning, redness, pain, bleeding, vaginal discharge, and large warts may cause obstructive symptoms in the anus (with defecation) or vaginal canal (with intercourse or childbirth).

PHYSICAL EXAM

- Lesions often have a typical rough, warty appearance with multiple fingerlike projections but may be soft, sessile, and smooth.
- Large lesions are cauliflower-like and may grow to >10 cm.
- Most common sites: penis, vaginal introitus, and perianal region
- May be seen anywhere on the anogenital epithelium or in the anogenital tract
- Warts often occur in clusters.

DIFFERENTIAL DIAGNOSIS

- Condylomata lata (flat warts of syphilis), lichen planus
- Normal sebaceous glands, seborrheic keratosis
- Molluscum contagiosum, keratomas, micropapillomatosis
- Scabies, skin tags, melanocytic nevi, psoriasis
- Vulvar intraepithelial neoplasia, squamous cell carcinoma (Bowen disease)

DIAGNOSTIC TESTS & INTERPRETATION

- Diagnosis is usually clinical, made by unaided visual examination of the lesions; biopsy if needed.
- Acetowhitening test: Subclinical lesions can be visualized by applying moistened gauze soaked with 5% acetic acid (vinegar) to the affected area for 5 minutes. Using a 10× hand lens or colposcope, warts appear as tiny white papules. A shiny white appearance of the skin represents foci of epithelial hyperplasia (subclinical infection), but because of low specificity, the CDC recommends against routine use of this test to screen for HPV mucosal infection.

Initial Tests (lab, imaging)

- Usually not required for diagnosis; serologic tests for syphilis may be helpful to rule out condylomata lata.
- Other testing for STIs; cervical and/or anal pap smear may be indicated.

Follow-Up Tests & Special Considerations

Because squamous cell carcinoma may resemble or coexist with condylomata, biopsy may be considered for lesions refractory to therapy.

Diagnostic Procedures/Other

Colposcopy, antroscopy, anoscopy, and urethroscopy may be required to detect anogenital tract lesions.

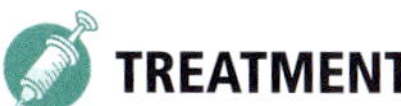

TREATMENT

GENERAL MEASURES

- Approximately, 30% resolve spontaneously in 4 months.
- Change therapy if no improvement after three treatments, clearance not complete after six treatments, or therapy's duration or dosage exceeds manufacturer's recommendations.
- Appropriate screening/counseling of partners
- HIV considerations: Treatment of external genital warts should not be different for HIV-infected persons.
  - Lesions may be larger or more numerous.
  - May not respond as well to therapy as immunocompetent persons

MEDICATION

First Line

- No single therapy for genital warts is ideal for all patients or clearly superior to other therapies.
- Recommendations for external genital warts, patient applied:
  - Podofilox (Condylox) (1)[C],(2)[A]: may be the most effective topical (2)[A]; Antimitotic action; apply 0.5% solution or gel to warts twice daily (allowing to dry) for 3 consecutive days at home followed by 4 days of no therapy; may repeat up to 4 total cycles; maximum of 0.5 mL/day or area <10 cm^2.
  - Imiquimod (Aldara) (1)[C],(2)[A]: immune enhancer; self-treatment with a 5% cream applied once daily at bedtime 3 times weekly until warts resolve for up to 16 weeks. Wash off with soap and water 6 to 10 hours after application. Imiquimod has been noted to weaken condoms and diaphragms; therefore, patients should refrain from sexual contact while the cream is on the skin.
  - Sinecatechins (Veregen) (1): immune enhancer and antioxidant, extract from green tea; apply a 0.5-cm strand of ointment 3 times daily for up to 16 weeks. Do not wash off after.
- Recommendations for external genital warts, provider applied:
  - Cryotherapy: liquid nitrogen applied to warts for two bursts of approximately 10 seconds (or whatever time is needed to freeze the wart without extension significantly deep or lateral to the wart) with thawing in between; usually requires 2 to 3 weekly sessions (1)[C],(2)[A]
  - TCA: 80% solution; apply only to warts; powder/talc to remove unreacted acid; repeat in office at weekly intervals; ideal for isolated lesions in pregnancy (1)[C],(2)[A]
- Recommendations for cervical warts: cryotherapy, surgical removal, TCA or bichloroacetic acid (BCA); for exophytic cervical warts: biopsy to exclude high-grade squamous intraepithelial lesion (HSIL) prior to starting treatment (1)[C],(2)[A]
- Recommendations for vaginal warts: cryotherapy, surgical removal, TCA or BCA 80–90% (1)[C],(2)[A]
- Recommendations for urethral meatus warts: cryotherapy or surgical removal (1)[C],(2)[A]
- Recommendations for anal warts: cryotherapy, TCA or BCA 80–90%, or surgery; specialty consultation for intra-anal warts (1)[C],(2)[A]

Pregnancy Considerations

Cryotherapy, surgery, or TCA; medications contraindicated in pregnancy: podophyllin, podophyllotoxin, sinecatechins, interferon, and imiquimod (1)[C],(2)[A]

Second Line

Podophyllin resin, intralesional interferon, photodynamic therapy, topical cidofovir (1)[C],(2)[A]

ISSUES FOR REFERRAL

Referrals should be considered for large condyloma impacting urinating, stooling or sexual function; intravaginal, cervical, or anal condylomata that require surgical excision

SURGERY/OTHER PROCEDURES

- Larger warts may require surgical excision, laser treatment, or electrocoagulation (including infrared therapy). Precaution: Laser treatment may create smoke plumes that contain HPV. CDC recommendation is for the use of a smoke evacuator no >2 inches from the surgical site. Masks are recommended; N95 is the most efficacious.
- Intraurethral, external (penile and perianal), anal, and oral lesions can be treated with fulgurating CO_2 laser. Oral or external penile/perianal lesions can also be treated with electrocautery or surgery.

ONGOING CARE

FOLLOW-UP RECOMMENDATIONS

No restrictions, except for sexual contact

Patient Monitoring

- Patients should be seen every 4 weeks until lesions resolve.
- Patients should follow up 3 months after completion of treatment.
- Persistent warts require biopsy.
- Sexual partners require monitoring.

PATIENT EDUCATION

- Discuss transmission. Provide information on HPV, STI prevention, and condom use.
- Explain to patients that it is difficult to know how or when a person acquired an HPV infection; a diagnosis in one partner does not prove sexual infidelity in the other partner.
- Emphasize the need for appropriate pap smears.

PROGNOSIS

- Asymptomatic infection persists indefinitely.
- It is unknown if current therapies for anogenital warts reduce the underlying HPV infection and treatment has not clearly been shown to decrease transmissible infectivity.
- Warts may clear with treatment or resolve spontaneously. However, recurrences are frequent, particularly in the first 3 months, and may necessitate repeated treatments.

COMPLICATIONS

- Malignant change: Progression of condylomata to cancer rarely, if ever, occurs, although squamous cell carcinoma may coexist in larger warts.
- Urethral, vaginal, or anal obstruction from treatment
- The prevalence of high-grade dysplasia and cancer in anal canal is higher in HIV-positive than in HIV-negative patients, probably because of increased HPV activity.

REFERENCES

1. Workowski KA, Bachmann LH, Chan PA, et al. Sexually transmitted infections treatment guidelines, 2021. *MMWR Recomm Rep*. 2021;70(4):1–187.
2. Barton S, Wakefield V, O'Mahony C, et al. Effectiveness of topical and ablative therapies in treatment of anogenital warts: a systematic review and network meta-analysis. *BMJ Open*. 2019;9(10):e027765. doi:10.1136/bmjopen-2018-027765.

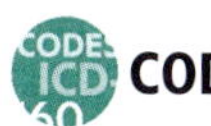

CODES

ICD10

A63.0 Anogenital (venereal) warts

CLINICAL PEARLS

- The majority of sexually active men and women will have acquired a genital HPV infection, usually asymptomatic, at some time.
- No single therapy for genital warts is ideal for all patients or clearly superior to other therapies.
- HPV vaccine is effective in preventing HPV infection, particularly if administered prior to the onset of engaging in sexual activity. Gardasil is approved and recommended for use in males and females aged 9 to 45 years.

CONJUNCTIVITIS, ACUTE

Virginia J. Van Duyne, MD

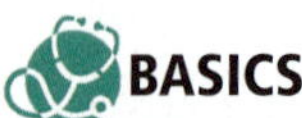

BASICS

Conjunctivitis (pink eye) is common in primary care; affects both children and adults; defined as an inflammation of the mucosal lining (conjunctiva) of the eye globe(s) and eyelid(s); it can be classified as infectious or noninfectious. Infectious causes can be bacterial or viral, and noninfectious causes can be caused by allergies, toxins, or nonspecific irritations of the membrane.

DESCRIPTION

Inflammation of the bulbar and/or palpebral conjunctiva of <4 weeks' duration

Geriatric Considerations

- Suspect bacterial, autoimmune, or irritative process.
- If purulent, risk of bacterial cause increases with age and long-term care facility residence, with age >65 years and bilateral lid adherence. Risk for bacterial infection is >70%.

Pediatric Considerations

Neonatal conjunctivitis may be gonococcal, chlamydial, irritative, or related to dacryocystitis. Children <5 years of age more likely to have bacterial involvement than adults, but most self-resolve in 2 to 5 days.

EPIDEMIOLOGY

- Bacterial conjunctivitis is more common in children and viral conjunctivitis is more common in adults.
- Infectious conjunctivitis occurs equally in females and males.

Incidence

- 1% of all visits in ambulatory primary care annually
- Affects 2% of the population (6 million individuals) annually in the United States

ETIOLOGY AND PATHOPHYSIOLOGY

- Viral
  - Adenovirus (common cold), coxsackievirus ; enterovirus (acute hemorrhagic conjunctivitis); herpes simplex; herpes zoster or varicella; measles, mumps, or influenza; SARS-CoV-2
- Bacterial
  - *Staphylococcus aureus*, MRSA, or *Staphylococcus epidermidis*; *Streptococcus pneumoniae*; *Haemophilus influenzae* (children); *Moraxella catarrhalis*
  - *Pseudomonas* spp. or anaerobes (contact lens users); *Acanthamoeba*-contaminated contact lens solution (rare; ~30 cases/year in United States); *Neisseria gonorrhoeae*; *Chlamydia trachomatis*: gradual onset 1 to 4 weeks
- Allergic
  - Hay fever, seasonal allergies, atopy
- Nonspecific
  - Irritative: topical medications, wind, dry eye, UV light exposure, smoke, chlorine
  - Autoimmune: Sjögren syndrome, etc.

RISK FACTORS

- History of contact with infected persons; sexually transmitted disease (STD) contact: gonococcal, chlamydial, syphilis, or herpes; contact lenses: pseudomonal or acanthamoeba keratitis
- Epidemic bacterial (streptococcal) conjunctivitis reported in school settings, epidemic adenoviral transmission in crowded settings, MRSA in long-term care facilities

GENERAL PREVENTION

- Wash hands frequently.
- Eyedropper technique: while eye is closed and head back, several drops over nasal canthus and then open eyes to allow liquid to enter; never touch tip of dropper to skin or eye.

COMMONLY ASSOCIATED CONDITIONS

Viral infection (e.g., common cold); possible sexually transmitted infection

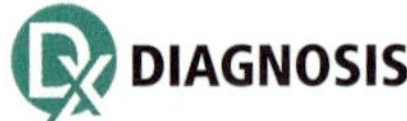

DIAGNOSIS

HISTORY

ALERT

Red flag: any decrease in visual acuity is not consistent with conjunctivitis alone; must document normal vision for diagnosis of true isolated conjunctivitis

- Viral: contact or travel; may start with one eye and then both; if herpetic, recurrences or vesicles on skin
- Bacterial: difficult to distinguish from viral; assume bacterial in contact lens wearer, unless cultures are negative. If recent STD or concurrent urethritis, suspect chlamydia/gonococcus. Gonococcal conjunctivitis is sight threatening and requires immediate ophthalmologic referral. Nursing home residents may have MRSA conjunctivitis—obtain culture.
- Allergic: itching, atopy, seasonal, dander
- Irritative: feels dry, exposure to wind, tear-film deficit may persist 30 days after acute conjunctivitis, chlorine from pools; medications: atropine, aminoglycosides, iodide, phenylephrine, antivirals among others
- Foreign body: Redness may persist 24 hours after removal.

PHYSICAL EXAM

- Must document normal visual acuity
- General: common to all types of conjunctivitis
  - Conjunctival injection; foreign body sensation
  - Eyelid sticking or crusting, discharge; normal visual acuity and pupillary reactivity
- Viral
  - Pharyngitis, preauricular lymphadenopathy and/or recent infectious contact make viral diagnosis much more likely.
  - Hemorrhagic coxsackievirus, adenoviral epidemics seen in health care facilities and community
  - Severe viral: herpes simplex or zoster burning sensation, rarely itching; unilateral, dermatomal distribution herpetic skin vesicles in zoster; palpable preauricular node
- Bacterial (non-STD): may be epidemic
  - Mucopurulent discharge or concomitant otitis media makes bacterial diagnosis twice as likely (1)[A].
  - Conjunctival chemosis/edema
  - If contact lens user, must rule out pseudomonal (or other bacterial) keratitis. If long-term care resident, culture to rule out MRSA.
- Bacterial: gonococcal (or meningococcal) hyperacute infection
  - Rapid onset 12 to 24 hours; severe purulent discharge; chemosis/conjunctival/eyelid edema
  - Rapid growth of superior corneal ulceration. Preauricular adenopathy; signs of STDs (chlamydia, GC, HIV, etc.)
- Allergic
  - Itching predominant, chemosis, edema; seasonal or animal dander allergies
- Nonspecific irritative
  - Dry eyes, intermittent redness, chemical/drug exposure
  - Foreign body: may have redness and discharge 24 hours after removal
- Cornea should be clear and without fluorescein uptake. Cloudy or ulcerated cornea signifies keratitis; consult ophthalmologist. Evert lid to inspect for foreign bodies.
- Skin: Look for herpetic vesicles, nits on lashes (lice), scaliness (seborrhea), lid inflammation (blepharitis, rosacea, or styes).
- Limbal flush at corneal margin if uveitis; if pupil is irregular (i.e., penetrating foreign body), emergent referral is warranted.
- Discharge on lid margin but no conjunctival injection: blepharitis

DIFFERENTIAL DIAGNOSIS

- Punctate keratitis due to prolonged contact lens wear
- Uveitis (iritis, iridocyclitis, choroiditis): limbal flush, hazy anterior chamber, and decreased visual acuity
- Acute glaucoma (emergency): headache, corneal clouding, poor visual acuity; corneal ulcer, keratitis, or foreign body: lesions or tear-film deficits on fluorescein exam; dacryocystitis: tenderness and swelling over tear sac (below medial canthus)
- Scleritis and episcleritis: red injected vessels radially oriented; pingueculitis: inflammation of a yellow nodular or wedge-like area of chronic conjunctival degeneration (pinguecula)
- Ophthalmia neonatorum: neonates in the first 2 days of life (gonococcal; 5 to 12 days of life): chlamydial, herpes simplex virus (HSV); blepharitis: Lid margins are inflamed producing itching, scale, or discharge but no conjunctival injection.
- Giant fornix syndrome: an elderly patient with recurrent or chronic conjunctivitis due to accumulation of infected material in enlarged fornices

DIAGNOSTIC TESTS & INTERPRETATION

Usually not needed initially for most common causes; culture swab if STD suspected, severe symptoms, contact lens user, or failed prior treatment.

Diagnostic Procedures/Other

Fluorescein exam to rule out corneal ulcer, herpes zoster, or abrasion; remove small, superficial foreign bodies with irrigation or moistened swab. Refer cases of prolonged symptoms (>7 days).

TREATMENT

GENERAL MEASURES

Viral conjunctivitis does not require antibiotics, most resolve spontaneously. Clean external eyelid with wet cloth up to 4 times per day. Stop use of contact lenses as long as eye is red. Eye patching is not beneficial.

MEDICATION

First Line

- Viral (nonherpetic)
  - Artificial tears for symptomatic relief; vasoconstrictor/antihistamine (e.g., naphazoline/pheniramine) QID for severe itch; may consider topical antibiotic (see bacterial below) if return to daycare requires treatment
  - Adenoviral conjunctivitis course may be shortened by one dose 5% povidone-iodine
- Viral (herpetic) (with ophthalmology consultation)
  - Ganciclovir gel: 0.15%, 5 times per day for 7 days
  - Acyclovir: PO 400 mg 5 times per day for HSV; 800 mg for zoster for 7 days
- Bacterial (nonsexually transmitted): 3 days of cool compresses to allow for self-resolution before starting antibiotic reduces unnecessary antibiotic use.
  - If preferred, may use topical antibiotics (NNT 7 by day 6) (immediate topical antibiotics may allow for earlier return to school for some children)
- Preferred agents: polymyxin B-trimethoprim solution 1 gtt 6 times per day for 5 to 7 days; erythromycin ophthalmic ointment: 1/2 inch 2 to 4 times per day for 5 days
- Alternatives: bacitracin ophthalmic ointment (over the counter [OTC]): apply 3 to 4 times per day for 5 to 7 days; fractional exhaled nitric oxide ophthalmic ointment; apply 0.5 inch to lid 4 times daily for 5 to 7 days; azithromycin 1% ophthalmic drops 1 drop 2 times daily for 2 days, then 1 drop daily for 5 days
- Bacterial (gonococcal)
  - Neonates: hospitalize for IV ceftriaxone or cefotaxime
  - Adults: ceftriaxone: 1 g IM as single dose and topical bacitracin ophthalmic ointment 0.5 inch QID; neonates 25 to 50 mg/kg IV or IM, not to exceed 125 mg, as a single dose; chlamydia in neonates requires oral erythromycin: 50 mg/kg/day divided q6h PO for 14 days, max 3 g/day
- Allergic and atopic: OTC medications are efficacious, no definitive evidence favoring one over another, cost varies widely.
  - Ketotifen (Zaditor, Alaway, and other OTC): 0.25% 1 drop 2 times per day; cetirizine (Zerviate): 0.24% 1 drop 2 times per day; olopatadine (Pataday, Patanol): 0.1% 1 drop 2 times per day or 0.2% 1 drop daily; cromolyn (Opticrom): 4% 1 drop 4 times per day; naphazoline (Vasocon-A, Naphcon-A, Opcon-A, Visine-A: OTC) 1 drop 4 times a day; azelastine (Astelin): 0.05% 1 drop 2 times per day; nedocromil (Alocril): 2% 1 drop 2 times per day
  - Alcaftadine (OTC): 0.25% 1 drop daily; epinastine 0.05% 1 drop 2 times per day; bepotastine (Bepreve) 1.5% 1 drop 2 times per day (2)
- Contraindications: Steroids are *not* beneficial in treatment of bacterial keratitis. Any topical steroid requires baseline and periodic specialist's exam. Topical immune modulators (tacrolimus, cyclosporine) are for specialist use only.
- Precautions
  - Do not allow dropper to touch the eye; case reports of eye irritation from gentamicin in infants, moxifloxacin in adults, sulfacetamide in allergic individuals

Second Line

- Viral and allergic: numerous OTC products, oral montelukast 10 mg daily
- Bacterial: second line (quinolones used as postoperative or for known resistant organisms)
  - Ofloxacin: 0.3% 1 gtt QID for 7 days; ciprofloxacin: 0.3% 1 gtt QID for 7 days
  - Levofloxacin: 0.3% 1 gtt QID for 7 days; azithromycin: 1.5% BID for 3 days

ISSUES FOR REFERRAL

Refer to ophthalmology for decreased visual acuity, suspected herpetic keratitis/contact lens–related conjunctivitis or immunocompromised (HIV), symptoms of acute angle closure glaucoma (fixed pupil, severe headache with nausea, ciliary flush). Suspicion for hyperacute bacterial conjunctivitis (gonococcal); refer for prolonged symptoms or worsening over 7 days (concern for severe adenoviral keratitis).

COMPLEMENTARY & ALTERNATIVE MEDICINE

Usually benign and self-limited; saline flushes, cool compresses, and similar treatments help.

ADMISSION, INPATIENT, AND NURSING CONSIDERATIONS

Acute gonococcal conjunctivitis (or very rare case of meningococcal conjunctivitis) requires inpatient treatment with ceftriaxone 50 mg/kg IV every day (pediatric), 1 g IM for one (adult) along with ophthalmologic consultation.

ONGOING CARE

FOLLOW-UP RECOMMENDATIONS

- If not resolved within 5 to 7 days, reconsider diagnosis or consult specialist.
- Allergic conjunctivitis (noncontagious) should return to school with doctor's note.

Patient Monitoring

Patient should follow up in 1 day if any worsening.

PATIENT EDUCATION

- No contact lenses until eyes are fully healed (~1 week). Discard current contact lenses.
- Adenovirus may persist on surfaces up to 28 days; practice soap hand washing and hypochlorite surface wipe use.
- Discard old eye makeup, especially mascara. Cool, moist compresses can ease irritation and itch.

PROGNOSIS

- Viral: 5 to 10 days of symptoms for pharyngitis with conjunctivitis, 2 weeks with adenovirus
- Herpes simplex: 2 to 3 weeks of symptoms
- Most common bacterial—*H. influenzae*, *Staphylococcus*, *Streptococcus*: self-limited; 74–80% resolution within 7 days, whether treated or not

COMPLICATIONS

- Corneal scars
- Corneal ulcers or perforation

REFERENCES

1. Johnson D, Liu D, Simel D. Does this patient with acute infectious conjunctivitis have a bacterial infection?: the rational clinical examination systematic review. *JAMA*. 2022:327(22):2231–2237.
2. Labib BA, Chigbu DI. Therapeutic targets in allergic conjunctivitis. *Pharmaceuticals (Basel)*. 2022;15(5):547.

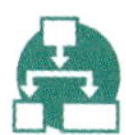

SEE ALSO

- Rhinitis, Allergic
- Algorithm: Eye Pain

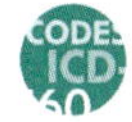

CODES

ICD10

- H10.30 Unspecified acute conjunctivitis, unspecified eye
- H10.33 Unspecified acute conjunctivitis, bilateral
- H10.32 Unspecified acute conjunctivitis, left eye

CLINICAL PEARLS

- Conjunctivitis does *not* cause decreased acuity or photophobia. If visual acuity is decreased or if there is pain with ocular movements, consider more serious ophthalmic disorders.
- Culture discharge in all *contact lens wearers and nursing home residents*. Consider referral, discard current lenses, and use spectacles for visual correction until eyes are fully healed.
- Antibiotics are of no value in viral conjunctivitis (most cases of infectious conjunctivitis).
- Cool compresses for 3 days before using any antibiotic is appropriate for treating conjunctivitis in healthy adults and children >1 month of age.

CONSTIPATION

Joseph Daniel Hogue, MD, MBA • Elizabeth L. Browning, DO • Francis Agama, MD, MS

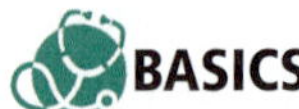

BASICS

- Unsatisfactory defecation characterized by infrequent bowel movements, difficult stool passage, or both.
- Characteristics may include <3 bowel movements a week, hard stools, excessive straining, a sense of incomplete evacuation, abdominal discomfort/bloating, painful bowel movements, and need for manual aid when defecating.

DESCRIPTION

Geriatric Considerations

Consider new-onset constipation after age 50 years a "red flag" for colorectal neoplasms that may require a colonoscopy. Use warm water enemas (instead of sodium phosphate enemas) for impaction in geriatric patients. Sodium phosphate enemas in older adults have been associated with hypotension, volume depletion, EKG changes (prolonged QT interval), and severe electrolyte disturbances.

Pediatric Considerations

Consider Hirschsprung disease in pediatric cases. This accounts for 25% of all newborn intestinal obstructions and can present as milder cases in older children with chronic constipation, abdominal distension, and decreased growth. Hirschsprung has a 5:1 male-to-female ratio and is associated with inherited conditions (e.g., Down syndrome).

Pregnancy Considerations

Constipation is common in pregnancy due to progesterone slowing GI motility, gravid pressure of uterus on colon, iron supplementation, and decreased physical activity.

EPIDEMIOLOGY

- More pronounced in children and elderly
- Predominant sex: female > male (2:1)
- Nonwhites > whites

Incidence

- 2.5 million office visits annually
- 92,000 hospitalizations annually

Prevalence

- 16% of adults >18 years of age, rising to 33% of adults >60 years of age
- 3% of pediatric visits relate to constipation.

ETIOLOGY AND PATHOPHYSIOLOGY

- Defecation reflex can be inhibited by voluntarily contracting the external sphincter or facilitated by straining to contract the abdominal muscles while voluntarily relaxing the anal sphincter. Rectal distention initiates the defecation reflex. The urge to defecate occurs with an increase in rectal pressure. Distention of the stomach also initiates rectal contractions and a desire to defecate (gastrocolic reflex).
- Constipation often runs in families, but no single gene has been identified. Identical twins are known to have higher concordance compared to nonidentical twins.

RISK FACTORS

- Extremes of age
- Female sex
- Polypharmacy
- Sedentary lifestyle or condition
- Low fiber diet and inadequate fluid intake
- Increased stress or history of abuse
- Depression
- Low calorie intake
- Low income and low educational status

GENERAL PREVENTION

High-fiber diet, adequate fluids, exercise, and training to "obey the urge" to defecate

COMMONLY ASSOCIATED CONDITIONS

- General debilitation (disease or aging)
- Dehydration
- Hypothyroidism, metabolic endocrinopathies
- Electrolyte abnormalities: hypokalemia, hypercalcemia
- Myopathies and neuropathies
- History of abdominal or pelvic surgery
- Down syndrome

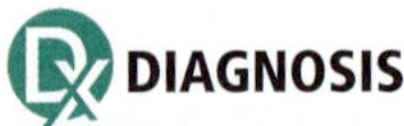

DIAGNOSIS

- Rome criteria (a.k.a. Rome IV criteria)
- Anorectal manometry (ARM)

ALERT

Red flags:

- New onset (especially after age of 50 years)
- Fever
- Nausea/vomiting
- Hematochezia/melena/rectal bleeding
- Unintentional weight loss >10 lb (4.5 kg)
- Change in bowel habits/narrowing diameter of the stool
- Family history of colon cancer or inflammatory bowel disease
- Abdominal pain
- Palpable masses in the abdomen and rectum
- Fatigue
- Iron deficiency anemia
- Neurologic deficits

HISTORY

- Assess onset of symptoms, number of bowel movements per week, straining, completeness of evacuation, and use of manual manipulation.
- Identify red flags; evaluate diet, lifestyle, prescription and OTC medication use; identify reversible causes; ask about history of sexual abuse, opioid use; identify any systemic or neurologic disorders that affect colonic motility.
- Bristol Stool Form Scale—seven categories of consistency (1)
- A diary of dietary intake and bowel patterns may help to identify causative agents, quantify the severity of the constipation, and measure treatment response.
- Rome IV criteria for primary constipation (1):
  - At least two of the following for 12 weeks in the previous 6 months:
    - <3 spontaneous stools per week
    - Straining at least 1/4 of the time
    - Hard stools (Bristol Stool Form Scale 1 to 2) at least 1/4 of time
    - Need for manual assist at least 1/4 of time
    - Sense of incomplete evacuation at least 1/4 of time
    - Sense of anorectal blockage at least 1/4 of time
  - Loose stools rarely seen without use of laxatives
  - Does not meet irritable bowel syndrome (IBS) criteria
  - Although there can be overlap, the history of primary constipation differs from constipation-predominant IBS.
    - In primary constipation, pain and bloating are relieved by adequate defecation. In IBS, pain and bloating predominate and are not readily relieved by defecation.
- Bowel Function Index—for opioid-induced constipation (OIC)
- Assessment tools such as the Constipation Assessment Scale, Constipation Scoring System, and Patient Assessment of Constipation-Symptoms questionnaire could be used to assess severity.

PHYSICAL EXAM

- Vital signs
- Abdominal exam, previous surgical scars, distention, hypoactive bowel sounds, tenderness, and masses
- Gynecologic exam: Evaluate for masses and rectocele.
- External anorectal examination: excoriations, scars, fistulas, fissures, hemorrhoids, rectal prolapse, and anal wink
- Digital rectal exam: Evaluate for structural lesions: masses, stool, fissures, and hemorrhoids; assess for pelvic floor dyssynergia and sphincter tone, strictures as noted by inability to insert, or difficulty inserting finger into anal canal.
- Neurologic exam

DIFFERENTIAL DIAGNOSIS

- Primary constipation (primary problem is within the GI tract) has four subtypes (2).
  - Normal colonic transit time most common subtype; can be difficult to differentiate from constipation-predominant IBS (IBS-C)
  - Slow colonic transit time
  - Pelvic floor/anal sphincter dysfunction (defecatory disorders)
  - Combination pelvic floor/anal sphincter dysfunction and slow transit
- Secondary constipation (outside the GI tract)
  - Endocrine dysfunction
    - Diabetes mellitus, hypothyroidism, hyperparathyroidism
  - Metabolic disorders
    - Chronic kidney disease and electrolyte abnormalities (hypercalcemia, hypokalemia, hypomagnesemia)
  - Mechanical disorders
    - Colonic stricture or obstruction: inflammation, ischemia, postradiation
  - Neurologic disorders
    - Central: multiple sclerosis, spinal cord injuries, Parkinson disease, dementia, traumatic brain injury
    - Peripheral: diabetes, Hirschsprung disease, Chagas disease
  - Myopathy
  - Pregnancy
  - Psychiatric/psychosocial
    - Abuse, anorexia nervosa, depression
  - Congenital
    - Hirschsprung disease/syndrome; hypoganglionosis; congenital dilation of the colon; small left colon syndrome
  - Medication effect
    - Opioids/NSAIDs; tricyclic antidepressants; antipsychotics; antacids (calcium, aluminum)
    - Calcium channel blockers: nifedipine and verapamil

- Iron and multivitamins with iron; diuretics
- Overuse of antidiarrheal medications
- 5-HT3 antagonists: ondansetron
- Antihistamines
- Chemotherapy agents: cyclophosphamide and vincristine

DIAGNOSTIC TESTS & INTERPRETATION

Identify red flags, secondary causes, and reversible conditions. If none present, go to first-line treatment. Routine use of lab studies or imaging, including colonoscopy, is not recommended in the absence of red flags.

Initial Tests (lab, imaging)

- CBC to screen for iron deficiency anemia
- Consider toxicology screen if illicit opioid use is suspected.
- Electrolytes, calcium, creatinine, glucose, and thyroid function testing (TSH) based on history and exam
- If red flags are present and due for colorectal cancer screening, should be referred for a colonoscopy

Diagnostic Procedures/Other

- ARM
- Balloon expulsion testing (BET)
- Surface electromyography
- Barium or magnetic resonance defecography
- Colonic transit time using radio-opaque markers and scintigraphy

Test Interpretation

- ARM and BET are recommended for all refractory cases; if negative, barium or magnetic resonance defecography to evaluate transit time
- Consider trial biofeedback with pelvic floor therapy.

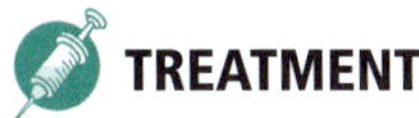

TREATMENT

GENERAL MEASURES

In patients with no known secondary causes, conservative nonpharmacologic treatment is recommended.

- Eliminate medications that cause constipation.
- Increase fluid intake.
- Increase soluble fiber (25 to 30 g/day) in diet.
- Encourage regular defecation attempts after eating.
- Regular exercise and/or increased physical activity

MEDICATION

First Line

Bulking agents (accompanied by adequate fluids) (2)

- Osmotic laxatives
  - Polyethylene glycol (PEG) (MiraLAX) 17 g/day PO dissolved in 4 to 8 oz of beverage (current evidence shows PEG to be superior to lactulose)
  - Lactulose (Chronulac, Enulose) 15 to 60 mL PO QHS (flatulence, bloating, cramping)
  - Sorbitol: 15 to 60 mL PO QHS (as effective as lactulose)
  - Magnesium salts (milk of magnesia): 15 to 30 mL PO once daily; avoid in renal insufficiency.
- Hydrophilic colloids (bulk-forming agents)
  - Psyllium (Konsyl, Metamucil, Perdiem Fiber): 1 tbsp (approximately 3.5 grams fiber) in 8-oz liquid PO daily up to TID
  - Methylcellulose (Citrucel): 1 tbsp (approximately 2 grams fiber) in 8-oz liquid PO daily up to TID
  - Polycarbophil (Mitrolan, FiberCon): 2 caplets (500 mg fiber per tab) with 8-oz liquid PO up to QID
  - Wheat dextrin (Benefiber): 2 tsp (1.5 gram fiber per tsp) up to TID

Second Line

- Stimulants (irritate bowel, causing muscle contraction; usually combined with a softener; work in 8 to 12 hours)
  - Senna/docusate (Senokot-S, Ex-lax, Peri-Colace): 1 to 2 tablets or 15 to 30 mL PO at bedtime
  - Bisacodyl (Dulcolax, Correctol): 1 to 3 tablets PO daily
- Stool softeners (less)
  - Docusate sodium (Colace)
- Suppositories
  - Osmotic: sodium phosphate
  - Lubricant: glycerin
  - Stimulatory: bisacodyl
  - Enemas: saline (Fleet enema)
- Long-term prescription agents
  - Lubiprostone (Amitiza)
  - Prucalopride (Motegrity); increased incidence of suicidal ideation reported in clinical trials
- Guanylate cyclase-C agonists (adult use only)
  - Plecanatide (Trulance): dose: 3 mg PO once daily
  - Linaclotide (Linzess): dose: 145 μg PO once daily; can use lower dose 72 μg once daily
- OIC (1)
- Trial of laxatives first followed by peripherally acting μ-opioid receptor antagonists
  - Methylnaltrexone (Relistor): dose: 38 to <62 kg: 8 mg; 62 to 114 kg: 12 mg SC every other day PRN
  - Naloxegol (Movantik): dose: 12.5 to 25.0 mg PO daily; discontinue other laxatives for 3 days when initiating naloxegol; avoid in patients on strong CYP3A4 inhibitors due to increased naloxegol levels and risk of opioid withdrawal.
  - Naldemedine (Symproic): dose: 0.2 mg PO daily; monitor for opioid withdrawal in patients on strong CYP3A4 inhibitors or P-gp inhibitors.
- Linaclotide (Linzess): dose 145 μg PO once daily; can use lower dose 72 μg once daily
- Prokinetic agents (partial 5-HT4 agonists): cisapride (Propulsid) has been withdrawn due to cardiac side effects; only available via IND protocols; tegaserod (Zelnorm) available for IBS-C; side effects include cardiac events, ischemic colitis and suicidal ideation.

ADDITIONAL THERAPIES

- Biofeedback and/or behavior therapy
- Acupuncture: initial randomized trial effective at 20 weeks; longer term trials needed

SURGERY/OTHER PROCEDURES

- Surgery rarely indicated; sometimes required for anatomic findings (rectocele or enterocoele) and in whom nonsurgical management has been ineffective.
  - Abdominal colectomy and ileorectal anastomosis

ADMISSION, INPATIENT, AND NURSING CONSIDERATIONS

- Toxic megacolon
- Manual disimpaction occasionally required in chronic refractory cases

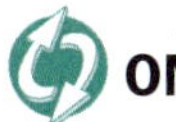

ONGOING CARE

DIET

Increase soluble fiber (bloating and gas can be problematic with insoluble fiber):

- Gradually increase intake to 25 g/day over a 6-week period.
- Oat bran, peas, onions, lentils, beans, seeds, nuts, and fruits- including bananas, apples, and strawberries
- Encourage liberal intake of fluids (1.5 to 2.0 L/day in adults).

PATIENT EDUCATION

- Occasional mild constipation is normal.
- Bowel training: The best time to move bowels is in the morning, after eating breakfast, when the normal bowel transit and defecation reflexes are functioning.

PROGNOSIS

- Occasional constipation responds well to simple measures.
- Habitual constipation can be a lifelong nuisance.
- Patients with neurologic compromise can suffer from obstipation, impaction, and toxic megacolon.
- No evidence for laxative dependence or harm from stimulant use; melanosis coli may develop but it is a benign condition.

COMPLICATIONS

- Volvulus; toxic megacolon
- Acquired megacolon in severe, long-standing cases
- Fluid and electrolyte depletion: laxative abuse
- Rectal ulceration (stercoral ulcer) related to recurrent fecal impaction; anal fissures; rectal prolapse; hemorrhoids

REFERENCES

1. Sadler K, Arnold F, Dean S. Chronic constipation in adults. *Am Fam Physician*. 2022;106(3):299–306.
2. Bharucha AE, Lacy BE. Mechanisms, evaluation, and management of chronic constipation. *Gastroenterology*. 2020;158(5):1232–1249.e3. doi:10.1053/j.gastro.2019.12.034.

ADDITIONAL READING

Staursky D, Shimoga D, Sharma A. Step on the accelerator: modern treatment of constipation. *Curr Opin Gastroenterol*. 2024;40(1):43–49. doi:10.1097/MOG.0000000000000982.

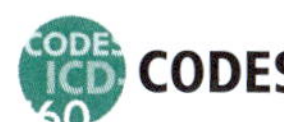

CODES

ICD10

- K59.00 Constipation, unspecified
- K59.01 Slow transit constipation
- K59.09 Other constipation

CLINICAL PEARLS

- Consider new-onset constipation after age 50 years a "red flag" for colorectal neoplasms.
- Consider Hirschsprung disease in cases of newborn/infant constipation.
- In patients with no known secondary causes, conservative nonpharmacologic treatment is recommended.
- Bulking agents and adequate hydration are important first-line steps in management.

CONTRACEPTION

Kristina Gracey, MD, MPH • Zoe Onion, MD

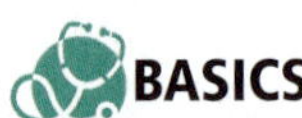

BASICS

DESCRIPTION

Medications or procedures that control timing of pregnancies and prevent unintended pregnancies; options are divided into two major categories: hormonal and nonhormonal.

EPIDEMIOLOGY

Incidence

42% of pregnancies in the United States are unintended. Unintended pregnancies are associated with increased risk of adverse maternal and infant outcomes.

RISK FACTORS

Unintended pregnancy: higher rates among patients ages 18 to 24 years and >40 years, unmarried patients, patients with less than a college education, and minority groups

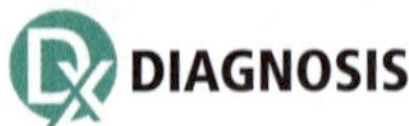

DIAGNOSIS

HISTORY

- Review past medical, family, social, obstetric, and gynecologic histories including menstrual history, prior contraceptive use, and prior sexually transmitted infections (STIs). Screen for hypertension.
- In family history of thrombophilia, consider testing before initiation of estrogen-containing contraception.
- Contraindications: See CDC medical eligibility criteria (MEC) (1) and chart or CDC Contraception app.
  - Estrogen-progestin contraceptives
    - Common absolute: age ≥35 years and smoking ≥15 cigarettes per day, <21 days postpartum, SBP ≥160 mm Hg or DBP ≥100 mm Hg, current/prior venous thromboembolism (VTE), thrombophilia, long-standing/complicated diabetes, ischemic heart disease, systemic lupus, migraine with aura, breast cancer, ESRD, decompensated cirrhosis
    - Common relative: age ≥35 years and smoking <15 cigarettes per day, breastfeeding <42 days postpartum, SBP 140 to 159 mm Hg or DBP 90 to 99 mm Hg (or well-controlled on medications), bariatric surgery, migraines without aura but age ≥35 years, breast cancer history, use of some anticonvulsants including topiramate and lamotrigine, use of rifampin
  - Progestin-only (pill/Depo-Provera/implant): absolute—current breast cancer
    - Common relative (Depo-Provera): heart disease, stroke, lupus, migraine with aura
    - Common relative (implant): liver cancer, unexplained vaginal bleeding
    - Common relative for insertion but do not require discontinuation (implant): ischemic heart disease, stroke, unexplained vaginal bleeding
    - Common relative (pill): bariatric surgery, ischemic heart disease, stroke, unexplained vaginal bleeding, use of some anticonvulsants including topiramate and lamotrigine, use of rifampin
- Levonorgestrel—intrauterine device (IUD)
  - Common absolute: postseptic abortion, postpartum sepsis, current breast cancer, distorted uterine cavity
  - Absolute contraindications for initiation but do not require discontinuation: cervical/endometrial cancer, PID, known untreated chlamydia or gonorrhea infection
  - Common relative: heart disease, lupus
- Copper IUD ("ParaGard," "Miudella")
  - Absolute: same as levonorgestrel IUD, ok to use in breast cancer
  - Absolute contraindications for initiation but not continuation: same as levonorgestrel IUD
  - Relative: thrombocytopenia, solid organ transplant

DIAGNOSTIC TESTS & INTERPRETATION

Initial Tests (lab, imaging)

Consider pregnancy test. Consider testing for gonorrhea and chlamydia prior to IUD insertion; Pap smear if indicated; contraception should not be withheld pending a Pap smear.

TREATMENT

GENERAL MEASURES

Method(s) should be selected based on patient's preference, effectiveness, need for STI prevention, side effects, and contraindications. It is essential to center patient autonomy in this discussion. Offer STI prevention measures to any patients at risk (PrEP, PEP).

MEDICATION

- Estrogen-progestin contraceptives
  - Mechanism of action: suppression of ovulation, thickening of cervical mucus, and endometrial changes
  - Efficacy: failure rate of 9% (approximately 8 pregnancies per 100 patients per year) with typical use and 0.3% with perfect use at 1 year
  - Side effects: irregular bleeding, nausea, headaches, mastalgia, depression; all estrogen-containing methods increase risk of venous thrombosis from ~2 per 10,000 users per year to 7 to 10 per 10,000 users per year (2).
  - Combined oral contraceptives (COCs)
    - COCs most contain ethinyl estradiol (EE) but differ in the amount (10 to 50 μg) and type of progestin; avoid estradiol >35 μg. Possible lower risk of VTE with estradiol 20 μg but not clearly proven. Start low, and escalate if breakthrough bleeding.
    - Dosing: Most have 21 active days and 7 placebo days. Alternatively, active pills can be taken continuously with scheduled withdrawal bleeds.
    - Initiation: recommended: "quick start" (begin pill on the day medication is obtained). Alternative: Begin the pill on the first day of menses or first Sunday. Note: If not starting pill within 5 days of start of menses, backup contraception is recommended for 7 days.
    - Nextstellis (estetrol 14.2 mg, drospirenone 3 mg): new plant-derived estrogen with mixed agonist/antagonist properties; similar efficacy to other COC; expensive (brand only); monitor potassium.
- Weekly hormonal patch: applied transdermally and changed weekly for 3 weeks; no patch worn during week 4 for withdrawal bleeding, unless user prefers fewer yearly periods (continuous cycling)
  - Ortho Evra, Xulane:
    - 20 μg/day EE and 150 μg/day norelgestromin
    - Produces higher serum estrogen levels than oral 20-μg pill (slightly increased risk of VTE)
    - Application site irritation; reduced efficacy in patients >90 kg
  - Twirla:
    - 30 μg/day of EE and 120 μg/day of levonorgestrel
    - Common adverse reactions: application site disorders, nausea, headache, weight gain
    - Contraindicated in patients with a BMI ≥30 kg/m^2; reduced effectiveness in patients with a BMI ≥25 to <30 kg/m^2
  - Vaginal contraceptive ring: Ring is inserted in the vagina and remains in place; adverse reactions: headaches, nausea and vomiting, vulvovaginal mycotic infection, vaginal discharge, UTI
    - NuvaRing: in vagina for 3 weeks followed by 1 week of ring-free interval; may also use continuous cycling for 4 weeks and then immediately replaced with a new ring (off-label)
      - 15 μg/day of EE and 120 μg/day of etonogestrel absorbed via vaginal wall
      - Although systemic exposure to estrogen is about 50% of exposure with COCs, the risk of VTE is similar.
    - Annovera: single ring is cleaned and used for up to 1 year; not adequately evaluated in patients with a BMI of >29 kg/m^2
- Progestin-only birth control
  - Mechanism of action: Primary mechanism is ovulation inhibition with possible secondary benefit from thickening of cervical mucus and thinning of endometrial lining.
  - Progestin-only pills (POPs)
    - Norethindrone 0.35 mg (MicroNor, etc.); efficacy: failure rate of about 0.3% with perfect use, 9% with typical use at 1 year; can be used in some patients with contraindications to estrogen, including (for example) breastfeeding patients; dosing: 1 pill at the same time daily, no placebo days; side effects: irregular/unscheduled bleeding (common)
    - Drospirenone 4 mg (Slynd); efficacy similar to COC; expensive (brand only); progestin with antiandrogen and antimineralocorticoid effect; may be particularly useful for PCOS and other high-androgen conditions; potassium levels may need to be monitored periodically if on another medication that increases potassium; 24 active pills, four placebo per pack; less menstrual irregularity than norethindrone
    - Norgestrel (Opill); first OTC contraceptive pill approved by FDA (2023); dosing: 1 pill at the same time daily, no placebo days; side effects: irregular/unscheduled bleeding (common); pregnancy rate is 2% in trials, likely >7 per 100 patient-years in real-world use.

- Injectable contraceptive (medroxyprogesterone acetate, DMPA) (Depo-Provera); efficacy: failure rate of 0.2% with perfect use, 6% with typical use at 1 year; dosing: one injection every 3 months; contraceptive levels of hormone persist for up to 4 months; side effects: irregular bleeding, weight gain (average of 5 lb per year of use), amenorrhea, depression
- LARCs: IUDs and implantable devices
- Mirena, Liletta, generics (52-mg levonorgestrel-releasing IUD):
  - Primary mechanism of action: produces sterile inflammatory reaction due to foreign body that is toxic to sperm and ova, thickens cervical mucus
  - Efficacy: failure rate of 0.2% with both perfect and typical use at 1 year (1 pregnancy per 400 to 500 users per year)
  - Release: 20 μg/day initially; reduces to 10 μg/day (FDA-approved for 8 years)
  - Safe and recommended in nulliparous patients/teenagers
  - Can be inserted immediately postpartum or immediately following D&C for miscarriage or abortion, although with higher rates of expulsion compared to delayed placement (6 to 10 weeks); may be used as postcoital contraception up to 5 days after intercourse (limited data)
  - Side effects: irregular bleeding for first 3 to 6 months that usually resolves; may see amenorrhea after 1 year
  - Side effect management: Consider NSAIDs, COCs, or POPs for spotting and cramps.
- Kyleena (19.5-mg levonorgestrel-releasing IUD): releases 17.5 μg/day initially; reduced to 7.5 μg/day (approved for 5 years)
- Skyla (13.5-mg levonorgestrel-releasing IUD): smaller insertion tube; more bleeding days than Mirena; release14 μg/day initially; reduces to 5 μg/day (approved for 3 years)
- ParaGard, Miudella (copper IUDs): ParaGard is a standard T-shaped device with more copper; Miudella has a flexible nickel/titanium frame with less copper and may adapt to a wider range of uterine shapes.
  - ParaGard approved for 10 years, effective for longer (especially in patients aged >30 years); Miudella approved for 3 years
  - Primary mechanism of action: produces sterile inflammatory reaction interfering with sperm transport and fertilization of an egg
  - Efficacy: failure rate with typical use at 1 year: 0.7% for ParaGard, 0.94% for Miudella
  - Side effects: increased menstrual bleeding and cramping (common), heavy bleeding (in the first year of use, discontinuation rates related to bleeding problems or pain are 12% for ParaGard users and 8.5% for Miudella)
  - ParaGard may be used as postcoital contraceptive within 120 hours of intercourse (Miudella not approved for this purpose)
- Nexplanon (etonogestrel implant):
  - Mechanism of action: inhibits ovulation
  - Efficacy: failure rate of 0.05% with perfect use, 0.3% with typical use at 1 year (1 pregnancy per 400 to 500 users per year)
  - Dosing: semirigid plastic rod containing 68 mg of etonogestrel; initially 60 to 70 μg/day; subsequently 25 to 30 μg/day
  - FDA-approved for 4 years, evidence-based efficacy to 5 years
  - Inserted only by certified providers, but technique is simple to learn
  - Side effects: menstrual irregularities (very common for 6 to 12 months, may persist for 3 years); if irregular bleeding, consider course of naproxen or exogenous estrogen (estradiol or COCs for 1 to 2 menstrual cycles)
- Emergency contraception: initiated as soon as possible after unprotected intercourse; copper IUD and levonorgestrel-IUD are the most effective, followed by ulipristal, levonorgestrel, and Yuzpe method.
  - Copper and 42-mg levonorgestrel-IUD (Mirena, Liletta) IUD: up to 5 days after intercourse; 0.04–0.19% failure rate
  - Ulipristal acetate (Ella): 30 mg once; selective progesterone modulator, up to 5 days after intercourse 2% failure rate
  - Levonorgestrel: 1.5 mg taken as two 0.75-mg tablets (plan B) or one 1.5-mg tablet (plan B one step); most effective within 72 hours; 1.1–2.4% failure rate; less nausea than "Yuzpe regimen"; available OTC; likely ineffective for people with BMI >30 kg/m^2
  - "Yuzpe regimen" 50 μg/0.25 mg, 2 tablets q12h (4 tablets total); any OCP may be used as long as the dose of estrogen component is ≥100 μg/dose; 3.2% failure rate; *note*: Antiemetic should be given 1 to 2 hours.

ADDITIONAL THERAPIES

- External condoms: failure rate of 2% with perfect use, 18% with typical use at 1 year
- Spermicides: All contain nonoxynol-9; may alter vaginal flora and mucosal barrier; failure rate: 28% with typical use at 1 year; may cause an increased risk of acquiring HIV infection
- Sponge (Today Sponge): Soft foam disk contains nonoxynol-9. Moisten with water before use; effective for 24 hours; must leave in for 6 hours after use; failure rate: 12–24% with typical use
- Diaphragm: latex or silicone dome-shaped device with flexible spring-activated rim, prevents sperm from entering cervix; used with spermicides; failure rate: 12% with typical use, 6% with perfect use at 1 year
- Phexxi: nonhormonal spermicidal prescription contraceptive; indicated as an on demand method of contraception; single-dose applicator vaginally immediately before or up to 1 hour prior to each episode of intercourse; avoid use in patients with a history of recurrent UTIs or urinary tract abnormalities; common side effects: discomfort, mycotic infection, UTI, and bacterial vaginosis; failure rate: 13.7%

SURGERY/OTHER PROCEDURES

Permanent sterilization

- Tubal ligation; failure rate: 0.5% at 1 year or salpingectomy
- Vasectomy; failure rate: 0.15% at 1 year

COMPLEMENTARY & ALTERNATIVE MEDICINE

- Fertility awareness methods: failure rate: 24% at 1 year typical use (~20 pregnancies per 100 patients per year)
- Withdrawal method: failure rate: 22% at 1 year
- Lactational amenorrhea method: effective only if the infant is <6 months old and exclusively breastfeeding, and mother has not resumed regular menses; failure rate: 7% at 1 year typical use

Pediatric Considerations

AAP and ACOG recommend LARCs as first-line agents.

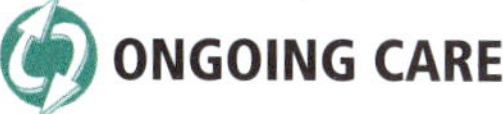

ONGOING CARE

FOLLOW-UP RECOMMENDATIONS

Patient Monitoring

1 to 3 months postinitiation to assess tolerance; consider IUD string-check 1 month after insertion; spontaneous expulsion rate highest in the first month; BP check within 3 months of initiating on estrogen-containing methods

PATIENT EDUCATION

Reproductive Health Access Project: https://www.reproductiveaccess.org/contraception/

COMPLICATIONS

- Estrogen-progestin contraceptives: serious (requires discontinuation): stroke, thromboembolism, hypertension, myocardial infarction, and cholestatic jaundice
- Injectable DMPA: decreased bone mineral density (BMD) if used for ≥2 years; mostly recovers after discontinuation; consider calcium/vitamin D supplementation if prolonged use.
- Nexplanon: insertion site reaction including pain, bleeding, paresthesias, and infection
- IUDs: uterine perforation (2); absolute risk of ectopic pregnancy is reduced with IUD, but if pregnancy does occur, there is a higher risk that it will be ectopic.
- Sponge and diaphragm: toxic shock syndrome

REFERENCES

1. Centers for Disease Control and Prevention. U.S. Medical Eligibility Criteria for Contraceptive Use, 2024. https://www.cdc.gov/contraception/hcp/usmec/. Accessed December 4, 2025.
2. Teal S, Edelman A. Contraception selection, effectiveness, and adverse effects: a review. *JAMA*. 2021;326(24):2507–2518.

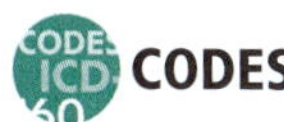

CODES

ICD10

- Z30.9 Encounter for contraceptive management, unspecified
- Z30.41 Encounter for surveillance of contraceptive pills
- Z30.431 Encounter for routine checking of intrauterine contracep dev

CLINICAL PEARLS

LARC methods provide very high efficacy and convenience for patients.

CORNEAL ABRASION AND ULCERATION

Jon S. Parham, DO, MPH, FAAFP

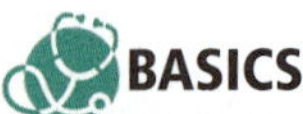

BASICS

As the most anterior eye structure, a cornea is unique: mechanical and immunologic eye protector, light refractor/transmitter, and conduit for nutrients and oxygen via tears to the eye. Cornea is the most sensitive tissue of the body.

DESCRIPTION

- Corneal traumatic injuries:
  - Corneal abrasions: result from any nonpenetrating violation of the exposed corneal epithelium
  - Superficial corneal ulcers, limited to partial loss of the corneal epithelium, with inflammation
  - Corneal stromal ulceration: violation of the epithelial and stromal layers, the inciting inflammation and possible infectious keratitis
  - Peripheral ulcerative keratitis (PUK) is a rare, noninfectious, serious corneal ulceration, complicating many autoimmune diseases, most commonly, systematic rheumatic tissue diseases.
- Photokeratitis of the cornea occurs when exposed to intense visible and/or ultraviolet light.
- Chemicals (acid or alkali [especially]) directly on the cornea may cause serious, corneal and anterior segment damage

EPIDEMIOLOGY

All unprotected eyes are vulnerable to corneal injuries.

Incidence

- Corneal abrasions:
  - Eight percent of total ER visits are eye trauma-related; 64% of these visits are corneal abrasions
  - Twelve percent of corneal abrasions relate to contact lenses, particularly in young people.
- Worldwide, infectious keratitis and ulceration is 6th leading cause of blindness.
- Chemical ocular injuries: 67% occur in young men at work

ETIOLOGY AND PATHOPHYSIOLOGY

- Corneal abrasions: caused by mechanical injury from inorganic or organic matter scratching corneal as eyes are rubbed with fingers or eyelid blinking or separately foreign matter impacting cornea with matter embedding in or perforating the cornea
- Acute severe or reoccurring corneal abrasion, keratitis, or ulceration can cause scarring with impairment or loss of vision
- Corneal ulcers: Injury precedes keratitis and infiltration, possibly causing infectious corneal ulceration.
- Pathogens causing ulcerations include:
  - Gram-positive bacteria ~20–69%, *Staphylococcus aureus* and coagulase-negative *Streptococcus* are common
  - Gram-negative bacteria ~21–35%, *Pseudomonas* spp. most common, (colonized contact lenses users)
  - Herpes simplex (most common viral cause)with or without bacterial superinfection; Herpes zoster
  - Fungal: Fusarium, Aspergillus, Curvularia, and Candida; rank order varies geographically
  - Parasites: Acanthamoeba is very, very rare in United States, but 85% are in contact lenses users.
- Photokeratitis from direct sunlight or that reflected off snow or water, tanning booth light, halogen lamp, welding torch, close lightening flash with unprotected or inadequate UV eye protection

RISK FACTORS

- Acute eye trauma: direct contact trauma, chemical burn, UV overexposure
- Contact lenses use:
  - The most common contributing factor for bacterial keratitis in the USA
  - Risky handling of contact lenses (poor hand and lenses hygiene)
  - Extended wear lenses, excessive wear times
- Autoimmune disorders: Sjögren, PUK, rheumatoid arthritis, inflammatory bowel disease
- Ocular surface diseases: chronic blepharitis, entropion, Graves eye disease, dry eyes/corneal dystrophy/bullous keratopathy/mucous membrane pemphigoid promote local edema and ulceration
- Lack of proper eye protection
- Males, age 20 to 34 years old
- Manufacturing, construction, agricultural work (equatorial especially)

GENERAL PREVENTION

- Strong, face/periorbital, skin contact-fitting eyewear during:
  - Work of hammering, grinding, sawing
  - Contact sports
- Occupational Safety and Health Administration mandates safety standards for at risk employees; see https://www.osha.gov/laws-regs/regulations/standardnumber/1926/1926.102.

COMMONLY ASSOCIATED CONDITIONS

- Xerophthalmia (common) or exophthalmos (occasional); allergic eye disease (common)
- Severe vitamin A deficiency (associated with corneal keratitis—rare)
- Neuropathy of cranial nerve V-1, the ophthalmic branch (rare)
- Critically ill or patients under anesthesia with impaired blink reflex or lagophthalmos and those on intermittent positive pressure ventilation (occasional)

DIAGNOSIS

Key historical questions and a systematic eye examination keenly focus the diagnosis

HISTORY

- Ask: when, where, engaged in what, and if wearing eye protection at or just prior to onset symptoms.
- Ask about recent significant ocular trauma, if so, consider penetrating injury (see "Additional Reading")
- Acute corneal foreign bodies: minor abrasions: abrupt foreign body (FB) sensation, severe photophobia/pain; but abrasions *without* FB sensation suggests acute keratitis or current erosion syndrome.
- Excessive UV or welding exposure: 1 to 12 hours *delay* in usually severe, *bilateral* symptoms: severe pain, scleral injection, photophobia, facial erythema
- Contact lenses misuse: pain and photophobia on awakening or interrupted sleep by searing eye pain: "classic" for recurrent erosion syndrome
- Other symptoms include: red eye, pain with extraocular muscle movement, eye twitching, excessive tearing, blurred or decreased vision, nausea, and headache.
- Past medical/surgical history: diabetes, immunosuppression, contact lenses use/misuse or refractive surgery, last tetanus shot date

PHYSICAL EXAM

- First step, document far or near visual acuity (VA) by Snellen chart: a two-line decrease is significant; if only hand motion or light is seen in a usually normal eye, then same day call to ophthalmologist.
- One drop ophthalmic topical ocular anesthetic (TOA) facilitates best exam; may place TOA before VA if too photophobic
- Survey: orbit (palpation), eyelids, globe surface, pupils, and extraocular muscles
- Slit lamp is ideal or otoscope or ophthalmoscope or even penlight for exam of cornea and associated structures.
- Evert the upper lid and then retract lower lid to inspect for FB; sweep with sterile, wet cotton swab for FB removal.
- Fluorescein stain cornea, examine with Wood light for corneal surface defects: retention of yellow or green color at abrasion or over full cornea in UV keratitis

DIFFERENTIAL DIAGNOSIS

- Corneal abrasion: acute angle-closure glaucoma, acute conjunctivitis, adult blepharitis, corneal ulcer, infective keratitis, uveitis, iritis, entropion, epidemic keratoconjunctivitis
- Corneal ulceration: contact lenses mechanical trauma; keratoconjunctivitis: atopic or sicca; keratitis: interstitial or infectious or neurotrophic or PUK; band keratopathy; and HLA-B27 syndromes

DIAGNOSTIC TESTS & INTERPRETATION

An "eye tray": instruments and meds

Initial Tests (lab, imaging)

- Corneal ulcer: uncommon to culture (corneal scrape) but need same day discussion with ophthalmologist
- Discuss topical antibiotics with eye specialist; may obscure true culture findings
- If suspicious for high-impact FB or direct injury: fluorescein (generous amount) stain exam with Wood lamp or slit lamp for ocular surface exam—if blue or diluted fluorescein color is flowing from surface, it indicates corneal or scleral penetration, a positive Siedel test.
- If penetrating injury suspicious for retained fb: acute transfer to emergency room for ophthalmology consult; do ocular CT scan if metallic or MRI if nonmetallic (1)[C].

Diagnostic Procedures/Other

- 1 to 2 drops 0.5% proparacaine or tetracaine ophthalmic solution topical anesthetic for pain control
- Tonometry for intraocular pressure testing (8 to 21 = normal) if need to rule out acute open angle glaucoma

- Slit or Wood lamp exam, after fluorescein stain identify:
  - Corneal trauma/fb/infection effects have planar geographic shape or more linear stains; simple corneal abrasions have uniform uptake, precise borders; several punctate or curvilinear shape stains from contact lenses; corneal ulcers positive uptake lesions with irregular borders; and herpetic dendrites with terminal bulb pattern (atypical herpetic lesion may appear as >4 mm abrasion) (2)[C]
- Abrasions, ulcerations, keratitis and infiltrates

Test Interpretation

Scraping culture: fungal, bacterial identifies bacteria, yeast to help identify specific infection

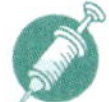

TREATMENT

Goals: Control pain, prevent infection, and teach patient daily self-monitoring (vision degradation, excess pain).

GENERAL MEASURES

- Normal saline (0.5 to 1.0 liter) irrigation of ocular surface and both fornices may flush away FB.
- If patient is cooperative, adherent epithelial FB without stain may be removed with sterile moist cotton swab or 25-gauge needle or syringe by experienced operator (see "Additional Reading")
- Give tetanus booster as indicated for eye abrasions/punctures (1)[C].
- Patching is *not* recommended (fails to reduce pain, delays healing, more risk of infection) (2)[C].

MEDICATION

- Oral analgesic: narcotics, acetaminophen, or NSAIDs
- Topical anesthetics include proparacaine hydrochloride 0.5%, tetracaine hydrochloride 0.5%.
  - Tetracaine does not require refrigeration; proparacaine does.
  - Patients should *not* use TOAs as overuse can cause superimposed infections or scaring, nor topical steroids.
- If photophobia and pain, miosis and limbal flush: topical cycloplegic agents like 1% cyclopentolate 1 drop q8h for 1 to 2 days
- Ophthalmic NSAIDs: Diclofenac 0.1%, 1 drop QID reduces moderate pain, limit to 1 to 2 day use as may impair healing or rarely damage cornea (3)[C].
- Caution: Frequent use of artificial tears may dilute other medications.

First Line

- Topical ophthalmic antibiotics to prevent corneal infection, especially in contact lenses users, fingernail, or plant matter involvement
- Some ophthalmic antibiotics include: polymyxin B/trimethoprim 1 drop q3h for 7 days for lower risk abrasions or erythromycin 0.5% ointment 1 ribbon q3h for 7 days.
  - Broad spectrum: polymyxin B/trimethoprim 1 drop q3h for 7 days or erythromycin ointment for lower risk abrasions
  - Higher risk abrasions (involving: contact lenses user, fingernail or plant matter) gram-negative coverage/antipseudomonal: ofloxacin 0.3% solution 1 to 2 drop q2–3h for 2 days, then same QID for 3 days or ciprofloxacin 0.3% solution, same dose/duration
- Fungal keratitis: if suspected, <24 hours referral to ophthalmologist for antifungal–topical antifungal agents
- Herpetic keratitis: <24 hours referral to ophthalmologist for confirmation; or may start (after phone consult ophthalmologist): trifluridine 1% solution 1 drop q2h while awake (2)[C]

ISSUES FOR REFERRAL

- Ophthalmology referral: timing
- Lack of improvement by 24 hours or worsening symptoms
- Any chemical burn or any penetrating globe or cornea injury: immediate referral to emergency room
- Any corneal ulcer or infiltrate: same day phone call
- Incomplete healing by 3 to 4 days
- Retained corneal fb or any stain/ring
- Any hyphema (blood) or hypopyon (pus): same day consult
- Anytime a vision loss of >2 lines on Snellen chart or abrupt decline hand or light recognition: same day consult (2)[C]

ADDITIONAL THERAPIES

Novel approaches: amniotic membrane/fluid, autogulous blood tears; proposed: topical insulin and substance P (3)[C]

ONGOING CARE

FOLLOW-UP RECOMMENDATIONS

Patient Monitoring

Follow up *all* corneal abrasions in 24 hours, especially lesions ≥4 mm, or decreased vision, or abrasions due to contact lenses.

PATIENT EDUCATION

Corneal Abrasion and Erosion (English and Spanish versions by American Academy Ophthalmology [AAO]) (https://www.aao.org/eye-health/diseases/what-is-corneal-abrasion); see if you qualify for a no-cost eye exam from AAO's EyeCare America program.

PROGNOSIS

- Minor corneal abrasions <4 mm heal within 24 to 72 hours; larger ones, maximum of 5 days
- Among extended wear contact lenses users, risk of microbial keratitis is 15 times higher than nonusers.
- Daily wear contact users occasionally wearing through the night have 9 times higher risk than nonusers for microbial keratitis (2)[C].

COMPLICATIONS

- Recurrence of abrasion or ulcer by reinjury or spontaneously
- Conversion of abrasion to keratitis or ulcer
- Scarring of the cornea may produce vision loss.
- Exogenous endophthalmitis, risk loss of vision or eye

REFERENCES

1. Ambikkumar A, Arthurs B, El-Hadad C. Corneal foreign bodies. *CMAJ*. 2022;194(11):E419.
2. Amed F, House RJ, Feldman BH. Corneal abrasions and corneal foreign bodies. *Prim Care*. 2015;42(3):363–375.
3. Dang DH, Riaz KM, Karamichos D. Treatment of non-infectious corneal injury: review of diagnostic agents, therapeutic medications, and future targets. *Drugs*. 2022;82(2):145–167.

ADDITIONAL READING

Xu P, Lim JK. Managing corneal foreign body injuries in a primary eye care setting. *Clin Exp Optom*. 2025;1–9. doi:10.1080/08164622.2025.2485237.

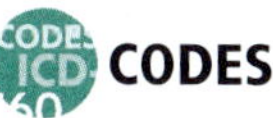

CODES

ICD10

- S05.00XA Inj conjunctiva and corneal abrasion w/o fb, unsp eye, init
- H16.009 Unspecified corneal ulcer, unspecified eye
- H16.049 Marginal corneal ulcer, unspecified eye

CLINICAL PEARLS

- VA testing is *the* vital sign at the beginning of every eye visit.
- When corneal abrasion is healed and asymptomatic, contact lenses use may restart.
- Eye patching is *not* recommended for corneal ulcerations or abrasions.
- Topical anesthetic drops are *not* recommended for use by patients.
- Consider topical NSAIDs and/or oral analgesics a maximum of 3 days for symptom control.
- Treatment usually involves frequent topical antimicrobial application.
- Referral to an ophthalmologist with timing (See also "Issues for Referral.")

CORNS AND CALLUSES

Jon S. Parham, DO, MPH, FAAFP • Sandra N. New, DNP

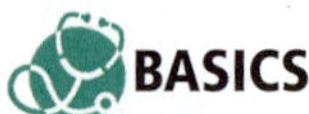

BASICS

Natural response of dermis to extraordinary contact stressors producing local hypertrophy of the epidermis and often pain

DESCRIPTION

- Corns and calluses are pressure-generated hyperkeratotic skin conditions of the feet or hands.
- A callus (tyloma [Greek]) is a diffuse area of hyperkeratosis, usually without a distinct border. Typically, callus is the result of exposure to repetitive forces, including friction and mechanical pressure. They tend to occur on the palms of hands and soles of feet. Calluses may or may not be painful.
- A corn (heloma [Greek]) is a circumscribed hyperkeratotic lesion with a central conical core of keratin that causes pain and inflammation. The conical core in a corn is a thickening of the stratum corneum. Corns typically occur at pressure points, or result from poor fitting shoes or an underlying bone lesion/spur.
- Hard corn or heloma durum (more common): often on toe surfaces, especially 5th toe (proximal interphalangeal [PIP] joint)
- Soft corn or heloma molle: commonly in the interdigital space
- Digital corns are also known as clavi or heloma durum.
- Intractable plantar keratosis (IPK) is a painful corn, usually located under a metatarsal head (1st and 5th most common), is typically more difficult to resolve, and often is resistant to usual conservative treatments.

EPIDEMIOLOGY

Corns and calluses are the most prevalent of all foot disorders. Palmar calluses at metacarpal heads are also common.

Incidence

- Incidence of corns and calluses are more common in elderly and less common in children.
- Women:men, 4:1; possibly due to ill-fitting fashionable shoes
- Blacks report corns and calluses 30% more often than whites.

Prevalence

- Corns and calluses represent 46% of foot disorders presenting to podiatric clinics and affect about 9.2 million Americans.
- About 38 per 1,000 people affected

ETIOLOGY AND PATHOPHYSIOLOGY

Common corns and calluses are skin signs and often produce symptoms, but are not a disease entity themselves. Repetitive, accumulated, or excessive friction and mechanical trauma on external skin produces a natural, protective dermal response of hyperkeratosis on hands and feet, particularly over bony prominences.

- Calluses typically form diffusely over bony prominences or deformities where there are repetitive forces and/or frequent weight-bearing forces. Examples include metatarsal head deformities or from ill-fitting shoes on normal bony anatomy. Although calluses may frequently form on palmar surfaces, symptoms are rare because these surfaces are nonweight bearing.
- Hard corns are an extreme form of callus with a keratin-based core, which in the case of IPK, may be derived from human papillomavirus (HPV), and extraordinary pressure. Corns are often found on the digital surfaces and commonly linked to bony protrusions, causing skin to rub against shoe surfaces. Corns rarely form on the hands (1).
- Soft corns arise from increased moisture from perspiration leading to skin maceration, along with mechanical irritation, especially between toes.

Genetics

No direct genetic basis

RISK FACTORS

- Extrinsic factors producing pressure, friction, moisture and local stress
  - Poorly fitting shoes with narrow toe box or with abrasive surfaces
  - Absence of socks or gloves for pressure mitigation or nonbreathable socks or gloves producing excess moisture
  - Repetitive activities: sports; guitar playing; manual labor; fingerstick testing; prolonged postures in prayer, gaming, or yoga
  - Walking barefoot or wearing thin-soled shoes offering no support
- Intrinsic factors
  - Bony malformations such as hammertoes, bunions
  - Neuropathy of distal extremities, such as frequently seen in diabetic patients
  - Gait disturbances

GENERAL PREVENTION

Reduce mechanical pressure or friction by wearing properly fitting shoes, gloves, and moisture wicking socks.

Geriatric Considerations

Regular foot exams, more frequently for diabetic and/or peripheral vascular disease patients, to assess for skin integrity, neuropathy, and pressure points are paramount.

COMMONLY ASSOCIATED CONDITIONS

- Foot ulcers in vascularly compromised individuals due to history of smoking and poor circulation or secondary to diabetes with microangiopathy and neuropathy
- Cellulitis, focal or regional symptoms/signs:
  - Pain, increasing size, redness, pain, or swelling
  - Purulent discharge
  - Fever
  - Color changes: pale, red, black
  - Excessive heat or coolness of skin to touch

DIAGNOSIS

- Visual examination of entire foot or hand and focal lesion(s)
- History of activities and particular shoes and socks (or gloves) that incite focal pain
- Examination of footwear or gloves typically worn for excessive wear areas

HISTORY

- Engage patient in identification of friction sites corresponding with pain.
- Inquire if patient has vascular or neurologic health issues such as smoking history, hyperlipidemia, or diabetes.
- Ask what has been done thus far to treat the thickened skin lesions.

PHYSICAL EXAM

- Calluses
  - Assess skin area of complaint for plantar and/or palmar hyperkeratosis and areas of pain.
  - Inspect feet and hands for areas of friction; palpate for focal, excessive hyperkeratosis, and tenderness.
  - Identify skin color changes.
  - Assess sensory response and vascular status in area of complaint.
- Corns
  - Hard corns
    - Assess dorsum of feet and toes for hard corns, note distinct, and circumscribed borders.
    - Identify central core mass and focal, marked tenderness to perpendicular pressure on direct palpation.
  - Soft corns
    - Inspect between toes for maceration and discoloration of hyperkeratotic lesion, commonly at the 4th to 5th intertriginous space.
    - Evaluate pain severity of corn—that are usually severely and focally painful (2).

DIFFERENTIAL DIAGNOSIS

- Plantar warts—viral (HPV) origin with blood capillary dots visible (often after débridement) and pain with bilateral compression to lesion (2)
- Porokeratosis (small nodule[s] from occluded sweat gland)
- Skin pressure (dark-colored) eschar overlying a pathologic wound, commonly affecting feet in diabetics and elderly

DIAGNOSTIC TESTS & INTERPRETATION

Rarely indicated

Initial Tests (lab, imaging)

- Radiographs are warranted if no external cause is found. Look for abnormalities in foot structure and bone spurs.
- Use of metallic radiographic marker (BB taped over skin lesion) and weight-bearing films often highlight the relationship between the callus and bony prominence.

Follow-Up Tests & Special Considerations

Evaluate chronic conditions: diabetes, vascular insufficiency, and recurrent infections (e.g., tinea pedis) that could worsen symptoms.

Diagnostic Procedures/Other

Biopsy with microscopic evaluation only in atypical appearing, persistent cases, such as IPK

Test Interpretation

Abnormal accumulation of keratin in epidermis, stratum corneum

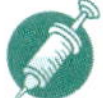

TREATMENT

Local débridement of hyperkeratosis and focal pressure/friction alleviation are foundational.

GENERAL MEASURES

- Management initially at home:
  - Soak affected skin areas in warm water until softened.
  - Use pumice stones or coarse sandpaper to reduce thickened soft skin.
  - Avoid chronic friction generating activities if possible.
- Management at office: Tangential-epidermal skin shaving to reduce stratum corneum thickness using size 15 (or 10 for larger areas) blade is temporarily very helpful. An 11-type scalpel is used to "core" out a corn's keratin center.
- Adding foam padding or silicon sleeve (1/8 to 1/4 inch thick) can reduce friction area over bony prominences.
- Wear socks or gloves (for hands) regularly.
- Cutouts of padding corresponding to pressure points placed in gloves or socks/shoes may off-load bony prominences
- Choose low-heeled shoes with soft uppers and deep, wide toe boxes.
- Shoe repair shops can stretch shoes made of certain materials to prevent friction point(s).
- Toe elevation via "figure-of-eight" strapping onto dorsal midfoot for corns or calluses on plantar toe surface
- The use of prefabricated or custom orthotics may be helpful in some cases.
- Silicone sleeves for toes, foam toe spacers, and small pieces of lamb's wool or adhesive felt strategically placed can significantly reduce "shoe to skin" friction areas, for example, dorsum and/or tip of hammer toes (2)[C]

MEDICATION

- Keratolytic agents may reduce pain, reoccurrence and corn size compared to scalpel débridement (3)[A]. Topical salicylic acid is usually well tolerated and safe with regular monitoring.
- Salicylic acid (40%) plasters and then blunt débridement may reduce time to multiple corn resolution by 3 months versus just débridement, but overall outcomes are equal (3)[B].

Geriatric Considerations

- The use of salicylic acid corn plasters can cause skin breakdown and ulceration in patients with thin-atrophic skin (diabetics and those with vascular compromise), so usually avoid this treatment.
- Aggressive use of pumice stones can also lead to excessive skin breakdown, especially surrounding the callus.

First Line

Off-loading of pressure points on hands or feet

Second Line

Chemical and/or surgical reduction of thickness of calluses and perhaps removal of the keratin core of corns

ISSUES FOR REFERRAL

If conservative treatments are not effective, a podiatrist or orthopedic referral is indicated for bony prominence debridement.

ADDITIONAL THERAPIES

Skin protection from excessive frictional shear forces and moisture using wicking sock material (merino wool or polyester)

SURGERY/OTHER PROCEDURES

- Surgical treatment of hammer toe, claw toe, or mallet toe to reduce bony abnormalities may correct stress friction points if reasonable conservative measures have failed.
- Modest evidence for surgical excision of foot IPK without boney excision and has stimulated research regarding viral presence (1)[A]

COMPLEMENTARY & ALTERNATIVE MEDICINE

- May benefit from urea-based lotions, creams, or ointments
- Warm water/Epsom salt soaks 20 minutes prior to pumice stone débridement

ADMISSION, INPATIENT, AND NURSING CONSIDERATIONS

- Admission very rarely indicated—unless progression to ulcerated lesion with signs of severe infection, gangrene, or sepsis
- Chronic venous-related edema or arterial insufficiency of feet requires a vascular surgery referral
- Nursing
  - Wound care, dressing changes for infected lesions, teaching signs and symptoms of infection to report
  - Shoe choice teaching: wide toe box, low-heel shoes with support, and wearing of diabetic socks by all at-risk persons

ONGOING CARE

Periodic assessment of feet for signs of corns or calluses, hyperkeratosis, and general skin/nail health by patient or professional

FOLLOW-UP RECOMMENDATIONS

Daily foot skin care with over-the-counter skin emollients can prevent dry skin that is more sensitive to pressure points.

PATIENT EDUCATION

- Mayo Clinic: http://www.mayoclinic.org/diseases-conditions/corns-and-calluses/symptoms-causes/syc-20355946
- American Academy of Dermatology: https://www.aad.org/public/everyday-care/injured-skin/burns/treat-corns-calluses
- American Podiatric Medical Association: https://www.apma.org/Patients/FootHealthList.cfm?navItemNumber=25223

PROGNOSIS

Complete cure is possible if all factors causing pressure or injury are eliminated.

COMPLICATIONS

Ulceration or infection (cellulitis) if simple calluses and corns are not properly addressed and sources of friction eliminated

REFERENCES

1. Reilly IN, Longhurst B, Vlahovic TC. Surgical excision of intractable plantar keratoses (corns) of the foot: a scoping review. *J Am Podiatr Med Assoc*. 2023;113(6):22–44.
2. Freeman DB. Corns and calluses resulting from mechanical hyperkeratosis. *Am Fam Physician*. 2002;65(11):2277–2280.
3. Stephenson J, Farndon L, Concannon M. Analysis of a trial assessing the long-term effectiveness of salicylic acid plasters compared with scalpel debridement in facilitating corn resolution in patients with multiple corns. *J Dermatology*. 2016;43(6):662–669.

ADDITIONAL READING

- American College of Foot and Ankle Surgeons: http://www.acfas.org/. Accessed October 30, 2024.
- Ashique KT, Srinivas CR, Sethy M. Toe elevation in corn management. *J Am Acad Dermatol*. 2020;83(5):e327–e328.
- Kumar S, Kapoor P, Brar AK, et al. Autoclavable metallic skin peeler: novel modality for paring of callosities. *J Am Acad Dermatol*. 2023;89(5):e205–e206.

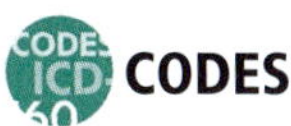

CODES

ICD10

L84 Corns and callosities

CLINICAL PEARLS

- Fundamental: Avoid ill-fitting shoes and wear moisture wicking socks.
- Most therapy for corns and calluses can be done as self-care at home using débridement, then padding over the affected area, and friction/pressure source-correction of the shoe.
- Cryotherapy may worsen discomfort and is not advised for treatment.

CORONARY ARTERY DISEASE AND STABLE ANGINA

Darnel Viray Dabu, MD, MPH, FAAFP, DipABLM • Wodwentzky Lefranc, MD

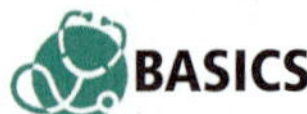

BASICS

Cardiovascular diseases are a major cause of death worldwide. Coronary artery disease (CAD) is a highly prevalent cardiovascular condition and a significant health burden for the population.

DESCRIPTION

- CAD is the pathologic process characterized by atherosclerotic plaque accumulation in the epicardial arteries, whether obstructive or nonobstructive.
- Stable angina is a chest discomfort due to myocardial ischemia that is reproducible at a certain level of exertion or emotional stress.
- Spectrum of acute coronary syndrome (ACS) includes unstable angina (UA), non–ST elevation myocardial infarction (NSTEMI), ST elevation myocardial infarction (STEMI) (See "Acute Coronary Syndromes: NSTE-ACS [Unstable Angina and NSTEMI].")
- Definitions
  - Chronic coronary syndromes is the term to describe the clinical presentations of CAD during stable periods, particularly those preceding or following an ACS.
  - Typical angina: three classical characteristics: (i) substernal chest pressure, pressure or heaviness that may radiate to the jaw, back, or arms and generally lasts from 2 to 15 minutes; (ii) occurs at a certain level of myocardial oxygen demand from exertion, emotional stress, or increased sympathetic tone; and (iii) relieved with rest or sublingual nitroglycerin
  - Atypical angina: exhibits two of the above typical characteristics
  - Noncardiac chest pain: exhibits ≤1 of the above typical characteristics
  - Anginal equivalent: Patients may present without chest discomfort but with nonspecific symptoms such as dyspnea, diaphoresis, fatigue, belching, nausea, light-headedness, or indigestion that occur with exertion or stress.
  - UA: anginal symptoms that are new or more frequent, more severe, or occurring with lessening degrees of myocardial demand; considered ACS but do not present with cardiac biomarker elevation
  - NSTEMI: elevation of cardiac biomarker (troponin) with either anginal symptoms, ischemic ECG changes other than ST elevation, or both
  - STEMI: presents with typical symptoms as mentioned above with ST elevations noted on ECG; generally caused by acute plaque rupture and complete obstruction of culprit vessel and may present prior to laboratory detection of troponin.

Geriatric Considerations

The elderly may present with atypical symptoms. Physical limitations may delay recognition of angina until it occurs with minimal exertion or at rest.

EPIDEMIOLOGY

- CAD causes about 1 in 5 deaths in the United States. Heart disease cost about $252.2 billion in 2019 to 2020 (Centers for Disease Control and Prevention) and $378 billion (American Heart Association [AHA]) annually for 2017 to 2019.
- ~80% of CAD is preventable with a healthy lifestyle.

Incidence

In the United States, the lifetime incidence risk of developing CAD in men and women after 40 years of age is 49% and 32%, respectively.

Prevalence

Approximately 20.1 million persons in the United States live with CAD, 11.1 million Americans have chronic stable angina pectoris, and 8.8 million persons with CAD had myocardial infarction (MI).

ETIOLOGY AND PATHOPHYSIOLOGY

Anginal symptoms occur during times of myocardial ischemia caused by a mismatch between coronary perfusion and myocardial oxygen demand. Atherosclerotic narrowing of the coronary arteries is the most common etiology of angina, but it may also occur in those with significant aortic stenosis, pulmonary hypertension, hypertrophic cardiomyopathy, coronary spasm, or volume overload.

Genetics

Many CAD-associated single-nucleotide polymorphisms have been identified, although many of their functions are not well characterized.

RISK FACTORS

- Classical risk factors: hypertension, ↑ LDL cholesterol, smoking, diabetes, premature CAD in first-degree relatives (men <55 years old; women <65 years old), age (>45 years for men; >55 years for women), ↓ HDL
- Other risk factors: obesity, sedentary lifestyle, chronic inflammation, abnormal ankle-brachial indices, renal disease

GENERAL PREVENTION

- Smoking cessation
- Regular aerobic exercise program and weight loss for obese patients (goal body mass index [BMI] <25 kg/m^2); a plant-based or Mediterranean-like diet is recommended.
- Blood pressure (BP) control (goal <140/90 mm Hg; consider <130/80 mm Hg for those with 10-year ASCVD risk ≥10%).
- Type 2 diabetes management: Consider more aggressive hemoglobin A1c (HbA1c) goal of 6.5–7% in younger, recently diagnosed individuals.
- At least moderate-intensity statin therapy for those with diabetes aged 40 to 75 years and those with 10-year ASCVD risk ≥7.5–20% (Recommendations of advisory organizations vary; caution: The older American College of Cardiology (ACC)/AHA risk calculator overestimates risk in many by as much as 50–100%. Newer calculators are available online and may be more accurate.)

COMMONLY ASSOCIATED CONDITIONS

Hyperlipidemia, peripheral vascular disease, cerebrovascular disease, hypertension, obesity, diabetes

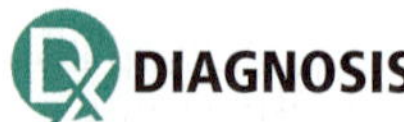

DIAGNOSIS

HISTORY

- Pain may be described with a clenched fist over the center of the chest (Levine sign). Episodes of angina are generally of the same character and in the same location as previous episodes. Dyspnea on exertion may present as the only symptom.
- May present with symptoms similar to gastric reflux or GI upset (indigestion, nausea, diaphoresis); atypical symptoms are more likely in women, the elderly, and diabetic patients.

PHYSICAL EXAM

Normal cardiac exam is possible, or cardiac exam may reveal dysrhythmias, heart murmurs indicative of valvular disease, gallops, or signs of congestive heart failure.

DIFFERENTIAL DIAGNOSIS

- Vascular: aortic dissection, pericarditis, myocarditis, MI, vasospasm
- Pulmonary: pleuritis, pulmonary embolism, pneumothorax
- Gastroesophageal: gastric reflux, esophageal spasm, peptic ulcer
- Musculoskeletal: costochondritis, arthritis, muscle strain, rib fracture
- Other: anxiety, psychosomatic, cocaine abuse

DIAGNOSTIC TESTS & INTERPRETATION

Initial Tests (lab, imaging)

- Serial cardiac troponins for those presenting acutely with symptoms
- Complete blood count, lipid profile, and HbA1c for risk stratification, Basic metabolic panel
- ECG—should be obtained unless there is a clearly noncardiac cause of the chest pain; may be normal or may show signs of ischemia; left bundle branch block or ventricular pacing makes interpretation for ischemia difficult.
- Chest x-ray may identify other causes of pain.

Follow-Up Tests & Special Considerations

- Stress testing is most helpful for patients at intermediate risk of CAD; exercise testing for those who can physically exercise (≥5 metabolic equivalents [METs]): standard exercise ECG for those with normal baseline ECG (i.e., without left bundle branch block or ventricular pacing); exercise stress testing with echo or perfusion imaging for those with abnormal baseline ECG, and for those with intermediate-high pretest probability; for those who cannot tolerate exercise, consider pharmacologic stress testing. Stress testing may also be useful to evaluate effectiveness of the therapeutic regimen.
- CT coronary angiography or cardiac MRI can be considered as a supplement/alternative to stress testing in patients with continued symptoms.

Diagnostic Procedures/Other

- Cardiac catheterization with coronary angiography: gold standard for confirmation and delineation of coronary disease and direction of interventional therapy or surgery
- Significant CAD is defined as ≥50% stenosis of the left main coronary artery or ≥70% stenosis of other major coronary arteries by angiography.

TREATMENT

GENERAL MEASURES

- AHA/ACC—recommended nonpharmacologic strategies as first-line therapy to lower the BP in those with elevated BP (120 to 129/<80 mmHg). BP control goal for patients with hypertension and CAD: <130/80 mm Hg.
- Smoking cessation goal: complete cessation, no exposure to secondhand smoke or e-cigarettes
- Physical activity goal: If no contraindications, an exercise regimen of 150 minutes/week of moderate-intensity aerobic activities or 75 minutes/week of higher-intensity aerobic activities.

MEDICATION

First Line

Recommendations based on AHA/ACC 2023 (1)[C]:

- β-Blockers: decrease myocardial oxygen demand, and decrease mortality in MI or heart failure; they are initial therapy. Metoprolol (25 to 400 mg daily [succinate] or divided BID [tartrate]) or carvedilol (3.125 to 25.000 mg BID) are preferred. Adjust doses according to clinical response.
- Calcium channel blockers (CCBs): cause arterial vasodilation, decreased myocardial oxygen demand, and improved coronary blood flow; only long-acting CCBs should be used:
  - Dihydropyridine CCBs: nifedipine (30 to 90 mg/day), amlodipine (5 to 10 mg/day), or felodipine (2.5 to 10.0 mg/day)
  - Nondihydropyridine CCBs: Diltiazem (120 to 480 mg/day) or verapamil (120 to 480 mg/day) also have negative inotropic effects and should not be used in those with ejection fracture <40% because they may precipitate heart failure.
- Nitrates: dilate systemic veins and arteries (including coronary vessels) and cause decreased preload
  - Sublingual nitroglycerin (0.4 mg every 5 minutes for up to 3 doses) used for acute anginal episodes
  - Long-acting nitrates such as isosorbide mononitrate (30 to 240 mg daily [extended release]) can be used for angina prophylaxis.
- Lipid-lowering agents:
  - High-intensity statin therapy is indicated for all patients with CAD regardless of lipid levels.
  - Atorvastatin (40 to 80 mg/day) and rosuvastatin (20 to 40 mg/day) are high-intensity statins.
  - Statins reduce risk of MI and revascularization need. Side effects include myalgias, transaminitis, rhabdomyolysis (rare), and impaired glucose tolerance. Evidence for benefit in primary prevention after age 75 years is sparse.
  - Ezetimibe may be added to statin therapy if LDL is not at goal.
  - Proprotein convertase subtilisin/kexin type 9 inhibitors further reduce LDL levels when used in combination with statins for high-risk patients and reduce cardiovascular events in highly selected patients but are expensive.
- Antiplatelets: decrease risk of thrombosis
  - Aspirin (75 to 162 mg/day) decreases risk of first MI and reduces adverse cardiovascular events in those with stable angina.
  - Clopidogrel (75 mg/day) may be used in patients with contraindications to aspirin.
  - Dual antiplatelet therapy with aspirin + clopidogrel, prasugrel, or ticagrelor is indicated after MI or percutaneous coronary intervention (PCI) (use prasugrel only after PCI. Do not use in patient with CVA history) for a period of time determined by the particular circumstances (2)[C].
- Angiotensin-converting enzyme inhibitors (ACEIs) act on the renin-angiotensin-aldosterone system to reduce BP and afterload. They also have effects on cardiac remodeling after MI.
  - ACEIs such as lisinopril (5 to 40 mg/day) and enalapril (2.5 to 20.0 mg BID) have been shown to reduce both cardiovascular death and MI in patients with CAD and left ventricular systolic dysfunction.
  - Angiotensin receptor blockers such as candesartan (4 to 32 mg daily) may be used in patients intolerant to ACEIs.
  - Side effects include cough (ACEIs predominantly), hyperkalemia, and angioedema.

Second Line

- Ranolazine (500 to 1,000 mg BID) decreases calcium overload in myocytes, acting as an antianginal/anti-ischemic agent. It does not affect HR or BP, and may be used as an adjunctive therapy when symptoms persist despite optimal dose of other antianginals.
- Low dose colchicine (0.5 to 0.6 mg/day) improves outcomes in those with established CAD, but should be reserved for those patients who remain at high risk despite maximal dose guideline-directed medical therapy.

ADDITIONAL THERAPIES

- If CAD associated with diabetes, an SGLT2 inhibitor or a GLP-1 agonist with proven cardiovascular benefit is recommended to reduce risk of MACE.
- Enhanced external counterpulsation may be considered for relief of symptoms if refractory angina.

SURGERY/OTHER PROCEDURES

- If optimal medical therapy is inadequate to control symptoms, consider coronary artery bypass graft (CABG) over PCI for those with severe left main coronary stenosis, significant lesions in ≥3 major coronary arteries, and for lesions not amenable to PCI.
- PCI with balloon angioplasty and/or stent placement is performed for significant lesions, especially if angina is not adequately controlled by optimal medical therapy. Additional techniques include laser therapy and atherectomy. PCI does not appear to decrease mortality or risk of MI versus aggressive medical management in those with stable angina (3)[A].

ONGOING CARE

FOLLOW-UP RECOMMENDATIONS

- Lifestyle modifications should be aggressively stressed at every visit. If stable, clinical follow-up should be at least annually to assess for symptoms, change in functional status, medical interventions, and monitoring for complications of CAD and its treatments.
- Vaccines: influenza, COVID-19 vaccines, and pneumococcal vaccine to reduce cardiovascular morbidity and mortality and all-cause death

DIET

Plant-based or Mediterranean-like diet is recommended and shown to lower all-cause mortality compared to standard diet. A diet emphasizing vegetables, fruits, legumes, nuts, whole grains, and lean protein is recommended. Reduce the percentage of calories from saturated fat (<6% of total calories) and replace with dietary monounsaturated and polyunsaturated fat.

PATIENT EDUCATION

Patient needs to receive ongoing therapeutic lifestyle interventions, individualized education on symptom management, social determinants of health risk factors, and medication adherence to improve knowledge and facilitate behavior change.

PROGNOSIS

Variable; depends on severity of symptoms, extent of CAD, and left ventricular function

COMPLICATIONS

ACS, arrhythmia, cardiac arrest, heart failure

REFERENCES

1. Virani SS, Newby LK, Arnold SV, et al. 2023 AHA/ACC/ACCP/ASPC/NLA/PCNA guideline for the management of patients with chronic coronary disease: a report of the American Heart Association/American College of Cardiology Joint Committee on clinical practice guidelines. *Circulation*. 2023;148(9):e9–e119. doi:10.1161/CIR.0000000000001168.
2. Lawton JS, Tamis-Holland JE, Bangalore S, et al; for Writing Committee Members. 2021 ACC/AHA/SCAI guideline for coronary artery revascularization: a report of the American College of Cardiology/American Heart Association Joint Committee on clinical practice guidelines. *J Am Coll Cardiol*. 2022;79(2):e21–e129.
3. Maron DJ, Hochman JS, Reynolds HR, et al; for ISCHEMIA Research Group. Initial invasive or conservative strategy for stable coronary disease. *N Engl J Med*. 2020;382(15):1395–1407.

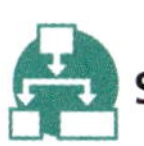

SEE ALSO

Algorithm: Chest Pain/Acute Coronary Syndrome

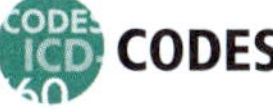

CODES

ICD10

- I25.119 Athscl heart disease of native cor art w unsp ang pctrs
- I25.118 Athscl heart disease of native cor art w oth ang pctrs
- I20.9 Angina pectoris, unspecified

CLINICAL PEARLS

- Maximize antianginal therapy combining β-blockers, CCBs, and nitrates as tolerated, along with high-intensity statin therapy and anti-platelet therapy.
- PCI may be considered for those with stable ischemic heart disease who continue to have angina on maximally tolerated medical therapy. PCI is first-line treatment for those with UA/NSTEMI/STEMI.

COSTOCHONDRITIS

Smriti Ohri, MD

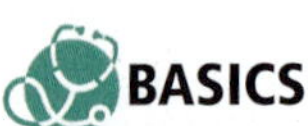

BASICS

DESCRIPTION

- Anterior chest wall pain and tenderness of the costochondral and costosternal regions, most often affecting the 2nd to the 5th costal cartilages
- System(s) affected: musculoskeletal
- Synonym(s): costosternal syndrome; parasternal chondrodynia; anterior chest wall syndrome

EPIDEMIOLOGY

- Predominant age: 40 to 50 years
- Predominant gender: female sex assigned at birth

Incidence

- Around one-third of noncardiac chest pain visits in emergency departments are of musculoskeletal origin.
- Around 10% of chest wall pain in primary care setting diagnosed with costochondritis.

ETIOLOGY AND PATHOPHYSIOLOGY

Although not fully understood, inflammation can be caused by pulling from adjoining muscles at costochondral or costosternal regions.

RISK FACTORS

- Unusual physical activity or upper extremity overuse
- Recent trauma (including motor vehicle accident, domestic violence) or new-onset physical activity
- Recent upper respiratory infection (URI) with coughing

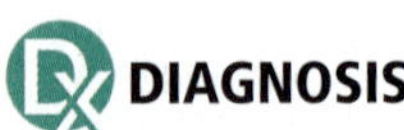

DIAGNOSIS

- Pain is usually sharp, achy, or pressure-like, involving multiple (and mostly unilateral 2nd to 5th) costal cartilages.
- Exacerbated by upper body movements and exertional activities
- Reproduced by palpation of the affected cartilage segments
- Chest tightness is often associated with the pain.

HISTORY

- A complete and thorough history (including a cardiac risk stratification with validated clinical prediction rules) is mandatory for an accurate diagnosis.
- Social history: careful screening and evaluation for domestic violence and substance abuse

PHYSICAL EXAM

- A thorough cardiopulmonary exam to exclude other conditions presenting with chest pain
  - Cardiac rhythm, murmurs, gallops, rubs
  - Adventitious lung sounds—rales, rhonchi, wheezes, rubs
- Tenderness over the costochondral junctions is necessary to establish the diagnosis but does not completely exclude other causes of chest pain.
- If swelling or redness of costal cartilage is present, the presentation is often termed Tietze syndrome (inflammatory condition generally involving single costal cartilage of ribs 2 or 3, typically unilateral presentation).
- Movement of upper extremity of the same side may reproduce the pain.

Pediatric Considerations

- Consider psychogenic chest pain in children who perceive family discord.
- Consider slipping rib syndrome in children with chronic chest and abdominal pain (1).

Geriatric Considerations

Consider herpes zoster in elderly patients.

DIFFERENTIAL DIAGNOSIS

- Consider alternate diagnosis if presence of other signs and symptoms, like shortness of breath, dyspnea on exertion, cough, fever, tachycardia and hypotension
- Cardiac
  - Coronary artery disease (CAD); acute coronary syndrome (ACS)
  - Cardiac contusion from trauma
  - Aortic aneurysm
  - Pericarditis
  - Myocarditis
- Gastrointestinal
  - Gastroesophageal reflux
  - Peptic esophagitis
  - Esophageal spasm
  - Cholecystitis
- Musculoskeletal
  - Fibromyalgia
  - Slipping rib syndrome
  - Costovertebral arthritis
  - Painful xiphoid syndrome
  - Rib trauma
- Psychogenic
  - Panic attacks
- Respiratory
  - Pulmonary embolism
  - Pneumonia
  - Chronic cough
  - Pneumothorax
- Other
  - Domestic violence and abuse
  - Herpes zoster
  - Spinal tumor
  - Metastatic cancer
  - Substance abuse (cocaine)

DIAGNOSTIC TESTS & INTERPRETATION

- Primarily a clinical diagnosis
- Laboratory exams and imaging to rule out other diagnoses

Initial Tests (lab, imaging)

Imaging is not indicated for the diagnosis of costochondritis.

Diagnostic Procedures/Other

None indicated for the diagnosis of costochondritis. Diagnostic tests should be directed toward ruling out other etiologies based on history and exam. For example:

- Consider ECG, particularly for patients with history of or risk factors for CAD.
- Consider chest x-ray in patients with appropriate cardiopulmonary symptoms.
- Consider CT imaging if high suspicion of aortic dissection, infectious or neoplastic process.
- Consider spiral CT for pulmonary embolism and D-dimer if history or risk factors are present.

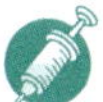

TREATMENT

Reassurance of benign nature of condition and potential for long, slow recovery from pain

GENERAL MEASURES

- Rest, local application of heat (or ice), massage
- Stretching exercises
- Minimize symptom-provoking activities (e.g., reduce frequency or intensity of exercise/work activity).

MEDICATION

- Pain relief with NSAIDs (oral or topical), acetaminophen, lidocaine patches, capsaicin cream
- The use of skeletal muscle relaxants may be beneficial if associated with muscle spasm.
- Refractory cases can be treated with local injections of combined lidocaine/corticosteroid into costochondral areas; rarely necessary

ISSUES FOR REFERRAL

- Consider referral to physical therapy for pain reduction and improvement in function in patients with prolonged symptoms (2)[B].
- Consider referral to gastroenterology or cardiology if an alternate diagnosis meriting special input is suspected.

COMPLEMENTARY & ALTERNATIVE MEDICINE

Limited data but may be safely tried if patient interested

- Chiropractic manipulation; exercise prescription
- Dry needling by properly trained providers
- Acupuncture
- Massage

ADMISSION, INPATIENT, AND NURSING CONSIDERATIONS

Only if cardiac or other serious etiology of chest pain is being considered

ONGOING CARE

FOLLOW-UP RECOMMENDATIONS

Follow-up within 1 week if diagnosis is unclear or symptoms do not abate with conservative treatment

PATIENT EDUCATION

- Educate regarding the self-limited (although potentially recurrent) nature of the illness.
- Instruct patient on proper physical activity regimens to avoid overuse syndromes.
- Avoid sudden, significant changes in activity.

PROGNOSIS

- Self-limited illness lasts for weeks to months and usually abates by 1 year.
- Often recurs

COMPLICATIONS

May be refractory or recurrent.

REFERENCES

1. Mott T, Jones G, Roman K. Costochondritis: rapid evidence review. *Am Fam Physician*. 2021;104(1):73–78.
2. Zaruba RA, Wilson E. Impairment based examination and treatment of costochondritis: a case series. *Int J Sports Phys Ther*. 2017;12(3):458–467.

ADDITIONAL READING

Collins RA, Ray N, Ratheal K, et al. Severe-post-COVID-19 costochondritis in children. *Proc (Bayl Univ Med Cent)*. 2021;35(1):56–57.

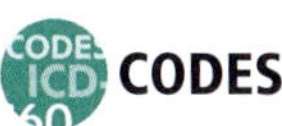

CODES

ICD10

M94.0 Chondrocostal junction syndrome [Tietze]

CLINICAL PEARLS

- A common disorder, accounting for up to 30% of all cases of chest pain
- Diagnosis is primarily clinical. Obtain lab and other testing to exclude other conditions based on patient risk.
- Self-limited (potentially recurrent) condition; activity modification helps prevent recurrence.

COUNSELING TYPES

Micheala Desere Davis, MD

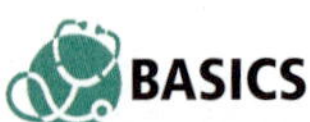

BASICS

DESCRIPTION

- Psychotherapeutic and counseling interventions play an important role in the management of chronic and acute-onset diseases and disorders. They are typically the primary initial mode of evaluation and/or treatment for most mild to moderate psychiatric disorders that reach the criteria using the *DSM-5* (1) or *ICD-11* diagnostic classification systems.
- Treatment and successful control of either medical or psychological conditions typically benefit from some form of professional counseling. Best outcomes occur when they are employed by a skilled practitioner. However, psychotherapy differs from generic counseling which can take many forms and is delivered commonly in nonmedical settings. In recent years, attempts to integrate counseling and psychotherapy within primary care practices have increased.
- Counseling approaches are usually tailored to the specific presenting problem or issue and serve educational and emotional support functions. Typically, counseling in medical settings will be time-limited and problem-focused and often not intended to lead to major medical symptom relief or major behavioral changes but to improve patient coping.
- The goals of psychotherapy range from increasing individual psychological insight and motivation for change to reduction of interpersonal conflict in the marriage or family, reduction of chronic or acute emotional suffering, or reversal of dysfunctional or habitual behaviors. There are several general classes of psychotherapy, starting with individual, marital, or family approaches. In addition, a number of psychological theories guide various methods and treatment philosophies. The following is a brief overview of commonly used psychotherapeutic and counseling methods.
- Psychodynamic therapy: Unconscious conflict manifests as patient's symptoms/problem behaviors:
  - Short term (4 to 6 months) and long term (≥1 year)
  - The focus is on increasing insight of underlying conflict or processes to initiate symptomatic change.
  - Therapist actively helps patient identify patterns of behavior stemming from existence of an unconscious conflict or beliefs and motivations that may not be accurately perceived by the individual.
- Cognitive-behavioral therapy (CBT): Patterns of thoughts and behaviors can lead to development and/or maintenance of symptoms. Thought patterns may not accurately reflect reality and may lead to psychological distress:
  - CBT aims at modifying thought patterns by increasing cognitive flexibility and changing dysfunctional behavioral patterns.
  - CBT encourages patient self-monitoring of symptoms and the precursors or results of maladaptive behavior
  - Uses therapist-assisted challenges to patient's basic beliefs/assumptions
  - May use *exposure*, a procedure derived from basic learning theories, which encourages gradual steps toward change, at a speed that is tolerated by the patient
  - CBT can be offered in group or individual formats, for adults or children.
  - A CBT practitioner attempts to combine practical interventions with emotional supports.
- Dialectical behavior therapy (DBT): Techniques such as social skills training, mindfulness, and problem solving are used to modulate impulse control and affect management:
  - DBT is a therapy approach that derives from CBT, but emphasizes emotional control in relationships.
  - Originally used in treatment of patients with self-destructive behaviors (e.g., cutting, suicide attempts)
  - Seeks to change rigid patterns of cognitions and behaviors that have been maladaptive
  - Uses both individual and group treatment modalities
  - The DBT therapist takes an active role in interpretation and support.
- Interpersonal psychotherapy: Interpersonal relationships in a patient's life are linked to symptoms. Therapy seeks to alleviate symptoms and improve social adjustment through exploration of patient's relationships and experiences. The focus is on one of four potential problem areas:
  - Grief or loss
  - Interpersonal role disputes
  - Role transitions
  - Interpersonal deficits: Therapist works with the patient in resolving the problematic interpersonal issues to facilitate change in symptoms.
- Family therapy: focuses on the family as a unit of intervention
  - Uses psychoeducation to increase patient's and family's insight
  - Teaches communication and problem-solving skills
- Motivational interviewing (MI): focuses on motivation as a key to successful change process
  - Short-term and problem-focused; many therapists use MI prior to initiating other therapies.
  - Focuses on identifying discrepancies between goals and behavior, and the patient's desire to change
  - "5 As" model is a brief counseling framework developed specifically for physicians to effect behavioral change in patients:
    - Assess for a problem.
    - Advise making a change.
    - Agree on action to be taken.
    - Assist with self-care support to make the change.
    - Arrange follow-up to support the change.
- Supportive and informational counseling (heterogeneous treatment)
  - Often focuses on situational factors maintaining symptoms
  - Often encourages the use of community resources
- Behavioral therapy: relatively nontheoretical approach to behavioral change or symptom reduction/eradication through application of principles of stimulus and response; MI is often performed at the onset of behavioral and parenting counseling or therapy.

Pediatric Considerations

- Important distinctions are made between psychotherapy and counseling for children/teens compared to adults/couples.
- The focus of evaluation must include attention to parent and family processes and factors. Interventions typically include interactions and sessions with parents as well as collateral work with teachers and other school personnel.
- Younger children will often be evaluated and diagnosed through behavioral descriptions provided by parents and other adults who know them well as through direct observation and/or play techniques. Children of all ages should be screened using behavioral checklists that are standardized and norm-referenced for age and gender.
- Any child or teenager who requests counseling should be interviewed initially by the primary care provider and referred appropriately. Most referrals will be in response to parental request, however.
- Psychotherapeutic interventions with the strongest empirical basis with children include behavior therapy/modification, CBT, and family/parenting therapy. Play therapy has the least empirical support, but has been found to be useful for developing rapport and for treating trauma in younger children. Insight-oriented therapies appear to be more effective with older children (age ≥10 years).
- There is controversy regarding the efficacy of psychopharmacologic treatment in preadolescents, although clear benefits have been demonstrated in some studies as well as clinical practice. Treatment guidelines for mild to moderate depressed mood and/or anxiety disorders typically recommend pediatric CBT initially, and studies have typically supported this approach in preteen and milder cases. Medications should be considered in more severe presentations.

EPIDEMIOLOGY

- 19 million adults suffer from clinical depression, and >20 million adults have a diagnosable anxiety disorder in the United States.
- One in four Americans report seeking some form of mental health treatment in their adult life. This includes generic counseling in nonmedical settings such as work, clergy, or school settings and also includes visits to primary care providers. It is estimated that between 3.5% and 5% of adults in the United States participate in formal mental health psychotherapy annually. Recent estimates emerging from the COVID-19 pandemic suggest these rates have increased since spring 2020.
- Public health experts report that the majority of those adults with diagnosable psychiatric disorders do not receive professional mental health services. This is due to multiple factors, including failure to identify, noncompliance with psychiatric referral, regional shortages of providers, economic or insurance barriers, and excessive time duration from referral to an available service.

RISK FACTORS

The need for psychotherapy or counseling services is associated with a host of socioeconomic and biogenetic factors, including the general effects of poverty, family or marital dysfunction, life stressors, medical diseases or conditions, and individual biologic predisposition to mental health disorders.

GENERAL PREVENTION

It is generally assumed that early identification and intervention of child and adolescent psychopathology increases the likelihood of reducing the risk for adult psychopathology, but this has not been sufficiently validated in all categories of psychological disorders. Data support such claims in disorders such as childhood ADHD, anxiety disorders, and habit disorders of childhood, however. A range of evidence-based therapies now exist that are designed for children and adults.

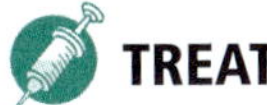

TREATMENT

GENERAL MEASURES

There is evidence of a "dose effect" in psychotherapy outcomes research, with some investigators suggesting that 6 to 8 sessions are necessary to yield positive initial effects in adults, and upward of 15 to 20 sessions for longer term, sustainable therapeutic effects. This dose effect may not be applicable to counseling services with primarily informational or emotional/supportive functions. Also, long-term therapy should be evaluated at 3- to 6-month intervals to determine efficacy.

MEDICATION

- Psychotherapy is most likely to be accompanied by use of pharmaceutical adjuncts in moderate to severe cases of psychological dysfunction that do not respond to other therapies or in cases of extremely poor quality of life or high risk. The most common examples are in cases of clinical depression or anxiety that clearly incapacitates the patient or significantly reduces his or her quality of life. Patients at risk for suicide or who represent a danger to others are also candidates for acute psychopharmacotherapy. Studies suggest that verbal and behaviorally oriented therapies can add efficacy to medication treatment in both depression and anxiety and reduce the risk of relapse.
- There is controversy in the research field regarding the efficacy of medication alone versus psychotherapy alone versus combined treatments. The most recent consensus has been that combined treatments in moderate to severe psychological dysfunction are most likely to render positive short-term results and increase the likelihood that such effects can be sustained over time. Many patients in mental health settings do not require psychotropic medications.

ADDITIONAL THERAPIES

- Anxiety disorders
  - Panic disorder with and without agoraphobia: CBT, psychodynamic therapy
  - Generalized anxiety disorder: CBT
  - Obsessive-compulsive disorder: CBT
  - Posttraumatic stress disorder: CBT, play therapy with children
  - Specific phobia: CBT
  - Social phobia: CBT
- Mood disorders
  - Unipolar depression: CBT, interpersonal therapy, psychodynamic therapy
  - Bipolar disorder: family therapy, interpersonal therapy, CBT/DBT
  - Schizophrenia: psychodynamic therapy, family therapy, CBT/DBT
- Eating disorders
  - Binge-eating disorder: CBT/DBT, interpersonal therapy, behavior modification
  - Bulimia nervosa: CBT/DBT, interpersonal therapy, behavior modification
- Personality disorders
  - Borderline: DBT, CBT
- Substance-use disorders
  - Alcohol: counseling, CBT, MI
  - Cocaine, heroin, opioids, cannabis: CBT, counseling
  - Smoking: MI, behavioral modification with evidence based medications

COMPLEMENTARY & ALTERNATIVE MEDICINE

A host of nonempirically based psychological and nutritional therapies can be found outside of mainstream medicine and psychological science. Very little or no evidence exists to support many experimental therapies, but all have the considerable power of the placebo effect fueling their anecdotal supports or claims. Placebo effects are also thought to be powerfully enhanced by the use of ingested or applied substances that create real physiologic, although not therapeutic, changes in the patient. If it makes them feel different, they are more likely to believe it helps. Placebo alone accounts for moderate amounts of perceived symptom improvement in a range of psychiatric medications, as well as nonregulated supplements.

ONGOING CARE

FOLLOW-UP RECOMMENDATIONS

Patient Monitoring

There is evidence of a "dose effect" in psychotherapy outcomes research, with investigators suggesting upward of 20 sessions for sustainable therapeutic effects. This dose effect may not be applicable to counseling services with primarily informational or emotional/supportive functions, because many patients cease attendance to psychotherapy sessions after one or a few sessions, most interventions of this type cannot be accurately evaluated by the referring provider. Long-term therapy should also be evaluated for effectiveness at regular periods. Patients at suicidal risk need to be monitored more often and in-person.

REFERENCES

1. American Psychiatric Association. *Diagnostic and Statistical Manual of Mental Disorders*. 5th ed. Arlington, VA: American Psychiatric Association; 2013.

ADDITIONAL READING

- Bortolotti B, Menchetti M, Bellini F, et al. Psychological interventions for major depression in primary care: a meta-analytic review of randomized controlled trials. *Gen Hosp Psychiatry*. 2008;30(4):293–302.
- Eddy KT, Dutra L, Bradley R, et al. A multidimensional meta-analysis of psychotherapy and pharmacotherapy for obsessive-compulsive disorder. *Clin Psychol Rev*. 2004;24(8):1011–1030.
- Furukawa TA, Watanabe N, Churchill R. Combined psychotherapy plus antidepressants for panic disorder with or without agoraphobia. *Cochrane Database Syst Rev*. 2007;2007(1):CD004364.
- Hunot V, Churchill R, Silva de Lima M, et al. Psychological therapies for generalised anxiety disorder. *Cochrane Database Syst Rev*. 2007;2007(1):CD001848.

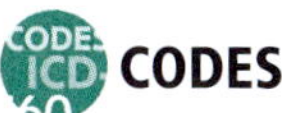

CODES

ICD10

- Z71.9 Counseling, unspecified
- Z71.89 Other specified counseling
- Z63.9 Problem related to primary support group, unspecified

CLINICAL PEARLS

- Combined medication and psychotherapeutic treatments in moderate to severe psychological dysfunction are most likely to render positive short-term results and increase the likelihood such effects can be sustained over time.
- Relapse is common over time and/or as treatments are discontinued or not reevaluated.
- Children <10 years may benefit significantly from counseling or behavior therapy alone for symptom relief.
- Older children and those with more severe symptoms typically require psychopharmacologic options in concert with counseling and/or CBT approaches.

CROHN DISEASE

Samir A. Shah, MD, AGAF, FACG, FASGE • Eric J. Mao, MD

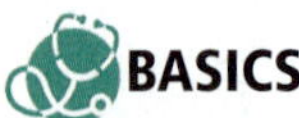

BASICS

DESCRIPTION

- A chronic, progressive inflammatory GI tract disorder, most commonly involving the terminal ileum (80%)
- Hallmark features:
  - Transmural inflammation that can result in strictures, fistulas, fissures, or abscesses; noncaseating granulomas (30%); skip lesions: diseased mucosa interspersed with normal mucosa; can be continuous, mimicking ulcerative colitis (UC); rectal sparing; diverse presentations: ileitis (1/3), ileocolitis (1/3); isolated colitis (1/3)

EPIDEMIOLOGY

Incidence

3 to 20 cases per 100,000 person-years in North America; incidence rising globally. Women are slightly more affected than men; increased incidence in northern climates

Prevalence

247 cases per 100,000 persons

ETIOLOGY AND PATHOPHYSIOLOGY

Genetics, environmental triggers, commensal microbial antigens, and immunologic abnormalities result in activation of inflammatory cells and subsequent tissue injury.

Genetics

- 15% of Crohn disease (CD) patients have a first-degree relative with inflammatory bowel disease (IBD); first-degree relative of an IBD patient has 3- to 30-fold increased risk of developing IBD by age 28 years.
- Associated genetic syndromes: Turner and Hermansky-Pudlak syndromes, glycogen storage disease type 1b

RISK FACTORS

Environmental factors:

- Cigarette smoking doubles the risk of CD; tobacco cessation reduces flares and relapses.
- Dietary factors: higher incidence if diet high in refined sugars, animal fat or protein, processed or ultraprocessed foods

COMMONLY ASSOCIATED CONDITIONS

- Extraintestinal manifestations
  - Arthritis (20%): skin disorders (10%): erythema nodosum, pyoderma gangrenosum, psoriasis; ocular disease (5%): uveitis (associated with HLA-B27), iritis, episcleritis
  - Kidney stones; osteopenia and osteoporosis; hypocalcemia; hypercoagulability: venous thromboembolism prophylaxis essential in hospitalized patients; gallstones: primary sclerosing cholangitis (PSC) (5%)
- Conditions that parallel disease activity
  - Peripheral arthropathy; episcleritis (not uveitis); oral aphthous ulcers and erythema nodosum

DIAGNOSIS

Must integrate history, symptoms, labs, radiology, endoscopic findings, histology preferably interpreted by a GI pathologist

HISTORY

Hallmarks: crampy abdominal pain (+/− bleeding), prolonged diarrhea, fatigue, weight loss, fever, perianal disease; children may present with failure to thrive or falling off growth curve.

- Factors exacerbating CD: concurrent infection, smoking, NSAIDs, antibiotics, stress

PHYSICAL EXAM

Presentation varies with location of disease and severity

- General: signs of sepsis/disease activity (fever, tachycardia, hypotension) or wasting/malnutrition
- Uveitis
- Abdominal: focal or diffuse tenderness, distension, rebound/guarding, rectal bleeding, palpable mass
- Perianal: fistula, fissures, abscess, skin tags
- Skin/joints: erythema nodosum, pyoderma gangrenosum; psoriasis; arthritis

DIFFERENTIAL DIAGNOSIS

- Acute, severe abdominal pain: perforated viscus, pancreatitis, appendicitis, diverticulitis, bowel obstruction, kidney stones, ovarian torsion
- Chronic diarrhea with crampy pain (colitis-like): UC, radiation colitis, infection, drugs, ischemia, microscopic colitis, celiac disease, malignancy (lymphoma, carcinoma), carcinoid, segmental colitis associated with diverticulosis, irritable bowel syndrome (IBS)
- Wasting illness: malabsorption, malignancy

DIAGNOSTIC TESTS & INTERPRETATION

Fecal calprotectin can help distinguish IBD from IBS and can be used to monitor IBD noninvasively.

Initial Tests (lab, imaging)

- CBC, serum chemistries, LFTs, erythrocyte sedimentation rate (ESR), C-reactive protein (CRP), serum iron, vitamin B_{12}, vitamin D-25 OH, fecal calprotectin
- If diarrhea, stool specimen for routine culture, *Clostridium difficile*, and ova and parasites in at risk populations
- With severe flares, KUB to rule out toxic megacolon
- Ileocolonoscopy provides the greatest diagnostic sensitivity and specificity and is considered the gold standard for visualization and obtaining biopsies. Capsule endoscopy allows small bowel visualization without biopsies (1)[C].
- Upper endoscopy for patients with upper GI signs or symptoms (1)[C]
  - Signs of upper GI CD: antral narrowing, segmental stricturing, inflammatory mucosa
- Cross-sectional imaging CT or magnetic resonance enterography (MRE) and ultrasound-evaluate transmural disease, strictures and fistulas
  - Signs of small bowel CD: narrowed lumen with nodularity (string sign); bowel loop separation (transmural inflammation); increased bowel wall enhancement or thickening suggests inflammation.
- Perianal disease: endoscopic ultrasound (EUS), MRI pelvis, exam under anesthesia
- Contraindications to endoscopy: perforated viscus, recent myocardial infarction, severe diverticulitis, toxic megacolon

Follow-Up Tests & Special Considerations

- Biosimilars equivalent to originator product in terms of safety, efficacy, and testing for therapeutic drug monitoring
- Treatment goals
  - Steroid-free clinical remission; biochemical (CRP and ESR) and biologic (calprotectin) remission
  - Radiologic response by cross-sectional or ultrasound imaging; endoscopic response and remission (2)
  - Symptoms may not correlate with disease activity, so objective testing (biomarkers, imaging, endoscopy) is crucial.

Diagnostic Procedures/Other

How to distinguish CD from UC:

- CD: small bowel or colonic disease, rectal sparing; skip lesions; granulomas, perianal disease; RLQ pain; rectal bleeding is uncommon.
- UC: continuous colonic involvement including the rectum; LLQ pain; rectal bleeding common

ALERT

CD can mimic UC with continuous bowel involvement; 10–15% of cases are difficult to differentiate.

TREATMENT

- Disease activity: Harvey-Bradshaw Index or Crohn's Disease Activity Index (CDAI)
- Disease severity: risk stratification for rapidly progressive disease
  - High-risk disease: age at diagnosis <30 years, extensive anatomic involvement, perianal or severe rectal disease, deep ulcers/severe endoscopic disease, prior surgical resection, stricturing/penetrating behavior, extraintestinal manifestation
- Disease severity considers longitudinal factors and prognosis, whereas disease activity is a one-time assessment of symptoms; disease severity/risk assessment should drive therapy decisions.
- Low-risk disease: budesonide or prednisone taper with advanced therapy or active monitoring
- Moderate-/high-risk disease: advanced therapy

GENERAL MEASURES
Step-wise approach and treat to target goals.

MEDICATION
- Mild to moderate CD
  - Asymptomatic with mild endoscopic disease: observation alone; no role for mesalamine in CD (1)[A]
  - Antibiotics not recommended (1)[C]
  - Induction: controlled ileal release budesonide (9 mg/day for 8 weeks and then discontinued over 2-week taper) for distal ileum and/or right colon involvement *or* prednisone taper
  - Maintenance: Stop therapy and observe or consider advanced therapy.
- Moderate to severe CD
  - Induction: biologic as initial induction agent to avoid corticosteroids; may need budesonide 6 to 9 mg or prednisone 40 to 60 mg/day for short-term to alleviate symptoms (1)[C]
  - Maintenance: no role for mesalamine. If steroids required for induction, consider advanced therapy.
- Immunomodulators:
  - Thiopurines: azathioprine or 6-mercaptopurine (6MP) for maintenance but not induction (1)[C]
  - Methotrexate (SC or IM): effective for induction and maintenance of steroid-dependent CD (1)[C]; take with folic acid 1 mg/day.
- Antitumor necrosis factor (anti-TNF): infliximab, adalimumab, certolizumab pegol for induction and maintenance (1)[C],(3)[A]
- Combination therapy: anti-TNF and immunomodulator
  - Combination therapy with standard dose immunomodulator is more effective than either alone. Combining anti-TNF with low-dose immunomodulator reduces immunogenicity.
- Anti-leukocyte trafficking: vedolizumab for induction and maintenance (1)[A],(3)[B]
- Anti-IL-12/IL-23: ustekinumab for induction and maintenance (1)[A],(3)[B]
- Anti-IL-23: guselkumab, mirikizumab, or risankizumab for induction and maintenance
- Janus kinase (JAK) inhibitor: upadacitinib 45 mg once a day for 12 weeks followed by maintenance dose of 30 or 15 mg daily. If no response at 12 weeks, extending another 12 weeks leads to response in just over 50% of the nonresponders.

First Line
- For moderate to severe CD patients naive to biologic drugs:
  - Infliximab, adalimumab, risankizumab, mirikizumab, guselkumab, or ustekinumab recommended over certolizumab (3)[A]
  - Vedolizumab recommended over certolizumab (3)[C]

Second Line
- For moderate to severe CD patients who never responded to anti-TNF (primary nonresponse):
  - Risankizumab is preferred over ustekinumab (3)[A]; unclear yet if mirikizumab, guselkumab equivalent to risankizumab
  - Vedolizumab is recommended over no therapy (3)[C].
  - Upadacitinib in recommended over no therapy
- For moderate to severe CD patients who previously responded to anti-TNF (secondary nonresponse):
  - Risankizumab is preferred over ustekinumab, but either therapy is recommended over no therapy (3)[A]; unclear yet if mirikizumab, guselkumab equivalent to risankizumab
  - Vedolizumab is recommended over no therapy (3)[C].
  - Upadacitinib in recommended over no therapy
  - If lost response due to antibody, can switch to a different anti-TNF (not a biosimilar of the previously failed drug) with an immunomodulator to prevent immunogenicity

ADDITIONAL THERAPIES
- Oral lesions: triamcinolone acetonide in benzocaine and carboxymethyl cellulose or topical sucralfate for aphthous ulcers, cheilitis
- Gastroduodenal CD: Case reports show success of anti-TNF therapy; symptomatic relief possible from proton pump inhibitors, H_2 receptor blockers, and/or sucralfate

SURGERY/OTHER PROCEDURES
Multidisciplinary care with colorectal surgery, gastroenterology, nutrition, radiology, pathology, etc., helps optimize outcomes.

ONGOING CARE

FOLLOW-UP RECOMMENDATIONS
- Monitor CBC, BMP, LFTs every 3 to 4 months.
- Actively monitor disease with CRP and calprotectin every 6 months.
- Goal of mucosal healing confirmed by endoscopy or imaging, or inflammatory markers
- Check TPMT/NUDT15 genotype/activity prior to thiopurine initiation and thiopurine metabolites 1 month afterwards
- With anti-TNF therapy, consider proactive therapeutic drug monitoring.

Patient Monitoring
- Vaccinations
  - Check titers; avoid live vaccines (MMR, varicella) in immunosuppressed patients.
  - Regardless of immunosuppression: HPV, influenza, COVID-19 vaccine, meningococcal, hepatitis A and B, Tdap, RSV (if ≥60 years)
  - Immunosuppressed patients ≥18 years: pneumococcal, recombinant zoster vaccine
- Cancer prevention
  - Colonoscopy with targeted biopsies every 2 to 5 years after 8 years of CD with at least 1/3 of colon involved; consider chromoendoscopy; in PSC patients, annual screening colonoscopy recommended.
  - Annual Pap smears if immunocompromised
  - Annual skin exam
- Bone health
  - Calcium and vitamin D supplementation with each course of corticosteroids or if vitamin D deficient
  - Bone density assessment if previous steroids, maternal history of osteoporosis, malnourished, amenorrheic, postmenopausal

DIET
Mediterranean diet

PATIENT EDUCATION
- Crohn's & Colitis Foundation: https://www.crohnscolitisfoundation.org/
- IBDandMe: https://ibdandme.org/

REFERENCES

1. Dolinger M, Torres J, Vermeire S. Crohn's disease. *Lancet*. 2024;403(10432):1177–1191. doi:10.1016/S0140-6736(23)02586-2.
2. Lichtenstein GR, Loftus EV, Afzali A, et al. ACG clinical guidelines: management of Crohn's disease in adults. *Am J Gastroenterol*. 2025;120(6):1225–1264.
3. Feuerstein JD, Ho EY, Shmidt E, et al. AGA clinical practice guidelines on the medical management of moderate to severe luminal and perianal fistulizing Crohn's disease. *Gastroenterology*. 2021;160(7):2496–2508.

ADDITIONAL READING

Ananthakrishnan AN, Adler J, Chachu KA, et al. AGA clinical practice guideline on the role of biomarkers for the management of Crohn's disease. *Gastroenterology*. 2023;165(6):1367–1399. doi:10.1053/j.gastro.2023.09.029.

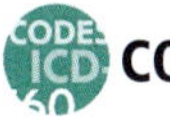

CODES

ICD10
- K50.0 Crohn's disease of small intestine
- K50.113 Crohn's disease of large intestine with fistula
- K50.011 Crohn's disease of small intestine with rectal bleeding

CLINICAL PEARLS
- Cigarette smoking doubles the risk of CD; tobacco cessation reduces flares and need for surgery.
- MRE allows assessment of luminal and extraluminal CD without radiation exposure.
- Assess for TB and HBV infection prior to initiating biologic therapy.
- Test for *Clostridium difficile* infection when evaluating diarrhea in all CD patients.
- Hospitalized CD patients require deep vein thrombosis prophylaxis.
- Any biologic or JAK inhibitor is effective in delaying or preventing postoperative recurrence in CD.
- Disease severity rather than disease activity should drive therapy decisions.

C

CROUP (LARYNGOTRACHEOBRONCHITIS)

Afsha Rais Kaisani, MD, FAAFP • Tasaduq Hussain Mir, MD, FAAFP

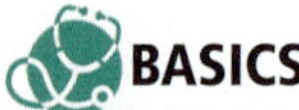

BASICS

Croup is a self-limited upper respiratory tract infection that affects 3% of children 6 months to 3 years of age. It results in inflammation of the larynx, trachea, and bronchi and presents with barking cough and inspiratory stridor. Although usually mild, croup can cause significant respiratory distress and even death.

DESCRIPTION

- The spectrum of croup includes laryngotracheitis (LT), laryngotracheobronchitis (LTB), and laryngotracheobronchopneumonitis.
- Mostly a viral infection and most common cause of airway obstruction in young children.
- May occur in absence of viral prodrome, known as spasmodic croup, occurring in older children; rapid onset and resolution and often has a recurrent course

EPIDEMIOLOGY

- Most commonly affects children aged 6 months to 3 years of age, peaks at 18 months; although rare, croup can affect children as young as 3 months and as old as 6 to 7 years.
- Sex: male > female.
- Most often occurs in the fall and early winter

Incidence

- Accounts for 1.3% of emergency department (ED) cases and 7% of hospitalizations for acute respiratory illness in children <5 years of age.
- <3% require laryngoscopic or airway procedures.
- 4.4% of children returned to the ED within 48 hours (1).

ETIOLOGY AND PATHOPHYSIOLOGY

- Infection of the larynx, trachea, and bronchi, causing narrowing of the airway secondary to inflammation and edema
- Narrow airway and negative-pressure inspiration pulls airway walls closer together creating inspiratory stridor.
- Typically caused by viruses; most common pathogen is parainfluenza virus, responsible for >80% of cases
  - Type 1 and 2 are the most common.
  - Type 3 is affiliated with bronchiolitis and pneumonia in young infants and children.
  - Type 4 (subtypes 4A and 4B), are associated with milder illness.
- Other viruses: RSV, paramyxovirus, influenza virus type A or B, adenovirus, rhinovirus, enteroviruses (coxsackie and echo), reovirus, measles virus where vaccination not common, and metapneumovirus
- *Mycoplasma pneumoniae* and *Corynebacterium diphtheriae* have been reported but are rare.
- Bacterial croup is commonly caused by *Staphylococcus aureus*, *Streptococcus pneumoniae*, *Haemophilus influenzae*, and *Moraxella catarrhalis*.
- Spasmodic croup cause is unclear, possibly allergy, airway hyperactivity, and gastroesophageal reflux.

Genetics

Congenital subglottic stenosis, which is a narrowing of the lumen of the cricoid region, can present as recurrent croup.

RISK FACTORS

Prior intubations, structural airway abnormality, prematurity, and age <3 years increase the risks for recurrent croup (more than two episodes per year) (2). Gastroesophageal reflux disease (GERD) and asthma are highly prevalent in patients with recurrent croup, however, neither are associated with significant bronchoscopy findings.

GENERAL PREVENTION

Croup spreads through droplets. Children should be considered contagious up to 3 days after the start of illness and/or until afebrile. There is no specific vaccine for croup, but seasonal influenza vaccine may contribute to decreased risk.

COMMONLY ASSOCIATED CONDITIONS

- Some evidence suggests croup hospitalization may be associated with future development of asthma.
- Underlying anatomic abnormality (e.g., subglottic stenosis, paradoxical vocal cord dysfunction)
- Consider GERD for patients with recurrent croup symptoms.
- COVID-19—a potential viral agent in patients with croup.

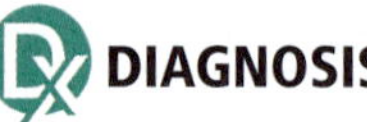

DIAGNOSIS

- Croup is a clinical diagnosis; most children present with acute onset of classic "seal-like" barking cough, inspiratory stridor, hoarseness, and chest wall indrawing.
- Low-to-moderate grade fever; absence of fever should not reduce suspicion for croup.
- Severity is determined by clinical inspection for signs of respiratory distress: nasal flaring, retractions, tripoding, sniffing position, abdominal breathing, and tachypnea. Although uncommon, hypoxia, cyanosis, and fatigue are late signs of severity.
- Consider SARS-CoV-2 testing in suspicious cases (3).
- Westley Croup Severity Score is the commonly used scoring system. It looks at five clinical features and scores are as follows: ≤2 mild; 3 to 7 moderate; 8 to 11 severe; ≥12 impending respiratory failure.
  - Level of consciousness: normal, including sleep = 0; disoriented = 5
  - Cyanosis: none = 0; with agitation = 4; at rest = 5
  - Stridor: none = 0; with agitation = 1; at rest = 2
  - Air entry: normal = 0; decreased = 1; markedly decreased = 2
  - Retractions: none = 0; mild = 1; moderate = 2; severe = 3

HISTORY

Croup is primarily a clinical diagnosis, characterized by abrupt onset of barking cough, inspiratory stridor, and hoarseness (2).

PHYSICAL EXAM

- Vital signs can demonstrate tachypnea and tachycardia.
- Pulse oximetry often is normal as there is no disturbance of alveolar gas exchange; however, oxygen saturation might be decreased in severe cases.
- Visual inspection of nasal flaring, retraction, and/or cyanosis indicate high suspicion for croup.
- Breathing sounds and voice are important for diagnosis; typically, the patient will present with hoarseness, stridor, and/or inspiratory wheezing to auscultation.
  - Stridor can be present at rest and aggravated by agitation.
  - Substantial wheezing, rhonchi, and rales should prompt alternative diagnosis.
- Decreased breath sounds and respiratory effort may indicate the child is progressing into respiratory failure and less able to mount an effort to move air (2).

DIFFERENTIAL DIAGNOSIS

- Foreign body aspiration
- Bacterial tracheitis: high fever, barking cough, respiratory distress, and rapid deterioration
- Retropharyngeal or peritonsillar abscess: similar septic appearance with dysphonia
- Allergic reaction (acute angioneurotic edema) includes spasmodic croup with classic nocturnal exacerbations.
- Epiglottitis: rapid onset, high fever, dysphonia, drooling, and prototypical posture of extended chin and leaning forward; the incidence of epiglottitis has significantly decreased with widespread vaccination against *H. influenzae*.
- Others: subglottic stenosis, thermal injury/smoke inhalation, hemangioma, airway anomalies (e.g., tracheomalacia/laryngomalacia), neoplasm, other anatomic obstructions (2)
- SARS-CoV-2 presents with more severe symptoms and response to treatment is not as rapid as expected (3).

DIAGNOSTIC TESTS & INTERPRETATION

- Croup does not require confirmatory testing.
- Blood work not required; if done, WBC counts may be mildly elevated with a predominance of lymphocytes.
  - An elevated WBC shift to the left (bandemia) would suggest bacterial etiology (epiglottitis, bacterial tracheitis, peritonsillar, and/or retropharyngeal abscess).
- Rapid antigen or viral culture tests should be reserved for patients in whom initial treatment is ineffective.
- If imaging were to be done, posteroanterior and lateral neck films will show funnel-shaped subglottic region with normal epiglottis: "steeple" or "pencil point" sign (present in 40–60% of children with croup).
  - A steeple sign can be seen in patients without croup warranting other considerations.
  - Monitor all patients during imaging as airway obstruction may occur rapidly.

- When suspecting an alternative diagnosis, the following findings can be appreciated:
  - Retropharyngeal abscess: bulging of posterior pharyngeal wall
  - Epiglottitis: "thumb sign," which is a thickened epiglottis
- Polymerase chain reaction testing from nasopharyngeal mucosa is used when SARS-CoV-2 is suspected as the cause of croup (3).

Initial Tests (lab, imaging)

Radiographic imaging is not routinely indicated. CT of the neck can be considered for patients with suspected abscess, tumor, or foreign body aspiration (2).

Follow-Up Tests & Special Considerations

Recurrent croup needs evaluation for other underlying conditions (e.g., asthma, GERD, anatomical airway abnormalities).

Diagnostic Procedures/Other

Laryngoscopy should be reserved for atypical presentations or when alternate diagnosis are suspected (2), such as those hospitalized but not intubated or those with a history of intubation and under 36 months of age.

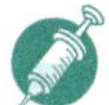

TREATMENT

- Treatment is supportive; severity of illness may dictate additional measurements.
- Outpatient patients with severe croup or impending respiratory failure should be transported via ambulance to the nearest hospital for management.
- The limited experience with COVID-19 croup suggests cases can present with severe pathology and may not improve as rapidly as with typical croup.

GENERAL MEASURES

- Symptomatic treatment
- Minimize lab tests, imaging, and procedures that upset the child; agitation worsens tachypnea and can be detrimental.
- Pulse oximetry and oxygen should be administered for hypoxemia or respiratory distress.
- Frequent clinical checks may be more sensitive in identifying worsening disease.
- Heliox is a helium and oxygen mixture used for respiratory conditions, and improves airflow resistance by decreasing gas density; data is limited on its benefits for croup (2)[B].

MEDICATION

Treatment is based on Wesley Croup Score: mild (0 to 2): one dose of dexamethasone; moderate to severe (≥3): dexamethasone and nebulized epinephrine; in patients with mild to moderate disease: single dose of dexamethasone and 3 daily doses of prednisolone showed no difference in symptom score.

First Line

- Corticosteroids: Oral corticosteroids should be used in patients with any severity to decrease laryngeal mucosa edema.
  - Dexamethasone 6 mg/kg is preferred due to its easy single dosing and ability to be given orally, intramuscular, and intravenous.
  - Other steroids (betamethasone, budesonide, prednisolone) are beneficial.
- Nebulized epinephrine; racemic or L-epinephrine (equal efficacy and side effect profiles); reserved for moderate-to-severe cases with stridor at rest
  - Racemic epinephrine is dosed at 0.05 mL/kg of 2.25% (max 0.5 mL) solution nebulized in normal saline to total volume of 3 mL.
  - L-epinephrine is dose at 0.5 mL/kg (max of 5 mL) of a 1:1,000 via nebulizer. Onset of action is within 1 to 5 minutes, and duration is of approximately 2 hours. Repeat as necessary as long as side effects are tolerated. Observe child for 2 hours to ensure no recurrence after epinephrine wears off.
- Antitussives and decongestants are not recommended.
- Antibiotics when suspecting a primary or secondary bacterial infection
- Oxygen as needed
- Humidified air without clinical benefit in croup (2)

SURGERY/OTHER PROCEDURES

Intubation is rarely required and may be need for fatigue due to increase work of breathing or obstruction; tube 0.5 to 1.0 mm smaller than normal

ADMISSION, INPATIENT, AND NURSING CONSIDERATIONS

- Outpatient care for mild cases
- In most cases, observation in the emergency room after medical management is sufficient.
- Admission criteria: poor response to therapy or recurrent stridor at rest after epinephrine wears off, increased oxygen requirement, pneumonia, or other serious conditions
- Discharge criteria
  - At least 2 hours since last epinephrine
  - Received dose of steroids
  - No stridor at rest, no difficulty breathing
  - Able to tolerate oral fluids
  - Normal air entry, color, and consciousness
  - Has home management and outpatient follow up established

ONGOING CARE

FOLLOW-UP RECOMMENDATIONS

If recurrent (>2 episodes in a year) or during first 90 days of life; consider host factors or allergic factors.

Patient Monitoring

60% of barking cough resolves within 48 hours and only 2% have symptoms persisting for longer than five nights (1).

DIET

- Cool, liquid diet is better tolerated.
- Frequent small feedings

PATIENT EDUCATION

- Croup is usually a self-limited and mild disease, but some will need hospital care.
- Avoid agitation, which may worsen symptoms; use antipyretics as needed. Keep hydrated with liquids, ice pops, etc.
- Emergency ambulance: cyanosis, lethargy, struggling to breathe, drooling and unable to swallow
- It is contagious in the first few days; good hand hygiene is very important.
- Cough may linger for a few weeks.
- Parents of patients with COVID-19–related croup should be counseled on quarantine guidelines.

PROGNOSIS

- Prognosis is usually good. The few cases that are severe respond to intensive respiratory management.
- Recurrence is rare in viral-mediated disease. If croup recurs, consider an anatomic, allergic, or obstructive etiology.

COMPLICATIONS

- Subglottic stenosis in intubated patients
- Bacterial tracheitis
- Cardiopulmonary arrest
- Pneumonia (2)

REFERENCES

1. Hanna J, Brauer PR, Morse E, et al. Epidemiological analysis of croup in the emergency department using two national datasets. *Int J Pediatr Otorhinolaryngol*. 2019;126:109641.
2. Smith DK, McDermott AJ, Sullivan JF. Croup: diagnosis and management. *Am Fam Physician*. 2018;97(9):575–580.
3. Venn AMR, Schmidt JM, Mullan PC. Pediatric croup with COVID-19. *Am J Emerg Med*. 2021;43:287.e1–e287.e3.

ADDITIONAL READING

Quraishi H, Lee DJ. Recurrent croup. *Pediatr Clin North Am*. 2022;69(2):319–328. doi:10.1016/j.pcl.2021.12.004.

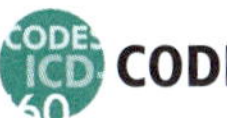

CODES

ICD10

- J05.0 Acute obstructive laryngitis [croup]
- J20.9 Acute bronchitis, unspecified
- J38.5 Laryngeal spasm

CLINICAL PEARLS

- Most common in fall and winter seasons in ages 6 months to 3 years
- Inspiratory stridor is clinically evident and should raise suspicion of croup.
- Symptoms often occur at night.
- Clinical diagnosis, medical management, and stabilization of the patient take priority over lab testing or imaging.
- Recurrence requires further evaluation.
- Consider other diagnoses in acute presentations with toxic appearance: epiglottitis, abscess, bacterial tracheitis.
- Be aware of severity if child becomes less noisy; less air movement can be sign of respiratory failure.
- Treatment: corticosteroid, supplemental oxygen as needed, and epinephrine for moderate to severe cases

CRYPTORCHIDISM

Pamela Ellsworth, MD

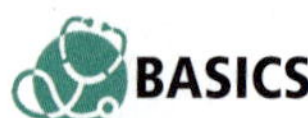

BASICS

DESCRIPTION

- Incomplete or improper descent of one or both testicles; also called *undescended testes* (1)
- Normally descent is in month 7 to 8 of gestation. The cryptorchid testis may be palpable or nonpalpable.
- Can be congenital or acquired
- Types of cryptorchidism
  - Prescrotal: at or above scrotal inlet
  - Abdominal: testis located inside the internal inguinal ring
  - Canalicular: testis located between the internal and external inguinal rings
  - Ectopic: located outside the normal path of testicular descent; may be ectopic to perineum, femoral canal, superficial inguinal pouch (most common), suprapubic area, or opposite hemiscrotum
  - Retractile: fully descended testis that moves freely between the scrotum and the groin
  - Iatrogenic: Previously descended testis becomes undescended due to scar tissue after inguinal surgery.
  - Also may be referred to as palpable versus nonpalpable (1)
- System(s) affected: reproductive
- Synonym(s): undescended testes (UDT)

EPIDEMIOLOGY

Incidence

Predominant age: newborn, more common in premature newborns

Prevalence

- In the United States, cryptorchidism occurs in 1–3% of full-term newborn males and 15–30% of premature newborn males (2).
- Spontaneous testicular descent occurs by age 1 to 3 months in 50–70% of full-term males.
- Descent at 6 to 9 months of age is rare (1).

ETIOLOGY AND PATHOPHYSIOLOGY

- Not fully understood, may involve alterations in
  - Mechanical factors (gubernaculum, length of vas deferens and testicular vessels, groin anatomy, epididymis, cremasteric muscles, and abdominal pressure), hormonal factors (gonadotropin, testosterone, dihydrotestosterone, müllerian-inhibiting substance [MIS]), and neural factors (ilioinguinal nerve and genitofemoral nerve)
  - Insulin-like growth factor 3 (IGF-3) or androgen receptor gene (1)
  - Environmental factors acting as endocrine disruptors
- Major regulators of testicular descent are the Leydig cell–derived hormones, testosterone, and IGF-3.
- Risk of ascent as high as 32% in retractile testis

Genetics

Increased risk of UDT in first-degree relatives suggests a genetic etiology.

RISK FACTORS

- Family history: highest risk if brother had UDT, followed by uncle and then father
- Low birth weight, prematurity, and small for gestational age (1)
- Retractile testes are at increased risk for ascent.
- Maternal smoking and diabetes during gestation

COMMONLY ASSOCIATED CONDITIONS

- Anatomic anomalies: inguinal hernia/hydrocele, abnormalities of vas deferens and epididymis, hypospadias, meningomyelocele
- Endocrine disorders: intersex abnormalities, hypogonadotropic hypogonadism, germinal cell aplasia
- Genetic disorders: Prune-belly syndrome, Prader-Willi syndrome, Kallmann syndrome, cystic fibrosis
- Wilms tumor

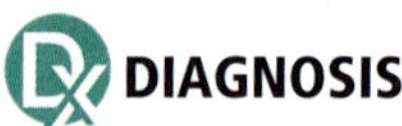

DIAGNOSIS

HISTORY

≥1 testicles in a site other than the scrotum

PHYSICAL EXAM

- Performed with warm hands, with child in sitting, standing, and squatting position
- A Valsalva maneuver and applied pressure to lower abdomen may help to identify the testes, especially a gliding testis.
- Failure to palpate a testis after repeated exams suggests an intra-abdominal or atrophic testis.
- An enlarged contralateral testis in the presence of a nonpalpable testis suggests testicular atrophy/absence.
- Testes should be palpated for quality and position at each recommended well-child visit (1)[B].

DIFFERENTIAL DIAGNOSIS

- Retractile testis (hypermobile testis): a normally descended testis that ascends into the inguinal canal because of an active cremasteric reflex (more common in males 4 to 6 years of age)
- Atrophic testis: may occur as a result of neonatal torsion
- Vanished testis may be the result of a lack of development or in utero torsion.

DIAGNOSTIC TESTS & INTERPRETATION

Initial Tests (lab, imaging)

- If only single testis not palpable in an otherwise normal male, no need for lab tests or imaging
- In phenotypic male newborn with bilateral, nonpalpable UDTs, hormone levels help determine whether the testes are ectopic or absent (1)[A].
  - Luteinizing hormone (LH), follicle-stimulating hormone (FSH), MIS, testosterone, serum electrolytes, karyotype
- If bilateral nonpalpable testes presents at >3 months of age, evaluate for disorders of sexual development (3) and evaluate for congenital adrenal hyperplasia.
- Ultrasound or other imaging should not delay referral to a specialist, as they are rarely needed in decision-making (1)[B].

Follow-Up Tests & Special Considerations

In infants <6 months of age, periodic examination to determine if testis becomes palpable prior to further intervention (1)

Pediatric Considerations

Without spontaneous testicular descent by 6 months, (gestational age adjusted) infant should be referred to urology, and surgery should be performed within 1 year (1)[B].

- In children with retractile testes, yearly examinations to rule out subsequent ascent (1)[B]

Diagnostic Procedures/Other

Laparoscopy can confirm presence or absence of testis when nonpalpable and determine the feasibility of performing a standard orchidopexy.

Test Interpretation

Higher incidence of carcinoma in UDT and alterations in spermatogenesis. Histologic changes occur by 1.5 years of age (4).

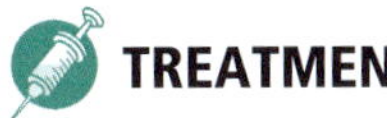

TREATMENT

GENERAL MEASURES

- Rule out retractile testis.
- American Urological Association (AUA) guidelines on cryptorchidism do not recommend use of hormonal therapy to induce testicular descent due to low response rate and lack of evidence for long-term efficacy (1).

MEDICATION

Medical therapy is not indicated in the United States per the AUA guidelines on cryptorchidism 2014 (1).

ISSUES FOR REFERRAL

- ≥1 testes not descended by 6 months age (1)[B]
- Bilateral nonpalpable UDTs (1)
- Newly diagnosed cryptorchidism after 6 months of age (1)[B]

SURGERY/OTHER PROCEDURES

- Benefits: avoids torsion, averts trauma, decreases but does not eliminate risk of malignancy, and prevents further alterations in spermatogenesis
- If no spontaneous testicular descent by 6 months of age (gestational age–adjusted), surgery should be performed within 1 year (1)[B].
- Prepubertal orchidopexy decreases risk of testicular cancer (1).
- Laparoscopy/abdominal exploration is performed first if testis is nonpalpable.
- If palpable, an inguinal approach is usually performed. If low lying, a single-incision scrotal approach can also be considered but may increase the risk of hernia.

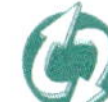

ONGOING CARE

FOLLOW-UP RECOMMENDATIONS

- Initial follow-up within 1 month of surgery and periodically thereafter to assess testicular size/growth
- Patients with retractile testes should be examined at least annually to monitor for secondary ascent until testis is no longer retractile (1)[B].

Patient Monitoring

- Patients should be followed after surgery to evaluate testicular growth.
- Testicular tumors occur mainly during or after puberty; thus, these children should be taught self-examination.

DIET

No restrictions

PATIENT EDUCATION

Discuss with parents about causes, treatments, patient's reproductive potential, and increased risk for testicular cancer.

PROGNOSIS

- Disorder is usually corrected with surgical therapy.
- If testicle is absent or orchiectomy is required, may consider placement of testicular prosthesis
- Early orchidopexy may decrease risk of testicular damage and risk of malignancy.

COMPLICATIONS

- Paternity rates are similar to the general population for men with a unilateral UDT; however, are lower (33–65%) for men with bilateral UDT
- Abnormalities also have been identified in the contralateral descended testis, suggesting that unilateral cryptorchidism is a bilateral disease.

REFERENCES

1. Kolon TF, Herndon CDA, Baker LA, et al. Evaluation and treatment of cryptorchidism. https://www.auanet.org/education/guidelines/cryptorchidism.cfm. Accessed October 3, 2017.
2. Sijstermans K, Hack WW, Meijer RW, et al. The frequency of undescended testis from birth to adulthood: a review. *Int J Androl*. 2008;31(1):1–11.
3. Docimo SG, Silver RI, Cromie W. The undescended testicle: diagnosis and management. *Am Fam Physician*. 2000;62(9):2037–2044, 2047–2048.
4. Park KH, Lee JH, Han JJ, et al. Histological evidences suggest recommending orchiopexy within the first year of life for children with unilateral inguinal cryptorchid testis. *Int J Urol*. 2007;14(7):616–621.

ADDITIONAL READING

- Fantasia J, Aidlen J, Lathrop W, et al. Undescended testes: a clinical and surgical review. *Urol Nurs*. 2015;35(3):117–126.
- Saylors S, Oyentunji TA. Management of undescended testis. *Curr Opin Pediatr*. 2024;36(5):554–561.

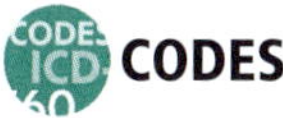

CODES

ICD10

- Q53.9 Undescended testicle, unspecified
- Q53.10 Unspecified undescended testicle, unilateral
- Q53.20 Undescended testicle, unspecified, bilateral

CLINICAL PEARLS

- If testicular descent does not occur by 6 months of age, it is unlikely to occur. Refer to urologist at 6 months.
- Children with bilateral, nonpalpable UDTs require laboratory evaluation to determine if viable testicular tissue is present and to rule out disorder of sexual differentiation.
- Radiologic imaging has no role in the initial evaluation of cryptorchidism.
- The risk of infertility is increased with bilateral UDTs.

CUSHING DISEASE AND CUSHING SYNDROME

Jennifer G. Foster, MD, MBA, FACP • Lisa C. Martinez, MD • Allison H. Ferris, MD

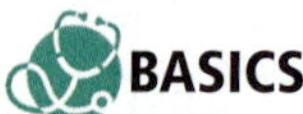

BASICS

DESCRIPTION

- Cushing syndrome is defined as excessive glucocorticoid exposure from exogenous sources (such as prednisone) or less commonly from endogenous sources (i.e., pituitary, adrenal, pulmonary, etc.).
- The most common cause of endogenous Cushing syndrome is Cushing disease, which is characterized by excessive adrenocorticotropic hormone (ACTH) secretion, typically from a benign pituitary adenoma.
  - Cushing syndrome from excess endogenous sources may also be caused by a benign or malignant nonpituitary corticotropin secreting tumor (known as ectopic Cushing syndrome).
- System(s) affected: endocrine/metabolic, musculoskeletal, skin/exocrine, cardiovascular, and neuropsychiatric

Pediatric Considerations

- Rare in infancy and childhood
- The most common presenting symptom is weight gain and lack of growth.

Pregnancy Considerations

- Women with Cushing syndrome have a risk of anovulatory infertility.
- Pregnancy may exacerbate the disease.

EPIDEMIOLOGY

Incidence

The estimated incidence of Cushing syndrome attributable to endogenous production of cortisol ranges from about 2 to 8 people per million annually.

Prevalence

- An estimated 10 to 15 cases per million people are affected yearly.
- Cushing disease most commonly affects adults 20 to 50 years old and is more prevalent in females.
- 2–5% prevalence reported in difficult-to-control diabetic patients with obesity and hypertension (HTN).

ETIOLOGY AND PATHOPHYSIOLOGY

- Cortisol is a steroid hormone produced by the zona fasciculata of the adrenal cortex. It is classically a catabolic hormone released during periods of stress. Excess levels of cortisol cause increased free glucose, insulin resistance, immunosuppression, neurocognitive changes, bone disorders (i.e., osteoporosis), mood disorders (e.g., depression), and protein catabolism.
- The most common cause of Cushing syndrome is prolonged glucocorticoid use from any route of administration (e.g., topical, inhaled, oral).
- Endogenous cause is either ACTH dependent or ACTH independent:
  - ACTH is typically secreted by the anterior pituitary gland and stimulates the adrenal glands to release cortisol. As such, release of ACTH from any source will result in increased cortisol levels.

Genetics

- Multiple endocrine neoplasia (MEN) syndrome
- McCune-Albright syndrome (mutation of *GNAS1* gene)

RISK FACTORS

Prolonged use of corticosteroids

GENERAL PREVENTION

Avoid corticosteroid exposure.

COMMONLY ASSOCIATED CONDITIONS

Psychiatric disorders, diabetes, HTN, hypokalemia, infections, dyslipidemia, and osteoporosis

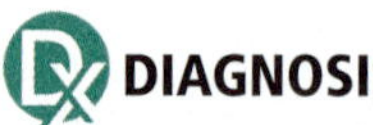

DIAGNOSIS

- The most common age at diagnosis ranges from age 30 to 49 years, but Cushing syndrome can be diagnosed from the ages, of 5 to 75 years.
- Symptoms may include facial plethora, round face, increased adiposity of dorsocervical fat pads, easy bruising, purple striae, thin skin, fragility fractures, and muscle weakness.

HISTORY

- Weight gain: 95%
- Easy bruising: 95%
- Diabetes or glucose intolerance: 90%
- Decreased libido: 90%
- Menstrual irregularity: 80%
- Depression/emotional lability: 50–80%

PHYSICAL EXAM

- Obesity (usually central): 95%
- Facial plethora: 90%
- Round or "moon" face (facial adiposity): 90%
- Proximal muscle weakness: 90%
- Thin skin: 85%
- HTN: 75%
- Hirsutism: 75%
- Purple striae on the skin, typically >1 cm
- Increased adipose tissue in neck and trunk: supraclavicular fat pads, dorsocervical fat pad
- Acne
- Skeletal growth retardation in children (epiphyseal plates remain open): 70–80%

DIFFERENTIAL DIAGNOSIS

- Obesity/Type 2 diabetes mellitus (T2DM)/HTN
- Polycystic ovarian syndrome
- Pseudo-Cushing (e.g., alcoholism, physical stress, severe major depression)

DIAGNOSTIC TESTS & INTERPRETATION

Initial testing includes midnight salivary cortisol measurement, 1 mg overnight dexamethasone suppression test, and 24-hour urinary free cortisol (UFC).

Initial Tests (lab, imaging)

- Guidelines recommend testing for Cushing syndrome after obtaining a detailed medication and drug history (excluding exogenous corticosteroid use) in patients with the following (1),(2)[C]:
  - Adrenal incidentaloma compatible with adenoma
  - Unusual features for age such as early osteoporosis and HTN
  - Abnormal growth and increased weight in children
- In patients suspected to have Cushing syndrome, one of the following screening tests can be performed:
  - 24-hour UFC (at least two measurements)
    - Measure concomitant 24-hour urinary creatinine excretion to verify adequacy of collection as results may be falsely low in the setting of renal impairment (GFR <60 mL/min).
    - Overall sensitivity and specificity: 90–97% and 85–99%, respectively.
  - Late night salivary cortisol (at least two measurements)
    - Cortisol secretion is highest in the morning and lowest between 11 PM and midnight.
    - Sensitivity and specificity are >90–95%.
    - May be inaccurate in patients who are night-shift workers
  - 1 mg overnight dexamethasone suppression test
    - Dexamethasone 1 mg given between 11 PM and midnight, and fasting plasma cortisol is measured between 8 and 9 AM the following morning.
    - A serum cortisol level <1.8 μg/dL excludes Cushing syndrome, but specificity is limited.
- A diagnosis of Cushing syndrome is made when two different tests above are unequivocally abnormal.
- Localization tests: Once the diagnosis of Cushing syndrome is confirmed:
  - Morning ACTH levels:
    - <10 pg/mL: ACTH-independent Cushing
    - >20 pg/mL: ACTH-dependent Cushing
    - 10 to 20 pg/mL: Corticotropin-releasing hormone stimulation test is recommended to differentiate between the two forms.
  - High-dose dexamethasone suppression test to determine source of ACTH: 8 mg of oral dexamethasone is given at 11 PM, with measurement of an 8-AM cortisol level the next day.
    - A baseline 8-AM cortisol measurement is also obtained the morning prior to ingesting dexamethasone. Suppression of serum cortisol level to <50% of baseline is suggestive of a pituitary source of ACTH rather than ectopic ACTH or primary adrenal disease. Sensitivity and specificity are 95% and 100%, respectively.
    - Another approach is to measure 8-AM cortisol after 8 mg dexamethasone given the night before: Cushing disease: cortisol suppressed to <5 μg/dL.

- Imaging:
  - Confirm Cushing diagnosis before imaging studies due to the possibility of both pituitary and adrenal incidentalomas.
    - Dotatate PET/CT, a high-resolution diagnostic tool, is quite useful in identifying tumors missed by other forms of imaging, with a sensitivity of around 90–91%.
    - Up to 19% of ectopic ACTH-secreting tumors can remain occult despite conventional body imaging and modalities of nuclear imaging such as scintigraphy/SPECT.
    - Octreotide scintigraphy to look for occult ACTH-secreting tumor
    - Chest CT scan if ectopic ACTH secretion is suspected
    - Abdominal CT scan if adrenal disease is suspected
    - Pituitary MRI if pituitary tumor is suspected (all patients with ACTH-dependent hypercortisolism)

ALERT

- Antiepileptic drugs, progesterone, oral contraceptives, rifampin, and spironolactone may cause a false-positive dexamethasone suppression test.
- Pregnancy: UFC is recommended instead of dexamethasone in the initial evaluation of pregnant women (or on birth control pills). Only UFC in the 2nd or 3rd trimester >3 times the upper limit of normal is suggestive of Cushing syndrome.

Diagnostic Procedures/Other

Testing for associated findings can be useful, including:

- Thyroid function, T2DM, osteoporosis
- Polycystic ovarian syndrome/hyperandrogenism
- Oligomenorrhea/hypogonadism
- Hypercoagulable state/venous thromboembolism
- Metastases from malignant tumors
- Atrial fibrillation
- Hypokalemia
- Growth hormone reduction

TREATMENT

- For patients with endogenous Cushing syndrome, the primary aim of therapy is complete resection of the underlying tumor.
- For patients with Cushing disease, the primary therapy is transsphenoidal pituitary surgery with selective adenomectomy.

MEDICATION

- It is important to manage the comorbidities associated with hypercortisolism such as diabetes mellitus or HTN.
- Medical therapy is usually ineffective for long-term treatment and is typically used in preparation for surgery or as adjunctive therapy after surgery or pituitary radiotherapy.
- Medical therapy prior to surgery can be indicated in those with very severe Cushing due to ectopic ACTH or Cushing disease requiring pharmacologi multitherapy to avoid rescue bilateral adrenalectomy (3).
- Medical therapy can be attempted either by targeting reduction of cortisol secretion or ACTH secretion (4):
  - Metyrapone, ketoconazole, and mitotane lower cortisol levels by directly inhibiting synthesis and secretion in the adrenal gland. Replacement glucocorticoid therapy is often required (5).
    - Metyrapone is notable for rapid onset of action as the nadir of cortisol levels after a single dose is 2 hours.
    - Mitotane inhibits steroidogenic enzymes in the adrenal gland inducing a chemical adrenalectomy. It has a long half-life due to accumulation in adipose tissue.
    - Ketoconazole and levoketoconazole inhibit enzymes in the adrenal gland, leading to a nadir of cortisol in 2 to 3 days of treatment.
    - Etomidate (IV) inhibits adrenal corticosteroid synthesis and is effective in rapidly lowering cortisol levels in severe Cushing syndrome.
  - Mifepristone is a potent glucocorticoid receptor antagonist. It is FDA approved to control hyperglycemia in adults with endogenous Cushing syndrome who have T2DM or glucose intolerance secondary to hypercortisolism that has not responded to (or who are not candidates for) surgery.
  - For Cushing disease, pituitary tumor–directed agents such as cabergoline or pasireotide may be effective as well.

SURGERY/OTHER PROCEDURES

Surgery is the preferred treatment for Cushing syndrome:

- Cushing disease is treated with transsphenoidal resection of pituitary adenomas.
  - Irradiation of pituitary can be used in patients in whom surgery is unsuccessful or not indicated.
- Adrenal tumor removal or unilateral or bilateral adrenalectomy are used for patients with primary adrenal disease.

ONGOING CARE

FOLLOW-UP RECOMMENDATIONS

Patient Monitoring

- Once treated, the physical signs/symptoms of Cushing disease/syndrome gradually disappear over a period of 2 to 12 months. Obesity, HTN, glucose intolerance, and osteoporosis may remain even after treatment. Treatment of these secondary signs/symptoms is recommended until complete resolution.
- Following surgery, patients may develop acute withdrawal of cortisol and should be monitored closely.
- In children, bone density and growth rate increase after treatment, although likely not to normal rates.

PATIENT EDUCATION

Education about diet and monitoring daily weight, early treatment of infections, and emotional lability

PROGNOSIS

- Generally chronic course with cyclic exacerbations and rare remissions
- Recurrence rate is 20% for adrenal tumors.
- Poor with small cell carcinoma of the lung (SCLC) producing ectopic ACTH hormone
- After surgery, a drop in cortisol level is a predictor.
- Some patients may need supraphysiologic steroid replacement postsurgery, tapered over months.

COMPLICATIONS

Untreated Cushing syndrome is often fatal secondary to cardiovascular, thromboembolic, and infectious causes.

REFERENCES

1. Nieman LK, Biller BMK, Findling JW, et al. Treatment of Cushing's syndrome: an Endocrine Society clinical practice guideline. *J Clin Endocrinol Metab*. 2015;100(8):2807–2831.
2. Fleseriu M, Auchus R, Bancos I, et al. Consensus on diagnosis and management of Cushing's disease: a guideline update. *Lancet Diabetes Endocrinol*. 2021;9(12):847–875. doi:10.1016/S2213-8587(21)00235-7.
3. Kamenický P, Droumaguet C, Salenave S, et al. Mitotane, metyrapone, and ketoconazole combination therapy as an alternative to rescue adrenalectomy for severe ACTH-dependent Cushing's syndrome. *J Clin Endocrinol Metab*. 2011;96(9):2796–2804.
4. Maness DL, Studebaker G, Knight CM. Cushing's syndrome: rapid evidence review. *Am Fam Physician*. 2024;110(3):270–280.
5. Nieman LK, Ilias I. Evaluation and treatment of Cushing's syndrome. *Am J Med*. 2005;118(12):1340–1346.

SEE ALSO

Algorithm: Cushing Syndrome

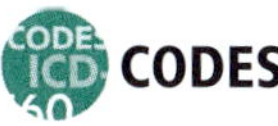

CODES

ICD10

- E24.9 Cushing's syndrome, unspecified
- E24.0 Pituitary-dependent Cushing's disease
- E24.2 Drug-induced Cushing's syndrome

CLINICAL PEARLS

- Cushing disease is due to excessive ACTH secretion from a pituitary tumor.
- Cushing syndrome is due to excessive corticosteroid exposure from exogenous sources (medications) or endogenous sources (pituitary, adrenal, pulmonary, etc.).
- Depression, alcoholism, medications, eating disorders, and other conditions can cause mild clinical and laboratory findings similar to those in Cushing syndrome (pseudo-Cushing syndrome).
- Symptoms may include facial plethora, round face, increased adiposity of dorsocervical fat pads, easy bruising, purple striae, thin skin, fragility fractures, and muscle weakness.

CUTANEOUS DRUG REACTIONS

Jennifer G. Foster, MD, MBA, FACP • Zoey Perham, MD • Allison H. Ferris, MD

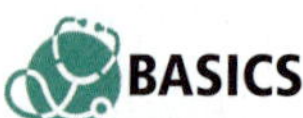

BASICS

DESCRIPTION

- Defined as an adverse cutaneous reaction in response to administration of a drug. Rashes are the most common form of adverse drug reaction (ADR) (1).
- Severity can range from mild eruption that resolves within 24 hours after the removal of the inciting agent, to severe skin damage with multiorgan involvement.
- Morbilliform and urticarial eruptions are most common, accounting for approximately 94% of cutaneous drug reactions
- Approximately 2% are life-threatening.

EPIDEMIOLOGY

- All ages are affected; immunosuppressed individuals are at increased risk
- Increased likelihood of severe cutaneous and systemic reactions in the geriatric population; unclear if due to polypharmacy or change in drug metabolism
- Difficult to distinguish from viral exanthems in pediatric patients

Incidence

In the United States, incidence of 1–3%; estimated 1/1,000 hospitalized patients has had a severe cutaneous reaction.

ETIOLOGY AND PATHOPHYSIOLOGY

Two classifications of ADR:

- Predictable (type A): dose dependent, known pharmacologic effect of drug, and drug–drug interaction. These make up the majority of cutaneous drug reactions.
- Unpredictable (type B): drug intolerance, drug idiosyncrasy (due to metabolism abnormality), drug allergy, and drug pseudoallergy
  - Immunologically mediated reaction: immunoglobulin (Ig) E–mediated reaction (type I hypersensitivity), cytotoxic/IgG/IgM induced (type II), immune complex reactions (type III), and delayed-type hypersensitivity (type IV) with T cells, eosinophils, neutrophils, and monocytes; immune mediated is the least common.
- Most common medications causing cutaneous drug reactions: carbamazepine and phenytoin.
- >700 drugs are known culprits.

Genetics

Genetics may play a role; certain HLA antigens have been associated with increased predisposition to specific drug eruptions:

- *HLA-B*5801*, *HLA-B*5701*, and *HLA-B*1502* have been linked to allopurinol-induced and carbamazepine-induced SJS/TEN, respectively. CYP2C9*3 variants linked to phenytoin-induced Stevens-Johnson syndrome (SJS)/toxic epidermal necrolysis (TEN).
- HLA-DQB1*0301 allele found in 66% of patients of erythema multiforme compared with 31% of control subjects

RISK FACTORS

The most common risk factor is immunosuppression; Genetic predisposition or autoimmunity are less frequent risk factors.

GENERAL PREVENTION

Always ask about prior adverse drug events. Be aware of medications with higher incidence of reactions as well as drug–drug reaction.

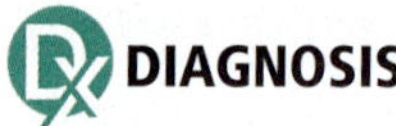

DIAGNOSIS

HISTORY

Develop a timeline outlining the onset of cutaneous eruption, and the onset and duration of all drugs and their dosages. Rule out other causes of the rash.

PHYSICAL EXAM

May present in different ways, including:

- Morbilliform eruption (exanthems)
  - Most frequent cutaneous reaction (75–95%); difficult to distinguish from viral exanthem; often secondary to antibiotics
  - Starts on trunk as pruritic red macules and papules, extending symmetrically to extremities in confluent fashion, sparing face, palms, soles, and mucous membranes
- Urticaria
  - Pruritic erythematous wheals distributed anywhere on the body, including mucous membranes
  - Lesions vary in size and shape (e.g., round, oval, rhomboid); may change over time.
  - Angioedema may appear as asymmetric soft tissue swelling which can compromise airway and be life-threatening.
  - Individual lesions usually fade within 24 hours, but new lesions may develop.
- Acneiform eruption
  - Folliculocentric, monomorphous pustules involving face, trunk, and proximal extremities; can also present in areas atypical of acne vulgaris such as forearms and legs.
  - Distinguished from acne vulgaris by absence of comedones
- Fixed drug eruption
  - Solitary/few, sharply demarcated, round/oval erythematous plaque with dusky center that may leave postinflammatory hyperpigmentation; may occur on skin or mucous membranes.
  - Onset is usually 30 minutes to 8 hours after administration of drug.
- Acute generalized exanthematous pustulosis (AGEP)
  - Rapidly appearing nonfollicular sterile pustules on an erythematous background, typically in intertriginous areas
  - Usually resolves within 1 to 3 days after removal of offending drug leaving a desquamation pattern.
  - Often causes fever and marked leukocytosis with neutrophilia and/or eosinophilia.
- Drug rash with eosinophilia and systemic symptoms (DRESS) syndrome
  - Drug-induced, multi-organ inflammatory response which may be life-threatening
  - Presentation can involve cutaneous eruptions (typically pruritic, erythematous papules, and patchy erythematous macules), fever, eosinophilia, hepatic dysfunction, renal dysfunction, and lymphadenopathy.
  - Onset usually 2 to 8 weeks after drug exposure
  - Symptoms and organ involvement may worsen after discontinuation of offending agent and then persist for months.
  - Mucosal involvement rare
- Erythema multiforme (EM)
  - Acute, immune-mediated, mucocutaneous condition
  - Most commonly associated with herpes simplex virus (HSV) and other viral/bacterial etiologies (i.e., *Mycoplasma*); less likely secondary to drug exposure (<10% of cases)
  - Palpable classic target lesions and/or two-zone atypical target lesions with localized erythema
  - Most commonly distributed symmetrically on extensor surfaces of acral extremities; may involve mucus membranes (25–60%)
- SJS/TEN
  - Classification and distinction between SJS and TEN determined by affected body surface area (BSA). SJS: <10% BSA; SJS–TEN overlap: 10–30% BSA; TEN: >30% BSA
  - TEN strongly associated with drug intake (>95%); SJS less strongly associated (~50%)
  - Onset usually 4 to 28 days; may be delayed up to 8 weeks after starting offending drug
  - Flat, atypical two-zone target lesions and erythematous macules are truncal and generalized with mucosal involvement
  - May develop confluent areas of bullae, erosions, and necrosis; significant risk for infection and sepsis
  - SJS: 1–5% mortality; TEN: 25–35% mortality
- Lichenoid eruption
  - Eruption of violaceous, pruritic, polygonal papules symmetrically distributed, favoring extensor surfaces/sun-exposed areas
  - Chronic lesions persist for weeks/months after the drug is discontinued.
- Photosensitivity reaction
  - Phototoxic reaction: usually occurs within minutes to hours after sunlight exposure with exaggerated sunburn-type reaction
  - Photoallergic reaction: more pruritic than painful; photodistributed but sparing scalp, submental, and periorbital areas
- Hypersensitivity vasculitis
  - Non-blanching petechiae/palpable purpura, commonly present on lower extremities
  - Onset usually 7 to 21 days after drug exposure
  - Biopsy reveals inflammation and necrosis of vessel walls.
- Sweet syndrome
  - Tender, edematous, violaceous papules, plaques, or nodules, with or without pustules/vesicles that spontaneously resolve; associated with fever and neutrophilia
  - Classically seen in young women after a mild respiratory illness or GI infection
- Exfoliative dermatitis/erythroderma
  - Severe end-stage dermatosis that develops from other drug reactions; commonly associated with systemic manifestations such as fever and chills
  - Generalized erythema with exfoliation and/or fine desquamation of large confluent areas
  - Increased risk of secondary infection and insensible fluid and temperature loss with hemodynamic instability

DIFFERENTIAL DIAGNOSIS

- Viral exanthem: Presence of fever, lymphocytosis, and other systemic findings may help in narrowing differential.
- Primary dermatosis (e.g., pustular psoriasis): Correlation of drug withdrawal to rash resolution may clarify diagnosis; skin biopsy can be helpful.
- Bacterial infection: Cultures of pustules may distinguish primary infection from AGEP and acneiform eruptions.

DIAGNOSTIC TESTS & INTERPRETATION

There are no specific tests available to confirm suspected drug reaction. Allergy testing may be able to identify the causal drug, however, the sensitivity of these tests vary and must be done at least 6 weeks after any topical corticosteroid or antihistamine treatment. Diagnosis relies on thorough history and physical exam with medication reconciliation.

Initial Tests (lab, imaging)

Selection of initial tests should be guided by clinical history and physical exam findings. CBC with differential; significant eosinophilia may be seen in DRESS and other drug-induced allergic reactions. LFT, urinalysis, and serum creatinine can assess for internal organ involvement; chest x-ray if suspected vasculitis

Diagnostic Procedures/Other

Special tests based on suspected mechanism:

- Type I: skin/intradermal testing, radioallergosorbent test (RAST)
- Type II: direct/indirect Coombs test
- Type III: ESR, C-reactive protein, ANA, complement components, cryoglobulin assays
- Type IV: patch testing, lymphocyte proliferation assay (investigational)
- Anaphylaxis/nonimmunologic mast and basophil cell reaction: plasma histamine, serum tryptase levels, 24-hour urine N-methylhistamine

Test Interpretation

SJS/TEN: partial or full-thickness necrosis of the epidermis, necrotic keratinocytes, vacuolization leading to subepidermal blister at basal membrane zone

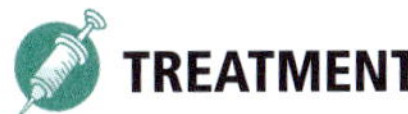

TREATMENT

GENERAL MEASURES

The most important initial treatment is to withdraw the offending agent. Do not rechallenge with drugs causing urticaria, bullae, angioedema, DRESS, anaphylaxis, or EM.

MEDICATION

- Depending on the type of eruption, symptomatic treatment may be useful but most require no additional therapy except cessation of offending agent.
- Anaphylaxis or widespread urticaria: epinephrine 0.1 to 0.5 mg (1:1,000 [1 mg/mL] solution) IM in mid-outer thigh every 5 to 15 min; prednisone PO 1 mg/kg in tapering doses may be given for severe refractory cases.
- Acute urticaria (<6 weeks) and chronic urticaria (>6 weeks): 2nd-generation antihistamines (preferred, less sedating): cetirizine 10 to 20 mg daily, loratadine 10 to 20 mg daily, fexofenadine 180 mg daily. H_2 antagonists: ranitidine 150 mg BID
- EM: Treatment is generally supportive with management of suspected underlying infection. Recurrent, HSV associated: prophylaxis with acyclovir 400 mg BID, valacyclovir 500 mg BID, or famciclovir 250 mg BID; "magic mouthwash" and oral antiseptic helpful for mucosal erosions; consider ophthalmology consult for ocular involvement.
- SJS/TEN: Treatment is supportive. Consult with a dermatologist, ophthalmologist, and gynecologist as applicable. Systemic corticosteroid use remains controversial. Consider IVIG 2 to 3 g/kg for severe disease, although limited studies have not shown survival benefits in adults. In pediatric SJS/TEN patients, IVIG and systemic glucocorticoids appear to improve outcome; varied success rates reported with use of antitumor necrosis factor-α agents, cyclosporine, cyclophosphamide, and plasmapheresis. Avoid débridement and consider using detached epidermis as natural biologic dressing to minimize risk for hypertrophic scars.
- DRESS: systemic corticosteroid therapy recommended in early stages of DRESS diagnosis with prednisolone 1 mg/kg/day. Abrupt discontinuation commonly induces relapse; therefore, tapering oral prednisolone should be done gradually for 6 to 8 weeks to 3 months. Topical corticosteroids, systemic antihistamines, and emollients for rashes reduce relapse and hospitalization in mild cases.
- AGEP: Topical corticosteroid use has been correlated with a decreased median duration of hospitalization; systemic steroid use generally not recommended given the benign course.

ADMISSION, INPATIENT, AND NURSING CONSIDERATIONS

Hospitalization is indicated with signs of severity present:

- Cutaneous: skin surface >60%, erythema confluence, facial edema, skin pain, palpable purpura, skin necrosis, bullae or epidermal detachment, positive Nikolsky sign, mucosal erosions, urticaria, and/or tongue edema
- General: high fever, lymphadenopathy, arthralgia or arthritis, dyspnea, hypotension
- Laboratory: eosinophilia >1,000/mm^3, lymphocytosis with atypical lymphocytes, abnormal liver function

ONGOING CARE

FOLLOW-UP RECOMMENDATIONS

Patient Monitoring

- Patients with anaphylaxis/angioedema should be given EpiPens to be kept at home, work, and in the car for secondary prevention as well as a Med-Alert bracelet; label the patient's medical record with the agent and reaction.
- If the patient needs to take the inciting drug (e.g., antibiotic) in the future, induction of drug tolerance or graded challenge procedures may be necessary.

PROGNOSIS

- Majority of cases are self-limited upon removal of offending drug.
- Anaphylaxis, angioedema, DRESS, SJS/TEN, and bullous reactions are potentially fatal.
- Severity-of-illness score for toxic epidermal necrolysis (SCORTEN), a prognostic scoring system, can be used to guide management of hospitalized patients of SJS/TEN; also, may be helpful when discussing prognosis

REFERENCES

1. Del Pozzo-Magaña BR, Liy-Wong C. Drugs and the skin: a concise review of cutaneous adverse drug reactions. *Br J Clin Pharmacol*. 2024;90(8):1838–1855. doi:10.1111/bcp.15490.

ADDITIONAL READING

- Ahmed AM, Pritchard S, Reichenberg J. A review of cutaneous drug eruptions. *Clin Geriatr Med*. 2013;29(2):527–545.
- Dodiuk-Gad RP, Chung WH, Valeyrie-Allanore L, et al. Stevens-Johnson syndrome and toxic epidermal necrolysis: an update. *Am J Clin Dermatol*. 2015;16(6):475–493.

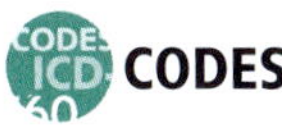

CODES

ICD10

- L27.1 Loc skin eruption due to drugs and meds taken internally
- L50.0 Allergic urticaria
- R21 Rash and other nonspecific skin eruption

CLINICAL PEARLS

- Virtually any drug can cause rash; antibiotics, anticonvulsants, and anti-inflammatories are the most common culprits for cutaneous drug reactions.
- Usually self-limited after withdrawal of offending agent
- Symptoms such as tongue swelling/angioedema, skin necrosis, blisters, high fever, dyspnea, and mucous membrane erosions signify more severe drug reactions.
- Useful resources: Drug Eruption Reference Manual by Jerome Litt; https://www.drugeruptiondata.com/

CYSTIC FIBROSIS

Saqeeb M. Ali, DO • Priscilla Becnel, MD, BS

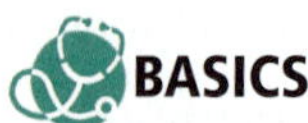

BASICS

DESCRIPTION

Cystic fibrosis (CF) is a chronic, multisystem autosomal recessive disorder due to CF transmembrane conductance regulator (CFTR) dysfunction which produces abnormally viscous secretions that impair organ function—predominantly in the lungs and pancreas. Presentation ranges from birth onward with chronic sinopulmonary disease, recurrent infections, pancreatic insufficiency, hepatobiliary disease, diabetes, and infertility. Diagnosis requires compatible features (or positive newborn screen) plus confirmatory sweat chloride, CFTR mutation analysis, or electrophysiology (EP) testing.

EPIDEMIOLOGY

Although most common in people with European ancestry, CF occurs in all racial groups.

Incidence

- 1 in 3,200 White people
- 1 in 10,000 Latin Americans
- 1 in 10,500 Native Americans
- 1 in 15,000 African Americans
- 1 in 30,000 Asian Americans

Prevalence

- ~35,000 in the United States and >180,000 worldwide (1),(2)
- U.S. median predicted survival ~53.1 years (95% CI, 51.6 to 54.7) (1),(2)

ETIOLOGY AND PATHOPHYSIOLOGY

Abnormal CFTR (7q31.2) alters epithelial chloride/sodium transport, creating dehydrated mucus, impaired mucociliary clearance, infection-driven neutrophilic inflammation, and airway damage leading to bronchiectasis and progressive lung failure.

Genetics

CF is autosomal recessive with >2,000 CFTR variants. F508del is most common in the United States (~85.5%), followed by G542X (~4.5%) and G551D (~4.2%) (1). Disease severity is modified by other genes (e.g., meconium ileus risk), infections, GERD, and environmental exposures (e.g., smoke).

GENERAL PREVENTION

Preconception counseling

- Preconception counseling: American College of Obstetricians and Gynecologists recommends universal preconception or early pregnancy CFTR carrier screening for all people, regardless of ancestry (3).
- Newborn screening detects most new cases and enables earlier care with better lung and nutritional outcomes.

COMMONLY ASSOCIATED CONDITIONS

- CF-related diabetes (CFRD): leading comorbidity (~29.2%) (1); progressive insulin deficiency with weight loss, declining lung function, or frequent exacerbations
- Upper airway: chronic rhinosinusitis (15.2%) (1), nasal polyps
- GI: pancreatic exocrine insufficiency with malabsorption of fat/protein/vitamins A, D, E, K; hepatobiliary disease (4.1%) (1); meconium ileus at birth; distal intestinal obstruction syndrome (DIOS); GERD.
- Endocrine/bone/joints: osteoporosis (4.1%) (1), arthropathy
- Reproductive: congenital bilateral absence of vas deferens (obstructive azoospermia) in males (9%) (1)
- Psychosocial: depression

Pregnancy Considerations

- Pulmonary disease may worsen during pregnancy.
- Increased risks of preterm delivery, intrauterine growth restriction, and cesarean delivery.
- Assisted reproductive technologies allow many men with CF to father children.

DIAGNOSIS

Criteria for diagnosis of CF

- At least one of the following:
  - ≥1 typical phenotypic features of CF: chronic pulmonary disease, chronic sinusitis, characteristic GI and nutritional abnormalities, salt loss syndromes, obstructive azoospermia
  - History of CF in a sibling
  - Positive newborn screening test
- *Plus* at least one of the following:
  - Elevated sweat chloride concentration on ≥2 occasions
  - Two mutations known to cause CF on separate alleles
  - Abnormalities in nasal potential difference (NPD) testing that are typical of CF

HISTORY

- History during prenatal period:
  - Routine prenatal ultrasonography indicates hyperechogenic bowel and/or bilateral absences of vas deferens (2)
    - Risk is the highest if there is evidence of meconium peritonitis, bowel dilatation, or absent gallbladder. Parents should be offered CF carrier screening if these findings are present.
- History during neonatal period:
  - Meconium ileus; generally considered pathognomonic for CF
  - Prolonged jaundice
- History during infancy:
  - Failure to thrive (6.9%) (1)
  - Chronic diarrhea and/or steatorrhea (7.7) (1)
  - Anasarca/hypoproteinemia
  - Pseudotumor cerebri (vitamin A deficiency)
  - Hemolytic anemia (vitamin E deficiency)
- History during childhood: recurrent endobronchial infection, bronchiectasis, chronic pansinusitis, steatorrhea, poor growth, DIOS, allergic bronchopulmonary aspergillosis (ABPA)
- History during adolescence and adulthood: recurrent endobronchial infection, bronchiectasis, ABPA, chronic sinusitis, hemoptysis, pancreatitis, portal hypertension, azoospermia, delayed puberty

PHYSICAL EXAM

- Vitals: tachypnea, hypoxia
- Respiratory: use of accessory muscles, rhonchi or crackles, hyperresonance on percussion, and nasal polyps
- GI: abdominal distension, hepatosplenomegaly if cirrhotic
- Other: digital clubbing (2.6%) (1), growth retardation, and pubertal delay

DIFFERENTIAL DIAGNOSIS

- Immunologic: immunodeficiency syndromes (e.g., common variable immunodeficiency [CVID], severe combined immunodeficiency [SCID])
- Pulmonary: asthma, chronic obstructive pulmonary disease (COPD), recurrent pneumonia, chronic/recurrent sinusitis, primary ciliary dyskinesia, bronchopulmonary dysplasia
- GI: celiac disease, inflammatory bowel disease, protein-losing enteropathy, pancreatitis of unknown etiology, Shwachman-Diamond syndrome, α-1 antitrypsin deficiency

DIAGNOSTIC TESTS & INTERPRETATION

Initial Tests (lab, imaging)

- Newborn screening tests blood levels of immunoreactive trypsin (IRT)
- Sweat chloride test (gold standard) (sensitivity: 99%; specificity: 93%) (1): performed after 2 weeks of age
- CFTR mutation analysis
  - Allele-specific PCR identifies >2,000 variants of mutations
  - Full-sequence testing is more costly and time-consuming.
- Electrophysiology (EP) testing (when sweat test and DNA testing inconclusive): NPD or intestinal current measurement (limited availability)
- Chest X-ray (CXR)

Follow-Up Tests & Special Considerations

To further investigate the presence of CF-related complications, these tests are generally ordered:

- Sputum culture (common CF organisms)
- Pulmonary function tests (PFTs)
- 72-hour fecal fat, stool elastase
- Liver function tests (LFTs)
- Oral glucose tolerance test
- Head CT: Abnormal sinus CT findings are nearly universal in CF.
- Chest CT: after abnormal CXR
- Referral to CF facility within first 24 to 72 hours of diagnosis recommended

Diagnostic Procedures/Other

Flexible bronchoscopy with bronchoalveolar lavage

Test Interpretation

- Clinical suspicion with symptoms of CF, positive newborn screening or siblings with CF
- Sweat chloride test
  - ≥ 60 mmol/L: confirmation of CF
  - 30 to 50 mmol/L: inconclusive test → follow up with CFTR mutation analysis
  - ≤29 mmol/L: CF unlikely → can follow up with genetic/EP testing if high clinical suspicion
- CFTR mutation analysis
  - Two CFTR variants: confirmation of CF
  - One CFTR variant or none: inconclusive → follow up with additional genetic tests or EP test if sweat chloride test is ≥ 60 mmol/L or inconclusive
- If additional genetic testing is positive for two CFTR variants or EP test results are in CF range: confirmation of CF (1),(2),(4)

TREATMENT

GENERAL MEASURES

- Cystic Fibrosis Foundation guidelines call for:
  - Quarterly visits with a multidisciplinary team, including dietitians, social workers, and physicians with PFTs and respiratory cultures done each visit (2)
    - Telehealth with home-based spirometry is a viable option for disease monitoring.
  - Chest imaging for monitoring: for adults, CXR every 2 to 4 years; for children, CXR every 2 years or low-dose chest CT every 2 to 3 years
  - PFT goals: >75% predicted for adults, >100% predicted for children <18-years-old
  - Annual screening for ABPA for patients aged >6 years with total serum IgE concentration and nontuberculous mycobacteria (NTM) cultures
  - Routine immunizations per national guidelines
  - Screen for osteoporosis all adults and children aged >8 years with a DEXA scan every 2 to 5 years.
  - Annual measurement of fat-soluble vitamins to rule out vitamin deficiencies
  - Annual diabetes screening with oral glucose test for patients aged ≥12 years
  - Annual LFTs, platelet counts abdominal exams and abdominal ultrasonography to assess liver and spleen every 2 years from childhood to late adolescence
  - Colorectal cancer screening with a colonoscopy every 5 years starting at 40 years of age
  - Avoidance of tobacco use and vaping
- All patients should be followed in a CF center (accredited sites listed at https://www.cff.org/)
- Infant care:
  - Monthly visits for first 6 months of life and then every 2 months until 1 year of life
  - Fecal elastase testing and salt supplementation
  - Consider palivizumab for RSV prophylaxis in infants with CF aged <2 years.

MEDICATION

- Pathogens for pulmonary infections: MRSA (~28%) and MSSA (~65%), *Stenotrophomonas maltophilia* (~5%), *Pseudomonas aeruginosa* (~30%), *Haemophilus influenzae* (~10%), NTM (2)
- For Pulmonary Exacerbations:
  - Antibiotics, oral
    - *Staphylococcus aureus*: Bactrim (MRSA), doxycycline (MRSA), or cephalexin
    - *P. aeruginosa*: fluoroquinolones
  - Antibiotics, IV
    - *S. aureus*: cefazolin or nafcillin
    - MRSA: vancomycin or linezolid
    - *P. aeruginosa*: Piperacillin/tazobactam or ceftazidime plus aminoglycoside (tobramycin)
  - Antibiotics should be targeted to most likely pathogen with most courses lasting 10 to 14 days.
  - Two IV antibiotics should be used if *Pseudomonas* is detected in pulmonary exacerbations.
  - Continue all chronic inhaled medications and airway clearance therapy during exacerbations.
- Medications recommended as long-term therapy in pulmonary disease:
  - Chronic pulmonary infections:
    - For chronic *P. aeruginosa* infections: tobramycin nebulizer 300 mg twice daily and/or aztreonam nebulizer 75 mg three times daily for 28 days; stop for 28 days and then resume use; can also consider oral azithromycin but patient must be screened for NTM (2),(4)
    - Chronic oral antibiotics are not recommended for prophylaxis.
  - Mucociliary clearance:
    - Nebulized dornase alfa 2.5 mg twice daily (2)
    - Hypertonic saline (7%) nebulizer 4 mL twice daily (4)
    - Inhaled mannitol 400 mg twice daily for patient aged ≥ 18 years (4)
  - Anti-inflammatories: high-dose ibuprofen (20 mg/kg to 30 mg/kg twice daily) in patients 6- to 17-years-old with FEV_1 ≥60 PPV (4)
  - CFTR modulator therapies:
    - Considered standard of care as it has shown to reduced pulmonary exacerbations, improve respiratory symptoms and delay disease manifestation
    - CFTR modulator drugs: ivacaftor, lumacaftor-ivacaftor, tezacaftor-ivacaftor, and elexacaftor-tezacaftor-ivacaftor (2)
    - Monitor for elevated creatine kinase, liver toxicity, cataracts, and hypertension.
  - Inhaled steroids are not recommended for chronic use in the absence of asthma or ABPA.
  - Insufficient evidence for chronic use of inhaled β agonist, inhaled anticholinergics, leukotriene modifiers, inhaled colistin
  - Pancreatic enzymes, often combined with H_2 blockers or PPI to increase effectiveness
  - Fat-soluble vitamin supplementation (A, D, E, and K)
  - Ursodeoxycholic acid is not recommended for the prevention of liver disease.

ADDITIONAL THERAPIES

- Airway clearance therapy with high-frequency chest wall oscillation vest, positive expiratory pressure devices, percussion, etc., to improve cough and mucus mobilization; aerobic exercise also recommended as an adjunct.
- CF-related osteoporosis: Start bisphosphonate therapy.
- CFRD: Start insulin therapy.

SURGERY/OTHER PROCEDURES

- Timing for lung transplantation (bilateral) is multifactorial. Key indications for referral are:
  - FEV_1 <50% predicted for those with a rapidly declining FEV_1 (>20% relative decline within 12 months) (1),(2)
  - FEV_1 <40% predicted with additional markers of shortened survival (1),(2)
  - FEV_1 <30% predicted for all others (1),(2)
- Liver transplantation is reserved for progressive liver failure ± portal hypertension with GI bleeding.
- Nasal polypectomy in some CF patients

ADMISSION, INPATIENT, AND NURSING CONSIDERATIONS

- Pulmonary exacerbation (most common reason for admission)
- Bowel obstruction
- Pancreatitis in pancreatic-sufficient patients
- Always admit on contact precautions and to private rooms.
- Increased salt loss increases risk of hyponatremic hypochloremic dehydration.
- Cautious use of IV fluids with worsening lung disease

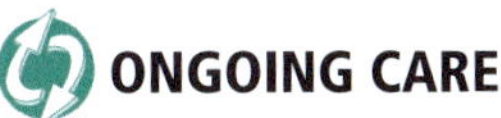

ONGOING CARE

FOLLOW-UP RECOMMENDATIONS

- Upon discharge for a pulmonary exacerbation, follow-up with CF specialist within 2 to 4 weeks
- Routine clinic visits every 3 months with airway cultures and PFTs as indicated
- Annual comprehensive nutritional evaluation

DIET

High-calorie, high-fat diet with BMI targets per CF Foundation. If goals unmet, involve dietitian; consider pancreatic enzymes and/or supplemental tube feeds.

PATIENT EDUCATION

Cystic Fibrosis Foundation: https://www.cff.org

PROGNOSIS

- Median survival is 53.1 years in the United States as of 2021 (1).
- Progression of lung disease usually determines length of survival.

REFERENCES

1. Ong T, Ramsey BW. Cystic fibrosis: a review. *JAMA*. 2023;329(21):1859–1871. doi:10.1001/jama.2023.8120.
2. Mall MA, Burgel PR, Castellani C, et al. Cystic fibrosis. *Nat Rev Dis Primers*. 2024;10(1):53. doi:10.1038/s41572-024-00538-6.
3. ACOG Committee Opinion No. 486: Update on carrier screening for cystic fibrosis. *Obstet Gynecol*. 2011;117(4):1028–1031. doi:10.1097/AOG.0b013e31821922c2.
4. Grasemann H, Ratjen F. Cystic fibrosis. *N Engl J Med*. 2023;389(18):1693–1707. doi:10.1056/nejmra2216474.

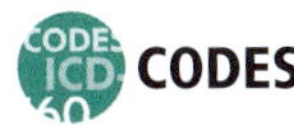

CODES

ICD10

- E84.9 Cystic fibrosis, unspecified
- E84.11 Meconium ileus in cystic fibrosis
- E84.0 Cystic fibrosis with pulmonary manifestations

CLINICAL PEARLS

- Meconium ileus is pathognomonic for CF.
- When sweat test is equivocal, CFTR genetic testing is diagnostic.
- Consider CF in any child with chronic diarrhea, especially with poor growth or failure to thrive.
- All children with nasal polyps, digital clubbing, or bronchiectasis should be evaluated.
- A rapid decline in pulmonary function suggests resistant organisms, CFRD, ABPA, or GERD.

DE QUERVAIN TENOSYNOVITIS

Michael J. Maddaleni, MD, CAQSM

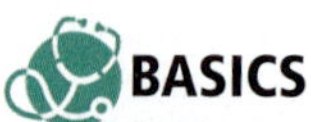

BASICS

DESCRIPTION

- First identified in 1895 by Fritz De Quervain, de Quervain tenosynovitis is a painful condition due to stenosis of the tendon sheath in the 1st dorsal compartment of the radial aspect of the wrist.
- Caused by repetitive motion of the extensor pollicis brevis (EPB) and abductor pollicis longus (APL) over the radial styloid with resultant metaplastic changes of the surrounding tendon sheath

EPIDEMIOLOGY

- The predominant age range is 30 to 50 years.
- Women are affected more commonly than men (1).
- With new occupational and professional demands, the prevalence of this condition is increasing gradually.

Incidence

- The overall incidence of de Quervain tenosynovitis is 0.9/1,000 person-years.
- For patients age >40 years, the incidence is 1.4/1,000 person-years compared with 0.6/1,000 person-years for those <20 years.
- Women have an incidence rate ratio of 2.8/1,000 person-years compared with 0.6/1,000 person-years in men.

Prevalence

Currently, estimated at 1.3% in females and 0.5% in males

ETIOLOGY AND PATHOPHYSIOLOGY

- Repetitive motions of the wrist and/or thumb result in microtrauma, metaplastic thickening of the tendons (EPB, APL), and narrowing of the surrounding tendon sheath.
- EPB and APL movement is resisted as they glide over the radial styloid causing pain with movements of the thumb and wrist.
- Among individual undergoing release of the 1st dorsal compartment, histopathology of the tendon sheaths was characterized by myxoid degeneration with dense fibrous tissue and mucopolysaccharide accumulation.
- Cadaveric analyses have identified an additional septum within the 1st dorsal compartment in 34–44% of individuals and subcompartmentalization has been reported in 86–94% of patients with de Quervain tenosynovitis.

RISK FACTORS

- Women age 30 to 50 years
- Pregnancy (primarily 3rd trimester and postpartum)
- Black race
- Systemic diseases (e.g., rheumatoid arthritis)
- Participation in activities that include repetitive motion or forceful grasping with thumb and wrist deviation such as golf, fly-fishing, racquet sports, rowing, or bicycling, video gaming, and more recently text messaging
- Repetitive movements with the hand/thumb requiring forceful grasping with wrist involving ulnar/radial deviation; dental hygienists, musicians, carpenters, assembly workers, and machine operators
- Recent analyses suggest anatomic variability including tendon insertion variation and subcompartmentalization of the 1st dorsal compartment may be the greatest risk factors.

GENERAL PREVENTION

Avoid overuse or repetitive movements of the wrist and/or thumb associated with forceful grasping and ulnar/radial deviation.

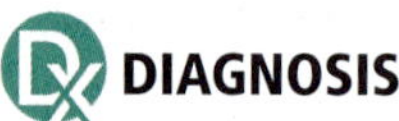

DIAGNOSIS

HISTORY

- Repetitive motion activity; overuse of wrist or thumb
- Gradually worsening pain along the radial aspect of the thumb and wrist with certain movements, particularly ulnar deviation of the wrist
- Pregnancy
- Sports, leisure, and occupational history
- Trauma (rare)

PHYSICAL EXAM

- Pain over the radial styloid exacerbated when patients move the thumb or make a fist
- Crepitus with movement of the thumb
- Swelling over the radial styloid and base of the thumb
- Decreased range of motion of the thumb
- Pain over the 1st dorsal compartment on resisted thumb abduction or extension
- Tenderness may extend proximally or distally along the tendons with palpation or stress.
- Finkelstein test: Ask the patient to actively ulnar deviate off the edge of a table and the examiner grasps the affected thumb and passively continues to deviate the hand in the ulnar direction. A positive test occurs when there is pain along the distal radius.
- Eichhoff test: Patient grasps a flexed thumb, and the examiner deviates the wrist in an ulnar direction.
- Finkelstein test is more sensitive for determining tenosynovitis of the APL and EPB tendons (2)[A].

DIFFERENTIAL DIAGNOSIS

- Scaphoid fracture
- Scapholunate ligament tear
- Dorsal wrist ganglion
- Osteoarthritis of the 1st carpometacarpal (CMC) joint
- Flexor carpi radialis tendonitis
- Infectious tenosynovitis
- Tendonitis of the wrist extensors
- Intersection syndrome
- Trigger thumb

DIAGNOSTIC TESTS & INTERPRETATION

Initial Tests (lab, imaging)

- Primarily a clinical diagnosis
- Radiographs of the wrist to rule out other pathology, such as CMC arthritis, if the diagnosis is in question
- MRI is the imaging test of choice to rule out coexisting soft tissue injury or wrist joint pathology.

Follow-Up Tests & Special Considerations

- Ultrasound can help to detect anatomic variations in the 1st dorsal extensor compartment of the wrist and target corticosteroid injections.
- Ultrasound imaging has been reported as 100% sensitive for detection of pathology.

Test Interpretation

Inflamed and thickened retinacular sheath of the tendon

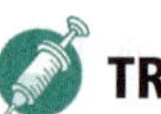

TREATMENT

- Most cases of de Quervain tenosynovitis are self-limited.
- Rest and NSAIDs (2)[A]
- Ice (15 to 20 minutes 5 to 6 times a day)
- Immobilization with a thumb spica splint (2)[A]
- Occupational therapy
- Acupuncture
- Corticosteroid injection (preferably ultrasound guided)
- Consider surgery if conservative measures fail >6 months.

GENERAL MEASURES

- If full relief is not achieved, a corticosteroid injection of the tendon sheath can improve symptoms.
- Anatomic variation, including subcompartmentalization of the 1st dorsal compartment or the EPB tendon traveling in a separate compartment, may complicate treatment. Ultrasound can distinguish these variants and improve anatomic accuracy of injections.
- Surgical release may be indicated after 3 to 6 months of conservative treatment if symptoms persist. Surgery is highly effective and has a relatively low rate of complications.

MEDICATION

First Line

Splinting, rest, and NSAIDs

Second Line

- Corticosteroid injection of the tendon sheath has shown significant cure rates. Additional injections are sometimes required.
- Corticosteroid injection plus immobilization is more effective than immobilization alone.
- Ultrasound-guided percutaneous tenotomy, retinaculum release, and/or injection of platelet-rich plasma are newer techniques that show promise for treatment of de Quervain tenosynovitis.

ISSUES FOR REFERRAL

Referral to a hand surgeon is indicated if there is no improvement with conservative therapy.

ADDITIONAL THERAPIES

- Hand therapy, along with iontophoresis/phonophoresis, may help improve outcomes in persistent cases.
- Patients may use thumb-stretching exercises as part of their rehabilitation.

SURGERY/OTHER PROCEDURES

- Indicated for patients who have failed conservative treatment
- Endoscopic release may provide earlier relief, fewer superficial radial nerve complications, and greater patient satisfaction with resultant scar compared to open release.

ADMISSION, INPATIENT, AND NURSING CONSIDERATIONS

Hospitalization for care associated with surgical treatment

ONGOING CARE

FOLLOW-UP RECOMMENDATIONS

- Additional corticosteroid injection may be performed at 4 to 6 weeks if symptoms persist. Caution with repeat steroid injections.
- Avoid repetitive motions and activities that cause pain.

DIET

As tolerated

PATIENT EDUCATION

Activity modification: Avoid repetitive movement of the wrist/thumb and forceful grasping.

PROGNOSIS

- Extremely good with conservative treatment
- Complete resolution can take up to 1 year.
- 95% success rates have been shown with conservative therapy >1 year.
- Up to 1/3 of patients will have persistent symptoms.

COMPLICATIONS

- Most complications are secondary to treatment. These include GI, renal, and hepatic injury secondary to NSAIDs use.
- Nerve damage may occur during surgery.
- Hypopigmentation, fat atrophy, bleeding, infection, and tendon rupture have been reported as potential adverse events from corticosteroid injection. Ultrasound guidance reduces the rate of complications.
- If not appropriately treated, thumb flexibility may be lost due to fibrosis.

REFERENCES

1. Wolf JM, Sturdivant RX, Owens BD. Incidence of de Quervain's tenosynovitis in a young, active population. *J Hand Surg Am*. 2009;34(1):112–115.
2. Huisstede BMA, Coert JH, Fridén J, et al; for European HANDGUIDE Group. Consensus on a multidisciplinary treatment guideline for de Quervain disease: results from the European HANDGUIDE study. *Phys Ther*. 2014;94(8):1095–1110.

ADDITIONAL READING

- Ali M, Asim M, Danish SH, et al. Frequency of de Quervain's tenosynovitis and its association with SMS texting. *Muscles Ligaments Tendons J*. 2014;4(1):74–78.
- Ashraf MO, Devadoss VG. Systematic review and meta-analysis on steroid injection therapy for de Quervain's tenosynovitis in adults. *Eur J Orthop Surg Traumatol*. 2014;24(2):149–157.
- Peters-Veluthamaningal C, van der Windt DAWM, Winters JC, et al. Corticosteroid injection for de Quervain's tenosynovitis. *Cochrane Database Syst Rev*. 2009;(3):CD005616.

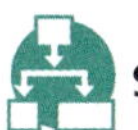

SEE ALSO

Algorithm: Pain in Upper Extremity

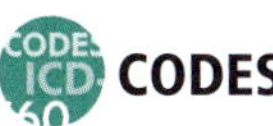

CODES

ICD10

M65.4 Radial styloid tenosynovitis [de Quervain]

CLINICAL PEARLS

- Repetitive movements of the wrist and thumb, and activities that require forceful grasping, are the most common causes of de Quervain tenosynovitis.
- Anatomic variations of the 1st dorsal compartment and metaplastic changes are identified in a majority of cases.
- Initial treatment is typically conservative.
- Corticosteroid injections are helpful and have lower complication rates if done under ultrasound guidance.
- Combined orthosis/corticosteroid injection approaches are more effective than either intervention alone.
- Ultrasound-guided percutaneous retinacular release and endoscopic surgery are helpful for recalcitrant cases.

DEEP VEIN THROMBOPHLEBITIS

Joshua T. Sutherland, MD, MS • Daniel Michniuk, MS, DO

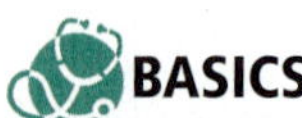

BASICS

DESCRIPTION

- An obstructive disease due to blood clots forming in the deep veins of the body (deep venous thrombosis [DVT]), most commonly in the lower extremities, and accompanied by inflammation of the vessel wall
- Classified as provoked or idiopathic

EPIDEMIOLOGY

- In United States: annually >200,000 people develop venous thrombosis
- ~1 in 5 cases are related to cancer and/or cancer treatment.
- Pregnancy, childbirth, or in the 3-months postpartum increases risk in women by 5-fold
- Age- and gender-adjusted incidence of venous thromboembolism (VTE) is 100 times higher in the hospital than in the community. Almost half of all VTEs occur either during or soon after discharge from a hospital stay or surgery.

Incidence

- United States: DVT incidence is ~80 cases per 100,000.
- Increased incidence in White and African American populations and with aging
- Incidence in pregnancy: ~0.5 to 3.0 cases per 1,000; 1–5% of central venous catheters are complicated by thrombosis.

Prevalence

- Prevalence of lower limb DVT is ~1 case per 1,000 population.
- At the time of DVT diagnosis, as many as 40% of patients also have asymptomatic pulmonary embolism (PE); conversely, 30% of patients diagnosed with PE do not a have demonstrable source.

ETIOLOGY AND PATHOPHYSIOLOGY

Virchow Triad: Factors involved may include venous stasis (due to venous obstrcution, shock, CHF), endothelial injury (due to trauma, inflammation, surgery), and hypercoagulability (due to malignancy, nephrotic syndrome, HRT); commonly due to mechanical injury to the vein, and increased venous pressure

Genetics

- Factor V Leiden, the most common thrombophilia, is found in 5% of the population and in 10–65% of all VTE events and increases VTE risk 3- to 6-fold.
- Prothrombin G20210A is found in 3% of whites; increases the risk of thrombosis ~3-fold

RISK FACTORS

- Constitutional: obesity, pregnancy, advanced age (>60 years), surgery, critical care admission
- Acquired: infections (e.g., COVID-19 up to 3 months after acute infection), disseminated intravascular coagulation, immobility (bed rest, surgical procedures, stroke, long-flights or drives), malignancy, previous DVT, pregnancy/puerperium, trauma, increased blood viscosity, medications (oral/transdermal contraceptives, hormonal therapies, chemotherapy), central venous catheters
- Hereditary: deficiencies of protein C, protein S, or antithrombin III; factor V Leiden mutation (R506Q), prothrombin G20210A mutation, dysfibrinogenemia, elevated factor VIII activity, hyperhomocysteinemia, sickle cell disease, polycythemia vera, autoimmune disease

GENERAL PREVENTION

- Early ambulation and avoidance of prolonged immobilization
- Mechanical thromboprophylaxis—particularly useful in high bleeding risk patients
- Prophylactic anticoagulation when appropriate (e.g., acutely ill, critical illness, debility)

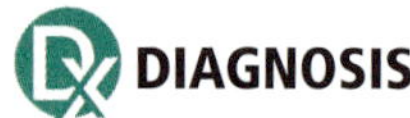

DIAGNOSIS

HISTORY

- Presenting symptoms vary; up to 50% of patients lack specific signs or symptoms.
  - Pain (~50% of patients), edema (~70% of patients, most specific)
  - Erythema, tenderness, prominent superficial veins
- Risk stratify using prediction models, (e.g., modified Wells criteria) (useful in determining pretest probability [PTP]) (1)
- Clinical assessment of bleeding risk (bleeding with the previous history of anticoagulation, history of liver disease, recent surgeries, history of GI bleed) is important prior to initiating treatment.

PHYSICAL EXAM

- Symptoms may present as pain, edema (most specific), tenderness, or discoloration; *Note*: Exam may be nonspecific or absent of findings.
- Resistance to passive dorsiflexion of the foot (Homan sign) is unreliable and nonspecific.
- Severe manifestation (phlegmasia cerulea dolens): Sudden and severe pain, massive edema, skin discoloration and diminished arterial flow can lead to limb ischemia and even death.

DIFFERENTIAL DIAGNOSIS

- Hypervolemia (when bilateral edema is present)
- Cellulitis
- Fracture +/− compartment syndrome
- Ruptured synovial cyst (Baker cyst)
- Extrinsic compression of vein (e.g., tumor, enlarged lymph node)
- Localized allergic reaction

DIAGNOSTIC TESTS & INTERPRETATION

Initial Tests (lab, imaging)

- Less valuable for diagnosis: CBC, metabolic panel
- Basic diagnostics:
  - D-dimer (high sensitivity and negative predictive value [NPV], low specificity)
    - Wells score is used for low to intermediate PTP (1 to 2); if negative, ruled out DVT
    - Potential for false-positives—inflammatory states, liver dysfunction, malignancy, pregnancy, trauma, recent surgery
    - Age-adjust as needed (>50 years) age (years) × 10 μg/L (using D-dimer assays with cutoff of 500 μg/L)
  - Gold standard: ultrasonography (compression or duplex)
  - Coagulation studies for bleeding risk
- Simplified testing based on Wells score
  - Score ≤0 = low PTP for DVT
    - Check high-sensitivity D-dimer
      - Negative = no further work-up, positive = do ultrasonography
  - Score 1 to 2 = intermediate PTP for DVT
    - Check high sensitivity D-dimer, follow-up with ultrasonography.
  - Score ≥3 = high PTP for DVT
    - Defer D-dimer, check ultrasonography.
    - *Note*: If initial ultrasound is negative, but clinical suspicion remains high, consider repeating interval ultrasound in 24 hours.
- If ultrasound is inconclusive, consider adjunctive imaging modalities.
  - CT venography, magnetic resonance venography. If these results are negative, diagnosis of DVT is excluded.

Follow-Up Tests & Special Considerations

- Determine provoked or unprovoked and additional evaluation (if indicated).
- Unprovoked DVT + family history of DVT (1st-degree relative) = consider testing for hereditary thrombophilia.
  - For example, factor V Leiden mutation, prothrombin G20210A genetic assay, antithrombin III functional assay, protein S antigen, functional assay, free protein S, protein C functional assay, phospholipid-dependent tests and anticardiolipin antibodies, lupus anticoagulant (check prior to starting heparin)
- Unprovoked DVT + contemplating stopping anticoagulation = delayed testing for antiphospholipid antibodies
- Perform sex-specific clinical exam and screening for malignancy rather than routine/extensive screening for malignancy.
  - Consider malignancy more likely as underlying cause if:
    - Recurrent VTE, unprovoked VTE, upper extremity DVT (not catheter-associated)
    - Abdominal DVT, bilateral lower extremity DVT

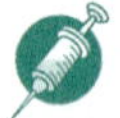

TREATMENT

Goal: Prevent recurrence, extension of the clot, and possible complications (e.g., PE).

GENERAL MEASURES

- National Institute for Health and Care Excellence (NICE) guidelines only treat proximal DVT (or extending distal thrombus on repeat imaging) and those with embolization (e.g., PE).
- Consider starting therapy before diagnosis confirmation in patients with high PTP and acceptable risk of bleeding.
- Isolated distal DVT
  - Benefits of anticoagulation are unclear. Treat if severely symptomatic or if there is thrombus extension on repeat imaging.
  - Treat for 3 months (if no contraindications).
  - Extend treatment if DVT is unprovoked or if provoked and persistent risk factor is present.
- Proximal/iliofemoral DVT
  - Treat with anticoagulation for ≥3 months alone unless contraindicated, rather than interventional approaches.
  - If high PTP and awaiting diagnostic tests, consider offering anticoagulation while awaiting results.
  - Initial bridging is not required for rivaroxaban (Xarelto) or apixaban (Eliquis).
  - Same indications for extended treatment as above

MEDICATION

First Line

- Unfractionated heparin
  - IV drip: initial dose of 80 U/kg followed by continuous infusion of 18 U/kg/hour; target aPTT ratio >1.5 to 2.0 times control.
  - Monitor aPTT q6h and adjust infusion rate accordingly until two successive values are within the therapeutic range.
- Low-molecular-weight heparin (LMWH)
  - Enoxaparin (Lovenox): 1 mg/kg/dose SC q12h or 1.5 mg/kg daily
  - Dalteparin (Fragmin): 200 U/kg SC q24h or 100 U/kg SC q12h
  - American College of Chest Physicians recommend that if LMWH is used, consider once daily dosing over twice daily dosing.
  - Consider reduced dosing in the setting of chronic kidney disease (CKD).
- Direct and indirect* factor Xa inhibitors (dual oral anticoagulants [DOACs])
  - Rivaroxaban (Xarelto): 15 mg PO twice daily with food for the first 3 weeks then 20 mg PO daily with food
  - Apixaban (Eliquis): 10 mg PO twice daily for 1 week followed by 2.5 to 5.0 mg PO twice daily: Consider reduced dosing in renal insufficiency.
  - Edoxaban (Savaysa): Initially give parenteral anticoagulants for 5 to 10 days and then transition to 60 mg PO daily (>60 kg), 30 mg PO daily (≤60 kg).
  - Fondaparinux* (Arixtra): 5 mg (body weight <50 kg), 7.5 mg (body weight = 50 to 100 kg), or 10 mg (body weight >100 kg) SC once daily. contraindicated with renal insufficiency (creatinine clearance [CrCl] <30 mL/min)
- Thrombin inhibitors: dabigatran (Pradaxa): Initially, give parenteral anticoagulants for 5 to 10 days and then transition to 150 mg PO twice daily for CrCl >30 mL/min.
- Vitamin K antagonists
  - Warfarin (Coumadin): Start with 2 to 5 mg/day. Adjust to a target INR of 2 to 3; overlap with a parenteral anticoagulant for a minimum of 5 days until therapeutic INR is sustained ≥24 hours.
  - DOACs preferred if possible
- Adverse effects
  - All anticoagulants increase risk of bleeding.
  - Heparin and LMWH can also cause heparin-induced thrombocytopenia (HIT) (LMWH has a lower risk) and injection site irritation.
  - Dosage adjustments may be required for patients with decreased CrCl.

Second Line

Pregnancy Considerations

- Offer LMWH rather than unfractionated heparin
- Warfarin (Coumadin) is contraindicated in pregnancy (teratogenic), but safe in breastfeeding.
- Avoid the use of oral direct thrombin inhibitors (e.g., Dabigatran) and anti-Xa inhibitors (e.g., Rivaroxaban, Apixaban).
- If on LMWH, discontinue ≥24 hours prior to induction of labor or cesarean delivery rather than continuing.
- Cancer associated DVT: Consider anticoagulation for at least 6 months with DOACs.

SURGERY/OTHER PROCEDURES

- Catheter-directed thrombolysis/open thrombectomy
  - Anticoagulation is preferred for iliofemoral DVT, symptoms <14 days, good functional status, low-bleeding risk, and life expectancy ≥1 year.
  - Thrombectomy is recommended for limb-threatening ischemia.
  - Note: can improve possibility of developing post-thrombotic syndrome after proximal (iliofemoral or femoral) DVT
- Inferior vena cava (IVC) filter
  - Consider for patients with proximal DVT and (absolute) contraindications for anticoagulation (e.g., high-bleeding risk).
  - Special consideration can be given to those who are chronically immobile, such as spinal cord injury patients.

ADMISSION, INPATIENT, AND NURSING CONSIDERATIONS

- Individualize:
  - Patients with concomitant low-risk PE, if the following criteria are met, can be considered for outpatient treatment.
    - Access to medications, ability to access outpatient care/follow-up, and home circumstances are adequate.
  - Clinical decision tool: PE Severity Index (PESI) can help determine if a patient can safely and adequately be treated in the outpatient setting (strong recommendation, low-certainty evidence).
  - Also consider the following in the decision: bleeding risk, clot burden, comorbid conditions requiring monitoring (e.g., severe renal or liver disease, thrombocytopenia, history of HIT).
- In patients with acute PE, if the following criteria are met, then hospital admission is not necessary:
  - The patient is clinically stable with good cardiopulmonary reserve.
  - No recent bleeding, severe renal or liver disease, or severe thrombocytopenia <70,000/μL
  - Expected to be compliant and feels well enough to be treated at home
- Admission for respiratory distress, elevated cardiac biomarkers, right ventricular dysfunction, candidate for thrombolysis, active bleeding, renal failure, phlegmasia alba dolens, phlegmasia cerulea dolens, history of HIT
- In medically stable and properly anticoagulated patients, an overlap of anticoagulation and warfarin monitoring may be done as an outpatient.
- Encourage ambulation, avoid bedrest, use limb elevation and graduated compression stockings for symptomatic patients.

ONGOING CARE

FOLLOW-UP RECOMMENDATIONS

Resumption of normal activity with avoidance of prolonged immobility

Patient Monitoring

Monitor platelet counts while on heparin, LMWH, and fondaparinux for HIT.

PATIENT EDUCATION

Dietary habits should be discussed when warfarin is initiated to ensure that intake of vitamin K-rich foods are monitored. Also, patients should avoid alcohol, cranberry juice, and grapefruit.

PROGNOSIS

- Most DVTs will resolve with the appropriate treatment without complication.
- Post-thrombotic syndrome occurs in approximately 43% of patients 2-years post-DVT.
- All-cause mortality varies at different time frames after DVT diagnosis: 30-day mortality: 3%; mortality between days 31 and 364: 13%; mortality between years 1 and 10: 42%
- DVT confined to the infrapopliteal veins has a small risk of embolization but can propagate proximally.

COMPLICATIONS

Major complications:

- Embolization (typically in the lungs in the form of a PE) can be fatal.
- Arterial embolism (paradoxical embolization) with AV shunting
- Chronic thromboembolic pulmonary hypertension
- Recurrence
- Chronic postthrombotic syndrome, chronic venous insufficiency, bleeding from the use of anticoagulants
- Phlegmasia cerulea dolens (rare but a surgical emergency)

REFERENCES

1. Modi S, Deisler R, Gozel K, et al. Wells criteria for DVT is a reliable clinical tool to assess the risk of deep venous thrombosis in trauma patients. *World J Emerg Surg*. 2016;11:24.

SEE ALSO

Antithrombin Deficiency; Factor V Leiden; Protein C Deficiency; Protein S Deficiency; Prothrombin 20210 (Mutation); Pulmonary Embolism

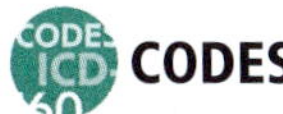

CODES

ICD10

- I80.209 Phlbts and thombophlb of unsp deep vessels of unsp low extrm
- I80.299 Phlebitis and thombophlb of deep vessels of unsp low extrm
- I80.10 Phlebitis and thrombophlebitis of unspecified femoral vein

CLINICAL PEARLS

- Patients may frequently present asymptomatic.
- Wells criteria help risk stratify.
- Early initiation of anticoagulation can improve outcomes.
- Recognize Virchow Triad: Virchovenous stasis (due to venous obstrcution, shock, CHF), endothelial injury (due to trauma, inflammation, surgery), and hypercoagulability (due to malignancy, nephrotic syndrome, HRT)

D

DEHYDRATION

Stephen W. Line, DO, CAQSM • July Jost, MD • Tanner J. Jennings, DO

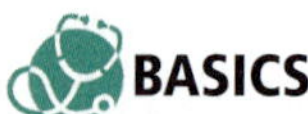

BASICS

DESCRIPTION

- Dehydration is defined as a deficiency in total body water (1).
- There are two types of dehydration:
  - Hypertonic: an uncompensated, predominant water deficit
  - Isotonic: a deficiency of water with an associated reduction in salt

EPIDEMIOLOGY

Dehydration is linked to higher mortality and morbidity, prevalent in many health care settings, and responsible for nearly 10% of pediatric hospitalizations in the United States (1),(2).

Incidence

Dehydration occurs in 17–28% of older adults in the United States.

Prevalence

Several retrospective studies have evaluated dehydration prevalence after hospital admission, estimating that 2.1–3.5% of patients meet dehydration criteria (1).

ETIOLOGY AND PATHOPHYSIOLOGY

- Body water can be lost through the skin (sweating, burns), lungs (pulmonary issues), kidneys (diuresis), and gastrointestinal tract (vomiting, diarrhea, bleeding).
- A negative fluid balance, where losses exceed intake, can cause hypovolemia and end-organ damage.
- "Third spacing" of fluids may occur with effusions, ascites, capillary leaks, or sepsis.

Geriatric Considerations

Elderly individuals face higher risks due to decreased kidney function, urine concentration, aldosterone secretion, vasopressin release, and renin activity. Increased immobility, fall risk, and impaired thirst mechanisms also contribute to these risks.

Genetics

Some dehydration cases are genetic (e.g., diabetes), whereas others are not (e.g., gastroenteritis).

RISK FACTORS

- Very young children and the elderly are most vulnerable.
- Acute or chronic illness
- Decreased cognition or mental status
- Lack of access to water
- Increased exertion (work or exercise) in hot or outdoor settings
- Medication exposure (e.g., diuretics)

GENERAL PREVENTION

- Educate patients/parents on early dehydration signs.
- Offer preferred beverages, especially during illness.
- Follow universal precautions (e.g., hand hygiene).
- Hydrate well before and after strenuous activity or extreme weather.

Clinical Finding	Mild	Moderate	Severe
Dehydration: children	5–10%	10–15%	>15%
Dehydration: adults	3–5%	5–10%	>10%
General condition: infants	Thirsty, alert, restless	Lethargic/drowsy	Limp, cold, cyanotic extremities, may be comatose
General condition: older children	Thirsty, alert, restless	Alert, postural dizziness	Apprehensive, cold, cyanotic extremities, muscle cramps
Quality of radial pulse	Normal	Thready/weak	Feeble or impalpable
Quality of respiration	Normal	Deep	Deep and rapid/tachypnea
Blood pressure	Normal	Normal to low	Low (shock)
Skin turgor	Normal skin turgor	Reduced skin turgor, cool skin	Skin tenting, cool, mottled, acrocyanotic skin
Eyes	Normal	Sunken	Very sunken
Tears	Present	Absent	Absent
Mucous membranes	Moist	Dry	Very dry
Urine output	Normal	Reduced	None passed in many hours
Anterior fontanelle	Normal	Sunken	Markedly sunken

COMMONLY ASSOCIATED CONDITIONS

- Hypernatremia/hyponatremia
- Hypokalemia
- Hyperglycemia
- Hypovolemic shock
- Renal failure
- Rhabdomyolysis
- Heat-related illness or injury

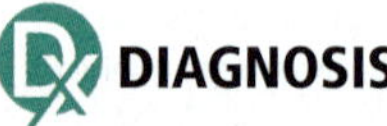

DIAGNOSIS

- Assessing hydration status involves evaluating the patient's history, clinical assessment, and laboratory values.
- Various clinical variables measure dehydration (see table).
- Percent dehydration is calculated as: (preillness weight − illness weight) / preillness weight × 100

HISTORY

- Fever
- Oral intake (amount and description)
- Diarrhea (duration, frequency, consistency, mucus/blood)
- Vomiting (duration, frequency, consistency, bilious/nonbilious)
- Urination pattern
- Sick contacts or recent illnesses
- Medication history (e.g., diuretics, laxatives, steroids)
- Heat exposure or recent exercise

PHYSICAL EXAM

- Vitals: blood pressure, pulse, temperature, respiratory rate
- Orthostatic vital signs
- Weight loss
- Mental status exam
- Sunken eyes and/or decreased tear production
- Dry or tacky mucous membranes
- Prolonged capillary refill (>3 seconds)
- Urine output: normal, reduced, or none for hours

Pediatric Considerations

In children, signs of dehydration include prolonged capillary refill, abnormal skin turgor, and unusual respiratory patterns. In infants, a sunken fontanelle is a warning sign. Tracking the number and weight of wet/soiled diapers helps assess hydration status.

DIFFERENTIAL DIAGNOSIS

- Decreased intake: ineffective breastfeeding, poor thirst response, anorexia, malabsorption, metabolic disorders, obtunded state
- Excessive losses: gastroenteritis, diarrhea, febrile illness, diabetic ketoacidosis, hyperglycemia, hyperosmolar hyperglycemic state, diabetes insipidus, intestinal obstruction, sepsis

DIAGNOSTIC TESTS & INTERPRETATION

Initial Tests (lab, imaging)

- Mild dehydration usually does not require serum or urine studies.
- For moderate to severe dehydration:
  - No single gold standard exists, but body mass changes and isotope dilution are reliable indicators.
  - Plasma/serum osmolality is the best test for identifying hypertonic dehydration.
  - Saliva osmolality shows moderate diagnostic accuracy in older populations.

- Urinalysis (specific gravity, hematuria, glucosuria) and urine osmolality are useful.
- Serum creatinine, BUN, and BUN/creatinine ratio are important tests.
- Imaging is generally unnecessary, but some patients might benefit from ultrasound assessment of inferior vena cava collapsibility and the diameter ratio of the inferior vena cava to the aorta (3). However, if used, ultrasound results should be used in conjunction with clinical assessments and lab results.

Follow-Up Tests & Special Considerations

Infants and the elderly may not concentrate urine maximally, making urinalysis and urine specific gravity less helpful.

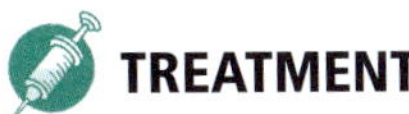

TREATMENT

GENERAL MEASURES

Oral rehydration therapy (ORT) is the first-line treatment for dehydration in both adults and children, with parenteral hydration and behavioral interventions as additional options.

MEDICATION

First Line

- If oral rehydration fails, IV rehydration is necessary while treating the underlying cause.
- For adults with moderate to severe hypovolemia:
  - Stage I: crystalloid fluid bolus, 20 mL/kg/hr until vital signs normalize
  - Stage II: Replace fluid deficit, start maintenance fluids, and account for losses.
    - Fluid deficit: (preillness weight – illness weight) × 1,000
    - 4-2-1 formula for maintenance:
      - 0 to 10 kg: +4 mL/kg/hr; 10–20 kg: +2 mL/kg/hr; 20 kg: +1 mL/kg/hr
      - Example for 50 kg: 90 mL/hr
- For children with moderate to severe dehydration:
  - Stage I: crystalloid fluid bolus, 10 to 20 mL/kg, may repeat up to 60 mL/kg
  - Stage II: Replace fluid deficit, start maintenance fluids, and account for losses over 24 to 48 hours.
- Alternative IV treatment for moderate dehydration in children:
  - Bolus with NS/lactated Ringer (LR) at 20 mL/kg for 1 hour
  - Replete deficit with D5 1/2 NS + 20 mEq KCl/L at 10 mL/kg for 8 hours
  - Maintenance with D5 1/4 NS + 20 mEq KCl for 16 hours
- IV fluid considerations
  - Choose crystalloid fluid based on the patient:
    - Common options: isotonic saline (0.9% NaCl), LR, D5 1/2 NS + 20 mEq KCl/L.
  - Rapid volume correction in severe hyponatremia can risk central pontine myelinolysis.
  - Use caution in older patients, those with heart failure, or advanced kidney disease; they need smaller boluses and frequent reassessment.
  - For young children, consider nasogastric fluid administration as an alternative to IV fluids.

Second Line

- Consider antiemetic/antidiarrheal medications when excessive vomiting or diarrhea is present.
- Ondansetron (PO, SL, IV): 4 to 8 mg every 4 to 8 hours as needed; reduces emesis frequency and improves oral hydration success. Risks include QT prolongation, constipation, and headaches.
- Promethazine (PO, PR, IM, IV): 12.5 to 25.0 mg every 4 to 6 hours as needed (max 50 mg/day); contraindicated in children <2 years of age due to fatal respiratory depression risk and caution needed with IM/IV administration due to severe soft tissue and vascular injury risk.
- Loperamide may shorten diarrhea duration in children with mild to moderate dehydration but is not recommended for children <3 years of age due to serious adverse event risks.

ISSUES FOR REFERRAL

- Severe dehydration may require critical care and ICU-level treatment.
- Consider surgical consultation for acute abdominal issues if necessary.

SURGERY/OTHER PROCEDURES

For causes like intestinal obstruction or appendicitis

ADMISSION, INPATIENT, AND NURSING CONSIDERATIONS

- Admission criteria:
  - Intractable vomiting/diarrhea
  - Severe electrolyte abnormalities
  - Hemodynamic instability
  - Inability to tolerate ORT
- Inpatient management:
  - Stabilize airway, breathing, and circulation.
  - Mild dehydration: Start ORT; if ineffective, use IV fluids.
    - The Holliday-Segar method helps determine maintenance ORT for children.
  - Moderate to severe dehydration or hemodynamic instability: Begin IV fluid resuscitation immediately.
    - Monitor strict inputs and outputs:
      - Input: oral intake, parenteral fluids and medications
      - Output: urine, stool, procedural fluid loss, body fluid drainage
- Discharge criteria:
  - Euvolemia and ability to tolerate oral diet/fluids
  - Successful treatment of underlying cause with clinical improvement

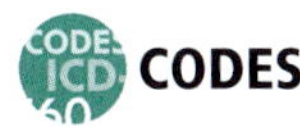

ONGOING CARE

DIET

- Bland foods: bananas, rice, applesauce, toast (BRAT diet)
- Small, frequent sips of room temperature liquids
- Oral rehydration salts or milk are better than water alone.
- Commercial oral rehydration solutions are available.

Pediatric Considerations

Continue breastfeeding ad lib. If diarrhea is present, lactose-free feeds may reduce the duration of diarrhea in children with mild to severe dehydration.

PATIENT EDUCATION

- Seek medical care if feeling faint, dizzy with positional changes, suddenly lethargic or confused, or experiencing a rapid heart rate.
- Call a physician if unable to tolerate fluids, vomiting persists >24 hours (adult) or >12 hours (child), diarrhea lasts >2 days, or if an infant/child is significantly less active or very irritable.

PROGNOSIS

Self-limited if treated early; potentially fatal if untreated and persistent

COMPLICATIONS

- Seizures
- Renal failure
- Cardiovascular arrest
- Mortality

REFERENCES

1. Frith J. New horizons in the diagnosis and management of dehydration. *Age Ageing*. 2023;52(10):afad193. doi:10.1093/ageing/afad193.
2. Gray M, Birkenfeld JS, Butterworth I. Noninvasive monitoring to detect dehydration: are we there yet? *Annu Rev Biomed Eng*. 2023;25:23–49. doi:10.1146/annurev-bioeng-062117-121028.
3. Kołodziej M, Jalali A, Łukasik J. Point-of-care ultrasound to assess degree of dehydration in children: a systematic review with meta-analysis. *Arch Dis Child*. 2024;109(4):275–281.

CODES

ICD10

- E86.0 Dehydration
- E87.1 Hypo-osmolality and hyponatremia
- E86.1 Hypovolemia

CLINICAL PEARLS

- Dehydration is the result of a deficiency in total body water leading to a negative fluid balance.
- Dehydration and its sequelae are a common cause of hospitalization in adults, children, and the elderly.
- Begin by assessing the level of dehydration, determining the underlying cause, and calculating necessary replacement needs.
- Treatment is directed at treating the underlying cause while restoring fluid balance via oral rehydration (preferred) or IV/IO/NG fluids (if necessary).

DELIRIUM

Dongsheng Jiang, MD, MSc • Juan Qiu, MD, PhD

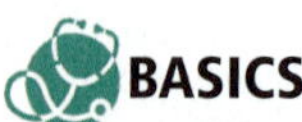

BASICS

DESCRIPTION

- A temporary neurocognitive complication of illness and/or medication(s) manifested by new confusion and impaired attention
- Requires evaluation to decrease morbidity and mortality

EPIDEMIOLOGY

- Predominant age: older persons
- Predominant sex: male = female

Incidence

- >50% in older ICU patients
- 11–51% in postoperative patients
- 19% after intracranial surgery and 42% after neurovascular surgery
- 10–40% in hospitalized older patients
- 20–22% in nursing home/post-acute care patients

Prevalence

- 1–2% in outpatients
- 8–17% in older ED patients

ETIOLOGY AND PATHOPHYSIOLOGY

- Multifactorial: believed to result from a decline in physiologic reserves with aging, resulting in a vulnerability to new stressors
- Often interaction between predisposing and precipitating risk factors

RISK FACTORS

- Two strongest predictors of delirium: ICU admission and history of dementia
- Predisposing risk factors
  - Advanced age, >70 years
  - Preexisting cognitive or functional impairment
  - Dehydration; malnutrition
  - History of alcohol abuse
  - Hearing or vision impairment
  - Multiple comorbidities
- Precipitating risk factors
  - Severe illness in any organ system
  - Medical devices (urinary catheter, restraints)
  - Polypharmacy (≥5 medications)
  - Medications, especially benzodiazepines, opioids, anticholinergics diphenhydramine, high-dose neuroleptics
  - Pain
  - Surgery
  - Sleep deprivation

COMMONLY ASSOCIATED CONDITIONS

Multiple but most common are the following:

- Medication changes
- Infections (especially lung, urine, and bloodstream, but consider meningitis as well)
- Toxic metabolic (especially low sodium, elevated calcium, renal failure, and hepatic failure)
- Heart attack or stroke
- Alcohol or drug withdrawal
- Preexisting cognitive impairment increases risk.

DIAGNOSIS

- Delirium is not just a diagnosis of exclusion—the diagnosis is made using a careful history, behavioral observation, and cognitive assessment.
- *Diagnostic and Statistical Manual of Mental Disorders*, 5th edition, diagnostic criteria include:
  - Disturbance in attention and awareness
  - Change in cognition not due to dementia or coma
  - Presence of an additional disturbance in cognition (e.g., memory deficit, language, visuospatial ability, disorientation, or perception)
  - Onset over short period (hours to days) and fluctuates during course of day
  - Evidence from history, exam, or lab that disturbance is caused by physiologic consequence of medical condition, intoxicating substance, medication use, or more than one cause.
- The Confusion Assessment Method (CAM) is the most well-validated and tested clinical tool (sensitivity 94–100% and specificity 90–95%) and has been adapted for ICU setting in adults (CAM-ICU) and children (pediatric CAM-ICU [pCAM-ICU]).
  - Four key diagnostic features of the CAM:
    - Acute change in mental status
    - Fluctuating course
    - Inattention
    - Disorganized thinking or altered level of consciousness
- Several nondiagnostic symptoms may be present:
  - Short- and long-term memory problems
  - Sleep–wake cycle disturbances
  - Hallucinations and/or delusions
  - Emotional lability
  - Tremors and asterixis
- Subtypes based on level of consciousness
  - Hyperactive delirium (15%): Patients are loud, agitated, restless, and disruptive.
  - Hypoactive delirium (20%): quietly confused; sleepy; may sit and not eat, drink, or move
  - Mixed delirium (50%): features of both hyperactive and hypoactive delirium
  - Normal consciousness delirium (15%): still displays disorganized thinking, along with acute onset, inattention, and fluctuating mental status
  - Subsyndromal delirium (23%): some delirium symptoms but does not progress to full delirium

HISTORY

- Time course of mental status changes
- Recent medication changes
- Symptoms of infection
- New neurologic signs
- Abrupt change in functional ability

PHYSICAL EXAM

- Comprehensive cardiorespiratory exam is essential.
- Focal neurologic signs are usually absent.
- Mini-Mental State Examination (MMSE) is the most well-known and studied cognitive screen, but it may not be the most appropriate in an acute care setting; shorter cognitive screens have been studied in delirious patients (i.e., Short Blessed Test [SBT], Brief Alzheimer Screen [BAS], and Ottawa 3DY) and may be helpful if performed serially over time.
- Gastrointestinal/genitourinary exam for constipation/urinary retention

DIFFERENTIAL DIAGNOSIS

- Depression (disturbance of mood, normal level of consciousness, fluctuates weeks to months)
- Acute stress disorder (disturbance of mood, normal level of consciousness, precipitated by traumatic event)
- Bipolar disorder, manic episode (pressured speech, impulsivity, fluctuates weeks to months, rarely sudden onset in older adults)
- Dementia (insidious onset, memory problems, normal level of consciousness, fluctuates days to weeks)
- Psychosis (rarely sudden onset in older adults)
- Seizure disorders (i.e., nonconvulsive status epilepticus)

DIAGNOSTIC TESTS & INTERPRETATION

Initial Tests (lab, imaging)

- Labs: guided by history and physical exam
  - CBC, CMP, TSH, UA, urine culture, blood culture, COVID-19 swab
  - Medication levels (digoxin, theophylline, antiepileptics) where applicable
- Chest radiograph
- Electrocardiogram as necessary

Follow-Up Tests & Special Considerations

- If preliminary lab tests do not indicate a precipitator of delirium, consider:
  - Venous blood gases
  - Troponin
  - Toxicology screen
  - Thiamine, B_{12}
  - HIV, syphilis, other infectious disease studies
  - Ammonia
  - CSF studies
- Noncontrast-enhanced head CT scan if
  - Recent fall
  - Receiving anticoagulants
  - New focal neurologic signs
  - Ruling out mass before lumbar puncture
- Brain MRI

Diagnostic Procedures/Other

- Lumbar puncture (rarely necessary)
- Electroencephalogram (rarely necessary)

TREATMENT

- Establish a comprehensive and well-coordinated multidisciplinary team to include physicians, nurses, pharmacists, psychologists, speech therapists, dieticians, physical/occupational therapists, spiritual/religious specialists, and social workers and to design and fine-tune treatment strategy according to each patient's unique situation.
- There is strong evidence for multicomponent nonpharmacologic interventions (1).
- Addressing any discomfort: pain, nausea, urinary or bowel retention, dehydration
- Keeping noise, alarms, and other disturbances to a minimum
- Maintenance of mobility
- Use eyeglasses, hearing aids, and other assistive devices.
- Family involvement/engagement
- Pharmacologic management of symptoms (reserve for severe circumstances)
- Addressing six risk factors (i.e., cognitive impairment, sleep deprivation, dehydration, immobility, vision impairment, and hearing impairment) in at-risk hospitalized patients can reduce the incidence of delirium by 33%.

GENERAL MEASURES

- De-escalation skill training for care staff
- Look for underlying causes: hypotension, hypoxia, hypoglycemia, drug overdose or withdrawal, and others.
- Remove unnecessary tubes/catheters.
- Actively involve family members in care
- Postoperative patients should be monitored for
  - Myocardial infarction/ischemia
  - Infection (i.e., pneumonia, urinary tract infection)
  - Pulmonary embolism
  - Urinary or stool retention (attempt catheter removal by postoperative day 2)
  - Anemia/bleeding
- Anesthesia route (general vs. epidural) may affect the risk of delirium. Depth of anesthesia likely affects risk of delirium.
- ICU sedation and avoidance of benzodiazepines may reduce risk.
- Multifactorial treatment: Identify contributing factors and provide preemptive care to avoid iatrogenic problems, with special attention to
  - CNS-oxygen delivery (attempt to attain):
    - SaO_2 >90% with goal of SaO_2 >95%
    - Systolic BP <2/3 of baseline or >90 mm Hg
    - Hematocrit >30%
  - Fluid/electrolyte balance
    - Sodium, potassium, and glucose normal (glucose <300 mg/dL in diabetics)
    - Treat fluid overload or dehydration.
  - Treat pain.
    - Scheduled acetaminophen with PRN morphine for breakthrough pain for example

ALERT

Any change with patient's medication can lead to delirium.

- Eliminate unnecessary medications.
  - Investigate new symptoms as potential medication side effects (i.e., Beers medications).
- Constipation and urinary retention can cause delirium, so monitor and regulate bowel/bladder function.
  - Bowel movement at least every 48 hours
  - Screen for urinary retention.
- Prevent major hospital-acquired problems.
  - Use a pressure-reducing mattress.
  - Avoid urinary catheters.
  - Encourage incentive spirometry.
  - Venous thromboembolism (VTE) prophylaxis if bedbound
  - Early mobilization
  - Environmental stimulation
    - Glasses and hearing aids
    - Clock and calendar
    - Soft lighting with curtains open during the day
    - Music and television, if desired
  - Sleep
    - Quiet and dark environment
    - Soft music
    - Therapeutic massage
- Restraints increase risk of delirium and falls/injury.
  - Use as a last resort for patients at risk for self-injury or risk for injuring caregivers. Remove as soon as possible.

MEDICATION

- Nonpharmacologic approaches are preferred for initial treatment, but medication may be needed for severe agitation and injurious behaviors, especially in the ICU setting.
- No FDA-approved medication for delirium treatment
- No medication can prevent delirium.

First Line

- For symptomatic management of intolerable agitation, delusion, or hallucinations:
  - Antipsychotics (in alphabetical order) have been used although their efficacy is unclear (2).
    - Haloperidol (Haldol): 1 to 2 mg PO; 1.0 to 2.5 mg IM; 0.5 to 1.0 mg IV
    - Olanzapine (Zyprexa) 2.5 to 5.0 mg PO
    - Quetiapine (Seroquel) 12.5 to 25.0 mg PO
    - Risperidone (Risperdal) 0.25 to 1.0 mg PO
- Precautions: Antipsychotics may cause extrapyramidal effects and increase fall risk, avoid in parkinsonism.
- Antipsychotics should not be used routinely to treat delirium in critically ill patients (3).
- For management of sedation in ICU patient
  - α_2-Agonist dexmedetomidine is preferred for sedation in ICU patients and is the only medication that has been found to possibly shorten delirium duration. The primary adverse effects of this medication include hypotension and bradycardia. Some studies have also found use of clonidine as an oral bridge off of dexmedetomidine.
- Melatonin and melatonin agonists are gaining interest as sleep aids in ICU patients.

Second Line

- Benzodiazepines should generally be avoided except in alcohol withdrawal, or if patient takes regularly at baseline, or when antipsychotic is contraindicated. Benzodiazepines can cause delirium. Lorazepam (Ativan): initially, 0.25 to 0.5 mg PO/IM/IV TID–QID PRN; may need to adjust to effect
- Cholinesterase inhibitors should be avoided.

REFERENCES

1. Fischer MA, Corsetti M. Geriatric psychiatric emergencies. *Emerg Med Clin North Am*. 2024;42(1):135–149. doi:10.1016/j.emc.2023.06.016.
2. Skains RM, Lee S, Han JH. Delirium prevention and management in older adults in the emergency department. *Emerg Med Clin North Am*. 2025;43(2):249–263. doi:10.1016/j.emc.2024.08.007.
3. Mart MF, Boehm LM, Kiehl AL, et al. Long-term outcomes after treatment of delirium during critical illness with antipsychotics (MIND-USA): a randomised, placebo-controlled, phase 3 trial. *Lancet Respir Med*. 2024;12(8):599–607. doi:10.1016/S2213-2600(24)00077-8.

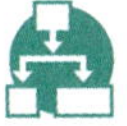

SEE ALSO

- Dementia; Depression; Substance Use Disorders
- Algorithm: Delirium

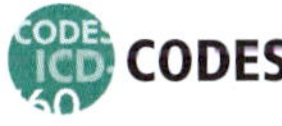

CODES

ICD10

- R41.0 Disorientation, unspecified
- F19.931 Oth psychoactive substance use, unsp w withdrawal delirium
- F10.231 Alcohol dependence with withdrawal delirium

CLINICAL PEARLS

- The criteria for delirium include an acute onset of fluctuating mental status, inattention, and either disorganized thinking or altered level of consciousness.
- Primary treatment for delirium is to identify and treat the underlying causes.
- Nonpharmacologic measures are preferable.
- Delirium may not resolve as soon as the treatable contributors resolve; may take weeks or months
- Team building and teamwork is critical in delirium prevention, early diagnosis, and treatment.

D

DEMENTIA

Hammad Mohsin, MD

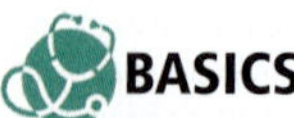

BASICS

DESCRIPTION

Dementia refers to cognitive decline from previous level of performance in various cognitive domains (attention, executive function perceptual-motor, social cognition, language, and memory) interfere significantly with ADLs in the absence of delirium or any other mental disorder.

- *DSM-5* classifies dementias under neurocognitive disorders (major and mild) and specifies the cause of neurocognitive decline secondary to the following:
  - Alzheimer dementia (AD)
  - Vascular dementia (VaD)
  - Lewy body dementia
  - Parkinson disease dementia
  - Frontotemporal dementia
  - Creutzfeldt-Jakob disease (CJD)
  - HIV dementia
  - Substance-induced/medication-induced neurocognitive disorder

EPIDEMIOLOGY

Prevalence

- In patients age ≥65 years
  - AD: 11.3% (5.3% in ages 65 to 74 years, 13.8% in ages 75 to 84 years, 34.6% in ages ≥85)
  - VaD: 1.6%
  - Other: 13%
- Estimated 5 to 6 million Americans living with dementia
- Annual incidence of Alzheimer and other dementias expected to double by 2050

ETIOLOGY AND PATHOPHYSIOLOGY

- AD: involves β-amyloid protein accumulation and/or neurofibrillary tangles (NFTs), synaptic dysfunction, neurodegeneration, and eventual neuronal loss
- Age, genetics, systemic disease, smoking, and other host factors may influence the β-amyloid accumulation and/or the pace of progression toward the clinical manifestations of AD.
- VaD
  - Cerebral atherosclerosis/emboli with clinical/subclinical infarcts

Genetics

- AD: positive family history in 50%, but 90% AD is sporadic; *APOE4* increases risk but full role unclear.
- Familial/autosomal dominant AD accounts for <5% AD: amyloid precursor protein (APP), presenilin-1 (PSEN-1), and presenilin-2 (PSEN-2).

RISK FACTORS

- Age is the strongest factor.
- Sex: female > male
- Genetic predisposition
- Hypertension: AD; VaD
- Hypercholesterolemia: AD; VaD
- Diabetes: VaD
- Obesity: VaD
- Cigarette smoking: VaD
- Endocrine/metabolic abnormalities:
  - Hypothyroidism, Cushing syndrome; thiamine and vitamin B_{12} deficiency
- Chronic alcoholism, other drugs
- Lower educational status
- Head injury early in life
- Sedentary lifestyle

GENERAL PREVENTION

- Treat reversible causes of dementia, such as drug-induced, alcohol-induced, and vitamin deficiencies.
- Treat hypertension, hypercholesterolemia, and diabetes.
- No evidence for statins (or any other specific medication) to prevent onset of dementia (1)[A]
- BP control and low-dose aspirin may prevent or lessen cognitive decline in VaD.
- Maintain or increase physical activity and exercise.
- Continue cognitively stimulating activities and social interactions.

COMMONLY ASSOCIATED CONDITIONS

- Anxiety and major depression
- Psychosis (delusions, delusions of persecution are common)
- Delirium
- Behavioral disturbances (agitation, aggression)
- Sleep disturbances

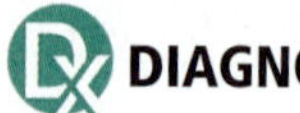

DIAGNOSIS

Clinical diagnosis

HISTORY

Requires a family member or someone who knows the patient well to describe changes in the patient's cognition and behavior.

- Probable diagnosis AD (2):
  - Age between 40 and 90 years (usually >65 years)
  - Progressive cognitive decline of insidious onset
  - No disturbances of consciousness
  - Deficits in areas of cognition
  - No other explainable cause of symptoms
  - Specifically rule out thyroid disease, vitamin deficiency (B_{12}), grief reaction, and depression.
  - Supportive factors: family history of dementia

PHYSICAL EXAM

Clinical assessment

- Physical exam to assess for neurologic deficits, motor and gait abnormalities, tremors, etc.
- No disturbances of consciousness
- Can start with brief initial screening tests for cognitive impairment
  - Mini-Cog test
  - General Practitioner Assessment of Cognition
  - Ascertain Dementia 8-Item Informant Questionnaire
- If screening is positive, should be screened for depression (such as with PHQ-2 and PHQ-9, and geriatric depression scale) and can be assessed by other cognitive assessment tools.
- Cognitive decline demonstrated by standardized instruments, including the following:
  - Mini-Mental State Examination (MMSE)
  - Montreal Cognitive Assessment (MoCA) test
  - ADAS-Cog
  - Use caution in relying solely on cognition scores, especially in those with learning difficulty, language barriers, or similar limitations.
- Neuropsychological testing extensively evaluates multiple cognitive domains and can help discriminate between normal aging and dementia. This may be useful in difficult situations when history and mental status examination do not agree and most useful when repeated over time.

DIFFERENTIAL DIAGNOSIS

- Major depression
- Medication side effect
- Chronic alcohol use
- Delirium
- Subdural hematoma
- Normal pressure hydrocephalus
- Brain tumor
- Thyroid disease
- Parkinson disease
- Vitamin B_{12} deficiency
- Toxins
  - Aromatic hydrocarbons, solvents, heavy metals, marijuana, opiates, sedative and hypnotics

DIAGNOSTIC TESTS & INTERPRETATION

Initial Tests (lab, imaging)

- Used to rule out causes
  - CBC, CMP
  - Thyroid-stimulating hormone
  - Vitamin B_{12} level
- Select patients based on clinical suspicion.
  - HIV, rapid plasma reagin (RPR)
  - Erythrocyte sedimentation rate (ESR)
  - Folate
  - Heavy metal and toxicology screen
- Research studies with cerebrospinal fluid (CSF) biomarkers in patient with confirmed AD have shown decreased β-amyloid (1 to 42) and increased τ and p-τ levels, which are specific features of AD, and CSF τ proteins are increased in CJD (3)[A].
- Neuroimaging (CT/MRI of brain):
  - Routine neuroimaging can help to distinguish specific types of dementia with structural imaging finding
  - Early age of onset (<65 years), rapid progression, focal neurologic deficits, cerebrovascular disease risk, or atypical symptoms: neuroimaging (MRI/CT) to rule out other causes
- Important findings
  - AD: diffuse cerebral atrophy starting in association areas, hippocampus (hippocampal atrophy may be the earliest sign), amygdala
  - VaD: old infarcts, including lacunar

Follow-Up Tests & Special Considerations

- Genetic testing for dementia is not recommended, such as testing for *APOE4* for Alzheimer, unless there are multiple family members diagnosed with AD at a young age.
- LP and CSF analysis can be considered in atypical presentations to identify infectious, inflammatory, or neoplastic etiologies.

Diagnostic Procedures/Other

PET scan not routinely recommended; has been approved to differentiate between Alzheimer disease and frontotemporal dementia

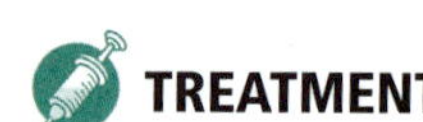

TREATMENT

GENERAL MEASURES

- Daily schedules and written directions
- Emphasis on nutrition, personal hygiene, accident-proofing the home, safety issues, sleep hygiene, and supervision
- Socialization (adult daycare)
- Sensory stimulation (display of clocks and calendars) in the early to middle stages

- Occupational training and structured physical exercise program
- Discussion with the family concerning support and advance directives

MEDICATION

- Cognitive dysfunction
- Medications for AD (4)[A] show a small improvement in some cognitive measures, but it remains unclear if the improvement is clinically significant and associated with side effects.
- Cognitive dysfunction, mild
  - Cholinesterase inhibitors: donepezil (Aricept), 5 to 10 mg/day; rivastigmine (Exelon), 1.5 to 6.0 mg BID, transdermal system 4.6 mg/24 hr and 9.5 mg/24 hr; galantamine (Razadyne), 4 to 12 mg BID, extended release 8 to 24 mg/day
    - Adverse events: nausea, vomiting, diarrhea, anorexia, nightmares, bradycardia/syncope
    - Galantamine warning: associated with mortality in patients with mild cognitive impairment in clinical trial
    - It is suggested to consider cholinesterase inhibitor for patients with mild to moderate dementia (MMSE 10 to 26). Responses may be quite variable.
    - Start drug with lowest acquisition cost; also consider adverse event profile, adherence, medical comorbidity, drug interactions, and dosing profiles.
- Cognitive dysfunction, moderate to severe
  - Cholinesterase inhibitors
  - Memantine (Namenda), NMDA receptor antagonist, 5 to 20 mg/day
    - Adverse events: dizziness, confusion, headache, constipation
    - Generally well tolerated with fewer side effects compared to cholinesterase inhibitors
    - Not shown to be beneficial in milder forms of AD
  - Combination cholinesterase inhibitor and memantine
    - The patients with moderate to advanced dementia (MMSE <17), recommendations are to add memantine (10 mg BID) to a cholinesterase inhibitor, or using memantine alone in patients who do not tolerate or benefit from a cholinesterase inhibitor.
    - In patients with severe dementia (MMSE <10), it is suggested to continue memantine. However, in advanced dementia, medications can be discontinued to maximize quality of life and patient comfort.
  - Monoclonal antibodies (MABs) (5)
  - Target amyloid deposits to slow the progression
  - Lecanemab and aducanumab are the only MABs approved by the FDA for treating Alzheimer disease.
  - MABs can slow the progression of Alzheimer disease and cognitive decline.
  - MABs can cause amyloid-related imaging abnormalities (ARIA), including ARIA-edema and ARIA-hemorrhage.
  - Patients should be closely monitored for ARIA and infusion reactions during the start of treatment.
- Commonly associated conditions
  - Psychosis and agitation/aggressive behavior:
    - Look for precipitating factors (infection, pain, depression, medications).
    - Nonpharmacologic therapies (behavioral interventions, music therapy, etc.) are preferred as first-line treatment.
    - Mood stabilizers (valproic acid, carbamazepine) have been used, although evidence is lacking.
    - For moderate to severe symptoms; antipsychotics: Initiate low doses, risperidone 0.25 to 1.00 mg/day; olanzapine 1.25 to 5.00 mg/day; quetiapine 12.5 to 50.0 mg/day; aripiprazole 5 mg/day; ziprasidone 20 mg/day
    - Atypical antipsychotic, quetiapine, is often first line due to decreased extrapyramidal side effect.
    - Novel antipsychotic, pimavanserin (selective 5-HT2A receptor inverse agonist) has shown to effectively treat Parkinson disease psychosis with minimal risk of worsening motor function associated with other treatment (6)[B].

ALERT

Black box warning on antipsychotics due to increased mortality in elderly with dementia

Geriatric Considerations

- Initiate pharmacotherapy at low doses and titrate slowly up if necessary.
- Benzodiazepines are potentially inappropriate for older adults, yet their use persists.

ALERT

- Benzodiazepine use is associated with increased fall risk (7)[A].

- Watch decreased renal function and hepatic metabolism.

First Line

Nonpharmacologic management: environmental modifications, caregiver training, music therapy, exercise, pet therapy

Second Line

- Cholinesterase inhibitors, memantine, atypical antipsychotics, antidepressants, mood stabilizers, methylphenidate, benzodiazepines, melatonin
- Antidepressants not clearly superior to placebo in treating depression (HTA-SADD)

ISSUES FOR REFERRAL

Neuropsychiatric evaluation helpful in early stages or mild cognitive impairment

ADDITIONAL THERAPIES

Behavioral modification

- Socialization, such as adult daycare, to prevent isolation and depression
- Sleep hygiene program as alternative to pharmaceuticals for sleep disturbance
- Scheduled toileting to prevent incontinence

ADMISSION, INPATIENT, AND NURSING CONSIDERATIONS

Psychiatry admission may be required because of safety concerns (self-harm/harm to others), self-neglect, aggressive behaviors, or other behavioral issues.

ONGOING CARE

FOLLOW-UP RECOMMENDATIONS

Patient Monitoring

- Progression of cognitive impairment by use of standardized tool (e.g., MMSE, ADAS-Cog)
- Development of behavioral problems
  - Sleep, depression, psychosis, aggression
- Adverse events of pharmacotherapy
- Nutritional status
- Caregiver evaluation of stress

PATIENT EDUCATION

- Advance care planning: Discuss safety, management of finances, medical decision-making, possible skilled facility placement; legal guardianship
- Advance directives, health care proxy should be established early on.
- National Institute on Aging: https://www.nia.nih.gov/health/topics/dementia

PROGNOSIS

- AD: usually steady progression leading to profound cognitive impairment; average survival about 10 years
- VaD: incrementally worsening dementia, but cognitive improvement is unlikely

COMPLICATIONS

- Wandering
- Sundowner syndrome is common in older people (who are sedated) and also in people who have dementia (can have adverse reaction to even small dose of psychoactive substances).
- Falls with injury
- Neglect and abuse
- Caregiver burnout

D

REFERENCES

1. McGuinness B, Craig D, Bullock R, et al. Statins for the prevention of dementia. *Cochrane Database Syst Rev*. 2009;(2):CD003160.
2. Blass DM, Rabins PV. In the clinic. Dementia. *Ann Intern Med*. 2008;148(7):ITC4-1–ITC4-16.
3. van Harten AC, Kester MI, Visser PJ, et al. Tau and p-tau as CSF biomarkers in dementia: a meta-analysis. *Clin Chem Lab Med*. 2011;49(3):353–366.
4. Birks J. Cholinesterase inhibitors for Alzheimer's disease. *Cochrane Database Syst Rev*. 2006;(1):CD005593.
5. Rabinovici GD, Lajoie R. Amyloid-targeting monoclonal antibodies for Alzheimer disease *JAMA*. 2023;330(6):507–509 doi:10.1001/jama.2023.11703.
6. Cummings J, Isaacson S, Mills R, et al. Pimavanserin for patients with Parkinson's disease psychosis: a randomised, placebo-controlled phase 3 trial. *Lancet*. 2014;383(9916):533–540.
7. Seppala LJ, Wermelink AMAT, de Vries M, et al; for EUGMS Task and Finish Group on Fall-Risk-Increasing Drugs. Fall-risk-increasing drugs: a systematic review and meta-analysis: II. psychotropics. *J Am Med Dir Assoc*. 2018;19(4):371.e11–371.e17.

SEE ALSO

Algorithm: Dementia

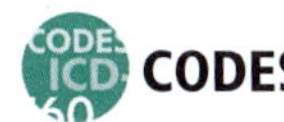

CODES

ICD10

- F03 Unspecified dementia
- G30.9 Alzheimer's disease, unspecified
- F01.50 Vascular dementia without behavioral disturbance

CLINICAL PEARLS

- Medications for AD show a small, statistically significant improvement in some cognitive measures, but it remains unclear if the improvement is clinically significant.
- Do not forget the role of adult protective services in case of elderly abuse—Elder Abuse hotline: 800-922-2275.
- A particular concern in nursing homes relates to finding alternatives to the use of physical restraints and antipsychotic medications.

DEMENTIA, VASCULAR

Birju B. Patel, MD, FACP, AGSF

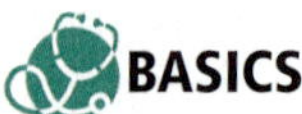

BASICS

Vascular dementia (also known as vascular cognitive impairment [VCI]) is a heterogeneous disorder caused by the sequelae of cerebrovascular disease that manifests in cognitive impairment affecting memory, thinking, learning, language, behavior, judgment, and executive dysfunction.

DESCRIPTION

- Vascular dementia (previously known as multi-infarct dementia) was first mentioned by Thomas Willis in 1672. Later, it was further described in the late 19th century by Binswanger and Alzheimer as a separate entity from dementia paralytica caused by neurosyphilis. This concept has evolved tremendously since the advent of neuroimaging modalities.
- Synonym(s): VCI; vascular cognitive disorder (VCD); Binswanger disease. *Diagnostic and Statistical Manual of Mental Disorders* (*DSM-5*) categorizes vascular dementia as mild or major VCD.

EPIDEMIOLOGY

Common cause of dementia in the elderly, and it frequently overlaps with Alzheimer dementia

Incidence

About 6 to 12 cases per 1,000/person age >70 years

Prevalence

- ~1.2–4.2% in those age >65 years
- 14–32% prevalence of dementia after a stroke

ETIOLOGY AND PATHOPHYSIOLOGY

No set pathologic criteria exist for the diagnosis of vascular dementia such as those that exist for Alzheimer dementia. Pathology includes the following:

- Large vessel disease: cognitive impairment that follows a stroke
- Small vessel disease (subcortical): includes white matter changes, subcortical infarcts, and incomplete infarction. This is usually the most common cause of multi-infarct dementia. Lacunar infarcts and deep white matter changes are typically included in this category.
- Transient ischemic attack (TIA)/stroke
- Vascular, demographic, genetic factors
  - Vascular disease (i.e., hypertension [HTN], peripheral vascular disease [PVD], atrial fibrillation, hyperlipidemia, diabetes, obstructive sleep apnea) (1)[B],(2)[C]

Genetics

- Cerebral autosomal dominant arteriopathy with subcortical infarcts and leukoencephalopathy (CADASIL) is caused by a mutation in the *NOTCH3* gene on chromosome 19 that results in leukoencephalopathy and subcortical infarcts. This is clinically manifested in recurrent strokes, migraine with aura, and vascular dementia.
- *Apolipoprotein E* gene type: Those with ApoE4 subtypes are at higher risk for developing both vascular and Alzheimer dementia.
- Amyloid precursor protein (APP) gene: leads to a form of vascular dementia called heritable cerebral hemorrhage with amyloidosis

RISK FACTORS

- Age (risk doubles every 5 years)
- Previous stroke
- Smoking
- Diabetes (especially with frequent hypoglycemia)
- Atherosclerotic heart disease; HTN; atrial fibrillation; PVD
- Hyperlipidemia
- Obstructive sleep apnea
- Low socioeconomic status (3)[C]

GENERAL PREVENTION

- Optimization and aggressive treatment of vascular risk factors, such as HTN, diabetes, and hyperlipidemia
- HTN is the single most modifiable risk factor and treatment for it must be optimized.
- Smoking is associated with white matter changes on imaging, which may be associated with small vessel disease and vascular dementia progression.
- Lifestyle modification: weight loss, physical activity, smoking cessation
- Hearing loss should be corrected.
- Depression and social isolation should be evaluated.
- Cognitively stimulating activity can be beneficial.
- Sleep apnea should be treated.
- Medication management for vascular risk reduction: aspirin usage, statin therapy for hyperlipidemia, antihypertensive therapy (4)[B]

COMMONLY ASSOCIATED CONDITIONS

- CADASIL
- Cerebral amyloid angiopathy (CAA) causes ischemic white matter damage due to amyloid deposition in penetrating cortical vessels.

DIAGNOSIS

Differentiation between Alzheimer dementia and vascular dementia can be difficult, and significant overlap is seen in the clinical presentation of these two dementias. The diagnosis of vascular dementia is a clinical diagnosis. Memory impairment is less prominent in vascular dementia versus Alzheimer dementia. The neuropsychological pattern observed in vascular dementia is impaired recall, relatively intact recognition, less severe forgetfulness with greater benefit from cues and more executive dysfunction.

HISTORY

- Gradual, stepwise progression is typical with multi-infarct dementia. This does not have to be present for all VCIs.
- Ask about onset and progression of cognitive impairment and the specific cognitive domains involved.
- Ask about vascular risk factors and previous attempts to control these risk factors.
- Ask about medication compliance.
- Ask about urinary incontinence and gait disturbances. Abnormal gait and falls are strong predictors of development of vascular dementia, particularly unsteady, frontal, and hemiparetic types of gait.
- Look for early symptoms, including difficulty performing cognitive tasks, memory, mood, and assessment of instrumental activities of daily living (IADLs).
- History may include TIAs, cerebrovascular accidents (CVAs), coronary atherosclerotic heart disease, atrial fibrillation, hyperlipidemia, and/or PVD. Small vessel disease usually presents with executive dysfunction. Large vessel disease usually presents with gait, visuospatial, and language dysfunction.

PHYSICAL EXAM

- Screen for HTN. Average daily home blood pressure (BP) is associated with progression of cerebrovascular disease and cognitive decline in the elderly.
- Focal neurologic deficits may be present.
- Gait assessment is important, especially looking at gait initiation, gait speed, and balance (5).
- Check for carotid bruits as well as abdominal bruits and assess for presence of PVD.
- Do a thorough cardiac evaluation that includes looking for arrhythmias (i.e., atrial fibrillation).

DIFFERENTIAL DIAGNOSIS

- Alzheimer dementia
- Depression
- Delirium
- CNS tumors
- Hypothyroidism/hyperthyroidism
- Vitamin B_{12} deficiency

DIAGNOSTIC TESTS & INTERPRETATION

- Cognitive testing, such as Saint Louis University Mental Status (SLUMS) and Montreal Cognitive Assessment (MoCA), provides more definitive information in terms of cognitive deficits, especially executive function, which may be lost earlier in vascular dementia.
- Neuropsychological testing may also be beneficial, especially in evaluating multiple cognitive domains and their specific involvements and deficits.

Initial Tests (lab, imaging)

As appropriate, consider complete blood count, comprehensive metabolic profile, lipid panel, thyroid function, hemoglobin A1C, and vitamin B_{12}.

- Cognitive deficits observed clinically do not always have to correlate with findings found on neuroimaging studies. White matter hyperintensities are frequently detected in patients with VCI.
- MRI is the gold standard of imaging (6).
- White matter changes and specific location of these changes can be associated with executive dysfunction and episodic memory impairment.

Follow-Up Tests & Special Considerations

Consider referral to a cognitive specialist for complex cases.

TREATMENT

Prevention is the real key to treatment:

- Control of risk factors, including HTN, hyperlipidemia, and diabetes
- Avoidance of tobacco and smoking cessation
- Healthy, low-cholesterol diet

MEDICATION

- Clinical evidence for use of acetylcholinesterase inhibitors and memantine reveals limited benefit in vascular dementia but may slow cognitive decline in patients with mixed Alzheimer and vascular dementia.
- Controlling BP with any antihypertensive medications, treatment of dyslipidemia (e.g., statins), and treatment of diabetes are very important.
- Selective serotonin reuptake inhibitors (SSRIs) may be of benefit for agitation and psychosis in vascular dementia.

ADDITIONAL THERAPIES

- Limit alcohol drink intake to $\leq$1/day in women and 2/day in men.
- Preventing new CVAs is key in managing vascular dementia; aspirin and other antiplatelet agents may be useful if no contraindications.

SURGERY/OTHER PROCEDURES

Patients with symptomatic carotid artery stenosis should be referred to a vascular surgeon to be evaluated for carotid endarterectomy. Carotid endarterectomy is recommended over carotid artery stenting in patients $>$70 years of age if perioperative morbidity/mortality are $<$6%.

COMPLEMENTARY & ALTERNATIVE MEDICINE

Ginkgo biloba should be avoided due to increased risk of bleeding, especially in CAA.

ADMISSION, INPATIENT, AND NURSING CONSIDERATIONS

- Remain sensitive to functional assessment and avoidance of pressure ulcers after CVAs.
- Avoid Foley catheter usage unless necessary due to increased risk of infection.
- Nonpharmacologic approaches to behavior management should be attempted prior to medication usage.
- Providing optimal sensory input to patients with cognitive impairment is important during hospitalizations to avoid delirium and confusion. Patients should be given frequent cues to keep them oriented to place and time. They should be informed of any changes in the daily schedule of activities and evaluations. Family and caregivers should be encouraged to be with patients with dementia as much as possible to further help them from becoming confused during hospitalization. Recreational, physical, occupational, and music therapy can be beneficial during hospitalization in avoiding delirium and preventing functional decline.
- Depression can present as "pseudodementia" with worsening confusion during hospitalization and is a treatable condition.

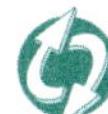

ONGOING CARE

Vascular dementia is a condition that should be followed with multiple visits in the office setting with goals of optimizing cardiovascular risk profiles for patients. Future planning and advanced directives should be addressed early. Family and caregiver evaluation and burden should also be evaluated.

FOLLOW-UP RECOMMENDATIONS

Perform regular follow-up with a primary care provider for risk factor modification and education on importance of regular physical and mental exercises as tolerated.

Patient Monitoring

Appropriate evaluation and diagnosis of this condition, need for future planning, optimizing vascular risk factors, lifestyle modification counseling, therapeutic interventions.

DIET

- The American Heart Association diet and Dietary Approaches to Stop Hypertension (DASH) diet is recommended for optimal BP and cardiovascular risk factor control.
- Low-fat, decreased concentrated sweets and carbohydrates, especially in those with metabolic syndrome

PATIENT EDUCATION

- Lifestyle modification is important in vascular risk reduction (smoking cessation, exercise counseling, dietary counseling, weight-loss counseling).
- Optimizing vascular risk factors via medications (i.e., HTN, diabetes, atrial fibrillation, PVD, heart disease)
- Avoiding smoking, including secondhand smoke
- Home BP monitoring and glucometer testing of blood sugars if HTN, impaired glucose tolerance, and/or diabetes is present
- Treat sleep apnea.

PROGNOSIS

- Vascular dementia results in shortened life expectancy and those with previous CVA have a worse prognosis.
- Lost cognitive abilities that persist after initial recovery of deficits from stroke do not usually return. Some individuals can have intermittent periods of self-reported improvement in cognitive function.
- Risk factors for progression of cognitive and functional impairment poststroke include age, prestroke cognitive abilities, depression, polypharmacy, and decreased cerebral perfusion during acute stroke.
- Unsteady or frontal gait can be a predictor for risk of development of vascular dementia.

COMPLICATIONS

- Behavioral abnormalities (delusions, hallucinations, etc.)
- Depression
- Falls
- Frequent hospitalizations
- Aspiration pneumonia
- Physical disability from stroke
- Severe cognitive impairment
- Caregiver stress and burnout

REFERENCES

1. Kalaria RN. The pathology and pathophysiology of vascular dementia. *Neuropharmacology*. 2018;134(Pt B):226–239.
2. Dichgans M, Leys D. Vascular cognitive impairment. *Circ Res*. 2017;120(3):573–591.
3. Sundbøll J, Horváth-Puhó E, Adelborg K, et al. Higher risk of vascular dementia in myocardial infarction survivors. *Circulation*. 2018;137(6):567–577.
4. White WB, Wolfson L, Wakefield DB, et al. Average daily blood pressure, not office blood pressure, is associated with progression of cerebrovascular disease and cognitive decline in older people. *Circulation*. 2011;124(21):2312–2319.
5. Montero-Odasso M, Verghese J, Beauchet O, et al. Gait and cognition: a complementary approach to understanding brain function and the risk of falling. *J Am Geriatr Soc*. 2012;60(11):2127–2136.
6. Iadecola C, Duering M, Hachinski V, et al. Vascular cognitive impairment and dementia: JACC scientific expert panel. *J Am Coll Cardiol*. 2019;73(25):3326–3344.

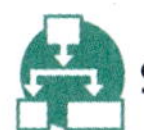

SEE ALSO

Alzheimer Disease; Depression; Mild Cognitive Impairment

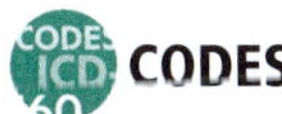

CODES

ICD10

- F01.50 Vascular dementia without behavioral disturbance
- F01.51 Vascular dementia with behavioral disturbance

CLINICAL PEARLS

- Executive dysfunction and gait abnormalities are often seen early and are more pronounced in vascular dementia as opposed to Alzheimer dementia.
- Memory is relatively preserved in vascular dementia when compared with Alzheimer dementia in the early stages of this disease.
- Stepwise progression, as opposed to progressive decline in Alzheimer dementia, is typical of multi-infarct dementia. History from a caregiver or family member is important in assessing this decline.
- Considerable overlap exists between vascular dementia and Alzheimer dementia in clinical practice, and classification into one of these categories is often difficult. Patients can have mixed etiologies as well.

DENTAL INFECTION

Bernadette Pendergraph, MD • Frances Leung, MD, MPH

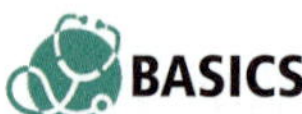

BASICS

Dental caries and periodontal disease are common dental infections.

DESCRIPTION

- Pain ± swelling in the head and neck region with odontogenic (teeth and supporting structures) origin of infection; if left untreated, can lead to serious and potentially life-threatening illnesses
- Assume any head and neck infection or swelling to be odontogenic in origin until proven otherwise.
- Antibiotics should be prescribed as an adjunct to proper dental intervention. Antibiotics should be prescribed for acute infections for 3 to 7 days.
- Gingivitis and periodontal disease may be treated with oral antibiotics. Soft tissue infections may require IV antibiotic treatment.

EPIDEMIOLOGY

~27% of Americans have untreated dental caries. 50% of children 6 to 8 years of age have dental caries and 85% of adults have at least one tooth with decay. 35% of Americans between the ages 30 and 90 years have periodontal disease. One in 2,600 hospital admissions are related to dental infection.

Incidence

- Overall incidence of dental caries in children is ~47%.
- Rates of untreated dental caries are highest in Latino and non-Latino Black individuals below the poverty line (up to 58%).

Prevalence

- Dental caries is the most common chronic disease worldwide with 2.44 billion people suffering permanent tooth decay.
- 90% of adults aged 20 to 64 years have had dental caries in their permanent teeth.

ETIOLOGY AND PATHOPHYSIOLOGY

- Caries are caused by a polymicrobial biofilm matrix (primarily *Streptococcus mutans*) that produces acid that damages the enamel, dentin, and cementum that is transmissible to household members.
- Caries progress to reversible pulpitis (intermittent pain), then irreversible pulpitis, followed by apical periodontitis (persistent tooth pain).

RISK FACTORS

- Low socioeconomic status/lack of dental insurance
- Smoking
- Household members with untreated dental caries (especially in past 12 months)
- Previous dental caries
- Gingival recession
- Poor oral hygiene; diet consisting of sugary foods and drinks, snacking without brushing; inadequate fluoride use
- Trauma to the teeth or jaw
- Physical and mental disabilities
- Poorly controlled systemic diseases (e.g., diabetes)
- Decreased salivary flow (e.g., use of anticholinergic medications, immunologic diseases, radiation therapy to head and neck, methamphetamine use)

GENERAL PREVENTION

- Most dental problems can be avoided through flossing/use of interdental brushes; brushing with fluoride toothpaste, systemic fluoride (fluoridated bottled water; fluoride supplements for high-risk patients and in nonfluoridated areas); fluoride varnish for all children age <6 years and moderate- to high-risk patients; regular dental cleanings
- Prevent transmission of *S. mutans* from mother/caregiver to infant by improving maternal dentition, chlorhexidine gluconate rinses, and use of xylitol products for mother especially during first 2 years of a child's life. Avoid smoking, which is linked to severe periodontal disease. Use of acid neutralization agents such as baking soda wiping after meals/snacks to decrease bacteria colonization.
- Good control of systemic diseases (e.g., diabetes) and changes in lifestyle (e.g., smoking cessation)
- Fluoride varnish provided by dental or medical primary care providers twice per year most cost-effective treatment for prevention of pit and fissure caries (1)[C]

COMMONLY ASSOCIATED CONDITIONS

- Extensive caries, crowding, multiple missing teeth
- Periapical and periodontal abscess
- Soft tissue cellulitis
- Periodontitis (deep inflammation ± infection of gingiva, alveolar bone support, and ligaments)

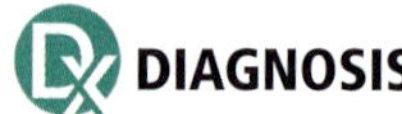

DIAGNOSIS

HISTORY

- Pain of involved tooth; may refer to ears, jaw, cheek, neck, or sinuses; unexplained headaches
- Hot/cold sensitivity
- Unprovoked, intermittent, and/or constant pain
- Pain with biting or chewing
- Trismus (inability to open mouth)
- Bleeding or purulent drainage from gingival tissues
- When severe infection (systemic): fever, difficulty breathing or swallowing, raspy voice, neck kept in flexed position, mental status changes

PHYSICAL EXAM

- Gingival edema and erythema
- Cheek (extraoral) or vestibular (intraoral) swelling
- Fluctuant mass at involved site
- Suppuration of gingival margin
- Submandibular or cervical lymphadenopathy
- Severe (systemic) infection signs include fever and airway compromise

DIFFERENTIAL DIAGNOSIS

- Bacterial or viral pharyngitis
- Pericoronitis (inflammation ± infection of gum flap over mandibular last molar, typically 3rd molars)
- Otitis media or externa; sinusitis
- Headache/migraine
- Viral (herpes simplex, herpangina, hand-foot-mouth disease) or aphthous stomatitis
- Temporomandibular joint (TMJ) dysfunction (myofascial pain, ± internal derangement of TMJ)
- Parotitis
- Retropharyngeal abscess

DIAGNOSTIC TESTS & INTERPRETATION

Initial Tests (lab, imaging)

- No initial labs needed unless patient looks acutely ill
- If acutely ill
  - Consider CBC with differential.
  - If abscess present, drain/aspirate pus and culture for aerobes and anaerobes.
- Individual films of suspected teeth, including root apices; test with palpation, percussion, and cold sensitivity.
- Panoramic film or CT scan of the teeth and jaw to evaluate the extent of infection

Follow-Up Tests & Special Considerations

- Panoramic radiograph, particularly if trismus present
- CT/MRI scan can be helpful if facial swelling extends below inferior border of mandible or into infraorbital space. This helps to locate for potential incision and drainage by oral and maxillofacial surgeon or ENT (1)[C],(2)[C].

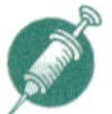

TREATMENT

- Early disease (gingivitis, periodontitis) does not typically warrant antibiotic use.
- Antibiotics should be prescribed for acute infections with local/systemic spread or when drainage/débridement is not possible.
- All antibiotics should be prescribed for the shortest duration possible, which is typically 3 to 7 days.
- Consider IV antibiotics only in the case of severe disease such as local infiltration or systemic infection.
- Appropriate pain control: anti-inflammatory agents are first line; short-course opioids in some cases
- Refer to oral health provider for definitive treatment: incision and drainage, root canal, extraction, pulpectomy, gum therapy
- If infection is severe (soft tissue infiltration, systemic symptoms), consider hospitalization with IV antibiotics until stable. It will likely require intraoral or extraoral incision and drainage; definitive treatment (extraction, pulpectomy, or root canal therapy) is necessary to prevent progression or recurrence.

GENERAL MEASURES

- NSAIDs typically provide appropriate analgesia; ibuprofen 400 mg (pediatrics: 10 mg/kg) q6h or naproxen 440 mg (pediatrics: 10mg/kg) q12h; if there is a contraindication or intolerance to NSAIDS, can use acetaminophen 650 to 1,000 mg (pediatrics: 10 to 15 mg/kg) q6–8h PRN for pain (3)[A].
- For more severe pain, consider adding acetaminophen to an NSAIDs (synergistic effect). On rare occasions, a short course of opioids may be necessary (3)[A].
- Local nerve block with long-acting anesthetic (0.5% bupivacaine plus 1:200,000 epinephrine) or local infiltration injection (0.5% bupivacaine plus 1:200,000 epinephrine or 4% articaine plus 1:100,000/1:200,000 epinephrine) may decrease need for rescue medications in the first 48 hours; avoid injecting through infection to avoid tracking infection (3)[A].

MEDICATION

First Line

- Amoxicillin: 500 mg PO TID, 1,000 mg IV BID; (pediatrics: 40 to 60 mg/kg/day PO divided q8h) *or*
- Penicillin: 500 mg PO QID, 1.2 to 2.4 million units IM/IV daily; pediatrics: 25 to 75 mg/kg/day PO divided q6–8h) *or*
- Metronidazole 500 mg PO/IV TID (penicillin allergy alternative or adjunct to above if infection is spreading); pediatrics: 30 mg/kg/day PO/IV divided q8h (2)[C]

Second Line

If no response to first-line treatment or inability to tolerate above medications

- Clindamycin 150 mg 4×/day; pediatrics: 10 to 25 mg/kg po divided q8h) *or*
- Amoxicillin/clavulanic acid: 500/125 mg PO TID or 875/125 mg PO BID, 1,000 to 2,000 mg IV TID *or*
- Clarithromycin 250 mg PO BID; pediatrics: 15 mg/kg/day po divided q12h (2)[C]

ISSUES FOR REFERRAL

Referral to oral health provider should be done in order to determine degree of infection, treat infection, and provide ongoing preventive dental cleanings and surveillance (1)[C].

SURGERY/OTHER PROCEDURES

- Incise and drain large, fluctuant abscesses.
- Root canal or extraction is definitive treatment.

ADMISSION, INPATIENT, AND NURSING CONSIDERATIONS

Criteria for hospital admission: swelling involving deep spaces of the neck, floor of the mouth, or infraorbital region; deviation of the airway; unstable vital signs; fever (>101°F); chills; raspy voice; confusion or delirium; or evidence of invasive infection (2)[C]

- Ensure secure airway.
- IV fluid resuscitation if necessary
- Initiate antibiotics as recommended above.
- Ensure good oral hygiene.
- Rinse or swab mouth with chlorhexidine gluconate BID.
- Use warm saltwater rinses several times per day, especially after incision and drainage; ice packs to decrease swelling and encourage drainage
- Discharge patient when
  - Airway not compromised
  - Abscess and sepsis eliminated
  - Able to take PO intake and ambulate

ONGOING CARE

Educate regarding proper oral hygiene, need for follow-up dental care, and potential medical complications that arise due to lack of dental care.

FOLLOW-UP RECOMMENDATIONS

- Follow up with oral health provider within 24 hours.
- Ensure adequate hydration, nutrition, and pain control (2)[C].

DIET

- Maintain a healthy diet; bacteria thrive on refined sugar and starch.
- Avoid sugary foods that stick between the teeth.
- Avoid the use of sugary/carbonated drinks throughout day; water as beverage of choice between meals

Pediatric Considerations

- Include oral health screening and exam at each well-child care visit.
- Limit frequency of sugary drinks, in-between meal snacks of sugary/sticky foods, and advise against sleeping with a bottle.
- Fluoride varnish twice a year (more for higher risk children) for children age <6 years; fluoride supplementation for children starting at 6 months of age if their primary water source is deficient in fluoride

PATIENT EDUCATION

- Control caries and periodontal disease.
- Brush at a minimum twice daily and use floss/interdental brush daily; brushing/flossing after every meal may further improve oral health. Children <2 years of age should use a smear of low fluoride toothpaste while those 2 to 5 years of age should use a pea sized amount of fluoride toothpaste.
- Fluoride supplementation is critical if primary water source is fluoride-deficient.
- Biannual dental visits at a minimum for oral care and fluoride varnish beginning when first primary tooth comes in (1)[C]
- Limit the frequency of sugar/carbonated drinks and sugary or sticky foods.
- Avoid milk, formula, or juice in bottles in children whose teeth have started to erupt; avoid sleeping with bottle.

PROGNOSIS

Prognosis is excellent with proper treatment.

COMPLICATIONS

- Ludwig angina
- Retropharyngeal and mediastinal infection
- Osteomyelitis
- Endocarditis/cardiac tamponade
- Submental or submandibular infection
- Can worse metabolic diseases including diabetes and atherosclerosis
- Brain abscess/death

REFERENCES

1. Cheng L, Zhang L, Yue L, et al. Expert consensus on dental caries management. *Int J Oral Sci*. 2022;14(1):17.
2. Jevon P, Abdelrahman A, Pigadas N. Management of odontogenic infections and sepsis: an update. *Brit Dent J*. 2020;229(6):363–370.
3. Carrasco-Labra A, Polk DE, Urquhart O, et al. Evidence-based clinical practice guidelines for the pharmacologic management of acute dental pain in adolescents, adults, and older adults: a report from the American Dental Association Science and Research Institute, the University of Pittsburgh, and the University of Pennsylvania. *J Am Dent Assoc*. 2024;155(2):102–117.e9.

ADDITIONAL READING

- Krol DM, Whelan K; and AAP Section on Oral Health. Maintaining and improving the oral health of young children. *Pediatrics*. 2023;151(1):e2022060417.
- Rajwani AR, Hawes SND, To A, et al. Effectiveness of manual toothbrushing techniques on plaque gingivitis: a systematic review. *Oral Health Prev Dent*. 2020;18(4): 843–854.
- Smiles for Life: A National Oral Health Curriculum. Society of Teachers of Family Medicine Group on Oral Health. http://www.smilesforlifeoralhealth.com/all-courses/. Accessed June 17, 2025.
- Stephens MB, Wiedemer JP, Kushner GM. Dental problems in primary care. *Am Fam Physician*. 2018;98(11):654–660.

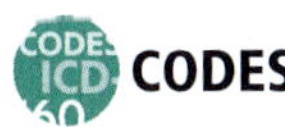

CODES

ICD10

- K02.9 Dental caries, unspecified
- K04.7 Periapical abscess without sinus
- K12.2 Cellulitis and abscess of mouth

CLINICAL PEARLS

- Dental related ED visits continue to rise, especially among the uninsured, underscoring the need for integrated oral health in primary care.
- Untreated dental infections can act as a nidus for systemic inflammation and are linked to adverse cardiovascular outcomes.
- Do not ignore tooth pain as it may be a sign of impending serious infection.
- Treat patients with local signs of soft tissue infection aggressively with an early referral to oral health professional and antibiotics as infections can spread quickly, leading to significant morbidity or even death.
- Prevention (oral hygiene, fluoride, dental visits) is the key to avoiding odontogenic infections.
- When indicated, amoxicillin and clindamycin are generally the antibiotics of choice for odontogenic infections.

DEPRESSION

Candace Ripperda, MD • Sarah Hovland, MD, MPH

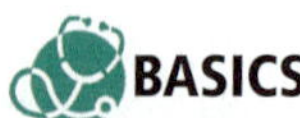

BASICS

DESCRIPTION

Primary mood disorder characterized by a sustained feeling of sadness and/or decreased interest in all or most activities once enjoyed, which represents a change from previous state

EPIDEMIOLOGY

Prevalence

- Lifetime prevalence of major depressive disorder (MDD) is 20% (1).
- Low risk before early teens; highest prevalence in teens and young adults (17% of adults 18 to 25 years old reporting a major depressive episode and 7.1% of ≥26 years old in 2020)

ETIOLOGY AND PATHOPHYSIOLOGY

Pathophysiology is poorly understood.

Genetics

Twin studies suggest 37% concordance.

RISK FACTORS

- Female > male (2:1)
- History of anxiety
- Substance abuse
- Adverse life events
- First-degree relative or spouse with depression, bipolar, suicide, substance abuse
- Presence of chronic medical conditions

GENERAL PREVENTION

Physical activity lowers risk for depression (2).

COMMONLY ASSOCIATED CONDITIONS

Bipolar disorder, cyclothymic disorder, grief reaction, anxiety disorders, somatoform disorders, schizophrenia/schizoaffective disorders, conduct disorder, substance abuse, PTSD, fibromyalgia, chronic pain, CAD, MS, diabetes, dementia

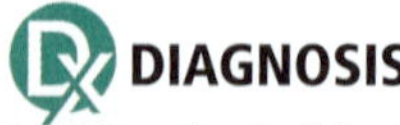

DIAGNOSIS

DSM-5 requires the following criteria for MDD (Criteria A, B, and C are met):

- Criterion A: ≥5 of the following symptoms present nearly every day during the same 2-week period, with at least 1 being either depressed mood or loss of interest or pleasure:
  - Dysphoria: subjective or observation by others of depressive mood most of the day
  - Anhedonia: decrease interest or pleasure in previously enjoyable activities most of the day either by subjective report or observation from other people
  - Notable change in appetite or unintentional significant weight loss
  - Insomnia or hypersomnia
  - Fatigue or energy loss
  - Agitation, restlessness, or slowed speech or body movements observable by others
  - Diminished thinking/concentration, poor memory
  - Worthlessness, inappropriate guilty feelings
  - Recurrent thoughts of death/harm, suicidal ideations, or suicide attempt or a devised plan for suicide
- Criterion B: Symptoms cause social, occupational, or functional distress.
- Criterion C: Symptoms are not attributable to substance effects or other medical conditions.
- Minor depression: 2 to 4 of the following symptoms of criteria A plus B and C as above and:
  - Persistent depressive disorder (dysthymia) and cyclothymic disorder not present
  - The mood disturbance does not occur exclusively during a psychotic disorder.

HISTORY

- The presence of four "SIGECAPS" symptoms plus depressed mood suggests depression.
  - Sleep: changes in sleep patterns
  - Interest: anhedonia
  - Guilt: guilt or feelings of worthlessness
  - Energy: fatigue
  - Concentration: impaired concentration
  - Appetite: changes in weight/appetite
  - Psychomotor: agitation or retardation
  - Suicidality: recurrent thoughts of death/homicidality
- Depression may present differently between genders; women may report physical ailments: headache, myalgias, GI distress; men may report aggression, substance use, risky behavior.

Pediatric Considerations

May present with somatic symptoms (headaches, GI upset), irritability, difficulty concentrating, frequent absences from school, or sudden change in grades

Geriatric Considerations

Difficult to diagnose due to medical comorbidities; may present as memory difficulties; Geriatric Depression Scale (GDS 15) improves rate of diagnosis.

PHYSICAL EXAM

Comprehensive physical and mental status examination

- Level of consciousness and orientation
- Appearance: hygiene, posture, clothing
- Attitude: hostility, apathy
- Behavior: eye contact, psychomotor agitation
- Mood: depressed, anxious, angry, tearful, etc.
- Affect: mood-congruent, flat, labile
- Memory: immediate, recent, and remote
- Speech: fluency, repetition, comprehension
- Thought content/process: delusions, hallucinations, suicidal/homicidal thoughts, flight of ideas, grandiosity, obsessions/compulsions
- Insight: understanding of own illness
- Judgment: ability to make rational decisions

DIFFERENTIAL DIAGNOSIS

- Depressed phase of bipolar disorder
- Adjustment disorder with depressed mood
- Medical comorbidity: adrenal disease, hypothyroidism, diabetes, liver or renal failure, malignancy, sleep disorders, chronic fatigue syndrome, fibromyalgia, vitamin deficiencies, anemia

DIAGNOSTIC TESTS & INTERPRETATION

- Patient Health Questionnaire-9 (PHQ-9); other tools: Beck Depression Inventory, Zung Self-Rating Depression Scale, or GDS 15
- Screen postpartum women using Edinburgh Postnatal Depression Scale (EPDS).
- Assess for suicidal/homicidal ideation; can use Columbia-Suicide Severity Rating Scale (C-SSRS)

Initial Tests (lab, imaging)

Laboratory test to exclude other conditions: compete blood count, electrolytes, kidney and liver function, thyroid-stimulating hormone, toxicology screen, vitamin levels (D, B_{12}, folate); consider pregnancy test. Rapid plasma reagin (RPR) and HIV test may be appropriate in treatment-resistant depression.

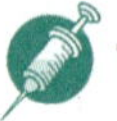

TREATMENT

- Psychotherapy and second-generation antidepressants are evidence-based first-line therapy, with similar efficacy in primary care setting (relative risk [RR] = 1.03; 95% CI, 0.88 to 1.22) (2)[A].
- Psychotherapy methods include:
  - Cognitive behavioral therapy (CBT): combines cognitive psychotherapy with behavioral therapy
  - Interpersonal psychotherapy (IPT): identifies a trigger of the depressive episode, focuses on improving relationships, social interactions, and builds social skills
  - Other therapies: psychodynamic psychotherapy, family and marital therapy, problem-solving therapy, supportive psychotherapy
- Acute phase (first 3 months of treatment):
  - Full evaluation, including risk to self and others, with selection of appropriate treatment setting
  - For mild to moderate symptoms, offer either psychotherapy or pharmacotherapy.
  - For moderate to severe symptoms, offer pharmacotherapy or combination therapy* (pharmacotherapy and psychotherapy [CBT or IPT]).
    - *May be more effective than either treatment alone for moderate to severe depression; reduces relapse rates and improves treatment adherence (2)[C]
  - Follow-up 2 to 4 weeks of starting medication
  - Increase dosage q2–4wk until remission; full effect is achieved at a given dose in 8 to 10 weeks.
  - Augmentation with a second medication warranted if response (benefit) but not remission
  - If no response at maximum tolerated FDA-approved dose to first antidepressant, switch antidepressants (and/or add psychotherapy).
- Continuation phase: Monitor for relapse.
  - Use depression rating scales and patient reports to monitor response.
  - Continue antidepressant for at least 6 to 9 months to reduce relapse once remission achieved.
  - In patients at high risk for relapse, longer courses or lifetime use may be needed.
- Discontinuation: Taper medication gradually at least over 2 weeks but may need months.
- Increased risk of relapse when an antidepressant is discontinued (2)[A]

MEDICATION

- First-line therapies are second-generation antidepressants. Selection should be guided by shared decision-making, along with provider familiarity, patient characteristics/preferences, comorbidities, known side effects, and cost (2)[C].
- Effectiveness is proven for individual medications versus placebo, but large direct head-to-head studies comparing medications is lacking. Synthesized head-to-head studies show amitriptyline, escitalopram, mirtazapine, paroxetine, venlafaxine, and vortioxetine were more effective than other antidepressants (ORs ranging between 1.19 and 1.96) (3)[A]

First Line

- Selective serotonin reuptake inhibitors (SSRIs)
  - Citalopram (Celexa): 20 to 40 mg/day; escitalopram (Lexapro): 10 to 20 mg/day (both with risk of QTc prolongation)
  - Fluoxetine (Prozac): 20 to 80 mg/day; paroxetine (Paxil): 20 to 40 mg/day or Paxil-CR 50.0 to 62.5 mg/day; avoid use of both in elderly (2).
  - Sertraline (Zoloft): 25 to 200 mg/day.
- Serotonin-norepinephrine reuptake inhibitors (SNRIs)
  - Desvenlafaxine (Pristiq): 50 to 100 mg/day; duloxetine (Cymbalta): 30 to 60 mg/day; venlafaxine XR (Effexor XR): 75 to 225 mg/day
  - Discontinuation symptoms: "Brain zap" headaches, myalgia, mood lability are common.
- Serotonin modulators
  - Vilazodone (Viibryd): 10 to 40 mg qHS (take with food); vortioxetine (Trintellix): 5 to 20 mg/day
- Adverse effects: SSRIs/SNRIs/serotonin modulators: sexual dysfunction and vivid dreams, GI upset, change in bowel movements, headache, dizziness, insomnia, weight gain
- Dopamine/norepinephrine reuptake inhibitor
  - Bupropion (Wellbutrin): 150 to 450 mg/day (lower rates of sexual dysfunction); although it does not treat anxiety like the SSRIs do, it is activating and helps with concentration (FDA approved for pediatric ADHD); less weight gain than SSRIs
  - Adverse effects: dose related increased risk of seizure, CNS stimulation, and anxiety
- Noradrenergic and specific serotonergic antidepressant
  - Mirtazapine (Remeron): 15 mg/day, 45 mg/day (max dose)(associated with weight gain, used off label for appetite stimulation)

Pregnancy Considerations

- Untreated depression has a higher incidence of preterm birth and low-birth-weight infants.
- In patients on antidepressants prior to pregnancy, a shared decision-making approach with the patient about risks/benefit of continuing medication during pregnancy should occur.
- SSRIs and psychotherapy are first line.
- Fluoxetine and sertraline have the most data in pregnancy and breastfeeding.
- Consider medication based on past treatments.
- Avoid paroxetine in pregnancy due to higher risk of cardiovascular defects in infants.
- The main concern with SSRIs and SNRIs in 3rd trimester of pregnancy is up to 1/3 of newborns experience neonatal adaptation syndrome (NAS).
  - NAS features jitteriness but can include increased crying, difficulty suckling, and rarely difficulty breathing; typically lasts 24 to 48 hours, is managed by close observation, but can last up to 2 weeks

Second Line

- Tricyclic (TCAs) antidepressants
  - Amitriptyline (Elavil): 25 to 50 mg bedtime (qHS); imipramine (Tofranil): 25 mg qHS or 150 mg/day (serotonin > norepinephrine reuptake inhibitor)
  - Desipramine (Norpramin): 25 mg/day; doxepin (Sinequan): 25 mg qHS up to 150 mg/day
  - Nortriptyline (Pamelor): 25 mg qHS; (norepinephrine > serotonin reuptake inhibitor)
  - Avoid use: arrhythmias, significant cardiac disease, seizures, osteoporosis, glaucoma
  - Common adverse effects: high risk of sedation, orthostatic hypotension, dry mouth, blurred vision, constipation, urinary retention, tachycardia, confusion/delirium, weight gain
- Other antidepressants
  - Dopamine/norepinephrine-reuptake inhibitor; *N*-Methyl-D-Aspartate (NMDA) receptor antagonist dextromethorphan/bupropion (Auvelity): 45 mg/105 mg to 90 mg/210 mg
- Augmentation/combination pharmacotherapies:
  - Can consider use of buspirone, L-thyroxine, triiodothyronine, atypical antipsychotics (especially aripiprazole and quetiapine)

ALERT

- Black box warning: increased risk of suicidality in children, adolescents, and young adults who are treated with antidepressants
- Serotonin syndrome: rare but potentially lethal complication from rapid increase in dose or addition of new medication with serotonergic effects
- Antidepressants can precipitate manic episodes in those with bipolar disorder.
- Antidepressant discontinuation syndrome: symptoms (FINISH pneumonic): flu-like symptoms, insomnia, nausea, imbalance, sensory disturbances, and hyperarousal; affects up to 50% of patients (2)

ISSUES FOR REFERRAL

Depression complicated by psychosis or treatment resistant depression

ADDITIONAL THERAPIES

Electroconvulsive therapy and ketamine for severe refractory depression; novel therapies being developed for major depression and treatment resistant depression: transcranial magnetic stimulation (TMS) therapy, and psilocybin

COMPLEMENTARY & ALTERNATIVE MEDICINE

- Exercise, good sleep hygiene, nutrition
- Full-spectrum bright light therapy
- St. John's wart

ADMISSION, INPATIENT, AND NURSING CONSIDERATIONS

Admit for risk of harm to self or others or inability to care for self.

ONGOING CARE

PATIENT EDUCATION

- Medications may take 2 to 4 weeks before beneficial effect is noted.
- Recommend exercise, good sleep hygiene, nutrition.
- Avoid alcohol, marijuana, and illicit substance use.
- The National Suicide Prevention Lifeline, 800-273-TALK (8255) or 988

PROGNOSIS

Complete remission 30% with first treatment; an additional 14.7–24.8% with switching antidepressant (1)[B]. Partial remission and remission without treatment occur commonly. Relapse risk increases with greater number of previous episodes.

REFERENCES

1. Gartlehner G, Dobrescu A, Chapman A, et al. Nonpharmacologic and pharmacologic treatments of adult patients with major depressive disorder: a systematic review and network meta-analysis for a clinical guideline by the American College of Physicians. *Ann Intern Med*. 2023;176(2):196–211.
2. Kovich H, Kim W, Quaste AM. Pharmacologic treatment of depression. *Am Fam Physician*. 2023;107(2):173–181.
3. Cipriani A, Furukawa TA, Salanti G, et al. Comparative efficacy and acceptability of 21 antidepressant drugs for the acute treatment of adults with major depressive disorder: a systematic review and network meta-analysis. *Lancet*. 2018;391(10128):1357–1366.

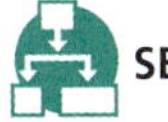

SEE ALSO

Depression, Geriatric; Depression, Pediatric; Depression, Postpartum; Depression, Treatment Resistant; Suicide; Suicide, Pediatric

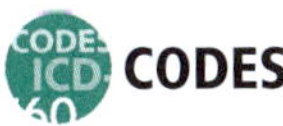

CODES

ICD10

- F32.9 Major depressive disorder, single episode, unspecified
- F33.9 Major depressive disorder, recurrent, unspecified
- F34.1 Dysthymic disorder

CLINICAL PEARLS

- Pharmacotherapy and psychotherapy, alone, can relieve depressive symptoms; however, combination therapy has higher and longer rates of improvement.
- Provide close follow-up and education for monitoring of depression.

DEPRESSION, ADOLESCENT

Janae Zolna Brill, MD, MPH

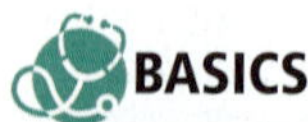

BASICS

DESCRIPTION

- Major depressive disorder (MDD) is a mood disorder characterized by sadness and/or irritable mood with impairment of functioning; abnormal psychological development; and a loss of self-worth, energy, and interest in typically pleasurable activities.
- Adolescents with depression are likely to suffer broad functional impairment across social, academic, family, and occupational domains, along with a high incidence of relapse and a high risk for substance abuse and other psychiatric comorbidity.

EPIDEMIOLOGY

- In 2022, 19.5% of US adolescents (ages 12 to 17 years) had a major depressive episode in the last year.
- The prevalence of depression in female adolescents is double that of male adolescents.

ETIOLOGY AND PATHOPHYSIOLOGY

- Early life adversities in the context of immune and brain abnormalities (blunted reward-related activity, altered volume of limbic brain regions, and white matter disruptions) are associated with increased risk of major depression.
- Neurobiologic changes (HPA axis overactivity, serotonergic modulation of emotional processing pathways, decreased dopaminergic reward processing) can contribute.
- External factors may contribute such as substance use, adverse childhood events, or inadequate social network.

Genetics

Offspring of parents with depression have 3 to 4 times increased rates of depression due to genetics as well as noninherited factors (increasing sensitivity to adversity and increasing exposure to risky environments).

RISK FACTORS

- Prior depressive episodes
- History of insomnia, anxiety disorders, attention deficit hyperactivity disorder (ADHD), high-functioning autism, early puberty in girls, chronic childhood illness, and/or learning disabilities
- Body dysmorphic disorder, dieting, and/or being overweight
- Increased screen time, particularly social media
- Female gender
- LGBTQ identified
- Substance use
- Low self-esteem, negative thinking, worry about school/grades
- Family history (having a parent or close relative with depression or bipolar)
- Academic difficulties, being bullied, witnessing violence, abuse, perceived discrimination, loss of a loved one, low socioeconomic status, poor family functioning, or low parental involvement

GENERAL PREVENTION

- Child and adolescent mental health may be improved by successfully treating maternal depression.
- Protective factors include:
  - Having positive social connections with family/peers
  - Participating in school and extracurricular activities
  - Avoiding cannabis, tobacco, and alcohol
  - Not dieting
  - Getting adequate sleep
  - Limiting social media
- The United States Preventive Services Task Force (USPSTF) recommends the screening of adolescents (12 to 18 years of age) for MDD with systems in place to ensure accurate diagnosis, appropriate treatment, and follow-up.

COMMONLY ASSOCIATED CONDITIONS

Generalized anxiety disorder, behavioral disorders, substance abuse, and eating disorders

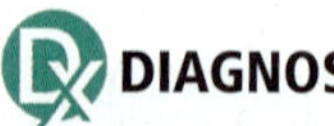

DIAGNOSIS

HISTORY

- Adolescents may present with medically unexplained somatic complaints (fatigue, irritability, headache).
- At least five symptoms have to be present with one being either a depressed mood or loss of pleasure or interest. These symptoms have to occur nearly every day during the same 2-week period.
  - Feeling sad or depressed mood
  - Loss of interest or pleasure in activities
  - Unintentional weight loss of >5% in 1 month
  - Insomnia or hypersomnia
  - Psychomotor retardation or agitation
  - Loss of energy
  - Feelings of rejection, worthlessness, or guilt
  - Decreased concentration
  - Recurrent thoughts of death, suicidal ideation or plan
- Above symptoms usually cause significant impairment in social or other areas of functioning.
- Symptoms when present should not be attributable to substance effects, medical conditions, schizophreniform, schizoaffective or delusional disorders, and no history of manic or hypomanic episodes.

PHYSICAL EXAM

Concentration, speech, affect, psychomotor activity, significant weight loss or gain, decline in personal hygiene, and other nonverbal cues may be assessed in clinical interview.

DIFFERENTIAL DIAGNOSIS

- Normal bereavement
- Substance-induced mood disorder
- Bipolar disorder
- Adjustment disorder with depressed mood
- Mood disorder secondary to a medical condition (thyroid, anemia, vitamin deficiency, diabetes)
- Mononucleosis or other viral diseases
- ADHD, posttraumatic stress disorder (PTSD), eating disorders, and anxiety disorders
- Sleep disorder

DIAGNOSTIC TESTS & INTERPRETATION

Initial Tests (lab, imaging)

May be used to rule out reversible or other underlying biologic diagnoses (consider CBC, TSH, CMP, ESR or CRP, B12, folate, mono spot, and urine drug testing)

Diagnostic Procedures/Other

- Depression is primarily diagnosed after a formal interview, with supporting information from caregivers and teachers.
- Standardized tests are useful as screening tools and to monitor response to treatment but should not be used as the sole basis for diagnosis:
  - Patient Health Questionnaire-9: modified for Teens (PHQ-A): ages 11 to 17 years
  - Beck Depression Inventory-II (BDI-II): ages ≥13 years
  - Children's Depression Inventory 2 (CDI 2): ages 7 to 17 years
- The evaluation of adolescents who screen positive for depression should include assessment of potential for harm to self and others using structured screening and interview tools, including Ask Suicide Screening or risk of suicide questionnaire.

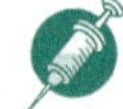

TREATMENT

GENERAL MEASURES

- Initial management should include education regarding the presentation, prognosis, and interpersonal impact of depression.
- Treatment should be considered based on the severity, duration, comorbidities, and biopsychosocial context of the depression. Consider initiating a period of active support and monitoring before prescribing formal treatment in the cases of mild depression.
- Psychological treatments for depression in adolescents show modest benefits compared to controlled conditions. However, >60% of youth receiving therapy do not respond and a small percentage (6%) deteriorate (1)[B].
- Social domains (family/school environments) can impact treatment efficacy and should therefore be incorporated into the patient's management plan (i.e., learning plans/accommodations, interpersonal family counseling).
- Patient's safety should also be addressed if there is concern for self-harm or suicidality. Assess home safety and access to weapons. Consider making a safety plan with the patient and family.
- A network meta-analysis showed that fluoxetine alone or combined with cognitive-behavioral therapy (CBT) was the most effective treatment for moderate to severe depression in adolescents (2)[A].

MEDICATION

First Line

- Fluoxetine: for depression in age >8 years; starting dose for age ≥12 years is 10 mg/day; usual effective dose 20 to 40 mg/day, max daily dose is 60 mg/day. The most studied selective serotonin reuptake inhibitors (SSRIs) and with the most favorable effectiveness and safety data has the longest half-life of the SSRIs and is not generally associated with withdrawal symptoms between doses and on discontinuation.
- Can titrate dose every 1 to 2 weeks if no significant adverse effects emerge (headaches, GI upset, insomnia, agitation, suicidal thoughts)

ALERT
SSRI black box warning to monitor for worsening condition, behavior changes, and suicidal thoughts in children, adolescents, and young adults (age <24 years).

- Closely monitor for suicidality and other adverse effects after initiating pharmacotherapy. Follow-up in 1 week is recommended.
- Given their rates of increased drug metabolism, adolescents may be at higher risk for withdrawal symptoms from SSRIs than adults; if these are present, twice-daily dosing may be considered.
- All other SSRIs except fluoxetine should be slowly tapered when discontinued.

Pediatric Considerations
- Venlafaxine was associated with an increased risk of suicidal ideation or behavior (2)[B].
- Paroxetine should be avoided due to short half-life, associated withdrawal symptoms, and higher association with suicidal ideation.
- Tricyclic antidepressants (TCAs) have not been proven to be effective in adolescents and should not be used.

Second Line
- Escitalopram: for depression in age ≥12 years; starting dose of 5 to 10 mg/day; may be increased by 5 mg every 3 weeks as needed, effective dose of 10 to 20 mg/day; considered the next preferred alternative if fluoxetine is not an option
- Sertraline: for depression in age ≥6 years; starting dose of 25 mg/day; may be increased by 12.5 to 25.0 mg every week as needed; effective dose of 50 to 200 mg/day
- Citalopram: for depression in age ≥7 years; starting dose of 10 mg/day; may be increased by 10 mg every 1 to 2 weeks as needed; effective dose of 20 to 40 mg/day; only one randomized controlled trial has shown benefit.

ISSUES FOR REFERRAL
Collaborative care interventions between mental health and primary care have a greater improvement in depressive symptoms after 12 months.

ADDITIONAL THERAPIES
- Transcranial magnetic stimulation is approved to treat adolescents ages ≥15 years with MDD. This noninvasive procedure uses magnetic fields to stimulate targeted brain regions. It is considered safe and well-tolerated, but the evidence for efficacy remains mixed.
- Treatment-resistant depression
  - Switching to another SSRI is preferred to switching drug classes (3)[A].
  - Electroconvulsive therapy (ECT) can be helpful for some adolescents with refractory depression (3)[B].
  - Ketamine infusion may be useful but currently lacks evidence (3)[C].

COMPLEMENTARY & ALTERNATIVE MEDICINE
Moderate intensity exercise shows benefit, but the study quality is low (3)[B]

ADMISSION, INPATIENT, AND NURSING CONSIDERATIONS
If severely depressed, psychotic, suicidal, or homicidal, inpatient management is indicated.

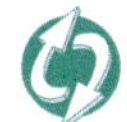 ONGOING CARE

- Antidepressant treatment should be continued for 6 to 12 months at full therapeutic dose after the resolution of symptoms at the same dosage.
- After resolution of symptoms, monitor monthly for 6 months, then regularly for the next 18 months.

FOLLOW-UP RECOMMENDATIONS
Patient Monitoring
- SSRI medications include black box warning to monitor for worsening condition, behavior changes, and suicidal thoughts.
- Systematic and regular tracking of goals and outcomes from treatment should be performed, including assessment of depressive symptoms and functioning in home, school, and peer settings.
- Diagnosis and initial treatment should be reassessed if no improvement is noted after 6 to 8 weeks of treatment.
- The goal of treatment should be sustained symptom remission and restoration of full function.

PATIENT EDUCATION
- Emphasize depression is a treatable condition.
- Explain how social media can increase feelings of isolation and depression.
- Encourage adolescents to talk to parents, guardians, teachers, or counselors about their feelings.
- Medications can be effective but need to be taken regularly, and it takes time for them to work.
- Discuss potential medication side effects including risk of suicidal thoughts and the need to report these symptoms immediately.

PROGNOSIS
- 60–90% of adolescent depressive episodes will remit within 1 year, but there is a 30–70% risk of recurrence within 5 years.
- Depression in adolescence predicts mental health disorders in adult life, substance use, psychosocial difficulties, long-term functional impairment, and chronic physical illness (including diabetes and heart disease).

COMPLICATIONS
- Treatment-induced mania, aggression, or lack of improvement in symptoms
- Poor academic performance, increased school absences, low self-esteem, and social isolation
- Risk of future mental health issues, suicidal thoughts and behaviors, eating disorders, and substance use disorders
- 1/3 of adolescents with suicidal ideation go on to make an attempt

REFERENCES

1. Cuijpers P, Karyotaki E, Ciharova M. et al. The effects of psychological treatments of depression in children and adolescents on response, reliable change, and deterioration: a systematic review and meta-analysis. *Eur Child Adolesc Psychiatry*. 2023;32(1):177–192.
2. Zhou X, Teng T, Zhang Y, et al. Comparative efficacy and acceptability of antidepressants, psychotherapies, and their combination for acute treatment of children and adolescents with depressive disorder: a systematic review and network meta-analysis. *Lancet Psychiatry*. 2020;7(7):581–601.
3. Hazell P. Updates in treatment of depression in children and adolescents. *Curr Opin Psychiatry*. 2021;34(6):593–599.

ADDITIONAL READING

- Cheung AH, Zuckerbrot RA, Jensen PS, et al; and GLAD-PC STEERING GROUP. Guidelines for Adolescent Depression in Primary Care (GLAD-PC): part II. treatment and ongoing management. *Pediatrics*. 2018;141(3):e20174082.
- Oberste M, Medele M, Javelle F, et al. Physical activity for the treatment of adolescent depression: a systematic review and meta-analysis. *Front Physiol*. 2020;11:185.
- Viswanathan M, Kennedy SM, McKeeman J, et al. *Treatment of Depression in Children and Adolescents: A Systematic Review*. Rockville, MD: Agency for Healthcare Research and Quality; 2020.

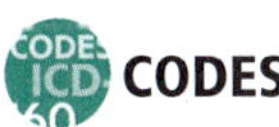 CODES

ICD10
- F32.9 Major depressive disorder, single episode, unspecified
- F33.9 Major depressive disorder, recurrent, unspecified
- F32.8 Other recurrent depressive disorders

CLINICAL PEARLS

- Adolescent depression is underdiagnosed and often presents with irritability and anhedonia.
- Use a collaborative, shared decision-making approach with adolescents and their families.
- Fluoxetine is the most studied FDA-approved for treatment of adolescent depression and is considered first-line treatment alone or combined with CBT.
- Initiate pharmacotherapy at a low dose and increase slowly to find an optimal dose and manage side effects.
- Referral to a child psychiatrist is appropriate for complex cases or treatment-resistant depression.
- Monitor for suicidality, especially during the 1st month of treatment.

D

DEPRESSION, GERIATRIC

Joseph Daniel Hogue, MD, MBA • Daniel J. Larez Solano, MD, MHA • Valencia L. Swims, MD

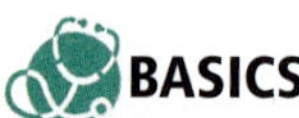

BASICS

DESCRIPTION

A primary mood disorder characterized by a depressed mood and/or a markedly decreased interest or pleasure in normally enjoyable activities most of the day, almost every day for at least 2 weeks, and causing significant distress or impairment in daily functioning. The geriatric population, typically defined as individuals aged ≥60 years, can have variable presentations and comorbid conditions that present different challenges than treating depression in the younger population.

EPIDEMIOLOGY

Incidence

- 2–5% of community-dwelling elderly
- 5–10% seen in primary care clinics
- 10–37% of hospitalized elderly patients
- 12–27% of nursing home residents

Prevalence

- The Global Burden of Disease Study (2021) estimated the prevalence of major depressive disorders among older adults (>60 years old) of 4.53% (95% uncertainty interval: 3.33 to 6.07).
- Suicide is the 11th leading cause of death in the United States for all ages. The elderly account for 24% of all completed suicides with the highest rates for males aged >85 years.

ETIOLOGY AND PATHOPHYSIOLOGY

- A complex interaction between heritable, biologic, psychological, and environmental factors
- Abnormalities in neurotrophins, neurogenesis, neuroimmune systems, and neuroendocrine systems

Genetics

Possible mechanisms, including genetic influences on monoamine transmission and associated transcriptional and translational activity and dysregulation in biologic processes and proteostasis involving C-peptide, FABP-liver, and ApoA-IV, APOE, and BDNF proteins

RISK FACTORS

- Female sex
- Lower socioeconomic status
- Widowed, divorced, or separated marital status
- Chronic physical health conditions
- History of mental health conditions
- Chronic or uncontrolled pain
- Family history of depression
- Death of a loved one
- Being a caregiver
- Functional/cognitive impairment
- Lack/loss of social support/social isolation
- Significant loss of independence
- Insomnia/sleep disturbance
- Personality traits
- Stressful life events

GENERAL PREVENTION

Limited but growing body of evidence suggest these interventions to prevent depression in the elderly:

- Following traditional dietary patterns (e.g., Mediterranean, Japanese, or Norwegian)
- Increasing the consumption of foods rich in omega-3 polyunsaturated fatty acids (e.g., salmon, tuna, sardine, mackerel)
- Engaging in regular physical activity and exercise
- Participation in social or group activities, including those focused on elderly populations

COMMONLY ASSOCIATED CONDITIONS

Chronic disease (e.g., coronary artery diseases [CAD], cerebrovascular diseases [CVD], diabetes, cancer, Parkinson disease, respiratory conditions, metabolic syndromes, cognitive impairment, sensory deficits)

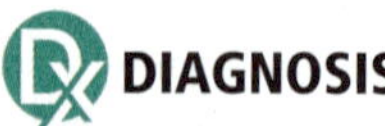

DIAGNOSIS

Refer to *Diagnostic and Statistical Manual of Mental Disorders*, 5th edition (DSM-5) criteria

HISTORY

- Depressed mood most of the day, nearly every day, and/or loss of interest/pleasure in life for at least 2 weeks
- Other common symptoms include the following:
  - Feeling hopeless, helpless, or worthless
  - Insomnia and loss of appetite/weight (alternatively, hypersomnia with increased appetite/weight in atypical depression)
  - Fatigue and loss of energy
  - Somatic symptoms (headaches, chronic pain)
  - Neglect of personal responsibility
  - Psychomotor retardation or agitation
  - Indecisiveness or diminished concentration
  - Thoughts of death or suicide
- Screening with "SIGECAPS"
  - **S**leep: changes in sleep habits from baseline, including excessive sleep, early waking, or inability to fall asleep
  - **I**nterest: loss of interest in previously enjoyable activities (anhedonia)
  - **G**uilt: excessive or inappropriate guilt that may or may not focus on a specific problem or circumstance
  - **E**nergy: perceived lack of energy
  - **C**oncentration: inability to concentrate on specific tasks
  - **A**ppetite: increase/decrease in appetite
  - **P**sychomotor: restlessness and agitation or the perception that everyday activities are too strenuous to manage
  - **S**uicidality: desire to end one's life or hurt oneself, harmful thoughts directed internally, recurrent thoughts of death or thoughts of homicide

PHYSICAL EXAM

Complete a thorough mental status examination, focused neurologic and physical examination to rule out other underlying conditions.

DIFFERENTIAL DIAGNOSIS

Concurrent medical conditions, cognitive disorders, and medications may cause symptoms that mimic depression:

- Medical conditions: hypothyroidism, vitamin B_{12} or folate deficiency, liver or renal failure, cancers, stroke, sleep disorders, electrolyte imbalances, Cushing disease, chronic fatigue syndrome
- Cognitive disorders: delirium, dementia, and other neurodegenerative disorders
- Medications: interferon-α, β_2-blockers, isotretinoin, benzodiazepines, glucocorticoids, GnRH agonists, levodopa, clonidine, H_2 blockers, baclofen, phenobarbital, topiramate, triptans, varenicline, metoclopramide, reserpine
- Other psychiatric disorders; caution should be taken to differentiate depression from bipolar disorder, as common treatments for depression (e.g., Selective serotonin reuptake inhibitors (SSRIs)) can trigger an episode of mania.

DIAGNOSTIC TESTS & INTERPRETATION

Initial Tests (lab, imaging)

Initial laboratory evaluation to rule out potential medical factors that could be causing symptoms

- Thyroid-stimulating hormone (hypothyroidism)
- CBC with differential (anemia, infection)
- Vitamin B_{12}, folic acid (deficiencies)
- Comprehensive metabolic panel
- Urine toxicology screen
- 24-hour urine free cortisol (Cushing disease)

Follow-Up Tests & Special Considerations

Additional testing for possible confounding medical disorders, as warranted (e.g., sleep study)

Diagnostic Procedures/Other

Validated screening tools and rating scales (1)[B]:

- Geriatric Depression Scale (GDS): 15- or 30-point scales
- Patient Health Questionnaire (PHQ-2 and PHQ-9)
- Hamilton Depression Rating Scale (HDRS): 17- or 21-item, clinician-administered scale
- Beck Depression Inventory (BDI): 21- or 13-item, self-report rating
- Cornell Scale for Depression in Dementia

Test Interpretation

Refer to appropriate scoring and interpretation instructions.

TREATMENT

Although 50% reduction in symptoms alone is considered clinically meaningful; the goal is to treat the patient to the point of remission (i.e., essentially the absence of depressive symptoms).

GENERAL MEASURES

- Lifestyle modifications:
  - Improve nutrition.
  - Encourage social interactions/activities.
  - Exercise and physical activity
- Psychotherapy:
  - Cognitive-behavioral therapy (CBT)
  - Psychodynamic psychotherapy

MEDICATION

Conservative initial dosing of antidepressants in the elderly, starting with 1/2 of the usual initiation dose for nonelderly adult and titrating dose every 2 to 4 weeks, as tolerated, to reach an adequate treatment dose

First Line

- SSRIs have been found to be effective in treating depression in the elderly and are considered first line for pharmacotherapy (2)[A].
- Choice of medication often reflects side effect profile or practitioner familiarity (2)[A]:
  - Citalopram: Start at 10 mg/day; treatment range is 10 to 20 mg/day.
  - Sertraline: Start at 25 mg/day; treatment range is 50 to 200 mg/day.
  - Escitalopram: Start at 5 to 10 mg/day; treatment range is 10 to 20 mg/day.

- SSRIs should not be used concomitantly with monoamine oxidase inhibitors (MAOIs).
- Common side effects: increased risk of falls, nausea, diarrhea, sexual dysfunction (2)[A]

Second Line

Atypical antidepressants: more effective than placebo in the treatment of depression in the elderly, although additional studies are needed to better delineate patient factors that determine response (2)[A]:

- Bupropion: Start at 100 to 150 mg/day for SR formulation or at 150 mg/day for XL formulation. Increase dose if appropriate in 3 to 4 days. Treatment range is from 150 to 400 mg/day for SR or 150 to 450 mg/day for XL. Avoid in patients with elevated seizure risk, tremors, anxiety, or psychosis (3)[C].
- Venlafaxine: Start at 75 mg/day XR and titrate weekly. Treatment range is 150 to 225 mg/day. Monitor for noradrenergic effects at higher doses (3)[C].
- Fluoxetine: Start at 10 mg/day; treatment range is 10 to 40 mg/day. Caution when using alongside drugs that affect cytochrome P450 (e.g., donepezil, risperidone) (3)[C].
- Paroxetine: Start at 10 mg/day; treatment range is 20 to 40 mg/day. Monitor for anticholinergic side effects (3)[C].
- Duloxetine: Start at 20 to 30 mg/day. Treatment range is from 60 to 120 mg/day; may also be associated with elevated BP; may help with chronic pain (3)[C]
- Mirtazapine: Start at 7.5 to 15.0 mg nightly. Treatment range is 15 to 45 mg/day; may be associated with dry mouth, weight gain, sedation, and cognitive dysfunction (3)[C]
- Desvenlafaxine: 50 mg/day in the morning; higher doses do not confer additional benefit; trial at 25 mg/day or at 50 mg every other day if CrCl <30 mL/min (3)[C]

ISSUES FOR REFERRAL

Depression with suicidal ideation, psychotic depression, bipolar disorder, comorbid substance abuse issues, polypharmacy, severe or refractory illness

ADDITIONAL THERAPIES

For patients who have not responded to initial SSRI trial:

- Try a different SSRI medication, switch to an atypical antidepressant, or augment initial antidepressant with bupropion.
- 2nd-generation antipsychotic agents (3)[C]:
  - Aripiprazole: Start at 2 to 5 mg/day. Treatment range is 5 to 15 mg/day; can produce sedation, weight gain
  - Used for augmentation in conjunction with other antidepressant medications
  - Note that these drugs carry a black box warning for increased risk of stroke and death in elderly with dementia.
- Tricyclic antidepressants (TCAs) (3)[C]:
  - Nortriptyline: Start at 25 mg nightly. Treatment aims for a plasma level of 50 to 150 ng/mL. Monitor for anticholinergic effects, weight gain, and increase risk of falls.
  - TCAs have been shown to be effective in treating depression. However, these are difficult for elderly patients to tolerate due to side effect profile and are potentially lethal in overdose, limiting their use as initial agents.
- MAOIs can be effective in the treatment of depression in the elderly. However, potential side effects and necessary dietary restrictions should be taken into consideration.
- Although not FDA-approved, buspirone, lithium, or triiodothyronine is used off-label to augment a primary antidepressant.
- Evidence for benefit of antidepressants in the treatment of depression in patients with dementia is equivocal. Consideration should be made for a limited trial with close monitoring for symptom improvement or side effects and used only in patients with severe symptoms.
- Electroconvulsive therapy (ECT) has been shown to produce remission of depressive symptoms in the elderly. However, due to lack of consistent evidence, it should only be considered as an option for patients with severe/psychotic depression or when there is a need for an urgent response.

COMPLEMENTARY & ALTERNATIVE MEDICINE

- St. John's wort may have minimal benefit but has many drug interactions to consider, especially with medications commonly prescribed for depression.
- Tryptophan and hydroxytryptophan: 150 to 300 mg/day; possible efficacy

ADMISSION, INPATIENT, AND NURSING CONSIDERATIONS

Inpatient care is indicated if imminent safety risk is present (e.g., acutely suicidal) or if unable to adequately care for themselves due to depression.

ONGOING CARE

FOLLOW-UP RECOMMENDATIONS

Due to the delay of benefit following the initiation of antidepressant therapy, it is necessary to ensure open communication with the patient to prevent premature discontinuation of therapy. An adequate explanation of potential side effects with instructions to call the office before discontinuing therapy is imperative.

Patient Monitoring

- A patient with severe depression who exhibits suicidality will require admission.
- Monitor for worsening anxiety symptoms or increase in suicidality especially in the week following initiation or switching of antidepressants.

DIET

Patients taking MAOIs need to avoid foods high in tyramine (i.e., certain cheeses and wines).

PATIENT EDUCATION

- Depression is a treatable illness.
- Medications need to be taken for 2 to 4 weeks before any beneficial effect is noted, and it may take 6 to 8 weeks to reach maximum efficacy.
- Depression is often a recurring illness.
- Stay active and connected with others.
- The Suicide and Crisis Lifeline is a free, national service available 24 hours a day by dialing 988.

PROGNOSIS

Estimates vary for initial clinical response and remission (between 30% and 70%).

COMPLICATIONS

- Impairment in social, occupational, or interpersonal functioning
- Difficulty performing activities of daily living and self-care
- Increase in medical services utilization and increased costs of care
- Increased risk of suicide

REFERENCES

1. Maurer DM, Raymond TJ, Davis BN. Depression: screening and diagnosis. *Am Fam Physician*. 2018;98(8):508–515.
2. Kok RM, Reynolds CF III. Management of depression in older adults: a review. *JAMA*. 2017;317(20):2114–2122.
3. Steffens DC. Treatment-resistant depression in older adults. *N Engl J Med*. 2024;390(7):630–639.

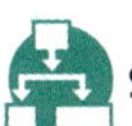

SEE ALSO

Algorithms: Depressed Mood Associated with Medical Illness; Depressive Episode, Major

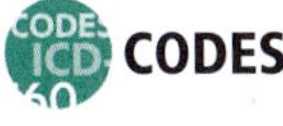

CODES

ICD10

- F32.9 Major depressive disorder, single episode, unspecified
- F03 Unspecified dementia
- F43.21 Adjustment disorder with depressed mood

CLINICAL PEARLS

- Late-life depression (LLD) is not a normal part of aging.
- Depression in the elderly may be difficult to diagnose due to medical and cognitive comorbidities.
- Depression may present primarily with cognitive dysfunction, and this may improve with treatment of the depression.
- SSRIs are considered first-line therapy. A full remission may take upward of 12 weeks of treatment.
- A multidisciplinary approach to the treatment of depression is often the most efficacious.

DEPRESSION, POSTPARTUM

Jennifer E. Cavin, MD

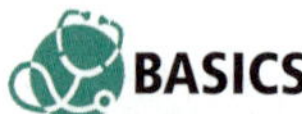

BASICS

DESCRIPTION

- Major depressive disorder (MDD) that recurs or has its onset most commonly in the early postpartum period but may occur prior to or within 12 months of delivery
- Postpartum depression (PPD) clinical manifestations are similar to nonperinatal depression (sleep disorders, anhedonia, psychomotor changes, etc.).
- Different from postpartum "blues" (sadness and emotional lability), a self-limited condition which is experienced by 30–70% of women and has an onset and resolution within first 10 days postpartum.

EPIDEMIOLOGY

Incidence

9–14% of women experience depression during the postpartum period (1).

Prevalence

>50% of women with PPD enter pregnancy depressed or have an onset during pregnancy.

ETIOLOGY AND PATHOPHYSIOLOGY

- May be related to sensitivity in hormonal fluctuations, including estrogen; progesterone; and other gonadal hormones as well as neuroactive steroids; cytokines; hypothalamic-pituitary-adrenal (HPA) axis hormones; altered fatty acid, oxytocin, and arginine vasopressin levels; and genetic and epigenetic factors
- Multifactorial including biologic-genetic predisposition in terms of neurobiologic deficit, destabilizing effects of hormone withdrawal at birth, inflammation, and psychosocial stressors

RISK FACTORS

- Previous episodes of PPD, history of MDD, or anxiety and depression during pregnancy
- History of premenstrual dysphoria
- Family history of depression
- Exposure to physical, sexual, or psychological violence (including intimate partner violence)
- Unintended or unwanted pregnancy, stressful life events, adolescent or single parenthood
- Low socioeconomic status, lack of social or financial support, lower educational attainment
- Gestational diabetes
- Complications during pregnancy or delivery, preterm birth, having a baby with a congenital abnormality
- Poor sleep quality, multiparity

GENERAL PREVENTION

- Universal screening, using validated rating scales, during pregnancy and postpartum year for better detection. Evidence suggests that screening pregnant and postpartum women for depression reduces depressive symptoms in women with depression and reduces the prevalence of depression in a given population. Evidence for pregnant women was less robust but is also consistent with the evidence for postpartum women regarding the benefits of screening, the benefits of treatment, and screening instrument accuracy (2)[A].
- Psychotherapy/counseling, particularly using cognitive behavioral therapy (CBT) and interpersonal therapy (IPT) based interventions, has been shown to be effective in small randomized trials in the prevention of PPD in at-risk individuals, but the USPSTF concludes that further research is needed (3)[A].
- Use of selective serotonin reuptake inhibitors (SSRIs), specifically sertraline, may be effective in preventing PPD in women at high risk for PPD (3)[A].

COMMONLY ASSOCIATED CONDITIONS

- Bipolar mood disorder, depressive disorder not otherwise specified, dysthymic disorder, cyclothymic disorder, MDD
- Postpartum blues

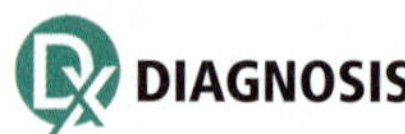

DIAGNOSIS

HISTORY

- Decreased interest in formerly compelling or pleasurable activities, depressed/low mood, guilt, low self-esteem
- Increased/decreased sleep, decreased energy, decreased concentration, increased/decreased appetite
- Psychomotor agitation or retardation, suicidal ideation

DIFFERENTIAL DIAGNOSIS

- Baby blues: not a psychiatric disorder; mood lability resolves within days
- Postpartum psychosis: a psychiatric emergency
- Postpartum anxiety/panic disorder
- Postpartum obsessive-compulsive disorder
- Hypothyroidism
- Postpartum thyroiditis: can occur in up to 5.7% of patients in the United States and can present as depression
- Bipolar disorder, depressive episode

DIAGNOSTIC TESTS & INTERPRETATION

Initial Tests (lab, imaging)

No blood testing is necessary, but selective tests based on history and symptoms might include complete blood count (CBC), thyroid-stimulating hormone (TSH), vitamin B_{12} level

Follow-Up Tests & Special Considerations

Urine analysis, urine drug screen

Diagnostic Procedures/Other

- Edinburgh Postnatal Depression Scale is a validated screening tool. A score of >11 indicates likely PPD.
- The Patient Health Questionnaire-9 (PHQ-9) is a validated commonly used screening tool.
- Edinburgh Postnatal Depression Scale (partner version): to be completed by mother's partner to obtain his or her view of mother's depression

TREATMENT

GENERAL MEASURES

- Assess for the presence of suicidal ideation.
- Assess for the presence of homicidal ideation and thoughts of harming the baby (infanticide).
- Assess for symptoms of psychosis including delusions and hallucinations.
- Suicidal ideation, homicidal ideation, or infanticide ideation may require immediate hospitalization.
- Psychotherapy is considered first-line treatment for mild depressive episodes.
- Strongly consider pharmacotherapy when symptoms of depression are moderate to severe.
- Outpatient individual psychotherapy in combination with pharmacotherapy may be beneficial.

MEDICATION

First Line

- For nonbreastfeeding women, selection of antidepressants is similar to nonpostpartum patients. Cochrane (2021) found low-certainty evidence that SSRI antidepressants may be more effective in treating postnatal depression than placebo as measured by response and remission rates (4)[A].
- SSRIs are generally safe. Paroxetine has been associated with fetal cardiac defects when used during pregnancy:
  - Sertraline (Zoloft): 50 to 200 mg/day PO, fluoxetine (Prozac): 20 to 60 mg/day PO
  - Paroxetine (Paxil): 20 to 50 mg/day; PO given at bedtime; (associated with very small increase in risk of cardiovascular defects with 1st trimester use), citalopram (Celexa): 20 to 40 mg/day PO, escitalopram (Lexapro): 10 to 20 mg/day PO
- Serotonin-norepinephrine reuptake inhibitors (SNRIs):
  - Venlafaxine (Effexor XR): 75 to 225 mg/day PO, desvenlafaxine (Pristiq): 50 to 100 mg/day PO
  - Duloxetine (Cymbalta): 60 to 120 mg/day PO
- Atypical antidepressants:
  - Bupropion (Wellbutrin): 150 to 450 mg/day PO (no sexual dysfunction, activating)
  - Mirtazapine (Remeron): 15 to 45 mg/day PO at bedtime; (increases appetite and is sedating at lower doses, no sexual dysfunction)
- Tricyclic antidepressants (TCAs), particularly nortriptyline, have been shown to be as effective as SSRIs, but are more lethal in overdose and have increased rates of unfavorable side effects; nortriptyline: 75 to 150 mg/day PO given at bedtime
- Bipolar disorder requires treatment with mood stabilizer.
- Among breastfeeding mothers: Breastfeeding should generally not preclude treatment with antidepressants.
  - SSRIs and some other antidepressants are considered a reasonable option during breastfeeding.
  - All antidepressants are excreted in breast milk but are generally compatible with lactation.
  - Sertraline has the lowest translactal passage and is considered most compatible with breastfeeding.
  - Avoid fluoxetine, citalopram, and venlafaxine due to increased translactal passage.

- Avoid bupropion due to case reports of infant seizures (5)[B].
- Start with low doses and increase slowly. Minimize polypharmacy. Attempt to maximize use of only one psychotropic medication at a time. Monitor infant for adverse side effects.
- Continuing an efficacious medication is preferred over switching antidepressants to avoid exposing the mother and infant to the risks of untreated PPD.
- Consider negative effects of untreated PPD on infant and child development.
- Discussions of the treatment options with the patient and her partner when possible. Take into account the patient's personal psychiatric history and previous response to treatment, the risks of no treatment or undertreatment, available data about the safety of medications during breastfeeding, and her individual expectations and treatment preferences.
- For further information: https://www.ncbi.nlm.nih.gov/books/NBK501922/?report=classic

Second Line

Consider switching to a different antidepressant if patient has a lack of response. Augmentation may be necessary in the setting of treatment-resistant PPD. Electroconvulsive therapy (ECT) is an option for depressed postpartum women who do not respond to antidepressant medications, have severe or psychotic symptoms, cannot tolerate antidepressant medications, are actively engaged in suicidal self-destructive behaviors, or have a previous history of response to ECT.

ISSUES FOR REFERRAL

- Obtain psychiatric consultation for patients with psychotic symptoms.
- Strongly consider immediate hospitalization if delusions or hallucinations are present.
- Hospitalization is indicated if mother's ability to care for self and/or infant is significantly compromised.

ADDITIONAL THERAPIES

- CBT and IPT are evidenced-based treatments shown to effectively treat PPD.
- Psychoeducation, listening visits (nondirective counseling), and psychodynamic psychotherapy may also improve symptoms of PPD.

SURGERY/OTHER PROCEDURES

Brexanolone was approved by the FDA in March 2019 for PPD. It is a rapidly acting steroid related to progesterone, with antidepressant effects. It is administered as a continuous IV infusion over a period of 60 hours. There is restricted access to this medication. It is only administered at sites enrolled in the Risk Evaluation and Mitigation Strategy Program, and it is very expensive (>$35,000 for a course of treatment). Consider in women with severe PPD who refuse or do not respond to ECT (5).

- Requires constant monitoring with pulse oximetry
- FDA recommends that providers monitor patient at least every 2 hours for excessive sedation and loss of consciousness.
- Side effects include dry mouth, hot flashes/flushing, diarrhea, dyspepsia, excessive sedation, loss of consciousness, dizziness.

COMPLEMENTARY & ALTERNATIVE MEDICINE

- Breastfeeding has been associated with reduced stress and improved maternal mood.
- Infant massage, infant sleep intervention, exercise, and bright light therapy may be beneficial.

ADMISSION, INPATIENT, AND NURSING CONSIDERATIONS

ALERT

Obtain psychiatric consultation for patients with refractory depression or psychotic symptoms. If delusions or hallucinations are present, strongly consider immediate hospitalization. The psychotic mother should *not* be left alone with the baby.

- Admission criteria/initial stabilization: presence of suicidal or homicidal ideation and/or psychotic symptoms and/or thoughts of harming baby and/or inability to care for self or infant, severe weight loss
- Discharge criteria: Absence of suicidal or homicidal ideation and/or psychotic symptoms and/or thoughts of harming the baby, mother must be able to care for self and infant.

 ONGOING CARE

FOLLOW-UP RECOMMENDATIONS

Patient Monitoring

- Collaborative care approach, including primary care visits and case manager follow-ups
- Consultation with the infant's doctor, particularly if the mother is breastfeeding while taking psychotropic medications

DIET

- Good nutrition and hydration, especially when breastfeeding
- Mixed evidence to support the addition of multivitamins with minerals and omega-3 fatty acids

PATIENT EDUCATION

- *This Isn't What I Expected: Overcoming Postpartum Depression* by Karen R. Kleiman and Valerie Davis Raskin
- Web resources: Postpartum Support International: https://www.postpartum.net/, La Leche League International: https://www.llli.org/, MGH Center for Women's Mental Health: https://www.womensmentalhealth.org/

PROGNOSIS

- Treatment of maternal depression to remission has been shown to have a positive impact on children's mental health.
- Some patients, particularly those with undertreated or undiagnosed depression, may develop chronic depression requiring long-term treatment.
- Untreated maternal depression is linked to impaired mother–infant bonding and cognitive and language development delay in infants and children.
- Postpartum psychosis is associated with tragic outcomes such as maternal suicide and infanticide.

COMPLICATIONS

- Suicide, self-injurious behavior, psychosis
- Neglect of baby, harm to the baby
- Preterm and low-birth-weight baby

REFERENCES

1. Liu X, Wang S, Wang G. Prevalence and risk factors of postpartum depression in women: a systematic review and meta-analysis. *J Clin Nurs*. 2022;31(19–20):2665–2677. doi:10.1111/jocn.16121.
2. O'Connor E, Rossom RC, Henninger M, et al. Primary care screening for and treatment of depression in pregnant and postpartum women: evidence report and systematic review for the US Preventive Services Task Force. *JAMA*. 2016;315(4):388–406.
3. O'Connor E, Senger CA, Henninger ML, et al. Interventions to prevent perinatal depression: evidence report and systematic review for the US Preventive Services Task Force. *JAMA*. 2019;321(6):588–601.
4. Brown JVE, Wilson CA, Ayre K, et al. Antidepressant treatment for postnatal depression. *Cochrane Database Syst Rev*. 2021;2(2):CD013560.
5. Leader LD, O'Connell M, VandenBerg A. Brexanolone for postpartum depression: clinical evidence and practical considerations. *Pharmacotherapy*. 2019;39(11):1105–1112.

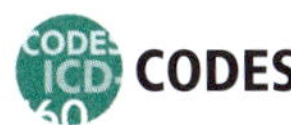 CODES

ICD10

- F53 Puerperal psychosis
- O90.6 Postpartum mood disturbance

CLINICAL PEARLS

- Universal screening for depression is recommended during the 1st and 3rd trimester and at regular intervals during the postpartum period.
- Early diagnosis and treatment are vital, as untreated PPD can lead to developmental difficulties for the infant and prolonged disability and suffering for the mother.
- Psychotherapy may be an effective monotherapy for mild to moderate depressive systems. In severe PPD, use of medications is strongly urged.
- Antidepressant treatment is safe during pregnancy and breastfeeding, and treatment should be individualized for each mom.

D

DEPRESSION, TREATMENT RESISTANT

Joseph Daniel Hogue, MD, MBA • Chad M. Ross, MD • Nadir Ebrahim, MD, MBA

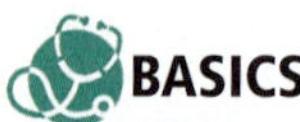

BASICS

DESCRIPTION

- Major depressive disorder (MDD) that has been unresponsive to treatment with at least ≥2 different classes of antidepressants is considered to be "treatment resistant."
- Individual antidepressants must be given for 6 to 8 weeks at standard doses before being considered a failure.

EPIDEMIOLOGY

- Depression affects >16 million people in the United States and >350 million people worldwide
- The average adult has a 16% lifetime risk of MDD, with majority experiencing onset before the age of 30 years.
- Approximately 1/3 of patients with MDD will develop treatment-resistant depression.

ETIOLOGY AND PATHOPHYSIOLOGY

Unclear; low levels of neurotransmitters (serotonin, norepinephrine, dopamine, and γ-aminobutyric acid [GABA]) have been indicated.

- Serotonin has been linked to irritability, hostility, and suicidal ideation.
- Norepinephrine has been linked to low energy.
- Dopamine may play a role in low motivation and depression with psychotic features.
- GABA can help with feelings of anxiety, stress, and fear.
- Growing evidence suggest that proinflammatory cytokine release in the brain has been linked to early uptake of serotonin, decrease dopamine release, and decrease effectiveness of SSRIs.

Genetics

A genetic abnormality in the serotonin transporter gene (5-HTTLPR) may increase risk for treatment-resistant depression.

RISK FACTORS

- Suicidal thoughts and behavior, severity of disease
- Early age of onset of major depression (<18 years of age)
- Recurrent depressive episodes
- Mislabeling bipolar patients as depressed
- Comorbid medical disease and chronic pain
- Comorbid personality, anxiety, and substance use disorder
- Adverse life events (childhood trauma or abuse, marital problems)
- Genetic familial predisposition to poor response to antidepressants
- Loss of employment and low socioeconomic status

GENERAL PREVENTION

- Medication adherence
- Maintenance electroconvulsive therapy (ECT) may prevent relapse.
- Adhering to psychotherapy

COMMONLY ASSOCIATED CONDITIONS

- Suicide
- Bipolar disorder, dysthymia, anxiety
- Substance use disorders
- Eating disorders
- Somatic symptom disorders

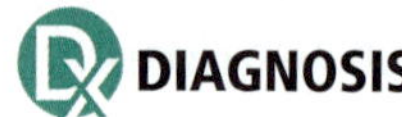

DIAGNOSIS

HISTORY

- Symptoms are the same as in MDD. However, patients do not respond to standard form of treatment.
- Important to screen for suicidality in treatment-resistant depression
- Screening with SIGECAPS
  - Sleep: too much or too little
  - Interest: inability to enjoy activities
  - Guilt: excessive and uncontrollable
  - Energy: poor
  - Concentration: inability to focus on tasks
  - Appetite: too much or too little
  - Psychomotor changes: restlessness/agitation or slowing/lethargy noted by others
  - Suicidality: desire to end life or feeling hopeless

PHYSICAL EXAM

Mental status exam may reveal poor hygiene, limited eye contact, poor relatedness, restricted affect, tearfulness, weight loss or gain, psychomotor retardation or agitation, and suicidal thoughts.

DIFFERENTIAL DIAGNOSIS

- Bipolar or personality disorder
- Persistent depressive disorder
- Posttraumatic stress disorder
- Dementia
- Early-stage Parkinson disease
- Medical illness such as malignancy, thyroid disease, HIV, anemia
- Substance use disorders

DIAGNOSTIC TESTS & INTERPRETATION

Initial Tests (lab, imaging)

Used to rule out medical factors that could be causing/contributing to treatment resistance

- CBC, complete metabolic profile
- Urine drug screen
- Thyroid-stimulating hormone (TSH)
- 25-OH vitamin D, Vitamin B_{12}, folate
- Urinalysis
- FSH, LH, HCG, testosterone, if applicable
- CT or MRI of the brain if neurologic disease, tumor, or dementia is suspected.

Follow-Up Tests & Special Considerations

Delirium and dementia often look like depression.

Diagnostic Procedures/Other

Depression is a clinical diagnosis and other diagnosis such as bipolar depression and dysthymic disorder should be ruled out. Use validated depression rating scales to assist:

- Beck Depression Inventory
- Hamilton Depression Rating Scale
- Patient Health Questionnaire 9 (PHQ-9)
- Edinburgh Postnatal Depression Scale if pregnant or postpartum

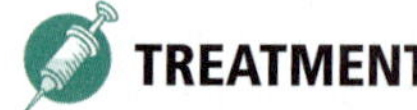

TREATMENT

MEDICATION

First Line

Please see "Depression" topic. When those fail, augmentation and combination strategies are as follows:

- Antidepressants in combination
  - Citalopram (start 20 mg/day; max dose 40 mg/day) + bupropion (start 100 mg BID; max dose 450 mg total) (1),(2)[B]
  - Tricyclic antidepressants (TCAs) and selective serotonin reuptake inhibitors (SSRIs) may be used in combination. Proceed with caution due to risk of serotonin syndrome; citalopram (start 20 mg/day; max dose 40 mg/day) + nortriptyline (start 25 mg at bedtime; max dose 150 mg at bedtime)
  - Serotonin and norepinephrine reuptake inhibitors (SNRI) and noradrenergic and specific serotonergic antidepressant (NaSSA) may also be used in combination, such as venlafaxine extended release (start 75 mg/day; max dose 225 mg/day) and mirtazapine (start 15 mg/day; max dose 45 mg/day).
- Antidepressants + antipsychotics
  - Citalopram (start 20 mg/day; max dose 40 mg/day) + aripiprazole (start 2 mg/day; up to 20 mg/day, different mechanism of action at higher doses) *or* + risperidone (start 0.5 to 1.0 mg at bedtime; max dose 6 mg/day) *or* + quetiapine (start 50 mg at bedtime; titrate to 100 to 300 mg at bedtime; max dose 600 mg/day) (1)[A],(2)
  - Olanzapine/fluoxetine combination (start 3 mg/25 mg to 12 mg/50 mg at bedtime) (1)[A],(2)
- Antidepressant + lithium
  - TCA: nortriptyline (start 25 mg at bedtime; max dose 150 mg at bedtime) + lithium (start 300 mg at bedtime; max dose 900 mg BID)
  - SSRI: citalopram (start 20 mg/day; max dose 40 mg QD) + lithium (start 300 mg at bedtime; max dose 900 mg BID) (1)[A],(2)
- In all combinations, citalopram (Celexa) can be replaced with other SSRIs such as fluoxetine (Prozac) 20 to 80 mg/day, sertraline (Zoloft) 50 to 200 mg/day, and escitalopram (Lexapro) 10 to 20 mg/day, vortioxetine (Trintellix) 5 to 20 mg/day or with SNRIs duloxetine (Cymbalta) 30 to 120 mg/day, venlafaxine XR (Effexor XR) 75 to 225 mg/day, or desvenlafaxine (Pristiq) 50 to 100 mg/day, or with a noradrenergic and specific serotonergic antidepressant (NaSSA) mirtazapine (Remeron) 15 to 45 mg at bedtime.

- Maximum doses for medication in treatment-resistant cases may be higher than in treatment-responsive cases.

Second Line

- Citalopram (start 20 mg/day; max dose 40 mg/day) + triiodothyronine (T3) (12.5 to 50 μg/day) (1),(2)[B]
- Citalopram (start 20 mg/day; max dose 40 mg/day) + buspirone (start 7.5 mg BID; max dose 30 mg BID) (1)[B],(2)
- Citalopram (start 20 mg/day; max dose 40 mg/day) + lisdexamfetamine (Vyvanse) (20 to 50 mg every morning) (1)[B],(2)
- Antidepressant in combination with therapy, particularly, cognitive-behavioral therapy (CBT) (3)[A]
- Monoamine oxidase inhibitor (MAOI)
  - Tranylcypromine (Parnate): Start 10 mg BID and increase 10 mg/day every 1 to 3 weeks; max dose 60 mg/day
  - Selegiline transdermal (Emsam patch): Apply 6 mg patch daily and increase 3 mg/day; max dose 12 mg/day
  - Side-effect profile (e.g., hypertensive crisis), drug-drug interactions, and dietary restrictions make MAOIs less appealing. Patch version does not require dietary restrictions at lower doses.
  - High risk of serotonin syndrome if combined with another antidepressant; 2-week washout period is advised.

ISSUES FOR REFERRAL

Psychiatric consultation recommended

ADDITIONAL THERAPIES

- First line
  - ECT: brief administration of electrical stimulation to the brain via superficial electrode placement
    - Safe and cost-effective option for treatment-resistant and life-threatening depression, with a 66.6% response rate (4)[A]
    - Known to rapidly relieve suicidality, psychotic depression, and catatonia
    - Cognitive side effects during treatment can occur but are more likely with bilateral lead placement.
- Second line
  - Deep brain stimulation (DBS): surgical implantation of intracranial electrodes, connected to an impulse generator implanted in the chest wall:
    - Reserved for those who have failed medications, psychotherapy, and ECT
    - Preliminary data is promising, showing 40–70% response rate and 35% remission rate. Further trials are being done.
  - Transcranial magnetic stimulation (TMS): noninvasive brain stimulation technique that is generally safe
    - Currently, only FDA-approved for less severe forms of the illness
  - Vagus nerve stimulation (VNS): surgical implantation of electrodes onto left vagus nerve
    - Use has become limited in recent years.
  - Ketamine (0.5 mg/kg single-dose infusion over 40 minutes): Studies show evidence of rapid improvement in mood and suicidal thinking. Currently, used off-label for treatment resistant depression (2)[B],(4). Esketamine, an intranasal spray, in conjunction with an oral antidepressant, has been FDA-approved for treatment-resistant depression. Dosing is 28 mg, 56 mg, or 84 mg twice a week for 1 to 4 weeks, followed by taper and/or maintenance treatment.
    - The effects of ketamine and esketamine appear temporary, usually lasting days to weeks (5). Continued studies are focusing on dosing and frequency of administration to maintain longer lasting response and remission.
  - Stanford Neuromodulation Therapy (SNT) (under investigation):
    - SNT: new TMS technique in which patients get 10 sessions daily of high-dose TMS for 5 consecutive days
    - 79% remission rate with SNT (n = 14) versus 13% remission rate with sham (n = 15)
  - Psilocybin (under investigation):
    - Psilocybin: psychedelic compound isolated from species of psilocybe mushrooms
    - 32.9% response rate and 26.6% remission rate at week 12 after a single dose of 25 mg psilocybin (n = 79).
    - 58% response rate up to 3 months after 2 doses, an initial low dose and a subsequent high dose of 25 mg psilocybin (n = 12).
  - Cytokine inhibitors/monoclonal antibody therapy (under investigation) (6)
    - Meta-analysis study in 2018 including 2370 participates suggested use of etanercept and infliximab had significant antidepressant qualifies
    - Another 2024 meta-analysis including 28 RCTs and 3,394 participates showed promising antidepressant effects of some NSAIDs such as celecoxib.

ADMISSION, INPATIENT, AND NURSING CONSIDERATIONS

- Inpatient care is indicated for severely depressed, psychotic, catatonic, or suicidal patients.
- Discharge criteria: symptoms improving, no longer suicidal, psychosocial stressors addressed

ONGOING CARE

FOLLOW-UP RECOMMENDATIONS

- Frequent visits (i.e., every month)
- During follow-up, evaluate side effects, dosage, and effectiveness of medication as well as need for referral to ECT or ketamine/esketamine treatment.
- Patients who have responded to ECT or ketamine/esketamine treatment may need maintenance treatments (q2–12 wk) to prevent relapse.
- Combination of lithium/nortriptyline after ECT appears to be as effective as maintenance ECT in reducing relapse.

DIET

Patients on MAOIs need dietary restriction of foods rich in tyramine.

PATIENT EDUCATION

- Educate patients that depression is a medical illness, not a character defect.
- Review signs and symptoms of worsening depression and when patient needs to come in for further evaluation.
- Discuss safety plan to address suicidal thoughts.

PROGNOSIS

With medication adherence, close follow-up, improved social support, and psychotherapy, prognosis improves.

COMPLICATIONS

- Suicide
- Disability
- Poor quality of life

REFERENCES

1. McIntyre RS, Filteau MJ, Martin L, et al. Treatment-resistant depression: definitions, review of the evidence, and algorithmic approach. *J Affect Disord*. 2014;156:1–7.
2. Taylor RW, Marwood L, Oprea E, et al. Pharmacological augmentation in unipolar depression: a guide to the guidelines. *Int J Neuropsychopharmacol*. 2020;23(9):587–625.
3. Wiles NJ, Thomas L, Turner N, et al. Long-term effectiveness and cost-effectiveness of cognitive behavioural therapy as an adjunct to pharmacotherapy for treatment-resistant depression in primary care: follow-up of the CoBalT randomised controlled trial. *Lancet Psychiatry*. 2016;3(2):137–144.
4. Ross EL, Zivin K, Maixner DF. Cost-effectiveness of electroconvulsive therapy vs pharmacotherapy/psychotherapy for treatment-resistant depression in the United States. *JAMA Psychiatry*. 2018;75(7):713–722.
5. Sanacora G, Frye MA, McDonald W, et al. A consensus statement on the use of ketamine in the treatment of mood disorders. *JAMA Psychiatry*. 2017;74(4):399–405.
6. Kajumba MM, Kakooza-Mwesige A, Naksujja N, et al. Treatment-resistant depression: molecular mechanisms and management. *Mol Biomed*. 2024;5(1):43. doi:10.1186/s43556-024-00205-y

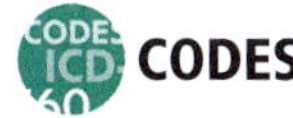

CODES

ICD10

- F32.9 Major depressive disorder, single episode, unspecified
- F33.9 Major depressive disorder, recurrent, unspecified

CLINICAL PEARLS

- Treatment-resistant depression is common, affecting 1/3 of those with MDD.
- Combination and augmentation strategies with antidepressants, antipsychotics, therapy, and mood stabilizers can be helpful.
- ECT and ketamine/esketamine should be considered in severe and life-threatening cases. DBS, TNS, and psilocybin are still experimental but showing excellent promise.

DERMATITIS HERPETIFORMIS

Nicholas Kidd, MD

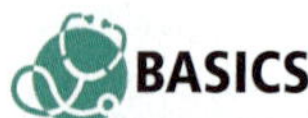

BASICS

DESCRIPTION

- Dermatitis herpetiformis (DH) is an autoimmune disease that presents as a chronic, relapsing, polymorphous, intensely pruritic, erythematous papulovesicular eruption with symmetrical distribution primarily involving extensor skin surfaces of the elbows, knees, buttocks, back, and scalp.
- DH is associated with autoimmune diseases, especially celiac disease, in addition to gluten sensitivity with genetic, environmental, and immunologic influences.
- DH is distinguished from other bullous diseases by characteristic histologic and immunologic findings as well as associated gluten-sensitive enteropathy (GSE).
- System(s) affected: skin
- Synonym(s): Duhring disease, Duhring-Brocq disease

EPIDEMIOLOGY

- Occurs most frequently in those of Northern European origin
- Rare in persons of Asian or African American origin
- Predominant age: most common in the 4th and 5th decades of life but may present at any age
- Slight male predominance, in comparison to celiac disease which is female dominant
- >90% have evidence of GSE, whereas only 20% are symptomatic of celiac disease (1).

Incidence

As high as 3.5/100,000 people per year

Prevalence

As high as 75/100,000 people (2)

ETIOLOGY AND PATHOPHYSIOLOGY

- Evidence suggests that epidermal transglutaminase (eTG) 3, is the autoantigen in DH. eTG is highly homologous with tissue transglutaminase (tTG), which is the antigenic target in celiac disease and GSE.
- The initiating event for DH is presumed to be the interaction of wheat peptides with tTGs, which results in the formation of an autoantigen with high affinity for particular class II major histocompatibility complex (MHC) molecules. Presentation of the autoantigen leads to activation of T cells and the humoral immune system.
- IgA antibodies against tTG cross-react with eTG and result in IgA-eTG immune complexes that are deposited in the papillary dermis. Subsequent activation of complement and recruitment of neutrophils to the area result in inflammation and microabscesses. Skin eruption may be delayed up to 5 to 6 weeks after exposure to gluten.
- Gluten applied directly to the skin does not result in eruption, whereas gluten taken by mouth or rectum does. This implies necessary processing by the GI system; thought to be immune complex-mediated disease.

Genetics

- High association with human leukocyte antigen (HLA)-DQ2 (95%), with remaining patients being positive for DQ8, DR4, or DR3 (1)
- Strong association with a combination of alleles DQA1*0501 and DQB1*0201/0202, DRB1*03 and DRB1*05/07, *or* DQA1*0301 and DQB1*0302 (3)

RISK FACTORS

- GSE: >90% of those with DH will have GSE, which may be asymptomatic (1),(4).
- Family history of DH or celiac disease

GENERAL PREVENTION

A gluten-free diet (GFD) results in the improvement of DH and reduces dependence on medical therapy. GFD also may reduce the risk of lymphomas associated with DH.

COMMONLY ASSOCIATED CONDITIONS

- Hypothyroidism, hyperthyroidism, thyroid nodules, thyroid cancer
- Celiac disease, GSE, gluten ataxia
- Gastric atrophy, hypochlorhydria, pernicious anemia
- GI lymphoma, non-Hodgkin lymphoma
- IgA nephropathy
- Autoimmune disorders, including systemic lupus erythematosus, dermatomyositis, Sjögren syndrome, rheumatoid arthritis, sarcoidosis, Raynaud phenomenon, insulin-dependent diabetes mellitus, myasthenia gravis, Addison disease, vitiligo, alopecia areata, primary biliary cirrhosis, and psoriasis

DIAGNOSIS

Diagnosis of DH involves a clinicopathologic correlation between clinical presentation, histologic and direct immunofluorescence (DIF) evaluation, serology, and response to therapy or dietary restriction (3),(4).

HISTORY

Waxing and waning, intensely pruritic eruption with papules and tiny vesicles; eruption may worsen with gluten intake. GI symptoms may be absent or may not be reported until prompted.

PHYSICAL EXAM

- The classic lesions of DH are described as symmetric, grouped, erythematous papules, and vesicles. Isolated vesicles are rarely seen due to intense itching.
- More commonly presents with erosions, excoriations, lichenification, hypopigmentation, and/or hyperpigmentation secondary to scratching and healing of old lesions
- Areas involved include extensor surfaces of elbows (90%), knees (30%), shoulders, buttocks, and sacrum. The scalp is also frequently affected. Oral lesions are rare.
- In children, purpura may be visible on digits and palmoplantar surfaces.
- Adults with associated enteropathy are most often asymptomatic, with about 20% experiencing steatorrhea and <10% with findings of bloating, diarrhea, or malabsorption. Children with associated enteropathy may present with abdominal pain, diarrhea, iron deficiency, and reduced growth rate.

DIFFERENTIAL DIAGNOSIS

- In adults
  - Bullous pemphigoid: linear deposition of C3 and IgG at the basement membrane zone
  - Linear IgA disease: homogeneous and linear deposition of IgA at the basement membrane zone, absence of GSE
  - Prurigo nodularis
  - Urticaria: wheals, angioedema, dermal edema
  - Erythema multiforme
- In children
  - Atopic dermatitis: face and flexural areas
  - Scabies: interdigital areas, axillae, genital region
  - Papular urticaria: dermal edema
  - Impetigo

DIAGNOSTIC TESTS & INTERPRETATION

Initial Tests (lab, imaging)

- Serum IgA tTG antibodies: Detection of tTG antibodies was noted to be up to 95% sensitive and >90% specific for DH in patients on unrestricted diets (3),(4).
- Serum IgA eTG antibodies: Antibodies to eTG, the primary autoantigen in DH, were shown to be more sensitive than antibodies to tTG in the diagnosis of patients with DH on unrestricted diets (95% vs. 79%) but are not widely available in all labs (3),(4).
- Serum IgA endomysial antibodies (EMA): Antibodies to EMA have a sensitivity between 50% and 100% and a specificity close to 100% in patients on unrestricted diets but are more expensive, time-consuming, and operator-dependent than tTG (3),(4).

Follow-Up Tests & Special Considerations

- Serologic assessment of anti-tTG and anti-eTG correlate with intestinal involvement of disease and in conjunction with anti-EMA may be useful in monitoring major deviations from GFD.
- Genetic testing for haplotypes HLA-DQ2 and HLA-DQ8 can also be offered to patients to determine genetic susceptibility, to screen patients with a high risk of CD, or if the diagnosis is not clear (3),(4).

Diagnostic Procedures/Other

- The gold standard test to establish a diagnosis of DH is DIF of the perilesional skin that demonstrate characteristic granular IgA deposits in dermal papillae and/or basement membrane. It is this key diagnostic feature that differentiates this blistering skin condition from all other dermatologic diseases (3),(4).
- DIF has a sensitivity and specificity of close to 100%. In patients with high suspicion for DH with a negative DIF, another perilesional skin biopsy should be obtained from a different site. Histopathology of these lesions with routine staining reveals neutrophilic microabscesses in the tips of the dermal papillae and may show subepidermal blistering.

TREATMENT

GENERAL MEASURES

GFD is the mainstay of treatment in DH and can lead to the complete resolution of symptoms (3),(4). Typically, requires 18 to 24 months of strict adherence to GFD prior to the resolution of skin lesions without any additional treatment. Lesions can recur within 12 weeks of reintroduction of gluten. Once prolonged remission has been obtained, some gluten may be tolerated in a subset of patients to build tolerance with immunologic response modification.

MEDICATION

Dapsone, sulfapyridine, and topical steroids are useful for immediate symptom management but should only be used as an adjunct to dietary modification.

First Line

- Dapsone, a sulfone, is a widely used FDA-approved medication.
- Initial dosing of 25 to 50 mg/day on a strict GFD typically results in improvement of symptoms within 24 to 72 hours (2).
- It is recommended to use a minimum effective dose with slow titration based on the patient's response and tolerability. The average maintenance dose is 1 mg/kg/day (50 to 150 mg/day) and can be increased up to 200 mg to obtain better symptom control (3).
- Minor outbreaks on the face and scalp are common even with treatment; not ideal for long-term use in DH
- Dapsone works by inhibiting neutrophil recruitment and IL-8 release, inhibiting the respiratory burst of neutrophils, and protecting cells from neutrophil-mediated injury, thereby suppressing the skin reaction. It has no role in preventing IgA deposition or mitigating the enteropathy (3).
- Precautions: See product labeling.
  - Common side effects include nausea, vomiting, headache, dizziness, weakness, and hemolysis.
  - A drop in hemoglobin of 1 to 2 g is characteristic with dapsone 100 mg/day.

ALERT

Monitor for potentially fatal dapsone-induced sulfone syndrome: fever, jaundice and hepatic necrosis, exfoliative dermatitis, lymphadenopathy, methemoglobinemia, and hemolytic anemia. Patients with glucose-6-phosphate dehydrogenase deficiency are at high risk for hemolytic anemia.

Pediatric Considerations

- <2 years: Dosing is not established.
- >2 years: 0.5 to 1.0 mg/kg/day

Pregnancy Considerations

- Category C: Safety during pregnancy is not established.
- Secreted in breast milk and will produce hemolytic anemia in infants
- Adherence to a strict GFD 6 to 12 months before conception should be considered with the hope of eliminating the need for dapsone during pregnancy due to its side effects profile (3).

Second Line

- High-potency topical steroids can be used acutely to control symptoms until dapsone becomes effective (3).
- The sulfonamides sulfapyridine (1 to 2 g/day) and sulfasalazine (2 to 4 g/day) are FDA-approved for use in DH. Common side effects include nausea, vomiting, and anorexia. The enteric-coated form may reduce side effects. Other side effects include agranulocytosis, hypersensitivity reactions, hemolytic anemia, proteinuria, and crystalluria (3).
- Topical steroids and 3rd-generation antihistamines can be used to provide relief from symptoms of pruritus and itching.
- Other medication such as rituximab or JAK inhibitors such as tofacitinib may improve DH (2).

ISSUES FOR REFERRAL

Over time, the management of DH warrants an interdisciplinary treatment that includes providing a referral to a dermatologist, gastroenterologist, and registered dietitian.

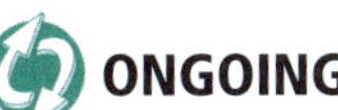

ONGOING CARE

FOLLOW-UP RECOMMENDATIONS

Patient Monitoring

- Every 6 to 12 months by a physician and a dietitian to evaluate GFD adherence and recurrence of symptoms
- Adherence to GFD can be monitored with serologic levels of anti-tTG, anti-eTG, and EMA levels.
- Patients on dapsone require lab monitoring weekly for the 1st month, biweekly for 2 months, and then every 3 months for the duration of medication use (3).

DIET

- Grains that should be avoided: wheat (including spelt, Kamut, semolina, and triticale), rye, and barley (including malt)
- Safe grains (gluten-free): rice, amaranth, buckwheat, corn, millet, quinoa, sorghum, teff (an Ethiopian cereal grain), and oats
- Care should be taken to avoid gluten-free grains that are contaminated with sources of gluten during processing such as oats.
- Sources of gluten-free starches that can be used as flour alternatives
  - Cereal grains: amaranth, buckwheat, corn, millet, quinoa, sorghum, teff, rice (white, brown, wild, basmati, jasmine), and Montina
  - Tubers: arrowroot, jicama, taro, potato, and tapioca
  - Legumes: chickpeas, lentils, kidney beans, navy beans, pea beans, peanuts, and soybeans
  - Nuts: almonds, walnuts, pistachios, chestnuts, hazelnuts, and cashews
  - Seeds: sunflower, flax, and pumpkin

PATIENT EDUCATION

- Although adherence to a GFD results in rapid improvement in GI symptoms, DH is slow to improve and in some cases may take more than a year (2).
- Patients started on dapsone should be made aware of potential hemolytic anemia and the signs associated with methemoglobinemia (3).
- The University of Chicago Celiac Disease Center: https://www.celiacdisease.net or http://www.cureceliacdisease.org/
- Gluten Intolerance Group of North America: https://www.gluten.org/
- Commercial source for gluten-free products: https://www.glutenfreemall.com

PROGNOSIS

- DH is a chronic disease with an excellent prognosis, provided strict adherence to a GFD which is the most sustainable method of eliminating cutaneous and GI disease.
- 10- to 15-year survival rates do not seem to differ from general population.
- Remission rates of 10–15%
- Skin disease responds readily to dapsone. Occasional new lesions (2 to 3 per week) are to be expected and are not an indication for altering the daily dosage (3).
- The risk of lymphoma may be decreased in those who maintain a GFD.

COMPLICATIONS

- The majority of complications are associated with GSE.
- Malnutrition, weight loss, anemia (folate, vitamin B_{12}, iron nutritional deficiencies)
- Abdominal pain, dyspepsia
- Osteoporosis, dental abnormalities
- Autoimmune diseases (especially hypothyroidism)
- Increased risk of enteropathy-associated T-cell lymphoma

REFERENCES

1. Bolotin D, Petronic-Rosic V. Dermatitis herpetiformis. Part I. Epidemiology, pathogenesis, and clinical presentation. *J Am Acad Dermatol*. 2011;64(6):1017–1024.
2. Reunala T, Hervonen K, Salmi T. Dermatitis herpetiformis: an update on diagnosis and management. *Am J Clin Dermatol*. 2021;22(3):329–338.
3. Bolotin D, Petronic-Rosic V. Dermatitis herpetiformis. Part II. Diagnosis, management, and prognosis. *J Am Acad Dermatol*. 2011;64(6):1027–1033.
4. Reunala T, Salmi TT, Hervonen K. Dermatitis herpetiformis: pathognomonic transglutaminase IgA deposits in the skin and excellent prognosis on a gluten-free diet. *Acta Derm Venereol*. 2015;95(8):917–922.

SEE ALSO

- Celiac Disease
- Algorithm: Rash

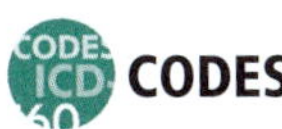

CODES

ICD10

L13.0 Dermatitis herpetiformis

CLINICAL PEARLS

DH is a chronic, relapsing, intensely pruritic rash that has a strong association with GSE.

DERMATITIS, ATOPIC

Dennis E. Hughes, DO, FACEP

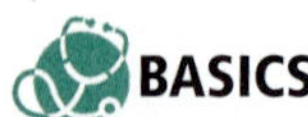

BASICS

DESCRIPTION

- A chronic, relapsing, inflammatory, intensely pruritic skin disease
- Early onset cases have coexisting allergen sensitization more often than late onset cases.
- Clinical phenotypical presentation is highly variable, suggesting multifactorial pathophysiology.
- May have significant effect on quality of life for patient and family-recurrent symptoms affect lifestyle and mental health

EPIDEMIOLOGY

- 45% of all cases begin in the first 6 months of life with 80–95% onset prior to age of 5 years.
- 50–66% of affected children will have a spontaneous remission before adolescence.
- Also, may have late-onset dermatitis in adults or relapse of childhood condition—primarily hand eczema
- Darker pigmented individuals are affected more often than whites.
- 60% incidence if one parent previously affected; rises to 80% if both parents previously affected; monozygotic twins have 80% concordance for the disorder.

Incidence

Varies worldwide, but all countries' populations are affected. The only consistent signal favored lower incidence in rural verses urban locations (exceptions are Canada and Mexico).

Prevalence

Approaching 20% prevalence in children and 10% in young adults; still present in later adulthood 2%

ETIOLOGY AND PATHOPHYSIOLOGY

- Current understanding is atopic dermatitis (AD) is a systemic T-helper cell driven disorder.
- Alteration in stratum corneum results in transepidermal water loss and defect in barrier function.
- Epidermal adhesion is reduced either as a result of (i) genetic mutation resulting in altered epidermal proteins or (ii) defect in immune regulation causing an altered inflammatory response.
- Interleukin-31 (IL-31) upregulation is thought to be a major factor in pruritus mediated by cytokines and neuropeptides rather than histamine excess.
- The damaged keratinocytes further released kinase inhibitors that result in a "skin dysbiosis" with overgrowth of staph and fungal species (1).

Genetics

- Recent discovery of association between AD and mutation in the filaggrin gene (*FLG*), which codes for a skin barrier protein
- Both epidermal and immune coding likely involved

RISK FACTORS

- "Itch–scratch cycle" (stimulates histamine release)
- Skin infections
- Emotional stress
- Irritating clothes and chemicals
- Excessively hot or cold climate
- Food allergies may be seen in association with AD, but there is no conclusive common origin. Studies of breastfeeding conveying decreased risk versus increased risk are mixed in conclusion.
- Exposure to tobacco smoke and other environmental pollutants (e.g., sulfur dioxide, nitrogen dioxide, carbon monoxide) (2)
- Some evidence suggests that repeated exposure to water high in mineral content may exacerbate condition.
- Family history of atopy
  - Asthma
  - Allergic rhinitis

COMMONLY ASSOCIATED CONDITIONS

- Food sensitivity/allergy in many cases; strong association with asthma and allergic rhinitis; "atopic march"—clinical succession of AD with subsequent development of allergic rhinitis followed by asthma
- Association with both cutaneous and extra-cutaneous infections: URI, OM, UTI, cellulitis, erysipelas, zoster, endocarditis, both methicillin-resistant and susceptible stains of *Staphylococcus aureus*, pharyngitis, and rarely sepsis
- Hyper-IgE syndrome (Job syndrome)
  - AD
  - Elevated IgE
  - Recurrent pyodermas
  - Decreased chemotaxis of mononuclear cells

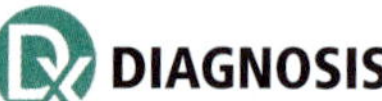

DIAGNOSIS

Clinical diagnosis

HISTORY

- Presence of major symptoms, including relapsing of condition, family history, typical distribution, and morphology necessary to make diagnosis of AD
- Most prevalent symptoms: itch (54%), dryness and scaling (19.6%), inflamed skin (7.2%), skin pain (8.2%), sleep disturbance (11.4%)

PHYSICAL EXAM

Primarily skin manifestations

- Distribution of lesions
  - Infants: trunk, face, and extensor surfaces; diaper-sparing
  - Children: antecubital and popliteal fossae, wrists and ankle locations
  - Adults: hands, feet, face, neck, upper chest, and genital areas as well as flexor surfaces
- Morphology of lesions
  - Infants: erythema and papules; may develop oozing, crusting vesicles
  - Children and adults: Lichenification and scaling are typical with chronic eczema as a result of persistent scratching and rubbing (lichenification is rare in infants).
- Associated signs
  - Facial erythema, mild to moderate
  - Perioral pallor
  - Infraorbital fold (Dennie–Morgan line)—atopic pleat
  - Dry skin progressing to ichthyosis
  - Increased palmar linear markings
  - Pityriasis alba (hypopigmented asymptomatic areas on face and shoulders)
  - Keratosis pilaris

DIFFERENTIAL DIAGNOSIS

- Photosensitivity rashes
- Contact dermatitis (especially if only the face is involved)
- Scabies
- Seborrheic dermatitis (especially in infants)
- Psoriasis or lichen simplex chronicus if only localized disease is present in adults
- Rare conditions of infancy
  - Histiocytosis X
  - Wiskott-Aldrich syndrome
  - Ataxia-telangiectasia syndrome
- Ichthyosis vulgaris

DIAGNOSTIC TESTS & INTERPRETATION

Initial Tests (lab, imaging)

- Serum IgE levels are elevated in as many as 80% of affected individuals, but test is not routinely ordered or indicated.
- Eosinophilia tends to correlate with disease severity.
- Scoring AD (SCORAD) is scoring system for AD comprising scores for area, intensity, and subjective symptoms.

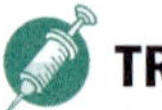

TREATMENT

The treatment of AD is an area of active research and many potential therapies are in states of development and testing.

GENERAL MEASURES

- Frequent systemic lubrication with thick emollient creams (e.g., Eucerin, Vaseline) over moist skin is the mainstay of treatment before any other intervention is considered. The "soak and seal" method is recommended.
- Minimize flare-ups and control the duration and intensity of flare-up.
- Avoid agents that may cause irritation (e.g., wool, perfumes).
- Minimize sweating.
- Lukewarm (not hot) bathing; no evidence significantly guides frequency of bathing but a minimum of twice weekly and when hygiene dictates for with post bath skin emollients.
- Avoid alkaline soaps; hypoallergenic cleansers with a slightly acidic (pH 5 to 6) with gentle mechanical removal of crusts, scale, and bacterial skin contaminants
- Sun exposure may be helpful.
- Humidify the house.
- Avoid excessive contact with water.
- Avoid lotions that contain alcohol.
- If very resistant to treatment, search for a coexisting contact dermatitis.

Pediatric Considerations

Chronic potent fluorinated corticosteroid use may cause striae, hypopigmentation, or atrophy, especially in children.

MEDICATION

First Line

- Infants and children: short-course moderate potency steroids such as hydrocortisone valerate 0.2% for flares followed by 0.5–1% topical hydrocortisone creams or ointments (use the "fingertip unit [FTU]" dosing)
- Adults: higher potency topical corticosteroids in areas other than face and skin folds; short-course, higher potency corticosteroids for flares; then, return to the lowest potency that will control dermatitis.
- Topical immunomodulators (tacrolimus or pimecrolimus) may be considered first-line therapy for AD in children aged >2 years. They may be used in combination with topical corticosteroids.
- Antihistamines for pruritus (e.g., hydroxyzine 10 to 25 mg at bedtime and as needed); limited benefit as sole treatment

Second Line

- Crisaborole, a PDE-4 inhibitor, decreases itching, inflammation, excoriation and lichenification. FDA-approved for mild to moderate AD in patients ≥3 months. It is a topical 2% ointment applied twice daily. It is very expensive and has moderate efficacy.
- Roflumilast, PDE-4 inhibitor, decreases itching, inflammation, excoriation and lichenification. It is FDA-approved for mild to moderate AD in patients ≥6 years. It is a topical 0.15% cream applied once daily. It is very expensive and has moderate efficacy.
- Plastic occlusion in combination with topical medication to promote absorption (not to be used on face)
- Topical tricyclic doxepin, as a 5% cream, may decrease pruritus.
- Modified Goeckerman regimen (tar and ultraviolet light)
- Topical antibiotics promptly at the first sign of secondary skin infection
- Dupilumab, a biologic drug that targets mediators of inflammation (IL-22, IL-17, IFN-γ), is FDA-approved for moderate-to-severe AD in patients ≥6 months of age. It is injected weekly. It is extremely expensive.
- Tralokinumab is a monoclonal antibody that specifically targets IL-13. It is approved for adults with moderate-to-severe AD who are candidates for systemic therapy. It is less effective than dupilumab but may be useful in those who do not tolerate dupilumab. It is extremely expensive.
- American Academy of Dermatology "choosing wisely" campaign recommends against routine antibiotic use unless clear evidence of secondary bacterial infection; use of oral/injectable corticosteroids; skin prick testing or radioallergosorbent blood testing

ISSUES FOR REFERRAL

- Ophthalmology evaluation for persistent vernal conjunctivitis
- If using topical steroids around eyes for extended periods, ophthalmology follow-up for cataract evaluation
- For consideration of systemic immunotherapy (cyclosporine, azathioprine, methotrexate) in the most severe cases and when associated mental health affects quality of life

ADDITIONAL THERAPIES

- Methods to reduce house mite allergens (micropore filters on heating, ventilation, and air-conditioning systems; impermeable mattress covers)
- Behavioral relaxation therapy to reduce scratching
- Bleach baths may reduce staph colonization, but definitive evidence for benefit in the condition is lacking. Recommend 1/2 cup of standard 6% household bleach for a full tub of water and soak for 5 to 10 minutes, blotting skin dry upon leaving the bath.

COMPLEMENTARY & ALTERNATIVE MEDICINE

- Evening primrose oil (includes high content of fatty acids)
  - May decrease prostaglandin synthesis
  - May promote conversion of linoleic acid to omega-6 fatty acid
- Probiotics may reduce the severity of the condition, thus reducing medication use.

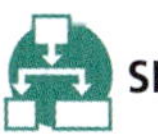

ONGOING CARE

FOLLOW-UP RECOMMENDATIONS

Patient Monitoring

Evaluate to ensure that secondary bacterial or fungal infection does not develop as a result of disruption of the skin barrier. Most patients with AD are colonized by *S. aureus*. There is a little evidence for the routine use of antimicrobial interventions to reduce skin bacteria, but treatment of clinical infection with coverage for *S. aureus* is recommended.

DIET

- Trials of elimination may find certain "triggers" in some patients.
- Breastfeeding in conjunction with maternal hypoallergenic diets may decrease the severity in some infants (varying opinions).

PATIENT EDUCATION

- American Academy of Dermatology Association: https://www.aad.org/skin-conditions/dermatology-a-to-z/atopic-dermatitis
- National Eczema Association: https://www.nationaleczema.org

PROGNOSIS

- Chronic disease
- Declines with increasing age
- 90% of pediatric patients have spontaneous resolution by puberty.
- Localized eczema (e.g., chronic hand or foot dermatitis, eyelid dermatitis, or lichen simplex chronicus) may continue in some adults.

COMPLICATIONS

- Cataracts are more common in patients with AD.
- Skin infections (usually *S. aureus*); sometimes subclinical
- Eczema herpeticum
  - Generalized vesiculopustular eruption caused by infection with herpes simplex or vaccinia virus
  - Causes acute illness requiring hospitalization
- Atrophy and/or striae if fluorinated corticosteroids are used on face or skin folds
- Systemic absorption may occur if large areas of skin are treated, particularly if high-potency medications and occlusion are combined.

REFERENCES

1. Meledathu S, Naidu MP, Brunner PM. Update on atopic dermatitis. *J Allergy Clin Immunol*. 2025;155(4):1124–1132. doi:10.1016/j.jaci.2025.01.013.
2. Schuler CF IV, Billi AC, Maverakis E, et al. Novel insights into atopic dermatitis. *J Allergy Clin Immunol*. 2023;151(5):1145–1154. doi:10.1016/j.jaci.2022.10.023.

SEE ALSO

Algorithm: Rash

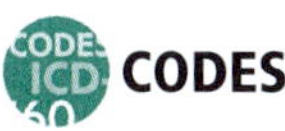

CODES

ICD10

- L20.9 Atopic dermatitis, unspecified
- L20.89 Other atopic dermatitis
- L20.83 Infantile (acute) (chronic) eczema

CLINICAL PEARLS

- Institute early and proactive treatment to reduce inflammation. Use the lowest potency topical steroid that controls symptoms.
- Monitor for secondary bacterial infection.
- Frequent systemic lubrication with thick emollient creams (e.g., Eucerin, Vaseline) over moist skin is the mainstay of treatment before any other intervention is considered.

DERMATITIS, CONTACT

Konstantinos E. Deligiannidis, MD, MPH, FAAFP • Christopher C. Paredes, MD • Stephen McCormick, MD, MPH

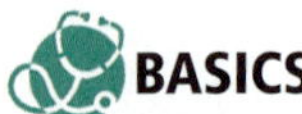

BASICS

DESCRIPTION

- A cutaneous reaction to an external substance in contact with the skin
- Each type has a different mechanism, whereas the clinical presentation is the same (1).
- Two main types with distinct mechanism and acuity, but similar presentation (2)
  - Irritant dermatitis (ID): chemical damage to stratum corneum causing inflammatory response; occurs 0 to 48 hours after exposure (3)
  - Allergic contact dermatitis (ACD): occurs after sensitization (first exposure) to a substance; delayed hypersensitivity reaction occurring over hours to days, representing immune cell response (2),(3)
- System(s) affected: skin/exocrine
- Synonym(s): dermatitis venenata

EPIDEMIOLOGY

Common

Incidence

Occupational contact dermatitis accounts for up to 70% of occupational skin disease occurrences and affects 20.5/100,000 workers per year in one Australian study. However, it is difficult to quantify due to diverse causes and manifestations; estimated 15% global lifetime incidence (4)

Prevalence

- Florists, hairdressers, cooks, beauticians, health care workers, and metal-working machine operators have the highest incidence.
- Predominant sex: male = female
  - Variations due to differences in exposure to offending agents as well as normal cutaneous variations between males and females (eccrine and sebaceous gland function and hair distribution) (5)

Geriatric Considerations

Increased incidence of ID secondary to skin dryness

Pediatric Considerations

Increased incidence of positive patch testing due to better delayed hypersensitivity reactions (2),(6)

ETIOLOGY AND PATHOPHYSIOLOGY

Hypersensitivity reaction to a substance generating cellular immunity response

- Plants
  - Urushiol (allergen): poison ivy, poison oak, poison sumac
  - Primary contact: plant (roots/stems/leaves)
  - Secondary contact: clothes/fingernails (not blister fluid—the established eruption is not itself contagious or transmissible)
- Chemicals
  - Nickel: jewelry, zippers, hooks, and watches (7)
  - Potassium dichromate: tanning agent in leather
  - Paraphenylenediamine: hair dyes, fur dyes, and industrial chemicals
  - Turpentine: cleaning agents, polishes, and waxes
  - Soaps and detergents
- Topical medicines
  - Neomycin: topical antibiotics
  - Thimerosal (Merthiolate): preservative in topical medications
  - Anesthetics: benzocaine
  - Parabens: preservative in topical medications
  - Formalin: cosmetics, shampoos, and nail enamel

Genetics

Increased frequency of ACD in families with allergies

RISK FACTORS

- Occupation
- Hobbies
- Travel
- Cosmetics
- Jewelry

GENERAL PREVENTION

- Identify and avoid causative agents.
- Use of protective gloves (with cotton lining) may be helpful.

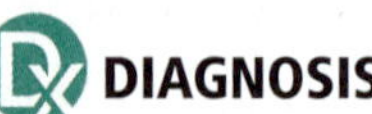

DIAGNOSIS

HISTORY

- Pruritic rash
- Assess for prior exposure to irritating substance.
- History suggestive of exposure (hiking, chemical use)

PHYSICAL EXAM

- Acute
  - Papules, vesicles, bullae with surrounding erythema
  - Crusting and oozing
  - Pruritus
- Chronic
  - Erythematous base
  - Thickening with lichenification
  - Scaling
  - Fissuring
- Distribution
  - Where epidermis is thinner (eyelids, genitalia)
  - Areas of contact with offending agent (e.g., nail polish)
  - Palms and soles are relatively more resistant, although hand dermatitis is common.
  - Deeper skin folds spared
  - Linear arrays of lesions
  - Lesions with sharp borders and sharp angles are pathognomonic.
  - Well-demarcated area with a papulovesicular rash

DIFFERENTIAL DIAGNOSIS

- Based on clinical impression
  - Appearance, periodicity, and localization
- Groups of vesicles
  - Herpes simplex
- Diffuse bullous or vesicular lesions
  - Bullous pemphigoid
- Photodistribution
  - Phototoxic/allergic reaction to systemic allergen
- Eyelids
  - Seborrheic dermatitis
- Scaly eczematous lesions
  - Atopic dermatitis
  - Nummular eczema
  - Lichen simplex chronicus
  - Stasis dermatitis
  - Xerosis
- Id reaction (See separate chapter "Id Reaction.")

DIAGNOSTIC TESTS & INTERPRETATION

Diagnostic Procedures/Other

Consider patch tests for suspected allergic trigger (systemic corticosteroids or recent, aggressive use of topical steroids may alter results).

Test Interpretation

- Intercellular edema
- Bullae

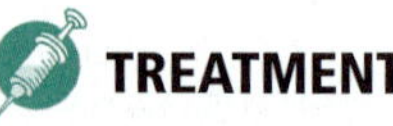

TREATMENT

GENERAL MEASURES

- Identify and remove offending agent (8)[C]:
  - Avoidance
  - Work modification
  - Protective clothing
  - Barrier creams, especially high-lipid content moisturizing creams (e.g., Keri lotion, petrolatum, coconut oil)
- Topical soaks with cool tap water, Burow solution (1:40 dilution), saline (1 tsp/pt water), or silver nitrate solution
- Lukewarm water baths
- Aveeno oatmeal baths
- Emollients (white petrolatum, Eucerin)

MEDICATION

First Line

- Topical medications (7)[C]
  - Lotion of zinc oxide, talc, menthol 0.15% (Gold Bond), phenol 0.5%
  - Corticosteroids for ACD as well as ID
    - High-potency steroids: fluocinonide (Lidex) 0.05% gel, cream, or ointment TID–QID
    - Use high-potency steroids only for a short time and then switch to low- or medium-potency steroid cream or ointment. Avoid long-term daily use (9)[C].
    - Caution regarding face/skin folds: Use lower potency steroids (7)[C] and avoid prolonged usage. Switch to lower potency topical steroid once the acute phase is resolved.
- Calamine lotion for symptomatic relief
- Topical antibiotics for secondary infection (bacitracin, erythromycin)

- Systemic
  - Antihistamine
    - Hydroxyzine: 25 to 50 mg PO QID, especially useful for itching
    - Diphenhydramine: 25 to 50 mg PO QID
    - Cetirizine: 10 mg PO BID–TID
- Corticosteroids
  - Prednisone: Taper starting at 60 to 80 mg/day PO, over 10 to 14 days, occasionally 21 days.
  - Used for moderate to severe cases, particularly involving face or genitals
  - Little published evidence to compare appropriate length of treatment, but clinical experience suggests that short courses of therapy (i.e., 5 to 7 days) are not adequate to prevent rebound dermatitis.
  - Treatment for up to 21 days for severe/extensive rash resulting from exposure to potent allergens like urushiol (e.g., poison ivy) is commonly recommended to prevent reemergence of dermatitis upon taper (rebound), although 14 days is usually adequate.
  - May use burst dose of steroids for up to 5 days for less persistent immunogens or less severe dermatitis
- Antibiotics for secondary skin infections
  - Dicloxacillin: 250 to 500 mg PO QID for 7 to 10 days
  - Amoxicillin-clavulanate: 500 mg PO BID for 7 to 10 days
  - Cephalexin: 500 mg PO QID for 7 to 10 days
  - Trimethoprim-sulfamethoxazole (Bactrim DS): 160 mg/800 mg (1 tablet) PO BID for 7 to 10 days (suspected resistant *Staphylococcus aureus*)
- Precautions
  - Antihistamines may cause drowsiness.
  - Prolonged use of potent topical steroids may cause local skin effects (atrophy, stria, telangiectasia).
  - Use tapering dose of oral steroids if using >5 days.

Second Line

Other topical or systemic antibiotics, depending on organisms and sensitivity

Pregnancy Considerations

Usual caution with medications

ISSUES FOR REFERRAL

May need referral to a dermatologist or allergist if refractory to conventional treatment

COMPLEMENTARY & ALTERNATIVE MEDICINE

The use of complementary and alternative treatment is a supplement and not an alternative to conventional treatment.

ADMISSION, INPATIENT, AND NURSING CONSIDERATIONS

Rarely needs hospital admission

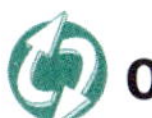

ONGOING CARE

FOLLOW-UP RECOMMENDATIONS

Stay active, but avoid overheating.

Patient Monitoring

- As necessary for recurrence
- Patch testing for etiology after resolved

DIET

No special diet

PATIENT EDUCATION

- Avoidance of irritating substance
- Cleaning of secondary sources (nails, clothes)
- Fallacy of blister fluid spreading disease

PROGNOSIS

- Self-limited
- Benign
- 55% of patients still had contact dermatitis at 2 years after diagnosis.
- Improvement in rash is less likely for those who remain in the same or similar profession.
- Increased length of exposure and atopy are poor prognostic indicators.

COMPLICATIONS

- Generalized eruption secondary to autosensitization
- Secondary bacterial infection

REFERENCES

1. Sultan TA, Hatem AMA. Management of contact dermatitis. *J Dermatol Dermatol Surg*. 2015;19(2):86–91.
2. Brar KK. A review of contact dermatitis. *Ann Allergy Asthma Immunol*. 2021;126(1):32–39. doi:10.1016/j.anai.2020.10.003.
3. Li Y, Li L. Contact dermatitis: classifications and management. *Clin Rev Allergy Immunol*. 2021;61(3):245–281. doi:10.1007/s12016-021-08875-0.
4. Johansen JD, Bonefeld CM, Schwensen JFB, et al. Novel insights into contact dermatitis. *J Allergy Clin Immunol*. 2022;149(4):1162–1171. doi:10.1016/j.jaci.2022.02.002.
5. Boonchai W, Likittanasombat S, Viriyaskultorn N, et al. Gender differences in allergic contact dermatitis to common allergens. *Contact Dermatitis*. 2024;90(5):458–465. doi:10.1111/cod.14479.
6. Admani S, Jacob SE. Allergic contact dermatitis in children: review of the past decade. *Curr Allergy Asthma Rep*. 2014;14(4):421.
7. Usatine RP, Riojas M. Diagnosis and management of contact dermatitis. *Am Fam Physician*. 2010;82(3):249–255.
8. Fonacier L, Bernstein DI, Pacheco K, et al. Contact dermatitis: a practice parameter-update 2015. *J Allergy Clin Immunol Pract*. 2015;3(Suppl 3):S1–S39. doi:10.1016/j.jaip.2015.02.009.
9. Nassau S, Fonacier L. Allergic contact dermatitis. *Med Clin North Am*. 2020;104(1):61–76.

ADDITIONAL READING

- Pelletier JL, Perez C, Jacob SE. Contact dermatitis in pediatrics. *Pediatr Ann*. 2016;45(8):e287–e292.
- Rashid RS, Shim TN. Contact dermatitis. *BMJ*. 2016;353:i3299.

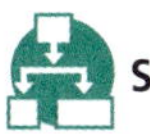

SEE ALSO

Algorithm: Rash

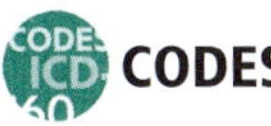

CODES

ICD10

- L25.9 Unspecified contact dermatitis, unspecified cause
- L23.9 Allergic contact dermatitis, unspecified cause
- L25.5 Unspecified contact dermatitis due to plants, except food

CLINICAL PEARLS

- Commonly occurs on hands and face
- Anyone exposed to irritants or allergic substances is predisposed to contact dermatitis, especially in occupations that have high exposure to chemicals.
- The most common allergens causing contact dermatitis are plants of the *Toxicodendron* genus (poison ivy, poison oak, poison sumac).
- Poison-ivy dermatitis typically requires 10 to 14 days (occasionally more) of topical or oral steroid therapy to prevent recurrent eruption.
- Worldwide, nickel is the number one patch-tested allergen causing ACD.
- The usual treatment for contact dermatitis is avoidance of the allergen or irritating substance and temporary use of topical steroids.
- A contact dermatitis eruption presents in a nondermatomal geographic fashion due to the skin being in contact with an external source.

DERMATITIS, DIAPER

Dennis E. Hughes, DO, FACEP

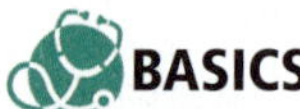

BASICS

DESCRIPTION
- Diaper dermatitis is a rash occurring under the covered area of a diaper (named for typical location, not etiology). It is usually initially a contact irritant dermatitis, but can be caused by or contributed by systemic conditions.
- Not usually a serious condition but patient discomfort and caregiver anxiety are considerations.
- System(s) affected: skin/exocrine
- Synonym(s): diaper rash; nappy rash; napkin dermatitis

Geriatric Considerations
Incontinence is a significant cofactor in the elderly population.

EPIDEMIOLOGY

Incidence
- The most common dermatitis is found in infancy.
- Peak incidence: 7 to 12 months of age and then decreases
- Lower incidence is reported in breastfed babies due to lower pH, urease, protease, and lipase activity.

Prevalence
Prevalence has been variably reported from 4–35% in children <2 years of age. Upward of 75% of infants will have episodes of varying duration and severity in the United States. Severity varies: 58% have slight symptoms; 34% moderate; 8% severe. Underreporting contributes to difficulty in determining impact of condition.

ETIOLOGY AND PATHOPHYSIOLOGY
- Immature infant skin with histologic, biochemical, functional differences compared to mature skin
- Wet skin is central in the development of diaper dermatitis, as prolonged contact with urine or feces results in susceptibility to chemical, enzymatic, and physical injury; wet skin is also penetrated more easily.
- Fecal proteases and lipases are irritants.
- Superhydrase urease enzyme found in the stratum corneum liberates ammonia from cutaneous bacteria
- Fecal lipase and protease activity is increased by acceleration of GI transit; thus, a higher incidence of irritant diaper dermatitis is observed in babies who have had diarrhea in the previous 48 hours.
- Once the skin is compromised, secondary infection by *Candida albicans* is common. 40–75% of diaper rashes that last >3 days are colonized with *C. albicans*.
- Bacteria may play a role in diaper dermatitis through reduction of fecal pH and resulting activation of enzymes.
- Allergy is exceedingly rare as a cause in infants.

RISK FACTORS
- Infrequent diaper changes
- Improper laundering (cloth diapers)
- Family history of dermatitis
- Hot, humid weather
- Recent treatment with oral antibiotics
- Diarrhea (>3 stools per day increases risk)
- Dye allergy
- Eczema may increase the risk.

GENERAL PREVENTION
Most effectively managed by prevention including rigorous attention to hygiene

COMMONLY ASSOCIATED CONDITIONS
- Contact (allergic or irritant) dermatitis
- Seborrheic dermatitis
- Psoriasis
- Candidiasis
- Atopic dermatitis

DIAGNOSIS

Correct diagnosis is key. The initial presentation of diseases other than contact irritant dermatitis may be in the diaper area. Avoid assuming that all diaper-area dermatitis is simple contact/irritant dermatitis by obtaining a comprehensive history and performing an appropriate general skin examination.

HISTORY
- Onset, duration, and change in the nature of the rash
- Presence of rashes outside the diaper area
- Associated scratching or crying
- Contact with infants with a similar rash
- Recent illness, diarrhea, or antibiotic use
- Fever
- Pustular drainage
- Lymphangitis

PHYSICAL EXAM
- Mild forms consist of shiny erythema ± scale.
- Margins are not always evident.
- Moderate cases have areas of papules, vesicles, and small superficial erosions.
- It can progress to well-demarcated ulcerated nodules that measure ≥1 cm in diameter.
- It is found on the prominent parts of the buttocks, medial thighs, mons pubis, and scrotum.
- Skin folds are spared or involved last (skin fold involvement suggests secondary infection with Candida sp. or *Staphylococcus aureus*).
- *Tidemark dermatitis* refers to the bandlike form of erythema of irritated diaper margins.
- Diaper dermatitis can cause an id reaction (autoeczematous) outside the diaper area.

DIFFERENTIAL DIAGNOSIS
- Contact dermatitis
- Seborrheic dermatitis
- Candidiasis
- Atopic dermatitis
- Scabies
- Acrodermatitis enteropathica (deficiency in zinc)
- Letterer-Siwe disease
- Congenital syphilis
- Child abuse
- Streptococcal/staphylococcal infection
- Kawasaki disease
- Biotin deficiency
- Psoriasis
- HIV infection

DIAGNOSTIC TESTS & INTERPRETATION

Initial Tests (lab, imaging)
Rarely needed

Follow-Up Tests & Special Considerations
- Consider a culture of lesions or a potassium hydroxide (KOH) preparation.
- The finding of anemia in association with hepatosplenomegaly and the appropriate rash may suggest a diagnosis of Langerhans cell histiocytosis or congenital syphilis.
- Finding mites, ova, or feces on a mineral oil preparation of a burrow scraping can confirm the diagnosis of scabies.

Test Interpretation

- The need for biopsy is rare.
- Histology may reveal acute, subacute, or chronic spongiotic dermatitis.

TREATMENT

Prevention is the key to treatment of this condition.

GENERAL MEASURES

- Expose the diaper area to air as much as possible.
- Use mild, slightly acidic or neutral pH cleanser with water; no rubbing and pat dry.
- Avoid impermeable waterproof pants during treatment (day or night); they keep the skin wet and subject to rash or infection.
- Change diapers frequently, even at night, if the rash is extensive.
- Superabsorbent diapers are beneficial (1), as they wick urine away from skin and still allow air to permeate. Manufacturer-associated data indicates diapers with a mesh-like top sheet construction may be superior in allowing stool to separate from skin.
- Discontinue using baby lotion, powder, ointment, or baby oil (except zinc oxide).
- The use of appropriately formulated baby wipes (alcohol and fragrance-free) is safe and as effective as water. Those baby wipes are commercially marketed as safe for sensitive skin appear to be generally equally effective.
- Apply zinc oxide ointment (1) or other barrier cream to the rash at the earliest sign and BID or TID (e.g., Desitin or Balmex). Thereafter, apply to clean, thoroughly dried skin.
- Cornstarch can reduce friction. Avoid talcum-containing products.

MEDICATION

First Line

- For a pure contact dermatitis, a low-potency topical steroid (hydrocortisone 0.5–1% TID for 3 to 5 days) and removal of the offending agent (urine, feces) should suffice.
- If candidiasis is suspected or diaper rash persists for >3 days, use an antifungal such as miconazole nitrate 2% cream, miconazole powder, econazole (Spectazole), clotrimazole (Lotrimin), or ketoconazole (Nizoral) cream at each diaper change. Candida superinfection is common in persistent dermatitis in the moist diaper area.
- If inflammation is prominent, consider a very low-potency steroid cream such as hydrocortisone 0.5–1% TID along with an antifungal cream ± a combination product such as clioquinol–hydrocortisone (Vioform–Hydrocortisone) cream.
- If a secondary bacterial infection is suspected, use an antistaphylococcal oral antibiotic or mupirocin (Bactroban) ointment topically.
- Precautions: Avoid high- or moderate-potency steroids often found in combination of steroid antifungal mixtures—these should never be used in the diaper area.

Second Line

- Sucralfate paste for resistant cases
- Recent study suggests that use of hydrocolloid dressings can speed healing of rash.
- Case reports support the use of immune modulators such as topical tacrolimus (0.03%) in refractory cases; however, it is not approved for children <2 years of age. Recent literature review by American Academy of Allergy and American College of Allergy found no findings to suggest harm.

ISSUES FOR REFERRAL

Consider if a systemic disease such as Langerhans cell histiocytosis, acrodermatitis enteropathica, or HIV infection is suspected.

ADMISSION, INPATIENT, AND NURSING CONSIDERATIONS

- Admission criteria/initial stabilization
  - Febrile neonates
  - Recalcitrant rash suggestive of immunodeficiency
  - Toxic-appearing infants
  - Abuse or neglect suspected
- Assist first-time parents with hygiene education.

ONGOING CARE

FOLLOW-UP RECOMMENDATIONS

Patient Monitoring

Recheck weekly until clear and then at times of recurrence.

PATIENT EDUCATION

Patient education is vital to the treatment and prevention of recurrent cases.

PROGNOSIS

- Quick, complete clearing with appropriate treatment
- Secondary candidal infections may last a few weeks after treatment has begun.

COMPLICATIONS

- Secondary bacterial infection (Consider community-acquired methicillin-resistant *S. aureus* [MRSA] in pustular dermatitis that does not respond to normal therapy.)
- Rare complication is inoculation with group A β-hemolytic *Streptococcus* resulting in necrotizing fasciitis.
- Secondary yeast infection

REFERENCES

1. Burdall O, Willgress L, Goad N. Neonatal skin care: developments in care to maintain neonatal barrier function and prevention of diaper dermatitis. *Pediatr Dermatol*. 2019;36(1):31–35.

ADDITIONAL READING

- Chadha A, Jahnke M. Common neonatal rashes. *Pediatr Ann*. 2019;48(1):e16–e22.
- Giacaman A, Boix-Vilanova J, Martín-Santiago A. Hydrocolloid dressing for the treatment of severe diaper dermatitis. *Pediatr Dermatol*. 2023;40(1):224–225. doi:10.1111/pde.15131.

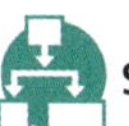

SEE ALSO

Algorithm: Rash

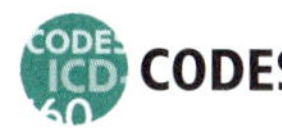

CODES

ICD10

- L22 Diaper dermatitis
- B37.2 Candidiasis of skin and nail

CLINICAL PEARLS

- Hygiene is the main preventative measure.
- Look for secondary infection in persistent cases (especially Candida, Staph spp.)
- Candida is present in most rashes that last more than a few days.

D

DERMATITIS, SEBORRHEIC

Briana Lindberg, MD, CAQSM

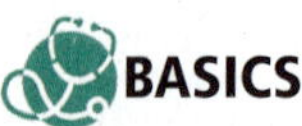

BASICS

DESCRIPTION

Chronic, superficial, recurrent inflammatory skin disorder affecting sebum-rich, hairy regions of the body, especially the scalp, eyebrows, and face and to lesser extent, chest, and back (1)

EPIDEMIOLOGY

Incidence

- Predominant age: adolescence, followed by infancy, and adulthood
- Predominant sex: male > female

Prevalence

- Affects 2–5% of the global population; up to 83% in immunosuppressed, HIV-positive individuals (2)
- Infantile seborrheic dermatitis (SD) is common in the first 3 months of life, affecting all ethnicities in all climates.

ETIOLOGY AND PATHOPHYSIOLOGY

- Skin surface yeast such as *Malassezia* may be a contributing factor.
- Genetic and environmental factors: Flares are common with stress/illness.
- Parallels increased sebaceous gland activity in infancy and adolescence or as a result of some acnegenic drugs.
- SD is more common in immunosuppressed patients, suggesting that immune mechanisms are implicated in the pathogenesis of the disease, although the mechanisms are not well-defined.

Genetics

Positive family history; no genetic markers have been identified to date.

RISK FACTORS

- Immunosuppressed conditions such as HIV/AIDS (2)
- Parkinson disease, neurologic disorders, facial paralysis
- Emotional stress (2)
- Obesity (2)
- Oily skin (2)
- Acne (2)
- Down syndrome
- Medications may cause flares/induce SD: buspirone, chlorpromazine, cimetidine, ethionamide, griseofulvin, haloperidol, interferon-α, methyldopa, psoralen, and IL-2 (2)

GENERAL PREVENTION

Seborrheic skin should be washed more often than usual to soften the affected areas.

COMMONLY ASSOCIATED CONDITIONS

- Parkinson disease
- HIV/AIDS
- Facial paralysis
- Down syndrome

DIAGNOSIS

Diagnosis of SD is usually made by history and physical exam. If unclear, a punch biopsy of the skin will confirm the diagnosis.

HISTORY

- Intermittent active phases manifest with burning, scaling, and itching, alternating with inactive periods; activity is increased in winter and early spring, with remissions commonly occurring in summer.
- Infants
  - Cradle cap: greasy scaling of the scalp with occasional erythema
  - Diaper and/or axillary rash
  - Age of onset: ~1 month
  - Usually self-resolves by 8 to 12 months
- Adults
  - Red, greasy, scaling rash consisting of macules and plaques with indistinct margins
  - Red, smooth, glazed appearance in skin folds
  - Hypopigmented, scaling macules on skin of color
  - Minimal pruritus
  - Chronic waxing and waning course
  - Bilateral and symmetric
  - Most commonly located in hairy skin areas: scalp and scalp margins, eyebrows and eyelid margins, nasolabial folds, ears and retroauricular folds, presternal area, middle to upper back, buttock crease, inguinal area, genitals, and armpits

PHYSICAL EXAM

- Scalp appearance varies from mild, patchy scaling to widespread, thick, adherent crusts. Plaques are rare.
- SD can spread onto the forehead, the posterior part of the neck, and the postauricular skin, as in psoriasis.
- Skin lesions manifest as brawny or yellow greasy scaling over red, inflamed skin.
- Hypopigmentation can be seen in skin tones of color.
- Infectious eczematoid dermatitis, with oozing and crusting, suggests secondary infection.
- Seborrheic blepharitis may occur independently.

DIFFERENTIAL DIAGNOSIS

- Atopic dermatitis: Distinction may be difficult in infants.
- Psoriasis
  - More common on the extensor surfaces of the knees, elbows, and the nail beds are usually involved.
  - Scalp psoriasis will be more sharply demarcated than SD with crusted, infiltrated plaques rather than mild scaling and erythema.
- *Candida*
- Tinea cruris/capitis: Suspect these when usual medications fail or hair loss occurs.
- Eczema of auricle/otitis externa
- Rosacea
- Discoid lupus erythematosus: Skin biopsy will be beneficial.
- Histiocytosis X: may appear as seborrheic-like eruption
- Dandruff: scalp only, non-inflammatory
- Drug eruption

DIAGNOSTIC TESTS & INTERPRETATION

Diagnostic Procedures/Other

- Consider biopsy if:
  - Usual therapies fail.
  - Petechiae are noted.
  - Histiocytosis X is suspected.
- Consider fungal cultures if:
  - Refractory to treatment
  - Pustules and alopecia are present.

Test Interpretation

Nonspecific changes

- Hyperkeratosis, acanthosis, accentuated rete ridges, focal spongiosis, and parakeratosis are characteristic.
- Parakeratotic scale around hair follicles and mild superficial inflammatory lymphocytic infiltrate

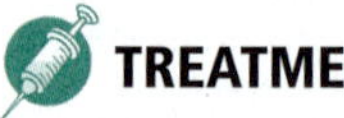

TREATMENT

GENERAL MEASURES

- Increase frequency of shampooing.
- Sunlight in moderate doses may be helpful.
- Infants (cradle cap) (3)[A]
  - As above, increasing frequency of shampooing with a mild, nonmedicated shampoo may help.
  - Remove thick scale by applying warm mineral oil and then wash off 1 hour later with a mild soap and a soft-bristle toothbrush or terrycloth washcloth.
- Adults
  - Wash all affected areas with antiseborrheic shampoos. Start with over-the-counter products (i.e., selenium sulfide), allowing shampoo/lotion to remain on the skin for several minutes before washing off, and increase to more potent preparations (those containing coal tar, sulfur, or salicylic acid) if no improvement is noted.
  - For dense scalp scaling, 10% liquor carbonic detergents in Nivea oil may be used at bedtime, covering the head with a shower cap. This should be done nightly for 1 to 3 weeks.

MEDICATION

First Line

- Cradle cap: Use a coal tar shampoo or ketoconazole shampoo if the nonmedicated shampoo is ineffective. Massage in, and keep on for several minutes before removing.

- Adults
  - Topical antifungal agents (1)[C],(2)[A]
    - Ketoconazole 2% or miconazole 2% shampoo twice a week (allow to remain on scalp for several minutes before washing off) for clearance and then once a week or every other week for maintenance (2)[A].
    - Ketoconazole 2% or sertaconazole 2% cream may be used to clear scales in other areas (2)[A].
    - Ciclopirox 1% shampoo twice weekly (2)[A].
    - Facial hair can also be treated with ketoconazole 2% shampoo.
  - Topical corticosteroids
    - Begin with 1% hydrocortisone and advance to more potent (fluorinated) steroid preparations daily for 2 to 4 weeks.
      - Avoid continuous use of potent steroids to reduce the risk of skin atrophy, hypopigmentation, and/or systemic absorption (especially in infants, children, and elderly).
      - Precautions: Fluorinated corticosteroids and higher concentrations of hydrocortisone (e.g., 2.5%) may cause atrophy or striae if used on the face or on skin folds.
  - Other topical agents
    - Coal tar 1% shampoo twice a week
    - Selenium sulfide 2.5% shampoo twice a week
    - Zinc pyrithione 1% shampoo twice a week
    - Lithium gluconate/succinate 8% ointment/gel twice a week
- Once controlled, washing with zinc soaps or selenium lotion with periodic use of steroid cream may help to maintain remission.

Second Line

- Calcineurin inhibitors (not linked to skin atrophy and hypopigmentation; just as effective as topical steroids; potentially more side effects)
  - Pimecrolimus 1% cream BID
  - Tacrolimus 0.1% ointment
- Systemic antifungal therapy
  - For severe or recalcitrant SD
    - Terbinafine: 250 mg/day × 4 to 6 weeks or pulse therapy 250 mg/day × 12 days/month for 3 months
    - Itraconazole: 200 mg/day, effective with good safety profile
      - Daily regimen for 1 week followed by two days per month for the following 2 months *or*
      - 150 to 200 mg/day once a week for a period of 2 to 3 months
    - Monitor potential hepatotoxic effects.
- Low-molecular-weight hyaluronic acid
  - Hyaluronic acid sodium salt gel 0.2% BID

ISSUES FOR REFERRAL

- No response to first-line therapy and concerns regarding systemic illness (e.g., HIV)
- Resistant SD in adults should prompt testing for HIV.

COMPLEMENTARY & ALTERNATIVE MEDICINE

- Honey, antifungal, antioxidant, and antibacterial: effective in remission of and prevention of relapses of SD
- Aloe vera, anti-inflammatory and antifungal: reduction in pruritus and scaling associated with SD
- Borage oil containing essential amino acid γ-lineolic acid (GLA): may be effective in infantile SD
- Tea-tree essential oil, antifungal, anti-inflammatory, and antioxidant: effective in mild to moderate cases
- Quassia amara extract, anti-inflammatory and antifungal, especially against *Malassezia* yeast: outperformed topical 2% ketoconazole and 1% ciclopiroxolamine

ONGOING CARE

Individuals with coiled hair or hair that is heat and/or chemically treated will need less drying agents to prevent hair breakage compared to those with straighter hair who may prefer drying agents. Applying shampoos and other topical treatments directly to scalp instead of hair shaft can decrease risk of hair damage.

FOLLOW-UP RECOMMENDATIONS

Patient Monitoring

Every 2 to 12 weeks depending on the disease severity and the patient's response to therapy

PATIENT EDUCATION

Seborrheic Dermatitis: https://familydoctor.org/familydoctor/en/diseases-conditions/seborrheic-dermatitis.html

PROGNOSIS

- In infants, SD usually remits after 6 to 8 months.
- In adults, SD is usually chronic and relapsing, with exacerbations and remissions. Disease is usually controlled with shampoos and topical steroids.
- Erythema or hypopigmentation typically resolves with treatment.

COMPLICATIONS

- Skin atrophy/striae are possible from fluorinated corticosteroids, especially if used on the face.
- Glaucoma and/or cataracts can result from use of fluorinated steroids around the eyes.
- Photosensitivity is caused occasionally by tar-containing products.
- Herpes keratitis is a rare complication of herpes simplex: Instruct patient to stop eyelid steroids if herpes simplex develops.

REFERENCES

1. LeFevre NM, Braudis K, Feigenbaum LS. Seborrheic dermatitis: diagnosis and treatment. *Am Fam Physician*. 2025;112(2):166–173.
2. Okokon EO, Verbeek JH, Ruotsalainen JH, et al. Topical antifungals for seborrhoeic dermatitis. *Cochrane Database Syst Rev*. 2015;(5):CD008138.
3. Victoire A, Magin P, Coughlan J, et al. Interventions for infantile seborrhoeic dermatitis (including cradle cap). *Cochrane Database Syst Rev*. 2019;3(3):CD011380.

ADDITIONAL READING

Kastarinen H, Oksanen T, Okokon EO, et al. Topical anti-inflammatory agents for seborrhoeic dermatitis of the face or scalp. *Cochrane Database Syst Rev*. 2014;(5):CD009446.

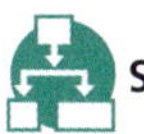

SEE ALSO

Algorithm: Rash

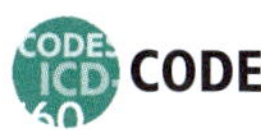

CODES

ICD10

- L21.9 Seborrheic dermatitis, unspecified
- L21.1 Seborrheic infantile dermatitis
- L21.0 Seborrhea capitis

CLINICAL PEARLS

- Search for an underlying systemic disease in a patient who is unresponsive to usual therapy.
- In infants, SD is usually self-limited.
- In adults, SD is usually chronic, with exacerbations and remissions. Disease is usually easily controlled with shampoos and topical steroids.

D

DERMATITIS, STASIS

Francesco Satriale, MD • Sarah A. Satriale, PA-C • Jessica A. Orner, MD

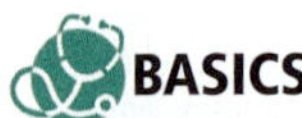

BASICS

DESCRIPTION

- Chronic, eczematous, scaling, erythematous plaques, and patches to the lower extremities accompanied by cycle of scratching, excoriations, weeping, crusting, and inflammation in patients with chronic venous insufficiency (CVI) and edema; clinical skin manifestation of CVI usually appears late in the disease; may present as a solitary lesion most often starting on medial ankle; can be associated with venous leg ulcers on bony prominences.
- System(s) affected: skin/exocrine
- Synonym(s): gravitational eczema; varicose eczema; venous dermatitis; stasis eczema

EPIDEMIOLOGY

Prevalence

- In the United States: common in patients age >50 years, estimating 15 to 20 million (6–7%); predominant age: adult, geriatric
- Predominant sex: female > male

ETIOLOGY AND PATHOPHYSIOLOGY

- Due to venous hypertension from venous incompetence (valve dysfunction and reflux) or obstruction (thrombosis or stenosis) of superficial, perforating, or deep veins
- Inflammatory changes include microvascular abnormalities (leaking capillaries with fibrin cuffs, thickened venules, microthrombosis) and increased leukocytes (macrophages, T lymphocytes, mast cells).
- Usually with chronic dependent edema; inflamed, edematous skin may be more susceptible to trauma.
- Itch may be caused by inflammatory mediators (from mast cells, monocytes, macrophages, or neutrophils) liberated in the microcirculation and endothelium. Abnormal leukocyte–endothelium interaction is proposed to be a major factor. A cascade of biochemical events leads to ulceration.

Genetics

Familial link probable

RISK FACTORS

- Atopy, chronic edema, superimposition of itch–scratch cycle
- Old age, obesity
- Cigarette use
- Previous DVT, previous pregnancy, hx vein stripping, vein harvesting for coronary artery bypass graft surgery
- Prolonged standing or sitting
- Hypertension, congestive heart failure
- Trauma
- Low-protein diet
- High-estrogen states
- Genetic propensity (familial history of congenital disease)

GENERAL PREVENTION

- Treat lower extremity edema with compression stockings, exercise, and leg elevation. This will mobilize the interstitial lymphatic fluid from the region of stasis dermatitis; also following DVT.
- Consider early treatment of venous insufficiency with specialist care and interventional procedures as indicated.
- Use topical emollients twice a day to prevent fissuring and itching.

COMMONLY ASSOCIATED CONDITIONS

Varicose veins, venous insufficiency, other eczematous disease, hyperhomocysteinemia, venous HTN

DIAGNOSIS

HISTORY

- Skin itching, pain, and burning may precede visible skin changes.
- Lower extremity edema (often initially around ankles) preceding skin eruption, insidious onset, usually bilateral
- Description may include aching/heavy legs.
- Erythema and scaling of lower extremities with later development of hyperpigmentation
- Symptoms may worsen in the evening with dependent edema.

PHYSICAL EXAM

- Evaluation of the lower extremities characteristically reveals:
  - Bilateral scaly, eczematous patches, papules, and/or plaques, hair loss
  - Violaceous (sometimes brown), erythematous lesions due to deoxygenation of venous blood (postinflammatory hyperpigmentation and hemosiderin deposition within the cutaneous tissue)
- Distribution: medial aspect of ankle, with frequent extension onto the foot and lower leg, occasionally lateral side of ankle, lower 1/3 of the extremity
- Early signs include prominent superficial veins and pitting ankle edema.
- Brawny induration, swelling, and warmth
- Venous ulcers (frequently accompany stasis dermatitis) often over bony prominences secondary to minor trauma; varicosities are often associated with ulcers.
- In later stages excoriations, weeping, and crusting
- May present as a solitary lesion mimicking a neoplasm
- Can present with comorbid atrophie blanche (hypopigmented patches with punctate red from microthrombosis) and/or lipodermatosclerosis (fibrosing panniculitis which can bind skin to subcutaneous tissues)
- May also develop contact sensitization to topical agents locally and/or autosensitization dermatitis (similar skin changes at a remote cutaneous site)

DIFFERENTIAL DIAGNOSIS

- Other eczematous diseases: atopic dermatitis, uremic dermatitis, contact dermatitis (due to topical agents used to self-treat), neurodermatitis, arterial insufficiency, sickle cell disease causing skin ulceration, cellulitis, erysipelas
- Tinea dermatophyte infection
- Pretibial myxedema
- Nummular eczema
- Lichen simplex chronicus
- Xerosis
- Asteatotic eczema
- Amyopathic dermatomyositis
- Psoriasis
- Actinic keratoses
- Skin cancer (squamous or basal cell carcinoma, rarely can mimic Kaposi sarcoma)

DIAGNOSTIC TESTS & INTERPRETATION

Initial Tests (lab, imaging)

Duplex ultrasound (US) imaging helps establish diagnosis and location(s) of venous insufficiency.

Follow-Up Tests & Special Considerations

- Can consider cross-sectional (CT or MR) venography if equivocal US results; be aware these are performed with contrast.
- Special consideration: Skin biopsy may help confirm stasis dermatitis in unclear cases; however, perform with extreme caution due to possibility of co-existing arterial insufficiency, which could result in nonhealing wound at biopsy site.

Diagnostic Procedures/Other

- Rule out arterial insufficiency. Check peripheral pulses; ankle brachial pressure index (ABPI or ABI)
- Screen for diabetes.
- Interventionalist may perform catheter-based venography to verify venous outflow obstruction prior to procedural management.

Test Interpretation

- Duplex US retrograde/reversed flow >0.5 second is diagnostic of reflux in superficial/perforating veins.
- Duplex US retrograde/reversed flow >1 second diagnostic of reflux in deep veins.
- ABPI <0.8 is suggestive of arterial insufficiency.
- ABPI can be elevated, >1.2 in diabetic patients and others with distal small vessel calcifications.
- Arterial duplex US and angiography are the gold standards for arterial insufficiency diagnosis.

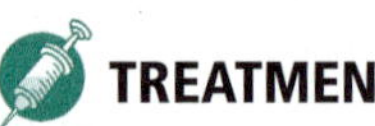

TREATMENT

GENERAL MEASURES

Primary role of treatment is to reverse effects of venous HTN. Appropriate care:

- Outpatient:
  - Reduce edema:
    - Leg elevation: legs above the level of heart for 30 minutes, 3 to 4 times daily; avoid prolonged dependent position.
    - Compression therapy: Mainstay of treatment of venous stasis ± ulcers (1),(2)[A]. Compression bandages can be safely applied in patients with ABI of 0.8 to 1.2.
    - Elastic bandage wraps: Ace bandages or Unna paste boot (zinc gelatin) or compression stockings
    - Graduated elastic compression of 30 to 40 mm Hg at the ankle improves ulcer healing rate and may prevent ulcer recurrence (2)[A].

  - Compression bandages containing both elastic and inelastic components (mixed component systems) are as effective as four-layer bandages, are easier to apply, and have less slippage, and associated with favorable quality of life outcomes.
  - High compression is contraindicated in arterial insufficiency.
  - Pneumatic compression devices are beneficial, especially in nonambulatory patients and those with a component of arterial insufficiency (3)[B].
- Improvement of lipodermatosclerosis:
  - Activity:
    - Avoid standing still for prolonged periods.
    - Stay active and exercise regularly.
    - Elevate foot of bed unless contraindicated.
- Inpatient, for endovascular radiofrequency ablation, vein stripping, sclerotherapy, or skin grafts:
  - Venous ulcer treatment: Treat infection: Débride the ulcer base of necrotic tissue (surgical necrotomy if possible, or enzymatic débridement with collagenase).
    - Autolytic: Modern wound dressings (hydrogel, hydrocolloids, alginate, foam bandages, plain nonadherent dressing) are better than traditional wet to dry dressing because they maintain moist wound environment, with less tissue damage on removal, and less frequent changing requirement (3)[A]. However, there is no difference in healing rate of venous stasis ulcers by use of hydrocolloid dressing versus simple nonadherent dressing when used beneath compression.
    - Biologic: Topical application of granulocyte-macrophage colony-stimulating factor promotes healing of ulcers (insufficient evidence).
    - Mechanical: wet to dry dressings, hydrotherapy, and irrigation
    - Surgical: modifying cause of venous HTN (by venous ligation, valvuloplasty, and endoscopic perforator vein surgery); treat ulcer by graft.

MEDICATION

First Line

- Pentoxifylline 400 mg TID is effective in treating venous leg ulcer.
- The use of low-dose aspirin as adjuvant treatment for venous leg ulcers is not supported.
- Avoid using neomycin, bacitracin, or other topical antiseptics due to lack of reliable evidence for efficacy (4)[A].
- If there is concern for secondary infection, treat with PO antibiotics for *Staphylococcus* or *Streptococcus* organisms (e.g., dicloxacillin 250 mg QID, cephalexin 500 mg QID, or levofloxacin 500 mg daily).
- If MRSA suspected, clindamycin 300 mg QID, doxycycline 100 mg BID, TMP/SMX or IV vancomycin.
- Uncomplicated stasis dermatitis can be treated with short courses (about 2 weeks) of topical steroids (3)[B] (topical triamcinolone 0.1% cream/ointment BID).
- Topical antipruritic: pramoxine, camphor, menthol, and doxepin
- Topical anesthetic (lidocaine/prilocaine) may reduce pain during débridement.
- Silver sulfadiazine (SSD) has a positive effect in wound healing (3)[A].
- Currently, insufficient evidence to recommend routine use of other phlebotonic medications to treat venous insufficiency.

Second Line

- Consider antibiotics on basis of culture results of exudate from infected ulcer craters.
- Lubricants when dermatitis is quiescent
- Chronic stasis dermatitis can be treated with topical emollients (e.g., white petroleum).
- Antipruritic medications (e.g., diphenhydramine, cetirizine hydrochloride)
- Hydrocolloid or a foam dressing may reduce ulcer pain; no evidence that ibuprofen dressings offer pain relief

ISSUES FOR REFERRAL

Consider referral for: nonhealing ulcer, arterial insufficiency, uncertain diagnosis, patch testing to evaluate for contact dermatitis, associated venous insufficiency disease (e.g., symptomatic varicose veins)

ADDITIONAL THERAPIES

Consider discontinuation of medications causing iatrogenic edema (such as amlodipine, gabapentin, etc.) as appropriate.

SURGERY/OTHER PROCEDURES

Sclerotherapy, ablation, valvuloplasty, or vein stripping, and skin grafting may be required for associated disease.

ADMISSION, INPATIENT, AND NURSING CONSIDERATIONS

- Encouraging elevation of the legs, physical activity, and wearing compression stockings.
- Cool compresses or colloidal oatmeal at night, followed by emollient application
- May apply dilute apple cider vinegar for 10 minutes 2 to 3 times weekly to decrease inflammation and reduce *Staphylococcus* colonization by acidifying the skin.

ONGOING CARE

FOLLOW-UP RECOMMENDATIONS

Patient Monitoring

- If Unna boot compression is used: Cut off and reapply boot once a week. Unna boots reduce edema by compression and prevent scratching.
- Regular use of high-compression stockings reduces chance of recurrent venous ulcer.

DIET

Lose weight, if overweight.

PATIENT EDUCATION

- Encourage staying active to keep circulation and leg muscles in good condition. Walking is ideal. Keep legs elevated while sitting or lying.
- Do not wear girdles, garters, or pantyhose with tight elastic tops. Do not scratch.
- Elevate foot of bed with 2- to 4-inch blocks. Apply compression stockings prior to getting out of bed when less edema is present. Regular use of high-compression stockings may prevent recurrence of venous ulcers.

PROGNOSIS

- Chronic course with intermittent exacerbations and remissions
- The healing process for ulceration is often prolonged and may take months.

COMPLICATIONS

- Sensations of itching, pain, and burning have negative impact on the quality of life.
- Secondary bacterial infection
- Contact sensitization to topical agents and superimposed contact dermatitis; auto sensitization rash in remote areas
- Bleeding at dermatitis sites
- Squamous cell carcinoma in edges of long-standing stasis ulcers
- Scarring, which in turn leads to further compromise to blood flow and increased likelihood of minor trauma

D

REFERENCES

1. Yosipovitch G, Nedorost ST, Silverberg JI, et al. Stasis dermatitis: an overview of its clinical presentation, pathogenesis, and management. *Am J Clin Dermatol*. 2023;24(2):275–286.
2. O'Meara S, Cullum N, Nelson EA, et al. Compression for venous leg ulcers. *Cochrane Database Syst Rev*. 2012;11(11):CD000265.
3. Evidence-based (S3) guidelines for diagnostics and treatment of venous leg ulcers. *J Eur Acad Dermatol Venereol*. 2016;30(11):1843–1875.
4. Agnihothri R, Shinkai K. Stasis dermatitis. *JAMA Dermatol*. 2021;157(12):1524.

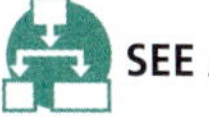

SEE ALSO

- Varicose Veins
- Algorithm: Rash

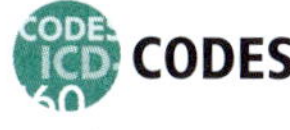

CODES

ICD10

- I83.10 Varicose veins of unsp lower extremity with inflammation
- I83.11 Varicose veins of right lower extremity with inflammation
- I83.12 Varicose veins of left lower extremity with inflammation

CLINICAL PEARLS

Treatment of edema associated with stasis dermatitis via elevation, exercise, and/or mechanical compression (stockings, bandages, or pneumatic devices) is essential for optimal results.

DIABETES MELLITUS, TYPE 1

Vicente T. San Martin, MD • Paloma Rodriguez, MD

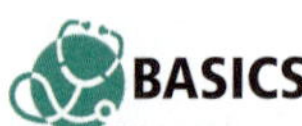

BASICS

DESCRIPTION

- Type 1 diabetes mellitus (T1D) is a chronic disease caused by insulin deficiency following autoimmune β-cell destruction.
- Three stages have been described:
  - 1: positive autoantibodies with normoglycemia
  - 2: positive autoantibodies with glucose intolerance
  - 3: positive autoantibodies with overt diabetes (autoantibodies may disappear over time) (1)[C]
- The velocity of presentation depends on the rate of β-cell destruction.
- Systems affected: endocrine, cardiovascular, nervous, renal, ocular

EPIDEMIOLOGY

- T1D accounts for 5–10% of all cases of diabetes.
- T1D can occur at any age (incidence peaks in puberty and early adulthood).

Incidence

The all-ages incidence for T1D is approximately 11.05 new cases per 100,000 people annually.

Prevalence

Global prevalence is 5.9 per 10,000 people (2)[C].

ETIOLOGY AND PATHOPHYSIOLOGY

There are two main categories of T1D (3)[C].

- Immune-mediated (90–95% of cases)
- Idiopathic: classic T1D presentation with no evidence of autoimmunity

Genetics

T1D has strong HLA associations, with linkage to the DQB1 and DRB1 haplotypes (3)[C].

RISK FACTORS

Increased susceptibility to T1D is inheritable.

GENERAL PREVENTION

Teplizumab is approved in individuals aged ≥8 years with stage 2 T1D, to delay the progression to stage 3 (3)[C].

COMMONLY ASSOCIATED CONDITIONS

Other autoimmune diseases (thyroid, celiac disease, primary adrenal insufficiency, atrophic gastritis)

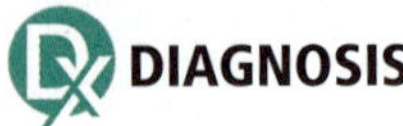

DIAGNOSIS

HISTORY

- Presentation depends on the rate of β-cell destruction and the degree of hyperglycemia.
- May present with mild symptoms or with symptoms of severe hyperglycemia and diabetic ketoacidosis (DKA): polyuria, polydipsia, weight loss, vision changes (blurriness), abdominal pain, nausea, vomiting

PHYSICAL EXAM

- Dehydration
- Kussmaul breathing, acetone odor, abdominal tenderness (in DKA)

DIFFERENTIAL DIAGNOSIS

- Type 2 diabetes
- Monogenic diabetes
- Secondary diabetes (pancreatic disease, drug-induced diabetes, other endocrine-associated diabetes)

DIAGNOSTIC TESTS & INTERPRETATION

Initial Tests (lab, imaging)

- Criteria for the diagnosis of diabetes in nonpregnant patients:
  - Fasting (>8 hours) glucose ≥126 mg/dL, *or*
  - Plasma glucose ≥200 mg/dL 2 hours after a glucose load of 1.75 g/kg (max dose 75 g), *or*
  - Glycated hemoglobin (A1c) ≥6.5%, *or*
  - Random glucose of ≥200 mg/dL in a patient with classic symptoms of hyperglycemia
    - In the absence of unequivocal hyperglycemia (glucose ≥200 mg/dL plus symptoms), the diagnosis requires two abnormal tests (3)[C].
- Other tests: Islet autoantibodies: GAD-65, IA2A, and ZnT8A (If T1D is suspected, assessment of antibodies is recommended as the primary investigation.) (2)[C]

Follow-Up Tests & Special Considerations

Screen for thyroid and celiac disease upon diagnosis and periodically thereafter (3)[C].

Test Interpretation

Any patient meeting diagnostic criteria for diabetes and testing positive for any of the recommended antibodies is considered to have T1D.

TREATMENT

GENERAL MEASURES

- Insulin replacement and education are the pillars of treatment.
- Glycemic goals:
  - Preprandial blood glucose (BG): 80 to 130 mg/dL
  - Peak postprandial BG: <180 mg/dL
  - Pediatric A1c goal: <7.5% (A1c <7% is reasonable if achieved without excessive hypoglycemia.)
  - Adult A1c goal: <7% (or <6.5%; less stringent A1c goals may be appropriate for elderly patients and other special populations.)
  - If using a continuous glucose monitor (CGM), most individuals should aim for a time in range (70 to 180 mg/dL) >70% (or >50% for those with frailty or high risk of hypoglycemia), with <4% time below 70 mg/dL, <1% time below 54 mg/dL and glycemic variability (%CV) ≤36% (2)[C].

MEDICATION

- The goal is to administer exogenous insulin to mimic physiologic insulin secretion, using a long acting insulin for basal replacement and short-acting insulin for mealtime replacement.
  - Basal insulin options:
    - Insulin analogs: insulin glargine, insulin degludec (longest duration of action)
    - Human insulin: NPH (has shorter duration of action and requires 2 or 3 injections per day when used as basal insulin)
  - Prandial insulin options:
    - Insulin analogs: lispro, aspart, glulisine (fastest onset of action and shortest duration of action)
    - Human insulin: regular

First Line

- Initial dose is 0.2 to 0.4 units/kg/day for insulin-naive patients (up to 1 unit/kg/day in puberty)
- ~50% of total dose given as basal and the rest as prandial insulin
- There are two main ways to deliver insulin:
  - Multiple daily injections (MDI) regimen consists of (3)[C]:
    - Basal dose: long-acting insulin once or twice a day
    - Prandial dose: short-acting insulin. Prandial dose has two components:
      - Carbohydrates intake component: an individualized insulin to carbohydrate ratio will be set *plus*
      - Correctional component: based on the individualized insulin sensitivity factor (ISF) and the BG goal (e.g., ISF 50 means that it's predicted that 1 U of insulin will decrease BG by 50 mg/dL)
    - Insulin analogs have the most physiologic profile for both basal and prandial replacement, and therefore are first-line options.
  - Continuous subcutaneous insulin infusion (CSII) of a rapid-acting insulin analog via a pump; this device delivers a continuous and hourly adjustable rate of basal insulin, combined with manual mealtime boluses (3)[C].
- CGM should be offered to all patients with T1D early in the disease.

Second Line

Due to a less physiologic pharmacokinetic profile, MDI using human insulins (NPH and regular) should be considered second line.

ISSUES FOR REFERRAL

All patients with T1D would benefit from endocrinology referral.

ADDITIONAL THERAPIES

- Inhaled rapid acting insulin may be used for mealtime coverage.
- Pancreatic and islet transplantation can potentially normalize glucose levels but require lifelong immunosuppression; allogeneic pancreatic islet cellular therapy (donislecel) is currently indicated for adults unable to reach A1C goals due to recurrent severe hypoglycemia, despite intensive management and education
- Pramlintide: delays gastric emptying, blunts glucagon secretion, and enhances satiety
- Investigational therapies (not yet FDA-approved): insulin icodec (weekly insulin), do-it-yourself automated insulin delivery systems (DIY AID) (3)[C]

SURGERY/OTHER PROCEDURES

- Patients should always have basal insulin continued if not eating prior to a procedure.
- If not eating prior to a procedure, prandial insulin should be held.

ADMISSION, INPATIENT, AND NURSING CONSIDERATIONS

Newly diagnosed patients with T1DM may require hospitalization during initiation of insulin therapy.

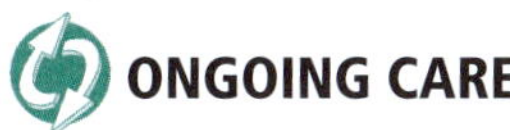

ONGOING CARE

FOLLOW-UP RECOMMENDATIONS

Regular exercise with insulin adjustments to avoid hypoglycemia

Patient Monitoring

- Blood pressure checks at every visit with a goal of <130/80 mm Hg
- Home BG monitoring or CGM are mandatory.
- A1c assessed quarterly
- If concomitant atherosclerotic cardiovascular disease (ASCVD), high-intensity statin therapy should be added.
- For patients aged >40 years, use moderate-intensity statin.
- Annual screenings (starting 5 years after diagnosis):
  - Albuminuria (urine albumin: creatinine ratio)
  - Dilated eye exam
  - Monofilament testing with pinprick, temperature, and vibration sensation
- Vaccines: influenza, pneumococcal pneumonia, hepatitis B, COVID-19

DIET

Carbohydrate counting using insulin-to-carbohydrate ratio with all meals and snacks allow patients flexibility in eating.

PATIENT EDUCATION

Patient education about diagnosis, carbohydrate counting, and nutritional recommendations is fundamental.

PROGNOSIS

Prognosis improves with appropriate glycemic control.

COMPLICATIONS

- Chronic:
  - Microvascular disease (retinopathy, nephropathy, neuropathy)
  - Macrovascular disease (coronary, peripheral, and cerebral artery disease)
- Acute:
  - Hypoglycemia
  - DKA

Pregnancy Considerations

- T1D confers maternal and fetal risk (spontaneous abortion, fetal demise, fetal anomalies, preeclampsia, macrosomia, neonatal hypoglycemia, and neonatal hyperbilirubinemia).
- Preconception counseling should address the importance of glycemic control to reduce risks.
- Glycemic targets: fasting <95 mg/dL, and 1-hour postprandial <140 mg/dL, or 2-hour postprandial <120 mg/dL; if using a CGM, a time in range (63 to 140 mg/dL) of >70% is recommended.
- A1c is lower during pregnancy due to increased RBC turnover; the target is <6% if achieved without hypoglycemia (3)[B].
- Dilated eye examinations should occur before pregnancy or in the 1st trimester, and monitored every trimester, as well as 1-year postpartum (3)[B].
- If no contraindication, women with T1D should start low-dose aspirin during the 1st trimester to lower the risk of preeclampsia (3)[C].

Pediatric Considerations

- In infants and toddlers, symptoms of T1D may be subtle or masquerade as an intercurrent illness.
- Polyuria may present as nocturia, bed-wetting, or incontinence in a previously continent child, and it may be difficult to recognize in diaper-clad children.

REFERENCES

1. Insel RA, Dunne JL, Atkinson MA, et al. Staging presymptomatic type 1 diabetes: a scientific statement of JDRF, the Endocrine Society, and the American Diabetes Association. *Diabetes Care*. 2015;38(10):1964–1974.
2. Holt RIG, DeVries JH, Hess-Fischl A, et al. The management of type 1 diabetes in adults. A consensus report by the American Diabetes Association (ADA) and the European Association for the Study of Diabetes (EASD). *Diabetes Care*. 2021;44(11):2589–2625.
3. American Diabetes Association Professional Practice Committee. 9. Pharmacologic approaches to glycemic treatment: standards of care in diabetes–2025. *Diabetes Care*. 2025;48(1 Suppl 1):S181–S206.

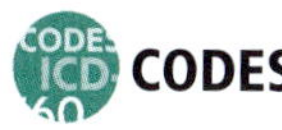

CODES

ICD10

- E10.319 Type 1 diabetes mellitus with unspecified diabetic retinopathy without macular edema
- E10.321 Type 1 diabetes mellitus with mild nonproliferative diabetic retinopathy with macular edema
- E10.351 Type 1 diabetes mellitus with proliferative diabetic retinopathy with macular edema

CLINICAL PEARLS

- T1D can occur at any age, but its incidence peaks in puberty and early adulthood.
- Any patient meeting diagnostic criteria for diabetes and testing positive for any of the recommended antibodies is considered to have T1D.
- A random C-peptide level, measured beyond 3 years of diabetes diagnosis, could be useful to differentiate from other types of diabetes if there is uncertainty (a C-peptide level <200 pmol/L is suggestive of T1D).
- Therapy with MDI or CSII and a multidisciplinary team care approach are associated with improved glycemic control, resulting in better long-term outcomes.
- Adult A1c goal is <7.0%; less stringent A1c goals may be appropriate for elderly patients and other special populations.

D

DIABETES MELLITUS, TYPE 2

Joseph Daniel Hogue, MD, MBA • Avinash Patel, MD • Mauro Amendola, MD, FAAFP

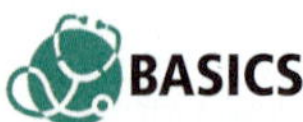

BASICS

DESCRIPTION

Diabetes mellitus (DM) type 2 is due to a progressive insulin secretory defect in the setting of insulin resistance.

Geriatric Considerations

Monitor for hypoglycemia; adjust doses for renal/hepatic dysfunction and cognitive function; less aggressive glucose targets than younger patients

Pediatric Considerations

Incidence is increasing and parallels obesity epidemic.

Pregnancy Considerations

- Diet, metformin, glyburide, and insulin are all options for treatment of gestational diabetes.
- In person with history of gestational diabetes, screen for diabetes/prediabetes with oral glucose tolerance test (OGTT) 6 to 12 weeks postpartum and every 3 years.

EPIDEMIOLOGY

Prevalence

Estimated 37.3 million Americans (11.3% of the population); 90–95% are likely type 2. Globally, prevalence is estimated to be 10.5% of adults.

ETIOLOGY AND PATHOPHYSIOLOGY

- Peripheral insulin resistance and defective insulin secretion with increased hepatic gluconeogenesis
- Obesity and visceral adiposity
- Associated with dyslipidemia, hypertension, and gut microbiome changes
- Drug or chemical induced (e.g., glucocorticoids, antiretroviral therapy, atypical antipsychotics, organ transplant immunosuppressants)

Genetics

- Family history is strongly predictive of risk.
- Polygenic; rarely monogenic (e.g., peroxisome proliferator-activated receptor [*PPAR*] γ and insulin gene mutations)

RISK FACTORS

- Parental history of type 2 diabetes: 2-fold to 3-fold increased risk
- Gestational diabetes or history of baby with birth weight ≥4 kg (≥9 lb)
- Polycystic ovarian syndrome (PCOS)
- Hypertriglyceridemia or low high-density lipoprotein (HDL)
- Ethnicity: African American, Latino, Native American, Asian, and Pacific Islander
- Sedentary lifestyle, visceral obesity

GENERAL PREVENTION

- Maintenance of normal weight, or weight loss of 7% body weight, decrease intake of carbohydrates and overall calories; moderate–intensity exercise (150 min/week)
- Metformin, α-glucosidase inhibitors, thiazolidinediones (TZDs), and glucagon-like peptide-1 receptor agonist (GLP-1 RA) in prediabetes

COMMONLY ASSOCIATED CONDITIONS

Hypertension, dyslipidemia, metabolic syndrome, fatty liver disease, PCOS, acanthosis nigricans, hemochromatosis

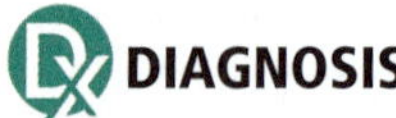

DIAGNOSIS

HISTORY

Polyuria, polydipsia, polyphagia, weight loss, fatigue, blurry vision, neuropathy, and frequent infections; many individuals are asymptomatic.

PHYSICAL EXAM

BMI, waist circumference, funduscopic exam, oral exam, cardiopulmonary exam, abdominal exam for hepatomegaly, focused neurologic exam, skin exam and diabetic foot exam

DIFFERENTIAL DIAGNOSIS

- Type 1 DM—low or absent insulin, C-peptide, positive β-cell autoantibodies, ketosis
- DM is one of the features of Cushing syndrome, acromegaly, pheochromocytoma, and glucagonoma
- Monogenic diabetes, latent autoimmune diabetes in adults (LADA), medication induced hyperglycemia

DIAGNOSTIC TESTS & INTERPRETATION

Initial Tests (lab, imaging)

Criteria for diagnosis

- HbA1c ≥6.5% *or*
- Hyperglycemic symptoms and random plasma glucose ≥200 mg/dL (11.1 mmol/L) *or*
- Fasting plasma glucose (FPG) ≥126 mg/dL (7 mmol/L) on two different occasions *or*
- 2-hour plasma glucose ≥200 mg/dL (11.1 mmol/L) during OGTT with 75-g glucose load
- If equivocal, perform different test on same sample or a repeat the test.

TREATMENT

Tight glucose control prevents long-term microvascular complications, but benefits on macrovascular outcomes are less apparent. Individuals likely to benefit from a more aggressive target are those without preexisting DM complications, with recent diagnoses of DM, and with long life expectancy.

- Use patient-centered approach.
- Dietary modification, regular exercise, control of cardiovascular risk factors (blood pressure [BP] and lipids)
- HbA1c targets—ADA recommendations and ACP targets differ.
  - HbA1c <7.0%: long life expectancy, no cardiovascular disease (CVD), short duration of DM, no history of hypoglycemia
  - HbA1c <8.0%: Limited life expectancy, advanced microvascular or macrovascular complications, extensive comorbidities, history of severe hypoglycemia or long-standing DM where lower goal is difficult to attain.
  - The ACP recommends an HbA1c between 7% and 8% in most patients.
  - ADA recommends preprandial glucose 80 to 130 mg/dL; postprandial glucose <180 mg/dL
- Continuous glucose monitoring (CGM) may be beneficial in patients using multiple-dose insulin (≥3 injections/day) or on an insulin pump, as well as those who have frequent or severe hypoglycemia, nocturnal hypoglycemia, or hypoglycemia unawareness (1).
- For patients not requiring insulin or insulin secretagogues, blood glucose monitoring may still be beneficial to provide feedback on lifestyle and pharmacologic therapy response.
- For cardiorenal risk reduction in high-risk patients, initiate therapy with GLP-1 RA or SGLT2 inhibitors with proven CVD benefit. SGLT2 inhibitors have proven benefit in patients with heart failure and CKD with GFR <60 or albuminuria >30 mg/g. Metformin to be used in combination to maintain HbA1c goal.
- Other alternatives include DPP-4i, TZD, sulfonyreas, and insulin.
- Always consider side effect profile, CV benefit, renal benefit, and cost.

GENERAL MEASURES

- Neuropathy: annual neurofilament foot exam
- Nephropathy: annual urine microalbumin-to-creatinine ratio and plasma creatinine (eGFR)
- Retinopathy: annual diabetic eye exam
- If 40 to 84 years old, prescribe moderate-to-high intensity statin.
- Hypertension: goal BP <130/80 mm Hg
- Pneumonia vaccine all diabetic patients aged ≥19 years; other age appropriate vaccines based on ACIP (1)

MEDICATION

First Line

Metformin—500 to 1,000 mg in divided doses BID or extended release QD (maximum 2,000 mg/day)

- Preferred due to high efficacy in lowering glucose, good safety profile, low hypoglycemia risk, low cost; weight neutral
- Avoid in severe acute illnesses (e.g., liver disease, cardiogenic shock, pancreatitis, hypoxia) due to risk of lactic acidosis.
- Caution with acute heart failure, alcohol abuse, elderly; associated with vitamin B_{12} deficiency
- Severe diarrhea in 10% of patients, requiring switch to another agent
- In CKD for eGFR 30 to 45 reduce dose to ≤1,000 mg, stop if eGFR <30.

Second Line

- General principles
  - If patient has CAD, heart failure, or CKD, consider drugs that improve outcomes with these conditions as first-line agents.
  - Consider drug-specific side effects such as weight gain, hypoglycemia.
  - Cost of drug is an important consideration.
- GLP-1 RA (incretins)
  - Exenatide (Byetta): 5 to 10 μg SC BID or exenatide ER (Bydureon) 2 mg/week
  - Liraglutide (Victoza): 0.6 to 1.8 mg/day; improved CV outcomes (2)

- Dulaglutide (Trulicity): 0.75 to 4.50 mg weekly; improved CV outcomes (2)
- Lixisenatide (Adlyxin): up to 20 μg SC QD
- Semaglutide injection (Ozempic): 0.25 to 2.00 mg weekly; improved CV outcomes (2); oral (Rybelsus) 3 to 14 mg daily neutral CV risk (1)
- Reduced risk of atherosclerotic CVD events
- Low hypoglycemia risk, promotes weight loss
- Small risk of acute pancreatitis, constipation, vitamin deficiency, gastroparesis
- Use cautiously in CKD $\geq$ stage 4.
- Contraindicated in personal or family history of medullary thyroid cancer or multiple endocrine neoplasia (MEN) type 2

• GLP-1/GIP RA—tirzepatide (Mounjaro): 2.5 to 15.0 mg weekly injection
  - Trials showed doses of 5 mg, 10 mg, 15 mg had clinically meaningful HbA1c reduction compared to placebo (3), superior HbA1c and weight reductions when compared to semaglutide and titrated insulin degludec
  - Similar side effect profile as GLP-1 RAs

• SGLT2 inhibitors
  - Canagliflozin (Invokana): 100 to 300 mg/day
  - Dapagliflozin (Farxiga): 5 to 10 mg daily
  - Empagliflozin (Jardiance): 10 to 25 mg daily
  - Ertugliflozin (Steglatro): 5 to 15 mg daily
  - Inhibit renal glucose reabsorption, cause weight loss, no hypoglycemia risk
  - Canagliflozin, dapagliflozin, and empagliflozin reduce CV mortality; slow progression of renal disease
  - Risk of genital mycotic infections and UTI; higher risk of euglycemic diabetic ketoacidosis (DKA); higher fracture risk; relatively expensive
    - Can be used in patients with GFR >20 mL/min up until dialysis or renal transplant
  - Dipeptidyl peptidase-4 (DPP-4) inhibitors
    - Alogliptin 25 mg daily
    - Saxagliptin 5 mg daily
    - Linagliptin 5 mg daily
    - Sitagliptin 100 mg daily
    - Inhibit DPP-4 enzyme, which deactivates endogenous GLP-1 and GIP
    - Low risk for hypoglycemia; reduce dose in renal impairment except linagliptin.
    - Weight neutral
    - No evidence for CV risk reduction
  - Sulfonylureas
    - Glipizide (Glucotrol): 2.5 to 40.0 mg/day
    - Glipizide extended-release: 5 to 20 mg/day
    - Glyburide (DiaBeta, Micronase): 1.25 to 20.00 mg/day, Glynase: 0.75 to 12.00 mg/day
    - Glimepiride (Amaryl): 1 to 8 mg/day
    - Stimulate β-cell production of insulin
    - Caution with renal or liver disease, sulfa allergy, creatinine clearance <50 mL/min.
    - Potentiate weight gain, high hypoglycemia risk especially when used with insulin
    - Inexpensive
  - TZD—pioglitazone (Actos): 15 to 45 mg/day; rosiglitazone (Avandia): 4 to 8 mg/day
    - Increases insulin sensitivity; activates PPARs
    - Pioglitazone reduces triglycerides; low cost
    - Can worsen heart failure symptoms
    - Increased risk of fractures/low bone mass
  - Insulin
    - Increases glucose disposal, inhibits hepatic glucose production
    - Consider as initial therapy if HbA1c >9%, catabolic symptoms, ketosis.
    - Use as additional therapy after dual/triple therapy has been tried.
    - Weight gain and hypoglycemia risk
    - Analogs have lower hypoglycemia risk than NPH and regular insulin but more expensive.
    - Basal insulin: Start with 0.1 to 0.3 U/kg/day. Titrate up every 2 days until achievement of desired result. Add mealtime (rapid/short-acting) insulin if post meal glucose is high. Mealtime starting dose can be 4 U or 10% of basal dose.
  - Rapid-acting analogs—lispro (Humalog), aspart (Novolog), glulisine (Apidra): duration of action 3 to 5 hours; ultrarapid (Fiasp and lispro-aabc) quicker onset
  - Inhaled insulin (Afrezza): rapid onset of action; duration of action 4.5 hours
  - Short-acting insulin—human regular (Humulin R/Novolin R/ReliOn R): duration of action 6 to 8 hours
  - Intermediate-acting insulin—human NPH (Humulin N/Novolin N/ReliOn N): duration 13 to 20 hours; human regular U-500 (Humulin R U-500): duration 6 to 10 hours
  - Basal insulin analogs—glargine U-100 (Lantus, Basaglar): duration 22 to 24 hours; glargine U-300 (Toujeo): duration 36 hours; degludec U-100, U-200 (Tresiba): duration 42 hours
  - Premixed insulin products—NPH/regular 70/30 (Novolin 70/30, Humulin 70/30), 70/30 and 50/50 aspart mix (Novolog mix), 75/25 and 50/50 lispro mix (Humalog mix)
  - Amylinomimetic—pramlintide (Symlin): 60 to 120 μg SC premeal
    - Delays gastric emptying, blunts glucagon, enhances satiety and weight loss
  - α-Glucosidase inhibitors—acarbose (Precose): 25 to 100 mg TID; miglitol (Glyset): 25 to 100 mg TID
    - Slows intestinal carbohydrate digestion, reduced post meal hyperglycemia
    - Avoid in renal insufficiency and bowel diseases.
  - Meglitinides—repaglinide (Prandin): 0.5 to 4.0 mg TID; nateglinide (Starlix): 60 to 120 mg TID
    - Take at beginning of meals.
    - Mechanism similar to SU but much shorter duration of action

• Combination therapy with drugs from different classes with complementary mechanisms of actions can be helpful.

SURGERY/OTHER PROCEDURES
Consider bariatric surgery if BMI >35 kg/m^2

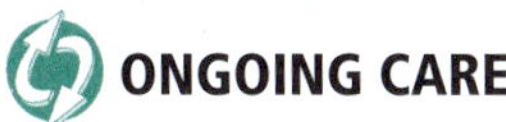

ONGOING CARE

PATIENT EDUCATION
Diabetes self-management

PROGNOSIS
Normal lifespan with good management

COMPLICATIONS
- ASCVD, peripheral vascular disease, stroke, foot ulcers, Charcot joints
- Microvascular: neuropathy, retinopathy, diabetic CKD
- GI: fatty liver disease, gastroparesis

REFERENCES

1. Samson SL, Vellanki P, Blonde L, et al. American Association of Clinical Endocrinology consensus statement: comprehensive type 2 diabetes management algorithm—2023 update. *Endocr Pract*. 2023;29(5):305–340.
2. Sim R, Chong CW, Loganadan NK, et al. Comparative effectiveness of cardiovascular, renal and safety outcomes of second-line antidiabetic drugs use in people with type 2 diabetes: a systematic review and network meta-analysis of randomised controlled trials. *Diabet Med*. 2022;39(3):e14780. doi:10.1111/dme.14780.
3. Min T, Bain SC. The role of tirzepatide, dual GIP and GLP-1 receptor agonist, in the management of type 2 diabetes: the SURPASS clinical trials. *Diabetes Ther*. 2021;12(1):143–157. doi:10.1007/s13300-020-00981-0.

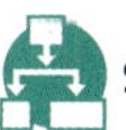

SEE ALSO

- Diabetes Mellitus, Type 1; Diabetic Ketoacidosis; Hypertension, Essential
- Algorithms: Type 2 Diabetes, Treatment; Weight Loss, Treatment

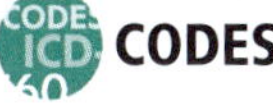

CODES

ICD10
- E11.329 Type 2 diabetes mellitus with mild nonproliferative diabetic retinopathy without macular edema
- E11.331 Type 2 diabetes mellitus with moderate nonproliferative diabetic retinopathy with macular edema
- E11.359 Type 2 diabetes mellitus with proliferative diabetic retinopathy without macular edema

CLINICAL PEARLS
- Individualize treatments and HbA1c targets based on life expectancy and comorbidities.
- Hypoglycemia poses more short-term danger than hyperglycemia.

DIABETIC KETOACIDOSIS

Daniel R. Matta, MD, DFPHM, FAAFP • Amanda Kimberley Davis, MD, MBBS

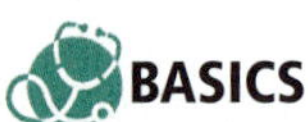

BASICS

DESCRIPTION

- A life-threatening medical emergency which most commonly occurs in patients with type 1 diabetes; however, it may occur in any type of diabetes mellitus and at any age.
- Characterized by a biochemical triad of hyperglycemia, ketosis, and high anion gap metabolic acidosis
- Rarely, it can occur in the absence of hyperglycemia (i.e., euglycemic diabetic ketoacidosis [DKA]) during pregnancy and in individuals taking sodium-glucose cotransporter-2 (SGLT2) inhibitors
- System(s) affected: endocrine/metabolic, neurology

EPIDEMIOLOGY

Incidence

Incidence by age group: 1 to 17 years (10.1%), 18 to 44 years (53.3%), 45 to 64 years (27.1%), 65 to 84 years (8.7%), and 85+ years (0.8%); most events occur in ages 17 to 44 years with type 1 diabetes mellitus (T1DM).

ETIOLOGY AND PATHOPHYSIOLOGY

- Impaired glucose utilization secondary to insulin deficiency leading to the activation of counter regulatory mechanisms (gluconeogenesis, glycogenolysis, proteolysis) which further increase blood glucose level and trigger ketone bodies production; resulting ketonemia and hyperglycemia lead to osmotic diuresis, dehydration, electrolytes disturbances and acidosis.
- Leading causes include infection, particularly UTI and pneumonia, and medication noncompliance. Other precipitating factors are:
  - First presentation of DM
  - Myocardial infarction (MI); cerebrovascular accident (CVA), pulmonary embolism (PE), pancreatitis
  - Medications (corticosteroids, sympathomimetics (e.g., dobutamine and terbutaline), atypical antipsychotics, SGLT2 inhibitors)
  - Alcohol and Illicit drugs (cocaine)
  - Trauma; surgery
  - Emotional stress, psychiatric comorbidities and social determinants of health
  - Pregnancy

RISK FACTORS

- Type 1 DM
- Ketosis-prone Type 2 DM (Hispanic and African American ethnicity, G6PD deficiency)
- Euglycemic ketoacidosis specially with SGLT2 inhibitor drug use
- Covid-19 infection
- Younger age at the time of DKA hospitalization, higher HbA1c, lower physical activity, lower socioeconomic status, and psychiatric symptoms have been associated with increased rates of DKA.

GENERAL PREVENTION

- Close monitoring of glucose during periods of stress, illness, and trauma with "sick day" management instructions
- Careful insulin control and regular monitoring of blood glucose levels along with education on symptom recognition

COMMONLY ASSOCIATED CONDITIONS

Over 30% of patients have features of both DKA and hyperosmolar hyperglycemic syndrome (HHS).

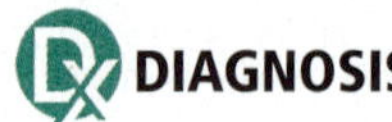

DIAGNOSIS

- Diagnostic criteria
  - Hyperglycemia >200 mg/dL or prior history of diabetes mellitus
  - Low bicarbonate (HCO_3) (usually ≤18 mEq/L)
  - Metabolic acidosis on arterial blood gases (ABGs) (pH <7.3)
  - Anion gap = serum sodium − (serum chloride + bicarbonate); >10 mmol
  - β-Hydroxybutyrate (β-HOB) ≥3 mmol/L or urine ketone ≥2+
- Diagnosis can be stratified into three levels of severity depending on laboratory findings and physical exam, most importantly the mental status.
  - Mild: pH >7.25 to <7.30; bicarbonate 15 to 18 mEq/L; alert; regular or observation nursing unit recommended moderate: pH 7.00 to 7.25; bicarbonate 10 to <15 mEq/L; alert or drowsy; intermediate care unit recommended
  - Severe: pH <7 bicarbonate and <10 mEq/L; stupor; ICU care required
- Individualization of treatment based on clinical and laboratory assessment is needed.

HISTORY

- Recent illness, injury, or surgery
- Changes in diet or medications; missed insulin doses/noncompliance, insulin pump failure
- Polyuria, polydipsia, polyphagia, weight loss, and dehydration
- Generalized weakness, malaise, fatigue, lethargy, nausea, vomiting, abdominal pain; develops over hours to days
- Anorexia or increased appetite

PHYSICAL EXAM

- Vital signs: hypotension, tachycardia, fever, or hypothermia
- Tachypnea, hyperpnea, Kussmaul respirations
- Fruity odor of ketotic breath (acetone smell)
- Abdominal tenderness, decreased bowel sounds
- Dry mucous membranes, poor skin turgor, dehydration
- Decreased reflexes
- Altered mental status, coma

DIFFERENTIAL DIAGNOSIS

- Hyperosmolar hyperglycemic state
- Alcoholic ketoacidosis, starvation ketosis, lactic acidosis
- Toxic ingestions (e.g., salicylates, methanol, ethylene glycol)
- Sepsis
- Acute pancreatitis

DIAGNOSTIC TESTS & INTERPRETATION

Initial Tests (lab, imaging)

ALERT

- Important labs:
  - β-HOB is the predominant ketone produced and is preferred over other serum ketones. β-HOB >3 mg/dL is abnormal and should be decreased to <1.5 mg/dL within 12 to 24 hours.
  - ABG or venous blood gases (VBG) for pH assessment: VBG pH correlates with 0.03 lower than ABG pH.
  - Urinalysis: ketonuria, glycosuria
  - Creatinine and BUN: Markedly increased serum ketones may cross-react and cause a falsely high serum creatinine.
  - Electrolytes derangements: hypomagnesemia, hypophosphatemia, base deficit with high anion gap
  - Decreased total body K^+: Severe acidosis causes an artificially elevated K^+ level.
  - Pseudohyponatremia secondary to hyperglycemia or hypertriglyceridemia: It is now accepted to correct Na+ concentration by adding 2.4 mmol/L to measured Na+ for every 100 mg/dL increase in serum glucose above 100 mg/dL.
  - Calculate serum osmolality: If calculated osmolality <320 mOsm/kg, consider etiologies other than DKA especially in patients with altered mentation.
  - Glycosylated hemoglobin (HbA1c) helps assess long-term history of diabetic control.
  - CBC: Consider DKA-related leukocytosis versus infection.
- Other tests
  - Blood and urine culture, chest x-ray, and lumbar puncture based on clinical suspicion for infection
  - ECG: frequently shows nonspecific sinus tachycardia, changes consistent with electrolyte abnormalities, and/or ischemic changes with MI as a precipitation factor
  - Troponin
  - Head CT scan if CVA or cerebral edema suspected

Follow-Up Tests & Special Considerations

Elevated lipase and amylase might not be reliable for diagnosis of pancreatitis in DKA.

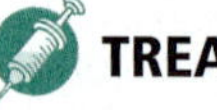

TREATMENT

- Restore circulatory volume and tissue perfusion.
- Gradual reduction of glucose level and osmolality
- Resolution of anion gap acidosis and ketosis
- Correction of electrolytes imbalance
- Identify and treat precipitating cause(s).

GENERAL MEASURES

- Severe DKA requires an ICU setting.
- Fluid resuscitation: Start isotonic crystalloid solution (e.g., 0.9% saline, or lactated Ringers bolus).
- Check serum glucose every hour along with serum electrolytes, BUN, creatinine, venous pH, and glucose every 2–4 hours until stable.
- Insulin infusion is the standard of care for critically ill and mentally obtunded patients. Subcutaneous (SC) insulin can be considered in uncomplicated DKA (1).

MEDICATION

First Line

- Intravenous fluid (IVF) is a priority.
  - Start fluid of choice at 15 to 20 mL/kg of body weight or 1,000 to 1,500 mL in the first hour of treatment.
  - After the first hour, IVF infusion rate should be adjusted based on hemodynamics and electrolytes (usually 250 to 500 mL/hr in patients without cardiac, renal, or hepatic compromise).
  - Consider use of 0.45% NaCl in patients with normal to high corrected Na+ concentration after initial fluid resuscitation. Although continuous 0.9% NaCl is not contraindicated, risk of hyperchloremic metabolic acidosis should also be considered.
  - When glucose is 200 mg/dL, change to 5% or 10% dextrose with 0.45% NaCl at same rate to prevent hypoglycemia.
    - In euglycemic DKA (glucose <200 with positive β-HOB) the 5% or 10% dextrose should be added to the 0.9% NaCl (or other chosen crystalloid) at the start of the insulin treatment (2).
- Insulin: Start IV infusion after initial IVF resuscitation and correction of hypokalemia (<3.3 mg/dL).
  - Optional initial bolus 0.1 U/kg IV and then continuous infusion at 0.1 U/kg/hr (do not use initial insulin bolus in children)
  - If bolus not given, 0.14 U/kg/hr continuous infusion is recommended.
  - Aim for rate of serum glucose reduction of 50 to 75 mg/dL/hr in the first hour; adjust infusion rate hourly until steady decline is achieved.
  - ADA recommends reducing infusion rate to 0.02 to 0.05 U/kg/hr IV to maintain serum glucose between 150 and 200 mg/dL until correction of acidosis.
  - Use of SC basal insulin (glargine 0.25 U/kg SC) within 12 hours of starting treatment may result in reduction of time to gap closure, shorter hospital stay, and less rebound hyperglycemia
  - Overlap and continue IV insulin infusion for 2 to 4 hours after SC insulin is initiated, to prevent recurrence of ketoacidosis and rebound hyperglycemia.
- Potassium: Establish adequate renal function (output ~0.5 mL/kg/hr). Start replacement with 10 to 20 mEq/L/hr of K^+ IV fluids when serum K^+ ≤5 mg/dL and continue to maintain K^+ between 4 and 5 (2).
  - Hold insulin if K^+ ≤3.3 mg/dL; give IV potassium 20 to 30 mEq/hr with fluids until >3.3 mg/dL to prevent cardiac arrhythmia. For each 0.1 unit of pH, serum K^+ will change by ~0.6 mEq in opposite direction.
- Phosphorus: Give only if there is muscle weakness, respiratory compromise and phosphorus <1 mg/dL. Dose: 20 to 30 mEq/L of K-Phos in fluids; may lead to hypocalcemia (2)
- Sodium bicarbonate: Use is not recommended.
- Magnesium: If Mg ≤1.2 mg/dL or ≤1.8 and patient is symptomatic, magnesium treatment should be considered.
- Precautions: If glucose does not fall by 10% in first hour, give regular insulin 0.14 U/kg IV bolus and then continuous infusion at previous rate.

Second Line

- In mild to moderate DKA, there is no significant difference in outcomes between the use of regular human IV insulin versus SC rapid acting analogs when combined with aggressive fluid administration (1).
- The use of SC insulin in uncomplicated DKA requires adequate fluid replacement, frequent POC blood glucose monitoring, treatment of concurrent infections, and adequate follow up to prevent recurrent DKA (1).
- Rapid acting SC insulin can be considered for patients who are alert, tolerating PO intake, serum bicarbonate >10 mEq/L, and pH >7.
- Load with 0.3 U/kg SC, followed by 0.1 to 0.2 U/kg q1–2h. Once glucose <200 mg/dL, reduce dosing to 0.05 to 0.10 U/kg q1–2 hours till resolution of ketoacidosis.

Pediatric Considerations

- Initial insulin infusion rates of 0.05 to 0.10 U/kg/hr are recommended (3)[C].
- Cerebral edema is a rare complication (~1%) but has a mortality of 20–50%. Treatment should be started as soon as suspected clinically and not delayed for neuroimaging.

Pregnancy Considerations

- DKA per se is not an indication for emergency delivery; imperative to stabilize mother first
- Euglycemic DKA

ADMISSION, INPATIENT, AND NURSING CONSIDERATIONS

- Admission criteria: blood glucose >250 mg/dL; pH <7.3; HCO_3 ≤15 mEq/L; ketones in urine; ICU setting for severe DKA
- Check renal function, electrolytes, venous pH, osmolality and glucose every 2 to 4 hours until stable (2).
- Discharge when DKA has resolved anion gap <12, glucose <200 mg/dL; pH >7.3; bicarbonate >18 mEq/L, plasma/capillary ketones <0.06 mmol/L. Patient must be tolerating PO intake and able to resume home medication regimen.

ONGOING CARE

FOLLOW-UP RECOMMENDATIONS

Follow up within 1 to 2 weeks for poorly controlled diabetics.

DIET

- NPO initially, advance diet when nausea and vomiting are controlled
- Avoid foods with high glycemic index (e.g., soft drinks, fruit juice, white bread, added sugar).

PATIENT EDUCATION

- Self-monitoring of glucose, glucose goals, and when to call PCP
- Recognition and prevention of hypoglycemia
- Early recognition and prevention of insulin pump failure
- Healthy nutritional choices
- Sick day management
- Proper use of insulin syringes/needles

PROGNOSIS

- Worse in the extremes of age and in the setting of coma and hypotension
- Overall DKA mortality of 0.5–2%; appropriate management has decreased mortality to <1% (2).

COMPLICATIONS

- Cerebral edema (most common cause of death in children with DKA)
- Pulmonary edema, respiratory distress, MI
- Vascular thrombosis
- Cardiac dysrhythmia (secondary to hypokalemia or acidosis)
- Acute renal failure

REFERENCES

1. American Diabetes Association Professional Practice Committee. 16. Diabetes care in the hospital: standards of care in diabetes—2025. *Diabetes Care*. 2025;48(1 Suppl 1):S321–S334.
2. Umpierrez GE, Davis GM, ElSayed NA, et al. Hyperglycemic crises in adults with diabetes: a consensus report. *Diabetes Care*. 2024;47(8):1257–1275. doi:10.2337/dci24-0032.
3. Cashen K, Petersen T. Diabetic Ketoacidosis. *Pediatric Rev*. 2019;40(8):412–420.

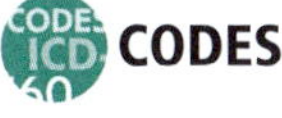

CODES

ICD10

- E10.11 Type 1 diabetes mellitus with ketoacidosis with coma
- E10.10 Type 1 diabetes mellitus with ketoacidosis without coma
- E13.11 Other specified diabetes mellitus with ketoacidosis with coma

CLINICAL PEARLS

- DKA is defined by a classic clinical triad of hyperglycemia, ketosis, and high anion gap metabolic acidosis.
- Admit if blood glucose >250 mg/dL, pH <7.3, HCO_3 ≤15 mEq/L, and ketones in urine.
- Potassium is falsely elevated due to acidosis; start replacement when K^+ ≤5.2 mg/dL and urine output is adequate.
- Resolution occurs when: venous pH >7.3, bicarb >18 mmol/L, plasma/capillary ketones <0.06 mmol/L. (2)

DIABETIC POLYNEUROPATHY

Madhavi Medipally, MD, FAAFP

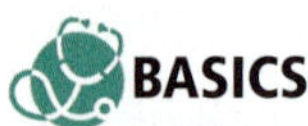

BASICS

DESCRIPTION

Peripheral nerve dysfunction seen in diabetes; several patterns described:

- Symmetric polyneuropathy: distal sensory or sensorimotor
- Mononeuropathy, radiculopathy, and polyradiculopathy
  - Cranial neuropathy
  - Focal limb or truncal neuropathy
  - Radiculoplexus neuropathy (diabetic amyotrophy)
- Acute painful small fiber neuropathy
- Autonomic neuropathies
- Chronic inflammatory demyelinating polyneuropathy (CIDP)

EPIDEMIOLOGY

Prevalence

Generalized polyneuropathy

- 10–30% at diabetes diagnosis
- 50% at 10 years
- Prevalence is higher in type 2 diabetes than type 1 diabetes.

ETIOLOGY AND PATHOPHYSIOLOGY

- Metabolic derangement due to hyperglycemia and dyslipidemia
  - Aldose reductase converts excess glucose to sorbitol, which causes nerve damage.
  - Nonenzymatic glycation of neural proteins and lipids forms damaging advanced glycosylation end products.
  - Protein kinase C activation causes vascular endothelial changes.
  - Oxidative stress from excessive production of reactive oxygen species
- Vasculopathy causing nerve ischemia: predominant factor in mononeuropathies

RISK FACTORS

- Poor glycemic control
- Duration of diabetes
- Hypertension
- Dyslipidemia
- Obesity
- Tobacco and alcohol consumption

GENERAL PREVENTION

- Maintenance of normal blood sugar
- Exercise and appropriate diet

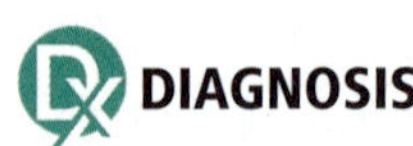

DIAGNOSIS

Individuals with type 1 diabetes duration >5 years and all individuals with type 2 diabetes should be assessed annually for diabetic polyneuropathy using history and clinical tests (1).

HISTORY

- Most common form (typical): symmetric distal sensory or sensorimotor polyneuropathy
  - Distressing numbness, tingling, pain of legs/feet, usually worse at night; allodynia; hyperalgesia
  - Silent sensory loss, patient unaware
  - Ataxia and falls due to proprioceptive loss
  - Neuropathic foot ulcers due to analgesia and repetitive injury
  - Neuropathic degeneration of foot joints
  - Hands involved late
  - Distal muscle involvement
- Symmetric proximal polyneuropathy
  - Proximal leg weakness and wasting
  - Muscles of shoulder girdle rarely involved
  - Pain and sensory changes less prominent
- Focal cranial or limb mononeuropathy
  - May involve 3rd, 4th, 6th, or 7th cranial nerve
  - Femoral, sciatic, or peroneal neuropathy: weakness or pain in nerve distribution
  - Any major peripheral nerve can be involved.
- Truncal neuropathies: painful radiculopathy over dermatomes
- Lumbar radiculoplexus neuropathy (diabetic amyotrophy)
  - Unilateral hip, thigh pain
  - Pelvic girdle and thigh weakness with atrophy
  - Recovery over months
- Diabetic autonomic neuropathy
  - GI: nocturnal diarrhea, sometimes alternating with constipation; gastroparesis with postprandial fullness; nausea and vomiting
  - Cardiovascular: postural dizziness, exercise intolerance
  - Urogenital: urinary hesitancy, overflow incontinence; erectile dysfunction; vaginal dryness; sexual dysfunction
  - Sudomotor: anhidrosis or hyperhidrosis; gustatory sweating of head and upper body
- CIDP: progressive, severe motor loss
- Diabetic cachexia: painful small fiber neuropathy with prominent weight loss and depression

PHYSICAL EXAM

- Symmetric distal polyneuropathy
  - "Stocking-and-glove" distal sensory loss
  - Large-fiber neuropathy: loss of vibration perception with 128-Hz tuning fork, absent ankle reflexes, balance issues and loss of protective sensation (LOPS) with 10-g monofilament
  - Small fiber involvement: loss of temperature and pinprick
  - Wasting, weakness of small muscles in foot; changes to arch of foot or clawing of toes
  - With small fiber involvement, there may be lack of objective sensory deficit despite pain.
- Symmetric proximal polyneuropathy
  - Proximal leg, arm wasting, and weakness
  - Loss of patellar reflexes
- Focal cranial or limb mononeuropathy
  - 3rd cranial nerve palsy: painful ophthalmoplegia and ptosis; preserved pupillary reflexes (in contrast to compressive palsies)
  - 6th cranial nerve: lateral gaze palsy
  - Femoral neuropathy: weakness of lower leg extension, hip flexion, quadriceps wasting, absent patellar reflex, sensory loss in anterior thigh
  - Sciatic neuropathy: pain or sensory loss in back of thigh and leg; weakness of hamstrings, lower leg muscles
  - Peroneal neuropathy: foot drop
- Truncal neuropathies: sensory loss along dermatome
- Lumbar radiculoplexopathy (amyotrophy)
  - Weakness and wasting pelvic girdle and thigh
  - Sensory loss in L2–L3
  - Absent patellar reflex
- Autonomic neuropathy
  - Cardiovascular: resting tachycardia; orthostatic hypotension, syncope
  - Gastroparesis: postprandial distension; gastric splash
- CIDP: motor weakness

DIFFERENTIAL DIAGNOSIS

- Metabolic
  - Uremia, hypothyroidism
- Drug induced
  - Antineoplastic drugs: cisplatin, vincristine
  - Antimicrobial drugs: metronidazole, nitrofurantoin and fluoroquinolones, isoniazid
  - Anticonvulsants: phenytoin
  - Immunosuppressants: tacrolimus, leflunomide
  - Statins
  - Alcohol
- Toxic
  - Heavy metals like lead, arsenic, and mercury
  - Industrial solvents like *n*-hexane, acrylamide
  - Occupational exposure: organophosphates, carbon disulfide
- Nutritional deficiency
  - B_{12}, B_1, B_6, folate, niacin, copper, and vitamin E; B_6 deficiency and toxicity causes neuropathic symptoms.
- Paraneoplastic polyneuropathy

DIAGNOSTIC TESTS & INTERPRETATION

Initial Tests (lab, imaging)

- Fasting plasma glucose, 2-hour glucose tolerance test (2-H GTT) or hemoglobin A1c for diagnosis and to assess glycemic control; may occur in "prediabetes"
- Serum vitamin B_{12}
- Thyroid function
- Creatinine and BUN
- Syphilis, HIV testing
- Serum protein electrophoresis
- In mononeuropathy/mononeuritis multiplex, test for vasculitis, paraproteinemia, lyme, and sarcoid.
- In radiculopathy or mononeuropathy, imaging studies to exclude compressive lesions

Diagnostic Procedures/Other

- Bedside testing of vibration perception with 128-Hz tuning fork, monofilament perception of 10-g filament, pinprick and temperature testing
- Quantitative sensory testing for vibratory and thermal thresholds
  - Standardized measures for assessing severity and risk of foot ulceration
- Electromyogram nerve conduction velocity
  - Useful to confirm mononeuropathy and entrapment syndromes
  - In small unmyelinated fiber painful neuropathy, test may be normal.
- Lumbar puncture
  - In CIDP, elevation of spinal fluid protein
- Skin biopsy with epidermal nerve fiber density
  - Enables direct study of small nerve fibers that are difficult to assess electrophysiologically
- Corneal confocal microscopy
  - Noninvasive approach; loss of corneal innervation correlates with neuropathy

Test Interpretation
- In nerve biopsy of peripheral nerve Wallerian degeneration, focal axonal swellings containing neurofilaments, axonal atrophy, and demyelination are seen.
- Obliterative microvascular lesions and perivascular inflammation

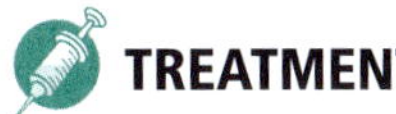

TREATMENT

GENERAL MEASURES
- Maintain blood glucose control.
- Treatment of other modifiable risk factors (including obesity, lipids and blood pressure) (1)
- Provide appropriate footwear to prevent pressure damage to insensate feet.

MEDICATION
Specific treatment to reverse nerve damage, other than improved glucose control, is not available. Initial treatment should focus on concurrent treatment of both sleep and mood disorders because of increased frequency of these problems in individuals with diabetic polyneuropathy (1). Current therapies target pain-relief. Combination of agents from different classes may be more effective when a single medication is ineffective.

First Line
- Management of pain and sensory neuropathy
  - Calcium channel modulators: pregabalin (1)
    - Binds same calcium channel as gabapentin
    - Linear pharmacokinetics and quicker onset of action compared to gabapentin
    - Usual dose: 150 to 600 mg/day; NNT ~4 to 10
    - Adverse effects are drowsiness, dizziness, and edema.
  - Selective serotonin: norepinephrine reuptake inhibitors (1)
    - Duloxetine has robust evidence of efficacy in the long term.
    - Usual dose 30 to 60 mg/day; NNT ~4 to 9
    - Adverse effects are nausea and dizziness.
- Management of autonomic neuropathy: very challenging and require both nonpharmacologic and pharmacologic measures
  - Orthostatic hypotension: adequate hydration, salt intake, compression garments over legs and abdomen, physical exercise, avoid medications aggravating hypotension (1)
    - Fludrocortisone (off-label)
    - Midodrine, droxidopa
  - Gastroparesis: foods with small particle size, withdrawing drugs with adverse effects on gastrointestinal motility (1)
    - Metoclopramide: Monitor for risk of extrapyramidal side effects; reserved for severe cases and short term only
    - Domperidone
    - Erythromycin (off-label): only effective for short-term use due to risk of tachyphylaxis
  - Diabetic diarrhea
    - Loperamide
    - Clonidine (off-label)
    - Octreotide (off-label)
    - Antibiotics for bacterial overgrowth
  - Hyperhidrosis
    - Propantheline (off-label)
    - Topical glycopyrrolate

Geriatric Considerations
Adverse effects may be more severe and may be attenuated by lower starting doses and more gradual titration. Anticholinergic effects of tricyclic antidepressants (TCAs) may cause urinary retention and cardiac arrhythmias.

Second Line
- Calcium channel modulators: gabapentin (1)
  - Binds Ca^{2+} channel–associated protein α_2-δ; inhibits neurotransmitter release
  - Dose range 300 to 1,200 mg TID; NNT ~4 to 8
  - Reduce dose in renal insufficiency.
  - Adverse effects: dizziness, fatigue, edema
- TCAs (1)
  - Analgesia may be related to effects on sodium channels.
  - Nortriptyline (25 to 150 mg); desipramine (25 to 200 mg) less sedating than amitriptyline but limited trial data
- Serotonin: norepinephrine reuptake inhibitor (1)
  - Venlafaxine at 75 to 225 mg daily
- Sodium channel blocker-lamotrigine, lacosamide, carbamazepine, oxcarbazepine, and valproic acid have been effective in five medium quality studies (1).
- Topical therapies
  - Capsaicin (1) 0.075% cream applied TID, 8% long-acting patch applied by health care professional in office
    - Depletes C fibers in skin of substance P
    - FDA approved and considered in individuals who prefer topical treatment
  - Lidocaine (1) 5% (700 mg) patches applied daily to feet (off-label);limited data
- Opiate analgesia: risks outweigh benefits and no evidence to support long-term use (1)
  - Tramadol and tapentadol (1)
    - Binds opiate receptors; also inhibits reuptake of norepinephrine and serotonin; fewer opiate side effects

ISSUES FOR REFERRAL
If CIDP is suspected, refer to neurologist for investigation/treatment.

ADDITIONAL THERAPIES
- Transcutaneous electrical nerve stimulation
- Percutaneous nerve stimulation
- Electrical spinal cord stimulation (1)
- Gastric electrical stimulation using surgical implantable device—FDA approved but limited data
- Actovegin, dextromethorphan with quinidine

COMPLEMENTARY & ALTERNATIVE MEDICINE
Acupuncture, Reiki, electromagnetic field treatment: no convincing trial data

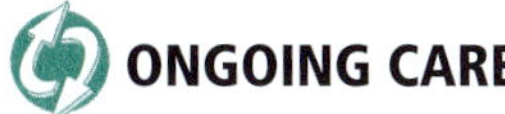

ONGOING CARE

PATIENT EDUCATION
Focus on glycemic control, weight management, cessation of tobacco and alcohol consumption, and sleep quality; requires multidisciplinary approach

PROGNOSIS
- Generalized symmetric polyneuropathies
  - Usually slow, chronic progression
  - Insensitive but painless foot as pain lessens
- Focal neuropathies
  - Recovery over months to years

COMPLICATIONS
- Claw foot deformity
- Neurotropic ulceration
  - Painless ulcers on weight-bearing area
  - Callus formation is a precursor to ulceration.
- Neuropathic arthropathy
  - Results in complete disorganization of joint structure in foot, Charcot joint

D

REFERENCES

1. Gandhi M, Fargo E, Prasad-Reddy L, et al. Diabetes: how to manage diabetic peripheral neuropathy. *Drugs Context*. 2022;11: 2021-10-2. doi:10.7573/dic.2021-10-2.

ADDITIONAL READING

- Elafros MA, Andersen H, Bennett DL, et al. Towards the prevention of diabetic peripheral neuropathy: clinical presentation, pathogenesis, and new treatments. *Lancet Neurol*. 2022;21(10):922–936.
- Patel K, Horak H, Tiryaki E. Diabetic neuropathies. *Muscle Nerve*. 2021;63(1):22–30.
- Vinik AI. Clinical practice. Diabetic sensory and motor neuropathy. *N Engl J Med*. 2016;374(15):1455–1464.

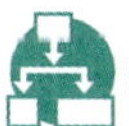

SEE ALSO

Diabetes Mellitus, Type 1; Diabetes Mellitus, Type 2

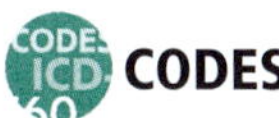

ICD10
- E10.42 Type 1 diabetes mellitus with diabetic polyneuropathy
- E11.42 Type 2 diabetes mellitus with diabetic polyneuropathy
- E13.42 Oth diabetes mellitus with diabetic polyneuropathy

CLINICAL PEARLS
- Occasionally, when glycemic control improves dramatically, as can occur when treatment for diabetes is initiated, there may be a worsening of neuropathy symptoms (described as treatment-induced neuropathy). Symptoms usually stabilize and gradually improve as glycemic control is maintained.
- It is common to combine agents with different mechanisms of action in the management of neuropathic pain. Topical therapies can be combined with systemic therapies. There is limited evidence-based data to support combination oral therapy.

DIARRHEA, ACUTE

Marie L. Borum, MD, EdD, MPH • Mason Eghbali, MD

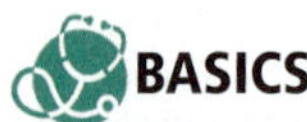

BASICS

DESCRIPTION

- An abnormal increase in stool water content, volume, or frequency (≥3 stools above baseline in 24 hours) for <14 days duration
- Most commonly secondary to infectious etiology; often self-limited
- Acute viral diarrhea (50–70%)
  - Most common cause of infectious diarrhea; noninflammatory (watery)
  - Frequently presents with associated nausea and/or vomiting
  - Symptoms usually develop after an incubation period of ~1 day and last for 1 to 3 days; typically self-limited
- Bacterial diarrhea (15–20%)
  - Most common infectious cause of inflammatory (bloody) diarrhea
  - Incubation period variable; diarrhea caused by preformed enterotoxin presents within 1 to 6 hours of contaminated food ingestion, whereas bacterial infection typically presents within 1 to 3 days.
  - Symptoms usually resolve in 1 to 7 days; antibiotic use attenuates length and/or severity of disease.
  - Suspect when concurrent illness in others who have shared potentially contaminated food.
- Protozoal infections (10–15%)
  - Typically, cause noninflammatory (watery) diarrhea
  - Long incubation period and prolonged disease course, symptoms develop approximately 7 days after exposure and commonly last >7 days.
  - Suspect when outbreaks of watery diarrhea in areas with contaminated water or food supply.
- Traveler's diarrhea (TD) typically begins 3 to 7 days after arrival in foreign location and resolves within 5 days; rapid onset, generally self-limited

EPIDEMIOLOGY

- In resource-limited countries, acute diarrhea is more common in children; no age predilection in resource-rich countries
- Acute diarrhea accounts for >128,000 U.S. hospital admissions and ~2.5 million annual deaths worldwide (1).
- The WHO categorizes acute diarrhea (symptoms <14 days) into watery and bloody (dysentery) subtypes.

Prevalence

- Fourth leading cause of death in children <5 years old and eighth leading cause of death among all ages worldwide
- Affects 11% of the general population
- In resource-rich countries, acute diarrhea is largely due to contaminated food and water.
- With improvements in sanitation and more widespread use of oral rehydration solution, death rates from diarrhea have declined. Nevertheless, nearly 7 billion cases of diarrheal disease occur worldwide each year.

ETIOLOGY AND PATHOPHYSIOLOGY

- Bacterial
  - *Escherichia coli*, *Salmonella*, *Shigella*, *Campylobacter jejuni* (most common bacterial causes)
  - *Vibrio parahaemolyticus*, *Vibrio cholerae*, *Yersinia enterocolitica*
  - *Clostridioides difficile*, *Staphylococcus aureus*
  - *Bacillus cereus*, *Clostridium perfringens*
  - *Listeria monocytogenes*
  - Aeromonas species
- Viral
  - *Norovirus* (most common overall cause of acute infectious diarrhea)
  - *Rotavirus* (children)
  - Adenovirus
  - Sapovirus
  - Cytomegalovirus (in immunocompromised)
  - Herpes simplex virus
- Protozoal
  - *Giardia lamblia*, *Entamoeba histolytica*
  - *Cryptosporidium* (in immunocompromised)
  - *Cyclospora*, *Microspora* (in immunocompromised)
- Pathophysiology (1)
  - Noninflammatory: most commonly viral; increased intestinal secretions without disruption of intestinal mucosa; watery character
  - Inflammatory: generally invasive or toxin-producing bacteria; disrupts mucosal integrity with subsequent tissue invasion/damage; bloody character
- Viral diarrhea: changes in small intestine cell morphology, including villous shortening, increased number of crypt cells, and increased cellularity of the lamina propria
- Bacterial diarrhea: Bacterial invasion of colonic wall leads to mucosal hyperemia, edema, and leukocytic infiltration.

RISK FACTORS

- Travel to resource-limited countries
- Failure to observe food/water precautions
- Immunocompromised host (HIV, malignancy, chemotherapy)
- Recent hospitalization
- Antibiotic use
- Proton pump inhibitor (PPI) use
- Daycare exposure
- Fecal-oral sexual contact
- Nursing home residence
- Pregnancy (12-fold increase for listeriosis) (1)

GENERAL PREVENTION

- Frequent handwashing reduces incidence of diarrhea by approximately 30%.
- Proper food and water precautions, particularly during foreign travel—"boil it, peel it, cook it, or forget it"
- Avoid undercooked meat, raw fish, unpasteurized milk.
- Rotavirus vaccine to all infants without a known contraindication
- Typhoid and cholera vaccine (for travel to endemic areas)
- TD prevention:
  - Pretravel counseling on high-risk food/beverage
  - Bismuth subsalicylate (BSS) may reduce the incidence of TD by up to 50%. Despite this, it is still not commonly used as prophylaxis (contraindicated in patients aspirin allergy, gout, renal insufficiency).
  - Routine antibiotic prophylaxis is not indicated in the vast majority of cases. Consider rifaximin and rifamycin SV in the rare case prophylaxis if indicated.
  - Probiotics, prebiotics, and synbiotics have unclear benefit as prophylaxis.

COMMONLY ASSOCIATED CONDITIONS

- Inflammatory bowel disease (IBD)
- Immunocompromised (HIV, malignancy, chemotherapy)

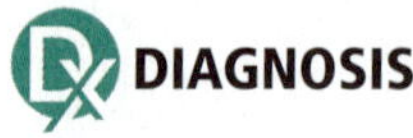

DIAGNOSIS

HISTORY

- Duration of symptoms <14 days
- Historical clues for dehydration: orthostatic hypotension, dizziness, increased thirst, decreased urine output, or altered mental status
- Description of stool—characteristics and output
  - Frequency; quantity; consistency; character: presence of mucus, blood, or fat; floating
  - *Giardia* associated with pale, greasy stools
- Weight loss
- Food history (unpasteurized dairy, raw or undercooked meat or fish)
- Associated symptoms: change in appetite, abdominal pain or bloating, nausea/vomiting, or fever
- Risk factors of acute diarrhea (see "Risk Factors")

PHYSICAL EXAM

- Assess degree of dehydration (1); ill-appearing, dry mucous membranes, tachycardia, orthostatic hypotension, decreased skin turgor, delayed capillary refill, altered mental status; can be absent in early dehydration
- Fever is more suggestive of inflammatory diarrhea.
- Thyroid: Assess for enlargement or nodules.
- Abdomen: Assess for distention, rigidity, rebound tenderness.
- Rectum: blood, tenderness, stool consistency

Geriatric Considerations

Fecal impaction or obstructing neoplasm can cause overflow diarrhea with chronic constipation.

DIFFERENTIAL DIAGNOSIS

- IBD; malabsorption
- Medications (cholinergic agents, magnesium-containing antacids, chemotherapy, antibiotics)
- Diverticulitis, ischemic colitis; spastic (irritable) colon
- Fecal impaction
- Endocrinopathies: thyroid disease
- Neoplasia
- Associated symptom of other systemic infections (influenza, HIV, dengue fever, and malaria)

DIAGNOSTIC TESTS & INTERPRETATION

Initial Tests (lab, imaging)

- Reserve laboratory testing for patients with persistent fever, moderate to severe disease characterized by passage of ≥6 stools per 24 hours, duration of >72 hours, dysentery, profuse watery diarrhea, immunosuppression, or if suspected outbreak (2).
- Complete blood count (CBC)
  - Leukocytosis, anemia (blood loss), eosinophilia (parasite infection), thrombocytopenia (hemolytic uremic syndrome [HUS])
- Basic metabolic panel (BMP)
  - Serum electrolytes, BUN, and creatinine (may elevate with volume depletion), non-anion gap metabolic acidosis

- Stool sample
  - Occult blood (IBD, bowel ischemia, and certain bacterial infections)
  - Fecal leukocytes: useful to distinguish inflammatory diarrhea from noninflammatory but should not be used to determine the infectious cause of diarrhea
  - Stool ova, parasites, and culture
  - Multiplex stool testing (PCR testing for bacterial, viral, and parasitic causes of diarrhea) if dysentery, moderate to severe disease, and symptoms lasting >7 days
  - *C. difficile* toxin (especially IBD, recently hospitalized or recent antibiotic use)
  - *Giardia* ELISA >90% sensitive in at-risk population
- Abdominal radiographs (flat plate and upright) if severe abdominal pain or concern for obstruction

Diagnostic Procedures/Other

- Abdominal imaging is not typically warranted. In patients with peritoneal signs, ileus, or well-localized lower quadrant pain, CT scan is the preferred modality to evaluate intra-abdominal disease (i.e., perforation, abscess, fulminant colitis, toxic megacolon)
- Consider sigmoidoscopy or colonoscopy in patients with persistent diarrhea, when there is no clear diagnosis after routine blood and stool tests, and if empiric or supportive therapy is ineffective.
- Consider colonoscopy in immunocompromised patients to evaluate for CMV colitis.

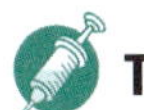

TREATMENT

GENERAL MEASURES

- Oral rehydration and electrolyte management are key to successful treatment.
  - Oral intake, as tolerated—"if the gut works, use it"
  - IV fluids if patient cannot tolerate oral rehydration or presents with severe dehydration
- Balanced electrolyte rehydration solutions recommended in elderly and profuse, watery TD (2)

MEDICATION

First Line

- For most patients with acute, nonbloody diarrhea (non-travel-associated), empiric antibiotic therapy is not recommended.
- Consider empiric antibiotics (macrolide: azithromycin or fluoroquinolone: ciprofloxacin) in patients with signs and symptoms of systemic infection, more severe disease, or clear cases of TD (2).
  - Fever; bloody diarrhea; fecal leukocytes
  - Immunocompromised host
  - Signs of severe volume depletion
- Tailor antibiotics to stool culture results.
  - *Giardia*: tinidazole 2 g PO once
  - *E. histolytica*: metronidazole 500 to 750 mg PO TID for 7 to 10 days, tinidazole 2 g PO daily for 3 to 5 days
  - *Shigella*: ciprofloxacin 500 mg PO BID for 3 to 5 days or ceftriaxone 1 to 2 g IM/IV daily for 5 days
  - *Campylobacter*: azithromycin 500 mg PO daily for 3 to 5 days or erythromycin 500 mg PO QID for 5 days
  - *C. difficile*: The Infectious Disease Society of America now recommends fidaxomicin 200 mg PO BID for 10 days as first-line therapy. Vancomycin 125 to 500 mg PO QID for 10 to 14 days can be used as alternative or for fulminant disease; consider fecal microbiota transplant in recurrent mild to moderate *C. difficile* infections.
  - TD: azithromycin (preferred) 1 g single dose or ciprofloxacin 500 mg PO BID for 3 days (or a 750 mg single dose), (or a 750-mg single-dose) azithromycin for 3 days (single-dose), rifamycin SV 388 mg PO BID for 3 days or rifaximin 200 mg PO TID for 3 days (noninvasive strains of *E.coli*); can combine with loperamide; loperamide or BSS may be used alone in cases of mild TD.
- General considerations
  - Antibiotics are not recommended in *Salmonella* infections unless caused by *Salmonella typhosa* or if the patient is febrile or immunocompromised.
  - Avoid antibiotics in patients with *E. coli* 0157:H7 due to risk of HUS.
  - Antibiotics are not indicated for foodborne toxigenic diarrhea.
  - Avoid antimotility agents (e.g., loperamide) in patients with febrile or bloody diarrhea or antibiotic-associated colitis due to risk of toxic megacolon.
  - Antimotility agents used with antibiotics may speed recovery from TD.
  - Antibiotics are not recommended for the treatment of mild TD.

COMPLEMENTARY & ALTERNATIVE MEDICINE

- BSS may help control rate of diarrhea stools (2).
- Probiotics are recommended for prevention of antibiotic-associated diarrhea and *C. difficile* infection recurrence and to treat acute infectious diarrhea in setting of symptomatic IBS; avoid in immunocompromised patients.
- Oral zinc supplementation reduces the duration of diarrhea in children 6 months to 5 years of age who reside in countries with a high prevalence of zinc deficiency or who have signs of malnutrition.

ADMISSION, INPATIENT, AND NURSING CONSIDERATIONS

Outpatient management, except for patients who are severely ill with signs of volume depletion

ONGOING CARE

DIET

- Early oral refeeding is encouraged. Regular diets are as effective as restricted diets.
- The traditional bananas, rice, applesauce, toast (BRAT) diet has little evidence-based support (despite heavy clinical use) and may result in suboptimal nutrition.

PATIENT EDUCATION

See "General Prevention."

PROGNOSIS

Acute diarrhea is rarely life-threatening if adequate hydration is maintained.

COMPLICATIONS

- Volume depletion, shock, sepsis
- HUS with *E. coli* 0157:H7
- Guillain-Barré syndrome with *C. jejuni*
- Reactive arthritis with *Salmonella*, *Shigella*, and *Yersinia*

REFERENCES

1. Hamilton KW, Cifu AS. Diagnosis and management of infectious diarrhea. *JAMA*. 2019;321(9):891–892.
2. Ferris A, Gaisinskaya P, Nandi N. Approach to diarrhea. *Prim Care*. 2023;50(3):447–459. doi:10.1016/j.pop.2023.03.010.

SEE ALSO

Botulism; Cholera; Food Poisoning, Bacterial

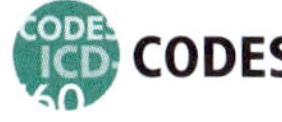

CODES

ICD10

- R19.7 Diarrhea, unspecified
- A09 Infectious gastroenteritis and colitis, unspecified
- A08.4 Viral intestinal infection, unspecified

CLINICAL PEARLS

- Viruses are the most common causes of acute diarrheal illness in the United States.
- Consider broad infectious etiologies if patients are immunocompromised (*Cytomegalovirus*, *Cryptosporidium*, *Cyclospora*, *Microspora*, *Mycobacterium avium* complex, and *Mycobacterium tuberculosis*).
- Oral rehydration is the most important and effective treatment for acute diarrhea.
- Avoid antimotility agents (e.g., loperamide) in febrile patients, bloody diarrhea, and antibiotic-associated colitis.
- Routine stool culture is not recommended, unless patients present with bloody diarrhea, fever, severe dehydration, signs of inflammatory disease, persistent symptoms >7 days, or have a history of immunosuppression.
- Start empiric antibiotics only in patients who are severely ill or immunocompromised.

DIARRHEA, CHRONIC

Marie L. Borum, MD, EdD, MPH • Beminet Kassaye, MD • Valerie Sarah Stark, MD, MPH

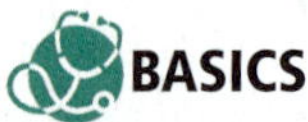

BASICS

DESCRIPTION

- Chronic diarrhea refers to an increased frequency of loose stools (Bristol types 5 to 7) and >3 loose stools per day for >4 weeks (1),(2).
- Etiologies: osmotic, secretory, malabsorptive, inflammatory, infectious, and hypermotility (2)

EPIDEMIOLOGY

Incidence

Varies by definition

Prevalence

Varies by etiology; worldwide prevalence is ~3–20% (2). U.S. prevalence is ~6.6%.

ETIOLOGY AND PATHOPHYSIOLOGY

Altered luminal water and electrolytes increases stool water volume.

- Osmotic (fecal osmotic gap >100 mOsm/kg) (3); resolves with fasting (2); less voluminous
  - Carbohydrate malabsorption: disaccharides, monosaccharides, and polyols; magnesium (Mg), citrates, phosphate, and sulfate ingestion
- Secretory (fecal osmotic gap <50 mOsm/kg) (1); persists with fasting (2) and overnight
  - Alcoholism, stimulant laxative ingestion; bacterial enterotoxins; postcholecystectomy/ileal resection <100 cm: excessive intestinal bile salts cause choleretic diarrhea.
  - Disordered motility: postvagotomy, autonomic neuropathy, hyperthyroidism
  - Neuroendocrine tumors: VIPoma; carcinoid syndrome, gastrinoma, somatostatinoma
  - Metastatic medullary thyroid cancer; adrenal insufficiency
  - Noninvasive infection: giardiasis, cryptosporidiosis
  - Microscopic colitis; protein-losing enteropathy
- Malabsorptive (1): increased stool volumes
  - Celiac disease, Whipple disease; tropical sprue, giardiasis, amyloidosis
  - Chronic mesenteric ischemia, lymphatic obstruction
  - Short bowel syndrome (>100 cm ileal resection)
  - Small intestinal bacterial overgrowth (SIBO); pancreatic exocrine insufficiency
- Inflammatory (1): liquid stool with occasional blood
  - Inflammatory bowel disease (IBD)—ulcerative colitis (UC); Crohn disease
  - Microscopic colitis; diverticulitis; vasculitis; radiation enterocolitis
  - Infections: *Clostridium difficile*, *Entamoeba histolytica*, cytomegalovirus (CMV), tuberculosis, *Salmonella*
  - Neoplasms: colon cancer, lymphoma
- Hypermotility (fecal osmotic gap 50 to 100 mOsm/kg) (1)
  - Irritable bowel syndrome (IBS); functional diarrhea (IBS distinguished by pain) (2),(3)
- Drugs (1): resolved with drug cessation
  - NSAIDs, PPIs, colchicine, metformin, digoxin, ACE inhibitors, β-blockers, gliptins, theophyllines, antibiotics, SSRIs, antineoplastic agents, excessive laxative use
  - Herbal: St. John's wort, echinacea, garlic, saw palmetto, ginseng, etc.
- Infectious
  - Bacterial: *C. difficile*, *Mycobacterium avium intracellulare*; viral: CMV; parasitic: *Giardia lamblia*, *Cryptosporidium*, *Isospora*, *E. histolytica*, *Strongyloides*
- Food allergies (1)

Genetics

- Celiac disease: HLA-DQ2 and HLA-DQ8 (3)
- IBD: polygenic (immediate family have 10× risk) (3)
- Cystic fibrosis (CF) transmembrane conductance regulator mutation

RISK FACTORS

- Osmotic
  - Excess nonabsorbable carbohydrates (i.e., artificial sweeteners); Mg-containing antacids (3), or poorly absorbed ions (phosphate, sulfate, Mg) (1)
  - Lactose intolerance, celiac disease
  - Medications (i.e., citrates, phosphates, sulfates, Mg-containing laxatives, sugar alcohols)
- Secretory
  - Postsurgical: small bowel resection/ileal surgery, vagotomy, bile acid malabsorption; neuroendocrine disease or stimulant laxative abuse; dysmotility syndromes
  - Medications (i.e., NSAIDs, caffeine, metformin, colchicine, carbamazepine, antibiotics, calcitonin) (3)
- Malabsorptive
  - CF; chronic alcohol abuse, celiac disease
  - Chronic pancreatitis/pancreatic insufficiency; medications (e.g., orlistat, acarbose, aminoglycosides, thyroid supplements)
- Inflammatory
  - IBD, NSAIDs use, antibiotics, radiation; HIV/AIDS, colorectal cancer, invasive infection (tuberculosis, *Yersinia*)
  - Pseudomembranous colitis (*C. difficile*)
  - Antineoplastic drugs (i.e., 5-fluorouracil, methotrexate, irinotecan), radiation
  - Immunosuppressants
- Hypermotility
  - Psychosocial stress, preceding infection
  - Stimulant medications (i.e., macrolides, metoclopramide, senna, bisacodyl [Dulcolax]) (3)
- Genetic predisposition

ALERT

Diabetes mellitus (DM) and cholecystectomy can cause secretory and osmotic diarrhea.

GENERAL PREVENTION

Varies by etiology; treat the underlying cause.

COMMONLY ASSOCIATED CONDITIONS

- IBD: arthralgias, aphthous stomatitis, uveitis/episcleritis, erythema nodosum, pyoderma gangrenosum, perianal fistulas, rectal fissures, ankylosing spondylitis, and PSC
- Celiac disease: dermatitis herpetiformis, type 1 DM, and IgA deficiency
- Latex-food allergy syndrome: latex, banana, avocado, kiwi, and walnut allergies (1)

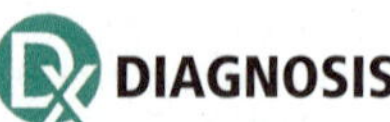

DIAGNOSIS

HISTORY

- Careful documentation of stool history: stooling onset, pattern, frequency, characteristics (greasy, floating, watery), volume, travel, diet, medications, family history, urgency, fecal incontinence
- Alarm features: rectal bleeding, weight loss, fever, nocturnal symptoms, onset after the age of 50 years
- Skin changes, arthritis, ocular problems, heat intolerance, polyuria/polydipsia, fever, flushing, alcohol use
- Food allergies (1)
- Flatus and bloating are predominant features of carbohydrate malabsorption (1).
- Fatty stools: foul smelling
- Risk factors: STIs, gastrointestinal surgeries, DM, radiation, family history of colorectal cancer (2)
- IBS or functional diarrhea by Rome IV criteria (2),(3):
  - IBS: recurrent abdominal pain ≥1 day/week in 3 months (symptoms >6 months) and ≥2 of the following criteria: defecation-related, change in stool frequency, or form
  - Functional diarrhea: ≥25% loose/watery stools without abdominal pain/bloating for >3 months (symptoms >6 months); normal abdominal, oral, and skin examinations; no alarm features

PHYSICAL EXAM

- General: volume depletion, nutritional status, recent weight loss, anasarca (1),(2)
- Skin: flushing (carcinoid), erythema nodosum or pyoderma gangrenosum (IBD), ecchymoses (vitamin K deficiency), dermatitis herpetiformis (celiac disease), hyperpigmentation (Addison disease) (1),(2)
- HEENT: iritis/uveitis/episcleritis, oral ulcerations, or aphthous stomatitis (IBD); lid lag, exophthalmos, or goiter (hyperthyroid); lymphadenopathy (Whipple disease)
- Cardiovascular: tachycardia (hyperthyroid), heart murmur (carcinoid syndrome) (2)
- Pulmonary: wheezing (carcinoid)
- Abdomen: hyperactive bowel sounds (IBD), distension and/or diffuse tenderness (IBD/IBS), anorectal fistulas or anal fissures (IBD), fecal impaction (overflow incontinence)
- Extremities: arthritis or spondylitis (IBD); tremor (hyperthyroid)

DIFFERENTIAL DIAGNOSIS

See "Etiology and Pathophysiology," "Commonly Associated Conditions," and "Risk Factors"

DIAGNOSTIC TESTS & INTERPRETATION

Initial Tests (lab, imaging)

Test patients with alarming or persistent symptoms and no identifiable cause.

- Blood: CBC, electrolytes (Mg, P, Ca), total protein, albumin, thyroid-stimulating hormone, free T_4, C-reactive protein, iron studies, anti-tissue transglutaminase IgA and total IgA
- Stool: fecal WBC, lactoferrin/calprotectin (preferred), culture, ova/parasite, *Giardia* antigen, *C. difficile* toxin, electrolytes, occult blood, osmolality, qualitative fecal fat (Sudan stain) (1), and total bile acids in a 48-hour stool collection

- Normal fecal calprotectin (<50 μg/g) or fecal lactoferrin (<7.25 μg/g) level rules out IBD for patients who meet Rome IV diagnostic criteria for IBS without alarm features (3)[A].
  - Fecal osmotic gap = 290 mOsm/kg—2 (Na[feces] + K[feces])
  - *C. difficile* testing only in diarrheal stools (3)[C]
  - Ova/parasite only in travelers to or from high-risk areas; perform *Giardia* antigen/PCR for all chronic watery diarrhea cases.
- CT or MRI to evaluate the GI tract structure (i.e., IBD, malignancy, chronic pancreatitis) (1)

Follow-Up Tests & Special Considerations

- Colonoscopy for any patients with alarm features (age, bleeding, cancer risk)
- Celiac disease: anti-TTG IgA plus total serum IgA (sensitivity/specificity >90%) in patients without IgA deficiency; 10% of celiac patients have IgA deficiency—may cause false-negative results so use IgG deamidated gliadin peptide (DGP) or IgG-TTG instead.
  - Confirm IgA TTG positive result by duodenal biopsy (2).
- Pancreatic insufficiency: fecal elastase, fecal chymotrypsin, serum trypsinogen
- Protein-losing enteropathy: fecal α_1-antitrypsin
- Microscopic colitis: colonic biopsy from normal-appearing mucosa (3)[C]
- Carbohydrate malabsorption: fecal pH (<7.0) and hydrogen breath test
- SIBO: hydrogen breath test and proximal jejunal aspirate with $>10^5$ CFU/mL coliform bacteria (3)
- Recent hospitalization or antibiotics: *C. difficile* toxin
- HIV ELISA, *Isospora*/*Cryptosporidium* stains
- Consider testing for protozoa, atypical infections, *Strongyloides*, *E. histolytica*, *Giardia*, *Cyclospora*, *Microsporidia*, and tropical sprue in travelers to or from a high-risk area.
- Allergy testing
- Laxative abuse: stool osmotic gap
- Neuroendocrine tumor: chromogranin A, somatostatin, VIP, gastrin, calcitonin; urine: 5-HIAA, histamine; CT or MRI abdomen (3)

Diagnostic Procedures/Other

- Colonoscopy with biopsies for IBD, microscopic or CMV colitis, and colorectal cancer
- Flexible sigmoidoscopy if pregnant, with comorbidities, or tenesmus/urgency predominate
- EGD with biopsies if malabsorption or small bowel enteropathy suspected
- MRCP if chronic pancreatitis is suspected
- CT or magnetic resonance enterography

Test Interpretation

- Celiac disease: intraepithelial lymphocytosis, crypt hyperplasia, villous atrophy
- Crohn disease: cobblestoning, creeping fat, strictures, linear ulcerations, skip lesions, noncaseating granulomas, lymphoid aggregates
- UC: crypt abscesses, continuous rectal lesion, loss of haustra ("lead pipe" sign)
- Lactose intolerance: normal-appearing villi, lactase deficiency
- Lymphocytic colitis: high intraepithelial lymphocytes, inflammatory cells in the lamina propria, normal mucosa
- Melanosis coli suggests laxative abuse.

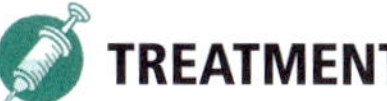

TREATMENT

GENERAL MEASURES

Fluids/electrolyte repletion; if stable, outpatient treatment

MEDICATION

First Line

- IBS-D/functional diarrhea: dietary modification (low FODMAP); antidiarrheals; bile acid sequestrants
- Lactose intolerance: lactose-free diet; postcholecystectomy, abdominal radiation therapy, or ileal resection: cholestyramine or colestipol 2 to 16 g/day PO split BID; DM: glucose control; hyperthyroidism: methimazole 5 to 20 mg/day PO, propylthiouracil (PTU) 100 to 150 mg/day PO divided; thyroid ablation; *C. difficile*: 10 days of vancomycin 125 mg PO q6h or metronidazole (Flagyl) 500 mg PO q8h or fidaxomicin 200 mg PO BID; *G. lamblia*: metronidazole 250 mg PO q8h × 5 to 7 days, nitazoxanide 500 mg PO q12h × 3 days
- Whipple disease: ceftriaxone 2 g IV for 14 days or penicillin 2 MU IV every 4 hours for 2 weeks and then trimethoprim/sulfamethoxazole [Bactrim] DS 160/800 mg PO BID for 1 to 2 years
- SIBO: rifaximin 550 mg PO BID, fluoroquinolones 250 to 750 mg PO BID, metronidazole 500 mg PO q6–8h
- Pancreatic insufficiency: pancrelipase; HIV/AIDS: antiretroviral therapy (HAART)
- Microscopic colitis: budesonide 9 mg/day PO, mesalamine 800 mg PO TID, bismuth subsalicylate (Pepto-Bismol) 786 mg PO TID; IBD: 5-ASA, short courses of corticosteroids and/or antibiotics, immunomodulators, anti-TNF therapy, cholestyramine; neuroendocrine tumor: octreotide 100 to 600 g/day SC (1)
- Celiac disease: gluten-free diet; IBS diarrhea predominant: rifaximin 550 mg PO TID × 14 days, alosetron 0.5 to 1.0 mg PO BID, peppermint oil, eluxadoline 100 mg PO BID; TCAs may also be considered (1).
- Symptom relief: loperamide 4 to 8 mg/day (if infection ruled out), diphenoxylate-atropine 1 to 2 tabs BID–QID, activated charcoal, fiber supplementation, bismuth subsalicylate 525 to 1,050 mg every 0.5 to 1.0 hour (1)

ISSUES FOR REFERRAL

GI referral for suspected inflammatory diarrhea or endoscopy/biopsy

SURGERY/OTHER PROCEDURES

- Resect neuroendocrine tumors; intestinal resection for refractory IBD
- Fecal transplant for recurrent *C. difficile*

ADMISSION, INPATIENT, AND NURSING CONSIDERATIONS

Hemodynamically unstable, severe electrolyte abnormalities, dehydration, malnutrition, AKI, or unable to tolerate oral intake

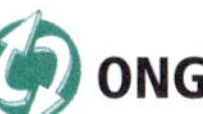

ONGOING CARE

DIET

Elimination diet: Avoid gluten-containing foods, nonabsorbable carbohydrates, lactose-containing products, and food allergens. Low FODMAP diet (avoid wheat/rye, onions, garlic, legumes, lactose dairy, artificial sweeteners) helps symptoms in up to 75% of IBS-D patients.

PATIENT EDUCATION

- Chronic diarrhea is generally defined as three or more loose bowel movements per day for >4 weeks.
- Wide variation in "normal" bowel habits; restrict colon stimulants.

PROGNOSIS

Varies according to etiology

COMPLICATIONS

- Fluid and electrolyte imbalances, AKI; malnutrition, anemia, weight loss
- Malignancy (colon cancer [IBD], lymphoma [IBD therapies], small bowel cancer [celiac, Crohn disease]); infection with immunosuppressive therapies for IBD

REFERENCES

1. Brenner DM, Domínguez-Muñoz JE. Differential diagnosis of chronic diarrhea: an algorithm to distinguish irritable bowel syndrome with diarrhea from other organic gastrointestinal diseases, with special focus on exocrine pancreatic insufficiency. *J Clin Gastroenterol*. 2023;57(7):663–670. doi:10.1097/MCG.0000000000001855.
2. Chu C, Rotondo-Trivette S, Michail S. Chronic diarrhea. *Curr Probl Pediatr Adolesc Health Care*. 2020;50(8):100841.
3. Burgers K, Lindberg B, Bevis ZJ. Chronic diarrhea in adults: evaluation and differential diagnosis. *Am Fam Physician*. 2020;101(8):472–480.

ADDITIONAL READING

Tripathi PR, Srivastava A. Approach to a child with chronic diarrhea. *Indian J Pediatr*. 2024;91(5):472–480. doi:10.1007/s12098-023-04587-9.

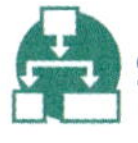

SEE ALSO

Algorithm: Diarrhea, Chronic

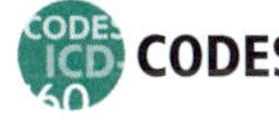

CODES

ICD10

K52.9 Noninfective gastroenteritis and colitis, unspecified

CLINICAL PEARLS

- A comprehensive medical history guides the appropriate workup and avoids unnecessary testing.
- Consider IBS-D, IBD, malabsorption syndromes, celiac disease, prescribed or OTC medication use, herbal product use, and chronic infections (immunocompromised) in the differential diagnosis.
- Treatment is based on the underlying cause.

D

DIVERTICULAR DISEASE

Amrutha Pavle, MD

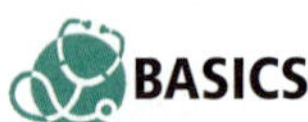

BASICS

DESCRIPTION

Diverticulum (single) or diverticula (multiple) are outpouchings of the colonic wall. Diverticular disease is a spectrum of diseases impacting the entire GI tract (except the rectum):

- Asymptomatic diverticulosis: common incidental finding on colonoscopy or imaging
- Symptomatic diverticulosis: also called symptomatic uncomplicated diverticular disease (SUDD); recurrent abdominal pain attributed to diverticulosis without colitis or diverticulitis (1)
- Acute diverticulitis: diverticular disease with associated inflammation and/or infection
  - Uncomplicated diverticulitis: abdominal pain and leukocytosis without peritoneal signs or systemic toxicity
  - Complicated diverticulitis: secondary abscess formation, bowel obstruction, perforation, peritonitis, fistula, or stricture in the setting of diverticular inflammation
- Diverticular bleeding: accounts for >40% of lower GI bleeds; often painless hematochezia unless accompanied by active diverticulitis; bleeding is more common with right-sided diverticula.

EPIDEMIOLOGY

Incidence

- Diverticular disease accounts for 500,000 hospitalizations per year in the United States.
- Diverticulitis occurs in 1–2% of the general population and in 4% of patients with diverticulosis (1). Diverticular bleeding occurs in 3–5% of patients with diverticulosis.

Prevalence

Prevalence of diverticulosis and the number of diverticula increase with age.

- Diverticulosis: 20% of people aged 40 years, 60% of people aged 60 years, and 70% by age of 80 years.
- Incidence of diverticulitis increased from 62 to 75/100,000 from 1998 to 2005; largest increase in patients <45 years of age—mostly due to changes in diet

ETIOLOGY AND PATHOPHYSIOLOGY

Diverticula form at points of weakness along the intestinal wall where small blood vessels (vasa recta) penetrate through the muscular layer of the colon.

- Age-related degeneration of the mucosal wall; increased intraluminal pressure from dense, fiber-depleted stools; and abnormal colonic motility contribute to diverticulosis.
- Most right-sided diverticula are true diverticula (involves all layers of the colonic wall).
- Most left-sided diverticula are pseudodiverticula (outpouchings of the mucosa and submucosa only).
- Diverticulitis occurs when local inflammation and infection contribute to tissue necrosis with risk for mucosal microperforation or macroperforation.
- Alterations in intestinal microbiota contribute to chronic inflammation (1).
- Thinning of the vasa recta over the neck of the diverticula increases susceptibility to bleeding.
- Diverticular disease and irritable bowel syndrome (IBS) may represent the same disease continuum.

Genetics

Although genetics may play a role, there is no known genetic pattern.

RISK FACTORS

- Age >40 years; low-fiber diet and high red-meat consumption
- Sedentary lifestyle, obesity, previous diverticulitis; risk rises with the number of diverticula.
- Smoking increases the risk of perforation (1).
- Risk of diverticular bleeding increases with NSAIDs, steroids, and opiate analgesics. Calcium channel blockers and statins protect against diverticular bleeding.

GENERAL PREVENTION

- High-fiber diet or nonabsorbable fiber (psyllium)
- Regular physical activity

COMMONLY ASSOCIATED CONDITIONS

Colorectal polyps, nonalcoholic fatty liver disease, hypothyroidism, arterial hypertension, colon cancer, connective tissue diseases, obesity, IBS, and inflammatory bowel disease

DIAGNOSIS

HISTORY

- Diverticulosis
  - 80–85% of patients are asymptomatic. Of the 15–20% with symptoms, 1–2% will require hospitalization, and 0.5% undergo surgery.
  - The most common symptom is dull, colicky abdominal pain, typically in the LLQ. Pain can be exacerbated by eating and by passing bowel movement or flatus. Diarrhea or constipation is common.
- Acute diverticulitis: uncomplicated (85%) and complicated (15%)
  - Abdominal pain: acute onset, typically in LLQ; fever and/or chills
  - Anorexia, nausea (20–62%), or vomiting; constipation (50%) or diarrhea (25–35%)
  - Dysuria and urinary frequency suggest bladder or ureteral irritation.
  - Pneumaturia and fecaluria if associated with a colovesical fistula
- Diverticular bleeding: melena, hematochezia (0.5/1,000 person-years); painless rectal bleeding
- Immunocompromised patients may not present with fever or leukocytosis and are at higher risk for perforation and abscess formation.

PHYSICAL EXAM

- Diverticulosis
  - Exam is usually normal.
  - May have intermittent distension or tympany
  - May have heme + stools
- Acute diverticulitis
  - Bowel sounds hypoactive (high-pitched/intermittent with obstruction); abdominal tenderness (usually LLQ); abdominal distension and tympany
  - Rebound tenderness, involuntary guarding, or rigidity suggests perforation and/or peritonitis; palpable mass in LLQ (20%)
  - Rectal exam may reveal tenderness or a mass.
  - Colovaginal, colovesical, and perirectal fistulae are rarely the initial presentation.

DIFFERENTIAL DIAGNOSIS

Urinary tract infection, nephrolithiasis, IBS, lactose intolerance, carcinoma, inflammatory bowel disease, fecal impaction, bowel obstruction, angiodysplasia, ischemic colitis, acute appendicitis, ectopic pregnancy

DIAGNOSTIC TESTS & INTERPRETATION

Initial Tests (lab, imaging)

- Diverticulosis: no labs or imaging needed
- Acute diverticulitis
  - WBC count is normal in up to 45% of cases. As diverticulitis worsens, WBC count becomes elevated with left shift.
  - Hemoglobin normal (unless bleeding); ESR elevated
  - Urinalysis may show microscopic pyuria or hematuria; urine culture: usually normal; persistent infection is suspicious for colovesical fistula.
  - Blood cultures positive in systemic cases
  - Plain films of the abdomen (acute abdominal series—supine and upright) to assess for free air under the diaphragm (bowel perforation) and signs of bowel obstruction (dilated loops of bowel)
  - CT scan with IV, oral, and/or rectal contrast (sensitivity: 98%, specificity: 99%) to stage disease and determine treatment plan (2)[A]
  - Ultrasound and MRI (sensitivity: 94%; specificity: 92%) are useful alternatives.
  - Barium enema is not recommended due to risk of peritoneal extravasation.
- Diverticular bleeding: anemia with bleeding; obtain coagulation panel.

Diagnostic Procedures/Other

Diverticular bleeding

- Endoscopy to evaluate GI bleeding; NG lavage to exclude upper GI bleeding
- Angiography if bleeding obscures endoscopy or when endoscopy cannot visualize a source; ^{99m}Tc-pertechnetate–labeled RBC scan (more sensitive) with follow-up angiography to localize bleeding

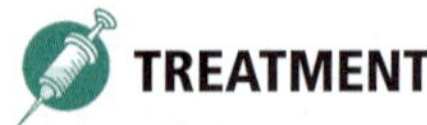

TREATMENT

GENERAL MEASURES

- Diverticulosis: outpatient therapy with fiber supplementation and/or bulking agents (psyllium) (>30 g/day) (2)[A]
- Uncomplicated diverticulitis: outpatient therapy (see exceptions below) with or without oral antibiotics; 1–2% of subjects require hospitalization for toxicity, septicemia, peritonitis, or failure of symptoms to resolve. Up to 30% of patients may require surgery at first episode of diverticulitis.
- Complicated diverticulitis: hospitalization, bowel rest, and IV antibiotics; Hinchey classification (severity):
  - Stage I: diverticulitis + confined paracolic abscess; stage II: diverticulitis + distant abscess; stage III: diverticulitis + purulent peritonitis; stage IV: diverticulitis + fecal peritonitis
- Symptomatic improvement is expected within 2 to 3 days. Antibiotics should be continued for 7 to 10 days.
- Diverticular bleeding: 80% of cases resolve spontaneously.

MEDICATION

First Line

- Symptomatic diverticulosis: cyclical rifaximin 400 mg PO BID for 7 days every month or continuous mesalamine 800 mg PO BID (2)[C]
- Acute diverticulitis
  - The routine use of antibiotics in uncomplicated diverticulitis is controversial (2),(3)[C].
  - Outpatient oral antibiotics: Cover for anaerobes and gram-negative bacteria with:
    - A fluoroquinolone (ciprofloxacin 750 mg BID or levofloxacin 750 mg QD) *plus* metronidazole 500 mg TID (may use clindamycin if metronidazole intolerant) or
    - Trimethoprim/sulfamethoxazole DS BID *plus* metronidazole 500 mg TID
    - Treat for 7 to 10 days.
  - Inpatient: Use IV antibiotics
    - Monotherapy with a β-lactam/β-lactamase inhibitor: piperacillin/tazobactam (3,375 g IV QID) or ampicillin/sulbactam 3 g IV q6h or ertapenem (1 g IV QD)
    - Penicillin-allergic patient: quinolone (levofloxacin 750 mg IV QD *plus* metronidazole 500 mg IV TID)
    - Unresponsive or severe disease: imipenem or meropenem
  - Recurrences of acute diverticulitis may be decreased by using mesalamine ± rifaximin or probiotics.
- Diverticular bleeding
  - Consider vasopressin 0.2 to 0.3 U/min through selective intra-arterial catheter.
- Precautions
  - Avoid morphine and other opiates that may increase intraluminal pressure or promote ileus.
  - Increased fiber intake is not recommended in the acute management of diverticulitis.

Second Line

- Outpatient: amoxicillin/clavulanate monotherapy (875/125 mg BID) (contraindicated in patients with clearance <30 mL/min) or moxifloxacin (400 mg PO QD) *plus* metronidazole (500 mg PO TID)
- Severely ill inpatients: ampicillin (500 mg IV q6h) + metronidazole (500 mg IV TID) + a quinolone *or* ampicillin + metronidazole + an aminoglycoside

ISSUES FOR REFERRAL

- Acute diverticulitis patients should follow up with a gastroenterologist or surgeon after resolution of diverticulitis (6 to 8 weeks) for colonoscopy to exclude malignancy, fistula, strictures, or inflammatory bowel disease (2).
- Acute complicated diverticulitis should have appropriate surgical and critical care/infectious disease consultations.

SURGERY/OTHER PROCEDURES

- Acute diverticulitis
  - Indications for emergent surgery: peritonitis, uncontrolled sepsis, perforation, obstruction
  - Hinchey I and II: consultation to interventional radiology to drain large abscesses (>4 cm)
  - Hinchey III or IV: frequently requires surgery during the same hospital admission
  - Elective colon resection in recurrent diverticulitis is a case-by-case decision and is typically performed during the quiescent phase following appropriate nonoperative treatment (2).
  - Immunocompromised patients are more likely to present with acute complicated diverticulitis, fail medical management, and have complications from elective surgery.
- Diverticular bleeding
  - Endoscopy and hemostasis via epinephrine injection, electrocautery, or clipping
  - Angiography is preferred over endoscopy in unstable patients to identify/embolize the bleeding source.
  - Massive or recurrent bleeding requires surgery to control hemorrhage.

COMPLEMENTARY & ALTERNATIVE MEDICINE

Probiotics have been used to prevent recurrence with mixed success.

ADMISSION, INPATIENT, AND NURSING CONSIDERATIONS

- Admit for systematic toxicity, sepsis, and/or peritonitis (complicated diverticulitis).
- Consider admitting patients with uncomplicated diverticulitis and the following: elderly, immunocompromised, evidence of microperforation, marked leukocytosis, temperature >39°C, intolerance of PO intake, severe abdominal pain, or unreliable follow-up.

ONGOING CARE

FOLLOW-UP RECOMMENDATIONS

Patient Monitoring

- Follow up outpatients 2 to 3 days after initiating antibiotic therapy and then weekly thereafter until symptom resolution.
  - Repeat imaging and/or inpatient therapy may be required if there is disease progression at follow-up.
- Colonoscopy should be performed in 6 to 8 weeks (unless done within the past year).

DIET

- Bowel rest with NPO during acute diverticulitis; advance diet as tolerated as bowel function returns
- Patients with known diverticulosis or a history of diverticulitis should consume a high-fiber diet to prevent recurrence (3).
- Avoiding nuts and popcorn is not necessary (3).

PROGNOSIS

- Good with early detection and prompt treatment
- After first episode of diverticulitis, there is a 33% chance of recurrence. After a second episode, there is a 66% chance of further recurrence. Rebleeding occurs in up to 6%.
- Most complications occur during first bout of diverticulitis. Younger patients are more likely to have recurrence.

COMPLICATIONS

Hemorrhage, perforation, peritonitis, obstruction, abscess, or colovesicular/colovaginal fistula

REFERENCES

1. Tursi A, Scarpignato C, Strate LL, et al. Colonic diverticular disease. *Nat Rev Dis Primers*. 2020;6(1):20.
2. Eckmann JD, Shaukat A. Updates in the understanding and management of diverticular disease. *Curr Opin Gastroenterol*. 2022;38(1):48–54.
3. Peery AF, Shaukat A, Strate LL. AGA clinical practice update on medical management of colonic diverticulitis: expert review. *Gastroenterology*. 2021;160(3):906–911.e1.

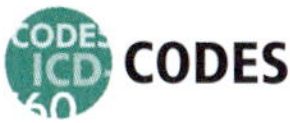

CODES

ICD10

- K57.92 Diverticulitis of intestine, part unspecified, without perforation or abscess without bleeding
- K57.13 Diverticulitis of small intestine without perforation or abscess with bleeding
- K57.21 Diverticulitis of large intestine with perforation and abscess with bleeding

CLINICAL PEARLS

- Diverticulosis is common in elderly patients with a sedentary lifestyle who consume a Western diet.
- Patients with diverticulosis benefit from a high-fiber diet.
- Antibiotics may not be necessary for low-risk patients with acute uncomplicated diverticulitis.
- Not all patients with recurrent diverticulitis require surgical intervention (colectomy).
- Dietary restrictions do not prevent recurrent diverticulitis.
- After an episode of diverticulitis, patients should undergo colonoscopy to rule out malignancy.
- Diverticular disease is a common cause of GI bleeding.

DOWN SYNDROME

Brian G. Skotko, MD, MPP • Michele Roberts, MD, PhD

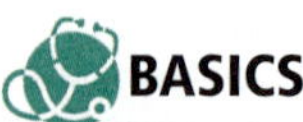

BASICS

DESCRIPTION

- Down syndrome (DS) is a congenital condition associated with intellectual disability and an increased chance of multisystem medical problems.
- Synonym: trisomy 21

Pediatric Considerations

A multidisciplinary evaluation is warranted (1).

Geriatric Considerations

Life expectancy has increased to ~60 years.

Pregnancy Considerations

The American College of Obstetricians and Gynecologists (ACOG) and the Society for Maternal-Fetal Medicine (SMFM) acknowledge that any women may choose noninvasive prenatal screening (NIPS). American College of Medical Genetics and Genomics (ACMG) recommends all women be offered NIPS (2),(3).

EPIDEMIOLOGY

Incidence

In the United States, 1/772 live births, ~5,100 births per year

Prevalence

~217,000 persons in the United States

ETIOLOGY AND PATHOPHYSIOLOGY

- Etiology: presence of all or part of an extra chromosome 21
- Trisomy 21: 95% of DS, an extra chromosome 21 is found in all cells due to nondisjunction, usually in maternal meiosis.
- Translocation DS: 3–4% of DS, extra chromosome 21q material is translocated to another chromosome (usually 13, 14, or 21); ~25% have parental origin.
- Mosaic DS: 1–2% of DS, manifestations may be milder.

Genetics

- Online Mendelian Inheritance in Man (OMIM) 190685
- Inheritance: most commonly sporadic nondisjunction resulting in trisomy 21
- Chance of having another child with DS is
  - 1% (or age risk, whichever is greater) after conceiving a pregnancy with nondisjunction trisomy 21
  - 10–15% for mothers/sisters and 3–5% for fathers/brothers who carry balanced translocation with chromosome 21
  - 100% if the parental balanced translocation is 21;21 (45,t[21;21])
  - Unclear after child with mosaic DS but ~1%

RISK FACTORS

- DS is believed to occur in all races and ethnicities with equal frequency, although live birth prevalence may differ based on different elective termination rates
- Chance of having an infant with DS increases with mother's age

GENERAL PREVENTION

Preimplantation diagnosis with in vitro fertilization (IVF), prenatal diagnosis followed by elective termination, and adoption are current options for expectant parents who do not wish to raise a child with DS.

COMMONLY ASSOCIATED CONDITIONS

- Cardiac
  - Congenital heart defects (40–50%)
- GI/growth
  - Feeding problems are common in infancy.
  - Structural defects (~12%)
  - Obesity
  - Gastroesophageal reflux
  - Constipation
  - Celiac disease (~5%)
- Pulmonary
  - Tracheal stenosis/tracheoesophageal fistula
  - Pulmonary hypertension
  - Obstructive sleep apnea (50–75%)
- Genitourinary
  - Cryptorchidism, hypospadias
- Hematologic/neoplastic
  - Transient abnormal myelopoiesis (~10%): generally resolves spontaneously; can be preleukemic (acute megakaryoblastic leukemia [AMKL]) in 20–30%
  - Leukemia (AMKL or acute lymphoblastic leukemia [ALL]) in 0.5–1%
  - Decreased risk of most solid tumors; increased risk of germ cell tumors/testicular cancer
- Endocrine
  - Hypothyroidism: congenital or acquired (13–63%)
  - Diabetes
- Skeletal
  - Atlantoaxial instability (15%): ~2% symptomatic
  - Short stature is common.
  - Scoliosis (Some cases have adult onset.)
  - Hip problems (1–4%)
- Immune/rheumatologic
  - Abnormal immune function with increased rate of respiratory infections
  - Increased risk of autoimmune disorders, including Hashimoto thyroiditis, celiac disease, and alopecia
- Neurologic
  - Intellectual ability ranging from mild to severe disability; average is moderate intellectual disability.
  - Autism spectrum disorder (<18%)
  - Hypotonia
  - Seizures (8%); typically occurring <1 year of age (infantile spasms) or >30 years of age
  - Alzheimer disease: At least 40% at age 40 years develop signs of dementia; percentage increases with age.
- Psychiatric
  - Attention deficit hyperactivity disorder (ADHD), obsessive-compulsive disorder (OCD), and autism spectrum disorder increased frequency in children.
  - Generalized depression and anxiety with increased frequency in young adults/adults
  - Down syndrome regression disorder is a very rare clinical regression syndrome that can occur in adolescents or young adults.
- Sensory
  - Hearing loss (75%): mostly conductive due to high frequency of asymptomatic middle ear effusion; otitis media (50–70%)
  - Visual impairment (60%): strabismus (refractive errors, 15%), myopia, hyperopia, nystagmus, cataracts (15%)
- Dermatologic
  - Xerosis, eczema, palmoplantar hyperkeratosis, atopic or seborrheic dermatitis, onychomycosis, syringomas, furunculosis/folliculitis, hidradenitis suppurativa

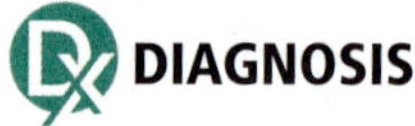

DIAGNOSIS

HISTORY

~85% of mothers of infants with DS learn of the diagnosis postnatally, although this is changing with the availability of prenatal screening such as NIPS.

PHYSICAL EXAM

- In November 2015, DS-specific growth charts were released. These charts do not represent "optimal" growth of children with DS; 50% BMI on the DS-specific growth curves corresponds to the 85% (overweight) on the standard NCHS growth curves (4).
- Infants and children
  - Brachycephaly (100%)
  - Hypotonia (80%)
  - Small ears, often low set and simplified
  - Upslanting palpebral fissure (90%)
  - Epicanthial folds (90%)
  - Brushfield spots
  - Depressed nasal bridge
  - Short neck, often with increased nuchal folds
  - Single palmar crease, single flexion crease on 5th finger
  - Increased space between toes 1 and 2, 5th finger clinodactyly, brachydactyly

DIAGNOSTIC TESTS & INTERPRETATION

Initial Tests (lab, imaging)

- Maternal prenatal screening includes the following:
  - 1st trimester: combined screen (maternal age, β-human chorionic gonadotropin [β-hCG], pregnancy-associated plasma protein A [PAPP-A], and nuchal translucency)
  - 2nd trimester: quad screen (α-fetoprotein, β-hCG, estriol, inhibin A)
  - Sequential screen (combined screen in 1st trimester, if abnormal, obtain amniocentesis *or* await 2nd trimester quad screening)
  - Integrated screen (combined screening in 1st trimester plus quad screen in 2nd trimester)
  - Prenatal cell-free DNA screening (beginning ~10 weeks' gestation) (2),(3)
- Prenatal diagnosis includes the following:
  - Chorionic villus sampling: 1st trimester, ~99% accurate, ~1% miscarriage
  - Amniocentesis: 2nd trimester, ~99% accurate, ~0.25% miscarriage rate
- Postnatal diagnosis
  - Fluorescence in situ hybridization (FISH) can be performed at time of clinical suspicion, but karyotype should always be done to differentiate genetic type of DS.
  - Karyotype of parents and adult siblings is indicated only if translocation DS is found in child.

- Workup for newborns (1)
  - Echo, with or without murmur
  - CBC with differential (to look for transient abnormal myelopoiesis)
  - Thyroid-stimulating hormone (TSH)
  - Audiogram
  - Ophthalmologic exam to assess for cataracts (Look for red reflex.)
  - Swallowing study for those with feeding difficulties
  - Car-seat test

Follow-Up Tests & Special Considerations

- After delivering a prenatal diagnosis, the clinician should offer "Understanding a Down Syndrome Diagnosis" (https://understandingdownsyndrome.org/).
- If the diagnosis is postnatal, the new parent and partner, if present, should be informed of the diagnosis promptly by a physician (preferably the obstetrician and pediatrician or family physician) on the basis of clinical observations and before the karyotype is available but with consideration of extenuating circumstances (e.g., birth parent's medical condition). The spouse/partner and infant should be present unless this would cause undue delay. The meeting should be private. Refer to the baby by name.
- In the postnatal setting, the clinician should be knowledgeable on the subject of DS and should conduct a discussion with content that is current, respectful, balanced, informative, and realistic but not overly pessimistic, concentrating on what is relevant to the 1st year of life.
- Cardiac follow-up, as indicated

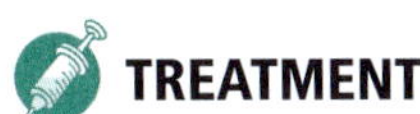

TREATMENT

ISSUES FOR REFERRAL

- Lactation consultant
- Physical/occupational/speech therapy (early intervention)
- Pediatric cardiologist, if indicated

SURGERY/OTHER PROCEDURES

Repair of congenital anomalies as needed.

COMPLEMENTARY & ALTERNATIVE MEDICINE

- There is no evidence to support the use of supplements in children with DS.
- Craniosacral manipulation is dangerous due to potential atlantoaxial instability.

ADMISSION, INPATIENT, AND NURSING CONSIDERATIONS

If the social situation indicates adoption, consider the National Down Syndrome Adoption Network (NDSAN) (https://www.ndsan.org/)—a national registry for families seeking to adopt a child with DS.

ONGOING CARE

FOLLOW-UP RECOMMENDATIONS

Patient Monitoring

- Children with DS: the American Academy of Pediatrics recommends ongoing assessment and review, at least annually, with the following surveillance (1):
  - Vision: Assess for strabismus, cataracts, and nystagmus by ophthalmologist by 6 months, annually between ages 1 and 5 years; every 2 years between ages 5 and 13 years; every 3 years between ages 13 and 21 years.
  - Hearing: neonatal screen with auditory brainstem response (ABR) or otoacoustic emissions (OAE), then audiogram every 6 months until age 3 years, and then annually
  - Thyroid: initial newborn screen; repeat TSH at 6 months, 12 months, and then annually (4)[C].
  - Screening for celiac disease (total IgA and tissue transglutaminase [tTG]-IgA) annually, if symptomatic
  - Three-view cervical spine films if patient symptomatic, beginning at 3 to 5 years of age
  - Hemoglobin test annually to screen for iron-deficiency anemia
  - Repeat echocardiogram in teens if with murmur or fatigue.
  - Sleep: Obtain a sleep study for everyone with DS between 3 and 5 years of age, given the high prevalence of obstructive sleep apnea
- Adults with DS: A comprehensive approach to medical care is also necessary (5). Monitor for obesity, hypothyroidism, and dementia.

DIET

- No special diet, but caloric needs are lower in adolescents/adults with DS than their peers.
- Obesity is prevalent at all ages.
- Dietary supplements targeting DS are of no benefit.

PATIENT EDUCATION

- Down Syndrome Clinic to You (DSC2U), an online health and wellness portal for patients with DS, their caregivers, and primary care providers; https://www.dsc2u.org
- National Down Syndrome Congress: 800-232-NDSC; https://www.ndsccenter.org/
- National Down Syndrome Society: 800-221-4602; https://ndss.org/
- The LuMind IDSC Down Syndrome Foundation provides information on the latest research for people with DS: https://lumindidsc.org/
- The National Center for Prenatal and Postnatal Resources provides peer-reviewed booklet for parents who have received a prenatal diagnosis of DS and have not yet made a decision about their pregnancy: https://www.lettercase.org/
- Down Syndrome Pregnancy provides free downloadable books and articles for expectant mothers who have decided to continue their pregnancies after a prenatal diagnosis of DS: https://downsyndromepregnancy.org/.
- Understanding a Down Syndrome Diagnosis provides an overview of DS and select resources: https://understandingdownsyndrome.org/

PROGNOSIS

- 99% of young adults/adults with DS report being happy with their lives.
- Life expectancy is ~60 years.

REFERENCES

1. Bull MJ, Trotter T, Santoro SL, et al; for Council on Genetics. Health supervision for children and adolescents with Down syndrome. *Pediatrics*. 2022;149(5):e2022057010. doi:10.1542/peds.2022-057010.
2. Rose NC, Kaimal AJ, Dugoff L, et al. Screening for fetal chromosomal abnormalities: ACOG Practice Bulletin, Number 226. *Obstetrics Gynecol*. 2020;136(4):e48–e69.
3. Dungan JS, Klugman S, Darilek S, et al. Noninvasive prenatal screening (NIPS) for fetal chromosome abnormalities in a general-risk population: an evidence-based clinical guideline of the American College of Medical Genetics and Genomics (ACMG). *Genet Med*. 2023;25(2):100336. doi:10.1016/j.gim.2022.11.004.
4. Zemel BS, Pipan M, Stallings VA, et al. Growth charts for children with Down syndrome in the United States. *Pediatrics*. 2015;136(5):e1204–e1211.
5. Tsou AY, Bulova P, Capone G, et al; for Global Down Syndrome Foundation Medical Care Guideline for Adults with Down Syndrome Workgroup. Medical care of adults with Down syndrome: a clinical guideline. *JAMA*. 2020;324(15):1543–1556.

ADDITIONAL READING

- Antonarakis SE, Skotko BG, Rafii MS, et al. Down syndrome. *Nat Rev Dis Primers*. 2020;6(1):9.
- Bull MJ. Down syndrome. *N Engl J Med*. 2020;382(24):2344–2352.

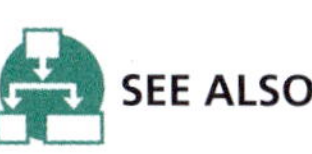

SEE ALSO

Algorithm: Intellectual Disability

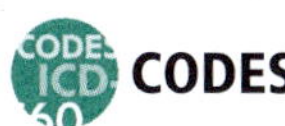

CODES

ICD10

- Q90.0 Trisomy 21, nonmosaicism (meiotic nondisjunction)
- Q90 Down syndrome
- Q90.1 Trisomy 21, mosaicism (mitotic nondisjunction)

CLINICAL PEARLS

- 99% of young adults/adults with DS report being happy with their lives.
- DS specialty clinics, including virtual ones like DSC2U, may improve medical outcomes.

D

DRUG ABUSE, PRESCRIPTION

Jeremy Golding, MD, FAAFP

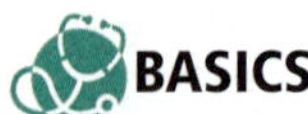

BASICS

Controlled substances are prone to misuse and diversion. Cautious prescribing should be considered in all cases, and monitoring all patients prescribed controlled substances to identify substance use disorder (SUD) is key. Patients with SUD should be offered treatment (and/or referred as needed).

DESCRIPTION

- Prescription drug abuse behaviors exist on a continuum and can include the following:
  - Use of medication for medical reasons other than what the prescriber intended
  - Use of medication for nonmedical reasons such as to get high (dissociative effects) or to enhance performance
  - Use of medication for any reason by someone other than the person it was intended for
- Commonly abused prescription medications include opioid analgesics, stimulants, central nervous system depressants, and barbiturates.
- *Diversion* is a term used to describe the rerouting of medications from prescriptions or other legitimate supplies for recreational use or criminal activity, such as selling prescription medication for personal profit.

EPIDEMIOLOGY

- From 2013 to 2018, substance use–related emergency department (ED) visits increased from 2.926 million to 4.132 million.
- The number of drug overdose deaths quadrupled from 1999 to 2019, and >932,000 deaths have been attributed to drug overdose.
- In 2020, >91,000 drug overdose deaths occurred in the United States in which opioids were responsible for 78.4% of those deaths.

Incidence

- Predominant sex: males > females
- 1 in 4 patients on long-term opioid therapy in primary care settings struggles with opioid addiction.
- Predominant age: highest among adults aged 18 to 25 years (mean 22 years), then adolescents and teens aged 12 to 17 years, followed by adults aged ≥26 years

Prevalence

In 2017, 191 million opioid prescriptions were issued and 11.5 million Americans reported misusing opioid medications.

ETIOLOGY AND PATHOPHYSIOLOGY

Opioids, benzodiazepines, stimulants, and barbiturates produce euphoria, tolerance, and dependence leading to misuse and addiction.

Genetics

Variant alleles affect the expression and function of opioid, dopamine, acetylcholine, serotonin, and γ-aminobutyric acid, helping to explain susceptibility to different forms.

RISK FACTORS

- Sociodemographic, psychiatric, pain, drug-related factors, genetics, sex, environment, and family history
- Ongoing opioid prescription (≥3 months) greatly increases risk of opioid-related overdose at 1 year (4-fold) and 5 years (30-fold).

GENERAL PREVENTION

- Try all available nonopioid treatments for pain before prescribing opioids for chronic pain.
- Limit/avoid prescribing controlled medications on the first visit and limit quantity of opioid pain medication prescribed to a few days.
- Screen by asking questions about unhealthy drug use (including prescription drugs, USPSTF-B recommendation).
- Conduct thorough history, review records (prescription monitoring programs [PMP]), and perform urine drug screens (UDSs) before deciding if a controlled substance is indicated.
- Avoid prescribing benzodiazepines in the treatment of anxiety. Try cognitive-behavioral therapy, mindfulness, selective serotonin reuptake inhibitors, PRN antihistamines (anti-H1), or buspirone.
- Support the use of CDC guidelines for prescribing controlled substances for chronic pain while integrating quality improvement measures, making these standard practice.
- Wean/stop prescription analgesics for chronic pain if ineffective for improving pain and function, if aberrant behaviors suggesting opioid use present, or if patient overdoses.
- Dose reduction of chronic opioids can decrease risk while improving pain, function, and quality of life.
- Prescribe intranasal naloxone to all patients prescribed chronic opioids, provide education to patient and family members on proper use in case of overdose and increase access to SUD services.
- Identify and treat underlying SUD.

COMMONLY ASSOCIATED CONDITIONS

- Opioids: tolerance, opioid-induced hyperalgesia, dependence, addiction (which can lead to loss of savings, job, close relationships and incarceration, hepatitis C virus or HIV infection, etc.), overdose/death, depression, constipation, low testosterone, and sexual dysfunction
- Benzodiazepines and barbiturates: dependence (withdrawal can cause seizures, delirium tremens, death), psychosis, anxiety, sleep driving, blackout states, cognitive impairment, impaired driving; increased fall risk and mortality in elderly patients
- Stimulants: dependence, hypertension, tachyarrhythmias, myocardial ischemia, seizures, hypothermia, psychosis, hallucinations, paranoia, anxiety

DIAGNOSIS

- Initial screening: "How many times in the past year have you used an illegal drug or used a prescription medication for nonmedical reasons?"; primary care setting sensitivity of 100% and specificity of ~75%
- Other screening tools: Drug Abuse Screening Test (DAST) helps determine involvement with drugs over the past year; assess alcohol use with CAGE or Alcohol Use Disorders Identification Test (AUDIT); SUD diagnostic criteria as per *DSM-5*

HISTORY

Patients may show hostile/threatening, impulsive or flattering behavior. Patients may ask for dose/quantity increase, fabricate false stories, ask for early refills, ask for specific drugs by name, make appointments near the end of the day and also try to establish care after clinic hours.

PHYSICAL EXAM

- Monitor patients for signs of sedation, confusion, or intoxication (can include slurred speech and unsteady gait in case of benzodiazepines). Patient may have unkept or disheveled appearance.
- Physical exam findings of opioid withdrawal including dilated pupils, frequent yawning, tachycardia, elevated blood pressure, and piloerection. In benzodiazepine withdrawal, symptoms include tachycardia, elevated blood pressure, and tremors.
- There are often no physical exam findings when a patient is misusing a prescription medication; other objective findings such as urine drug testing should be used in monitoring.

DIFFERENTIAL DIAGNOSIS

Depression, anxiety, mania, psychosis

DIAGNOSTIC TESTS & INTERPRETATION

UDSs are recommended to ensure safe use of medication and prevent diversions. Assessing baseline CBC, electrolytes, renal function, liver function, thyroid function, fasting plasma glucose, lipid panel along with testing for communicable diseases (HIV, hepatitis, and syphilis) may help rule out other pathologic states.

Initial Tests (lab, imaging)

- UDSs: Ensure the panel includes semisynthetics (hydrocodone, hydromorphone, oxycodone) and synthetics (methadone, fentanyl, propoxyphene, meperidine) along with tramadol and buprenorphine. Test for other drugs of abuse such as benzodiazepines (clonazepam, alprazolam, lorazepam are ordered individually), cocaine, amphetamine, alcohol metabolites, marijuana and consider other drugs that may be highly prevalent in your area (e.g., gabapentin, PCP, barbiturates).
- Codeine will be positive for codeine plus morphine.
- Morphine will be positive for morphine.
- Oxycodone (OxyContin) will be positive for oxycodone and oxymorphone.
- Hydrocodone will be positive for hydrocodone and hydromorphone.
- Buprenorphine will be positive for buprenorphine and norbuprenorphine.
- Diazepam will be positive for nordiazepam, oxazepam, and temazepam.
- Chlordiazepoxide will be positive for nordiazepam and oxazepam.
- Alprazolam will be positive for α-hydroxyalprazolam.
- Clonazepam will be positive for 7-aminoclonazepam.
- Lorazepam will be positive for lorazepam-glucuronide.

Follow-Up Tests & Special Considerations

Random pill counts are useful for identifying patients taking more controlled substance than prescribed. Random urine drug testing can also be concurrently collected. Ancillary services such as rehab may help improve outcomes.

Test Interpretation

- Screening drug tests (by enzyme-linked immunosorbent assay method) may result in false positives from interactions with other commonly prescribed medications or substances people are frequently exposed to (e.g., poppy seeds [opioid], hemp food products [marijuana], diet pills, and energy drinks [amphetamines]); treatment decisions should be based on highly specific confirmation testing (e.g., by gas chromatography/mass spectrometry).
- Results are positive if drugs (or metabolites of drugs) that are not prescribed are present; positive in presence of illicit drugs (e.g., cocaine)
- Suspect diversion when negative for prescribed drug at a time when the patient reported taking it.

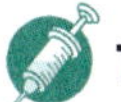

TREATMENT

The general approach to treatment includes inpatient, residential, or outpatient detoxification as required; counseling and intensive counseling as needed; and ongoing medication-assisted treatment (MAT) with buprenorphine or injectable naltrexone. Several interventions for treatment and prevention of opioid use disorder (OUD) are likely cost-effective, but the research base for other drugs is less robust (1)[A].

- Buprenorphine/naloxone: Begin taper to initiate discontinuation whenever there is evidence of prescription opioid abuse. Some situations indicate immediate discontinuation rather than taper (e.g., diversion or plan to switch to buprenorphine/naloxone treatment).
- Opioid discontinuation through interdisciplinary pain care programs, buprenorphine-assisted or methadone programs, and detoxification programs have achieved opioid discontinuation rates >85%.
- Effective medications to treat OUD include methadone hydrochloride, buprenorphine, and naltrexone hydrochloride, but these medications are underused, and the risk of relapse is still high (2).
- Benzodiazepines cannot be stopped abruptly for risk of seizures and death, therefore discontinue via slow taper.
- Amphetamines can be stopped abruptly without risk of severe withdrawal or death.

GENERAL MEASURES

Multiple treatments are available including inpatient programs (detoxification and induction into MAT), outpatient programs (MAT and behavioral health), and peer-led support services.

MEDICATION

Short-term opioid detoxification programs use clonidine, buprenorphine, or methadone under the direction of an addiction specialist. Long-term MAT with buprenorphine/naloxone, methadone, or naltrexone is more effective than short-term detoxification.

- Buprenorphine and naloxone MAT
  - Any provider (MD, DO, NP, or PA) may prescribe buprenorphine/naloxone after completing training.
  - Buprenorphine/naloxone titrated to the maximum of 24 mg/day for patients who continue to use opioids.
  - Naloxone-based formulations discourage misuse (such as by sniffing or IV) because naloxone displaces buprenorphine binding to opioid receptors when taken parenterally.
  - Buprenorphine available as monthly long-acting injectable administered by a nurse at clinic, eliminating the need for daily dosing and diversion-related issues while creating an opportunity to offer support.
  - Naltrexone (oral or long-acting injectable), an opioid antagonist, reduces cravings for opioids and opioid-euphoria when ingested; started after a person has been off opioids for 7 days to avoid acute, severe withdrawal.
  - Buprenorphine/naloxone and methadone are similarly effective when used in long-term opioid maintenance therapy.
- Methadone: dispensed by addiction specialists for treatment of OUD at a certified opioid treatment program

First Line

Multiple modalities including MAT, support groups, etc. tailored to specific patient needs

ISSUES FOR REFERRAL

Enlist the help of chemical dependency groups/addiction specialists/pain management and psychiatry/psychology when polysubstance abuse suspected and to treat underlying psychiatric disorders.

ADDITIONAL THERAPIES

- Behavioral health support or SMART Recovery and 12-step programs such as AA and NA
- Residential treatment programs (short-term vs. long-term rehabilitation, transitional support programs, crisis stabilization units)
- Al-Anon/Alateen and Learn to Cope provide helpful free support groups for family members.

COMPLEMENTARY & ALTERNATIVE MEDICINE

Mindfulness and meditation, acupuncture, or yoga may help with stress reduction.

ADMISSION, INPATIENT, AND NURSING CONSIDERATIONS

Consider additional support if continued use of opioids despite outpatient treatment, concomitant alcohol and benzodiazepine dependence (increased risk of seizures), mental confusion/delirium, history of seizures, psychosis, suicidal ideation, serious, or absence of social support.

ONGOING CARE

Treatment with MAT should continue for as long as the patient benefits from it.

FOLLOW-UP RECOMMENDATIONS

Expert opinion suggests high-frequency visits (such as weekly) when a patient begins MAT.

Patient Monitoring

Monitor patients with in-person check-ins, drug testing, and review of the PMP.

DIET

If concern for opioid-induced constipation, tapering dose to complete cessation with increase in high-fiber diet, stool softeners, stimulant laxative, and increased hydration

PATIENT EDUCATION

- Controlled medication should be inaccessible to others (ideally in locked box/bag). Diverting medication may result in legal charges.
- Address "red flags"; dose escalation when necessary; provide support and strategies for managing stress, cravings, preoccupation about the next dose and abuse identification.

PROGNOSIS

The majority of patients with SUD are able to achieve remission.

COMPLICATIONS

Misuse of opioids and benzodiazepines may lead to overdose and death. Misuse of stimulants may lead to psychosis and cardiac conditions such as myocardial infarction and arrhythmias.

REFERENCES

1. Rodríguez-Tanta LY, Summers A, Shaya FT. Cost-effective interventions to prevent prescription drug misuse: a systematic review. *Front Public Health*. 2025;13:1514851.
2. Volkow ND, Jones EB, Einstein EB, et al. Prevention and treatment of opioid misuse and addiction: a review. *JAMA Psychiatry*. 2019;76(2):208–216.

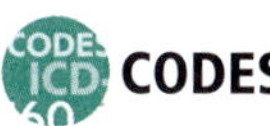

CODES

ICD10

- F19.10 Other psychoactive substance abuse, uncomplicated
- F11.10 Opioid abuse, uncomplicated
- F15.10 Other stimulant abuse, uncomplicated

CLINICAL PEARLS

- Addiction is a treatable chronic disease. Most licensed physicians and nurse practitioners may now provide MAT with buprenorphine without the requirement of special certification.
- Discontinue prescription opioid analgesics if pain or functionality does not improve or if there is evidence of abuse or diversion (e.g., positive UDSs, driving while intoxicated [DWI], overdose, early refills).
- PMPs reduce doctor shopping but not ED visits for overdose and prescription drug abuse–related deaths.

DUCTAL CARCINOMA IN SITU

Andrew Timothy Ng, MBBS • Prarthna V. Bhardwaj, MD

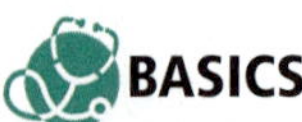

BASICS

DESCRIPTION

- Ductal carcinoma in situ (DCIS) is a heterogeneous group of malignant lesions with neoplastic, clonal proliferation of noninvasive epithelial cells confined to the milk ducts.
- Comprises 1 in 4 cases of all newly diagnosed breast cancers
- Mortality from DCIS with subsequent progression to invasive breast carcinoma (IBC) is low (<1%), regardless of histologic type or treatment.

EPIDEMIOLOGY

Incidence

- Estimated 59,080 new diagnoses of DCIS for US women in 2025 (1)
- DCIS accounts for ~80–85% of in situ breast carcinomas (lobular carcinoma in situ [LCIS] accounts for approximately 15–20%) and ~25% of all new breast cancers.
- Increase in incidence with increase in age; rate of DCIS doubles from age range of 40 to 49 years to 70 to 84 years.

ETIOLOGY AND PATHOPHYSIOLOGY

Genetics

BRCA1 and *BRCA2* has been associated with DCIS, but with a lower strength of association compared to invasive breast cancer.

RISK FACTORS

- Female sex, nulliparity, late age at first birth or menopause, older age, first-degree relative with breast cancer, long-term use of postmenopausal combined estrogen and progestin therapy, history of atypical ductal hyperplasia (ADH), obesity, alcohol use, dense breast tissue
- Associations with age at menarche, lactation history, oral contraceptive use, and smoking remain unclear.

GENERAL PREVENTION

- Screening may result in overdiagnosis with little or no reduction in the incidence of advanced cancers.
- General screening guidelines—U.S. Preventive Services Task Force (USPSTF):
  - Biennial mammography (MMG) for women aged 40 to 74 years (B recommendation)
  - Insufficient evidence regarding benefits and harms of screening MMG if ≥75 years old
  - Current evidence suggests that both digital MMG and digital breast tomosynthesis (DBT) are effective primary screening modalities.
  - Insufficient evidence to assess the balance of benefits and harms of adjunctive screening using breast ultrasonography, magnetic resonance imaging (MRI), DBT, or other methods in women identified to have dense breasts on an otherwise negative screening mammogram
- Clinical breast exam (CBE):
  - USPSTF does not address the CBE in its most recent 2024 screening guideline, but previous 2019 guidelines stated that there is insufficient evidence to assess benefits and harms when added to MMG screening for women aged ≥ 40 years.
  - WHO states CBE may be beneficial in settings with weak health settings (MMG not accessible) for women 50 to 69 years old.
- Risk reduction:
  - Limit alcohol intake to <1 drink per day, exercise, maintain a healthy diet, and weight control.
  - Hormonal risk reduction agents recommended in certain high-risk women ≥35 years old; tamoxifen for premenopausal women and raloxifene for postmenopausal women
  - Anastrozole (an aromatase inhibitor) significantly decreases incidence of DCIS in postmenopausal women.

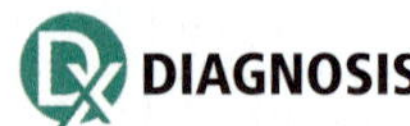

DIAGNOSIS

PHYSICAL EXAM

- CBE with patient in upright and supine position; evaluating for asymmetry, spontaneous discharge, skin changes, nipple retraction/excoriation (Paget disease)
- Palpation of all breast quadrants, including lymph nodes (axillary, supraclavicular, and cervical)
- Positive clinical findings: Refer for diagnostic imaging and/or surgical evaluation unless <30 years old with a low clinical suspicion (observe 1 to 2 menstrual cycles; refer if clinical findings persist).

DIFFERENTIAL DIAGNOSIS

Usual ductal hyperplasia, columnar cell changes, flat epithelial atypia, ADH, LCIS, microinvasive carcinoma, intraductal papilloma, mucinous breast lesions

DIAGNOSTIC TESTS & INTERPRETATION

Initial Tests (lab, imaging)

- MMG breast imaging–reporting and data system (BI-RADS): BI-RADS is a quality assurance (QA) method published by the American Radiology Society.
  - BI-RADS has been extended to breast US and MRI interpretation as well.
  - Components of BI-RADS report:
    - Indication for study and type of examination
    - Overall breast composition, including breast density
      - A—Breasts are almost entirely fatty tissue.
      - B—scattered areas of fibroglandular density
      - C—heterogenously dense
      - D—extremely dense
- DCIS most often seen as clustered microcalcifications.

Follow-Up Tests & Special Considerations

- Sensitivity of breast MRI screening > MMG; with decreased specificity resulting in an increased number of false positives
- Specific recommendations vary by organization, but screening MRI is only recommended in certain women with higher-than-average risk per consensus recommendations:
  - *BRCA* mutation—commence at ages 25 to 29 years
  - First-degree relative of *BRCA* carrier
  - ≥20% lifetime risk of breast cancer defined by models that are largely based on family history (commonly used models include Gail Model and Tyrer-Cuzick model)
  - Thoracic radiation between the ages of 10 and 30 years—annual breast MRI to begin 10 years after radiation therapy but not prior to age 25 years
  - Presence of Li-Fraumeni, *PTEN*, or Bannayan-Riley-Ruvalcaba syndrome in patient or first-degree relative
  - ≥20% risk of breast cancer based on gene and/or risk level: ATM, CDH1, CHEK2, PALB2, PTEN, STK11, TP53
- Pathology
  - Tissue is necessary for diagnosis: typically core needle (CN) or vacuum-assisted (VA) biopsy (mammographic/stereotactic, US, or MRI guided).
  - Fine-needle aspiration (FNA) is not adequate for specific diagnosis of DCIS; however, it can suggest the presence of neoplastic cells.
  - Histologic classification
    - Classification is subjective; however, traditionally classified as either low, intermediate, or high grade based on architectural patterns (comedo, solid, cribriform, clinging, papillary, and micropapillary), nuclear grade (I, II, or III), and the absence or presence of necrosis
    - Ductal intraepithelial neoplasia (DIN) is an alternative histologic classification incorporating size as a discriminating factor.
    - Grade is more important for prognosis, risk for progression, and local recurrence.
    - Comedo-type necrosis (necrosis filling central portion of involved duct) is typically seen in high-grade DCIS, with varying degrees of necrosis in other types of DCIS.
  - Determination of ER and PR status

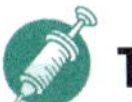

TREATMENT

MEDICATION

- For patients undergoing bilateral mastectomy for other reasons, chemoprevention is *not* required for DCIS.
- Secondary chemoprevention following breast-conserving surgery for ER+ DCIS:
  - Tamoxifen for premenopausal patients or tamoxifen or an aromatase inhibitor for postmenopausal patients for 5 years
  - There may be some advantage for aromatase inhibitor therapy in patients <60 years old or patients with concerns for thromboembolism.
  - Considered in lumpectomy patients with or without whole breast radiation
  - Adjuvant chemotherapy is not indicated.

SURGERY/OTHER PROCEDURES

- Surgery is the primary treatment option.
  - Options for surgery are based on risk of recurrence, anatomic location, extent of disease, and the ability to achieve "negative" margins.
- Surgical options include the following:
  - Breast conservation (lumpectomy) without lymph node procedure, with or without breast radiation therapy
  - A sentinel lymph node biopsy may be considered if the lumpectomy is in an anatomic location compromising the performance of a future sentinel lymph node procedure.
  - Patients not amenable to margin-free lumpectomy should have total mastectomy.
  - Mastectomy with or without sentinel node biopsy plus optional breast reconstruction
  - A complete axillary lymph node dissection should not be performed in the absence of evidence of invasive cancer and proven axillary metastatic disease.
  - Long-term cause-specific survival with mastectomy seems to be equivalent to lumpectomy with whole breast radiation.
- Radiation considerations:
  - Radiation decreases recurrence rates by about 50% but with no overall survival benefit.
  - Side effects include burden of daily treatments, slight increase in secondary cancers, inability to receive radiation therapy again in ipsilateral breast.
- DCIS recurrence considerations:
  - Recurrence generally requires mastectomy; rates of recurrence for DCIS and IBC are similar:
    - ~50% of recurrences are pure DCIS; ~50% are IBC.

ONGOING CARE

FOLLOW-UP RECOMMENDATIONS

- History and physical exam should occur every 6 to 12 months for the first 5 years and then annually after that.
- MMG every 12 months (first mammogram 6 to 12 months after breast conservation therapy)
- If treated with tamoxifen or an aromatase inhibitor, monitor per consensus guidelines for breast cancer risk reduction.

PROGNOSIS

- 10-year breast cancer–specific survival of around 98%
- Risk of local recurrence after mastectomy 1–2%
- Higher risk of local recurrences after breast-conserving therapy occurs in:
  - Age <40 years, larger tumor size, high nuclear grade, comedo-type necrosis, close/positive margin status (related to DCIS volume)
- ER+ tumors are associated with lower risk for recurrence.
- There is interest in identifying subsets of patients who have low rates of ipsilateral breast tumor recurrence such that they might safely forgo radiation.
  - The Oncotype DX DCIS test may help clinicians in selecting which patients with DCIS might safely forgo radiation therapy after breast-conserving surgery.
    - The test results in an Oncotype DX DCIS score, with the following risk categories:
      - *DCIS score <39*—low risk of recurrence
        - Radiation therapy benefits likely to be small and will not outweigh the risks of side effects
      - *DCIS score 39 to 54*—intermediate risk of recurrence
        - Radiation therapy benefits unclear relative to the risks of side effects
      - *DCIS score 55 to 100*—high risk of recurrence
        - Radiation therapy benefits are likely to be greater than the risks of side effects.

REFERENCES

1. American Cancer Society. *Cancer Facts & Figures 2025*. Atlanta, GA: American Cancer Society; 2025.

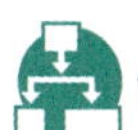

SEE ALSO

Breast Cancer

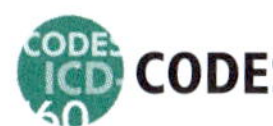

CODES

ICD10

- D05.10 Intraductal carcinoma in situ of unspecified breast
- D05.11 Intraductal carcinoma in situ of right breast
- D05.12 Intraductal carcinoma in situ of left breast

CLINICAL PEARLS

- DCIS is a heterogeneous group of *noninvasive* neoplastic breast ductal epithelial cell lesions.
- The incidence of DCIS has continued to increase in women with increase in age; more stable incidence in women >50 years of age
- Increased incidence, including for women <50 years of age, attributable to advancements in screening MMG.
- The primary goal of DCIS treatment is to prevent recurrence and progression to IBC.
- The Oncotype DX DCIS score may help clinicians in selecting which patients with DCIS who may safely forgo radiation therapy after breast-conserving surgery.
- Current standard of care is local treatment with breast-conserving therapy or mastectomy, with consideration for postoperative whole breast radiation therapy and/or postsurgical tamoxifen or aromatase inhibitor therapy, unless otherwise contraindicated.
- With appropriate therapy, the overall prognosis of pure DCIS is excellent.

D

DUPUYTREN CONTRACTURE

Karl T. Clebak, MD, MHA, FAAFP • Morris K. Taylor, MD

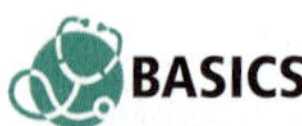

BASICS

DESCRIPTION

- Palmar fibromatosis is caused by progressive fibrosis of the palmar fascia, leading to flexion deformities and functional loss.
- Distinct from "trigger finger," which results from thickening of the distal flexor tendon.
- Similar change rarely occurs in plantar fascia, usually appearing simultaneously.
- System(s) affected: musculoskeletal
- Dupuytren diathesis is an aggressive heritable form associated with age of onset <40 years, bilateral presentation to include radial digits, plantar fibromatosis (Ledderhose disease), and penile fibromatosis (Peyronie disease) (1).
- Synonyms: morbus Dupuytren; Dupuytren disease; "Celtic hand"; Viking disease; palmar fascial fibromatosis, contracture of palmar fascia

EPIDEMIOLOGY

Prevalence

- Increases with age; mean prevalence in western countries: 12%, 21%, and 29% at ages 55, 65, and 75 years, respectively; Norway: 30% of males aged >60 years; Spain: 19% of males aged >60 years
- More common in Caucasian men of Scandinavian or Northern European ancestry
- Mean age of onset is 60 years with typical age-range of onset between 40 and 80 years.

ETIOLOGY AND PATHOPHYSIOLOGY

- Definitive etiology unknown; possibly oxidative stress, altered wound repair, and/or abnormal immune response
- Progresses through three stages (Luck classification) (1):
  - Proliferative phase: proliferation of myofibroblasts with thickening of the palmar fascia and nodule development on palmar surface
  - Involutional stage: Myofibroblasts spread along palmar fascia to fingers with cord development via production of more type 3 collagen.
  - Residual phase: Fibroblasts are predominant with dense collagen leading to cord tightening and contracture flexion formation.

Genetics

- Autosomal dominant inheritance with incomplete penetrance:
  - Siblings with 3-fold risk
- 68% of male relatives of affected patients develop disease at some time.
- Possible association with HLA alleles

RISK FACTORS

- Smoking (mean 16 pack-years, odds ratio: 2.8)
- Increasing age
- Male/Caucasian; male > female (range 3.5:1 to 9:1)
- Vibration exposure and manual work—risk doubles if regular (weekly) exposure
- Diabetes mellitus (DM) (increases with duration of DM, usually mild; middle and ring fingers are involved)
- Excessive alcohol consumption
- Cirrhosis
- Northern European ethnicity
- Family history
- Hand trauma
- Low body weight and BMI

COMMONLY ASSOCIATED CONDITIONS

- Alcoholism
- Epilepsy (inconstant data)
- DM, particularly type 1 DM
- Chronic lung disease
- Occupational hand trauma (vibration)
- Hypercholesterolemia
- Carpal tunnel syndrome
- Peyronie disease
- HIV
- Cancer
- Adhesive capsulitis of shoulder

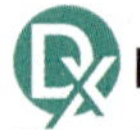

DIAGNOSIS

Diagnosis is primarily clinical, relying on history and physical examination.

HISTORY

- Caucasian male aged 40 to 80 years
- Family history and additional risk factors as listed above.
- Commonly report loss of ability to complete iADLs (1)
- Gradual onset of a painless palmar nodule.
- Progression to include:
  - Pain of palpable nodule
  - Loss of function of affected finger
- Ring finger or middle finger is the most common, but any digit can be involved (1).
- Metacarpophalangeal (MCP) joint is most commonly affected; proximal and distal interphalangeal joints are rarely affected (1).

PHYSICAL EXAM

- Visual inspection and palpation of the affected region of the palm to assess for nodule or cordlike band
- Earliest sign is triangular "puckering" over the flexor tendon proximal to flexor crease. Palmar nodules, adjacent to distal palmar crease present early and are pathognomonic.
- Assess for contracture of the affected finger.
  - More common in ulnar digits
  - Hueston table top test—ask patient to lay hands flat on table, positive if patient is unable to lie fingers flat
  - Garrod nodes—callous over knuckles, associated with severe disease progression
- Tubiana staging (2)
  - 0: no extension deficit, no disease
  - N: no extension deficit, nodule present on exam
  - I: 1 to 45 degrees of extension deficit (surgical referral warranted)
  - II: 46 to 90 degrees of extension deficit
  - III: 91 to 135 degrees of extension deficit
  - IV: >135 degrees of extension deficit

DIFFERENTIAL DIAGNOSIS

- Camptodactyly: early teens; tight fascial bands on ulnar side of small finger
- Diabetic cheiroarthropathy: all four fingers
- Volkmann ischemic contracture
- Trigger finger (thickening of the distal flexor tendon)
- Ganglion cyst
- Claw hand deformity from proximal ulnar nerve lesion

DIAGNOSTIC TESTS & INTERPRETATION

Initial Tests (lab, imaging)

Diagnosis is based on history and physical; testing is not routinely indicated. MRI can assess cellularity of lesions that correlate with recurrence after surgery. Ultrasound of palm can assess nodules and cords.

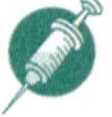

TREATMENT

No definitive cure exists and all treatments are palliative. Patients must be educated that risk for recurrence exists with all treatment, surgical and non-surgical (3).

GENERAL MEASURES

- Observation for mild disease is reasonable.
- Use of extension splints
- Physical therapy for range of motion
- See indications for surgical referral below.

MEDICATION

Repeat collagenase treatment can yield similar deformity correction but may lead to a higher risk of adverse events.

First Line

- Clostridial collagenase injections (FDA-approved 2010):
  - Degrades collagen to allow manual rupture of diseased cord
  - Best for isolated cord of MCP joint
  - 5-year recurrence rate of 47%; comparable with surgical recurrence rates
  - More rapid recovery of hand function compared to limited fasciectomy with fewer serious adverse events
  - Complications: injection site reaction, skin tear
  - Can do two cords concurrently
  - Can be effective for postsurgical recurrence
- Steroid injection:
  - Can treat acute nodules or painful knuckle pads
  - Serial triamcinolone injections improved long-term outcomes when combined with needle aponeurotomy.
  - Steroid alone is associated with 50% recurrence in 1 to 3 years.

Second Line

Extracorporeal shockwave treatment

ISSUES FOR REFERRAL

Indications for orthopedic surgery referral:

- Any involvement of PIP joints
- MCP joints contracted >30 degrees
- Impaired function
- Disabling deformity

ADDITIONAL THERAPIES

Percutaneous and needle fasciotomy:

- Best for MCP joint; improvement of 93% versus improvement of 57% for PIP joint
- Recurrence common; 50%
- Shown to be effective for recurrent disease
- Better for MCP joints in patients with comorbid conditions; lower complication rate but higher recurrence
- At 3 months and 1 year, outcomes of needle fasciotomy and collagenase injections are the same.

SURGERY/OTHER PROCEDURES

- Dermofasciectomy/limited fasciectomy/segmental aponeurectomy:
  - Greater initial correction over nonincisional treatment; higher complication rates; superior long-term advantages over collagenase injections and needle fasciotomy
  - Percutaneous aponeurotomy and lipofilling (PALF) is a new, minimally invasive procedure that appears to have shorter convalescence, less long-term complications, similar operative contraction correction, and no significant difference at 1 year in results versus limited fasciectomy.
- Indications:
  - Any involvement of the PIP joints
  - MCP joints contracted at least 30 degrees
  - Positive Hueston table top test (Patient is unable to lay palm flat on a table.)
- May require skin grafts for wound closure with severe cutaneous shrinkage
- 80% have full range of movement with early surgery.
- Amputation of 5th digit if severe and deforming
- MCP joints respond better to surgery than PIP joints, especially if contracted >45 degrees.

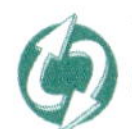

ONGOING CARE

FOLLOW-UP RECOMMENDATIONS

Patient Monitoring

Regular follow-up every 6 months to 1 year

PATIENT EDUCATION

- Avoid risk factors (alcohol, vibratory exposure, etc.), especially if strong family history.
- For mild disease: Stretch digits passively twice daily and avoid repeated tool gripping.

PROGNOSIS

- Unpredictable but usually slowly progressive; without any treatment, progression is observed in about 50% over 6 years.
- 10% may regress spontaneously.
- Dupuytren diathesis predicts aggressive course. Features include ethnicity (Nordic), family history, bilateral lesions outside of palm, age <50 years—all factors with 71% risk of recurrence compared to baseline 23% without any risk factors.
- MCP joints have better prognosis than PIP joints after surgery and collagenase injection.

COMPLICATIONS

- Complex regional pain syndrome
- Operative nerve injury
- Postoperative recurrence in 46–80%
- Postoperative hand edema and skin necrosis
- Digital infarction
- Limited hand function

REFERENCES

1. Dutta A, Jayasinghe G, Deore S, et al. Dupuytren's contracture—current concepts. *J Clin Orthop Trauma*. 2020;11(4):590–596.
2. Mella JR, Guo L, Hung V. Dupuytren's contracture: an evidence based review. *Ann Plast Surg*. 2018;81(6S Suppl 1):S97–S101.
3. Wong CR, Huynh MNQ, Fageeh R, et al. Outcomes of management of recurrent Dupuytren contracture: a systematic review and meta-analysis. *HAND (NY)*. 2022;17(6):1104–1113.

ADDITIONAL READING

- Eaton C. Evidence-based medicine: Dupuytren contracture. *Plast Reconstr Surg*. 2014;133(5):1241–1251.
- Lanting R, Broekstra DC, Werker PMN, et al. A systematic review and meta-analysis on the prevalence of Dupuytren disease in the general population of Western countries. *Plast Reconstr Surg*. 2014;133(3):593–603.
- Obed D, Salim M, Schlottmann F, et al. Short-term efficacy and adverse effects of collagenase clostridium histolyticum injections, percutaneous needle fasciotomy and limited fasciectomy in the treatment of Dupuytren's contracture: a network meta-analysis of randomized controlled trials. *BMC Musculoskelet Disord*. 2022;23(1):939.

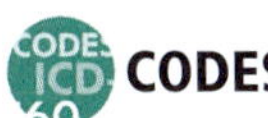

CODES

ICD10

M72.0 Palmar fascial fibromatosis [Dupuytren]

CLINICAL PEARLS

- Dupuytren contracture is a fixed flexion deformity of (most commonly) the 4th and 5th digits due to palmar fibrosis. 90% of cases are progressive; not "trigger finger" which is due to thickening of the distal flexor tendon
- Refer patients with involvement of the PIP joints or MCP joints involvement with contractures of >30 degrees.
- Both surgical and enzymatic fasciotomy have high rate of recurrence.

DYSHIDROSIS

Robyn Lee Reese, DO • Adrianna D. M. Clapp, MD, BSc

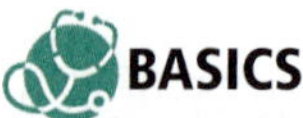

BASICS

DESCRIPTION

- Common, chronic or recurrent dermatitis involving the palms and soles. The precise definition is not well-settled, with many terms used interchangeably.
- Nonerythematous; symmetric, fluid filled, deep vesicular eruption primarily of the palms, soles, and interdigital areas
- Associated with burning, itching, and pain
- System(s) affected: dermatologic, exocrine, immunologic
- Synonym(s): dyshidrotic eczema, pompholyx (from Greek "bubble"), lamellar dyshidrosis, acute palmoplantar eczema, cheiropompholyx, keratolysis exfoliativa, vesicular palmoplantar eczema, desquamation of interdigital spaces pompholyx, acute and recurrent vesicular hand dermatitis, recurrent vesicular palmoplantar dermatitis

EPIDEMIOLOGY

Incidence

- Mean age of onset is ≤40 years.
- Male < female
- Comprises 5–20% of hand eczema cases

Prevalence

20 cases/100,000 people

ETIOLOGY AND PATHOPHYSIOLOGY

- Exact mechanism is unknown; thought to be multifactorial (allergies, genetics, and dermatophyte infection implicated)
- Dermatopathology: intraepidermal spongiosis without effect on eccrine sweat glands
- Vesicles remain intact due to thickness of stratum corneum of palmar/plantar skin (1).
- Immunologic reaction: theorized that rapid rise in immunoglobulin levels may precipitate vesicle formation

Genetics

- Atopy: 50% of patients with dyshidrotic eczema have atopic dermatitis (1). Transcriptome analysis results in a large overlap between vesicular hand eczema and atopic dermatitis.
- Hypothesized that overexpression of 2 water/glycerol channel proteins (aquaporin-3 and aquaporin-10) may alter the function of the epidermal water permeability barrier.
- Rare autosomal dominant form of pompholyx found in Chinese population maps to chromosome 18q22.1–18q22.3 (2)

RISK FACTORS

- Many risk factors and aggravating factors are disputed in the literature, with none being consistently associated.
- Atopy
- Other dermatologic conditions
  - Atopic dermatitis (early in life)
  - Contact dermatitis (later in life)
  - Dermatophytosis (present in 10% of patients with the condition) (2)
  - Hyperhidrosis (present in 40% of patients with the condition)
  - Contact sensitivity present in 30–67% patients (2)
- Sensitivity to
  - Foods
  - Drugs: neomycin, quinolones, acetaminophen, oral contraceptives, and IV immunoglobulin therapy
  - Metals: nickel (more common in young women), cobalt, and chromate (more common in men) sensitivity which may include implanted orthopedic or orthodontic metals (1)
  - Smoking
  - Detergents/solvents
  - Increased water exposure (e.g., florists, hair stylists, health care workers)
  - Cement exposure (construction/industrial workers)
  - Climate: hot/cold weather; humidity
  - Stress
  - Prolonged wear of occlusive gloves
  - Sunlight/UVA radiation

GENERAL PREVENTION

- Control emotional stress.
- Avoid excessive sweating.
- Avoid exposure to irritants.
- Avoid diet high in metal salts (chromium, cobalt, nickel).
- Avoid smoking.

COMMONLY ASSOCIATED CONDITIONS

- Atopic dermatitis
- Allergic contact dermatitis
- Parkinson disease
- HIV (2)

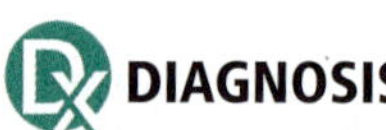

DIAGNOSIS

HISTORY

- Episodes of pruritic rash
- Recent emotional stress
- Familial or personal history of atopy
- Exposure to allergens or irritants
  - Occupational, dietary, or household
  - Cosmetic and personal hygiene products
  - Vesicular eruption typically occurs 24 hours after allergen challenge (1).
- Costume jewelry use
- IV immunoglobulin therapy
- HIV
- Smoking

PHYSICAL EXAM

- Transient, often recurrent, symmetrical vesicular eruptions located on plantar surface of the foot and volar hand and lateral fingers; lesions may not heal completely between flares (1).
- Prodrome: Intense pruritus may occur prior to vesicular eruption.
- Early findings:
  - 1 to 2 mm, clear, nonerythematous, deep-seated vesicles (lasting 2 to 3 weeks)
  - Has a "tapioca pudding" appearance
- Late findings:
  - Unroofed vesicles with inflamed bases
  - Desquamation (terminal phase)
  - Peeling, rings of scale, or lichenification is common

DIFFERENTIAL DIAGNOSIS

- Vesicular tinea pedis/manuum
- Vesicular id reaction/dermatophytid
- Contact dermatitis (allergic or irritant)
- Scabies
- Chronic vesicular hand dermatitis
- Drug reaction
- Bullous disorders: dyshidrosiform bullous pemphigoid, pemphigus, bullous impetigo, epidermolysis bullosa
- Pustular psoriasis
- Acrodermatitis continua
- Erythema multiforme
- Herpes simplex infection
- Pityriasis rubra pilaris
- Vesicular mycosis fungoides
- Palmoplantar pustulosis

DIAGNOSTIC TESTS & INTERPRETATION

Diagnosis is based on clinical exam.

Follow-Up Tests & Special Considerations

- Skin culture in suspected secondary infection (most commonly, *Staphylococcus aureus*) (3)
- Consider antibiotics based on culture results and severity of symptoms.

Diagnostic Procedures/Other

- Potassium hydroxide (KOH) wet mount (if concerned about dermatophyte infection)
- Patch test (if suspecting allergic cause) (3)

Test Interpretation

- Fine, 1- to 2-mm spongiotic, intraepidermal vesicles with little to no inflammatory change
- No eccrine glandular involvement
- Thickened stratum corneum
- Pompholyx may be confused with PPP but will contain the following distinguishing histopathologic features that PPP will not: vesicles with spongiosis and neutrophils only on the top, without microabscesses on the edges of vesicles.

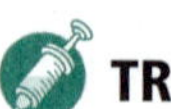

TREATMENT

GENERAL MEASURES

- Avoid possible inciting factors: stress, direct skin contact with irritants, nickel, occlusive gloves, household cleaning products, smoking, sweating.
- Use moisturizers/emollients for symptomatic relief and to maintain effective skin barrier (3).
- Skin care
  - Avoid shoes with known irritants (e.g., leather, rubber soles).
  - Wear socks and gloves made of cotton and change frequently.
  - Wash infrequently in lukewarm water, carefully dry, and then apply emollient.
  - Avoid direct contact with fresh fruit.

MEDICATION

First Line

- Mild cases: topical steroids (high potency) (2)[C]
  - Ointment preferred
  - Considered cornerstone of therapy but limited published evidence
  - Steroid use limited to 2 weeks each episode due to risk of infection (3)[C]
- Moderate to severe cases
  - Ultra high-potency topical steroids with occlusion over treated area (3)[C]
  - Prednisone 40 to 100 mg/day tapered after blister formation ceases (2)[C]. Limited use due to significant side effects (3)[B]
  - Psoralens plus ultraviolet (UV)-A (PUVA) therapy, either systemic/topical or immersion in psoralens (2)[C]
- Recurrent cases (3)[C]
  - Systemic steroids at onset of itching prodrome
  - Prednisone 60 mg PO for 3 to 4 days

Second Line

- Topical calcineurin inhibitors (Mitigate the long-term risks of topical steroid use.): Topical tacrolimus, pimecrolimus; may not be as effective on plantar surface
- Other therapies
  - Oral cyclosporine (3)[C]; monitor for hypertension and renal injury.
  - Systemic alitretinoin (teratogenic)
  - Topical bexarotene (a teratogenic retinoid X receptor agonist approved for use in cutaneous T-cell lymphoma)
  - Methotrexate (significant side effects including GI intolerance and hepatotoxicity) (3)[C]
  - Azathioprine (1)[C] (6- to 8-week onset of action; must monitor for GI side effects, liver toxicity, blood dyscrasia)
  - Disulfiram or sodium cromoglycate in nickel-allergic patients (1)[C]
  - Mycophenolate mofetil (2)[C] (GI side effects; benefit: no hepatotoxicity with long-term use) (3)[B]
  - Tap water iontophoresis (2)[C]

ISSUES FOR REFERRAL

- Dermatologist (if moderate to severe)
- Allergist (if allergen testing required)
- Psychologist (if stress modification needed)

ADDITIONAL THERAPIES

- Other oral agents:
  - Thalidomide (do not use in pregnancy/no available studies on efficacy)
  - Dapsone 100 to 150 mg daily (also limited literature on efficacy; may be used in combination with steroids) both significant side effects; very limited use (3)[C]
- High-dose UVA1 radiation therapy (1)[C]
- UV-free phototherapy
- Treat underlying dermatophytosis (1).
- BTXA in those in which hyperhidrosis is an exacerbating factor
- Monoclonal antibody therapy (i.e., tralokinumab, dupilumab) has shown promising results in recent case studies (4).

COMPLEMENTARY & ALTERNATIVE MEDICINE

- Conservative management:
  - Antihistamines: hydroxyzine, cetirizine, loratadine
  - Soaks/cold compresses of weak solutions of potassium permanganate, Burow solution (aluminum acetate), or vinegar 15 minutes, 4 times daily (3)[C]
- Exposure to sunlight as maintenance therapy, 12 minutes every other day, 10 to 15 exposures
- Dandelion juice (not for atopic patients)
- Cognitive relaxation techniques (3)[C]

ONGOING CARE

FOLLOW-UP RECOMMENDATIONS

Patient Monitoring

- Dyshidrotic Eczema Area and Severity Index (DASI); useful in assessing severity and effect of therapy, but not studied in large cohorts (1)
- Parameters used in the DASI score:
  - Number of vesicles per square centimeter
  - Erythema
  - Desquamation
  - Severity of itching
  - Surface area affected
- Grading: mild (0 to 15), moderate (16 to 30), severe (31 to 60)
- Monitor BP and glucose in patients receiving systemic corticosteroids.
- Monitor for adverse effects of medications.

DIET

- Consider diet low in metal salts if history of nickel sensitivity (3)[B].
- Updated recommendations for low-cobalt diet are available (1).

PATIENT EDUCATION

- Instructions on self-care, complications, and avoidance of triggers/aggravating factors
- American Academy of Dermatology: dyshidrotic eczema at https://www.aad.org/public/diseases/eczema/types/dyshidrotic-eczema

PROGNOSIS

- Condition is benign and usually heals without scarring.
- Lesions may spontaneously resolve.
- Recurrence is common.

COMPLICATIONS

- Quality of life impact: skin tightening, pain, and decreased dexterity
- Secondary bacterial infections with or without steroid use (*S. aureus* most common)
- Dystrophic nail changes
- Fissures and ulcerations
- Psychological distress
- Lymphedema

REFERENCES

1. Veien NK. Acute and recurrent vesicular hand dermatitis. *Dermatol Clin*. 2009;27(3):337–353.
2. Wollina U. Pompholyx: a review of clinical features, differential diagnosis, and management. *Am J Clin Dermatol*. 2010;11(5):305–314.
3. Lofgren SM, Warshaw EM. Dyshidrosis: epidemiology, clinical characteristics, and therapy. *Dermatitis*. 2006;17(4):165–181.
4. Parmar NV, Hammadi AA. Successful treatment of dyshidrotic palmoplantar eczema with tralokinumab [published online ahead of print April 14, 2024]. *Australas J Dermatol*. doi:10.1111/ajd.14268.

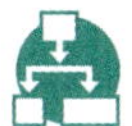

SEE ALSO

Algorithm: Rash

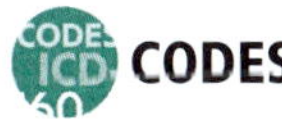

CODES

ICD10

L30.1 Dyshidrosis [pompholyx]

CLINICAL PEARLS

- Dyshidrosis is a transient, recurrent, vesicular eruption, most commonly of the palms, soles, and interdigital areas.
- Etiology and pathophysiology are unknown but are most likely related to a combination of genetic and environmental factors.
- Best prevention is effective skin care and limiting exposure to irritating agents.
- Treatment is based on disease severity; preferred treatments include topical steroids, oral steroids, and calcineurin inhibitors.
- Although benign and self-healing, this condition can be chronic and debilitating with major concern for superimposed bacterial infection that may be avoided by preventive measures, early treatment, and recognition.

DYSMENORRHEA

Maggie C. Wertz, MD

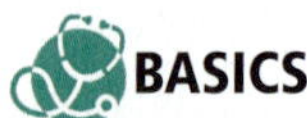

BASICS

DESCRIPTION

- Pelvic pain occurring at/around time of menses; a leading cause of absenteeism for women <30 years old
- Primary dysmenorrhea: pelvic pain without pathologic physical findings; diagnosis of exclusion
- Secondary dysmenorrhea: often more severe, results from specific pelvic pathology; often resistant to typical treatments for dysmenorrhea; severity based on activity impairment
- Mild: painful, rarely limits daily function, rarely requires analgesics
- Moderate: daily activity affected, rare absenteeism, requires analgesics
- Severe: daily activity affected, likelihood of absenteeism increased, limited benefit from analgesics
- System affected: reproductive
- Synonym(s): menstrual cramps

EPIDEMIOLOGY

- Predominant age
  - Primary: onset 6 to 12 months after the start of menarche, teens to early 20s
  - Secondary: 20s to 30s
- Predominant sex: women only

Prevalence

- Up to 90% of menstruating females have experienced primary dysmenorrhea (1).
- Up to 42% lose days of school/work monthly due to dysmenorrhea
- Up to 20% reported impairment in daily activities and/or sleep

ETIOLOGY AND PATHOPHYSIOLOGY

- Primary: Elevated prostaglandin (PGF2α) production through indirect hormonal control (decrease in progesterone at start of menses leads to increase in prostaglandins) causes nonrhythmic hypercontractility and increased uterine muscle tone with vasoconstriction and resultant uterine ischemia. Ischemia results in hypersensitization of type C pain nerve fibers; intensity of cramps is directly proportional to amount of PGF2α released (1).
- Secondary: endometriosis (most common cause); adenomyosis; congenital abnormalities of uterine/vaginal anatomy; cervical stenosis; pelvic inflammatory disease; ovarian cysts; pelvic tumors, especially leiomyomata (fibroids) and uterine polyps

Genetics

Not well studied

RISK FACTORS

- Primary (1),(2)
  - Cigarette smoking
  - Alcohol use
  - Early menarche (age <12 years)
  - Age <30 years
  - Family history of dysmenorrhea
  - Irregular/heavy menstrual flow
  - Nonuse of oral contraceptives
  - Sexual abuse/history of sexual assault
  - Psychological symptoms (depression, anxiety, increased stress, etc.)
  - Nulliparity
- Secondary
  - Pelvic infection
  - Use of intrauterine device (IUD) in the few months following insertion
  - Structural pelvic malformations
  - Family history of endometriosis in first-degree relative

GENERAL PREVENTION

- Primary: regular exercise; early childbirth and higher parity; use of hormonal contraceptives
- Secondary: Reduce risk of sexually transmitted infections (STIs)

Pediatric Considerations

Onset with first menses raises probability of genital tract anatomic abnormality (i.e., transverse vaginal septum, imperforate or minimally perforated hymen, uterine anomalies).

COMMONLY ASSOCIATED CONDITIONS

- Irregular/heavy menstrual periods
- Longer menstrual cycle length/duration of bleeding
- Anxiety/depression
- Decreased quality of life

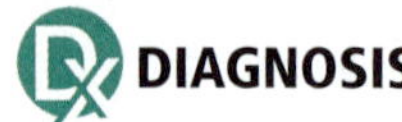

DIAGNOSIS

Typically, a clinical diagnosis is based on characteristic symptom history of suprapubic/low back cramping/pain occurring at or near menstrual flow onset lasting for 8 to 72 hours (2).

HISTORY

- Primary: onset once ovulatory cycles are established in adolescents; 6 to 12 months after menarche on average
- Patients may have associated nausea, vomiting, diarrhea, headache, fatigue, insomnia, pain radiating into the low back or inner thighs, and rarely syncope and fever. These are all considered to be secondary to prostaglandin release.
- Recurrence at or just before the onset of the menstrual flow
  - Pelvic pain occurring between menstrual periods is not likely to be dysmenorrhea.
  - Present with most menstrual periods (cyclic)
- Acute relief associated with the following:
  - Use of analgesics, especially NSAIDs
  - Local topical heat application
  - Orgasm
- Response to NSAIDs helps confirm diagnosis.
- Impact of symptoms on daily activities can help determine severity.
- Secondary: can be associated with chronic pelvic pain, midcycle pain, dyspareunia, abnormal uterine bleeding, typical onset after age 25 years, nonmidline pain, progression of severity, lack of response to NSAIDs/hormonal treatment and infertility.

PHYSICAL EXAM

- Primary: Physical exam is typically normal. Examine to rule out secondary dysmenorrhea only if the history is inconsistent with primary dysmenorrhea. Pelvic exam is recommended if patient is sexually active to rule out infection.
- Secondary: Evaluate for cervical discharge, uterine enlargement, tenderness, irregularity, or fixation.

DIFFERENTIAL DIAGNOSIS

- Primary: History is characteristic.
- Secondary: Endometriosis (most common), pelvic/genital infection; complication of pregnancy; missed/incomplete abortion; ectopic pregnancy; uterine/ovarian neoplasm; UTI; complication with IUD use; congenital uterine or cervical anomaly; adenomyosis; leiomyomata (fibroids); pelvic adhesions; inflammatory bowel disease; irritable bowel syndrome; chronic pelvic pain (idiopathic)

DIAGNOSTIC TESTS & INTERPRETATION

Initial Tests (lab, imaging)

All tests should only be performed if indicated based on history or if patient has symptoms refractory to first-line therapies; most cases of primary dysmenorrhea can be diagnosed on history alone.

- Pregnancy test
- Urine testing for infection
- Gonorrhea/chlamydia cervical testing, especially in women aged <25 years and in high-prevalence areas
- Primary: Consider pelvic ultrasound to rule out secondary abnormalities.
- Secondary: ultrasound and/or laparoscopy to define anatomy for severe/refractory cases. MRI may be useful as second-line noninvasive imaging if ultrasound is nondiagnostic and fibroids, ovarian torsion, deep endometriosis, or adenomyosis is suspected.

Follow-Up Tests & Special Considerations

Counsel regarding appropriate preventive measures for STI and pregnancy.

Diagnostic Procedures/Other

Laparoscopy is rarely needed and is usually only considered in cases of suspected endometriosis or pelvic adhesions not definitively identified on transvaginal ultrasound.

Test Interpretation

- Primary: none
- Secondary: Specific anatomic abnormalities may be noted (see "Differential Diagnosis").

Pregnancy Considerations

Consider ectopic pregnancy when pelvic pain occurs with vaginal bleeding in a patient with a positive pregnancy test.

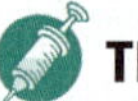

TREATMENT

- Reassure the patient that treatment success is very likely with adherence to recommendations.
- Relief may require the use of several treatment modalities at the same time.

GENERAL MEASURES

- Regular exercise (1),(3)[A] and topical local heat (1)[C] are noninvasive general measures to relieve pain. Local heat in conjunction with the use of an NSAID is superior to an NSAID alone (1)[C].
- High-frequency transcutaneous electrical nerve stimulation (TENS) has been found to be beneficial (1),(4). Low-frequency TENS is not recommended because it is not superior to placebo.
- Secondary dysmenorrhea: treatment of suspected/confirmed underlying cause of pain

MEDICATION

First Line

- NSAIDs: inhibit the peripheral production of prostaglandins. No NSAID has been found to be superior to others. Medication should be taken on scheduled dosing starting 1 to 2 days prior to onset of menses and continued for 2 to 3 days (1),(2). If one NSAID preparation does not work, another NSAID preparation should be tried. Each preparation should be taken as prescribed for at least 3 menstrual cycles prior to determining effectiveness.
  - Ibuprofen 400 mg PO q8h
  - Naproxen sodium 500 mg PO q12h
  - Celecoxib 400 mg PO × 1 and then 200 mg PO q12h
  - Mefenamic acid 500 mg PO × 1 and then 250 mg PO q6h (not to exceed 3 days)
- Hormonal contraceptives: recommended for primary dysmenorrhea in women desiring contraception (2)[C]. Directly suppresses ovulation and limits endometrial growth resulting in reduced prostaglandin production, intrauterine pressure, and uterine contractions. Continuous rather than cyclic dosing has been found to be superior for pain control (4). Amenorrhea by any means can improve symptoms of dysmenorrhea. Estrogen-containing contraceptives are recommended first-line medications for secondary dysmenorrhea due to endometriosis, although progestin-only methods have been shown to be just as or even more effective (5).
  - Low- and high-dose combined oral contraceptives (COCs) along with transdermal and intravaginal combined contraceptives have all been found to be superior to placebo (1)[C].
  - Levonorgestrel IUDs are just as effective as COCs (4)[C].
  - Progestin-only contraceptives including subcutaneous and subdermal preparations appear to decrease primary dysmenorrhea but to a lesser extent than combined options and IUDs (1),(2)[B].
- Potential contraindications to NSAIDs and COCs
  - Platelet disorders
  - Gastric ulceration or gastritis
  - Personal and family history of thromboembolic disorders
  - Vascular disease
  - Migraines with aura
  - Active smoking
- Precautions for first-line options
  - GI irritation
  - Lactation
  - Coagulation disorders
  - Impaired renal function
  - Heart failure
  - Liver dysfunction
  - Pregnancy
  - Hypertension
- Significant possible interactions
  - Coumadin-type anticoagulants
  - Aspirin with other NSAIDs

Second Line

- Acetaminophen and acetaminophen with caffeine are superior to placebo and have less potential side effects than NSAIDs (1)[B].
- Behavioral interventions, such as relaxation exercises including yoga, may help alleviate pain in primary dysmenorrhea (5).
- Nifedipine may be effective in some women and may be used in women trying to conceive (pregnancy Category C).

SURGERY/OTHER PROCEDURES

Laparoscopic uterosacral nerve ablation and presacral neurectomy have been shown to relieve pain at 6 and 12 months, respectively, but are still reserved for patients with pain resistant to all other first- and second-line treatments (1),(4)[B]. Hysterectomy is effective for dysmenorrhea but should only be considered in very rare occasions and when all desired childbearing is complete (1).

COMPLEMENTARY & ALTERNATIVE MEDICINE

- Chinese herbal medicine shows promising evidence of decreasing pain, but more evidence is needed.
- Acupuncture treatments have been shown to decrease pain in dysmenorrhea, but further randomized, well-designed studies are needed. Additionally, these treatments must be frequent and timely for effectiveness.
- Acupoint stimulation, particularly noninvasive stimulation (acupressure), has been found to reduce pain scores but is inferior to NSAIDs (5).
- Aromatherapy abdominal massage performed daily for 10 minutes, 7 days prior to onset of menses can decrease primary dysmenorrhea.
- Further research needed to determine benefit and safety for regular use of oral fennel, oral ginger, oral fenugreek, oral valerian, extracorporeal magnetic innervation, vitamin K_1 injection into the spleen-6 acupuncture point, use of high-frequency vibratory stimulation tampon, transdermal nitroglycerin, and vaginal sildenafil.

ADMISSION, INPATIENT, AND NURSING CONSIDERATIONS

Both primary and secondary dysmenorrhea are usually managed in the outpatient setting.

- Primary: outpatient care
- Secondary: usually outpatient care

ONGOING CARE

FOLLOW-UP RECOMMENDATIONS

Normal

DIET

Insufficient evidence for any specific dietary changes

PATIENT EDUCATION

Reassure the patient that primary dysmenorrhea is treatable with the use of NSAIDs, COCs, IUDs, exercises, or local heat and that it will usually abate with age and parity.

PROGNOSIS

- Primary: reduced with age and parity
- Secondary: likely to require therapy based on underlying cause

COMPLICATIONS

- Primary: anxiety and/or depression
- Secondary: infertility from underlying pathology

REFERENCES

1. Burnett M, Lemyre M. No. 345—primary dysmenorrhea consensus guideline. *J Obstet Gynaecol Can*. 2017;39(7):585–595.
2. Osayande AS, Mehulic S. Diagnosis and initial management of dysmenorrhea. *Am Fam Physician*. 2014;89(5):341–346.
3. Brown J, Brown S. Exercise for dysmenorrhoea. *Cochrane Database Syst Rev*. 2010;(2):CD004142.
4. Oladosu FA, Tu FF, Hellman KM. Nonsteroidal antiinflammatory drug resistance in dysmenorrhea: epidemiology, causes, and treatment. *Am J Obstet Gynecol*. 2018;218(4):390–400.
5. McKenna KA, Fogleman CD. Dysmenorrhea. *Am Fam Physician*. 2021;104(2):164–170.

ADDITIONAL READING

- Ryan SA. The treatment of dysmenorrhea. *Pediatr Clin North Am*. 2017;64(2):331–342.
- Woo HL, Ji HR, Pak YK, et al. The efficacy and safety of acupuncture in women with primary dysmenorrhea: a systematic review and meta-analysis. *Medicine (Baltimore)*. 2018;97(23):e11007.

SEE ALSO

- Dyspareunia; Endometriosis; Menorrhagia (Heavy Menstrual Bleeding); Premenstrual Syndrome (PMS) and Premenstrual Dysphoric Disorder (PMDD)
- Algorithm: Pelvic Pain

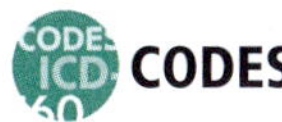

CODES

ICD10

- N94.6 Dysmenorrhea, unspecified
- N94.4 Primary dysmenorrhea
- N94.5 Secondary dysmenorrhea

CLINICAL PEARLS

- Dysmenorrhea is a leading cause of absenteeism for women aged <30 years.
- In women who desire contraception, hormonal contraceptives are the preferred treatment.
- All NSAIDs studied have been found to be equally effective in the relief of dysmenorrhea and should be initiated 1 to 2 days prior to onset of menses with scheduled dosing for at least 2 to 3 days with each menstrual cycle.

DYSPAREUNIA

Leah N. Delfinado, MD • Sonia Gilani, MD

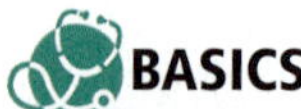

BASICS

The information presented in this chapter pertain to genito-pelvic pain and penetration disorder (GPPPD).

DESCRIPTION

- Recurrent and persistent genital or pelvic pain associated with sexual activity, which is not exclusively due to intensity of intercourse, lack of lubrication or vaginismus, an involuntary contraction of vaginal muscles
  - May be superficial, causing pain with attempted vaginal insertion, or deep
  - Complex, multifactorial disorder involving psychosocial and physical conditions (1)
  - Comprised of a marked anxiety or fear of vulvovaginal pain either in anticipation of or resulting from pain with penetration
- Dyspareunia and vaginismus were previously viewed as separate conditions but are now combined into GPPPD as described by the *DSM-5* (1).
- Individuals whose sexual activity do not involve penetration can still have this disorder if they have pain interfering with sexual function.

EPIDEMIOLOGY

- Predominant age: all ages
- Predominant sex: female > male

Incidence

>50% of all sexually active women will report GPPPD at some time.

Geriatric Considerations

Up to 50% of menopausal women are affected by symptoms associated with genitourinary syndrome of menopause which includes a constellation of genital, sexual, and urinary symptoms associated with decreased androgen and estrogen levels thus decreasing blood supply to the area.

Prevalence

10–20% of US women are affected varying by age and population (2).

ETIOLOGY AND PATHOPHYSIOLOGY

Female

- Vulva and vagina
  - Dermatologic diseases: Lichen sclerosus, lichen planus, contact dermatitis
  - Inadequate lubrication: premature ovarian failure, bilateral oophorectomy, menopause, pituitary tumors, postpartum status, diabetes mellitus, chemotherapy/radiation therapy, and medications (See "Medication.")
  - Pelvic floor dysfunction
  - Vaginal atrophy
  - Vaginismus
  - Vaginitis
  - Vulvodynia
- Bladder
  - Interstitial cystitis
- Uterus and adnexa
  - Ovarian masses
  - Uterine retroversion
- Pelvis
  - Adhesions or chronic pelvic inflammatory disease
  - Endometriosis
- Iatrogenic
  - Hysterectomy
  - Dilation and curettage
- Postpartum
  - Obstetric trauma—perineal tears, episiotomy, instrumented delivery, cesarean delivery
  - Breastfeeding atrophy
- Genitourinary syndrome of menopause
- Medications such as gonadotropin-releasing hormone agonists, selective estrogen receptor modulators, tamoxifen, aromatase inhibitors, progestogens, and danazol
- Female genital mutilation
- Trauma
- Psychological disorders
  - Anxiety
  - Depression
  - PTSD
  - History of sexual abuse

RISK FACTORS

- Demographic risk factors: younger age, minority racial groups (3), lower socioeconomic status, and being in postpartum, perimenopausal, or postmenopausal period
- Psychosocial risk factors: depression, anxiety, low sexual satisfaction, and history of sexual abuse
- Other etiologies: irritable bowel syndrome, musculoskeletal disorders, and fibromyalgia

Pregnancy Considerations

- GPPPD is common in late pregnancy and postpartum.
  - Breastfeeding atrophy, perineal pain, fatigue, and stress can be risk factors in postpartum period.
- Vacuum-assisted or forceps vaginal delivery or history of pelvic floor surgery increases risk.
- Women who experience delivery interventions including episiotomy are at greater risk than women who deliver over an intact perineum or who have an unrepaired laceration.

COMMONLY ASSOCIATED CONDITIONS

- Vaginismus: involuntary contraction of pelvic floor muscles with attempted vaginal penetration
- Vulvodynia: chronic genital pain of at least 3 months duration with no known etiology
  - Vestibulodynia: vulvar vestibule pain lasting >3 months unrelated to infection, skin disorders, or other identifiable factors
  - Clitorodynia: Form of vulvodynia localized to the clitoris associated with frequent and intense pain episodes may cause significant impairment.

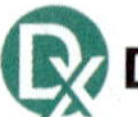

DIAGNOSIS

- For women, the diagnosis of GPPPD is made with the persistent or recurrent presence (at least 6 months) of ≥1 of the following symptoms per the *DSM-5*:
  - Recurrent difficulty having intercourse
  - Marked vulvovaginal or pelvic pain during intercourse or penetration attempts
  - Marked fear or anxiety about vulvovaginal or pelvic pain anticipating, during, or resulting from vaginal penetration
  - Marked tensing or tightening of the pelvic floor muscles during attempted vaginal penetration
- Symptoms have persisted for a minimum of 6 months and cause clinically significant distress in the individual not better explained by nonsexual mental health disorder, medical disorders, intimate partner violence, or substance/medications (4).

HISTORY

Obtain a detailed sexual history including, but not limited to, number of partners and their gender; temporality of symptoms and their evolution with time; presence and degree of personal distress; alleviating factors; personal health problems; medication use; substance use; past or current abuse or violence experienced; number of pregnancies; menstrual status; physical activity; and injuries related to genito-pelvic area.

PHYSICAL EXAM

- A complete exam, including a focused pelvic exam, to identify pathology
  - Exam must include inspection and palpation of urethra, vulva, and vaginal areas; palpation of the uterine, bladder, and adnexal structures; rectovaginal exam; penis, scrotum, pelvic floor muscles and digital rectal exam.
  - Assess for atrophy, discoloration, lesions, or trauma.
  - Sensory mapping with a cotton-tipped applicator to localize sensitive and painful areas. Document location with reference to the "clock face" by starting on vestibule.
  - It may be beneficial for patients to contribute to the exam with the use of a mirror (2).
  - Musculoskeletal evaluation will help rule out associated etiologies such as pelvic muscle overactivity or myofascial disorders (4). Palpation of pelvic floor muscles: levator ani, obturator internus, and piriformis can help localize.
    - Tenderness of vaginal muscles during single digit exam can indicate pelvic floor dysfunction (2).
- Because examination often reproduces the pain, examiner should be cautious and sensitive to patient's anxiety.

DIFFERENTIAL DIAGNOSIS

- Refer to section on etiology.
- Many conditions can cause GPPPD and individuals can experience >1 type of sexual dysfunction.

DIAGNOSTIC TESTS & INTERPRETATION

- Typically, not necessary for diagnosis unless an undiagnosed, underlying medical condition is suspected.
- Cultures, biopsy, or microscopy can be considered as indicated based on history and exam findings to rule out organic causes of pain.

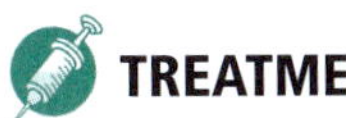

TREATMENT

GENERAL MEASURES

- Initiate specific treatment when initial evaluation identifies an organic cause (2).
- Once organic causes are ruled out, treatment is a multidimensional and multidisciplinary approach.
- Nonpharmacologic measures
  - Psychologic interventions
    - Sexual skills training
    - Cognitive-behavioral therapy
    - Mindfulness
    - Couples therapy
  - Pelvic floor physical therapy
  - Self-dilation enabled by prescription and OTC-based products can alleviate vaginismus and pelvic floor trigger points (1).
  - Education on genital hygiene, avoidance of harsh detergents or perfumed products (2)
- Lubricants and vaginal moisturizers reduce pain associated with vaginal dryness but do not treat the underlying causes of sexual pain; several times per week with lubricants during intercourse
- Genitourinary syndrome of menopause: Vaginal estrogen is most effective if symptomatic.
- Breastfeeding associated vulvovaginal atrophy: topical estrogen

MEDICATION

First Line

Depends on the etiology (2)

- Antibiotics, antifungals, or antivirals, as indicated, for infection
- Water and silicone based vaginal lubricants or moisturizers containing hyaluronic and polycarbophil products can be used several times per week for vaginal dryness.
- Low dose vaginal estrogen as cream, rings, and tablets is preferred for genitourinary syndrome of menopause; they have been shown to provide faster relief than systemic estrogen.
- Nonestrogen intravaginal treatments like ospemifene or prasterone can be recommended as an alternative for women with history of breast cancer (2).
- SSRIs to treat underlying depression
- Analgesics like NSAIDs and topical anesthetics for pain
- Neuropathic pain associated with vulvar vestibulitis/vulvodynia may respond to tricyclic antidepressants (amitriptyline or nortriptyline) or gabapentin.
- Trigger point injections with local anesthetics or botox

ISSUES FOR REFERRAL

Referral for long-term therapy with consultants with expertise in treating sexual dysfunction should be considered such as pelvic floor physical therapy.

SURGERY/OTHER PROCEDURES

- Consideration of surgical interventions for GPPPD due to altered anatomy, uterine position, fibroids, or prior pelvic surgery
  - Laparoscopic excision of endometriotic lesions or pelvic adhesions
  - Surgical vestibulectomy can be considered if medical measures fail with vulvar vestibulitis.
- U.S. Food and Drug Administration (FDA) warns against the use of medical devices for unapproved uses including "vaginal rejuvenation" procedures.

COMPLEMENTARY & ALTERNATIVE MEDICINE

- Sitz baths may relieve painful inflammation.
- Perineal massage
- Antioxidants may improve symptoms associated with endometriosis.

ONGOING CARE

FOLLOW-UP RECOMMENDATIONS

Patient Monitoring

- Outpatient follow-up depends on therapy.
- Every 6 to 12 months once resolved

DIET

A high-fiber diet may help if constipation is a contributing cause.

PATIENT EDUCATION

- Boston Women's Health Book Collective and Judy Norsigian. *Our Bodies, Ourselves*. New York, NY: Touchstone; 2011.
- Kegel exercise information
- Provide couples with information about sexual arousal techniques.

PROGNOSIS

Depends on underlying cause, but most patients will respond to treatment

REFERENCES

1. American College of Obstetricians and Gynecologists' Committee on Practice Bulletins—Gynecology. Female sexual dysfunction: ACOG practice bulletin clinical management guidelines for obstetrician-gynecologists, number 213. *Obstet Gynecol*. 2019;134(1):e1–e18. doi:10.1097/AOG.0000000000003324.
2. Hill DA, Taylor CA. Dyspareunia in women. *Am Fam Physician*. 2021;103(10):597–604.
3. Azim KA, Happel-Parkins A, Moses A, et al. Racialized differences across experiences and measurements of pain in genitopelvic pain/penetration disorder. *J Sex Med*. 2023;20(2):224–228. doi:10.1093/jsxmed/qdac028.
4. American College of Obstetricians and Gynecologists' Committee on Gynecologic Practice; American Society for Colposcopy and Cervical Pathology. Committee Opinion No. 673: persistent vulvar pain. *Obstet Gynecol*. 2016;128(3):e78–e84. doi:10.1097/aog.0000000000001645.

ADDITIONAL READING

Sorensen J, Bautista KE, Lamvu G, et al. Evaluation and treatment of female sexual pain: a clinical review. *Cureus*. 2018;10(3):e2379.

SEE ALSO

- Endometriosis; Pelvic Inflammatory Disease; Sexual Dysfunction in Women; Vulvovaginitis, Estrogen Deficient; Vulvovaginitis, Prepubescent
- Algorithms: Discharge, Vaginal; Dyspareunia

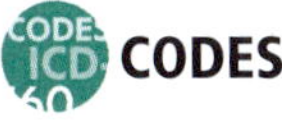

CODES

ICD10

- N94.1 Dyspareunia
- F52.6 Dyspareunia not due to a substance or known physiol cond

CLINICAL PEARLS

- Thorough history to determine if patient feels pain before, during, or after intercourse will help identify cause.
- GPPPD includes ≥1 of the following symptoms: tightening of the vaginal muscle with decreased ability or inability to accommodate penetration; tension, pain, or burning felt when penetration is attempted; a decrease in or no desire to have intercourse; avoidance of sexual activity; intense phobia or fear of pain (2)
- A complete history and pelvic exam is needed for appropriate diagnosis.
- Low dose vaginal estrogen is the preferred hormonal treatment for female sexual dysfunction (1).
- Psychologic interventions are recommended as part of treatment (1).
- Pelvic floor physical therapy is recommended to restore muscle function (1).
- Episiotomy does not offer any benefit in the prevention of GPPPD; an episiotomy in fact may cause more future discomfort.

DYSPEPSIA, FUNCTIONAL

Ricardo David Espinosa, MD

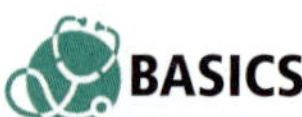

BASICS

DESCRIPTION

- Dyspepsia is defined as the presence of postprandial fullness, early satiety, and epigastric or burning pain for the last 6 months in the absence of systemic, structural, or organic disease.
- Rome IV criteria divides patients into two subtypes:
  - Postprandial distress syndrome (PDS): which is defined as the feelings of fullness that interferes with the ability of intake of a normal-sized meal; more common
  - Epigastric pain syndrome (EPS): which is defined as recurrent burning epigastric pain or discomfort
- System(s) affected: gastrointestinal (GI)
- Synonym(s): idiopathic dyspepsia; nonulcer dyspepsia; nonorganic dyspepsia; PDS; and EPS

EPIDEMIOLOGY

Prevalence

- 5–20% prevalence worldwide (varies based on criteria)
- Overall more common in Western cultures, women, and younger adults
- PDS subtype may be more common in Eastern cultures.

ETIOLOGY AND PATHOPHYSIOLOGY

Unknown but proposed mechanisms or associations include gastric motility disorders including abnormal gastric emptying and accommodation, vagal sensory dysfunction, eosinophilic duodenitis, *Helicobacter pylori* infection, alteration in upper GI microbiome, postinfectious complications, immune activation, inflammation, and gut-brain axis disorders

Genetics

Possible link to G-protein β_3 subunit 825 CC genotype, serotonin transport genes, and/or cholecystokinin-A-receptor gene polymorphisms

Geriatric Considerations

Patients age >60 years with new-onset dyspepsia should undergo endoscopy.

Pediatric Considerations

Be alert for family system dysfunction.

Pregnancy Considerations

Pregnancy may exacerbate symptoms.

RISK FACTORS

- Other functional disorders: fibromyalgia, temporomandibular joint pain, chronic fatigue syndrome, irritable bowel syndrome.
- Anxiety/depression, psychosocial stressors (e.g., divorce, unemployment; history of physical, sexual or emotional trauma/abuse)
- Infection with *H. pylori*
- Smoking
- Female gender
- NSAIDs use
- Gastroparesis
- Gastroesophageal reflux disease (GERD)

GENERAL PREVENTION

Avoid modifiable risk factors.

COMMONLY ASSOCIATED CONDITIONS

Other functional bowel disorders (common)

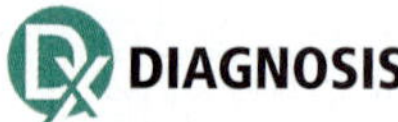

DIAGNOSIS

HISTORY

- Postprandial fullness or early satiety following meals at least 1 time/week
- Epigastric pain or burning pain at least three times/week
- Belching
- Bloating
- Nausea
- Heartburn
- Symptoms for 3 months with an onset of 6 months before diagnosis (Rome IV criteria)
- Alarm features include (1),(2):
  - Unintended weight loss
  - Progressive dysphagia
  - Odynophagia
  - Persistent vomiting
  - GI bleeding
  - Family history of upper GI cancer
  - Age ≥60 years
  - Feeling nodules on neck, armpits, breasts
  - Upper abdominal masses
- The presence of the above of alarm features are enough indication to get an upper GI endoscopy.

PHYSICAL EXAM

- Document weight status and vital signs.
- Check for lymph nodes.
- Examine for signs of systemic illness.
  - Murphy sign for cholecystitis
  - Rebound and guarding for ulcer perforation
  - Palpate during muscle contraction to assess for abdominal wall pain (Carnett sign).
  - Palpate abdominal wall for masses.
  - Succussion splash may indicate mechanical obstruction or gastroparesis.
  - Jaundice
  - Thyromegaly

DIFFERENTIAL DIAGNOSIS

- Peptic ulcer disease; GERD
- Cholecystitis; choledocholithiasis
- Gastric or esophageal cancer; esophageal spasm
- Malabsorption syndromes; celiac disease
- Pancreatic cancer; pancreatitis
- Inflammatory bowel disease; carbohydrate malabsorption; gastroparesis
- Ischemic bowel disease
- Intestinal parasites
- Irritable bowel syndrome
- Ischemic heart disease
- Diabetes mellitus; thyroid disease; connective tissue disorders
- Medication effects

DIAGNOSTIC TESTS & INTERPRETATION

Initial Tests (lab, imaging)

- Functional dyspepsia is a diagnosis of exclusion. Order labs based on clinical suspicion.
- Test for *H. pylori* (stool antigen or urea breath test) in areas of high *H. pylori* prevalence (2)[A].
- CBC (if anemia or infection are suspected)
- Liver-associated enzymes/right upper quadrant ultrasound (if hepatobiliary disease is suspected)
- Pancreatic enzymes (if pancreatic disease is suspected)
- Upper endoscopy for patients age 45 to 60 years or with alarm symptoms to rule out malignancy (2)[C]
- Self-report questionnaires can track symptoms (1).

Diagnostic Procedures/Other

- Esophageal manometry or gastric accommodation studies are infrequently needed (1)[C].
- Motility studies are unnecessary, unless gastroparesis is strongly suspected (2)[C].

Test Interpretation

None (By definition, this a functional disorder.)

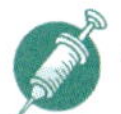

TREATMENT

GENERAL MEASURES

- Reassurance/physician support is helpful (1)[C].
- Treatment is based on presumed etiologies.
- Discontinue offending medications (1)[C].
- Routine endoscopy not recommended in dyspeptic patients age <60 years without alarm features (2)[B]
- In younger patients with no alarm symptoms, "test and treat" for *H. pylori* is appropriate.

MEDICATION

First Line

- Treat *H. pylori* if confirmed on testing (1),(2)[A].
- Trial of once daily proton pump inhibitor (PPI) medication (e.g., omeprazole 20 mg PO QD) or H_2 receptor antagonist for up to 8 weeks in patients without alarm symptoms—most effective for patients with EPS (1),(2),(3)
- Prokinetics have been proposed as first-line agents in PDS, although efficacy data for metoclopramide, 5 to 10 mg PO TID 30 minutes before meals (only agent approved in United States) are limited. Prokinetics should be prescribed at the lowest effective dose to avoid potential side effects (2)[C]. Use with caution due to side effects of tardive dyskinesia, parkinsonian symptoms, and QT prolongation.

Second Line

- Trial of tricyclic antidepressant (TCA) medication is more helpful for EPS than PDS (e.g., amitriptyline 25 mg PO QD, can up-titrate to 50 mg PO QD), with a NNT of 6 (2)[A]; caution in elderly; there is insufficient data to support the use of SSRIs/SNRIs.
- Trazodone 25 mg at bedtime is an alternative (3). Consider buspirone or mirtazapine if no response or if contraindications to TCA.
- Gabapentin 300 mg twice daily can be a useful adjunct, particularly for treatment of GI pain symptoms.

ADDITIONAL THERAPIES

- Stress reduction (3)
- Psychotherapy and/or cognitive-behavioral therapy effective in some patients (1),(2)[B]
- Patients should be given a positive diagnosis and reassured of benign prognosis.

COMPLEMENTARY & ALTERNATIVE MEDICINE

Alternative medicine approaches show promise but need further study and are not currently recommended (2)[C].

- STW 5 (Iberogast) shown to be helpful in some studies.
- Probiotics have theoretical benefit but lack consistent trial data to support routine use.
- Hypnotherapy may help.
- Transcutaneous electroacupuncture may help (1)[B].

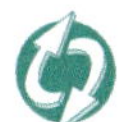

ONGOING CARE

FOLLOW-UP RECOMMENDATIONS

Patient Monitoring

- Provide ongoing support and reassurance.
- Consider upper endoscopy if persistent symptoms.
- Change medications if no difference in symptoms after 4 weeks (1)[C].
- Discontinue medications once symptoms resolve (1)[C].

DIET

- Limited data to support dietary modification, including restricting high fermentable oligosaccharides, disaccharides, monosaccharides and polyols (FODMAP) foods
- Consider limiting fatty foods (3).
- Avoid foods that exacerbate symptoms: wheat and cow milk proteins, peppers or spices, coffee, tea, and alcohol (3).

PATIENT EDUCATION

Reassurance and stress reduction techniques

PROGNOSIS

Long-term/chronic symptoms with symptom-free periods

COMPLICATIONS

Iatrogenic, from evaluation to rule out serious pathology

REFERENCES

1. Lacy BE, Cangemi DJ. Updates in functional dyspepsia and bloating. *Curr Opin Gastroenterol*. 2022;38(6):613–619. doi:10.1097/MOG.0000000000000882.
2. Moayyedi PM, Lacy BE, Andrews CN, et al. ACG and CAG clinical guideline: management of dyspepsia. *Am J Gastroenterol*. 2017;112(7):988–1013.
3. Gwee KA, Lee YY, Suzuki H, et al. Asia-Pacific guidelines for managing functional dyspepsia overlapping with other gastrointestinal symptoms. *J Gastroenterol Hepatol*. 2023;38(2):197–209.

ADDITIONAL READING

Jamshidfar N, Hamdieh M, Eslami P, et al. Comparison of the potency of nortriptyline and mirtazapine on gastrointestinal symptoms, the level of anxiety and depression in patients with functional dyspepsia. *Gastroenterol Hepatol Bed Bench*. 2023;16(1):468–477. doi:10.22037/ghfbb.v16i1.2513.

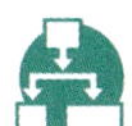

SEE ALSO

- Irritable Bowel Syndrome
- Algorithm: Dyspepsia

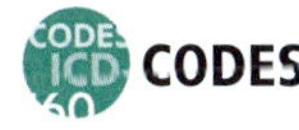

CODES

ICD10

K30 Functional dyspepsia

CLINICAL PEARLS

- Dyspepsia without underlying organic disease is classified as functional or idiopathic.
- Consider empiric acid suppression therapy as first line for functional dyspepsia.
- Test and treat approach to *H. pylori* appropriate in younger patients with no alarm symptoms.
- Extensive diagnostic testing is not recommended unless alarm symptoms are present.

DYSPHAGIA

Felix B. Chang, MD, DABMA, DABIHM, DABIM, FAAMA

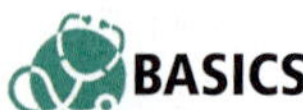

BASICS

Subjective sensation of difficulty or abnormality of swallowing

DESCRIPTION

- Oropharyngeal: difficulty transferring food bolus from oropharynx to proximal esophagus
- Esophageal: difficulty moving food bolus through the body of the esophagus to the pylorus

EPIDEMIOLOGY

5–8% of the general population >50 years of age

Incidence

- Esophageal food impaction 25 per 100,000 persons per year
- Males to female (1.5:1)

Prevalence

- 10–30% among community-dwelling individuals ≥65 years old
- Up to 40% in hospital settings
- ~30% of patients in nursing homes
- ~40% in patients in geriatrics acute care
- 60% in older patients that are institutionalized
- ~20% in postextubation patients in ICU

ETIOLOGY AND PATHOPHYSIOLOGY

- Oropharyngeal (transfer) dysphagia—difficulty initiating swallowing; coughing; aspiration
  - Functional motor disordered in the oropharynx
  - Mechanical: pharyngeal and laryngeal cancer, acute epiglottitis, carotid body tumor, pharyngitis, tonsillitis, strep throat, lymphoid hyperplasia of lingual tonsil, lateral pharyngeal pouch, hypopharyngeal diverticulum
  - Neuromyogenic: stroke, head trauma, Parkinson disease, amyotrophic lateral sclerosis (ALS), myasthenia, polymyositis, dermatomyositis, muscular dystrophies, thyrotoxicosis, hypothyroidism, amyloidosis, Cushing syndrome
- Esophageal dysphagia—sensation of food getting stuck
  - Mechanical: carcinomas, diverticula, webs, Schatzki ring, structures (peptic, chemical, trauma, radiation), foreign body; eosinophilic esophagitis
  - Extrinsic mechanical: peritonsillar abscess, thyroid disorders, tumors, vascular compression (enlarged left atrium, aberrant subclavius, aortic aneurysm), adenopathy, duplication cyst
- Neuromuscular: achalasia, spasm, hypertonic sphincter, scleroderma, CVA, Alzheimer disease, Huntington chorea, Parkinson disease, multiple sclerosis, polymyositis, dermatomyositis, neuromuscular junction, (myasthenia gravis, Lambert-Eaton syndrome, botulism), hyperthyroidism and hypothyroidism, Guillain-Barré syndrome, SLE, ALL, amyloidosis, diabetic neuropathy, brainstem tumors, Chagas disease
  - Infections: diphtheria, meningitis, tertiary syphilis, Lyme disease, rabies, poliomyelitis, CMV, esophagitis (*Candida*, herpetic)

Genetics

Charge syndrome:

- 22q11.2 (diGeorge Syndrome)
- Microduplication of 11q13.3–FGF3 and FGF4 genes
- Germline gain of function mutation in KIT gene
- Polymorphisms of COMT and BDMF genes can contribute to dysphagia in older adults

RISK FACTORS

- Children: hereditary and/or congenital malformations
- Adults: age >50 years; elderly: GERD, stroke, COPD, chronic pain
- Medications: quinine; potassium chloride; vitamin C; tetracycline; trimethoprim (Bactrim); clindamycin; NSAIDs; procainamide; anticholinergics; bisphosphates; seizure meds: phenobarbital, carbamazepine, and phenytoin; antihistaminics, TCAs: amitriptyline, imipramine; antipsychotics: haloperidol, phenothiazine, butyrophenone, thioxanthene; xybutynin; opiates; rizatriptan; ACE; ARB; calcium channel blockers; β-blockers; α_2-agonist; HCTZ and chlorothiazide; cytotoxic; antineoplastics: interferon-α, ribavirin; sibutramine; β_2-agonist bronchodilators, muscle relaxants
  - Xerostomia: ACE inhibitors, antiarrhythmics, antiemetics, diuretics, SSRI; cytotoxic, sunitinib, everolimus
  - Neurologic: CVA, myasthenia gravis, multiple sclerosis, Parkinson disease, ALS, Huntington chorea, dementia; HIV patients with CD4 cell count <100 cells/mm^3
- Trauma or irradiation of head, neck, and chest; mechanical lesions; extrinsic mechanical lesions: lung, thyroid tumors, lymphoma, metastasis; iron deficiency
- Smoking, excess alcohol intake, obesity

GENERAL PREVENTION

Liquid and soft food diet as appropriate

COMMONLY ASSOCIATED CONDITIONS

Peptic structure, esophageal webs and rings, carcinoma, history of stroke, dementia, pneumonia

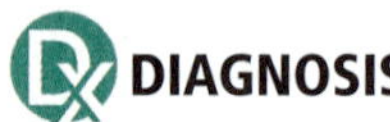

DIAGNOSIS

History and physical exam identify the anatomical site and likely cause of dysphagia in 80% of causes. To assess the swallowing anatomy and physiology for diagnosis of dysphagia, videofluoroscopy or fiber endoscopy are helpful.

HISTORY

- Oropharyngeal dysphagia presents as difficulty initiating the swallowing process. Dysphagia for solids that progresses to involve liquids more likely reflects mechanical obstruction.
- Progressive dysphagia is usually caused by cancer or a peptic stricture. Intermittent dysphagia is most often related to a lower esophageal ring.
- Inquire about heartburn, weight loss, hematemesis, coffee ground emesis, anemia, regurgitation of undigested food particles, and respiratory symptoms.
- Inquire about regurgitation, aspiration, or drooling immediately after swallowing as this may represent oropharyngeal dysphagia, smoking, alcohol abuse.
- Does the food bolus feel stuck?
  - Upper sternum or back of throat may represent oropharyngeal dysphagia, whereas sensation over the lower sternum is typical of esophageal dysphagia.
- Is odynophagia (pain) present?
  - Inflammation, achalasia, diffuse esophageal spasm, esophagitis, pharyngitis, pill-induced esophagitis, cancer
  - Globus sensation ("lump in the throat")?
    - Cricopharyngeal or laryngeal disorders
  - History of sour taste in the back of the throat or chronic heartburn suggests GERD.
- Symptoms: weight loss or chest pain? Double aortic arch, right aortic arch with retroesophageal left subclavian artery and left ligamentum arteriosum
- Halitosis: Rule out diverticulum, tissue disorder.
- Changes in speech, hoarseness, weak cough, dysphonia? Rule out neuromuscular dysfunction.

PHYSICAL EXAM

- Skin: telangiectasia, sclerodactyly, calcinosis (rule out autoimmune disease); Raynaud phenomenon, sclerodactyly may be found in CREST syndrome or systemic scleroderma; stigmata of alcohol abuse (palmar erythema; telangiectasia)
- Head, eye, ear, nose, throat (HEENT):
  - Oropharyngeal: pharyngeal erythema/edema, tonsillitis, pharyngeal ulcers or thrush, odynophagia (bacterial, viral, fungal infections); tongue fasciculations (ALS)
  - Neck: masses, lymphadenopathy, neck tenderness (thyroiditis), goiter
- Neurologic:
  - Cranial nerve exam: sensory: cranial nerves V, IX, and X; motor: cranial nerves V, VII, X, XI, and XII
  - CNS, mental status exam, strength testing, Horner syndrome, ataxia, cogwheel rigidity

DIFFERENTIAL DIAGNOSIS

First step is to distinguish between oropharyngeal and esophageal pathology.

DIAGNOSTIC TESTS & INTERPRETATION

Diagnosis of oropharyngeal dysphagia starts with a thorough clinical assessment. One of the following four symptoms suggest oropharyngeal dysphagia: delayed or absent oropharyngeal swallow initiation; deglutitive postnasal regurgitation or egress of fluids through the nose during swallowing; deglutitive cough (suggests aspiration); repetitive swallowing to achieve clearance of material from the hypopharynx.

- EGD is recommended for the initial assessment of patient with esophageal dysphagia; barium esophagography is recommended as an adjunct if EGD findings are negative (1)[C].
- For accurate diagnosis of eosinophilic esophagitis, biopsies from normal-appearing mucosa in the midthoracic and distal esophagus should be requested for all patients with unexplained solid food dysphagia (1)[B].
- If the etiology of dysphagia is not determined by an endoscopy or a barium swallow study, use manometry to assess for esophageal motility disorders suggested by a dilated esophagus, a spastic esophagogastric junction, infrequent or impaired esophageal contractions, sigmoid esophagus.
- Older patients with chronic illness or recent pneumonia should be screened for dysphagia; if it is present, the physician and patient should discuss goals of care (1)[C]. The diagnosis of eosinophilic esophagitis is established by upper endoscopy and esophageal biopsy, with and increase of eosinophils >15 per high-power field. Biopsies from normal-appearing mucosa in the mid thoracic and distal esophagus should be requested (1).

Initial Tests (lab, imaging)

- CBC (infection and inflammation); antiacetylcholine antibodies (myasthenia); TSH, free T_4 cobalamin levels, LFT
- In esophageal dysphagia, an upper gastrointestinal endoscopy is preferred particularly if structural causes are suspected, or a barium swallow if an upper endoscopy is contraindicated.

Diagnostic Procedures/Other

The Chicago classification is an accepted framework for interpreting high-resolution manometry (HRM) studies to aid in the diagnosis of esophageal motility disorders. Functional lumen imaging probe (FLIP) measures esophageal distensibility and contractile response during endoscopy and is helpful if HRM is inconclusive. It is helpful as an adjunct to HRM.

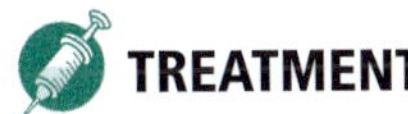

TREATMENT

The goal of treatment is to improve food transfer and to prevent aspiration.

GENERAL MEASURES

- Exclude cardiac disease.
- Ensure airway patency and adequate pulmonary function.
- Assess nutritional status; speech therapy

MEDICATION

Modify medications taken by patient according to patient functional swallowing ability.

First Line

Patients with GERD symptoms, esophagitis, or peptic stricture should undergo acid suppression therapy with standard doses of proton pump inhibitors for 8 to 12 weeks (1)[A].

- Older patients with chronic illness or recent pneumonia should be screened for dysphagia; if it is present, the physician and patient should discuss goals of care (1)[C].

ISSUES FOR REFERRAL

Swallow and speech, nutritional evaluation, cancer

ADDITIONAL THERAPIES

Self-expanded metal stent is safe, effective, and quicker in palliation.

SURGERY/OTHER PROCEDURES

- Esophageal dilatation (pneumatic or bougie) for achalasia; esophageal stent; laser for cancer palliation
- Need for enteral feeding; hospitalization with total or near-total obstruction of esophageal lumen
- Stenting and thermal ablative therapy are options for palliative treatment in esophageal cancer patients.
- Neuromuscular electrical stimulation (NMES) coupled with traditional swallowing therapy may improve swallowing after stroke (2)[C].

ONGOING CARE

Swallow therapy may reduce the incidence of chest infections or pneumonia after stroke

FOLLOW-UP RECOMMENDATIONS

In patients with progressive conditions goal is to maintain current state.

Patient Monitoring

Medications should be reviewed.

DIET

See "General Prevention."

PATIENT EDUCATION

- Drink using small sips of liquids, without any gulping.
- Sit upright at 90 degrees and avoid drinking or eating when lying down or slouched.
- Eat slowly, small bites of food, chew food completely before swallowing.

PROGNOSIS

- 45% reported mortality within 12 months in nursing home residents with oropharyngeal dysphagia and aspiration.
- Swallowing treatment reduced incidence of pneumonia, no difference in swallow quality of life (QOL) scores
- Screening for dysphagia its impact on symptoms and QOL domains is important in palliative care (3)[C].

COMPLICATIONS

Pneumonia, lung abscess, aspiration pneumonia, airway obstruction; malnutrition and dehydration

REFERENCES

1. Wilkinson JM, Codipilly DC, Wilfahrt RP. Dysphagia: evaluation and collaborative management. *Am Fam Physician*. 2021;103(2):97–106.
2. Alamer A, Melese H, Nigussie F. Effectiveness of neuromuscular electrical stimulation on post-stroke dysphagia: a systematic review of randomized controlled trials. *Clin Interv Aging*. 2020;15:1521–1531.
3. Tan LLC, Lim Y, Ho P, et al. Understanding quality of life for palliative patients with dysphagia using the swallowing quality of life (SWAL-QOL) questionnaire. *Am J Hosp Paliat Care*. 2021;38(10):1172–1176.

ADDITIONAL READING

- Radhakrishnan C, Forough AS, Cichero JAY, et al. A difficult pill to swallow: an investigation of factors associated with medication swallowing difficulties. *Patient Prefer Adherence*. 2021;15:29–40.
- Thiyagalingam S, Kulinski AE, Thorsteinsdottir B, et al. Dysphagia in older adults. *Mayo Clin Proc*. 2021;96(2):488–497.

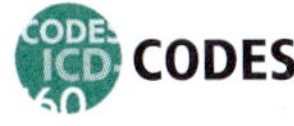

CODES

ICD10

- R13.10 Dysphagia, unspecified
- R13.12 Dysphagia, oropharyngeal phase
- R13.14 Dysphagia, pharyngoesophageal phase

CLINICAL PEARLS

- Dysphagia is relatively common in older adults, particularly in the nursing home setting.
- Targeted studies (instrumental evaluation) using videofluoroscopic swallowing studies, fiberoptic endoscopy, and EGD help identify specific causes of dysphagia.
- A careful history helps distinguish oropharyngeal dysphagia from esophageal dysphagia
- Treatment should be targeted to the specific cause of dysphagia (e.g., behavioral modification, dietary texture changes, swallowing exercises for oropharyngeal; acid suppression, dilatation for esophageal).

ECTOPIC PREGNANCY

Kristina Gracey, MD, MPH

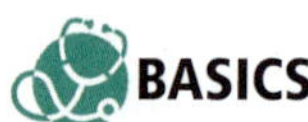

BASICS

DESCRIPTION

Ectopic: pregnancy implanted outside the uterine cavity; subtypes include:

- Tubal: pregnancy implanted in the fallopian tube
- Abdominal: pregnancy implanted intra-abdominally, usually after tubal abortion or rupture of tubal ectopic pregnancy
- Heterotopic pregnancy: implanted intrauterine pregnancy (IUP) and a separate pregnancy outside the uterine cavity
- Ovarian: implantation of pregnancy in ovarian tissue
- Cervical: implantation of pregnancy in cervix
- Intraligamentary: implantation of pregnancy within the broad ligament

EPIDEMIOLOGY

Prevalence

- Ectopic pregnancy occurs in about 2% of all pregnancies (1), and about 1 in 10 first-trimester pregnancies presenting to the emergency department with pain and/or bleeding. In the United States, ectopic pregnancy is the leading cause of first-trimester maternal deaths.
- Heterotopic pregnancy, although very rare, occurs with greater frequency in women undergoing in vitro fertilization (IVF); increasing incidence of nontubal, and particularly cesarean scar ectopic pregnancies, due in part to more cesarean sections and more IVF

ETIOLOGY AND PATHOPHYSIOLOGY

Most ectopic pregnancies occur in the fallopian tube, followed by the ampulla, isthmus, and then the fimbria. One cause of tubal pregnancy is impaired movement of the fertilized ovum to the uterine cavity due to dysfunction of the tubal cilia, scarring, or narrowing of the tubal lumen.

RISK FACTORS

- History of pelvic inflammatory disease (PID), endometritis, or current gonorrhea/chlamydia infection, pelvic adhesive disease (infection or prior surgery), tobacco use, and patients with disorders that affect ciliary motility may be at increased risk (e.g., endometriosis).
- Previous ectopic pregnancy, history of tubal surgery
- Use of an intrauterine device (IUD): IUD reduces absolute risk (and therefore number) of ectopic pregnancies, but in a patient with an IUD in place presenting with a pregnancy, there is an increased likelihood that the pregnancy is ectopic, compared with a patient without an IUD.
- Use of assisted reproductive technologies

GENERAL PREVENTION

Screen for and treat STIs (i.e., gonorrhea, chlamydia) that can cause PID and tubal scarring that increase the risk for an ectopic pregnancy.

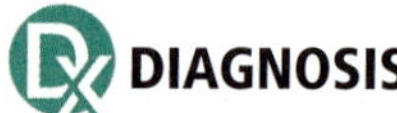

DIAGNOSIS

HISTORY

Classically sudden-onset abdominal pain following cessation of/or irregular menses and acute vaginal bleeding; other common symptoms include nausea and/or vomiting, and pain referred to the shoulder (from hemoperitoneum); ectopic pregnancies can also be asymptomatic.

PHYSICAL EXAM

- Abdominal tenderness ± rebound tenderness
- Vaginal bleeding may be present.
- Palpable mass on pelvic exam (adnexal or cul-de-sac fullness), cervical motion tenderness
- In cases of rupture and significant intraperitoneal bleeding, signs of shock such as pallor, tachycardia, and hypotension may be present.

DIFFERENTIAL DIAGNOSIS

Missed, threatened, inevitable, or completed abortion (miscarriage), gestational trophoblastic neoplasia ("molar pregnancy"), appendicitis, salpingitis, PID, ruptured corpus luteum or hemorrhagic cyst, ovarian tumor, benign or malignant, ovarian torsion, cervical polyp, cancer, trauma, or cervicitis

DIAGNOSTIC TESTS & INTERPRETATION

Initial Tests (lab, imaging)

- CBC and ABO type and antibody screen
- Transvaginal ultrasound (TVUS) is the gold standard for diagnosis:
  - Failure to visualize a normal intrauterine gestational sac when serum human chorionic gonadotropin (hCG) is above the discriminatory level (>1,500 to 2,000 IU/L) suggests (but is not definitively diagnostic of) an abnormal pregnancy. TVUS is often inconclusive, and the pregnancy is then called "pregnancy of unknown location" (PUL).
  - An hCG level of 3,500 IU/L is associated with a 99% probability of detecting a normal intrauterine gestational sac in clinical practice.
  - These values are not validated for multiple gestations.
- If TVUS unavailable or inconclusive for IUP, check serial hCG levels (1). Serial quantitative serum levels normally increase by at least 35% every 48 hours. Higher initial hCG levels increase less than lower initial hCG levels (1). Abnormal rise (<35%) should prompt workup for gestational abnormalities. Clinical impression of acute abdomen/intraperitoneal bleeding concurrent with a positive hCG level is indicative of ectopic pregnancy until proven otherwise.
- MRI may also be useful but costly and rarely used if TVUS is available; benefits particularly for abdominal or cesarean scar pregnancy

Follow-Up Tests & Special Considerations

hCG levels should be carefully monitored and followed. All patients should receive counseling about return precautions (severe abdominal pain, heavy vaginal bleeding, nausea or vomiting).

Diagnostic Procedures/Other

In the setting of an undesired pregnancy, uterine aspiration or D&C can identify the presence/absence of intrauterine chorionic villi. When an IUP has been evacuated, hCG levels should drop by 50% within 48 hours.

Test Interpretation

Products of conception (POC; especially chorionic villi) outside the uterine cavity

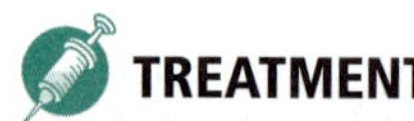

TREATMENT

GENERAL MEASURES

Management of ectopic pregnancy usually requires medical management or surgery with comparable efficacy from either in appropriately chosen candidates. A very few patients with low and declining hCG levels and meeting other criteria may be managed expectantly (2)[A]. Patients who are diagnosed early can often be managed with medication. However, those who have concern for tubal rupture with signs of hemodynamic instability will require surgical intervention.

MEDICATION

First Line

- Medication therapy with methotrexate is the preferred treatment if the patient is hemodynamically stable and is able to comply with follow-up.
  - Methotrexate: treatment for unruptured tubal pregnancy or for remaining POCs after laparoscopic salpingostomy. If TVUS is suggestive but not diagnostic, in the hemodynamically stable patient who qualifies for medical management, confirm suspected US findings with 2 hCG levels drawn 48 hours apart. Rise <35% is consistent with nonviable pregnancy. Methotrexate is most effective when pregnancy is <3 cm diameter, hCG <5,000 mIU/mL, and no fetal heart activity is seen. Success rate is 88% if hCG <1,000 mIU/mL, 71% if hCG 1,000 to 2,000 mIU/mL, and 38% if 2,000 to 5,000 mIU/mL. All regimens require following quantifying hCG to 0. Contraindications: hemodynamic instability or any evidence of rupture, moderate to severe anemia, severe hepatic or renal dysfunction, immunodeficiency; relative contraindications: fetal heart activity seen, large gestational sac (>3 to 4 cm), noncompliance or limited access to hospital or transportation, hCG >5,000 mIU/ml; precautions immunologic, hematologic, renal, GI, hepatic, and pulmonary disease, or interacting medications
- Three main dosage regimens exist and for use, require a reliable, hemodynamically stable patient (1).
  - Single: IM methotrexate 50 mg/m^2 of body surface area (BSA); may repeat once if <15% decline in hCG between day 4 and 7; if there is a decrease in hCG by at least 15% between day 4 and 7, adequate treatment occurred; follow hCG weekly. The single-dose regimen is preferred for simplicity, safety, lower adverse effect rate and comparable effectiveness to multidose regimens (3).

- Two dose: methotrexate 50 mg/m^2 of BSA once and then repeated on day 4; if <15% decline in hCG between day 4 and 7, may repeat third dose on day 7 (not needed if hCG decrease is 15% or more). Repeat hCG as needed on days 11 and 14 until decreases >15% in the interval and then weekly. If not dropping by day 14, refer for surgical management; may be somewhat more effective for higher initial hCG levels than is the single dose regimen
- Multidose (fixed dose with frequent injections): methotrexate 1 mg/kg IM/IV every other day on days 1, 3, 5, and 7, with leucovorin 0.1 mg/kg IM rescue in between on days 2, 4, 6, and 8 (counteracts effects of methotrexate); maximum 4 doses until hCG drop below 15%; course may be repeated 7 days after last dose if necessary.
- Pretreatment testing: serum hCG, CBC, liver and renal function tests, blood type and screen
- Patient counseling: During therapy, refrain from use of alcohol, aspirin, NSAIDs, and folate supplements (decreases efficacy of methotrexate); avoid excessive sun exposure due to risk of sensitivity. Adherence to scheduled follow-up appointments is critical. Increased abdominal pain may occur during treatment; however, severe pain, nausea, vomiting, bleeding, dizziness, or light-headedness may indicate treatment failure and require urgent evaluation. Rupture of ectopic pregnancy during methotrexate treatment ranges from 7% to 14%.
- Adverse reactions of methotrexate include nausea, diarrhea, abdominal cramping, cough, and the rare risk of neutropenia and leukopenia
- Systemic methotrexate may be offered in some kinds of nontubal ectopic pregnancies, but data is limited.

ISSUES FOR REFERRAL

Consider gynecologic consultation if not experienced in medical management and for surgical care.

ADDITIONAL THERAPIES

- Physician or patient may elect for surgical treatment as primary method and then postop hCG should guide need for supplemental methotrexate.
- After evidence of medical failure or tubal rupture, surgery is necessary.
- Treatment of cervical, ovarian, abdominal, or other ectopic pregnancy is complicated and requires immediate specialist referral.
- Offer anti-D Rh prophylaxis at a dose of 50 μg to all Rh-negative women who have a surgical procedure to manage an ectopic pregnancy or if there has been significant bleeding or abdominal pain.
- Expectant management to allow for spontaneous resolution of PUL is acceptable in asymptomatic patients with no evidence of rupture or hemodynamic instability coupled with an appropriately low and decreasing hCG levels (<1,500 mIU/mL) and no extrauterine mass suggestive of ectopic. Ruptured tubal pregnancies may occur even with extremely low hCG levels (<100 mIU/mL) (4).
- With expectant management of PUL, repeat TVUS weekly (or when hCG above discriminatory zone) until location is confirmed or clinical picture is unstable.

SURGERY/OTHER PROCEDURES

- Indications include hemodynamic instability, ruptured ectopic pregnancy, inability to comply with medical follow-up, previous tubal ligation, known tubal disease, current heterotopic pregnancy, desire for permanent sterilization at time of diagnosis.
- Laparoscopy is the first-line surgical management (4).
- Salpingectomy (tubal removal) is preferred and is indicated for uncontrolled bleeding, recurrent ectopic pregnancy, severely damaged tube, large gestational sac, or patient's desire for sterilization (4). Salpingostomy (preservation of tube) is considered in patients who wish to maintain fertility particularly if contralateral tube is damaged/absent. No difference in recurrence rate compared to salpingectomy.

ADMISSION, INPATIENT, AND NURSING CONSIDERATIONS

- Admission if a patient does not meet criteria for methotrexate management, if there is a high suspicion of rupture or signs/symptoms of hemodynamic instability including orthostasis, shock, and severe abdominal pain or inability to tolerate oral intake.
- Inpatient observation in the setting of an uncertain diagnosis, particularly with an unreliable patient, may be appropriate.
- Surgical emergency: Two large-bore IV access lines should be placed in case immediate aggressive resuscitation as needed; blood product transfusion if necessary en route to the operating room; in cases of shock, pressors and cardiac support may be necessary.
- Strict input/output, hourly vitals, orthostatics if mobile, frequent abdominal exams, serial hematocrit, pad counts if heavy vaginal bleeding
- Discharge criteria: afebrile, abdominal pain resolving or resolved, diagnosis established, surgical treatment, and recovery is complete

ONGOING CARE

FOLLOW-UP RECOMMENDATIONS

Patient Monitoring

- Serial serum quantitative hCG until level drops to zero. After methotrexate administration, strict monitoring protocol should be followed. Following salpingostomy, weekly hCG levels are appropriate.
- Pelvic US for persistent or recurrent masses
- Pain control: brief course of narcotics usually necessary with medical or surgical management
- Liver and renal function tests weekly following methotrexate administration if repeat dosing is required.
- Some clinicians recommend delaying subsequent pregnancy for at least 3 months after treatment with methotrexate due to risk for teratogenicity (4).

DIET

During treatment, avoid alcohol and foods and vitamins high in folate due to interaction with methotrexate efficacy.

PATIENT EDUCATION

- Signs and symptoms of ectopic pregnancy should be reviewed.
- Patients should be encouraged to plan subsequent pregnancies and seek early medical care on discovery of future pregnancies.

PROGNOSIS

- Chronic ectopic pregnancies are rare and treated with surgical removal of the fallopian tube.
- Future fertility depends on fertility prior to ectopic pregnancy and degree of tubal compromise. In women with normal fertility, treatment options make no differences in future fertility rates. In women with subfertility, expectant or medical treatments confer better future fertility (4).
- If infertility persists beyond 12 months, the fallopian tubes should be evaluated.

COMPLICATIONS

Hemorrhage and hypovolemic shock, persistent trophoblastic tissue after medical or surgical management, infection, infertility, blood transfusions with associated infections/transfusion reaction, disseminated intravascular coagulation in the setting of massive hemorrhage.

REFERENCES

1. Tonick S, Conageski C. Ectopic pregnancy. *Obstet Gynecol Clin North Am*. 2022;49(3):537–549.
2. Al Wattar BH, Solangon SA, de Braud LV, et al. Effectiveness of treatment options for tubal ectopic pregnancy: a systematic review and network meta-analysis. *BJOG*. 2024;131(1):5–14.
3. Yuk JS, Lee JH, Park WI, et al. Systematic review and meta-analysis of single-dose and non-single-dose methotrexate protocols in the treatment of ectopic pregnancy. *Int J Gynaecol Obstet*. 2018;141(3):295–303.
4. Diagnosis and management of ectopic pregnancy: Green-top Guideline No. 21. *BJOG*. 2016;123(13):e15–e55.

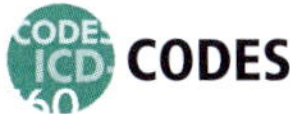

CODES

ICD10

- O00.0 Abdominal pregnancy
- O00.8 Other ectopic pregnancy
- O00.1 Tubal pregnancy

CLINICAL PEARLS

- Diagnosis requires high clinical suspicion in the setting of abdominal pain and a positive pregnancy test until IUP is confirmed.
- Monitoring patients carefully with a combination of TVUS, serial hCG levels, and clinical status is essential to help prevent poor outcomes in patients with suspected or confirmed ectopic pregnancy.

EJACULATORY DISORDERS

Payam Sazegar, MD

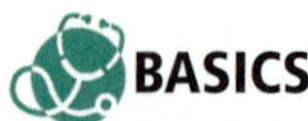

BASICS

DESCRIPTION

- Group of dysfunctions involving altered time and control (premature ejaculation [PE], delayed ejaculation [DE]), presence (anejaculation [AE]), direction (retrograde ejaculation [RE]), volume (perceived ejaculate volume reduction [PEVR]), or force (decreased force of ejaculation [DFE]) of ejaculation
- PE is defined as a persistent/recurrent pattern of ejaculation occurring during partnered sexual activity within 1 minute following vaginal penetration and before the individual wishes it + present for 6 months + causing significant distress for individual.
  - Natural biologic response is to ejaculate within 2 to 5 minutes after vaginal penetration.
  - Ejaculatory control is an acquired behavior that increases with experience.
  - Comorbidities common (diabetes, hypertension, sexual desire disorder, erectile dysfunction [ED])
- DE: prolonged time to ejaculate (>30 minutes) despite desire, stimulation, and erection
- Aspermia (lack of sperm in the ejaculate):
  - AE: lack of emission or contractions of bulbospongiosus muscle
  - RE: partial or complete ejaculation of semen into the bladder
  - Obstruction: ejaculatory duct obstruction or urethral obstruction
- Also:
  - Painful ejaculation: genital or perineal pain during or after ejaculation
  - Ejaculatory anhedonia: normal ejaculation lacking orgasm or pleasure
  - Hematospermia: presence of blood in the ejaculate (often not a serious condition)

EPIDEMIOLOGY

Prevalence

- PE is common; reported prevalence in American males is 5–20%.
- DE is reported in 5–8% of men aged 18 to 59 years, but <3% have the problem for >6 months.
- Predominant age: all sexually mature age groups

ETIOLOGY AND PATHOPHYSIOLOGY

Male sexual response:

- Erection mediated by parasympathetic nervous system
- Normal ejaculation consists of three phases:
  - Emission phase: Semen is deposited into urethra by contraction of prostate, seminal vesicles, vas deferens; under autonomic sympathetic control
  - Ejaculation phase: semen forcibly propelled out of urethra by rhythmic contractions of the bulbospongiosus and ischiocavernosus muscles; this is mediated by the somatic nervous system on the motor branches of the pudendal nerve. Bladder neck contracture by α-adrenergic receptors ensures anterograde ejaculation.
  - Orgasm: the pleasurable sensation associated with ejaculation (cerebral cortex); smooth muscle contraction of accessory sexual organs; release of pressure in posterior urethra
- PE:
  - Hypersensitivity/hyperexcitability of glans penis
  - 5-hydroxytryptamine (5-HT) receptor sensitivity
  - Psychogenic (inexperience, anxiety/guilt, low frequency of sex, relationship problems)
  - Urologic (ED, prostatitis, urethritis)
  - Endocrine (hyperthyroid, obesity, diabetes)
  - Lack of physical or sexual activity
  - Withdrawal or detox from prescription or illicit drugs (e.g., opioids)
- DE:
  - Rarely due to underlying painful disorder (e.g., prostatitis, seminal vesiculitis)
  - Often has a psychogenic component
  - Sometimes associated with low testosterone levels
  - Sexual performance anxiety and other psychosocial factors
  - Drugs or medications may impair ejaculation (e.g., MAOIs, SSRIs, α-blockers and β-blockers, thiazides, antipsychotics, tricyclic antidepressants, NSAIDs, opiates, alcohol, cannabis).
- AE:
  - Never has ejaculate: congenital structural disorder (müllerian duct cyst, Wolffian abnormality)
  - Acquired causes: surgery (radical prostatectomy, retroperitoneal lymph node dissection), spinal cord injury or other sympathetic nerve injury (especially T10–T12 level), diabetes mellitus (DM) with neuropathy, and medications (α-blockers and β-blockers, benzodiazepines, SSRIs, MAOIs, TCAs, antipsychotics, aminocaproic acid)
- RE:
  - Transurethral resection of the prostate (25%) or other prostate resection procedures
  - Surgery on the neck of the bladder
  - Extensive pelvic surgery
  - Retroperitoneal LN dissection for testicular cancer (also may produce failure of emission)
  - Neurologic disorders (multiple sclerosis [MS], DM)
  - Medications (tamsulosin, other α-blockers, SSRIs, antipsychotics)
  - Urethral stricture (may be posttraumatic)
- Painful ejaculation:
  - Infection or inflammation (orchitis, epididymitis, prostatitis, urethritis)
  - Ejaculatory duct obstruction
  - Seminal vesicle calculi
  - Obstruction of the vas deferens
  - Psychological/functional
- Hematospermia (often unable to find cause):
  - Usually not a serious condition
  - Inflammation/infection
  - Calculi: bladder, seminal vesicle, prostate, urethra
  - Trauma to genital area (cycling, constipation, masturbation)
  - Obstruction
  - Cyst
  - Tumor (1–3% prostate cancers present with hematospermia)
  - Arteriovenous malformations
  - Iatrogenic
  - Hypertension

RISK FACTORS

ED: pudendal neuralgia, substance use, psychotropic medications, psychological distress, or relationship issue

GENERAL PREVENTION

Screen for sexually transmitted infections (STIs).

COMMONLY ASSOCIATED CONDITIONS

- Neurologic disorders (e.g., multiple sclerosis)
- Diabetes
- Prostatitis
- Ejaculatory duct obstruction
- Urethral stricture
- Psychological disorders
- Endocrinopathies
- Relationship/interpersonal difficulties

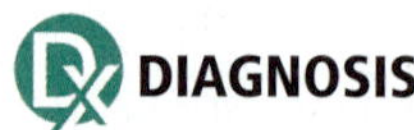

DIAGNOSIS

HISTORY

Detailed sexual history, including:

- Time frame of the problem
- Quality of patient's sexual response
- Sense of ejaculatory control and sexual distress
- Overall assessment of the relationship
- Detailed history of recent and current medications
- History of past trauma or recent infections
- Past surgical history with particular attention to genitourinary (GU) surgeries
- Supplements and alternative therapies tried
- Many men do not distinguish initially between problems related to erection and ejaculation.
- Include the sexual partner in the interview, especially if the patient expresses a belief that he is not meeting his partner's needs.
- In review of systems, elicit any evidence of testosterone deficiency or prolactin excess, especially if anhedonia present.

PHYSICAL EXAM

- Check vitals. Look for focal neurologic signs (MS, spinal cord injury) and psychiatric disorders.
- Thorough GU exam, including:
  - Size and texture of testes and epididymis
  - Verification of the presence of the vas deferens
  - Location and patency of urethral meatus
  - Digital rectal examination to evaluate prostate consistency, size, and possible midline lesions

DIAGNOSTIC TESTS & INTERPRETATION

- Fasting glucose or HbA1c to rule out diabetes
- Postorgasmic urinalysis will confirm RE. Semen fructose level, sperm count, and viscosity can be measured.
- AE will have fructose negative, sperm negative, and nonviscous postorgasmic urinalysis.
- In painful ejaculation, urinalysis and urine culture needed to rule out infection
- If prostate cancer is considered, check prostate-specific antigen (PSA).
- In anhedonia, consider checking testosterone, prolactin, glucose, TSH.
- In hematospermia, painful ejaculation, or if ejaculatory duct obstruction is considered, transrectal ultrasound (TRUS)
- TRUS-guided seminal vesicle aspiration if ejaculatory duct obstruction is present
- If suspicious of anatomic abnormality, can get scrotal US and/or MRI

Initial Tests (lab, imaging)

Consider CBC, HbA1c, PSA, TSH, testosterone, and urine studies. Often, no workup is needed for PE. For hematospermia, check CBC, coagulation tests, urine culture, chem panel, STI screening, semen analysis, and, condom test.

Follow-Up Tests & Special Considerations

Scrotal US or MRI TRUS; most patients do not require these tests.

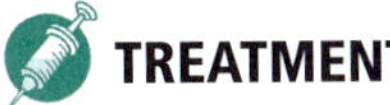

TREATMENT

GENERAL MEASURES

- Identifying any medical cause (even if not reversible) helps patient accept condition.
- Improve partner communication.
- Psychological counseling for patient and partner
- Reduce performance pressure through reassurance.
- PE:
  - Use sensate focus therapy (gradual progression of nonsexual contact to sexual contact).
  - Quiet vagina: Female partner stops moving just prior to ejaculation.
  - Techniques to learn ejaculatory control (e.g., coronal squeeze technique [squeezing the glans penis until ejaculatory urge ceases] or start-and-stop technique [cessation of penile stimulation when ejaculation approaches and resumption of stimulation when ejaculatory feeling ends])
- DE:
  - Change to antidepressant less likely to cause DE (citalopram, fluvoxamine, nefazodone) (1)[C]
- AE/RE:
  - Discontinue offending medications.
  - Improve diabetic control.
  - If urethral obstruction present, refer to urology.
  - RE may be helped if intercourse occurs when bladder is full.
  - Consider penile vibratory stimulation (effective in spinal cord injuries >T10) or electroejaculation (place on monitor if lesions above T6 because autonomic dysreflexia may result) to collect sperm in AE cases.
- Painful ejaculation:
  - Rule out infection. Counseling may be beneficial.
  - If seminal vesicle stones are possible, refer to urology.
- Hematospermia:
  - Often benign and resolves spontaneously, without known cause. Reassure initially.
  - May try empiric antibiotic, but little evidence to support
  - If persistent or high degree of suspicion for abnormality, refer to urologist.

MEDICATION

- PE:
  - Treat underlying erectile dysfunction (a common comorbidity) with PDE5 inhibitors.
  - First line:
    - Antidepressants "on-demand": clomipramine 20 to 50 mg 4 to 24 hours before intercourse, sertraline 50 mg 4 to 8 hours before intercourse, and paroxetine 20 mg 3 to 4 hours before intercourse (1)[A]
    - Daily dosing of clomipramine 20 to 50 mg, sertraline 25 to 200 mg, fluoxetine 5 to 20 mg, or paroxetine 10 to 40 mg can delay ejaculation within 1 to 3 weeks of starting (1)[A].
    - PDE5 inhibitor with or without SSRI
  - Second line:
    - Topical anesthetic gel (e.g., 2.5% prilocaine ± 2.5% lidocaine [EMLA]) 2.5 g applied under a condom for 30 minutes prior to intercourse (2)[B]
    - Tramadol 5 to 50 mg used "on demand" 2 hours before sex; also, available in spray form (2)[B]
    - Modafinil, behavioral/sex therapy, pelvic floor muscle therapy (1),(3)[B]
- DE:
  - No FDA-approved pharmacotherapy
  - Patients who must continue SSRIs may respond to bupropion and buspirone (2)[C].
  - Sex therapy, self-stimulation therapies (2)[C]
  - Consider oxytocin, pseudoephedrine, and midodrine (1),(2)[C].
- AE and RE:
  - First line: sympathomimetics (pseudoephedrine 60 mg PO daily to QID) or anticholinergics (imipramine 25 to 75 mg PO BID) that enhance bladder outlet resistance (2)[B]
  - Second line: for RE, can try postejaculation bladder harvest of sperm (if fertility desired); for AE, can try midodrine, penile vibratory stimulation, or electroejaculation
  - α-Agonists and antihistamines can be helpful but are not approved by the FDA.
- Painful ejaculation:
  - Treat underlying infection/inflammatory process.
  - No specific pharmacotherapy (2)[C]

ISSUES FOR REFERRAL

Refer to a urologist:

- Ejaculatory duct obstruction
- Seminal vesicle or prostatic stones
- Urethral obstruction
- Vas deferens obstruction
- Calculi
- Persistent or severe hematospermia

SURGERY/OTHER PROCEDURES

Transurethral resection of the ejaculatory ducts (if duct obstruction present)

COMPLEMENTARY & ALTERNATIVE MEDICINE

Daily caffeine consumption and folic acid supplementation may be beneficial.

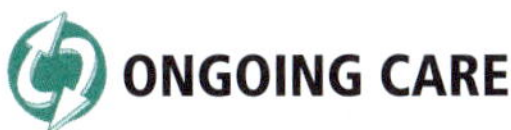

ONGOING CARE

PATIENT EDUCATION

See "General Measures."

PROGNOSIS

PE often improves with therapy and counseling

COMPLICATIONS

Psychological impact on some males: signs of severe inadequacy, self-doubt, additional anxiety, and guilt

REFERENCES

1. Shindel AW, Althof SE, Carrier S, et al. Disorders of ejaculation: an AUA/SMSNA guideline. *J Urol*. 2022;207(3):504–512.
2. Chen T, Mulloy EA, Eisenberg ML. Medical treatment of disorders of ejaculation. *Urol Clin North Am*. 2022;49(2):219–230.
3. Haghighi M, Jahangard L, Meybodi AM, et al. Influence of modafinil on early ejaculation—results from a double-blind randomized clinical trial. *J Psychiatr Res*. 2022;146:264–271.

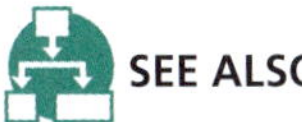

SEE ALSO

Erectile Dysfunction

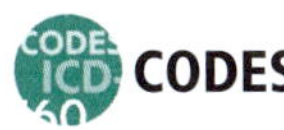

CODES

ICD10

- F52.4 Premature ejaculation
- N53.11 Retarded ejaculation
- N53.14 Retrograde ejaculation

CLINICAL PEARLS

- If erectile dysfunction is contributing to ejaculatory difficulty, management of erectile dysfunction should precede attempted management of ejaculatory disorders.
- Medications should always be thoroughly reviewed because they may be the primary cause of ejaculatory disorders.
- PE and DE generally have both psychogenic and physical causes, whereas AE and RE are due to organic neurogenic/autonomic dysfunction.
- A multidisciplinary approach, including the primary care physician, urologists, psychologists, and other appropriate health care professionals, is essential to the proper treatment of ejaculatory disorders.

ELDER ABUSE

Thomas Triantafillou, MD • Naisargi Modi, MD

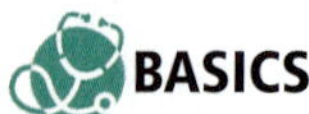

BASICS

DESCRIPTION

- Elder abuse (EA) includes failing to meet an older adult's needs or intentional financial, physical, or emotional actions causing risk of or actual harm. EA is often underrecognized.
- Clinicians can use the Age-Friendly Health System (AFHS) model, focusing on Matters Most, Mentation, Medications, and Mobility (4Ms). EA can be framed by societal influences (provider/caregiver education), individual factors (history of abuse), and the nature of the abuse.
- AFHS and Geriatric Emergency Department Accreditation (GEDA) frameworks can inform one's strategy or cycles of improvement on EA.
- Extensions of such approaches can link to collaborations with first responders (police, fire department) or older adult services Department of Aging (DOA), Adult Protective Services (APS), Program of All-inclusive Care of the Elderly (PACE).

EPIDEMIOLOGY

Incidence

Incidence is ~11% to 21% over 10 years (1),(2). Higher rates occur in nursing homes.

Prevalence

Prevalence is ~21% (2).

ETIOLOGY AND PATHOPHYSIOLOGY

The etiology of EA involves biopsychosocial factors in combination with increased dependence on a caregiver.

RISK FACTORS

- Risk factors include female sex, cognitive impairment (memory, executive), disability, and age >74 years (Reis da Silva, 2024).
- Unclear advance directives
- Caregivers burnout
- Medical factors: delirium (e.g., from electrolyte imbalance), anemia, traumatic brain injury (TBI), infection, myocardial ischemia, urinary retention, constipation, end-of-life delirium, mood disorders, cognitive impairment, medication issues (polypharmacy), or movement disorders (e.g., parkinsonism).
- EA is associated with poorer outcomes and higher resource use (e.g., rehab, nursing home care).

GENERAL PREVENTION

- Complete annual wellness visits to discuss advanced care plan, power of attorney for health or finances, goals of care (GOC), degree of self-sufficiency, the role of the caregiver, the risk of caregiver burnout, and use an EA screening tool.
- Assess caregiver stress and burden (meet without patient). Screen for risk or presence of mood disorders (depression: PHQ-2 or PHQ-9; anxiety: General Anxiety Disorder-7 (GAD-7); loneliness: 3-item UCLA) or cognitive impairment (Folstein Mini-Mental State Examination [MMSE]), Montreal Cognitive Assessment [MoCA], Saint Louis University Mental Status [SLUMS]).
- Encourage socialization. Refer to community programs: DOA, Alzheimer's Association, programs at a municipality.

COMMONLY ASSOCIATED CONDITIONS

Social isolation, increased dependence for activities of daily living/instrumental activities of daily living (ADLs/IADLs), depression, cognitive impairment, and aggressive behavior

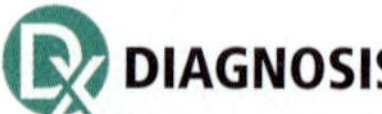

DIAGNOSIS

- Types of EA: physical or sexual, violation of personal rights, material exploitation, neglect (includes abandonment), financial, and psychological
- The context can vary from self-neglect, institutional (nursing home, assisted living), or domestic (home). Use a validated screening tool.

HISTORY

- Advance care plan
- Review of living arrangements, degree of physical or cognitive function, who the caregivers are, and is there evidence of caregiver burnout.

PHYSICAL EXAM

- Assess frailty, weight loss, general appearance including hygiene or clothing.
- Assess mentation (progressive memory loss, depression, anxiety, suicidal ideation).
- Check for evidence suggesting an unexplained injury: falls, burns, bruises (consider the effect of antiplatelets or anticoagulants or conditions associated with bruising or change in skin condition), fractures (consider the expected effect of osteopenia or osteoporosis).
- Skin exam
  - Large bruises (>5 cm) located at the face, lateral arm, back, or inner thighs
  - Patterned injury suggesting inappropriate restraint such as bite marks, ligature marks
  - Burn marks in patterns inconsistent with unintentional injury, for example, stocking and glove pattern suggesting forced immersion.
  - Open wounds, cuts, punctures, tissue swelling, untreated injuries in various stages of healing
  - Check for pressure ulcers on the bony prominences of the patient

DIFFERENTIAL DIAGNOSIS

- Dementia (FAST 6 or 7), or dementia in a withdrawn or malnourished patient
- Elderly with Alzheimer, vascular, or Lewy body dementia (LBD) can present with delusions.
- Psychosis
- Substance use disorders or exposure to toxins
- Parkinson disease resulting in fractures or bruises
- Coagulopathy with malignancy or other conditions
- Antiplatelet therapy associated with bruising
- Wasting from malignancy (cachexia), infections, or chronic disease
- Delirium due to electrolyte (sodium), TBI, infection, heart disease, urine retention, constipation, end-of-life
- Thyroid disorder associated with altered mental status, delirium, depression, frailty, or anxiety
- Fixed drug reaction, fragile photo-aged skin, steroid purpura, allergic reaction

DIAGNOSTIC TESTS & INTERPRETATION

Initial Tests (lab, imaging)

- CBC, CMP; vitamin B_{12}, folic acid, RPR, TSH (if forgetful); PT/INR (if bruising)
- CT brain (non-contrast) for moderate to severe TBI; x-ray of areas with pain or suspected fracture

Follow-Up Tests & Special Considerations

- Anemia: iron, TIBC, ferritin
- Change in mental status: vitamin B_1, vitamin B_6; consider toxicology; consider encephalopathy panel.
- Delirium: post-void residual
- Anti-amyloid medications for Alzheimer dementia: Update radiology if patient is on treatment and can be associated with brain bleeding or swelling.

Diagnostic Procedures/Other

- Interview a patient in private. Obtain collateral history including risk for substance use disorders, falls.
- Use tools to assess cognition, such as MoCA (forgetfulness, MCI), SLUMS, MMSE (proprietary), or Mini-Cog.
- Use mood screening tools for depression (Geriatric Depression Scale (GDS), PHQ2 or PHQ9), for anxiety GAD-7, or somatization (PHQ-15).
- Assess the patient's capacity (for example, use Aid to Capacity Evaluation).
- Documentation
  - Can document "suspect mistreatment" but avoid making a definitive diagnosis of EA in an initial assessment; include the abuser's name/relationship/contact, if known.
  - Pictures need to include the patient's name, medical number, date and time taken. Take pictures of torn clothes.
  - Document that a call was made to APS.
- Some states require reporting only if the patient cannot do so. Reporters in good faith are protected.

TREATMENT

Consider the use of the abuse intervention model (3)[B]

- Domain I—vulnerable older adult (victim): Address physical needs (physical therapy, assist devices); cognition (nutritious diet, activity, sleep); mental health (screen/treat depression; involve social work); and determinants of health (DOH) (housing, warmth, nutrition, social support).
- Domain II—trusted others (perpetrator): Educate about EA; offer financial planning support; treat perpetrator's substance/mood issues (refer to care); if elder's safety is at risk, involve law enforcement and APS.
- Domain III—context of abuse (circumstances): Reduce isolation (community resources, consider assisted living, involve social work); address relationship conflict (counseling); respect cultural values when discussing dementia.

ISSUES FOR REFERRAL

- Ethical concerns due to secondary gain (ethics consult)
- Mood or behavior concern (behavioral health services, social work consult)
- Cognitive assessment (neuropsychology, neurology, geriatrics consult)
- Social services assessment (DOA referral [patient can self-refer])

ADDITIONAL THERAPIES

Physical and occupational therapy for mobility/safety, strength and balance physical therapy referral, cognitive therapy, a pharmacist for medication review, and a geriatric consult (comprehensive assessment).

COMPLEMENTARY & ALTERNATIVE MEDICINE

Relaxation or wellbeing techniques for caregivers or patients; support groups

ADMISSION, INPATIENT, AND NURSING CONSIDERATIONS

- Ensure victims are discharged with follow-up care.
- Report to APS (or facility ombudsman/regulator) and law enforcement if injuries are present.
- Provide mental health follow-up and treat neglect injuries (wound care).
- Notify security if limiting visitors.
- Disposition options: safe caregiver/family, assisted living, or nursing home

ONGOING CARE

FOLLOW-UP RECOMMENDATIONS

- Educate caregivers on burnout signs and home support resources. Review state reporting laws: http://www.napsa-now.org/wp-content/uploads/2014/11/Mandatory-Reporting-Chart-Updated-FINAL.pdf.
- Contact the APS. A helpful resource is http://www.napsa-now.org/get-help/help-in-your-area/.
- Contact the DOA to request an assessment at home.
- ED providers should notify the Long-Term Care Ombudsman for nursing home residents.

Patient Monitoring

Frequent home or clinic visits.

DIET

Mediterranean diet; MIND diet for cognitive health

PATIENT EDUCATION

- For EA resources in your state, https://ncea.acl.gov, or call 800-677-1166
- Elder care locator, 800-677-1116, https://eldercare.acl.gov/Public/Index.aspx
- Alzheimer's Association, 800-272-3900; Alzheimer's Association. Abuse. https://www.alz.org/help-support/caregiving/safety/abuse
- National Organization for Victim Assistance, https://www.trynova.org/

PROGNOSIS

EA and self-neglect are associated with an overall increased risk of mortality.

COMPLICATIONS

Higher mortality, hospitalizations, functional decline, loneliness, and depression

REFERENCES

1. Burnes D, Hancock DW, Eckenrode J, et al. Estimated incidence and factors associated with risk of elder mistreatment in New York State. *JAMA Netw Open*. 2021;4(8):e2117758. doi:10.1001/jamanetworkopen.2021.17758.
2. Marrs SA, Yelvington M, Rhodes A, et al. An exploration of the knowledge and current practices of frontline workers regarding elder abuse. *J Appl Gerontol*. 2025;44(3):473–485. doi:10.1177/07334648241274906.
3. Mosqueda L, Burnight K, Gironda MW, et al. The abuse intervention model: a pragmatic approach to intervention for elder mistreatment. *J Am Geriatr Soc*. 2016;64(9):1879–1883. doi:10.1111/jgs.14266.

ADDITIONAL READING

Van Royen K, Van Royen P, De Donder L, et al. Elder abuse assessment tools and interventions for use in the home environment: a scoping review. *Clin Interv Aging*. 2020;15:1793–1807. doi:10.2147/CIA.S261877.

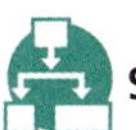

SEE ALSO

National Adult Protective Services Association (NAPSA) Resources: https://www.napsa-now.org/resources/

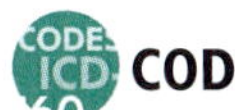

CODES

ICD10

- T74.11XA Adult physical abuse, confirmed, initial encounter
- T74.21XA Adult sexual abuse, confirmed, initial encounter
- T74.01XA Adult neglect or abandonment, confirmed, initial encounter

CLINICAL PEARLS

- Have a high clinical suspicion of EA.
- If a systematic process is developed, adopt tools to proactively screen for EA risk factors.
- Patient with capacity: The APS cannot act if a patient does not agree.
- Patient with impaired capacity: A medicolegal process, along with guidance from the APS, can lead to temporary guardianship (probate court).

ENCOPRESIS

Parul Chaudhri, DO

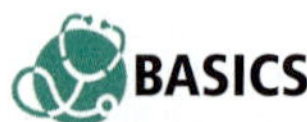

BASICS

DESCRIPTION

- Defined by *DSM-5* and Rome IV diagnostic criteria, as repetitive and inappropriate passage of feces
- Diagnostic criteria: chronologic and developmental age of at least 4 years of age; repeated passage of stool in inappropriate places—floors, clothes; symptoms mostly involuntary but may be intentional; at least one event per month for 3 months; behavior can't be explained by other medical conditions or use of substances (e.g., laxatives); excludes mechanisms involving constipation
- Categories:
  - With constipation and overflow incontinence (functional constipation or retentive encopresis)—more common
  - Without constipation (nonretentive fecal soiling or nonretentive fecal incontinence)
- Constipation is passing delayed or infrequent hard stools with pain and straining.

EPIDEMIOLOGY

Incidence

There is no clear difference in the incidence of functional constipation between women and men. Constipation in children accounts for 3% of primary care visits and 25% referrals to pediatric gastroenterology. Functional constipation is the cause of 95% of all constipation in children and adolescents with median age of onset ~2.3 years of age and often coinciding with transition to solid foods, toilet training, or start of school.

Prevalence

- Occurs in 4% of children 5 to 6 years of age and 1–2% of children aged 11 to 12 years; more frequent in boys
- 25% of children with functional constipation will have adult GI issues.

ETIOLOGY AND PATHOPHYSIOLOGY

- In 90% of cases, encopresis develops as a consequence of chronic constipation, with resulting overflow incontinence (retentive encopresis). The other 10% are caused by specific organic etiologies.
- Constipation causes pain with defecation which causes further stool withholding. Stool withholding increases colonic water absorption, making stools harder and more difficult to pass.
- Withholding behaviors such as hiding, rocking back and forth, or fidgeting when feeling the urge to defecate can be confused with signs of straining to defecate. Many children voluntarily withhold stool for fear of pain or a preoccupation with not interrupting social activities.
- Chronic constipation with irregular and incomplete evacuation results in progressive rectal distension and stretching of the internal/external anal sphincters.
- Chronic rectal distension causes habituation, leading to the loss of sensing the normal urge to defecate causing abdominal pain, nausea, and bloating. Eventually, soft or liquid stool leaks around the retained fecal mass.
- Psychological: stool withholding, fear, anxiety; difficulty with toilet training, including unusual anxiety or conflict with parent; resistance to using public toilet facilities, such as school bathrooms or outdoor toilets; associated with abuse; developmental delay
- Anatomic: rectal distension and desensitization, anal fissure or painful defecation; muscle hypotonia, slow intestinal motility; Hirschsprung disease, cystic fibrosis; spinal cord defects (e.g., spina bifida), congenital anorectal malformations; anal stenosis, anterior displacement of the anus, postoperative stricture of anus or rectum; pelvic mass, neurofibromatosis
- Dietary or metabolic: inadequate dietary fiber; excessive protein or milk intake; inadequate water intake; hypothyroidism; hypercalcemia; hypokalemia; diabetes insipidus; diabetes mellitus; food allergy; gluten enteropathy
- Medication side effects

Genetics

None known; although incidence may be higher in children with family history of constipation

RISK FACTORS

Transition of foods: breast milk to formula or cow's milk or start of solid foods; parental conflicts or divorce; new sibling; history of constipation; painful defecation; difficulty with bowel training, including social pressure related to early daycare placement; organic/anatomic causes; anxiety and depression; insufficient fluid or fiber intake; fear of using bathrooms/public restrooms; attention deficit; history of abuse; medications (particularly opiates, ADD/ADHD medications, antidepressants)

GENERAL PREVENTION

Family education: toilet training when ready; optimize fluid and fiber intake.

COMMONLY ASSOCIATED CONDITIONS

Constipation, developmental and behavioral diagnoses, urinary incontinence, cow's milk protein allergy, autism and ADHD, psychosocial or neurologic conditions—especially nonretentive fecal incontinence, UTI

DIAGNOSIS

Functional constipation is a clinical diagnosis based on above criteria. No additional testing or labs in children with no red flag symptoms.

HISTORY

- Stool pattern, consistency, and interval; abdominal pain that improves with stool passage; hiding while defecating before child is toilet-trained; avoiding use of the toilet
- Signs/symptoms of constipation: hard, large caliber stools <3 defecations per week, pain or discomfort with stool passage, withholding stool, blood on stool or in diaper/toilet bowl
- Diet low in fiber or fluids, high in dairy products
- No stool passage in the first 48 hours of life
- Urinary symptoms: recurrent UTIs or enuresis
- General symptoms: decreased appetite fevers/chills
- Stressors, family, social and family history of constipation or medication use: opiates or antidepressants
- Abrupt onset after age 5 years is more likely to be associated with psychological trauma.

PHYSICAL EXAM

- Neurologic exam of lower extremities and perineal area, with attention to S1–S4 distribution, perineal sensation, cremasteric reflex, anal sphincter tone, and evidence of neural tube defects
- Genital examination and digital rectal exam: assess for anal fissures, sphincter tone, rectal distension/impaction, and occult or visible blood.
- Abdominal exam: bowel sounds, percussion note (tympany), abdominal distension; palpate for stool (most common in left lower quadrant) strength/laxity of abdominal musculature
- Growth parameters: height, weight, head circumference
- Insufficient evidence of doing digital rectal exam in the absence of specific clinical indications

DIFFERENTIAL DIAGNOSIS

Irritable bowel syndrome, celiac disease, hypothyroidism, Down syndrome, anal fissures, trauma, Hirschsprung disease, cerebral palsy, hypercalcemia, neuromuscular disease

DIAGNOSTIC TESTS & INTERPRETATION

Most cases diagnosed by history and physical

Initial Tests (lab, imaging)

Used only to rule out organic causes: UA/urine culture: UTI/glucosuria; thyroid function tests: hypothyroidism; electrolyte panel, including calcium: hypokalemia, hypercalcemia, or hyperglycemia; abdominal plain films if impaction is suspected and otherwise not confirmed by physical exam

Follow-Up Tests & Special Considerations

Failure to pass meconium within 48 hours of birth, failure to thrive, bloody diarrhea, or bilious vomiting in a neonate should be promptly evaluated to exclude aganglionic megacolon; constipation and diarrhea, rash, failure to thrive, or recurrent pneumonia—consider cystic fibrosis; patients with abdominal distension or ileus should be evaluated for possible obstruction.

TREATMENT

GENERAL MEASURES

- Four key elements: dietary modification, behavior modification, medications, disimpaction (if needed)
- Anticipatory toilet training advice about when children should reduce reliance on diapers or use pull-ups during the daytime hours (average age for toilet training in girls is 29 months; 31 months for boys)
- Eliminate impaction prior to initiating any maintenance therapy.
- Once stools are regular in frequency, child should sit on toilet BID at the same time each day for 10 to 15 minutes and for 10 to 15 minutes after meals. Incorporate positive reinforcement for successful bowel movements.

- Juices containing sorbitol (e.g., apple, pear, prune) increase water content and promote stool softness.
- Recommended daily fluid intake: ages 1 to 3 years: 4 cups; ages 4 to 8 years: 5 cups; age >8 years: 7 to 8 cups
- Recommended fiber intake: A rough guide in children is to add 5 g to child's age in years.
- Children may experience shame, bullying, and rejection. Adolescents may have depression, anxiety, and social problems.
- Parents of children with these issues may need extra education. They may also feel shame, blame, and/or dismissal.
- 50%–60% recovery rate after 1 year of intensive treatment.

MEDICATION

- Remove impaction and start maintenance treatment.
- No RCTs have compared methods of disimpaction: can use oral agents, enemas, and rectal suppositories; oral agents are least traumatic. Glycerin suppositories are the best option for infants.

First Line

- Disimpaction with polyethylene glycol (PEG): Give 17 g (240 mL) water or juice: 1 to 1.5 g/kg/day for 3 days for disimpaction (may occasionally need higher doses via NG in hospital setting if at home treatment fails). Use 0.4 to 0.8 g/kg/day for maintenance.
- Disimpaction with mineral oil for child aged >1 year; give 15 to 30 mL/year of age to maximum of 240 mL; for maintenance: 1 to 3 mL/kg/day or divided BID; may mix with orange juice to make palatable; avoid in infants to avoid aspiration pneumonia.
- Disimpaction with saline enema: 5 to 10 mL/kg once/day for 3 to 6 days up to 5 yo, adult dose
- Other maintenance regimens include the following: Milk of Magnesia (MOM) 400 mg (5 mL): 1 to 2 mL/kg/day BID; magnesium citrate: 4 mL/kg/day; lactulose 10 g (15 mL): 1 to 3 mL/kg/day divided BID; Senna syrup 8.8 g sennoside (5 mL): ages 2 to 6 years: 2.5 to 7.5 mL/day divided BID; age 6 to 12 years: 5 to 15 mL/day divided BID; bisacodyl suppository 10 mg: 0.5 to 1.0 suppository once or twice per day—children >2 years old; sorbitol containing juices: 1 to 3 mL/kg BID in infants
- Continue maintenance medications for 1 to 2 months after symptom resolution or until after toilet training is achieved.

ISSUES FOR REFERRAL

- No improvement after 6 months of treatment; refer to pediatric gastroenterology.
- Refer to psychologist or use combination medical and behavior therapy if no improvement in 3 months.

ADDITIONAL THERAPIES

Behavioral treatment and counseling; caregiver education

SURGERY/OTHER PROCEDURES

If refractory symptoms, consider anorectal manometry to evaluate for internal anal sphincter achalasia (or ultrashort-segment Hirschsprung disease). If present, this condition can be treated successfully in most patients with an internal sphincter myectomy.

COMPLEMENTARY & ALTERNATIVE MEDICINE

- Children who receive combination of behavioral and medication treatment are more likely to have resolution of encopresis at 3 and 6 months than with medication alone.
- No evidence that biofeedback training adds benefit to conventional treatment.
- Behavioral interventions combined with laxative therapy (rather than laxative therapy alone) improve continence in children with functional fecal incontinence associated with constipation.
- No evidence for effectiveness of either probiotics or increased physical activity

ADMISSION, INPATIENT, AND NURSING CONSIDERATIONS

- Admission criteria/initial stabilization: continued soiling and recurrent impaction on outpatient medical therapy; decreased intake leading to malnutrition or dehydration, recalcitrant vomiting or concern for obstruction; involve appropriate agencies if concern for abuse; hospital admission and abdominal films may be necessary to ensure complete removal of impaction. This may include direct gastric administration of balanced electrolyte–PEG solutions if the patient cannot tolerate by mouth. Serial abdominal films and observation of rectal effluent can help determine treatment adequacy.
- IV fluids if the patient is dehydrated and has difficulty tolerating oral intake
- Nursing to document stool output and character
- Discharge criteria: Stools that are looser in consistency and clearer are a successful inpatient end point; abdominal radiograph showing less fecal loading (compared with a pretreatment x-ray) with improving serial abdominal exams

ONGOING CARE

Record bowel movements successfully passed as well as soiling episodes as well as incorporating a reward system to promote continued efforts at sitting on the toilet regularly. Open communication and close follow-up are essential in the long run.

FOLLOW-UP RECOMMENDATIONS

Follow-up monthly at first with clinician to review the patient's stooling regimen, conduct a physical exam, and re-adjust the home regimen as needed to ensure continued progress and remission of symptoms.

Patient Monitoring

- Continue maintenance treatment for 6 months to 2 years with visits every 4 to 10 weeks for support and to ensure compliance; more frequent visits with oppositional or anxious children
- Treat recurrences of impaction promptly and emphasize compliance with medication and regular bathroom visits.
- Refer children for mental health evaluation and counseling if no progress with comprehensive behavior plan.

DIET

Adequate fluid and fiber intake; reduce cow's milk products. Avoid excessive consumption of bananas, rice, apples, and gelatin.

PATIENT EDUCATION

- Demystify defecation.
- Carefully explain the treatment plan including medications and dietary changes.
- Avoid punishment for inadvertent soiling.
- In children >4 years of age, explain to parents how overreliance on diapers and pull-ups (while convenient) can prolong the problem.
- Always attempt to use positive reinforcement for successful toilet sits and medication compliance.
- If positive approach is unsuccessful, consider removing desired privileges (e.g., TV, video games) for noncompliance with behavioral plan. Some children respond well to a token economy (earned privileges) to promote desired behavior.
- Encourage regular physical activity.

PROGNOSIS

- Many children exhibit a good response and relapse due to parental noncompliance.
- From 30% to 50% of children may still have encopresis after 5 years of treatment.
- Children with psychosocial or emotional problems preceding the encopresis are more recalcitrant to treatment.

COMPLICATIONS

- Colitis due to excessive enema/suppository
- Perianal dermatitis
- Anal fissure

ADDITIONAL READING

- Baird DC, Bybel M, Kowalski AW. Toilet training: common questions and answers. *Am Fam Physician*. 2019;100(8):468–474.
- Constipation Guideline Committee of the North American Society for Pediatric Gastroenterology, Hepatology and Nutrition. Evaluation and treatment of constipation in infants and children: recommendations of the North American Society for Pediatric Gastroenterology, Hepatology and Nutrition. *J Pediatr Gastroenterol Nutr*. 2006;43(3):e1–e13.
- LeLeiko NS, Mayer-Brown S, Cerezo C, et al. Constipation. *Pediatr Rev*. 2020;41(8):379–392.
- Lu PL, Mousa HM. Constipation: beyond the old paradigms. *Gastroenterol Clin North Am*. 2018;47(4):845–862.

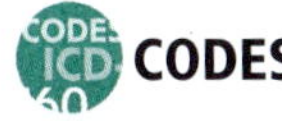

CODES

ICD10

- R15.9 Full incontinence of feces
- R15.1 Fecal smearing
- F98.1 Encopresis not due to a substance or known physiol condition

CLINICAL PEARLS

- 90% of encopresis results from chronic constipation.
- Address toddler constipation early by decreasing excessive milk intake, increasing fruits/vegetables intake, and ensuring adequate fluid and fiber intake.
- Eliminate fecal impaction before initiating maintenance therapy.

ENDOCARDITIS, INFECTIVE

Theodore B. Flaum, DO • Alexa Finkelstein, BS

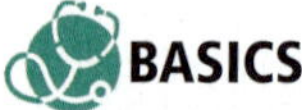

BASICS

Infective endocarditis (IE) is an infection of the inner layer of the heart including the valves (native/prosthetic), interventricular septum, intracardiac devices, chordae tendineae, and mural endocardium. IE occurs worldwide and is generally fatal if left untreated.

DESCRIPTION

- An infection of the valvular (primarily) and/or mural (rarely) endocardium
- System(s) affected: cardiovascular, endocrine/metabolic, hematologic/lymphatic, immunologic, pulmonary, renal/urologic, skin/exocrine, neurologic
- Synonym(s): bacterial endocarditis; subacute bacterial endocarditis (SBE); acute bacterial endocarditis (ABE)

EPIDEMIOLOGY

More common in males (range is 3:2 to 9:1.); >50% of cases in the United States occur in individuals >60 years of age.

Incidence

- Incidence at ~15 in 100,000, increasing from previous years
- The predominant form of IE is community associated. Up to 1/3 of cases are health care acquired in resource-rich countries.
- Increasing incidence of cardiovascular device-related infections due to a higher frequency of implantable devices
- Can be community- or hospital-acquired
- Most commonly affects the mitral valve and aortic valve (increased left-sided pressures and turbulent flow)

ETIOLOGY AND PATHOPHYSIOLOGY

IE is most commonly caused by a nonbacterial thrombus that adheres to an endocardial surface, coupled with a bacterial source sufficient to seed the thrombus. This can occur from direct bacterial invasion or valvular trauma:

- Native valve endocarditis
  - Acute: *Staphylococcus aureus* (most common); *Streptococcus* groups A, B, C, G; *Streptococcus pneumoniae*; *Staphylococcus lugdunensis*; *Enterococcus* spp.; *Haemophilus influenzae* or *parainfluenzae*; *Neisseria gonorrhoeae*
  - Subacute: α-hemolytic streptococci, *Streptococcus bovis*, *Enterococcus* spp., *S. aureus*, *Staphylococcus epidermidis*; HACEK organisms
- Intravenous drug abuse endocarditis (IVDA) (most commonly tricuspid valve): *S. aureus*, *Enterococcus* spp.; *Pseudomonas aeruginosa*, *Burkholderia cepacia*, other bacilli (gram-negative); *Candida* spp.
- Prosthetic valve endocarditis
  - Early (≤12 months after valve implantation): *S. aureus*, *S. epidermidis*; gram-negative bacilli; *Candida* spp., *Aspergillus* spp.
  - Late (>12 months after valve implantation): α-hemolytic streptococci, *S. aureus*, *Enterococcus* spp., *S. epidermidis*, *Candida* spp., *Aspergillus* spp.
- Culture-negative endocarditis: 10% of cases; *Bartonella quintana* (homeless), *Brucella* spp., fungi, *Coxiella burnetii* (Q fever), *Chlamydia trachomatis*, *Chlamydophila psittaci*, HACEK organisms
- Device-related endocarditis: coagulase-negative staphylococci or *S. aureus*

RISK FACTORS

- Injection drug use, IV catheterization, certain malignancies (colon cancer), poor dentition/infection, chronic hemodialysis, age >60 years, male sex, implantable cardiac devices
- Highest risk with (1):
  - Previous IE
  - Prosthetic cardiac valves (including transcatheter-implanted prostheses and homografts)
  - Cardiac transplant with valvular regurgitation
  - Prosthetic material used for cardiac valve repair (such as annuloplasty rings or chords)
  - Congenital heart disease (CHD): unrepaired cyanotic CHD or repaired CHD residual shunts of valvular regurgitation at the site of or adjacent to the site of a prosthetic patch or prosthetic device

GENERAL PREVENTION

- Good oral hygiene
- Antibiotic prophylaxis is only recommended in patients with a high risk of adverse outcomes if IE were to occur (see "Risk Factors"). Administer 30 to 60 minutes prior to the procedure (exception vancomycin which should be administered 120 minutes prior to the procedure).
- In high-risk patients, consider antibiotic prophylaxis for dental procedures involving manipulation of gingival tissue, manipulation of the periapical region of teeth, or perforation of the oral mucosa.
- Prophylaxis is not recommended for EGD, TEE, colonoscopy, or cystoscopy in absence of evidence for active/ongoing infection.

COMMONLY ASSOCIATED CONDITIONS

Most patients with IE have preexisting conditions (see "Risk Factors" above).

DIAGNOSIS

The 2023 Duke-International Society for Cardiovascular Infectious Diseases (ISCVID) revised guidelines for diagnosis of IE:

- Major criteria
  - Blood culture/microbiology:
    - Typical microorganisms for IE identified in ≥2 separate blood cultures. This includes *S. aureus*, viridans group streptococci, *Streptococcus gallolyticus* (formerly *S. bovis*), HACEK group organisms, and community-acquired enterococci.
    - Persistently positive blood cultures for an organism consistent with IE
    - A single positive blood culture for *C. burnetii* or an anti–phase-1 IgG antibody titer >1:800
    - Positive molecular tests (such as PCR) for specific pathogens like *Tropheryma whipplei* or *Bartonella* spp. from a blood sample.
  - Imaging:
    - Echocardiogram findings consistent with IE, including:
      - Vegetation (a mass on a heart valve or supporting structures)
      - Abscess, pseudoaneurysm, or intracardiac fistula
      - New valvular regurgitation (leaky heart valve)
      - New partial dehiscence of a prosthetic valve
    - Advanced imaging findings are now included as major criteria:
      - Positron emission tomography (PET)/CT scan showing abnormal activity around the site of a prosthetic valve (implanted >3 months prior) or other intracardiac devices
      - Cardiac CT scan demonstrating specific signs of IE such as valvular vegetations, perforations, or abscesses
  - Surgical: Direct evidence of endocarditis found during surgery, such as vegetations or an abscess
- Minor criteria
  - Predisposing heart condition or injection drug use
    - Fever with a temperature of ≥38°C (100.4°F)
    - Vascular phenomena, including major arterial emboli, septic pulmonary infarcts, mycotic aneurysm, intracranial hemorrhage, conjunctival hemorrhages, and Janeway lesions
    - Immunologic phenomena, such as glomerulonephritis, Osler nodes, Roth spots, and a positive rheumatoid factor
    - Microbiologic evidence that does not meet a major criterion (e.g., a single positive blood culture of a typical organism)
    - Imaging evidence that is suggestive but not definitive for IE on echocardiogram, PET/CT scan, or cardiac CT scan; diagnostic classification
- Three or four minor criteria
  - Rejected IE if:
    - A firm alternative diagnosis is established.
    - There is resolution of symptoms with antibiotic therapy for ≤4 days.
    - There is no pathologic evidence of IE at surgery or autopsy after antibiotic therapy for ≤4 days.
    - The criteria for "possible" or "definite" IE are not met.
    - The diagnosis of IE is categorized based on the combination of these criteria.
  - Definite IE is diagnosed with:
    - Two major criteria
    - One major criterion and three minor criteria
    - Five minor criteria
    - Pathologic confirmation of IE from a vegetation or abscess specimen
  - Possible IE is diagnosed with: one major criterion and one or two minor criteria.

HISTORY
- Fever (>38°C), chills, cough, dyspnea, orthopnea; especially in subacute endocarditis: night sweats, weight loss, fatigue
- Review risk factors
- Symptoms of transient ischemic attack, cerebrovascular accident (CVA), or myocardial infarction (MI) on presentation

PHYSICAL EXAM
- Most patients with IE have new murmur or change to an existing murmur. Signs of heart failure are common if valve function is compromised.
- Peripheral stigmata of IE: splinter hemorrhages in fingernail beds, Osler nodes, Roth spots, Janeway lesions, palatal/conjunctival petechiae, splenomegaly, hematuria
- Neurologic findings consistent with CVA

DIFFERENTIAL DIAGNOSIS
Vasculitis, temporal arteritis, fever of unknown origin, infected central venous catheter, marantic endocarditis, connective tissue diseases, intra-abdominal infections, rheumatic fever, salmonellosis, brucellosis, Lyme disease, malignancy, tuberculosis, atrial myxoma, septic thrombophlebitis

DIAGNOSTIC TESTS & INTERPRETATION
Follow-Up Tests & Special Considerations
If indicated, follow-up imaging to evaluate for secondary system involvement or to rule out other causes:
- Chest x-ray: may reveal evidence of septic pulmonary emboli or signs of congestive heart failure
- CT chest/abdomen/pelvis: Evaluate distal sites of infections and/or infarction.

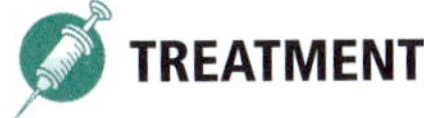

TREATMENT

GENERAL MEASURES
In general, antibiotic therapy for IE should be targeted to the organism isolated from blood cultures. The duration of therapy should be calculated from the first day of the negative blood cultures.

MEDICATION
First Line
- Start empiric treatment after three sets of blood cultures have been drawn. Results guide treatment.
  - Native valves: ampicillin-sulbactam IV with gentamicin IV/IM; if penicillin-allergic, use vancomycin IV with gentamicin IV/IM and with ciprofloxacin PO/IV.
  - Prosthetic valves: vancomycin IV with gentamicin IV/IM and rifampin PO, if <12 months postsurgery; if >12 months, use native valve regimen.
- Penicillin-susceptible viridans streptococci or *S. bovis*
  - Native valve: penicillin G IV continuously or ceftriaxone IV/IM for 4 weeks
  - Prosthetic valve: penicillin G IV for 6 weeks or ceftriaxone IV/IM ± gentamicin IV/IM for 2 weeks
- Penicillin-resistant viridans streptococci or *S. bovis*
  - Native valve: penicillin G IV + gentamicin IV/IM
  - Prosthetic valve: penicillin G IV or ceftriaxone IV/IM for 6 weeks + gentamicin IV/IM for 2 weeks
- Penicillin-susceptible *Staphylococcus*
  - Native valve: oxacillin or nafcillin IV for 6 weeks; for oxacillin-resistant strains, use vancomycin IV for 6 weeks.
  - Prosthetic valve: oxacillin or nafcillin IV + rifampin IV/PO for 6 weeks + gentamicin IV for first 2 weeks; for oxacillin-resistant strains, use vancomycin IV + rifampin IV/PO both for 6 weeks + gentamicin IV/IM for the first 2 weeks
- Penicillin-resistant *Staphylococcus*
  - Native valve: vancomycin for 6 weeks or daptomycin IV for 6 weeks
  - Prosthetic valve: vancomycin + rifampin IV/PO + gentamicin IV/IM for 2 weeks
- Penicillin-sensitive *Enterococcus*
  - Native or prosthetic valve: ampicillin IV or penicillin G IV + gentamicin IV for 4 to 6 weeks.
- HACEK organisms: ceftriaxone IM or IV for 4 weeks *or* ampicillin-sulbactam IV for 4 weeks *or* ciprofloxacin PO or IV for 4 weeks

SURGERY/OTHER PROCEDURES
Surgery is required in 50% of IE cases; indications:
- Heart failure due to aortic or mitral valve disease
- Prevention of embolism: aortic or mitral valve vegetations >10 mm with prior embolic episodes; isolated very large vegetation >15 mm; in patients with major ischemic stroke, surgery is delayed for at least 4 weeks, if possible.
- Uncontrolled infection: persistent fever and positive cultures >7 to 10 days; infection caused by fungi or resistant organism; presence of abscess, fistula, false aneurysm, or enlarging vegetations
- Early prosthetic valve IE

ADMISSION, INPATIENT, AND NURSING CONSIDERATIONS
- Need for IV antibiotics
- Hemodynamic or clinical instability
- Monitoring and adjusting therapy if there is antibiotic resistance

ONGOING CARE

FOLLOW-UP RECOMMENDATIONS
Patient Monitoring
- Baseline ECG; monitor ECG for conduction disturbances/MI in initial weeks of therapy.
- TTE at the conclusion of therapy
- Blood cultures q48h until negative

DIET
Heart-healthy diet low in sodium, saturated fats and cholesterol, with emphasis on fruits, vegetables, whole grains, and lean protein

PATIENT EDUCATION
- Practice excellent dental hygiene: brush 2x/day, floss daily, regular cleanings
- Smoking cessation and avoid IV drug use

PROGNOSIS
The 1-year mortality of IE is 30%. Late complications contribute to poor prognosis. These include heart failure, reinfection, and cerebral emboli. The 10-year survival is 60–90%.

COMPLICATIONS
- Cerebral complications are the most frequent and severe, occurring in 15–20% of patients. Neurologic events are the most frequent complications in patients with IE requiring ICU admission. Ischemic stroke is the presenting symptom of IE in 20% of cases.
- Emboli: arterial, infectious (e.g., abscesses of heart, lung, brain, meninges, bone, pericardium)
- Inflammatory/immune disorders (e.g., arthritis, myositis, glomerulonephritis)
- Other complications: congestive heart failure, ruptured valve cusp, sinus of Valsalva aneurysm, arrhythmia, and mycotic aneurysms

E

REFERENCES

1. Miao H, Zhang Y, Zhang Y, et al. Update on the epidemiology, diagnosis, and management of infective endocarditis: a review. *Trends Cardiovasc Med*. 2024;34(8):499–506. doi:10.1016/j.tcm.2024.01.001.

ADDITIONAL READING
- Fowler VG, Durack DT, Selton-Suty C, et al. The 2023 Duke-International Society for cardiovascular infectious diseases criteria for infective endocarditis: updating the Modified Duke Criteria. *Clin Infect Diseases*. 2023;77(4):518–526. doi:10.1093/cid/ciad271.
- Mulliken JS, Bainbridge ED. Infective endocarditis. *Med Clin North Am*. 2025;109(3):667–681. doi:10.1016/j.mcna.2024.12.009.
- Patel SK, Hassan SMA, Côté M, et al. Current trends and challenges in infective endocarditis. *Curr Opinion Cardiol*. 2025;40(2):75–84. doi:10.1097/HCO.0000000000001192.

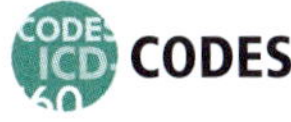

CODES

ICD10
- I33.0 Acute and subacute infective endocarditis
- I39 Endocarditis and heart valve disord in dis classd elswhr
- A54.83 Gonococcal heart infection

CLINICAL PEARLS
- Preprocedural antibiotic prophylaxis is recommended for patients with artificial heart valves, a previous history of IE, CHD, and cardiac transplants with valvulopathy.
- TEE/TTE and blood cultures are the mainstays for diagnosing IE.
- The most commonly identified organisms are viridans *Streptococcus* spp. and *Staphylococcus*.
- Valves most commonly involved: (i) mitral valve, (ii) aortic valve, (iii) combination of aortic and mitral valves, (iv) tricuspid valve, (v) pulmonic valve

ENDOMETRIOSIS

Kenneth A. Ballou, MD

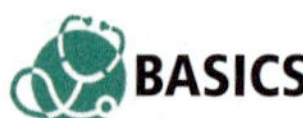

BASICS

DESCRIPTION

- Endometriosis is a common and potentially painful, debilitating estrogen-dependent gynecologic condition predominately affecting women of reproductive age.
- Symptoms and signs generally consist of pelvic and/or abdominal pain, pelvic mass, and/or decreased fertility.
- Manifests as estrogen-dependent implants of endometrial tissue found outside the uterus. Although endometriomas have been recorded in liver, bowel, umbilicus, lung, and other tissue, the most common pathologic sites are:
  - Peritoneum (bladder, cul-de-sac, pelvic walls, ligaments, and fallopian tubes)
  - Ovaries
  - Rectovaginal septum
- Ectopic endometrial implants proliferate and slough with the menstrual cycle.
- Stage I (minimal) to IV (severe); staging is useful in therapeutic planning but does not correlate with pain severity.

EPIDEMIOLOGY

Prevalence

- Biologic females only; affects 190 million worldwide (1), or about 1 in 10 women (2)
- Affects 6–10% of fertile women
- Found in 9–50% of infertile women
- Found in 12–70% of women with chronic pelvic pain

Pediatric Considerations

Endometriosis may begin with puberty, as endometrial implants are dependent on ovarian hormones. This can lead to debilitating pelvic pain and severe dysmenorrhea associated with missed school, and family/social activities.

Pregnancy Considerations

The presence of endometriosis decreases fecundability from 15–20% per month to 2–10% per month. 9–50% of infertile women have endometriosis. However, pelvic endometriosis symptoms generally improve during pregnancy.

Geriatric Considerations

Although menopause often results in a resolution of symptoms, pelvic endometriosis may extend into menopause and may be exacerbated by hormone replacement therapy (HRT).

ETIOLOGY AND PATHOPHYSIOLOGY

- Not fully understood; several factors are believed to play a role, including immunologic changes and genetic predisposition in the presence of abnormal proliferating endometrial tissue implants causing chronic peritoneal inflammation.
- Theories include:
  - Sampson theory: Retrograde menstruation results in peritoneal implantation and disease.
  - Halban theory: Distant disease is probably caused by hematogenous/lymphatic dissemination or metaplastic transformation.
  - Coelomic metaplasia: Coelomic epithelium remains undifferentiated in the peritoneal cavity and differentiates to form functioning endometrium.
- Endometrial-associated infertility is multifactorial:
  - Pelvic inflammation
  - Anatomic disruption of pelvic structures (Involvement of the fallopian tube may cause isthmic tubal obstruction.)
  - Proliferation and activation of peritoneal macrophages (may predispose to gamete phagocytosis)
  - Alteration in eutopic endometrium

Genetics

Women with a first-degree relative with endometriosis have a 7- to 10-fold increase in the risk of developing endometriosis themselves. Those with affected first-degree relatives have a 26% chance of severe manifestations versus 12% if no first-degree affected relatives.

RISK FACTORS

- Family history
- Prolonged lifetime exposure to menstruation and ovulation (early menarche, late menopause)
- Delayed childbirth/nulliparity
- Low body mass index, white race
- Prolonged menstruation (>5 days)/shorter menstrual cycles (<28 days)

GENERAL PREVENTION

- Suppression of heavy menstruation and ovulation with oral contraceptives during adolescence may delay sequelae.
- Some factors are considered protective:
  - Fruits, green vegetables, n-3 long-chain fatty acids
  - Regular aerobic exercise (>4 hours per week)
- Early diagnosis and treatment might help prevent sequelae.

COMMONLY ASSOCIATED CONDITIONS

Infertility, dysmenorrhea, ovarian cysts, dyspareunia, chronic abdominal/pelvic pain syndrome, pelvic inflammatory disease, and irritable bowel disease

DIAGNOSIS

HISTORY

- Dysmenorrhea (50–90% of cases) due to deep infiltrating endometrial implants
- Dyspareunia with or without postcoital bleeding due to lesions of the cul-de-sac, uterosacral ligaments, and posterior vaginal fornix
- Dyschezia due to involvement of the rectosigmoid colon and rectovaginal regions
- Chronic pelvic pain (≥6 months) that worsens with time and begins 1 to 2 days prior to menstrual cycles
- Hematochezia, suggesting colorectal involvement
- Cyclic nausea, abdominal distention
- Infertility (late finding)
- History of pelvic pain, infertility, and hysterectomy in first- or second-degree relative

PHYSICAL EXAM

- Focal pain/tenderness on pelvic exam is associated with endometriosis in 66% of patients.
- Pelvic mass may be present.
- Immobile pelvic organs (frozen pelvis)
- Rectovaginal exam revealing uterosacral nodules, beading, or tenderness
- Exquisite tenderness in the region of the uterosacral ligament is found in severe cases.

DIFFERENTIAL DIAGNOSIS

Differential diagnosis of pelvic pain includes all causes of acute abdomen and

- Pelvic adhesions
- Nonspecific dysmenorrhea
- Acute salpingitis/pelvic inflammatory disease
- Ovarian cyst/hydrosalpinges
- Uterine leiomyomas
- Adenomyosis
- Irritable bowel syndrome
- Inflammatory bowel disease
- Intraabdominal adhesions
- Pelvic malignancy
- Complications of intrauterine/ectopic pregnancy
- Urinary tract infection/interstitial cystitis
- Anal fissures
- Psychosexual pain syndrome, vaginal atrophy, vulvodynia, infectious vaginitis, or cervicitis
- Chronic pain syndrome

DIAGNOSTIC TESTS & INTERPRETATION

Initial Tests (lab, imaging)

- Initial diagnosis is primarily clinical.
- Labs are only useful to rule out other diagnoses; there are no reliable labs to rule in endometriosis.
- CA-125 levels are not recommended due to low specificity.
- If history and physical exam reveal adnexal pain or tenderness with/without fullness on pelvic exam
  - Transvaginal ultrasound (US) is the modality of choice; transabdominal pelvic US is less sensitive. MRI may be useful for evaluating deeper retrosigmoid and ureteral infiltrating lesions but generally has lower sensitivity.
  - Both modalities are poor in detecting peritoneal implants and adhesions.

Diagnostic Procedures/Other

Definitive diagnosis is made only by microscopic characteristics of tissue biopsied during laparoscopy or laparotomy.

Test Interpretation

- Laparoscopically visualized red and blue-black lesions described as "powder-burns," adhesions, and "chocolate cysts" on the ovarian and peritoneal surfaces
- Histologically described endometrial glands and stroma on analysis of biopsied lesions

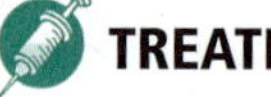

TREATMENT

GENERAL MEASURES

Management is dependent on multiple factors:

- Age and reproductive desires of the patient
- The certainty of the diagnosis
- The degree of degradation on quality of life due to pain and infertility
- The threat to other organ systems: GI tract, bladder

MEDICATION

Medications are used to improve the patient's quality of life through symptom relief and to prevent progression of the disease and its potential to cause organ dysfunction. Unfortunately, few studies of medical therapy report patient-relevant outcomes. Many patients gain only limited or intermittent benefit from medical therapies.

First Line

Patients found to have endometriomas during incidental surgery or studies may not need any treatment. Others with minimal symptoms may find sufficient relief with NSAIDs medications begun just before onset of menses. Increased exercise, especially aerobic, may help others. Medication therapy should be individualized, with recognition that persistence and recurrence despite treatment is common.

- Combined oral contraceptives and progestins are considered first line. Cyclic combined oral contraceptive pills (OCPs) suppress ovulation; combination OCPs or low-dose progestin-only medications prescribed as continuous combined contraception for 3 to 6 months if symptoms persist despite cyclic OCP use, or if there is chronic, noncyclic pelvic pain
- Medroxyprogesterone acetate 150 mg IM q 3 months; prolonged use may lead to loss of bone mineral density of uncertain clinical significance.
- Levonorgestrel intrauterine device (IUD) (Mirena) found to decrease recurrence of painful menstruation.

Second Line

- Gonadotropin-releasing hormone (GnRH) agonists: inhibit pituitary gonadotropin synthesis and induce a hypoestrogenic state; norethindrone acetate 5 mg PO once daily plus conjugated equine estrogen 0.625 mg PO once daily may be used as "add-back" therapy.
  - Leuprolide acetate (Lupron Depot) 3.75 mg IM each month or 11.25 mg IM every 3 months (gluteal)
  - Nafarelin (Synarel) intranasal one spray (200 μg) in one nostril each morning and the other nostril each evening (start between days 2 and 4 of menstrual cycle)
  - Goserelin (Zoladex) implant 3.6 mg SC in upper abdominal wall every 28 days
  - Aromatase inhibitors (anastrozole and letrozole) prolong the remission induced by GnRH medications.
- Danazol: also effective, with side effects similar to GnRH analogs

ALERT

Calcium (1,000 to 1,500 mg/day) with vitamin D 1,000 to 2,000 IU daily or low-dose estrogen with progestogen is recommended when using GnRH agonists to prevent calcium loss.

ISSUES FOR REFERRAL

- Refer early to a gynecologist with expertise in medical and surgical treatment of endometriosis, especially if the patient desires to conceive in the future.
- Indications for referral to include the following:
  - Need for definitive diagnosis
  - Failure to respond to a conservative or first-line therapy
  - Chronic pelvic pain
  - Delayed fertility

ADDITIONAL THERAPIES

Regular exercise and counseling for pain-management strategies; narcotics are contraindicated for chronic pain.

SURGERY/OTHER PROCEDURES

Surgery (laparoscopy or laparotomy) is both diagnostic and therapeutic (first line or when conservative measures fail):

- Peritoneal endometriosis: laser ablation/excision/fulguration
- Ovarian endometriosis (endometriomas) >3 to 4 cm: ablation, excision, drainage
- Lysis of adhesions (LOA)
- Hysterectomy with bilateral salpingo-oophorectomy may be considered for debilitating symptoms refractory to other medical or surgical treatments in patients who do not desire pregnancy:
  - Relieves pain in 80–90%, but pain recurs in 10% within 1 to 2 years after surgery
  - Postoperative HRT should include estrogen and progestogen or progesterone.
- Interruption of nerve pathways: Laparoscopic ablations and presacral neurectomy improve dysmenorrhea.
- Fertility procedures: Ablation or excision of lesions with LOA is recommended to treat infertility in stages I and II disease:
  - Spontaneous conception should be attempted for 1 year prior to assisted reproduction techniques.
  - Disease does not endanger in vitro fertilization (IVF) pregnancies.

ALERT

Surgery for endometriomas may decrease ovarian reserve in advanced disease.

COMPLEMENTARY & ALTERNATIVE MEDICINE

- Osteopathic manipulative therapy found to improve quality of life.
- Postsurgical use of Chinese herbal medicine has been found to be effective.
- Acupuncture may be effective in relieving pain (3).
- Botulinum toxin injections have been used to control pain.

ONGOING CARE

FOLLOW-UP RECOMMENDATIONS

Routine gynecologic care

Patient Monitoring

Symptomatic and asymptomatic pelvic masses (https://www.acog.org/)

PROGNOSIS

- Excellent, especially if diagnosis and treatment plans are initiated early in disease course
- Poor for recovery of fertility if the disease has progressed to stage III/IV
- Symptoms and signs improve after bilateral oophorectomy.

COMPLICATIONS

Sequelae include chronic pelvic pain, reduced quality of life, repetitive surgical intervention, depression, medication side effects and costs, and infertility.

REFERENCES

1. Horne AW, Missmer SA. Pathophysiology, diagnosis, and management of endometriosis. *BMJ*. 2022;379:e070750. doi:10.1136/bmj-2022-070750.
2. Zondervan KT, Becker CM, Missmer SA. Endometriosis. *N Engl J Med*. 2020;382(13):1244–1256.
3. Li PS, Peng XM, Niu XX, et al. Efficacy of acupuncture for endometriosis-associated pain: a multicenter randomized single-blind placebo-controlled trial. *Fertil Steril*. 2023;119(5):815–823. doi:10.1016/j.fertnstert.2023.01.034.

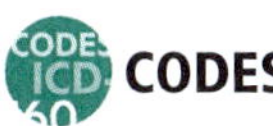

CODES

ICD10

- N80.2 Endometriosis of fallopian tube
- N80.5 Endometriosis of intestine
- N80.0 Endometriosis of uterus

CLINICAL PEARLS

- Endometriosis should be considered in patients of reproductive age with chronic pelvic/abdominal pain, dysmenorrhea, and/or decreased fertility.
- Initial diagnosis is clinical; no absolutely reliable diagnostic lab tests other than tissue biopsy evaluation are available, although transvaginal US may be helpful.
- First-line treatments include NSAIDs and oral birth control medications.
- Refer to an experienced gynecologist if fertility is desired, or if symptoms refractory to first-line treatments.

E

ENDOMETRITIS AND OTHER POSTPARTUM INFECTIONS

Rashmi Rode, MD, FAAFP • Chelsea Mendonca, MD

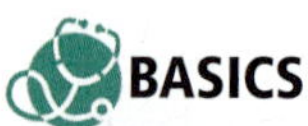

BASICS

DESCRIPTION

- Endometritis—a polymicrobial infection of the uterine lining (decidua)—is the most common postpartum infection.
- It usually presents around postpartum day 7 but in 15% of cases, it can occur as late as 6 weeks postpartum (1).
- Less common but significant infections include those involving the myometrium, parametrial tissues, cervix, vagina, or perianal areas; these may lead to serious complications such as pelvic cellulitis, abscesses, septic pelvic vein thrombophlebitis, or parametrial phlegmon.
- System(s) affected: reproductive
- Synonym(s): postpartum infection; endometritis; myometritis; metritis; endomyometritis; endoparametritis, puerperal endometritis

EPIDEMIOLOGY

Prevalence

- Affects 1–3% of all births
- Route of delivery is a strong predictor of the likelihood of developing endometritis, with rates reported after vaginal delivery (<3%), nonlaboring cesarean (7%), and cesarean delivery after trial of labor (30%) (2).
- 30–35% of postpartum infections occur after labor without prophylaxis; 2–15% occur with prophylaxis.
- One of the top five causes of maternal mortality, contributing to 11% of maternal deaths globally

ETIOLOGY AND PATHOPHYSIOLOGY

Postpartum endometritis often follows chorioamnionitis or mechanical trauma. It is typically polymicrobial:

- Aerobes (70%): *Streptococcus agalactiae*, *Staphylococcus aureus*, *Escherichia coli*
- Anaerobes (80%): *Bacteroides*, *Clostridium*, *Fusobacterium*, *Peptostreptococcus*
- *Mycoplasma* and *Ureaplasma* species may also contribute.
- Viral causes (e.g., herpes simplex virus [HSV], cytomegalovirus [CMV]) should be considered in immunocompromised patients.
- Severe cases may involve septic pelvic vein thrombosis or parametrial phlegmon.

RISK FACTORS

- Cesarean delivery (especially without antibiotic prophylaxis)
- Chorioamnionitis, prolonged labor, preterm prelabor rupture of membranes, multiple vaginal exams
- Genital tract colonization (e.g., group B *Streptococcus* [GBS], bacterial vaginosis [BV])
- Meconium-stained amniotic fluid
- Operative delivery, perineal trauma, internal fetal monitoring
- HIV, obesity, maternal diabetes, anemia, low socioeconomic status
- Nasal colonization with *S. aureus*
- Immunosuppression

GENERAL PREVENTION

- Intrapartum prophylaxis for GBS colonization of genital tract
- Vaginal delivery
  - Avoid unnecessary vaginal examinations.
  - Treat chorioamnionitis during labor.
  - Avoid manual placental extraction and retained placental products.
  - Aseptic technique for operative vaginal delivery
  - Antibiotic prophylaxis for manual removal of the placenta has not been demonstrated to be effective.
- Cesarean delivery
  - Preoperative paint and scrub with 10% povidone-iodine or an alcohol-based solution decreases puerperal infection by up to 38% (1).
  - Prophylactic antibiotics before both emergency and scheduled cesarean deliveries prior to skin incision reduce postpartum infection (1).
    - Administer antibiotics within 1 hour of the start of surgery. Repeat for lengthy procedures or excessive blood loss.
    - Weight-based intravenous (IV) cefazolin is recommended 60 minutes before skin incision: 1 to 2 g IV for patients without obesity and 2 g for patients with obesity or weight ≥80 kg (1),(2)
    - Adjunctive azithromycin 500 mg IV is recommended for patients with labor or rupture of membranes (1).
- Vaginal preparation with povidone-iodine solution or chlorhexidine-alcohol solutions immediately before cesarean delivery reduces the risk of postoperative endometritis.

COMMONLY ASSOCIATED CONDITIONS

- Intra-amniotic infection (IAI)/chorioamnionitis
- Wound infection

DIAGNOSIS

- Diagnosis is made clinically.
- The Infectious Diseases Society of America (IDSA) defines endometritis as a fever >38°C on >2 occasions >6 hours apart after the first 24 hours postpartum and up to 10 days postdelivery, in association with the following (3):
  - Uterine tenderness
  - Abdominal pain
  - Foul-smelling lochia and exclusion of other sites of infection

HISTORY

- History of cesarean delivery or chorioamnionitis
- Fever and chills
- Malaise
- Headache
- Anorexia
- Abdominal pain
- Heavy vaginal bleeding or foul smelling lochia

PHYSICAL EXAM

- Temperature >38°C (100.4°F), tachycardia
- Uterine tenderness (hallmark)
- Purulent or malodorous lochia, ileus, diffuse abdominal pain

DIFFERENTIAL DIAGNOSIS

- "5 Ws": wind (pneumonia); water (UTI/pyelonephritis); wound infection; walking (deep venous thrombosis, pulmonary embolus); wonder drug (medication-related fever)
- Infections unrelated to pregnancy: influenza, COVID-19, appendicitis, *C. difficile*, gastritis
- Septic pelvic thrombophlebitis

DIAGNOSTIC TESTS & INTERPRETATION

Initial Tests (lab, imaging)

- CBC (WBC may be physiologically elevated postpartum)
- CMP, blood cultures if systemic infection suspected
- Diagnosis often made on clinical grounds; potential testing includes: genital tract cultures and rapid test for GBS (may be done during labor)
- If the patient meets criteria for SIRS and or suspected sepsis, follow institution guidelines (i.e., serum lactate, fluid resuscitation, two sets of blood cultures, and timely administration of broad spectrum antibiotics).
- If patient not responding to antibiotics in 24 to 48 hours:
  - Ultrasound for retained products of conception, pelvic abscess, or mass
  - CT scan or MRI looking for pelvic vein thrombophlebitis, abscess, or deep-seated wound infection
  - Echocardiogram to rule out infective endocarditis

Follow-Up Tests & Special Considerations

Other, less typical causes of endometritis can be potentially lethal. These include group A strep infection, staph toxic shock syndrome (TSS), and *Clostridium*. These tend to have onset within 24 to 48 hours of delivery, and require aggressive fluid resuscitation, antibiotics, and source control.

- Group A strep endometritis/sepsis is typically associated with high fever, hypotension, and multi-organ failure.
- Staph TSS is characterized by high fever, hypotension, and diffuse rash and desquamation. It is often accompanied by multi-organ involvement.
- *Clostridium sordelli* is often rapid in onset of shock with progressive refractory hypotension, generalized massive edema and evidence of hemoconcentration, in the absence of fever.
- *Clostridium perfringens* can be considered in a severely ill person with evidence of intravascular hemolysis. It may cause myonecrosis ("gas gangrene") which can be identified on imaging.

Diagnostic Procedures/Other

Paracentesis/culdocentesis with culture rarely necessary

Test Interpretation

Histologic endometritis: >5 neutrophils/high-power field (HPF) ≥1 plasma cell in stroma

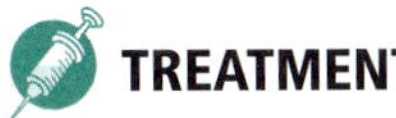

TREATMENT

GENERAL MEASURES

- Hospitalization for moderate to severe cases
- IV fluids, analgesia, and hemodynamic support

MEDICATION

Broad spectrum coverage is recommended, to include gram-positive, gram-negative, and anaerobic bacteria. Recent antibiotic exposure should also be taken into account.

First Line

- Clindamycin 900 mg IV q8h *plus* gentamicin 5 mg/kg IV q24h *plus* ampicillin 2 g IV q6h (if suspected *Enterococcus* or GBS colonization with clindamycin-resistant organism) until the patient is afebrile for 24 hours. Potential side effects include nephrotoxicity, ototoxicity, pseudomembranous colitis, or diarrhea (in up to 6%) (4).
- For monotherapy, cefoxitin 2 g IV q6h may be considered until the patient is afebrile for 24 to 48 hours (5).
- Penicillin allergy:
  - Clindamycin 900 mg IV q8h *plus* gentamicin (5 mg/kg IV q24h) *plus* vancomycin 1.5 gm IV q12h (for GBS colonization with clindamycin-resistant organism or suspicion of methicillin-resistant *S. aureus* [MRSA])

Second Line

- Ampicillin/sulbactam 3 g IV q6h
- Cefotetan 2 g IV q12h ± ampicillin 2 g IV q6h if no improvement in 48 hours
- Consider adding a macrolide (for chlamydia).
- Contraindications
  - Drug allergy, renal failure (aminoglycosides)
  - Avoid sulfa, tetracyclines, and fluoroquinolones before delivery and if breastfeeding. Metronidazole is relatively contraindicated if breastfeeding.
- Precautions:
  - Clindamycin and other antibiotics occasionally cause pseudomembranous colitis.
  - Antibiotic-associated diarrhea (*C. difficile*)
  - Gentamicin can cause renal injury.
- Note: heparin typically indicated for septic pelvic vein thrombophlebitis; requires 10 days of full anticoagulation

ISSUES FOR REFERRAL

Infectious disease referral for renal dysfunction

SURGERY/OTHER PROCEDURES

- Ultrasound to look for retained products of conception if not responsive to initial therapy
- Curettage for retained products of conception
- Surgery or image-guided drainage to drain abscess

ADMISSION, INPATIENT, AND NURSING CONSIDERATIONS

- Inpatient care is recommended for postpartum infections.
- Many infections occur after hospital discharge. Therefore, education regarding the importance of fever, pain, heavy vaginal bleeding, foul smelling lochia, or other signs of infection should occur prior to discharge.
- IV antibiotics and close observation for severe infections
- Open and drain infected wounds.
- Optimize fluid status.

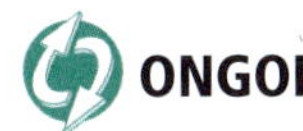

ONGOING CARE

FOLLOW-UP RECOMMENDATIONS

Patient Monitoring

- Individualize according to severity.
- IV antibiotics can be stopped when the patient is afebrile for 24 to 48 hours.
- Oral antibiotics on discharge are not necessary, unless patient was bacteremic; then, continue oral antibiotics to complete a 7-day course.

DIET

As tolerated, although may be limited by ileus

PATIENT EDUCATION

- Advise patient to contact physician with fever >38°C (100.4°F) postpartum, heavy vaginal bleeding, foul-smelling lochia, or other symptoms of infection.
- Information available at https://www.healthline.com/health/pregnancy/complications-postpartum-endometritis

PROGNOSIS

With supportive therapy and appropriate antibiotics, most patients improve quickly and recover without complication.

COMPLICATIONS

- Resistant organisms, peritonitis, pelvic abscess
- Septic pelvic thrombophlebitis, ovarian vein thrombosis
- Sepsis, death

REFERENCES

1. Mackeen AD, Sullivan MV, Berghella V. Evidence-based cesarean delivery: preoperative management (part 7). https://www.ajogmfm.org/article/S2589-9333(24)00088-0/fulltext. Accessed July 23, 2025.
2. Committee on Practice Bulletins-Obstetrics. ACOG Practice Bulletin No. 199: use of prophylactic antibiotics in labor and delivery. *Obstet Gynecol*. 2018;132(3):e103–e119.
3. Miller JM, Binnicker MJ, Campbell S, et al. Guide to utilization of the microbiology laboratory for diagnosis of infectious diseases: 2024 update by the Infectious Diseases Society of America (IDSA) and the American Society for Microbiology (ASM). *Clin Infect Dis*. 2024;ciae104. doi:10.1093/cid/ciae104.
4. World Health Organization. *WHO Recommendations for Prevention and Treatment of Maternal Peripartum Infections*. Geneva: World Health Organization; 2016.
5. Bailey P, Schacht L, Pazienza G, et al. Cefoxitin for intra-amniotic infections and endometritis: a retrospective comparison to traditional antimicrobial therapy regimens within a healthcare system. *Clin Infect Dis*. 2024;79(1):247–254. doi:10.1093/cid/ciae042.

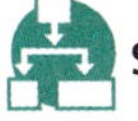

SEE ALSO

Algorithm: Pelvic Pain

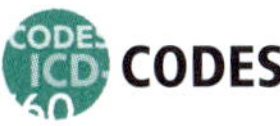

CODES

ICD10

- O86.12 Endometritis following delivery
- O86.4 Pyrexia of unknown origin following delivery
- O86.13 Vaginitis following delivery

CLINICAL PEARLS

- Postpartum endometritis is more common after cesarean delivery, particularly if unscheduled.
- The infection is usually polymicrobial.
- Treat base on clinical findings (e.g., unexplained postpartum fever, fundal tenderness, and foul-smelling lochia), using broad-spectrum antibiotics.
- Endometrial and blood cultures are not routinely done.
- For cesarean delivery, give prophylactic antibiotics within 60 minutes before surgery.

ENURESIS

Nancy V. Nguyen, DO • Hermione Gaw, MD

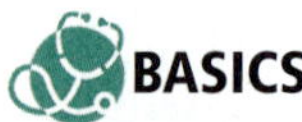

BASICS

DESCRIPTION

- Classification
  - Primary nocturnal enuresis (NE): 80% of all cases; person who has never established urinary continence on consecutive nights for a period of ≥6 months
  - Secondary NE: 20% of cases; resumption of enuresis after at least 6 months of urinary continence
- NE: intermittent nocturnal incontinence after the anticipated age of bladder control (age 5 years)
  - Primary monosymptomatic NE (PMNE): bed-wetting with no history of bladder dysfunction or other lower urinary tract (LUT) symptoms
  - Nonmonosymptomatic NE (NMNE): bed-wetting with LUT symptoms (LUTS) such as frequency, urgency, daytime wetting, hesitancy, straining, weak or intermittent stream, post-urination dribbling, lower abdominal or genital discomfort, or sensation of incomplete emptying

ALERT

Adult-onset NE with absent daytime incontinence is a serious symptom; complete urologic evaluation and therapy are warranted.

- System(s) affected: nervous, renal/urologic
- Synonym(s): bed-wetting; sleep enuresis; nocturnal incontinence; primary NE

EPIDEMIOLOGY

Incidence

- Depends on family history
- Spontaneous resolution: 15% per year

Prevalence

- Very common; 5 to 7 million children in the United States
- 10% of 7-year-olds; 3% of 11- to 12-year-olds; 0.5–1.7% at 16- to 17-year-olds (1)
- Two times more common in males than females
- Nocturnal > daytime (3:1)

Geriatric Considerations

Infrequent; often associated with daytime incontinence (formerly referred to as diurnal enuresis)

ETIOLOGY AND PATHOPHYSIOLOGY

- A disorder of sleep arousal, a low nocturnal bladder capacity, and nocturnal polyuria are the three factors that interrelate to cause NE.
- Both functional and organic causes (below); many theories, none absolutely confirmed
- Detrusor instability
- Deficiency of arginine vasopressin (AVP); decreased nocturnal AVP or decreased AVP stimulation secondary to an empty bladder (Bladder distension stimulates AVP.)
- Maturational delay of CNS
- Severe NE with some evidence of interaction between bladder overactivity and brain arousability: association with children with severe NE and frequent cortical arousals in sleep
- Organic urologic causes in 1–4% of enuresis in children: urinary tract infection (UTI), occult spina bifida, ectopic ureter, lazy bladder syndrome, irritable bladder with wide bladder neck, posterior urethral valves, neurologic bladder dysfunction
- Organic nonurologic causes: epilepsy, diabetes mellitus, food allergies, obstructive sleep apnea, chronic renal failure, hyperthyroidism, pinworm infection, sickle cell disease
- NE occurs in all stages of sleep.

Genetics

Most commonly, NE is an autosomal-dominant inheritance pattern with high penetrance (90%).

- 1/3 of all cases are sporadic.
- 75% of children with enuresis have a first-degree relative with the condition.
- Higher rates in monozygotic versus dizygotic twins (68% vs. 36%)
- If both parents had NE, risk in child is 77%; 44% if one parent is affected. Parental age of resolution often predicts when child's enuresis should resolve.

RISK FACTORS

- Family history
- Stressors (emotional, environmental) common in secondary enuresis (e.g., divorce, death)
- Constipation and/or encopresis
- Organic disease: 1% of monosymptomatic NE (e.g., urologic and nonurologic causes)
- Psychological disorders
  - Comorbid disorders are highest with secondary NE: depression, anxiety, social phobias, conduct disorder, hyperkinetic syndrome, internalizing disorders.
  - Association with ADHD; more pronounced in ages 9 to 12 years
- Altered mental status or impaired mobility

COMMONLY ASSOCIATED CONDITIONS

- Obstructive sleep apnea syndrome (10–54%) (2): Atrial natriuretic factor inhibits renin-angiotensin-aldosterone pathway leading to diuresis.
- Constipation (33–75%) (2)
- Behavioral problems (specifically ADHD in 12–17%) (2)
- Overactive bladder or dysfunctional voiding (up to 41%) (2)
- UTI (18–60%) (2)

DIAGNOSIS

HISTORY

- If the child ever had a prolonged period of dryness
- LUTS
- Fluid intake diary
- Voiding and stooling patterns (voiding diary); constipation issues
- Sleep history (sleep apnea, sleep disturbances)
- Psychosocial history (patient, parental, school/bullying, etc.)
- Family history of enuresis

PHYSICAL EXAM

- Poor growth and/or hypertension suggests renal disease.
- ENT: evaluation for adenotonsillar hypertrophy (associated with sleep apnea)
- Abdomen: enlarged bladder, kidneys, fecal masses
- Back: dimpling, tufts of hair on sacrum
- Genitourinary exam
  - Males: meatal stenosis, hypospadias, epispadias, phimosis
  - Females: vulvitis, vaginitis, labial adhesions, ureterocele at introitus; evidence of abuse
- Rectal exam: tone, fecal soiling, fecal impaction; in adult males, DRE for prostate enlargement
- Neurologic exam, especially lower extremity muscle tone and coordination, deep tendon reflexes, and sensation

DIFFERENTIAL DIAGNOSIS

- Primary NE
  - Delayed physiologic urinary control
  - UTI (both primary and secondary)
  - Spina bifida occulta
  - Obstructive sleep apnea (both primary and secondary)
  - Idiopathic detrusor instability
  - Previously unrecognized myelopathy or neuropathy (e.g., multiple sclerosis, tethered cord, epilepsy)
  - Anatomic urinary tract abnormality (e.g., ectopic ureter)
- Secondary NE
  - Acute situational stress (most common cause)
  - Bladder outlet obstruction
  - Neurologic disease, neurogenic bladder (e.g., spinal cord injury)

DIAGNOSTIC TESTS & INTERPRETATION

Initial Tests (lab, imaging)

- Only obligatory test in children is urinalysis.
- Urinalysis and urine culture: UTI, pyuria, hematuria, proteinuria, glycosuria, and poor concentrating ability (low specific gravity) may suggest organic etiology, especially in adults.
- Urinary tract imaging is usually not necessary.
- If abnormal clinical findings: renal and bladder ultrasound
- IV pyelogram, voiding cystourethrogram (VCUG), or retrograde pyelogram is rarely indicated.
- MRI if spinal dysraphism is suspected

Follow-Up Tests & Special Considerations

- Secondary enuresis: (if no psychosocial factors identified) serum glucose, BUN, creatinine, thyroid-stimulating hormone (TSH), urine culture
- In children, imaging and urodynamic studies are helpful for significant daytime symptoms, history of UTIs, suspected structural abnormalities, and in refractory cases.

Diagnostic Procedures/Other

Urodynamic studies may be beneficial.

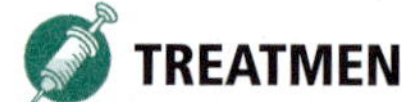

TREATMENT

GENERAL MEASURES

- Use nonpharmacologic approaches as first line before prescribing medications (2)[A].
- Simple behavioral interventions (e.g., scheduled wakening, positive reinforcement, bladder training, diet changes) are effective, although less than alarms or medications (2)[B]; found to achieve dryness in 15–20% of cases (1)
  - Patient education (fragmented sleep, low nocturnal bladder capacity, and increased nocturnal urine production)

- – Encourage normal daytime drinking and reduction of intake 2 hours prior to sleep.
- – Voiding before bed and scheduled waking for nighttime voiding
- – Nightlights to light the way to the bathroom
- – Reward system for dry nights
- – Use pull up over regular underwear or cloth underwear with built in waterproof barrier.
- – "Cleanliness training": child helps with changing wet bedding
- – Do not shame or punish bed-wetting; have child participate in removing/laundering soiled bedding.
- – Treat underlying constipation.
- Secondary enuresis:
  - – Referral for behavioral counseling if suspicion
  - – Stool softeners and cathartics if constipation present
- If behavioral interventions alone have no success, combined therapy (e.g., enuresis alarm, bladder training, motivational therapy, and pelvic floor muscle training) is more effective than each component alone or than pharmacotherapy (2)[A].
- Enuresis alarms (bells or buzzers)
  - – 66–70% success rate; must be used nightly for 2 to 4 months; offers cure; significant parental involvement
  - – If successful, it should be used until 14 consecutive dry nights achieved.

MEDICATION

First Line

Desmopressin (DDAVP): synthetic analogue of vasopressin that decreases nocturnal urine output (1)[A]

- Intranasal DDAVP: adults only, 20 mg (2 sprays) intranasally at bedtime
  - – U.S. Food and Drug Administration (FDA) recommends against use in children due to reports of severe hyponatremia resulting in seizures and deaths in children using intranasal formulations of desmopressin.
- Oral DDAVP: safe in children, available in tablet or fast-melting oral form (not available in United States); begin with 0.2 mg tablet taken at bedtime on empty stomach; after 14 days of inefficient treatment, can titrate up to 0.4 mg (1)
  - – Maximally effective in 1 hour; effect lasts 8 to 10 hours.
  - – If treatment is successful, can be continued for 3 months, then stop for 2 weeks for test of dryness.
  - – High relapse rate after discontinuation without a structured withdrawal program. If relapse occurs, oral desmopressin can continue to be prescribed in 3-month blocks.
  - – Important side effects: water intoxication and hyponatremia, presenting as headache, nausea, vomiting, convulsions; fluid intake in the evening can be restricted to 200 to 250 mL and no drinks during the night to avoid excessive fluid intake. Suspend the dose in children who display symptoms.
  - – 60–70% success; 30% of children have full response and 40% have partial response.
  - – Long-lasting curative effect is low.

Pediatric Considerations

U.S. FDA recommends against using intranasal formulations of desmopressin in children due to reports of severe hyponatremia resulting in seizures and deaths (2)[A].

Second Line

- Anticholinergics: Monotherapy is not recommended in children. Before considering, screen for constipation and residual urine.
  - – Oxybutynin (Ditropan, Ditropan XL, Oxytrol patch): anticholinergic; smooth muscle relaxant, antispasmodic; may increase functional bladder capacity and aids in timed voiding
    - ○ 30–50% success; 50% relapse after stopped
    - ○ Ditropan: adults: 5 mg PO TID–QID; children >5 years old with overactive bladder who have failed alarm therapy and desmopressin can try 5 mg at bedtime.
    - ○ Ditropan XL: adults: 5 mg/day PO; increase to 30 mg/day PO (5- to 10-mg tablet).
    - ○ Oxytrol patch: 1 patch every 3 to 4 days (3.9 mg/patch) (Periodic trials of the medication, that is, weekends or weeks at a time, will help determine efficacy and resolution of primary disturbance.)
  - – Other anticholinergics (may be used in adults; not yet approved for label use in children): tolterodine 2 to 4 mg/day, fesoterodine 4 to 8 mg/day, solifenacin 5 to 10 mg/day
- Imipramine (Tofranil): tricyclic antidepressant, anticholinergic effects; increases bladder capacity, antispasmodic properties
  - – Dose: adults, 25 to 75 mg and children aged >6 years, 10 to 25 mg PO given 1 hour before bedtime; increase by 10 to 25 mg at 1- to 2-week intervals; treat for 2 to 3 months and consider drug holiday for 2 weeks before restarting. When discontinuing, taper by halving dosage every 1 to 2 weeks
  - – Desmopressin may be added if the effect is incomplete.
  - – 40% success rate but relapses after discontinuation are high (1).
  - – Pretreatment ECG recommended identifying underlying rhythm disorders such as long QT syndrome.
- Precautions
  - – Oxybutynin: glaucoma, myasthenia gravis, GI or genitourinary obstruction, ulcerative colitis, constipation, megacolon; use a decreased dose in the elderly.
  - – Tolterodine: urinary retention, gastric retention, constipation, uncontrolled narrow-angle glaucoma; significant drug interactions with CYP2D6, CYP3A3/4 substrates
  - – Desmopressin: Avoid in patients at risk for electrolyte changes or fluid retention (congestive heart failure [CHF], renal insufficiency). Stop during gastroenteritis or other acute illness with risk of dehydration.
  - – Imipramine: Do not use with monoamine oxidase inhibitors (MAOIs), hypotension, and arrhythmias; low-toxic therapeutic ratio; in pediatrics, generally reserved for older children recalcitrant to other treatments who have no cardiac history and are not taking medications that may predispose them to arrhythmias (3).
- Combination therapy with DDAVP and oxybutynin has better results than individual use.

ISSUES FOR REFERRAL

- Primary NE: persistent enuresis despite nonpharmacologic and pharmacologic therapies
- Diurnal incontinence or NMNE with voiding dysfunction or underlying medical condition

COMPLEMENTARY & ALTERNATIVE MEDICINE

Acupuncture with limited data

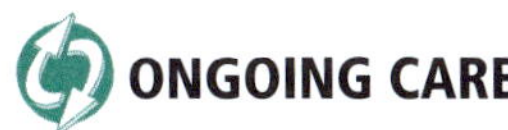

ONGOING CARE

FOLLOW-UP RECOMMENDATIONS

Patient Monitoring

- With nonpharmacologic treatment, reassess every 1 to 3 months.
- With enuresis alarm, reassess in 1 to 3 weeks.
- With DDAVP, reassess in 1 to 2 weeks, then every 3 months.
- With imipramine, reassess in 1 month (monitor for UTI or constipation).

DIET

Limit fluid and caffeine intake 1 to 2 hours before sleep.

PATIENT EDUCATION

- https://www.hypnoticworld.com/hypnosis-scripts/habits-disorders/enuresis; https://wetstop.com; https://www.dri-sleeper.com; https://www.nitetrain-r.com; https://bedwettingstore.com
- App store for free bed-wetting diary apps (e.g., My Dryness Tracker, Bedwetting Tracker, HapPee Time)

PROGNOSIS

In children, NE is usually self-limiting; 1% will persist as adult; evaluate for organic causes.

COMPLICATIONS

UTI, perineal excoriation, psychological disturbance (especially in children)

REFERENCES

1. Kuwertz-Bröking E, von Gontard A. Clinical management of nocturnal enuresis. *Pediatr Nephrol*. 2018;33(7):1145–1154.
2. Baird DC, Seehusen DA, Bode DV. Enuresis in children: a case based approach. *Am Fam Physician*. 2014;90(8):560–568.
3. Guzman JA, Palmer LS. Nocturnal enuresis. *Pediatr Rev*. 2024;45(8):479–481. doi:10.1542/pir.2023-006166.

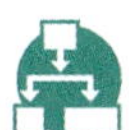

SEE ALSO

- Incontinence, Urinary Adult Female; Incontinence, Urinary Adult Male
- Algorithms: Enuresis, Secondary

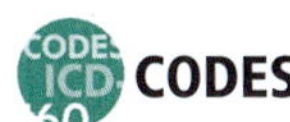

ICD10

- N39.44 Nocturnal enuresis
- R32 Unspecified urinary incontinence
- F98.0 Enuresis not due to a substance or known physiol condition

CLINICAL PEARLS

- Behavioral and lifestyle interventions are the first-line treatment for PMNE; alarms and desmopressin are the most effective treatments.
- Secondary enuresis: most often due to psychosocial factors

EPICONDYLITIS

Caleb Weiss Kiesow, MD, BS • Anthony Lloyd Overfield, MD

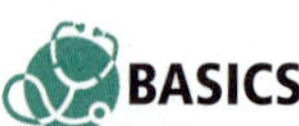

BASICS

DESCRIPTION
- Tendinopathy of the elbow characterized by pain and tenderness at the myotendinous junctions or tendinous insertions of the wrist flexor/extensor tendons at the humeral epicondyles
- Although commonly known as medial and lateral epicondylitis, without microscopic histologic examination, the more appropriate term is medial epicondyle tendinopathy (MET) and lateral epicondyle tendinopathy (LET).
- Most commonly secondary to chronic (overuse) pathology, although acute (traumatic) etiology can occur.
- Two types
  - MET/common flexor tendinopathy (CFT) ("golfer's elbow")
    - Involves the wrist flexor and pronator teres tendons, which have proximal attachment at the medial epicondyle
  - LET/common extensor tendinopathy (CET) ("tennis elbow")
    - Involves the wrist extensor and supinator tendons, which have proximal attachment at the lateral epicondyle
    - Most commonly involves the extensor carpi radialis brevis (ECRB) tendon
- May be caused by various different athletic or occupational activities
- Common in carpenters, plumbers, gardeners, and overhead athletes
- 75% of cases involve the dominant arm.

EPIDEMIOLOGY
- Predominant age: >40 years
- Predominant sex: male = female

Incidence
- Common overuse injury
- Lateral (80–90%) > medial (10–20%)
- Estimated between 1% and 3%
- Dominant extremity > nondominant

Prevalence
- MET: 0.4%
- LET: 1.3%

ETIOLOGY AND PATHOPHYSIOLOGY
- Acute (tendonitis, tear)
  - Rare, uncommon pathology
  - Inflammatory response to injury or sudden, violent contraction
- Chronic (tendinosis or tendinopathy)
  - Overuse injury
  - Repetitive wrist flexion (MET) or extension (LET) places strain across enthesis of flexor or extensor group, respectively.
  - Degeneration, calcium deposition, fibroblast proliferation, microvascular proliferation, hyaline cartilage destruction, diminished restorative inflammatory response
- Aggravating activities
  - Tool/racquet griping
  - Shaking hands, picking up a beverage
  - Occupational (painters, mechanics, cooks)
  - Sports (golf, tennis, archery, throwing)

Genetics
There are no known genetic components to LET or MET.

RISK FACTORS
- Repetitive wrist motions
  - Flexion/pronation: MET
  - Extension/supination: LET
- Smoking
- Obesity
- Forceful activities of the upper extremity

GENERAL PREVENTION
- Limit overuse of the wrist flexors, extensors, pronators, and supinators.
- Proper technique when working with hand tools or playing racquet sports
- Lighter tools and smaller grips

COMMONLY ASSOCIATED CONDITIONS
- Ipsilateral metacarpal osteoarthritis (common)
- Rotator cuff tendinopathy (common)
- Carpal tunnel syndrome (rare)
- Contralateral and MET (rare)

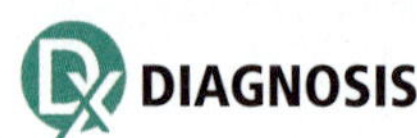

DIAGNOSIS

HISTORY
- Insidious onset
- Pain localized to lateral or medial elbow, at or just distal to bony epicondyle
- Aching pain, often radiates from epicondyle to forearm or wrist
- Pain with gripping
- Sensation of mild forearm weakness

PHYSICAL EXAM
- Localized pain at or just distal to the affected epicondyle
- MET
  - Tenderness at origin of wrist flexor tendons
  - Increased pain with resisted wrist flexion and pronation
  - Normal elbow range of motion
  - Increased pain with gripping/handshake
- LET
  - Tenderness at origin of wrist extensors
  - Increased pain with resisted wrist extension and forearm supination
  - Normal elbow range of motion
  - Increased pain with gripping

DIFFERENTIAL DIAGNOSIS
- Osteoarthritis, such as posterior osteophytes
- Epicondylar fractures
- Posterior interosseous nerve entrapment (lateral elbow pain)
- Radial tunnel syndrome (lateral elbow pain)
- Ulnar neuropathy (medial elbow pain)
- Pronator syndrome (anteromedial elbow pain)
- Synovitis
- Thoracic outlet syndrome
- Medial collateral ligament injury
- Referred pain from shoulder or neck

DIAGNOSTIC TESTS & INTERPRETATION

Initial Tests (lab, imaging)
Imaging is not required for initial evaluation and treatment of a classic overuse tendinopathy. Diagnosis remains clinical.

Follow-Up Tests & Special Considerations
- Anterior-posterior (A-P)/lateral radiographs:
  - If decreased range of motion, trauma, or no improvement with initial conservative therapy; assess for fractures or signs of arthritis.
- For recalcitrant cases
  - Musculoskeletal ultrasound (US) reveals abnormal tendon appearance (e.g., hypoechoic, tendon thickening, partial tear at tendon origin, calcifications, hyperemia). US can also guide injections of prolotherapy, platelet-rich plasma (PRP), steroid and/or anesthetic.
  - MRI remains the gold standard and can show intermediate or high T2 signal intensity within the common flexor or extensor tendon or the presence of peritendinous soft tissue edema.
  - Shear wave elastography can evaluate tissue stiffness and elasticity providing objective data to distinguish normal and pathologic tendons.
    - Diagnostic accuracy is comparable to superior to conventional gray-scale US.

Diagnostic Procedures/Other
Infiltration of local anesthetic at the point of maximal tenderness under US guidance with subsequent resolution of symptoms supports the diagnosis if clinically in doubt.

Test Interpretation
Positive test: temporary near complete relief after local anesthetic injection

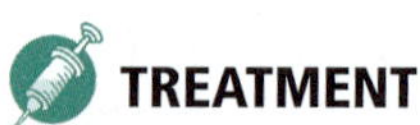

TREATMENT

GENERAL MEASURES
Initial treatment consists of activity modification, counterforce bracing, oral or topical NSAIDs, ice, and physical therapy.
- If left untreated, symptoms typically last between 6 months and 2 years. For patients with good function and minimal pain, consider conservative management using a "wait and see" approach based on patient preference.
- Modify activity, encourage relative rest, and correct faulty biomechanics.
- Bracing
  - Splinting is not recommended except for severe cases, as it is associated with higher rates of limited duty, more medical visits, higher charges, and longer duration of treatment than those managed without splints.
  - Counterforce bracing with a forearm strap is easy and inexpensive. Systematic reviews are inconclusive about overall efficacy, but initial bracing may improve the ability to perform daily activities in the first 6 weeks.
- Ice frequently after activities
- Physical therapy
  - Infiltration of local anesthetic can reduce pain and may permit better participation in physical therapy.
  - Eccentric strength training and stretching program
  - Therapeutic US
  - Corticosteroid iontophoresis
  - Dry needling

MEDICATION

First Line

- Topical NSAIDs: Evidence suggests topical NSAIDS are significantly more effective than placebo with respect to pain and number needed to treat (NNT) to benefit (NNT = 7) in the short term (up to 4 weeks) with minimal adverse effects (1)[A].
- Oral NSAIDs: unclear efficacy with respect to pain and function, but may offer short-term pain relief; associated with adverse GI effects (1)[A]

Second Line

- Corticosteroid injections provide consistent short-term relief (<6 weeks), with improvement in pain and grip strength with limited benefit at intermediate and long-term follow-up.
- Overall effectiveness is inconclusive due to low validity across studies
- In direct comparison, corticosteroid injections demonstrated favorable outcomes to PRP in treatment of LET in the short term (<2 months); but less effective with regard to pain and function 6 months after injection (2)[A]

ISSUES FOR REFERRAL

Failure of conservative therapy

ADDITIONAL THERAPIES

Given the mechanism of injury, many new treatments are targeted at strengthening the underlying tendon rather than strict palliation of pain. High-quality evidence is limited for many of these interventions.

- Glyceryl trinitrate (GTN) transdermal patch
  - Nitric oxide (NO) is a small free radical generated by NO synthesis. 1/4 of a 5-mg/24-hour GTN transdermal patch is applied once daily for up to 24 weeks.
  - Significant decreases in pain are seen at 3 weeks and 6 months compared to placebo patch.
- Extracorporeal shock wave therapy (ESWT) is a noninvasive, nonelectrical therapy found to be 89% effective in treating LET in some studies and is noted to be as effective as splinting (3)[A].
- Prolotherapy
  - Injection of a dextrose solution into the tendon attachment stimulates a localized inflammatory response, leading to increased blood flow to stimulate healing (4)[A].
- PRP injections
  - Injection of supraphysiologic autologous PRP leads to a local inflammatory response. Platelets degranulate, release growth factors, and stimulate the physiologic healing cascade.
  - PRP treatment of chronic LET significantly reduces pain and increases function. The benefit exceeds that of corticosteroid injection even after a follow-up of 1 year (5)[A].
- US-guided percutaneous needle tenotomy
  - Injection of a local anesthetic followed by US-guided tendon fenestration, aspiration, and abrasion of the underlying bone; thought to break apart scar tissue and stimulate inflammation and healing
- Botulinum toxin A for chronic LET
  - Injections into the forearm extensor muscles (60 units) can be performed in the outpatient setting.

SURGERY/OTHER PROCEDURES

- Surgical tenotomy is required in only 4–11% of patients.
- Can be completed open, arthroscopically, percutaneous, and/or US assisted
- Above methods have similar outcomes overall, but varying relative benefits that should be individualized to patients goals (4)[A]
- Improvements in VAS, DASH scores, and grip strength seen in 5-year study (4)[A]
- Denervation of the lateral humeral epicondyle
  - Transection of the posterior cutaneous nerve of the forearm with implantation into the triceps may help with chronic symptoms and pain.

COMPLEMENTARY & ALTERNATIVE MEDICINE

Acupuncture: effective for short-term pain relief for lateral epicondyle pain

ADMISSION, INPATIENT, AND NURSING CONSIDERATIONS

May rarely be necessary after surgical intervention

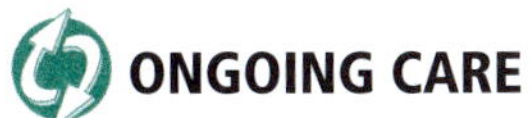

ONGOING CARE

FOLLOW-UP RECOMMENDATIONS

No specific guidelines, consider medium (4 to 6 weeks) and longer term (12 week) follow-up to assess intervention efficacy.

Patient Monitoring

- Symptom progression
- Activity level
- Functional ability

DIET

No specific dietary recommendations

PROGNOSIS

- Good: Majority resolve with conservative care.
- Natural history of disease is 6 to 12 months without intervention

COMPLICATIONS

- Chronic pain, weakness
- Rare tendon rupture

REFERENCES

1. Pattanittum P, Turner T, Green S, et al. Non-steroidal anti-inflammatory drugs (NSAIDs) for treating lateral elbow pain in adults. *Cochrane Database Syst Rev*. 2013;2013(5):CD003686.
2. Li A, Wang H, Yu Z, et al. Platelet-rich plasma vs corticosteroids for elbow epicondylitis: a systematic review and meta-analysis. *Medicine (Baltimore)*. 2019;98(51):e18358.
3. Zhang L, Zhang X, Pang L, et al. Extracorporeal shock wave therapy versus local corticosteroid injection for chronic lateral epicondylitis: a systematic review with meta-analysis of randomized controlled trials. *Orthop Surg*. 2024;16(11):2598–2607.
4. Ansari A, Shoaib D, Tanbour Y, et al. The Efficacy of different tenotomies in the treatment of lateral epicondylitis: a systematic review. *J Clin Med*. 2024;13(22):6764.
5. Xu Y, Li T, Wang L, et al. Platelet-rich plasma has better results for long-term functional improvement and pain relief for lateral epicondylitis: a systematic review and meta-analysis of randomized controlled trials. *Am J Sports Med*. 2024;52(10):2646–2656.

ADDITIONAL READING

- Barreto ESR, Antunes Júnior CR, Alencar VB, et al. The efficacy of botulinum toxin in tennis elbow: a meta-analysis of randomized clinical trials. *Int Orthop*. 2024;48(12):3139–3149.
- Cullinane FL, Boocock MG, Trevelyan FC. Is eccentric exercise an effective treatment for lateral epicondylitis? A systematic review. *Clin Rehabil*. 2014;28(1):3–19.
- Dingemanse R, Randsdorp M, Koes BW, et al. Evidence for the effectiveness of electrophysical modalities for treatment of medial and lateral epicondylitis: a systematic review. *Br J Sports Med*. 2014;48(12):957–965.
- Green S, Buchbinder R, Barnsley L, et al. Acupuncture for lateral elbow pain. *Cochrane Database Syst Rev*. 2002;2002(1):CD003527.
- Kim JH, Hoy JF, Smith SR, et al. Recalcitrant lateral epicondylitis: a systematic review on current nonoperative and operative treatment modalities. *JBJS Rev*. 2024;12(8).
- Lin YC, Wu WT, Hsu YC, et al. Comparative effectiveness of botulinum toxin versus non-surgical treatments for treating lateral epicondylitis: a systematic review and meta-analysis. *Clin Rehabil*. 2018;32(2):131–145.
- Mattie R, Wong J, McCormick Z, et al. Percutaneous needle tenotomy for the treatment of lateral epicondylitis: a systematic review of the literature. *PM R*. 2017;9(6):603–611.
- Ozden R, Uruç V, Doğramaci Y, et al. Management of tennis elbow with topical glyceryl trinitrate. *Acta Orthop Traumatol Turc*. 2014;48(2):175–180.

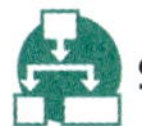

SEE ALSO

Algorithm: Pain in Upper Extremity

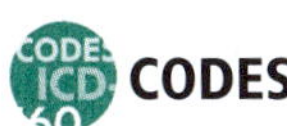

CODES

ICD10

- M77.00 Medial epicondylitis, unspecified elbow
- M77.10 Lateral epicondylitis, unspecified elbow
- M77.01 Medial epicondylitis, right elbow

CLINICAL PEARLS

- MET (golfer's elbow) is characterized by pain and tenderness at the tendinous origins of the wrist flexors on the medial epicondyle.
- LET (tennis elbow) is characterized by pain and tenderness at the tendinous origins of the wrist extensors on the lateral epicondyle.
- Left untreated, symptoms typically last between 6 months and 2 years.
- Most patients improve using conservative treatment with oral NSAIDs, activity modification, and physical therapy.
- Newer therapies such as ESWT, PRP, prolotherapy, and tenotomy are directed toward tendon regeneration.

EPIDIDYMITIS

Jarrett Keller Sell, MD, FAAFP, AAHIVS • Kendal Schaetzle, DO

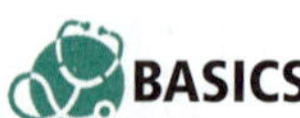

BASICS

DESCRIPTION

- Inflammation of the epididymis resulting in scrotal pain and swelling, induration of the posterior epididymis, involvement of the adjacent testicle, and possible hydrocele formation
- Acute epididymitis: scrotal pain for <6 weeks
- Chronic epididymitis: scrotal pain for ≥6 weeks
- Epididymitis with involvement of the testis is named epididymo-orchitis.
- Classification: infectious (bacterial, viral, fungal, parasitic) versus noninfectious (chemical, traumatic, autoimmune, idiopathic, industrial, vaso-epididymal reflux syndrome)
- System(s) affected: reproductive

EPIDEMIOLOGY

- Predominant age: generally younger, sexually active men or older men with UTIs and bladder outlet obstruction (e.g., benign prostatic hyperplasia [BPH])
- Predominant sex: male only

Pediatric Considerations

Epididymitis is the most common cause of acute scrotal pain in prepubertal boys—more common than testicular torsion.

Incidence

- Common (600,000 cases annually in the United States) (1)
- 1 in 1,000 adult males per year
- 1.2 in 1,000 boys aged 2 to 13 years per year (2),(3)

Prevalence

Common

ETIOLOGY AND PATHOPHYSIOLOGY

- Infectious epididymitis
  - Retrograde passage of urinary bacteria from the prostate or urethra to the epididymis via the ejaculatory ducts and the vas deferens; rarely, hematogenous spread
  - Causative organism is identified in 80% and varies according to age.
- Noninfectious epididymitis
  - Often no etiology is found; however, can be instigated by trauma, autoimmune disease, or vasculitis
  - Likely secondary to reflux of sterile urine causing a chemical inflammation
  - Can develop with strenuous exercise with a full bladder when urine is pushed through internal urethral sphincter (located at proximal end of prostatic urethra) or prolonged periods of sitting
  - Reflux of urine through orifice of ejaculatory ducts at verumontanum may occur with history of urethritis/prostatitis because inflammation may produce rigidity in musculature surrounding orifice to ejaculatory ducts, holding them open.
  - Exposure of epididymis to foreign fluid may produce inflammatory reaction within 24 hours.
- <14 years of age
  - Cause largely unknown, although likely from anatomic abnormalities resulting in urine reflux such as vesicoureteral reflux, ectopic ureter, or anorectal malformation (rectourethral fistula)
  - May also result from postinfectious syndrome from *Mycoplasma pneumoniae*, enterovirus, or adenovirus
- 14 to 35 years of age
  - Usually *Chlamydia trachomatis*, *Neisseria gonorrhoeae*, or *Mycoplasma genitalium* in sexually active males
  - With anal intercourse, likely enteric pathogens (e.g., *Escherichia coli*)
- >35 years of age
  - Commonly enteric bacteria, but occasionally *Staphylococcus aureus* or *Staphylococcus epidermidis*
  - In elderly men, often with distal urinary tract obstruction, BPH, UTI, or catheterization
  - Tuberculosis (TB), if sterile pyuria, nodularity of vas deferens (hematogenous spread), and recent infection. TB is the most common granulomatous disease affecting the epididymitis.
  - Sterile urine reflux after transurethral prostatectomy
  - Granulomatous reaction following BCG intravesical therapy for bladder cancer
- Amiodarone may cause a dose-dependent noninfectious epididymitis; usually resolves with decreasing drug dosage (<200 mg/day)
- Syphilis, blastomycosis, coccidioidomycosis, and cryptococcosis are rare causes, but brucellosis can be a common cause in endemic areas.

RISK FACTORS

- UTI
- Prostatitis
- Urethral catheter
- Urethral instrumentation or transurethral surgery
- Urethral or meatal stricture
- Prostate biopsy
- Prostate brachytherapy for prostate cancer
- Anal intercourse
- High-risk sexual activity
- Strenuous physical activity
- Prolonged sedentary periods
- Bladder obstruction (BPH, prostate cancer)
- HIV-immunosuppressed patient
- Severe Behçet disease
- Presence of foreskin
- Constipation
- Increased intra-abdominal pressure (due to frequent physical strain)

GENERAL PREVENTION

- Safer sexual practices
- Mumps vaccination
- Antibiotic prophylaxis for urethral manipulation
- Early treatment of prostatitis/BPH
- Vasectomy or vasoligation during transurethral surgery
- Avoid vigorous rectal exam with acute prostatitis.
- Emptying the bladder prior to physical exertion
- Physical conditioning prior to intense physical exertion
- Treat constipation.

COMMONLY ASSOCIATED CONDITIONS

- Prostatitis/urethritis/orchitis
- Hematospermia
- Constipation
- UTI

DIAGNOSIS

HISTORY

- Gradual onset of scrotal pain, radiating to the groin region over 1 to 2 days
- Urethral discharge or symptoms of UTI, such as urinary frequency, dysuria, cloudy urine, or hematuria
- Detailed sexual history
- Fever only in 11–19% (3)
- Progresses from the posterior-lying epididymis to the body/head of epididymis
- Entire hemiscrotum may become swollen and red; the testis becomes indistinguishable from the epididymis; the scrotal wall becomes thick and indurated, and reactive hydrocele may occur.
- Noninfectious epididymitis
  - Unilateral scrotal pain/swelling preceded by prolonged intense physical exertion with full bladder
  - No symptoms of infection

Pediatric Considerations

- Bacteremia from *Haemophilus influenzae* infection may produce acute epididymitis.
- Must rule out testicular torsion (with scrotal ultrasound [US]) in adolescent males particularly those aged >13 years
- History not helpful in distinguishing epididymitis from testicular torsion

Geriatric Considerations

Patients with diabetic neuropathy may have no pain despite severe infection/abscess.

PHYSICAL EXAM

- Epididymis is markedly tender to palpation.
- The tail of the epididymis is larger in comparison with the contralateral side.
- Elevation of the testis in epididymis reduces the discomfort (Prehn sign).
- Absence of a cremasteric reflex should raise suspicion for testicular torsion.

DIFFERENTIAL DIAGNOSIS

- Testicular/testicular appendage torsion
- Urethritis/orchitis
- Testicular trauma
- Epididymal congestion following vasectomy
- Testicular malignancy
- Epididymal cyst
- Inguinal hernia
- Spermatocele
- Hydrocele
- Hematocele
- Varicocele
- Epididymal adenomatoid tumor or rhabdomyosarcoma
- Vasculitis (Henoch-Schönlein purpura)

DIAGNOSTIC TESTS & INTERPRETATION

Initial Tests (lab, imaging)

- All suspected cases should be evaluated for objective evidence of inflammation by one of the following:
  - Urinalysis/urine culture preferably on first-void urine to evaluate for leukocyte esterase and bacteriuria
  - Gram stain urethral discharge; ≥2 WBC per oil immersion field; evaluate for gonococcal infection.
  - Microscopic examination of sediment from a spun first-void urine with ≥10 WBC per high-power field
- Urine gonorrhea and chlamydia testing for all suspected cases

- Sexually active patients with acute epididymitis should also be tested for HIV and syphilis (4).
- Elevated CRP level can help distinguish epididymitis from testicular torsion (2)
- A clear urinalysis and negative culture suggest noninfectious epididymitis.
- If testicular torsion/mass cannot be excluded (especially in children), Doppler US is test of choice (2),(3).
- US is not necessary for diagnosis in those with high clinical suspicion for epididymitis and low concern for torsion.

Pediatric Considerations

Further radiographic imaging in children should be done to rule out anatomic abnormalities or torsion.

Diagnostic Procedures/Other

This is a clinical diagnosis.

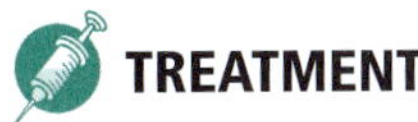

TREATMENT

GENERAL MEASURES

- Bed rest or restriction of activity
- Scrotal elevation, athletic scrotal supporter
- Ice pack
- Avoid constipation.
- Spermatic cord block with local anesthesia in severe cases
- If noninfectious epididymitis:
  - No strenuous physical activity and avoidance of Valsalva maneuvers for several weeks
  - Empty bladder prior to strenuous exercises.

MEDICATION

First Line

- Empiric treatment for all sexually active adults at time of clinical diagnosis and before all test results are complete is recommended (4).
- Sexually active adults $<$35 years: doxycycline 100 mg PO BID for 10 days (*C. trachomatis* coverage) *plus* ceftriaxone 500 mg IM $\times$ 1 or 1 g IM if weigh $>$150 kg (*N. gonorrhoeae* coverage). Treat all sexual partners within last 60 days (2)[C],(4).
- $\geq$35 years of age, not suspecting STD with enteric etiology (i.e., bacteriuria due to bladder outlet obstruction, prostate biopsy, urinary instrumentation, systemic disease, and/or immunosuppression)
  - Levofloxacin 500 mg/day PO for 10 days (4)
  - Note: 2016 FDA black box warning on fluoroquinolones due to disabling and potentially permanent side effects. Consider trimethoprim-sulfamethoxazole for milder infections.
- Men who practice insertive anal intercourse: ceftriaxone 500 mg IM $\times$ 1 plus fluoroquinolone as above. If HIV positive, usually there is no difference in treatment (2)[C].
- Analgesia:
  - NSAIDs (e.g., naproxen or ibuprofen) for mild to moderate pain
  - Consider steroid if patient cannot tolerate NSAIDs.
  - Acetaminophen with codeine or oxycodone for moderate to severe pain
- Septic or toxic patient
  - 3rd-generation cephalosporin or aminoglycoside
- For Behçet, sarcoid, Henoch-Schönlein purpura
  - Steroids, such as methylprednisolone, 40 mg/day recommended
- Chronic epididymitis: 2-week course of NSAIDs, scrotal icing/elevation; if no improvement, may add TCA or neuroleptic (2)

Second Line

- Trimethoprim-sulfamethoxazole (Bactrim, Septra) double strength PO BID for 10 to 14 days; increasing bacterial resistance may limit effectiveness.
- Add rifampin (rifampicin) or vancomycin, as required.

Pediatric Considerations

- May be postinfectious inflammatory condition; treat with anti-inflammatories and analgesics.
- Antibiotic therapy can be reserved for young infants until positive urine cultures (2).

ISSUES FOR REFERRAL

- If suspicion is high for testicular torsion, then urgent US or referral to emergency department for possible surgery (1)[C].
- Epididymitis in age $<$14 years requires a urology referral due to high incidence of associated urogenital abnormalities.
- If medical management fails, should be referred to urologist to rule out anatomic abnormality
- If HIV positive, CMV, *Salmonella*, toxoplasmosis, *Ureaplasma urealyticum*, *Corynebacterium* sp., *Mycoplasma* sp., and *Mima polymorpha* may also be considered.

SURGERY/OTHER PROCEDURES

- Vasostomy to drain infected material if severe or refractory case
- Scrotal exploration if unable clinically to distinguish between epididymitis and testicular torsion
- Drainage of abscesses, epididymectomy, or epididymo-orchidectomy in severe cases refractory to antibiotics
- Surgery to correct underlying anatomic abnormality or obstruction

ADMISSION, INPATIENT, AND NURSING CONSIDERATIONS

- Intractable pain
- Sepsis
- Abscess
- Persistent vomiting
- Scheduled surgery
- Purulent drainage
- Most can be managed as an outpatient.

ONGOING CARE

FOLLOW-UP RECOMMENDATIONS

Patient Monitoring

- Routine follow-up in 1 week. Follow up within 72 hours if symptoms fail to improve with treatment for reevaluation of diagnosis and therapy.
- Swelling and tenderness after antibiotic course should be evaluated for other infections, abscess, tumor, infarction, cancer, TB, and fungal epididymitis.
- Consider nucleic acid amplification test (NAAT) testing for less common sexually transmitted pathogens such as *Mycoplasma genitalium* and *Ureaplasma*.
- In noninfectious epididymitis, follow up in 4 weeks to assess efficacy of NSAIDs and lifestyle changes.

DIET

Consider constipation prevention (high-fiber diet) and/or treatment.

PATIENT EDUCATION

- Stress completing course of antibiotics, even when asymptomatic
- Early recognition and treatment of UTI or prostatitis
- Safer sexual practices; avoid sex until antibiotic course completed and partner treated.
- Repeat STI testing in 3 months to evaluate for reinfection if STI identified.
- If treated for STI, refer sexual partners for evaluation and empirically treat sexual contacts within 60 days preceding onset of symptoms.
- If noninfectious epididymitis, then educate on etiology and proper lifestyle changes.

PROGNOSIS

- Pain improves within 1 to 3 days, but induration may take several weeks/months to completely resolve.
- If bilateral involvement, sterility may result.
- In noninfectious epididymitis, symptoms usually resolve in $<$1 week.

COMPLICATIONS

- Recurrent epididymitis
- Infertility
- Oligospermia
- Testicular necrosis or atrophy
- Secondary abscess formation
- Fournier gangrene (necrotizing synergistic infection)

REFERENCES

1. Trojian TH, Lishnak TS, Heiman D. Epididymitis and orchitis: an overview. *Am Fam Physician*. 2009;79(7):583–587.
2. McConaghy JR, Panchal B. Epididymitis: an overview. *Am Fam Physician*. 2016;94(9):723–726.
3. European Association of Urology, European Society for Paediatric Urology. *EAU Guidelines on Paediatric Urology*. Arnhem, Netherlands: European Association of Urology; 2016.
4. Workowski KA, Bachmann LH, Chan PA, et al. Sexually transmitted infections treatment guidelines, 2021. *MMWR Recomm Rep*. 2021;70(4):1–187. doi:10.15585/mmwr.rr7004a1.

ADDITIONAL READING

Somekh E, Gorenstein A, Serour F. Acute epididymitis in boys: evidence of a post-infectious etiology. *J Urol*. 2004;171(1):391–394.

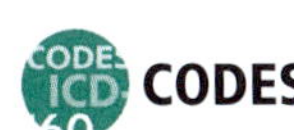

CODES

ICD10

- N45.1 Epididymitis
- N45.2 Orchitis
- N45.3 Epididymo-orchitis

CLINICAL PEARLS

- With epididymitis, pain is gradual in onset, and the tenderness is mostly posterior to the testis. With testicular torsion, the symptoms are quite rapid in onset, the testis will be higher in the scrotum and may have a transverse lie, and the cremasteric reflex will be absent. The absence of leukocytes on urine analysis and decreased blood flow on scrotal US with Doppler will suggest torsion.
- Prostatic massage is contraindicated in epididymitis because of the risk for worsening local infection. The potential for sepsis is increased with acute prostatitis.
- Noninfectious epididymitis is a clinical diagnosis of exclusion, because infectious causes are much more common, but must be considered in certain occupations, such as soldiers and laborers.

EPISCLERITIS

Dongsheng Jiang, MD, MSc

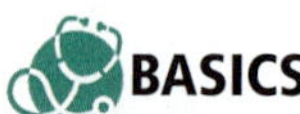

BASICS

- Episcleritis is irritation and inflammation of the episclera, a thin layer of vascular connective tissue between the conjunctiva and sclera.
- Usually a benign self-limited condition, typically resolving without treatment within 3 weeks
- Topical lubricants and/or topical corticosteroid treatment may relieve symptoms while awaiting spontaneous resolution.

DESCRIPTION

- Edema and injection confined to the episcleral tissue
- Two types
  - Simple episcleritis: diffuse scleral involvement—more common
  - Nodular episcleritis: focal area(s) of involvement—less common

EPIDEMIOLOGY

Slight female predominance (~60–65%)

Incidence

- May occur at any age
- Peak incidence in 40s to 50s
- Community incidence not well-known (~20 to 50 cases per 100,000 person-years)

Prevalence

Not historically well-known; a recent community study found a prevalence of 53 cases per 100,000 person-years.

ETIOLOGY AND PATHOPHYSIOLOGY

- Etiology: usually idiopathic, but up to 1/3 of the patients can have systemic autoimmune conditions (1)
- Pathophysiology:
  - Nonimmune (e.g., dry eye syndrome, with histology showing widespread vasodilation, edema, lymphocytic infiltration)
  - Immune (systemic vasculitis or rheumatologic disease)

COMMONLY ASSOCIATED CONDITIONS

- Usually not associated with another condition
- One-third of the cases have a systemic autoimmune disease (2):
  - Rheumatoid arthritis
  - Vasculitis
  - Inflammatory bowel disease
  - Ankylosing spondylitis
  - Psoriatic arthritis
  - Systemic lupus erythematosus
  - Gout
  - Herpes zoster
  - Hypersensitivity disorders
    - Rosacea
    - Contact dermatitis
    - Penicillin sensitivity
    - Erythema multiforme
- It can be an uncommon manifestation of other ocular infectious conditions

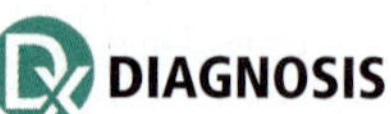

DIAGNOSIS

Episcleritis is a clinical diagnosis.

HISTORY

- History should elicit potential causative factors, recurrence, or associated systemic disease.
- A detailed reviewed of systems should be performed on all patients on the first visit
- Vision is usually normal (2).
- Pain: absent or mild and localized to the eye
- Mild tearing may be present.
- 80% unilateral; bilateral suggests systemic disease (2).

PHYSICAL EXAM

- Check visual acuity; decreased vision is very unusual with episcleritis, and its presence should raise suspicion for another condition such as scleritis.
- The white sclera will have a pink or purplish hue.
- Focal hyperemia
- Pupils are equal and reactive.
- Superficial episcleral vascular dilation
- Episcleral edema
  - Diffuse in simple episcleritis
  - Focal in nodular episcleritis
- Tenderness over involved area may be present but is usually absent.
- Phenylephrine test (3):
  - It is used to differentiate episcleritis from scleritis.
  - Apply 10% phenylephrine drops.
    - Blanching = episcleritis (superficial blood vessels)
    - Nonblanching = scleritis (deeper vessels

ALERT

Recurrent episodes, difficulty confirming the diagnosis, or worsening symptoms should prompt an ophthalmology referral.

DIFFERENTIAL DIAGNOSIS

- Scleritis
- Bacterial or viral conjunctivitis
- Uveitis
- Herpes (ulcerative) keratitis
- Superficial keratitis
- Increased intraocular pressure (ocular hypertension)

DIAGNOSTIC TESTS & INTERPRETATION

First episode typically does not require extensive lab work or diagnostic studies unless episcleritis is recurrent or with no known associated systemic disease (2). May consider:

- Labs: CBC, CMP, ESR, CRP, RF, ANA, ANCAs, complement 3 and 4, RPR, HLA B27, ACE, UA
- TB screening: PPD or T Spot
- Imaging: CXR, chest CT

TREATMENT

- Simple episcleritis is usually self-limited (up to 21 days), but it can recur.
- Nodular type can be prolonged and painful.

MEDICATION

Treatment for episcleritis typically consists of symptomatic relief. The goal is to suppress the inflammation, which will, in turn, relieve the discomfort or pain.

First Line

Topical lubricants such as artificial tears are typically used for initial management of symptomatic episcleritis.

Second Line

- Topical NSAIDs such as Diclofenac 0.1% and Ketorolac 0.5%
- Topical corticosteroids are useful when discomfort is not sufficiently controlled by conservative measures (1).
  - Fluorometholone 0.1% drops 4 times daily; if not effective, may increase frequency
  - Prednisolone 0.5–1% eye drops
- Refractory episcleritis may be treated with oral NSAIDs or COX inhibitors such as Indomethacin or Ketorolac (1).

ISSUES FOR REFERRAL

Ophthalmology referral advised:

- If prescribing corticosteroid eye drops
- Recurrent episodes, uncertain diagnosis, and/or worsening symptoms
- If concern for progression to scleritis.

ADDITIONAL THERAPIES

- Topical NSAIDs have not been shown to have a significant benefit over artificial tears.
- When episcleritis results from viral infection, appropriate antiviral therapy is indicated.

ONGOING CARE

FOLLOW-UP RECOMMENDATIONS

Episcleritis is usually self-limited (up to 21 days) and does not typically require follow-up.

PROGNOSIS

Most patients have no ocular complications and make a full recovery.

COMPLICATIONS

Associated complications are rare.

- Anterior uveitis may occur in 4–16% of cases.
- Decreased vision may occur in 0–4% of cases.
- Ocular hypertension has been reported in 0–3.5% of cases.

REFERENCES

1. Daniel Diaz J, Sobol EK, Gritz DC. Treatment and management of scleral disorders. *Surv Ophthalmol*. 2016;61(6):702–717. doi:10.1016/j.survophthal.2016.06.002.
2. Woodward R, Konda SM, Grewal DS. Autoimmune inflammatory eye disease: demystifying clinical presentations for the internist. *Curr Allergy Asthma Rep*. 2023;23(8):471–479. doi:10.1007/s11882-023-01088-9.
3. Miller JR, Hanumunthadu D. Inflammatory eye disease: an overview of clinical presentation and management. *Clin Med (Lond)*. 2022;22(2):100–103. doi:10.7861/clinmed.2022-0046.

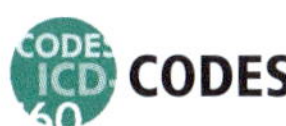

CODES

ICD10

- H15.109 Unspecified episcleritis, unspecified eye
- H15.129 Nodular episcleritis, unspecified eye
- H15.102 Unspecified episcleritis, left eye

CLINICAL PEARLS

- Episcleritis is the irritation and inflammation of the episclera, a thin layer of vascular connective tissue between the conjunctiva and sclera.
- A benign, self-limited disorder, usually resolving within 3 weeks of symptom onset
- Often not painful and presents without decrease in visual acuity.
- Although treatment is often not needed, when employed, the goal is symptomatic relief while awaiting spontaneous resolution.
- Topical lubricants and/or topical corticosteroid treatment may relieve symptoms.
- Associated complications are uncommon and not severe but may include anterior uveitis, decreased vision, and ocular hypertension.
- Episcleritis can be an early presentation of scleritis, which is more severe. Accurate diagnosis of episcleritis is important.

EPISTAXIS

Stacy E. Potts, MD, MEd • Cailee A. Dean, DO

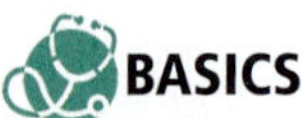

BASICS

DESCRIPTION

- Hemorrhage from the nares, nasal cavity, or nasopharynx involving either the anterior or posterior mucosal surfaces
- Intractable or refractory epistaxis: recurrent or persistent despite appropriate packing or multiple episodes during a short period, each requiring medical attention
- Synonym(s): nosebleed

EPIDEMIOLOGY

Incidence

- Bimodal, with peaks in children up to 15 years old and in adults >50 years old, particularly ages 70 to 79 years
- Most common in males age <49 years
- Rare in children age <2 years
- ~6% of patients seek medical attention; accounts for ~1 in 200 ER visits

Prevalence

Estimated lifetime prevalence: ~60%

ETIOLOGY AND PATHOPHYSIOLOGY

- Most nosebleeds are due to local causes as opposed to systemic disease.
- Anterior: 80–90% of all cases (Kiesselbach plexus)
- Posterior: 10–20% of cases (Woodruff plexus); usually branches of sphenopalatine arteries: may be asymptomatic or may present with other symptoms (hematemesis, hemoptysis)
- Trauma
  - Epistaxis digitorum (nose picking); foreign bodies; septal perforation; nasal fracture; nasal surgery; barotrauma
- Local inflammation, irritation, and insult
  - Infection (viral URI, sinusitis, TB, syphilis); irritant inhalation (smoking, rhinitis, current or past cocaine use)
  - Topical steroid or antihistamine use; chronic and excessive use of nasal vasoconstrictors
  - Septal deviation (disproportionate, unilateral air movement)
  - Low humidity, nasal oxygen use, CPAP
  - Tumors: benign, malignant
  - Vascular malformations, especially in context of prior trauma (e.g., carotid artery aneurysm)
- Systemic
  - Thrombocytopenia; congenital or acquired coagulopathies; liver or renal disease; chronic alcohol abuse
  - Leukemia; anticoagulant drug use; CHF; hereditary hemorrhagic telangiectasia (HHT)
  - Collagen abnormalities; mitral valve stenosis; multiple myeloma; polycythemia vera; HIV

Genetics

Multifactorial

RISK FACTORS

- Local irritation from multiple causes
- Medications/supplements including aspirin, clopidogrel, sildenafil, warfarin, ginseng, garlic, ginkgo biloba, and other anticoagulants
- History of septoplasty/turbinate procedures, anemia, and thrombocytopenia are risk factors for recurrent epistaxis.

GENERAL PREVENTION

- Humidification at night
- Cut fingernails and minimize picking
- For topical-nasal medication users, direct spray laterally away from septum; use opposite hand to spray (i.e., right hand to spray in left nostril).
- Petroleum jelly to prevent anterior mucosal drying

COMMONLY ASSOCIATED CONDITIONS

- Vascular malformation/telangiectasia (HHT)
- Neoplasm (rare; consider if persistent and unilateral)
- Systemic conditions:
  - Coagulopathy: primary or iatrogenic; thrombocytopenia
  - Cirrhosis; renal failure; alcohol misuse
- No proven association with hypertension but may make control of bleeding more difficult

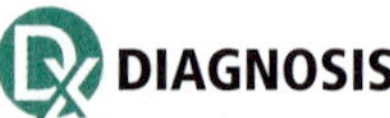

DIAGNOSIS

HISTORY

- Assess for symptoms of anemia and cardiovascular compromise.
- Assess for nausea, hematemesis, and hemoptysis, which may indicate a posterior and more severe bleed.
- Determine the side on which bleeding began, as well as its severity and duration.
- Identify and define trauma (including nose picking) and other possible precipitants (e.g., cocaine use).
- Ask about previous episodes of epistaxis and their frequency (if applicable).
- Identify comorbid conditions (e.g., cardiovascular compromise symptoms, cirrhosis, primary coagulopathies).
- Review current medications, including nasal sprays, anticoagulants, antiplatelets, and attempted treatments.
- Review family history of recurrent nose bleeds or bleeding disorders.

PHYSICAL EXAM

- Assess for airway patency and cardiovascular stability.
- Focus on localizing site of bleeding to anterior versus posterior nasal cavity. Most cases are due to anterior nasal septal bleeding.
- When formally examining the nasal cavity, have patient seated in an upright or semi-upright position.
- Use a nasal speculum, if available, with a reliable light source to increase visualization of the nasal cavities.
- Between exams, have the patient lean forward and pinch their nose (or use nasal clips) to avoid blood from draining into the posterior pharynx.

DIFFERENTIAL DIAGNOSIS

- Diagnosis usually apparent; the differential diagnosis for the etiology is key.
- Posterior bleeding should be included in the differential for any chronic blood loss anemia.

DIAGNOSTIC TESTS & INTERPRETATION

Lab testing and imaging are not indicated in most uncomplicated cases in which bleeding is easily controlled.

Initial Tests (lab, imaging)

- Mild cases, responsive to pressure: no labs
- For recurrent or intractable cases
  - CBC, PT/PTT, BMP
  - PT/PTT if on warfarin or other medications affecting coagulation
  - Cross-match when appropriate.
- Toxicology screen when nasal use of illicit drugs is suspected
- For most cases, imaging is not indicated.

Follow-Up Tests & Special Considerations

Consider evaluation for neoplasia if recurrent unilateral epistaxis, especially if not responding to treatment.

Diagnostic Procedures/Other

Nasal endoscopy (1)

Pediatric Considerations

More likely anterior, idiopathic, and recurrent

Geriatric Considerations

More likely to be posterior bleed; more likely to use predisposing medications

TREATMENT

- Most cases are managed as outpatient (1).
- Step 1: direct pressure
- Patient applies direct pressure by pinching the lower part of the nose (nasal ala) for 5 to 20 minutes without a break. This stops bleeding in most patients. Advise patient to position head slightly flexed forward in "sniffing" position.
- An ice pack placed over the dorsum of the nose may help with hemostasis.
- Inspect the nasal septum for the bleeding site.

GENERAL MEASURES

Resuscitation, as indicated. Use universal "circulation, airway, breathing (CAB)" approach.

MEDICATION

First Line

If general measures fail, affected naris may be sprayed with topical vasoconstrictor, as follows (2):

- Oxymetazoline: 0.05%
- Phenylephrine: 0.5–1%
- Epinephrine: 1:1,000
- Cocaine: 4%

Second Line

- Chemical (silver nitrate) or electrical cautery
- Nasal packing: ribbon gauze, nasal tampons, nasal balloon catheter
- For intractable/refractory: Consider surgical ligation, endoscopic ligation/cautery, and endovascular embolization.

ISSUES FOR REFERRAL

- Posterior bleeding frequently requires an otolaryngology (ENT) consultation.
- Anterior bleeding that fails conservative measures, packing, and cauterization
- Recurrent episodes
- HHT patients should establish care with ENT.
- Concurrent anticoagulation
  - If bleeding stops with packing and INR is therapeutic, may continue same dose of warfarin. If INR supratherapeutic, manage appropriately.
  - If bleeding persists despite packing, stop anticoagulation and administer vitamin K (10 mg IV ×1), recheck INR in 30 minutes. If still >1.5, give prothrombin complex concentrate (PCC).
  - Novel anticoagulation agents may be associated with lower rates of epistaxis than warfarin. When epistaxis occurs, it may be harder to control.

ADDITIONAL THERAPIES

- Nasal packing: Either with ribbon gauze or preformed nasal tampons; systemic prophylactic antibiotics are unnecessary in the majority of patients with nasal packs; topical antibiotics may be as effective and cheaper (3).
- FloSeal: A biodegradable hemostatic sealant (a thrombin-type gel) in one study is more effective and better tolerated than packing (2).
- Local application of tranexamic acid may reduce bleeding time as compared to anterior packing.
- If an actively bleeding anterior septal site is visualized, this may be treated with gentle silver nitrate cautery for ~10 seconds for definitive treatment. 75% silver nitrate is preferred. Apply in a spiral fashion, starting around the bleeding vessel, moving inward.
- Limit cautery (silver nitrate) to one side of septum, or wait 4 to 6 weeks in between treatments to reduce risk of perforation.
- Posterior: Posterior packing or tamponade with balloon devices (Foley catheters have been used); inpatient monitoring is generally required in these cases.
- Recurrent epistaxis: Cochrane review in children shows no difference in effectiveness between antiseptic nasal cream, petroleum jelly, silver nitrate cautery, or no treatment.

SURGERY/OTHER PROCEDURES

- Packing, anterior bleed
  - Layering of Vaseline ribbon gauze (1/2 inch)
    - For gauze packing, be certain that both ends of the ribbon gauze protrude from the nostril.
    - Packing is layered from the floor upward.
    - Secure packing with gauze across the outside of the nostril.
  - Nasal tampon may be used after lubricating the tip with KY Jelly or antibiotic cream or ointment.
  - Additional saline may be needed to expand the tampon if the bleeding has slowed.
  - Merocel and Rapid Rhino packs are easier to use than gauze packing and are usually well tolerated.
- Packing, posterior bleed
  - In the emergent setting, this may be attempted using a Foley catheter or a specific posterior packing balloon.
  - With both methods, the tubing is introduced through the nose similar to the passage of a nasogastric tube. Once it reaches the posterior oral pharynx, the balloon is inflated and the tubing is pulled back outward to tamponade the posterior bleeding source.
    - If using a Foley catheter (10 to 14F catheter), the balloon can be inflated with 10 mL of saline.
    - Traction is maintained with an umbilical cord clamp with adequate padding between the clip and the nose to avoid injury.

ADMISSION, INPATIENT, AND NURSING CONSIDERATIONS

- Consider hospitalization for elderly or for patients with posterior bleeding or coagulopathy; may also consider if significant comorbidities
- Admission criteria/initial stabilization
  - Posterior bleed
  - Intractable vomiting
  - Hemodynamic changes
  - Clotting dysfunction
  - Universal ABC approach; stop blood loss.

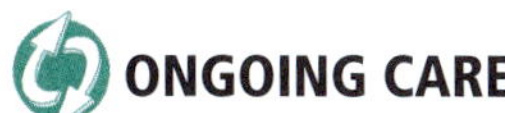

ONGOING CARE

FOLLOW-UP RECOMMENDATIONS

Patient Monitoring

- Hemodynamic monitoring if severe blood loss
- 24-hour minimum for leaving packing in place; some recommend 3 to 5 days. Rebleed usually occurs between 24 and 48 hours. Longer durations of packing have increased risk of mucosal injury and toxic shock syndrome.

PATIENT EDUCATION

- Demonstrate proper pinching pressure techniques.
- Avoidance of trauma or irritants is key.
- Management of systemic illness and proper use of medication

PROGNOSIS

- Most are self-limited.
- Good results with proper treatment.

COMPLICATIONS

- Septal perforation
- Pressure-induced tissue necrosis of the nasal mucosa
- Toxic shock syndrome with packing
- Arrhythmias triggered by packing (particularly posterior)

REFERENCES

1. Tunkel DE, Anne S, Payne SC, et al. Clinical practice guideline: nosebleed (epistaxis) executive summary. *Otolaryngol Head Neck Surg*. 2020;162(1):8–25.
2. Gottlieb M, Long B. Managing epistaxis. *Ann Emerg Med*. 2023;81(2):234–240.
3. Tunkel DE, Holdsworth SM, Alikhaani JD, et al. Plain language summary: nosebleed (epistaxis). *Otolaryngol Head Neck Surg*. 2020;162(1):26–32. doi:10.1177/0194599819889945.

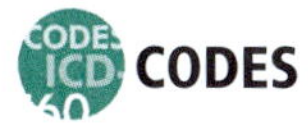

CODES

ICD10

R04.0 Epistaxis

CLINICAL PEARLS

- Most epistaxis is anterior and responds well to timed pressure over the anterior nares for 5 to 20 minutes.
- Most nosebleeds are idiopathic or as a result of digital trauma.
- Posterior nosebleeds can be asymptomatic or present with nausea, hematemesis, or heme-positive stool. Posterior bleeds are often more severe and can require specialist intervention.
- Consider evaluation for neoplasm in cases of recurrent unilateral epistaxis.

E

ERECTILE DYSFUNCTION

Zakary S. Newberry, MD • Roland W. Newman II, DO

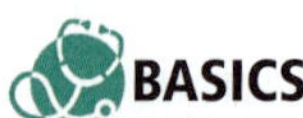

BASICS

DESCRIPTION

- Erectile dysfunction (ED): the consistent or recurrent inability to acquire and/or sustain an erection of sufficient rigidity and duration for sexual intercourse
- ED was previously assumed to be a symptom of aging in men. It is more often the result of concurrent medical conditions of the patient or from medications used to treat those conditions.
- Sexual problems are frequent among older men and have a detrimental effect on their quality of life but are infrequently discussed with their physicians.
- Synonym(s): impotence

EPIDEMIOLOGY

Incidence

In the United States, the incidence is 25.9/1,000 people and increases with age.

Prevalence

Overall prevalence for some degree of ED:

- 52% in men aged 40 to 70 years
- Age-related increase ranges from 12.4% in men aged 40 to 49 years to >70% of men over 70.
- Prevalence is likely underestimated due to underreporting.

ETIOLOGY AND PATHOPHYSIOLOGY

- Erections are neurovascular events.
  - With stimulation, nitrous oxide is released, which increases production of cyclic guanosine 3′,5′-monophosphate (cGMP).
  - This leads to relaxation of cavernous smooth muscle, increasing blood flow to penis.
  - As cavernosal sinusoids distend with blood, there is passive compression of subtunical veins, which decreases venous outflow, leading to an erection.
- ED may result from problems with systems required for normal penile erection.
  - Vascular: diseases that compromise blood flow (peripheral vascular disease, diabetes, arteriosclerosis, essential hypertension, and some medications that treat hypertension)
  - Neurologic: diseases that impair nerve conduction to brain or penile vasculature (spinal cord injury, stroke, diabetes)
  - Endocrine: diseases associated with changes in testosterone, luteinizing hormone, prolactin levels
  - Structural: phimosis, lichen sclerosis, congenital curvature
  - Psychological: patients suffering from depression, performance anxiety, premature ejaculation

RISK FACTORS

- Advancing age
- Cardiovascular disease (CVD)
- Diabetes mellitus (DM)
- Metabolic syndrome
- Sedentary lifestyle
- Cigarette smoking
- Pelvic surgery, radiation, trauma/injury to pelvic area or spinal cord
- Medications, including SSRIs, β-blockers, clonidine, digoxin, spironolactone, antiandrogens, corticosteroids, H_2 blockers, or anticonvulsants
- Central neurologic and endocrinologic conditions
- Alcohol, cocaine, opioid, or marijuana abuse
- Psychological conditions including stress, anxiety, depression, sexual abuse, or relationship problems

GENERAL PREVENTION

- Lifestyle interventions, including exercise, limiting alcohol, and smoking cessation.
- Treating the above risk factors.

COMMONLY ASSOCIATED CONDITIONS

- CVD:
  - There is a documented two-way relationship between ED and CVD. ED has been identified as an independent risk marker for CVD with ED found to confer a 25% increased 10-year risk of CVD in the QRISK model (1). Men with ED have a greater likelihood of having angina, myocardial infarction, stroke, transient ischemic attack, congestive heart failure, or cardiac arrhythmia compared to men without ED.
- DM and metabolic syndrome
- Neurologic and psychiatric conditions

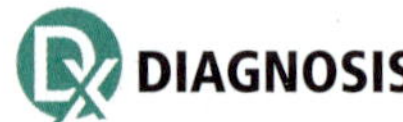

DIAGNOSIS

HISTORY

- Review past medical history thoroughly, including chronic conditions, surgeries, trauma, and medications.
- Review a detailed social history, including substance use and sexual history, with attention to presence of nocturnal erections, premature ejaculation, and libido.
- Discuss speed of onset and duration of symptoms
- International Index of Erectile Function (IIEF) patient questionnaire is a useful tool in the clinical assessment and measurement of effectiveness of ED treatments.
- Erection Hardness Scale (EHS) also can be helpful in self-assessment (2).

PHYSICAL EXAM

- Signs and symptoms of hypogonadism, including gynecomastia, small testicles, or decreased body hair
- Penile plaques (Peyronie disease)
- Detailed examination of the cardiovascular, neurologic, and genitourinary systems
  - Blood pressure, waist circumference, BMI
  - Check femoral and lower extremity pulses to assess vascular supply to genitals.
  - Check anal sphincter tone and genital reflexes, including cremasterics and bulbocavernosus.
    - Note: Absence of the bulbocavernosus reflex can be present in up to 30% of normal patients.
  - Digital rectal exam (DRE) is not required, but should be considered as BPH/LUTS can be comorbid with ED and considered before testosterone supplementation (1).

DIFFERENTIAL DIAGNOSIS

- Premature ejaculation
- Decreased libido
- Anorgasmia
- Acute versus chronic ED

DIAGNOSTIC TESTS & INTERPRETATION

Initial Tests (lab, imaging)

- HbA1c, lipid panel, CBC, CMP, TSH
- Morning total and free testosterone level (1)[C]; if low, obtain FSH and LH to determine primary (testicular) versus secondary (hypothalamic/pituitary) etiology
- Specialized testing may be indicated in men with ED who have a more complex history (young, lifelong dysfunction, prior pelvic trauma, etc.)
  - Doppler, angiogram, and cavernosogram are available radiologic modalities but not recommended in routine practice for the diagnosis of ED.

Diagnostic Procedures/Other

Questionnaires to assess the severity of ED, including the IIEF, EHS, and the Sexual Health Inventory for Men (SHIM).

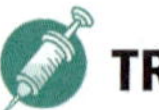

TREATMENT

- Lifestyle modifications and managing contributing medications is first-line therapy.
- Cardiovascular risk stratification and risk-factor management is recommended in all men with vasculogenic ED (1).
- Current smoking is significantly associated with ED, and smoking cessation has a beneficial effect on the restoration of erectile function (3)[A].
- Men should be counseled on all options for management of ED, including phosphodiesterase type 5 (PDE-5) inhibitors, vacuum erection devices (VEDs), intraurethral alprostadil, intracavernosal injections, and penile prosthesis implantation (1).

GENERAL MEASURES

- Psychosexual therapy alone or in combination with psychoactive drugs may be helpful in men whose ED is related to depression or anxiety.
- Weight loss and physical activity for men with metabolic syndrome with ED is recommended (3)[B].

MEDICATION

First Line

PDE-5 inhibitors are effective in ED, including those with DM, spinal cord injury, and sexual dysfunction associated with antidepressants.

- Shared decision-making should include discussion on cost, ease of use, and adverse effects
  - Sildenafil (Viagra): usual daily on-demand dose: 50 to 100 mg at least 1 hour and up to 4 hours prior to sexual intercourse
  - Vardenafil (Levitra): usual daily on-demand dose: 10 mg within at least 1 hour prior to sexual intercourse
  - Vardenafil (Staxyn): (oral-dissolving tablet) usual daily on-demand dose: 10 mg within at least 1 hour prior to sexual intercourse

– Tadalafil (Cialis): usual daily dose 2.5 to 5.0 mg/day regardless of activity or on-demand dosing 5 to 20 mg at least 30 minutes and up to 36 hours prior to sexual intercourse
– Avanafil (Stendra): usual daily on-demand dose: 50 to 200 mg at least 15 to 30 minutes prior to sexual intercourse, no more than once daily
  ○ Avanafil may have better effect with fewer side effects than sildenafil (4)[B].
- Adverse effects of PDE-5 inhibitors: headache, facial flushing, dyspepsia, nasal congestion, dizziness, hypotension, increased sensitivity to light (sildenafil), vision changes, lower back pain (tadalafil), and priapism
- Sildenafil and vardenafil should be taken on an empty stomach for maximum effectiveness. Tadalafil can be taken with or without food.

Geriatric Considerations

Use doses at the lower end of the dosing range for elderly patients and evaluate exercise tolerance before prescribing.

- Sildenafil 25 mg/day
- Vardenafil 5 mg/daily

Second Line

Intraurethral and intracavernosal injectables are shown to be effective and should be administered based on patient's preference (1),(3)[B]. Intraurethral suppositories are a less invasive treatment option than intracavernosal injections; however, they are not as effective. Alprostadil, also known as prostaglandin E1, causes smooth muscle relaxation of the arterial blood vessels and sinusoidal tissues in the corpora:

- Intraurethral alprostadil (Muse): Intraurethral suppository: 125- and 250-μg pellets; administer 5 to 50 minutes before intercourse. ≤2 doses in 24 hours are recommended.
- Intracavernosal alprostadil (available in 2 formulations):
  – Alprostadil (Caverject): usual dose: 10 to 20 μg, max dose of 60 μg; inject at right angles into one of the lateral surfaces of the proximal 3rd of the penis using a 0.5-inch, 27- or 30-gauge needle. Do not use >3 times a week or more than once in 24 hours.
  – Alprostadil may also be combined with papaverine (Bimix) plus phentolamine (Trimix), plus atropine (Quadmix).
- VED: noninvasive option, available over-the-counter
- Penile prosthesis

ALERT

- Initial trial dose of intracavernosal therapies should be administered under supervision of a provider with expertise in these therapies.
- Patient should notify physician if erection lasts >4 hours.
- Do not use vacuum devices in men with sickle cell anemia or blood dyscrasias.
- Testosterone supplementation in men with hypogonadism improves ED and libido.
  – Do not prescribe testosterone to men with ED who have normal testosterone levels (3).

- Contraindications: Nitroglycerin (or other nitrates) and phosphodiesterase inhibitors: theoretical potential for severe hypotension
- Precautions/side effects:
  – Testosterone: *precautions*: Exogenous testosterone reduces sperm count and thus do not use in patients wishing to keep fertility; *side effects*: acne, sodium retention
  – Intraurethral suppository: local penile pain, urethral bleeding, dizziness, and dysuria
  – Intracavernosal injection: penile pain, edema and hematoma, palpable nodules or plaques, and priapism
  – PDE-5 inhibitors: Use caution with congenital prolonged QT syndrome, class Ia or II antiarrhythmics, nitroglycerin, α-blockers (e.g., terazosin, tamsulosin), retinal disease, unstable cardiac disease, liver and renal failure.
- Significant possible interactions
  – PDE-5 inhibitor concentration is affected by CYP3A4 inhibitors (e.g., erythromycin, indinavir, ketoconazole, ritonavir, amiodarone, cimetidine, clarithromycin, delavirdine, diltiazem, fluoxetine, fluvoxamine, grapefruit juice, itraconazole, nefazodone, nevirapine, saquinavir, and verapamil). Serum concentrations and/or toxicity may be increased. Lower starting doses should be used in these patients.
  – PDE-5 inhibitor concentration may be reduced by rifampin and phenytoin.

ADDITIONAL THERAPIES

- Men with relationship difficulties who received therapy plus sildenafil had more successful intercourse than those who received only sildenafil (5)[A].
- A topical over-the-counter therapy, composed of a hydroalcoholic gel (MED3000) was recently FDA approved for treatment of ED. It is already available in the United Kingdom over-the-counter.

SURGERY/OTHER PROCEDURES

Penile prosthesis (inflatable and malleable/semirigid options)

COMPLEMENTARY & ALTERNATIVE MEDICINE

- Trazodone, yohimbine, and herbal therapies have not proven to be efficacious and are not recommended.
- Low-intensity shock wave treatment is not FDA approved but may be effective.

ONGOING CARE

FOLLOW-UP RECOMMENDATIONS

Patient Monitoring

Treatment should be assessed at baseline and after at least 1 to 3 weeks of treatment; monitor the quality and quantity of penile erections as well as the level of satisfaction achieved.

DIET

- Diet and exercise to achieve a normal BMI.
- Limit alcohol.

PROGNOSIS

- In the presence of sexual stimulation, PDE-5 inhibitors are 55–80% effective.
  – Lower success rates with DM and radical prostatectomy patients who suffer from ED
- Overall effectiveness is 70–90% for intracavernosal alprostadil and 43–60% for intraurethral alprostadil.
- Penile prostheses are associated with an 85–90% patient satisfaction rate.

REFERENCES

1. Burnett AL, Nehra A, Breau RH, et al. Erectile dysfunction: AUA guideline. *J Urol*. 2018;200(3):633–641.
2. Irwin GM. Erectile dysfunction. *Prim Care*. 2019;46(2):249–255.
3. Rew KT, Heidelbaugh JJ. Erectile dysfunction. *Am Fam Physician*. 2016;94(10):820–827.
4. Kumar M, Pathade AD, Gupta SV, et al. Efficacy and safety of avanafil as compared with sildenafil in the treatment of erectile dysfunction: a randomized, double blind, multicenter clinical trial. *Int J Urol*. 2022;29(4):351–359. doi:10.1111/iju.14785.
5. Melnik T, Soares BGO, Nasselo AG. Psychosocial interventions for erectile dysfunction. *Cochrane Database Syst Rev*. 2007;2007(3):CD004825.

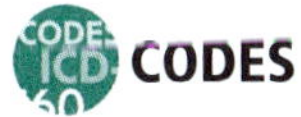

CODES

ICD10

- N52.03 Combined arterial insufficiency and corporo-venous occlusive erectile dysfunction
- N52.2 Drug-induced erectile dysfunction
- F52.21 Male erectile disorder

CLINICAL PEARLS

- Nitrates should be withheld for 24 hours after sildenafil or vardenafil administration and for 48 hours after use of tadalafil. PDE-5 inhibitors are contraindicated in patients taking concurrent nitrates of any form, as it can lead to severe hypotension and syncope.
- Reserve surgery for those who do not respond to drug treatment.
- The use of PDE-5 inhibitors with α-adrenergic antagonists may increase the risk of hypotension. Tamsulosin is the least likely to cause orthostatic hypotension.
- ED may be a marker for subclinical CVD. Thoroughly assess patients with nonpsychogenic ED for cardiovascular risks.

ERYSIPELAS

Barbara M. Kiersz Mueller, DO, CFMDL1, AIT, IEC

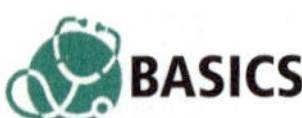

BASICS

DESCRIPTION

- Distinct form of cellulitis: an acute, well-demarcated, superficial bacterial skin infection (most commonly on face or leg) with lymphatic involvement almost always caused by *Streptococcus pyogenes*
- Usually acute, but a chronic recurrent form can also exist
- Nonpurulent
- System(s) affected: skin, exocrine

EPIDEMIOLOGY

- Predominant age: infants, children, and adults >45 years
- Greatest in elderly (aged >75 years)
- No gender/racial predilection

Incidence

- Erysipelas occurs in ~24/1,000 persons-years (1).
- Incidence on the rise since the 1980s

Prevalence

Unknown

ETIOLOGY AND PATHOPHYSIOLOGY

- Group A streptococci induce inflammation and activation of the contact system, a proinflammatory pathway with antithrombotic activity, releasing proteinases and proinflammatory cytokines.
- The generation of antibacterial peptides and the release of bradykinin, a proinflammatory peptide, increase vascular permeability and induce fever and pain.
- The M proteins from the group A streptococcal cell wall interact with neutrophils, leading to the secretion of heparin-binding protein, an inflammatory mediator that also induces vascular leakage.
- This cascade of reactions leads to the symptoms seen in erysipelas: fever, pain, erythema, and edema.
- Group A β-hemolytic streptococci primarily; commonly *S. pyogenes*, occasionally, other *Streptococcus* groups C/G
- Rarely, group B streptococci/*Staphylococcus aureus* may be involved.

RISK FACTORS

- Disruption in the skin barrier (surgical incisions, insect bites, eczematous lesions, local trauma, abrasions, dermatophytic infections, intravenous drug user [IVDU])
- Chronic diseases (diabetes, malnutrition, nephrotic syndrome, heart failure)
- Immunocompromised (HIV)/debilitated
- Fissured skin (especially at the nose and ears)
- Toe-web intertrigo and lymphedema
- Leg ulcers/stasis dermatitis
- Venous/lymphatic insufficiency (saphenectomy, varicose veins of leg, phlebitis, radiotherapy, mastectomy, lymphadenectomy)
- Alcohol abuse
- Morbid obesity
- Recent streptococcal pharyngitis
- Varicella

GENERAL PREVENTION

- Good skin hygiene
- It is recommended that predisposing medical conditions, such as tinea pedis and stasis dermatitis, be appropriately managed first.
- Men who shave within 5 days of facial erysipelas are more likely to have a recurrence.
- With recurrences, search for other possible sources of streptococcal infection (e.g., tonsils, sinuses).
- Compression stockings should be encouraged for patients with lower extremity edema.
- Consider suppressive prophylactic antibiotic therapy, such as penicillin, in patients with >2 episodes in a 12-month period.

Pediatric Considerations

Group B *Streptococcus* may be a cause of erysipelas in neonates/infants.

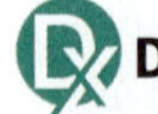

DIAGNOSIS

Prodromal symptoms before the skin eruption of erysipelas may include:

- Moderate- to high-grade fever
- Chills
- Headache
- Malaise
- Anorexia, usually in the first 48 hours
- Vomiting
- Arthralgias

ALERT

It is important to differentiate erysipelas from a methicillin-resistant *S. aureus* (MRSA) infection, which usually presents with an indurated center, significant pain, and later evidence of abscess formation.

PHYSICAL EXAM

- Vital signs: moderate- to high-grade fever with resultant tachycardia; hypotension may occur.
- The presence of a fever in erysipelas can be considered a differentiating factor from other skin infections.
- Headache and vomiting may be prominent.
- Acute onset of intense erythema; well-demarcated painful plaque (2)
- Peau d'orange appearance
- Milian ear sign (Erythema involves skin of ear as well as face implies erysipelas.)
- Vesicles and bullae may form but are not uniformly present.
- Desquamation may occur later.
- Lymphangitis
- Location (most commonly unilateral; bilateral presentation should prompt consideration of alternative diagnosis)
  - Lower extremity 70–80% of cases
  - Face involvement is less common (5–20%), especially nose and ears.
  - Chronic form usually recurs at site of the previous infection and may recur years after initial episode.
- Patients on systemic steroids may be more difficult to diagnose because signs and symptoms of the infection may be masked by anti-inflammatory action of the steroids.
- Systemic toxicity resolves rapidly with treatment; skin lesions desquamate on days 5 to 10 but usually heal without scarring.
- In geriatric patients, facial involvement presents in a butterfly pattern. Pustules characteristically absent and regional lymphadenopathy with lymphangitic streaking is seen.

Pediatric Considerations

- Abdominal involvement is more common in infants, especially around umbilical stump.
- Face, scalp, and leg involvement are common in older children due to the excoriations when scratching in atopic dermatitis, allowing an easy port of entry.

Geriatric Considerations

- Fever may not be as prominent.
- 80% of cases affect the lower extremities. The rest are usually on the face.
- High-output cardiac failure may occur in debilitated patients with underlying cardiac disease.
- More susceptible to complications

DIFFERENTIAL DIAGNOSIS

- Cellulitis (Margins are less clear and do not involve ear.)
- Necrotizing fasciitis (systemic illness and more pain)
- Skin abscess (feel for area of fluctuance)
- DVT (needs to rule out if clinically suspected)
- Acute gout (Check patient history.)
- Insect bite (Check patient history.)
- Dermatophytes
- Impetigo (blistered/crusted appearance; superficial)
- Ecthyma (ulcerative impetigo)
- Herpes zoster (dermatomal distribution)
- Erythema annulare centrifugum (raised pink-red ring/bull's-eye marks)
- Contact dermatitis (no fever, pruritic, not painful)
- Giant cell urticaria (transient, wheal appearance, severe itching)
- Angioneurotic edema (no fever)
- Scarlet fever (widespread rash with indistinct borders and without edema; rash is most common early in skin folds; develops generalized "sandpaper" feeling as it progresses)
- Toxic shock syndrome (diffuse erythema with evidence of multiorgan involvement)
- Lupus (of the face; less fever, positive antinuclear antibodies)
- Polychondritis (common site is the ear)
- Other bacterial infections to consider:
  - Meat, shellfish, fish, and poultry workers: *Erysipelothrix rhusiopathiae* (known as erysipeloid)
  - Human bite: *Eikenella corrodens*
  - Cat/dog bite: *Pasteurella multocida*/*Capnocytophaga canimorsus*
  - Salt water exposure: *Vibrio vulnificus*
  - Fresh/brackish water exposure: *Aeromonas hydrophila*

DIAGNOSTIC TESTS & INTERPRETATION

Reserve diagnostic tests for severely ill, toxic patients, patients who failed initial antibiotic therapy, or those who are immunosuppressed.

Initial Tests (lab, imaging)

- Leukocytosis
- Blood culture (<5% positive)
- Elevated erythrocyte sedimentation rate (ESR) and C-reactive protein (CRP)
- Streptococci may be cultured from exudate/noninvolved sites.

Test Interpretation

Biopsy is not needed; however, skin findings would show.

- Dermal and epidermal edema, extending into the SC tissues
- Peau d'orange appearance caused by edema in the superficial tissue surrounding the hair follicles
- Vasodilation and enlarged lymphatics
- Mixed interstitial infiltrate mainly consisting of neutrophils and mononuclear cells
- Endothelial cell swelling
- Gram-positive cocci in lymphatics and tissue with rare invasion of local blood vessels
- Fibrotic thickening of lymphatic vessel walls with possible luminal occlusion may be seen in recurrent erysipelas.

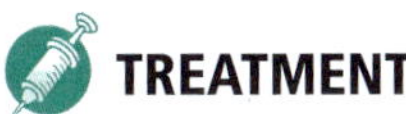

TREATMENT

GENERAL MEASURES

- Symptomatic treatment of myalgias and fever
- Adequate fluid intake
- Local treatment with cold compresses
- Elevation of affected extremity
- Appropriate therapy for any underlying predisposing condition

MEDICATION

- Antibiotics cure 50–100% of infections, but which regimen is most successful is unclear.
- Antibiotics may be as effective when given orally versus intravenously unless systemic symptoms are present (fever, chills).
- A 5-day course of antibiotics may be as effective as a 10-day course at curing.

First Line

- Adults
  - Extremities, total 5 days, nondiabetic
    - Primary
      - Penicillin G: 1 to 2 million U IV q6h *or* cefazolin 1 g IV q8h
    - Alternative (if penicillin allergic)
      - Vancomycin 15 mg/kg IV q12h
      - When afebrile, change to oral regimen of Trimethoprim-sulfamethoxazole (TMP-SMX) or clindamycin
  - Total 10 days, diabetics
    - Early mild:
      - TMP-SMX DS: 1 to 2 tabs PO BID and penicillin VK 500 mg PO QID *or* cephalexin 500 mg PO QID
  - Severe disease, 5 to 10 days
    - MP or MER or ERTA IV and linezolid 600 mg IV/PO BID *or* vancomycin IV or daptomycin 4 mg/kg IV q24h
  - Facial
    - Primary
      - Vancomycin: 15 mg/kg (actual weight) IV q8–12h with target trough 15 to 20 mg/L
    - Alternative
      - Daptomycin 4 mg/kg IV q24h or linezolid 600 mg IV q12h
- Children
  - Penicillin G
    - 0 to 7 days, <2,000 g = 50,000 U/kg q12h
    - 8 to 28 days, <2,000 g = 75,000 U/kg q8h
    - 0 to 7 days, >2,000 g = 50,000 U/kg q8h
    - 8 to 28 days, >2,000 g = 50,000 U/kg q6h
    - >28 days = 50,000 U/kg/day
  - Cefazolin
    - 0 to 7 days, <2,000 g = 25 mg/kg q12h
    - 8 to 28 days, <2,000 g = 25 mg/kg q12h
    - 0 to 7 days, >2,000 g = 25 mg/kg q12h
    - 8 to 28 days, >2,000 g = 25 mg/kg q8h
    - >28 days = 25 mg/kg q8h
- No reported group A streptococci resistance to β-lactam antibiotics
- In chronic recurrent infections, prophylactic treatment after the acute infection resolves:
  - Penicillin G benzathine: 1.2 million U IM q4wk *or* penicillin VK 500 mg PO BID or azithromycin 250 mg PO QD
- If staphylococcal infection is suspected or if patient is acutely ill, consider a β–lactamase-stable antibiotic.
- Consider community-acquired MRSA, and depending on regional sensitivity, may treat MRSA with TMP-SMX DS 1 tab PO BID *or* vancomycin 1 g IV q12h *or* doxycycline 100 mg PO BID.

ISSUES FOR REFERRAL

Recurrent infection, treatment failure

ADDITIONAL THERAPIES

For patients with worsening skin symptoms after initiation of antibiotics, a trial of topical 1% hydrocortisone may be considered.

ADMISSION, INPATIENT, AND NURSING CONSIDERATIONS

- Admission criteria/initial stabilization
  - Patient with systemic toxicity
  - Patient with high-risk factors (e.g., elderly, lymphedema, postsplenectomy, diabetes)
  - Failed outpatient care
- IV therapy if systemic toxicity/unable to tolerate PO
- Discharge criteria: no evidence of systemic toxicity with resolution of erythema and swelling

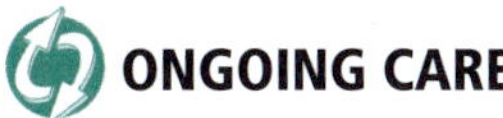

ONGOING CARE

FOLLOW-UP RECOMMENDATIONS

Bed rest with elevation of extremity during acute infection and then activity as tolerated

PROGNOSIS

- Patients should recover fully if adequately treated.
- May experience deepening of erythema after initiation of antibiotics
- Most respond to therapy after 24 to 48 hours.
- Mortality is <1% in patients receiving appropriate treatment.
- Bullae formation suggests longer disease course and often indicates a concomitant *S. aureus* infection that may require antibiotic coverage for MRSA.
- Chronic edema/scarring may result from chronic recurrent cases.
- Rarely, obstructive lymphadenitis may result from chronic recurrent cases.

COMPLICATIONS

- Recurrent infection
- Abscess (suggests staphylococcal infection)
- Necrotizing fasciitis
- Lymphedema (most prominent risk factor for recurrence) (3)
- Bacteremia, which may lead to sepsis
- Pneumonia (due to sepsis/toxin-producing organism)
- Meningitis (due to sepsis/toxin-producing organism)
- Embolism
- Gangrene
- Bursitis, septic arthritis, tendinitis, or osteitis

REFERENCES

1. Jendoubi F, Rohde M, Prinz JC. Intracellular streptococcal uptake and persistence: a potential cause of erysipelas recurrence. *Front Med (Lausanne)*. 2019;6:6. doi:10.3389/fmed.2019.00006.
2. Breen JO. Skin and soft tissue infections in immunocompetent patients. *Am Fam Physician*. 2010;81(7):893–899.
3. Inghammar M, Rasmussen M, Linder A. Recurrent erysipelas—risk factors and clinical presentation. *BMC Infect Dis*. 2014;14:270.

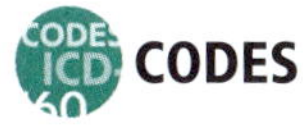

CODES

ICD10

A46 Erysipelas

CLINICAL PEARLS

- Athlete's foot is the most common portal of entry.
- Erysipelas is distinguished from cellulitis by its sharp, shiny, fiery-red, raised border.
- In recurrent cases, search for other possible source of streptococcal infection (e.g., tonsils, sinuses, intertrigo).
- Most erysipelas infections now occur on the legs, rather than the face.

ERYTHEMA MULTIFORME

D. Melessa Phillips, MD, MPH • Anthony Jay Carter, MD

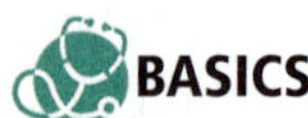

BASICS

DESCRIPTION

- An acute, uncommon, and usually self-limiting inflammatory skin condition that presents with discrete targetoid lesions; cutaneous and/or mucosal sites can be involved.
  - 90% of cases triggered by infectious agents (1).
  - 10% are drug associated.
- 3 clinically recognized erythema multiforme (EM) subtypes:
  - Acute EM:
    - EM minor (EMm)—predominantly cutaneous involvement
    - EM major (EMM)—predominantly mucosal involvement, often severe
  - Recurrent EM—frequent occurrences over a period of years
  - Persistent EM—continuous EM lesions, marked resistance to therapy

EPIDEMIOLOGY

Incidence

Annual U.S. incidence <1% (1)

Prevalence

- Most common in adults aged 20 to 40 years; rare <3 years old and >50 years of age
- >20% of cases occur in children >3 years old and in adolescents, associated with *Mycoplasma pneumoniae* infection
- Recurs in 37% of cases, usually in spring and autumn (2)

ETIOLOGY AND PATHOPHYSIOLOGY

- Etiology (2),(3)
  - Viral infections: herpes simplex virus (HSV-1 most common and HSV-2), SARS-CoV-2, Epstein-Barr, hepatitis C, coxsackievirus, varicella, mumps, poliovirus, cytomegalovirus, HIV, parvovirus B19
  - Bacterial infections: *M. pneumoniae, Yersinia enterocolitica, Mycobacterium tuberculosis, Streptococcus*
  - Fungal infections: *Histoplasma*, *Candida*
  - Drugs: NSAIDs, anticonvulsants, antibiotics (penicillin, sulfonamides, erythromycin, nitrofurantoin, tetracyclines), statins allopurinol, tumor necrosis factor (TNF)-α inhibitors, barbiturates
  - Vaccines: stronger association with HPV, MMR, and small pox vaccines, infrequently associated with hepatitis B, meningococcal, pneumococcal, varicella, influenza, diphtheria-pertussis-tetanus, *Haemophilus influenzae*, and COVID-19
  - Other: inflammatory bowel disease, autoimmune diseases, malignancies (lymphoma, leukemia, solid organ tumors), high benzoic acid (a food preservative) consumption, polymorphous light eruption
  - Idiopathic: no identifiable cause
- Pathophysiology: (1)
  - Herpes-associated EM (HAEM): HSV antigens incite a cell-mediated delayed hypersensitivity reaction, generating cytotoxic T-cells, cytokines, and cell death
  - Drug-induced EM: keratinocytes positive for TNF-α toxic cell injury and necrosis

Genetics

- Familial tendency documented in EMm
- HLA-B62 found in patients with recurrent EM and in patients with recurrent HSV infection
- HAEM: strong association with the HLA-DQB1*0301 allele

RISK FACTORS

Age 20 to 40 years or >65 years, prior EM, immunosuppression, prior acute or recurrent HSV-1 or HSV-2 infection, current infection with known associated pathogens, drug-induced

GENERAL PREVENTION

- Safe sex practice, good handwashing hygiene, sun protection on exposed areas, avoidance of flare-causing drugs
- Suppression of HSV with oral acyclovir or valacyclovir may help prevent herpes-related recurrent EM episodes (2).

COMMONLY ASSOCIATED CONDITIONS

See "Etiology and Pathophysiology."

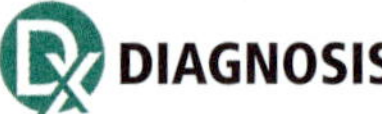

DIAGNOSIS

- Diagnosis is based on clinical history and physical examination findings.
- No specific objective or laboratory criteria exist for diagnosis.

HISTORY

- Most useful is a detailed history of acute or recurrent symptoms of a viral infection or use of a new medication.
  - Acute cutaneous involvement (EMm): typical three-zone lesions (see below) confined to the skin with minimal or no mucosal involvement
    - Lesions most often develop 10 days after HSV infection or outbreak.
    - Lesions appear initially on the extremities over 48 to 72 hours; spread centripetally
    - Cutaneous lesions usually resolve spontaneously within 1 to 3 weeks.
    - Postinflammatory hyperpigmentation may remain for months, especially in dark-skinned patients.
  - Acute mucosal involvement (EMM):
    - Prodromal symptoms of malaise, fever, and fatigue common.
    - Characterized by superficial erosions/ulcerations and pseudomembranous formation on mucosal surfaces
    - Oral mucosal (labial, buccal, and vermillion lip) surfaces are affected in up to 70% of patients; classic cutaneous lesions may or may not occur simultaneously.
    - Genital (25%) and ocular (17%) mucosa less commonly involved
- Recurrent EM:
  - History of ≥3 EM episodes a year (average 6 episodes a year), mean duration 6 to 10 years.
    - Clinical severity increases with each recurrence (2).
    - HSV strongly associated with recurrent EM subtype
    - Persistent EM: the continuous appearance of EM lesions without interruption, marked resistance to therapy. Mucosal involvement is not required for the diagnosis (2).

PHYSICAL EXAM

- Complete skin and mucous membrane exam for typical/atypical EM lesions:
  - Skin (cutaneous) lesions (EMm):
    - Begin peripherally on the extremities, preferentially on extensor surfaces and in areas of previous physical trauma and sunburn.
    - Typical "target" lesions are distinct, targetoid papules with three zones surrounding a dusky-appearing central area of epidermal necrosis: a dark red inflammatory zone encompassed by a lighter edematous ring and an erythematous zone on the extreme periphery.
    - Atypical lesions are those with only two concentric rings and may be concurrent with typical lesions (3).
  - Mucosal lesions (EMM):
    - Bullous lesions that quickly evolve into painful erosions and pseudomembranes
- At least two mucosal sites involved:
  - Eyes (conjunctivitis, keratitis)
  - Mouth (stomatitis, cheilitis, characteristic blood-stained crusted erosions on lips)
  - Urogenital (balanitis, urethritis, vulvitis) involvement more common in recurrent EM
- Look for physical findings of concurrent systemic infection and/or malignancy, vaccine injection sites

DIFFERENTIAL DIAGNOSIS

Stevens-Johnson syndrome/toxic epidermal necrolysis (SJS/TEN): SJS/TEN no longer considered part of the same disease spectrum as EM

Geriatric Considerations

- In contrast with EM that affects 20- to 40-year-olds, SJS/TEN are most likely to occur in elderly, clinically unwell patients with multiple medical comorbidities who are at risk of being administered new or cross-reacting drugs from multiple clinicians.
- Careful history of recent office or emergency room visits and/or hospital discharge may reveal a newly prescribed medication as the etiology.
- Unlike EM, 90% of patients have severe mucosal involvement, most commonly at 2 or more sites.
- Unlike EM, SJS/TEN are commonly preceded by vague prodromal constitutional symptoms (malaise, flu-like syndrome, with fever >38.5°C
- SJS/TEN lesions can be generalized but are often concentrated on the face and trunk.
- SJS/TEN lesions are flat, macular lesions with ill-defined borders that progress to bullae followed by painful skin sloughing and detachment, (<10% [SJS] to >30% [TEN] of total body surface area)
- SJS/TEN can rapidly become life-threatening with a 10–50% mortality rate due to significant risks of sepsis, pulmonary edema, cardiac disease, and coagulopathies
- Urticaria: transient (<24 hours) pruritic wheal-and-flare skin lesions, each lasting <24 hours

- Fixed drug eruption: a distinctive cutaneous allergic reaction, usually a single lesion, recurring at the same site upon reexposure to a drug or other chemical agent
- Other differential diagnosis considerations: bullous pemphigoid, paraneoplastic pemphigus, Rowell syndrome, polymorphous light eruption, cutaneous small-vessel vasculitis, meningococcemia, recurrent aphthous ulcers, herpetic gingivostomatitis, necrotizing gingivitis

DIAGNOSTIC TESTS & INTERPRETATION

In unclear cases, histopathologic analysis via skin/punch biopsy of lesions may assist in making a diagnosis (2).

Initial Tests (lab, imaging)

EM patients should be evaluated for underlying HSV infection with polymerase chain reaction (PCR) testing of active HSV lesions and/or serologic testing for HSV IgG antibodies (1).

Follow-Up Tests & Special Considerations

- Consider antinuclear antibodies, rheumatoid factor, and anti-Ro and anti-La antibodies to rule out various autoimmune diseases.
- Antibody staining to interferon (IFN)-γ and TNF-α may help differentiate between HAEM and drug-associated EM.
- Erythrocyte sedimentation rate, white blood cell count, and liver function enzymes can be checked in severe EMM cases to assess for secondary infection or suspicion of SJS/TEN.

Test Interpretation

- HSV IgG antibody serology is preferred over HSV IgM testing for accuracy
- Histopathology of both cutaneous and mucous membrane EM lesions show similar pathology (1):
  - Liquefactive degeneration of basal epidermal cells, necrotic keratinocytes, and exocytosis of lymphocytes
  - Epidermal necrosis and subepidermal bulla formation is seen in lesions undergoing evolution that develop in the dusky central portion of targetoid lesions and bulla.
  - Direct immunofluorescence of tissue may help distinguish EM from other diseases considered in the differential diagnosis.

TREATMENT

GENERAL MEASURES

- Management depends on the subtype and severity of the disease, identification of an underlying cause, and the clinician's observed and anticipated course of the disease.
- Most cases of EMm without mucosal involvement are self-limiting and can be treated symptomatically in the outpatient setting.
- Severe cases of EMM with extensive, painful oral mucosal involvement causing poor oral intake may warrant inpatient admission for fluid, nutritional, and pain management.
- Any drug suspected as a cause of EM should be immediately discontinued.

MEDICATION

First-line treatment (3)[C]:

- Acute EM minor: cutaneous
  - First-line: topical steroids, topical anesthetics, oral antihistamines
    - Medium-potency topical steroids for lesions on trunk and extremities
    - Low-potency topical steroids for lesions on the face and intertriginous skin
    - Oral antihistamines for pruritic lesions
    - HAEM: Antiviral therapy with oral acyclovir (400 mg BID), valacyclovir (500 mg BID), or famciclovir (250 mg BID) can be used but may not affect clinical course of disease.
    - Symptomatic *M. pneumoniae* infection: Treat with antibiotics (azithromycin, clarithromycin, doxycycline, minocycline) in adults and children >8 years old; fluoroquinolone (not routinely used in children) if previous antibiotics fail
    - SARS-CoV-2–related EM: has been associated with use of hydroxychloroquine to treat COVID-19
- Acute EM major: mucosal involvement (3)[C]
  - First-line therapy: high-potency corticosteroid gel, oral antiseptic or anesthetic solutions, tapered systemic glucocorticoid therapy
    - Oral mucous membranes: mild to moderate disease
      - High-potency topical corticosteroid gel (e.g., fluocinonide 0.05% gel applied 2 to 3 times per day)
      - Mouthwashes that contain a combination of lidocaine 2%, antacids, and diphenhydramine 12.5 mg/5 mL (e.g., Maalox, swish and spit as needed up to 4 times per day)
    - Oral mucous membranes: severe disease:
      - Systemic corticosteroids (prednisone 40 to 60 mg/day, tapered over 2 to 4 weeks) may be used for severe symptoms; controlled studies have not been done to validate efficacy.
    - Ocular involvement (uveitis, keratitis):
      - Immediate ophthalmology consultation
      - Ophthalmic preparations (antibiotics, nonpreserved dexamethasone 0.1%, lubricants such as nonpreserved hyaluronate) can be used at ophthalmologist's discretion.
    - Genital involvement: treatment of active or inactive HSV-2 infection, topical antibiotics, low-medium potency topical steroids
- Recurrent EM:
  - Most difficult type to treat, refractory to known treatments
  - First-line therapy: prophylactic topical, continuous oral or intermittent antiviral prophylaxis for at least 6 to 12 months with oral acyclovir, valacyclovir, or famciclovir. If the patient is unresponsive to one antiviral, consider doubling the dose or switching to a different antiviral regimen. Continuous oral acyclovir is only treatment for recurrent EM assessed by a randomized controlled trial (3)[C].

Second Line

- Second-line therapy for recurrent and persistent EM should be managed by a dermatologist.
- Azathioprine, dapsone, mycophenolate mofetil, cyclosporine levamisole, rituximab, and apremilast treatments are reported in the literature.

ISSUES FOR REFERRAL

- If ocular mucosal involvement is suspected, early ophthalmologic consultation is imperative to prevent long-term visual consequences.
- Consultation with infectious disease or intensivist is warranted if secondary infection or sepsis is likely.
- Dermatology consultation should be promptly obtained if the diagnosis of EM is in doubt, SJS/TEN is a possible consideration, or second-line therapy is warranted for recurrent and persistent disease.

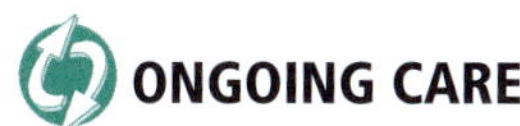

ONGOING CARE

COMPLICATIONS

Secondary infection, scarring, eye damage

REFERENCES

1. Sokumbi O, Wetter DA. Clinical features, diagnosis, and treatment of erythema multiforme: a review for the practicing dermatologist. *Int J Dermatol*. 2021;51(8):889–902.
2. Shrihari TG, Shetty SR. Erythema multiforme: a mysterious lesion! *Indian J Med Paediatr Oncol*. 2018;39(3):363–367.
3. Soares A, Sokumbi O. Recent updates in the treatment of erythema multiforme. *Medicina*. 2021;57(9):921.

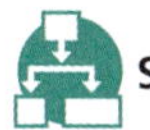

SEE ALSO

Cutaneous Drug Reactions; Dermatitis Herpetiformis; Pemphigoid Gestationis; Stevens-Johnson Syndrome; Toxic Epidermal Necrolysis; Urticaria

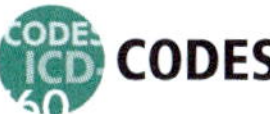

CODES

ICD10

- L51.0 Nonbullous erythema multiforme
- L51.1 Stevens-Johnson syndrome
- L51.3 Stevens-Johnson syndrome-toxic epidermal necrolysis overlap syndrome

CLINICAL PEARLS

- EM is diagnosed by history and physical exam. Skin/punch biopsy may be helpful in when clinical diagnosis is unclear.
- 90% of cases are caused by infectious agents with HSV predominant, and 10% are drug-induced.
- Most EM treatment recommendations are based on small case series or expert opinion; very few randomized controlled studies are available (3).

ERYTHEMA NODOSUM

Melissa J. Wilcox, MD

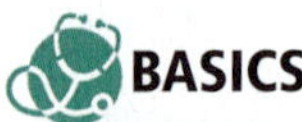

BASICS

DESCRIPTION

- A delayed-type IV hypersensitivity reaction to various antigens, or an autoimmune reaction presenting as a panniculitis (1) that affects subcutaneous fat
- The clinical pattern of multiple, bilateral, erythematous, tender nodules in a typically anterior pretibial distribution that undergo a characteristic pattern of color changes, similar to that seen in bruises. Unlike erythema induratum, the lesions of erythema nodosum (EN) do not typically ulcerate.
- Occurs most commonly on the shins; less commonly on the thighs, forearms, trunk, head, or neck
- Often associated with nonspecific prodrome including fever, weight loss, and arthralgia
- Often idiopathic but may be associated with a number of clinical entities
- Usually remits spontaneously in weeks to months without scarring, atrophy, or ulceration
- Uncommon to have recurrences after the initial presentation
- Divided into acute (more common) and chronic (rare)

Pregnancy Considerations

May have repeat outbreaks during pregnancy

Pediatric Considerations

A rare pediatric variant has lesions only on palms or soles, often unilateral; typically has a shorter duration in children than in adults

EPIDEMIOLOGY

Frequently observed in women aged 18 to 34 years

Incidence

- 1 to 5/100,000/year
- Predominant age: 20 to 30 years
- Predominant sex: female > male (6:1) in adults

Prevalence

- Varies geographically depending on the prevalence of disorders associated with EN
- Reported 1 to 5/100,000

ETIOLOGY AND PATHOPHYSIOLOGY

- Idiopathic: up to 55%
- Infectious: 44%; streptococcal pharyngitis (most common), mycobacteria, mycoplasma, chlamydia, mycoplasma, coccidioidomycosis, rarely can be caused by *Campylobacter* spp., *Rickettsiae*, *Salmonella* spp., psittacosis, syphilis
- Sarcoidosis: 11–25%
- Drugs: 3–10%; sulfonamides, amoxicillin, oral contraceptives, bromides, azathioprine, vemurafenib
- Pregnancy: 2–5%
- Enteropathies: 1–4%; ulcerative colitis, Crohn disease, Behçet disease, celiac disease, diverticulitis
- Rare causes: <1% (2)
  - Fungal: dermatophytes, coccidioidomycosis, histoplasmosis, blastomycosis, Kerion of Celso
  - Viral/chlamydial: infectious mononucleosis; lymphogranuloma venereum; paravaccinia; HIV; hepatitis B, C
  - Malignancies: lymphoma/leukemia, sarcoma, myelodysplastic syndrome
  - Vasculitis: Takayasu arteritis
  - Sweet syndrome (acute febrile neutrophilic dermatosis)
  - Sorafenib, pembrolizumab, dupilumab
  - COVID-19 virus, SARS-CoV-2 vaccine (3)

Genetics

A positive family history is usually associated with infectious etiologies.

RISK FACTORS

See "Etiology and Pathophysiology."

COMMONLY ASSOCIATED CONDITIONS

See "Etiology and Pathophysiology."

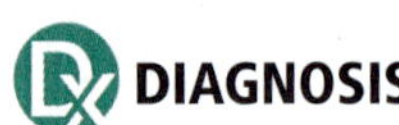

DIAGNOSIS

HISTORY

- Often a prodrome 1 to 3 weeks prior to the onset of lesions; can consist of malaise, fever, weight loss, cough, and arthralgia
- Increasingly tender nodules on the legs, usually over the shins
- Fever, malaise, chills, fatigue
- Headache
- Can precede systemic process by weeks

PHYSICAL EXAM

- Lesions initially present as warm, tender, erythematous firm nodules and plaques and become fluctuant, gradually fading to resemble a bruise >1 to 2 months (erythema contusiformis).
- Classically on anterior pretibial, although can extend proximally to involve thighs or trunk (atypically can involve extensor surface of forearms), rarely on the face
- Diameter varies from 1 to 10 cm with poor demarcation.

DIFFERENTIAL DIAGNOSIS

- Nodular vasculitis or erythema induratum (warm ulcerating calf nodules)
- Superficial thrombophlebitis
- Cellulitis
- Weber-Christian disease (violaceous, scarring nodules)
- Lupus panniculitis
- Cutaneous polyarteritis nodosa
- Sarcoidal granulomas
- Cutaneous T-cell lymphoma
- EN leprosum (clinically similar to EN but shows vasculitis on histopathology)
- Subcutaneous infection (including *Staphylococcus*, *Sporothrix schenckii*, *Nocardia brasiliensis*, *Mycobacterium marinum*, *Leishmania braziliensis*)

DIAGNOSTIC TESTS & INTERPRETATION

Diagnosis is made clinically, with support of testing (4)[C].

- ESR or C-reactive protein (CRP): often elevated, but can be normal in up to 40% (5)[C]
- CBC: mild leukocytosis (5)
- Urine pregnancy test (5)
- Throat culture, antistreptolysin O titer (5)
- Blood and/or stool culture, stool ova and parasites (O&P)
- Tuberculin skin testing (5)
- Seronegative rheumatoid factor

Follow-Up Tests & Special Considerations

Consider CXR for hilar adenopathy or infiltrates related to sarcoidosis or tuberculosis (4).

Diagnostic Procedures/Other

- Deep-incisional or excisional skin biopsy including subcutaneous tissue; rarely necessary except in atypical cases with ulceration, duration >12 weeks, or absence of nodules overlying lower limbs (4)
- Histology commonly reveals acute inflammation of the dermo-hypodermic junction and interlobular septa of the subcutaneous fat, developing without signs of necrosis or sequelae. Tissue culture should be considered in biopsy cases.
- Recently, cutaneous ultrasound can also be used to detect mixed lobular/septal panniculitis (6).

Test Interpretation
- Septal panniculitis without vasculitis
- Neutrophilic infiltrate in septa of fat tissue early in course
- Thickened, hyperechoic subcutaneous tissue with septal inflammation (blurry/hypoechoic septa) (6)
- Actinic radial (Miescher) granulomas, consisting of collections of histiocytes around a central stellate cleft, may be seen.

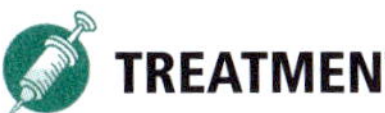

TREATMENT
- Condition is usually self-limited within 1 to 2 months
- All medications listed as treatment for EN are off-label uses of the medications. There are no specific FDA-approved medications.

GENERAL MEASURES
- Mild compression bandages and leg elevation may reduce pain (wet dressings, hot soaks, and topical medications are not useful).
- Discontinue potentially causative drugs.
- If specific cause is identified, treatment of the condition typically leads to resolution of EN.
- Indication for treatment is poorly defined in literature; hence, therapy specifically for EN is directed toward symptom management.

MEDICATION
First Line
- NSAIDs:
  - Ibuprofen 400 mg PO q4–6h (not to exceed 3,200 mg/day)
  - Indomethacin 25 to 50 mg PO TID
  - Naproxen 250 to 500 mg PO BID
- Precautions
  - GI upset/bleeding (avoid in Crohn or ulcerative colitis)
  - Fluid retention
  - Renal insufficiency
  - Dose reduction in elderly, especially those with renal disease, diabetes, or heart failure
  - May mask fever
  - NSAIDs can increase cardiovascular (CV) risk.
- Significant possible interactions
  - May blunt antihypertensive effects of diuretics and β-blockers
  - NSAIDs can elevate plasma lithium levels.
  - NSAIDs can cause significant elevation and prolongation of methotrexate levels.

Second Line
- Potassium iodide 400 to 900 mg/day divided BID or TID for 3 to 4 weeks (for persistent lesions); need to monitor for hyperthyroidism with prolonged use; pregnancy class D (7)[B]
- Corticosteroids for severe, refractory, or recurrent cases in which an infectious workup is negative. Prednisone 1 mg/kg/day for 1 to 2 weeks is the recommended dose/duration. Potential side effects include hyperglycemia, hypertension, weight gain, worsening gastroesophageal reflux disease, mood changes, bone loss, osteonecrosis, and proximal myopathy (2).
- For EN related to Behçet disease, one can also consider colchicine 0.6 to 1.2 mg BID. Potential side effects include GI upset and diarrhea (8)[B].
- A small retrospective case series supported using colchicine 0.6 mg BID for recurrent or severely symptomatic EN (9)[B]

ADMISSION, INPATIENT, AND NURSING CONSIDERATIONS
Occasionally, admission may be needed for the antecedent illness (e.g., tuberculosis).

ONGOING CARE

FOLLOW-UP RECOMMENDATIONS
- Keep legs elevated.
- Elastic wraps or support stockings may be helpful when patients are ambulating.

Patient Monitoring
Monthly follow-up or as dictated by underlying disorder

DIET
No restrictions

PATIENT EDUCATION
- Lesions will resolve over a few weeks to months.
- Scarring is unlikely.
- Joint aches and pains may persist.
- <20% recur.

PROGNOSIS
- Individual lesions resolve generally within 2 weeks.
- Total time course of 6 to 12 weeks but may vary with underlying disease
- Joint aches and pains may persist for years.
- Lesions do not scar.
- Recurrences: occurs over variable periods, averaging several years; seen most often in sarcoid, streptococcal infection, pregnancy, and oral contraceptive use; if medication induced, avoid recurrent exposure.

COMPLICATIONS
- Vary according to underlying disease
- None expected from lesions of EN

REFERENCES

1. Chowaniec M, Starba A, Wiland P. Erythema nodosum—review of the literature. *Reumatologia*. 2016;54(2):79–82.
2. Schwartz RA, Nervi SJ. Erythema nodosum: a sign of systemic disease. *Am Fam Physician*. 2007;75(5):695–700.
3. Xie Y, Yin B, Shi X. Erythema nodosum following SARS-CoV-2 vaccine. *J Eur Acad Dermatol Venereol*. 2022;36(10):e752–e753. doi:10.1111/jdv.18304.
4. Pérez-Garza DM, Chavez-Alvarez S, Ocampo-Candiani J, et al. Erythema nodosum: a practical approach and diagnostic algorithm. *Am J Clin Dermatol*. 2021;22(3):367–378. doi:10.1007/s40257-021-00592-w.
5. Cribier B, Caille A, Heid E, et al. Erythema nodosum and associated diseases. A study of 129 cases. *Int J Dermatol*. 1998;37(9):667–672.
6. Nazzaro G, Maronese CA, Passoni E. Ultrasonographic diagnosis of erythema nodosum. *Skin Res Technol*. 2022;28(2):361–364. doi:10.1111/srt.13112.
7. Horio T, Imamura S, Danno K, et al. Potassium iodide in the treatment of erythema nodosum and nodular vasculitis. *Arch Dermatol*. 1981;117(1):29–31.
8. Yurdakul S, Mat C, Tüzün Y, et al. A double-blind trial of colchicine in Behçet's syndrome. *Arthritis Rheum*. 2001;44(11):2686–2692.
9. Hrin ML, Patel PV, Jorizzo JL, et al. Colchicine for erythema nodosum: a retrospective case series. *J Cutan Med Surg*. 2023;27(6):662–663.

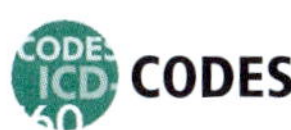

CODES

ICD10
- L52 Erythema nodosum
- A18.4 Tuberculosis of skin and subcutaneous tissue

CLINICAL PEARLS
- Lesions of EN appear to be erythematous patches, but when palpated, their underlying nodularity is appreciated.
- Evaluation for a concerning underlying etiology is necessary in EN, but most cases are idiopathic.
- EN generally follows a self-limited course with spontaneous resolution in 4 to 8 weeks, however, symptomatic therapy with anti-inflammatories can be considered for patient comfort.

E

ESOPHAGEAL VARICES

Maximos Attia, MD, FAAFP • Marcelle Meseeha, MD, FACP

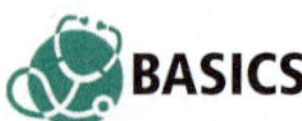

BASICS

DESCRIPTION

- Dilated submucosal esophageal veins connecting the portal and systemic circulations
- Most commonly results from portal hypertension (usually a result of cirrhosis)
- Variceal rupture: most common fatal complication of cirrhosis; severity of liver disease correlates with presence of varices and risk of bleeding.

EPIDEMIOLOGY

Incidence

- 50% of cirrhotic patients have varices; 5–10% annual progression rate such that 90% of cirrhotic patients will have varices at 10 years following diagnosis
- 1-year rate of first variceal bleeding is 5% for small varices and 15% for large varices.

Prevalence

- 50% of patients with esophageal varices experience bleeding at some point.
- Variceal bleeding: 10–20% mortality in the 6 weeks following the episode

ETIOLOGY AND PATHOPHYSIOLOGY

- Portal hypertension causes the formation of portacaval anastomoses to decompress the portal circulation. This leads to a congested submucosal venous plexus with tortuous dilated veins, particularly in the distal esophagus. Variceal rupture results in hemorrhage.
- Pathophysiology of portal hypertension:
  - Increased resistance to portal flow at the level of hepatic sinusoids caused by:
    - Intrahepatic vasoconstriction due to decreased nitric oxide production and increased release of endothelin-1 (ET-1), angiotensinogen, and eicosanoids
    - Sinusoidal remodeling causes disruption of blood flow.
  - Increased portal flow caused by hyperdynamic circulation due to splanchnic arterial vasodilation through mediators such as nitric oxide, prostacyclin, and TNF
- Causes of portal hypertension:
  - Prehepatic:
    - Extrahepatic portal vein obstruction
    - Massive splenomegaly with increased splenic vein blood flow
  - Posthepatic:
    - Severe right-sided heart failure, constrictive pericarditis, and hepatic vein obstruction (Budd-Chiari syndrome)
  - Intrahepatic:
    - Cirrhosis (accounts for most cases of portal hypertension)
  - Less frequent causes are schistosomiasis, massive fatty change, diseases affecting portal microcirculation as nodular regenerative hyperplasia, and diffuse fibrosing granulomatous disease as sarcoidosis.

Genetics

Cirrhosis is rarely hereditary.

RISK FACTORS

- Cirrhosis. In cirrhotic patients, thrombocytopenia and splenomegaly are independent predictors of esophageal varices.
- Noncirrhotic portal hypertension. Increased bleeding risk for known varices is associated with varix size, endoscopic signs (red wale marks, cherry-red spots), vessel wall thickness, and abrupt increase in variceal pressure (i.e., Valsalva maneuver).
- MELD/Child-Pugh score; presence of portal vein thrombosis; high hepatic venous pressure gradient (HVPG)

GENERAL PREVENTION

Prevent underlying causes: Prevent alcohol abuse, administer hepatitis B vaccine (HBV), needle hygiene, IV drug use (needle exchange programs reduce risk of hepatitis); specific screening and therapy for hepatitis B and C, hemochromatosis

COMMONLY ASSOCIATED CONDITIONS

- Portal hypertensive gastropathy; varices in stomach, duodenum, colon, rectum (causes massive bleeding, unlike hemorrhoids); rarely at umbilicus (caput medusae) or ostomy sites
- Isolated gastric varices can occur due to splenic vein thrombosis/stenosis from hypercoagulability/contiguous inflammation (most commonly, chronic pancreatitis).
- Other complications of cirrhosis: hepatic encephalopathy, ascites, hepatorenal syndrome, spontaneous bacterial peritonitis, hepatocellular carcinoma

DIAGNOSIS

- First indication of varices is often GI bleeding: hematemesis, hematochezia, and/or melena
- Occult bleeding (anemia): uncommon

HISTORY

- Underlying history of cirrhosis/liver disease. Variceal bleed can be initial presentation of previously undiagnosed cirrhosis.
- Alcohol abuse, exposure to blood-borne viruses through intravenous drug use or sexual practices
- Hematemesis, melena, or hematochezia
- Rapid upper GI bleed can present as rectal bleeding.

PHYSICAL EXAM

- Assess hemodynamic stability: hypotension, tachycardia (active bleeding).
- Abdominal exam—liver palpation/percussion (often small and firm with cirrhosis)
- Splenomegaly, ascites
- Visible abdominal periumbilical collateral circulation (caput medusae)
- Peripheral stigmata of alcohol abuse: spider angiomata on chest/back, palmar erythema, testicular atrophy, gynecomastia
- Rectal varices
- Hepatic encephalopathy; asterixis
- Blood on rectal exam

DIFFERENTIAL DIAGNOSIS

- Upper GI bleeding: 10–30% are due to varices.
  - In patients with known varices, as many as 50% bleed from nonvariceal sources.
  - Peptic ulcer; gastritis; gastric/esophageal malignancy
  - Congestive gastropathy of portal hypertension; arteriovenous malformation
  - Mallory-Weiss tears; aortoenteric fistula
  - Hemoptysis; nosebleed
- Lower GI bleeding
  - Rectal varices; hemorrhoids
  - Colonic neoplasia
  - Diverticulosis/arteriovenous malformation
  - Rapidly bleeding upper GI site
- Continued/recurrent bleeding risk: actively bleeding/large varix, high Child-Pugh severity score, infection, renal failure

DIAGNOSTIC TESTS & INTERPRETATION

Initial Tests (lab, imaging)

- Anemia: Hemoglobin may be normal in active bleeding; may require 6 to 24 hours to equilibrate
- Thrombocytopenia: most sensitive and specific parameter
- Aspartate aminotransferase (AST), alanine aminotransferase (ALT), alkaline phosphatase, bilirubin; prolonged PT; albumin
- BUN, creatinine
- Sodium level; may drop in patients treated with terlipressin
- Noninvasive tests are preferred to rule out high-risk varices (HRVs) (1)[B].
- Esophagogastroduodenoscopy

Diagnostic Procedures/Other

- Transient elastography (TE) for identifying CLD patients at risk for developing clinically significant portal hypertension (CSPH)
- HVPG >10 mm Hg: gold standard to diagnose CSPH (normal: 1 to 5 mm Hg)
- HVPG response of ≥10% or to ≤12 mm Hg to IV propranolol identifies responders to nonselective β-blocker (NSBB) and is linked to a decreased risk of variceal bleeding (2)[A].
- Video capsule endoscopy screening
- Doppler sonography
- CT- or MRI-angiography (second line, not routine)
  - Venous-phase celiac arteriography: demonstrates portal vein and collaterals; hepatic vein occlusion
  - Portal pressure measurement using retrograde catheter in hepatic vein

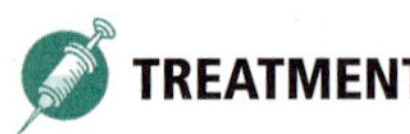

TREATMENT

GENERAL MEASURES

- Treat underlying cirrhotic comorbidities.
- Variceal bleeding is often complicated by hepatic encephalopathy and infection.
- Active bleeding (1)
  - IV access, hemodynamic resuscitation
  - Type and crossmatch packed RBCs; overtransfusion increases portal pressure and increases rebleeding risk.

- – Treat coagulopathy as necessary. Fresh frozen plasma may increase blood volume and increase rebleeding risk.
- – Avoid sedation, monitor mental status, and avoid nephrotoxic drugs and β-blockers acutely.
- – IV octreotide to lower portal venous pressure as adjuvant to endoscopic management; IV bolus of 50 μg followed by drip of 50 μg/hr
- – Terlipressin (alternative): 2 mg q4h IV for 24 to 48 hours and then 1 mg q4h
- – Erythromycin 250 mg IV 30 to 120 minutes before endoscopy
- – Urgent upper GI endoscopy for diagnosis and treatment
  - ○ Variceal band ligation preferred to sclerotherapy for bleeding varices; also for nonbleeding medium-to-large varices to decrease bleeding risk
  - ○ Ligation: lower rates of rebleeding, fewer complications, more rapid cessation of bleeding, higher rate of variceal eradication
- Repeat ligation/sclerosant for rebleeding.
- If endoscopic treatment fails, consider self-expanding esophageal metal stents or per oral placement of Sengstaken-Blakemore–type tube up to 24 hours to stabilize patient for TIPS.
- As many as 2/3 of patients with variceal bleeding develop an infection, most commonly spontaneous bacterial peritonitis, UTI, or pneumonia; antibiotic prophylaxis with oral norfloxacin 400 mg or IV ceftriaxone 1 g q24h for up to a week
- In active bleeding, avoid β-blockers, which decrease BP and blunt the physiologic increase in heart rate during acute hemorrhage.
- Prevent recurrence of acute bleeding.
  - – Vasoconstrictors: terlipressin, octreotide (reduce portal pressure)
  - – Endoscopic band ligation (EBL): if bleeding recurs or pressure measurement shows portal pressure remains >12 mm Hg
  - – TIPS: second-line therapy if above methods fail; TIPS decreases portal pressure by creating communication between hepatic vein and an intrahepatic portal vein branch.

MEDICATION

Primary prevention of variceal bleeding

- Endoscopy: assesses variceal size, presence of red wale sign (longitudinal variceal reddish streak that suggests either a recent bleed or a pending bleed) to determine risk stratification
  - – Primary prophylaxis: (i) NSBB, (ii) endoscopic variceal ligation (EVL)
  - – Endoscopy every 2 to 3 years if cirrhosis but no varices; every 1 to 2 years if small varices and not receiving β-blockers (2)[A]

First Line

- Not actively bleeding; NSBBs reduce portal pressure and decrease risk of first bleed from 25% to 15% when used as primary prophylaxis; beneficial in cirrhosis with small varices and increased hemorrhage risk as well as cirrhosis with medium-to-large varices (2)
- Carvedilol: 6.25 mg daily (2)[A] is more effective than NSBB in dropping HVPG.
  - – Propranolol: 20 mg BID increase until heart rate decreased by 25% from baseline
  - – Nadolol 80 mg daily; increase as above
  - – Contraindications: severe asthma
- Chronic prevention of rebleeding (secondary prevention): NSBBs and EBL reduce rate of rebleeding to a similar extent, but β-blockers reduce mortality, whereas ligation does not.

Second Line

Obliterate varices with esophageal ligation if not tolerant of medication prophylaxis.

- During ligation: proton pump inhibitors, such as lansoprazole 30 mg/day, until varices obliterated
- Management of Budd-Chiari syndrome: anticoagulation, angioplasty/thrombolysis, TIPS, and orthotopic liver transplantation
- Management of EHPVO: anticoagulation; mesenteric-left portal vein bypass (Meso-Rex procedure) (2)

ISSUES FOR REFERRAL

Refer for endoscopy, liver transplant, and interventional radiology for TIPS.

ADDITIONAL THERAPIES

Pneumococcal and A vaccine (HAV)/HBV

SURGERY/OTHER PROCEDURES

- Esophageal transection: in rare cases of uncontrollable, exsanguinating bleeding
- Liver transplantation

ONGOING CARE

FOLLOW-UP RECOMMENDATIONS

Patient Monitoring

- EVL, every 1 to 4 weeks, until varices eradicated
- Endoscopic screening in patients with known cirrhosis every 2 to 3 years; yearly in patients with decompensated cirrhosis
- Patients with a liver stiffness <20 kPa and with platelets >150,000 can avoid endoscopic screening and may follow up by annual TE and platelet count.

PATIENT EDUCATION

National Digestive Diseases Information Clearinghouse (https://www.niddk.nih.gov/health-information/digestive-diseases) or American Liver Foundation (http://www.liverfoundation.org/)

PROGNOSIS

- In cirrhosis, 1-year survival is 50% for those who survive at least 2 weeks following a variceal bleed.
- In-hospital mortality remains high and is related to severity of underlying cirrhosis, ranging from 0% in Child-Pugh class A disease to 32% in Child-Pugh class C disease.
- Prognosis in noncirrhotic portal fibrosis is better than for cirrhotic portal fibrosis.

COMPLICATIONS

- Formation of gastric varices after eradication of esophageal varices
- Esophageal varices can recur.
- Hepatic encephalopathy, renal dysfunction, hepatorenal syndrome
- Infections after banding/ligation of varices

REFERENCES

1. Jakab SS, Garcia-Tsao G. Evaluation and management of esophageal and gastric varices in patients with cirrhosis. *Clin Liver Dis*. 2020;24(3):335–350.
2. Kaplan DE, Ripoll C, Thiele M, et al. AASLD practice guidance on risk stratification and management of portal hypertension and varices in cirrhosis. *Hepatology*. 2024;79(5):1180–1211. doi:10.1097/HEP.0000000000000647.

ADDITIONAL READING

Jothimani D, Rela M, Kamath PS. Liver cirrhosis and portal hypertension: how to deal with esophageal varices? *Med Clin North Am*. 2023;107(3):491–504. doi:10.1016/j.mcna.2023.01.002.

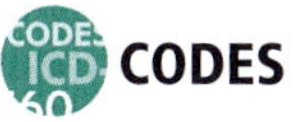

CODES

ICD10

- I85.0 Esophageal varices
- I85 Esophageal varices
- I85.1 Secondary esophageal varices

CLINICAL PEARLS

- Thrombocytopenia is the most sensitive marker of increased portal pressure and large esophageal varices.
- Roughly half of all patients with cirrhosis will have esophageal varices. One in three of those patients with varices will experience a variceal bleed. The risk of bleeding relates directly to the size and appearance of the esophageal varices.
- NSBB (nadolol, propranolol, carvedilol) act to reduce pressure in the portal circulation and are the preferred pharmacologic choice for primary prevention of variceal bleeding
- In acute bleeding, avoid β-blockers, and overtransfusion can elevate portal pressure and increase bleeding risk.

ESSENTIAL TREMOR SYNDROME

Jennifer E. Svarverud, DO • Briana D. Krewson, DO, MPH

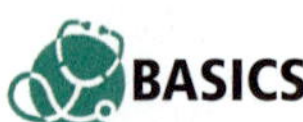

BASICS

DESCRIPTION

- Essential tremor is a postural (occurring with voluntary maintenance of a position against gravity) or kinetic (occurring during voluntary movement) flexion–extension tremor that is slow and rhythmic and primarily affects the hands, forearms, head, or voice with a frequency of 4 to 12 Hz. Symptoms must be present for ≥3 years for a formal diagnosis of essential tremor.
- Older patients tend to have lower frequency tremors, whereas younger patients exhibit frequencies in the higher range.
- The tremor occurs in the absence of other neurologic signs such as dystonia, ataxia, or parkinsonism. The disease may be familial, sporadic, or associated with other movement disorders. Incidence and prevalence increase with age, but symptom onset can occur at any age. The tremor can be intermittent and exacerbated by emotional or physical stressors, fatigue, and caffeine.
- Systems affected include neurologic, musculoskeletal, ear/nose/throat (ENT) (voice).

EPIDEMIOLOGY

Essential tremor is the most common pathologic tremor in humans.

Incidence

Can occur at any age, but bimodal peaks exist in the 2nd and 6th decades. Incidence rises significantly after age 49 years.

Prevalence

The overall prevalence for essential tremor has been estimated between to be about 1%, but is increased in older patients with an estimated prevalence of >5% at age 60 years and up to 22% at age 95 years. The prevalence of essential tremor is similar in males and females.

ETIOLOGY AND PATHOPHYSIOLOGY

- Suspected to originate from an abnormal oscillation within thalamocortical and cerebello-olivary loops, as lesions in these areas tend to reduce essential tremor
- Essential tremor is not a homogenous disorder; many patients have other motor manifestations and nonmotor features, including cognitive and psychiatric symptoms.

Genetics

- Positive family history in 30–70% of patients; autosomal dominant inheritance is demonstrated in many families with poor penetrance. Twin studies suggest that environmental factors are also involved.
- A link to genetic loci exists on chromosomes 2p22–2p25, 3q13, and 6p23. In addition, a Ser9Gly variant in the dopamine D_3 receptor gene on 3q13 has been suggested as a risk factor.

COMMONLY ASSOCIATED CONDITIONS

- Can be present in 10% of patients with Parkinson disease (PD); characteristics of PD that distinguish it from essential tremor include 3- to 5-Hz resting tremor; accompanying rigidity, bradykinesia, or postural instability; and no change with alcohol consumption
- Patients with essential tremor have a 4% risk of developing PD.
- Resting tremor, typically of the arm, may be seen in up to 20–30% of patients with essential tremor. Although action tremor is the hallmark feature of essential tremor, it is commonly found in patients with PD as well.

DIAGNOSIS

Essential tremor is a clinical diagnosis.

HISTORY

- Core criteria for diagnosis:
  - Bilateral action postural or kinetic tremor (occurs with voluntary muscle contraction) of the hands and forearms
  - Absence of other neurologic signs with the exception of cogwheel phenomenon
  - May have tremor in other locations to include head, voice, or lower limbs
  - Symptoms must be present for at least 3 years' duration.
- Secondary criteria include positive family history and beneficial response to alcohol.
- The tremor is slowly progressive; it is usually intermittent in onset and becomes persistent over time.

PHYSICAL EXAM

- Tremor can affect upper limbs (~95% of patients).
- Less commonly, the tremor affects head (~34%), lower limbs (~30%), voice (~12%), tongue (~7%), face (~5%), and trunk (~5%).
- The tremor is worsened by voluntary movements, caffeine consumption, fatigue, or stress and improves with alcohol consumption.

DIFFERENTIAL DIAGNOSIS

- PD
- Enhanced physiologic tremor
- Wilson disease
- Hyperthyroidism
- Multiple sclerosis
- Dystonic tremor
- Cerebellar tremor
- Asterixis
- Psychogenic tremor
- Orthostatic tremor
- Drug-induced or enhanced physiologic tremor (amiodarone, cimetidine, lamotrigine, itraconazole, valproic acid, SSRIs, steroids, lithium, cyclosporine, β-adrenergic agonists, ephedrine, theophylline, tricyclic antidepressants [TCAs], antipsychotics)

DIAGNOSTIC TESTS & INTERPRETATION

Initial Tests (lab, imaging)

- No specific biologic marker or diagnostic test is available.
- Ceruloplasmin and serum copper to rule out Wilson disease
- Thyroid-stimulating hormone to rule out thyroid dysfunction
- Serum electrolytes, BUN, creatinine
- Brain MRI usually is not necessary or indicated unless Wilson disease is found or exam findings imply central lesion.

Diagnostic Procedures/Other

- Accelerometry evaluates tremor frequency and amplitude; >95% of PD cases exhibit frequencies in the 4- to 6-Hz range, and 95% of essential tremor cases exhibit frequencies in the 5- to 8-Hz range.
- Surface electromyography is less helpful in distinguishing essential tremor from PD.

Test Interpretation

Posture-related tremor seen on exam

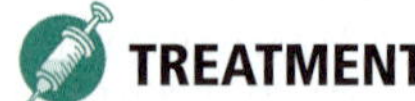

TREATMENT

GENERAL MEASURES

Stress management, decreased caffeine consumption, and adequate sleep

MEDICATION

Pharmacologic treatment should be considered when tremor interferes with activities of daily living (ADLs) or causes psychological distress. Increased doses of first-line therapies and initiation of second-line therapies that are often required to mitigate symptoms.

First Line

- Propranolol (a nonselective β-andrenergic receptor antagonist) is used as the first-line treatment for essential tremor for both exclusively situational essential tremor, and frequent or daily essential tremor.
  - For situational essential tremor, low-dose propranolol at 10 or 20 mg taken 1 hour prior to the event is recommended.
  - For frequent essential tremor, propranolol is started at 60 to 80 mg once daily if extended release or can be divided 2 to 4 times daily for immediate release per panel. The medication is titrated overtime as needed, with a maximum dose of 360 mg/day.
  - Propranolol 60 to 360 mg/day in divided doses or in long-acting formulation reduces limb tremor magnitude by ~50%, and almost 70% of patients experience improvement in clinical rating scales. Starting dose is 60 to 80 mg once daily if extended-release formulation or divided 2 to 4 times per day if immediate release. There is insufficient evidence to recommend propranolol for vocal tremor. Single doses of propranolol, taken before social situations that are likely to exacerbate tremor, are useful for some patients.

- Primidone (a barbiturate) is preferred in patients who have a contraindication to β-blocker usage, including home morbidities like asthma or heart block. Primidone is initiated at 25 to 50 mg nightly before bed, with dose increases of 25 mg every 3 to 7 days as needed for symptom control. It is recommended that older adults start at a dose of 25 mg nightly, whereas most other adults should be initiated at 50 mg nightly. The maximum dose is 750 mg/day; however, benefit is unlikely if there is no effect of the medication at a dose of 250 mg/day.
- Propranolol and primidone have similar efficacy when used as initial therapy for limb tremor; both carry a level A recommendation (1)[A]. Propranolol and primidone monotherapies can remain effective for essential tremor reduction for about 1 year, at which point doses of these medications may need to be increased.
- 30–50% of patients will not respond to either propranolol or primidone.
- If the essential tremor does not respond adequately to monotherapy with the first-line medication options, they may be used together or switched from one to the other first-line option.

Second Line

- Topiramate is recommended to start as a dose of 25 mg BID and can increase to up to 150 to 400 mg daily (1)[B].
- Gabapentin starting at 100 to 300 mg TID and can be titrated up to 1,200 mg daily (1)[B].
- Atenolol is considered the best alternative to propranolol for patients with a contraindication to a nonselective β-blocker. Sotalol, nadolol, and atenolol are alternative β blockers; each has less evidence than propranolol to support use. Metoprolol is not currently recommended as treatment for essential tremor.
- Clonazepam and alprazolam should be used with caution because of potential abuse.
- Clozapine has shown efficacy at doses of 6 to 75 mg/day but is recommended only for refractory cases of limb tremor because of a 1% risk of agranulocytosis. The American Academy of Neurology (AAN) indicates that insufficient evidence exists to support or refute the efficacy of clozapine for chronic use (1)[A].
- Levetiracetam and 3,4-diaminopyridine are probably ineffective at reducing limb tremor and should not be considered according to the AAN (1)[A].
- Other medications that have been evaluated for treatment of essential tremor, with limited data to support their use, include acetazolamide, clonidine, flunarizine, methazolamide, nimodipine, olanzapine, phenobarbital, pregabalin, quetiapine, sodium oxybate, and zonisamide (1)[A].

ADDITIONAL THERAPIES

- Current research is exploring vibration therapy, T-type calcium channel blockers, and GABA-A receptors modulators.
- Alcohol (even in modest amounts) may provide transient improvement in symptoms, but brief duration of action, subsequent rebound, and associated risk of developing alcohol addiction make it a less attractive option for long-term treatment; recommended against long-term use.
- Botulinum toxin A injections should be offered as a treatment option for cervical dystonia (level A recommendation from AAN) and may be offered medically refractory cases (1)[B].

SURGERY/OTHER PROCEDURES

- Deep brain stimulation provides a magnitude of benefit that is superior to all available medications and may be used to treat medically refractory limb tremor; it has fewer adverse effects than thalamotomy.
- Bilateral thalamic ventral intermediate nucleus stimulation is effective in reducing tremor and functional disability; however, paresthesias and dysarthria are possible complications.
- Unilateral thalamotomy may be used to treat limb tremor that is refractory to medical management.
- Bilateral thalamotomy is not recommended because of adverse side effects.
- There is growing interest in development of external neuromodulator devices for the treatment of essential tremor to include exoskeletons, orthosis, and biomechanical loading. Currently, evidence for these devices is limited and of low quality, and further research is needed.

COMPLEMENTARY & ALTERNATIVE MEDICINE

Physical therapy may be considered for strengthening and training in use of weighted devices (writing utensils, phone, computer mouse) and noninvasive handheld devices to help offset tremor. Although strength training has not been shown to have improvement in functional ability, no negative effects have been reported.

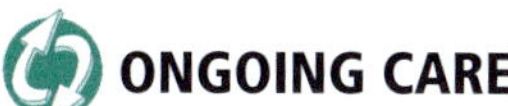

ONGOING CARE

DIET

Avoid caffeine.

PATIENT EDUCATION

Although essential tremor can cause significant impairment in daily functioning, it does not decrease life expectancy.

PROGNOSIS

Tremor tends to worsen with age, increasing in amplitude.

REFERENCES

1. Zesiewicz TA, Elble RJ, Louis ED, et al. Evidence-based guideline update: treatment of essential tremor: report of the Quality Standards Subcommittee of the American Academy of Neurology. *Neurology*. 2011;77(19):1752–1755.
2. Okelberry T, Lyons KE, Pahwa R. Updates in essential tremor. *Parkinsonism Relat Disord*. 2024;122:106086
3. Shanker V. Essential tremor: diagnosis and management. *BMJ*. 2019;366:14485.

ADDITIONAL READING

- Buijink AW, Contarino MF, Koelman JH, et al. How to tackle tremor—systematic review of the literature and diagnostic work-up. *Front Neurol*. 2012;3:146.
- Deuschl G, Raethjen J, Hellriegel H, et al. Treatment of patients with essential tremor. *Lancet Neurol*. 2011;10(2):148–161.

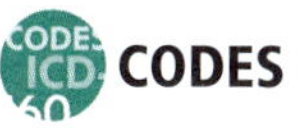

CODES

ICD10

G25.0 Essential tremor

CLINICAL PEARLS

- Core criteria for diagnosis of essential tremor include bilateral action or postural tremor of the hands, forearm, and/or head without a resting component present for at least 3 years.
- Beneficial response to alcohol and positive family history help to differentiate essential tremor from PD (PD is characterized by tremor at rest, bradykinesia, and rigidity, and it does not improve with alcohol use.).
- 10% of patients with PD will have both resting tremors of PD and essential tremor.
- Wilson disease, thyroid disease, and medication effect should be ruled out.
- Brain MRI is usually not necessary or indicated.
- First-line treatments include propranolol and primidone. 30–50% of patients will not benefit from these first-line treatments (2),(3).

E

EUSTACHIAN TUBE DYSFUNCTION

Nida Zahra, MD, FAAFP • Zaiba Jetpuri, DO, MBA, FAAFP

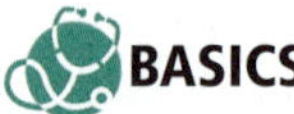

BASICS

The eustachian tube (ET) connects the posterior nasopharynx to the middle ear. The proximal two-thirds of the ET is composed of cartilage, while the distal third closest to the middle ear is made of bone. Its primary function is to equilibrate pressure within the middle ear to atmospheric pressure. It also ventilates and drains the middle ear space which prevents and clears infection and debris. When the ET malfunctions by either becoming too dilated (patulous dysfunction) or occluded (obstructive dysfunction), it results in ET dysfunction (ETD).

DESCRIPTION

- A spectrum of disorders involving impairment of the functional valve of the ET
- ETD can be classified as *patulous dysfunction*, in which the ET is excessively open, or *dilatory dysfunction*, in which there is failure of the tubes to dilate (i.e., open) appropriately.
- Pathophysiology related to pressure dysregulation, impaired protection secondary to reflux of irritating material into the middle ear, or impaired clearance by the mucociliary system
- May occur in the setting of pressure changes (e.g., scuba diving or air travel) or acute upper airway inflammation (e.g., allergic or infectious rhinosinusitis, acute otitis media [OM])
- Chronic ETD may lead to a retracted tympanic membrane, recurrent serous effusion, recurrent OM, adhesive OM, chronic mastoiditis, or cholesteatoma.
- Synonym(s): auditory tube dysfunction; ET disorder; blocked ET; patulous ET

ALERT

Sudden sensorineural hearing loss (SSNHL) can be misdiagnosed as ETD.

- A simple 512-Hz tuning fork test lateralizes to the opposite ear in SSNHL and to the affected ear in ETD with conductive hearing loss.
- Any SSNHL is a medical emergency and should be referred to an otolaryngologist immediately.

EPIDEMIOLOGY

Adults: >2 million health care visits annually

- Median age: 48
- Females > males
- Most common comorbidity is acute rhinitis.

Prevalence

Greater in children than in adults due to shorter, more horizontal tubes, immature floppy elastic cartilage, and larger adenoids than adults (0.77 adult visits to every one pediatric visit) (1)

ETIOLOGY AND PATHOPHYSIOLOGY

- Under normal circumstances, the ET is closed, opening to release a small amount of air to equilibrate middle ear pressure with surrounding atmospheric pressure.
- ETD is failure of the ET, palate, nasal cavities, and nasopharynx to regulate middle ear and mastoid pressure.
- ET functions:
  - Ventilation/regulation of middle ear pressure
  - Protection from nasopharyngeal (NP) secretions
  - Drainage of middle ear fluid
  - ET is closed at rest and opens with yawning, swallowing, and chewing.
- Cycle of dysfunction: structural or functional obstruction of the ET:
  - Negative pressure develops in middle ear.
  - Serous exudate is drawn to the middle ear by negative pressure or refluxed into the middle ear if the ET opens momentarily.
  - Infection of static fluid causes edema and release of inflammatory mediators, exacerbating the cycle of inflammation and obstruction.
- In children, a horizontal and shorter ET predisposes to difficulties with ventilation and drainage.
- Adenoid hypertrophy can block the torus tubarius (proximal opening of the ET).
- In adults, paradoxical closing of the ET with swallowing occurs in a majority of affected patients.
- Tumors that impair/occlude the ET or that invade the tensor veli palatini to impair normal swallow regulation can also lead to dysfunction.

Genetics

Twin studies show a genetic component. Specific genetic cause is undefined.

RISK FACTORS

Adult and pediatric:

- Allergic rhinitis, tobacco exposure, GERD, chronic sinusitis, adenoid hypertrophy or NP mass, neuromuscular disease, altered immunity
- Prematurity and low birth weight, young age, daycare, crowded living conditions, low socioeconomic status, prone sleeping position, prolonged bottle use, craniofacial abnormalities (e.g., cleft palate, Down syndrome)

Pregnancy Considerations

ETD may be exacerbated by rhinitis of pregnancy; symptoms resolve postpartum.

GENERAL PREVENTION

- Control of upper airway inflammation: allergies, infectious rhinosinusitis, GERD
- Autoinsufflation of middle ear (i.e., blow gently against pinched nostril and closed mouth)
- Avoid atmospheric pressure changes (e.g., plane flight, scuba diving) in the setting of acute allergy exacerbation or URI.
- Avoid exposure to environmental irritants: tobacco smoke and pollutants.

COMMONLY ASSOCIATED CONDITIONS

- Hearing loss
- OM: acute, chronic, and serous; chronic mastoiditis; cholesteatoma
- Allergic rhinitis, chronic sinusitis/URI, adenoid hypertrophy
- GERD
- Cleft palate, Down syndrome
- Obesity
- NP or other tumor

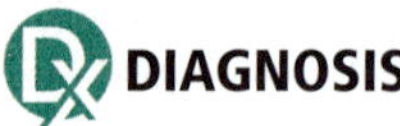

DIAGNOSIS

HISTORY

- Symptoms of ear pain, fullness, "plugging," hearing loss, tinnitus, popping or snapping noises, and vertigo
  - Unilateral or bilateral; evaluate adults with persistent unilateral symptoms for NP tumor.
  - History of previous ear infections, surgeries, head trauma, recent flying or diving
  - Voice change (hyponasal or hypernasal voice, consider NP mass or palatal dysfunction)
  - Differentiate patulous dysfunction, in which patient's own voice and breath sounds are amplified (autophony), from dilatory dysfunction, in which patient complains more of ear pain, "plugged" ear, hearing loss, and tinnitus.
- ETDQ-7 is a questionnaire that attempts to quantify ETD in adult patients. Based on presence and intensity of symptoms in past 1 month, severity is rated on 1 to 7 scale. A total score >14.5 categorizes patient as having ETD (2).
  - Pressure in ears in past 1 month?
  - Pain in ears in past 1 month?
  - A feeling that ears are clogged or "underwater?"
  - Ear symptoms when you have cold or sinusitis?
  - Crackling or popping sounds in the ears?
  - Ringing in ears?
  - A feeling that your hearing is muffled?

PHYSICAL EXAM

- Pneumatic otoscopy: retracted tympanic membrane, effusion, decreased drum movement
- Toynbee maneuver: View changes of the drum while patient autoinsufflates against closed lips and pinched nostrils; may show various degrees of retraction
  - Entire drum may be retracted and "lateralize" with insufflation.
  - Posterosuperior quadrant (pars flaccida) may form a retraction pocket.
- Tuning fork tests: 512-Hz fork placed on the forehead lateralizes to affected ear (Weber test); the fork will be louder behind the ear on the mastoid than in front of the ear (bone conduction > air conduction, Rinne test) in conductive hearing loss.
- Nasopharyngoscopy: adenoid hypertrophy or NP mass
- Anterior rhinoscopy: deviated nasal septum, polyps, mucosal hypertrophy, turbinate hypertrophy

DIFFERENTIAL DIAGNOSIS

- SSNHL (a medical emergency)
- Tympanic membrane perforation
- Barotrauma
- Temporomandibular joint disorder
- Ménière disease
- Otic capsule dehiscence
- Superior semicircular canal dehiscence

DIAGNOSTIC TESTS & INTERPRETATION

Initial Tests (lab, imaging)

- ETD is a generally a clinical diagnosis. Diagnosis can be confirmed by nasal endoscopy and audiology studies.
- No routine radiologic studies needed unless unilateral symptoms are persistent for >3 months. CT scan (not necessary) may show changes related to OM or middle ear/mastoid opacification.
- MRI might determine cause of ETD (in recalcitrant cases), as the ET opening can be visualized during Valsalva.

Diagnostic Procedures/Other

- Audiogram may show conductive hearing loss.
- Tympanometry: Type B or C tympanograms indicates fluid or retraction, respectively; negative middle ear peak pressures seen even with normal (type A) tympanograms
- Nasal endoscopy is helpful in patients with severe ear complaints (e.g., severe hearing loss, recurrent OM with effusion) to evaluate nasopharynx as well as ET anatomy and function.

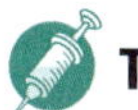

TREATMENT

- Due to limited high-quality evidence, it is difficult to recommend any one treatment option/intervention as superior.
- Use of a "nasal balloon" shown effective for clearing OM with effusion; unclear of benefit for ETD
- General principle is to remove or fix the underlying cause (e.g., infection, tumor, perforation of TM; restore tensor palatini muscle) and reduce or eliminate the cycle of infection/inflammation
- Although no evidence exists, some consider antibiotics for AOM and rhinosinusitis; decongestants, nasal steroids, intranasal/sinus rinses, antihistamines (if allergic rhinitis is present), and surgery/procedures for recalcitrant cases
- Tympanostomy tubes ± adenoidectomy when indicated for recurrent ear infections or severe progressive retractions

MEDICATION

- Antibiotics only if infection is suspected as cause of ETD especially moderate to severe cases of bacterial rhinosinusitis
- Few data support pharmacologic treatments such as decongestants, nasal steroids, or antihistamines for ETD.
- Medications treat comorbid conditions.
- Decongestants, topical, oral
  - Avoid prolonged use (>3 days); can cause rhinitis medicamentosa
  - Decongestants are most useful for acute ETD related to a resolving URI.
  - Decongestants are not typically used for relief of chronic ETD in children.
    - Phenylephrine
    - Pseudoephedrine
    - Oxymetazoline
- Nasal steroids (may be beneficial for those with allergic rhinitis)
  - Beclomethasone (Beconase, Vancenase)
  - Budesonide (Rhinocort)
  - Fluticasone propionate (Flonase)
  - Mometasone (Nasonex)
  - Triamcinolone (Nasacort)
- 2nd-generation H1 antihistamines (may be beneficial for those with ETD and chronic rhinitis)
  - Cetirizine (Zyrtec) (tablets, chewable tablets, liquid)
  - Desloratadine (Clarinex) (tablets, RediTabs, liquid)
  - Fexofenadine (Allegra) (tablets, RediTabs, liquid)
  - Levocetirizine (Xyzal) (tablets, liquid)
- Antihistamine nasal sprays (may be beneficial for those with ETD and chronic rhinitis)
  - Azelastine (Astepro or Astelin)
  - Olopatadine (Patanase)

ADDITIONAL THERAPIES

- Any activity that promotes swallowing, such as chewing gum, eating, or drinking, can open the ET and promote relief of symptoms.
- Patients with ETD should refrain from flying during times of nasal congestion or ear infection. If the patient must fly, advise them to take oral and intranasal decongestants an hour prior to take off.
- Patients should refrain from scuba diving.

SURGERY/OTHER PROCEDURES

- Myringotomy and pressure equalization tube placement to ventilate middle ear, relieve pressure, and prevent sequelae of chronically retracted drum
- Patients with ETD during pressure changes may benefit from minimally invasive laser eustachian tuboplasty.
- Balloon tuboplasty (limited data in terms of efficacy, safety, and long-term outcomes)
- Microwave ablation (MWA) targeting hypertrophic tissue at the orifice of the ET (3)
- Adenoidectomy if hypertrophied tissue is present
  - In children, first set of tubes are typically placed alone. Adenoidectomy is performed with second set of tubes if problems recur.
  - Some advocate adenoidectomy even in absence of excess tissue; reduces frequency and number of subsequent tubes

COMPLEMENTARY & ALTERNATIVE MEDICINE

Osteopathic manipulative treatment (OMT) can be used in the treatment of ETD.

- Galbreath technique
- Modified Muncie technique

ONGOING CARE

FOLLOW-UP RECOMMENDATIONS

- Monitor pressure equalization tubes every 6 to 8 months in children and every 6 to 12 months in adults.
- Monitor tympanic membrane retraction pocket for progression every 6 to 12 months to allow for early intervention for progression in hearing loss, obvious ossicular erosion, or cholesteatoma.

DIET

Breastfeeding is associated with lower incidence of ETD and OM.

PROGNOSIS

If symptoms of ETD persist beyond age 7 years, patient is more likely to have long-term problems and require regular monitoring.

COMPLICATIONS

Morbidity related to hearing compromise or associated sequela of chronic ear infections

E

REFERENCES

1. Anastasiadou S, Bountzis P, Gkogkos DE, et al. Eustachian tube dysfunction diagnostic pathway—what is the current state of the art and how relevant is chronic nasal disease? *J Clin Med*. 2024;13(13):3700. doi:10.3390/jcm13133700.
2. Alper CM, Teixeira MS, Mandel EM, et al. Dissecting eustachian tube dysfunction: from phenotypes to endotypes. *PloS One*. 2023;18(4):e0283885. doi:10.1371/journal.pone.0283885.
3. Bal R, Deshmukh P. Management of eustachian tube dysfunction: a review. *Cureus*. 2022;14(11):e31432. doi:10.7759/cureus.31432.

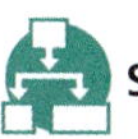

SEE ALSO

Algorithm: Ear Pain/Otalgia

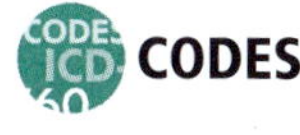

CODES

ICD10

- H69.90 Unspecified Eustachian tube disorder, unspecified ear
- H69.00 Patulous Eustachian tube, unspecified ear
- H68.109 Unspecified obstruction of Eustachian tube, unspecified ear

CLINICAL PEARLS

- ETD can be acute or chronic. Treatment is based on the underlying etiology.
- Rule out SSNHL (medical emergency), which can be misdiagnosed as ETD, especially in patients with unilateral symptoms.

FACTOR V LEIDEN

Kevin Gray, MD • Daniel Chilcote, DO

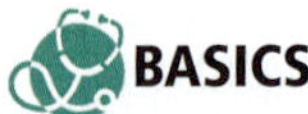

BASICS

DESCRIPTION

- Factor V Leiden (FVL) is a genetic point mutation in the F5 gene at the activated protein C (APC) cleavage site on the factor V and Va molecule leading to increase in thrombin and as a result leads to clot formation. This is the most common form of inherited thrombophilia.
- System(s) affected: cardiovascular, gastrointestinal, hemo/lymphatic/immunologic, nervous, pulmonary, reproductive
- Synonym(s): FVL thrombophilia; FVL mutation, hereditary APC resistance

Pediatric Considerations

- The incidence of venous thrombosis in healthy children is extremely low (0.07/100,000 per year).
- There is a weak, however significant, association between procoagulant states (including FVL) and coronary events in younger patients.

Pregnancy Considerations

- Recurrent pregnancy loss is a possible complication.
- Increased thrombotic risk in pregnancy and postpartum (additive) especially in homozygous state
- Possible increased risk of IUGR, preeclampsia, placental abruption: evidence mixed
- Women with a history of adverse pregnancy outcomes should be tested for thrombophilia if they are planning a future pregnancy (1).

EPIDEMIOLOGY

Prevalence

- ~5–8% occurrence of heterozygosity in Caucasians, Hispanic Americans ~2%, African Americans ~1%, and Asian Americans ~0.45% of those heterozygous for FVL small percentage of individuals develop venous thromboembolism (VTE), estimated 5–10%
- General population 4–5% without history of VTE; 12–14% reported in parts of Greece, Sweden, and Lebanon. No reports seen in Chinese or Japanese.

ETIOLOGY AND PATHOPHYSIOLOGY

- Factor V is a protein that is part of the clotting cascade that circulates in the plasma. When exposed to tissue factor, factor V amplifies the production of thrombin, which further promotes clotting by activating factor V into procoagulant factor Va.
- For balance, thrombin also promotes APC production, which will cleave and inactivate factor V, Va, and VIII, thereby keeping the clotting cascade in check (negative feedback loop).
- In FVL, a point mutation at the binding site of APC (Arg506Glu) renders it less able to cleave factor V or Va. This reduces the anticoagulant role of factor V as a cofactor to APC and increases the *procoagulant* role of activated factor V because there is now 20-fold slower degradation of factor Va.

RISK FACTORS

- Risk for VTE is ~7-fold in heterozygous and ~80-fold in homozygous FVL individuals, compared with individuals without the mutation. This risk is compounded/increased by the presence of the following:
  - Having non-O blood type (A, B, or AB): 2- to 4-fold
  - Oral contraceptives: homozygotes up to 100-fold; heterozygotes, 35-fold. The increased risk is halved when the patient uses desogestrel-containing oral contraceptives.
  - Hormone replacement therapy (HRT) and selective estrogen receptor modulators (SERMs) both increase the risk of thrombosis; in patients with FVL, that risk is compounded.
  - In men with an underlying thrombophilia, testosterone therapy can promote VTE.
  - Pregnancy and *homozygous* FVL increase the risk of thrombosis 7- to 16-fold during pregnancy and the puerperium.
  - Those with combined thrombophilias and end-stage renal disease are at risk for developing calciphylaxis.
  - 30% of patients with VTE is attributed to FVL and prothrombin G2021A mutation; however the risk is weaker compared to antithrombin III, protein C, and protein S deficiency, which is around 1% in the general population.
- FVL versus general population, a modest increase in the recurrence risk of VTE is seen.

GENERAL PREVENTION

ALERT

Patients with FVL without thrombosis do not require prophylactic anticoagulation.

COMMONLY ASSOCIATED CONDITIONS

Venous thrombosis

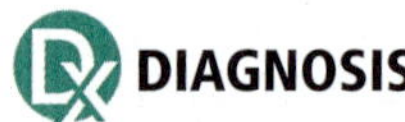

DIAGNOSIS

HISTORY

- It is critical to differentiate between provoked and unprovoked VTE and determine family history, risk factors, and detailed symptoms.
- In up to 70% of patients suffering from VTE, a provoking factor is present.
- Isolated pulmonary embolism (PE) without evidence of deep vein thrombosis (DVT), however, is less common than general population; this phenomenon is known as "FVL paradox."
- There is no clinical feature specific for FVL; most patient are asymptomatic until they develop thrombosis.
- Recurrent pregnancy loss
- Family history of thrombosis
- Family history of FVL mutation

PHYSICAL EXAM

- Findings suggestive of VTE in any form (DVT, PE, cerebral thrombosis): 10–26% of patients with VTE are carriers of the FVL mutation.
- Test individuals who develop VTE in unusual location (e.g., portal vein, cerebral vein, or recurrent VTE) especially <50 years old.

DIFFERENTIAL DIAGNOSIS

- Protein C deficiency
- Protein S deficiency
- Antithrombin deficiency
- Other causes of APC resistance (e.g., antiphospholipid antibodies)
- Dysfibrinogenemia
- Dysplasminogenemia
- Homocystinemia
- Prothrombin G20210A mutation
- Elevated factor VIII levels

DIAGNOSTIC TESTS & INTERPRETATION

Initial Tests (lab, imaging)

- For VTE diagnosis, tests, and imaging, refer to DVT/PE chapters.
- NICE guidelines specifies the only clear indication for thrombophilia testing including FVL is when the consideration is being given to discontinuing anticoagulation therapy after an unprovoked VTE event.
- FVL thrombophilia should be suspected in individuals with the following:
  - A history of first and recurrent VTE manifest as DVT or PE, especially in women with a history of VTE during pregnancy or in association with use of estrogen-containing contraceptives; more particular in 3rd generation
  - A family history of recurrent thrombosis
- Functional assay for APC resistance: plasma-based coagulation assay using factor V–deficient plasma to which patient plasma is added along with purified APC. The relative prolongation of the aPTT is used to assay for the defect. Heparin, direct thrombin inhibitors, and factor Xa inhibitor may cause false-negative results. In the absence of exposure to anticoagulants, functional testing is preferred to genetic testing due to cost and time to diagnosis.
- FVL molecular genetic test: DNA-based for factor V mutation, will be unaffected by anticoagulation and other drugs; recommended in individuals on direct thrombin inhibitors or direct factor Xa inhibitors, those with strong lupus inhibitors, and significantly prolonged baseline aPTT

Follow-Up Tests & Special Considerations

- For individuals with family history of FVL, genetic testing is preferred, especially if they have concomitant antiphospholipid syndrome or who are receiving anticoagulant—this will elucidate potential source of test interference for direct thrombin inhibitor or direct factor Xa inhibitor.
- Inherited genetic factors such as FVL, prothrombin mutation 20210A, antithrombin, protein C or protein S deficiencies, non-O blood group, as well as CYP2C9*2 and the rs4379368 mutations, have been shown to be genetic predictive risk factors for VTE in women. Therefore, consider testing for mutations prior implementing combined oral contraception and monitor for potential thrombogenicity induced by COC therapy.

Diagnostic Procedures/Other

- Thrombophilia testing in pediatric patients with recurrent central venous catheter (CVC)-related VTE.
- If thrombophilia is suspected in children with VTE, include testing: FVL mutation, prothrombin mutation G20210A, antithrombin deficiency, protein C deficiency, protein S deficiency, and antiphospholipid
- The thrombophilia screen consists of antithrombin III, protein C and S deficiency, PCR for FVL mutation and prothrombin G2021A mutation, testing for antiphospholipid antibodies and homocysteine level.

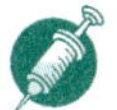

TREATMENT

Only indicated if with thrombotic event. For asymptomatic patients (no thrombotic event), prophylaxis is not recommended.

GENERAL MEASURES

- Initiation of anticoagulation therapy for acute venous thrombosis should be the same in patients with and without FVL or other inherited thrombophilia.
- The treatment for first VTE in patients with FVL or any other thrombophilias does not differ from those without it.
- VTE treatment should be a minimum of 3 months for the first episode.
- For those patients with recurrence, the risks and benefits of indefinite anticoagulation need to be assessed and considered.

MEDICATION

First Line

- First-line treatment for first VTE is the same for a patient with and a patient without FVL.
- In patients with proximal DVT or PE, anticoagulation therapy is recommended over no therapy (Grade 1B).
- In patients with DVT or PE and no cancer, anticoagulation suggested are dabigatran, rivaroxaban, apixaban, or edoxaban over vitamin K antagonist (all Grade 2B).
- In patients with cancer-associated thrombosis, low molecular weight heparin (LMWH) is recommended.
- LMWH:
  - Enoxaparin (Lovenox): SubQ: 1 mg/kg every 12 hours (preferred) or 1.5 mg/kg once every 24 hours; note: in select low-risk patients, may consider outpatient treatment using 1 mg/kg every 12 hours for the remainder of the course after first dose administered in hospital or urgent care center.
  - Fondaparinux (Arixtra): 5 mg (body weight <50 kg), 7.5 mg (body weight 50 to 100 kg), or 10 mg (body weight >100 kg) SC daily
  - Tinzaparin (Innohep): 175 anti-Xa IU/kg SC daily for minimum of 5 days and patient is adequately anticoagulated with warfarin (INR of >2 for 2 consecutive days)
  - Dalteparin (Fragmin): 200 IU/kg SC daily
- Oral anticoagulant
  - Apixaban (Eliquis): treatment dose: 10 mg BID × 7 days and then 5 mg BID × 3 to 6 months
  - Rivaroxaban (Xarelto): treatment dose: 15 mg BID × 7 days and then 20 mg daily × 3 to 6 months
  - Dabigatran (Pradaxa): After at least 5 days of initial therapy with a parenteral anticoagulant, transition to dabigatran in hemodynamically stable patients: 150 mg BID
- Contraindications
  - Active bleeding precludes anticoagulation.
  - Risk of bleeding is a relative contraindication to long-term anticoagulation.
- Precautions
  - Observe patient for signs of embolization, further thrombosis, or bleeding.
  - Avoid IM injections. Periodically check stool and urine for occult blood; monitor CBCs, including platelets.
  - LMWH: adjust dosage in renal insufficiency; may also need dose adjustment in pregnancy
- Significant possible interactions
  - Agents that intensify the response to oral anticoagulants: alcohol, allopurinol, amiodarone, anabolic steroids, androgens, many antimicrobials, cimetidine, chloral hydrate, disulfiram, famotidine, NSAIDs, sulfinpyrazone, tamoxifen, thyroid hormone, vitamin E, salicylates, acetaminophen
  - Agents that diminish the response to anticoagulants: aminoglutethimide, antacids, barbiturates, carbamazepine, cholestyramine, diuretics, griseofulvin, rifampin, oral contraceptives

Second Line

- Heparin 80 mg/kg IV bolus followed by 18 g/kg/hr continuous infusion
- Oral anticoagulant
  - Warfarin (Coumadin) PO with dose adjusted to an INR of 2.0 to 3.0
  - Contraindications
    - Active bleeding precludes anticoagulation.
    - Risk of bleeding is a relative contraindication to long-term anticoagulation.
    - Warfarin is contraindicated in patients with history of warfarin skin necrosis.
    - Warfarin is contraindicated in pregnancy.
  - Precautions
    - Heparin: thrombocytopenia and/or paradoxical thrombosis with thrombocytopenia
    - Warfarin: necrotic skin lesions (typically breasts, thighs, or buttocks

ISSUES FOR REFERRAL

- Recurrent thrombosis on anticoagulation
- Difficulty anticoagulating
- Genetic counseling
- Homozygous state in pregnancy

SURGERY/OTHER PROCEDURES

Recommendations are against routine use of inferior vena cava filter in addition to anticoagulation, except when there is contraindication for anticoagulation.

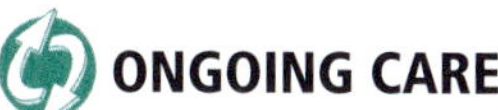

ONGOING CARE

FOLLOW-UP RECOMMENDATIONS

Patient Monitoring

Warfarin use requires periodic (~monthly after initial stabilization) INR measurements, with a goal of 2.0 to 3.0

DIET

Large amounts of foods rich in vitamin K may interfere with anticoagulation with warfarin.

PATIENT EDUCATION

- Patients should be educated about the following:
  - Use of oral anticoagulant therapy
  - Avoidance of systemic NSAIDs while on anticoagulation
- The role of family screening is unclear because most patients with this mutation do not have thrombosis. In a patient with a family history of FVL, consider screening during pregnancy or if considering oral contraceptive use.

PROGNOSIS

- Most patients heterozygous for FVL do not have thrombosis.
- Homozygotes have about a 50% lifetime incidence of thrombosis.
- Recurrence rates after a first thrombosis are not clear; some estimate as high as 5%.
- FVL does not increase overall mortality.

COMPLICATIONS

- Recurrent thrombosis
- Bleeding on anticoagulation

REFERENCES

1. Dłuski D, Mierzyński R, Poniedziałek-Czajkowska E, et al. Adverse pregnancy outcomes and inherited thrombophilia. *J Perinat Med*. 2018;46(4):411–417.

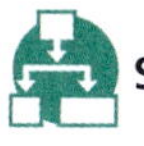

SEE ALSO

Deep Vein Thrombophlebitis

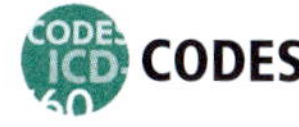

CODES

ICD10

D68.51 Activated protein C resistance

CLINICAL PEARLS

- Extremely rare in Asian and African populations
- Asymptomatic patients with FVL do not need anticoagulation.
- For pregnant women homozygous for FVL but no prior history of VTE, postpartum prophylaxis with prophylactic or intermediate-dose LMWH or vitamin K antagonists with target INR 2.0 to 3.0 for 6 weeks is recommended. Antepartum prophylaxis is added if there is positive family history of VTE.

F

FAILURE TO THRIVE

Durr-e-Shahwaar Sayed, DO

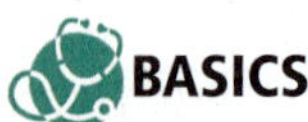

BASICS

DESCRIPTION

- Failure to thrive (FTT), now growth faltering, is not a diagnosis but a sign of inadequate nutrition in young children manifested by a failure of physical growth, usually affecting weight. In severe cases, decreased length and/or head circumference may develop.
- It is suspected when either weight or BMI for age fall below the 5th percentile or weight drops two or more percentile lines on standard growth charts *or* weight-for-length falls below the 5th percentile.
- Diagnosis should be confirmed by calculating a Z-score rather than relying on weight/BMI measurements alone. A negative Z-score implies some degree of malnutrition.
- A combination of anthropometric criteria rather than one criterion should be used to identify children at risk of FTT.

Pediatric Considerations

- Children with genetic syndromes, intrauterine growth restriction (IUGR), or prematurity follow different growth curves
- 25% of children will decrease their weight or height crossing ≥2 major percentile lines in the first 2 years of life. These children are failing to reach their genetic potential or demonstrating constitutional growth delay (slow growth with a bone age < chronologic age). After shifting down, these infants grow at a normal rate along their new percentile and do not have FTT.

EPIDEMIOLOGY

Incidence

- Predominant age: 6 to 12 months; 80% <18 months
- Predominant sex: male = female

Prevalence

- As many as 10% of children seen in primary care have signs of growth failure.
- 1–5% of pediatric inpatient admissions are for FTT.
- Occurs more frequently in children living in poverty

ETIOLOGY AND PATHOPHYSIOLOGY

- Often grouped into four major categories:
  - Inadequate caloric intake (most frequent)
  - Inadequate caloric absorption
  - Excessive caloric expenditure
  - Defective utilization
- Causes of FTT can be grouped by pathophysiology (including examples):
  - Inadequate intake: breastfeeding difficulty, incorrect formula preparation, poor transition to food (6 to 12 months), poor feeding habits (e.g., excess juice, restrictive diet), mechanical problems (e.g., oromotor dysfunction, congenital anomalies, GERD, CNS, or PNS anomalies), oral aversion, poverty, neglect/abuse, poor parent–child interaction, caregiver feeding style
  - Inadequate absorption: necrotizing enterocolitis, short gut syndrome, biliary atresia, liver disease, cystic fibrosis, celiac disease, milk protein allergy, vitamin/mineral deficiency, environmental enteric dysfunction
  - Increased expenditure: hyperthyroidism, congenital/chronic cardiopulmonary disease, HIV, immunodeficiencies, malignancy, renal disease, obstructive sleep apnea
  - Defective utilization: metabolic disorders, congenital infections (TORCH: toxoplasmosis, other agents, rubella, cytomegalovirus, herpes simplex)

RISK FACTORS

- Psychosocial risks (1)
  - Poverty, parent(s) with mental health disorder or cognitive impairment, ineffective parenting skills or hypervigilant parents, families with unique health/nutritional beliefs, physical or emotional abuse, substance abuse, social isolation
- Medical risks (1)
  - Intrauterine exposures, history of IUGR, congenital abnormalities, oromotor dysfunction, premature or sick newborn, infant with physical deformity, acute or chronic medical conditions, developmental delay, lead poisoning, anemia

GENERAL PREVENTION

- Educate parents on normal feeding and parenting skills.
- Access to supplemental feeding programs (Women, Infants, and Children [WIC])

DIAGNOSIS

HISTORY

- Successful treatment of FTT is almost always accomplished by a careful and detailed history because most cases are due to underfeeding or inappropriate feeding.
- Prenatal and developmental history/prenatal exposures
- Past medical history: acute/chronic disease affecting caloric intake, digestion, absorption, or causing increased energy need or defective utilization
- Medication history, including complementary and alternative medications
- Family history: stature of parents and growth trajectories of siblings, chronic diseases, genetic disorders, developmental delay, consanguinity
- Diet history from birth: breast/formula feeding; timing and introduction of solids; who feeds the child, when, and how often; placement of child during feeds; amounts consumed/caloric intake; beverages consumed; snacking; vomiting or stooling associated with feeds; oral aversions or unusual behaviors during feeding
- Social history: family composition, socioeconomic status, hygiene practices, child-rearing beliefs, stressors, parental depression, parental substance abuse, caretaker personal history of abuse/neglect
- Review of systems: anorexia, activity level, mental status, fevers, dysphagia, vomiting, gastroesophageal reflux, stool pattern/consistency, dysuria, urinary frequency

PHYSICAL EXAM

- A combination of anthropometric criteria, rather than one criterion, should be used.
- In addition to percentiles for growth measurement, Z-score should be calculated to assess how far a child's measurements deviate from expected mean; a negative score implies malnutrition
- Accurate measurement of height, weight, and head circumference from the National Center for Health Statistics (NCHS) (https://www.cdc.gov/growthcharts/)
- The World Health Organization (WHO) growth charts may be more appropriate for breastfed infants (http://www.who.int/childgrowth/standards/en/).
- Exam should assess for the following:
  - Signs of dehydration or severe malnutrition
    - Severity of malnutrition estimated via Gomez classification: Compare current weight for age with expected weight for age (50th percentile): severe, <60% of expected; moderate, 61–75%; mild, 76–90%
  - Dysmorphic features
  - Mental status (alert, responsive to stimuli)
  - Any signs of physical abuse and neglect
- Observe interaction with caregivers and feeding techniques, specifically bonding and social/psychological cues.

DIFFERENTIAL DIAGNOSIS

Differentiate based on growth patterns.

- FTT classically is low weight for age, with normal linear growth and head circumference *or* low weight for age, followed by decreased linear growth *or* low weight for age, leading to decreased linear growth and decreased head circumference (without neurologic signs).
- If low linear growth with normal weight for length *or* low linear growth and proportionately low weight and decreased head circumference:
  - Consider genetic potential (constitutional short stature or growth delay), genetic syndromes, teratogens, and endocrine disorders.
- If microcephaly with prominent neurologic signs, with poor growth secondary to presumed neurologic disorder:
  - Consider TORCH infections, genetic syndromes, teratogens, and brain injury (i.e., hypoxic/ischemic).

DIAGNOSTIC TESTS & INTERPRETATION

- Labs useful only in ~1% of cases and generally not recommended
- A period of addressing nutritional causes preferred prior to extensive labs or other workup

Initial Tests (lab, imaging)

- Tests considered in initial evaluation:
  - CBC with differential, ESR, lead level
  - Electrolytes, BUN/creatinine, liver function tests, TSH, free T4, glucose
  - Urinalysis and urine culture
- Other tests as dictated by history and exam:
  - Amylase/lipase, serum zinc level, iron studies, IGF-1, karyotype, genetic testing, sweat chloride test, stool for ova and parasite or fat/reducing substances, guaiac, α_1-antitrypsin and elastase, radioallergosorbent test for IgE food allergies, tissue transglutaminase and total IgA (celiac sprue), p-ANCA and fecal calprotectin (for inflammatory bowel disease), TB test, HIV, hepatitis A and B, other infections
  - X-ray of hand/wrist to assess bone age and for skeletal dysplasia

Follow-Up Tests & Special Considerations

- Prospective 3-day food diary for accurate record of caloric intake should be obtained.
- Home visit by a clinician to observe infant feeding, interaction of caretakers, and home environment
- Observe breastfeeding and/or formula preparation to ensure adequacy and offer instruction.

Diagnostic Procedures/Other

Can consider

- Skeletal survey if suspicion of physical abuse
- Bone age if possible endocrine disorder/ constitutional growth delay
- Swallow study, small bowel follow-through if possible oromotor dysfunction, GERD, structural abnormalities
- Brain imaging if microcephalic or neurologic findings on examination
- Echocardiogram if murmur auscultated

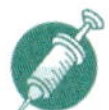

TREATMENT

GENERAL MEASURES

- Caregiver and infant interaction should be evaluated in infants and children with FTT.
- Age-appropriate nutritional counseling should be provided.
  - The goal is to improve nutrition to allow catch-up growth (weight gain 2 to 3 times > average for age).
- Calculate energy needs based on recommended energy intake for age and then increase by 50%.
- Alternatively, may calculate caloric requirements for infants to achieve catch-up growth
  - kcal/kg/day required = RDA for age (kcal/kg) × ideal weight for height/actual weight, where ideal weight for height is the median weight for the patient's height.
- Try various strategies to increase caloric intake, such as the following:
  - Optimize breastfeeding support; consider supplementation.
  - Higher calorie formulas
  - Addition of rice cereal or fats to current foods
  - Limit intake of milk to 24 to 32 oz/day.
  - Avoid juice/soda.
  - Vitamin and/or nutritional supplements
  - Take into account cultural differences in food preparation.
  - Assist with social determinants of health and offer referrals to address poverty/food insecurity (WIC, food stamps, and other transitional assistance).
- Rapid high-calorie intake can cause diarrhea, malabsorption, hypokalemia, and hypophosphatemia. Therefore, increasing formulas >24 kcal/oz is not recommended.
- The target energy intake should be slowly increased to goal over 5 to 7 days.
- Catch-up growth should be seen in 2 to 7 days.
- Accelerated growth should be continued for 4 to 9 months to restore weight and height.
- Consider visiting nurse referral, early childhood intervention referral, and social services evaluation.

MEDICATION

No specific medication recommended

ISSUES FOR REFERRAL

Multidisciplinary clinics may be of benefit for children with complicated situations, failure to respond to initial treatment, or when the PCP does not have access to specialized services such as nutrition, psychology, PT/OT, and speech therapy.

SURGERY/OTHER PROCEDURES

In severe cases, nasogastric tube feedings/gastrostomy considered.

ADMISSION, INPATIENT, AND NURSING CONSIDERATIONS

- Hospitalization should be considered if:
  - Outpatient management fails.
  - There is evidence of severe dehydration or malnutrition.
  - There are signs of abuse or neglect.
  - There are concerns that the psychosocial situation presents harm to child.
  - During catch-up growth, some children will develop nutritional recovery syndrome:
    - Symptoms include sweating, increased body temperature, hepatomegaly (increased glycogen deposits), widening of cranial sutures (brain growth > bone growth), increased periods of sleep, fidgetiness, and mild hyperactivity.
  - There may also be an initial period of malabsorption with resultant diarrhea.
- Catch-up growth should be seen in 2 to 7 days. If this is not seen, reevaluate cause.

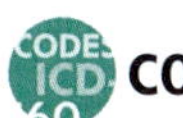

ONGOING CARE

FOLLOW-UP RECOMMENDATIONS

- Close (every 2 to 4 weeks at first, then 1 to 2 months if improving); long-term follow-up with frequent visits
- Children with history of FTT are at increased risk of recurrent FTT.
- If the family fails to comply, notify child protection authorities.

DIET

Nutritional requirements for a "normal" child:

- Infant
  - 120 kcal/kg/day, decreased to 95 kcal/kg/day at 6 months; if breastfed, ensure appropriate frequency and duration of feeding
  - Between 6 to 12 months continue same amount of breast milk and/or formula, with puréed foods consumed several times a day.
- Toddler
  - Three meals plus two nutritional snacks, 16 to 32 oz of whole milk per day; stop all juice/soda; feed in a social environment.
- Rate of weight gain expected for age:
  - 0 to 3 months: 26 to 31 g/day
  - 3 to 6 months: 17 to 18 g/day
  - 6 to 9 months: 12 to 13 g/day
  - 9 to 12 months: 9 g/day
  - 1 to 3 years: 7 to 9 g/day

PATIENT EDUCATION

- Counsel parents regarding need to avoid "food battles," which can worsen the problem.
- Educate parents regarding infant social and physiologic cues, formula/food preparation, proper feeding techniques, and importance of relaxed and social mealtimes.
- "Failure to thrive: What this means for your child," available from AAFP at: https://www.aafp.org/afp/2011/0401/p837.html
- WIC provides grants to states for supplemental foods, health care referrals, and nutrition education for low-income pregnant, breastfeeding, and nonbreastfeeding postpartum women and to infants and children up to age 5 years at nutritional risk: https://www.fns.usda.gov/wic/women-infants-and-children-wic

PROGNOSIS

- Most show improvement in dietary intake with intervention (1)[B].
- Children with FTT are at increased risk for future undernutrition, overnutrition, and eating disorders.

COMPLICATIONS

- Complications can be related to underlying cause, thus identifying and treating growth failure early is important.
- Developmental delays, behavioral problems, problems in school, and shorter stature later in life are potential complications.

REFERENCES

1. Black MM, Tilton N, Bento S, et al. Recovery in young children with weight faltering: child and household risk factors. *J Pediatr*. 2016;170:301–306.

CODES

ICD10

- R62.7 Adult failure to thrive
- R62.51 Failure to thrive (child)
- P92.6 Failure to thrive in newborn

CLINICAL PEARLS

- FTT is a sign of inadequate nutrition. It is rarely due to a medical condition.
- Medical and/or social issues are suggested by history and physical exam; extensive lab or imaging tests rarely needed
- A multidisciplinary team approach for treatment is critical to help children with FTT.

FEVER OF UNKNOWN ORIGIN (FUO)

Alexandra Renee Zaballa, MD • Jenny T. Giang-Griesser, MD

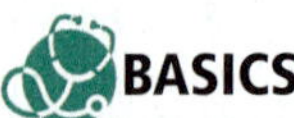

BASICS

DESCRIPTION

- Classic definition
  - Repeated fever >38.3°C (>100.9°F)
  - Fever duration >3 weeks in adults or ≥8 days among children.
  - Diagnosis remains uncertain despite thorough inpatient or outpatient evaluation (1).
- Categories of fever of unknown origin (FUO): infection, malignancy, noninfectious inflammatory diseases (rheumatologic or connective tissue disease), miscellaneous disease, and undiagnosed illness
- Often an atypical presentation of a common disease versus a rare disease; 75% of cases resolve without reaching a definitive diagnosis.

EPIDEMIOLOGY

Incidence

The exact incidence is not known.

Prevalence

The definition of fever with unresolved cause (true FUO) is difficult, as it is a moving target, given the constant advancement of imaging and biomarker analysis. Therefore, the prevalence of FUO is unknown.

ETIOLOGY AND PATHOPHYSIOLOGY

- True FUO are uncommon; most frequently, FUO is an atypical presentation of a common condition.
- Spectrum of causes varies widely:
  - Higher percentage of infectious causes in developing countries compared to developed countries.
  - Although infection is the most common cause of FUO in developed countries, there is a higher incidence of noninfectious inflammatory disease when compared to developing countries.
- Infection
  - Abdominal or pelvic abscesses; amebic hepatitis
  - Catheter-associated infections
  - Dental abscesses
  - Endocarditis/pericarditis
  - HIV (acute and/or advanced stage)
  - Mycobacterial infection (often with advanced HIV)
  - Osteomyelitis
  - Prostatitis
  - Pyelonephritis or renal abscess
  - Sinusitis
  - Tuberculosis
  - Other pathogens (brucellosis, cytomegalovirus, disseminated fungal infections, enteric fever, Epstein-Barr virus, malaria, toxoplasmosis)
  - Wound infections
  - Other miscellaneous infections
- Neoplasms
  - Atrial myxoma
  - Colorectal cancer and other GI malignancies
  - Hepatoma
  - Lymphoproliferative diseases (e.g., lymphoma; leukemia)
  - Myelodysplastic syndromes
  - Multiple myeloma
  - Solid tumors (e.g., renal cell carcinoma, neuroblastoma, sarcomas)
- Noninfectious inflammatory disease
  - Autoimmune/connective tissue diseases
    - Adult still disease
    - Juvenile idiopathic arthritis (JIA)
    - Rheumatoid arthritis
    - Systemic lupus erythematosus
  - Granulomatous disease
    - Crohn disease
    - Granulomatosis with polyangiitis (GPA)
    - Sarcoidosis
  - Vasculitis syndromes
    - Antiphospholipid syndrome
    - Giant cell arteritis
    - Kawasaki disease
    - Panarteritis nodosa (PAN)
    - Polymyalgia rheumatica
- Other causes
  - Alcoholic hepatitis
  - Castleman syndrome
  - Cerebrovascular accident
  - Cirrhosis
  - Medications
    - Allopurinol, captopril, carbamazepine, cephalosporins, cimetidine, clofibrate, erythromycin, heparin, hydralazine, hydrochlorothiazide, isoniazid, meperidine, methyldopa, nifedipine, nitrofurantoin, penicillin, phenytoin, procainamide, quinidine, sulfonamides
    - Medication reactions include hypersensitivity, serotonin syndrome, adrenergic fever, neuroleptic malignant syndrome, malignant hyperthermia, anticholinergic fever, DRESS syndrome, chemotherapy/infusion-related reaction, mitochondrial uncoupling (pesticides/toxins) (1).
  - Endocrine disease
  - Familial Mediterranean fever
  - Factitious/fraudulent fever
  - Occupational causes
  - Periodic fever
  - Pulmonary emboli/deep vein thrombosis
  - Sarcoidosis
  - Thermoregulatory disorders
  - Thyroid disease
- In up to 20–30% of cases, the cause of the fever is never identified despite a thorough workup.

RISK FACTORS

- Travel (e.g., malaria, enteric fevers, tick-borne illness) and immigration
- Exposure to biologic or chemical agents
- HIV infection (particularly in acute infection and advanced stages)
- Elderly
- History of substance use,

Geriatric Considerations

In geriatric populations aged >65 years, noninfectious multisystem diseases, such as polymyalgia rheumatica, giant cell arteritis, and other vasculitides have a higher incidence than infection. Common infectious causes in the elderly are intra-abdominal abscess, urinary tract infections, tuberculosis, and endocarditis. Other common causes of FUO in patients aged >65 years include malignancies (particularly hematologic cancers) and drug-induced fever.

Pediatric Considerations

- 1/3 are self-limited undefined viral syndromes. 1/2 of FUO in pediatric cases are infectious. Collagen vascular disease and malignancy are the next most common. Inflammatory bowel disease is a more common cause of FUO in older children and adolescents.
- If the child is well-appearing, outpatient observation with serial evaluations and monitoring is reasonable.
- In ill-appearing children, admission in indicated for closer monitoring, expedited evaluation, and supportive therapies.

DIAGNOSIS

The initial approach should include a comprehensive history and physical examination, as well as laboratory testing. The decision of what further testing should be gathered should be guided by the resulting information (2).

HISTORY

- Onset and pattern of fever
- Constitutional symptoms:
  - Chills, night sweats, myalgias, weight loss with an intact appetite (infectious etiology)
  - Arthralgias, myalgias, fatigue (inflammatory etiology)
  - Fatigue, night sweats, weight loss with loss of appetite (neoplastic etiology)
- Past medical history: chronic infections, abdominal diseases, transfusion history, malignancy, psychiatric illness, and recent hospitalization
- Past surgical history: type of surgery performed, postoperative complications, and any indwelling foreign material
- Comprehensive medication history, including over-the-counter and herbal products
- Family history, such as, hereditary causes, periodic fever syndromes and recent febrile illnesses in close contacts
- Social history: travel, animal exposure (e.g., pets, exotic animals, occupational, farms), dietary habits, living environment, sexual activity, sick contacts, recreational or illicit drug use, homelessness, incarceration

ALERT

Obtain a thorough travel, psychosocial, occupational, sexual, medication, and recreational drug use history.

PHYSICAL EXAM

- Vital signs: Temperature, heart rate, blood pressure, and height/weight measurements particularly in comparison to previous measurements can point to certain etiologies.
- Physical findings with high diagnostic yield generally involve skin, eyes, lymph nodes, liver and spleen. Helpful clues can be found with:
  - Funduscopic exam for choroid tubercles or Roth spots
  - Temporal artery tenderness
  - Oral-mucosal lesions
  - Cardiac auscultation for bruits and murmurs
  - Pulmonary exam: consolidation or effusion
  - Abdominal palpation for masses or organomegaly and tenderness or peritoneal signs
  - Rectal examination for blood, fluctuance, and/or tenderness
  - Testicular examination
  - Lymph node examination for evolving lymphadenopathy
  - Skin and nail bed exam for rashes, clubbing, nodules, lesions, and erosions
  - Focal neurologic signs
  - Musculoskeletal exam for tenderness or effusion
  - Serial exams help identify evolving physical signs (e.g., findings associated with endocarditis).

DIAGNOSTIC TESTS & INTERPRETATION

Thorough history and examination typically guides ordered tests and imaging.

Initial Tests (lab, imaging)

- CBC, C-reactive protein, ESR, PCT, ANA, peripheral blood smear, ferritin
- Comprehensive metabolic panel (electrolytes, BUN, creatinine, LFTs), calcium, lactate dehydrogenase, creatine phosphokinase
- Heterophile antibody testing
- Hepatitis, RPR, and HIV testing
- ≥2 blood cultures drawn from different sites, within hours, without administering antibiotics
- Urinalysis and urine culture
- Chest x-ray, ultrasound (US)/CT/MRI of abdomen and pelvis (with directed biopsy, if indicated)

Follow-Up Tests & Special Considerations

- Rheumatoid factor and antinuclear antibody test
- Serologies: Epstein-Barr, Lyme disease, Q fever, cytomegalovirus, brucellosis, amebiasis, coccidioidomycosis, histoplasmosis
- Serum ferritin; serum protein electrophoresis
- TB testing
  - Tuberculin skin test
    - May not be helpful if anergic or acute infection
    - If test negative, repeat in 2 weeks.
  - Interferon-γ release assay (IGRA)
    - Preferred in those likely to be infected with TB and/or who are BCG-vaccinated
  - AFB smear; sputum and urine cultures for TB
- Thyroid function tests
- Technetium-based scan (Infection tumor)
- FDG-PET/CT scan if infectious process, inflammatory process, or tumor suspected; PET scans have a high negative predictive value and good sensitivity (but may have false positives).
- US of abdomen and pelvis (with directed biopsy, if indicated) if renal obstruction or biliary pathology suspected
- Echocardiogram if endocarditis, atrial myxomas, or pericardial effusion is suspected
- Lower extremity Doppler if deep vein thrombosis/pulmonary embolism suspected
- CT scan of chest if pulmonary embolism suspected
- Indium-labeled leukocyte scanning if inflammatory process or occult abscess suspected
- Bone scan if osteomyelitis or metastatic disease suspected

Diagnostic Procedures/Other

- Liver biopsy if granulomatous disease suspected
- Temporal artery biopsy, particularly in the elderly
- Lymph node, muscle, or skin biopsy, if clinically indicated
- Bone marrow aspiration biopsy with smear, culture, histologic examination, and flow cytometry
- Lumbar puncture, if clinically indicated
- Endoscopy procedures can be helpful for IBD or sarcoidosis.

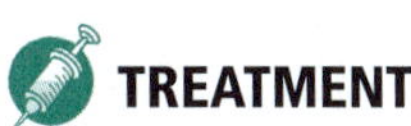

TREATMENT

GENERAL MEASURES

- Treatment depends on the specific etiology.
- Consider discontinuation of recently started or potentially offending medications.
- Empiric therapy is not recommended in patients with prolonged fever, because it may camouflage and therefore delay diagnosis, and subsequently also hamper correct treatment decisions (3).
- Therapeutic trials are a last resort and should be as specific as possible based on available clinical evidence. Avoid "shotgun" approaches because they obscure the clinical picture, have untoward effects, and do not provide a diagnostic solution.
- Empiric therapy is prudent in a few difficult-to-diagnose life-threatening cases, for example, CNS or miliary tuberculosis, or giant cell arteritis/temporal arteritis.

MEDICATION

First Line

- Antipyretic therapy as a symptomatic approach is a special form of empiric therapy, as it does not necessarily require understanding the cause of fever.
- First-line drugs depend on the diagnosis.
- Evidence does not support isolated treatment of fever.

Second Line

Consider a therapeutic trial only if the patient has localizing symptoms associated with the fever or continues to decline. Consultation with appropriate specialists (infectious disease, rheumatology) is recommended in this case (3).

- Antibiotic trial based on patient's history and suspected culture negative endocarditis
- Antituberculous therapy if there is a high risk for TB pending definitive culture results
- Corticosteroid trial based on patient's history (once occult malignancy is ruled out) if temporal arteritis is suspected

ALERT

- Empiric antibiotic therapy has not been shown to be effective unless the patient is neutropenic, immunocompromised, or critically ill (2).
- If a steroid trial is initiated, patient may have a relapse after treatment or if certain conditions (e.g., TB) have been undiagnosed.

ADDITIONAL THERAPIES

Febrile patients have increased caloric and fluid demands.

SURGERY/OTHER PROCEDURES

The need for exploratory laparotomy has been largely eliminated with the advent of more sophisticated tests and imaging modalities.

ADMISSION, INPATIENT, AND NURSING CONSIDERATIONS

- Reserved for the ill and debilitated
- Consider if factitious fever has been ruled out or an invasive procedure is indicated.

ONGOING CARE

FOLLOW-UP RECOMMENDATIONS

Patient Monitoring

If the etiology of the fever remains unknown, repeat the history, physical exam, and screening lab studies.

DIET

No specific dietary recommendations have been shown to ameliorate undiagnosed fever.

PATIENT EDUCATION

Maintain an open line of communication between physician and patient/family as the workup progresses:

- The extended time required in establishing a diagnosis can be frustrating.

PROGNOSIS

- Depends on etiology, age, and time to diagnosis
  - Patients with HIV have the highest mortality.
- Spontaneous remission is not uncommon in patients with unknown cause of FUO after a thorough workup including a negative FDG-PET/CT scan
- 1-year survival rates (reflecting deaths due to all causes)
  - <35 years of age is 91%, 35 to 64 years of age is 82%, >64 years of age is 67%

COMPLICATIONS

Pregnancy Considerations

Fever increases the risk of neural tube defects in pregnancy and can also trigger preterm labor.

REFERENCES

1. Antoniadou C, Gavriilidis E, Chatzopoulos P, et al. Fever and inflammation of unknown origin in the 21st century. *Eur J Intern Med*. 2025;142:106443. doi:10.1016/j.ejim.2025.106443.
2. Xie N, Zhang W, Tian F, et al. Fever of unknown origin: clinical significance of the etiology and common inflammatory parameters. *Diagn Microbiol Infect Dis*. 2025;112(3):116801. doi:10.1016/j.diagmicrobio.2025.116801.
3. Trapani S, Fiordelisi A, Stinco M, et al. Update on fever of unknown origin in children: focus on etiologies and clinical approach. *Children (Basel)*. 2023;11(1):20.

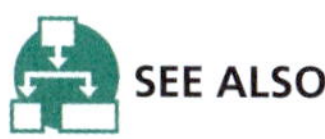

SEE ALSO

Algorithms: Fever in First 60 Days of Life; Fever of Unknown Origin (FUO)

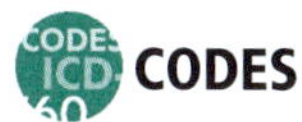

CODES

ICD10

R50.9 Fever, unspecified

CLINICAL PEARLS

- A sequential approach to FUO based on a careful history, physical examination, with targeted testing and imaging typically yields an appropriate diagnosis and avoids excessive nontargeted testing. With repeat examination and questioning, causes often become clear over time.
- Empiric therapy is indicated only for carefully defined circumstances.
- FUO cases that defy precise diagnosis after intensive investigation and prolonged observation generally have a favorable prognosis.
- FUO in older persons often presents as an atypical presentation of a common disease.
- The most common causes of FUO in high-income countries are noninfectious inflammatory diseases and idiopathic causes.

FIBROCYSTIC CHANGES OF THE BREAST

Sharon Koehler, DO, FACS

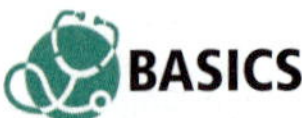

BASICS

Fibrocystic changes (FCC) of the breast are commonly described as benign breast lesions. Often, the role of the clinician is to rule out other more worrisome findings. These findings generally affect premenopausal women and require no specific treatment.

DESCRIPTION

- Benign epithelial lesions are common findings in women and can be divided into nonproliferative and proliferative and with and without atypia.
- FCC are not a disease but refers to a group of benign, nonproliferative histologic findings. It is the most frequent female benign epithelial lesion.
- FCC are seen clinically in up to 50% and histologically in up to 90% of women.
- FCC may also be described as aberrations of normal development and evolution.
- The most common symptoms are cyclic pain, tenderness, swelling, and fullness.
- The breast tissue may feel dense with areas of thicker tissue having an irregular, nodular, or ridge-like surface.
- Women may experience sensitivity to touch with a burning sensation. For some, the pain is so severe that it limits exercise or the ability to lie prone.
- Sensitivity often associated with monthly hormonal fluctuations.
- Histologically, FCC may contain solid elements including adenosis, sclerosis, apocrine metaplasia, stromal fibrosis, and epithelial metaplasia and hyperplasia.
  - Depending on the presence of epithelial hyperplasia, FCC is classified as nonproliferative, proliferative without atypia, or proliferative with atypia (1).
  - Nonproliferative lesions are generally not associated with an increased risk of breast cancer.
- System(s) affected: endocrine/metabolic, reproductive
- Synonym(s): diffuse cystic mastopathy; fibrocystic disease; chronic cystic mastitis; or mammary dysplasia

EPIDEMIOLOGY

FCC occurs with great frequency in the general population. It affects women between the ages of 25 and 50 years, and it is rare below the age of 20 years.

Incidence

Unknown but very frequent

Prevalence

Up to 1/3 of women aged 30 to 50 years have cysts in their breasts (1). It most commonly presents in the 3rd decade, peaks in the 4th decade when hormonal function is at its peak, and sharply diminishes after menopause. With hormone replacement therapy, FCC may extend into menopause.

ETIOLOGY AND PATHOPHYSIOLOGY

- FCC originates from an exaggerated response of breast stroma and epithelium to a variety of circulating and locally produced hormones (mainly estrogen and progesterone) and growth factors.
- Cysts may form due to dilatation of the lobular acini possibly due to imbalance of fluid secretion and resorption or due to obstruction of the duct leading to the lobule.

Genetics

No known genetic risk factors are defined but there are familial tendencies.

RISK FACTORS

- In many women, methylxanthine-containing substances (e.g., coffee, tea, cola, and chocolate) can potentiate symptoms of FCC, although a direct causality has not been established.
- Diet high in saturated fats may increase risk of FCC.

COMMONLY ASSOCIATED CONDITIONS

FCC categorized as proliferative with atypia confers a higher risk of breast cancer.

DIAGNOSIS

HISTORY

- Obtain personal history of breast biopsy and family history of breast disease (benign or malignant).
- Determine (if known) if there is a family history of deleterious mutations: *BRCA1, BRCA2, PALB2, CHEK2, CDH1, PTEN, STK11, PT53, ATM, BARD1, BRIP1, CASP8, CTLA4, CYP19A1, FGFR2, H19, LSP1, MAP3K1, MRE11A, NBN, RAD51*, and *TERT*.
- Inquire regarding pertinent signs/symptoms, such as breast pain, swelling, nipple discharge, palpable lumps, retractions, skin changes, and tenderness. Symptomatically, the condition is manifested as premenstrual cyclic mastalgia, with pain and tenderness to touch.

PHYSICAL EXAM

- The patient should be examined in the following positions while disrobed down to the waist:
  - With the patient standing with arms at sides, observe for elevation of the level of a nipple, dimpling, bulging, and peau d'orange.
  - With the patient's arms raised above her head, observe for dimpling and elevation/retraction of the nipple (may accentuate a mass fixed to the pectoral fascia). If so, have the patient push her hands down against her hips to flex and tense the pectoralis major muscles; move the mass to determine fixation to the underlying fascia.
  - If the patient has large and pendulous breasts, ask her to lean forward, so that her breasts hang free from the chest wall (retraction and masses may become more evident).
  - Axillary lymph nodes are evaluated with the patient sitting up, the arm supported by the examiner's arm while finger pads gently palpate the axilla from the posterior axillary line to the pectoralis.
  - With the patient lying supine, palpate with the pads of the three middle fingers (with varying pressures from light, to medium, to deep), rotating the fingers in small circular motions and moving in vertical overlapping passes from rostral to caudal and then back caudal to rostral in the next pass. The entire breast from the 2nd to 6th rib and from the left sternal border to the midaxillary line must be palpated against the chest wall.
- Be certain to examine the creases under and between the breasts. If the patient has noted a lump, ask her to point it out; always palpate the opposite breast first.
- Patients with FCC have clinical breast findings that range from mild alterations in texture to dense, firm breast tissue with palpable masses.

DIFFERENTIAL DIAGNOSIS

- Pain
  - Mastitis
  - Costochondritis
  - Pectoralis muscle strain
  - Neuralgia
  - Breast cancer
  - Angina pectoris
  - Gastroesophageal reflux disease (GERD)
  - Superficial phlebitis of the thoracoepigastric vein (Mondor disease)
- Masses
  - Breast cancer
  - Sebaceous cyst
  - Fibroadenoma
  - Lipoma
  - Fat necrosis
  - Phyllodes tumor
  - Granuloma
- Skin changes
  - Breast cancer (peau d'orange: thickened skin similar to peel of an orange)
  - Eczema
  - Infection
  - Fungus
  - Paget disease

DIAGNOSTIC TESTS & INTERPRETATION

- Evaluation should focus on excluding breast cancer.
- Testing may be conducted based on a level of clinical suspicion.
- FCC can be evaluated with mammogram, although dense breast tissue may appear normal in women <35 years of age.
- Ultrasound (US) is the most useful method for assessing a cyst.

Initial Tests (lab, imaging)

- On mammogram, FCC appears as nodular densities of breast tissue; solitary cysts can appear as round or ovoid or well-circumscribed masses, usually with low to intermediate density. FCC may also contain calcifications.
- On US, if a simple cyst is demonstrated as an anechoic structure with imperceptible wall and posterior acoustic enhancement, benign diagnosis is confirmed and no further imaging or intervention is indicated.
- MRI is indicated in patients with *BRCA1*, *BRCA2*, or other related deleterious mutation, or in any woman with ≥25% lifetime risk for breast cancer. Additionally, MRI may be indicated for extremely dense breasts as well as inconclusive findings on other breast imaging.
- On MRI, cystic changes are well-circumscribed lesions of high-signal intensity on T2-weighted sequences and of low-signal intensity on T1-weighted images (1).

Diagnostic Procedures/Other
- Fine-needle aspiration (FNA) biopsy:
  - Allows differentiation of cystic and solid lesions
  - Aspirate may be straw-colored, dark brown, or green.
  - Cells sent for cytology can reveal cancer with high accuracy.
  - Low morbidity
- If the lesion disappears, no further evaluation is necessary (including cytologic evaluation of aspirated fluid).
- On the basis of the presence and degree of epithelial hyperplasia, FCC is comprised of nonproliferative (approximately 65% of the total), proliferative without atypia (approximately 30% of the total), and proliferative with atypia (approximately 5–8% of the total) (2).

Test Interpretation
Certain histologic changes in the setting of FCC confer an increased risk for breast cancer:
- Nonproliferative changes: relative risk of 1.2 to 1.4
- Proliferative disease (PD) without atypia: relative risk of 1.7 to 2.1
- PD with atypia: relative risk ≥4

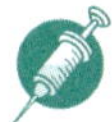

TREATMENT
- After ruling out malignancy by means of examination and/or imaging and diagnostic procedures, FCC may not require treatment and often resolves with time.
- Cool compresses, avoiding trauma, and around-the-clock wearing of a well-fitting, supportive brassiere may be useful for symptom relief.
- Reduction in caffeine, additional supplementation with vitamin E, and/or evening primrose oil have been advocated. Trials have not proven benefit (1).

MEDICATION
First Line
Analgesics and anti-inflammatory drugs are used to reduce cyclic breast pain and swelling. This includes oral and topical NSAIDs or acetaminophen.
- Acetaminophen: 1,000 mg every 6 to 8 hours; maximum daily dose of 3,000 mg unless directed by health care provider
- Ibuprofen: 400 mg every 4 to 6 hours as needed
- Naproxen: 500 mg every 12 hours as needed

Second Line
- Oral contraceptives (OCPs) may be useful in modulating symptoms or in preventing the development of new changes in females with cyclic symptoms.
- For severe pain, consider the following (3)[A]:
  - Danazol is effective for reducing breast pain and tenderness but has androgenic effects and is associated with hepatotoxicity and teratogenicity, which limits its use. This drug is administered orally at a dosage of 100 to 400 mg/day in 2 divided doses.
  - Tamoxifen 10 mg/day for 3 to 6 months; along with teratogenicity, this selective estrogen receptor modulator (SERM) can increase the risk of thromboembolism and endometrial carcinoma in treated females.
  - Several other medications, such as bromocriptine and GnRH agonists have been studied, but are associated with toxicities.

ISSUES FOR REFERRAL
- If discrete palpable lesion in a woman aged <30 years: US, then consider referral to a breast surgeon, especially if not a simple cyst/lesion resolving at follow-up in a different phase of menstrual cycle
- If discrete palpable lesion in a woman aged >30 years: diagnostic mammography ± US, and refer to a breast surgeon

SURGERY/OTHER PROCEDURES
- Breast cyst aspiration can be both diagnostic and therapeutic.
- Core-needle biopsies performed under stereotactic guidance with vacuum assistance has similar accuracy in distinguishing between malignant and benign lesions compared to open surgical biopsy (4)[A].
- Biopsy results must be assessed for concordance.

COMPLEMENTARY & ALTERNATIVE MEDICINE
- The use of vitamin E has shown effectiveness in treating breast pain due to FCC.
- Anecdotal evidence supports the use of evening primrose oil for FCC.

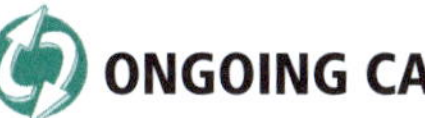

ONGOING CARE

FOLLOW-UP RECOMMENDATIONS
Condition is benign, chronic, and recurrent.

Patient Monitoring
- Follow-up times are variable, depending on the clinical situation and pertinent family history.
- US is useful to differentiate cysts from solid lesions and in evaluating women <35 years of age for FCC but is not useful for screening.
- Screening mammograms: Refer to the USPSTF, ACOG, or ACS recommendations for screening schedules.

DIET
The role of caffeine consumption in the development and treatment of FCC has never been proven; however, some patients report relief of symptoms after abstinence from coffee, tea, and chocolate.

PATIENT EDUCATION
- Patient information on fibrocystic breasts from the Mayo Foundation for Medical Education and Research: http://www.mayoclinic.com/health/fibrocystic-breasts/DS01070
- Information on breast cancer prevention from the National Cancer Institute: https://www.cancer.gov/
- Information on fibrocystic breasts from the American Cancer Society: https://www.cancer.org/cancer/types/breast-cancer/non-cancerous-breast-conditions/fibrosis-and-simple-cysts-in-the-breast.html

PROGNOSIS
Prognosis is generally excellent and symptoms tend to resolve after menopause.

REFERENCES

1. Pearlman M, Griffin J, Swain M, et al; for American College of Obstetricians and Gynecologists' Committee on Practice Bulletins—Gynecology. Practice bulletin no. 164: diagnosis and management of benign breast disorders. *Obstet Gynecol*. 2016;127(6):e141–e156.
2. Hartmann LC, Sellers TA, Frost MH, et al. Benign breast disease and the risk of breast cancer. *N Engl J Med*. 2005;353(3):229–237.
3. Srivastava A, Mansel RE, Arvind N, et al. Evidence-based management of mastalgia: a meta-analysis of randomised trials. *Breast*. 2007;16(5):503–512.
4. Bruening W, Fontanarosa J, Tipton K, et al. Systematic review: comparative effectiveness of core-needle and open surgical biopsy to diagnose breast lesions. *Ann Intern Med*. 2010;152(4):238–246.

ADDITIONAL READING

- Ali AA, Faraj FH. Clinicopathological profile of mastalgia in females: incidence, types, and pathological correlations. a cross-sectional study. *Ann Med Surg (Lond)*. 2023;85(10):4764–4772. doi:10.1097/MS9.0000000000001159.
- Hafiz SP, Barnes NLP, Kirwan CC. Clinical management of idiopathic mastalgia: a systematic review. *J Prim Health Care*. 2018;10(4):312–323.
- Salzman B, Collins E, Hersh L. Common breast problems. *Am Fam Physician*. 2019;99(8):505–514.

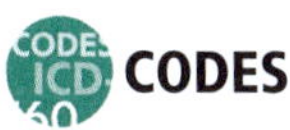

CODES

ICD10
- N60.19 Diffuse cystic mastopathy of unspecified breast
- N60.09 Solitary cyst of unspecified breast
- N60.29 Fibroadenosis of unspecified breast

CLINICAL PEARLS
- FCC of the breast comprise a spectrum of histopathologic changes are a common finding in reproductive-aged women. The former term of fibrocystic disease is a misnomer.
- Atypia, as demonstrated histopathologically, confers an increased cancer risk and may require additional diagnostic workup.
- NSAIDs are the first-line treatment.
- OCPs, danazol, and tamoxifen are second-line treatments, the latter two with considerable adverse effects.
- Consultation with a breast specialist is recommended for symptomatic disease refractory to simple measures or for diagnostic issues.

FIBROMYALGIA

Frederic Stuart Leeds, MD, MS, FAAFP

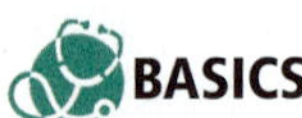

BASICS

DESCRIPTION

- Chronic, widespread noninflammatory musculoskeletal pain syndrome with multisystem manifestations; although the specific pathophysiology has not been fully elucidated, it is generally thought to be a disorder of altered "pain gating."
- Synonym(s): FMS; fibrositis, fibromyositis (misnomers)

EPIDEMIOLOGY

Incidence

- Predominant sex: female (70–90%) > male
- Predominant age range: 20 to 65 years

Prevalence

2–5% of adult U.S. population; 8% of primary care patients

ETIOLOGY AND PATHOPHYSIOLOGY

- Fibromyalgia is a primary pain disorder characterized by an underlying mechanism of mixed central and peripheral sensitization—resulting in pathologic sensitivity to multiple classes of noxious sensation (nociceptive, nociplastic, and neuropathic).
- Alterations in neuroendocrine, neuromodulation, neurotransmitter, neurotransporter, biochemical, and neuroreceptor function/physiology
- Sleep abnormalities—α-wave intrusion
- Systemic inflammation is not a feature of fibromyalgia, although localized immunologic and inflammatory processes in the CNS may play a role. There may be a distinctive cytokine profile in patients with fibromyalgia.

Genetics

- Genetics
  - High familial aggregation
  - Inheritance is unknown but likely polygenic.
  - Odds ratio may be as high as 8.5 for a first-degree relative of a familial proband.
- Environmental—several triggers have been described:
  - Physical trauma or severe illness
  - Stressors (e.g., work, family, life events, and physical or sexual abuse)
  - Viral and bacterial infections

RISK FACTORS

- Female gender
- Poor functional status
- Negative/stressful life events
- Low socioeconomic status

GENERAL PREVENTION

No known strategies for prevention

COMMONLY ASSOCIATED CONDITIONS

- Often a comorbid condition with other rheumatologic or neurologic disorders
- Psychiatric comorbidities, including depression, anxiety, and posttraumatic stress disorder (PTSD) occur in 2/3 of patients—similar to findings in other chronic pain conditions.
- Obesity is common and associated with increased severity of symptoms.

DIAGNOSIS

- ACR criteria, revised in 2016 (1)
  - Based on Widespread Pain Index (WPI) and Symptom Severity Scale (SSS); the WPI assesses pain in each of 19 body regions over the past week (range: 0 to 19). The SSS assesses three elements—fatigue, waking unrefreshed, and cognitive symptoms—each rated on a scale from 0 (no problem) to 3 (severe, pervasive, life-disturbing). Additionally, the SSS includes a score (0 to 3) for the extent of other somatic symptoms (such as headache, abdominal pain, depression, or irritable bowel symptoms). The total score ranges from 0 to 12.
    - Generalized pain present in 4/5 body regions; and
    - Must have WPI $\geq$7 + SS $\geq$5, or WPI 4 to 6 and SS $\geq$9; *and*
    - Symptoms for >3 months
    - Fibromyalgia may be diagnosed irrespective of other active disease entities (i.e., it need not be the only explanation for the patient's symptoms).
- The revised Fibromyalgia Impact Questionnaire (FIQr) or the simpler Visual Analogue Scale Fibromyalgia Impact Questionnaire (VASFIQ) should be used for initial and serial assessments of patient's functional status and response to therapy.

HISTORY

- Invariant symptoms include
  - Chronic widespread pain $\geq$3 months: bilateral limbs and in the axial skeleton
  - Fatigue and sleep disturbances
- Often present:
  - Mood disorders, including depression, anxiety, panic symptoms, and PTSD
  - Cognitive impairment: qualitatively different from that seen in isolated mood disorders ("fibro fog")
  - Headaches: typically tension and migraine types
  - Other regional pain syndromes, such as irritable bowel syndrome, chronic pelvic pain, vulvodynia, and interstitial cystitis
  - Small-fiber neuropathies and "nonanatomic" paresthesias
  - Exercise intolerance, dyspnea, and palpitations
  - Sexual dysfunction
  - Ocular dryness
  - "Multiple chemical sensitivity" and an increased tendency to report drug reactions
  - Impaired social/occupational functioning
  - Symptoms can wax and wane on a day-to-day basis, varying in quality, intensity, and location. Emotional distress can both trigger and aggravate symptoms.

PHYSICAL EXAM

- Classic fibromyalgia tender points (TPs): 9 symmetric pairs (5 anterior, 4 posterior)
- The presence of $\geq$11 TPs carries a sensitivity of 88% and specificity 81% for the disease.
- TPs in fibromyalgia are distinct from the "trigger points" found in myofascial pain syndromes and are not sites for therapeutic injection.
- Examine joints for swelling, tenderness, erythema, decreased range of motion, crepitus, and cystic or mass lesions. These are typically absent in fibromyalgia.
- Document absence of inflammatory features (e.g., no synovitis, enthesopathy, dermatologic or ocular findings).
- Neurologic exam: may demonstrate generalized or "nonanatomic" dysesthesia, hyperesthesia or hypesthesia; focal neurologic findings suggest alternative or additional diagnoses.

DIFFERENTIAL DIAGNOSIS

- RA, SLE, sarcoidosis, and other inflammatory connective tissue disorders
- Diffuse/advanced OA, seronegative spondyloarthropathies (AS, psoriatic arthritis, etc.)
- Polymyalgia rheumatica; drug-induced endocrine and inflammatory myopathies
- Post–COVID-19 conditions (PCC) ("long COVID") viral/postviral polyarthralgia syndromes
- Anemia and iron deficiency, sickle cell disease and variants
- Electrolyte disturbances: magnesium (Mg), Na, K, Ca; vitamin deficiencies: D, B_{12}, B_6
- Obstructive sleep apnea, restless leg syndrome, joint hypermobility syndromes (Ehlers-Danlos et al.)
- Complex regional pain syndromes (CRPS), opioid-induced hyperalgesia
- Hypothyroidism, hyperparathyroidism
- Lyme disease, hepatitis B and C (chronic)
- Generalized muscular deconditioning, peripheral vascular disease
- Central poststroke pain syndromes
- Multiple sclerosis, spinal cord syndromes, inflammatory polyneuropathies (AIDP, CIDP, etc.)
- Malignancies: metastatic and paraneoplastic syndromes
- Somatic symptom disorder and other psychiatric conditions with associated somatization symptoms
- Overlap syndromes
  - Myalgic encephalomyelitis/chronic fatigue syndrome/chronic fatigue immune dysfunction syndrome (ME/CFS/CFIDS)
  - Myofascial pain syndrome (more anatomically localized than fibromyalgia, but these may co-occur)

DIAGNOSTIC TESTS & INTERPRETATION

Initial Tests (lab, imaging)

- CBC with differential, ESR or CRP, CPK, TSH, comprehensive metabolic profile; consider 25-OH vitamin D, Mg, vitamin B_{12}, folate, and urine drug screen.
- ANA, RF, Lyme titers, and other rheumatologic labs generally unnecessary, unless there are specific or localizing symptoms suggestive of inflammatory or infectious disease.
- Imaging is not generally indicated, except to exclude other specific diagnoses.

Diagnostic Procedures/Other

- Sleep studies may be indicated to rule out obstructive sleep apnea or narcolepsy.
- Consider psychiatric or neuropsychiatric evaluation for comorbid mood disorders and cognitive disturbances.

TREATMENT

Evidence-based interventions:

- Includes both medication and nonpharmacologic interventions (2); a multimodal approach using safe combinations of mutually reinforcing therapies, both pharmacologic and nonpharmacologic, provides the best results. In general, a partial or complete remission can only be achieved with committed changes in lifestyle, including regular exercise, proper sleep hygiene, and smoking cessation.
- Nonpharmacologic
  - Educate about diagnosis, signs, symptoms, and treatment options: online resources include:
    - https://www.fmaware.org
    - https://www.fibromyalgiaforums.org/
    - https://www.moregooddays.com/fibromyalgia
  - VASFIQ for initial assessment and interval evaluation during treatment
  - Cognitive-behavioral therapy (CBT) improves mood, energy, pain, and functional status (2)[A].
  - Acceptance and commitment therapy (ACT)
  - Aerobic exercise: moderately intense, with gradual titration to minimize symptom exacerbation ("start low and slow") (2)[A]
  - Strength/resistance training—mild to moderate; tai chi—equal or superior to aerobic exercise
  - Aquatic exercise training; mixed exercise training (combined aerobic, resistance, flexibility)
  - Weight loss may augment the benefits of exercise.
  - Sleep hygiene
  - Mitigate/eliminate tobacco, alcohol, and substance use.
  - There is a growing body of evidence supporting the use of transcranial direct current stimulation (tDCS) as a safe and effective alternative to drug therapy.
- Pharmacologic
  - Three U.S. Food and Drug Administration (FDA)-approved drugs: duloxetine, milnacipran, and pregabalin; others are off-label. Recent studies suggest that these agents, when used as monotherapy, only benefit a minority of responders.
  - **Caution**: Fibromyalgia patients are frequently treated with multidrug regimens; monitor closely for drug interactions, and especially for "stacked" sedative, serotonergic, and anticholinergic effects.

MEDICATION

First Line

- Duloxetine initially 30 mg/day for 1 week and then increase to 60 mg/day as tolerated; taper if discontinued (2)[A].
- Milnacipran day 1: 12.5 mg/day; days 2 to 3, begin dividing doses: 12.5 mg BID; days 4 to 7: 25 mg BID; after day 7: 50 mg BID; max dose 100 to 200 mg BID; taper if discontinued (2)[A].
- Pregabalin: Start with 75 mg BID, titrate over 1 week to 150 mg BID; max dose 450 mg/day (some authorities recommend up to 600 mg daily) divided BID to TID (2)[A]
- Cyclobenzaprine 5 mg qHS; titrate to 10 mg BID to TID as tolerated; a new sublingual form was FDA approved for use in fibromyalgia in August 2025 (2)[A].

Second Line

- Gabapentin: Start at 300 mg HS, titrate to 1,200 to 2,400 mg/day divided BID to TID; max dose of 3,600 mg daily
- Amitriptyline 10 to 50 mg PO HS to treat pain, fatigue, and sleep disturbances; TCAs that are secondary amines (e.g., desipramine, nortriptyline) may be similarly effective and less sedating.
- Venlafaxine XR 37.5 to 225.0 mg; likely to be as effective as other SNRIs (duloxetine, milnacipran)
- Tramadol 50 to 100 mg q6h; likely more effective in combination with acetaminophen (2)[B]
- Quetiapine 25 to 100 mg qHS
- Low-dose naltrexone 4.5 mg qHS
- Several agents have shown some promise of benefit, albeit with limited evidence, including pramipexole, memantine, low-dose naltrexone, medical cannabis (especially with higher CBD:THC ratios), and hyperbaric O_2 therapy.
- Cholecalciferol may be beneficial in patients with low 25-OH vitamin D levels.

ISSUES FOR REFERRAL

In cases of unclear diagnosis or poor response to therapy, refer to rheumatology, neurology, and/or pain management.

ADDITIONAL THERAPIES

- Trigger point (not tender point) injections for regional myofascial dysfunction may provide relief.
- Multidisciplinary rehab (specialized clinic with physical medicine and therapy, occupational therapy, and integrated pain management)
- Ineffective or dangerous treatment modalities (2)
  - NSAIDs, full-agonist opioids (except in refractory cases), benzodiazepines, SSRIs (although may have efficacy in combination therapy with TCAs or pregabalin), Mg, guaifenesin, thyroxine, corticosteroids, DHEA, growth hormone, valacyclovir, interferon, calcitonin, nabilone, and antiepileptic agents (other than those listed above)
  - *Fibromyalgia often presents concurrently with other pain syndromes that may respond to NSAIDs, corticosteroids, opioids, and other agents.*

COMPLEMENTARY & ALTERNATIVE MEDICINE

- The following have evidence-based support for their efficacy and safety:
  - Acupuncture and electroacupuncture, biofeedback, hypnotherapy
  - Balneotherapy (mineral-rich baths)
  - Yoga, tai chi, and qi gong
  - Mindfulness-based meditation
- Low-level laser therapy (LLLT)
- Limited double-blind trials have shown effectiveness of supplementation with S-adenosyl-L-methionine and acetyl-L-carnitine.
- Likely to be ineffective: chiropractic treatment, multivitamin therapy, homeopathy, massage therapy

ONGOING CARE

FOLLOW-UP RECOMMENDATIONS

Patient Monitoring

- For efficacy of initial therapy: at 2- to 4-week intervals, then every 1 to 6 months, tailored to patient's needs
- Advance exercise gradually and as tolerated.

DIET

Patient should make healthy choices and address negative dietary habits. Caloric or carbohydrate restriction may be helpful in obese patients. Reduction in pain has been reported in patients following hypocaloric and vegan diets, as well as a diets low in fermentable oligosaccharides, disaccharides, monosaccharides and polyols (FODMAPs).

PATIENT EDUCATION

It is important to make a clear diagnosis of fibromyalgia and communicate it to the patient (1).

PROGNOSIS

- A chronic, fluctuating course is characteristic of the disease; 50% with partial remission after 2 to 3 years of therapy; complete remission possible but uncommon
- Poorer outcomes tied to greater duration and severity of symptoms, depression, obesity, insufficient engagement and "ownership" of the treatment plan, advanced age, and lack of social support

REFERENCES

1. Winslow BT, Vandal C, Dang L. Fibromyalgia: diagnosis and management. *Am Fam Physician*. 2023;107(2):137–144.
2. Filipovic T, Filipović A, Nikolic D, et al. Fibromyalgia: understanding, diagnosis and modern approaches to treatment. *J Clin Med*. 2025;14(3):955. doi:10.3390/jcm14030955.

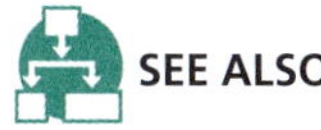

SEE ALSO

Algorithm: Fatigue

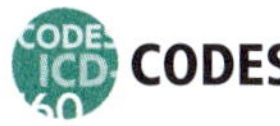

CODES

ICD10

M79.7 Fibromyalgia

CLINICAL PEARLS

- Fibromyalgia is a diagnosis of inclusion (not exclusion).
- Screen for comorbid sleep and mood disorders.
- Normal lab and imaging studies support the diagnosis of fibromyalgia if clinical criteria are satisfied.
- The most effective first-line treatments are exercise and psychosocial interventions.
- Reserve pharmacotherapy for refractory symptoms.
- Patient-centered management with multiple modalities improves outcomes (Isolated, single-modality therapy is rarely effective.).

FOLLICULITIS

David C. Cadena Jr., MD • Mayra A. Perez, DO

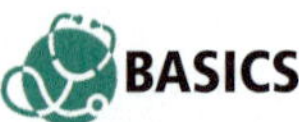

BASICS

DESCRIPTION

- Common skin condition involving inflammation of the hair follicle
- Most frequent symptom is pruritus.
- Painless or tender pustules, vesicles, or pink/red papulopustules up to 5 mm in size
- Most commonly infectious in etiology:
  - *Staphylococcus aureus* bacteria
  - *Pseudomonas aeruginosa* infects areas of the body exposed to poorly sanitized hot tubs, pools, or contaminated water.
  - Fungal (dermatophytic, *Pityrosporum*, *Candida*)
  - Viral (VZV, herpes simplex virus [HSV])
  - Parasitic (*Demodex* mites, schistosomes)
- Noninfectious types
  - Acneiform folliculitis
  - Actinic superficial folliculitis
  - Acne vulgaris
  - Keloidal folliculitis
  - Folliculitis decalvans
  - Perioral dermatitis
  - Fox-Fordyce disease
  - Pruritus folliculitis of pregnancy
  - Toxic erythema of the newborn
  - Eosinophilic folliculitis (seen in HIV positive/immunocompromised)
  - Follicular mucinosis
- Skin disorders that may produce a follicular eruption:
  - Pseudofolliculitis barbae: similar in appearance; occurs after shaving; commonly known as razor bumps, occurs more frequently in black men
  - Atopic dermatitis
  - Follicular psoriasis
  - Rosacea

EPIDEMIOLOGY

Affects persons of all ages, gender, and race; those who shave or have chronic conditions such as diabetes or those who are immunocompromised are at increased risk.

Incidence

Superficial folliculitis is most commonly a self-limited condition; therefore, the exact incidence is not known.

Prevalence

Folliculitis is a relatively common skin condition; prevalence rate in the United States is 8 per 1,000.

ETIOLOGY AND PATHOPHYSIOLOGY

Predisposing factors to folliculitis

- Chronic staphylococcal carrier
- Diabetes mellitus
- Malnutrition
- Pruritic skin disease (e.g., scabies, eczema)
- Exposure to poorly chlorinated swimming pools/hot tubs
- Occlusive corticosteroid use (for multiple hours)
- Bacteria
  - Most frequently due to *S. aureus* (increasing number of methicillin-resistant *S. aureus* [MRSA] cases)
  - Also due to *Streptococcus* species, *Pseudomonas* (following exposure to water contaminated with the species), or *Proteus*
  - May progress to furuncle and carbuncle
- Fungal
  - Dermatophytic (tinea capitis, tinea corporis, tinea pedis)
  - *Pityrosporum* (Pityrosporum orbiculare) commonly affecting teenagers and men, predominantly on upper chest and back
- Viral
  - HSV
  - Molluscum contagiosum
- Parasitic
  - *Demodex* mites (commonly *Demodex folliculorum*), common around nasolabial area
  - Schistosomes (swimmer's itch)
- Acneiform type commonly drug induced (systemic and topical corticosteroids, lithium, isoniazid, rifampin), EGFR inhibitors
- Severe vitamin C deficiency
- Actinic superficial type occurs within 24 to 48 hours of exposure to the sun, resulting in multiple follicular pustules on the shoulders, trunk, and arms.
- Acne vulgaris
- Keloidal folliculitis is a chronic condition affecting mostly black patients; involves the neck and occipital scalp, resulting in hypertrophic scars and hair loss; usually consequence of uncontrolled folliculitis barbae
- Folliculitis decalvans is a chronic folliculitis that leads to progressive scarring and alopecia of the scalp.
- Rosacea consists of papules, pustules, and/or telangiectasias of the face; individuals are genetically predisposed; *can be confused with folliculitis*
- Fox-Fordyce disease affects the skin containing apocrine sweat glands (i.e., axillae), resulting in follicular papules.
- Eosinophilic pustular folliculitis has three variants: classic (Ofuji disease), associated with HIV infection, and infantile.
- Toxic erythema of the newborn is a self-limiting pustular eruption usually appearing during the first 3 to 4 days of life and subsequently fading in the following 2 weeks.
- *Malassezia* infections

Genetics

No known genetic predisposition

RISK FACTORS

- Hair removal (shaving, plucking, waxing, epilating agents)
- Other pruritic skin conditions: eczema, scabies
- Occlusive dressing or clothing
- Sweating
- Personal carrier or contact with MRSA-infected persons
- Diabetes mellitus
- Immunosuppression (medications, chemotherapy, HIV)
- Use of hot tubs or saunas
- Use of EGFR inhibitors
- Chronic antibiotic use (gram-negative folliculitis)
- Tattoo recipient

GENERAL PREVENTION

- Good hygiene practices
  - Wash hands frequently with antimicrobial soap.
  - Wash towels, clothes, and linens frequently with hot water to avoid reinfection.
- Good hair removal practices
  - Exfoliate beforehand.
  - Use witch hazel, alcohol, or Tend Skin afterward.
  - Shave in direction of hair growth; use shaving gel and moisturizer.
  - Decrease frequency of shaving.
  - Use clippers primarily or single-blade razors if straight shaving is desired.

COMMONLY ASSOCIATED CONDITIONS

Impetigo, scabies, acne, follicular psoriasis, eczema, xerosis, *Staphylococcus*/MRSA colonization

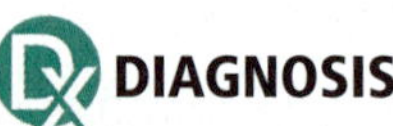

DIAGNOSIS

HISTORY

- Recent use of hot tubs, swimming pools, topical corticosteroids, certain hairstyling and shaving practices, antibiotics or systemic steroids
- HIV status
- History of STDs (specifically syphilis)
- MRSA exposures/carrier status
- Home and work environment (risk/exposure potential)
- Pityrosporum folliculitis occurs more often in warm, moist climates.
- Inquire about the timeline in which the lesions have occurred, including previous similar episodes.

PHYSICAL EXAM

- Characteristic lesions are 1- to 5-mm–wide vesicles, pustules, or inflamed papules with surrounding erythema.
- Rash occurs on hair-bearing skin, especially the face (beard), proximal limbs, scalp, and pubis.
- Pseudomonal folliculitis appears as a widespread rash, mainly on the trunk and limbs.
- In pseudofolliculitis barbae, the growing hair curls around and penetrates the skin at shaved areas.

DIFFERENTIAL DIAGNOSIS

- Acne vulgaris/acneiform eruptions
- Arthropod bite
- Contact dermatitis
- Perioral dermatitis
- Cutaneous candidiasis
- Milia
- Atopic dermatitis
- Follicular psoriasis
- Hidradenitis suppurativa

DIAGNOSTIC TESTS & INTERPRETATION

Initial Tests (lab, imaging)

- Diagnosis can be made clinically, taking risk factors, history, and locations of lesions into account.
- Culture and Gram stain may be done for larger lesions lancing or unroofing the pustule.

- KOH preparation as well as Wood lamp fluorescence to identify *Candida* or yeast
- Tzanck smear where suspicion of herpetic simplex viral folliculitis is high
- Ultrasound can be performed for questionably deeper seeding infections.

Follow-Up Tests & Special Considerations

- If risk factors or clinical suspicion exist, consider serologies for HIV or syphilis.
- If recurrent, consider HIV testing and A1C/fasting blood sugar testing to evaluate for diabetes.
- Consider punch biopsy with uncertain diagnosis.
- Treat positive bacterial culture according to sensitivities.
- Positive HIV serology: Follow up with CD4 count and punch biopsy to rule out eosinophilic folliculitis.

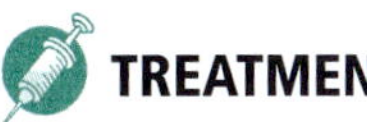

TREATMENT

GENERAL MEASURES

- Lesions usually resolve spontaneously.
- Avoid shaving or waxing affected areas (1)[C].
- Warm compresses may be applied TID.
- Systemic antibiotics are typically unnecessary.
- Topical mupirocin may be used in presumed *S. aureus* infection (2).
- Topical antifungals for fungal folliculitis
- Preventive measures:
  - Antibacterial soaps (Dial soap, chlorhexidine, or benzoyl peroxide wash when showering/bathing)
  - Bleach baths (1/2 cup of 6% bleach per standard bathtub and soak for 5 to 15 minutes followed by water, rinse 1 to 2 times a week)
  - Keep skin intact; daily skin care with noncomedogenic moisturizers; avoid scratching.
  - Avoid trauma to skin: Use an electric razor as able.
  - Clean shaving instruments daily or use disposable razor, disposing after one use (1).
  - Change washcloths, towels, and sheets daily.

MEDICATION

Antiseptic and supportive care is usually enough. Systemic antibiotics may be used for severe or persistent infection but have questionable efficacy, and available evidence is of generally low quality (3)[A].

First Line

- Staphylococcal folliculitis
  - Topical mupirocin ointment applied TID for 10 days
  - Cephalosporin (cephalexin): 250 to 500 mg PO QID for 7 to 10 days
  - Dicloxacillin: 250 to 500 mg PO QID for 7 to 10 days
- For MRSA
  - Bactrim DS: 1 to 2 tablets (160 mg/800 mg) BID PO for 5 to 10 days
  - Clindamycin: 300 mg PO TID for 10 to 14 days
  - Minocycline: 200 mg PO initially and then 100 mg BID for 5 to 10 days
  - Doxycycline: 50 to 100 mg PO BID for 5 to 10 days
- *Pseudomonas* folliculitis
  - Topical dilute acetic acid baths
  - Ciprofloxacin: 500 to 750 mg PO BID for 7 to 14 days for severe infections
- Eosinophilic folliculitis/eosinophilic pustular folliculitis
  - HAART treatment for HIV-positive–related causes
  - High-potency topical corticosteroids for inflammation
  - Antihistamines (hydroxyzine, cetirizine) to control itching
  - Can consider: tacrolimus topically BID *or*
  - Isotretinoin 0.5 mg/kg/day PO with caution
  - Itraconazole or metronidazole
- Fungal folliculitis
  - Topical antifungals: ketoconazole 2% cream or shampoo or selenium sulfide shampoo daily *or*
  - Econazole cream applied to affected area BID for 2 to 3 weeks
    - Systemic antifungals for relapses fluconazole (100 to 200 mg/day for 3 weeks) *or* itraconazole (200 mg/day for 1 week) *or* griseofulvin (500 mg/day for 2 to 4 weeks)
    - Do not use oral ketoconazole due to risk of liver failure.
- Parasitic folliculitis
  - 5% permethrin: Apply to affected area, leave on for 8 hours, and wash off.
  - Ivermectin: 200 μg/kg PO and repeat in 1 to 2 weeks if topical application unsuccessful
- Herpetic folliculitis
  - Valacyclovir: 500 mg PO TID for 5 to 10 days or
  - Famciclovir: 500 mg PO TID for 5 to 10 days or
  - Acyclovir: 200 mg PO 5 times daily for 5 to 10 days

ISSUES FOR REFERRAL

Unusual or persistent cases should be biopsied and referred to dermatology.

ADDITIONAL THERAPIES

- Stay informed: Testing strips can be used to test hot tubs and pools. This will help determine proper chlorine levels.
- Both hot tubs and pools should have a pH level of 7.2 to 7.8.

SURGERY/OTHER PROCEDURES

Incision and drainage are unlikely to be necessary and typically not preferred due to potential for scar formation unless secondary abscess has formed. If isolated abscess has developed, it may be treated with incision and drainage alone.

ONGOING CARE

FOLLOW-UP RECOMMENDATIONS

Patient Monitoring

- Resistant cases should be followed every 2 weeks until cleared.
- Consider prompt system therapy for worsening cases.

DIET

Caloric monitoring for obese patients; weight reduction will decrease risk of skin trauma and distension.

PATIENT EDUCATION

- Avoid shaving in involved areas.
- Monitor hot tub and pools.

PROGNOSIS

- Usually resolves with treatment; however, *S. aureus* carriers may experience recurrences.
- Mupirocin nasal treatment for carrier status and for family/household members might be helpful.
- Resistant or severe cases may warrant testing for diabetes mellitus or immunodeficiency (HIV).

COMPLICATIONS

- Primary complication is recurrent folliculitis.
- Extensive scarring with hyperpigmentation
- Progression to furunculosis or abscess

REFERENCES

1. Khanna N, Chandramohan K, Khaitan BK, et al. Post waxing folliculitis: a clinicopathological evaluation. *Int J Dermatol*. 2014;53(7):849–854.
2. Sartelli M, Guirao X, Hardcastle TC, et al. 2018 WSES/SIS-E consensus conference: recommendations for the management of skin and soft-tissue infections. *World J Emerg Surg*. 2018;13:58.
3. Lin HS, Lin PT, Tsai YS, et al. Interventions for bacterial folliculitis and boils (furuncles and carbuncles). *Cochrane Database Syst Rev*. 2021;2(2):CD013099.

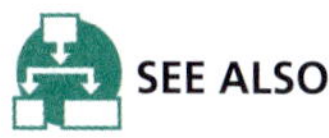

SEE ALSO

Algorithm: Rash

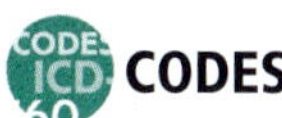

CODES

ICD10

- L73.9 Follicular disorder, unspecified
- L66.2 Folliculitis decalvans
- L73.8 Other specified follicular disorders

CLINICAL PEARLS

- Folliculitis lesions are typically 1- to 5-mm clusters of pruritic erythematous papules and pustule surrounding hair follicles.
- Most commonly due to *S. aureus*; if community has increased incidence of MRSA, consider anti-MRSA treatment.
  - It is extremely important to educate patients on proper hygiene and skin care techniques to prevent chronic or recurrent cases.
- If not improving after 2 weeks, consider oral antibiotics or biopsy for confirmation.

F

FOOD ALLERGY

Idil D. Ezhuthachan, MD, MS • Melinda M. Rathkopf, MD, MBA • Brian Vickery, MD

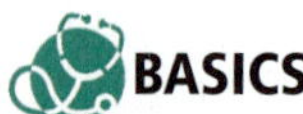

BASICS

Food allergies are adverse health effects arising from a specific immune response that occurs reproducibly on exposure to a given food. Immune responses can be IgE-mediated or non-IgE-mediated. This chapter focuses on IgE-mediated food allergy.

DESCRIPTION

- A reproducible hypersensitivity reaction related to specific food exposures mediated by IgE
- System(s) affected: gastrointestinal (GI), heme/lymphatic/immunologic, pulmonary, skin, cardiovascular
- Synonym(s): IgE-mediated food reactions, food hypersensitivity, anaphylaxis, allergic reaction

EPIDEMIOLOGY

- Found at all ages
- Traditionally felt more common in infants and young children
- Increasing prevalence in adults (1)
- Predominant sex: male > female in children, female > male in adults
- May disproportionately impact in underserved and minority populations

Incidence

Egg allergy incidence has been reported as 1.23% in infants, whereas this number for cow's milk allergy was 0.54%.

Prevalence

- 3% prevalence of IgE-mediated food allergy as assessed by an oral food challenge (OFC) the diagnostic gold standard.
- Self-reported prevalence of food allergy is >10%: with 1 in 10 adults and 1 in 12 children.
- In children, the most common food allergies are cow's milk (2%), egg (0.6–0.8%), peanut (1.2–2%), and tree nuts (approximately 1%) (2).
- Adults more commonly have allergies to shellfish (2.9%), milk (1.9%), peanuts (1.8%), tree nuts (1.2%), and fish (0.9%) (3).
- Most children outgrow milk and egg allergy; 30% of children with peanut allergy outgrow by school age.

ETIOLOGY AND PATHOPHYSIOLOGY

- Allergic reactions to food are a result of incomplete of immunologic tolerance to protein-based allergens in food, resulting in immune-mediated systemic responses.
- Any ingested substance can cause allergic reactions:
  - 90% of food allergies in the United States involve cow's milk, egg white, wheat, soy, peanut, tree nuts (e.g., walnut, pecan, cashew, and pistachio), fish, shellfish, and sesame.
  - Food dyes and additives are rare causes of allergy.

Genetics

- HLA alleles have been identified as genetic determinants for peanut allergy.
- Food allergy screening is currently not recommended for siblings of food allergy patients.

RISK FACTORS

- Sex (male children, female adults)
- Race/ethnicity (Asian and Black children at higher risk)
- Allergic or atopic predisposition (particularly eczema)
- Family history of food hypersensitivity

GENERAL PREVENTION

- High-risk infants who are regularly fed peanut protein (6 g/week) have 80% risk reduction in developing peanut allergy by age 5 years
- Current recommendations for food allergy prevention through nutrition include:
  - Introduce peanut and egg to all infants around 6 months of age, but not before 4 months.
  - Do not deliberately delay the introduction of other allergenic foods.
- Have epinephrine autoinjectors for patients at risk for anaphylaxis.

COMMONLY ASSOCIATED CONDITIONS

- Food protein-induced enterocolitis syndrome (FPIES); eosinophilic esophagitis
- Atopic dermatitis; asthma; allergic rhinitis

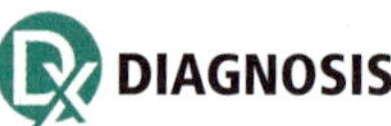

DIAGNOSIS

HISTORY

- Symptoms after food ingestion/exposure—usually within minutes
  - GI: nausea, vomiting, diarrhea, abdominal pain
  - Skin: urticaria/angioedema, pallor, flushing, contact rashes
  - Respiratory: allergic rhinitis, asthma, bronchospasm, stridor, cough
  - Other: anaphylaxis, ocular injection
- Document a temporal relationship between symptoms and suspected food.
- Differentiate true food allergy/hypersensitivity from food intolerance.
- Inquire about cofactors—exercise, sleep deprivation, NSAIDs use, alcohol consumption, and illness.

PHYSICAL EXAM

- Vital signs; growth parameters
- Signs of allergic disease—pulmonary, skin exam in particular
- Other exam findings based on clinical presentation

DIFFERENTIAL DIAGNOSIS

- Nonimmune food intolerance such as enzyme deficiencies (e.g., lactose intolerance)
- Toxic food exposures (e.g., scombroid fish, bacterial food poisoning)
- GI: irritable bowel syndrome, celiac disease, dumping syndrome, inflammatory bowel diseases
- Dermatologic: chronic/recurrent urticaria
- Psychiatric: generalized anxiety disorder, psychosomatic manifestations
- Other immune-mediated reactions to food:
  - Oral allergy syndrome
    - Commonly causes oral pruritus and possibly edema, rarely progresses or causes anaphylaxis.
  - Galactose-α-1,3-galactose (α-gal)
    - Following a lone star tick bite, susceptible patients may develop an IgE hypersensitivity to α-gal manifesting as a delayed anaphylactic reaction 3 to 6 hours after mammalian meat ingestion; confirmed by IgE specific to α-gal
  - Food-dependent exercise-induced anaphylaxis
    - Ingestion of certain foods results in anaphylaxis if followed by exercise; diagnosed through history and food-specific IgE (skin or serum IgE test)
  - Eosinophilic esophagitis
    - Chronic inflammation of the esophagus leading to feeding difficulties, dysphagia, chest pain, food impaction, and possibly poor growth
  - FPIES
    - A GI food hypersensitivity presenting with lethargy, repetitive vomiting, diarrhea; symptoms usually occur within 1 to 4 hours of food ingestion.
  - Food protein-induced allergic proctocolitis
    - Allergic inflammation of the distal colon in infants; presents in the first months of life with rectal bleeding, most commonly associated with cow's milk and soy proteins

DIAGNOSTIC TESTS & INTERPRETATION

Initial Tests (lab, imaging)

- OFCs are the gold standard in food allergy diagnosis.
  - Delay OFC in patients with history of anaphylaxis until IgE sensitivity declines or disappears.
  - Most allergic reactions occur within 30 minutes to 2 hours after OFC.
- Allergy tests are confirmatory (not diagnostic). Interpretation depends on the history of exposure and specific symptoms.
- Epicutaneous (prick or puncture) allergy skin tests document IgE-mediated immunologic hypersensitivity.
- Food-specific IgE assays (fluorescent enzyme immunoassay [FEI]) detect specific IgE antibodies to offending foods and may help in diagnosis.
  - The term RadioAllergoSorbent Test (RAST) is outdated and no longer used. ImmunoCAP is the standard method for measuring allergen-specific IgE in the blood. Although "RAST" is still used informally, the current terminology is serum-specific IgE testing via ImmunoCAP.
- Both skin and serum IgE testing have a high sensitivity (low false-negative rate) *but* a low specificity (high false-positive rate).
  - If positive without a history suggestive of an IgE-mediated reaction, an OFC may be necessary to clarify diagnosis. If negative, food allergy is unlikely.
  - Test only for specific IgE to foods based on patient history.

- Component-resolved diagnosis measures specific allergenic food proteins to identify specific IgE and can be helpful in predicting clinical reactivity.
- Widespread allergy skin testing or serum IgE tests, such as food panels, are *not* recommended (2).

Follow-Up Tests & Special Considerations

Periodic monitoring of food-specific IgE levels every 1 to 2 years may be helpful. If the levels are decreasing over time, this may be indicative of remission. A supervised oral challenge can help confirm resolution.

Diagnostic Procedures/Other

Other emerging test include component-resolved diagnostics and basophil activation. Other biomarkers and use of artificial intelligence in diagnostic interpretation are on the horizon but not accepted as standard of care.

Test Interpretation

Both skin and serum IgE tests should be evaluated in the context of patient's clinical history and symptoms.

- A positive test in the absence of relevant symptoms may not indicate a true allergy.
- A patient with strong history may have an allergy even if the test results are negative.

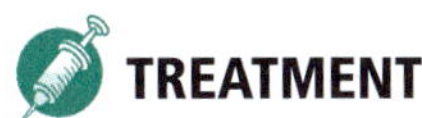

TREATMENT

GENERAL MEASURES

- Food avoidance is the mainstay of treatment. Patients with severe food allergy should meticulously avoid their offending foods and carry an epinephrine auto-injector.
- Immunotherapy may be effective for certain food allergies.
- Subcutaneous immunotherapy or hyposensitization (e.g., "allergy shots") with food extracts are not recommended.

MEDICATION

- Patients with significant type 1, IgE-mediated hypersensitivity should have epinephrine available.
- Monitor patients receiving epinephrine for a systemic anaphylactic reaction to a food (~20% may require another dose).
- Symptomatic treatment for milder reactions with non-sedating antihistamines is generally adequate but use of epinephrine should not be delayed.
- Omalizumab, a monoclonal antibody against IgE, is approved for ages 1 year and up to reduce allergic reactions in food allergic patients.
- For patients aged 1 to 17 years with allergic sensitivity to peanut protein, oral immunotherapy with peanut allergy powder (Palforzia) is available to reduce the risk for anaphylaxis after accidental peanut protein exposure.

ISSUES FOR REFERRAL

Infants and toddlers with food allergy-related concerns should be promptly referred instead of waiting and watching in order not to delay allergen introduction.

ADDITIONAL THERAPIES

Self-injectable epinephrine for anaphylaxis; adjunct therapy with corticosteroids and/or antihistamines as indicated

COMPLEMENTARY & ALTERNATIVE MEDICINE

Benefits of herbal medicines, probiotics, and prebiotics in food allergy are inconclusive.

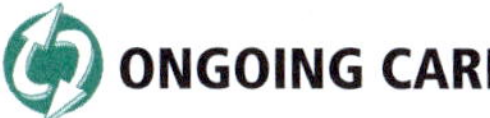

ONGOING CARE

FOLLOW-UP RECOMMENDATIONS

Patient Monitoring

Follow-up skin prick tests and/or serum IgE studies as clinically indicated to monitor for resolution

DIET

- Strict avoidance of offending food
- Dietary counseling to maintain a nutritionally sound diet while avoiding offending foods

PATIENT EDUCATION

- Food Allergy Research & Education: 800-929-4040; https://www.foodallergy.org
- Allergy & Asthma Network: http://www.allergyasthmanetwork.org; American College of Allergy Asthma and Immunology: https://college.acaai.org; and American Academy of Allergy, Asthma & Immunology: https://www.aaaai.org

PROGNOSIS

- Food allergy is frequently a transient phenomenon:
  - Many children will outgrow food hypersensitivity within the 1st or 2nd decade of life
  - ≥50% of the children diagnosed with milk, egg, or wheat allergy have resolution of their allergy later on in childhood; up to 30% of peanut allergy may resolve by 6 years of age.
  - Significant reductions in skin prick test wheal size and serum specific IgE level can indicate the development of tolerance.
- Adults with food hypersensitivity (particularly to nuts, fish, or shellfish) tend to maintain their allergy (2).

COMPLICATIONS

- Anaphylaxis; angioedema; asthma; environmental allergies
- Decreased quality of life; anxiety; depression

REFERENCES

1. Boyd H, Santos AF. Novel diagnostics in food allergy. *J Allergy Clin Immunol*. 2025;155(2):275–285. doi:10.1016/j.jaci.2024.12.1071.
2. Nsouli TM. New insights in the optimal diagnosis and management of food allergy. *Allergy Asthma Proc*. 2023;44(5):306–314. doi:10.2500/aap.2023.44.230046.
3. Sindher SB, Long A, Chin AR, et al. Food allergy, mechanisms, diagnosis and treatment: innovation through a multi-targeted approach. *Allergy*. 2022;77(10):2937–2948. doi:10.1111/all.15418.

ADDITIONAL READING

- Bright DM, Stegall HL, Slawson DC. Food Allergies: Diagnosis, Treatment, and Prevention. *Am Fam Physician*. 2023;108(2):159–165.
- Tilles SA, Adelman DC, Greenhawt M, et al. Barriers and solutions to optimal food allergy prevention, diagnostic, and management strategies. *J Allergy Clin Immunol Pract*. 2025;13(8):1928–1934. doi:10.1016/j.jaip.2025.04.030.

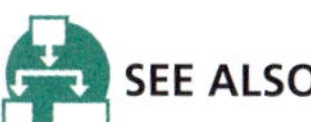

SEE ALSO

Anaphylaxis; Celiac Disease; Irritable Bowel Syndrome

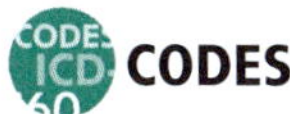

CODES

ICD10

- T78.1XXA Oth adverse food reactions, not elsewhere classified, init
- T78.00XA Anaphylactic reaction due to unspecified food, init encntr
- L27.2 Dermatitis due to ingested food

CLINICAL PEARLS

- Many common childhood food allergies are outgrown by adulthood. Up to 30% of children with peanut allergy may outgrow their sensitivity. Tree nut, fish, and shellfish allergies are less likely to be outgrown.
- Oral itching following ingestion of fresh fruits and vegetables suggests oral allergy syndrome, which is commonly not associated with anaphylaxis.
- Maternal dietary restrictions during pregnancy and lactation do not prevent atopic disease in infants.
- Breastfeeding is recommended for the first 6 months of life, particularly with a family history of atopy or food allergy.
- Delaying introduction of solid foods beyond 6 months does not prevent development of allergies.
- Introduce peanut and egg around 6 months of age (not before 4 months).
- OFCs remains the diagnostic gold standard.

FOOD POISONING, BACTERIAL

Ethan J. Anderson, DO • Meghana Doniparthi, MD

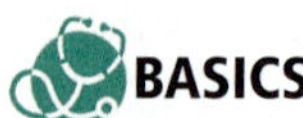

BASICS

DESCRIPTION

- Food poisoning or foodborne illness is caused by the consumption of food or water that is contaminated with bacterial, parasitic, or viral pathogens; less commonly molds, toxins, contaminants and/or allergens
- Symptoms are most commonly gastrointestinal in nature and are typically self-limited. Some cases can lead to severe dehydration and critical illness.

EPIDEMIOLOGY

- The cause is unclear in up to 80% of cases. Most foodborne illnesses are secondary to viral causes, *Norovirus* being the most common. Other viral causes include hepatitis A, rotavirus, and adenovirus.
- *Campylobacter* and nontyphoidal *Salmonella* are the most common causes of bacterial foodborne illness in the United States. Other pathogens include Shiga toxin-producing *Escherichia coli* (STEC), *Shigella*, *Cyclospora*, *Yersinia*, *Listeria*, and *Vibrio*.
- *Salmonella* (nontyphoidal) infections are the bacterial foodborne illnesses most commonly associated with hospitalizations and deaths.

Incidence

There are approximately 4.5 million cases of major foodborne illness in the United States each year, leading to approximately 40,000 hospitalizations and 600 deaths (1). Per World Health Organization, 1 in 10 people experience foodborne illness worldwide, accounting for approximately 420,000 deaths annually.

Prevalence

Due to the acute nature of food poisoning, the prevalence and incidence are similar as above.

ETIOLOGY AND PATHOPHYSIOLOGY

- Invasive pathogens:
  - *Campylobacter jejuni*: timing: 2 to 5 days; symptoms: diarrhea (bloody), cramps, vomiting, fever; food sources: raw and undercooked poultry, unpasteurized milk, and contaminated meats
  - *Salmonella*, nontyphoidal: timing: 6 to 48 hours; symptoms: small volume, mucopurulent/bloody diarrhea, fever, cramps, vomiting; food sources: contaminated eggs, poultry; unpasteurized milk or juice, cheese; contaminated raw fruit and vegetables; and contaminated peanut butter
  - *Clostridium perfringens*: timing: 8 to 16 hours; symptoms: watery diarrhea, nausea, cramps; sources: dry/precooked or undercooked meats, poultry, home-canned goods
  - Enterohemorrhagic *E. coli* (ETEC): timing: 1 to 8 days; symptoms: severe diarrhea often becoming bloody, abdominal pain, vomiting; sources: undercooked ground beef, juice, unpasteurized milk, raw produce, and contaminated water
  - *Shigella*: timing: 4 to 7 days; symptoms: abdominal cramps, fever, mucopurulent and bloody diarrhea; food sources: contaminated water, raw produce, uncooked foods, foods handled by infected food workers
  - Shiga toxin-producing *E. coli* (STEC); may present with hemolytic uremic syndrome
  - *Yersinia enterocolitica*: timing: 4 to 7 days; symptoms: abdominal pain, fever, diarrhea (possibly bloody), vomiting; food sources: undercooked beef and pork, unpasteurized dairy products, tofu, contaminated water; additionally, can be due to exposure to house pets with diarrhea
  - *Vibrio parahaemolyticus*: timing: 4 to 96 hours; symptoms: nausea, vomiting, diarrhea, abdominal pain; food source: undercooked or raw seafood, especially shellfish
  - *Vibrio vulnificus*: timing: 1 to 7 days; symptoms: vomiting, diarrhea, abdominal pain, bacteremia, wound infections; can be fatal in patients with liver disease or those who are immunocompromised; food source: undercooked or raw seafood, particularly oysters
  - Enterotoxigenic *E. coli* ("traveler's diarrhea"): timing: 1 to 3 days; symptoms: watery diarrhea, abdominal cramps, tenesmus, fecal urgency, and vomiting; sources: food or water contaminated by human feces
  - *Listeria monocytogenes*: timing: 4 to 48 hours; symptoms: nausea, vomiting, fever, watery diarrhea; pregnant women may have a flu-like illness leading to premature delivery or stillbirth; immunocompromised patients may develop meningitis and bacteremia; food sources: unpasteurized/contaminated milk, soft cheese, and processed deli meats
- Preformed enterotoxin syndromes:
  - *Staphylococcus aureus*: timing: 1 to 6 hours; symptoms: sudden onset of severe nausea and vomiting; abdominal cramps and fever; sources: improperly refrigerated meats and potato, mayonnaise, and egg salads
  - *Bacillus cereus*: timing: symptom onset: 10 to 16 hours; symptoms: sudden onset of severe nausea, vomiting and watery diarrhea, nausea and cramps; sources: soil, improperly cooked rice/fried rice and red meats
  - *Clostridium botulinum*: timing: 12 to 72 hours; symptoms: vomiting, diarrhea, slurred speech, diplopia, dysphagia, and descending muscle weakness/flaccid paralysis; source: improperly canned foods

RISK FACTORS

Recent travel to developing countries; food handlers, daycare attendees, nursing home residents, recently hospitalized patients, or patients recently exposed to antibiotics; altered immunity due to underlying disease or use of certain medications, including antacids, H_2 blockers, and proton pump inhibitors; cross-contamination and subsequent ingestion of improperly prepared and stored foods; pregnancy; children aged <5 years and adults aged >65 years; immunocompromised patients

GENERAL PREVENTION

- Food preparation: Wash hands, cutting boards, and preparation surfaces. Wash fresh produce thoroughly before consuming. Keep raw meat, poultry, fish, and their juices away from other food (e.g., salad). Wear gloves when handling raw meat. Thoroughly cook the meat. Refrigerate leftovers within 2 to 3 hours in clean, shallow, covered containers. If the temperature is >90°F, refrigerate within 1 hour.
- Travel to underdeveloped countries: Eat only freshly prepared food and avoid beverages and foods prepared with nonpotable water. Bottled, carbonated, and boiled beverages are safe to drink.
- Chemoprophylaxis with bismuth subsalicylates reduces risk over 3-week period. Short-term prophylactic antibiotics are indicated for high-risk traveler's (e.g., immunocompromised) (2).

COMMONLY ASSOCIATED CONDITIONS

- Botulism: symmetric neurologic deficits and changes in mental status due to ingestion of toxin types A, B, and E produced by *C. botulinum*; outbreaks typically involve home-canned foods such as fruits, vegetables and meats.
- Neonatal meningitis: Immunocompromised hosts, particularly neonates (<29 days old), can contract meningitis from systemic *L. monocytogenes* infection.
- Hemolytic uremic syndrome: microangiopathic hemolytic anemia, renal impairment and thrombocytopenia caused by *Shigella* and STEC
- Guillain-Barré syndrome: ascending paralysis strongly associated with *C. jejuni* infection
- Reactive arthritis: can occur after severe infections with *Salmonella*, *Shigella*, *Yersinia*, or *Campylobacter* species
- Irritable bowel syndrome: can occur after infections with *Campylobacter*, *Salmonella*, *Shigella*, STEC, and *Giardia*.

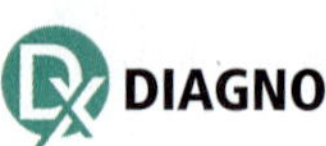

DIAGNOSIS

HISTORY

- Onset, duration, frequency, severity, and character (i.e., watery, bloody, mucus-filled, etc.) of diarrhea (>3 unformed stools daily or the passage of >250 g of unformed stool per day)
- Suspect bacterial food poisoning when multiple persons have rapid onset of symptoms after eating the same meal; fever, blood or mucus in stool; abdominal pain; dehydration; or recent travel to a foreign country
- Further evaluation and treatment of patients with high fever (≥101.3°F), ≥6 stools per day, blood in the stools, elevated white blood cell count, signs of dehydration, or diarrheal illness that lasts >2 to 3 days

PHYSICAL EXAM

- Signs of dehydration: delayed capillary refill, decreased skin turgor, dry mucous membranes, and orthostatic hypotension
- Fever may suggest invasive or toxin-producing bacteria.
- Abdominal exam: Assess for pain, peritoneal signs, and bowel activity to differentiate from other acute abdominal processes; rectal exam for blood, rectal pain, stool consistency

DIFFERENTIAL DIAGNOSIS

- Inflammatory/autoimmune: inflammatory bowel disease (Crohn disease, ulcerative colitis, microscopic colitis); celiac disease; eosinophilic gastroenteritis
- Infectious: cholecystitis, choledocholithiasis, cholangitis, hepatitis; small intestinal bacterial overgrowth, diverticulitis, *Helicobacter pylori*, appendicitis, Whipple's disease, parasitic infection
- Other: short bowel syndrome, tube feeding, mesenteric ischemia

DIAGNOSTIC TESTS & INTERPRETATION

Initial Tests (lab, imaging)

- For mild, self-limiting illness, a stool culture is unlikely to change management unless there are signs of fever, blood, or severe diarrhea. However, diagnostic stool studies are recommended for moderate to severe disease with symptoms >7 days. These studies include bacterial culture along with culture-independent molecular nucleic acid amplification test (NAAT) testing (2)[C].
- Testing for fecal leukocytes, lactoferrin, calprotectin, and fecal occult blood is not indicated in acute diarrhea.
- Abdominal CT may be helpful when suspecting possible intra-abdominal pathology with unclear presentation.

Follow-Up Tests & Special Considerations

Traditional culture should accompany positive molecular testing to aid in reporting to the public health department. Reporting requirements vary by state and organism. Serologic and endoscopic evaluation is not generally recommended.

Diagnostic Procedures/Other

Consider endoscopic evaluation for persistent, unexplained symptoms in patients with AIDS.

Test Interpretation

Clinical correlation is needed with molecular testing as DNA is detected and reported, not organism viability (3)[C].

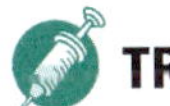

TREATMENT

Most cases of food poisoning are self-limited.

MEDICATION

First Line

- Oral rehydration with fluids and salt (2)[C]: weight based in children; approximately 2 L/day in adults (3)[C]; prioritize balanced electrolytes in elderly with severe disease
- Empiric antibiotic therapy is not recommended unless diarrhea is present in infants <3 months, immunocompromised individuals, travelers with fever >38.5°C with bloody diarrhea, and signs of sepsis (3)[C].

Second Line

- Consider antibiotics with severe illness requiring hospitalization, fever (>101.3°F), and signs of invasive disease (hematochezia, fecal WBC), symptoms lasting >1 week, or >8 liquid stools a day.
- Pathogen-specific therapy (3)[C]:
  - *B. cereus*: supportive care only
  - *C. jejuni*: mild: supportive care only; severe: erythromycin 500 mg BID for 5 days or azithromycin 500 mg on day 1, with 250 mg/day for days 2 to 5; resistant to most fluoroquinolones (2)[C]
  - *C. botulinum*: supportive care only; antitoxin can be helpful early during illness.
  - *C. perfringens*: supportive care only
  - ETEC (e.g., 0157:H7): supportive care; closely monitor renal function, hemoglobin, and platelets. Antibiotics may increase risk of HUS.
  - Enterotoxigenic *E. coli* (common cause of traveler's diarrhea): generally self-limited; antibiotics shorten course of illness; azithromycin 500 mg daily on day 1 with 250 mg daily for days 2 to 5 (preferred); ciprofloxacin 500 mg BID for 3 days; or trimethoprim/sulfamethoxazole 160/800 mg BID for 3 to 7 days
  - *Salmonella* (nontyphoidal): no therapy for mild disease; for individuals at increased risk for invasive disease (i.e., <3 months old, immunocompromised, joint disease), treat with ciprofloxacin, ceftriaxone, or amoxicillin.
  - *Shigella*: azithromycin (drug of choice secondary to quinolone resistance) 500 mg on day 1 and then 250 mg daily on days 2 to 5 or ciprofloxacin 500 mg BID 3 days
  - *S. aureus*: supportive care only
  - Noncholera *Vibrio*: not indicated in mild, noninvasive, disease; severe ceftriaxone and doxycycline
  - *Vibrio cholerae*: doxycycline 300 mg 1-time dose in most cases; alternative treatment includes azithromycin 1,000 mg as single dose or 500 mg/day for 3 days, ceftriaxone, or ciprofloxacin.
  - *Yersinia*: usually, supportive care only; trimethoprim/sulfamethoxazole 160/800 mg BID for 5 days; or ciprofloxacin 500 mg BID for 7 to 10 days

ADDITIONAL THERAPIES

- For severe nausea/vomiting, ondansetron is effective in children. Promethazine or ondansetron are effective for adults.
- Loperamide 4 mg initially and then 2 mg after each loose/watery stool to a maximum of 8 mg in a 24-hour period may be used when adequately hydrated *unless* high fever, bloody diarrhea, and/or severe abdominal pain present (signs of enteroinvasion).
- Bismuth subsalicylate 525 mg QID is moderately effective in traveler's diarrhea.
- Evidence for the effectiveness of probiotics and prebiotics is limited and inconsistent. Recommendation only for postantibiotic-associated disease (2).

ADMISSION, INPATIENT, AND NURSING CONSIDERATIONS

Consider admission for IV fluids if patient failed oral rehydration.

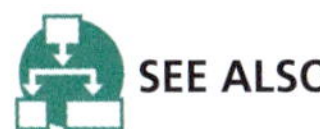

ONGOING CARE

FOLLOW-UP RECOMMENDATIONS

Patient Monitoring

- Report applicable infections to the CDC's National Notifiable Disease Monitoring System; this includes but is not limited to botulism, campylobacteriosis, cholera, listeriosis, salmonellosis, shigellosis, and STEC (3).
- Monitor hemoglobin, platelets, electrolytes, creatinine, and blood urea nitrogen in patients diagnosed with enterohemorrhagic *E. coli* (e.g., 0157:H7) and other STEC.

DIET

- Modify food intake when nausea is present or vomiting prevents intake. As nausea subsides, drink adequate fluids; following rehydration, add in bland, low-fat meals; and rest. Avoid alcohol, coffee, nicotine, and spicy foods.
- Breastfeed nursing infants on demand; older children should be offered usual food.

PATIENT EDUCATION

When traveling to regions with high incidence of foodborne illness, do not drink local water nor ice that was not purified before drinking. Thoroughly cook food and avoid reheated rice.

PROGNOSIS

Most infections are self-limited. Antibiotics for moderate to severe traveler's diarrhea shorten duration by several days.

COMPLICATIONS

Although generally self-limited, complications range by species, including bacteremia, reactive arthritis, and toxic megacolon. Guillain-Barré disease is associated with recent *C. jejuni* infection.

REFERENCES

1. Fleckenstein JM, Kuhlmann FM, Sheikh A. Acute bacterial gastroenteritis. *Gastroenterol Clin North Am*. 2021;50(2):283–304.
2. Shah HJ, Jervis RH, Wymore K, et al. Reported incidence of infections caused by pathogens transmitted commonly through food: impact of increased use of culture-independent diagnostic tests—foodborne diseases active surveillance network, 1996–2023. *MMWR Morb Mortal Wkly Rep*. 2024;73(26):584–593.
3. Shane AL, Mody RK, Crump JA, et al. 2017 Infectious Diseases Society of America Clinical Practice Guidelines for the diagnosis and management of infectious diarrhea. *Clin Infect Dis*. 2017;65(12):1963–1973

SEE ALSO

Appendicitis, Acute; Botulism; Brucellosis; Dehydration; Diarrhea, Acute; Guillain-Barré Syndrome; Hypokalemia; Intestinal Parasites; Salmonella Infection; Typhoid Fever

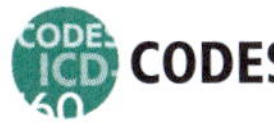

CODES

ICD10

- A05.9 Bacterial foodborne intoxication, unspecified
- A02.0 Salmonella enteritis
- A04.5 Campylobacter enteritis

CLINICAL PEARLS

- Consider bacterial food poisoning when multiple patients present with fever and blood/mucus in stool after recent travel or ingesting the same food.
- Testing generally does not change management. Consider stool culture and molecular testing with moderate to severe symptoms or persistent symptoms >7 days.
- Mainstay of treatment remains oral hydration.
- Consider empiric antibiotics for traveler's diarrhea in cases of moderate to severe disease.
- Withhold antispasmodics and antidiarrheal agents if there is concern for enteroinvasion (high prolonged fever, bloody diarrhea, severe pain, septicemia).

FROSTBITE

Frank J. Domino, MD

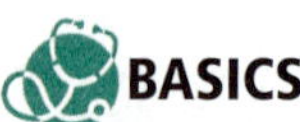

BASICS

DESCRIPTION

- A severe localized injury due to cold exposure, causing tissue to freeze, resulting in direct cellular injury and progressive dermal ischemia (most commonly of exposed hands, feet, face, and ears)
- Systems affected: integumentary, vascular, muscular, skeletal, nervous
- Synonym: dermatitis congelationis; freezing cold injury (FCI)

EPIDEMIOLOGY

- Predominantly adults but can affect all ages
- Predominant sex: male ≤ female, potentially more common in females due to increased surface area in conjunction with less body mass although exposure rates in males may be higher (1)

ETIOLOGY AND PATHOPHYSIOLOGY

- Prolonged exposure to cold
- Ice crystals form intracellularly and extracellularly. Vasoconstriction reduces blood flow and microvascular endothelial injury leads to ischemia. Cellular dehydration leads to abnormal electrolyte concentrations and cell death.
- In severe cases, tissue injury extends to muscle and bone leading to necrosis and mummification. Rewarming injured endothelium results in edema and bullae as the ice crystals melt. Inflammatory mediators such as prostaglandins and thromboxane A2 induce vasoconstriction and platelet aggregation, worsening ischemia.
- In severe frostbite, the chronic inflammation can result in an imbalance of proinflammatory and antiinflammatory macrophages, which can lead to delayed healing (2).
- If refreezing occurs after thawing, cascade of events are more extreme (1).

RISK FACTORS

- Prolonged exposure to below freezing temperatures, especially combined with wind and/or water exposure
- High-altitude activities, such as mountaineering
- Military operations in cold environments
- Constricting or wet clothing with inadequate insulation
- Altered mental status due to alcohol, drugs, or psychiatric illness
- The experience of homelessness
- Previous cold-related injury
- Dehydration and/or malnutrition
- Conditions that interfere with total heat production and/or thermoregulation (i.e., endocrine abnormalities) (1)
- Conditions that promote loss of body heat including chronic skin conditions, hyperhidrosis, burns (including sunburns) (1)
- Hypothermia
- Any condition that results in decreased vasoconstriction and/or vascular pathology as in (1):
  - Smoking; Raynaud phenomenon; peripheral vascular disease; diabetes

GENERAL PREVENTION

- Dress in layers with appropriate cold weather gear and avoid clothing that is too constricting.
- Cover exposed areas and extremities appropriately.
- Stay dry; avoid alcohol and minimize wind exposure.
- Ensure adequate hydration and caloric intake.
- Use supplemental oxygen at very high altitudes (>7,500 meters).
- Exercise can protect against frostbite by increasing core and peripheral temperatures. Note: Caution should be made that the exercise will not lead to exhaustion and inability to seek for shelter/warmth.
- Appropriate use of chemical or electric hand and foot warmers can help maintain peripheral warmth.
- Recognize expected temperatures and take into consideration wind chills prior to exposure and if possible avoid exposure.
- Avoid emollients on the skin as they can lead to a false sense of protection (1).
- Avoid alcohol, caffeine, and other medications that can cause vasoconstriction (1).

COMMONLY ASSOCIATED CONDITIONS

- Hypothermia
- Alcohol or drug abuse

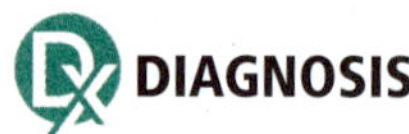

DIAGNOSIS

HISTORY

- Significant cold exposure—determine length and severity.
- Throbbing pain
- Paresthesias
- Numbness
- Loss of coordination and dexterity

PHYSICAL EXAM

- Hands, feet, face, and ears are most commonly affected.
- Before rewarming, skin may be insensate, white or grayish-yellow in color, cyanotic, or hard and waxy to touch.
- After rewarming, immediate physical exam findings can be categorized as:
  - Grade 1: no cyanosis on the extremity
  - Grade 2: cyanosis isolated to the distal phalanx
  - Grade 3: intermediate and proximal phalangeal cyanosis
  - Grade 4: cyanosis over the carpal or tarsal bones
- Frostbite can alternatively be categorized into four degrees (similar to burn injuries):
  - 1st degree: numbness and erythema; a white or yellow, firm, slightly raised plaque develops; no gross tissue infarction occurs; there may be slight epidermal sloughing. Mild edema is common.
  - 2nd degree: superficial skin vesiculation; a clear or milky blisters, surrounded by erythema and edema
  - 3rd degree: deeper hemorrhagic blisters
  - 4th degree: extends through the dermis to involve subcutaneous tissues, with necrosis extending into muscle and bone
  - 1st- and 2nd-degree injuries are superficial.
  - 3rd- and 4th-degree injuries are deep (3)[C].

DIFFERENTIAL DIAGNOSIS

- Frostnip: a superficial cold injury that resolves spontaneously without tissue loss
- Chilblains (pernio): a localized inflammatory reaction to cold and wet exposure without tissue freezing; typically presents as edematous, erythematous to violaceous skin lesions
- Immersion foot (trench foot): inflammatory reaction of the feet to prolonged exposure to cold and moisture
- COVID-toes, a SARS-CoV-2 phenomenon related to pernio/chilblains (4)

DIAGNOSTIC TESTS & INTERPRETATION

Initial Tests (lab, imaging)

- Baseline labs: CBC, CMP, UA for myoglobinuria, culture wound if suspected infection
- Radiography can be an initial imaging to identify extent of soft tissue involvement versus bone involvement (2).
- Technetium (Tc)-99m scintigraphy can identify tissue viability at early stage and identify candidates for thrombolytic therapy.
- MRI/MRA, duplex ultrasonography, and standard or digital subtraction angiography are occasionally used.
- Consider serial photographs at time of injury, at 24 hours, and every several days until hospital discharge.
- For severe frostbite especially, angiography and bone scans, as well as MRI/MRA, US, and infrared thermal imaging, are useful to determine need for thrombolysis versus amputation (2).
- Angiography and bone scans can be used to determine effectiveness of thrombolysis if done before and after treatment (2).
- There is some evidence that angiography has been shown to accurately determine the need for amputation whereas bone scans cannot reveal this information (caution with angiography with renal insufficiency).
- SPECT/CT should be used to reveal clinical prognosis (2).

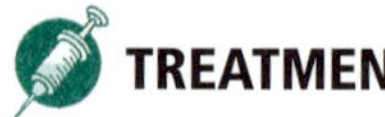

TREATMENT

GENERAL MEASURES

- Correct hypothermia.
- Assess for additional injuries.
- Remove jewelry from affected extremities.
- Initiate rewarming of affected body part only if there is no risk of refreezing. Warm affected parts of body in 37–39°C water for approximately 30 minutes until the involved part takes on a red or purple appearance and becomes pliable to touch. A whirlpool bath can help with rewarming and antiseptic. Avoid using other heat sources, such as a fire or space heater to rewarm affected parts avoided.
- Apply topical aloe vera gel before dressing.
- Selectively drain clear or cloudy blisters; leave hemorrhagic blisters intact.
- Splint and elevate affected extremity.

- Tetanus prophylaxis
- Oral hydration if patient is alert and has no GI symptoms; otherwise, IV hydration with warm normal saline in small boluses
- Daily bathing in warm water with active and passive mobilization
- Dry, loose bulky dressings, including in between fingers/toes (3)[C]
- Pain control (1)
- Antibiotics only if infectious complications become apparent (1)

ALERT
- Avoid rubbing the affected area as this can lead to further tissue damage.
- Patients should avoid weight-bearing on frostbitten limbs prior to definitive care.

MEDICATION

First Line

- Tissue plasminogen activator (tPA) for deep injury (grade 3 and 4) (5), administered (either IV or intra-arterially) within 24 hours of injury may prevent damage from microvascular thrombosis and reduce amputation rates; if administered, should be done so immediately after rewarming (5)
- **Precaution**: tPA should not be used with history of recent bleeding, stroke, peptic ulcer, or recent surgery.
- Heparin is recommended as adjunctive therapy in tPA protocols. Heparin is not recommended as monotherapy.
- Consider low-molecular-weight dextran in patients not given other systemic treatments (e.g., tPA) (3)[C].
- Iloprost is indicated for severe frostbite if tPA is contraindicated (5).
- Update tetanus toxoid (3)[C].
- Ibuprofen 400 mg q12h (inhibit prostaglandins) (3)[C]
- NSAIDs for mild to moderate pain; narcotic analgesia for moderate to severe pain
- Use systemic antibiotics for proven infection. Prophylactic antibiotics are not recommended (3)[C].

Second Line

Pentoxifylline 400 mg q8h

ADDITIONAL THERAPIES

- Heated oxygen
- Warm IV fluids
- Botulinum toxin injections to improve sequelae including chronic pain

SURGERY/OTHER PROCEDURES

- Urgent surgery is rarely needed.
- Fasciotomy is indicated if the patient develops elevated compartment pressures (3)[C].
- Surgical débridement, as needed, to remove necrotic tissue
- Amputation only if tissues are necrotic: may take 4 to 12 weeks for the demarcation of tissue necrosis to become definitive
- Consider imaging with 99mTc bone scan and/or MRA in severe cases to determine extent of injury; assess viability of surrounding tissue and determine need for surgery.

ADMISSION, INPATIENT, AND NURSING CONSIDERATIONS

- Hospitalization is generally recommended unless no blisters are present after rewarming (e.g., grade 1/1st-degree frostbite) (3)[C].
- Patients are typically best cared for in a hospital with experience treating frostbite injuries (trauma center or burn unit).
- Administer tPA in intensive care setting.
- Ensure proper hydration and nutrition.
- Treat pain (often requires narcotic analgesia).
- Wound care—clean dressings and twice daily whirlpool baths
- Apply aloe vera gel q6–8h through resolution of blisters.
- Elevate injured extremities above heart level to minimize edema.
- Physical therapy and early mobilization
- If patient cannot tolerate oral fluids or has altered mental status, give warmed normal saline in small boluses (3)[C].

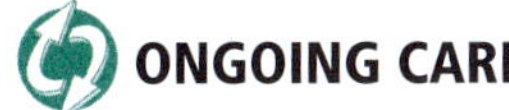

ONGOING CARE

FOLLOW-UP RECOMMENDATIONS

- Protect injured body parts.
- Continue physical therapy.
- Avoid smoking and alcohol.
- Avoid recurrent cold exposure.
- Ensure properly fitting clothing and footwear.

Patient Monitoring

Monitor growth of affected extremity in pediatric patients.

DIET

- As tolerated
- Warm oral fluids

PATIENT EDUCATION

Provide education on:

- Protection from cold injuries
- Risk factors for frostbite
- Early signs and symptoms of frostbite
- Field treatment of cold injuries
- Wound care

PROGNOSIS

- Grade 1: no amputation and no sequelae
- Grade 2: potential soft tissue amputation and nail sequelae
- Grade 3: potential bone amputation of the digit and functional sequelae
- Grade 4: potential bone amputation of the limb with functional sequelae
- Other factors that attribute to poor prognosis include:
  - Severity of injury as seen above
  - Longer duration of exposure
  - Concomitant substance abuse

COMPLICATIONS

- Tissue loss: Distal parts of an extremity may undergo spontaneous amputation; tissue necrosis requiring amputation
- Gangrene; hyperhidrosis due to nerve injury; decreased hair and nail growth
- Raynaud phenomenon
- Frostbite arthropathy and osteoarthritis
- Chronic regional pain; neuropathy
- Localized osteoporosis
- Premature closure of epiphyses in pediatric patients

REFERENCES

1. Fudge J. Preventing and managing hypothermia and frostbite injury. *Sports Health*. 2016;8(2):133–139.
2. Gao Y, Wang F, Zhou W, et al. Research progress in the pathogenic mechanisms and imaging of severe frostbite. *Eur J Radiol*. 2021;137:109605.
3. McIntosh SE, Hamonko M, Freer L, et al. Wilderness Medical Society practice guidelines for the prevention and treatment of frostbite. *Wilderness Environ Med*. 2011;22(2):156–166.
4. Volansky R. Diagnosing "COVID toes" and other challenges in the derm-rheum overlap. Healio 2021. https://www.healio.com/news/rheumatology/20210818/diagnosing-covid-toes-and-other-challenges-in-the-dermrheum-overlap. Accessed October 25, 2025.
5. Hickey S, Whitson A, Jones L, et al. Guidelines for thrombolytic therapy for frostbite. *J Burn Care Res*. 2020;41(1):176–183.

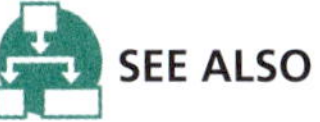

SEE ALSO

- Hypothermia
- Algorithm: Hypothermia

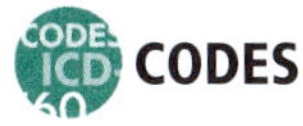

CODES

ICD10

- T33.90XA Superficial frostbite of unspecified sites, init encntr
- T34.90XA Frostbite with tissue necrosis of unsp sites, init encntr
- T33.829A Superficial frostbite of unspecified foot, initial encounter

CLINICAL PEARLS

- Frostbite is a tetanus-prone injury. Provide appropriate tetanus prophylaxis.
- Avoid rewarming en route to the hospital if there is a chance of refreezing; rewarm only with water.
- Assess for additional injuries to areas which may be insensate.
- tPA can reduce amputation rates. Use within 24 hours of injury in appropriate clinical settings.
- Early assessment of the degree of tissue involvement is difficult. Delay surgery until a definite tissue demarcation of necrosis occurs (may take 4 to 12 weeks).

FURUNCULOSIS

Zoltan Trizna, MD, PhD

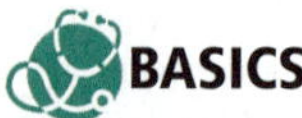

BASICS

DESCRIPTION

- Acute bacterial abscess of a hair follicle (often *Staphylococcus aureus*)
- System(s) affected: skin/exocrine
- Synonym(s): boils; carbuncles (clusters of boils)

EPIDEMIOLOGY

Incidence

- Predominant age
  - Adolescents and young adults
  - Clusters have been reported in teenagers living in crowded quarters, within families, or in high school athletes.
- Predominant sex: male = female

Prevalence

Exact data are not available. In US military settings approximately 5% of the skin infections were carbuncles or furuncles.

ETIOLOGY AND PATHOPHYSIOLOGY

- Infection spreads away from hair follicle into surrounding dermis.
- Pathogenic strain of *S. aureus* (usually); most cases in United States are now due to community-acquired methicillin-resistant *S. aureus* (CA-MRSA), whereas methicillin-sensitive *S. aureus* (MSSA) is most common elsewhere (1)[A].

Genetics

Unknown

RISK FACTORS

- Carriage of pathogenic strain of *Staphylococcus* spp. in nares, skin, axilla, and perineum
- Rarely, polymorphonuclear leukocyte defect or hyperimmunoglobulin E–*Staphylococcus* spp. abscess syndrome
- Diabetes mellitus, malnutrition, alcoholism, obesity, atopic dermatitis
- Primary immunodeficiency disease and AIDS (common variable immunodeficiency, chronic granulomatous disease, Chédiak–Higashi syndrome, C3 deficiency, C3 hypercatabolism, transient hypogammaglobulinemia of infancy, immunodeficiency with thymoma, Wiskott-Aldrich syndrome)
- Secondary immunodeficiency (e.g., leukemia, leukopenia, neutropenia, therapeutic immunosuppression)
- Medication impairing neutrophil function (e.g., omeprazole)
- The most important independent predictor of recurrence is a positive family history.

GENERAL PREVENTION

Patient education regarding self-care (see "General Measures"); treatment and prevention are interrelated.

COMMONLY ASSOCIATED CONDITIONS

- Usually normal immune system
- Diabetes mellitus
- Polymorphonuclear leukocyte defect (rare)
- Hyperimmunoglobulin E–*Staphylococcus* sp. abscess syndrome (rare)
- See "Risk Factors."

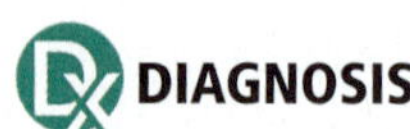

DIAGNOSIS

HISTORY

- Located on hair-bearing sites, especially areas prone to friction or repeated minor traumas (e.g., underneath belt, anterior aspects of thighs, nape, buttocks)
- No initial fever or systemic symptoms
- The folliculocentric nodule may enlarge, become painful, and develop into an abscess (frequently with spontaneous drainage).

PHYSICAL EXAM

- Painful erythematous papules/nodules (1 to 5 cm) with central pustules
- Tender, red, perifollicular swelling, terminating in discharge of pus and necrotic plug
- Lesions may be solitary or clustered.

DIFFERENTIAL DIAGNOSIS

- Folliculitis
- Pseudofolliculitis
- Carbuncles
- Ruptured epidermal cyst
- Myiasis (larva of botfly/tumbu fly)
- Hidradenitis suppurativa
- Atypical bacterial or fungal infections

DIAGNOSTIC TESTS & INTERPRETATION

Initial Tests (lab, imaging)

Obtain culture if with multiple abscesses marked by surrounding inflammation, cellulitis, systemic symptoms such as fever, or if immunocompromised.

Follow-Up Tests & Special Considerations

- Immunoglobulin levels in rare (e.g., recurrent or otherwise inexplicable) cases
- If culture grows gram-negative bacteria or fungus, consider polymorphonuclear neutrophil leukocyte functional defect.

Test Interpretation

Histopathology (although a biopsy is rarely needed)

- Perifollicular necrosis containing fibrinoid material and neutrophils
- At deep end of necrotic plug, in SC tissue, is a large abscess with a Gram stain positive for small collections of *S. aureus*.

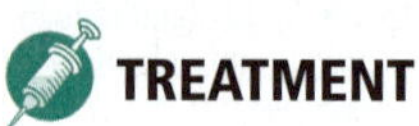

TREATMENT

GENERAL MEASURES

- Moist, warm compresses (provide comfort, encourage localization/pointing/drainage) 30 minutes QID
- If pointing or large, incise, and drain: Consider packing if large or incompletely drained.
- Routine culture is not necessary for localized abscess in nondiabetic patients with normal immune system.
- Sanitary practices: Change towels, washcloths, and sheets daily; clean shaving instruments; avoid nose picking; change wound dressings frequently; do not share items of personal hygiene (2)[B].

MEDICATION

First Line

- Systemic antibiotics are usually not necessary, unless there is extensive surrounding cellulitis or fever. Other indications include a single abscess >2 cm, immunocompromise.
- No important differences were found in comparative trials regarding efficacy or safety outcomes between different oral antibiotics for the treatment of boils or bacterial folliculitis (1)[A].

- Resistant strains of *S. aureus* (MRSA): clindamycin 300 mg q6h or doxycycline 100 mg q12h or trimethoprim-sulfamethoxazole (TMP-SMX DS) 1 tab q8–12h or minocycline 100 mg q12h
- If multiple abscesses, lesions with marked surrounding inflammation, cellulitis, systemic symptoms such as fever, or if immunocompromised: Place on antibiotic therapy directed at *S. aureus* for 7 to 14 days, and consider >1 antibiotic to cover MRSA and streptococci. Dicloxacillin (Dynapen, Pathocil) 500 mg PO QID *or* cephalexin 500 mg PO QID *or* clindamycin 300 mg TID may be added to TMP-SMX, for example.

Second Line

- Antibiotic therapy selected by confirmed bacterial sensitivity (culture and sensitivity [C&S]). Rarely, IV antibiotics may be indicated if cellulitis is present or large abscess requiring significant surgical procedure. Treatments for MRSA include linezolid PO or IV and IV vancomycin.
- If known or suspected impaired neutrophil function (e.g., impaired chemotaxis, phagocytosis, superoxide generation), add vitamin C 1,000 mg/day for 4 to 6 weeks (prevents oxidation of neutrophils).
- If antibiotic regimens fail:
  - May try PO pentoxifylline 400 mg TID for 2 to 6 months (inhibits neutrophil activation and adhesion)
  - Contraindications: recent cerebral and/or retinal hemorrhage; intolerance to methylxanthines (e.g., caffeine, theophylline); allergy to the particular drug selected
  - Precautions: prolonged prothrombin time (PT) and/or bleeding; if on warfarin, frequent monitoring of PT

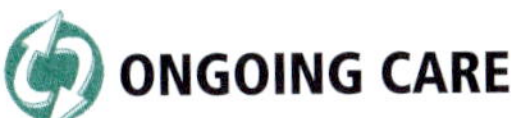

ONGOING CARE

FOLLOW-UP RECOMMENDATIONS

Patient Monitoring

Instruct patient to see physician if compresses are unsuccessful.

DIET

Unrestricted

PROGNOSIS

- Self-limited: usually drains pus spontaneously and will heal with or without scarring within several days
- Recurrent/chronic: may last for months or years
- If recurrent, usually related to chronic skin carriage of staphylococci (nares or on skin). Treatment goals are to decrease or eliminate pathogenic strain *or* suppress pathogenic strain.
  - Culture nares, skin, axilla, and perineum (culture nares of family members)
  - Mupirocin 2%: Apply to both nares BID for 5 days each month.
  - Consider a course of rifampin (600 mg daily for 1 to 2 weeks), especially in recurrent cases in which first-line decolonization has failed. Always use in combination with an oral antibiotic with established effectiveness against MRSA. Use with clindamycin or doxycycline may be particularly effective.
  - Culture anterior nares every 3 months; if failure, retreat with mupirocin or consider clindamycin 150 mg/day for 3 months.
  - Long-term efficacy of strategies to eliminate carrier state (decolonization) remains unclear.
- Especially in recurrent cases, wash entire body and fingernails (with nailbrush) daily for 1 to 3 weeks with povidone-iodine (Betadine), or chlorhexidine (Hibiclens), although all can cause dry skin and irritation. Diluted bleach baths may be helpful as well (¼ cup of 6% household bleach in a full bathtub, 15 minutes daily for 5 days).

COMPLICATIONS

- Scarring
- Bacteremia
- Seeding (e.g., septal/valve defect, arthritic joint)

REFERENCES

1. Lin HS, Lin PT, Tsai YS, et al. Interventions for bacterial folliculitis and boils (furuncles and carbuncles). *Cochrane Database Syst Rev*. 2021;2(2):CD013099.
2. Fritz SA, Camins BC, Eisenstein KA, et al. Effectiveness of measures to eradicate *Staphylococcus aureus* carriage in patients with community-associated skin and soft-tissue infections: a randomized trial. *Infect Control Hosp Epidemiol*. 2011;32(9):872–880.

ADDITIONAL READING

- Ibler KS, Kromann CB. Recurrent furunculosis—challenges and management: a review. *Clin Cosmet Investig Dermatol*. 2014;7:59–64.
- Nowicka D, Grywalska E. *Staphylococcus aureus* and host immunity in recurrent furunculosis. *Dermatology*. 2019;235(4):295–305.
- Stahlman S, Williams VF, Oh GT, et al. Skin and soft tissue infections, active component, U.S. Armed Forces, January 2016–September 2020. *MSMR*. 2021;28(4):27–38.

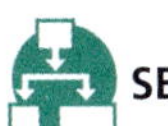

SEE ALSO

Folliculitis; Hidradenitis Suppurativa

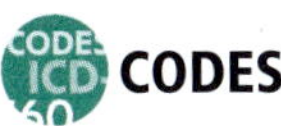

CODES

ICD10

- L02.92 Furuncle, unspecified
- L02.12 Furuncle of neck
- L02.429 Furuncle of limb, unspecified

CLINICAL PEARLS

- Pathogens may be different in different localities. Keep up-to-date with the locality-specific epidemiology.
- If few, furuncles/furunculosis do not need antibiotic treatment. If systemic symptoms (e.g., fever), cellulitis, or multiple lesions occur, oral antibiotic therapy is used.
- Folliculitis, furunculosis, and carbuncles are parts of a spectrum of pyodermas.
- Other causative organisms include aerobic (e.g., *Escherichia coli*, *Pseudomonas aeruginosa*, and *Streptococcus faecalis*), anaerobic (e.g., *Bacteroides*, *Lactobacillus*, and *Peptostreptococcus*), and *Mycobacteria*.
- Decolonization (treatment of the nares with topical antibiotic) is only recommended if the colonization was confirmed by cultures because resistance is common and treatment is of uncertain efficacy.

F

GALACTORRHEA

Kelley V. Lawrence, MD, NABBLM-C • Cecile T. Robes, DO • Elizabeth Joyce Trout, MD, FAAFP, MLS (ASCP)

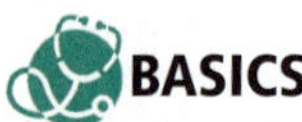

BASICS

DESCRIPTION

- Milky nipple discharge not associated with lactation, defined as >1 year after pregnancy or cessation of breastfeeding
- Does not include serous, purulent, or bloody nipple discharge
- System(s) affected: endocrine/metabolic, nervous, reproductive

Pediatric Considerations

Can occur in infants secondary to maternal estrogen exposure; advise parents not to palpate and not to express milk (colloquially called "witches milk").

Pregnancy Considerations

Milk production often begins during the 2nd trimester; milk leakage that occurs during pregnancy is not pathophysiologic galactorrhea.

EPIDEMIOLOGY

- Predominant age: 15 to 50 years (reproductive age), most commonly ages 20 to 35 years
- Third most common breast complaint in women
- Men with prolactinomas may present with shorter duration of symptoms, higher prolactin levels, and larger more resistant tumors.

Incidence

- Marked variability reported
- Specific data in pediatric population limited

Prevalence

Approximately 20–25% of women experience galactorrhea in their lifetime.

ETIOLOGY AND PATHOPHYSIOLOGY

- Oxytocin stimulates the anterior pituitary to secrete prolactin, which induces lactation.
- Prolactin secretion is inhibited by dopamine produced in the hypothalamus.
- Galactorrhea results either from prolactin overproduction or loss of inhibitory regulation by dopamine.
- Physiologic galactorrhea can be due to pregnancy, nipple stimulation, nipple piercing, exercise, or sexual activity.
- Hyperprolactinemia can be due to overproduction by malignancy or mass effect, most commonly prolactinoma.
- Hyperprolactinemia secondary to systemic diseases:
  - Hypothyroidism
  - Chronic renal failure (reduced clearance of prolactin leading to elevated serum levels)
  - Cirrhosis
  - Adrenal insufficiency
- Acupuncture has also been shown to cause galactorrhea.
- Medications/substances:
  - Cardiovascular (α-methyldopa, reserpine, verapamil, spironolactone)
  - GI (domperidone, metoclopramide, rabeprazole)
  - Herbal (anise [licorice], barley, blessed thistle, fenugreek seed, fennel, goat's rue)
  - Illicit (cocaine, marijuana)
  - Antimicrobials (isoniazid, protease inhibitors)
  - Opioids
  - Psych/neuro (neuroleptics, antipsychotics [notably risperidone], stimulants, SSRIs, tricyclic antidepressants, MAOIs)
  - Reproductive (estrogens depot-medroxy-progesterone acetate [DMPA], copper IUD)
  - DMARDs (azathioprine)
- Rarely associated with adrenal insufficiency, post-breast reduction surgery, acromegaly, or wall conditions (such as trauma, burns, herpes simplex virus [HSV] pain in nipple/areolar dermatome); infiltrative diseases of the pituitary gland can also rarely lead to galactorrhea.

Genetics

Multiple endocrine neoplasia type 1 increases risk for pituitary adenomas, of which prolactinomas make up approximately 40%.

RISK FACTORS

- Hypothyroidism
- Use of medications that cause galactorrhea (see above list)

GENERAL PREVENTION

- Avoid frequent nipple stimulation.
- Avoid medications that can suppress dopamine.

COMMONLY ASSOCIATED CONDITIONS

Commonly associated with hypothyroidism, chronic kidney disease, hypogonadism, and pituitary adenoma

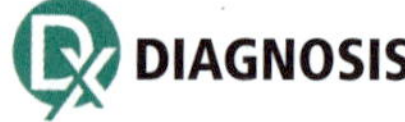

DIAGNOSIS

HISTORY

- Usually bilateral milky nipple discharge that may be spontaneous or induced by stimulation
- Determine possibility of pregnancy or recent discontinuation of lactation.
- Association with initiation of new medication or supplement
- Signs of hypogonadism related to hyperprolactinemia (oligomenorrhea, amenorrhea, anovulation, infertility, decreased libido, erectile dysfunction, hot flashes)
- Mass effects from pituitary enlargement (headache, vision changes)

PHYSICAL EXAM

- Breast examination should be performed both seated while leaning forward and laying back on exam table with attention to the presence of spontaneous or induced nipple discharge (with gentle hand expression); technique for hand expression is the same as for a lactating person—one documented approach is called the Marmet technique (see "Additional Reading").
- Should observe bilateral, milky white, or brown nipple discharge
- Perform formal visual field testing if pituitary adenoma suspected.

DIFFERENTIAL DIAGNOSIS

- Pregnancy-induced lactation or recent weaning (Average duration of lactation after weaning is 40 days, but can be longer in cases of prolonged duration of breastfeeding.)
- Nonmilky (straw colored, gray, yellow, green, brown) nipple discharge: intraductal papilloma, fibrocystic disease
- Purulent breast discharge: typically due to infection; may see breast redness, pain, warmth, and edema; possible diagnoses include mastitis, breast abscess, impetigo, eczema.
- Bloody breast discharge: If palpable mass, edema, or axillary lymphadenopathy, consider malignancy (Paget disease, breast cancer).

DIAGNOSTIC TESTS & INTERPRETATION

Initial Tests (lab, imaging)

- Rule out physiologic lactation (urine hCG testing, breastfeeding within past year).
- If negative hCG, measure prolactin (normal prolactin level in nonpregnant women is up to 30 ng/mL, although values may vary with different laboratories. During pregnancy, serum prolactin ranges 200 to 500 ng/mL) (1)[C].
- If prolactin is elevated, evaluate thyroid, liver, and renal function (TSH, free T4, hepatic panel, BMP) for possible underlying etiology.
- Prolactin levels fluctuate (highest in early morning) and may be falsely elevated by a recent breast examination, vigorous exercise, or sexual activity. Elevated and borderline levels should be confirmed with repeat level drawn in a fasting, nonexercised state, with no breast stimulation (2)[C].
- If a breast mass is palpated, consider evaluation with mammogram and/or ultrasound.

Follow-Up Tests & Special Considerations

- Follicle-stimulating hormone and luteinizing hormone if amenorrheic
- Growth hormone levels if acromegaly suspected
- Measure adrenal steroids if signs of Cushing disease present.
- Consider formal visual field testing.

- Pituitary MRI with gadolinium if the serum prolactin level is significantly elevated (>200 ng/mL and outside of physiologic breastfeeding/lactation) or if a tumor is otherwise suspected
- Although not part of a routine workup, if it remains unclear whether breast discharge is milk, the Sudan IV Stain test that can be done on the breast discharge to evaluate for fat droplets.

Test Interpretation

Falsely normal or mildly elevated prolactin levels can be seen sometimes in the setting of very high prolactin levels. This is called the "hook effect" of the antibody/antigen interaction of ELISA testing. If suspicion for elevated prolactin remains, request a diluted sample for testing (1:100 dilution).

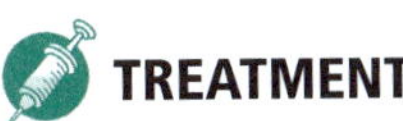

TREATMENT

GENERAL MEASURES

- Identify and treat the underlying cause.
- Idiopathic galactorrhea (normal prolactin levels) does not require treatment (3)[C].
- As long as pituitary and thyroid function are normal, galactorrhea does not require treatment if the discharge is not troublesome to the patient (4).
- Avoid excess nipple stimulation, include nursing pads to manage nipple discharge.
- Discontinue causative medications, if possible.

MEDICATION

- Dopamine agonists (cabergoline and bromocriptine) are first-line therapy for hyperprolactinemia, whether idiopathic or caused by prolactinoma (3)[C].
  - Dopamine agonists work to reduce prolactin levels and shrink tumor size. Therapy is not curative (3)[C].
  - If patient is attempting conception, bromocriptine is preferred, as cabergoline must be stopped 1 month prior to conception.
- Contraindications are similar for all and include the following:
  - Uncontrolled hypertension
  - Sensitivity to ergot alkaloids
- Precautions
  - Dopamine agonists may cause nausea, vomiting, psychosis, or dyskinesia.
  - Discontinue therapy if a patient becomes pregnant (bromocriptine hasn't been associated with increased risk of congenital malformations or abortions, however still recommended to stop per Endocrine Society).
- Significant possible drug interactions: serotonergic agents, ergot derivatives, antipsychotic agents
- Therapy should be continued for at least 2 years. If prolactin level has normalized, can consider tapering treatment at that time.

First Line

Cabergoline (Dostinex)

- Start at 0.25 mg PO twice weekly and increase by 0.25 mg monthly until prolactin levels normalize. Usual dose ranges from 0.25 to 3.00 mg PO weekly.
- More efficacious and better tolerated than bromocriptine (3)[C]
- Check ESR and serum creatinine at baseline and every 6 to 12 months.
- Monitor prolactin monthly until normalized, and then every 3 months during treatment.
- If patients require >3.5 mg cabergoline weekly, recommend annual echocardiogram to monitor for valvular disease/damage.

Second Line

Bromocriptine

- Start at 1.25 mg QHS PO with food and increase every 3 to 7 days by 2.5 mg/day until therapeutic response achieved (usually 2.5 to 15.0 mg/day).
- Check creatinine, CBC, hepatic panel, HbA1c, at least twice yearly. Pregnancy test every 4 weeks during amenorrheic periods.
- Monitor prolactin monthly until normalized and then every 3 months during treatment.

ISSUES FOR REFERRAL

Dependent on underlying pathology; neurology, endocrinology, neurosurgeon, and/or breast surgeon as indicated

SURGERY/OTHER PROCEDURES

For tumors >10 mm, patients may require pituitary surgery or radiotherapy.

COMPLEMENTARY & ALTERNATIVE MEDICINE

Alternative modalities used to cease milk production include ingestion of peppermint, parsley, and/or sage on a regular basis and topical application of cabbage leaves over the breast tissue.

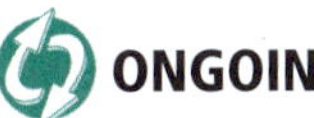

ONGOING CARE

FOLLOW-UP RECOMMENDATIONS

Patient Monitoring

- Check prolactin levels every month until normalized. After levels normalize, check again every 3 months while on dopamine agonist therapy. After discontinuation, prolactin should be checked every 3 months for the 1st year and then yearly discontinuation of therapy (3)[C].
- Monitor visual fields and/or MRI at least yearly until stable for prolactinoma.

DIET

No restrictions; may include peppermint, parsley, and sage in diet for symptom management

PATIENT EDUCATION

- Caution patient about symptoms of mass enlargement in pituitary (vision changes, headaches).
- Inform patient that offending medications should be discontinued long-term.
- Educate new moms that this condition can be normal in infants due to exposure to maternal hormones.

PROGNOSIS

- Symptoms can recur after discontinuation of a dopamine agonist (risk of recurrence is as high as 66%).
- 5 years after transsphenoidal surgery 76% of patients are disease free.
- Prolactinomas <10 mm can resolve spontaneously.

COMPLICATIONS

- If enlarging pituitary adenoma, risk of permanent visual field loss
- Surgery carries risk of hypopituitarism, diabetes insipidus, CSF leak, and local infection.
- Osteoporosis if amenorrhea persists without estrogen replacement (1)[C]
- Hyperprolactinemia does not increase breast cancer risk.

REFERENCES

1. Majumdar A, Mangal NS. Hyperprolactinemia. *J Hum Reprod Sci*. 2013;6(3):168–175.
2. Huang W, Molitch ME. Evaluation and management of galactorrhea. *Am Fam Physician*. 2012;85(11):1073–1080.
3. Melmed S, Casanueva FF, Hoffman AR, et al. Diagnosis and treatment of hyperprolactinemia: an Endocrine Society clinical practice guideline. *J Clin Endocrinol Metab*. 2011;96:273–288.
4. Bruehlman RD, Winters S, McKittrick C. Galactorrhea: rapid evidence review. *Am Fam Physician*. 2022;106:695–700.

ADDITIONAL READING

DiVasta AD, Weldon CB, Labow BI. The breast: examination and lesions. In: Emans SJ, Laufer MR, DiVasta AD, (eds). *Emans, Laufer, Goldstein's Pediatric & Adolescent Gynecology*. 7th ed. Philadelphia, PA: Wolters Kluwer, 2020:781.

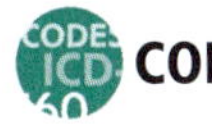

CODES

ICD10

- N64.3 Galactorrhea not associated with childbirth
- N64.52 Nipple discharge

CLINICAL PEARLS

- Galactorrhea is a common disorder, affecting up to 50% of reproductive-age women.
- Galactorrhea is defined as bilateral milk production, usually whitish in appearance but can be varied.
- Common causes include idiopathic, nipple stimulation, dopamine-suppressing medications, systemic disease, or pituitary prolactinoma.
- Evaluate prolactin >200 ng/mL (or signs of suspicion for a pituitary macroadenoma) with a gadolinium-enhanced MRI focused on the pituitary.
- If treatment is desired, first-line medication is cabergoline; second-line is bromocriptine.

G

GASTRITIS

Marie L. Borum, MD, EdD, MPH • Abdelrhman Refaey, MD

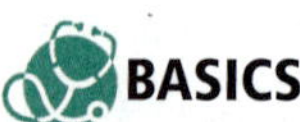

BASICS

DESCRIPTION

- Inflammation of the gastric mucosa
- Classified as:
  - Acute: neutrophilic infiltration on histology
  - Chronic: mixture of mononuclear cells lymphocytes, macrophages on histology
- Subtypes:
  - Erosive gastritis
    - Mucosal injury by a noxious agent (especially nonsteroidal anti-inflammatory drugs [NSAIDs] or alcohol)
    - Vascular congestion due to portal hypertension (HTN) or gastric antral vascular ectasia (GAVE)
  - Reflux gastritis—reaction to prolonged biliary/pancreatic fluid reflux
  - Hemorrhagic gastritis (stress ulceration)—a reaction to hemodynamic disorder (e.g., hypovolemia or hypoxia [shock]); common in intensive care unit (ICU) patients, especially post burn/trauma
  - Infectious/environmental gastritis
    - *Helicobacter pylori* infection (most common cause of gastritis); *H. pylori* has been linked with gastric cancer.
    - Viral systemic infection caused by cytomegalovirus (CMV) or Epstein-Barr virus (EBV)
  - Atrophic gastritis
    - Metaplastic atrophic gastritis: autoimmune primary (pernicious) anemia
    - Frequent in elderly and prolonged proton pump inhibitor (PPI) use (chronic *H. pylori*)
    - Major risk factor for gastric cancer

Geriatric Considerations

Persons aged >60 years often harbor *H. pylori* infection.

Pediatric Considerations

Gastritis is rare in infants or children. Most common etiology for pediatric gastritis is *H. pylori* infection.

EPIDEMIOLOGY

- Prevalence increases with age (more common in elderly).
- Affects both sexes; autoimmune gastritis is more common in women.
- *H. pylori* is common.

Incidence

~2 million annual visits in the United States

Prevalence

- ~50% of people >60 years of age are infected with *H. pylori* versus 20% of people <40 years of age.
- 1/4 to 1/3 of U.S. adults are infected with *H. pylori*. The prevalence increases with age.
- Rates of infection are higher in minority groups, immigrants, and lower socioeconomic status.

ETIOLOGY AND PATHOPHYSIOLOGY

- Noxious agents damage the gastric mucosal barrier, exposing underlying epithelial tissue.
- Infection: *H. pylori*, *Staphylococcus aureus* exotoxins, and viral infections (EBV, CMV)
- Alcohol via cell DNA damage and subsequent pyroptosis
- Aspirin and other NSAIDs through inhibition of protective prostaglandin synthesis
- Emotional stress due to cortisol production

Genetics

Potential role of toll-like receptor 1 (TLR1) in *H. pylori*-associated gastritis

RISK FACTORS

- Age >60 years and exposure to noxious drugs/chemicals (e.g., alcohol, NSAIDs, tobacco)
- Hypovolemia, hypoxia (shock), burns, head injury, complicated postoperative course
- Autoimmune diseases (thyroiditis, type 1 diabetes mellitus, Addison disease, vitiligo, erosive oral lichen planus)

GENERAL PREVENTION

- Avoid injurious drugs or chemical agents, alcohol, and tobacco.
- Patients with hypovolemia or hypoxia (especially ICU patients) should receive prophylaxis with H_2 antagonists, PPIs, prostaglandins, or sucralfate.
- Consider testing for *H. pylori* in patients on long-term NSAID therapy, with idiopathic thrombocytopenic purpura (ITP), or unexplained iron deficiency anemia.
- Test and treat *H. pylori* in individuals at increased risk of gastric cancer, those with atrophic gastritis or gastric intestinal metaplasia, and adult household contacts of *H. pylori*-positive patients (1).

COMMONLY ASSOCIATED CONDITIONS

- Gastric or duodenal peptic ulcer
- Primary (pernicious) anemia—atrophic gastritis
- Portal HTN, hepatic failure
- Mucosa-associated lymphoid tissue (MALT) lymphoma

DIAGNOSIS

HISTORY

- Burning epigastric pain or discomfort, often aggravated by eating
- Unintentional weight loss, anorexia
- Nausea, with or without vomiting
- Significant bleeding is unusual except in hemorrhagic gastritis.
- Rectal bleeding/melena
- Hiccups, belching, bloating or fullness
- Neurologic symptoms related to vitamin B_{12} deficiency if atrophic gastritis
- History of smoking, alcohol, NSAID, radiotherapy, gallbladder disorders, autoimmune disorders, IBD, vasculitis or eosinophilic disorders
- Can be asymptomatic

PHYSICAL EXAM

- Vital signs to assess hemodynamic stability
- Abdominal exam often normal; mild epigastric tenderness
- May have heme-positive stool
- Stigmata of chronic alcohol use
- Pallor, delayed capillary refill if anemic or hypovolemic

DIFFERENTIAL DIAGNOSIS

- Functional abdominal pain (dyspepsia)
- Peptic ulcer disease, viral gastroenteritis
- Gastric cancer (elderly), cholecystitis
- Pancreatic disease (inflammation vs. tumor)

DIAGNOSTIC TESTS & INTERPRETATION

Initial Tests (lab, imaging)

Usually normal

- Evaluate for iron deficiency anemia (CBC, ferritin).
- Stool analysis for fecal *H. pylori* antigen
  - 95% specificity and sensitivity
  - Can be used for diagnosis and eradication
- ^{13}C-urea breath test for *H. pylori*—95% specificity and sensitivity
- *H. pylori*, serology serum IgG
  - Inexpensive; 85% sensitivity, 79% specificity
  - Positive in history of colonization or prior infections; *cannot be used to assess eradication*
- Patients with autoimmune chronic gastritis may have antibodies to intrinsic factor (IF) or parietal cells, elevated serum fasting gastrin, decreased serum pepsinogen 1 (PGI) and PGI-to-PGII ratio.
- Patients with pernicious anemia may have macrocytic anemia with low serum vitamin B_{12} levels and IF autoantibodies.
- Drugs that may alter lab results: Antibiotics, PPIs, and bismuth-containing compounds may affect urea breath test for *H. pylori*.
  - Hold PPIs for 2 weeks, H_2 antagonists for 24 hours, and antibiotics for 4 weeks prior to stool or breath tests (2)[B].

Follow-Up Tests & Special Considerations

Endoscopy for *H. pylori:* Obtain multiple biopsies in body and antrum for culture; polymerase chain reaction (PCR); histology with H&E plus second staining; rapid urease testing

Diagnostic Procedures/Other

- Gastroscopy with biopsy is first line in:
  - Age >50 years with new-onset symptoms
  - Weight loss, persistent vomiting, or GI bleed
- Consider for patients <50 years of age who are *H. pylori*-negative.
- Gastric biopsies recommended if there is a poor response to treatment. *Patients must discontinue PPIs for 2 weeks prior to improve diagnostic accuracy.*

TREATMENT

GENERAL MEASURES

- *H. pylori* treatment is required to relieve symptoms.
- Parenteral fluid and electrolyte supplements if unable to tolerate oral intake
- Discontinue NSAID use. Abstinence from alcohol; smoking cessation

MEDICATION

First Line

- Antacids: liquid form, 30 mL 1 hour after meals and at bedtime
- H_2 receptor antagonists oral cimetidine (Tagamet) 300 mg q6h or famotidine (Pepcid) 20 mg BID or nizatidine (Axid); 150 mg BID not shown to be clearly superior to antacids
- Sucralfate (Carafate): 1 g q4–6h on an empty stomach; rationale uncertain but empirically helpful
- Prostaglandins (misoprostol [Cytotec]): can help allay gastric mucosal injury; dosage 100 to 200 μg QID
- PPIs if no response to antacids or H_2 antagonists (omeprazole or esomeprazole 20 mg daily or BID)
- *H. pylori* (1)
  - First line in treatment-naive patients:
    - Bismuth quadruple therapy (BQT) for 14 days—85% eradication (especially in areas with high or unknown rates of clarithromycin resistance)
      - PPI standard dose BID (e.g., omeprazole 20 mg BID)
      - Bismuth subsalicylate 300 or 524 mg or Bismuth subcitrate 120 to 300 mg QID
      - Tetracycline 500 mg QID
      - Metronidazole 500 mg TID or QID
  - Alternative:
    - Rifabutin triple therapy: rifabutin 50 mg, amoxicillin 1 g, and omeprazole 40 mg 3 times daily for 14 days (available as the combination pill Talicia)
    - Vonoprazan-based therapies: 14 days
      - vonoprazan-amoxicillin dual (Voquezna DualPak): vonoprazan 20 mg BID plus amoxicillin 1 g TID
      - Vonoprazan-amoxicillin-clarithromycin triple (Voquezna TriplePak): vonoprazan 20 mg, amoxicillin 1 g, clarithromycin 500 mg BID
  - Clarithromycin triple therapy (CTT)
    - Avoid clarithromycin triple therapy empirically unless clarithromycin susceptibility is confirmed.
    - Short course (14 days) of amoxicillin 1 g BID, PPI BID (omeprazole 20 mg BID, etc.), and clarithromycin 500 mg BID
    - *If PCN allergy*: Use metronidazole 500 mg TID instead of amoxicillin.
    - Alternative: Prevpac combination pill (lansoprazole, amoxicillin, and clarithromycin)
- *H. pylori* treatment failure: Use a different regimen; avoid clarithromycin (unless confirmed susceptibility).
  - Optimized BQT for 14 days if not previously used
  - If optimized BQT has already been used, the next option is rifabutin triple therapy for 14 days (PPI + amoxicillin + rifabutin), especially if antibiotic susceptibility unknown or testing is not available.
- Levofloxacin triple therapy (high-dose PPI BID, amoxicillin 1 g TID, levofloxacin 500 mg once daily) should only be used if *H. pylori* is known to be levofloxacin-sensitive, or if BQT and rifabutin triple therapy have failed or unavailable.
- Clarithromycin-based regimens should be avoided unless clarithromycin susceptibility is confirmed.
- Probiotics are considered as adjuncts in symptomatic *H. pylori* infection; may decrease severity of gastritis, peptic ulcers; and possibly slow progression toward atrophic gastritis and gastric adenocarcinoma (3)[A]:
  - Probiotics alone likely do not eradicate *H. pylori*.
  - Possible regimens as used in trials: *Bifidobacterium spp.* BID × 14 days
  - Contraindications: hypersensitivity
- Precautions: Bismuth may turn stool black.

Pregnancy Considerations

- Avoid sodium carbonate and magnesium trisilicate containing antacids.
- Women with hyperemesis gravidarum (HG) have a higher prevalence of *H. pylori* infection. Treatment can be deferred until after delivery. Routine testing for *H. pylori* is not recommended in those with HG.

SURGERY/OTHER PROCEDURES

Surgical intervention is not necessary, except in the case of phlegmonous gastritis or gastritis with high-grade dysplasia.

COMPLEMENTARY & ALTERNATIVE MEDICINE

Studies suggest cranberry, garlic, curcumin, ginger, and Pistacia gum may prevent and/or reduce *H. pylori* infection due to anti-inflammatory properties.

ADMISSION, INPATIENT, AND NURSING CONSIDERATIONS

Prophylaxis in ICU patients

ONGOING CARE

FOLLOW-UP RECOMMENDATIONS

Confirm *H. pylori* eradication >4 weeks after treatment.

Patient Monitoring

- Consider repeat endoscopy after 6 weeks if gastritis was severe or poor treatment response.
- Surveillance endoscopy in patients with mild to moderate atrophic gastritis not recommended; patients with advanced atrophic gastritis should obtain endoscopy with biopsy sampling every 3 years.
- Surveillance may be suspended when two or more endoscopies are negative for dysplasia.

DIET

Diet restrictions (e.g., bland, light, soft foods) depend on symptom severity. In general, avoid caffeine, spicy foods, alcohol, peppermint, carbonated beverages, and high-fat-content food.

PATIENT EDUCATION

- Quit smoking; limit alcohol; adjust diet.
- Relaxation; avoid NSAIDs.

PROGNOSIS

Phlegmonous gastritis has a 40–50% mortality even with treatment.

COMPLICATIONS

- Bleeding from extensive mucosal erosion or ulceration
- Gastric outlet obstruction due to edema
- Gastric intestinal metaplasia, which puts patient at a 10- to 15-fold increase of developing gastric cancer
- Clearing *H. pylori* before the development of chronic gastritis may prevent development of gastric cancer.
- Chronic autoimmune gastritis has increased risk of development of gastric neuroendocrine tumors and adenocarcinoma due to dysplasia.

REFERENCES

1. Chey WD, Howden CW, Moss SF, et al. ACG clinical guideline: treatment of *Helicobacter pylori* infection. *Am J Gastroenterol*. 2024;119(9):1730–1753. doi:10.14309/ajg.0000000000002968.
2. Yang H, Guan L, Hu B. Detection and treatment of *Helicobacter pylori*: problems and advances. *Gastroenterol Res Pract*. 2022;2022:4710964. doi:10.1155/2022/4710964.
3. Buzás GM, Birinyi P. Newer, older, and alternative agents for the eradication of *Helicobacter pylori* infection: a narrative review. *Antibiotics (Basel)*. 2023;12(6):946. doi:10.3390/antibiotics12060946.

ADDITIONAL READING

Rugge M, Genta RM, Malfertheiner P, et al. RE.GA.IN.: the Real-world Gastritis Initiative—updating the updates. *Gut*. 2024;73(3):407–441. doi:10.1136/gutjnl-2023-331164.

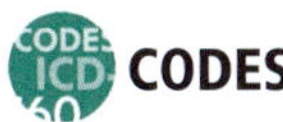

CODES

ICD10

- K29.5 Unspecified chronic gastritis
- K29.40 Chronic atrophic gastritis without bleeding
- K29.50 Unspecified chronic gastritis without bleeding

CLINICAL PEARLS

- *H. pylori* is the most common cause of gastritis; >50% of adult patients are colonized with *H. pylori* by age 60 years.
- *H. pylori* antibodies decline in the year after treatment and should not be used to determine eradication.
- *H. pylori* stool antigen tests can be used before and after therapy to assess for eradication and reinfection.
- Several courses of therapy may be necessary to eradicate *H. pylori*.
- In cases of suspected gastritis, discontinue PPI 2 weeks prior to endoscopy to improve diagnostic accuracy.

GASTROESOPHAGEAL REFLUX DISEASE

Frank J. Domino, MD • Liana C. Brooks, MD

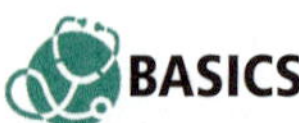

BASICS

DESCRIPTION
- Changes of the esophageal mucosa resulting from reflux of gastric contents into the esophagus
- Often described as "heartburn," "acid indigestion," and "acid reflux"

EPIDEMIOLOGY

Incidence
5/1,000 person-years

Prevalence
- The prevalence of GERD in North America is ~15% (95% CI, 10.7–20.9%) (1).
- There is no association between gender and symptoms of GERD in North America.
- Advanced age increases risk of GERD; >50 years old, odds ratio (OR) of 1.32 (95% CI, 1.46–2.06) (1)
- Pediatric population: Regurgitation occurs in nearly 50% of newborn infants, resolving spontaneously in 90% of children by age 1 year (1).

ETIOLOGY AND PATHOPHYSIOLOGY
- Stomach acid contacts the squamous mucosal lining of the esophagus, which is less acid resistant than gastric columnar mucosa, followed by release of chemokines and cytokines causing symptoms and disease.
- GERD can be the result of one or a combination of the following: lower esophageal sphincter (LES) dysfunction, esophageal hypersensitivity, delayed gastric emptying, and increased gastroesophageal junction distensibility.
- Patients with severe GERD often have evidence of a hiatal hernia which can trap acid, impair acid emptying, reduce LES pressure, and increase retrograde acid flow.

Genetics
Genetic heterogeneity may account for 31–43% of the predisposition to develop GERD (2).

RISK FACTORS
- Obesity; OR of 1.7 (95% CI, 1.4–2.1) (1): higher prevalence of hiatal hernia, increased intra-abdominal pressure, bile, and pancreatic enzymes
- Tobacco use; OR of 1.2 (95% CI, 1.04–1.5) (1)
- Hiatal hernia
- Pregnancy
- Diet; alcohol use
- Scleroderma; neuromuscular disorders

GENERAL PREVENTION
- Weight loss (1)[A],(2)[A]
- Tobacco cessation (1)[B]
- Decrease consumption of spicy, acidic and fatty foods, alcoholic and carbonated beverages, chocolate, and caffeine (2)[C].
- Elevate head of bed at night for selected patients (2)[C].
- Avoid meals within 2 to 3 hours of bedtime (2)[C].
- Smaller portions
- Remain upright during and after meals.
- Infants: use of car seat for 2 to 3 hours after meals, thickened feedings, burp frequently while feeding

COMMONLY ASSOCIATED CONDITIONS
- Erosive esophagitis occurs in 18–25% of patients with GERD (1).
- Barrett esophagus: prevalence of 7% (95% CI, 5%–9%) in patients with GERD (1)
- Esophageal adenocarcinoma
- Peptic ulcer disease (PUD)
- Peptic esophageal stricture
- Extraesophageal reflux: asthma, aspiration, chronic cough, laryngitis, vocal cord granuloma, sinusitis, otitis media
- Halitosis

DIAGNOSIS

HISTORY
- Typical symptoms: acid regurgitation, heartburn, dysphagia (mostly postprandial)
- Extraesophageal signs and symptoms: chronic cough, bronchospasm, wheezing, hoarseness, sore throat, throat clearing; conditions such as laryngitis, pharyngitis, and pulmonary fibrosis
- Atypical symptoms: epigastric fullness/pressure/pain, dyspepsia, nausea, bloating, belching, odynophagia (sometimes reflective of ulcer), chest pain, lump in throat, hypersalivation (water brash)
- Heartburn: retrosternal burning sensation
- Regurgitation; sour or acid taste in mouth
- Symptoms worse with bending or lying down
- Diet, alcohol and tobacco use

PHYSICAL EXAM
Often benign but look for potential
- Epigastric tenderness or palpable epigastric mass
- Dental erosions

DIFFERENTIAL DIAGNOSIS
- Angina/coronary artery disease
- Infectious esophagitis (*Candida*, herpes, HIV, cytomegalovirus)
- Chemical esophagitis; pill-induced esophagitis; eosinophilic esophagitis
- PUD
- Biliary tract disease
- Achalasia or other upper gastrointestinal motility disorders
- Esophageal stricture or anatomic defect (ring, sling, paraesophageal hernia)
- Irritable bowel syndrome
- Gastrointestinal malignancy
- Functional heartburn
- Rumination

DIAGNOSTIC TESTS & INTERPRETATION
Society of American Gastrointestinal and Endoscopic Surgeons diagnose GERD with one or greater of the following (1)[A]:
- A mucosal break >5 mm (Los Angeles [LA] grade B/C/D) observed on endoscopy in a patient with typical symptoms (please note that esophagogastroduodenoscopy [EGD] must be performed after cessation of PPI for 2 to 4 weeks)
- Barrett esophagus (>3 cm) on biopsy
- Abnormal reflux monitoring off therapy

Initial Tests (lab, imaging)
- For patients with typical GERD symptoms, an EGD with biopsy and pH probe is not required for a formal diagnosis, and instead, a trial of PPI is recommended (2)[B].
- PPI is given daily for 8 weeks (30 to 60 minutes before a meal) and symptoms are monitored. If symptoms completely resolve, most likely diagnosis is GERD with a sensitivity of 78% and specificity of 54% (2).
- Patients presenting with alarm symptoms such as weight loss and GI bleeding, dysphagia, or multiple risk factors for Barrett esophagus should undergo EGD as first test for evaluation.
- No lab studies are needed for initial workup of GERD (1).
- Appropriately evaluate patients who present with symptoms suspicious for cardiac disease.

Follow-Up Tests & Special Considerations
- In patients who fail initial PPI challenge, or have symptoms that recur after discontinuation following 8-week PPI trial, endoscopy is recommended (ideally 2 to 4 weeks after PPIs are stopped).
- In patients for whom diagnosis of GERD is suspected but not clear, and endoscopy shows no evidence of GERD, reflux monitoring is recommended off therapy to establish diagnosis.

Diagnostic Procedures/Other
- Upper endoscopy
  - Recommended for those with alarm signs such as dysphagia, bleeding, anemia, weight loss, recurrent vomiting
  - Recommended if uncontrolled persistent symptoms after twice-daily PPI for 4 to 8 weeks.
  - Recommended if at risk for Barrett esophagus (or with known history requiring surveillance)
- High-resolution manometry (HRM)
  - Helpful in refractory cases, can evaluate peristaltic function, record LES pressure, and diagnose motility disorders
  - HRM helps with placement of pH probes, operative planning for surgical or endoscopic anti-reflux procedures.
  - Used for patients unresponsive to PPI with inconclusive pH monitoring or those with noncardiac chest pain especially those not responsive to PPI trial to assess motility abnormalities.
- Ambulatory reflux (pH) monitoring
  - Evaluate excessive acid exposure in those with GERD symptoms, normal endoscopy, and no response to PPI.
  - Used to document acid exposure time, frequency of reflux, and symptom correlation.
  - Discontinue PPI for 7 days prior to test.
  - Measured for 24 to 96 hours depending on placement technique
  - Calculate SI or SAP; both are a ratio of event to time to objectify GERD. If SAP >95% or SI >50%, test is positive (2).
- Barium swallow: not used for GERD diagnosis; used to evaluate complaints of dysphagia or to outline anatomic abnormalities (hiatal hernia)

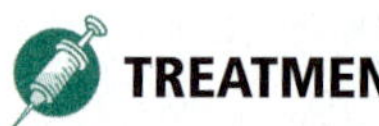

TREATMENT

GENERAL MEASURES
Lifestyle changes are first-line intervention, reviewed in the "General Prevention" section.
- Stepwise approach to therapy
  - Phase I: lifestyle and diet modifications, antacids plus H_2 blockers or PPIs (PPI > H_2 blockers > placebo) (1)[A]
  - Phase II: If symptoms persist, consider endoscopy.
  - Phase III: If symptoms still persist, consider surgery: laparoscopic preferred over open fundoplication (1)[A].

MEDICATION

First Line
- Antacids are used exclusively for on-demand symptom relief with little evidence to favor one type over another.
- Alginates (sodium alginate), usually combined with antacid, alleviate mild reflux symptoms, especially postprandial.

- H_2 blockers in equipotent oral doses (e.g., famotidine 20 mg BID, nizatidine 150 mg BID, cimetidine 400 mg BID); ranitidine pulled from U.S. market.
  - Block histamine receptors in parietal cells of stomach to reduce acid production
  - Renally excreted—adjust dose in chronic kidney disease.
  - Less effective than PPIs (1),(2)
  - Can be used in conjunction to PPI for bedtime relief (2)[C]
  - For individuals with partial response to intermittent H2RA therapy, institute standard dose therapy for 2 to 4 weeks. Stopping H2RA and starting PPI is reasonable alternative.
- PPIs in equipotent oral doses (e.g., pantoprazole 40 mg/day, dexlansoprazole 30 mg/day, esomeprazole 40 mg/day, lansoprazole 30 mg/day, omeprazole 20 mg/day, rabeprazole 20 mg/day)
  - Irreversibly bind proton pump (H^+/K^+ ATPase), effective onset within 4 days
  - Complete symptom relief at 4 weeks in 70–80% of patients with EE (2).
  - PPIs are more effective than H_2 blocker and prokinetics for healing erosive and nonerosive esophagitis (2)[A].
  - PPIs increase risk of *Clostridium difficile* infections and have a theoretical risk of hypomagnesemia, bone fracture, vitamin B_{12} deficiency, and community-acquired pneumonia (2).
  - Dose 30 to 60 minutes before meals except dexlansoprazole (2)
  - GERD relief and healing rates vary minimally among PPIs (2)
- Reevaluate symptoms after 4 to 8 weeks of treatment (1).
- Discontinuation of long-term PPI can cause potential rebound acid hypersecretion due to high levels of gastrin which can be reduced by tapering PPI dose before stopping (2)[C]. This has been primarily demonstrated to occur in health controls, strong evidence for increase in symptoms after abrupt PPI withdrawal is lacking.
- Blood dyscrasias and anemia may occur with PPIs and H_2 blockers.
- Tachyphylaxis may occur with H_2 blockers.
- Vonoprazan (a potassium-competitive acid blocker [PCAB]) has been recently approved for treatment of erosive esophagitis.
- A trial of baclofen at a dosage of 5 to 20 mg 3 times a day can be considered in patients with objective documentation of continued symptomatic reflux despite optimal PPI therapy.

Pregnancy Considerations

- Trial lifestyle changes first; if that fails, antacids and sucralfate are first-line options (2).
- H_2 blockers (category B) and all PPIs are category B except omeprazole (category C) (2).

Pediatric Considerations

Antacids or liquid H_2 blockers and PPIs are available. Prokinetics have a minimal role due to safety concerns and limited efficacy.

Second Line

- Sucralfate is a mucosal barrier agent.
  - Limited data, could be as efficacious as H2RA (2)[C]
  - Dose: 1 g PO QID 1 hour before meals and at bedtime for 4 to 8 weeks
- Prokinetics: metoclopramide
  - Increase LES pressure, esophageal peristalsis, and gastric emptying
  - Can be used as adjunct, limited data (2)[C]
  - Dose: 5 to 10 mg before meals
  - Metoclopramide is a dopamine blocker; risk of dystonia and tardive dyskinesia
- Baclofen is a GABA B receptor agonist.
  - Inhibits transient relaxations of LES
  - Rarely used to treat GERD in children without underlying neurologic problems

ISSUES FOR REFERRAL

Treatment resistant, persistent, severe disease or advanced esophageal disease (e.g., dysplasia, Barrett esophagus) should be referred to a specialist.

SURGERY/OTHER PROCEDURES

- Laparoscopic fundoplication, wrapping gastric fundus around distal esophagus, decreases reflux into esophagus by improving function of GE junction.
  - Partial and total fundoplications have similar outcomes, but partial has fewer complications (1).
  - GERD remission is similar between PPI and fundoplication although recent systemic reviews suggest more significant patient reported outcome satisfaction in comparison with long-term use of PPIs (1).
  - Surgery has higher risk of severe adverse events (1).
  - Surgery is a recommended option for long-term treatment of patients with objective evidence of GERD, especially those who have severe reflux esophagitis (LA grade C or D), large hiatal hernias, and/or persistent, troublesome GERD symptoms.
- Bariatric surgery
  - BMI >35 kg/m^2; prevalence of GERD increases up to 6-fold (2)
  - Obesity increases risk of complications or failure of fundoplication.
  - Gastric sleeve or Roux-en-Y gastric bypass are beneficial for the obese patient with GERD (1),(2).
  - Manometry to rule out esophageal dysmotility, achalasia, or scleroderma prior to surgery
- Ablative endoscopic techniques, radiofrequency ablation to levels below and above the LES, results in thickening of the sphincter, decreases transient relaxation rate, and reduces esophageal exposure to gastric acid (1) (contradicting results in multiple studies) (2).
- Transoral incisionless fundoplication (TIF), endoscopically suturing serosa to serosa creating a valve around esophagogastric junction, reducing acid reflux (contradicting results in multiple studies) (1),(2)

ONGOING CARE

FOLLOW-UP RECOMMENDATIONS

Patient Monitoring

- Monitor symptoms over time. Consider additional workup and/or treatment if symptoms fail to improve after 8 weeks of PPI treatment.
- Repeat endoscopy in 4 to 8 weeks if there is a poor symptomatic response to medical therapy, especially in older patients.
- Monitoring recommendations changes depending on level of disease and dysplasia.

PATIENT EDUCATION

Lifestyle and dietary modifications per "General Prevention" section

PROGNOSIS

- 2/3 of patients with nonerosive esophagitis have symptomatic relapse when PPI stopped (2)
  - Consider maintenance PPI for patients with GERD complications as relapse is common.
  - LA classification is endoscopic scoring system: mild (grades A and B) and severe (grades C and D). Patients with LA grade C or D will need long-term PPI therapy to heal (2)[A].
- Intermittent PPI therapy or as needed can successfully manage noncomplicated GERD (2)[C].
- Medical and surgical therapy are equally effective for symptom reduction (1).
- Laparoscopic fundoplication has a 6.9% reoperation rate within 10 years (1).

COMPLICATIONS

- Peptic stricture: 10–15%
- Risk of Barrett esophagus, progression to adenocarcinoma:
  - Men are at greater risk than women.
  - Annual incidence of adenocarcinoma with Barrett esophagus and low-grade dysplasia is 0.54% (95% CI, 0.32–0.76%) (1).
  - Annual incidence of adenocarcinoma with Barrett esophagus and high-grade dysplasia is 1.73% (95% CI, 0.99–2.47%) (1).
- Bleeding due to mucosal injury

Geriatric Considerations

- Complications from PPI use more likely (e.g., enteric infection), higher risk for side effects from medical management
- Increased risk of adenocarcinoma

REFERENCES

1. Maret-Ouda J, Markar SR, Lagergren J. Gastroesophageal reflux disease: a review. *JAMA*. 2020;324(24):2536–2547. doi:10.1001/jama.2020.21360.
2. Katz PO, Dunbar KB, Schnoll-Sussman FH, et al. ACG clinical guideline for the diagnosis and management of gastroesophageal reflux disease. *Am J Gastroenterol*. 2022;117(1):27–56. doi:10.14309/ajg.0000000000001538.

ADDITIONAL READING

- Abdel-Aziz Y, Metz DC, Howden CW. Review article: potassium-competitive acid blockers for the treatment of acid-related disorders. *Aliment Pharmacol Ther*. 2021;53(7):794–809.
- Kasugai K, Ogasawara N. Gastroesophageal reflux disease: pathophysiology and new treatment trends. *Intern Med*. 2024;63(1):1–10. doi:10.2169/internalmedicine.1551-23.

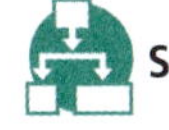

SEE ALSO

Algorithms: Abdominal Pain, Upper; Dyspepsia

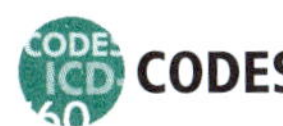

CODES

ICD10

- R12 Heartburn
- K21.9 Gastro-esophageal reflux disease without esophagitis
- K21.0 Gastro-esophageal reflux disease with esophagitis

CLINICAL PEARLS

- Formal diagnosis of GERD requires a combination of endoscopy, biopsy, and pH monitoring.
- Consider GERD in nonsmokers with a chronic cough (>3 weeks).
- PPIs provide the most rapid symptomatic relief and healing of esophagitis.
- Consider additional workup and/or treatment if symptoms fail to improve after 8 weeks of PPI treatment.
- Endoscopy is recommended for patients with alarm symptoms, risk factors for Barrett esophagus, or continued symptoms despite adequate PPI trial.
- PCABs are an emerging option for treating patients with esophageal reflux disease.

G

GAY HEALTH

Stacy P. Rubin, MD

BASICS

- Men who have sex with men (MSM) is a clinical term that refers to sexual behavior alone, regardless of sexual orientation, as MSM may include men who identify as gay, bisexual, or heterosexual. Sexual orientation is independent of gender identity.
- MSM are less likely to access health care and are disproportionately impacted by mental health issues, substance use and abuse, and sexually transmitted infections (STI).

DESCRIPTION

- LGBTQ individuals report structural barriers within the health care system, as well as fear, stigma, and internalized homophobia as contributing factors to health disparities when compared to non-LGBTQ counterparts.
- LGBTQ individuals may hide their sexual orientation out of fear of stigma and discrimination, so it is important to ask all patients about sexual orientation and behavior in a nonjudgmental environment.
- Although this chapter reviews the important topics that affect this population disproportionately, primary care of MSM foremost is about delivering the same level of care to all patients, regardless of sexual orientation.

GENERAL PREVENTION

- The majority of screening guidelines are the same for MSM as they are for non-MSM age- and sex-matched populations.
- Centers for Disease Control and Prevention (CDC) and the United States Preventative Services Task Force (USPSTF) suggest at least annual screening for HIV, syphilis, gonorrhea, and chlamydia as detailed below, with increased frequency and other screening tests based on the level of risk of the patient's behavioral practices.
- CDC recommends testing for hepatitis B serology at least at the initial visit, and vaccination for MSM who are seronegative or for whom vaccination status cannot be ascertained (1)[A]. However, in 2022, the Advisory Committee on Immunization Practices (ACIP) expanded hepatitis B vaccination recommendations to include all adults aged 19 to 59 years.
- Screening for hepatitis C is recommended in all patients between the ages of 18 and 79 years at least once in a lifetime. Annual screening for hepatitis C is only recommended in MSM with HIV.
- Screening for hepatitis A is not recommended. However, hepatitis A vaccination is recommended for MSM.
- Annual digital anorectal examination (DARE) is recommended as a screening for anal cancer, but there is insufficient evidence to recommend obtaining anal cytology in all MSM patients.
- The ACIP recommends routine vaccination schedules be followed for MSM patients, including vaccination against: (i) hepatitis A and B viruses; (ii) human papillomavirus (HPV) for all patients between 11 and 26 years old with additional consideration for MSM patients outside this age category; and (iii) smallpox monkeypox virus, live nonreplicating, especially if there is high prevalence in geographical area. ACIP recommends using shared decision-making for serogroup B meningococcal vaccine (MenB) and quadrivalent meningococcal vaccine against serogroups A, C, W, and Y (MenACWY) in MSM.
- Cultivating a welcoming environment is the cornerstone of prevention of disease for the LGBTQ community. Consider accessing community or web-based resources for more information on creating an LGBTQ safe zone for clinical practice sites.

DIAGNOSIS

- STI
  - Taking a detailed sexual history is of paramount importance in LGBTQ individuals. The CDC suggest the 5Ps approach (partners, practices, protection from STI, past history of STI, and pregnancy intention) when obtaining a patient's sexual history.
  - Physicians should screen for behaviors placing patients at increased risk of STI such as:
    - Anonymous sexual encounters
    - Multiple active sex partners (or partners with multiple active partners or a history of multiple partners)
    - Inconsistent barrier protection (condom) use
    - Substance use during and around sex, including exchanging sex for drugs or money
    - History of or current STI
    - Receptive and insertive anal intercourse, with receptive having higher risk of STI transmission
  - Screening of all sexually active MSM should include at least annual screening for HIV, syphilis, chlamydia, and gonorrhea at all sites of contact (urethra, rectum, and pharynx if applicable). Screening for hepatitis C should be performed at the initial visit and conducted annually in HIV-infected patients. Screening for STI can be performed more frequently (every 3 to 6 months) based on risk of sexual practices.
  - MSM are at risk of sexual transmission of enteric pathogens such as *Shigella*, *E. coli*, *Campylobacter*, hepatitis A, and parasitic infections such as *Giardia lamblia* and *Entamoeba histolytica* through oral-anal contact or through contact with fecally-contaminated fingers or objects.
  - MSM continue to be at risk for monkeypox infections in the United States. In 2022, outbreaks were identified in the MSM community almost exclusively.
  - Pre-exposure prophylaxis (PrEP) and post-exposure prophylaxis (PEP) regimens for non-HIV STI are on the horizon, such as Doxy PEP (doxycycline 200 mg once, 24 to 72 hours after intercourse) for chlamydial and syphilitic infections, but none have been approved by the FDA or recommended in CDC guidelines yet due to limitations in sample size of studies (2)[C].
- HIV
  - 69% of new cases of HIV diagnosed in 2018 were among MSM. These disproportionately affected Black and Latinx MSM, young MSM, and transgender women. Up to 44% of MSM may not know their HIV status (1).
  - When patients are adherent to drug regimens, PrEP has a >90% efficacy in preventing HIV transmission in patients with detectable drug levels.
  - Indications for PrEP:
    - HIV negative (confirm with RNA viral load if exposed within last 4 weeks)
    - Sexually active, but not with a monogamous HIV-negative partner
    - Male sex partner within last 6 months
    - And at least one of the following: (i) insertive or receptive anal sex without condoms in the past 6 months; (ii) any STI in the last 6 months; or (iii) in a sexual relationship with an HIV-positive partner
  - Prior to initiating PrEP, clinicians must exclude acute or chronic HIV infection, assess renal function, and screen for hepatitis B and C. Patients should be vaccinated for hepatitis B virus if appropriate.
  - There are three FDA-approved regimens for PrEP in MSM patients, two oral and one injection-based (3)[A]. The oral regimens are daily, fixed-dose single-pill combinations and have similar efficacy.
  - Combination tenofovir disoproxil fumarate (TDF)/emtricitabine (FTC); should not be used if creatinine clearance (CrCl) <60 mL/min
  - Combination tenofovir alafenamide (TAF)/FTC (only FDA-approved for MSM and transgender women); TAF is a version of tenofovir with less impact on bone and renal integrity than TDF; should not be used with CrCl <30 mL/min
  - Cabotegravir (CAB) intramuscular injection once every 2 months, with or without oral lead-in therapy, was FDA-approved in late 2021; may be used in renal impairment with CrCl ≥15 mL/min
  - Alternative dosing, "on-demand" dosing, or "2-1-1 PrEP" means patients take 2 doses of TDF/FTC within 2 to 24 hours before sex and 1 dose daily for 2 days afterward. Presently, this regimen is not approved by FDA or recommended by CDC. On-demand use of TAF/FTC has not been studied.
  - Patients need follow-up while on PrEP to screen for HIV and other STI every 3 months. CrCl should be monitored every 6 months, and lipids and weight should be reviewed annually (3)[A].
  - PEP is indicated after exposure to a known HIV-positive partner ≤72 hours prior through mucous membranes, which includes sexual exposure via oral, anal, and vaginal sex.
  - PEP generally involves a 28-day course of highly active antiretroviral therapy (HAART) in a three-drug combination of two nucleoside reverse transcriptase inhibitors (NRTI) and an integrase strand transfer inhibitor (INSTI) or a protease inhibitor (PI).
  - Selection of medications is based on side effect profiles, patient adherence, and patient convenience.

- Preferred PEP regimens are TDF/FTC *or* TDF/lamivudine (3TC) *plus* raltegravir *or* dolutegravir in patients with CrCl ≥60 mL/min. Adjust dose of TDF/FTC or TDF/3TC for patients with CrCl <60 mL/min.
- Alternative PEP regimens include:
  - Combination elvitegravir/cobicistat/emtricitabine/tenofovir disoproxil fumarate (EVG/COBI/FTC/TDF) fixed-dose; cannot use with CrCl <70 mL/min
  - TDF/FTC *plus* darunavir *and* ritonavir in patients with normal renal function; provide renally adjusted dose of TDF-containing medication for CrCl <60 mL/min.
- Counsel on safer sex and risk reduction for repeated exposures, including immediate transition to PrEP after completing PEP.

- Hepatitis C
  - MSM have a slightly higher prevalence of hepatitis C infection than the general population. However, MSM who are HIV-positive are at much higher risk of hepatitis C infection compared to both MSM who are HIV-negative and patients who are not MSM.
  - Screening for hepatitis C is recommended in all MSM patients at initial visit and then more frequently based on risk assessments.
  - Annual screening for hepatitis C is recommended in MSM with HIV.
- Anal cancer
  - The annual incidence of anal cancer is five times higher in MSM who are HIV-negative than the general population. This risk increases to between 78- and 168-times higher in MSM who are HIV-positive.
  - Anal carcinoma has been linked to certain high-risk subtypes of HPV, specifically types 16 and 18.
  - Screening for anal dysplasia with anal cytology may be considered for at-risk populations, especially HIV-infected MSM, but further research is needed for appropriate screening intervals. Anal cytology only should be performed if there is the potential for referral for high-resolution anoscopy and subsequent treatment, if indicated.
  - HPV vaccine is recommended for all patients age 11 to 26 years (can start at age 9 years) to reduce the risk of HPV-related cancer. Providers can consider giving HPV vaccination above age 26 years given high incidence and prevalence of HPV-related anal cancers in MSM patients.
- Substance use and substance use disorders
  - MSM have significantly higher rates of use of nearly all substances as well as higher rates of substance use disorders than men who do not identify as MSM.
  - "Chem sex" refers to use of drugs in conjunction with sexual intercourse by MSM. Inhaled nitrites ("poppers"), stimulants (methamphetamine and cocaine), GHB, ketamine, and alcohol are often used during or around sexual encounters to increase pleasure and performance.
  - Chem sex may be associated with unprotected intercourse and other high-risk sexual behaviors, which may increase risk of HIV and STI transmission.
- Substance abuse treatment programs implementing cognitive behavioral intervention from a harm reduction perspective are beneficial in reducing stimulant use and sexual risk-taking behavior.
  - Most MSM do not report substance use or abuse. It is important to avoid inadvertently introducing or contributing to stigma in the clinical environment by not assuming that all MSM engage in high-risk behaviors.
- Mental health
  - Rates of mental illness or serious mental illness among MSM are 2 to 3 times as high as rates among other men.
  - Risk of deliberate self-harm is also increased especially among MSM youth due to stressors such as having an identity different from family and peers, isolation, bullying, family rejection, and self-nonacceptance.
- Intimate partner violence (IPV) and domestic violence (DV)
  - A recent study reported ~21% of sexual minority men have a history of physical abuse and ~50% have a history of psychological abuse; the highest rates were reported among bisexual men.
  - Providers can stigmatize same-gender IPV as not being serious, especially when wounds may not be overt or physical strength of both partners may be considered equal.
  - Clinicians should screen for IPV and DV with patients alone and respond with compassion and connection to local LGBTQ-welcoming resources.

Pediatric Considerations

- Normalizing nonheterosexual identities and behaviors during regular screening of sexual development during adolescent well-visits may reduce stigma and decrease risk for negative mental health outcomes.
- Regular assessments of mental health and suicide risk should include questions about family and peer support, experiences of stigma, connection to an LGBTQ community, and self-acceptance.
- Same-gender parenting
  - There is no causal relationship between parents' sexual orientation and children's emotional, psychosocial, and behavioral development.
  - Pathways to parenting for same-gender couples include adoption, fostering, IVF, and surrogacy.

ONGOING CARE

- Establish with patients that information related to sexual orientation is asked confidentially of all patients to provide them with the best care.
- Take an inclusive and complete sexual history, and individualize regular discussions about substance abuse, HIV/STI, mental health, and IPV/DV.
- Create a welcoming environment by displaying LGBTQ-friendly symbols and using intake forms and waiting room and marketing materials inclusive of same-gender couples and sexual identities.
- Avoid labeling patients as gay, lesbian, bisexual, or transgender unless prompted by the patients. Many patients may not choose to label at all.
- Understand the significance of terms used in LGBTQ communities, such as "bottom" partner (receptive sex) and "top" partner (insertive sex) and use that language with patients.

PATIENT EDUCATION

- Educate patients on risk-reduction strategies for safer sex such as condoms, PrEP, and PEP, and avoiding or limiting substance use around sex.
- Educate patients on LGBTQ-specific or welcoming resources in your community for substance use and abuse, IPV/DV, mental health, and suicide prevention.

REFERENCES

1. Workowski KA, Bachmann LH, Chan PA, et al. Sexually transmitted infections treatment guidelines, 2021. *MMWR Recomm Rep*. 2021;70(4):1–187. doi:10.15585/mmwr.rr7004a1.
2. Centers for Disease Control and Prevention. Men who have sex with men (MSM). https://www.cdc.gov/std/treatment-guidelines/msm.htm. Accessed June 16, 2025.
3. Centers for Disease Control and Prevention. US Public Health Service: Preexposure prophylaxis for the prevention of HIV infection in the United States—2021 Update: a clinical practice guideline. https://stacks.cdc.gov/view/cdc/112360. Accessed June 16, 2025.

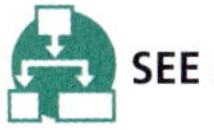

SEE ALSO

- GLAAD: https://www.glaad.org/
- The Safe Zone Initiative: https://www.theszinitiative.org/

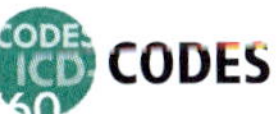

CODES

ICD10

- Z11.59 Encounter for screening for other viral diseases
- Z11.4 Encounter for screening for human immunodeficiency virus
- Z72.52 High risk homosexual behavior

CLINICAL PEARLS

- Provide MSM patients with the same comprehensive primary care delivered to all patients.
- Screen all sexually active MSM annually (https://stacks.cdc.gov/view/cdc/112360) for HIV, syphilis, rectal and urethral gonorrhea, chlamydia, and pharyngeal gonorrhea.
- Screen for hepatitis C virus annually in HIV-positive MSM.
- Counsel patients on risk-reduction strategies for safer sex such as condoms, PrEP, and PEP, and avoiding or limiting substance use around sex.

G

GENITO-PELVIC PAIN/PENETRATION DISORDER (VAGINISMUS)

Jeffrey D. Quinlan, MD, FAAFP

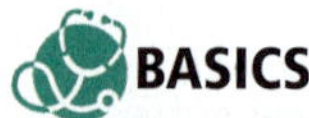

BASICS

Genito-pelvic pain/penetration disorder is the name of the conditions formerly known as vaginismus and dyspareunia. Vaginismus results from involuntary contraction of the vaginal musculature. Primary vaginismus occurs in women who have never been able to have penetrative intercourse. Women with secondary vaginismus were previously able to have penetrative intercourse but are no longer able to do so.

DESCRIPTION

- Persistent or recurrent difficulties for 6 months or more with at least one of the following:
  - Inability to have vaginal intercourse/penetration on at least 50% of attempts
  - Marked genito-pelvic pain during at least 50% of vaginal intercourse/penetration attempts
  - Marked fear of vaginal intercourse/penetration or of genito-pelvic pain during intercourse/penetration on at least 50% of vaginal intercourse/penetration attempts
  - Marked tensing or tightening of the pelvic floor muscles during attempted vaginal intercourse/penetration on at least 50% of occasions
- The disturbance causes marked distress or interpersonal difficulty.
- Dysfunction is not as a result of:
  - Nonsexual mental disorder
  - Severe relationship stress
  - Other significant stress
  - Substance or medication effect
- Specify if with a general medical condition (e.g., lichen sclerosus, endometriosis).

Pregnancy Considerations

May first present during evaluation for infertility

- Pregnancy can occur in patients with genito-pelvic pain/penetration disorder when ejaculation occurs on the perineum.
- Vaginismus may be an independent risk factor for cesarean delivery.

EPIDEMIOLOGY

Incidence

The incidence of vaginismus is thought to be about 1–17% per year worldwide. In North America, 12–21% of women have genito-pelvic pain of varying etiologies (1).

Prevalence

- True prevalence is unknown due to limited data/reporting.
- Population-based studies report prevalence rates of 0.5–30.0%.
- Affects women in all age groups
- Approximately 15% of women in North America report recurrent pain during intercourse.

ETIOLOGY AND PATHOPHYSIOLOGY

Most often multifactorial in both primary and secondary vaginismus

- Primary
  - Psychological and psychosocial issues
    - Negative messages about sex and sexual relations in upbringing may cause phobic reaction.
    - Poor body image and limited understanding of genital area
    - History of sexual trauma
  - Abnormalities of the hymen
  - History of difficult gynecologic examination
- Secondary
  - Often situational
  - Often associated with dyspareunia secondary to:
    - Vaginal infection
    - Inflammatory dermatitis
    - Surgical or postdelivery scarring
    - Endometriosis
    - Inadequate vaginal lubrication
    - Pelvic radiation
    - Estrogen deficiency
  - Conditioned response to pain from physical issues previously listed

RISK FACTORS

- Most often idiopathic
- Although the exact role in the condition is unclear, many women report a history of abuse or sexual trauma.
- Often associated with other sexual dysfunctions

COMMONLY ASSOCIATED CONDITIONS

- Marital stress, family dysfunction
- Anxiety
- Vulvodynia/vestibulodynia

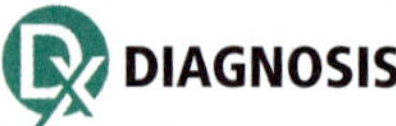

DIAGNOSIS

DSM-5-TR has combined vaginismus and dyspareunia in a condition called genito-pelvic pain/penetration disorder.

HISTORY

- Complete medical history
- Full psychosocial and sexual history, including the following:
  - Onset of symptoms (primary or secondary)
  - If secondary, precipitating events, if any
  - Relationship difficulty/partner violence
  - Inability to allow vaginal entry for different purposes
    - Sexual (penis, digit, object)
    - Hygiene (tampon use)
    - Health care (pelvic examination)
  - Infertility
  - Traumatic experiences (exam, sexual, etc.)
  - Religious beliefs
  - Views on sexuality

PHYSICAL EXAM

- Pelvic examination is necessary to exclude structural abnormalities or organic pathology.
- Educating the patient about the examination and giving her control over the progression of the examination is essential because genital/pelvic examination may induce varying degrees of anxiety in patients.
- Referral to a gynecologist, family physician, or other provider specializing in the treatment of sexual disorders may be appropriate.
- Contraction of pelvic floor musculature in anticipation of examination may be seen.
- Lamont classification system aids in the assessment of severity:
  - First degree: perineal and levator spasm relieved with reassurance
  - Second degree: perineal spasm maintained throughout the pelvic exam
  - Third degree: levator spasm and elevation of buttocks
  - Fourth degree: levator and perineal spasm and elevation with adduction and retreat

DIFFERENTIAL DIAGNOSIS

- Vaginal infection
- Vulvodynia/vestibulodynia
- Vulvovaginal atrophy
- Urogenital structural abnormalities
- Interstitial cystitis
- Endometriosis

DIAGNOSTIC TESTS & INTERPRETATION

No laboratory tests indicated unless signs of vaginal infection are noted on examination. When diagnosing of this disorder has been conducted, five factors should be considered.

- Partner factors
- Relationship factors
- Individual vulnerability factors
- Cultural/religious factors
- Medical factors

Test Interpretation

Not available; may be needed to check for secondary causes

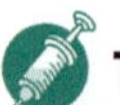

TREATMENT

- Genito-pelvic pain/penetration disorder may be successfully treated (1)[B],(2)[A]. Integrative, multidisciplinary approaches appear to be the most effective in managing vaginismus, particularly when psychological and physical therapies are combined (2)[A].
- Meta-analysis of RCTs documented a trend toward higher efficacy of active treatment versus controls, whereas the meta-analysis of observational studies indicated that women with vaginismus benefit from a range of treatments in almost 80% of cases (3)[A].
- Another meta-analysis of level 1 evidence found that 2/3 of the treatment effect for female sexual dysfunction may be accounted for by placebo (4)[A].

- Outpatient care is appropriate.
- Treatment of physical conditions, if present, is first line (see "Secondary" under "Etiology and Pathophysiology").
- Most begin with pelvic floor physical therapy and myofascial release.
- Evidence suggests that cognitive-behavioral therapy may be effective, including desensitization techniques, such as gradual exposure, aimed at decreasing avoidance behavior and fear of vaginal penetration (5).
- Evidence suggests that sex therapy may be effective (6)[A].
  - Involves Kegel exercises to increase control over perineal muscles
  - Stepwise vaginal desensitization exercises
    - With vaginal dilators that the patient inserts and controls
    - With woman's own finger(s) to promote sexual self-awareness
    - Advancement to partner's fingers with patient's control
    - Coitus after achieving largest vaginal dilator or three fingers; important to begin with sensate-focused exercises/sensual caressing without necessarily a demand for coitus
    - Female superior at first; passive (nonthrusting); female-directed
    - Later, thrusting may be allowed.
- Topical anesthetic or anxiolytic with desensitization exercises may be considered.
- Patient education is an essential component of treatment (see "Patient Education" section).

MEDICATION

- Antidepressants and anticonvulsants have been used with limited success. Low-dose tricyclic antidepressant (amitriptyline 10 mg) may be initiated and titrated as tolerated.
- Topical anesthetics or anxiolytics may be used in combination with either cognitive-behavioral therapy or desensitization exercises as noted above (6)[B].
- Botulinum neurotoxin type A injections may improve vaginismus in patients who do not respond to standard cognitive behavioral and medical treatment for vaginismus.
  - Dosage: 20, 50, and 100 to 400 U of botulinum toxin type A injected in the levator ani muscle have been shown to improve vaginismus (6)[B].
- Intravaginal botulinum neurotoxin type A injection (100 to 150 U) followed by bupivacaine 0.25% with epinephrine 1:400,000 intravaginal injection (20 to 30 mL) while the patient is anesthetized may facilitate progressive placement of dilators and ultimately resolution of symptoms.

ISSUES FOR REFERRAL

For diagnosis and treatment recommendations, the following resources may be consulted:

- Obstetrics/gynecology
- Pelvic floor physical therapy
- Psychiatry
- Sex therapy
- Hypnotherapy

SURGERY/OTHER PROCEDURES

Contraindicated

COMPLEMENTARY & ALTERNATIVE MEDICINE

- Biofeedback
- Functional electrical stimulation

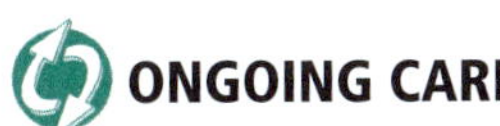

ONGOING CARE

FOLLOW-UP RECOMMENDATIONS

Desensitization techniques of gentle, progressive, patient-controlled vaginal dilation

Patient Monitoring

General preventive health care

PATIENT EDUCATION

- Education about pelvic anatomy, nature of vaginal spasms, normal adult sexual function
- Handheld mirror can help the woman to learn visually to tighten and loosen perineal muscles.
- Important to teach the partner that spasms are not under conscious control and are not a reflection on the relationship or a woman's feelings about her partner.
- Instruction in techniques for vaginal dilation
- Resources
  - American College of Obstetricians and Gynecologists: https://www.acog.org/
  - Valins L. *When a Woman's Body Says No to Sex: Understanding and Overcoming Vaginismus*. New York, NY: Penguin; 1992.

PROGNOSIS

Favorable, with early recognition of the condition and initiation of treatment

REFERENCES

1. Landry T, Bergeron S. How young does vulvovaginal pain begin? Prevalence and characteristics of dyspareunia in adolescents. *J Sex Med*. 2009;6(4):927–935.
2. Zulfikaroglu E. Vaginismus treatment: a systematic review and meta-analysis of contemporary therapeutic approaches. *J Sex Med*. 2026;23(1):qdaf295. doi:10.1093/jsxmed/qdaf295.
3. Maseroli E, Scavello I, Rastrelli G, et al. Outcome of medical and psychosexual interventions for vaginismus: a systematic review and meta-analysis. *J Sex Med*. 2018;15(12):1752–1764.
4. Weinberger JM, Houman J, Caron AT, et al. Female sexual dysfunction and the placebo effect: a meta-analysis. *Obstet Gynecol*. 2018;132(2):453–458.
5. Mestre-Bach G, Blycker GR, Potenza MN. Behavioral therapies for treating female sexual dysfunctions: a state-of-the-art review. *J Clin Med*. 2022;11(10):2794.
6. Melnik T, Hawton K, McGuire H. Interventions for vaginismus. *Cochrane Database Syst Rev*. 2012;12(12):CD001760.

SEE ALSO

Dyspareunia; Sexual Dysfunction in Women

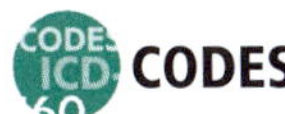

CODES

ICD10

- N94.2 Vaginismus
- N94.1 Dyspareunia

CLINICAL PEARLS

- In a patient with suspected genito-pelvic pain/penetration disorder, a complete medical history, including a comprehensive psychosocial and sexual history and a patient-centric, patient-controlled educational pelvic exam should be conducted.
- This condition can be treated effectively. Further research into the most effective methods is needed.
- Cognitive-behavioral therapy may be effective for the treatment of this condition.
- Botox injection therapy is in the experimental stages but looks promising for the treatment of vaginismus. Bupivacaine and dilation under general anesthesia has also been tried as a treatment for vaginismus.

GERIATRIC CARE: GENERAL PRINCIPLES

Muneeza Khan, MD, FAAFP

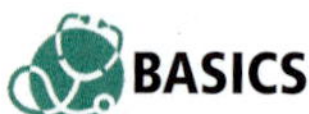

BASICS

DESCRIPTION
"First do no harm"; many well-intended diagnostic and therapeutic interventions with efficacy established in younger patients may not benefit the elderly. Geriatric care, more than many other medical specialties, focuses on preserving and improving function and comfort, rather than on life extension.

EPIDEMIOLOGY
By 2050, the U.S. population anticipated to be >65 years old will be 22%, and those >85 years old may reach 4.5%. The geriatric population is projected to be 83.7 million.

ETIOLOGY AND PATHOPHYSIOLOGY
Physiology of aging
- The aging process is not pathologic but part of the developmental continuum. Physiologic changes associated with aging tend to diminish the body's compensatory reserve and increase susceptibility to disease.
  - Aging increases body fat and decreases total body water and lean body mass. This results in hydrophilic drugs having a smaller apparent volume of distribution. Lipophilic drugs will have an increased volume of distribution and longer half-life.
  - Aging decreases renal elimination of drugs.
  - Declining lung capacity, oxygen uptake, cardiac output, muscle mass, glomerular filtration rate, as well as blood flow to the brain, liver, and kidneys are associated with aging and must be considered in the diagnosis and treatment of elderly patients.

RISK FACTORS
Access to care
- Despite Medicare, persistent barriers to care include but not limited to lack of provider responsiveness, medical bills, and transportation; barriers more prevalent in female population and with increasing age
- Telemedicine could enhance access to care via the following:
  - Encrypted email or home telehealth for those who are technologically equipped
  - Phone visits for those with adequate hearing
  - Nurse visits at home to evaluate and plan care by reporting to provider

GENERAL PREVENTION
- Vaccination schedule for seniors: https://www.cdc.gov/vaccines/hcp/imz-schedules/adult-age.html
- Function is the heart of geriatric care. Assess and promote function at each encounter as changes in functional independence are common. Assess: activities of daily living (ADLs), instrumental ADLs (IADLs) (ability to use equipment such as a phone).
- Hearing assessment via hearing
  - Handicapped inventory
- Depression via Geriatric Depression Scale: https://consultgeri.org/try-this/general-assessment/issue-4.pdf
- Cognition via Mini Cognitive Assessment Instrument (https://www.alz.org/media/Documents/mini-cog.pdf) and Montreal Cognitive Assessment (https://www.mocatest.org/)
- Falls: Those with two or more falls in the past year, fall with injury requiring medical treatment, or fear of falling due to difficulty with gait or balance require a full fall risk assessment: https://www.cdc.gov/steadi/
- Urinary incontinence: Inquire if patient has lost urine >5 times in past year.
- Polypharmacy (≥5 medications)
  - Use pill bottles, pharmacy records, and patient and caregiver input to reconcile medication lists.
  - Query OTC and CAM medications.
  - Reconcile medications at each visit
  - Attempt to simplify medications at each encounter.
- Substance use: CAGE criteria: https://www.mdcalc.com/cage-questions-alcohol-use
- Advanced care planning

ALERT
Completion of an advanced directive is critically important

- Definition: Advanced directives are documents a person completes while still in possession of decisional capacity to ensure their values are reflected when considering how treatment decisions should be made on her or his behalf in the event she or he loses the capacity to make such decisions.
- Instruments:
  - Durable power of attorney: Patient (called the principal) appoints an agent to handle specific health, legal, and financial responsibilities.
  - Health care proxy: a durable power of attorney specifically for health care decisions; their role is to express the patient's wishes and make health care decisions if the patient cannot speak for themselves.
  - Living will: a legal document that allows patients to express their wishes for end-of-life medical care in case they become unable to communicate their decisions
  - Discussions and completion of orders pertaining to end of life care, referred to as POLST (physician order for life-sustaining treatment) in most states and MOLST (medical orders for life-sustaining treatment) in some northeastern states

DIAGNOSIS

HISTORY
Optimizing communication
- Speak directly to your patient unless directed toward their surrogate.
- Assess and manage emotionally charged interactions. Refrain from taking negative energy personally.
- Assess patient and caregiver health literacy and adjust explanations accordingly.
- Gauge the degree of social and financial support.
- Establish patient's values, preferences, and goals of care.

PHYSICAL EXAM
Geriatric-specific considerations:
- Orthostatic hypotension: contributes to poor energy, diminished functional status, increased risk of falls, and decline in renal function due to ineffective organ perfusion
- Hypothermia/hyperthermia: increased susceptibility in the elderly; less likely to mount a fever in the setting of infection; consider thyroid derangement.
- Weight loss: Assess access to food; may be presenting feature in mood disorder, thyroid derangement, dementia, malignancy
- Hearing: Check for cerumen impaction; perform Whisper Test: https://www.youtube.com/watch?v=PzRzpW6JKzQ
- Gait, balance, and proximal muscle strength: assessed via Timed Get up and Go Test (https://www.cdc.gov/steadi/hcp/clinical-resources/index.html), functional reach test and Tinetti balance assessment tool (https://neurotoolkit.com/tinetti/)

DIFFERENTIAL DIAGNOSIS
Geriatric-specific presentations:
- Coronary artery disease: Elderly patients with coronary heart disease often present with atypical symptoms, including exertional dyspnea. Silent myocardial ischemia is also common.
- Constipation: Constipation due to slow transit is very common and may be associated with fecal impaction and overflow fecal incontinence.
- Delirium: Nearly 30% of older patients experience delirium at some time during hospitalization.
- Urinary tract infection (UTI): UTI is the most common infectious illness in adults aged ≥65 years, but diagnosis of UTI is fraught with difficulty because of the high prevalence of asymptomatic bacteriuria and pyuria, neither of which should be treated unless symptomatic. Asymptomatic bacteriuria is a marker for debility, but treatment does not improve outcomes and may cause harm.
- Depression: It is more common in elderly females. If left untreated, it is often the precursor of overt dementia.
- Insomnia: Late-life insomnia is often persistent and may prompt self-medication with over-the-counter sleep aids or alcohol.
- Hearing difficulties: Some studies showed increased incidence of dementia in patient with hearing difficulties.
- Visual Impairment: Macular degeneration, glaucoma, and cataracts are the most commonly encountered causes and a yearly eye exam is important.

DIAGNOSTIC TESTS & INTERPRETATION

Informed decision-making

- Decision-making capacity: Evaluate in four areas: ability to understand information about treatment, ability to appreciate how that information applies to their situation, ability to reason with that information, and ability to make a choice and express it (https://www.aafp.org/pubs/afp/issues/2018/0701/p40.html).
- Surrogate decision maker
  - Patient-identified agent (durable power of attorney for health care, medical power of attorney, health care agent)
  - Court-appointed surrogate (legal guardian or conservator)

Diagnostic Procedures/Other

- Avoid unnecessary patient/caregiver burden if results will not significantly enhance the plan of care.
- Take into consideration renal function for imaging studies involving contrast.

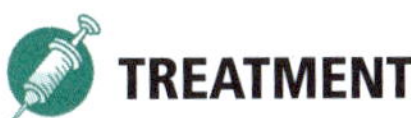

TREATMENT

GENERAL MEASURES

- Align with patients' goals of care and optimize nonpharmacologic options first.
- Feasibility for patient and caregivers: Assess cost, availability, travel burden, and adherence.
- Nonpharmacologic (1)
  - Occupational therapy, physical therapy, speech therapy, hearing aids
  - Walking assist devices
  - Nonpharmacologic treatment of depression and insomnia
- Pharmacologic
  - Start low and go slow.
  - Adjust dose for renal and hepatic function, volume of distribution, decreased protein binding (more free/active drug available), drug–drug interactions.
  - Anticoagulants and hypoglycemic medication (insulin and sulfonylureas) are high risk.
  - Beers criteria: medications with the best geriatric benefit-to-risk ratio; https://geriatricscareonline.org/ProductAbstract/american-geriatrics-society-updated-beers-criteria-for-potentially-inappropriate-medication-use-in-older-adults/CL001#
- Deprescribing: AGA and Choosing Wisely suggest:
  - Don't recommend percutaneous feeding tubes in patients with dementia; they do not prolong life and may worsen suffering and thirst.
  - Avoid antipsychotics as the first choice to treat behavioral and psychological symptoms of dementia.
  - Nonpharmacologic interventions are more efficacious than pharmacologic interventions for reducing aggression and agitation in adults with dementia. Antipsychotic medications increase risk of death. They may have a role in a palliative plan that focuses on nonpharmacologic means of soothing agitation.
  - In diabetes care, meticulously avoid hypoglycemia, which is of far greater potential harm to the patient than is hyperglycemia. Metformin is generally safe. The major goal, especially in care of the older or more debilitated population, is maintenance of glucose levels below those that cause symptomatic polyuria and polydipsia. This is not a specific A1c target.
  - Don't use benzodiazepines or other sedative hypnotics in older adults for insomnia, agitation, or delirium.
  - Don't use antimicrobials to treat bacteriuria in older adults unless specific urinary tract symptoms are present. Delirium in patients seen in the ED and hospital is not likely caused by bacteruria or lower UTI, but usually by other causes.
  - Don't prescribe cholinesterase inhibitors for dementia without periodic assessment for perceived cognitive benefits and adverse gastrointestinal effects.
  - Don't recommend screening for breast, colorectal, prostate, or lung cancer without considering life expectancy and the risks of testing, overdiagnosis, and overtreatment.
  - Avoid using prescription appetite stimulants or high-calorie supplements for treatment of anorexia or cachexia in older adults; instead, optimize social supports, discontinue medications that may interfere with eating, provide appealing food and feeding assistance, and clarify patient goals and expectations.
  - Don't prescribe any medication without conducting a drug regimen review. Deprescribe when possible.
  - Don't use physical restraints to manage behavioral symptoms of hospitalized older adults with delirium.
- Geriatric pain management:
  - Stepwise care, nonpharmacologic interventions (PT, massage, environmental changes [e.g., music and aromatherapy], followed by cautious use of medication as necessary). NSAIDs involve significant risks in the elderly (renal, GI, cardiovascular). Use low doses of naproxen or ibuprofen preferentially, with GI-protective medication (e.g., omeprazole) if chronic therapy is needed.
  - Pharmacologic: Consider Beers criteria. Many commonly used medications (e.g., gabapentin) offer little benefit and significant potential for harm.
- Assess the home environment: Visiting Nurse Association (VNA) evaluation (social worker, PT/OT). Home visitation, social activity, and group support may be of particular value. Consider adult day program enrollment.

MEDICATION

First Line

Acetaminophen is the safest when used in <3 g dose over 24 hours.

Second Line

Use caution with tramadol, narcotics, and NSAIDs.

ADMISSION, INPATIENT, AND NURSING CONSIDERATIONS

Inpatient prevention measures:

- Falls, acute delirium, skin breakdown, pain management, infections
- Encourage physical activity and avoid sedentary behavior.

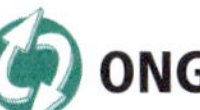

ONGOING CARE

FOLLOW-UP RECOMMENDATIONS

- Realistic expectations
- Carefully review medications, eliminate hospital-prescribed unnecessary medications.

Patient Monitoring

Use team members optimally: home health/VNA, social services

DIET

A well-balanced diet should be encouraged and caloric intake should be optimal.

PATIENT EDUCATION

- Resources for caregivers:
  - Support group: Alzheimer's Association 800-272-3900
  - Respite care: It is important for caregivers to seek occasional respite from their responsibilities.
  - Local agency on aging (Councils on Aging)
- Elder mistreatment: Be aware of warning signs such as bruises and lacerations, fractures, malnutrition, and dehydration; can also screen using:
  - Brief Abuse Screen for the Elderly (BASE)
  - Elder Assessment Instrument (EAI): pressure ulcers, signs of sexual abuse, change in the ability to manage and control finances (be alert for signs of financial exploitation)
- Consider referral for palliative care, a philosophy of care for those with serious illnesses that focuses on symptom, pain and stress relief with the goal of optimizing functional status and quality of life.
- Consider referral for hospice, a model of end-of-life care that provides physical, emotional, and spiritual support to patients with <6 months life expectancy to maintain optimal quality of life and death with dignity. Hospice extends support to the patient's family and caregivers.

REFERENCES

1. Abraha I, Cruz-Jentoft A, Soiza RL, et al. Evidence of and recommendations for non-pharmacological interventions for common geriatric conditions: the SENATOR-ONTOP systematic review protocol. *BMJ Open*. 2015;5(1):e007488.

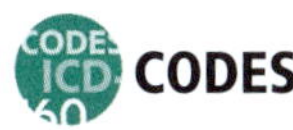

CODES

ICD10

Z71.89 Other specified counseling

CLINICAL PEARLS

- Use a patient-centered approach using shared decision-making to establish goals of care and align all clinical decisions within the context of these goals.
- Use an interdisciplinary team approach to optimize holistic care for elders and their caregivers.

G

GIARDIASIS

Marie L. Borum, MD, EdD, MPH • Maxwell Shayan Madani, MD

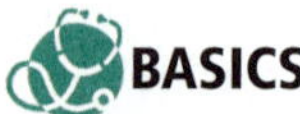

BASICS

DESCRIPTION

- *Giardia lamblia* (also known as *Giardia duodenalis* or *Giardia intestinalis*) is a protozoan pathogen that leads to intestinal infection and is one of the most common causes of diarrhea worldwide.
- The life cycle consists of cysts and trophozoite stages. Transmission occurs via ingestion of infective cysts, followed by excystation in the duodenum with the release of trophozoites, leading to symptoms.
  - Trophozoites pass to the large intestine, where they revert to the infectious cyst form, which are excreted in the stool back into the environment.
- Most infections result from ingestion of unfiltered surface water (e.g., contaminated swimming areas) or fecal-oral transmission; less commonly acquired through contaminated food

EPIDEMIOLOGY

- Age: most commonly children <5 years old and adults aged 25 to 44 years (1)
- Gender: more common in males
- Minimal seasonal variability: slight increase in cases reported in summer and early fall
- The highest risk areas include South and Southeast Asia, North Africa, the Caribbean, and South America (1).

Pediatric Considerations

- Most common in early childhood
- Chronic infection in children can lead to intestinal malabsorption (may also be associated with growth restriction/failure to thrive).

Incidence

- Estimated to cause 280 million diarrheal infections annually (2)
- In 2019, 14,887 cases were reported in the United States (~6 cases per 100,000).
- In the United States, giardiasis affects 1.2 million individuals annually, resulting in 3,584 hospitalizations per year (3).
- The actual rate of giardiasis infection is likely much higher due to underreporting.

Prevalence

Occurs in about 2% of adults and 6–8% of children in developed countries, whereas 33% of people in developing countries have had giardiasis (3).

ETIOLOGY AND PATHOPHYSIOLOGY

Giardia trophozoites colonize the surface of the proximal small intestine.

- Cellular attachment to host enterocytes via the ventral suction disc and the excretion of parasite products results in structural damage compromising intestinal epithelial cells and inhibiting the function of brush border enzymes. This causes electrolyte imbalances and increased intestinal permeability, leading to the production of diarrhea (2).

Genetics

G. lamblia has eight defined genotypes (referred to as assemblages A–H), but only A and B are known to infect humans (2).

RISK FACTORS

- Daycare centers
- Anal intercourse
- Wilderness camping
- Travel to developing countries
- Children adopted from developing countries
- Drinking untreated water from lakes, streams, or wells
- Swimming in contaminated recreational water (pools, lakes, streams, rivers)
- Pets with *Giardia* infection/diarrhea
- Eating raw produce

GENERAL PREVENTION

- Hand hygiene
- Water purification when camping and when traveling to developing countries. Boiling is the most effective.
- Properly cook all foods.
- Protect public water supply from fecal contamination.
- Sanitary disposal of feces
- Barrier protection during anal intercourse

COMMONLY ASSOCIATED CONDITIONS

Hypogammaglobulinemia, common variable immunodeficiency, IgA deficiency, and immunosuppression are associated with prolonged course of the disease and treatment failures.

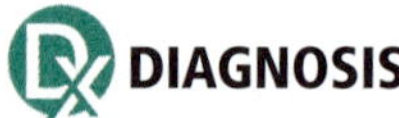

DIAGNOSIS

HISTORY

- Acute giardiasis
  - 50–75% of infected people are asymptomatic (3).
  - Symptomatic infections occur more frequently in children than adults (3).
  - Symptoms usually appear 1 to 2 weeks after exposure and may last 1 to 4 weeks.
  - Diarrhea (90%); malaise (86%)
  - Foul-smelling and fatty stools (75%); flatulence (75%)
  - Abdominal cramps and bloating (71%)
  - Nausea (69%); weight loss (66%); vomiting (23%)
  - Fever (15%); constipation (13%); urticaria (10%)
- Chronic giardiasis
  - Loose stools, steatorrhea
  - Profound weight loss, malabsorption, stunted growth
  - Malaise, fatigue
  - Depression
  - Abdominal cramping, borborygmi, flatulence, burping

PHYSICAL EXAM

- Vital signs are typically normal.
- Nonspecific; abdominal exam; may have bloating, tenderness, or increased bowel sounds
- Assess for weight loss, signs of dehydration, malabsorption, or failure to thrive in children.

DIFFERENTIAL DIAGNOSIS

- Cryptosporidiosis, microsporidiosis, strongyloidiasis, cyclosporiasis, amebiasis, *Dientamoeba fragilis* infection
- Viral gastroenteritis or traveler's diarrhea is caused by a range of pathogens, including *Escherichia coli* and *Campylobacter* spp.
- Other causes of malabsorption include lactose intolerance, celiac sprue, tropical sprue, bacterial overgrowth syndromes, and Crohn disease.
- Irritable bowel syndrome (diarrhea without weight loss)

DIAGNOSTIC TESTS & INTERPRETATION

Initial Tests (lab, imaging)

- Light microscopy of stool for ova and parasites:
  - Three serial stool specimens over 2 to 3 days; single stool specimen examination has 50–70% sensitivity; three serial specimens increases to >90% (3).
  - Cysts in fixed or fresh stools, and occasionally trophozoites are found in fresh diarrhea stools.
  - Test limitations: labor-intensive; experienced operator for interpretation; intermittent shedding means that ova may not be present in the stool sample.
- Direct fluorescent antibody (DFA) testing, nucleic acid amplification testing (NAAT) and ELISA testing have >95% sensitivity, specificity, and faster turnaround time compared to stool microscopy.
- Serologic tests for circulating IgG and IgM antibodies to *Giardia* are not appropriate for clinical diagnosis (1).

Follow-Up Tests & Special Considerations

String test is largely of historical interest.

Diagnostic Procedures/Other

Esophagogastroduodenoscopy (EGD) with biopsy and a sample of small intestinal fluid

Test Interpretation

Intestinal biopsy shows flattened, mild lymphocytic infiltration and trophozoites on the surface.

TREATMENT

Outpatient for mild cases; inpatient if symptoms are severe enough to cause dehydration warranting parenteral fluid replacement

GENERAL MEASURES

- No treatment is required in asymptomatic patients.
- Prophylactic therapy is indicated for asymptomatic patients in close contact with pregnant or immunocompromised individuals and asymptomatic food handlers.
- Fluid replacement is the first line for dehydration.

MEDICATION

First Line

- Drugs of choice
  - Tinidazole: 2 g PO single dose (3)[A] and for ages ≥3 years: 50 mg/kg PO single dose
  - Nitazoxanide: 500 mg PO BID for 3 days for ages ≥12 years (3)[A]
    - 200 mg PO BID for 3 days for ages 4 to $<$12 years
    - 100 mg PO BID for 3 days for ages 1 to $<$4 years

Second Line

Alternative agents

- Metronidazole: 250 mg PO TID for 5 to 7 days or 500 mg PO BID for 5 to 7 days (3)[A]
- Albendazole: 400 mg PO daily for 5 days
- Mebendazole 200 mg PO TID for 5 days
- Paromomycin: 10 mg/kg PO TID for 5 to 10 days
- Furazolidone: 100 mg PO QID for 7 to 10 days
- Quinacrine: 100 mg PO TID for 5 days for nitroimidazole-refractory cases (4)

Precautions

- Consumption of alcohol while on treatment with tinidazole or metronidazole has been associated with a disulfiram-like effect (diaphoresis, palpitations, facial flushing, nausea, vertigo, hypotension, and tachycardia) (3).
- Patient with refractory giardiasis who fail monotherapy may warrant combination therapy, high-dose therapy, and/or longer courses of therapy (3).
  - Confirmation of treatment failure is best provided by PCR (1).
  - Treatment failure might be due to host factors or to true drug resistance, which is increasingly common, particularly in travelers returning from South and Southeast Asia (1).

Pregnancy Considerations

- For patients with mild giardiasis, delay of treatment until second trimester may be reasonable to avoid adverse drug effects to the fetus.
- Medications to treat giardiasis are relatively contraindicated during pregnancy.
- Paromomycin is a nonaminoglycoside recommended in pregnancy due to lower risk of teratogenicity because systemic absorption is low; cure rate, however, is about 60%, which is lower than most other agents (3).

Pediatric Considerations

- For children $<$12 months of age, metronidazole is the drug of choice.
- For children 12 to 36 months of age, nitazoxanide is preferred.
- For children ≥36 months of age, tinidazole is preferred.

ISSUES FOR REFERRAL

Patients with treatment failure should be discussed with or referred to a specialist, who should exclude underlying problems such as celiac disease, inherited disaccharidase deficiency, and immunodeficiency disorders, particularly of total and IgA antibody production (1).

ADDITIONAL THERAPIES

Fluids to prevent dehydration

SURGERY/OTHER PROCEDURES

There have been no cases recorded in literature in which giardiasis has required surgical intervention.

COMPLEMENTARY & ALTERNATIVE MEDICINE

Zinc and vitamin A have been associated with protective effect against giardiasis among children.

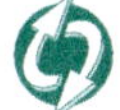

ONGOING CARE

FOLLOW-UP RECOMMENDATIONS

Patient Monitoring

Monitor symptoms, weight, and stool exams, particularly if patients fail to improve.

DIET

Low-lactose/lactose-free for at least 1 month; low-fat diet is generally helpful.

PATIENT EDUCATION

- Handwashing is more important than water purification to prevent transmission in outdoor enthusiasts.
- Lactose intolerance may follow *Giardia* infection and cause persistent diarrhea posttreatment. Recommend patients adhere to a low-lactose/lactose-free diet to mitigate symptoms.
- CDC facts about *Giardia* and swimming pools: http://www.cdc.gov/healthywater/pdf/swimming/resources/giardia-factsheet.pdf
  - Don't swim if you have diarrhea.
  - Wash hands with soap after changing diapers before returning to the pool.
  - Do not ingest pool, lake, or river water.
  - Use chlorine to kill *Giardia* in water used for recreational activities.

PROGNOSIS

- Generally, prognosis is excellent; most patients are asymptomatic.
- Majority of infections resolve within a few weeks; occasionally may last for months and persist as chronic infections; patients with underlying immunodeficiency may experience more severe and prolonged illness.
- Mortality is rare, except in those cases of extreme dehydration that are untreated or inadequately treated, which occurs mainly in infants or malnourished children (3).

COMPLICATIONS

Malabsorption, impaired growth development, hypersensitivity reactions, weight loss, postinfectious IBS, and lactose intolerance; more rarely cholecystitis, cholangitis, granulomatous hepatitis, impaired exocrine pancreatic function

ALERT
Reportable disease to the CDC

REFERENCES

1. Mørch K, Hanevik K. Giardiasis treatment: an update with a focus on refractory disease. *Curr Opin Infect Dis*. 2020;33(5):355–364. doi:10.1097/QCO.0000000000000668.
2. Adam RD. *Giardia duodenalis*: biology and pathogenesis. *Clin Microbiol Rev*. 2021;34(4):e0002419. doi:10.1128/CMR.00024-19.
3. Leung AKC, Leung AAM, Wong AHC, et al. Giardiasis: an overview. *Recent Pat Inflamm Allergy Drug Discov*. 2019;13(2):134–143.
4. Ydsten KA, Hellgren U, Asgeirsson H. Quinacrine treatment of nitroimidazole—refractory giardiasis. *J Infect Dis*. 2022;225(10):1773–1776.

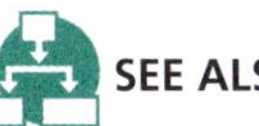

SEE ALSO

Algorithm: Diarrhea, Chronic

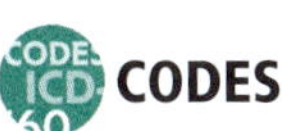

CODES

ICD10

A07.1 Giardiasis [lambliasis]

CLINICAL PEARLS

- Daycare facilities and public swimming pools are common sources of *Giardia* transmission (a history of camping or recent travel is not required for the diagnosis).
- Abdominal bloating and loose, foul-smelling stool are common presenting symptoms.
- First-line treatment is tinidazole and nitazoxanide. Metronidazole is also highly effective (but less well tolerated).
- Most treatment failures may warrant combination therapy, high-dose therapy, and/or longer courses of therapy.
- NAAT and ELISA testing are preferred for diagnosis.

G

GILBERT SYNDROME

Jared Morphew, MD • Astrud San Antonio Villareal, MD, FAAFP

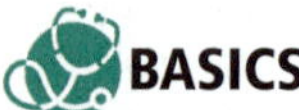

BASICS

Also known as Meulengracht disease

DESCRIPTION

A benign, inherited syndrome in which mild, intermittent unconjugated hyperbilirubinemia occurs in the absence of hemolysis or liver dysfunction

Pediatric Considerations

- Rare for the disorder to be diagnosed before puberty
- May contribute to prolongation of neonatal jaundice, especially in breastfed infants or infants with other hemolytic disorders

Pregnancy Considerations

The relative fasting that may occur with morning sickness can elevate bilirubin level.

EPIDEMIOLOGY

- Predominant age: present from birth but most often presents in the 2nd or 3rd decade of life
- Predominant sex: male > female (2 to 7:1)

Prevalence

The reported prevalence of Gilbert syndrome (GS) is between 2% and 20% in different populations (with the highest prevalence in the Middle Eastern population), with most presentations during or after adolescence.

ETIOLOGY AND PATHOPHYSIOLOGY

Indirect hyperbilirubinemia in GS results from impaired hepatic bilirubin clearance (~30% of normal) due to decreased levels of the enzyme uridine diphosphoglucuronate-glucuronosyltransferase (UDPGT). Hepatic bilirubin conjugation (glucuronidation) is thus reduced, although this may not be the only defect.

Genetics

- Inherited defects within the promoter region of the gene that encodes the enzyme UDPGT yields reduced conjugation of bilirubin with glucuronic acid. In particular, patients with GS have a mutation in the UGT1A1 gene.
- Once considered as an autosomal dominant condition, GS is now thought to be inherited in an autosomal recessive manner.

RISK FACTORS

- Male gender
- Family history; particularly first-degree relatives

GENERAL PREVENTION

Avoidance of known triggers (dehydration, prolonged fasting, intense exercise)

COMMONLY ASSOCIATED CONDITIONS

GS is part of a spectrum of hereditary disorders that includes types I and II Crigler-Najjar syndrome. However, bilirubin levels in these cases will be >6 mg/dL. There is an associated increased risk of cholelithiasis in certain populations. A neonatal presentation may lead to prolonged jaundice.

DIAGNOSIS

HISTORY

- In patients with GS, a nonpruritic jaundice can occur in the setting of stressors like fasting, dehydration, infection, lack of sleep, physical exertion or overexertion, menstruation, or surgery. Other symptoms that may present during an episode of jaundice, including fatigue, are caused by the triggering factor and are not directly a result of GS.
- Some medications may also trigger episodes of jaundice in patients with GS due to abnormal metabolism. Because patients with GS have reduced UGT1A1 activity, using medications that are metabolized by UGT1A1 increases the risk of drug inducted toxicity. Examples of these medications are irinotecan (chemotherapeutic agent) and antivirals (atazanavir, indinavir), rifampin, and cyclosporine. Other medications that may compete or suppress with UGT1A1 activity include but are not limited to nonsteroidal anti-inflammatory drugs, acetaminophen, statin, ezetimibe, lamotrigine, lorazepam, oxazepam, ethinylestradiol, buprenorphine, menthol, tyrosine kinase inhibitors.

PHYSICAL EXAM

The physical exam is usually normal. Occasional mild jaundice and mild scleral icterus precipitated by the aforementioned triggers may be seen. Careful attention should be paid for the stigmata of chronic liver disease, which should be absent.

DIFFERENTIAL DIAGNOSIS

- Hemolysis or hemolytic anemias
- Hemolytic disorders (autoimmune hemolytic anemia, sickle cell disease, G6PD deficiency, hereditary spherocytosis)
- Ineffective erythropoiesis (megaloblastic anemias, certain porphyrias, thalassemia major, sideroblastic anemia, severe lead poisoning, congenital dyserythropoietic anemias)
- Crigler-Najjar syndrome type I or type II
- Drug-induced unconjugated hyperbilirubinemia
- Acute severe viral hepatitis
- Hepatic failure
- Biliary tract disease

DIAGNOSTIC TESTS & INTERPRETATION

Initial Tests (lab, imaging)

- Bilirubin: elevated but <4 mg/dL (103 μmol/L) and usually <3 mg/dL (51 μmol/L), virtually all unconjugated (indirect), with conjugated bilirubin within the normal range and/or <20% of the total bilirubin
- CBC with peripheral smear is normal.
- Reticulocyte count, haptoglobin, and lactate dehydrogenase levels are normal.
- Liver function tests (LFTs) (aspartate aminotransferase [AST], alanine transaminase [ALT], alkaline phosphatase, and γ-glutamyl transpeptidase [GGT]) are normal.
- Direct Coombs test is normal.
- Up to 60% of patients with GS have a clinically insignificant mild hemolysis that frequently can only be detected with sophisticated red cell survival studies.
- Drugs that may alter lab results: Bilirubin level may be raised by nicotinic acid and some other medications and lowered by phenobarbital. Administration of corticosteroids can reduce the plasma bilirubin concentrations as steroids increase the hepatitic uptake of bilirubin.
- Disorders that may alter lab results: Bilirubin levels increase during fasting and may increase during a febrile illness.

Follow-Up Tests & Special Considerations

GS should be suspected if unconjugated hyperbilirubinemia persists in the absence of hemolysis or other liver dysfunction. A definitive diagnosis may be reported after 3 to 12 months of follow-up if the exam and diagnostic workup is otherwise normal.

Diagnostic Procedures/Other

- A presumptive diagnosis can be made in patients who have:
  - – Unconjugated hyperbilirubinemia on repeated testing
  - – Normal CBC, blood smear, and reticulocyte count
  - – Normal plasma aminotransferases and alkaline phosphatase
- Confirmatory testing is rarely necessary. When patients continue to have normal lab studies apart from the plasma bilirubin elevation in the next 12 to 18 months, GS can be definitively diagnosed; regarding possible additional testing:
  - – A 48-hour fast is impractical and nonspecific for GS.
  - – Provocation testing with rifampin could be employed if there is significant diagnostic doubt:
    - ○ After 12 hours of fasting, an increase of total bilirubin to >1.9 mg/dL 2 hours after an oral dose of 900 mg distinguishes patients with GS with a sensitivity of 100% and a specificity of 100%.
  - – Genetic testing is available in the form of polymerase chain reaction (PCR) or DNA-fragment sequencing for DNA mutations in the *UGT1A1* gene.

ALERT
A liver biopsy is not usually needed to exclude other diagnoses unless concomitant liver disease is present.

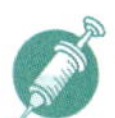

TREATMENT

- Outpatient
- Avoid unnecessary testing and procedures. Genetic testing is reserved for atypical cases.
- Specific treatment is not necessary.
- It is essential to discuss the mode of inheritance with patients and their family members to avoid unnecessary testing and alleviate undue concern.

MEDICATION

- There are no medications indicated for GS.
- Exercise caution when using medications that are metabolized by UGT1A1.

ISSUES FOR REFERRAL

If there is concern for findings consistent with another liver disease, referral to liver disease specialist for additional evaluation and treatment is warranted.

SURGERY/OTHER PROCEDURES

There is no indication for any procedure or surgery to treat GS.

COMPLEMENTARY & ALTERNATIVE MEDICINE

Complementary and alternative medicine (CAM) strategies aim to minimize triggers that may elevate bilirubin levels, such as stress, dehydration, illness, and excessive physical exertion.

ADMISSION, INPATIENT, AND NURSING CONSIDERATIONS

Exercise caution when using medications that are metabolized by UGT1A1 while admitted. Avoid dehydration while admitted.

ONGOING CARE

FOLLOW-UP RECOMMENDATIONS

Patient Monitoring

Once GS has been diagnosed, no further monitoring is required.

DIET

There are no specific foods to avoid. Avoid any extreme dieting or irregular eating schedules. Remain hydrated.

PATIENT EDUCATION

- Reassure patients that GS is benign.
- Educate patients on common triggers for jaundice.
- Recommend patients to inform medical providers of their diagnosis.
- Instruct patients to seek medical help if severe or prolonged jaundice occurs because these may be signs of a separate disease process.

PROGNOSIS

- GS is benign with an excellent prognosis.
- Patients with GS are able to serve as donors for right lobe of liver for transplantation.
- Preliminary evidence suggests that patients with GS may have protective properties against cardiovascular disease, type 2 diabetes mellitus, some cancers such as Hodgkin lymphoma, and all-cause mortality.

COMPLICATIONS

Patients are at risk for more severe drug interaction development of pigmented gallstones and worse presentation of neonatal jaundice.

ALERT
The impact of UGT1A1 mutations on the metabolism of medications should be taken into consideration in patients with known or suspected GS.

ADDITIONAL READING

Grant LM, Faust TW, Thoguluva Chandrasekar V, et al. *Gilbert Syndrome*. Treasure Island (FL): StatPearls Publishing; 2025. https://www.ncbi.nlm.nih.gov/books/NBK470200/. Accessed December 12, 2025.

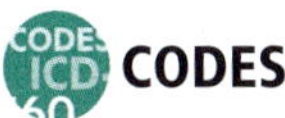

CODES

ICD10

- E80.4 Gilbert syndrome
- E80.6 Other disorders of bilirubin metabolism

CLINICAL PEARLS

- GS is a benign, inherited syndrome, in which mild, intermittent unconjugated hyperbilirubinemia causing jaundice occurs with otherwise normal liver function.
- Reduced hepatic bilirubin conjugation (glucuronidation) occurs due to altered UGT1A1 gene promotion.
- GS is diagnosed when a mild, persistent, or recurrent elevation in unconjugated hyperbilirubinemia persists in the absence of hemolysis or other liver dysfunction.
- Confirmatory tests are not frequently needed, and a liver biopsy is not recommended unless there is serious concern for concomitant liver disease.
- Patient education and reassurance is essential, and unnecessary testing and procedures should be avoided.

GINGIVITIS

Karlynn Sievers, MD • Stephanie Vaux Voyles, MD

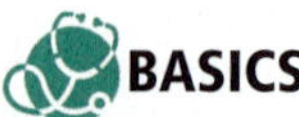

BASICS

DESCRIPTION

Gingivitis is a reversible form of inflammation of the gingiva. It is a mild form of periodontal disease. Classification includes the following:

- Plaque induced
- Not plaque induced (bacterial, viral, or fungal; e.g., necrotizing ulcerative gingivitis, Vincent disease ["trench mouth"], denture related)
- Modified by systemic factors (e.g., pregnancy, puberty, HIV, diabetes, smoking, leukemia)
- Modified by medications (calcium channel blockers, antipsychotics, antiepileptics, antirejection medications, hormones)
- Modified by malnutrition (vitamin deficiencies)
- Acute or chronic
- System(s) affected: gastrointestinal; ears, nose, throat; dental
- Synonym(s): mild periodontal disease; gum disease

Geriatric Considerations

More frequent in this age group

Pediatric Considerations

Cases of plaque-induced gingivitis are common in children (most common form of pediatric periodontal disease) and usually require no specific interventions other than improved oral hygiene.

Pregnancy Considerations

- Very common in pregnant women; hormonal effect
- Self-limited

EPIDEMIOLOGY

- Predominant age: children, teenagers, and young adults
- 42% of adults in the United States have periodontal diseases.

ETIOLOGY AND PATHOPHYSIOLOGY

Inflammation of the marginal gingiva; this can progress to deeper, destructive inflammation; if involving supporting bone, classified as periodontitis, not gingivitis

- Inadequate plaque removal
- Medication induced (e.g., oral contraceptives, antiepileptics)
- Nutritional deficiencies
- Vasoconstriction (nicotine, methamphetamine)
- Endocrine/hormonal variations
  - Pregnancy, menses, menarche
- Chronic debilitating disease
- Vincent disease, necrotizing ulcerative gingivitis
  - Synergistic infection with fusiform bacillus (*Fusobacterium* spp.) and spirochete (*Borrelia vincentii*)
- Pathology
  - Acute or chronic inflammation
  - Hyperemic capillaries
  - Polymorphonuclear infiltration
  - Papillary projections in subepithelial tissue
  - Fibroblasts

Genetics

Possible genetic link (up to 30% of population); rare condition called hereditary gingival fibromatosis, where severe gingival hyperplasia covers teeth, associated with hirsutism

RISK FACTORS

- Poor dental hygiene/plaque formation
- Pregnancy
- Uncontrolled diabetes mellitus
- Malocclusion, dental crowding, faulty dental restorations
- Smoking
- Mouth breathing
- Xerostomia
- HIV positive; AIDS
- Vitamin C deficiency; coenzyme Q10 deficiency
- Dental appliances (dentures, braces)
- Necrotizing ulcerative gingivitis
  - Stress
  - Lack of sleep
  - Malnutrition
  - Viral illness
  - Typically, teens and young adults
- Bronchial asthma and other respiratory diseases
- Rheumatoid arthritis
- Epilepsy

GENERAL PREVENTION

- Good oral hygiene
  - Adults
    - Regular twice-daily brushing with fluoride toothpaste
    - Powered toothbrushes, especially the oscillating-rotating type, improve gingivitis.
    - Daily "high-quality" flossing (studies show that flossing only helps when it is done correctly), water jets, and interdental brushes (1)
    - Chlorhexidine with oral hygiene (2)
      - Use in acute phase.
  - Pediatrics
    - Regular twice-daily brushing with fluoride toothpaste under parental supervision until full manual dexterity (~8 years of age)
    - Regular flossing if no spaces between teeth
- Cleaning by a dentist or hygienist every 6 months or more frequently, as indicated
- Mouth rinse with essential oils (menthol, thymol, eucalyptol; e.g., Listerine) combined with brushing (2)

COMMONLY ASSOCIATED CONDITIONS

- Periodontitis
- Glossitis
- Pedunculated growths (pyogenic granulomata)

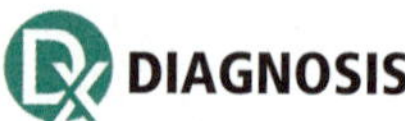

DIAGNOSIS

HISTORY

- Gingival erythema, edema, and bleeding
- Gingiva is tender to touch but otherwise painless.
- Bleeding of gingiva when brushing, flossing, or eating
- Inquire about HIV risk, pregnancy, nutritional deficiencies, diabetes, and other risk factors as indicated (see "Risk Factors").
- Smoking history
- Poor oral hygiene, infrequent dental visit history

PHYSICAL EXAM

- Normal gums should appear pink, firm, stippled, and scalloped.
- Gingivitis—marginal gingiva edematous with blunted papilla (usually painless, except to touch)
- Gingiva erythema: bright red or red-purple appearance
- Bleeding with manipulation of gingiva
- Biofilm of plaque (soft) and calculus (calcified, not easily removed)
- Edema of interdental papillae
- HIV gingivitis
  - Also called linear gingival erythema
  - Narrow band of bright red inflamed gum surrounding neck of tooth
  - Painful
  - Bleeds easily
  - Rapid destruction of gingival tissue and can progress to periodontitis with destruction of underlying support tissues (periodontal ligament, supporting alveolar bone)
- Vincent disease/necrotizing ulcerative gingivitis
  - Ulcers
  - Fever
  - Malaise
  - Regional lymphadenopathy
  - Pain
  - Mouth odor

DIFFERENTIAL DIAGNOSIS

- Periodontitis (deeper inflammation, causing destruction to connective tissue, ligaments, and alveolar bone)
- Glossitis
- Desquamative gingivitis (painful, persistent, usually middle-aged women)
- Pericoronitis (gum flap traps food and plaque over partially erupted 3rd molar), common in adolescence
- Gingival ulcers (aphthous, herpetic, malignancy, TB, syphilis)
- Specific forms of gingivitis: See "Description," including acute necrotizing ulcerative gingivitis (Vincent disease) and HIV gingivitis (linear gingival erythema), adrenal crisis, leukemia.

DIAGNOSTIC TESTS & INTERPRETATION

Initial Tests (lab, imaging)

- No tests usually needed
- Possible smear or culture to identify causative agent (HIV gingivitis includes gram-negative anaerobes, enteric strains, and yeast—*Candida*.)
- Labs for contributing conditions (HIV, pregnancy, diabetes, nutritional deficiencies)
- Increase in C-reactive protein

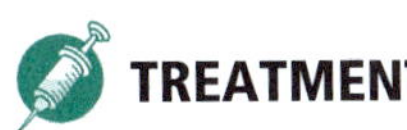

TREATMENT

GENERAL MEASURES

- Stop any contributing medications.
- Remove irritating factors (plaque, calculus, faulty dental restorations, or partial dentures).
- Good oral hygiene (see "General Prevention")
- Regular dental checkups (for scaling and polishing if plaque and/or tartar are present)
- Smoking cessation
- Special needs patients: use of tray-applied 10% carbamide peroxide gels

MEDICATION

First Line

- Chlorhexidine rinses or varnishes may be used. (Note: Prolonged use of chlorhexidine can lead to blackening of the tongue and taste alterations/metallic.) (3)
- Essential oil mouthwash (EOMW) may be equally effective to chlorhexidine for reduction of gingival inflammation (2),(3).
- Antibiotics indicated *only* for acute necrotizing ulcerative gingivitis (Vincent disease):
  - Penicillin V: pediatric dose, 25 to 50 mg/kg/day divided q6h; adult dose, 250 to 500 mg q6h, *or*
  - Metronidazole: pediatric dose, 30 mg/kg/day PO/IV divided q6h; maximum 4 g/day; adult dose, 500 mg BID or TID for 10 days, *or*
  - Amoxicillin/clavulanic acid: pediatric dose, 30 mg/kg/day PO divided q12h; information: use 125 mg/31.25 mg/5 mL suspension; adult dose, 875 mg/125 mg PO BID for 10 days
  - Erythromycin: pediatric dose, 30 to 40 mg/kg/day divided q6h; adult dose, 250 mg q6h
  - Clindamycin: penicillin allergy; pediatric dose, 8 to 20 mg/kg/day in 3 to 4 divided doses as hydrochloride; adults, 300 mg q6h (maximum 1.8 g/day)
  - Doxycycline: adult dose, 100 mg BID 1st day and then QD for 10 days
- Topical corticosteroids
  - Triamcinolone 0.1% in Orabase (spray or ointment), applied locally TID, QID
- Precautions
  - Erythromycin frequently causes GI issues.

Second Line

- Acetaminophen or ibuprofen for pain
- Other antibiotics or antifungal rinses or systemic according to culture or smear
- Decapinol oral rinse (surfactant that acts as a physical barrier, making it harder for bacteria to stick to the polysaccharide pellicle on tooth and mucosal surfaces) to reduce bacteria (not recommended for pregnant women or children aged <12 years); should be used in conjunction with traditional oral hygiene practices when those practices alone are not enough

ISSUES FOR REFERRAL

- Dental referral for acute gingivitis and routine cleanings and further treatment, as needed
- If gingivitis becomes periodontitis, deep root scaling, root planing, and antibiotics may be indicated.

SURGERY/OTHER PROCEDURES

- Débridement for acute necrotizing gingivitis
- Minor surgery may be necessary to correct tissue overgrowth for gingivitis caused by medicines/hereditary gingival fibromatosis.

COMPLEMENTARY & ALTERNATIVE MEDICINE

- Bilberry: potentially helpful in reducing inflammation and stabilizing collagen tissue
- Coenzyme Q10: topically, to restore coenzyme Q10 deficiency
- Replace any nutritional deficiencies (e.g., vitamins A, B_{12}, C).

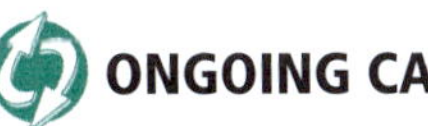

ONGOING CARE

FOLLOW-UP RECOMMENDATIONS

Patient Monitoring

Until clear; dental follow-up for continued cleanings and secondary prevention

DIET

- Well-balanced diet that includes fruits, vegetables, vitamin C
- Avoid sugary snacks and drinks, which contribute to plaque formation.
- Soft foods during flare, if significant inflammation/bleeding

PATIENT EDUCATION

- Good oral hygiene, including twice-daily brushing with circular oscillating electric brush, fluoridated toothpaste, and daily flossing or dental water jet treatment (1); regular dental visits
- Printable and viewable patient information available from the American Dental Association at http://www.mouthhealthy.org/en.org/en/ and the American Academy of Periodontology under "patient resources" at http://www.perio.org/ and NIDCR at http://www.nidcr.nih.gov/oralhealth/Topics/GumDiseases/PeriodontalGumDisease.htm

PROGNOSIS

- Usual course: acute, relapsing, intermittent; chronic
- Prognosis: generally favorable, responds well to appropriate treatment
- Left untreated, may progress to periodontitis (controversial), which is a major cause of tooth loss

COMPLICATIONS

Severe periodontal disease (which is associated with supporting bone loss, tooth loss, heart disease, diabetes, dementia, and preterm birth)

REFERENCES

1. Badahdah A, Hariri MA, Aljohani MS, et al. Alleviation of plaque and gingivitis with dental water jet in regular and orthodontic patients: a systematic review and meta-analysis. *Healthcare (Basel)*. 2025;13(4):396. doi:10:3390/healthcare13040396.
2. Karamani I, Kalimeri E, Seremidi K, et al. Chlorhexidine mouthwash for gingivitis control in orthodontic patients: a systematic review and meta-analysis. *Oral Health Prev Dent*. 2022;20:279–294. doi:10.3290/j.ohpd.b3170043.
3. Figuero E, Roldan S, Serrano J, et al. Efficacy of adjunctive therapies in patients with gingival inflammation: a systematic review and meta-analysis. *J Clin Periodontol*. 2020;47(Suppl 22):125–143.

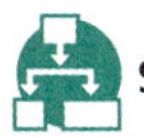

SEE ALSO

- Dental Infection; Glossitis
- Algorithm: Bleeding Gums

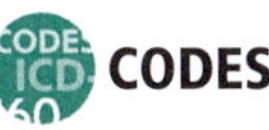

CODES

ICD10

- K05.10 Chronic gingivitis, plaque induced
- K05.11 Chronic gingivitis, non-plaque induced
- K05.00 Acute gingivitis, plaque induced

CLINICAL PEARLS

- Gingivitis may be prevented and treated with regular dental cleanings, good oral hygiene, and use of certain mouth rinses including chlorhexidine.
- Untreated, gingivitis may progress to periodontitis, a possible contributor to systemic inflammation and its consequences (e.g., coronary artery disease and uncontrolled diabetes).
- New-onset or difficult-to-treat gingivitis, consider differential of etiology: pregnancy, HIV, diabetes, medications, and vitamin deficiencies.

GLAUCOMA, PRIMARY CLOSED-ANGLE

Bethany Marshall, PharmD • Catherine Schaefer, MD, MS, BS

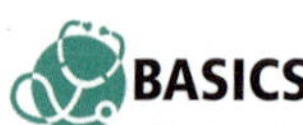

BASICS

DESCRIPTION

- Glaucoma is a progressive decline in vision from damage to the optic nerve and is usually associated with elevated intraocular pressure (IOP).
- Angle-closure is a mechanical blockage of the trabecular meshwork (TM) by the peripheral iris, causing increase in IOP.
- In primary angle-closure (PAC), there is an anatomical predisposition with no identifiable secondary pathologic condition.
- In secondary angle-closure, there is an identifiable pathologic cause, such as iris neovascularization or an enlarged cataractous lens.
- Angle-closure can be classified as the following:
  - Primary angle-closure suspect (PACS) is >180 degrees of iridotrabecular contact (ITC), but no evidence of TM or optic nerve damage
  - PAC is >180 degrees of ITC with peripheral anterior synechiae (PAS) or elevated IOP but with no optic neuropathy.
  - Primary angle-closure glaucoma (PACG) is PAC with glaucomatous optic neuropathy.
  - Acute primary angle-closure (APAC) or acute angle-closure crisis (AACC) is when the angle is occluded with symptomatic high IOP. It is a medical emergency requiring prompt treatment.
  - Chronic angle-closure (CAC) may develop after APAC in which synechial closure persists. It can also develop when the angle gradually closes and the angle function becomes progressively compromised leading to a slow rise in IOP. Vision loss may be the presenting complaint because of the asymptomatic nature of the condition.

Geriatric Considerations

Increased risk with age and cataracts.

Pregnancy Considerations

Majority of IOP-lowering medications are within class C, and the risk of adverse effects to the fetus must be balanced with risk of vision loss in the mother.

EPIDEMIOLOGY

- Female sex. PAC is 2 to 4 times more common in women than in men. Women tend to have smaller anterior segments and shorter axial lengths.
- More likely in those of Inuit and East or South Asian descent

Prevalence

The prevalence of PACG in patients >40 years varies depending on race and ethnicity. The burden of PACG is greater in Asian countries. The prevalence is as follows:

- Black: 0.1–0.2%
- White: 0.1–0.6%
- Japanese: 0.3%
- Other East Asian: 0.4–1.4%
- Inuit: 2.1%

ETIOLOGY AND PATHOPHYSIOLOGY

- PAC happens when the iris touches the TM in the anterior chamber angle. ITC obstructs aqueous humor outflow through the TM, increasing IOP. Prolonged ITC can cause scarring, with formation of PAS.
- The most common underlying mechanism of angle-closure is pupillary blockage of the aqueous flow from posterior to anterior chamber. This causes increase in pressure in the posterior chamber as compared to the anterior chamber. The buildup of pressure in the posterior chamber leads to anterior bowing of the iris and closing of the angle.
- One of the most important factors in closing the angle in an anatomically predisposed eye is dilation of the pupil. Dilation may occur as a result of a variety of causes including darkness, emotion, and medications that can cause the pupil to dilate. Pupillary block is maximal when the pupil is in the mid-dilated position.
- Plateau iris syndrome is an atypical configuration of the anterior chamber angle that can result in acute or chronic PAC. Angle-closure in plateau iris is most often caused by anteriorly positioned ciliary processes that narrow the anterior chamber recess by pushing the peripheral iris forward. A component of pupillary block is often present.

Genetics

First-degree relatives have a 1–12% increased risk in whites; 6 times greater risk in Chinese patients with positive family history

RISK FACTORS

- Age >50 years
- Female gender
- Family history of angle-closure
- Hyperopia
- Anterior positioned lens
- Medications that can induce angle-closure by dilating the pupil include:
  - Adrenergic agonists (albuterol, phenylephrine)
  - Anticholinergics (oxybutynin, atropine), antihistamines, antidepressants including selective serotonin reuptake inhibitors (SSRIs)
  - Tricyclic antidepressants (TCAs)
  - Cocaine
- Medications that can induce angle-closure by causing an uveal effusion include:
  - Topiramate
  - Sulfonamides

GENERAL PREVENTION

- Routine eye exam with gonioscopy for high-risk populations
- Prophylactic laser peripheral iridotomy (LPI) may be considered in PACS patients for preventing PACG
- Argon laser peripheral iridoplasty for plateau iris syndrome

COMMONLY ASSOCIATED CONDITIONS

- Cataract
- Hyperopia

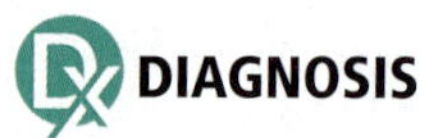

DIAGNOSIS

HISTORY

- Patient may be asymptomatic, have subacute symptoms or have compromised peripheral vision.
- Acute symptoms commonly include unilateral:
  - Severe eye pain
  - Blurred vision
  - Eye redness
  - Halos around lights/objects
  - Headache
  - Nausea and vomiting
- Family history of acute angle-closure glaucoma
- Obtain history of prescription, over-the-counter, and herbal medications.

PHYSICAL EXAM

Includes, but is not limited to, the following in the undilated eye:

- Visual field testing
- Visual acuity with refractive error (hyperopic eyes especially in older phakic patients)
- Pupil examination (reactivity and relative defects)
- Slit-lamp examination demonstrates conjunctival hyperemia (in acute cases), central and peripheral anterior chamber shallowing, corneal edema, iris abnormalities (diffuse and focal iris atrophy, posterior synechiae), lens changes (cataract and glaukomflecken-patchy localized anterior subcapsular lens opacities).
- IOP elevation.
- Gonioscopy allows visualization of the anatomy of the angle of both eyes. Look for ITC and PAS.
- Anterior segment imaging with ultrasound (US) biomicroscopy
- Anterior segment optical coherence tomography (AS-OCT) to understand the angle anatomy

DIFFERENTIAL DIAGNOSIS

- Secondary angle closure due to iris membranes
- Secondary pupillary block due to the following:
  - Uveitis with secondary posterior synechiae leading to iris bombe
  - Lens-related disorders, such as ectopia lentis or malpositioned intraocular lenses.
- Retinal conditions leading to the forward shift of the lens-iris diaphragm
- Topiramate induced myopic shift with acute bilateral angle closure.
- Malignant glaucoma (also called aqueous misdirection)

DIAGNOSTIC TESTS & INTERPRETATION

Initial Tests (lab, imaging)

- Gonioscopy
- US biomicroscopy
- AS-OCT

Diagnostic Procedures/Other

Diagnosis is done by gonioscopy

Test Interpretation

Narrow or closed anterior chamber angle

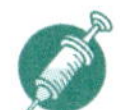

TREATMENT

ALERT

For patients with acute symptoms (severe eye pain, blurred vision, eye redness, halos around lights/objects, headache, nausea and vomiting) and asymmetric pupillary response, obtain immediate consultation with ophthalmology.

GENERAL MEASURES

Goals of treatment are to reverse or prevent angle-closure process, control IOP, and prevent damage to the optic nerve.

MEDICATION

During acute attack, medical therapy lowers IOP to relieve symptoms and clear corneal edema so that LPI can be performed as soon as possible.

First Line

Prostaglandin inhibitors (latanoprost 0.005%, bimatoprost 0.01%, travoprost 0.004%): increase TM outflow; relatively safe and most effective (1)[A]

Second Line

- β-Antagonists (timolol 0.5%): decrease aqueous production; caution in patients with lung disease
- α-Antagonists (brimonidine 0.2%): improve aqueous outflow; do not use in combination with MAOis.
- Carbonic anhydrase inhibitors (CAIs) (dorzolamide 2%, acetazolamide): decrease aqueous production; available topically and systemically; do not use in patients with sulfonamide allergy or thrombocytopenia.
- Hyperosmotic agents (glycerin 5%, mannitol 20%): decrease viscosity of aqueous humor; contraindicated in renal or heart failure.

SURGERY/OTHER PROCEDURES

- Definitive therapy for PAC, PACG, and AACC is Nd:YAG or argon LPI. LPI can be performed temporally or superiorly. Location of the LPI, does not seem to influence the occurrence of new postoperative dysphotopsias.
- Surgical iridectomy may be performed if cornea is cloudy and laser iridotomy cannot be performed.
- Plateau iris syndrome may be initially treated by either LPI or lensectomy if a cataract is present. Eyes with plateau iris syndrome remain predisposed to angle closure despite a patent iridotomy or lensectomy.
  - Argon laser peripheral iridoplasty may be needed to flatten and thin the peripheral iris.
- Growing evidence shows cataract extraction alone can lower IOP and reduce the risk of lens-induced angle closure. This can be considered as a treatment option in appropriate cases. Other procedures to reduce IOP include argon laser peripheral iridoplasty (especially for plateau iris syndrome), anterior chamber paracentesis, goniosynechialysis, and trabeculectomy.
  - APAC patients who underwent phacoemulsification with an IOL had better IOP control, deeper anterior chambers and required less glaucoma medications than those who underwent LPI alone. Performing phacoemulsification weeks to months after the initial LPI did not appear to adversely affect outcomes compared to early phacoemulsification (1)[B].
  - Clear lens extraction (CLE) can be considered for first-line treatment of eyes with more advanced angle closure disease, such as APAC eyes with an IOP >30 mm Hg (2)[C].

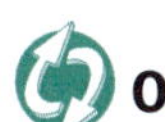

ONGOING CARE

FOLLOW-UP RECOMMENDATIONS

Patient Monitoring

- Evaluate fellow eye due to high risk of similar event.
- Prophylactic LPI may be scheduled if angle is anatomically narrow.

PATIENT EDUCATION

- Advise patient to seek emergency attention if experiencing a change in visual acuity, blurred vision, eye pain, or headache.
- PACS patients and no LPI; avoid use of decongestants, motion sickness medications, adrenergic agents, antipsychotics, antidepressants, and anticholinergic agents.

PROGNOSIS

- Prognosis depends on ethnicity, underlying eye disease, and time to treatment.
- After LPI, most PACS subjects can be expected to have no further treatment.
- Many PAC and APAC eyes, and most PACG eyes are given additional treatment to control IOP after LPI.

COMPLICATIONS

- Chronic angle closure
- Iris atrophy
- Cataracts
- Optic atrophy
- Malignant glaucoma
- Central retinal artery/vein occlusion
- Permanent decrease in visual acuity and/or blindness
- Fellow (contralateral) eye attack

REFERENCES

1. Lin Y-H, Wu C-H, Huang S-M, et al. Early versus delayed phacoemulsification and intraocular lens implantation for acute primary angle-closure. *J Ophthalmol*. 2020;2020:8319570.
2. Tanner L, Gazzard G, Nolan WP, et al. Has the EAGLE landed for the use of clear lens extraction in angle-closure glaucoma? And how should primary angle-closure suspects be treated? *Eye (Lond)*. 2020;34(1):40–50.

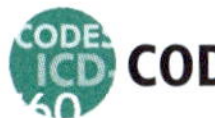

CODES

ICD10

- H40.20X0 Unsp primary angle-closure glaucoma, stage unspecified
- H40.219 Acute angle-closure glaucoma, unspecified eye
- H40.2290 Chronic angle-closure glaucoma, unsp eye, stage unspecified

CLINICAL PEARLS

For patients with acute symptoms (severe eye pain, blurred vision, eye redness, halos around lights/objects, headache, nausea and vomiting) and asymmetric pupillary response, obtain immediate consultation with ophthalmology.

GLAUCOMA, PRIMARY OPEN-ANGLE

Bethany Marshall, PharmD • Catherine Schaefer, MD, MS, BS

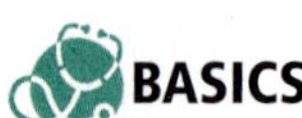

BASICS

DESCRIPTION

Primary open-angle glaucoma (POAG) is a chronic, progressive optic neuropathy which causes loss of the optic nerve rim and retinal nerve fiber layer (RNFL) with associated visual field defects. POAG is associated with increased intraocular pressure (IOP). Normal IOP is 10 to 21 mm Hg. However, early glaucoma can be present even with normal IOP, which can make early detection very difficult.

Pregnancy Considerations

Prostaglandins should be avoided during pregnancy in the treatment of POAG.

EPIDEMIOLOGY

Prevalence

- Prevalence in persons >40 years of age is ~3.5%.
- POAG is the second leading cause of blindness and the leading cause of blindness of people of African descent in the United States.

ETIOLOGY AND PATHOPHYSIOLOGY

- Aqueous humor is produced by the ciliary epithelium of the ciliary body and is secreted into the posterior chamber of the eye. The purpose of aqueous humor is to maintain the shape and function of the eye as well as provide nourishment. Aqueous humor then flows through the pupil and enters the anterior chamber to be drained by the trabecular meshwork (TM) in the iridocorneal angle of the eye. It then drains into the Schlemm canal and passes into the episcleral venous system. 5–10% of the total aqueous humor outflow leaves via the uveoscleral pathway.
- IOP is maintained by a balance of aqueous humor production in the ciliary body and drainage by the TM.
- Impaired aqueous humor outflow through the TM leads to greater resistance in the aqueous humor drainage system and causes an increase in IOP.
- IOP varies with blood pressure and respirations as well as throughout the day with lower IOP observed in the evenings.
- Increase in IOP above normal values over time can damage the optic nerve, eventually leading to vision loss. Typically, peripheral vision is lost before central vision, which allows POAG to go undiagnosed for longer.

Genetics

- TMCO1 genotype has been found to increase the risk of developing glaucoma among non-Hispanic whites.
- The myocilin (MYOC) gene was the first gene associated with POAG.

RISK FACTORS

- Myopia
- Diabetes mellitus, hypothyroidism, hypertension
- African descent
- Positive family history
- Prolonged use of corticosteroids
- Systemic calcium channel blockers
- High coffee consumption
- Prior history of pars plana vitrectomy
- Obstructive sleep apnea

GENERAL PREVENTION

Higher dietary nitrate and green leafy vegetable intake has been associated with a lower POAG risk. Evidence suggests that nitrate, a precursor of nitric oxide, is beneficial for blood circulation.

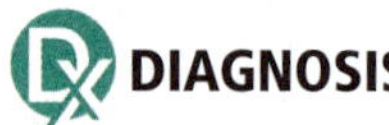

DIAGNOSIS

HISTORY

Painless, slowly progressive visual loss; patients are generally unaware of the visual loss until late in the disease. Central visual acuity remains unaffected until late in the disease.

PHYSICAL EXAM

- Visual acuity and visual field assessment
- Ophthalmoscopy to assess optic nerve for glaucomatous damage
- Tonometry to measure IOP; the IOP may be elevated or within the normal range.
- CDR score of >0.5: Normal eyes show a characteristic configuration for disc rim thickness of inferior ≥ superior ≥ nasal ≥ temporal (ISNT rule).
- Earliest visual field defects are paracentral scotomas and peripheral nasal steps.

DIFFERENTIAL DIAGNOSIS

- Normal-tension glaucoma
- Optic nerve pits
- Anterior ischemic optic neuropathy
- Compressive lesions of the optic nerve or chiasm

DIAGNOSTIC TESTS & INTERPRETATION

Initial Tests (lab, imaging)

Optical coherence tomography (OCT) can be useful in the detection of glaucoma.

- The RNFL is thinner in patients with glaucoma.
- OCT angiography (OCTA) demonstrates a decrease in macular vessel density in eyes with POAG. OCTA shows that parapapillary choroidal microvasculature dropout (MvD) is associated with progressive RNFL thinning in POAG. Macular, peripapillary, and choroidal vessel density measurements may complement visual field and structural OCT measurements (1)[A].

Diagnostic Procedures/Other

- Visual field testing: perimetry
- Tonometry to measure IOP: Thicker corneas resist the deformation inherent in most methods of tonometry, which may result in an overestimation of the IOP. Thinner corneas may give an artificially low reading.

Test Interpretation

- Atrophy and cupping of optic nerve
- Macular ganglion cell-inner plexiform layer (mGCIPL) OCT thickness is effective for predicting glaucoma progression regardless of the presence of high myopia (2)[B]. The peripapillary RNFL of highly myopic eyes tends to be thinner than that of normal eyes.

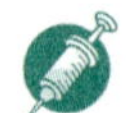

TREATMENT

GENERAL MEASURES

- Early Manifest Glaucoma Trial compared observation to treatment with betaxolol combined with argon laser trabeculoplasty (ALT) and found that early treatment delays progression, with the magnitude of initial IOP reduction influencing disease progression.
- Ocular Hypertension Treatment Study of patients with increased IOP of 24 to 32 mm Hg were treated with topical ocular hypotensive medication with a ~20% reduction in IOP. At 5 years, treatment reduced the incidence of POAG by >50%: 9.5% in the observation group versus 4.4% in the medication-treated group.
- Advanced Glaucoma Intervention Study randomized patients to laser trabeculoplasty or filtering surgery when medical therapy failed. In follow-up, if IOP was always <18 mm Hg, visual fields tended to stabilize. When IOP was >17 mm Hg, more than half of the time, patients tended to have worsening of visual fields.
- Collaborative Initial Glaucoma Treatment Study demonstrated that both initial medical and surgical (trabeculectomy) treatment achieved significant IOP reduction, and both had little visual field loss over time.
- The selective laser trabeculoplasty (SLT) versus eye drops for first-line treatment of ocular hypertension and glaucoma trial showed a reduction in IOP in SLT compared to medical treatment over a 3-year period.

MEDICATION

More than one medication, with different mechanisms of action, may be needed. Categories include the following:

- Prostaglandin analogues: generally used as first-line treatment; enhance uveoscleral outflow and increase aqueous humor outflow through the TM: latanoprost 0.005% 1 drop at bedtime; travoprost 0.004% 1 drop at bedtime; bimatoprost 0.01% 1 drop at bedtime
  - Latanoprostene bunod, 0.024% solution; this is a combination drug with one of the actions being the release of nitric oxide. Instill 1 drop at bedtime.
  - Contraindications/precautions
    - Prostaglandin analogues may cause increased pigmentation of the iris and periorbital tissue.
    - Increased pigmentation and growth of eyelashes
    - Should be used with caution in active intraocular inflammation (iritis/uveitis)
    - Caution is also advised in eyes with risk factors for herpes simplex, iritis, and cystoid macular edema.
    - Macular edema may be a complication associated with treatment.
    - Avoid during pregnancy.

- β-Adrenergic antagonists (nonselective and selective): decrease aqueous humor formation; best when used as an add-on therapy: timolol 0.25% (initial) to 0.5% 1 drop in affected eye q12h; gel-forming solution (0.25% or 0.5%) 1 drop in affected eye once daily (nonselective); betaxolol 0.5% 1 drop in affected eye BID (selective)
  - Nonselective β-adrenergic antagonists: Avoid in asthma, chronic obstructive pulmonary disease (COPD), 2nd- and 3rd-degree atrioventricular (AV) block, and decompensated heart failure. Betaxolol is a selective β-adrenergic antagonist and is safer in patients with pulmonary disease.
  - β-Adrenergic antagonists: caution in patients taking calcium antagonists because of possible AV conduction disturbances, left ventricular failure, or hypotension
- Adrenergic agonists (selective α_2-adrenergic agonists)
  - Brimonidine tartrate 0.2%: 1 drop TID (α_2-adrenergic agonist) decreases aqueous humor formation and increases uveoscleral outflow.
    - Brimonidine should not be used in infants and young children because of the risk of CNS depression, apnea, bradycardia, and hypotension.
    - Monoamine oxidase inhibitors and tricyclic antidepressants may interfere with the metabolism of brimonidine and result in toxicity.
- Carbonic anhydrase inhibitors (oral, topical) decrease aqueous humor formation.
  - Acetazolamide: 250 mg PO 1 to 4 times per day
  - Dorzolamide 2%: 1 drop TID
  - Brinzolamide 1%: 1 drop TID
  - Carbonic anhydrase inhibitors
    - Do not use with sulfa drug allergies.
    - Do not use if patient has cirrhosis because of the risk of hepatic encephalopathy.
- Rho kinase (ROCK) inhibitors increase aqueous humor outflow through the trabecular outflow pathway by decreasing actomyosin-driven cellular contraction and reducing production of fibrotic extracellular matrix proteins.
  - Netarsudil 0.02%: 1 drop once daily in the evening
  - Corneal verticillata, or whorl keratopathy, can occur with its usage.
- Parasympathomimetics (miotics) including direct-acting cholinergic agonists increase aqueous humor outflow.
  - Pilocarpine 1–4%: 1 drop in affected eye BID–QID (direct-acting cholinergic agonist)
  - Parasympathomimetics (miotics): cause pupillary constriction and may cause decreased vision in patients with a cataract; may cause eye pain or myopia due to increased accommodation; all miotics break down the blood–aqueous humor barrier and may induce chronic iridocyclitis.
- Hyperosmotic agents: increase blood osmolality, drawing water from the vitreous cavity; these can be especially helpful in acute emergencies when awaiting evaluation by specialist or awaiting surgical intervention.
  - Mannitol 20% solution is administered IV at 0.5 to 2 g/kg of body weight over a period of 45 minutes.
  - Glycerin 50% solution is administered orally; dosage is 1.0 to 1.5 g/kg, this is usually 4 to 7 oz. To improve the taste, the solution may be mixed with a small amount of orange juice and poured over crushed ice.
  - Hyperosmotic agents: caution in diabetics; dehydrated patients; and those with cardiac, renal, and hepatic disease
- Contact lens wearers: Many glaucoma drops contain benzalkonium chloride; remove contact lens prior to administration and wait 15 minutes before reinsertion.

SURGERY/OTHER PROCEDURES

- ALT
  - Improves aqueous humor outflow
- Selective 532-nm Nd:YAG laser trabeculoplasty (SLT)
  - As effective as ALT in lowering IOP
  - May be repeated if necessary
- Trabeculectomy (glaucoma filtering surgery)
  - Usually reserved for patients needing better IOP control after maximal medical therapy and who may have previously undergone an ALT/SLT
- Shunt (tube) surgery (e.g., Molteno, Ahmed devices)
  - Reserved for difficult glaucoma cases in which conventional filtering surgery has failed or is likely to fail
  - Tube Versus Trabeculectomy (TVT) study showed after 5 years of follow-up, both procedures were associated with similar IOP reduction and the number of glaucoma medications needed.
- Ciliary body ablation: indicated to lower IOP in patients with poor visual potential or those who are poor candidates for filtering or shunt procedures
- Minimally invasive glaucoma surgery (MIGS) is frequently combined with cataract surgery; currently targeted at patients with mild to moderate glaucoma
  - Schlemm canal, suprachoroidal, or subconjunctival stents
  - The Kahook Dual Blade performs an excisional goniotomy by removing a strip of TM.
  - Cataract extraction can decrease IOP in patients with ocular hypertension.

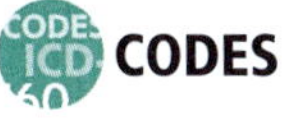

ONGOING CARE

FOLLOW-UP RECOMMENDATIONS

Patient Monitoring

- Monitor vision and IOP every 3 to 6 months.
- Optic nerve evaluation every 3 to 18 months, depending on POAG control
- A worsening of the mean deviation by 2 dB on the Humphrey field analyzer and confirmed by a single test after 6 months had a 72% probability of progression.

PATIENT EDUCATION

POAG is a silent robber of vision, and patients may not appreciate the significance of their disease until much of their visual field is lost. Patients should ensure compliance with any prescribed medications if diagnosed with POAG.

PROGNOSIS

- With standard glaucoma therapy, the rate of visual field loss in POAG is slow.
- Patients still may lose vision and develop blindness, even when treated appropriately.
- The structure of the mGCIPL was better preserved in surgically treated eyes than in medically treated eyes, even when the IOPs were similar during follow-up in cases of advanced glaucoma.

COMPLICATIONS

Blindness

REFERENCES

1. WuDunn D, Takusagawa HL, Sit AJ, et al. OCT angiography for the diagnosis of glaucoma: a report by the American Academy of Ophthalmology. *Ophthalmology*. 2021;128(8):1222–1235.
2. Shin JW, Song MK, Sung KR. Longitudinal macular ganglion cell-inner plexiform layer measurements to detect glaucoma progression in high myopia. *Am J Ophthalmol*. 2021;223:9–20.

ADDITIONAL READING

Weinreb RN, Khaw PT. Primary open-angle glaucoma. *Lancet*. 2004;363(9422):1711–1720.

G

CODES

ICD10

H40.1190 Primary open-angle glaucoma, unspecified eye, stage unspecified

CLINICAL PEARLS

- Painless, slowly progressive visual loss; patients generally are unaware of the visual loss until late in the disease. Central visual acuity remains unaffected until late in the disease.
- Patients still may lose vision and develop blindness, even when treated appropriately.
- Topical or system steroids can cause the IOP to increase.

GLOMERULONEPHRITIS, ACUTE

Tove Martine Goldson, MD, PhD • Nida Ali Sajan, DO

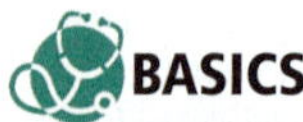

BASICS

DESCRIPTION

- Acute glomerulonephritis (GN) is an inflammatory or immune-mediated process involving the glomerulus of the kidney, resulting in a clinical syndrome consisting of sudden onset of hematuria, proteinuria, and renal insufficiency (1).
- Acute GN may be caused by primary glomerular disease or secondary to systemic disease.
- Clinical severity ranges from self-limited asymptomatic microscopic or gross hematuria to a rapidly progressive loss of kidney function over days to weeks.

ALERT

Urgent investigation and treatment are required to avoid irreversible loss of kidney function and subsequent progression to chronic kidney disease and end-stage renal disease.

EPIDEMIOLOGY

- Infection-related GN
  - Acute postinfectious GN (APSGN) most commonly manifests children and occurs about 2 weeks after resolution of group A β-hemolytic *Streptococcus* infection. This occurs in high frequency in highly populated and economically disadvantaged communities around the world. As APSGN has sharply declined in the Western world, the number of *Staphylococcus* infection–associated glomerulonephritis (SAGN) cases has increased in patients aged 50 to 80 years (2).
  - Can also occur as a result of other bacterial infections, such as infective endocarditis, VP shunt nephritis, or less commonly with viral, helminthic, or parasitic infections
- IgA nephropathy
  - Most common primary GN in the world
  - Median age at diagnosis is 40 to 45 years in Western nations.
  - Incidence differs geographically: Asia > United States.
  - HSP, the form with extrarenal manifestations, typically occurs in children <10 years old.
- Anti-GBM disease
  - Goodpasture syndrome: a notable cause of pulmonary-renal syndrome
  - Peak distribution in 3rd and 6th to 7th decades
- ANCA-associated GN:
  - Often has a relapsing and remitting course
  - Four disease presentations:
    - Granulomatosis with polyangiitis (GPA), formerly Wegener granulomatosis
    - Microscopic polyangiitis (MPA)
    - Isolated pauci-immune GN—when isolated to kidneys
    - Eosinophilic GPA, formerly Churg-Strauss disease—GN relatively common but renal involvement rarely severe
- MPGN
  - May be primary or secondary to systemic diseases
  - Epidemiology varies depending on the mechanism of injury and is more often a subacute or chronic presentation.
- Lupus nephritis (LN)
  - About 20–60% of systemic lupus patients will have renal involvement.
  - Incidence of lupus nephritis is higher among Black and Hispanic populations in comparison to White populations.
  - Six classes
    - Minimal mesangial LN
    - Mesangial proliferative LN
    - Focal LN (can be proliferative [active] and/or sclerosing [chronic] disease)
    - Diffuse LN (can be proliferative [active] and/or sclerosing [chronic] disease)
    - Membranous LN
    - Advanced sclerotic LN
- Cryoglobulin-associated vasculitis
  - 80% of cases with hepatitis C virus (HCV) infection
  - May also be associated with autoimmune disease or dysproteinemia

Prevalence

- In patients >65 years of age, with an average age of 75 years, about 1.2% of people are affected by either primary or secondary GN.
- In patients between the ages of 37 and 65 years of age, GN was much less commonly seen, with only about 0.12% of people affected by either primary or secondary GN (3).
- The incidence and prevalence of GN in children is unknown. Acute postinfectious GN is the most common type but has diminished over the years.

ETIOLOGY AND PATHOPHYSIOLOGY

- Systemic and/or local immune activation causes glomerular injury.
- Immune-complex mediated: antigen-antibody formation and deposition in the kidneys. Immune complexes are seen on immunofluorescence.
  - APSGN
  - SAGN
  - IgA nephropathy
  - MPGN
    - Cryoglobulin-associated GN
  - LN
- Direct antibody-mediated injury, linear staining on immunofluorescence
  - Anti-GBM disease
- Pauci-immune GN, not seen on immunofluorescence staining
  - ANCA-associated GN
- Alternative complement pathway dysregulation
  - C3 glomerulopathy

RISK FACTORS

- Epidemics of nephritogenic strains of streptococci are triggers for APSGN.
- Anti-GBM disease has been associated with prior pulmonary injury and inhalation exposures, such as hydrocarbon solvents.
- ANCA-associated GN may be drug induced (e.g., hydralazine, levamisole-contaminated cocaine) and is also associated with environmental exposures such as silica.
- Hepatitis B is associated with MPGN. Hepatitis C is associated with both MPGN and cryoglobulinemic GN.

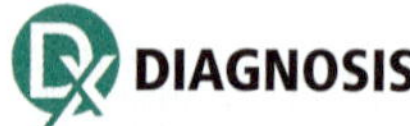

DIAGNOSIS

HISTORY

- Symptoms: cola- or tea-colored urine, decreased urine volume, blurry vision, dizziness, light-headedness, headache, altered mentation, edema, dyspnea, generalized malaise
- Timing
  - APSGN typically occurs 1 to 3 weeks after pharyngitis or 2 to 6 weeks after skin infection.
  - SAGN typically develops while the infection is ongoing.
  - IgA nephropathy may present within several days after an acute infection.
- Patients may also present with complaints more specific to the associated disease:
  - LN: joint pain or rash
  - Pulmonary-renal syndromes: hemoptysis (see "Physical Exam")
  - ANCA-associated GN: sinusitis, pulmonary infiltrates, arthralgias
  - IgA-HSP: abdominal or joint pain and purpura
  - Cryoglobulinemia-associated GN: purpura and skin vasculitis

PHYSICAL EXAM

- Majority of patients will have normal exam but can often present with hypertension and signs of fluid overload.
- Sinus disease: ANCA-associated GN/GPA
- Pharyngitis or impetigo: APSGN or IgA nephropathy
- Pulmonary hemorrhage (pulmonary-renal syndrome): anti-GBM disease/Goodpasture syndrome, ANCA-associated GN, or LN
- Hepatomegaly or liver tenderness: cryoglobulinemia-associated GN or IgA nephropathy
- Purpura: ANCA-associated GN or HSP/IgA nephropathy

DIFFERENTIAL DIAGNOSIS

Nonglomerular hematuria: trauma, prostate diseases, urologic cancer, cystitis, nephrolithiasis, renal cysts, thrombotic microangiopathy

DIAGNOSTIC TESTS & INTERPRETATION

Initial Tests (lab, imaging)

- Urinalysis
  - Dysmorphic red blood cells (RBCs) or RBC casts on urine microscopy indicate glomerular hematuria and strongly suggest the diagnosis of an acute GN.
  - Pyuria and white blood cell casts may also be present.
- Proteinuria: 24-hour collection or random urine protein/creatinine ratio
- Electrolytes, blood urea nitrogen, creatinine, complete blood count
- Blood cultures, followed by echocardiogram if endocarditis is suspected
- Serologies may help clarify etiology:
  - Antistreptolysin O titer, streptozyme
  - Complement levels (C3, C4)
  - Antinuclear antibody (ANA) to rule out LN
  - ANCA screen: myeloperoxidase and antiproteinase 3 antibodies
  - Anti-GBM antibody

  - Hepatitis B surface antigen and antibody
  - Hepatitis C antibody
  - Cryoglobulins
  - Rheumatoid factor
  - HIV testing
  - Serum free light chain to assess for monoclonal gammopathies
- Renal ultrasound to rule out structural causes of glomerular disease
- Chest x-ray in the setting of hemoptysis or a suspected infiltrate

Diagnostic Procedures/Other

Definitive diagnosis is made via renal biopsy.

Test Interpretation

Renal biopsy

- Light microscopy
  - Diffuse hypercellularity suggests a proliferative disease such as IgA nephropathy, LN, or APSGN.
  - Presence of glomerular crescents correlates with RPGN and disease severity.
  - Significant overlap between endothelial, mesangial, and epithelial cell proliferation
- Immunofluorescence
  - Pattern of IgG, IgA, IgM, C3, C4, C1q, fibrin, lambda and kappa light chains staining may aid in characterizing the GN.
  - LN typically positive for all immunoglobulins and complements
  - Isolated mesangial IgA staining is pathognomonic for IgA nephropathy.
  - Crescentic GN in absence of immune complex staining suggests ANCA-associated GN.
  - Crescentic GN with linear staining of IgG is characteristic of anti-GBM.
- Electron microscopy: The location of immunoglobulin deposits is useful in pointing to a particular diagnosis.

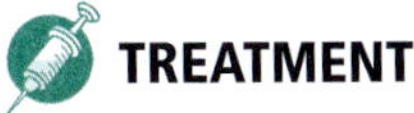

TREATMENT

GENERAL MEASURES

Treat the underlying condition if able.

MEDICATION

First Line

- Diuretics
- Calcium channel blockers
- Avoid ACE inhibitors or ARBs if acute renal dysfunction is present.
- Treatment of underlying infection, if appropriate

Second Line

- Supportive care is typically adequate in APSGN.
- Crescents on renal biopsy may be an indication for steroids in APSGN and, in other cases, are often an indication for additional potent immunosuppressive medications.
- Treatment with antiviral therapy for nephritic syndromes that have been shown to be secondary to underlying viral infections such as HCV and hepatitis B virus (HBV)
- Commonly used immunosuppressive medications include:
  - Corticosteroids—may consider initiation in high doses even prior to kidney biopsy
  - Cyclophosphamide
  - Mycophenolate-mofetil (MMF)
  - Calcineurin inhibitors (cyclosporine, tacrolimus)
  - Rituximab
- Choice of immunosuppressive agent depends on patient characteristics and the disease process.
- Plasmapheresis may also be considered in some cases for RPGN or ANCA-associated renal disease with diffuse pulmonary hemorrhage.
- Dialysis may be needed for uremia, hyperkalemia refractory to medical management, intractable acidosis, and diuretic-resistant pulmonary edema.

ISSUES FOR REFERRAL

- Consultation with a nephrologist is usually required to assist with renal biopsy to confirm diagnosis and assist with management.
- Consultation with a rheumatologist may also be helpful in cases with systemic manifestations.

ADMISSION, INPATIENT, AND NURSING CONSIDERATIONS

- Consider admission for patients with no urine output, rapidly deteriorating renal function, significant hypertension, and suspicion of pulmonary hemorrhage or fluid overload that is compromising heart or respiratory function.
- Hemodynamically stable patients without complications may be managed as outpatients.

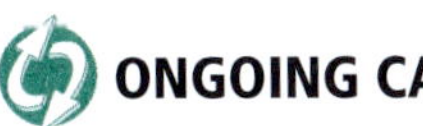

ONGOING CARE

FOLLOW-UP RECOMMENDATIONS

Patient Monitoring

- Regular blood pressure checks and urinalysis to detect recurrence, assessment of renal function to detect acute or follow chronic renal disease as a result of the primary event, and regular clinical assessment to detect suspicious symptoms that may herald a recurrence (i.e., rash, joint complaint, hemoptysis)
- Periodic reassessment of serology tests to follow asymptomatic individuals

DIET

- Salt-restricted diet (<2 g/day) and fluid restriction until edema and hypertension clear
- Avoid foods that are high in potassium and phosphorus if significant renal dysfunction is present.

PATIENT EDUCATION

National Kidney Foundation: https://www.kidney.org/kidney-topics/glomerulonephritis

PROGNOSIS

- The GN may be self-limited or part of a chronic disease that makes the possibility of recurrence of acute disease likely, with the potential for progressive loss of renal function over time.
- Some forms of acute GN (including ANCA-associated and severe lupus) require long-term immunosuppression to prevent recurrence.

COMPLICATIONS

- Hypertensive retinopathy and encephalopathy
- Microscopic hematuria may persist for years.
- Chronic kidney disease
- Nephrotic syndrome (~10%)

REFERENCES

1. Kidney Disease: Improving Global Outcomes (KDIGO) Glomerular Diseases Work Group. KDIGO 2021 clinical practice guideline for the management of glomerular diseases. *Kidney Int*. 2021;100(4S):S1–S276.
2. Satoskar AA, Parikh SV, Nadasdy T. Epidemiology, pathogenesis, treatment and outcomes of infection-associated glomerulonephritis. *Nat Rev Nephrol*. 2020;16(1):32–50. doi:10.1038/s41581-019-0178-8.
3. Wetmore JB, Guo H, Liu J, et al. The incidence, prevalence, and outcomes of glomerulonephritis derived from a large retrospective analysis. *Kidney Int*. 2016;90(4):853–860.

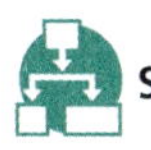

SEE ALSO

- Glomerulonephritis, Postinfectious; Henoch-Schönlein Purpura; Hyperkalemia; Hypertensive Emergencies; IgA Nephropathy; Lupus Nephritis; Nephrotic Syndrome; Vasculitis
- Algorithms: Acute Kidney Injury (Acute Renal Failure); Hematuria

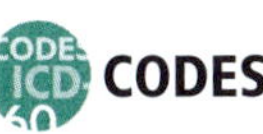

CODES

ICD10

- N00.9 Acute nephritic syndrome with unsp morphologic changes
- N00.2 Acute nephritic syndrome w diffuse membranous glomrlneph
- N00.8 Acute nephritic syndrome with other morphologic changes

CLINICAL PEARLS

- Dysmorphic RBCs and RBC casts are a key component of the urinalysis in GN.
- APSGN in children is typically a self-limited disease, whereas SAGN is more likely to cause persistent kidney damage.
- Searching for other organ involvement is useful in establishing a definitive diagnosis.
- With the discovery of a GN, monitor the initial renal function labs frequently to identify an RPGN.
- Clinical course and treatment strategies depend on the underlying disease process.

GLOMERULONEPHRITIS, POSTINFECTIOUS

Theodore B. Flaum, DO • Alexa Finkelstein, BS

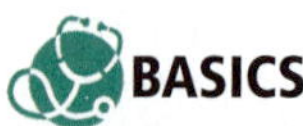

BASICS

DESCRIPTION

Postinfectious glomerulonephritis (PIGN) is an immune complex disease associated with nonrenal infection by certain strains of bacteria, most commonly *Streptococcus* and *Staphylococcus*. The most common form of PIGN, poststreptococcal glomerulonephritis (PSGN), is preceded by infection with *Streptococcus* species and predominantly affects children. The clinical presentation can be asymptomatic or with an acute nephritic syndrome, characterized by gross hematuria, proteinuria, edema, hypertension (HTN), and acute kidney injury.

EPIDEMIOLOGY

PIGN is declining globally, especially in developed countries, in large part due to better hygiene and a decreased incidence of streptococcal skin infections. There are an estimated 470,000 new cases per annum of PSGN worldwide, and it remains the most common cause of acute nephritis in children globally, with 97% of cases occur in developing countries. PSGN is primarily a pediatric disease, but a recent increase in cases has been seen in nonstreptococcal GN in adults.

Incidence

Based on a review of 11 population-based studies published between 1988 and 2000, the estimated incidence of infection related glomerulonephritis is 2 cases per 100,000 person-years in adults in developing countries and 0.3 cases per 100,000 in developed countries, compared to 24.3 and 6 cases per 100,000 person-years, respectively, in children.

Prevalence

PIGN has a low prevalence in developed countries, about 0.13 cases per 100,000 people in the United States, but its prevalence is significantly higher in low-income regions.

ETIOLOGY AND PATHOPHYSIOLOGY

- Glomerular immune complex disease induced by specific nephritogenic strains of bacteria:
  - >95% of cases are caused by group A β-hemolytic *Streptococcus* (GAS) (1)
  - *Staphylococcus* (predominantly *Staphylococcus aureus*; more commonly methicillin-resistant *S. aureus* [MRSA], occasionally coagulase-negative *Staphylococcus*)
  - Gram-negative bacteria including *Escherichia coli*, *Yersinia*, *Pseudomonas*, and *Haemophilus* (2)
  - Occasionally viral, fungal, helminthic or protozoal causes
- Proposed mechanisms for the glomerular injury (3) are related to the deposition of circulating immune complexes with streptococcal or staphylococcal antigens—while these complexes can be detected in patients with streptococcal- or staphylococcal-related GN they do not correlate to disease activity. IgG is the most frequent immunoglobulin in PSGN (2).
- These glomerular immune complexes result in complement activation and inflammation:
  - Nephritis-associated plasmin receptor (NAPlr): activates plasmin; contributes to activation of the alternative complement pathway
  - Streptococcal pyrogenic exotoxin B (SPE B): binds plasmin and acts as a protease; promotes the release of inflammatory mediators
- Activation of the alternative complement pathway causes initial glomerular injury as evidenced by C3 deposition and decreased levels of serum C3. The lectin pathway of complement activation has also been recently implicated in glomerular injury (1).

RISK FACTORS

- Children 5 to 12 years of age
- Older patients (>65 years of age) with immunocompromising comorbid conditions such as diabetes and alcohol abuse

GENERAL PREVENTION

- Early antibiotic treatment for streptococcal and staphylococcal infections, although efficacy in preventing GN is uncertain
- Improved hand hygiene and respiratory etiquette
- Prophylactic penicillin treatment to be used in closed communities and household contacts of index cases in areas where PIGN is prevalent

COMMONLY ASSOCIATED CONDITIONS

Group A streptococcal pharyngitis or skin infections are classic triggers or other bacterial infections such as staphylococcal aureus or pneumococcal infections.

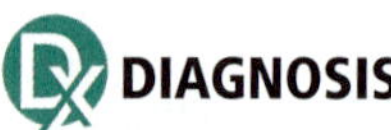

DIAGNOSIS

HISTORY

- Usually history of antecedent GAS skin/throat infection
- Patients present with acute nephritic syndrome, characterized by sudden onset of hematuria associated with edema and HTN for 1 to 2 weeks after an infection.
- A triad of edema (usually generalized), gross hematuria, and HTN is classic, but not always seen.
- Urine described as "tea-colored" or "cola-colored"
  - Gross hematuria: present in 25–60% of patients
  - Microscopic hematuria: subclinical cases of PIGN
  - Oliguria: present in 18–51% of patient
- The latent period between GAS infection and PIGN depends on the site of infection: 1 to 3 weeks following GAS pharyngitis and 3 to 6 weeks following GAS skin infection.
- Adult PIGN most commonly follows staphylococcal infections (three times more common than streptococcal infections) of the upper respiratory tract, skin, heart, lung, bone, or urinary tract. Studies show 7–16% of cases of adult PIGN have no preceding evidence of infection and, in 24–59%, the offending microorganism cannot be identified.

PHYSICAL EXAM

- Constitutional:
  - Fever: 40–50% of patients
- Cardiovascular:
  - Edema: present in ~2 of 3 adult patients due to sodium and water retention; less common in pediatric patients
  - HTN: present in 80–90% of patients and varies from mild to severe; secondary to fluid retention; hypertensive encephalopathy is an uncommon but serious complication.
- Pulmonary:
  - Respiratory distress: due to pulmonary edema (rare)
- Neurologic:
  - Encephalopathy and seizures are rare.

DIFFERENTIAL DIAGNOSIS

The diagnosis of PIGN is generally accomplished by history once the diagnosis of acute nephritis is made, with documentation of a recent infection and nephritis beginning to resolve 1 to 2 weeks after presentation. However, with progressive disease (>2 weeks, persistent hematuria/HTN >4 to 6 weeks, or no adequate documentation of a GAS or other infection) the differential diagnosis of GN needs to be considered and renal biopsy performed:

- Membranoproliferative glomerulonephritis (MPGN): Patients with MPGN have persistent nephritis and hypocomplementemia beyond 4 to 6 weeks. Patients with PIGN tend to have resolution of their disease and a return to normal C3 and CH50 levels within 2 to 4 weeks.
- Secondary causes of GN: Lupus nephritis and Henoch-Schönlein purpura nephritis have similar features to PIGN. Hypocomplementemia is not characteristic of Henoch-Schönlein purpura, and the hypocomplementemia that occurs in lupus nephritis usually results in reductions in both C3 and C4, whereas C4 levels are normal in PIGN.
- IgA nephropathy often presents after an upper respiratory infection. It can be distinguished from PIGN based on a shorter time frame between the upper respiratory illness and onset of hematuria, as well as history of gross hematuria, as PIGN recurrence is rare. IgA nephropathy is a chronic illness and will recur. Patients with IgA nephropathy have normal C3/C4 levels.
- IgA-dominant acute PIGN: a recently recognized form of PIGN occurring in poststaphylococcal GN; this differs from primary IgA nephropathy in that these patients do not have a history of renal disease (2)[A].
- Pauci-immune crescentic GN: In elderly with severe renal failure and active urine sediment, this is much more common, so antineutrophil cytoplasmic antibody (ANCA) testing should be done (2)[A].

DIAGNOSTIC TESTS & INTERPRETATION

Initial Tests (lab, imaging)

- Urinalysis
  - Hematuria with possible dysmorphic red cells
    - Gross hematuria: present in 25–60% of patients
    - Microscopic hematuria: subclinical cases of PIGN
  - +/− RBC casts and pyuria
  - Proteinuria ~90% of patients (nephrotic range proteinuria is uncommon in children)
- Renal function
  - Decreased GFR with elevated creatinine to the point of renal insufficiency in 25–83% of cases, more commonly in adults (83%)

Follow-Up Tests & Special Considerations

- Culture: PSGN usually presents weeks after a GAS infection; only ~25% of patients will have either a positive throat or skin culture.
- Complement: 90% of pediatric patients (slightly fewer adult patients) will have depressed C3 and CH50 levels in the first 2 weeks of the disease, whereas C2 and C4 levels remain normal. C3 and CH50 levels return to normal within 4 to 8 weeks after presentation.
- Serology: Elevated titers of antibodies support evidence of a recent GAS infection. Streptozyme test measuring antistreptolysin O (ASO), antihyaluronidase (AHase), antistreptokinase (ASKase), anti–nicotinamide-adenine dinucleotidase (anti-NAD), and anti-DNAse B antibodies: positive in >95% of patients with PSGN due to pharyngitis and 80% with skin infections. In pharyngeal infection, ASO, anti-DNAse B, anti-NAD, and AHase titers are elevated. In skin infections, only the anti-DNAse and AHase titers are typically elevated.

Diagnostic Procedures/Other

Renal biopsy is rarely done in children; recommended in most adults to confirm the diagnosis and rule out other glomerulopathies

Test Interpretation

- Light microscopy: diffuse proliferative glomerulonephritis with prominent endocapillary proliferation and numerous neutrophils within the capillary lumen. Deposits may also be found in the mesangium ("starry sky"). Severity of involvement varies and correlates with clinical findings. Crescent formation is uncommon and is associated with a poor prognosis.
- Immunofluorescence microscopy: deposits of C3 and IgG distributed in a diffuse granular pattern
- Electron microscopy: dome-shaped subepithelial electron-dense deposits that are referred to as "humps;" these deposits are immune complexes, and they correspond to the deposits of IgG and C3 found on immunofluorescence. Rate of clearance of these deposits affects recovery time.

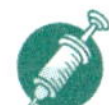

TREATMENT

MEDICATION

- No specific therapy exists for PIGN, and no randomized controlled trials indicate that aggressive immunosuppressive therapy has a beneficial effect in patients with rapidly progressive crescentic disease. Despite this, patients with >30% crescents on renal biopsy are often treated with steroids.
- Older patients often require hospitalization to treat complications of heart failure (HF) from volume overload (2).
- Management is mainly supportive, with focus on treating the clinical manifestations of PIGN (HTN; pulmonary edema):
  - Salt and water restriction and loop diuretics
  - Calcium channel blockers/angiotensin-converting enzyme (ACE) inhibitors may be used in cases of severe HTN.
- Patients with evidence of persistent bacterial infection should be given a course of antibiotic therapy.

ISSUES FOR REFERRAL

Consider referral to nephrology if poor recovery, worsening renal function, or complications develop.

SURGERY/OTHER PROCEDURES

Acute dialysis is required in approximately 50% of elderly patients (1),(2).

ADMISSION, INPATIENT, AND NURSING CONSIDERATIONS

Admission may be necessary for elderly at risk for complications such as new onset or exacerbation of preexisting CHF (2).

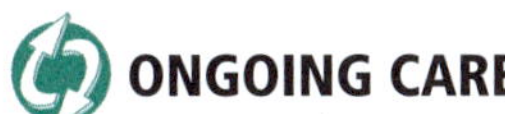

ONGOING CARE

FOLLOW-UP RECOMMENDATIONS

Patient Monitoring

- Repeat urinalysis to check for clearance of hematuria and/or proteinuria.
- Monitor blood pressure, kidney function, and for signs of fluid overload.
- Consider other diagnosis if no improvement within 2 weeks.

DIET

Renal diet if requiring instances of dialysis

PATIENT EDUCATION

Educate patient/family about signs of relapse or complications.

PROGNOSIS

- Most children with PIGN have an excellent outcome, with >90% of cases achieving full recovery of renal function.
- Elderly patients, especially adults, develop HTN, recurrent proteinuria, and renal insufficiency long after the initial illness. Adults with multiple comorbid factors have the worst prognosis and highest incidence of chronic renal injury following PIGN (2).
- Complete remission in adult PIGN is only 26–56%. This has declined since the 1990s, suggesting prognosis is worsening.
- The presence of diabetes, higher creatinine levels, and more severe glomerular disease (e.g., crescents) on biopsy are all risk factors for developing end-stage renal disease (2).

COMPLICATIONS

Complications related to PIGN are primarily due to volume overload. These complications can include HTN and, less commonly, pulmonary edema. Patients may also develop recurrent proteinuria and renal insufficiency; however, this is rare.

REFERENCES

1. Hunt EAK, Somers MJG. Infection-related glomerulonephritis. *Pediatr Clin North Am*. 2019;66(1):59–72.
2. Nasr SH, Radhakrishnan J, D'Agati VD. Bacterial infection-related glomerulonephritis in adults. *Kidney Int*. 2013;83(5):792–803.
3. Nadasdy T, Hebert LA. Infection-related glomerulonephritis: understanding mechanisms. *Semin Nephrol*. 2011;31(4):369–375.

ADDITIONAL READING

- Balasubramanian R, Marks SD. Post-infectious glomerulonephritis. *Paediatr Int Child Health*. 2017;37(4):240–247.
- Ramdani B, Zamd M, Hachim K, et al. Acute postinfectious glomerulonephritis [in French]. *Nephrol Ther*. 2012;8(4):247–258.
- Wen YK. Clinicopathological study of infection-associated glomerulonephritis in adults. *Int Urol Nephrol*. 2010;42(2):477–485.

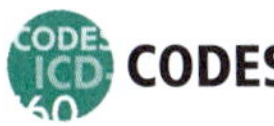

CODES

ICD10

- N05.9 Unsp nephritic syndrome with unspecified morphologic changes
- N00.9 Acute nephritic syndrome with unsp morphologic changes

CLINICAL PEARLS

- PIGN is an immune complex disease occurring after infection with certain strains of bacteria, most commonly group A *Streptococcus pyogenes*.
- The clinical presentation can be asymptomatic or with an acute nephritic syndrome, characterized by gross hematuria, proteinuria, edema, HTN, and acute kidney injury.
- Treatment is primarily supportive and includes treating HTN and edema, along with antibiotics for any ongoing bacterial infection.
- Persistent nephritis and low C3 levels for >2 weeks should prompt evaluation for other causes of GN, such as MPGN or systemic lupus erythematosus nephritis.

GLUCOSE INTOLERANCE

Joseph Daniel Hogue, MD, MBA • Kayla Sweeten, MD • Christopher McDaniel, MD

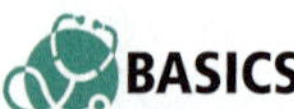

BASICS

DESCRIPTION

- Glucose intolerance is an intermediate stage between a normal glucose metabolism and diabetes. It occurs due to a gradual decline in β-cell function.
- Individuals with impaired fasting glucose (IFG) and/or impaired glucose intolerance (IGT) have been referred to as having prediabetes:
  - IFG: 100 to 125 mg/dL
  - IGT: 140 to 199 mg/dL 2 hours after ingestion of 75 g oral glucose load
  - Hemoglobin A1c (HbA1c) 5.7–6.4%

EPIDEMIOLOGY

- An estimated 97.6 million adults aged ≥18 years old had prediabetes in 2021 (1)
- In the United States, an estimated 88 million people ≥18 years old, are living with prediabetes as of 2020, based on the National Diabetes Statistics Report.
- Only 11% of people with prediabetes are aware of their condition.
- Among all US adults aged ≥18 years old, crude estimates for 2017 to 2020 was 38% of all US adults had prediabetes, based on their fasting glucose or HbA1c level.
- Prediabetes has a 34.5% prevalence among adults >18 years old and 51% of adults ≥65 years old in the United States (2).

Incidence

- Systematic review indicates a 5-year cumulative incidence of developing diabetes of 9–25% for people with an HbA1c of 5.5–6% and 25–50% with an HbA1c of 6–6.5%.
- Highest incidence in American Indians/Alaska Natives, non-Hispanic blacks, and Hispanics (2)

Prevalence

- As of 2020, prevalence of prediabetes in the United States was 34.5% in adults >20 years old and 51% in adults >65 years old. According to ADA, in 2015 84.1 million Americans >18 years old had prediabetes.
- As of 2021, the US prevalence was 8.9%.

ETIOLOGY AND PATHOPHYSIOLOGY

Progressive loss of insulin secretion on the background of insulin resistance

Genetics

- Genetic heterogeneity is established by family, twin, immunologic, and HLA disease association studies.
- Variants in 11 genes have been shown to be significantly associated with future development of type 2 diabetes and IFG. Variants in eight of these genes have been associated with impaired β-cell function.

RISK FACTORS

- Body mass index (BMI) ≥25: overweight
- History of gestational diabetes mellitus (GDM)
- Sedentary lifestyle
- Medications

GENERAL PREVENTION

- Lifestyle modification with weight reduction, smoking cessation, dietary therapy (DASH or Mediterranean diet) and increased physical activity (150 min/week of moderate-intensity aerobic exercise).
- A decrease in excess body fat provides the greatest risk reduction.

Pregnancy Considerations

- Screening for diabetes in pregnancy is based on risk factor analysis:
  - High risk: first prenatal visit
  - Average risk: 24 to 28 weeks' gestation
- Women with GDM should be screened for diabetes 6 to 12 weeks' postpartum with 75-g OGTT and then every 1 to 3 years via any method.

COMMONLY ASSOCIATED CONDITIONS

- Obesity (abdominal and visceral obesity)
- Dyslipidemia with high triglycerides (TG)
- PCOS
- GDM
- Congenital diseases (Down, Turner, Klinefelter, and Wolfram syndromes)

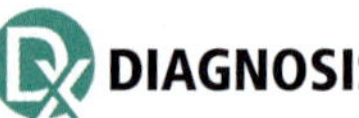

DIAGNOSIS

Who to screen

- BMI ≥25 or ≥23 for Asian Americans
- Age >35 years
- First-degree relative with diabetes
- High TG >250 mg/dL
- Low HDL <35 mg/dL
- HTN: BP >130/80 Hg or on treatment
- History of GDM
- History of cardiovascular disease
- Ethnic group at increased risk (African American, Native American, Hispanics, Asian American, Pacific Islander)
- PCOS
- Conditions associated with insulin resistance such as severe obesity or acanthosis nigricans
- Patients with prediabetes (HbA1c >5.7) (2)
- Patients with history of GDM should have lifelong testing at least every 3 years.
- Persons with HIV, exposure to high-risk medicines, or history of pancreatitis

HISTORY

- No clear symptoms
- Polyuria
- Polydipsia
- Weight loss
- Blurred vision
- Polyphagia

PHYSICAL EXAM

- General physical exam
- BMI assessment

DIFFERENTIAL DIAGNOSIS

- Type A insulin resistance
- Leprechaunism
- Rabson-Mendenhall syndrome
- Lipoatrophic diabetes
- Pancreatitis
- Cushing syndrome
- Glucagonoma
- Pheochromocytoma
- Hyperthyroidism
- Somatostatinoma
- Aldosteronoma
- Drug-induced hyperglycemia
  - Thiazide diuretics (high doses)
  - β-Blockers
  - Corticosteroids (including inhaled corticosteroids)
  - Thyroid hormone
  - α-Interferon
  - Pentamidine
  - Protease inhibitors
  - Atypical antipsychotics
  - Selective serotonin reuptake inhibitors

DIAGNOSTIC TESTS & INTERPRETATION

Initial Tests (lab, imaging)

- Fasting glucose, 2-hour OGTT, or HbA1c is equally appropriate.
- Repeat screen at 3-year intervals with normal results, sooner depending on risk status.

Follow-Up Tests & Special Considerations

- Fasting lipid profile
- Creatinine and GFR
- Urinalysis
- Microalbumin-to-creatinine ratio
- Thyroid-stimulating hormone with free T_4
- Periodic measurement of vitamin B_{12} levels for patients on long-term metformin therapy especially those with anemia or peripheral neuropathy

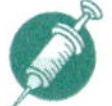

TREATMENT

- ADA recommends lifestyle modification as the primary intervention which can include physical activity focused on weight loss and medical nutrition therapy (preferably via a registered dietitian).
- Mediterranean diet and diets high in fiber-rich foods such as vegetables, fruits, whole grains, seeds, and nuts plus white meat sources are protective against type 2 diabetes.
- Consider referring patients with prediabetes to an intensive diet and physical activity behavioral counseling program adhering to the tenets of the Diabetes Prevention Program targeting a loss of 7% of body weight and should increase their moderate-intensity physical activity (such as brisk walking to at least 150 min/week).
- Resistance training and endurance exercise both reduce diabetes risk.
- Interrupt prolonged sitting every 30 minutes with short bouts of physical activity.
- Diabetes prevention programs are cost-effective and often covered by third-party payers.
- Screen and treat modifiable risk factors for cardiovascular disease.
- Diabetes self-management education and support systems are appropriate venues for people with prediabetes to receive education and support to develop and maintain behaviors that can prevent or delay the onset of diabetes.
- Technology-assisted tools including internet-based social networks, distance learning, DVD-based content, and mobile applications can be useful elements of effective lifestyle modification to prevent diabetes.

MEDICATION

Consider metformin therapy for prevention of type 2 diabetes, especially in those with BMI >35, those aged <60 years, HbA1c >6% and women with prior GDM and/or rising HbA1c despite lifestyle intervention.

First Line

Metformin (drug of choice): started at 850 mg once daily for 1 month; if tolerating, increase to 850 mg twice daily. Observational data suggest it can be used safely down to GFR of 30 to 45 but may require dose adjustments.

Second Line

GLP-1 agonists: Recent clinical trials in primarily obese patients, GLP-1 agonists have shown various benefits including weight loss, improvement in β-cell function, and a return to a normal glycemic state. Overall prediabetes incidence decreased by 84–96% (1)[A]. Semaglutide and tirzepatide have been shown to delay or prevent progression to diabetes in 1.0 to 3.5 years studies (3).

ISSUES FOR REFERRAL

- Diabetes educator/registered dietitian upon diagnosis
- Exercise physiologist
- Lifestyle coaching
- Obesity specialist

ADDITIONAL THERAPIES

Alternative/botanical therapy:

- In individuals with prediabetes, vitamin D may reduce the risk of progression to type 2 diabetes. As it is inexpensive and confers little risk, empiric vitamin D supplementation in people with prediabetes is reasonable.
- Although studies lack large sample size and ideal design, there is some evidence that fenugreek, bitter melon, and cinnamon can reduce hyperglycemia and improve insulin sensitivity (1).

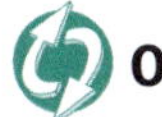

ONGOING CARE

FOLLOW-UP RECOMMENDATIONS

Patient Monitoring

- At least annual monitoring for development of diabetes with HbA1c, 2-hour OGTT, or fasting glucose
- BP should be routinely measured.
- Annual testing for lipid abnormalities and microalbuminuria (for detection and therapy modification of incipient diabetic nephropathy)
- Monitoring of BMI

DIET

- Mediterranean diet has been shown to be beneficial. One small cohort study showed that the addition of about 10 g of extra virgin olive oil to meals improved postprandial glucose by reducing DPP4 activity and increasing insulin and GLP-1. It also showed a significant decrease in TG and apolipoprotein B-48.
- Limit high glycemic carbohydrates and sucrose-containing foods.
- Diets high in fiber, vegetables, nuts, seeds, and whole grains
- Intermittent fasting has shown benefit in improving fasting glucose as well as postprandial hyperglycemia (4)[C].

PROGNOSIS

- Individuals with IFG and/or IGT have high risk for the future development of diabetes.
- Prediabetes increases the risk of developing type 2 diabetes, heart disease, and stroke.
- 20–70% of individuals with prediabetes who do not lose weight, change their dietary habits, and/or engage in moderate physical activity will progress to type 2 diabetes within 3 to 6 years.
- Lifestyle intervention reduced 3-year diabetes incidence by 58% compared to 31% with metformin.

COMPLICATIONS

- Cardiovascular and peripheral artery disease
- Stroke: 2 to 4 times higher risk
- Ketoacidosis
- Sexual dysfunction
- Gastroparesis
- Nephropathy and potential for renal failure
- Retinopathy and potential for loss of vision
- Peripheral and autonomic neuropathy

REFERENCES

1. Deng R. A review of the hypoglycemic effects of five commonly used herbal food supplements. *Recent Pat Food Nutr Agric*. 2012;4(1):50–60.
2. American Diabetes Association. Standards of medical care in diabetes—2017. *Diabetes Care*. 2017;40(Suppl 1):S11–S119.
3. Papaetis GS. Incretin-based therapies in prediabetes: current evidence and future perspectives. *World J Diabetes*. 2014;5(6):817–834.
4. Arnason TG, Bowen MW, Mansell KD. Effects of intermittent fasting on health markers in those with type 2 diabetes: a pilot study. *World J Diabetes*. 2017;8(4):154–164.

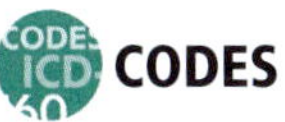

CODES

ICD10

- E74.39 Other disorders of intestinal carbohydrate absorption
- R73.09 Other abnormal glucose
- R73.01 Impaired fasting glucose

CLINICAL PEARLS

- Patient education and lifestyle reinforcement should be emphasized in all clinical encounters as lifestyle optimization is essential for all patients with prediabetes.
- Research shows that you can lower your risk for type 2 diabetes by 58% by losing 7% of your body weight (or 15 lb if you weigh 200 lb).
- Recommend exercising moderately (such as brisk walking) 30 min/day, 5 days a week.
- Consider concurrent cardiovascular risks and further workup as indicated clinically.

GONOCOCCAL INFECTIONS

Rashmi Rode, MD, FAAFP • Adam Mendonca, MD

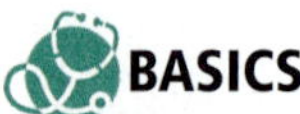

BASICS

DESCRIPTION

- *Neisseria gonorrhoeae*, a gram-negative intracellular diplococcus, causes a sexually and vertically transmitted bacterial infection. It typically presents in the urogenital tract, pharynx, rectum, or conjunctiva. Urogenital infection is most common. Disseminated infections can lead to arthritis, tenosynovitis, rash, endocarditis, or meningitis. Asymptomatic carriers are common, especially among women.
- In neonates, *N. gonorrhoeae* causes ophthalmia neonatorum after vaginal delivery, which can lead to blindness if untreated.

EPIDEMIOLOGY

- Age: 15 to 49 years; highest in 20 to 24 years age group
- Sex: global incident rate of 19 (11 to 29) per 1,000 women and 23 (10 to 43) per 1,000 men (1)
- Concern: Extended-spectrum cephalosporin (ESC) resistance is growing worldwide.

Incidence

- Annual incidence noted in 2020 was 82.4 million new cases per year (1).
- In the United States, the rate of gonorrhea increased by 60.6% among men and 43.6% among women, with the highest rates observed in adolescents, young adults, and certain racial and ethnic minorities (2).

Prevalence

- Incidence and prevalence are roughly equal. The true prevalence is higher due to asymptomatic cases
- The incidence in men is higher than in women.

ETIOLOGY AND PATHOPHYSIOLOGY

- Only *N. gonorrhoeae* and *Neisseria meningitidis* are pathogenic.
- Infection progresses through:
  - *Neisseria* strains produce pili, which are critical for host cell attachment, genetic transfer, and motility.
  - The outer membrane contains three proteins—PorB, Opa, and Rmp—that assist in acquiring nutrients, facilitate attachment, and prevent bacterial destruction.
  - Colonization and invasion of epithelial cells.
  - Transcellular transcytosis occurs, leading to the release of the bacteria into the subepithelial layer and intracellular proliferation.
  - The host response features leukocyte infiltration, epithelial sloughing, formation of microabscesses in the submucosa, and the production of purulent pus.

Genetics

Deficiency of late components of complement cascade (C7–C9) predisposes to disseminated disease.

RISK FACTORS

- Age ≤25 years
- Prior or current STI or partner with STI
- Inconsistent condom use
- Multiple/new sexual partners
- Men who have sex with men (MSM)
- Commercial sex work or substance use
- Infants born to infected mothers
- Children: Suspect sexual abuse.
- Autoinoculation (e.g., conjunctivitis)

GENERAL PREVENTION

- Consistent condom use during all forms of sexual activities
- Partner treatment; consider expedited partner therapy (EPT)
- Routine STI screening in high-risk populations
- All newborns should receive ocular erythromycin 0.5% ointment to prevent gonococcal ophthalmia neonatorum.

COMMONLY ASSOCIATED CONDITIONS

Other STIs:

- *Chlamydia trachomatis*
- Syphilis
- HIV
- Hepatitis B and C
- Herpes

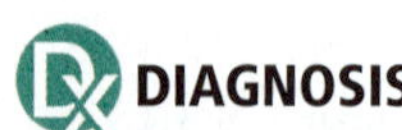

DIAGNOSIS

HISTORY

Sexual history:

- Number and gender of partners
- Sexual practices
- Use of barrier protection
- STI history
- Future or current pregnancy plans
- Onset: Symptoms occur 1 to 14 days post-exposure
- Up to 10% of men and 20–40% of women are asymptomatic.
- In men, common symptoms
  - White, yellow, or greenish discharge from the penis
  - Pain or burning when urinating
  - Painful or swollen testes
- In Women, mostly asymptomatic; when symptoms present, they are
  - Vaginal discharge
  - Pain or burning when urinating
  - Vaginal bleeding between periods or during sexual intercourse
- Pharynx: often asymptomatic, sore throat possible
- Rectum: bleeding, discharge, tenesmus, itching, often asymptomatic
- Disseminated gonococcal infection: fever, rash, arthritis, tenosynovitis, endocarditis, meningitis
- Infants with eye infection: redness, pain, soreness, ulcers, and tearing

PHYSICAL EXAM

- Genitourinary (GU): urethral or cervical discharge, tenderness on exam in both males and females
- Pharynx: exudative pharyngitis (rare)
- Rectum: discharge or normal exam
- Disseminated: pustular rash, large joint arthritis, tenosynovitis, meningeal signs

DIFFERENTIAL DIAGNOSIS

C. trachomatis, UTIs, other vaginitis, or urethritis (bacterial, viral, or parasitic)

DIAGNOSTIC TESTS & INTERPRETATION

Initial Tests (lab, imaging)

- Recommended test: nucleic acid amplification testing (NAAT) most sensitive
- Specimens
  - First-stream urine sample without urethral cleansing (preferred in men)
  - Clinician- or patient-collected vaginal or endocervical swabs
  - Pharyngeal and rectal swabs for MSM with a history of unprotected anal or oral sex
  - Urethral swab
- Other options:
  - Genital culture—specific and less expensive, but has lower sensitivity
  - Gram stain (diagnostic for symptomatic urethritis in men) but only 50–70% of asymptomatic infections in men are detected and it is less reliable in women
  - Polymerase chain reaction (PCR)-based rapid diagnostic tests (RDT), or point of care (POC) NAATs—decreases loss to follow-up, and reduces overtreatment
  - Blood culture is 50% sensitive in disseminated disease. Joint fluid culture is 50% sensitive in septic arthritis. Screen for additional STIs, especially chlamydia, syphilis, and HIV.
  - Imaging is not recommended.

Follow-Up Tests & Special Considerations

- In cases of suspected or documented treatment failure, clinicians should perform both culture and antimicrobial susceptibility testing (AST). The minimum inhibitory concentration (MIC) gradient strip test method is the preferred method.
- AST measures the MIC of an antimicrobial agent required to inhibit growth.
- A test of cure is not routinely recommended for persons with uncomplicated urogenital or rectal gonorrhea who are treated with any of the recommended or alternative regimens. However, any person with pharyngeal gonorrhea should return 7 to 14 days after initial treatment for a test of cure by using either culture or NAAT. A test of cure is also recommended for special circumstances such as pregnancy, persistent symptoms, or suspected treatment failure.
- Because of the risk of reinfection, routine repeat testing is recommended 3 months after initial treatment, regardless of whether sexual partners have been treated.

Diagnostic Procedures/Other

- Culdocentesis may demonstrate free purulent exudate and provide material for Gram staining and culture. Gram staining material from unroofed skin lesions may show typical organisms.
- Pelvic ultrasound or CT scan may demonstrate thick, dilated fallopian tubes or abscess formation.

Test Interpretation

- Gram-negative intracellular diplococci
- Nonpathologic gram-negative diplococci may be found in extragenital locations. For this reason, Gram stain of pharyngeal or rectal swabs is not recommended.

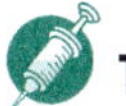

TREATMENT

GENERAL MEASURES

- Annual screening for *N. gonorrhoeae* infection is recommended for all sexually active women aged <25 years and for older women at increased risk for infection (e.g., those aged ≥25 years who have a new sex partner, >1 sex partner, a sex partner with concurrent partners, or a sex partner who has an STI) (3)
- Annual screening is also recommended for all MSM, with more frequent screening (every 3 to 6 months) for MSM at higher risk (multiple or anonymous partners, substance use, or recent STI) (3).
- STI counseling and condom use
- In children and adolescents, suspect sexual abuse.

MEDICATION

- Dual therapy for gonococcal infection with ceftriaxone and azithromycin is no longer recommended.
- Fluoroquinolones not considered as treatment option
- Clinicians who diagnose *N. gonorrhoeae* infection with suspected cephalosporin treatment failure should perform culture and AST of relevant clinical specimens, and report the case to CDC through state and local public health authorities within 24 hours.

First Line

- Uncomplicated urogenital, anorectal, and pharyngeal gonorrheal infection
  - Ceftriaxone 500 mg IM in a single dose; for persons weighing ≥150 kg (300 lbs), use 1 gram IM in a single dose.
    - If IM ceftriaxone is not available, cefixime 800 mg PO once is an alternative. Cefixime has limited treatment efficacy for pharyngeal gonorrhea.
  - If chlamydial infection has not been excluded, also give doxycycline 100 mg PO twice a day for 7 days.
  - Alternative (e.g., severe cephalosporin allergy): gentamicin 240 mg IM once *plus* azithromycin 2 g PO once
  - Conjunctivitis: ceftriaxone, 1 g IM single dose; consider saline solution lavage of infected eye.
- Meningitis and endocarditis: ceftriaxone 1 to 2 g IV every 12 to 24 hours 10 to 14 days for meningitis; 4 weeks for endocarditis
- Contraindications: Doxycycline is contraindicated in pregnancy and young children.

Pediatric Considerations

- Children >45 kg: same dosing as adults
- Children <45 kg: uncomplicated urethral, cervical, rectal, or pharyngeal gonococcal infections
  - Ceftriaxone 25 to 50 mg/kg IV or IM in a single dose, not to exceed 125 mg IM
  - Disseminated infections: ceftriaxone 50 mg/kg IV or IM daily (max dose 1 g) in single dose; bacteremia or arthritis: 7 days; meningitis: 10 to 14 days; endocarditis: 4 weeks
- Ophthalmic neonatorum prophylaxis: single application of erythromycin 0.5% ophthalmic ointment to each eye immediately after delivery
- Neonatal conjunctivitis: ceftriaxone 25 to 50 mg/kg IV or IM in a single dose (not to exceed 125 mg)
- *Conjunctival exudates should be cultured for definitive diagnosis.*
- Asymptomatic infants born to mothers with untreated gonorrhea: ceftriaxone 25 to 50 mg/kg IV or IM, not to exceed 125 mg in a single dose

Pregnancy Considerations

- Pregnant women should be treated with the same treatments as listed above. For uncomplicated urogenital, anorectal, and pharyngeal gonorrheal infection, if chlamydial infection has not been excluded add azithromycin 1 g single dose PO or add alternative of amoxicillin 500 mg PO 3 times daily for 7 days.
- An alternative is treatment with spectinomycin. If spectinomycin or other regimens are not possible, consultation with an infectious disease specialist is recommended.

Second Line

See CDC STD treatment guidelines: https://www.cdc.gov/std/treatment-guidelines/default.htm

ISSUES FOR REFERRAL

Infectious disease specialist should be consulted for the following conditions.

- Suspected cephalosporin treatment failure
- Gonococcal conjunctivitis in adults
- Cephalosporin allergy in pregnancy
- Disseminated gonococcal infection

ADDITIONAL THERAPIES

Where permissible by state law, gonorrhea EPT may be given with ceftriaxone 500 mg IM in a single dose or a single 800 mg oral dose of cefixime.

ADMISSION, INPATIENT, AND NURSING CONSIDERATIONS

- Hematogenously disseminated infection
- Pneumonia or eye infection in infants

ONGOING CARE

FOLLOW-UP RECOMMENDATIONS

Testing for reinfection 3 months after initial treatment

Patient Monitoring

- Advise patients and sex partners to abstain for 7 days after single-dose treatment.
- Retest all pregnant women 4 weeks after treatment and again in 3rd trimester
- CDC: Screen all MSM annually at sites of contact (urethra, rectum, pharynx), regardless of condom use. Increase screening to every 3 to 6 months if at increased risk.

PATIENT EDUCATION

- Counseling concerning risk reduction, condom use, future fertility, and full STI testing
- Encourage patient to notify partners (from past 60 days); consider EPT.
- Recommend that patient to abstain from sex until 7 days after patient and all partners have been treated.
- Recommend retesting 3 months after treatment given high prevalence of reinfection.

PROGNOSIS

Complete cure with return to normal function with adequate and timely treatment

COMPLICATIONS

Pelvic inflammatory disease, infertility, ectopic pregnancy, urethral stricture, corneal scarring, destruction of joint articular surfaces, cardiac valvular damage

Pediatric Considerations

Vertical transmission is a significant risk among patients with gonococcal infection at the time of delivery.

REFERENCES

1. World Health Organization. Global progress report on HIV, viral hepatitis and sexually transmitted infections, 2021. https://www.who.int/publications/i/item/9789240027077. Accessed on August 28, 2025.
2. Davidson KW, Barry MJ, Mangione CM, et al; for US Preventive Services Task Force. Screening for chlamydia and gonorrhea: US Preventive Services Task Force recommendation statement. *JAMA*. 2021;326(10):949–956. doi:10.1001/jama.2021.14081.
3. Workowski KA, Bachmann LH, Chan PA, et al. Sexually Transmitted Infections Treatment Guidelines, 2021. *MMWR Recomm Rep*. 2021;70(4):1–187. doi:10.15585/mmwr.rr7004a1.

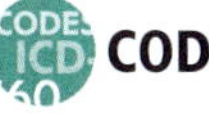

SEE ALSO

Chlamydia Infection (Sexually Transmitted); HIV/AIDS; Pelvic Inflammatory Disease; Syphilis

CODES

ICD10

- A54.9 Gonococcal infection, unspecified
- A54.03 Gonococcal cervicitis, unspecified
- A54.31 Gonococcal conjunctivitis

CLINICAL PEARLS

- Gonococcal antibiotic resistance is a significant clinical problem.
- Screen patients with gonorrhea for chlamydia, syphilis, HIV, and hepatitis.
- Expedited partner treatment should be offered where feasible

GOUT

Sangili Chandran, MD • Janki Majithia, DO • Rakan Al-Adwan, MD

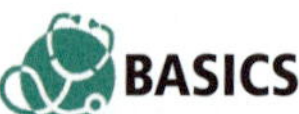

BASICS

DESCRIPTION

- An inflammatory arthritis caused by the accumulation of uric acid crystals in the joints. It often presents as sudden, severe pain, swelling, redness, and warmth in a joint.
- Characterized by deposition of monosodium urate (MSU) crystals in joints and soft tissues, resulting in arthritis, soft tissue masses called tophi, urate nephropathy, and uric acid nephrolithiasis
- The long limb, foot, ankle, and knee are preferentially involved, with the 1st metatarsophalangeal joint (podagra) characteristically affected.
- Flares are usually monoarticular. Polyarticular flares can be associated with pronounced systemic symptoms, including fever, chills, and delirium.
- Gout is related to a hyperuricemia (serum uric acid level >6.8 mg/dL).

EPIDEMIOLOGY

Prevalence

- Gout affects about 1–4% of the global population, with higher rates in developed countries due to dietary and lifestyle factor.
- Gout has a higher incidence in males (6%) than females (2%).

ETIOLOGY AND PATHOPHYSIOLOGY

Four pathophysiological stages:

- Development of hyperuricemia (from uric acid overproduction and/or renal underexcretion)
- Deposition of MSU crystals in joints and soft tissues (changes in uric acid solubility is caused by low temperature, trauma, or acidosis)
- MSU crystals are phagocytosed by synovial macrophages and monocytes resulting in an inflammatory response. The inflammatory response will present clinically as intense pain, swelling, erythema, and warmth.

Genetics

Consider *HLA-B*5801* mutation genotyping for people in Asian origin.

RISK FACTORS

- Age >40 years
- Excessive purine consumption from diet (alcohol [especially beer], red meat, seafood, sugar-sweetened beverages)
- Diabetes mellitus, metabolic syndrome, obesity
- Congestive heart failure, chronic kidney disease (CKD), dyslipidemia, hypertension
- Smoking
- Urate-elevating medications: thiazide diuretics, loop diuretics (less of a risk vs. thiazides), niacin, aspirin
- High ambient and humid temperatures
- Transplant-associated gout can happen in immunosuppressed solid organ transplant recipients on low-dose prednisolone and calcineurin inhibitors (cyclosporine and tacrolimus) as these medications increase uric acid (1).
- Hyperuricemia from rapid cell turnover/tumor lysis syndrome (e.g., hemolysis, chemotherapy)

GENERAL PREVENTION

- Diet modification: Avoid purine-rich foods like red meat and shellfish. Reduce alcohol consumption (beer and liquor).
- Maintain fluid intake and avoid dehydration.

COMMONLY ASSOCIATED CONDITIONS

- Nontraumatic joint disorders
- Renal disease

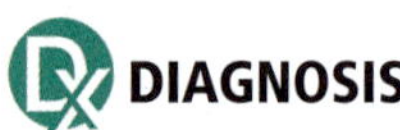

DIAGNOSIS

HISTORY

- Typical first presentation of gout:
  - Intensely painful acute inflammatory arthritis, usually a gout flare, affecting a lower limb joint, which can be self-limited over a period of 7 to 14 days if goes untreated
  - Lower limb and monoarticular arthritis are common early in course of disease—gout flares can occur in the joints or periarticular tissues (e.g., bursae, tendons, and entheses), whereas upper extremity and polyarticular presentations are usually seen in chronic cases.
  - Joint may be swollen, warm, erythematous and exquisitely tender to touch. The pain can be described as stabbing, gnawing, burning, or throbbing.
  - There is substantial limitation in using the affected areas, difficulty walking, and fear of even minimal physical contact.
  - Often awakes patients from sleep due to an intolerance to contact with clothing or bedsheets
  - There is a rapid onset of intense pain, often progressing rapidly over 12 to 24 hours.
  - Acute attacks are usually precipitated by infection, injury, dehydration, or excess alcohol or purine intake.
  - Fever can be present.
  - Subcutaneous or intraosseous nodules, referred to as tophi, can be seen after many recurrent attacks.
- Chronic manifestations of gout:
  - Subcutaneous tophi located in joints, ears, olecranon bursae, finger pads, tendon
  - Tophi are firm and hard, vary in size, can become acutely inflamed, but usually not tender.
  - Can ulcerate with thick/white discharge and superimposed infections

PHYSICAL EXAM

- Examine joint(s) for tenderness, swelling, and range of motion (ROM).
- Tophi can be found in the affected joints, the helix of the ear, over the olecranon process, or on the Achilles tendon.

DIFFERENTIAL DIAGNOSIS

Septic arthritis, calcium pyrophosphate deposition disease (formerly "pseudogout"), hydroxyapatite deposition disease, cellulitis, osteoarthritis, rheumatoid or psoriatic arthritis

DIAGNOSTIC TESTS & INTERPRETATION

- Diagnostic compound score for patients presenting with monarthritis in primary care settings (Janssens criteria) (2):
  - Male sex (2 points)
  - Previous patient-reported arthritis attack (2 points)
  - Onset within 1 day (0.5 point)
  - Joint redness (1 point)
  - 1st metatarsophalangeal joint involvement (2.5 points)
  - Hypertension or cardiovascular disease (1.5 points)
  - Serum uric acid >5.88 (3.5 points)
- Score interpretations:
  - <4 points (unlikely gout)
  - 4 to 8 points (possible gout)
  - >8 points (likely gout)
- Initial acute gout episode
  - Uric acid (may be normal or low), CBC (WBC maybe elevated), ESR/CRP, and CMP (creatinine may be elevated)
  - Synovial fluid analysis: urate crystals (negatively birefringent under polarizing microscopy), cell count (WBC usually 2,000 to 5,000 cells/mm^3); gram stain and culture to rule out infection
  - 24-hour urine to screen for uric acid overproduction (>800 mg/24 hr) in those with onset before the age of 25 years or with a history of urolithiasis

Follow-Up Tests & Special Considerations

- Plain x-rays are normal early in disease but can reveal periarticular erosions with periosteum overgrowth in chronic gout.
- Ultrasonography can show a double contour sign (reflecting monosodium urate crystal deposition on the surface of hyaline articular cartilage), intra-articular or intrabursal tophi, and a snowstorm appearance.
- Dual-energy CT (DECT) imaging can show urate deposition at articular or periarticular sites.

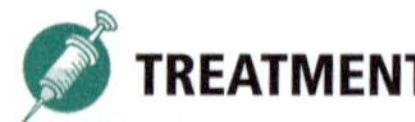

TREATMENT

GENERAL MEASURES

Supportive care—ice packs, rest, mobility assistance, and adequate nutrition and hydration

MEDICATION

First Line

- Treatment should be initiated within 12 to 24 hours of acute gout attack and continued for 1 to 2 days after attack has subsided (1).
  - Urate-lowering therapy should not be interrupted during an acute gout attack.
  - Mild/moderate gout severity (≤6 of 10 on visual analog pain scale, particularly for an attack involving only one or a few small joints or one to two large joints)
  - NSAIDs:
    - Naproxen: 500 mg BID
    - Meloxicam: 7.5 to 15 mg/day
    - Indomethacin: 50 to 150 mg/day (generally less well tolerated than others)
    - Diclofenac: 75 mg BID
    - Ibuprofen: 800 mg every 8 hours

- Oral/intra-articular/intramuscular/intravenous corticosteroids
  - Corticosteroids are useful in patients with acute gout flare who cannot tolerate NSAIDs or have contraindications to NSAIDs and colchicine such as CKD.
  - When monotherapy is insufficient for acute flares, a combination of NSAIDs with either intra-articular corticosteroid, oral steroid, or colchicine may be used.
    - Oral corticosteroids—medium dose (15 to 20 mg/day) to high dose (30 to 35 mg/day) for 5 days
- Intra-articular/intramuscular/intravenous preparation—triamcinolone acetonide, dexamethasone, methylprednisolone
- Colchicine: used for gout attacks where the onset was <36 hours prior to treatment initiation
  - Begin a loading dose of 1.0 to 1.2 mg followed by 0.5 to 0.6 mg 1 hour later, after 12 hours, resume 0.5 to 0.6 mg every 8 hours with no more than 6 mg per course and at least 3 days between courses.
- Severe gout (≥7 of 10 pain scale, involving ≥4 joints with arthritis involving >1 region, or involving three separate large joints)
  - Initial combination therapy is an option and includes the use of full doses of the following:
    - Colchicine and NSAIDs
    - PO corticosteroids and colchicine
    - Intra-articular steroids

- Chronic treatment includes using urate-lowering therapies (3) for a serum uric acid <6 mg/dL (may need <5 mg/dL to improve symptoms). Titrate medication to a goal uric acid level of <6 g/dL.
  - Urate-lowering agents can be prescribed during an acute attack provided that effective anti-inflammatory prophylaxis has been initiated first such as:
    - Low-dose NSAIDs: naproxen 250 mg PO BID
    - Low-dose colchicine: 0.5 to 0.6 mg once or twice daily
    - If colchicine and NSAIDs, contraindicated, or ineffective:
      - Low-dose prednisone at ≤10 mg/day
    - Treatment duration of at least 6 months *or* 3 months after achieving serum urate target.
  - Urate-lowering agents:
    - Allopurinol: xanthine oxidase inhibitor—does not reduce number of acute attacks
      - Start no higher than 100 mg/day (50 mg/day in stage 4 or 5 CKD).
      - Titrate dose upward q2–5wk to maximum dose.
      - Monitor serum uric acid level and renal function 3 months in the 1st year and annually thereafter.
      - Monitor for allopurinol hypersensitivity syndrome (AHS), pruritus, rash, elevated hepatic transaminases, and eosinophilia. *HLA-B*5801* allele for AHS should be performed in those of Korean, Chinese, or Thai.
    - Febuxostat: selective xanthine oxidase inhibitor
      - Start 40 mg/day; titrate to 80 mg/day.
    - Probenecid: uricosuric agent
      - Alternative if xanthine oxidase inhibitor is contraindicated
      - May be used in addition to allopurinol or febuxostat if serum urate target not achieved
      - Increased risk of urolithiasis with this agent
      - Not recommended if CrCl is <50 or if there is history of urolithiasis
      - Start 250 mg BID; titrate to 2,000 mg/day.

Second Line

- If not responding to initial pharmacologic monotherapy, add a second agent.
- IL-1 inhibitors: for patients who have intolerable side effects or have contraindications to first-line anti-inflammatory therapy
  - Anakinra 100 mg SQ daily for 5 days
  - Canakinumab 150 mg SQ × 1 dose (Monitor for adverse events, including serious infections.)

ADDITIONAL THERAPIES

- Losartan possesses uricosuric properties; consider for hypertensive patients.
- Fenofibrate possesses uricosuric properties and may be useful with lipid disorders.

SURGERY/OTHER PROCEDURES

Large tophi may need to be surgically removed.

COMPLEMENTARY & ALTERNATIVE MEDICINE

Vitamin C (>500 mg QD) has been shown to reduce serum uric acid levels (1)[C].

ONGOING CARE

FOLLOW-UP RECOMMENDATIONS

Patient Monitoring

- Serum uric acid measurements q2–5wk while titrating urate-lowering treatment to goal
- Regularly monitor CBC, renal function, liver function test, and urinalysis.

DIET

- Avoid:
  - Organ meats high in purine content (sweetbreads, liver, kidney)
  - High-fructose corn syrup
- Limit:
  - Beef, lamb, pork, and seafood with high purine content
  - Servings of sugar, sweetened beverages, and desserts
  - Table salt
  - Alcohol (particularly beer)
- Encourage:
  - Coffee intake of >4 cups per day
  - Foods rich in dietary fiber, folate, vitamin C
  - Dairy products (4)
  - Cherry consumption may be of benefit in gout prophylaxis (5)[C]
  - Weight loss if overweight

PATIENT EDUCATION

- Explain that there may be increased flare-ups with the initiation of urate-lowering therapy.
- Advise patient symptoms of nephrolithiasis and importance of hydration.

PROGNOSIS

Usually successfully managed with treatment and lifestyle modifications

COMPLICATIONS

- Inflammatory arthritis and joint destruction
- Uric acid nephropathy and renal stones

REFERENCES

1. Abhishek A, Roddy E, Doherty M. Gout—a guide for the general and acute physicians. *Clin Med (Lond)*. 2017;17(1):54–59.
2. Neogi T, Jansen TLTA, Dalbeth N, et al. 2015 Gout classification criteria: an American College of Rheumatology/European League Against Rheumatism collaborative initiative. *Arthritis Rheumatol*. 2015;67(10):2557–2568.
3. Zhang W, Doherty M, Bardin T, et al. EULAR Standing Committee for International Clinical Studies Including Therapeutics. EULAR evidence based recommendations for gout. Part II: Management. Report of a task force of the EULAR Standing Committee for International Clinical Studies Including Therapeutics (ESCISIT). *Ann Rheum Dis*. 2006;65(10):1312–1324. doi:10.1136/ard.2006.055269.
4. da Silva MT, Diniz MFHS, Coelho CG, et al. Intake of selected foods and beverages and serum uric acid levels in adults: ELSA-Brasil (2008–2010). *Public Health Nutr*. 2020;23(3):506–514.
5. Lamb KL, Lynn A, Russell J, et al. Effect of tart cherry juice on risk of gout attacks: protocol for a randomised controlled trial. *BMJ Open*. 2020;10(3):e035108.

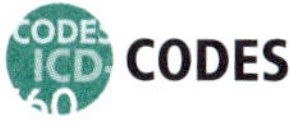

CODES

ICD10

- M10.269 Drug-induced gout, unspecified knee
- M10.161 Lead-induced gout, right knee
- M10.221 Drug-induced gout, right elbow

CLINICAL PEARLS

- Acute gouty arthritis can affect ≥1 joint; the 1st metatarsophalangeal joint is most commonly involved at presentation (podagra).
- MSU crystals found in synovial fluid aspirate are pathognomonic for gout.
- Pharmacologic treatment should begin within 24 hours of acute gout flare. NSAIDs and/or corticosteroids are effective for mild/moderate attacks.
- Asymptomatic hyperuricemia does not require treatment.

G

GRANULOMA ANNULARE

Niloufar Akhavan Tabib, DO • Laura J. Schoerning, DO

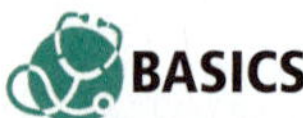

BASICS

DESCRIPTION

Granuloma annulare (GA) is a benign skin condition characterized by groups of skin-colored to erythematous papules that are usually in an annular (ring-like) pattern and typically located on the dorsal aspects of the hands and feet. There are five types of GA: localized, generalized, subcutaneous (SC), patch, and perforating.

EPIDEMIOLOGY

Incidence

- GA is a relatively common, noninfectious granulomatous disease. Incidence is reported to be 0.04% per year within the United States (1).
- Although most lesions resolve spontaneously within 2 years, some persist for ≥10 years.
- Predominant sex: female > male (3:1) (1)
- Onset of symptoms occurs at <30 years old in 2/3 of all patients. Typical ages for onset of each subtype are:
  - Localized: <30-years-old
  - Generalized: bimodal: <10-years-old, 30 to 60-years-old
  - SC: 2 to 14-years-old
  - Patch: >30-years-old
  - Perforating: children and young adults
- Distribution of subtypes:
  - Localized: 75%
  - Generalized: 10–15%
  - SC: <5%
  - Patch type: <5%
  - Perforating: <5%

Prevalence

Prevalence is reported to be highest in the 5th decade of life (1).

ETIOLOGY AND PATHOPHYSIOLOGY

The etiology of GA remains unknown; however, recent studies have helped to further elucidate its underlying cause. It is hypothesized to be related to upregulation of T-helper (Th) 1 and Th2 pathways in GA lesions. Increased cytokine expression was subsequently noted to include tumor necrosis factor-α (TNF-α), interleukin (IL)-1β, IL-4, interferon (IFN)-γ, IL-12/23p4, and IL-31. Janus kinase-signal transducer and activator of transcription (JAK-STAT) pathways were also found to be activated in GA. Response by "M1" and "M2" macrophages was described, which can be related to histopathologic findings of collagen degradation followed by tissue remodeling and mucin deposition, respectively.

Genetics

There is some evidence for a genetic predisposition. Two studies reported an increased frequency of HLA-Bw35 in patients with generalized GA. Of note, HLA-Bw35 has also been associated with thyroid disease.

RISK FACTORS

No definite risk factors have been identified. There are reported associations between GA and diabetes mellitus (DM), autoimmune thyroid disease, dyslipidemia, human immunodeficiency virus, Epstein-Barr virus, herpes simplex virus, tuberculosis, hepatitis B and C, and other autoimmune disorders among others. There have also been associations with certain drug exposures, trauma, sun exposure, and malignancies (most commonly lymphoma).

GENERAL PREVENTION

There are no known preventive measures for GA.

COMMONLY ASSOCIATED CONDITIONS

- DM: The association between GA and DM remains controversial but there is increasing evidence of an association. Early studies from the 1980s showed a possible link and a recent large, retrospective cohort study (51,169 patients with GA) showed that 21% of patients had both GA and DM while 13.3% of matched controls had DM (1).
- Autoimmune thyroid disease: Multiple case reports have linked thyroid disease with both generalized and localized GA. In one case-control study, 24 women with localized GA were compared to 100 age-matched women with non-GA dermatologic disease. A statistically significant increase in the incidence of autoimmune thyroid disease among those with localized GA as compared with those with other non-GA cutaneous disease was identified (12% vs. 1%, $p = .022$) (2),(3).
- Malignancy: There is no definitive relationship between GA and malignancy. A review of the literature found 14 case reports and 2 correlation studies in which patients who had ≥1 malignancies also had GA. In a majority of these cases, the malignancies were hematologic, primarily lymphoma (2),(3).
- Dyslipidemia: Dyslipidemia may be associated with GA. A single case-control study ($n = 140$) demonstrated a statistically significant increase in hyperlipidemia among patients with GA compared to controls (79.3% vs. 51.9%, $p = <.001$). Further studies, including the large, retrospective cohort study noted above, have demonstrated significant associations with GA and hyperlipidemia.
- Infectious: Among patients with GA, those who also have HIV appear more likely to have the generalized subtype. In one study of 34 patients with GA and HIV, 20 (59%) had generalized GA (2). Additional viral triggers have been suggested to include SARS-CoV-2, Epstein Barr virus, and varicella zoster virus. There has been recent data showing evidence of potential bacterial triggers to include *Chlamydiales* spp. and *Borrelia* spp. (1).
- Iatrogenically-induced: Several drugs have been implicated in triggering GA: acetazolamide, anti-TNF-α agents, amlodipine, allopurinol, botulinum toxin, desensitization injections, immune checkpoint inhibitors, immunizations, levetiracetam, paroxetine, topiramate, and phototherapy (1).
- Note: Conclusions regarding associations between GA and various diseases, including those listed above, are limited by both design and power. Consequently, in the absence of new research, definitive associations between GA and other diseases cannot be made.

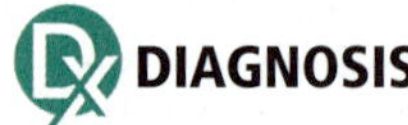

DIAGNOSIS

HISTORY

Cutaneous lesions of GA are generally asymptomatic. Lesions often persist for months or years, especially in patients who have generalized GA. In most cases, regardless of subtype, GA resolves spontaneously but may thereafter recur without obvious trigger.

PHYSICAL EXAM

- Localized: asymptomatic, flesh-colored or erythematous annular, or arciform plaque with a moderately firm, rope-like border and central clearing, ranging from 5 mm to 5 cm in diameter. Small 1- to 2-mm papules may be noted peripheral to the primary lesion. The most common locations are the dorsal aspects of the distal upper and lower extremities; involvement of palms is rare. It is common to have multiple lesions at the time of presentation.
- Generalized: Lesions have the same morphology as localized GA lesions, but tend to be larger, greater in number (usually >10), persist for a longer period of time, and are more widespread.
- SC: firm, nontender nodules that tend to grow rapidly; usually solitary but may occur in groups; most common location is scalp and/or anterior aspect of the lower extremities, followed by upper extremities and buttocks.
- Patch: Erythematous macules and patches are distributed symmetrically on the extremities and trunk. The typical annular configuration may or may not be present; often involves proximal extremities
- Perforating: Damaged collagen from dermis is extruded onto skin surface. Papules may be up to 4 mm in diameter and display yellowish umbilication, crusting, or scale. Lesions are often widely distributed on the body and cause scaring.

DIFFERENTIAL DIAGNOSIS

- Localized: tinea corporis, annular lichen planus, nummular eczema, pityriasis rosea, erythema migrans, leprosy, annular psoriasis
- Generalized: sarcoidosis, lichen planus, cutaneous metastases, mycosis fungoides (cutaneous T-cell lymphoma), pityriasis rosea, secondary syphilis
- Patch type: erythema migrans
- SC: rheumatoid nodules, SC sarcoidosis
- Perforating: molluscum contagiosum, sarcoidosis, insect bites, reactive perforating dermatoses

DIAGNOSTIC TESTS & INTERPRETATION

Initial Tests (lab, imaging)

- Diagnosis is typically established by history and physical examination; laboratory investigations are rarely needed. Microscopic evaluation of skin cells using potassium hydroxide (KOH) preparation may be useful to exclude a fungal process.
- Consider laboratory testing to evaluate comorbid dyslipidemia, DM, thyroid disease, HIV, hepatitis B/C, and malignancy as clinically indicated.

Diagnostic Procedures/Other

Punch biopsy and histologic evaluation may aid in confirming the diagnosis and identifying the subtype. Immunohistochemical streptavidin-biotin–horseradish peroxidase (HRP) analysis for CD68/KP-1 (a marker for histiocytic differentiation) may also aid in the diagnosis. Ultrasound evaluation has been shown to assist in diagnosis of SC GA, which may be beneficial in the pediatric population (1).

Test Interpretation

Dermal infiltrate demonstrating foci of degenerative collagen associated with palisading granulomas around an anuclear dermis with mucin deposition. Mucin deposition is a strong indicator of a GA diagnosis. Histologic variants include interstitial (histiocytic infiltrate between collagen fibers), classic (palisading dermal granulomas), and epithelioid (tuberculoid and sarcoidal granulomas).

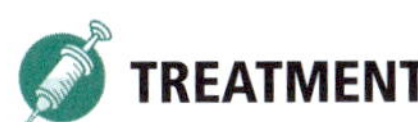

TREATMENT

GENERAL MEASURES

GA is a self-limited condition that is likely to regress spontaneously. The clinician's primary role after making the diagnosis is to educate the patient about the natural history of GA and to consider screening for conditions that may be associated with this disease. No specific treatment has been satisfactorily studied in reliable randomized controlled trials with most recommendations based upon case reports, case series, and retrospective reviews.

MEDICATION

- The trauma induced by biopsy alone can cause involution of lesions through an unknown mechanism.
- Given the self-limited nature of the disease, it is incumbent on providers to assess the risk/benefit ratio of treatment. Reassurance is often all that is required for localized, asymptomatic disease.
- The following therapies have been tried with variable success. Duration of therapy is often undefined and is based on clinical response.

First Line

Topical and intralesional corticosteroids

- High-potency topical (class I or II), with or without occlusion (1)[C],(3)[C]
- Intralesional triamcinolone: concentration of 2.5 to 5.0 mg/mL (3)[C]; technique: Insert the needle into the dermis at the elevated border and slowly inject while withdrawing the needle, with enough volume to cause the lesion to begin to blanch. Take care to avoid allowing the tip of the needle to push through to inserting the needle through the lesion.

Second Line

- Doxycycline: 100 mg/day for 8 to 10 weeks (1)[C],(3)[C]
- Pimecrolimus cream: 1% BID (3)[C]
- Tacrolimus ointment: 0.1% BID (3)[C]
- Chloroquine: 250 mg/day (1)[C],(3)[C]
- Hydroxychloroquine: 9 mg/kg/day for 2 months, 6 mg/kg/day for month 3, 2 mg/kg/day for month 4 (3)[C]
- Isotretinoin: 0.50 to 0.75 mg/kg/day (3)[C]
- Rifampin 600 mg, ofloxacin 400 mg, with minocycline 100 mg once daily (1)[C],(3)[C]
- Dapsone: 100 mg/day for mean duration of 9.8 months (1)[C],(3)[C]
- Cyclosporine: 3 to 4 mg/kg/day (3)[C]
- Methotrexate: 10 mg IM weekly for 11 months (1)[C]
- Niacinamide: 500 mg TID (3)[C]
- Fumaric acid esters: variable dosing schemes (3)[C]
- Interferon-γ 1b: intralesional injection, 2.5×10^5 IU/lesion for 7 consecutive days followed by 3 times per week for 2 weeks (3)[C]
- TNF-α inhibitors, such as infliximab 5 mg/kg IV weeks 0, 2, and 6, then variable or adalimumab 80 mg SC at week 0, and then 40 SC at week 1 and every other week, or etanercept 50 mg twice weekly (3)[C]
- Photodynamic therapy (1)[C]
- Pentoxifylline 400 mg TID (1)[C]

ADDITIONAL THERAPIES

- Cryotherapy (one 10- to 60-second freeze thaw cycle) (3)[C]
- Fractional thermolysis (e.g., YAG fractionated laser) (3)[C]
- 585- to 595-nm pulsed dye laser (3)[C]
- Narrowband ultraviolet B (NBUVB)
- Psoralen ultraviolet A (PUVA)
- Surgical excision (for SC GA) (2)[C]
- Apremilast: phosphodiesterase-4 inhibitor (1)[C]
- Tofacitinib: JAK inhibitor (1)[C]
- Control of comorbidities, such as DM and hyperlipidemia (1)[C]

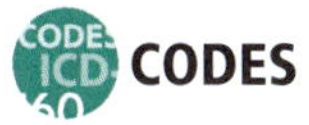

ONGOING CARE

FOLLOW-UP RECOMMENDATIONS

Routine follow-up is not required unless treatment is initiated. In such situations, follow-up is recommended to monitor for possible adverse effects of treatment. Referral to a dermatologist is prudent for patients who have generalized GA, cosmetic concerns, and for patients whose lesions persist despite conservative therapy.

PATIENT EDUCATION

Patients should be educated that GA is a benign, self-limited condition that may persist for months to years, spontaneously resolve, and spontaneously recur. Additionally, patients may benefit from knowing that GA is not thought to be of an infectious etiology and is not transmissible to others.

PROGNOSIS

>50% of cases resolve spontaneously within 2 months to 2 years after onset, although recurrence, typically at the original site, is common (>40%). Patients aged <39 years tend to have a shorter duration of illness.

COMPLICATIONS

Complications of treatment are much more likely than complications from GA.

REFERENCES

1. Joshi TP, Duvic M. Granuloma annulare: an updated review of epidemiology, pathogenesis, and treatment options. *Am J Clin Dermatol*. 2022;23(1):37–50. doi:10.1007/s40257-021-00636-1.
2. Piette EW, Rosenbach M. Granuloma annulare: pathogenesis, disease associations and triggers, and therapeutic options. *J Am Acad Dermatol*. 2016;75(3):467–479.
3. Keimig EL. Granuloma annulare. *Dermatol Clin*. 2015;33(3):315–329.

CODES

ICD10

L92.0 Granuloma annulare

CLINICAL PEARLS

- GA is benign, self-limited condition. Consider risk-to-benefit ratio when partnering with patients to determine treatment.
- When initiating therapy for localized GA, start with high-dose topical corticosteroids or intralesional corticosteroids followed by cryotherapy or other listed topical therapies. For widespread disease, consider initiating treatment with antimalarials or phototherapy.
- Consider GA in the differential diagnosis of lesions that appear to be tinea, especially when these lesions lack scale and are KOH negative.
- Consider fasting lipid panel, fasting blood glucose or HbA1C, TSH, free T4, thyroid antibodies, hepatitis B and C panel, HIV screening test, and age-appropriate cancer screening, especially in those with generalized or atypical presentations of GA.

G

GRANULOMA, PYOGENIC

Michelle Moran McDonough, MD

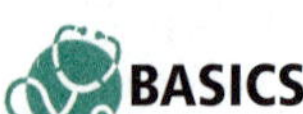

BASICS

DESCRIPTION
- Pyogenic granulomas (PGs) are benign vascular proliferations that appear most commonly on the skin and mucous membranes as rapidly growing erythematous to violaceous nodules that develop into pedunculated masses with an erosive surface that is friable and tends to bleed profusely due to the vascular nature of the lesion.
- Most common sites are the head, neck, lips, oral cavity, trunk, and extremities (1).
- Less commonly presents as a sessile lesion
- Rarely regress completely without intervention (1)
- Synonyms: lobular capillary hemangioma, granuloma telangiectaticum, granuloma gravidarum

EPIDEMIOLOGY
- The peak incidence of PG occurs in children and young adults (1).
- Commonly seen in early pregnancy
- Male predominance in childhood through adolescence and female predominance during reproductive years before age 50 years

Incidence
Unknown

Prevalence
- Up to 1 in 25,000 adults are diagnosed with an intraoral PG in their lifetime (1).
- Cutaneous PGs account for 0.5% of childhood skin nodules (1).

ETIOLOGY AND PATHOPHYSIOLOGY
- Definitive cause remains under investigation.
- Initially thought to be associated with capillary proliferation resulting from aberrant healing response to minor trauma
- More recent studies are showing involvement in oncogenic mutations of the MAPK pathway and showing no left to right laterality bias challenging the trauma-induced hypothesis.
- Some medications are associated with higher risk of development such as retinoids, progesterone and estrogen, protease inhibitors, and antineoplastics such as epidermal growth factor receptor inhibitors.
- Likely also related to hormonal changes in pregnancy by inducing swelling of endothelial cells, releasing vasoactive mediators from damaged mast cells, and increasing vascular permeability
- Not considered a hemangioma or neoplasm; no true granulomatous histology present. Instead, PGs manifest as plump endothelial cells with significant mitotic activity.

RISK FACTORS
- Pregnancy
- Possibly trauma
- Inflammatory systemic diseases
- Medications such as retinoids, hormone therapy containing progesterone or estrogen, protease inhibitors, and neoplastics such as epidermal growth factor receptor inhibitors

GENERAL PREVENTION
Good oral hygiene may be helpful. Avoid medications implicated in increased risk where possible.

COMMONLY ASSOCIATED CONDITIONS
- Pregnancy—common
- Cancer with antineoplastic treatment—common
- Inflammatory dermatoses or inflammatory systemic diseases—rare

DIAGNOSIS

HISTORY
- Solitary lesion that develops rapidly from days to weeks possibly after minor trauma; develops an erosive surface and bleeds easily
- Grows early in pregnancy and partially regresses postpartum

PHYSICAL EXAM
- Most commonly located on the head, neck, mouth, lips, and upper extremities, especially in children
- Among oral lesions, gingiva is the most common location.
- Usually a bright red, friable papule; can also be purple, yellow, or brown
- Moist and sometimes scaly-appearing surface with serosanguineous crusting and sharp demarcation
- Usually <1 cm but ranges from a few millimeters to 2 to 3 cm in diameter
- Giant lesions may occur on areas such as the foot (rare).
- Soft; pedunculated or sessile
- Solitary red papule, grows rapidly, forming a stalk, may bleed, and ulcerate
- Dermoscopy exam: red structureless, homogenous area surrounded by a white collarette intersected by white lines

DIFFERENTIAL DIAGNOSIS
- Benign lesions
  - Cherry/infantile hemangioma
  - Fibrous papule
  - Bacillary angiomatosis due to *Bartonella*
  - Carbuncle or furuncle
- Malignant lesions
  - Basal cell carcinoma
  - Squamous cell carcinoma
  - Amelanotic melanoma
  - Kaposi sarcoma
  - Cutaneous metastases

DIAGNOSTIC TESTS & INTERPRETATION

Initial Tests (lab, imaging)
No labs are necessary for the diagnosis.

Diagnostic Procedures/Other
Excisional/shave biopsy with pathology interpretation

Test Interpretation
Microscopic examination reveals the following:
- Small, endothelial-lined vascular spaces
- Loose/dense connective tissue stroma
- Acute and chronic inflammatory cells
- No true granuloma formation
- Abundant mitotic activity
- Resembles granulation tissue in an edematous matrix, showing immature capillaries with interspersed tissue

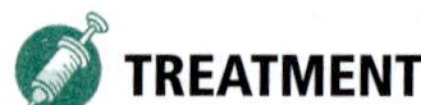

TREATMENT

Full-thickness surgical excision is best to yield material for histopathologic analysis and avoid recurrence (2)[C]. Excision must be adequate to avoid recurrence. Even a small fragment of tissue left behind may lead to recurrence.

GENERAL MEASURES
Consider discontinuing medications implicated with increased risk where possible such as retinoids, protease inhibitors, hormonal therapy with estrogen and/or progesterone, and antineoplastics such as vascular endothelial growth factor receptor inhibitors.

MEDICATION

First Line
- Topical 5% imiquimod once daily for up to 17 weeks (2)[C]
- Silver nitrate
- Topical timolol (especially for lesions on the eyelid) or propranolol applied 1 to 2 times daily with occlusive dressing for up to 2 months (2)[C]
- Topical 1.5% phenol solution may be used for periungual lesions.

ISSUES FOR REFERRAL
May consider referral to ear, nose, and throat (ENT) specialist or dermatologist for surgical excision or laser therapy

ADDITIONAL THERAPIES
- Sclerotherapy with injection of monoethanolamide oleate achieved 100% remission in a small study but was painful upon injection and had postinflammatory hyperpigmentation (3)[C]
- Sclerotherapy with injection of ethanol had 100% resolution in a small study with short-term follow up (3)[C]
- Intralesional injection of triamcinolone 2 mg weekly for 8 weeks has been successful in some case studies (2)[C].

SURGERY/OTHER PROCEDURES
- Surgical excision is the most effective with a 98% resolution rate (3)[C].
- Shave biopsy can be used for pedunculated lesions and is more effective if combined with cautery or silver nitrate leading to a resolution rate of 90% (3)[C].
- Punch biopsy acceptable for small lesions
- Electrosurgery: Electrodesiccation and curettage has a 97% resolution rate (3)[C].
- Cryotherapy with liquid nitrogen requires more sessions and a lower rate of resolution at 67% (3)[C].
- Nd:YAG, pulsed dye, or CO_2 laser can be effective but often require more than one treatment (3)[C].
- Diode laser therapy may be more effective than surgical excision with faster healing times but needs more research (3)[C].

COMPLEMENTARY & ALTERNATIVE MEDICINE
There are several case studies of utilization of sodium chloride directly applied to the lesion with paraffin protecting the surrounding healthy skin and applying an occlusive dressing with reapplication of sodium chloride daily for up to 1 month with mixed results of improvement or resolution, but evidence is lacking.

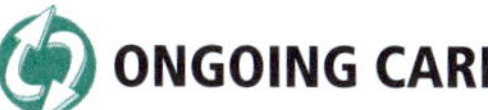

ONGOING CARE

FOLLOW-UP RECOMMENDATIONS
Patients should be counseled to return if receiving treatment and lesion does not resolve or if it recurs.

PATIENT EDUCATION
Patient should avoid trauma to area following excision.

PROGNOSIS
- Some lesions spontaneously resolve on their own (usually within 6 months).
- With treatment, recurrence rates are between 4% and 5% (1).

COMPLICATIONS
- Recurrence: After removal or destruction of solitary lesion, multiple satellite lesions can form around original treatment site.
- Without removal, lesions can continue to bleed as they are friable.

REFERENCES

1. Borden A, Harrington JW. Pyogenic granuloma: an overview of pathogenesis, diagnosis, and management. *Consultant*. 2018;58(6):e181.
2. Plachouri KM, Georgiou S. Therapeutic approaches to pyogenic granuloma: an updated review. *Int J Dermatol*. 2019;58(6):642–648. doi:10.1111/ijd.14268.
3. Kaleeny JD, Janis JE. Pyogenic granuloma diagnosis and management: a practical review. *Plast Reconstr Surg Glob Open*. 2024;12(9):e6160.

ADDITIONAL READING

- Gilmore A, Kelsberg G, Safranek S. Clinical inquiries. What's the best treatment for pyogenic granuloma? *J Fam Pract*. 2010;59(1):40–42.
- Hinen HB, Boccuto L, Trenor CC III, et al. Corrigendum: childhood vascular tumors. *Front Pediatr*. 2020;8:573023. doi:10.3389/fped.2020.573023. Erratum in: *Front Pediatr*. 2021;9:649610.
- Koo MG, Lee SH, Han SE. Pyogenic granuloma: a retrospective analysis of cases treated over a 10-year. *Arch Craniofac Surg*. 2017;18(1):16–20. doi:10.7181/acfs.2017.18.1.16.
- Losa Iglesias ME, Becerro de Bengoa Vallejo R. Topical phenol as a conservative treatment for periungual pyogenic granuloma. *Dermatol Surg*. 2010;36(5):675–678.
- Zaballos P, Llambrich A, Cuéllar F, et al. Dermoscopic findings in pyogenic granuloma. *Br J Dermatol*. 2006;154(6):1108–1111. doi:10.1111/j.1365-2133.2006.07193.x.

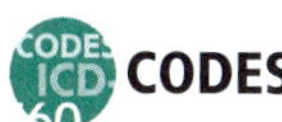

CODES

ICD10
- L98.0 Pyogenic granuloma
- K06.8 Oth disrd of gingiva and edentulous alveolar ridge
- K13.4 Granuloma and granuloma-like lesions of oral mucosa

CLINICAL PEARLS
- Benign, vascular tumor, usually rapidly growing, that involves exposed areas, such as distal extremities and face, as well as in the oral cavity
- Excision must be adequate to avoid recurrence.
- Excisional biopsy is recommended to ensure proper diagnosis and rule out malignancy.
- Excision with primary closure is superior to shave excision with cautery in terms of recurrence risk, but both are effective.

GRAVES DISEASE

Juan Perez, DO

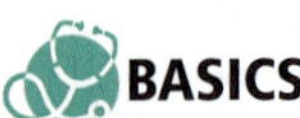

BASICS

DESCRIPTION

Autoimmune disease in which thyroid-stimulating hormone receptor (TSHR) activation by thyrotropin receptor antibodies (TRAb) cause increased thyroid hormone secretion; most common cause of hyperthyroidism; classic findings are thyrotoxicosis, diffuse goiter, ophthalmopathy (orbitopathy), and occasionally localized dermopathy (pretibial myxedema).

EPIDEMIOLOGY

Incidence

- Annual incidence of 20 to 50 cases per 100,000 persons
- Peaks between 30 and 50 years of age
- Hyperthyroidism occurs in 0.2% of pregnancies, of which 95% is due to Graves disease.
- Graves disease accounts for 60–80% of all cases of hyperthyroidism.

ETIOLOGY AND PATHOPHYSIOLOGY

- Excessive production of thyroid-stimulating hormone (TSH) receptor antibodies from B cells primarily within the thyroid, likely due to genetic clonal lack of suppressor T cells
- Binding of these antibodies to TSH receptors in the thyroid activates the receptor, stimulating thyroid hormone synthesis and secretion as well as thyroid growth (leading to goiter).
- Binding to similar antigen in retro-orbital connective tissue causes ocular symptoms.

Genetics

Higher risk with personal or family history of any autoimmune disease, especially Hashimoto thyroiditis

RISK FACTORS

- Female gender (5 to 10 times more than men)
- Postpartum period
- Family history (15% of patients with Graves disease have an affected relative.)
- Medications: iodine, selenium, amiodarone, lithium, highly active antiretroviral therapy (HAART); rarely, immune-modulating medications (e.g., interferon therapy)
- Smoking (higher risk of developing ophthalmopathy)
- Low vitamin D levels
- Bacterial/viral infections

GENERAL PREVENTION

Screening TSH in asymptomatic patients not recommended.

COMMONLY ASSOCIATED CONDITIONS

- Mitral valve prolapse
- Type 1 diabetes mellitus
- Addison disease, hypokalemic periodic paralysis
- Vitiligo, alopecia areata

DIAGNOSIS

HISTORY

- Tachycardia, palpitations
- Tremor, restlessness
- Hyperactivity, anxiety, emotional lability, insomnia, poor concentration
- Sweating, heat intolerance
- Pruritus, skin changes
- Weight loss with increased appetite
- Fatigue, dyspnea (due to muscle weakness)
- Oligomenorrhea/amenorrhea (women), loss of libido, erectile dysfunction (men), gynecomastia
- Loose, frequent stools
- Blurred vision or diplopia, lacrimation, photophobia, gritty sensation in eyes (ocular dryness), retro-orbital discomfort, painful eye movement, loss of color vision or visual acuity
- Worsening of chronic medical conditions (anxiety, bipolar disorder, glucose intolerance, heart failure, or angina)

Geriatric Considerations

Elderly may present with atrial fibrillation, weight loss, or dyspnea.

PHYSICAL EXAM

- Ophthalmologic (present in 50% of cases): Grittiness/discomfort in the eyes, retrobulbar pressure/pain, lid lag/retraction, proptosis, ophthalmoplegia, papilledema, and loss of color vision may signify optic neuropathy.
- Thyroid: enlarged (goiter), nontender, and without nodules; possible bruit (increased blood flow)
- Integumentary: fine hair, warm skin, onycholysis, palmar erythema, brittle nails, clubbing of fingers, possible pretibial myxedema (orange peel appearance), possible hyperpigmented plaques (dermopathy)
- Cardiac: resting tachycardia, hyperdynamic circulation, possible atrial fibrillation
- Extremities: fine tremor, hyperreflexia, proximal myopathy; rarely, soft tissue edema of extremities and clubbing of digits (acropachy)

DIFFERENTIAL DIAGNOSIS

- Hashimoto thyroiditis, toxic multinodular goiter, or toxic adenoma
- Iatrogenic: iodine, medications (amiodarone) induced, or thyroid hormone overreplacement
- Tumors: adenoma, human chorionic gonadotropin (hCG)-producing tumors, struma ovarii, or metastatic thyroid cancer

DIAGNOSTIC TESTS & INTERPRETATION

Initial Tests (lab, imaging)

- TSH is initial test: suppressed (low or undetectable).
- TSH <0.1 mU/L has $>98\%$ sensitivity and $>92\%$ specificity in confirming suspected thyroid disease. Elevated free T_4 with low TSH confirms hyperthyroidism.
- T_3 maybe elevated as well in conjunction with free T_4 or isolated elevation, known as T_3 toxicosis.

Follow-Up Tests & Special Considerations

Thyroid peroxidase (TPO) antibodies present in nearly all Hashimoto thyroiditis patients and in 70–80% of patients with Graves disease. TSHR antibodies (TRAb) are specific to Graves disease. In cases where TRAb are normal, but TPO antibodies are elevated, Hashitoxicosis may be the cause of the hyperthyroidism. If both TRAb and TPO antibodies are absent, then non-autoimmune causes such as nodular thyroid disease are likely.

Pregnancy Considerations

Increase in serum T_4-binding globulin concentration and initial stimulation of TSH by hCG results in a total T_4 and T_3 rise during first half of pregnancy. The TSH level is decreased throughout pregnancy and should be compared to the trimester-specific ranges for pregnancy. Measurement of TRAb is positive in 95% of patients with Graves and should be used if diagnosis is unclear in pregnancy (1)[A].

Diagnostic Procedures/Other

- In cases where thyroid antibodies are negative or where there is nodularity of the thyroid gland to palpation, imaging should be pursued.
- After confirming suppressed TSH and high T_4, perform radioactive iodine uptake (RAIU) and scan. Patients with Graves disease will have diffuse, elevated RAIU (vs. localized/nodular elevated uptake in adenoma and multinodular goiter and decreased uptake in thyroiditis or exogenous thyroid hormone).

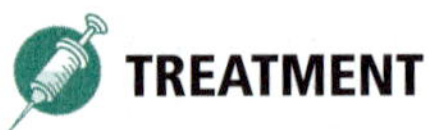

TREATMENT

GENERAL MEASURES

The goal is to correct the hypermetabolic state with the fewest side effects and lowest incidence of posttreatment hypothyroidism.

MEDICATION

First Line

- Antithyroid drugs: methimazole (MMI) and propylthiouracil (PTU)
  - Compete with the thyroid for iodine, thereby decreasing the synthesis of thyroid hormone; PTU blocks peripheral conversion of T_4 to T_3.
  - Treatment of choice for children and for adults who refuse RAI
  - May use as pretreatment for older or cardiac patients before RAI or surgery
  - MMI is now almost exclusively used except during the 1st trimester of pregnancy. It has longer duration of action, allowing for once daily dosing, more rapid efficacy, and lower incidence of side effects (2)[A].
  - Lowest effective dose of MMI should be used (1)[B].
  - Major side effects necessitating change in treatment: polyarthritis (1–2%), idiopathic granulocytopenia (0.5%), and cholestasis/jaundice (rare)

- After 12 to 18 months of therapy, measure TRAbs and TSH. Patients with normal levels have a greater chance of remission once thionamides are discontinued. Thus, MMI can be discontinued if TRAbs and TSH levels are normal. Monitor for recurrence (3).
- Relapse rates up to 50% in patients who respond initially; higher rates if smoker, large goiter, or positive thyroid-stimulating antibodies at end of treatment

- Radioactive iodine (RAI)
  - Concentrates in the thyroid gland and destroys thyroid tissue
  - Treatment of choice for definitive therapy of hyperthyroidism, in the absence of moderate or severe orbitopathy (1)[A]
  - Risks: side effects (neck soreness, flushing, decreased taste); worsening ophthalmopathy (15% incidence, higher in smokers); posttreatment hypothyroidism (80% incidence, not dosage dependent); radiation thyroiditis (1% incidence); need to adhere to safety precautions until radiation is eliminated from the body
  - Pretreatment with antithyroid medication should be considered in patients with severe disease and the elderly to reduce risk of posttreatment transient hyperthyroidism and posttreatment radiation thyroiditis.
  - May be repeated in as soon as 3 months if minimal response or after 6 months if not euthyroid (2)[A]

Second Line

Thyroidectomy is indicated with relapsed thyrotoxicosis, in the presence of goiter, when orbitopathy is present, when thyroid cancer is suspected, or in pregnant women in the 2nd trimester of pregnancy.

ISSUES FOR REFERRAL

- Endocrinologist for RAI therapy; if patient is pregnant or breastfeeding
- Ophthalmologist for Graves ophthalmopathy
- Surgeon if failed drug therapy or refusing RAI; obstruction or cosmesis

ADDITIONAL THERAPIES

- Graves hyperthyroidism
  - β-Blockers provide prompt control of adrenergic symptoms; start while workup is in progress (2)[A]. Long-acting propranolol is used most commonly and titrated to symptom control (40 to 160 mg/day).
  - Symptom control may be achieved with iodides, which block the conversion of T_4 to T_3 and inhibit TSH release; use for pregnant patients who do not tolerate antithyroid medication or in conjunction with antithyroid medications; should not be used long term (may cause a paradoxical increase in TSH release) or in combination with RAI
  - IV corticosteroids are used when rapid control of thyrotoxicosis is needed, they inhibit deiodinase type 2 thereby inhibiting conversion of T_4 to T_3 (4).
  - Bile acid sequestrants are used as adjuncts with antithyroid drugs; their mechanism is binding of thyroid hormones in the enterohepatic circulation (4).
- Graves ophthalmopathy
  - For corneal protection: tinted glasses when outdoors, artificial tears, patching/taping the lids at night
  - For orbitopathy: Mild cases can be treated with lubricants, nocturnal ointments, botulinum toxin injection for upper lid retraction, and smoking cessation. Moderate to severe cases should be treated with pulse-dose IV glucocorticoid if no contraindications. Alternative is PO steroid (prednisone 60 to 80 mg/day for 2 to 4 weeks and then taper off).
  - Newly approved by the FDA is the use of teprotumumab, which is a fully humanized monoclonal antibody inhibitor of insulin-like growth factor 1 receptor in patients with moderate to severe ophthalmopathy (4),(5).
  - Compressive optic neuropathy is a medical emergency managed with a combination of IV glucocorticoid, orbital irradiation, and surgical decompression (4),(5).
- Graves dermopathy: Medium- to high-potency topical corticosteroids with occlusive dressing.

SURGERY/OTHER PROCEDURES

Indications for thyroidectomy include persistent or recurrent thyrotoxicosis, diffusely enlarged thyroid with compressive symptoms, concurrent hyperparathyroidism or thyroid cancer, nodular thyroid, active Graves ophthalmopathy, and 2nd-trimester pregnancy (4),(5).

ADMISSION, INPATIENT, AND NURSING CONSIDERATIONS

ICU for severe thyrotoxicosis with hemodynamic compromise (thyroid storm)

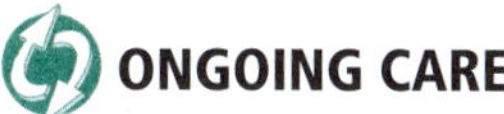

ONGOING CARE

FOLLOW-UP RECOMMENDATIONS

Patient Monitoring

TSH and T_4 levels every 1 to 2 months for first 6 months, then every 3 months for a year, and then every 6 to 12 months thereafter. For patients on treatment with PTU and MMI, check CBC and liver function yearly. Also, check anti-TSH receptor antibodies at 12 months of treatment to determine possibility of discontinuing medication. Remission is much more likely in the context of a normal value for anti-TSH receptor antibodies.

Pregnancy Considerations

- RAI is contraindicated in pregnancy and during breastfeeding.
- PTU is preferred in 1st trimester of pregnancy due to teratogenic effects of MMI. Switch to MMI in 2nd and 3rd trimesters due to risk of PTU-induced hepatotoxicity.
- Postpartum exacerbation of hyperthyroidism is common for women not currently under treatment, so TSH and symptoms should be monitored.

PROGNOSIS

Generally good with treatment, although may have irreversible ocular, cardiac, and psychiatric consequences

COMPLICATIONS

Increased morbidity due to osteoporosis, atherosclerotic disease, insulin resistance and obesity, and endothelial cell dysfunction (thromboembolic risk)

REFERENCES

1. Ren Z, Qin L, Wang JQ, et al. Comparative efficacy of four treatments in patients with Graves' disease: a network meta-analysis. *Exp Clin Endocrinol Diabetes*. 2015;123(5):317–322.
2. Bahn Chair RS, Burch HB, Cooper DS, et al; for American Thyroid Association and American Association of Clinical Endocrinologists. Hyperthyroidism and other causes of thyrotoxicosis: management guidelines of the American Thyroid Association and American Association of Clinical Endocrinologists. *Thyroid*. 2011;21(6):593–646.
3. Ross DS, Burch HB, Cooper DS, et al. 2016 American Thyroid Association guidelines for diagnosis and management of hyperthyroidism and other causes of thyrotoxicosis. *Thyroid*. 2016;26(10):1343–1421.
4. Kotwal A, Stan M. Current and future treatments for Graves' disease and Graves' ophthalmopathy. *Horm Metab Res*. 2018;50(12):871–886.
5. Dosiou C, Kossler AL. Thyroid eye disease: navigating the new treatment landscape. *J Endocr Soc*. 2021;5(5):bvab034.

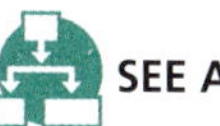

SEE ALSO

Algorithms: Anxiety; Cardiac Arrhythmias; Weight Loss, Unintentional

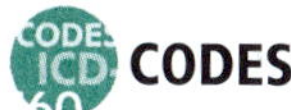

CODES

ICD10

- E05.00 Thyrotoxicosis w diffuse goiter w/o thyrotoxic crisis
- E05.01 Thyrotoxicosis w diffuse goiter w thyrotoxic crisis or storm
- E05.20 Thyrotoxicosis w toxic multinod goiter w/o thyrotoxic crisis

CLINICAL PEARLS

- Graves disease accounts for 60–80% of all cases of hyperthyroidism.
- Potential morbidities of hyperthyroidism include ophthalmopathy, atrial fibrillation, congestive heart failure (CHF), stroke, seizure, and osteopenia/osteoporosis.

G

GYNECOMASTIA

Muneeza Khan, MD, FAAFP

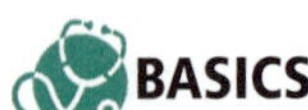

BASICS

DESCRIPTION

- Benign glandular proliferation of male breast tissue
- Increase in estrogen activity relative to androgen leads to the development of gynecomastia.
- Gynecomastia can be transient and may represent the normal physiologic changes that occur in utero or in adolescence. However, gynecomastia presenting or persisting in adulthood is typically pathologic in nature.
- Pseudogynecomastia which is lipomastia (subareolar fat)

EPIDEMIOLOGY

- 60–90% of infants and 50–60% of pubertal males have transient gynecomastia.
- Up to 70% of men between 50 and 69 years of age report gynecomastia.

Incidence

A study out of Bulgaria in 2007 put the incidence of pubertal gynecomastia at 3.9% in Caucasian boys ages 10 to 19 years.

Prevalence

Prevalence in adolescents varies from 22% to 69% and in adult males ranges from 36% to 57% (1).

ETIOLOGY AND PATHOPHYSIOLOGY

Multiple factors can alter the estrogen to androgen ratio and precipitate gynecomastia:

- Decrease in androgen production
- Increase in estrogen production
- Increase in peripheral conversion to estrogen
- Inhibition of the androgen receptor
- Increase in the level of sex hormone–binding globulin (SHBG) or the affinity of androgens to SHBG (decreases free or bioavailable testosterone)
- Displacement of estrogen relative to testosterone from SHBG due to medications

RISK FACTORS

Gynecomastia can be physiologic or pathologic in nature.

- Physiologic gynecomastia presents in infants and adolescent boys and resolves spontaneously.
  - Neonatal gynecomastia: The placenta converts dehydroepiandrosterone (DHEA) and dehydroepiandrosterone sulfate (DHEA-S) to estrone and estradiol resulting in transient gynecomastia.
  - Adolescent gynecomastia: Transient increases in estradiol levels at the onset of puberty lead to gynecomastia.
- Pathologic gynecomastia: persistent or adult-onset gynecomastia; 25% of cases are idiopathic, most secondary to age-associated decline in free testosterone and adipose tissue–mediated aromatase activity.

ALERT

- Illicit drugs: marijuana, heroin, methadone, alcohol, amphetamines, and over-the-counter bodybuilding supplements
- Hormones: androgens, anabolic steroids, estrogens, estrogen agonist, and human chorionic gonadotropin (hCG)
- Antiandrogens or inhibitors of androgen synthesis: bicalutamide, flutamide, nilutamide, cyproterone, and GnRH agonists (leuprolide and goserelin)
- Anti-infectives: metronidazole, ketoconazole, minocycline, isoniazid
- Antiulcer medications: cimetidine, ranitidine, metoclopramide, and proton pump inhibitors
- Cytotoxic agents: methotrexate, alkylating agents, and vinca alkaloids
- Cardiovascular drugs: Digoxin, spironolactone, calcium channel blockers, ACE inhibitors, amiodarone, methyldopa, reserpine, minoxidil, and recently statins can be added to this list.
- Psychoactive drugs: antidepressants, benzodiazepines, phenothiazines, antipsychotics (typical and atypical) (i.e., haloperidol and risperidone)
- Medications: HIV medications like efavirenz, phenytoin, penicillamine, sulindac, or theophylline
- Causes to rule out:
  - Primary hypogonadism: androgen insensitivity syndromes (defect in the androgen receptor), Klinefelter syndrome
  - Testicular tumor: germ cell (secretes hCG), Leydig cell (secretes estrogen), Sertoli cell (excessive aromatization to estrogens)
  - Adrenal tumors (secrete DHEA-S and estrogens)
  - Ectopic hCG tumors (hepatoblastoma, gastric tumors, renal cell carcinomas)
  - Cirrhosis
  - Secondary hypogonadism: Kallmann syndrome or prolactinemia, which can also stimulate milk production in breast tissue
  - Hyperthyroidism
  - Renal disease or dialysis
  - Malnutrition/starvation
  - Rare (true hermaphroditism [both testicular and ovarian tissue present])

Pediatric Considerations

Transient gynecomastia is seen in neonates or pubertal boys; typically resolves within 6 to 24 months

Geriatric Considerations

Medications and age-associated decline in testosterone production and increase in SHBG production leads to low free testosterone levels. The increased ratio of fat mass to lean mass leads to adipose tissue–mediated peripheral conversion of androgens to estrogen.

COMMONLY ASSOCIATED CONDITIONS

- Prostate carcinoma—treatment estrogen and antiandrogen leads to gynecomastia in 50–75% of patients.
- Cirrhosis
- Primary hypogonadism; especially Klinefelter syndrome—primary hypogonadism; at risk for breast cancer
- Testicular tumors; Leydig or Sertoli cell tumors especially when associated with Peutz-Jeghers syndrome or Carney complex

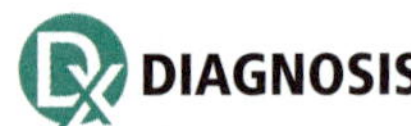

DIAGNOSIS

HISTORY

- If suspicious of hypogonadism, ask about erectile dysfunction, muscle mass, and decreased shaving frequency and libido.
- Obtain a family history including Carney complex and Peutz-Jeghers syndrome.
- Review medication list extensively and inquire about the use of illicit substances.
- Herbal supplements, marijuana use, and over-the-counter cimetidine or other H_2 antagonist use

PHYSICAL EXAM

- Careful breast exam to evaluate characteristics:
  - Firm, concentric glandular tissue beneath the nipple and areola palpable by pinching the thumb and forefinger together from either side of the breast toward the nipple. Diameter of this tissue for diagnostic purposes ranges from >0.5 to >2 cm, but the most recent large study recommended 1 cm as the diagnostic criteria. Patients are most often classified using Simon's or similar criteria.
  - Grade I: small visible breast enlargement, no skin redundancy
  - Grade IIa: moderate breast enlargement without any skin redundancy
  - Grade IIb: moderate breast enlargement with skin redundancy
  - Grade III: marked breast enlargement with marked skin redundancy (i.e., pendulous female breasts) (2)
  - May involve one or both breasts
  - Usually asymptomatic but may be painful or tender if it is of recent onset
  - Off center, hard, fixed mass is concerning for malignancy, although palpation of subareolar fat is more consistent with pseudogynecomastia.
  - Breast discharge should raise concern for malignancy or prolactinemia. In the latter, the discharge is typically clear or milky.
- Thyroid exam

- Abdominal exam (Evaluate for masses and liver size.)
- Genitourinary exam (Evaluate for testicular size, hair pattern, and presence of ovary or uterus.)
- Visual field exam (Evaluate for peripheral field defect.)

DIFFERENTIAL DIAGNOSIS

- Pseudogynecomastia—fat deposition without glandular proliferation often seen in obesity
- Breast cancer—typically unilateral; firm; eccentric to the nipple; skin dimpling, nipple retraction/discharge, and lymphadenopathy
- Lipomas, sebaceous cyst, dermoid cyst, mastitis, hematoma, hamartoma

DIAGNOSTIC TESTS & INTERPRETATION

Laboratory and radiologic investigations should be tailored to fit history and physical exam findings.

Initial Tests (lab, imaging)

- Luteinizing hormone (LH) and follicle-stimulating hormone (FSH)—elevated in primary hypogonadism and decreased in secondary hypogonadism
- Morning total and free testosterone—decreased testosterone level in hypogonadism
- hCG—elevated in germ cell tumors and ectopic hCG tumors
- Estradiol—elevated in Leydig cell tumors, Sertoli cell tumors, adrenal tumors, and with increased aromatase activity
- DHEA-S levels, which can be increased in adrenal tumors
- Urine for drugs of abuse (UDA)
- Other tests to consider include creatinine, liver function test, TSH, and prolactin.

Diagnostic Procedures/Other

Consider biopsy to rule out malignancy (i.e., off center, hard, fixed, discharge).

Test Interpretation

- Elevated hCG: Check testicular ultrasound; if positive for a mass, likely a testicular germ cell tumor. If the ultrasound is negative, consider extragonadal germ cell tumor or hCG-secreting neoplasm and order a CXR and CT abdomen.
- Elevated LH: if in relation to low testosterone, likely primary hypogonadism. If elevated in relation to high testosterone, check thyroid-stimulating hormone (TSH) and free thyroxine (FT_4). If FT_4 is elevated and TSH is suppressed, likely hyperthyroidism; if TSH and FT_4 are normal, likely androgen resistance
- Normal or decreased LH in relation to low testosterone: Check prolactin level. If prolactin is elevated, likely due to a prolactin-secreting pituitary tumor (need MRI); if normal, likely due to secondary hypogonadism
- Normal or decreased LH in relation to increased estradiol: Check testicular ultrasound. If positive for a mass, likely Leydig or Sertoli cell tumor. If negative for mass, check CT abdomen to evaluate the adrenals. If mass is present, possible adrenal neoplasm versus adenoma; if no mass is detected, then likely due to increased aromatase activity in extraglandular tissue

TREATMENT

GENERAL MEASURES

- Gynecomastia usually regresses spontaneously within 6 months of onset. Monitor for the first 6 months.
- Neonatal and pubertal gynecomastia spontaneously resolves within 6 to 24 months. Persistent pubertal gynecomastia (>24 months) occurs in 8% of pubertal boys. In adult males, 75% of gynecomastia is secondary to persistent pubertal gynecomastia, medications, and idiopathic conditions. Only 25% is related to an underlying medical condition.
- All illicit drug use and offending medications should be stopped if appropriate.
- Treat underlying medical conditions (i.e., testosterone replacement for hypogonadal men, dopamine agonist for prolactinoma, appropriate treatment for thyrotoxicosis, and tumor resection).

MEDICATION

There are no U.S. Food and Drug Administration–approved medications for the treatment of gynecomastia.

- SERMs: Clinical trials of both tamoxifen (10 to 20 mg/day) and raloxifene (60 mg/day) showed partial reduction in pubertal gynecomastia and successful resolution of idiopathic gynecomastia in 90% of study participants after 3 to 9 months.
- Aromatase inhibitors block peripheral conversion of androgens to estrogens. In prostate cancer patients, anastrozole prevented the development of gynecomastia in patients undergoing androgen deprivation therapy.

ADDITIONAL THERAPIES

In clinical trials, prophylactic radiotherapy prevented the development of gynecomastia in prostate cancer patients on androgen deprivation therapy.

SURGERY/OTHER PROCEDURES

Surgery can be recommended if gynecomastia does not regress within 12 months either spontaneously or after medical therapy, significant discomfort (i.e., pain, tenderness), it causes embarrassment or anxiety, or if biopsy is suspicious for malignancy. Multiple surgical techniques are available and studies indicate good patient satisfaction overall (2).

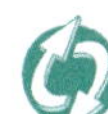

ONGOING CARE

FOLLOW-UP RECOMMENDATIONS

Patient Monitoring

Every 3 to 6 months for 24 months; consider medical therapy (i.e., tamoxifen) if severe, painful symptoms persist after 6 to 12 months and surgery if symptoms persist after 12 to 24 months. In individuals with asymptomatic or mild disease, routine yearly breast and physical exam is recommended.

PATIENT EDUCATION

Patients should be reassured of the benign nature of gynecomastia in almost all cases.

PROGNOSIS

- Good in physiologic cases because they often regress spontaneously within 3 to 6 months
- Majority of patients experience regression once underlying disorder is treated or offending agents are eliminated.
- The majority of patients, who undergo surgery, are satisfied with the postoperative cosmetic appearance.

REFERENCES

1. Kanakis GA, Nordkap L, Bang AK, et al. EAA clinical practice guidelines—gynecomastia evaluation and management. *Andrology*. 2019;7(6):778–793.
2. Burger A, Sattler A, Grünherz L, et al. Scar versus shape: patient-reported outcome after different surgical approaches to gynecomastia measured by modified BREAST Q®. *J Plast Surg Hand Surg*. 2023;57(1–6):1–6. doi:10.1080/2000656X.2021.1981349.

SEE ALSO

Algorithm: Gynecomastia

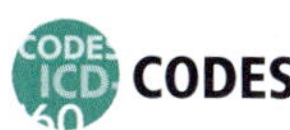

CODES

ICD10

N62 Hypertrophy of breast

CLINICAL PEARLS

- Gynecomastia can be transient and may represent normal physiologic changes in neonates or adolescents. Gynecomastia presenting or persisting in adulthood is pathologic.
- Lab and radiologic studies associated with gynecomastia including thyrotoxicosis, prolactinemia, hypogonadism, testicular tumors, adrenal tumors, and ectopic hCG tumors.
- ~25% of gynecomastia is idiopathic in nature, and treatment should focus on symptom control.
- Clinical trials of SERMs, aromatase inhibitors, and radiation therapy seem promising. Surgery is the treatment of choice for refractory gynecomastia.

G

HAMMER TOES

Neil J. Feldman, DPM

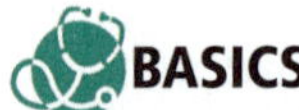

BASICS

Contraction deformities of the toes

DESCRIPTION

- Hammer toes include three distinct types of deformity.
  - Hammer toe (as defined) involves a plantar flexion deformity of the proximal interphalangeal (PIP) joint with varying degrees of hyperextension of the metatarsophalangeal (MTP) and distal interphalangeal (DIP) joint, primarily in sagittal plane (1).
  - Claw toe involves a plantar flexion deformity of the PIP and DIP joint with varying degrees of hyperextension of the MTP.
  - Mallet toe involves a plantar flexion deformity of the DIP joint only.
- Each can be flexible, semirigid, or fixed.
  - Flexible: passively correctable to neutral position
  - Semirigid: partially correctable to neutral position
  - Fixed: not correctable to neutral position without intervention

EPIDEMIOLOGY

Most common deformity of lesser digits, typically affecting only one or two toes:

- Second toe is the most commonly involved.
- Hallux malleus is term used when the great toe (hallux) is involved.

Incidence

- Undefined
- Increases with age, duration of deformity (from flexible to rigid)

Prevalence

- Predominant sex: female > male (2)
  - Female predominance from 2.5:1 to 9.0:1, depending on age group
- Can range from 1% to 20% of population studied
- Blacks are more often affected than whites (2).

ETIOLOGY AND PATHOPHYSIOLOGY

- Can be congenital or acquired
- Three categories of acquired hammer toes:
  - Flexor stabilization (most common cause and occurs in pronated foot/foot with pes planus). The flexor digitorum longus (FDL) muscle remains overactive, overusing the toes to assist in relative foot instability.
  - Extensor substitution (most common with pes cavus)—occurs during the swing phase of gait. The extensor digitorum longus (EDL) muscle remains overactive, substituting for dysfunctional hip and ankle extensors.
  - Flexor substitution—the least common cause and seen commonly with pes cavus. The FDL muscle remains overactive with relative weakness/dysfunction to the Achilles and flexor hallucis longus (FHL), which are the main plantar flexors of the foot.
- Biomechanical dysfunction results in muscle/tendon imbalance between the EDL tendon at the PIP joint and the FDL tendon at the MTP joint; the imbalance at the MTP joint level leads to the altering of the stabilizing force of the intrinsic muscles inserting into the extensor sling and wing apparatus of the MTP joint. In the case of classic hammer toes, the toe(s) sublux dorsally as the MTP hyperextends. This results in plantar flexion of the PIP joint and hyperextension of the MTP joint (2).
- Specific pathomechanics vary by etiology:
  - Toe length discrepancy or narrow footwear toe box induces PIP joint flexion by forcing digit to accommodate shoe.
    - May also lead to MTP joint synovitis secondary to overuse, with elongation of plantar plate and MTP joint hyperextension
    - 4th and 5th toes commonly assume an adductovarus attitude, which can make the toes appear to sit on their side and in advanced cases, can cause one toe to sit directly under another toe.
  - Rheumatoid arthritis (RA) causes MTP joint destruction and resultant subluxation.
  - Any condition that compromises intra-articular and periarticular tissues, first ray instability with or without a bunion deformity, an anatomically long 2nd metatarsal, inflammatory joint disease, neuromuscular conditions, improper-fitting shoes, and trauma.
  - Damage to joint capsule, collateral ligaments, or synovia leads to unstable PIP joint or MTP joint.

Genetics

- Significant heritability rates of 49–90%
- Specific genetic markers are not identified.

RISK FACTORS

- Pes cavus, pes planus
- Hallux valgus
- Metatarsus adductus
- Ankle equinus
- Neuromuscular disease (rare)
- Trauma; improperly fitted shoes (narrow toe box) and/or tight hosiery
- Abnormal metatarsal and/or digit length
- Inflammatory joint disease (e.g., RA)
- Connective tissue disease
- Diabetes mellitus

GENERAL PREVENTION

- Proper fitting of shoes. Use of pressure-dispersive footwear, shoes with soft uppers, and extra-depth toe boxes can help reduce pain and irritation from rubbing.
- Foot orthoses modulate biomechanical dysfunction and muscular imbalance, preventing progression (2).
- Limiting use of shoes in the growing foot. Use of zero drop shoes when necessary. Traditional shoes have an elevated heel relative to the ball of the foot (MTP joints). Therefore, at rest, the toes are positioned in dorsal subluxation at the MTP joints and forced to be contracted (termed toe spring).
- Perform toe strengthening exercises, which will help with prevention of imbalance between the extrinsic muscles of the calf and the intrinsic muscles of the foot.
- Control of predisposing factors (e.g., inflammatory joint disease) may also slow progression.
- Use of toe separators could aid in improved function of all of the lesser toes limiting the overuse of a particular toe and the development and/or worsening of that particular toe and subsequent deformity.

COMMONLY ASSOCIATED CONDITIONS

- Hallux valgus
- Cavus foot (pes cavus)
- Flat foot (pes planus)
- Metatarsus adductus
- Dorsal callus

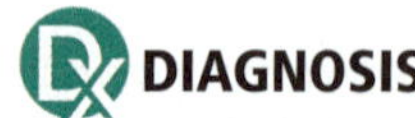

DIAGNOSIS

History and physical exam are typically sufficient for diagnosis of hammer toes. Additional tests are available to exclude other conditions.

HISTORY

- Location, duration, severity, and rate of progression of foot deformity
- Type, location, duration of pain
  - Patients often relate sensation of lump on plantar aspect of MTP joint.
- Degree of functional impairment
- Improving/exacerbating factors
- Type of footwear and hosiery worn
- Peripheral neurologic symptoms
- Any prior treatment rendered

PHYSICAL EXAM

- Note MTP joint hyperextension, PIP joint flexion, and DIP joint extension or flexion.
- Observe any adjacent toe deformities (e.g., hallux valgus, flexion contractures).
- Assess degree of flexibility and reducibility of deformity in both weight-bearing and non–weight-bearing positions (2).
- Note any hyperkeratosis over the joint, ulcers, clavi (dorsal PIP joint, metatarsal head), adventitious bursa, erythema, or skin breakdown or ulceration (2).
- Palpate for pain over dorsal aspect of PIP joint or MTP joint.
- Drawer test of MTP joint
- Palpate web spaces to exclude interdigital neuroma.
- Neurovascular evaluation (e.g., pulses, sensation, muscle bulk)

DIFFERENTIAL DIAGNOSIS

- Hammer toe: hyperextension of the MTP and DIP joints and plantar flexion of the PIP joint
- Claw toe: dorsiflexion of MTP joint and plantar flexion of the DIP joint
- Mallet toe: fixed or flexible deformity of the DIP joint of the toe
- Overlapping 5th toe
- Interdigital neuroma
- Plantar plate rupture
- Nonspecific synovitis of MTP joint
- Fracture; exostosis
- Arthritis (e.g., rheumatoid, psoriatic)

DIAGNOSTIC TESTS & INTERPRETATION

Initial Tests (lab, imaging)

- Not required unless clinically indicated to rule out suspected metabolic or inflammatory arthropathies (2)[C]: rheumatoid factor, antinuclear antibodies (ANA), HLA-B27 serologies for inflammatory disease
- Weight-bearing x-rays of affected foot in anteroposterior (AP), lateral, and oblique views (2)[C]:
  - AP view superior for assessing transverse plane MTP subluxation or dislocation
  - Lateral view is best for the evaluation of hammer toe.

Follow-Up Tests & Special Considerations

MRI or bone scan if osteomyelitis is suspected

Diagnostic Procedures/Other

- Nerve conduction studies or EMG if neurologic disorder is suspected
- Doppler or plethysmography if impaired circulation and surgery is considered
- Computerized weight-bearing pressure testing is indicated only in setting of neuromuscular deficiencies.

Test Interpretation

Histologic evaluation is not necessary before treatment.

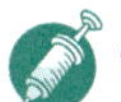

TREATMENT

- Goal of treatment is to relieve symptoms and help patients return to their normal activity level.
- Surgical and nonsurgical interventions are available.
- Mild and asymptomatic cases may not require treatment.

GENERAL MEASURES

Nonsurgical (conservative) treatments include

- Shoe modifications (wider and/or deeper toe box) to accommodate the deformity and decrease the pressure over osseous prominences. Avoid high-heeled shoes (2)[C].
- Toe sleeve or orthodigital padding of the hammer toe prominence
- Metatarsal pads in reducible deformities and crest pads in nonreducible deformities
- Dynamic toe splints for MTP joint subluxations or dislocations with (semi)reducible deformity
- Hammer toe–straightening orthotics or taping to reduce flexible deformities
- Débridement of hyperkeratotic lesions can reduce symptoms. Topical keratolytics may be helpful (2)[C].
- In-shoe foot orthotics can mitigate abnormal biomechanics.
- Physical therapy for stretching and strengthening of the toes helps preserve flexibility, which include intrinsic muscle strengthening (short foot exercises).
- Use of toe separators can be of benefit with some hammer toe deformities.

MEDICATION

First Line

NSAIDs may be helpful in managing symptoms of pain and joint inflammation.

ISSUES FOR REFERRAL

If nonsurgical (conservative) treatment is unsuccessful and/or impractical or patient has combined deformity of MTP joint, PIP joint, and/or DIP joint, refer to podiatric physician/surgeon or orthopedic surgeon.

SURGERY/OTHER PROCEDURES

- Surgical procedures for the correction of hammer toes depend on the degree and flexibility of the contracture(s) and related abnormalities.
- Surgical interventions for *flexible* hammer toes include (1)
  - PIP joint arthroplasty or arthrodesis (most common)
  - Flexor tenotomy for reducible or mallet toe deformities with distal ulceration
  - Extensor tendon lengthening/tenotomy/MTP joint capsulotomy
  - Flexor tendon transfer with digital arthrodesis
  - Exostosectomy
  - Implant arthroplasty
- Surgical interventions for semirigid/rigid hammer toes include (1)
  - PIP joint resection arthroplasty or arthrodesis
  - Girdlestone-Taylor flexor-to-extensor transfer
  - Metatarsal shortening (Weil osteotomy)
  - Exostosectomy
  - Middle phalangectomy (more common in 5th toe)
  - Soft tissue releases/lengthening
  - Diaphysectomy of the proximal phalanx (less common)
  - Phalangeal base resection as part of Hoffman-Clayton procedure for RA mutilans

ONGOING CARE

FOLLOW-UP RECOMMENDATIONS

- Obtain radiographs immediately following surgery or at the first postoperative visit; subsequent x-rays as needed
- Full weight-bearing in a postoperative (surgical) shoe or other device based on the procedure(s) performed and the individual patient
- Pinning often used across the MTP joint, which often requires patient to be non–weight-bearing to the forefoot for 3 to 5 weeks
- Elevate the foot to minimize swelling.
- Return to regular shoe wear after pain is controlled, swelling has subsided, and wounds have healed.
- Role and efficacy of postoperative physical therapy is unclear.

PATIENT EDUCATION

- Patients should be aware of mild to moderate swelling and plantar foot discomfort that may persist for many (1 to 6) months after surgery and may limit footwear options until resolved.
- MTP joint and PIP joint may remain stiff for extended periods of time.
- "Molding" of the operative toe (assuming the contours of adjacent toes) is common.
- Encourage patients to wear shoes of adequate size with "roomy" (rounded or squared) toe box.

PROGNOSIS

- Nonoperative (conservative) treatment in mild deformities usually alleviates pain; however, the deformity may progress.
- Surgical treatment of flexible hammer toe deformity reliably corrects the deformity and alleviates pain. Recurrence and progression are common, especially if the patient continues to wear ill-fitting shoes.
- Surgical treatment of fixed hammer toe deformity provides reliable deformity correction and pain relief. Recurrence is less common; however, adjacent toes can subsequently develop deformities.

COMPLICATIONS

- Common complications specific to digital surgery include but are not limited to
  - Persistent edema
  - Recurrence of deformity
  - Residual pain
  - Excessive stiffness
  - Metatarsalgia
- Less common complications include
  - Numbness (e.g., digital nerve palsy)
  - Flail toe
  - Symptomatic osseous regrowth
  - Malposition of toe
  - Malunion/nonunion
  - Infection
  - Sausage toe
  - Vascular impairment (e.g., toe ischemia, gangrene)

REFERENCES

1. Shirzad K, Kiesau CD, DeOrio JK, et al. Lesser toe deformities. *J Am Acad Orthop Surg*. 2011;19(8):505–514.
2. Thomas JL, Blitch EL IV, Chaney DM, et al; and Clinical Practice Guideline Forefoot Disorders Panel. Diagnosis and treatment of forefoot disorders. Section 1: digital deformities. *J Foot Ankle Surg*. 2009;48(3):418.e1–418.e9.

ADDITIONAL READING

Richie D. Exposing the Myths about Metatarsalgia. *Podiatry Management*. 2022;57–63. https://podiatrym.com/pdf/2022/9/Richie922web.pdf. Accessed September 13, 2025.

SEE ALSO

Algorithm: Foot Pain

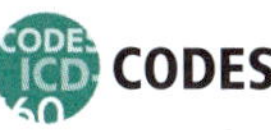

CODES

ICD10

- M20.40 Other hammer toe(s) (acquired), unspecified foot
- M20.41 Other hammer toe(s) (acquired), right foot
- M20.42 Other hammer toe(s) (acquired), left foot

CLINICAL PEARLS

- Hammer toe is a plantar flexion deformity of the PIP joint. Claw toe and mallet toe are additional types of hammer toes.
- Initial management of hammer toe deformity is conservative. Consider surgery if pain persists or the deformity worsens.
- Properly fitting footwear helps minimize recurrence. Patients should be aware of mild to moderate swelling and plantar foot discomfort that may persist for months after surgery and may limit footwear options until resolved.

HAND-FOOT-AND-MOUTH DISEASE

Sahil Mullick, MD, FAAFP • Sneha K. Patel, MD, MS • Harmeet Wadhawan, MD

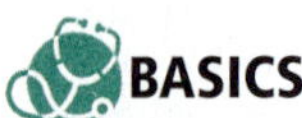

BASICS

DESCRIPTION

- Common clinical syndrome caused by several coxsackie and enterovirus serotypes
- Classic appearance of oral enanthem along with exanthem of hands and feet (classically) and potentially located elsewhere
- Exanthem (rash) may be macular, maculopapular, and/or vesicular.
- Synonym(s): herpangina (when affecting oral mucosa and posterior pharynx)

EPIDEMIOLOGY

- Self-limiting illness resolves in 7 to 10 days
- Moderately contagious
- Infection is spread by direct contact with nasal secretions, saliva, blister fluid, or stool.
- Infected individuals are most contagious during the 1st week of the illness but may continue to spread illness for days to weeks after. Some exposed individuals (especially adults) may be asymptomatic but still contagious.
- The viruses that cause hand-foot-and-mouth disease (HFMD) can persist for weeks after symptoms have resolved, most commonly in stool, allowing transmission following resolution of symptoms.
- The incubation period is 3 to 7 days.

Incidence

- Children <5 years of age are most commonly affected, especially in daycare facilities.
- Can occur as isolated cases, outbreaks, or epidemics
- Occurs worldwide
- Vertical transmission is possible.
- Most large outbreaks occur in Southeast Asia.

ETIOLOGY AND PATHOPHYSIOLOGY

- HFMD is not the same as foot (hoof) and mouth disease found in cattle, and there is no cross species infectious concern.
- Transmission by the fecal–oral route or contact with skin lesions or oral secretions; caused by viruses that belong to the enterovirus genus and replicated in the GI tract, most commonly coxsackievirus A16 and enterovirus 71 (previously caused outbreaks)
- Also coxsackie viruses A5, A7, A9, A10, B2, B5
- More severe cases are associated with enterovirus 71 (1).

GENERAL PREVENTION

- Handwashing is effective in reducing transmission, specifically before food handling or after diaper changes and toileting.
- Disinfect surfaces and fomites, avoiding close contact and sharing of personal items with infected persons.
- Exclusion of children from group settings during the first few days of the illness in the presence of open lesions in the mouth or on the skin may reduce the spread of infection.
- Pregnant woman should avoid contact with infected individuals.
- Work continues on multivalent vaccine development.

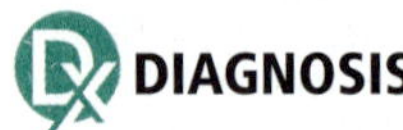

DIAGNOSIS

HISTORY

- 1- to 2-day prodrome of fever, anorexia, malaise, abdominal pain, upper respiratory symptoms
- Fever may last 3 to 4 days followed by sore throat.
- Progression of disease divided into five stages: rash, neurologic dysfunction, early cardiopulmonary failure, cardiopulmonary failure, recovery; most patients only develop rash (2)[C]
- Maculopapular rash on hands, feet, and mouth; oral lesions may precede skin findings.
- Often history of sick contacts

PHYSICAL EXAM

- Oral enanthem along with tender vesicles becoming ulcers on buccal mucosa, sides of tongue, and palate
- May persist for up to 1 week
- Cutaneous vesicles 3 to 5 mm in diameter start as painful maculopapular eruptions, occur typically on dorsal aspect of fingers and toes.
- May also occur on the palms, soles, buttocks, and groin
- Adults are less likely to have cutaneous findings.
- Nail dystrophies are not uncommon and may persist for weeks following the acute infection.
- Be mindful of central nervous system (CNS) symptoms. Although rare, CNS involvement is possible.

DIFFERENTIAL DIAGNOSIS

- Herpetic gingivostomatitis
- Aphthous stomatitis
- Scabies
- Chickenpox
- Measles
- Rubella
- Scarlet fever
- Roseola infantum
- Fifth disease
- Other enteroviral infections
- Kawasaki disease
- Viral pharyngitis
- Varicella
- Rickettsial infection (RFSF)
- Behcet syndrome
- Pemphigus vulgaris
- Stevens-Johnson syndrome
- HIV

DIAGNOSTIC TESTS & INTERPRETATION

Clinical diagnosis is typically adequate.

Initial Tests (lab, imaging)
Although not typically performed, culture for responsible virus (virus isolation) can be obtained from oral lesions, cutaneous vesicles, nasopharyngeal swabs, stool, and CSF. Polymerase chain reaction (PCR) of throat swabs and vesicle fluid is the most efficient test if enterovirus 71 is suspected.

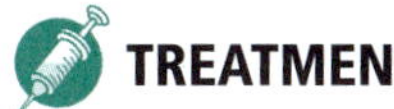

TREATMENT

- Symptomatic
- No current specific antiviral treatments
- Avoid spicy or acidic foods to limit oral pain.
- Encourage adequate oral hydration, although IV fluids may be required in more severe cases of dehydration.

GENERAL MEASURES
Isolation of patients to avoid cross-infection

MEDICATION
- Symptomatic care using ibuprofen or acetaminophen for pain from oral ulcers or fever
- Soothing mouthwashes ("magic mouthwash") containing lidocaine are not recommended as they do not appear to be superior to placebo and have risk of side effects when absorbed systemically.
- Antiviral treatments are not available.

Pediatric Considerations
Avoid aspirin use in treating febrile illness in children due to concern of Reye syndrome—an encephalopathy associated with aspirin use in viral illness in children.

ADMISSION, INPATIENT, AND NURSING CONSIDERATIONS
- Patients with CNS manifestations or autonomic dysregulation may require hospitalization.
- Admit those with dehydration unable to maintain adequate oral hydration.
- IV immunoglobulin is not recommended.
- Indicators of HFMD severity include high fever, nervous system involvement, abnormal respiratory rate and rhythm, circulatory dysfunction, increased white blood cell count, increased blood glucose, and increased blood lactate.

ONGOING CARE

DIET
- Encourage cold liquids (e.g., ice cream, popsicles) to prevent dehydration.
- Avoid acidic, salty, and spicy foods, as they will increase pain.

COMPLICATIONS
- Dehydration most common due to painful oral ulcerations
- CNS involvement (i.e., aseptic meningitis) is a rare complication, although it is on the rise globally, particularly in severe cases.
- Enterovirus 71 has caused outbreaks and has been implicated in more severe disease associated with CNS infection.
- Cardiopulmonary complications include myocarditis, pneumonitis, and pulmonary edema.
- HFMD eye involvement is only observed in young adult patients, some cases may have residual visual loss.
- Fever >3 days and lethargy are associated with CSF pleocytosis.

REFERENCES

1. Saguil A, Kane SF, Lauters R, et al. Hand-foot-and-mouth disease: rapid evidence review. *Am Fam Physician*. 2019;100(7):408–414.
2. Zhu P, Ji W, Li D, et al. Current status of hand-foot-and-mouth disease. *J Biomed Sci*. 2023;30(1):15. doi:10.1186/s12929-023-00908-4.

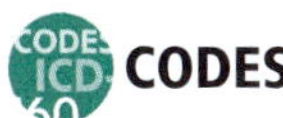

CODES

ICD10
- B08.4 Enteroviral vesicular stomatitis with exanthem
- B34.1 Enterovirus infection, unspecified
- B08.5 Enteroviral vesicular pharyngitis

CLINICAL PEARLS

- Most common: May to October
- Children <5 years of age tend to have worse symptoms than older children.
- HFMD is the most common cause of mouth sores in pediatric patients.
- Typical symptoms include low-grade fever, maculopapular rash on hands and soles of the feet, and painful oral ulcers.
- Dehydration is a common problem secondary to swallowing aversions.
- Usually self-limiting, resolving in 7 to 10 days
- Careful handwashing to limit dissemination

H

HEADACHE, CLUSTER

Samuel C. Wang, MD

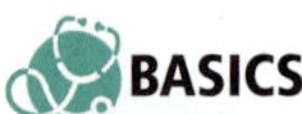

BASICS

DESCRIPTION

- A primary headache disorder characterized by circadian and circannual episodes consisting of multiple attacks of severe, unilateral sharp, searing, or piercing pain typically localized to the periorbital and/or temporal areas
- It is the most common headache among trigeminal autonomic cephalgias (TACs)
- Accompanied by signs of ipsilateral parasympathetic autonomic activation as well as restlessness or agitation
- Autonomic symptoms: signs of parasympathetic hyperactivity (ipsilateral lacrimation, eye redness, nasal congestion) and sympathetic hypoactivity (ipsilateral ptosis and miosis)
- Individual attacks occur from once every other day up to 8 times per day and can last 15 to 180 min/day if untreated.
- Attacks usually occur in series (cluster periods) that are often seasonal, lasting for weeks or months, and are separated by remission periods usually lasting months to years.
- About 10–15% of patients have chronic symptoms without remission periods (i.e., chronic cluster headache [cCH]).

EPIDEMIOLOGY

Prevalence

1-year prevalence: 53/100,000

- Gender: male > female; 4.3:1 overall
- Mean age of onset: 30 years; women often develop cluster headache (CH) earlier in life (20s).

ETIOLOGY AND PATHOPHYSIOLOGY

Complex and incompletely understood; possible mechanisms include the following:

- Activation of the trigeminovascular and parasympathetic system which leads to the release of neurokinins and vasodilatory peptides including vasoactive intestinal peptide (VIP), and calcitonin gene-related peptide (CGRP)
- Posterior hypothalamus activation; hypothalamic-midbrain-brainstem interconnections may trigger an attack by activating trigeminal nociceptive pathways through increased parasympathetic outflow.
- Alterations in the descending pain modulation network and disordered pain modulation during cluster periods
- Dysregulation of areas of the brain related to circadian rhythm and chronobiology, including the pineal gland, suprachiasmatic nucleus, and other "clock" areas

Genetics

- Autosomal dominant in 5% of cases; otherwise, recessive or multifactorial
- First-degree relatives are 5 to 18 times more likely, and second-degree relatives are 1 to 3 times more likely to be affected by cluster headaches.
- >50% with migraine and 18% with CH in family history
- Association of core circadian genes and other clock-controlled genes (CCGs), which have a circadian pattern of expression

RISK FACTORS

- Age: 70% onset before age 30 years
- Cigarette smoking or childhood exposure to cigarette smoke
- History of head trauma

COMMONLY ASSOCIATED CONDITIONS

- Depression (24%) with increased risk of suicide
- History of migraine, frequently in female patients; medication-overuse headache
- Asthma (9%)
- Sleep apnea (30–80%)

DIAGNOSIS

International Classification of Headache Disorders (3rd edition, 2018) criteria

- At least five attacks of severe or very severe unilateral orbital, supraorbital, and/or temporal pain lasting 15 to 180 minutes if untreated
- Either one or both of the following:
  - At least one of the following symptoms ipsilateral to the headache:
    - Conjunctival injection and/or lacrimation
    - Nasal congestion and/or rhinorrhea
    - Eyelid edema
    - Forehead and/or facial sweating/flushing
    - Miosis and/or ptosis
  - Restlessness or agitation during an acute attack
- Attack frequency: once every other day to eight times per day for more than half of the time during cluster periods
- Episodic CH (eCH): at least two cluster periods lasting 7 days to 1 year, separated by a pain-free interval of ≥3 months (80–90% of cases)
- cCH: occurring for ≥ 1 year without remission period, or remission period lasting <3 months, for at least one year

HISTORY

- Episodic periods of recurring headaches, described as excruciating, unilateral, sharp, searing, or piercing pain typically localized to the periorbital and/or temporal area
- Conjunctival injection, tearing, nasal congestion, rhinorrhea, sweating on the ipsilateral side
- Timing of headaches is diurnal in nature, often occurring at the same time each day (mostly at night).
- Patients are often restless and pace the floor during an acute attack because lying down seems to exacerbate the pain.
- Presence of triggers such as vasodilators (e.g., alcohol, nitroglycerin, sildenafil), histamine, certain foods, or strong odors
- Circadian or circannual rhythm of cluster periods, often recurring around the same time of the year, with spring and fall being the most common

PHYSICAL EXAM

Exam is often unremarkable, unless performed during an acute attack:

- Distress, crying spells, restlessness, agitation
- Ipsilateral lacrimation, conjunctival injection, eyelid edema, ptosis, and miosis
- Edematous nasal mucosa or rhinorrhea

DIFFERENTIAL DIAGNOSIS

- Other TACs (e.g., paroxysmal hemicrania, short-lasting unilateral neuralgiform headache attacks with conjunctival injection and tearing [SUNCT], hemicrania continua), hypnic headaches, trigeminal and other facial neuralgias, migraine, temporal arteritis, herpes zoster, acute angle closure glaucoma
- Secondary CH:
  - Vascular causes: vertebral or carotid artery dissection, brain arteriovenous malformations, intracranial artery aneurysms
  - Tumors: pituitary tumors/meningiomas/carcinomas, cavernous hemangioma
  - Infections/inflammation: sinusitis, herpes zoster ophthalmicus, inflammation of the cavernous sinus (i.e., Tolosa-Hunt syndrome)
  - Ophthalmic causes: glaucoma, orbital pseudotumor

DIAGNOSTIC TESTS & INTERPRETATION

Diagnosis is primarily clinical and often delayed (>40% report 5-year delay in diagnosis).

Initial Tests (lab, imaging)

Neuroimaging (MRI/CT head with detailed study of pituitary and cavernous sinus) is recommended at least once for all patients diagnosed with TACs in order to exclude other intracranial conditions that may mimic TACs.

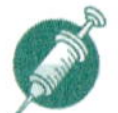

TREATMENT

Many of the medications discussed are used off-label in the treatment of CH (1).

GENERAL MEASURES

- Avoid major changes in sleep habits.
- Stop smoking.
- Avoid use of alcohol during cluster period.
- Avoid exposure to known triggers.

MEDICATION

- Avoid opioid analgesics for treatment of acute attacks.
- Goal is abortion of acute attacks and concomitant use of transitional and preventive treatments for the duration of the cluster period.
- Long-term prophylaxis should be used for chronic CH
- Assess cardiovascular risk before instituting vasoactive drugs, such as triptans or ergot derivatives.

First Line

- Abortive therapy:
  - Oxygen: 100% at 12 to 15 L/min via nonrebreather mask or demand valve oxygen mask while in an upright position provides relief within 15 minutes; higher flow used if resistant to lower-flow oxygen; excellent side effect profile (2)[A]
  - Sumatriptan
    - SC: 6 mg, up to 12 mg/24 hr with at least 1 hour between injections is the most effective medication for acute attacks; NNT = 2.4 and 3.3 for headache relief and pain free in 15 minutes, respectively
    - Intranasal: 20 mg once in single nostril contralateral to the side of the headache; may repeat in 2 hours, max dose 40 mg/24 hr; NNT = 3.2 for headache relief at 30 minutes (2)[A]

- Zolmitriptan
  - Intranasal: 5- and 10-mg dosage both effective; may repeat in 2 hours, max 2 times per day; NNT = 12 and 4.9 for headache relief in 15 minutes for 5 and 10 mg, respectively (2)[A]
- Noninvasive vagus nerve stimulation (nVNS):
  - FDA-approved durable medical device that delivers electrical stimulation while positioned on the neck overlying the vagus nerve. Modest efficacy in short-term pain reduction for eCH was demonstrated in two double-blind, sham controlled trials ACT-1 and ACT-2; NNT = 5 and 3 respectively

- Transitional therapy:
  - May be used to rapidly reduce attack frequency until the effectiveness of longer term prophylactic treatment is reached; longer-term preventive agents should be started concurrently.
    - Suboccipital nerve or greater occipital nerve steroid injections (preferred option): 3.75 mg of cortivazol injected into the suboccipital area on the ipsilateral side of the headache; single injection or series of 3 injections, given 48 to 72 hours apart, reduces attack frequency during cluster period when used as add-on therapy to verapamil; NNT = 2.5 (3)[A]
    - Steroids: prednisone 60 to 100 mg daily for 5 days with a taper no longer than 18 days to avoid side effects; several open studies suggested benefit but no rigorous trials to prove efficacy; adverse effects for short-term use: hyperglycemia, insomnia, psychosis, hyponatremia, edema, elevated blood pressure, peptic ulcer
- Preventive therapy:
  - Should be initiated at the start of a cluster period
  - Verapamil: Start at 80 mg TID and increase by 80 mg/wk to 480 mg and then 80 mg every 2 weeks if needed; short- or long-acting equivalent; most patients respond to daily dose of 240 to 480 mg, but up to 960 mg/day may be needed; NNT = 1.2 (2)[A] baseline ECG and ECG monitoring during treatment is required.
  - Galcanezumab: 300 mg SC injection every month until cluster period ends; only FDA-approved medication for eCH prophylaxis; has not been shown to be effective for cCH; most common side effects are nasopharyngitis, hepatic enzyme elevation, and local injection site reaction and pain; NNT = 5.2 (4)[B]
  - nVNS: FDA approved for preventive treatment of cCH and eCH; one prospective, open-label RCT (PREVA study) showed greater reduction from baseline in number of CH per week in nVNS + standard of care compared to standard of care alone; NNT = 4

ALERT

Triptans are contraindicated in ischemic cardiac disease, stroke, uncontrolled hypertension, Prinzmetal angina, basilar migraine, hemiplegic migraine, ischemic bowel disease, and peripheral vascular disease.

Second Line

- Abortive treatment:
  - Lidocaine: 1 mL of 4–10% lidocaine solution administered intranasally on ipsilateral side of symptoms; no well-controlled randomized controlled trials (RCTs) done
  - Octreotide: 100 μg injected SC; can be considered in patients when triptans are contraindicated; main side effect is GI upset.
- Preventive treatment:
  - Lithium: Start 300 mg BID; titrate to therapeutic range of 600 to 1,500 mg/day. In a head-to-head trial with verapamil, lithium was shown to be comparable; must monitor drug levels and liver, renal, and thyroid function; caution with nephrotoxic drugs, diuretics; monitor for CNS side effects.
  - Topiramate: 25 to 100 mg BID showed efficacy in several small, open-label trials; can be used as an add-on therapy with verapamil

ADDITIONAL THERAPIES

Pregnancy Considerations

- Collaboration between headache specialist, obstetrician, and lactation specialist is recommended (5)[C].
- For acute treatment, oxygen is most appropriate first-line therapy. Intranasal triptans (pregnancy Category C), intranasal lidocaine (pregnancy Category B), and/or subcutaneous sumatriptan (pregnancy Category C) can be used as second-line therapy.
- For transitional therapy, steroids (pregnancy Category C/D) can be used, but systemic use should be avoided in 1st trimester.
- As preventive therapy, verapamil (pregnancy Category C) remains the preferred option. There are no studies on the safety of galcanezumab use in pregnancy. Avoid ergotamines (pregnancy Category X).

SURGERY/OTHER PROCEDURES

- No evidence for hyperbaric oxygen treatment or CPAP
- Botox shows conflicting results in two small open-label trials. An RCT is ongoing.
- Surgery or Gamma Knife radiation may be considered for refractory CH patients.
- Neuromodulation: Although a promising area of continuing research, it is invasive, expensive, and should be considered only for refractory patients.

COMPLEMENTARY & ALTERNATIVE MEDICINE

For prophylaxis: Melatonin 10 mg in late evening has shown reduction in headache frequency versus placebo in a small RCT.

ADMISSION, INPATIENT, AND NURSING CONSIDERATIONS

Intractable, severe pain; suicidal ideation

ONGOING CARE

FOLLOW-UP RECOMMENDATIONS

Patient Monitoring

- Anticipate cluster bouts and initiate prophylaxis early.
- Monitor for depression and suicidal ideation, especially in those with cCH.

DIET

Avoid alcohol consumption.

PROGNOSIS

- Unpredictable but often chronic course
- Attack frequency often decreases with increasing age.
- Possibility of transformation of eCH to cCH

COMPLICATIONS

Depression and suicide

REFERENCES

1. Diener HC, May A. Drug treatment of cluster headaches. *Drugs*. 2022;82(1):33–42.
2. Robbins MS, Starling AJ, Pringsheim TM, et al. Treatment of cluster headache: the American Headache Society evidence-based guidelines. *Headache*. 2016;56(7):1093–1106.
3. Gordon A, Roe T, Villar-Martinez MD, et al. Effectiveness and safety profile of greater occipital nerve blockade in cluster headache: a systematic review. *J Neurol Neurosurg Psychiatry*. 2023;95(1):73–85. doi:10.1136/jnnp-2023-331066.
4. Yuan H, Spare NM, Silberstein SD. Targeting CGRP for the prevention of migraine and cluster headache: a narrative review. *Headache*. 2019;59(Suppl 2):20–32.
5. Bjørk MH, Kristoffersen ES, Tronvik E, et al. Management of cluster headache and other trigeminal autonomic cephalalgias in pregnancy and breastfeeding. *Eur J Neurol*. 2021;28(7):2443–2455.

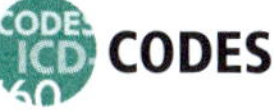

CODES

ICD10

- G44.009 Cluster headache syndrome, unspecified, not intractable
- G44.019 Episodic cluster headache, not intractable
- G44.029 Chronic cluster headache, not intractable

CLINICAL PEARLS

- Patients are often agitated and restless during acute attacks.
- High-flow oxygen and triptans are first-line therapy for acute attacks.
- Among triptans, injected forms are more effective than nasal sprays, which are more effective than oral forms.
- Galcanezumab is FDA approved for prophylaxis of eCH.
- nVNS is FDA approved for prophylaxis of both eCH and cCH.
- Abortive, transitional, and prophylactic treatments must all be considered.

HEADACHE, MIGRAINE

Seniha Ozudogru, MD • Karly Pippitt, MD

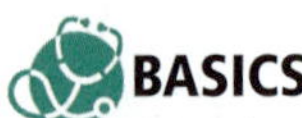

BASICS

DESCRIPTION

Recurrent headache disorder manifesting in attacks lasting 4 to 72 hours; typically: unilateral, pulsating, moderate to severe intensity, and associated nausea and/or photo/phonophobia (1)

- Most frequent subtypes of migraine (1):
  - Without aura: >80% of migraines; vomiting, photophobia, and/or phonophobia
  - With aura: visual or other (motor, sensory or brainstem symptoms, including previously known as basilar or hemiplegic migraine); fully reversible neurologic phenomenon, develop gradually over 5 minutes and last up to 60 minutes
  - Chronic migraine: >15 migraine days/month, >4 hours/attack, for ≥3 months
  - Menstrual migraine: migraine attacks in a menstruating person, onset 1 to 2 days prior to menses or up to day 3 of menstruation, occurring in 2 of 3 menstrual cycles and at no other time during cycle
  - Menstrually related migraine: menstrual migraine plus migraine attacks at other times during cycle
- Rare but important subtypes (1):
  - Status migrainosus: migraine lasting >72 hours
  - Prolonged aura: aura symptoms >60 minutes (can last up to 7 days); should consider secondary causes
  - Ocular: repeated attacks of monocular visual disturbance, scintillations, scotomata, or blindness, with migraine
  - Vertiginous: migraine with vertigo or dizziness
  - Acephalgic migraine (migraine aura without headache): typical aura symptoms not followed by a migraine headache

EPIDEMIOLOGY

- Female > male (3:1)
- Affects >28 million Americans

ETIOLOGY AND PATHOPHYSIOLOGY

- Neurogenic theory: Activation of hypothalamus and brainstem nuclei; trigeminal vascular system activation and release of neuropeptides (CGRP, PACAP)
- Cortical spreading depression: main hypotheses for migraine with aura; change in electrical activity with reduced blood flow, leading to aura

Genetics

>80% have a family history

RISK FACTORS

- Female sex (menstrual cycle)
- Family history of migraine
- Triggers include sleep disruption and diet influences (skipped meals, alcohol, chocolate, cheese, caffeine overuse, monosodium glutamate [MSG], and artificial sweeteners)

GENERAL PREVENTION

- Lifestyle modifications are cornerstone: sleep hygiene, stress management, healthy diet, adequate hydration, and regular exercise
- Prophylactic medication for frequent attacks

COMMONLY ASSOCIATED CONDITIONS

- Depression, anxiety, PTSD
- Sleep disturbance (sleep apnea)
- IBS
- Other pain syndromes (cervical spine disease, endometriosis)

DIAGNOSIS

Clinical diagnosis; recommend thorough history and neurologic examination.

HISTORY

- Validated migraine screening tool: ID migraine (2)
  - In the last 3 months did you have the following symptoms with headaches: Nauseated or sick to stomach? Light bothered you? Headaches limited ability to work/study/do what you needed for a day?
    - Yes to 2 questions: 81% migraine probability; yes to 3 questions increases migraine probability to 93% (2)
- Headache usually begins with mild pain escalating to unilateral (30–40% bilateral) throbbing (40% nonthrobbing) pain lasting 4 to 72 hours.
  - If side-locked headache or potential secondary causes (tumor, systemic illnesses), evaluate for alternative diagnosis.
- Pain intensified by movement; can be associated with: nausea, vomiting, diarrhea, photophobia, phonophobia, muscle tenderness, light-headedness, vertigo
- May be preceded by aura; visual disruptions most common: scotoma, hemianopsia, fortification spectra, geometric visual patterns, and occasionally hallucinations; somatosensory disruption in face/arms; speech difficulties
- Headache diary: episodes/month, HA days/month, frequency, amount and effect of medications
- Identify possible triggers (stress, sleep disturbance, food, caffeine, alcohol).
- Migraine disability assessment (MiDAS) is useful to assess disability and correlates with headache diaries

PHYSICAL EXAM

Neurologic exam, including fundoscopy, to rule out other causes

DIFFERENTIAL DIAGNOSIS

- Other primary headache syndromes (idiopathic intracranial hypertension [IIH], trigeminal autonomic cephalgia [TAC])
- Secondary headaches: medication overuse headache (MOH), tumor, infection, vascular pathology, drug use

DIAGNOSTIC TESTS & INTERPRETATION

- Neuroimaging appropriate with suspicious symptoms and/or abnormal exam (3)[C]. Red flags include the following:
  - New onset >50 years old
  - Change in usual headache pattern
  - Atypical pattern/unremitting/progressive neurologic symptoms
  - Prolonged/different/change in typical aura
- Workup
  - Consider systemic disease (hypothyroidism, SLE) in appropriate clinical scenario and evaluate accordingly.

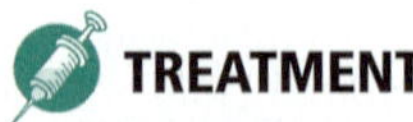

TREATMENT

GENERAL MEASURES

- Consistent sleep hours and eating habits
- Cold compresses

MEDICATION

- Abortive treatments
  - Mild to moderate attacks:
    - Acetaminophen; when combined with metoclopramide relief rates similar to triptans (4)[A]
    - NSAIDs effective in up to 60% (4)[B]
    - Aspirin-acetaminophen–caffeine (Excedrin Migraine) (4)[B]
  - Moderate to severe attacks:
    - Triptans when OTC agents fail *or* first line for moderate to severe attacks (4)[C]
      - Sumatriptan 100 mg PO; can repeat in 2 hours; max 200 mg/24 hr; sumatriptan 3 or 4 or 6 mg SC; can repeat in 1 hour; max 12 mg/24 hr; rapid onset, should consider for wakeup headache, migraine with severe GI upset; sumatriptan intranasal 20 mg; can repeat in 2 hours; max 40 mg/24 hr
      - Rizatriptan 10 mg PO (5 mg if using propranolol for prophylaxis); can repeat in 2 hours; max 30 mg/24 hr
      - Naratriptan 2.5 mg PO; can repeat in 4 hours; max 5 mg/24 hr
      - Zolmitriptan 2.5 mg PO; 5 mg intranasal; can repeat in 2 hours; max 5 mg for oral, 10 mg for nasal spray/24 hr
      - Frovatriptan 2.5 mg PO; can repeat in 4 hours; max 5 mg/24 hr
      - Eletriptan 40 mg PO; can repeat in 2 hours; max 80 mg/24 hr
        - Frovatriptan and naratriptan have slow onset but long half-lives—ideal for long migraine duration and menstrual migraine.
    - Antiemetics: dopamine antagonists (4)[B]
  - Contraindications: Avoid triptans and ergots in coronary artery disease (CAD) or uncontrolled HTN.
  - Precautions
    - Frequent use of rescue drugs can result in MOH
    - Triptan common adverse reactions: chest pain, flushing, weakness, dizziness, paresthesias; recommend trying >1 triptan before consider class failure.

- Other abortive treatment (5)
  - Ubrogepant 50 and 100 mg: can repeat in 2 hours; max 200 mg/24 hr
  - Rimegepant 75 mg ODT: 1 daily PRN; max 75 mg/24 hr
  - Dihydroergotamine: status migrainosus and triptan resistance/failure drug of choice; ergotamine oral tabs and dihydroergotamine nasal sprays are convenient and safer than IM injections.
  - Lasmiditan 50 and 100 mg: 5-HT1F receptor agonist; schedule V; do not drive for 8 hours; safe with CV risk factors
  - Zavegepant intranasal 10 mg/spray: 1 spray in 1 nostril/24 hr
- First-line preventive (6)[A]: lifestyle modifications, trigger reduction, CBT
  - Consider prophylaxis:
    - Quality of life severely impaired
    - ≥6 headache days/month, ≥4 headache days/month of moderate severity, or ≥2 headache days/month of severe impairment
    - Frequent, long, or uncomfortable auras
- Preventive treatment of migraine: divalproex, topiramate, metoprolol, and propranolol to reduce frequency; amitriptyline, venlafaxine, lisinopril, and candesartan are options (6)[A].
  - NSAIDs can be effective prevention if predictable triggers (menses)
  - CGRP monoclonal antibodies:
    - Erenumab 70 and 140 mg, full CGRP receptor antagonist; 1 SC/month
    - Fremanezumab partial CGRP receptor antagonist; 225 mg monthly SC injections or 675 mg quarterly SC injections
    - Galcanezumab partial CGRP receptor antagonist; 240 mg loading dose, then 120 mg monthly SC injections
    - Eptinezumab 100 mg/mL: Dilute with 0.9% NaCl; infuse over 30 minutes. If not enough benefit can increase the dose to 300 mg for the second cycle.
  - CGRP small molecule antagonists:
    - Rimegepant 75 mg ODT: 1 tab every other day
    - Atogepant 10, 30, and 60 mg: 1 tab daily
  - *Chronic migraine*: onabotulinumtoxinA (Botox) injections every 3 months (6)[A]

Pregnancy Considerations

New-onset headaches in pregnancy, consider preeclampsia and venous sinus thrombosis.

- Acetaminophen, antiemetics, and short-acting opioids can be considered acutely.
- No data for increased teratogenicity with triptans, acceptable when compellingly needed.
- Ergotamines contraindicated
- Avoid herbal remedies.
- β-Blockers and calcium channel blockers: safe and effective prophylaxis
- Occipital nerve blocks and trigger point injections (lidocaine and bupivacaine) are considered safe.

Pediatric Considerations

- NSAIDs first line; triptans are effective for acute treatment.
- Rizatriptan FDA-approved for >6 years old; sumatriptan succinate, almotriptan, zolmitriptan nasal spray FDA-approved for >12 years old (7)[A]

ISSUES FOR REFERRAL

Obscure diagnosis, unresponsive to usual treatment

COMPLEMENTARY & ALTERNATIVE MEDICINE

- Riboflavin (vitamin B_2): 400 mg/day (6)[B]
- Magnesium: 400 mg/day (6)[B]
- MIG-99 (feverfew): 6.25 mg TID (6)[B]
- Acupuncture

ONGOING CARE

FOLLOW-UP RECOMMENDATIONS

Patient Monitoring

- Monitor attack frequency and medication use via headache diary.
- Migraine (especially with aura) is risk factor for stroke; consider lipids and risk reduction like tobacco cessation. In migraine with aura, avoid estrogen due to increased stroke risk (2)[A].

PATIENT EDUCATION

- Trigger identification and modification can significantly improve frequency.
- Setting expectations is critical, especially with prophylactic medications where success is 50% reduction in severity of headaches or decrease in disability from headaches.
- Benefits from prophylactic medications take time.

PROGNOSIS

- With increasing age, typically reduction in severity, frequency, and disability
- Most attacks subside within 72 hours

COMPLICATIONS

- Status migrainosus (>72 hours)
- MOH: headache ≥10 days/month for >3 months due to regular overuse of a rescue headache medication; likelihood with butalbital > opiates > triptans > NSAIDs
- Cerebral ischemic events (rare)

REFERENCES

1. Headache Classification Committee of the International Headache Society (IHS). The International Classification of Headache Disorders, 3rd edition. *Cephalalgia*. 2018;38(1):1–211.
2. Sacco S, Merki-Feld GS, Ægidius KL, et al. Hormonal contraceptives and risk of ischemic stroke in women with migraine: a consensus statement from the European Headache Federation (EHF) and the European Society of Contraception and Reproductive Health (ESC). *J Headache Pain*. 2017;18(1):108.
3. Loder E, Weizenbaum E, Frishberg B, et al; for American Headache Society Choosing Wisely Task Force. Choosing wisely in headache medicine: the American Headache Society's list of five things physicians and patients should question. *Headache*. 2013;53(10):1651–1659.
4. Becker WJ. Acute migraine treatment in adults. *Headache*. 2015;55(6):778–793.
5. Charles AC, Digre KB, Goadsby PJ, et al. Calcitonin gene-related peptide-targeting therapies are a first-line option for the prevention of migraine: An American Headache Society position statement update. *Headache*. 2024;64(4):333–341. doi:10.1111/head.14692.
6. Loder E, Burch R, Rizzoli P. The 2012 AHS/AAN guidelines for prevention of episodic migraine: a summary and comparison with other recent clinical practice guidelines. *Headache*. 2012;52(6):930–945.
7. Patterson-Gentile C, Szperka CL. The changing landscape of pediatric migraine therapy: a review. *JAMA Neurol*. 2018;75(7):881–887.

SEE ALSO

Algorithm: Headache, Chronic

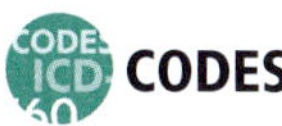

CODES

ICD10

- G43.909 Migraine, unsp, not intractable, without status migrainosus
- G43.109 Migraine with aura, not intractable, w/o status migrainosus
- G43.409 Hemiplegic migraine, not intractable, w/o status migrainosus

CLINICAL PEARLS

- Migraine is a chronic headache disorder of unclear etiology often characterized by unilateral, throbbing pain that may be associated with additional neurologic symptoms.
- Consider OTC analgesics for mild attacks; migraine-specific treatments for more severe attacks or those not responding to OTC medications
- Avoid opiates and barbiturates or frequent (>8/month) triptan or NSAIDs use to minimize MOH
- Counsel on lifestyle modifications and trigger identification.
- Prophylactic treatment if frequent/debilitating migraines

HEADACHE, TENSION

Madhavi Medipally, MD, FAAFP

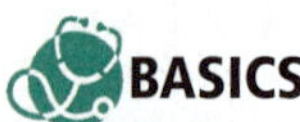

BASICS

DESCRIPTION

- A bilateral mild to moderate, nonthrobbing head pain or pressure, without other associated symptoms
- Tension-type headache (TTH) replaced the older terms muscle contraction headache; stress, ordinary, or essential headache; idiopathic headache; and psychogenic headache

EPIDEMIOLOGY

It is the most common type of primary headache and the second-most prevalent headache disorder in the world.

Prevalence

- Peak age of prevalence in the United States is in the 4th decade.
- Prevalence of episodic TTH decreases with age, whereas the prevalence of chronic TTH increases with age.

ETIOLOGY AND PATHOPHYSIOLOGY

- Not well understood, multifactorial etiology with both peripheral and central nervous system mechanisms triggering TTH
- Activation of peripheral nociceptors leads to myofascial pain in episodic TTH.
- Prolonged stimulation of nociceptors sensitizes the central pain pathways leading to chronic TTH.
- Nitric oxide may play an important role in TTH.

RISK FACTORS

Associated with triggers/precipitating factors:

- Stress (mental or physical)
- Change in sleep regimen
- Skipping meals, dehydration
- Certain foods (caffeine, alcohol, chocolate)
- Environmental factors (sun glare, odors, smoke, noise, lighting)
- Female hormonal changes
- Medications (e.g., nitrates, SSRIs, antihypertensives)
- Overuse of abortive headache medication

GENERAL PREVENTION

Lifestyle factors to promote headache prevention include avoiding triggers, increasing exercise, keeping regular sleep patterns, decreasing caffeine and alcohol, and staying adequately hydrated.

COMMONLY ASSOCIATED CONDITIONS

- 83% of patients with migraine headaches also suffer from TTHs.
- Possible increased prevalence of comorbid anxiety and depression

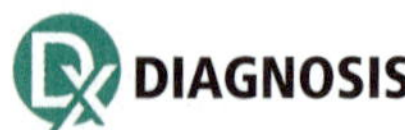

DIAGNOSIS

HISTORY

Obtain a thorough pain history to rule out other headache disorders, including onset, location, radiation, quality of pain, severity, associated symptoms; concurrent medical conditions and medications; and recent trauma or other procedures.

- Diagnosis is based on clinical assessment.
- Pain may be described in many ways, such as "dull," "band-like," and "pressure."
- Diagnostic criteria by the International Headache Society (ICHD-3) (1):
  - Episodic TTH: ≥10 headache episodes that meet all of the following criteria:
    - Headache lasting 30 minutes to 7 days
    - At least two of the following:
      - Bilateral location
      - Pressing/tightening (nonpulsating) quality
      - Mild or moderate intensity
      - Not aggravated by routine physical activity
    - Not associated with:
      - Nausea or vomiting
      - No more than one of photophobia or phonophobia
    - Headache not due to another ICHD-3 diagnosis
  - Chronic TTH: ≥15 days/month (on average) for >3 months that meet all of the following criteria:
    - Headache lasting hours to days, or unremitting
    - At least two of the following:
      - Bilateral location
      - Pressing/tightening (nonpulsating) quality
      - Mild or moderate intensity
      - Not aggravated by routine physical activity
    - Both of the following:
      - No more than one of photophobia, phonophobia, or mild nausea
      - Neither moderate or severe nausea nor vomiting
- Must assess and rule out "red flag" symptoms that suggest secondary headache causes as follows:
  - Thunderclap headache, fever, meningismus, focal neurologic deficit, pregnancy, age >50 years, neoplasm history, positional exacerbation of headache, worsened by sneezing/coughing, painful eye, and vision changes

PHYSICAL EXAM

- Assess vital signs looking for elevated blood pressure.
- Usually unremarkable clinical exam
- Head and neck: palpation of myofascial tissues for pericranial muscle tenderness including the cervical paraspinal muscles, trapezius, muscles of mastication, and for pain near the jaw around the temporomandibular joint
- Neurologic exam: mental status, pupillary responses, motor-strength testing, deep tendon reflexes, sensation, cerebellar function, gait testing, signs of meningeal irritation

DIFFERENTIAL DIAGNOSIS

- Migraine or cluster headache
- Ischemic cerebrovascular disease, cerebral venous thrombosis, intracranial hemorrhage
- Temporal arteritis
- Arterial hypertension (HTN), benign intracranial HTN
- Intracranial neoplasm
- Infection such as meningitis, encephalitis, sinusitis, and acute otitis media
- Medication (nonprescription analgesic dependency, nitrates)
- Caffeine dependency
- Metabolic disorders (hypoxia, hypercapnia, hypoglycemia)
- Temporomandibular joint syndrome
- Eyes: glaucoma, refractive errors
- Cervical spondylosis
- Severe anemia or polycythemia
- Paget disease of bone

DIAGNOSTIC TESTS & INTERPRETATION

- Most primary headaches with typical features do not require lab testing or diagnostic imaging and recommendations regarding TTH and neuroimaging are not well-defined.
- MRI/CT imaging is rarely revealing for chronic or recurrent headaches with normal neurologic findings (see "Additional Reading").

Initial Tests (lab, imaging)

Labs and neuroimaging (CT or MRI) should be considered when a secondary cause is suspected:

- Atypical pattern of headache (does not fit specific category such as migraine, cluster, or tension)
- Rapid increase in frequency
- Unexplained focal neurologic findings
- New onset after age 35 years
- Sudden onset or worsening with exertion

Follow-Up Tests & Special Considerations

Some may find that a headache diary is useful to track symptoms, triggers, and response to treatment.

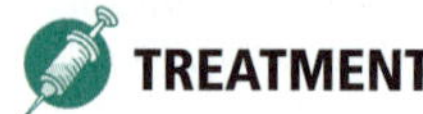

TREATMENT

GENERAL MEASURES

Relief measures include relaxation routines; rest in quiet, dark room; hot bath or shower; massage of back of neck and temples

MEDICATION

- Nonsteroidal anti-inflammatory drugs (NSAIDs), aspirin, or acetaminophen are effective for short-term relief of episodic TTH (2)[B].
- Amitriptyline (10 to 25 mg nightly) should be considered first line for prophylaxis of chronic TTH (2)[B].

First Line

- For acute treatment in episodic TTH:
  - NSAIDs:
    - Ibuprofen (Motrin, Advil): 400 mg; may repeat q8h PRN (max 3.2 g/day)
    - Naproxen sodium (Naprosyn): 220 to 550 mg BID PRN (max 1,250 mg base/day)
    - Contraindications: aspirin or NSAIDs allergy or bronchospasm, renal disease, bleeding disorders, increased risk of cardiovascular events (myocardial infarction [MI], stroke, new onset or worsening of HTN)
    - Drug interactions: antihypertensives, anticoagulants, antiplatelet drugs, aspirin, lithium, methotrexate
    - Adverse effects: epigastric distress, peptic ulcer
  - Aspirin: 650 to 1,000 mg; may repeat q6h PRN (max 4 g/day):
    - Contraindication: aspirin or NSAIDs allergy or bronchospasm, bleeding disorders, peptic ulcer
    - Drug interactions: anticoagulants, antiplatelet drugs, ACE inhibitors, β-blockers, corticosteroids, NSAIDs, sulfonylureas
    - Adverse effects: GI irritation/bleeding, thrombocytopenia
  - Acetaminophen (Tylenol): 1,000 mg; may repeat q6h PRN (max 3 to 4 g/day):
    - Adverse effects (rare): rash, pancytopenia, liver damage
    - Precaution: hepatic impairment, consumption of ≥3/day alcoholic beverages

- For prophylaxis in frequent episodic and chronic TTH:
  - Tricyclic antidepressants (TCAs): amitriptyline (Elavil): Start at 10 mg, may slowly up-titrate to 100 mg QHS.
    - Not FDA-approved for chronic TTH, but there is high quality evidence that TCAs have moderate benefit and are superior to placebo (3)[A]. Benefits are observed after 3 months of use.
    - Consider if patient has depression, anxiety, or insomnia; efficacy is observed in patients without comorbid depression.
    - Mechanism is thought to involve both central and peripheral pathways, including inhibition of norepinephrine reuptake and modulation of pain pathways.
    - Contraindications: acute recovery phase (within 30 days) of MI, use of monoamine oxidase inhibitors (MAOIs) within 14 days
    - Drug interactions: clonidine, MAOIs, quinolone antibiotics, SSRIs, sympathomimetics, azole antifungals, valproic acid
    - Adverse effects: weight gain, drowsiness, dry mouth, tachycardia, heart block, blurred vision, urinary retention, seizure

Second Line

- For acute treatment in episodic TTH:
  - Caffeine combinations: 130 mg caffeine with 500 mg acetaminophen and/or 500 mg aspirin q6h PRN (2)[C]
  - Ketorolac: 60 mg IM once, for severe episodes
  - Opioids (e.g., codeine), butalbital, or their combination are not recommended. Consider secondary causes of headache or secondary gain such as drug-seeking behavior for personal use or diversion/sale.
- For prophylaxis in frequent episodic and chronic TTH:
  - Mirtazapine: 15 to 30 mg/day (not FDA-approved for chronic TTH) (2)[B]
  - Venlafaxine 150 mg/day (2)[B]

ALERT

Use of abortive agents >2 days/week may lead to medication-overuse headaches; must withdraw acute treatment to diagnose.

ADDITIONAL THERAPIES

- The combination of stress management therapy and a TCA (amitriptyline) may be most effective for chronic TTH.
- Topiramate: 100 mg/day (limited clinical evidence for prevention of chronic TTH; not FDA-approved for chronic TTH)
- Alternative TCAs with evidence of benefit (3)[B]:
  - Nortriptyline (Pamelor): 25 to 50 mg/day (mild to moderately sedating, causes weight gain)
  - Protriptyline (Vivactil): 25 mg/day (nonsedating, causes weight loss)
- Tizanidine has conflicting clinical evidence for use in chronic TTH, thus should not be considered.

SURGERY/OTHER PROCEDURES

Trigger point lidocaine injections may reduce headache frequency, while botulinum toxin type a (Botox) injections have conflicting evidence to support their use in TTH.

COMPLEMENTARY & ALTERNATIVE MEDICINE

Many complementary and alternative medicine treatment modalities have been investigated with varying degrees of success, although quality evidence remains limited (4). Some modalities include the following:

- Tiger Balm or peppermint oil applied topically to the forehead
- Biobehavioral therapies including cognitive-behavioral therapy and biofeedback therapy
- Electromyography (EMG) biofeedback with or without relaxation therapy
- Physical therapy, including positioning, ergonomic instruction, massage, transcutaneous electrical nerve stimulation, application of heat/cold, manual joint mobilization techniques
- Exercise, primarily upper-limb resistance training (5)
- Chiropractic spinal manipulation has equivocal evidence in the management of episodic and chronic TTH.
- Cervical manual therapy, particularly soft-tissue and trigger-point therapies
- Acupuncture (6)
- Intraoral splinting, particularly with a stabilization splint (SS) or a nociceptive trigeminal inhibition splint (NTIS) (7)

ONGOING CARE

DIET

- Identify and avoid dietary triggers.
- Regulate meal schedule.

PATIENT EDUCATION

- National Headache Foundation: https://www.headaches.org/resources
- Family Doctor by American Academy of Family Physicians: https://familydoctor.org/condition/headaches

PROGNOSIS

Most cases are intermittent and decrease with age.

COMPLICATIONS

- Medication-overuse headache
- GI bleeding from NSAIDs use
- Dependence/addiction to narcotic analgesics

REFERENCES

1. Headache Classification Committee of the International Headache Society (IHS). The international classification of headache disorders, 3rd edition. *Cephalalgia*. 2018;38(1):1–211.
2. Becker WJ, Findlay T, Moga C, et al. Guideline for primary care management of headache in adults. *Can Fam Physician*. 2015;61(8):670–679.
3. Jackson JL, Mancuso JM, Nickoloff S, et al. Tricyclic and tetracyclic antidepressants for the prevention of frequent episodic or chronic tension-type headaches in adults: a systematic review and meta-analysis. *J Gen Intern Med*. 2017;32(12):1351–1358.
4. Sun-Edelstein C, Mauskop A. Complementary and alternative approaches to the treatment of tension-type headache. *Curr Pain Headache Rep*. 2012;16(6):539–544.
5. Varangot-Reille C, Suso-Martí L, Dubuis V, et al. Exercise and manual therapy for the treatment of primary headache: an umbrella and mapping review. *Phys Ther*. 2022;102(3):pzab308.
6. Linde K, Allais G, Brinkhaus B, et al. Acupuncture for the prevention of tension-type headache. *Cochrane Database Syst Rev*. 2016;4(4):CD007587.
7. Martínez-Álvarez O, Wojtovicz E, De la Hoz JL, et al. Effectiveness of intraoral splints in the treatment of migraine and tension-type headache: a systematic review. *Clin Exp Dent Res*. 2023;9(6):1180–1190.

ADDITIONAL READING

Viera AJ, Antono B. Acute headache in adults: a diagnostic approach. *Am Fam Physician*. 2022;106(3):260–268.

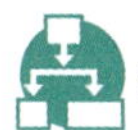

SEE ALSO

Algorithm: Headache

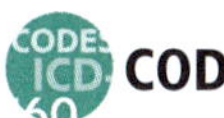

CODES

ICD10

- G44.209 Tension-type headache, unspecified, not intractable
- G44.219 Episodic tension-type headache, not intractable
- G44.229 Chronic tension-type headache, not intractable

CLINICAL PEARLS

- Typical characteristics include bilateral mild to moderate, nonthrobbing head pain or pressure, without other associated symptoms.
- First-line therapy for TTH includes NSAIDs or acetaminophen. For preventive therapy, TCAs have benefit, but they are not FDA-approved for this indication.
- Consider secondary causes and obtain further testing, such as neuroimaging, if there are unexplained focal neurologic signs, atypical presentation, late onset (>50 years of age), or when usual treatment fails.
- Chronic TTH is difficult to treat, and it can lead to medication-overuse headaches if abortive therapy is used >2 days/week.
- Avoid the use of opioids or butalbital-containing medications as first-line treatment for recurrent headaches.

HEARING LOSS

Laura Torrico Brusky, MD

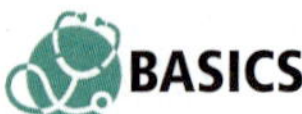

BASICS

Hearing loss (HL) is one of the most common conditions that interfere with a person's ability to work and lead a normal life; when occurring at birth, can limit child development and speech; when onset occurs in childhood, can lead to poor literacy; when occurs later in life, can contribute to the development of dementia

DESCRIPTION

- HL is the inability to perceive sound. Divided by different levels of severity:
  - Mild (>25 dB): difficult to understand speech in a loud environment.
  - Moderate (>40 dB): affects speech development in children
  - Severe (>60 dB): able to hear only loud sounds; no speech
  - Profound (>80 dB): unable to hear any sound
- Also distinguished as conductive or sensory neural:
  - Conductive hearing loss (CHL): external and middle ear
  - Sensorineural hearing loss (SNHL): inner ear (cochlea) and/or acoustic nerve/acoustic central nuclei

EPIDEMIOLOGY

>1.5 billion people live with HL, 403 million (26%) of whom have moderate-to-complete HL in their better ear.

Prevalence

Hearing impairment is the third cause of disability worldwide. WHO estimates that 60% of HL in children is due to preventable causes. In the United States, the prevalence doubles with every 10-year increase in age.

ETIOLOGY AND PATHOPHYSIOLOGY

- Causes in children:
  - Infections
    - Middle ear infections (otitis media [OM])
    - Mumps, rubella measles, meningitis (cochlea)
  - Birth related causes (ototoxic meds, low birth, prematurity)
  - Genetic
    - >100 mutations: congenital HL in newborns
    - Syndromes (e.g., Stickler syndrome, Alport syndrome)
  - Other causes
    - Impacted cerumen
    - Perforation of tympanic membrane (TM), Cholesteatoma (chronic OM)
- Causes in adults:
  - CHL
    - Impacted cerumen
    - External ear infection (swimmer's ear)
    - Cholesteatoma and chronic OM
    - Barotrauma
    - Radiotherapy (damage to middle ear and TM)
    - Otosclerosis
  - SNHL
    - Acoustic neuroma compression of 8th nerve.
    - Cholesteatoma invading the inner ear/cochlea
    - Ménière disease with cochlear hydrops
    - Chronic diseases
  - Diabetes, HTN: microvascular/macrovascular changes in inner ear and auditory system
  - Autoimmune diseases: hypothesized that autoantibodies destroy hair cells of the inner ear and vestibular nerve; common in lupus, Cogan disease, vitiligo, sarcoidosis, rheumatoid arthritis
  - Ototoxic drugs: damage to hair cells
    - Aminoglycosides
    - Cisplatin
    - Radiotherapy: damages inner ear, auditory, and vestibular nerve pathways
    - Macrolides: caution in individuals with personal/family history of HL
  - Substance use disorder: permanent HL (opioids) or temporary (cocaine, heroin)
- Environmental exposure
  - Noise: permanent damage to hair cells
  - Tobacco exposure
- COVID-19 infection: caused by the inflammation or autoimmune process
- Age-related HL
  - Gradual and progressing degeneration of inner ear but also of the central auditory nerve pathways; worsening with age; starts with high frequencies; worsening speech intelligibility
    - Sudden HL is often associated with tinnitus and vertigo.
      - Possible causes: viral, vascular (brainstem stroke), illicit drugs, COVID-19, autoimmune

RISK FACTORS

- Lifestyle
  - Smoking 2.8% incidence
  - Chronic conditions 3.8% incidence (metabolic syndrome, diabetes, HTN)
- Leisure
  - Loud prolonged noise exposure (hunting, playing music through headphones, attending concerts)
  - Illicit drug use
- Genetic susceptibility
- Infections

GENERAL PREVENTION

Based on reduction of risk factors

- Noise induced HL is 16% of the disabling HL in adults worldwide accounting for 4 million daily is attributable to occupational noise exposure.
  - Hearing conservation program: required for work exposure >85 dB; includes noise exposure monitoring; personal hearing protection; audiometric evaluations; employee education
  - Antioxidant drugs may help the regeneration of hair cells of organ of Corti (unclear mechanism).
  - Hearing protection during leisure activity noise exposure (appropriate headphones while attending concerts, play music, hunting)
- Nutrition
  - Balanced and adequate nutrition during pregnancy and childhood, reduces HL in adult life and overall life span.
  - Supplements
- Antioxidants, carotenoids, folate, maintenance of antioxidants homeostasis
- Vitamin A and zinc: decrease frequency of OM episodes

COMMONLY ASSOCIATED CONDITIONS

Tinnitus and vertigo are common in SNHL.

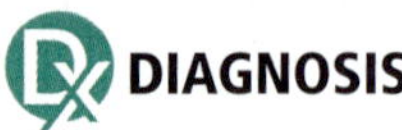

DIAGNOSIS

HISTORY

Attention to:

- Family history of HL
- Prior history of ear infections or ear infections as a child
- Associated symptoms: tinnitus, otalgia, otorrhea, vertigo
- Loud noise exposure
- Substance use disorder (opioids)
- History of surgery on skull base/ear

PHYSICAL EXAM

- External exam: Determine if there are deformities of external ear; facial asymmetry, and facial nerve paralysis.
- Otoscopy: Determine possible cause of CHL.
  - Hyperemia of TM; effusion in middle ear; evidence of TM rupture; visible cholesteatoma; chronic infection; impacted cerumen
- Pneumoscopy: to evaluate if the TM is hypomobile (effusion in middle ear), hypermobile (otosclerosis), or normally mobile

- Finger rub test: can rule out profound or severe HL
- Whispered voice test: A whisper heard from ~2 feet away is a good screen for intact hearing.
- Tuning fork test: 256 Hz if cannot hear, HL is about 10 to 15 dB. Use 512 Hz if failed in 256 Hz tuning fork test; if failed in this too, HL is about 20 to 30 dB.
- Weber test: tuning fork placed in midline of forehead
  - Normal: sound heard in both ears
  - CHL: sound louder in affected ear
  - SNHL: sound louder in normal ear
  - HL: Sound louder in affected ear
- Rinne test: tuning fork near ear, then mastoid
  - Normal: sound louder with fork near ear
  - CHL: sound louder with fork on mastoid
  - SNHL: sound louder in contralateral ear

DIAGNOSTIC TESTS & INTERPRETATION

- Pure Tone audiometry:
  - Determine the severity of HL if CHL or SNHL or mixed, unilateral, or bilateral. 2021 WHO standards: Normal hearing is defined as an average value for the air and bone conduction curve evaluated at 4 octave frequencies (0.5 kHz, 1 kHz, 2 kHz, 4 kHz) that is below 20 dB.
- Speech audiometry: consists of speech reception threshold and words discrimination score; it is useful to determine prognosis of hearing aids.
- Impedance audiometry
  - Tympanometry: abnormal in middle ear effusion, otosclerosis
- Auditory brainstem response (ABR): Assess auditory central pathways; used when failed otoacoustic emissions (OAE).
- OAE: valid newborn screening
- Imaging
  - CT head without contrast: Evaluate fractures of temporal bone and inner ear.
  - MRI skull base: to evaluate for acoustic neuroma

TREATMENT

- Amplification options/treatment
  - Even though treatment of HL has clear benefits on quality of life (QOL), access is still low and cost remains the main barrier.
- External ear hearing aids
  - In moderate HL, studies show benefit in QOL in using hearing aids.
- Implantable hearing aids
  - In moderate to severe HL.
- Cochlear implants
  - In bilateral profound to severe HL since birth, the earlier the implantation the better as it will influence speech development.

MEDICATION

- Oral antibiotic therapy
  - In acute OM
- Oral corticosteroid therapy: first line in sudden HL
  - In viral stroke related HL
  - Ménière disease hydrops

ISSUES FOR REFERRAL

- Failed newborn screening
- Speech therapist: if speech delay or speech impediment is present
- Neurology and neurosurgery: intracranial masses, complications

ADDITIONAL THERAPIES

Aural rehabilitation optimizes auditory function through an integration of sensory management, perceptual training, and counseling.

SURGERY/OTHER PROCEDURES

Surgical options for CHL:

- Cholesteatoma débridement and removal *plus* mastoidectomy
- Myringotomy with ear tubes placement
- Tympanoplasty with or without ossicula chain reconstruction (otosclerosis)

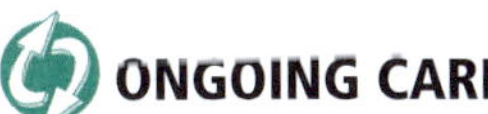

ONGOING CARE

FOLLOW-UP RECOMMENDATIONS

Patient Monitoring

Audiogram and clinical exam are the primary means of monitoring patients.

DIET

- Salt restriction to 2 g/day is helpful for patients with Ménière disease.
- Balanced diet can be helpful in pregnancy and childhood and in slowing progression of HL related to chronic disease.

PATIENT EDUCATION

- Avoid excessive and prolonged noise exposure and use protective equipment.
- Limit use of ototoxic medicine to strictly necessary.

PROGNOSIS

- SNHL is usually permanent and may be progressive.
- Idiopathic sudden SNHL (ISSNHL) may recover spontaneously in 32–70% of cases, but urgent referral and treatment is recommended to maximize recovery.

COMPLICATIONS

Chronic OM can involve the inner ear and lead to serious complications if not treated in time.

ADDITIONAL READING

- Hu S, Sun Q, Xu F, et al. Age-related hearing loss and its potential drug candidates: a systematic review. *Chinese Med*. 2023;18:121. doi:10.1186/s13020-023-00825-6.
- Hughes ML, Rodriguez AI, Hatch J, et al. Hearing and vestibular loss with misuse of opioids and illicit drugs: a review of the literature. *Audiol Neurootol*. 2022;27(4):271–281. doi:10.1159/000521965.

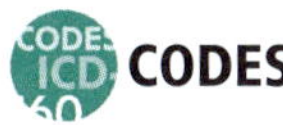

CODES

ICD10

- H91.11 Presbycusis, right ear
- H91 Other and unspecified hearing loss
- H91.09 Ototoxic hearing loss, unspecified ear

CLINICAL PEARLS

- Diagnose/treat sudden HL as soon as possible because it can possibly be reversible with early treatment.
- Encourage discussion about prevention of risk factors of HL and screen annually at any age to detect early HL and recommend treatment when available.

HEART FAILURE, ACUTELY DECOMPENSATED

Jeffrey Shih, MD • Alexandre J. Wenk-Bodenmiller, MD

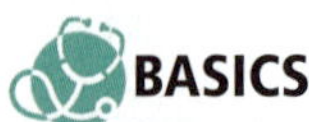

BASICS

DESCRIPTION

Acute decompensated heart failure (ADHF) is a clinical syndrome of worsened signs and symptoms of heart failure (HF). It is a heterogenous group of syndromes presenting with different phenotypes. The worsened symptoms of ADHF are due to a rise in cardiac filling pressures. This can be due to worsening dysfunction of the myocardium or heart valves; however, it can also arise from complications related to the pericardium or endocardium. The pathophysiology is characterized by either impaired ventricular filling or decreased ejection of blood resulting in pulmonary vascular and/or systemic venous congestion. In severe cases, it can cause tissue hypoperfusion and present as cardiogenic shock. ADHF can be a new diagnosis or represent worsening of preexisting HF. A number of terms have been used to describe this pathology including acute HF and acute decompensation of chronic HF.

EPIDEMIOLOGY

Incidence

HF is one of the most common causes of admission and readmission in the United States in those >65 years of age, responsible for >1 million annual hospitalizations.

Prevalence

HF is primarily a disease of the elderly. About half of people who have HF die within 5 years of diagnosis, and 90% of patients who have HF die within 10 years.

ETIOLOGY AND PATHOPHYSIOLOGY

- Two main pathophysiologic conditions lead to the clinical findings of HF, namely systolic and/or diastolic dysfunction. Systolic dysfunction is an inotropic abnormality, whereas diastolic dysfunction is a compliance abnormality.
  - The terms HF with reduced, mid-range, or preserved LVEF (HFrEF, HFmrEF, HFpEF, respectively) describe the HF phenotypes.
  - HF guidelines have also described three clinical profiles of patients with ADHF that take into account the patient's clinical manifestations, hemodynamics, and systemic perfusion:
    - Patients with volume overload: evidenced by pulmonary vascular and/or systemic venous congestion and often triggered by an acute hypertensive crisis
    - Patients with depression of cardiac output: evidenced by hypotension, renal hypoperfusion, and/or shock
    - Patients with signs and symptoms of both volume overload and shock
- ADHF can result from the following:
  - Myocardial disease: Exacerbation of preexisting chronic HF can be triggered by medication noncompliance, diet, infection, or some other acute insult such as coronary artery disease (CAD) and myocardial infarction (MI), immune-mediated and inflammatory damage, infiltrative diseases, metabolic derangements, toxins, and genetic abnormalities.
  - Valvular disease: progressive or acute regurgitant or stenotic valvular lesions
  - Abnormal ventricular filling: elevated afterload and hypertension (HTN), valvular and myocardial structural defects, pericardial and endomyocardial pathologies, high-output states, volume overload
  - Arrhythmias: atrial fibrillation, tachyarrhythmias, high-grade heart block, bradyarrhythmias
- Approximately 70% of patients with ADHF have worsening chronic HF, 25% present with HF for the first time, and 5% present with advanced or end-stage HF.

Genetics

HF may be secondary to dilated cardiomyopathy (DCM). In patients with a family history of DCM, genetic variants have been implicated in 25–40% of patients. With no recognized family history of DCM, variants can be found in 10–30% of patients.

COMMONLY ASSOCIATED CONDITIONS

Patients with HF commonly have comorbid conditions; commonly include CAD, HTN, obesity, diabetes mellitus, chronic kidney disease

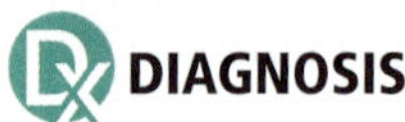

DIAGNOSIS

HISTORY

The most common presenting symptom is dyspnea. Patients may also present with orthopnea, paroxysmal nocturnal dyspnea, edema, or fatigue.

PHYSICAL EXAM

- An S_3 gallop has high positive predictive value of elevated filling pressures. An S_3 gallop combined with jugular venous distension has high sensitivity for identifying patients with elevated pulmonary capillary wedge pressure.
- Rales (crackles) and sometimes wheezing can be present but are an insensitive sign of ADHF.
- Edema, hepatomegaly, and ascites are non-specific signs of elevated filling pressures.
- Tachycardia and low pulse pressure may be present and can signify a low cardiac output state.

DIFFERENTIAL DIAGNOSIS

The diagnosis of ADHF can at times be challenging or may be secondary to another issue. The differential diagnosis includes: pulmonary embolism, MI, tamponade, pneumothorax, acute respiratory distress syndrome (ARDS), sepsis, chronic obstructive pulmonary disease (COPD), pneumonia, constrictive pericarditis, high-output states (anemia, hyperthyroidism).

DIAGNOSTIC TESTS & INTERPRETATION

Laboratory data are adjunctive and help with prognostication and clinical course.

Initial Tests (lab, imaging)

- Assess blood pressure (BP), heart rate, and other signs and symptoms of hypoperfusion to rule out hemodynamic instability and signs of cardiogenic shock. A lactic acid level may help to identify those who are in cardiogenic shock.
- ECG and cardiac troponins to evaluate for acute coronary syndrome (ACS). Note that elevated troponins can be found in many HF patients in the absence of ACS.
- BUN, creatinine, electrolytes, liver function tests, TSH (new onset), UA, iron studies (new onset), glucose, and CBC.
- Transthoracic echocardiogram: recommended immediately in hemodynamically unstable ADHF patients and within 48 hours when cardiac structure and function are either not known or may have changed since previous studies.
- BNP and/or N-terminal fragment pro-BNP (NT-proBNP): Measurement of BNP or NT-proBNP is recommended in all patients with acute dyspnea and suspected ADHF when the cause of dyspnea is unclear. BNP <100 essentially will rule out HF. BNP >400 is suggestive of ADHF as a cause of dyspnea. BNP 100 to 400 is an intermediate range and may indicate HF but also other cardiac, noncardiac (e.g., pulmonary), or multiple conditions.
- NT-proBNP values >450 pg/mL for people age <50 years, >900 pg/mL ages 50 to 75 years, and >1,800 pg/mL ages >75 years are highly suggestive of ADHF as a cause of dyspnea.
- Chest x-ray: to assess for pulmonary congestion and to detect other cardiac or noncardiac diseases that may cause or contribute to the patient's symptoms
- Lung ultrasound (LUS): emerging as a recommended diagnostic tool for ADHF (1) with a positive LUS defined by the presence of >3 B lines in two bilateral lung zones yielding a specificity of 92.7% and LR of 7.4%

Diagnostic Procedures/Other

Cardiac catheterization may be considered when CAD is suspected. Pulmonary artery catheterization is not recommended for the routine management of ADHF but has growing evidence of benefit in the management of cardiogenic shock.

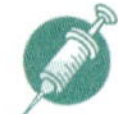

TREATMENT

The initial goals of treatment are to improve hemodynamics and organ perfusion, alleviate symptoms, limit cardiac and renal damage, and to restore oxygenation. Once stabilized, the goal is to identify the inciting cause or precipitating factors, decrease hospital length of stay, and to optimize as well as educate the patient to prevent future exacerbations. Below recommendations are all derived from the 2022 AHA/ACC/HFSA guideline for the management of HF (2)[C] and its 2024 update (3)

GENERAL MEASURES

- There is no definitive evidence that sodium and fluid restriction improves outcomes. However, it is reasonable to include restrictions on both to facilitate decongestion.
- Monitoring daily weights and intake and output balance can help guide treatment.

MEDICATION

ALERT

- Although many therapies in the acute phase do not improve long-term mortality, prompt and evidence-based treatment of ADHF leads to improved patient centered outcomes including avoidance of mechanical ventilation, symptomatic and functional improvement, and decreased length of stay. Vital signs and physical exam should guide the initial triage and resuscitation of critically ill patients with suspected ADHF. Critically ill, hypertensive patients (typically SBP >180) in ADHF may benefit from afterload reduction with vasodilators such as nitrates, whereas those who are hypotensive or demonstrating signs of shock may benefit from the addition of vasopressors and/or inotropes. In either case, respiratory support with the early use of noninvasive positive pressure ventilation (NIPPV) such as CPAP/BiPAP has been associated with improved outcomes.
- Once stabilized, diuretics are given for symptom control in parallel to guideline directed medical therapies (GDMT) that have been shown to improve long-term survival. As tolerated, a full GDMT regimen includes four components: ACE inhibitors (also, ARBs/ARNIs), β-receptor blockers, mineral corticoid receptor antagonists (MRA), and SGLT2 inhibitors. It should be noted that there are no class IA drug recommendations for ADHF. SGLT2 inhibitors and mineralocorticoid antagonists have little effect to reduce BP and in the absence of contraindications, can be initiated at any time during hospitalization and continued at discharge if feasible.
- In conjunction with GDMT, risk factor modification with antihypertensives, statins, and glycemic agents should be considered.
- Early follow-up within 7 days is recommended as part of a transition-of-care plan on discharge.

First Line

- Vasodilators: Consider in ADHF with systolic BP (SBP) >90 mm Hg. Patients with hypertensive ADHF should receive IV vasodilators as initial therapy to improve hemodynamics if no contraindications exist. Vasodilators lower ventricular filling pressure and systemic vascular resistance to indirectly improve cardiac function. Use in chronic HF is not effective.
  - IV nitroglycerin decreases preload and afterload by relaxing the smooth muscle in peripheral venous capacitance and arterial resistance vessels, respectively (IV 10 to 20 μg/minute, increase up to 200 μg/minute).
  - IV nitroprusside: Administer with caution, start with 0.3 μg/kg/minute, and increase up to 5 μg/kg/minute.
- IV loop diuretics are recommended for all patients with ADHF and symptoms of fluid overload in hemodynamically stable patients; be cautious of electrolyte abnormalities and if kidney disease is present. Diuresis should be instituted early in ADHF, continuous infusion is no better than bolus. Give an adequate dose that results in sodium loss and enhanced urine output. Furosemide is the most commonly used diuretic but bumetanide is also available in IV form.
  - Furosemide: New-onset ADHF patients should get boluses of 20 to 40 mg IV if their renal function is normal. Consider higher doses if there is chronic kidney disease even if the patient is loop diuretic-naive. If on furosemide chronically, initial IV dose should be equal or exceed chronic oral daily dose (1.0 to 2.5 times home dose). Monitor for appropriate urine output.
  - Torsemide is not available in IV formulation in all countries.
  - Bumetanide can be given at 0.5 to 1.0 mg IV for patients without chronic use of loop diuretics.
  - When congestion fails to improve with initial diuretic therapy, consideration should be given to addition of second type of diuretic orally (metolazone) or intravenously (chlorothiazide).
- Patients with renal insufficiency or renal hypoperfusion may have diuretic resistance. If diuresis is refractory to single agent loop agents, then a thiazide and an MRA can be considered. Common thiazides for this indication include: hydrochlorothiazide 25 to 50 mg PO or metolazone 2.5 to 20.0 mg/day PO. MRAs include spironolactone or eplerenone (25 to 50 mg PO).
- Acetazolamide 500 mg IV daily in combination with a loop diuretic can achieve better decongestion than a loop diuretic alone.
- NIPPV with BIPAP or CPAP decreases symptom severity, rate of intubation, and early mortality in ADHF.

Second Line

- Tolvaptan is approved for use in hypervolemic hyponatremia and increases free water loss. It can be used as an adjunct in those with ADHF with hyponatremia. Tolvaptan can result in risk of hepatotoxicity and can result in too rapid correction of sodium.
- Inotropes: reserved for patients with a low cardiac output phenotype or cardiogenic shock
  - Phosphodiesterase inhibitors (milrinone, enoximone) decrease pulmonary resistance; may be used for patients on β-blockers but may increase medium-term mortality in CAD patients. Hypotension can occur.
  - Dobutamine infusion 2.5 to 20.0 μg/kg/minute can be used in cardiogenic shock.
  - Low-dose dopamine infusion may be considered (3 to 5 μg/kg/minute).
  - No clear differences in efficacy and adverse effects based on one randomized trial comparing dobutamine and milrinone
- Vasopressors: Consider in patients with cardiogenic shock and low mean arterial pressure below 60 mm Hg despite treatment with another inotrope.
- Mechanical circulatory support (MCS) should be considered in patients who do not respond favorably to single inotropic support.

SURGERY/OTHER PROCEDURES

Heart valve surgery if valvular disease is responsible, PCI/CABG for patients with CAD/MI if applicable. For more rare diagnosis, consider disease specific approaches such as pericardiectomy for constrictive pericarditis.

ADMISSION, INPATIENT, AND NURSING CONSIDERATIONS

- Admission criteria considerations:
  - Evidence of severely decompensated HF: hypotension, worsening renal function, altered mental status, dyspnea at rest, concomitant arrhythmia, ACS, decreased functional status
  - Consider observation unit stay for stable patients with preexisting HF and the following: no acute interventions needed for comorbid condition, SBP >120 mm Hg, RR <32 breaths/minute, BUN <40 mg/dL, creatinine <3 mg/dL, no evidence of ischemia or elevated troponins, and BNP <1,000, N-type pro-BNP <5,000, and the clinical impression that the patient could be discharged in the next 24 hours.
- Discharge criteria: improved symptoms, SBP normalized at 100 to 120 mm Hg, good urine output, serum sodium >135 mEq/L, HF outpatient education

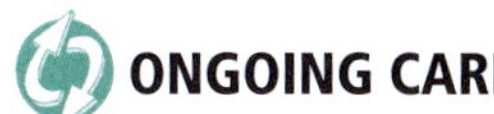

ONGOING CARE

FOLLOW-UP RECOMMENDATIONS

Patient Monitoring

Early follow-up and multidisciplinary care to reduce hospitalization and mortality

PATIENT EDUCATION

Monitoring and self-care; teach: medication, activity, daily weight (and how to adjust diuretic)

COMPLICATIONS

Arrhythmia, pulmonary edema, hyponatremia, death

REFERENCES

1. Silvers SM, Gemme SR, Hickey S, et al. Clinical policy: critical issues in the evaluation and management of adult patients presenting to the emergency department with acute heart failure syndromes: approved by ACEP Board of Directors, June 23, 2022. *Ann Emer Med*. 2022;80(4):e31–e59.
2. Heidenreich PA, Bozkurt B, Aguilar D, et al. 2022 AHA/ACC/HFSA guideline for the management of heart failure: a report of the American College of Cardiology/American Heart Association joint committee on clinical practice guidelines. *Circulation*. 2022;145(18):e895–e1032.
3. Hollenberg SM, Stevenson LW, Ahmad T, et al. 2024 ACC expert consensus decision pathway on clinical assessment, management, and trajectory of patients hospitalized with heart failure focused update: a report of the American College of Cardiology solution set oversight committee. *J Am Coll Cardiol*. 2024;84(13):1241–1267.

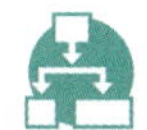

SEE ALSO

Heart Failure, Chronic

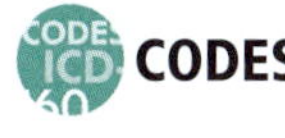

CODES

ICD10

- I50.9 Heart failure, unspecified
- I50.21 Acute systolic (congestive) heart failure
- I50.31 Acute diastolic (congestive) heart failure

CLINICAL PEARLS

Look for an underlying cause of each episode of ADHF.

HEART FAILURE, CHRONIC

Jeffrey Shih, MD

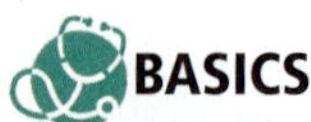

BASICS

DESCRIPTION

Heart failure (HF) results from inability of the heart to fill and/or pump blood sufficiently to meet tissue metabolic needs. Adequate cardiac output can be achieved only at the expense of elevated filling pressures. It is the principal complication of heart disease. For acute HF, see "Heart Failure, Acutely Decompensated."

- Can involve the left heart, the right heart, or be biventricular; it is progressive and manifested by remodeling (a complex process involving changes in the heart's structure and function due to abnormalities in hemodynamic loading, neurohormones, and other contributing factors). The AHA/ACC uses a staging system to delineate the one-way progression of HF: stage A: at risk for HF, no structural disease; stage B: structural disease, no HF symptoms; stage C: structural disease, HF symptoms; stage D: end-stage disease.
- The New York Heart Association (NYHA) classification is a subjective grading scale used for classifying a patient's functional status: NYHA I: asymptomatic; NYHA II: symptomatic with moderate exertion; NYHA III: symptomatic with mild exertion and may limit activities of daily living; NYHA IV: symptomatic at rest.

EPIDEMIOLOGY

HF accounts for close to 1 million hospitalizations a year, with 25% readmission in 30 days.

Incidence

In the United States, 550,000 new cases are diagnosed annually with >250,000 deaths/year. Incidence of HF with preserved ejection fraction (HFpEF) continues to rise accounting for >50% of HF cases.

Prevalence

Estimated 64 million individuals with HF worldwide; ~6.2 million people in the United States; prevalence increases with age; primarily a disease of the elderly; 75% of hospital admissions for HF are for persons >65 years of age.

ETIOLOGY AND PATHOPHYSIOLOGY

- Two physiologic components explain the clinical findings of HF and result in four categories:
  - HF with reduced ejection fraction (HFrEF): an *inotropic* abnormality, often from myocardial infarction (MI) or dilated cardiomyopathy (CM), resulting in diminished systolic emptying (ejection fraction [EF] ≤40%)
  - HF with mid-range EF (HFmEF): mild systolic dysfunction with EF of 41–49%, clinically behaves like HFpEF
  - HFpEF: a *compliance* abnormality, often due to hypertensive CM, in which the ventricular relaxation is impaired (EF ≥50%)
- Most common etiologies: coronary artery disease (CAD)/MI and hypertension (HTN). Others include myocarditis and CM (alcoholic, viral, drugs, muscular dystrophy, infiltrative [e.g., amyloidosis, sarcoidosis], postpartum, infectious [e.g., Chagas disease, HIV], hypertrophic CM [HCM], inherited familial dilated CM); valvular and vascular abnormalities (valvular stenosis or regurgitation, rheumatic heart; renal artery stenosis, usually bilateral, may cause recurrent "flash" pulmonary edema); chronic lung disease and pulmonary HTN; arrhythmias (atrial fibrillation [AFib], other tachyarrhythmias, high-grade heart block, frequent PVCs); other (high-output states: hyperthyroidism, anemia, dialysis fistulas; cardiac depressants [β-blocker overdose], stress-induced; iatrogenic volume overload [extreme overload in patients with normal hearts and kidneys]; idiopathic: 20–50% of idiopathic dilated CM are familial.)

Genetics

Multiple genetic abnormalities responsible for a variety of phenotypes have been identified. The TTN gene, which encodes the titin protein, is one of the most recognized causes of familial CM.

RISK FACTORS

CAD/MI, HTN, obesity, valvular heart disease, diabetes, cardiotoxic medications, older age, cigarette smoking

GENERAL PREVENTION

Address the common risk factors for HF including HTN, CAD, and obesity.

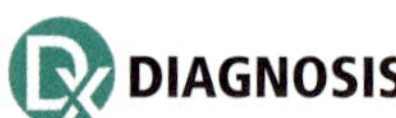

DIAGNOSIS

The Framingham criteria can be used during initial evaluation of suspected HF. Two major criteria or one major and two minor criteria must be met. Major criteria include acute pulmonary edema, cardiomegaly, hepatojugular reflex, neck vein distension, paroxysmal nocturnal dyspnea (PND)/orthopnea, rales or S3. Minor criteria include ankle edema, dyspnea on exertion (DOE), hepatomegaly, nocturnal cough, pleural effusion or HR >120. The H_2FPEF score may help determine the likelihood diagnosis of HFpEF (1). In clinical practice, signs and symptoms of HF are combined with diagnostic testing to confirm the clinical suspicion.

HISTORY

- DOE: *cardinal sign of left-sided HF*; deteriorating exercise capacity: easy fatigued, general weakness; nocturnal nonproductive cough, orthopnea, and PND; sometimes frothy or pink sputum; wheezing, especially nocturnal, in absence of an alternative cause; Cheyne-Stokes respirations.
- Anorexia and/or fullness or dull pain in right upper quadrant (hepatic congestion); nausea and poor appetite may indicate right-sided HF or advanced HF.

PHYSICAL EXAM

- Increased filling pressures: rales and sometimes wheezing, peripheral edema, S_3 gallop, hepatomegaly, jugular venous distention, hepatojugular reflux, ascites
- Remodeling: enlarged or displaced point of maximal impulse
- Poor cardiac output: hypotension, pulsus alternans, tachycardia, narrow pulse pressure, cool extremities, cyanosis

DIFFERENTIAL DIAGNOSIS

Simple dependent edema, pulmonary embolism, exertional asthma, cardiac ischemia, asthma/chronic obstructive pulmonary disorder, constrictive pericarditis, nephrotic syndrome, cirrhosis, venous occlusive disease

DIAGNOSTIC TESTS & INTERPRETATION

Diagnosis based on a combination of clinical findings, laboratory data, cardiac imaging

Initial Tests (lab, imaging)

- β-Type natriuretic peptide (BNP) and N-terminal pro-BNP (NT-BNP): helpful in acute setting to differentiate the cause of dyspnea (BNP <100 essentially rules out HF, >400 confirms HF); elevated BNP: pulmonary embolism, renal failure, and acute coronary syndromes; sacubitril/valsartan can raise BNP levels a modest amount. Obesity may lower BNP levels. BNP-guided therapy in chronic HF is not well established.
- Lab findings often nonspecific abnormalities: respiratory alkalosis, azotemia, elevated creatinine (cardiorenal syndrome), dilutional hyponatremia (poor prognosis), hyperbilirubinemia or cholestatic hepatic abnormalities, electrolyte imbalance
- Chest x-ray (CXR): increased heart size, vascular redistribution (cephalization) with "butterfly" pattern of pulmonary edema, interstitial and alveolar edema, Kerley B lines, and pleural effusions. CXR is relatively insensitive for the diagnosis of HF.
- Echocardiogram: evaluates heart function and structural abnormalities. Critical for proper diagnosis and characterization of HF, RV function, diastolic dysfunction, ventricular size, wall thickness, and valvular abnormalities; repeat if change suspected in underlying cardiac status; usually transthoracic, but transesophageal is possible for evaluation.
- Cardiac magnetic resonance imaging: useful when echocardiographic images are suboptimal or to assess for specific causes of a CM (amyloidosis, HCM, sarcoidosis, arrhythmogenic RV CM, hemochromatosis, etc.)
- 12-lead ECG: Evaluate for underlying causes.

Follow-Up Tests & Special Considerations

Modify and treat comorbidities. Screen first-degree relatives of patients with a heritable CM.

Diagnostic Procedures/Other

Nuclear imaging: estimates ventricular size, assess for ischemia or infarction, amyloidosis, and systolic function; cardiac catheterization: important for excluding CAD as etiology considering risk factors; endomyocardial biopsy: for special circumstances (e.g., suspected giant cell myocarditis)

Test Interpretation

Echo LVEF: HFrEF <40%; HFmEF 40–49%; HFpEF >50%

TREATMENT

GENERAL MEASURES

Focus on comorbidities and risk stratification, improving hemodynamics, nonpharmacologic management, and blocking neurohormonal response to improve survival and symptoms (1).

MEDICATION

Summary: Diuretics are used for decongestion to improve symptoms. Renin-angiotensin-aldosterone system (RAAS) inhibition (ACEi)/angiotensin receptor inhibitors, angiotensin receptor blockers (ARB), or angiotensin receptor neprilysin inhibitors (ARNI), and mineralocorticoid receptor antagonists (MRA) plays an important role in neurohormonal blockade. Start β-blocker once acute HF resolved. Sodium-glucose cotransporter-2 inhibitors (SGLT2i): reduce hospitalization and cardiovascular (CV) death across all HF subgroups; avoid nonsteroidal anti-inflammatory drugs, which worsens HF; avoid nondihydropyridine calcium channel blockers (diltiazem and verapamil) with HFrEF due to possible increased mortality.

First Line

Consists of ACEi/ARB/ARNI, β-blocker, MRA, and SGLT2i (all [A]-level evidence); loop diuretics as needed for decongestion (2)[C]

- ACEis: decrease afterload, increase survival (HFrEF), improve symptoms, and exercise capacity in all NYHA classifications; greatest benefit for patients with HFrEF and post-MI. All ACEis are considered equally effective. Initiate at low doses, titrate as tolerated to targeting doses: enalapril: 2.5 mg PO BID; lisinopril: 2.5 to 5.0 mg daily; and others. Maximum mortality benefit is achieved at low doses.
- ARBs: indicated if intolerant to ACEi. Avoid combination of ACEi and ARB; (starting dose) candesartan: 4 to 8 mg PO daily; losartan: 25 to 50 mg PO daily; valsartan: 20 to 40 mg PO BID. Maximum mortality benefit is achieved at low doses also.
- β-Blockers: Initiate in hemodynamically stable/compensated patients at low dose, titrate upward slowly; decrease mortality in HFrEF; evidence for titration to heart rate (HR) rather than specific dose; (starting dose) carvedilol: 3.125 mg PO BID; metoprolol succinate ER: 12.5 mg/day PO; bisoprolol: 1.25 to 10 mg once daily; titrate to maximally tolerated doses.
- ARNIs (sacubitril/valsartan): reduces the risk of CV death and HF hospitalizations in patients with HFrEF. Recommended dose: 49/51 mg PO BID to a target of 97/103 PO BID; in patients with HFrEF and NYHA class II to III who tolerate an ACEi or ARB with CrCl >30, replacement by an ARNI is recommended to reduce morbidity and mortality (NNT to prevent one CV death over 3.5 years: 31). ACEi should be discontinued at least 36 hours prior to starting ARNIs due risks of angioedema.
- SGLT-2is (e.g., dapagliflozin and empagliflozin): show improvement in worsening HF and CV death in patients with EF ≤40% and NYHA II to III, irrespective of diabetes; may decrease overall death (NNT 50 to 60 per year); recommended dose: empagliflozin or dapagliflozin 10 mg PO daily; also, recommended in HFpEF due to improvement in morbidity
- Diuretics help manage volume overload/reduce preload.
  - Torsemide (Demadex): 10 to 200 mg/day PO; furosemide (Lasix): 40 to 120 mg/day PO; bumetanide (Bumex): 0.5 mg to 10.0 mg/day IV/PO. There is likely no difference in efficacy of the loop diuretics.
  - Metolazone (Zaroxolyn): 2.5 to 20.0 mg/day PO; hydrochlorothiazide: 12.5 to 100.0 mg/day PO; chlorothiazide (Diuril): 250 to 2,000 mg/day IV/PO
- MRA: spironolactone, eplerenone (improve mortality when added to standard therapy in NYHA class II to IV + EF ≤35%): spironolactone 12.5 to 25.0 mg/day PO; max 50 mg/day PO; eplerenone 25 to 50 mg/day; caution regarding hyperkalemia and chronic kidney disease (CKD); eplerenone less likely to cause gynecomastia; finerenone, a nonsteroidal MRA, shows promise in HFmEF and HFpEF.
- Combination of isosorbide dinitrate and hydralazine (20.0 mg/37.5 mg PO TID): effective for improving survival and reducing hospitalizations in African Americans; can be used if the patient is unable to take an ACEi/ARB

Second Line

- Vericiguat, a guanylate cyclase simulator, shown to reduce the risk of death from CV causes or hospitalization for HF. Starting dose 2.5 mg QD; FDA-approved in patients with an EF ≤45%, recent HF hospitalization, or need for IV diuretics
- Ivabradine (Corlanor): considered in NYHA II and III HF, EF ≤35%, on maximally tolerated β-blockers with HR >70 to reduce hospitalization; do not give to patients currently in AFib and discontinue if AFib develops.
- Digoxin: reduces symptoms, without positive effect on mortality; considered as an add-on strategy at low doses, in patients with preserved renal function (CrCl >50 mL/min)
- Glucagon-like peptide-1 (GLP-1) receptor agonist and glucose-dependent insulinotropic polypeptide (GIP) receptor agonist (tirzepatide) may reduce the risk of worsening HF and CV death in obese patients with HFpEF.

ISSUES FOR REFERRAL

Cardiology referral: patients who remain symptomatic despite maximal standard HF regimen

ADDITIONAL THERAPIES

Device therapy including implantable cardioverter-defibrillators (ICDs) and cardiac resynchronization therapy (CRT) are shown to improve outcomes.

- CRT recommended: sinus rhythm with a QRS width ≥150 ms due to left bundle branch block (LBBB), LVEF ≤35%, persistent NYHA II to IV HF despite guideline-directed medical therapy (GDMT), chronic RV pacing or bradyarrhythmias, and anticipated need for pacemaker
- Consider CRT: LVEF ≤35%, sinus rhythm, QRS width >150 ms, non-LBBB pattern
- ICD recommended: primary prevention in patients with *nonischemic* and *ischemic* CM, at least 40 days post-MI; LVEF ≤35% and NYHA class II or III HF. or LVEF ≤30% if NYHA I, on optimal medical therapy and >1 year estimated survival; contraindicated in end-stage HF or NYHA IV HF

SURGERY/OTHER PROCEDURES

Mitral valve edge-to-edge repair is a consideration for those with functional mitral regurgitation and without severe left ventricular dilation. Cardiac transplantation or left ventricular assist device (LVAD) implantation is a consideration for those with persistent NYHA III to IV symptoms refractory to medical therapy. Refer to an advanced HF specialist.

COMPLEMENTARY & ALTERNATIVE MEDICINE

A formal cardiac rehabilitation program has been shown to improve quality of life and is approved for those with an EF ≤35%, NYHA II to IV despite being on optimal HF therapy for at least 6 weeks.

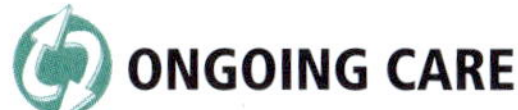

ONGOING CARE

FOLLOW-UP RECOMMENDATIONS

Every 6 to 12 months if stable and closer follow-up depending on clinical situation

Patient Monitoring

Patient instruction on monitoring weight; consideration for remote monitoring programs utilizing invasive and noninvasive modalities

DIET

Reduce sodium load; no clear evidence of an optimal sodium intake; fluid restriction: 2,000 mL but no clear evidence of optimal fluid restriction level

PATIENT EDUCATION

Educate patient on management of weight gain or new edema. Have patients weigh themselves and report weight gains of >2 lb in a day or 5 lb above dry weight. Recommend lifestyle modifications to reduce common conditions associated with HF.

PROGNOSIS

After diagnosis: 1-year survival ~75%, 5-year survival <50%, 10-year survival <25%

COMPLICATIONS

Sudden death, progressive pump failure

REFERENCES

1. Kittleson MM, Panjrath GS, Amancherla K, et al. 2023 ACC expert consensus decision pathway on management of heart failure with preserved ejection fraction: a report of the American College of Cardiology Solution Set Oversight Committee. *J Am Coll Cardiol*. 2023;81(18):1835–1878.
2. Heidenreich PA, Bozkurt B, Aguilar D, et al. 2022 AHA/ACC/HFSA guideline for the management of heart failure: a report of the American College of Cardiology/American Heart Association Joint Committee on clinical practice guidelines. *J Am Coll Cardiol*. 2022;79(17):e263–e421.

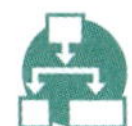

SEE ALSO

Algorithm: Congestive Heart Failure: Differential Diagnosis

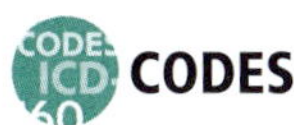

CODES

ICD10

- I50.9 Heart failure, unspecified
- I50.1 Left ventricular failure
- I50.22 Chronic systolic (congestive) heart failure

CLINICAL PEARLS

Core medications for management: β-blockers, ACEi/ARB/ANRI, MRA, and SGLT2i

HEAT ILLNESS: HEAT EXHAUSTION AND HEAT STROKE

Sean C. Robinson, MD, CAQSM • Alexandra Bray, MD

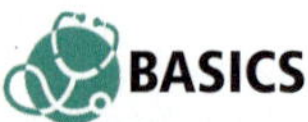

BASICS

DESCRIPTION

- A continuum of increasingly severe illness caused by dehydration, electrolyte losses, and failure of thermoregulatory mechanisms when exposed to elevated environmental temperatures
  - Heat exhaustion is a mild to moderate form of heat illness displaying dehydration type symptoms with a normal to elevated temperature (1).
  - Heat stroke is characterized by an elevated core temperature >104°F with central nervous system (CNS) abnormalities and is a true medical emergency (1),(2).
- Can be exertional (related to activity) or nonexertional
- System(s) affected: endocrine/metabolic, nervous, hepatic, hematologic
- Synonym(s): heat illness; heat injury; hyperthermia; heat collapse; heat prostration

Geriatric Considerations

Elderly persons are more susceptible.

Pediatric Considerations

Children are more susceptible.

Pregnancy Considerations

Pregnant women may be more susceptible to volume depletion with heat stress.

EPIDEMIOLOGY

- Predominant age: more likely in children or elderly
- Predominant sex: male = female

Incidence

- Depends on intensity of heat; estimate of 20/100,000 persons per season
- Concern for increasing incidence because ambient environmental temperatures continue to rise

Prevalence

- Depends on predisposing conditions in combination with environmental factors
- Roughly 600 deaths per year in the United States

ETIOLOGY AND PATHOPHYSIOLOGY

- Excess heat has direct cellular toxicity. Excess heat also leads to an imbalance between inflammatory and anti-inflammatory cytokines, vascular endothelial damage, and end-organ dysfunction.
- Interplay between failure of heat-dissipating mechanisms, an overwhelming heat stress, and an exaggerated acute-phase inflammatory response

RISK FACTORS

- Poor acclimatization to heat
- Poor physical conditioning
- Salt or water depletion
- Obesity
- Acute febrile or GI illnesses
- Chronic illnesses: uncontrolled diabetes mellitus, hypertension, cardiac disease
- Alcohol and other substance abuse
- High heat and humidity, poor environmental air circulation
- Heavy, restrictive clothing
- Nutritional supplements (e.g., ephedra) (2)
- Medications (α-adrenergics, anticholinergics, antihistamines, antipsychotics, benzodiazepines, β-blockers, calcium channel blockers, clopidogrel, diuretics, laxatives, neuroleptics, phenothiazines, thyroid agonists, tricyclic antidepressants) (1)

GENERAL PREVENTION

- The most important factor in preventing heat illness is prevention. Activity modification and adequate fluid replacement are key preventive measures.
- Allow acclimatization through proper conditioning and activity modification.
- Dress appropriately with loose-fitting, open-weave, light-colored clothing.
- Consume a proper volume of fluids, particularly during physical activity in hot environments.
- Never leave children (or pets) unattended in cars during hot weather.
- Try to gain access to air-conditioned environments during hot weather.

DIAGNOSIS

- Heat exhaustion: Symptoms are milder than in heat stroke, and there are no CNS derangements:
  - Fatigue, lethargy, weakness, dizziness, nausea, vomiting, myalgias, headache, profuse sweating, tachycardia, hypotension, thirst, hyperventilation
  - Core temperature usually elevated but can be normal; if elevated, <104°F (40°C)
- Heat stroke: marked by mental status changes and elevated core temperature
  - *Classic (nonexertional)*: caused by environmental exposure, primarily in elderly or chronically ill patients, and may develop gradually over days
    - Delirium
    - Confusion
    - Coma
    - Core temperature >104°F (>40°C)
    - Hot, flushed, dry skin
  - *Exertional*: typically younger, active patients; rapid onset
    - Exhaustion
    - Confusion, disorientation
    - Delirium
    - Coma
    - Hot, flushed skin, typically with sweating
    - Core temperature >104°F (>40°C) (1),(2)

HISTORY

- Heat cramps: sweating; muscle cramps/spasms
- Heat exhaustion: sweating; fatigue, light-headedness/dizziness; cramping; nausea, vomiting; headache
- Heat stroke: altered mental status

PHYSICAL EXAM

- Rectal temperature (*Don't rely on oral temperature.*)
- Heat exhaustion: tachycardia; cool/clammy skin
- Heat stroke: rectal (core temperature) elevated (>104°F); hot/dry skin (compensatory sweating impaired)

DIFFERENTIAL DIAGNOSIS

- Febrile illnesses, sepsis
- Drug-induced fluid loss
- Cardiac arrhythmia or infarction
- Acute cocaine intoxication
- Neuroleptic malignant syndrome
- Malignant hyperthermia (an autosomally inherited disorder of skeletal and cardiac muscle in which patients have abnormal muscle metabolism on exposure to halothane or skeletal muscle reactants)

DIAGNOSTIC TESTS & INTERPRETATION

Detect end-organ damage.

Initial Tests (lab, imaging)

- Creatinine, BUN, electrolytes (sodium in particular)
- Liver enzymes, muscle enzymes (creatine phosphokinase)
- CBC—hemoconcentration
- Urinalysis: increased urine specific gravity
- Drugs that may alter lab results: diuretics

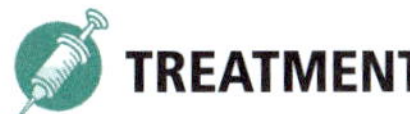

TREATMENT

GENERAL MEASURES

- For heat stroke: immediate body immersion in ice water to cool core temperature. Monitor hemodynamics and airway status (1). Admit to monitor for complications.
- Careful fluid and electrolyte replacement with normal saline; avoid hypotonic fluids. Follow serum sodium (1),(2)[C].
- Consider CVP monitoring.
- For heat exhaustion, consider:
  - Evaporative cooling: spraying water over the patient and using fans to facilitate evaporative and convective heat loss (1)
  - Immerse hands and forearms in cold water.
  - Ice or cold packs on the neck, groin, and axillae (1),(2)[C]
- No clear superiority of any one method for heat exhaustion (1)

MEDICATION

First Line

- No medications are required in the initial management. Use isotonic saline solution to rehydrate
- Do not use antipyretics to lower core temperature in heat illness.

Second Line

- For severely ill, consider immunomodulators such as corticosteroids (patients in ICU setting).
- Iced gastric, bladder, or peritoneal lavage
- If disseminated intravascular coagulation (DIC), consider appropriate replacement therapy.

ADMISSION, INPATIENT, AND NURSING CONSIDERATIONS

- *Cool patient immediately* (prior to transport) if heat stroke is suspected or once diagnosed.
- Rapid cooling: Remove clothing, wet patient down, and apply ice packs.
- Emergency treatment; best in a hospital setting

ONGOING CARE

FOLLOW-UP RECOMMENDATIONS

Rest with legs elevated.

Patient Monitoring

- Rectal temperature monitoring: Cooling may be discontinued when the core temperature drops to 102°F (38.9°C) and stabilizes.
- Heat stroke patients may require airway management, hemodynamic monitoring, and careful fluid and electrolyte administration and monitoring.
- Consider CVP monitoring.

DIET

- Cool or cold clear liquids only (noncarbonated)
- Avoid caffeine.
- Unrestricted sodium

PATIENT EDUCATION

- Proper hydration is the key to prevention.
- Proper conditioning and acclimatization
- Recognize signs and symptoms of heat stress—fatigue and headache.
- Skin exposure facilitates heat loss in hot, humid conditions (use proper sun protection).

PROGNOSIS

- If mental function is not altered and serum chemistries are normal, the prognosis is good and recovery within 24 to 48 hours is typical.
- The mortality rate for heat stroke (10–80%) is directly related to the duration and intensity of hyperthermia as well as to the speed and effectiveness of diagnosis and treatment.
- The priority in heat-related illness is early recognition and intervention. The faster the patient is cooled to below 40°C, the lower the patient mortality (3).

COMPLICATIONS

- May involve failure of any major organ system
- Cardiac arrhythmias or infarction
- Pulmonary edema, acute respiratory distress syndrome
- Coma, seizures
- Acute renal failure
- Rhabdomyolysis
- DIC
- Hepatocellular necrosis

REFERENCES

1. Roberts WO, Armstrong LE, Sawka MN, et al. ACSM expert consensus statement on exertional heat illness: recognition, management, and return to activity. *Curr Sports Med Rep*. 2023;22(4):134–149. doi:10.1249/JSR.0000000000001058.
2. Eifling KP, Gaudio FG, Dumke C, et al. Wilderness Medical Society clinical practice guidelines for the prevention and treatment of heat illness: 2024 update. *Wilderness Environ Med*. 2024;35(Suppl 1):112S–127S. doi:10.1177/10806032241227924.
3. Bouchama A, Abuyassin B, Lehe C, et al. Classic and exertional heatstroke. *Nat Rev Dis Primers*. 2022;8(1):8. doi:10.1038/s41572-021-00334-6.

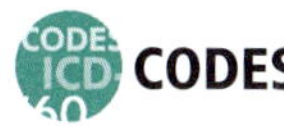

CODES

ICD10

- T67.5XXA Heat exhaustion, unspecified, initial encounter
- T67.0XXA Heatstroke and sunstroke, initial encounter
- T67.3XXA Heat exhaustion, anhydrotic, initial encounter

CLINICAL PEARLS

- Exertional heat stroke is a life-threatening medical emergency that requires immediate whole body cooling (cold/ice water immersion preferred).
- The diagnosis of heat stroke includes an elevated core temperature and signs of CNS dysfunction (e.g., mental status changes, irritability, ataxia, confusion, seizures, or coma).
- Start the cooling process immediately when heat exhaustion is recognized, beginning with wetting the skin with a cool mist and giving oral rehydration solutions if the patient is alert and oriented.
- If in the field (e.g., sporting events, wilderness), cooling should begin immediately (prior to transport if possible).
- Do not rely on oral temperature—a rectal temperature is always preferred.

HEMATURIA

Sahil Mullick, MD, FAAFP • Anysha K. Mattu, MD

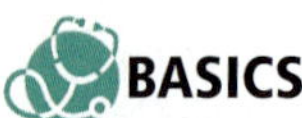

BASICS

DESCRIPTION

Gross (visible) or microscopic (nonvisible) blood in urine, either symptomatic or asymptomatic

EPIDEMIOLOGY

Prevalence

Children: gross: 0.13%; asymptomatic microscopic hematuria (AMH): 0.4–4.1%; adults: AMH: 0.9–17%

ETIOLOGY AND PATHOPHYSIOLOGY

- Trauma
  - Exercise-induced (resolves within 24 hours of ceasing activity)
  - Abdominal trauma or pelvic fracture with renal, bladder, or ureteral injury
  - Iatrogenic from abdominal or pelvic surgery, indwelling catheters, or foreign body
  - Physical/sexual abuse
- Neoplasms
  - Urologic malignancies or benign tumors
  - Endometriosis of the urinary tract (suspect in females with cyclic hematuria)
- Inflammatory/infectious causes
  - UTI: most common cause in adults
  - Renal diseases: radiation nephritis and cystitis, acute/chronic tubulointerstitial nephritis (due to drugs, infections, systemic disease)
  - Glomerular disease
    - Goodpasture syndrome (antiglomerular basement membrane disease; autoimmune; associated pulmonary hemorrhage)
    - IgA nephropathy
    - Lupus nephritis
    - Henoch-Schönlein purpura
    - Membranoproliferative, poststreptococcal, or rapidly progressive glomerulonephritis (GN)
    - Wegener granulomatosis
  - Endocarditis/visceral abscesses
  - Infections: schistosomiasis, tuberculosis (TB), syphilis
- Metabolic causes
  - Stones (85% have hematuria)
    - Hypercalciuria: a common cause of gross and microscopic hematuria in children
    - Hyperuricosuria
    - Drugs that cause calculi such as acyclovir
- Congenital/familial causes
  - Cystic disease: polycystic kidney disease, solitary renal cyst
  - Benign familial hematuria or thin basement membrane nephropathy (autosomal dominant)
  - Alport syndrome (X-linked in 80%; hematuria, proteinuria, hearing loss, corneal abnormalities)
  - Fabry disease (X-linked recessive inborn error of metabolism; vascular kidney disease)
  - Nail–patella syndrome (autosomal dominant; nail and patella hypoplasia; hematuria in 33%)
  - Renal tubular acidosis type 1 (autosomal dominant or autoimmune)
- Hematologic causes
  - Bleeding dyscrasias (e.g., hemophilia)
  - Sickle cell anemia/trait (renal papillary necrosis)
- Vascular causes
  - Hemangioma
  - Arteriovenous malformations (rare)
  - Nutcracker syndrome: compression of left renal vein, renal parenchymal congestion
  - Renal artery/vein thrombosis
  - Arterial emboli to kidney
- Chemical causes
  - Aminoglycosides, cyclosporine, analgesics, oral contraceptives, Chinese herbs, cyclophosphamide, anticoagulants (Coumadin, Eliquis, Xarelto), sulfa drugs, penicillins
- Obstruction
  - Strictures or posterior urethral valves
  - Hydronephrosis from any cause
  - Benign prostatic hyperplasia: Rule out other causes of hematuria.
- Other causes: loin pain hematuria (most often in young women on oral contraceptives)

RISK FACTORS

- Smoking
- Occupational exposures (dyes, paints, printer, rubber, or tire manufacturing, petrochemicals)
- Medications (e.g., cyclophosphamide, pioglitazone therapy >1 year)
- Pelvic irradiation
- Chronic infection, especially with calculi
- Recent upper respiratory infection (URI)
- Positive family history of stones, GN, or cancer
- Chronic indwelling foreign body

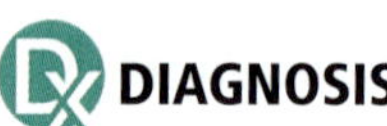

DIAGNOSIS

HISTORY

Considerations

- Burning, urgency, frequency: UTI
- Dark cola-colored urine: glomerular origin
- Clots: extraglomerular bleeding
- Arthritis/arthralgias/rash: lupus, vasculitis, Henoch-Schönlein purpura
- Flank pain: stones, infarction, pyelonephritis
- Recent URI: poststreptococcal GN, membranoproliferative GN
- Concurrent URI: IgA nephropathy
- Excessive vitamin intake: stones
- Marathon runner: traumatic, rhabdomyolysis
- Travel: schistosomiasis, TB
- Painless hematuria, smoking history, weight loss: malignancy
- Family history: Alport disease (hereditary nephritis), sickle cell, polycystic, IgA nephropathy, thin basement membrane disease, von Willebrand
- Any episode of visible hematuria (VH) in the urine, even if transient, is associated with an OR of 7.2 for urologic cancers.

PHYSICAL EXAM

Considerations

- Elevated BP, edema, and weight gain: glomerular disease
- Fever: infection
- Costovertebral angle tenderness
- Palpable kidney: neoplasm, polycystic
- Genitalia: meatal erosion, lesions

DIFFERENTIAL DIAGNOSIS

UTI, BPH, rhabdomyolysis, vaginal bleeding, rectal bleeding, drugs (rifampin and phenazopyridine) can turn urine orange/red mistaking for hematuria.

DIAGNOSTIC TESTS & INTERPRETATION

A hematuria risk index may assist in stratifying patients at risk for urothelial malignancies requiring intensive testing. High-risk indicators are VH, age >50 years, male gender, family history of urological malignancies, and smoking.

Initial Tests (lab, imaging)

- If acute cystitis/UTI is ruled out, guidelines recommend evaluating AMH with upper urinary tract imaging and cystoscopy; none recommend cytology or urine markers for initial AMH evaluation (1)[C].
- Urine dipstick (sensitivity 91–100%; specificity 65–99%)
  - False negatives are rare but can be caused by high-dose vitamin C.
  - False positives: oxidizers used to cleanse the perineum, alkaline urine (>9), semen; free hemoglobin (hemolysis) and myoglobin (rhabdomyolysis)
  - Heme-negative red urine: Food dyes, beets, blackberries, rhubarb, porphyria, rifampin, phenytoin, phenazopyridine may discolor the dipstick, making interpretation difficult.
  - Any proteinuria >2+ raises concern for glomerular disease.
- Microscopic urinalysis should always be done to confirm dipstick findings and quantify RBCs (1)[C].
  - American Urological Association (AUA) defines clinically significant microscopic hematuria as ≥3 RBCs/HPF on a properly collected urinary specimen when there is not an obvious benign cause (1).
  - Positive dipstick, but a negative microscopic exam should be followed by three repeat tests. If anyone is positive, proceed with a workup (1).
  - Exclude factitious or nonurinary causes, such as menstruation, mild trauma, exercise, poor collection technique, or chemical/drug causes by cessation of activity/cause and a repeat urinalysis (1)[C].
  - RBC casts are pathognomonic for glomerular origin; dysmorphic cells are suggestive.
- Renal function tests (eGFR, BUN, creatinine), albumin, and electrolytes to differentiate intrinsic renal disease and to evaluate for risks for imaging with contrast (1)[C]
  - Indicators of renal disease are significant (>500 mg/day) proteinuria, red cell casts, dysmorphic RBCs, increased creatinine, and albumin:creatinine ratio ≥30 mg/mmol (1).
- Urine culture if suspected infection/pyuria
- Multidetector CT urography (MDCTU); sensitivity 95%, specificity 92%
  - The initial imaging of choice in nonpregnant adults without contraindications to contrast or radiation with unexplained hematuria per the AUA and the American College of Radiology (ACR) (1)
  - Normal does not obviate the need for cystoscopy, particularly in high-risk patients
  - Presence of calculi on noncontrast does not exclude another diagnosis or need for contrast phase.

- CT
  - Noncontrast CT is preferred first line in adult patients with acute flank pain suspicious of stones.
  - Perform unenhanced helical CT for suspected stone disease in children if US is negative.
  - Perform CT abdomen and pelvis with contrast in children with traumatic hematuria.
- Renal and bladder US (RBUS)
  - Best for differentiating cystic from solid masses
  - Sensitive for hydronephrosis; point of care US may help avoid CT with suspected stones.
  - No radiation or iodinated contrast exposure and cost-efficient
  - US can be used first line in patients with contraindications to CTU or at low risk of malignancy.
  - Sensitivity and NPV: for renal cancer = 85.7% and 99.9% and for upper tract urothelial cancer = 14.3% and 99.7%
  - Poor sensitivity for renal masses <3 cm
  - Main disadvantage is inability to fully evaluate the urothelium for transitional cell cancer.
- Magnetic resonance urography (MRU)
  - High sensitivity/specificity for renal parenchyma; less useful for collecting system or stones
  - Can be used in patients with contraindications to MDCTU
- MRI
  - Similar to CT in sensitivity for renal masses
  - No radiation exposure but least cost-efficient
  - Limited ability to reliably detect urinary tract calcifications
  - Can be combined with retrograde pyelogram (RPG) for patients who cannot tolerate MDCTU or MRU

Follow-Up Tests & Special Considerations

- Other tests depend on suspected etiology: STD testing, antineutrophil cytoplasmic antibody (ANCA), C3, C4, antistreptolysin O (ASO) titer, hemoglobin electrophoresis, prothrombin time (PT)/international normalized ratio (INR) for patients on warfarin.
- Consider genetic testing in patients suspected of having familial hematuria.
- Voided urine cytology (sensitivity 43.5%; specificity 95.7%; positive predictive value 47.6%; negative predictive value 94.9%)
  - Not recommended for routine evaluation of AMH; consider in those with significant risk factors for urinary malignancy (1)
- Insufficient evidence to recommend routine use of urinary tumor markers
- Malignancies are more likely in patients with VH than in patients with nonvisible hematuria (13.8% vs. 3.1%).
- Summary positive predictive value of VH for bladder/renal cancer in age >15 years is 5.1%; risk increases with age and male gender.
- VCUG in children with frequent UTIs

Diagnostic Procedures/Other

- Flexible cystoscopy (sensitivity 62%; specificity 43–98%)
  - Best for evaluation of bladder, prostate and urethra; NPV for bladder tumors is 99%.
  - AUA recommends all patients with hematuria who are ≥35 years of age and all patients with risk factors for bladder cancer regardless of age to receive cystoscopy in addition to imaging (1).
- Renal biopsy
  - Not routine but may be necessary to diagnose GN or in the face of increasing renal insufficiency
- RPG
  - Reserved when MDCTU equivocal or in addition to US or noncontrast studies in patients who are contraindicated for contrast or MRI
  - Sensitive for small lesions of supravesicular collecting system
  - Requires cystoscopy
- Ureteroscopy/pyeloscopy
  - For visualization of suspected supravesical collecting system lesions
  - Biopsy, excision, fulguration, or extraction of lesions/stones possible
  - Requires anesthesia and cystoscopy
  - Risk of injury to collecting system

Pregnancy Considerations

US is initial imaging choice for pregnant patients. MRU or RPG combined with either MRI or US are alternatives.

Pediatric Considerations

- Consider UTI, GN, Wilms tumor, child abuse, hyperuricemia, hypercalciuria, familial causes.
- The AAP recommends workup for hematuria should not be initiated for hematuria in a pediatric patient before repeating a dipstick urinalysis. In patients with persistent ASM, most common diagnoses on renal biopsy are hypercalciuria (30–35%), hyperuricemia (5–20%), and glomerulonephritides, such as IgAN and thin basement membrane disease.
- Gross or symptomatic hematuria needs a full workup.
  - If eumorphic RBCs, consider UTI, hypercalciuria, familial causes, or masses, stones or cysts. Obtain a family history, urine culture, US and urinary Ca:Cr ratio. Urine Ca:Cr ratio >0.2 (mg/mg) is suggestive of hypercalciuria in children >6 years of age.
  - If dysmorphic RBCs, with proteinuria, elevated blood pressure, edema, or a positive family history, consider renal consult.
- Renal US identifies most congenital and malignant conditions; CT is reserved for cases of suspected trauma (with contrast) or stones (without contrast).

TREATMENT

MEDICATION

First Line

Treatment of the underlying cause of hematuria; discontinue drugs that cause hematuria.

ISSUES FOR REFERRAL

- Nephrology referral for proteinuria, red cell casts, elevated serum creatinine, and albumin:creatinine ratio ≥30 mg/mmol
- Urology referral for stones, vascular/anatomic anomalies, or nutcracker syndrome

ADDITIONAL THERAPIES

Surgery for removal of endometriosis if causing hematuria with symptoms

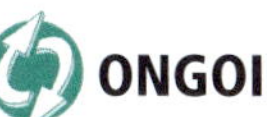

ONGOING CARE

Close follow-up by specialists indicated based on the underlying cause

FOLLOW-UP RECOMMENDATIONS

May repeat urinalysis in 12 months if initial testing is negative (2). If repeat is positive, then may need further evaluation.

Patient Monitoring

Recent literature suggests that, after thorough initial negative investigations (imaging, cystoscopy), no follow-up is indicated for the patient with AMH unless symptoms or frank hematuria develop. AUA recommends annual urinalyses in these patients, until two consecutive are negative and consideration for repeat workup if hematuria persists for 3 to 5 years (1).

DIET

Increased fluids for stones or clots

PROGNOSIS

- Excellent for common causes of hematuria
- Poorer for malignant tumors and certain types of nephritis
- Persistent AMH is associated with an increased risk of end-stage renal disease in patients aged 16 to 25 years.

REFERENCES

1. Linder BJ, Bass EJ, Mostafid H, et al. Guideline of guidelines: asymptomatic microscopic haematuria. *BJU Int*. 2018;121(2):176–183.
2. Barocas DA, Boorjlan SA, Alvarez RD, et al. Microhematuria: AUA/SUFU guideline. *J Urol*. 2020;204(4):778–786.

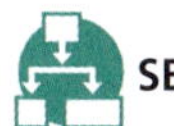

SEE ALSO

Algorithm: Hematuria

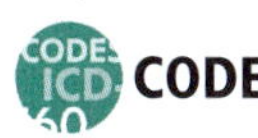

CODES

ICD10

- R31.9 Hematuria, unspecified
- R31.1 Benign essential microscopic hematuria
- R31.0 Gross hematuria

CLINICAL PEARLS

- Screening patients for AMH is an "I" recommendation from the USPSTF.
- AMH and hematuria persisting after treatment of UTIs must be evaluated.
- Patients with bladder cancer can have intermittent microscopic hematuria; a thorough evaluation in high-risk patients is needed after just one episode.
- In patients with AMH, a history of anticoagulant use does not preclude the need for an evaluation and any new hematuria in patients on anticoagulants requires full evaluation including imaging and cystoscopy (1)[C].
- Signs of underlying renal disease indicate the need for a nephrologic workup, but a urologic evaluation is still needed in the presence of persistent hematuria.

H

HEMOCHROMATOSIS

Alethea Y. Turner, DO, FAAFP • Kaleb R. Ward, DO

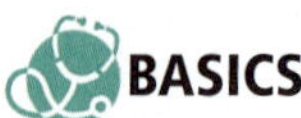

BASICS

DESCRIPTION

Hereditary hemochromatosis (HH) is a genetic disease with autosomal recessive inheritance that results in iron overload and subsequent deposition into various tissues.

- HH includes at least four types of iron overload conditions, which involve gene mutations that alter iron metabolism.
- There is no mechanism to excrete excess iron, so the surplus is stored in tissue, eventually resulting in severe damage to the affected organ(s).
- Patients are often asymptomatic, but late effects may include diabetes, liver cirrhosis, hypermelanotic pigmentation of the skin, cardiac issues and other complications.
- Synonym(s): bronze diabetes; Troisier-Hanot-Chauffard syndrome

EPIDEMIOLOGY

Incidence

- Predominant age: Metabolic abnormality is congenital, but symptoms typically present between the 3rd and 5th decades for HH types 1, 3, and 4; type 2 juvenile hemochromatosis typically presents between the 1st and 3rd decades of life, and neonatal presentation is rare.
- Predominant sex: Gene frequency is equal between male and female, although clinical signs are more frequent in men.

Prevalence

- Prevalence in the United States for carrying an *HFE* gene mutation (type 1 HH) is 5.4% for the *C282Y* gene and 13.5% for the *H63D* gene; prevalence for homozygosity is 0.3% for *C282Y* and 1.9% for *H63D* (1).
- Type 1 accounts for >90% of HH cases in the United States and primarily occurs in people of northern European descent; ~1 in 200 white adults in the United States are *C282Y* homozygous (1).

Pediatric Considerations

Juvenile (type 2) HH is rare but can present in young patients as hypogonadism and cardiomyopathy.

ETIOLOGY AND PATHOPHYSIOLOGY

- HH type 1 is caused by mutations in the *HFE* gene (most frequently *C282Y* and/or *H63D*), and is the most common form. Other variations include type 2 which is caused by mutations in either the *HJV* or *HAMP* gene, type 3 by mutations in the *TFR2* gene, and type 4 by mutations in the *SLC11A3* gene.
- Types 1 to 3 involve a deficiency in an iron-regulating hormone named hepcidin, which causes increased intestinal absorption of iron through excessive expression of ferroportin (a transmembrane protein that transports iron out of the cell and into the bloodstream).
- Type 4 is caused by an insensitivity of ferroportin to hepcidin (4a) or an inactivity of ferroportin itself (4b); the latter leads to iron accumulation within mesenchymal tissue.
- Other rare types of HH exist as a result of different gene mutations.
- Increased plasma iron and transferrin saturation (TS) leads to elevated levels of unbound iron, which are then absorbed into various tissue, eventually causing organ dysfunction.

Genetics

- Genetically heterogeneous disorder of iron overload; types 1, 2, and 3 are autosomal recessive; type 4 is autosomal dominant.
- Biochemical penetrance is incomplete and expressivity is variable; in type 1 HH the penetrance for developing clinically significant iron overload is rare, but approximately 75% of men with type 1 HH and 50% of women will have an increase in TS (with or without elevated serum ferritin [SF]) (2).
- Factors contributing to variable expressivity include different mutations in the same gene, mitigating or exacerbating genes, and environmental factors.

RISK FACTORS

- Family history
- White men between the ages of 30 and 50 years (particularly for HFE-related HH)
- Loss of blood, such as that which occurs during menstruation and pregnancy, delays the onset of symptoms in women
- Alcohol consumption because it increases the absorption of iron and damages the liver along with the oxidative effects of iron

GENERAL PREVENTION

- First-degree relatives of those with HH should be screened; typically, with fasting TS and ferritin levels.
- Children of a diagnosed parent, HFE testing of the other parent is recommended with no further testing required if the results are normal.

ALERT

Screening of the general population is *not* recommended because only a small subset of patients with HH will develop symptoms or advanced disease (2).

COMMONLY ASSOCIATED CONDITIONS

See "Complications."

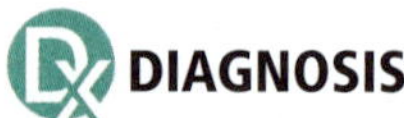

DIAGNOSIS

HISTORY

- Fatigue, weakness
- Arthralgias
- Abdominal pain
- Loss of libido or impotency
- Symptoms of diabetes
- Skin pigmentation or blistering

PHYSICAL EXAM

- Hepatomegaly
- Increased skin pigmentation
- Hepatic tenderness and/or jaundice
- Peripheral edema and/or ascites
- Gynecomastia
- Testicular atrophy

DIFFERENTIAL DIAGNOSIS

- Inflammatory syndromes
- Various causes of hepatitis
- Biliary or alcoholic cirrhosis
- Repeated transfusions
- Sideroblastic anemia
- β-Thalassemia major

DIAGNOSTIC TESTS & INTERPRETATION

Initial Tests (lab, imaging)

There is currently no evidence to support a concrete relationship between symptoms and the degree of iron overload (1).

- SF: ≥300 μg/L for men and postmenopausal women and 200 μg/L for premenopausal women (2); may be elevated for a number of other reasons including but not limited to inflammation (consider checking inflammatory markers); if elevated with suspicion of hemochromatosis, obtain fasting TS.
- Fasting TS (serum iron concentration ÷ total iron-binding capacity × 100) is the earliest biochemical marker to be increased in HH: ≥45% is suspicious for HH but warrants further evaluation because it can be elevated in other disease processes including chronic anemias.
- Confirmatory testing should be done through HFE gene mutation analysis.

Follow-Up Tests & Special Considerations

- After diagnosis, check ALT, AST, hematocrit, and hemoglobin to determine the need for phlebotomy.
- Test for other causes of hepatitis if transaminitis exists to rule out concomitant disease.
- Hepatic MRI should be done to measure liver iron content if hepatomegaly is present; SF is >1,000 μg/L and/or ALT/AST are elevated.
- Monitor for liver lesions with an abdominal ultrasound every 6 months if severe liver fibrosis or cirrhosis is present.
- Assess for complications of HH and order appropriate testing when necessary.
- Cardiac MRI can assess degree of myocardial iron overload when indicated.
- Consider screening for osteoporosis in patients >50 years with additional risk factors (i.e., alcohol or tobacco use).

Diagnostic Procedures/Other

Consider liver biopsy if there is a need to determine the degree of liver fibrosis for staging or to confirm the etiology of liver damage (2).

Test Interpretation

- Hepatic MRI without contrast (T2-weighted imaging) can rule out iron overload within the liver (negative predictive value 0.88) and diagnose it as well but with slightly less accuracy (positive predictive value 0.74) (2)[B].
- Liver biopsy will reveal increased hepatic parenchymal iron stores and evidence of any fibrosis or cirrhosis.

TREATMENT

GENERAL MEASURES

Due to a lack of evidence, there is debate regarding when treatment should be initiated (particularly in asymptomatic patients) as well as what the target serum indices and frequency of phlebotomy should be. American and European liver associations recommend initiating treatment when SF is above the normal limit (see "Initial Tests [lab, imaging]"). The American College of Gastroenterology further outlines their recommendations regarding initiation of treatment based on whether the patient is *C282Y* homozygote or *C282Y/H63D* heterozygote (2). If HH diagnosis is confirmed, there is no liver involvement, SF remains normal, and the patient is asymptomatic, it is reasonable to monitor SF at least annually.

- Phlebotomy (~500 mL per session) is the mainstay of therapy and is performed once or twice weekly in the initial treatment phase and may take up to 2 to 3 years to deplete iron stores (1),(2).
- When the patient finally becomes iron deficient, a lifelong maintenance program of ~2 to 6 phlebotomies a year is required to keep iron storage normal or below normal (2).
- Erythrocytapheresis (~600 mL per session) is an alternative to phlebotomy and only removes red cells from the blood; it is expensive and not widely available. However, there is limited evidence that erythrocytapheresis in the maintenance phase of treatment can reduce the frequency of treatments (1.9 vs 3.3 treatments annually when compared to phlebotomy) (2)[B].
- Adverse effects of phlebotomy and erythrocytapheresis are mild and are typically secondary to hypovolemia, so prehydration is recommended.

MEDICATION

- If phlebotomy is not feasible or if it is contraindicated (severe anemia or heart failure), a second-tier option is chelation therapy with parenteral deferoxamine (monitor patients for auditory or visual changes), oral deferasirox (contraindicated in renal or hepatic failure, and can increase risk of gastrointestinal hemorrhage in some patients) or oral deferiprone (can cause agranulocytosis and neutropenia); of these options, deferoxamine is preferred in most patients (2)[C].
- Proton pump inhibitor (PPI) use for a minimum of one year may reduce the absorption of iron in patients with HH and decrease the overall number of phlebotomies needed. Consider adding a PPI as adjunct therapy to phlebotomy.
- Testosterone replacement in men with HH may improve symptoms of erectile dysfunction and decreased libido, but risks of hepatotoxicity must be considered.
- Hepatitis A and hepatitis B immunizations should be provided if there is no evidence of previous exposure.
- Pneumococcal vaccination should be given if cirrhosis is present.

ALERT

Caution is advised for prescribing androgens in the setting of hypogonadism secondary to risk of hepatotoxicity.

ISSUES FOR REFERRAL

- Hematology referral to assist with scheduled phlebotomy and monitoring.
- Refer to a gastroenterologist if liver biopsy is indicated and for the management of concomitant liver disease.
- Referrals to cardiology, endocrinology, and/or orthopedics may be indicated depending on system involvement.

ADDITIONAL THERAPIES

Experimental treatments with hepcidin mimetics to decrease intestinal iron absorption and to reduce levels of iron from the reticuloendothelial system are being researched.

SURGERY/OTHER PROCEDURES

Liver transplant is indicated in end-stage liver disease.

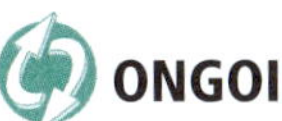

ONGOING CARE

FOLLOW-UP RECOMMENDATIONS

Patient Monitoring

- Measure hemoglobin and hematocrit before each phlebotomy; skip phlebotomy if hemoglobin is <11 g/dL (2).
- During the initiation phase of treatment, check SF every 1 to 3 months (2).
- Once iron stores are depleted, the maintenance phase of treatment should include phlebotomy every 1 to 6 months (adjusted based on patient's need) to maintain SF levels near 50 μg/L (2).
- During maintenance therapy, measure TS and SF yearly.

DIET

- Avoid consumption of iron-fortified foods, oysters, uncooked shellfish, vitamin C supplements, and iron-containing supplements. Natural food sources of vitamin C and iron are considered safe.
- Black tea chelates iron and may be consumed with meals.
- Minimize alcohol use; consumption of >60g/day increases the risk of developing cirrhosis by 9-fold (2).

PATIENT EDUCATION

- Adequate hydration prior to phlebotomy is recommended.
- Blood collected through phlebotomy may be donated.
- http://www.hemochromatosis.org/

PROGNOSIS

- The presence or absence of cirrhosis is a critical factor for prognosis (2).
- Type 2 HH is associated with earlier onset and increased disease severity than type 1 HH (2).
- SF <1,000 μg/L, normal AST, and the absence of hepatomegaly have a negative predictive value of 95% for severe fibrosis or cirrhosis (2).
- Patients diagnosed and treated before the development of cirrhosis or diabetes have a normal life expectancy.
- Cirrhosis is associated with an increased risk of hepatocellular carcinoma (annual incidence of 3–4%) and mortality.
- Cirrhosis is irreversible; diabetes, arthralgias and symptoms of hypogonadism may not improve with phlebotomies, but other complications and symptoms may be averted with successful management (2).

COMPLICATIONS

Complications develop as a result of untreated HH.

- Arthritis and chondrocalcinosis sometimes requiring joint replacement surgery
- Osteoporosis
- Diabetes mellitus
- Hypogonadism
- Arrhythmia
- Congestive heart failure
- Cirrhosis (prevalence of 20–45% in *C282Y* homozygotes with SF >1,000 μg/L)
- Hepatocellular carcinoma (one study suggests carcinoma risk is higher in men with p.C282y homozygosity).
- Infection from *Listeria monocytogenes*, *Escherichia coli*, *Yersinia enterocolitica*, or *Vibrio vulnificus* is rare, but those with iron overload are at increased risk (2).

REFERENCES

1. Buzzetti E, Kalafateli M, Thorburn D, et al. Interventions for hereditary haemochromatosis: an attempted network meta-analysis. *Cochrane Database Syst Rev*. 2017;3(3):CD011647.
2. Kowdley KV, Brown KE, Ahn J, et al. ACG clinical guideline: hereditary hemochromatosis. *Am J Gastroenterol*. 2019;114(8):1202–1218.

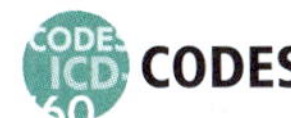

CODES

ICD10

- E83.110 Hereditary hemochromatosis
- E83.118 Other hemochromatosis
- E83.111 Hemochromatosis due to repeated red blood cell transfusions

CLINICAL PEARLS

- Screening of the general population for hemochromatosis is not recommended, but testing is recommended if there is clinical suspicion or family history.
- Many patients with iron overload remain asymptomatic.
- An elevated TS is the earliest abnormality in hemochromatosis. Ferritin is a sensitive measure of iron overload but can be elevated in a variety of infectious and inflammatory conditions without iron overload being present. Genetic testing is recommended to confirm HH.
- Patients with HH who have hepatomegaly, transaminitis, and/or serum transferrin >1,000 μg/L should be evaluated for liver iron content via hepatic MRI or sometimes liver biopsy.
- Initiate once or twice weekly phlebotomy when SF levels are elevated, especially when symptoms or clinical findings are present and recommend hydration prior to phlebotomy.
- Goal is to achieve and then maintain SF levels near 50 μg/L without causing anemia below a hemoglobin of 11 g/dL.

HEMORRHOIDS

Donna I. Meltzer, MD

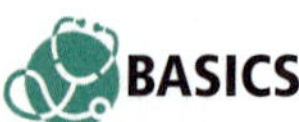

BASICS

DESCRIPTION

- Varicosities of the hemorrhoidal venous plexus
- External hemorrhoids
  - Located below (distal to) the dentate line; somatic innervation (painful)
  - Covered by squamous epithelium
- Internal hemorrhoids
  - Located above (proximal to) the dentate line; visceral innervation (painless)
  - Covered by columnar epithelium
  - Classification of internal hemorrhoids (1)
    - Grade I: Hemorrhoid vessel bulges without prolapse.
    - Grade II: Hemorrhoid prolapses with straining but reduces spontaneously.
    - Grade III: Hemorrhoid prolapses with straining and requires manual reduction.
    - Grade IV: chronically prolapsed—cannot be reduced
- Internal and external hemorrhoids often coexist.
- Although often asymptomatic, hemorrhoids can present with itching, bleeding, soilage, prolapse, or pain.
- Pain and thrombosis more common with external than internal hemorrhoids

Geriatric Considerations

Hemorrhoids and rectal prolapse are more common in elderly.

Pediatric Considerations

- Uncommon in infants and children; most common cause is chronic liver failure; other findings (rectal polyps, skin tags, condyloma) often misdiagnosed as hemorrhoids
- In adolescents, chronic constipation and prolonged toilet time can result in hemorrhoids.

Pregnancy Considerations

- Common in pregnancy
- Often resolve after delivery
- No treatment required, unless extremely painful

EPIDEMIOLOGY

- Predominant age: adults; peak from 45 to 65 years (2)
- Predominant sex: male = female

Incidence

Common; >3.5 million office visits in United States per year are related to hemorrhoidal disease (1).

Prevalence

- ~4–5% in general population in the United States
- 39% prevalence on routine screening colonoscopy (2)

ETIOLOGY AND PATHOPHYSIOLOGY

- Exact pathophysiology is unknown.
- There are three primary hemorrhoidal cushions—typically located in left lateral, right anterior, and right posterior positions. Hemorrhoidal cushions augment anal closing pressure and protect the anal sphincter during stool passage. During Valsalva, increased intra-abdominal pressure raises pressure within the hemorrhoidal cushions. Mechanisms implicated in symptomatic hemorrhoidal disease include the following:
  - Dilated veins of hemorrhoidal plexus
  - Tight internal anal sphincter
  - Abnormal distention of the arteriovenous anastomosis
  - Prolapse of the cushions and the surrounding connective tissues

Genetics

No known genetic pattern

RISK FACTORS

- Pregnancy
- Pelvic space-occupying lesions
- Liver disease; portal HTN
- Constipation (prolonged straining)
- Occupations that require prolonged sitting
- Loss of perianal muscle tone due to old age, rectal surgery, birth trauma/episiotomy, anal intercourse
- Obesity
- Chronic diarrhea

GENERAL PREVENTION

- Avoid constipation by consuming high-fiber diet (>30 g/day) and ensuring proper hydration.
- Avoid prolonged sitting or straining on the toilet.

COMMONLY ASSOCIATED CONDITIONS

- Liver disease; cirrhosis, ascites
- Pregnancy
- Constipation

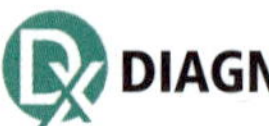

DIAGNOSIS

Diagnosis is typically straightforward through history and inspection of the perineum, rectal exam, and anoscopy.

HISTORY

- Symptoms
  - Bleeding (~60%)
  - Classically, bright red blood per rectum, may range from scant blood on toilet paper to copious blood in the toilet bowl
  - Pruritus (~55%)
  - Perianal discomfort (~20%)
  - Soiling (~10%)
  - Constipation or diarrhea
  - Straining with defecation
- More extensive internal hemorrhoids
  - Feeling of incomplete evacuation
- External hemorrhoids
  - Episodic bleeding on stool or toilet paper, pruritus, and irritation from compromised hygiene and pain
- Thrombosed hemorrhoids present as acute painful mass.
- Ask about diet (fiber, fluid intake), bowel patterns (frequency, consistency, incontinence), bowel habits (prolonged sitting), change in stools, and systemic symptoms (weight loss, pain, fever).
- Ask about past medical history and family history (gastrointestinal disease, colorectal cancer).

PHYSICAL EXAM

- Visual anorectal inspection at rest and with Valsalva maneuver in left lateral or lithotomy or knee-chest position
- Digital rectal exam: Check sphincter tone and tenderness.
- Anoscopy
  - Internal hemorrhoid appears as purple mass on lumen wall.
  - Examine for additional anorectal pathology (skin tags, mass, abscess, fissure, fistula).
- Attempt to reduce prolapsed hemorrhoids.
- Abdominal exam to exclude mass
- Peripheral stigmata of cirrhosis and portal HTN (caput, telangiectasias, palmar erythema)

DIFFERENTIAL DIAGNOSIS

- Rectal or anal neoplasia
- Condyloma
- Skin tag
- Inflammatory bowel disease
- Anal fistula, fissure, or abscess
- Rectal polyp
- Rectal prolapse

DIAGNOSTIC TESTS & INTERPRETATION

Initial Tests (lab, imaging)

Not indicated unless anemia is suspected

Diagnostic Procedures/Other

Sigmoidoscopy or colonoscopy depending on risk factors for malignancy in patients with rectal bleeding

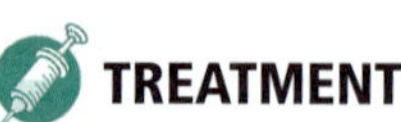

TREATMENT

Prevention

- Fiber supplements and adequate fluid intake
- Stool softeners
- Anal hygiene

GENERAL MEASURES

- Hemorrhoids are a recurrent disease, even after surgical excision. Preventive measures should be continued indefinitely.
- For mild symptoms or prevention
  - Avoid prolonged sitting during bowel movements; effect of squatting is unknown.
  - Avoid straining.
  - Avoid constipation by eating a high-fiber diet or by taking fiber supplements (psyllium husk); if necessary, take regular stool softeners.
  - Regular exercise, weight loss if indicated
- Pruritus or mild discomfort after stooling might respond to topical corticosteroid ointment, anesthetic ointments or sprays, and warm sitz baths.
- Constipation relief, anal hygiene, local ointments, and sitz baths are effective through the stage of easy reduction (grade II). More severe stages often require ligation or surgery.

MEDICATION

First Line

- Dietary modification with adequate fluid and high fiber (25 to 35 g/day) is first-line, nonoperative therapy for symptomatic hemorrhoids (2).
- Fiber supplementation (psyllium husk) helps relieve overall symptoms and bleeding (3)[A].
- Stool softener or bulk-forming laxative to soften stool

- Sitz bath with warm water for pain relief
- Topical anesthetics (benzocaine, lidocaine, pramoxine), steroids, emollients; these over-the-counter (OTC) products have been traditionally used but lack strong evidence for long-term use (3).
  - Local anesthetics for relief of pain and itch; applied to perianal area (not inserted into rectum)
  - Dibucaine 1% ointment (Nupercainal), lidocaine 5% (Preparation H, Tucks), pramoxine 1% foam, ointment, wipe (Proctofoam); benzocaine 20% spray, ointment. Use sprays with caution as alcohol in product may cause burning sensation.
- Anti-inflammatory agents (corticosteroids) to decrease swelling, discomfort, and itch
  - Hydrocortisone ointment, cream (0.25–2.5%) (Anusol HC, Cortifoam); rectal suppositories are for short-term use only.
- Astringents to help dry skin
  - Witch hazel solution, wipes, pads (Preparation H, Tucks) after stooling
- Vasoconstrictors to shrink hemorrhoids and ameliorate bleeding, pain, itch
  - 0.25% phenylephrine ointment, suppository, gel (Preparation H, Rectacaine)

Second Line

Treatment for special cases

- Acute thrombosed external hemorrhoids: If present within 72 hours after pain onset, recommend incision and clot evacuation or excision of hemorrhoid complex. Early surgical excision may resolve symptoms faster and lower incidence of recurrence (3)[C].
- Strangulated hemorrhoid: Untreated irreducible hemorrhoid can progress to thrombosis and necrosis. Treatment requires urgent or emergent hemorrhoidectomy.
- Acute hemorrhoidal bleeding associated with portal HTN: Treatment depends on degree of hemorrhoids and amount of bleeding. Differentiate from more serious anorectal varices which require medical management (correct coagulopathy) and surgical interventions (suture ligation and shunts if necessary).

SURGERY/OTHER PROCEDURES

- Indications: failure of medical and nonoperative therapy, symptomatic grade III or IV hemorrhoids in presence of a concomitant anorectal condition requiring surgery, or patient's preference
- Office-based procedures for patients with grade I or II (or III) internal hemorrhoids who have failed conservative management
  - Rubber band ligation (RBL) most common and most effective office-based procedure for symptomatic internal (not external) hemorrhoids. Consider pausing antiplatelet and anticoagulation therapy (3)[A].
  - Infrared photocoagulation: Infrared light waves cause necrosis within hemorrhoid; similar or slightly higher recurrence rates compared to RBL; less postoperative pain and fewer complications (1),(2)[A],(3)[A]
  - Sclerotherapy: submucosal injections causing local thrombosis; might be best for patients at increased bleeding risk (anticoagulated, advanced liver disease); care must be taken to inject proper site; not for advanced disease or if evidence of infection, inflammation, or ulceration
  - Cryotherapy is no longer recommended due to high rate of complications.
- Surgery for patients with symptomatic grade III or IV disease (internal or external hemorrhoids) or for those who have failed nonoperative treatments (3)[A]
  - Closed hemorrhoidectomy—closure of mucosal defect; less postoperative pain and bleeding compared to open approach (3)[A]
  - Open hemorrhoidectomy—tissue removed and mucosal defect left open
  - Different technologies are available to excise hemorrhoidal tissue: diathermy, lasers, ultrasonic dissectors; associated with less pain.
- Other techniques reduce surgical time, early postoperative pain, urinary retention, and time to return to normal activity.
  - Doppler guided hemorrhoidal artery ligation (HAL): anoscope or proctoscope with Doppler probe to identify and ligate hemorrhoidal artery; less pain but higher recurrence rates (3)[A].
  - Stapled hemorrhoidopexy: excises submucosa; shorter recovery but more recurrent disease than conventional hemorrhoidectomy; not for initial treatment given risk of complications (2),(3)[A]
  - LigaSure hemorrhoidectomy: electrosurgical technique to coagulate vessels; reduces operating time, is superior in terms of patient tolerance, and is equal to conventional hemorrhoidectomy in long-term symptom control (2)[A],
  - Laser treatment for Grade II and III hemorrhoids; more long term outcome studies are needed.
- No gold standard surgical treatment; need to individualize based on symptoms and risks/benefits of each procedure

COMPLEMENTARY & ALTERNATIVE MEDICINE

- Oral bioflavonoids have shown beneficial effect on bleeding, pruritus, and recurrence (1),(3)[A].
- Topical nifedipine (compounded by pharmacist) can relieve pain of thrombosed hemorrhoids.
- Topical nitroglycerin (0.4%) has been used to decrease anal sphincter spasm in thrombosed hemorrhoids; headache is the primary side effect.
- Botulinum toxin injection into anal sphincter to relieve spasm and pain of thrombosed hemorrhoid

ONGOING CARE

FOLLOW-UP RECOMMENDATIONS

- Encourage physical fitness, weight management, and dietary compliance.
- Avoid prolonged sitting and straining on the toilet.

Patient Monitoring

As needed, depending on treatment

DIET

High fiber with a target of 30 g of insoluble fiber per day through sources such as wheat bran cereals, oatmeal, peanuts, artichokes, beans, corn, peas, spinach, potatoes, apples, apricots, blackberries, raspberries, prunes, pears, bananas; adequate fluids (6 to 8 glasses of water per day); avoid excessive caffeine.

PATIENT EDUCATION

Increasing dietary fiber: https://familydoctor.org/fiber-how-to-increase-the-amount-in-your-diet/

PROGNOSIS

- Spontaneous resolution
- Recurrence

COMPLICATIONS

- Thrombosis
- Ulceration
- Anemia (rare)
- Incontinence
- Pelvic sepsis following hemorrhoidectomy

REFERENCES

1. Cengiz TB, Gorgun E. Hemorrhoids: a range of treatments. *Cleve Clin J Med*. 2019;86(9):612–620.
2. Mott T, Latimer K, Edwards C. Hemorrhoids: diagnosis and treatment options. *Am Fam Physician*. 2018;97(3):172–179.
3. Hawkins AT, Davis BR, Bhama AR, et al. The American Society of Colon and Rectal Surgeons clinical practice guidelines for the management of hemorrhoids. *Dis Colon Rectum*. 2024;67(5):614–623.

ADDITIONAL READING

- Aibuedefe B, Kling SM, Philp MM, et al. An update on surgical treatment of hemorrhoidal disease: a systematic review and meta-analysis. *Int J Colorectal Dis*. 2021;36(9):2041–2049.
- Gardner IH, Siddharthan RV, Tsikitis VL. Benign anorectal disease: hemorrhoids, fissures, and fistulas. *Ann Gastroenterol*. 2020;33(1):9–18.
- Sandler RS, Peery AF. Rethinking what we know about hemorrhoids. *Clin Gastroenterol Hepatol*. 2019;17(1):8–15.

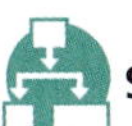

SEE ALSO

Colon Cancer; Portal Hypertension; Rectal Cancer

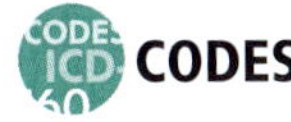

CODES

ICD10

- K64.9 Unspecified hemorrhoids
- K64.4 Residual hemorrhoidal skin tags
- K64.1 Second degree hemorrhoids

CLINICAL PEARLS

- Hemorrhoids are common. Internal hemorrhoids are typically painless. External hemorrhoids are typically painful.
- Many cases can be managed conservatively.
- All patients should be encouraged to consume 25 to 35 g of fiber per day.
- More advanced hemorrhoidal disease requires intervention with ligation or surgery.

HENOCH-SCHÖNLEIN PURPURA

Janki Majithia, DO

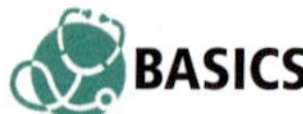

BASICS

Also known as Immunoglobulin-A Vasculitis (IgAV)

DESCRIPTION

- Henoch-Schönlein purpura (HSP) is a nonthrombocytopenic, predominantly IgA-mediated, small vessel vasculitis that affects multiple organ systems and occurs in both children and adults.
- HSP is often self-limited, with the greatest morbidity and mortality attributable to long-term renal damage.
- Characterized by a tetrad of purpuric skin lesions, arthralgia, abdominal pain, and nephropathies

EPIDEMIOLOGY

Most common vasculitis in children, with a marked seasonal pattern and frequent association with preceding upper respiratory tract infections.

Incidence

- Annual incidence for children is estimated to be 20/100,000 children <17 years of age with peak incidence of 70/100,000 in children between the ages of 4 and 6 years.
- Annual incidence for adults is estimated to be 5/100,000.
- Gender: Male-to-female ratio is between 1.2:1 and 1.8:1
- Race/ethnicity: most common in White and Asian, less common among African American

Prevalence

Annual prevalence: 10 to 22/100,000 persons; more common in fall and winter

ETIOLOGY AND PATHOPHYSIOLOGY

- Autoimmune disorder in which IgA production is increased in response to trigger(s), IgA1 immune complexes then activate the complement pathway, leading to production of inflammatory cytokines and chemokines.
- IgA-containing immune complex deposition results in small vessel inflammation which leads to fibrosis and necrosis within skin, intestinal mucosa, joints, and kidneys.
- No single etiologic agent has been identified; however there are some associations (listed below) and a popular theory is one of a multihit model leading to HSP-associated glomerulonephropathy.
  - Infections are suggested by prevalence in the fall/winter and a common upper respiratory infection (URI) prodrome. Associated pathogens include (but are not limited to) group A *Streptococcus* (may be present in up to 30% of HSP-associated nephritis), parvovirus B19, *Bartonella henselae*, *Helicobacter pylori*, *Haemophilus parainfluenzae*, coxsackievirus, adenovirus, hepatitis A and B viruses, *Mycoplasma*, Epstein-Barr virus, herpes simplex, varicella, *Campylobacter*, methicillin-resistant *Staphylococcus aureus*.
  - Drugs are most often associated with adults with HSP: acetaminophen, angiotensin-converting enzyme inhibitors (ACEI), angiotensin II receptor antagonists (ARB), some antibiotics including clarithromycin quinolones, etanercept, codeine, nonsteroidal anti-inflammatory drugs (NSAIDs).
  - Vaccinations are rarely associated with HSP; MMR, pneumococcal, meningococcal, influenza and hepatitis B

Genetics

Associated with α_1-antitrypsin deficiency, familial Mediterranean fever, HLA-A2, HLA-A11, HLA-B35, HLA-DRB1, renin-angiotensin and nitric oxide synthetase polymorphisms

RISK FACTORS

- Age peak in children 3 to 10 years
- Male > female
- Recent infections
  - Group A *Streptococcus*, parainfluenza, parvovirus B19, mycoplasma, adenoviruses, EBV, VZV, *H. pylori* and COVID-19
- Medications and vaccines
  - β-Lactam/macrolide antibiotics, NSAIDs, ACEI inhibitors/ARBs. Vaccines include influenza, hepatitis B, and MMR.
- Genetic and familial factors
  - HLA associations (HLA-DRB1-01, HLA-B35)

COMMONLY ASSOCIATED CONDITIONS

- Rare association is with solid tumors, lymphoma, prostate cancer, non–small cell lung cancer, multiple myeloma.
- Possible relationship with *H. pylori* infection and immune-related disorders (food allergy, drug allergy, inflammatory bowel disease)

DIAGNOSIS

Palpable purpura/petechiae (mandatory criteria)—without thrombocytopenia or coagulopathy and *at least one* of the following:

- Diffuse abdominal pain
- Biopsy with predominant IgA deposition
- Arthralgia or arthritis (acute onset)
- Renal involvement (hematuria or proteinuria)
- Direct immunofluorescence showing IgA deposition (negative staining does not exclude IgAV)

HISTORY

- Exposure to possible trigger, including recent infection (particularly URI) or offending drug
- Rash (most common presenting symptom): purpuric, palpable; predominant distribution often symmetric on dependent areas (lower extremities and buttocks); may spread elsewhere, typical duration 3 to 10 days with no definitive temporal association with other symptoms
- Gastrointestinal (GI) (about 50–75% of cases)
  - Nausea/vomiting
  - Abdominal pain (diffuse, colicky, may be transient or constant)
  - Hematochezia/melena
- Polyarthritis (about 75% of cases)
  - Often symmetric involvement of knees and ankles
- Renal (about 20–55% of cases)
  - Gross hematuria (higher in adults than children)
  - Oliguria or anuria
- Fatigue
- Low-grade fever
- Rare symptoms: periorbital or scrotal swelling, headache, seizures, neuropathy, behavioral changes, hemoptysis

PHYSICAL EXAM

- Classic tetrad of IgAV includes: palpable purpura without thrombocytopenia and coagulopathy, arthritis/arthralgia, abdominal pain, and kidney disease.
- Rash (96% of cases, 74% primary presenting symptom):
  - May start as urticaria, develops into nonblanching, palpable purpura, with or without petechiae, ecchymoses and bullae
  - Distribution usually symmetric, most commonly involving the lower extremities but may involve the face and trunk
- Abdominal tenderness (66% of cases, 12% primary presenting symptom):
  - Evidence of GI hemorrhage (28% of cases), recommend rectal examination to assess for hematochezia.
- Joint tenderness (64% of cases, 15% primary presenting symptom):
  - Mainly affects knees or ankles; may have associated warmth and limited range of motion, less commonly effusion; erythema is absent; nonmigratory, transient; lower extremity edema
- Orchitis (5%): presents as scrotal swelling and tenderness, may have associated torsion
- Renal disease(<1% primary presenting symptom): Hypertension (HTN) may be present.
- Rarely, patients present with central nervous system (CNS) or pulmonary involvement

DIFFERENTIAL DIAGNOSIS

- Infection:
  - Meningococcemia
  - Rocky Mountain spotted fever
  - Bacterial endocarditis
  - Rheumatic fever
  - Epstein-Barr virus
  - Sepsis
- Vasculitides:
  - Polyarteritis nodosa
  - Granulomatosis with polyangiitis
  - Microscopic polyangiitis
  - Systemic lupus erythematosus
  - Kawasaki disease
  - Urticarial vasculitis
  - Cryoglobulinemia-associated vasculitis

- Other:
  - Acute post-streptococcal glomerulonephritis
  - Inflammatory bowel disease
  - Idiopathic thrombocytopenic purpura/thrombotic thrombocytopenic purpura
  - Juvenile idiopathic arthritis/mixed connective tissue disease/juvenile dermatomyositis
  - Leukemia/lymphoma
  - Hereditary hemorrhagic telangiectasia
  - Acute surgical abdomen
  - Child abuse

DIAGNOSTIC TESTS & INTERPRETATION

- Histologic analysis of skin/renal biopsies, revealing leukocytoclastic vasculitis of postcapillary venules
- Labs directed toward excluding other illnesses and assessing degree of renal involvement

Initial Tests (lab, imaging)

- Complete blood count: Leukocytosis and thrombocytosis may occur. Eosinophilia is common. Thrombocytopenia indicates an alternative cause of purpura; anemia if GI hemorrhage occurs
- Blood culture if sepsis is a concern
- Basic serum chemistry panel: evaluate renal function
- Urinalysis/estimated glomerular filtration rate, hematuria
- Prothrombin time/international normalized ratio and partial thromboplastin time: normal in HSP; abnormal coagulation studies may indicate an alternative cause of purpura.
- Acute phase reactants (erythrocyte sedimentation rate [ESR]/C-reactive protein)
- IgA level: often elevated, nonspecific and nonsensitive
- Complement levels: normal; sometimes decreased
- Antistreptolysin O titer: evaluates for preceding streptococcal infection
- Imaging not routine for HSP but may be performed to rule out alternative etiologies or complications
  - Abdominal radiographs for free air and US intussusception (most serious and common GI manifestation)
  - CT arteriography may be necessary to identify the location of bleeding in patients with GI hemorrhage.

Diagnostic Procedures/Other

- Renal biopsy: obtain if diagnosis is uncertain or if urinalysis shows nephrotic range proteinuria; biopsy may show mesangial IgA deposition, mesangial proliferation, or, in severe cases, crescentic glomerulonephritis.
- Skin biopsy of purpura: IgA deposition in the dermis on immunofluorescence
- Endoscopy for hemorrhage as symptomatic overlap of HSP with inflammatory bowel disease
- Barium enema may be therapeutic for intussusception.

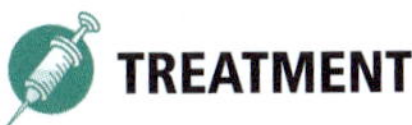

TREATMENT

GENERAL MEASURES

Rest and elevation of affected areas may limit purpura. Hydration and nutrition play a supportive role in treatment.

MEDICATION

- In the absence of renal dysfunction or complication, HSP is usually self-limited and best managed with supportive care as it resolves in 94% of children and 89% of adults.
- NSAIDs effective for symptomatic joint pain. Caution is advised in cases of renal involvement and consider acetaminophen as an alternative.
- Steroids are useful early in disease for patients with severe joint and abdominal pain, cerebral vasculitis, pulmonary hemorrhage, orchitis and in those with glomerulonephritis with severe renal involvement. Oral prednisone (1 to 2 mg/kg/day) or pulsed intravenous methylprednisolone (10 to 30 mg/kg/day) may decrease both duration of abdominal pain and severity of joint pain. This may have benefit in preventing GI bleeding and causes of surgical abdomen, including intussusception; may benefit dermatologic and renal complications
  - Early steroids have no effect on prevention or development of renal involvement after 1 year.
- Immunosuppressive (cyclosporine [Sandimmune] and mycophenolate [CellCept]) therapy may be beneficial for patients with evidence of severe renal involvement and those with steroid-resistant disease. There have been many small case studies and case reports showing benefit in these patients. High-dose IV pulse steroids, cyclophosphamide, rituximab, mycophenolate, and plasmapheresis, have all been described in small studies. Consensus for when to definitively use these agents is still controversial and the subject of further research (1)[B].
- ACEI or ARB may be helpful in patients with HSP and persistent proteinuria.

ISSUES FOR REFERRAL

Nephrology referral for renal biopsy if nephrotic range proteinuria at any time or proteinuria >100 mg/mmol for 3 months after diagnosis

ADMISSION, INPATIENT, AND NURSING CONSIDERATIONS

Admission criteria/initial stabilization

- Insufficient oral intake, renal insufficiency
- Severe abdominal pain, severe GI bleeding
- Altered mental status
- Mobility restriction due to arthritis
- HTN, nephrotic syndrome

ONGOING CARE

FOLLOW-UP RECOMMENDATIONS

Patient Monitoring

- Seen weekly during the acute illness with history, physical exam (include BP measurement), and urinalysis.
- Because ~100% of patients who develop renal involvement will do so within 6 months of HSP diagnosis, all patients should be followed at least monthly with BP and urinalysis for a duration of at least 6 months.
- Women with a history of HSP should be monitored for proteinuria and HTN during pregnancy.
- Consider work-up for occult malignancy in patients with adult-onset HSP.

PATIENT EDUCATION

National Kidney and Urologic Diseases Information Clearinghouse (NKUDIC): IgAV

PROGNOSIS

- Long-term prognosis heavily dependent on presence and severity of nephritis
- HSP is self-limited in 94% of children and 89% of adults.
- Most cases of HSP resolve within 4 weeks of diagnosis. Recurrence rate within 6 months of diagnosis is 33%.
- Factors associated with poorer prognosis include age >8 years, fever at presentation, purpura above the waist, elevated ESR or IgA concentration, low initial proteinuria, and increasing severity of renal histology grade.
- Chronic renal disease occurs in up to 20% of children with nephritic and nephrotic syndrome compared with 50% of adults who had any renal involvement. Risk of long-term renal failure is ≤5%.
- Risk factors that may result in renal failure include old age, HTN, elevated serum creatinine, and nephrotic and mixed nephritic–nephrotic syndrome at the onset of disease.

COMPLICATIONS

- Nephrotic/nephritic syndrome and renal failure, HTN
- Hemorrhagic cystitis, ureteral obstruction
- Intestinal infarction, perforation, obstruction, stricture
- GI hemorrhage, intussusception
- Alveolar hemorrhage
- CNS complications, including cerebral hemorrhage and seizure
- Anterior uveitis
- Myocarditis
- Orchitis, testicular torsion

H

REFERENCES

1. Pohl M. Henoch-Schönlein purpura nephritis. *Pediatr Nephrol*. 2015;30(2):245–252.

ADDITIONAL READING

Kawasaki Y. The pathogenesis and treatment of pediatric Henoch-Schönlein purpura nephritis. *Clin Exp Nephrol*. 2011;15(5):648–657.

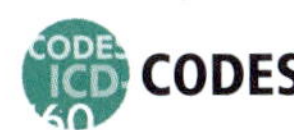

CODES

ICD10

D69.0 Allergic purpura

CLINICAL PEARLS

- HSP is a systemic small vessel vasculitis characterized by clinical tetrad of palpable purpura, abdominal pain, arthralgia, and renal dysfunction.
- The main form of treatment is supportive care, but oral corticosteroids may be beneficial if there appears to be severe renal involvement.
- In all patients with HSP, regardless of renal involvement at presentation, it is reasonable to check BP and urinalysis at weekly to monthly intervals for at least 6 months after diagnosis to monitor for developing renal dysfunction.

HEPATIC ENCEPHALOPATHY

Walter M. Kim, MD, PhD • Mehak Riaz, MBBS, MSc

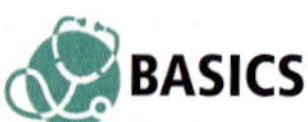

BASICS

DESCRIPTION

- Altered mental and neuromotor functioning in association with acute or chronic liver disease and/or portosystemic shunting
- Wide spectrum of reversible neurologic/psychiatric abnormalities ranging from subclinical alterations to coma: Prominent features are confusion, impaired arousability, and a "flapping tremor" (asterixis).

EPIDEMIOLOGY

Male = female (reflects prevalence of underlying liver disease)

Incidence

- Risk of first episode of overt hepatic encephalopathy (HE) is 5–25% within 5 years of cirrhosis diagnosis.
- Posttransjugular intrahepatic portosystemic shunt (TIPS), median cumulative 1-year incidence of overt HE is 10–50%

Prevalence

- May occur at any age; parallels the age predominance of fulminant liver disease: peaks in the 40s (Cirrhosis peaks in the late 50s.)
- ~50% of patients with decompensated cirrhosis demonstrate features of HE (1)
- Occurs in all cases of fulminant hepatic failure or acute liver failure (ALF).

ETIOLOGY AND PATHOPHYSIOLOGY

- There is no defined pathophysiology for the development of HE. However, elevated serum levels of ammonia (hyperammonemia) correlate with the severity of HE, suggesting a central role of ammonia as a neurotoxin. Inflammation and gut dysbiosis have also been implicated in the disease pathophysiology.
- Classifications based on 4 factors have been proposed:
  - According to the underlying disease:
    - Type A: resulting from ALF
    - Type B: resulting from portosystemic bypass or shunting in absence of inherent liver disease
    - Type C: resulting from cirrhosis
  - According to severity of manifestation:
    - West Haven classification: Covert to grades I–IV (see "Physical Exam" section).
  - According to time course:
    - Episodic HE
    - Recurrent HE: >1 episode occurring within 6 months
    - Persistent HE: persistent behavioral alterations interspersed with relapses of overt HE
  - According to precipitating factors: Non-precipitated or precipitated
- HE presents most commonly in patients with long-standing cirrhosis and spontaneous shunting of intestinal blood through collateral vessels or surgical portacaval shunts.
- Asterixis is the inability to maintain a particular posture due to metabolic encephalopathy. Abnormal diencephalic function leads to the characteristic liver flap noted when the arms and wrists are held in extension.
- Several metabolic factors are implicated in HE based on the failure of the liver to detoxify noxious CNS agents (e.g., ammonia, mercaptan, tyramine, fatty acids, lactate, manganese)
- Ammonia is considered to act as a false neurotransmitter by inducing effects on inhibitory and excitatory neurotransmission through alteration of membrane potential.
- Increased ammonia production leads to astrocyte swelling that can lead to fatal cerebral edema and death.

Genetics

- Unknown/unclear
- Conditions that predispose an individual to developing chronic liver disease such as cystic fibrosis, α_1-antitrypsin deficiency, hemochromatosis, and Wilson disease can contribute to the development of HE.

RISK FACTORS

In patients with underlying liver disease, precipitating factors include:

- Electrolyte disturbance (Na^+, K^+, Mg^{2+} most common); infection (overt or occult, including spontaneous bacterial peritonitis [SBP]); GI hemorrhage
- Use of sedative (e.g., benzodiazepines) or opiate drugs; fluid abnormalities including from diuretic overuse
- TIPS—a radiologically inserted shunt to lower portal pressure—elderly patients and those with worse liver function are at increased risk of developing HE following TIPS.

GENERAL PREVENTION

- Recognize early signs (e.g., asterixis, disorientation) and seek prompt treatment. Avoid nonessential medications, particularly opiates, benzodiazepines, and sedatives. Consider lactulose therapy as secondary prevention for recurrence of overt HE.
- For patients who have already experienced bouts of overt HE while on lactulose monotherapy, lactulose + rifaximin is the best-documented agent to maintain remission (2).

COMMONLY ASSOCIATED CONDITIONS

- Cirrhosis; portal hypertension; may occur as a complication of acute fatty liver of pregnancy
- Occurs rarely in patients with a portacaval shunt accompanied by normal liver function

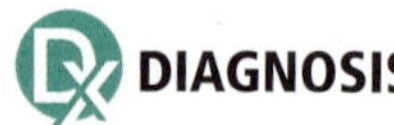

DIAGNOSIS

HISTORY

Preexisting liver disease; altered mental status, confusion; impaired arousability; constipation

PHYSICAL EXAM

- Age <10 years
  - Signs of underlying liver disease are prominent; fulminant hepatic failure or advanced cirrhosis; progression is very rapid, often over hours. Wilson disease can imitate HE.
- Ages 10 to 60 years
  - Five grades of confusion and degree of obtundation (West Haven classification)

West Haven Grade	Clinical Features
0	No apparent abnormality without mental status changes
I	Difficulty in concentration, short-term memory loss, altered sleep rhythm
II	Asterixis, lethargy, disorientation in time, personality change, and inappropriate behavior
III	Somnolence, stupor, marked confusion, and bizarre behavior
IV	Coma

- Prominent signs of underlying liver disease (50%); jaundice is most common; ascites is second most common.
- GI bleeding with hematemesis or melena (20%)
- Systemic infection, urinary tract infection, or pulmonary infection (20%)
- Age >60 years
  - Signs of underlying liver disease diminish (25%); configure confusion more prominent
  - Precipitating GI hemorrhage or infection is less often identified. Progression is slower
- Vital signs:
  - Bradycardia; increased blood pressure suggestive of increased intracranial pressure (ICP)
- Jaundice, ascites, other correlates of liver disease (e.g., spider telangiectasias, muscle wasting)
- CNS exam: Assess short-term memory and presence of asterixis ("liver flap"—a flapping of the wrist when arms and wrists are extended). Use Glasgow Coma Scale in patients with grades III–IV West Haven criteria of HE severity (2)
- Pupillary reaction regresses from normal to sluggish and then absent with worsening HE

DIFFERENTIAL DIAGNOSIS

- Metabolic encephalopathy related to anoxia, hypoglycemia, hypokalemia, hypo- or hypercalcemia, or uremia
- Head trauma, concussion, subdural hematoma; transient ischemic attack (TIA), ischemic stroke
- Increased intracranial pressure (ICP), intracranial hemorrhage (ICH)
- Alcohol intoxication; alcohol withdrawal syndrome, confusion due to medications or illicit drugs
- Meningitis, encephalitis; Wilson disease without cirrhosis; Reye syndrome; Wernicke-Korsakoff syndrome

DIAGNOSTIC TESTS & INTERPRETATION

- Clinical findings are diagnostic in 80% of cases.
- Response to treatment often confirms the diagnosis.
- EEG (limited utility): symmetric slowing of basic (α) rhythm (also common with other metabolic encephalopathies)
- Number connection test (NCT), line drawing test, critical flicker frequency (CFF) test, digit symbol test (DST), continuous reaction time (CRT) test, inhibitory control test (ICT), repeatable battery for the assessment of neuropsychological status (RBANS), and other psychometric tests may be used to assess minimal HE
- Use Glasgow Coma Scale in patients with more severe HE (grades III-IV)

Initial Tests (lab, imaging)

- Serum ammonia level is elevated in 90% of patients with HE and appears to correlate with HE severity (3), however, is not diagnostic for HE.
- Liver function tests, including aspartate aminotransferase (AST); alanine aminotransferase (ALT); and serum albumin
- Prothrombin time (PT) and international normalized ratio (INR) often elevated reflecting liver dysfunction
- Complete blood count (CBC): anemia and leukocytosis; complete metabolic profile (CMP) to identify hypokalemia, hyperbilirubinemia, altered calcium concentration, hypomagnesemia, and hypoglycemia; BUN: Creatinine >20 suggests dehydration or GI bleeding.
- Diagnostic paracentesis to rule out SBP in setting of ascites
- Blood, urine, sputum, and ascitic fluid cultures to identify infection, ABG to assess acid-base as clinically indicated
- Toxicology screen; head CT to identify frontal cortical atrophy and/or edema as well as to rule out other causes of altered mental status
- MRI is more sensitive than CT.

Follow-Up Tests & Special Considerations

- Serial neurocognitive assessment to determine progression or regression of severity/grading of HE
- Clinicians should not rely on serial monitoring of serum ammonia levels when evaluating severity of HE

Test Interpretation

- Cerebral edema is seen in 100% of fatal cases.
- Glial hypertrophy is observed in chronic encephalopathy

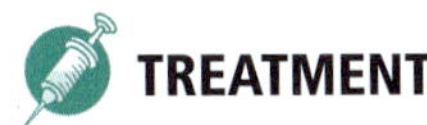

TREATMENT

GENERAL MEASURES

- Identify and treat precipitating causes: electrolyte imbalance, GI bleeding, infection
- Avoid sedatives, benzodiazepines, opiates, diphenoxylate, and atropine.
- Grade I or higher: Ensure adequate fluid and caloric ≥1,000 kcal (4.19 MJ) intake; avoid hypoglycemia
- If clumsiness and poor judgment are prominent, institute fall precautions.

MEDICATION

First Line

- Lactulose syrup (nonabsorbable disaccharide with laxative action that decreases colonic transit time and bacterial digestion that acidifies the colon to promote conversion of ammonia [NH_3] to ammonium [NH_4^+] which decreases ammonia absorption and reduces serum ammonia levels): 30 to 45 mL PO up to every hour for goal of 3 to 6 bowel movements per day; decrease to 15 to 30 mL BID when ≥3 bowel movements per day are observed.
- Lactulose enema (for patients who cannot tolerate oral lactulose or have suspected ileus): 300 mL lactulose plus 700 mL tap water, retained for 1 hour
- If worsening HE occurs acutely or there is no improvement in 2 days, add rifaximin: 400 mg PO TID or 550 mg PO BID (nonabsorbable antibiotic); highly effective in reversing minimal HE
- Contraindications: total ileus; hypersensitivity reaction; precautions: hypokalemia; other electrolyte imbalance; dehydration and renal failure

Second Line

- Neomycin: 1 to 2 g/day PO divided q6–8h, if renal function is within normal limits
- Polyethylene glycol as an alternative to lactulose
- Metronidazole and vancomycin are alternative antibiotics, although use is limited by adverse side effect profile and risk of anti-microbial resistance.
- Flumazenil may be of benefit in select patients.

ISSUES FOR REFERRAL

Refer early to experienced transplant center, especially if refractory to drug therapies.

ADDITIONAL THERAPIES

Fecal microbiota transplantation (FMT), probiotics, branched-chain amino acids, and IV L-ornithine L–aspartate; supporting evidence is preliminary

SURGERY/OTHER PROCEDURES

- Artificial liver perfusion devices are useful in fulminant hepatic failure as a bridge to transplantation
- Liver failure with recurrent, intractable overt HE is indication for liver transplant
- Consider liver transplant in patients with grade II to IV HE

COMPLEMENTARY & ALTERNATIVE MEDICINE

Probiotics and prebiotics have been associated with improvement of HE through modulation of gut flora.

ADMISSION, INPATIENT, AND NURSING CONSIDERATIONS

- Monitor clinical status closely in grades I and II when diagnosis is clear and watch for progression
- Evaluate patients with grades II to IV HE in fulminant hepatic failure for liver transplantation.

ONGOING CARE

FOLLOW-UP RECOMMENDATIONS

Activity as tolerated once resolved. After the first episode of HE, start secondary prophylaxis with nonabsorbable disaccharides (lactulose) at 20 mL of syrup twice daily and modulate dose for a goal of 2 to 3 soft bowel movements per day. If HE recurs (one or more HE episodes within 6 months), then add rifaximin

Patient Monitoring

- Asterixis and using the trail-making test (ask patient to connect-the-dots according to numbers) helps monitor HE patients. Periodic evaluation helps determine maintenance treatment and diet. Test daily at first and then at each visit when changes in drugs and diet are made.
- See patients biweekly if there are changes on the trail-making test. Stable patients should be seen monthly.
- NCT or line drawing test at each office visit can also help with patient monitoring.
- In cirrhosis, evaluate for transplantation and periodically monitor Model for End-Stage Liver Disease (MELD) score.
- Uncontrolled diabetes and malnutrition are associated with precipitation of overt HE in cirrhotic patients.

DIET

- Weight loss with sarcopenia may worsen HE.
- Regular protein diet (1.2 to 1.5 g/kg/day); protein-limited diets are avoided as patients are typically malnourished. Vegetable protein diets are better tolerated than animal protein diets in patients with advanced cirrhosis; special IV/enteral formulations with increased branched chain amino acids are available.
- Patients with grade III to IV HE require nutritional support by parenteral nutrition or jejunal feeds.

PATIENT EDUCATION

American Association for the Study of Liver Diseases: https://www.aasld.org/

PROGNOSIS

- With appropriate treatment and monitoring, acute HE often resolves.
- Chronic liver disease
  - HE recurs with variable frequency. With each recurrence, HE is more difficult to treat—the degree of improvement with treatment is reduced, and the mortality rate approaches 80%.

COMPLICATIONS

- Recurrence; with many recurrences, permanent basal ganglion injury (non-Wilsonian hepatolenticular degeneration)
- Hepatorenal syndrome

REFERENCES

1. Orman ES, Roberts A, Ghabril M, et al. Trends in characteristics, mortality, and other outcomes of patients with newly diagnosed cirrhosis. *JAMA Netw Open*. 2019;2(6):e196412.
2. European Association for the Study of the Liver. EASL clinical practice guidelines on the management of hepatic encephalopathy. *J Hepatol*. 2022;77(3):807–824.
3. Ntuli Y, Shawcross DL. Infection, inflammation and hepatic encephalopathy from a clinical perspective. *Metab Brain Dis*. 2024;39(8):1689–1703. doi:10.1007/s11011-024-01402-y.

ADDITIONAL READING

Chen A, Tait C, Minacapelli C, et al. Pathophysiology of hepatic encephalopathy: a framework for clinicians. *Clin Liver Dis*. 2024;28(2):209–224. doi:10.1016/j.cld.2024.01.002.

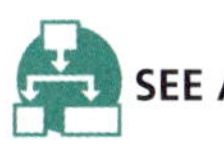

SEE ALSO

Algorithm: Delirium

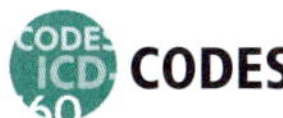

CODES

ICD10

- K72.91 Hepatic failure, unspecified with coma
- K72.11 Chronic hepatic failure with coma
- K70.40 Alcoholic hepatic failure without coma

CLINICAL PEARLS

- HE includes a spectrum of neuropsychiatric findings that occur in patients with significant alterations in hepatic function.
- Lactulose remains the cornerstone of therapy for HE.
- Asterixis ("liver flap") is the classic physical finding associated with HE.
- Elevated serum ammonia level is not diagnostic for HE; it may, however, correlate with disease severity.

HEPATITIS A

Marie L. Borum, MD, EdD, MPH • Pavan S. Vemulakonda, MD

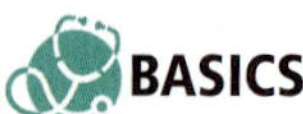

BASICS

DESCRIPTION

Hepatotropic infection caused by the hepatitis A virus (HAV), a small RNA virus

EPIDEMIOLOGY

Incidence

- The most common acute viral hepatitis worldwide with 150 million cases globally each year (1)
- Since the release of the HAV vaccine in 1995, incidence in the United States has decreased significantly. Regional outbreaks in people experiencing homelessness, in health care workers, and due to contaminated food contribute to ongoing disease.
- As many as 1/2 of current HAV infections in the United States are acquired during travel to endemic countries.

Prevalence

- Serologic evidence of prior HAV infection is present in approximately 1/3 of the US population.
- Seroprevalence for HAV has been decreasing in many parts of the world but remains high in developing nations where HAV tends to occur within the first few years of life.

Pediatric Considerations

Often, milder or asymptomatic in children; severity increases with age; asymptomatic infections occur in 70% of children <6 years of age.

Pregnancy Considerations

Increased risk of complications; vertical transmission has been reported; fecal-oral transmission during birth is possible. Breastfeeding is not contraindicated.

ETIOLOGY AND PATHOPHYSIOLOGY

- HAV is a single-stranded positive-sense linear RNA enterovirus of the Picornaviridae family. Infection is primarily within hepatocytes. HAV is excreted into the bile and then stool, providing major route of spread. Humans are the only known natural reservoir. Transmitted primarily through fecal-oral route (contaminated food); transmission is also possible sexually and parenterally. Incubation is 15 to 50 days with a mean of 28 days.
- Disease course is divided into four phases: incubation phase (asymptomatic); prodromal phase (fever, malaise, anorexia, nausea, vomiting); icteric phase (presence of dark-colored urine, pale-colored stools, jaundice and right upper quadrant pain); convalescent phase (resolution of symptoms). It does not cause chronic disease.
- Greatest infectivity period is 2 weeks before the appearance of jaundice or elevation of liver enzymes when HAV concentration is highest in the stool. HAV excretion can persist for up to 3 weeks after symptom onset.
- Virus is stable in water and on surfaces for months but is easily killed with high heat or cleaning agents.

Genetics

Autoimmune hepatitis is rarely associated with HLA class II DR3, DR13, and DR4 after HAV infection.

RISK FACTORS

- Person-to-person contact: intimate exposure, particularly anal-oral contact; residential institutions; employment in health care; household exposure; child care centers, schools
- Consumption of improperly handled food or water: Travel to developing countries accounts for >50% of cases in North America and Europe; consumption of raw/undercooked shellfish, vegetables, or other foods
- Other modes of transmission: injection of illicit drugs, blood exposure, or transfusion (rare); no identifiable risk factor in 60% of cases

GENERAL PREVENTION

- Proper sanitation and personal hygiene (handwashing), especially for food handlers, health care, and daycare workers
- HAV vaccination provides protection for 20+ years (2).
- Vaccine is recommended for:
  - All children aged 12 to 23 months, with catch-up administration until 18 years old; all travelers to countries with high endemic rate of hepatitis A (parts of Africa, Central and South America, and South and Southeast Asia)
  - Men who have sex with men; individuals using (primarily illicit) injection and noninjection drugs; individuals with occupational risks; pregnant women, if risk of infection or severe outcomes is present; all individuals ≥1 year of age with HIV
  - Chronic liver disease (including pre-liver and post-liver transplant patients); household members and close contacts of children adopted from countries with a high HAV prevalence (prior to arrival); individuals experiencing homelessness or unstable housing; unvaccinated individuals exposed during an outbreak
- Routine vaccination no longer recommended for those receiving blood products to treat clotting disorders
- HAV is *not* killed by freezing; HAV is killed by heating surfaces, supplies, or food to >185°F for 60 seconds; direct contact with chlorine is also virucidal.
- Eligible patients should receive postexposure prophylaxis (PEP) within 14 days of exposure.

DIAGNOSIS

Case definition for acute hepatitis A (2)

- Clinical criteria
  - An acute illness with a discrete onset of any sign or symptom consistent with acute viral hepatitis (e.g., fever, headache, malaise, anorexia, nausea, vomiting, diarrhea, abdominal pain, or dark urine) *and* (i) jaundice or elevated total bilirubin levels ≥3 mg/dL, *or* (ii) elevated serum alanine aminotransferase (ALT) levels >200 IU/L, *and* (iii) the absence of a more likely diagnosis
- Laboratory criteria for diagnosis
  - Confirmatory laboratory evidence: immunoglobulin M (IgM) antibody to HAV (anti-HAV) positive *or* nucleic acid amplification test (NAAT; such as polymerase chain reaction [PCR] or genotyping) for HAV RNA positive
- Case classification—meets the clinical criteria and is IgM anti-HAV positive *or* a case that has HAV RNA detected by NAAT (such as PCR or genotyping) *or* a case that meets the clinical criteria and occurs in a person who had contact (e.g., household or sexual) with a laboratory-confirmed hepatitis A case 15 to 50 days prior to onset of symptoms

HISTORY

- Onset often abrupt; common initial symptoms include nausea, emesis, diarrhea, and headache; symptom severity increases with age; pediatric cases (<6 years) frequently asymptomatic
- Other presenting historical findings: fever, malaise, fatigue, myalgias, anorexia, joint pain, dark urine (bilirubinuria), right upper abdominal pain, pruritus (can suggest cholestasis)

PHYSICAL EXAM

- Fever (variable); jaundice and icterus present in >70% of adults and older children
- Hepatomegaly and right upper quadrant tenderness are common.
- Rare symptoms include lymphadenopathy (especially cervical), arthritis, rash.
- Asterixis suggests acute hepatic failure.

DIFFERENTIAL DIAGNOSIS

- Hepatitis B, C, D, E; HIV infection, drug/toxin-induced hepatitis; hepatic steatosis, alcoholic hepatitis; autoimmune hepatitis; hemochromatosis (adults); Wilson disease
- Malaria and adenovirus infection; Epstein-Barr virus (EBV), cytomegalovirus (CMV), herpes simplex virus, yellow fever; primary or secondary hepatic malignancy, ischemic hepatitis, or Budd-Chiari syndrome

DIAGNOSTIC TESTS & INTERPRETATION

Initial Tests (lab, imaging)

- Anti-HAV IgM (blood and stool): positive at time of onset of symptoms sensitivity and specificity >95%; primary test used to diagnose acute infection; anti-HAV IgG: appears soon after IgM and may persist from years to lifetime
- AST/ALT elevated ~500 to 5,000: ALT usually > AST; alkaline phosphatase: mildly elevated
- Bilirubin typically elevated ≤10 mg/dL and typically rises following rise in ALT/AST, consistent with hepatocellular injury pattern.
- Prothrombin time and partial thromboplastin time usually remain normal or near normal. Significant rises should raise concern for acute hepatic failure or coexisting chronic liver disease.
- Mild leukocytosis; aplasia and pancytopenia; thrombocytopenia may predict illness severity.
- Albumin, electrolytes, and glucose to evaluate for hepatic and renal function (rare renal failure)
- Urinalysis (not clinically necessary): bilirubinuria
- Consider ultrasound (US) to rule out biliary obstruction only if lab pattern is cholestatic.

Follow-Up Tests & Special Considerations

Illness usually resolves within 4 weeks of onset. Lab recovery is observed by 6 months in 85% of patients. Repeat labs are not indicated unless new or persistent symptoms.

Diagnostic Procedures/Other

Abdominal ultrasonography can rule out biliary obstruction, thrombosis, cirrhosis, and other intra-abdominal pathology.

Test Interpretation

Positive serum markers in hepatitis A

- Acute disease: anti-HAV IgM only; recent disease (last 6 months): anti-HAV IgM and IgG
- Previous disease or prior vaccination: anti-HAV IgM negative and IgG positive

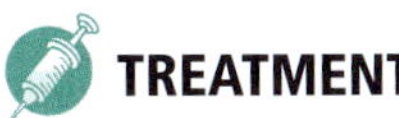

TREATMENT

GENERAL MEASURES

- Maintain appropriate nutrition/hydration; avoid alcohol.
- Universal precautions to prevent spread (e.g., washing hands, proper handling of food and water)
- Monitor coagulation defects, fluid, electrolytes, acid-base imbalance, hypoglycemia, and renal function; laboratory evaluation including coagulation factors to rule out hepatic failure; refer to liver transplant center for fulminant failure (rare).
- Report cases to public health department.

MEDICATION

- Preexposure vaccination
- Travelers: first dose as soon as possible in travelers to endemic areas
  - For unvaccinated or partially vaccinated healthy individuals aged 12 months and older, administer a single dose as soon as possible and complete the series within the recommended time frame. In addition, consider concurrent immunoglobulin (GamaSTAN) administration to those >40 years of age, with chronic liver disease, or with immunosuppression if <2 weeks from planned departure.
  - Patients with contraindications, those refusing vaccination, and those <6 months of age should receive immunoglobulin therapy (IG).
- PEP: Give PEP to persons who have not previously received HAV vaccine within 2 weeks of exposure to HAV.
  - Administer hepatitis A vaccine series as soon as possible to healthy persons aged 12 months and older (Twinrix is not recommended for PEP). Consider IG co-administration for individuals >40 years of age. A second dose of vaccine is not needed if patient has previously received at least 1 dose of vaccine. Administer IG (0.1 mL/kg) to persons <1 year of age.
  - Administer vaccine and IG to individuals with significant comorbidities (immunosuppression, liver disease) not previously vaccinated. A second dose of vaccine is not needed if the patient has previously received at least 1 dose of vaccine.
- Vaccination with same manufacturer is preferred.
- >95% of adults achieve protective antibodies after first vaccine administration and most achieve 100% after receiving their second dose.
- Hepatitis A vaccination is safe during pregnancy.

First Line

No antiviral medications available; spontaneous resolution occurs in ~99% of patients; symptom management recommend; use caution with acetaminophen; if used, limit to ≤2 g/day. Avoid hepatotoxic agents.

Second Line

- Antiemetics (e.g., ondansetron); IV fluids if patient is presenting with signs of dehydration
- Pruritus: diphenhydramine 50 mg PO IM q6h; consider cholestyramine 4 g BID if cholestasis is present.

ISSUES FOR REFERRAL

Dictated by severity of illness; for hepatic failure, refer to liver transplant program.

SURGERY/OTHER PROCEDURES

Liver transplant in fulminant hepatic failure—only rare indications

COMPLEMENTARY & ALTERNATIVE MEDICINE

Avoid hepatotoxic botanicals including barberry, comfrey, golden ragwort, groundsel, huang qin, kava kava, pennyroyal, sassafras, senna, valerian, wall germander, and wood sage.

ADMISSION, INPATIENT, AND NURSING CONSIDERATIONS

Dictated by severity of illness; usually outpatient unless signs of liver failure; treat dehydration and electrolyte imbalances; enteric isolation; private rooms, gowns, and masks are not necessary. 1:100 bleach dilution can be used to clean surfaces; frequent handwashing; use gloves when handling potentially contaminated material.

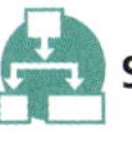

ONGOING CARE

FOLLOW-UP RECOMMENDATIONS

Return to work/school 10 to 14 days after onset of symptoms. Maintain hygiene as patients remain infectious for up to 3 weeks from symptom onset.

Patient Monitoring

Coagulation defects, fluid and electrolytes, acid–base imbalance, hypoglycemia, renal function

DIET

Adequate balanced nutrition with increased fluid intake; avoid alcohol.

PATIENT EDUCATION

Segregate food handlers with HAV. HAV immunity persists after infection.

PROGNOSIS

- Excellent; case-fatality ratio ranges from 0.3% to 0.6% for all ages; increased risk in elderly and those with chronic liver disease
- The most important prognostic factor is age; the greater the age, the more likely chance of adverse reactions.

COMPLICATIONS

- Risk of liver failure higher in patients >50 years of age and those with preexisting liver diseases
- Relapsing hepatitis—patient can experience symptoms during the 6 months following initial infection; can last between 3 weeks and 12 months; present with elevated aminotransferases and persistence of serum anti-HAV IGM antibodies.
- Prolonged cholestasis: characterized by prolonged periods of jaundice, malaise, and pruritus (>3 months); resolves spontaneously
- Autoimmune hepatitis: can be seen after HAV infection; however, responds well to steroids

REFERENCES

1. Van Damme P, Pintó RM, Feng Z, et al. Hepatitis A virus infection. *Nat Rev Dis Primers*. 2023;9(1):51. doi:10.1038/s41572-023-00461-2.
2. Nelson NP, Weng MK, Hofmeister MG, et al. Prevention of hepatitis A virus infection in the United States: recommendations of the Advisory Committee on Immunization Practices, 2020. *MMWR Recomm Rep*. 2020;69(5):1–38. doi:10.15585/mmwr.rr6905a1.

ADDITIONAL READING

Yang J, Wang D, Li Y, et al. Metabolomics in viral hepatitis: advances and review. *Front Cell Infect Microbiol*. 2023;13:1189417. doi:10.3389/fcimb.2023.1189417.

SEE ALSO

- Hepatitis B; Hepatitis C
- Algorithms: Cirrhosis; Hyperbilirubinemia and Jaundice

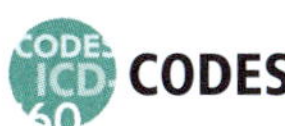

CODES

ICD10

B15.9 Hepatitis A without hepatic coma

CLINICAL PEARLS

- HAV vaccine is indicated for all children, travelers, those at elevated risk of disease, and patients with liver impairment.
- Screen all HIV-positive patients with HAV IgG and vaccinate those with negative results.
- HAV disease severity directly correlates with age; children are often asymptomatic.
- Treatment is supportive.

HEPATITIS B

Kento Sonoda, MD • Ryunosuke Hisatomi, MD

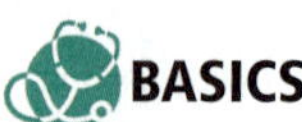

BASICS

DESCRIPTION

Hepatitis B virus (HBV) infection, caused by a DNA virus, is often transmitted by body fluids (blood, semen, and vaginal secretions). HBV is a serious global health care concern due to the spectrum of liver disease. It can cause ranging from acute hepatitis to cirrhosis and/or hepatocellular carcinoma (HCC).

EPIDEMIOLOGY

Incidence

- The highest HBV infection rate by age group is among adults aged 30 to 49 years, accounting for 46% of newly reported chronic cases (1).
- Predominant sex: fulminant HBV: male > female (2:1)
- Around 2,000 confirmed new cases of hepatitis B in the United States every year. Many more (>10,000) are believed to go unconfirmed each year.
- Lower incidence in the United States compared to Asia and Africa due to better access to health care, use of vaccinations, and preventive measure.

Prevalence

- In 2023, 17,650 newly identified cases of chronic hepatitis B were reported to CDC (~6.1/100,000).
- New cases of chronic hepatitis B among non-Hispanic Asians/Pacific Islanders (19/100,000) 10× greater than identified cases among non-Hispanic White persons (1.9/100,000)

ETIOLOGY AND PATHOPHYSIOLOGY

DNA virus of the Hepadnaviridae family; two modes of transmission:

- Horizontal: mucosal surface contact with infectious bodily fluids
- Vertical: maternal-to-newborn perinatal

Genetics

Family history of HBV and/or HCC

RISK FACTORS

- Universal one time screening in all patients aged >18 years (regardless of risk)
- Universal screening in pregnancy
- Screen the all high-risk groups.
- Household or sexual contacts with hepatitis B; persons born in regions with increase (>2%) prevalence (Asia, Africa, Eastern Europe); HIV- and HCV-positive patients; persons born in the United States who were not vaccinated as infants or whose parents are from regions of high prevalence; individuals with chronic liver disease; pregnant persons; persons with a history of incarceration
- Additional risk factors:
  - Donors and recipients of blood/products; persons on hemodialysis or immunosuppressive therapy; needle stick/occupational exposure; intranasal drug use; body piercing/tattoos; survivors of sexual assault; infants born to mothers positive for hepatitis B surface antigen (HbsAg)
- If HBsAg screening is positive, test for antibodies to HBsAg (anti-HBs) and hepatitis B core antigen (anti-HBc) to distinguish between infection and immunity. Vaccinate if seronegative.

Pediatric Considerations

- Shorter acute course; fewer complications
- 90% of vertical/perinatal infections become chronic.

Pregnancy Considerations

- Screen for HBsAg at first prenatal visit.
- If HBsAg positive, obtain HBV DNA.
- Consider treating patients with high viral load at 28 weeks or history of previous HBV-positive infant with oral nucleoside/nucleotide medication beginning at 28 to 32 weeks to reduce perinatal transmission. Infants born to HBV-infected mothers require hepatitis B immune globulin (HBIG) and HBV vaccine within 12 hours of birth.
- Breastfeeding safe if HBIG and HBV vaccines are administered and the areolar complex is without fissures or open sores. Avoid oral nucleoside/nucleotide medications during lactation.
- Continue treatment while pregnant to decrease viral load and decrease the chances of vertical transmission.

GENERAL PREVENTION

- Vaccination
  - Three IM injections at 0, 1, and 6 months in infants or healthy adults
  - Indicated for all medically stable infant weighing 2,000 g (4 lb, 6 oz) or more within 24 hours of birth; unvaccinated children and adolescents aged <19 years; all adults aged 19 to 59 years; adults aged ≥60 years with risk factors or who request vaccination; health care and public safety workers, sexual contacts, and household contacts of HBsAg carriers
  - CDC does not recommend administration of more than 2 complete hepatitis B series except for certain cases related to patients on hemodialysis.
- Other preventive measures
  - Proper hygiene/sanitation by health care workers, intravenous drug users, and tattoo/piercing artists
  - Safe sexual practices (condoms)
  - HBsAg carriers cannot donate blood or tissue.
  - Postexposure (e.g., needle stick):
    - HBIG 0.06 mL/kg in <24 hours in addition to vaccination (no more than 7 days after exposure)
    - Second dose of HBIG should be administered 30 days after exposure.

COMMONLY ASSOCIATED CONDITIONS

- HIV, hepatitis C coinfection
- Extrahepatic manifestations:
  - Serum sickness-like syndrome (fever, erythematous rash, myalgias, arthralgias, fatigue); glomerulonephritis (membranous or membranoproliferative glomerulonephritis, IgA-mediated nephropathy)
  - Polyarteritis nodosa (primary systemic necrotizing vasculitis, high fever, weakness, malaise, loss of weight and appetite); cryoglobulinemia (Raynaud phenomenon, arthritis, sicca syndrome)
  - Neurologic/psychological condition (Guillain-Barré syndrome, altered mental status, depression/psychosis)

DIAGNOSIS

HISTORY

Exposure: detailed family history, such as HBV infection and liver disease, vaccination status and social history including alcohol use, drug use, and sexual history

- Acute HBV
  - Fever, fatigue, arthralgias, myalgias, anorexia, nausea, vomiting, right upper quadrant (RUQ) abdominal pain
  - Jaundice/scleral icterus, dark urine, pale stools
- Chronic HBV: typically asymptomatic

PHYSICAL EXAM

Evaluate for stigmata of chronic liver disease: jaundice/scleral icterus, RUQ tenderness, hepatomegaly, palmar erythema, ascites, spider nevi, hepatic encephalopathy.

DIFFERENTIAL DIAGNOSIS

- Epstein-Barr virus (EBV); cytomegalovirus (CMV); hepatitis A, C, D, or E
- Drug-induced, alcoholic, or autoimmune hepatitis
- Wilson disease; hemochromatosis; HIV

DIAGNOSTIC TESTS & INTERPRETATION

Diagnosis of HBV infection is based on serologic testing (HBsAg, anti-HBs, anti-HBc); HBV DNA quantification and evaluation of liver function; acute infection indicated if IgM anti-HBc is positive; chronic infection determined by persistence of HBsAg for >6 months

Initial Tests (lab, imaging)

- AST/ALT: markedly elevated in acute HBV, ALT typically higher than AST
  - Transaminases may be normal or mildly elevated in chronic HBV; may increase before bilirubin
- Bilirubin (conjugated/unconjugated): normal to markedly elevated in acute HBV; last test to normalize as acute infection resolves
- Alkaline phosphatase: mild elevation
- HBcAb IgM may be the only early finding ("window period" before HBsAg is positive).
- For acute hepatitis: PT/INR, albumin, electrolytes, glucose, CBC; if severe acute HBV, check for superinfection with hepatitis D (HDV Ag and HDV Ab); hepatitis B serologic markers
- Hepatitis B e-antigen (HBeAg+) indicates high replication/infectivity; confirmed with high HBV DNA (≥10^5 copies/mL); benefit from medical therapy
- Screen for HDV, HIV, HCV, and immunity to hepatitis A virus (HAV Ab total/IgG).
  - Acute HBV and HDV coinfection tends to be more severe than acute HBV infection alone.
- Ultrasound to document ascites, organomegaly, signs of portal hypertension, hepatic or portal obstruction, and screen for HCC

Follow-Up Tests & Special Considerations

- Chronic HBV: HBsAg+ persistence >6 months; has five distinct phases based on HBsAg, HBeAg, HBV DNA, ALT, liver inflammation: immune-tolerant, immune-reactive HBeAg positive, inactive carrier, HBeAg negative, and occult hepatitis B.
  - Measure HBV DNA level and ALT q3–6mo.
  - If age >40 years and ALT borderline or mildly elevated, consider liver biopsy.
  - Measure baseline AFP.
  - Follow HBeAg for elimination every 6–12 mo.
- Screening for HCC (1)
  - HCC surveillance recommended for all patients with viral load >100,000 copies/mL
  - Abdominal ultrasound and α-fetoprotein testing every 6 months as screening for HCC; if ultrasound is abnormal, CT or MRI of the liver is recommended.
  - Continue surveillance even after treatment.

Diagnostic Procedures/Other

- Liver biopsy is diagnostic.
- Noninvasive tests (Hepascore, FibroTest) or elastography (FibroScan) can be used to assess fibrosis.

Marker	Acute Infection	Chronic Infection	Inactive Carrier	Resolved Infection	Susceptible to Infection	Vaccinated
HBsAg	+	+	+	−	−	−
Anti-HBs	−	−	−	+	−	+
Anti-HBc	+IgM	−IgM; +total/IgG	+	+	−	−
HBeAg	+	±	−	−	−	−
Anti-HBe	−	±	+	±	−	−
HBV DNA	Present	Present	Low negative	−	−	−
ALT	Marked elevation	Normal to mildly elevated	Normal	Normal	Normal	Normal

Test Interpretation

Liver biopsy in chronic HBV may show interface hepatitis and inflammation, necrosis, cholestasis, fibrosis, cirrhosis, or chronic active hepatitis.

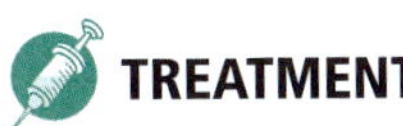

TREATMENT

GENERAL MEASURES

- Vaccinate for HBV if seronegative.
- Monitor CBC, coagulation, electrolytes, glucose, renal function. Monitor ALT and HBV DNA; increased ALT and reduced DNA imply response to therapy. Screen for HCC if HBsAg positive.
- High risk for developing HCC with chronic HBV infection—needs routine monitoring

MEDICATION

- First-line therapy for chronic HBV is use of nucleoside/nucleotide analogues (tenofovir or entecavir) or pegylated interferon. Treat patients with cirrhosis, high HBV DNA (>2,000 IU/mL), and/or active/advanced liver disease.
- Goals of therapy: loss of HBsAg with sustained HBV DNA suppression, improvement in patient-oriented outcomes, HBeAg loss/seroconversion and ALT normalization

First Line

- Acute HBV
  - Supportive care; spontaneously resolves in 95% of immunocompetent adults
  - Antiviral therapy not indicated except: fulminant liver failure or immunosuppressed
  - Treat patients with severe or protracted course and those with acute liver failure.
  - Treatment options include monotherapy with tenofovir or entecavir.
- Chronic HBV: treatment per HBeAg status.
  - FDA-approved drugs: lamivudine 100 mg, adefovir 10 mg, entecavir* 0.5 to 1 mg, telbivudine 600 mg, or tenofovir alafenamide* 25 mg, all given PO every day (dose based on renal function and age); pegylated interferon (peg-IFN) α2a (Pegasys)*, α2b SC weekly for 48 weeks (1)[A]
  - *Recommended as first-line treatment options for chronic hepatitis B
- Extended oral regimens are indicated (1)[A]
  - HBeAg positive: Treat 6 to 12 months post disappearance of antigen and gain of antibody.
  - HBeAg negative: Treat indefinitely or until clearance of antigen with antibody development.
- Change/add drug based on resistance; confirm medication adherence prior to assuming drug resistance.
- Precautions:
  - Oral drugs: renal insufficiency
  - Peg-IFN: coagulopathy, myelosuppression, depression/suicidal ideation

ISSUES FOR REFERRAL

- Referral to hepatology and transplant for all persistent HBsAg positive, fulminant acute hepatitis, end-stage liver disease or HCC
- Chronic hepatitis B therapy (1)

SURGERY/OTHER PROCEDURES

Liver transplantation, operative resection, radiofrequency ablation for HCC

ADMISSION, INPATIENT, AND NURSING CONSIDERATIONS

Worsening course (marked increase in bilirubin, transaminases, or symptoms); hepatic failure (high PT, encephalopathy)

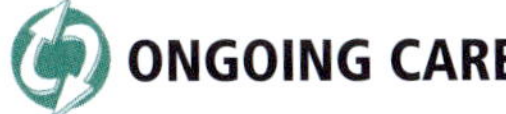

ONGOING CARE

FOLLOW-UP RECOMMENDATIONS

Patient Monitoring

- Serial ALT and HBV DNA: high ALT + low HBV DNA associated with favorable therapy response
- Monitor HBV DNA q3–6mo during therapy: undetectable DNA at week 24 of oral therapy associated with low resistance at year 2.
- Ultrasound q6–12mo to screen for HCC starting at age 40 years in men and 50 years in women (1)[B]

HBeAg	HBV DNA Viral Load	ALT[a]	Recommend
+	≥20,000 IU/mL	Elevated	Treat with antiviral or interferon.
+	≥20,000 IU/mL	Elevated but <2× ULN	Monitor every q3–6mo; treat if biopsy shows moderate fibrosis
+	≥20,000 IU/mL	Normal	Observe q6mo, consider treatment if ALT elevated. Biopsy if age >40 years or ALT is high normal to mild elevation.
−	≥2,000 IU/mL	Elevated	Treatment indicated
−	≥2,000 IU/mL	Elevated but <2× ULN	Consider biopsy or serum fibrosis marker, treatment if findings concerning.
−	≥2,000 IU/mL	Normal	Monitor q3mo.
−	≤2,000 IU/mL	Normal	Monitor q3–6mo.
Cirrhosis	Any	Any	Treat with mono or combination treatment.
Liver failure	Any	Any	Treat and refer for transplant.

[a]ALT elevated if >2× ULN; ULN for male = 30 IU/mL and for female = 19 IU/mL.

DIET

Alcohol increases risk of cirrhosis or HCC.

PATIENT EDUCATION

https://www.cdc.gov/hepatitis-b/about/index.html

PROGNOSIS

Chronic hepatitis B

- Once HBV is diagnosed, the 5-year cumulative incidence of developing cirrhosis is ~8–20% in those with untreated chronic HBV. Of patients with chronic HBV, 2–5% will progress to HCC with or without presence of cirrhosis.

COMPLICATIONS

- Hepatic necrosis; cirrhosis; hepatic failure; HCC
- Severe flare of chronic HBV with corticosteroids and other immunosuppressants
- Reactivation of infection if immunosuppressed; premedicate prophylactically if HBsAg positive or if HBcAb positive and receiving systemic chemotherapy.

REFERENCES

1. Conners EE, Panagiotakopoulos L, Hofmeister MG, et al. Screening and testing for Hepatitis B virus infection: CDC recommendations—United States, 2023. *MMWR Recomm Rep*. 2023;72(1):1–25.

ADDITIONAL READING

- Dusheiko G, Agarwal K, Maini MK. New approaches to chronic hepatitis B. *N Engl J Med*. 2023;388(1):55–69. doi:10.1056/NEJMra2211764.
- Rajbhandari R, Nguyen VH, Knoble A, et al. Advances in the management of hepatitis B. *BMJ*. 2025;389: e079579. doi:10.1136/bmj-2024-079579.

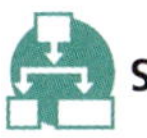

SEE ALSO

Cirrhosis of the Liver; Hepatitis A; Hepatitis C

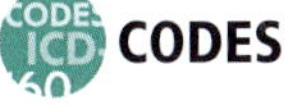

CODES

ICD10

- B19.10 Unspecified viral hepatitis B without hepatic coma
- B16.9 Acute hepatitis B w/o delta-agent and without hepatic coma
- B18.1 Chronic viral hepatitis B without delta-agent

CLINICAL PEARLS

- Screen all patients born in countries with endemic disease for HBV infection using HBsAg.
- Chronic HBV is present if HBsAg persists >6 months. Patients with chronic HBV need lifetime monitoring for disease progression and HCC.
- Acute HBV is diagnosed with HBsAg and IgM anti-HBc; treatment is supportive.
- Antiviral therapy is based on the presence or absence of cirrhosis, the ALT level, and HBV DNA levels.

H

HEPATITIS C

Tiffany Yu, MD

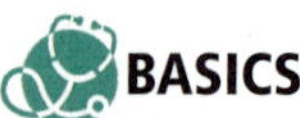

BASICS

DESCRIPTION

Systemic viral infection involving the liver

EPIDEMIOLOGY

Geriatric Considerations

Patients >60 years of age may be less responsive to therapy (1).

Pregnancy Considerations

- Routine prenatal hepatitis C virus (HCV) testing
- For HCV-infected mothers, retest HCV RNA postpartum to evaluate for spontaneous clearance.

Pediatric Considerations

- Test children born to HCV-positive mothers (ideally at 2 to 6 months of age).
- Treatment starts ≥3 years of age (1).

Incidence

- Incidence of acute hepatitis C has more than doubled since 2013.
- IV drug use accounts for ~60–70% of new cases.
- Universal screening now recommended for all adults (at least once); annual screening for high-risk groups

Prevalence

HCV is the most common bloodborne infection in the United States.

ETIOLOGY AND PATHOPHYSIOLOGY

- Enveloped, single-stranded RNA virus
- Seven known genotypes (GT) with 86 subtypes
- GT 1 is the predominant form in US (1).

Genetics

- No known predisposing genetic factors
- Transmission occurs primarily via parenteral exposure to infected blood.

RISK FACTORS

- IV drug use, HIV infection, chronic hemodialysis
- Blood/blood product transfusion or organ transplantation before July 1992
- Household or health care–related exposure
- Children born to HCV-positive mothers

GENERAL PREVENTION

- Do not share hygiene products.
- Use clean needles and dispose of needles properly. Do not share needles; cover cuts and sores.
- Practice safe sex (condoms).

COMMONLY ASSOCIATED CONDITIONS

- Hepatitis B coinfection, HIV coinfection
- Mixed cryoglobulinemia
- HCV-related renal disease—most commonly membranoproliferative glomerulonephritis

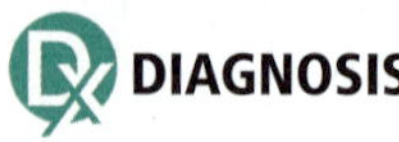

DIAGNOSIS

HISTORY

- Determine exposure risk: detailed social history, alcohol and injection drug use, history of transfusions before 1992; prior incarceration; birth cohort (1945 to 1965), history of hemodialysis
- Chronic HCV: Most cases are mildly symptomatic (nonspecific fatigue, depression) or asymptomatic (isolated elevation in ALT, AST) until advanced liver disease has developed.
- Acute HCV: typically asymptomatic but may result in mild illness
  - Average onset of symptoms (if present) is 2 to 12 weeks postexposure
  - Fatigue, jaundice, dark urine, steatorrhea, nausea, abdominal pain, low-grade fevers, myalgias, arthralgias (1)

PHYSICAL EXAM

- RUQ tenderness/hepatomegaly and/or jaundice
- Signs of advanced fibrosis/cirrhosis: spider angioma, caput medusa, palmar erythema, jaundice, gynecomastia, Terry nails
- HCV-associated conditions with pertinent physical exam findings: arthralgias/myalgias, neuropathy, livedo reticularis, lichen planus

DIFFERENTIAL DIAGNOSIS

Hepatitis A or B; EBV, CMV; alcoholic hepatitis; nonalcoholic steatohepatitis (NASH); hemochromatosis; Wilson disease, α_1-antitrypsin deficiency; ischemic, drug-induced, or autoimmune hepatitis

DIAGNOSTIC TESTS & INTERPRETATION

Initial Tests (lab, imaging)

Screening

- One-time, routine HCV antibody (Ab) screening for all adults aged 18 to 79 years of age. Follow up HCV RNA to confirm active infection.

Follow-Up Tests & Special Considerations

- Anti-HCV Ab
  - If nonreactive, no further action unless exposure within the last 6 months (test with HCV RNA.)
  - If reactive, test for HCV RNA.
    - If not detected, no current HCV infection and no further action required
    - If detected, current HCV infection confirmed
- Anti-HCV Ab detected 4 to 10 weeks after infection
  - ~97% of patients with HCV will develop Abs by 6 months after exposure.
  - Consider HCV RNA testing in immunocompromised.
- HCV RNA detected 2 weeks after infection
- Pretreatment testing and assessment
  - Recommend CBC, liver function tests, INR, eGFR within 6 months of starting HCV treatment
  - Non-invasive liver fibrosis assessment (elastography; Fibrosis-4 (FIB-4); APRI—AST to Platelet Ratio Index)
  - Screening for HIV coinfection
  - Hepatitis B serologies

Diagnostic Procedures/Other

Evaluate for hepatic fibrosis:

- FIB-4 score prior to initiation of treatment.
- Liver imaging: ultrasound (US), CT scan, MRI, transient US elastography, MR elastography
- Liver biopsy (gold standard)

Test Interpretation

- FIB-4 scoring: https://www.hepatitisc.uw.edu/page/clinical-calculators/fib-4
  - Score >3.25 indicates advanced fibrosis.

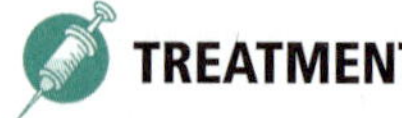

TREATMENT

GENERAL MEASURES

- Goal is to achieve sustained virologic response (SVR), reduce adverse events and all-cause mortality.
- Report acute HCV to state health department.
- Treat all patients with virologic evidence of HCV.
- Exceptions: children <3 years of age, pregnancy, short life expectancy

MEDICATION

First Line

- Patients are first divided into those without cirrhosis and those with compensated cirrhosis.
- Simplified treatment does not require a genotype.
- Simplified treatment guidelines for patients without cirrhosis (https://www.hcvguidelines.org/treatment-naive/simplified-treatment) and with compensated cirrhosis (https://www.hcvguidelines.org/treatment-naive/simplified-treatment-compensated-cirrhosis)
- For all treatments, review all patient medications (including over-the-counter medications and supplements) for drug interactions with HCV treatment (https://www.hep-druginteractions.org/)
- Screen for hepatitis B infection as all medications for hepatitis C carry a black box warning for hepatitis B reactivation.

Second Line

If a patient fails initial treatment, alternative regimens include:

- Sofosbuvir (400 mg)/velpatasvir (100 mg)/voxilaprevir (100 mg) (SOF/VEL/VOX) +/− weight-based ribavirin
- Glecaprevir (300 mg)/pibrentasvir (120 mg) plus daily sofosbuvir (400 mg) and weight-based ribavirin

ISSUES FOR REFERRAL

- Referral to gastroenterology, hepatology or infectious disease specialists if a patient fails to achieve SVR with initial first-line treatment
- Refer to liver transplant program if fulminant acute hepatitis, complication of end-stage disease, decompensated cirrhosis or HCC.

ADDITIONAL THERAPIES

Chronic HCV treatment with traditional agents, pegylated interferon (PEG-IFN) and ribavirin, is often poorly tolerated and less effective than DAA treatments, which limits consideration as first-line treatment. Patients previously treated with PEG-IFN and ribavirin can be treated with first-line options.

SURGERY/OTHER PROCEDURES

See "Follow-up Recommendations."

COMPLEMENTARY & ALTERNATIVE MEDICINE

- No strong evidence or guidelines to support effective complementary/alternative therapy.
- Avoid supplements and over-the-counter medications during hepatitis C treatments.

ADMISSION, INPATIENT, AND NURSING CONSIDERATIONS

Standard precautions

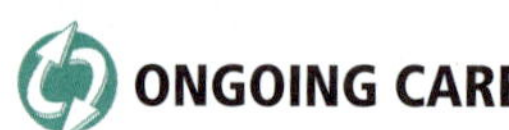

ONGOING CARE

FOLLOW-UP RECOMMENDATIONS

- All patients treated should have a viral load 12 weeks after therapy completion.
- AASLD and IDSA recommend an abdominal US every 6 months for patients with cirrhosis, to monitor for HCC.
- If cirrhosis is present, patients need endoscopic screening for varices.

Medications*	Abbreviation	Standard Dose	Common Side Effects (>10%); Contraindications
A: Elbasvir-grazoprevir (Zepatier)	ELB/GZR	50 mg/100 mg daily	Fatigue, headaches; avoid with OATP1B1/3 inhibitors or CYP3A inducers.
B: Glecaprevir-pibrentasvir (Mavyret)	GLEC/PIB	300 mg/120 mg daily	Fatigue, headaches, nausea, diarrhea, pruritus; must take with food; take 3 tablets at the same time each day.
C: Ledipasvir-sofosbuvir (Harvoni)	LED/SOF	90 mg/400 mg daily	Fatigue, headaches, weakness, irritability, insomnia, dizziness, depression, nausea, diarrhea, myalgias, cough
D: Sofosbuvir-velpatasvir (Epclusa)	SOF/VEL	400 mg/100 mg daily	Fatigue, headaches, irritability, insomnia, depression, rash, nausea, weakness

Simplified regimen for non-cirrhotic patients:

- B for 8 weeks *or* D for 12 weeks

Simplified regimen for compensated cirrhotic patients:

- For GT 1–6: regimen B for 8 weeks

or

- For GT 1, 2, 4, 5, 6: regimen D for 12 weeks
- For GT 3: NS5A RAS testing results dictate treatment regimen:
  – If NO Y93H: can be treated with regimen D for 12 weeks

Genotype Directed Non-Simplified Treatment Regimens for Treatment Naive Patients (Genotype, Regimen, Duration, Evidence):

Without Cirrhosis

Genotype 1a	Genotype 1b	Genotype 2	Genotype 3	Genotype 4	Genotype 5 or 6
GLEC/PIB × 8 weeks (1A)	GLEC/PIB × 8 weeks (1A)	GLEC/PIB × 8 weeks (1A)	GLEC/PIB × 8 weeks (1A)	GLEC/PIB × 8 weeks (1A)	GLEC/PIB × 8 weeks (1A)
LED/SOF × 12 weeks (1A)	SOF/VEL × 12 weeks (1A)	SOF/VEL × 12 weeks (1A)	SOF/VEL × 12 weeks (1A)	SOF/VEL × 12 weeks (1A)	SOF/VEL × 12 weeks (1B)
SOF/VEL × 12 weeks (1A)	ELB/GZR × 12 weeks (1A)			ELB/GZR × 12 weeks (1A)	LED/SOF × 12 weeks (IIa, B)
LED/SOF × 8 weeks (HIV-uninfected, HCV viral load <6 million IU/mL) (1B)	LED/SOF × 12 weeks (1A)			LED/SOF × 12 weeks (1A)	
	LED/SOF × 8 weeks (HIV-uninfected, HCV viral load <6 million IU/mL) (1B)				

With Compensated Cirrhosis

Genotype 1a	Genotype 1b	Genotype 2	Genotype 3	Genotype 4	Genotype 5 or 6
SOF/VEL × 12 weeks (1A)	SOF/VEL × 12 weeks (1A)	SOF/VEL × 12 weeks (1A)	SOF/VEL × 12 weeks (1A)†	SOF/VEL × 12 weeks (1A)	GLEC/PIB x 8 weeks (1A)
LED/SOF × 12 weeks (1A)	ELB/GZR × 12 weeks (1A)	GLEC/PIB × 8 weeks (1B)	GLEC/PIB × 8 weeks (1B)	GLEC/PIB × 8 weeks (1B)	SOF/VEL × 12 weeks (1B)
GLEC/PIB × 8 weeks (1B)	LED/SOF × 12 weeks (1A)			ELB/GZR × 12 weeks (IIa, B)	LED/SOF × 12 weeks (IIa, B)
	GLEC/PIB × 8 weeks (1B)			LED/SOF × 12 weeks (IIa, B)	

†Must complete NS5A resistance-associated substitutions (RASs) for Y93H

Patient Monitoring

- Assess medication adherence
- SVR12: Undetectable HCV RNA 12 weeks after therapy translates to long-term cure.
- If no evidence of cirrhosis, once SVR is achieved there is no need for continued surveillance.
- SVR decreases risk of portal hypertension, hepatic decompensation, and HCC.
- Monitor for HBV reactivation while on medication if the patient has history of HBV infection.

DIET

- Low-fat, high-fiber diet, and exercise
- Avoid alcohol.

PATIENT EDUCATION

- Avoid alcohol, tobacco, and illicit drugs.
- Education on risk of transmission to sexual partners
- Caution with nutritional supplements and herbal medications

PROGNOSIS

- Modern treatment regimens have SVR of >95% in most circumstances.
- Approximately 5–25% of patients with chronic HCV develop cirrhosis in 10 to 20 years.
- Patients with HCV and cirrhosis have a 1–4% annual risk of HCC and 3–6% annual risk of hepatic decompensation.
- Following successful SVR, there is ~70% reduction in risk of HCC and 90% reduction in risk of liver-related mortality (1).

COMPLICATIONS

- Fibrosis and cirrhosis typically develop within the first 5 to 10 years of infection if untreated.
- Risk factors for cirrhosis: age, white race, hypertension, alcohol use, anemia; risk for decompensation: diabetes, hypertension, anemia

REFERENCES

1. Benjaram S, Kapur S, Mckay A, et al. Hepatitis C—everything a primary care physician needs to know about diagnosis, management and follow-up. *J Clin Med*. 2025;14(13):4801. doi:10.3390/jcm14134801.

ADDITIONAL READING

Fricker GP, Ghany MG, Mera J, et al. Tools needed to support same-day diagnosis and treatment of current hepatitis C virus infection. *J Infect Dis*. 2024;229 (Suppl 3):S362–S369. doi:10.1093/infdis/jiad177.

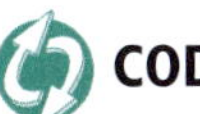

CODES

ICD10

- B19.20 Unspecified viral hepatitis C without hepatic coma
- B17.10 Acute hepatitis C without hepatic coma
- B18.2 Chronic viral hepatitis C

CLINICAL PEARLS

- HCV is the most common cause of HCC in the western world. GT 1 is most common in the US.
- 1 of 10 patients with HCV has no identifiable risk factors; 15–25% of HCV-infected persons clear the infection without specific treatment.
- One-time routine HCV screening in all adults aged 18 to 79 years and HCV testing as part of routine prenatal care are recommended. Screen others if high risk.
- Half of all patients with acute HCV develop chronic HCV, 25% of those develop cirrhosis over time.
- Use noninvasive fibrosis testing for staging.
- Sustained virologic response is associated with reduced morbidity and mortality.

H

HERNIA

Frank B. Beacham, MD, MEHP

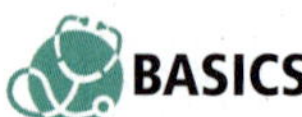

BASICS

DESCRIPTION

Areas of weakness through which structures can pass

- Types
  - Inguinal
    - Direct: acquired; herniation through defect in transversalis fascia of abdominal wall medial to inferior epigastric vessels; increased frequency with age as fascia weakens
    - Indirect: congenital; herniation lateral to the inferior epigastric vessels through internal inguinal ring into inguinal canal; a "complete hernia" descends into the scrotum, an "incomplete hernia" remains in the inguinal canal.
  - Pantaloon: combination of direct and indirect inguinal hernia with protrusion of abdominal wall on both sides of the epigastric vessels
  - Femoral: herniation descending through the femoral canal deep to the inguinal ligament; has a narrow neck and is especially prone to incarceration and strangulation
  - Incisional or ventral: herniation through a defect in the anterior abdominal wall at the site of a prior surgical incision
  - Congenital: herniation through defect in abdominal wall fascia due to collagen deficiency disease
  - Umbilical: defect at umbilical ring
  - Epigastric: protrusion through the middle line above the level of the umbilicus
  - Spigelian hernia: herniation through Spigelian line (lateral border of the rectus abdominis) for a lateral ventral hernia result
  - Sports hernia (not a true hernia): strain or tear of soft tissue of groin or lower abdomen
  - Others: obturator, sciatic, perineal
- Definitions
  - Reducible: Extruded sac and its contents can be returned to intra-abdominal position spontaneously or with gentle manipulation.
  - Irreducible/incarcerated: Extruded sac and its contents cannot be returned to original intra-abdominal position.
  - Strangulated: Blood supply to hernia sac contents is compromised.
  - Richter: Partial circumference of the bowel is incarcerated or strangulated. Partial wall damage may occur, increasing potential for bowel rupture and peritonitis.
  - Sliding: Wall of a viscus forms part of the wall of the inguinal hernia sac (i.e., right side–cecum, left side–sigmoid colon).

Geriatric Considerations

Abdominal wall hernias increase with advancing age, with significant increase in risk during surgical repair.

Pregnancy Considerations

- Increased intra-abdominal pressure and hormone imbalances with pregnancy may contribute to increased risk of abdominal wall hernias.
- Umbilical hernias are associated with multiple, prolonged deliveries.

EPIDEMIOLOGY

Incidence

- 75–80% groin hernias: inguinal and femoral
- 2–20% incisional/ventral, depends if prior surgery was associated with infection or contamination
- 3–10% umbilical, considered congenital
- Groin
  - Cumulative incidence of 25% in males; 3% in females
  - Two peaks: most inguinal hernias present between the ages of 0 to 5 and 75 to 80 years of age
  - ~50% of children aged <2 years have a patent processus vaginalis (this decreases to 40% after the age of 2 years). Only between 25% and 50% are clinically significant.
  - Inguinal hernia in <5% of newborns male-to-female ratio 10:1
  - Increased incidence in premature infants
  - Increased incidence in patients with abdominal aortic aneurysms
  - Femoral <10% of all groin hernias, 40% present as a surgical emergency
- Incisional/ventral: ~10–23% of abdominal surgeries complicated by an incisional hernia, most common in upper midline incisions; females have a higher risk of strangulation and incarceration.
- Incidence ratio: male = female
- Umbilical: 10–20% of newborns; most close by age 5 years

Prevalence

- Groin and inguinal hernias are more prevalent in men; femoral and umbilical more prevalent in women
- Most inguinal hernias are indirect in men and women.
- Incisional/ventral hernias (IVH) are more prevalent in smokers and obese individuals.

ETIOLOGY AND PATHOPHYSIOLOGY

Loss of tissue strength and elasticity (especially with aging or congenital defect in abdominal fascia) results in a fascial defect of the abdominal wall. Most pediatric hernias are congenital (e.g., patent processus vaginalis). Most adult hernias are a result of acquired weakness in the tissues of the anterior abdominal wall.

Genetics

No known genetic pattern

RISK FACTORS

- Increased abdominal pressure, coughing, heavy lifting, constipation, pregnancy, ascites, prostatism, open prostatectomy (carries 4 times risk), obesity, advancing age (loss of tissue turgor), smoking, steroid use, low birth weight, prematurity
- Age: Femoral and scrotal hernias, along with recurrent groin hernias, are associated with increased risk for acute hernia surgery.

COMMONLY ASSOCIATED CONDITIONS

Obesity, chronic obstructive pulmonary disease, multiple abdominal surgeries, pregnancy, advanced age, Ehlers-Danlos syndrome, Marfan syndrome, polycystic kidney disease (PKD), osteogenesis imperfecta, Down syndrome, abdominal aortic aneurysm

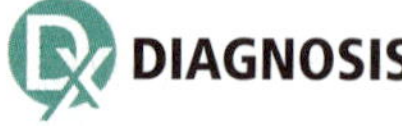

DIAGNOSIS

HISTORY

- May observe protrusion through abdominal wall during increased intra-abdominal pressure (Valsalva maneuver or cough)
- Pain, nausea, vomiting, bloating; relieved with reclining; may signal complication (e.g., strangulation)

PHYSICAL EXAM

- Examine initially with patient standing. During palpation, the patient should cough, strain, or perform Valsalva maneuver to determine the extent of intracavitary content movement. Repeat exam with patient in supine position.
- Inguinal (superior to inguinal ligament)
  - Direct inguinal hernia: Finger in inguinal canal finds defect of the transversalis fascia as a deep (posterior to anterior) bulge palpated with increased intra-abdominal pressure.
  - Indirect inguinal hernia: Finger in inguinal canal finds a persistent process vaginalis as a bulge (lateral to medial) that may extend into scrotum.
- Femoral (inferior to inguinal ligament): bulge in upper middle thigh; neck of the sac protrudes lateral to and below a finger placed on the pubic tubercle.
- Umbilical: palpable protrusion at umbilicus
- Incisional/ventral: palpable protrusion at site of prior abdominal incision or midline superior to the umbilicus
- Epigastric: palpable protrusion off midline above umbilicus

DIFFERENTIAL DIAGNOSIS

Lymphadenopathy, hydrocele, lipoma, varices, cryptorchidism, abscess, tumor, sports hernia (athletic pubalgia), pelvic fractures, adductor tears, omphalomesenteric duct, urachal cyst

DIAGNOSTIC TESTS & INTERPRETATION

Imaging rarely required; reserve for suspected abdominal hernia or unclear diagnosis; plain radiographs to rule out obstruction

- Ultrasound (US) is the best initial imaging modality for identifying occult inguinal hernia.
- CT or tangential radiography for incisional and abdominal wall hernias and postsurgical patients with complaints of abdominal pain
- If there is difficulty with routine imaging, MRI with Valsalva is an option.
- Herniography is no longer recommended.

Follow-Up Tests & Special Considerations

Patients in whom an occult inguinal hernia is suspected should undergo MRI definitive examination (1)[A].

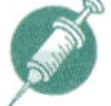

TREATMENT

- Elective repair
- Three options for elective inguinal hernia repair: open, laparoscopic, robotic
- Elective surgical repair is associated with significantly lower morbidity and mortality.

- Acute setting
  - Pain management for symptomatic hernias
  - Strangulated hernias should be surgically repaired early to prevent complications such as necrosis and viscus perforation.
  - Manual reduction of incarcerated hernias improves outcomes by allowing for elective repair after swelling and inflammation subside.
  - Complication rate is greater with emergent pediatric inguinal hernia repairs compared to elective procedures.
  - Acute hernia repair carries a higher morbidity and lower survival rate.
  - Laparoscopic repair of IVH is safe, has fewer complications, shorter hospital stays, and possibly a shorter surgical time. Postoperative pain and recurrence rates are similar to open repair.
  - For patients undergoing repair, operative times are shorter for extraperitoneal laparoscopic repair compared to open mesh repair with no difference in complication rates (2)[B].
  - Mesh is generally preferred for hernia repairs; there have been numerous FDA product recalls in the past—primarily related to complications of bowel perforation and obstruction (https://www.fda.gov/medicaldevices/productsandmedicalprocedures/implant).

MEDICATION

- Antibiotics: Prophylaxis does not reduce wound infections after groin hernia repairs.
- Antibiotics are recommended for uncomplicated inguinal or femoral hernia repairs using mesh or if there are other risks for infection.
- Pain: Local anesthetic during surgical repair results in significant reduction of postoperative pain. Tension-free procedures (e.g., Lichtenstein) may be performed under local anesthesia.

ISSUES FOR REFERRAL

Warn patients of symptoms or signs of incarceration or strangulation (acute abdominal pain, fever, bloody bowel movements), which mandate immediate evaluation.

ADDITIONAL THERAPIES

Geriatric Considerations

Use of a truss (external supportive device) for direct inguinal hernias is common; this is primarily for pain control.

SURGERY/OTHER PROCEDURES

Inguinal hernias should be surgically repaired. Watchful waiting in asymptomatic patients is safe if the patient has significant comorbidities that may compromise urgent repair.

- Incarceration and strangulation are absolute indications for hernia repair.
- Contraindications: patients who are not surgical candidates based on risk factors
  - Avoid elective repair in pregnant patients or patients with active infections.
- Special considerations
  - Umbilical hernias <0.5 cm can usually be followed clinically.
  - Umbilical hernias in children age 2 to 4 years typically close spontaneously.
  - Operative times and complication rates are similar when comparing single-incision laparoscopic inguinal hernia repair versus traditional multiport laparoscopic repair.
  - "Watchful waiting" is recommended in pregnancy. Elective postpartum repair has similar outcomes and no increased risk of incarceration or strangulation before or during delivery.
  - Women have lower recurrence rates using laparoscopic compared with open method.
  - Ascites is not a strict contraindication for repair.
- Gold standard
  - Inguinal hernia
    - Open: Lichtenstein with mesh (37%): decreased recurrence rates
    - Laparoscopic (14%) with mesh: decreased hospital stay and postoperative pain
      - Requires general anesthesia
      - Transabdominal preperitoneal (TAPP) versus total extraperitoneal (TEP)
      - Robotic repair can be a consideration although the procedure is longer than open or laparoscopic and may have 30-day operative complications of ~5% versus ~1% for other techniques (3)[B].
    - Pediatric: Laparoscopic percutaneous repair is an efficient, safe, and effective alternative to open repair. It is associated with reduced operative times and no increase in complication or recurrence rates. Avoid mesh in pediatric patients (3)[B].
  - Incisional/ventral
    - Laparoscopic repair is effective for most patients with primary or recurrent ventral hernias; there is <10% recurrence rate.
  - Umbilical
    - Pediatric: open excision with suture closure
    - Adult: Open repair with mesh may reduce hernia recurrence.
- Complications
  - Recurrence
  - Seromas
  - Postoperative pain, temporary or chronic: less with laparoscopic versus open technique
  - Wound infection
  - Injury to cord structures in inguinal herniorrhaphy; with nerve injury, most symptoms will resolve.

ONGOING CARE

PATIENT EDUCATION

Cleveland Clinic: http://my.clevelandclinic.org/disorders/hernia/hic_hernia.aspx

PROGNOSIS

- Groin (pediatric): low recurrence rates (<3%) with surgery; may spontaneously resolve in infants
- Groin (adult): ≥1% per year risk of bowel strangulation without surgical treatment; 0–10% postoperative recurrence rates, depending on surgeon experience and procedure type
- Incisional/ventral: 3–5% postoperative occurrence: 2–17% postrepair recurrence, increased to 20–46% in larger hernias
- Umbilical (pediatric)
  - High rate of spontaneous resolution
  - Hernia is less likely to close further in older children and in children with larger defects.
- Umbilical (adult): up to 11% postoperative recurrence
- Epigastric: most ultimately become incarcerated and/or strangulated without surgical treatment; recurrence is high due to frequency of missed defects during repair.

REFERENCES

1. Hope WW. State of the art: advances in hernia care. *Am Surg*. 2024;90(8):1983–1989.
2. Shakil A, Aparicio K, Barta E, et al. Inguinal hernias: diagnosis and management. *Am Fam Physician*. 2020;102(8):487–492.
3. Aiolfi A, Cavalli M, Ferraro SD, et al. Treatment of inguinal hernia: systematic review and updated network meta-analysis of randomized controlled trials. *Ann Surg*. 2021;274(6):954–961.

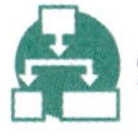

SEE ALSO

Algorithms: Abdominal Pain, Lower; Intestinal Obstruction; Pelvic Pain

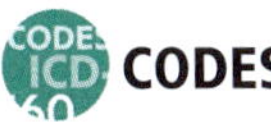

CODES

ICD10

- K46.9 Unspecified abdominal hernia without obstruction or gangrene
- K40.90 Unil inguinal hernia, w/o obst or gangr, not spcf as recur
- K41.90 Unil femoral hernia, w/o obst or gangrene, not spcf as recur

CLINICAL PEARLS

- Inguinal hernias are either direct or indirect:
  - Direct: acquired herniation through defect in transversalis fascia of abdominal wall medial to inferior epigastric vessels
  - Indirect: congenital herniation lateral to the inferior epigastric vessels; a "complete hernia" descends into the scrotum; an "incomplete hernia" remains within the inguinal canal.
- Femoral: descends through the femoral canal deep to the inguinal ligament
- Umbilical: Defect occurs at umbilical ring tissue. Most pediatric umbilical hernias close spontaneously within the first few years of life.
- Incarceration and strangulation are the primary complications associated with hernias.
- For hernias in women, and bilateral hernias, a laparoscopic endoscopic procedure is preferable.

H

HERPES EYE INFECTIONS

Stephanie L. Conway-Allen, PharmD, RPh • Kathleen A. Barry, MD

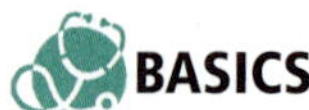

BASICS

DESCRIPTION

- Eye infection (blepharitis, conjunctivitis, keratitis, stromal keratitis, uveitis, retinitis, glaucoma, or optic neuritis) caused by herpes simplex virus (HSV) types 1 or 2 or varicella-zoster virus (VZV, also known as human herpes virus type 3 [HHV3]).
  - HSV: most often affects the cornea (herpes keratoconjunctivitis); HSV1 > HSV2; can be further divided into primary and recurrent
  - VZV: When VZV is reactivated and affects the ophthalmic division of the 5th cranial nerve, this is known as herpes zoster ophthalmicus (HZO), a type of shingles.
- System(s) affected: eye, skin, central nervous system (CNS) (neonatal)

EPIDEMIOLOGY

Predominant age: HSV—mean age of onset 37.4 years but can occur at any age, including primary infection in newborns; VZV usually advancing age (>50 years)

Incidence

- HSV keratitis: In Europe, North America, and South America, approximated at 12.5 to 31.5 new or recurrent cases per 100,000 person-years (1).
- VZV: 1 million new cases of shingles per year in the United States; 25–40% develop ophthalmic complications. Temporary keratitis is most common.

Prevalence

VZV: Prevalence of herpes zoster infection is 20–30%; ocular involvement in 50% if not treated with antivirals; overall lifetime prevalence of HZO: 1%

ETIOLOGY AND PATHOPHYSIOLOGY

- HSV and VZV are Herpesviridae dsDNA viruses.
- HSV: primary infection from direct contact with infected person via saliva, genital contact, or birth canal exposure (neonates)
  - Primary infection may lead to severe disease in neonates, including eye, skin, CNS, and disseminated disease.
  - Recurrent infection is more common overall cause of herpetic eye infections.
- VZV: Primary infection from direct contact with infected person may cause varicella ("chickenpox") and/or lead to a latent state within trigeminal ganglia.
  - Reactivation of the virus may affect any dermatome (resulting in herpes zoster or "shingles"), including the ophthalmic branch (HZO).

RISK FACTORS

- HSV: personal history of HSV or close contact with HSV-infected person
  - General risk factors for reactivation: stress, trauma, fever, UV light exposure, other viral infections
  - Risk factors for HSV keratitis: UV laser eye treatment, some topical ocular medications such as prostaglandin analogues and primary/secondary immunosuppression
- HZO
  - History of varicella infection, advancing age (>50 years), sex (female > male), acute/painful prodrome, trauma, stress, immunosuppression (2)

ALERT
Consider primary/secondary immunodeficiency disorders in all zoster patients <40 years of age (e.g., AIDS, malignancy).

GENERAL PREVENTION

- Contact precautions with active lesions (HSV and VZV).
- VZV can be spread to those who have not had chickenpox, are not immunized, or are not immune.
- Varicella recombinant zoster vaccine (Shingrix) (VZV only): 2 doses 2 to 6 months apart recommended by the CDC for all persons age 50 years and older.
  - Do not give varicella vaccine during an acute infection.
- Acyclovir can be used prophylactically to prevent recurrence of ocular HSV.

Pregnancy Considerations

- Pregnant women without history of chickenpox should avoid contact with persons with active zoster.
- Pregnancy increases risk of recurrence of HSV/VZV.
- Shingrix is contraindicated during pregnancy.

COMMONLY ASSOCIATED CONDITIONS

Primary and secondary immunocompromised states

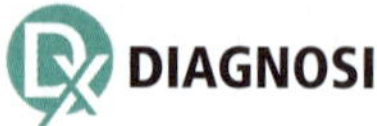

DIAGNOSIS

HISTORY

- Varies according to the virus and the ocular structures involved
- History of varicella or herpes simplex infection
- Acute onset, eye pain, headache, photophobia, tearing, ocular redness, decreased or blurry vision (2)
- May present with a prodromal period of fever, malaise, headache, and eye pain before skin eruptions and eye lesions (HZO) (2)

PHYSICAL EXAM

- Varies according to the virus and ocular structures involved
  - HSV most commonly affects the corneal epithelium.
  - VZV most commonly affects corneal stroma and uvea (2).
- Typically unilateral in presentation
  - HZO presents as early as 1 to 2 days after unilateral vesicular eruption in a dermatomal pattern (2).
- Decreased visual acuity
- Conjunctival injection near the limbus
- Decreased corneal sensation
- Dendritic pattern seen with conjunctival florescence staining

ALERT
Unilateral dermatomal vesicular rash most commonly in ophthalmic branch (V_1) of trigeminal nerve (VZV).

- Hutchinson sign: Vesicular lesion on nose from VZV indicates an increased risk of HZO due to involvement of nasociliary branch of trigeminal nerve, which also innervates the eye (2)[A].

DIFFERENTIAL DIAGNOSIS

- Any other cause of red, painful eye
  - Bacterial, fungal, allergic, or other viral conjunctivitis
  - Acute angle-closure glaucoma
- Corneal abrasion, recurrent corneal erosion, toxic conjunctivitis
- Temporal arteritis; trigeminal neuralgia

DIAGNOSTIC TESTS & INTERPRETATION

Initial Tests (lab, imaging)

Typically none needed, as diagnosis is based on history and physical exam (2)[C]

- Corneal swab for HSV DNA by polymerase chain reaction (PCR) (PPV = 96%)
- If vesicle present, can perform a Tzanck smear for VZV or HSV (multinucleated giant cells)
- Antibody titers to assess exposure only; direct fluorescent antibody (DFA); tissue culture

ALERT
Urgent ophthalmology referral for slit-lamp exam, dilated fundus exam, and intraocular pressure measurement

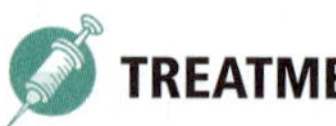

TREATMENT

GENERAL MEASURES

- Avoid contact with nonimmune people.
- No contact lenses should be worn during treatment period.
- Cool compresses; artificial tears; oral pain medications

MEDICATION

First Line

- HSV corneal epithelial disease
  - Trifluridine 1%: Apply 1 drop q2h while awake to a max of 9 drops daily until reepithelialization occurs and then 1 drop q4h for an additional 7 days.
  - Acyclovir: 400 mg PO 5 times/day for 10 days
  - Ganciclovir: 0.15% gel: Apply 1 drop in eye q3h while awake, ~5 times daily, until reepithelialization occurs, and then 1 drop q8h for 7 days.
  - Trifluridine and acyclovir cure about 90% of treated eyes within 2 weeks with no significant differences in effectiveness (3)[A].
  - Evidence is conflicting whether ganciclovir is as good as or better than acyclovir (3)[A].
  - Epithelial débridement by an ophthalmologist may accelerate healing in combination with treatment as above (3)[A].
  - Avoid topical steroids.
- Utility of PO antivirals unclear HSV stromal keratitis or uveitis (without epithelial disease): combination of antiviral and steroid treatment; requires ophthalmology evaluation
  - Prednisolone acetate: 1% drops QID with slow taper (1)[A]
  - Consider systemic steroids in severe uveitis (1)[A].
  - Trifluridine: 1% drops QID for prophylaxis while on topical steroids

- HZO
  - Valacyclovir (Valtrex) 1 g PO TID for 7 to 10 days or famciclovir (Famvir) 500 mg PO TID for 7 to 10 days or acyclovir 800 mg PO 5 times a day for 7 to 10 days
  - Valacyclovir and famciclovir result in significant reduction in PHN compared to acyclovir (number needed to treat [NNT] = 3) with equivalent efficacy (4)[A].
  - Topical antibiotic ophthalmic ointment to protect ocular surfaces (e.g., bacitracin, polymyxin B): 0.5-inch ribbon BID to TID for 7 to 10 days (5)[C]
  - If immunocompromised: acyclovir 10 to 15 mg/kg IV q8h for 10 days
  - Prednisolone acetate: 1% drops QID with slow taper with an ophthalmologist (5)[C]
- Cycloplegic agent if anterior uveitis present; intraocular pressure-lowering agent if necessary

Second Line

- HSV: acyclovir 2 g/day PO in divided doses over 10 days in patients intolerant of topical antivirals
- Topical idoxuridine, acyclovir, brivudine, although approved internationally, are not approved for use in the United States.
- Concomitant treatment with interferon may also improve outcomes but is not currently available.

ALERT

HZO: Antiviral therapy is most effective within the first 72 hours of rash onset but should still be initiated >72 hours after onset because of the possible complications of HZO (6)[C].

- Topical antiviral agents
  - Toxic to corneal epithelium, especially after 10 to 14 days of continuous use
- Acyclovir: Reduce dosage in renal insufficiency.
- Topical steroids
  - Prescribe only in consultation with an ophthalmologist.
  - Contraindicated with active corneal epithelial disease, which is best monitored with a slit lamp
  - Can increase intraocular pressure; cause corneal thinning; and, with long-term use, cause cataracts
- Prednisone: caution in immunocompromised patients

ISSUES FOR REFERRAL

Emergent or urgent ophthalmology referral, depending on severity of disease

ADDITIONAL THERAPIES

- Recurrent HSV requires suppressive therapy.
- HZO leading to PHN is common and can be treated with gabapentin or pregabalin, TCAs, opioids, and/or lidocaine gel.

SURGERY/OTHER PROCEDURES

Corneal transplantation for severe scarring or perforation

ADMISSION, INPATIENT, AND NURSING CONSIDERATIONS

- Severe systemic VZV disease
- Systemic HSV in neonates—see "Herpes Simplex Virus, Pediatric."

ONGOING CARE

FOLLOW-UP RECOMMENDATIONS

Patient Monitoring

Monitor with slit-lamp exam q1–2d until improvement and then q3–4d until epithelial defect resolves. After epithelial disease resolves, can monitor weekly until off topical antivirals

PATIENT EDUCATION

Educate about the importance of early recognition of recurrent symptoms and need for prompt evaluation and treatment.

PROGNOSIS

- Many cases are self-limited but, depending on the ocular structure involved, can lead to permanent blindness, especially in the setting of recurrent disease.
- Ocular HSV is the number one cause of infectious blindness worldwide.
- Recurrent ocular HSV
  - HSV epithelial disease without treatment.
  - Without sequelae, 40% resolve.
  - With treatment, 90–95% resolve without complication.

Pediatric Considerations

- Neonatal primary HSV often disseminated, with high mortality rate; 37% develop vision worse than 20/200.
- Pediatric cases more likely to be bilateral (26%), recurrent (48% in 15 months), and may cause amblyopia.

COMPLICATIONS

- Recurrence
- Corneal neovascularization and scarring resulting in poor vision
- Neurotrophic ulcer with perforation
- Secondary bacterial or fungal infection
- Secondary glaucoma in 10%
- PHN in 20–40% with VZV, typically longer lasting in older patients
- Vision loss from optic neuritis or chorioretinitis

REFERENCES

1. Knickelbein JE, Hendricks RL, Charukamnoetkanok P. Management of herpes simplex virus stromal keratitis: an evidence-based review. *Surv Ophthalmol*. 2009;54(2):226–234.
2. Liesegang TJ. Herpes zoster ophthalmicus natural history, risk factors, clinical presentation, and morbidity. *Ophthalmology*. 2008;115(Suppl 2):S3–S12.
3. Wilhelmus KR. Antiviral treatment and other therapeutic interventions for herpes simplex virus epithelial keratitis. *Cochrane Database Syst Rev*. 2015;1(1):CD002898.
4. McDonald EM, de Kock J, Ram FS. Antivirals for management of herpes zoster including ophthalmicus: a systematic review of high-quality randomized controlled trials. *Antivir Ther*. 2012;17(2):255–264.
5. Dworkin RH, Johnson RW, Breuer J, et al. Recommendations for the management of herpes zoster. *Clin Infect Dis*. 2007;44(Suppl 1):S1–S26.
6. Carter WP III, Germann CA, Baumann MR. Ophthalmic diagnoses in the ED: herpes zoster ophthalmicus. *Am J Emerg Med*. 2008;26(5):612–617.

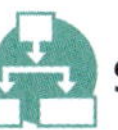

SEE ALSO

- Herpes Simplex; Herpes Simplex Virus, Pediatric; Herpes Zoster (Shingles)
- Algorithm: Eye Pain

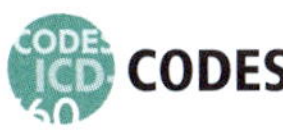

CODES

ICD10

- B00.50 Herpesviral ocular disease, unspecified
- B02.30 Zoster ocular disease, unspecified
- B00.52 Herpesviral keratitis

CLINICAL PEARLS

- HSV and VZV can lead to a wide array of ocular manifestations, ranging from self-limited disease to potentially vision-threatening disease and complications.
- An exam with fluorescein stain should be performed on all patients with possible HSV keratitis or HZO.
- Topical antiviral treatment is appropriate for HSV, but systemic PO antiviral treatment is necessary for HZO.
- Consult ophthalmology before prescribing topical steroids and for patients with HZO.
- Hutchinson sign (vesicular lesion on nose from VZV) is a strong indicator of HZO.
- Varicella recombinant zoster vaccine (Shingrix) is effective at preventing zoster and HZO as well as decreasing the duration of PHN.

HERPES SIMPLEX

Frances J. Boly, DO • Laura Mallinger, DO

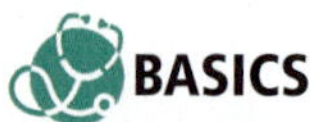

BASICS

DESCRIPTION

Herpes simplex virus (HSV) infections, caused by HSV-1 and HSV-2, are highly prevalent worldwide, with most adults carrying antibodies. After primary infection, the virus establishes latency in ganglia and may reactivate with stress, trauma, or immune compromise. Mucocutaneous disease presents as painful vesicles on an erythematous base, most often oral or genital, while less common forms involve the central nervous system (CNS) or eyes. Diagnosis is clinical, supported by polymerase chain reaction (PCR) or culture when needed, and treatment relies on antivirals and supportive care.

EPIDEMIOLOGY

- All ages are affected. HSV-1 is typically acquired in childhood whereas HSV-2 is acquired in young-middle adulthood.
- HSV-1 was once mainly oral/ocular and HSV-2 genital; now HSV-1 causes genital infection as often as HSV-2.
- Incidence and prevalence are declining in high-income countries (1)[C].

Incidence

$>$1 million new U.S. cases annually

Prevalence

- 45% of the US is estimated to be infected with HSV-1 and 14.4% with HSV-2
- $>$90% of adults worldwide have HSV antibodies by the age of 40 years
- 20% of pregnant women are seropositive for HSV-2.

ETIOLOGY AND PATHOPHYSIOLOGY

- Enveloped, dsDNA viruses from the family *Herpesviridae*
- Transmission occurs via direct mucosal/skin contact, saliva, sexual contact, vertical (during delivery), rarely transplacentally.
- Primary infection: The virus enters through mucosa and replicates at the site of contact; replication leads to cell lysis resulting in characteristic vesicles.
- Latency: Virus enters sensory nerve endings and via retrograde transport, establishes latency in sensory ganglion neurons.
- Reactivation: The virus is reactivated and transported to epithelial cells where it continues to replicate and shed, with or without characteristic ulcerations.
  - Triggered by stress, acute illness, trauma, immunodeficiency, etc.
- Dissemination: spreads to atypical sites, including lungs, gastrointestinal tract, CNS, and eyes
  - May occur during pregnancy or severely immunocompromised states

RISK FACTORS

- Unprotected sexual activity
- Immunocompromised states: advanced age, malignancy, AIDS, diabetes
- Atopic eczema, especially in children
- Occupational exposure (herpetic whitlow in dental professionals)
- High-contact sports (herpes gladiatorum)
- Vertical transmission to the neonate; greatest risk during primary genital infection of the mother

GENERAL PREVENTION

- Avoid contact of active lesions.
- Hand hygiene
- Avoid kissing, sharing beverages, sharing utensils, and sharing toothbrushes when lesions present.
- Genital herpes: Avoid sexual contact if active lesions, but consistent barrier protection use is advised with known limitations; antiviral therapy to reduce viral shedding
- Adult male circumcision reduces transmission to partners.

COMMONLY ASSOCIATED CONDITIONS

- Erythema multiforme: 50% of cases associated with HSV
- Herpetic whitlow, Herpes gladiatorum, Bell palsy
- Screen severe, treatment-resistant, or unusual HSV for concurrent HIV infection.

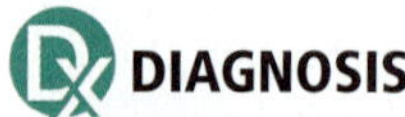

DIAGNOSIS

HISTORY

- Many patients are unaware of exposure and primary infection is usually subclinical or asymptomatic.
- Prodrome of flu-like symptoms, and itching or tingling in the area for several days prior to primary outbreak and 6 to 48 hours in subsequent outbreaks.
- Outbreak precipitated by sunlight, fever, trauma, menses, and stress

PHYSICAL EXAM

- Vesicles cluster and become painful ulcerated lesions with erythematous base.
- Primary herpetic gingivostomatitis and pharyngitis: early childhood; incubation 2 to 12 days, followed by fever, sore throat, edema, and erythema
  - Vesicles on pharynx ulcerate and multiply to involve mucosa of entire mouth; bleeding gums; cervical adenopathy; fever, poor oral intake, and excess salivation; autoinoculation of other sites may occur; resolves in 10 to 14 days
- Herpes keratoconjunctivitis: unilateral with regional adenopathy; blepharitis; lasts 2 to 3 weeks; systemic involvement prolongs course
- Eczema herpeticum: painful, diffuse, pox-like eruption, complicating atopic dermatitis; sudden appearance of lesions in typically atopic areas; high fever, localized edema, adenopathy
- Herpetic whitlow: localized painful/itchy infection of finger, followed by vesicles that coalesce with swelling and erythema; mimics pyogenic paronychia; neuralgia and axillary adenopathy are possible; heals in 2 to 3 weeks
- Congenital: jaundice, hepatosplenomegaly, disseminated intravascular coagulation, encephalitis, seizures, temperature instability, chorioretinitis, and conjunctivitis with or without vesicles.
- Recurrent diseases from reactivation:
  - Herpes labialis: recurrent lesions with HSV-1; usually $<$1 recurrence/6 months, but 5–25% have $>$1 attack/month; vesicles with vermilion border, ulcerate and crust within 48 hours; heal 8 to 10 days; may have local adenopathy
  - Ocular herpes: keratitis, blepharitis, or keratoconjunctivitis; dendritic ulcers, decreased corneal sensation and visual acuity; uveitis may cause permanent visual loss.

DIFFERENTIAL DIAGNOSIS

Impetigo, aphthous stomatitis, herpes zoster, folliculitis, herpangina, Stevens-Johnson syndrome, secondary fungal or bacterial infection, lymphogranuloma venereum

DIAGNOSTIC TESTS & INTERPRETATION

Initial Tests (lab, imaging)

- Clinical diagnosis; testing reserved for atypical and immunocompromised patients
- Tzanck smear: multinucleated giant cells with eosinophilic intranuclear inclusions (fix slide with ethanol/methanol, stain with Giemsa or Wright stain); does not distinguish serotypes and has a low sensitivity (84%), requiring follow-up testing
- HSV culture is most common; high yield if swab collected within 48 hours of outbreak, but can take 6 days to be positive; highly specific, but 20% false-negative rate
  - 3 weeks after infection, 50% test positive; 6 weeks after infection, 70%; 16 weeks, nearly 100%
- Nucleic acid amplification test (NAAT) distinguishes between serotypes and may be preferable due to DNA stability, speed, increased reliability in older/ulcerated lesions, and higher sensitivity compared to culture.
- Serologic testing may be necessary in patients with recurrent or atypical presentation or in patients participating in high-risk sex. HSV IgM can be positive during initial or recurrent infection. IgG can take 2 weeks to 6 months to develop. Western blot IgG is not widely available. ELISA testing is highly variable depending on immunoassay used.

Follow-Up Tests & Special Considerations

- No follow-up needed if adequately treated
- Screen for other sexually transmitted infections in patients with primary genital herpes.

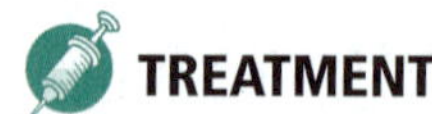

TREATMENT

GENERAL MEASURES

- Symptom management
- Cool dressings moistened with aluminum acetate solution
- Genital lesions: pour a cup of warm water over genitals or sit in a warm bath (sitz bath) while urinating if lesions cause urinary difficulty
- Children with gingivostomatitis who resist oral intake or have extensive skin disease (eczema herpeticum) may require IV hydration.

MEDICATION

First Line

- Treat promptly, preferably in prodrome.
- For episodic treatment of recurrent infection, start treatment within 1 day of symptoms.
- Suppressive therapy to those with severe psychological distress or pain or pregnant women after 36 weeks' gestation
- Topical therapy: Penciclovir (Denavir): 1% cream; apply to oral lesions q2h while awake for 4 days.

- Acyclovir (generic)
  - Mucocutaneous (or genital) HSV
    - Primary infection: 400 mg 3 times per day for 7 to 10 days. If severe, start with 5 to 10 mg/kg IV q8h for the first few days and then complete 10-day PO course.
    - Recurrence 800 mg PO BID for 5 days, or 800 mg PO TID for 2 days
    - Suppression: 400 mg BID
  - Keratitis HSV: 400 mg PO 5 times per day; topical treatment is preferred as first line.
  - Pediatric dosing:
    - <3 months, <35 weeks' gestation, 40 mg/kg/day IV q12h for 14 to 21 days
    - <3 months, >35 weeks' gestation, 60 mg/kg/day IV q8h for 14 to 21 days
    - >3 months, weight-based dosing, 40 to 80 mg/kg/day (max 1,000 mg/day) q8h for 5 to 7 days
    - Suppression: <3 months, 900 mg/m^2/day PO q8h for 6 months (max 3,200 mg/day)
  - Safe in pregnancy and lactation—Category B (2),(3)[B]
- Valacyclovir (Valtrex)
  - Herpes labialis: 2,000 mg PO q12h for 1 day
  - Primary genital herpes: 1 g PO BID for 7 to 10 days, started within 48 to 72 hours of symptoms
  - Recurrent genital herpes: 500 mg PO BID for 3 days, started within 24 hours of symptoms or 1 g PO QD for 5 days
  - Suppression: 1 g PO daily and decrease to 500 mg QD if <10 outbreaks/year, 500 mg BID in pregnancy starting at 36 weeks
- Famciclovir (Famvir)
  - Primary genital herpes: 250 mg PO TID for 7 to 10 days
  - Recurrence: 1 g PO BID for 1 day within 6 hours of symptoms, 500 mg PO for 1 day then 250 mg BID for 2 days, or 125 mg PO BID for 5 days
  - Suppression: 250 mg PO BID
- Precautions
  - Renal dosing for all oral antivirals
  - Significant interactions: Probenecid with IV acyclovir or valacyclovir may reduce renal clearance and elevate antiviral levels.

Second Line

- Foscarnet
  - Drug of choice for acyclovir resistance in immunocompromised persons with systemic HSV; assume valacyclovir and famciclovir resistance also.
  - 40 mg/kg IV q8h–q12h, requires adequate hydration, or 1% cream 5 times per day but requires pharmacy compounding
- Other topicals
  - Ophthalmic preparations: acyclovir, vidarabine (Vira-A), ganciclovir, trifluridine
  - Topical acyclovir and penciclovir improve recurrent herpes labialis healing times by ~10% (2)[B].
  - Topical analgesics: Lidocaine 2% or 5% helps reduce pain associated with vulvar and penile outbreaks.
- Over-the-counter topical antivirals: docosanol

ISSUES FOR REFERRAL

Refer recurrent cases of herpes keratoconjunctivitis to an ophthalmologist.

ADMISSION, INPATIENT, AND NURSING CONSIDERATIONS

Pregnancy Considerations

- Cesarean section and/or acyclovir are indicated if active genital lesions or prodrome present at time of delivery; consider cesarean if primary genital herpes is suspected within previous 4 weeks.
- Daily PO antivirals after 36 weeks with history of genital herpes to prevent outbreak at time of delivery
- Avoid fetal scalp electrodes, forceps, vacuum extractor, and artificial rupture of membranes if mother has history of genital HSV.
- Risk of viral shedding at delivery from asymptomatic recurrent genital HSV is low (~1.6%).
- Primary maternal infection carries a 60% risk of neonatal infection at time of delivery.

Pediatric Considerations

Neonates with likely exposure or those who exhibit signs of infection should be cultured and immediately start treatment (IV acyclovir).

ONGOING CARE

FOLLOW-UP RECOMMENDATIONS

- Follow-up not necessary; lesions and symptoms resolve within 10 days.
- Extensive cases should be rechecked in 1 week; monitor for secondary bacterial infections.
- Consider long-term suppression. Reassess annually the need for continued treatment.

DIET

If oral lesions are present, avoid salty, acidic, or sharp foods.

PATIENT EDUCATION

- Discuss viral course, that timing of exposure is difficult to determine, and that HSV will remain in the body indefinitely. Acknowledging psychological impact helps reduce stigmatization.
- Emphasize hygiene to avoid self-spreading or exposing others. Frequent hand washing; avoid scratching; cover active, moist lesions.
- Reinforce safe sexual practices. Transmission is possible even when disease appears inactive. Condoms do not protect against exposed or oral lesions.
- Inform sex partners of infection before starting having sex.

PROGNOSIS

- Duration of primary disease is 5 days to 2 weeks.
- Treatment shortens duration, reduces complications, and mitigates recurrences (if used for suppression).
- Viral shedding during recurrence is briefer; frequency of recurrence varies depending on individual host factors.
- Newborns/immunocompromised are at highest risk for morbidity/mortality.
- HSV remains dormant in dorsal root ganglia and can reactivate, causing recurrent symptoms.

COMPLICATIONS

- People with genital HSV have a higher risk of HIV infection due to open ulcers.
- Herpes encephalitis; herpes pneumonia, pneumonitis
- Hepatitis; disseminated herpes; acute urinary retention; neonatal infection

REFERENCES

1. Omarova S, Cannon A, Weiss W, et al. Genital herpes simplex virus—an updated review. *Adv Pediatr*. 2022;69(1):149–162.
2. Rahimi H, Mara T, Costella J, et al. Effectiveness of antiviral agents for the prevention of recurrent herpes labialis: a systematic review and meta-analysis. *Oral Surg Oral Med Oral Pathol Oral Radiol*. 2012;113(5):618–627.
3. Sawleshwarkar S, Dwyer DE. Antivirals for herpes simplex viruses. *BMJ*. 2015;351:h3350.

ADDITIONAL READING

Groves MJ. Genital herpes: a review. *Am Fam Physician*. 2016;93(11):928–934.

SEE ALSO

- Herpes, Genital
- Algorithm: Genital Ulcers

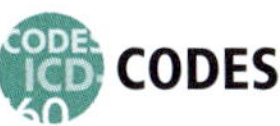

CODES

ICD10

- B00 Herpesviral [herpes simplex] infections
- B00.0 Eczema herpeticum
- B00.1 Herpesviral vesicular dermatitis

CLINICAL PEARLS

- Characteristic vesicular, ulcerative rash with lifelong infection and commonly reoccurs
- 25–30% of the U.S. population has serologic evidence of genital herpes (HSV-2), and >80% is seropositive for HSV-1.
- Most individuals are unaware they are infected, allowing for asymptomatic viral transmission.
- Viral suppression for patients with frequent recurrences reduces transmission and decreases outbreak frequency.

H

HERPES ZOSTER (SHINGLES)

Marium Palur Afzal, MD

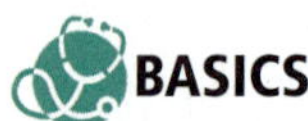

BASICS

DESCRIPTION

- Results from reactivation of latent varicella-zoster virus (VZV) (human herpesvirus type 3) infection
- Postherpetic neuralgia (PHN) is defined as pain persisting at least 1 month after rash has healed. The term *zoster-associated pain* is more clinically useful.
- Herpes zoster ophthalmicus (HZO) is an important complication involving the ophthalmic (V1) branch of the trigeminal nerve.
- Zoster usually presents as a painful unilateral vesicular eruption with a dermatomal distribution.
- System(s) affected: nervous; integumentary; exocrine
- Synonym(s): shingles

EPIDEMIOLOGY

Incidence

- Incidence increases with age—2/3 of cases occur in adults aged ≥50 years. Incidence is increasing overall as the US population ages.
- Herpes zoster: 4/1,000 persons per year with higher rates in older adults and women
- PHN: 18% in adult patients with herpes zoster; 33% in patients ≥79 years of age
- Individual lifetime risk of 30% in the United States

Prevalence

~1 million new cases of herpes zoster annually in the United States

Pregnancy Considerations

May occur during pregnancy; defer vaccination until after pregnancy.

Geriatric Considerations

- Increased incidence of zoster outbreaks
- Increased incidence of PHN

Pediatric Considerations

- Occurs less frequently in children
- Has been reported in newborns infected in utero

ETIOLOGY AND PATHOPHYSIOLOGY

Reactivation of VZV from dorsal root/cranial nerve ganglia; on reactivation, the virus replicates within neuronal cell bodies, and virions are carried along axons to dermatomal skin zones, causing local inflammation and vesicle formation.

RISK FACTORS

- Increasing age
- Immunosuppression (malignancy or chemotherapy)
- Physical trauma
- Female
- HIV infection
- Spinal surgery
- Family history

GENERAL PREVENTION

- Shingrix (recombinant herpes zoster vaccine) is the preferred vaccine. It is recommended for immunocompetent adults aged ≥50 years. It is also recommended for adults who previously received zostavax.
- Consider 2 doses of Shingrix for adults aged ≥19 years who are or will be immunodeficient or immunosuppressed.
  - 2 doses separated by 2 to 6 months
  - Those who would benefit from completing the series in a shorter period, the second dose can be administered 1 to 2 months after the first.
- No specific amount of time to wait before giving Shingrix to patients who have had herpes zoster. Do not give Shingrix to patients with acute episode of herpes zoster.
- Patients with active zoster may transmit disease-causing varicella virus—typically through direct contact.

COMMONLY ASSOCIATED CONDITIONS

Immunocompromised states, HIV infection, posttransplantation, immunosuppressive drugs, and malignancy

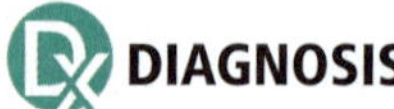

DIAGNOSIS

HISTORY

- Prodromal phase (sensory changes over involved dermatome occurs 48 to 72 hours prior to rash)
  - Constitutional symptoms (e.g., fatigue, malaise, headache, low-grade fever) are variable.
  - Tingling, paresthesias
  - Itching
  - Boring "knife-like" pain
  - Allodynia and hyperalgesia
- Acute phase
  - Dermatomal rash

PHYSICAL EXAM

- Acute phase
  - Rash: initially erythematous and maculopapular; evolves to characteristic grouped vesicles usually in one dermatome but may affect two to three adjacent dermatomes; thoracic and cervical dermatomes are most commonly involved sites.
  - Vesicles become pustular and/or hemorrhagic in 3 to 4 days.
  - The lesions typically do not cross the midline, although bilateral herpes zoster could be an atypical clinical presentation.
  - Rash crusts and resolves by 14 to 21 days. Patients are most infectious in the crusting stage before the lesions dry out.
  - Weakness in distribution of rash (1%)
- Possible zoster sine herpete (zoster without rash) and other chronic disorders associated with VZV without the typical rash
- Ramsay Hunt syndrome presents with ipsilateral facial paralysis, auricular pain (with or without hearing loss), and vesicular rash in the external auditory canal or outer ear.
- HZO: Vesicles on tip of the nose (Hutchinson sign) indicate involvement of the external branch of cranial nerve V and are associated with increased incidence of HZO.
- Chronic phase
  - PHN is the most common complication (15% overall; increases with age).
  - 1–5% of cases may affect the motor nerves, causing weakness (*zoster motorius*), facial nerve involvement (Ramsay Hunt syndrome), spinal motor radiculopathies.
  - Lesions usually heal 2 to 4 weeks after onset, but scarring and pigmentation changes are common (1).

DIFFERENTIAL DIAGNOSIS

Rash

- Herpes simplex virus
- Dermatitis herpetiformis
- Coxsackievirus
- Contact dermatitis
- Impetigo
- Superficial pyoderma

DIAGNOSTIC TESTS & INTERPRETATION

Initial Tests (lab, imaging)

Rarely necessary; clinical appearance is distinct.

Follow-Up Tests & Special Considerations

- Viral culture
- Consider intact skin scraping sample from the affected area for VZV DNA polymerase chain reaction (PCR) to confirm zoster sine herpete.
- Tzanck smear (does not distinguish from herpes simplex, and false-negative results occur)
- PCR of vesicular fluid
- Immunofluorescent antigen staining
- Varicella-zoster–specific IgM

Test Interpretation

- Multinucleated giant cells with intralesional inclusion (on Tzanck smear)
- Lymphatic infiltration of sensory ganglia with focal hemorrhage and nerve cell destruction

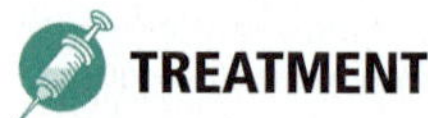

TREATMENT

GENERAL MEASURES

- Treat to control symptoms and prevent complications.
- Antiviral therapy decreases viral replication, lessens inflammation and nerve damage, and reduces the severity and duration of long-term pain.
- Prompt analgesia may shorten the duration of zoster-associated pain.
- Calamine and colloidal oatmeal may help reduce itching and burning.

MEDICATION

First Line

- Acute treatment
  - Antiviral agents initiated within 72 hours of skin lesions help relieve symptoms, speed resolution, and prevent or mitigate PHN (2).
  - Antivirals do not significantly reduce the incidence of PHN (3).
  - Valacyclovir: 1,000 mg PO TID for 7 days
  - Famciclovir: 500 mg PO TID for 7 days
  - Acyclovir: 800 mg q4h (5 doses daily) for 7 days
  - In children, oral acyclovir is the drug of choice.
- Analgesics (acetaminophen, NSAIDs)
- Corticosteroids do not prevent PHN but may accelerate resolution of acute neuritis.
  - Tricyclic antidepressants (TCAs); amitriptyline 10 to 25 mg at bedtime and other low-dose TCAs relieve pain acutely and may reduce pain duration; dose may be titrated up to 75 to 150 mg/day as tolerated.
  - Lidocaine patch 5% (Lidoderm) applied over painful areas (limit three patches simultaneously or trim a single patch) for up to 12 hours may be effective.
  - Gabapentin: 300 to 600 mg TID for pain; limited by adverse effects
  - Capsaicin cream and other analgesics may be useful adjuncts. Use opioids sparingly.
  - Pregabalin: 150 to 300 mg/day divided BID or TID reduces pain; use is limited by side effects.
- Prevention of PHN and zoster-associated pain: There are no treatments to prevent PHN. Treatment may, however, shorten duration and/or reduce severity of symptoms.
  - Antiviral therapy with valacyclovir, famciclovir, or acyclovir given during acute skin eruption may decrease the duration of pain.
  - Low-dose amitriptyline (25 mg at bedtime) started within 72 hours of rash onset and continued for 90 days may reduce PHN incidence/duration.
  - Paravertebral blockade: Nerve blocks during the acute phase shorten the duration of pain; somatic blocks, paravertebral blocks, and repeated/continuous epidural blocks can be used to prevent PHN (1).
  - Insufficient evidence to suggest that corticosteroids reduce incidence, severity, or duration of PHN
- Precautions
  - Assess renal function prior to using valacyclovir, famciclovir, acyclovir, gabapentin, and pregabalin.
  - Valacyclovir, famciclovir, and acyclovir are pregnancy Category B.

COMPLEMENTARY & ALTERNATIVE MEDICINE

Cupping therapy (traditional Chinese medicine) shows potential benefit. Definitive evidence is lacking.

ADMISSION, INPATIENT, AND NURSING CONSIDERATIONS

- Outpatient treatment, unless disseminated or occurring as complication of serious underlying disease requiring hospitalization
- Consultation with ophthalmology for ophthalmic involvement (VZO)

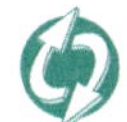

ONGOING CARE

Recommend vaccine administration after the current episode has resolved. Studies are now showing that the zoster vaccine may lower the risk for future dementia.

FOLLOW-UP RECOMMENDATIONS

Refer to ophthalmology if concern that ophthalmic branch of the trigeminal nerve is involved.

Patient Monitoring

Follow duration of symptoms—particularly PHN. Consider hospitalization if symptoms are severe; patients are immunocompromised; >2 dermatomes are involved; serious bacterial superinfection, disseminated zoster, ophthalmic involvement, or meningoencephalitis develops.

DIET

No special diet

PATIENT EDUCATION

- The rash typically lasts 2 to 3 weeks.
- Encourage good hygiene and proper skin care.
- Warn of potential for dissemination (dissemination must be suspected with constitutional illness signs and/or spreading rash).
- Warn of potential PHN.
- Warn of potential risk of transmitting illness (chickenpox) to susceptible persons.
- Seek medical attention if any eye involvement.

PROGNOSIS

- Immunocompetent individuals should experience spontaneous and complete recovery within a few weeks.
- Acute rash typically resolves within 14 to 21 days.
- PHN may occur in patients despite antiviral treatment.

COMPLICATIONS

- PHN
- HZO: 10–20%
- Superinfection of skin lesions
- Meningoencephalitis
- Disseminated zoster
- Hepatitis; pneumonitis; myelitis
- Cranial and peripheral nerve palsies
- Acute retinal necrosis

REFERENCES

1. Patil A, Goldust M, Wollina U. Herpes zoster: a review of clinical manifestations and management. *Viruses*. 2022;14(2):192. doi:10.3390/v14020192.
2. Tsatsos M, Athanasiadis I, Myrou A, et al. Herpes zoster ophthalmicus: a devastating disease coming back with vengeance or finding its nemesis? *J Ophthalmic Vis Res*. 2022;17(1):123–129. doi:10.18502/jovr.v17i1.10177.
3. Harbecke R, Cohen JI, Oxman MN. Herpes zoster vaccines. *J Infect Dis*. 2021;224(12 Suppl 2):S429–S442.

ADDITIONAL READING

Lim DZJ, Tey HL, Salada BMA, et al. Herpes zoster and post-herpetic neuralgia-diagnosis, treatment, and vaccination strategies. *Pathogens*. 2024;13(7):596. doi:10.3390/pathogens13070596.

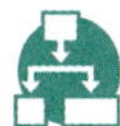

SEE ALSO

- Bell Palsy; Chickenpox (Varicella Zoster); Herpes Eye Infections; Herpes Simplex
- Algorithm: Genital Ulcers

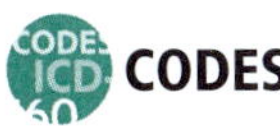

CODES

ICD10

- B02.9 Zoster without complications
- B02.29 Other postherpetic nervous system involvement

CLINICAL PEARLS

- Initiate antiviral therapy within 72 hours of rash onset for maximal effect.
- Patients with active herpes zoster can transmit clinically active disease (chickenpox) to susceptible individuals.
- Shingrix (recombinant) is the recommended vaccine for healthy adults age ≥50 years, including those who previously received zostavax (live attenuated) to prevent shingles and related complications.
- HZO is a potentially debilitating complication.

HERPES, GENITAL

Deyanna M. Boston, MD • William B. Meier, MD

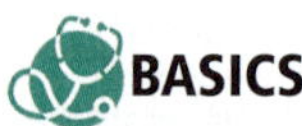

BASICS

DESCRIPTION

- Chronic, recurrent herpes simplex virus (HSV) type 1 (HSV-1) or 2 (HSV-2) infection of any area innervated by the sacral ganglia
- HSV-1 primarily causes anogenital and orolabial lesions; HSV-2 typically causes anogenital lesions. However, HSV-1 is now the leading cause of new genital infections (1).
- Primary episode: initial infection, no preexisting antibodies to HSV-1 or HSV-2 (may be asymptomatic)
- First episode, nonprimary: initial genital eruption; preexisting antibodies are present.
- Reactivation: recurrent episodes
- Synonym(s): herpes genitalis

EPIDEMIOLOGY

- Most commonly infected from age 15 to 30 years; prevalence increases with age due to cumulative exposure.
- HSV-2: females infected 2 to 3× > males
- United States: HSV-1 infectivity highest in Mexican Americans and HSV-2 highest in non-Hispanic Black individuals

Incidence

- Incidence in the United States is estimated to be ~572,000 to 1.6 million new cases per year; highest in 18- to 24-year-olds.
- Incident genital HSV infections globally in 2020 among individuals aged 15 to 49 years was estimated at 42.4 million.

Prevalence

- Globally, in 2020, genital HSV-1 and HSV-2 infections were estimated at 846.1 million people aged 15 to 49 years.
- HSV-1 infects an estimated 3.7 billion people, and HSV-2 infects about 491 million people globally, representing 67% and 13% of the population between 15 and 49 years old, respectively (1).
- Between ages 14 and 49 years, the prevalence of HSV-1 in the United States is ~48% and the prevalence of HSV-2 is ~12%.
- HSV-2 prevalence is estimated at 60–95% in the HIV-positive population (2).
- Up to 90% of those who are seropositive lack formal diagnosis.

ETIOLOGY AND PATHOPHYSIOLOGY

- HSV is a double-stranded DNA virus of the Herpetoviridae family (2).
- Spread via genital-to-genital contact, oral-to-genital contact, and via maternal–fetal transmission.
- Incubation is 4 to 7 days after exposure.
- Risk of transmission highest when lesions are present.
- Viral shedding is possible in the absence of lesions, increasing the risk of transmission due to inadequate barrier/abstinence precautions.
- Viral shedding occurs intermittently, unpredictably, and more commonly with HSV-2.
- HSV infection increases the risk of HIV.

RISK FACTORS

- Risk increases with age, number of lifetime partners, history of sexually transmitted infections (STIs—particularly HIV), sexual encounters before the age of 17 years, and partner with HSV-1 or HSV-2.
- Infection with HSV-1 confers 3-fold risk of infection with HSV-2.
- Immunosuppression, fever, stress, hormonal shifts, sun exposure, dietary intake and trauma increase risk of reactivation.

GENERAL PREVENTION

- Barrier contraception and avoiding sexual contact when symptoms/lesions are present.
- Abstinence is the only means of complete protection.

COMMONLY ASSOCIATED CONDITIONS

Syphilis, HIV, chlamydia, gonorrhea, other STIs

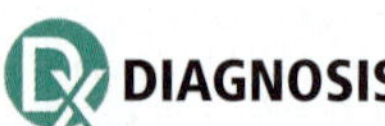

DIAGNOSIS

HISTORY

- Majority are asymptomatic (74% for HSV-1, 63% for HSV-2) or do not recognize clinical manifestations of infection.
- Symptoms present during primary episode are often more severe, last longer , and are associated with constitutional symptoms.
- Common presenting symptoms (primary episode): multiple genital ulcers, dysuria, pruritus, fever, tender inguinal lymphadenopathy, headache, malaise, myalgias, cervicitis/dyspareunia, urethritis (watery discharge)
- Common presenting symptoms for recurrent episodes: prodrome of tingling, burning, or shooting pain (2 to 24 hours before lesion appears); single ulcer/lesion; dysuria; pruritus (lasting 4 to 6 days on average)
- Recurrent episodes are more frequent with HSV-2, especially the 1st year after infection. Recurrences are less frequent over time. An increasing proportion of anogenital herpetic infections have been attributed to HSV-1, especially prevalent among young women and men who have sex with men.
- Less common presentations: tenesmus from anal involvement, proctitis, stomatitis, pharyngitis, sacral paresthesias

PHYSICAL EXAM

- Lesions around groin/perineum and within anus, vagina, and on cervix
- Lesion may appear in various stages as papular, vesicular, pustular, ulcerated, or crusted.
- Inguinal lymphadenopathy
- Extragenital manifestations include meningitis, recurrent meningitis (Mollaret syndrome), sacral radiculitis/paresthesias, encephalitis, transverse myelitis, and hepatitis.

Pediatric Considerations

- Neonatal infection occurs in ~10/100,000 live births; 80% of infections result from asymptomatic maternal viral shedding during an undiagnosed primary infection in the 3rd trimester.
- Transmission ranges from 30% to 50% if the primary episode is near time of delivery. Risk is higher with HSV-1. Neonatal disease is associated with high morbidity and mortality.
- Suspect sexual abuse with genital lesions in children.

DIFFERENTIAL DIAGNOSIS

- HIV; syphilis; chancroid, herpes zoster
- Ulcerative balanitis, granuloma inguinale; lymphogranuloma venereum
- Cytomegalovirus, Epstein-Barr virus
- Drug eruption, trauma
- Behçet syndrome
- Ulcus vulvae acutum (Lipschütz ulcer)
- Neoplasia

DIAGNOSTIC TESTS & INTERPRETATION

Initial Tests (lab, imaging)

- Testing can confirm clinical diagnosis via microscopy, culture, serologic assays, molecular assays or point of care testing.
- Culture by unroofing vesicle to obtain fluid sample. Specificity >99%; sensitivity of 50%.
- PCR-rapid, high sensitivity and specificity of 100%
- Serologic assays (particularly if lesions are absent)
  - Seroconversion occurs 10 days to 4 months after infection. *Antibody testing is not necessary if a positive culture or PCR has been obtained.*
  - *IgM antibody testing to determine a primary episode (especially during pregnancy) if IgM is positive and IgG is negative.*
- Western blot and type-specific IgG antibody (glycoprotein G) enzyme-linked immunosorbent assay (ELISA) are used to discriminate between HSV-1 and HSV-2 (2).
  - Western blot: >97–99% sensitive and specific but labor intensive and not readily available
  - ELISA: 81–100% sensitive; 93–100% specific for HSV-2 but lower for HSV-1 detection. False positives are possible.

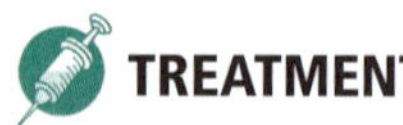

TREATMENT

GENERAL MEASURES

- Ice packs to perineum, sitz baths, topical anesthetics
- Analgesics, NSAIDs

MEDICATION

Start antiviral medication within 72 hours of symptom onset (including prodrome). After 3 days, antivirals may help if new lesions form or for significant pain. Persons with HIV will require higher doses for longer duration.

First Line

- Valacyclovir (Valtrex): prodrug of acyclovir, improved bioavailability, requires less frequent dosing (3)
  - Primary episode
    - 1 g PO BID for 7 to 10 days, extend duration if lesions persist at 10 days
  - Episodic therapy
    - 500 mg PO BID for 3 days
    - 1 g PO daily for 5 days
    - For immunocompromised persons and those with HIV, 1 g PO daily for 5 to 10 days

- Daily suppression
  - 500 mg PO daily
  - 1 g PO daily
  - For immunocompromised persons and those with HIV, 500 mg PO BID
- Acyclovir: most studied, least expensive antiviral in genital herpes; decreases pain, duration of viral shedding, and time to resolution
  - Primary episode
    - 400 mg PO TID for 7 to 10 days, extend duration if lesions persist at 10 days
  - Episodic therapy
    - 800 mg BID for 5 days
    - 800 mg TID for 2 days
    - For immunocompromised persons and those with HIV, 400 mg TID for 5 to 10 days
  - Daily suppression (>6 episodes per year)
    - 400 mg BID
    - For immunocompromised persons and those with HIV, 400 to 800 mg 2 to 3 times per day
  - Severe, complicated infections (IV therapy)
    - 5 to 10 mg/kg per dose q8h until clinical improvement; switch to PO therapy to complete a 10-day course (14 days for CNS involvement).
  - Precautions
    - Modify dose in renal insufficiency.
- Famciclovir (Famvir)
  - Primary episode
    - 250 mg PO TID for 7 to 10 days, extend duration if lesions persist at 10 days
  - Episodic therapy
    - 125 mg PO BID for 5 days
    - 1 g PO BID for 1 day
    - 500 mg PO once, followed by 250 mg PO BID for 2 days
    - For immunocompromised persons and those with HIV, 500 mg PO BID for 5 to 10 days
  - Daily suppression 250 mg PO BID
    - 250 mg PO BID
    - For immunocompromised persons and those with HIV, 500 mg PO BID

ISSUES FOR REFERRAL

For acyclovir-resistant HSV, in consultation with infectious disease specialist:

- Foscarnet: 40 to 80 mg/kg per dose IV q8h until clinical resolution
  - First-line treatment
  - Associated with significant nephrotoxicity
- Cidofovir: 5 mg/kg IV once weekly

Pregnancy Considerations

ACOG clinical management guidelines:

- Pregnant women with a history of genital herpes should be offered suppressive therapy starting at 36 gestational weeks until delivery to decrease reactivation rate and reduce the risk of neonatal infection:
  - Acyclovir 400 mg PO TID
  - Valacyclovir 500 mg PO BID
- Monitor for outbreaks during pregnancy. Caesarean delivery is recommended if prodromal symptoms or lesions are present at onset of labor.

Pediatric Considerations

- High-risk infants include those with active symptoms or lesions, those delivered vaginally with maternal lesions present, and those born during a primary maternal episode. Monitor closely; obtain diagnostic laboratory specimens (HSV PCR and ocular, nasal, anal, and oral cultures). If symptomatic, require prolonged treatment:
  - Acyclovir 20 mg/kg IV q8h for 14 days if skin or mucosal lesions, 21 days if disseminated or CNS disease
- Low-risk infants who are asymptomatic can be observed while obtaining serum HSV PCR and ocular, nasal, anal, and oral cultures.
- Infants with possible HSV infection should be isolated from other neonates; maternal separation is not necessary, and breastfeeding is not contraindicated.

COMPLEMENTARY & ALTERNATIVE MEDICINE

Zinc-based creams and supplements may reduce pain.

ONGOING CARE

Counsel persons with genital herpes and their sex partners with goal of helping patients cope with the infection and preventing sexual and perinatal transmission.

FOLLOW-UP RECOMMENDATIONS

Patient Monitoring

Test for HIV and other STIs.

PATIENT EDUCATION

- Patient education helps in treatment of subsequent outbreaks and reduces transmission risk:
  - Options include daily suppressive therapy and episodic therapy.
  - Alert partners of history prior to sexual activity.
  - Avoid sexual contact when symptoms or lesions are present.
  - Viral shedding and transmission can occur when symptoms/lesions are *not* present.
    - Shedding increased with HSV-2 and HIV.
  - 100% condom use reduces HSV-2 transmission risk by 30%.
  - Sexual activity between concordant couples (i.e., both partners with the same type of HSV) does not increase risk of outbreaks.
  - Ensure maternity care team knows HSV status.
- Herpes resource center: http://www.ashasexualhealth.org/stdsstis/herpes/
- Centers for Disease Control and Prevention: https://www.cdc.gov/herpes/about/?CDC_AAref_Val

PROGNOSIS

- Resolution of signs/symptoms: 3 to 21 days
- Average recurrence rate is one to four episodes per year.
- Antivirals can reduce transmission, shedding, and frequency of outbreaks.

Pediatric Considerations

Neonatal infection survival rates: localized >95%, CNS 85%, systemic 30%

COMPLICATIONS

- Lowered self-esteem, guilt, anger, depression, fear of rejection, and fear of transmission to partner
- The risk of being infected with HIV is 2- to 3-fold with HSV-2.
- Hepatitis with disseminated HSV, especially in pregnancy
- HSV-2 meningitis is a rare complication of HSV-2 genital herpes infection that affects women more than men.

REFERENCES

1. Harfouche M, AlMukdad S, Alareeki A, et al. Estimated global and regional incidence and prevalence of herpes simplex virus infections and genital ulcer disease in 2020: mathematical modelling analyses. *Sex Transm Infect*. 2025;101(4):214–223.
2. Nath P, Kabir MA, Doust SK, et al. Diagnosis of herpes simplex virus: laboratory and point-of-care techniques. *Infect Dis Rep*. 2021;13(2):518–539.
3. Plunkett M, Neville CT, Chang JG. Genital herpes: rapid evidence review. *Am Fam Physician*. 2024;110(5):487–492.

ADDITIONAL READING

- Management of genital herpes in pregnancy: ACOG Practice Bulletin, Number 220. *Obstet Gynecol*. 2020;135(5):e193–e202.
- Mangione CM, Barry MJ, Nicholson WK, et al. Serologic screening for genital herpes infection: US Preventive Services Task Force reaffirmation recommendation statement. *JAMA*. 2023;329(6):502–507. doi:10.1001/jama.2023.0057.

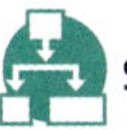

SEE ALSO

Algorithm: Genital Ulcers

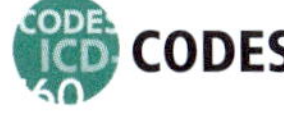

CODES

ICD10

- A60 Anogenital herpesviral [herpes simplex] infections
- A60.02 Herpesviral infection of other male genital organs
- A60.0 Herpesviral infection of genitalia and urogenital tract

CLINICAL PEARLS

- HSV-1 and/or HSV-2 cause genital herpes.
- Many seropositive individuals are unaware that they are infected.
- Most primary episodes are asymptomatic.
- Viral shedding occurs in the absence of lesions.
- Meticulous (100%) condom use decreases (but does not eliminate) transmission of HSV.

H

HICCUPS

Katherine R. Baldwin, MD

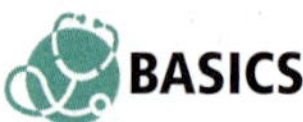

BASICS

DESCRIPTION

- Hiccups are caused by a repetitive sudden involuntary contraction of the inspiratory muscles (predominantly the diaphragm) with the abrupt closure of the glottis, which stops the inflow of air and produces a characteristic sound.
- Hiccups are classified based on their duration: Hiccup bouts last up to 48 hours; persistent hiccups last >48 hours but <1 month; intractable hiccups last for >1 month.
- System(s) affected: nervous, pulmonary
- Synonym(s): hiccoughs; singultus

Geriatric Considerations

Can be a serious problem, particularly among the elderly

Pregnancy Considerations

- Fetal hiccups are rhythmic fetal movements (confirmed sonographically) that can be confused with contractions.
- Fetal hiccups are a sign of normal neurologic development.

EPIDEMIOLOGY

- Predominant age: all ages (including fetus)
- Predominant sex: male > female (4:1)

Incidence

Overall incidence in the general population is uncertain.

Prevalence

Self-limited hiccups are extremely common, as are intraoperative and postoperative hiccups.

ETIOLOGY AND PATHOPHYSIOLOGY

- Results from stimulation of ≥1 limbs of the hiccup reflex arc (vagus and phrenic nerves) with a "hiccup center" located in the upper spinal cord and brain (1)
- In men, >90% have an organic basis; in women, psychogenic causes are more common.
- Specific underlying causes include:
  - CNS disorders: vascular lesions (AV malformation), infectious causes (meningitis, encephalitis), structural lesions (intracranial/brainstem mass lesions, multiple sclerosis, hydrocephalus, syringomyelia), posterior inferior cerebellar artery (PICA) aneurysm; seizure disorder
  - Diaphragmatic irritation (tumors, pericarditis, eventration, splenomegaly, hepatomegaly, peritonitis)
  - Irritation of the tympanic membrane
  - Nerve irritation: pharyngitis, laryngitis, neck tumors
  - Mediastinal and other thoracic lesions (pneumonia, aortic aneurysm, tuberculosis [TB], myocardial infarction [MI], lung cancer, rib exostoses)
  - Esophageal lesions (reflux esophagitis, achalasia, *Candida* esophagitis, carcinoma, obstruction)
  - Gastrointestinal (GI) disorders (gastritis, GERD, PUD, distention, cancer)
  - Hiccups have been reported as an initial presentation of COVID-19.
  - Cardiovascular disorders (MI, pericarditis)
  - Hepatic lesions (hepatitis, hepatoma); pancreatic lesions (pancreatitis, pseudocysts, cancer)
  - Inflammatory bowel disease; cholelithiasis, cholecystitis
  - Prostatic disorders
  - Appendicitis; postoperative, particularly with abdominal procedures
  - Metabolic causes (uremia, hyponatremia, gout, diabetes)
  - Drug-induced (dexamethasone, methylprednisolone, anabolic steroids, benzodiazepines, α-methyldopa, propofol, levofolinate, oxaliplatin, fluorouracil, carboplatin, cisplatin, tramadol)
  - Toxic (alcohol-induced)
  - Psychogenic causes (anorexia, conversion, grief, malingering, schizophrenia, stress)
  - Idiopathic

RISK FACTORS

- GI disease (PUD; GERD; GI surgeries)
- Metabolic disease (electrolyte disorders; renal failure)
- CNS disease (cerebrovascular accident; brain tumors; head trauma)
- Medications (anesthetic agents; steroids; dopamine agonists)
- Other: carbonated beverages; excess alcohol; stress

GENERAL PREVENTION

- Identify and correct relevant underlying cause(s).
- Avoid gastric distention.
- Acupuncture shows promise compared to chronic drug therapy for controlling hiccups.

DIAGNOSIS

- Hiccup attacks usually occur at brief intervals and last seconds or minutes. Persistent bouts lasting >48 hours often imply an underlying physical or metabolic disorder.
- Intractable hiccups may occur continuously for months or years (2).
- Hiccups usually have a frequency of 4 to 60 per minute (2).
- Persistent and intractable hiccups warrant further evaluation.

HISTORY

- Severity and duration of hiccup bouts
- Associated medical conditions that could be causative—GI, cardiac, neurologic, or pulmonary disorders
- Recent surgery (especially genitourinary)
- Behavioral health history
- Review of medications
- Alcohol and illicit drug use

PHYSICAL EXAM

- Correlate exam with potential etiologies (e.g., rales with pneumonia; organomegaly with splenic or hepatic disease)
- Examine the ear canal for foreign bodies.
- Head and neck masses and lymphadenopathy
- Complete neurologic exam

DIFFERENTIAL DIAGNOSIS

Hiccups are rarely confused with burping (eructation).

DIAGNOSTIC TESTS & INTERPRETATION

- When an underlying etiology is suspected, consider condition-specific testing (e.g., CBC, electrolytes, BUN, creatinine, LFTs, amylase/lipase, metabolic panel, chest x-ray) for hiccups lasting longer than 48 hours.
- Fluoroscopy can evaluate hemidiaphragm movement.

Diagnostic Procedures/Other

- Upper endoscopy; CT scan (or other imaging) of brain, thorax, abdomen, and pelvis to look for underlying causes
- Head MRI with contrast, lumbar puncture
- The extent of the workup is often in proportion to the duration and severity of the hiccups (1).

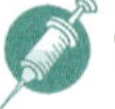

TREATMENT

- Outpatient (usually)
- Inpatient (if elderly, debilitated, or intractable hiccups)
- Many hiccup treatments are purely anecdotal.

GENERAL MEASURES

- Evaluate frequent bouts or persistent hiccups.
- Treat underlying cause when identified (1),(2)[C].
  - Dilate esophageal stricture or obstruction.
  - Treat ulcers or reflux disease.
  - Correct electrolyte abnormalities.
  - Remove hair or foreign body from ear canal.
  - Bitters for alcohol-induced hiccups
  - Catheter stimulation of pharynx for operative and postoperative hiccups
  - Antifungal treatment for *Candida* esophagitis
- Medical measures
  - Relieve gastric distention (gastric lavage, nasogastric aspiration, induced vomiting).
  - Cautious counterirritation of the vagus nerve (supraorbital pressure, carotid sinus massage, digital rectal massage)
  - Respiratory center stimulants (breathing 5% CO_2)
  - Behavioral health modification (hypnosis, meditation, paced respirations)
  - Phrenic nerve block or electrical stimulation (or pacing) of the dominant hemidiaphragm
  - Acupuncture
  - Miscellaneous (cardioversion)

MEDICATION

First Line

- Physical maneuvers: breath holding, Valsalva maneuver, breathing into a bag, fright, ice water gargles
- Others: swallowing granulated sugar, hard bread, or peanut butter; biting on a lemon, pulling knees to chest, or leaning forward to compress chest
- Drug therapy if physical maneuvers have failed or treatment is directed toward a specific cause of hiccups
- Pharmacologic therapy
  - Baclofen: 5 to 10 mg PO TID (1),(2)[B]
- Gabapentin (Neurontin): 300 mg PO HS; may increase up to 1,800 mg/day PO in divided doses (2)[B]; 1,200 mg/day PO for 3 days and then 400 mg/day PO for 3 days in patients undergoing stroke rehabilitation or in the palliative care setting where chlorpromazine adverse effects are undesirable (2)
- Chlorpromazine (FDA-approved for hiccups): 25 to 50 mg PO/IV TID
- Metoclopramide: 5 to 10 mg PO QID
- Haloperidol: 2 to 5 mg PO/IM followed by 1 to 2 mg PO TID
- Phenytoin: 200 to 300 mg PO HS
- Nifedipine: 10 to 20 mg PO daily to TID
- Amitriptyline: 10 mg PO TID
- Viscous lidocaine 2%: 5 mL PO daily to TID
- Combination of lansoprazole 15 mg PO daily, clonazepam 0.5 mg PO BID, and dimenhydrinate 25 mg PO BID
- Contraindications: Refer to manufacturer's literature.
  - Chlorpromazine is not recommended in elderly patient with dementia.
- Baclofen is not recommended in patients with stroke or other cerebral lesions or in severe renal impairment. Avoid abrupt withdrawal of baclofen.
- Other possible drug therapies (1)
  - Amantadine, carbidopa, and levodopa in Parkinson disease
  - Steroid replacement in Addison disease
  - Antifungal agent in *Candida* esophagitis
  - Ondansetron in carcinomatosis with vomiting
  - Nefopam (a nonopioid analgesic with antishivering properties related to antihistamines and antiparkinsonian drugs) is available outside the United States in both IV and oral formulations.
  - Olanzapine 10 mg QHS or chlorpromazine 25 mg PO TID in combination with olanzapine 5 mg PO daily (3)
  - Pregabalin 375 mg/day

ISSUES FOR REFERRAL

For acupuncture or phrenic nerve crush, block, or electrostimulation; continuous cervical epidural block; cardioversion

SURGERY/OTHER PROCEDURES

- Phrenic nerve crush or transaction or electrostimulation of the dominant diaphragmatic leaflet
- Resection of rib exostoses

COMPLEMENTARY & ALTERNATIVE MEDICINE

- Acupuncture is increasingly used to manage persistent or intractable hiccups, especially in cancer patients (2)[A].
- Home remedies (none of which are universally effective) (1)
  - Swallowing a spoonful of sugar
  - Sucking on hard candy or swallowing peanut butter
  - Holding breath and increasing pressure on diaphragm (Valsalva maneuver)
  - Tongue traction
  - Lifting the uvula with a cold spoon
  - Inducing fright
  - Smelling salts
  - Rebreathing into a paper (not plastic) bag
  - Sipping ice water
  - Rubbing a wet cotton-tipped applicator between hard and soft palate for 1 minute

ADMISSION, INPATIENT, AND NURSING CONSIDERATIONS

Most patients can be managed as outpatients; those with severe intractable hiccups may require rehydration, pain control, IV medications, or surgery.

ONGOING CARE

FOLLOW-UP RECOMMENDATIONS

Patient Monitoring

Until hiccups cease

DIET

Avoid gastric distension from overeating, carbonated beverages, and aerophagia.

PATIENT EDUCATION

See "General Measures."

PROGNOSIS

- Hiccups often cease during sleep.
- Most acute benign hiccup bouts resolve spontaneously or with home remedies.
- Intractable hiccups may last for years or decades.
- Hiccups have persisted despite bilateral phrenic nerve transection.

COMPLICATIONS

- Inability to eat
- Weight loss
- Exhaustion, debility
- Insomnia
- Cardiac arrhythmias
- Wound dehiscence
- Death (rare)

REFERENCES

1. Leung AKC, Leung AAM, Wong AHC, et al. Hiccups: a non-systematic review. *Curr Pediatr Rev*. 2020;16(4):277–284. doi:10.2174/1573396316666200508112951.
2. Thompson DF, Brooks KG. Gabapentin therapy of hiccups. *Ann Pharmacother*. 2013;47(6):897–903.
3. Srinivasan M, Yadav G, Singh Y, et al. Comparison of efficacy of combination therapy with chlorpromazine and olanzapine with chlorpromazine alone for treatment of hiccups in traumatic brain injury patients—a randomised control trial. *J Clin Diagn Res*. 2022;16(9):28–31.

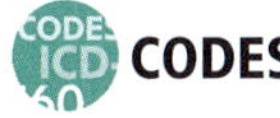

CODES

ICD10

- R06.6 Hiccough
- F45.8 Other somatoform disorders

CLINICAL PEARLS

- Most hiccups resolve spontaneously.
- An organic cause is more likely in men and individuals with intractable hiccups.
- Rule out foreign body in the ear canal as a trigger.
- Baclofen and gabapentin are the only pharmacologic agents proven to be clinically effective.
- Acupuncture may be effective for persistent hiccups.

H

HIDRADENITIS SUPPURATIVA

Tharani Ravi, MD • Madeline Hazle, MD

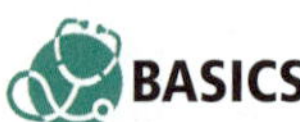

BASICS

DESCRIPTION

- Chronic inflammatory skin disease manifested as recurrent inflammatory nodules, abscesses, sinus tracts, and complex scar formation
- Areas affected are tender, malodorous, often with exudative drainage.
- Has higher risk of concomitant decrease in quality of life secondary to physical, emotional, and psychological stress.
- Common in intertriginous skin regions: axillae, groin, perianal, perineal, inframammary skin
- System affected: skin, psychosocial
- Synonym(s): acne inversa; Verneuil disease; apocrinitis; hidradenitis axillaris

EPIDEMIOLOGY

- Predominant sex: female > male (3:1)
- African Americans

Incidence

Peak onset during 2nd and 3rd decades of life but can be found from puberty until age 40 years

Prevalence

1–4%

ETIOLOGY AND PATHOPHYSIOLOGY

- Not fully understood; previously considered a disorder of apocrine glands but more recently thought to be due to a follicular epithelium defect.
- Pathogenesis is multifactorial with immunologic, hormonal, genetic, and environmental factors playing a role.
- The primary events are follicular hyperkeratosis and occlusion of terminal hair follicle.
- Mechanical stress on skin (intertriginous regions) precipitates follicular rupture and immune response.
- Bacterial involvement is a secondary event.
- Rupture and reepithelialization cause sinus tracts to form.

Genetics

- Familial occurrences suggest single gene transmission (autosomal dominant), but the condition may also be polygenic.
- Estimated 40% of patients have an affected first-degree family member.

RISK FACTORS

- Obesity
- Smoking
- Hyperandrogenism
- Drugs: oral contraceptives, IM medroxyprogesterone acetate, levonorgestrel, lithium

GENERAL PREVENTION

- Lose weight if overweight or obese.
- Smoking cessation
- Avoid constrictive clothing/synthetic fabrics, frictional trauma, heat exposure, excessive sweating, shaving, depilation, and deodorants.
- Use of antiseptic soaps

COMMONLY ASSOCIATED CONDITIONS

- Acne vulgaris, acne conglobate
- Perifolliculitis capitis abscedens et suffodiens (dissecting cellulitis of scalp)
- Pilonidal disease
- Metabolic syndrome/obesity
- Polycystic ovary syndrome (PCOS) and androgen dysfunction
- Thyroid disease
- Arthritis and spondyloarthritis (seronegative)
- Inflammatory bowel disease
- Squamous cell carcinoma
- PAPASH syndrome (pyogenic arthritis, pyoderma gangrenosum, acne, and suppurative hidradenitis)
- Type 2 diabetes mellitus

DIAGNOSIS

HISTORY

- Diagnostic criteria adopted by the 2nd International Conference on Hidradenitis Suppurativa, 2009
- All three criteria (morphology, location, progression) must be present for diagnosis:
  - Typical lesions: painful nodules, abscesses, draining sinus, bridged scars, and "tombstone" double-ended pseudocomedones in secondary lesions
  - Typical topography: axillae, groins, perineal and perianal region, buttocks, infra- and intermammary folds
  - Chronicity and recurrences, commonly refractory to initial treatments

PHYSICAL EXAM

- Tender dome-shaped nodules 0.5 to 3.0 cm in size are present.
  - Location corresponds with the distribution of apocrine-related mammary tissue and terminal hair follicles dependent on low androgen concentrations.
  - Sites ordered by frequency of occurrence: axillary, inguinal, perianal and perineal, mammary and inframammary, buttock, pubic region, chest, scalp, retroauricular, eyelid
  - Large lesions are often fluctuant; comedones may be present.
- Possible malodorous discharge
- Hurley clinical staging system
  - **Stage I**: nodule/abscess formation without sinus tracts or scarring
  - **Stage II**: more than one lesion widely spaced with tract and scar formation
  - **Stage III**: diffuse, multiple interconnected tracts and abscesses with scarring
- Sartorius clinical staging system (points attributed)
  - Anatomic region involved
  - Quantity and quality of lesions
  - Distance between lesions
  - Presence or absence of normal skin between lesions
- Other scoring tools include: IHS4, HiSCR, and HASI-R which include more information including response to treatment and changes in severity.

DIFFERENTIAL DIAGNOSIS

- Acne vulgaris, conglobate
- Furunculosis/carbuncles
- Infected Bartholin or sebaceous cysts
- Lymphadenopathy/lymphadenitis
- Cutaneous Langerhans cell histiocytosis
- Actinomycosis
- Granuloma inguinale
- Lymphogranuloma venereum
- Apocrine nevus
- Crohn disease with anogenital fistula(s) (may coexist with hidradenitis suppurativa [HS])
- Fox-Fordyce disease

DIAGNOSTIC TESTS & INTERPRETATION

Initial Tests (lab, imaging)

- Cultures of skin or aspirates of boils are most commonly negative. When positive, cultures are often polymicrobial and commonly grow *Staphylococcus aureus* and *Staphylococcus epidermidis*.
- May note increased erythrocyte sedimentation rate (ESR), leukocytosis, decreased serum iron, normocytic anemia, or changes in serum electrophoresis pattern

Follow-Up Tests & Special Considerations

- Consider biopsy of concerning lesions due to increased risk of squamous cell carcinoma.
- If the patient is female, overweight, and/or hirsute, consider evaluating for polycystic ovary syndrome
- Incidence is rare after menopause and before puberty (consider premature adrenarche).
- If pregnant, do not use isotretinoin or tetracyclines for teratogenicity.

Diagnostic Procedures/Other

- Incision and drainage, culture and biopsy
- Ultrasound may be useful in planning an excision to identify the full extent of sinus tracts.

Test Interpretation

- Dermis shows granulomatous inflammation and inflammatory cells, giant cells, sinus tracts, subcutaneous abscesses, and extensive fibrosis.
- Hair follicular dilatation and occlusion by keratinized stratified squamous epithelium

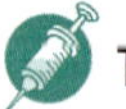

TREATMENT

Despite the prevalence of this condition, most trials have been small and underpowered. Evidence is therefore generally of poor quality. Treatment goals: Reduce extent of disease, prevent new lesions, remove chronic disease, and limit scar formation.

- Conservative treatment includes all items under "General Prevention," plus use of warm compresses, sitz baths, topical antiseptics for inflamed lesions, and nonopioid analgesics.
- Weight loss and smoking cessation result in marked improvement (1).
- Corticosteroids, isotretinoin, and zinc gluconate
- For stages I and II, attempt medical treatment.
- Short medical trial may be appropriate in stage III prior to moving on to surgical therapies.
- Adalimumab (anti-TNF-α antibody) and anti-IL-17 secukinumab are the only two FDA-approved biologics for HS, demonstrating moderate efficacy (2).
- No medications are curative; relapse is almost inevitable, but the disease may be controlled; usually must fail other treatments before starting biologics; they can be a costly option.

GENERAL MEASURES

- Education and psychosocial support
- Appropriate hygiene including avoidance of shearing stress to skin (light clothing), daily cleansing with antibacterial soap
- Diet: Avoid dairy, high glycemic loads.
- Pain control
- Improve environmental factors that cause follicular blockage (See "General Prevention").
- Smoking cessation and weight loss

MEDICATION

First Line

- Stage I disease (mild-to-moderate disease): Consider either systemic or topical antibiotics.
  - Skin cleansers (i.e., chlorhexidine 4% solution) are part of first line; however, no data exists on efficacy for specific agents and have very limited data, mostly expert opinion.
  - Keratolytic agents could be considered; however, it can cause irritant dermatitis.
  - Topical antibiotics (clindamycin was studied in clinical trials) (1)[B]
    - Clindamycin 0.1% solution BID for 12 weeks with benzoyl peroxide 5–10% solution was shown to reduce the rates of *S. aureus* resistance.
    - Topical 15% resorcinol could be a well-tolerated alternative to patients with resistance to topical clindamycin (1),(3)
  - Systemic antibiotics: tetracyclines are first line for patients demonstrating no response to topical treatments.
    - For mild-to-moderate HS, tetracycline medications were recommended for a 12-week course for maintenance (i.e., doxycycline 100 mg q12h or clindamycin 300 mg BID)
    - Dapsone 50 to 150 mg daily (recommended for 3-month course, not as effective in Hurley stage III disease) (1)[C]
  - Intralesional corticosteroids: limited evidence; possible reduction in pain, erythema, edema, and lesion size (1) (triamcinolone acetonide 10 mg/mL usually 0.2 to 2.0 mL injection)
- Stage II and III disease
  - Should be treated with first-line interventions to decrease severity; consider immediate referral to dermatology if disease is severe.
  - Biologic medications: TNF-α inhibitors such as adalimumab 40 mg weekly, can improve disease severity and quality of life in those with moderate-to-severe HS (1),(2)[A]. Secukinumab (IL-17A inhibitor) was FDA approved in 2023 for treatment of moderate-to-severe HS; other anti-TNF agents such as infliximab have been tested and there is ongoing study on other potential biologics such as IL-1 inhibitors, anti-IL 12/23 agents, JAK inhibitors (2),(3).
  - Minor surgical procedures (punch débridement, local unroofing) to treat individual lesions or sinus tracts

Second Line

- Clindamycin and rifampin combination treatment could be effective in Hurley stage I to II with inadequate response to tetracyclines or as adjunct in severe disease
- Spironolactone has been shown to help in hormonal cases for women.
- Retinoids should be used as a second- or third-line medication due to the limited and mixed result data.
- Limited and weak evidence for immunosuppressants such as methotrexate, azathioprine, colchicine/minocycline, cyclosporine.
- Short courses of pulse steroids can be considered for acute flares or long term (the lowest appropriate dose) corticosteroids for severe HS treatment.
- IV ertapenem 1 g for 6-week course has been shown to be highly effective; however, should only be used as a bridge to surgery, given concern for antibiotic resistance and cost prohibitive home infusion costs (1).

ISSUES FOR REFERRAL

- Lack of response to treatment, stages II and III disease, or concern for malignancy
- If significant psychosocial stress exists secondary to disease, refer for stress management or psychiatric evaluation.
- Suspicion of hyperandrogenic states (e.g., PCOS) should prompt investigation or referral.
- Severe perianal/perivulvar disease or otherwise very extensive disease may prompt referral to plastic surgeon or reconstructive urologist.

SURGERY/OTHER PROCEDURES

- Important mode of treatment; necessary to remove tunnels and scarring
- Incision and drainage and deroofing are preferred in acute phase, while more extensive surgical procedures are typically deferred until the remission phase.
- Could be used in conjunction with antibiotics or if first-line therapy fails
- Various surgical approaches have been used for stages II and III disease (e.g., skin-tissue-sparing excision with electrosurgical peeling [STEEP])
- Laser therapy for Hurley stages I and II disease (rarely used); no consensus on the benefit
- Cryotherapy and photodynamic therapy have shown variable results; they are not routinely recommended.

ONGOING CARE

FOLLOW-UP RECOMMENDATIONS

Follow-up monthly or sooner to evaluate progress and to assist with symptom management.

DIET

- Avoid dairy and high glycemic loads.
- Healthy diet that promotes weight loss
- May benefit from zinc supplementation

PATIENT EDUCATION

- Severity can range from only two to three papules per year to extensive draining sinus tracts.
- Medications are temporizing measures, rarely curative. Attempts at local surgical "cures" do not affect recurrence at other sites.
- Smoking cessation and weight loss can improve symptoms significantly.
- Hidradenitis Suppurativa Foundation: https://www.hs-foundation.org/

PROGNOSIS

- Individual lesions heal slowly in 10 to 30 days.
- Recurrences may last for several years.
- Relentlessly progressive scarring and sinus tracts are likely with severe disease.
- Radical wide-area excision, with removal of all hair-bearing skin in the affected area, shows the greatest chance for cure.
- Increased all-cause mortality

COMPLICATIONS

- Contracture and stricturing of the skin after extensive abscess rupture, scarring, and healing; or at sites of surgical excisions
- Lymphatic obstruction, lymphedema
- Psychosocial: anxiety, malaise, depression, self-injury
- Anemia, amyloidosis, and hypoproteinemia (due to chronic suppuration)
- Lumbosacral epidural abscess, sacral bacterial osteomyelitis
- Squamous cell carcinoma may develop in indolent sinus tracts.
- Disseminated infection or septicemia (rare)
- Urethral, rectal, or bladder fistula (rare)

REFERENCES

1. Saunte DML, Jemec GBE. Hidradenitis suppurativa: advances in diagnosis and treatment. *JAMA*. 2017;318(20):2019–2032.
2. Lim SYD, Oon HH. Systematic review of immunomodulatory therapies for hidradenitis suppurativa. *Biologics*. 2019;13:53–78.
3. Billewicz M, Wojtania J, Woźniacka A. Hidradenitis suppurativa: a new therapeutic approach for an old disease. *Postepy Dermatol Alergol*. 2024;41(4):350–356.

ADDITIONAL READING

Jemec GBE. Clinical practice. Hidradenitis suppurativa. *N Engl J Med*. 2012;366(2):158–164.

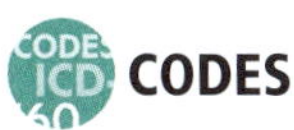

CODES

ICD10

L73.2 Hidradenitis suppurativa

CLINICAL PEARLS

- Chronic inflammatory disease of the skin, often difficult to control with behavior changes and medication alone
- First-line treatment for mild disease is topical and/or systemic antibiotics.
- For patients with refractory or severe disease, wide local excision provides the only chance at a cure. Success rates depend on the location and extent of excision.
- This is a difficult to treat disease that can greatly affect the patient's quality of life.

HIRSUTISM

Jarrett Keller Sell, MD, FAAFP, AAHIVS • Kendal Schaetzle, DO

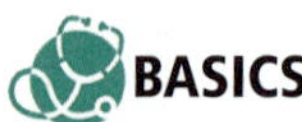

BASICS

DESCRIPTION

- Presence of excessive terminal (coarse, pigmented) hair of body and face, in a masculine pattern
- May be present as an ethnic characteristic or may develop as a result of androgen excess
- Most often seen in polycystic ovary syndrome (PCOS), which is characterized by hirsutism, acne, menstrual irregularities, and obesity
- System(s) affected: dermatologic, endocrine, metabolic, reproductive

EPIDEMIOLOGY

Prevalence

5–10% of reproductive age cisgender women

ETIOLOGY AND PATHOPHYSIOLOGY

- Due to increased androgenic hormones, either from increased peripheral binding (idiopathic) or increased production from the ovaries, adrenals, or body fat
- Exogenous medications
- Can be a symptom of PCOS, androgen-secreting tumors, virilizing disorders, or androgenic medication use

Genetics

Multifactorial

RISK FACTORS

- Family history/ethnicity (e.g., Ashkenazi Jewish and Mediterranean ethnicities)
- Obesity

GENERAL PREVENTION

Women with late-onset congenital adrenal hyperplasia (CAH) should be counseled that they may be carriers for the severe early-onset childhood disease.

COMMONLY ASSOCIATED CONDITIONS

- PCOS: the most common cause of premenopausal hirsutism
- Prolonged amenorrhea and anovulation, common
- Acne, common
- Central obesity
- Virilization (rapid onset, clitoromegaly, balding, deepening voice) (1)

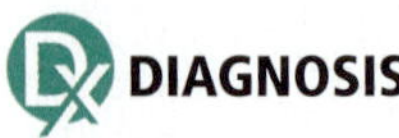

DIAGNOSIS

HISTORY

- Severity, time course, and age of onset of hirsutism
- Weight, BMI
- Psychosocial impact on patient
- Pubertal, menstrual and fertility history, anovulation (defined as ovulatory cycle >35 days)
- Severe acne, especially if treatment resistant
- Presence of virilization
- Medication history: Look for use of valproic acid, testosterone, danazol, glucocorticoids, topical androgen use by partner, and athletic performance drugs.
- The presence of galactorrhea

PHYSICAL EXAM

- Increased hair growth in premenopausal women, particularly over the chin, neck, sideburns, lower back, sternum, areola, abdomen, shoulders, buttocks, perineal area, and inner thighs
- Check skin for acne, striae, acanthosis nigricans (velvety black skin in the axillae or neck).
- Virilization: deep voice, male pattern balding, increased muscle mass, and clitoromegaly
- The Ferriman-Gallwey scale (an instrument that rates hair growth in nine areas on a scale of 0 to 4, with >8 being positive) may be used for diagnosis and to monitor response to therapy, but it may underrate patient's perception of hirsutism and can be altered by previous cosmetic treatment. Scores between 8 and 15 are considered to be mild hirsutism, 16 to 25 moderate, and >25 severe (1),(2).

DIFFERENTIAL DIAGNOSIS

- PCOS (72–82%)—irregular menses, elevated androgens, polycystic ovaries on US, infertility, insulin resistance
- Idiopathic hyperandrogenemia (6–15%)—hirsutism with normal ovaries on US, elevated androgen levels, no other explainable cause
- Idiopathic hirsutism (4–7%)—hirsutism with normal menses, androgen levels, and ovaries on ultrasonography, no other explainable cause
- Late-onset or nonclassic CAH (2–4%), a genetic enzyme deficiency, which typically presents in adolescence with severe hirsutism and irregular menses
- Androgen-secreting tumor (0.2%)—ovaries (benign or malignant) or adrenals (commonly malignant)
- Thyroid dysfunction, most commonly presents with menstrual irregularity and not commonly as isolated hirsutism
- Hyperprolactinemia, if accompanied by galactorrhea and/or amenorrhea
- Rare endocrine disorders—Cushing (hypercortisolism), acromegaly
- Medication side effects (e.g., cyclosporine, danazol, glucocorticoids, minoxidil, testosterone)

DIAGNOSTIC TESTS & INTERPRETATION

- Assess androgen levels. Guidelines recommend screening hyperandrogenemic women for CAH due to 21-hydroxylase deficiency by measuring early morning 17α-hydroxyprogesterone (17α-OHP) levels (1).
- PCOS diagnosed with two out of three signs: oligo-anovulation, clinical and/or biochemical hyperandrogenemia, polycystic ovaries on US (1)[C]
- Lab testing can be considered to rule out underlying tumor and pituitary diseases (rare) if suggested by history, physical, or initial testing.

Initial Tests (lab, imaging)

- Random total testosterone level is usually sufficient as an initial screen (1)[C].
- Normal upper limit for serum total testosterone in adult women is approximately 40 to 60 ng/dL (1.4 to 2.1 nmol/L). Patients who have clinical features consistent with PCOS but have normal total testosterone should have repeat testing, with an early morning serum free testosterone level calculated from sex hormone-binding globulin (SHBG). A morning free testosterone is 50% more sensitive (3).
- If testosterone is >150 (some use 200) ng/dL, ultrasound for ovarian and CT scan for adrenal tumor (1).
- The workup for PCOS recommended by the American College of Obstetricians and Gynecologists (ACOG) includes the above plus:
  - Screening for metabolic syndrome with a fasting and 2-hour glucose after 75-g glucose load, lipid panel, waist circumference, and blood pressure (4)
- Ovarian US to look for polycystic ovaries
- If the patient is amenorrheic, check prolactin, FSH, LH, TSH, and a pregnancy test (5). An LH/FSH ratio >2 is consistent with PCOS.

Follow-Up Tests & Special Considerations

- 17α-OHP
  - Best evaluated during the follicular phase or on a random day in women with infrequent menses or amenorrhea
  - Elevations of 17α-OHP (>300) can indicate late-onset CAH.
  - Consider in patients with onset in early adolescence or high-risk group (Ashkenazi Jewish) (1)[C].
  - If elevated, order corticotropin stimulation test.
- If prolactin level is high, consider MRI of the pituitary if medication causes not suspected.
- If PCOS is diagnosed, ACOG recommends screening for dyslipidemia and diabetes mellitus type 2 (4).
- Suggest against testing for elevated androgen levels in eumenorrheic women with unwanted local hair growth.
- Dehydroepiandrosterone sulfate (DHEA-S) should be checked in virilization (2).
  - Levels >700 ug/dL may indicate adrenal tumor.

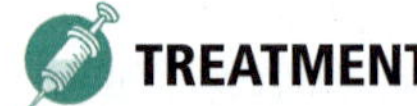

TREATMENT

GENERAL MEASURES

- Treatment depends on patient preference and psychosocial effect.
- Treatment goal is to decrease new hair growth and improve metabolic disorders.
- If patient desires pregnancy, induction of ovulation may be necessary.
- Provide contraception, as needed.
- A calorie-restricted diet is recommended in all overweight patients with PCOS. Weight loss has positive effects on fertility, metabolic profile, and may improve hirsutism (5).
- Treat accompanying acne.

MEDICATION

First Line

- Direct hair removal or pharmacologic therapy recommended for mild hirsutism (1)[B]
- Oral contraceptives are first line to manage menstrual abnormalities and hirsutism/acne (2),(3); they will suppress ovarian androgen production and increase SHBG, improve metabolic syndrome, and slow but not reverse hair growth.
  - Doses of 20 to 35 μg ethinyl estradiol effectively decrease ovarian androgen production. The progestins norgestimate, desogestrel, and drospirenone are the least androgenic, but they are associated with a higher VTE risk, especially in severely obese patients (3).

- They take 6 months to show effect and are continued for years.
- Oral preparations, compared to vaginal or transdermal, are better at controlling hirsutism and acne; by passing through the liver, they induce SHBG production.
- For patients with high risk for VTE, it is recommended to use the lowest dose of an ethinyl estradiol based oral contraceptive and a low-risk progesterone-based oral contraceptive (1).

- Progesterone (depot or intermittent oral) can be used if estrogens are contraindicated.
- Eflornithine (Vaniqa) HCl cream: Apply BID at least 8 hours apart; reduces facial hair in 40% of women (must be used indefinitely to prevent regrowth); only FDA-approved hirsutism treatment, may be costly and not covered by insurance
- Laser therapy with eflornithine cream shown to have a more rapid response
- Combination oral contraceptives and antiandrogen is contraindicated first line unless those with severe hirsutism and significant emotional distress or no success with oral contraceptives alone (failure of therapy after 6 months) (1)[B].

Second Line

- Antiandrogenic drugs will further reduce hirsutism by 15–25%. Usually begun 6 months after first-line therapy if results are suboptimal. Must be used in combination with oral contraceptives to prevent menorrhagia and potential fetal toxicity. All should be avoided in pregnancy (1).
  - Spironolactone, 50 to 200 mg/day: Onset of action is slow; use with oral contraceptives to prevent menorrhagia. Watch for hyperkalemia, especially with drospirenone-containing OCP (e.g., Yaz, Yasmin); avoid use in pregnancy.
  - Finasteride: 2.5 to 7.5 mg/day decreases androgen binding; not approved by FDA. Use with contraception (pregnancy Category X).
  - Cyproterone, not available in the United States: 12.5 to 100 mg/day for days 5 to 15 of cycle combined with ethinyl estradiol 20 to 50 μg for days 5 to 25 of cycle
  - Leuprolide, 3.75 mg IM monthly, can cause bone loss, vaginal dryness, and hot flashes; avoid use in pregnancy.
  - Flutamide or bicalutamide are not commonly recommended due to potential hepatotoxicity (1)[C].
  - Topical antiandrogen therapy is not clearly effective and not recommended.
- Insulin-lowering drugs are not recommended alone for treating hirsutism (1),(2).
  - Metformin, which should not be used as monotherapy for hirsutism, is likely less effective than oral contraceptives, especially in those with PCOS and a BMI of 25 to 30 kg/m^2 (5).
- Steroids: used in late-onset CAH
  - Dexamethasone: 2 mg/day
- Cosmetic treatment: includes many methods of hair removal
  - Temporary: shaving, chemical depilation, plucking, waxing
  - Permanent: Laser epilation and photoepilation are preferred to electrolysis (2).
  - For direct hair removal, electrolysis rather than photoepilation is recommended in women with blonde or white hair (2).
  - Pharmacologic therapy is suggested to minimize regrowth.

Pregnancy Considerations

- May have related infertility
- As hormone balance improves, fertility may increase; provide contraception, as needed.
- Several medications used for treatment are contraindicated in pregnancy.

COMPLEMENTARY & ALTERNATIVE MEDICINE

Small trials may indicate some benefit in the treatment of hirsutism for the following herbal therapies: fennel, licorice, spearmint, saw palmetto, green tea, combination of Zingiber and neem, curcumin, and teupolioside (6).

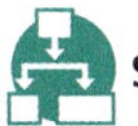

ONGOING CARE

FOLLOW-UP RECOMMENDATIONS

Patient Monitoring

Monitor for known side effects of medications.

DIET

Diet consisting of low-calorie, low-glycemic index foods improve fertility and metabolic parameters in patients with PCOS who are overweight (5).

PATIENT EDUCATION

- Hormonal treatment stops further hair growth and will improve but not reverse present hair.
  - Treatment takes 6 months to take effect and may need to be lifelong.
- Cosmetic measures may be needed for the already present hair.

PROGNOSIS

- Good (with long-term therapy) for halting further hair growth
- Moderate to poor for reversing current hair growth

COMPLICATIONS

- If PCOS is present, dysfunctional uterine bleeding may lead to anemia.
- If PCOS is present, anovulation may increase endometrial hyperplasia and uterine cancer risk.
- Androgenic excess may adversely affect lipid status, cardiac risk, and bone density.

REFERENCES

1. Martin KA, Anderson RR, Chang RJ, et al. Evaluation and treatment of hirsutism in premenopausal women: an Endocrine Society clinical practice guideline. *J Clin Endocrinol Metab*. 2018;103(4):1233–1257.
2. Matheson E, Bain J. Hirsutism in women. *Am Fam Physician*. 2019;100(3):168–175.
3. Teede HJ, Misso ML, Costello MF, et al; for the International PCOS Network. Recommendations from the international evidence-based guideline for the assessment and management of polycystic ovary syndrome. *Fertil Steril*. 2018;110(3):364–379. doi:10.1016/j.fertnstert.2018.05.004.
4. American College of Obstetricians and Gynecologists' Committee on Practice Bulletins—Gynecology. ACOG practice bulletin no. 194: polycystic ovary syndrome. *Obstet Gynecol*. 2018;131(6):e157–e171. doi:10.1097/AOG.0000000000002656.
5. Williams T, Moore JB, Regehr J. Polycystic ovary syndrome: common questions and answers. *Am Fam Physician*. 2023;107(3):264–272.
6. Ghanbarian R, Ranjbai M, Babaeian M, et al. A narrative review of herbal remedies for managing hirsutism. *Int J Prev Med*. 2024;15:17. doi:10.4103/ijpvm.ijpvm_62_23.

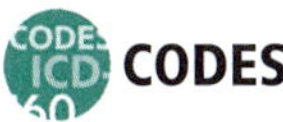

SEE ALSO

Acne Vulgaris; Infertility; Polycystic Ovarian Syndrome (PCOS)

CODES

ICD10

- L68.0 Hirsutism
- E28.2 Polycystic ovarian syndrome

CLINICAL PEARLS

- PCOS is the most common cause of hirsutism (diagnosed with two out of three: oligoanovulation, clinical and/or biochemical hyperandrogenemia, polycystic ovaries on US).
- Diagnosis is based on androgen level in all women with abnormal hirsutism score; total testosterone for initial testing
- Virilization (clitoromegaly, balding, deepening voice): Suspect if testosterone >150 ng/dL; look for adrenal or ovarian tumors.
- Lifestyle modification and OCPs are first-line therapy for hirsutism, menstrual irregularities, and acne.

H

HIV/AIDS

Manju Mahajan, MD, FAAFP • Philip J. Bolduc, MD

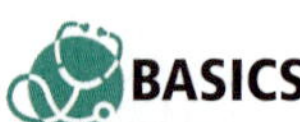

BASICS

DESCRIPTION

HIV is a retrovirus that integrates into CD4 T lymphocytes, altering cell-mediated immunity and causing cell death, severe immunodeficiency, opportunistic infections, and malignancies if not treated. Untreated HIV infection typically advances through several stages: viral transmission, acute retroviral syndrome, recovery, seroconversion, and then chronic infection, leading (an average of 8 to 10 years later) to AIDS.

EPIDEMIOLOGY

Incidence

There were approximately 1.3 million new cases of HIV worldwide in 2022, including an estimated 31,800 new infections in the United States, the latter reflecting a 12% decrease from 2018. The year 2022 saw 37,981 individuals aged ≥13 years diagnosed with HIV in the United States and its territories, comprising both new and preexisting infections.

Prevalence

There were approximately 1.2 million persons with HIV (PWH) in the United States in 2022: ~13% unaware of their status. HIV continues to disproportionately affect certain populations, particularly racial and ethnic minorities and men who have sex with men (MSM). Globally, there were an estimated 38 million PWH in 2022.

ETIOLOGY AND PATHOPHYSIOLOGY

HIV is a single-stranded, positive-sense, enveloped RNA lentivirus that primarily infects CD4+ cells. After entering target cells, viral RNA is transcribed to DNA through reverse transcription, imported into the host cell nucleus, and integrated into host DNA. The virus can become latent for many years, or when the CD4+ cell is activated, produce new viral RNA and proteins that are packaged and released to infect other CD4+ cells. Of its two subtypes, HIV-1 causes most infections, whereas HIV-2 primarily found in West Africa.

RISK FACTORS

Most people acquire HIV through anal or vaginal sex or by sharing needles, syringes, or other drug injection equipment. Only certain body fluids can transmit HIV, primarily semen, blood, human milk, vaginal or rectal fluids, and cerebrospinal fluid (CSF). Urine, feces, saliva, and sweat do not transmit HIV unless visibly contaminated with blood. Perinatal transmission can occur during pregnancy, childbirth, and nursing (breastfeeding).

GENERAL PREVENTION

- Everyone aged 13 to 64 years (CDC) or 15 to 65 years (USPSTF) once in a lifetime (more often if risk factors). All pregnant people should be screened at the first prenatal visit and again in the 3rd trimester if at high risk or in a high-prevalence area. STIs increase susceptibility to HIV infection, so testing for HIV must be considered whenever diagnosing and treating STIs.
- Behavioral interventions, including counseling for at-risk populations, are recommended to reduce high-risk behaviors. Consistent and correct use of condoms during sexual activity reduces transmission.
- Harm reduction strategies for people who inject drugs, such as needle and syringe exchange programs and use of sterile injection equipment, are effective.
- Treatment as prevention (TasP): PWH with viral suppression on antiretroviral therapy (ART) are not infectious to their sexual partners. Early diagnosis and initiation of ART in PWH reduces community viral load and transmission risk.
- Preexposure prophylaxis (PrEP) with antiretroviral medications are highly effective and recommended by USPSTF for individuals at substantial risk, including MSM, transgender women, heterosexuals with high-risk exposures, and people who inject drugs.
- Postexposure prophylaxis (PEP): Taking 28 days of full ART after an HIV exposure is highly effective at preventing HIV transmission.

DIAGNOSIS

- Acute HIV: onset in 2 to 6 weeks, symptomatic in 40–90%, lasts 1 to 3 weeks; 60–90% have fever, maculopapular rash, adenopathy, sore throat (FRAT); 30–50% have nausea, vomiting, diarrhea, headache, myalgias/arthralgias; <30% have weight loss, thrush, neurologic symptoms (aseptic meningitis), mucosal ulcers, hepatosplenomegaly; generally absent: cough, rhinorrhea, nasal or chest congestion; this resembles mononucleosis (think dry) more than colds/flu (wet).
- Initial screening HIV test 4th generation HIV test algorithm: This set of tests can detect the HIV-1 p-24 antigen, antibodies to HIV-1 and HIV-2, and, if needed, HIV-1 RNA. It is usually positive within 2 weeks of infection and is the preferred method to screen for HIV beyond this window period. Rapid antibody-only HIV testing is useful in some situations (such as on labor and delivery or in community settings) but requires confirmatory testing.
- AIDS: To be diagnosed with AIDS, a person must have both HIV and either an AIDS-defining condition or an absolute CD4 count less than 200 cells/mm^3 (or <14% if <18 years old).
- AIDS-defining conditions include both opportunistic infections (such as *Pneumocystis jiroveci* pneumonia (PJP), cryptococcal meningitis, candida esophagitis, others), certain cancers (such as non-Hodgkin lymphoma, Kaposi sarcoma and invasive cervical cancer), and AIDS wasting syndrome.

HISTORY

- HIV remains a stigmatizing condition; focus on establishing rapport, developing trust, and putting the patient at ease. Assess the patient's knowledge about HIV and their readiness to begin ART. Discuss case management, insurance, housing, transportation, and food access.
- HIV-specific history: Ascertain the date of diagnosis and infection risk factor; lowest CD4 and highest viral load; prior ART regimens, reasons for stopping, and any known resistance; and use of PrEP or PEP medications prior to infection.
- Additional history: past medical, surgical, social, substance use and mental health history; past hospitalizations, transfusions, or blood product receipt, especially during 1975–1985 or outside the United States and Canada; immunization history, travel history, current medications, allergies. Determine if sexual or drug use partners are at risk of infection and offer to link them to care if possible.

PHYSICAL EXAM

Findings suggestive of chronic HIV infection include generalized lymphadenopathy, wasting, seborrheic dermatitis, herpes zoster, psoriasis, molluscum contagiosum, extensive condylomata, thrush, genital candidiasis, aphthous ulcers, oral hairy leukoplakia, recurrent herpes simplex.

DIAGNOSTIC TESTS & INTERPRETATION

Initial Tests (lab, imaging)

- CD4 cell count and percentage, plasma HIV RNA viral load and genotype
- CBC with differential, lipids, A1c, complete metabolic panel, urinalysis, urine HCG for people with childbearing potential
- Screen for hepatitis A/B/C, chlamydia, gonorrhea, syphilis; MMR and varicella IgG; HLA-B5701 (if using abacavir), glucose-6-phosphate dehydrogenase (G6PD) (if African or Mediterranean descent); cryptococcal antigen, toxoplasma, and CMV IgG if CD4 <100 or if have suspicion for clinical disease; PPD or interferon-γ release assay (IGRA) to screen for latent TB infection; eye exam to screen for CMV and toxoplasma retinochoroiditis if CD4 <100.

TREATMENT

GENERAL MEASURES

- Initiation of ART is recommended as soon as possible. Create a patient-centered, stigma-free care environment and address barriers to care. The goal of ART is to reduce the HIV viral load (ideally to nondetectable levels) but at least to <200 copies/mL.
- It is more common for viremia to reflect incomplete ART adherence without resistance than true development of drug resistance.

MEDICATION

Six classes of antiretroviral medications are available which target specific points in the multistep HIV life cycle: entry inhibitors, nucleoside reverse transcriptase inhibitors (NRTIs), nonnucleoside reverse transcriptase inhibitors (NNRTIs), integrase strand transfer inhibitors (INSTIs), protease inhibitors (PIs), and capsid inhibitors.

First Line

- ART should ideally be initiated within 7 days of diagnosis (same-day initiation encouraged if clinically appropriate and no contraindications exist). Initial regimens with an INSTI plus two NRTIs are recommended because of high efficacy, tolerability, and limited resistance. Recommended first-line regimens and dosages:
  - Bictegravir/tenofovir alafenamide/emtricitabine: 50 mg/25 mg/200 mg PO once daily (single-tablet regimen)
  - Dolutegravir 50 mg PO once daily plus either:
    - Tenofovir alafenamide 25 mg/emtricitabine 200 mg PO once daily, or
    - Tenofovir disoproxil fumarate 300 mg/emtricitabine 200 mg PO once daily, or
    - Tenofovir disoproxil fumarate 300 mg/lamivudine 300 mg PO once daily.
  - Dolutegravir/lamivudine: 50 mg/300 mg PO once daily (for select patients without hepatitis B and with viral load <500,000 copies/mL)

- Long-acting injectable therapy is available for select patients: cabotegravir 600 mg IM plus rilpivirine 900 mg IM every 2 months (after oral lead-in) for those who are virologically suppressed and prefer nondaily therapy
- Boosted protease inhibitor regimens (e.g., darunavir/ritonavir or atazanavir/ritonavir plus two NRTIs) reserved for patients unable to take INSTI-based regimens

- Ongoing monitoring of viral load, CD4 count, and safety labs is recommended throughout therapy.

ADDITIONAL THERAPIES

Opportunistic infection prophylaxis:

- If CD4 <200: PJP sulfamethoxazole/trimethoprim (Bactrim DS) 1 tablet daily
- If CD4 <100: toxoplasmosis: Bactrim DS 1 tablet daily.
- If CD4 <50 and not on suppressive ART: mycobacterium avium complex (MAC): azithromycin 1200 mg once a week.

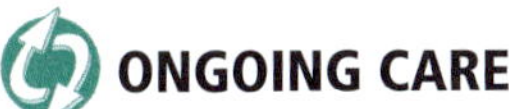

ONGOING CARE

FOLLOW-UP RECOMMENDATIONS

- PrEP:
  - Indicated for patients without HIV who may be exposed to HIV, including MSM, transgender women, commercial sex workers, persons who inject drugs and share needles, and persons whose partner is HIV positive with detectable or unknown viral load. PrEP is 99% effective in preventing HIV transmission via sexual route and >74% effective via needle sharing.
  - Prior to providing PrEP: Ensure patient does not have HIV through confirmatory testing, screen for chlamydia, gonorrhea, syphilis, HCV, and HBV, and obtain baseline kidney function.
  - Medication regimens approved by the U.S. Food and Drug Administration (FDA):
    - Emtricitabine 200 mg + tenofovir disoproxil fumarate 300 mg PO daily (F/TDF)
    - Emtricitabine 200 mg + tenofovir alafenamide 25 mg PO daily (F/TAF)
    - Cabotegravir 600 mg IM every 2 months
- PEP
  - Occupational or nonoccupational postexposure prophylaxis (PEP/nPEP) is recommended ideally within 24 hours but not <72 hours after exposure to the blood, semen, vaginal or rectal secretions, CSF, or breast milk of a known HIV-positive source person, whether occupational (health care workers, first responders, etc.) or nonoccupational (such as through sex or needle sharing) exposures. Counsel patients with more than one course of PEP on prevention and consider PrEP.
  - PEP/nPEP comprises 28 days of a three-drug ART regimen: Bictegravir/emtricitabine/tenofovir alafenamide (BIC 50 mg/FTC 200 mg/TAF 25 mg PO once daily) *or* dolutegravir 50 mg PLUS (tenofovir alafenamide 25 mg *or* tenofovir disoproxil fumarate 300 mg) PLUS (emtricitabine 200 mg *or* lamivudine 300 mg)
  - Complete HIV, hepatitis B, and hepatitis C testing at baseline, 4 to 6 weeks, 3 months, and 6 months after exposure. For sexual exposures, test for syphilis, gonorrhea, and chlamydia at presentation and 4 to 6 weeks after exposure, plus again for syphilis 6 months postexposure

Patient Monitoring

- CD4 count–q3–6mo in first 2 years after initiation of ART; after 2 years with viral suppression: CD4 >300 to 500 cells/mm^3 monitor annually; >500 cells/mm^3, monitoring is optional; viral load: 2 to 8 weeks after ART initiation and then every 4 to 8 weeks until suppressed. First 2 years of ART: q3–4 mo; after 2 years virally suppressed: q6mo
- Cr, LFTs, CBC with differential: q3–6mo; UA for proteinuria q6–12mo if on TDF or TAF; fasting lipid panel: annually, 2 months after ART start or change; fasting glucose or HbA1c: annually (if not diabetic); TB screen: annual IGRA or PPD for patients at risk for TB exposure
- Health care maintenance
  - HCV, HBV (HBsAg, HBsAb, HBcAb) testing per risk factors
  - Breast, colon, prostate, lung cancer, and AAA screening recommendations are same as for people without HIV.
  - Dual-energy X-ray absorptiometry (DEXA) for postmenopausal women and men with HIV aged ≥50 years
  - Cervical cancer screening: abnormal cytology is 11× higher in cisgender females with HIV. Begin Pap smears within 1 year of sexual activity onset, but no later than age 21 years, or at the time of HIV diagnosis if later. For those aged 21 to 29 years, an annual Pap test (liquid-based cytology) is recommended. After three consecutive annual normal results, the screening interval may be extended to every 3 years. For individuals aged ≥30 years, either annual Pap testing or co-testing with Pap and HPV testing is appropriate; after three consecutive normal results (with or without HPV testing), the interval can be extended to every 3 years. Screening should continue regardless of age.
  - Anal cancer screening: Assess for anal symptoms (e.g., unexplained itching, bleeding, perianal lesions) and perform digital anorectal examination (DARE) annually. Anal Pap yearly in all HIV-positive MSM and transgender women aged ≥35 years and others aged ≥45 years.
- Review contraception with people of child bearing potential
- Vaccinations:
  - Influenza (inactivated) and COVID: yearly; PCV20 once; tetanus-diphtheria (Td) every 10 years (substitute Tdap once); hepatitis A and B if nonimmune; HEPLISAV-B preferred over Engerix, Twinrix; MMR/varicella (MMRV): can give to nonimmune, nonpregnant PWH with CD4 >200; do not give quadrivalent MMRV; Shingrix: Give to all PWH ≥18 years old 2 doses 0 and 2 to 6 months; HPV for all nonpregnant PWH 9 to 26 years old at 0, 1 to 2, 6 months; if 27 to 45 years old, benefit is uncertain.
  - Mpox vaccine: for MSM/transgender women who have sex with men (TGW): JYNNEOS 2 doses SC 4 weeks apart. RSV single dose for PWH ≥75 years or 60 to 74 years old with CD4 <200 or with conditions, with risk for severe RSV; meningococcal: MenACWY every 5 years; if first time, give 2 doses at least 8 weeks apart (may also give MenB to 16- to 23-years-olds based on individual risk) (1)

PATIENT EDUCATION

Patient education and counseling on medication adherence, sexual health, and risk reduction should be ongoing. Discuss complexities, difficulty, and yet importance of communicating HIV status to sexual partners if safe to do so.

PROGNOSIS

- The prognosis of HIV infection is now excellent for individuals who are diagnosed early and have uninterrupted access to and adherence with ART. The survival remains vastly improved for all PWH who successfully maintain viral suppression.
- Despite advances, disparities in outcomes persist due to barriers in access to care, social determinants of health, and comorbidities.

REFERENCES

1. Horberg M, Thompson M, Agwu A, et al. Primary care guidance for providers of care for persons with human immunodeficiency virus: 2024 update by the HIV Medicine Association of the Infectious Diseases Society of America. *Clin Infect Dis*. 2024;ciae479. doi:10.1093/cid/ciae479.

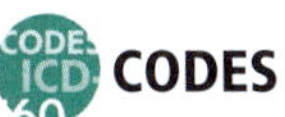

CODES

ICD10

- Z21 Asymptomatic human immunodeficiency virus infection status
- B20 Human immunodeficiency virus [HIV] disease
- R75 Inconclusive laboratory evidence of human immunodef virus

CLINICAL PEARLS

- Initiate ART as soon as possible after diagnosis; do not delay for baseline labs unless an acute opportunistic infection is present.
- Long-acting injectable ART is now available for select patients.
- Screening and management of comorbidities (metabolic syndrome, behavioral health, substance use) are a central part of routine HIV care as is addressing health disparities and access to care.
- Oral and injectable PrEP prevention strategies are available for at-risk individuals.

H

HODGKIN LYMPHOMA

Darnel Viray Dabu, MD, MPH, FAAFP, DipABLM • Taras Memko, MD

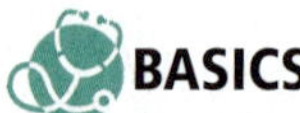

BASICS

Hodgkin Lymphoma (HL) is a neoplasm of the lymphatic system representing one of the common cancers in young adults; characterized by a low number of malignant cells deriving from B lymphocytes and an extensive inflammatory microenvironment

DESCRIPTION

- Historical background:
  - Described first in 1832 by Thomas Hodgkin who noted differences in patients from tuberculosis and syphilis
  - Carl Sternberg (1898) and Dorothy Reed (1902) independently identified the hallmark Reed-Sternberg (RS) cells—the microscopic hallmarks of Hodgkin disease.
  - Initially treated with herbs, surgery, and arsenic in the 19th century; HL showed sensitivity to X-rays in the beginning of the 20th century. Chemotherapy is instituted as first-line treatment in the early 1970s.
- Subtypes:
  - Classical HL (cHL)—95% of cases; includes nodular sclerosing 70%, mixed cellularity 20–25%, lymphocyte rich 5% and lymphocyte depleted <5%
  - Nodular lymphocyte predominant HL (NLPHL)—5% of cases

EPIDEMIOLOGY

- Incidence: 2 to 3 per 100,000 per year
- 11% of all lymphoid malignancies
- Bimodal age distribution peaks at 20 to 40 years and around 55 years, typically, diagnosed at median age of 39 years
- 1.3:1 male-to-female ratio

ETIOLOGY AND PATHOPHYSIOLOGY

- cHL is a B-cell lymphoma of germinal center origin that has lost its B-cell phenotype.
- RS cells have clonal rearrangements of immunoglobulin genes resulting in nonfunctional immunoglobulins and expression of apoptosis through oncogenic events.
- NLPHL lacks typical RS cells but has lymphocytic and histiocytic cells, characterized by larger cells with folded multilobulated nuclei ("popcorn cells" or LP cells)
- Genome-wide association studies identified 19p13.3 at intron 2 of *TCF3*.

Genetics

- First-degree relative: 3 to 9 times risk
- Siblings of younger patients: 7 times risk
- Weak correlation with certain HLA alleles

RISK FACTORS

- HIV: increased risk of HL in patients who are HIV positive
- Epstein-Barr virus (EBV): detected in nearly 45% of HL cases
- Genetic predisposition: significantly in identical twins

GENERAL PREVENTION

Avoid exposure to chemicals such as pesticides, herbicides, and benzene.

COMMONLY ASSOCIATED CONDITIONS

HIV infection, geography, socioeconomic factors and family history

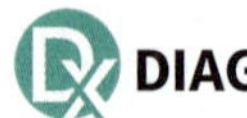

DIAGNOSIS

HISTORY

- Painless lymphadenopathy (cervical/supraclavicular)
- Pel-Ebstein (cyclic) fever—high-grade fever every 7 to 10 days
- Constitutional symptoms or "B symptoms": drenching night sweats, profound weight loss, fatigue, anorexia
- Chronic pruritus may be encountered.
- If mediastinal lymphadenopathy is large, it can cause chest pain and shortness of breath.
- Can present with a mass on chest radiograph

PHYSICAL EXAM

- Lymphadenopathy 70% (cervical > supraclavicular > axillary)—firm, rubbery consistency
- PET/CT or MRI are reliable for evaluating splenic involvement. Splenomegaly may be present.
- Hepatomegaly may be present.
- Tonsillar enlargement may be present.

DIFFERENTIAL DIAGNOSIS

Non-HL, solid tumor metastases, sarcoidosis, autoimmune disease, drug reaction and infections like HIV, syphilis, tuberculosis.

DIAGNOSTIC TESTS & INTERPRETATION

Initial Tests (lab, imaging)

- CBC with differential—may show eosinophilia, ESR
- Comprehensive metabolic panel, LDH
- HIV, EBV, HCV
- Pregnancy test for women of childbearing age
- Echocardiogram—in anticipation of treatment with anthracycline
- Pulmonary function tests (PFTs)—DLCO measurement in anticipation of treatment with bleomycin
- Chest x-ray
- Computed tomography (CT) with contrast of chest, abdomen, and pelvis
- Positron emission tomography (PET): for initial staging, midtreatment decision-making, and end-of-treatment evaluation

Follow-Up Tests & Special Considerations

- Fertility considerations include semen cryopreservation and ovarian tissue/oocyte preservation.
- Splenic RT: pneumococcal, *Haemophilus influenzae*, meningococcal vaccine

Geriatric Considerations

Poorer prognosis if present at age ≥60 years: less likely to tolerate intensive chemotherapy or be included in a trial

Pediatric Considerations

Young females (<30 years of age) treated with thoracic radiation are at high risk for breast cancer, and early breast cancer screening is recommended.

Pregnancy Considerations

Abdominal ultrasonography to detect subdiaphragmatic disease

- Delay until after delivery if asymptomatic and early stage
- ABVD is more likely to cause fetal malformations in 1st trimester; malformation risk is lower when used in 2nd and 3rd trimesters.
- Vinblastine monotherapy to control symptoms

Diagnostic Procedures/Other

- Excisional/incisional lymph node biopsy
- Immunohistochemistry
- Bone marrow biopsy if cytopenia with negative PET
- Lumbar puncture and MRI of the brain if neurologic symptoms

Test Interpretation

- Morphology: RS cells in cHL described as "owl eye" appearance—two nucleoli in two separate nuclear lobes, abundant slightly basophilic cytoplasm; popcorn cells noted in NLPHL
- Immunophenotype: CD15+, CD30+, CD45−, CD3− (T-cell marker), and typically CD20−
- Cytogenetics: no consistent or specific karyotypic findings

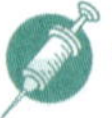

TREATMENT

- Ann Arbor staging with Cotswold modification
- Intent of treatment: curative
- All subsequent treatment and follow-up care recommendations are based on consensus guidelines.
- Recent advancements: Brentuximab vedotin, etoposide, cyclophosphamide, doxorubicin, dacarbazine, and dexamethasone (BrECADD) regimen has outperformed the traditional bleomycin, etoposide, doxorubicin, cyclophosphamide, vincristine, procarbazine, and prednisone (BEACOPP) regimen; progression-free survival rate (94.3% vs. 90.9%) and reduces disease progression risk by 34%; additionally, BrECADD demonstrated better fertility preservation, with improved follicle-stimulating hormone (FSH) recovery rates in both men and women.

MEDICATION

First Line

- Early stage disease: combined modality chemotherapy/radiotherapy *or* chemotherapy
- Advanced stage disease: chemotherapy
- PET/CT used after cycle 2 (PET-2) to guide either escalation or de-escalation of therapy (1)
- Chemotherapy:
  - ABVD (doxorubicin, bleomycin, vinblastine, dacarbazine):
    - Severe phlebitis—need for central line to administer treatment
    - Highly emetogenic
    - Vinblastine: risk of neuropathy
    - Bleomycin: risk of pulmonary toxicity, death; test dose may be administered prior to first cycle.
    - Doxorubicin: risk of cardiotoxicity; monitor LVEF.
  - AAVD (doxorubicin, brentuximab vedotin [anti-CD30 chimeric antibody conjugated to synthetic antimicrotubule agent monomethyl auristatin E], vinblastine, dacarbazine):
  - Superior to ABVD per ECHELON-1 trial in terms of PFS as well as OS
  - Preferred especially if abnormal PFTs
  - Brentuximab vedotin: peripheral neuropathy, nausea, fatigue, neutropenia, diarrhea
  - AAVD now deemed to be preferred front-line therapy for patients with Stage III or IV HL.

Second Line

- Reserved for patients with relapsed/refractory (R/R) disease
- Therapeutic strategy and sequencing of treatment influenced by: eligibility for ASCT, functional response to salvage chemotherapy, duration of remission, prior therapy and co-morbidities
- Standard: chemotherapy agents not used for initial treatment followed by high-dose therapy with autologous stem cell transplant (HDT/ASCT).
- Pembrolizumab (anti-PD1) FDA-approved for patients with R/R cHL who have failed 2 or more lines of therapy
- Nivolumab (anti-PD1) in a phase 2 study of R/R cHL showed ORR 69% with durable response and favorable safety profile.
- Third-line novel agents undergoing studies: proteosome inhibitors (bortezomib), mammalian target of rapamycin (mTOR) inhibitors (everolimus), immunomodulators (lenalidomide); CAR T-cell therapy directed to CD30 noted high rates of durable response in heavily pretreated patients.
- Median survival <3 years if failed second-line therapy, including HDT/ASCT
- NLPHL
  - Treated with rituximab + CHOP (CD20 positive)
- Allogeneic stem cell transplant (alloSCT) remains a curative-intent treatment option for patients with R/R cHL, including those who have failed an autologous transplantation.

ADDITIONAL THERAPIES

Radiotherapy is used postsalvage chemotherapy or ASCT.

ONGOING CARE

Patients treated with ABVD become neutropenic. Treatment is continued despite neutropenia with no clear increased risk of infection with or without growth factors.

FOLLOW-UP RECOMMENDATIONS

Patient Monitoring

- During therapy: CBC, nutrition, and hydration
- Restage with PET after 2 cycles of chemotherapy: sensitive prognostic indicator
- Posttreatment surveillance:
  - History and physical: q3–6mo for the first 2 years, then q6–12mo for the next 1 year, and then annually
  - Laboratory studies
    - CBC, platelets, BMP, ESR (if elevated at time of diagnosis), as indicated clinically
    - Thyroid-stimulating hormone (TSH) annually if radiation to neck
  - Imaging:
    - PET-CT to demonstrate negativity within 3 months following completion of treatment to document "complete response"; no role for annual surveillance PET
    - CT scans no more often than every 6 months for the first 2 years or as clinically indicated
    - Annual breast mammogram beginning 8 to 10 years after therapy or at age 40 years (whichever first) if chest or axillary irradiation (annual breast MRI as well if initially radiated between ages 10 and 30 years) according to the American Cancer Society
  - Annual influenza vaccine and *Streptococcus pneumoniae* vaccine
  - Referral for cancer survivorship with psychosocial support
  - Smoking cessation: Combination of smoking and chest irradiation dramatically increases risk of lung cancer.

PATIENT EDUCATION

- Reproductive impact
- Risks of secondary malignancy

PROGNOSIS

- Cure rate for cHL is 85%; survival rates: 1-year, 92%; 5-year, 87%; 10-year, 80%; factors like age, gender, and lymphocyte count influence prognosis.
- International prognostic score for advanced disease:
  - Age >45 years
  - Male gender
  - Albumin <4 g/dL
  - Hemoglobin <10.5 g/dL
  - Lymphocytopenia: <600 lymphocyte cells/dL or lymphocytes <8% of WBC
  - WBC ≥15,000 cells/dL
  - Stage IV disease

COMPLICATIONS

Late complications: peripheral neuropathy, cardiovascular risks from treatment, and secondary malignancies

REFERENCES

1. Barrington SF, Kirkwood AA, Franceschetto A, et al. PET-CT for staging and early response: results from the response-adapted therapy in advanced Hodgkin lymphoma study. *Blood*. 2016;127(12):1531–1538.

ADDITIONAL READING

Borchmann P, Moccia AA, Greil R, et al. Tolerability and efficacy of BrECADD versus BEACOPP in advanced-stage classical Hodgkin lymphoma: GHSG HD21, a randomized study. *J Clin Oncol*. 2024;42(suppl 17):LBA7000–LBA7000.

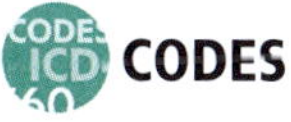

ICD10

- C81.96 Hodgkin lymphoma, unspecified, intrapelvic lymph nodes
- C81.44 Lymphocyte-rich Hodgkin lymphoma, lymph nodes of axilla and upper limb
- C81.75 Other Hodgkin lymphoma, lymph nodes of inguinal region and lower limb

CLINICAL PEARLS

- HL mainly affects young people.
- Treatment includes chemotherapy +/− RT.
- If patient develops neutropenia during treatment of HL with ABVD regimen, chemotherapy should be continued provided there is no concern for an infection without delays.
- Long-term effects of chemotherapy should be discussed with patients.
- Close collaboration between oncologist and PCP is required for future monitoring.

HOMELESSNESS

Dana Sprute, MD, MPH, FAAFP • Madeline Elaine Huff, MD, MS

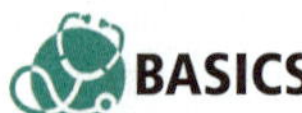

BASICS

DESCRIPTION

- Lacking a fixed, regular, and adequate nighttime residence.
- Chronic homelessness: lacking fixed, regular housing for at least 1 year, or at least four episodes of being unhoused in the past 3 years for a combined length of at least 1 year.
- People struggling with homelessness often have complex and chronic medical illnesses such as mental illness, substance use disorders, and physical disabilities (1).

EPIDEMIOLOGY

Incidence

- Increasing since 2017 nationwide; 6% overall increase year-to-year, expect for this past year which showed >12% increase over the previous year. This marked the largest increase since data collection began in 2007.
- The COVID-19 pandemic disrupted accounting of unsheltered people, but conditions during the pandemic may have increased the incidence (1).

Prevalence

In 2023, 0.19% of the U.S. population (approximately 653,100 individuals) experienced homelessness on any given night: 61% in sheltered locations and 39% in unsheltered locations (1).

- 5% are veterans, 28% are families with children, 5% are unaccompanied youth (age <25 years) and 22% are chronically homeless individuals.
- 50% of the homeless population is white.
- Veterans: decreasing due to policy changes; decreased by 50% over a decade (2010 to 2020) (2)
- Transgender individuals: 0.6% identify as transgender and 0.6% as gender nonconforming (2)
- Addiction disorders: 46% report substance use as a major factor contributing to homelessness (1).
- Psychiatric illness: 25% of adults experiencing homelessness (1)
- Postincarceration: 50,000 people each year enter homeless shelters from jails/prisons (1).

RISK FACTORS

- Poverty
  - 2024 federal poverty level: $31,200 annual income for four-person household in the lower 48 states and District of Columbia, slightly higher in Alaska and Hawaii (2)
  - In 2022, 11.5% of U.S. population below federal poverty line
- Unemployment: U.S. rate 4.3% in July 2024 (U.S. Bureau of Labor Statistics)
- Lack of affordable health care: In 2023, 7.7% of U.S. population (334 million) were uninsured for the entire calendar year (3).
- Lack of affordable housing: <30% of gross income for housing costs, including utilities; roughly 40.9 million U.S. households spend >30% on housing costs; 19 million households spend ≥50% of income on housing.
- Intimate partner violence (IPV): 12% of overall persons experiencing homelessness and about 20% of families experiencing homelessness report IPV; IPV often involves exertion of psychological and financial control that leaves survivors with poor credit, limited support, and few resources.

GENERAL PREVENTION

- Policy and funding for community programs to provide emergency/rapid housing, housing stabilization, and case management services; the CARES Act of 2020 and the American Rescue Plan Act of 2021 provide funding for permanent housing. Over the past 5 years, the fastest growing forms of assistance include rapid rehousing and "other permanent housing."
- Increased Medicaid eligibility, expanded home- and community-based services, and case management for people experiencing homelessness.
- HUD: increasing permanent supportive housing units; increasing services for veterans, families with children, and those with disabilities
- Social justice policy recommendations: permanent affordable housing; foreclosure and homelessness prevention; increased funds for HUD McKinney-Vento programs (emergency, transitional, and permanent housing) and National Housing Trust Fund, rural homeless assistance, universal health care, universal livable income, employment/workforce services; prevention of hate crimes against the homeless, decriminalization of homelessness

COMMONLY ASSOCIATED CONDITIONS

- Hunger and malnutrition
- Exposure-related conditions (frostbite, heatstroke)
- Substance use disorders and their associated conditions
  - Liver disease (alcohol, hepatitis B and C)
  - Abscesses (intravenous drug use)
  - Overdose
- Dental problems
- Psychiatric illness
- Trauma (increased risk of assault, victims of hate crime)
- Infectious diseases
  - Skin/nail infection and infestation (lice, bedbugs, and scabies)
  - Tuberculosis, HIV/AIDS, STI
- Worsening of chronic medical conditions; lack of healthy food, places to store medications, or medical equipment; lack of restful sleep; decreased health literacy; limited transportation to appointments

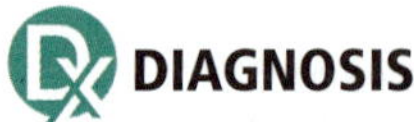

DIAGNOSIS

HISTORY

- Living conditions: location, access to food, restrooms, place to store medicines, safety
- Prior homelessness: causes and circumstances
- Family members, especially dependent children
- Medications: OTC medication, dietary supplements, medication "borrowed" from others
- Prior providers: oral health, primary and specialty care, current medical home
- Mental health: stress, anxiety, appetite, sleep, concentration, mood, speech, memory, thought process and content, auditory/visual hallucinations, suicidal/homicidal ideation, insight, judgment, impulse control, social interactions; symptoms of brain injury (headaches, seizures, memory loss, irritability, dizziness, insomnia, poor organizational/decision-making skills), trauma history
- Alcohol/nicotine/drug use: amount, frequency, duration
- Gender identity/orientation, behaviors, rape, pregnancies, hepatitis, HIV/AIDS, other STIs
- History of or current abuse: emotional, physical, sexual; patient safety
- Legal problems/violence: history of incarceration
- Activities: routines (treatment feasibility); level of strenuous activity
- Work: previous types of jobs, length held, veteran status, occupational injuries/toxic exposures; vocational skills, interest
- Education: highest level; ever in special education; assess ability to read/language skills/English fluency.
- Nutrition/hydration: diet, food resources, preparation skills, liquid intake
- Cultural heritage/affiliations: family, friends, faith community, other sources of support
- Strengths: coping skills, job skills, resourcefulness, abilities, interests

PHYSICAL EXAM

- Comprehensive exam: height, weight, BMI, especially abdominal, cardiopulmonary, dermatologic, oral, feet, neurologic, mental status
- Focused exams: for patients uncomfortable with full-body, unclothed exam at first visit
- Dental assessment: age-appropriate teeth, obvious caries, dental/referred pain, diabetes, CVD

DIAGNOSTIC TESTS & INTERPRETATION

Initial Tests (lab, imaging)

- Mental health: Patient Health Questionnaire (PHQ-9, PHQ-2), MHS-III, MDQ, GAD-7
- Cognitive assessment: Mini-Mental State Examination (MMSE), Montreal Cognitive Assessment (MOCA), Traumatic Brain Injury Questionnaire (TBIQ), Repeatable Battery for the Assessment of Neuropsychological Status (RBANS)

- Developmental assessment: Ages & Stages Questionnaires, Parents' Evaluation of Developmental Status (PEDS), Denver II, or other screening tool
- Interpersonal violence: IPV, sexual assault, TBI
- Forensic evaluation: if indicated by history
- Baseline labs: as needed to address suspected medical concerns
- TB screening: PPD or T-SPOT.TB/QuantiFERON-TB Gold if available
- STI screening: HIV/AIDS, chlamydia, gonorrhea, syphilis, hepatitis B, hepatitis C, trichomonas
- Substance abuse: Simple Screening Instrument for Alcohol and Other Drugs (SSI-AOD), urine drug screen

Follow-Up Tests & Special Considerations

- Reproductive health care and STIs: Obtain detailed sexual history (sexual identity, orientation, behaviors/sexual practices, number of partners). Consider patient exploitation, especially if mental illness/developmental disability suspected. Communicate willingness to initiate contraception first visit without exam. Genital exam recommended, but be sensitive to patient, especially if there is a possible sexual abuse history. If pelvic exam is refused, consider self-collected testing and/or empiric treatment for STI (and possibility of multiple orifice infection). Dispense medications on site; facilitate partner treatment.
- Consider access to facilities, even if residing at a shelter. For example, patient may not have access to restroom for colonoscopy bowel prep.
- Pediatric care: complete exam every visit; use each visit to identify/address problems and provide vaccinations because homeless families may not see a medical provider unless child is sick. Vision and hearing screening at every visit. Facilitate referrals as able.

TREATMENT

- Enlist community resources: mental health and substance abuse programs, free clinics, case management.
- Health care maintenance: vaccinations (hepatitis A and B, pneumococcal, Tdap, influenza, SARS-CoV2), cancer and chronic disease screening for adults; Early and Periodic Screening, Diagnosis, and Treatment (EPSDT) program screening and vaccinations for children
- Care plan
  - Basic needs: Food, clothing, and housing
  - Patient goals and priorities: immediate/long-term health needs; address patient's concerns first.
  - Action plan: simple language, pocket card
  - After hours: extended clinic hours and access
  - Safety plan: violence and abuse; mandatory reporting requirements
  - Emergency plan: location of nearest emergency department (ED), preparation for evacuation
  - Adherence plan: use of interpreter; identification of potential barriers

MEDICATION

- Simple regimen: low pill count, once-daily dosing
- Dispensing: small amounts on site to promote follow-up, decrease loss/theft/misuse; determine resources for written prescriptions.
- Storage of medications: If no access, avoid medications requiring refrigeration.
- Patient assistance: free/low-cost drugs depending on available local options
- Aids to adherence: harm reduction, outreach/case management, directly observed therapy
- Side effects: Primary reason for medication nonadherence are drugs causing diarrhea, polyuria, nausea, and/or disorientation.
- Analgesia/symptomatic treatment: Consider pain contract, single provider for pain medication refills.
- Dietary supplements: multivitamins with minerals, nutritional supplements
- Managed care: generics, if possible; assistance getting prescription filled.
- Lab monitoring: Monitor patients on antipsychotic medications for metabolic disorders using available laboratory resources.

ADDITIONAL THERAPIES

- Associated problems/complications
  - Fragmented care: multiple providers; use electronic medical record (EMR) as possible; list prescribed medication on wallet-sized card.
  - Masked symptoms/misdiagnosis: for example, weight loss, dementia, edema, lactic acidosis
  - Focus on immediate concerns, not possible future consequences.
  - Integrated treatment for concurrent mental illness/substance use disorders
  - Support for parent of child abused by others and for abused parent
  - Large appointment burdens: specialty care may be difficult to obtain.
- Follow-up
  - Reliable phone/email contact for patient/friend/family/case manager
  - Frequent follow-up, incentives, nonjudgmental care regardless of adherence
  - Anticipate/accommodate unscheduled clinic visits.
  - Provide car fare, tokens, and help with transportation services.
  - Monitor school attendance and address health/developmental problems with family/school.

ADMISSION, INPATIENT, AND NURSING CONSIDERATIONS

- Admission is beneficial if living conditions are not conducive to treatment of medical, psychiatric, and substance use disorders.
- Discharge considerations:
  - Acute or chronic wound care: Bed rest, extended periods of elevation, rest, or icing are not feasible in most instances.
  - Need for durable medical equipment (DME): Portable oxygen tanks and nebulizers may not be covered by the hospital and may be cumbersome to use in absence of stable housing.
  - Medications: It is preferable to fill prescriptions at hospital outpatient pharmacy.
  - Outpatient follow-up: Transportation to appointments should be arranged if possible.

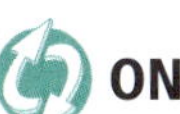

ONGOING CARE

FOLLOW-UP RECOMMENDATIONS

- Patients with a history of nonadherence need additional support (e.g., case manager, outreach) to succeed in ongoing care after hospital discharge.
- Limited telephone access to schedule appointments; may be unable to receive telephone messages with test results or rescheduled appointment times; some social service agencies will provide phone, mail, email, Internet, and laundry services.
- Arrange appointments prior to discharge.
- Document the best way to contact the individual.
- Work with experienced health care agency designed to address physical/mental health services and substance use treatment.

PATIENT EDUCATION

- National Health Care for the Homeless Council: https://nhchc.org/
- National Alliance to End Homelessness: https://endhomelessness.org/

PROGNOSIS

Mortality rates are 3 to 4 times higher than general U.S. population.

REFERENCES

1. National Alliance to End Homelessness. State of homelessness: 2024 edition. https://endhomelessness.org/homelessness-in-america/homlessness-statistics/state-of-homelessness/. Accessed August 27, 2024.
2. U.S. Department of Health and Human Services. Annual update of the HHS poverty guidelines. https://aspe.hhs.gov/topics/poverty-economic-mobility/poverty-guidelines. Accessed August 27, 2024.
3. de Sousa T, Andrichik A, Prestera E, et al; for Abt Associates. *The 2023 Annual Homeless Assessment Report (AHAR) to Congress. Part 1: Point-in-Time Estimates of Homelessness*: December 2023. U.S. Department of Housing and Urban Development, Office of Community Planning and Development; 2023.

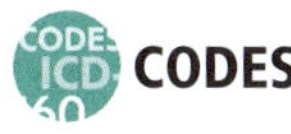

CODES

ICD10

- Z59.0 Homelessness
- Z59.1 Inadequate housing
- Z59.8 Other problems related to housing and economic circumstances

CLINICAL PEARLS

- Permanent supportive housing is an important step toward ending homelessness, in accordance with a Housing First approach.
- Assistance in gaining access to benefits or providing help to support basic needs decreases stress, improves therapeutic relationship, and allows individuals to focus on physical and mental health.

HORDEOLUM (STYE)

Konstantinos E. Deligiannidis, MD, MPH, FAAFP • Christopher C. Paredes, MD

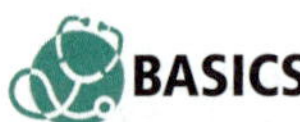

BASICS

DESCRIPTION
- An acute inflammation or infection of the eyelid margin involving the sebaceous gland of an eyelash (external hordeolum) or a meibomian gland (internal hordeolum)
- System(s) affected: skin/exocrine
- Synonym(s): internal hordeolum; external hordeolum; zeisian stye; meibomian stye; stye

EPIDEMIOLOGY
- Predominant age: none
- Predominant sex: male = female

Incidence
Unknown: Although external hordeolum is common; internal hordeolum is rare.

ETIOLOGY AND PATHOPHYSIOLOGY
- Bacterial infection of sweat or sebaceous glands, causing an acute inflammatory reaction
- In an internal hordeolum, the meibomian gland may become obstructed, leading to a pustule on the conjunctival surface as opposed to the margin of the eyelid.
- Most commonly caused by *Staphylococcus aureus* (~90–95% of all cases) or by *Staphylococcus epidermidis*
- Seborrhea can predispose to infections of the eyelid.

Genetics
No known genetic pattern

RISK FACTORS
- Poor eyelid hygiene
- Previous hordeolum
- Contact lens wearers
- Application of old or contaminated makeup
- Seborrheic dermatitis
- Predisposing blepharitis (low-grade infections of the eyelid margin)
- Ocular rosacea
- Diabetes
- Immunodeficiency

GENERAL PREVENTION
- Good personal hygiene with attention to cleansing the eyelids on a daily basis helps to prevent recurrent infections
- Avoidance of old or contaminated makeup

COMMONLY ASSOCIATED CONDITIONS
- Acne
- Seborrhea
- An association may exist between hordeolum during childhood and developing rosacea in adulthood.

DIAGNOSIS

HISTORY
- Localized inflammation (vs. involvement of the entire eyelid or surrounding skin)
- Foreign body sensation in the eye
- Symptoms may start as vague eyelid pain and inflammation, and then localize 1 to 2 days later.
- Prior episodes are common.

PHYSICAL EXAM
- Localized inflammation of the eyelashes or a small pustule at the margin of the eyelid
- Localized swelling and tenderness on the internal or external aspect of the eyelid with an opening to either side
- To determine if an internal hordeolum is obstructed, the eyelid should be gently everted to examine for a pustule on the tarsal conjunctiva.
- Itching or scaling of the eyelids; collection of discharge, redness, and irritation leading to localized tenderness and pain
- The size of the swelling usually correlates to the severity of the hordeolum.

DIFFERENTIAL DIAGNOSIS
- Chalazion
- Blepharitis
- Eyelid neoplasms
- Periorbital cellulitis
- Dacryocystitis
- Squamous cell carcinoma

DIAGNOSTIC TESTS & INTERPRETATION
Culture of the eyelid margins usually is not necessary.

Diagnostic Procedures/Other
History and eye exam

Test Interpretation
Bacterial contamination and white cells in eyelid discharge

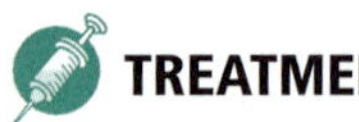

TREATMENT

GENERAL MEASURES
- The hordeolum should not be expressed.
- Warm compresses to the area of inflammation can help increase blood supply and encourage spontaneous drainage.

MEDICATION

First Line
- A Cochrane review found no evidence for or against nonsurgical treatment of internal hordeolum. External hordeola were not considered (1)[A].
- Usually, a hordeolum spontaneously drains within 1 to 2 weeks, aided by warm compresses to the area.
- Also, lid scrubs, digital massage, and alternative medicine have been used to reduce healing time and to relieve symptoms.
- Application of an antibiotic ointment (e.g., erythromycin) to the margin of the eyelid after proper cleansing (except in children age <12 years, in whom there is a risk of blurred vision and amblyopia) helps reduce bacterial proliferation. There is little evidence that any topical therapy is effective. Erythromycin ophthalmic ointment may be applied up to 6 times per day for 7 to 10 days or an antibiotic ointment containing bacitracin (2).
- Treat underlying dry eye with artificial tears.

Second Line

- Occasionally, the use of an aminoglycoside ophthalmic ointment, such as gentamicin or tobramycin, may be necessary if condition is refractory to simpler treatment (case reports).
- Oral dicloxacillin, cephalexin, or doxycycline for 2 weeks if refractory to topical antibiotics

ISSUES FOR REFERRAL

Consider ophthalmology referral if unresponsive to oral antibiotics.

SURGERY/OTHER PROCEDURES

- If the infection becomes localized to a single gland, incision, drainage, or curettage sometimes is necessary. This is an in-office procedure with a local anesthetic: Exercise caution because ocular perforation has been reported with the injection of an anesthetic to an infected lid.
- Use of combined antibiotic ointment (neomycin sulfate, polymyxin B sulfate, and gramicidin) after surgery was not shown to have any statistically significant benefit compared with artificial tears.

COMPLEMENTARY & ALTERNATIVE MEDICINE

A Cochrane review found low-quality evidence that acupuncture (with or without antibiotics and/or warm compresses) may increase the chance of improvement of hordeolum compared to antibiotics and/or warm compresses (3)[A].

ADMISSION, INPATIENT, AND NURSING CONSIDERATIONS

Outpatient

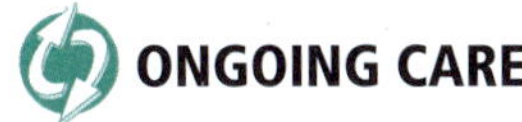

ONGOING CARE

FOLLOW-UP RECOMMENDATIONS

No restrictions

Patient Monitoring

The patient should be seen within several weeks to assess the effectiveness of therapy or should at least call the physician's office with a progress report.

DIET

No special diet

PATIENT EDUCATION

- The patient should be instructed in proper cleansing of the eyelids using a solution of tap water and baby shampoo or a commercially prepared hypoallergenic cleanser.
- The stye should not be squeezed or incised.

PROGNOSIS

- Usually responds well to good hygiene and warm compresses
- Inflammation usually improves within 1 to 2 weeks.
- Hordeolum tends to recur in some patients, usually due to incomplete elimination of bacteria.

COMPLICATIONS

An internal hordeolum, if untreated, may lead to chalazion, infections of adjacent glands, or generalized cellulitis of the lid.

REFERENCES

1. Lindsley K, Nichols JJ, Dickersin K. Non-surgical interventions for acute internal hordeolum. *Cochrane Database Syst Rev*. 2017;1(1):CD007742.
2. Alsoudi AF, Ton L, Ashraf DC, et al. Efficacy of care and antibiotic use for chalazia and hordeola. *Eye Contact Lens*. 2022;48(4):162–168.
3. Cheng K, Law A, Guo M, et al. Acupuncture for acute hordeolum. *Cochrane Database Syst Rev*. 2017;(2):CD011075.

ADDITIONAL READING

- Bamford JTM, Gessert CE, Renier CM, et al. Childhood stye and adult rosacea. *J Am Acad Dermatol*. 2006;55(6):951–955.
- Hirunwiwatkul P, Wachirasereechai K. Effectiveness of combined antibiotic ophthalmic solution in the treatment of hordeolum after incision and curettage: a randomized, placebo-controlled trial: a pilot study. *J Med Assoc Thai*. 2005;88(5):647–650.
- Kim JH, Yang SM, Kim HM, et al. Inadvertent ocular perforation during lid anesthesia for hordeolum removal. *Korean J Ophthalmol*. 2006;20(3):199–200.
- Nakatani M. Treatment of recurrent hordeolum with Broncasma Berna. *Eye (Lond)*. 1999;13(Pt 5):692.
- Wald ER. Periorbital and orbital infections. *Infect Dis Clin North Am*. 2007;21(2):393–408, vi.

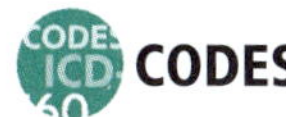

CODES

ICD10

- H00.019 Hordeolum externum unspecified eye, unspecified eyelid
- H00.029 Hordeolum internum unspecified eye, unspecified eyelid
- H00.039 Abscess of eyelid unspecified eye, unspecified eyelid

CLINICAL PEARLS

- A hordeolum should not be expressed.
- Warm compresses to the area of inflammation can encourage spontaneous drainage.
- Application of an antibiotic ointment (e.g., erythromycin) to the margin of the eyelid after proper cleansing helps reduce bacterial proliferation but may have no effect on the healing of the stye.
- Good personal hygiene with attention to cleansing the eyelids on a daily basis can prevent recurrent infections.

HORNER SYNDROME

Betty Brenda Yue, MPA • Grace Shih, MD, MAS

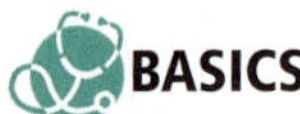

BASICS

DESCRIPTION

- A constellation of neurologic signs and symptoms manifested as a classic triad of ipsilateral miosis, eyelid ptosis, and anhidrosis of the ipsilateral face and/or neck (with iris heterochromia in children).
- System(s) affected: nervous, skin/exocrine
- Synonym(s): Bernard syndrome, Bernard-Horner syndrome (HS); or oculosympathetic palsy, oculosympathoparesis, and Von Passow syndrome (triad with heterochromia iridis)

EPIDEMIOLOGY

Incidence

- Estimated incidence of pediatric HS is 1.42 per 100,000 in patients <19 years of age, with a birth prevalence of 1 in 6,250 for those with congenital onset of HS.
- Incidence in adults is not known in United States but reported as 2.95 per 100,000 in South Korea (1).

ETIOLOGY AND PATHOPHYSIOLOGY

- Disruption of the sympathetic chain (first, second, or third order) may produce signs and symptoms of HS as a result of loss of sympathetic innervation to the eye and/or face.
  - Ptosis: Sympathetic innervation to the Müller muscle in the upper eyelid and the lower eyelid retractors helps to maintain normal eyelid position. When sympathetic innervation to these structures is interrupted, a subtle ptosis of both the upper lid (ptosis) and lower lid (reverse ptosis) may result and may persist with downward gaze. This ptosis may be subtle, often ≤2 mm. Lower lid may become elevated, which narrows the palpebral fissure or pseudo-enophthalmos.
  - Miosis: The radially oriented pupillary dilator muscle produces pupillary dilation in response to stimulation by the sympathetic nervous system. Anisocoria will be more pronounced in dim lighting, reflecting impairment of dilation in the affected eye. The affected eye will constrict normally in response to light but will be slower to dilate than the unaffected pupil.
  - Anhidrosis: When present, anhidrosis may assist in localizing a lesion; sympathetic fibers innervating sweat glands of the lower face and vasodilatory muscles branch off before the superior cervical sympathetic ganglion and travel along the external carotid artery; lesions affecting primary and secondary neurons are more likely to produce anhydrosis of both the upper and lower face.
- Etiologies in adults:
  - Arnold-Chiari malformation, basal meningitis (e.g., syphilis), cerebral vascular accident: lateral medullary (Wallenberg) syndrome, cervical cord trauma, cervical spondylosis, demyelinating disease (multiple sclerosis), intrapontine hemorrhage, neck trauma, syringomyelia/syringobulbia, tumor (basal skull, pituitary), unintended subdural placement of lumbar epidural catheter
  - Aneurysm/dissection of aorta, central venous catheterization, chest tubes, 1st rib fracture, lymphadenopathy (Hodgkin, leukemia, tuberculosis, sarcoid), mandibular tooth abscess, neuroblastoma, Pancoast tumor or infection of lung apex, proximal common carotid artery dissection, thoracic outlet obstruction (cervical rib, subclavian artery aneurysm), trauma/surgical injury, tumor (thyroid, mediastinum)
  - Carotid cavernous fistula or other pathology, carotid endarterectomy or carotid artery stenting, cluster headaches/paroxysmal hemicrania, internal carotid artery dissection, herpes zoster, lesions of the middle ear (acute otitis media), Lyme disease, tumor (nasopharyngeal, pituitary, paratrigeminal, metastasis, skull base), tonsillectomy, trauma/surgical injury, Raeder paratrigeminal syndrome
- Etiologies in children: perinatal injury to the brachial plexus—most common: brainstem glioma, neuroblastoma, vascular anomalies, surgical interventions in the neck/chest, idiopathic

Genetics

Rare autosomal dominant inheritance

RISK FACTORS

- Recent trauma to the head/neck/thorax (e.g., motor vehicle accident [MVA])
- Smoking (Pancoast tumor)
- Known aneurysm of the carotid or subclavian arteries
- Known malignancy/tumor/mass
- Previous surgery (neck/thoracic)
- Cluster headache

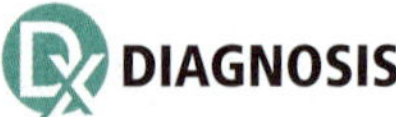

DIAGNOSIS

HISTORY

- When did symptoms begin? (acute vs. chronic?)
- Any visual symptoms? (blurred vision, field loss, transient visual loss, diplopia)
- Previous ophthalmic history? (eye trauma, surgery, etc.)
- Are symptoms associated with pain? (ipsilateral head/neck/face)
- Recent head/neck trauma or surgical procedures?
- Any associated headaches or other neurologic signs?
- Does the degree of ptosis vary over the course of the day or with fatigue?
- Any sweating abnormalities or flushing on one side of the face?

Pediatric Considerations

- Congenital HS will affect iris color as iris melanocytes require sympathetic innervation to produce melanin, if the innervation is not present at birth a lighter iris will occur resulting in heterochromia prior to age 2 years.
- Loss of facial flushing can be appreciated (harlequin sign—affected side will appear pale secondary to denervation supersensitivity to circulating adrenaline). This flushing occurs with nursing or crying.
- New onset, nontraumatic HS in a child necessitates workup for neuroblastoma.

ALERT

HS in the presence of pain merits urgent evaluation.

- Acute-onset, ipsilateral facial or neck pain: Consider carotid artery dissection until proven otherwise, even in the absence of obvious head/neck trauma. Pain from dissection is usually located around the temple and orbit. Patients may also experience amaurosis fugax and dysgeusia. If missed, stroke is a potential complication.
- Axial, shoulder, scapula, arm, or hand pain may be related to Pancoast tumor or cervical cord lesion.

- Paratrigeminal syndromes:
  - Raeder paratrigeminal syndrome type I: orbital pain, miosis, ptosis, with associated ipsilateral lesions of CN III to VI; suspect middle cranial fossa mass or cavernous sinus lesion.
  - Raeder paratrigeminal syndrome type II: episodic retrobulbar or orbital pain, miosis, ptosis with no CN lesions; suspect migraine variant.

PHYSICAL EXAM

- Measure pupillary diameter under both dim and bright lighting to determine presence of anisocoria. In HS, anisocoria will be greater in dim/dark lighting conditions.
- Evaluate pupil reactivity to light and accommodative response.
- A pupillary dilation lag may be present and the affected pupil may gradually dilate 5 to 15 seconds after exposure to light.
- Examine the upper lids for ptosis (often <2 mm).
- A slight elevation of the lower lid relative to unaffected eye may be present.
- Additional acute features of sympathetic disruption may include ipsilateral conjunctival injection, conjunctival chemosis and nasal congestion.
- Biomicroscopic/slit-lamp exam of the eye, including iris structure and color (if available)
- Observe for the presence of nystagmus, facial swelling, lymphadenopathy, or vesicular eruptions.
- A full cranial nerve exam with special attention to extraocular movements
- Palpation and inspection of the neck for any masses or evidence of trauma
- Neurologic and chest exams for associated physical findings

DIFFERENTIAL DIAGNOSIS

- Physiologic anisocoria (~20% population) = varies by <1 mm and may fluctuate throughout the day.
- Neurologic diseases (myasthenia gravis, botulinum toxin)

- 3rd nerve palsy
- Pharmacologic causes including unilateral use of miotics or mydriatics, acetophenazine, alseroxylon, bupivacaine, butaperazine, carphenazine, chloroprocaine, deserpidine, diacetylmorphine, diethazine, ethopropazine, etidocaine, guanethidine, influenza virus vaccine, levodopa, lidocaine, mepivacaine, mesoridazine, methdilazine, methotrimeprazine, oral contraceptives, perazine, prilocaine, procaine, prochlorperazine, promazine, propoxycaine, reserpine, thioproperazine, thioridazine, trifluoperazine

DIAGNOSTIC TESTS & INTERPRETATION

Initial Tests (lab, imaging)

- Lab: CBC, FTA-ABS, VDRL, purified protein derivative; vanillylmandelic acid, homovanillic acid to rule out neuroblastoma in pediatric patients
- Imaging considerations are unique because of the long pathway traveled by the sympathetic nervous system. A lesion at any point along this pathway, extending from the hypothalamus down to T2 may contribute to the onset of HS. Recommended imaging includes the following:
  - In the chronic setting, a CTA head and neck with IV contrast is appropriate.
  - Acute setting (or for patients unable to tolerate MRI), an initial CT head without contrast and CTA of the head/neck with IV contrast by HS MRI cervical and thoracic spine without and with contrast (2)[A].
  - Consider carotid angiogram if MRA or CTA yield equivocal results.

Pediatric Considerations

In a child of any age without contributory history, MRI brain, neck, and chest as outlined above is appropriate. Clinicians may consider MRI abdomen as well if clinical suspicion of neuroblastoma is high.

Pregnancy Considerations

Most authors believe that pregnant patients may undergo MRI safely, but it should be noted that contrast material (e.g., gadolinium) is FDA category C.

Diagnostic Procedures/Other

To diagnose HS, apraclonidine test is the gold standard with specificity 95% and sensitivity 93%. Cocaine test is largely historical. Note that bilateral HS may result in a false negative assessment due to lack of asymmetry (3)[B].

- Topical 0.5% apraclonidine drops: (3)[B],(4)[B]
  - Apraclonidine is a strong α-2 agonist and weak α-1 agonist with little to no effect on the normal pupil. To test for HS, 1 drop of apraclonidine is placed in each eye, and reassess after 60 minutes. The miotic eye with HS should dilate and the anisocoria reverses.
  - A positive test result occurs when both pupils become equally sized, or if the affected pupil becomes the larger one. *Note*: The apraclonidine test may be negative in cases of acute trauma, as there has not been enough time for denervation hypersensitivity to develop (2 to 5 days).
- Topical 1% hydroxyamphetamine drops
  - Used to differentiate between preganglionic (first- and second-order neurons) and postganglionic (third-order neuron) HS.
  - 1 hour after instillation of 1% hydroxyamphetamine drops, the pupils should be evaluated. Dilation of both pupils indicates a lesion of the first- or second-order neurons. Failure of the pupil to dilate, or poor dilation, indicates a third-order neuron lesion (test considered positive when anisocoria increases by $\geq$1 mm).
- Digital pupillometry: objectively measures pupil size and dilation lag, characteristic of HS; pupillometry can reliably distinguish HS from physiologic anisocoria and may obviate the need for pharmacologic testing in some cases specificity 68–93%, sensitivity 95% (5)[B]

Pediatric Considerations

Due to transsynaptic degeneration in children, the hydroxyamphetamine test is not reliable.

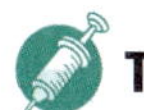

TREATMENT

GENERAL MEASURES

Once life-threatening etiologies have been excluded, cosmesis or functional vision impairment due to ptosis may be addressed if symptoms have persisted for 12 months.

MEDICATION

- Carotid artery dissection: Pharmacologic treatment options include thrombolysis, antithrombotic therapy with anticoagulation, or antiplatelet therapy (6)[C].
- For mild ptosis, oxymetazoline hydrochloride 0.1% can be used. Oxymetazoline is an α-adrenergic receptor agonist and selectively activates α-adrenergic receptors in the Müller muscle. This can raise the ptotic eyelid by 1.0 to 1.3 mm. Some patients may get more dramatic effect than others. Oxymetazoline reaches peak effect ~2 hours post-instillation and can last up to 8 hours. In two clinical trials oxymetazoline significantly improved superior visual field deficits. Common side effects include instillation site discomfort, headache, and dry eye (7).

ISSUES FOR REFERRAL

Depending on etiology of HS, referrals may include neurosurgery, oncology, interventional radiology, pulmonology, neurology/neuro-ophthalmology, and oculoplastic surgery.

SURGERY/OTHER PROCEDURES

- Surgical intervention depending on etiology.
- Consider ptosis repair for cosmesis or functional vision impairment secondary to ptosis if symptoms have persisted for 12 months (oculoplastics).

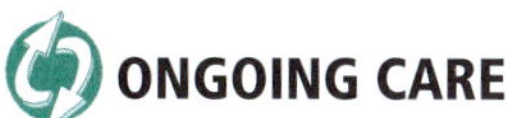

ONGOING CARE

PROGNOSIS

- Postganglionic: usually benign
- Central and preganglionic: poorer prognosis

COMPLICATIONS

- Chronic pupillary constriction
- Cosmesis

REFERENCES

1. Han J, Park SY, Lee JY. Nationwide population-based incidence and etiologies of pediatric and adult Horner syndrome. *J Neurol*. 2021;268(4):1276–1283.
2. American College of Radiology. ACR Appropriateness Criteria® Horner Syndrome. American College of Radiology. https://www.acr.org/Clinical-Resources/Clinical-Tools-and-Reference/Appropriateness-Criteria. Accessed December 12, 2025.
3. Bremner F. Apraclonidine is better than cocaine for detection of Horner syndrome. *Front Neurol*. 2019;10:55.
4. Chen PL, Chen JT, Lu DW, et al. Comparing efficacies of 0.5% apraclonidine with 4% cocaine in the diagnosis of Horner syndrome in pediatric patients. *J Ocul Pharmacol Ther*. 2006;22(3):182–187.
5. Disse LR, Bockisch CJ, Weber KP, et al. Differentiation of Horner syndrome and physiological anisocoria by automated pupillometry. *J Neuro-ophthalmol*. 2025;00:1–6.
6. Sadaka A, Schockman SL, Golnik KC. Evaluation of Horner syndrome in the MRI era. *J Neuroophthalmol*. 2017;37(3):268–272.
7. Slonim CB, Foster S, Jaros M, et al. Association of oxymetazoline hydrochloride, 0.1%, solution administration with visual field in acquired ptosis: a pooled analysis of 2 randomized clinical trials. *JAMA Ophthalmol*. 2020;138(11):1168–1175.

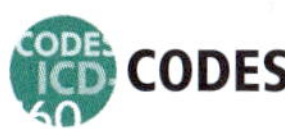

CODES

ICD10

- G90.2 Horner's syndrome
- S14.5XXA Injury of cervical sympathetic nerves, initial encounter

CLINICAL PEARLS

- HS triad: ipsilateral miosis, eyelid ptosis, and anhidrosis caused by a lesion of the oculosympathetic pathway
- Red flag: HS in the presence of acute-onset, ipsilateral facial or neck pain: Consider carotid artery dissection until proven otherwise.
- Ptosis is mild, usually <2 mm.

H

HYDROCELE

Tomas P.J. Reilly, MD

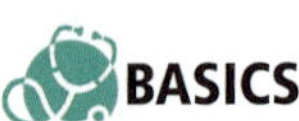

BASICS

DESCRIPTION

A hydrocele is a collection of serous fluid between the parietal and visceral layers of the tunica vaginalis within the scrotum.

- Communicating hydrocele (patent processus vaginalis)
  - Direct communication between the hydrocele sac and the peritoneal cavity
  - Contains peritoneal fluid
  - Almost always with associated indirect inguinal hernia
  - Can fluctuate in size; increase in size when upright or during straining; decreases in size with recumbent position
- Noncommunicating hydrocele (processus vaginalis is not patent)
  - No direct connection between the hydrocele sac and the peritoneal cavity
  - Fluid contained is from the mesothelial lining.
  - Can be isolated to the cord with the distal and proximal portions of the processus vaginalis closed
  - Tend to stay the same size or slowly increase in size over time
- Acute hydrocele: fluid collection resulting from an acute process within the tunica vaginalis, typically involving only the scrotum
- Although this disorder is found nearly exclusively in male patients, there are rare hydroceles into the canal of Nuck in females which result from a fluid collection in an abnormal open pouch of peritoneum extending into the labia majora.
- System(s) affected: urogenital

Pediatric Considerations

Most congenital communicating hydroceles resolve spontaneously by 2 years of age.

EPIDEMIOLOGY

Predominant age: childhood (congenital); adulthood (acquired)

Incidence

Estimated at 0.7–4.7% of male infants

Prevalence

- 1,000/100,000
- Estimated at 1% of adult men

ETIOLOGY AND PATHOPHYSIOLOGY

- Congenital
  - Incomplete closure of the processus vaginalis trapping peritoneal fluid anywhere along the length of the tunica vaginalis
  - Failure of closure of the processus vaginalis maintains a communication to the peritoneal cavity
- Acquired
  - Secondary to inflammation, infection, trauma or obstruction of lymphatic or venous drainage
  - Idiopathic in which hydrocele can develop without any clearly identifiable cause

RISK FACTORS

- For adult acquired hydroceles:
  - Imbalance of the secretion and reabsorption of fluid from the lining of the tunica vaginalis
  - Infection
  - Tumors
  - Trauma
  - Ipsilateral renal transplantation (due to disruption of the spermatic cord during the procedure)
  - Ventriculoperitoneal shunt
  - Ehlers-Danlos syndrome
  - Peritoneal dialysis
  - History of scrotal surgery (to include varicocelectomy)
- For congenital hydroceles:
  - Exstrophy of the bladder
  - Cloacal exstrophy
  - Prematurity
  - Low birth weight
  - Patent processus vaginalis

COMMONLY ASSOCIATED CONDITIONS

For adult acquired hydroceles:

- Testicular tumors
- Scrotal trauma
- Ventriculoperitoneal shunt
- Nephrotic syndrome
- Renal failure with peritoneal dialysis
- Epididymitis or orchitis

DIAGNOSIS

HISTORY

- Acute, subacute, or chronic swelling of the scrotum or inguinal canal
- Frequent changes in size of the hydrocele with position change or activity (indicative of a communicating hydrocele)
- Usually painless unless acute onset
- Sensation of heaviness or pressure in the scrotum
- Pain radiating to the flank/back

PHYSICAL EXAM

- Swelling in the scrotum or inguinal canal
- Scrotal mass (usually fluctuant)
- Fluctuation in size with change of position (communicating hydrocele)
- Scrotal mass that transilluminates
- A fluctuant mass that is reducible with gentle pressure can identify a communicating hydrocele versus noncommunicating.

DIFFERENTIAL DIAGNOSIS

- Indirect inguinal hernia
- Orchitis
- Epididymitis
- Varicocele
- Traumatic testicular injury
- Testicular torsion or torsion of appendix testes
- Testicular neoplasm

DIAGNOSTIC TESTS & INTERPRETATION

Initial Tests (lab, imaging)

- Inguinoscrotal ultrasound (US) can demonstrate the presence of bowel (e.g., distinguish incarcerated hernia from a hydrocele of the cord) as well as the presence of testicular torsion.
- Testicular MRI when US is unable to distinguish etiology
- Doppler US or testicular nuclear scan can identify testicular torsion.

ALERT

Aspiration of a hydrocele for diagnosis is not indicated and may lead to severe complications if herniated bowel is present.

Diagnostic Procedures/Other

Transillumination of the hemiscrotum along with history and exam are usually sufficient in making the diagnosis, but a formal US should be obtained prior to treatment to verify scrotal contents.

TREATMENT

ISSUES FOR REFERRAL

- Urology referral for symptomatic adults or if underlying diagnosis is unclear
- Pediatric urology/surgery referral for children with symptomatic noncommunicating hydrocele
- Pediatric urology/surgery referral if not resolved by 2 years of age

SURGERY/OTHER PROCEDURES

- Children: For congenital hydrocele, surgical treatment is generally deferred until 2 years of age because many hydroceles will spontaneously resolve. Some evidence shows that delaying longer than 2 years may be appropriate and decreases unnecessary surgery (1)[C]. When surgery is indicated, children with communicating hydroceles may undergo either open or laparoscopic approach.
  - Laparoscopic repair offers the benefit of contralateral exploration which may reveal additional defects. It also may have diminished postoperative pain and a lower rate of complications.
  - Open scrotal approach involves ligation and removal of the processus vaginalis. The benefit of this approach is improved cosmesis and decreased operative time (2)[B].
  - Open inguinal approach involves ligation of the processus vaginalis and excision, distal splitting, or drainage of hydrocele sac (in a hydrocele of the cord, the sac can be completely removed).
- Adults: No therapy is needed unless the hydrocele causes discomfort or unless there is a significant underlying cause such as a tumor.
  - Aspiration of the hydrocele with instillation of a sclerosing agent has been successfully used in adults.
  - If resection is indicated, all the open surgical techniques have the same 6% rate of recurrence; however, the overall rate of complications and the rate of postoperative hematoma were lowest with the Lord's repair (3)[B].
  - Postoperative complications as well as cost and time to work resumption can be less in treatment by aspiration and sclerotherapy versus resection, but the recurrence rate may be higher.

ADMISSION, INPATIENT, AND NURSING CONSIDERATIONS

- Open inguinal or scrotal approach is typically performed as an outpatient.
- Laparoscopic approach in pediatric patients may require 24-hour admission for postoperative monitoring.
- Sclerotherapy is a same-day office procedure.

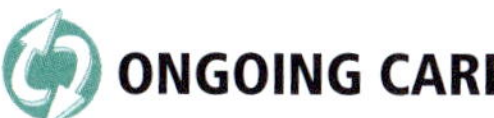

ONGOING CARE

FOLLOW-UP RECOMMENDATIONS

Patient Monitoring

- Depending on method of treatment, initial follow-up is generally in the first 4 to 6 weeks.
- With sclerotherapy, follow-up is for confirmation of resolution or to proceed with retreatment.
- Postoperative follow-up at 2 to 4 weeks and subsequent 2- to 3-month intervals until resolution of any postoperative complications

PROGNOSIS

- Children/infants: As stated above, most congenital hydroceles resolve spontaneously with no intervention by age 2 years. For those who do need treatment, nearly all patients have resolution of symptoms after surgical intervention with very low long-term morbidity.
- Adults: low risk of long-term morbidity with either treatment method with eventual resolution of symptoms in nearly all cases depending on the underlying etiology (e.g., peritoneal dialysis)

COMPLICATIONS

- Complication rate for a scrotal approach may reach 30%.
- Postoperative traumatic hydrocele is common and usually resolves spontaneously.
- Injury to testicle, epididymis, vas deferens, or spermatic vessels
- Suture granuloma
- Pain and swelling
- Hematoma
- Wound infection
- Recurrence

REFERENCES

1. Hall NJ, Ron O, Eaton S, et al. Surgery for hydrocele in children—an avoidable excess? *J Pediatr Surg*. 2011;46(12):2401–2405.
2. Alp BF, Irkilata HC, Kibar Y, et al. Comparison of the inguinal and scrotal approaches for the treatment of communicating hydrocele in children. *Kaohsiung J Med Sci*. 2014;30(4):200–205.
3. Tsai L, Milburn PA, Cecil CL IV, et al. Comparison of recurrence and postoperative complications between 3 different techniques for surgical repair of idiopathic hydrocele. *Urology*. 2019;125:239–242.

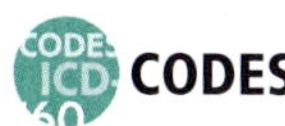

CODES

ICD10

- N43.0 Encysted hydrocele
- N43.3 Hydrocele, unspecified
- N43.2 Other hydrocele

CLINICAL PEARLS

- A hydrocele can usually be diagnosed by physical exam and transillumination. If there is any concern for other underlying process, a formal US is recommended.
- Aspiration alone is not indicated as the primary treatment of a hydrocele due to high recurrence rate.
- Attempted aspiration of an unconfirmed hydrocele could lead to bowel injury in an undiagnosed inguinal hernia and should not be attempted.
- Expectant management of children with hydrocele until >2 years of age is acceptable to allow sufficient time for spontaneous resolution, decreasing the likelihood of an unnecessary procedure.
- In adults, surgical resection costs more and has more complications than aspiration and sclerotherapy but has a much lower recurrence rate and a much higher patient satisfaction rate.

HYDRONEPHROSIS

Megan Mendez Miller, DO

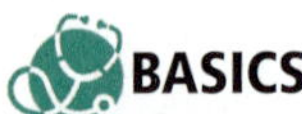

BASICS

DESCRIPTION

- Hydronephrosis refers to a structural finding: dilatation of the renal calyces and pelvis.
- Can be accompanied with hydroureter (dilatation of the ureter)
- Hydronephrosis should not be used interchangeably with obstructive uropathy, which refers to the damage to renal parenchyma resulting from urinary tract obstruction (UTO).

EPIDEMIOLOGY

- More common in children than adults due to congenital anomalies.
- Hydronephrosis is more common in women for adults <60 years old and in men for adults >60 years old.

ETIOLOGY AND PATHOPHYSIOLOGY

- Hydronephrosis develops with increased pressure in the urinary collecting system, most commonly from some form of obstruction.
- Nonobstructive hydronephrosis can occur in the setting of very high urinary output such as with diabetes insipidus or as a physiologic change in pregnancy.
- Hydronephrosis may be acute/chronic, partial/complete, and uni-/bilateral.
- Obstruction may occur at an level of the GU system:
  - Kidney: nephrolithiasis, transitional cell carcinoma, sloughed renal papillae, congenital ureteropelvic junction (UPJ) obstruction, blood clot, fungal ball
  - Ureter: nephrolithiasis, transitional cell carcinomas, strictures, sloughed renal papillae, retroperitoneal fibrosis, extrinsic compression
  - Bladder: neurogenic bladder, extrinsic compression, posterior urethral valves
  - Urethra: prostatic hypertrophy or cancer, strictures
- Hydronephrosis in a transplanted kidney is more common than in native kidneys, due to ureteral reflux, strictures, ureteral compression (from peritransplant lymphoceles, hematomas) and bladder dysfunction.

Pediatric Considerations

- Antenatal hydronephrosis is diagnosed in 1–5% of pregnancies, usually by US, as early as the 12th to 14th week of gestation.
- Children with antenatal hydronephrosis are at greater risk of postnatal pathology.
- Postnatal evaluation begins with US exam; further studies, such as voiding cystourethrogram (VCUG), based on the severity of postnatal hydronephrosis
- In neonates, it is the most common cause of abdominal mass.
- Common etiologies in children are VUR, congenital UPJ obstruction, neurogenic bladder, and posterior urethral valves.
- Pediatric diagnostic algorithm differs from adult due to different differential diagnosis necessitating age-appropriate testing.

Pregnancy Considerations

- Physiologic hydronephrosis in pregnancy is more prominent on the right than left and can be seen in up to 80% of pregnant women.
- Dilatation is caused by hormonal effects, external compression from expanding uterus, and intrinsic changes in the ureteral wall.
- Despite high incidence, most cases are asymptomatic.
- If symptomatic and refractory to medical management, ureteric calculus should be considered and urinary infection must be excluded.

DIAGNOSIS

HISTORY

- Symptoms vary according to cause, chronicity, location, and degree of obstruction.
- Although often asymptomatic, hydronephrosis can be associated with pain ranging from vague, intermittent discomfort to severe renal colic.
- Can be associated with hematuria
- Nausea and vomiting may be associated with pain or infection.
- Fever and chills suggest coexisting urinary infection.
- Anuria suggests complete obstruction bilaterally or unilateral obstruction of a solitary kidney.
- Polyuria may occur due to impaired urinary concentration in partial obstruction.
- Symptoms of chronic kidney disease (CKD): anorexia, malaise, weight gain, edema, shortness of breath, mental state changes, tremors from long-standing obstruction
- Symptoms of bladder outlet obstruction: weak urine stream, nocturia, straining to void, overflow incontinence, urgency, and frequency
- General medical and surgical history: malignancy (extrinsic compression), radiotherapy (ureteric stricture/fibrosis), surgery (iatrogenic obstruction), trauma hematoma or fibrosis), gynecologic disease (extrinsic compression from endometriosis, ovarian masses, uterine prolapse), smoking (urothelial cancer), drugs (methysergide-induced retroperitoneal fibrosis)

PHYSICAL EXAM

- General signs
  - Volume overload (edema, rales, hypertension [HTN]) from renal failure
  - Diaphoresis, tachycardia, tachypnea with pain
  - High-grade fever, if infection
- Abdominal exam: CVA tenderness, palpable bladder, rarely palpable abdominal mass (may be visible, particularly in thin children)
- Pelvic exam: pelvic mass, uterine prolapse, palpable enlarged prostate (cancer or benign), urethral meatal stenosis, phimosis

DIAGNOSTIC TESTS & INTERPRETATION

- Urinalysis with microscopy: hematuria, proteinuria, crystalluria, pyuria
- Midstream urine culture and sensitivity: Exclude UTI.
- Basic metabolic panel: Elevated urea and creatinine may indicate obstructive uropathy. Hyperkalemic nonanion gap metabolic acidosis may indicate type 4 distal RTA due to obstruction.
- CBC: anemia of CKD, leukocytosis; if infection, check platelet count prior to considering ureteral instrumentation.
- Prostate-specific antigen (PSA): adult males age >50 years or with abnormal digital rectal exam or bladder outlet obstruction signs or symptoms
- Urine cytology: for malignant cells in urothelial malignancies
- US and noncontrast CT scanning are effective in diagnosing presence and cause of obstruction in most cases.
- US: screening test of choice for hydronephrosis
  - Sensitivity 90%, specificity 84.5%. Does not assess function and rarely detects cause and level of obstruction. Degree of hydronephrosis does not correlate with duration or severity of the obstruction.
  - Advantages: detects renal parenchymal disease (decreased renal size, increased cortical echogenicity, cortical thinning, cysts); no exposure to radiation or contrast; safe in pregnancy, contrast allergy, and renal dysfunction
  - False-positive findings 15.5%: normal extrarenal pelvis, parapelvic cysts, VUR, excessive diuresis
  - False-negative findings 10%: dehydration, acute obstruction, calyceal dilatation misinterpreted as renal cortical cysts, and retroperitoneal fibrosis
- Noncontrast helical CT (NHCT): test of choice for suspected nephrolithiasis
  - Reported sensitivity 94–96%, specificity 94–100%. Stone is most commonly found at levels of ureteric luminal narrowing: UPJ, pelvic brim, and the vesicoureteric junction.
  - Typical findings in acute obstruction are hydronephrosis with hydroureter proximal to the level of obstruction, perinephric stranding, and renal swelling. If chronic, renal atrophy may be noted.
  - Advantages: no contrast exposure, time-saving, cost-effective, identifies extraurinary pathology (1)
  - Disadvantages: does not assess function or degree of obstruction; higher radiation exposure, although low radiation dose protocols have shown comparable accuracy
- DTPA or MAG-3 radionuclide renal scan (diuretic renal scintigraphy)
  - Indicated only for evaluation of hydronephrosis without apparent obstruction
  - Determines presence of true obstruction as well as total and split (right vs. left) renal function
  - Furosemide is given 20 minutes after the tracer and the T1/2 for the tracer's washout is measured. T1/2; <10 minutes is unobstructed, >20 minutes

is obstructed, and 10 to 20 minutes is equivocal; some experts consider <15 minutes normal.
  - Advantages: no contrast exposure, safe in contrast allergy and renal dysfunction
  - False-positive findings: delayed excretion due to renal failure, massive dilatation causing a water-reservoir effect of delayed excretion without obstruction
  - False-negative findings: dehydration or inadequate diuretic challenge
- Multiphase contrast-enhanced CT
  - Nonenhanced phase detects stones and swelling.
  - Parenchymal phase demonstrates decreased enhancement of renal parenchyma with acute obstruction; can identify extraurinary causes of obstruction and determine the relative glomerular filtration rate (GFR) of each kidney with accuracy equal to radionuclide renal scan
  - Delayed phase allows visualization of the collecting system and soft tissue filling defects (e.g., urothelial cancer).
- Magnetic resonance urography (MRU): indicated when US and NHCT are nondiagnostic
  - Provides anatomic, functional, and prognostic information; sensitivity not superior to US or NHCT for nephrolithiasis (70%) but superior for soft tissue causes including strictures
  - Advantages: no radiation exposure, safe in pregnancy
  - Disadvantages: more expensive and time-consuming (35 minutes vs. 5 minutes) and less available compared with CT. Gadolinium is contraindicated in renal failure especially when GFR is <30 mL/min due to risk of nephrogenic systemic fibrosis.

Follow-Up Tests & Special Considerations

The presence of fever in the setting of hydronephrosis should be considered a medical emergency due to the risk of bacteremia from urinary infection in an obstructed urinary system.

Diagnostic Procedures/Other

Cystoscopy, retrograde pyelogram ± ureteroscopy, and biopsy are occasionally used to determine the cause of obstruction (e.g., small urothelial cancer missed on imaging) or to confirm a normal distal ureter prior to pyeloplasty. In addition, such procedures are often needed to establish a definitive pathologic diagnosis for mass lesions.

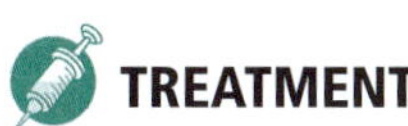

TREATMENT

GENERAL MEASURES

- Medical treatment: correction of fluid and electrolyte abnormalities, pain control, antibiotics as an adjunct to drainage if infection present
- Relief of obstruction: prompt drainage indicated in the presence of UTI, compromised renal function, or uncontrollable/persistent pain
  - Bladder outlet obstruction: urethral or suprapubic catheter
  - Ureteric obstruction: retrograde (cystoscopic) or antegrade (percutaneous) stenting (2)
- VUR is often managed conservatively with antibiotics; surgical management may be required in severe cases in children or women of childbearing age.
- Medical expulsive therapy (MET) with α-blockers or calcium channel blockers indicated for urethral stones <10 mm in patients with controlled pain, no signs of sepsis, with good renal function (3)[C]

SURGERY/OTHER PROCEDURES

- Hydronephrosis due to obstruction
  - Congenital UPJ obstruction: Pyeloplasty (open or laparoscopic) and minimally invasive stricture incision (endopyelotomy) are used with comparable results.
  - Nephrolithiasis: Extracorporeal shock wave lithotripsy (ESWL) is the initial treatment of choice for management of impacted upper urethral stones ≤2 cm. Ureteroscopy with or without intracorporeal lithotripsy has lower retreatment but higher complication rates and longer hospital stay; ureteral stenting pre-ESWL or postureteroscopy associated with no additional benefit and more discomfort and morbidity (4)[A],(5)
  - Transitional cell cancer: nephroureterectomy
  - Idiopathic retroperitoneal fibrosis: ureterolysis (frees ureters from inflammatory mass)
  - Prostate disorders: various treatment modalities, including transurethral resection of the prostate (TURP) and radical prostatectomy
- Nonobstructed hydronephrosis
  - VUR: ureteric reimplantation, endoscopic subureteral injection

ADMISSION, INPATIENT, AND NURSING CONSIDERATIONS

Obstruction coexisting with infection (pyonephrosis) is a true urologic emergency requiring urgent drainage. Typically, this requires placement of percutaneous nephrostomy tube(s) because retrograde (cystoscopic) stenting is often difficult, but both are equally effective.

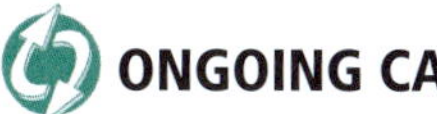

ONGOING CARE

FOLLOW-UP RECOMMENDATIONS

- Serial monitoring of kidney function (electrolytes, BUN, and creatinine) and BP until renal function stabilizes. Frequency of monitoring depends on severity of renal dysfunction.
- Follow-up US after stabilization of renal function to assess for resolution of hydronephrosis. If hydronephrosis persists, consider diuretic radionuclide study to rule out persistent obstruction.

PROGNOSIS

- Recovery of renal function depends on etiology, presence or absence of UTI, and degree and duration of obstruction.
- Significant recovery can occur despite days of complete obstruction, although some irreversible injury may develop within 24 hours. Delays in therapy can lead to irreversible renal damage (6).
- Diagnostic testing is of poor predictive value. Course of incomplete obstruction is highly unpredictable.

COMPLICATIONS

- Urine stasis: increased risk of infection and stones formation
- Obstruction causes progressive atrophy of kidney with irreversible loss of function.
- Spontaneous rupture of a calyx may occur with urine extravasation in the perinephric space.
- Postobstructive diuresis: marked polyuria after relief of obstruction:
  - Caused mostly by fluid and solute overload but may be exacerbated by impaired renal tubular concentrating ability. Urine output may be >500 mL/hr.
  - Replace urine losses with hypotonic fluid (usually with 0.45% NaCl) and only enough to avoid volume depletion. Replacement of urine output with equal amounts of saline will perpetuate the diuresis.

REFERENCES

1. Worster A, Preyra I, Weaver B, et al. The accuracy of noncontrast helical computed tomography versus intravenous pyelography in the diagnosis of suspected acute urolithiasis: a meta-analysis. *Ann Emerg Med*. 2002;40(3):280–286.
2. Ramsey S, Robertson A, Ablett MJ, et al. Evidence-based drainage of infected hydronephrosis secondary to ureteric calculi. *J Endourol*. 2010;24(2):185–189.
3. Seitz C, Liatsikos E, Porpiglia F, et al. Medical therapy to facilitate the passage of stones: what is the evidence? *Eur Urol*. 2009;56(3):455–471.
4. Aboumarzouk OM, Kata SG, Keeley FX, et al. Extracorporeal shock wave lithotripsy (ESWL) versus ureteroscopic management for ureteric calculi. *Cochrane Database Syst Rev*. 2011;(12):CD006029.
5. Shen P, Jiang M, Yang J, et al. Use of ureteral stent in extracorporeal shock wave lithotripsy for upper urinary calculi: a systematic review and meta-analysis. *J Urol*. 2011;186(4):1328–1335.
6. Cohen EP, Sobrero M, Roxe DM, et al. Reversibility of long-standing urinary tract obstruction requiring long-term dialysis. *Arch Intern Med*. 1992;152(1):177–179.

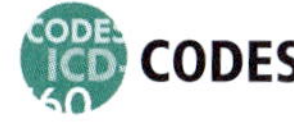

CODES

ICD10

- N13.2 Hydronephrosis with renal and ureteral calculous obstruction
- N13.30 Unspecified hydronephrosis
- Q62.0 Congenital hydronephrosis

CLINICAL PEARLS

- US and noncontrast CT identify most causes of hydronephrosis.
- Relief of obstruction, when present, is the primary treatment.

HYPERCHOLESTEROLEMIA

Michelle Nelson, MD, FAAFP

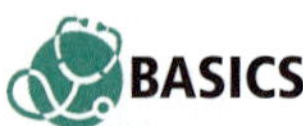

BASICS

DESCRIPTION

- Elevated cholesterol is a significant risk factor for atherosclerotic cardiovascular disease (ASCVD).
- Lipoprotein subtypes:
  - Low-density lipoproteins (LDL): atherogenic; primary target of therapy
  - High-density lipoproteins (HDL): atheroprotective
  - Triglycerides (TGs)
- System(s) affected: cardiovascular (CV)

EPIDEMIOLOGY

According to the CDC, 10% of U.S. adults aged ≥20 years have hypercholesterolemia, and 7% of U.S. children and adolescents between the ages of 6 and 19 years have hypercholesterolemia.

Prevalence

Disease incidence and prevalence increases with age.

ETIOLOGY AND PATHOPHYSIOLOGY

- Pathophysiology
  - Deposition of cholesterol in vascular walls creates fatty streaks that become fibrous plaques.
  - Inflammation causes plaque instability, leading to plaque rupture.
  - Atherosclerosis, inflammation, and vascular reactivity have a multifactorial etiology.
- Etiology of hypercholesterolemia
  - Primary: genetic causes (familial dyslipidemia)
  - Secondary: obesity, diet, excessive alcohol intake, hypothyroidism, diabetes mellitus (DM), inflammatory disease, liver disease, nephrotic syndrome, chronic renal failure, medications (thiazide diuretics, carbamazepine, cyclosporine, progestins, anabolic steroids, corticosteroids, protease inhibitors, antipsychotics, isotretinoin)

Genetics

- Familial hypercholesterolemia (FH)
  - Elevated LDL levels from birth
  - Prevalence is 1:300 worldwide for heterozygous FH.
  - Predisposition to atherosclerotic disease in early adulthood and high coronary heart disease risk at younger ages; individuals with homozygous FH typically die before 20 years old.
  - Early lipid-lowering drug therapy has been shown to reduce ASCVD risk.
- Early lipid screening of first-degree relatives is recommended.

RISK FACTORS

Obesity, physical inactivity, family history, cigarette smoking, excessive alcohol use; the relationship between dietary saturated fat and hypercholesterolemia and coronary artery disease is complex.

GENERAL PREVENTION

Regular physical activity, weight control (see "Ongoing Care"), diet lower in saturated fats (grade 1B); giving specific, targeted goals for exercise is more effective than a general recommendation.

COMMONLY ASSOCIATED CONDITIONS

Hypertension, DM, obesity

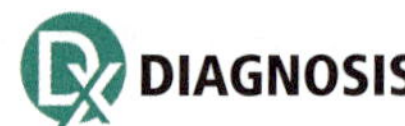

DIAGNOSIS

Screening recommendations:

- U.S. Preventive Services Task Force (USPSTF) (1)[C]: total cholesterol and HDL cholesterol (HDL-C) every 5 years
  - Adults ≥40 years of age
  - No recommendation for or against screening in adults aged 21 to 39 years
  - No recommendation for or against screening in children and adolescents
- American Diabetes Association: at least yearly dyslipidemia screening for patients with DM

Pediatric Considerations

- National Heart, Lung, and Blood Institute: Recommends universal lipid screening on all children between 9 and 11 years and between 17 and 21 years old. This was endorsed by the American Academy of Pediatrics (2), although pros and cons should be discussed with patients and family as more research is needed on population cost and harms vs benefit of screening.
- Screening recommended for children with a family history of premature coronary artery disease or familial hypercholesterolemia.

HISTORY

Review possible secondary etiologies and assess other ASCVD risk factors

PHYSICAL EXAM

Nonspecific findings; may calculate BMI and examine for xanthomas

DIAGNOSTIC TESTS & INTERPRETATION

Initial Tests (lab, imaging)

- Lipid panel (nonfasting preferred); LDL is usually a calculated value and is accurate if TG is <350 mg/dL. Perform fasting labs in hypertriglyceridemia (TG >440 mg/dL) or conditions that can elevate TG such as pancreatitis.
- Consider genetic etiology in very high LDL (>190 mg/dL) or TG (>500 mg/dL).

TREATMENT

ALERT

Multiple guidelines exist. The 2018 American College of Cardiology/AHA (ACC/AHA) cholesterol guidelines return to targeting LDL goals. Risk stratifying patients should be reserved for primary prevention as patients with established CV disease should be considered high-risk (secondary prevention).

- United States: ACC/AHA cholesterol guidelines (3)
  - According to the ACC/AHA, four groups benefit from statin therapy:
    - Primary elevation of LDL-C ≥190 mg/dL: high-intensity statin
    - Patients with DM aged 40 to 75 years with LDL-C >70 mg/dL: moderate-intensity statin
    - ASCVD risk based on PREVENT Risk Calculator: https://professional.heart.org/en/guidelines-and-statements/prevent-calculator
      - 10-year ASCVD risk <5%: lifestyle modifications with Mediterranean diet and exercise
      - 10-year ASCVD risk 5–7.5%: lifestyle modifications, with Mediterranean diet and exercise; discuss potential benefits and harms of moderate intensity statin with patient.
      - 10-year ASCVD risk 7.5–10%: lifestyle modifications, with Mediterranean diet and exercise; ACC recommends moderate-intensity statin; USPSTF recommends just shared decision making regarding statin
      - 10-year ASCVD risk ≥100%: moderate to high-intensity statin
    - Secondary ASCVD prevention
      - Age ≤75 years: high-intensity statin with goal to reduce LDL-C >50%; add ezetimibe if LDL is >70 mg/dL after maximal statin therapy in very high-risk ASCVD patients.*
      - Age >75 years: moderate- or high-intensity statin as tolerated
  - *Definition of very high-risk ASCVD is at least one major ASCVD event and multiple high-risk conditions:
    - Major ASCVD events: acute coronary syndrome or history of myocardial infarction, history of ischemic stroke, symptomatic peripheral arterial disease
    - High-risk conditions: age >65 years, heterozygous FH, history of CABG or PCI, DM, HTN, chronic kidney disease, current smoker, history of congestive heart failure, LDL-C >100 mg/dL despite maximum medical therapy
    - Controversy exists regarding the threshold calculated risk with which to treat patients: The Pooled Cohort Equations calculator significantly *overestimates* 10-year ASCVD risk (by ≥50%). Therefore, discuss with patients the benefits and harms of statin therapy—factors in patient longevity.

- United States: USPSTF 2022 statin recommendations (1)[C]
  - Adults aged 40 to 75 years with no history of CVD, one or more CVD risk factors (dyslipidemia, hypertension, DM, or smoking), and a calculated 10-year CVD event risk of ≥10%: low- to moderate-intensity statin (grade B recommendation)
  - Adults aged 40 to 75 years with no history of CVD, one or more CVD risk factors, and a calculated 10-year CVD event risk of 7.5–10%: low- to moderate-dose statin (grade C recommendation)
  - Adults aged ≥76 years with no history of CVD: insufficient evidence to make recommendation

ALERT
In hypertriglyceridemia with TG>500 mg/dL, TG lowering becomes the primary goal until <500 mg/dL to prevent acute pancreatitis. Statin therapy is usually recommended as first line unless TGs remain >500. Fibrates may be used cautiously with statins (increased risk of rhabdomyolysis).

MEDICATION

- Therapeutic lifestyle changes are cornerstone therapies to be attempted before drug therapy.
- Available data do not support initiation of statin therapy for primary prevention in most adults aged >75 years (ALLHAT-LLT).
- Check a lipid panel 4 to 12 weeks after starting medication to evaluate response and/or adherence. Subsequent monitoring is not generally indicated unless there is a question of patient adherence.

First Line

HMG-CoA reductase inhibitors (statins)

- Categorized based on intensity
  - High intensity (reduces LDL-C by >50%): atorvastatin 40 to 80 mg/day, rosuvastatin 20 to 40 mg/day
  - Moderate intensity (reduces LDL-C by 30%–49%): atorvastatin 10 to 20 mg/day, rosuvastatin 5 to 10 mg/day, simvastatin 20 to 40 mg/day, pravastatin 40 to 80 mg/day, lovastatin 40 mg/day, fluvastatin XL 80 mg/day, fluvastatin 40 mg BID, pitavastatin 2 to 4 mg/day
  - Low intensity (reduces LDL-C by <30%): simvastatin 10 mg/day, pravastatin 10 to 20 mg/day, lovastatin 20 mg/day, fluvastatin 20 to 40 mg/day, pitavastatin 1 mg/day
- Effect is greatest in lowering LDL-C; shown to decrease coronary heart disease incidence and all-cause mortality (1).
- Contraindications: pregnancy, lactation, or active liver disease
- Adverse reactions:
  - Mild myalgia is common.
  - Liver transaminase elevations: alanine aminotransferase (ALT) before therapy to establish baseline; if ALT >3 times upper limit of normal, do not start statin; routine monitoring is not recommended.
  - Association with increased cases of DM: 0.1 excess cases of DM per 100 persons on moderate-intensity statin and 0.3 excess cases per 100 persons on high-intensity statin
  - Myopathies (considered rare but not well studied)
  - Statin intolerance strategies: Consider using a different statin (pravastatin, simvastatin, dose reduction, or alternate day therapy. A majority of patients who had previously discontinued statins due to side effects are able to restart the same or another statin and tolerate them.

ALERT
U.S. Food and Drug Administration alert: Do not prescribe simvastatin at 80 mg/day due to increased myopathy risk. Patients who have been at this drug dosage for >1 year can continue if no signs of myopathy. Dose restrictions to reduce myopathy risk include the following: Do not exceed simvastatin 10 mg/day with amiodarone, verapamil, and diltiazem Do not exceed simvastatin 20 mg/day with amlodipine and ranolazine.

Pregnancy Considerations

Statins contraindicated during pregnancy, possibly unsafe with lactation

Second Line

- Second-line drugs are now recommended as primary prevention if LDL-C is >70 mg/dL on maximal statin therapy.
- Ezetimibe: can be taken by itself or in combination with a statin: monotherapy (10 mg/day) or ezetimibe/simvastatin; effect: lowers LDL-C; one randomized controlled trial shows combination therapy with statin has small benefit in reducing CV events and CV-related mortality after acute coronary syndromes.
- Fibrates gemfibrozil, fenofibrate; effect: most effective in lowering TG with moderate effect in lowering LDL and raising HDL. More recent studies fail to show mortality benefit in most patients.
- Bempedoic acid is recommended to lower total cholesterol and LDL-C in statin-intolerant patients preferably in combination with ezetimibe if LDL-C goals are not reached with ezetimibe alone.
- Niacin raises HDL but no evidence for improved outcomes; should not be used routinely
- PCSK9 inhibitors (e.g., alirocumab, evolocumab): monoclonal antibodies; current evidence shows decreased incidence of CVD in secondary prevention without affecting incidence of all-cause mortality; VERY expensive medications
- Icosapent ethyl, an omega-3 fatty acid as adjunct to statin for hypertriglyceridemia treatment and CV risk reduction
- In patients with ASCVD risk factors, the American Heart Association (AHA) released a statement in 2022 recommending sodium glucose cotransporter 2 inhibitors and glucagon-like peptide-1 receptor agonists (GLP1-RA), regardless if the patient has DM or not.

ADDITIONAL THERAPIES

Antithrombotic therapies for patients with type 2 DM and risk factors for CVD

COMPLEMENTARY & ALTERNATIVE MEDICINE

Omega-3 fatty acids and fish oil intake: sources—fatty fish, plants (flaxseed, canola oil, soybean oil, nuts); they decrease TG and LDL level, and increases HDL. Overall CV benefit and mortality reduction is uncertain.

ADMISSION, INPATIENT, AND NURSING CONSIDERATIONS

If lipid panel was checked while inpatient due to a myocardial infarction, a fasting lipid panel recheck in 4 to 12 weeks is recommended after discharge as the first lab may not be accurate.

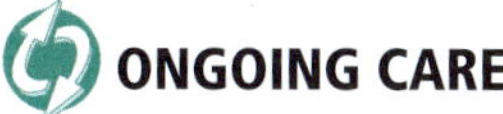

ONGOING CARE

FOLLOW-UP RECOMMENDATIONS

Moderate-intensity exercise for 150 minutes per week: increases HDL, lowers TC, and helps control weight

Patient Monitoring

Routine monitoring of liver function tests is not recommended if initial ALT is within normal range.

DIET

Plant-based diets and the Mediterranean diet, which are high in legumes, fruits, vegetables, nuts, fish, and olive oil reduce the risk of CV disease.

PATIENT EDUCATION

AHA: https://www.heart.org/en/healthy-living/healthy-eating/eat-smart/nutrition-basics/mediterranean-diet

COMPLICATIONS

Myocardial infarction, peripheral artery disease, cerebrovascular accident

REFERENCES

1. Mangione CM, Barry MJ, Nickolson WK, et al; for US Preventive Services Task Force. Statin use for the primary prevention of cardiovascular disease in adults: US Preventive Services Task Force recommendation statement.
2. Berger JH, Chen F, Faerber J, et al. Adherence with lipid screening guidelines in standard- and high-risk children and adolescents. *Am Heart J*. 2021;232:39–46.
3. Grundy SM, Stone NJ, Bailey AL, et al. 2018 AHA/ACC/AACVPR/AAPA/ABC/ACPM/ADA/AGS/APhA/ASPC/NLA/PCNA guideline on the management of blood cholesterol: executive summary: a report of the American College of Cardiology/American Heart Association Task Force on clinical practice guidelines. 2019;73(24):3168–3209.

SEE ALSO

Diabetes Mellitus, Type 2; Hypertension, Essential; Obesity

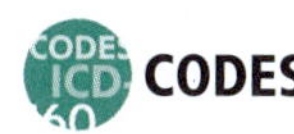

CODES

ICD10

E78.0 Pure hypercholesterolemia

CLINICAL PEARLS

- A plant-based diet (Mediterranean diet) and exercise should be tried before pharmaceutical interventions for most with hypercholesterolemia
- It is not generally recommended to start statins in patients ≥75 years of age for primary prevention. Statins can be continued if already initiated previously, but benefits and harms should be reconsidered regularly as patients age

H

HYPEREMESIS GRAVIDARUM

Jeremy Golding, MD, FAAFP

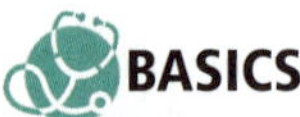

BASICS

- Nausea and vomiting in pregnancy is a common condition that affects approximately 70–80% of pregnancies.
- Hyperemesis gravidarum (HG) is a severe form of nausea and vomiting in pregnancy that affects 0.5–2% of pregnancies and can have significant adverse physical and psychological sequela.
- HG is a diagnosis of clinical judgement and is one of the most common indications for hospitalization during pregnancy.
- HG is associated with several adverse fetal outcomes including preterm delivery, low birth weight, small for gestation age, low 5-minute Apgar scores, and neurodevelopmental delay.

DESCRIPTION

- Although morning sickness is common during pregnancy, HG is a rare condition.
- Intractable vomiting in a pregnant woman that interferes with fluid and electrolyte balance as well as nutrition:
  - Usually associated with the first 8 to 20 weeks of pregnancy
  - Associated with high estrogen and human chorionic gonadotropin (hCG) levels
  - Symptoms usually begin ~2 weeks after first missed period, peak around the 12th week, and resolve by the 20th week
- System(s) affected: endocrine/metabolic, gastrointestinal, reproductive

EPIDEMIOLOGY

- Generally affects young women, primiparous, nonsmokers, and nonwhite people
- Other risk factors: prior history of hyperemesis, preexisting diabetes, hyperthyroid disorder, psychiatric illness, asthma, and GI disorders

Incidence

HG occurs in 0.5–2% of pregnancies.

Prevalence

The most common cause of hospitalization in the first half of pregnancy; the second most common cause of hospitalization of all pregnant women

ETIOLOGY AND PATHOPHYSIOLOGY

Etiology is unknown; proposed influences include the following:

- Hyperthyroidism
- Hyperparathyroidism
- Pregnancy hormones
- Liver dysfunction
- Autonomic nervous system dysfunction
- CNS neoplasm
- Addison disease
- Possible psychological factors

Genetics

Increased risk if maternal family history of HG

RISK FACTORS

Nulliparity; multiple gestations; history of migraines; history of motion sickness; black or Asian women; gestational trophoblastic disease; fetus with trisomy 21; female fetus; possible association with *Helicobacter pylori* infection

GENERAL PREVENTION

Guidance regarding dietary habits to avoid dehydration and nutritional depletion

- Small, frequent meals
- Avoid an overly empty or full stomach.
- Avoid greasy, spicy, and fatty foods.
- Eat bland, low-fiber, high-protein snacks.

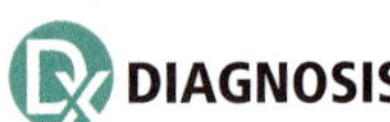

DIAGNOSIS

Intractable nausea and vomiting in pregnancy leading to dehydration and electrolyte imbalances after the exclusion of other causes of severe nausea and vomiting

HISTORY

- Nausea
- Vomiting with retching >3 times per day
- Decreased urine output
- Fatigue
- Dizziness with standing
- Poor appetite

PHYSICAL EXAM

- >5% weight loss from prepregnancy weight
- Thyroid evaluation
- Signs of dehydration, such as orthostatic hypotension, large ketonuria, high urine specific gravity

DIFFERENTIAL DIAGNOSIS

Other common causes of vomiting must be considered: gastroenteritis, gastritis, reflux esophagitis, peptic ulcer disease, cholelithiasis, cholecystitis, pyelonephritis, appendicitis, pancreatitis, anxiety, hyperparathyroidism, hypercalcemia, thyrotoxicosis, *H. pylori* infection

DIAGNOSTIC TESTS & INTERPRETATION

Initial laboratory studies for HG are used to evaluate maternal clinical status and rule out other possible causes of nausea and vomiting.

Initial Tests (lab, imaging)

- Urinalysis: may see glucosuria, albuminuria, granular casts, and hematuria (rare); ketosis more common
- Thyroid-stimulating hormone (TSH), free T_4
- Electrolytes, BUN, creatinine
- Liver enzymes and bilirubin levels
- Hematocrit
- Hepatitis panel
- Calcium
- Albumin

Diagnostic Procedures/Other

Indicated only if it is necessary to rule out other diagnoses, as listed in the following section:

- Upper abdominal ultrasound if pancreatitis or cholecystitis are suspected
- Abdominal MRI if appendicitis is suspected
- Ultrasound if hydatidiform mole or multiple gestation is suspected

Test Interpretation

- Urinalysis: When positive for ketones and high specific gravity indicate starvation ketosis and volume depletion
- TSH, free T_4: A transient hyperthyroidism (suppressed TSH with normal free T_4) may be present in approximately 50% of HG. If TSH is suppressed with elevated free T_4, further investigation is needed for overt hyperthyroidism.
- Electrolytes, BUN, creatinine: Dehydration can cause low potassium, low sodium, and elevated BUN and creatinine.
- Liver enzymes and bilirubin levels: Mild elevation of AST and ALT occurs in approximately 50% of cases and self-resolves.
- Hematocrit: Dehydration causes increase (volume contraction).
- Hepatitis panel: Hepatitis A, B, and C may present similarly to hyperemesis; consider and rule out.
- Calcium: Hypercalcemia resulting from hyperparathyroidism occurs rarely.
- Albumin: Decreased albumin may indicate malnutrition secondary to nausea and vomiting.

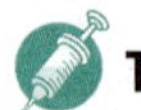

TREATMENT

Pyridoxine and doxylamine (pregnancy Category A) are first-line treatments for HG (1)[C]. This is followed by metoclopramide or ondansetron (pregnancy Category B) and then prochlorperazine (pregnancy Category C), methylprednisolone (pregnancy Category C), or promethazine (pregnancy Category C).

GENERAL MEASURES

- First, treat dehydration and electrolyte imbalances and then treat nausea.
- IV fluids, either normal saline or 5% dextrose normal saline (with consideration for potential thiamine deficiency)
- For severe cases, consider PO thiamine 25 to 50 mg TID or IV 100 mg in 100 mL of normal saline over 30 minutes once weekly and potential parental nutrition if needed.
- Ondansetron carries an FDA warning for QT prolongation. It has unclear risk in the setting of pregnancy. The majority of the current studies shows no increased fetal risk.

MEDICATION

- Pyridoxine (vitamin B_6) 25 mg PO or IV q8h, max dose of 200 mg/day
- Antihistamines (e.g., diphenhydramine [25 to 50 mg q4–6h], doxylamine [12.5 mg PO BID], meclizine [25 mg PO q4–6h], and dimenhydrinate [25 to 50 mg PO q4–6h]) (2)[C]
- Combination product Diclegis (sustained-release pyridoxine 10 mg and doxylamine 10 mg) dosed (start 2 tabs PO QHS; if symptoms persist, increase to 1 tab in AM and 2 QHS; if symptoms still persist, take 1 tab every AM, 1 midday, and 2 QHS; max of 4 tablets/day) or doxylamine 12.5 mg and pyridoxine 25 mg
- Phenothiazines (e.g., promethazine or prochlorperazine): associated with prolonged jaundice, extrapyramidal effects, and hyper- or hyporeflexia in newborns
- Metoclopramide 10 mg PO q6–8h

- Methylprednisolone 16 mg PO/IV q8h for 2 to 3 days and then taper over 2 weeks if initial 3-day treatment is effective; reserved for severe cases with unclear benefit
- Ondansetron 4 to 8 mg PO q8h

First Line

- For women with mild to moderate nausea, pyridoxine (vitamin B_6) 10 to 25 mg PO or IV q8h can improve symptoms and has a good safety profile. Maximum dose is 200 mg/day.
- If nausea and vomiting continue, combination doxylamine succinate 12.5 mg and pyridoxine 25 mg PO q8h; this combination is more effective than either drug alone.
- Ginger capsules 350 mg PO TID can be added with refractory vomiting.

Second Line

- Antihistamines such as diphenhydramine, meclizine, and dimenhydrinate; doxylamine-pyridoxine should be discontinued before starting a different antihistamine.
- Metoclopramide 10 mg PO q8h
- Promethazine 12.5 mg PO or rectally q8h
- Ondansetron 4 to 8 mg PO or IV q8h

ISSUES FOR REFERRAL

- Inpatient management required for IV antiemetics and fluids for symptoms refractory to outpatient management
- May also consider psychiatry or psychology referral if psychological assessment is warranted

ADDITIONAL THERAPIES

- Glucocorticoids (methylprednisolone 16 mg IV q8h for 48 to 72 hours) of uncertain benefit but may be considered for severe and refractory cases
- H_2 receptor antagonists (cimetidine and ranitidine) as adjunctive therapy to reduce heartburn/acid reflux

SURGERY/OTHER PROCEDURES

Rarely, if all pharmacologic and nonpharmacologic interventions fail and weight loss continues, tube feeding or parenteral nutrition is required. Enteral nutrition, either through a gastric or duodenal route, is preferred to the parenteral route as it may relieve nausea and vomiting.

COMPLEMENTARY & ALTERNATIVE MEDICINE

- Ginger 350 mg PO q6h may help (3)[A].
- Mixed evidence for acupressure and acupuncture; acupressure bands at the Neiguan point are effective adjuvant treatment in severe hyperemesis (4)[A].
- Medical hypnosis may be a helpful adjunct to the typical medical treatment regimen, but further study is needed.

ADMISSION, INPATIENT, AND NURSING CONSIDERATIONS

- In some severe cases, parenteral therapy in the hospital or at home may be required.
- Enteral volume and nutrition repletion may be indicated, but early enteral tube feeding does not improve maternal or perinatal outcomes (5)[A].

ONGOING CARE

Approximately 10% of patients with HG will be affected throughout the pregnancy.

FOLLOW-UP RECOMMENDATIONS

Overall quality of life and future fertility plans can be impacted by severity of nausea and vomiting (6)[B].

Patient Monitoring

- In severe cases, follow-up on a daily basis for weight monitoring
- Special attention should be given to monitor for ketosis, hypokalemia, or acid–base disturbances due to hyperemesis.

DIET

- Bland or liquid diet as tolerated
- For outpatient: a diet rich in carbohydrates and protein, such as fruit, cheese, cottage cheese, eggs, beef, poultry, vegetables, toast, crackers, rice; patients should avoid spicy meals and high-fat foods. Encourage small amounts at a time every 1 to 2 hours.

PATIENT EDUCATION

- Attention should be given to psychosocial issues, such as possible ambivalence about the pregnancy.
- Patients should be instructed to take small amounts of fluid frequently to avoid volume depletion.
- Avoid individual foods known to be irritating to the patient.
- Wet-to-dry nutrients (sherbet, broth, gelatin to dry crackers, toast)

PROGNOSIS

- Self-limited illness with good prognosis if patient's weight is maintained at >95% of prepregnancy weight.
- With complication of hemorrhagic retinitis, mortality rate of pregnant patient is 50%.

COMPLICATIONS

- Maternal complications:
  - Vitamin deficiency, dehydration, and malnutrition
  - In severe cases, Wernicke encephalopathy secondary to thiamine deficiency, coma, and even death
- Fetal complications:
  - Patients with >5% weight loss are associated with intrauterine growth retardation and fetal anomalies.
  - Poor weight gain is associated with slightly increased risk for small for gestational age infant <2,500 g and premature birth <37 weeks (7)[A].
  - Hemorrhagic retinitis
  - Liver damage

REFERENCES

1. Maltepe C, Koren G. The management of nausea and vomiting of pregnancy and hyperemesis gravidarum—a 2013 update. *J Popul Ther Clin Pharmacol*. 2013;20(2):e184–e192.
2. Boelig RC, Barton SJ, Saccone G, et al. Interventions for treating hyperemesis gravidarum. *Cochrane Database Syst Rev*. 2016;2016(5):CD010607.
3. Viljoen E, Visser J, Koen N, et al. A systematic review and meta-analysis of the effect and safety of ginger in the treatment of pregnancy-associated nausea and vomiting. *Nutr J*. 2014;13:20.
4. Adlan AS, Chooi KY, Mat Adenan NA. Acupressure as adjuvant treatment for the inpatient management of nausea and vomiting in early pregnancy: a double-blind randomized controlled trial. *J Obstet Gynaecol Res*. 2017;43(4):662–668.
5. Grooten IJ, Koot MH, van der Post JA, et al. Early enteral tube feeding in optimizing treatment of hyperemesis gravidarum: the Maternal and Offspring outcomes after Treatment of HyperEmesis by Refeeding (MOTHER) randomized controlled trial. *Am J Clin Nutr*. 2017;106(3):812–820.
6. Heitmann K, Nordeng H, Havnen GC, et al. The burden of nausea and vomiting during pregnancy: severe impacts on quality of life, daily life functioning and willingness to become pregnant again—results from a cross-sectional study. *BMC Pregnancy Childbirth*. 2017;17(1):75.
7. Veenendaal MVE, van Abeelen AFM, Painter RC, et al. Consequences of hyperemesis gravidarum for offspring: a systematic review and meta analysis. *BJOG*. 2011;118(11):1302–1313.

ADDITIONAL READING

- Boelig RC, Barton SJ, Saccone G, et al. Interventions for treating hyperemesis gravidarum: a Cochrane systematic review and meta-analysis. *J Matern Fetal Neonatal Med*. 2018;31(18):2492–2505.
- McParlin C, O'Donnell A, Robson SC, et al. Treatments for hyperemesis gravidarum and nausea and vomiting in pregnancy: a systematic review. *JAMA*. 2016;316(13):1392–1401.

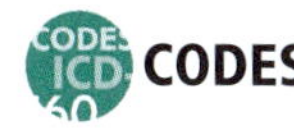

CODES

ICD10

- O21.9 Vomiting of pregnancy, unspecified
- O21.0 Mild hyperemesis gravidarum
- O21.1 Hyperemesis gravidarum with metabolic disturbance

CLINICAL PEARLS

- Do not allow patients to become volume depleted. Once this occurs, it is more difficult to treat.
- Do not be hesitant to use medications for nausea/vomiting, as this may help avoid volume depletion.
- Consider secondary causes of hyperemesis if it develops after 12 weeks of gestation.

HYPERKALEMIA

Bhavin Bharat Patel, DO

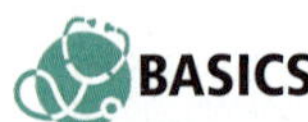

BASICS

DESCRIPTION

- An electrolyte disorder defined as a plasma potassium (K) concentration >5.5 mEq/L (>5 mmol/L)
- Hyperkalemia depresses cardiac conduction and can lead to fatal arrhythmias.
- Normal K regulation involves tightly coordinated mechanisms:
  - After ingestion, K enters the portal circulation, stimulating pancreatic insulin release, which promotes entry of K into cells.
  - In the kidneys, K stimulates renin release from juxtaglomerular cells, activating the renin-angiotensin-aldosterone system (RAAS). Angiotensin II in the lungs stimulates aldosterone secretion from the adrenal zona glomerulosa. Aldosterone acts on the renal collecting ducts to enhance K excretion and sodium reabsorption.
- Four major causes
  - Increased load: either endogenous from tissue breakdown (i.e., rhabdomyolysis or hemolysis) or exogenous (dietary or iatrogenic), usually in association with impaired renal function due to chronic kidney disease (CKD)
  - Decreased excretion (most common): due to reduced glomerular filtration rate or impaired aldosterone secretion
  - Cellular redistribution: shifts from intracellular space (majority of K is intracellular) to extracellular space (as in metabolic acidosis, tissue injury)
  - Pseudohyperkalemia: artificial elevation of K due to hemolysis of blood sample, thrombocytosis, or leukocytosis

Geriatric Considerations

Increased risk for hyperkalemia because of decline in renin and aldosterone production with age, which impairs renal K excretion, especially in the setting of comorbid conditions

EPIDEMIOLOGY

Prevalence

- 5–9% of hospitalized patients (1)
- 1–2% in general population but as high as 34% in patients with CKD

ETIOLOGY AND PATHOPHYSIOLOGY

- Impaired K excretion (most common)
  - Renal insufficiency/failure, obstructive uropathy
  - Addison disease
  - Mineralocorticoid deficiency
  - Type IV renal tubular acidosis
  - Cirrhosis
  - Congestive heart failure
  - Sickle cell disease
  - Amyloidosis
  - Systemic lupus erythematosus
- Increased K intake (2)
  - Bananas, potatoes, melons, citrus juice, avocados, red meat, nuts, and dried fruits
  - Salt substitutes given to CKD patients
- Transcellular shift (redistribution)
  - Metabolic acidosis
  - Insulin deficiency
  - Hyperglycemia (diabetic ketoacidosis or hyperosmolar hyperglycemic state)
  - Tissue damage (rhabdomyolysis, tumor lysis syndrome, burns, trauma)
- Medication-induced (3)
  - RAAS inhibitors
  - K-sparing diuretics
  - NSAIDs
  - Heparin
  - Trimethoprim
  - β-Blockers
- Pseudohyperkalemia
  - Hemolysis of blood sample (artifactual)
  - Thrombolysis, thrombocytosis, leukocytosis
  - Hereditary spherocytosis
  - Infectious mononucleosis
  - Familial pseudohyperkalemia

Genetics

Associated with some inherited diseases and conditions

- Familial hyperkalemic periodic paralysis
- Congenital adrenal hyperplasia
- Gordon syndrome

RISK FACTORS

- Impaired renal excretion of K
- Acidemia
- Massive cell breakdown (rhabdomyolysis, burns, trauma)
- Use of K-sparing diuretics
- Excess K supplementation
- Comorbid conditions: CKD, diabetes, heart failure, liver disease

GENERAL PREVENTION

Low K diet and oral supplement compliance in those at risk

COMMONLY ASSOCIATED CONDITIONS

- Acute kidney injury (AKI) or CKD, typically with GFR <30 mL/min
- Congestive heart failure; myocardial infarction
- Rhabdomyolysis
- Liver disease
- Use of offending medications

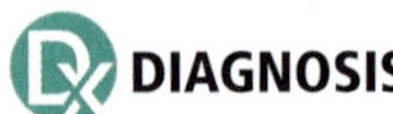

DIAGNOSIS

Serum K level greater than the normal range (3.5 to 5.0 mEq/L); patients may be asymptomatic until >6 mEq/L.

HISTORY

- Neuromuscular cramps, myalgias, muscle weakness or paralysis
- Abdominal pain
- Palpitations, arrhythmia, or cardiac arrest
- Numbness

PHYSICAL EXAM

- Decreased deep tendon reflexes
- Muscle weakness or flaccid paralysis of extremities

DIAGNOSTIC TESTS & INTERPRETATION

- Serum electrolytes
- Renal function: BUN, creatinine
- Urinalysis: K, creatinine, osmoles (to calculate fractional excretion of K and transtubular K gradient; both assess renal handling of K)
- Disorders that may alter lab results
  - Acidemia: K shifts from the intracellular to extracellular space
  - Insulin deficiency
  - Hemolysis of sample
- Cortisol, aldosterone, and renin levels to check for mineralocorticoid deficiency when other causes are ruled out

Diagnostic Procedures/Other

ECG abnormalities usually occur when K ≥7 mEq/L.

- Peaked T wave with shortened QT interval in precordial leads (most common, usually the earliest ECG change; however, neither sensitive nor specific) (4)[C].
- Progressive changes include lengthening of the PR interval, loss of the P wave, and widening of the QRS.
- Sine wave pattern may develop at very high K >8 mEq/L.
- Can eventually lead to arrhythmias including bradycardia, ventricular fibrillation, and asystole

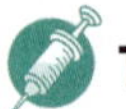

TREATMENT

MEDICATION

- Stabilization of myocardial membranes:
  - Initial treatment with calcium gluconate IV 1,000 mg over 2 to 3 minutes with cardiac monitoring (5)[A]
    - Can repeat after 5 minutes if needed
    - Effect begins within minutes, but only lasts 30 to 60 minutes and should be used in conjunction with definitive therapies.
    - Can also administer IV calcium chloride (3 times as concentrated; however, central or deep vein administration is necessary due to risk of tissue necrosis if extravasation occurs).
- If suspected, stop offending agent and address any reversible causes
- Shifting K intracellularly
  - Regular insulin 10 U IV with dextrose (25 to 50 g) may drive K intracellularly but does not decrease total body K and may result in hypoglycemia (close monitoring advised, especially 1 to 2 hours postinjection) (5)[B].
  - Nebulized albuterol (at 10 to 20 mg/4 mL saline >10 minutes—4 to 8 times bronchodilation dose) and other β-agonists have an additive effect with insulin and glucose (5)[B].
  - Sodium bicarbonate is not routinely recommended but some possible benefits in severe metabolic acidosis (6)[C].
- Remove K from body
  - Cation exchange resins definitive treatment but require several doses and best used with rapidly acting transient therapies above and when dialysis not readily available
  - Gastrointestinal cation exchangers, patiromer calcium (Veltassa), sodium polystyrene sulfonate (Kayexalate), and sodium zirconium cyclosilicate (Lokelma) bind K in the intestinal tract. Patiromer in particular is favored for improved tolerance and decreased side effects in both acute and chronic settings (7)[C].

 - Patiromer calcium (Veltassa): 8.4 g PO daily (dose may vary 4.2 to 16.8 g BID in studies)
   - This requires $\sim$7 to 24 hours to lower K. This may be repeated q12h, if necessary (8)[C].
 - Lokelma: 10 mg PO TID for up to 48 hours
   - This can take effect as early as in 1 hour, but typically within 2 to 4 hours (9)[C].
 - Sodium polystyrene sulfonate (Kayexalate): 15 g PO or 30 g rectally
   - This requires 1 to 4 hours to lower K and may be repeated q6h, if necessary.
   - Enema has faster effect than PO (5)[C].
 - Loop diuretics (furosemide): 20 to 40 mg IV × 1 (dose can be repeated as needed); may need to give isotonic fluids as well if patient is euvolemic or hypovolemic prior to furosemide
 - Hemodialysis is the definitive therapy when other measures are not effective. This may be required particularly when conditions, such as digitalis toxicity, rhabdomyolysis, end-stage renal disease, or severe AKI, are present; should watch for post-dialysis rebound (5)[A]
 - Little clinical evidence for the use of diuretics (loop and thiazides); however, can consider for control of chronic hyperkalemia (5)[B]
- Chronic hyperkalemia treatment
 - Review medication and discontinue those that can be contributing to hyperkalemia.
 - Dietary counseling of K-rich food
 - Diuretic therapy using thiazide and loop diuretics

ALERT
- Sodium polystyrene sulfonate (Kayexalate) provides a sodium load that may exacerbate fluid overload in patients with cardiac or renal failure.
- Avoid sodium polystyrene sulfonate use in patients who are postoperative or with a bowel obstruction or ileus due to high risk of intestinal necrosis.
- Rapid administration of calcium in patients with suspected digitalis toxicity may result in a fatal dysrhythmia. Calcium should be administered slowly over 20 to 30 minutes in 5% dextrose with extreme caution. Preferred therapy is digoxin-specific antibody fragments.

ADDITIONAL THERAPIES
Mineralocorticoid replacement (10)
- If the patient does not have a contraindication (greater than stage 1 HTN, volume overload, history of heart failure) to mineralocorticoid administration then
 - Consider a trial of fludrocortisone 0.1 mg daily × 3 to 5 days (10) (in patients with moderately advanced CKD, consider maintaining or increasing diuretics in tandem with the assistance of nephrology consulting service).

ADMISSION, INPATIENT, AND NURSING CONSIDERATIONS
- If hyperkalemia is severe, treat first, and then do diagnostic investigations.
- IV calcium to stabilize myocardium (caution in setting of digoxin toxicity/digoxin induced hyperkalemia, as this treatment can induce heart block)
- Regular insulin (usually 10 U IV, given with 50 mL of 50% glucose [if serum glucose $<$250 mg/dL] to avoid hypoglycemia); consider repeating if elevation persists.
- Inhaled β_2-agonist (nebulized albuterol)
- Discontinue any medications that may increase K (e.g., K-sparing diuretics, exogenous K).
- Admit for cardiac monitoring if ECG changes are present or if K is $>$6 mEq/L (6 mmol/L).
- Consider if patient meets criteria for emergent hemodialysis.

ONGOING CARE

FOLLOW-UP RECOMMENDATIONS
Patient Monitoring
Serum K levels rechecked every 2 to 4 hours until stabilized.

DIET
Dietary K intake is rarely the only culprit, even in CKD. Recommend $\leq$80 mEq ($\leq$80 mmol) of K per 24 hours if difficult to control hyperkalemia or symptoms (11).

PATIENT EDUCATION
Consult with a dietitian about a low-K diet.

PROGNOSIS
- Associated with poor prognosis in patients with heart failure and CKD
- Associated with poor prognosis in disaster medicine, with trauma, tissue necrosis, K supplementation, metabolic acidosis, if calcium gluconate administered for treatment of hyperkalemia, if AKI, or if prolonged duration of hyperkalemia (6)

COMPLICATIONS
- Life-threatening cardiac arrhythmias
- Potential complications of the use of ion-exchange resins for the treatment of hyperkalemia include volume overload and intestinal necrosis (7)[C].

REFERENCES

1. Betts KA, Woolley JM, Mu F, et al. The prevalence of hyperkalemia in the United States. *Curr Med Res Opin*. 2018;34(6):971–978. doi:10.1080/03007995.2018.1433141.
2. Palmer BF, Clegg DJ. Diagnosis and treatment of hyperkalemia. *Cleve Clin J Med*. 2017;84(12):934–942.
3. Ben Salem C, Badreddine A, Fathallah N, et al. Drug-induced hyperkalemia. *Drug Saf*. 2014;37(9):677–692. doi:10.1007/s40264-014-0196-1.
4. Wong R, Banker R, Aronowitz P. Electrocardiographic changes of severe hyperkalemia. *J Hosp Med*. 2011;6(4):240.
5. Viera AJ, Wouk N. Potassium disorders: hypokalemia and hyperkalemia. *Am Fam Physician*. 2015;92(6):487–495.
6. Khanagavi J, Gupta T, Aronow WS, et al. Hyperkalemia among hospitalized patients and association between duration of hyperkalemia and outcomes. *Arch Med Sci*. 2014;10(2):251–257.
7. Ingelfinger JR. A new era for the treatment of hyperkalemia? *N Engl J Med*. 2015;372(3):275–277.
8. Bushinsky DA, Williams GH, Pitt B, et al. Patiromer induces rapid and sustain potassium lowering in patients with chronic kidney disease and hyperkalemia. *Kidney Int*. 2015;88(6):1427–1433.
9. Peacock WF, Rafique Z, Vishnevskiy K, et al. Emergency potassium normalization treatment including sodium zirconium cyclosilicate: a phase II, randomized, double-blind, placebo-controlled study (ENERGIZE). *Acad Emerg Med*. 2020;27(6):475–486. doi: 10.1111/acem.13954.
10. Mantford JR, Linas S. How dangerous is hyperkalemia? *J Am Soc Nephrol*. 2017;28(11):3155–3165.
11. Ramos CI, González-Ortiz A, Espinosa-Cuevas A, et al. Does dietary potassium intake associate with hyperkalemia in patients with chronic kidney disease? *Nephrol Dial Transplant*. 2021;36(11):2049–2057. doi:10.1093/ndt/gfaa232.

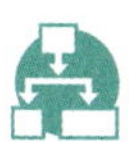

SEE ALSO

- Addison Disease; Hypokalemia
- Algorithm: Hyperkalemia

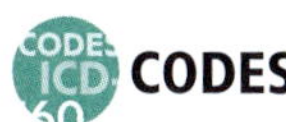

CODES

ICD10
E87.5 Hyperkalemia

CLINICAL PEARLS

- Urgent management of hyperkalemia takes precedence to a thorough diagnostic workup. Urgent treatment includes stabilization of the myocardium with calcium gluconate to protect against arrhythmias and pharmacologic strategies to move K from the extracellular (vascular) space into cells.
- Calcium and dextrose/insulin are only temporizing measures and do not lower total body K levels. Definitive treatment with either dialysis or cation exchange resin (sodium polystyrene sulfonate) is necessary.
- To lower a patient's risk of developing hyperkalemia, recommend a low-K diet, use selective β_1-blockers, such as metoprolol or atenolol, instead of nonselective β-blockers such as carvedilol. Avoid NSAIDs. Concomitant use of kaliuretic loop diuretics may be useful.

HYPERNATREMIA

Katherine Shoemaker Chu, MD • Jane J. Kim, MD

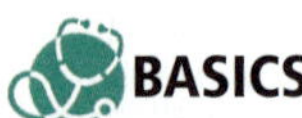

BASICS

DESCRIPTION

- Defined as serum sodium (Na) concentration >145 mEq/L, which usually represents a state of hypertonicity (1),(2)
- Na concentration reflects balance between total body water (TBW) and total body Na. Hypernatremia occurs from deficit of water relative to Na.
- Dehydration refers to hypernatremia from water loss.
- Hypovolemia refers to concomitant water and salt loss.
- Hypernatremia commonly results from net water loss or, more rarely, from primary Na gain.
- Hypernatremia will not develop in patients with intact thirst mechanisms who are able to access and consume water (2).

EPIDEMIOLOGY

Incidence

- More common in elderly and very young due to dependence on others for water access
- Seen in 1–2% of adults with normal kidney function presenting to the emergency department (1).
- Between 4–26% of patients in the ICU will develop hypernatremia during their stay, this has been associated with increased in-hospital mortality (3)

ETIOLOGY AND PATHOPHYSIOLOGY

- Due to the powerful effect of the thirst mechanism, hypernatremia typically occurs in patients who cannot readily access water such as infants, intubated patients, and those with altered mental status or patients with hypodipsia (1).
- Water loss out of proportion to salt loss is the most common cause of hypernatremia. The following conditions lead to excessive water loss (1),(2),(4):
  - Transdermal loss such as burns or excessive sweating (e.g., fever, infants under radiant heaters, heat exposure, extreme exercise)
  - Urinary loss
    - Nephrogenic diabetes insipidus (DI): medication-related, congenital or due to renal dysfunction, hypercalcemia, hypokalemia
    - Central DI: due to head trauma, stroke, meningitis, neoplasm, pituitary infiltration, etc.
    - Osmotic diuresis: glucose, urea, and mannitol
    - Renal losses: loop diuretic use, post-obstructive diuresis, intrinsic kidney disease
  - Gastrointestinal loss
    - Osmotic diarrhea: lactulose, malabsorption, and some types of infectious diarrhea
    - Enterocutaneous fistula
    - Vomiting, NG suction
- Disorders of the thirst mechanism can result in hypernatremia due to reduced water intake (e.g., intracranial lesions, primary hypodipsia, chronic volume expansion in mineralocorticoid excess).
- Excess Na (increase in total body Na) less commonly leads to hypernatremia. The following condition as may result in excessive total body Na:
  - IV infusion of hypertonic NaCl or $NaHCO_3$ during treatment of brain injury, metabolic acidosis, or hyperkalemia
  - Sea water ingestion
  - Excessive use of $NaHCO_3$ antacid
  - Incorrect infant formula preparation, tube feeding
  - Excessive Na in dialysate solutions
- With acute hypernatremia, the rapid decrease in brain volume can cause vascular injury leading to intracranial hemorrhage and possibly irreversible neurologic damage (2),(4).

Genetics

Some forms of DI may be hereditary (see "Diabetes Insipidus" for more information).

RISK FACTORS

- Infants/children
- Elderly patients (may also have a diminished thirst response to osmotic stimulation via an unknown mechanism)
- Patients who are intubated/have altered mental status
- Acute gastrointestinal illness
- Poorly controlled diabetes mellitus
- Prior brain injury
- Surgery
- Diuretic therapy, especially loop diuretics
- Iatrogenic (hypertonic fluids, $NaHCO_3$, etc.)

GENERAL PREVENTION

- Treatment/prevention of underlying cause
- Properly prepare infant formula and never add salt to any commercial infant formula.
- Ensure patients have access to water when appropriate

COMMONLY ASSOCIATED CONDITIONS

- Gastroenteritis
- Altered mental status
- Burns
- Head injury
- High fever

DIAGNOSIS

HISTORY

- History of conditions leading to water loss or impaired thirst: nausea, vomiting, diarrhea, polyuria, fever, heat exposure, extreme exercise, brain injury
- Neurologic symptoms are common:
  - Mild: thirst, anorexia
  - Moderate: altered mental status, myalgia, muscle weakness, twitching, lethargy, irritability, fatigue
  - Severe: seizure (especially if rapid development of hypernatremia), coma, death
- Severity of symptoms correlate with rapidity of the increase in Na as well as the degree of hypernatremia.
- Severe symptoms are likely to occur with sudden increases in plasma Na levels or at concentrations >160 mEq/L.

PHYSICAL EXAM

- Signs of water or volume loss: tachycardia, hypotension, orthostatic hypotension, dry mucous membranes, poor skin turgor
- Neurologic abnormalities: lethargy, weakness, tremor, brisk reflexes/clonus, focal deficits (in cases of intracerebral bleeding/lesion), confusion, coma, seizures

DIFFERENTIAL DIAGNOSIS

- DI (central vs nephrogenic)
- Salt ingestion
- Hypertonic dehydration
- Diabetic crises
- Impaired thirst mechanism
- GI losses (vomiting, diarrhea, NG suction)
- Renal losses (loop diuretics, osmotic diuresis, etc.)

DIAGNOSTIC TESTS & INTERPRETATION

Initial Tests (lab, imaging)

- Serum Na, potassium, BUN, creatinine, glucose, calcium, and osmolality
- Hemoglobin/hematocrit (may be elevated above baseline due to hemoconcentration)
- Urine Na and osmolality (4)
  - Low urine osmolality: urine osmolality (usually <300 mOsm/kg) < serum osmolality suggests DI
  - Intermediate urine osmolality (400 to 800 mOsm/kg) may be from hypovolemia, osmotic diuresis, partial DI
  - High urine osmolality (>800 mOsmol/kg) suggests extrarenal water loss or, rarely, salt ingestion

Follow-Up Tests & Special Considerations

- Special tests for DI
  - Water deprivation test: have patient refrain from drinking water for extended period of time with close sodium, vitals, and urine output monitoring. Patients with DI will continue to have a large output of dilute urine despite deprivation (1).
  - Following this, to distinguish between nephrogenic DI and central DI, desmopressin can be administered.
    - Urine osmolality does not increase after desmopressin administration in nephrogenic DI. Patients with central DI will experience a >50% increase in urine osmolality and decrease in urine volume after desmopressin administration (4).
- Head CT/MRI in patients with central DI or hypodipsia to rule out intracranial lesions

TREATMENT

GENERAL MEASURES

- The treatment of hypernatremia involves treating the underlying cause and correcting the water deficit.
- Determine the duration of hypernatremia because speed of correction depends on symptom severity and rate of development of hypernatremia.
- Acute hypernatremia: relatively uncommon, may occur in acute DI, severe hyperglycemia, or salt ingestion
  - Consider nephrology and/or ICU consultation to aid in management
  - In hypernatremia that developed over minutes to hours: administer D5W to achieve normonatremia, consider emergent dialysis (2)
  - If the hypernatremia developed over 1 to 2 days: D5W infusion with the goal of lowering the serum Na by 2 mEq/L/hr; when serum Na decreases to 145 mEq/L, stop the infusion or continue at a rate aimed at replacing ongoing fluid losses (2).
  - Overcorrection has not been shown to be harmful in these cases (2).
- Chronic hypernatremia (>48 hours): Avoid rapid correction to prevent development of cerebral edema. This risk is greatest in infants and children.
- Correcting hypernatremia through oral/enteral feeding is preferred whenever possible (1)
- If IVF is needed, D5W infusion aimed at correcting the calculated free water deficit (available through MDCalc) in 24 to 48 hours, at a rate of no greater than 10 to 12 mEq/L/day. The rate of the D5W infusion will often need to be adjusted for ongoing water losses (1)[C]
- Check serum Na q4–6 hours to determine correction at desired rate.
- Correct at maximum of 0.5 mEq/L/hr or 10 to 12 mEq/L/day
- There is currently no evidence to support increasing Na in overcorrection of hypernatremia in adults (2)[B]
- Hypernatremia with hypervolemia: can treat hypervolemia with diuretics while simultaneously correcting hypernatremia
  - Concomitant diuretic treatment will increase urinary water losses and may necessitate increased water repletion.
- High infusion rates of D5W may cause hyperglycemia.
- Hyperglycemia-induced osmotic diuresis will increase urinary water losses and necessitate increased water repletion.
- Dialysis can be considered in cases of acute kidney injury and/or oliguria, or after conventional treatment has failed.

MEDICATION

First Line

- See "General Measures" for overall approach because treatment generally includes free water or hypotonic IV fluids rather than medication.
- May use medication in treatment of DI (see "Diabetes Insipidus" for more information).

Second Line

Continuous renal replacement therapy (CRRT): Used in emergent situations including severe, acute hypernatremia with AKI, and/or oliguria, or following failure of treatments outlined above.

ISSUES FOR REFERRAL

Underlying renal involvement associated with hypernatremia would benefit from a nephrology referral.

ADMISSION, INPATIENT, AND NURSING CONSIDERATIONS

- Decision to admit will depend on severity of hypernatremia, access to close follow-up, etiology of hypernatremia, ability to hydrate, acuity of hypernatremia, and comorbidities.
- Consider ICU admission for acute, severe, or symptomatic hypernatremia.
- Will likely need nephrology consultation for oliguria, severe hypernatremia, hypernatremia associated with kidney injury, or if dialysis will be needed.
- Discharge criteria: stabilization of serum Na level and resolution of symptoms

ONGOING CARE

FOLLOW-UP RECOMMENDATIONS

Patient Monitoring

- Frequent neurologic checks during acute correction
- q4–6 hours labs for chronic hypernatremia correction
- Daily weight, electrolytes, and blood glucose throughout hospitalization
- Periodic monitoring of urine osmolality and urine output in DI.

DIET

- Ensure proper nutrition during acute phase.
- After resolution of acute phase, may consider Na-restricted diet for patient depending on etiology of hypernatremia
- Low-salt, low-protein diet in nephrogenic DI

PATIENT EDUCATION

Ensure patients have access to water and are staying hydrated. Ensure infant formulas are mixed appropriately.

PROGNOSIS

Overall prognosis is good as long as hypernatremia is caught and addressed early. Studies have shown that failure to correct hypernatremia in 72 hours is associated with increased mortality in hospitalized patients (1). Acute, severe hypernatremia that is not treated emergently can cause permanent neurologic impairment or even death.

COMPLICATIONS

- More common if rapid development of hypernatremia
- CNS thrombosis/hemorrhage
- Seizures
- Demyelination can occur with rapid increase in serum sodium (2)
- Serum Na >180 mEq/L (>180 mmol/L): often results in residual CNS damage

REFERENCES

1. Miller NE, Rushlow D, Stacey SK. Diagnosis and management of sodium disorders: hyponatremia and hypernatremia. *Am Fam Physician*. 2023;108(5):476–486.
2. Sterns RH. Disorders of plasma sodium—causes, consequences, and correction. *N Engl J Med*. 2015;372(1):55–65.
3. Olsen MH, Møller M, Romano S, et al. Association between ICU-acquired hypernatremia and in-hospital mortality: data from the Medical Information Mart for Intensive Care III and the Electronic ICU Collaborative Research Database. *Crit Care Explor*. 2020;2(12):e0304. doi:10.1097/CCE.0000000000000304.
4. Muhsin SA, Mount DB. Diagnosis and treatment of hypernatremia. *Best Pract Res Clin Endocrinol Metab*. 2016;30(2):189–203. doi:10.1016/j.beem.2016.02.014.

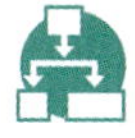

SEE ALSO

- Diabetes Insipidus
- Algorithm: Hypernatremia

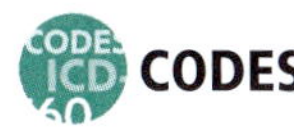

CODES

ICD10

- P74.21 Hypernatremia of newborn
- E87.0 Hyperosmolality and hypernatremia

CLINICAL PEARLS

- Occurs from water deficit in comparison to total body Na stores
- Common causes include dehydration, DI, impaired access to fluids.
- Avoid rapid correction of chronic hypernatremia to prevent development of cerebral edema (goal rate is 10 mEq/L in 24 hours).
- Monitor serum Na and adjust water repletion to achieve desired rate of correction as available formulas for calculating water deficit and estimating ongoing water losses have limited accuracy.

H

HYPERPARATHYROIDISM

Juan Perez, DO

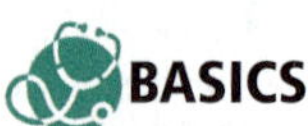

BASICS

DESCRIPTION

Excess production of parathyroid hormone (PTH)

- Primary hyperparathyroidism (HPT): intrinsic parathyroid gland dysfunction resulting in excessive secretion of PTH with a lack of response to feedback inhibition by elevated calcium
- Secondary HPT: appropriate increased secretion of PTH in response to hypocalcemia and/or hyperphosphatemia; can be caused by vitamin D deficiency, kidney dysfunction, decreased calcium intake or absorption, and/or phosphate loading
- Tertiary HPT: autonomous hyperfunction of the parathyroid gland in the setting of long-standing secondary HPT

EPIDEMIOLOGY

Prevalence

- Primary HPT is 1 in 500 to 1 in 1,000 in the United States.
- Primary HPT and malignancies are the etiology for 90% of patients with hypercalcemia.
- Neoplasia is the most frequent cause of hypercalcemia in hospitalized and emergency room patients and primary HPT is responsible for most cases outside the hospital setting (1),(2).
- Predominantly postmenopausal females

ETIOLOGY AND PATHOPHYSIOLOGY

PTH is synthesized by the four parathyroid glands, which are located behind the thyroid gland, and mostly regulated by calcium levels.

- Ectopic (abnormal locations and most common is the thymus) or supernumerary glands (more than four glands)
- PTH releases calcium from bone by osteoclastic stimulation (increasing bone resorption).
- PTH increases reabsorption of calcium in the distal tubules of the kidneys.
- PTH increases phosphorus excretion by decreasing reabsorption in the proximal tubules of the kidneys.
- PTH stimulates conversion of 25-hydroxycholecalciferol (25[OH]D) to 1,25-dihydroxycholecalciferol (1,25[OH]$_2$D or active vitamin D) in the kidneys. 1,25(OH)$_2$D increases calcium and phosphate absorption from the GI tract and kidneys, and stimulates osteoclastic activity and bone resorption.
- Primary HPT: unregulated PTH production and release due to the loss of normal feedback control by extracellular calcium, causing increase in serum calcium
  - Solitary adenoma (80–85%)
  - Diffuse parathyroid gland hyperplasia (10–15%), either sporadically or in association with multiple endocrine neoplasia
  - Parathyroid carcinoma (<1%)
- Secondary HPT: adaptive parathyroid gland hyperplasia and hyperfunction from decreased calcium
  - Dietary from vitamin D deficiency causes decreased calcium absorption or calcium deficiency
  - Chronic renal disease including renal parenchymal loss causing hyperphosphatemia; impaired calcitriol production causing hypocalcemia
- Tertiary HPT: autonomous oversecretion of PTH following prolonged parathyroid stimulation

Genetics

- A genetic basis of primary HPT identified in about 10% of all cases
- Patients with multiple gland hyperplasia in the absence of renal disease should be screened for MEN-I gene mutation.
- Neonatal severe primary HPT: Infants born without both calcium-sensing receptor (CaSR) gene alleles
- HPT—jaw tumor syndrome
- Familial hypocalciuric hypercalcemia (FHH): loss of one CaSR gene alleles

RISK FACTORS

Chronic kidney disease, increasing age, poor nutrition, radiation, and/or family history

GENERAL PREVENTION

Adequate intake of calcium and vitamin D may help prevent secondary HPT.

COMMONLY ASSOCIATED CONDITIONS

- Vitamin D deficiency
- Chronic renal failure

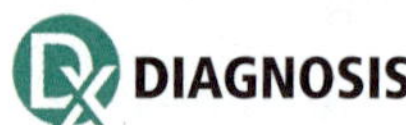

DIAGNOSIS

HISTORY

- History of present illness
  - Almost 80% of patients are asymptomatic.
  - Kidney stones (15–20%)
  - Symptoms due to hypercalcemia like mental fogginess, memory impairment, polyuria, polydipsia, constipation, nausea, anorexia, bone pain, decreased concentration, altered mental status, fatigue, and muscle weakness
  - Higher PTH levels are associated with more features such as renal disease and fragility fractures.
- Past medical history
  - The following conditions may be associated with HPT:
    - MEN syndromes, nephrolithiasis (in 20–30%), nephrocalcinosis, pancreatitis, gastroduodenal ulcer, hypertension, short QT interval, left ventricular hypertrophy, osteitis fibrosa cystica, cystic bone lesions, spontaneous fracture, vertebral collapse, osteoporosis, gout, pseudogout, anxiety, depression, psychosis, coma, conjunctivitis, band keratopathy, conjunctival calcium deposits
- Medications: hydrochlorothiazide or lithium (decreases parathyroid sensitivity to calcium in small subset of patients)

PHYSICAL EXAM

- 70–80% of patients have no obvious symptoms or signs of disease.
- Physical findings related to the underlying cause of HPT may be found.

DIFFERENTIAL DIAGNOSIS

- Increased PTH: Ectopic PTH production is rare, but first rule out:
  - FHH: Rule out FHH with a 24-hour urine calcium:creatinine ratio.
  - Drug side effect (thiazide diuretics and lithium)
- Nonparathyroid causes
  - Malignancy: lung (squamous cell) carcinoma, breast carcinoma, multiple myeloma, lymphoma, leukemia, prostate cancer
  - Granulomatous diseases: sarcoidosis, tuberculosis, berylliosis, histoplasmosis, coccidioidomycosis
  - Drugs: vitamin D intoxication, milk-alkali syndrome, thiazide diuretics
  - Endocrine: hyperthyroidism, acute adrenal insufficiency
  - High bone turnover: immobilization, Paget disease

DIAGNOSTIC TESTS & INTERPRETATION

Initial Tests (lab, imaging)

- Often detected by incidental hypercalcemia on routine labs
- Calculate corrected calcium: [serum calcium in mg/dL + 0.8 × (4 − patient's albumin in g/dL)]; alternatively, order an ionized calcium level.
- If hypercalcemia is confirmed, follow with intact PTH level (3)[B].
  - PTH-dependent: High or (abnormally) normal PTH suggests primary HPT.
  - PTH-independent: Undetectable or low PTH suggests PTH-independent hypercalcemia.
- Other findings may include low serum phosphate and high 24-hour urine calcium excretion.
- In secondary HPT, an elevated phosphorus suggests chronic renal failure; a low phosphorus suggests another cause, commonly 25(OH)D deficiency. Both are common causes of elevated PTH levels while having normal corrected calcium levels.

Follow-Up Tests & Special Considerations

- A 24-hour urine calcium concentration to creatinine clearance ratio >0.02 suggests primary HPT; a ratio <0.01 may be normal or indicate FHH; an important finding because FHH does not require surgery (3)[B]
- Routine measurement of 25(OH)D levels is recommended in all patients with primary HPT. In case of vitamin D deficiency (<20 ng/mL or <50 nmol/L), defer management decisions until levels are maintained >20 ng/mL (50 nmol/L) (3)[B].

Diagnostic Procedures/Other

- Imaging is not required for diagnosis. It is required for surgical planning, especially for minimally invasive parathyroidectomy (MIP).
  - Imaging is also indicated to localize hyperplasia or an ectopic parathyroid gland in repeat surgery.
- Imaging options for presurgical localization
  - Technetium-99m sestamibi with or without single-photon emission computed tomography (SPECT): it has the greatest reported success in localizing single parathyroid adenomas but often inaccurate in multigland disease.
  - Neck ultrasound (US): painless, noninvasive, and does not expose the patient to radiation; however, its accuracy is operator-dependent (4)[C].
  - Four-dimensional CT (4D-CT) may be more effective for primary localization than both US and sestamibi-SPECT (4)[B].

– Positron emission tomography (PET) using C-methionine (MET-PET) is comparable to US and technetium-99m sestamibi with SPECT in terms of diagnostic use.
– CT and MRI are mostly used to localize ectopic mediastinal glands.

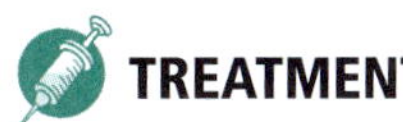

TREATMENT

MEDICATION

- Primary HPT: Operative management is curative; indications for surgical intervention are mentioned below. For those awaiting or unable to have surgery:
  - Bisphosphonates (alendronate): reduce bone turnover and help to maintain bone density; avoid in kidney disease (GFR ≤35).
  - Calcimimetics (cinacalcet) (3)[B]: activates CaSR in parathyroid gland thereby inhibiting PTH secretion; FDA-approved for symptomatic patients who are unfit for surgery; no long-term data on its effect on constitutional, neuropsychologic symptoms, or fractures
  - Selective estrogen receptor modulator therapy (raloxifene): antagonizes PTH-mediated bone resorption
    - Hormone replacement therapy with estrogens is not recommended as first-line treatment; must weigh benefit with risks of known systemic effects; can be used in postmenopausal women who do not undergo or refuse surgery
- Secondary HPT: Treatment is often aimed at underlying etiology.
  - Calcium replacement
  - Vitamin D analogues (paricalcitol and calcitriol)
  - Phosphorus-binding agents (sevelamer)
  - Calcimimetic (cinacalcet)
- Tertiary HPT
  - Medical treatment is not curative and generally not indicated.

SURGERY/OTHER PROCEDURES

- Operative management is curative for patients with primary HPT in 95–98% of patients. It is the first-line treatment for pediatrics. It is also usually the first-line treatment for young adults up ot 50 years of age (5)[C].
- Indications for parathyroidectomy
  - Symptomatic primary HPT
    - Nephrolithiasis
    - Fragility fractures
    - Osteitis fibrosa cystica
  - Asymptomatic primary HPT (6)[C]
    - Serum Ca^+ level >1 mg/dL above normal
    - Age <50 years
    - Creatinine clearance <60 mL/min
    - 24-hour urine for calcium >400 mg/day (>10 mmol/day) and increased stone risk by biochemical stone risk analysis
    - Presence of nephrolithiasis or nephrocalcinosis by x-ray, US, or CT
    - Bone density loss with a T-score <−2.5 at the lumbar spine, femoral neck, total hip, or distal 1/3 radius
- Surgical removal of diseased gland or tissue is only proven curative therapy for HPT; options include:
  - Bilateral open neck exploratory surgery
  - MIP using preoperative sestamibi scan with SPECT/US/4D-CT and intraoperative PTH levels (high sensitivity 79–95% to predict location of single parathyroid adenoma) (7), which result in decreased pain, smaller incisions, improved cosmetic results, lower morbidity, and decreased length of hospital stay when compared with open neck exploratory surgery
- Follow postoperative serum calcium, magnesium, and phosphorus levels; monitor closely for hypocalcemia "hungry bone" syndrome.
- Patients may need IV calcium infusion postoperatively with oral calcitriol and calcium supplementation initially. Hungry bone pain syndrome can be severe, although less common now.

ADMISSION, INPATIENT, AND NURSING CONSIDERATIONS

Critical hypercalcemia requires IV fluid rehydration, saline diuresis with IV saline and loop diuretics, IV bisphosphonate therapy, and SC calcitonin (4 U/kg q12h), corticosteroids, and hemodialysis (8) for severe symptoms.

ONGOING CARE

FOLLOW-UP RECOMMENDATIONS

Patient Monitoring

In patients with primary HPT who are asymptomatic, measurement of serum calcium and creatinine annually and bone density scan every 1 to 2 years is sufficient (6)[C].

DIET

- In the presence of hypercalciuria or elevated $1,25(OH)_2D$ levels, dietary calcium restriction is recommended. Otherwise, daily calcium intake should be maintained at up to 1,000 mg.
- Restrict dietary phosphate in secondary HPT.

PATIENT EDUCATION

Signs of severe hypercalcemia

PROGNOSIS

Prognosis after surgery is excellent in primary HPT, with resolution of many of the preoperative symptoms.

COMPLICATIONS

Related to high levels of PTH and/or elevated calcium

REFERENCES

1. Jacobi J. Management of endocrine emergencies in the ICU. *J Pharm Pract*. 2019;32(3):314–326.
2. Endres DB. Investigation of hypercalcemia. *Clin Biochem*. 2012;45(12):954–963.
3. Silva BC, Cusano NE, Bilezikian JP. Primary hyperparathyroidism. *Best Pract Res Clin Endocrinol Metab*. 2024;38(1):101247. doi:10.1016/j.beem.2018.09.013.
4. Cheung K, Wang TS, Farrokhyar F, et al. A meta-analysis of preoperative localization techniques for patients with primary hyperparathyroidism. *Ann Surg Oncol*. 2012;19(2):577–583.
5. Markowitz ME, Underland L, Gensure R. Parathyroid disorders. *Pediatr Rev*. 2016;37(12):524–535.
6. Bilezikian JP, Brandi ML, Eastell R, et al. Guidelines for the management of asymptomatic primary hyperparathyroidism: summary statement from the Fourth International Workshop. *J Clin Endocrinol Metab*. 2014;99(10):3561–3569.
7. Kunstman JW, Kirsch JD, Mahajan A, et al. Clinical review: parathyroid localization and implications for clinical management. *J Clin Endocrinol Metab*. 2013;98(3):902–912.
8. Kulkarni P, Tucker J, King T, et al. Symptomatic versus asymptomatic primary hyperparathyroidism: a systematic review and meta-analysis. *J Clin Transl Endocrinol*. 2023;32:100317.

ADDITIONAL READING

Salvatore M, Arnold A, Belaya Z, et al. Epidemiology, pathophysiology, and genetics of primary hyperparathyroidism. *J Bone Miner Res*. 2022;37(11):2315–2329.

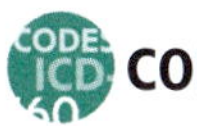

CODES

ICD10

- E21.3 Hyperparathyroidism, unspecified
- N25.81 Secondary hyperparathyroidism of renal origin
- E21.1 Secondary hyperparathyroidism, not elsewhere classified

CLINICAL PEARLS

- 80% of patients with primary HPT are asymptomatic.
- HPT is often detected by an incidental finding of hypercalcemia on a routine serum chemistry analysis.
- Classic symptoms of HPT include painful bones, renal stones, abdominal pain, and behavioral changes (stones, bones, moans, and groans).
- Repeat calcium (elevated), correct for serum albumin, and obtain intact PTH levels to make an initial diagnosis.
- Secondary HPT is due to excessive secretion of PTH in response to hypocalcemia, which can be caused by vitamin D deficiency or renal failure.
- In patients with primary HPT who are asymptomatic, measurement of serum calcium and creatinine annually and bone density scan every 1 to 2 years is sufficient.

H

HYPERPROLACTINEMIA

D'Ann Wilson Somerall, FAANP, FNP-BC, DNP, CRNP, MAEd • William E. Somerall Jr., MD, MAEd

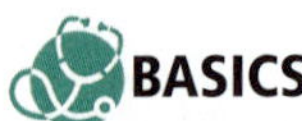

BASICS

DESCRIPTION

Hyperprolactinemia is an abnormal elevation in the serum prolactin (PRL) level from either physiologic or pathologic influences of the lactotroph cells of the pituitary gland.

EPIDEMIOLOGY

Incidence

In the general population, hyperprolactinemia affects 5 to 20 people per 100,000 per year.

Prevalence

- Predominant age: reproductive age
- Predominant sex: female (70%) > male (30%)
- More readily detected in females because a slight elevation in PRL causes changes in menstruation and galactorrhea; men present with headache, visual disturbances, and erectile dysfunction (1).
- Adenomas in men are typically larger because of delayed onset of symptoms (1).

ETIOLOGY AND PATHOPHYSIOLOGY

- PRL, which is produced by lactotrophs in the anterior pituitary, is regulated by:
  - Inhibitory factors, primarily dopamine, are produced in the hypothalamus and delivered via the hypothalamic-pituitary vessels in the pituitary stalk.
  - Stimulatory factors, primarily thyrotropin-releasing hormone (TRH)
- Causes of hyperprolactinemia include the following:
  - Physiologic
    - Pregnancy due to increased estrogen
    - Breastfeeding or nipple stimulation
    - Stress, including postoperative state
    - Medications—concentrations are typically in the 25 to 100 ng/mL range (2)[A].
      - Dopamine (D_2) blockers: prochlorperazine, metoclopramide
      - Dopamine depleting: α-methyldopa, reserpine
      - Antidepressants: tricyclic antidepressants (TCAs); paroxetine (an SSRI) causes transient hyperprolactinemia—usually resolves in 7 to 10 days
      - Gastric motility drugs: metoclopramide and domperidone
      - Verapamil (but no other calcium channel blockers; thought to decrease the hypothalamic synthesis of dopamine)
      - Older antipsychotics (category is the most common cause of medication-induced): haloperidol, fluphenazine, risperidone (level of elevation with risperidone greater than with other antipsychotics)
      - Newer antipsychotics (asenapine, iloperidone, lurasidone) may cause elevation but less than the older antipsychotics (1).
  - Pathologic
    - Hypothyroidism (due to elevated TRH)
    - Chest wall conditions such as herpes zoster, trauma, or postthoracotomy
    - PRL-secreting adenoma in the anterior pituitary (microadenoma: <1 cm; macroadenoma: >1 cm)
    - Pituitary stalk compression/disruption:
      - Craniopharyngioma, Rathke cleft cyst
      - Meningioma, astrocytoma
      - Metastases
      - Head trauma
      - Infiltrative/inflammatory disorders
    - Diminished PRL clearance (chronic renal failure, cirrhosis, cocaine)
  - Idiopathic hyperprolactinemia—a substantial number of cases where the serum levels are between 20 and 100 ng/mL the cause cannot be found (3)[A].

Genetics

Unknown

RISK FACTORS

See causes in "Etiology and Pathophysiology" section.

GENERAL PREVENTION

Avoid offending medications.

COMMONLY ASSOCIATED CONDITIONS

- Infertility
- Osteoporosis
- Amenorrhea
- Gynecomastia

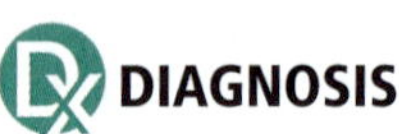

DIAGNOSIS

Based on clinical history, physical exam, and laboratory findings; symptoms listed below are typically found in premenopausal women. Postmenopausal women are typically diagnosed due to headaches, or impaired vision where an incidental finding of a lactotroph adenoma via MRI.

HISTORY

- Galactorrhea
- Amenorrhea or oligomenorrhea
- Infertility
- Osteoporosis/osteopenia
- Decreased libido, impotence
- Weight gain
- Pregnancy
- Chronic kidney disease
- Also, may have signs and symptoms of pituitary enlargement:
  - Headache
  - Visual field impairment (bitemporal hemianopia)
  - Hypopituitarism (secondary to tumor pressure on surrounding structures)
- Also, may have signs and symptoms of associated conditions:
  - Hypothyroidism
  - Cushing disease
  - Acromegaly
  - Multiple endocrine neoplasia (MEN)-1 syndrome

PHYSICAL EXAM

- Visual field testing (bitemporal field loss)
- Cranial nerve exam
- Examination of chest wall for lesions
- Signs of hypothyroidism

DIFFERENTIAL DIAGNOSIS

Macroprolactinemia: Macroprolactin, a polymer of several units of PRL, is detected by immunologically based lab tests but is not biologically active. If the patient is asymptomatic but found to have elevated PRL, consider this diagnosis and notify the lab. No treatment is required.

DIAGNOSTIC TESTS & INTERPRETATION

- Serum PRL (most accurate results if checked fasting, in morning; food only has a small effect on concentrations, thus fasting is not required, but if elevated levels, repeat on a fasting specimen)
  <25 μg/L normal; >25 μg/L abnormal; >30 in postmenopausal women; >250 μg/L often indicates a prolactinoma (4)[A].
- Pregnancy test
- Thyroid-stimulating hormone (TSH)
- Luteinizing hormone (LH)/follicle-stimulating hormone (FSH) if amenorrheic
- Chem panel

Initial Tests (lab, imaging)

A single measurement of serum PRL (levels drawn prior to a breast exam)—a level above the upper limit of normal confirms the diagnosis

- Pituitary MRI: single best imaging

Follow-Up Tests & Special Considerations

Formal visual field testing if pituitary adenoma is suspected

Diagnostic Procedures/Other

CT scan if MRI is contraindicated

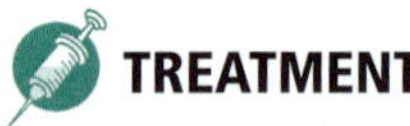

TREATMENT

GENERAL MEASURES

- Discontinue offending medications, if any (4)[A].
- Treat underlying causes (4)[A].
- For asymptomatic patients with mild PRL elevations, observation alone may be considered (4)[A],(5)[A].
- Medications indicated for (4)[A]:
  - Symptoms of hypogonadism, such as decreased libido
  - Galactorrhea (if bothersome to patient)
  - Restoration of fertility
  - Pituitary adenoma
  - Prevention of osteoporosis

MEDICATION

First Line

- Dopamine agonists: Decrease serum PRL concentrations and decrease the size of the most lactotroph adenomas.
- Cabergoline (Dostinex): This is now the first-line choice due to efficacy and favorable side effect profile (4)[A],(6)[A]: dosed 0.25 mg twice weekly or 0.5 once a week. Although more expensive, cabergoline was more effective than bromocriptine in reducing persistent hyperprolactinemia, galactorrhea, and amenorrhea/oligomenorrhea (5)[A]; has recently been reported to be associated with significant improvements in the body mass index, total HDL and LDL cholesterol levels, and insulin sensitivity (7); decrease in proinflammatory markers; and carotid intima-media thickness, indicated with bromocriptine failure or resistance; has been shown to reduce erectile dysfunction in hyperprolactinemic men (4)[A]
- Adverse effects (better tolerated if start with low dose, slow titration, given at night with food):
  - Nausea/vomiting
  - Headache, dizziness, fatigue
  - Postural hypotension (5)[A]
- Contraindications
  - Uncontrolled hypertension
  - Cardiac valvular disorders
  - Pulmonary, pericardial, or retroperitoneal fibrotic disorders
- Bromocriptine (Parlodel): This has the longest clinical history: dosed BID; begin at 1.25 mg once at bedtime or after dinner for 1 week then increase to BID; preferred by some clinicians when infertility is an indication for treatment (2)[A],(5)[A]
- Both are effective for reducing tumor size and improving symptoms (5)[A].
- SE less with cabergoline than bromocriptine (5)[A]

Second Line

Pergolide (Permax) is no longer used in the United States. If patient is still on this medication, do not withdraw abruptly.

ADDITIONAL THERAPIES

Patients with medically and surgically refractory prolactinomas; radiotherapy produced a reduction in PRL levels in nearly all patients and normalization in over a quarter of patients with low complication rates (5)[A].

SURGERY/OTHER PROCEDURES

- For adenomas, medical treatment will be successful in 80–90% of patients. In some cases, surgery is indicated (4):
  - Intolerance or resistance to medical treatment
  - Headache
  - Visual field loss
  - CSF leak due to tumor apoplexy or shrinkage
  - Cranial nerve deficit
- Risks include a high recurrence rate (up to 40%), CSF leakage, meningitis, pituitary insufficiency, and transient diabetes insipidus (6).

ONGOING CARE

FOLLOW-UP RECOMMENDATIONS

Reevaluate lab levels after 1 month; if normal, continue the initial dose. If lab levels do not decrease, but patient experiences no side effects increase cabergoline to 1.25 mg 2 to 3 times per week or bromocriptine to 5 mg twice a day.

Patient Monitoring

- After at least 2 years of treatment, no tumor and PRL levels normal may consider decreasing and stopping medication; must be followed closely, as the tumor may grow back (4)
- Consider:
  - Formal visual field testing yearly (2)[A]
  - Serial MRIs if clinically indicated (2)[A]

Pregnancy Considerations

- If pregnancy is desired in a woman with hyperprolactinemia, dopamine agonists are not approved during pregnancy and should be discontinued once pregnancy is confirmed, but their use is recommended if neurologic findings are present (4)[A].
- With microprolactinoma: Treat with bromocriptine if symptomatic; monthly pregnancy tests; discontinue bromocriptine when pregnancy is confirmed.
- With macroprolactinomas: A definitive, individualized plan is made. Options include discontinuation of bromocriptine at conception and careful monitoring of PRL levels and VS, with or without MRI scan evidence of tumor enlargement; prepregnancy transsphenoidal surgery with debulking of tumor; continuation of bromocriptine throughout gestation, with a risk to the fetus.
- Careful monitoring of visual fields in each trimester; no need to monitor PRL levels, as they are normally high due to pregnancy (4)[A].

PATIENT EDUCATION

Discuss risks of untreated hyperprolactinemia:

- Headache
- Visual field loss
- Decreased bone density
- Infertility

PROGNOSIS

- Following treatment for 1 to 2 years, if PRL levels have remained normal, consider stopping meds.
- 5–10% of microadenomas may progress to macroadenomas.
- Follow-up imaging not needed unless signs or symptoms of enlarging tumor
- >10 years, 7% chance of progression of PRL-secreting microadenoma (2)

COMPLICATIONS

- If pituitary adenoma, risk of permanent visual field loss
- For patients with high doses of cabergoline, suggest cardiac US every 2 years.

REFERENCES

1. Somerall WE Jr, Somerall DW. Hyperprolactinemia: the ABCs of diagnosis and management. *Women's Healthcare*. 2020;8(6):6–12.
2. Casanueva FF, Molitch ME, Schlechte JA, et al. Guidelines of the Pituitary Society for the diagnosis and management of prolactinomas. *Clin Endocrinol (Oxf)*. 2006;65(2):265–273.
3. Inder WJ, Castle D. Antipsychotic-induced hyperprolactinaemia. *Aust N Z J Psychiatry*. 2011;45(10):830–837.
4. Hoffman AR, Melmed S, Schlechte J. Patient guide to hyperprolactinemia diagnosis and treatment. *J Clin Endocrinol Metab*. 2011;96(2):35A–36A.
5. Wang AT, Mullan RJ, Lane MA, et al. Treatment of hyperprolactinemia: a systematic review and meta-analysis. *Syst Rev*. 2012;1:33.
6. Bloomgarden E, Molitch ME. Surgical treatment of prolactinomas: cons. *Endocrine*. 2014;47(3):730–733.
7. Inancli SS, Usluogullari A, Ustu Y, et al. Effect of cabergoline on insulin sensitivity, inflammation, and carotid intima media thickness in patients with prolactinoma. *Endocrine*. 2013;44(1):193–199.

ADDITIONAL READING

- Das L, Dutta P. Association of primary hyperparathyroidism with pituitary adenoma and management issues. *Best Pract Res Clin Endocrinol Metab*. 2025;39(2):101978. doi:10.1016/j.beem.2025.101978.
- Klibanski A. Clinical practice. Prolactinomas. *N Engl J Med*. 2010;362(13):1219–1226.

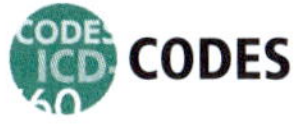

CODES

ICD10

E22.1 Hyperprolactinemia

CLINICAL PEARLS

- If a cause for hyperprolactinemia cannot be found by history, examination, and routine laboratory testing (>250 μg/L often indicates a prolactinoma), an intracranial lesion might be the cause and brain MRI with specific pituitary cuts and intravenous contrast media should be performed.
- Treatment of hyperprolactinemia should be targeted at correcting the cause (hypothyroidism, discontinuation of offending medications, etc.).
- There is a difference among antipsychotics in influencing PRL levels. In general, those with the highest potency D_2 antagonism are most likely to elevate PRL levels. Among the newer atypical antipsychotics, risperidone has been identified as more likely to elevate PRL.
- High PRL levels decrease testosterone by inhibiting gonadotropin-releasing hormone (GnRH), LH, and FSH secretion and by decreasing central dopamine activity, both of which are important in mediating sexual arousal.

H

HYPERSENSITIVITY PNEUMONITIS

Anna Brickell, MD • Brittany Lauren Carmack, MD

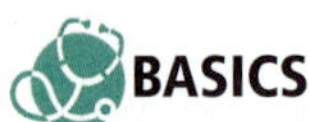

BASICS

DESCRIPTION

- Hypersensitivity pneumonitis (HP) is also called extrinsic allergic alveolitis (EAA).
- HP is a diffuse inflammatory disease of the lung parenchyma caused by an immunologic reaction to aerosolized antigenic particles found in a variety of environments. Classification depends on time frame involved:
  - Acute: fever, chills, diaphoresis, myalgias, nausea; cough and dyspnea are common but not necessarily present. Occurs 4 to 12 hours after heavy exposure to an inciting agent. Symptoms subside within 12 hours to several days after removal from exposure. Complete resolution occurs within weeks.
  - Subacute: mainly caused by continual low-level antigen exposure, could have a low-grade fever in the 1st week; cough, dyspnea, fatigue, anorexia, weight loss—develop over days to weeks
  - Chronic: from recurrent exposure either acute or subacute cases; prolonged and progressive cough, dyspnea, fatigue, weight loss; could lead to fibrosis and respiratory failure
- Farmer's lung is an old term of this disease, a type of HP, particular to the farmer population; causative agent is a bacterium found in moldy hay or straw. Farmer's lung now has new and different etiologies due to modernization of farming practices.

EPIDEMIOLOGY

- Not well-defined; tends to occur in adults as a result of occupation-related exposure, but some home environmental exposures are also seen
- HP is increasingly recognized as an important cause of fibrotic interstitial lung disease (1).

Incidence

0.9/100,000

Prevalence

- Farmers: 1–19% exposed farmers
- Bird fanciers: 6–20% exposed individuals
- Others: 1–8% exposed

ETIOLOGY AND PATHOPHYSIOLOGY

- Hypersensitivity reaction involving immune complexes: Inhaled antigens bind to IgG, triggering complement cascade (types III and IV immunologic reactions) (1).
- Cellular-mediated reaction: T cell–mediated immune inflammatory response
- Farming, vegetable, or dairy cattle workers
  - Moldy hay, grain, silage: thermophilic actinomycetes, such as *Faenia rectivirgula*
  - Mold on pressed sugar cane: *Thermoactinomyces sacchari*, *Thymus vulgaris*
  - Tobacco plants: *Aspergillus* sp., *Scopulariopsis brevicaulis*
  - Mushroom worker's lung: *Saccharopolyspora rectivirgula*, *T. vulgaris*, *Aspergillus* spp.
  - Potato riddler's lung: thermophilic actinomycetes, *T. vulgaris*, *F. rectivirgula*, *Aspergillus* sp.
  - Wine maker's lung: *Mucor stolonifer*
  - Cheese washer's lung: *Penicillium caseifulvum*, *Aspergillus clavatus*
  - Coffee worker's lung: coffee bean dust
  - Tea grower's lung: tea plants
- Ventilation and water-related contamination
  - Contaminated humidifiers and air conditioners: amoebae, nematodes, yeasts, bacteria
  - Unventilated shower: *Epicoccum nigrum*
  - Hot-tub lung: *Cladosporium* sp., *Mycobacterium avium complex*
  - Sauna taker's lung: *Aureobasidium* sp.
  - Summer-type pneumonitis: *Trichosporon cutaneum*
  - Swimming pool lifeguard's lung: aerosolized endotoxin and *M. avium complex*
  - Contaminated basement pneumonitis: *Cephalosporium* and *Penicillium* spp.
- Bird and poultry handling
  - Bird fancier's lung: droppings, feathers, serum proteins
  - Poultry worker's lung: serum proteins
  - Turkey-handling disease: serum proteins
  - Canary fancier's lung: serum proteins
  - Duck fever: feathers, serum proteins
- Veterinary work and animal handling
  - Laboratory worker's lung: urine, serum, pelts, proteins
  - Pituitary snuff taker's disease: dried, powdered neurohypophysis
  - Furrier's lung: animal pelts
  - Bat lung: bat serum protein
  - Fish meal worker's lung: fish meal
  - Coptic lung: cloth wrapping of mummies
  - Mollusc shell HP: sea-snail shell
  - Pearl oyster shell pneumonitis: oyster shells
- Grain and flour
  - Grain measurer's lung: cereal grain, grain dust
  - Miller's lung: *Sitophilus granarius*
  - Malt worker's disease: *Aspergillus fumigatus*, *A. clavatus*
- Lumber milling, construction, wood stripping, paper, wallboard manufacture
  - Wood dust pneumonitis: *Alternaria* sp., *Bacillus subtilis*
  - Sequoiosis: *Graphium*, *Pullularia*, *Trichoderma* sp., *Aureobasidium pullulans*
  - Maple bark disease: *Cryptostroma corticale*
  - Wood trimmer's disease: *Rhizopus* sp., *Mucor* sp.
  - Wood pulp worker's disease: *Penicillium* sp.
  - Suberosis: *Trogon viridis*, *Penicillium glabrum*
- Plastic manufacturing, painting, electronics, chemicals
  - Chemical HP: diphenyl diisocyanate, toluene diisocyanate
  - Detergent worker's lung: *B. subtilis* enzymes
  - Pauli reagent alveolitis: sodium diazobenzene sulfate
  - Vineyard sprayer's lung: copper sulfate
  - Pyrethrum pneumonitis: *pyrethroids*
  - Epoxy resin lung: phthalic anhydride
  - Bible printer's lung: moldy typesetting water
  - Machine operator's lung: *Pseudomonas fluorescens*, aerosolized metal working fluid
- Textile workers
  - Byssinosis: cotton mill dust
  - Velvet worker's lung: nylon, tannic acid, potato starch
  - Upholstery fabric: aflatoxin-producing fungus, *Fusarium* sp.
  - Lycoperdonosis: puffball spores

Genetics

No evidence of clear genetic susceptibility; possible genetic predisposition involving tumor necrosis factor alpha (TNF-α) and major histocompatibility complex (MHC) class II genes (1)[B]

RISK FACTORS

- Contact with organic antigens increases risk of developing HP. Viral infection at time of exposure may increase risk.
- Nonsmokers have an increased incidence of HP compared with smokers. The mechanisms that account for the "protective" effect of smoking are poorly understood, but nicotine is thought to inhibit macrophage activation and lymphocyte proliferation and function (1).
  - Smokers have a diminished antibody response to inhaled antigens.
  - However, smokers who develop disease tend to have the chronic form, and mortality is higher.

GENERAL PREVENTION

Avoidance of offending antigen and/or use of protective equipment

COMMONLY ASSOCIATED CONDITIONS

Constrictive bronchiolitis

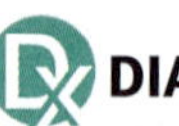

DIAGNOSIS

- Diagnosis criteria most widely used but not validated: (i) history and physical and pulmonary function tests (PFTs) indicating restriction or diffusion disease; DL_{co} is the most frequently affected lung parameter, but may be normal in up to 22% of patients; (ii) radiologic imaging consistent with interstitial lung disease; (iii) exposure to a recognized cause; (iv) proof of sensitization in bronchoalveolar lavage (BAL) fluids (serum precipitins and/or lymphocytosis)
- Six significant predictors: exposure to a known antigen, positive antibodies precipitating, (if identified) recurrent episodes of symptoms, inspiratory crackles, symptoms 4 to 8 hours after exposure, weight loss (1)
- Acute form: develops 4 to 12 hours following exposure; cough, dyspnea without wheezing, fever, chills, diaphoresis, headache, nausea, malaise, chest tightness; symptoms last hours to days.
- Sequela (prior subacute, chronic): gradual or progressive productive cough, dyspnea, fatigue, anorexia, weight loss can lead to respiratory failure; develops over days, weeks to months
- Symptomatic improvement when away from work or home

PHYSICAL EXAM

- Acute: fever, tachypnea, diffuse fine rales
- Sequela or chronic: inspiratory crackles, progressive hypoxia, weight loss, diffuse rales, clubbing, rarely wheezing

DIFFERENTIAL DIAGNOSIS

- Acute: acute infectious pneumonia: influenza (or other viral pneumonia), mycoplasma, *Pneumocystis jiroveci* pneumonia, asthma, aspiration
- Chronic: sarcoidosis, chronic bronchitis, chronic obstructive pulmonary disease, tuberculosis, collagen vascular disease, idiopathic pulmonary fibrosis, lymphoma, fungal infections, *P. jiroveci* pneumonia

DIAGNOSTIC TESTS & INTERPRETATION

- Testing for positive precipitating antibodies is NOT diagnostic because up to 40% may have positive antibody without disease; antigens that cover most cases: pigeon and parakeet sera, dove feather, *Aspergillus* sp., *Penicillium*, *S. rectivirgula*, and *Thalassomonas viridans*
- PFTs: Typical profile is a restrictive pattern with low diffusing capacity; could also have an obstructive pattern
- BAL with serum precipitins and lymphocytosis (>50%) and a relative predominance of CD8—low CD4-to-CD8 ratio; findings not unique to HP
- Positive antigen–specific inhalation challenge testing: reexposure to the environment, inhalation challenge to the suspected antigen in a hospital setting, but it lacks standardization (1)
- Chest x-ray (CXR): used to rule out other diseases
  - Acute: ground-glass infiltrates, nodular or striated patchy opacities, interstitial pattern in a variety of distributions in lung field; up to 20% could be normal.
  - Sequela/chronic: upper lobe fibrosis, nodular or ground-glass opacities, volume loss, emphysematous changes
- CT scan of chest; patterns not specific to HP:
  - Acute: ground-glass opacities, poorly defined centrilobular nodules, and ground-glass opacities and air trapping on expiratory images (1),(2)
  - Chronic: fibrosis, ground-glass attenuation, irregular opacities, bronchiectasis, loss of lung volume, honeycombing, emphysematous changes (1),(2)
- High-resolution CT (HRCT) mid-to-upper zone predominance of centrilobular ground glass or nodular opacities with signs of air trapping (1)
- Usually start with CXR; may progress to HRCT based on findings (1)

Diagnostic Procedures/Other

Lung biopsy:

- Transbronchial: reveals small, poorly formed noncaseating granulomas near respiratory or terminal bronchioles, large foam cells, peribronchial fibrosis
- Open lung biopsy: highest yield in advanced disease; reveals varying patterns of organizing pneumonia, centrilobular and perilobular fibrosis, multinucleated giant cells with clefts

ALERT

HP in farmers must be distinguished from febrile, toxic reactions to inhaled dusts (organic dust toxic syndrome [ODTS]). Nonimmunologic reactions occur 30–50% more commonly than HP in farmers. ODTS is associated with intense exposure occurring on a single day.

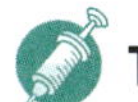

TREATMENT

GENERAL MEASURES

- Outpatient, except for acute pneumonitis cases and admission for workup (BAL, lung biopsy)
- Every effort should be made to remove the patient completely from repeated exposure to the causative antigen. This action offers the best outcome of disease.

MEDICATION

First Line

- Avoidance of offending antigen is primary therapy and results in disease regression (1).
- Corticosteroids: help control the symptoms of exacerbations but do not improve long-term outcomes
  - Prednisone: 20 to 50 mg daily (1)
  - For severe symptomatic patients, initial course of 1 to 2 weeks with taper (1)

Second Line

- Bronchodilators and inhaled corticosteroids may symptomatically improve patients with wheeze and chest tightness.
- Oxygen may be needed in advanced cases.
- Lung transplantation may be the last resort in severe cases unresponsive to therapy.

ISSUES FOR REFERRAL

Referral to pulmonologist/immunologist

ADMISSION, INPATIENT, AND NURSING CONSIDERATIONS

Supportive management, as needed, to maintain oxygenation and ventilation:

- Unstable ventilation, oxygen requirement, mental status changes
- Need for invasive evaluation (lung biopsy)

ONGOING CARE

FOLLOW-UP RECOMMENDATIONS

Patient Monitoring

- Initial follow-up should be weekly to monthly, depending on severity and course.
- Follow treatments with serial CXR, PFTs, and circulating antibody levels.

DIET

No dietary restrictions

PATIENT EDUCATION

Note that chronic exposure may lead to a loss of acute symptoms with exposure (i.e., the patient may lose awareness of exposure–symptom relationship).

PROGNOSIS

- Presence of fibrosis is a poor prognosis factor (1).
- Acute: good prognosis with reversal of pathologic findings if elimination of offending antigen early in disease
- Sequela/chronic: Corticosteroids have been found to improve lung function acutely but offer no significant difference in long-term outcome (1)[C].

COMPLICATIONS

- Progressive interstitial fibrosis with eventual respiratory failure
- Cor pulmonale and right-sided heart failure

REFERENCES

1. Spagnolo P, Rossi G, Cavazza A, et al. Hypersensitivity pneumonitis: a comprehensive review. *J Investig Allergol Clin Immunol*. 2015;25(4):237–250.
2. D'souza RS, Donato A. Hypersensitivity pneumonitis: an overlooked cause of cough and dyspnea. *J Community Hosp Intern Med Perspect*. 2017;7(2):95–99.

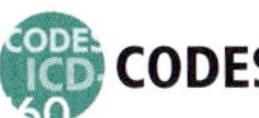

CODES

ICD10

- J67.9 Hypersensitivity pneumonitis due to unspecified organic dust
- J67.0 Farmer's lung
- J67.2 Bird fancier's lung

CLINICAL PEARLS

- Skin testing is not useful for the diagnosis of HP.
- Diagnosis should be suspected in every patient with unexplained cough and dyspnea on exertion, functional impairment (restriction or diffusion defect), and unclear fever, especially if exposure to potential antigens is known (workplace, domestic bird keeping, moldy walls in the home).
- HP may mimic viral upper respiratory illness or asthma exacerbation. Misdiagnosis has critical therapeutic and prognostic implications because it may delay proper treatment, result in significant morbidity, unnecessary hospitalizations, and irreversible fibrosis to the lungs (1).
- Once the disease is established, smoking does not appear to attenuate its severity, and it may predispose to more chronic and severe course.
- Use of protective gear on individuals with high-risk exposure occupations can prevent HP.
- Chronic HP is increasingly recognized as an important mimic of other fibrotic lung diseases (1).

HYPERTENSION, ESSENTIAL

Valerie Coppenrath, PharmD • Beth K. Mazyck, MD • Laquita Morris, MD

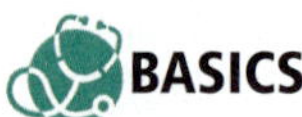

BASICS

DESCRIPTION

- Primary hypertension (HTN) is HTN without an identifiable cause; also known as essential HTN; an important risk factor for cardiovascular disease (CVD), and other comorbidities much controversy regarding recommended thresholds for diagnosis and treatment remains
- HTN is defined (Joint National Committee [JNC] 8 and the International Society of Hypertension) as (all pressures in mm Hg) (1):
  - Age <60 years: systolic BP (SBP) ≥140 and/or diastolic BP (DBP) ≥90 at ≥2 visits
  - Age ≥60 years: SBP ≥150 and/or DBP ≥90 at ≥2 visits
  - With diabetes or chronic kidney disease (CKD): SBP ≥140 and/or DBP ≥90
- The American College of Cardiology (ACC)/ American Heart Association (AHA) designates SBP ≥130 and/or DBP ≥80 as "stage 1 hypertension" which should be treated with exercise and lifestyle modification, reserving medication for patients at "higher risk" (defined as age ≥65, CKD, diabetes, or known CVD).

Geriatric Considerations

Isolated systolic HTN is common. Therapy is effective at preventing stroke, CVD, and all-cause mortality (2)[A]. Optimal targets for blood pressure can remain the same, but adverse reactions to medications are more frequent, which may change treatments targets. ACC/AHA does not make specific recommendations regarding choice of antihypertensive in older adults. Individualize target and treatment based on patient risks, preferences, and medication tolerance.

Pediatric Considerations

HTN in children is defined as SBP or DBP ≥95th percentile on repeated measurements. Measure BP during routine exams beginning at age 3 years; pre-HTN: SBP or DBP between 90th and 95th percentile

Pregnancy Considerations

Elevated BP during pregnancy may represent chronic HTN, pregnancy-induced HTN, or preeclampsia. Preferred agents: labetalol, nifedipine, methyldopa, or hydralazine (see "Preeclampsia and Eclampsia [Toxemia of Pregnancy]").

EPIDEMIOLOGY

Prevalence

Almost half of adults (48.1%) in the United States have HTN by ACC/AHA guideline; prevalence is higher in men.

ETIOLOGY AND PATHOPHYSIOLOGY

>90% of cases of HTN have no identified cause. For differential diagnoses and causes of secondary HTN, see "Hypertension, Secondary and Resistant."

RISK FACTORS

Family history, obesity, alcohol use, excess dietary sodium, stress, physical inactivity, tobacco use, insulin resistance, obstructive sleep apnea (OSA), and other causes of sleep disruption

DIAGNOSIS

- Despite more aggressive guidelines issued by the ACC/AHA in 2017, many experts consider recommendations from JNC 8 (1) and NICE (3) to retain primacy.
- Critics of the ACC/AHA guidelines note multiple methodologic concerns. Thresholds of <130/80 (as endorsed by ACC/AHA) compared to JNC 8 would result in the diagnosis of and treatment for HTN of millions more people, with unclear benefits and some inevitable harms.
- This chapter uses JNC 8 as its basis, but recommendations are relevant regardless of the specific guideline being applied. We recommend assessment of overall CV risk and joint decision-making regarding BP target.

HISTORY

HTN is asymptomatic except in extreme cases or after related CV complications develop. Headache can be seen with higher BP, often present on awakening and occipital in location.

PHYSICAL EXAM

- Weight assessment and waist circumference should be measured. Measure BP in both arms (correct technique is essential to accurate diagnosis and treatment). Incorrect BP determination is a common cause of overdiagnosis.
- Complete cardiac and peripheral pulse exam: Compare radial and femoral pulse for differences in volume and timing (evaluation for aortic coarctation [especially in young persons], subclavian stenosis); funduscopic exam for arteriolar narrowing, AV compression, hemorrhages, exudates, and papilledema

DIFFERENTIAL DIAGNOSIS

- Secondary HTN: Consider workup only if the history, physical exam, or basic laboratory evaluation suggest a higher likelihood. Also consider for patients who prove nonresponsive to treatment (see "Hypertension, Secondary and Resistant").
- White coat HTN: elevation of BP in office setting and normal BP outside office

DIAGNOSTIC TESTS & INTERPRETATION

ALERT

- Measuring BP: caffeine, exercise, and smoking avoided >30 minutes before measurement. Patient should be seated with back supported quietly for at least 5 minutes with feet on floor and patient's arm supported at heart level. Use correct cuff size. Deflate cuff slowly or use an automated device. Average two or more measurements. May leave patient alone to obtain in-office readings using an automated or patient-activated cuff.
- 2021 United States Preventive Services Taskforce (USPSTF) statement (4)[A]: A diagnosis of HTN should be confirmed with BP measurements outside the clinical setting. Home BP measurements (HBPM) correlate better with CV outcomes than office values and also help to mitigate the errors of clinic measurement. HBPM for diagnosis and for monitoring should be encouraged. For HBPM results, ≥135/85 should be used as a diagnostic threshold, and <135/85 should be the treatment target.
- Ambulatory BP monitoring (ABPM) is the ideal method, but this is not widely available in the US.

Initial Tests (lab, imaging)

- Complete blood count, basic metabolic panel, urinalysis, lipids, fasting glucose or hemoglobin A1c
- Estimate 10-year ASCVD risk using a calculator. Consider possibility of sleep apnea particularly in patients with excess weight (2).
- ECG to evaluate possible presence of left ventricular hypertrophy (LVH) or rhythm abnormalities

Follow-Up Tests & Special Considerations

- ABPM or HBPM if "white coat" or masked HTN is suspected, episodic HTN, or autonomic dysfunction; ambulatory measurement may be especially helpful if there is suspected autonomic dysfunction.
- Perform CV risk assessment. The AHA/ACC risk tool overestimates risk (by 50% or more, especially in older patients). A definition of "low risk" excludes patients with a history of CVD, diabetes mellitus, CKD, and familial hypercholesterolemia or familial premature coronary artery disease.

TREATMENT

GENERAL MEASURES

- The treatment discussed follows JNC 8 guidelines. Recent systematic reviews and meta-analyses of randomized trials do not support recommendations for lower-than-standard targets for the average-risk population. Weigh potential harms of therapy against potential benefits, ideally through shared decision-making.
- Treatment goals:
  - Age <60 years: SBP <140 and DBP <90 (for HBPM <135/85)
  - Age ≥60 years: SBP <150 and DBP <90 (for HBPM <140/90)
  - Age ≥60 years with CKD or diabetes: SBP <140 and DBP <90 (for HBPM <135/85)
  - More aggressive treatment may be considered in high-risk patients meeting enrollment criteria for SPRINT because aggressive treatment shows improvement in outcomes, but 61 nondiabetic patients would need to be treated (NNT) for 3 years to a goal SBP of <120 to prevent one major cardiovascular outcome and NNT is 90 over 3 years to prevent one death.
  - In secondary prevention, no firm conclusions can yet be drawn regarding the comparative effectiveness of intensive versus standard therapy.
  - Individual treatment goals should be established with patients after discussion of the potential benefits and harms (shared decision-making) (2).
- Treatment considerations:
  - Review current medications and supplements for potential contributors to HTN.
  - Recommend lifestyle improvements, including diet, exercise, and reducing or eliminating tobacco/ alcohol.
  - Benefit of pharmacologic treatment of low-risk patients with class I HTN (140 to 150/90 to 99) remains uncertain, with harms including syncope, kidney injury, and electrolyte abnormalities. Individualize decisions.

- Treating patients with CKD or diabetes to lower-than-standard BP targets, <140/90, does not appear to further reduce mortality or morbidity. Individualize goal BP based on risk factors and patient preferences.
- The majority of treatment benefit is attained by lowering very high SBP (e.g., from 190 to 150, as compared with the benefit of lowering from 150 to 136). Striving for small additional drops in BP by adding fourth or fifth medications to achieve a "target" is less clinically beneficial and more likely to cause adverse effects. Lower than standard JNC-8 DBP targets are not associated with decreased morbidity/mortality.

MEDICATION

- For initial monotherapy, choose from angiotensin II receptor blockers (ARBs), angiotensin-converting enzyme inhibitors (ACEI), dihydropyridine (DHP) calcium channel blockers (CCBs), or thiazide diuretics. ARBs are preferred over ACEI due to fewer side effects. Amlodipine is the preferred CCB. There is no significant difference between hydrochlorothiazide (HCTZ) and chlorthalidone.
- Many patients require multiple medications—especially those presenting with BP >20/10 mmHg above target, for whom it may be appropriate to begin with combination therapy.
- Multiple drugs at submaximal dose may achieve target BP with fewer side effects. However, these benefits must be balanced against adherence challenges associated with increased pill burden and more complicated dosing regimens. Consider combination pills in these scenarios.
- Taking medication at bedtime improves BP control compared to morning administration but does not improve CV or mortality outcomes.
- ARBs or ACEI should be used in patients with diabetes, proteinuria, atrial fibrillation, or heart failure with reduced ejection fraction (HFrEF) but *not in pregnancy*.
- α-Adrenergic blockers are not first choice for monotherapy but are suitable as combination therapy for males with benign prostatic hypertrophy (BPH).
- Non-DHP CCB could be considered in patients with isolated systolic HTN, atherosclerosis, angina, migraine, or asthma; well documented to reduce risk of stroke
- β-Blockers should be prioritized in patients with ischemic heart disease, atrial fibrillation, CHF, migraine, and with history of ST-segment elevation myocardial infarction (STEMI).

First Line

- ARBs losartan: 25 to 100 mg in 1 or 2 doses; has unique but modest uricosuric effect; valsartan: 80 to 320 mg/day; irbesartan: 75 to 300 mg/day; candesartan: 4 to 32 mg/day; renin inhibitor: aliskiren 150 to 300 mg daily
- ACEI: lisinopril: 5 to 40 mg/day; enalapril: 5 to 40 mg/day; ramipril: 2.5 to 20 mg/day
- Thiazide diuretics may not be effective with creatinine clearance <30 mL/min. Chlorthalidone: 12.5 to 25.0 mg/day (longer half-life and more potent than HCTZ but causes more hyponatremia and hypokalemia); HCTZ: 12.5 to 50.0 mg/day
- DHP CCB: amlodipine: 2.5 to 10.0 mg/day; nifedipine (sustained release): 30 to 90 mg/day; non-DHP: diltiazem CD: 180 to 360 mg/day; verapamil (sustained release): 120 to 480 mg/day
- Contraindications: Thiazide diuretics may worsen gout. β-Blockers (relative) in asthma, heart block, diabetes, and peripheral vascular disease; likely avoid in patients with metabolic syndrome or insulin-requiring diabetes. Diltiazem or verapamil: Do not use with systolic dysfunction or heart block.

Second Line

- Before escalating therapy, ensure that patient is adherent to prescribed regimen. Choose additional medications with complementary effects (i.e., ACEI/ARBs with diuretic or a vasodilator with a diuretic or β-blocker). Don't combine ACEI and ARB.
- Evidence from the ACCOMPLISH trial suggests that the combination of ACEI/CCB should be prioritized over ACEI/HCTZ to achieve better CV outcomes.
- Medication-refractory HTN (see "Hypertension, Secondary and Resistant"): spironolactone 25 to 100 mg/day or eplerenone 50 mg once to twice daily
- β-Blockers may be effective in patients with resting tachycardia. Metoprolol succinate allows for once-daily dosing over a wide dosage range (25 to 400 mg daily). Carvedilol and labetalol combine α- and β-blockade.
- Centrally acting α_2-agonists: clonidine 0.1 to 1.2 mg BID or weekly patch 0.1 to 0.3 mg/day, guanfacine 1 to 3 mg daily, or methyldopa 250 to 2,000 mg BID
- α-Adrenergic antagonists: prazosin 1 to 10 mg BID, terazosin 1 to 20 mg/day, or doxazosin 1 to 16 mg/day
- Vasodilators: hydralazine 10 to 25 mg TID; minoxidil 2.5 mg BID; risk of tachycardia and fluid retention, so generally combined with β-blocker and/or diuretic; minoxidil: rarely used due to adverse effects; may be more effective than other medications in renal failure and refractory HTN
- Metolazone and loop diuretics may be used with more severe renal impairment, but outcomes data are absent; loop diuretics (for volume overload): furosemide 20 to 320 mg/day or torsemide 5 to 100 mg/day
- K^+-sparing diuretics in patients with hypokalemia while taking thiazides: amiloride 5 to 10 mg/day or triamterene 50 to 150 mg/day

COMPLEMENTARY & ALTERNATIVE MEDICINE

Biofeedback and relaxation exercises

ONGOING CARE

FOLLOW-UP RECOMMENDATIONS

Patient Monitoring

ALERT

Repeat electrolytes, BUN/creatinine 3 to 6 weeks after initiating thiazide diuretics, ARB, or ACE-I. Reevaluate patients q3–6mo until stable and then q6–12mo. Consider BP self-monitoring; monitor quality-of-life issues including sexual function. Poor medication adherence is a leading cause of apparent medication failure. At least annual creatinine and K^+ for patients on diuretics, ARBs, and ACEIs.

DIET

- ~20% of patients respond to reduced-salt diet (<6 g NaCl or <2.4 g Na/day). Using salt substitutes may decrease all-cause mortality and cardiovascular mortality. Limit alcohol consumption to <1 oz/day.
- Consider Dietary Approaches to Stop Hypertension (DASH) diet; longer-term studies are required to determine the diet's effects on major cardiovascular outcomes.

COMPLICATIONS

Heart and renal failure, LVH, MI, retinal hemorrhage, stroke, dementia or cognitive decline, drug side effects, erectile dysfunction, all-causing mortality

REFERENCES

1. James PA, Oparil S, Carter BL, et al. 2014 Evidence-based guideline for the management of high blood pressure in adults: report from the panel members appointed to the Eighth Joint National Committee. *JAMA*. 2014;311(5):507–520.
2. Qaseem A, Wilt TJ, Rich R, et al. Pharmacologic treatment of hypertension in adults aged 60 years or older to higher versus lower blood pressure targets: a clinical practice guideline from the American College of Physicians and the American Academy of Family Physicians. *Ann Intern Med*. 2017;166(6):430–437.
3. *Hypertension in Adults: Diagnosis and Management*. National Institute for Health and Care Excellence; 2023.
4. Krist AH, Davidson KW, Mangione CM, et al; for US Preventive Services task Force. Screening for hypertension in adults: US Preventive Services Task Force reaffirmation recommendation statement. *JAMA*. 2021;325(16):1650–1656.

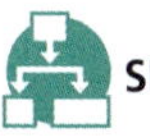

SEE ALSO

Hypertension, Secondary and Resistant; Hypertensive Emergencies; Polycystic Kidney Disease

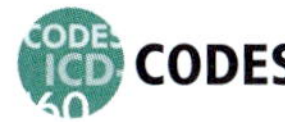

CODES

ICD10

I10 Essential (primary) hypertension

CLINICAL PEARLS

- NNT to prevent a major adverse CV events (MACE) ranges from 10 to 50 per year in patients with severe HTN to 100s or 1,000s per year for patients with mild HTN. Overly aggressive treatment may cause significant harms, especially in the elderly.
- Measure BP outside the office.
- For nonresponders to specific medication classes, consider sequential monotherapy instead of combination therapy—especially for those within 20/10 mm Hg of target.

HYPERTENSION, SECONDARY AND RESISTANT

George Maxted, MD

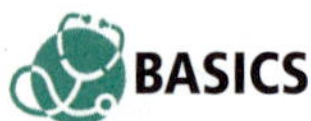

BASICS

DESCRIPTION

Uncontrolled hypertension (HTN) comprises the following entities (see "Alert"):

- Resistant HTN: blood pressure (BP) that remains above goal in spite of the concurrent use of three antihypertensive agents of different classes; ideally, one of the three agents should be a diuretic, and all agents should be prescribed at optimal dose amounts. The diagnosis does not include "white coat effect" or medication nonadherence, although consideration of these is part of the evaluation.
- Secondary HTN: elevated BP that results from an identifiable underlying mechanism
- The 2017 revised ACC/AHA guideline recommends a change in the classification of HTN. For the purposes of this chapter, we are considering stage 2 HTN: systolic BP (SBP) ≥140 mm Hg or diastolic BP (DBP) ≥90 mm Hg (1)[C].

Geriatric Considerations

- Onset of HTN in adults >60 years of age is a strong indicator of secondary HTN.
- In patients >80 years of age, consider a higher target SBP of ≥150 mm Hg. Be cautious to avoid excessive diastolic lowering. A recent Cochrane review, considering studies of patients with average age of 70 years, concluded that a target BP of 140/90 or lower reduces the risk of stroke and cardiovascular outcomes, although the effect on mortality is unclear (2)[A].
- Secondary causes more common in the elderly include sleep apnea, renal disease, atherosclerotic renal artery stenosis (ARAS), and primary aldosteronism (PA).
- Noncompressible arteries (Osler phenomenon)—mostly in elderly with arteriosclerosis: Brachial and radial artery pulsations are present at high cuff pressures.

ALERT

- Pseudoresistance: inaccurate measurement of BP (cuff too small, patient not at rest; sitting quietly for 5 minutes)
- Poor adherence: In primary care settings, this has been estimated to occur in 40–60% of patients with HTN.
- White coat effect: prevalence 20–40%; do not make clinical decisions about HTN based solely on measurement in the clinic setting. Home BP monitoring (HBPM), self-BP monitoring (SBPM), remote monitoring, or ambulatory BP monitoring (ABPM) are more reliable.

EPIDEMIOLOGY

- Predominant age: In general, HTN has its onset between ages 30 and 50 years. Patients with resistant HTN are more likely to experience the combined outcomes of death, myocardial infarction, congestive heart failure (CHF), stroke, or chronic kidney disease.
- Depending on etiology, age of onset can vary. Age of onset <20 or >50 years increases likelihood of a secondary cause for HTN.

Prevalence

- Prevalence of resistant HTN is estimated to be 10–15% (3). NHANES: 53% of adults are controlled to a BP of <140/90 mm Hg. The most common cause of apparently resistant HTN is likely medication nonadherence.
- Secondary HTN occurs in about 5–10% of adults with chronic HTN.
- A recent study of secondary HTN among otherwise healthy children with a diagnosis of HTN indicated a prevalence of 3.7%.

ETIOLOGY AND PATHOPHYSIOLOGY

- Obstructive sleep apnea (OSA) (25–50%)
- Primary hyperaldosteronism (8–20% of resistant HTN cases)
- Chronic renal disease (1–2% of hypertensives)
- Renovascular disease (0.2–0.7%, up to 35% of elderly, 20% of patients undergoing cardiac catheterization)
- Cushing syndrome (<0.1%)
- Pheochromocytoma (0.04–0.1% of hypertensives)
- Other rare causes: hyperthyroidism, hyperparathyroidism, aortic coarctation, intracranial tumor
- Drug-related causes (many)
  - Medications, especially NSAIDs (may also blunt effectiveness of ACE inhibitors), decongestants, stimulants, anorectic agents including herbals (e.g., guarana, ma huang, bitter orange), natural licorice (in some chewing tobacco), glucocorticoids
  - Oral contraceptives (OCP): Cessation of OCP may result in normalization of the BP. Postmenopausal estrogen does not appear to correlate as strongly (3).
  - Cocaine, amphetamines, other illicit drugs; drug and alcohol withdrawal syndromes
- Lifestyle factors: obesity, dietary salt, excessive alcohol, physical inactivity

Genetics

Genetic variants have been detected in patients with resistant HTN, but are estimated to account for <3% of BP variance (3).

RISK FACTORS

A large cohort study revealed that those with resistant HTN (16.2%) were more likely to be male, white, older, and diabetic; factors predictive of resistant or secondary HTN: obesity, diabetes, worsening of control in previously stable hypertensive patient, onset in patients age <20 years or >50 years, lack of family history of HTN, significant target end-organ damage, stage 2 HTN (SBP >160 mm Hg or DBP >100 mm Hg), renal disease, and alcohol or drug use

GENERAL PREVENTION

The prevention of resistant and secondary HTN is thought to be the same as for primary or essential HTN: a Dietary Approaches to Stop Hypertension (DASH) diet, a low-sodium diet, weight loss in obese patients, exercise, limitation of alcohol intake, and smoking cessation. Relaxation techniques may be of help.

COMMONLY ASSOCIATED CONDITIONS

Sleep disorders; obesity

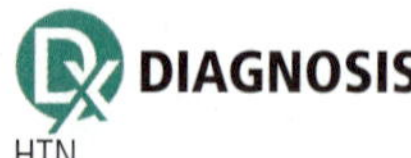

DIAGNOSIS

HTN

HISTORY

- Ask or review at every visit: SANS mnemonic: (i) Salt intake, (ii) Alcohol intake, (iii) NSAIDs use, (iv) Sleep. These identify the most common causes of poorly controlled HTN.
- Ask about medication adherence. Estimates are that during the 1st year of treatment for HTN, only 20% of patients have sufficiently high adherence to achieve clinical benefit (3).
- Review home BP readings; consider ABMP.
- History varies with etiology of secondary HTN; OSA: loud snoring while asleep, daytime somnolence; pheochromocytoma: episodes of headache, palpitations, sweating; Cushing syndrome: weight gain, fatigue, weakness, easy bruising, amenorrhea; increased intravascular volume: swelling

PHYSICAL EXAM

- Ensure that the BP is measured correctly. The patient should be sitting quietly with back supported for at least 5 minutes before measurement; proper cuff size: bladder encircling at least 80% of the arm; support arm at heart level; minimum of two readings at least 1 minute apart; check BP in both arms. Also check standing BP for orthostasis.
- The USPSTF recommends "obtaining measurements outside the clinical setting for diagnostic confirmation"; attention to findings related to possible etiologies: renovascular HTN: systolic/diastolic abdominal bruit; pheochromocytoma: diaphoresis, tachycardia; Cushing syndrome: hirsutism, moon facies, dorsal hump, purple striae, truncal obesity; thyroid disease: enlarged thyroid, tremor, exophthalmos, tachycardia; coarctation of the aorta: upper limb HTN with decreased or delayed femoral pulses

DIFFERENTIAL DIAGNOSIS

Pseudoresistance

DIAGNOSTIC TESTS & INTERPRETATION

- ECG performed as part of the initial workup; LVH is an important marker of resistant HTN.
- Sleep study if history and physical indicate; the Epworth Sleepiness Scale and other tools may be helpful.
- Home-based polysomnography has been shown to be accurate in screening for OSA. Overnight oximetry is not helpful.

Initial Tests (lab, imaging)

Initial limited diagnostic testing should include urinalysis, CBC, potassium, sodium, glucose, creatinine, lipids, thyroid-stimulating hormone (TSH), and calcium. 50% of patients with hyperaldosteronism may have normal potassium levels; urine spot test for microalbuminuria, an important marker of ASCVD risk

- Imaging tests listed are necessary only if history, physical, or lab data indicate.
- Abdominal US: if renal disease is suspected
- Duplex ultrasonography may be the preferred test for renovascular disease. MR angiography (MRA) of renal vasculature is sensitive but has low specificity and potentially more harmful. Conventional catheter angiography or CT angiography may be required to confirm the diagnosis.

Follow-Up Tests & Special Considerations

Further testing for PA may be considered.

- Empiric treatment with an aldosterone antagonist may be preferable and more clinically relevant.
- Plasma aldosterone-to-renin ratio (ARR) is the preferred lab test, but the test is difficult to perform and interpret properly. Consult your reference lab and interpret results with caution.
  - Further testing (screening) for pheochromocytoma: 30-minute supine plasma (or 24 hours urinary) metanephrines (consult lab for best local option)
  - Other tests to consider for resistant or secondary HTN: 24-hour urine for free cortisol, calcium, parathyroid hormone (PTH), overnight 1-mg dexamethasone suppression test, urine toxicology screen

Diagnostic Procedures/Other

Consider 24-hour ABPM, especially if white coat effect is suspected. HBPM results predict mortality, stroke, and other target organ damage better than office BP. Optimal protocol involves two paired measurements: morning and evening (four measurements) over 4 to 7 days.

- Oscillometric, electronic, upper arm, fully automatic device with memory: average multiple readings over several days
- Remote BP monitoring devices may be useful in the clinical management of HTN, but thus far have not been shown to be more effective than standard monitoring.

TREATMENT

- Treatment modality depends on etiology of HTN. Please see each etiology listed for information on proper treatment. Empiric trial of aldosterone antagonist is a commonly used initial medication strategy if diagnostic workup does not reveal a specific cause.
- The National Institute for Health Care and Excellence (3) offers a useful management algorithm emphasizing lifestyle modification: diet, less sodium, exercise, and alcohol in moderation.
- Emphasize adherence to JNC 8 and/or AHA/ACC guidelines, with emphasis on lifestyle modification. Obese patients and elderly may be particularly responsive to diuretics. Tolerance to diuretics may occur: long-term adaptation to thiazides or the "braking effect." Consider increasing the dose of thiazide, switching to longer-acting diuretic (e.g., chlorthalidone), or adding an aldosterone inhibitor.
- Treatment specific to certain secondary etiologies
  - PA: aldosterone receptor antagonist: spironolactone or eplerenone (latter has less estrogenic effect); a new agent, lorundrostat is under study—an aldosterone synthetase inhibitor.
  - Cushing syndrome: aldosterone receptor antagonist
  - OSA: continuous positive airway pressure (CPAP) ± oxygen, surgery, weight loss, upper airway nerve stimulation; a mandibular advancement device (MAD) may be as effective as CPAP for OSA for some.
  - Nocturnal hypoxia: oxygen supplementation
  - Renal sympathetic denervation: Cochrane review: There is low-certainty evidence that renal denervation (RDN) does not improve major cardiovascular outcomes and renal function. Conversely, moderate-certainty evidence exists that it may improve 24-hour ABPM and diastolic office-measured BP. Two catheter-based devices have been approved for RDN (Paradise and Symplicity). AHA recommends considering for very select patients.
- The treatment of ARAS is controversial. Percutaneous stenting may not be effective. ACEi and ARB medications may confer long-term mortality benefit (3)[C].
- A dual endothelin antagonist (aprocitentan [Tryvio]) lowers SBP about 4 mm Hg in resistant HTN, but is expensive and lacks evidence of improved outcomes.

MEDICATION

- Follow treatment guidelines and algorithms by JNC 8 and AHA/ACC/CDC, understanding the differences between them.
- Adding a medication to the regimen may have greater efficacy than increasing the dose of medications.
- Chlorthalidone may be more effective than HCTZ. Empiric use of aldosterone antagonists (low-dose spironolactone, eplerenone) is often very effective. Amiloride, a potassium sparing diuretic, has been shown to have similar benefits. If addition of aldosterone antagonist to a multi-drug regimen is not effective, initiate workup for secondary causes.

ALERT

- Agents specific for treatment of HTN emergencies should be initiated in those situations, in which immediate BP reduction will prevent or limit end-organ damage (see "Hypertensive Emergencies").
- Renovascular HTN: Angioplasty is the treatment of choice for fibromuscular dysplasia of a renal artery.
- CORAL study: In patients with atherosclerotic renovascular disease and HTN, renal artery stenting did not improve outcomes over medical therapy alone.
- Referral to an HTN specialist or clinic: Retrospective studies indicate improved control rates for patients with resistant HTN referred to special HTN clinics.

First Line

- ARB, CCB, ACEi, and thiazide diuretics are first-line medications for HTN. Combinations of medicines or changing medicines is recommended for BP nonresponsiveness.
- Note: People of African descent may not respond fully to ACEi or ARB medications.

Second Line

Add an aldosterone antagonist as above. β-Blockers, α-blocker, or combined α/β blocker (e.g., labetolol)—especially if another compelling indication such as ischemic heart disease, heart failure, migraine, or tachyarrhythmia is present.

Third Line

Addition of central agents (clonidine or guanfacine), direct vasodilators (hydralazine isosorbide mononitrate or dinitrate, minoxidil) are options with adequate diuretic.

ISSUES FOR REFERRAL

If control is not successful, consider referral to a HTN center or nephrology.

SURGERY/OTHER PROCEDURES

See "renal sympathetic denervation" on "Treatment."

ADMISSION, INPATIENT, AND NURSING CONSIDERATIONS

Hypertensive urgency or emergency general measures

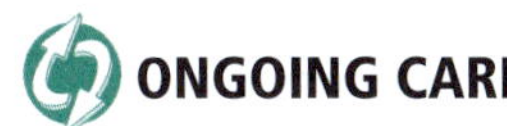

ONGOING CARE

FOLLOW-UP RECOMMENDATIONS

Encourage aerobic activity of 30 minutes/day, depending on patient's condition.

Patient Monitoring

Remote BP monitoring may be useful in a clinical setting.

DIET

Reduced salt may lower BP in some patients. Recommend the Mediterranean diet or DASH.

PATIENT EDUCATION

HBPM predicts outcomes better than office monitoring of BP.

REFERENCES

1. James PA, Oparil S, Carter BL, et al. 2014 Evidence-based guideline for the management of high blood pressure in adults: report from the panel members appointed to the Eighth Joint National Committee (JNC 8). *JAMA*. 2014;311(5):507–520.
2. Falk JM, Froentjes L, Kirkwood JE, et al. Higher blood pressure targets for hypertension in older adults. *Cochrane Database Syst Rev*. 2024;12(12):CD011575.
3. Carey RM, Calhoun DA, Bakris GL, et al. Resistant hypertension: detection, evaluation, and management: a scientific statement from the American Heart Association. *Hypertension*. 2018;72(5):e53–e90.

SEE ALSO

Aldosteronism, Primary; Coarctation of the Aorta; Cushing Disease and Cushing Syndrome; Hyperparathyroidism; Hypertension, Essential; Hyperthyroidism; Pheochromocytoma

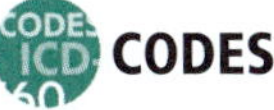

ICD10

- I15.9 Secondary hypertension, unspecified
- I15.8 Other secondary hypertension
- I15.0 Renovascular hypertension

CLINICAL PEARLS

Aldosterone inhibitors should be considered in all cases of resistant HTN.

HYPERTHYROIDISM

Vicente T. San Martin, MD • Claudia Guzman, MD

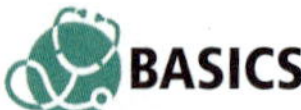

BASICS

Hyperthyroidism and thyrotoxicosis result from an excess of thyroid hormone (TH); the former refers to hormone overproduction by the thyroid gland, whereas the latter may arise from either thyroidal or nonthyroidal sources (1).

DESCRIPTION

- Hyperthyroidism is most commonly caused by Graves disease (GD), toxic multinodular goiter (TMNG), and toxic adenoma (TA) (1),(2).
- Patients can develop thyrotoxicosis from other causes, such as subacute thyroiditis and drug-induced thyroiditis.
- Subclinical hyperthyroidism: suppressed thyroid-stimulating hormone (TSH) with normal thyroxine (T_4) and triiodothyronine (T_3)
- Thyroid storm: extreme manifestation of hyperthyroidism with acute, severe symptoms affecting multiple organ systems; up to 50% mortality (2)

EPIDEMIOLOGY

Incidence

- Approximately 0.5 to 1.5 cases per 1,000 person-years globally
- GD: most common cause in iodine-sufficient areas; peak incidence: 2nd and 3rd decades of life
- TMNG: more frequent in iodine-deficient areas; most common cause in patients aged >65 years (1)

Prevalence

The global prevalence is 0.2–1.3% (1).

ETIOLOGY AND PATHOPHYSIOLOGY

- GD: autoimmune disease; characterized by autoantibodies that activate the TSH receptor (TSHr)
- TMNG: autonomous production and release of T_3 and T_4 due to constitutive activation of TSHr or somatic mutations in Gsα (1)
- TA: thyroid nodule with a somatic activating mutation in the TSHr gene, leading to autonomous overproduction of THs
- TSH-producing pituitary adenoma: rare benign pituitary tumor that secretes excess TSH, causing elevated TH (should be distinguished from TH resistance, which can show similar labs) (1)
- Gestational transient thyrotoxicosis: results from the thyroid-stimulating activity of human chorionic gonadotropin (hCG); serum hCG peaks at 9 to 12 weeks of gestation, with higher risk in twin pregnancy and in hyperemesis gravidarum.
- Iodine-induced hyperthyroidism: occurs after exposure to high iodine doses, most often from iodinated contrast media but also from seaweed or potassium iodide tablets; typically develops 3 to 10 weeks after exposure (1)
- Subacute/de Quervain thyroiditis: granulomatous giant cell thyroiditis, often preceded by an upper respiratory tract infection; viruses such as coxsackievirus, adenovirus, echovirus, and influenza have been implicated; typically benign and self-limited course
- Postpartum thyroiditis: occurs in 8–11% of pregnancies; the thyrotoxic phase is usually asymptomatic and is associated with a high risk of permanent hypothyroidism.
- Drug-induced thyroiditis: amiodarone, interferon-α, interleukin-2, lithium, immune check point inhibitors (anti-CTLA-4, anti-PD-1 antibodies), tyrosine-kinase inhibitors (sorafenib, vandetanib) (1),(2)

Genetics

- GD: concordance rate of GD among monozygotic twins is 30%
- Polymorphisms involved in immune checkpoints and immune response (FOXP3, PTPN22, CTLA4, CD40, FCRL3) (1)

RISK FACTORS

- Female sex, iodine excess, irradiation, infections, postpartum period, drugs
- Positive family history, especially in maternal relatives
- Other autoimmune disorders
- Perturbation of gut microbiota
- Use of alemtuzumab (30% of patients develop GD)

GENERAL PREVENTION

- Hyperthyroidism cannot usually be fully prevented, especially autoimmune forms
- Risk can be reduced by maintaining adequate iodine intake.

COMMONLY ASSOCIATED CONDITIONS

- Autoimmune diseases occur in 9.7% of patients with GD (rheumatoid arthritis, pernicious anemia, systemic lupus, celiac disease, Addison disease, vitiligo) (1)
- Down syndrome

DIAGNOSIS

HISTORY

Hypermetabolic state that may involve several organ systems (1),(2):

- Constitutional: fatigue, weakness, increased appetite, weight loss
- Neuropsychiatric: agitation, anxiety, emotional lability, psychosis, coma, poor concentration and memory
- Gastrointestinal: increased appetite, hyperdefecation
- Gynecologic: irregular menses
- Cardiovascular: palpitations and chest discomfort that mimics angina

PHYSICAL EXAM

- Skin: warm, moist, pretibial myxedema (GD only), localized dermopathy, onycholysis
- Eyes: exophthalmos (GD only), upper lid retraction
- Endocrine: hyperhidrosis, heat intolerance, goiter, gynecomastia, subfertility in women
- Cardiovascular: tachycardia, systolic hypertension, atrial fibrillation (AF)
- Musculoskeletal: clubbing, proximal muscle weakness, osteoporotic fractures
- Neurologic: tremor, anxiety, brisk deep tendon reflexes

Geriatric Considerations

Classic symptoms and signs may be absent.

DIFFERENTIAL DIAGNOSIS

- Anxiety
- Pregnancy, menopause
- Pheochromocytoma, carcinoid syndrome

DIAGNOSTIC TESTS & INTERPRETATION

- 95% have suppressed TSH and elevated free T_4 and T_3.
- TSH, T_4, and T_3 can all be elevated in case of a TSH-producing pituitary adenoma.
- Presence of TSHr antibody or thyroid-stimulating immunoglobulin is diagnostic of GD.

Initial Tests (lab, imaging)

- TSH, free T_4, total T_4, and T_3 will establish the diagnosis.
- TSHr antibodies
- Nuclear medicine uptake and scanning:
  - Increased thyroid iodine uptake is seen with TMNG, TA, and GD.
  - GD shows a diffuse uptake.
  - TMNG will show a heterogeneous uptake, whereas TA will show a "hot" nodule.
  - Decreased or absent iodine uptake is characteristic of thyroiditis and extrathyroidal sources of TH.
  - Ultrasound is not diagnostic of hyperthyroidism itself, but it may be useful to determine the cause.

Follow-Up Tests & Special Considerations

TSH may remain low in the early period after initiating treatment, even when T_4 and T_3 levels have decreased.

Test Interpretation

Thyroid function tests can be affected by analytical interference from antibodies or by biotin supplementation.

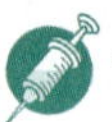

TREATMENT

- Observation may be appropriate for patients with mild hyperthyroidism (TSH >0.1 or no symptoms), especially those who are young and with low risk of complications.
- Subclinical hyperthyroidism should be treated in patients who are at high risk for cardiovascular disease and osteoporosis, especially those aged > 65 years (3).
- GD can be managed by either antithyroid drugs (ATD), radioactive iodine therapy (RAIT), or thyroidectomy; due to the chance of remission, 12- to 18-month trial of ATD may be considered prior to offering RAIT or surgery.
- For TMNG and TA, the treatment of choice is RAIT. Medical therapy with ATD can be used but has shown a high recurrence rate. Surgery is considered in special cases. Radiofrequency ablation is a minimally invasive alternative to RAIT in younger patients with small nodules (2).
- Treatment of subacute thyroiditis is supportive with NSAIDs and β-blockers; steroids may be used in refractory cases.

GENERAL MEASURES
Focus on symptom control, minimizing complications, and supporting overall health.

MEDICATION
First Line
- ATD: Methimazole and propylthiouracil (PTU) are thioamides that inhibit iodine oxidation, organification, and iodotyrosine coupling. PTU can block peripheral conversion of T_4 to T_3. Both can be used as primary treatment for GD and prior to RAIT or surgery.
- Duration of treatment: 12 to 18 months; 50–60% relapse after stopping. Long-term methimazole (5 to 10 years) is feasible with a recurrence rate of 15% (1). The most serious side effects are hepatitis (0.1–0.2%), vasculitis, and agranulocytosis.
  - Methimazole (preferred): adults: 10 to 30 mg PO daily (can be divided in 2 to 3 doses if needed); children: 0.2 to 0.5 mg/kg/day PO daily (max 30 mg/day) (3)
  - PTU: adults (preferred in thyroid storm and 1st trimester of pregnancy): 100 to 150 mg PO q8h; in thyroid storm, higher doses are often used; children: 5 to 7 mg/kg/day PO divided q8h (max 300 mg/day)

Pediatric Considerations
In children, hyperthyroidism is usually treated first with weight-based methimazole, avoiding PTU due to liver risks.

Pregnancy Considerations
PTU is currently the drug of choice during 1st trimester, and methimazole is preferred in the 2nd and 3rd trimester. Treat with lowest effective dose (PTU can cross the placenta and put the fetus at risk for goiter). RAIT is contraindicated.

Second Line
- β-Adrenergic blocker: Propranolol in high doses (>160 mg/day) inhibits T_3 activation by up to 30%. Atenolol, metoprolol, and nadolol can be used.
- Glucocorticoids: reduce the conversion of T_4 to T_3. In TED, the use of steroids before and after RAIT helps prevent disease worsening
- Cholestyramine: binds TH in the gut during their enterohepatic recirculation (3)
- Other agents:
  - Lithium: inhibits TH secretion and iodotyrosine coupling; use is limited by toxicity
  - Lugol solution or saturated solution of potassium iodide (SSKI); blocks release of TH from the gland but should be administered at least 1 hour after thioamide; otherwise, acts as a substrate for TH production (Jod-Basedow effect)

ISSUES FOR REFERRAL
- Referral is indicated for severe or uncontrolled disease, thyroid storm, large goiters, or adverse reactions to ATD.
- Refer patients with TED to an experienced ophthalmologist.

ADDITIONAL THERAPIES
Teprotumumab: IGF-1 receptor monoclonal antibody approved for active TED

SURGERY/OTHER PROCEDURES
Thyroidectomy is indicated when there is a large or compressive goiter, suspicion of malignancy, failure or contraindication to ATD or RAIT, severe ophthalmopathy, or special circumstances such as pregnancy.

COMPLEMENTARY & ALTERNATIVE MEDICINE
Selenium is an adjunctive therapy in mild GD or early TED, acting as an antioxidant.

ADMISSION, INPATIENT, AND NURSING CONSIDERATIONS
Some patients require inpatient management due to severity, complications, or risk of thyroid storm.

ONGOING CARE

FOLLOW-UP RECOMMENDATIONS
Smoking cessation in GD patients as this is a risk factor for TED

Patient Monitoring
- While on ATD, check thyroid tests, CBC, and liver function tests q3mo.
- After RAIT, check thyroid tests at 6 to 12 weeks, 6 months, and annually thereafter if euthyroid; TSH may remain undetectable for months even after patient is euthyroid.

DIET
Sufficient calories to prevent weight loss

PROGNOSIS
Depends on the underlying cause, severity, patient age, comorbidities, and response to treatment:
- GD: Some patients achieve remission, although relapses are common.
- TMNG: usually requires definitive treatment (RAIT or surgery) for cure
- Thyroid storm: life-threatening if untreated; prompt recognition and management significantly reduce mortality.

COMPLICATIONS
TED, heart failure, AF, muscle wasting, proximal muscle weakness, increased risk of cerebrovascular accident (CVA), and cardiovascular mortality

REFERENCES

1. Wiersinga WM, Poppe KG, Effraimidis G. Hyperthyroidism: aetiology, pathogenesis, diagnosis, management, complications and prognosis. *Lancet Diabetes Endocrinol*. 2023;11(4):282–298.
2. Lee SY, Pearce EN. Hyperthyroidism: a review. *JAMA*. 2023;330(15):1472–1483.
3. Ross DS, Burch HB, Cooper DS, et al. 2016 American Thyroid Association guidelines for diagnosis and management of hyperthyroidism and other causes of thyrotoxicosis. *Thyroid*. 2016;26(10):1343–1421.

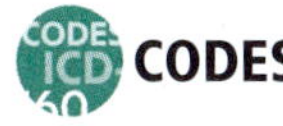

CODES

ICD10
- E05.81 Other thyrotoxicosis with thyrotoxic crisis or storm
- E05.80 Other thyrotoxicosis without thyrotoxic crisis or storm
- E05.1 Thyrotoxicosis with toxic single thyroid nodule

CLINICAL PEARLS
- Hyperthyroidism is most commonly caused by GD, TMNG, and TA.
- GD is common in young adults, whereas TMNG is common in patients aged >65 years.
- ATD can be used as the primary treatment for GD and prior to RAIT or surgery.
- TSH may remain low in the early period after initiating ATD, even when euthyroid. Follow up with T_4 and T_3.
- RAIT is the first-line treatment in TMNG and TA; contraindicated in pregnancy
- Thyroid storm is a medical emergency that needs hospitalization and aggressive treatment.

HYPERTRIGLYCERIDEMIA

S. Lindsey Clarke, MD, FAAFP • Katherine G. W. Johnson, MD

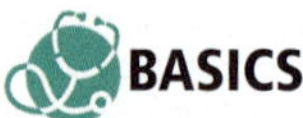

BASICS

DESCRIPTION

- Hypertriglyceridemia (HTG) is a common form of dyslipidemia characterized by an excess fasting plasma concentration of triglycerides (TGs).
  - TGs are fatty molecules that occur naturally in vegetable oils and animal fats and are major sources of dietary energy.
  - Absorbed TGs are packaged into very low-density lipoproteins (VLDL) and chylomicrons.
  - The liver also converts excess carbohydrates to TGs. This is a major contributor to HTG for most patients.
- HTG is a risk factor for acute pancreatitis at levels ≥500 mg/dL and especially ≥1,000 mg/dL.
  - Risk is 10–20% at these TG levels.
  - Third leading cause of acute pancreatitis
- HTG is also independently associated with cardiovascular disease (atherosclerotic cardiovascular disease [ASCVD]) at levels ≥175 mg/dL.
  - The American Heart Association (AHA) and the American College of Cardiology (ACC) consider persistent HTG as a risk-enhancing factor.
  - A large Danish population study in 2018 showed that TG ≥264 mg/dL conferred a 10-year risk of major adverse cardiovascular events comparable to that of statin eligible individuals.
  - However, a causal relationship between HTG and ASCVD has not been firmly established.
  - Moreover, lowering TG has not been proven to reduce cardiovascular risk.
- AHA and ACC classify HTG into two categories:
  - Moderate: 175 to 499 mg/dL (2.0 to 5.6 mmol/L), characterized mainly by excess VLDL
  - Severe: ≥500 mg/dL (≥5.6 mmol/L), characterized by excess VLDL and chylomicrons

EPIDEMIOLOGY

- Predominant gender: male > female
- Predominant race: Hispanic, white > black

Prevalence

- 25–33% of U.S. population has TG levels ≥150 mg/dL.
- 1.7% has TG levels ≥500 mg/dL.
- Highest prevalence at age 50 to 70 years
- The most common genetic syndromes with HTG, familial combined hyperlipidemia and familial HTG, each affect ≤1% of general population.

ETIOLOGY AND PATHOPHYSIOLOGY

- Primary
  - Familial
  - Acquired (sporadic)
- Secondary
  - Lifestyle factors
    - Diet high in refined carbohydrates or excess calories
    - High intake of ultra-processed foods
    - Excess alcohol intake
    - Physical inactivity
    - Obesity and overweight
  - Medical conditions
    - Type 2 diabetes mellitus
    - Metabolic syndrome/insulin resistance
    - Hypothyroidism
    - Chronic liver disease
    - Chronic kidney disease, nephrotic syndrome
    - Autoimmune disorders (e.g., systemic lupus erythematosus)
    - Paraproteinemias (e.g., macroglobulinemia, myeloma, lymphoma, lymphocytic leukemia)
    - Pregnancy (usually physiologic and transient)
  - Medications
    - Acitretin
    - β-blockers
    - Bile acid sequestrants
    - Cyclophosphamide
    - Cyclosporine
    - Glucocorticoids
    - Isotretinoin
    - Oral estrogens
    - Protease inhibitors
    - Second-generation antipsychotics
    - Tamoxifen and raloxifene
    - Thiazides

Genetics

- Familial chylomicronemia (type 1 dyslipidemia): autosomal recessive inheritance of lipoprotein lipase deficiency; 0.0001% population prevalence
- Familial combined hyperlipidemia (type IIb): usually autosomal dominant, caused by overproduction of apolipoprotein (APO) B-100; approximately 1% prevalence
- Familial dysbetalipoproteinemia (type III): usually autosomal recessive, caused by lipoprotein overproduction due to inheritance of two APOE2 variants; 0.01% prevalence
- Familial HTG (type IV): autosomal dominant, caused by an inactivating mutation of the lipoprotein lipase gene; 1% prevalence
- Primary mixed HTG (type V)

RISK FACTORS

- Genetic susceptibility
- Obesity, overweight
- Lack of exercise
- Type 2 diabetes mellitus
- Alcoholism
- Certain medical conditions and drugs (see "Etiology and Pathophysiology")

GENERAL PREVENTION

- Maintain healthy body weight.
- Moderation of dietary fat and refined carbohydrates
- Regular aerobic exercise
- Avoid excess alcohol.

COMMONLY ASSOCIATED CONDITIONS

- Pancreatitis
- Coronary artery disease
- Type 2 diabetes mellitus and insulin resistance
- Dyslipidemias
- Metabolic syndrome
- Nonalcoholic steatohepatitis (NASH)
- Polycystic ovary syndrome

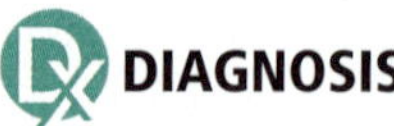

DIAGNOSIS

HISTORY

- Usually asymptomatic
- Patients with chylomicronemia syndrome can have memory loss, headache, vertigo, dyspnea, and paresthesias.
- Pancreatitis: epigastric pain, nausea, and vomiting
- Assess for other cardiac risk factors.
- Family history of coronary artery disease

PHYSICAL EXAM

- Obesity, overweight (body mass index ≥25 kg/m^2)
- Eruptive cutaneous, tuberous, and striate palmar xanthomas
- Lipemia retinalis
- Epigastric tenderness in pancreatitis
- Hepatomegaly in NASH and chylomicronemia

DIFFERENTIAL DIAGNOSIS

Primary and secondary HTG

DIAGNOSTIC TESTS & INTERPRETATION

Initial Tests (lab, imaging)

- Serum: turbid with milky supernatant
- Fasting (12 hours) or nonfasting lipid profile
  - USPSTF recommends screening adults aged 40 to 75 years to identify dyslipidemia and to calculate 10-year ASCVD risk; repeat every 5 years.
  - American Academy of Pediatrics recommends screening all children for dyslipidemia at 9 to 11 years and 17 to 21 years of age, but USPSTF found insufficient evidence for screening in children and adolescents.
  - Statin therapy may be indicated for LDL and ASCVD risk reduction in some adults (e.g., clinical ASCVD, diabetes) regardless of lipid levels.
  - Confirm severe HTG with fasting measurement.
- Evaluation for secondary causes
  - Glycosylated hemoglobin A1c (HbA1c), fasting or postprandial glucose for type 2 diabetes mellitus
  - Creatinine, urinary protein measurement for nephrotic syndrome, renal failure
  - Thyroid-stimulating hormone for hypothyroidism
- Pancreatitis: serum lipase; US and/or CT scan of pancreas
- Atherosclerosis: cardiac stress testing, coronary CT angiography, cardiac catheterization, and coronary angiography

Follow-Up Tests & Special Considerations

- Repeat lipid panel after 1 to 3 months of therapy.
- High levels of apolipoprotein B (apoB >130 mg/dL) predict ASCVD in patients whose LDL cannot be calculated due to HTG. But evidence for routine clinical measurement of apoB in patients with HTG is lacking.

TREATMENT

GENERAL MEASURES

- Cardiovascular risk reduction through LDL lowering should be prioritized over TG lowering unless patient is at risk for pancreatitis due to severe HTG (TG ≥500 mg/dL) (1)[C].
- Therapeutic lifestyle changes are first-line interventions for all patients and can reduce TG by as much as 50%:
  - Dietary modification (limit carbohydrate intake to 50–60% of calories; restrict sugars and alcohol)
  - Moderate-intensity physical activity can reduce TG by 20–30%.
  - Weight loss of 5–10% can reduce TG by as much as 20%.
  - Persons with severe HTG should abstain from alcohol.
- Address secondary causes and remove offending drug when possible.
- Improve glycemic control if diabetic.
- Control other cardiac risk factors, such as hypertension, diabetes mellitus, and smoking.
- Primary HTG: Screen other family members.

MEDICATION

First Line

- Statins: preferred for ASCVD risk reduction; primarily affect LDL but also may lower TG 15–30%; USPSTF recommends statins for primary prevention of ASCVD in adults aged 40 to 75 years who have clinical risk factors and 10-year ASCVD risk ≥10%. Dosing depends on intensity of statin desired based on ASCVD risk. See "Coronary Artery Disease and Stable Angina" and "Hypercholesterolemia."
  - Atorvastatin: 10 to 80 mg/day
  - Rosuvastatin: 5 to 40 mg/day
  - Adverse reactions: myalgias, myopathy, rhabdomyolysis (especially if combined with fibrates); contraindicated in pregnancy and lactation
- Fibrates: preferred for reducing risk of pancreatitis in severe HTG; may lower TG up to 50% and may decrease cardiovascular and coronary events but not all-cause mortality (2)[A]:
  - Adverse reactions: GI upset, hepatotoxicity, cholelithiasis, myalgias, rhabdomyolysis (when combined with a statin), gemfibrozil-warfarin interaction (enhanced anticoagulation)
  - Fenofibrate: 30 to 200 mg daily (preferred, may be used with statins)
  - Gemfibrozil: 600 mg BID; avoid in combination with statins due to high risk of muscle injury

Second Line

- Icosapent ethyl (Vascepa) 2 g BID: preferred add-on therapy for ASCVD risk reduction in patients with known ASCVD or diabetes mellitus plus additional risk factors and persistent HTG despite statin therapy (3)[C],(4).
  - 2019 REDUCE-IT trial showed 25% reduction in major adverse cardiovascular events in this high-risk population.
  - Adverse reactions: atrial fibrillation/flutter, major bleeding (caution with coagulopathy, anticoagulation or antiplatelet therapy)
- Other marine omega-3 fatty acids
  - Omega-3-acid ethyl esters (Lovaza, other fish oils): 4 g daily or 2 g BID
  - Appropriate for reducing pancreatitis risk but do not improve ASCVD risk
  - May lower TG 30–50%
  - Limited tolerability due to adverse GI effects (diarrhea, nausea, abdominal pain, eructation)

ISSUES FOR REFERRAL

- Severe HTG refractory to treatment
- Familial HTG syndromes

ADDITIONAL THERAPIES

Apolipoprotein C3 inhibitors olezarsen and plozasiran, now in phase 3 clinical trials, show promise for substantial TG reduction.

ADMISSION, INPATIENT, AND NURSING CONSIDERATIONS

- Acute pancreatitis
- In acute hypertriglyceridemic pancreatitis with TG $>$1,000 mg/dL, the following interventions can be used to lower TG rapidly and safely to $<$500 mg/dL:
  - Plasmapheresis for 1 to 3 days
  - Insulin infusion
    - Regular insulin 0.1 to 0.3 U/kg/hr IV for 2 to 4 days
    - Administer separate infusion of dextrose 5% if blood glucose $<$200 mg/dL.
    - Non-inferior to plasmapheresis in 2024 meta-analysis of five studies
- Discharge criteria: stabilization of acute complicating illness

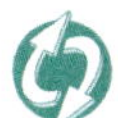

ONGOING CARE

FOLLOW-UP RECOMMENDATIONS

1 to 3 months after initiation or modification of therapy (repeat fasting lipid profile)

Patient Monitoring

- Fasting lipid profile every 6 to 12 months
- Maintain TG $<$500 to 1,000 mg/dL to reduce risk of acute pancreatitis.
- Hepatic transaminases
- Creatine phosphokinase if patient has myalgias

DIET

- Limit carbohydrates to 50–60% of total caloric intake.
- Increase dietary fiber.
- Avoid sugars and refined carbohydrates.
- Moderate alcohol intake ($<$1 oz/day) or complete abstinence if TGs are very high.
- Restrict dietary fat to 30% of total caloric intake; restrict further to 15% of caloric intake if TG ≥1,000 mg/dL.
- Increase marine-derived omega-3 polyunsaturated fatty acids. Eat fatty fish such as salmon, mackerel, sardines, and trout.
- Eliminate trans-fatty acids.
- Mediterranean-style diet reduces TG 10–15% more than a low-fat diet.

PATIENT EDUCATION

Smoking cessation for cardiovascular risk reduction

PROGNOSIS

- Good with correction of TG levels
- Patients with primary HTG usually require lifelong treatment.

COMPLICATIONS

- Atherosclerosis
- Chylomicronemia syndrome
- Pancreatitis

REFERENCES

1. Grundy SM, Stone NJ, Bailey AL, et al. 2018 AHA/ACC/AACVPR/AAPA/ABC/ACPM/ADA/AGS/APhA/ASPC/NLA/PCNA guideline on the management of blood cholesterol: executive summary: a report of the American College of Cardiology/American Heart Association Task Force on clinical practice guidelines. *J Am Coll Cardiol*. 2019;73(24):3168–3209.
2. Jakob T, Nordmann AJ, Schandelmaier S, et al. Fibrates for primary prevention of cardiovascular disease events. *Cochrane Database Syst Rev*. 2016;11(11):CD009753.
3. Orringer CE, Jacobson TA, Maki KC. National Lipid Association scientific statement on the use of icosapent ethyl in statin-treated patients with elevated triglycerides and high or very-high ASCVD risk. *J Clin Lipidol*. 2019;13(6):860–872.
4. Wright J, Subramanian S. Therapy for hyperlipidemia. *Med Clin North Am*. 2024;108(5):881–894.

ADDITIONAL READING

- Simha V. Management of hypertriglyceridemia. *BMJ*. 2020;371:m3109.
- Virani SS, Morris PB, Agarwala A, et al. 2021 ACC expert consensus decision pathway on the management of ASCVD risk reduction in patients with persistent hypertriglyceridemia: a report of the American College of Cardiology Solution Set Oversight Committee. *J Am Coll Cardiol*. 2021;78(9):960–993.

SEE ALSO

- Hypercholesterolemia; Pancreatitis, Acute
- Algorithm: Hypertriglyceridemia

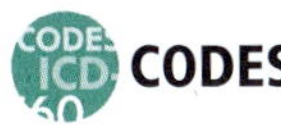

CODES

ICD10

E78.1 Pure hyperglyceridemia

CLINICAL PEARLS

- HTG is likely a risk factor for atherosclerosis at levels ≥175 mg/dL and for acute pancreatitis at levels ≥500 to 1,000 mg/dL.
- Therapeutic lifestyle interventions (diet and exercise) are recommended for all patients who have HTG and for all patients at risk for ASCVD.
- Address reversible secondary causes of HTG such as uncontrolled diabetes and medications that raise TGs.
- In patients with TG levels $<$500 mg/dL, the main pharmacologic strategy for cardiovascular risk reduction is statins. Icosapent ethyl can further reduce cardiovascular events in high-risk patients.
- For patients with TG levels ≥500 mg/dL, the greatest amount of TG lowering is achieved with fibrates. But, the magnitude of clinical benefit is uncertain, so statin use is generally recommended first for cardiovascular risk reduction, with cautious addition of fibrates, if needed.

HYPOGLYCEMIA, DIABETIC

Afsha Rais Kaisani, MD, FAAFP • Tasaduq Hussain Mir, MD, FAAFP

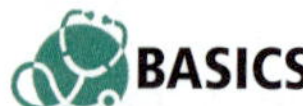

BASICS

Hypoglycemia is defined as a low plasma glucose level in an individual with or without symptoms that may cause them harm. According to American Diabetic Association (ADA), hypoglycemia is defined as any blood sugar level <70 mg/dL.

DESCRIPTION

- Abnormally low concentration of glucose in circulating blood of a patient with diabetes mellitus (DM); often referred to as an *insulin reaction*, as classified by the ADA:
  - Level 1: hypoglycemia alert value; <70 mg/dL (3.9 mmol/L) but ≥54 mg/dL (3.0 mmol/L); may or may not be accompanied by symptoms; asymptomatic hypoglycemia if symptoms not present; should alert patients to ingest carbohydrate (CHO) to prevent progressive hypoglycemia
  - Level 2: clinically significant hypoglycemia; <54 mg/dL (3.0 mmol/L)
  - Level 3: severe hypoglycemia; this involves cognitive impairment requiring external assistance for recovery.
  - Pseudohypoglycemia: typical symptoms but glucose ≥70 mg/dL (3.9 mmol/L)
- Hypoglycemia is the leading limiting factor in the glycemic management of Type 1 DM (T1DM) and Type 2 DM (T2DM). Severe or frequent hypoglycemia requires modification of treatment regimens with higher treatment goals.

EPIDEMIOLOGY

Incidence

- Common in patients with long-standing T1DM and children age <7 years or individuals age >75 years with long-standing T2DM
- Nearly 3/4 of severe hypoglycemic episodes occur during sleep.
- RECAP-DM study: Hypoglycemia was reported in 35.8% of patients with T2DM who added sulfonylurea or thiazolidinedione to metformin therapy during the past year.

ETIOLOGY AND PATHOPHYSIOLOGY

- Loss of hormonal counterregulatory mechanism in glucose metabolism
- Impaired insulin, glucagon, and epinephrine secretion

RISK FACTORS

- Taking medications known to cause hypoglycemia (e.g., insulin, insulin secretagogues: sulfonylureas [SU] [glyburide, glimepiride, glipizide, etc.] and glinide derivatives [repaglinide, nateglinide])
- Intensive insulin therapy (further lowering HbA1c from 7% to 6%)
- Comorbidities: renal/liver disease, congestive heart failure, hypothyroidism, hypoadrenalism, gastroenteritis, gastroparesis (unpredictable CHO delivery), autonomic neuropathy, pregnancy, anxiety, depression, polypharmacy
- Patient characteristics: advance age, young children with T1DM, reduced cognitive function (including dementia) and those with intellectual disability
- Longer duration of DM (including those using insulin for >5 years)
- Lifestyle and social factors: irregular eating schedules, starvation, prolonged fasting, weight loss, food insecurity, eating disorder, elevated stress or unplanned life events, current smokers with T1DM, individuals fasting for religious or cultural reasons
- Alcohol consumption, especially if on insulin or insulin secretagogues; evening consumption of alcohol is associated with an increased risk of nocturnal and fasting hypoglycemia, especially in patients with T1DM.
- History of severe hypoglycemia (especially recent within the past 3 to 6 months)
- Other antidiabetes medications such as dipeptidyl peptidase 4 inhibitors, glucagon-like peptide-1 receptor agonists (GLP-1RA), and sodium-glucose contransporter-2 inhibitors agents carry a lower but present risk of hypoglycemia, which may increase when combining agents from different categories.

Geriatric Considerations

- American Geriatric Society Beers Criteria recommend avoiding long-acting SU (e.g., glyburide) due to prolonged half-life in older adults and risk for prolonged hypoglycemic episodes. Medications should be dosed for age and renal function.
- Individualize pharmacologic therapy in older adults to reduce the risk of hypoglycemia, avoid overtreatment, and simplify complex regimens if possible while maintaining the HbA1c target.

Pediatric Considerations

Children may not realize when they have hypoglycemia, needing increased supervision during times of higher activity such as competitive sports. Children may have higher glycemic goals for this reason. Caregivers should be instructed in use of glucagon.

Pregnancy Considerations

Hypoglycemia management and avoidance education should be reemphasized and blood glucose monitoring increased due to more stringent glycemic goals and increased risk in early pregnancy.

GENERAL PREVENTION

- Maintain routine schedule of diet (consistent CHO intake), medication, and exercise.
- Self-monitoring of blood glucose (SMBG) or continuous glucose monitoring (CGM) (1)[A]
  - Particularly helpful for asymptomatic hypoglycemia and if taking insulin or secretagogue
  - Consider CGM rather than SMBG with T1DM or those requiring multiple injections of insulin, insulin pump therapy, or pregnant diabetic.
- Diabetes treatment and teaching programs (DTTPs) especially for high-risk type 1 patients, which teach flexible insulin therapy to enable dietary freedom
- Hypoglycemia may be decreased with use of insulin analogs, automated insulin delivery systems, and CGM.

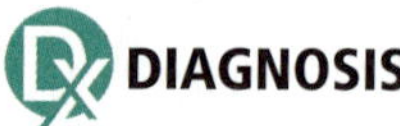

DIAGNOSIS

HISTORY

Discuss timing of episodes, awareness, frequency, and causes. Symptoms vary considerably between individuals.

- Adrenergic symptoms: hunger, trembling, pallor, sweating, shaking, pounding heart, anxiety, urinary incontinence
- Neurologic symptoms: altered cognition, dizziness, poor concentration, drowsiness, weakness, confusion, light-headedness, slurred speech, vision changes, unsteadiness, poor coordination
  - Hypoglycemia causes deterioration in reading span and subject-verb agreement, demonstrating that language processing is impaired during hypoglycemia.
- Behavioral symptoms: tearfulness, confusion, fatigue, irritability, aggressiveness
- Surgical history (e.g., bariatric procedures [gastric sleeve or Roux-en-Y gastric bypass])

PHYSICAL EXAM

- General: confusion, lethargy
- HEENT: diplopia
- Coronary: tachycardia
- Neurologic: tremulousness, weakness, paresthesia, stupor, seizure, or coma
- Mental status: irritability, anxiety, inability to concentrate, or short-term memory loss
- Skin: pale, diaphoresis
- End-organ damage: microvascular, macrovascular, ophthalmologic, neurologic, renal

DIFFERENTIAL DIAGNOSIS

Hypoglycemia not associated with DM may be seen in:

- Chronic alcoholics and binge drinkers
- GI dysfunction causing postprandial hypoglycemia or alimentary reactive hypoglycemia
- Hormonal deficiency states (hormonal reactive hypoglycemia)
- Hypoglycemia of sepsis
- Islet cell tumors
- Factitious hypoglycemia from surreptitious injection of insulin

DIAGNOSTIC TESTS & INTERPRETATION

- Plasma, serum, or whole-blood glucose
- SMBG and CGM are especially useful for asymptomatic hypoglycemia (1)[A].
- Low HbA1c level may be due to chronic hypoglycemia.
- Disorders that may alter lab results: Conditions that affect erythrocyte turnover, such as hemolysis or blood loss, renal disease, and hemoglobin variants may alter HbA1c. Consider using fructosamine and glycated albumin as alternatives to monitoring glycemic status, specifically in the past 2 to 4 weeks (2)[A].

Follow-Up Tests & Special Considerations

Hypoglycemic reading from a CGM sensor should be verified by SMBG fingerstick glucose testing prior to treatment, unless specific device is approved otherwise.

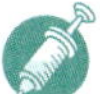

TREATMENT

Fast-acting CHO at the hypoglycemia alert value of ≤70 mg/dL. Individuals should recheck their glucose 15 minutes after ingesting CHO and repeat ingestion as needed.

GENERAL MEASURES

- Oral glucose: pure glucose preferred; any form of CHO that contains glucose should be effective, avoid CHO high in protein for acute treatment or prevention of hypoglycemia.
- Glucagon should be prescribed to patients at risk of clinically significant hypoglycemia. People in close contact with these individuals should be instructed in how to use an emergency glucagon kit.
- Insulin-treated patients with hypoglycemia unawareness or an episode of clinically significant hypoglycemia should have glycemic targets raised to strictly avoid hypoglycemia.
- α-Glucosidase inhibitors (acarbose) prevent digestion of complex CHOs; therefore, hypoglycemia must be treated with monosaccharides, such as glucose tablets.
- Patients with T1DM should use insulin analogs to reduce hypoglycemia risk.
- Address medications (i.e., insulin, SU, GLP-1RA, thiazolidinediones) that may induce hypoglycemia.
- CGM-augmented CSII with automated insulin suspension when blood glucose falls below a threshold value reduces the combined rate of severe and moderate hypoglycemia in T1DM and reduces nocturnal hypoglycemia without increasing HbA1c levels in patients >16 years old (3)[A].

MEDICATION

- Conscious patients (2)[A]
  - Glucose (15 to 20 g) is preferred, although any form of CHO may be used.
    - Any sugar-containing food or beverage that can be rapidly absorbed: honey, juice, or non-diet soda (4 to 5 oz), candy (5 to 6 pieces of hard candy), or glucose tablets (4 tablets = 16 g CHO)
    - Takes ~15 minutes to be digested and enter bloodstream as glucose
    - "Rule of 15": 15 to 20 g CHO (~60 to 80 calories simple CHO) repeated q15min until blood sugar is ≥70 mg/dL
- Loss of consciousness at home or people unable or unwilling to consume CHO by mouth—administer glucagon.
  - IM or SC in the deltoid or anterior thigh; forms include injection powder requiring reconstitution prior to injection, prefilled pen, and/or syringe.
    - Age <6 years and/or weight <20 to 25 kg: 0.50 mg
    - Age ≥6 years and/or weight >20 to 25 kg: 1 mg
    - May repeat dose in 15 minutes if needed
  - Intranasal glucagon—comes in a ready-to-use fixed-dose autoinjector; does not require active participation from the patient. Place the device in one nostril followed by pressing a plunger.
    - Age ≥ 4 years: 3 mg initial dose; may repeat dose in 15 minutes if needed
- In unconscious, with emergency medical personnel present or patient hospitalized (3)[A]:
  - Give 25 g IV 50% dextrose q5–10min until patient awakens.
  - Then, feed orally and/or administer 5% dextrose IV at level that will maintain blood glucose >100 mg/dL.
  - Patients with hypoglycemia secondary to oral hypoglycemics should be monitored for 24 to 48 hours because hypoglycemia may recur after clinical recovery.

ADMISSION, INPATIENT, AND NURSING CONSIDERATIONS

Admission criteria/initial stabilization

- Any doubt of cause
- Expectation of prolonged hypoglycemia (e.g., caused by SU drug)
- Inability to drink/eat
- Treatment has not resulted in prompt sensory recovery.
- Seizures, coma, or altered behavior (e.g., ataxia, disorientation, unstable motor coordination, dysphasia) secondary to documented or suspected hypoglycemia
- Discharge criteria: Normoglycemia and risk of severe hypoglycemia are negligible.

ONGOING CARE

FOLLOW-UP RECOMMENDATIONS

Discuss hypoglycemia prevention at all visits.

DIET

- Alcohol consumption may place patients with diabetes at increased risk for delayed hypoglycemia.
- CHO sources high in protein should not be used to treat or prevent hypoglycemia.
- Fats may slow absorption of CHOs and may prolong the acute glycemic response.
- Food insecurity increases risk of hypoglycemia due to inadequate or erratic CHO consumptions following administration of SU or insulin.

PATIENT EDUCATION

- Always have access to quick-acting CHO.
- Consider ingestion of added CHO if pre-exercise blood sugar <100 mg/dL or a reduced insulin dose.
- Educate patients, their relatives, close friends, teachers, and supervisors of DM diagnosis and signs/symptoms of hypoglycemia and treatment.
- Teach SMBG/CGM and self-adjustment for insulin therapy, diet control, and exercise regimen.
- Wear medical alert identification bracelet or necklace.

COMPLICATIONS

- Coma, seizure, myocardial infarction, stroke (especially in elderly)
- Prolonged or severe hypoglycemia may cause permanent neurologic damage and/or cognitive impairment.
- Children with T1DM have a greater vulnerability to neurologic manifestations of hypoglycemia.

ALERT

Intensively lowering blood glucose below current recommendations increased the risk of death versus standard treatment strategy.

REFERENCES

1. McCall AL, Lieb DC, Gianchandani R, et al. Management of individuals with diabetes at high risk for hypoglycemia: an Endocrine Society clinical practice guideline. *J Clin Endocrinol Metab*. 2023;108(3):529–562. doi:10.1210/clinem/dgac596.
2. American Diabetes Association Professional Practice Committee. 6. Glycemic goals and hypoglycemia: standards of care in diabetes—2025. *Diabetes Care*. 2025;48(Suppl 1):S128–S145.
3. Cryer PE, Axelrod L, Grossman AB, et al; for Endocrine Society. Evaluation and management of adult hypoglycemic disorders: an Endocrine Society clinical practice guideline. *J Clin Endocrinol Metab*. 2009;94(3):709–728.

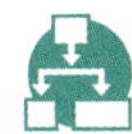

SEE ALSO

- Diabetes Mellitus, Type 1
- Algorithm: Hypoglycemia

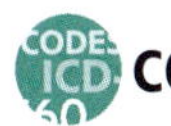

CODES

ICD10

- E11.649 Type 2 diabetes mellitus with hypoglycemia without coma
- E10.649 Type 1 diabetes mellitus with hypoglycemia without coma
- E13.649 Oth diabetes mellitus with hypoglycemia without coma

CLINICAL PEARLS

- Abnormally low concentration of glucose in patients with DM; often referred to as an *insulin reaction*
- Treatment includes:
  - Immediate administration of glucose—in form of CHO (oral), IM, IV or intranasal glucagon
  - Patient education and empowerment—address hypoglycemia in every visit with patients at risk.
  - Frequent SMBG or CGM with flexible insulin (or other drug) regimens
  - Individualized glycemic goals based in part on the risk of hypoglycemia
- "Rule of 15" is an easy way to teach patients to manage hypoglycemia at home: 15 to 20 g CHO (~60 to 80 calories simple CHO) SMBG, repeat q15min until blood sugar is ≥70 mg/dL.

HYPOGLYCEMIA, NONDIABETIC

Matthew A. Silva, PharmD, RPh, BCPS • Pablo I. Hernandez Itriago, MD, MHCM, FAAFP

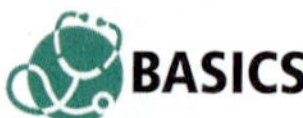

BASICS

DESCRIPTION

- Hypoglycemia is defined by the Whipple triad as low plasma glucose level (≤60 mg/dL) with hypoglycemic symptoms that are relieved when glucose is corrected.
- Occurs commonly in patients with diabetes receiving insulin secretagogues (sulfonylureas, meglitinides) or insulins; is less common in patients without diabetes
- Hypoglycemia is also seen after GI or bariatric surgery (in association with dumping syndrome).
- Postprandial or reactive hypoglycemia is insulin dependent and occurs in response to a meal, nutrients, drugs, or herbal substances and may occur 2 to 3 hours postprandially or later.
- Spontaneous (fasting) hypoglycemia may be associated with primary conditions including hypopituitarism, Addison disease, myxedema, rare metabolic diseases and inborn errors of metabolism such as glycogen storage disease, critical illness, heart failure, hepatic or renal failure, and sepsis

EPIDEMIOLOGY

Incidence

0.5–8.6% of hospitalized patients ≥65 years without diabetes

ETIOLOGY AND PATHOPHYSIOLOGY

- Reactive, postprandial, insulin dependent
  - Alimentary hyperinsulinism
  - Meals including refined or processed carbohydrates, liquid forms of fructose, sucrose, or glucose
  - Certain nutrients, including galactose, leucine
  - Glucose intolerance (prediabetes)
  - GI surgery, especially bariatric surgery (i.e., Roux-en-Y gastric bypass)
- Spontaneous
  - Fasting
  - Restricted food access (i.e., unhoused persons, persons in hospitals, prisons)
  - Alcohol or prescription medication–associated (insulin, sulfonylureas, meglitinides, thiazolidinediones, incretin mimetics, sodium-glucose cotransporter-2 (SGLT-2) inhibitors, DPP-IV inhibitors, angiotensin-converting enzyme-inhibitors, β-blockers, salicylates, methimazole, quinine, hydroxychloroquine, fluoroquinolones, doxycycline and tetracycline derivatives, linezolid, sertraline, disopyramide, pentamidine, gabapentin, tramadol) (1)
  - Consider medication administration errors as a source of unexplained hypoglycemia in persons without diabetes, especially those with polypharmacy.
  - Poisoning (ethanol, wild-mushroom, β-adrenergic receptor antagonists) and toxidromes (salicylates, NSAIDs, oral hypoglycemics)
  - Nonprescription over-the-counter (OTC) agents, including performance-enhancing agents; adulterated versions of phosphodiesterase inhibitors and performance-enhancing agents are routinely imported and adulterated, containing sulfonylureas and other hypoglycemic agents.
  - Natural medicines or herbs (bitter melon, caffeine, cassia cinnamon, chromium, fenugreek, ginseng, guarana, mate, stevia, vanadium)
  - Physiologic stress and postsurgical (e.g., Roux-en-Y bariatric surgery, gastrectomy) hypoglycemia, dumping syndrome
  - Islet cell hyperplasia or tumor (insulinomas), leukemia or other neoplasia-related process (tumor mediated insulin like growth factor-2 [IGF-2]) and insulin receptor upregulation
  - Extrapancreatic insulin-secreting tumors and other large tumors secreting IGF-2
  - Autoimmune hypoglycemia (Hirata disease) and insulin receptor mutations
  - Heart failure with or without SGLT-2 inhibitors (empagliflozin, dapagliflozin, canagliflozin)
  - Infectious or inflammatory hepatic disease or failure; renal disease or failure
  - Renal glycosuria
  - Glucagon deficiency
  - Adrenal insufficiency
  - Catecholamine deficiency
  - Hypopituitarism
  - Hypothyroidism
  - Eating disorders
  - Exercise or physical activity (i.e., manual labor)
  - Pregnancy
  - Severe nutrient deficiencies (i.e., selenium)
  - Ketotic hypoglycemia of childhood
  - Congenital disorders and errors of inborn metabolism, glycogen storage disease
  - Sepsis, cachexia, anorexia

Genetics

Monogenic and congenital hyperinsulinism (i.e., channelopathies, enzyme and transport anomalies, transcription factor or enzyme abnormalities) (2)

RISK FACTORS

Prolonged fasting or inability to consume food and nutrition orally, alcohol, medications, pregnancy, critical illness or surgery, endocrine diseases or tumors, excess caffeine, a family history of congenital disorders of inborn metabolism or glycogen storage diseases

GENERAL PREVENTION

- Follow dietary and exercise guidelines.
- Patient recognition of early symptoms and knowledge of corrective action

Pediatric Considerations

- Usually divided into two syndromes:
  - Transient neonatal hypoglycemia
  - Hypoglycemia of infancy and childhood
- Screening infants for hypoglycemia is appropriate when pregnancy was complicated by maternal diabetes.
- Cases of hypoglycemia observed in children taking propranolol for infantile hemangioma
- Associated with indomethacin when treating patent ductus arteriosus
- Consider errors of inborn metabolism, galactosemia, fructose intolerance and glycogen storage disease in children and young adults.

Geriatric Considerations

- More likely to have underlying disorders or be caused by medications
- Iatrogenic hypoglycemia is common in the hospitalized elderly with renal insufficiency.

COMMONLY ASSOCIATED CONDITIONS

- Heart failure; severe, chronic hepatic and renal disease; alcoholism
- Addison disease; adrenocortical insufficiency
- Myxedema
- Malnutrition (patients with renal failure)
- GI and bariatric surgery
- Panhypopituitarism
- Insulinoma and other neoplastic process

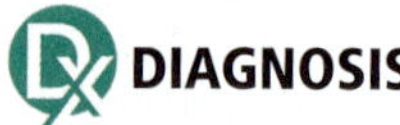

DIAGNOSIS

HISTORY

- Adrenergic symptoms are prominent with acute drop in glucose ≤60 mg/dL
  - Anxiety, tremulousness, dizziness
  - Diaphoresis, flushing
  - Heart palpitations
  - Adrenergic symptoms may be masked by β-receptor antagonists (i.e., metoprolol, propranolol, bisoprolol, carvedilol) or rate-blocking calcium channel antagonists (verapamil, diltiazem)
- CNS (neuroglycopenic) symptoms appear at a serum glucose ≤50 mg/dL
  - Headache
  - Light-headedness, fatigue, and weakness
  - Visual disturbances
  - Changes in personality, confusion
- GI and cholinergic symptoms
  - Hunger, nausea, belching
  - Diaphoresis, palmar sweating

PHYSICAL EXAM

- CNS (neuroglycopenic) symptoms predominate with gradual glucose reduction:
  - Convulsions, coma
  - Hypotension
- Adrenergic and cholinergic symptoms: more prominent in acute drop in glucose
  - Tremulousness
  - Diaphoresis, flushing
  - Heart palpitations

DIFFERENTIAL DIAGNOSIS

- CNS disorders
- Psychogenic/pseudohypoglycemia: Symptoms of hypoglycemia or self-diagnosis in patients in whom low blood glucose may not be detectable and may be impossible to convince that they do not suffer from hypoglycemia after all tests are found to be normal.

DIAGNOSTIC TESTS & INTERPRETATION

Initial Tests (lab, imaging)

- Blood glucose ≤45 mg/dL (≤2.5 mmol/L) when symptomatic followed by symptom resolution with feeding (3)[C]
- Plasma glucose overnight fasting: ≤60 mg/dL (≤3.33 mmol/L); confirm on ≥2 occasions (3)[C].

- Plasma glucose 72-hour fasting: ≤45 mg/dL (≤2.5 mmol/L) for females; ≤55 mg/dL (≤3.05 mmol/L) for males; fasting may be ended when Whipple triad is achieved or hypoglycemia is demonstrated (3)[C].
- Imaging (abdominal) using transabdominal ultrasound, CT, MRI, or PET (2)[C]

Follow-Up Tests & Special Considerations

- Misinterpretation of glucose tolerance tests may lead to misdiagnosis of hypoglycemia; ≥1/3 of normal patients have hypoglycemia, with or without symptoms, during the 4-hour glucose tolerance test. These patients may be at future risk for type 2 diabetes.
- If hypoglycemia presents as a primary disorder, consider hyperinsulinism and extrapancreatic tumors.
- C-peptide measurement (3)[C]
- Check liver studies, serum insulin, adrenocorticotropic hormone (ACTH), and cortisol. Serum insulin should be suppressed when glucose is <60 mg/dL (2)[C].
- Serum β-hydroxybutyrate <2.7 mg/dL in the presence of high-serum insulin, C-peptide, and low-serum glucose suggests excessive insulin production (3)[C].
- Insulin radioimmunoassay: Elevated insulin levels suggest islet cell hyperplasia or tumor.
- Drugs that may alter lab results: Many drugs can affect glucose levels. Review drugs individually and refer to drug or laboratory reference.
- Ensure comprehensive medication reconciliation to address medication, supplements, recreational substances, and consider toxicology workup (i.e., salicylates, NSAIDs, β-receptor antagonists).

Diagnostic Procedures/Other

For definitive diagnosis (2),(3)[C]:

- Document low glucose levels and symptoms with low levels.
- Evidence that symptoms are relieved by ingestion of glucose or food
- Identify the specific type of hypoglycemia (2),(3)[C].

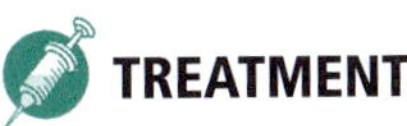

TREATMENT

GENERAL MEASURES

- Oral carbohydrate for alert patient without drug overdose (2 to 3 tbsp of sugar in glass of water or fruit juice, 1 to 2 cups of milk, piece of fruit, or several soda crackers)
- If unable to swallow: Use glucagon IM or SC.
- Discontinue, avoid, or control causative medications/agents.
- Avoid alcohol.
- If triggered by meals: Try high-protein diet with carbohydrate restriction.
- Nonhypoglycemic hypoglycemia or pseudohypoglycemia
- Symptoms may pertain to chronic fatigue and somatic complaints.
- Management difficult; listening is important. Try 120 g carbohydrate diet.
- Counseling may be useful for stress and other problems.
- CGM sensors and devices sampling interstitial fluid may identify patterns of post-prandial or fasting-associated hypoglycemia allowing for 15% variance between interstitial and blood glucose and a lag between blood and interstitial spaces. CGM can be considered educational for self-management, not diagnostic.

MEDICATION

- Once diagnosis is established, begin therapy that is appropriate for underlying disorder (3)[C].
- If unable to swallow: glucagon 1 mg (1 unit) IV, IM, or SC; if no response, give IV bolus of 25 to 50 g of 50% glucose solution followed by continuous infusion until patient able to take by mouth; intranasal glucagon is 3 mg (one actuation per device) into a single nostril; may repeat 1 time after 15 minutes if there is no response using a second intranasal device (2)[C].
- Postsurgical gastrectomy patients unresponsive to dietary changes may benefit from propantheline, psyllium, fiber, or oat bran to delay gastric emptying.

ISSUES FOR REFERRAL

Refer if suspecting rare inborn errors of metabolism, genetic disorders, fructose intolerance, galactosemia or glycogen storage disease, or refractory to usual treatments

SURGERY/OTHER PROCEDURES

If islet cell tumor (insulinoma) or other insulin-secreting tumor, surgery is treatment of choice; if inoperable, diazoxide may relieve symptoms (2)[C].

ADMISSION, INPATIENT, AND NURSING CONSIDERATIONS

Persistent hypoglycemia unresponsive to oral intake of glucose

ONGOING CARE

FOLLOW-UP RECOMMENDATIONS

Patient Monitoring

Hypoglycemia from sulfonylureas can last for hours to days depending on half-life and renal function.

DIET

- High protein, high fiber, complex carbohydrates from plant and multigrain sources (whole food) with some fat
- Frequent small feedings (six daily); avoid liquid calories (2)[C]
- Avoid fasting

PATIENT EDUCATION

- Recognition of early symptoms of hypoglycemia and how to take corrective action
- Exercise routine or daily activity may need to be adjusted.
- Patients with recurrent hypoglycemia should have glucose source at hand for immediate ingestion during symptoms.

PROGNOSIS

Favorable, with appropriate treatment

COMPLICATIONS

- Insulinoma: If tumor is identified and removed, some surgical risk is involved.
- Organic brain syndrome: may occur with extensive, prolonged hypoglycemia

REFERENCES

1. Palani G, Stortz E, Moheet A. Clinical presentation and diagnostic approach to hypoglycemia in adults without diabetes mellitus. *Endoc Pract*. 2023;29(4):286–294.
2. Kittah NE, Vella A. Management of endocrine disease: Pathogenesis and management of hypoglycemia. *Euro J Endocrinol*. 2017;177(1):R37–R47.
3. Cryer PE, Axelrod L, Grossman AB, et al. Evaluation and management of adult hypoglycemic disorders: an Endocrine Society clinical practice guideline. *J Clin Endocrinol Metab*. 2009;94(3):709–728.

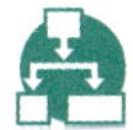

SEE ALSO

- Hypoglycemia, Diabetic; Insulinoma
- Algorithm: Hypoglycemia

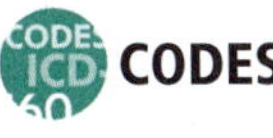

ICD10

- E16.2 Hypoglycemia, unspecified
- E16.1 Other hypoglycemia
- P70.4 Other neonatal hypoglycemia

CLINICAL PEARLS

- Symptoms coincide with low blood glucose levels and resolve with PO/IV glucose or glucagon.
- Avoid known agents/nutrients that trigger hypoglycemia.
- Treat the underlying cause.

H

HYPOKALEMIA

Anush Pillai, DO, FAAFP

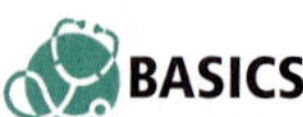

BASICS

DESCRIPTION

A serum potassium concentration <3.5 mEq/L (normal range, 3.5 to 5 mEq/L)

- Mild: 3 to 3.5 mEq/L
- Moderate: 2.5 to 3 mEq/L
- Severe: <2.5 mEq/L

EPIDEMIOLOGY

Predominant sex: male = female

Prevalence

- >20% of hospitalized patients, >10% with alcoholism
- 80% of patients receiving diuretics
- 12–18% of patients with chronic kidney disease
- Higher (5–20%) in individuals with eating disorders
- Associated risk after bariatric surgery

ETIOLOGY AND PATHOPHYSIOLOGY

Most common causes:

- Decreased intake: deficient diet in alcoholics and elderly; anorexia nervosa; patients receiving TPN or enteral nutrition; starvation
- GI loss: vomiting, diarrhea, nasogastric tubes, laxative abuse, malabsorption, chemotherapy, radiation enteropathy, bulimia, etc.
- Intracellular shift of potassium: metabolic alkalosis, insulin excess, β-adrenergic catecholamine excess (acute stress, β_2-agonists), thyrotoxicosis, hypokalemic periodic paralysis, intoxications (theophylline, caffeine, barium, risperidone, quetiapine, verapamil, toluene), refeeding syndrome, intensive exercise
- Renal potassium loss
  - Drugs: diuretics especially loop and thiazides, amphotericin B, aminoglycosides, antipseudomonal penicillins (carbenicillin), high-dose penicillin, clay (bentonite)
  - Mineralocorticoid excess: primary hyperaldosteronism (Conn syndrome); secondary hyperaldosteronism (congestive heart failure, cirrhosis, nephrotic syndrome, malignant hypertension, renin-producing tumors); renovascular hypertension
  - Exogenous mineralocorticoids (glycyrrhizic acid in licorice, carbenoxolone, nasal steroids)
  - Osmotic diuresis (e.g., poorly controlled diabetes)
  - Types I and II renal tubular acidosis
- Magnesium depletion
- Glucocorticoid excess: Cushing syndrome, exogenous steroids, ectopic adrenocorticotrophic hormone production, refeeding syndrome
- Diabetic ketoacidosis (DKA) treatment with delayed/inadequate potassium replenishment

Genetics

Some rare, familial disorders associated with hypokalemia

- 11-β-Hydroxysteroid dehydrogenase deficiency
- Fanconi syndrome
- Geller syndrome
- Sodium channel mutations: Bartter, Gitelman, Liddle syndrome

RISK FACTORS

- Higher systolic BP
- Thiazide/loop diuretic use
- Low serum cholesterol/low BMI
- Higher albumin-to-creatinine ratio

GENERAL PREVENTION

When initiating a diuretic, monitor potassium level.

COMMONLY ASSOCIATED CONDITIONS

- Acute GI illnesses with severe vomiting or diarrhea
- Increased risk of cardiac arrhythmias
- Predictor of development of severe alcohol withdrawal syndrome

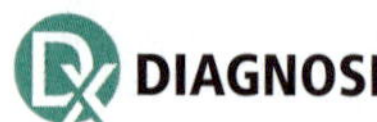

DIAGNOSIS

- Usually asymptomatic until serum potassium is <3.0 mEq/L, unless it falls rapidly or patient has potentiating factor, for example, disposition to arrhythmia
- Signs and symptoms mainly involve neuromuscular, cardiovascular, renal, and endocrine system.

HISTORY

- Diuretic use, malnutrition, vomiting, diarrhea
- Easy fatigability, leg cramps, muscle weakness
- Polyuria, polydipsia, nocturia; hyperglycemia, alkalosis/acidosis
- Heart failure, shortness of breath

PHYSICAL EXAM

- Neuromuscular—skeletal muscle weakness (proximal > distal), ascending paralysis
  - Smooth muscle—GI hypomobility
  - Respiratory muscle—respiratory acidosis, respiratory arrest
- Cardiovascular—hypotension, orthostasis, peripheral edema; auscultate for arrhythmias and rales.
- Renal—metabolic acidosis, rhabdomyolysis, myoglobinuria; chronic kidney disease (tubulointerstitial nephritis, nephrogenic diabetes insipidus, renal cyst)

DIFFERENTIAL DIAGNOSIS

Hypokalemia is a laboratory diagnosis that does not require distinction from other entities once laboratory error has been excluded.

DIAGNOSTIC TESTS & INTERPRETATION

- Serum potassium <3.5 mEq/L (<3.5 mmol/L)
- Disorders that may alter lab results: leukemia and leukocytosis

Initial Tests (lab, imaging)

- ECG
- Start workup if history rules out GI or iatrogenic causes (1).
  - Serum and urinary potassium level to evaluate the severity of hypokalemia
  - Basic metabolic panel (serum sodium, potassium, glucose, chloride, bicarbonate, BUN, creatinine); serum magnesium, calcium, and/or phosphorus to exclude associated electrolyte abnormality especially if alcoholism is suspected.
  - Spot urine electrolytes (potassium and chloride) to differentiate renal versus nonrenal cause.
  - Arterial blood gas to detect metabolic acidosis or alkalosis
  - Urinalysis and urine pH for renal tubular acidosis
  - Serum digoxin level for patient on digitalis
  - Creatinine kinase for rhabdomyolysis in severe hypokalemia
  - Clinical suspicion is high: urine/serum drug screen for amphetamines and other sympathomimetic stimulants; TSH in case of tachycardia or suspicion of hypokalemic periodic paralysis

Follow-Up Tests & Special Considerations

- Two major components (1)
  - Urine potassium excretion to distinguish renal loss versus other causes
  - Acid–base status
- 24-hour urinary potassium excretion (best method): >15 mEq/day = inappropriate renal loss; if unavailable:
  - Spot urine potassium-to-creatinine ratio >13 mEq/g (1.5 mEq/mmol) can indicate inappropriate renal loss; or
  - Transtubular potassium gradient (TTKG) > 4 can also suggest renal loss. In renal loss, 24-hour urine K > 30 mEq
    - TTKG = (urine K^+/plasma K^+) / (urine Osm/plasma Osm)
- Metabolic acidosis + low urinary excretion → GI loss (laxative abuse, villous adenoma). In GI loss, kidneys will preserve potassium (K) and 24-hour urine K < 30 mEq.
- Metabolic acidosis + urinary potassium wasting → DKA, renal tubular acidosis type 1 or 2
- Metabolic alkalosis + low urinary excretion → vomiting, bulimic, or diuretic use
- Metabolic alkalosis + urine potassium wasting →
  - Normotensive: vomiting (low urine chloride); Gitelman/Bartter syndrome (normal urine chloride), diuretics (Urine chloride varies with types.)
  - Hypertensive: primary aldosteronism, Liddle syndrome, Geller syndrome, glucocorticoid resistance
- If excessive renal potassium loss (>20 mEq/day) and hypertension, obtain plasma renin and aldosterone levels to differentiate adrenal from nonadrenal causes of hyperaldosteronism.

Diagnostic Procedures/Other

Consider imaging in cases with high clinical index of suspicion (1)

- MRI/CT of adrenal gland with suspicion of mineralocorticoid, glucocorticoid, or catecholamine excess
- MRI of pituitary gland to exclude Cushing syndrome
- Abdominal CT for VIPoma

Test Interpretation

ECG (2)

- T-wave flattening, ST-segment changes
- U waves (small, positive deflection after T wave, best seen in V_2 and V_3)
- Arrhythmias include sinus bradycardia, PAC/PVC, paroxysmal atrial or junctional tachycardia, atrioventricular block, ventricular tachycardia or fibrillation.

TREATMENT

- Determine cause.
- Reduce potassium loss; replenish stored potassium.

GENERAL MEASURES

Manage underlying disease or eliminate causative factor.

- Discontinue laxative, use potassium-neutral or potassium-sparing diuretics.
- Treat diarrhea and vomiting.
- Use H_2 blockers in patient with nasogastric suction.
- Control hyperglycemia if glucosuria is present.

MEDICATION

- Nonemergent conditions (serum potassium >2.5 mEq/L [>2.5 mmol/L], no cardiac manifestations)
  - Oral therapy preferred: 40 to 120 mEq/day (40 to 120 mmol/day) in divided doses
  - Ensure adequate hydration (100 to 250 mL of water), better if given with or after meal.
  - IV potassium only when oral administration is not feasible (e.g., vomiting, postoperative state)
    - Rate should not exceed 10 mEq/hr, and concentration should not exceed 40 mEq/L to lessen burning and discomfort at IV site and to avoid phlebitis.
    - A central line is recommended for rate >10 mEq/hr; up to 40 mEq in 100 mL can be safely given via central access.
    - Potassium chloride (KCl) is suitable for all forms of hypokalemia.
    - Potassium bicarbonate or precursor (gluconate, acetate, or citrate) in metabolic acidosis
    - Potassium phosphate in phosphate deficiency as in DKA (3)[C]
- Emergent situations (serum potassium <2.5 mEq/L [<2.5 mmol/L], arrhythmias) (1)[A]
  - IV replacement—standard infusion rate: 10 mmol/hr; maximum infusion rate: 20 mmol/hr
  - Central line preferred. Normal saline is preferred because D5W can cause transcellular shift of potassium into cells. D5W will cause insulin release and worsen hypokalemia.
- If patient is hypomagnesemic (1)[A]
  - First, give 4 mL MgSO4 50% (8 mmol) in 10 mL of NaCl 0.9% >20 minutes and then start first 40 mmol KCl infusion followed by magnesium replacement.
- Precautions
  - Any form of potassium replacement carries the risk of hyperkalemia.
  - Serum potassium should be checked more frequently in groups at higher risk: the elderly, diabetic patients, and patients with renal insufficiency.
  - Patients receiving insulin for DKA require more timely and aggressive potassium replacement in order to account for the intracellular shift (4)[A].
  - Dietary potassium is almost entirely coupled to phosphate, rather than chloride, and does not correct potassium loss from chloride depletion (e.g., diuretics or vomiting).
- Significant possible interactions: Concomitant administration of potassium-sparing diuretics (spironolactone, triamterene, amiloride, ACE inhibitors) magnifies risk of hyperkalemia.

Geriatric Considerations

- Younger patient has a higher prevalence for hypokalemia, but elderly develop hypokalemia more rapidly.
- Low serum potassium can induce limb paralysis, myonecrosis, and increase fall risk.

ISSUES FOR REFERRAL

Patient with unexplained hypokalemia, refractory hyperkalemia, or features suggesting alternative diagnosis (e.g., aldosteronism or hypokalemic periodic paralysis) should be referred to endocrinology or nephrology.

ADMISSION, INPATIENT, AND NURSING CONSIDERATIONS

- Outpatient follow-up is sufficient for asymptomatic patients treated with oral replacement.
- Patients with cardiac manifestations require IV replacement with continuous cardiac monitoring in an inpatient setting.
- Patient with life-threatening complications such as arrhythmias or respiratory failure requires ICU admission.

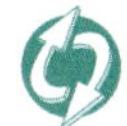

ONGOING CARE

FOLLOW-UP RECOMMENDATIONS

Patient Monitoring

Patients receiving IV therapy should have continuous cardiac monitoring and serum potassium levels monitored.

DIET

- Ensure adequate intake: potassium-rich food including oranges, bananas, cantaloupes, kiwi, prunes, raisins, dried beans, dried apricots, mangos, avocado, dates, figs, spinach, and squash.
- Reduce sodium intake: High-sodium diet can cause urinary potassium loss.

PATIENT EDUCATION

- Instructions for appropriate diet
- Potassium Fact Sheet for Consumers: https://ods.od.nih.gov/pdf/factsheets/Potassium-Consumer.pdf

PROGNOSIS

- Most hypokalemia will correct with replacement after 24 to 72 hours.
- If primary cause is eliminated, hypokalemia will likely resolve with no further treatment needed.
- Associated with higher morbidity and mortality because of cardiac arrhythmias

COMPLICATIONS

- Hyperkalemia during the course of treatment
- Increased risk of digoxin toxicity
- Increased risk of arrhythmias by increasing myocyte's resting potential and in turn its refractory period

REFERENCES

1. Kardalas E, Paschou SA, Anagnostis P, et al. Hypokalemia: a clinical update. *Endocr Connect*. 2018;7(4):R135–R146.
2. Skogestad J, Aronsen JM. Hypokalemia-induced arrhythmias and heart failure: new insights and implications for therapy. *Front Physiol*. 2018;9:1500.
3. Asmar A, Mohandas R, Wingo CS. A physiologic-based approach to the treatment of a patient with hypokalemia. *Am J Kidney Dis*. 2012;60(3):492–497.
4. Kovesdy CP, Matsushita K, Sang Y, et al. Serum potassium and adverse outcomes across the range of kidney function: a CKD Prognosis Consortium meta-analysis. *Eur Heart J*. 2018;39(17):1535–1542.

ADDITIONAL READING

Viera AJ, Wouk N. Potassium disorders: hypokalemia and hyperkalemia. *Am Fam Physician*. 2015;92(6):487–495.

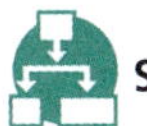

SEE ALSO

- Hyperkalemia
- Algorithm: Hypokalemia

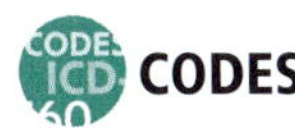

CODES

ICD10

E87.6 Hypokalemia

CLINICAL PEARLS

- In patients with cardiac ischemia, heart failure, or left ventricular hypertrophy, even mild to moderate hypokalemia can cause arrhythmias.
- Uncorrected hypomagnesemia can hinder the correction of hypokalemia.
- Hypokalemia in an otherwise healthy young woman should prompt evaluation for bulimia nervosa.
- Supplement potassium (via dietary intake or supplements) when prescribing drugs that cause hypokalemia; minimize dosage of non–potassium-sparing diuretics.

HYPONATREMIA

Vikas Gupta, MD, MPH

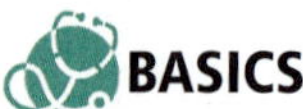

BASICS

Think about hyponatremia as a water problem, rather than a true sodium (Na^+) problem.

DESCRIPTION

- Hyponatremia is a plasma Na^+ concentration of <135 mEq/L.
- In healthy individuals, the excess water is renally excreted in due to suppression of antidiuretic hormone (ADH) to maintain homeostatic state.

EPIDEMIOLOGY

Prevalence

- Most common electrolyte disorder seen in the general hospital population, affecting 2%.
- 7.7% outpatients (1)

Geriatric Considerations

Elderly patients have decreased renal mass placing them at risk for decreased urinary concentration and decreased response to ADH. Presenting symptoms may be frequent falls and gait disturbances. Clinicians should also consider the impact of comorbidities and acute disease.

Pediatric Considerations

Children are at increased risk of brain herniation from cerebral edema.

ETIOLOGY AND PATHOPHYSIOLOGY

- Volume status and serum osmolality must be ascertained to determine etiology in order to direct management.
- Normal serum osmolality is 280 to 295 mOsm/kg.
- Serum osmolality (Osm) (mmol/kg) = (2 × serum [Na]) + (serum [glucose]/18) + (blood urea nitrogen (BUN)/2.8)
- Hypertonic hyponatremia: serum Osm >295 mOsmol/kg
  - Accumulation of solutes that are osmotically active, causing water shifts from intracellular fluid (ICF) to extracellular fluid (ECF), resulting in dilution.
    - Causes: hyperglycemia, mannitol, sorbitol, radiologic contrast
- Isotonic hyponatremia ("pseudohyponatremia"): serum Osm 275 to 295 mOsm/kg
  - Falsely low levels of sodium; actual levels are normal.
  - Osmolality is normal; usually euvolemic
  - Unchanged TBW and Na^+
  - Causes: hyperlipidemia, hyperproteinemia (e.g., multiple myeloma), jaundice (caused by elevated lipoprotein X levels), laboratory artifact, hyperglycemia
- Hypotonic hyponatremia: serum Osm <275 mOsmol/kg
  - Subdivided by volume status into hypovolemic, euvolemic, or hypervolemic
  - Hypovolemic hyponatremia: low TBW and low Na^+
    - Signs include orthostatic hypotension, decreased skin turgor, dry mucous membranes.
    - If urine Na^+ <30 mmol/L, it indicates extrarenal loss such as GI loss (vomiting, diarrhea), third-spacing (pancreatitis, burns), skin loss (burns, cystic fibrosis, sweating), and heat-related illnesses.
    - If Urine Na^+ >30 mmol/L, it indicates renal loss such as cerebral salt wasting, adrenal insufficiency, diuretics, and osmotic diuresis.
- Euvolemic hyponatremia: mild to moderate increase in TBW, normal Na^+ (most common subtype)
  - Signs include a nonedematous state.
  - If urine Osm >100 mOsm/kg, causes include syndrome of inappropriate antidiuretic hormone (SIADH), hypothyroidism, adrenal insufficiency, and medications (e.g., thiazide diuretics, loop diuretics, carbamazepine, clofibrate, cyclosporine, levetiracetam, oxcarbazepine, SSRIs, TCAs, vincristine, barbiturates, chlorpropamide, opioids).
  - If urine Osm <100 mOsm/kg, causes include primary polydipsia, beer potomania, and exercise-induced hyponatremia.
- Hypervolemic hyponatremia: increased TBW and Na^+
  - Signs include edematous state.
  - Urine Na^+ <30 mmol/L
  - Causes include congestive heart failure (CHF), cirrhosis, nephrotic syndrome, hypoalbuminemia, psychogenic polydipsia, renal failure.

Genetics

Mutations have been associated with nephrogenic syndrome of inappropriate antidiuresis (NSAID; SIADH).

GENERAL PREVENTION

Maintain appropriate hydration.

COMMONLY ASSOCIATED CONDITIONS

- Hypothyroidism, hypopituitarism
- Cirrhosis, CHF, nephrotic syndrome
- Adrenocortical hormone deficiency
- SIADH is associated with cancers, pneumonia, tuberculosis, encephalitis, meningitis, head trauma, cerebrovascular accident, and HIV infection.
- Medications: thiazide diuretics, SSRIs, carbamazepine
- Marathon runners in hot environments
- Beer potomania
- Tea-and-toast diet
- Ecstasy use

DIAGNOSIS

- Symptoms are related to the rate of fall in serum Na^+, onset, and degree of hyponatremia (1)[C],(2)[C].
- Acute (≤48 hours): no time for full adaptation, more likely to present with moderate or severe symptoms
- Chronic (>48 hours): develops gradually, organ systems adapt to Na^+ concentration, associated with minimal symptoms
- Mild (serum Na^+ 130 to 134 mEq/L): usually asymptomatic, fatigue, loss of appetite
- Moderate (serum Na^+ 120 to 129 mEq/L): nausea, vomiting, lethargy
- Severe (serum Na^+ 115 to 119 mEq/L): headache, lethargy, restlessness, disorientation
- Severe/rapid decrease in serum Na^+ can cause seizures, coma, brain herniation, respiratory arrest, and may be fatal.
- Other signs and symptoms: headache, dizziness, ataxia, weakness, muscle cramps, anorexia, hiccups, depressed deep tendon reflexes, hypothermia, positive Babinski responses, cranial nerve palsies, orthostatic hypotension

> **ALERT**
>
> Low Na^+ creates an osmotic gradient between plasma and cells, resulting in fluid shift into cells. This causes cerebral edema and increased intracranial pressure; eventually, this can lead to hyponatremic encephalopathy and brain herniation.

HISTORY

- Symptoms include headache, nausea, vomiting, muscle cramps.
- Can progress to lethargy or restlessness and disorientation

PHYSICAL EXAM

- Volume status: skin turgor, jugular venous pressure, heart rate, peripheral edema, orthostatic blood pressure measurement
- Evaluate for underlying illness: signs of dehydration, volume overload, CHF, cirrhosis, hypothyroidism
- Decreased reflexes may be seen.
- Evaluate patient's gait for unsteadiness and ataxia. Perform a complete neurologic exam.

DIAGNOSTIC TESTS & INTERPRETATION

Initial Tests (lab, imaging)

- BUN, creatinine, glucose, electrolytes, liver function studies
- Thyroid-stimulating hormone (TSH)
- Lipid panel
- Serum Osm
- Urine Osm
- Urine Na^+
- Chest x-ray to rule out pulmonary pathology if SIADH is diagnosed

Follow-Up Tests & Special Considerations

MRI brain/pituitary if pituitary problem is suspected or if SIADH from CNS problem is suspected.

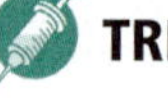

TREATMENT

GENERAL MEASURES

- Assess all medications that patient is taking.
- Institute seizure precautions.
- Institute fluid restriction for hypervolemic patients.
- Fluid resuscitation in hypovolemic patients. Indications for 3% hypertonic saline versus normal saline solution include: acute hyponatremia, symptomatic hyponatremia, association with intracranial pathology already at risk for cerebral edema (1)[C],(2)[C].

MEDICATION

ALERT

Rapid correction of severe symptomatic hyponatremia has been associated with osmotic demyelination syndrome (ODS). This results in irreversible injury. Symptoms are apparent 2 to 6 days after injury and include seizure, coma, spastic paraparesis, dysarthria, and dysphagia. Patients at increased risk are those with Na^+ <105 mEq/L, alcoholism, hypokalemia, and malnutrition. MRI brain may not be positive until 4 weeks after symptom onset

- Treatment is tailored to etiology, degree of hyponatremia, onset, and symptomatology:
  - TBW = a coefficient × weight (kg) as in the following table:

	Total Body Water
Children and men	0.6 × weight
Women and elderly men	0.5 × weight
Elderly women	0.45 × weight

- Asymptomatic, euvolemic patients can be treated with fluid restriction; etiology must be addressed.
- Below is an example demonstrating how to calculate the amount of fluids in a patient who needs hyponatremia correction:
  - In a 50-year-old female who weighs 70 kg, and you need to correct Na^+ at a rate of 8 mEq/24 hr, first calculate the TBW (70.0 × 0.5 = 35.0).
  - Then, calculate Na^+ deficit needed to achieve desired level = TBW × correction rate in 24 hours = 35 × 8 = 280 mEq.
  - This means that you need to give 280 mEq of Na^+ to the patient in 24 hours to achieve a correction rate of 8 mEq/24 hr.
  - 1 L of 3% hypertonic saline contains 513 mEq of Na^+. This means that you need to give (280 mEq × 1,000 mL) / 513 mEq = 546 mL/24 hr (approximately 23 mL/hr).
  - 1 L of 0.9% normal saline contains 154 mEq of Na^+. This means that you need to give (280 mEq × 1,000 mL) / 154 mEq = 1,818 mL/24 hr (approximately 75 mL/hr).
- For severe hyponatremia (<125 mEq/L), 3% hypertonic saline should be given.
  - Done as a 50 to 100 mL bolus, with the goal increasing the serum Na^+ 2 to 3 mEq/L. The bolus may be given twice if symptoms have not resolved.
  - Done as a continuous infusion of 3% to increase the serum Na^+ 6 to 8 mEq/L, with the goal to not exceed correction of 10 to 12 mEq/L in the first 24 hours.
  - Desmopressin can also be considered, given 1 to 2 μg every 4 to 6 hours.
  - Serum Na^+ should be checked every 2 hours. The infusion rate and fluids should be changed to isotonic saline when appropriate.
  - In patients who do not respond to the aforementioned approach, consider the use of vasopressin V2-receptor antagonists, such as tolvaptan or conivaptan. This class of medications should not be used in patients with liver disease.
  - For mild to moderate hyponatremia, use isotonic saline solution (0.9%).
  - In patients with severe hyponatremia (euvolemic and hypervolemic state) who do not respond to the aforementioned approach, consider the use of vasopressin V2-receptor antagonists, such as tolvaptan or conivaptan (3)[A]. This class of medications should not be in used in patients with liver disease.
  - Patients with hypervolemic hyponatremia caused by cirrhosis, heart failure, or kidney disease benefit from restriction of Na^+ and fluids, diuretic therapy, and management of the underlying etiology.
  - Treat underlying etiology.
  - Chronic hyponatremia resulting from SIADH (4)[A]: demeclocycline (inhibits ADH action at the collecting duct) if fluid restriction alone is not effective.
    - Contraindications: drug allergy, pregnancy, children <8 years old; caution in renal and hepatic disease
    - In doses of 600 to 1,200 mg/day, the drug produces nephrogenic diabetes insipidus.
    - Significant possible interactions: oral anticoagulants, oral contraceptives, penicillin
    - In case of overcorrection, relower Na^+ concentration. Begin with infusion of 3 mL/kg of 5% dextrose in water over 1 hour. Repeat Na^+ measurement. Be cautious, dextrose infusion rates >250 to 300 mL/hr can cause significant hyperglycemia in both diabetic and nondiabetic patients and may lead to osmotic diuresis and subsequent free water loss with increased serum Na^+ concentration. Consider 2 to 4 μg IV desmopressin every 8 hours to prevent overcorrection.

ALERT

Caution: If severe hyponatremia, consider hypertonic saline (3% Na^+ chloride) with central line access, exercise extreme caution, and monitor serum Na^+ as frequently as every 1 to 2 hours.

First Line

- Fluid resuscitation (hypovolemia)
- Fluid restriction (euvolemia/hypervolemia)

Second Line

Vasopressin V2-receptor antagonists

ADMISSION, INPATIENT, AND NURSING CONSIDERATIONS

- Admission is mandatory if the patient is symptomatic or has acute hyponatremia (developing over <48 hours), which increases the risk of cerebral edema.
- Admission is advised if patient is asymptomatic and has a serum Na^+ <125 mEq/dL.

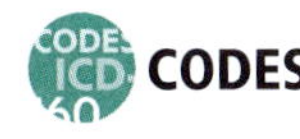

ONGOING CARE

DIET

- Euvolemic hyponatremia: Restrict water to 1.0 to 1.5 L/day.
- Hypervolemic hyponatremia: water and Na^+ restriction

PROGNOSIS

- In hospitalized patients, hyponatremia is associated with an elevated risk of adverse clinical outcomes and higher mortality (1).
- In community-dwelling, middle-aged, and elderly adults, mild hyponatremia has been shown to be an independent predictor of death.
- Associated with poor prognosis in patients with acute pulmonary embolism.
- Associated with poor prognosis in patients with liver cirrhosis and those waiting for liver transplant; it is associated with significant postoperative risk and short-term graft loss.

COMPLICATIONS

- Occult tumor may be present if SIADH is identified.
- Hypervolemia if isotonic saline solution is used.
- Osmotic demyelination syndrome (central pontine and extrapontine irreversible myelinolysis) if the Na^+ is corrected too quickly
- Hyponatremia is the cause of 30% new-onset seizures in intensive care settings.
- Chronic hyponatremia is associated with increased risk of osteoporosis, attention deficit, gait disturbances, falls, and fractures.

REFERENCES

1. Rondon-Berrios H, Agaba EI, Tzamaloukas AH. Hyponatremia: pathophysiology, classification, manifestations and management. *Int Urol Nephrol*. 2014;46(11):2153–2165.
2. Williams DM, Gallagher M, Handley J, et al. The clinical management of hyponatraemia. *Postgrad Med J*. 2016;92(1089):407–411.
3. Rozen-Zvi B, Yahav D, Gheorghiade M, et al. Vasopressin receptor antagonists for the treatment of hyponatremia: systematic review and meta-analysis. *Am J Kidney Dis*. 2010;56(2):325–337.
4. Basu A, Ryder RE. The syndrome of inappropriate antidiuresis is associated with excess long-term mortality: a retrospective cohort analyses. *J Clin Pathol*. 2014;67(9):802–806.

CODES

ICD10

E87.1 Hypo-osmolality and hyponatremia

CLINICAL PEARLS

- Assess all medications patient is taking because many are associated with hyponatremia.
- Alcohol-dependent individuals with vitamin deficiencies, elderly women taking thiazide diuretics, and people with hypokalemia or burns are at increased risk of ODS from too rapid correction of hyponatremia. Chronic hyponatremia is also a risk factor.
- Bronchogenic carcinoma and pancreatic, duodenal, and prostate cancer, as well as thymoma, lymphoma, and mesothelioma, are neoplastic diseases associated with SIADH.

HYPOPARATHYROIDISM

Rashida Adenwala, MD

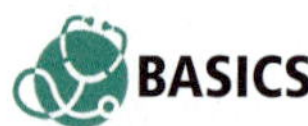

BASICS

DESCRIPTION

- Deficient or absent secretion of parathyroid hormone (PTH) (1)
- Acute hypoparathyroidism: mild tetany (muscle cramps, perioral numbness, paresthesias of hands and feet) or severe (carpopedal spasm, laryngospasm, heart failure, cardiac arrhythmias, seizures, stridor)
- Chronic: often asymptomatic; lethargy, anxiety/depression, urolithiasis and renal impairment, dementia, blurry vision, parkinsonism or other movement disorders, dental abnormalities, and dry, puffy, coarse skin, ischemic heart disease
- System(s) affected: endocrine/metabolic, musculoskeletal, nervous, ophthalmologic, renal, cardiac, psychiatric

Pediatric Considerations

- May occur in premature infants
- Maternal hypercalcemia can result in infantile hypocalcemia with suppressed parathyroid development.
- Infants of mothers with hypocalciuric hypercalcemia can also have hypoparathyroidism (hypoPTH).
- Congenital absence of parathyroids
- Autoimmune hypoparathyroidism appears later in childhood

Pregnancy Considerations

- For women with hypoparathyroidism, calcium and calcitriol requirements may change, so close monitoring of serum calcium adjusted for albumin q3–4wk during pregnancy
- Hypocalcemia in pregnancy is associated with uterine contractions and an increased risk of preterm labor or miscarriage.
- Maternal hypocalcemia can be associated with secondary fetal hyperparathyroidism (hyperPTH) causing skeletal complications and fractures.

EPIDEMIOLOGY

More common in women; affects all ages

Incidence

- Chronic hypoPTH—0.8 to 2.3/100,000 per person-years
- Transient/temporary after total thyroidectomy—20–30%
- Most common after anterior neck surgery, particularly when the surgeon performs few anterior neck dissections (<50 to 100 per year)
- Transient hyperPTH is common (6.9–46% of thyroidectomies).

Prevalence

- Affects 24 to 37/100,000 persons per year in the United States (1)
- Genetic disorders account for <10% of all hypoparathyroidism, but represent a large proportion of cases in children.

ETIOLOGY AND PATHOPHYSIOLOGY

- PTH aids in regulating calcium homeostasis; reduced or absent PTH results in hypocalcemia, hyperphosphatemia, and hypercalciuria.
- Acquired hypoparathyroidism
  - Surgical: removal or damage to parathyroid glands during neck surgery (2) (hungry bone syndrome)
  - Autoimmune: isolated/acquired disease or combined with other endocrine deficiencies in polyglandular autoimmune (PGA) syndrome
  - Deposition of heavy metals in gland: copper (Wilson disease) or iron (hemochromatosis, thalassemias), aluminium, radiation-induced destruction, and infiltration (metastatic, granulomatous, inflammatory or amyloid protein)
  - Functional/transient hypoparathyroidism: may result from hypomagnesemia or hypermagnesemia because magnesium is crucial for PTH secretion and activation of the PTH receptor
  - Congenital
- Infiltrative: metastatic carcinoma, hemochromatosis, Wilson disease, granulomas

Genetics

- X-linked or in autosomal recessive mutations in the transcription factor glial cell missing B (GCMB)
- Mutations in transcription factors or regulators of parathyroid gland development

RISK FACTORS

Neck surgery and neck trauma, neck malignancies, family history of hypocalcemia, PGA syndrome

GENERAL PREVENTION

Intraoperative identification and preservation of parathyroid tissue

COMMONLY ASSOCIATED CONDITIONS

DiGeorge syndrome; Bartter syndrome; PGA syndrome type I; Multiple endocrine deficiency autoimmune candidiasis (MEDAC) syndrome; Juvenile familial endocrinopathy; Addison disease; Moniliasis (HAM) syndrome: a polyglandular deficiency syndrome, possibly genetic, characterized by hypoparathyroidism

DIAGNOSIS

HISTORY

Often asymptomatic; ask about previous neck trauma or surgery, head or neck irradiation, family history of hypocalcemia, or presence of other autoimmune endocrinopathies.

- Cardinal clinical feature: neuromuscular hyperexcitability
- Also includes: fatigue, circumoral or distal extremity paresthesias, muscle spasm, seizures, neuropsychiatric symptoms

PHYSICAL EXAM

- Surgical scar on neck
- Chvostek sign: ipsilateral twitching of the upper lip on tapping the facial nerve on the cheek; 15% of normocalcemic people have positive sign (1).
- Trousseau sign: painful carpal spasm after 3-minute occlusion of brachial artery with BP cuff; BP cuff inflation to above systolic BP for 3 minutes leads to carpal spasm (flexion of metacarpophalangeal [MCP] joints, extension of interphalangeal [IP] joints, adduction of fingers and thumb).
- Tetany, laryngospasm or bronchospasm, cardiac arrhythmias, refractory heart failure, dyspnea, edema
- Dry, coarse, puffy hair; brittle nails; vitiligo; tooth enamel defects
- Loss of deep tendon reflexes
- Cataracts or ectopic calcifications

DIFFERENTIAL DIAGNOSIS

- Vitamin D deficiency/resistance
- Pseudohypoparathyroidism, presents in childhood; kidney and bone unresponsiveness to PTH; characterized by hypocalcemia, hyperphosphatemia, and, in contrast to hypoparathyroidism, elevated PTH concentrations
- Hypoalbuminemia, renal failure, malabsorption, familial hypocalcemia, hypomagnesemia

DIAGNOSTIC TESTS & INTERPRETATION

Initial Tests (lab, imaging)

- Calcium: low ionized and total (correct serum calcium level for albumin)
- Phosphorus: high
- Intact or "whole" PTH: low; distinguish from pseudohypoparathyroidism or secondary causes
- Magnesium: low or normal
- BUN, creatinine (Cr): monitor renal function, especially in the elderly
- 1,25-OH vitamin D level: low can worsen hypoparathyroidism
- Urinary calcium: normal or high
- Calcium should be monitored after thyroid or parathyroid surgery, including intraoperatively
- Radiographs/MRI may show absent tooth roots, calcification of cerebellum, choroid plexus, or cerebral basal ganglia.

Follow-Up Tests & Special Considerations

- ECG: prolongation of ST and QTc intervals, nonspecific repolarization changes, dysrhythmias
- Urine calcium: Cr ratio (normal 0.1 to 0.2) may be low before treatment; monitor to prevent stones.
- Osteoblastic metastasis of prostate, breast, or lung cancer; consider appropriate imaging.
- Use PTH measurement early (12 to 24 hours post total thyroidectomy) to predict which patients will *not* develop postsurgical hypoPTH. A value >10 pg/mL means permanent hypoPTH is unlikely.
- Genetic testing for patients with nonsurgical hypoPTH with positive family history, syndromic features, or age <40 years

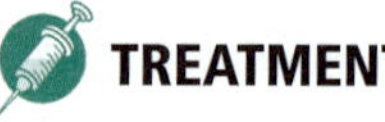

TREATMENT

GENERAL MEASURES

- Monitor ECG during calcium repletion.
- Maintenance therapy: may require lifelong treatment with calcium and calcitriol; maintain serum calcium in low normal range: 8 to 8.5 mg/dL (2.00 to 2.12 mmol/L).
- Thiazide diuretics with a low-salt diet to prevent hypercalciuria, nephrocalcinosis, and nephrolithiasis
- Oral calcium and vitamin D supplementation after thyroidectomy may reduce the risk for symptomatic hypocalcemia.

MEDICATION

Acute hypoparathyroidism

- Hypoparathyroid with severe symptoms (tetany, seizures, cardiac failure, laryngospasm, bronchospasm)
  - IV calcium gluconate: 1 or 2 g, each infused over 10 minutes; central venous catheter preferred; follow with infusion of 10 g calcium gluconate in 1 L 5% dextrose water at a rate of 1 to 3 mg calcium gluconate per kg body weight per hour (2)[B].
- Hypomagnesemia: acutely: 1 to 2 g IV q6h; long-term magnesium oxide tablets (600 mg) once or twice per day

First Line

Chronic hypoparathyroidism

- Calcium:
  - Oral calcium carbonate preferred; take with meals and stop PPI for better absorption.
  - Oral calcium citrate: preferred for patients on PPI therapy and those with constipation on calcium carbonate
  - Starting dose: 1 to 3 g/day of elemental calcium; divided doses preferred
  - Aim for low normal plasma calcium.
  - Children: oral elemental calcium: 25 to 50 mg/kg daily
- Calcitriol
  - Vitamin D 1, 25-dihydroxycholecalciferol preferred form of vitamin D replacement; start at 0.25 μg/day; usual doses 0.5 to 2.0 μg/day (3)[A].
  - Children: Calcitriol: 0.25 μg daily for age >1 year
- If hyperphosphatemia level well above normal (>6.5 mg/dL): low phosphate diet or phosphate binder

Second Line

Palopegteriparatide (Yorvipath)

- Drug class: PTH analog; first and only PTH replacement therapy; FDA approved in August 2024
  - Not first line due to cost, injection delivery, monitoring needs, and limited long-term safety data
  - Use if unable to adequately control with standard therapy or have complications from conventional treatment.
- Mechanism: long-acting PTH analog (prodrug releasing PTH[1 to 34]) via daily subcutaneous injection
  - Available as prefilled injection pens, delivering 6 to 30 μg of PTH(1 to 34) per day
  - Dosing:
    - 18 μg once daily; titrated in 3 μg increments/decrements based on serum calcium levels; range: 6 to 30 μg/day, though up to 60 μg/day may be used with supplemental calcium or vitamin D if needed
    - For doses >30 μg/day, 2 separate injections given sequentially at distinct injection sites
  - Monitoring: Check serum calcium 7 to 10 days after initiating or changing dose; then every 4 to 6 weeks once stable
  - Safety and warnings
    - Common side effects: injection site reactions, orthostatic hypotension, headache, diarrhea, back pain, hypercalcemia, sore throat
    - Serious risks: hypercalcemia (especially early or after dose changes),hypocalcemia (particularly if abruptly discontinued), orthostatic hypotension, digoxin toxicity
    - Osteosarcoma risk: observed in rats; not confirmed in humans, but caution advised in high-risk patients

ISSUES FOR REFERRAL

Endocrinologist for long-term management; nephrologist for renal impairment/recurrent stones; ophthalmologist for eye involvement; geneticist if concern for inherited syndrome; cardiologist for ischemic heart disease/arrhythmias

SURGERY/OTHER PROCEDURES

Autotransplantation of cryopreserved parathyroid tissue: restores normocalcemia in 23% of cases

ADMISSION, INPATIENT, AND NURSING CONSIDERATIONS

Admission criteria/initial stabilization: laryngospasm, seizures, tetany, QT prolongation

ONGOING CARE

FOLLOW-UP RECOMMENDATIONS

Patient Monitoring

- Total corrected serum calcium level in low normal range (8.0 to 8.5 mg/dL or 2.00 to 2.12 mmol/L), 24-hour urine calcium <300 mg, and calcium-phosphate product <55. If Ca <2 mmol/L or <8 mg/dL, then treat even if asymptomatic (4)[B].
- Measurement of serum calcium, phosphate, magnesium, and Cr weekly to monthly during initial management when stable, measure every 6 months (4)[B]
- 24-hour urine for calcium and Cr secretion yearly
- If symptoms of renal stone disease or increasing Cr, get renal imaging every 5 years (4)[B].
- Annual slit-lamp and ophthalmologic evaluations are recommended.
- DEXA scan: standard monitoring recommended (4)[B]

DIET

Low-phosphate diet in patients with hyperphosphatemia

PATIENT EDUCATION

https://www.hypopara.org/

PROGNOSIS

Hypoparathyroidism following neck surgery is often transient. Length of required treatment may vary depending on origin.

COMPLICATIONS

- Reversible: due to low calcium levels, most likely to improve with adequate treatment
  - Neuromuscular symptoms: paresthesias (circumoral, fingers, toes), tetany, seizures, parkinsonian symptoms; pseudotumor cerebri
  - Renal: hypercalciuria, nephrocalcinosis, nephrolithiasis
  - Cardiovascular: heart failure, arrhythmias
- Irreversible: when condition starts early in childhood and will not improve with calcium and vitamin D treatment
  - Stunting of growth
  - Enamel defects and hypoplasia of teeth
  - Atrophy, brittleness, and ridging of nails
  - Cataracts and basal ganglia calcifications

REFERENCES

1. Abate E, Clarke B. Review of hypoparathyroidism. *Front Endocrinol (Lausanne)*. 2017;7:172.
2. Al-Azem H, Khan A. Hypoparathyroidism. *Best Pract Res Clin Endocrinol Metab*. 2012;26(4):517–522.
3. Bilezikian JP, Khan A, Potts JT Jr, et al. Hypoparathyroidism in the adult: epidemiology, diagnosis, pathophysiology, target-organ involvement, treatment, and challenges for future research. *J Bone Miner Res*. 2011;26(10):2317–2337.
4. Brandi M, Bilezikian D, Shoback D, et al. Management of hypoparathyroidism: summary statement and guidelines. *J Clin Endocrinol Metab*. 2016;101(6):2273–2283.

ADDITIONAL READING

Bollerslev J, Rejnmark L, Marcocci C, et al. European Society of Endocrinology clinical guideline: treatment of chronic hypoparathyroidism in adults. *Eur J Endocrinol*. 2015;173(2):G1–G20.

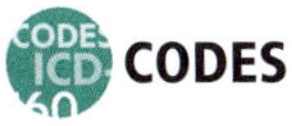

CODES

ICD10

- E20 Hypoparathyroidism
- E20.8 Other hypoparathyroidism
- E20.0 Idiopathic hypoparathyroidism

CLINICAL PEARLS

Often asymptomatic; consider if hypocalcemic with fatigue and circumoral or distal extremity paresthesias

- Correct the serum calcium level for albumin level.
- Monitor calcium after thyroid or parathyroid surgery.
- Distinguish hypoparathyroidism from pseudohypoparathyroidism and secondary causes by PTH level.
- Serum levels of magnesium and 25-OH should be measured to rule out deficiency that could contribute to reduced serum calcium levels.

HYPOTHERMIA

Corey J. Costanzo, DO, MPH, MS • Matthew Morrow, DO

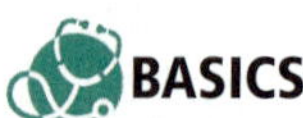

BASICS

DESCRIPTION

- Accidental hypothermia is the result of an unanticipated environmental exposure to cold temperatures. It is manifested as a core temperature of <35°C (95°F), and it may take hours to days to develop (1).
- Although patients with cold-water immersion may appear dead, they can sometimes be resuscitated; therefore, it is important to evaluate, treat as indicated, rewarm, and reassess.
- System(s) affected: all body systems
- Synonym(s): accidental hypothermia

EPIDEMIOLOGY

- Predominant age: young children and elderly
- Predominant sex: male > female

Geriatric Considerations

More common in elderly due to lower metabolic rate, impaired ability to maintain normal body temperature, and impaired ability to detect temperature changes (2)

Incidence

From 1999 to 2011, the CDC reported 16,911 deaths due to hypothermia.

Prevalence

Estimates vary widely; typically a secondary issue

ETIOLOGY AND PATHOPHYSIOLOGY

Core temperature is typically tightly maintained between 36.5°C and 37.5°C (97.7°F and 99.5°F). Accidental hypothermia is most often the result of overwhelming environmental cold stress. Other contributing factors include (1):

- Decreased heat production (e.g., hypopituitarism; hypothyroidism; adrenal insufficiency) (1)
- Increased heat loss (e.g., immersion—this is the most commonly encountered form of hypothermia in emergency situations—or burns) (1)
- Alcohol consumption (contributes in up to 68% of cases) (1)
- Impaired thermoregulation (e.g., stroke, central nervous system (CNS) tumors) (1)

Pediatric Considerations

- Children are at greater risk for hypothermia due to a larger ratio of surface area to body mass (2).
- Young infants cannot increase heat production through shivering and children have limited glycogen stores to maintain heat production.
- Children and infants have a decreased ability to recognize, avoid, or escape hypothermic exposure. Also, the history may not suggest hypothermia. Hypothermia does not require extreme exposure in children. Nonaccidental trauma may contribute.

RISK FACTORS

- Alcohol consumption; drug intoxication
- Bronchopneumonia
- Cardiovascular disease; cardiac arrest
- Cold-water immersion; prolonged environmental exposure
- Dermal dysfunction (burns, erythrodermas)
- Endocrinopathies (myxedema, severe hypoglycemia)
- Excessive fluid loss, malnutrition
- Hepatic failure; renal failure/uremia; sepsis
- Hypothalamic and CNS dysfunction
- Mental illness; Alzheimer disease
- Trauma (especially head) (1),(2)

GENERAL PREVENTION

- Appropriate clothing, with particular attention to head, feet, and hands (1)
- For outdoor activities, carry survival bags with rescue foil blanket and dry clothes for use if stranded or injured.
- Avoid alcohol.
- Remain alert to early symptoms and initiate preventive steps (e.g., drinking warm fluids; getting out of the cold) (1).
- Identify medications that may predispose to hypothermia (e.g., neuroleptics, sedatives, hypnotics, tranquilizers) (1).

COMMONLY ASSOCIATED CONDITIONS

- Addison disease; hypothyroidism; hypopituitarism; diabetes; ketoacidosis
- CNS dysfunction
- Congestive heart failure
- Pulmonary infection; sepsis
- Uremia

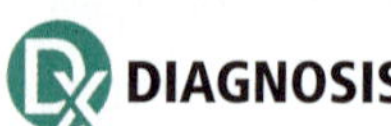

DIAGNOSIS

HISTORY

- Presentation varies with temperature of patient.
- The history is often apparent in the setting of outdoor environmental exposures. It may be less clear with cold indoor environments. Patients can present with confusion, dizziness, dyspnea, altered mental status. Taking a careful history is particularly important in cases of "indoor hypothermia."

ALERT

History of prolonged exposure to cold may make the diagnosis obvious, but hypothermia may be overlooked in other situations, especially in comatose patients. Always obtain a core temperature if hypothermia is suspected.

PHYSICAL EXAM

- Esophageal temperature is most accurate, minimally invasive method of assessing core temperature (1).
  - Must have secure airway
  - Probe inserted into lower third of esophagus
  - Peripheral thermometers are associated with reduced accuracy. The use of rectal thermometers is more accurate.
- Exam findings vary with the temperature of the patient at the time of presentation (2).
  - Mild (32–35°C/89.6–95°F)
    - Lethargy, shivering, mild confusion
    - Tachypnea, tachycardia, elevated BP
    - Hyperventilation
    - Loss of fine motor coordination
    - Peripheral vasoconstriction
    - Hyperactive reflexes
  - Moderate (28–32°C/82.4–89.6°F)
    - Delirium
    - Hypotension, hypoventilation
    - Cyanosis
    - Arrhythmias (bradycardia, prolonged PR interval, AV junctional rhythm, accelerated idioventricular rhythm, prolonged QT interval, altered T waves)
    - CNS depression, slowed reflexes
    - Muscular rigidity
    - Generalized edema
  - Severe (<28°C/<82.4°F)
    - Very cold skin
    - Rigidity, areflexia, unresponsive
    - Apnea
    - Bradycardia, hypotension
    - No pulse: ventricular fibrillation, asystole
    - Pupils (dilated <27°C; fixed and dilated <27°C)

ALERT

Use specially designed thermometers that can record low temperatures and measure core temperatures.

Pediatric Considerations

- Infants may present with bright red, cold skin, and lethargy.
- A child's body temperature drops faster than an adult does when immersed in cold water.
- Altered mental status is the most important clue to significant hypothermia in children (2).

DIFFERENTIAL DIAGNOSIS

- Cerebrovascular accidents
- Intoxication, drug overdose
- Complications of diabetes, hypothyroidism, hypopituitarism

DIAGNOSTIC TESTS & INTERPRETATION

Initial Tests (lab, imaging)

- Arterial blood gases (correct for temperature)
- CBC with platelet counts
- Serum electrolytes; BUN/creatinine; glucose; calcium; magnesium
- Urinalysis
- Coagulation studies; fibrinogen level
- Blood culture
- Liver function studies; amylase
- Cardiac enzymes
- Alcohol level and toxicology screen
- Cervical spine, chest, and abdomen x-rays, if appropriate
- Bedside ultrasound to assess hemodynamics
- CT of the head for any concern regarding mental status

Follow-Up Tests & Special Considerations

Serum cortisol and TSH if underlying endocrine dysfunction (hypothalamus stimulates release of hormones in response to hypothermia)

Diagnostic Procedures/Other

ECG

Test Interpretation

Serum potassium >12 mmol/L in adults is associated with nonsurvival.

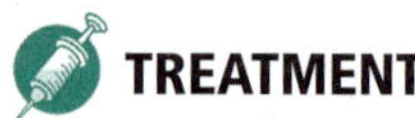

TREATMENT

GENERAL MEASURES

- Prehospital (2),(3)
  - Factors to guide treatment (Although helpful, core temperature should not be the sole basis to guide treatment.)
    - Level of consciousness
    - Shivering intensity
    - Cardiovascular stability based on blood pressure and cardiac rhythm

- Treatment (1),(3)
  - Basic life support (1)
  - Remove wet garments; dry the patient (3).
  - Protect against heat loss and wind chill.
  - If mildly hypothermic, passive rewarming with insulation, a vapor barrier; warm environment is generally sufficient.
  - For colder, nonshivering patients, add active rewarming—a nonshivering patient will not rewarm spontaneously (1).
    - Warm intravenous fluids before infusion (3).
    - Active rewarming can include warm blankets, heating pads, radiant heat, and forced warm air (3).
    - Give warm, humidified oxygen if available.
    - If far from definitive care, begin active rewarming but do not delay transport.
  - Active core rewarming for severely hypothermic patients
- See "Admission, Inpatient, and Nursing Considerations."

MEDICATION

- For sepsis or bacterial infections, begin antibiotics.
- For hypoglycemia: D50W at a dose of 1 mg/kg
- Thiamine: 100 mg, if alcoholic or cachectic
- Naloxone: 2 mg if opioid use suspected
- Levothyroxine: 150 to 500 μg for myxedema
- Severe acidosis: Consider sodium bicarbonate.
- Precautions (2)
  - Medications including epinephrine, lidocaine, and procainamide can accumulate to toxic levels if used repeatedly; avoid until core temperature is >30°C (>86°F):
    - When temperature reaches >30°C, IV medications are indicated. Administer slowly.
  - Consider vasopressors according to standard ACLS algorithm with concurrent rewarming in setting of cardiac arrest.
  - Use all drugs cautiously due to impaired metabolism and renal elimination. Once rewarming has occurred, there is mobilization of depot stores.
  - Routine use of steroids or antibiotics does not increase survival or decrease postresuscitative damage.

ADMISSION, INPATIENT, AND NURSING CONSIDERATIONS

- Rewarming depends on severity of hypothermia and presence of cardiac arrest (1),(2),(3).
  - If no cardiac arrest, consider active external rewarming.
  - If cardiac arrest is present, consider active internal rewarming.
- Warm core first.
  - Don't rewarm frostbitten extremities until core temperature is >34°C (93.2°F) (2).
- The rate of rewarming is determined by whether perfusing cardiac output is present.
  - If a perfusing cardiac output is present, 1–2°C/hr is appropriate. If not, use a faster rate of >2°C/hr.
- Monitor core temperature, BP, cardiac rhythm.
- Correct metabolic acidosis.
- Evaluate for frostbite and other trauma.
- Mild hypothermia
  - Passive rewarming
  - Administration of heated IV solutions
  - Provide warm fluids by mouth if fully alert.
- Moderate hypothermia
  - Active external rewarming
  - Administration of heated IV solutions
- Severe hypothermia (active internal [core] rewarming) (2)
  - Heated IV fluids
  - Heated humidified oxygen
  - Extracorporeal life support (preferred method in cardiac arrest)
    - Cardiopulmonary bypass, extracorporeal membrane oxygenation
  - Body cavity lavage (second options)
    - Thoracic cavity lavage, peritoneal lavage (40–45°C/104–113°F)
    - Continuous arteriovenous rewarming
    - Hemodialysis and hemofiltration
- Cardiac arrhythmias
  - Atrial fibrillation and sinus bradycardia are common—patients usually convert to NSR with rewarming.
  - If ventricular fibrillation is present, treat with one shock. If patient does not respond, consider deferring further attempts until rewarm has occurred.
  - Do not treat transient ventricular arrhythmias.
  - If cardiac pacing required, preferable to use external noninvasive pacemaker
- Admit patients, preferably to the ICU, with underlying disease, physiologic abnormalities, or core temperature <32°C (89.6°F).
- Normal saline is preferred as fluid of choice, AND IV bolus preferred over infusion when practical.
- Heat IVs from 40–42°C (104–107.6°F) if possible—should be no colder than core temperature.

ALERT

- Avoid overheating dextrose solutions; dextrose caramelizes at 60°C (140°F).
- Avoid fluid overload. Avoid lactated Ringer solution because of decreased lactate metabolism (2).
- Heart is irritable and susceptible to arrhythmias; take care transporting.
- Electrolytes may fluctuate with rewarming, check electrolytes (particularly potassium) frequently.
- Monitor blood pressure frequently with rewarming as hypotension can develop from severe dehydration and fluid shifts.
- Discharge from emergency department once normothermic, if mild hypothermia and no predisposing conditions or complications and has suitable place to go. All others require admission.

ONGOING CARE

FOLLOW-UP RECOMMENDATIONS

Patient Monitoring

- During acute episode: Monitor cardiac rhythm, urinary output, check electrolytes, blood gases, and glucose frequently.
- Following acute episode: continued therapy for underlying disorder

DIET

Warm fluids only if alert and able to swallow

- Alcohol intake increases risk of becoming hypothermic in cold conditions.
- Refer to social service agency for help with housing, heat, and/or clothing, if appropriate.

PATIENT EDUCATION

Persons with known cardiovascular disease should use caution when exercising outdoors in cold weather.

PROGNOSIS

- Mortality rates are decreasing due to increased recognition and advanced therapy (2).
- Mortality usually depends on age and the severity of underlying cause and comorbidities.
  - Mortality rate in healthy patients is <5%, those with coexisting illness is >50%.
  - Mortality rates increase with age. Over half of deaths are seen in patients >65 years.

COMPLICATIONS

- Core temperature after drop (2)
- Cardiac arrhythmias
- Hypotension, sepsis
- Hyperkalemia, hypoglycemia, metabolic acidosis
- Rhabdomyolysis
- Pneumonia, pulmonary edema, ARDS
- Pancreatitis, peritonitis, GI bleeding, ileus
- Acute tubular necrosis, bladder atony
- Intravascular thromboses/DIC
- Gangrene of extremities
- Compartment syndrome
- Seizures, cerebral ischemia, delirium

REFERENCES

1. Dow J, Giesbrecht GG, Danzl DF, et al. Wilderness Medical Society clinical practice guidelines for the out-of-hospital evaluation and treatment of accidental hypothermia: 2019 update. *Wilderness Environ Med*. 2019;30(4S):S47–S69.
2. Paal P, Pasquier M, Darocha T, et al. Accidental hypothermia: 2021 update. *Int J Environ Res Public Health*. 2022;19(1):501.
3. Haverkamp FJC, Giesbrecht GG, Tan ECTH. The prehospital management of hypothermia—An up-to-date overview. *Injury*. 2018;49(2):149–164.

H

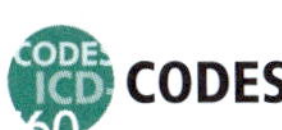

CODES

ICD10

- T68.XXXA Hypothermia, initial encounter
- T68.XXXD Hypothermia, subsequent encounter
- T68.XXXS Hypothermia, sequela

CLINICAL PEARLS

- The most common cause of hypothermia in the United States is inadvertent cold exposure associated with alcohol intoxication.
- With a severely decreased core temperature, begin resuscitation (if possible) unless there are obvious lethal injuries. Continue resuscitation and rewarm to 33–35°C and reassess.
- Hypothermia, coagulopathy, and acidosis are the trauma triad associated with higher rates of death (3).

HYPOTHYROIDISM, ADULT

Theresa Yurkonis, DO, MHSA • Alvin Soto Soto, MD • Francisco Vizcaino, MD

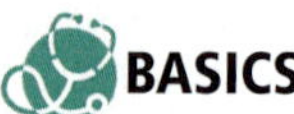

BASICS

DESCRIPTION
- Metabolic state resulting from decreased levels of free thyroid hormone or from resistance to hormone action
- Subclinical: elevated TSH, normal free T_4
- Overt: elevated TSH, subnormal free T_4

EPIDEMIOLOGY
Incidence
- Women: 3.5/1,000 person-years
- Men: 0.6/1,000 person-years

Prevalence
- Overt hypothyroidism: 11.7% of the U.S. population
- Subclinical hypothyroidism 4–20% of adults

ETIOLOGY AND PATHOPHYSIOLOGY
- Primary: abnormality at the thyroid gland (>95% of cases)
  - Most common cause worldwide: environmental iodine deficiency
  - Most common cause in the United States: Hashimoto thyroiditis (chronic autoimmune thyroiditis)
  - Postablative/posttherapeutic
  - Transient hypothyroidism: de Quervain syndrome (viral), postpartum
  - Drug use: propylthiouracil, methimazole, lithium, amiodarone, antiepileptic drugs, tyrosine kinase inhibitors (sunitinib), interleukin-2, or interferon-α, and possibly GLP-1/GIP receptor agonist
- Secondary is deficiency of TSH from pituitary gland, tertiary deficiency of TRH from hypothalamus
- Peripheral: T_3 and T_4 excessively degraded by ectopically produced type 3 iodothyronine deiodinase (rare)

Genetics
- TSH levels and T_4 levels have a genetic factor with a chance of 40–60% being transferred from parent to child (1).
- Hashimoto thyroiditis patients have a 4.9% change of having a first-degree relative with the same diagnosis.

RISK FACTORS
- Personal or family history of autoimmune diseases
- External head or neck irradiation
- Treatment with amiodarone, lithium, interferon-α, sunitinib, or sorafenib
- Down syndrome or Turner syndrome

GENERAL PREVENTION
- Iodized salt has significantly decreased iodine-deficient causes of hypothyroidism in western countries.
- Those needing additional supplementations include people consuming unbalanced vegetable-based or salt-restricted diets as well as young females and those pregnant or lactating.

COMMONLY ASSOCIATED CONDITIONS
Autoimmune disorders if applicable

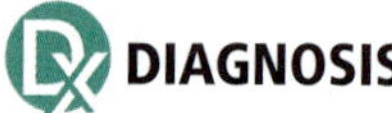

DIAGNOSIS

HISTORY
Symptoms can vary and can be nonspecific.
- Lethargy
- Cold intolerance
- Constipation
- Dry skin
- Muscle cramps, arthralgias, paresthesias
- Modest weight gain (4 to 11 lbs [2.0 to 4.5 kg])
- Menstrual disturbances, infertility, subfertility
- Depression
- Change in voice (hoarseness)
- Sleep apnea
- Carpal tunnel syndrome

PHYSICAL EXAM
- Dry, thickened skin
- Hair loss/brittle hair
- Periorbital edema
- Non-pitting swelling of hands and feet (myxedema)
- Bradycardia; reduced systolic blood pressure, increased diastolic blood pressure
- Delayed deep tendon reflex relaxation
- Macroglossia
- Goiter

Geriatric Considerations
Frequently nonspecific signs and symptoms

DIFFERENTIAL DIAGNOSIS
- Chronic fatigue syndrome, depression
- Anemia
- Congestive heart failure
- Primary adrenal insufficiency

DIAGNOSTIC TESTS & INTERPRETATION
Initial Tests (lab, imaging)
- Primary hypothyroidism
  - Elevated TSH (nonpregnant adult >4.5 mIU/L)
  - Decreased serum free T_4
- Central (secondary or tertiary) hypothyroidism
  - Decreased TSH and decreased serum free T_4
  - TRH stimulation test if suspecting hypothalamo-pituitary cause
- Subclinical hypothyroidism
  - Elevated serum TSH
  - Normal serum free T_4
- Note: Serum free triiodothyronine (T_3) or total T_3 should not be done to diagnose hypothyroidism.

Follow-Up Tests & Special Considerations
- Antithyroid antibodies (thyroid peroxidase antibodies and antithyroglobulin antibodies) if autoimmune suspected
- Drugs that decrease TSH: glucocorticoids, dopamine agonists, octreotide
- Drugs that increase TSH: phenytoin, amiodarone, dopamine antagonist (metoclopramide/domperidone), oral cholecystographic dyes (sodium ipodate), or estrogen or androgen in excess
- Drugs that increase free T_4: heparin, high intake of biotin
- TSH has circadian fluctuations, particularly higher levels in the evening and may be influenced by acute illness, inflammation, pregnancy, chronic protein malnutrition, hepatic failure or nephrotic syndrome

Test Interpretation
Screening
- Patient with symptoms specific to hypothyroidism, imaging abnormalities of thyroid, or laboratory abnormalities including:
  - Substantial hyperlipidemia or change in lipid pattern
  - Hyponatremia
  - High serum muscle enzyme concentrations
  - Macrocytic anemia
  - Pericardial or pleural effusion
  - Pituitary or hypothalamic disorder
- Pregnant women
  - Personal or family history of thyroid disease
  - Diabetes mellitus type 1
  - History of recurrent miscarriage, morbid obesity, or infertility; TPO Ab should be considered.
  - Universal screening not recommended for pregnant patients or planning pregnancy
- U.S. Preventive Services Task Force found insufficient evidence for or against screening nonpregnant, asymptomatic children or adults (2)[A].
- ACOG recommends women with history of autoimmune disease or strong family history of thyroid disease should be screened at age 19 years.

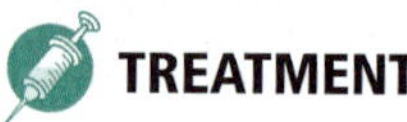

TREATMENT

GENERAL MEASURES
Patients with hypothyroidism should not be treated with iodine supplementation unless they are from an area with known iodine insufficiency (3)[B].

MEDICATION
First Line
- Levothyroxine (Synthroid, Levothroid)
  - 1.5 to 1.8 μg/kg/day (use ideal body weight) (2)[A]; titrate by 12.5 to 25.0 μg/day every 4 to 8 weeks until TSH in normal range.
  - For patients with CAD, multiple comorbidities, or elderly, 12.5 to 25.0 μg is the recommended starting dose despite ideal body weight, titrating as above.
  - Elderly patients may require 2/3 of dose used in young adults because clearance is decreased.

- – Use caution when changing between capsule, tablet, and liquid because formulations may be absorbed differently.
- – Levothyroxine should be taken on an empty stomach, ideally an hour before breakfast.
- – Medications that interfere with its absorption should be taken 4 hours after; these include ferrous sulfate, proton pump inhibitors, calcium carbonate, bile acid resins.
- Contraindications
- Uncorrected adrenocorticoid insufficiency
- MI, acute
- Precautions
  - – Diabetic patients may need readjustment of hypoglycemic agents with institution of T_4.
  - – Dosage of vitamin K antagonists may need adjustment; monitor prothrombin time while initiating treatment.
  - – Patients on digoxin may need close monitoring.
  - – Patients requiring doses that are higher than expected should be evaluated for GI disorders that may lead to decrease thyroid hormone absorption (*Helicobacter pylori*, celiac disease).
- Subclinical hypothyroidism treatment is directed by the following criteria:
  - – TSH >10 mU/L treatment indicated due to increased risk of coronary artery disease and conversion to overt hypothyroidism is elevated
  - – TSH 7.0 to 9.9 mU/L treat patients aged <65 years due to evidence of increased cardiovascular events.
  - – TSH <6.9 mU/L treat patients with convincing symptoms, high titers of anti-TPO, or goiter as they may quickly progress to overt hypothyroidism.
- If elective surgery: achieve euthyroid state prior to procedure if possible; risk overall not significantly elevated
- If urgent surgery: Proceed with individualized replacement therapy preoperatively and postoperatively.

Pregnancy Considerations

- Replacement therapy may need adjustment; average dose increases from 25% to 50% (4)[A].
- TSH levels should be monitored monthly during first half of pregnancy and at least once in second half; goal TSH of 2.0 to 2.5 mIU/L for 1st trimester and <3 mIU/L for 2nd and 3rd trimester (4)[A]
- Postpartum: Check TSH levels at 6 weeks (4)[A].

Second Line

Liothyronine (T_3) or desiccated thyroid hormone (T_3 and T_4) may be an alternative for patients who do not tolerate T_4 alone.

ISSUES FOR REFERRAL

- Pregnant patients or women planning on becoming pregnant should see an OB provider comfortable with management or be referred to endocrinology.
- Presence of goiter, nodule, or other structural changes in the thyroid gland
- Presence of adrenal or pituitary disorders

COMPLEMENTARY & ALTERNATIVE MEDICINE

Vitamin D deficiency may play a role in immune-mediated hypothyroidism and severity of disease.

ADMISSION, INPATIENT, AND NURSING CONSIDERATIONS

IV formulation is only indicated if patient is unable to tolerate oral medication for >1 week or myxedema coma is expected. Dose should be 70–80% expected dose as this is amount absorbed.

ONGOING CARE

FOLLOW-UP RECOMMENDATIONS

Patient Monitoring

- Monitor TSH every 4 to 8 weeks after initiating treatment or after change in dose. Once stabilized, periodic TSH level should be done after 6 months and then at 12-month intervals or more frequently if clinically indicated.
- T_4 measurements not routinely needed unless central hypothyroidism
- Monitor cardiac function in older patients.
- Check TSH more frequently during pregnancy, initiation of estrogen supplementation, or after large changes in body weight.

DIET

Iodine content is found highest in fish and marine plants naturally.

PATIENT EDUCATION

- Describe signs of thyrotoxicity
- Counsel on importance of taking on empty stomach.

PROGNOSIS

- Normalization of TSH results in symptoms improvement and no additional risks.
- Relapses will occur if treatment is interrupted.
- Myxedema coma has a 25–60% mortality rate.

COMPLICATIONS

- Complications only present if unable to achieve and maintain an euthyroid state.
- Increased susceptibility to infection
- Megacolon
- Sexual dysfunction, infertility
- Organic psychosis, depressed mood
- Hypersensitivity to opiates
- Treatment over long periods can lead to decreased bone mineral density.
- Can precipitate adrenal crisis if levothyroxine initiated prior to steroids in patients with untreated adrenal insufficiency
- Treatment-induced congestive heart failure in people with coronary artery disease (small risk)

REFERENCES

1. Zamwar UM, Muneshwar KN. Epidemiology, types, causes, clinical presentation, diagnosis, and treatment of hypothyroidism. *Cereus*. 2023;15(9):e46241.
2. Chaker L, Bianco AC, Jonklaas J, et al. Hypothyroidism. *Lancet*. 2017;390(10101):1550–1562.
3. Wilson SA, Stem LA, Bruehlman RD. Hypothyroidism: diagnosis and treatment. *Am Fam Physician*. 2021;103(10):605–613.
4. Alexander EK, Marqusee E, Lawrence J, et al. Timing and magnitude of increases in levothyroxine requirements during pregnancy in women with hypothyroidism. *N Engl J Med*. 2004;351(3):241–249.

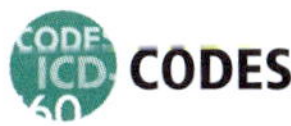

CODES

ICD10

- E03.9 Hypothyroidism, unspecified
- E06.3 Autoimmune thyroiditis
- E89.0 Postprocedural hypothyroidism

CLINICAL PEARLS

- Screening test: Order TSH levels; serum free T_4 should be obtained only if TSH is abnormal.
- Monitor TSH every 4 to 8 weeks after initiating treatment or after change in dose, then every 6 to 12 months or as needed.

ID REACTION

Sahil Mullick, MD, FAAFP • Idorenyin Emmanuel Udoeyop, MD

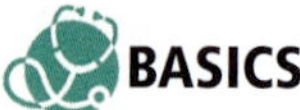

BASICS

DESCRIPTION

- A generalized skin reaction associated with various infectious (fungal, bacterial, viral, or parasitic) or inflammatory cutaneous conditions distant from the primary disease site (1).
- Autoeczematization is another name for id reaction and is described as a widespread skin response that appears at a distance from the primary skin infection or stimulus (2).
  - Dermatophytid is the most frequently referenced id reaction. A dermatophytid is an autosensitization reaction in which a secondary cutaneous reaction occurs at a site distant to a primary fungal infection. The eruption typically begins within 1 to 2 weeks of the onset of the main lesion or following exacerbation of the main lesion.
  - Most commonly, id reactions are characterized by localized vesicular lesions, erythema nodosum, and erythema multiforme.
  - System(s) affected: skin/exocrine
  - Synonym(s): dermatophytid, trichophytid, autoeczematization, secondary cutaneous reaction

EPIDEMIOLOGY

- Predominant age: all ages
- Predominant sex: male = female
- Predominant race: all races

Incidence

Unknown

ETIOLOGY AND PATHOPHYSIOLOGY

- Precise pathophysiology is uncertain. Circulating antigens may react with antibodies at sensitized areas of the skin. An abnormal immune recognition of autologous skin antigens may also occur. Inflammation may lower the irritation threshold of the skin, and hematogenous spread of cytokines from the primary site of inflammation may also play a role (1).
- It is believed that T lymphocytes and keratinocytes play a role in the development of id reaction (2)
  - Etiology
    - Infectious
      - Fungal infections: *Trichophyton mentagrophytes*, *Trichophyton rubrum*, *Epidermophyton floccosum*, and *Candida* spp.
      - Bacterial infections: Most commonly *Streptococcus pyogenes*, *Staphylococcus aureus*, and *Mycobacterium tuberculosis* ("tuberculid")
      - Viral infections: HSV, *Molluscum contagiosum*, orf, and milker's nodules
      - Parasitic infections: *Sarcoptes scabiei*, *Leishmania* spp., and *Pediculus humanus capitis*.
    - Allergic
      - Id reactions occur in patients with nickel and aluminum allergy or, less commonly, second to concurrent treatment with antibacterial agent and terbinafine.
    - Miscellaneous
      - Id reaction rarely develops due to retained postoperative sutures, cyanoacrylate application, ionizing radiation, blunt trauma, red tattoo ink, post-picosecond laser tattoo removal.
      - Rarely, id reaction has been documented in patients receiving intravesical BCG live therapy for transitional cell carcinoma.

RISK FACTORS

- Fungal infection of the skin, especially tinea pedis
- Stasis dermatitis

GENERAL PREVENTION

- Good skin hygiene (particularly in intertriginous areas) to minimize risk of developing fungal infections
- Promptly treat any developing fungal infection.

COMMONLY ASSOCIATED CONDITIONS

- Primary fungal infection
- Stasis dermatitis

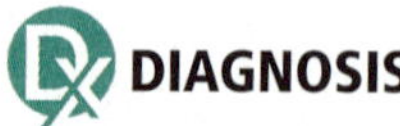

DIAGNOSIS

HISTORY

Itchy rash: Inquire about presence of lesions (typically fungal or bacterial) that could have incited the id reaction in the preceding days to weeks.

PHYSICAL EXAM

- Common
  - Symmetric, pruritic vesicles on the palms, and most commonly on lateral aspects of fingers
  - Tinea infection on the feet; contact or other eczematous dermatitis; bacterial, fungal, or viral infection of the skin
- Less common
  - Papules
  - Lichenoid eruption
  - Erythema nodosum
- Eczematoid eruption

DIFFERENTIAL DIAGNOSIS

- Pompholyx (dyshidrotic eczema)
- Contact dermatitis
- Drug eruptions
- Pustular psoriasis
- Folliculitis
- Scabies

DIAGNOSTIC TESTS & INTERPRETATION

- Potassium hydroxide (KOH) or fungal culture of primary lesion
- No fungal elements are present at the site of the id reaction.
- Special tests: Skin shows a positive trichophyton reaction. A wheal >10 mm at 20 minutes and induration >5 mm at 72 hours is a positive response.

Follow-Up Tests & Special Considerations

- The id reaction resolves with successful eradication of the primary skin condition.
- It is important to distinguish dermatophytids from drug-induced allergic reactions because continued treatment is essential to clear the underlying infection.

Test Interpretation

Histology

- Vesicles in the upper dermis
- Superficial perivascular lymphohistiocytic infiltrate with small numbers of eosinophils and increased granular cell layer
- No infectious agents present in biopsy specimen.

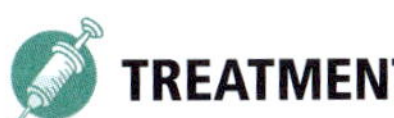

TREATMENT

GENERAL MEASURES

- Outpatient treatment of the underlying infection or eczematous dermatitis
- Symptomatic treatment of pruritus with antihistamines and/or topical steroids if needed (may require class 1 or 2 steroid)
- Treatment for secondary bacterial infection
- Stopping causative agent
- Compression stocking and leg elevation is recommended if stasis dermatitis is responsible for the id reaction (2).

MEDICATION

First Line

- PO antihistamines for pruritus (3)
  - Chlorpheniramine: 4 mg PO q4–6h PRN; max 24 mg/24 hr (pediatric: 6 to 11 years 2 mg PO q4–6h PRN; max 12 mg/24 hr; ≥12 years, refer to adult dosing)
  - Diphenhydramine: 25 to 50 mg PO q4–6h PRN; max 400 mg/24 hr (pediatric: 5 mg/kg/24 hr divided q6h PRN; 2 to 5 years max 37.5 mg/24 hr; 6 to 11 years max 150 mg/24 hr; ≥12 years, refer to adult dosing)
  - Hydroxyzine: 25 to 100 mg PO q6–8h PRN; max 600 mg/24 hr (pediatric: 2 mg/kg/24 hr divided q6h PRN)
- Topical treatments for pruritus
  - Triamcinolone 0.1% ointment TID
  - Hydrocortisone 0.5%, 1%, 2.5%: up to QID
  - Capsaicin 0.025%, 0.075% cream: Apply TID–QID; EMLA (2.5% lidocaine + 2.5% prilocaine) applied 30 to 60 minutes prior to capsaicin may minimize burning.
  - Doxepin 5% cream: Apply QID for up to 8 days (to max of 10% of the body).
  - White petroleum emollients: Apply after short bath/shower in warm (not hot) water.
- Systemic steroids only if reaction is severe or generalized (e.g., prednisone 20 mg)

Second Line

- Topical and/or systemic antifungals for identified associated fungal infection (common)—(see "Tinea" [Capitis, Corporis, Cruris])
- Topical or systemic antibiotics for any secondary bacterial infection
- Treatment with antiviral agents for erythema multiforme associated with HSV is required.

ISSUES FOR REFERRAL

Consider referral to allergist for possible allergic cause if no clear infectious trigger is identified.

ONGOING CARE

PATIENT EDUCATION

Avoid hot, humid conditions that promote fungal growth. Aerate susceptible body areas (e.g., wear sandals or open footwear). If possible, wear loose-fitting clothing and undergarments, dry wet skin after bathing, and use powders and antiperspirants to discourage fungal growth. Treat primary dermatitis promptly.

PROGNOSIS

After appropriate treatment, complete resolution in days to weeks

COMPLICATIONS

- Secondary bacterial infection (cellulitis)
- After resolution of dermatophytid, postinflammatory hyperpigmentation is common and disappears without treatment in 1 month.

REFERENCES

1. Ilkit M, Durdu M, Karakaş M. Cutaneous id reactions: a comprehensive review of clinical manifestations, epidemiology, etiology, and management. *Crit Rev Microbiol*. 2012;38(3):191–202.
2. Bertoli MJ, Schwartz RA, Janniger CK. Autoeczematization: a strange id reaction of the skin. *Cutis*. 2021;108(3):163–166.
3. Cotes MES, Swerlick RA. Practical guidelines for the use of steroid-sparing agents in the treatment of chronic pruritus. *Dermatol Ther*. 2013;26(2):120–134.

ADDITIONAL READING

- Elmariah SB, Lerner EA. Topical therapies for pruritus. *Semin Cutan Med Surg*. 2011;30(2):118–126.
- Yosipovitch G, Bernhard JD. Clinical practice: chronic pruritus. *N Engl J Med*. 2013;368(17):1625–1634.

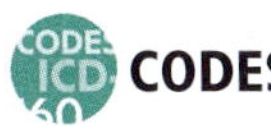

CODES

ICD10

- L30.2 Cutaneous autosensitization
- B35.9 Dermatophytosis, unspecified

CLINICAL PEARLS

- When one skin eruption follows another closely in time, consider an id reaction.
- When assessing an itchy rash, inquire about potential fungal or bacterial lesions in the preceding days to weeks as a potential prelude to the id reaction.

IMMUNE THROMBOCYTOPENIA (ITP)

Tara Baney, MS, CRNP • Allison Holmes, DO

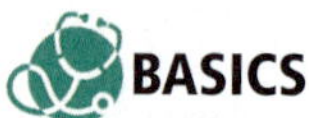

BASICS

DESCRIPTION

- Immune thrombocytopenia (ITP) is a condition characterized by the destruction of normal platelets due to auto-antibodies against platelet antigens and/or impaired thrombopoiesis in response to an unknown stimulus.
- ITP is defined as platelet count $<100 \times 10^9$/L, once other causes of thrombocytopenia have been ruled out (1).
- ITP nomenclature:
  - Newly diagnosed (<3 months), persistent (3 to 12 months), and chronic (>12 months)
  - Primary ITP due to autoimmune mechanisms, due to platelet destruction, and/or platelet underproduction with no other cause
  - Secondary ITP is caused by other disorders.
  - Drug-induced ITP caused drug dependent platelet antibodies that cause platelet destruction
- ITP is a common disease of childhood that typically follows a viral infection. Onset is within 1 week, and spontaneous resolution occurs within 2 months in >80% of patients.
- In adults, ITP is usually a chronic disease and spontaneous remission is rare.
- Synonym(s): idiopathic thrombocytopenic purpura; immune thrombocytopenic purpura; and Werlhof disease

EPIDEMIOLOGY

- Peak age: pediatric ITP: 2 to 4 years; chronic ITP: >50 years with incidence 2 times higher in persons aged 60 years than those <60 years of age
- Predominant gender: pediatric ITP: male = female; chronic ITP: female > male (1.2 to 1.7:1)

Incidence

- Pediatric acute ITP: 1.9 to 6.4/100,000 children per year; adult ITP: 1.6/100,000 per year (1)
- Peak incidence of ITP is in the spring and early summer in temperate climates. This observation supports the notion that viral triggers are an important cause of ITP.

Prevalence

Limited data; 12/100,000 persons

ETIOLOGY AND PATHOPHYSIOLOGY

- Infection/immune changes are the most common cause of ITP.
- Accelerated platelet uptake/destruction by reticuloendothelial phagocytes results from action of IgG autoantibodies against platelet membrane glycoproteins IIb/IIIa, GP Ib/IX, GP Ia/IIa, and GP VI. There is also cell-mediated platelet destruction by autoreactive cytotoxic T cells.
- Humoral and cellular immunity interfere with megakaryocyte maturation, causing decreased production.
- Fc-independent desialylated platelet clearance has been proposed as the mechanism of refractoriness to therapies that target the classic FC-dependent pathway.
- Association in patients receiving immune checkpoint inhibitor therapy

RISK FACTORS

- Autoimmune thrombocytopenia (e.g., Evans syndrome)
- Common variable immunodeficiency (CVID)
- Drug side effect (e.g., quinidine, vancomycin, penicillin, sulfonamides)
- Infections: *Helicobacter pylori*, hepatitis C, HIV, CMV, varicella zoster, measles, rubella, influenza, EBV, Whipple disease
- Vaccinations: Live virus vaccinations carry a lower risk than natural viral infection: 2.6/100,000 cases MMR vaccine doses versus 6 to 1,200/100,000 cases of natural rubella or measles infections. Vaccine-induced immune thrombotic thrombocytopenia (VITT) is more like autoimmune heparin-induced thrombocytopenia (HIT) than ITP.
- Bone marrow transplantation
- Autoimmune disease, such as systemic lupus erythematosus, antiphospholipid antibody syndrome
- Lymphoproliferative disorders

DIAGNOSIS

A careful history, physical exam, and review of CBC and peripheral blood smear remain the key components of the diagnosis of ITP.

HISTORY

- Often asymptomatic; found incidentally on routine CBC
- Posttraumatic bleeding occurs at counts of 40 to 60×10^9/L.
- With counts $<30 \times 10^9$/L, bruising tendency, epistaxis, menorrhagia, and gingival bleeding are common.
- Spontaneous bleeding may occur with platelet count $<20 \times 10^9$/L.
- Intracerebral bleeding is rare (1.4%) and may occur with counts $<20 \times 10^9$/L and associated trauma or vascular lesions.
- Female gender and NSAIDs use have been associated with bleeding.
- Fatigue
- Normal white blood cell and red blood cell unless secondary ITP and cause effects these cell lines also.

PHYSICAL EXAM

- Bleeding tends to occur in skin and mucosal membranes causing ecchymoses, petechiae, purpura, epistaxis, and gingivorrhagia.
- Abnormal uterine bleeding
- Hemorrhagic bullae on buccal mucosa due to acute, severe thrombocytopenia.
- No splenomegaly, hepatomegaly, lymphadenopathy

DIFFERENTIAL DIAGNOSIS

- Acute leukemia
- Thrombotic thrombocytopenic purpura, hemolytic uremic syndrome, disseminated intravascular coagulopathy (ITP)
- Factitious: platelet clumping on peripheral smear
- Thrombocytopenia secondary to sepsis
- Myelodysplastic syndrome, particularly in older patients
- Decreased marrow production: malignancy, drugs, viruses, megaloblastic anemia
- Posttransfusion
- Gestational thrombocytopenia
- Isoimmune neonatal purpura
- Congenital thrombocytopenias
- Alcohol-induced thrombocytopenic purpura

DIAGNOSTIC TESTS & INTERPRETATION

Diagnosis of ITP is often a diagnosis of exclusion. Other more worrisome or pathologic causes of thrombocytopenia need to be ruled out.

Initial Tests (lab, imaging)

- CBC with differential and peripheral smear:
  - Isolated decreased platelet count $<100 \times 10^9$/L
  - Giant platelets often present.
  - Normal red blood cell/white blood cell
- For patients with history, exam, CBC, and peripheral smear typical of ITP, consider the following:
  - PT/PTT is normal.
  - In adults, serologies for hepatitis B, hepatitis C, and HIV infections are recommended (1)[C].
  - In pediatric ITP, immunoglobulin levels to exclude CVID are commonly obtained (1)[C].
  - Other tests are not necessary for patients with typical ITP presentation: antiplatelet, antinuclear, antiphospholipid antibodies; *H. pylori* testing; thrombopoietin; platelet parameters; direct antiglobulin test; reticulocyte count; urinalysis; and thyroid function tests (1)[C].
- Further studies should be considered if the patient with thrombocytopenia also presents with: fever, arthralgia, lymphadenopathy, family history of bleeding disorder, risk factors for HIV, or abnormalities in other cell lines.
- Other tests not currently recommended in the guidelines:
  - Reticulated platelets or immature platelet function (RP/IPF) to make a differential diagnosis in cases of ITP yields a sensitivity and specificity of 83% and 75%, respectively.
  - Testing for platelet antibodies such as GPIIb/IIIa and GPIb/IX yield sensitivity and specificity of 90% and 78%, respectively.

Follow-Up Tests & Special Considerations

- Hepatitis B testing if Ritxuan is considered for therapy.
- Bone marrow biopsies is no longer recommended.
- Blood type in case of need for transfusion

Diagnostic Procedures/Other

Imaging is not necessary. Bone marrow aspiration/biopsy: is not necessary for diagnosis in children/adults (1)[C]; consider if other cause is being ruled out (1).

Test Interpretation

- Peripheral smear: normal red blood cell/white blood cell with large or giant platelets but diminished number
- Marrow reveals normal to abundant megakaryocytes with normal erythroid/myeloid precursors.

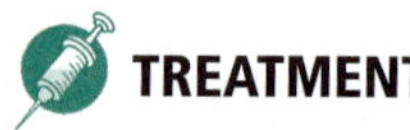

TREATMENT

GENERAL MEASURES

- Management is based on platelet count and hemorrhagic manifestations.
  - Critical bleeding, hemodynamically unstable, or cardiopulmonary/neurologic compromise
  - Severe bleeding hemoglobin drops ≥2 g/dL, requires ≥2 transfusions of packed red blood cells (PRBCs) but does not fit critical bleeding.
  - Minor bleeding does not fit critical or severe bleeding.

- Risk of bleeding is greatest in the following:
  - Prior bleeding
  - Platelet count <10,000/microL
  - >60 years of age
- Recommend treatment for newly diagnosed patients with a platelet count $<30 \times 10^9$/L (1).
- The main goal is a platelet count associated with adequate hemostasis, rather than normal count (1).
- Outpatient management unless patient has platelet count $<20 \times 10^9$/L and is at risk for bleeding or has bleeding

MEDICATION

First Line

- Pediatric
  - First-line treatment
    - Significant bleeding
      - Single-dose IV immunoglobulin (IVIG) 0.8 to 1.0 g/kg, especially when a more rapid increase in platelet count is desired (1)[C]; do not administer in patients with IgA deficiencies because of anaphylaxis risk.
      - A short course of corticosteroids (e.g., PO prednisone 2 mg/kg/day for 2 weeks with 3 weeks taper) (1)[C]
      - Single-dose of anti-Rho(D) immunoglobulin (anti-D), 50 to 75 g/kg for non-splenectomized children who are Rh-positive, with negative direct antiglobulin test (1); do not use in children with hemoglobin <9 g/dL or evidence of hemolysis (1)[C].
  - For children with no/mild bleeding (bruising and petechiae only with no mucosal bleeding), observation alone regardless of platelet count (1)[C]
  - Secondary for pediatric/adolescent
    - Rituximab (Rituxan) 375 mg/m^2 weekly for 4 weeks (1)
    - High-dose dexamethasone 0.6 mg/kg/day for 4 days every 4 weeks (1)
    - Inadequate data: azathioprine, cyclosporin A, danazol, mycophenolate mofetil, anti-CD52 monoclonal antibody, and interferon
    - Thrombopoietin receptor agonist newer second-line therapy to stimulate platelet production (2)
    - Splenectomy for chronic or persistent ITP; completed if all other therapies have failed (1)[C],(2)
- Adult
  - First line
    - Treatment is recommended for newly diagnosed patients with platelet count $<30 \times 10^9$/L (1).
    - Dexamethasone 40 mg/day for 4 days is preferred over longer courses of steroids or IVIG, as shorter course has equivalent efficacy without as many adverse effects.
    - Corticosteroids contraindicated:
      - IVIG: 1 to 2 g/kg once, repeating as necessary (1), *or*
      - Anti-D: 50 to 75 µg/kg once, RhD positive, but many clinicians are hesitant to use because of risk of severe hemolytic transfusion reaction; do not use anti-D in patients with low hemoglobin or evidence of hemolysis (1).
  - Second line, adult ITP: Romiplostim appears to be the best option for patients who fail to respond to prior treatment or relapse thereafter, although avatrombopag and eltrombopag are reasonable alternatives (2)[A].
    - If splenectomy is contraindicated/have risk of bleeding, thrombopoietin receptor agonists: eltrombopag (Promacta), 50 mg/day PO *or* romiplostim (Nplate), 1 µg/kg SC weekly
    - Rituximab, 375 mg/m^2 IV weekly for 4 weeks, for patients at high risk of bleeding who have failed first-line therapy or postsplenectomy (1)
    - Others to consider: azathioprine, cyclosporine A, cyclophosphamide, danazol, dapsone, mycophenolate mofetil, and vincristine
    - Asymptomatic postsplenectomy, with platelet counts $>30 \times 10^9$/L, no treatment is required (1)[C].
    - Avatrombopag (Doptelet), 5 daily doses (60 mg if baseline platelet count $<40 \times 10^9$/L or 40 mg if 40 to $<50 \times 10^9$/L) and fostamatinib (Tavalisse), 100 mg twice daily
- ITP in pregnancy
  - Preeclampsia/gestational thrombocytopenia may cause thrombocytopenia unrelated to ITP.
  - Corticosteroids or IVIG are considered safe and first line (1)[C].
  - ITP management at time of delivery is based on maternal bleeding risks and mode of delivery based on obstetric indications. Platelet autoantibodies can cross the placenta and cause neonatal thrombocytopenia.
  - Cesarean section can be considered if platelet count $>50 \times 10^9$/L.
  - Prednisone and/or IVIG may be considered 2 to 3 weeks prior to delivery.
- ITP secondary to HIV: Antivirals should be considered before other treatment (1)[C]. If treatment is required, corticosteroids, IVIG, or anti-D are first-line options. Splenectomy is a second-line option (1).
- ITP secondary to HCV: Antivirals should be considered before other treatment (1). If treatment required, IVIG is initial treatment (1). Based on recent studies, TPO mimetics are approved for HCV-related ITP because they increase platelets to a level required to initiate antiviral therapy.
- ITP and *H. pylori*: Screen for *H. pylori* in patients in whom eradication therapy would be considered if result is positive (1).
- ITP secondary to immune checkpoint inhibitor therapy: Stop the offending agent and treat with first-line therapy for ITP in adults.
- Emergency treatment
  - Intracranial or GI bleeding, massive hematuria, internal hematoma, or emergent surgery required
  - IV corticosteroids (e.g., IV methylprednisolone, 1 g/day for 3 doses) with caution in patients with GI bleeding and/or IVIG 1 g/kg; repeat the following day for count $<50 \times 10^9$/L (1)[C].
  - Platelet transfusions may also be considered with IVIG for significant bleeding (1)[C].
  - Recombinant factor VIIa not only promotes hemostasis but also increases risk of thrombosis. Efficacy of antifibrinolytic agents, aminocaproic acid, and tranexamic acid, is unproved in randomized trials; use as adjunctive treatments only.

ISSUES FOR REFERRAL

Hematology consultation is recommended for acute bleeding or for those who fail first-line therapies.

SURGERY/OTHER PROCEDURES

Splenectomy

- Mortality rate is low (<1%) even in patients with severe thrombocytopenia. Laparoscopic splenectomy has similar long-term outcomes vs. open splenectomy and has better short-term outcomes in medically suitable patients. The reported 5- to 10-year efficacy is ~65% for all patients.
- Necessary vaccinations prior to splenectomy: polyvalent pneumococcal vaccine and quadrivalent meningococcal vaccine every 3 to 5 years and one-time *Haemophilus influenzae type b* (Hib)
- Raise the platelet count to at least 20×10^9/L prior to surgery.

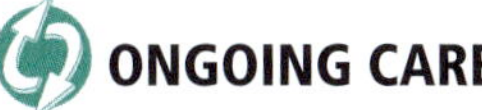

ONGOING CARE

FOLLOW-UP RECOMMENDATIONS

Patient Monitoring

Platelet counts weekly for patients on steroids then monthly if stable; if on short-course of dexamethasone platelet counts are recommended after 10 days of therapy. A second course is recommended if platelet count increment is below target goal.

DIET

Some following foods and supplements can cause significant bleeding: garlic, ginger, *Ginkgo biloba*, and saw palmetto (not comprehensive list).

PATIENT EDUCATION

Modify activity to prevent injury or bruising; avoid contact sports. Avoid anticoagulants, aspirin and other platelet-inhibiting drugs, and NSAIDs.

PROGNOSIS

- Acute ITP: ~80–85% of patients complete recover within 2 months. 15% proceed to chronic ITP.
- Chronic ITP: ~10–20% of the patients recover spontaneously; remainder with diminished platelets for months to years; may see spontaneous remissions (5%) and relapses
- ~10% are refractory (fail therapy/splenectomy).

COMPLICATIONS

- Related to thrombocytopenia: 1% mortality due to intracranial hemorrhage/severe blood loss
- Related to treatment: adverse effects from medications

REFERENCES

1. Neunert C, Terrell DR, Arnold DM, et al. American Society of Hematology 2019 guidelines for immune thrombocytopenia. *Blood Adv*. 2019;3(23):3829–3866.
2. Yang R, Lin L, Yao H, et al. Therapeutic options for adult patients with previously treated immune thrombocytopenia—a systematic review and network meta-analysis. *Hematology*. 2019;24(1):290–299.

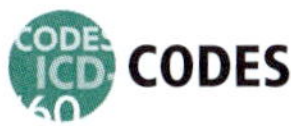

CODES

ICD10

D69.3 Immune thrombocytopenic purpura

CLINICAL PEARLS

ITP is defined as platelet count $<100 \times 10^9$/L, once other causes of thrombocytopenia have been ruled out.

IMPETIGO

Rade N. Pejic, MD

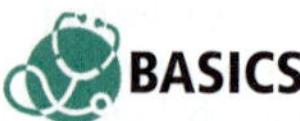

BASICS

DESCRIPTION

- A contagious, superficial, intraepidermal infection occurring prominently on exposed areas of the face and extremities, most often seen in children
- Primary impetigo (pyoderma): invasion of previously normal skin
- Secondary impetigo (impetiginization): invasion at sites of minor trauma (abrasions, insect bites, underlying eczema)
- Infected patients usually have multiple lesions.
- Cultures are positive in >80% cases for *Staphylococcus aureus* either alone or combined with group A β-hemolytic streptococci; *S. aureus* is the more common pathogen since the 1990s.
- Nonbullous impetigo: most common form of impetigo; formation of vesiculopustules that rupture, leading to crusting with a characteristic golden appearance; local lymphadenopathy may occur.
- Bullous impetigo: staphylococcal impetigo that progresses from small to large flaccid bullae (newborns/young children) caused by epidermolytic toxin release; ruptured bullae leaving brown crust; less lymphadenopathy; trunk more often affected; <30% of patients
- Folliculitis: considered by some to be *S. aureus* impetigo of hair follicles
- Ecthyma: a deeper, ulcerated impetigo infection often with lymphadenitis
- System(s) affected: skin/exocrine
- Synonym(s): pyoderma; impetigo contagiosa; impetigo vulgaris

EPIDEMIOLOGY

Incidence

- Predominant sex: male = female
- Predominant age: children aged 2 to 5 years

Prevalence

In the United States: not reported but common

Pediatric Considerations

- Poststreptococcal glomerulonephritis may follow impetigo (in young children).
- Impetigo neonatorum may occur due to nursery contamination.

ETIOLOGY AND PATHOPHYSIOLOGY

- Coagulase-positive staphylococci: pure culture ~50–90%; more contagious via contact
- β-Hemolytic streptococci: pure culture only ~10% of the time (primarily group A)
- Mixed infections of streptococci and staphylococci are common; data suggest increasing importance of staphylococci over the past decades.
- Methicillin-resistant *S. aureus* (MRSA) detected in some cases
- Direct contact or insect vector
- Can result from contamination at trauma site
- Regional lymphadenopathy

RISK FACTORS

- Warm, humid environment
- Tropical or subtropical climate
- Summer or fall season
- Minor trauma, insect bites, breaches in skin
- Poor hygiene, poverty, crowding, epidemics, wartime
- Familial spread
- Poor health with anemia and malnutrition
- Complication of pediculosis, scabies, chickenpox, eczema/atopic dermatitis
- Contact dermatitis (*Rhus* spp.)
- Burns
- Contact sports
- Children in daycare
- Carriage of group A *Streptococcus* and *S. aureus*

GENERAL PREVENTION

- Close attention to family hygiene, particularly hand washing among children
- Covering of wounds
- Avoidance of crowding and sharing of personal items
- Treatment of atopic dermatitis

COMMONLY ASSOCIATED CONDITIONS

- Malnutrition and anemia
- Crowded living conditions
- Poor hygiene
- Neglected minor trauma
- Any chronic/underlying dermatitis
- Can occur as coinfection with scabies

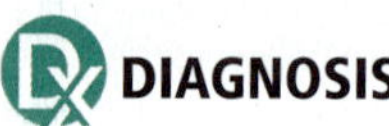

DIAGNOSIS

HISTORY

- Lesions are often described as painful.
- May be slow and indolent or rapidly spreading
- Most frequent on face around mouth and nose or at site of trauma

PHYSICAL EXAM

- Tender red macules or papules as early lesions (contact dermatitis presents with pruritic lesions)
- Thin-roofed vesicles to bullae: usually nontender
- Pustules
- Weeping, shallow, red ulcers
- Honey-colored crusts
- Satellite lesions
- Often multiple sites
- Bullae on buttocks, trunk, face

DIFFERENTIAL DIAGNOSIS

- Nonbullous
  - Contact dermatitis
  - Chickenpox
  - Herpes
  - Folliculitis
  - Erysipelas
  - Insect bites
  - Severe eczematous dermatitis
  - Scabies
  - Tinea corporis
- Bullous
  - Burns
  - Pemphigus vulgaris
  - Bullous pemphigoid
- Stevens-Johnson syndrome

DIAGNOSTIC TESTS & INTERPRETATION

Initial Tests (lab, imaging)

- None usually necessary in typical presentations; cultures of pus/bullae fluid may be helpful if no response to empiric therapy.
  - Culture: taken from the base of lesion after removal of crust; will grow both staphylococci and group A streptococci
  - Antistreptolysin-O (ASO) titer: can be weak positive for streptococci but overall not useful
  - Antideoxyribonuclease B (anti-DNase B) and antihyaluronidase (AHT) response more reliable than ASO response.
  - Streptozyme: positive for streptococci
- Disorders that may alter lab results: Streptococcal pharyngitis will alter streptococcal enzyme tests.

Follow-Up Tests & Special Considerations

- Monitor for spread of disease and systemic manifestations.
- Serologic testing is helpful in context of impetigo with subsequent poststreptococcal glomerulonephritis.

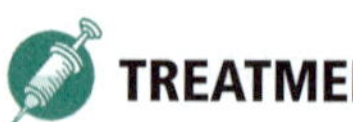

TREATMENT

GENERAL MEASURES

- Treatment speeds healing, improves cosmetic appearance, and avoids spread of disease.
- Prevent with mupirocin ointment TID to sites of minor skin trauma.
- Remove crusts; clean with gentle washing 2 to 3 times daily; and clean with antibacterial soap, chlorhexidine, or Betadine (povidone iodine).
- Washing of entire body may prevent recurrence at distant sites.

MEDICATION

- In 2014, the Infectious Diseases Society of America (IDSA) recommended topical treatment for limited lesions and oral medication when the disease is more severe/extensive (1)[C]. A 2017 Canadian systematic review found that topical mupirocin is equally or more effective than oral treatments for nonextensive impetigo (2)[A]. Penicillin and macrolide therapy is no longer recommended. Fluoroquinolones are not indicated due to resistance patterns and risk of serious adverse events.
- Consult the local hospital or health department for microbial resistance information.
- Nonbullous (minor spread, treat 7 days; widespread, treat 10 days); bullous (treat 10 days)
  - Mupirocin (Bactroban) 2% topical ointment applied TID for 5 to 7 days (nonbullous only); not as effective on scalp as around mouth
  - Retapamulin 1% ointment to be applied BID for 5 days (very expensive) (3)[A]
  - Ozenoxacin 1% cream applied BID for 5 days (very expensive) (3)[A]
  - Dicloxacillin: adult 250 mg PO QID; pediatric <40 kg: 12 to 25 mg/kg/day divided q6h; >40 kg: 125 to 250 mg/kg/day divided q6h
- Dicloxacillin, cephalexin, topical mupirocin, and fusidic acid are effective, unless local staphylococcal strains are resistant. For MRSA infections, treatment options include clindamycin, tetracyclines, or trimethoprim-sulfamethoxazole. Oral doses given for 7 days are usually sufficient (4)[C].
- 1st-generation cephalosporins
  - Children
    - Cephalexin 25 to 50 mg/kg/day divided, q6–12h
    - Cefaclor 20 to 40 mg/kg/day divided q8h
    - Cephradine 25 to 50 mg/kg/day divided q6–12h
    - Cefadroxil 30 mg/kg/day divided BID
  - Adults
    - Cephalexin 250 mg up to QID
    - Cefaclor 250 mg TID
    - Cephradine 500 mg BID
    - Cefadroxil 1 g/day in divided doses
- Clindamycin 300 mg q6–8h
- Severe bullous disease may require IV therapy such as nafcillin or cefazolin.

ISSUES FOR REFERRAL

If resistant or extensive infections occur, especially in immunocompromised patients

ADDITIONAL THERAPIES

Monitor for microbial resistance patterns.

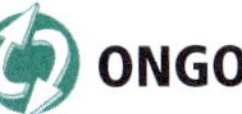

ONGOING CARE

FOLLOW-UP RECOMMENDATIONS

- Athletes are restricted from contact sports.
- School and daycare contagious restrictions
- Children can return to school 24 hours after initiation of antimicrobial treatment.

Patient Monitoring

If not clear within 7 to 10 days, culture the lesions.

PATIENT EDUCATION

Avoidance of infection spread is the key; hand washing is vital, especially for reducing spread in children.

PROGNOSIS

- Complete resolution in 7 to 10 days with treatment
- Antibiotic treatment will not prevent or halt glomerulonephritis, as it will in rheumatic fever.
- If not clear within 7 to 10 days, culture is necessary to find resistant organism.
- Recurrent impetigo: Evaluate for carriage of *S. aureus* in nares (also perineum, axillae, toe web). Apply mupirocin ointment to nares BID for 5 days for decolonization.

COMPLICATIONS

- Ecthyma
- Erysipelas
- Poststreptococcal acute glomerulonephritis
- Cellulitis
- Bacteremia
- Osteomyelitis
- Septic arthritis
- Pneumonia
- Lymphadenitis

REFERENCES

1. Stevens DL, Bisno AL, Chambers HF, et al. Practice guidelines for the diagnosis and management of skin and soft tissue infections: 2014 update by the Infectious Diseases Society of America. *Clin Infect Dis*. 2014;59(2):147–159.
2. Edge R, Argáez C. *Topical Antibiotics for Impetigo: A Review of the Clinical Effectiveness and Guidelines*. Ontario, Canada: Canadian Agency for Drugs and Technologies in Health; 2017.
3. Gahlawat G, Wubshet T, Bushell M, et al. Emerging treatment strategies for impetigo in endemic and nonendemic settings: a systematic review. *Clin Ther*. 2021;43(6):986–1006. doi:10.1016/j.clinthera.2021.04.013.
4. Del Giudice P, Hubiche P. Community-associated methicillin-resistant *Staphylococcus aureus* and impetigo. *Br J Dermatol*. 2010;162(4):905–906.

ADDITIONAL READING

- Clebak KT, Malone MA. Skin infections. *Prim Care*. 2018;45(3):433–454. doi:10.1016/j.pop.2018.05.004.
- Koning S, van der Sande R, Verhagen AP, et al. Interventions for impetigo. *Cochrane Database Syst Rev*. 2012;1(1):CD003261.

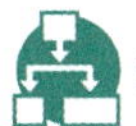

SEE ALSO

Algorithm: Rash

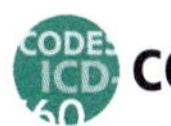

CODES

ICD10

- L01.01 Non-bullous impetigo
- L01.03 Bullous impetigo
- L01.00 Impetigo, unspecified

CLINICAL PEARLS

- Superficial, intraepidermal infection
- Predominantly staphylococcal in origin
- Microbial resistance patterns need to be monitored.
- Topical treatment is recommended for limited lesions and oral medication only when the disease is more severe/extensive.

I

INCONTINENCE, FECAL

Kalyanakrishnan Ramakrishnan, MD, FRCS

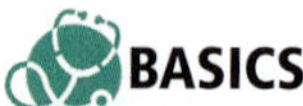

BASICS

Continuous or recurrent involuntary passage of feces through the anal canal for >1 month in an individual who has previously achieved continence

- Recurrent, involuntary loss of stool
- Assess rectal tone and voluntary squeeze and differentiate overflow incontinence from fecal impaction.
- Endorectal ultrasound (EUS) is the simplest, most reliable, and least invasive method to detect anal sphincter defects.
- The goal of treatment is to restore continence and/or improve quality of life.

DESCRIPTION

Major incontinence is the involuntary evacuation of feces. Minor incontinence includes passage of flatus and/or occasional seepage of liquid stool. Categories include urge and passive incontinence.

Geriatric Considerations

- Fecal incontinence increases with age and is an important cause for nursing home placement among the elderly.
- Idiopathic fecal incontinence is more common in older women.

EPIDEMIOLOGY

Incidence

Patients are often embarrassed and do not report fecal incontinence unless specifically queried ("silent affliction").

Prevalence

- 7% of adults; 15% of adults age >90 years; women > men
- 56–66% of hospitalized older patients and >50% of nursing home residents
- 50–70% of patients who have urinary incontinence also suffer from fecal incontinence.

Pregnancy Considerations

Obstetric injury to the pelvic floor may result in either temporary or persistent fecal incontinence.

Geriatric Considerations

Fecal impaction with overflow diarrhea is common in older patients.

ETIOLOGY AND PATHOPHYSIOLOGY

- Continence requires the complex orchestration of pelvic musculature, nerves, and reflex arcs.
- Stool volume/consistency, colon transit time, anorectal sensation, rectal compliance, anorectal reflexes, external/internal sphincter muscle tone, puborectalis muscle function, and mental capacity all play a role in maintaining continence.
- Congenital: spina bifida and myelomeningocele with spinal cord damage
- Trauma: anal sphincter damage from vaginal delivery or surgical procedures
- Medical: diabetes mellitus (most common metabolic disorder causing incontinence through pudendal nerve neuropathy), stroke, spinal cord trauma, neurodegenerative disorders, inflammatory bowel disease (IBD), rectal neoplasia

Genetics

No clear genetic association detected in the genome-wide association study.

RISK FACTORS

- Poor functional status—older age, female sex, obesity, limited physical activity
- Potential association with child abuse and adult sexual abuse
- Neurologic/neuropsychiatric conditions—multiple sclerosis, spinal cord injury, stroke, diabetic neuropathy (dementia, depression)
- Trauma: pelvic surgery, vaginal delivery, radiation. Risk factors during vaginal delivery include occipitoposterior presentation, prolonged second stage of labor, assisted vaginal delivery (forceps or vacuum-assist), and episiotomy.
- Diarrhea, IBD, irritable bowel syndrome (IBS), menopause, smoking, constipation, fecal impaction
- Congenital abnormalities, such as imperforate anus/rectal prolapse

GENERAL PREVENTION

- Behavioral/lifestyle changes: Obesity, limited physical activity/exercise, poor diet, and smoking are modifiable risk factors.
- Post meal bowel regimen—defecate regularly after meals to maximize positive impact of gastrocolic reflex.
- Pelvic floor muscle training during and after pregnancy and pelvic surgery; increase fiber intake (>30 g/day).

COMMONLY ASSOCIATED CONDITIONS

- Increasing age (>65 years)
- Chronic medical conditions—diabetes mellitus, dementia, stroke, spinal cord compression, depression, immobility, chronic obstructive pulmonary disease, IBS, and IBD
- Perineal trauma (obstetric); anorectal surgery; history of pelvic/rectal irradiation; urinary incontinence/pelvic organ prolapse

DIAGNOSIS

Diagnosis is based on history and physical findings.

HISTORY

- Patients seldom volunteer information about fecal incontinence. Direct questioning is important.
- Problem-specific history includes (1)[C]
  - Severity of soiling by liquid stool or gross incontinence of solid stool
  - Onset and duration (recent onset vs. chronic); frequency, presence of constipation/diarrhea
  - Bristol stool form scale (consistency, character, appearance of stool)
- Review diet; medical, surgical, and obstetric history; lifestyle; and mobility; thorough medication review
- Evaluate for social withdrawal and depression.

PHYSICAL EXAM

- Inspect perineum for dermatitis, hemorrhoids, fistula, surgical scars, skin tags, rectal prolapse, soiling, and ballooning of the perineum (sarcopenia of pelvic musculature). A patulous anal orifice may indicate myopathy or a neurologic disorder.
- Evaluate the external sphincter response to perineal skin stimulation (anal wink). Absence suggests neuropathy.
- Ask the patient to bear down, preferably in standing position, to assess for rectal prolapse.
- Digital rectal exam to assess anal canal pressure sphincter tone, rectal bleeding, hemorrhoids, neoplasm, fecal consistency, and diarrhea/distal fecal impaction
- General neurologic examination, including perianal sensation and mental status evaluation (1)[C]

DIFFERENTIAL DIAGNOSIS

- Anorectal disorders
  - Prolapsed internal hemorrhoids; rectal prolapse
  - Trauma: obstetric, surgical, accidental, sexual
  - Inflammatory/infectious gastrointestinal disorders, ischemic colitis, fistulas, bowel neoplasms, radiation proctitis
- Neurologic disorders
  - Stroke, dementia, neoplasms, spinal cord injury, and/or diseases causing altered level of consciousness
  - Pudendal neuropathy, neurosyphilis, multiple sclerosis, diabetes mellitus
- Miscellaneous causes
  - Infectious diarrhea, fecal impaction and overflow, IBS, laxative abuse, IBD, short bowel syndrome, myopathies, senescence and frailty, collagen vascular disease, psychological and behavioral problems

DIAGNOSTIC TESTS & INTERPRETATION

Diagnostic approach should be individualized, minimally invasive, practical and feasible. History and physical examination are generally sufficient for diagnosis. If uncertainty remains, consider:

- Plain abdominal x-ray (fecal impaction, constipation)
- Sigmoidoscopy/anoscopy/colonoscopy (hemorrhoids, colitis, neoplasm)

Initial Tests (lab, imaging)

- Stool studies (culture, ova and parasites, *Clostridium difficile* toxin assay)—if travel, antibiotic use, tube feedings, or sepsis
- Thyroid-stimulating hormone (TSH), electrolytes, and BUN in elderly patients
- EUS—most reliable and least invasive test for defining anatomic defects in the external and internal anal sphincters, rectal wall, and the puborectalis muscle (1)[B]. EUS can reliably predict therapeutic response to sphincteroplasty.

Follow-Up Tests & Special Considerations

- Defecography measures anorectal angle, evaluates pelvic descent, and detects occult/overt rectal prolapse. MRI defecography (dynamic MRI) further defines pelvic floor anatomy.
- Anorectal manometry measures maximal resting anal pressure, amplitude/duration of squeeze, rectoanal inhibitory reflex, threshold of conscious rectal sensation, rectal compliance, and anorectal pressures during straining.
- Pudendal nerve terminal motor latency (PNTML) measures neuromuscular integrity between the pudendal nerve and the anal sphincter; is operator-dependent and has poor correlation with clinical and histologic findings
- Electromyography can assess neurogenic/myopathic damage.

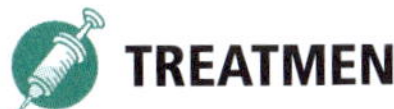

TREATMENT

GENERAL MEASURES

- In ambulatory patients, scheduled (or prompted) defecation is effective, particularly in those with overflow incontinence.
- Kegel exercises to strengthen pelvic floor
- If bed bound, scheduled osmotic or stimulant laxatives and suppositories promote evacuation and minimize fecal leakage.
- Use of stool deodorants (Peri-Wash, Derifil, Devrom), barrier creams to prevent/treat associated dermatitis.

MEDICATION

Limited evidence that antidiarrheals (loperamide, codeine) and drugs enhancing sphincter tone (phenylephrine gel, sodium valproate) are of benefit (2)[B]. Cholestyramine, colestipol useful in diarrhea following malabsorption or cholecystectomy; alosetron in diarrhea associated with IBS; amitriptyline in idiopathic fecal incontinence

First Line

Specific treatment of underlying disorder (e.g., infectious diarrhea/IBD) may improve fecal continence.

Second Line

- Stool-bulking agents: high-fiber diet, psyllium products, methylcellulose useful in milder forms of incontinence (1),(3)[B]
- Antidiarrheal agents, such as adsorbents or opium derivatives, may reduce diarrhea-associated incontinence (1),(3)[C].
- Disimpacting patients with fecal impaction/overflow incontinence and using bowel regimens prevent recurrence.

ADDITIONAL THERAPIES

- Biofeedback: initial treatment modality in motivated patients with some voluntary sphincter control (1)[C]; teaches patients to recognize rectal distension and contract the external anal sphincter, keeping intra-abdominal pressure low
- Biofeedback plus electrical stimulation of the anal sphincters is more effective than either measure. Patients with systemic neurologic disorders, anal deformities, or frequent episodes of incontinence respond poorly.

SURGERY/OTHER PROCEDURES

- Surgery should be considered only when nonsurgical approaches have failed. Sphincter repair offered in highly symptomatic patients with a well-defined defect of external anal sphincter (1),(3)[A].
- Tissue-bulking agent such as silicone elastomer or polysaccharide gel injected into the anorectal mucosa or the intersphincteric space in patients with internal anal sphincter dysfunction is no longer recommended as first-line treatment modality in view of diminishing long-term efficacy and cost.
- Artificial anal sphincter implantation/dynamic graciloplasty (gracilis muscle transposed into anus as modified sphincter) considered in patients with severe fecal incontinence and irreparable sphincter damage (1)[B]
- Colostomy/ileostomy appropriate in patients with disabling fecal incontinence and failed multiple therapeutic options (1)[B]; continent stomas created using the appendix/cecum as entry points enables flushing the colon in these patients.
- Anal plugs minimize fecal leakage in patients who do not benefit from other treatment modalities, especially immobilized, institutionalized, or neurologically disabled patients; plugs are often poorly tolerated (1),(3)[B].
- Sacral nerve stimulation (neuromodulation) via implantation of electrodes delivering low-amplitude electrical stimulation to sphincter muscles improves rectal tone, especially in those with a coexistent sphincter defect (3)[B].
- SECCA procedure—temperature-controlled radiofrequency energy delivered to the anorectal junction distal to the dentate line to cause scarring, and anal canal narrowing is no longer recommended.
- Magnetic anal sphincter (MAS) devices—series of 14 to 20 interlinked titanium beads with magnetic cores forming a flexible ring encircling the external anal sphincter 3 to 5 cm from the anal verge. During defecation, the beads separate allowing evacuation after which the beads approximate closing the canal (4)[C], useful in moderate/severe incontinence.
- A vaginally placed bowel control device that the patient inflates to control leakage and deflates to defecate (Eclipse System) is well tolerated and effective (4)[B].
- Percutaneous posterior tibial nerve stimulation at the ankle for 30 minutes weekly for 12 weeks (50% efficacy) and the TOPAS pelvic floor repair system (polypropylene mesh placed behind the anorectum to support the puborectalis) (55% efficacy) are other recent advances in controlling fecal incontinence (4)[B].

COMPLEMENTARY & ALTERNATIVE MEDICINE

Ten acupuncture sessions per week did improve quality of life, but this modality has not been studied in detail (3)[C].

ADMISSION, INPATIENT, AND NURSING CONSIDERATIONS

- If secondary to fecal impaction, manual evacuation of fecal mass (after lubrication with lidocaine jelly)
- Avoid hot water, soap, or hydrogen peroxide enemas.

ONGOING CARE

FOLLOW-UP RECOMMENDATIONS

Periodic rectal exam

Patient Monitoring

Consider impaction if there is <1 bowel movement every other day in patients with fecal incontinence.

DIET

High fiber (20 to 30 g/day) and at least 1.5 L fluid daily; avoid precipitants (caffeine).

PATIENT EDUCATION

Kegel/sphincter training exercises are helpful but not sufficient for treating fecal incontinence.

PROGNOSIS

- Reimpaction likely if bowel regimen discontinued
- 50% failure rate over 5 years following overlapping sphincteroplasty

COMPLICATIONS

- Depression and social isolation, skin ulcerations
- Artificial bowel sphincter: infection, erosion, mechanical failure

REFERENCES

1. Bordeianou LG, Thorsen AJ, Keller DS, et al. The American Society of Colon and Rectal Surgeons clinical practice guidelines for the management of fecal incontinence. *Dis Colon Rectum*. 2023;66(5):647–661.
2. Mack I, Hahn H, Gödel C, et al. Global prevalence of fecal incontinence in community-dwelling adults: a systematic review and meta-analysis. *Clinical Gastroenterol Hepatol*. 2024;22(4):712–731.e8. doi:10.1016/j.cgh.2023.09.004.
3. Assmann SL, Keszthelyi D, Kleijnen J, et al. Guideline for the diagnosis and treatment of faecal incontinence—a URG/ESCP/ESNM/ESPCC collaboration. *United European Gastroenterol J*. 2022;10(3):251–286.
4. Menees S, Chey WD. Fecal incontinence: pathogenesis, diagnosis, and updated treatment strategies. *Gastroenterol Clin North Am*. 2022;51(1):71–91. doi:10.1016/j.gtc.2021.10.005.

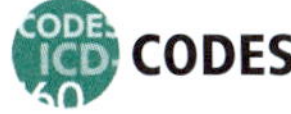

CODES

ICD10

- R15.9 Full incontinence of feces
- R15.2 Fecal urgency
- R15.0 Incomplete defecation

CLINICAL PEARLS

- Scheduled defecation after meals, bulking agents, and scheduled enemas minimize impaction and are helpful in managing mild/moderate fecal incontinence.
- Differentiate true incontinence from pseudoincontinence (overflow or functional incontinence).
- New-onset fecal incontinence may indicate spinal cord compression

I

INCONTINENCE, URINARY ADULT FEMALE

Vanessa Joyce M. Evardone, MD, BSMT

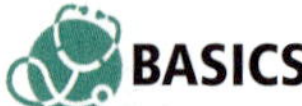

BASICS

- Urinary incontinence (UI): involuntary urine (ur) loss; common in women; few seek care despite effective options; may affect quality of life (QoL)
- UI: transient (acute, <6 months, and reversible if cause addressed) or chronic (have subtypes)

DESCRIPTION

- Stress UI: increased intra-abdominal pressure (coughing, exertion); most common in younger women
- Urge UI: sudden uncontrollable ur loss, preceded or accompanied by urgency; from overactive bladder (OAB) or detrusor overactivity (DO); most common in older adults
- Mixed UI: >1 type of UI, often a combo (stress and urge UIs); overall most common type
- Overflow UI: high-residual volume from inadequate bladder emptying (chronic ur retention), causing frequent dribbling; predisposes to recurrent infections, vesicoureteral reflux, autonomic dysreflexia
- Functional UI: ur loss due to deficits in cognition or mobility with normal ur system function
- Continuous UI: sustained slow leakage in between regular voiding; may have no awareness nor bladder fullness

EPIDEMIOLOGY

Prevalence

- Overall prevalence in women: 10–20% (up to 77% in nursing homes)
- In women, stress UI decreases with age, whereas urge UI increases.

ETIOLOGY AND PATHOPHYSIOLOGY

- Stress UI: 2 types—anatomic (urethral hypermobility from lack of pelvic support) and intrinsic sphincter deficiency (impaired urethral closure); stress UI is secondary to surgical scarring, radiation, hormonal, or age-related changes.
- Urge UI: DO (usual cause) or OAB from neuro causes (SCI), abd trauma, infection, Rx, certain fluids, or idiopathic; DO could be idiopathic or neurogenic (MS).
- Overflow UI: detrusor underactivity ("neurogenic bladder"), increased bladder ur volume (DM or Rx), or bladder outlet obstruction (fibroids, pelvic organ prolapse [POP], masses)
- Mixed UI: aggregate of etiologies from each type of UI present.
- Functional UI: cognitive impairment (dementia, delirium, intellectual disabilities) unable to recognize need for toilet; psych issues and mental illness (decreased awareness); medical conditions (arthritis) and physical disability impairing mobility; poor vision; and environmental barriers
- Continuous UI: constant involuntary ur loss; ectopic ureters in females usually open in urethra distal to sphincter or in the vagina, causing sustained leakage through the urethra or extra-urethral (urogenital fistulas: vesicovaginal [most common], ureterovaginal, and urethrovaginal).

RISK FACTORS

Advanced age, vaginal atrophy (menopause), impaired cognition-function, obesity (BMI >30), medical conditions (DM, chronic obstructive pulmonary disease [COPD]), multiparity, pelvic floor dysfunction (vaginal birth, pelvic surgery or radiation), urethral diverticula, POP, neuro diseases (stroke, MS, Parkinson disease), smoking, constipation, caffeine, and high-impact exercises

DIAGNOSIS

HISTORY

- Age: Onset in childhood indicates congenital cause (ectopic ureter); stress UI is common in women 19 to 64 years old; mixed UI is common in women >65 years old.
- Nature-duration: Stress UI presents with small spurts of ur loss, typically dry at night in bed, and may have pelvic floor Sx (bulging, dyspareunia, pressure). Urge UI have sudden urge followed by large amounts of ur leakage (use pads), frequency, nocturia, and maybe triggered by sensory stimuli (cold).
- Suprapubic pain with dysuria: infection, interstitial cystitis
- Surgical Hx: Pelvic surgery (gynecologic or bowel) can injure the pelvic floor and affect neuro function.
- Comorbidities: constipation, DM, CHF, COPD, sleep apnea, neuro dysfunction (cognition), depression
- Medication that decrease bladder contractility ⇒ ur retention and overflow (antidepressants, antihistamines, antimuscarinics, anti-Parkinson, antipsychotics, β-adrenergic agonists, CCBs, opioids, sedative-hypnotics, skeletal muscle relaxants); detrusor irritability or increased Cr clearance (EtOH, caffeine, diuretics); increased urethral sphincter tone ⇒ ur retention and overflow (α-adrenergic agonists, TCAs, amphetamines); and decreased urethral sphincter tone ⇒ stress UI (α-adrenergic antagonists); ACEi ⇒ chronic dry cough (stress UI)
- Tobacco smoking
- 3-day voiding diary (fluid-caffeine intake, ur Sx, situations and timing of UI, patient habits)
- The International Consultation on Incontinence Questionnaire (ICIQ)

PHYSICAL EXAM

- Neuro exam (sensation deficit in perineal–sacral area) and cognitive-functional evaluation.
- Pelvic exam: perineum and external genitalia (vaginal atrophy), half speculum vaginal exam (POP), bimanual pelvic exam (masses-cystocele, pelvic floor resting tone-function based on ability to isolate-contract pelvic floor using Oxford scale), and anorectal exam (fecal impaction, rectocele or posterior vaginal wall prolapse).
- CST: immediate ur leakage on coughing and Valsalva with comfortably full bladder; excellent reliability, sensitivity, and specificity for stress UI versus urodynamics (UDS); increased sensitivity performed in standing position but can be done in supine lithotomy position; PPV: 78–97%
- Cotton swab test (urethral hypermobility): Little diagnostic utility to UDS; may predict response to midurethral sling (MUS) surgery.
- UDS testing: unnecessary in uncomplicated UI; postvoid residual (PVD) if patient reports incomplete voiding, POP past introitus, or for stress UI surgery; PVR (catheterization or sonography) within 10 minutes postmeasured void (normal: <100 mL for adults and <150 mL for older adults for voided volume >200 mL, or 1/3 of total voided volume)

DIFFERENTIAL DIAGNOSIS

- Nocturnal enuresis: idiopathic, DO, neurogenic, cardiogenic, sleep apnea
- Continuous leakage: ectopic ureter, fistulas
- Postvoid dribbling: urethral diverticulum, idiopathic, iatrogenic, surgical
- Pain (dyspareunia): interstitial cystitis, STI
- POP
- Hematuria, recurrent UTIs, or pelvic mass: malignancy
- Functional UI: neurologic, cognitive, psychological, physical impairment
- Mnemonic for causes of UI: TOILETED (DIAPPERS) Thin dry vaginal-urethral epithelium (atrophic urethritis-vaginitis), Obstruction (stool impaction/ constipation), Infection, Limited (restricted) mobility, Emotional (psychological, depression), Therapeutic medications (pharmacologic), Endocrine disorders (excessive urine), Delirium

DIAGNOSTIC TESTS & INTERPRETATION

Initial Tests (lab, imaging)

- UA: in all patients (infection, hematuria, proteinuria, glycosuria)
- Ur Cx: if suspicious for infection (Tx of asymptomatic bacteriuria will not improve UI in elderly.)
- Renal function: if concern for renal impairment or obstruction
- TSH: if with constipation
- Imaging is unnecessary in uncomplicated UI; renal US for hydronephrosis if suspicious for obstruction (microhematuria)
- Urodynamic testing: for complicated UI or if surgery considered.
- Bladder scan if overflow UI suspected (PVR >200 mL)

Diagnostic Procedures/Other

UDS and cystoscopy: after failing conservative Tx; include cystometric study of detrusor function, pressure flow studies (bladder emptying), and cystoscopy (women with microhematuria or recurrent UTIs).

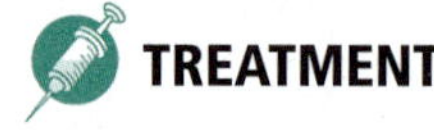

TREATMENT

GENERAL MEASURES

- Stepwise approach: conservative (first line), Rx-mechanical devices (second line), invasive interventions (third line).
- Tx correctable causes (infection, constipation).

- Stress UI: 6- to 8-week trial of behavioral modification and pelvic floor training; if no improvement, refer to urology.
- Urge UI: behavior modification, pelvic floor muscle training (PFMT), and medication; behavior modification plus medication: more effective versus medication alone
- Mixed UI: directed at predominant Sx (stress or urge UI)

MEDICATION

First Line

Conservative management

- I. Behavioral Techniques: (i) bladder training (resist and expanding intervals between voiding); more benefit if supervised by health care provider; (ii) double voiding (voiding then waiting few minutes before trying again to empty bladder completely); (iii) toileting assistance (scheduled q2–4 hours); (iv) fluid-diet management: less EtOH, caffeine (<1 cup/day), or acidic food; less fluid intake before sleep and <2 L/day; diet changes; and weight loss (moderate weight loss improves UI in BMI ≥30 kg/m^2); (v) lifestyle changes (more active, stop smoking)
- II. PFMT (Kegel): effective for stress UI (may help urge UI); ± bladder training, manual feedback (palpating pelvic muscle during exercise), biofeedback (vaginal-anal device for visual-audio feedback on pelvic muscle contraction), or electrical stimulation. Pelvic floor therapists improve technique or use of weighted intravaginal cones. Home electrode stimulation Tx (vagina, anus) is a Medicare-covered option (if unable to voluntarily contract pelvic muscle).

Second Line

- I. Medications
  - Stress UI: no FDA-approved Rx.
  - Topical estrogen may be beneficial for urgency and frequency Sx in postmenopausal women with vaginal atrophy (transdermal or oral may worsen UI).
  - Urge UI: if behavior Tx is unsuccessful, antimuscarinic agents (selective: darifenacin, solifenacin; nonselective: oxybutynin, tolterodine, trospium) and β3-AR agonists (mirabegron, vibegron) are FDA-approved. Dual Tx (mirabegron and low-dose anticholinergic agents) can be considered.
  - Anticholinergic agents inhibit involuntary detrusor contractions; effective for urge UI and OAB (significant clinical improvement with modest improvement in QoL)
  - No single anticholinergic shown to be overall superior (higher doses: more effective but more side effects); extended-release and transdermal prep have fewer side effects (dry mouth and eyes, constipation, impaired cognition). Avoid in narrow-angle glaucoma, ur retention, impaired gastric emptying, long QT (worsening of arrhythmias), and frailty.
  - β3-AR agonists: no associated significant cognitive decline; avoided in ESRD, ESLD and uncontrolled HTN (BP check weeks postinitiation)
  - Rx: can be used for both urge and mixed UIs; combo Tx (Rx-behavior) is more effective than either modality alone.
  - OnabotulinumtoxinA for urge UI: similar Sx reduction as antimuscarinic (anticholinergic agents) options, with more Sx resolution; risk of ur retention, incomplete bladder emptying, and UTI
- II. Mechanical
  - Vaginal inserts (pessaries, tampons): option for stress UI in pregnancy, in nonsurgical candidates, and in those unresponsive to prior surgeries; compress bladder neck and/or urethra leading to decreased ur loss; pessaries: low-cost, low-risk, quick results
  - Urethral plugs: prevent UI during activities (running); limited evidence; associated with ADRs (UTI, hematuria, device migration into bladder)

Third Line

Individualized: based on Sx, goals, and expectations. Surgery may be used as first line for moderate to severe stress UI.

- Stress UI
  - Sling procedures: Mesh is the most common and studied for stress UI; better outcomes at 1 year than PFMT. Other options: autologous fascia pubovaginal sling (PVS), Burch colposuspension. POP may unmask UI in 40% of women (repair both during same surgery).
  - Intravesical balloons: more effective than sham Tx; more effective than behavior Tx with neuromodulation.
  - Periurethral injections (bulking agents: silicone polymers, collagen) leads to increased periurethral resistance (recurrent UI postsurgery or cannot tolerate surgery but often require injections); low-quality evidence: improved outcomes versus no Tx
- Urge UI
  - Neuromodulation (sacral nerve stimulation): invasive (surgically implanted), expensive, frequent complications, and inferior to onabotulinumtoxinA and posterior tibial nerve stimulation (PTNS)
  - OnabotulinumtoxinA (intravesical injection to detrusor via cystoscopy): FDA approved, well tolerated, and significant improvement in overall OAB and QoL (prior inadequately treated with anticholinergic agents).
  - Bladder augmentation: complex reconstructive surgery procedure leads to increased bladder size and elasticity; after failing all other Tx

Geriatric Considerations

- UI: not a normal part of aging
- Anticholinergic agents used with caution; can worsen cognition and delirium (cumulative effects with use)
- Urethral sling
- Medication list review
- β3-AR agonists increase BP; not used in ESRD or ESLD

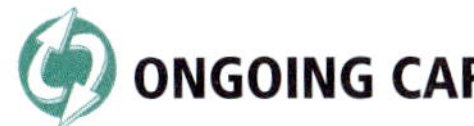

ONGOING CARE

COMPLICATIONS

Skin maceration (nursing home admissions), social isolation and depression, fear of leakage, impaired sexual function/QoL, risk of falls and fractures.

ADDITIONAL READING

Riemsma R, Hagen S, Kirschner-Hermanns R, et al. Can incontinence be cured? A systematic review of cure rates. *BMC Med*. 2017;15(1):63.

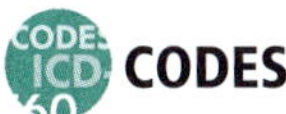

CODES

ICD10

- R32 Unspecified urinary incontinence
- N39.3 Stress incontinence (female) (male)
- N39.41 Urge incontinence

CLINICAL PEARLS

- Most UI: diagnosed with Hx and PE in conjunction with CST, PVR, and UA; UDS does not add value in uncomplicated UI.
- Rule out infection (UTI, STI), hematuria.
- Try lifestyle changes first for all types of UI.
- Pelvic floor training: safe effective first line Tx for stress and urge UI; can improve QoL; if no improvement in stress UI: mesh sling has high success rates; if no improvement in urge UI, anticholinergic agents (antimuscarinics) and β3-ARs could be used.

INCONTINENCE, URINARY ADULT MALE

Laura Bujold, DO, MS

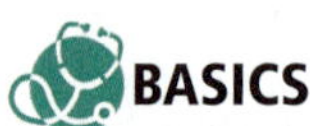

BASICS

DESCRIPTION

- Urinary incontinence (UI) is a pathologic condition of an acute or chronic nature that refers to the involuntary loss of urine leading to medical, financial, social, or hygienic problems. Five main types of UI have been described: stress, urge, mixed, overflow (urinary retention), and functional UI (1).
- Stress incontinence: involuntary urine leaks secondary to increased intra-abdominal pressure being greater than the sphincter can control; may be precipitated by sneezing, laughing, coughing, exertion
- Urge incontinence: Involuntary leakage of urine associated with urgency is believed to be secondary to uncontrolled contraction of the urinary bladder. It is also called detrusor overactivity.
- Mixed incontinence: involuntary leakage of urine with urgency and with stress, such as sneezing, laughing, coughing, exertion
- Overflow incontinence: also known as urinary retention; this occurs with bladder overdistention due to impaired detrusor contraction or bladder outlet obstruction (due to benign prostatic hyperplasia [BPH], bladder stones, bladder tumors, pelvic tumors, urethral strictures, or spasms).
- Functional UI: urine leakage variable, often due to environmental or physical barriers to toileting (i.e., reduced mobility)
- Polyuria is defined by excessive amounts of urine (≥2.5 to 3 L) >24 hours.
- Nocturnal polyuria is where >33% of total daily urine output occurs during sleeping hours.

EPIDEMIOLOGY

- Stress incontinence in men is rare and is often attributable to prostate surgery, neurologic disease, or trauma.
- Reported rates of incontinence range from 1% after transurethral resection to 2–66% after radical prostatectomy and 1–15% following transvesical prostatectomy, although rates decline with time (1).

Prevalence

- 12.4% prevalence of UI in community-dwelling adult men in the United States
- 4.5% reported moderate to severe UI, of which 48.6% experienced urge, 23.5% experienced other UI, 15.4% experienced mixed, and 12.5% experienced stress incontinence per the NHANES report in 2010 (1).

ETIOLOGY AND PATHOPHYSIOLOGY

- Incontinence secondary to bladder abnormalities
  - Detrusor overactivity results in urge incontinence.
  - Detrusor overactivity commonly is associated with bladder outlet obstruction from BPH.
  - Medications that increase bladder contractility or exacerbate obstructive effects
- Incontinence secondary to outlet abnormalities
  - Sphincteric damage secondary to pelvic surgery or radiation
  - Sphincteric dysfunction secondary to neurologic disease
  - Commonly associated with BPH due to compression of the urethra, affecting urinary flow
- Mixed incontinence is caused by abnormalities of both the bladder and the outlet overflow or by enlarged prostate/bladder neck contracture from prostate surgery.
- Stress incontinence is caused by weakened urethral sphincter and/or pelvic floor weakness.

RISK FACTORS

- Age
- Diseases: diabetes, BPH, hypertension (HTN), major depression, neurologic disease
- History of urinary tract infections (UTIs)
- Pelvic trauma, including prostate surgery
- Polypharmacy

GENERAL PREVENTION

Proper management of conditions, such as symptomatic bladder outlet obstruction caused by BPH early in the course, may prevent continence problems later in life.

COMMONLY ASSOCIATED CONDITIONS

Male UI often has a negative impact in both mental and physical aspects of quality of life. It is an independent risk factor for depression and anxiety, and it may significantly reduce work productivity.

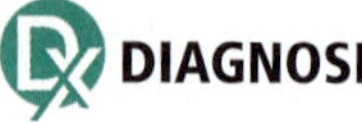

DIAGNOSIS

HISTORY

- 3 Incontinence Questions tool questionnaire:
  - During the last 3 months, have you leaked urine (even a small amount)? If no, end quiz.
  - During the last 3 months, did you leak urine (check all that apply):
    - When you were performing some physical activity, such as coughing, sneezing, lifting, or exercise?
    - When you had the urge or the feeling that you needed to empty your bladder, but you could not get to the toilet fast enough?
    - Without physical activity and without a sense of urgency?
  - During the last 3 months, did you leak urine most often (check only one):
    - When you were performing some physical activity, such as coughing sneezing, lifting, or exercise?
    - When you had the urge or the feeling that you needed to empty your bladder, but you could not get to the toilet fast enough?
    - Without physical activity and without a sense of urgency?
    - About equally as often with physical activity as with a sense of urgency?
- Voiding symptoms
  - Duration and characteristics of incontinence
  - Precipitants, severity, timing, and associated symptoms (BPH, fluid intake, etc.)
  - Use of pads, briefs, diapers.
  - Alteration in bowel habits
  - Previous treatments and effect on incontinence
- Transient causes: UTI, delirium, medications, constipation, immobility
- Geriatric patients: Assess cognitive levels (dementia/delirium), psychological disorders, mobility problems.
- Medication use: diuretics, drugs for BPH, opioids, muscle relaxants, anticholinergics, antidepressants
- Alcohol and drug use, including caffeine
- Surgery: pelvic surgery or radiation, bowel, back, genitourinary procedures, abdominoperineal resection, prostatectomy: radical for cancer, open/transurethral for benign disease
- Red flag symptoms requiring rapid referral to specialist management
  - Pain, hematuria, recurrent UTI, history of prostate irradiation, history of radical pelvic surgery (i.e., prostate surgery), constant leakage suggesting fistula, voiding difficulty, suspected neurologic disease

PHYSICAL EXAM

- Abdominal examination
  - Suprapubic tenderness suggests UTI.
  - Surgical scars suggesting prior pelvic surgery
  - Suprapubic mass may be a palpable bladder and suggest retention.
  - Suprapubic mass may also be an abdominal mass applying pressure on a normal bladder.
  - Increased abdominal girth
- Genitourinary examination: external genitalia, DRE (prostate)
- Musculoskeletal (look for neurogenic or functional causes.)
  - Extremities, spine, skeletal deformities, scars from previous spinal surgery
  - Sacral abnormalities may be associated with neurogenic bladder dysfunction.
- Neurologic
  - Motor, sensory, reflexes

DIFFERENTIAL DIAGNOSIS

- Transient (infections, meds, constipation, etc.)
- Chronic
  - Urge incontinence
  - Stress incontinence
  - Mixed incontinence
  - Overflow incontinence
  - Functional UI

DIAGNOSTIC TESTS & INTERPRETATION

Initial Tests (lab, imaging)

- Urinalysis and urine culture to check for glucosuria, pyuria, proteinuria, and/or blood
  - If UTI is present, treat and then reassess need for further workup because this frequently causes UI.
- Voiding diary, the 3 Incontinence Questions (1)[C]
- Pad test if quantity of leakage or objective outcome measure is desired (low sensitivity)
- Postvoid residual (PVR) volume if difficulty voiding or other lower urinary tract symptoms using ultrasound (US) to measure PVR: PVR persistently ≥100 mL indicates voiding dysfunction (1)[C].
- PVR >200 mL suggests overflow incontinence. A patient whose PVR is <200 mL does not have overflow incontinence.
- Uroflowmetry
- PSA only if diagnosis of prostate cancer will influence treatment or if levels can help decision-making for patients at risk for BPH
- Renal function
- Voiding cystogram in select cases

Diagnostic Procedures/Other

- Prostate US and biopsy if indicated by physical exam or PSA level
- Urethrocystoscopy to exclude suspected bladder or urethral pathology or before invasive therapies
- Imaging of upper and lower urinary tract is not routinely indicated as part of UI assessment.

TREATMENT

Conservative, nonmedication interventions, such as behavioral modification, timed voiding, bladder training, and pelvic floor muscle training, should be considered *first-line therapies*, prior to initiating any pharmacologic therapy.

GENERAL MEASURES

- Bladder diaries
- Bladder training and timed voiding are effective.
- Pelvic floor muscle training speeds recovery of continence following radical prostatectomy
- Weight loss may improve UI symptoms.
- Constipation is associated with UI, but treatment may not improve UI.
- Reduction in caffeine intake does not improve UI but may improve urgency and frequency.
- Pads may be used for urine containment in UI as well as external sheaths (1)[B]—external sheaths may have similar rates of UTIs with indwelling catheters but result in better QoL (1)[B].
  - Men with UI should be counseled that leakage is not a normal part of aging and that goals of treatment include elimination of the need for these.

MEDICATION

First Line

- Urge incontinence: There is no consistent evidence that drug therapy is better than behavioral therapy in UUI (1)[B], and behavioral therapy results in higher patient satisfaction (1)[B].
- Antimuscarinic agents are first-line drug therapy in UUI (1)[B], and there is no evidence that any one agent is superior for UUI (1)[A].
- Oxybutynin (Ditropan XL) 5 to 15 mg PO every day
- Tolterodine (Detrol LA) 2 to 4 mg PO every day
- Darifenacin (Enablex) 7.5 to 15 mg PO every day
- Solifenacin (Vesicare) 5 to 10 mg PO every day
- Trospium chloride (Sanctura XR) 60 mg PO every day
- Transdermal oxybutynin (Gelnique) 10% apply daily (EAU Grade B)—no dry mouth
- Fesoterodine (Toviaz) 4 to 8 mg PO every day
- Mirabegron, a β_3-agonist, has been shown in some trials and systematic reviews to be as efficacious as antimuscarinics.
- Mirabegron (Myrbetriq): 25 to 50 mg PO daily; *caution*: HTN
- Review efficacy and side effects 4 to 6 weeks after treatment initiation.
- Most patients will stop antimuscarinic therapy within 3 months due to adverse effects, nonefficacy, or cost.
- Caution in those with bladder outlet obstruction and PVR >250 to 300 mL: In men with urgency associated with BPH, consider α-blockers (i.e., tamsulosin, alfuzosin, silodosin) as monotherapy or in combination with antimuscarinic for residual overactive bladder.
- Stress incontinence
  - No generally accepted drug therapy
  - Mixed stress and urge incontinence; ER formulations are preferred due to reduced side effects.

Second Line

- Urge incontinence
- Tricyclic antidepressants
  - Imipramine 10 to 25 mg PO BID/TID
- Desmopressin (DDAVP) for occasional short-term relief of UI
  - 25 to 50 μg PO or intranasal at bedtime
- Intradetrusor botulinum toxin injections 100 U intravesical injections (not FDA-approved)
- Duloxetine for temporary improvements of incontinence with dose titration (mixed stress/urge)

Geriatric Considerations

Anticholinergics and tricyclics may result in significant cognitive impairment in elderly patients.

ISSUES FOR REFERRAL

- Prior pelvic surgery/invasive procedure or radiation of the prostate or urethra
- PVR >300 mL
- Neurologic disease
- Recurrent bladder or prostate infections
- Pelvic pain
- Severe incontinence requiring multiple heavy pads or diapers each day

ADDITIONAL THERAPIES

- Pelvic floor rehabilitation (Kegel exercises) may significantly reduce both stress and urge incontinence in male patients and should be considered a part of initial management for stress UI.
- Overflow incontinence is usually caused by poor bladder contractility with urinary retention.
  - Indwelling or intermittent catheterization, evaluate for outlet obstruction.

SURGERY/OTHER PROCEDURES

- Urge incontinence
  - Sacral nerve stimulation with behavioral therapy
  - Augmentation cystoplasty and urinary diversion
  - Botulinum toxin injection via cystoscopy
- Stress incontinence
  - Urethral bulking agents: modest success rates with low cure rates
  - Male sling procedures: promising short-term and intermediate results but no long-term studies
  - Artificial urinary sphincter implant has excellent long-term continence rates and is considered gold standard.
    - Success rates have been defined as use of ≤1 pad/day and have ranged from 59% to 90% at follow-up intervals from 1 to 8 years. Surgical intervention has very high patient satisfaction rate, but revision is often required due to urethral erosion, infection, or atrophy. Foley catheter trauma is a common cause of late urethral erosion.

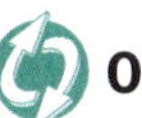

ONGOING CARE

FOLLOW-UP RECOMMENDATIONS

- To assess associated symptoms, severity, and hassles of incontinence, there are:
  - Michigan Incontinence Symptom Index (M-ISI)
- International Consultation on Incontinence Questionnaire-Urinary Incontinence Short Form
- To assess severity of UI, there are:
  - Sadvik questionnaire—used to assess frequency and amount of leakage
  - 24-hour pad weight
  - Bladder diary

COMPLICATIONS

- Dermatitis, candidiasis, skin breakdown
- Social isolation
- Avoidance of sex
- Weight gain

REFERENCES

1. Khandelwal C, Kistler C. Diagnosis of urinary incontinence. *Am Fam Physician*. 2013;87(8):543–550.

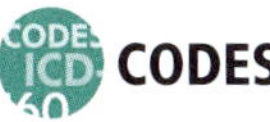

CODES

ICD10

- R32 Unspecified urinary incontinence
- N39.3 Stress incontinence (female) (male)
- N39.41 Urge incontinence

CLINICAL PEARLS

- Think "outside" the lower urinary tract: Comorbid medical illness and impairments are independently associated with UI; treat contributing comorbidities and rule out secondary causes.
- Always check PVR: PVR ≥100 mL indicates voiding dysfunction; ≥200 mL suggests overflow incontinence.

INFECTIOUS MONONUCLEOSIS, EPSTEIN-BARR VIRUS INFECTIONS

Dennis E. Hughes, DO, FACEP

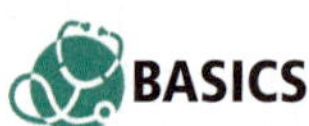

BASICS

DESCRIPTION

- Epstein-Barr virus (EBV) is a member of the γ-herpes virus family; human herpes virus 4
  - Two subtypes: ST1 predominates in Western hemisphere, Southeast Asia; ST1 and ST2 equally prevalent in Africa
- Primary infection typically occurs in childhood. The majority of individuals seroconvert by 2 years of age with little clinical manifestation of illness. A second peak occurs in adolescence and young adulthood—this group commonly manifests initial infection as infectious mononucleosis (IM) (1).
- WHO classified EBV as "tumor virus" (group I carcinogen) due to cancer association.

EPIDEMIOLOGY

Incidence

- Military recruits, college students, and others living in cloistered and crowded populations have highest symptomatic infection rate. Overall rate in the United States is 500/100,000.
- Predominant age of symptomatic primary infection is 15 to 24 years; 200 to 800/100,000 affected
- Incidence increases during the summer months.

Prevalence

- Worldwide 95% of population has been infected by adulthood. By age of 5 years, 50% of children have been infected; the vast majority of those without manifesting symptoms.
- Seroconversion occurs later in childhood in developed countries; there is suggestion of race/ethnicity disparity in the United States with higher seroprevalence in non-Hispanic black, Asian, and Hispanic populations; also, higher prevalence in larger households and lower levels of parental education

ETIOLOGY AND PATHOPHYSIOLOGY

- After inoculation, the virus replicates in the nasopharyngeal epithelium with resulting cell lysis, virion spread, and viremia. EBV exhibits dual tropism for B-cells and epithelial cells. The reticuloendothelial system is affected, resulting in a host response and the appearance of atypical lymphocytes in the peripheral blood. Viral genome can be detected in the oral cavity 1 week prior to symptoms.
- A polyclonal B-cell proliferative response follows. Relatively few (<0.1%) of circulating lymphocytes are infected by EBV in the acute illness.
- A persistent (asymptomatic) state ensues with the EBV genome invisible to the immune system. The maintenance of the invisible state (to host immunity) is thought to be due to EBV particles wrapping themselves in host cell-derived membranes and a low rate of viral reproduction (1).
- Either through B-cell stimulation or diminished EBV-specific immune modulation, the previously latent EBV-infected B cells replicate and enter a "lytic" phase, allowing clinical expression of the EBV genome. Risk of this occurring may be linked to host genetic factors, smoking, increased BMI, and low vitamin D/sunlight exposure. The proteins produced may either modify host response to or contribute directly to malignancy.
- Immunosuppression (organ transplant/acquired immune deficiency) can result in transformation and lymphoproliferative disorders.

RISK FACTORS

- Age (highest incidence of symptomatic infection in adolescent, young adults)
- Socio-hygienic level ("crowded conditions")
- Geographic location
- Close, intimate contact; especially "deep kissing" in adolescents and young adults
- Immunosuppression
- Possibly some risk of transmission by fomites (e.g., shared toys)

GENERAL PREVENTION

- Avoid close physical contact with symptomatic EBV/IM patients.
- Meticulous handwashing and hygiene to reduce transmission
- General precautions with potential blood exposure (EBV can be transmitted via blood contamination as well as hematopoietic cell and solid organ transplant.).
- EBV vaccines under investigation (lack of intimate knowledge of mechanism of immune response has impaired ability to develop an effective vaccine).

COMMONLY ASSOCIATED CONDITIONS

- IM: Symptomatic primary EBV infection is common in otherwise healthy adolescents and young adults.
  - Clinical features vary in severity and duration: In children age <10 years, generally mild; in adolescents and adults, symptoms can be more severe and protracted (are dependent on intensity of T-cell response).
  - Incubation period is 30 to 50 days (extremely long for a viral infection).
- X-linked lymphoproliferative syndrome (XLP—rare, inherited extreme vulnerability to EBV infection)
- Lymphoproliferative syndromes due to EBV infections in transplant recipients
- Lymphomas (B-cell lymphoblastic, T-cell)
- Lymphocytic interstitial pneumonitis
- Hairy leukoplakia of the tongue, leiomyosarcoma, and CNS lymphomas in patients with AIDS
- Burkitt lymphoma (most common childhood tumor in Africa and Papua New Guinea where malaria is also endemic and may be a cofactor); much higher prevalence than other areas of the world
- Nasopharyngeal carcinoma (seen worldwide, but highest prevalence in Africa and Asia)
- Parotid gland carcinoma
- Hodgkin lymphoma (most common EBV-associated malignancy in the United States, European Union)
- Postulated to be associated with multiple sclerosis (two to three times incidence in EBV-positive individuals)
- Chronic active EBV (CAEBV) due to loss of host control of viral replication

DIAGNOSIS

Diagnostic accuracy of clinical signs and symptoms varies.

HISTORY

- May be either abrupt or insidious in onset
- IM syndrome of fatigue, malaise, and sore throat
- In adults, temperature may rise to 103°F (39.4°C) and gradually fall over a variable period of 7 to 10 days; in severe cases, temperature elevations of 104 to 105°F (40.0 to 40.6°C) may persist for 2 weeks.
- Children typically have low-grade fever or are afebrile.
- Rash, conjunctivitis
- Chest pain (myocarditis and pericarditis)

PHYSICAL EXAM

- Fever, lymphadenopathy, pharyngitis in >50%, with palatal petechiae and hepatosplenomegaly in ~10%
- Diffuse hyperemia and hyperplasia of oropharyngeal lymphoid tissue
- Gelatinous, grayish-white exudative tonsillitis persists for 7 to 10 days in 50%.
- Petechiae at border of hard and soft palates in 60% (LR+1.32 to 11.40)
- Bilateral upper eyelid edema (Hoagland sign)
- Axillary, epitrochlear, popliteal, inguinal, mediastinal, and mesenteric lymphadenopathy (95% of patients; LR+1.85 to 4.70).
- Lymph node enlargement subsides over days/weeks.
- Tender lymphadenopathy (cervical nodes are most commonly enlarged); absence of any lymphadenopathy LR-0.37
- Splenomegaly in 50% (LR+1.9 to 6.6)
- Skin manifestations in 3–16%
  - Erythematous macular/maculopapular rash
  - Petechial and purpuric exanthems reported
  - Rash typically on trunk and upper arms; occasionally, the face and forearms are involved.

DIFFERENTIAL DIAGNOSIS

- Streptococcal pharyngitis and tonsillitis
- Diphtheria
- Blood dyscrasias
- Rubella, measles, viral hepatitis, cytomegalovirus
- Toxoplasmosis
- Acute HIV infection

DIAGNOSTIC TESTS & INTERPRETATION

Initial Tests (lab, imaging)

- CBC with differential
- Lymphocytes and atypical lymphocytes (2)
  - Increased numbers of lymphocytes (especially atypical lymphocytes; may be up to 70% of leukocytes) in peripheral blood
  - In 1st week after onset, WBC count is normal/moderately decreased. Due to EB-related neutrophil fragility, automated processing can result in pseudoneutropenia.
    - By week 2, atypical lymphocytosis develops.
  - During early illness, atypical lymphocytes are B cells transformed by the EBV; later, atypical cells are activated CD8 T lymphocytes.
- Antibodies
  - Heterophile antibodies in 80–90% of adults; monospot (latex agglutination) test highly specific, but sensitivity varies from 70% to 90%.
  - Heterophile antibody is an IgM response, which appears during the first 2 weeks of illness; disappears in 4 to 6 weeks (higher false negative rate in children <4 years of age).
  - In general, agglutinin titer is higher in IM than other disorders; an unabsorbed heterophile titer >1:128 and ≥1:40 is significant.

- Specific antibodies to EBV-associated antigens (2)
  - Develop regularly in IM
  - Viral capsid-specific IgM and IgG are present early in illness.
  - Viral capsid-IgM disappears after several weeks; viral capsid-IgG persists for life.
- Liver tests: Transaminitis, hyperbilirubinemia are common; jaundice is rare.
- Atypical lymphocytes are not specific for EBV infections and may be present in other clinical conditions, including rubella, infectious hepatitis, allergic rhinitis, asthma, and atypical pneumonia.
- Routine abdominal ultrasound to monitor for splenic enlargement is not necessary.
- Consider abdominal ultrasound for those wishing to return to strenuous activity/contact sports at day 21 of illness to exclude splenomegaly.

Follow-Up Tests & Special Considerations

- Abnormal hepatic enzymes persist in 80% of patients for several weeks; hepatomegaly in 15–20%
- In transplant recipients, quantitative polymerase chain reaction (PCR) used to monitor EBV loads

Diagnostic Procedures/Other

Chest x-ray

- Hilar adenopathy may be observed in IM cases with extensive lymphoid hyperplasia.
- Cardiomegaly with "water bottle" appearance suggestive of pericardia effusion (echocardiogram for confirmation) (3)

Test Interpretation

- Mononuclear infiltrations of lymph nodes, tonsils, spleen, lungs, liver, heart, kidneys, adrenal glands, skin, and CNS
- Bone marrow hyperplasia with small granuloma formation may be present; these findings are nonspecific and have no prognostic significance.

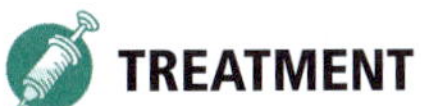

TREATMENT

- Treatment is primarily supportive.
- NSAIDs or acetaminophen
- During acute stage, limit activity for 4 weeks to reduce potential complications (e.g., splenic rupture) (2).
- Transplant recipients who develop EBV infection may require alteration of immunosuppressive therapy and administration of monoclonal anti-CD20 (rituximab).

MEDICATION

- In primary infections:
  - Antimicrobial agents (usually penicillin) only if throat culture is positive for group A β-hemolytic streptococci; incidence of rash following β-lactam antibiotic therapy previously is much lower than historically thought.
  - Warm saline gargles for oropharyngeal pain
  - Corticosteroids
    - May provide some symptomatic relief but no improvement in resolution of illness; a recent Cochrane review of seven studies provided no support for routine use.
    - Consider in severe pharyngotonsillitis with oropharyngeal edema and airway encroachment. Dexamethasone 0.3 mg/kg/day may be used for 1 to 3 days.
- Antiviral medications (acyclovir) have been found to shorten recovery time and improve subjective symptoms in acute EBV infection in small studies.

SURGERY/OTHER PROCEDURES

- Splenectomy may be necessary with profound thrombocytopenia that is refractory to corticosteroids.
- Only current effective treatment for XLP is hematopoietic stem cell transplantation. There is some use of monoclonal antibody to delay progression pre-HST or treat relapse posttransplant.
- Splenic rupture may necessitate emergent surgical intervention.

ONGOING CARE

FOLLOW-UP RECOMMENDATIONS

Patient Monitoring

- Avoid contact sports, heavy lifting, and excess exertion until spleen and liver have returned to normal size (ultrasound can verify). Current consensus is that if after 3 weeks and normal exam, no fever, and no constitutional symptoms, patients may return to contact sport activities (Guidelines suggest a shared decision-making approach with patients and family on return to play.).
- Eliminate alcohol/exposure to other hepatotoxic drugs until LFTs return to normal.
- Rates of complications are highest during the first 3 weeks of illness.
- Symptoms (malaise, fatigue, intermittent sore throat, lymphadenopathy) may persist for months.

PROGNOSIS

- Most recover in ~4 weeks.
- Fatigue may persist for months.

COMPLICATIONS

- Neurologic (rare)
  - Aseptic meningitis, meningoencephalitis
  - Bell palsy, Guillain-Barré syndrome
  - Transverse myelitis, cerebellar ataxia, acute psychosis
- Hematologic (rare)
  - Thrombocytopenia, early in illness
  - Hemolytic anemia with neutropenia (early), hemophagocytic syndrome (splenomegaly, fever, cytopenia)
  - Agammaglobulinemia
- Pneumonitis
- Airway obstruction
- Cardiovascular
  - Primarily myocarditis and pericarditis with acute EBV; CEBV can result in coronary artery lesions (dilatation and aneurysm formation) (3).
- Splenic rupture
- Transformation into a chronic state (persistent mono-like symptoms and systemic inflammation) (4)

REFERENCES

1. Yu H, Robertson ES. Epstein-Barr virus history and pathogenesis. *Viruses*. 2023;15(3):714. doi:10.3390/v15030714.
2. Leung AKC, Lam JM, Barankin B. Infectious mononucleosis: an updated review. *Curr Pediatr Rev*. 2024;20(3):305–322. doi:10.2174/1573396320666230801091558.
3. Chen X, Li Y, Deng L, et al. Cardiovascular involvement in Epstein-Barr virus infection. *Front Immunol*. 2023;14:1188330. doi:10.3389/fimmu.2023.1188330.
4. Kawada JI, Ito Y, Ohshima K, et al; for Committee for Guidelines for the Management of Chronic Active EBV Disease, Related Disorders (the MHLW Research Team in Japan). Updated guidelines for chronic active Epstein-Barr virus disease. *Int J Hematol*. 2023;118(5):568–576. doi:10.1007/s12185-023-03660-5.

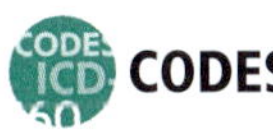

CODES

ICD10

- B27.00 Gammaherpesviral mononucleosis without complication
- B27.09 Gammaherpesviral mononucleosis with other complications
- B27.01 Gammaherpesviral mononucleosis with polyneuropathy

CLINICAL PEARLS

- 98% of patients with acute IM present with some combination of fever, sore throat, cervical node enlargement, and tonsillar hypertrophy.
- False-negative monospot (heterophile antibody) is common in the first 10 to 14 days of illness. 90% will have heterophile antibodies by week 3 of illness.
- Lymphocytosis (not monocytosis) is common in IM.
- Treatment of IM is primarily supportive.

INFERTILITY

Daniela Diaz Rubayo, MD

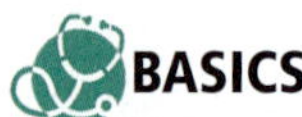

BASICS

DESCRIPTION

Definition: failure to conceive after 12 months of regular unprotected intercourse. Earlier evaluation can be considered based on medical history and physical findings. Evaluation at 6 months is warranted for women >35 years of age. More immediate evaluation is recommended in women >40 years of age. Primary infertility: Couple has never been pregnant. Secondary infertility: Couple has had at least one conception.

EPIDEMIOLOGY

Incidence

The incidence of infertility increases with age, with a decline in fertility in the early 30s, accelerating in the late 30s. ~85% of couples will conceive within 12 months of unprotected intercourse. ~95% of couples will conceive within 24 months of unprotected intercourse.

Prevalence

- Infertility affects 8.8% of U.S. women between the ages of 15 and 49 years (1).
- ~9% of couples between age 15 and 34 years, 25% between age 35 and 39 years, and ~30% between age 40 and 44 years meet the criteria for being infertile, according to the National Survey of Family Growth. This may increase as more women delay childbearing.

ETIOLOGY AND PATHOPHYSIOLOGY

- Most cases are multifactorial: Approximately 85% are due to identifiable causes such as tubal disease, ovulatory dysfunction, and male factor infertility (due to abnormal sperm production or delivery). The other 15% have unexplained causes of infertility.
- Acquired: The most common cause of infertility in the United States is pelvic inflammatory disease (PID) secondary to sexually transmitted infections (STIs), followed by endometriosis, polycystic ovary syndrome (PCOS), premature ovarian failure, and increased maternal age. ~25% of infertility diagnoses are due to ovulatory disorders (e.g., PCOS, hyperprolactinemia, hypothyroidism or hyperthyroidism, primary ovarian insufficiency, ovarian dysgenesis/agenesis, exposure to chemo or radiotherapy, eating disorder, tumors, prior surgery). 70% of women with anovulation have PCOS.
- Diminished ovarian reserve (DOR): low fertility due to insufficient quantity or functional quality of oocytes
- Congenital abnormalities: anatomic (e.g., undescended testicles, bicornuate uterus) and genetic

Genetics

There is a higher incidence of genetic abnormalities among the infertile population, including Klinefelter syndrome (47, XXY), Turner syndrome (45X or mosaic), and fragile X syndrome. Y chromosomal microdeletions are associated with isolated defects of spermatogenesis → found in 16% of men with azoospermia or severe oligospermia.

RISK FACTORS

- Female
  - Gynecologic history: irregular/abnormal menses, STIs, dysmenorrhea, fibroids
  - Medical history: advanced age, endocrinopathy, autoimmune disease, undiagnosed celiac disease, collagen vascular diseases, thrombophilia, obesity, and cancer
  - Surgical history: appendicitis, pelvic surgery, intrauterine surgery, tubal ligation
  - Social history: smoking, alcohol/substance abuse, eating disorders, exercise, advanced maternal age
- Male
  - Medical history: STI, prostatitis, medication use (i.e., β-blockers, calcium channel blockers, antiulcer medication), endocrinopathy, cancer
  - Surgical history: orchiopexy, hernia repair, vasectomy with/without reversal
  - Social: smoking, alcohol/substance abuse, anabolic steroids, environmental exposures, occupations leading to increased scrotal temperature (frequent use of saunas, hot tubs, or tight underwear), prescription drugs that impair male potency

COMMONLY ASSOCIATED CONDITIONS

Pelvic pathology, endocrine dysfunction, and anovulation (hyperandrogenism, PCOS)

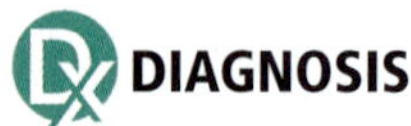

DIAGNOSIS

HISTORY

Complete reproductive history including the age of partners; history of abortion, dilation and curettage, bilateral tubal ligation, vasectomy, or other pelvic/abdominal surgery; age at menarche; regularity of menstrual cycle (i.e., every 21 to 35 days); physical development (Tanner stages), previous methods of contraception, history of abnormal Pap smears and treatment; coital frequency and timing; history of sexual dysfunction; history of STI, endocrine abnormalities, malignancy or chronic illness; family history of reproductive issues; medications: drug abuse, allergies, and exposure to environmental hazards

PHYSICAL EXAM

- Body mass index (BMI), distribution of body fat, and waist circumference
- Female
  - Signs of PCOS: androgen excess, obesity, signs of insulin resistance like acanthosis nigricans
  - Vaginal exam: Describe rugation, discharge, and anatomic variation.
  - Uterine size/shape, mobility, tenderness
- Male: Abnormalities of the penis or urethral meatus, testes: volume, symmetry, masses (varicocele, hydrocele), presence/absence of vas deferens

DIFFERENTIAL DIAGNOSIS

Kallman syndrome, idiopathic hypogonadotropic hypogonadism, luteinizing hormone (LH) deficiency, follicle-stimulating hormone (FSH) deficiency, growth hormone deficiency, hemochromatosis, endometriosis, thyroid disease, prolactinoma, obesity, PCOS

DIAGNOSTIC TESTS & INTERPRETATION

Initial Tests (lab, imaging)

Evaluation is directed by history:

- Assessment of ovulation
  - Irregular or infrequent menses
  - High LH to FSH ratio suggests PCOS.
  - Basal body temperature (BBT) charting to confirm ovulation is low cost and may be helpful for some couples to guide the timing of intercourse.
  - LH surge happens 12 to 36 hours before ovulation. Testing usually starts 2 days before expected ovulation.
  - Follicle size can guide timing of artificial insemination and intercourse.
  - Elevated progesterone level in the blood retrospectively indicates ovulation.
  - Cervical mucosal change (thin mucosa in the proliferative phase versus clear, slippery and stretchy mucosa during ovulation vs. thick mucosa in the luteal phase)
  - Endometrial biopsy (invasive procedure) is occasionally used to determine ovulation.
- Assessment of ovarian reserve
  - Women >35 years old need to have ovarian reserve assessed. On day 3 of menses, an FSH >15 to 20 IU/L and estradiol >60 pg/mL (1) is suggestive of the impaired reserve.
  - Elevated FSH and LH and low estradiol indicate ovarian insufficiency.
  - Anti-müllerian hormone (AMH) and antral follicle counts (AFCs): The number of antral follicles measured by transvaginal ultrasound (US) is termed the "antral follicle count," and a low count is defined as <4 follicles that are between 2 and 10 mm in both ovaries. AMH decreases as a woman approaches menopause. AMH can be measured at any time during the cycle and is not affected by hormones.
  - Clomiphene challenge test: After administration of clomiphene from day 5 to 9, measure FSH of ≥10 mIU/mL on day 10 to help confirm the diagnosis of DOR.
- Semen analysis is warranted in all infertile couples. Semen analysis alone is not used to predict male fertility potential.
  - Semen collection: collected after 2 to 7 days of abstinence. Repeat the test 2 to 3 times due to inherent variability within the same individual. A repeat analysis with at least a 1-month interval is required to diagnose "abnormal" semen analysis (1).
  - Parameters for normal male values: semen volume 1.5 mL or more, pH 7.2 to 7.8, sperm concentration 15 million spermatozoa per milliliter or more, total sperm number 39 million spermatozoa per ejaculate or more, motility 40% or more forward progressions, sperm morphology (percentage of normal forms) 4% or more, white blood cell count <1 million/μL
  - Additional labs
    - Prolactin, thyroid-stimulating hormone, 17-hydroxyprogesterone, androgen levels
    - HIV, herpes simplex virus 1 and 2, chlamydia, gonorrhea, rapid plasma reagin, hepatitis B and CMV
    - Genetic testing based on family history

- Transvaginal US for anatomic abnormality
- Hysterosalpingogram (HSG) to evaluate patency of tubes and contour of the cavity may be both diagnostic and therapeutic.

Follow-Up Tests & Special Considerations

Abnormal imaging may need surgical evaluation.

Diagnostic Procedures/Other

Hysteroscopy is the gold standard used to visualize the endometrial cavity directly; may be indicated to evaluate filling defects on HSG or SHG. Laparoscopy is used to directly visualize the peritoneal cavity and may be done to evaluate abnormal findings on HSG such as suspected adhesions causing fallopian tube abnormality. Laparoscopy is the only way to diagnose endometriosis definitively.

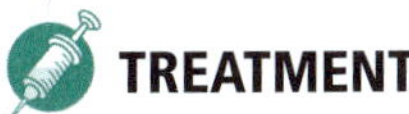

TREATMENT

GENERAL MEASURES

- Lifestyle changes that may improve fertility: achieving an ideal BMI, cessation of smoking, limiting exposure to caffeine and alcohol, coital frequency and timing (every 1–2 days around the expected ovulation period)
- BBT tracking and detection of LH surge may be helpful for some couples. BBT is not as reliable as other methods for ovulation prediction.
- Be mindful of the couple's emotional state: Depression, anger, anxiety, and marital discord are common.
- All female fertility patients should be given folate supplementation of 0.4 to 0.8 mg/day by mouth. Dietary carotenoids in males may improve sperm quality.
- In vitro fertilization (IVF) is the most effective infertility treatment available for women with unexplained infertility who have not conceived after 2 years of regular unprotected sexual intercourse:
  - Eggs are removed from the female and fertilized outside the body. The embryo is monitored for 3 to 5 days and then implanted into the uterus on day 3 or 5.
  - Anatomic causes should be referred for IVF. A surgical consult may be required.
  - Fewer complications have been reported for individuals undergoing IVF for anatomic causes rather than ovulatory dysfunction (low APGAR scores, diabetes mellitus).
  - Compared to the general population, an increased risk of preterm birth and low birth weight has also been seen among subfertile women who conceived naturally without IVF.
  - Donor eggs may be obtained.
  - Women <40 years of age or those who have not conceived after 2 years of unprotected intercourse or 12 cycles of artificial insemination should be offered three complete cycles of IVF.
  - Women aged 40 to 42 years with no evidence of previous IVF or low ovarian reserve should be offered one complete cycle of IVF.
- Intrauterine insemination (IUI) without ovarian stimulation can be considered in special circumstances: physical disabilities limiting vaginal intercourse or psychosexual issues, people in same-sex relationships, etc.
- Male factors
  - IUI: Sperm is placed via a catheter directly in the uterus. IUI effectively increases sperm count to have successful fertilization, but IUI success rate is only 7 to 10% in each cycle.
  - Intracytoplasmic sperm injection (ICSI) is performed in conjunction with IVF for males with severe abnormalities (i.e., <5 million sperm) or those who have failed to conceive with IUI. A single sperm is injected directly into the cytoplasm of the egg. Fertilization occurs ~70% of the time.
  - Donor sperm may be obtained.

MEDICATION

First Line

- Treatment of infertility depends on etiology.
- Women:
  - Anovulation: must determine if HYPOgonadotropic or NORMOgonadotropic
    - Hypogonadotropic patients: Standard treatment to induce ovulation consists of daily injections of both FSH and LH, which need to be carefully monitored to avoid ovarian hyperstimulation syndrome (OHSS).
    - Normogonadotropic patients: most commonly due to PCOS. Ovulation induction with letrozole (aromatase inhibitor) is first-line therapy and found to be superior to clomiphene for patients with PCOS (1)
    - Unexplained infertility: Controlled OHSS, as with clomiphene citrate and IUI. IVF may be recommended as the second line.
  - Coital or cervical problems: IUI
  - Endometriosis: either IVF or surgery
- Male:
  - Lifestyle changes: increasing frequency and timing of intercourse
  - Medication changes to improve sperm count, testicular function, sperm production, and quality by discontinuing or changing certain selective serotonin reuptake inhibitors, calcium channel blockers, and highly active antiretroviral therapy medications. Various studies have shown the effectiveness of clomiphene citrate in improving the sperm count.
  - Surgery: reversal of sperm blockage (e.g., vasectomy, varicocele)
  - Sperm retrieval if ejaculation is problematic.

Second Line

If clomiphene and letrozole fail to induce ovulation:

- Metformin is beneficial in anovulatory women with PCOS and glucose intolerance; start with 500 mg daily and increase to ~1,500 mg/day; monitor renal function; may take up to 3 months to be effective
- Consider oral contraceptive pills (OCPs) for ≥2 cycles and then retry clomiphene immediately after stopping OCPs.
- Cabergoline or bromocriptine is used if prolactin is elevated or if there is no withdrawal bleeding after progesterone administration. Once pregnancy has occurred, the medication can be stopped.
- Human menopausal gonadotropins (HMG) or recombinant FSH is indicated if there is resistance to clomiphene or hypogonadotropic.

ISSUES FOR REFERRAL

Reproductive endocrinology and urology; consider using surrogate pregnancy if the female cannot conceive.

SURGERY/OTHER PROCEDURES

Reproductive surgery may be necessary for those with anatomic causes of infertility. Consider treatment of varicocele and aspiration of sperm. Ovarian drilling/wedge resection in patients with PCOS for reducing ovarian androgen production.

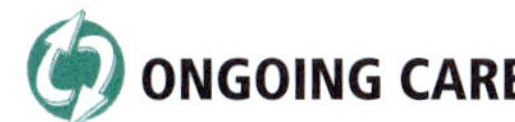

ONGOING CARE

FOLLOW-UP RECOMMENDATIONS

Specialist, if not successful after 3 to 6 cycles of oral ovulation induction

DIET

Limit caffeine and alcohol intake.

PATIENT EDUCATION

American Society for Reproductive Medicine (http://www.asrm.org); Resolve: patient advocacy group (http://www.resolve.org)

PROGNOSIS

Most couples (80–90%) will achieve a pregnancy within 12 months of attempting pregnancy with regular unprotected sexual intercourse. Fecundability progressively decreases over time.

COMPLICATIONS

Anxiety, multiple pregnancies, OHSS, and a slightly increased risk of congenital abnormalities; women diagnosed with infertility and women receiving fertility treatment are at a higher risk of maternal morbidity than are fertile women.

REFERENCES

1. Carson SA, Kallen AN. Diagnosis and management of infertility: a review. *JAMA*. 2021;326(1):65–76. doi:10.1001/jama.2021.4788.

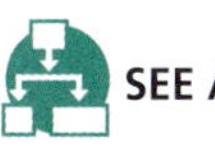

SEE ALSO

- Amenorrhea; Endometriosis; Metabolic Syndrome; Polycystic Ovarian Syndrome (PCOS); Pelvic Inflammatory Disease
- Algorithm: Infertility

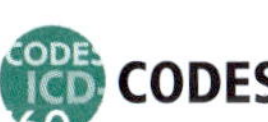

CODES

ICD10

- N97.9 Female infertility, unspecified
- N46.9 Male infertility, unspecified
- N97.1 Female infertility of tubal origin

CLINICAL PEARLS

Infertility is often multifactorial.

I

INFLUENZA

Susan McDiarmid, EdD, MS, PA-C • Michelle E. Duffelmeyer, MD

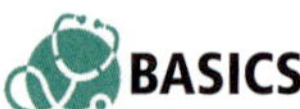

BASICS

DESCRIPTION

Acute, typically self-limited, febrile infection caused by orthomyxovirus influenza types A and B marked by inflammation of nasal mucosa, pharynx, conjunctiva, and respiratory tract

EPIDEMIOLOGY

- Outbreaks of influenza occur annually during the fall–winter months in the Northern and Southern Hemispheres.
- Influenza virus can undergo antigenic shift (abrupt change) leading to viral strains with little immunologic resistance in a population, resulting in pandemic outbreaks. Minor seasonal variations are called *antigenic drift*.
- Persons of all ages are susceptible to infection. Higher concern for:
  - Those <2 and >65 years of age
  - Immunocompromised states, including pregnancy and up to 2 weeks postpartum
  - Individuals with cardiovascular or pulmonary disease, Addison disease, or diabetes
  - Residents of nursing homes or other long-term care facilities

Incidence

Incidence is difficult to ascertain as most individuals do not seek medical care and are therefore not diagnosed.

Prevalence

Preliminary data for the United States 2024 to 2025 season reveals an estimated 47 to 82 million influenza cases requiring 21 to 37 million medical visits, 610,000 to 1.3 million hospitalizations, and 27,000 to 130,000 deaths, which is trending higher than the 2023 to 2024 season. Predominant strains include influenza A (H1N1 and H1N2). Final end of season estimates will be available in November 2025.

ETIOLOGY AND PATHOPHYSIOLOGY

Orthomyxovirus (influenza types A [majority] and B); influenza A virus subtypes HxNx based on hemagglutinin and neuraminidase

- Incubation is 1 to 4 days; infected persons are most contagious during peak symptoms. Spread by aerosolized droplets or contact with respiratory secretions, hemagglutinin binds to columnar respiratory epithelium where replication occurs, and neuraminidase protein facilitates spread along respiratory epithelium (1).

RISK FACTORS

- For contracting disease:
  - Crowded environments such as nursing homes, barracks, schools, and correctional facilities
- For complications:
  - Neonates, infants, elderly; pregnancy (including 2 weeks postpartum) especially in 3rd trimester
  - Chronic pulmonary diseases; cardiovascular diseases, including valvular pathology and congestive heart failure
  - Metabolic disease, morbid obesity; hemoglobinopathies; malignancy
  - Immunosuppression; neuromuscular diseases that limit respiratory function and ability to handle secretions

GENERAL PREVENTION

- All persons ≥6 months should be vaccinated annually unless contraindicated.
- Live attenuated influenza vaccine (LAIV) is a quadrivalent intranasal vaccine approved for healthy, nonpregnant individuals between 2 and 49 years of age.
- Inactivated influenza vaccine (IIV) is available either as trivalent (IIV3) or quadrivalent (IIV4) with either three or four strains of influenza. IIV also is available as high-dose, intradermal, cell culture–based (ccIV3), MF59-adjuvanted (aIIV3), and recombinant hemagglutinin vaccine (RIV3).
- IIV is recommended annually for all persons aged ≥6 months. Protection occurs 1 to 2 weeks after immunization. Mild side effects include low-grade fever and local reaction at the vaccination site. Inactivated IM dose: ≥3 years of age: 0.5 mL; children 6 to 35 months of age: 0.25 mL Intradermal formulation for 18- to 64-year-olds uses a short 30-gauge needle in a single-use prefilled syringe with 0.1 mL vaccine; somewhat higher local reactions when given intradermal; single annual dose except for children <9 years of age, who should receive 2 doses (4 weeks apart) the 1st year they receive influenza vaccine
- Vaccine contraindication: Severe allergy such as anaphylaxis to IIV components, allergies from eggs are not considered a contraindication; observe all patients for 15 minutes after vaccination; no skin testing with influenza vaccine is needed in egg-allergic patients. RIV is safe in patients with an egg allergy.
- IIV-HD: High-dose quadrivalent IIV contains 4 times the antigen concentration of IIV. Licensed for persons ≥65 years of age. Results in higher antibody levels but somewhat higher rates of local reactions. Advisory Committee on Immunization Practices does not express a preference for/against IIV-HD.
- Antiviral prophylaxis depends on current resistance patterns each year; see https://www.cdc.gov/flu/ for patterns or check with local health department.
- Prophylaxis is not a substitute for vaccination but consider in high-risk groups that have not been vaccinated or need additional control measures during epidemics. Consider in staff and residents in nursing home outbreaks, immune-deficient persons who are expected not to respond to immunization after viral exposure.

Pediatric Considerations

Vaccinate children aged ≥6 months annually. Recommend all household members with children aged <6 months be vaccinated. For children who need 2 doses, administer first dose as soon as available, second dose to be given before the end of October. For prophylaxis, oseltamivir dosage varies by weight and is recommended by the CDC for prophylaxis for children aged ≥3 months; zanamivir is approved for prophylaxis for children ≥5 years of age at a dosage of 2 inhalations per day. Prophylaxis treatment duration is 7 days.

Pregnancy Considerations

- The CDC recommends vaccinating all women who will be pregnant during influenza season. If unvaccinated at the time of flu season, pregnant women should receive IIV or RIV.
- Oseltamivir, zanamivir, peramivir, rimantadine, and amantadine are pregnancy Category C. Baloxavir not recommended in pregnant patients due to lack of data.

COMMONLY ASSOCIATED CONDITIONS

Pneumonia, cardiac complications, central nervous system involvement, myositis, rhabdomyolysis, multisystem organ failure

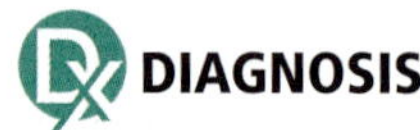

DIAGNOSIS

HISTORY

Sudden onset of:

- Fever (37.7 to 40.0°C), especially within 3 days of illness onset
- Anorexia; chills, sweats, malaise, myalgia, arthralgia
- Headache; sore throat/pharyngitis
- Nonproductive cough; rhinorrhea, nasal congestion
- Gastrointestinal symptoms of nausea, vomiting, and diarrhea (occur in up to 20% of children)
- Altered mental status (especially in the elderly or immunosuppressed)

PHYSICAL EXAM

- Physical exam is not specific for influenza.
- Exclude complications (otitis media, pneumonia, pharyngitis, sinusitis, and tracheobronchitis)

DIFFERENTIAL DIAGNOSIS

- Respiratory viral infections including, SARS-CoV-2, respiratory syncytial virus, parainfluenza, adenovirus, enterovirus ("influenza-like illness")
- Infectious mononucleosis; coxsackievirus infections; viral/streptococcal tonsillitis
- Atypical mycoplasmal pneumonia; *Chlamydia pneumoniae*; Q fever
- Less likely possibilities include severe acute respiratory syndrome, primary HIV infection, acute myeloid leukemia, tuberculosis, anthrax, and malaria.

DIAGNOSTIC TESTS & INTERPRETATION

Initial Tests (lab, imaging)

During influenza season, decision to pursue diagnostic testing is based on clinical findings; various testing modalities:

- Antigen detection; rapid influenza diagnostic tests (RIDTs); outpatient office based testing detects viral antigens within 10 to 15 minutes; moderate sensitivity (80%), high specificity
- Molecular assay
  - Reverse transcription polymerase chain reaction (RT-PCR); high sensitivity (90–95%) and specificity
- Immunofluorescence
  - Commercial rapid enzyme-linked immunosorbent assay antigen tests are available. Some rapid tests diagnose influenza A, whereas others diagnose A and B. Sensitivity and specificity vary by manufacturer, strain of influenza, and age of patient. False-negative results are common, particularly during peak influenza activity.

Follow-Up Tests & Special Considerations

The influenza severity scale stratifies patients into low, medium, and high risk based on 10 variables: age, sex, smoking status, chronic pulmonary disease, diabetes mellitus, influenza vaccination status, cough, sputum production, shortness of breath, and need for regular support for activities of daily living.

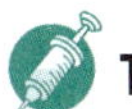

TREATMENT

- Symptomatic treatment (saline nasal spray, analgesic gargle, antipyretics, analgesics, expectorants, suppressants)
- Cool-mist or ultrasonic humidifier to increase moisture of inspired air
- Counsel on droplet precautions: wearing a disposable surgical mask around others. 5 days is the average period of viral shedding in immunocompetent hosts. Hospitalized patients may require oxygen or ventilatory support.
- Tobacco cessation

MEDICATION

- Antiviral treatment depends on yearly resistance patterns; check https://www.cdc.gov/flu/ or with local health department. Antivirals are most effective if administered within first 48 hours. Antivirals are recommended for patients at risk of complications (i.e., diabetes, CHD, COPD, asthma, etc.) or were hospitalized.
- Antivirals include baloxavir, oseltamivir, zanamivir, and peramivir. Amantadine *and* rimantadine are currently *not recommended due to resistance*. IV zanamivir is no longer available.
- Consider antivirals for patients whose onset of symptoms is within the past 48 hours and who wish to shorten the duration of illness and further reduce their relatively low risk of complications.
- Symptomatic treatment is preferred for those patients *without risk factors* and *without* signs of lower respiratory tract infection.
- Antiviral effect is 24-hour reduction of symptoms and a reduction in complication rates.
  - Baloxavir dose: oral, 1-time dose
    - 40 to <80 kg, 40 mg; >80 kg, 80 mg; for children aged >12 years, use adult dosing.
    - Children aged ≥5 years and adolescence <20 kg: oral suspension: oral: 2 mg/kg once as a single dose
    - Contraindicated in severe infection, immunocompromised, and pregnant patients
    - Similar reduction in symptoms as oseltamivir but greater reduction in viral shedding and superior for influenza B (2)
  - Zanamivir dose: 2 inhalations BID for 5 days (age ≥7 years)
    - Contraindicated in patients with asthma, COPD, and patients with severe infection
  - Oseltamivir dose: 75 mg PO BID for 5 days (age ≥13 years)
  - Oseltamivir for children ≥1 year of age
    - <15 kg, 30 mg BID; >15 to 23 kg, 45 mg BID; >23 to 40 kg, 60 mg BID; >40 kg, 75 mg BID
  - Oseltamivir for children <1 year of age: 3 mg/kg/dose BID
  - Peramivir dose: 600 mg IV infusion over 15 to 30 minutes for adults ≥18 years of age
- Antipyretics
  - Acetaminophen: in children
- Precautions
  - Zanamivir bronchospasm if the patient has COPD or asthma; have a bronchodilator available
  - Amantadine has anticholinergic properties.
  - Rimantadine may increase the risk of seizures in those with an underlying seizure disorder.
  - Oseltamivir may cause nausea and vomiting; may be less severe if taken with food
  - Peramivir may cause serious skin reactions.
  - Baloxavir may cause diarrhea and hypersensitivity reactions.
- Adjust dose of antivirals if creatinine clearance <60 mL/min.
- Ibuprofen or other NSAIDs for symptomatic relief; aspirin: should not be used in children aged <16 years due to risk of Reye syndrome; outpatient treatment except for cases with severe complications or in high-risk groups

ADMISSION, INPATIENT, AND NURSING CONSIDERATIONS

- Initiate droplet precautions for confirmed or suspected influenza.
- Initiate prompt antiviral therapy for patients hospitalized with influenza related illness, regardless of prior duration of symptoms.

ONGOING CARE

FOLLOW-UP RECOMMENDATIONS

Mild cases: follow-up typically not required; moderate/severe: Follow up until symptoms and secondary sequelae resolve.

PROGNOSIS

Good

COMPLICATIONS

- Sepsis; pneumonia (primary viral or secondary bacterial)
- Apnea in neonates; Reye syndrome

Geriatric Considerations

Complications requiring hospitalization are more likely in elderly patients.

REFERENCES

1. Sriwilaijaroen N, Vavricka CJ, Kiyota H, et al. Influenza A virus neuraminidase inhibitors. *Methods Mol Biol*. 2022;2556:321–353. doi:10.1007/978-1-0716-2635-1_21.
2. Committee on Infectious Diseases. Recommendations for prevention and control of influenza in children, 2024–2025: policy statement. *Pediatrics*. 2024;154(4):e2024068507. doi:10.1542/peds.2024-068507.

ADDITIONAL READING

Centers for Disease Control and Prevention. Preliminary Estimated Flu Disease Burden 2024-2025 Flu Season. https://www.cdc.gov/flu-burden/php/data-vis/2024-2025.html. Accessed October 12, 2025.

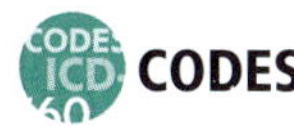

CODES

ICD10

- J10.08 Influenza due to other identified influenza virus with other specified pneumonia
- J11.89 Influenza due to unidentified influenza virus with other manifestations
- J10.81 Influenza due to other identified influenza virus with encephalopathy

CLINICAL PEARLS

- Influenza is an acute, (typically) self-limited, febrile infection caused by influenza virus types A and B.
- All persons aged >6 months should be vaccinated against influenza on an annual basis (there are rare exceptions).
- Recommend concurrent administration of pneumonia vaccine if indicated per CDC guidelines.
- Complications from influenza are most common in the very young, very old, and individuals with comorbid disease.
- Hand hygiene either with soap and water (slightly superior) or with alcohol-based hand rubs and covering coughs are simple ways to reduce the spread of influenza.

INGROWN TOENAIL

Daniel Scott Morrison, MD • Chirag N. Shah, MD

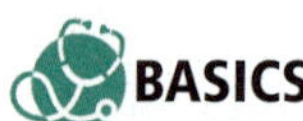

BASICS

DESCRIPTION

- In an ingrown toenail, the distal margin of the nail plate grows into the lateral nail fold, causing irritation, inflammation, and sometimes bacterial or fungal infection:
  - Stage 1 (inflammation): erythema, edema, tenderness of lateral nail fold
  - Stage 2 (abscess): granuloma (inflamed tissue) at edges, drainage (serous or purulent)
  - Stage 3 (chronic inflammation): chronic inflammation with continued purulence with granulation tissue growing over the nail plate and significant nail fold hypertrophy
- Can reoccur
- Synonym(s): onychocryptosis, unguis incarnatus

EPIDEMIOLOGY

- Great toenail is most often affected.
- Lateral edge of nail is affected about twice as much as the medial edge.
- Most common in males aged 14 to 25 years
- Infrequent, but more often in elderly females than in elderly males
- More common in those with lower incomes

Prevalence

- 2.5–5.0% of total population
- 5% of population aged >65 years
- 2:1 male-to-female ratio

ETIOLOGY AND PATHOPHYSIOLOGY

- Nail plate penetrates the nail fold, causing a foreign body reaction (inflammation).
- Bacteria or fungi may enter through the opening in the nail fold, causing infection and abscess formation.
- The inflamed and infected area leads to granulation tissue and hypertrophy of the nail fold.

RISK FACTORS

- Genetic factors
  - Increased nail fold width
  - Decreased nail thickness
  - Medial rotation of the toe
- Factors that may increase risk:
  - Distorted, thickened nail (onychogryphosis)
  - Fungal infection (onychomycosis)
  - Hyperhidrosis
  - Obesity
  - Improper trimming of the lateral nail plate
  - Poorly fitting shoes
  - Trauma to nail or nail fold
  - Conditions that predispose to pedal edema (i.e., thyroid dysfunction, diabetes, obesity, heart failure, renal disease)

GENERAL PREVENTION

- Properly fitting shoes
- Proper nail trimming (see "Patient Education")

DIAGNOSIS

HISTORY

- Patients most often present with pain, redness, and swelling in the toe along edge(s) of nail.
- Drainage can occur as inflammation and/or infection develop.

PHYSICAL EXAM

- Nail fold tenderness
- Erythema and edema
- Drainage (serous or purulent)
- Granulation tissue
- Lateral nail fold hypertrophy

DIFFERENTIAL DIAGNOSIS

- Cellulitis
- Felon (pulp abscess on plantar aspect of toe)
- Onychogryphosis (gross thickening and hardening of the nail)
- Onycholysis (separation of nail from nail bed)
- Onychomycosis (fungal infection of the nail)
- Osteomyelitis
- Paronychia (infection or inflammation around the nail fold)
- Subungual exostosis (bony projection from distal phalanx)
- Subungual osteochondroma (benign bone tumor)

DIAGNOSTIC TESTS & INTERPRETATION

Initial Tests (lab, imaging)

None usually needed

- Consider x-ray, MRI, or bone scan if osteomyelitis is suspected.
- Consider x-ray if subungual exostosis or osteochondroma is suspected.

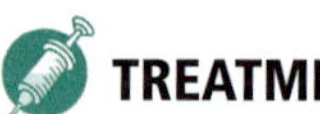

TREATMENT

GENERAL MEASURES

- Majority of mild cases (stage 1) respond well to conservative therapy.
- Soaking the toe (1)[C]
- Bluntly insert a cotton wisp or dental floss underneath the ingrown portion of the nail (1)[C].
- Splint to separate nail edge from lateral fold; can also make a cotton nail case from cotton and cyanoacrylate adhesive, tape the lateral nail fold, or use a brace or wire to lift the edge of the nail (1)[C]
- Stage 2 ingrown nails without significant pain or erythema often respond to conservative treatment, as above, especially cotton wool, or a trial of cryotherapy.

MEDICATION

- NSAIDs are usually adequate for analgesia.
- Topical antibiotic can be applied after soaking.
- Oral antibiotics are not useful as an adjunct to surgical treatment (2)[B].

SURGERY/OTHER PROCEDURES

- No favorable effect was observed between chemical or surgical versus conservative management (3)[A].
- Nail avulsion techniques include:
  - Partial avulsion of the nail with phenol nail matrix ablation may reduce the risk of recurrence versus just nail avulsion alone (3)[A].
    - Obtain surgical consent after explaining the risks, benefits, and alternatives.
    - Achieve local anesthesia with a digital wing or ring block.
    - May consider placing a tourniquet around the base of the toe to assist with hemostasis (caution in patients with diabetes or peripheral vascular disease)
    - Elevate the ingrown part of the nail from the nail bed with a periosteal (Freer) elevator or hemostat.
    - Incise the nail longitudinally with scissors or a nail splitter a few millimeters from the ingrown border, starting at the distal edge and proceeding to the matrix.
    - Grasp, down to the cuticle, the avulsed fragment with a hemostat, and pull this portion gently out with a hemostat, using longitudinal traction, as well as rotation to the lateral nail fold if needed.
    - Remove the tourniquet once hemostasis is attained.
    - Dip a swab in 80–88% phenol solution (phenol use is contraindicated in pregnancy).
    - Apply the phenol for 30 to 60 seconds to the nail matrix under the proximal nail fold. Wash the area with 70% isopropyl (rubbing) alcohol to neutralize phenol.
- Nonsurgical interventions, such as a flexible gutter splint, are another option for treatment of stage 2 or 3 ingrown nails (1)[A].
  - J flexible gutter splint
    - Cut a 1- to 2-cm long piece of sterilized plastic tube, such as IV tubing, 2 to 3 mm in diameter (alternatively, you may use a cap from a 29-gauge needle).
    - Make a slit in the tubing lengthwise and cut the end off at an angle.
    - Apply local anesthesia with a digital wing or ring block.
    - Release the ingrown edge of the nail from the nail fold with a hemostat.

  - Slide the tube, angled end first, along the ingrown edge of the nail.
  - Consider fixing the tube in place with self-curing formable acrylic resin (used for dentures and sculptured nails), tape, or a single suture through the nail plate.
  - Leave the tube in place until nail has grown beyond the nail fold.
- Bilateral partial matricectomy should be considered in patients with severe ingrown toenail or recurrence.
- Permanent destruction of the germinal matrix can be used to prevent recurrence. The use of phenol for nail bed ablation is probably more effective than nail avulsion alone in preventing recurrence (3)[A].
  - Other options for nail bed ablation:
    - Sodium hydroxide (NaOH)
    - Cryotherapy
    - Electrocautery with a special flattened tip coated with Teflon on one side to protect the proximal nail fold
    - Carbon dioxide laser
    - Surgical excision of the nail matrix

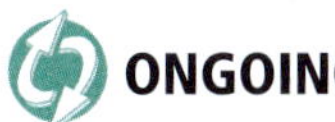

ONGOING CARE

FOLLOW-UP RECOMMENDATIONS

- Dress with antibiotic ointment or sterile petroleum jelly; cover with sterile gauze and tube gauze.
- Postop instructions should include the following:
  - Rest and elevate the foot for 12 to 24 hours.
  - Take NSAIDs for discomfort.
  - Change dressing and wash with soap and water at least daily for 1 to 2 weeks following the procedure.
  - Expect a sterile exudate for 2 to 6 weeks.
  - Avulsed nails may take 6 to 12 months to grow completely out (if no matrix ablation).
  - Call for increasing pain, redness, or swelling.
  - Average time to return to normal activities is 2 weeks.
- Patients treated conservatively should be followed up in the office every 7 to 10 days until marked improvement is noted.

PATIENT EDUCATION

- Trim nails straight across perpendicular to long axis of the nail (do not round corners) and not too short.
- Wear properly fitting, comfortable shoes.

COMPLICATIONS

- Cellulitis after surgical procedure (uncommon)
- Damage to fascia or periosteum from overly aggressive matrix ablation
- Damage to nail bed
- Distal toe ischemia due to prolonged use of a tourniquet during surgery (rare)
- Nail plate deformity (due to nail matrix damage)
- Osteomyelitis (rare)
- Permanent narrowing of nail (if partial matrix ablation is performed)
- Persistent postoperative wound drainage particularly with excessive phenolization of adjacent tissues
- Recurrence (40–80% with avulsion alone, 0.6–14% with matrix ablation, 6–13% with gutter splint)

REFERENCES

1. Huang S, Wang J, Chen Z, et al. Surgical interventions for ingrown toenail. *Foot Ankle Surg*. 2024;30(3):181–190. doi:10.1016/j.fas.2023.12.003.
2. Sargin S, Gulcu A, Aslan A. Does the type of surgical technique and the use of prophylactic antibiotics affect the clinical results in symptomatic ingrown toenail patients? *Int J Low Extrem Wounds*. 2024;23(1):124–132. doi:10.1177/15347346211043602.
3. Exley V, Jones K, O'Carroll G, et al. A systematic review and meta-analysis of randomised controlled trials on surgical treatments for ingrown toenails part I: recurrence and relief of symptoms. *J Foot Ankle Res*. 2023;16(1):35. doi:10.1186/s13047-023-00631-1.

ADDITIONAL READING

- Bryant A, Knox A. Ingrown toenails: the role of the GP. *Aust Fam Physician*. 2015;44(3):102–105.
- Eekhof JAH, Van Wijk B, Knuistingh Neven A, et al. Interventions for ingrowing toenails. *Cochrane Database Syst Rev*. 2012;2012(4):CD001541. doi:10.1002/14651858.CD001541.pub3.
- Mayeaux EJ Jr, Carter C, Murphy TE. Ingrown toenail management. *Am Fam Physician*. 2019;100(3):158–164.
- Thakur V, Vinay K, Haneke E. Onychocryptosis—decrypting the controversies. *Int J Dermatol*. 2020;59(6):656–669. doi:10.1111/ijd.14769.

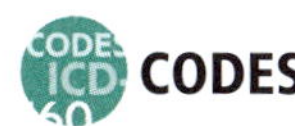

CODES

ICD10

L60.0 Ingrowing nail

CLINICAL PEARLS

- Nonsurgical interventions are appropriate for patients with stage 1 and mild stage 2 ingrown toenails.
- The most common surgical intervention for treatment of an ingrown toenail is partial nail avulsion with phenol matrix ablation.
- Patients can prevent ingrown toenails by trimming nails properly and wearing properly fitting shoes.
- Oral and topical antibiotics are not useful in the treatment of ingrown nails in conjunction with surgical treatment.

I

INJURY AND VIOLENCE

Emily Ann Gorman, DO • Naomi Kasturiarachi, DO

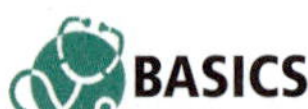

BASICS

DESCRIPTION

- Injury, intentional or not, is often predictable and preventable. Unintentional injuries are no longer considered "accidents" given that most injuries are preventable.
- As of 2020, unintentional injury is the 4th leading cause of death in the United States. Injury is the leading cause of death for people aged 1 to 44 years, accounting for some 80,000 deaths in 2020. It is also a leading cause of disability for people of all ages, regardless of sex, race/ethnicity, or socioeconomic status. Violence-related deaths accounted for >58,000 deaths in the United States in 2020 (>36,000 suicides and >21,000 homicides).

EPIDEMIOLOGY

Incidence

- Children mostly die of unintentional injuries: motor vehicle traffic (MVT), drowning, poisoning, and suffocation.
- MVT is the most common type of unintentional injury deaths in adolescents.

ALERT

Poisoning, which includes drug overdose, has been the leading cause of injury deaths in the United States overall since 2011 and is particularly deadly for persons ages 15 to 64 years, as the leading cause of injury deaths among ages 25 to 64 years and the second leading cause of unintentional injury deaths for ages 15 to 24 years.

- Approximately 4.4 million people worldwide die yearly from injuries, of which all forms of violence combine to cause nearly 1/3 of these deaths (World Health Organization [WHO]).
- Unintentional MVT deaths rank third in the United States for overall injury deaths, first in those aged 5 to 24 years and third in those aged 1 to 4 years and aged 25 to >65 years.
- Among leading causes of injury deaths in the United States, unintentional falls rank third overall. Firearms are related to the fourth and fifth leading causes of injury deaths in the United States, suicide and homicide, respectively.
- Homicide is the second leading cause of death in 2020 for persons aged 15 to 24 years in the United States.

ALERT

Consider homicide as cause of unexplained death in young children.

ETIOLOGY AND PATHOPHYSIOLOGY

Multifactorial

RISK FACTORS

- Motor vehicle accident (MVA):
  - MVT deaths accounted for 40,698 deaths in 2020 with an age-adjusted rate of 11.9 deaths per 100,000 persons (CDC). Each year, approximately 3 million people are nonfatally injured in the United States from motor vehicle crashes (CDC). The leading cause of death for U.S. teens is MVAs (CDC). In the United States, 1 in 3 deaths involved drunk driving and almost 1 in 3 deaths implicated speeding (CDC).
  - Motorcyclists are more likely to die in a motor vehicle crash than car occupants. The risk of death is reduced by 37% with helmets (CDC).
  - Risk factors for involvement in an MVA include high speed, teenage drivers, consumption of alcohol or drugs affecting the central nervous system, fatigue, and distracted driving (handheld mobile phones and inadequate visibility).
  - Increased risk of death by MVA in the United States: not using seat belts, car seats, and booster seats; drunk driving; speeding (CDC)
- Pedestrians:
  - >7,000 pedestrians were killed by motor vehicles and an estimated 104,000 were treated in EDs for nonfatal injuries in the United States (2020; CDC, National Center for Injury Prevention and Control [NCIPC]).
- Bicycles:
  - In the United States, >800 bicyclists died and nearly 357,000 bicycle-related injuries occurred in 2020 (CDC, NCIPC).
  - Risk factors for cyclist injury include age (5 to 19 years for nonfatal injury, 50 to 59 years highest bicycle death rates), male sex, urban area at nonintersection location, and alcohol involvement.
- Sports- and recreation-related injury (CDC):
  - >2.6 million children (0 to 19 years old) treated in EDs each year
  - Prevention tips include: Use protective gear that is in good condition, fits properly, and worn correctly; sports program and/or school has instituted action plan to teach athletes ways to lower risk of getting a concussion and other injuries; monitor temperature to prevent heat-related injuries; and serve as a role model of safe behavior.
- Drowning: a leading cause of unintentional injury death among all children, particularly those 1 to 4 years of age
  - Children at increased risk include African Americans and those unattended in bathtubs, swimming pools, and recreational water activities (CDC, NCIPC).
- Suffocation: increased risk for children aged <1 year, unsafe sleeping environments (CDC)
- Falls (CDC, NCIPC):
  - The leading cause of nonfatal injuries accounting for >6.5 million nonfatal injuries in the United States in 2020
  - Most common cause of traumatic brain injuries (TBIs)
  - Risk factors for falls include lower body weakness, vitamin D deficiency, difficulties with walking and balance, use of medications (tranquilizers, sedatives, antidepressants, some over-the-counter medicines), vision problems, foot pain or poor footwear, home hazards (broken/uneven steps, throw rugs, clutter).
- **Violence**: Risk factors include adverse childhood exposures (ACEs); lack of access to social, capital, community organization, and economic resources; familial instability; community and family violence; access to firearms; mental health; personal or household member alcohol and drug use; exposure to suicidal behavior; history of aggressive behavior; cognitive deficits; poor supervision; poor peer-to-peer interaction; academic failure; poverty; and lower socioeconomic class (CDC).
- Homicide and gun violence: Homicide is the second leading cause of death for persons aged 15 to 34 years in the United States (CDC). Most common victims are young males. Firearms are used in more than half of U.S. homicides.
- Suicide: Females are more likely to have suicidal thoughts, but males are 4 times more likely to complete suicide. Most common methods are firearms for males and poisoning for females (CDC, NCIPC).
- Adolescent violence (CDC):
  - In 2019, nearly 8% of students participated in a physical fight at school in the last year.
  - >9% of high schoolers reported not going to school on ≥1 day(s) in the last 30 days because they felt unsafe at school or on their way to or from school.
  - 4% of students have carried a weapon to school; >7% of students have been threatened or injured by a weapon at school.
- Bullying (CDC):
  - In 2020, 20% of students report being bullied on school property in the last year.
  - >15% of students report cyberbullying.
  - Bullying is associated with social, emotional, and academic difficulties.
- Interpersonal and intimate partner violence (IPV):
  - WHO reports about 38% of female homicides globally were killed by male partners, similar to CDC reports of nearly half of female homicide victims in the United States are killed by a current or former male intimate partner.
  - Approximately 1 in 4 women and almost 1 in 10 men have experienced sexual violence, physical violence, and/or stalking in their lifetime from an intimate partner (CDC).
  - Dating violence among teens:
    - Almost 1 in 11 female and approximately 1 in 15 male high school students report physical dating violence in the last year (CDC).
    - Approximately 1 in 9 female and 1 in 36 male high school students report sexual dating violence in the last year (CDC).
  - Risk factors include individual risk factors (such as low income, young age, heavy alcohol and drug use, depression and suicide attempts, unemployment, being a victim of physical or psychological abuse, witnessing IPV between parents as child, unplanned pregnancy), relationship factors (such as marital conflict, economic stress, association with antisocial and aggressive peers), community factors (such as poverty, low social capital), and societal factors (such as traditional gender norms or gender inequality, societal income inequality).
  - Protective factors include high friendship quality, social support, neighborhood collective efficacy (community cohesiveness, mutual trust, willingness to intervene for the common good), coordination of resources, and services among community agencies.

ALERT

Poisonings (CDC):

- The U.S. epidemic of drug overdoses (poisonings) includes >898,000 deaths from 2001 to 2020 from an overdose involving any opioid (prescription and illicit).
- In 2021, >107,500 drug overdose deaths occurred in the United States.

- Opioids, primarily synthetic fentanyl and fentanyl derivatives, are the main cause of drug overdose deaths. In 2021, opioids were involved in 75% of all drug overdose deaths; two out of three opioid-involved overdose deaths involved synthetic opioids.
- Preventive measures of opioid deaths include improve opioid prescribing, reduce exposure to opioids, prevent misuse, and access to naloxone and treat opioid use disorder.

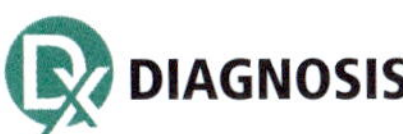

DIAGNOSIS

HISTORY

- Mechanism, timing, and location of injury:
  - Blunt versus penetrating; intentional versus unintentional; others injured versus isolated injury; circumstances (weather, substance use, restrained vs. unrestrained)
  - Does history correlate with level of injury (i.e., level of suspicion for abuse [elderly, child, or partner])?
  - Is further evaluation required (blood and/or urine testing, response to opioid receptor antagonists, imaging)?
- IPV: neurologic deficits, seizures, chronic pain, GI, STI, pregnancy, psychiatric presentations
  - Screen women of childbearing age for IPV and intervene if screening results are positive.

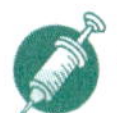

TREATMENT

- Prevention: The primary focus for reducing injury and violence is individually tailored prevention based on risk factors combined with population-level prevention (1).
- Primary (i.e., prevent crash), secondary (i.e., prevent injury from crash), and tertiary (i.e., prevent poor outcomes from injury) prevention (1)[C]
- Motor vehicle injuries (CDC) (2):
  - Infants, toddlers, and children: age-appropriate child safety seats and passenger restraints with distribution programs, education programs for parents and caregivers, safety seat checkpoints, penalties for drivers transporting children under the influence of drugs and/or alcohol, legislation regarding restraint of motor vehicle occupants
  - Adolescents and adults: seat belts, airbags, graduated driver licensing programs, blood alcohol concentration laws, minimum drinking age laws, sobriety checkpoints, ignition interlocks, programs for alcohol servers, zero-alcohol tolerance laws for young drivers, school-based education programs on drinking and driving; emergency medical services (EMS) response times, engineering cars for rapid extraction, organized trauma systems; collapsible automobile steering columns have been shown to decrease injury mortality and morbidity; texting and driving penalties
  - Older adults: alternative transportation programs, screening for high-risk drivers, gradual curtailment of driving privileges, more frequent license renewal process
  - Bicycle helmets can reduce risk of head injury by 63–88%. Canadian helmet legislation decreased mortality by 52%.
  - Pedestrian injury: pedestrian safety education, reflective clothing, use of crosswalks, limit mobile phone use while crossing roads, street lighting for pedestrians, fluorescent clothing for pedestrians and cyclists
  - Cyclists injury: flashing lights and reflectors at night (1)[B], helmet use and laws, cyclists separation for motor vehicles
- Sports-related injuries: proper equipment: Helmets can prevent bicyclist head injuries and mortality; plan of action for dealing with concussion and head injury in young athletes, with guidelines regarding if or when it is safe to return to play (CDC)
- Drowning: Improved supervision of young children, especially for those with epilepsy; swimming lessons; trained lifeguard supervision; fencing; locked gates and pool alarms; no use of alcohol in recreation aquatic activities; personal flotation devices and boating safety awareness; parental and caregiver certification in CPR
- Falls:
  - Home safety assessments, installation of handrails and grab bars, removal of tripping hazards, nonslip mats, exercise programs such as tai chi to improve strength and balance, night lights, cataract surgery, gradual withdrawal of psychotropic medication
  - In 2018, United States Preventive Services Task Force (USPSTF) recommends exercise interventions to prevent falls in community-dwelling adults aged ≥65 years who are at increased risk for falls.
- Violence (homicide, suicide, assaults) (CDC):
  - Primary prevention: Most effective strategies focus on younger age groups to change individual attitudes and behaviors.
  - Secondary prevention: Detect and identify violence in early stages. The USPSTF recommends that clinicians screen women of childbearing age for IPV, such as domestic violence, and provide or refer women who screen positive to intervention services.
  - Gun and school violence prevention among youth: social and emotional learning via CDC Whole School, Whole Community, Whole Child Model (CDC)
  - Tertiary prevention: IPV reduced by alcoholism treatment for partner; intense advocacy interventions of >12 hours.
  - Suicide: access to mental health services, improved family and community support, development of healthy coping and problem-solving skills, reduced access to lethal means (CDC)
  - USPSTF recommends screening adults for depression when depression care supports are in place to assure accurate diagnosis, effective treatment, and follow-up.

ALERT

Poisonings (CDC): In response to the opioid epidemic, the *CDC Guideline for Prescribing Opioids for Chronic Pain—United States, March 2016* was released to **improve prescribing practices**, to aid in early identification of those at high risk for addiction, and to prevent opiate and heroin addiction and deaths.

- Prevent and treat opioid abuse: prescribing practice quality improvement programs; substance abuse counseling and medication for the treatment of opioid use disorders (MOUD) such as buprenorphine and methadone
- In April 2018, the U.S. Surgeon General issued an advisory emphasizing the importance of the overdose-reversing drug naloxone. *Consider use of* naloxone *to counter the effects of opioid overdose. Multiple doses of* naloxone *may be required because the duration of many opioids is greater than that of* naloxone.
- Follow acute care guidelines and call 911; may contact Poison Control Center hotline after discovered ingestion of toxin for recommendations (3)

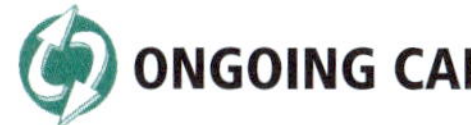

ONGOING CARE

COMPLICATIONS

Social burden of injury: loss of productivity, emotional loss, nonmedical expenditures, reduced quality of life, litigation, rehabilitation, mental health costs, altered family and peer relationships, chronic pain, substance use and abuse, changes in lifestyle (CDC)

REFERENCES

1. Sleet DA, Dahlberg LL, Basavaraju SV, et al; for Centers for Disease Control and Prevention (CDC). Injury prevention, violence prevention, and trauma care: building the scientific base. *MMWR Suppl*. 2011;60(4):78–85.
2. National Center for Injury Prevention and Control: https://www.cdc.gov/injury. Accessed 11/21/2024.
3. Mowry JB, Spyker DA, Brooks DE, et al. 2015 Annual report of the American Association of Poison Control Centers' National Poison Data System (NPDS): 33rd annual report. *Clin Toxicol (Phila)*. 2016;54(10):924–1109.

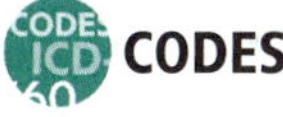

CODES

ICD10

- T14.90 Injury, unspecified
- T14.8 Other injury of unspecified body region
- R29.6 Repeated falls

CLINICAL PEARLS

- Injury and violence are predictable and preventable.
- Unintentional injury is a leading cause of death in the United States.

INSOMNIA

Susanne Wild, MD

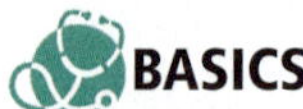

BASICS

DESCRIPTION

Difficulty initiating or maintaining sleep or nonrestorative sleep despite adequate opportunity and circumstances for sleep, resulting in at least one of the following forms of daytime impairment:

- Fatigue or malaise
- Attention, concentration, or memory impairment
- Social or vocational dysfunction or poor school performance
- Mood disturbance or irritability
- Daytime sleepiness
- Motivation, energy, or initiative reduction
- Proneness for errors or accidents at work or while driving
- Tension, headaches, or GI symptoms in response to sleep loss
- Concerns or worries about sleep

EPIDEMIOLOGY

- Predominant age: increases with age
- Predominant sex: female > male (5:1)

Prevalence

- Most common sleep disorder
- Insomnia (transient and chronic): 5–35% of the population; 10–15% associated with daytime impairment
- Chronic insomnia: 10% middle-aged adults; 1/3 of people >65 years

ETIOLOGY AND PATHOPHYSIOLOGY

- Transient/intermittent (<30 days) and short term (<3 months)
  - Usually caused by an identifiable stressor
  - Stressor can be:
    - Physical (e.g., medical illness, high altitude)
    - Psychological (e.g., stress, excitement, bereavement)
    - Psychosocial (e.g., work deadlines, housing insecurity)
    - Interpersonal (e.g., arguments)
- Usually resolves when stressor is removed
- Chronic (>3 months)
  - Usually not due to one single cause
  - Possible contributing factors:
    - Medical (e.g., gastroesophageal reflux disease, sleep apnea, chronic pain)
    - Psychiatric (e.g., mood, anxiety, psychotic disorders)
    - Primary sleep disorder (e.g., idiopathic, psychophysiologic [heightened arousal and learned sleep-preventing associations], paradoxical [sleep state misperception])
    - Circadian rhythm disorder (e.g., irregular pattern, jet lag, delayed/advanced sleep phase, shift work)
    - Environmental (e.g., lights, noises, movements [partner/young children/pets])
    - Behavioral (e.g., poor sleep hygiene, adjustment sleep disorder)
    - Substance induced
    - Medications (e.g., antihypertensives, antidepressants, corticosteroids, levodopa-carbidopa, phenytoin, quinidine, theophylline, thyroid hormones)

Genetics

No known factors

RISK FACTORS

- Age
- Female gender
- Medical comorbidities
- Unemployment
- Psychiatric illness
- Impaired social relationships
- Shift work
- Separation from spouse or partner
- Drug and substance abuse
- Family or personal history of insomnia

GENERAL PREVENTION

- Practice consistent sleep hygiene:
  - Fixed wake-up times and bedtimes regardless of amount of sleep obtained (weekdays and weekends)
  - Avoid naps; go to bed only when sleepy.
  - Sleep in a cool, dark, quiet environment.
  - No activities in bedroom associated with anything but sleep or sex
  - 30-minute wind-down time before sleep
  - If unable to sleep within 20 minutes, move to another environment and engage in quiet activity until sleepy.
- No alcohol, caffeine, or nicotine within 4 hours of bedtime
- Fixed eating times
- Avoid medications that interfere with sleep.
- Regular moderate exercise; avoid within 4 hours of bedtime.

COMMONLY ASSOCIATED CONDITIONS

- Psychiatric disorders
- Painful musculoskeletal conditions
- Obstructive sleep apnea
- Restless leg syndrome
- Drug or alcohol addiction/dependence

DIAGNOSIS

HISTORY

- Daytime sleepiness and napping
- Unintended sleep episodes (e.g., dozing at a stoplight while driving)
- Insomnia history
  - Duration, time of problem
  - Sleep latency, difficulty in maintaining sleep (repeated awakening), early morning awakening, nonrestorative sleep, or patterns (weekday vs. weekend, with or without bed partner, home vs. away)
- Sleep hygiene
  - Bedtime/wakening time
  - Physical environment of sleep area: LED clocks, TV, room lighting, ambient noise
  - Activity: nighttime eating, exercise, sexual activity
  - Intake: caffeine, alcohol, herbal supplements, diet pills, illicit drugs, prescriptions, over-the-counter (OTC) sleep aids
- Symptoms or history of depression, anxiety, obsessive-compulsive disorder, or other major psychological symptomatology
- Symptoms of restless leg syndrome and periodic limb movement disorder
- Snoring and other symptoms of sleep apnea
- Symptoms of drug or alcohol abuse
- Current medication use
- Chronic medical conditions
- Acute change or stressors such as travel or shift work
- Sleep diary: sleep log for 7 consecutive days

PHYSICAL EXAM

No association with specific findings on physical examination

DIFFERENTIAL DIAGNOSIS

- Obstructive sleep apnea
- CNS hypersomnias (e.g., narcolepsy)
- Circadian rhythm sleep disturbances
- Sleep-related movement disorders (e.g., restless leg syndrome)
- Insomnia due to medical or neurologic disorder
- Mood and anxiety disorders such as depression or anxiety

DIAGNOSTIC TESTS & INTERPRETATION

Diagnostic testing usually not required; consider polysomnography if sleep apnea or periodic limb movement disorder is suspected by history (1)[C].

Initial Tests (lab, imaging)

Testing based on history and exam to evaluate for comorbid conditions

Diagnostic Procedures/Other

Polysomnography or multiple sleep latency test not routinely indicated but may be considered if initial diagnosis is uncertain and interventions have proven unsuccessful.

TREATMENT

- Transient and short-term insomnia
  - May use medications for short-term use only
  - Self-medicating with alcohol can increase awakenings and sleep-stage changes.
- Chronic insomnia
  - Treatment of underlying condition (major depressive disorder, generalized anxiety disorder, medications, pain, substance abuse)
  - Advise good sleep hygiene.
  - Cognitive-behavioral therapy is first-line treatment for chronic insomnia (CBT-I) (2).
  - Behavioral therapy is an effective treatment for insomnia and a potentially more effective long-term treatment than pharmacotherapy (3)[B].
  - Ramelteon and doxepin are the only agents without known abuse potential.

MEDICATION

- Reserved for transient and short-term insomnia such as with jet lag, stress reactions, transient medical condition
- Short-term pharmacologic intervention can also be offered if CBT-I is not effective or not available
- No consistent advantage of using medication in addition to CBT-I
- Recommendation to limit use of benzodiazepine receptor agonists to up to 4 weeks, dual orexin receptor antagonists to up to 3 months (4)
- Benzodiazepine receptor agonists
  - Nonbenzodiazepine hypnotics
    - Act on benzodiazepine receptor, so have abuse potential
      - Zaleplon (Sonata) 5 to 20 mg; half-life 1 hour
      - Zolpidem (Ambien) 5 to 10 mg (males); 5 mg (females); half-life 2.5 to 3 hours
      - Zolpidem (Ambien CR) 6.25 to 12.5 mg (males); 6.25 mg (females); half-life 2.5 to 3 hours
      - Eszopiclone (Lunesta) 1 to 3 mg; half-life 6 hours
  - Benzodiazepine hypnotics
    - Short acting
      - Triazolam (Halcion) 0.125 to 0.5 mg; half-life 1.5 to 5.5 hours
    - Intermediate acting
      - Lorazepam (Ativan) 2 to 4 mg; half-life 12 hours
      - Temazepam (Restoril) 7.5 to 30 mg; half-life 8.8 hours
      - Estazolam (Prosom) 1 to 2 mg; half-life 10 to 24 hours
    - Long acting
      - Flurazepam (Dalmane) 15 to 30 mg; half-life 40 to 100 hours
      - Quazepam (Doral) 7.5 to 15 mg; half-life 39 hours (parent drug), 73 hours (active metabolite)
  - Contraindications/precautions are as follows:
    - Not indicated for long-term treatment due to risks of tolerance, dependency, daytime attention and concentration compromise, incoordination, rebound insomnia
    - Long-acting benzodiazepines associated with higher incidence of daytime sedation and motor impairment
    - Avoid in elderly, pregnant, breastfeeding, substance abusers, and patients with suicidal or parasuicidal behaviors.
    - Avoid in patients with untreated obstructive apnea and chronic pulmonary disease.
- Nonbenzodiazepine receptor agonists may occasionally induce parasomnias (sleepwalking, sleep eating, sleep driving).
- Melatonin receptor agonist
  - Ramelteon (Rozerem) 8 mg; half-life 1 to 2.6 hours
    - Effective to reduce sleep time onset for short- and long-term use in adults, without abuse potential. Onset may take up to 3 weeks.
- Sedating antidepressants
  - Doxepin (Silenor) 3 to 6 mg; half-life 15 hours (the only antidepressant with FDA approval for insomnia)
  - Trazodone (Oleptro) 25 to 200 mg; half-life 3 to 9 hours
  - Mirtazapine (Remeron) 7.5 to 15 mg; half-life 20 to 40 hours
  - Amitriptyline (Elavil) 25 to 100 mg; half-life 10 to 26 hours
- Orexin receptor agonists
  - Suvorexant (Belsomra) 10 to 20 mg; half-life 12 hours
  - Lemborexant (Dayvigo) 5 to 10 mg; half-life 17 to 19 hours
  - Daridorexant (Quviviq) 25 to 50 mg; half-life 8 hours
- Sedating antihistamines are not recommended.
- Antipsychotics should only be prescribed if the patient has a concurrent psychiatric diagnosis warranting their use.

Geriatric Consideration

Caution (risk of falls and confusion) when prescribing benzodiazepines or other sedative hypnotics; if absolutely necessary, use short-acting nonbenzodiazepine agonists at half the dosage or melatonin agonists for short-term treatment.

COMPLEMENTARY & ALTERNATIVE MEDICINE

- Melatonin: particularly effective in patients with delayed sleep phase disorder (e.g., due to jet lag of shift work); decreases sleep latency when taken 30 to 120 minutes prior to bedtime, but there is no good evidence for efficacy in insomnia, and long-term effects are unknown (5)[B].
- Valerian: inconsistent evidence supporting efficacy, and its slow onset of action (2 to 3 weeks) makes it unsuitable for the acute treatment of insomnia
- CBT (including relaxation therapy): effective and considered more useful than medications; recommended initial treatment for patients with chronic insomnia; no improvement of efficacy when combined with medication
- Mindfulness awareness practices: improved sleep quality and sleep-related daytime impairment for older adults per small randomized trial
- Behavioral interventions such as stimulus control therapy, sleep restriction, and relaxation training may all be effective.

ONGOING CARE

FOLLOW-UP RECOMMENDATIONS

- Daily exercise improves quality of sleep and may be more effective than medication.
- Avoid exercise within 4 hours of bedtime.

Patient Monitoring

- Reassess need for medications periodically; avoid standing prescriptions. Treatment response should be measured by using patient self-report (e.g., sleep diary); wearable sleep monitors are often inaccurate.
- Caution patients that nonbenzodiazepine agonists (zolpidem, zaleplon, eszopiclone), as well as benzodiazepines, can be habit forming.

DIET

- Avoid caffeine or reserve for morning only.
- Avoid heavy late-night snacks (light snack at bedtime may help).
- Avoid alcohol within 4 hours of bedtime.

PROGNOSIS

Situational insomnia should resolve with time.

COMPLICATIONS

- Daytime sleepiness, cognitive dysfunction
- Pulmonary hypertension if chronic sleep apnea left untreated
- Sleep apnea may lead to hypertension, stroke, or cardiac ischemia.

REFERENCES

1. Kushida CA, Littner MR, Morgenthaler T, et al. Practice parameters for the indications for polysomnography and related procedures: an update for 2005. *Sleep*. 2005;28(4):499–521.
2. Quaseem A, Kansagara D, Forciea MA, et al; for the Clinical Guidelines Committee of the American College of Physicians. Management of chronic insomnia disorder in adults: a clinical practice guideline from the American College of Physicians. *Ann Intern Med*. 2016;165(2):125–133.
3. Ebben MR, Spielman AJ. Non-pharmacological treatments for insomnia. *J Behav Med*. 2009;32(3):244–254.
4. Matheson EM, Brown BD, DeCastro AO. Treatment of chronic insomnia in adults. *Am Fam Physician*. 2024;109(2):154–160.
5. Verster GC. Melatonin and its agonists, circadian rhythms and psychiatry. *Afr J Psychiatry (Johannesbg)*. 2009;12(1):42–46.

SEE ALSO

- Anxiety (Generalized Anxiety Disorder); Depression; Fibromyalgia; Sleep Apnea, Obstructive
- Algorithms: Anxiety; Insomnia, Chronic; Restless Legs Syndrome

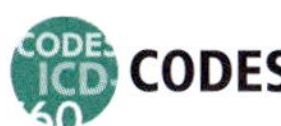

CODES

ICD10

- G47.00 Insomnia, unspecified
- F51.02 Adjustment insomnia
- F51.01 Primary insomnia

CLINICAL PEARLS

- CBT-I is the first-line treatment for insomnia.
- Treatment of underlying etiology of the insomnia and consistent sleep hygiene are key.
- Most medications are indicated for short-term use only.
- Sedative hypnotics are not recommended in the elderly because risks may outweigh benefits.

INTERSTITIAL CYSTITIS/PAINFUL BLADDER SYNDROME

Dmitry Bisk, MD • An-Thu N. Nguyen, DO

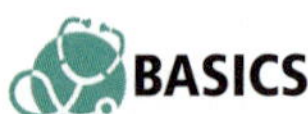

BASICS

DESCRIPTION

- A condition characterized by pain, pressure or discomfort of the bladder or pelvic region associated with one or more of the following urinary symptoms: increased frequency, urgency, or nocturia
- A chronic inflammatory disease of unknown etiology, with associated urinary symptoms for >6 weeks without other identifiable causes such as infection or other pathology
- The symptoms in many patients are insidious, and the disease progresses for years with relapsing and remitting symptoms often before diagnosis is established.
- Types include interstitial cystitis/bladder pain syndrome without Hunner lesions and interstitial cystitis/bladder pain syndrome with Hunner lesions.
- System(s) affected: renal/urologic
- Synonym(s): urgency frequency syndrome; IC/bladder pain syndrome; chronic cystitis; Hunner ulcer

Pregnancy Considerations

Unpredictable symptom improvement or exacerbation during pregnancy; may be associated with increased risk of preeclampsia and preterm birth, but further prospective studies are needed; usual problems of unknown effect on fetus with medications taken during pregnancy

EPIDEMIOLOGY

- Occurs predominantly among white patients
- Predominant sex: female > male (5:1) in patients 25 to 80 years of age
- Most common in adults >30 years of age and diagnosis increases with age

Incidence

Difficult to estimate due to different diagnostic criteria and regional differences, but 1-year incidence has been reported as:

- 21 per 100,000 female patients
- 4 per 100,000 male patients

Prevalence

In the United States:

- Prevalence is variable.
- Up to 1.2 million female and 82,000 male patients affected, but many cases likely are undiagnosed.
- 0.052% but may be ≥10%

ETIOLOGY AND PATHOPHYSIOLOGY

- Etiology is unclear, and pathophysiology is likely multifactorial.
- Potential causes include:
  - Disruption of urothelium, production of antiproliferative factor, and diminished glycosaminoglycan layer
  - Afferent nerve plasticity
  - Pelvic floor dysfunction
  - Mast cell infiltration, bladder nitric oxide
  - Reduced vascularization
  - Neurogenic inflammation
  - Autoimmune

RISK FACTORS

Unclear but some reported risks include the following:

- Female
- Recent urinary tract infection (UTI)
- Irritable bowel syndrome (IBS)
- Allergies
- History of sexual abuse

COMMONLY ASSOCIATED CONDITIONS

- Fibromyalgia/Chronic fatigue syndrome
- Allergies
- Depression and panic disorder
- Vulvodynia
- Sexual dysfunction
- Sleep disturbance
- Migraines
- Chronic prostatitis
- Chronic pelvic pain and pelvic floor dysfunction
- IBS
- Anal/rectal disease
- Chronic scrotal pain
- Trauma
- Autoimmune conditions such as systemic lupus erythematosus (SLE) and Sjögren syndrome

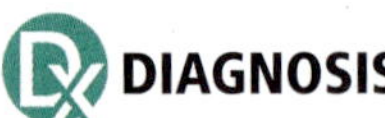

DIAGNOSIS

- A clinical diagnosis in uncomplicated cases can be characterized by symptoms that have been present for >6 weeks without other causes such as infection or other disorders.
  - Pain, pressure, or discomfort of the bladder or pelvic area and at least one of the following urinary symptoms:
    - Increased daytime frequency, urgency, or nocturia
- Cystoscopy with hydrodistension or urodynamic studies should not be used to establish a diagnosis in uncomplicated presentations but can be considered if diagnosis is unclear or the presentation is complex. Cystoscopy can help identify Hunner lesions (painful lesions within the dome or lateral wall of the bladder) which could change management options (1).

HISTORY

- Thorough history detailing baseline bladder/pelvic pain and urinary symptoms (with voiding patterns)
- Common urinary symptoms at presentation are urgency and frequency with small void volumes.
- Symptoms can be variable with flares and remission.
- Episodes may be related to menses, stress, sexual activity, IBS, endometriosis, vulvodynia, fibromyalgia, chronic fatigue syndrome, and autoimmune conditions.
- Common food triggers: caffeine, sodas and other carbonated drinks, alcohol, acidic foods (citrus, tomatoes), vinegar, and hot peppers
- Use of validated questionnaires:
  - O'Leary/Sant Voiding and Pain Indices (http://www.ichelp.org/wp-content/uploads/2015/06/OLeary_Sant.pdf)

PHYSICAL EXAM

- Exams findings can be nonspecific; most common: dysphoric mood, bladder neck tenderness, suprapubic tenderness, and levator ani tenderness.
- Abdominal exam: evaluate for masses, hernias, suprapubic tenderness, costovertebral tenderness.
- Female pelvic exam
  - Findings suggesting interstitial cystitis can include pelvic floor spasms, suprapubic tenderness, rectal spasms, urethral tenderness, and bladder base tenderness when examining the anterior vaginal wall.
- Male digital rectal exam
  - Tenderness of the prostate can occur, but it may lead to a false diagnosis of chronic prostatitis.
  - Findings suggesting interstitial cystitis can include spasms of the sphincter.

DIFFERENTIAL DIAGNOSIS

- UTI
- Acute and chronic prostatitis
- Overactive bladder
- Urge incontinence
- Bladder neoplasm
- Bladder or ureteral stone
- Chronic pelvic pain
- Urogenital prolapse
- Urethral diverticulum
- Neurologic bladder disease
- Nonurinary pelvic disease (STIs, endometriosis, pelvic relaxation, pudendal neuralgia)

DIAGNOSTIC TESTS & INTERPRETATION

Initial Tests (lab, imaging)

- Voiding diary to record symptoms and to establish baseline symptoms when evaluating treatment
- Urinalysis and urine culture to rule out infection
- Gonorrhea and chlamydia testing
- Urine biomarkers and cytology are not recommended unless at increased risk.

Diagnostic Procedures/Other

- Cystoscopy with hydrodistension to differentiate other pathology if necessary (1).
- Urodynamic studies are not recommended for routine evaluation but can be used to differentiate other coexisting disorders (overactive bladder, stress urinary incontinence, or voiding dysfunction) (1).
- Intravesical lidocaine (anesthetic bladder challenge) can help to pinpoint the bladder as the source of pain in patients with pelvic pain.
- Potassium sensitivity test and bladder biopsy are not recommended in routine cases.

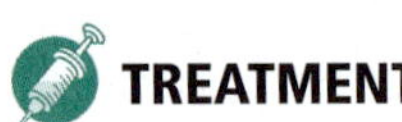

TREATMENT

GENERAL MEASURES

- The goal of treatment should be to control symptoms and to increase patient's quality of life.
- There is no universally effective treatment plan. There is also no strong evidence that any treatment method is effective and more large trials are needed. However, conservative general measures should be tried first for all patients and include the following (1)[C]:
  - Patient education on normal bladder function, disease course, lack of cure, expectant management

- Diet changes (elimination diets such as caffeine, alcohol, other carbonated beverages, high citrus foods, tomatoes, and bananas)
- Meditation, counseling, and stress management
- Regular exercise
- Manual physical therapy maneuvers by a trained clinician that improve pelvic, abdominal, and/or hip muscular trigger points; lengthen muscle contractures; and release painful scars should be offered to patients with pelvic floor tenderness. Kegel exercises should be avoided.
- Avoidance of activity that exacerbates the pain
- Efficacy of treatment should be periodically reassessed, and infective treatments should be stopped.

MEDICATION

- Randomized controlled trials of most medications for interstitial cystitis demonstrate limited benefit over placebo; there are no clear predictors of what will benefit an individual. Prepare the patient that treatment may involve trial and error.
- A systemic review of treatment options including antidepressants, pentosan polysulfate sodium, and neuromuscular blockade did not demonstrate conclusive evidence that they are effective for the treatment of symptoms (2)[A].
- Conservative therapies should be trialed first and more aggressive therapies can be started based on patient's symptoms and quality of life (1)[C].
- Treatments should be based on symptoms, symptom severity, and patient preferences (1)[C].
- Multiple simultaneous treatments may be considered if it is in the patient's best interest, and patient's symptoms are followed and assessed carefully (1)[C]

First Line

Note: AUA consensus states that patient education, pain management, general relaxation, stress reduction, behavior modification, and self-care are first-line therapy (1)[C].

Second Line

- Patients can be prescribed analgesic medications (e.g., acetaminophen, NSAIDs) with proper indications and discussion of risks and benefits (1).
- Medication choice (listed below in alphabetical order) should be based on patient's symptoms and preferences (1)[C].
  - Amitriptyline: 25 to 100 mg daily, most effective at ≥50 mg/day; initiate with lower dose and titrate.
  - Cimetidine 400 mg BID. Side effects are rare (1)[C].
  - Hydroxyzine 25 to 75 mg QHS; common side effects include drowsiness and xerostomia (1)[C].
  - Pentosan polysulfate 100 mg TID on empty stomach; may take several months (3 to 6) to become effective; (only FDA-approved treatment for interstitial cystitis); side effects can include headache, nausea, diarrhea, dizziness, rash, edema, and hair loss. Patients may need to be counseled on routine eye exams and increased rare atypical maculopathy risk (1)[C].
- Treatment of Hunner lesions if found with laser, electrocautery, and/or injection of triamcinolone

Third Line

Intravesical treatment (listed in alphabetical order) (1)[C]

- Dimethyl sulfoxide (DMSO) q2wk for 6 weeks and then PRN (only FDA-approved intravesical treatment); side effects include pain with instillation, unpleasant odor, and exacerbation of long-term pain.
- Heparin 10 to 20,000 units in 2 to 5 mL of solution, 3 times a week.
- Lidocaine 1% 20 to 30 mL considered a short-term treatment option.

ADDITIONAL THERAPIES

- Oral cyclosporine A for Hunner lesions refractory to triamcinolone injection, intravesical hyaluronic acid, and/or intravesical chondroitin sulfate may be offered as a treatment option if other therapies outline above have not been effective in improving symptoms and quality of life (1)[C].
- Sildenafil 25 mg; small randomized trial demonstrated urinary symptom improvement after 3 to 6 months.
- Long-term antibiotics and/or long-term systemic oral glucocorticoid should not be used (1).

SURGERY/OTHER PROCEDURES

- Cystoscopy under anesthesia with low-pressure hydrodistention (1)[C].
- Transurethral laser fulguration and/or injection of triamcinolone (effective for Hunner lesion) (1)[C].
- Intradetrusor onabotulinumtoxinA may be administered if other treatments have not provided improvement of quality of life. Patients need to be counseled on the possibility of intermittent self-catheterization risk (1)[C].
- Neurostimulation: After a trial of neurostimulation, a permanent neurostimulation device can be placed if other treatments have not been effective in providing the patient with improvement of symptoms or quality of life (1)[C].
- Major surgery such as urinary diversion with or without cystectomy can be considered in carefully selected patients who have failed all other therapies and need improvement with quality of life (1)[C].

COMPLEMENTARY & ALTERNATIVE MEDICINE

One small trial of 21 patients undergoing hyperbaric oxygen therapy showed a 28% decrease in pain at 3 months.

ONGOING CARE

DIET

Dietary modification, elimination diet (caffeine, chocolate, citrus, tomatoes, carbonated beverages, potassium-rich foods, soybean, spicy foods, acidic foods, and alcohol)

PATIENT EDUCATION

- Interstitial Cystitis Association, 110 Washington St. Suite 340, Rockville, MD 20850; 1-800-HELPICA: http://www.ichelp.org/
- Given overlap with chronic pelvic pain syndrome, patients may benefit from home exercises—examples: https://youtu.be/NnqAkM9r2a8 or https://youtu.be/R3Rydb1nZU4

PROGNOSIS

- Patients often report decreased quality of life.
- Potential symptom plateau after approximately 5 years of symptoms

REFERENCES

1. Hanno PM, Erickson D, Moldwin R, et al; for American Urological Association. Diagnosis and treatment of interstitial cystitis/bladder pain syndrome: AUA guideline amendment. *J Urol*. 2015;193(5):1545–1553.
2. Imamura M, Scott NW, Wallace SA, et al. Interventions for treating people with symptoms of bladder pain syndrome: a network meta-analysis. *Cochrane Database Syst Rev*. 2020;7(7):CD013325.

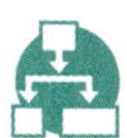

SEE ALSO

- Urinary Tract Infection (UTI) in Women
- Algorithm: Pelvic Girdle Pain (Pregnancy or Postpartum Pelvic Pain)

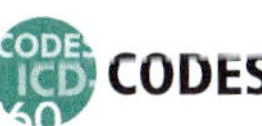

CODES

ICD10

- N30.10 Interstitial cystitis (chronic) without hematuria
- N30.11 Interstitial cystitis (chronic) with hematuria

CLINICAL PEARLS

- In most cases, this is a clinical diagnosis that is characterized by symptoms that have been present for >6 weeks without other underlying causes. Symptoms include pain, pressure, or discomfort of the bladder or pelvic area and at least one of the following urinary symptoms: increased daytime frequency, urgency, or nocturia.
- At present, there is no definitive treatment for interstitial cystitis.
- Most patients with severe disease receive multiple treatment approaches. Regular multidisciplinary follow-up, pharmacologic therapy, avoidance of symptom triggers, and psychological and supportive therapy are all important because this disease tends to wax and wane. Monitor patients for comorbid depression.
- Empower patients to manage their symptoms, communicate regularly with their physicians, and learn as much as they can about this disease, which may help them to optimize their outcome.

INTERSTITIAL NEPHRITIS

Nawal Aamir, MD • Amar Pandit, MD

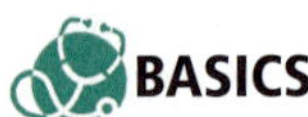

BASICS

DESCRIPTION

- Acute and chronic tubulointerstitial diseases result from interactions between renal and inflammatory cells.
- Injury to renal cells triggers new antigen expression, inflammatory cell infiltration, and proinflammatory activation. The outcome is acute interstitial nephritis (AIN) or chronic interstitial nephritis (CIN).
- In AIN, altered tubular function precedes decreased glomerular filtration rate.
- AIN typically presents as acute kidney injury (AKI) after exposure to offending drugs or agents (OFA), often with predominantly non-albumin, that is, tubular proteinuria, sterile pyuria, microscopic hematuria, and white cell casts.

EPIDEMIOLOGY

Incidence

- AIN accounts for 15–20% of patients with AKI.
- Peak incidence is in women aged 60 to 70 years. Tubulointerstitial nephritis with uveitis (TINU) typically presents in adolescent females IgG4-related disease occurs more commonly in men >50 years.

Pediatric Considerations

Children with prior lead poisoning are at higher risk for CIN as young adults.

Geriatric Considerations

Older patients (≥65 years) typically have more severe disease, higher risk of permanent damage, especially from drug-induced AIN (87% vs. 64%), and more proton pump inhibitor-induced AIN (18% vs. 6%), but less AIN from autoimmune or systemic causes (7% vs. 27%).

ETIOLOGY AND PATHOPHYSIOLOGY

- AIN
  - T cell activation by an antigen leads to delayed drug hypersensitivity reactions, which leads to interstitial inflammatory infiltrates that damage tubules.
  - Renal dysfunction generally is partially or completely reversible.
  - Hypersensitivity to drugs (75%): not dose dependent; the top three were omeprazole (12%), amoxicillin (8%), and ciprofloxacin (8%) (1)[C]; many implicated; NSAIDs, antibiotics, proton pump inhibitors, diuretics, AEDs, antivirals, anticancer drugs, allopurinol, H_2 blockers, diphenylhydantoin, sulfasalazine, and mesalamine
  - Infections (10–15%): *Streptococci*, *Legionella*, *Leptospira*, *Leishmania*, *Escherichia coli*, *Campylobacter*, *Salmonella*, *Treponema pallidum*, *Mycobacterium tuberculosis*, *Histoplasma*, *Coccidioides*, *Toxoplasma*, CMV, EBV, HSV, HIV, and perhaps the SARS-CoV-2 (COVID-19) virus (2)
  - Autoimmune (10–15%): sarcoidosis, SLE, Sjögren syndrome, granulomatosis with polyangiitis, cryoglobulinemia
  - Toxins (e.g., snake bite venom)
  - Idiopathic (5–10%): TINU syndrome and anti-tubular basement membrane (anti-TBM) disease
- CIN
  - Characterized by interstitial scarring, fibrosis, and tubular atrophy, resulting in progressive CKD
  - Often follows long-term exposure to OFA (e.g., heavy metals, especially lead); long-term exposure to agents that cause AIN (PPIs, NSAIDs) can also cause CIN.
  - CIN in agricultural communities (CINAC) or Mesoamerican nephropathy or CKD of unknown etiology (CKDu): In farming communities from Central America (mainly Nicaragua and El Salvador); etiology is not known but could be related to pesticide exposure, heat stress, and genetic predisposition.
  - May be found incidentally on routine labs

Genetics

Significant associations have been reported between certain HLA genotypes and AIN, especially drug-induced AIN. These genetic associations influence susceptibility to AIN, disease severity, and treatment response. In the future, HLA typing may help stratify risk in patients prescribed high-risk medications (PPIs, antibiotics, ICIs). Discussion of these genetic associations is beyond the scope of this chapter.

GENERAL PREVENTION

- Review need for medication (e.g., PPIs) at every visit and discontinue when not needed or when safer alternatives are available (e.g., H2 receptor blockers).
- Ask for over-the-counter medications especially "herbal supplements" and "alternative/natural/holistic medications" as these may contain heavy metals or other chemicals with potential to cause AIN.
- Early recognition and prompt discontinuation of OFA

COMMONLY ASSOCIATED CONDITIONS

- Chronic pyelonephritis
- Abuse of analgesics
- Lithium use
- Gout and gout therapy
- Immune disorders
- Malignancy (lymphoma, multiple myeloma)
- Amyloidosis
- Exposure to heavy metals (e.g., lead, cadmium)
- Renal papillary necrosis
- Uveitis

DIAGNOSIS

- History and clinical presentation
  - Medication exposure: AIN onset ranges from 3 to 5 days up to several weeks to months (longer with NSAIDs). ICI-induced AIN can rarely occur a few months after the medication has been discontinued.
  - Suspect in patients with nonspecific symptoms (malaise, fatigue, fever, nausea, vomiting, rash) plus AKI and abnormal urinalysis; patients can be asymptomatic, and AKI may be detected incidentally.
  - Systemic signs: fever (27%), maculopapular rash (15%), peripheral eosinophilia (23%), arthralgias (45%); less common when NSAIDs and PPIs are the OFA.
  - Drug Reaction with Eosinophilia and Systemic Symptoms (DRESS): severe idiosyncratic drug reaction; potentially life-threatening; lymphadenopathy often present
  - Eye pain and redness: Suspect TINU.
  - Infections, exposure to heavy metals or herbal supplements
  - Oliguria (~50%) and signs of volume overload in those with severe AKI
- CIN
  - Hypertension (HTN), oliguria or polyuria (due to impaired ability to concentrate urine), polydipsia
  - Patients may be asymptomatic early in the course of disease.

PHYSICAL EXAM

- Increased BP
- Fluid retention/extremity swelling/weight gain
- Rash accompanying renal findings in acute AIN
- Lung crackles/rales
- Pericardial rub in uremic pericarditis

DIFFERENTIAL DIAGNOSIS

- AKI secondary to other causes:
  - Prerenal, intrarenal, postrenal
  - Aminoglycosides can cause acute tubular necrosis.
  - NSAIDs can exacerbate prerenal disease.
- CKD secondary to long-standing HTN, diabetes, and chronic pyelonephritis

DIAGNOSTIC TESTS & INTERPRETATION

Most of these tests are nonspecific and may only be positive in a minority of cases on AIN. Definitive diagnosis requires a kidney biopsy.

Initial Tests (lab, imaging)

- Serum chemistries
  - Elevated creatinine (40% may eventually require dialysis) and BUN
  - Hypokalemia or hyperkalemia, hyponatremia, hyperchloremic metabolic acidosis
- CBC
  - Eosinophilia (80%; lower in NSAID-induced AIN ~15%)
  - Anemia
- Urinalysis:
  - Normal urinalysis does not rule out AIN.
  - Sterile pyuria, that is, pyuria without bacteruria.
  - Microscopic hematuria
  - Urine sediment may show WBC casts.
  - Eosinophiluria: low sensitivity for AIN
  - Decreased tubular function may be indicated by isosthenuria, that is, decreased ability to concentrate urine. Urine SG will be ~1.01.
  - Fanconi syndrome: glycosuria (even in the absence of hyperglycemia), phosphaturia
- Proteinuria:
  - Low grade (<1 g/24 hr) but can be higher in NSAID-induced kidney injury.
  - Proteinuria is predominantly non-albumin (urine albumin to creatinine ratio is <50% of urine protein to creatinine ratio).
- Urinary biomarkers:
  - Urinary $\alpha 1$- and $\beta 2$-microglobulin, immunoglobulins, TNF-α, CXCL9, IL-9 may aid diagnosis and monitoring
- Chest x-ray (CXR): to evaluate for TB, sarcoidosis, infections

- Serologies for autoimmune (e.g., sarcoidosis, Sjögren, GPA, Behçet) and infectious diseases:
  - Sarcoidosis: ACE, calcium, 1,25-dihydroxyvitamin D
  - SLE: ANA, anti-dsDNA, anti-Smith, C3, C4
  - IgG4-related disease: low C3 and C4, high IgG4 levels, eosinophilia
  - Sjögren syndrome: anti-Ro/SSA, anti-La/SSB
  - ANCA vasculitis: ANCA, anti-proteinase-3, and anti-MPO
  - Serum protein electrophoresis
  - Urinary legionella antigen
- Liver function tests: may be elevated with drug-induced liver injury
- Renal ultrasound: There are no reliable confirmatory ultrasound findings for AIN. Ultrasound may be done to rule out obstruction as a cause of AKI.
- IV contrast studies (IVP, CT) relatively contraindicated; gallium-67 scan has limited utility.

Diagnostic Procedures/Other

- Renal biopsy: gold standard for AIN diagnosis; contraindicated in bleeding diathesis, solitary kidney (relative contraindication), uncontrolled HTN, sepsis, or renal parenchymal infection
- Indications: AKI in patients on an OFA is known to cause AIN but with normal UA; persistent AKI after OFA withdrawal; consideration for steroids; advanced renal failure with <3 months onset; high-grade proteinuria

Test Interpretation

- AIN: Biopsy shows interstitial infiltrate consisting of T lymphocytes and monocytes; however, may include eosinophils, plasma cells, and neutrophils.
- CIN: Tubular atrophy, fibrosis, and mononuclear cell infiltration; storiform fibrosis seen in IgG4-related disease

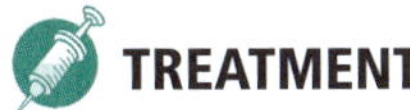

TREATMENT

GENERAL MEASURES

- Discontinue OFA, including topical NSAIDs; If multiple potential OFA, discontinue one at a time if mild AKI or discontinue all if severe AKI.
- Reduce exposure to nephrotoxins.
- Supportive care: maintain hydration; manage fever/rash; control BP; correct anemia; correct acidosis and electrolyte imbalances
- Short-term dialysis as needed
- Renally dose medications; consider renal biopsy at 4 to 7 days or sooner if patient has severe AKI.
- Document drug allergy in medical record.

MEDICATION

- No evidence-based guidelines for AIN management; withdrawal of OFA is first step.
- Consider medication therapy if AKI is severe at presentation, especially if dialysis appears imminent, or if AKI persists for 5 to 7 days after OFA withdrawal

First Line

- Steroid regimen:
  - Prednisone 0.5 to 1.0 mg/kg/day for 1 to 2 weeks; close monitoring of kidney function is essential. In the event of delayed recovery, this dose may be extended to no more than 6 weeks
  - Taper prednisone over 2 to 6 weeks. Taper may need to be slower for patients with TINU (4 to 6 months) and other autoimmune conditions.
  - Pulse dosing with IV methylprednisolone 125 to 250 mg/day for 3 days may be considered in those with severe AKI (those with imminent need for dialysis).
- Steroids started within 7 days of OFA withdrawal have better outcomes.
- NSAID-induced AIN generally does not respond to steroids.

Second Line

- Limited evidence with treating AIN in patients who are steroid-dependent
- Mycophenolate mofetil (MMF) may be considered in biopsy-proven AIN patients. Prescription may need to be continued for 1 to 3 years (3)[C].
- Lead toxicity: chelation (succimer, EDTA)
- SLE nephritis: steroids + MMF or cyclophosphamide or azathioprine
- Urate nephropathy:
  - Urate-lowering agents (allopurinol, dose-adjusted for renal function).
  - Note: Allopurinol can itself cause AIN.
  - Discontinue thiazides.
- Lithium-induced nephritis: Use amiloride as adjunct.
- Indinavir-induced nephritis: Use probenecid as adjunct.

ISSUES FOR REFERRAL

Nephrology referral for patients with AKI, proteinuria, acid-base, or electrolyte disorders

ADMISSION, INPATIENT, AND NURSING CONSIDERATIONS

Hospitalization required for AKI and/or serious electrolyte or acid-base disturbances

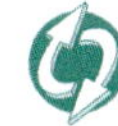

ONGOING CARE

FOLLOW-UP RECOMMENDATIONS

Patient Monitoring

If nephrotoxic agents cannot be discontinued, monitor renal function, electrolytes, and phosphorus frequently.

DIET

- Customize based on presentation: low potassium (<2 g/day) if patients have hyperkalemia; low sodium diet; moderate protein intake
- High fiber, consider DASH diet.

PATIENT EDUCATION

Refer to National Kidney Disease Education Program. (866) 4-KIDNEY; http://www.niddk.nih.gov/healthinformation/health-communication-programs/nkdep/Pages/default.aspx.

PROGNOSIS

- Early detection (within 1 week of creatinine rise) and prompt OFA discontinuation lead to favorable long-term outcomes. Unfortunately, recovery is often incomplete with persistent elevation in serum creatinine in up to 40%, especially in those with NSAID-induced AIN.
- Renal biopsy reveals degree of inflammation and extent of chronicity (fibrosis, global glomerulosclerosis). Renal prognosis is worse in those with advanced chronicity.
- AIN: recovery in weeks to months; 65% recover, 23% have long-term impairment.
- 1/3 require acute dialysis before resolution.
- 12% progress to ESRD; more common in older patients with underlying chronic kidney disease
- CIN may progress to ESRD.
- Untreated severe AKI: 45–70% mortality.

COMPLICATIONS

- Chronic tubulointerstitial disease may progress to ESRD, requiring dialysis or transplant.
- Analgesic use increases risk of transitional cell carcinoma of the uroepithelium.

REFERENCES

1. Muriithi AK, Leung N, Valeri AM, et al. Biopsy-proven acute interstitial nephritis, 1993–2011: a case series. *Am J Kidney Dis*. 2014;64(4):558–566.
2. Ng JH, Zaidan M, Jhaveri KD, et al. Acute tubulointerstitial nephritis and COVID-19. *Clin Kidney J*. 2021;14(10):2151–2157.
3. Preddie DC, Markowitz GS, Radhakrishnan J, et al. Mycophenolate mofetil for the treatment of interstitial nephritis. *Clin J Am Soc Nephrol*. 2006;1(4):718–722.

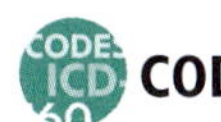

CODES

ICD10

- N12 Tubulo-interstitial nephritis, not spcf as acute or chronic
- N10 Acute tubulo-interstitial nephritis
- N11.9 Chronic tubulo-interstitial nephritis, unspecified

CLINICAL PEARLS

- First treatment step: Remove offending agents.
- Most common in older patients on NSAIDs, PPIs, and antibiotics
- Renal biopsy is gold standard for AIN diagnosis.
- Immunosuppressive therapy is considered if no improvement within 3 to 7 days after stopping the OFA.

I

INTIMATE PARTNER VIOLENCE

Rhonda A. Faulkner, PhD • Alyssa Jeanne Vest Hart, DO • Zehra Khan, MD

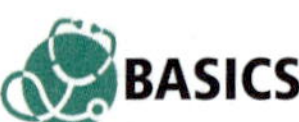

BASICS

DESCRIPTION

- Intimate partner violence (IPV) is abuse or aggression that occurs in a romantic relationship between a former or current partner.
- May include physical, sexual, and/or emotional abuse; economic or psychological actions; stalking; or threats of actions that influence another person
- Although women are at greater risk of experiencing IPV, it occurs among patients of any race, age, sexual orientation, religion, gender, and socioeconomic background.
- Synonym(s): domestic violence (DV); spousal abuse; partner abuse; family violence

EPIDEMIOLOGY

Incidence

- In the United States, women experience 4.8 million incidents of physical or sexual assault annually.
- It is estimated that the COVID-19 pandemic has increased the incidence of IPV due to exacerbations of the risk factors that influence perpetrators of IPV.

Prevalence

- About 1 in 4 women and nearly 1 in 10 men experience a form of IPV in their lifetime.
- Over 43 million women and 38 million men have experienced a form of IPV in their lifetime.
- IPV is estimated to cost the U.S. economy >$10.4 billion annually (1).

Geriatric Considerations

About 1 to 2 million U.S. citizens aged >65 have been injured, exploited, or mistreated by someone caring for them.

Pediatric Considerations

- IPV can occur in adolescence, known as teen dating violence (TDV). TDV affects millions of U.S. teens each year.
- Approximately 1 in 5 female high school students report being physically and/or sexually abused by a dating partner; female between 16 and 24 years of age are more vulnerable to IPV than any other age group.
- About 11 million women and 5 million men reported experiencing IPV before the age of 18 years.
- Children living in violent homes are at increased risk of physical, sexual, and/or emotional abuse; anxiety and depression; decreased self-esteem; emotional, behavioral, social, and/or physical disturbances; and lifelong poor health.

Pregnancy Considerations

- IPV leads to unintended pregnancies, induced abortions, and sexually transmitted infections (STIs). Pregnant women who experience IPV are twice as likely to have an abortion.
- IPV in pregnancy also increases the likelihood of miscarriage, stillbirth, preterm delivery, and low-birth-weight babies.

RISK FACTORS

- Patient/victim risk factors
  - Substance abuse (drug or alcohol), high-risk sexual behavior
  - Poverty/financial stressors/unemployment/less education
  - Recent loss of social support, family disruption and life cycle changes, social isolation
  - Prior history of abusive relationships or experiencing abuse as child
  - Mental or physical disability in family
  - Pregnancy
  - Transgender-identifying women
  - Attempting to leave the relationship
- Perpetrator risk factors
  - Substance abuse, depression, personality disorders
  - Young age
  - Unemployment, recent job loss or instability, low academic achievement
  - Witnessing/experiencing violence as child
  - Threatening to self or others, violence to children or outside the home
  - Owns weapons
- Relational risk factors
  - Marital conflict or instability, economic stress, traditional gender role norms, poor family functioning, obsessive/controlling relationship

Geriatric Considerations

Factors associated with IPV in geriatric populations: female gender, immigration stress, fear, social isolation, low income, poor physical health, low cognitive functioning, absence of social support, depressive symptoms, neglect, caregiver stress, and burden

Pediatric Considerations

Factors associated with IPV in pediatric populations: transgender, adverse childhood experiences, trauma symptoms, depression, gender attitudes, and economic hardship (1)

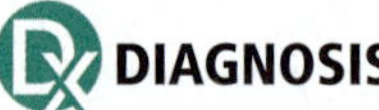

DIAGNOSIS

- The U.S. Preventive Services Task Force (USPSTF) in 2013 issued guidelines recommending that clinicians screen all women of reproductive age for IPV and provide or refer women to ongoing support services when appropriate (2)[A].
- The U.S. Department of Health and Human Services has recommended that IPV screening and counseling be a core part of women's preventive health visits.

Pregnancy Considerations

The American College of Obstetrics and Gynecologists (ACOG) recommends that physicians screen all women for IPV at periodic intervals, including during obstetric care (at the first prenatal visit, at least once per trimester, at the postpartum checkup), offer ongoing support, and review prevention and referral options.

HISTORY

- Physicians should introduce the subject of IPV in a general way (i.e., "I routinely ask all patients about intimate partner violence. Have you ever been in a relationship where you were afraid?").
- Address patient confidentiality prior to screening (i.e., "I want you to know everything you say here is confidential, meaning that I will not talk to anyone else about what is said unless you tell me [insert laws in your state about what is necessary to disclose].").
- Screen patient alone, without partner, parent, or others present.
- Ask screening questions in patient's primary language; do not use children or other family members as interpreters.
- HITS questions: Each HITS question is scored on a 5-point scale (never, rarely, sometimes, fairly often, and frequently, with a score of >10 indicating likely victimization; sensitivity 30–100% and specificity 86–99%). "How often does your partner:
  - **H**urt you physically?; **I**nsult or talk down to you?; **T**hreaten you with harm?; **S**cream or curse at you?" (3)
- Partner Violence Scale (sensitivity 35–71%; specificity 80–94%)
  - "Have you ever been hit, kicked, punched, or otherwise, hurt by someone within the past year? If so, by whom?"
  - "Do you feel safe in your current relationship?"
  - "Is there a partner from a previous relationship who is making you feel unsafe now?"
- SAFE questions
  - **S**tress/safety: "Do you feel safe in your relationship?"
  - **A**fraid/abused: "Have you ever been in a relationship where you were threatened, hurt, or afraid?"
  - **F**riends/family: "Are your friends or family aware that you have been hurt? Could you tell them, and would they be able to give you support?"
  - **E**mergency plan: "Do you have a safe place to go and the resources you need in an emergency?"
- Assess pregnancy difficulties such as poor/late prenatal care, low-birth-weight babies, and perinatal deaths as well as repeat abortions (unplanned pregnancy may be a result of sexual assault or reproductive coercion).
- Pelvic and abdominal pain, chronic without demonstrable pathology, gynecologic disorders
- Headaches, back pain
- STIs
- Depression, suicidal ideation, anxiety, fatigue, eating disorders, substance abuse
- Overuse of health services/frequent emergency room visits
- Nonadherence with medication/treatment plan and/or missed appointments

PHYSICAL EXAM

- Clinical presentation/psychological signs and symptoms
  - Delay in seeking treatment, inconsistent explanation of injuries, reluctance to undress
  - Signs of battered woman syndrome and/or posttraumatic stress disorder (PTSD) (flat affect/avoidance of eye contact, evasiveness, heightened startle response, sleep disturbance, traumatic flashbacks)
  - Suspicious partner accompaniment at appointment; overly solicitous partner and/or refusal to leave exam room
- Physical signs and symptoms
  - Tympanic membrane rupture
  - Rectal or genital injury (centrally located injuries with bathing-suit pattern of distribution—concealable by clothing)

- Head and neck injuries (site of 50% of abusive injuries)
- Scrapes, loose or broken tooth, bruises, cuts, or fractures to face or body
- Knife wounds, cigarette burns, bite marks, welts with outline of weapon (such as belt buckle)
- Defensive posture injuries
- Injuries inconsistent with explanation or in various stages of healing
- Malnutrition or pressure ulcers in the elderly

DIAGNOSTIC TESTS & INTERPRETATION

Initial Tests (lab, imaging)

Liver function tests (LFTs), amylase, lipase if abdominal trauma is suspected, BUN and creatinine if malnutrition/dehydration is suspected, pregnancy test and STI testing (HIV Ab/Ag, syphilis screen, gonorrhea and chlamydia NAAT, trichomonas) in cases of sexual abuse, X-ray if suspected fracture, radiographic skeletal survey for children <2 years old if physical abuse is suspected

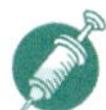

TREATMENT

- Treatment includes initial diagnosis; ongoing medical care; emotional support, counseling, and patient education regarding the DV cycle; referrals to community and supportive services as needed.
- On diagnosis, use the SOS-DoC intervention:
  - **S**: Offer *S*upport and assess *S*afety:
    - Support: "You are not to blame. I am sorry this is happening to you. There is no excuse for you to be treated this way."
    - Remind patient of your commitment to confidential communication.
    - The objective is to maximize safety as IPV can result in death. Making a safety plan can decrease the risk of mortal harm.
    - Safety assessment involves inquiring patients about their concerns and fears.
    - Victim factors associated with increased risk of danger:
      - Attempting to leave the relationship
      - Seeking outside intervention
      - Suicidal
      - Homicidal
    - Safety: Listen and respond to safety issues for the patient: "Do you feel safe going home?"; "Are your children safe?"
  - **O**: Discuss *O*ptions, including safety planning and follow-up:
    - Provide information about IPV and help when needed. Make referrals to local resources.
    - "Do you need or want to access a safety shelter or IPV service agency?"
    - "Do you want police intervention and if so, would you like me to call the police, so they can make a report with you?"
    - Offer numbers to local resources and National IPV Hotline: 1-800-799-SAFE (open 24/7; can provide physicians in every state with information on local resources)
  - **S**: Validate patient's *S*trengths: It is crucial that providers affirm understanding of the patient's difficulty.
    - "It took courage for you to talk with me today. You have shown great strength in very difficult circumstances."
  - **Do**: *Do*cument observations, assessment, and plans:
    - Use patient's own words regarding injury and abuse. Language should be chosen carefully; "patient reports" as opposed to "patient denies/claims," which may suggest the clinician does not believe the patient
    - Legibly document injuries: Use a body map.
    - If possible, photograph patient's injuries if given consent. Photographs must include the patient's face or identifying features with the injury in order to be useful as legal evidence.
    - Make patient safety plan. Prepare patient to get away in an emergency:
    - Encourage patient to prepare an emergency kit to keep in a safe place: keys (house and car); important papers (Social Security card, birth certificates, photo ID/driver's license, passport, green card); cash, food stamps, credit cards; medication for self and children; children's immunization records; important phone numbers/addresses (friends, family, local shelters); personal care items (e.g., extra glasses)
    - Encourage patient to arrange a signal with someone to let that person know when she or he needs help
  - **C**: Offer *C*ontinuity:
    - Offer a follow-up appointment and assess barriers to access.

GENERAL MEASURES

- Reporting child and elder abuse to protective services is mandatory in most states. Several states have laws requiring mandatory reporting of IPV.
- National Domestic Violence Hotline: 1-800-799-SAFE (7233)
- Post resources and posters in both English and Spanish in exam rooms, bathrooms, waiting rooms; available at https://www.thehotline.org/stakeholders/download-and-request-materials/

ADDITIONAL THERAPIES

Rape Abuse & Incest National Network (RAINN) Hotline: 1-800-656-HOPE (4673)

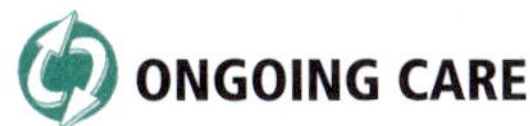

ONGOING CARE

FOLLOW-UP RECOMMENDATIONS

Schedule prompt follow-up appointment. Inquire about what occurred since last visit. Offer ongoing support and resources.

PATIENT EDUCATION

- Counsel patients about nonviolent ways to resolve conflict and about the cycle of violence
- CDC: https://www.cdc.gov/intimate-partner-violence/about/index.html
- National Domestic Violence Hotline: thehotline.org
- National Coalition Against Domestic Violence: ncadv.org
- National Resource Center on Domestic Violence: nrcdv.org

PROGNOSIS

Victims of IPV can suffer from PTSD, anxiety, and depression. Counseling, support, and resources can improve their prognosis.

REFERENCES

1. Kyle J. Intimate partner violence. *Med Clin North Am*. 2023;107(2):385–395.
2. Moyer VA; for U.S. Preventive Services Task Force. Screening for intimate partner violence and abuse of elderly and vulnerable adults: U.S. Preventive Services Task Force recommendation statement. *Ann Intern Med*. 2013;158(6):478–486.
3. Dicola D, Spaar E. Intimate partner violence. *Am Fam Physician*. 2016;94(8):646–651.

ADDITIONAL READING

- Thackeray JD, Hibbard R, Dowd MD; for Committee on Child Abuse and Neglect, Committee on Injury, Violence, and Poison Prevention. Intimate partner violence: the role of the pediatrician. *Pediatrics*. 2010;125(5):1094–1100.
- Perone HR, Dietz NA, Belkowitz J, et al. Intimate partner violence: analysis of current screening practices in the primary care setting. *Fam Pract*. 2022;39(1):6–11.

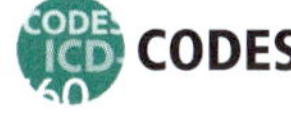

CODES

ICD10

- T74.91XA Unspecified adult maltreatment, confirmed, initial encounter
- T74.11XA Adult physical abuse, confirmed, initial encounter
- T74.31XA Adult psychological abuse, confirmed, initial encounter

CLINICAL PEARLS

- Display resource materials in the office (e.g., posting abuse awareness posters/National Domestic Violence Hotline, 1-800-799-SAFE, in both English and Spanish, in all exam rooms and restrooms).
- Given the high prevalence of IPV and the lack of harm and potential benefits of screening, routine screening is recommended.
- For those who screened positive, offer resources, reassure confidentiality, and provide close follow-up.

IRRITABLE BOWEL SYNDROME

Marie L. Borum, MD, EdD, MPH • Mrudula Bandaru, MD, BS

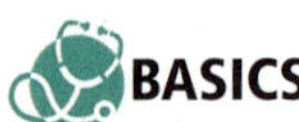

BASICS

DESCRIPTION

- A chronic functional brain-gut disorder characterized by chronic and recurrent abdominal pain and altered bowel habits in the absence of an organic cause; more common in patients aged <50 years and in women
- May be characterized as diarrhea-predominant (IBS-D), constipation-predominant (IBS-C), mixed (IBS-M), or unclassified (IBS-U); may alternate between symptoms

EPIDEMIOLOGY

Irritable bowel syndrome (IBS) accounts for 25–50% of visits to gastroenterologists and ~2 million primary care visits annually in United States with estimated cost of $1.5 to 10 billion/year.

Incidence

1–2% per year

Prevalence

- Pooled estimate of ~4% globally using Rome IV criteria or 10% globally using Rome III criteria
- Predominant age: 20 to 39 years. If age >50 years, consider other diagnoses. In the United States, affects 10–15% of the population. In the United States, female > male (3:1). Females more likely to have IBS-C as compared to males.
- More common in low socioeconomic communities

ETIOLOGY AND PATHOPHYSIOLOGY

- IBS pathophysiology is multifactorial and complex; linked to abnormal motility, inflammation, alterations in the gut microbiome, and increased visceral sensitivity. Triggers may include luminal contractions, delayed transit, or environmental factors.
- Postinfectious IBS (PI-IBS) occurs in ~10% after infectious enteritis. Risk is 6 times higher postinfection. Causes may include malabsorption, increased enteroendocrine cells/lymphocytes or antibiotic use.
- Food sensitivity, microbiome dysbiosis, genetic, and psychosocial causes including early childhood stress are under study. Biopsies show increased mast cell and lymphocyte activity in the ileum, jejunum, and colon, possibly tied to visceral hypersensitivity (1).
- Elevated pro-inflammatory cytokines are observed and may reflect gut inflammation.
- Ongoing studies are exploring low-grade mucosal/neural inflammation and its role in "brain-gut" axis dysfunction (1).

Genetics

Unknown; some studies suggest a genetic susceptibility relatives of someone with IBS are 2 to 3 times more likely to have IBS. Further research is still required.

RISK FACTORS

Female sex (odds ratio 1.67), other family members with similar GI disorder; psychological factors: stress, abuse history, anxiety, depression, or somatization; somatic factors: GI infection, pain syndromes, obesity, antibiotic use, and abdominal surgery; social factors: socioeconomic status in childhood

Pediatric Considerations

No risk to mother or fetus

GENERAL PREVENTION

See "Diet" section.

COMMONLY ASSOCIATED CONDITIONS

- Other functional GI disorders (heartburn, dyspepsia, GERD, nausea, diarrhea, incontinence, pelvic floor dyssynergia, and constipation)
- Chronic conditions including migraines, fibromyalgia, chronic pelvic pain, temporomandibular joint dysfunction, chronic fatigue syndrome, sleep disorders, noncardiac chest pain, and overactive bladder
- Psychiatric disorders: major depression, anxiety, and somatoform disorders

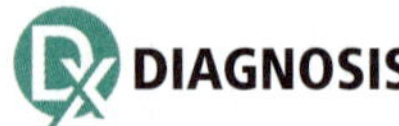

DIAGNOSIS

HISTORY

- Rome IV criteria: recurrent abdominal pain >1 day/week, on average, in the previous 3 months with an onset >6 months before diagnosis associated with at least two of the following:
  - Related to defecation
  - Change in frequency of stools
  - Change in form (appearance) of stools
- Four bowel patterns in the Rome IV classification:
  - IBS-D: >25% diarrhea with Bristol stool type 6 or 7 and <25% constipation
  - IBS-C: >25% constipation with Bristol stool types 1 or 2 and <25% diarrhea
  - IBS-M: >25% constipation and >25% diarrhea
  - IBS-U: meets Rome IV criteria but not subtypes
- Patient has no warning signs (red flags).

PHYSICAL EXAM

- Complete exam to exclude other causes including digital rectal exam. Vital signs and physical exam typically unremarkable, but patients may have mild abdominal tenderness.
- There is an absence of peritoneal signs, ascites, lymph node enlargement, jaundice, and organomegaly.

DIFFERENTIAL DIAGNOSIS

- Differential diagnosis consideration in IBS is broad. With IBS-D symptoms, consider celiac disease, small intestinal bacterial overgrowth (SIBO), pancreatic insufficiency, inflammatory bowel disease (IBD), and microscopic colitis; endocrine disorders (hyperthyroidism/hypothyroidism, Addison disease, diabetes mellitus); lactose intolerance; fructose malabsorption; infections (*Giardia lamblia, Entamoeba histolytica, Salmonella, Campylobacter, Yersinia, Clostridium difficile*)
- Medication induced: opioid constipation, laxative abuse; magnesium antacids; somatization; depression; villus adenoma, endocrine tumors (gastrinoma or carcinoid); radiation damage to colon or small bowel

DIAGNOSTIC TESTS & INTERPRETATION

- No definitive diagnostic laboratory test for IBS; use a positive diagnostic strategy, not diagnosis of exclusion. With a typical history and no warning signs (e.g., anemia, weight loss, nocturnal diarrhea, family history of colorectal cancer/IBD/celiac sprue), obtain CBC and age-appropriate colorectal cancer screening
- For IBS-D evaluation: fecal calprotectin or lactoferrin, basic metabolic profile; stool O&P; *Giardia* antigen; *Clostridium difficile* toxin)
- For IBS-C evaluation: Consider abdominal to assess stool burden.
- Plasma anti-cytolethal distending toxin B (anti-CdtB) and anti-vinculin antibodies may be elevated in IBS-D and IBS-M but not in IBS-C. Diagnostic value is still under investigation.

Initial Tests (lab, imaging)

Rule out pathology specific to the patient's symptoms:

- IBS-D: CRP, IgA tissue transglutaminase (rule out celiac disease) with IgA level, fecal calprotectin or fecal lactoferrin, thyroid-stimulating hormone (TSH), and stool for ova and parasites
- IBS-C: TSH, electrolytes, calcium (hyperparathyroidism); abdominal pain: LFTs, lipase or amylase
- In the absence of alarm symptoms, labs such a fecal calprotectin (<40 μg/g) are considered sufficient to effectively rule out IBD. CRP (<0.5 mg/dL) and fecal lactoferrin (<7 μg/g) can be used as an alternative (2).
- Consider hydrogen breath testing to exclude bacterial overgrowth. In patients who do not respond to treatment consider further evaluation with imaging (ultrasound or CT), endoscopy, video capsule endoscopy, or sitz marker study.

Follow-Up Tests & Special Considerations

- Consider lactulose breath test to assess for SIBO associated with IBS.
- Consider colonoscopy in patients at high risk for microscopic colitis (female gender, >60 years old, and more intense diarrhea).

Diagnostic Procedures/Other

- In patients with diarrhea, sigmoidoscopy/colonoscopy with biopsies may be used to rule out IBD or microscopic colitis.
- Abdominal radiograph to assess for severity of stool burden in IBS-C or if concern for a structure lesion. Additional imaging may be considered including pelvic imaging and/or abdominal CT scan.
- Physiologic testing (anorectal manometry and balloon expulsion) to rule out dyssynergic defecation in patients with severe constipation refractory to dietary change and osmotic laxative therapy

ALERT

- Screen all persons >45 years of age (or those with warning signs/red flags) for colorectal cancer.
- Red flag signs: age of onset >50 years, rectal bleeding or melena, nocturnal diarrhea, progressive abdominal pain, unexplained weight loss, laboratory abnormalities

TREATMENT

- Main goals: Relieve symptoms and improve quality of life (3). Therapy should be aimed at specific subtype of IBS. Establishing a productive clinician–patient relationship aids in the management of all patients with IBS.
- Low fermentable oligosaccharides, disaccharides, mono saccharides, and polyps (FODMAP) diet is recommended.
- Soluble fiber helpful (particularly if constipation)
- Psychosocial therapy: Goal should be to decrease stress and anxiety.
- Lifestyle modification
  - Exercise 3 to 5 times per week decreases severity (3).
  - Food diary to determine triggers (3)

MEDICATION

- Soluble fiber (psyllium 3 to 4 g/day) increases stool bulk; in all types of IBS helps both constipation and diarrhea but not abdominal pain (2)[B]; has been shown to improve both constipation and diarrhea in patients with all types of IBS
- For all types of IBS:
  - Antispasmodics: hyoscyamine 0.125 to 0.250 mg PO/SL q4h PRN and dicyclomine 20 to 40 mg PO BID
    - Side effects: dry mouth, dizziness, and blurred vision; used as needed
  - Tricyclic antidepressants (TCAs): Start at the lowest dose; mainly used for IBS-D due to ability to slow intestinal transit time; multimodal mechanism of action in IBS.
    - Side effects: dry mouth, insomnia, flushing, and palpitations; Numbers needed to treat (NNT) is 4.5. Numbers needed to harm (NNH) ranges from 9 to 18.
- IBS-D
  - Loperamide (4 to 8 mg/day up to TID PRN) decreases stool frequency and increase stool consistency (use in limited doses and as needed for patients with IBS-M); may also use diphenoxylate and atropine
  - Bile acid sequestrants (cholestyramine, colestipol, and colesevelam) for suspected bile acid malabsorption
  - Rifaximin (2-week course) improves bloating, pain, and stool consistency; favorable safety profile with an NNH of 8,971; reserved for patients who failed to respond to other therapies
  - Alosetron (Lotronex; 0.5 to 1.0 mg PO BID) is a 5-HT_3 antagonist; slows gut transit; indicated for women with IBS-D ≥6 months unresponsive to standard therapy
  - Ondansetron reduces stool consistency, frequency and urgency; no significant effect on pain
  - Eluxadoline (75 to 100 mg BID) is a mixed opioid receptor agonist and antagonist; used for severe IBS-D refractory to all other agents; side effect: acute pancreatitis
- IBS-C
  - Laxatives such as polyethylene glycol (17 g of powder dissolved in 8 oz of water, daily) may improve stool frequency and constipation but not pain.
  - Antibiotics such as neomycin
  - Lubiprostone (8 μg BID with meals) is a prostaglandin E1 analog; increases intestinal secretion and peristalsis; NNT of 12.5; side effects: nausea and diarrhea
  - Linaclotide (290 μg QD) is a guanylate cyclase 2C agonist; improves bowel function and reduces abdominal pain and overall severity in adults only; NNT of 6
  - Plecanatide (3 mg QD) approved for IBS-C; increases intestinal transit and fluid content; comparable to linaclotide; NNT of 9
  - Tenapanor (50 mg BID) is a sodium/hydrogen exchanger 3 (NHE3) inhibitor; reduces absorption of sodium and phosphate and increases intestinal fluid volume and transit
- Mixed: Use medications to match symptoms.

First Line

- IBS-D: trial loperamide with dose titrated based on response
- IBS-C: Modify lifestyle and diet habits and slowly introduce fiber supplementation (percutaneous endoscopic gastrostomy [PEG]).

Second Line

- If loperamide fails for IBS-D: trial bile acid sequestrants, rifaximin, alosetron
- If PEG fails for IBS-C: trial guanylate cyclase agonists (linaclotide, plecanatide) or NH3 inhibitors (tenapanor)

ISSUES FOR REFERRAL

- If recurring symptoms, dietician can evaluate for triggers.
- Behavioral health referral may help with management of affective, mood or personality disorders.
- Brain-gut behavioral therapies (gut-directed hypnotherapy, cognitive-behavioral therapy [CBT], mindfulness) may improve symptoms in those with mood disturbances.
- Gastroenterology referral for difficult to control cases

ADDITIONAL THERAPIES

Probiotics are not routinely recommended, although they have been associated with an improvement in symptoms.

COMPLEMENTARY & ALTERNATIVE MEDICINE

Herbal/natural remedies: widely marketed, but no clear evidence of benefit

ONGOING CARE

FOLLOW-UP RECOMMENDATIONS

Patient Monitoring

The IBS Severity Scoring System is validated to assess severity response to treatment.

DIET

- A low FODMAP diet; avoid large meals, fatty foods, gas-producing foods, and caffeine, which can exacerbate symptoms.
- Increase fiber slowly.
- Initially, consider 2 weeks of lactose-free diet to rule out lactose intolerance.
- A gluten-free diet may resolve symptoms for some patients despite negative testing for celiac disease (nonceliac gluten sensitivity). However, studies have shown inconclusive evidence.

PATIENT EDUCATION

IBS is not a psychiatric illness but is a chronic condition with no increased risk of malignancy. A broad approach is necessary to ensure all potential causes are evaluated.

PROGNOSIS

- IBS is a chronic relapsing disorder that reduces quality of life but does not increase mortality.
- Evidence suggests that "symptom shifting" occurs in some patients, whereby resolution of functional bowel symptoms is followed by the development of functional symptoms in another system.

REFERENCES

1. Lacy BE, Pimentel M, Brenner DM, et al. ACG clinical guideline: management of irritable bowel syndrome. *Am J Gastroenterol*. 2021;116(1):17–44.
2. Lembo A, Sultan S, Chang L, et al. AGA Clinical practice guideline on the pharmacological management of irritable bowel syndrome with diarrhea. *Gastroenterology*. 2022;163(1):137–151. doi:10.1053/j.gastro.2022.04.017.
3. Jayasinghe M, Damianos JA, Prathiraja O, et al. Irritable bowel syndrome: treating the gut and brain/mind at the same time. *Cureus*. 2023;15(8):e43404. doi:10.7759/cureus.43404.

ADDITIONAL READING

Greer KB, Sultan S. Irritable bowel syndrome. *Ann Intern Med*. 2025;178:ITC113-ITC128. doi:10.7326/ANNALS-25-01965.

SEE ALSO

Algorithm: Diarrhea, Chronic

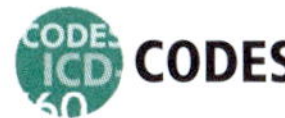

CODES

ICD10

- K58.9 Irritable bowel syndrome without diarrhea
- K58.0 Irritable bowel syndrome with diarrhea
- K58 Irritable bowel syndrome

CLINICAL PEARLS

- Use Rome IV criteria to establish the diagnosis of IBS.
- Goals of treatment are to relieve symptoms and improve quality of life.
- Many patients can successfully manage their symptoms with attention to their dietary triggers. IBS subtype directed medical therapy is indicated if lifestyle/diet modifications do not improve symptoms.
- If patients do not respond to initial treatment, consider further evaluation (including imaging and/or referral for endoscopy) to exclude organic pathology.

KAWASAKI SYNDROME

Khadija Kabani, DO, FAAFP • Caroline Kelley, DO

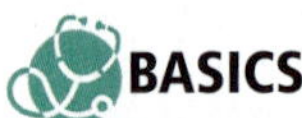

BASICS

DESCRIPTION

- Kawasaki syndrome (KS) is a self-limited acute, febrile, systemic vasculitis of small- and medium-sized arteries that predominantly affects patients aged 6 months to 5 years.
- The most prominent cause of acquired coronary artery disease in children in developed countries (1)
- Vasculitis of coronary arteries results in aneurysms/ectasia, myocardial infarction (MI)/ischemia or sudden death.
- System(s) affected: cardiovascular, gastrointestinal, hematologic/lymphatic/immunologic, musculoskeletal, nervous, pulmonary, renal/urologic, skin/exocrine

ALERT

Consider in any child with extended high fever unresponsive to antibiotics or antipyretics, rash, and nonexudative conjunctivitis.

EPIDEMIOLOGY

Incidence

- Worldwide: affects all races but most prevalent in Asia; Japan annual incidence rate 265/100,000 in children <5 years old
- In the United States, annual incidence in children aged <5 years is 20/100,000 with the highest prevalence observed among children of Asian and Pacific Islander heritage.
- Leading cause of acquired heart disease in children in developed countries
  - Predominant age: 1 to 5 years; median age of diagnosis is 1.5 years.
  - 85% of cases are children <5 years of age and 50% <2 years of age.

Prevalence

- Highest to lowest prevalence: Asian > African American > Hispanic > White
- Seasonal variation: peaks in winter and early spring (January to March) in temperate places; peaks in summer in Asia
- Outbreaks at 2- to 3-year intervals

ETIOLOGY AND PATHOPHYSIOLOGY

- Etiology is largely unknown; however, recent studies have shown specific genetic markers may predispose some children.
- Infectious agent triggers abnormal inflammatory reaction in children with genetic predisposition.
- Acute KS causes a necrotizing arteritis in the smooth muscle layer of medium extraparenchymal arteries, destroying arterial walls into the adventitia, especially in coronary arteries.

Genetics

- Populations at higher risk and family link suggest a genetic predisposition.
- Siblings of patients in Japan have a 10- to 30-fold increased risk, and >50% develop KS within 10 days of first case; increased occurrence of KS in children whose parents also had illness in childhood
- Single-nucleotide polymorphisms in six different genes have been implicated in KS (Fcγ receptor 2A, CASP3, HLA class II, B-cell lymphoid kinase, ITPKC, CD40).
- Coronary aneurisms are associated with variants in TGF-β signaling pathways.

RISK FACTORS

- Male to female prevalence 1.5:1 in the United States
- African Americans at 1.5 times risk; Asian Americans at 2.5 times risk
- Sibling with Kawasaki

DIAGNOSIS

- ≥5 days of fever and ≥4 of the following five principal clinical features (1); *or* <4 features and presence of coronary artery disease on 2D echocardiography:
  - Bilateral, nonpurulent conjunctival injection with limbic sparing
  - Erythematous changes to mouth, pharynx, tongue, and lips
  - A polymorphous, generalized, erythematous rash
  - Changes in the skin of the peripheral extremities (edema of hands/feet; erythema of palms/soles; desquamation of fingers/toes)
  - Cervical lymphadenopathy (>1 node >1.5 cm in diameter)
- Note: Diagnosis can be made at day 4 of fever in a patient with >4 principal clinical features, especially if redness/swelling of hands/feet is present.

Pediatric Considerations

- Prolonged fever without rash that is treated with antibiotics and followed by a rash may appear to be a drug reaction.
- Incomplete KS (atypical KS)
  - ≥5 days of fever, two to three principal clinical features, labs indicating systemic inflammation, and exclusion of other diseases
  - Incomplete cases with <4 clinical criteria often occur in infants ≤6 months of age or older children/adolescents. The frequency of coronary artery aneurysms (CAAs) is higher in patients with missed diagnosis/delayed treatment. Therefore, in infants with prolonged fever and few clinical features, consider echocardiography and inflammatory labs.

HISTORY

- Fever is the first sign during the acute phase.
- Symptoms may not occur all at once but usually occur in close proximity.

PHYSICAL EXAM

- High-spiking and remittent fever for ≥5 days
  - Fever is high (102 to 105 °F [39.4 to 40.5 °C]) and unresponsive to antibiotics/antipyretics.
  - May be prolonged up to 10 to 12 days with more rare cases lasting 3 to 4 weeks (1)
- Bilateral, painless, nonpurulent, conjunctival injection without corneal ulceration or edema; limbic sparing
- Changes in lips and oral cavity: redness and swelling of lips in the acute stage; cracking, fissuring, bleeding in subacute phase; strawberry/erythematous tongue
- Extensive erythematous polymorphous rash: within 5 days of fever
  - Morbilliform is most common; may be maculopapular, scarlatiniform; can resemble erythema multiforme, erythroderma, urticarial exanthem; rarely micropustular
  - Perineal desquamation, especially in skin folds
- Extremity changes: reddened palms and soles on days 3 to 5; edema of hands and feet on days 4 to 7; painful induration; desquamation of fingers and toes that begins in periungual area at 2 to 3 weeks
- Acute, unilateral cervical lymphadenopathy (least common symptom): ≥1 lymph nodes >1.5 cm, firm, nonfluctuant, and slight tenderness
- Cardiac exam: tachycardia, gallop rhythms, hyperdynamic precordium, innocent flow murmurs, depressed contractility
- Other organ system involvement
  - Cardiovascular: myocarditis; pericarditis (often subclinical), CAAs, and other medium-sized arterial aneurysms
  - Gastrointestinal: anorexia, abdominal pain, vomiting/diarrhea, acute gallbladder hydrops, hepatic enlargement, jaundice
  - Renal: proteinuria, sterile pyuria
  - Joints: polyarthritis of small joints in acute phase; weight-bearing joints affected after 10th day from onset of fever
  - Neurologic: aseptic meningitis, peripheral neuropathy (unilateral facial palsy), transient high-frequency hearing loss

DIFFERENTIAL DIAGNOSIS

- Bacterial: scarlet fever, bacterial cervical lymphadenitis, *Mycoplasma* infection, leptospirosis, Lyme disease, Rocky Mountain spotted fever
- Toxin mediated: staphylococcal scalded-skin syndrome, streptococcal scarlet fever, toxic shock syndrome (1)
- Viral: measles, adenovirus, Epstein-Barr virus, SARS-CoV-2; multisystem inflammatory syndrome in children (MIS-C) is a rare but serious complication of COVID-19 (2).
- Toxoplasmosis
- Reiter syndrome
- Hypersensitivity drug reactions (erythema multiforme minor, Stevens-Johnson syndrome)
- Juvenile rheumatoid arthritis
- Acrodynia (mercury poisoning)

DIAGNOSTIC TESTS & INTERPRETATION

- Initial workup: CBC with differential, urinalysis (UA)/culture, liver function tests including AST, ALT, and albumin, blood culture; lumbar puncture if signs of meningitis or if <90 days old
  - Leukocytosis with immature and mature granulocytes
  - Anemia: normochromic, normocytic
  - Thrombocytosis (500,000 to >1,000,000/mm^3) in 2nd and 3rd week; thrombocytopenia during acute phase is associated with CAA and MI.
- Elevated C-reactive protein (CRP) (>35 mg/L in 80% cases), erythrocyte sedimentation rate (ESR) (>60 mm/hour in 60% cases), and α1-antitrypsin
- Normal ESR, CRP, and PLTs after day 7 suggest diagnosis other than KS.
- ESR can be artificially high after intravenous immunoglobulin (IVIG) therapy.

- Hyponatremia
- Moderately elevated AST, ALT, GGT, and bilirubin
- Decreased albumin and protein
- CSF pleocytosis may be seen.
- Nasal swab to rule out adenovirus, coronavirus (SARS-CoV-2)

Initial Tests (lab, imaging)

- If KS is suspected, obtain ECG and echocardiogram (3)[B].
  - ECG may show arrhythmias, prolonged PR interval, and ST/T wave changes.
  - Echocardiography detects abnormalities of vessels and aneurysm.
  - Cardiac stress test if CAA seen on echocardiogram
- Baseline chest x-ray may show pleural effusion, atelectasis, and congestive heart failure.

Diagnostic Procedures/Other

- No laboratory study is diagnostic; diagnosis rests on constellation of clinical features and exclusion of other illnesses.
- Magnetic resonance coronary angiography is noninvasive modality to visualize coronary arteries for stenosis, thrombi, and intimal thickening.
- Patients with complex coronary artery lesions (CALs) may benefit from coronary angiography after the acute inflammatory process has resolved; generally recommended in 6 to 12 months

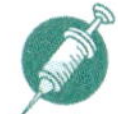

TREATMENT

GENERAL MEASURES

Use antibiotics until bacterial etiologies are excluded (e.g., sepsis or meningitis).

MEDICATION

- Optimal therapy is IVIG 2 g/kg IV >10 to 12 hours with high-dose aspirin preferably within 7 to 10 days of fever (3)[A], followed by low-dose aspirin until follow-up echocardiograms indicate a lack of coronary abnormalities.
  - IVIG lowers the risk of CAA, can shorten fever duration, and improve irritability.
  - CALs develop in 3–5% of children treated with IVIG. CALs develop in up to 25% of untreated children (1).
- Retreatment with IVIG if clinical response is incomplete or fever persists/returns >36 hours after start of IVIG treatment
  - 2/3 of nonresponders respond to the second dose of IVIG.
- Aspirin 80 to 100 mg/kg/day in 4 doses beginning with IVIG administration (3)[C]; switch to low-dose aspirin (3 to 5 mg/kg/day) when afebrile for 48 to 72 hours. Maintain low dose for 6 to 8 weeks until follow-up echocardiogram is normal and CRP and/or ESR are normal.
- Children with larger aneurysms may necessitate both aspirin and anticoagulant therapy (2).
- Aspirin does not appear to reduce CAA.
- Corticosteroids have conflicting evidence for use and:
  - Should not be used as first-line agent in all KS patients; reserve for IVIG resistant cases
  - Longer course of corticosteroids together with IVIG and aspirin can be used for highest risk of IVIG failure (3)[B].
- Contraindications
  - IVIG: documented hypersensitivity, IgA deficiency, anti-IgE/IgG antibodies, severe thrombocytopenia, coagulation disorders
  - Aspirin: vitamin K deficiency, bleeding disorders, liver damage, documented hypersensitivity, hypoprothrombinemia
- Precautions
  - High-dose aspirin therapy can result in tinnitus, decreased of renal function, and increased transaminases.
  - Do not use ibuprofen in children with CAAs who are taking aspirin for antiplatelet effects.
  - Yearly influenza vaccination is recommended for children requiring long-term treatment with aspirin. Delay any live vaccines for 11 months after IVIG treatment.

First Line

High dose IVIG and aspirin should be instituted promptly upon established diagnosis (1).

Second Line

- In patients refractory to IVIG, consider a second dose of IVIG in patients with persistent fever at least 36 hours after first IVIG dose or high-dose pulse steroids (3)[B].
- Infliximab and/or cyclosporin (3)[C]
- Immunomodulatory monoclonal antibody therapy (except TNF-α blockers), cytotoxic agents, or rarely plasma exchange in highly refractory patients (3)[C].

ISSUES FOR REFERRAL

- Pediatric cardiologist if abnormalities on echo or if extensive stenosis
- Pediatric hematology if anticoagulant therapy could be of benefit

ADDITIONAL THERAPIES

Antiplatelet agents (clopidogrel, dipyridamole), heparin, low-molecular-weight heparin, or warfarin are sometimes added to the low-dose aspirin regimen, depending on severity of CAAs.

SURGERY/OTHER PROCEDURES

- Rarely needed; coronary artery bypass grafting for severe obstruction/recurrent MI
- Coronary revascularization via percutaneous coronary intervention for patients with evidence of ischemia on stress testing

ADMISSION, INPATIENT, AND NURSING CONSIDERATIONS

Consider discharge if afebrile after IVIG treatment for >24 hours and clinical improvement.

ONGOING CARE

FOLLOW-UP RECOMMENDATIONS

With aneurysms, contact and high-risk sports should be avoided.

Patient Monitoring

- Follow up with primary care physician within 1 week of discharge. Follow up with cardiology within 2 weeks of discharge.
- Patients with complex CALs may require a combination of β-blockers to decrease oxidative stress and antithrombotic therapy (1). These patients may benefit from coronary angiography at 6 to 12 months.
- Patients receiving long-term ASA should be fully immunized (1).

PROGNOSIS

- Usually self-limited
- Relates entirely to the extent and severity of cardiac disease (1)
- Moderate-sized aneurysms usually regress in 1 to 2 years, resolving in 50–66% of cases.
- Recurrence (3% in Japan, <1% in the United States)
- Sudden death in early adulthood (rare)

COMPLICATIONS

- 15–25% of untreated patients develop CAAs in convalescent phase.
- 2–7% of treated patients develop aneurysms. 1% develop giant aneurysms.
- Risk factors for aneurysm: male, <1 year of age, ↑ ESR >4 weeks, fever >2 weeks, fever >48 hours after IVIG treatment
- Mortality of 0.08–0.17% is due to cardiac disease.

REFERENCES

1. Son MBF, Newburger JW. Kawasaki disease. *Pediatr Rev*. 2018;39(2):78–90.
2. Selmek K, Harding M. Kawasaki disease. *Pediatr Rev*. 2024;45(7):425–427.
3. McCrindle BW, Rowley AH, Newburger JW, et al. Diagnosis, treatment, and long-term management of Kawasaki disease: a scientific statement for health professionals from the American Heart Association. *Circulation*. 2017;135(17):e927–e999. doi:10.1161/CIR.0000000000000484.

ADDITIONAL READING

- Jone PN, Tremoulet A, Choueiter N, et al. Update on diagnosis and management of Kawasaki disease: a scientific statement from the American Heart Association. *Circulation*. 2024;150(23):e481–e500.
- Most ZM, Hendren N, Drazner MH, et al. Striking similarities of multisystem inflammatory syndrome in children and a myocarditis—like syndrome in adults: overlapping manifestations of COVID-19. *Circulation*. 2021;143(1):4–6. doi:10.1161/CIRCULATIONAHA.120.050166.
- Rife E, Gedalia A. Kawasaki disease: an update. *Curr Rheumatol Rep*. 2020;22(10):75. doi:10.1007/s11926-020-00941-4.

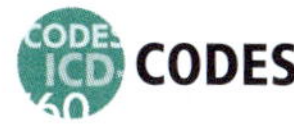

CODES

ICD10

M30.3 Mucocutaneous lymph node syndrome [Kawasaki]

CLINICAL PEARLS

- The diagnosis of KS rests on a constellation of clinical features.
- Once KS is suspected, all patients need an inpatient cardiac evaluation, including ECG and echocardiogram.
- Optimal therapy is IVIG 2 g/kg IV over 8 to 12 hours, with high-dose aspirin 80 to 100 mg/kg/day until patient afebrile 48 to 72 hours (3).

KERATOACANTHOMA

Emily M. Meara, MD • Ryan Svoboda, MD, MS

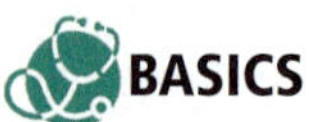

BASICS

DESCRIPTION

- Most commonly presents as a solitary, rapidly proliferating, dome-shaped, erythematous or flesh-colored papule or nodule with a central keratinous plug, typically reaching 1 to 2 cm in diameter
- Clinically and microscopically resembles squamous cell carcinoma (SCC)
- Considered by some to be a low-grade variant of SCC
- Other presentations include grouped, multiple, keratoacanthoma (KA) centrifugum marginatum, intraoral, subungual, regressing, nonregressing, and generally eruptive (1).
- Some lesions may resolve spontaneously, but lesions do have the potential for invasion and metastasis; therefore, treatment is required.
- Three clinical stages of KAs (1):
  - Proliferative: rapid growth of the lesion over weeks to several months
  - Maturation/stabilization: Lesion stabilizes and growth subsides.
  - Involution: spontaneous resolution of the lesion, leaving a hypopigmented, depressed scar; most but not all lesions will enter this stage.
- System(s) affected: integumentary

EPIDEMIOLOGY

- Greatest incidence age >50 years but may occur at any age.
- Presentation increases during summer and early fall seasons.
- Most frequently on sun-exposed and hair-bearing skin, but may occur anywhere
- Predominant sex: male > female (2:1)
- Most commonly in fair-skinned individuals; highest rates in Fitzpatrick skin type I to III
- 104 cases per 100,000 individuals

ETIOLOGY AND PATHOPHYSIOLOGY

- Derived from an abnormality causing hyperkeratosis within the follicular infundibulum
- Squamous epithelial cells proliferate to extend upward around the keratin plug and proceed downward into the dermis. This process is followed by invasion of elastic and collagen fibers.
- Cellular mechanism responsible for the hyperkeratosis is currently unknown. The role of human papillomavirus (HPV) has been discussed but has no established causality (2).
- Regression may be due to immune cytotoxicity or terminal differentiation of keratinocytes.
- Multiple etiologic factors have been implicated:
  - UV radiation
  - May be provoked by surgery, cryotherapy, chemical peels, or laser therapy
  - Viral infections: HPV or Merkel cell polyomavirus
  - Genetic predisposition: Muir-Torre syndrome, xeroderma pigmentosum, Ferguson-Smith syndrome
  - Immunosuppression
  - BRAF inhibitors (1)
  - Chemical carcinogen exposure

Genetics

- Mutation of *p53* or *H-ras*
- Ferguson-Smith (AD)
- Witten-Zak (AD)
- Muir-Torre (AD)
- Xeroderma pigmentosum (AR)
- Gzybowski (sporadic)
- Incontinentia pigmenti (XLD)

RISK FACTORS

- UV exposure/damage: outdoor and/or indoor tanning
- Fitzpatrick skin type I to III
- Trauma (typically appears within 1 month of injury): laser resurfacing, surgery, cryotherapy, tattoos
- Chemical carcinogens: tar, pitch, and smoking
- Immunocompromised state (e.g., solid organ transplant)
- Discoid lupus erythematosus lesions/burn scars
- HPV infection

GENERAL PREVENTION

Multimodal ultraviolet protection measures

COMMONLY ASSOCIATED CONDITIONS

- Frequently, the patient has concurrent sun-damaged skin and other conditions associated with heavy sun exposure: solar elastosis, solar lentigines, actinic keratosis, nonmelanoma skin cancers (basal cell carcinoma, SCC).
- In Muir-Torre syndrome, patients have an increased risk of developing KAs, sebaceous neoplasms, and malignancy of the GI and GU tracts; may have sebaceous differentiation (seboacanthoma)

DIAGNOSIS

HISTORY

- Lesion typically begins as a small, solitary, pink papule that undergoes a rapid growth phase, classically reaching a diameter of 1 to 2 cm, although size may vary.
- Once the proliferative stage has subsided, the lesion size generally remains stable.
- May decrease in size, indicating regression
- Usually asymptomatic, although occasionally tender
- If multiple lesions present, important to elicit a family history and recent therapies or treatments
- If sebaceous neoplasms present, must review history for signs/symptoms of GI or GU malignancies (e.g., Mayo Muir-Torre syndrome risk score)

PHYSICAL EXAM

- Firm, solitary, erythematous or flesh-colored, dome-shaped papule or nodule with a central keratin plug, giving a crateriform appearance
- Surrounding skin and borders of lesion may show telangiectasia, atrophy, or dyspigmentation.
- Usually solitary; multiple lesions can occur.
- Most commonly seen on sun-exposed areas: face, neck, scalp, dorsum of upper extremities, and posterior legs
- May also be seen on areas without sun exposure: buttocks, anus, subungual, mucosal surfaces
- Subungual KAs are typically very painful and seen on the first 3 digits of the hands.
- Examine for regional lymphadenopathy due to risk of metastasis.
- Dermoscopy (3)
  - Central keratin highest sensitivity to distinguish from SCC
  - White circles, blood spots; white circles highest specificity
  - Cannot reliably distinguish between KA and classic SCC

DIFFERENTIAL DIAGNOSIS

- SCC
- Nodular or ulcerative basal cell carcinoma
- Cutaneous horn
- Hypertrophic actinic keratosis
- Amelanotic melanoma
- Merkel cell carcinoma
- Cutaneous metastasis of carcinoma
- Molluscum contagiosum
- Prurigo nodularis
- Verruca vulgaris
- Verrucous carcinoma
- Sebaceous adenoma
- Hypertrophic lichen planus
- Hypertrophic lupus erythematosus
- Deep fungal infection
- Atypical mycobacterial infection
- Nodular Kaposi sarcoma

DIAGNOSTIC TESTS & INTERPRETATION

- Excisional biopsy, including the center of the lesion as well as the margin, is the best diagnostic test but may be impractical depending on clinical setting and scheduling constraints (2)[C].
- A shave biopsy may be insufficiently deep to distinguish a KA from an SCC.
- If unable to perform an excisional biopsy, a deep shave (saucerization) of the entire lesion, extending into the subcutaneous fat, can be performed.
- Punch biopsies should be avoided because they give an insufficient amount of tissue to represent the entire lesion.

Initial Tests (lab, imaging)

- Subungual KA: radiograph of the digit to monitor for osteolysis (cup-shaped radiolucent defect)
- Tumors with aggressive features such as perineural invasion may benefit from advanced imaging (e.g., ultrasound, CT, or MRI) to assess for regional lymphadenopathy.
- Most lesions do not require imaging.

Follow-Up Tests & Special Considerations

In most cases, follow-up testing is not required.

Diagnostic Procedures/Other

A deep shave (saucerization) or excisional biopsy is commonly sufficient for diagnosis.

Test Interpretation

- Pathology of biopsy: well-demarcated central core of keratin surrounded by well-differentiated, mildly pleomorphic, atypical squamous epithelial cells with a characteristic glassy eosinophilic cytoplasm
- Histopathology: keratin-filled crater encompassed with epithelial lips
- May see elastic and collagen fibers invading into the squamous epithelium
- Histologic differentiation of a KA from an SCC may be difficult and unreliable, although immunochemical staining for cellular protein Ki-67 may help do this.
- KAs have a greater tendency than SCCs to display fibrosis and intraepidermal abscesses of neutrophils and eosinophils.
- Regressing KA shows flattening and fibrosis at base of lesion.

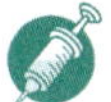

TREATMENT

- Treatment of choice is a surgical excision; however, there are several treatment options available (2)[C].
- For aggressive tumors (>2 cm) or lesions in cosmetically sensitive areas (face, digits, genitalia) that require tissue sparing, consider Mohs micrographic surgery. Mohs micrographic surgery is the treatment of choice in cases with perineural or perivascular invasion.
- Small lesions (<2 cm) of the extremities may undergo electrodesiccation and curettage (ED&C).
- Immunocompromised patients should receive expedited surgical treatment.

MEDICATION

- Nonsurgical management is a viable and relatively cost-effective option in select cases not amenable to surgery due to lesion number, size, or location; may also consider for patients with multiple comorbidities who are unwilling or unable to undergo surgery
- Evidence for the following treatments is based on case reports and retrospective reviews:
  - Intralesional methotrexate 12.5 to 25.0 mg in 0.5 mL normal saline every 2 to 3 weeks for 1 to 4 treatment sessions (4)[B]
    - Monitor for pancytopenia with complete blood count (4)[C].
  - 5% imiquimod cream 3 times per week for 11 to 13 weeks (4)[B]
  - Topical 5% 5-fluorouracil cream twice daily, 61–92% cure rate (4)[B]
  - Intralesional 5-fluorouracil of 50 mg/mL on a weekly basis for 3 to 8 treatment sessions—98% cure rate (4)[B]
  - Intralesional IFN α-2a or α-2b (83%, 100% cure rate, respectively) (4)[B]
  - Intralesional bleomycin—100% cure rate (4)[B]
  - Isotretinoin oral 0.5 to 1.0 mg/kg/day

ISSUES FOR REFERRAL

Dermatology referral if lesions are >2 cm, numerous, mucosal, or subungual

ADDITIONAL THERAPIES

- Photodynamic therapy with methyl aminolevulinic acid and red light; successful case reports (1)[B] but also reported aggravation following treatment
- Cryotherapy (1)
- Argon or YAG lasers
- Radiotherapy, primary or adjuvant: KAs may regress with low doses of radiation but may require doses up to 25 to 50 Gy in low-dose (5 to 10 Gy) fractions for possible SCC (1)[B].
- Erlotinib (EGFR inhibitor) 150 mg daily for 21 days, single case report (1)[B]

SURGERY/OTHER PROCEDURES

Excisional and office-based procedures as discussed above.

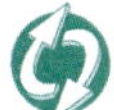

ONGOING CARE

FOLLOW-UP RECOMMENDATIONS

After the surgical site has healed or lesion has resolved, patient should initially be seen every 6 months due to increased risk of developing new lesions or skin cancers; monitor annually at minimum going forward (3)[C].

Patient Monitoring

- Skin self-exams should be routinely performed with detailed instructions (see "Additional Reading").
- If multiple KAs are present in patient or family members, evaluate for Muir-Torre syndrome and obtain a colonoscopy beginning at age 25 years, as well as testing for genitourinary cancer (3)[C].

PATIENT EDUCATION

- Sun protection measures: sun block with SPF >30, wide-brimmed hats, long sleeves, dark clothing, avoiding indoor tanning
- Arc welding may produce harmful UV radiation and skin should not be exposed.
- Tar, pitch, and smoking should be avoided.

PROGNOSIS

- Atrophic scarring and hypopigmentation can occur with self-resolution but may be significantly reduced by intervention.
- 52 of 445 cases (12%) spontaneously regressed without treatment and none of these recurred (2).
- 393 cases (88%) regressed following medical or excisional treatment (2).
- 445 cases are reported with no metastases or deaths attributable to the KA (2).
- 4–8% recurrence
- Mucosal and subungual lesions do not regress; must undergo treatment

REFERENCES

1. Kwiek B, Schwartz RA. Keratoacanthoma (KA): an update and review. *J Am Acad Dermatol*. 2016;74(6):1220–1233.
2. Savage JA, Maize JC Sr. Keratoacanthoma clinical behavior: a systematic review. *Am J Dermatopathol*. 2014;36(5):422–429.
3. Cavicchini S, Tourlaki A, Lunardon L, et al. Amelanotic melanoma mimicking keratoacanthoma: the diagnostic role of dermoscopy. *Int J Dermatol*. 2013;52(8):1023–1024.
4. Chitwood K, Etzkorn J, Cohen G. Topical and intralesional treatment of nonmelanoma skin cancer: efficacy and cost comparisons. *Dermatol Surg*. 2013;39(9):1306–1316.

ADDITIONAL READING

- The American Academy of Dermatology: https://www.aad.org/spot-skin-cancer/learn-about-skincancer/types-of-skin-cancer
- The Skin Cancer Foundation: https://www.skincancer.org/

SEE ALSO

Squamous Cell Carcinoma, Cutaneous

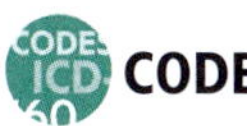

CODES

ICD10

- D23.9 Other benign neoplasm of skin, unspecified
- D48.5 Neoplasm of uncertain behavior of skin
- L85.8 Other specified epidermal thickening

CLINICAL PEARLS

- Suspect KA with a solitary, dome-shaped, erythematous or flesh-colored papule or nodule with a central keratinous plug.
- If KA is in the differential diagnosis, elicit time frame of onset during patient encounter; rapid onset supports diagnosis.
- Due to the broad differential diagnosis of a suspected KA and unreliable clinical differentiation between these, strongly consider surgical excision as first-line therapy.
- Medical and radiation therapies are reasonable and effective options available for patients who are not surgical candidates or for lesions that are not amenable for surgery.

KERATOSIS, ACTINIC

Jennifer M. Corliss, MD, FAAFP

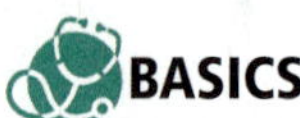

BASICS

DESCRIPTION
- Common, usually multiple, premalignant lesions on sun-exposed areas of the skin. Many resolve spontaneously, but a small proportion progress to squamous cell carcinoma (SCC).
- Common consequence of excessive cumulative ultraviolet (UV) light exposure
- Synonym(s): solar keratosis

Geriatric Considerations
Frequent problem

Pediatric Considerations
Rare (if child, look for freckling and other stigmata of xeroderma pigmentosum)

EPIDEMIOLOGY

Incidence
- Rates vary with age and exposure to sun.
- Predominant age: ≥40 years; progressively increases with age
- Predominant sex: male > female
- Common in those with blonde and red hair; rare in darker skin types

Prevalence
- Age-adjusted prevalence rate for actinic keratoses (AKs) in U.S. Caucasians is 6.5%.
- For 65- to 74-year-old males with high sun exposure: ~55%; low sun exposure: ~18%

ETIOLOGY AND PATHOPHYSIOLOGY
- The epidermal lesions are characterized by atypical keratinocytes at the basal layer with occasional extension upward. Mitoses are present. The histopathologic features resemble those of SCC in situ or SCC (the distinction depends on the extent of epidermal involvement).
- Cumulative UV exposure

Genetics
The *p53* chromosomal mutation has been shown consistently in both AKs and SCCs. Many new genes have been shown recently to have similar expression profiles in AKs and SCCs.

RISK FACTORS
- Exposure to UV light (especially long-term and/or repeated exposure due to outdoor occupation or recreational activities, indoor or outdoor tanning)
- Skin type: burns easily, does not tan
- Immunosuppression, especially organ transplantation

GENERAL PREVENTION
Sun avoidance and sun protective techniques are helpful.

COMMONLY ASSOCIATED CONDITIONS
- SCC
- Other features of chronic solar damage: lentigines, elastosis, and telangiectasias

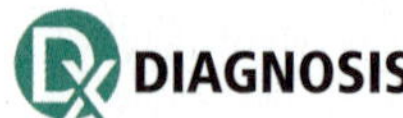

DIAGNOSIS

HISTORY
- The lesions are frequently asymptomatic; symptoms may include pruritus, burning, and mild hyperesthesia.
- Lesions may enlarge, thicken, or become more scaly. They also may regress or remain unchanged.
- Most lesions occur on the sun-exposed areas (head and neck, hands, forearms).

PHYSICAL EXAM
- Usually small (<1 cm), often multiple red, pink, or brown macules, papules, or plaques that are rough to palpation, sometimes more easily felt than seen.
- Yellow or brown adherent scale is often present on top of the lesion.
- Several clinical variants exist.
  - Atrophic: dry, scaly macules with indistinct borders and an erythematous base
  - Hypertrophic: Overlying hyperkeratosis (in an extreme form, cutaneous horn) may be impossible to differentiate from SCC clinically.
  - Pigmented: smooth tan/brown plaque, spreading centrifugally
  - Bowenoid: red scaly plaques with distinct borders
  - Actinic cheilitis: inflammatory lesion involving usually the lower lip

DIFFERENTIAL DIAGNOSIS
- SCC (hypertrophic type)
- Keratoacanthoma
- Bowen disease
- Basal cell carcinoma
- Verruca vulgaris
- Less likely: verrucous nevi, warty dyskeratoma, lichenoid keratoses, seborrheic keratoses, porokeratoses, seborrheic dermatitis or psoriasis (near hairline), lentigo maligna, solar lentigo, discoid lupus erythematosus

DIAGNOSTIC TESTS & INTERPRETATION

Diagnostic Procedures/Other
- The diagnosis is usually made clinically, unless there is a suspicion of carcinoma.
- Skin biopsy is especially recommended if large, ulcerated, indurated, or bleeding, or if the lesions are nonresponsive to treatment.

Test Interpretation
- Dysplastic keratinocytes in lower levels of epidermis with a dermal lymphocytic infiltrate
- Neoplastic cells, mostly found in the lower epidermal layers, are cytologically identical to those of SCCs.
- If neoplastic cells extend throughout entire epidermis or into the dermis, the lesions will qualify as an SCC in situ or invasive SCC, respectively.
- Malignant cells are sparse except of the bowenoid variety.
- Hypertrophic, atrophic, bowenoid, acantholytic, and pigmented varieties show the corresponding epidermal findings.

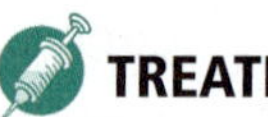

TREATMENT

- First-line treatment is cryotherapy (technically, this is considered a surgical procedure, especially by insurance companies). Medical therapy is usually reserved for multiple or extensive AKs ("field therapy").
- Cryotherapy combined with a topical approach resulted in significantly higher complete clearance rates than monotherapy (1)[A].
- A variety of topical therapies and cryosurgery are associated with long-term cure (2)[A].

GENERAL MEASURES

- Sun-protective techniques
- Sunscreens and physical sun protection recommended

MEDICATION

First Line

- Topical treatments target both visible and subclinical lesions.
- With the exception of generic 5-fluorouracil, medication cost is high ($600 to $1,200 per course).
- Topical fluorouracil (Efudex, Carac, Fluoroplex cream, Fluoroplex solution)
  - Daily or BID for 3 to 6 weeks, depending on the brand, concentration, and formulation
  - Can be very irritating
  - Likely the most effective of the topical treatments listed in this section (1)[A]
- Topical imiquimod (Aldara) 5% cream
  - Apply 2 days per week at night for up to 16 weeks to an area not larger than the forehead or one cheek.
  - Can be irritating
- Topical imiquimod (Zyclara) 3.75% cream
  - Apply once a day for 2 weeks, followed by 2 weeks of no treatment, and then apply once a day for another 2 weeks
  - Can be irritating
- Diclofenac (Solaraze) 3% gel
  - Apply BID for 60 to 90 days
  - The least irritating of the topical AK treatments, therefore patients tend to be more compliant with it

Second Line

- Topical tretinoin (Retin-A) or tazarotene (Tazorac): may be used to enhance the efficacy of topical fluorouracil
- Systemic retinoids: used infrequently
- δ-Aminolevulinate and methyl aminolevulinate combined with laser (photodynamic therapy) (see below)

ADDITIONAL THERAPIES

Close monitoring with no treatment is an appropriate option for mild lesions.

SURGERY/OTHER PROCEDURES

- Cryosurgery ("freezing," liquid nitrogen)
  - Most common method for treating AK
  - Cure rate: 75–98.8%
  - May cause atrophy and hypopigmentation
  - May be superior to photodynamic therapy for thicker lesions
- Photodynamic therapy with a photosensitizer (e.g., aminolevulinic acid) and "blue light"
  - May clear >90% of AKs
  - Less scarring than cryotherapy
  - May be superior to cryotherapy, especially in the case of more extensive skin involvement
- Curettage and electrocautery (electrodesiccation and curettage [ED&C]; "scraping and burning")
- Medium-depth peels, especially for the treatment of extensive areas
- CO_2 laser therapy
- Dermabrasion
- Surgical excision (excisional biopsy)

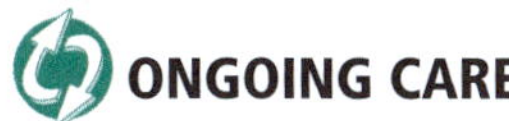

ONGOING CARE

FOLLOW-UP RECOMMENDATIONS

Patient Monitoring

Depends on associated malignancy and frequency with which new AKs appear

PATIENT EDUCATION

- Teach sun-protective techniques.
  - Limit outdoor activities between 10AM and 4PM.
  - Wear protective clothing and wide-brimmed hat.
  - Proper use (including reapplication) of sunscreens with SPF >30, preferably a preparation with broad-spectrum (UV-A and UV-B) protection
- Teach self-examination of skin (melanoma, squamous cell, basal cell).
- Patient education materials
  - http://dermnetnz.org/lesions/solar-keratoses.html

PROGNOSIS

Very good; a significant proportion of the lesions may resolve spontaneously (3), with regression rates of 20–30% per lesion per year.

COMPLICATIONS

- AKs are premalignant lesions that may progress to SCCs. The rate of malignant transformation is unclear; the reported percentages vary but range from 0.1% to a few percent per year per lesion.
- Patients with AKs are at increased risk for other cutaneous malignancies.
- Approximately 60% of SCCs arise from an AK precursor.

REFERENCES

1. Heppt MV, Steeb T, Ruzicka T, et al. Cryosurgery combined with topical interventions for actinic keratosis: a systematic review and meta-analysis. *Br J Dermatol*. 2019;180(4):740–748. doi:10.1111/bjd.17435.
2. Steeb T, Wessely A, Petzold A, et al. Evaluation of long-term clearance rates of interventions for actinic keratosis: a systematic review and network meta-analysis. *JAMA Dermatol*. 2021;157(9):1066–1077.
3. Criscione VD, Weinstock MA, Naylor MF, et al; for Department of Veterans Affairs Topical Tretinoin Chemoprevention Trial Group. Actinic keratoses: natural history and risk of malignant transformation in the veterans affairs topical tretinoin chemoprevention trial. *Cancer*. 2009;115(11):2523–2530.

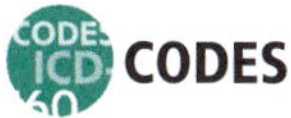

CODES

ICD10

L57.0 Actinic keratosis

CLINICAL PEARLS

- AKs are premalignant lesions, although most will not progress to SCC and many will regress with time.
- Often more easily felt than seen
- Therapy-resistant lesions should be biopsied, especially on the face.

KERATOSIS, SEBORRHEIC

Karl T. Clebak, MD, MHA, FAAFP • Michael T. Partin, MD • Christopher R. Davis, MD, MPH

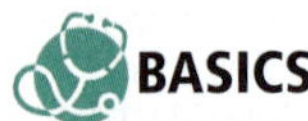

BASICS

DESCRIPTION

- Common benign tumor of the epidermis formed from proliferation of keratinocytes
- Frequently appears in multiples on the head, neck, and trunk (sparing the palms and soles) of older individuals but may occur on any hair-bearing area of the body
- Typically presents as multiple, well circumscribed, yellow to brown raised lesions that feel greasy, velvety, or warty; usually described as having a "stuck-on" appearance
- Clinical variants include the following:
  - Common seborrheic keratosis
  - Dermatosis papulosa nigra
  - Stucco keratosis
  - Flat seborrheic keratosis
  - Pedunculated seborrheic keratosis
- Synonym(s): SK, verruca seborrhoica; seborrheic wart; senile wart; basal cell papilloma; verruca senilis; benign acanthokeratoma; barnacles of aging

EPIDEMIOLOGY

Incidence

- Predominant age: appear most commonly in those aged 31 to 50 years, and incidence increases with age, peaking at age 60 years
- Predominant sex: slightly more common and more extensive involvement in males
- Most common among white people, except for the dermatosis papulosa nigra variant, which usually presents in darker skinned individuals

Prevalence

- 69–100% in patients >50 years of age
- The prevalence rate increases with age.

ETIOLOGY AND PATHOPHYSIOLOGY

- Etiology remains largely unclear with ultraviolet (UV) light and genetics thought to be involved.
- The role of human papillomavirus is uncertain.
- There have been rare reports of malignant transformation into squamous cell carcinoma (1).

Genetics

An autosomal dominant inheritance pattern is suggested

RISK FACTORS

- Advanced age
- Exposure to UV light and genetic predisposition are possible risk factors.

GENERAL PREVENTION

Sun protection methods may help prevent seborrheic keratoses from developing.

COMMONLY ASSOCIATED CONDITIONS

- Sign of Leser-Trélat: a paraneoplastic syndrome characterized by a rapid outbreak of multiple seborrheic keratoses often associated with an internal malignancy, most commonly adenocarcinoma; seborrheic keratosis may resolve with treatment of the malignancy and reappear with neoplasm recurrence.
- Documentation of other cutaneous lesions, such as basal cell carcinoma, malignant melanoma, or squamous cell carcinoma, growing adjacent to or within a seborrheic keratosis, has been reported. The exact relationship between lesions is unclear.

DIAGNOSIS

HISTORY

Generally asymptomatic, but trauma or irritation of the lesion may result in pruritus, erythema, bleeding, pain, and/or crusting

PHYSICAL EXAM

- Typically begin as oval- or round-shaped, flat, dull, sharply demarcated patches
- As they mature, may develop into thicker, elevated, uneven, verrucous-like papules, plaques, or peduncles with a waxy or velvety surface, and appear "stuck on" to the skin
- Commonly appear on sun-exposed areas of the body, predominately the head, neck, or trunk but may appear on any hair-bearing skin
- Surface tends to crumble when scratched.
- Vary in color (black, brown, tan, gray to white, or skin-colored) as well as size, ranging from several millimeters to several centimeters, but the average diameter is 0.5 to 1.0 cm
- Usually occur as multiples; patients having >100 is not uncommon
- Common clinical variants include:
  - Common seborrheic keratoses: on hair-bearing skin, usually on the face, neck, and trunk; verrucous-like, waxy, or velvety lesions that appear "stuck on" to the skin
  - Dermatosis papulosa nigra: small black papules that usually appear on the face, neck, chest, and upper back; symmetric distribution most common in darker skinned individuals, more common in females; most have a positive family history
  - Stucco keratoses: small gray-white, rough, verrucous papules; usually occur in large numbers on the lower extremities or forearms; more common in men
  - Flat seborrheic keratoses: oval-shaped, tan to brown patches or macules on face, chest, and upper extremities; increases with age
  - Pedunculated seborrheic keratoses: Hyperpigmented peduncles appear on areas of friction (neck, axilla).

DIFFERENTIAL DIAGNOSIS

Consider the following diagnoses if the seborrheic keratosis is:

- Pigmented
  - Malignant melanoma
  - Melanocytic nevus
  - Angiokeratoma
  - Pigmented basal cell carcinoma
- Lightly pigmented
  - Basal cell carcinoma
  - Bowen disease
  - Condyloma acuminatum
  - Fibroma
  - Verruca vulgaris
  - Eccrine poroma
  - Invasive squamous cell carcinoma
  - Acrochordon (skin tag)
  - Acrokeratosis verruciformis of Hopf
  - Follicular infundibulum tumor
- Flat
  - Solar lentigo
  - Verrucae planae juveniles
- Hyperkeratotic
  - Actinic keratosis

DIAGNOSTIC TESTS & INTERPRETATION

Initial Tests (lab, imaging)

Testing is generally not indicated unless diagnosis is unclear or malignancy is suspected.

Diagnostic Procedures/Other

- Diagnosis is generally made clinically.
- Biopsy should be performed if the seborrheic keratosis is atypical or has recently been inflamed or changed in appearance.
- Dermoscopy can assist in confirmation if diagnosis is uncertain. Common findings are pigment networks, pigmented globules, streaks, homogenous blue patterns, milia-like cysts, blotches, blue-whitish veils, and hairpin vessels (2).

Test Interpretation

Several histologic variants exist and can include the following:

- Acanthosis and papillomatosis due to basaloid cell proliferation
- "Squamous eddies" or squamous epithelial cell clusters
- Hyperpigmentation
- Hyperkeratosis
- Horn cysts
- Pseudocysts

TREATMENT

- Treatment is typically performed for cosmetic concerns but is usually not required
- Removal of seborrheic keratoses may be indicated if:
  - They are aesthetically displeasing or undesirable (common patient concern, although removal for this reason is not always covered by insurance).
  - They are symptomatic (e.g., easily irritated, gets caught on clothing or jewelry).
  - There is a concern for their association with malignancy.

MEDICATION

- Generally medical therapies are not considered first line, with surgical approaches being favored
- HP40 (Eskata) is an FDA-approved topical treatment for raised seborrheic keratosis, consisting of a 40% hydrogen peroxide solution. The treatment may require two office visits for application, may be less effective than other treatment methods, and has not shown better cosmetic results than other treatments.
- Some reports exist regarding successful treatment of seborrheic keratoses using tazarotene, diclofenac gel, imiquimod, calcitriol, and dobesilate.
- Topical vitamin D analogs do not seem to be effective.

ISSUES FOR REFERRAL

- New seborrheic keratoses that appear abruptly, particularly if many occur within a short time frame concerning for Leser-Trélat sign
- A seborrheic keratosis becomes inflamed or changes in appearance

SURGERY/OTHER PROCEDURES

- A surgical approach to treatment is generally preferred with the selected therapy depending upon physician preference and availability of the treatment.
- The following procedures can be used in practice:
  - Cryotherapy (liquid nitrogen)
    - Spray flat lesions for 5 to 10 seconds; may require more time or additional treatments if the seborrheic keratosis is thicker
    - Possible complications include scarring, hypopigmentation, recurrence.
  - Curettage
    - Curette (metal hand tool with small scoop at the tip) is used to scrape off the lesion.
    - Requires local anesthesia
  - Electrodessication
    - Tool with needle-like metal tip that uses electric current to destroy affected tissue
    - Requires local anesthesia
  - Shave excision
    - Scalpel or flexible razor blade is used to remove lesion.
    - Requires local anesthesia
  - Laser
    - Intense beams of light are used to burn and vaporize the lesion.
    - Requires local anesthesia
  - Chemical peel
    - An application of chemical solution (e.g., Trichloroacetic acid) is used to remove the top layer of skin.
- In a small study ($n = 25$), a majority of patients preferred cryotherapy over curettage due to decreased wound care after the procedure with no statistically significant differences in patient's ratings of cosmetic appearance between curettage and cryotherapy (3)[B].

ONGOING CARE

FOLLOW-UP RECOMMENDATIONS

Patient Monitoring

After initial diagnosis, follow-up is not usually required unless:

- Inflammation or irritation develops.
- There is a change in appearance.
- New seborrheic keratoses suddenly appear.

PATIENT EDUCATION

- Sun-protective methods may help reduce seborrheic keratosis development.
- Patient education materials
  - http://www.aad.org/public/diseases/bumps-and-growths/seborrheic-keratoses
  - https://www.cdc.gov/skin-cancer/prevention/

PROGNOSIS

- Seborrheic keratoses generally do not become malignant, although there are some reports of this occurring in rare situations.
- Sign of Leser-Trélat usually represents a poor prognosis.

COMPLICATIONS

- Irritation and inflammation due to mechanical irritation (e.g., from clothing, jewelry)
- Possible complications of surgical treatment include hypopigmentation, hyperpigmentation, scarring, incomplete removal, and recurrence.
- Misdiagnosis (rare)

REFERENCES

1. Nozaki H, Ishida-Yamamoto A, Nakagawa T, et al. Malignant transformation from seborrheic keratosis to squamous cell carcinoma is more likely to occur in nonexposed areas: a single-center retrospective study. *J Dermatol*. 2025;52(7):e618–e619. doi:10.1111/1346-8138.17756.
2. Marghoob AA, Usatine RP, Jaimes N. Dermoscopy for the family physician. *Am Fam Physician*. 2013;88(7):441–450.
3. Wood LD, Stucki JK, Hollenbeak CS, et al. Effectiveness of cryosurgery vs curettage in the treatment of seborrheic keratoses. *JAMA Dermatol*. 2013;149(1):108–109.

ADDITIONAL READING

Higgins JC, Maher MH, Douglas MS. Diagnosing common benign skin tumors. *Am Fam Physician*. 2015;92(7):601–607.

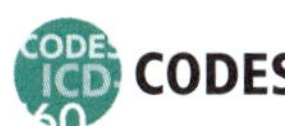

CODES

ICD10

- L82.1 Other seborrheic keratosis
- L82.0 Inflamed seborrheic keratosis

CLINICAL PEARLS

- Seborrheic keratoses are one of the most common benign tumors of the epidermis, and frequency increases with age.
- Although seborrheic keratoses do not need to be removed, there are many options for doing so if patients request this (with surgical methods generally being preferred).
- Underlying internal malignancy should be considered if large numbers of seborrheic keratoses appear suddenly.

KNEE PAIN

*Lee A. Mancini, MD, CAQSM, CSCS*D, CSN*

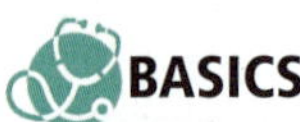

BASICS

DESCRIPTION

A common outpatient complaint with a broad differential

- Knee pain may be acute, chronic, or an acute exacerbation of a chronic condition.
- Trauma, overuse, and degenerative change are frequent causes.
- A detailed history, including patient's age, pain onset and location, mechanism of injury, and associated symptoms can help narrow the differential diagnosis.
- A thorough and focused examination of the knee (as well as the back, hips, and ankles) helps to establish the correct diagnosis and appropriate treatment.

EPIDEMIOLOGY

Incidence

- Knee complaints account for 12.5 million primary care visits annually.
- The incidence of knee osteoarthritis (OA) is 240 cases per 100,000 person-years.

Prevalence

- The knee is a common site of lower extremity injury.
  - Patellar tendinopathy and patellofemoral syndrome are the most common causes of knee pain in runners.
- OA of the hip/knee is 11th cause of global disability and 38th most common cause of disability-adjusted life years (DALYs).

ETIOLOGY AND PATHOPHYSIOLOGY

- Trauma (ligament or meniscal injury, fracture, dislocation)
- Overuse (tendinopathy, patellofemoral syndrome, bursitis, apophysitis)
- Age (arthritis, degenerative conditions in older patients; apophysitis in younger patients)
- Rheumatologic (rheumatoid arthritis [RA], systemic lupus erythematosus [SLE])
- Crystal arthropathies (gout, pseudogout)
- Infectious (bacterial, postviral, Lyme disease)
- Referred pain (hip, back)
- Vascular (popliteal artery aneurysm, deep vein thrombosis)
- Others (tumor, cyst, plica)

RISK FACTORS

- Obesity
- Malalignment
- Poor flexibility, muscle imbalance, or weakness
- Rapid increases in training frequency and intensity
- Improper footwear, training surfaces, technique
- Activities that involve cutting, jumping, pivoting, deceleration, kneeling
- Previous injuries

GENERAL PREVENTION

- Maintain body mass index <25 kg/m^2.
- Proper exercise technique, volume, and equipment; avoid overtraining.
- Correct postural strength and flexibility imbalances.

COMMONLY ASSOCIATED CONDITIONS

- Fracture, contusion
- Effusion, hemarthrosis
- Patellar dislocation/subluxation
- Meniscal or ligamentous injury
- Tendinopathy, bursitis
- Osteochondral injury
- OA, septic arthritis
- Muscle strain

DIAGNOSIS

HISTORY

- Pain location, quality, and mechanism of injury guide diagnostic reasoning (also see "Differential Diagnosis"):
  - Diffuse pain: OA, patellofemoral pain syndrome, chondromalacia
  - Pain ascending/descending stairs: meniscal injury, patellofemoral pain syndrome
  - Pain with prolonged sitting, standing from sitting: patellofemoral pain syndrome
  - Mechanical symptoms (locking): meniscal injury
- Mechanism of injury:
  - Hyperextension, deceleration, cutting: anterior cruciate ligament (ACL) injury
  - Hyperflexion, fall on flexed knee, "dashboard injury": posterior cruciate ligament (PCL) injury
  - Lateral force (valgus load): medial collateral injury
  - Twisting on planted foot: meniscal injury
- Effusion:
  - Rapid onset (2 hours): ACL tear, patellar subluxation/dislocation, large meniscal tear, tibial plateau fracture; hemarthrosis is common.
  - Slower onset (24 to 36 hours), smaller: meniscal injury, ligament sprain, arthritis
  - Swelling behind the knee: popliteal (Baker) cyst

PHYSICAL EXAM

- Observe gait (antalgia); patellar tracking
- Inspect for malalignment, atrophy, swelling, ecchymosis, or erythema.
- Palpate for effusion, warmth, and tenderness.
- Evaluate active and passive range of motion (ROM) and flexibility of quadriceps and hamstrings.
- Evaluate strength and muscle tone.
- Note joint instability, locking, and catching.
- Evaluate hip ROM, strength, and stability.
- Special tests:
  - Patellar apprehension test: patellar instability; patellar grind test: patellofemoral pain or OA (1)
  - Lachman test (more sensitive and specific), pivot shift, anterior drawer, lever sign: ACL integrity
  - Posterior drawer, posterior sag sign: PCL integrity
  - Valgus/varus stress test: medial collateral ligament (MCL)/lateral collateral ligament (LCL) integrity
  - McMurray test, Apley grind test, Thessaly test: meniscal injury
  - Ober test: iliotibial band (ITB) tightness
  - Dial test: positive with posterolateral corner laxity
  - Patellar tilt test and squatting may help suggest patellofemoral pain syndrome.
  - Patella facet tenderness suggests OA or patellofemoral pain syndrome (1).

DIFFERENTIAL DIAGNOSIS

- Acute onset: fracture, contusion, cruciate or collateral ligament tear, meniscal tear, patellar dislocation/subluxation; if systemic symptoms: septic arthritis, gout, pseudogout, Lyme disease, osteomyelitis
- Insidious onset: patellofemoral pain syndrome/chondromalacia, ITB syndrome, OA, RA, bursitis, tumor, tendinopathy, loose body, bipartite patella, degenerative meniscal tear
- Anterior pain: patellofemoral pain syndrome, patellar injury, patellar tendinopathy, Prepatellar or suprapatellar bursitis, tibial apophysitis, fat pad impingement, quadriceps tendinopathy, OA (1)
- Posterior pain: PCL injury, posterior horn meniscal injury, popliteal cyst or aneurysm, hamstring or gastrocnemius injury, deep venous thrombosis (DVT)
- Medial pain: MCL injury, medial meniscal injury, pes anserine bursitis, medial plica syndrome, OA
- Lateral pain: LCL injury, lateral meniscal injury, ITB syndrome, OA

DIAGNOSTIC TESTS & INTERPRETATION

Initial Tests (lab, imaging)

- Suspected septic joint, gout, pseudogout:
  - Arthrocentesis with cell count, Gram stain, culture, synovial fluid analysis, erythrocyte sedimentation rate (ESR), CRP
- Suspected RA:
  - CBC, ESR, rheumatoid factor
- Consider Lyme titer.
- Radiographs to rule out fracture in patients with acute knee trauma (Ottawa Rules):
  - Age >55 years *or*
  - Tenderness at the patella or fibular head *or*
  - Inability to bear weight four steps *or*
  - Inability to flex knee to 90 degrees
- Radiographs help diagnose OA, osteochondral lesions, patellofemoral pain syndrome:
  - Weight-bearing, upright anteroposterior, lateral, merchant/sunrise, notch/tunnel views

Follow-Up Tests & Special Considerations

- MRI is "gold standard" for soft tissue imaging.
- Ultrasound may help diagnose tendinopathy, effusions, ligamentous tears, among other diagnostic findings.
- CT can further elucidate fracture.

Diagnostic Procedures/Other

Arthroscopy may be beneficial in the diagnosis of certain conditions, including meniscus and ligament injuries.

Geriatric Considerations

OA, degenerative meniscal tears, and gout are more common in middle-aged and elderly populations.

Pediatric Considerations

- 3 million pediatric sports injuries occur annually.
- Look for physeal/apophyseal and joint surface injuries in skeletally immature:
  - Acute: patellar subluxation, avulsion fractures, ACL tear
  - Overuse: patellofemoral pain syndrome, apophysitis, osteochondritis dissecans, patellar tendonitis, stress fracture
  - Others: neoplasm, juvenile RA, infection, referred pain from slipped capital femoral epiphysis

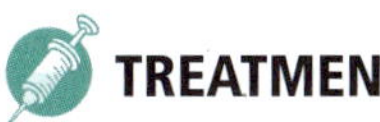

TREATMENT

GENERAL MEASURES

Acute injury: PRICEMM therapy (**p**rotection, **r**elative rest, **i**ce, **c**ompression, **e**levation, **m**edications, **m**odalities)

MEDICATION

First Line

- Oral medications:
  - Acetaminophen: up to 3 g/day; safe and effective in OA
  - Nonsteroidal anti-inflammatory drugs (NSAIDs):
    - Ibuprofen: 200 to 800 mg TID
    - Naproxen: 250 to 500 mg BID.
      - Useful for acute sprains, strains
      - Useful for short-term pain reduction in OA. Long-term use is not recommended due to side effects.
      - Not recommended for fracture, stress fracture, chronic muscle injury; may be associated with delayed healing; low dose and brief course only if necessary
  - Celecoxib: 200 mg QD may be effective in OA with less GI side effects than NSAIDs (2)[A].
- Topical medications:
  - Topical NSAIDs provide pain relief in OA and may be more tolerable than oral medications (3)[A].
  - Topical capsaicin may be an adjuvant for pain management in OA.
- Injections:
  - Intra-articular corticosteroid injection will likely provide short-term benefit in knee OA stage 2 or 3.
  - Viscosupplementation may reduce pain and improve function in patients with OA. Peak effectiveness is 4 to 6 weeks from 3rd injection.
  - Platelet-rich plasma (PRP) and prolotherapy injections can provide long term relief.
  - Stem cell therapy with insufficient data

Second Line

Tramadol/opioids: not recommended; can be used with acute injuries for severe pain

ISSUES FOR REFERRAL

- Acute trauma, young athletic patient
- Joint instability
- Lack of improvement with conservative measures
- Salter-Harris physeal fractures (pediatrics)

ADDITIONAL THERAPIES

- Physical therapy is recommended as initial treatment for patellofemoral pain and tendinopathies.
- Muscle strengthening improves outcome in OA.
- Foot orthoses, taping, acupuncture
- May need bracing for stability

SURGERY/OTHER PROCEDURES

- Surgery may be indicated for certain injuries (e.g., ACL tear in competitive athletes or grade IV OA).
- Chronic conditions refractory to conservative therapy may require surgical intervention.

COMPLEMENTARY & ALTERNATIVE MEDICINE

May reduce pain and improve function in early OA:

- Glucosamine sulfate (500 mg TID)
- Chondroitin (400 mg TID)
- Turmeric or curcumin 1,000 mg/day
- Collagen hydrolysates 10 g daily
- S-adenosyl-L-methionine (SAMe), ginger extract, methylsulfonylmethane: less reliable improvement with inconsistent supporting evidence
- Acupuncture: need to do 4 weeks or 10 sessions

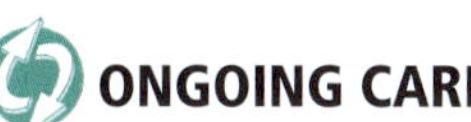

ONGOING CARE

FOLLOW-UP RECOMMENDATIONS

- Activity modification in overuse conditions
- Rehabilitative exercise in OA:
  - Low-impact exercise: walking, swimming, cycling
  - Strength, ROM, and proprioception training

Patient Monitoring

- Rehabilitation after initial treatment of acute injury
- In chronic and overuse conditions, assess functional status, rehabilitation adherence, and pain control at follow-up visit.

DIET

Weight reduction by 10% improved function by 28%.

PATIENT EDUCATION

- Review activity modifications.
- Encourage active role in the rehabilitation process.
- Review medication risks and benefits.

PROGNOSIS

Varies with diagnosis, injury severity, chronicity of condition, patient motivation to participate in rehabilitation, and whether surgery is required

COMPLICATIONS

- Disability
- Arthritis
- Chronic joint instability
- Deconditioning

REFERENCES

1. Hong E, Kraft MC. Evaluating anterior knee pain. *Med Clin North Am*. 2014;98(4):697–717.
2. Bijlsma JW, Berenbaum F, Lafeber FP. Osteoarthritis: an update with relevance for clinical practice. *Lancet*. 2011;377(9783):2115–2126.
3. Zeng C, Wei J, Persson MSM, et al. Relative efficacy and safety of topical non-steroidal anti-inflammatory drugs for osteoarthritis: a systematic review and network meta-analysis of randomised controlled trials and observational studies. *Br J Sports Med*. 2018;52(10):642–650.

ADDITIONAL READING

Collins NJ, Bisset LM, Crossley KM, et al. Efficacy of nonsurgical interventions for anterior knee pain: systematic review and meta-analysis of randomized trials. *Sports Med*. 2012;42(1):31–49.

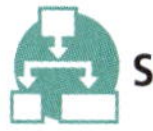

SEE ALSO

Algorithms: Knee Pain; Popliteal Mass

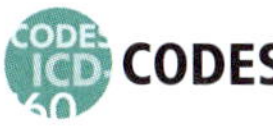

CODES

ICD10

- M25.569 Pain in unspecified knee
- M17.9 Osteoarthritis of knee, unspecified
- M76.50 Patellar tendinitis, unspecified knee

CLINICAL PEARLS

- A careful history (location/quality of pain and mechanism of injury) targets diagnosis for most causes of knee pain.
- Consider ligamentous injury, meniscal tear, and fracture for patients presenting with acute knee pain.
- Consider OA, patellofemoral pain syndrome, tendinopathy, bursitis, and stress fracture in patients presenting with more chronic symptoms.
- Consider physeal, apophyseal, or articular cartilage injury in young patients presenting with knee pain.
- The presence of an effusion in a patient <30 years of age indicates a significant injury, infection, or inflammatory diagnosis.
- Referred pain from the hip (slipped capital femoral epiphysis, Legg-Calvé-Perthes disease) can present as knee pain.

LABYRINTHITIS

Joseph Daniel Hogue, MD, MBA • Karah A. Snider, DO • Scott Rosen, MD

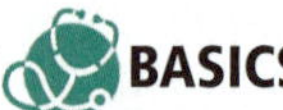

BASICS

- Inflammation of the membranous labyrinth of the inner ear that often leads to impaired hearing and balance.
- May also be referred to as vestibular neuritis, vestibular neuronitis, neurolabyrinthitis, or acute peripheral unilateral vestibuloplasty

DESCRIPTION

- Typically presents as a sudden onset of room-spinning vertigo that lasts for hours to days; may also be accompanied by unilateral sensorineural hearing loss and tinnitus
- Can be categorized as suppurative or serous/toxic labyrinthitis (1)
- Labyrinthitis is a clinical diagnosis in the absence of neurologic deficits.
- Often associated with vestibular hypofunction of the involved ear; peripheral vertigo improves over time with central compensation. Hearing loss generally improves in the case of serous labyrinthitis but is permanent in the case of suppurative labyrinthitis.
- System(s) affected: nervous, special sensory (auditory and vestibular)
- Key symptoms: vertigo, nausea, vomiting, gait impairment

ALERT

- "Vertigo" and "dizziness" are commonly used terms. Clarify symptoms by giving options of alternative descriptions such as light-headedness, disequilibrium, room-spinning vertigo, or imbalance.
- Hearing loss and duration of symptoms can help narrow the differential diagnosis in patients with vertigo.
- Vestibular neuritis/neuronitis occurs due to inflammation of the vestibular nerve causing vertigo lasting hours to days without the auditory symptoms of labyrinthitis (2).

EPIDEMIOLOGY

- Most common in 30 to 50 years of age
- 10% of all patients seen for dizziness, if vestibular neuritis is included

Incidence

Estimated incidence of 3.5 per 100,000 if including vestibular neuritis

Prevalence

Unclear due to limited data; increases with age.

ETIOLOGY AND PATHOPHYSIOLOGY

- Viral labyrinthitis is the most common etiology with acute inflammation and damage to the labyrinth, involving both the vestibular apparatus and cochlea.
  - Common viral causes: *cytomegalovirus*, mumps, varicella zoster, rubeola, influenza, parainfluenza, herpes simplex, adenovirus, *coxsackievirus*, respiratory syncytial virus, HIV
- Bacterial invasion of the inner ear, either from a middle ear infection or meningitis, occurs in suppurative labyrinthitis (1).
  - Common bacterial causes: *Streptococcus pneumoniae, Haemophilus influenzae, Moraxella catarrhalis, Neisseria meningitidis, Streptococcus* spp., *Staphylococcus* spp., *Borrelia burgdorferi*

RISK FACTORS

- Viral upper respiratory infection
- Otitis media
- Cholesteatoma
- Head trauma
- Meningitis

GENERAL PREVENTION

- Early treatment of acute otitis media to prevent complications
- Scheduled immunizations (to prevent common viral pathogens)
- Prevent maternal transmission of pathogens, including syphilis and HIV.

COMMONLY ASSOCIATED CONDITIONS

- Viral upper respiratory infection
- Otitis media
- Cholesteatoma
- Head injury

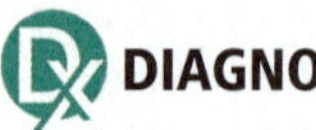

DIAGNOSIS

Clinical diagnosis based on history and physical examination

HISTORY

- Acute onset vertigo *and* sensorineural hearing loss in one ear that lasts hours to days
- Nausea and vomiting are common.
- Affected ear may have a fullness sensation or tinnitus (roaring, ringing).
- Upper respiratory tract infection symptoms
- Otorrhea or otalgia (not common with viral causes)
- Severe headache, fever, and nuchal rigidity in the setting of meningitis

PHYSICAL EXAM

- Fast-beating unilateral nystagmus toward affected ear during the acute phase and away from affected ear during the convalescent phase, 48 to 72 hours later
- Nystagmus does not change direction with gaze.
- Symptoms abate with eyes open and visual fixation.
- Gait instability with preserved ability to ambulate; if patient sways or falls, it is towards affected ear.
- Serous/purulent effusion may be present in the middle ear.
- Otologic exam may be unremarkable in the setting of viral labyrinthitis.
- Retraction of the tympanic membrane and keratinaceous debris may be present with cholesteatoma.

DIFFERENTIAL DIAGNOSIS

- Benign paroxysmal positional vertigo (BPPV) is the most common cause of vertigo. Unlike labyrinthitis, BPPV is episodic, with severe symptoms lasting <1 minute. BPPV is diagnosed using the Dix-Hallpike maneuver. Unlike labyrinthitis, it is not associated with hearing loss.
- Ménière disease is more episodic than labyrinthitis; it comes and goes, rather than remaining continuous, and is associated with the triad of episodic vertigo, tinnitus, and hearing loss.
- Vestibular migraine is the second most common cause of recurrent vertigo, lasting hours and usually with a history of migraine. Up to 10% of cases can occur without headaches.
- Autoimmune inner ear disease
- Cardiovascular accident (CVA): cerebellar or brainstem infarct
- Cerebellopontine-angle tumors (e.g., vestibular schwannoma, acoustic neuroma)
- Temporal bone fracture
- Less common etiologies: parainfectious encephalomyelitis or cranial polyneuritis, Ramsay Hunt syndrome, HIV infection, syphilis, temporal lobe epilepsy, perilymphatic fistula, superior canal dehiscence, idiopathic sudden single-sided deafness, multiple sclerosis, vasculitis (cerebral or systemic)

DIAGNOSTIC TESTS & INTERPRETATION

- Routine lab studies are not helpful unless an autoimmune cause is suspected.
- CT of the temporal bone may be indicated in the setting of complicated otitis media or cholesteatoma.
- Consider lumbar puncture only if meningitis is suspected.
- Consider screening for syphilis or HIV when clinically indicated by risk factors or clinical history.
- Imaging is not required for the diagnosis of acute labyrinthitis.
- With acute sensorineural hearing loss or other associated neurologic symptoms, an MRI of the IACs and/or MRA of the brain and brainstem are recommended.

Initial Tests (lab, imaging)

- Labs and/or imaging is not recommended.
- Profound imbalance or associated focal neurologic signs are not typical and should prompt imaging.

Follow-Up Tests & Special Considerations

Labyrinthitis ossificans is fibrosis of the internal auditory canal following bacterial meningitis and is thought to occur due to a suppurative labyrinthitis. This can occur rapidly, especially after *S. pneumoniae* meningitis.

Diagnostic Procedures/Other

- Audiogram may show varying degrees of both sensorineural hearing loss and discrimination loss.
- Vestibular tests are not typically indicated in the acute setting. If vertigo and dizziness persist after expected resolution of symptoms, videonystagmography should be used.

Test Interpretation

Caloric testing may show relative weakness of the horizontal semicircular canal of the affected side. Sensitivity and specificity of this test are variable within literature.

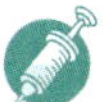

TREATMENT

- Considered a self-limited disorder; symptom management and reassurance in the acute phase
- Vestibular suppressants as needed (see "Medication") for severe acute attacks of vertigo only. Patients should be advised *not* to use these medications as scheduled medications or for prophylaxis without symptoms because this can delay central compensation (2)[B].
- Sudden single-sided sensorineural hearing loss should be managed with high-dose steroids as soon as possible, ideally within 2 weeks. Steroids have not been found to definitively improve vestibular symptoms (3)[B].
- Vestibular rehabilitation is the mainstay of treatment for persistent vertigo and dizziness and has been shown to be safe and effective management for unilateral peripheral vestibular dysfunction.
- Patients should begin exercises as soon as the acute phase resolves and movement is tolerable, generally within 2 to 3 days of onset.
- For suppurative labyrinthitis, appropriate antibiotics to eradicate infection. Surgical intervention may also be required with tympanostomy tubes or mastoidectomy, depending on the extent of middle ear involvement.

GENERAL MEASURES

Vestibular exercises for prolonged symptoms and unilateral vestibular loss have been shown to alleviate postural control.

MEDICATION

Use of the following drugs should be on a PRN basis. Benzodiazepines can also assist with the anxiety associated with vertigo. No patient should take vestibular suppressants as a chronic medication because they can block central compensation.

- Vestibular suppressants
  - Lorazepam (Ativan): 0.5 to 2.0 mg SL/PO BID PRN or diazepam (Valium) 2 to 5 mg QID PO PRN
  - Meclizine (Antivert, Bonine, Zentrip [dissolvable]) 12.5 to 25.0 mg PO BID–TID PRN
  - Dimenhydrinate (Dramamine) 25 to 50 mg PO q4–6h PRN
- Antiemetics
  - Ondansetron (Zofran) 4 to 8 mg PO TID PRN or granisetron (Kytril) 1 mg PO TID PRN
  - Meclizine (Antivert, Bonine) 12.5 to 25.0 mg PO q4h PRN
  - Promethazine (Phenergan) 12.5 to 25.0 mg PO/PR QID PRN or prochlorperazine (Compazine) 25 mg PR BID PRN
  - Metoclopramide (Reglan) 10 mg PO TID PRN
- Antivirals
  - Acyclovir 800 mg PO 5 times/day for 7 days can be used in cases associated with herpes.
- Steroids
  - Prednisone 1 mg/kg/day up to maximum 60 mg daily for 1 week, followed by 1 week taper
  - Methylprednisolone initially 100 mg PO daily and then tapered to 10 mg PO daily over 3 weeks
  - Dexamethasone 0.4 to 0.8 mL of 24 mg/mL strength given via transtympanic injection for three to four sessions; can be used for salvage therapy
  - Given early in the setting of bacterial meningitis, may decrease the otologic sequelae, specifically labyrinthitis ossificans
  - Used in treatment of labyrinthitis for associated sudden sensorineural hearing loss, ideally within the first 2 weeks

Geriatric Considerations

- Avoid excessive use of scopolamine, meclizine, and other vestibular suppressants following the initial event because this will delay central compensation.
- Benzodiazepines are the preferred vestibular suppressant treatment but do increase the risk of falls in older persons.

Pregnancy Considerations

Dimenhydrinate, diphenhydramine, ondansetron, granisetron, and metoclopramide are pregnancy Category B.

First Line

- Benzodiazepines, which are better vestibular suppressants, are preferred over antihistamine/anticholinergics such as meclizine. Sublingual benzodiazepines are very effective for vertigo and should be considered first-line therapy.
- Urgent steroid treatment in acute setting

ISSUES FOR REFERRAL

- Consider neurology referral for suspected central causes.
- Consider otolaryngology/neurotology referral for progressive hearing loss and vertigo, or in cases of suppurative labyrinthitis requiring surgical intervention.

ADDITIONAL THERAPIES

Vestibular rehabilitation may be considered.

ADMISSION, INPATIENT, AND NURSING CONSIDERATIONS

Patients with systemic infection or intractable nausea and vomiting may need to be hospitalized.

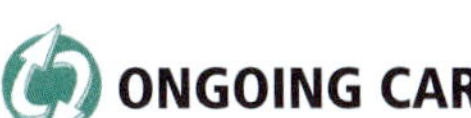

ONGOING CARE

FOLLOW-UP RECOMMENDATIONS

Patient Monitoring

Follow hearing loss weekly with audiograms until hearing stabilizes. Acute vertiginous symptoms may last up to 6 weeks. Residual symptoms have been documented to last years.

DIET

Alcohol may exacerbate symptoms.

PATIENT EDUCATION

Opening eyes with visual fixation should improve symptoms, whereas closing eyes may make symptoms worse. Minimize rapid head movement until symptoms resolve. Avoid vestibular suppressants long term because this can inhibit central compensation.

PROGNOSIS

Typically, self-limited with complete recovery; not likely to reoccur; some studies suggest there may be a correlation with development of BPPV and panic disorder.

COMPLICATIONS

- Permanent hearing loss, more common with bacterial causes, and chronic impairment of balance
- If bacterial labyrinthitis is not treated sufficiently, there is increased risk of developing into mastoiditis.

REFERENCES

1. Kaya S, Schachern PA, Tsuprun V, et al. Deterioration of vestibular cells in labyrinthitis. *Ann Otol Rhinol Laryngol*. 2017;126(2):89–95.
2. Sandhu JS, Rea PA. Clinical examination and management of the dizzy patient. *Br J Hosp Med (Lond)*. 2016;77(12):692–698.
3. Yoo MH, Yang CJ, Kim SA, et al. Efficacy of steroid therapy based on symptomatic and functional improvement in patients with vestibular neuritis: a prospective randomized controlled trial. *Eur Arch Otorhinolaryngol*. 2017;274(6):2443–2451.

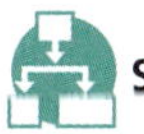

SEE ALSO

Ménière Disease; Postconcussion Syndrome (Mild Traumatic Brain Injury); Tinnitus

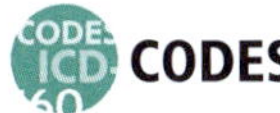

CODES

ICD10

- H83.02 Labyrinthitis, left ear
- H83.01 Labyrinthitis, right ear
- H83.09 Labyrinthitis, unspecified ear

CLINICAL PEARLS

- Episodic vertigo tends to be caused by BPPV or Ménière disease, whereas persistent vertigo with sensorineural hearing loss and tinnitus is more consistent with labyrinthitis.
- Ask patients to describe symptoms in their own words; alternative symptoms include light-headedness, vertigo, disequilibrium, or imbalance.
- Benzodiazepines are better vestibular suppressants and are preferred over antihistamine/anticholinergics such as meclizine. Vestibular suppressants should be used for short duration only because these will delay central compensation.
- Vestibular neuritis would be considered if there was no hearing involvement.

LACTOSE INTOLERANCE

Nihal K. Patel, MD

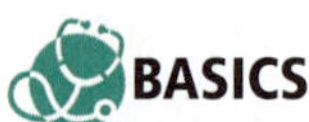

BASICS

DESCRIPTION

- Lactose intolerance is a syndrome of abdominal pain, bloating, and flatulence after the ingestion of lactose.
- Lactose malabsorption results from a reduction in lactase activity in the brush border of the small intestinal mucosa.
- Lactase activity peaks at birth then decreases after the first few months of life, declining continuously throughout life. 75% of adults worldwide exhibit a decline in lactase activity after birth. *Only 50% of lactase activity is needed to digest lactose without causing symptoms of lactose intolerance*.
  - Congenital lactose intolerance is very rare
  - Primary lactose intolerance is relatively common in adults who develop low lactase levels after childhood
  - Secondary lactose intolerance: inability to digest lactose caused by any condition injuring the intestinal mucosa (e.g., infectious enteritis, celiac disease, eosinophilic gastroenteritis, or inflammatory bowel disease) or a reduction of available mucosal surface (e.g., resection)
- Lactose malabsorption may be asymptomatic and is equally common in healthy patients and in those with functional bowel disorders.
- System(s) affected: endocrine/metabolic, gastrointestinal

Pediatric Considerations

- Primary lactose intolerance begins in late childhood.
- No consensus on whether young children (<5 years of age) should avoid lactose following diarrheal illness
- Lactose-free formulas are available.
- Exclude milk protein allergy.

EPIDEMIOLOGY

Incidence

- ≥50% of infants with acute or chronic diarrheal disease have lactose intolerance; particularly common with rotavirus infection
- Lactose intolerance is also common with giardiasis, ascariasis, irritable bowel syndrome (IBS), tropical and nontropical sprue, and AIDS malabsorption syndrome.

Prevalence

- In South America, Africa, and Asia, rates of lactose intolerance are >50%.
- In the United States, the prevalence is 15% among whites, 53% among Hispanics, and 80% among African Americans.
- In Europe, lactose intolerance varies from 15% in Scandinavian countries to 70% in Italy.
- Predominant age:
  - Primary: teenage and adult
  - Secondary: depends on underlying condition
- Predominant sex: male = female

ETIOLOGY AND PATHOPHYSIOLOGY

- Primary lactose intolerance: The normal decline in lactase activity in the intestinal mucosa is genetically determined and permanent after weaning from breast milk.
- Secondary lactose intolerance: associated with gastroenteritis in children; also associated with any gastrointestinal infection or inflammation of the small intestine with resultant lactose malabsorption in both adults and children

Genetics

- In whites, lactase deficiency is associated with a single nucleotide polymorphism (SNP) consisting of a nucleotide switch of T for C 13910 bp on chromosome 2. This results in variants of CC-13910 (lactase nonpersistence) *or* CT-13910/TT-13910 (lactase persistence) (1). SNP (C/T-13910) is associated with lactase persistence in northern Europeans.
- Other SNPs (G/C-14010, T/G-13915, and C/G-13907) linked to lactase persistence in some of African descent.

RISK FACTORS

- Adult-onset lactase deficiency has wide geographic variation.
- Age:
  - Signs and symptoms usually do not become apparent until after age 6 to 7 years.
  - Symptoms may not be apparent until adulthood, depending on dietary lactose intake and rate of decline of intestinal lactase activity.
  - Lactase activity correlates with age, regardless of symptoms.

GENERAL PREVENTION

Lactose avoidance relieves symptoms. Patients can learn what level of lactose is tolerable in their diet.

COMMONLY ASSOCIATED CONDITIONS

- Tropical or nontropical sprue
- Giardiasis
- IBS or other functional bowel disorders
- Small intestinal bacterial overgrowth (SIBO)
- Celiac disease

DIAGNOSIS

- Lactose intolerance can be presumed in patients manifesting mild symptoms after ingestion of significant amounts of lactose (such as >2 servings of dairy per day), with resolution of symptoms after avoidance of lactose-containing foods for 1 week.
- A positive lactose hydrogen breath test is confirmatory.
- Lactose intolerance can mimic symptoms of functional gastrointestinal disorders. Lactose intolerance can also be a coexisting condition.

HISTORY

- Assess daily lactose consumption.
- A single dose of lactose (12 g, equivalent to 1 cup of milk) consumed alone typically produces no or only minor symptoms in persons with lactose intolerance.
- Lactose doses of 15 to 18 g are well tolerated with other nutrients. Doses >18 g cause progressively more symptoms, and quantities >50 g elicit symptoms in most individuals with bona fide lactose intolerance.
- Symptoms arise 30 minutes to 2 hours after consumption of lactose-containing products.
- Symptoms include bloating, flatulence, cramping abdominal discomfort, and diarrhea or loose stools. Vomiting may be noted in adolescents.
- Abdominal pain may be crampy in nature and often is localized to the periumbilical area or lower quadrant.
- Stools usually are bulky, frothy, and watery, although diarrhea may be rare in adults.
- Only 20–30% of individuals with lactose malabsorption develop symptoms.

PHYSICAL EXAM

- Vital signs and general appearance are typically normal.
- Audible bowel sounds (borborygmi) on physical examination (may be particularly bothersome to the patient). The exam is otherwise typically normal or nonspecific.

DIFFERENTIAL DIAGNOSIS

- Functional GI disorder (e.g., IBS)
- SIBO
- Celiac disease
- Inflammatory bowel disease
- Infectious enteritis (e.g., giardiasis)
- Drug or radiation induced enteritis
- Sucrase deficiency
- Cow's milk protein allergy

DIAGNOSTIC TESTS & INTERPRETATION

Initial Tests (lab, imaging)

- The lactose breath test (LBT) is a confirmatory for lactose intolerance. It is noninvasive and easy to perform (sensitivity 78%; specificity 98%) (2).
- Intestinal bacteria digest carbohydrates and produce measurable hydrogen and methane in expired breath:
  - Administer lactose when fasting (2 g/kg; max dose 25 g in children; 50 g in adults). Note any symptoms; sample breath hydrogen at baseline and at 30-minute intervals for 3 hours. Compare postlactose and baseline values. A rise in hydrogen concentration value of 20 ppm over baseline is diagnostic for lactose malabsorption. An early peak (15 to 30 minutes) suggests SIBO.

- Small bowel biopsy for histology and direct measurement of lactase activity (rarely needed).
- A positive LBT confirms lactose malabsorption but does not determine etiology.

Diagnostic Procedures/Other

- Lactose tolerance test is an alternative to LBT in adults and measures lactose absorption through serum glucose measurements. Following oral administration of a 50-g test dose in adults (2 g/kg in children), blood glucose levels are monitored at 0, 60, and 120 minutes. An increase in blood glucose of $<$20 mg/dL (1.1 mmol/L) with the concurrent development of symptoms is diagnostic. False-negative results may occur in patients with diabetes or bacterial overgrowth.
- Stool electrolyte testing, if done, may indicate a stool osmotic gap $>$125 mOsm/kg, (not specific for lactose intolerance).

Test Interpretation

Low lactase enzyme activity in intestinal mucosa, tested by small bowel biopsy, may be patchy or focal.

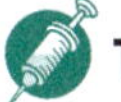

TREATMENT

There is insufficient evidence to recommend any particular treatment (including probiotics, colonic adaptation, and other supplements) as definitive first line.

- In the absence of a correctable underlying disease, there are four general treatment principles (3).
  - Avoid milk/dairy products to improve symptoms.
  - Up to 12 to 15 g of lactose can be tolerated without significant symptoms (1 cup of milk).
  - Gradually reintroduce lactose as symptoms allow. Spreading lactose servings throughout the day improves tolerance.
  - If symptoms persist, substitute fermented and matured milk products for lactose.
- Certain strains, concentrations, and preparations of probiotics may alleviate symptoms.
- Incrementally increasing doses of lactose to induce adaptation have limited success.
- Insufficient evidence to routinely recommend lactose-reduced or hydrolyzed milk, lactase supplements consumed with milk or probiotics
- Maintain calcium and vitamin D intake.

MEDICATION

First Line

Lactase (Lactaid, Lactrase): Effectiveness varies.

- Commercially available "lactase" preparations are bacterial or yeast β-galactosidases.
- Take 1 to 2 capsules or tablets prior to ingesting dairy products.
- Can add tablets or contents of capsules to milk (1 to 2 caps/tabs per quart of milk) before drinking; also commercially available in milk in some areas
- Not effective for all people with lactose intolerance

COMPLEMENTARY & ALTERNATIVE MEDICINE

Certain probiotic formulations taken with meals may alleviate some symptoms of lactose intolerance (4)[B].

ONGOING CARE

DIET

- Reduce or restrict dietary lactose to control symptoms—patient-specific "trial and error."
- Yogurt and fermented products such as hard cheese are often better tolerated than milk.
- Supplement calcium (e.g., calcium carbonate)
- Prehydrolyzed milk (Lactaid) is available.

PATIENT EDUCATION

- Read labels on commercial products—milk sugar is used in many products and may cause symptoms.
- Patients may tolerate whole milk or chocolate milk better than skim milk (slower rate of gastric emptying).
- Lactose consumed with other food products is better tolerated than when milk is consumed alone.
- Primary lactase deficiency is permanent; secondary lactose intolerance usually is temporary, although it may persist for months after the inciting event.
- 20% of prescription drugs and 6% of over-the-counter (OTC) medicines may contain lactose as a base.
- Most patients with lactose intolerance or malabsorption can tolerate 12 to 15 g of lactose per day.

PROGNOSIS

- Normal life expectancy
- Symptoms can be controlled through diet alone if lactase tablets are ineffective.

COMPLICATIONS

Calcium deficiency: Avoidance of milk and other dairy products can lead to reduced calcium intake, which may increase the risk for osteoporosis and fracture.

REFERENCES

1. Jansson-Knodell CL, Krajicek EJ, Savaiano DA, et al. Lactose intolerance: a concise review to skim the surface. *Mayo Clin Proc*. 2020;95(7):1499–1505. doi:10.1016/j.mayocp.2020.04.036.
2. Ghafoor A, Karunaratne T, Rao SSC. Bacterial overgrowth and lactose intolerance: how to best assess. *Curr Opin Clin Nutr Metab Care*. 2022;25(5):334–340. doi:10.1097/MCO.0000000000000861.
3. Zingone F, Bertin L, Maniero D, et al. Myths and facts about food intolerance: a narrative review. *Nutrients*. 2023;15(23):4969. doi:10.3390/nu15234969.
4. Deng Y, Misselwitz B, Dai N, et al. Lactose intolerance in adults: biological mechanism and dietary management. *Nutrients*. 2015;7(9):8020–8035.

ADDITIONAL READING

Facioni MS, Raspini B, Pivari F, et al. Nutritional management of lactose intolerance: the importance of diet and food labelling. *J Trans Med*. 2020;18(1):260. doi:10.1186/s12967-020-02429-2.

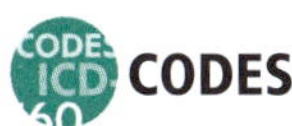

CODES

ICD10

- E73.9 Lactose intolerance, unspecified
- E73.1 Secondary lactase deficiency
- E73.8 Other lactose intolerance

CLINICAL PEARLS

- The diagnosis of lactose intolerance is based on clinical history and confirmed by hydrogen breath testing.
- Most lactose-intolerant patients can tolerate up to 12 to 15 g of lactose per day (equivalent to 1 cup of milk).
- Lactose-intolerant patients may tolerate yogurt and fermented products better than milk and cheese.
- A diary helps identify problematic foods. Patients should read ingredient labels to look for milk, lactose, whey, and curd.
- Lactose-intolerant patients may tolerate whole milk or chocolate milk better than skim milk due to slower gastric emptying.
- Many patients with lactose intolerance unnecessarily avoid all dairy products, potentially causing inadequate intake of calcium and vitamin D.

L

LARYNGITIS

Karlynn Sievers, MD • Bethany Price, DO

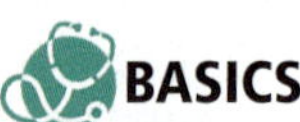

BASICS

DESCRIPTION

- Laryngitis is inflammation, erythema, and edema of the mucosa of the larynx and/or vocal cords characterized by hoarseness, loss of voice, throat pain, coughing, and often a negative impact on a person's quality of life and daily activities.
- There is a range of severity, but most cases are acute and are associated with viral upper respiratory infection, irritation, or acute vocal strain.
- System(s) affected: pulmonary; ears, nose, throat (ENT)
- Synonym(s): acute laryngitis; chronic laryngitis; croup or laryngotracheitis (in children)

EPIDEMIOLOGY

Children are more susceptible than adults due to increased risk of symptomatic inflammation from smaller airway.

Prevalence

Common; approximately 1.7% of population have dysphonia with 50% of this being caused by acute laryngitis. Prevalence rates are increasing but difficult to calculate because many patients do not seek medical attention.

ETIOLOGY AND PATHOPHYSIOLOGY

- Misuse or abuse of voice
- Infectious
  - Viral: influenza A, B; parainfluenza; adenovirus; coronavirus; rhinovirus; human papillomavirus; cytomegalovirus; varicella-zoster virus; herpes simplex virus; respiratory syncytial virus; coxsackievirus, COVID-19 (SARS-CoV-2)
  - Fungal: uncommon but thought to be underdiagnosed, potentially accounting for up to 10% of presentations in both immunocompromised and immunocompetent patients; risk factors include recent antibiotic or inhaled corticosteroid use : histoplasmosis, blastomycosis, *Coccidioides*, *Cryptococcus*, and *Candida*.
  - Bacterial (uncommon): β-hemolytic *Streptococcus*, *Streptococcus pneumoniae*, *Haemophilus influenzae*, tuberculosis (TB), leprosy, *Moraxella catarrhalis*, *Mycoplasma pneumoniae*, *Chlamydophila pneumoniae*. In patients with chronic laryngitis, methicillin-resistant *S. aureus* (MRSA) should be considered as a potential cause.
  - Secondary syphilis if left untreated
  - Leprosy (in 30–55% of those with leprosy, larynx is affected; in tropical and warm countries)
- Irritants
  - Inhalation of irritating substances (e.g., air pollution, cigarette smoke)
  - Aspiration of caustic chemicals
  - Gastroesophageal reflux disease (GERD)/ laryngopharyngeal reflux disease (LPRD)
  - Excessively dry environment
  - Allergy exposures (including pollens)
- Anatomic
  - Aging changes: muscle atrophy, loss of moisture in larynx, and bowing of vocal cords
  - Vocal cord nodules/polyps ("singer's nodes")
  - Local cancer
- Iatrogenic: inhaled steroids such as those used to treat asthma, surgical injury, endotracheal intubation injury
- Neuromuscular disorder (e.g., myasthenia gravis); stroke
- Rheumatoid arthritis
- Trauma (e.g., blunt or penetrating trauma to neck)

RISK FACTORS

- Acute:
  - Infection or trauma
  - Upper respiratory tract viral infection (e.g., influenza, rhinovirus, adenovirus, parainfluenza)
  - Voice overuse—excess talking, singing, or shouting
  - Pneumonia—viral or bacterial
  - Coughing
  - Lack of immunization against pertussis or diphtheria
  - Immunocompromised
- Chronic (persists beyond 3 weeks):
  - Allergic laryngitis
  - Chronic rhinitis/sinusitis with postnasal drip (PND)
  - Voice abuse
  - GERD/LPRD
  - Smoking: primary or secondhand
  - Excessive alcohol use
  - Autoimmune disorders (e.g., rheumatoid arthritis)
  - Granulomatous diseases (e.g., sarcoidosis)
- Environmental pollution; constant exposure to dust or other irritants such as chemicals at workplace
- Medications: inhaled steroids, anticholinergics, antihistamines, anabolic steroids

Geriatric Considerations

May be more ill, slower to heal; need to consider neoplasm

Pediatric Considerations

- Common
- Consider congenital/anatomic causes.

GENERAL PREVENTION

- Avoid overuse of voice (speech therapy/voice training is helpful for vocal musicians/public speakers).
- Influenza virus vaccine is recommended, as well as other routine vaccines.
- Quit smoking and avoid secondhand smoke.
- Limit or avoid alcohol/caffeine/acidic foods.
- Control GERD/LPRD.
- Maintain proper hydration status.
- Avoid allergens.
- Wear mask around chemical/environmental irritants.
- Good handwashing (infection prevention)

COMMONLY ASSOCIATED CONDITIONS

- Viral pharyngitis
- Diphtheria (rare): Membrane can descend into the larynx.
- Pertussis: larynx involved as part of the respiratory system
- Bronchitis; pneumonitis
- Croup, epiglottitis, in children

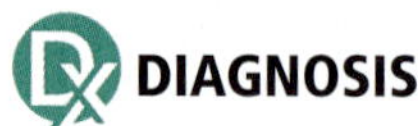

DIAGNOSIS

HISTORY

- Hoarseness, throat "tickle," dry cough, and rawness
- Dysphonia (abnormal-sounding voice)
- Constant urge to clear the throat
- Possible fever
- Malaise
- Dysphagia/odynophagia
- Regional cervical lymphadenopathy
- Stridor or possible airway obstruction in children
- Cough may be worse at night in children.
- Hemoptysis
- Laryngospasm or sense of choking
- Allergic rhinitis/rhinorrhea/PND
- Occupation or other reasons for voice overuse
- Smoking history
- Blunt or penetrating trauma to neck
- GERD/LPRD

PHYSICAL EXAM

- Head and neck exam, including airway patency, cervical nodes; cranial nerve exam
- Visualization of the larynx: preferably with a flexible or rigid endoscope or with an indirect mirror examination as a screening technique to dictate further appropriate testing
- Note quality of voice (i.e., hoarse, breathy, wet, "hot potato like," asthenic [weak], strained).

DIFFERENTIAL DIAGNOSIS

- Diphtheria
- Vocal nodules or polyps
- Laryngeal malignancy
- Thyroid malignancy
- Upper airway malignancy
- Epiglottitis
- Pertussis
- Laryngeal nerve trauma/injury
- Foreign body (in children)
- Autoimmune (rheumatoid arthritis)

DIAGNOSTIC TESTS & INTERPRETATION

- Rarely needed
- WBCs elevated in bacterial laryngitis
- Viral culture (seldom necessary)

Follow-Up Tests & Special Considerations
- Barium swallow, only if needed for differential diagnosis
- CT scan if foreign body suspected
- Do not offer CT imaging before visualization of the larynx with laryngoscopy (1).

Diagnostic Procedures/Other
- Fiber optic or indirect laryngoscopy: Look for red, inflamed, and occasionally hemorrhagic vocal cords; rounded edges and exudate (Reinke edema)
- Consider otolaryngologic evaluation and biopsy: laryngitis lasting >2 weeks in adults with history of smoking or alcohol abuse to rule out malignancy.
- pH probe (24-hour): no difference in incidence of pharyngeal reflux as measured by pH probe between patients with chronic reflux laryngitis and healthy adults
- Fiberoptic laryngoscopy for diagnosis of subtle lesions (e.g., vocal cord nodules or polyps)

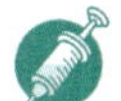

TREATMENT
- Limited but good evidence that treatment beyond supportive care is ineffective.
- Supportive care consists of hydration, voice rest, humidification, and limitation of caffeine.
- Antibiotics appear to have no benefit in acute laryngitis because etiologies are predominantly viral. In chronic laryngitis, consider bacterial sources such as MRSA (1),(2),(3).
- Corticosteroids in severe cases of laryngitis to reduce inflammation such as croup
- May need voice training, if voice overuse (1)
- Nebulized epinephrine reduces croup symptoms 30 minutes posttreatment; evidence does not favor racemic epinephrine or L-epinephrine or IPPB over simple nebulization. Racemic epinephrine reduces croup symptoms at 30 minutes, but effect lasts only 2 hours.
- Botulinum toxin injections for spasmodic dysphonia (1)

GENERAL MEASURES
- Acute:
  - Usually a self-limited illness lasting <3 weeks and not severe
  - Antibiotics of no value
  - Avoid excessive voice use, including whispering.
  - Steam inhalations or cool-mist humidifier
  - Increase fluid intake, especially in cases associated with excessive dryness.
  - Avoid smoking (or secondhand exposure).
  - Warm saltwater gargles
- Chronic:
  - Symptomatic treatment as above
  - Voice therapy (for patients with intermittent dysphagia and vocal abuse)
  - Smoking cessation
  - Reduction or cessation of alcohol intake
  - Occupational change or modification, if exposure driven
  - Allergen avoidance
  - Consider discontinuing offending medication (e.g., inhaled steroids).
- Reflux laryngitis:
  - Elevate head of bed
  - Diet changes
  - Other antireflux lifestyle change management
  - H_2 blockers or proton pump inhibitors (4)

MEDICATION
Usually none

First Line
- Analgesics
- Antipyretics (rare)
- Cough suppressants
- Throat lozenges
- Plenty of fluids

Second Line
- Inhaled corticosteroids (consider only if allergy induced)
- Oral corticosteroids: only if urgent need in adults (presenter, singer, actor)
- Oral corticosteroids: Evidence of benefit has been studied with single-dose dexamethasone in children ages 6 months to 5 years for moderate-severity croup; reduces symptoms within 6 hours; reduces hospitalizations, hospital length of stay, and revisits to office
- Standard of care is to prescribe proton pump inhibitors for chronic laryngitis if GERD or LPRD is suspected; however, evidence suggests only a modest benefit, if any (4).
- Treat nonviral infectious underlying causes.
- Candidal laryngitis:
  - Mild cases: oral antifungal (fluconazole)
  - Amphotericin B or echinocandin can be given in life-threatening cases.

ISSUES FOR REFERRAL
- Immediate ENT referral for patients with stridor or respiratory distress
- The novel SARS-CoV-2 (COVID-19 pandemic) has become a significant cause of acute viral laryngitis. Case reports have shown higher rates of severe laryngitis with the newer omicron variant, including reports of fatal upper airway stenosis (5).
- Referral to ENT for persistent symptoms (>2 to 3 weeks) especially in those with history of smoking or alcohol abuse to rule out malignancy; or concern for foreign body
- Consider GI consult to rule out GERD/LPRD.

SURGERY/OTHER PROCEDURES
- Vocal cord biopsy of hyperplastic mucosa and areas of leukoplakia if cancer or TB is suspected
- Removal of nodules or polyps if voice therapy fails

COMPLEMENTARY & ALTERNATIVE MEDICINE
Some experts, although not well studied, have recommended barberry, black currant, *Echinacea*, *Eucalyptus*, German chamomile, goldenrod, goldenseal, warmed lemon and honey, licorice, marshmallow, peppermint, saw palmetto, slippery elm, vitamin C, and zinc.

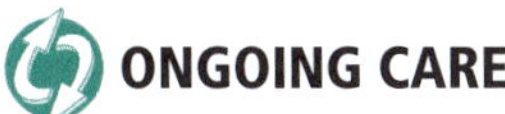

ONGOING CARE

PATIENT EDUCATION
- Educate on the importance of voice rest, including whispering.
- Provide assistance with smoking cessation.
- Help the patient with modification of other predisposing habits or occupational hazards.

PROGNOSIS
Complete clearing of the inflammation without sequelae

COMPLICATIONS
Chronic hoarseness

REFERENCES

1. Francis DO, Smith LJ. Hoarseness guidelines redux: toward improved treatment of patients with dysphonia. *Otolaryngol Clin North Am*. 2019;52(4):597–605.
2. Reveiz L, Cardona AF. Antibiotics for acute laryngitis in adults. *Cochrane Database Syst Rev*. 2015;(5):CD004783.
3. Carpenter PS, Kendall KA. MRSA chronic bacterial laryngitis: a growing problem. *Laryngoscope*. 2018;128(4):921–925.
4. Durazzo M, Lupi G, Cicerchia F, et al. Extra-esophageal presentation of gastroesophageal reflux disease: 2020 update. 2020;9(8):2559.
5. Kimura Y, Hirabayashi E, Yano M, et al. COVID-19 Omicron variant-induced laryngitis. *Auris Nasus Larynx*. 2023;50(4):637–640. doi:10.1016/j.anl.2022.08.007.

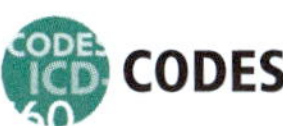

CODES

ICD10
- J37.0 Chronic laryngitis
- J04.0 Acute laryngitis
- J05.0 Acute obstructive laryngitis [croup]

CLINICAL PEARLS
- Laryngitis is usually self-limited and needs only comfort care. Standard treatment is voice rest, hydration, humidification, and limit caffeine intake.
- Refer to ENT for direct visualization of vocal cords for prolonged laryngitis.
- Corticosteroids have some benefits for children with moderately severe croup.
- Voice training useful for chronic laryngitis

LEAD POISONING

Jason Chao, MD, MS

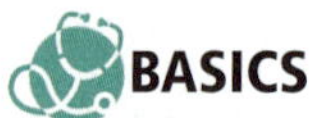

BASICS

DESCRIPTION
- Results from a high body burden of lead (Pb)—an element with no known physiologic purpose
- Synonym(s): Pb poisoning, inorganic

EPIDEMIOLOGY
- Predominant age: 1 to 5 years, adult workers
- Predominant sex: male > female (1:1 in childhood)

Prevalence
- Half of US children have detectable blood Pb levels, and ~2% have blood Pb levels >5 μg/dL
- Centers for Disease Control and Prevention (CDC) estimates 2.5% of U.S. children aged 1 to 5 years have blood Pb levels ≥3.5 μg/dL

ETIOLOGY AND PATHOPHYSIOLOGY
- Inhalation of Pb dust or fumes, or ingestion of Pb
- Pb replaces calcium in bones. Pb interferes with heme synthesis, causes interstitial nephritis, and interferes with neurotransmitters, especially glutamine. High Pb levels can lead to encephalopathy, seizures, and coma.
- Pb crosses blood–brain barrier by displacing calcium ions. Pb exposure early in life causes methylation changes leading to epigenetic alterations that may predispose to brain dysfunction.

RISK FACTORS
- Children with pica or with iron-deficiency anemia
- Residence in or frequent visitation to deteriorating pre-1978 housing with Pb-painted surfaces or recent renovation
- Soil/dust exposure near older homes, Pb industries, or urban roads
- Sibling or playmate with current or past Pb poisoning
- Dust from clothing of Pb worker or hobbyist
- Pb dissolved in water from Pb or Pb-soldered plumbing
- Pb-glazed ceramics leachate (especially with acidic food or drink)
- Folk remedies, spices, and cosmetics
  - Latin America: azarcon, greta, litargirio (a topical agent)
  - Asia and Middle East: chuifong tokuwan, pay-loo-ah, ghasard, bali goli, kandu, ayurvedic herbal medicine from South Asia, kohl (alkohl, ceruse), surma, saoott, cebagin
- Hobbies: target shooting, glazed pottery making, Pb soldering, preparing Pb shot or fishing sinkers, stained-glass making, car/boat repair, home remodeling
- Occupational exposure: plumbers, pipe fitters, Pb miners, auto repairers, glass manufacturers, ship builders, printer operators, plastic manufacturers, Pb smelters and refiners, steel welders or cutters, construction workers, rubber product manufacturers, battery manufacturers, bridge reconstruction workers, firing range workers, military and law enforcement
- Dietary: zinc or calcium deficiency
- Imported toys or jewelry with Pb
- Retained bullet fragments, especially if multiple fragments, associated with fracture, or in joints

Pediatric Considerations
- Children are at increased risk because of incomplete development of the blood–brain barrier prior to 3 years of age (allowing more Pb into the CNS).
- Ingested Pb 40% bioavailable in children (10% in adults)
- Common childhood behaviors such as frequent hand-to-mouth activity and pica (repeated ingestion of nonfood products) increase the risk of Pb ingestion.

Pregnancy Considerations
Cross-sectional studies suggest an association between elevated blood Pb and preeclampsia.

GENERAL PREVENTION
- Counsel families on sources of Pb and how to decrease exposure.
- Screen high-risk children.
  - Medicaid requires children to receive blood Pb screening at ages between 12 and 24 months.
- Warn parents about unsafe home renovations.
- Wet mopping and dusting with a high-phosphate solution (e.g., powdered automatic dishwasher detergent with 1/4 cup per gallon of water) helps control Pb-bearing dust. High-phosphate detergent is no longer available in some states.
- If tap water is potentially Pb contaminated, use cold water instead of hot water and run for 30 to 60 seconds to flush pipes. Use Pb-free water source if possible (bottled or distilled water).

COMMONLY ASSOCIATED CONDITIONS
Iron-deficiency anemia

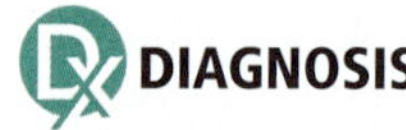

DIAGNOSIS

HISTORY
- Often asymptomatic
- Mild-to-moderate toxicity
  - Myalgias, paresthesias, fatigue, irritability, lethargy
  - Abdominal discomfort, arthralgia, difficulty concentrating, headache, tremor, vomiting, weight loss, muscular exhaustibility
- Severe toxicity: three major clinical syndromes:
  - Alimentary type: anorexia, metallic taste, constipation, severe abdominal cramps due to intestinal spasm and sometimes associated with abdominal wall rigidity
  - Neuromuscular type (characteristic of adult plumbism): peripheral neuritis, usually painless and limited to extensor muscles
  - Cerebral type or Pb encephalopathy (more common in children): seizure, coma, and long-term sequelae, including neurologic defects, delayed mental development, and chronic hyperactivity (or other behavioral changes)
- Chronic exposure may cause renal failure.

PHYSICAL EXAM
Often normal but abdominal tenderness may be severe. Neurologic exam may reveal neuropathy or encephalopathy.

DIFFERENTIAL DIAGNOSIS
- Alimentary type may present as acute abdomen.
- Neuromuscular type presents similar to other polyneuropathies.
- May be confused with ADD, intellectual disability, autism, dementia, and other causes of seizures
- Elevated erythrocyte protoporphyrin may be caused by iron-deficiency anemia or (less commonly) hemolytic anemia.
- Erythropoietic protoporphyria produces a very high erythrocyte protoporphyrin level.

DIAGNOSTIC TESTS & INTERPRETATION
- Venous blood Pb reference value >3.5 μg/dL (0.17 μmol/L); CDC lowered the reference value from >5 μg/dL (0.24 μmol/L) in 2021 (1)[C].
- Confirm screening capillary Pb levels >3.5 μg/dL (0.17 μmol/L) with a venous sample.
- Hemoglobin and hematocrit slightly low; eosinophilia; basophilic stippling on peripheral smear (not diagnostic)
- Renal function is decreased in late stages.
- Abdominal radiograph for Pb particles in gut if recent ingestion is suspected.
- Radiograph of long bones may show metaphyseal changes (resulting from growth arrest). Films are not routinely recommended.

Initial Tests (lab, imaging)
Screening questionnaires are only 60% sensitive to identify children with elevated blood levels.

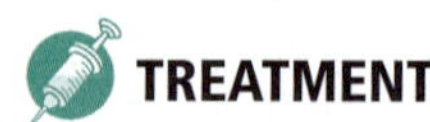

TREATMENT

Blood Level (μg/dL)	Time to Confirmation Testing	Early Follow-up Testing	Later Follow-up Testing after BLL Declining
≥ref value–9	3 mo	3 mo	6–9 mo
10–19	1 mo	1–3 mo	3–6 mo
20–44	2 wk	2–4 wk	1–3 mo
45–59	48 hr	As soon as possible	As soon as possible
60–69	24 hr	As soon as possible	As soon as possible
≥70	Urgently as emergency test	As soon as possible	As soon as possible

Source: Centers for Disease Control and Prevention. https://www.cdc.gov/lead-prevention/hcp/clinical-guidance/index.html. Accessed October 17, 2024.

ALERT
- For Pb levels >3.5 μg/dL, confirm with repeat testing according to the table.
- For blood Pb levels persistently >15 μg/dL, contact local public health department for home inspection.
- For any elevated level, educate on sources of Pb exposure.
- Pb level 3.5 to 15 μg/dL: complete history and physical exam, follow-up Pb monitoring—annually for 6 years; complete inspection of home or workplace to determine source of Pb and Pb-hazard reduction; neurodevelopmental monitoring: iron status, hemoglobin, or hematocrit
- Pb level 15 to 44 μg/dL: Confirm with venipuncture. Consider abdominal radiography if pica (with GI decontamination if "flecks" noted on radiograph).

- Pb level 45 to 69 μg/dL: treatment to lower level plus free erythrocyte protoporphyrin, oral chelation therapy, or hospitalization if Pb-safe environment cannot be ensured
- Pb >70 μg/dL: Hospitalize for chelation therapy (2)[C].

GENERAL MEASURES
Remove child from source of exposure.

MEDICATION
- Consider oral chelation for asymptomatic and Pb >45 and <70; chelation (preferably parenteral) for Pb >70 or symptomatic Pb <70 (2)[C]
- If evidence of Pb in GI tract, withhold chelation until bowel is decontaminated, because all chelating agents increase absorption of lead by the gut

First Line
- Oral chelation: succimer (Chemet), dimercaptosuccinic acid (DMSA) 350 mg/m^2 or 10 mg/kg q8h for 5 days and then q12h for 2 weeks; this may be repeated after 2 weeks off if Pb levels are not stabilized at <15 μg/dL (<0.72 μmol/L).
- Parenteral (IV) chelation (begin after establishment of adequate urine output):
  - Dimercaprol (if available, British anti-Lewisite [BAL] is no longer manufactured) (BAL) 75 mg/m^2 given deep IM, then BAL 450 mg/m^2/day divided q4h for 5 days plus Ca edetate calcium disodium (Ca EDTA) 1,500 mg/m^2/day continuous IV infusion for 5 days. If rebound Pb level ≥45 μg/dL (≥2.17 μmol/L), chelation may be repeated after 2-day interval if symptomatic or after 5-day interval if asymptomatic.
  - Calcium disodium edetate ($CaNa_2EDTA$) 1,000 mg/m^2/day (35 to 50 mg/kg/d) for 5 days; may be repeated after 5 to 7 days
  - In adults, dimercaprol had greater impact on reducing Pb levels than $CaNa_2EDTA$.
  - Contraindications: Do not give BAL to patients with a peanut allergy (the drug solution contains peanut oil).
- Diazepam for initial control of seizures; further control maintained with paraldehyde
- Precautions
  - Succimer: GI upset, rash, nasal congestion, muscle pains, elevated liver function tests
  - BAL: nausea, vomiting, fever, headache, transient hypertension, hepatocellular damage
  - Ca EDTA: renal failure; increased excretion of zinc, copper, and iron
    - Do not confuse Ca EDTA with Na EDTA
- Significant possible interactions
  - Do not give vitamins with minerals while giving chelation.
  - BAL may precipitate hemolytic crisis in a patient with glucose-6-phosphate dehydrogenase deficiency.

Second Line
Oral chelation with penicillamine (D-penicillamine, Depen, Cuprimine)
- Penicillin-allergic patient should not receive penicillamine (cross-sensitivity is common).
- 10 to 15 mg/kg/day given BID mixed in apple juice/sauce on empty stomach (*not* FDA-approved)
- Penicillamine may cause GI upset, renal failure, granulocytopenia, liver dysfunction, iron deficiency, and drug-induced lupus-like syndrome.

ISSUES FOR REFERRAL
Involve health department with any elevated levels. Consult experienced clinician for chelation.

ADDITIONAL THERAPIES
- Remove patient from potential source of Pb if Pb level >45 μg/dL until complete home inspection is performed.
- If desired medication is not available due to drug shortage or cost, alternatives include compounded drugs and consulting a poison center or medical toxicologist.

SURGERY/OTHER PROCEDURES
- Remove retained bullets if Pb poisoning present.
- Consider prophylactic bullet removal, especially if intraarticular.

COMPLEMENTARY & ALTERNATIVE MEDICINE
Garlic has been used to treat mild-to-moderate Pb poisoning in adults.

ADMISSION, INPATIENT, AND NURSING CONSIDERATIONS
- Blood Pb level >70 μg/dL
- If symptomatic, blood Pb level >35 μg/dL
- Contact Poison Control center (1-800-222-1222) or Pediatric Environmental Health Specialty Unit (https://www.pehsu.net/health_professionals_families/ for guidance).
- Outpatient care unless parenteral chelation or immediate removal from contaminated environment is required.
- If Pb source is in the home, the patient must reside elsewhere until the abatement process is completed.
- Avoid visit to any site of potential contamination.

ONGOING CARE
Early intervention (before age 3) programs for elevated lead levels improve standardized test performance in elementary school

FOLLOW-UP RECOMMENDATIONS
Patient Monitoring
- Expect rebound after chelation due to release of Pb from bone stores.
- Check for rebound Pb level 7 to 10 days after chelation therapy. Monitor biweekly or monthly thereafter.
- Correct iron or other detected nutritional deficiencies.
- Once Pb <35 μg/dL, repeat testing every 1 to 3 months until level <25 μg/dL is achieved. Then, monitor every 3 to 6 months until level <10 μg/dL. Once <9 μg/dL, test every 6 to 9 months.
- Consider surveillance for Pb level if retained bullets are present.

DIET
- Avoid pica.
- Adequate calcium, iron, zinc, magnesium, and vitamins C and D to reduce absorption of Pb.

PATIENT EDUCATION
- National Lead Information Center: https://www.epa.gov/lead/forms/lead-hotline-national-lead-information-center
- Centers for Disease Control and Prevention, Lead Poisoning Prevention Program: https://www.cdc.gov/lead-prevention/about/?CDC_AAref_Val=https://www.cdc.gov/nceh/lead/default.htm

PROGNOSIS
- Symptomatic Pb poisoning without encephalopathy generally improves with chelation, but subtle CNS toxicity may be long-lasting or permanent.
- Preschool children with higher Pb levels have lower reading and math scores in elementary school.
- Early childhood high body lead burden is correlated with higher risk of juvenile delinquency and arrest as an adult.
- Children with high Pb levels at age 11 years have lower IQ score and socioeconomic status in adulthood.
- With Pb encephalopathy, permanent sequelae (e.g., mental retardation, seizure disorder, blindness, and hemiparesis) occurs in 25–50%.

COMPLICATIONS
- CNS toxicity may be long-lasting or permanent.
- Long-term Pb exposure may cause chronic renal failure (Fanconi-like syndrome), gout, or Pb line (blue–black) on gingival tissue.
- Pb exposure in pregnancy is associated with reduced birth weight and premature birth.

REFERENCES

1. Ruckart PZ, Jones RL, Courtney JG, et al. Update of the blood lead reference value—United States, 2021. *MMWR Morb Mortal Wkly Rep*. 2021;70(43):1509–1512.
2. Centers for Disease Control and Prevention. Recommended actions based on blood lead levels. https://www.cdc.gov/lead-prevention/hcp/clinical-guidance/index.html. Accessed 23 August 2024.

ADDITIONAL READING

Jenkins D, Grossman D, Slusky D, et al. Blood lead testing in flint before and after water contamination. *Pediatrics*. 2022;150(6):e2022056541.

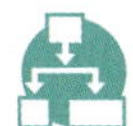

SEE ALSO

Anemia, Iron Deficiency

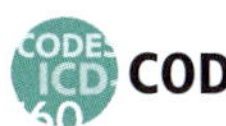

CODES

ICD10
- T56.0X4A Toxic effect of lead and its compounds, undetermined, init
- T56.0X1A Toxic effect of lead and its compounds, accidental, init

CLINICAL PEARLS
- Screen children 6 to 11 months of age with ≥1 risk factors.
- Children living in high-risk communities (>12% elevated Pb) should be tested annually from 1 to 5 years of age.
- CDC lowered the blood lead reference value (BLRV) from 5 μg/dL to 3.5 μg/dL in 2021.
- There is no safe Pb level.
- There are no studies that show consistent benefit for chelation in asymptomatic children with Pb <45 μg/dL. Environmental removal of Pb sources is critical.

LEGIONNAIRES' DISEASE

Kenneth A. Ballou, MD

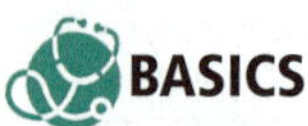

BASICS

DESCRIPTION

- *Legionnaires' disease* was named for an epidemic of lower respiratory tract disease at the 1976 American Legion convention in Philadelphia. The previously unrecognized causative bacterium was isolated, identified, and named *Legionella pneumophila*. The organism primarily causes pneumonia and flulike illness. *Legionella* preferentially colonizes commercial water systems (e.g., hotels, hospitals, apartment buildings, air conditioning cooling towers).
  - It is one of the three most common causes of pneumonias and the most common atypical pneumonia.
- System(s) affected: pulmonary, gastrointestinal (GI)
- Synonym(s): *Legionella* pneumonia; legionellosis; Pontiac Fever (self-limited flulike illness without pneumonia caused by *Legionella* spp.)

EPIDEMIOLOGY

- Predominant age: 15 months to 84 years; 74–91% of patients are >50 years old (1).
- Predominant gender: male > female

Incidence

- Cases of Legionnaires' disease have increased 4-fold in the United States since 2000; almost 10,000 cases are reported in 2018.
- Outbreaks are most common in late summer/early fall.
- ~2–9% of all cases of pneumonia in the United States. Legionnaires' disease is fatal in one of every 10 cases.

ETIOLOGY AND PATHOPHYSIOLOGY

- *L. pneumophila* is a weak gram-negative aerobic saprophytic freshwater bacterium. It is widely distributed in soil and water. Bipolar flagella provide motility; grow optimally at 40–45°C
- Exists in nature as a protozoan parasite, often within fresh water biofilms
- Serogroups 1 to 6 account for clinical disease.
- Serogroup 1 represents 70–92% of all clinical cases of *Legionella* in the United States.
- In the lung, *Legionella* infects alveolar macrophages.
- The organism is transmitted by breathing in contaminated water droplets or by aspiration of contaminated water (e.g., contaminated shower water was responsible for the inaugural Philadelphia outbreak).
- Community outbreaks have been associated with whirlpools, spas, fountains, and aboard cruise ships.

RISK FACTORS

- Impaired cellular immunity (*Legionella* are intracellular pathogens.)
- Male gender
- Smoking; alcohol abuse
- Immunosuppression; HIV; diabetes; organ transplant recipients; chronic or high-dose corticosteroid use
- Chronic cardiopulmonary disease
- Advanced age
- Use of antimicrobials within the past 3 months

GENERAL PREVENTION

- *Not transmitted person to person* (Respiratory isolation is unnecessary.)
- Superheat and flush water systems: Heat water to at least 158°F and flush for 30 minutes.
- Ultraviolet light and copper-silver ionization are bactericidal.
- Monochloramine disinfection of municipal water supplies decreases risk for *Legionella* infection.
- 0.2 micron water filters—must change regularly
- Keep water heaters >140°F; cold water <68°F.

DIAGNOSIS

- Illness ranges from asymptomatic seroconversion and mild febrile illness to severe pneumonia.
- Wound infections with *Legionella* also reported.
- Incubation period is 2 to 14 days.

HISTORY

- Signs and symptoms (with associated percentage):
  - Cough: 92% (typically dry; rarely productive)
  - Fever/chills: 90%
  - Dyspnea: 62%
  - Pleuritic chest pain: 35%
  - Headache: 48%
  - Myalgia/arthralgia: 40%
  - Watery diarrhea: 50%
  - Nausea and vomiting: 49% (2)
  - Neuropsychiatric symptoms include encephalopathy, confusion, disorientation, obtundation, depression, hallucinations, insomnia, and seizure: 53%.
- History of immunosuppression increases risk.

PHYSICAL EXAM

- Fever
- Relative bradycardia (key sign)
  - Temperature ≥102°F with an inappropriately low pulse rate of <100 beats/min (normal compensatory reaction to fever is >110 beats/min.)
- Rales and signs of consolidation (e.g., pectoriloquy, egophony, or tactile fremitus)

DIFFERENTIAL DIAGNOSIS

- Other bacterial pneumonias, especially atypical pneumonias: *Mycoplasma pneumoniae*, Q fever (*Coxiella burnetii*), *Chlamydophila pneumoniae*, *Chlamydophila psittaci*, *Francisella tularensis*
- Viral pneumonias, such as adenovirus, influenza (human, avian, swine), cytomegalovirus (CMV)
- Must be differentiated from COVID-19 pulmonary disease; COVID-19 testing recommended

DIAGNOSTIC TESTS & INTERPRETATION

Indications for *Legionella* testing:

- Failed outpatient antibiotic treatment for community-acquired pneumonia (CAP)
- Severe pneumonia, particularly those requiring intensive care
- Immunocompromised patients with pneumonia
- Patients with a history of traveling away from their home within 10 days of illness onset, especially with a history of commercial lodging such as hotel or cruise-ship stay within the last 2 weeks
- Pneumonia in the setting of a known Legionnaires' disease outbreak
- Pneumonia beginning ≥48 hours after hospital admission

Initial Tests (lab, imaging)

Diagnosis:

- *Legionella* PCR detects ~100% of all *Legionella* spp. from lower respiratory secretions.
- Urinary antigen test (UAT) detects serogroup 1 (which causes 80% of disease). UATs are highly specific (95–100%) but of variable sensitivity.
- *Legionella* culture (gold standard) requires an adequate sputum sample and special media (buffered charcoal yeast extract [BCYE] agar). Culture has variable sensitivity (10–80%) and time delays of up to 7 days for results.
- Other lab abnormalities:
  - Hyponatremia; hypophosphatemia (transient)
  - Lymphopenia
  - Mildly elevated serum transaminases; elevated LDH; elevated creatine kinase
  - Microscopic hematuria
  - Highly elevated C-reactive protein (CRP) (>30)
  - Highly elevated ferritin (≥2 times normal)
- Chest radiograph
  - Not specific for *Legionella*; commonly shows unilateral lower lobe patchy alveolar infiltrate with consolidation
  - Cavitation and abscess formation are more common in immunocompromised patients.
  - Pleural effusion occurs in up to 50%.
  - May take 1 to 4 months for radiographic findings to resolve. Progression of infiltrate on x-ray can be seen despite antibiotic therapy.

Diagnostic Procedures/Other

Transtracheal aspiration/bronchoscopy occasionally necessary to obtain sputum/lung samples

Test Interpretation

- Multifocal pneumonia with alveolitis and bronchiolitis and fibrinous pleuritis; may have serous or serosanguineous pleural effusion
- Abscess formation occurs in up to 20% of patients.
- Progression of infiltrates on x-ray (despite appropriate therapy) suggests Legionnaires' disease. Radiographic improvement may not correlate with clinical findings (longer lag times).
- Use of procalcitonin levels of limited value as it is not as sensitive in atypical pathogens such as *Legionella*

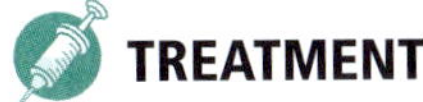

TREATMENT

GENERAL MEASURES

- Supportive care:
  - Oxygenation, hydration, and electrolyte balance with antibiotic therapy
- Extrapulmonary complications and higher mortality may be seen in patients with AIDS and other immunosuppressive conditions.
- In severe pneumonia, start empiric antibiotics to include coverage for *Legionella*.

MEDICATION

First Line

- Antibiotics that achieve high intracellular concentrations (e.g., macrolides, fluoroquinolones) are most effective; first-line treatment is either macrolide (azithromycin preferred) or quinolone (levofloxacin or moxifloxacin);
- Start antibiotics parenterally if unable to tolerate orally:
  - Levofloxacin is the preferred agent (3):
    - Levofloxacin 750 mg/day IV daily (switch to PO when patient is afebrile and tolerating PO meds) for 7 to 14 days
    - Moxifloxacin 400 mg/day IV daily (switch to PO when patient is afebrile and tolerating PO meds) for 7 to 14 days
  - Azithromycin may also be used first line. It requires a shorter duration of treatment than levofloxacin due to a longer half-life:
    - Azithromycin 500 mg/day IV daily (switch to PO when afebrile/tolerating PO meds) for 7 to 10 days
    - Clarithromycin 500 mg PO twice a day for 14 to 21 days
- Contraindications: hypersensitivity reactions
- Precautions: liver disease
- Significant drug interactions:
  - Can increase theophylline, carbamazepine, and digoxin levels; can increase activity of oral anticoagulants
  - May decrease the effectiveness of digoxin, quinidine, oral contraceptives, and hypoglycemic agents
- Longer courses of treatment (up to 21 days) may be needed in immunocompromised patients or valvular heart disease.

Second Line

- Doxycycline 100 mg IV/PO as a loading dose, then 100 mg q12h for 14 to 21 days
- Doxycycline should not be used in pregnant patients and is not approved for children aged <8 years.
- Tetracycline 500 mg PO q6h for 14 to 21 days
- Minocycline 100 mg PO q12h for 14 to 21 days
- Caution when using tetracyclines as there are increased rates of resistance in some species of *Legionella* organisms

ADMISSION, INPATIENT, AND NURSING CONSIDERATIONS

- Inability to tolerate oral antibiotics
- Hypoxemia
- Criteria for direct admission to the ICU:
  - Any major criteria for severe CAP:
    - Septic shock requiring vasopressor support
    - Acute respiratory failure requiring intubation and/or mechanical ventilation
  - Three or more minor criteria for severe CAP:
    - RR ≥30 breaths/min, PaO_2:FiO_2 ratio ≤250, multilobular infiltrates, confusion/disorientation, uremia (BUN ≥20 mg/dL), leukopenia (WBC <4,000 cells/mm^3), thrombocytopenia (PLT <100,000 cells/mm^3), hypothermia (temperature <36°C), hypotension requiring aggressive fluid resuscitation
- Discharge criteria: afebrile; able to tolerate oral antibiotics; return to normal/baseline room-air oxygen saturation

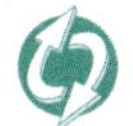

ONGOING CARE

FOLLOW-UP RECOMMENDATIONS

Patient Monitoring

- Monitor respiratory status, hydration, and electrolyte status closely.
- Chest radiography lags behind the clinical status and may not help with monitoring clinical response.

PATIENT EDUCATION

- Disease prevention: Eliminate pathogens from water supplies; low-emission cleaning of cooling towers with control measurements of water and air samples.
- *Legionella* is not spread from person to person.

PROGNOSIS

- Improved prognosis when appropriate antibiotics are started early in the disease course
- Recovery is variable:
  - Patients may clinically worsen despite appropriate initial treatment (first 1 to 2 days of therapy).
  - Improvement with defervescence in 3 to 5 days and complete recovery in 6 to 10 days is typical. Some have a more protracted course.
- Mortality in nosocomial infections as high as 15–34%

COMPLICATIONS

- Dehydration; hyponatremia; respiratory insufficiency requiring ventilator support
- Bacteremia/lung abscess formation in up to 20%
- Extrapulmonary diseases:
  - Endocarditis (most common extrapulmonary site); cellulitis; sinusitis; pancreatitis; pyelonephritis; encephalitis; pericarditis; perirectal abscess
- Renal failure; disseminated intravascular coagulation; multiple organ dysfunction syndrome (MODS); coma
- Death occurs in 8–12% of treated immunocompetent patients and in up to 80% of untreated immunocompromised patients.

REFERENCES

1. Viasus D, Gaia V, Manzur-Barbur C, et al. Legionnaires' disease: update on diagnosis and treatment. *Infect Dis Ther*. 2022;11(3):973–986.
2. Jomehzadeh N, Moosavian M, Saki M, et al. Legionella and Legionnaires' disease: an overview. *J Acute Dis*. 2019;8(6):221–232.
3. Metlay JP, Waterer GW, Long AC, et al. Diagnosis and treatment of adults with community-acquired pneumonia. An official clinical practice guideline of the American Thoracic Society and Infectious Diseases Society of America. *Am J Respir Crit Care Med*. 2019;200(7):e45–e67.

ADDITIONAL READING

Bellew S, Grijalva CG, Williams DJ, et al. Pneumococcal and Legionella urinary antigen tests in community-acquired pneumonia: prospective evaluation of indications for testing. *Clin Infect Dis*. 2019;68(12):2026–2033.

SEE ALSO

Pneumonia, Bacterial

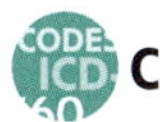

CODES

ICD10

- A48.2 Nonpneumonic Legionnaires' disease [Pontiac fever]
- A48.1 Legionnaires' disease

CLINICAL PEARLS

- Consider Legionnaires' disease in patients with pneumonia who have GI and other extrapulmonary findings (atypical CAP) and a relative bradycardia. Relative lymphopenia, mildly elevated serum transaminases (aspartate aminotransferase/alanine aminotransferase), highly increased ferritin levels, or hypophosphatemia are other laboratory clues to *Legionella* infection.
- Serology is not useful in early stages of the disease (an increase in *Legionella* antibody titers cannot be detected until 3 to 4 weeks after symptom onset).
- Urine antigen testing and *Legionella* sputum PCR are the most sensitive and practical initial tests. Sputum culture is definitive but can take up to 7 days.
- Consider Legionnaires' disease in cases of nosocomial pneumonia and in any community acquired pneumonia requiring inpatient treatment.
- Macrolides and quinolones are first-line agents.

LESBIAN HEALTH

Tina D'Amato, DO

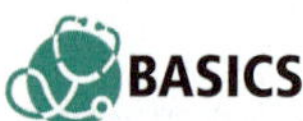

BASICS

DESCRIPTION

- A lesbian is a woman who has her primary emotional and sexual relationships with women.
- Sexual behaviors
  - May be celibate, sexually active only with women or with men, women and/or nonbinary partners
  - ~75% of self-reported lesbians have reported prior or ongoing sexual contact with men.
- Sexual orientation and gender are complex concepts and defining them can be challenging.

EPIDEMIOLOGY

Prevalence

- Estimated to be between 1% and 5%
- Approximately 1.4 million women living in the United States identify as lesbians; another 2.6 million women identify as bisexual
- 2022 Gallup Poll results had 1% of women identifying as lesbian.
- 2022 Gallup Poll shows 2.2% of generation Z and 1.5% of millennials identify as lesbian compared to 0.5% of generation X, 0.7% of boomers, and 0.2% of silent generation.
- 2021 American Community Survey from United States Census Bureau estimates 631,900 households are headed by female same-sex couples.

RISK FACTORS

Higher incidence for the following risk factors compared to heterosexual women:

- Elevated BMI
  - Lesbian women have a higher prevalence of overweight/obesity than all other female sexual orientation groups.
  - Higher prevalence rates of obesity have been found among lesbians who are African American, who live in urban or rural areas, who have lower levels of education, or who have lower socioeconomic status.
- Alcohol use
  - More common use than reported in heterosexual women
  - Age 20 to 34 years is at highest risk for daily use and heavy use of alcohol. Those numbers decline in older age groups, but even one drink per day can increase risks for cancer, hepatic, and heart disease.
- Tobacco use
  - 1.5 to 2 times more likely to smoke than heterosexual women
  - Aggressive marketing by tobacco industry to LGBT individuals
- Sexual minority stress (1)
  - Increased risk for health issues secondary to greater exposure to social stresses related to prejudice and stigma
  - Many of the increased health risks in lesbians can be attributed to behaviors that are the result of dealing with the stress and stigma of homophobia and discrimination.
- The above factors can increase risks for cardiovascular disease (CVD), type 2 diabetes, hepatic disease, and cancers.

GENERAL PREVENTION

Health Access and Outcomes

- Between 2013 and 2018, heterosexual women had significant reductions in delayed/absent medical care due to costs that was not seen in their lesbian peers.
- During 2016 and 2018, lesbian and bisexual women had significantly higher odds of undesirable health outcomes and access to health care compared to their heterosexual peers.

COMMONLY ASSOCIATED CONDITIONS

- Cervical cancer
  - Lesbians are equally at risk for developing cervical cancer compared to heterosexual women.
  - HPV can be transmitted genitally skin to skin, oral to genitals, and digital to genitals.
  - The risk of cervical cancer is highest in lesbians:
    - With prior HPV infection/abnormal Pap smear
    - Who have had a history of heterosexual intercourse
  - Lesbian and bisexual women are 10 times less likely to have adequate cervical cancer screening compared to heterosexual women.
  - Tobacco use influences cervical cell atypia.
- Breast cancer
  - Risk factors same as heterosexual women
    - Moderate or heavy alcohol consumption
    - Obesity
    - Nulliparity or first child born after age 30 years
  - Mammogram screening rates lower among lesbians
  - Data suggest lesbians have increased mortality rate compared to heterosexual women.
- Ovarian cancer
  - Elevated BMI and tobacco use increase risks.
  - Lesbians less likely to have been on hormonal contraception for ≥5 years
  - Lesbians less likely to have been pregnant or breastfed an infant before age 30 years
  - Lesbians at increased risk for ovarian cancer may want to explore potential benefits of long-term progestin-containing contraception to reduce risk.
- Endometrial cancer
  - Elevated BMI and tobacco use increases risks.
  - Lesbians less likely to have been pregnant
  - Lesbians with polycystic ovarian syndrome should be asked about sustained amenorrhea and consider use of progestin-containing contraception or regular schedule of induced "withdrawal bleeds" to reduce risks.
- CVD
  - Lesbians have higher rates of obesity, alcohol use, smoking, and stress, which increase risks for CVD.
  - A study of French population published in the May 17, 2023 Journal of The American Heart Association identified lesbian and bisexual women as having lower cardiovascular health scores compared to their heterosexual peers
- Mental health diagnoses
  - 2 times more likely to see general physician for mental/emotional complaint compared to heterosexual women
  - More likely to seek care if physician is aware of their sexual orientation
    - Depression
      - Discrimination stress proposed factor
      - Double the rate compared to heterosexual women
    - Suicide
      - "Out" lesbian women are 2 to 2.5 times more likely to have had suicidal ideation in the last 12 months compared to heterosexual women.
      - Lesbian women who were not "out" were more likely to have attempted suicide compared to heterosexual women.
    - Anxiety disorders
      - 3 times risk, multiple diagnoses
      - Higher rates of PTSD, panic, phobia, and 2- to 4-fold higher rate of generalized anxiety disorder
    - Alcohol abuse
      - Greatest in lesbians ages 20 to 34 years
      - Bar culture
      - May not feel comfortable in traditional Alcoholics Anonymous environment
      - Sexual minority females are more likely than heterosexual counterparts to be current alcohol users, binge drinkers, and heavy drinkers.
    - Substance abuse
      - Sexual minority women are at higher rates of all substance abuse compared to heterosexual counterparts.
        - Bisexual women have highest rates of substance abuse compared to lesbian and heterosexual women.
      - Higher levels of socioeconomic instability were associated with increased odds for substance abuse.
        - Household Pulse Survey from United States Census Bureau showed how COVID-19 pandemic impacted the LGBTQ population significantly greater than heterosexual counterparts.
- Sexually transmitted infections (STIs)
  - Many lesbians underestimate their STI risks.
  - Difficult to ascertain accurate statistics because of lack of research and the confounding factors of relying on identifiers of sexual orientation versus sexual behaviors
  - Increased risk during menstruation and activities causing friction
  - Lesbian sexual practices include the following:
    - High risk: oral–vaginal contact, genital–genital contact, oral–anal contact, digital stimulation/penetration, and sharing of sex toys
    - Lower risk: kissing, rubbing genitals against partner's body/clothing
- Bacterial vaginosis
  - Higher rate than heterosexual women; estimated 25–52% prevalence
  - Increased incidence with smoking, receptive oral sex, symptomatic partner, and new partner
  - Often found in monogamous lesbian couples suggesting it can be sexually transmitted; consider treating asymptomatic partner especially in recurrent cases.

- Chlamydia, gonorrhea, hepatitis B, syphilis, trichomonas, and herpes can all be transmitted woman to woman (WTW).
- HPV
  - Can be transmitted WTW
  - Up to 30% of women who have sex with women (WSW) have genital HPV.
  - 12% of WSW report genital warts.
  - 25% of WSW report cervical abnormalities.
  - Vaccine rates in WSW have improved significantly but still well below the 80% goal of Healthy People 2020 target. WSW may not get vaccine due to perceived decreased risks.
- HIV—transmission between women is rare but possible. WSW are more likely to have sexual contact with men having sex with men (MSM) than heterosexual women.
- STI screening and prevention
  - Screen based on woman's history.
  - Encourage safer sex practices:
    - Avoid menstrual blood/open sores.
    - Dental dams for oral sex, condoms on sex toys, and cleaning immediately after use
    - Vinyl/latex gloves for manual sex, limit friction with lubricants
- Psychosocial considerations
  - Sexual abuse
    - 3 times more likely than heterosexual women to report having been sexually assaulted
    - 43% of lesbians reported at least one sexual assault in their lifetime.
    - History of childhood sexual abuse can be associated with more complicated and difficult "coming out."
  - Intimate partner violence: National Coalition Against Domestic Violence reports 43.8% of lesbians have experienced rape, physical violence, and/or stalking by an intimate partner.
  - Parenthood: A reported 41% of lesbians desire to have a child. Perinatal depression is common and may be more common than in heterosexual women.
    - >30% have biologic children.
      - Often from previous heterosexual relationship
      - Adoption
      - Assisted reproductive technology/donor insemination
      - Some will engage in high-risk sexual behaviors (MSM, "one-night stand") in an attempt to get pregnant.
      - Providers should discuss parenting with their lesbian patients.
      - Encourage both partners or nonbiologic parent to adopt child to ensure permanent legal relationship to child.
      - Discuss durable power of attorney for health care and finances in the event of death or separation.
      - Adolescents who have been reared in lesbian mother families since birth demonstrate healthy psychological adjustment.
      - Children raised by same-sex parents have similar academic performance levels as their peers raised by different-sex parents.
  - Adolescent lesbians
    - Increased risk for eating disorders
    - Higher rates of substance use particularly polysubstance abuse
    - If also having sexual contact with males, higher rates of pregnancy compared to heterosexual counterparts due to (2)
      - High rates of early sexual initiation
      - Greater number of partners
      - Less contraceptive use
    - Higher rates of physical and/or sexual abuse—childhood sexual abuse does not cause children to become LGBTQ.
  - Aging lesbians
    - Elders aging "back into the closet"
      - Discrimination by religious and other groups that own nursing homes
      - Fear of discrimination by caregivers/health care workers
      - Few elder care programs specifically directed at LGBT persons

TREATMENT

GENERAL MEASURES

- Create a safe practice environment for lesbian patients.
  - Have nondiscrimination policy posted where it is visible to patients.
  - Educate staff to be comfortable dealing with the needs of lesbian patients and their families.
  - Brochures/photos should feature both same-sex and heterosexual couples.
  - Intake forms should include options for patient to indicate sexual preference and include options for partnered status.
  - Use "gender-neutral" language. For example, "Do you have a significant other?"
  - Avoid heterosexist assumptions ("What do you use for birth control?" asking instead "Do you plan to become pregnant or have a child? Do you need birth control?").
- Ask about sexual orientation.
  - Many physicians do not ask.
  - Intake/annual physical forms should include questions about orientation/activity.
  - Twice as likely to identify as a sexual minority if questions asked in an indirect way
- Take a detailed sexual history.
  - Sexual identity and sexual behaviors are not always strongly correlated.
  - Ask about behaviors ("Do you have sex with women, men, or both?"); do not just assume current/past sexual activity with women.
  - STI screening based on reported history/activity
  - Address contraception when appropriate.
  - Some physicians may create barriers by believing a patient's sexual self-identity and behaviors are not pertinent to competent care (3).
- Respect the partners.
  - Treat them as you would to any other spouse/partner.
  - Assure access if partner is hospitalized.
  - Recommend durable power of attorney if couple is not legally married.
- Follow same preventive screening guidelines and lifestyle recommendations as for heterosexual women (Pap smear, mammography, colonoscopy screening, safer sex, exercise, diet, alcohol moderation, and tobacco avoidance).
- Legal/U.S. government
  - Healthy People 2010 identified lesbian/gay Americans as 1 of 6 population groups affected by health care disparities.
  - Healthy People 2020 goals are to increase routine data collection efforts on LGBT populations via health care surveys
    - Questions about sexual orientation and gender identity were added to many population surveys.
  - Healthy People 2030 focus is on collecting data on specific health needs of LGBT population and improving health in LGBT adolescents.
    - The goal is to add questions about gender and sexual identity on more state and national surveys.
- Access to health insurance was increased with supreme court decisions on *United States v. Windsor* in 2013 and *Obergefell v. Hodges* in 2015. Some states still recognize same-sex civil union, but access to health insurance varies by state.
- Affordable Care Act (ACA): prohibits discrimination based on sexual orientation in any program receiving federal funds (Medicare/Medicaid); increased emphasis on research and data collections in LGBT population; National Health Interview Survey (NHIS); In 2013, the survey added a question about sexual orientation.

REFERENCES

1. Frost DM, Lehavot K, Meyer IH. Minority stress and physical health among sexual minority individuals. *J Behav Med*. 2015;38(1):1–8.
2. Committee on Adolescence. Office-based care for lesbian, gay, bisexual, transgender, and questioning youth. *Pediatrics*. 2013;132(1):198–203.
3. Knight DA, Jarrett D. Preventive health care for women who have sex with women. *Am Fam Physician*. 2017;95(5):314–321.

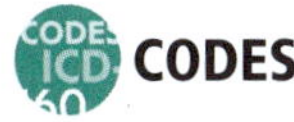

CODES

ICD10

- E66.3 Overweight
- Z72.0 Tobacco use
- F10.10 Alcohol abuse, uncomplicated

CLINICAL PEARLS

Create a safe health care environment for all patients. Use gender-neutral language. Do not assume heterosexuality or sexual practices.

LEUKEMIA, ACUTE LYMPHOBLASTIC (ALL) IN ADULTS

Sarah E. Nickolich, MD • Myles Stanley Nickolich, MD

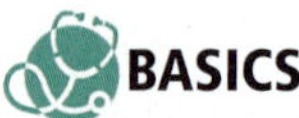

BASICS

Acute lymphoblastic leukemia (ALL) results from abnormal proliferation of hematopoietic stem cells in the bone marrow or extramedullary tissue.

DESCRIPTION

ALL in adults is the result of a clonal proliferation, of lymphocyte progenitor cells which are also known as lymphoblasts.

- ALL is defined by the presence of ≥20% lymphoblasts in the bone marrow (1).
- ALL subdivided based on the type of white blood cell (WBC) affected: T cell ALL or B cell ALL.
- B cell ALL is further separated into two major categories based on Philadelphia chromosome status:
  - Philadelphia chromosome negative (Ph−) ALL: further defined by molecular characteristics and subdivided into an additional category called Philadelphia chromosome-like (Ph-like) ALL which carries a poor prognosis.
  - Philadelphia chromosome positive (Ph+) ALL: characterized by the presence of Philadelphia chromosome and classically carried a poor prognosis but now has significant improvement in survival with the advent of treatment regimens incorporating tyrosine kinase inhibitors (TKIs) (often used in chronic myeloid leukemia) (1).
- Acute lymphoblastic lymphoma (LBL) is a related disease, arising from lymphoblasts. ALL and acute LBL are often managed similarly.
  - LBL presents as a mass, often in the mediastinum, with <20% blasts in the bone marrow.
  - ALL may present with a mass lesion but contains ≥20% blasts in the bone marrow (2).

Pregnancy Considerations

Many chemotherapy (CTX) drugs are teratogenic. Risk/benefit discussions are necessary if diagnosis is made during pregnancy.

Pediatric Considerations

ALL is the most common malignancy in children: accounting for 30% of all pediatric malignancies and 80% of pediatric leukemias (See "Acute Coronary Syndromes: NSTE-ACS [Unstable Angina and NSTEMI]; Acute Coronary Syndromes: STEMI.") (2).

Geriatric Considerations

- Geriatric-aged patients can experience decreased tolerance for classic CTX-based regimens, often have high-risk disease features, and have higher rates of developing treatment-related myeloid neoplasms such as myelodysplastic syndrome and acute myeloid leukemia.
- Recent advancements in chemo-immunotherapy treatment options for ALL have dramatically improved the tolerability of treatment and survival rates for patients aged >60 years. 4-year survival rates have improved to 80–85% among patients able to receive newer chemo-immunotherapy-based treatments (1).

EPIDEMIOLOGY

Bimodal distribution: early peak around age 5 years, second peak at around age 50 years (2). 80% of cases occur in children, 20% in adults.

Incidence

- Incidence of ALL is 1.7/100,000 per year (2).
- In 2024, there were 6,800 new cases of ALL in the United States (1).
- Higher incidence in older age, males, whites, those with history of radiation, CTX, or certain genetic disorders.

ETIOLOGY AND PATHOPHYSIOLOGY

The pathophysiology of ALL involves the abnormal proliferation and differentiation of clonal lymphoid cells. These malignant cells proliferate and replace the bone marrow cells that would normally create red blood cells, normal WBCs, and platelets. Therefore, resulting in anemia, neutropenia, and thrombocytopenia.

Genetics

There is increased risk of ALL in patients with genetic disorders such as trisomy 21, Klinefelter syndrome, and Fanconi anemia (2).

RISK FACTORS

- Age >70 years
- History of ionizing radiation exposure
- Human T-cell lymphotropic virus (HTLV) type 1 is associated with adult T-cell ALL.
- Epstein-Barr virus (EBV) is associated with mature B-cell ALL (2).

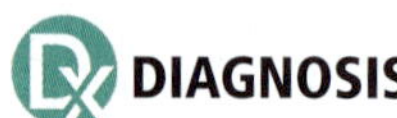

DIAGNOSIS

HISTORY

- Symptoms arise from sequelae of bone marrow suppression and/or from leukemic cell organ infiltration.
- B symptoms: fever, weight loss, night sweats
- Anemia: fatigue, shortness of breath, lightheadedness, angina, headache, palpitations
- Thrombocytopenia: easy bruising or bleeding
- Neutropenia: fever, infection
- Lymphocytosis: joint pain
- CNS: confusion; meningeal infiltration and cranial nerve involvement occurs in 5–8% of adults (2).

PHYSICAL EXAM

- Thrombocytopenia: petechiae, ecchymoses, epistaxis, retinal hemorrhages
- Anemia: pallor, flow murmur
- Neutropenia: fever, infections
- Lymphocytosis: lymphadenopathy; hepatosplenomegaly occurs in approximately 20% of adults.
- CNS: cranial nerve palsies, meningeal signs
- Extramedullary presentations in testis, skin or mediastinum (thymic area).

DIFFERENTIAL DIAGNOSIS

- Malignant disorders: other leukemias, acute myeloid leukemia, chronic myeloid leukemia in lymphoid blast phase, lymphomas; multiple myeloma, and myelodysplastic syndromes
- Nonmalignant disorders: aplastic anemia, myelofibrosis, autoimmune diseases (Felty syndrome, lupus), infectious mononucleosis, immune thrombocytopenic purpura, leukemoid reaction to infection

DIAGNOSTIC TESTS & INTERPRETATION

Initial Tests (lab, imaging)

- CBC with platelets and differential: evidence of leukocytosis (or more rarely, leukopenia); may also present with anemia and thrombocytopenia
- Coagulation studies (PT, PTT, fibrinogen)
- Peripheral blood smear: lymphoblasts (B cell or T cell)
- Pregnancy test in female patients
- CT/MRI of head with contrast if neurologic symptoms are present
- Blood cultures in patients with fever or suspected infection

Follow-Up Tests & Special Considerations

- Hepatitis C, HIV, EBV, HTLV 1, HTLV 2, HSV testing—all are potential precursors conditions that can cause oncogenic transformation.
- Hepatitis B testing—a pretreatment consideration
- CT of the neck, chest, abdomen, and pelvis with IV contrast and PET/CT if suspicion of lymphomatous involvement.
- Flow cytometry for immunophenotyping of marrow/blood lymphoblasts: B lineage (CD19, CD20, CD22, CD24), T lineage (CD2, CD3, CD5, CD7), common ALL antigen (CD10); human leukocyte antigen (HLA)-DR, terminal deoxynucleotidyl transferase (TdT), aberrant myeloid antigens (CD13, CD33), and stem cell antigen (CD34) (1)
- Cytochemical stains: myeloperoxidase negative; Sudan black B usually negative; TdT positive; periodic acid–Schiff ± is variable, depending on subtype.
- Cytogenetics: Specific chromosomal abnormalities have independent diagnostic and prognostic significance.
- Reverse transcription polymerase chain reaction (RT-PCR) or fluorescence in situ hybridization (FISH) for rapid diagnosis of BCR/ABL1+ ALL
- Genomic analysis by next-generation sequencing: detection of mutations associated with Ph-like ALL
- In consultation with a hematopoietic stem cell transplant center: HLA typing of patient and siblings.

Diagnostic Procedures/Other

- Bone marrow aspiration and biopsy with immunohistochemistry, immunophenotyping, cytogenetics, and molecular diagnostics
- Lymph node biopsy, if applicable
- Lumbar puncture (LP) for CNS involvement and for intrathecal (IT) CTX.

Test Interpretation

Diagnosis is based on the presence of lymphoblasts (>20%) in the bone marrow. In some cases, the diagnosis can be made based on the presence of certain molecular abnormalities, even if the percentage of blasts is lower. Bone marrow biopsy typically shows diffuse replacement of marrow, T-cell or B-cell lineage determined by CD expression.

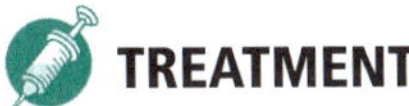

TREATMENT

GENERAL MEASURES

- Treatment of ALL is determined by patient's age and presence of Philadelphia chromosome.
- Three phases to CTX: induction, consolidation, and maintenance

MEDICATION

- Induction; goal: Achieve complete remission and restore normal hematopoiesis.
- Induction therapies may be recommended based on disease characteristics, patient age, comorbidities, and preferences/availability of options at the treating center. Additionally, treatment regimens may vary between countries. Currently, CTX-based treatment regimens approved in the United States for induction regimens include hyperfractionated cyclophosphamide, vincristine, anthracycline, and dexamethasone (hyper-CVAD), Cancer and Leukemia Group-B (CALGB) 8811 (Larson) protocol, and CALGB 10403. Of note, chemo-immunotherapy based regimens (including agents blinatumomab or inotuzumab) are currently in clinical trial for use as first-line agents and, although not FDA-approved, are being used in clinical practice due to their improved tolerability compared to combination CTX-based regimens (1).
- Following induction, measurable residual disease (MRD) status and molecular characteristics of the leukemia itself are the most important factors for consideration of treatment options in consolidation and maintenance.
- Should MRD-negative status not be achieved in induction, a repeat induction regimen would be considered (which could be a second cycle of induction therapy or transition to a completely different treatment course).
- Should MRD-negative remission be achieved following induction, the disease characteristics identified from molecular studies and patient age/comorbidity status are the primary drivers of consolidation and maintenance strategies (1).
- Consolidation; goal: Eliminate residual leukemic cells after induction therapy.
- The exact treatment course would be determined based on the induction regimen chosen. Allogeneic (from another donor) hematopoietic stem cell transplant may be considered during consolidation therapy.
- Maintenance; goal: Prevent relapse and prolong remission
- Although the exact maintenance regimen would be based on the overall treatment protocol chosen, many maintenance strategies include a steroid, vincristine, and 6-mercaptopurine (6-MP) based treatment. A common maintenance strategy is POMP: daily 6-MP, weekly methotrexate, monthly vincristine, with pulses of prednisone for 2 to 3 years. Ph+ ALL may also incorporate TKI use into maintenance strategies for up to 5 years post consolidation therapy (1).

ISSUES FOR REFERRAL

Suspicion for acute leukemia requires urgent referral to a hematologist-oncologist for diagnosis confirmation and management.

SURGERY/OTHER PROCEDURES

In some centers, patients may undergo surgical placement of a port for CTX. PICC lines are preferred due to easy removal after treatment to decrease the risk of infections.

ADMISSION, INPATIENT, AND NURSING CONSIDERATIONS

- Consider hospital admission in patients with febrile neutropenia.
- Hospital admission is required for most CTX inductions

ONGOING CARE

- Patients on CTX and radiation should receive annual physical, eye, dental, and dermatologic exams.
- Cancer survivorship is a partnership between patient, primary care physician, and oncologist who outlines ongoing surveillance needs for the patient.

FOLLOW-UP RECOMMENDATIONS

- Age-appropriate vaccinations (avoid live vaccines during CTX); age and sex appropriate cancer screenings
- Timings of vaccinations should be discussed with the transplant physician for patients who have undergone allogeneic hematopoietic stem cell transplant, particularly in the first year after transplant.

Patient Monitoring

Specialized monitoring may be required depending on the treatment regimen.

DIET

Nutritional support including neutropenic diet while neutropenic; avoid alcohol; calcium/vitamin D for steroid-induced osteoporosis

PATIENT EDUCATION

Neutropenic precautions; physical rehabilitation for deconditioning; smoking cessation.

PROGNOSIS

Prognosis is based on age, comorbidities, clinical presentation at time of diagnosis and cytogenetic findings. Presence of MRD after induction is an independent marker of poor prognosis (2). Only 40–50% of adults achieve long-term survival (1).

COMPLICATIONS

- Hyperleukocytosis: WBC >50,000 to 100,000 can lead to leukostasis, a medical emergency with microvascular white cell plugs; presents with neurologic deficits or respiratory distress, treated with fluids, and cytoreductive therapy
- Tumor lysis syndrome (high uric acid, potassium, phosphate, decreased calcium, leads to renal failure, and cardiac arrhythmias) may be prevented by administering allopurinol prior to CTX. Increase fluids; IV urate oxidase (rasburicase) can be used to treat hyperuricemia rapidly (if not G6PD deficient).
- Neutropenia from myelosuppression
- High-dose cyclophosphamide: severe nausea and vomiting; use appropriate antiemetic regimen.
- Vincristine can cause neurotoxicity and ileus.
- Alkylating agents and corticosteroids can cause avascular necrosis or osteonecrosis.
- Steroid-induced hyperglycemia
- Anthracyclines causes cardiotoxicity.
- Asparaginase therapy increases risks for deep vein thromboses and veno-occlusive disease.
- Opportunistic infections (*Pneumocystis carinii* pneumonia, bacterial and fungal pneumonia or sepsis)
- CTX can cause sterility, pancreatitis and liver dysfunction, arachnoiditis and CNS effects.
- Relapse of ALL in marrow or extramedullary sites (CNS, testis)

REFERENCES

1. Kantarjian H, Jabbour E. Adult acute lymphoblastic leukemia: 2025 update on diagnosis, therapy, and monitoring. *Am J Hematol*. 2025;100(7):1205–1231. doi:10.1002/ajh.27708.
2. Gbenjo JTC, McCrary GLM, Wilson SE. Leukemia: what primary care physicians need to know. *Am Fam Physician*. 2023;107(4):397–405.

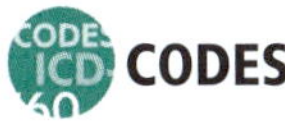

CODES

ICD10

- C91.00 Acute lymphoblastic leukemia not having achieved remission
- C91.01 Acute lymphoblastic leukemia, in remission
- C91.02 Acute lymphoblastic leukemia, in relapse

CLINICAL PEARLS

- ALL diagnosis is based on the presence of ≥20% lymphoblasts or characteristic mutations in the bone marrow.
- Treatment should be at an appropriate cancer center for tailored therapy based on mutations in ALL cells.
- Patients need to be monitored closely for CTX toxicities and progression of disease.

LEUKEMIA, ACUTE MYELOID

Jan Cerny, MD, PhD

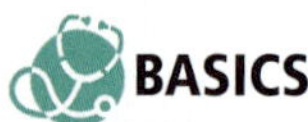

BASICS

DESCRIPTION

- Acute myeloid leukemia (AML) is characterized by proliferation of abnormal immature myeloid progenitors (blasts) with reduced capacity to differentiate leading to bone marrow failure and a variety of systemic symptoms.
- Historically, the French–American–British (FAB) classification system divided AML based on the cell morphology with the addition of cytogenetics (subtypes M0 to M7).
- The World Health Organization (WHO) classifications attempt to provide more meaningful prognostic information.
  - AML with defining genetic abnormalities:
    - Translocation in t(8;21) RUNX1::RUNX1T1 fusion, t(9;11) KMT2A, t(6;9) DEK::NUP214, t(1;22) RBM15::MRTFA, t(15;17) APL with PML::RARA fusion
    - Inversion in chromosome 16 inv(16) CBFB::MYH11, inv(3) MECOM
    - Other defined genetic alterations
  - AML, myelodysplasia related: presence of a prior myelodysplastic syndrome (MDS) or myeloproliferative neoplasm (MPN) that transformed into AML
  - Myeloid neoplasms postcytotoxic therapy: AML, MDS, and MDS/MPN exposed to cytotoxic therapy
  - Myeloid neoplasms associated with germline predisposition: Down syndrome, Fanconi anemia, RASopathies
  - Acute leukemias of mixed or ambiguous lineage (*biphenotypic acute leukemia*)
  - Myeloid sarcoma

EPIDEMIOLOGY

- New cases in men and women is 4.1 per 100,000 men and women per year.
- Male ≥ female

Incidence

The incidence of AML increases with age, and median age is 67 years.

Prevalence

~20,050 cases estimated in 2022 making it the most common type of leukemia in adults

ETIOLOGY AND PATHOPHYSIOLOGY

Genetics

- Three risk groups
  - Good risk: inv(16), t(8;21), t(15;17)
  - Standard risk: normal karyotype
  - Poor risk: monosomy 5 and 7 (typically secondary AML), deletion 5q, abnormalities of 11q23, or complex karyotype
- *FLT3* gene mutations, especially internal tandem duplications (FLT3-ITD), have been associated with poor survival in AML. These and growing list of (onco)gene (e.g., *NPM1, IDH1/2, DNMT3A*, and *P53*) mutations have been studied to further risk-stratify patients (1).

RISK FACTORS

- Genetic predisposition (e.g., Down syndrome); Bloom syndrome (~25% develop AML), Fanconi anemia (52%), neurofibromatosis, Li-Fraumeni syndrome, Wiskott-Aldrich syndrome, Kostmann syndrome, and Diamond-Blackfan anemia
- Radiation exposure
- Immunodeficiency states
- Chemical and drug exposure (nitrogen mustard and alkylating agents; benzene)
- MDS
- Cigarette smoking

GENERAL PREVENTION

Treatment of high-risk MDS with hypomethylating agents (5-azacitidine [Vidaza]) may prolong time to transformation from MDS into AML

COMMONLY ASSOCIATED CONDITIONS

- Disseminated intravascular coagulopathy (DIC) especially in acute promyelocytic leukemia (APL) but may be seen in any AML
- Leukostasis (high blast number and increased adhesive ability of blasts)
- Tumor lysis syndrome (TLS): spontaneous or in response to chemotherapy

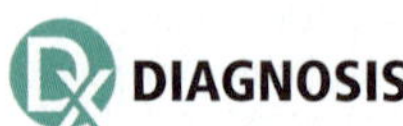

DIAGNOSIS

HISTORY

Fatigue (anemia or tumor burden); bleeding (low platelets or DIC); difficulty clearing infections (neutropenia or immune dysregulation)

PHYSICAL EXAM

- Mostly nonspecific and related to marrow or tissue infiltration
  - Fever, bleeding, pallor, splenomegaly, hepatosplenomegaly
  - Lymphadenopathy (usually reactive)
- If CNS is involved, symptoms of increased intracranial pressure can be present.
- Occasionally, patients will present with prominent extramedullary sites of leukemia (e.g., skin infiltration or ultimately as a myeloid sarcoma).

DIFFERENTIAL DIAGNOSIS

- Virus-induced cytopenia, lymphadenopathy, and organomegaly
- Immune cytopenias (including systemic lupus erythematosus [SLE])
- Drug-induced cytopenias
- Other marrow failure and infiltrative diseases (e.g., aplastic anemia, paroxysmal nocturnal hemoglobinuria, MDS, Gaucher disease)

DIAGNOSTIC TESTS & INTERPRETATION

- CBC shows subnormal RBCs, neutrophils, and platelets.
- Bone marrow for histology, flow cytometry, and cytogenetics to establish diagnosis and prognosis
- ESR
- Lactate dehydrogenase (LDH) and uric acid can be elevated (e.g., TLS).
- Coagulation profil e can be normal or prolonged (e.g., DIC).
- Lumbar puncture for leukemic cells.
- Ultrasonography or CT scan of the abdomen may discover organomegaly.

Diagnostic Procedures/Other

Bone marrow studies are usually necessary to make the diagnosis.

- Aspirates: for cell morphology, cytochemistries, immunophenotyping (can confirm differentiation stage of AML); cytogenetics: chromosomal aberration (prognostic value; see "Genetics")

Test Interpretation

- Marrow is usually hypercellular and the normal architecture effaced; leukemic blast count is 20% or more. Newer updates no longer require >20% blast count for AML type with defining genetic abnormalities.
- Liver and spleen may be infiltrated with leukemic cells.

TREATMENT

- Classical (cytotoxic) chemotherapy has been the backbone of AML therapy; it consists of induction and consolidation phase ± maintenance (APL), but more recently, other transplant-ineligible AML patients can be treated with hypomethylating agent (oral) azacytidine.
- Bone marrow transplantation (BMT) for high-risk AML
- Relatively modest improvements have been made in AML induction chemotherapy. Supportive care had improved significantly.

GENERAL MEASURES

- Close monitoring of bone marrow, liver, heart, renal function, and coagulation parameters (risk for DIC)
- Supportive therapy with
  - Good hydration
  - Transfusions of packed RBCs and platelets based on patient's needs (threshold as for platelets as low as 5,000); use leukoreduced, irradiated blood products because all patients can be considered for BMT.
  - Avoid antiplatelet agents (e.g., aspirin products).
  - Follow febrile neutropenic guidelines in neutropenic patient who becomes febrile (even low-grade fever).

Geriatric Considerations

- Older patients (>60 to 65 years of age) remain a therapeutic challenge. These patients are offered so-called reduced-intensity or nonmyeloablative BMT.
- Adding growth factors (granulocyte colony-stimulating factor [G-CSF]) may reduce toxicity in older patients (but is not broadly accepted).
- Hypomethylating agent, such as 5-azacitidine or decitabine, with or without Venetoclax have been broadly adopted and prolong survival in older adults ineligible for classical chemotherapy.

Pregnancy Considerations

Chemotherapy is a viable option in the 2nd and 3rd trimesters.

MEDICATION

First Line

- APL (APL, AML with t[15;17])
  - All-trans retinoic acid (ATRA) and arsenic trioxide both promote maturation to granulocytes. Their combination can be used in low and intermediate risk APL for (chemotherapy) free treatment.
  - Idarubicin is often added to induction therapy, in high risk group.
  - Monoclonal anti-CD33 (Mylotarg) is being added as well in order to minimize chemotherapy use in this curable leukemia.

- Treatment of AML in younger adults: AML (other than APL)
  - Induction (daunorubicin or idarubicin [anthracycline and cytarabine]): The generally accepted combination is 3 + 7 (anthracycline is given for 3 days and cytarabine for 7 days) or more intensive regimens with high-dose cytarabine (HiDAC) or high dose of anthracycline.
  - Liposomal preparation of daunorubicin and cytarabine (Vyxeos) is now available for AML with MDS changes or therapy-related AML.
- Remission is typically consolidated in younger patients by the following:
  - In good-risk AML, 3 to 4 cycles of HiDAC and BMT is reserved for time of recurrence.
  - In poor-risk patients, 1 to 2 cycles of HiDAC (until donor is identified) are followed by allogeneic BMT.
  - Intermediate-risk AML should be treated based on individual patient's features, donor availability, and access to clinical trials. A meta-analysis showed that even intermediate-risk patients benefit from allogeneic BMT.
- Treatment of AML in older adults (>65 years of age) remains a challenge. These patients have poor performance status, more likely secondary AML, higher incidence of unfavorable cytogenetics, comorbidities, shorter remissions, and shorter overall survival. Liposomal daunorubicin and cytarabine is an agent approved for secondary and therapy related AML.
  - Intensive chemotherapy may be feasible for patients with good performance status; alternative regimens with mitoxantrone, fludarabine, and clofarabine
  - Newly diagnosed patients who are 75 years or older or who have conditions that preclude them from receiving intense induction therapy have following options of novel (targeted) agents
    - Low-dose cytarabine with glasdegib (DAURISMO, Pfizer Labs)
    - Hypomethylating agents (azacytidine, Vidaza; decitabine, Dacogen) with ivosidenib (Tibsovo; IDH1 inhibitor)
    - Hypomethylating agents (azacytidine, Vidaza; decitabine, Dacogen) with venetoclax (Venclexta; BCL-2 inhibitor)
- FLT-3 inhibitors such as midostaurin (Rydapt) are approved as addition to induction and consolidation chemotherapy, and gilteritinib (Xospata) is approved for relapsed/refractory AML.
- Ivosidenib (Tibsovo; IDH1 inhibitor) and enasidenib (Idhifa; IDH2 inhibitor) are approved for relapsed/refractory AML. Both of these agents can cause differentiation syndrome similar to the one seen in ATRA or arsenic treated APL patients.
- Precautions
  - If organ failure, some drugs may be avoided or dose reduced (e.g., no anthracyclines in patients with preexisting cardiac problems).
  - Patients will be immunosuppressed during treatment. Avoid live vaccines. Administer varicella-zoster or measles immunoglobulin as soon as exposure of patient occurs.
- Significant possible interactions: Allopurinol accentuates the toxicity of 6-mercaptopurine.
- Targeted therapies: midostaurin for AML with FLT3 mutations (both ITD and TKD). Ivosidenib (IDH1 inhibitor) and enasidenib (IDH2 inhibitor) for relapsed/refractory AML with respective IDH mutations; gemtuzumab ozogamicin (anti-CD33 monoclonal antibody) for relapsed/refractory AML with CD33 expression

Second Line

- Healthy, younger patients are usually offered reinduction chemotherapy and allogeneic BMT.
- Older patients would receive hypomethylating agent with or without venetoclax or targeted agent (FLT3 or IDH 1/2 inhibitor).

SURGERY/OTHER PROCEDURES

- BMT: Decision between myeloablative and nonmyeloablative approach should be based on patient's performance status, comorbidities, and AML risk factors.
  - Allogeneic BMT is usually indicated in first remission in intermediate- or high-risk AML or in second remission in all other AML patients. Matched related donor used to be preferred over matched unrelated donor (lower risk of graft vs. host disease); recent data suggest equal outcomes because allogeneic transplant regimens and post-transplant care have improved significantly.
- Haploidentical transplants and cord blood have emerged as alternative sources of hematopoietic stem cells for adults that show comparable outcomes as well.
- Autologous BMT may be acceptable in specific situations (e.g., no donor is available).

ADMISSION, INPATIENT, AND NURSING CONSIDERATIONS

- Induction treatment for AML requires inpatient care, usually on a specialized ward. Episodes of febrile neutropenia typically require admission and IV antibiotics.
- Appropriate hydration to prevent TLS
- IV may lead to chemical burns in the event of extravasation.

ONGOING CARE

FOLLOW-UP RECOMMENDATIONS

Patient Monitoring

- Repeat bone marrow studies to document remission and also if a relapse is suspected.
- Follow CBC with differential, coagulation studies, uric acid level, and other chemistries related to TLS (creatinine, potassium, phosphate, calcium); monitor urinary function at least daily during induction phase and less frequently later.
- Physical evaluation, including weight and BP, should be done frequently during treatment.

DIET

Total parenteral nutrition (TPN) in case of severe mucositis

PATIENT EDUCATION

Leukemia Society of America: https://www.lls.org/leukemia

PROGNOSIS

AML remission rate is 60–80%, with only 20–40% long-term survival. The wide variable prognosis is due to prognostic group (age, cytogenetics, and genetics).

COMPLICATIONS

- Acute side effects of chemotherapy, including febrile neutropenia
- TLS
- DIC
- Late-onset cardiomyopathy in patients treated with anthracyclines
- Chronic side effects of chemotherapy (secondary malignancies)
- Graft versus host disease in patients who have received allogeneic BMT

REFERENCES

1. Döhner H, Wei AH, Appelbaum FR, et al. Diagnosis and management of AML in adults: 2022 recommendations from an international expert panel on behalf of the ELN. *Blood*. 2022;140(12):1345–1377.

SEE ALSO

Disseminated Intravascular Coagulation; Leukemia, Acute Lymphoblastic (ALL) in Adults; Leukemia, Chronic Myelogenous; Myelodysplastic Syndromes (MDS); Myeloproliferative Neoplasms

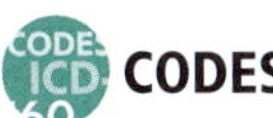

ICD10

- C92.00 Acute myeloblastic leukemia, not having achieved remission
- C92.01 Acute myeloblastic leukemia, in remission
- C92.02 Acute myeloblastic leukemia, in relapse

CLINICAL PEARLS

- AML is a proliferation and accumulation of abnormal immature myeloid progenitors (blasts) with reduced capacity to differentiate into more mature cellular elements. This leads to bone marrow failure and results in a variety of systemic symptoms.
- AML is the most common leukemia in adults.
- Prognosis of leukemia depends on the cytogenetic and molecular profile of the disease.
- Allogeneic transplant remains the only therapy with curative potential for patients with intermediate- and high-risk AML.

LEUKEMIA, CHRONIC LYMPHOCYTIC

Jan Cerny, MD, PhD • Geoffrey Matthes, MD, MSc

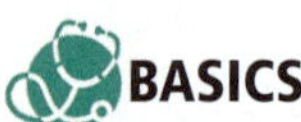

BASICS

DESCRIPTION

- Chronic lymphocytic leukemia (CLL) is a monoclonal disorder characterized by a progressive accumulation of mature but functionally incompetent lymphocytes.
- Based on percentage of prolymphocytes, the disease may be regarded as CLL (<10% prolymphocytes), prolymphocytic leukemia (PLL; >55%), or CLL/PLL (>10% and <55%).
- Small lymphocytic lymphoma is a lymphoma variant of CLL.
- System(s) affected: hematologic, lymphatic, immunologic

EPIDEMIOLOGY

Incidence

- CLL represents the most common form of leukemia in adults in the United States (2021 incidence 21,050).
- Second leading cause of death among adults with leukemia in the United States after acute myeloid leukemia
- CLL primarily affects elderly individuals, with median age of diagnosis being 70 years.
- Predominant sex: male > female (1.6:1); higher among white people

ETIOLOGY AND PATHOPHYSIOLOGY

- The cell of origin in CLL is a clonal B cell arrested in the B-cell differentiation pathway, intermediate between pre–B cells and mature B cells. In the peripheral blood, these cells resemble mature lymphocytes.
- Genetic mutations leading to disrupted function and prolonged survival of affected lymphocytes are suspected, but not well known. The BCL2 proto-oncogene (suppressor of apoptosis or programmed cell death) is overexpressed in CLL.

Genetics

Familial cases are rare. CLL does occur at higher frequency among first-degree relatives of patients with the disease, and several somatic gene mutations have been identified at significantly higher rates among CLL patients (1).

RISK FACTORS

Uncertain; possible chronic immune stimulation is suspected; monoclonal B-cell lymphocytosis: 1% risk progression to CLL

COMMONLY ASSOCIATED CONDITIONS

- Immune system dysregulation is common.
- Autoimmune hemolytic anemia (AIHA)
- Immune thrombocytopenia purpura (ITP)
- Pure red cell aplasia (PRCA)

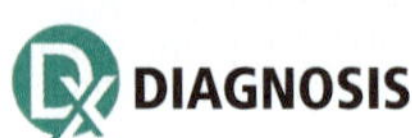

DIAGNOSIS

HISTORY

- CLL is often discovered incidentally (up to 40% of patients are asymptomatic at the time of diagnosis).
- Others may have the following symptoms:
  - B symptoms: fevers, night sweats, >10% weight loss
  - Fatigue and/or other symptoms of anemia
  - Enlarged lymph nodes (lymphadenopathy = LAD)
  - Mucocutaneous bleeding and/or petechiae
  - Early satiety and/or abdominal discomfort related to an enlarged spleen, rarely enlarged liver
  - Recurrent infection(s)

PHYSICAL EXAM

- Lymphadenopathy (localized or generalized)
- Organomegaly (splenomegaly, hepatomegaly)
- Mucocutaneous bleeding (thrombocytopenia)
- Skin: petechiae (thrombocytopenia), pallor (anemia), rash (leukemia cutis)

DIFFERENTIAL DIAGNOSIS

- Infectious:
  - Bacterial (tuberculosis, pertussis)
  - Viral (mononucleosis)
- Neoplastic:
  - Leukemic phase of non-Hodgkin lymphomas
  - Hairy cell leukemia
  - PLL
  - Large granular lymphocytic leukemia
  - Waldenstrom macroglobulinemia

DIAGNOSTIC TESTS & INTERPRETATION

Initial Tests (lab, imaging)

- CBC with differential: B cell absolute lymphocytosis with >5,000 B lymphocytes/μL; often also shows anemia and/or thrombocytopenia in advanced stage
- Blood smear: ruptured lymphocytes ("smudge" cells) and morphologically small mature-appearing lymphocytes
- Confirm with immunophenotyping on peripheral blood via flow cytometry or lymph node biopsy: CLL cells are positive for CD19, CD20 (dim), CD23, and CD5; low levels of surface membrane immunoglobulin (Ig)—either IgM or IgM&D; only a single Ig light chain is expressed (κ or λ) confirming monoclonality. CLL cells are also negative for Cyclin-D1.
- Additional labs:
  - Hemolysis labs (in cases associated with high disease activity or AIHA): high LDH and indirect bilirubin, low haptoglobin, +/− elevated reticulocyte count (bone marrow infiltration)
  - High plasma β_2-microglobulin (poor prognosis)
  - Hypogammaglobulinemia, low IgG level
- Liver/spleen ultrasound: not required for initial workup
- CT scan of chest/abdomen/pelvis: not necessary for staging but may identify compression of organs or internal structures from enlarged lymph nodes
- Positron emission tomography (PET) scan: not recommended unless Richter transformation (RT) is suspected

Diagnostic Procedures/Other

- Bone marrow biopsy: not performed routinely but may be helpful to assess etiology of cytopenia found in conjunction with CLL diagnosis
- Lymph node biopsy: Consider if lymph node(s) begins to rapidly enlarge in a patient with known CLL to assess for transformation to a high-grade lymphoma (RT), especially with fever, weight loss, and painful lymphadenopathy.

Test Interpretation

- Bone marrow biopsy aspirate usually shows >30% lymphocytes.
- Cytogenetics (fluorescence in situ hybridization) may show chromosomal changes, which are prognostic:
  - Unfavorable: del(17p) or TP53 mutation, del(11q), unmutated immunoglobulin heavy-chain variable (IGHV)
  - Neutral: normal, trisomy 12
  - Favorable: del(13q), mutated IGHV

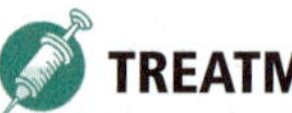

TREATMENT

GENERAL MEASURES

- Patients with frequent infections due to hypogammaglobulinemia likely to benefit from infusions of intravenous immunoglobulin (IVIG).
- Genetic risk stratification in therapy selection for advanced or symptomatic CLL
  - Very high-risk disease: del(17p) and/or TP53 mutations
  - High-risk disease: IGHV unmutated (without 17p del or TP53 mutation)
  - Standard risk disease: IGHV mutated (without 17p del or TP53 mutation)
- Indications for treatment include: constitutional (B) symptoms, cytopenias (thrombocytopenia or anemia), or AIHA and/or thrombocytopenia poorly responsive to corticosteroids, progressive symptomatic organomegaly (splenomegaly or lymphadenopathy), absolute lymphocyte doubling time (<6 months), or rarely extranodal involvement.

MEDICATION

First Line

- Standard of care for new diagnosis with no symptoms or early-stage disease: observation
- Low-risk disease, Rai stage 0: observation with periodic follow-up
- Intermediate-risk group, Rai stages I and II: Observe until evidence of disease progression or development of symptoms.
- High-risk patients, Rai stage III and IV: Initiate treatment. Selection of first-line therapy depends on patient functional status (age, performance status, and medical comorbidities) as well as genetic risk stratification of their CLL (above).
- Main groups of therapeutic agents:
  - Targeted therapies: preferred especially for very high–risk and high-risk patients
    - Bruton tyrosine kinase (BTK) inhibitor: ibrutinib, acalabrutinib, and zanubrutinib
    - BCL2 inhibitor venetoclax
  - Immunotherapy:
    - Monoclonal anti-CD20 antibodies (immunotherapy): rituximab (R), obinutuzumab, ofatumumab
  - Chemotherapy:
    - Alkylators: cyclophosphamide (C), chlorambucil, and bendamustine (B)
    - Purine analogs: fludarabine (F) cladribine, and pentostatin (P)
- Ibrutinib or acalabrutinib (Newer agents have fewer side effects.) (2)

- First generation BTK inhibitor (Ibrutinib) is known for a wide variety of cardiac and pulmonary complications and increased risk of bleeding.
- Venetoclax in combination with obinutuzumab offer very effective regimens; fixed duration
- Combinations of BTK inhibitor and venetoclax are being evaluated for the possibility of time-limited treatment for CLL patients that achieved complete response at the molecular level.
- Combination regimens: FC, FR (lower toxicity), BR, PCR, and FCR are used less often, but FCR can offer time-limited and highly effective therapy in IGHV-mutated CLL; such chemotherapy agents increase the risk of myeloid malignancies in the long term.
- Steroids, high dose: useful in autoimmune manifestations of CLL (AIHA, ITP)

Second Line

- Second-line therapy depends on time to progression and previous therapy.
- Early relapse (within 1 year after chemoimmunotherapy, 2 to 3 years after FCR), treatment with targeted therapy is favored.
  - Alternative BTK inhibitor
  - Venetoclax: as monotherapy and with rituximab in relapsed/refractory CLL and in patients with 17p deletion (2)
  - PI3K kinase inhibitors: idelalisib (PI3Kδ) with rituximab in patients with comorbidities. Duvelisib (PI3Kδ and PI3Kγ): approved as single agent for patients (PJP prophylaxis is recommended.) (2)
    - PI3K Inhibitors are known for many adverse events, and are rarely used; hyperglycemia, hepatotoxicity, pneumonitis, and diarrhea; these agents received initially an accelerated approval, and they are currently intensively scrutinized for their safety and long-term outcome.
  - Obinutuzumab alone or with chlorambucil in patients with comorbidities and previously untreated CLL
- Other options:
  - Lenalidomide, a thalidomide derivative, can be useful in some situations.
- Allogenic (nonmyeloablative conditioning) stem cell transplant (hSCT) may be considered in high-risk and younger patients, particularly those with refractory or RT.
- On the contrary to other non-Hodgkin lymphoma, chimeric antigen receptor T (CAR-T) cells are still in investigational phase as therapies for CLL.

ISSUES FOR REFERRAL

- Surgical consultation for splenectomy in patients with progressive splenomegaly +/− refractory cytopenias
- Radiation oncology consultation for large or bulky lymphadenopathy, particularly those causing compressive symptoms

ADDITIONAL THERAPIES

- Patients at high risk for tumor lysis syndrome (TLS) should be given allopurinol to prevent uric acid nephropathy.
- Patients would require prophylactic antibiotics when they start treatment; PJP and HSV prophylaxis
- Rapid reduction in white blood cell count is sometimes warranted in cases of leukostasis (WBC $>400 \times 10^9$/L).
- Vaccinations (avoid live vaccines):
  - Annual influenza vaccine
  - Pneumococcal vaccine every 5 years
  - Zoster vaccine recombinant, adjuvanted for treatment-naïve patients, or those treated with BTK inhibitor
  - COVID-19 vaccination

ADMISSION, INPATIENT, AND NURSING CONSIDERATIONS

Complications of disease (AIHA) or of therapy (febrile neutropenia, TLS); venetoclax can be associated with TLS and monitoring inpatient may be needed.

ONGOING CARE

FOLLOW-UP RECOMMENDATIONS

Patient Monitoring

Patients with low-risk CLL and/or patients in remission:

- CBC with differential (lymphocytosis), LDH, and β_2-microglobulin every 3 to 6 months
- Physical exam (lymphadenopathy, organomegaly)

PATIENT EDUCATION

Leukemia and Lymphoma Society has educational pamphlets: https://www.lls.org/resource-center/download-or-order-free-publications?language=English&category=Leukemia&sortby=alpha

PROGNOSIS

- Rai system used in the United States and Binet system in Europe; International Prognostic Score for early stage CLL (IPS-E) for predicting time to first treatment.
- Rai staging system:
  - Stage 0: lymphocytosis only; low-risk status
  - Stage I: lymphocytosis and adenopathy; intermediate-risk status
  - Stage II: lymphocytosis +/− adenopathy and splenomegaly and/or hepatomegaly; intermediate-risk status
  - Stage III: lymphocytosis and anemia (hemoglobin <11 g/dL); high-risk status
  - Stage IV: lymphocytosis and thrombocytopenia (platelets $<100 \times 10^9$/L); high-risk status
- IPS-E is helpful to identify patients who are at risk of needed therapy sooner.
  - The IPS-E score is calculated by giving one point for each of the following:
    - Unmutated IGHV
    - Lymphocytes $>15 \times 10^9$/L
    - Palpable lymph nodes
    - A score of 0 indicated low risk, 1 intermediate risk, and 2 to 3 high risk of progressing to symptomatic disease requiring treatment. More than half of the high-risk group would require treatment within 5 years of their diagnosis.
- Adverse risk factors:
  - Advanced stage, peripheral lymphocyte doubling time <12 months, diffuse marrow infiltration, increased number of prolymphocytes or cleaved cells, poor response to chemotherapy, high β_2-microglobulin and thymidine kinase levels and low micro RNAs (miRNAs), abnormal karyotyping: del(17p) and del(11q), mutated IGHV genes (expression of ZAP-70 $>20\%$ or CD38 $>30\%$ evaluated by immunophenotyping are surrogate markers.), NOTCH1 mutation (associated with unmutated IGVH), increased Cumulative Illness Rating Scale (CIRS)

COMPLICATIONS

Acute or long-term effects of chemotherapy and targeted therapy, RT, AIHA (fludarabine) slightly increased risk of solid tumors (Kaposi sarcoma, malignant melanoma, laryngeal, lung and colon cancer), increased risk of infections, impaired immune system, membranoproliferative glomerulonephritis (MPGN), leukostasis, and TLS.

REFERENCES

1. Yan H, Tian S, Kleinstern G, et al. Chronic lymphocytic leukemia (CLL) risk is mediated by multiple enhancer variants within CLL risk loci. *Hum Mol Genet*. 2020;29(16):2761–2774.
2. Burger JA. Treatment of chronic lymphocytic leukemia. *N Engl J Med*. 2020;383(5):460–473.

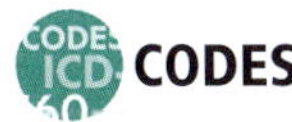

CODES

ICD10

- C91.12 Chronic lymphocytic leukemia of B-cell type in relapse
- C91.11 Chronic lymphocytic leukemia of B-cell type in remission
- C91.10 Chronic lymphocytic leukemia of B-cell type not having achieved remission

CLINICAL PEARLS

- CLL is the most common form of leukemia in adults in the United States.
- CLL primarily affects elderly individuals, median age of diagnosis being 70 years. Incidence continues to rise in those aged >55 years.
- Clinical monitoring of asymptomatic and low-risk patients is a reasonable approach ("watch and wait").
- CLL patients needs to be up-to-date with vaccines for immunocompromised patients and need annual skin surveillance.
- High-risk patients, patients with bulky disease, and patients who fail their first line of treatment typically have a poorer prognosis and may require intensive therapies, including allogeneic hematopoietic stem cell transplantation.
- Several novel agents are being developed to improve therapeutic approaches to CLL.

L

LEUKEMIA, CHRONIC MYELOGENOUS

Jan Cerny, MD, PhD

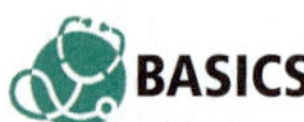

BASICS

DESCRIPTION

- Chronic myelogenous leukemia (CML) is a myeloproliferative neoplasm characterized by clonal proliferation of myeloid precursors in the bone marrow with continuing differentiation into mature granulocytes.
- The hallmark of CML is Philadelphia chromosome (translocation t[9;22]).
- Natural history of the disease evolves in three clinical phases: a chronic phase, an accelerated phase, and a blast phase or crisis (can transform to acute myeloid leukemia [80%] or acute lymphoblastic leukemia [20%]).

EPIDEMIOLOGY

Incidence

- Per year, 1.9 cases/100,000 persons
- Median age at diagnosis: 65 years
- Predominant sex: male > female (1.7:1)

Prevalence

Accounts for 15–20% of adult leukemias

ETIOLOGY AND PATHOPHYSIOLOGY

Philadelphia chromosome is a balanced translocation between *BCR* (on chromosome 22) and *ABL* (on chromosome 9) genes t(9;22)(q34;q11). This fusion gene, *BCR-ABL*, codes for an abnormal, constitutively active tyrosine kinase that affects numerous signal transduction pathways, resulting in uncontrolled cell proliferation and reduced apoptosis.

Genetics

Acquired genomic changes

RISK FACTORS

Ionizing radiation exposure (uncommon)

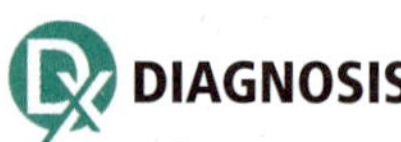

DIAGNOSIS

85–90% of patients present in the chronic phase, and the disease can be found incidentally during routine screening (up to 50%).

HISTORY

- Chronic phase: fatigue, weight loss, night sweats, abdominal fullness owing to enlarged spleen, early satiety, dyspnea, and bleeding; rare: bruising, left upper quadrant abdominal pain, sternal pain (owing to expanding bone marrow), and gouty arthritis; up to 30% of patients are asymptomatic.
- Accelerated phase: progressive splenomegaly and left upper quadrant abdominal pain occasionally referred to the left shoulder (owing to splenic infarction or rupture), progressive weight loss and sweats, unexplained fever or bone pain, chloromas (extramedullary tumors)
- Blast phase: bleeding, bruising, infections, lymphadenopathy, prominent constitutional symptoms

PHYSICAL EXAM

- Splenomegaly (50–90%), hepatomegaly (<10%)
- Less common: splenic friction rub, lymphadenopathy, lower sternal tenderness

DIFFERENTIAL DIAGNOSIS

- Chronic myelomonocytic leukemia, chronic neutrophilic leukemia, chronic eosinophilic leukemia, juvenile myelomonocytic leukemia, infectious mononucleosis, leukemoid reaction, polycythemia vera, and treatment with granulocyte-stimulating factors
- Acute myelogenous leukemia resembles blast crisis with myeloid blasts, and acute lymphoblastic leukemia resembles blast crisis with lymphoid blasts.
- Atypical CML is a chronic myeloproliferative disorder with a clinical hematologic picture similar to CML, but it lacks the Philadelphia chromosome and *BCR-ABL* rearrangement. A hallmark feature is dysplastic granulopoiesis.

DIAGNOSTIC TESTS & INTERPRETATION

- CBC
  - WBC count: markedly increased (50,000 to 100,000/μL), with granulocytes in all stages of maturation, including occasional (<10%) blasts in chronic phase, basophilia, eosinophilia
  - Hematocrit: may be normal, slightly increased, or decreased
  - Platelets: may be normal, elevated, or occasionally low
  - In accelerated phase: anemia, >20% basophils, thrombocytopenia
- Bone marrow biopsy: hypercellular marrow, myeloid hyperplasia; in accelerated phase: 10–19% blasts, ≥20% blasts in blood or marrow indicates blast phase
- Genetics
  - Demonstration of the Philadelphia chromosome, t(9;22), by cytogenetic techniques, fluorescence in situ hybridization (FISH), or reverse transcription-polymerase chain reaction (RT-PCR)
  - Additional cytogenetic abnormalities occur in the accelerated and blast phases (monosomy 7; t[3,21]; trisomies 8 and 19; Philadelphia chromosome duplication; abnormalities of chromosome 17 such as monosomy, trisomy, and isochromosome mutations). These may contribute to resistance to tyrosine kinase inhibitors (TKIs; e.g., imatinib). Further molecular testing (mutations within *BCR-ABL*) is suggested in case of loss of response to therapy.
- Others:
  - Low or absent leukocyte alkaline phosphatase in neutrophils
  - High lactate dehydrogenase (LDH)
  - Elevated uric acid

Initial Tests (lab, imaging)

- CBC, LDH, uric acid, LFTs, bone marrow biopsy and aspiration, cytogenetics on bone marrow, FISH for *BCR-ABL*, and baseline RT-PCR (quantitative as well as qualitative analysis to identify BCR-ABL transcript type)
- Abdominal ultrasound or CT scan shows splenomegaly; not mandatory

Follow-Up Tests & Special Considerations

- Routine CBC with differential until complete hematologic response (CHR)
- Serial monitoring of *BCR-ABL* by RT-PCR every 3 months to evaluate response to treatment
- Mutation analysis of tyrosine kinase domain of *ABL* kinase can predict resistance to therapy with TKIs.
- HLA-A*02 positive is associated with CML, and a protective effect is seen with the HLA-B*35 allele (pooled odds ratio 0.64, 95% CI 0.48–0.86).

Diagnostic Procedures/Other

Bone marrow aspiration and biopsy

Test Interpretation

Myeloid hyperplasia with elevated myeloid: erythroid ratio, normal maturation, marrow basophilia, and increased reticulin fibrosis

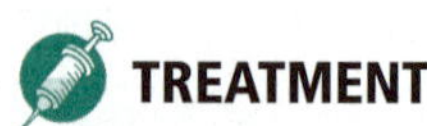

TREATMENT

MEDICATION

- TKIs (e.g., imatinib) provide durable, long-term control of disease.
- The response to TKIs is assessed at specific time points from the beginning of treatment and is categorized as follows:
  - CHR: normalization of peripheral counts, no disease symptoms, no immature cells
  - Complete cytogenetic response (CCR): no Philadelphia-positive metaphases on chromosome analysis
  - Major molecular response (MMR): decreased level of *BCR-ABL* transcript by PCR 3-log
  - Complete molecular response (CMR): *BCR-ABL* transcript is undetectable by PCR.
  - Failure to achieve CHR in 3 months is an indication to change therapy.
  - Hematologic, cytogenetic, and molecular response to TKIs are the most important prognostic indicators or predictors of outcome.

First Line

- Imatinib mesylate (Gleevec), an oral TKI, 400 mg/day
- Side effects: thrombocytopenia, anemia, elevated liver enzymes, edema, GI disturbances, rash
- International Randomized Study of Interferon versus STI571 (IRIS) established imatinib as first-line therapy, and it has shown long term efficacy after 10-year follow-up (1)[A].
- Imatinib dose can be increased to 600 and 800 mg/day if only suboptimal response is achieved with standard dose.
- 2nd-generation TKIs have shown higher efficacy and fewer side effects and are approved for first-line therapy of chronic phase CML: nilotinib (Tasigna), dasatinib (Sprycel), and bosutinib (Bosulif).

Second Line

- 2nd-generation TKIs; active against most of *BCR-ABL* mutants; not active in *T315I* mutation
  - Dasatinib
    - 100 mg/day in patients resistant or intolerant to imatinib and 70 mg BID or 140 mg/day for patients in accelerated or blastic phase
    - Side effects: pleural effusions, QTc prolongation, cytopenias, pulmonary arterial hypertension
  - Nilotinib
    - 400 mg PO BID in patients resistant or intolerant to imatinib in chronic or accelerated phase
    - Side effects: cytopenias, QTc prolongation, pancreatitis, hyperglycemia, risk of thrombotic events
  - Bosutinib
    - 400 mg PO daily, 500 mg in patients resistant or intolerant to prior therapy in chronic or accelerated phase
    - Side effects: GI toxicity, myelosuppression, hepatotoxicity, fluid retention, pancreatitis
- 3rd-generation TKI
  - Ponatinib has restricted approval due to the risk of thrombotic events, but in addition to omacetaxine (below), they are the only effective agents in patients with *T315I* mutation approved by the FDA.
  - Olverembatinib is showing promise in TKI-resistant chronic phase and accelerated phase patients with *T315I* mutation.
  - Vodobatinib is part of an ongoing phase 2 study for patients refractory to ≥3 TKI including ponatinib.
- Other approved agents or in development:
  - Omacetaxine (protein synthesis inhibitor) is approved for patient with resistance or intolerance to two or more TKIs.
  - Asciminib (a STAMP inhibitor, specifically targeting the ABL myristoyl pocket) is approved for patients with chronic phase CML who have been treated previously with two or more TKIs, or who have the *T315I* mutation.
  - If active treatment is required during pregnancy, interferon-α can be used in any trimester without significant risk to the fetus.

ISSUES FOR REFERRAL

All patients with CML should be referred to a hematologist. Patients with inadequate response to TKIs or with *T315I* mutation should consult with a bone marrow transplant (BMT) physician.

ADDITIONAL THERAPIES

Agents targeting leukemic stem cells are being developed for clinical use; emerging agents being studied: PF-114 (4th-generation oral TKI), HQP1351 (3rd-generation oral TKI)

SURGERY/OTHER PROCEDURES

Allogeneic BMT

- It is the only known cure; however, 71% of patients who achieve CCR with imatinib maintain that response beyond 7 years, and no patient progressed on the trial between years 5 and 6 of treatment.
- Most effective in patients <50 years of age who are in the chronic phase
- Initial mortality is higher (related to the use of myeloablative regimens) than medical management but provided higher rates of survival in pre-TKI era.
- Significant improvement in transplant techniques leading to better outcomes, such as alternative sources of stem cells; nonmyeloablative regimens have shown improvements in transplant-related mortality.
- Transplant option should be thoroughly discussed with young patients in chronic phase and considered an alternative to TKIs, especially if the patient does not tolerate TKIs or disease is not responding.
- Can be considered in blast phase CML patients in remission, accelerated phase CML with suboptimal or resistant response to TKIs, and chronic phase patients who fail to achieve CHR by 3 months, have no cytogenetic response or cytogenetic relapse, have *T315I* mutation, or have extramedullary disease with chronic phase CML cells

ADMISSION, INPATIENT, AND NURSING CONSIDERATIONS

- Acute abdominal symptoms (infarcted or ruptured spleen); tumor lysis syndrome owing to initial therapy; complications of BMT
  - Hydroxyurea might be given, with the goal of reduction of the WBC count, but it has minimal impact on patient response to TKIs.
  - Induction chemotherapy (for acute leukemia) in setting of blastic phase
  - Allopurinol to prevent tumor lysis syndrome in patients with very high counts; however, probably not necessary when TKIs are used
- Discharge criteria: abatement of acute symptoms

ONGOING CARE

FOLLOW-UP RECOMMENDATIONS

- Frequency depends on disease risk at presentation and response to first-line therapy.
- Although splenomegaly persists, avoid contact sports or trauma to abdomen.

Patient Monitoring

- CBC with differential: weekly until blood counts are stable and then every 2 to 4 weeks during CHR; once in CCR and stable, patient can be followed less frequently (3-month intervals).
- Bone marrow cytogenetics (evaluation for clonal evolution) every 6 months while in CHR; every 12 to 18 months while in CCR, MMR, CMR
- Quantitative RT-PCR every 3 months (peripheral blood)
- ECGs (concern for QT prolongation), LFTs while on TKIs; nilotinib, bosutinib, and ponatinib can cause pancreatitis.
- Blood pressure monitoring because several TKIs have been associated with elevated blood pressure and related cardiovascular complications

PROGNOSIS

- With treatment and good response, the survival is similar to the normal population.
- Without treatment: CML invariably will progress to accelerated phase within 2 to 5 years and blast phase within several months of the accelerated phase.
- Poor prognosis: patients presenting in accelerated or blastic phase or presenting with very large spleen size, platelets >700,000/μL, and patients resistant to TKIs (*T315I* mutation)

COMPLICATIONS

- Splenic infarct or rupture
- Progression to accelerated or blastic phase
- Thrombotic events owing to elevated platelets
- Bleeding owing to low or dysfunctional platelets
- Sequelae of anemia

REFERENCES

1. Hochhaus A, Larson RA, Guilhot F, et al. Long-term outcomes of imatinib treatment for chronic myeloid leukemia. *N Engl J Med*. 2017;376(10):917–927.

ADDITIONAL READING

- Jabbour E, Kantarjian H. Chronic myeloid leukemia: 2022 update on diagnosis, therapy, and monitoring. *Am J Hematol*. 2022;97(9):1236–1256.
- Senapati J, Sasaki K, Issa GC, et al. Management of chronic myeloid leukemia in 2023—common ground and common sense. *Blood Cancer J*. 2023;13(1):58. doi:10.1038/s41408-023-00823-9.

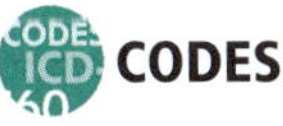

CODES

ICD10

- C92.2 Atypical chronic myeloid leukemia, BCR/ABL-negative
- C92.12 Chronic myeloid leukemia, BCR/ABL-positive, in relapse
- C92.22 Atypical chronic myeloid leukemia, BCR/ABL-negative, in relapse

CLINICAL PEARLS

- CML belongs to the myeloproliferative disorders group.
- The gold standard for diagnosis of CML is detection of the Philadelphia chromosome or its products, *BCR-ABL* mRNA, and fusion protein.
- TKIs provide durable, long-term control of the disease and have dramatically altered treatment.
- Atypical CML is a form of clinically typical CML but without the presence of the typical *BCR-ABL* translocation.
- Blastic phase (a.k.a. blast crisis) is a form of acute leukemia that is a possible complication of CML.

L

LEUKOPLAKIA, ORAL

Sawyer J. Sparks, DO • Scott Michael Dickson, MD

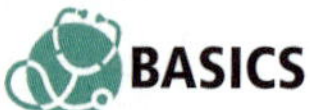

BASICS

DESCRIPTION

- Leukoplakia is defined by the World Health Organization (WHO) as "a white plaque of questionable risk having excluded (other) known diseases or disorders that carry no increased risk for cancer."
- Characterized by asymptomatic, well-demarcated white plaques that cannot be wiped away, this condition requires a biopsy for histopathologic evaluation to assess for premalignant or malignant changes, or to rule out other differential diagnoses.
- System(s) affected: gastrointestinal (GI)

EPIDEMIOLOGY

Most common in individuals who use tobacco (smoking and especially smokeless), heavy alcohol use, and areca nuts (Asian populations).

Incidence

250,000 annual cases worldwide

Prevalence

- Age of onset is >40 years old with peak in the 60s.
- Males are 3 times more likely to be affected than females.
- Smokers are 6 times more likely to be affected than nonsmokers.
- Higher prevalence in Asian and Oceanic populations.

Geriatric Considerations

Malignant transformation to carcinoma is more common in older patients.

ETIOLOGY AND PATHOPHYSIOLOGY

Hyperkeratosis or dyskeratosis of the oral squamous epithelium; tissue cell exposure to carcinogens spurs adaptive changes including hyperplasia. Continued irritant exposure can lead to cellular degeneration of the epithelium and eventually apoptosis or malignant transformation.

- Tobacco use in any form
- Alcohol consumption
- Dental restorations/prosthetic appliances/periodontitis
- *Candida albicans* infection
- Human papillomavirus, types 16 and 18
- Vitamin and combined micronutrient deficiencies
- Syphilis
- Chronic trauma or irritation
- Epstein-Barr virus (oral hairy leukoplakia)
- Areca/betel nut (Asian populations)
- Mouthwash/toothpaste containing the herbal root extract sanguinaria
- Hormonal disturbances/estrogen therapy
- Ultraviolet exposure

Genetics

- Dyskeratosis congenital and epidermolysis bullosa increase the likelihood of oral malignancy.
- p53 overexpression; PTEN allelic loss correlates with leukoplakia and particularly squamous cell carcinoma.
- Changes in expression of p53, FGFR1, p16INK4a, and 3p, 9p, and 17 (especially TP53) gene mutations can have greater cancer risk. Decreased expression of E-cadherin, hMLH1, and CD1a.
- Biomarkers: IL-6, IL-8, and TNF-α have been detected in leukoplakia, and there is new research showing possible use of Hsp27 and PTHRP/PTHLH as biomarkers.

RISK FACTORS

- 70–90% of oral leukoplakia is related to tobacco, particularly smokeless tobacco or areca/betel nut use.
- Alcohol increases risk 1.5-fold.
- Repeated or chronic mechanical trauma from dental appliances or cheek biting
- Chemical irritation to oral regions
- Diabetes
- Risk factors for malignant transformation of leukoplakia:
  - Female
  - Long duration of leukoplakia
  - Nonsmoker (idiopathic leukoplakia)
  - Located on tongue or floor of mouth
  - Size >200 mm^2
  - Nonhomogenous type
  - Presence of epithelial dysplasia
  - Presence of *C. albicans*
  - Possible shift of oral microbiome in those with malignant transformation.

GENERAL PREVENTION

- Avoid tobacco of any kind, alcohol, habitual cheek biting, tongue chewing, areca/betel nut chewing/ingestion.
- Use well-fitting dental equipment.
- Regular dental check-ups to avoid bad restorations
- Diet rich in fresh fruits and vegetables may help to prevent cancer.
- HPV vaccination may be preventive.

COMMONLY ASSOCIATED CONDITIONS

- Oral hairy leukoplakia; Epstein-Barr virus-induced lesion that occurs primarily in HIV patients
- Erythroplakia in association with leukoplakia, "speckled leukoplakia," or erythroleukoplakia is a marker for underlying dysplasia.

DIAGNOSIS

Leukoplakia is an asymptomatic white patch or patches on the oral mucosa that cannot be wiped off with gauze.

HISTORY

- History of tobacco or alcohol use or oral exposure to irritants
- Elicit timing of onset, progression, and presence of pain or sensitivity.
- Identify sources of friction or chronic irritation.

PHYSICAL EXAM

- Location
  - Can develop on any oral mucosal surface
  - Floor of mouth, ventrolateral tongue, and soft palate complex are more likely to have dysplastic lesions.
- Appearance
  - Varies from homogeneous, nonpalpable, faintly translucent white areas to thick, with or without fissuring, papillomatous, indurated plaques
  - May feel rough or leathery
  - Lesions can become exophytic or verruciform.
  - Color may be white, gray, yellowish white, or brownish gray.
  - Cannot be wiped or scraped off
- WHO classification
  - Homogeneous refers to color.
    - Flat, corrugated, wrinkled, or pumice
  - Nonhomogeneous refers to color and texture (more likely to be dysplastic or malignant).
    - Erythroleukoplakia (mixture of red and white)
    - Proliferative verrucous leukoplakia (PVL) (multifocal, mostly women)

DIFFERENTIAL DIAGNOSIS

- Geographic tongue
- Developmental/genetic (rare):
  - Cannon white sponge nevus (diffuse bilateral white plaques of buccal mucosa, tongue)
  - Hereditary benign intraepithelial dyskeratosis
  - Pachyonychia congenita; Genodermatoses; Darier-White disease
- Reactive/frictional:
  - Leukoedema (delicate gray-white lines, disappear with stretching)
  - Contact desquamation
  - Morsicatio mucosae oris (cheek/gum biting)
  - Benign alveolar ridge keratosis (ill-fitting dentures)
  - Hairy tongue (elongated filiform papillae, may become pigmented from food/bacteria)
  - Nicotinic stomatitis and smokeless tobacco keratosis (South Asian "paan" or "gutka"; American/Swedish snuff; Ethiopian "toombak")
  - Glassblower white patch
  - Actinic cheilitis
  - Aspirin burn
  - Cinnamon-induced contact stomatitis
  - Epithelial peeling
  - Keratotic lesions
  - Linea alba
- Infectious:
  - Candidiasis
  - Hairy leukoplakia (associated with EBV and HIV-infected individuals)
  - Syphilis
- Immune-mediated:
  - Lichen planus (typically symmetric, bilateral, reticular white lesions)
  - Lichenoid lesions
  - Benign migratory glossitis
- Autoimmune:
  - SLE
  - Chronic graft versus host disease

DIAGNOSTIC TESTS & INTERPRETATION

Biopsy with histopathologic examination to assess presence and grade of dysplasia is the gold standard.

Initial Tests (lab, imaging)

Consider saliva culture if *C albicans* infection is suspected.

Follow-Up Tests & Special Considerations

- Biopsy is necessary to rule out carcinoma if lesion is persistent, changing, or unexplained.
- Consider CBC, rapid plasma reagin (RPR).

Diagnostic Procedures/Other

- Oral cytology is superior to conventional oral examination.
- Noninvasive brush biopsy and analysis of cells with DNA–image cytometry constitute a sensitive and specific screening method.
- Patients with dysplastic or malignant cells on brush biopsy should undergo more formal excisional biopsy.
- Excisional biopsy is a definitive procedure.

Test Interpretation

- Biopsy specimens range from hyperkeratosis to keratosis of unknown significance (KUS) to dysplasia to invasive carcinoma.
- At initial biopsy, 6% are invasive carcinoma.
- 0.13–6% subsequently undergo malignant transformation.
- Location is important: 60% on floor of mouth or lateral border of tongue are cancerous; buccal mucosal lesions are generally not malignant but require biopsy if not resolving.

TREATMENT

- All oral leukoplakias should be treated because they are potentially malignant.
- Treatment may include the following:
  - Some small lesions may respond to cryosurgery.
  - For 2 to 3 circumscribed lesions, surgical excision is treatment of choice.
  - For multiple or large lesions where surgery would cause unacceptable deformity, consider cryosurgery or laser surgery.
- Complete excision is standard treatment for dysplasia or malignancy.
- After treatment, up to 30% of leukoplakia recurs, and some leukoplakia still transforms to squamous cell carcinoma.
- Oral hairy leukoplakia may be treated with podophyllin with acyclovir cream.

GENERAL MEASURES

- Abstinence from predisposing habits; alcohol and tobacco (smoked and smokeless).
- Eliminate habitual lip biting.
- Correct ill-fitting dental appliances, bad restorations, or sharp teeth.
- β-Carotene, lycopene, retinoids, and cyclooxygenase-2 (COX-2) inhibitors may cause partial regression.
- For hairy tongue: tongue brushing

MEDICATION

Carotenoids; vitamins A, C, and K; topical bleomycin; NSAIDs, and photodynamic therapy are ineffective to prevent malignant transformation and recurrence. No generally approved standard systemic pharmacotherapy regimen at this time, but there is a new research being done on chemoprevention.

ISSUES FOR REFERRAL

Consider otolaryngologist or oral surgery referral for extensive disease.

ADDITIONAL THERAPIES

Systemic therapies that may reduce progression include retinoids, COX-2 inhibitors, epidermal growth factor inhibitors, and peroxisome proliferator-activated receptor-γ agonists.

SURGERY/OTHER PROCEDURES

- Scalpel excision, laser ablation, electrocautery, or cryoablation
- Cryotherapy slightly less effective than photodynamic therapy response and recurrence
- Biopsy/excision algorithm:
  - KUS that is poorly demarcated and likely frictional: Rebiopsy and follow up.
  - KUS that is well demarcated and >3 cm: Follow up every 3 months; rebiopsy every 12 months.
  - KUS that is <3 cm: Excise/ablate with narrow margins; follow up every 3 months; if recurs, excise with wider margins.
  - PVL: Follow up every 3 months; excise verrucous or nodular areas.
  - Dysplastic/SCC: Excise.

COMPLEMENTARY & ALTERNATIVE MEDICINE

Low or very low evidence for systemic β-carotene, herbal extracts, freeze-dried black raspberry gel, and Bowman-Birk inhibitor

ONGOING CARE

FOLLOW-UP RECOMMENDATIONS

Patient Monitoring

- Follow-up appointments every 3 to 6 months during the 1st year following surgical removal and then annually thereafter based on anticipated risk and patient preference
- Biopsy as needed

DIET

Regular

PATIENT EDUCATION

- If biopsy is negative, stress importance of periodic and careful follow-up.
- Initiate a dental referral to eliminate dental factors.
- Stress importance of stopping tobacco and alcohol use.
- Encourage participation in smoking cessation program.

PROGNOSIS

- Most leukoplakia is benign.
- Leukoplakia may regress, remain stable, or progress.
- 0.13–6% of initially benign lesions subsequently develop into cancer. Most important predictor of transformation into squamous cell carcinoma is degree of epithelial dysplasia.
- Lack of treatment generally results in malignant development at an annual rate of 2–4%.
- 5-year survival rate of oral cancer is 50%.

COMPLICATIONS

- New lesions may develop after treatment.
- Larger lesions and nonhomogeneous leukoplakia are associated with higher rates of malignant transformation.

ADDITIONAL READING

Reamy BV, Derby R, Bunt CW. Common tongue conditions in primary care. *Am Fam Physician*. 2010;81(5):627–634.

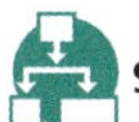

SEE ALSO

HIV/AIDS; Infectious Mononucleosis, Epstein-Barr Virus Infections

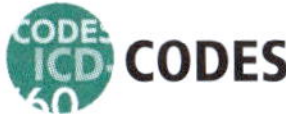

CODES

ICD10

- K13.21 Leukoplakia of oral mucosa, including tongue
- K13.3 Hairy leukoplakia

CLINICAL PEARLS

- White plaque or patches on the oral mucosa that cannot be rubbed or easily scrapped off
- Excisional biopsy is indicated for any undiagnosed leukoplakia.
- After treatment, up to 30% of leukoplakia recurs, and some leukoplakia still transforms to squamous cell carcinoma; thus, long-term surveillance is essential.
- To lessen risk of malignant transformation, encourage tobacco and alcohol cessation, HPV vaccination, and consider *C. albicans* eradication.

L

LICHEN PLANUS

Dongsheng Jiang, MD, MSc • Juan Qiu, MD, PhD

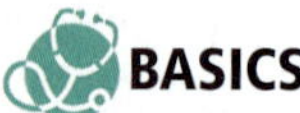

BASICS

Lichen planus (LP) is an idiopathic eruption with characteristic shiny, flat-topped (Latin: *planus*, "flat") purple (violaceous) papules and plaques on the skin, often accompanied by characteristic mucous membrane lesions. Itching may be severe.

DESCRIPTION

- Classic (typical) LP is a relatively uncommon inflammatory disorder of the skin and mucous membranes; hair and nails may also be affected.
  - Skin lesions are small, flat, angular, red-to-violaceous, shiny, pruritic papules and/or plaques with overlying fine, white lines (called Wickham striae), or gray-white puncta; most commonly seen on the flexor surfaces of the upper extremities, extensor surfaces of the lower extremities, the genitalia, and on the mucous membranes
  - On the oral mucosa, lesions typically appear as raised white lines in a lacelike pattern seen most often on the buccal mucosa.
  - Onset is abrupt or gradual. Course is unpredictable; may resolve spontaneously, recur intermittently, or persist for many years
- Drug-induced LP
  - Clinical and histopathologic findings may mimic those of classic LP. Lesions usually lack Wickham striae (see in the following text) and oral involvement is rare.
  - There is generally a latent period of months from drug introduction until lesions appear.
  - Lesions resolve when the inciting agent is discontinued, often after a prolonged period.
- LP variants
  - Follicular: also called lichen planopilaris; typically seen on the scalp, can lead to scarring alopecia
  - Annular: papules spread centrifugally as central area resolves; occur on glans penis, axillae, and oral mucosa
  - Linear: may be an isolated finding
  - Hypertrophic: itchy, hyperkeratotic, thick plaques on dorsal legs and feet
  - Atrophic: rare, most often the result of resolved lesions
  - Bullous LP: Intense inflammation in the dermis leads to blistering of epidermis.
  - LP pemphigoides: a combination of LP and bullous pemphigoid (IgG autoantibodies to collagen 17)
  - Nail LP: affects the nail matrix, lateral thinning, longitudinal ridging, and fissuring
- System(s) affected: skin/exocrine
- Synonym(s): lichenoid eruptions

EPIDEMIOLOGY

- Predominant age: 30 to 60 years old; rare in children and the geriatric population
- Predominant sex: female > male

Prevalence

In the United States, 450/100,000

ETIOLOGY AND PATHOPHYSIOLOGY

LP is considered to be a T cell–mediated autoimmune response to self-antigens on damaged keratinocytes.

RISK FACTORS

Exposure to certain drugs or chemicals

- Thiazides, furosemide, β-blockers, sulfonylureas, antimalarials, penicillamine, gold salts, and angiotensin-converting enzyme inhibitors, NSAIDs, isoniazid, tetracyclines, allopurinol

COMMONLY ASSOCIATED CONDITIONS

- Hepatitis C virus infection, particularly in certain geographic regions (Asia, South America, the Middle East, Europe). Hepatitis should be considered in patients with widespread presentations of LP and those with primarily oral disease.
- Chronic active hepatitis, lichen nitidus, and primary biliary cirrhosis
- Dyslipidemia
- Others:
  - Bullous pemphigoid
  - Alopecia areata
  - Myasthenia gravis
  - Vitiligo
  - Ulcerative colitis
  - Graft-versus-host reaction
  - Lupus erythematosus (lupus erythematosus–LP overlap syndrome)
  - Morphea and lichen sclerosis et atrophicus

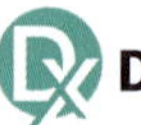

DIAGNOSIS

- LP is most commonly diagnosed by its appearance despite its range of clinical presentations.
- Dermoscopy: Most common findings are polymorphic pearly white structures, radial capillaries, and blue-gray granules.
- A skin/mucosal biopsy is recommended.

HISTORY

A minority of patients have a family history of LP. Affected families have an increased frequency of human leukocyte antigen B7 (HLA-B7). A thorough drug history should be performed.

PHYSICAL EXAM

- Skin (often severe pruritus)
  - Papules: 1 to 10 mm, shiny, flat-topped (planar) lesions that occur in crops; lesions may have a fine scale.
  - Evidence of scratching (i.e., crusts and excoriations) is usually absent.
  - Color: violaceous, with white lacelike pattern (Wickham striae) on surface of papules. Wickham striae are best seen after topical application of mineral oil and, if present, are virtually pathognomonic for LP.
  - Shape: polygonal or oval. Annular lesions may appear on trunk and mucous membranes. Various shapes and sizes may be noted (polymorphic).
  - Arrangement: may be grouped, linear, or scattered individual lesions
  - Koebner phenomenon (isomorphic response): New lesions may be noted at sites of minor injuries, such as scratches or burns.
  - Distribution: ventral surface of wrists and forearms, dorsa hands, glans penis, dorsa feet, groin, sacrum, shins, and scalp. Hypertrophic (verrucous) lesions may occur on lower legs and may be generalized.
  - Postinflammatory hyperpigmentation: Lesions typically heal, leaving darkly pigmented macules in their wake.
- Mucous membranes (40–60% of patients with skin lesions; 20% have mucous membrane lesions without skin involvement.)
  - Most commonly asymptomatic, nonerosive, milky-white lines with an elegant, lacy, netlike streaked pattern
  - Usually seen on buccal mucosa but may appear on tongue, gingiva, palate, or lips
  - Less commonly, LP may be erosive; rarely bullous
  - Painful, especially if ulcers present
  - Lesions may develop into squamous cell carcinoma (1–3%).
  - Glans penis, labia minora, vaginal vault, and perianal areas may be involved.
- Hair/scalp
  - LP of the hair follicle (lichen planopilaris) presents with keratotic plugs at the follicle orifice with a violaceous rim; may result in atrophy and permanent destruction of hair follicles (scarring alopecia)
- Nails (10%)
  - Involvement of nail matrix may cause proximal-to-distal linear grooves and partial or complete destruction of nail bed with pterygium formation.

DIFFERENTIAL DIAGNOSIS

- Skin
  - Lichen simplex chronicus
  - Eczematous dermatitis
  - Psoriasis
  - Discoid lupus erythematosus
  - Other lichenoid eruptions (those that resemble LP)
  - Pityriasis rosea
  - Lichen nitidus
  - Self-induced dermatoses
- Oral mucous membranes
  - Leukoplakia
  - Oral hairy leukoplakia
  - Candidiasis
  - Squamous cell carcinoma (particularly in ulcerative lesions)
  - Aphthous ulcers
  - Herpetic stomatitis
  - Secondary syphilis
- Genital mucous membranes
  - Psoriasis (penis and labia)
  - Nonspecific balanitis, Zoon balanitis
  - Fixed drug eruption (penis)
  - Candidiasis (penis and labia)
  - Pemphigus vulgaris, bullous pemphigoid, and Behçet disease (all rare)
- Hair and scalp
  - Scarring alopecia (central centrifugal cicatricial alopecia)

DIAGNOSTIC TESTS & INTERPRETATION

If suggested by history
- Serology for hepatitis
- Liver function tests

Diagnostic Procedures/Other
- Skin biopsy
- Direct immunofluorescence helps to distinguish LP from discoid lupus erythematosus.

Test Interpretation
- Dense, bandlike (lichenoid) lymphocytic infiltrate of the upper dermis
- Vacuolar degeneration of the basal layer
- Hyperkeratosis and irregular acanthosis, increased granular layer
- Basement membrane thinning with "saw-toothing"
- Degenerative keratinocytes, known as colloid or Civatte bodies, are found in the lower epidermis.
- Melanin pigment in macrophages

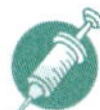

TREATMENT

Although LP can resolve spontaneously, treatment is usually requested by patients who may be severely symptomatic or troubled by its cosmetic appearance.

GENERAL MEASURES
- Goal is to relieve itching and resolve lesions.
- Discontinue potentially causative medications
- Asymptomatic oral lesions require no treatment.
- For oral LP:
  - No treatment is curative.
  - Goal of treatment is to resolve pain, heal ulcerative lesions, decrease the risk for oral cancer.

MEDICATION

First Line
- Skin (1),(2)
  - Ultra-high-potency and high-potency topical steroids: 0.05% clobetasol propionate or 0.1% betamethasone valerate BID for 2 to 4 weeks
  - Triamcinolone acetonide 0.1% or fluocinonide 0.05% under occlusion
  - Intralesional corticosteroids (e.g., triamcinolone [Kenalog] 5 to 10 mg/mL) for recalcitrant and hypertrophic lesions
  - "Soak and smear" technique: can lead to a rapid improvement of symptoms in even 1 to 2 days and may obviate the need for systemic steroids. Soaking allows water to hydrate the stratum corneum and allows the anti-inflammatory steroid in the ointment to penetrate more deeply into the skin. Smearing of the ointment traps the water in the skin because water cannot move out through greasy materials.
    - Soaking is done in a bathtub using lukewarm plain water for 20 minutes and then, without drying the skin, the affected area is immediately smeared with a thin film of the steroid ointment containing clobetasol or another superpotent topical steroid.
    - Soak and smear may be done for 4 to 5 days or longer, if necessary. The treatments are best done at night because the greasy ointment applied to the skin gets on pajamas (instead of on daytime clothes) and the ointment is on the skin during sleep. A topical steroid cream is applied thereafter during the daytime hours, if necessary.
- Oral LP (3):
  - Clobetasol propionate cream 0.05% (1 to 2 applications daily)
  - Erosive and/or extensive multisite: systemic corticosteroids (prednisone, prednisolone) are recommended as first-line therapy in European guidelines: (0.5 to 1.0 mg/kg tapered over a short period of time, usually 4 to 6 weeks)
  - Intralesional injection of triamcinolone acetonide or betamethasone may be considered in refractory erosive lesion.

Pediatric Considerations
Children may absorb a proportionally larger amount of topical steroid because of larger skin surface-to-weight ratio.

Second Line
Skin and mucous membranes
- Oral steroids: reserved for acute exacerbation, severe or widespread, or unresponsive to topical steroids; prednisone at 0.5 to 1.0 mg/kg body weight/day (30 to 60 mg/day) for 3 to 6 weeks, taper over 4 to 6 weeks
- Isotretinoin 10 mg, or acitretin 30 mg, or alitretinoin 30 mg PO daily in some refractory cases; observe carefully for resultant dyslipidemia.
- Topical calcineurin inhibitors: 0.1% tacrolimus (Protopic ointment) BID or 1% pimecrolimus (Elidel) cream BID
- Topical retinoids: tretinoin 0.05% BID; isotretinoin 0.1% BID
- Topical calcipotriol
- Other medications used occasionally: metronidazole, sulfasalazine, methotrexate, cyclosporine, hydroxychloroquine, dapsone, thalidomide, griseofulvin, azathioprine, mycophenolate mofetil
- Methotrexate: dosage range from 2.5 to 20.0 mg per week (4)
- Narrow-band UVB (NBUVB) and broad-band UVB (BBUVB): especially when systemic steroids and immunosuppressive drugs are contraindicated
- Psoralen plus ultraviolet A (PUVA) therapy
- Low-level laser therapy and photodynamic therapy

ALERT
Avoid oral and topical retinoids during pregnancy.

ADDITIONAL THERAPIES
Antihistamines (e.g., hydroxyzine 25 mg PO q6h) have limited benefit for itching but may be helpful for sedation at bedtime.

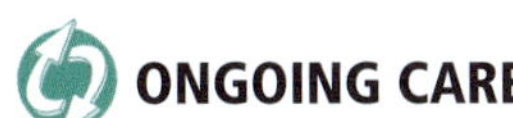

ONGOING CARE

FOLLOW-UP RECOMMENDATIONS

Patient Monitoring
Serial oral examinations for erosive/ulcerative lesions

PATIENT EDUCATION
- Oral, erosive, or ulcerative LP: annual follow-up to screen for malignancy
- Maintain good oral hygiene and dental status.
- Avoid hot, salty, acidic or spicy foods, alcohol, smoking and use of tobacco products especially in patients with atrophic and erosive lesions.
- Avoid mucosal trauma: Avoid dry, crispy foods such as corn chips, pretzels, and toast.

PROGNOSIS
- Spontaneous resolution in weeks is possible, but disease may persist for years, especially oral lesions and hypertrophic lesions on the shins.
- There is a tendency toward relapse.
- Recurrence in 12–20%, especially in those with generalized involvement

COMPLICATIONS
- Alopecia
- Nail destruction
- Squamous cell carcinoma of the mouth or genitals

REFERENCES

1. Thandar Y, Maharajh R, Haffejee F, et al. Treatment of cutaneous lichen planus (part 1): a review of topical therapies and phototherapy. *Cogent Med*. 2019;6(1).
2. Thandar Y, Maharajh R, Haffejee F, et al. Treatment of cutaneous lichen planus (part 2): a review of systemic therapies. *J Dermatolog Treat*. 2019;30(7):633–647. doi:10.1080/09546634.2018.1544411.
3. Louisy A, Humbert E, Samimi M. Oral lichen planus: an update on diagnosis and management. *Am J Clin Dermatol*. 2024;25(1):35–53. doi:10.1007/s40257-023-00814-3.
4. Tekin B, Xie F, Lehman JS. Lichen planus: what is new in diagnosis and treatment? *Am J Clin Dermatol*. 2024;25(5):735–764. doi:10.1007/s40257-024-00878-9.

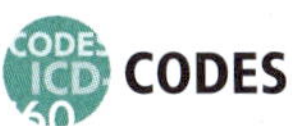

CODES

ICD10
- L43.9 Lichen planus, unspecified
- L43.0 Hypertrophic lichen planus
- L43.1 Bullous lichen planus

CLINICAL PEARLS
- 7 *P*'s of LP: **p**urple, **p**lanar, **p**olygonal, **p**olymorphic, **p**ruritic (not always), **p**apules that heal with **p**ostinflammatory hyperpigmentation.
- Serial oral or genital exams are indicated for erosive/ulcerative LP lesions to monitor for the development of squamous cell carcinoma.
- The "soak and smear" technique can lead to a rapid improvement of symptoms in 1 to 2 days and may obviate the need for systemic steroids.

L

LICHEN SIMPLEX CHRONICUS

Dongsheng Jiang, MD, MSc • Juan Qiu, MD, PhD

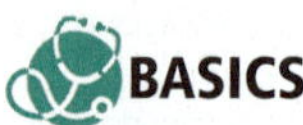

BASICS

DESCRIPTION

- Lichen simplex chronicus (LSC) is a chronic dermatitis resulting from chronic, repeated rubbing or scratching of the skin. Skin becomes thickened with accentuated lines ("lichenification").
- Definition/terminology (1):
  - LSC: localized lichenified plaques often with excoriations
  - Prurigo nodularis (PN): a chronic pruritic condition which is frequently more broadly distributed across multiple regions as nodules
  - Neurodermatitis: include other chronic itchy conditions, such as PN and atopic dermatitis

EPIDEMIOLOGY

Geriatric Considerations

Most common in middle age and elderly

Pediatric Considerations

Rare in preadolescents

Incidence

- Peak incidence: ages 35 to 50 years
- Predominant sex: females > males (2:1)

Prevalence

Common—affects 12% of the population

ETIOLOGY AND PATHOPHYSIOLOGY

- Itch–scratch cycle leads to a chronic dermatosis. Repeated scratching or rubbing causes inflammation and pruritus, which leads to continued scratching.
- Primary LSC: scratching secondary to nonorganic pruritus, habit, or a conditioned response to stress/anxiety
- Common triggers are excess dryness of skin, heat, sweat, and psychological stress.
- Secondary LSC: begins as a pruritic skin disease that evolves into neurodermatitis, which persists after resolution of the primary condition; precursor dermatoses include atopic dermatitis, contact dermatitis, lichen planus, stasis dermatitis, psoriasis, tinea, and insect bites.
- There is a possible relation between disease development and underlying neuropathy, particularly radiculopathy or nerve root compression.
- Pruritus-specific C neurons are temperature sensitive, which may explain itching that occurs in warm environments.

RISK FACTORS

- Anxiety disorders
- Dry skin
- Insect bites
- Pruritic dermatosis

GENERAL PREVENTION

Avoid common triggers such as psychological distress, environmental factors such as heat and excessive dryness, skin irritation, and the development of pruritic dermatoses.

COMMONLY ASSOCIATED CONDITIONS

- PN is a nodular variety of the same disease process.
- Atopic dermatitis
- Anxiety, depression, and obsessive-compulsive disorders

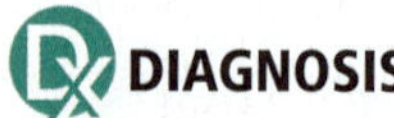

DIAGNOSIS

HISTORY

- Gradual onset
- Begins as a localized area of pruritus
- Most patients acknowledge that they respond with vigorous rubbing, itching, or scratching, which brings temporary satisfaction.
- Pruritus is typically paroxysmal, worse at night, and may lead to scratching during sleep.
- Can be asymptomatic with patient scratching at night while asleep

PHYSICAL EXAM

- Well-circumscribed lichenified plaques with varying amounts of overlying excoriation or scaling
- Lichenification: accentuation of normal skin lines
- Hyperpigmentation or hypopigmentation can be seen.
- Scarring is uncommon with typical LSC; can be seen following ulcer formation or secondary infection
- Most commonly involves easily accessible areas
  - Lateral portions of lower legs/ankles
  - Nape of neck (lichen simplex nuchae)
  - Vulva/scrotum/anus
  - Extensor surfaces of forearms
  - Palmar wrist
  - Scalp
- Dermoscopic criteria: (in genital disease)
  - Rich vascularization, linear, serpentine, and dotted in shape
  - Diffuse arrangement
  - White-grayish background

DIFFERENTIAL DIAGNOSIS

- Lichen sclerosis
- Psoriasis
- Atopic dermatitis
- Contact, irritant, or stasis dermatitis
- Extramammary Paget disease
- Lichen planus
- Lichen amyloidosis
- Tinea
- Nummular eczema
- Other systemic disease:
  - T-cell lymphoma
  - Lymphoma
  - Multiple myeloma
  - Lung cancer
  - Leukemia
  - GI tract cancer

DIAGNOSTIC TESTS & INTERPRETATION

Initial Tests (lab, imaging)

- No specific diagnostic test
- Microscopy (i.e., KOH prep) and culture preparation may be helpful in identifying possible bacterial or fungal infection.

Diagnostic Procedures/Other

- Skin biopsy if diagnosis is in question
- Patch testing may be used to rule out a contact dermatitis.

Test Interpretation

- Hyperkeratosis
- Acanthosis
- Lengthening of rete ridges
- Hyperplasia of all components of epidermis
- Mild to moderate lymphohistiocytic inflammatory infiltrate with prominent lichenification

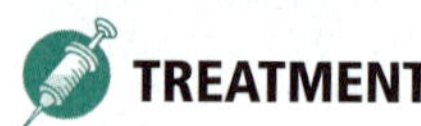

TREATMENT

GENERAL MEASURES

- Treat underlying causes
- Patient education is critical.
- Low likelihood of resolution if patient is unable to avoid scratching/rubbing. SSRIs may be effective in controlling compulsive scratching resulting from a psychiatric diagnosis such as anxiety disorder or OCD.
- Treatment aimed at reducing inflammation and pruritus

MEDICATION

Treatment is based on disease severity (1):

- Mild disease—options include:
  - Emollients
  - High-potency topical steroids
  - Topical calcineurin inhibitors
  - Combination of topical steroids and salicylates
  - Menthol
  - Pramoxine
  - Topical doxepin
  - Topical aspirin with dichloromethane
  - Topical ketamine/amitriptyline/lidocaine
- Moderate disease—below usually combined with a first-line treatment
  - Antidepressants (SSRIs, tricyclic antidepressants [TCAs], i.e., imipramine)
  - Gabapentin
  - For nighttime itch: mirtazapine, sedating antihistamines
  - Topical acetaminophen
  - Cyclosporine
  - Methotrexate
  - Narrowband ultraviolet B
- Severe disease:
  - Nemolizumab
  - Dupilumab
  - Janus kinase inhibitors (i.e., tofacitinib)
  - Transcutaneous electrical nerve stimulation
  - Focused ultrasound (in vulvar areas)

First Line

ALERT

High-dose and prolonged treatment with topical steroids can cause dermal/epidermal atrophy as well as pigmentary changes and should not be used on the face, intertriginous areas, or anogenital region. Duration of treatment on other parts of the body should not exceed 3 weeks without close physician supervision.

ISSUES FOR REFERRAL

- No response to treatment
- Presence of signs and symptoms suggestive of a systemic cause of pruritus
- Consultation with a psychiatrist for patients with severe stress, anxiety, or compulsive scratching
- Consultation with an allergist for patients with multisystem atopic symptoms

ADDITIONAL THERAPIES

- Psychotherapy
- Cooling of the skin with ice or cold compresses
- Soaks and lubricants to improve barrier layer function
- Occlusion of lesion with bandages or Unna boots
- Nail trimming
- Silk underwear to decrease friction in genital LSC

COMPLEMENTARY & ALTERNATIVE MEDICINE

- Wet cupping can be as effective as high-potency steroids (2). Wet cupping is to use a needle or scalpel to make a small skin incision then place the cup to draw out a small amount of blood or extracellular fluid.
- Acupuncture is effective.
- Cognitive-behavioral therapy may improve awareness and help to identify coping strategies.
- Hypnosis may be beneficial in decreasing pruritus and preventing scratching.
- Homeopathic remedies (i.e., thuja and graphite) have been used.

ONGOING CARE

FOLLOW-UP RECOMMENDATIONS

Patient Monitoring

Patients should be followed for response to therapy, complications from therapy (especially topical steroids), and secondary infections.

DIET

Regular balanced diet

PATIENT EDUCATION

- Patients should understand the cause of this disease and the critical role they play in its resolution. Emphasize that scratching and rubbing must stop for lesions to heal; medications ineffective if scratching continues
- Stress reduction techniques can be useful for patients for whom stress plays a role.
- Avoid exposure to known triggers.

PROGNOSIS

- Often chronic and recurrent, can be persistent on genitals
- Good prognosis if the itch–scratch cycle can be broken.
- After healing, the skin should return to normal appearance but may also retain accentuated skin markings or post inflammatory pigmentary changes that may be slow to resolve.

COMPLICATIONS

- Secondary infection
- Scarring is rare without ulceration or secondary infection.
- Complications related to therapy, as mentioned in medication precautions
- Squamous cell carcinoma within affected regions is rare.

REFERENCES

1. Ju T, Vander Does A, Mohsin N, et al. Lichen simplex chronicus itch: an update. *Acta Derm Venereol*. 2022;102:adv00796. doi:10.2340/actadv.v102.4367.
2. Zhai Y, Hui YY, Jiang ZF, et al. Efficacy and safety of wet cupping in the treatment of neurodermatitis: a systematic review and meta-analysis. *Front Med (Lausanne)*. 2024;11:1478073. doi:10.3389/fmed.2024.1478073.

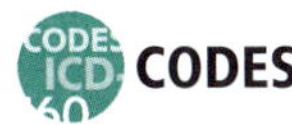

CODES

ICD10

L28.0 Lichen simplex chronicus

CLINICAL PEARLS

- LSC is a chronic inflammatory condition that results from repeated scratching and rubbing.
- Primary LSC originates de novo, whereas secondary LSC occurs in the setting of a preexisting pruritic dermatologic condition.
- LSC is a clinical diagnosis based on history and skin examination with biopsy only indicated in difficult or unclear cases.
- Stopping the itch–scratch cycle through patient education, skin lubrication, and topical medications is key.
- Treatment is based on disease severity.

L

LONG QT INTERVAL

Caitlyn M. Rerucha, MD, MSEd, FAAFP, CAQSM • Matthew J. Kenney, DO • Andrew Collyer, DO

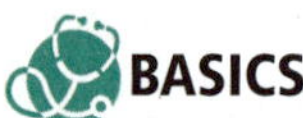

BASICS

DESCRIPTION

- QT interval: the interval from the beginning of the QRS complex to the end of the T wave on the surface electrocardiogram (ECG). This represents the period from the onset of ventricular depolarization to completion of repolarization of the ventricular myocardium, or ventricular systole. The QT interval is normal if it is <50% of the RR interval.
- Corrected QT interval (QTc): The QT interval has an inverse relationship with heart rate. The QTc is the QT interval corrected for heart rate, and it estimates the QT interval at a heart rate of 60 beats/min. See formulas.
- Prolonged QTc is generally defined as >470 ms for adult males and >480 ms for adult females:
  - 460 to 469 ms considered borderline in men
  - 470 to 479 ms considered borderline in women (1)
  - 450 to 459 ms considered borderline in children aged 1 to 15 years old
- Most cases of prolonged QT are acquired, but several genetic mutations cause inherited long QT syndrome (LQTS) (1).
- Prolonged QTc from any cause can precipitate polymorphic ventricular tachycardia (VT) called torsade de pointes (TdP), leading to dizziness, syncope, syncope with generalized seizures, and sudden cardiac arrest from ventricular arrhythmias (VA).

EPIDEMIOLOGY

A more common channelopathy; it may be congenital (2) or acquired; congenital often presents in childhood, but may present as early as newborn period or go undiagnosed until middle age; the mean onset is 14 years of age.

Incidence

Incidence of medication-induced QTc prolongation and TdP varies with medication and a host of other factors. Exact incidences are difficult to estimate but may be 1/2,000 to 1/2,500. The incidence of congenital infantile phenotype positive/genotype positive is 1/2,000 and it is suspected that genotype positive/phenotype negative may be as high as 1/1,000.

Prevalence

Congenital LQTS is estimated to occur in 1/2,500 to 1/7,000 births. The true incidence of mutations in the population is likely much higher.

ETIOLOGY AND PATHOPHYSIOLOGY

- Acquired
  - Demographics: increasing age, female sex
  - Electrolyte abnormalities: hypokalemia, hypocalcemia, and hypomagnesemia
  - Noncardiac disease: hypothyroidism, renal impairment, and hepatic impairment
  - Cardiac disease: heart failure, LVH, and myocardial ischemia
  - Scenarios: rapid increase in the QT interval >60 ms, conversion from atrial fibrillation/bradycardia
  - Medications (*denote "high-risk" medication for TdP 25) (1)
    - Antiarrhythmic medications (quinidine, procainamide, dronedarone, dofetilide, sotalol, disopyramide, and amiodarone)
    - Antipsychotic medications: especially if given IV (haloperidol*, chlorpromazine*, thioridazine*, pimozide*)
    - Antidepressants: most commonly used drugs responsible (SSRIs, SNRIs, trazodone, TCAs)
    - Antibiotics/antivirals/antifungals/antiprotozoals/antimalarials: macrolides (clarithromycin*, erythromycin*, also CYP3A4 inhibitors), fluoroquinolones, quinine, and chloroquine
    - Antiemetics: metoclopramide, ondansetron, promethazine
    - Opioids: methadone*, buprenorphine
    - Antihistamines: cetirizine, hydroxyzine, diphenhydramine
    - Decongestants: pseudoephedrine, phenylephrine
    - Stimulants: albuterol, phentermine
    - Misc: chloroquine*, pentamidine*, various antimuscarinics, and anticonvulsants
- Congenital
  - >13 genes have been identified that encode for subunits of various ion membrane channels
  - Mutations of KCNQ1 (LQTS1), KCNH2 (LQTS2), and SCN5A (LQTS3) account for over 90% of cases.
  - Loss of function mutations in several potassium ion membrane channels or gain of function mutations in the sodium or calcium ion membrane channels in cardiac myocytes
- Pathophysiology
  - Depolarization (phase 0) of the myocardium results from the rapid influx of sodium through sodium channels (I_{Na}) causing myocyte contraction during systole; seen on ECG as the QRS complex
  - Repolarization occurs through the efflux of potassium from the cell (phases 2 and 3) by rapid (I_{Kr}) and slow (I_{Ks}) components of the delayed rectifier; represented by the T wave on an ECG
  - Drug-induced QT prolongation most often due to blockade of the I_{Kr} channel leading to delay in phase 3 rapid repolarization.
  - In both cases, deviation from normal ion channel function leads to transmural dispersion of repolarization currents across the myocardium, triggering early after depolarizations which may devolve into TdP (1).
  - Prolonged QT interval alone does not denote imminent risk for TdP; TdP is often self-limited, but TdP can cause syncope or degrade to VF.

Genetics

- >12 distinct genotypes are linked to LQTS (2). LQT1 is most common cause of congenital LQTS.
- Penetrance is highly variable making both diagnosis and management challenging (1).

RISK FACTORS

For the feared complication, TdP, risk factors include the following:

- Female (~2 times increased risk), QTc >500 ms (2 to 3 times increased risk), QTc >60 ms over previous baseline (for every 10 ms increase in the QTc, there is a 5–7% increased risk for developing TdP), history of syncope or presyncope, history of TdP, bradycardia, liver or kidney disease (by increasing blood levels of QT-prolonging medications), medications that cause QTc prolongation (high doses, fast infusions, combination of medications), medications that inhibit CYP3A4, electrolyte abnormalities (hypokalemia, hypomagnesemia, hypocalcemia)
- For congenital LQTS: catecholamine surges from exercise, emotional stress, loud noises, postpartum depression.

GENERAL PREVENTION

- Avoid (or use with caution) causative medications, including combinations with potentially additive effects.
- Replete electrolytes (goal: Mg >2 mg/dL, K = 4.5 to 5.0 mEq/L).
- Treat underlying diseases.
- Avoid strenuous sports and other stimulating activities, like amusement park rides or jumping into cold water, in LQTS.
- Avoid sudden loud noises in LQTS (alarm clocks, doorbells, telephones).

COMMONLY ASSOCIATED CONDITIONS

- Illnesses with associated severe vomiting and/or diarrhea leading to electrolyte disturbances
- Eating disorders—anorexia nervosa, bulimia
- Andersen-Tawil syndrome (LTQS type 7)—prolonged QT interval, muscle weakness, facial dysmorphism
- Timothy syndrome (LQTS type 8)—prolonged QT interval, hand/foot, facial, and neurodevelopment
- Jervell and Lange-Nielsen syndrome (JLNS)—associated with profound sensorineural hearing loss

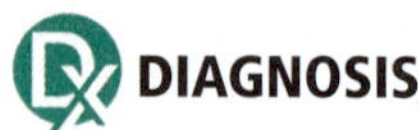

DIAGNOSIS

HISTORY

- Incidental finding on ECG in asymptomatic patients
- Evaluate for syncope, presyncopal episodes, palpitations, and associated precipitating events (emotional triggers, swimming, diving).
- Key family history items that increase the likelihood of congenital LQTS include:
  - History of syncope, sudden cardiac death, or other arrhythmic disorders
  - Premature sudden deaths (<40 years of age and autopsy negative)
  - Unexplained motor vehicle accidents
  - Unexplained drownings
  - Generalized seizures (frequently, patients with LQTS have been misdiagnosed with and treated for epilepsy)
- History of seizures in patient or family members (tonic–clonic movement may be due to cerebral hypoperfusion during episodes of ventricular arrhythmia or syncope)
- Detailed medication history
- Congenital deafness

PHYSICAL EXAM

- The physical exam is typically unremarkable because patients with QT syndrome typically have structurally normal hearts.
- May include signs of underlying cardiac disease, hypothyroidism, liver, or renal impairment
- Congenital deafness present in many forms of congenital LQTS

DIFFERENTIAL DIAGNOSIS

When evaluating long QT interval, differential should include causes of acquired LQTS: QT-prolonging drugs, hypokalemia, hypomagnesemia, hypocalcemia, neurologic conditions leading to subarachnoid bleed, structural heart disease.

DIAGNOSTIC TESTS & INTERPRETATION

Initial Tests (lab, imaging)

- ECG
- Electrolyte panel: especially calcium, magnesium, and potassium.
- TSH with reflex T4

Follow-Up Tests & Special Considerations

- Echocardiogram to evaluate for cardiomyopathy
- Outpatient cardiac rhythm monitoring (Holter, event, or implantable monitoring)
- Genetic testing for LQTS mutations is available. Indications to pursue testing include family history of early, unexplained cardiac death, family history of LQTS, or clinical suspicion based on patient's history or examination.

Test Interpretation

- The QT interval is best measured from the onset of the QRS to the completion of the T wave; most commonly measured in lead II or V_2
- QTc calculation can be performed in several ways using RR interval immediately preceding the QT interval for calculation. The Bazett formula is most commonly used method.

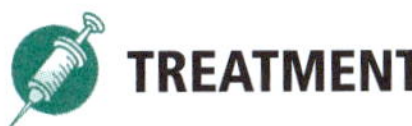

TREATMENT

GENERAL MEASURES

- Treat VT, TdP, and VF emergently per ACLS guidelines.
- Withdraw offending agents and correct electrolytes.
- Treat underlying disorder in the setting of gastrointestinal illness, eating disorder, or neurologic conditions involving subarachnoid bleed.
- Avoid triggers, if known.

MEDICATION

First Line

- For TdP: magnesium sulfate 2 g infused over 2 to 5 minutes, followed by continuous infusion of 2 to 4 mg/min if needed. Flushing is a normal side effect of bolus injections. Monitor for magnesium toxicity in those with renal insufficiency.
- For congenital LQTS, to prevent life-threatening arrhythmias: propranolol or nadolol generally regarded as the best β-blockers for management of LQTS, although rigorous studies are lacking.
- β-Blockers are effective in decreasing, but not eliminating the risk of fatal arrhythmias. Patients receiving metoprolol had significantly more breakthrough clinical events (e.g., syncope, aborted cardiac arrest, implantable cardiac defibrillator [ICD] shock, or sudden cardiac death [SCD]) compared with those receiving propranolol or nadolol (3)[A].

Second Line

- For high-risk patients who remain symptomatic on a β-blocker, ICDs with or without pacemaker may be indicated.
- If no medications are available, an automated external defibrillator is the most useful treatment for any patient with LQTS who converts into a life-threatening arrhythmia.

ISSUES FOR REFERRAL

Refer to cardiologist or electrophysiologist to establish diagnosis, especially for congenital LQTS.

ADDITIONAL THERAPIES

Trials are currently being conducted on medicines that block cardiac sodium channels for LQTS type 3.

SURGERY/OTHER PROCEDURES

- ICD for those with a history of major cardiac events (whether treated with appropriate medical therapy or not).
  - ICDs do not prevent TdP, so patients should continue optimal medical therapy in conjunction to ICD.
- Left cervical—thoracic sympathetic denervation was used for symptomatic LQTS prior to the advent of β-blockers. It is still an option for those patients with LQTS who are refractory to β-blocker therapy (1)[B].

ADMISSION, INPATIENT, AND NURSING CONSIDERATIONS

- Treat TdP, VT, and VF promptly as per ACLS guidelines. Correct electrolytes on an emergent basis. Evaluate for acquired QT prolongation. If no cause is found, consider congenital LQTS.
- Patients with prolonged QTc and syncope/near syncope should be monitored on telemetry.
- Obtain a baseline ECG if initiating or combining medications with QT-prolonging medications, then when the drug reaches steady state, at 30 days, and annually thereafter.
- Avoid QT-prolonging medications in patients with congenital LQTS.
- Monitor electrolytes, urgently treat hypomagnesemia and hypokalemia, and discontinue/change offending medications.

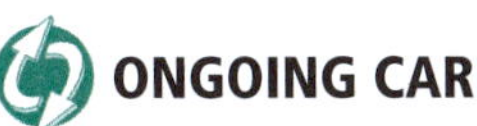

ONGOING CARE

FOLLOW-UP RECOMMENDATIONS

All patients with LQTS should follow regularly with a cardiologist or electrophysiologist. Classically, patients were limited to low static and low dynamic stresses in the activities they participated in. In 2015, the AHA and ACC released new participation guidelines that allow participation in competitive sports if they meet certain criteria.

Patient Monitoring

- On routine visits, ask about syncope, presyncope, and palpitations in those who have QTc prolongation.
- For pre-participation examinations, ask all participants about these similar symptoms and family history. In individuals responding yes to these questions, have a low threshold to evaluate their QTc with ECG.
- Consider ECG and/or outpatient cardiac rhythm monitoring with medication additions or dosage changes.
- Prompt evaluation is warranted for symptomatic QTc prolongation of any cause.
- Check and correct for electrolyte imbalances.

DIET

- Those with known LQTS often benefit from additional potassium in their diet, whether through diet or supplementation.
- Avoiding caffeinated products, supplements with stimulant properties (such as ginseng), alcohol, and illicit/recreational drugs is also recommended as these can all increase the risk of life-threatening arrhythmias.
- QT prolongation noted in the setting of ketogenic diet and diabetic ketoacidosis irrespective of electrolyte disturbances.

PATIENT EDUCATION

- Educate patients with QTc prolongation about medications side effects and medication interactions.
- Patients with congenital forms of LQTS should be aware of and avoid triggers (depending on their specific gene mutation).
- Consider the emotional and psychological impacts.

PROGNOSIS

Acquired LQTS will resolve after withdrawal of offending agents and normalization of metabolic abnormalities. Patients with underlying cardiovascular disease may be at increased risk of mortality and require further intervention. Prognosis for congenital LQTS if untreated is quite poor.

COMPLICATIONS

TdP resulting in ventricular fibrillation, sudden cardiac death, seizures, loss of consciousness, drowning, and other accidents

REFERENCES

1. Abrams DJ, Macrae CA. Long QT syndrome. *Circulation*. 2014;129(14):1524–1529.
2. Groffen AJ, Bikker H, Christiaans I. Long QT syndrome overview. In: Adam MP, Feldman J, Mirzaa GM, Pagon RA, Wallace SE, Amemiya A, eds. *GeneReviews*. Seattle (WA): University of Washington; 1993.
3. Went TR, Sultan W, Sapkota A, et al. A systematic review on the role of beta-blockers in reducing cardiac arrhythmias in long QT syndrome subtype 1–3. *Cureus*. 2021;13(9):e17632.

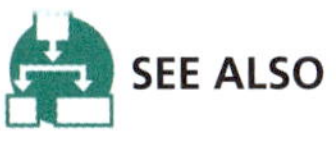

SEE ALSO

Algorithms: Cardiac Arrhythmias; Torsade de Pointes (TdP): Variant Form of Polymorphic Ventricular Tachycardia (VT)

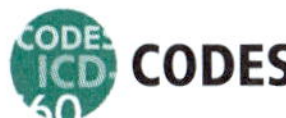

CODES

ICD10

I45.81 Long QT syndrome

CLINICAL PEARLS

- Evaluate for acquired causes before making a diagnosis of congenital LQTS.
- Any patient with symptoms of palpitations, syncope, presyncope, any collapse, or with family history of sudden cardiac death should be evaluated with appropriate initial work up, including ECG with QTc evaluation.
- For accurate diagnosis, calculate QTc manually.
- Magnesium sulfate is the treatment of choice during ACLS for TdP.

LUNG, PRIMARY MALIGNANCIES

Samantha Howard Caldwell, MD

BASICS

Primary lung cancers are the leading cause of cancer-related deaths in the United States (~estimated 130,180 deaths in 2021 which accounts for 25% of all cancer-related deaths). Lung cancer is mainly diagnosed in older people at average age of diagnosis at 70 years. It has the lowest 5-year survival rate (~18% vs breast cancer at 91%, prostate cancer at 99%, and colorectal cancer at 65%). 85% of lung cancer is due to smoking; remaining 15% is caused by radon exposure, genetics, second-hand smoke, asbestos, and other air pollution.

DESCRIPTION

- Two broad categories
  - Non–small cell lung cancer (NSCLC) accounts for 85% of all lung cancers.
    - Adenocarcinoma (~40% of NSCLC): most common type in the United States and occurs in both smokers and nonsmokers; metastasizes earlier than squamous cell; usually starts from peripheral lung tissue
    - Squamous cell carcinoma (SCC): accounts for 30% of NSCLC; usually occurs close to large airways
    - Large cell (~10% of NSCLC): named because of the cells, large nuclei
  - Small cell lung cancer (SCLC): accounts for 15% of all lung cancers; centrally located, aggressive and metastasizes very easily through the blood seeding lymph nodes, bones, brain, adrenals, and liver
- Others: mesothelioma, carcinoid tumor

EPIDEMIOLOGY

Incidence

- There were 209,500 new cases of lung cancer in 2021 and 131,888 deaths in the United States in 2022 (CDC).
- Male patients had both higher rates (54.1 versus 45.5 per 100,000) and higher chance of death (35.2 versus 25.9 per 100,000) compared to females.
- Overall, lung cancer causes more deaths than breast, prostate, colorectal, and brain cancers combined.
- Average age of diagnosis: 70 years old
- Due to decreases in smoking, lung cancer deaths are declining in the United States.

ETIOLOGY AND PATHOPHYSIOLOGY

Genetics

- Genetics accounts for approximately 8% of lung cancers.
- NSCLC
  - Oncogenes: Ras family (H-ras, K-ras, N-ras), EGFR, NTRK, ALK, etc.
  - Tumor suppressor genes: retinoblastoma (Rb), *p53*
- SCLC
  - Oncogenes: Myc family
  - Tumor suppressor genes: *p53* mutation, Rb inactivation

RISK FACTORS

- Smoking
- Secondhand smoke exposure
- Radon
- Environmental/occupational exposures
  - Air pollution
  - Asbestos exposure (synergistic increase in risk for smokers)
  - Ionizing radiation
  - Mutagenic gases (halogen ethers, mustard gas, aromatic hydrocarbons)
  - Metals (inorganic arsenic, chromium, nickel)
- Lung scarring from tuberculosis
- Radiation therapy to breast or chest

GENERAL PREVENTION

- Smoking cessation and prevention programs
- USPSTF recommends annual screening for lung cancer with low-dose computed tomography (LDCT) in adults aged 50 to 80 years who have a 20 pack-year smoking history and currently smoke or have quit within the past 15 years (1).
- Screening should be discontinued once a person has not smoked for 15 years or develops a health problem that substantially limits life expectancy or the ability or willingness to have curative lung surgery.

COMMONLY ASSOCIATED CONDITIONS

- Paraneoplastic syndromes: hypertrophic pulmonary osteoarthropathy, Lambert-Eaton syndrome (LES), Cushing syndrome, hypercalcemia from ectopic parathyroid-releasing hormone (PTHrP), syndrome of inappropriate antidiuretic hormone (SIADH)
- Hypercoagulable state
- Pancoast syndrome
- Superior vena cava (SVC) syndrome
- Pleural effusion
- Chronic obstructive pulmonary disease (COPD), other sequelae of cigarette smoking

DIAGNOSIS

HISTORY

- May be asymptomatic
- Respiratory
  - Cough (new/change in chronic cough)
  - Wheezing and stridor
  - Dyspnea
  - Hemoptysis
  - Pneumonitis (fever, productive cough)
- Constitutional
  - Malaise
  - Bone pain (metastatic disease)
  - Fatigue
  - Weight loss, anorexia
  - Fever
  - Anemia
- Other presentations
  - Chest pain (dull, pleuritic), shoulder/arm pain (Pancoast tumors), dysphagia
  - Plethora (redness of face or neck), hoarseness (involvement of recurrent laryngeal nerve)
  - Horner syndrome, neurologic abnormalities (e.g., headaches, syncope, weakness, cognitive impairment)
  - Pericardial tamponade (pericardial invasion)

PHYSICAL EXAM

- General: fever, chills, night sweats, weight loss
- Head, eye, ear, nose, throat (HEENT) : Horner syndrome, dysphonia, stridor, scleral icterus, dysphagia
- Neck: supraclavicular/cervical lymph nodes, mass
- Lungs: effusion, wheezing, airway obstruction, dyspnea
- Abdomen/groin: hepatomegaly or lymphadenopathy
- Extremities: signs of hypertrophic pulmonary osteoarthropathy, deep venous thrombosis (DVT), fingernail clubbing
- Neurologic: headache, syncope, weakness, cognitive impairment

DIFFERENTIAL DIAGNOSIS

COPD (may coexist), asthma, granulomatous (tuberculosis, sarcoidosis), cardiomyopathy/congestive heart failure (CHF)

DIAGNOSTIC TESTS & INTERPRETATION

Initial Tests (lab, imaging)

- Serum
  - Complete blood count (CBC)
  - Comprehensive metabolic panel (CMP)—check for hyponatremia (SIADH).
  - Serum calcium—check for hypercalcemia (paraneoplastic syndrome).
- Sputum cytology
- Chest x-ray (CXR): Nodule or mass, especially if calcified, persistent infiltrate, atelectasis, mediastinal widening, Hilar enlargement, pleural effusion
- CT scan of chest (with IV contrast): nodule or mass (central or peripheral), lymphadenopathy
- Biopsy and cytology are definitive diagnosis.
- Evaluation for metastatic disease
  - Positron emission tomography (PET) scan to evaluate metastasis mediastinal lymphadenopathy
  - MRI and CT can also be used to detect metastases.

Follow-Up Tests & Special Considerations

Staging

- Both NSCLC and SCLC: staged from I to IV based on: primary tumor (T), lymph node status (N), and presence of metastasis (M)
- SCLC further staged by:
  - Limited disease: confined to ipsilateral hemithorax
  - Extensive disease: beyond ipsilateral hemithorax (stages IIIB and IV), which may include malignant pleural or pericardial effusion or hematogenous metastases (stage IV)
  - Most commonly metastasize to lymph nodes (pulmonary, mediastinal), then liver, adrenal glands, bones, brain

Diagnostic Procedures/Other

- Biopsy with pathology review using
  - Bronchoscopy with transbronchial biopsy (WANG needle); usually for centrally located tumors
  - CT-guided biopsy of lung mass or metastatic site; usually for peripherally located tumors
  - Endobronchial ultrasound (EBUS)-guided fine-needle aspiration
  - Enlarged mediastinal lymph nodes necessitate staging by mediastinoscopy, video-assisted thoracoscopy, and EBUS-guided fine-needle aspiration

- Video-assisted thoracoscopy (associated pleural disease and suspected mediastinal nodal spread)
- In patients with advanced NSCLC, screening for mutations in EGFR, BRAF, *KRAS G12C*, NTRK, *ALK, ROS1, MET exon 14, and RET* non-SCC (NSCC) or mixed squamous histology
- PD-L1 testing
- Bone marrow aspirate (SCLC)

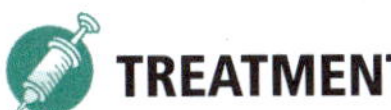

TREATMENT

After diagnosis of a suspicious nodule, patient will undergo a multidisciplinary evaluation to determine the optimal diagnostic, treatment, and follow up strategy.

GENERAL MEASURES

- NSCLC
  - Stage I, stage II, and selected stage III tumors are surgically resectable. Neoadjuvant or adjuvant therapy is recommended for select patients with high risk IB, II, and IIIA NSCLC. Patients with resectable disease but who are not surgical candidates may receive radiation therapy.
  - Patients with unresectable or N2, N3 disease are treated with concurrent chemoradiation followed by maintenance immunotherapy. Select patients with T3 or N2 disease can be treated effectively with surgical resection and either pre- or postoperative chemotherapy or chemoradiation therapy.
  - Patients with distant metastases (M1B) can be treated with chemotherapy, targeted therapy, immunotherapy, or radiation therapy for palliation or supportive care alone
- SCLC
  - Limited stage: concurrent chemoradiation
  - Extensive stage: combination of chemotherapy and immunotherapy
  - Consider prophylactic cranial irradiation (PCI) in patients achieving a complete or partial response.
- Quality-of-life assessments: Karnofsky Performance Status (KPS) scale; Eastern Cooperative Oncology Group (ECOG)
- Discussions with patient and family about end-of-life care

MEDICATION

- Adjuvant chemotherapy following surgery improves survival in patients with fully resected stages II and III NSCLC.
- Comfort measures: oxygen and morphine for shortness of breath, antibiotics for lung infections, diuretics for pulmonary edema, benzodiazepines for anxiety, and corticosteroids for lung obstruction

First Line

- NSCLC
  - Stages II and III: neoadjuvant or adjuvant chemotherapy
    - Cisplatin-based doublets (combination with paclitaxel, etoposide, vinorelbine, docetaxel, gemcitabine)
    - Carboplatin alternative for patients unlikely to tolerate cisplatin
    - Cisplatin plus pemetrexed (NSCC)
  - Unresectable stages IIA and IIIB
    - Concurrent chemoradiation
      - Cisplatin plus etoposide, vinblastine, or pemetrexed (NSCC) plus concurrent radiation
      - Carboplatin plus paclitaxel plus concurrent radiation
      - Carboplatin plus pemetrexed (NSCC) plus concurrent radiation
    - Durvalumab consolidation post chemoradiation for stage III
  - Stage IV
    - No chemotherapy regimen can be recommended for routine use.
    - Cisplatin- or carboplatin-based doublets are standard of care in the absence of targetable mutations.
    - Pembrolizumab with pemetrexed and carboplatin for adenocarcinoma without EGFR, ROS, or ALK mutations regardless of PD-L1 expression
    - Pembrolizumab, atezolizumab, or cemiplimab monotherapy for NSCLC with PD-L1 expression ≥50% of tumor cells
    - Osimertinib first line for most patients with EGFR mutations
    - Dabrafenib with trametinib for untreated patients with BRAF V600E mutations
    - Alectinib, lorlatinib, crizotinib, brigatinib, ceritinib, or crizotinib for untreated ALK-positive NSCLC
    - Crizotinib, ceritinib, or entrectinib for patients with ROS1-positive NSCLC
    - Sotorasib for KRAS G12C mutated tumors
    - Larotrectinib or entrectinib for NTRK fusion positive tumors
    - Capmatinib, crizotinib, or tepotinib for tumors with MET exon 14 skipping mutations
    - Selpercatinib, pralsetinib, cabozantinib, or vandetanib for tumors with RET rearrangements
- SCLC
  - Cisplatin or carboplatin plus etoposide with addition of atezolizumab in extensive stage disease

Second Line

- NSCLC
  - Cisplatin-based doublets +/− bevacizumab (NSCC) if not previously used
  - Docetaxel +/− ramucirumab, pemetrexed if not previously used (NSCC), gemcitabine, or nivolumab (squamous cell)
  - Immunotherapy may be considered if progressed during or after first-line platinum-based drug.
- SCLC
  - Lurbinectedin, topotecan, or clinical trial; alternatives include CAV (cyclophosphamide, doxorubicin, vincristine), gemcitabine, docetaxel, paclitaxel, nivolumab, and temozolomide

ADDITIONAL THERAPIES

- Smoking cessation counseling
- Consider IV bisphosphonates or denosumab in patients with bone metastases to reduce skeletal-related events.

SURGERY/OTHER PROCEDURES

Resection for NSCLC, for stages I, II, and IIIA, if medically fit to undergo surgery

COMPLEMENTARY & ALTERNATIVE MEDICINE

Mind–breathing-body therapies: creative outlets (i.e., music, art, dance), Tai chi, meditation, biofeedback, hypnosis, yoga

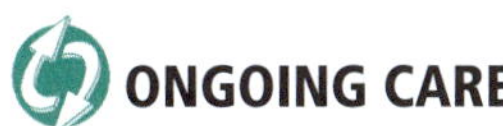

ONGOING CARE

FOLLOW-UP RECOMMENDATIONS

Patient Monitoring

Visits every 3 to 6 months in the first 2 years after surgery with physical exam and CT scan

PATIENT EDUCATION

- National Cancer Institute: https://www.cancer.gov/
- Smokefree.gov: https://smokefree.gov/

PROGNOSIS

- NSCLC 5-year survival
  - Localized disease: for stages IA1, IA2, and IA3 is 92%, 83%, and 77%, respectively; stages IB and IIA is 68% and 60%, respectively
  - Regional disease: for stages IIIA, IIIB, and IIIC is 36%, 26%, and 13%, respectively
  - Distant metastatic disease: for stages IVA and IVB is 10% and <1%, respectively
- SCLC
  - Without treatment: median survival from diagnosis of only 2 to 4 months
  - 5-year survival rate: ranges from 2% (stage IV) to 31% (stage I)
  - Extensive-stage disease: median survival of 6 to 12 months; long-term disease-free survival is rare.

COMPLICATIONS

- Thrombosis
- Paraneoplastic syndromes
- Fatigue, anorexia, weight loss
- Chemotherapy-induced nausea/vomiting
- Neutropenia, anemia
- Neurotoxicities, nephrotoxicities

REFERENCES

1. Krist AH, Davidson KW, Mangione CM, et al; for US Preventive Services Task Force. Screening for lung cancer: US Preventive Services Task Force recommendation statement. *JAMA*. 2021;325(10):962–970.

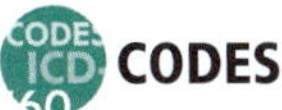

CODES

ICD10

- C34.90 Malignant neoplasm of unsp part of unsp bronchus or lung
- C34.10 Malignant neoplasm of upper lobe, unsp bronchus or lung
- C34.30 Malignant neoplasm of lower lobe, unsp bronchus or lung

CLINICAL PEARLS

- NSCLC (>85% of all lung cancers); normally originate in periphery; adenocarcinoma (~40% of NSCLC); SCC (~25% of NSCLC); large cell (~10% of NSCLC)
- SCLC centrally located, early metastases, aggressive
- Smoking cessation reduces morbidity/mortality. Smoking cessation interventions should be offered to all patients with lung cancer.

LUPUS ERYTHEMATOSUS, SYSTEMIC (SLE)

Sahil Mullick, MD, FAAFP • Syed Murtaza Haider Zaidi, MD, MBBS

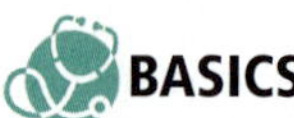

BASICS

DESCRIPTION

- Multisystem autoimmune inflammatory disorder with variable presentation, disease course, and prognosis
- Can manifest in any organ system, especially dermatologic, renal, hematologic, musculoskeletal, cardiovascular
- Synonyms: lupus; SLE

EPIDEMIOLOGY

Incidence

- 5 to 12 per 100,000 person-years in United States
- Significant variation based on ethnicity: Black 16, American Indian/Alaska Native 7.4, Hispanic 5.6, Asian/Pacific Islander 4.6, White 3.3 per 100,000 person-years
- Strong female predominance: 9.8 versus 0.8 per 100,000 person-years (~12× higher)
- Peak incidence: 3rd to 7th decades of life for females, 5th to 7th decades for males

Prevalence

- Ranges from 20 to 150 cases per 100,000 in United States
- Strong female predominance: 179 versus 21 cases per 100,000 (~9× higher) with highest in Black women: 498 per 100,000

ETIOLOGY AND PATHOPHYSIOLOGY

Genetic, environmental, immunoregulatory, hormonal, and epigenetic factors all play a role.

Genetics

Over 100 gene loci susceptible for SLE in genome-wide association studies (1)[C].

RISK FACTORS

- Ethnicity: highest risk in Black populations; intermediate risk in Asian, Hispanic, and American Indian/Alaska Native populations
- Hormonal: female sex, early menarche/menopause, endometriosis, surgical menopause
- Family history of SLE or autoimmune disease
- Environmental: cigarette smoking, crystalline silica exposure, exogenous female hormones, certain medications (drug-induced lupus), UV light, viral infections, vitamin D deficiency, alfalfa sprouts, foods containing canavanine

COMMONLY ASSOCIATED CONDITIONS

Antiphospholipid syndrome, depression, fibromyalgia, thyroid disease, connective tissue disease syndromes (such as rheumatoid arthritis, Sjögren syndrome, systemic sclerosis)

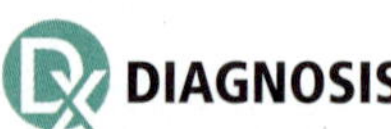

DIAGNOSIS

- Suspect in multisystem disease including fever, fatigue, and signs of inflammation.
- Classification criteria from European League Against Rheumatism/American College of Rheumatology (EULAR/ACR) in 2019: sensitivity 96%, specificity 93% (2)[C]
- Each criterion is assigned points, from 2 to 10. Patients with 10 or more points and at least one clinical criterion are classified as having SLE.
- Do not exclude clinically appropriate patients from treatment solely based on classification criteria (2)[C].
- Previous criteria from ACR and Systemic Lupus International Collaborating Clinics (SLICC) still used widely in clinical practice

HISTORY

- Common symptoms: fatigue, arthralgia, fever, oral ulcers, hair loss, rash, photosensitivity, myalgias
- Presentations that may raise suspicion: unprovoked venous thromboembolism (VTE), cerebrovascular accident at young age, acute pericarditis, recurrent pregnancy loss, new-onset seizure or psychosis, unexplained cytopenias or renal failure

PHYSICAL EXAM

- Constitutional (common): weight loss, fever, lymphadenopathy, fatigue
- Skin (common)
  - Nonspecific: nonscarring alopecia, painless oral or nasal ulcers, photosensitivity, vasculitis, Raynaud phenomenon
  - Acute cutaneous lupus erythematosus (ACLE) (malar/butterfly rash that spares the nasolabial folds, photodistributed maculopapular rash)
  - Subacute cutaneous lupus erythematosus (SCLE) (annular or papulosquamous, photodistributed lesions), chronic cutaneous lupus erythematosus (CCLE) (discoid lesions with scarring and dyspigmentation)
- Musculoskeletal (common):
  - Synovitis, especially symmetric polyarthritis, periarticular involvement (tendons, joint capsule), leading to nonerosive joint deformities (Jaccoud arthropathy)
- Pericarditis/pneumonitis, pleural effusion, VTE
- Edema or anasarca in advanced renal disease; pallor, jaundice, splenomegaly in hematologic disease; seizures, psychosis, delirium, mononeuritis multiplex, peripheral or cranial neuropathies, and cognitive impairment in CNS disease

DIFFERENTIAL DIAGNOSIS

- Extremely broad due to variable presentation and widespread disease manifestations
- Consider other conditions like thyroid disease, fibromyalgia, mixed connective tissue disease, Sjögren syndrome, systemic sclerosis, and organ-specific diagnoses based on presentation.
- Consider drug-induced lupus (hydralazine, procainamide, isoniazid, methyldopa, quinidine, chlorpromazine).

DIAGNOSTIC TESTS & INTERPRETATION

Initial Tests (lab, imaging)

- Based on presentation and level of suspicion
- Low suspicion: Limited initial laboratory evaluation may include complete blood count (CBC), complete metabolic panel (CMP), thyroid-stimulating hormone (TSH), ESR/CRP, and urinalysis; imaging based on signs/symptoms
- Higher suspicion: immunologic testing
  - Lupus specific
    - ANA (titer ≥1:80 by immunofluorescence); sensitivity 97.8%, specificity 74.7%
    - Anti-dsDNA (sensitivity 70%, specificity 96%)
    - Anti-Smith (sensitivity 39.7%, specificity 98.6%)
  - Supporting:
    - Complement levels (low C3 and/or C4)
    - Anti-cardiolipin, anti-β2GP1, lupus anticoagulant

Follow-Up Tests & Special Considerations

- 24-hour urine collection or spot protein/creatinine ratio to quantify proteinuria (2)[C]
- Anemia (hemolysis evaluation): reticulocyte count, indirect bilirubin, haptoglobin, direct Coombs (2)[C]
- Screen for antiphospholipid syndrome at diagnosis if not already done (3)[C]
- Baseline metabolic labs: lipid panel, fasting glucose or HbA1c, vitamin D level, TSH
- Special tests: Chest CT, ECHO, MRI, lumbar puncture, renal biopsy (if lupus nephritis is suspected)

Diagnostic Procedures/Other

- Renal biopsy: urine protein >500 mg/24 hr (2)[C]
- Skin biopsy if necessary to confirm clinical findings of cutaneous lupus (2)[C]

Test Interpretation

- Skin biopsy: interface vacuolar dermatitis consisting of perivascular lymphohistiocytic infiltrate with dermal mucin; may have immune-complex deposition at dermoepidermal junction
- Renal biopsy: per International Society of Nephrology/Renal Pathology Society

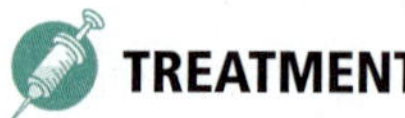

TREATMENT

GENERAL MEASURES

- Requires a multidisciplinary, individualized approach to treatment
- General treatment goals: achieving remission or low disease activity, preventing flares and end-organ damage, increasing survival, improving quality of life (3)[C]
- Supportive measures include sun protection, smoking cessation, adequate exercise, managing cardiovascular risk factors (lipids, glucose, blood pressure, weight).
- Preconception counseling, family planning
- Immunizations: 2019 EULAR guidelines for vaccination

MEDICATION

First Line

- Hydroxychloroquine
  - Recommended for all patients with SLE, unless contraindicated
  - Reduces flares, improves skin/musculoskeletal manifestations, reduces thrombosis and bone mass loss, prevents organ damage, increases survival; safe in pregnancy

- Dosing: 200 to 400 mg/day as single daily dose or 2 divided doses; limit to 5 mg/kg/day (actual body weight) (3)[C]
- Most common adverse reactions are gastrointestinal (nausea, vomiting, diarrhea, abdominal pain) and cutaneous (rash) and usually mild.
- Retinal damage:
  - Less common at doses <5 mg/kg/day
  - Risk factors: high doses, renal insufficiency, macular disease, tamoxifen use
  - Ophthalmologic screening at baseline (3)[C]
  - Yearly screening after 5 years in absence of other risk factors (3)[C].
- Cardiomyopathy: conduction abnormalities including prolonged QT interval
- Other adverse reactions include proximal myopathy and neuropathy, neuropsychiatric changes, hypoglycemia.
- Caution in hepatic and/or renal disease, with insulin, antidiabetic medications medication that affects cardiac conduction, especially QT prolonging agents

- Glucocorticoids
  - Dose and route of administration depend on organ involvement and severity.
    - Topical steroids used in cutaneous disease.
    - Oral steroids used for initial management, flares, and/or maintenance therapy
    - Life/organ-threatening flares frequently require pulsed IV methylprednisolone (250 to 1,000 mg/day for 1 to 3 days) (3)[C]
  - Dose of chronic maintenance therapy should be minimized to <7.5 mg/day and discontinued if possible (3)[C].
  - Early immunomodulatory therapy may help minimize glucocorticoid needs (3)[C].

Second Line

- Choice of agent depends on disease manifestations, patient characteristics (e.g., age and childbearing potential), safety, and cost.
- Consider methotrexate, azathioprine, or mycophenolate for patients not controlled on hydroxychloroquine, unable to adequately taper glucocorticoids, or for initial treatment in more severe disease. Consider anifrolumab, belimumab, voclosporin add-on for high residual disease activity or frequent flares despite standard treatments. Consider cyclophosphamide or rituximab for severe life/organ-threatening or refractory disease (3)[C].

ISSUES FOR REFERRAL

Mild disease without significant end-organ involvement may be appropriate for treatment in primary care; generally requires multidisciplinary team in coordination with rheumatology; severe disease best managed in dedicated lupus center

ADDITIONAL THERAPIES

IVIG has shown to successfully treat cutaneous and neuropsychiatric symptoms of SLE, with reduction in disease activity, reduction daily steroid requirement. Agents in late phase trials or early clinical use include obinutuzumab (anti-CD20), deucravacitinib (TYK2 inhibitor), litifilimab (anti-BDCA 2), and chimeric antigen receptor (CAR) T-cell therapies targeting B cells.

SURGERY/OTHER PROCEDURES

Renal transplant for end-stage renal disease

COMPLEMENTARY & ALTERNATIVE MEDICINE

Supplements with some evidence of benefit: vitamin D, omega-3 fatty acids, *N*-acetylcysteine, turmeric (4)[C]

ADMISSION, INPATIENT, AND NURSING CONSIDERATIONS

Difficult to differentiate SLE flare from infection; may need to treat both pending full evaluation. IV pulse methylprednisolone (250 to 1,000 mg/day for 1 to 3 days) for organ-threatening flares.

ONGOING CARE

FOLLOW-UP RECOMMENDATIONS

Patient Monitoring

- Intensity of monitoring depends on manifestations, severity, medication regimen, comorbidities.
- Stable, inactive disease without significant organ involvement or comorbidities may be followed every 6 to 12 months.
- Evaluation should include at least one validated measure of disease activity (i.e., Systemic Lupus Erythematosus Disease Activity Index).
- Vigilant monitoring of kidney function (i.e., every 3 months) in high-risk ethnicity, male sex, juvenile-onset, high serologic activity, positive anti-C1q antibodies (3)[C]
- Atherosclerotic cardiovascular disease (ASCVD)
  - Manage as per established guidelines.
  - Standard ASCVD risk calculators may underestimate risk in SLE—take into account SLE-specific factors (i.e., high disease activity, high doses of glucocorticoids, lupus nephritis, antiphospholipid antibodies).
- Osteoporosis
  - Adequate calcium/vitamin D intake, smoking cessation, weight-bearing exercise, limited alcohol intake
  - Long-term glucocorticoid use: clinical fracture risk assessment +/− bone mineral density measurement
  - 2017 ACR guideline for prevention and treatment
- Ophthalmologic evaluation with hydroxychloroquine (retinal damage) and/or glucocorticoids (cataracts, glaucoma)
- Malignancy: Follow routine cancer-screening guidelines for general population.
- Neuropsychiatric: Consider screening for mood disorders and cognitive impairment

DIET

Avoid alfalfa sprouts and echinacea D.

PATIENT EDUCATION

- Centers for Disease Control and Prevention: https://www.cdc.gov/lupus
- Lupus Foundation of America: https://www.lupus.org/

PROGNOSIS

Permanent, treatment-free remission is rare; 10-year survival ~90%; increased all-cause mortality in SLE compared to general population with standardized mortality ratio (SMR) of 2.6; despite advances in the treatment, SLE remains a chronic relapsing-remitting disease with variable prognosis.

COMPLICATIONS

Medication toxicity (including osteoporosis and osteonecrosis), obstetric complications, malignancy (especially hematologic, cervical, breast, lung), renal failure, cardiovascular and thromboembolic events, infections, and death

REFERENCES

1. Ameer MA, Chaudhry H, Mushtaq J, et al. An overview of systemic lupus erythematosus (SLE) pathogenesis, classification, and management. *Cureus*. 2022;14(10):e30330. doi:10.7759/cureus.30330.
2. Aringer M, Costenbader K, Daikh D, et al. 2019 European League Against Rheumatism/American College of Rheumatology classification criteria for systemic lupus erythematosus. *Arthritis Rheumatol*. 2019;71(9):1400–1412. doi:10.1002/art.40930.
3. Fanouriakis A, Kostopoulou M, Alunno A, et al. 2019 update of the EULAR recommendations for the management of systemic lupus erythematosus. *Ann Rheum Dis*. 2019;78(6):736–745. doi:10.1136/annrheumdis-2019-215089.
4. Furer V, Rondaan C, Heijstek MW, et al. 2019 update of EULAR recommendations for vaccination in adult patients with autoimmune inflammatory rheumatic diseases. *Ann Rheum Dis*. 2020;79(1):39–52. doi:10.1136/annrheumdis-2019-215882.

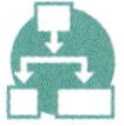

SEE ALSO

Antiphospholipid Antibody Syndrome

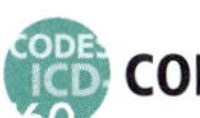

CODES

ICD10

- M32.0 Drug-induced systemic lupus erythematosus
- M32.14 Glomerular disease in systemic lupus erythematosus
- M32.19 Other organ or system involvement in systemic lupus erythematosus

CLINICAL PEARLS

- Multisystem disease, variable presentation—maintain high index of suspicion for diagnosis.
- Increased all-cause mortality, particularly with renal disease, infections, cardiovascular disease
- Low threshold for renal biopsy—lupus nephritis is a major risk factor for poor outcomes.
- Aggressiveness of therapy should reflect intensity of disease.

LUPUS NEPHRITIS

Neena R. Gupta, MD

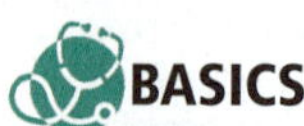

BASICS

DESCRIPTION

- Renal disease associated with systemic lupus erythematosus (SLE)
- A kidney biopsy is necessary to confirm the diagnosis (1).
- Clinical manifestations primarily due to immune complex–mediated glomerular disease; tubulointerstitial and vascular involvement often coexist. Diagnosis is based on clinical findings, urine abnormalities, autoantibodies, and renal biopsy.
- Treatment and prognosis depend on severity of disease
- Early diagnosis improves renal outcomes.

EPIDEMIOLOGY

- Peak incidence of SLE is 15 to 45 years of age. Mean age of diagnosis is between 25 and 30 years of age.
- The lifetime incidence of lupus nephritis (LN) in patients with SLE is 20–60%.
- Predominant sex: female > male (10:1)
- Once SLE develops, LN affects both genders equally; it is more severe in children and men and less severe in older adults.
- More common in African American and Asian populations.

Incidence

- SLE: 1 to 22/100,000
- Up to 60% of SLE patients develop LN over time; 25–50% of SLE patients have nephritis as the initial presentation.

Pediatric Considerations

LN is more common and more severe in children: 60–80% of children have LN at or soon after SLE onset.

Prevalence

SLE: 7 to 159/100,000

ETIOLOGY AND PATHOPHYSIOLOGY

- Immune complex–mediated inflammation injures glomeruli, tubules, interstitium, and vasculature.
- Glomeruli: Varying degrees of mesangial proliferation, crescent formation, and fibrinoid necrosis cause reduced glomerular filtration rate (GFR).
- Persistent inflammation (chronicity) leads to sclerosis and glomerular loss.
- Tubulointerstitial injury (edema, inflammatory cell infiltrate acutely; tubular atrophy in chronic phase) with or without tubular basement membrane immune complex deposition leads to reduced renal function.
- Vascular lesions: immune complex deposition and noninflammatory necrosis in arterioles
- SLE is a multifactorial disease, with multigenic inheritance; exact etiology remains unclear.
- Defective T-cell autoregulation and polyclonal B-cell hyperactivity contribute to dysregulated apoptosis. Impaired clearance of apoptotic cells inhibits self-tolerance to nuclear antigen.
- Anti-DNA, anti-C1q, anti–α-actin, and other nuclear component autoantibodies develop.
- Deposition of circulating immune complexes or autoantibodies attaching to local nuclear antigens leads to complement activation, inflammation, and tissue injury.
- Interaction of genetic, hormonal, and environmental factors leads to great variability in LN severity.

Genetics

- Polygenic inheritance; clustering in families, ~25% concordance in identical twins
- Interaction of general SLE susceptibility genes with more renal-specific genes and epigenetic changes

RISK FACTORS

Younger age, African American or Hispanic race, more ACR criteria for SLE, longer disease duration, hypertension, lower socioeconomic status, family history of SLE, anti-dsDNA antibodies, low albumin to globulin ratio

COMMONLY ASSOCIATED CONDITIONS

Other organ systems often involved in SLE.

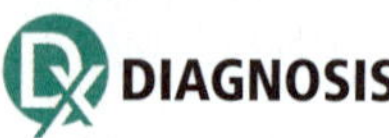

DIAGNOSIS

HISTORY

- Assess for signs/symptoms of SLE.
- Active nephritis is often accompanied by fever, peripheral edema, nausea, vomiting, headache and dizziness.

PHYSICAL EXAM

- Hypertension, fever
- Pleural/pericardial rub (serositis)
- Skin rash
- Edema
- Arthritis
- Alopecia
- Oral ulcers
- Signs of synovitis

DIFFERENTIAL DIAGNOSIS

- Primary glomerular disease
- Secondary renal involvement in other systemic disorders such as antineutrophil cytoplasmic antibody (ANCA)-associated vasculitis, Henoch-Schönlein purpura (HSP), antiglomerular basement membrane disease, polyarteritis nodosa, and viral infections

DIAGNOSTIC TESTS & INTERPRETATION

- Renal biopsy is the gold standard for diagnosing and classifying LN.
- Active urine sediment suggests nephritis with no attributable cause other than SLE.
- Autoantibodies, low C3, C4, and CH50 complement levels support LN.
- Emerging non-invasive biomarkers: Serum anti-C1q; Urinary neutrophil gelatinase-associated lipocalin (NGAL); monocyte chemoattractant protein 1 (MCP1); can be helpful in monitoring disease progression and response to treatment.

Initial Tests (lab, imaging)

Urinalysis (dipstick and sediment), spot urine protein to creatinine ratio, serum, creatinine, eGFR, serologic markers, anti-dsDNA, C3, C4, CH50 (1)

Follow-Up Tests & Special Considerations

- Monitor disease activity every 3 months (1): urinalysis for hematuria and proteinuria; blood for C3, C4, anti-dsDNA, serum albumin, and creatinine.
- Manage patients with estimated GFR (eGFR) of <60 mL as per National Kidney Foundation guidelines for chronic kidney disease (CKD): https://kdigo.org/guidelines/ckd-evaluation-and-management/.
- Biomarker panel: α_1-acid glycoprotein (AGP); ceruloplasmin; lipocalin-like prostaglandin synthase (LPGDS); transferring correlates with disease activity in children.

Pregnancy Considerations

- Pregnancy leads to worsening of renal function. Risk factors include renal impairment at baseline, active disease, hypertension, and proteinuria.
- Risk factors for fetal loss include elevated serum creatinine, heavy proteinuria, hypertension, and anticardiolipin antibodies.
- Renin-angiotensin system blockade and mycophenolate mofetil (MMF) are contraindicated in pregnancy; azathioprine can be used, U.S. FDA pregnancy Category D.

Test Interpretation

- On renal biopsy immunofluorescence microscopy: Immune complex deposits consisting of IgG, IgA, IgM, C1q, and C3 ("full house") are highly suggestive of LN.
- Revised ISN/RPS 2003 histologic classification guides therapeutic decisions: https://www.kidney-international.org/article/S0085-2538(15)52418-6/fulltext. Revised 2008 classification awaits endorsement.
- LN is classified as purely mesangial (class I-minimal mesangial LN and II-mesangial proliferative LN), focal proliferative LN: <50% glomeruli (class III), diffuse proliferative LN: ≥50% (class IV), membranous LN (class V), and advanced sclerosis LN (class VI); subdivisions for activity (A) and chronicity (C) in class III/IV and for segmental (S) or global (G) glomerular involvement in class IV (class III A, C, A/C and class IV S[A], G[A], S[A/C], S[C], G[C]); LN class may change with or without therapy.
- Focal and diffuse proliferative LN (classes III and IV) are common and most likely to progress to ESRD.

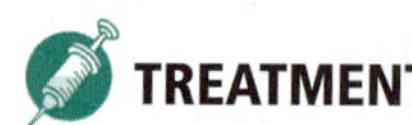

TREATMENT

GENERAL MEASURES

- Monitor bone density; optimize vitamin D and calcium intake, BMI, and regular exercise.
- Low-salt diet, blood pressure control, dyslipidemia management
- Avoid sun or ultraviolet light exposure, use broad-spectrum sunscreen.

MEDICATION

Note: Other than methylprednisolone, prednisone, and belimumab, no other medications listed below are FDA-approved for LN.

First Line

- Class I + II LN: no specific therapy; monitor urine protein-to-creatinine ratio (UPCR); renin-angiotensin system blockade (ACEI or ARB) to manage BP and proteinuria (e.g., lisinopril 5 to 40 mg/day PO, losartan 25 to 100 mg/day PO)
- Proliferative LN (class III or IV [±V])
- Principles of treatment:
  - Avoid delay; proteinuria reduction of at least 25% by 3 months, 50% by 6 months and UPCR target below 0.5 to 0.7 by 12 months
  - Patients with baseline nephrotic range proteinuria may need an additional 6 to 12 months.
- INDUCTION: steroids + immunosuppressive agent (for mild class III, high-dose steroids may be sufficient):
  - Glucocorticoids: methylprednisolone pulses, 0.25 to 0.50 g/day up to 3 days followed by oral prednisone 0.5 to 1.0 mg/kg/day with max of 80 mg for up to 2 weeks, tapered to <5 mg/day by week 25 (1) *and*
  - Cyclophosphamide: IV cyclophosphamide (low dose = 0.5 g every 2 weeks for total of 6 doses) (1) *or*
  - MMF: Target dose of 2 to 3 g/day for 6 months; MMF is as effective as cyclophosphamide in achieving remission with fewer side effects (1).
  - MMF (target dose 1 to 2 g/day) with calcineurin inhibitor (CNI) is an alternative to patients with nephrotic range proteinuria
  - High dose IV cyclophosphamide (0.50 to 0.75 g/m^2) monthly for 6 doses is an option for patients at high risk for kidney failure.
  - In Asian population, combination of tacrolimus, MMF, and glucocorticoids is found to be superior to cyclophosphamide and glucocorticoids.
- MAINTENANCE:
  - Glucocorticoids: low dose oral prednisone (2.5 to 5.0 mg/day) (1) *and*
  - MMF 1.5 to 2.0 g/day *or* azathioprine: 2 mg/kg/day PO if MMF is not tolerated (1)
  - Optimum duration is unclear but gradual withdrawal (glucocorticoids first) after at least 3 years therapy in complete clinical response (1).
- Pure class V LN: good prognosis, no standardized treatment
  - MMF (2 to 3 g/day) with IV methylprednisolone pulse (500 to 2,500 mg) followed by oral prednisone (20 mg/day tapered to ≤5 mg/day by 3 months) (1),(2)
  - Options for nephrotic range proteinuria patients include CNI (especially tacrolimus) or IV cyclophosphamide, either as monotherapy or in combination with MMF (1),(2).
- New guidelines include the use of voclosporin in combination with MMF and steroids for patients with active LN. 23.7 mg BID on an empty stomach (caution with reduced GFR).
- Belimumab (a B-cell activating factor inhibitor) in combination with standard initial and subsequent therapy as 10 mg/kg IV every 2 weeks for 3 doses followed by maintenance dosing every 4 weeks for total of 100 weeks has been shown to improve outcome.
- Hydroxychloroquine: all LN of any class unless contraindicated; maximum daily dose not to exceed 5 mg/kg/day and adjust for GFR with regular ophthalmologic follow-up

Second Line

Refractory LN: no response to initial treatment within 3 to 4 months; multitarget therapy recommended; change either cyclophosphamide to MMF or vice versa, rituximab, obinutuzumab; CNI (tacrolimus, voclosporin), belimumab, stem cell transplantation, IVIG, or plasma exchange (3)[C].

ISSUES FOR REFERRAL

Nephrology consults for initial management and relapses.

ADDITIONAL THERAPIES

- RAS blockade is beneficial because of antiproteinuric and antihypertensive effects.
- Vaccination review
- Treat hypertension, dyslipidemia, and other modifiable cardiovascular risk factors.
- Low-dose aspirin for high-risk aPL profile

SURGERY/OTHER PROCEDURES

- Renal transplant for ESRD when indicated
- Patient and graft survival rates similar to non-SLE patients
- Recurrent LN ranges between 0% and 30%; graft loss due to recurrence is rare.

ADMISSION, INPATIENT, AND NURSING CONSIDERATIONS

Admission criteria/initial stabilization

- Uncontrolled hypertension, acute kidney injury
- Severe extrarenal manifestation
- Nephrology input for management and renal biopsy

ONGOING CARE

FOLLOW-UP RECOMMENDATIONS

Patient Monitoring

- UPCR, urine microscopy, serum albumin, creatinine, antibody titers (especially anti-dsDNA), C3, C4, BP at least every 3 months for first 2 to 3 years followed by 6 to 12 months if no active disease
- CBC, LFT, and hydration per immunosuppressive regimen

DIET

Low-salt diet. For eGFR <60 mL: Follow National Kidney Foundation guidelines for CKD.

PATIENT EDUCATION

- Medication adherence and self-monitoring for relapse.
- Preconception counseling
- Smoking cessation

PROGNOSIS

- 10-year survival of 88% and 94% in SLE patients with and without renal involvement, respectively
- Relapse rate is ~35%; 10–20% of patients progress to ESRD within 10 years.
- 5-year renal survival of class IV LN <30% before 1970 has improved to >80% in last 2 decades.
- Remission of proteinuria is the best prognostic factor. Others include low baseline proteinuria, normal creatinine, white race, and treatment initiated within 3 months of diagnosis.
- Poor prognosis: crescentic diffuse proliferative LN, higher activity/chronicity index, APOL 1 risk alleles, African American race, lower socioeconomic status, poor response to treatment, high creatinine at baseline, uncontrolled hypertension, and relapse

COMPLICATIONS

- Risks of immunosuppressive therapy: infections, malignancy, GI upset, primary amenorrhea with cyclophosphamide, teratogenic effect of MMF
- Vascular thromboses with aPL antibodies
- About 10–20% of patients develop ESRD requiring dialysis/kidney transplantation.

REFERENCES

1. Kidney Disease: Improving Global Outcomes. KDIGO 2024 Clinical Practice Guideline for the Management of Lupus Nephritis. https://kdigo.org/wp-content/uploads/2024/01/KDIGO-2024-Lupus-Nephritis-Guideline.pdf. Accessed November 26, 2024.
2. Fanouriakis A, Kostopoulou M, Cheema K, et al. 2019 Update of the Joint European League Against Rheumatism and European Renal Association-European Dialysis and Transplant Association (EULAR/ERA-EDTA) recommendations for the management of lupus nephritis. *Ann Rheum Dis*. 2020;79(6):713–723.
3. Roveta A, Parodi EL, Brezzi B, et al. Lupus nephritis from pathogenesis to new therapies: an update. *Int J Mol Sci*. 2024;25(16):8981. doi:10.3390/ijms25168981.

ADDITIONAL READING

Alforaih N, Whittall-Garcia L, Touma Z. A review of lupus nephritis. *J Appl Lab Med*. 2022;7(6):1450–1467. doi:10.1093/jalm/jfac036.

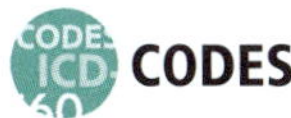

CODES

ICD10

M32.14 Glomerular disease in systemic lupus erythematosus

CLINICAL PEARLS

- Early diagnosis, correct classification (based on renal biopsy), and rapid treatment improve renal survival.
- Treat proliferative/progressive LN with a short induction course followed by maintenance therapy using glucocorticoids and immunosuppressants. There is an emerging role for biologics as well.
- Due to advances in diagnosis and treatment, survival rates for patients have improved dramatically over the past several decades.

L

LYME DISEASE

Mario P. DeMarco, MD, MPH

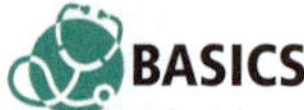

BASICS

Lyme disease is caused by the bacterium *Borrelia burgdorferi*.

DESCRIPTION

- An infection caused by *Borrelia* spirochetes, transmitted primarily by ixodid ticks
- *Ixodes scapularis* (deer ticks) in the Northeast and Great Lakes areas
- *Ixodes pacificus* in the West (black-legged ticks and Western black-legged ticks)

EPIDEMIOLOGY

In 2023, >89,000 cases of Lyme disease were reported to the Centers for Disease Control and Prevention. Approximately 476,000 people may get Lyme disease each year in the United States.

Incidence

High incidence U.S. states: Connecticut, Delaware, Maine, Maryland, Massachusetts, Minnesota, New Hampshire, New Jersey, New York, Pennsylvania, Rhode Island, Vermont, Virginia, West Virginia, and Wisconsin

Prevalence

Predominant age: most common in children aged 5 to 14 years and in adults aged 50 to 69 years

ETIOLOGY AND PATHOPHYSIOLOGY

- Average incubation period 7 to 10 days after tick bite
- Transmission is greatest in May to October with peak incidence in June and July.
- Climate change is contributing to expanded range for the vector and has potential to widen time window for transmission.
- If a tick is infected, the chance of transmission increases with time attached: 0% at 24 hours, 12% at 48 hours, 79% at 72 hours, and 94% at 96 hours of attachment.
- The primary animal reservoir is the white-footed mouse.
- Spirochetes multiply and spread within dermis, resulting in characteristic (erythema multiforme [EM]) rash. Hematogenous dissemination results in involvement of central nervous system (CNS), cardiovascular, or other organ stems.

Genetics

Human leukocyte antigen haplotype DR4 or DR2 increases susceptibility to prolonged arthritis.

RISK FACTORS

Lyme endemic area; ixodid ticks are common on deer; hunters, hikers, gardeners at increased risk

GENERAL PREVENTION

- Wear appropriate clothing when outdoors in endemic areas during times of high tick activity. Clothing should cover the ankles, and pretreat clothes, shoes, and tents with 0.5% permethrin.
- "Tick checks": Examine skin after outdoor activities.
- Remove ticks as soon as possible to limit transmission.
- To prevent of tick bites: *N,N*-diethyl-meta-toluamide (DEET), picaridin ethyl-3-(N-n-butyl-N-acetyl) aminopropionate (IR3535), oil of eucalyptus (OLE), p-menthane-3,8-diol (PMD), 2-undecanone
- Prophylactic treatment with 1 dose of 200 mg of doxycycline within 72 hours of a tick that has been attached for at least 36 hours is indicated in endemic areas; number needed to treat = 50

COMMONLY ASSOCIATED CONDITIONS

- Coinfection with other tick-borne illness (e.g., babesiosis, ehrlichiosis, anaplasmosis)
- Comorbid human granulocytic anaplasmosis and/or babesiosis in patients living in endemic regions

DIAGNOSIS

- Test with a sensitive enzyme immunoassay (EIA) or immunofluorescence assay, which quantifies antibodies against *B. burgdorferi*, and then follow this test with a Western immunoblot assay for specimens yielding either a positive or equivocal results in the EIA.
- Both the EIA test needs to be positive (or equivocal) and the Western blot needs to be positive (or in some cases equivocal) for the diagnosis of Lyme disease.
- Of note, antibodies can take from 2 to 6 weeks to develop, so if there is a high suspicion for Lyme disease, serum testing can be repeated several weeks following initial presentation.

HISTORY

- History of a tick bite followed by EM and/or illness (fever, fatigue, headache, myalgias)
- EM—round, flat or raised, erythematous bull's-eye lesion that expands in diameter over days to weeks that has an area of central clearing
  - Common sites: axilla, back, abdomen, groin, or popliteal fossa
  - 75–80% presenting with EM have a single lesion.
- Early Lyme disease: incubation period 3 to 30 days; patients may be asymptomatic; fever; headache; myalgias; arthralgias, regional lymphadenopathy
- Early disseminated Lyme disease:
  - Carditis: pleuritic chest pain, palpitations, light headaches, fainting, shortness of breath
  - Facial palsies or other cranial neuropathies
  - Joint pain (polyarthritis/polyarthralgia)
  - Late disease: monoarthritis, iritis, conjunctivitis, migratory musculoskeletal pain
- Late Lyme disease arises months after exposure.
  - Recurrent synovitis; recurrent tendonitis and bursitis
  - Encephalopathic symptoms: severe headaches and neck stiffness; confusion; facial palsy on one or both sides of the face
  - Peripheral nerve involvement: radiculoneuropathy, numbness, tingling, shooting pain/weakness in the arms or legs
  - Symptoms mimicking CNS diseases: multiple sclerosis–like symptoms; stroke-like symptoms; transverse myelitis

PHYSICAL EXAM

- Early Lyme disease:
  - EM in 70–80% of patients; expanding erythema arises 3 to 30 days, average is about 7 days, after tick detaches. Lesions are often >5 cm, flat or raised, may be homogeneous or have an area of central clearing (classic target session).
- Disseminated Lyme disease:
  - Skin: multiple EM lesions
  - Neurology: facial palsies (unilateral- or bilateral) or other cranial neuropathies
  - Cardiovascular: irregular pulse, bradycardia (heart block); friction rub (pericarditis)

DIFFERENTIAL DIAGNOSIS

- Other tick-borne illnesses: Rocky Mountain spotted fever (RMSF), ehrlichiosis, babesiosis, anaplasma, Southern tick–associated rash illness (STARI)
- Autoimmune process: juvenile rheumatoid arthritis (RA); systemic lupus erythematosus (SLE); RA
- Viral syndromes
- Contact dermatitis, cellulitis
- Granuloma annulare (mimic EM)
- Syphilis

DIAGNOSTIC TESTS & INTERPRETATION

- A tick bite is considered to be high risk only if the tick bite was from an identified *Ixodes* spp. vector species, it occurs in a highly endemic area, and the tick was attached for ≥36 hours (1)[A].
- Patients who have a typical EM lesion and who live in or have traveled to a Lyme-endemic area can be diagnosed with acute Lyme disease without laboratory testing.
- Serologic testing of patients presenting with EM lesions is not recommended due to insensitivity of serologic assays during the acute stage of infection.
- Health care providers should order Lyme testing only when there is existing clinical and epidemiologic support for diagnosis.

Initial Tests (lab, imaging)

- Potential tick exposure in a Lyme disease endemic area who have ≤1 skin lesions compatible with EM, recommended clinical diagnosis rather than laboratory testing
- Testing for IgM or IgG-class antibodies to *B. burgdorferi* solely by immunoblot, without a prior positive or equivocal first-tier immunoassay, is strongly discouraged due to an increase frequency of false-positive result.
- CDC recommends two-tier testing.
  - Tier 1 is an antibody screening assay.
  - Tier 2 is an immunoblot.
    - If the immunoassay(s) are negative, no further test is necessary.
    - If the immunoassays are positive or equivocal, reflex testing by immunoblot is required.
    - For patients with symptoms lasting ≤30 days, both IgM and IgG specific anti-*B. burgdorferi* immunoblots should be performed.
    - For patients with symptoms over 30 days, only anti-*B. burgdorferi* IgG immunoblot should be performed.
- Modified two-tiered Lyme disease serologic testing
  - Both tiers are immunoassays, done concurrently or sequentially.
  - Results are faster and simpler to interpret.

Follow-Up Tests & Special Considerations

- Arthritis: Serology + PCR of synovial fluid is both sensitive and specific.
- Neuroborreliosis: serology + CSF pleocytosis (PCR of CSF has a very low sensitivity.)

Diagnostic Procedures/Other

Synovial fluid when arthritis symptoms are present; lumbar puncture (CSF) when neurologic findings are present

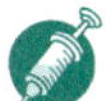

TREATMENT

Prophylactic antibiotic therapy should be given only to adults and children within 72 hours of removal of an identified high-risk tick bite—not for bites that are equivocal risk or low risk (1)[A]; doxycycline 200 mg PO for adults and 4.4 mg/kg up to 200 mg for children (1)[A]

MEDICATION

For people intolerant of amoxicillin, doxycycline, and cefuroxime, macrolides (azithromycin, clarithromycin, or erythromycin) may be used. Macrolides have lower efficacy, so patients treated with them should be monitored to ensure that symptoms resolve.

First Line

- Early Lyme disease (1)[A]: doxycycline 100 mg PO BID for 10 days (use with caution in children <8 years or in pregnant women); *or* amoxicillin 500 mg PO TID for 14 days (pediatric dose 50 mg/kg/day); *or* cefuroxime axetil 500 mg PO BID for 14 days; alternative: azithromycin 500 mg QD for 7 to 10 days or clarithromycin 500 mg BID for 14 to 21 days
- Early disseminated Lyme disease
  - Neurologic disease:
    - In patients aged ≤16 years with acute facial nerve palsy but without other evidence of Lyme disease, corticosteroid treatment should be administered within 72 hours. Treat with appropriate Lyme therapy.
    - Adults: doxycycline 100 mg PO for 14 to 21 days
    - Children: doxycycline 4.4 mg/kg/day divided into 2 doses; 14 to 21 days
    - Lyme meningitis or radiculoneuritis: adults doxycycline 200 mg PO divided into 1 or 2 doses for 14 to 21 days or ceftriaxone 2 g IV once a day for 14 to 21 days, or cefotaxime 2 g IV every 8 hours for 14 to 21 days
  - Cardiac disease:
    - Mild (asymptomatic, first-degree AV block, PR <300 ms): adults doxycycline 100 mg PO BID or amoxicillin 500 mg PO TID for 14 to 21 days; children: doxycycline 4.4 mg/kg/day PO, divided BID for 14 to 21 days or amoxicillin 50 mg/kg/day PO, divided TID for 14 to 21 days or cefuroxime 30 mg/kg/day PO, divided BID for 14 to 21 days
    - Severe (symptomatic, first-degree AV block with PR interval ≥300 ms, second- or third-degree AV block): adults: ceftriaxone 2 g IV QD for 14 to 21 days; children: ceftriaxone 50 to 75 mg/kg IV QD for 14 to 21 days
  - Arthritis:
    - Adults: doxycycline 100 mg BID PO for 28 days or amoxicillin 500 mg TID PO for 28 days or cefuroxime 500 mg BID PO for 28 days
    - Children ≥8 years old: doxycycline 4.4 mg/kg/day PO, divided BID for 28 days, or amoxicillin 50 mg/kg PO daily divided TID for 28 days or cefuroxime 30 mg/kg/day PO, divided BID for 28 days
    - Children <8 years old: amoxicillin 50 mg/kg/day PO for 28 days or cefuroxime 30 mg/kg/day PO, divided into 2 doses for 28 days
    - Parenteral treatment: adults: ceftriaxone 2 g IV QD for 14 to 28 days; children: ceftriaxone 50 to 75 mg/kg IV QD for 14 to 28 days
- Contraindications:
  - Allergies to specific medications
  - Doxycycline should be used with caution in children and in women who are pregnant or breastfeeding and can be avoided if other treatment options are available.
- Precautions:
  - In ~15% of patients treated with IV therapy, a Jarisch-Herxheimer–type reaction develops within 24 hours.
  - Significant interactions: oral anticoagulants and oral contraceptives

Pregnancy Considerations

Because *B. burgdorferi* can cross the placenta, pregnant patients with active disease should be treated with parenteral antibiotics.

SURGERY/OTHER PROCEDURES

Temporary pacemaker with carditis and high-grade heart block

ADMISSION, INPATIENT, AND NURSING CONSIDERATIONS

Admit patients with Lyme carditis and symptoms of chest pain, syncope, or dyspnea and those with second- or third-degree heart block or first-degree heart block of ≥300 ms or symptoms of meningitis.

ONGOING CARE

FOLLOW-UP RECOMMENDATIONS

Do not retest patient to determine whether antibody titers have declined after treatment because seroreactivity often persists for months after treatment of early infection and years after treatment of late infection.

PATIENT EDUCATION

- In endemic areas, protect against tick exposure. Avoid "painting" the tick with nail polish or petroleum jelly, or using heat, detach ticks from skin.
- Prevention: Use repellents that contain 20–30% DEET. Bathe as soon as possible after coming indoors (within 2 hours) and perform regular tick checks.

PROGNOSIS

Early treatment with antibiotics can shorten the duration of symptoms and prevent later disease. Late-stage disease response to treatment is variable. Symptoms may take weeks to resolve. Untreated rash usually resolves in 3 to 4 weeks. Excellent long-term prognosis with early antibiotics. Neurologic symptoms arise in about 15% of untreated Lyme disease patients.

COMPLICATIONS

- Posttreatment Lyme disease syndrome (PTLDS): pain, fatigue, or difficulty thinking that last for >6 months after they finish treatment; no proven treatment for PTLDS
- PTLDS: 10–20% lingering symptoms of fatigue, pain, or joint and muscle aches; can last for 6 months
- Lyme carditis >40% syncopal presentation

REFERENCES

1. Lantos PM, Rumbaugh J, Bockenstedt LK, et al. Clinical practice guidelines by the Infectious Diseases Society of America (IDSA), American Academy of Neurology (AAN), and American College of Rheumatology (ACR): 2020 guideline for the prevention, diagnosis, and treatment of Lyme disease. *Arthritis Care Res (Hoboken)*. 2021;73(1):1–9.

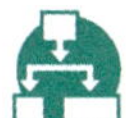

SEE ALSO

https://www.cdc.gov/lyme/index.html

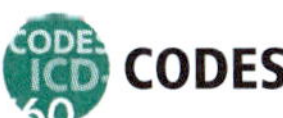

CODES

ICD10

- A69.20 Lyme disease, unspecified
- A69.2 Lyme disease

CLINICAL PEARLS

- Time of diagnosis and treatment varies by patient race with Black patients less likely to be diagnosed in the early stage and nearly 5 times the odds of disseminated disease at diagnosis compared to White patients.
- Steps to prevent Lyme disease include using insect repellent, removing ticks promptly, applying pesticides, and reducing tick habitat. There is no test that can "prove cure." Antibodies can persist long after the infection is gone.

L

LYMPHANGITIS

Kirby W. Curtis, DO • Grace H. Chiu, MD, FAAFP

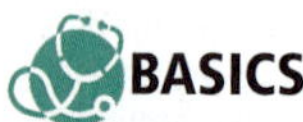

BASICS

DESCRIPTION

- Acute or chronic inflammation of lymphatic vessels that typically presents as red, tender streaks rapidly extending proximally to regional lymph nodes
- May be infectious or noninfectious; commonly occurs on an extremity due to skin infection
- Lymphatic filariasis (elephantiasis) most common cause worldwide; bacterial infection most common cause in North America

EPIDEMIOLOGY

Prevalence

~51 million cases of lymphatic filariasis worldwide each year

ETIOLOGY AND PATHOPHYSIOLOGY

- Acute infectious lymphangitis
  - Most commonly caused by skin breakdown with secondary infection, typically bacterial
  - *Streptococcus pyogenes* (group A β-hemolytic *Streptococcus*) most common cause in immunocompetent
  - Consider gram-negative bacteria or fungi in immunocompromised patients
  - Less commonly caused by: *Staphylococcus aureus, Pasteurella multocida* (cat, dog, or other animal bite), *Bartonella henselae* (cat bite, cat scratch disease), *Erysipelothrix* (fish exposure), *Spirillum minus* (rat bite disease), *Pseudomonas* spp., other *Streptococcus* spp., *Aeromonas hydrophila* (fresh water exposures), *Bacillus anthracis* (cutaneous anthrax), Parapoxvirus (occupational milker's nodule), herpes simplex virus (herpetic whitlow), *Chlamydia trachomatis* (lymphogranuloma venereum), *Rickettsia africae* and *Rickettsia sibirica* (spotted fever rickettsial infections)
- Chronic lymphangitis
  - Filarial lymphangitis-typically affects extremities but can result in genital lymphatic involvement
    - Lymphatic filariasis (elephantiasis) most common cause of lymphangitis worldwide
    - Inflammation of lymph vessels due to presence and death of parasite transmitted via mosquito bite
    - Usually caused by nematodes (helminth) *Wuchereria bancrofti*; less commonly, *Brugia malayi* and *Brugia timori*
    - Endemic areas: Asia, Africa, the Western Pacific, the Caribbean, and South America
  - Nodular lymphangitis
    - Also known as sporotrichoid lymphangitis or lymphocutaneous syndrome
    - Painful or painless nodular subcutaneous swellings along lymphatic vessels
    - Lesions may ulcerate with accompanying regional lymphadenopathy
    - Usually does not develop as rapidly as acute lymphangitis and may not present with systemic symptoms
    - Typical of infections from: *Sporothrix schenckii, Nocardia brasiliensis, Mycobacterium marinum, Leishmania* sp., *Francisella tularensis*, and systemic mycoses (coccidioidomycosis, blastomycosis, histoplasmosis)
    - Pathology may show granulomas.
  - Granulomatous intestinal lymphangitis: rare; associated with Crohn disease
  - Lymphangitis secondary to compromised lymphatic drainage
    - Following surgical procedures, trauma, malignancy, or radiation
    - Congenital or acquired anatomic abnormalities-elephantiasis nostras verrucosa (in setting of congestive heart failure and obesity)
  - Cutaneous lymphangitis carcinomatosa or neoplastic lymphangitis: rare presentation of skin metastasis—~5% of all skin metastases; caused by neoplastic occlusion of dermal lymphatic vessels
    - Associated cancers include breast (most common), lung, stomach, pancreas, and rectal.
- Acute noninfectious lymphangitis
  - Sclerosing lymphangitis of the penis: swelling around coronal sulcus of penis as a result of vigorous sexual activity or masturbation
  - Arthropod bites such as tick, mite, or spider

RISK FACTORS

- Skin infection—bacterial, viral, fungal
- Impaired lymphatic drainage
- Peripheral venous catheter; IV drug abuse
- Skin trauma including human, animal, insect, or spider bites
- Diabetes mellitus
- Immunocompromising condition
- Residence in filariasis endemic areas

GENERAL PREVENTION

- Proper wound and skin care
- Reduce chronic lymphedema with compression devices or by treating underlying processes
- Insect repellant; arthropod bite precautions
- Chemoprevention (albendazole, ivermectin, diethylcarbamazine citrate) in endemic areas for lymphatic filariasis

COMMONLY ASSOCIATED CONDITIONS

- Cellulitis, erysipelas
- Lymphedema
- Filarial infection (*W. bancrofti*)
- Prior lymph node dissection
- Tinea pedis (athlete's foot)
- Sporotrichosis

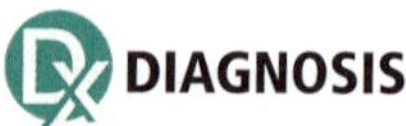

DIAGNOSIS

HISTORY

- Skin breakdown or trauma
- Erythematous streaks that can spread within a few hours
- Systemic symptoms: fever, chills, malaise, loss of appetite, headache, muscle aches
- Travel to filariasis endemic areas

PHYSICAL EXAM

- Erythematous, linear streaks from site of infection proximally toward regional lymph nodes
- Tenderness and warmth over affected skin and/or lymph nodes (lymphadenitis)
- Blistering of affected skin
- Fluctuance, swelling, or purulent drainage
- Nodular lymphangitis can present with subcutaneous swellings along the lymphatic channels
- Sporotrichosis may present with papulonodular lesions that may ulcerate
- Sites may be painless

DIFFERENTIAL DIAGNOSIS

- Superficial thrombophlebitis: thrombus or infection within the thrombosis (septic thrombophlebitis) (1)[C]
- Contact dermatitis
- Cellulitis
- Erysipelas
- Allergic reaction: less likely to be allergic if >24 hours after exposure (e.g., insect bite)

DIAGNOSTIC TESTS & INTERPRETATION

Initial Tests (lab, imaging)

- CBC may show leukocytosis
- Microbiologic investigations—identify potential underlying infectious agent to guide treatment
  - Swab, aspirate, and/or biopsy of primary site, nodule, or distal ulcer for histology and culture
  - Blood cultures if systemic symptoms present
  - Serology (*F. tularensis*, Histoplasma)
  - Blood smear (filaria)
  - FNAC for filariasis of testiculoscrotal swelling but not for other superficial locations

Follow-Up Tests & Special Considerations

Imaging: rarely used but can help in identifying anatomic abnormalities in lymphatic vessels—lymphangiography and lymphoscintigraphy

Diagnostic Procedures/Other

For challenging cases, dynamic contrast-enhanced MR lymphangiography (DCMRL) and central lymphangiography (CL) are available

TREATMENT

GENERAL MEASURES

- Hot, moist compresses to affected area
- Elevate affected extremity
- Compression devices and weight loss may help lymphedema.
- Abstinence from sexual activity for sclerosing lymphangitis

MEDICATION

- Treat common organisms empirically. Use culture and susceptibility to guide antibiotic treatment (1)[C].
- If mild disease, outpatient oral antibiotics
- If no improvement after 48 hours of oral antibiotics, reassess and consider IV antibiotics and/or hospitalization.
- IV antibiotics if systemically ill
- If necrotizing fasciitis is suspected, treat aggressively with IV antibiotics and surgical intervention.

First Line

- *Streptococcus pyogenes* (group A strep)
  - Amoxicillin—oral antibiotic therapy
    - Adults and children ≥40 kg: mild to moderate: 500 mg PO q12h; severe: 875 mg PO q12h or 500 mg PO q8h
    - Children <3 months: 30 mg/kg/day PO divided q12h
    - Children ≥3 months, ≤40 kg: mild to moderate: 25 mg/kg/day PO divided q12h or 20 mg/kg/day divided q8h; severe: 45 mg/kg/day PO divided q12h or 40 mg/kg/day divided q8h
    - Adverse effects:
      - Common: nausea, vomiting, diarrhea
      - Serious: anaphylaxis, Stevens-Johnson syndrome (SJS), toxic epidermal necrolysis (TEN)
    - Drug interactions: methotrexate, venlafaxine, warfarin, hormonal contraceptives
    - Contraindications: hypersensitivity to penicillin
  - Ampicillin/sulbactam-IV antibiotic therapy
    - Adults and children ≥40 kg: 1.5 to 3.0 g IV/IM q6h
    - Children <40 kg: 200 mg/kg/day IV infusion, in divided doses q6h; maximum 8 g ampicillin per day
    - Adverse effects:
      - Common: diarrhea, injection site pain and reactions
      - Serious: anaphylaxis, SJS, TEN, *Clostridium difficile* diarrhea, pseudomembranous enterocolitis
    - Drug interactions: hormonal contraceptives
    - Contraindications: hypersensitivity to penicillin
- Lymphatic filariasis: diethylcarbamazine, ivermectin, albendazole, and doxycycline
- Acetaminophen or ibuprofen (NSAIDs) for pain and fever

Second Line

- *Streptococcus pyogenes* (group A strep)
  - Oral therapy: cephalexin, macrolides for penicillin and cephalosporin allergic (azithromycin, clarithromycin, erythromycin), clindamycin (for penicillin allergic patients)
  - IV therapy: ceftriaxone, clindamycin (for penicillin allergic patients)
- *S. aureus*: consider risk for methicillin-resistant *S. aureus* (MRSA)
  - Oral therapy: amoxicillin, cephalexin, sulfamethoxazole-trimethoprim, doxycycline, clindamycin, linezolid
  - IV therapy: nafcillin, oxacillin, cefazolin, vancomycin, daptomycin, linezolid

SURGERY/OTHER PROCEDURES

- Incision and drainage (I&D) of abscess if present
- Necrotizing fasciitis requires surgical evaluation and likely débridement
- Nodular lymphangitis may benefit from I&D

ADMISSION, INPATIENT, AND NURSING CONSIDERATIONS

- Admit for signs of serious systemic illness (i.e., sepsis): fluids if in hypotensive shock
- IV antibiotics, ICU, or surgery as indicated
- Discharge on oral antibiotics after systemic symptoms resolve. Home IV antibiotics are an option depending on clinical setting.

ONGOING CARE

- Routine use of compression devices to reduce lymphedema
- Lymphedema physical therapy

FOLLOW-UP RECOMMENDATIONS

- Elevate affected area
- 48-hour follow-up to ensure improvement
- Work up recurrent lymphangitis to ascertain underlying cause (other infectious organism, anatomic abnormality, etc.)

Patient Monitoring

Close follow-up to ensure response to treatment and decreasing inflammation

PATIENT EDUCATION

- Instruct patients on proper wound and skin care
- Elevate affected extremity
- Use compression devices as recommended

PROGNOSIS

- Good prognosis for uncomplicated cases
- Antimicrobial therapy is effective in 90% of patients
- Untreated, can spread rapidly, especially group A *Streptococcus*

COMPLICATIONS

Sepsis, cellulitis, necrotizing fasciitis, myositis, lymphedema

REFERENCES

1. Kano Y, Momose T. Acute lymphangitis. *Cleve Clin J Med*. 2020;87(3):129–130.

ADDITIONAL READING

Benjamin J, O'Leary C, Hur S, et al. Imaging and interventions for lymphatic and lymphatic-related disorders. *Radiology*. 2023;307(3):e220231. doi:10.1148/radiol.220231.

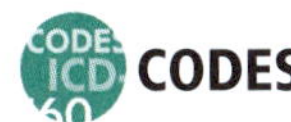

CODES

ICD10

- I89.1 Lymphangitis
- L03.91 Acute lymphangitis, unspecified
- N48.29 Other inflammatory disorders of penis

CLINICAL PEARLS

- Lymphangitis classically presents with erythematous linear streaks of the skin from site of entry (e.g., bite, cut, abrasion) proximally to regional lymph nodes.
- Patients with prior surgical lymph node dissection are predisposed to lymphangitis.
- Patients with severe systemic symptoms should be admitted for treatment with IV antibiotics.
- Parasitic or fungal infections can cause acute or chronic lymphangitis.
- Treatment of underlying skin infection (such as tinea pedis) may prevent recurrence.

LYMPHEDEMA

Erin W. DeLaney, MD • Matthew Delaney, MD

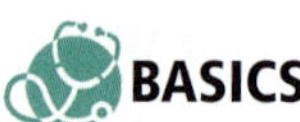

BASICS

DESCRIPTION

- Accumulation of lymphatic fluid in the interstitial tissue causing swelling
- Lymphedema can develop when lymphatic vessels are missing or impaired (primary) or when lymph vessels are damaged or lymph nodes are removed (secondary).
- Most commonly occurs in the lower limb(s) (80% of cases) but also can occur in the arm(s), face, trunk, and external genitalia

EPIDEMIOLOGY

Incidence

- More common in females than in males
- Commonly seen in patients with breast cancer:
  - Occurs in 13% of patients with breast cancer treated with surgery and 42% of those treated with surgery and radiation therapy
- Occurs in 25% of patients after gynecologic cancer surgery.

Prevalence

- 120 million people worldwide are affected with primary lymphatic filariasis.
- 10 million people are affected by nonfilarial secondary lymphedema in the United States.

ETIOLOGY AND PATHOPHYSIOLOGY

- Primary lymphedema results from inherited conditions affecting the lymph nodes or lymphatic vessels.
- Secondary lymphedema:
  - Postoperative: gradual failure of distal lymphatics, which have to "pump" lymph at a greater pressure through damaged proximal ducts; risk is higher with postoperative radiation because radiation reduces regrowth of ducts due to fibrous scarring.
  - Other causes include trauma, recurrent infection, malignancy (including metastatic disease), and marked obesity.
  - Most common cause in developing countries is filariasis (*Wuchereria bancrofti*).

Genetics

- Milroy disease is autosomal dominant and is diagnosed either at birth or within the 1st year of life.
- Lymphedema praecox has onset between the ages of 1 and 35 years.
- Lymphedema tarda occurs in those >35 years of age.
- Genetics referral is indicated with primary lymphedema and lymphedema tarda.

RISK FACTORS

- Filariasis: most common cause worldwide
- Lymphadenectomy or radiation therapy of lymph nodes, especially nodes of the underarm, groin, pelvis, and neck regions in cancer treatment (mastectomy, melanoma)
- Prior trauma, serious burns, infection of affected limb
- Obesity (body mass index: >50 kg/m^2)
- Inflammatory disorders: arthritis, sarcoidosis, dermatitis

GENERAL PREVENTION

Maintenance of healthy body weight, treatment of congestive heart failure, and early recognition of infection, cancer, and venous insufficiency

COMMONLY ASSOCIATED CONDITIONS

Venous disease, morbid obesity, regional cancer, filarial disease (Africa and Asia)

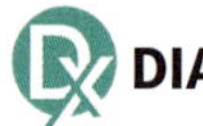

DIAGNOSIS

HISTORY

- First symptom is often painless swelling
- Feeling of heaviness in the limb, especially at the end of the day and in hot weather

PHYSICAL EXAM

- Initial: pitting edema, can spread proximally or distally
- Later: nonpitting; after 1st year, does not spread proximally/distally, but spreads radially
- Hyperkeratosis (thicker skin)
- Papillomatosis (rough skin)
- Increase in skin turgor
- Positive Stemmer sign (inability to pinch the skin of the dorsum of the second toe between the thumb and forefinger); false positives are rare.

DIFFERENTIAL DIAGNOSIS

- CHF, renal failure, lipedema
- Hypoalbuminemia, protein-losing nephropathy
- DVT, chronic venous disease
- Postoperative complications following ipsilateral surgery
- Cellulitis, Baker cyst, idiopathic edema

DIAGNOSTIC TESTS & INTERPRETATION

- Lack of response to elevation or diuretic therapy may indicate a lymphatic insufficiency.
- Diuretics increase excretion of salt and water, thereby decreasing plasma volume, venous capillary pressure, and filtration.
  - Diuretics improve filtration edema but do not improve lymph drainage over the long term.
- Some relevant protein biomarkers for lymphedema have been identified and show promise for early- and latent-stage diagnosis although routine lab testing is not necessary for the majority of patients

Initial Tests (lab, imaging)

- Comprehensive chemistry panel to evaluate for hepatic or renal impairment
- TSH to evaluate for hypothyroidism
- Urinalysis to evaluate for protein-losing nephropathy
- Ultrasound evaluates for acute/chronic DVT; also gives information about soft tissue changes but does not inform about truncal anatomy of the lymphatics

Follow-Up Tests & Special Considerations

- For most patients, a detailed history, physical and ultrasound are all the steps that are needed to confirm the diagnosis. There are several options for the subset of patients who may need additional imaging.
  - Lymphangiogram: direct cannulation of lymphatics through the skin; rarely used and has risk for infection and local inflammation
  - Fluorescence microlymphography may be highly sensitive (91.4%) and specific (85.7%), atraumatic, and is without radiation.
  - Lymphoscintigraphy: radiolabeled protein technetium-99m–labeled colloid
    - Measures lymphatic function, lymph movement, lymph drainage, and response to treatment
    - Sensitivity, 73–97%; specificity, 100%
    - Best to use 1 hour and delayed images together
  - Indocyanine green lymphography: reported
    - Superior to lymphoscintigraphy in early diagnosis of lymphedema of the arm
    - Accurately screens postsurgically for subclinical lymphedema (1)[B]
  - CT scan: calf skin thickening, thickening of the SC compartment, increased fat density, thickened perimuscular aponeurosis; typical honeycomb appearance
  - MRI: circumferential edema, increased volume of SC tissue, honeycomb pattern above the fascia between the muscle and subcutis; cannot differentiate primary from secondary lymphedema

Test Interpretation

Lymphedema stages:

- Stage 0: no swelling, but can feel that the affected area is heavy or full, or skin is tight
- Stage 1: has swelling of the affected area; will notice increase in size or stiffness of affected area; will notice swelling improves when affected area is raised
- Stage 2: more swelling than stage 1, which does NOT improve when affected area is elevated; will notice that affected area is hard and larger in size than stage 1
- Stage 3: increased swelling compared with stage 2; may be to the point that you cannot lift or move the arm or leg on your own; affected skin can become dry and thick. Fluid can leak from the skin, or blisters can form.

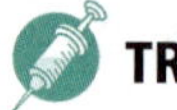

TREATMENT

GENERAL MEASURES

- Seek optimal weight; early treatment of cellulitis; avoid trauma to the affected area (direct injury, venipunctures, inept nail care, extreme heat/cold).
- Achieve mechanical reduction and maintenance of limb size: compression garments or compression pumps.
- Elevate affected limb/area, but avoid stasis.
- Avoid BP cuffs and other focal constriction in affected limbs.

- Prevent skin infection with daily cleansing, inspection, and skin care (with emollients).
- Nonsurgical treatment (compression therapy) of varicose veins
- Doubtful that air travel is associated with increased limb volumes

MEDICATION

ALERT

No medications, including diuretics, have been shown to be effective to treat lymphedema.

ISSUES FOR REFERRAL

- Refer to physical therapist with lymphedema training for manual decongestive therapy.
  - In patients with recurrent or metastatic disease, discuss with oncologist prior to initiation of complete decongestive therapy in order not to promote the spread of cancer.
- Provide education for patient/family for self-administration of therapy.
- Education for family about bandaging
- Fitting for compression garments (2)[A]

ADDITIONAL THERAPIES

- Exercise: Lymph flow occurs as a result of inspiratory reduction in the intrathoracic pressure associated with inspiration. The best results are achieved with combination of flexibility, strength, and aerobic training.
- Compression with custom-made elastic stocking (Minimum pressure is 40 mm Hg.)
  - Protection against external incidental trauma
  - Decreases the intrinsic trauma on the skin due to chronically increased interstitial pressures, which cause stretch of the skin and SC tissues
  - No data on preference of custom-made versus prefabricated
  - Replace every 3 to 6 months or when starting to lose elasticity.
- Multilayer bandaging: inner layer of tubular stockinette followed by foam and padding to protect the joint flexures and to even out the contours of the limb so that pressure is distributed evenly; outer layer of at least two short-stretch extensible bandages; more effective than hosiery alone
- From a resource utilization standpoint pneumatic devices may be preferable to bandages as they are reusable and can easily be applied by the patient.
  - Pneumatic pumps develop high pressures like systolic BP and can reduce limb girth significantly; wear a compression sock afterward (2)[A].
  - Advanced pneumatic compression devices (APCDs) are programmable, offer a more individualized fit, reduced rates of cellulitis by at least 75%, and reduce early treatment costs by 37–54% depending on health care setting (3)[B].

SURGERY/OTHER PROCEDURES

- Bypass procedures: Creation of lymphatic–venous anastomosis or lymph node transplantation (most effective) via microsurgery showed a reduction in use of conservative compression therapy (4)[C]; reserved for refractory cases only.
- Low-level laser therapy in smaller studies was shown to be noninferior to manual lymphatic drainage or in combination in arm volume reduction among breast cancer patients in half the treatment time (4)[C]. This treatment uses lasers to stimulate lymphatic vessel growth, improve lymph fluid flow, and repair skin damage.
- Thoracic sympathetic ganglion block for breast cancer–related lymphedema showed better life quality and arm size reduction >50%, especially in patients with high-grade lymphedema (5).
- Debulking procedures (Charles procedure): radical excision of SC tissue with primary or staged skin grafting
  - Men had less improvement than women.
  - Main risk is infection and necrosis of the skin graft.
  - Liposuction is cosmetically preferred to debulking (4)[C].

COMPLEMENTARY & ALTERNATIVE MEDICINE

Osteopathic manipulative treatment can be helpful in treatment of lymphedema by removing myofascial and skeletal restrictions to lymphatic flow and also by providing direct encouragement of lymphatic drainage.

ADMISSION, INPATIENT, AND NURSING CONSIDERATIONS

- Systemic signs of infection
  - May admit to specialized rehabilitation unit for combination treatment in patients with heart failure or severe pulmonary disease
  - IV antibiotics for infection; cellulitis is most common.
- Affected extremity positioning with some distal elevation
- Encourage patient mobilization/exercise.
- Patient education for bandaging/wound care
- Discharge criteria
  - Improved signs/symptoms of infection (e.g., elevated WBC count, fever, abnormal vital signs)
  - Clinical improvement in wound appearance

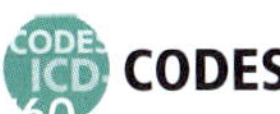

ONGOING CARE

FOLLOW-UP RECOMMENDATIONS

Lymphedema will return in several days if patient stops wearing compression garments during the day and bandaging at night.

Patient Monitoring

- Daily visit to therapist for acute treatment
- Monthly visits for maintenance care

DIET

Lower sodium, healthy protein, and weight loss-oriented (if needed)

PATIENT EDUCATION

- Use compression garments, especially when exercising.
- Avoid affected limb(s) being dependent for long period of time: Patient should perform daily skin examination.
- National Library of Medicine: https://medlineplus.gov/lymphaticdiseases.html

PROGNOSIS

No cure but treatment can produce good results with daily care

COMPLICATIONS

- Infection (local vs. systemic): common
- Risk of wound formation (punctures/abrasions) that are difficult to heal: common
- Lymphangiosarcoma: found in lymphedematous arms of patients following radical mastectomy, also in patients with Milroy disease; treatment is radiotherapy with surgery; reserved for patients with discrete nonmetastatic disease.

REFERENCES

1. Keo HH, Husmann M, Groechenig E, et al. Diagnostic accuracy of fluorescence microlymphography for detecting limb lymphedema. *Eur J Vasc Endovasc Surg*. 2015;49(4):474–479.
2. Rogan S, Taeymans J, Luginbuehl H, et al. Therapy modalities to reduce lymphoedema in female breast cancer patients: a systematic review and meta-analysis. *Breast Cancer Res Treat*. 2016;159(1):1–14.
3. Karaca-Mandic P, Hirsch AT, Rockson SG, et al. The cutaneous, net clinical, and health economic benefits of advanced pneumatic compression devices in patients with lymphedema. *JAMA Dermatol*. 2015;151(11):1187–1193.
4. Merchant SJ, Chen SL. Prevention and management of lymphedema after breast cancer treatment. *Breast J*. 2015;21(3):276–284.
5. Choi E, Nahm FS, Lee PB. Sympathetic block as a new treatment for lymphedema. *Pain Physician*. 2015;18(4):365–372.

CODES

ICD10

- I89.0 Lymphedema, not elsewhere classified
- I97.2 Postmastectomy lymphedema syndrome
- Q82.0 Hereditary lymphedema

CLINICAL PEARLS

- Affected skin has a heavy feeling, with painless swelling initially, later nonpitting swelling.
- No medications, including diuretics, are useful.
- Rule out DVT if unilateral limb affected or CHF if bilateral.
- Early referral to lymphedema therapist for manual therapy and placement of compression devices/wrappings
- Aggressive weight loss and health promotion as needed
- High risk for cutaneous-sourced infections, so promote therapeutic skin care
- Lymphoscintigraphy is standard diagnostic measure if clinical diagnosis is uncertain.
- Refer primary lymphedema and lymphedema tarda to genetics.

MACULAR DEGENERATION, AGE-RELATED

Jennifer Bustamante, DO • Chanel M. Lear, DO, MBS

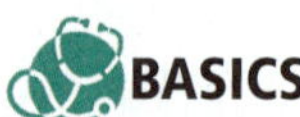

BASICS

DESCRIPTION

- Age-related macular degeneration (AMD) is a progressive eye disease that damages the macula, the part of the retina responsible for sharp central vision.
- AMD is the leading cause of central vision loss in older adults worldwide.
- Classified as:
  - "Dry"/nonexudative or atrophic/geographic atrophy, such as drusen or macular pigmentary changes
  - "Wet"/exudative or neovascular AMD (nAMD)

EPIDEMIOLOGY

- nAMD form is more common in white people.
- Predominant sex: female

Prevalence

- 6–9% of global legal blindness
- Worldwide, AMD cases are projected to rise from 196 million in 2020 to 288 million by 2040.
- People 65 to 74 years old: 11%
- People ≥75 years old: 27.9%

ETIOLOGY AND PATHOPHYSIOLOGY

- Atrophic/nonexudative
  - Drusen and/or pigmentary changes in the macula is "hallmark." Drusen are deposits of hyaline material between the retinal pigment epithelium (RPE) (a pigment layer underneath the retina that normally helps remove metabolic by-products from the retina) and Bruch membrane (the limiting membrane between the RPE and the choroid).
  - Visible light can result in the formation and accumulation of metabolic by-products in the RPE, a pigment layer underneath the retina that normally helps remove metabolic by-products from the retina. Excess accumulation of these metabolic by-products interferes with the normal metabolic activity of the RPE and can lead to the formation of drusen.
  - Drusen enlargement and pigmentary changes mark progression from early to intermediate AMD.
  - Aging leads to vessel resistance, choriocapillaris thinning, lipid accumulation, and reduced photoreceptors.
- nAMD
  - nAMD generally arises from the atrophic stage.
    - Type 1 neovascularization (occult choroidal neovascular membrane [CNVM]): CNVM grows into the sub-RPE space through breaks in Bruch membrane, causing serous or fibrovascular RPE detachment.
    - Type 2 (classic CNVM): CNVM penetrates the RPE into the subretinal space; appears as lacy gray-green lesions
    - Type 3 (retinal angiomatous proliferation): originates from retinal deep capillary plexus, growing downward toward the RPE
    - Polypoidal choroidal vasculopathy (PCV): subtype of nAMD with recurrent serosanguineous pigment epithelial detachment (PED); optical coherence tomography (OCT) shows multiple, sharply peaked or notched PED with hyperreflective ring and hyporeflective lumen.

Genetics

Complement factor H (CFH) on chromosome 1q32 and ARMS2/HTRA1 region on chromosome 10q26 are important susceptibility genes for AMD.

RISK FACTORS

- Advanced age
- Obesity
- Hypertension
- Hyperlipidemia
- Cigarette smoking
- *Chlamydia pneumoniae* infection
- Family history
- Excess sunlight exposure
- Blue or light iris color
- Hyperopia
- Short stature
- Chronic Inflammation

GENERAL PREVENTION

- Antioxidants, zinc, omega-3 and omega-6 fatty acids
- Ultraviolet (UV) protection for eyes
- Routine ophthalmologic visits

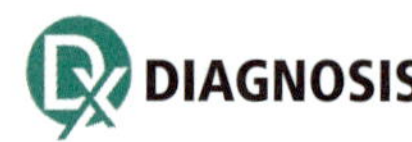

DIAGNOSIS

HISTORY

- Primary visual symptoms (e.g., blurred vision, metamorphopsia, difficulty reading, loss of central vision, difficulty in low light)
- Associated symptoms: photopsia, scotomas, and visual field loss

PHYSICAL EXAM

- Best corrected visual acuity testing (Snellen or Early Treatment Diabetic Retinopathy Study chart)
- On Amsler grid testing, the horizontal or vertical lines may become broken, distorted, or missing.
- Atrophic/nonexudative stage: drusen (small yellowish white lesions)
- nAMD
  - Blood vessels growing underneath the retina from the choroid are called CNVMs or subretinal neovascularization (SRN). The choroid is the vascular layer underneath the RPE.
  - Subretinal fluid or hemorrhage, exudates
- Disciform scar: an advanced stage resulting in a fibrovascular scar

DIFFERENTIAL DIAGNOSIS

- Diabetic macular edema
- Hypertensive retinopathy
- Central retinal artery occlusion
- Topiramate can cause a macular neurosensory retinal detachment.
- Pentosan polysulfate sodium, which is FDA approved for the treatment of interstitial cystitis, may be associated with the development of a pigmentary maculopathy.

DIAGNOSTIC TESTS & INTERPRETATION

Diagnostic Procedures/Other

- Biomicroscopy of the ocular fundus through a dilated pupil with a slit lamp
- Color fundus photography for documentation
- Fundus autofluorescence for geographic atrophy assessment
- Fundus fluorescein angiography (FFA): differentiates between atrophic and nARMD; gold standard
- Indocyanine green video angiography: may identify occult or hidden CNVMs
- OCT is the primary imaging tool for AMD, detecting subretinal fluid, retinal thickening, and PED. Advanced modalities like SD-OCT, SS-OCT, and OCTA offer improved evaluation of AMD.
- Near-infrared imaging
- Adaptive optics

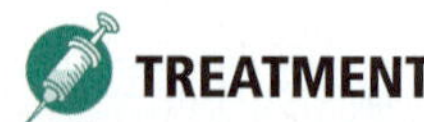

TREATMENT

GENERAL MEASURES

Low-vision aids may be helpful.

MEDICATION

First Line

- Nonneovascular (dry) AMD
  - Lifestyle changes and daily AREDS2 supplements (vitamins C, E, zinc, copper, lutein, zeaxanthin) to slow progression; smoking cessation, blood pressure control, and a healthy diet are essential. Complement inhibitors may benefit select patients with geographic atrophy.
- Neovascular (wet) AMD
  - Ranibizumab (Lucentis)
    - A recombinant, humanized monoclonal antibody that inhibits all active forms of vascular endothelial growth factor (VEGF)
    - Administered via intravitreal injection at a dose of 0.5 mg every 4 weeks
    - After 1 year of treatment, up to 40% of patients gained ≥3 lines, and approximately 95% maintained vision.
    - The PrONTO study showed that an OCT-guided variable-dosing regimen achieved outcomes comparable to monthly dosing in the MARINA and ANCHOR trials.
    - In a multicenter comparison, ranibizumab and bevacizumab both effectively stabilized vision, with no significant difference in visual outcomes.
    - The 2-year CATT study found that fixed-interval dosing produced slightly better visual outcomes than as-needed (PRN) dosing.
  - Aflibercept (Eylea)
    - A VEGF trap fusion protein that binds both VEGF-A and placental-like growth factor
    - Injected intravitreally, at a dose of 2 mg, every 4 weeks for 12 weeks and then every 8 weeks
    - Dosed as needed after the 12-week fixed dosing schedule resulted in a 5.3-letter gain in best corrected visual acuity at 52 weeks.
    - May be beneficial in patients who are not responding to ranibizumab or bevacizumab
    - Anti-VEGF treatment with either ranibizumab or aflibercept has limited efficacy for the complete resolution of PEDs.
      - Patients with a PED tend to have worse outcomes when switched from a fixed regimen to a PRN strategy.

- Brolucizumab (Beovu)
  - It is a humanized single-chain antibody fragment that inhibits all isoforms of VEGF-A. It is the smallest of the anti-VEGF antibodies.
  - Injected intravitreally, at a dose of 6 mg monthly for the first 3 doses, followed by one dose every 8 to 12 weeks
  - A 12-week treatment cycle may be a viable option, which would help reduce the frequency of IVIs. Greater than 50% of brolucizumab treated eyes were maintained on every 12 weeks of dosing.
  - There have been some reports of retinal vasculitis and/or retinal vascular occlusion after Beovu was approved by the FDA. There have been cases reported with severe visual loss with brolucizumab treatment.
- Faricimab (Vabysmo) neutralizes angiopoietin-2 and VEGF-A. It has the potential advantage of being administered every 16 weeks. It has recently been approved by the FDA for the treatment of nAMD.
  - 6 mg injected intravitreally, every 4 weeks for the first 4 doses. Then based on clinical outcomes, patients may receive subsequent treatments every 2, 3, or 4 months. Faricimab was noninferior to aflibercept (1)[A].

Second Line

- Nonneovascular (dry) AMD
  - Recently approved therapies include complement cascade inhibitors.
  - Complement is believed to play an important role in retinal degeneration secondary to AMD.
  - Pegcetacoplan (C3 inhibitor) and avacincaptad pegol (C5 inhibitor)
  - These injectable drugs can slow the progression of geographic atrophy by up to 20%, but do not restore lost vision.
- Neovascular (wet) AMD
  - Bevacizumab (Avastin) is a full-length antibody to VEGF, administered intravitreally at a dose of 1.25 mg; widely used off-label because of its lower cost

SURGERY/OTHER PROCEDURES

- Laser treatment for CNVMs located ≥200 microns from the center of the macula has been evaluated in the Macular Photocoagulation Study (MPS). Anti-VEGF treatment is the first-line therapy for subfoveal CNVMs.
- Vitrectomy has been used to remove CNVMs, but this is generally not recommended.
- CNVMs can cause subretinal hemorrhage. Vitrectomy within 7 days may help. Tissue plasminogen activator (tPA) can assist in clot removal, and intravitreal gas (with or without tPA) may displace submacular blood.
  - Intravitreal anti-VEGF monotherapy may be helpful in the treatment of nAMD associated with a submacular hemorrhage.
- Photodynamic therapy (PDT) with verteporfin is not frequently used anymore.
  - Patients should be informed of a <4% risk of acute, severe vision loss after PDT.
  - Ranibizumab has greater clinical efficacy than PDT.
  - Combination treatment with intravitreal ranibizumab and PDT appears to offer similar gain in visual acuity when compared with ranibizumab monotherapy.

COMPLEMENTARY & ALTERNATIVE MEDICINE

The Age-Related Eye Disease Study (AREDS) found that a high-dose regimen of antioxidant vitamins and mineral supplements reduced progression of AMD in some cases.

- The AREDS2 found the addition of lutein with zeaxanthin alone or in combination with omega-3 fatty acids had no overall effect in further reducing the risk of progression to advanced AMD. The recommended daily doses: vitamin C 500 mg, vitamin E 400 IU, lutein 10 mg, zeaxanthin 2 mg, zinc 80 mg. Original formulation included β-carotene, but it was removed from the AREDS2 due to increased risk of lung cancer in smokers.
- Dietary supplements are not universally approved; not recommended for AMD prophylaxis

ONGOING CARE

DIET

- Eating dark green, leafy vegetables (spinach/collard greens), which are rich in carotenoids, may decrease the risk of developing the nAMD.
- Fish consumption with omega-3 fatty acid intake may reduce the risk of AMD.
- A Mediterranean-type diet may reduce the risk of developing AMD (2)[A].

PROGNOSIS

- Patients with bilateral soft drusen and pigmentary changes in the macula, but no evidence of exudation, have an increased likelihood of developing nAMD and subsequent visual loss.
- Patients with bilateral drusen carry a cumulative risk of 14.7% over 5 years of suffering significant visual loss in one eye from nAMD.
- Patients with nAMD in one eye and drusen in the opposite eye are at an annual risk of 5–14% for developing nAMD in the opposite eye with drusen.
- Patients with nAMD with stable preoperative fluid on OCT generally do not have worsening of their nAMD after cataract surgery.
- Aspirin use is not significantly associated with progression to late AMD. When aspirin is medically indicated, patients with ARMD do not need to avoid taking it.
- Anti-VEGF treatment for nAMD was associated with preserved useful vision in almost 20% of patients over their average remaining lifetime (3)[B].

COMPLICATIONS

- Blindness
- The intraocular pressure should be monitored in eyes receiving intravitreal anti-VEGF injections.

REFERENCES

1. Heier JS, Khanani AM, Quezada Ruiz C, et al. Efficacy, durability, and safety of intravitreal faricimab up to every 16 weeks for neovascular age-related macular degeneration (TENAYA and LUCERNE): two randomised, double-masked, phase 3, non-inferiority trials. *Lancet*. 2022;399(10326):729–740. doi:10.1016/S0140-6736(22)00010-1.
2. Keenan TD, Agrón E, Mares J, et al. Adherence to the Mediterranean diet and progression to late age-related macular degeneration in the Age-Related Eye Disease Studies 1 and 2. *Ophthalmology*. 2020;127(11):1515–1528.
3. Finger RP, Puth M-T, Schmid M, et al. Lifetime outcomes of anti-vascular endothelial growth factor treatment for neovascular age-related macular degeneration. *JAMA Ophthalmol*. 2020;138(12):1234–1240.

ADDITIONAL READING

- Fleckenstein M, Schmitz-Valckenberg S, Chakravarthy U. Age-related macular degeneration: a review. *JAMA*. 2024;331(2):147–157.
- Thomas CJ, Mirza RG, Gill MK. Age-related macular degeneration. *Med Clin North Am*. 2021;105(3):473–491. doi:10.1016/j.mcna.2021.01.003.

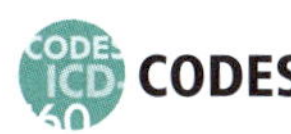

CODES

ICD10

- H35.32 Exudative age-related macular degeneration
- H35.31 Nonexudative age-related macular degeneration
- H35.3290 Exudative age-related macular degeneration, unspecified eye, stage unspecified

CLINICAL PEARLS

- Patients may notice straight lines appear crooked (e.g., telephone poles).
- The AREDS found that a high-dose regimen of antioxidant vitamins and mineral supplements reduces progression of AMD in some cases.
- Adults >55 years old should undergo a dilated funduscopic exam to screen for AMD.

M

MARFAN SYNDROME

Karl T. Clebak, MD, MHA, FAAFP • Makayla B. Lagerman, MD

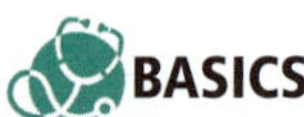

BASICS

DESCRIPTION

- Marfan syndrome (MFS) is an inherited disorder of connective tissue.
- Because many features of MFS appear in the general population, diagnostic criteria (Ghent nosology) are useful for diagnosis including features with major and minor criteria (1).
- System(s) affected: musculoskeletal, cardiovascular, ocular, pulmonary, skin/integument, connective tissue (dura)

Pediatric Considerations

Early surgical intervention may reduce the degree of scoliosis. Pectus excavatum deformities can worsen during adolescent growth and may require surgical evaluation for symptomatic or cosmetic concerns.

Pregnancy Considerations

- Consider pregnancy in MFS high risk and consult with a cardiologist; screening transthoracic echocardiogram with serial monitoring.
- Consider β-blockers in all pregnancies to minimize risk of aortic dilation.
- Consider elective surgery before pregnancy if aortic root diameter is >47 mm.
  - Type A aortic dissection may require urgent surgical repair; Type B aortic dissection may require medical management over surgical intervention, but treatment should be individualized.
  - Prepartum aortic root diameter 40 to 45 mm may remain stable during pregnancy (2).
- Avoid spinal anesthesia due to risk of dural ectasia.

EPIDEMIOLOGY

- Congenital; although clinical manifestations may be apparent in infancy, affected individuals may not present until adolescence or young adulthood.
- No gender, ethnic, or racial predilection; with advanced paternal age, a slightly increased risk of de novo mutation resulting in MFS in offspring

Incidence

1/5,000 to 1/10,000 live births

ETIOLOGY AND PATHOPHYSIOLOGY

Genetic abnormality; mutations of the fibrillin-1 (*FBN1*) gene

Genetics

- MFS is an autosomal dominant condition with complete penetrance and variable expressivity.
- *FBN1* mutations have been identified in 92% of patients with MFS.
- Each child of an affected parent has a 50% chance of inheriting MFS and may be more or less severely affected. 25% of cases result from de novo mutation, most of which result from de novo *FBN1* mutation.

RISK FACTORS

Hypertension and increased BMI may increase risk of acute aortic dissection.

GENERAL PREVENTION

Prenatal diagnosis in families with a known mutation

COMMONLY ASSOCIATED CONDITIONS

- Ligamentous laxity, crowded teeth, cataracts, glaucoma, mitral valve prolapse (MVP), aortic regurgitation, and palpitations
- High prevalence of migraines, obstructive sleep apnea in MFS; may be a risk factor for aortic root dilatation.

DIAGNOSIS

- In the revised Ghent (Ghent II) nosology: Diagnosis is made in a person without known family history of MFS, who has at least one of the following:
  - An *FBN1* pathogenic variant known to be associated with MFS and aortic root enlargement (Ao) (Z-score ≥2) or ectopia lentis (EL) *Z*-score calculator for aortic root enlargement: http://www.marfan.org/
  - Demonstration of Ao (Z-score ≥2) and EL or a defined combination of features yielding a systemic score ≥7
- Systemic features, scoring system (see "Physical Exam"):
  - Wrist *and* thumb sign +3; wrist *or* thumb sign +1
  - Pectus carinatum deformity +2; pectus excavatum or chest asymmetry +1
  - Hindfoot deformity +2; pes planus +1
  - Pneumothorax +2; dural ectasia +2
  - Protrusio acetabuli +2 by x-ray, CT, or MRI; reduced elbow extension +1
  - Reduced upper-to-lower segment (US/LS) ratio *and* increased arm/height *and* no severe scoliosis +1
  - Scoliosis or thoracolumbar kyphosis +1
  - Facial features (3/5) +1; myopia >3 diopters +1
  - Skin striae +1
  - MVP (all types) +1
- Maximum: 20 points; score ≥7 indicates systemic involvement. In adults with suggestive findings but who do not meet Ghent criteria, consider alternative diagnoses: EL syndrome, MVP syndrome, MASS (**M**VP, **A**ortic dilation, **S**kin, and **S**keletal) phenotype, nonspecific connective tissue disorder. In potential MFS diagnoses, close follow-up is recommended.

PHYSICAL EXAM

- Facial features: dolichocephaly (head length longer than expected compared with width), enophthalmos, down-slanting palpebral fissures, malar hypoplasia, micrognathia; high-arched, narrow palate
- Thumb sign: Distal phalanx of thumb protrudes from clenched fist. Wrist sign: Thumb and 5th digit overlap when circling wrist.
- Pectus carinatum deformity: pectus excavatum or chest asymmetry beyond normal variation.
- Hindfoot valgus with forefoot abduction and lowering of the midfoot
- Height may be normal or may be ≥3.3 *SD* > mean. Increased arm span to height ratio >1.05.
- Reduced US/LS ratio: US is measured from the top of the head to the top of the midpubic bone; LS is measured from the top of the pubic bone to the sole of the foot.
- Scoliosis or thoracolumbar kyphosis is diagnosed if, on bending forward, there is a vertical difference ≥1.5 cm between the ribs of the left and right hemithorax.
- Reduced elbow extension if angle between upper and lower arm measures ≤170 degrees on full extension
- Skin: Striae atrophicae are significant if not associated with significant weight changes (or pregnancy) and if located on mid-back, lumbar region, upper arm, axilla, or thigh.
- Joint hypermobility, high-arched palate, and recurrent or incisional herniae were removed from diagnostic criteria (1).

DIFFERENTIAL DIAGNOSIS

Clinical manifestations overlapping with MFS in cardiovascular, ocular, and skeletal systems:

- EL syndrome: no aortic root dilatation
- MVP syndrome: Limited systemic features may include pectus excavatum, scoliosis, mild arachnodactyly; aortic enlargement and EL preclude this diagnosis.
- MASS phenotype (also *FBN1* mutation): MVP; myopia; borderline, nonprogressive aortic enlargement, nonspecific *s*keletal and *s*kin involvement; aortic involvement is usually nonprogressive; some risk for more severe vascular involvement; may be impossible to differentiate from MFS before age 20 years
- Shprintzen-Goldberg, Loeys-Dietz, Ehlers-Danlos, and Stickler syndrome; congenital contractural arachnodactyly; Weill-Marchesani syndrome, multiple endocrine neoplasia type 2B, fragile X syndrome
- Homocystinuria: marfanoid habitus, thrombosis, mental retardation; urine amino acid analysis is diagnostic; lens dislocates downward
- Familial thoracic aortic aneurysm
- Aortopathy next generation sequencing (NGS) panel is likely to play a more prominent role, especially as variant of unknown significance (VUS) are classified

DIAGNOSTIC TESTS & INTERPRETATION

- Sequencing of *FBN1* is the preferred method for molecular diagnosis. Mutations are found in 95% of patients meeting diagnostic criteria for MFS (1).
- Echocardiography: Measure aortic root at the level of sinuses of Valsalva; check for MVP. Consider CT or MRI to confirm accuracy of echocardiogram.
- Urinary homocysteine to rule out homocystinuria
- Anteroposterior (AP) radiograph: protrusio acetabuli
- Scoliosis: Cobb angle ≥20 degrees on radiographs
- Hindfoot valgus with forefoot abduction and lowering of the midfoot: anterior and posterior views
- MRI or CT to evaluate for dural ectasia if symptomatic (symptoms highly variable, nonspecific, and include lower back pain)

Diagnostic Procedures/Other

- EL is diagnosed on slit-lamp examination after maximal dilatation of the pupil (60%); lens dislocation is most often upward and temporal.
- Myopia: >3 diopters contributes to MFS systemic score.

Test Interpretation

- Cystic medial necrosis of the aorta: descriptive, not pathognomonic
- Myxomatous degeneration of cardiac valves

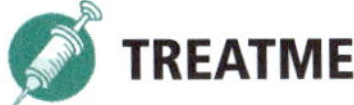

TREATMENT

MEDICATION

- Prevention of aortic complications: β-blockers; dosage is adjusted to target heart rate (resting heart rate is rate 60 beats/min, <100 beats/min after submaximal exercise) (1)[C].
- The evidence for β-blocker therapy to reduce morbidity and mortality in MFS is limited to a single, small, prospective randomized, and nonblinded clinical trial.
- If β-blockers contraindicated: ARBs may slow aortic dilation in children and adolescents.
- Losartan plus β-blockers has been suggested to prevent progressive aortic root dilatation, but clinical trials needed to assess improved outcomes with medication.
- Preliminary evidence suggests calcium channel blockers may increase risk of aortic complications.
- Genetic and molecular factors are likely to influence drug effects but remain unknown. Medical treatment should be individualized, with careful monitoring.

ISSUES FOR REFERRAL

Multidisciplinary management: clinical geneticist, cardiologist, ophthalmologist, orthopedist, cardiothoracic surgeon, pediatric surgery (pectus carinatum deformities)

SURGERY/OTHER PROCEDURES

- When cardiac symptoms develop or aortic root diameter is ≥5 cm, consider surgical intervention. Many patients will ultimately require cardiovascular surgery:
  - Dissection of ascending aorta (type A) is a surgical emergency. Consider prophylactic surgery when diameter of sinus of Valsalva approaches 5 cm, rate of change approaches 1 cm/year, and with progressive aortic regurgitation; other risk factors: family history, other cardiac pathology, pregnancy
  - Dissection of descending thoracic aorta (type B): Surgical indications include intractable pain, limb or organ ischemia, and aortic diameter >5.5 cm (or rapidly increasing) (1).
- Mitral valve repair: for severe mitral valve regurgitation or progressive LV dilatation or dysfunction, or in patients undergoing valve-sparing root replacement (1)
- Lens subluxation: Incidence of glaucoma is high; surgery is performed only if untreatable with corrective lenses; surgical removal of lens for opacity, impending complete luxation, lens-induced glaucoma or uveitis, or anisometropia or refractive error not amenable to optical correction (1).
- Severe pectus excavatum may interfere with pulmonary or cardiac function. Refer for surgery prior to end of adolescent age.
- Scoliosis: bracing for curves 20 to 40 degrees until growth is complete or surgery if >40 degrees.
- Surgery for only most severe cases of dural ectasia
- Hip replacement in middle age or later if protrusio acetabuli has led to severe arthritic change.

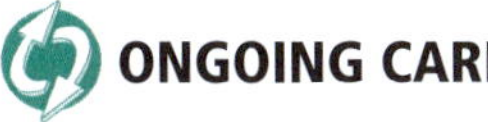

ONGOING CARE

FOLLOW-UP RECOMMENDATIONS

Exercise restrictions: Avoid sports that can increase aortic root enlargement or pneumothorax. Follow recommendation from the National Marfan Foundation and guidelines from the American Heart Association/American College of Cardiology Task Forces.

Patient Monitoring

Exams at least twice per year while patient is growing, with attention to the cardiovascular system and to scoliosis

- Cognitive ability is usually normal, but visual and medical difficulties may interfere with learning (3)[C].
- Cardiac
  - Aortic root dilatation usually progressive; age <20 years, echocardiogram yearly; adults with repeatedly normal aortic root measurements, echocardiogram every 2 to 3 years (1)[C]
  - Consider 6-month repeat imaging following initial surveillance to assess rate of dilatation, more frequent if aortic diameter is increasing rapidly (≥5 cm/year) or approaching surgical threshold (≥4.5 cm in adults)
  - Regular imaging after surgical repair of aorta
- Musculoskeletal
  - Excessive linear growth of long bones, extremities disproportionately long, paucity of muscle mass, peak growth velocity 2 years early; growth curves for MFS are available (3)[C].
  - Evaluate for scoliosis, joint laxity, and pectus deformity every visit to age 1 year, annually for ages 1 to 5 years, semiannually for ages 6 to 18 years, and yearly thereafter.
  - Bone age in preadolescence: Consider hormonal therapy for large discrepancy (3)[C].
  - Scoliosis or pectus deformity may progress more rapidly than in those without MFS.
  - Excellent prognosis for scoliosis curves <30 degrees; bracing may be effective for curves <35 degrees; rapid progression is likely if curve is >50 degrees (3)[C].
- Annual ophthalmologic evaluation: EL, myopia, cataract, glaucoma, and retinal detachment; myopia is very common with early onset, rapid progression, and high degree of severity; early monitoring and aggressive refraction to prevent amblyopia (1)[C]
- Respiratory: pulmonary function tests (PFTs) with symptoms
- Provide genetic counseling at diagnosis, discuss pregnancy risks in adolescence, and discuss activity restrictions starting age 6 years. Review symptoms of potential catastrophic events: aortic dissection, vision changes, and pneumothorax starting age 6 years.

DIET

Early diagnosis of homocystinuria is important because clinical complications can be minimized with appropriate diet and medication.

PROGNOSIS

Life-threatening complications involve cardiovascular dysfunction. With appropriate diagnosis, treatment, and monitoring, lifespan is nearly normal.

COMPLICATIONS

Bacterial endocarditis, aortic dissection, aortic or mitral valve insufficiency, dilated cardiomyopathy, retinal detachment, glaucoma, pneumothorax

REFERENCES

1. Loeys BL, Dietz HC, Braverman AC, et al. The revised Ghent nosology for the Marfan syndrome. *J Med Genet*. 2010;47(7):476–485.
2. Narula N, Devereux RB, Malonga GP, et al. Pregnancy-related aortic complications in women with Marfan syndrome. *J Am Coll Cardiol*. 2021;78(9):870–879.
3. Tinkle BT, Saal HM; for Committee on Genetics. Health supervision for children with Marfan syndrome. *Pediatrics*. 2013;132(4):e1059–e1072.

ADDITIONAL READING

Isselbacher EM, Preventza O, Hamilton Black J III, et al; for Writing Committee Members. 2022 ACC/AHA guideline for the diagnosis and management of aortic disease: a report of the American Heart Association/American College of Cardiology Joint Committee on clinical practice guidelines. *J Am Coll Cardiol*. 2022;80(24):e223–e393.

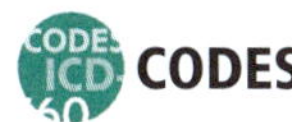

CODES

ICD10

- Q87.40 Marfan's syndrome, unspecified
- Q87.43 Marfan's syndrome with skeletal manifestation
- Q87.418 Marfan's syndrome with other cardiovascular manifestations

CLINICAL PEARLS

- Because many features of MFS appear in the general population, diagnostic criteria have been established. Molecular diagnostic testing for *FBN1* genetic mutations plays an increasing role.
- Screen very tall athletes for aortic root dilatation.
- EL and aortic root dilatation are the best discrimination features; height ≥3.3 *SD* above the mean is a simple discriminant in primary care.

MASTITIS

Amena Payami, DO

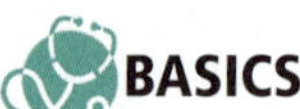

BASICS

DESCRIPTION

- Mastitis is an inflammation of the breast tissue and can include the mammary glands, areola, nipple, and subcutaneous fat.
- Usually associated with bacterial infection and milk stasis in the postpartum mother
- It can be lactational or nonlactational.
- It is usually an acute condition but can become chronic cystic mastitis.

EPIDEMIOLOGY

- It predominantly affects females, mostly in the puerperium period.
- The epidemic form is rare in the age of reduced hospital stays for mothers and newborns, and antibiotic use.
- Posttraumatic mastitis can be due to ornamental nipple piercing increasing risk of transmission of bacteria to deeper breast structures, *Staphylococcus aureus* is the predominant organism.

Incidence

- 3–20% of breastfeeding mothers develop nonepidemic mastitis, with greatest incidence among breastfeeding mothers 2 to 6 weeks postpartum.
- Neonatal form occurs at 1 to 5 weeks of age, with equal gender risk and unilateral presentation.
- Pediatric form occurs at around or after puberty, with 82% of cases in girls.

ETIOLOGY AND PATHOPHYSIOLOGY

- Microabscesses along milk ducts and surrounding tissues
- Inflammatory cell infiltration of breast parenchyma and surrounding tissues
- Nonpuerperal (infectious) *S. aureus* (including methicillin-resistant *S. aureus* [MRSA]), *Bacteroides* spp., *Peptostreptococcus*, *Staphylococcus* (coagulase negative), *Enterococcus faecalis*, *Histoplasma capsulatum*, *Salmonella enterica*, rare case of *Actinomyces europaeus*
- Puerperal (infectious) *Staphylococcus aureus* (including MRSA), *Streptococcus pyogenes* (group A or B), *Enterobacteriaceae*, *Corynebacterium* spp., *Bacteroides* spp., *Staphylococcus* (coagulase negative), *Escherichia coli*, *Salmonella* spp. (1)
- Rare secondary site for tuberculosis in endemic areas (1% of mastitis cases in these areas): single breast nodule with mastalgia
- Tuberculosis mastitis in nonendemic areas has also been reported in patients with exposure to TNF-α inhibitors and other immunomodulating compounds.
- *Corynebacterium* spp. associated with greater risk for development of chronic cystic mastitis
- Granulomatous mastitis
  - Idiopathic: predilection for Asian and Hispanic women
    - Association with α_1-antitrypsin deficiency, hyperprolactinemia with galactorrhea, oral contraceptive use, *Corynebacterium* spp. infection, and breast trauma
    - Most women have a history of lactation in previous 5 years.
    - New cases have been reported in male-to-female transgender patients in setting of exogenous progesterone and estrogen treatment.
  - Lupus; autoimmune
- Puerperal: retrograde migration of surface bacteria up milk ducts, bacterial trapping behind plugged milk in the ductal outflow tracts; bacterial migration from nipple fissures to breast lymphatics; occasionally, secondary monilial infection in the face of recurrent mastitis or diabetes; seeding from mother to neonate in cyclical fashion may occur.
- Nonpuerperal: a variety of causes including: ductal ectasia, breast carcinoma, inflammatory cysts, chronic recurring SC or subareolar infections, parasitic infections (*Echinococcus*; filariasis; guinea worm in endemic areas), herpes simplex, cat-scratch disease, and in older patients, smoking; lupus is a rare cause.

RISK FACTORS

- Milk stasis: inadequate emptying of breast (scarring due to previous breast surgery [breast reduction, biopsy, or partial mastectomy], scarring of breast due to prior mastitis), breast engorgement: interruption of breastfeeding, milk oversupply, plugged ducts
- Nipple trauma increases risk of transmission of bacteria to deeper breast structures: *S. aureus* predominant organism.
- Neonatal colonization with epidemic *Staphylococcus*
- Neonatal—occurs more commonly in bottle-fed babies.
- Maternal diabetes
- Maternal HIV
- Smoking

GENERAL PREVENTION

Regular emptying of both breasts and nipple care to prevent fissures when breastfeeding; also good hygiene including handwashing and washing breast pumps after each use

COMMONLY ASSOCIATED CONDITIONS

Breast abscess

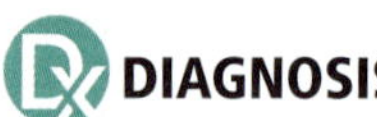

DIAGNOSIS

- Fever >38.5°C, malaise, and myalgia
- Nausea $\pm$ vomiting
- Localized breast tenderness, firmness, heat, swelling, and redness
- Possible breast mass

HISTORY

Breast pain, "hot cords burning in chest wall"

PHYSICAL EXAM

- Breast tenderness
- Localized breast induration, redness, and warmth
- Peau d'orange appearance to overlying skin

DIFFERENTIAL DIAGNOSIS

- Abscess (bacterial, idiopathic granulomatous mastitis, fungal, tuberculosis)
- Tumor, including inflammatory breast cancer
- Idiopathic granulomatous mastitis
- Wegener granulomatosis
- Sarcoidosis
- Foreign body granuloma
- Vasospasm (may be presentation for Raynaud): Consider yeast infection if nipple pain and burning and/or infant with thrush.
- Ductal cyst (ductal ectasia)
- Consider monilial infection in lactating mother, especially if mastitis is recurrent.
- Mondor disease—thrombophlebitis of the superficial veins of the breast and anterior chest wall

DIAGNOSTIC TESTS & INTERPRETATION

Initial Tests (lab, imaging)

Mastitis is typically a clinical diagnosis and labs are rarely needed. In those ill enough to need hospitalization, consider the following:

- CBC, blood culture
- In epidemic puerperal mastitis: milk leukocyte count, milk culture (or if recurrent outpatient mastitis), neonatal nasal culture
- No imaging required for postpartum mastitis in a breastfeeding mother that responds to antibiotic therapy
- Mammography for women with nonpuerperal mastitis
- Breast ultrasound (US) to rule out abscess formation in women with a mass or fluctuance on palpation; special consideration for this in women with breast implants who have mastitis

Follow-Up Tests & Special Considerations

Lactating mothers produce salty milk from affected side (higher Na and Cl concentrations) as compared with unaffected side. Consider breast milk culture if suspect MRSA. Also consider testing for tuberculosis as may be initial presentation.

Diagnostic Procedures/Other

Options if further progression to abscess formation: needle aspiration, incision and drainage, excisional biopsy, US-guided core needle biopsy is diagnostic method of choice for idiopathic granulomatous mastitis.

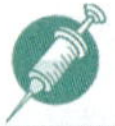

TREATMENT

- A Cochrane review found that insufficient evidence exists to confirm or refute the effectiveness of antibiotic therapy for the treatment of lactational mastitis (2)[A]. If present <24 hours and symptoms are mild, conservative management with milk removal and supportive measures is recommended.
- For patients with early idiopathic granulomatous mastitis and mild symptoms or those concerned for surgical scarring, close surveillance or observation alone is acceptable nonsurgical management.

GENERAL MEASURES

- Supportive care including analgesia, warm compress and effective, frequent milk removal from the affected breast via breastfeeding, pumping, or hand expression
- Smoking cessation for patients with periductal mastitis

MEDICATION

- Prioritized on the basis of likelihood of MRSA as etiologic factor and clinical severity of condition; treat for 10 to 14 days.
- For idiopathic granulomatous mastitis and localized infection, usually resolves with antibiotics and drainage

First Line

- Outpatient
  - Effective milk removal is most important management step.
  - Dicloxacillin 500 mg QID *or* cephalexin 500 mg QID
  - Trimethoprim/sulfamethoxazole (TMP/SMX) 800 mg/160 mg BID (If mastitis not improving within 48 hours after starting first-line treatment, consider MRSA.)

- Doxycycline 100 mg BID; consider MRSA (if clinical course <3 weeks).
- *Lactobacillus fermentum* or *Lactobacillus salivarius* 9 log 10 CFU/day

- Inpatient
  - Nafcillin 2 g q4h *or* oxacillin 2 g q4h *or* Vancomycin 1 g q12h (MRSA possible)
  - Daptomycin 1 g q24h
- If idiopathic granulomatous mastitis, consider corticosteroids ± methotrexate; may consider mycophenolate mofetil in patient refractory to treatment with antibiotics, steroids, and methotrexate

Pediatric Considerations

- TMP/SMX given to breastfeeding mothers with mastitis can potentiate jaundice for neonates.
- Treatment with doxycycline is limited to <3 weeks; long-term theraphy (over 3 to 4 weeks) is not recommended because it may cause damage to infant's growth cartilage, teeth discoloration, and imbalance of intestinal flora.

Second Line

- If mastitis is odoriferous and localized under areola, add metronidazole 500 mg TID IV or PO.
- If yeast is suspected in recurrent mastitis, add topical and oral nystatin. Consider testing nipple tissue and milk for presence of yeast. Oral treatment can be considered for mother as well.

ISSUES FOR REFERRAL

- Abscess formation
- Need for breast biopsy (suspected abscess or IGM)

ADDITIONAL THERAPIES

- Warm packs to improve blood flow and milk letdown and/or ice packs to reduce inflammation to affected breast for comfort
- The use of a breast pump may aid in breast emptying, especially if the infant is unable to assist in doing this.
- Wear supporting bra that is not too tight.

SURGERY/OTHER PROCEDURES

In cases of biopsy-proven idiopathic granulomatous mastitis, the most effective and fastest way for complete eradication is surgical removal. The addition of steroids increases the rate of complete remission and decreases remission rate compared to surgery alone; NNT 3.84

COMPLEMENTARY & ALTERNATIVE MEDICINE

- Breast lift technique for lymphatic breast drainage (can reduce engorgement and relieve plugging)
- Cold cabbage leaf compress to be applied up to 15 minutes twice per day (Avoid long or frequent application of cabbage leaves as milk production can be diminished with this.)
- To prevent recurring plugs and mastitis, can use sunflower lecithin 1,200 mg 3 to 4 times/day

ADMISSION, INPATIENT, AND NURSING CONSIDERATIONS

- If a new mother is admitted to the hospital for treatment of her mastitis, rooming-in of the infant with the mother is highly recommended so that breastfeeding can continue. In some hospitals, rooming-in may require hospital admission of the infant.
- Admission criteria/initial stabilization: failure or outpatient/oral therapy (patient unable to tolerate oral therapy, nonadherent to oral therapy, or severe illness without adequate supportive care at home); neonatal mastitis also requires admission.
  - Administer antibiotics.
  - Empty breasts frequently, if breastfeeding.
  - Give analgesics for pain: ibuprofen or acetaminophen.
  - Breastfeeding/pumping of breasts encouraged baby and/or breast pump to bedside
- Start infant with feedings on affected side.
- Abscess drainage is not a contraindication for breastfeeding.
- Massage in direction from blocked area toward nipple.
- Positioning the infant at breast with chin or nose pointing to blockage might help drain affected area.
- Discharge criteria: Patients should be afebrile and tolerating oral antibiotics well.

ONGOING CARE

FOLLOW-UP RECOMMENDATIONS

Patient Monitoring

- Rest for lactating mothers, up to bathroom; admit to medical floor. If concern for sepsis or hemodynamic instability, admit to intermediate level of care or ICU.
- Follow up with breast imaging such as mammography or US in women >40 years of age after resolution of acute pathology to exclude underlying breast cancer.

DIET

- Encourage oral fluids.
- Multivitamin, including vitamin A

PATIENT EDUCATION

- Encourage oral fluids. Rest is essential.
- Regular emptying/draining of both breasts with breastfeeding
- Nipple care (simply with breast milk or with hypoallergenic nipple balm) to prevent fissures
- Best nipple/areola health comes with optimized latch—seek help with latch if needed from a lactation professional.

PROGNOSIS

- Puerperal
  - Good with prompt (within 24 hours of symptom onset) antibiotic treatment and breast emptying; 96% success rate
  - 11% risk of abscess if left untreated with antibiotics
  - Antibodies develop in breast glands within first few days of infection, which may provide protection against infection or reinfection.
- Rare risk of abscess formation beyond 6 weeks postpartum if no recurrent mastitis
- Idiopathic granulomatous mastitis recurrence rates high; encourage close follow-up.

COMPLICATIONS

Breast abscess 3% of women with puerperal mastitis; recurrent mastitis with resumption of breastfeeding or with breastfeeding after next pregnancy; cessation of breastfeeding; bacteremia; sepsis

REFERENCES

1. Wilson E, Woodd SL, Benova L. Incidence of and risk factors for lactational mastitis: a systematic review. *J Hum Lact*. 2020;36(4):673–686.
2. Jahanfar S, Ng CJ, Teng CL. Antibiotics for mastitis in breastfeeding women. *Cochrane Database Syst Rev*. 2013. 2013(2):CD005458. doi:10.1002/14651858.CD005458.pub3.

SEE ALSO

Algorithms: Breast Discharge; Breast Pain

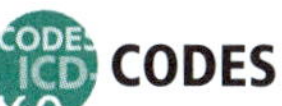

CODES

ICD10

- O91.11 Abscess of breast associated with pregnancy
- O91.211 Nonpurulent mastitis associated with pregnancy, first trimester
- O91.113 Abscess of breast associated with pregnancy, third trimester

CLINICAL PEARLS

- Emptying/draining of the breasts on a regular schedule (recommend following baby's cues, but going no more than 3 to 4 hours between feeds), avoiding constrictive clothing or bras that might obstruct breast ducts, attention to good latch technique for mom and baby, "adequate rest," and a liberal intake of oral fluids for the mother can all reduce the risk of a breastfeeding mother developing mastitis.
- Reassure mothers that it is safe (and imperative for healing) to feed baby and/or pump the affected breast.
- Among breastfeeding mothers, if the symptoms of mastitis fail to resolve within several days of appropriate management, including antibiotics, NSAIDs, and breast emptying, further investigations may be required to confirm resistant bacteria, abscess formation, an underlying mass, or inflammatory or ductal carcinoma.
- >2 recurrences of mastitis in the same location or with associated axillary lymphadenopathy warrant evaluation with US and/or mammography to rule out an underlying mass.

MASTOIDITIS

Samantha Carroll, MD

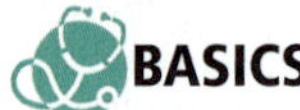

BASICS

Mastoiditis is an inflammatory process of the mastoid bone. It is the most frequent serious complication seen from acute otitis media (AOM).

DESCRIPTION

- Clinical manifestations of mastoiditis typically appear days to weeks after the first middle ear symptoms.
- Subdivided according to pathologic stage:
  - Acute mastoiditis with periostitis (incipient mastoiditis): purulent material in the mastoid cavities; symptom duration typically ≤1 month
  - Coalescent mastoiditis (acute mastoid osteitis): destruction of the thin bony septae between air cells; followed by the formation of abscess cavities with pus dissecting into adjacent areas
- Masked mastoiditis (subacute mastoiditis): low grade, persistent infection with destruction of the bony septae between air cells; occurs in patients with persistent middle ear effusion or recurrent episodes of inadequately treated AOM
- Chronic mastoiditis: associated with failed treatment of chronic otitis media; often associated with cholesteatoma; symptoms last months to years

EPIDEMIOLOGY

The highest incidence in children aged <2 years

- Similar to population susceptible to AOM (male, daycare attendance)
- Less common if immunizations up-to-date and antibiotics used to treat suppurative AOM

Incidence

1.2 to 6.1 per 100,000 children per year in United States (1)

ETIOLOGY AND PATHOPHYSIOLOGY

- Subclinical stage begins with AOM and inflammation of mastoid air cells.
- Mastoid is part of petrous temporal bone composed of air-filled cells.
- Mastoid aditus and antrum form a narrow connection between middle ear and mastoid air cells.
  - Fluid in the middle ear can cause obstruction at aditus or antrum, blocking outflow tract of mastoid air cells.
  - Edema and accumulation of purulent material most commonly spreads from mastoid air cells to periosteum via mastoid emissary veins with penetration of periosteum (acute mastoiditis with periosteitis).
- Acute mastoid osteitis can spread to adjacent areas in head and neck with abscess formation: subperiosteal abscess (most common complication), Bezold abscess, suppurative labyrinthitis, suppurative CNS complications (2)
- AOM: *Streptococcus pneumoniae*, nontypeable *Haemophilus influenzae*
- Acute mastoiditis: *S. pneumoniae* (most common), group A *Streptococci—Streptococcus pyogenes*, *Staphylococcus aureus* (including methicillin-resistant *S. aureus* [MRSA]), *H. influenzae*, *Fusobacterium necrophorum*
- Chronic mastoiditis: *Pseudomonas aeruginosa*, *S. aureus*, anaerobic bacteria, polymicrobials (organisms present in external ear canal), rarely *Mycobacterium tuberculosis*
- Abscess: *S. aureus*, mycobacteria, *Aspergillus*
- Increased incidence of penicillin-resistant *S. pneumoniae* infections has gradually led to higher incidence of mastoiditis as complication of AOM.

RISK FACTORS

- Cholesteatoma appears as squamous pearl in anterosuperior area of middle ear near tympanic membrane.
- Recurrent AOM or chronic suppurative otitis media
- Immunocompromised state

GENERAL PREVENTION

- Ensure immunizations (particularly pneumococcal vaccine) are up-to-date.
- Referral to ENT for chronic otitis media
- Appropriate diagnosis and treatment of AOM; prevent recurrent AOM.
- Wear ear plugs when swimming or showering to keep water out of the ears with AOM.
- Treat chronic eustachian tube dysfunction (pressure equalization tubes).
- Early diagnosis of cholesteatoma

COMMONLY ASSOCIATED CONDITIONS

AOM

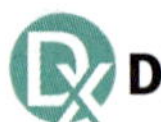

DIAGNOSIS

Mastoiditis is a clinical diagnosis. Clinical findings including redness of the mastoid area, with anterior protrusion of the affected ear, ear drainage, fever, irritability. Laboratory and imaging, such as a CT scan, are adjunct tests used if the clinical exam is uncertain.

HISTORY

- Most common symptoms in infancy
  - Lethargy/malaise/irritability
  - Fever
  - Poor feeding/decreased appetite
- Recent ear infection
- Otorrhea (drainage from an ear infection)
- Otalgia and/or pain on mastoid bone behind the ear
- Swelling or redness over mastoid
- Swelling of the ear lobe
- Headache
- Hearing loss
- Chronic: persistent ear drainage, persistent ear pain
- Chronic: AOM nonresponsive to antibiotic
- Suspicion for mastoiditis increases when symptoms of AOM persist >2 weeks.

PHYSICAL EXAM

- Acute:
  - Fever
  - Erythema, tenderness, and/or edema overlying mastoid (postauricular)
  - Palpable postauricular fluctuance (later finding): most commonly postauricular in children aged >1 year and above ear in children aged <1 year
  - Protrusion of the pinna upward and outward in children aged >1 year or down and outward in children aged <1 year
  - Otoscopic exam: AOM present; may have perforation of TM with or without purulent discharge
- Chronic mastoiditis:
  - Persistent or intermittent mucopurulent drainage
  - Decreased hearing
  - May be painless from chronic process
  - Otoscopic exam: may have mucopurulent discharge, perforation of TM

DIFFERENTIAL DIAGNOSIS

- Mumps, parotitis
- Severe otitis externa
- Periauricular cellulitis
- Benign neoplasm: aneurysmal bone cyst, fibrous dysplasia
- Malignant neoplasm: acute lymphocytic leukemia, acute myelogenous leukemia, Burkitt lymphoma, non-Hodgkin lymphoma, rhabdomyosarcoma, neuroblastoma
- Deep neck space infections

DIAGNOSTIC TESTS & INTERPRETATION

Initial Tests (lab, imaging)

- CBC with differential: elevated WBC count
- Elevated erythrocyte sedimentation rate (ESR) and C-reactive protein (CRP) in acute but may be normal in chronic
- Blood cultures
- Myringotomy/tympanocentesis: send for cultures, Gram stain, acid-fast stain
- Aspiration if postauricular fluctuance is present: Send for cultures.
- Plain films of mastoid has low diagnostic yield but may show loss of sharpness of mastoid outline, clouding of mastoid air cells, or demineralization of bony septa (3). These changes are not diagnostic and can also be seen in AOM.
- Preferred: CT scan of the temporal bone (97% sensitivity; 94% positive predictive value for identifying intracranial complications)
  - Clouding/opacification of air cells (also in AOM)
  - Mastoid air cell coalescence
  - Cortical bone erosion
  - Absence of mastoid opacification excludes the diagnosis
- Use CT scan with contrast if complications are suspected (suppurative extension)
- Due to radiation, CT scan in children should be performed when clinically appropriate. Indications include neurologic signs; vomiting/lethargy; suspected cholesteatoma; fever after 48 to 72 hours of therapy
- Technetium-99m bone scan is more sensitive to osteolytic changes than CT scan.
- Ultrasound may be considered in the future, initial literature shows that ultrasound was able to successfully identify 9 out of 10 patients with complications from mastoiditis.
- MRI: partial-to-complete opacification of the mastoid air cells ± middle ear cleft
  - Needed to evaluate for intracranial complications if clinical or radiographic suspicion
- Consider MRA if venous sinus thrombosis suspected.

Follow-Up Tests & Special Considerations

- Send all cultures for aerobic and anaerobic growth.
- Interpret normal WBC with caution in symptomatic, immunocompromised patients.
- Lumbar puncture if meningitis suspected
- Consider immunologic evaluations in children with recurrent episodes of OM leading to mastoiditis.

Diagnostic Procedures/Other

- Tympanocentesis to obtain middle ear fluid for culture and sensitivity
- Myringotomy with culture (also therapeutic)
- Audiography if hearing loss suspected
- Obtain CSF if intracranial extension suspected.
- Biopsy tissue protruding through TM or tympanostomy tube

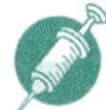

TREATMENT

- IV antibiotics and myringotomy (± tympanostomy tubes) are the preferred treatment for uncomplicated acute mastoiditis (reflecting a shift away from more invasive surgical treatment).
- To avoid intracranial complications, simple mastoidectomy is recommended if patients do not respond to treatment after 48 hours.
- Myringotomy or incision and drainage may be necessary if an abscess is present in mastoid air cells.

GENERAL MEASURES

Inpatient care during acute phase for IV antibiotics

MEDICATION

First Line

- Empiric antibiotics against most common organisms: *S. pneumoniae* (including multiple resistant strains), *S. pyogenes*, *S. aureus* (including MRSA), *P. aeruginosa*
- Use combination therapy with 3rd-generation cephalosporin (ceftriaxone or cefotaxime) plus clindamycin with coverage for resistant strains.
- Ceftriaxone 2 g IV q24h
  - Pediatric dosing: 50 to 100 mg/kg/day IV divided q12–24h
  - Precaution: Adjust dose with renal impairment.
  - Consider levofloxacin 750 mg IV q24h if severe β-lactam allergy.
- Ampicillin-sulbactam 200 to 300 mg/kg/d IV
- Clindamycin for coverage of ceftriaxone-resistant *S. pneumoniae* in pediatric patients: clindamycin pediatric dosing: 20 to 40 mg/kg/day IV divided q6–8h
- Cefotaxime 1 to 2 g IV q4–8h, depending on severity
  - Pediatric dosing: 100 to 200 mg/kg/day q6–8h
- Add vancomycin 30 to 60 mg/kg/day divided q8–12h if concerned for MRSA or acute on chronic exacerbation:
  - Pediatric dosing: 15 mg/kg/dose q6–8h
  - Precaution: Adjust dose with renal impairment.
- For patients with a history of recurrent AOM or recent antibiotic administration, treat with piperacillin and tazobactam 3.375 g IV q6h: pediatric dosing: 300 mg/kg/day based on piperacillin component divided q6–8h
- Once culture results are available, target treatment based on antibiotic sensitivities.

Second Line

- Oral antibiotics after 7 to 10 days of IV antibiotics and once myringotomy/blood cultures identify pathogen and sensitivities. Common oral antibiotics: Amoxicillin-clavulanate (Augmentin) or clindamycin + 3rd-generation cephalosporin for 3 weeks or total treatment duration of ≥4 weeks for intracranial complications (4)
- For chronic mastoiditis: Use topical drops, ofloxacin otic solution (0.3%) or neomycin, polymyxin B, hydrocortisone 3 drops, 3 to 4 times/day.

ISSUES FOR REFERRAL

- Consult ENT for mastoiditis in adults and children.
- Consult neurosurgery for intracranial complications.
- Consider infectious disease consult for assistance with antibiotic management.

SURGERY/OTHER PROCEDURES

- Perform tympanocentesis to obtain cultures and guide antibiotic choice.
- Myringotomy and tympanostomy tubes allow for middle ear drainage.
- Clean ear canal under microscopic guidance to ensure pressure-equalization tube patency and adequate drainage of middle ear.
- Simple mastoidectomy is most effective for management of subperiosteal abscesses, bony erosion, or other complications or if trial of conservative therapy (drainage, myringotomy, and IV antibiotics) fails.

ADMISSION, INPATIENT, AND NURSING CONSIDERATIONS

- Admission criteria/initial stabilization
  - Clinical or imaging evidence of acute mastoiditis
  - Hospitalize patients with acute mastoiditis and start IV antibiotics immediately.
- Avoid getting affected ear wet.
- Discharge criteria
  - Afebrile for 48 hours before IV antibiotics are discontinued
  - Clinical improvement
  - Able to tolerate oral antibiotics

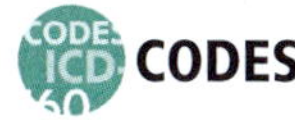

ONGOING CARE

FOLLOW-UP RECOMMENDATIONS

- Oral antibiotics for 3 weeks following course of IV antibiotics (total duration of antibiotics is ≥4 weeks for intracranial complications)
- For chronic mastoiditis, consider several months of antimicrobial prophylaxis with amoxicillin.

Patient Monitoring

- Assess for hearing loss postoperatively (audiogram) after acute condition has subsided.
- Follow-up with ENT and/or neurosurgery, particularly patients with hearing loss and/or intracranial complications

PATIENT EDUCATION

- Avoid getting the affected ear wet.
- Complete full course of antibiotics.

PROGNOSIS

- Depends on severity and stage of disease
- Most cases of mastoiditis recover fully if diagnosis is made early and treated appropriately.
- Conductive hearing loss may require reconstructive surgery; hearing loss may be permanent.

COMPLICATIONS

Complication rate 5–29% (4)

- Extracranial: subperiosteal abscess; osteomyelitis of the temporal bone; suppurative labyrinthitis; permanent hearing loss; facial nerve paralysis
- Intracranial
  - Intracranial abscess: epidural/subdural/cerebral
  - Meningitis/cerebritis/periosteitis

REFERENCES

1. Bridwell RE, Koyfman A, Long B. High risk and low prevalence diseases: acute mastoiditis. *Am J Emerg Med*. 2024;79:63–69. doi:10.1016/j.ajem.2024.02.009.
2. Kaufmann MR, Shetty K, Camilon PR, et al. Management of acute complicated mastoiditis: a systematic review and meta-analysis. *Pediatr Infect Dis J*. 2022;41(4):297–301.
3. Loh R, Phua M, Shaw CL. Management of paediatric acute mastoiditis: systematic review. *J Laryncgol Otol*. 2018;132(2):96–104.
4. Mansour T, Yehudai N, Tobia A, et al. Acute mastoiditis: 20 years of experience with a uniform management protocol. *Int J Pediatr Otorhinolaryngol*. 2019;125:187–191.

CODES

ICD10

- H70.90 Unspecified mastoiditis, unspecified ear
- H70.009 Acute mastoiditis without complications, unspecified ear
- H70.099 Acute mastoiditis with other complications, unspecified ear

CLINICAL PEARLS

- Suspect mastoiditis if symptoms of AOM persist >2 weeks despite a normal-appearing TM.
- Temporal bone CT is the best diagnostic tool; use only when mastoiditis is suspected to limit radiation exposure in children.
- Hospitalize patients with acute mastoiditis for IV antibiotics. Consult ENT for drainage procedure.
- Treat with broad-spectrum IV antibiotics; collect middle ear fluid cultures to guide-specific therapy. Total duration of antibiotics is ≥4 weeks for intracranial complications.
- If conservative treatment fails after 3 to 5 days, perform mastoidectomy to avoid intracranial complications.

MEDIAL TIBIAL STRESS SYNDROME (MTSS)/SHIN SPLINTS

Shane L. Larson, MD • Briana Lindberg, MD, CAQSM

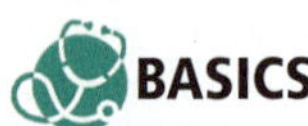

BASICS

DESCRIPTION

The term medial tibial stress syndrome (MTSS) is preferred to "shin splints." MTSS is an aching pain along the inner edge of the tibial shaft that develops when the musculature and/or periosteum in the (lower) leg become irritated by repetitive activity. The condition is part of a continuum of stress-related injuries to the lower leg and is not related to pain from ischemia (compartment syndrome) or stress fractures.

- Related pathology: tendonitis/periostitis of the medial soleus muscles, anterior tibialis, and posterior tibialis muscles
- Synonyms: tibial stress reaction, anterior muscle syndrome, tibial periostitis, perimyositis, soleus syndrome, shin splints

EPIDEMIOLOGY

Incidence

Common, can account for 4–35% of reported running injuries; frequently occurs bilaterally (1)

Pediatric Considerations

MTSS may account for up to 31% of all overuse injuries in high school athletes.

ETIOLOGY AND PATHOPHYSIOLOGY

- Multifactorial anatomic and biomechanical factors
  - Overuse injuries caused or limited by
    - Microtrauma from repetitive motion leading to periosteal inflammation
    - Overpronation of the subtalar joint and tight gastrocnemius/soleus complex with increased eccentric loading of musculature inserting along the medial shin
    - Interosseous membrane pain
    - Periostitis
    - Tears of collagen fibers
    - Enthesopathy
  - Anatomic structures affected include the following:
    - Flexor hallucis longus
    - Tibialis anterior
    - Tibialis posterior
    - Soleus
    - Crural fascia
- Pathogenesis is theorized to be due to the following:
  - Calf muscle traction on periosteum
  - Persistent repetitive loading on tibia, which leads to inadequate bone remodeling with subsequent tibial cortex changes
  - Possible microfissures causing pain without evidence of fracture or ischemia

RISK FACTORS

- Intrinsic (personal) risk factors (1):
  - Greater ranges of internal and external (>65 degrees) hip rotation
  - Significant overpronation at the ankle
  - Imbalance of musculature of the ankle and foot (inversion/eversion misbalance)
  - Female gender
  - Lean calf girth
  - Femoral neck anteversion
  - Navicular drop
  - Genu varum
  - History of previous MTSS
- External (environmental) risk factors (1):
  - Lack of physical fitness
  - Inexperienced runners—particularly those with rapid increases in mileage and inadequate prior conditioning
  - Excessive overuse or distance running, particularly on hard or inclined (crowned) surfaces
  - Prior injury
  - Equipment (shoe) failure
- Other risk factors:
  - Elevated BMI
  - Lower bone mineral density
  - Tobacco use
- Those typically affected by MTSS include the following:
  - Runners
  - Military personnel—common in recruit/boot camp
  - Gymnasts, soccer, and basketball players
  - Ballet dancers

GENERAL PREVENTION

- Proper technique for guided calf stretching and lower extremity strength training, although supplementary gastrocnemius and soleus stretching has no statistical significance in reducing risk of shin splints
- Rehabilitate prior injuries adequately.
- Other recommendations
  - Gait analysis and retraining, particularly for overpronation
  - Orthotic footwear inserts were found to be preventative in naval recruits.

COMMONLY ASSOCIATED CONDITIONS

Pes planus (flat feet)

ALERT

Rule out stress fracture and compartment syndrome where pain often persists at rest.

DIAGNOSIS

HISTORY

- Patients typically describe dull, sharp, or deep pain along the lower leg that is resolved with rest.
- Patients are often able to run through the pain in early stages.
- Pain is commonly associated with exercise (also true with compartment syndrome), but in severe cases, pain may persist with rest.

PHYSICAL EXAM

- Tenderness to palpation is typically elicited along the posteromedial border of the middle-to-distal 3rd of the tibia.
- Pain with plantar flexion
- Preservation of neurovascular integrity via palpable distal pulses, intact sensation, reflexes, and muscular strength

DIFFERENTIAL DIAGNOSIS

- Bone
  - Tibial stress fractures
    - Typically, pain persists at rest or with weight-bearing activities.
    - Focal tenderness over the anterior tibia
    - Hopping on involved leg will reproduce pain (less likely with MTSS).
- Muscle/soft tissue injury
  - Strain, tear, tendinopathy
  - Muscle hernia
- Fascial
  - Chronic exertional compartment syndrome (1)
    - Pain without direct tenderness on exam
    - Pain increases with exertion and resolves at rest.
    - Pain is described as cramping or squeezing.
    - Pain with possible weakness or paresthesias on exam
  - Interosseous membrane tear
- Nerve
  - Spinal stenosis
  - Lumbar radiculopathy
  - Common peroneal nerve entrapment
- Vascular
  - DVT
  - Popliteal arterial entrapment
    - Rare but limb-threatening disease
    - History of intermittent unilateral claudication
    - MRI reveals compression of the artery by the medial head of the gastrocnemius muscle.
- Infection
  - Osteomyelitis
- Malignancy
  - Bone tumors

DIAGNOSTIC TESTS & INTERPRETATION

Clinical history and exam are considered gold standard in diagnosing MTSS (1).

Initial Tests (lab, imaging)

- Plain radiographs help rule out stress fractures if >2 weeks of symptoms.
- Bone scintigraphy
  - Diffuse linear vertical uptake in the posterior tibial cortex on the lateral view
  - Stress fractures demonstrate a focal ovoid uptake.
- High-resolution MRI reveals abnormal periosteal and bone marrow signals, which are useful for early discrimination of tibial stress fractures.

Follow-Up Tests & Special Considerations

Increased pain and localized tenderness warrant further imaging with MRI due to concern for tibial stress fracture (1).

Diagnostic Procedures/Other

Exclude compartment syndrome using intracompartmental pressure testing.

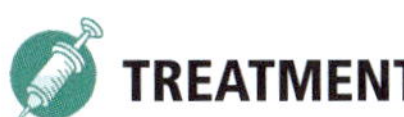

TREATMENT

GENERAL MEASURES

- Activity modification with a gradual return to training based on improvement of symptoms
- Running on flat and firm surfaces can help minimize pain.
- Patients should maintain fitness with low-impact activities such as swimming and cycling.
- Continue activity modification until pain free on ambulation.

MEDICATION

- Analgesia with acetaminophen or oral nonsteroidal anti-inflammatory agent
- Cryotherapy (ice massage) is also advised to relieve acute-phase symptoms (1)[C].

ADDITIONAL THERAPIES

- Orthotics may be beneficial.
- Calf stretch, peroneal stretch, TheraBand exercises, and eccentric calf raises may improve endurance and strength (2)[A].
- Compression stockings have been used to treat MTSS with mixed results.
- Structured running programs with warm-up exercises have not been demonstrated to reduce pain in young athletes (3)[B].
- CAM boot for people with significant pain with weight-bearing

SURGERY/OTHER PROCEDURES

- Surgical intervention includes a posterior medial fascial release in individuals with both
  - Severe limitation of physical activity and
  - Failure of 6 months of conservative treatment
    - Counsel patients that complete return of activity to sport may not be always achieved postoperatively. Surgical risks include infection and hematoma formation.
- Extracorporeal shock wave therapy (ESWT) may decrease recovery time when added to a running program (2)[A].

COMPLEMENTARY & ALTERNATIVE MEDICINE

- Individualized polyurethane orthoses may help chronic running injuries.
- Special insoles, low-energy laser treatment, pulsed electromagnetic field, and knee braces have not been shown to improve outcomes (2)[A].
- Ultrasound, acupuncture, aquatic therapy, electrical stimulation, whirlpool baths, cast immobilization, taping, and steroid injection may help improve pain.
- Physical therapy approaches including Kinesio tape and fascial distortion massage may yield quicker return to activity.
- Osteopathic manipulative treatment may yield quicker return to athletic/activity as well.

ONGOING CARE

FOLLOW-UP RECOMMENDATIONS

Patient Monitoring

- Once well, recommend gradual return to preinjury running pace.
- Maintain stretching and strengthening exercises.
- Identify and correct preinjury training errors.
- Good supportive footwear is recommended as is replacing running shoes every 350 to 450 miles.
- Allow a gradual return to activity dictated by symptoms (pain).

PROGNOSIS

The condition is usually self-limiting, and most patients respond well with rest and nonsurgical intervention.

COMPLICATIONS

- Stress fractures and compartment syndrome
- Undiagnosed MTSS or chronic exertional compartment syndrome can lead to a complete fracture or tissue necrosis, respectively.

REFERENCES

1. Moen MH, Tol JL, Weir A, et al. Medial tibial stress syndrome: a critical review. *Sports Med*. 2009;39(7):523–546.
2. Winters M, Eskes M, Weir A, et al. Treatment of medial tibial stress syndrome: a systematic review. *Sports Med*. 2013;43(12):1315–1333.
3. Moen MH, Holtslag L, Bakker E, et al. The treatment of medial tibial stress syndrome in athletes; a randomized clinical trial. *Sports Med Arthrosc Rehabil Ther Technol*. 2012;4:12.

ADDITIONAL READING

- Abelson B. Tibialis anterior–effective stretching technique. https://www.youtube.com/watch?v=6Z6XM63x2TM. Accessed August 23, 2023.
- Fields KB, Sykes JC, Walker KM, et al. Prevention of running injuries. *Curr Sports Med Rep*. 2010;9(3):176–182.
- Hamstra-Wright KL, Bliven KCH, Bay C. Risk factors for medial tibial stress syndrome in physically active individuals such as runners and military personnel: a systematic review and meta-analysis. *Br J Sports Med*. 2015;49(6):362–369.
- Reinking MF, Austin TM, Richter RR, et al. Medial tibial stress syndrome in active individuals: a systematic review and meta-analysis of risk factors. *Sports Health*. 2017;9(3):252–261.
- Reshef N, Guelich DR. Medial tibial stress syndrome. *Clin Sports Med*. 2012;31(2):273–290.
- Yeung SS, Yeung EW, Gillespie LD. Interventions for preventing lower limb soft-tissue running injuries. *Cochrane Database Syst Rev*. 2011;(7):CD001256.

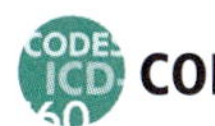

CODES

ICD10

- S86.899A Other injury of other muscle(s) and tendon(s) at lower leg level, unspecified leg, initial encounter
- S86.891A Other injury of other muscle(s) and tendon(s) at lower leg level, right leg, initial encounter
- S86.892A Other injury of other muscle(s) and tendon(s) at lower leg level, left leg, initial encounter

CLINICAL PEARLS

- MTSS is the preferred term for "shin splints."
- Diagnosis is based on a reliable history of repetitive overuse accompanied by characteristic shin pain; imaging only if strong suspicion for stress fracture
- MTSS pain is typically along the middle and distal 3rd of the posteromedial tibial surface, worsened with activity, and relieved with rest (vs. compartment syndrome or stress fracture, where pain persists with rest).
- Treatment includes ice, activity modification, analgesics, eccentric stretching, gait retraining, and a gradual return to activity.
- Symptoms recur if return to activity is "too much too fast."

MEDICAL MARIJUANA

Alex Kipp, MD, MALS

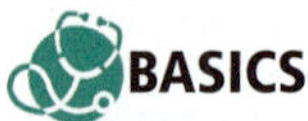

BASICS

Medical marijuana, also known as medicinal cannabis, refers to the use of natural chemicals derived from the leaves, flower, stems, seeds of the flowering plant, *Cannabis sativa*, used to treat symptoms of various diseases.

DESCRIPTION

- "*Cannabis*" refers to the genus which has two main subspecies, *Cannabis sativa* and *Cannabis indica*. "Marijuana" is a term popularized in the 1930s by officials seeking to dissuade people from using cannabis by making it sound foreign and dangerous.
- Cannabis interacts with the endocannabinoid system (ECS) in our bodies.
  - The ECS has two main receptors that, when activated, decrease neurotransmitter release:
    - CB1—expressed in the central nervous system
    - CB2—expressed in the periphery including the immune system
- These receptors are activated by endocannabinoids or exogenous cannabinoids originating from cannabis.
- It is believed that endocannabinoids are related to help us forget pain, such as during childbirth.
- The best studied cannabinoids are δ-9-tetrahydrocannabinol (THC) and cannabidiol (CBD). Most of the psychoactive properties come from THC acting on CB1 receptors. CBD acts on the CB2 receptors and initiates more anxiolytic and sedative properties (1).

EPIDEMIOLOGY

As of June 2025, 40 states, 3 territories (Guam, Puerto Rico, U.S. Virgin Islands), and the District of Columbia have legalized the use of cannabis for medical purposes.

- At the federal level, cannabis continues to be a Schedule 1 substance and federal funding for research of cannabis can only be done studying harms or abuse potential.

Prevalence

- Cannabis use is becoming more common, with 13% of those surveyed report use in the last month, and 18.7% in the past year. Differentiating cannabis use for recreational versus medicinal purposes is more difficult as more states legalize recreational use (2).
- The most common indications for medical cannabis use were surveyed to be anxiety, insomnia, and chronic pain. Medical marijuana licenses obtained from various states has decreased with the increase of cannabis becoming legalized for recreational purposes.

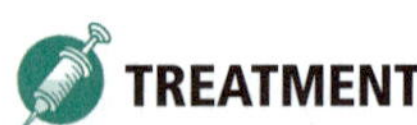

TREATMENT

Conditions that qualify for medical cannabis vary by state. The most common conditions approved by states include chronic pain, cancer-related weight loss/cachexia, chemotherapy-induced nausea and vomiting (CINV), and epilepsy (3).

- Chronic pain
  - Cannabinoids may benefit patients with chronic nociceptive and neuropathic pain, pain associated with cancer, and fibromyalgia.
    - Suggested number needed to treat (NNT) for neuropathic and palliative pain reduction is 5.6 with inhaled cannabis (4)
    - In a systematic review, there is moderate to high certainty evidence that noninhaled medical cannabis or cannabinoids results in a small improvement in pain relief, physical functioning, and sleep quality among patients with chronic pain.
  - In studies of Medicare Part D data from 2010 to 2015, states with active cannabis dispensaries saw 3.472 million fewer doses of opioids dispensed, predominantly hydrocodone and morphine, indicating that cannabis use can help to reduce opioid prescribing for chronic pain (5).
  - Studies have shown that medicinal cannabis use is associated with a reduction in death from opioids (6).
- CINV
  - Variable evidence of efficacy of cannabis-based medications for CINV.
    - Suggested NNT for improvement in CINV is 3 (4).
  - A 2023 clinical trial showed benefit of oral THC: CBD extract in the prevention of CINV
- Multiple sclerosis muscle spasticity
  - Substantial evidence that oral cannabinoids may be an effective treatment for spasticity
    - The American Academy of Neurology gives cannabis a level A for effectiveness.
    - Suggested NNT for 30% improvement in clinician evaluated spasticity is 7 to 10 with low-strength evidence (4).
- Posttraumatic stress disorder (PTSD)
  - A 2022 prospective study showed that participants who used cannabis were 2.57 times more likely to no longer meet *DSM-5* criteria for PTSD than control (7).
  - In a small crossover study, there was improvement in self-reported nightmares with use of medical cannabis.
    - Overall, there is insufficient high-quality evidence to recommend medical cannabis for PTSD.
- Epilepsy
  - In 2018, FDA-approved cannabinoid oral solution (cannabidiol [Epidiolex]) for treatment of seizures related to two rare childhood conditions: Lennox-Gastaut syndrome and Dravet syndrome.
  - For adult epilepsy, most studies focus on nonmedical marijuana (CBD) instead of medical marijuana (THC) due to anxiolytic and sedating effects.
    - The data for CBD continues to be low quality and strength, although patients may show perceived reduction in seizure.

MEDICATION

- FDA-approved products (8)
  - Cannabis-derived compounds (extracted directly from plant)
    - Cannabidiol (Epidiolex)—purified form of CBD; cannot be prescribed off-label
      - Indicated for seizures associated with Lennox-Gastaut syndrome or Dravet syndrome in patients aged ≥2 years
      - Obtain liver function tests
        - Can cause dose-related elevations in transaminases
        - Resolution occurred with discontinuation or dose reduction.
        - The most common adverse reactions (≥10%) are somnolence; decreased appetite; diarrhea; transaminase elevations; fatigue, malaise, and asthenia; rash; insomnia, sleep disorder, and poor quality sleep; and infections.
  - Cannabis-related compounds (synthesized in lab)
    - Dronabinol (synthetic THC): Marinol (capsule) and Syndros (oral solution)
      - Indicated for
        - CINV
        - Anorexia in patients with AIDS
      - Most common adverse reactions (≥3%) are abdominal pain, dizziness, euphoria, nausea, paranoid reaction, somnolence, thinking abnormal, and vomiting.
    - Nabilone (similar to THC, synthetic): Cesamet (capsule)
      - Indicated for CINV
- *Not* FDA-approved but approved in other countries in North America and Europe
  - Nabiximols (Sativex)
    - Oromucosal spray containing THC and CBD in 1:1 ratio, directly extracted
      - Indicated for moderate to severe spasticity due to multiple sclerosis

ONGOING CARE

Pediatric Considerations

- Pediatric cannabis exposure is associated with potentially serious symptoms:
  - Respiratory depression or failure
  - Tachycardia
  - Temporary coma
- Adolescents have increased vulnerability to adverse long-term outcomes given the impact cannabis has on the adolescent brain.
- Association with tobacco, alcohol, and other substance use in adulthood (9)

Pregnancy and Lactation Considerations

- Pregnant women should be discouraged from using medical cannabis in any form, around conception, during pregnancy and throughout breastfeeding.
- Potential effects on fetal development as THC crosses the fetal-placental barrier and significantly impacts fetal brain development
- American College of Obstetricians and Gynecologists (ACOG) and American Academy of Pediatrics (AAP) have recommended that marijuana use be discouraged for breastfeeding mothers (10).

COMPLICATIONS

- Short-term complications
  - Intoxication may cause:
    - Acute physiologic effects: conjunctival injection, orthostatic hypotension, tachycardia, dry mouth, and poor motor coordination
    - Acute psychologic effects: relaxation, euphoria, altered sensory perception
  - Withdrawal may cause (mainly psychological symptoms, no physical dependence has been documented):
    - Irritability, depression, restlessness, insomnia
- Long-term complications
  - Respiratory
    - With limited data, it is unclear if there is association between regular cannabis use and increased risk of developing COPD. Regular cannabis smoking may be less significant than regular tobacco smoking in development of COPD. This is dependent on how a patient takes in cannabis. Vaping is less damaging than smoking.
  - Cardiovascular risk
    - Limited studies and cases of marijuana precipitating arrhythmias, stress cardiomyopathy, and arteritis
  - Cancer risk
    - Limited quality evidence that shows no statistical evidence of association between cannabis smoking and incidence of lung cancer.
  - Psychological
    - Cannabis use disorder
      - Cannabis use leading to clinically significant impairment or distress over a period of 12 months that can include:
        - Consuming cannabis in significant amounts or for prolonged periods more than intended
        - Spending a great deal of time in activities related to cannabis
        - Unable to fulfill obligations relating to work, school, home
      - Increased association with anxiety, psychosis, and depression
      - Increased risk of schizophrenia in early chronic users, likely reflecting unmasking of individual susceptibility to psychotic illness
      - Associated with higher rate of suicide among users with bipolar disorder
  - Gastrointestinal
    - Cannabis-induced hyperemesis syndrome
      - Occurs in chronic users (likely >1 year of daily use), suggested to be due to downregulation of CB1; similar to cyclical vomiting syndrome, although without association of other psychological conditions such as anxiety
      - Emesis episodes are episodic and may stop after a hot shower.
      - Alternatively, TCAs have been used as long term therapy.
      - For acute management, haloperidol, benzodiazepines, and topical capsaicin have been used.

REFERENCES

1. Hameed M, Prasad S, Jain E, et al. Medical cannabis for chronic nonmalignant pain management. *Curr Pain Headache Rep*. 2023;27(4):57–63. doi:10.1007/s11916-023-01101-w.
2. Jeffers AM, Glantz S, Byers A, et al. Sociodemographic characteristics associated with and prevalence and frequency of cannabis use among adults in the US. *JAMA Netw Open*. 2021;4(11):e2136571. doi:10.1001/jamanetworkopen.2021.36571.
3. U.S. Department of Health and Human Services. Cannabis (marijuana) and cannabinoids: What you need to know. National Center for Complementary and Integrative Health. https://www.nccih.nih.gov/health/cannabis-marijuana-and-cannabinoids-what-you-need-to-know. Accessed 16 September 2024.
4. Andreae MH, Carter GM, Shaparin N, et al. Inhaled cannabis for chronic neuropathic pain: a meta-analysis of individual patient data. *J Pain*. 2015;16(12):1221–1232. doi:10.1016/j.jpain.2015.07.009.
5. Bradford AC, Bradford WD, Abraham A, et al. Association between US state medical cannabis laws and opioid prescribing in the medicare part D population. *JAMA Intern Med*. 2018;178(5):667–672. doi:10.1001/jamainternmed.2018.0266.
6. Bachhuber MA, Saloner B, Cunningham CO, et al. Medical cannabis laws and opioid analgesic overdose mortality in the United States, 1999–2010. *JAMA Intern Med*. 2014;174(10):1668–1673.
7. Bonn-Miller MO, Brunstetter M, Simonian A, et al. The long-term, prospective, therapeutic impact of cannabis on post-traumatic stress disorder. *Cannabis Cannabinoid Res*. 2022;7(2):214–223. doi:10.1089/can.2020.0056.
8. U.S. Food and Drug Administration. FDA and cannabis: research and drug approval process. https://www.fda.gov/news-events/public-health-focus/fda-and-cannabis-research-and-drug-approval-process. Accessed 16 September 2024.
9. Dharmapuri S, Miller K, Klein JD. Marijuana and the pediatric population. *Pediatrics*. 2020;146(2):e20192629. doi:10.1542/peds.2019-2629.
10. Matson TE, Carrell DS, Bobb JF, et al. Prevalence of medical cannabis use and associated health conditions documented in electronic health records among primary care patients in Washington state. *JAMA Netw Open*. 2021;4(5):e219375.

ADDITIONAL READING

- Bell AD, MacCallum C, Margolese S, et al. Clinical practice guidelines for cannabis and cannabinoid-based medicines in the management of chronic pain and co-occurring conditions. *Cannabis Cannabinoid Res*. 2024;9(2):669–687. doi:10.1089/can.2021.0156.
- Sazegar P. Cannabis essentials: tools for clinical practice. *Am Fam Physician*. 2021;104(6):598–608.

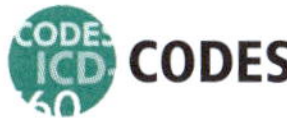

CODES

ICD10

F12.90 Cannabis use, unspecified, uncomplicated

CLINICAL PEARLS

- The clinical evidence supporting benefits of medical cannabis are suboptimal. Current evidence shows limited benefit in a number of conditions, including CINV, chronic pain, and epilepsy.
- Counseling of medical cannabis users will need to include advice to safeguard against accidental pediatric ingestion as well as short and long term potential complications.

M

MELANOMA

Ravjot Kaur Virdi, DO, MPH • Jon Richards, MD, PhD

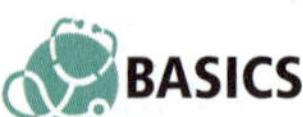

BASICS

DESCRIPTION

- Melanoma is a malignancy arising from melanocytes, the melanin-producing cells found throughout the body. Although melanocytes are widely distributed, malignant transformation commonly occurs in the skin. Therefore, melanoma is classified into the following categories:
  - Cutaneous melanoma: arises from melanocytes in the stratum basale of the epidermis
  - Noncutaneous melanoma
    - Mucosal melanoma: originates from melanocytes in the mucosal membrane, most commonly in the head, neck, anorectal, and genitourinary regions
    - Uveal melanoma: originates from melanocytes in the uvea
    - Melanoma of unknown primary: likely originates from a less common site of melanocytes
- Because cutaneous melanoma constitutes the vast majority of melanoma, this review focuses on cutaneous melanoma.
- Major histologic subtypes
  - Superficial spreading melanoma (70%): occurs on sun-exposed trunk/extremities, often from preexisting nevus; irregularly pigmented macule/plaques
  - Nodular melanoma (15–30%): occurs on sun-exposed trunk/extremities; blue-black or pink nodules; smooth, ulcerate/bleed easily
  - Lentigo maligna melanoma (<10%): occur on chronically sun-damaged face/forearms in elderly
  - Acral lentiginous melanoma (<5%): occurs on palms, soles, nails; variegated macules; more common in darker-skinned or Asian patients
- Uncommon subtypes
  - Amelanotic melanoma (2–10%): mimics benign skin conditions ("great pretender")
  - Spitzoid melanoma: resembles Spitz tumors; amelanotic or blue-black papules/nodules
  - Desmoplastic melanoma: occurs on sun-damaged skin in elderly; scar-like or mimics nonmelanoma cancers
  - Pigment synthesizing (animal-type) melanoma: slow-growing blue-black nodules; usually on extremities

EPIDEMIOLOGY

Incidence

- From 2018 to 2022, U.S. melanoma incidence was 21.9/100,000 men and women per year, with a median diagnosis age of 66 years.
- Rates rose ~1.2% annually between 2013 and 2022.
- Higher incidence in non-Hispanic White men >75 years of age

Prevalence

- Melanoma is the 5th most common U.S. cancer.
- In 2022, ~1.5 million people were living with melanoma.
- 2.2% lifetime risk of developing melanoma based on 2018–2021 data.

ETIOLOGY AND PATHOPHYSIOLOGY

- Etiology: UV damage (sunburns, tanning beds, poor photoprotection), dysplastic/giant congenital nevi, and genetic mutations
- Pathophysiology: genetic or UV injury drives uncontrolled melanocyte proliferation, progressing from radial to vertical growth with deeper invasion and metastasis

Genetics

- Predisposing inherited skin conditions: familial atypical multiple mole melanoma syndrome, xeroderma pigmentosum
- 50% of melanomas harbor BRAF mutations (most often V600E).
- CDKN2A mutations raise risk by 35 to 70 times.
- BRCA2 mutation increases risk by 2.5%.

RISK FACTORS

- Personal/family history of melanoma or other skin cancers
- Fair skin, freckles, light eyes, red/blond hair
- >50 melanocytic nevi or >5 cm congenital nevi
- Indoor tanning (WHO class 1 carcinogen)
- Chronic immunosuppression (leukemia, lymphoma, AIDS, posttransplant)
- Occupational ionizing radiation exposure

GENERAL PREVENTION

- Regular sunscreen (SPF 15 to 30+), protective clothing, sun avoidance
- Avoid tanning beds.
- For high-risk adults: periodic total-body skin exams
- Biopsy suspicious lesions (narrow excision, 1 to 3 mm margins)

COMMONLY ASSOCIATED CONDITIONS

- Other skin cancers: basal cell, squamous cell
- Autoimmune diseases: rheumatoid arthritis, lichen planus, lupus, scleroderma
- Parkinson disease

DIAGNOSIS

HISTORY

- Onset and changes in lesion (size, shape, color, bleeding, itching)
- Personal/family history of skin cancer
- Sunburns, tanning bed use, chronic sun exposure
- Immunosuppression
- Occupational exposures

PHYSICAL EXAM

- ABCDE: asymmetry, border irregularity with indistinct margins, color variegation, diameter ≥6 mm, evolution over time
- Ugly duckling sign: lesion unlike patient's other nevi
- Bleeding, ulceration, sensory change/itch
- Location: sun-exposed sites (White people); palms/soles/nails (African Americans)
- Ocular exams (iris/retina)

DIFFERENTIAL DIAGNOSIS

- Benign lesions: seborrheic keratosis, angiomas, dermatofibroma, irritated benign nevi, solar lentigo
- Precancerous lesions: actinic keratosis, dysplastic nevi, Bowen disease
- Other skin cancers: basal cell, squamous cell

DIAGNOSTIC TESTS & INTERPRETATION

Initial Tests (lab, imaging)

- Total body skin exam for suspicious lesions
- Dermoscopy: first-line diagnostic tool; increases sensitivity and specificity of clinical diagnosis (1)
  - Features: irregular pigment network, atypical dots/streaks, multiple asymmetric colors, blue-white veil, atypical vessels

Follow-Up Tests & Special Considerations

- Excisional biopsy (preferred): full thickness with 1 to 3 mm margin
- Incisional/partial biopsy: if complete excision is not feasible (face, palms/soles, nails, large lesions)

Diagnostic Procedures/Other

- Sentinel lymph node biopsy (SLNB) (1)
  - Indicated if ≥1 mm depth
  - Consider if 0.8 to 1.0 mm or <0.8 mm with high-risk features (ulceration, high mitotic rate, positive margin, lymphovascular invasion, age <40 years)
- Advanced workup if metastatic or positive SLNB
  - Labs: CBC, CMP, LDH
  - Imaging: CT/PET-CT chest, abdomen, pelvis, MRI brain, lymph node US, bone scan

Test Interpretation

- Diagnosis is based on architectural and cytologic features; immunohistochemistry/molecular tests if results are unclear
  - Poor prognosis features: increased Breslow depth, ulceration, high mitotic rate, microsatellitosis, positive margins, lymphovascular invasion
- American Joint Committee on Cancer tumor-node-metastasis (TNM) criteria for staging: considers tumor thickness (mm) and ulceration, nodal involvement, and distant metastasis

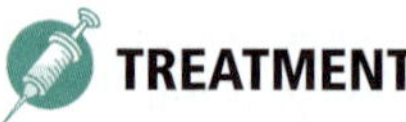

TREATMENT

GENERAL MEASURES

- Educate on self-skin exams, lymph node checks, photoprotection.
- Counsel increased risk of melanoma in family members.

MEDICATION

First Line

- Primary treatment: full surgical excision; curative in most stage I to II cases
- For high-risk (stage IIIB and C) melanoma: adjuvant nivolumab or pembrolizumab (anti-PD-1 monoclonal antibody) for 1 year

- For unresectable or metastatic melanoma, regimens include either/both of the following (2):
  - Immunotherapy combination therapy
    - Ipilimumab (anti-CTLA-3 monoclonal antibody) + nivolumab or pembrolizumab (anti-PD-1 monoclonal antibody)
    - Contraindications: severe asthma, unstable cardiovascular disease, prior anaphylaxis, autoimmune disease
    - Adverse effects: dermatitis, colitis, pneumonitis, endocrinopathies—managed with glucocorticoids
  - Targeted combination therapy for BRAF-mutated melanoma (BRAF + MEK inhibitors)
    - Vemurafenib (BRAF inhibitor) + cobimetinib (MEK inhibitor)
      - Contraindications: known hypersensitivity reaction
      - Adverse effects: diarrhea, nausea, rash, arthralgia, cardiomyopathy, hepatotoxicity, ocular toxicity, severe cutaneous reactions
    - Dabrafenib (BRAF inhibitor) + trametinib (MEK inhibitor)
      - Contraindications: known hypersensitivity reaction
      - Adverse effects: nausea, fatigue, hypertension, dermatologic reactions, fever, hemorrhage, thromboembolic events, pneumonitis, interstitial lung disease

Second Line

- Nivolumab and relatlimab (Opdualag): combination anti-PD-1 and anti-LAG-3 inhibitor
  - 18–20% overall response rate
  - Contraindications: known hypersensitivity reaction
  - Adverse effects: dermatitis, colitis, pneumonitis, endocrinopathies
- High-dose interleukin-2:
  - 10–15% durable response rate
  - Contraindications: significant cardiovascular, pulmonary, renal, hepatic, or CNS disease; poor performance status
  - Adverse effects: severe hemodynamic instability, renal/hepatic disease, infections
- Chemotherapy: various agents (dacarbazine, cisplatin, carboplatin/paclitaxel, etc.)
  - <20% overall response with median duration of 4 to 6 months
  - Contraindications: severe bone marrow suppression, uncontrolled infection, poor performance status, pregnancy
  - Adverse effects: myelosuppression, nausea/vomiting, alopecia, fatigue, neuropathy

ISSUES FOR REFERRAL

- Dermatology: lifelong follow-up for all patients
- Oncology: referral for high-risk stage II and all stage III to IV melanomas

ADDITIONAL THERAPIES

Talimogene laherparepvec (T-VEC): intralesional oncolytic HSV-1 expressing GM-CSF

- Mechanism of action: direct tumor lysis + immune activation
- Indication: unresectable, injectable cutaneous, subcutaneous, or nodal melanoma with limited visceral disease

SURGERY/OTHER PROCEDURES

- Surgical excision (standard of care) (1)
  - In situ: 0.5 cm margin
  - ≤1 mm thickness: 1 cm margin
  - 1.01 to 2.00 mm thickness: 1 to 2 cm margins
  - 2.01 to 4.00 mm thickness: 2 cm margins
  - ≥4 mm thickness: 2 cm margins
- Mohs surgery: sometimes utilized for in situ, but not routine for melanoma
- Radiation: palliative for localized disease, stereotactic radiosurgery for brain mets

COMPLEMENTARY & ALTERNATIVE MEDICINE

- Mind-body: Meditation, yoga, acupuncture improve quality of life, reduce stress, and manage side effects.
- Psychosocial: support groups, counseling, and integrative care teams enhance coping

ADMISSION, INPATIENT, AND NURSING CONSIDERATIONS

- Most patients are managed outpatient, but admit if:
  - Patient factors: advanced age, comorbidities, poor support, hospice needs
  - Clinical instability: sepsis/bleeding, neurologic compromise, organ dysfunction
  - Lab/radiology: severe hypercalcemia, cytopenias, liver failure, cord compression, brain edema/metastasis, malignant effusions
  - Toxicity: severe immune-related or BRAF/MEK inhibitor adverse effects
  - Perioperative: wide excisions, lymph node dissection, surgical complications
- Inpatient care: stabilization, targeted medications (IV steroids if immunotherapy is used, antiepileptics, bisphosphonates, antibiotics, analgesics), imaging (brain MRI to evaluate for metastasis), procedures as needed
- Nursing: Monitor vitals/neurologic status, manage symptoms, medications, and adherence.
- Discharge: instructions on medications, follow-ups, red flag symptoms (dyspnea, diarrhea, fever, bleeding, neurologic changes)

ONGOING CARE

FOLLOW-UP RECOMMENDATIONS

Patient Monitoring

- Stage IA: skin/lymph node exam every 6 month × 2 years and then annually
- Stage IB to IIA: exam every 4 to 6 months × 2 years and then annually
- Stage IIB to IIIA: exam every 3 to 4 months × 2 to 3 years, then every 6 months up to 5 years, and then annually; CT scan of chest/abdomen/pelvis every 6 months × 3 years and then annually; nodal US if SLNB + without complete dissection
- Stage IIC to IIID: exam every 3 months × 3 years and then every 6 months up to 5 years; CT scan of chest/abdomen/pelvis on same schedule; nodal US as above
- Metastatic disease: surveillance tailored to treatment response

DIET

- No melanoma-specific diet guidelines
- For patients on immunotherapy: Mediterranean diet may improve response rates and progression-free survival.

PATIENT EDUCATION

- Photoprotection: sunscreen, protective clothing, no tanning beds
- Skin checks: regular full-body exams monitoring for lesions using ABCDE criteria

PROGNOSIS

- Older age and male sex are associated with worse outcomes.
- Increased Breslow depth, higher number of positive lymph, elevated LDH predict poorer prognosis
- 5-year relative survival (2015 to 2021) in the United States: 94.7%
- Median age at death: 72 years

COMPLICATIONS

Metastatic spread to lymph nodes, liver, lung, brain, and bone

REFERENCES

1. Swetter SM, Tsao H, Bichakjian CK, et al. Guidelines of care for the management of primary cutaneous melanoma. *J Am Acad Dermatol*. 2019;80(1):208–250.
2. Seth R, Agarwala SS, Messersmith H, et al. Systemic therapy for melanoma: ASCO guideline update. *J Clin Oncol*. 2023;41(30):4794–4820. doi:10.1200/JCO.23.01136.

ADDITIONAL READING

National Cancer Institute. Cancer Stat Facts: Melanoma of the Skin. Surveillance, Epidemiology, and End Results Program. https://seer.cancer.gov/statfacts/html/melan.html.

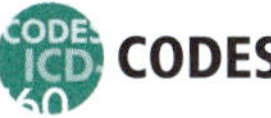

CODES

ICD10

- C43.9 Malignant melanoma of skin, unspecified
- C43.30 Malignant melanoma of unspecified part of face
- C43.4 Malignant melanoma of scalp and neck

CLINICAL PEARLS

- UV exposure and tanning beds are key modifiable risk factors. Use of sunscreen, protective clothing, and regular skin exams is proven preventive strategies.
- Superficial spreading melanoma accounts for ~70% of cases. Nodular, acral lentiginous, and amelanotic subtypes present atypically (pink nodules, nail lesions, "scar-like" plaques).
- In situ or thin (<1 mm) melanomas are often curable with surgical excision. Delayed diagnosis increases risk of nodal spread and mortality. Use ABCDE criteria for early identification.
- SLNB is indicated for melanomas ≥1 mm thick, or thinner lesions (<0.8 to 1.0 mm) with high-risk features. Early detection of nodal involvement guides staging and adjuvant therapy.
- Immunotherapy and BRAF/MEK inhibitors are frontline treatments that markedly improve survival but require vigilant monitoring for severe adverse effects.

MÉNIÈRE DISEASE

Sangili Chandran, MD • Mohammed Mirza, MD

BASICS

- An inner ear (labyrinthine) disorder characterized by recurrent attacks of hearing loss, tinnitus, vertigo, and sensations of aural fullness
- Ménière disease (MD) is a condition with at least two spontaneous episodes of vertigo lasting longer than 20 minutes but <12 hours, an audiogram showing evidence of low to medium frequency sensorineural hearing loss in one ear at any point in time, and fluctuating aural symptoms such as hearing loss, tinnitus, or aural fullness (1).
- Clinically, it involves the triad of:
  - Vertigo lasting 20 minutes to 12 hours
  - Audiometrically documented sensorineural hearing loss (predominantly low frequency)
  - Fluctuating aural symptoms (tinnitus or aural fullness)

DESCRIPTION

- Often unilateral initially; nearly half become bilateral over time.
- Severity and frequency of vertigo may diminish with time, but hearing loss is often progressive and/or fluctuating.
- Usually idiopathic (Ménière disease) but may be secondary to another condition causing endolymphatic hydrops (Ménière syndrome).
- There are five clinical subtypes of both unilateral and bilateral disease (1).
  - Type 1: refers to classic unilateral MD and metachronic bilateral MD (symptom onset in one ear followed by the other)
  - Type 2: refers to delayed unilateral MD (hearing loss onset preceding vertigo onset by months or years) or synchronic bilateral MD (simultaneous symptom onset in both ears)
  - Type 3: familial MD (most families have bilateral hearing loss, but unilateral patient may coexist in the same family)
  - Type 4: sporadic MD with migraine
  - Type 5: sporadic MD with an autoimmune disease
- System(s) affected: nervous
- Synonym(s): Ménière syndrome; endolymphatic hydrops

EPIDEMIOLOGY

- Predominant age of onset: 40 to 60 years
- Predominant gender: female > male, but overall fairly equal
- Race/ethnicity: White, Northern European > Black
- Incidence up to 150/100,000 per year

ETIOLOGY AND PATHOPHYSIOLOGY

- May be secondary to injury or other disorders (e.g., reduced middle ear pressure, allergy, endocrine disease, lipid disorders, vascular, viral, syphilis, autoimmune)
- Theories include increased pressure of the endolymph fluid due to increased fluid production or decreased resorption. This may be caused by endolymphatic sac pathology, abnormal development of the vestibular aqueduct, or inflammation caused by circulating immune complexes. Increased endolymph pressure may cause rupture of membranes and changes in endolymphatic ionic gradient.
- Others include vascular compromise, cochlear trauma, and viral infection or reactivation

Genetics

Family history in 10% of cases with an autosomal dominant inheritance pattern (2).

RISK FACTORS

May include

- Stress
- Allergy
- Increased salt, caffeine, alcohol, or nicotine
- Chronic exposure to loud noise
- Vascular abnormalities (including migraines)
- Viral exposures (herpes simplex virus)

GENERAL PREVENTION

Reduce known risk factors.

COMMONLY ASSOCIATED CONDITIONS

- Anxiety (secondary to the disabling symptoms)
- Migraines
- Hyperprolactinemia
- Hypothyroidism

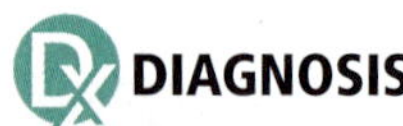

DIAGNOSIS

HISTORY

- Symptomatic episodes are typically spontaneous but may be preceded by an aura of increasing fullness in the ear and tinnitus. These may occur in clusters, with long periods of symptom-free remissions.
- Formal criteria for diagnosis from American Academy of Otolaryngology–Head and Neck Surgery:
  - At least two episodes of vertigo >20 minutes to 12 hours in duration (usually described as rotatory spinning or rocking sensations)
  - Tinnitus or aural fullness; symptoms can fluctuate.
  - Hearing loss: Audiometric testing shows low- to mid-frequency (sensorineural) hearing loss in affected ear on at least one occasion in correlation with an episode of vertigo (3).
  - During severe attacks pallor, sweating, nausea, vomiting, falling, prostration may occur (3).

PHYSICAL EXAM

- Physical exam rules out other conditions; no finding is unique to MD.
- Horizontal nystagmus may be seen during attacks.
- Otoscopy is typically normal.
- Triggering of attacks in the office with Dix-Hallpike maneuver suggests diagnosis of benign paroxysmal positional vertigo (BPPV), not MD as vertigo is typically of shorter duration and triggered by head movements in BPPV.

DIFFERENTIAL DIAGNOSIS

- Acoustic neuroma or other CNS tumor
- Multiple sclerosis
- Autoimmune inner ear disease
- Temporal bone fractures
- Syphilis
- Viral labyrinthitis
- Transient ischemic attack (TIA), migraine
- Diabetes or thyroid dysfunction
- Medication side effects

DIAGNOSTIC TESTS & INTERPRETATION

Testing to rule out other conditions

Initial Tests (lab, imaging)

- Consider serologic tests specific for *Treponema pallidum* in at-risk populations.
- Thyroid, fasting blood sugar, and lipid studies
- Consider MRI to rule out acoustic neuroma or other CNS pathology, including tumor, aneurysm, and multiple sclerosis.

Diagnostic Procedures/Other

- Audiometry using pure tone and speech to show low-frequency sensorineural (nerve) loss and impaired speech discrimination; usually shows low-frequency sensorineural hearing loss
- Tuning fork tests (i.e., Weber and Rinne), ABR, or MRI to rule out acoustic neuroma
- Electrocochleography may be useful to confirm etiology.
- Caloric testing: Reduced activity on either side is consistent with Ménière diagnosis but is not itself diagnostic.
- Head-impulse testing (4)[C]

Test Interpretation

- Cytochemical analysis can reveal altered AQP4 and AQP6 expression in the supporting cell, altered cochlin, and mitochondrial protein expression (5)[B].
- Familial MD has been associated with DTNA and FAM136A genes (6)[B].

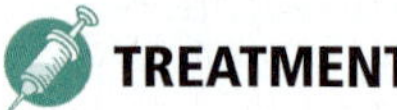

TREATMENT

- Medications are primarily for symptomatic relief of vertigo and nausea.
- During attacks, bed rest with eyes closed prevents falls. Attacks rarely last >4 hours.

GENERAL MEASURES

Salt restriction diet has remained the primary first-line treatment, although evidence of its validity remains inconclusive (7).

MEDICATION

First Line

- Acute attack: Initial goal is stabilization and symptom relief; for severe episodes
  - Benzodiazepines (such as diazepam): decrease vertigo and anxiety
  - Antihistamines (meclizine/dimenhydrinate): decrease vertigo and nausea
  - Anticholinergics (transdermal scopolamine): reduce nausea and emesis associated with motion sickness
  - Antidopaminergic agents (metoclopramide, promethazine): decrease nausea, anxiety
  - Rehydration therapy and electrolyte replacement
  - Steroid taper for acute hearing loss
- Maintenance (goal is to prevent/reduce attacks)
  - Lifestyle changes (e.g., low-salt diet) are needed.
  - Diuretics may help reduce attacks by decreasing endolymphatic pressure and volume; there is insufficient evidence to recommend routine use:
    - Hydrochlorothiazide; hydrochlorothiazide/triamterene (Dyazide, Maxzide)
    - Acetazolamide (Diamox)
  - Contraindications/warnings:
    - Atropine: cardiac disease, especially supraventricular tachycardia and other arrhythmias, prostatic enlargement
    - Scopolamine: children and elderly, prostatic enlargement
    - Diuretics: electrolyte abnormalities, renal disease
  - Precautions:
    - Sedating drugs should be used with caution, particularly in the elderly. Patients are cautioned not to operate motor vehicles or machinery. Atropine and scopolamine should be used with particular caution.
    - Diuretics: Monitor electrolytes.

Second Line

- Steroids, both intratympanic and systemic (PO or IV), have been used for longer treatment of hearing loss:
  - Addition of prednisone 30 mg/day to diuretic treatment reduced severity and frequency of tinnitus and vertigo in one pilot study.
  - Dexamethasone is practical to use due to better tolerance by patients, as methylprednisolone creates burning sensation in the middle ear mucosa.
- Evidence is lacking for routine use of famciclovir (Famvir); may improve hearing more than balance.

ISSUES FOR REFERRAL

- Consider ear, nose, throat/neurology referral.
- Patients should have formal audiometry to confirm hearing loss.

ADDITIONAL THERAPIES

- Application of intermittent pressures via a myringotomy using a Meniett device has been shown to relieve vertigo (8)[B]: safe; requires a long-term tympanostomy tube
- Vestibular rehabilitation may be beneficial for patients with persistent vestibular symptoms: safe and effective for unilateral vestibular dysfunction
- International consensus on treatment of MD suggests that vestibular rehabilitation should be offered as treatment option for patients between vertigo crises (9).

SURGERY/OTHER PROCEDURES

- Interventions that preserve hearing:
  - Endolymphatic sac surgery shown to be effective in controlling vertigo in 75% of patients with MD who failed medical therapy
  - Vestibular nerve section (intracranial procedure)
    - More invasive
    - Decreases vertigo and preserves hearing
    - Tympanostomy tube: may decrease symptoms by decreasing the middle ear pressure
- Interventions for patients with no serviceable hearing:
  - Labyrinthectomy: very effective at controlling vertigo but causes deafness
  - Vestibular neurectomy
  - Endoscopic vestibular nerve section
  - Cochlear implantation

ONGOING CARE

FOLLOW-UP RECOMMENDATIONS

Patient Monitoring

Due to the possibility of progressive hearing loss despite decrease in vertiginous attacks, it is important to monitor changes in hearing and to monitor for more serious underlying causes (e.g., acoustic neuroma).

DIET

Diet is usually not a factor, unless attacks are brought on by certain foods. Consider salt restriction.

PROGNOSIS

- Alert patients about the nature of alternating attacks and remission.
- Between attacks, patient may be fully active but is often limited due to fear or lingering symptoms. This can be severely disabling.
- 50% resolve spontaneously within 2 to 3 years.
- Some cases last >20 years.
- Severity and frequency of attacks diminish, but hearing loss is often progressive.
- 90% can be treated successfully with medication; 5–10% of patients require surgery for incapacitating vertigo.

COMPLICATIONS

Loss of hearing; injury during attack; inability to work

REFERENCES

1. Borowiec E, Crossley J, Hoa M. Understanding fluctuating hearing loss. *Hear J*. 2020;73(6):12–13.
2. Perez-Carpena P, Lopez-Escamez JA. Current understanding and clinical management of Ménière's disease: a systematic review. *Semin Neurol*. 2020;40(1):138–150.
3. Basura GJ, Adams ME Monfared A, et al. Clinical practice guideline: Ménière's disease executive summary. *Otolaryngol Head Neck Surg*. 2020;162(4):415–434.
4. Lee SU, Kim HJ, Koo JW, et al. Comparison of caloric and head-impulse tests during the attacks of Meniere's disease. *Laryngoscope*. 2017;127(3):702–708.
5. Ishiyama G, Lopez IA, Sepahdari AR, et al. Meniere's disease: histopathology, cytochemistry, and imaging. *Ann N Y Acad Sci*. 2015;1343:49–57.
6. Frejo L, Giegling I, Teggi R, et al. Genetics of vestibular disorders: pathophysiological insights. *J Neurol*. 2016;263(Suppl 1):S45–S53.
7. Shim T, Strum DP, Mudry A, et al. Hold the salt: history of salt restriction as a first-line therapy for Menière's disease. *Otol Neurotol*. 2020;41(6):855–859.
8. Ahsan SF, Standring R, Wang Y. Systematic review and meta-analysis of Meniett therapy for Meniere's disease. *Laryngoscope*. 2015;125(1):203–208.
9. Dunlap PM, Holmberg JM, Whitney SL. Vestibular rehabilitation: advances in peripheral and central vestibular disorders. *Curr Opin Neurol*. 2019;32(1):137–144.

SEE ALSO

- Hearing Loss; Labyrinthitis; Tinnitus
- Algorithm: Dizziness

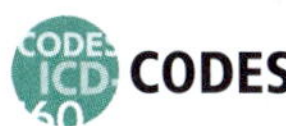

CODES

ICD10

- H81.03 Ménière's disease, bilateral
- H81.09 Ménière's disease, unspecified ear
- H81.0 Ménière's disease

CLINICAL PEARLS

- MD is characterized by vertigo (lasting 20 minutes to 12 hours), with associated hearing loss, tinnitus +/− aural fullness.
- There is a wide differential diagnosis for MD; therefore, one must fully investigate symptoms.
- Multiple medical, surgical, and rehabilitative treatments are available to decrease the severity and frequency of attacks.

M

MENINGITIS, BACTERIAL

Dylan G. Fedor, DO, BSc • Samuel Douglas Stringfellow, DO, BSc

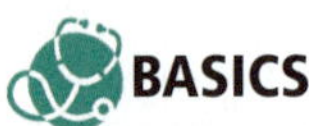

BASICS

DESCRIPTION
Bacterial infection of the meninges resulting in inflammation, pain, and systemic illness

EPIDEMIOLOGY
Predominant age: neonates, infants, and elderly; predominant sex: male = female

Incidence
- Varies by age and pathogen
- Overall incidence of bacterial meningitis ranges from ~1/100,000 in affluent countries to 80/100,000 in poorer countries. Incidence rises with age.

Prevalence
15,000 to 25,000 cases occur annually in the United States.

ETIOLOGY AND PATHOPHYSIOLOGY
Community-acquired bacterial meningitis in adults is most commonly due to *Streptococcus pneumoniae* and *Neisseria meningitidis*. Nosocomial or postsurgical meningitis occurs after manipulation of the central nervous system (CNS).

- Newborns (<2 months): *Escherichia coli*, *Streptococcus agalactiae s*
- Infants and children: *S. pneumoniae*, *N. meningitidis*, *Haemophilus influenzae*
- Adolescents and young adults: *N. meningitidis*, *S. pneumoniae*
- Immunocompromised adults: *S. pneumoniae*, *Listeria monocytogenes*, gram-negative bacilli such as *Pseudomonas aeruginosa*; mixed bacterial infection in <1% of cases
- Older adults: *S. pneumoniae*, *N. meningitidis*, *L. monocytogenes*
- Gram-negative bacilli: *E. coli*, *Klebsiella*, *Enterobacter*, *P. aeruginosa*

Genetics
Some Native American populations appear to have genetic susceptibility to invasive disease.

RISK FACTORS
Those at risk include:

- Household or close contacts of case patients; immunocompromised (including HIV, asplenia, or patients taking eculizumab, ravulizumab), alcohol use disorder, diabetes, pregnancy, elderly; neurosurgical procedure/head injury; close living quarters (dormitories or military barracks); and work exposures
- Neonates: prematurity, low birth weight, premature rupture of membranes, maternal peripartum infection, and urinary tract abnormalities, untreated maternal group B *Streptococcus*; anatomical abnormality of nasopharynx and subarachnoid space (congenital, trauma), dural fistula
- Parameningeal source: otitis, sinusitis, mastoiditis, skull fracture; complement deficiencies, properdin, factor H, and factor D

GENERAL PREVENTION
Vaccines play a crucial part in meningitis and overall disease prevention. Meningitis caused by *H. influenzae* type B has decreased following routine vaccination. Meningococcal conjugate vaccine (MenACWY) with booster has decreased meningococcal disease 4-fold. The pneumococcal conjugate vaccine has decreased incidence rates of *S. pneumoniae* by 41–97% in children and older adults. Chemoprophylaxis is recommended for close contacts of meningococcal meningitis. Aseptic techniques for head wounds, skull fractures, and surgeries that could infect the cerebrospinal fluid (CSF).

COMMONLY ASSOCIATED CONDITIONS
Alcohol use disorder, elderly, infancy, diabetes mellitus, multiple myeloma, head trauma, immunocompromise, coma, seizures, sepsis, sinusitis, CSF shunt/drain, asplenia, cancer, sickle cell anemia

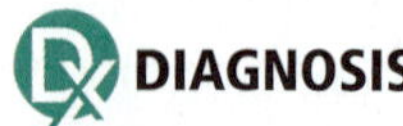

DIAGNOSIS

HISTORY
- Antecedent upper respiratory infection, sinusitis, and some sort of head trauma.
- Review of systems (ROS): fever, headache, vomiting, photophobia, seizures, confusion, nausea, rigors, sweats, and weakness
- Elderly: Findings often subtle—often includes confusion.
- Infants: irritability, lethargy, poor feeding; food exposures, and birth history

PHYSICAL EXAM
95% of patients will present with at least two of the following: headache, fever, neck stiffness, and altered mental status (1)

- Meningismus; focal neurologic deficits and papilledema
- Meningococcal rash: starts off as macular and erythematous then progresses to petechial or purpuric; purpura fulminans lesions should raise suspicion for meningococcus.
- Brudzinski sign: Passive flexion of neck elicits involuntary flexing of knees in supine position (sensitivity 5%).
- Kernig sign: resistance or pain with passive knee extension following 90-degree hip flexion in supine position (sensitivity 30%)
- Late signs and symptoms: hemiparesis, stroke, cognitive impairment, coma, epilepsy, hearing loss, and permanent visual impairment

DIFFERENTIAL DIAGNOSIS
- Bacteremia, sepsis, brain abscess, seizure disorder, other nonbacterial meningitides; aseptic meningitis, stroke, Lyme disease, leptospirosis, subarachnoid hemorrhage, central nervous vasculitides
- Inflammatory noninfectious: Behçet disease, systemic lupus erythematosus (SLE), sarcoidosis, migraine

DIAGNOSTIC TESTS & INTERPRETATION
CSF analysis (culture, PCR) are gold standard.

Initial Tests (lab, imaging)
- Obtain a head CT scan before lumbar puncture (LP) if there are focal neurologic findings, papilledema, or altered mentation. This helps to assess the risk for herniation.
- If signs of elevated intracranial pressure (ICP) is not present, waiting for head CT scan head before LP can lead to patient harm (1).
- CSF should be sent for Gram stain and culture, cell count with differential, protein, and glucose and lactate concentration if obtained before antibiotics (2).
- Complete blood count (CBC), complete metabolic panel (CMP), blood cultures, coagulation studies, chest radiograph, C-reactive protein (CRP)

Follow-Up Tests & Special Considerations
Do not delay initiation of empiric antibiotics and dexamethasone once blood cultures are obtained. There is a 13–30% increase in mortality every hour antibiotics are delayed (1).

Diagnostic Procedures/Other
- Prompt LP and empiric antibiotics.
- LP contraindications: signs of increased ICP (decerebrate posturing, papilledema), skin infection at site of LP, CT or MRI evidence of obstructive hydrocephalus, cerebral edema, herniation

Test Interpretation
- Bacterial meningitis: opening pressure >200 mm H_2O; CSF protein is usually high; CSF glucose is usually low; cell counts >1,000 cells/μL, predominantly neutrophils (neutrophilic pleocytosis)
- Suspect ruptured brain abscess when WBC count is usually high (>100,000).
- Reserve bacterial antigen tests for cases where initial CSF Gram stain is negative and CSF culture is negative at 48 hours.

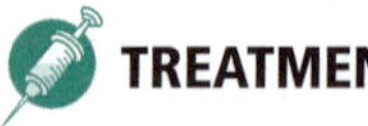

TREATMENT

GENERAL MEASURES
Initiate empiric antibiotic therapy immediately after LP (goal is <1 hour after presentation). If head CT scan is needed, initiate antibiotic therapy immediately after blood cultures (blood cultures > antibiotics > CT > LP) (1). Watch for seizures and aspiration precautions.

MEDICATION
Empiric antibiotic IV therapy with dexamethasone for known or suspected *S. pneumoniae* or *H. influenzae* type b meningitis until culture results are available (2)

First Line
- Neonates (3): ampicillin: 150 mg/kg/day divided q8h and cefotaxime: 100 mg/kg/day divided q8h
- Infants >4 weeks of age: ceftriaxone: 100 mg/kg/day divided q12–24h or cefotaxime 300 mg/kg/day divided q6–8h and vancomycin: 60 mg/kg/day divided q6h

- Adults (1),(3)
  - Immunocompetent: cefotaxime: 2 g IV q4–6h or ceftriaxone: 2 g IV q12h
    - In countries with ceftriaxone resistance rates >1%, add vancomycin 15 to 20 mg/kg IV q8–12h (target trough level 15 to 20 mcg/ml).
    - In adults over >50 years of age, add ampicillin 2 g IV q4h or meropenem 2 g IV q8h.
  - Immunocompromised: vancomycin 15 to 20 mg/kg IV q8–12h, plus ampicillin 2 g IV q4h, plus either cefepime 2 g IV q8h or meropenem 2 g IV q8h.
  - If meropenem is used, ampicillin is not needed. If *Listeria* is identified then ampicillin/penicillin and gentamicin should be used. If there is a severe allergy to ampicillin/penicillin then meropenem can be used.
  - Penicillin-allergic patients:
    - If penicillin reaction was mild, can consider ceftriaxone; if there is a cephalosporin reaction and there were no signs of anaphylaxis, can consider meropenem.
    - Severe allergy: vancomycin: 15 to 20 mg/kg q8–12h (goal trough of 15 to 20) plus moxifloxacin 400 mg IV daily
- Treatment duration (2):
  - *S. pneumoniae*: 10 to 14 days
  - *N. meningitidis*, and *H. influenzae*: 7 days
  - Group B *Streptococcus*, *E. coli*, *L. monocytogenes*: 14 to 21 days
  - Neonates: 12 to 21 days or at least 14 days after sterile CSF culture
- Corticosteroids:
  - Early treatment with dexamethasone 0.15 mg/kg IV q6h for 2 to 4 days given with or up to 20 minutes before antibiotics; continue in adults if CSF Gram stain is gram-positive diplococcus, if cultures are growing *S. pneumoniae*, or *H. influenzae* type B (3)[A]. Discontinue if *Listeria* is identified.
  - Dexamethasone has shown decreased hearing loss and neurologic sequela. It is questionable if it helps with mortality, and more research is needed. It is recommended in patients over 6 weeks given at the same time antibiotics are given (1).

Second Line

- Antipseudomonal penicillins should be given in combination with other appropriate agents.
- Aztreonam 2 g IV q6–8h; fluoroquinolones (e.g., moxifloxacin or levofloxacin) IV 400 mg q24h or 750 IV q24h; meropenem IV 2 g q8h

ISSUES FOR REFERRAL

Consultation from infectious disease and/or critical care specialist

ADDITIONAL THERAPIES

Chemoprophylaxis in close contacts include household members, roommates/dorm mates, intimate contacts, contacts at a childcare center, exposed military recruits; travelers who had direct contact with respiratory or oral secretions from an index patient

SURGERY/OTHER PROCEDURES

Postsurgical bacterial meningitis, or associated with head trauma or shunt: empiric cover for MRSA and aerobic gram-negative organisms, such as *Pseudomonas* spp. and *Enterobacteriaceae*.

ADMISSION, INPATIENT, AND NURSING CONSIDERATIONS

- Bacterial meningitis requires hospitalization. ICU monitoring may be needed. Patients with suspected meningococcal infection require respiratory isolation for 24 hours.
- Droplet precautions of hospitalized patients as soon as diagnosis is suspected through the first 24 hours of antimicrobial therapy.

ONGOING CARE

FOLLOW-UP RECOMMENDATIONS

Patient Monitoring

- Brainstem auditory—evoked response hearing test for infants before hospital discharge
- Vaccinations per CDC recommendations:
  - **Meningococcal vaccination**:
    - All 11 to 12 years old should get a MenACWY vaccine, with a booster dose at 16 years old. Teens and young adults (16 to 23 years old) may get a MenB vaccine.
    - A MenABCWY vaccine is now available but should only be given if MenACWY and MenB would be given at the same visit.
  - Pneumococcal vaccination:
    - PCV15 or PCV20: Infants and young children need 4 doses of pneumococcal conjugate vaccine, at 2, 4, 6, and 12 to 15 months of age.
    - Between 2 and 65 years of age: may qualify for additional vaccinations with PCV20, PCV21, or PPSV23 depending on their condition; qualifying conditions include smoking, chronic lung disease, alcoholism, injection drug use, homelessness, and immunocompromised status.
    - Age >49 years: should receive a PCV15, PCV20, or PCV21 if they have never been vaccinated or vaccination status is unknown; if PCV15 is used will need PPSV23 1 year later.
    - Age > 65 years: If patient has received PCV13 or PPSV23 (over 1 year ago) they would qualify for PCV20 or PCV21. If they have received PCV15, PCV20, or PCV21 they do not need an additional booster.
- Prophylaxis: During 2019 to 2020, 11 meningococcal isolates from United States patients had mutations conferring penicillin or ciprofloxacin resistance.
  - Per CDC recommendations chemoprophylaxis for close contacts of patient with confirmed meningococcal meningitis (please use local antibiotic gram for choosing agent if available):
    - Rifampin: 600 mg PO BID for 2 days
    - Ciprofloxacin: 500 mg PO for 1 dose
    - Ceftriaxone: 250 mg IM for 1 dose
    - Azithromycin: 500 mg PO single dose for ciprofloxacin-resistance *N. meningitidis* exposure (not first line)

DIET

Regular, as tolerated, except with syndrome of inappropriate secretion of antidiuretic hormone (SIADH).

PROGNOSIS

- Mortality: pneumococcal meningitis as high as 30%, and meningococcal meningitis as high as 10% (1)
- Mortality rate of untreated disease approaches 100%.

COMPLICATIONS

- Complications depend on available resources, bacteria, and if dexamethasone was used.
- Up to 50% in children and up to 32% of adults develop long-term neurologic complications (cognitive impairment) after bacterial meningitis.
- Cerebrovascular complications: subdural effusion or empyema, stroke, septic sinus thrombosis, intracranial hypertension, cerebral edema, temporal lobe or cerebellar herniation, obstructive hydrocephalus, visual impairment, learning deficits, sensorineural hearing loss cranial nerve palsies
- Other: septic shock, microvascular thrombosis, DIC, depression, SIADH, purpura fulminans

REFERENCES

1. Pajor MJ, Long B, Koyfman A, et al. High risk and low prevalence diseases: adult bacterial meningitis. *Am J Emerg Med*. 2023;65:76–83. doi:10.1016/j.ajem.2022.12.042.
2. World Health Organization. Who guidelines on meningitis diagnosis, treatment and care. Geneva: World Health Organization; 2025. https://www.who.int/publications/i/item/9789240108042. Accessed October 2, 2025.
3. Hasbun R. Progress and challenges in bacterial meningitis: a review [published correction appears in *JAMA*. 2023;329(6):515. doi:10.1001/jama.2023.0570]. *JAMA*. 2022;328(21):2147–2154. doi:10.1001/jama.2022.20521.

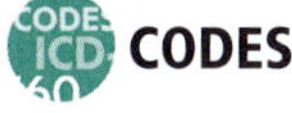

CODES

ICD10

- G00.9 Bacterial meningitis, unspecified
- G00.2 Streptococcal meningitis
- G00.8 Other bacterial meningitis

CLINICAL PEARLS

- Initiate empiric antibiotic therapy as soon as possible (<1 hour after presentation is goal).
- If LP is delayed, draw blood cultures, start antibiotics and dexamethasone.
- Tailor antibiotics once microbiologic diagnosis is established.

M

MENINGITIS, VIRAL

Zoe J. Foster, MD, FAAFP • Jeffrey Wisinski, DO

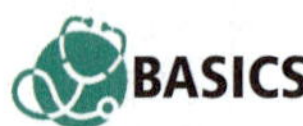

BASICS

DESCRIPTION

- A clinical syndrome characterized by fever and signs/symptoms of acute meningeal inflammation (including but not limited to headache, photophobia, neck stiffness, and/or nausea and vomiting)
- Viral meningitis (VM) is the most common cause of aseptic (nonbacterial) meningitis.

EPIDEMIOLOGY

Incidence

- Most common form of meningitis
- Peaks summer to fall in temperate climates (but is year round in subtropical or tropical climates)
  - Nonpolio enteroviruses are the most common cause of VM; estimated 75,000 VM cases caused by enterovirus annually in the United States
  - Herpes simplex-2 and varicella zoster virus (VZV) are important causes in adults (particularly immunosuppressed individuals).

Prevalence

Varies by geographical location and causative pathogen

ETIOLOGY AND PATHOPHYSIOLOGY

- In immunocompetent hosts, VM is a rare complication of an acute viral infection like gastroenteritis, mumps, adenovirus, coxsackievirus, herpes simplex virus (HSV), VZV, and arthropod-borne viruses.
  - Case reports indicate that SARS-CoV-2, rotavirus A, and hepatitis E can cause VM.
  - In immunocompromised hosts, viral pathogens may include cytomegalovirus (CMV) and Epstein-Barr virus (EBV).
- 25–60% of VM cases are caused by nonpolio human enteroviruses, typically transmitted via the fecal-oral route.
- Mosquito-borne viruses include West Nile, Zika, Chikungunya, dengue, St. Louis encephalitis virus, and Eastern equine encephalitis virus; tick-borne viruses include: Powassan virus, Colorado tick fever virus, tick-borne encephalitis virus
- Recurrent benign lymphocytic (Mollaret) meningitis is generally associated with HSV-2 (80% of cases).

Genetics

None identified

RISK FACTORS

- Age (most common in children <5 years)
  - Babies <1 month of age are more likely to have severe disease.
- Immunocompromised host (patients more susceptible to CMV, HSV, and EBV)
- Diabetes, chronic renal failure (patients more susceptible to VZV)
- Close contacts of people with VM are unlikely to get VM, but may get the primary viral syndrome.

Geriatric Considerations

Cases of VM in the elderly are rare (most common cause is VZV, HSV); consider alternative diagnoses (e.g., cancer, medication-induced aseptic meningitis) (1).

GENERAL PREVENTION

- Handwashing and general hygiene procedures
- Avoid sharing drinks/cups and silverware with others, especially those who are ill.
- Avoid exposure to mosquitos and ticks; if outdoors, recommend use of appropriate clothing, DEET, and mosquito nets.
- Ensure immunizations are up-to-date.

COMMONLY ASSOCIATED CONDITIONS

Encephalitis; myopericarditis; neonatal enteroviral sepsis; meningoencephalitis; flaccid paralysis

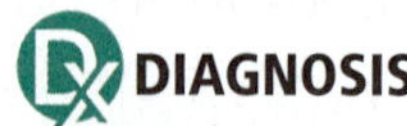

DIAGNOSIS

HISTORY

- Predominant adult symptoms include acute onset (hours to days) of:
  - Fever (incidence varies by virus; 65–83% in enterovirus, 54–98% in mumps, 6–52% in HSV)
  - Headache (prominent early symptom); photophobia (mainly with enterovirus, 79–85% of cases; 33–64% in HSV; 7% in mumps)
  - Myalgias/arthralgias (88% in enterovirus; 50% in HSV; 14–21% in mumps)
  - Nausea/vomiting, malaise
  - Nuchal rigidity (55–69% in enterovirus; 22–71% in HSV; 8–85% in mumps)
    - Altered mental status, seizure, or focal neurologic deficits should prompt consideration of alternative diagnoses.
- "Classic triad" (headache, neck stiffness, photophobia) is present in <1/3 of cases.
- In infants, nonspecific symptoms are more common, including poor feeding, vomiting, lethargy, fever (most common), and irritability (most common).
- Additional historical elements:
  - Travel history and outdoor activities; sexual history (e.g., HSV, HIV); immunocompromised host, including solid-organ transplant and HIV (CMV, HSV, adenovirus, West Nile virus); history of VZV infection; immunization status (mumps, influenza, VZV)

PHYSICAL EXAM

- Vital signs: fever, tachycardia, tachypnea, hypotension
- Neurologic:
  - Lack of mental status changes (if present, consider alternative diagnoses)
  - Photophobia
  - Meningeal signs (neither sensitive nor specific)
    - Nuchal rigidity; Brudzinski sign (neck flexion elicits involuntary hip and knee flexion in supine patient) and Kernig sign (resistance to knee extension following flexion of hips to 90 degrees) are poorly sensitive (~5%) in patients with meningitis.
    - Jolt accentuation test: rapid horizontal rotation of the head accentuates headache (of questionable utility in diagnosis of meningitis given low sensitivity and specificity) (2)[C]
  - Asymmetric flaccid paralysis is seen in West Nile virus infection (1)[C].
- HEENT:
  - Parotitis (in mumps infection); herpangina (coxsackievirus A); bulging fontanelle (in infants); generalized lymphadenopathy (EBV, HIV)
- Dermatology:
  - Vesicular rash of hand, foot and mouth disease (coxsackievirus)
  - Generalized maculopapular rash
    - Presence of a palpable petechial/purpuric rash should prompt consideration of bacterial meningitis (BM).
- Abdomen: splenomegaly (in EBV); abdominal pain

DIFFERENTIAL DIAGNOSIS

- BM; fungal meningitis (consider if immunocompromised; agents include *Coccidioides* and *Cryptococcus neoformans*) (3)[C]
- Other infectious agents (tuberculosis; syphilis; leptospirosis; Lyme disease; ehrlichiosis; amebiasis) (3)[C]
- Parameningeal infections (e.g., subdural empyema), encephalitis, postinfectious encephalomyelitis, viral syndrome (e.g., influenza)
- Leukemia, lymphoma, or other neoplastic disease (including metastasis)
- Migraine/tension headache, acute metabolic encephalopathy, postoperative aseptic meningitis
- Drug-induced (chemical) meningitis (NSAIDs, TMP/SMX, amoxicillin, TNF-α inhibitors, lamotrigine, IVIG, and monoclonal antibodies) (1)[C]
- Brain/epidural abscess, inflammatory disorders (e.g., Behçet, sarcoidosis, SLE) (1)[C]

DIAGNOSTIC TESTS & INTERPRETATION

Initial Tests (lab, imaging)

- Serum labs: CBC, BMP, procalcitonin (PCT)/C-reactive protein, blood cultures (3)[C]
  - CBC: normal or mildly elevated WBC
  - BMP: CSF glucose levels should be compared to plasma levels.
  - PCT/C-reactive protein: should be normal in VM (Consider BM in adults when serum PCT is elevated.)
  - Blood cultures: should be negative in VM
- Lumbar puncture (LP):
  - LP differentiates VM from BM
    - Do not delay empiric antibiotics if there is concern for BM. Consider validated clinical decision-making tool (e.g., BM score) in children to calculate risk of BM.
  - Contraindications/risks:
    - Signs/symptoms of increased intracranial pressure (focal neurologic findings, papilledema, altered mental status, new-onset seizure), impaired cellular immunity, local infection over potential LP site, suspected epidural abscess, use of anticoagulation or potential coagulopathy, and possibility of cardiorespiratory compromise due to patient positioning during procedure
      - Consider CT scan if clinical concern for increased intracranial pressure.
    - Procedural risks include cerebral herniation, post-LP headache, bleeding, infection, and pain.

- CSF analysis:
  - Opening pressure: should be normal
  - Ensure enough CSF volume is drawn and saved so that additional workup (i.e., PCR, NAAT) can be done if preliminary CSF analysis is not diagnostic.
  - Cell count/differential:
    - 100 to 1,000 WBC/μL (can be higher in enteroviral meningitis)
    - Lymphocyte predominance (in early infection, may be PMN predominance)
    - RBCs suggest traumatic tap, but may be seen in HSV meningitis/encephalitis.
  - CSF glucose: usually normal (may have mild decrease in mumps or HIV)
  - CSF protein: normal to mildly elevated
  - CSF lactate: normal (if elevated >4.2 mmol/L, highly suggestive of BM; levels less reliable if antibiotics have been started prior to LP)
- Gram stain: should be negative for bacteria
- CSF culture:
  - Gold standard for diagnosis of BM; should be negative for bacterial pathogens in VM
- PCR/NAAT and metagenomic next-generation sequencing (mNGS) (3)[C]:
  - Improved sensitivity/specificity
  - Useful for rapid identification of multiple possible pathogens (bacteria, viruses, fungi)—sensitivity for pathogens varies by test; may allow early discontinuation of empiric therapies
  - Results of mNGS should be interpreted in the context of traditional microbiology results. Some mNGS may not reliably detect RNA viruses. There is a risk for false positive results.
- CSF IgM antibodies for arboviruses (4)[C]

Follow-Up Tests & Special Considerations

Disorders that may alter lab results:

- Diabetes: Consider current blood sugar level to correlate with CSF glucose level.
- Neurologic diseases (e.g., history of stroke or transient ischemic attack, intracranial neoplasm, demyelinating disease)

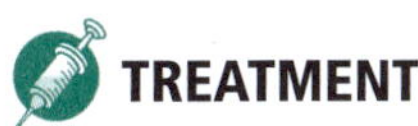

TREATMENT

GENERAL MEASURES

Management includes supportive care (e.g., pain control, IV fluids) and low threshold for empiric antibiotics for BM pending laboratory results (2)[C].

MEDICATION

First Line

- Antipyretics/analgesics (Adult doses are presented; titrate doses to pain relief.)
  - Acetaminophen (Tylenol) 500 to 1,000 mg PO q8h; 325 to 650 mg PR q4–6h (limit 3 g/24 hours)
  - Ibuprofen 400 to 800 mg PO q8h
  - Naproxen 550 mg PO BID
  - Consider short term opioids if pain uncontrolled.
- Antiemetics
  - Ondansetron (Zofran) 4 to 8 mg IV q8h
  - Promethazine (Phenergan) 12.5 to 25.0 mg PO/PR/IM/IV q4–6h (Consider maximum dose of 50 mg/24 hours to limit side effects.)
- Antiviral agents (2)[C]
  - Empiric acyclovir at 10 mg/kg IV q8h (adult dose) for patients with CSF pleocytosis, negative Gram stain, and suspicion for HSV while awaiting results of definitive (e.g., HSV or VZV PCR) testing
    - Immunocompetent patients with HSV meningitis improve with or without antiviral therapy and can be treated with supportive care alone.
    - VM due to HIV will resolve with supportive care alone.
- Antibiotics (targeted to most likely pathogen)
  - Not indicated for treatment of VM
  - Empiric treatment is reasonable while ruling out BM. Initiate following blood cultures and LP if possible. Consider, especially in elderly, those pretreated with antibiotics, ill appearing, and immunocompromised patients.
    - If very low risk for BM, treat symptomatically and observe in the inpatient setting pending laboratory results.
- Corticosteroids (2)[C]
  - Not recommended in VM (recommended as adjunctive treatment in BM)

ISSUES FOR REFERRAL

For patients with known CSF shunts/drains, recent neurosurgery/trauma, or intrathecal pumps in the setting of possible VM or BM, an emergent neurosurgical referral is warranted (3)[C].

ADMISSION, INPATIENT, AND NURSING CONSIDERATIONS

- Initial inpatient management includes pain management and empiric antibiotics (pending lab results); IV fluids (based on hydration status and clinical presentation); neurologic monitoring for changes in mental status, fever, neck stiffness, headache; contact precautions and private room until BM ruled out
- Discharge depends on clinical parameters (dehydration, emesis, pain control, functional level, social circumstances, and ability to follow up). VM in stable patients can be managed in the outpatient setting.

ONGOING CARE

FOLLOW-UP RECOMMENDATIONS

- Close follow-up to ensure resolution of all symptoms.
  - A small portion of adults suffer from ongoing neuropsychological morbidities (cognitive dysfunction, sleep disturbances, decreased psychomotor speed, impaired visuoconstructive functions, and impaired executive functioning) following VM, with the degree of disability dependent on the causative virus.
- Developmental surveillance after VM in children as children are more likely to have severe complications of disease.

Patient Monitoring

- Residual symptoms (subjective cognitive impairment, fatigue, excessive sleepiness) are common following VM.
- Monitor for neurologic complications:
  - Seizures, altered mental status, new onset weakness; assess ability to have companion monitor change in mental/neurologic status if patient discharged.

DIET

Push fluids; diet as tolerated

PATIENT EDUCATION

- Discuss very low probability of transmission to close contacts. Encourage handwashing.
- Recurrence of headache, myalgia, and weakness is possible over 2 to 3 weeks.

PROGNOSIS

- Recovery generally within 7 to 10 days
  - In some patients, return to work may be delayed and quality of life may take months to return to baseline, as headaches and other neurologic symptoms may intermittently persist for weeks to months.
- There is a low mortality rate from VM.
- Very young children and some adults suffer from prolonged neuropsychological disabilities as a result of VM.

COMPLICATIONS

- Common: fatigue, irritability, muscle weakness
- Rare: neuropsychological problems and developmental delay

REFERENCES

1. Gundamraj V, Hasbun R. Viral meningitis and encephalitis: an update. *Curr Opin Infect Dis*. 2023;36(3):177–185. doi:10.1097/QCO.0000000000000922.
2. Kohil A, Jemmieh S, Smatti MK, et al. Viral meningitis: an overview. *Arch Virol*. 2021;166(2):335–345.
3. Poplin V, Boulware DR, Bahr NC. Methods for rapid diagnosis of meningitis etiology in adults. *Biomark Med*. 2020;14(6):459–479.
4. Xu H, Chen P, Guo S, et al. Progress in etiological diagnosis of viral meningitis. *Front Neurol*. 2023;14:1193834. doi:10.3389/fneur.2023.1193834.

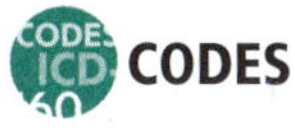

CODES

ICD10

- A87.9 Viral meningitis, unspecified
- A87.1 Adenoviral meningitis
- A87.0 Enteroviral meningitis

CLINICAL PEARLS

- VM cannot be reliably distinguished from BM based on clinical findings alone.
- Hospitalize potential meningitis cases for evaluation and treatment with broad-spectrum antibiotics until BM has been ruled out.
- VM is more common than BM, especially when vaccination rates are high.
- Morbidity and mortality with VM is low.

M

MENINGOCOCCAL DISEASE

Clare Donahue, DO • Hieu Nguyen, DO

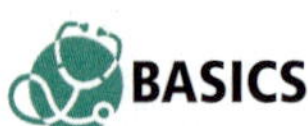

BASICS

DESCRIPTION

- Acute, rapidly progressive (within hours) infection caused by *Neisseria meningitidis*, presenting as meningitis and/or meningococcemia
- Can affect young, previously well individuals, including infants
- Fever, nausea, vomiting, headache, decreased ability to concentrate, and myalgias are common early symptoms.
- Petechial rash on the trunk/lower extremities occurs in >50% of cases.
- High morbidity and mortality, especially for meningococcemia, if not promptly recognized and treated; case fatality rate is 10–15%. Patients who survive have long-term sequelae in 10–20% of cases.

EPIDEMIOLOGY

Incidence

- 0.1–1.5/100,000 in developed countries; higher in endemic regions
- Most common in adolescents and young adults, followed by infants aged <1 year
  - 35–40% of cases occur in children aged <5 years.
- Outbreaks occur in close-contact settings (daycare, dormitories, military barracks).
- Disease occurs year round, but in temperate climates, will peak in winter/early spring

ETIOLOGY AND PATHOPHYSIOLOGY

- *N. meningitidis* is a fastidious, aerobic, gram-negative diplococcus with at least 13 serotypes.
- Virulence factors (polysaccharide capsule, lipooligosaccharide endotoxin, pili) enable epithelial invasion, bloodstream dissemination, and blood-brain barrier penetration. Virulence factors (polysaccharide capsule, lipooligosaccharide endotoxin, pili) enable epithelial invasion, bloodstream dissemination, and blood-brain barrier penetration.
- Humans are the only known reservoir for *N. meningitidis*.
- Nasopharyngeal colonization is a prerequisite for the development of systemic infection.
- Six serogroups in the United States are responsible for most cases of clinical disease: A, B, C, W, X, and Y.
  - B: predominant in infants and young adults
  - Y: resurgence in United States since 2021

RISK FACTORS

- <1 year of age
- Immunocompromised states
  - Complement deficiency
  - Asplenia
  - HIV
  - Solid organ transplant
  - Patients on immunosuppressive therapies
- Crowded living conditions (e.g., dormitories, military barracks, daycare)
- Exposure to active/passive tobacco smoke

GENERAL PREVENTION

- Vaccines (1)[A]
- Meningococcal ACWY (MenACWY):
  - All adolescents should be vaccinated at age 11 to 12 years, with a booster at age 16 years.
  - Children (2 months and older) and adults at increased risk should receive a 2 to 4 dose primary series and regular boosters.
  - People exposed to outbreaks or traveling to areas with high rates of serogroups A, C, W, or Y should also be vaccinated.
  - Protective antibody levels achieved within 7 to 10 days of immunization
- Meningococcal B (MenB):
  - Recommended for individuals 10 years and older at increased risk, including those with occupational exposure
  - Shared decision-making advised for healthy teens and young adults aged 16 to 23 years (preferred vaccination at ages 16 to 18 years)
  - Required for Hajj pilgrims age >2 years
  - Recommended for travelers to sub-Saharan Africa's "meningitis belt"
- Pentavalent vaccine (MenABCWY) can be used if an individual ≥10 years of age requires MenACWY and MenB vaccination at the same visit.

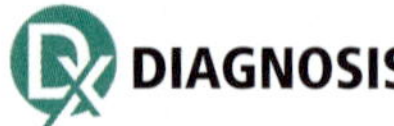

DIAGNOSIS

HISTORY

Symptoms

- Early symptoms (first 6 to 9 hours): flulike illness (sudden onset of fever, chills, nausea, vomiting, myalgias, and/or nonsuppurative sore throat) (2)[C]
- Sore throat may be mistaken for streptococcal disease (strep throat).
- Myalgias, fever, and chills may be mistaken for influenza.
- Meningitis symptoms: headache, neck stiffness, photophobia, altered mental status (3)[A]
  - Classic meningitis triad (fever, neck stiffness, altered mental status) present in less than half of cases.
- Meningococcemia symptoms: fever, early signs of sepsis, and nonblanching hemorrhagic rash (i.e., petechiae, purpura) (2)[C]
- Inquire about possible sick contacts, living conditions, and other exposures

PHYSICAL EXAM

- Vitals: fever, hypotension, tachycardia
- Neuro: focal neurologic deficits, nuchal rigidity, photophobia, bulging fontanelles, coma, seizure
- Focal neurologic deficits and seizures are more commonly seen with *Haemophilus influenzae* or *Streptococcus pneumoniae*.
- Onset of specific meningitis symptoms (e.g., neck stiffness, photophobia, bulging fontanelle) can occur within 12 to 15 hours.
- Late signs of meningitis (e.g., unconsciousness, delirium, or seizures) occur after ~15 hours in infants <1 year and after ~24 hours in older children.
- Cardiologic/pulmonary: S3 gallop, rales
- Dermatologic: ecchymosis, petechiae, purpura (can occur anywhere but often prominent in the extremities). Rash is 80–90% specific for meningococcal disease (and present in 60–80% of cases).

DIFFERENTIAL DIAGNOSIS

- Other bacterial/viral meningitis
- Toxic shock syndrome (TSS)
- Steven-Johnson syndrome (SJS)
- Acute endocarditis
- Rocky Mountain spotted fever
- Hemolytic uremic syndrome
- Kawasaki disease
- Measles
- Influenza

DIAGNOSTIC TESTS & INTERPRETATION

ALERT

- Isolation of *N. meningitidis* from sterile body fluid culture is the gold standard (2)[C],(3)[A].
- Antibiotics may sterilize cultures within 2 hours; send samples before therapy if possible but *do not* delay treatment.

Initial Tests (lab, imaging)

- Definitive diagnosis is through culture (blood, CSF, or other sterile body fluid) (2)[C],(3)[A].
- PCR can identify bacterial DNA in CSF or blood for select organisms, even after antibiotic administration in some cases, but should not replace culture at this time (3)[A].
- Lumbar puncture (LP)/CSF:
  - Gram stain showing gram-negative diplococci
  - Increased WBCs with polymorphonuclear predominance
  - CSF glucose–to–serum glucose ratio <0.4 (i.e., very low)
  - Protein concentration >2,200 mg/L (i.e., elevated)
  - Positive for *N. meningitidis* antigen
  - CSF culture positive in 80–90% of cases
- Head CT prior to LP only if focal neurologic signs or concern for space-occupying lesions
- CBC with differential
  - Leukocytosis (left shift; toxic granulation) or leukopenia; thrombocytopenia
- Coagulation studies
  - Prolonged PT/PTT; low fibrinogen; elevated fibrin degradation products

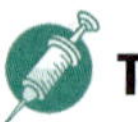

TREATMENT

MEDICATION

Begin empiric IV antibiotics immediately upon suspicion; do not delay for labs, imaging, or LP (2),(3).

First Line

- Antibiotics (2)[C],(3)[A]
  - Preterm to <1 month: ampicillin plus cefotaxime *or* ampicillin plus gentamicin
    - Cefotaxime
      - 0 to 7 days: 50 mg/kg q12h
      - 8 to 28 days: 50 mg/kg q8h
    - Ampicillin
      - >2,000 g
        - 0 to 7 days: 50 mg/kg q8h
        - 8 to 28 days: 50 mg/kg q6h
      - <2,000 g
        - 0 to 7 days: 50 mg/kg q12h
        - 8 to 28 days: 50 mg/kg q8h

- 1 month to 50 years: Third-generation cephalosporins (cefotaxime *or* ceftriaxone) are first line.
  - If severe penicillin allergy: chloramphenicol plus trimethoprim-sulfamethoxazole (TMP-SMX) plus vancomycin
  - Ceftriaxone:
    - Adults: 1 to 2 g IV once daily (maximum 4 g/day).
    - Children (excluding neonates): 100 mg/kg IV once daily (maximum 4 g/day).
  - Cefotaxime:
    - Adults: 1 to 2 g IV every 6 to 8 hours (total daily dose 4 to 6 g).
    - Children: 50 mg/kg IV every 6 hours
- >50 years of age or patients with significant comorbidity, alcohol abuse, or impaired immunity: ampicillin plus ceftriaxone plus vancomycin
  - Ampicillin: 2 g IV q4h
  - Ceftriaxone: 2 g IV q12h
  - Vancomycin: 30 to 45 mg/kg/day IV divided q6h
  - If severe penicillin allergy: TMP-SMX plus vancomycin
- Penicillin G
  - Effective if the isolate is penicillin-sensitive (MIC <0.1 μg/mL).
  - Penicillin G 4 million units IV q4h (pediatric dose: 0.25 mU/kg/day IV divided q4–6h) × 7 days

- For isolates with a penicillin MIC of 0.1 to 1 μg/mL, a 3rd-generation cephalosporin is preferred.
  - Ampicillin 2 g IV q4h (pediatric dose: 200 to 300 mg/kg/day IV divided q6h) × 7 days
- Dexamethasone (2)[C], (3)[A]
  - Often given initially in immunocompetent adults and children >6 weeks of age (10 to 20 minutes before or with the first dose of antibiotics) with suspected bacterial meningitis while awaiting microbiologic study results
    - Most effective for *S. pneumoniae* meningitis with uncertain benefit in meningococcal meningitis
  - Dosage
    - Infants and children >6 weeks: IV 0.15 mg/kg per dose q6h for the first 2 to 4 days of antibiotic treatment
- Chemoprophylaxis (2)[C]
  - Indicated for close contacts (<3 ft and >8 hours exposure) *or* direct contact with oral secretions from 1 week before onset until 24 hours after effective therapy regardless of vaccination status
    - Ideally given within 24 hours of case identification
    - Not indicated >14 days postexposure or for casual contacts, including most health care workers
  - Consider antimicrobial susceptibility testing on meningococcal isolates to inform prophylaxis decisions due to rising ciprofloxacin-resistant, beta-lactamase-producing *N. meningitidis* serogroup Y in the United States.
  - Prophylactic regimens
    - Ceftriaxone
      - <15 years of age: 125 mg IM as a single dose
      - Adults: 250 mg IM as a single dose
      - Recommended for pregnant women
    - Rifampin
      - Pediatric
        - <1 month: 10 mg/kg/day in divided doses q12h × 2 days
        - Infants and children: 20 mg/kg/day in divided doses q12h × 2 days (max 600 mg/dose)
      - Adult: 600 mg IV or PO q12h × 2 days
    - Ciprofloxacin
      - Adults: 500 mg PO as a single dose
- Vaccination (1)[A]
  - Offer to household contacts if case due to vaccine-preventable serogroup
- Precautions
  - Adjust the dosage of medications in patients with severe renal dysfunction.
  - Additional treatment may be needed to eliminate nasopharyngeal colonization.

Second Line

- For meningitis
  - Chloramphenicol: 1 g IV q6h (pediatric dose: 75 to 100 mg/kg/day divided q6h)
    - Use in cases of severe β-lactam allergy or when first-line agents are contraindicated.
    - Can cause aplastic anemia
  - Ceftriaxone 2 g IV q12h (pediatric dose: 80 to 100 mg/kg/day divided q12–24h)
    - 2nd line if severe penicillin allergy (do not use if history of anaphylactic reaction to penicillin)
  - In large outbreaks, a single dose of long-acting chloramphenicol has been used. Single-dose ceftriaxone shows equal efficacy in one randomized controlled trial.
- Precautions
  - Ceftriaxone should not be used in patients with a history of anaphylactic reactions to penicillin (e.g., hypotension, laryngeal edema, wheezing, hives).
  - Chloramphenicol may cause aplastic anemia.

ISSUES FOR REFERRAL

Consider infectious disease consultation for outbreaks and infectious disease and critical care consultation for complicated cases.

ADMISSION, INPATIENT, AND NURSING CONSIDERATIONS

- Begin antibiotics promptly; if meningitis suspected, consider corticosteroids and obtain LP immediately.
- Droplet isolation until 24 hours after antibiotics

ONGOING CARE

PATIENT EDUCATION

Educate family and close contacts on risk of contracting meningococcal infection, chemoprophylaxis, vaccine protection, and need for prompt evaluation if symptomatic.

PROGNOSIS

- Mortality is ~10–15% despite prompt antibiotic therapy.
- Poor prognostic factors: hypotension, thrombocytopenia, altered mental status, leukopenia, young age
- Up to 20% of survivors develop long-term sequelae including sensorineural hearing loss, cognitive deficits, or limb loss.

COMPLICATIONS

- Immediate: septic shock, DIC, renal failure, adrenal failure (Waterhouse-Friderichsen syndrome), purpura fulminans, seizures, cerebral edema
- Long term: hearing loss, amputation, chronic pain, neurological deficits, PTSD, depression

REFERENCES

1. Mbaeyi SA, Bozio CH, Duffy J, et al. Meningococcal vaccination: recommendations of the Advisory Committee on Immunization Practices, United States, 2020. *MMWR Recomm Rep*. 2020;69(9):1–41.
2. Cejin MC, Koyfman A, Long B. High risk and low incidence diseases: meningococcal disease. *Am J Emerg Med*. 2026;99:114–122. doi:10.1016/j.ajem.2025.09.031.
3. van de Beek D, Brouwer MC, Koedel U, et al. Community-acquired bacterial meningitis. *Lancet*. 2021;398(10306):1171–1183. doi:10.1016/S0140-6736(21)00883-7.

ADDITIONAL READING

- Centers for Disease Control and Prevention. Clinical overview of meningococcal disease. https://www.cdc.gov/meningococcal/clinical-info.html.
- Deghmane AE, Taha S, Taha MK. Global epidemiology and changing clinical presentations of invasive meningococcal disease: a narrative review. *Infect Dis (Lond)*. 2022;54(1):1–7.
- Hasbun R. Progress and challenges in bacterial meningitis: a review. *JAMA*. 2022;328(21):2147–2154. doi:10.1001/jama.2022.20521.

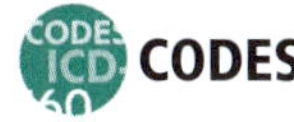

CODES

ICD10

- A39.4 Meningococcemia, unspecified
- A39.0 Meningococcal meningitis
- A39.2 Acute meningococcemia

CLINICAL PEARLS

- Invasive meningococcal disease can be rapidly fatal.
- Petechial/purpuric rash is highly specific for meningococcal disease.
- Early identification and treatment with antibiotics is essential to promote good clinical outcomes (treat and then test in suspected cases).
- Close contacts should receive chemoprophylaxis (even if vaccinated).
- All adolescents and children in high-risk groups should receive the MenACWY vaccine; MenB vaccines are recommended for high-risk individuals aged ≥10 years

MENISCAL INJURY

Jennifer Schwartz, MD

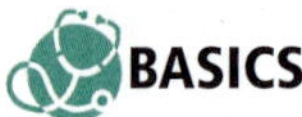

BASICS

DESCRIPTION

- The menisci are fibrocartilaginous structures between the femoral condyles and the tibial plateaus.
- The menisci help to stabilize the knee (with the anterior cruciate ligament [ACL]) and distribute forces across the joint to provide shock absorption.
- Meniscal tears can lead to knee pain and disability and, ultimately, are a risk factor for the development of knee osteoarthritis (OA).

Pediatric Considerations

- Meniscal injuries are less common in children aged <10 years. In this population, they are often due to a discoid meniscus.
- MRI is still the study of choice but is less sensitive and specific for diagnosing meniscal tears in children aged <12 years.
- Increased BMI in pediatric patients correlates with more complex tears and lower repair success rates.

EPIDEMIOLOGY

Bimodal age distribution—young athletes (traumatic) and older patients (degenerative)

Incidence

Medial meniscus more commonly injured

Prevalence

- One of the most common musculoskeletal injuries
- Meniscal surgery is the most common type of orthopedic surgery performed in the United States.

ETIOLOGY AND PATHOPHYSIOLOGY

- Traumatic tears are acute. They generally occur due to a twisting motion of the knee with foot planted.
  - Common in younger patients (aged <40 years) without underlying knee OA
  - Manifests with sudden pain
- Degenerative tears are chronic. They generally occur with overuse and minimal trauma.
  - There is an age related increase in prevalence, and they are often comorbid with knee OA.
  - Symptoms evolve slowly.

Genetics

No specific gene locus has been identified.

RISK FACTORS

- Nonmodifiable risk factors: male, discoid meniscus, ligamentous laxity
- Traumatic tear:
  - High degree of physical activity (especially cutting sports)
  - ACL insufficiency
- Degenerative tear:
  - Increased age (>60 years)
  - Obesity
  - Work-related kneeling/squatting/climbing stairs

GENERAL PREVENTION

- Treatment and rehabilitation of previous knee injuries, particularly ACL injuries
- Strengthening and increased flexibility of quadriceps and hamstring muscles
- Weight management

COMMONLY ASSOCIATED CONDITIONS

- Traumatic tear: ACL concomitantly torn in 1/3 of cases
- Degenerative tear: OA, Baker cyst (greater association with medial meniscal tears)

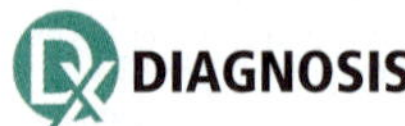

DIAGNOSIS

HISTORY

- Medial or lateral knee pain and swelling (increased with knee flexion)
- Noncontact twisting mechanism of injury (if trauma present)
- ±Mechanical symptoms (i.e., locking, catching)
  - In young patients, it is often due to entrapped meniscal tissue after a trauma; in older patients, may also be due to degenerative factors or OA

PHYSICAL EXAM

- Effusion—typically >24 hours postinjury
- Joint line tenderness (medial and/or lateral)
- Decreased range of motion of knee, pain with full flexion (posterior horn tear) or extension (anterior horn tear)
- Accuracy of special tests (McMurray test, Apley grind test) varies.

DIFFERENTIAL DIAGNOSIS

- ACL or collateral ligament tear
- Pathologic plica
- Osteochondritis dissecans
- Loose body or fracture
- OA
- Patellofemoral syndrome

DIAGNOSTIC TESTS & INTERPRETATION

- Plain radiographs can detect fractures, loose bodies, or arthritic changes.
- Ultrasound may help to identify meniscal tears.
- MRI is the primary imaging test for detecting meniscal tears.

Follow-Up Tests & Special Considerations

Meniscal tears are often found incidentally on MRI and may not always be the cause of a patient's symptoms—important to correlate history, physical exam, and imaging findings.

- Asymptomatic tears are more common in middle-aged/older patients and those with OA.

Diagnostic Procedures/Other

Arthroscopy may be needed if the MRI is indeterminate.

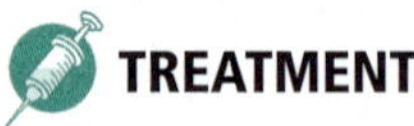

TREATMENT

GENERAL MEASURES

- Nonoperative management is recommended as first-line treatment for most meniscal tears. This includes the following:
  - Rest, ice, activity modification
  - OTC medication
  - Physical therapy (PT)
  - Intra-articular corticosteroid injections
- Multiple trials have shown no increased benefit to surgery versus PT in patients aged >40 years with degenerative meniscal tears (1)[A].
- In young/active patients with meniscal tears, early surgery is not always superior to PT.

MEDICATION

First Line

- NSAIDs (i.e., ibuprofen up to 800 mg PO TID, naproxen [Naprosyn] 500 mg PO BID) or acetaminophen (Tylenol)
- Corticosteroid injection (5 cc lidocaine plus 1 cc methylprednisolone acetate [Depo-Medrol] [80 mg/mL] or equivalent)

ISSUES FOR REFERRAL

Surgical consultation for patients not improving with PT or wishing surgical repair

ADDITIONAL THERAPIES

- Weight control
- Platelet-rich plasma (PRP) injections may improve symptoms from degenerative meniscal tears.

SURGERY/OTHER PROCEDURES

- Consider surgical intervention if:
  - Concurrent injuries (i.e., ACL tear)
  - Mechanical symptoms (knee "catching" or "locking")
    - Early surgery may be most effective in alleviating subjective mechanical symptoms in patients aged <40 years (2)[B].
    - No benefit to early surgery for alleviating mechanical symptoms in older patients.
  - No improvement with conservative treatment
- Meniscal preservation surgery (i.e., meniscal repair or replacement) is preferred in older patients and may have better outcomes than meniscectomy (3)[B].
  - Will better preserve knee biomechanics and delay progression of OA
- Meniscectomy (removal of injured portion of meniscus) can lead to articular cartilage degeneration and OA.

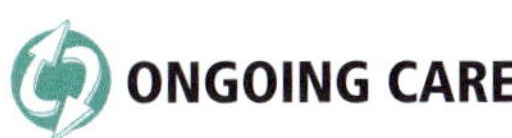

ONGOING CARE

FOLLOW-UP RECOMMENDATIONS

Return to play requires the athlete to be pain free, have full range of motion, and have full strength.

PATIENT EDUCATION

Patients should be aware of the risks and benefits of surgery compared with conservative treatment.

PROGNOSIS

Following meniscal repair, patients can generally return to activities in 3 to 6 months. Prognosis is better if tear is peripheral/lateral and <2.5 cm.

COMPLICATIONS

Meniscectomies increase the risk of developing OA.

REFERENCES

1. Rotini M, Papalia G, Setaro N, et al. Arthroscopic surgery or exercise therapy for degenerative meniscal lesions: a systematic review of systematic reviews. *Musculoskel Surg*. 2023;107(2):127–141.
2. Damsted C, Thorlund JB, Hölmich P, et al. Effect of exercise therapy versus surgery on mechanical symptoms in young patietns with a meniscal tear: a secondary analysis of the DREAM trial. *Br J Sports Med*. 2023;57(9):521–527.
3. Husen M, Kennedy NI, Till S, et al. Benefits of meniscal repair in selected patients aged 60 years and older. *Orthop J Sports Med*. 2022;10(9).

ADDITIONAL READING

- Noorduyn JCA, van de Graaf VA, Willigenburg NW, et al. Effect of physical therapy vs arthroscopic partial meniscectomy in people with degenerative meniscal tears: five-year follow-up of the ESCAPE randomized clinical trial. *JAMA Netw Open*. 2022;5(7):e2220394.
- Rohde MS, Shea KG, Dawson T, et al. Age, sex, and BMI differences related to repairable meniscal tears in pediatric and adolescent patients. *Am J Sports Med*. 2023;51(2):389–397.
- Sihvonen R, Paavola M, Malmivaara A, et al; for FIDELITY (Finnish Degenerative Meniscus Lesion Study) Investigators. Arthroscopic partial meniscectomy for a degenerative meniscus tear: a 5-year follow-up of the placebo-surgery controlled FIDELITY (Finnish Degenerative Meniscus Lesion Study) trial. *Br J Sports Med*. 2020;54(22):1332–1339.

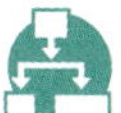

SEE ALSO

Algorithm: Knee Pain

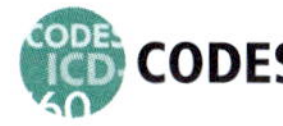

CODES

ICD10

- S83.209A Unsp tear of unsp meniscus, current injury, unsp knee, init
- S83.249A Oth tear of medial meniscus, current injury, unsp knee, init
- S83.289A Oth tear of lat mensc, current injury, unsp knee, init

CLINICAL PEARLS

- Chronic/degenerative meniscal tears are common in patients >40 years old and are associated with knee OA.
- Acute/traumatic meniscal tears are more common in young athletes.
- Conservative management is generally preferred as first-line treatment for meniscal tears. This includes PT/education with the option of later surgery.
- MRI is imaging modality of choice to identify meniscal tears.
- In patients opting for surgery, meniscal repairs have a better functional outcome and a decreased risk of OA compared with meniscectomy.

M

MENOPAUSE

Madeline Taskier, MD • Emmeline Ha, MD

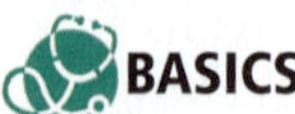

BASICS

DESCRIPTION

- Natural menopause: 12 consecutive months of amenorrhea in a nonpregnant person with a uterus ≥40 years old; mean age of 51 years; resulting from cessation of ovarian hormonal activity
- Perimenopause/menopausal transition (MT): the onset of irregular menses to the final menstrual cycle; begins on average of 4 years before menopause; mean age of 47 years
- Postmenopause: usually >1/3 of a woman's life
- Primary ovarian insufficiency: irregularity or cessation of ovulatory cycles before age 40 years
- Surgical menopause: removal of hormone-producing ovaries leading to immediate menopause

EPIDEMIOLOGY

- The median age of menopause is 51 years in the United States.
- 5% of people undergo menopause after age 55 years; 5% between 40 and 45 years
- Earlier onset in Hispanic patients and later onset in Japanese American patients compared with White patients

ETIOLOGY AND PATHOPHYSIOLOGY

- As women age, the number of ovarian follicles decreases. Ovarian production of estrogen varies and then decreases. Follicle-stimulating hormone (FSH) production varies and then increases.
- Insufficient estradiol production leads to the absence of the luteinizing hormone (LH) surge, resulting in anovulation. Anovulation causes lack of progesterone production.
- Failure to produce estradiol leads to thinning of endometrial lining and eventually menstruation ceases.
- Estrone (produced by adipose tissue) becomes the dominant form of estrogen during menopause.

RISK FACTORS

Oophorectomy/hysterectomy; sex chromosome abnormalities (e.g., Turner syndrome and fragile X syndrome); family history of early menopause; smoking (earlier age of onset by 2 years); chemotherapy and/or pelvic radiation; low body mass index (BMI)

GENERAL PREVENTION

Menopause is a physiologic event and cannot be prevented. It is associated with increased risk of medical issues, including cardiovascular disease (CVD) and osteoporotic fractures.

- Decrease risk of CVD by increasing exercise, maintaining healthy diet and weight, avoiding tobacco use, treating hypertension, hyperlipidemia, and diabetes mellitus.
- Decrease risk of osteoporotic fractures with weight-bearing exercise and fall prevention, avoidance of smoking and excessive alcohol intake, dietary calcium of 1,200 mg/day, adequate vitamin D intake

DIAGNOSIS

12 consecutive months of amenorrhea in a nonpregnant woman ≥40 years of age

HISTORY

- Cessation of menses: Generally preceded by irregular cycles with heavy bleeding followed by diminished bleeding
- Vasomotor symptoms reported by 80%:
  - Sudden unpleasant feeling of heat and sweating, most commonly over face, neck, and chest, typically lasting 1 to 5 minutes; intervals unpredictable (1)
  - Associated with clamminess, anxiety, and heart palpitations
  - Generally begin 2 years before the final menstrual period, peak during 1 year after the final menstrual period, and then diminish
  - Frequency and duration varies: 87% of women who report flushes experience them daily; ~33% have >10 per day. Mean duration of symptoms lasts 4 to 10.2 years and may begin during MT and extend well past menopause.
  - Varies with ethnicity: greatest in Black and Hispanic women; least in Asian women
  - More common in patients with comorbid obesity
- Genitourinary syndrome of menopause:
  - Vulvovaginal atrophy in 50%:
    - Vaginal/vulvar dryness, itching, dyspareunia, and possible sexual dysfunction
    - Increases risk of vaginal infections and urinary tract infections
- Anxiety/depression: new diagnosis of depression is 2.5 times more likely during the MT as compared to premenopause.
- Sleep disturbance: arousal from sleep, chronic sleep disruption, and chronic insomnia
- Change in intensity and severity of migraines
- Skin thinning, mild hirsutism, brittle nails

Geriatric Considerations

Vaginal bleeding in postmenopausal patients is abnormal; endometrial cancer must be ruled out.

PHYSICAL EXAM

- Decrease in breast size and change in breast texture
- Genitourinary exam: atrophic vulva and vaginal mucosa; possible signs of uterine prolapse with Valsalva maneuvers

DIFFERENTIAL DIAGNOSIS

Pregnancy, thyroid diseases, pituitary adenoma, Sheehan syndrome, hypothalamic dysfunction, anorexia nervosa, Asherman syndrome, and obstruction of uterine outflow tract

DIAGNOSTIC TESTS & INTERPRETATION

Initial Tests (lab, imaging)

- Lab testing for menopause is not required; age and symptoms establish the diagnosis.
- Lab tests appropriate in age <45 years if premature/early menopause suspected or to rule out other causes of oligomenorrhea/amenorrhea:
  - Elevated serum FSH level >30 mIU/mL indicates ovarian failure.
  - Symptoms may precede lab changes.
- Infertility evaluation: may use elevated day 3 FSH, decreased anti-müllerian hormone levels, and decreased antral follicle count to predict decreased ovarian reserve
- Estrogens, androgens, and oral contraceptive pills (OCPs) may alter lab results.

Follow-Up Tests & Special Considerations

- Pregnancy test
- TSH and prolactin level if pituitary disease is suspected
- Abnormal uterine bleeding, including postmenopausal bleeding, should be evaluated by TVUS and/or EMB. If endometrial stripe is <5 mm on TVUS, EAC is unlikely.
- Breast cancer screening: U.S. Preventive Services Task Force (USPSTF) recommends mammogram every 2 years from ages 40 to 75 years. Women with a strong family history of breast cancer in a first-degree relative may warrant earlier screening. The American College of Obstetricians and Gynecologists (ACOG) recommends mammogram every 1 to 2 years from ages 40 to 75 years. The American Cancer Society recommends annual mammogram for ages 40 to 54 and then every other year for ages 55 years and older until life expectancy is <10 years.
- Osteoporosis screening: USPSTF recommends bone mineral density (BMD) screening with dual energy x-ray absorptiometry (DEXA) scan in women aged >65 years or <65 years if the risk for fracture is equivalent to that of a 65-year-old woman (using the FRAX tool to assess, https://www.sheffield.ac.uk/FRAX/). Risk factors include a previous history of fractures, low body weight, cigarette smoking, and family history of osteoporotic fracture.

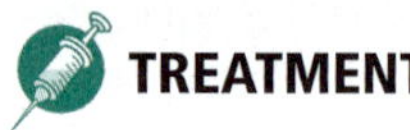

TREATMENT

GENERAL MEASURES

Behavioral modifications to manage vasomotor symptoms including lowering ambient temperature, layered clothing, and avoiding possible triggers (heat, stress, caffeine, alcohol, tobacco, spicy foods); during vasomotor episodes, portable fans or ice packs and relaxation techniques have also been shown to be helpful.

MEDICATION

First Line

Hormone therapy (HT): most effective treatment for vasomotor symptoms and has been shown to prevent bone loss and fracture (2). Developing an individual risk-benefit profile is essential, factoring in age, time from menopause, severity of symptoms, and CVD risk factors. For patients <60 years old or within 10 years of menopause onset, the risk-benefit profile is favorable. Treatment goal is to minimize menopausal symptoms to improve quality of life (2).

- HT can reduce weekly hot flush frequency by ~75%.
- HT may also help with disrupted sleep and urogenital atrophy
- Long-term use of hormone replacement therapy has more risks than benefits, including breast, ovarian, and endometrial cancer; venous thromboembolism; CVD; and gallbladder disease.

- Less worrisome side effects include breast tenderness, vaginal bleeding, bloating, headaches.
- HT should be individualized with the lowest effective dose for the shortest duration of time needed to relieve vasomotor symptoms (1). Lower doses have similar symptom reduction profiles for many patients. Results of ultra-low-dose regimens are mixed.
- Estrogen is available orally, transdermally (patch, gel, or spray), intravaginally (rings), or intramuscularly. Treatment regimens include but are not limited to:
  - Low dose: conjugated equine estrogen (CEE) 0.3 to 0.45 mg/day *or* micronized estradiol 17β 0.5 mg/day *or* transdermal estradiol 17β 0.025 mg/day
  - Max dose: CEE 0.625 mg/day *or* micronized estradiol 17β 1.0 mg/day *or* transdermal estradiol 17β 0.10 mg/day
  - Transdermal estradiol spray: 1.53 mg per spray, start at 1 spray per day and increase to 3 sprays per day. Transdermal estradiol gel should be applied on a large area of skin.
  - Intravaginal estradiol: vaginal ring inserted every 3 months releases 0.05 to 0.10 mg/day.
  - Injectable estrogen: estradiol cypionate 1 to 5 mg or estradiol valerate 10 to 20 mg every 4 weeks
- In patients with an intact uterus, give estrogen with progestin because unopposed estrogen carries an increased risk of EAC. Micronized progesterone 100 to 200 mg/day can be used as progestin. Alternative: medroxyprogesterone acetate (MPA) 2.5 mg/day.
- Combination forms are available as oral pills or transdermally. Oral pills are available with CEE, estradiol, or micronized estradiol as the estrogen source and drospirenone, MPA, norethindrone, or norgestimate as the progestin source. Combination estradiol/progestin transdermal treatments have either levonorgestrel or norethindrone as progestin source.
- Tissue-selective estrogen complex: bazedoxifene (selective estrogen receptor modulator [SERM])+ conjugated estrogens; provides endometrial protection without need for progesterone for relief of vasomotor symptoms and bone loss prevention
- Precautions:
  - The Women's Health Initiative (WHI) study demonstrated that women who take CEE with MPA versus placebo had increased CHD events, invasive breast cancer, stroke, pulmonary embolism, dementia, gallbladder disease, urinary incontinence; benefits included decreased hip fractures, diabetes, and vasomotor symptoms.
  - Breast cancer risk not seen until 5 years of use
  - Women on estrogen alone had no increased risk of invasive breast cancer but did increase abnormal mammograms requiring follow-up investigations.
  - HT should *not* be used for cardioprotective benefit as risk outweighs benefit.
  - Higher doses of estrogen can cause hypercoagulability, breast tenderness, gallbladder disease, and hypertension.
  - Contraindications to HT: estrogen-dependent malignancies; unexplained uterine bleeding or untreated endometrial hyperplasia; history of thromboembolism, stroke, or other coagulopathy; coronary artery disease; active liver disease; untreated hypertension; current or past breast cancer; smoking
- For genitourinary syndrome of menopause:
  - Topical estrogen reverses vaginal atrophy, enhances blood flow, and reduces urinary tract infections. Continue for as long as distressing symptoms remain. Initiate treatment daily for 1 to 2 weeks and then decrease to 2 times weekly. Comes as estradiol cream, tablet, or ring. No evidence of difference in efficacy between various intravaginal estrogenic preparations. Apply vaginally:
    - Ospemifene: 60 mg PO daily; SERM for moderate to severe dyspareunia associated with vaginal atrophy
    - Estradiol cream 0.01% (1 g), conjugated estrogen 0.625 mg/g (0.5 g), vaginal tablet (10 μg) used twice weekly, or vaginal ring (7.5 μg daily lasting for 3 months)
    - Nonestrogen vaginal lubricant may be as effective as topical estrogen for some.

Second Line

Nonhormonal treatments may be helpful to treat vasomotor symptoms (3):

- Paroxetine (7.5 mg/day): approved for treatment of vasomotor symptoms; shows modest decrease in hot flushes.
- Other SSRI/SRNIs: Venlafaxine (37.5 to 100 mg/day) or fluoxetine (20 mg/day) and citalopram (20 mg/day) reduce hot flushes compared to placebo.
- Gabapentin (300 to 900 mg/day) decreases hot flushes compared to placebo.
- Clonidine (0.05 mg BID) may be used to treat mild hot flashes, less effective than SSRI/SRNIs.
- Fezolinetant (45 mg/day): first-in-class approved neurokinin 3 receptor antagonist; acts on the hypothalamic thermoregulatory center to reduce vasomotor symptoms. Liver function must be evaluated before and during treatment.

COMPLEMENTARY & ALTERNATIVE MEDICINE

- Phytoestrogens, herbs, and other supplements do not have clear benefit in relieving menopause symptoms compared to placebo. Some may interact with anticoagulants, like warfarin, so should be used with caution.
- Hypnotherapy and mindfulness meditation may provide relief for some.
- Acupuncture has not been shown to be more effective than simulated acupuncture for relieving hot flashes.
- Yoga has not been shown to relieve hot flashes but may be helpful for some symptoms associated with menopause.
- Compounded bioidentical HT should be avoided, given concerns about safety, including possibility of overdosing or underdosing, lack of efficacy and safety studies, and lack of a label providing risks (2).
- Overall, most data involves short-term trials, so little is known about their long-term safety. But, mind-body practices such as acupuncture, hypnosis, meditation, and yoga generally have good safety records (3).

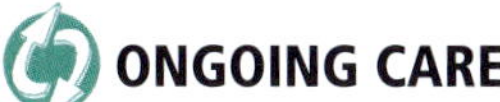

ONGOING CARE

FOLLOW-UP RECOMMENDATIONS

Patient Monitoring

If HT initiated, consider decrease or discontinuation after 3 to 5 years to minimize risks.

DIET

Calcium-rich diet and vitamin D supplementation (800 to 1,000 IU/day) to prevent osteoporosis

PATIENT EDUCATION

- Smoking cessation, reducing alcohol intake
- Exercise >30 minutes, 3 times weekly
- Healthy nutrition to prevent cardiovascular and maintain healthy BMI

PROGNOSIS

If untreated, vasomotor symptoms will resolve but vaginal/vulvar atrophy will worsen.

COMPLICATIONS

- Osteoporosis: accelerated bone loss up to 3–5% per year for 5 to 7 years
- Increased risk of CVD following menopause

REFERENCES

1. American College of Obstetricians and Gynecologists. ACOG practice bulletin no. 141: management of menopausal symptoms. *Obstet Gynecol*. 2014;123(1):202–2016. doi:10.1097/01.AOG.0000441353.20693.78.
2. Faubion SS, Crandall CJ, Davis L, et al; for The North American Menopause Society. The 2022 hormone therapy position statement of the North American Menopause Society. *Menopause*. 2022;29(7):767–794. doi:10.1097/GME.0000000000002028.
3. Shufelt CL, Brown VV, Carpenter JS, et al; for The North American Menopause Society. The 2023 nonhormone therapy position statement of The North American Menopause Society. *Menopause*. 2023;30(6):573–590. doi:10.1097/GME.0000000000002200.

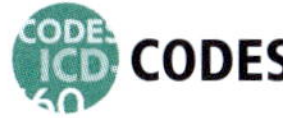

CODES

ICD10

- E28.310 Symptomatic premature menopause
- N95.1 Menopausal and female climacteric states
- Z78.0 Asymptomatic menopausal state

CLINICAL PEARLS

- Menopause is usually diagnosed by history alone.
- HT can be used short term for relief of moderate to severe vasomotor symptoms. Use the lowest effective dose for the shortest duration of time.
- In patients with a uterus, give estrogen with progestin because unopposed estrogen increases the risk of endometrial hyperplasia or cancer.

MESOTHELIOMA

William Edwin Martin, MD, MBA, MPH • Kristen EB Said, MD, MPH

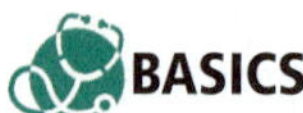

BASICS

DESCRIPTION

- Mesothelioma is a rare, insidious, and aggressive malignancy of the mesothelial or serous tissues primarily found in the pleura (80–95%), peritoneum (5–20%), and rarely, the tunica vaginalis and pericardium (1–2%).
- Inhalation of asbestos is the predominant cause of mesothelioma, most often from remote occupational exposure (≥20 years earlier).
- Histologically, there are three types of malignant mesothelioma: epithelioid type (most common and least aggressive), sarcomatoid type (most aggressive), and biphasic type.
- Mesothelioma has a rapidly fatal course (median survival 17 to 25 months for resectable pleural mesothelioma) (1).

EPIDEMIOLOGY

Incidence

- The incidence in the United States has recently begun to decline, a trend attributable to the delayed effects of the asbestos ban initiated in the 1970s.
- Globally, areas of endemic clustering persist, typically in regions with high levels of ongoing asbestos-related industry. Incidence rates are not available, however, due to lack of quality reporting data.
- Incidence increases with age, peaking in the 5th and 6th decade of life, with 70% of pleural disease occurring in males. Peritoneal involvement is slightly higher in women.
- There are 3,000 cases of mesothelioma diagnosed in the United States annually (1).

Prevalence

In the United States, 1 case per 100,000 persons without asbestos industry exposure and 2 to 3 per 100,000 persons with asbestos exposure (1).

ETIOLOGY AND PATHOPHYSIOLOGY

- The predominant cause of mesothelioma is exposure to asbestos (hydrated magnesium silicate fibrous minerals).
- The majority of asbestos fibers are either amphibole (needle-like) or serpentine (curved). All types are capable of causing mesothelioma, although amphiboles (particularly crocidolite and amosite) are more carcinogenic. Serpentine fibers, the predominant fiber type in the United States, are mostly found in ships, buildings, brake lining, and ceiling tiles (2).
- There is a long latent period, typically 20 to 50 years, between exposure and the development of mesothelioma (3).
- The pathogenesis of mesothelioma is multifactorial and not fully understood, but the predominant cause is via inhaled or ingested asbestos fibers becoming trapped in pleural or peritoneal membranes, causing irritation and inflammation. This continued tissue damage and inflammation leads to tumor formation (3).
- Tumors coalesce with a gradual progression from the parietal to visceral pleura and eventual invasion of surrounding structures (2).
- In addition to asbestos, tumors have arisen after prior radiation or exposure to talc, erionite, or mica or in patients with familial Mediterranean fever and diffuse lymphocytic leukemia.

Genetics

- A substantial percentage (>10%) of patients harbor germline mutations in cancer predisposition genes, notably BAP1. BAP1 mutations are linked to an inherited susceptibility to mesothelioma and a pattern of familial cancers. Patients may report an elevated personal or familial history of cancers, especially mesothelioma and uveal melanoma (1),(4).
- In addition to BAP1, other mutations have been associated with genetic predisposition, including MLH1, MLH3, TP53, BRAC2 (1),(4).

RISK FACTORS

- The predominant risk factor is exposure to asbestos with a dose-dependent risk.
- Occupational exposures involve mining or milling of fibers; work with textiles, cement, friction materials, or insulation; or shipbuilding.
- Nonoccupational exposures include renovation or destruction of asbestos-containing buildings, exposure to industrial sources in the community or natural geologic sources, or exposure to soiled clothing of asbestos workers.
- Radiation exposure, proximity to naturally occurring asbestos deposits, or inhalation of other fibrous silicates can contribute to malignant mesothelioma.
- In contrast to lung cancer and asbestosis, it appears to be no synergistic effect between smoking and the development of mesothelioma.

GENERAL PREVENTION

- Avoidance of asbestos exposure
- Strict adherence to protective protocols for workers in buildings where asbestos is found
- Continued aggressive remediation of asbestos-affected buildings and homes

DIAGNOSIS

Most often presenting symptoms are nonspecific; so, a thorough exposure history supported by imaging is most helpful.

HISTORY

- Symptoms are usually nonspecific and occur when disease is advanced, leading to delays in presentation.
- Pleural mesothelioma presents with gradual onset of pulmonary symptoms, such as, chest pain (chest wall invasion), breathlessness (pleural infusion), and cough. Fatigue, night sweats, anorexia, and weight loss may also be present and worsen with disease progression (3).
- Peritoneal disease presents with vague abdominal pain, increased abdominal girth, nausea, anorexia, and weight loss.
- Establishing a history of asbestos exposure is a challenge as patients may not remember potential exposure events 30 years prior. Asbestos-specific questionnaires may be helpful (2).
- Community and paraoccupational exposures must also be included. Questions pertaining to household contacts from workers, home renovations, nonindustrial settings (e.g., schools), and nearby asbestos industries (e.g., mines and factories) (2),(3).

PHYSICAL EXAM

- Pulmonary findings consistent with pleural effusion, including decreased breath sounds, dullness to percussion, and asymmetric chest wall expansion
- Abdominal findings consistent with ascites, including abdominal distension, fluid wave, and tenderness are found in cases involving the peritoneum.
- Clubbing may be found in extremities.
- Neurologic findings consistent with spinal cord compression are possible.

DIFFERENTIAL DIAGNOSIS

- Pleural mesothelioma's differential diagnosis includes inflammatory reactions (empyema, pleural effusion), metastatic tumor from other sites, fibrosarcoma, malignant fibrous histiocytoma, sarcomatoid carcinoma, and synovial sarcoma.
- Peritoneal mesothelioma's differential diagnosis includes peritoneal carcinomatosis, serous peritoneal carcinoma, ovarian carcinoma in women, lymphomatosis, and tuberculous peritonitis.

DIAGNOSTIC TESTS & INTERPRETATION

Initial Tests (lab, imaging)

- Biomarkers may be elevated in mesothelioma, such as mesothelin; however, they require further study and do not have an established routine use in diagnosis or monitoring response to therapy (3).
- Chest x-ray is insensitive and nonspecific. Further imaging is often required (3).
- Pleural mesothelioma diagnosis requires tissue. Thoracentesis for cytology and closed pleural biopsy may be adequate, but often, more invasive procedures such as video-assisted thoracoscopic surgery (VATS) is needed to obtain an adequate specimen (1).

Follow-Up Tests & Special Considerations

- Seeding of biopsy sites and tracks may occur in mesothelioma. The usage of prophylactic radiotherapy has largely been discontinued in the wake of negative results from randomized controlled studies (3).
- Immunohistochemical panels help support the histopathologic diagnosis (3).

Diagnostic Procedures/Other

- Chest x-ray is insensitive and nonspecific. Common findings include unilateral pleural effusion, thickening, or calcifications. Further imaging is often required, with CT of the chest and abdomen being the initial test of choice (2),(3).
- CT, MRI, PET, or integrated PET-CT helps with clinical staging in pleural and peritoneal disease (2),(3).
- Mediastinoscopy and thoracoscopy can assist when diagnostic uncertainty remains and in the full surgical staging of pleural disease (3).
- Pleural mesothelioma diagnosis requires tissue. Thoracentesis for cytology and closed pleural biopsy may be adequate, but often, more invasive procedures such as VATS is needed to obtain an adequate specimen (4).

Test Interpretation

- Initial clinical staging is conducted through imaging. However, as evidenced by postmortem studies, clinical staging frequently underrepresents the actual extent of the disease (3).
- The tumor, node, metastasis (TNM) staging system is widely used, although alternative staging systems are adopted by some centers. The TNM system facilitates treatment selection by quantifying the progression of the disease based on the extent of pleural infiltration, the level of lymph node involvement, and the existence of metastases (3).
- The Butchart staging system, being the oldest, continues to be employed in certain regions of the world. The system seeks to define the resectability and the degree of lymph node involvement.

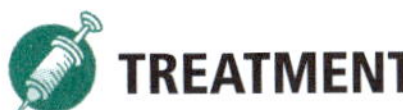

TREATMENT

Treatment is generally ineffective with a median survival of 9 to 12 months. However, multidisciplinary approaches are essential to prolonging life and palliation.

GENERAL MEASURES

- A multidisciplinary team is important in management and should include thoracic surgery, oncology, pathology, pulmonary, and radiology for patient-specific planning of management.
- Pain assessment and control should follow principles of cancer pain management.

MEDICATION

First Line

- Chemotherapy remains the mainstay treatment in pleural disease; combined therapy with cisplatin + gemcitabine, pemetrexed, or raltitrexed are all associated with longer median survival than cisplatin alone (1),(3),(5).
- Addition of bevacizumab to cisplatin and pemetrexed in pleural disease showed a small survival advantage but was never filed for licensing, and doubt remains on its value (3).
- Hyperthermic intraoperative or early postoperative intraperitoneal chemotherapy can increase drug concentration in the peritoneum and decrease systemic side effects. Use cisplatin, mitomycin C, fluorouracil, doxorubicin, and/or paclitaxel (1).

Second Line

- Palliative benefit in pleural disease with mitomycin C, vinblastine, cisplatin, and pemetrexed alone or in combination with carboplatin (1)
- Radiation therapy continues to evolve as part of the multidisciplinary approach to mesothelioma and may also be considered for palliation or as an adjunct to surgery. However, survival benefits have not been demonstrated in randomized controlled studies (3),(6).

ISSUES FOR REFERRAL

- Pulmonary, oncology, and surgical follow-up after discharge as indicated
- Psychological services and support should be offered.

ADDITIONAL THERAPIES

- Nivolumab and ipilimumab combined immunotherapy have shown superiority as a front-line treatment when compared to standard chemotherapy and is the first systemic therapy approved for pleural mesothelioma since 2004 (3).
- Gene therapy, photodynamic therapy, noninvasive delivery of alternating electric fields

SURGERY/OTHER PROCEDURES

- For pleural mesothelioma, the role of surgery remains controversial due to its modest amount of data, lack of standardization, and no proven survival benefit for aggressive surgical treatments. Most patients are not offered surgery due to their degree of disease progression and functional status. Instead, most are offered palliative chemotherapy (1).
- Pleurectomy/decortication (P/D) and extrapleural pneumonectomy (EPP) does reduce tumor load, but there remains no clear effect on mortality (1).
- Surgical multimodality therapy remains a common approach for stages I to III pleural mesothelioma. The surgery for mesothelioma after radiation therapy (SMART), which has promising results, combines radiation therapy and surgery. The most common multimodal approach combines P/D or EPP and intraoperative lavage of chemotherapeutic agents (1),(6).
- For aggressive treatments, the first prospective randomized control trial, mesothelioma and radical surgery (MARS), failed to demonstrate any added survival benefit with the addition of surgery to chemotherapy. However, the trial was criticized for its design, which the ongoing MARS 2 trial aims to address (1),(3).

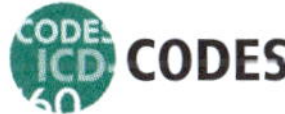

ONGOING CARE

FOLLOW-UP RECOMMENDATIONS

- Smoking cessation
- Immunization for pneumococcal pneumonia and influenza

Patient Monitoring

Monitor for paraneoplastic phenomenon, including fever, thrombocytosis, malignancy-related thrombosis, hypoglycemia, and rare Coombs-positive hemolytic anemia.

PROGNOSIS

- Prognosis must be individualized and is based on gender, stage, histology, and level of completeness of cytoreduction. Stage and histology are the most important predictors in prognosis (1),(2).
- Poorly differentiated tumor grade, advanced age, and male gender are all independent predictors of poorer prognosis (1),(2).

COMPLICATIONS

Relapses and progression, infection and dysphagia

Geriatric Considerations

Age >65 years is associated with significantly increased morbidity and mortality.

REFERENCES

1. Carbone M, Adusumilli PS, Alexander HR Jr, et al. Mesothelioma: scientific clues for prevention, diagnosis, and therapy. *CA Cancer J Clin*. 2019;69(5):402–429.
2. Brims F. Epidemiology and clinical aspects of malignant pleural mesothelioma. *Cancers (Basel)*. 2021;13(16):4194.
3. Janes SM, Alrifai D, Fennell DA. Perspectives on the treatment of malignant pleural mesothelioma. *N Engl J Med*. 2021;385(13):1207–1218.
4. Panou V, Gadiraju M, Wolin A, et al. Frequency of germline mutations in cancer susceptibility genes in malignant mesothelioma. *J Clin Oncol*. 2018;36(28):2863–2871.
5. Scagliotti GV, Gaafar R, Nowak AK, et al. Nintedanib in combination with pemetrexed and cisplatin for chemotherapy-naive patients with advanced malignant pleural mesothelioma (LUME-Meso): a double-blind, randomised, placebo-controlled phase 3 trial. *Lancet Respir Med*. 2019;7(7):569–580.
6. Gomez DR, Rimner A, Simone CB, et al. The use of radiation therapy for the treatment of malignant pleural mesothelioma: expert opinion from the National Cancer Institute Thoracic Malignancy Steering Committee, International Association for the Study of Lung Cancer, and Mesothelioma Applied Research Foundation. *J Thorac Oncol*. 2019;14(7):1172–1183.

CODES

ICD10

- C45.1 Mesothelioma of peritoneum
- C45.2 Mesothelioma of pericardium
- C45.0 Mesothelioma of pleura

CLINICAL PEARLS

- Mesothelioma remains a rare but universally fatal disease in part due to long latency.
- Multimodal treatment has decreased recurrence rates and has extended survival time.
- The main risk factor is asbestos exposure.

M

METABOLIC DYSFUNCTION-ASSOCIATED STEATOTIC LIVER DISEASE (MASLD)

Jill T. Wei Doherty, MD • Daniel T. Lee, MD, MA

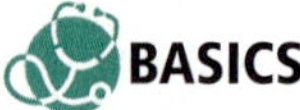

BASICS

- A spectrum of fatty liver diseases ranging from metabolic dysfunction-associated steatotic fatty liver disease (MASLD), to metabolic dysfunction-associated steatohepatitis (MASH), to fibrosis and cirrhosis, not due to other causes of fatty infiltration of liver (such as alcohol use).
- Defined as hepatic steatosis plus at least one cardiometabolic risk factor (obesity, hyperlipidemia, prediabetes, diabetes, hypertension (HTN))
- Most common chronic liver disease in the United States and worldwide

DESCRIPTION

- MASLD: previously referred to as NAFLD
  - Reversible condition in which large vacuoles of triglyceride fat accumulate in hepatocytes
  - Liver biopsy: fatty deposits in cells without hepatocellular injury (no hepatocyte ballooning, no necrosis, no fibrosis)
  - ALT and AST normal or <3 to 4 times upper limit of normal (ULN)
  - Possible risk of progressing to cirrhosis or liver failure
  - Synonym: steatosis
- MASH: progressive form of MASLD
  - Liver biopsy: fatty deposits in cells with hepatocellular injury (ballooning, acute/chronic inflammation, ± fibrosis)
  - ALT and AST elevated, but generally <3 to 4 times ULN
  - 30% with MASH may progress to fibrosis over 5 years, may progress to cirrhosis, liver failure, and rarely hepatocellular cancer
- MASH cirrhosis: presence of cirrhosis with current or previous histologic evidence of steatosis or steatohepatitis

EPIDEMIOLOGY

- Most common chronic liver disease in industrialized Western countries
- Predominant age: 40s to 50s; can occur in children
- Predominant sex: male > female (40% vs. 26%)
- Leading indication for liver transplantation in women and those >65 years old (1)

Prevalence

- United States estimate: 30% but often is undiagnosed (1)
- Present in 58–74% of obese (BMI ≥30 kg/m^2); 90% of morbidly obese (BMI ≥40 kg/m^2); 69–87% with type 2 diabetes mellitus (DM); 50% with dyslipidemia

ETIOLOGY AND PATHOPHYSIOLOGY

Primary mechanism is thought to be *insulin resistance*, leading to increased lipolysis, triglyceride synthesis, increased hepatic uptake of free fatty acids, accumulation of hepatic triglyceride, oxidative stress, inflammation and fibrosis with result.

- MASLD: excessive triglyceride accumulation in the liver and impaired ability to remove fatty acids
- MASH: multiple hit theory (insulin resistance, adipose tissue hormones, oxidative stress damage, genetic factors, intestinal bacteria) that causes inflammation and acts on liver parenchymal cells leading to steatohepatitis

Genetics

- Largely unknown: some familial clustering and increased heritability
- MASLD: more first-degree relatives with cirrhosis than matched controls
- MASH: 18% with affected first-degree relative

RISK FACTORS

- Type 2 DM, cardiovascular disease (CVD), and chronic kidney disease (CKD)
- Metabolic risk factors: HTN, hyperlipidemia, obesity, visceral fat
- Protein–calorie malnutrition; total parenteral nutrition (TPN) >6 weeks
- Severe weight loss (starvation, bariatric surgery)
- Organic solvent exposure (e.g., chlorinated hydrocarbons, toluene); vinyl chloride; hypoglycin A
- Gene for hemochromatosis/other conditions with increased iron stores
- Smoking
- Drugs: tetracycline, glucocorticoids, tamoxifen, methotrexate, amiodarone, antiretroviral agents for HIV, valproic acid, fialuridine, many chemotherapy regimens, nucleoside analogues
- History of cholecystectomy
- Increasing age associated with increased prevalence, severity, advanced fibrosis, and mortality

Pregnancy Considerations

Acute fatty liver of pregnancy: rare but serious complication in 3rd trimester—50% of cases are associated with preeclampsia

Pediatric Considerations

- Pediatric MASLD
  - Increasing prevalence of MASLD among children parallels rise in pediatric obesity, with prevalence of 9.6%
  - Vitamin E of possible benefit
- Reye syndrome: fatty liver syndrome with encephalopathy usually following viral illness and aspirin use

GENERAL PREVENTION

- Avoid excess alcohol: ≤2 units per day (men); ≤1 unit per day (women)
- Maintain appropriate BMI.
- Prevention and optimal management of diabetes
- Avoid hepatotoxic medications.

COMMONLY ASSOCIATED CONDITIONS

Central obesity; HTN; type 2 diabetes; insulin resistance; hyperlipidemia; preeclampsia in pregnancy; CVD and arrhythmias; hypothyroidism; hypogonadism; OSA; CKD; growth hormone deficiency; polycystic ovary syndrome (PCOS)

DIAGNOSIS

- Routine screening not recommended because of lack of effective drug treatment and unclear long-term benefits of screening (1)
  - Consider MASLD in patients with asymptomatic aminotransferase elevations.
  - MASLD has no distinguishing historical/lab features to differentiate from other chronic liver disorders.
  - May present as cryptogenic cirrhosis
- Often found incidentally on routine imaging (ultrasound or CT)

HISTORY

- Typically asymptomatic
- Possible fatigue and/or abdominal fullness
- Vague right upper quadrant pain
- History of medications, family history

PHYSICAL EXAM

Usually normal, but signs may include:

- Liver tenderness
- Mild to marked hepatomegaly
- Splenomegaly
- In advanced cases: cutaneous stigmata of chronic liver disease or portal HTN (e.g., palmar erythema, spider angiomata, ascites); jaundice

DIFFERENTIAL DIAGNOSIS

- Viral hepatitis; drug- or toxin-induced hepatitis; autoimmune hepatitis
- Alcoholic liver disease
- Celiac disease
- Muscle disease, if nonhepatic cause of elevated enzymes is possible
- Hemochromatosis; Wilson disease; lipodystrophy

DIAGNOSTIC TESTS & INTERPRETATION

MASLD: positive criteria for diagnosis

- Presence of hepatic steatosis detected by imaging, biomarkers or histology *and* at least one of the following metabolic syndrome traits in the absence of secondary causes of steatosis (2):
  - Insulin resistance (either prediabetes or DM)
  - Abdominal obesity or BMI ≤25 (or ethnicity adjusted equivalent)
  - HTN (BP ≥130/85 mm Hg or on medication for HTN)
  - Plasma triglycerides ≥150 mg/dL or on lipid-lowering medication
  - Plasma HDL ≤40 mg/dL (male), ≤50 mg/dL (female), or on lipid-lowering medication
- No history of significant alcohol consumption and exclusion of other causes of hepatic steatosis

Initial Tests (lab, imaging)

- ALT and AST may be elevated
  - Nonalcoholic, usually AST/ALT <1
  - Level of enzyme elevation does NOT correlate with degree of fibrosis.
- Elevated ferritin (1.5 times normal)
- Elevated alkaline phosphatase, total/direct bilirubin
- Lipid abnormalities: elevated total cholesterol, elevated LDL, elevated triglycerides, decreased HDL
- If cirrhosis present: decreased serum albumin, elevated PT, thrombocytopenia
- Serum labs to exclude other causes of liver disease: celiac, α_1-antitrypsin, iron, copper, hepatitis serologies, anti-smooth muscle antibody, ANA, serum γ-globulin
- Ultrasound (US) is first-line imaging: Fatty liver appears hyperechogenic.

Follow-Up Tests & Special Considerations

- Use of noninvasive tests (NITs) in the evaluation and management of MASLD to quantify fibrosis by estimating liver stiffness (3)
- Risk stratification with fibrosis-4 (FIB-4) index score: classify as low, intermediate, high risk
  - Low risk (<1.3): primary care management

- Intermediate risk (1.30 to 2.67): Consider NITs (e.g., vibration controlled transient elastography [VCTE] or enhanced liver fibrosis [ELF] test).
- High risk ($>$2.67): referral to hepatology
- Serum biomarkers: ELF panel
- Serial monitoring of NITs is used to assess disease progression and response to lifestyle modification or treatments (3).
- A combination of $\geq$2 NITs, combining serum and/or imaging-based biomarkers, is preferred for staging and risk stratification of patients with MASLD.

Diagnostic Procedures/Other

- Liver stiffness measurement: VCTE or FibroScan
- MRI-derived proton density fat fraction (PDFF): gold standard for noninvasive confirmation of steatosis (reserved for cases where precise quantification of liver fat is needed to resolve diagnostic ambiguity or guide management)
- Liver biopsy should only be considered for patients with NIT results that are indeterminant or discordant, conflict with clinical findings, or if there is concern for an alternative cause of liver disease (3).

Test Interpretation

MASLD activity score (MAS): used to grade diagnosis mostly for research and clinical trials, based on three histologic features: steatosis (0 to 3), inflammation (0 to 3), and hepatocyte ballooning (0 to 2), for score between 0 and 8. NASH is very likely with scores $\geq$5.

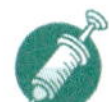

TREATMENT

Emphasis on early management of metabolic risk factors, MASLD associated with increased cardiovascular morbidity and mortality, type 2 diabetes (if not at baseline), CKD (stage 3 or higher), and extra hepatic cancers

GENERAL MEASURES

- Weight loss for those who are overweight or obese is the only therapy that has good evidence of benefits and safety. Aim for sustained weight loss (5–10% body weight) (1).
- Diet modification: Mediterranean diet has been shown to reduce liver fat (3). Limit carbohydrates and saturated fats (1). Abstinence from alcohol or at least limit alcohol consumption.
- Aerobic exercise 5 times per week for a total of 150 minutes per week
- Tight diabetes control
- Treat metabolic syndrome—HTN, dyslipidemia, and obesity
- Vaccination for hepatitis A and hepatitis B for those nonimmune
- Pneumococcal and annual influenza vaccination; COVID-19 and RSV vaccinations if indicated
- Avoid hepatotoxic medications.

MEDICATION

- Currently, no definitively effective medication treatment to treat MASLD or MASH
- Some promising agents include:
  - Thiazolidinediones (pioglitazone) (1)
    - Can use in patients with and without type 2 DM, but preferentially use only with type 2 DM
  - GLP-1 receptor agonists (semaglutide, liraglutide, tirzepatide, survodutide, retatrutide)
    - Histologic reduction in steatosis, less progression to fibrosis, and helps with weight loss
    - Can use in patients with and without type 2 DM
  - Resmetirom: thyroid hormone receptor β-agonist (2)
    - MASH resolution and fibrosis reduction in phase 3 RCT
    - FDA-approved for adults with noncirrhotic MASH and moderate to advanced fibrosis (F2 to F3)
  - Vitamin E 800 IU daily
    - Only use with biopsy proven MASH and those without diabetes
    - Long-term safety concerns at high does; avoid in patients at higher risk for prostate cancer or hemorrhagic stroke.
  - Statins (1)
    - Improve cardiovascular risk and decrease fatty infiltration
    - Benefits outweigh minimal risk of liver failure even in patients with compensated cirrhosis.
  - SGLT2 inhibitors (1)
    - Show reduction in steatosis by imaging, unclear effect on progression to fibrosis
    - Use in patients with type 2 DM
  - Lanifibranor: pan-peroxisome proliferator-activated receptor (PPAR) agonist (2)
    - MASH resolution and fibrosis improvement although with some weight gain in phase 2b RCT

ISSUES FOR REFERRAL

Refer to hepatology if persistent AST/ALT elevations, advanced fibrosis (stage F3 or greater) on liver scan, or fibrosis on liver biopsy.

SURGERY/OTHER PROCEDURES

- Bariatric surgery: may be considered in obese patients with MASLD, MASH, or advanced fibrosis who do not achieve weight loss goals after adequate trial of lifestyle modifications (1)
- Liver transplant: MASLD is second most common cause for liver transplant; however, MASLD will recur in the transplanted liver in 80–100% of patients (1).

ONGOING CARE

FOLLOW-UP RECOMMENDATIONS

- Annual monitoring of LFTs
- Surveillance with NITs to evaluate for disease progression every 2 to 4 years or sooner if increasing metabolic risk factors (3)
- Routine liver biopsy is not recommended but may be repeated 5 years after baseline biopsy if progression of fibrosis is suspected (1).
- Hepatic fibrosis staging is the strongest predictor for mortality in patients with histologically confirmed MASLD.
- Screening for hepatocellular carcinoma (HCC) in non-cirrhotic MASLD is yet to be determined.

DIET

Low in saturated and trans fat; low in simple carbohydrates; avoid excessive alcohol or abstinence preferred; coffee consumption of at least two cups daily (avoiding extra sugar/cream) may reduce the risk of fibrosis progression.

PATIENT EDUCATION

Extensive counseling on sustained lifestyle changes in nutrition, exercise, and alcohol use.

PROGNOSIS

Within the spectrum of MASLD, only MASH has been shown to be progressive, potentially leading to cirrhosis, HCC, cholangiocarcinoma, and/or liver failure.

- Cirrhosis develops in up to 20% of patients. Up to 42% of patients develop HCC without showing cirrhosis (1).
- Transplantation is effective, but MASH often recurs after due to ongoing risk factors.

COMPLICATIONS

Progressive disease may lead to decompensated cirrhosis and portal HTN with complications such as ascites, encephalopathy, bleeding varices, and hepatorenal or hepatopulmonary syndromes.

REFERENCES

1. Rinella ME, Neuschwander-Tetri BA, Siddiqui MS, et al. AASLD practice guidance on the clinical assessment and management of nonalcoholic fatty liver disease. *Hepatology*. 2023;77(5):1797–1835.
2. Targher G, Valenti L, Byrne CD. Metabolic dysfunction-associated steatotic liver disease. *N Engl J Med*. 2025;393(7):683–698.
3. Wattacheril JJ, Abdelmalek MF, Lim JK, et al. AGA clinical practice update on the role of noninvasive biomarkers in the evaluation and management of nonalcoholic fatty liver disease: expert review. *Gastroenterology*. 2023;165(4):1080–1088.

ADDITIONAL READING

Gofton C, Upendran Y, Zheng MH, et al. MAFLD: how is it different from NAFLD? *Clin Mol Hepatol*. 2023;29(suppl):S17–S31.

SEE ALSO

Algorithm: Weight Loss, Treatment

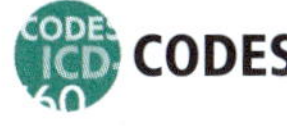

CODES

ICD10

K76.0 Fatty (change of) liver, not elsewhere classified

CLINICAL PEARLS

- MASLD is a major cause of liver disease and is increasing every year with increasing rates of overweight and obesity.
- Elevated ALT suggests steatohepatitis—does not correlate with fibrosis severity.
- Spectrum ranges from MASLD to MASH, advanced fibrosis, and cirrhosis.
- High prevalence in patients with prediabetes and diabetes.
- FIB-4 is initial noninvasive risk tool.
- Mediterranean diet and structured exercise are the cornerstones of therapy for MASLD.

METABOLIC SYNDROME

Naomi Parrella, MD, Dipl. ABOM, FOMA, FAAFP • Sylvia M. Robinson, MD

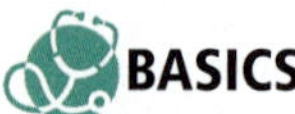

BASICS

DESCRIPTION

Metabolic syndrome (MetS) is a cluster of progressive abnormalities—central adiposity with insulin resistance, atherogenic dyslipidemia, elevated BP, dysglycemia, and a proinflammatory/prothrombotic milieu—associated with higher risk of ASCVD, heart failure, chronic kidney disease (CKD), stroke, T2DM, MASLD (formerly NAFLD), select cancers, depression/cognitive decline, and all-cause mortality (1).

EPIDEMIOLOGY

Incidence

Parallels obesity and T2DM trends: rising with ultraprocessed dietary patterns, inactivity and sleep disruption.

Prevalence

U.S. adult prevalence remains high (≈1/3 to 2/5 depending on definition). Global estimates ~25–35%, varying by cohort/criteria.

ETIOLOGY AND PATHOPHYSIOLOGY

Visceral adipose expansion leading to ectopic lipid deposition, lipotoxicity, impaired adipokines (↓ adiponectin), leptin/insulin resistance (IR); endothelial dysfunction; oxidative stress; prothrombotic state (↑ PAI-1); RAAS/sympathetic activation. MASLD/MASH both reflect and worsen systemic IR; fibrosis severity predicts outcomes. Circadian misalignment, sleep restriction, ultraprocessed foods (UPFs), and physical inactivity exacerbate IR and appetite regulation.

Genetics

Polygenic susceptibility (small individual effects, large aggregate risk); epigenetic programming (e.g., maternal hyperglycemia, small for gestational age [SGA]/large for gestational age [LGA]); environmental exposures ("obesogens"); family history of MetS/T2DM/ASCVD increases risk

RISK FACTORS

Perinatal (SGA/LGA, maternal GDM), premature pubarche/adrenarche, aging, certain ancestries, family history; ultraprocessed diet, sugar-sweetened beverages, inactivity/sedentary time, alcohol and tobacco use, poor sleep/obstructive sleep apnea (OSA), chronic stress; weight-promoting meds (e.g., antipsychotics, glucocorticoids, some β-blockers/anticonvulsants).

GENERAL PREVENTION

Healthy weight maintenance; regular physical activity; minimize UPFs; emphasize Mediterranean/DASH-like/low insulin diet patterns; adequate protein and fiber; limit added sugars/refined starches; alcohol moderation; tobacco cessation; sufficient sleep; stress management

COMMONLY ASSOCIATED CONDITIONS

Obesity; hypertension; atherogenic dyslipidemia; hypertriglyceridemia; hyperinsulinemia; acanthosis/skin tags; GERD, gallstones, MASLD/MASH; OSA; osteoarthritis, PCOS; CKD; hyperuricemia; hypogonadism; erectile dysfunction, mood/cognitive disorders.

DIAGNOSIS

Harmonized (Joint Interim Statement [JIS] 2009) criteria—any 3 of 5 (*pediatrics: use ≥90th percentile waist circumference and adolescent lipid thresholds):

- Waist circumference* (ethnicity-specific; e.g., non-Hispanic White and Black males ≥94 cm, females ≥80 cm; ATP III legacy males ≥102 cm, females ≥88 cm; International Diabetes Federation (IDF) recommends Hispanic/Latino and South/East Asian males ≥ 90 cm, females ≥ 80 cm)
- Triglycerides* ≥150 mg/dL (or on therapy)
- HDL-C* <40 mg/dL (males) or <50 mg/dL (females) (or on therapy)
- Blood pressure* ≥130/85 mm Hg (or on therapy)
- Fasting glucose ≥100 mg/dL (or on therapy)

HISTORY

Dietary pattern (UPF load, sugary beverages, alcohol), sleep/OSA symptoms, activity and sedentary time, medications, family history (MetS/T2DM/ASCVD/CKD), reproductive/PCOS history, mental health, weight trajectory/attempts

PHYSICAL EXAM

Waist circumference; BMI (appreciating limitations of BMI, see "Obesity"); properly measured BP (consider out-of-office); signs of IR (acanthosis nigricans, skin tags), hirsutism; hepatomegaly; edema; features of secondary hypertension

DIFFERENTIAL DIAGNOSIS

Hypothyroidism; Cushing syndrome; medication-induced metabolic derangements (antipsychotics, anticonvulsants, glucocorticoids, select β-blockers, thiazides); familial dyslipidemias; lipodystrophy; secondary causes of hypertension; alcohol-related fatty liver disease

DIAGNOSTIC TESTS & INTERPRETATION

Initial Tests (lab, imaging)

- Fasting lipid panel; fasting glucose and/or HbA1c
- ALT/AST and MASLD case finding with FIB-4 first line (thresholds: <1.3 low risk; ≥2 rule in age >65 years) → elastography (VCTE) or ELF if indeterminate/high (details in MASLD chapter)
- Estimated glomerular filtration rate (eGFR) and urine albumin-creatinine ratio (UACR) (CKD risk)
- Consider apoB when low-density lipoprotein cholestrol (LDL-C) discordant; optional hs-CRP; optional fasting insulin for counseling

Follow-Up Tests & Special Considerations

- 75-g OGTT if glycemic status uncertain
- OSA assessment (STOP-Bang; sleep study if indicated)
- CAC scoring for ASCVD risk refinement when it will change management
- Periodic FIB-4 in steatosis-at-risk patients; reflex to VCTE/ELF per MASLD chapter

Diagnostic Procedures/Other

- VCTE (elastography) or ELF for secondary liver fibrosis risk assessment
- Sleep study when high suspicion for OSA
- CAC scoring for borderline/intermediate ASCVD risk

Test Interpretation

MetS is present with ≥3 criteria. Use apoB to capture atherogenic particle burden when LDL-C appears "normal" but risk is high. FIB-4 low (<1.3) usually rules out advanced fibrosis; indeterminate/high warrants elastography/ELF or hepatology referral.

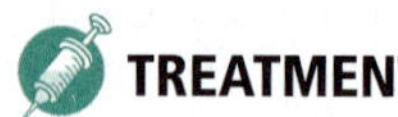

TREATMENT

GENERAL MEASURES

- Nutrition: Mediterranean/DASH-like; minimize UPFs; adequate protein and fiber; limit added sugars/refined starches.
- Time-restricted eating (TRE) (8 to 10 hours window) can modestly improve weight/glycemia (2).
- Physical activity: ≥150 to 300 minutes/week moderate-intensity aerobic + 2 days/week resistance; break up sitting.
- Sleep/behavior: Treat OSA; regular sleep/wake; stress management; tobacco abstinence; alcohol moderation
- Weight targets: Weight loss of 5–10% yields meaningful risk reduction; ≥10–15% amplifies benefit (T2DM remission odds, ASCVD risk).

MEDICATION

First Line

- GLP-1 RA/dual GIP–GLP-1 (e.g., semaglutide 2.4 mg; tirzepatide) for obesity phenotypes: large weight loss; semaglutide lowered MACE by ~20% in adults with obesity without diabetes and established ASCVD (3). Growing class-level evidence for kidney and cardiovascular protection (4). Tirzepatide for moderate-to-severe OSA in adults with obesity reduced apnea-hypopnea index (AHI) and body weight and improved sleep-related outcomes. Coordinate with sleep medicine for selection and monitoring (5). (See "Obesity" and OSA sections.)
- SGLT2i in T2DM/CKD/HF phenotypes: robust HF hospitalization and kidney protection; MACE reduction present overall, strongest with higher baseline risk (6)
- Metformin for dysglycemia/IR (weight-neutral, prediabetes prevention benefit); monitor vitamin B_{12}.

Second Line
- Lipid management per CVD chapter: high-intensity statin ± ezetimibe/PCSK9 pathway; consider apoB target.
- Blood pressure per CVD chapter: often <130/80 mm Hg (consider 120 to 129 mm Hg SBP if tolerated); favor RAAS blockers with albuminuria
- MASLD/MASH: consider resmetirom for noncirrhotic MASH F2–F3 as adjunct to lifestyle/risk-factor control.

ISSUES FOR REFERRAL
Hepatology (high/indeterminate FIB-4, suspected advanced fibrosis, imaging concerns, resmetirom candidacy); sleep medicine (suspected OSA); cardiology (ASCVD risk refinement/HF/CKD overlap); obesity medicine/endocrinology (pharmacotherapy escalation); bariatric surgery evaluation; mental health (mood disorders, disordered eating, trauma)

ADDITIONAL THERAPIES
Supplements/herbals show heterogeneous and mostly low-certainty effects; may be considered as adjuncts via shared decision-making; avoid substituting for proven therapies.

SURGERY/OTHER PROCEDURES
Metabolic-bariatric surgery for eligible patients (see "Obesity"): durable improvement/remission of MetS; optimize peri-op nutrition, OSA, glycemia, BP, and thrombosis prophylaxis.

COMPLEMENTARY & ALTERNATIVE MEDICINE
Evidence mixed and generally low certainty (7); discuss risks, interactions, and expectations; integrate only as adjuncts (7).

ADMISSION, INPATIENT, AND NURSING CONSIDERATIONS
For planned procedures/surgery: Optimize weight, glycemia, BP, OSA, lipids, and nutrition to reduce complications/readmissions. Screen for alcohol use disorder and depression/anxiety when relevant.

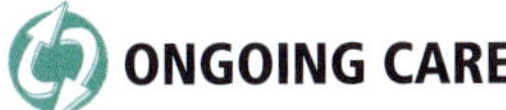

ONGOING CARE

FOLLOW-UP RECOMMENDATIONS

Patient Monitoring
Track weight, waist, BP each visit. Recheck TG/HDL-C, glucose/HbA1c, eGFR/UACR, ALT/AST per risk; repeat FIB-4 in steatosis-at-risk; consider apoB and CAC if it will change management. Document CKM stage to align therapy (e.g., add SGLT2i for CKD/HF; GLP-1/GIP–GLP-1 for ASCVD risk/weight) (1).

DIET
- See "Treatment."
- Whole-food pattern with minimal UPFs; adequate protein; high fiber; omega-3 fats; limit added sugars/refined starches; tailor to cultural preferences and sustainability.

PATIENT EDUCATION
MetS is modifiable. Combining lifestyle, appropriate pharmacotherapy, and, if needed, surgery reverses many components and reduces events (2),(3),(4),(6).

PROGNOSIS
Persistent MetS increases all-cause and CV mortality; partial or full remission of MetS components reduces CVD, stroke, and mortality risk. CKM stage correlates with graded increases in adverse outcomes (1).

COMPLICATIONS
Progression of ASCVD and T2DM; MASLD progression to MASH and cirrhosis; stroke; CKD/ESKD; cognitive decline; increased risk of select cancers (e.g., postmenopausal breast, pancreatic, colorectal)

REFERENCES

1. Ndumele CE, Rangaswami J, Chow SL, et al; for the American Heart Association. Cardiovascular-kidney-metabolic health: a presidential advisory from the American Heart Association. *Circulation*. 2023;148(20):1606–1635.
2. Manoogian ENC, Wilkinson MJ, O'Neal M, et al. Time-restricted eating in adults with metabolic syndrome: a randomized controlled trial. *Ann Intern Med*. 2024;177(11):1462–1470.
3. Lincoff AM, Brown-Frandsen K, Colhoun HM, et al; for the SELECT Investigators. Semaglutide and cardiovascular outcomes in obesity without diabetes. *N Engl J Med*. 2023;389(24):2221–2232.
4. Badve SV, Bilal A, Lee MMY, et al. Effects of GLP-1 receptor agonists on kidney and cardiovascular outcomes: systematic review and meta-analysis of randomised trials. *Lancet Diabetes Endocrinol*. 2025;13(1):15–28.
5. Malhotra A, Grunstein RR, Fietze I, et al; for the SURMOUNT-OSA Investigators. Tirzepatide for the treatment of obstructive sleep apnea and obesity. *N Engl J Med*. 2024;391(13):1193–1205.
6. Patel SM, Kang YM, Im K, et al. Sodium-glucose cotransporter-2 inhibitors and major adverse cardiovascular outcomes: a collaborative trial-level meta-analysis. *Circulation*. 2024;149(23):1789–1801.
7. Abdulghani MF, Al-Fayyadh S. Natural products for managing metabolic syndrome: a scoping review. *Front Pharmacol*. 2024;15:1366946.

ADDITIONAL READING

- Świątkiewicz I, Woźniak A, Taub PR. Time-restricted eating and metabolic syndrome: current status and future perspectives. *Nutrients*. 2021;13(1):221.
- European Association for the Study of the Liver (EASL), European Association for the Study of Diabetes (EASD), European Association for the Study of Obesity (EASO). EASL-EASD-EASO Clinical Practice Guidelines on the management of metabolic dysfunction-associated steatotic liver disease (MASLD). *J Hepatol*. 2024;81(3):492–542.
- Koskinas KC, Van Craenenbroeck EM, Antoniades C, et al; for the ESC Scientific Document Group. Obesity and cardiovascular disease: an ESC clinical consensus statement. *Eur Heart J*. 2024;45(38):4063–4098.
- Lane MM, Gamage E, Du S, et al. Ultra-processed food exposure and adverse health outcomes: an umbrella review of epidemiological meta-analyses. *BMJ*. 2024;384:e077310.
- American Diabetes Association Primary Care Advisory Group. Standards of care in Diabetes—2025 abridged for primary care. *Clin Diabetes*. 2025;43(2):182.

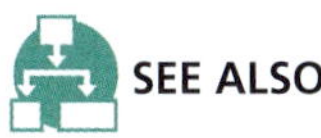

SEE ALSO

Diabetes Mellitus, Type 2; Hypertension, Essential; Obesity; Sleep Apnea, Obstructive; Polycystic Ovarian Syndrome (PCOS); Metabolic Dysfunction-Associated Steatotic Liver Disease (MASLD)

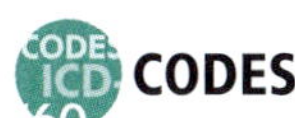

CODES

ICD10
E88.81 Metabolic syndrome

CLINICAL PEARLS
- Measure waist every visit; a rising TG:HDL-C ratio (>2) or waist-to-height ≥0.5 should trigger full MetS workup and counseling.
- Stage CKM in the note and set targets (A1c, BP, LDL-C/apoB, eGFR/UACR, weight); re-stage at follow-ups to guide therapy intensity (1).
- Case-find MASLD in all MetS/T2DM/obesity with FIB-4 → elastography/ELF; refer high fibrosis risk. (See MASLD chapter for cutoffs and resmetirom criteria.)
- In MetS + established ASCVD—even without diabetes—offer semaglutide 2.4 mg to reduce MACE (~20%) and address adiposity (3).
- Layer therapies by phenotype: Use SGLT2i for CKD/HF protection; GLP-1/GIP–GLP-1 for ASCVD/CKD risk and weight; many patients benefit from both (4),(6).
- Prescribe an 8- to 10-hour TRE window for patients who prefer structure; pair with protein-forward, minimally processed meals for adherence (2).
- Minimize UPFs; anchor Mediterranean/DASH variants; add fiber and adequate protein to curb appetite and improve lipids.
- Review meds for weight gain (e.g., antipsychotics, steroids); switch to weight-neutral alternatives when feasible.
- Escalate early if <5% weight loss at 3 to 6 months on lifestyle alone, add obesity management medications, and consider metabolic-bariatric surgery when criteria are met.
- Use apoB to adjudicate discordant lipids and CAC to guide preventive intensity when decisions are uncertain.
- Screen and treat OSA; therapy augments BP/glycemic control and weight efforts.

METATARSALGIA

Ammar Shahid, MD • Marc McKenna, MD, CAQSM

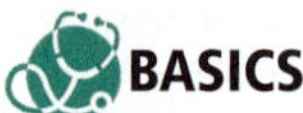

BASICS

DESCRIPTION

- Metatarsalgia is defined as pain in the forefoot under one or more metatarsal heads.
- There are three groups:
  - Primary: due to anatomic issues between the metatarsal and other parts of the foot
  - Secondary: due to conditions that increase metatarsal loading via indirect mechanisms, such as chronic synovitis or fracture or injury to the metatarsophalangeal (MTP) joint
  - Iatrogenic usually after a prior forefoot surgery, such as with halux valgus surgery

EPIDEMIOLOGY

Incidence

The overall incidence in the general population is 5–36%; especially common in athletes engaging in high-impact sports (running, jumping, dancing), in rock climbers (12.5%), and in older active adults; most common in women aged 3 to 60 years.

Prevalence

Common

ETIOLOGY AND PATHOPHYSIOLOGY

- The 1st metatarsal head bears significant weight when walking or running. A normal metatarsal arch ensures this balance. The 1st metatarsal head normally has adequate padding to accommodate increased forces.
- Reactive tissue can build a callus around the metatarsal head, compounding the pain.
  - Excessive or repetitive stress; Forces are transmitted to the forefoot during several stages (midstance and push off) of walking and running. These forces are translated across the metatarsal heads at nearly 3 times the body weight.
  - A pronated splayfoot disturbs this balance, causing equal weight-bearing on all metatarsal heads.
  - Any foot deformity changes distribution of weight, impacting areas of the foot that do not have sufficient padding.
  - Soft tissue dysfunction: intrinsic muscle weakness, laxity in the Lisfranc ligament
  - Abnormal foot posture: forefoot varus or valgus, cavus or equinus deformities, loss of the metatarsal arch, splayfoot, pronated foot, inappropriate footwear
  - Dermatologic: warts, calluses (1)[C]
- Great toe
  - Hallux valgus (bunion), either varus or rigidus
- Lesser metatarsals
  - Freiberg infraction (i.e., aseptic necrosis of the metatarsal head usually due to trauma in adolescents who jump or sprint)
  - Hammer toe or claw toe
  - Morton syndrome (i.e., long 2nd metatarsal)

RISK FACTORS

- Obesity
- Forefoot surgery or trauma
- High heels, narrow shoes, or overly tight-fitting shoes (rock climbers typically wear small shoes)
- Competitive athletes in weight-bearing sports (e.g., ballet, basketball, running, soccer, baseball, football)
- Foot deformities or changes in range of motion (ROM) (e.g., pes planus, pes cavus, tight Achilles tendon, tarsal tunnel syndrome, hallux valgus, prominent metatarsal heads, excessive pronation, hammer toe deformity, tight toe extensors) (1)[C]

Geriatric Considerations

- Concomitant arthritis
- Metatarsalgia is common in older athletes.
- Age-related atrophy of the metatarsal fat pad may increase the risk for metatarsalgia.

Pediatric Considerations

- Muscle imbalance disorders (e.g., Duchenne muscular dystrophy) causing foot deformities in children.
- In adolescent girls, consider Freiberg infraction.
- Salter-Harris type I injuries may affect subsequent growth and healing of the epiphysis.

Pregnancy Considerations

- Forefoot pain during pregnancy usually results from change in gait, center of mass, and joint laxity.
- Wear properly fitted low-heeled shoes.

GENERAL PREVENTION

- Wear properly fitted shoes with good padding.
- Start weight-bearing exercise programs gradually.
- Adequate stretching, particularly of the calf muscles
- Weight loss, if overweight

COMMONLY ASSOCIATED CONDITIONS

- Arthritis
- Morton neuroma
- Sesamoiditis
- Plantar keratosis—callus formation

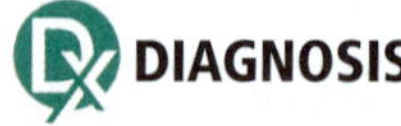

DIAGNOSIS

HISTORY

- Pain gradually develops and persists over the heads of one or more metatarsals. Pain is usually on the plantar surface and worsen during midstance gait phase.
- Pain is often chronic.
- Predisposition with pes cavus and hyperpronation
- Pain often described as walking with a pebble in the shoe; aggravated during midstance or propulsion phases of walking or running

PHYSICAL EXAM

- Point tenderness over plantar metatarsal heads
- Pain in the interdigital space or a positive metatarsal squeeze test suggests Morton neuroma.
- Plantar keratosis
- Tenderness of the metatarsal head(s) with pressure applied by the examiner's finger and thumb
- Erythema and swelling (occasionally)

DIFFERENTIAL DIAGNOSIS

- Stress fracture (most commonly 2nd metatarsal)
- Morton neuroma (i.e., interdigital neuroma)
- Tarsal tunnel syndrome
- Sesamoiditis or sesamoid fracture
- Salter-Harris type I fracture in children
- Arthritis (e.g., gouty, rheumatoid, inflammatory, osteoarthritis, septic, calcium pyrophosphate dihydrate crystal deposition disease [CPPD])
- Lisfranc injury
- Avascular necrosis of the metatarsal head
- Ganglion cyst
- Foreign body
- Vasculitis (diabetes)
- Bony tumors

DIAGNOSTIC TESTS & INTERPRETATION

Often a clinical diagnosis; testing is not always required

Initial Tests (lab, imaging)

- Weight-bearing radiographs: anteroposterior, lateral, and oblique views:
  - Occasionally, metatarsal or sesamoid axial films (to rule out sesamoid fracture) or skyline view of the metatarsal heads to assess the plantar declination of the metatarsal heads: obtained with the MTP joints in dorsiflexion (to evaluate alignment)
- Ultrasound and MRI in recalcitrant cases especially if concern for stress fracture (2)[C]
- MR arthrography of the MTP joint can delineate capsular tears, typically of the distal lateral border of the plantar plate (an often underrecognized cause of metatarsalgia).
- Only if diagnosis is in question
  - Erythrocyte sedimentation rate or C-reactive protein
  - Rheumatoid factor
  - Uric acid
  - Glucose
  - CBC with differential

Diagnostic Procedures/Other

Plantar pressure distribution analysis may help distinguish pressure distribution patterns due to malalignment.

TREATMENT

Treatment for metatarsalgia is typically conservative.

- Relieve pain
- Ice initially
- Rest: temporary alteration of weight-bearing activity; use of cane or crutch; for more physically active patients, suggest an alternative exercise or cross-training:
  - Moist heat later
  - Taping or using gel metatarsal cushion
  - Stiff-soled shoes will act as a splint.
  - Gastrocnemius stretching exercises
- Relieve the pressure beneath the area of maximal pain by redistributing the pressure load of the foot, which can be achieved through orthotics.
- Weight loss, if overweight

MEDICATION

Nonsteroidal anti-inflammatory medications for 7 to 14 days if no contraindications

ISSUES FOR REFERRAL

High-level athletes may benefit from early podiatric or orthopedic evaluation.

ADDITIONAL THERAPIES

- Physical therapy to restore normal foot biomechanics
- Low-heeled (<2 cm height) wide-toe-box shoes
- Metatarsal bars, pads, and arch supports; metatarsal bars are often more effective than pads; if hallux valgus present, may try a valgus splint
- Orthotics/rocker bar (Prescriptive orthotics have been shown to be an effective treatment.)
- Thick-soled shoes
- Shaving the callus may provide temporary relief. Callus excision is not recommended.
- Corticosteroid injection may benefit interdigital neuritis but should be used with caution because it may cause MTP instability and fat pad atrophy.
- Improve flexibility and strength of the intrinsic muscles of the foot with:
  - Exercises (e.g., towel grasps, pencil curls)
  - Physical therapy to maintain ROM and restore normal biomechanics

SURGERY/OTHER PROCEDURES

- If no improvement with conservative therapy for 3 months, refer to foot/ankle orthopedic surgeon or podiatrist.
- Surgery may help correct anatomic abnormality: bunionectomy, partial osteotomy, or foot fusion surgery (arthrodesis). Success rates vary depending on procedure.
- Direct plantar plate repair (grade II medial collateral ligament tear) combined with Weil osteotomy can restore normal alignment of the MTP joint, leading to diminished pain with improved functional scores.
- Callus removal is generally not recommended.
- Morton neurectomy and ultrasound-guided alcohol ablation of Morton neuroma are options (3)[C].
- Surgery only as a last resort if no anatomic abnormality is present.

COMPLEMENTARY & ALTERNATIVE MEDICINE

Magnetic insoles are not effective for chronic nonspecific foot pain.

ADMISSION, INPATIENT, AND NURSING CONSIDERATIONS

Patients generally admitted only for surgery

ONGOING CARE

FOLLOW-UP RECOMMENDATIONS

Patient Monitoring

If stress fracture has been ruled out and patient's condition has not improved >3 months of conservative treatment, consider surgical evaluation or corticosteroid injection (depending on the condition).

PATIENT EDUCATION

- Instruct about wearing proper shoes and gradual return to activity.
- Cross-training until symptoms subside. Goal is to restore normal foot biomechanics, relieve abnormal pressure on the plantar metatarsal heads, and relieve pain (4)[C].

PROGNOSIS

Outcome depends on the severity of the problem and whether surgery is required to correct it.

COMPLICATIONS

- Back, knee, and hip pain due to change in gait
- Transfer metatarsalgia following surgical intervention, which subsequently transfers stress to other areas.

REFERENCES

1. DiPreta JA. Metatarsalgia, lesser toe deformities, and associated disorders of the forefoot. *Med Clin North Am*. 2014;98(2):233–251.
2. Besse JL. Metatarsalgia. *Orthop Traumatol Surg Res*. 2017;103(1S):S29–S39.
3. Musson RE, Sawhney JS, Lamb L, et al. Ultrasound guided alcohol ablation of Morton's neuroma. *Foot Ankle Int*. 2012;33(3):196–201.
4. Espinosa N, Brodsky JW, Maceira E. Metatarsalgia. *J Am Acad Orthop Surg*. 2010;18(8):474–485.

ADDITIONAL READING

- Birbilis T, Theodoropoulou E, Koulalis D. Forefoot complaints—the Morton's metatarsalgia. The role of MR imaging. *Acta Medica (Hradec Kralove)*. 2007;50(3):221–222.
- Burns J, Landorf KB, Ryan MM, et al. Interventions for the prevention and treatment of pes cavus. *Cochrane Database Syst Rev*. 2007;2007(4):CD006154.
- Deshaies A, Roy P, Symeonidis PD, et al. Metatarsal bars more effective than metatarsal pads in reducing impulse on the second metatarsal head. *Foot (Edinb)*. 2011;21(4):172–175.
- Pace A, Scammell B, Dhar S. The outcome of Morton's neurectomy in the treatment of metatarsalgia. *Int Orthop*. 2010;34(4):511–515.
- Park CH, Chang MC. Forefoot disorders and conservative treatment. *Yeungnam Univ J Med*. 2019;36(2):92–98.
- Thomas JL, Blitch EL IV, Chaney DM, et al; for Clinical Practice Guideline Forefoot Disorders Panel. Diagnosis and treatment of forefoot disorders. Section 2. Central metatarsalgia. *J Foot Ankle Surg*. 2009;48(2):239–250.
- Cooke R, Manning C, Palihawadana D, et al. Metatarsalgia: anatomy, pathology and management. *Br J Hosp Med (Lond)*. 2021;82(9):1–8.

SEE ALSO

Morton Neuroma (Interdigital Neuroma)

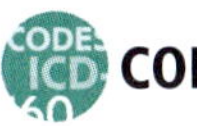

CODES

ICD10

- M77.40 Metatarsalgia, unspecified foot
- G57.60 Lesion of plantar nerve, unspecified lower limb
- M77.42 Metatarsalgia, left foot

CLINICAL PEARLS

- Metatarsalgia refers to pain of the plantar surface of the forefoot in the region of the metatarsal heads.
- Metatarsalgia is common in athletes who participate in high-impact sports involving the lower extremities.
- Patients describe as "walking with a pebble in the shoe." Pain is worse during midstance or propulsion phases of walking or running. The most common physical finding is point tenderness over the plantar metatarsal heads.
- Typical treatment is conservative, including rest and ice, activity modification, and ensuring proper padding under the foot.
- Pregnant patients should wear properly fitted, low-heeled shoes to reduce incidence of metatarsalgia.

MILD COGNITIVE IMPAIRMENT

Birju B. Patel, MD, FACP, AGSF

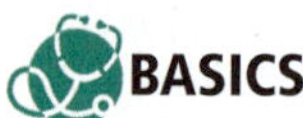

BASICS

DESCRIPTION

- Mild cognitive impairment (MCI) is defined as significant cognitive impairment in the absence of dementia, as measured by standard memory tests:
  - Subjective memory concerns
  - Preservation of independence in functional activities of daily living (ADLs)
  - Impairment in ≥1 cognitive domains (attention, executive dysfunction, memory, learning, visuospatial, language)
  - Other terms used in the literature relating to MCI: cognitive impairment not dementia (CIND); mild cognitive disorder; some of these conditions do not progress to dementia. *DSM-5* mentions "mild neurocognitive disorder" (mNCD), which may be a precursor to Alzheimer disease and has many of the same features as MCI.
- Older adults with MCI are three times more likely to progress to dementia in 2 to 5 years than age matched cohorts (1)[A].

EPIDEMIOLOGY

Incidence

- Predominant sex: male > female
- Predominant age:
  - Higher in older persons and in those with less education
  - 12 to 15/1,000 person-years in those age ≥65 years
  - 50 to 75/1,000 person-years in those age ≥75 years

Prevalence

- MCI is more prevalent than dementia in the United States.
- 12–18% for those age ≥60 years; ~25% for age 80 to 84 years; prevalence increases with age and for those with lower educational level (2).

ETIOLOGY AND PATHOPHYSIOLOGY

- Subtypes of MCI:
  - Single-domain amnestic
  - Multiple-domain amnestic
  - Nonamnestic single domain
  - Nonamnestic multiple domain
- The amnestic subtypes are higher risk for progression to Alzheimer disease.
- Vascular, neurodegenerative, traumatic, metabolic, psychiatric, or a combination

Genetics

In certain subsets of MCI where the disease will progress to Alzheimer disease one must consider apolipoprotein (APO) E4 genotype: Various pathways exist leading to amyloid accumulation and deposition thought to be associated with Alzheimer disease.

RISK FACTORS

- Diabetes; hypertension; hyperlipidemia; cerebrovascular disease
- Smoking
- Sleep apnea
- APO E4 genotype
- Low educational levels
- Depression
- Sedentary lifestyle
- Hearing loss

GENERAL PREVENTION

Optimize vascular risk factors and focus on a healthy, active lifestyle.

COMMONLY ASSOCIATED CONDITIONS

See "Risk Factors."

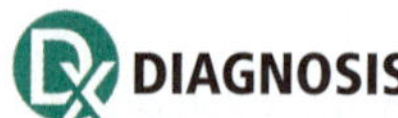

DIAGNOSIS

HISTORY

- Focus on cognitive deficits and impairment. MCI is meant to reflect a change in cognition and not lifelong impaired cognition.
- Review all medications that may affect cognition with emphasis given to anticholinergic medications (patients on these may mistakenly be classified as having MCI).
- Rule out depression. The prevalence of depression in patients with MCI is higher than age-matched cohorts.
- Assess function (ADLs, instrumental ADLs) and subtle changes in daily function (e.g., in the workplace).
- Impact on interpersonal relationships and caregiver stress
- Assess vascular risk factors (hypertension, diabetes, hyperlipidemia, and cerebrovascular disease).
- Assess behavioral changes (agitation, aggression, impulsivity, disinhibition, apathy, and others).
- Olfactory dysfunction may be associated with amnestic MCI and progression to Alzheimer disease. This can be easily evaluated in patients with memory impairment (3).

PHYSICAL EXAM

- A general exam focusing on clinical clues to identifying vascular disease (e.g., bruits, abnormal BP)
- Neurologic exam to rule out reversible CNS causes cognitive impairment or other causes of cognitive impairment.
- Office measures of cognitive function, depression, and functional status

DIFFERENTIAL DIAGNOSIS

- Normal aging (age-related cognitive impairment, age-associated memory impairment)
- Early Alzheimer disease
- Delirium; dementia; depression
- "Reversible" cognitive impairment
  - Medications (anticholinergics and medications with anticholinergic properties)
  - Hypothyroidism
  - Vitamin B_{12} deficiency
- Give consideration to sleep conditions, especially sleep apnea, that can contribute to cognitive deficits.

DIAGNOSTIC TESTS & INTERPRETATION

- Formal screening with standardized cognitive tests is important (e.g., Montreal Cognitive Assessment [MoCA] and Saint Louis University Mental Status [SLUMS]); MoCA may be more sensitive for detecting and following MCI.
- Neuropsychological testing should be considered for all patients with presumed MCI, as a follow-up after any failed screening methods

Initial Tests (lab, imaging)

- Complete blood count
- Comprehensive metabolic profile
- Thyroid-stimulating hormone
- Vitamin B_{12}
- Syphilis and HIV testing
- Cerebrospinal fluid (CSF) biomarkers can be used to assess for Alzheimer disease, if available. Blood based biomarker tests are being evaluated.
- Imaging tests are helpful when there are focal neurologic deficits or rapid or atypical presentations:
  - CT scan can detect structural CNS conditions leading to cognitive impairment:
    - Subdural hematoma; normal pressure hydrocephalus; metastatic disease; cerebrovascular accident
  - MRI further evaluates vascular, infectious, neoplastic, and inflammatory conditions.
  - Amyloid PET scans can be used to assess for amyloid in those felt to be high risk for Alzheimer disease.

Follow-Up Tests & Special Considerations

- Document progression of functional impairment, cognitive decline, concurrent depression, and comorbid conditions.
- Advanced care planning while patient is competent
- Early education of caregivers on safety, maintaining structure, managing stress, support, and future planning
- Focus on driving ability and safety.
- Work-related issues should be explored and optimized as best possible.
- Neuropsychological testing should be done at 1- to 2-year intervals depending on subjective concerns and ongoing diagnosis of MCI.
- If early Alzheimer disease is being considered and anti-amyloid therapies are being considered, confirmatory testing is needed (lumbar puncture for CSF biomarkers, blood biomarkers, amyloid specific scans, ApoE testing, etc.) This workup may not be readily available and referral to specialized centers may be necessary.

Test Interpretation

- Little is known about MCI pathology due to a lack of longitudinal studies and heterogeneity of population studied.
- Alzheimer disease pathophysiology:
  - Neurofibrillary tangles in hippocampus
  - Senile plaques (amyloid deposition)
  - Neuronal degeneration

- Those with MCI have intermediate amounts of pathologic findings of Alzheimer disease with amyloid deposition and neurofibrillary tangles in the mesial temporal lobes compared with those with dementia.
- Amnestic MCI is associated with white matter hyperintensity volume on MRI, whereas nonamnestic MCI is associated with infarcts.

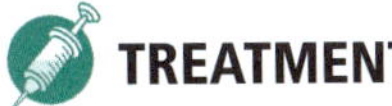

TREATMENT

GENERAL MEASURES

Atherosclerotic risk factors should be treated aggressively.

MEDICATION

The use of cholinesterase inhibitors (ChEIs) in MCI is not associated with any delay in the onset of Alzheimer disease or dementia. Moreover, the safety profile showed that the risks associated with ChEIs are significant. Therefore, ChEIs are not routinely recommended (1)[B]. Anti-amyloid therapies require confirmatory diagnosis of Alzheimer disease and should not be used in MCI.

ISSUES FOR REFERRAL

Consider referral to a memory specialist (i.e., geriatrician, neurologist, geropsychiatric, neuropsychologist) to evaluate and differentiate subtypes of MCI and specific cognitive deficits.

ADDITIONAL THERAPIES

There may be benefit in terms of improvement in performance on tests for global cognitive functioning with cognitive training and physical exercise.

COMPLEMENTARY & ALTERNATIVE MEDICINE

- No evidence suggests the efficacy of vitamin E in the prevention or treatment of people with MCI.
- Long-term use of *Ginkgo biloba* extract has shown to have no benefit in the treatment of MCI and in terms of progression to dementia. In addition, *Ginkgo biloba* can be associated with increase in bleeding risk including CNS bleeds (4)[B].

ADMISSION, INPATIENT, AND NURSING CONSIDERATIONS

Delirium is more common in patients hospitalized with all forms of cognitive impairment.

- Avoid medications that may worsen or precipitate cognitive decline (e.g., anticholinergics, antihistamines, and sedatives).
- Patients may be extremely sensitive to the hospital environment:
  - Moderate level of stimulation is best.
  - Avoid sensory deprivation. Make sure that patients have access to hearing aids and eyeglasses.
  - Use frequent cueing and have caregivers or family in the room whenever possible with patient.
  - Frequently orient patients to date and time.

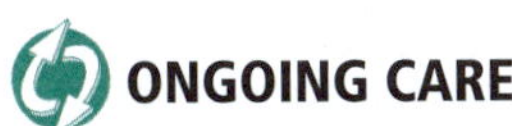

ONGOING CARE

FOLLOW-UP RECOMMENDATIONS

Reevaluate every 6 to 12 months to determine if symptoms are progressing.

Patient Monitoring

Appropriate cognitive and functional testing should be used to evaluate progression, along with clinical history and exam. If a medication is started, patients need to be followed more frequently to evaluate for efficacy, side effects, dose titration, and so forth. Declining executive function may be an early marker to progression of MCI to dementia, and clinicians should monitor and advise patients and families proactively to look for this. Impairments in ADL function is a good clue to progression to dementia from MCI. Attempts should be made to wean medications that can impact cognition.

DIET

Diet to minimize atherosclerotic risk factors should be emphasized.

PATIENT EDUCATION

- Long-term planning topics should be discussed including advanced directives, firearm safety, driving safety, finances, and estate planning.
- Encourage lifestyle changes:
  - Physical activity, such as walking 30 minutes daily on most days of the week, as exercise modestly improved some measures of cognition in some studies
  - Mental activity that stimulates language skills and psychomotor coordination should be encouraged. Computer activities, reading books, crafts, crossword puzzles, and games may be linked to decreased risk of development of MCI (5)[C].
- Cognitive rehabilitation strategies may be beneficial in helping with daily activities relating to memory tasks in MCI.
- Treatment of vascular risk factors (hypertension, diabetes, cerebrovascular disease, and hyperlipidemia) is important in lowering risk of progression to dementia (e.g., intensive blood pressure lowering in the Sprint Mind study reduced incidence of MCI with target SBP of 120 mm Hg).
- There are no FDA-approved medications or dietary agents currently for MCI shown to have benefit.
- In those with sleep apnea, compliance with CPAP improves cognition.
- Good dental hygiene and regular dental evaluation must be maintained. Significant periodontal disease is associated with MCI.
- Excessive alcohol consumption, above recommended limits, worsens cognition.
- Treat hearing loss.

PROGNOSIS

- Older adults with MCI have three times higher risks of progression to dementia in 2 to 5 years.
- Amnestic subtypes of MCI are most likely to progress to dementia.
- Neuropsychological testing measures, CSF biomarkers, and neuroimaging studies are being used in specialty settings to predict conversion to dementia. These are not widely available or cost-effective and are not used in general use.
- Women are more likely to progress to dementia.
- Olfactory dysfunction can be higher risk for progression to dementia.
- Patients with neuropsychiatric symptoms, such as anxiety or depression, are higher risk for progression to Alzheimer disease. This may be helpful in identifying higher risk MCI patients (6)[C].

REFERENCES

1. Petersen RC, Lopez O, Armstrong MJ, et al. Practice guideline update summary: mild cognitive impairment [RETIRED]: report of the Guideline Development, Dissemination, and Implementation Subcommittee of the American Academy of Neurology. *Neurology*. 2018;90(3):126–135.
2. Petersen RC. Mild cognitive impairment. *Continuum (Minneap Minn)*. 2016;22(2 Dementia):404–418.
3. Roberts RO, Christianson TJH, Kremers WK, et al. Association between olfactory dysfunction and amnestic mild cognitive impairment and Alzheimer disease dementia. *JAMA Neurol*. 2016;73(1):93–101.
4. Vellas B, Coley N, Ousset PJ, et al; for GuidAge Study Group. Long-term use of standardised Ginkgo biloba extract for the prevention of Alzheimer's disease (GuidAge): a randomised placebo-controlled trial. *Lancet Neurol*. 2012;11(10):851–859.
5. Marshall GA, Rentz DM, Frey MT, et al. Executive function and instrumental activities of daily living in mild cognitive impairment and Alzheimer's disease. *Alzheimers Dement*. 2011;7(3):300–308.
6. Roberto N, Portella MJ, Marquié M, et al. Neuropsychiatric profiles and conversion to dementia in mild cognitive impairment, a latent class analysis. *Sci Rep*. 2021;11(1):6448.

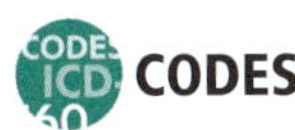

CODES

ICD10

G31.84 Mild cognitive impairment, so stated

CLINICAL PEARLS

- Amnestic MCI affects primarily memory and is more likely to progress to Alzheimer disease.
- Screen for reversible factors, particularly anticholinergic medications, depression, and sleep disorders.
- Look closely at vascular risk factors and optimize them.
- Memory disorders clinics use neuropsychiatric testing and newer modalities to further rule out Alzheimer disease (blood biomarkers, amyloid PET, Tau PET scans)
- ChEIs should not be used routinely unless memory complaints are affecting quality of life in patients. Potential side effects of these medications should be thoroughly discussed with patients and their families. A baseline ECG should be done prior to initiation of ChEIs due to risk of bradycardia and syncope.
- Neuropsychological testing is recommended in individuals suspected of having MCI. Patients with MCI and with prominent subjective complaints should have follow-up testing to evaluate for progression between 1 and 2 years after the initial assessment.

M

MISCARRIAGE (EARLY PREGNANCY LOSS)

Clara M. Keegan, MD

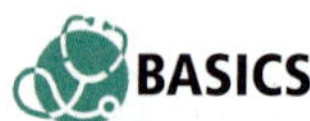

BASICS

DESCRIPTION

- Miscarriage, also known as early pregnancy loss (EPL) or spontaneous abortion (SAb), is the failure or loss of a pregnancy before 13 weeks' gestational age (WGA).
- Related terms
  - Anembryonic gestation: gestational sac on ultrasound (US) without visible embryo after 6 WGA
  - Complete abortion: entire contents of uterus expelled
  - Ectopic pregnancy: pregnancy outside the uterus
  - Embryonic or fetal demise: cervix closed; embryo or fetus present in the uterus without cardiac activity
  - Incomplete abortion: abortion with retained products of conception, generally placental tissue
  - Induced or therapeutic abortion: evacuation of uterine contents or products of conception medically or surgically
  - Inevitable abortion: cervical dilatation or rupture of membranes in the presence of vaginal bleeding
  - Recurrent abortion: three or more consecutive pregnancy losses at <15 WGA
  - Threatened abortion: vaginal bleeding in the 1st trimester of pregnancy
  - Septic abortion: a spontaneous or therapeutic abortion complicated by pelvic infection; common complication of illegally performed induced abortions
- Synonym(s): SAb
  - Missed abortion and blighted ovum are used less frequently in favor of terms representing the sonographic diagnosis.

EPIDEMIOLOGY

Predominant age: increases with advancing age, especially >35 years; at age 40 years, the loss rate is twice that of age 20 years.

Incidence

- Threatened abortion (1st-trimester bleeding) occurs in 20–25% of clinical pregnancies.
- Between 10% and 15% of all clinically recognized pregnancies end in EPL, with 80% of these occurring within 12 weeks after last menstrual period (LMP) (1).
- When both clinical and biochemical (β-hCG detected) pregnancies are considered, about 30% of pregnancies end in EPL.
- One in four people with a uterus will have an EPL during their lifetime (1).

ETIOLOGY AND PATHOPHYSIOLOGY

Chromosomal anomalies (50% of cases), congenital anomalies, trauma, maternal factors: uterine abnormalities, infection (toxoplasma, other viruses, rubella, cytomegalovirus, herpesvirus), maternal endocrine disorders, hypercoagulable state

Genetics

Approximately 50% of 1st-trimester EPLs have significant chromosomal anomalies, with 50% of these being autosomal trisomies and the remainder being triploidy, tetraploidy, or 45X monosomies.

RISK FACTORS

Most cases of EPL occur in patients without identifiable risk factors; however, risk factors include the following: chromosomal abnormalities, advancing maternal age, uterine abnormalities, and maternal chronic disease (antiphospholipid antibodies, uncontrolled diabetes mellitus, polycystic ovarian syndrome, obesity, hypertension, thyroid disease, renal disease); other possible contributing factors include smoking, alcohol intake, cocaine use, infection, and luteal phase defect.

GENERAL PREVENTION

- Insufficient evidence supports the use of aspirin and/or other anticoagulants, bed rest, hCG, immunotherapy, uterine muscle relaxants, or vitamins for general prevention of EPL, before or after threatened abortion is diagnosed.
- By the time the hemorrhage begins, half of pregnancies complicated by threatened abortion already have no fetal cardiac activity.
- In threatened abortion, oral progestogens may reduce the risk of EPL (RR 0.73, 95% CI 0.59–0.92) and possibly increase the rate of live birth (RR 1.07, 95% CI 1–1.15).
- Antiphospholipid syndrome: The combination of unfractionated heparin and aspirin reduces risk of EPL in women with antiphospholipid antibodies and a history of recurrent abortion.

DIAGNOSIS

HISTORY

- The possibility of pregnancy should be considered in a reproductive-aged person with a uterus who presents with nonmenstrual vaginal bleeding.
- Vaginal bleeding
  - Characteristics (amount, color, consistency, associated symptoms), onset (abrupt or gradual), duration, intensity/quantity, and exacerbating/precipitating factors
  - Document LMP if known: It allows calculation of estimated gestational age.
- Abdominal pain/uterine cramping, as well as associated nausea/vomiting/syncope
- Rupture of membranes
- Passage of products of conception
- Prenatal course: toxic or infectious exposures, family or personal history of genetic abnormalities, past history of ectopic pregnancy or EPL, endocrine disease, autoimmune disorder, bleeding/clotting disorder

PHYSICAL EXAM

- Orthostatic vital signs to estimate hemodynamic stability
- Abdominal exam for tenderness, guarding, rebound, bowel sounds (Peritoneal signs are more likely with ectopic pregnancy.)
- Speculum exam for visual assessment of cervical dilation, blood, and products of conception (confirms diagnosis of EPL)
- Bimanual exam to assess for uterine size–dates discrepancy and adnexal tenderness or mass

DIFFERENTIAL DIAGNOSIS

- Ectopic pregnancy: potentially life-threatening; must be considered in any woman of childbearing age with abdominal pain and vaginal bleeding
- Physiologic bleeding in normal pregnancy (implantation bleeding)
- Subchorionic bleeding
- Cervical polyps, neoplasia, and/or inflammatory conditions
- Hydatidiform mole pregnancy
- hCG-secreting ovarian tumor

DIAGNOSTIC TESTS & INTERPRETATION

Initial Tests (lab, imaging)

- Quantitative hCG
  - Particularly useful if intrauterine pregnancy (IUP) has not been documented by US
  - Serial quantitative serum hCG measurements can assess viability of the pregnancy. Serum hCG should rise at least 53% every 48 hours through 7 weeks after LMP. An inappropriate rise, plateau, or decrease of hCG suggests abnormal IUP or possible ectopic pregnancy.
- Complete blood count (CBC) with differential
- Cultures: gonorrhea/chlamydia
- US exam to evaluate fetal viability and to rule out ectopic pregnancy
  - hCG >2,000 mIU/mL necessary to detect IUP via transvaginal US (TVUS), >5,500 mIU/mL for abdominal US
  - TVUS criteria for nonviable intrauterine gestation: 7-mm fetal pole without cardiac activity or 25-mm gestational sac without a fetal pole, IUP with no growth over 1 week, or previously seen IUP no longer visible
  - Structures and timing: with TVUS, gestational sac of 2 to 3 mm generally seen around 5 WGA; yolk sac by 5.5 WGA; fetal pole with cardiac activity by 6 WGA

Follow-Up Tests & Special Considerations

- In the case of vaginal bleeding with no documented IUP and hCG <2,000 mIU/mL, follow serum hCG levels weekly to zero.
- If levels plateau, consider ectopic pregnancy or retained products of conception. If levels are very high, consider gestational trophoblastic disease.
- If initial hCG level does not permit documentation of IUP by TVUS, follow serum hCG in 48 hours to document appropriate rise.
- Repeat US once hCG is at a level commensurate with visualization on US (see above).
- Provide the patient with ectopic precautions in interim: worsening abdominal pain, dizziness/syncope, nausea/vomiting.
- In a pregnancy of unknown location with hCG rise <53% in 48 hours, offer methotrexate for treatment of presumed ectopic pregnancy.

Diagnostic Procedures/Other

- Fetal heart tones can be auscultated with Doppler US. starting between 10 and 12 WGA in a viable pregnancy.
- In threatened abortion, fetal cardiac activity at 7 to 11 WGA is 90–96% predictive of continued pregnancy (1).

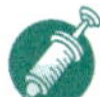

TREATMENT

GENERAL MEASURES

- Discuss contraception plan at the time of diagnosis of EPL, as ovulation can occur prior to resumption of normal menses.
- Expectant management ("watchful waiting") is 90% effective for incomplete abortion, although it may take several weeks for the process to be complete (1). This approach is only recommended in the 1st trimester and is more effective in women with symptoms of impending pregnancy loss.

MEDICATION

- Rates of complete miscarriage and of need for surgical evacuation are equivalent with expectant management and medication.
- Long-term conception rate and pregnancy outcomes are similar for women who undergo expectant management, medical treatment, or surgical evacuation.
- Infection rates are lower with medical versus surgical management.

First Line

- Misoprostol: most common agent for inducing passage of tissue in incomplete abortion or embryonic demise
  - Off-label use; has not been submitted to the FDA for consideration for use in treatment of early pregnancy failure; recognized by the World Health Organization (WHO) as a life-saving medication for this indication
  - Efficacy: Complete expulsion of products of conception in 71% by day 3 and 84% by day 8.
  - Efficacy depends on route of administration, gestational age of pregnancy, and dose.
  - Recommended dose is 800 mcg vaginally; alternate regimens include the WHO regimen of 600 mcg sublingually q3h for up to 3 doses; multidose regimens and oral dosing (including buccal and sublingual) may result in increased side effects.
  - The addition of mifepristone 200 mg, if available, given 24 hours before misoprostol increases the efficacy to 83.8% (ARR 16.7%, 95% CI 7.1–26.3%) (2)[A].
- Common adverse effects include abdominal pain/cramping, nausea, and diarrhea. Pain increases at higher doses but is manageable with oral analgesia.
- Recommended for stable patients who decline surgery but do not want to wait for spontaneous passage of products of conception.

Second Line

Patients with evidence of anemia should receive iron supplementation.

ISSUES FOR REFERRAL

Patients should be monitored for up to 1 year for the development of pathologic grief. There is an insufficient evidence to support counseling to prevent development of anxiety or depression related to grief following EPL.

ADDITIONAL THERAPIES

Rh immunoglobulin is not required for Rh-negative patients with EPL in the 1st trimester.

SURGERY/OTHER PROCEDURES

- Uterine aspiration (suction dilation and curettage [D&C] or manual uterine aspiration [MUA], also known as manual vacuum aspiration [MVA]) is the conventional treatment.
- Indications: septic abortion, heavy bleeding, hypotension, persistent IUP after medical or expectant management, patient's choice
- Risks (all rare): anesthesia (usually local), uterine perforation, intrauterine adhesions, cervical trauma, infection that may lead to infertility or increased risk of ectopic pregnancy
- When compared with expectant management, surgical intervention leads to fewer days of vaginal bleeding, with a lower risk of incomplete abortion and heavy bleeding and a similar risk of infection, but with a higher cost. It is appropriate to prioritize the patient's preference in determining management.
- Vacuum aspiration (manual or electric) is considered preferable to sharp curettage, as aspiration is less painful, takes less time, involves less blood loss, and does not require general anesthesia. The WHO supports use of suction curettage over rigid metal curettage.
- Although data from induced abortions suggest that antibiotic prophylaxis with doxycycline 200 mg in a single dose reduces the already rare risk of postprocedure infection, data are insufficient to support use of antibiotics before aspiration for EPL.

COMPLEMENTARY & ALTERNATIVE MEDICINE

A systematic review of Chinese herbal medicine alone and in conjunction with Western medicine showed benefit over Western medicine alone in achieving continued viability at 28 weeks (number needed to treat [NNT] = 4.8 pregnancies with combined therapy). However, the available studies did not meet international standards for reporting quality.

ADMISSION, INPATIENT, AND NURSING CONSIDERATIONS

- If the patient has orthostatic vital signs, initiate resuscitation with IV fluids and/or blood products, if needed.
- Hemodynamically unstable patients may require IV fluids and/or blood products to maintain BP.

ONGOING CARE

FOLLOW-UP RECOMMENDATIONS

All patients should be offered follow-up in 2 to 6 weeks to monitor for resolution of bleeding, return of menses, and symptoms related to grief, as well as to review the contraception plan.

Patient Monitoring

- If EPL occurs in setting of previously documented IUP and abortion is completed with resumption of normal menses, it is not necessary to check or follow serum hCG to 0.
- After medical management, confirm complete expulsion with US or serial serum β-hCG.
- If pregnancy is not immediately desired, offer effective contraception. Immediate insertion of an intrauterine device is both acceptable and safe.
- If pregnancy is desired, provide preconception counseling. There is no evidence that it is necessary to wait a certain number of cycles before attempting conception again.

DIET

NPO if patient will undergo D&C under general anesthesia

PATIENT EDUCATION

- Pelvic rest for 1 week after D&C or MUA; advise the patients to call if there is an excessive bleeding (soaking two pads per hour for 2 hours), fever, pelvic pain, or malaise, which could indicate retained products of conception or endometritis.
- A patient fact sheet on miscarriage is available through the American Academy of Family Physicians: https://www.aafp.org/afp/2011/0701/p85.html
- Additional patient references are available through the Reproductive Health Access Project:
  - https://www.reproductiveaccess.org/resource/what-is-a-miscarriage
  - https://www.reproductiveaccess.org/resource/miscarriage-treatment-options/

PROGNOSIS

- Prognosis is excellent once bleeding is controlled.
- Recurrent miscarriage: prognosis depends on etiology; up to 70% rate of success with subsequent pregnancy

COMPLICATIONS

- D&C or MUA: uterine perforation, bleeding, adhesions, cervical trauma, and infection that may lead to infertility or increased risk of ectopic pregnancy. Bleeding and adhesions are more common with D&C than with MUA; all complications are rare.
- Retained products of conception

REFERENCES

1. Prine LW, MacNaughton H. Office management of early pregnancy loss. *Am Fam Physician*. 2011;84(1):75–82.
2. Schreiber CA, Creinin MD, Atrio J, et al. Mifepristone pretreatment for the medical management of early pregnancy loss. *N Engl J Med*. 2018;378(23):2161–2170.

ADDITIONAL READING

American College of Obstetricians and Gynecologists. ACOG practice bulletin No. 200; early pregnancy loss. *Obstet Gynecol*. 2018;132(5):e197–e207.

SEE ALSO

- Ectopic Pregnancy
- Algorithm: Recurrent Pregnancy Loss

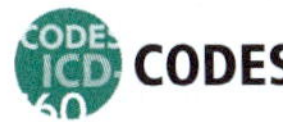

CODES

ICD10

- O03.9 Complete or unspecified spontaneous abortion without complication
- O03.4 Incomplete spontaneous abortion without complication
- O02.1 Missed abortion

CLINICAL PEARLS

- Any pregnant woman with abdominal pain and/or vaginal bleeding must be evaluated to rule out ectopic pregnancy, which is potentially life-threatening.
- As all options have similar long-term outcomes, patient's preference should determine whether management is expectant, medical, or procedural.

M

MITRAL REGURGITATION

Yongkasem Vorasettakarnkij, MD, MSc

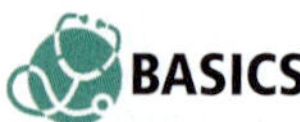

BASICS

DESCRIPTION

- Disorder of mitral valve (MV) closure, either primary, secondary (functional), or mixed, resulting in a backflow of the left ventricular (LV) stroke volume into the left atrium (LA); uncompensated, this leads to LV and LA enlargement, elevated pulmonary pressures, atrial fibrillation (AF), heart failure (HF), and sudden cardiac death.
- Types of mitral regurgitation (MR):
  - Acute versus chronic
  - Primary versus secondary (functional) and mixed
    - Primary: abnormalities at any level of the MV structures (annulus, leaflets, chordae tendineae, and papillary muscles)
    - Secondary: No valvular abnormalities are found. The abnormal and dilated LV causes papillary muscle displacement, resulting in leaflet tethering with annular dilatation that prevents coaptation.
    - Mixed: mixed abnormalities of both primary and secondary types
- System(s) affected: cardiac; pulmonary

EPIDEMIOLOGY

Moderate to severe MR affects 2.5 million people in the United States (2000 data). It is the most common valvular disease and is expected to double by 2030.

Prevalence

- By severity on echocardiography:
  - Mild MR: 19% (up to 40% if trivial jets included)
  - Moderate MR: 1.9%
  - Severe MR: 0.2%
- By category: degenerative (myxomatous disease, annular calcification): 60–70%, ischemic: 20%, endocarditis: 2–5%, rheumatic: 2–5%

ETIOLOGY AND PATHOPHYSIOLOGY

- Acute MR
  - Leaflet perforation: infective endocarditis, trauma
  - Chordae tendineae rupture: trauma, spontaneous rupture, infective endocarditis, or rheumatic fever
  - Papillary muscle rupture or dysfunction: acute myocardial infarction (MI), severe myocardial ischemia, or trauma
- Chronic MR
  - Primary—degenerative (mitral annular calcification, MV prolapse [MVP]), infective endocarditis, rheumatic heart disease (RHD), inflammatory diseases (lupus, eosinophilic endocardial disease), toxin-induced (anorectic drugs), congenital
  - Secondary (functional)
    - Ischemic: coronary artery disease (CAD)/MI
    - Nonischemic: cardiomyopathy from any cause, annular dilatation from chronic AF, dyssynchrony from right ventricular pacing
- Acute MR: Acute MV damage leads to sudden LA and LV volume overload. Sudden rise in LV volume load without LV remodeling results in impaired forward cardiac output and possible cardiogenic shock.
- Chronic MR: LV eccentric hypertrophy compensates for increased regurgitant volume to maintain forward cardiac output and alleviate pulmonary congestion. However, LV remodeling can result in LV dysfunction. LA compensatory dilatation for the larger regurgitant volume predisposes patients to develop AF.
- Ischemic MR: papillary muscle rupture, ischemia during acute MI, and incomplete coaptation of leaflets or restricted valve movement from chronic ischemia

RISK FACTORS

Age, hypertension, RHD, endocarditis, anorectic drugs, radiation

GENERAL PREVENTION

- Risk factor modification for CAD
- Antibiotic prophylaxis for poststreptococcal RHD
- Routine dental endocarditis prophylaxis is no longer recommended.

COMMONLY ASSOCIATED CONDITIONS

MVP with MR common in Marfan syndrome

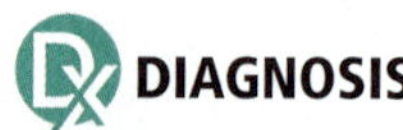

DIAGNOSIS

HISTORY

- Associated conditions: RHD, prior MI, connective tissue disorder
- Acute MR; sudden onset of dyspnea; orthopnea, paroxysmal nocturnal dyspnea
- Chronic MR; exertional dyspnea, fatigue; palpitation: paroxysmal/persistent AF

PHYSICAL EXAM

- Acute MR
  - Rapid and thready pulses
  - Signs of poor tissue perfusion with peripheral vasoconstriction
  - Hyperdynamic precordium without apical shift
  - S_3 and S_4 (if in sinus rhythm)
  - Systolic murmur at left sternal border and base: early, middle, or holosystolic murmur; often soft, low-pitched decrescendo murmur
  - Rales
- Chronic MR
  - Brisk upstroke of arterial pulse; leftward displaced LV apical impulse
  - Systolic thrill at the apex (suggests severe MR); soft S_1 and widely split S_2, S_3 gallop; loud P_2 (if pulmonary hypertension)
  - Holosystolic murmur at apex that radiates to axilla or to left parasternal border
  - Ankle edema, jugular venous distension, and ascites, if development of right-sided HF

DIFFERENTIAL DIAGNOSIS

- Aortic stenosis (AS): usually midsystolic but can be long; difficult to distinguish from holosystolic, at apical area, and radiating to the carotid arteries (unlike MR)
- Tricuspid regurgitation: holosystolic but at left lower sternal border, does not radiate to axilla, and may increase in intensity with inspiration (unlike MR)
- Ventricular septal defect (VSD): harsh holosystolic murmur at lower left sternal border but radiates to right sternal border (not axilla)

DIAGNOSTIC TESTS & INTERPRETATION

Initial Tests (lab, imaging)

- Chest x-ray (CXR)
  - Acute MR: pulmonary edema, normal heart size
  - Chronic MR: LA and LV enlargement
- ECG
  - Acute MR: varies depending on etiologies (e.g., AMI)
  - Chronic MR
    - P mitrale from LA enlargement, AF
    - LV hypertrophy
    - Q waves from prior MI
- Cardiac enzymes: brain natriuretic peptide, if appropriate
- Transthoracic echocardiogram (TTE)
  - Indications for TTE
    - Baseline evaluation of LV size and function, right ventricular function, LA size, pulmonary artery pressure, and severity of MR
    - Delineation of the mechanism of MR
    - Surveillance of asymptomatic moderate to severe LV dysfunction (ejection fraction [EF] and end-systolic dimension [ESD])
    - Evaluate MV apparatus and LV size and function after a change in sign/symptom in MR patient.
    - Evaluate after MV repair or replacement.
  - Findings in acute MR
    - Evidence of etiology: flail leaflet or vegetations
    - Normal LA and LV size
  - Findings in chronic MR
    - Evidence of degenerative, rheumatic, ischemic, congenital, and other causes
    - Enlarged LA and LV

Follow-Up Tests & Special Considerations

- Intervals for follow-up TTE: See "Follow-Up Recommendations."
- Cardiovascular magnetic resonance (CMR):
  - TTE results are not satisfactory to assess LV and right ventricular volumes, function, or MR severity.
- Transesophageal echocardiogram (TEE)
  - Intraoperatively to define the anatomic basis of MR and to guide repair
  - Nondiagnostic information about severity, mechanism of MR, and/or status of LV function from noninvasive imaging
- Exercise hemodynamics with either Doppler echocardiography or cardiac catheterization.
  - Discrepancy between symptoms and the severity of MR from resting TTE in symptomatic patients with chronic primary MR
- Exercise treadmill testing
  - To establish symptom status and exercise tolerance in asymptomatic patients with chronic primary MR
- Noninvasive imaging (stress nuclear/positron emission tomography, CMR, stress echocardiography, cardiac CT angiography)
  - To establish etiology of chronic secondary MR and/or to assess myocardial viability

Diagnostic Procedures/Other

Cardiac catheterization

- Left ventriculography and hemodynamic measurement
  - Noninvasive tests are inconclusive regarding the severity of MR, LV function, and the need for surgery.
- Coronary angiography: prior to MV surgery in patients at risk for CAD

Test Interpretation

Quantification of severe MR requires an integration of the following structural parameters:

- LA size: dilated, unless acute
- LV size: dilated, unless acute
- MV morphology: flail leaflet, ruptured papillary muscle, large perforation, severe retraction, poor leaflet coaptation
- Doppler parameters: large central jet (>50% of LA), pulmonary vein systolic flow reversal, vena contracta ≥0.7 cm
- Quantitative parameter: effective regurgitant orifice area ≥0.4 cm^2, regurgitation volume ≥60 mL, regurgitation fraction ≥50%

TREATMENT

MEDICATION

- Acute, severe MR
  - Medical therapy has a limited role and is aimed to stabilize hemodynamics preoperatively.
  - Vasodilators (nitroprusside, nicardipine): to improve hemodynamic compensation but is often limited by systemic hypotension (1),(2)
- Chronic MR
  - Primary
    - Asymptomatic and normal LV systolic function: no proven long-term medical therapy
    - Symptomatic or asymptomatic with LV systolic dysfunction: diuretics, β-blockers, angiotensin-converting enzyme inhibitors (ACEIs) or angiotensin receptor blockers (ARBs) or angiotensinreceptor-neprilysin inhibitor (ARNI), mineralocorticoid receptor antagonists (MRAs), and sodium-glucose cotransporter 2 inhibitors (SGLT2i) as indicated in standard therapy for HF (1),(2)
  - Secondary: LV dysfunction or symptomatic (stages B to D): ACEIs or ARBs or ARNI, β-blockers, MRAs, and SGLT2i as indicated in standard therapy for HF (1)

SURGERY/OTHER PROCEDURES

- Isolated MV surgery is not indicated for patients with mild to moderate MR.
- Acute, severe MR secondary to acute MI
  - Acute rupture of papillary muscle: emergency MV repair/replacement
  - Papillary muscle displacement: aggressive medical stabilization and intra-aortic balloon pump; valve surgery is usually required in addition to revascularization.
- Chronic severe MR
  - Severe primary MR
    - MV surgery
      - Symptomatic patients (stage D) who are operable and not high risk (1),(2)
      - Asymptomatic patients
        - LV systolic dysfunction (EF ≤60% and/or ESD ≥40 mm, stage C2) (1),(2).
        - Preserved LV systolic function (EF ≥60% and ESD ≤40 mm, stage C1):
          - MV repair is reasonable if the likelihood of a successful and durable repair without residual MR is >95% and expected mortality is <1% (1).
          - MV surgery should be considered if concomitant with AF secondary to MR or resting pulmonary hypertension (pulmonary artery systolic pressure >50 mm Hg) (2).
          - MV repair should be considered if significant LA dilatation (volume index ≥60 mL/m^2 or diameter ≥55 mm) when an enduring repair is likely and performed at a heart valve center (2).
          - MV surgery may be considered if progressive increase in LV size or decrease in EF on ≥3 serial imaging studies (1).
      - MV repair is recommended over MV replacement in patients with MR from degenerative disease, when a successful and durable repair can be accomplished (1),(2).
    - Transcatheter edge-to-edge repair (TEER): may be considered for symptomatic patients (stage D), who have favorable anatomy for the repair and inoperable or at high surgical risk (1),(2).
  - Severe secondary MR
    - MV surgery
      - Undergoing coronary artery bypass graft (CABG) (1),(2) or other cardiac surgery (2)
      - Severely symptomatic patients (NYHA classes III and IV) despite optimal GDMT for HF (1),(2)
      - Chordal-sparing MVR is preferred over downsized annuloplasty repair in ischemic MR patients (1).
    - Cardiac resynchronization therapy is recommended for symptomatic patients (stages B to D) who meet the indications for device therapy (1),(2).
    - TEER: is reasonable for persistent symptoms despite maximally tolerated GDMT, who have LVEF 20%–50%, LV end-systolic diameter ≤7.0 cm, pulmonary artery systolic pressure ≤70 mm Hg, and favorable anatomy for the repair (1).

Geriatric Considerations

Medical therapy alone for patients >75 years of age with MR is preferred, owing to increased operative mortality and decreased survival (compared with those with AS), especially with preexisting CAD or need for MV replacement. MV repair is preferable than MV replacement.

ADMISSION, INPATIENT, AND NURSING CONSIDERATIONS

Acute MR: Stabilize airway, breathing, circulation (ABCs). Obtain urgent surgical consultation.

ONGOING CARE

FOLLOW-UP RECOMMENDATIONS

- Chronic MR with new-onset or changing symptoms: TTE
- Chronic MR: asymptomatic patients with normal LV function
  - Mild MR with normal LV size and no pulmonary hypertension: annual clinical evaluation and TTE every 3 to 5 years or more frequently depending on course
  - Moderate MR: annual clinical evaluation and TTE every 1 to 2 years
  - Severe MR: clinical evaluation and TTE every 6 to 12 months; biomarkers and/or global longitudinal strain may be considered.
  - Consider serial CXRs and ECGs and consider stress test if exercise capacity is doubtful.

PATIENT EDUCATION

- Exercise after MV repair: Avoid sports with risk for bodily contact or trauma. Low-intensity competitive sports are allowed.
- Competitive athletes with MR: asymptomatic with normal LV size and function, normal pulmonary artery pressures, and sinus rhythm: no restrictions; mildly symptomatic and those with LV dilatation: activities with low to moderate dynamic and static cardiac demand allowed; AF and anticoagulation: no contact sports

PROGNOSIS

- Acute, severe MR: Mortality risk with surgery is 50%; mortality risk with medical therapy alone is 75% in the first 24 hours and 95% at 2 weeks.
- Chronic MR: asymptomatic severe MR with normal LVEF: 10% yearly rate of progression to symptoms and subnormal resting LVEF; symptomatic severe MR: 8-year survival rate, 33% without surgery; mortality rate, 5% yearly

Pregnancy Considerations

MR with NYHA functional classes III and IV at high risk for maternal and/or fetal risk

COMPLICATIONS

Acute pulmonary edema, CHF, AF, bleeding risk with anticoagulation, endocarditis, sudden cardiac death

REFERENCES

1. Otto CM, Nishimura RA, Bonow RO, et al. 2020 ACC/AHA guideline for the management of patients with valvular heart disease: a report of the American College of Cardiology/American Heart Association Joint Committee on clinical practice guidelines. *Circulation*. 2021;143(5):e72–e227.
2. Vahanian A, Beyersdorf F, Praz F, et al; for ESC/EACTS Scientific Document Group. 2021 ESC/EACTS guidelines for the management of valvular heart disease. *Eur Heart J*. 2022;43(7):561–632.

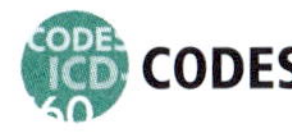

CODES

ICD10

- I34.0 Nonrheumatic mitral (valve) insufficiency
- I05.1 Rheumatic mitral insufficiency
- Q23.3 Congenital mitral insufficiency

CLINICAL PEARLS

Follow-up for mild to moderate MR: serial exam and/or echo (mild, every 3 to 5 years; moderate, 1 to 2 years) unless LV structural changes; severe primary MR is usually managed with MV repair.

MITRAL STENOSIS

Sahil R. Bharwani, DO, MPH

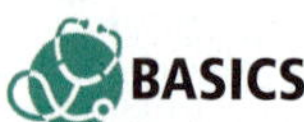

BASICS

DESCRIPTION

- Mitral stenosis (MS) is narrowing of the mitral valve area (MVA) causing obstruction of left ventricular (LV) inflow, resulting in increased left atrial (LA) pressures and consequent elevation of pulmonary venous pressure. The most common etiology for MS is rheumatic heart disease (RHD).
- Normal valve orifice is 4 to 6 cm^2; symptoms typically seen when orifice is <2.5 cm^2.
- Staging of the disease is used to guide appropriate treatment regimen.
  - Stage A, "at risk of MS": mild valve doming with normal flow velocity and *no* hemodynamic obstruction or symptoms; no symptoms or echocardiographic changes
  - Stage B, "progressive MS": increased diastolic doming, increased flow velocity, but MVA >1.5 cm^2, diastolic pressure 1/2 time <150 ms; no symptoms; mild to moderate LA enlargement and normal pulmonary pressures at rest on echo
  - Stage C, "asymptomatic severe MS": diastolic doming, MVA <1.5 cm^2, diastolic pressure half time >150 ms, severe LA enlargement, pulmonary artery systolic pressure (PASP) >30 mm Hg, but *no* symptoms; severe LA enlargement and elevated PASPs >50 mm Hg on echo
  - Stage D, "symptomatic severe MS": stage C with dyspnea on exertion and decreased exercise tolerance; severe LA enlargement and elevated PASPs >50 mm Hg on echo.

EPIDEMIOLOGY

Global prevalence of RHD is 40.5 million cases. There are 305,000 deaths attributed to RHD annually. Incidence of rheumatic disease in the continental United States remains low (<2 per 100,000 school-aged children).

ETIOLOGY AND PATHOPHYSIOLOGY

- Narrowing of the mitral valve orifice leads to obstruction of blood flow between LA and LV. This impairs LV filling during diastole and causes increased LA pressure.
- Increased LA pressure is transmitted passively ("back pressure") to the pulmonary circulation causing pulmonary hypertension (HTN) and pulmonary congestion over time leading to right-sided failure.
- Chronic LA pressure overload results in atrial dilation and fibrosis, resulting in atrial fibrillation.
- Rheumatic fever: most common cause (see "Risk Factors")
  - Pathognomonic commissural fusion, leaflet thickening, and "fish mouth appearance" seen with RHD
  - The anatomic changes of severe MS is thought to be secondary to recurrent episodes of ARF as well as a chronic autoimmune process caused by cross-reactivity between a streptococcal protein and valve tissue.
- Aging (extension of mitral annular calcification)
- Rare causes: congenital (associated with mucopolysaccharidoses); autoimmune: systemic lupus erythematosus (SLE), rheumatoid arthritis, malignant carcinoid, Whipple disease, methysergide therapy; and other acquired: LA myxoma, LA thrombus, endomyocardial fibrosis

RISK FACTORS

- ARF and RHD are the greatest risk factors. ARF occurs 2 to 3 weeks after an episode of untreated pharyngitis caused by rheumatogenic group A streptococci (GAS) organism in a genetically susceptible host.
  - 30–40% of rheumatic fever patients eventually develop MS, presenting 20 years after diagnosis of ARF.
  - Recurrent infections can accelerate the progression of the disease.
  - Low socioeconomic status (i.e., crowded conditions) favors the spread of streptococcal infection
- Aging (increasing valvular calcification)
- Chest irradiation (increasing tissue fibrosis)
- Use of drugs—MDMA (ecstasy), ergot alkaloids

GENERAL PREVENTION

- Prompt recognition and treatment of GAS infection in at-risk populations; recognition of cardinal signs and symptoms of ARF via Jones criteria
- Transthoracic echo (TTE) screening has been shown to increase diagnosis of RHD in asymptomatic patients residing in areas of high prevalence.

COMMONLY ASSOCIATED CONDITIONS

Atrial fibrillation (30–40% of symptomatic patients), other valvular problems (aortic stenosis and insufficiency), pulmonary HTN and right heart failure, systemic embolism, infective endocarditis

DIAGNOSIS

HISTORY

- History of ARF or RHD
- Severity depends on valve area; most early cases will be asymptomatic.
- Mean age of symptom onset in rheumatic valvular disease is in the late 30s to 40s. Latent period 20 to 40 years after infection. Rapid progression can be seen in some high prevalence areas.
- Presenting features usually include dyspnea on exertion, decrease exercise tolerance, chest pain, palpitations, hoarseness, hemoptysis, fatigue, paroxysmal nocturnal dyspnea, orthopnea, atrial fibrillation, and embolic events.
- In advanced disease, symptoms of pulmonary HTN and right heart failure predominate: jugular venous distention, hepatomegaly, ascites, and peripheral edema.
- Not infrequently, symptoms are first noted in pregnancy: mitral facies, plethoric cheeks, and bluish patches.

PHYSICAL EXAM

- Elevated jugular venous pressure, diastolic thrill in the left lateral decubitus position. A right ventricle lift may be felt in the left parasternal area in patients with pulmonary HTN.
- Auscultation
  - Classic murmur: accentuated S_1, opening snap (OS), apical early decrescendo diastolic rumble with presystolic accentuation (presystolic accentuation of murmur is lost with atrial fibrillation). Murmur is low pitch and best heard at the apex in the left lateral decubitus position.
  - Murmur is accentuated with exercise and decreased with rest and Valsalva. With mobile, noncalcified valve, murmur persists throughout diastole and S_1, and the OS remains loud. With increasing severity of MS, murmur often is difficult to hear. Duration of murmur reflective of severity. S_1 and the OS may be soft to absent. A shorter S_2 to OS interval indicates more severe MS (<70 ms).
- If pulmonary HTN is present: Increased P_2, high-pitched decrescendo diastolic murmur of pulmonic insufficiency is heard (Graham Steell murmur); may have signs of right heart failure; RV lift can also be seen.
- May also find associated aortic or tricuspid murmurs due to involvement from RHD

DIAGNOSTIC TESTS & INTERPRETATION

Initial Tests (lab, imaging)

- ECG: LA enlargement ("P mitrale"), atrial fibrillation, and right ventricular hypertrophy may be seen.
- Chest radiograph: LA enlargement, straightening of the left heart border, a "double density" on right, and elevation of the left main stem bronchus; prominent pulmonary arteries at the hilum with rapid tapering, RVH, and edema pattern with Kerley A and B lines (late presentation)
- TTE recommended in all patients with signs of symptoms of MS. It is used to diagnose and assess for concomitant valvulopathies
- Transesophageal echocardiogram (TEE) should be performed if TTE images are nondiagnostic or if being considered for a percutaneous mitral balloon commissurotomy (PMBC) or valvuloplasty (PMBV) to exclude thrombus in LA and evaluate severity of MR.
- Exercise stress testing with Doppler echocardiography can also be considered in patients with MS who have a discrepancy in their symptoms and signs and resting echo findings.
- Cardiac catheterization and use of Gorlin formula to assess LA and LV pressures is indicated when echo is inconclusive or there is discrepancy between the echo, symptoms and severity (Class I).
- CT imaging: provides MVA estimates, LA cavity size; useful prior to surgery, to evaluate for concomitant coronary artery disease (CAD)

Follow-Up Tests & Special Considerations

- If valve area >1.5 cm^2 and mean pressure gradient <5 mm Hg, clinical follow-up in 3 to 5 years is recommended.
- Otherwise, follow-up is usually symptom based. Symptomatic patients with severe MS need further evaluation for interventional/surgical treatment.
- Holter monitor placement to rule out paroxysmal atrial fibrillation

Diagnostic Procedures/Other

- Exercise testing is recommended for those with clinical discrepancy.
- Wilkins score evaluates valvular anatomy from a TTE in order to see if patient is a candidate for surgery.

Test Interpretation

- Rheumatic fever–induced pathologic changes: leaflet thickening, leaflet calcification, commissural fusion, chordal shortening
- MV area defined: normal: 4 to 6 cm^2, progressive MS: >1.5 cm^2, asymptomatic severe MS: <1.5 cm^2, severe MS: <1.5 cm^2, very severe MS: <1.0 cm^2

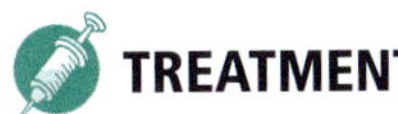

TREATMENT

GENERAL MEASURES

- Treatment is dependent on severity of stenosis and symptoms.
- Patients who have a valvular area >1.5 cm^2 and no symptoms can be managed medically.
- MS is generally progressive, and medical therapy only delays the need for definitive therapy. It entails:
  - Treatment to prevent recurrence of rheumatic fever
  - Treatments aimed at improving dyspnea and exercise tolerance
  - Controlling the ventricular rate whether in sinus rhythm or atrial fibrillation
  - Anticoagulation for prevention of thromboembolic events

MEDICATION

First Line

- Use of anticoagulation for prevention of thromboembolism
  - Class I recommendations: MS and atrial fibrillation or history of atrial fibrillation, MS and prior embolic event, or MS and LA thrombus
  - Class IIB recommendations: patients with enlarged LA and spontaneous contrast on echo
- Warfarin is the accepted modality for anticoagulation in patients with rheumatic mitral valve disease (international normalized ratio range 2 to 3). Factor Xa inhibitors and direct thrombin inhibitors are not approved for use in atrial fibrillation with patients that have moderate-to-severe MS (1),(2).
- Heparin is used for anticoagulation with atrial fibrillation.
- Antibiotic prophylaxis against rheumatic fever and/or carditis is recommended for patients with history of rheumatic fever. Secondary prophylaxis is dependent on many factors: number of previous attacks, time since previous infection, risk for getting GAS, age of patient, and absence or presence of cardiac involvement.
- Diuretics for congestive symptoms and symptomatic heart failure
- β-Blockers or nondihydropyridine calcium channel blockers used for controlling heart rate both in sinus rhythm and atrial fibrillation to allow adequate diastolic filling and decrease LA diastolic pressure, tachycardia, or exertional symptoms (class IIa)
- Ivabradine can be helpful because it doesn't affect myocardial contraction.
- Consider cardioversion, especially in patients with mild MS and recent diagnosis of atrial fibrillation (<6 months).

Second Line

Consider amiodarone or digoxin if β-blockers and calcium channel blockers are not beneficial in controlling rapid ventricular rate. Consider digoxin in patients with symptomatic systolic dysfunction.

SURGERY/OTHER PROCEDURES

- Surgical techniques include percutaneous balloon valvotomy open mitral commissurotomy, or closed mitral commissurotomy and mitral valve replacement.
- Patients with severe MS and symptoms consistent with NYHA classes III and IV are candidates for surgery.
- Any patient with a valve area >1.5 cm^2, LA thrombus, moderate or severe MR, severe or bicommissural calcifications, severe aortic valve disease, moderate TR or TS, and concomitant CAD requiring bypass surgery are *not* candidates for PMBC or PMBV.
- Transcatheter balloon mitral valvuloplasty is considered the first-line treatment for patients with rheumatic mitral valve stenosis and favorable valve anatomy (3).
- Per the 2014 AHA/ACC Valvular Heart Disease Guidelines (which is similar to the 2017 European Society of Cardiology Guidelines), PMBC or PMBV is recommended for patients with the following: symptomatic severe MS (MVA <1.5 cm^2) and favorable valve morphology; symptomatic severe MS with severe (NYHA III/IV) symptoms who have suboptimal valve anatomy and are not candidates or are high risk for surgery; asymptomatic very severe MS (MVA <1 cm^2) and favorable valve anatomy in the absence of contraindications; asymptomatic very severe MS (MVA <1 cm^2) and favorable valve anatomy in the absence of contraindications; asymptomatic severe MS and favorable valve morphology with new-onset atrial fibrillation in absence of contraindications; symptomatic patients with MVA >1.5 cm^2 if there is evidence of hemodynamically significant MS during exercise
- Patient's age, bleeding risk, and other comorbidities prior to deciding if patient should have a prosthetic versus mechanical valve

Pregnancy Considerations

- Volume expansion during pregnancy can exacerbate heart failure symptoms. Patients with known severe MS, prepregnancy discussions should be pursued with a cardiologist.
- Warfarin (Coumadin) is considered relatively safe in the 2nd and 3rd trimesters if anticoagulation is required. However, unfractionated heparin is preferred prior to labor and delivery.

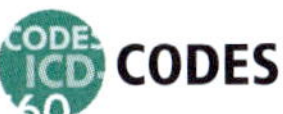

ONGOING CARE

FOLLOW-UP RECOMMENDATIONS

- Counsel patients that MS usually is slowly progressive but can have sudden onset of atrial fibrillation, which could become rapidly fatal. Call 911 for marked worsening of symptoms.
- Echocardiographic surveillance in asymptomatic patients in any degree of MS: very severe (MVA <1 cm^2) MS: yearly, severe (MVA ≤1.5 cm^2) MS: every 1 to 2 years, mild or moderate MS (MVA >1.5 cm^2): every 3 to 5 years
- Follow-up will depend on the severity of the MS and the patient's symptoms. Asymptomatic patients will need annual history and examination. Symptomatic patients are followed closely based on clinical response to adjust therapy and plan definitive treatment.

DIET

Salt restriction for pulmonary congestion

PROGNOSIS

- Asymptomatic latent period after rheumatic fever for 10 to 30 years. 10-year survival for asymptomatic or minimally symptomatic patients is 80%. 10-year survival after onset of debilitating symptoms is only 0–15%. Mean survival with significant pulmonary HTN is <3 years.
- Commissurotomy is an effective means of reducing stenosis but is not curative. Restenosis sometimes occurs and can be early (<5 years) or late (>20 years).

COMPLICATIONS

Left and right heart failure, atrial fibrillation and systemic embolic events, pulmonary HTN, hepatic congestion, and infective endocarditis

REFERENCES

1. Otto CM, Nishimura RA, Bonow RO, et al. 2020 ACC/AHA Guideline for the management of patients with valvular heart disease: executive summary: a report of the American College of Cardiology/American Heart Association Joint Committee on Clinical Practice Guidelines. *Circulation*. 2021;143(5):e35–e71.
2. January CT, Wann LS, Calkins H, et al. 2019 AHA/ACC/HRS focused update the management of patients with atrial fibrillation: a report of the American College of Cardiology/American Heart Association Task Force on Clinical Practice Guidelines and the Heart Rhythm Society. *J Am Coll Cardiol*. 2019;74(1):104–132.
3. Praz F, Beyersdorf F, Haugaa K, et al. Valvular heart disease: from mechanisms to management. *Lancet*. 2024;403(10436):1576–1589.

CODES

ICD10

- I01.1 Acute rheumatic endocarditis
- Q23.2 Congenital mitral stenosis
- I34.2 Nonrheumatic mitral (valve) stenosis

CLINICAL PEARLS

- Asymptomatic patients may be followed clinically with yearly exams for development of symptoms with periodic echo to evaluate valve area and PA systolic pressure
- Once symptoms of MS develop, initiate appropriate medical therapy and advise patient that surgical therapy may be needed to prolong survival. Almost all cases of MV stenosis progress in severity over time.

MITRAL VALVE PROLAPSE

Justin T. Ertle, MD

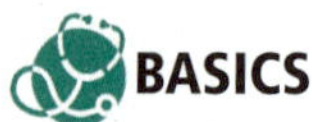

BASICS

DESCRIPTION

- Mitral valve prolapse (MVP) is the billowing of one or both mitral valve leaflets into the left atrium (LA) during ventricular systole.
- MVP can be classified in different ways, including by etiology (primary or secondary; see "Etiology and Pathophysiology") or by morphology (classic MVP and nonclassic MVP; see "Test Interpretation").
- MVP is often asymptomatic and often has a benign clinical course; however, it may occasionally be associated with symptoms such as palpitations, or more serious complications, such as mitral regurgitation (MR) (see "Complications") or even sudden cardiac death (1)[A].
- Synonyms include systolic click-murmur syndrome; billowing mitral cusp syndrome; myxomatous mitral valve; floppy valve syndrome; redundant cusp syndrome; Barlow syndrome.

EPIDEMIOLOGY

Prevalence

- Estimated 1–3% of the population (2),(3)
- Equally distributed by gender (2),(3).
- Typically found in adults, though not at a certain stage of adulthood (2),(3)

ETIOLOGY AND PATHOPHYSIOLOGY

- The pathophysiology of MVP typically involves myxomatous degeneration of the mitral valve leaflets, characterized by expansion of the valve spongiosa layer, structural alterations in collagen, and structurally abnormal chordae (2),(3).
- Papillary muscle or chordae disruption, dysfunction, or rupture may also cause MVP; this can occur without a process causing myxomatous degeneration or as part of the natural history of a process causing myxomatous degeneration.
- The etiology of MVP is multifactorial and includes the following (2):
  - Primary MVP: sporadic or familial
  - Secondary MVP
    - "Syndromic" MVP: myxomatous degeneration associated with connective tissue disorders, for example, Marfan syndrome, Ehlers-Danlos syndrome, osteogenesis imperfecta, pseudoxanthoma elasticum, Loeys-Dietz syndrome
    - Associated with congenital heart disease: atrial septal defect, Ebstein anomaly
- Papillary/chordae disruption, dysfunction or rupture: infarction, endocarditis, rheumatic fever, trauma, hypertrophic cardiomyopathy

Genetics

- In primary MVP, both autosomal dominant and X-linked instances have been found.
  - Autosomal dominant: variable penetrance; several genetic loci so far identified (2)
    - *MMVP1*: chromosome 16 p11.2–p12.1
    - *MMVP2*: chromosome 11 p15.4
    - *MMVP3*: chromosome 13 q31.3–q32.1
  - X-linked: One gene identified, filamin A gene, Xq28 (2)
- Connective tissue disorders, which often have a genetic basis, are associated with secondary MVP (see "Etiology and Pathophysiology").

RISK FACTORS

- Medical conditions implicated in the development of MVP include both heritable and sporadic congenital abnormalities as well as other disease processes. (See "Etiology and Pathophysiology.")
- MVP is more common with leaner BMI (2)

COMMONLY ASSOCIATED CONDITIONS

- Conditions implicated in the development of MVP include both heritable and sporadic congenital abnormalities, as well as other disease processes. (See "Etiology and Pathophysiology.")
- MVP is implicated in the development of other medical conditions/complications, such as MR and stroke. (See "Complications.")
- Some associated conditions that are less clearly either (i) a cause of MVP or (ii) caused by MVP include von Willebrand disease; primary hypomastia; thoracic skeletal abnormalities; prolapse of the tricuspid, pulmonic, or aortic valves.

DIAGNOSIS

HISTORY

- Most patients with MVP are asymptomatic.
- Symptoms that occur may be related to MVP itself, to MR as a result of MVP, or to other complications of MVP such as stroke, arrhythmia, etc.
- Symptoms related to MVP include: palpitations (most commonly associated symptom), atypical chest pain, fatigue, exercise intolerance, orthostasis/presyncope, and neuropsychiatric symptoms such as panic attacks.
- Symptoms related to progression of MR: fatigue, dyspnea, exercise intolerance, orthopnea, paroxysmal nocturnal dyspnea

PHYSICAL EXAM

- The principal auscultatory finding is a midsystolic click, though not heard in all cases (2).
- This may also be followed by mid- to late-systolic murmur, loudest at the apex (2).
- Dynamic auscultation may help differentiate between similar systolic sounds.
  - Maneuvers that decrease end-diastolic volume move the click and murmur toward S1: standing up, Valsalva.
    - Note: Valsalva maneuver may help differentiate hypertrophic obstructive cardiomyopathy (HOCM) from MVP as it increases the intensity of the murmur in HOCM, whereas it increases the duration of the murmur in MVP.
  - Maneuvers that increase end-diastolic volume move the click and murmur toward S2: squatting, leg raise.
- Exam findings may also reflect the presence of MR as a result of MVP.
  - MR holosystolic murmur best heard at the apex, with radiation to the left axilla
  - The duration of the murmur corresponds with the severity of MR. Presence of an S3 may indicate severe regurgitation.

DIFFERENTIAL DIAGNOSIS

- Ejection clicks (do not change timing with systole)
- Papillary muscle dysfunction
- MR
- Tricuspid regurgitation
- Hypertrophic cardiomyopathy

DIAGNOSTIC TESTS & INTERPRETATION

Initial Tests (lab, imaging)

- Transthoracic echocardiogram (TTE) is the diagnostic modality of choice after an appropriate physical exam; echocardiogram is required for definitive diagnosis.
  - In asymptomatic patients with physical signs of MVP, echocardiography is indicated for the diagnosis of MVP and assessment of MR, leaflet morphology, and ventricular compensation.
  - Echocardiography is not indicated to exclude MVP in asymptomatic patients with ill-defined symptoms in the absence of a constellation of clinical symptoms or physical findings suggestive of MVP, or a positive family history.
- Electrocardiogram (EKG) may be considered but is not required in the workup of MVP, without other indication.
  - Palpitations are a common symptom, which should prompt EKG.
  - EKG in MVP is typically normal; however, EKG findings in MVP can include nonspecific ST-T wave changes, T-wave inversions, prominent Q waves, even prolonged QT.

Follow-Up Tests & Special Considerations

- Ambulatory heart rhythm monitor should be considered if patient has palpitations but is not indicated for asymptomatic MVP.
- Transesophageal echocardiography (TEE), particularly with 3D imaging, may be considered to further visualize anatomy if intervention is planned or there is limited visibility of the mitral valve on TTE.
- Angiography is rarely used for diagnostic purposes but may be recommended for hemodynamic assessment when noninvasive options are inconclusive.
- Patients with MVP and severe MR may require coronary angiography and TEE if cardiac surgical referral is planned (see "Issues for Referral").
- Cardiac MRI and/or electrophysiology studies may be indicated in patients with findings that may indicate an elevated risk of sudden cardiac death (SCD) (see "Complications") (3)[C].

Test Interpretation

MVP is defined as anterior, posterior, or bileaflet prolapse of at least 2-mm superior displacement into the LA during systole on the parasternal long-axis annular plane of the valve on echocardiogram, with or without associated leaflet thickening (2).

- Morphologic Classification (2):
  - Classic MVP (a.k.a. Barlow syndrome): prolapse with >5 mm of leaflet thickening
  - Nonclassic MVP (fibroelastic deficiency): prolapse with <5 mm of leaflet thickening
- "Flail" mitral prolapse is the term for a severe form in which a segment or segments of a leaflet protrude into the left atrium during systole; typically, this is associated with torn chordae or ruptured papillary muscle.

TREATMENT

GENERAL MEASURES

- Reassurance is appropriate for patients with milder forms of prolapse and low symptom burden; normal lifestyle and regular exercise is encouraged.
- If MVP is associated with palpitations, fatigue, or anxiety, patients are encouraged to limit alcohol, cigarettes, and caffeine.
- MVP with orthostatic symptoms may be managed by liberalizing fluid and salt intake. Support stockings may also be beneficial.

MEDICATION

- Aspirin (75 to 325 mg daily) may be considered for MVP with "high-risk" echocardiographic features (thickening >5 mm or valve redundancy).
- Aspirin (75 to 325 mg daily) is recommended for patients with MVP and transient ischemic attacks (TIAs).
- Warfarin may be considered for patients with MVP and (TIA) who continue to experience TIAs despite aspirin.
- Aspirin (75 to 325 mg daily) is considered for patients with MVP and history of stroke, without high-risk echocardiographic features (thickening >5 mm or valve redundancy), MR, atrial fibrillation, or left atrial thrombus.
- Warfarin is considered for patients with MVP and history of stroke, who do have either high-risk echocardiographic features (thickening >5 mm or valve redundancy), MR, atrial fibrillation, or left atrial thrombus.
- Patients with MVP and palpitations may be treated with β-blockers.

ISSUES FOR REFERRAL

- Cardiology referral is indicated in MVP with significant symptoms, high-risk features, or concomitant cardiac diagnoses. Electrophysiologist referral would be recommended for significant arrhythmia.
- Cardiothoracic surgery referral is indicated in patients with indication for surgical repair.
- Genetic counselling is considered when a heritable condition is suspected.

SURGERY/OTHER PROCEDURES

MVP and myxomatous valve degeneration is the most common cause of chronic primary MR requiring surgery in high-income countries.

- Referral for consideration of mitral valve surgery is indicated for the following:
  - Severe primary MR with symptoms
  - Asymptomatic MR patients with LV systolic dysfunction (LVEF ≤60%, LVESD ≥40 mm)
- Minimally invasive surgery and surgery for asymptomatic patients without LV systolic dysfunction is an area of ongoing research.
  - Asymptomatic patients with atrial fibrillation or pulmonary hypertension may be considered for surgical intervention.
- In general, if surgery is indicated for MR, mitral valve repair is preferred over replacement when possible, due to lower rates of operative mortality and long-term complications.

ONGOING CARE

FOLLOW-UP RECOMMENDATIONS

Periodic monitoring with TTE is recommended in asymptomatic patients with known valvular heart disease, at intervals depending on valve lesion, severity, ventricular size, and ventricular function.

- Asymptomatic MVP with no significant MR can be followed every 3 to 5 years.
- Patients who are symptomatic or have high-risk features on initial echocardiogram, including moderate to severe MR, may need serial echocardiograms and should be followed clinically at least once per year.

PATIENT EDUCATION

- Patients can be counselled that MVP is often a benign condition.
- Patients should be counselled that there is no contraindication to pregnancy based on the diagnosis of MVP alone.
- Patients should be counselled to promptly report any change in symptom status, which may require repeat echocardiography.
- Educate patients on occasional familial MVP occurrence.
- Restriction from high-intensity competitive sports is recommended if a patient has MVP with any one of the following features:
  - Moderate LV enlargement or LV dysfunction
  - Uncontrolled tachyarrhythmias
  - Prolonged QT interval
  - Unexplained syncope
  - Prior resuscitation from cardiac arrest
  - Aortic root enlargement

PROGNOSIS

- Prognosis is excellent for asymptomatic patients without complications; MVP is often benign with a normal life expectancy.
- Overall, the prognosis of MVP is closely tied to whether MR develops and how it progresses as well as occurrence of other serious complications (2).
- Ventricular arrhythmias and SCD both occur more often with MVP that in the general population but are still rare. ECG T-wave inversions and prolonged QT may be predictors of more serious arrhythmia (1)[A] (see "Complications"). SCD occurs in the community at 0.06–0.08% per year; in MVP, this appears to be 1.75 to 2.3 times higher; per 100 patient-years there is an estimated 0.14 SCD events in patients with MVP (3).

COMPLICATIONS

- MR — MVP and myxomatous valve degeneration is the most common cause of chronic primary MR in high-income countries.
  - Many additional complications may arise as a consequence of severe MR:
    - Heart failure
    - Pulmonary hypertension with associated RV dysfunction
    - Left atrial dilatation with associated paroxysmal supraventricular tachycardias (including atrial fibrillation)
- Arrhythmias, including premature atrial complexes, supraventricular tachycardias, ventricular ectopy, and ventricular arrhythmias in general (3)
- SCD occurs more often with MVP than in the general population; still very rare (See "Prognosis.")
  - Patients with MVP who have bileaflet prolapse, cardiac fibrosis, ST-T wave abnormalities, complex ventricular ectopy, or ventricular arrhythmias seem to specifically have elevated risk of SCD (3).
- Cerebrovascular ischemia (stroke and TIAs)
- Infective endocarditis

REFERENCES

1. Oliveri F, Kakargias F, Panday P, et al. Arrhythmic mitral valve prolapse: diagnostic parameters for high-risk patients: a systematic review and meta-analysis. *Pacing Clin Electrophysiol*. 2021;44(10):1746–1755.
2. Delling FN, Vasan RS. Epidemiology and pathophysiology of mitral valve prolapse: new insights into disease progression, genetics, and molecular basis. *Circulation*. 2014;129(21):2158–2170.
3. Nalliah CJ, Mahajan R, Elliott AD, et al. Mitral valve prolapse and sudden cardiac death: a systematic review and meta-analysis. *Heart*. 2019;105(2):144–151.
4. Otto CM, Nishimura RA, Bonow RO, et al. 2020 ACC/AHA guideline for the management of patients with valvular heart disease: a report of the American College of Cardiology/American Heart Association Joint Committee on clinical practice guidelines. *Circulation*. 2021;143(5):e72–e227.

ADDITIONAL READING

- Guy TS, Hill AC. Mitral valve prolapse. *Annu Rev Med*. 2012;63:277–292.
- Nishimura RA, Vahanian A, Eleid MF, et al. Mitral valve disease—current management and future challenges. *Lancet*. 2016;387(10025):1324–1334.

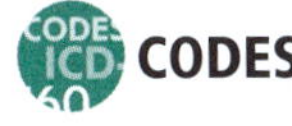

CODES

ICD10

- I34.1 Nonrheumatic mitral (valve) prolapse
- I05.8 Other rheumatic mitral valve diseases

CLINICAL PEARLS

- MVP is the billowing of one or both mitral valve leaflets into the LA during ventricular systole.
- The principal auscultatory finding is a midsystolic click, although this is not heard in all cases; the click may also be followed by mid- to late-systolic murmur, loudest at the apex.
- Echocardiogram is required for definitive diagnosis.
- The etiology of MVP is multifactorial and can be secondary to a diverse range of other conditions such as connective tissue disorders, congenital heart disease, infarction, endocarditis, rheumatic fever, and trauma.

MOLLUSCUM CONTAGIOSUM

Dongsheng Jiang, MD, MSc

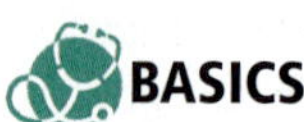

BASICS

DESCRIPTION

Molluscum contagiosum is a common, benign, viral (poxvirus) skin infection, characterized by small (2 to 5 mm), waxy white or flesh-colored, dome-shaped papules often with central umbilication. Lesions contain a cheesy grayish white material. Molluscum contagiosum is highly contagious and spreads by autoinoculation, skin-to-skin contact, sexual contact, and shared clothing/towels. Molluscum contagiosum is a self-limited infection in immunocompetent patients but can be difficult to treat and disfiguring in immunocompromised patients.

EPIDEMIOLOGY

Prevalence

- 1% in the United States, occurring mainly in children aged 2 to 15 years and sexually active young adults
- 5–18% HIV population

ETIOLOGY AND PATHOPHYSIOLOGY

- DNA virus; Poxviridae family
- Four genetic virus types, clinically indistinguishable
- Virions invade and replicate in cytoplasm of epithelial cells causing abnormal cell proliferation.
- Genome encodes proteins to evade host immune system.
- Incubation period: 2 to 6 weeks
- Time to resolution: 6 to 24 months
- Not associated with malignancy
- No cross-hybridization or reactivation by other poxviruses

RISK FACTORS

- Skin-to-skin contact with infected person
- Contact sports
- Swimming
- Atopic dermatitis
- Sexual activity with infected partner
- Immunocompromised: HIV, chemotherapy, corticosteroid therapy, transplant patients, patients on biologics

GENERAL PREVENTION

- Avoid skin-to-skin contact with host (e.g., contact sports, sexual activity).
- Avoid sharing clothing and towels.

COMMONLY ASSOCIATED CONDITIONS

- Atopic dermatitis
- Immunosuppression medications: corticosteroids, biologics, chemotherapy, etc.
- HIV/AIDS

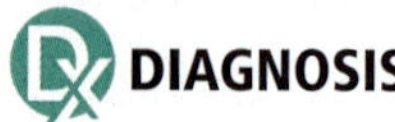

DIAGNOSIS

HISTORY

- Contact with known infected person
- Participation in contact sports
- Sexual activity

PHYSICAL EXAM

- Perform thorough skin exam including conjunctiva and anogenital area.
- Discrete, firm papules with a central umbilication
- White curd-like core under umbilicated center
- Lesions are flesh-colored, pearly, or red in color and frequently located in intertriginous areas.
- May have surrounding erythema or dermatitis
- Immunocompetent hosts: average of 11 to 20 lesions, 2 to 5 mm diameter (range: 1 to 10 mm)
- Immunocompromised hosts may have hundreds of widespread lesions or "giant" molluscum (lesions >1 cm)
- Sexually active: inner thighs, anogenital area

Pediatric Considerations

- Infants <3 months: Consider vertical transmission. If vertical transmission, lesions often located on scalp
- Children: fever, >50 lesions, limited response to therapy; consider immunodeficiency.
- Children: anogenital lesions; most likely autoinoculation if lesions present elsewhere on body. However, provider should consider possible sexual abuse.

DIFFERENTIAL DIAGNOSIS

- Verruca vulgaris
- Chickenpox
- Milia
- AIDS patients: *Cryptococcus neoformans*, penicilliosis, histoplasmosis, coccidioidomycosis
- Basal cell carcinoma
- Benign appendageal tumors: syringomas, hidrocystomas, ectopic sebaceous glands
- Condyloma acuminatum
- Dermatofibroma
- Eyelid: abscess, chalazion, foreign-body granuloma
- Folliculitis/furunculosis
- Keratoacanthoma
- Oral squamous cell carcinoma
- Trichoepithelioma
- Warty dyskeratoma
- Amelanotic melanoma
- Papular urticaria

DIAGNOSTIC TESTS & INTERPRETATION

Initial Tests (lab, imaging)

- Virus cannot be cultured.
- Culture lesion if concern is secondary infection.
- Sexual transmission: Test for other sexually transmitted infections, including HIV.
- Microscopy: scrape lesion
  - Core material has characteristic Henderson-Paterson intracytoplasmic viral inclusion bodies.
  - Crush prep with 10% potassium hydroxide will show characteristic inclusion bodies as well.
  - Alternatively, hematoxylin-eosin-stained formalin-fixed tissue shows same confirmatory features.

Diagnostic Procedures/Other

Clinical exam generally diagnostic, but dermatoscopy can be helpful.

Test Interpretation

Characteristic dermoscopic findings:

- Central pore or umbilication, white-to-yellow polylobular structure, and crown vessels

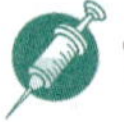

TREATMENT

GENERAL MEASURES

- In healthy patients, molluscum contagiosum is generally self-limited and resolves spontaneously; therefore, treatment is optional (1)[A].
- No single intervention is shown to be convincingly more effective than any other in treating molluscum contagiosum (1)[A].
- There are no FDA-approved treatments for molluscum contagiosum.
- Treatment decision is typically based on patient's age, location, number of lesions, comorbidities, availability, and cost.
- Three categories of treatment: destructive, immune-enhancing, and antiviral

MEDICATION

First Line

Cantharidin 0.7–0.9% solution: In office application to lesions, cover with dressing; wash off in 2 to 6 hours or sooner if blistering. Repeat treatment every 2 to 4 weeks until lesions resolve (1)[A].

- Not commercially available in the United States but may be prepared in the United States by compounding pharmacy from powder; might be available as solution from Canada
- Adverse effects: blistering, erythema, pain, pruritus develop after the office visit. Initially no discomfort, so this medication may be particularly useful in children.
- Precautions: Do not use on face or on genital mucosa.

Second Line

- Benzoyl peroxide 10% cream: Apply to each lesion twice daily for 4 weeks (1)[A].
  - Inexpensive, available over the counter
  - Adverse effects: mild dermatitis
- Imiquimod 5% cream: 3–5 times per week for 12 weeks
  - Adverse effects: mucositis, leukopenia, vitiligo (2)
- Other topicals reported: podophyllotoxin, trichloroacetic acid, salicylic acid, lactic acid, glycolic acid, and tretinoin (3)
- Cimetidine: oral; 25–40 mg/kg/day (3)
- For immunocompromised patients (including HIV) with refractory lesions, consider
  - Cidofovir: topical cream or IV

ISSUES FOR REFERRAL

Immunocompromised patients not responding to first- or second-line treatment

SURGERY/OTHER PROCEDURES

- Cryotherapy: 1 or 2 cycles of 10 to 20 seconds (3); repeat every 3 to 4 weeks as needed until lesions disappear.
  - Adverse effects: erythema, edema, pain, blistering
  - Contraindications: cryoglobulinemia, Raynaud disease
- Curettage under local or topical anesthesia (1)[A]
  - Adverse effects: pain, scarring
- Intralesional immunotherapy:
  - Candida antigen, PPD, vitamin D, MMR
  - Benefits: low to no recurrence
  - Adverse effects: erythema, edema, allergic reaction, anaphylaxis

COMPLEMENTARY & ALTERNATIVE MEDICINE

- Australian lemon myrtle oil: Apply 10% solution once daily for 21 days (1)[A].
- Potassium hydroxide 5–10% solution: Apply 1 to 2 times a day until the lesions disappeared completely (1)[A].

Pediatric Considerations

- Treatment is optional for immunocompetent children.
- Surgical interventions: second line in small children due to associated pain
- Pain control: Pretreat with topical lidocaine or EMLA before surgical treatment.
- Note: adverse effect: lidocaine or EMLA over large body surface area: methemoglobinemia and CNS toxicity. Refer to manufacturer's recommendations on dosing and use in children.

Pregnancy Considerations

Treatments safe in pregnancy: curettage, cryotherapy, incision, and expression

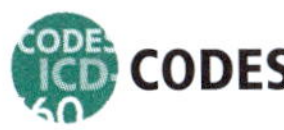

ONGOING CARE

FOLLOW-UP RECOMMENDATIONS

Patient Monitoring

Depends on type of treatment

PATIENT EDUCATION

- Cover lesions to prevent spread.
- Avoid scratching to prevent autoinoculation.
- Avoid sharing towels and clothing.
- Practice safe sex or avoid sexual activity when lesions present.

PROGNOSIS

- Immunocompetent: self-limited, resolves in 3 to 12 months (range: 2 months to 4 years)
- Immunocompromised: lesions difficult to treat; may persist for years

COMPLICATIONS

- Secondary infection
- Scarring, hyper-/hypopigmentation (generally only occurs as a result of treatment, not when lesions resolve spontaneously)

REFERENCES

1. van der Wouden JC, van der Sande R, Kruithof EJ, et al. Interventions for cutaneous molluscum contagiosum. *Cochrane Database Syst Rev*. 2017;5(5):CD004767.
2. DiBiagio JR, Pyle T, Green JJ. Reviewing the use of imiquimod for molluscum contagiosum. *Dermatol Online J*. 2018;24(6):13030/qt3b4606qt.
3. Meza-Romero R, Navarrete-Dechent C, Downey C. Molluscum contagiosum: an update and review of new perspectives in etiology, diagnosis, and treatment. *Clin Cosmet Investig Dermatol*. 2019;12:373–381.

ADDITIONAL READING

- Clebak KT, Malone MA. Skin Infections. *Prim Care*. 2018;45(3):433–454.
- Nowicka D, Bagłaj-Oleszczuk M, Maj J. Infectious diseases of the skin in contact sports. *Adv Clin Exp Med*. 2020;29(12):1491–1495.

CODES

ICD10

B08.1 Molluscum contagiosum

CLINICAL PEARLS

- Observation is preferred treatment in healthy patients as lesions will spontaneously resolve.
- Reassure parents that a child's lesions will heal naturally and generally resolve without scarring.
- No specific treatment has been identified as superior to any other, and no treatment is FDA approved.
- Consider topical corticosteroids for pruritus or associated dermatitis.

M

MORTON NEUROMA (INTERDIGITAL NEUROMA)

Lee A. Mancini, MD, CAQSM, CSCS*D, CSN

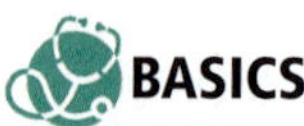

BASICS

DESCRIPTION

- Painful condition of the webbed spaces of the toes
- Features perineural fibrosis of the common digital nerve as it passes between metatarsals
  - The interspace between the 3rd and 4th metatarsals is most commonly affected.
  - The interspace between the 2nd and 3rd metatarsals is the next most common site.
- Systems affected: musculoskeletal, nervous
- Synonyms: plantar digital neuritis; Morton metatarsalgia; intermetatarsal neuroma

EPIDEMIOLOGY

Prevalence

- Unknown
- Mean age: 45 to 50 years
- Predominant sex: female > male (8:1)

ETIOLOGY AND PATHOPHYSIOLOGY

- Lateral plantar nerve joins a portion of medial plantar nerve, creating a nerve with a larger diameter than those going to other digits.
- Etiology not fully understood; four main theories:
  - Chronic traction damage
  - Inflammatory environment due to intermetatarsal bursitis
  - Compression by the deep transverse intermetatarsal ligament
  - Ischemia of vasa nervorum
- Nerve lies in SC tissue, deep to the fat pad of foot, just superficial to the digital artery and vein.
- Superficial to the nerve is the strong, deep transverse metatarsal ligament that holds the metatarsal bones together.
- With each step the patient takes, the inflamed nerve becomes compressed between the ground and the deep transverse metatarsal ligament. This can generate perineural fibrotic reaction with subsequent neuroma formation.

RISK FACTORS

- High-heeled shoes
  - Transfer more weight to the forefoot.
- Shoes with tight toe boxes
  - Cause lateral compression
- Pes planus (flat feet)
  - Pulls nerve medially, increasing irritation
- Obesity
- Female gender
- Ballet dancing, particularly associated with the demi-pointe position
- Basketball, aerobics, tennis, running, and similar activities
- Hyperpronation

GENERAL PREVENTION

- Wear properly fitting shoes.
- Avoid high heels and shoes with narrow toe boxes.

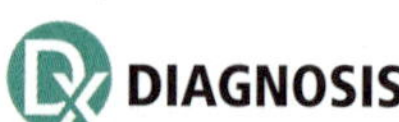

DIAGNOSIS

HISTORY

- Most common complaint is pain localized to interspace between 3rd and 4th toes.
- Pain is less severe when not bearing weight.
- Pain, cramping, or numbness of the forefoot during weight-bearing or immediately after strenuous foot exertion
- Radiation of pain to the toes
- Pain is relieved by removing shoes and massaging the foot.
- Patients often complain of "walking on a marble."
- Burning pain in the ball of the foot radiating to the toes
- Tingling or numbness in the toes
- Aggravated by wearing tight or narrow shoes

PHYSICAL EXAM

- Intense pain when pressure applied between metatarsal heads, sometimes with a palpable nodule
- Assess midfoot motion and digital motion to determine if arthritis or synovitis.
- Palpate along metatarsal shafts to assess for metatarsalgia or stress fractures.
- Special testing (See "Diagnostic Procedures/Other.")

DIFFERENTIAL DIAGNOSIS

- Stress fracture
- Hammer toe
- Metatarsophalangeal synovitis
- Metatarsalgia
- Arthritis
- Traumatic neuroma
- Osteomyelitis
- Bursitis
- Foreign body
- Freiberg infraction (avascular necrosis of the metatarsal head, most commonly in adolescent females at the 2nd metatarsal)
- Neoplasm (malignancy, osteochondroma, neurofibroma)
- Gout

DIAGNOSTIC TESTS & INTERPRETATION

Initial Tests (lab, imaging)

- Predominantly a clinical diagnosis; imaging should be reserved for when the diagnosis is unclear.
- Imaging may be helpful if more than one web space is involved.
- Radiographs may help to rule out osseous pathology if diagnosis is in question, but plain films usually are normal in patients with a Morton neuroma.
- Ultrasound (US) has 79% specificity and 99% sensitivity for Morton neuromas but is poor at assessing the size of the lesion. Specificity declines to 50% for lesions <6 mm.
- MRI can rule out an osseous tumor and help with surgical planning; MRI has a sensitivity of 83% and a specificity of 99% for diagnosis of Morton neuroma.

Diagnostic Procedures/Other

- Five special tests have been described: thumb index finger squeeze test, Mulder sign, foot squeeze test, plantar percussion test, and toe tip sensation deficit.
  - Thumb index finger squeeze test is the most sensitive and specific (96% and 96%, respectively); positive when pain elicited by squeezing the symptomatic intermetatarsal space between the index finger and thumb
  - Mulder sign is a painful "click" produced by squeezing the metatarsal heads together while compressing the neuroma between the thumb and index finger of the other hand; sensitivity 40–84%
  - Foot squeeze test is positive when pain is induced in the symptomatic web space when the metatarsal heads are compressed by grasping the foot; sensitivity 40%
  - Plantar and dorsal percussion tests are positive when percussion of the affected web space elicits pain.
  - Toe tip sensation deficit exists when the sensation of the toe distal to the affected web space is decreased relative to the other toes.
- More than one of the above tests being positive increases the diagnostic accuracy.

Test Interpretation

Pathologic examination shows chronic fibrosis and thickening within and around the digital nerve. Arterial thickening and thrombosis of the common digital artery are sometimes present.

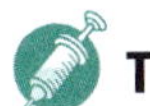

TREATMENT

GENERAL MEASURES

- Stepwise treatment, with typical progression from conservative measures followed by infiltrative treatment and ultimately surgical treatment
- Surgical treatments are the most successful (89%) followed by infiltrative (84%) then conservative (48%) as assessed by patient satisfaction with pain reduction at ≥6 months.
- Conservative treatments include the following:
  - Flat shoes with a roomy toe box
  - Plantar pads or metatarsal bar may help with alignment of metatarsal heads to provide relief.
  - There is no role for varus or valgus footwear padding.
  - There is no role for extracorporeal shock wave therapy (ESWT).
- NSAIDs for temporary symptom relief (1)[A]

MEDICATION

First Line

- Injectable steroids (e.g., betamethasone phosphate/acetate or methylprednisolone): number needed to treat (NNT) for significant benefit over conservative measures at 6 months = 2.3 (2)[A]
- One study demonstrated clinically significant improvement in use of US guidance versus palpation for corticosteroid injection.

Second Line

US-guided alcohol ablation therapy to sclerose the nerve is effective and has a lower complication rate than surgery.

ISSUES FOR REFERRAL

- Continued pain despite conservative treatments and injections
- Large interdigital neuromas (>5 mm diameter) or young patients who may benefit from earlier operative intervention
- One study demonstrated a cut-off value of 6.3 mm or larger Morton neuroma was associated with failure of corticosteroid injection.

SURGERY/OTHER PROCEDURES

- Surgical removal of the neuroma or shortening of the metatarsals, with or without release of the transverse metatarsal ligament, have an 89% success rate at 6 months defined by satisfaction scores.
- Small trials have been conducted using other invasive, nonsurgical techniques including injection with botulinum toxin, cryoablation, radiofrequency ablation, and platelet-rich plasma, but evidence is limited at this time.

ONGOING CARE

FOLLOW-UP RECOMMENDATIONS

At diagnosis or if no improvement after 3 months of conservative treatment, consider corticosteroid injection.

- May repeat injection if no improvement after 2 to 4 weeks or consider referring for surgical management
- 21–51% of patients receiving a single corticosteroid injection require surgical intervention within 2 to 4 years.
- Size >5 mm and younger patients are more likely to undergo invasive treatment.

PATIENT EDUCATION

Wear properly fitting comfortable shoes.

PROGNOSIS

- 48% satisfaction rate with conservative treatment
- 85% satisfaction rate with infiltrative treatment
- 89% satisfaction rate with operative treatment

COMPLICATIONS

- Hip and knee pain can develop secondary to gait changes.
- Complications vary by treatment type.
- Failure rate is 47% with conservative treatment; 9–23% with invasive, nonsurgical treatment; and 4% with surgical treatment.
- Surgical complications vary by specific procedure and include keloid, CRPS, and stiffness. There was a global complication rate of 21% with operative treatment.

REFERENCES

1. Thomson CE, Gibson JNA, Martin D. Interventions for the treatment of Morton's neuroma. *Cochrane Database Syst Rev*. 2004;2004(3):CD003118.
2. Saygi B, Yildirim Y, Saygi EK, et al. Morton neuroma: comparative results of two conservative methods. *Foot Ankle Int*. 2005;26(7):556–559.

ADDITIONAL READING

Jain S, Mannan K. The diagnosis and management of Morton's neuroma: a literature review. *Foot Ankle Spec*. 2013;6(4):307–317.

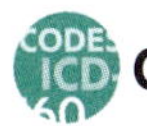

CODES

ICD10

- G57.60 Lesion of plantar nerve, unspecified lower limb
- G57.61 Lesion of plantar nerve, right lower limb
- G57.62 Lesion of plantar nerve, left lower limb

CLINICAL PEARLS

- Morton neuroma is usually a clinical diagnosis but can be further evaluated with US or MRI.
- Typical treatment is stepwise with conservative, then infiltrative, and then operative treatment.
- Morton neuromas with >5 mm diameter are more likely to require operative treatment.
- Younger patients are more likely to require operative treatment.
- Neurectomy is the definitive treatment. Patients should be aware of surgical complications.

MOTION SICKNESS

Robert B. Bonanno, MD

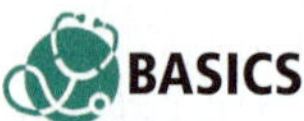

BASICS

DESCRIPTION

- Motion sickness is a physiologic response in affected individuals to a situation in which sensory conflict about body motion exists among visual receptors, vestibular receptors, and body proprioceptors.
- Often induced when patterns of motion differ from those previously experienced or expected
- Differs from "cybersickness" or "virtual reality sickness" (symptoms, including dizziness, that result from exposure to computer-based stimuli) in the fact that some form of actual movement is generally required to diagnose motion sickness
- Systems affected: nervous, gastrointestinal (GI)
- Synonym(s): car sickness; sea sickness; air sickness; space sickness; physiologic vertigo; kinetosis

EPIDEMIOLOGY

- Females more likely to be affected than males (1)[C].
- Pregnancy increases risk (possibly secondary to hormonal changes).
- Children <2 years of age unlikely to be affected, although highest incidence in children 6 to 12 years of age

Prevalence

Estimation is complex although motion sickness is a common physiologic phenomenon that can develop in any individual with the right conditions. Estimations of prevalence vary widely by activity, from <1–1% of those riding in cars, trains or pressurized commercial aircraft to 25% of those traveling on large ships to up to 80% of astronauts during their first 3 days of space travel (1)[C].

ETIOLOGY AND PATHOPHYSIOLOGY

- Precise etiology unknown; thought to be due to a mismatch of vestibular and visual sensations, particularly those to which an individual has not been habituated
- Rotary, vertical, and low-frequency motions produce more symptoms than linear, horizontal, and high-frequency motions (2)[C].

Genetics

Heritability estimates range from 55% to 75% (1)[C].

RISK FACTORS

- Motion (auto, plane, boat, amusement rides)
- Visual stimuli (e.g., moving horizon)
- Poor ventilation (fumes, smoke, carbon monoxide)
- Emotions (fear, anxiety)
- Zero gravity
- Pregnancy, menstruation, oral contraceptive use
- History of migraine headaches, especially vestibular migraine

GENERAL PREVENTION

See "General Measures."

Pediatric Considerations

- Rare in children <2 years of age
- Incidence peaks between 6 and 12 years of age.
- Antihistamines may cause paradoxical agitation in children.
- Scopolamine should be avoided in children.

Geriatric Considerations

- Age confers some resistance to motion sickness.
- Elderly are at increased risk for anticholinergic side effects from treatment.

Pregnancy Considerations

- Pregnant patients are more likely to experience motion sickness.
- Scopolamine should be avoided in patients with severe preeclampsia due to increased risk of eclamptic seizures.

COMMONLY ASSOCIATED CONDITIONS

- Migraine headache
- Vestibular syndromes

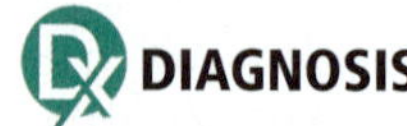

DIAGNOSIS

HISTORY

Presence of the following signs and symptoms in the context of a typical stimulus (3):

- Nausea
- Vomiting
- Stomach awareness (feeling of fullness in epigastrium)
- Diaphoresis
- Facial and perioral pallor
- Hypersalivation
- Yawning, hyperventilation
- Anxiety, panic
- Malaise/fatigue/lethargy
- Weakness
- Confusion
- Dizziness

PHYSICAL EXAM

No specific findings

DIFFERENTIAL DIAGNOSIS

- Mountain sickness
- Vestibular disease, central and peripheral
- Gastroenteritis
- Metabolic disorders
- Toxin exposure
- Concussion
- Hypoglycemia
- Nausea and vomiting of pregnancy

DIAGNOSTIC TESTS & INTERPRETATION

None usually indicated

Initial Tests (lab, imaging)

Can consider pregnancy test or fingerstick glucose to rule out hypoglycemia

Follow-Up Tests & Special Considerations

Multiple online questionnaires (such as the Motion Sickness Susceptibility Questionnaire) are available to help patients recognize their susceptibility to motion sickness and what situations are most likely to cause symptom development.

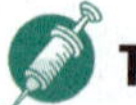

TREATMENT

- Follow guidelines under "General Measures" section to prevent motion sickness (3)[C].
- Premedicate before travel with anticholinergic or antihistamine agents (3)[A]:
  - For extended travel, consider treatment with scopolamine transdermal patch.
- Serotonin receptor agonist (rizatriptan) may be effective for migraineurs with motion sickness (2)[C].

GENERAL MEASURES

- Avoid noxious types of motions; travelling in inclement weather may exacerbate symptoms.
- Improve ventilation; avoid noxious stimuli.
- Eat before travel (light, soft, bland, low-fat, and low-acid foods); avoid alcohol; avoid traveling on an empty stomach.
- Increase airflow around face.
- Use semirecumbent seating or lay supine.
- Fix vision on horizon; avoid fixation on moving objects; keep eyes fixed on still, distant objects.
- Avoid reading while actively traveling.
- Frequent and graded exposure to stimulus that triggers nausea (habituation)
- Counsel patient on choosing location within the mode of transportation that minimizes motion (over the wing in airplanes, driver or front passenger seat in automobiles, facing the waves away from the rocking bow in boats, near the front on buses).

MEDICATION

First Line

First-generation antihistamines

- Drug interactions: increased risk of adverse CNS reactions (drowsiness/dizziness) when use with other drugs with anticholinergic properties or CNS effects (sedatives, hypnotics, opiates, anxiolytics, alcohol)
- Adverse effects: drowsiness, dizziness, impaired coordination, headache, urinary retention

- Use with caution in elderly patients and patients with asthma, glaucoma or enlarged prostate
  - Meclizine (Antivert): Take 60 minutes before travel.
    - Contraindications: not recommended in patients with a hypersensitivity to meclizine
    - Adults and adolescents >12 years of age: 25 to 50 mg PO q24h starting 1 hour before travel
    - Children <12 years of age: not recommended
  - Promethazine (Phenergan): Take 30 to 60 minutes before travel.
    - Contraindicated in children <2 years of age and use with caution in children >2 years of age due to risk of respiratory depression (FDA boxed warning).
    - Use in caution in patients with seizure disorders.
    - Adults: 25 mg PO q12h (also available as IM injection or rectal suppository)
  - Dimenhydrinate (Dramamine): Take 30 to 60 minutes before travel.
    - Adults and adolescents: 50 to 100 mg PO q4–6h, maximum 400 mg/day
    - Children 6 to 12 years of age: 25 to 50 mg PO q6–8h, maximum 150 mg/day
    - Children 2 to 6 years of age: 12.5 to 25.0 mg PO q6–8h, maximum 75 mg/day
  - Diphenhydramine (Benadryl): Take 30 minutes before travel.
    - Adults and adolescents over 12 years of age: 25 to 50 mg PO q6–8h, maximum 300 mg/day
    - Children 6 to 12 years of age: 12.5 to 25.0 mg PO q4–6h, maximum 150 mg/day
- Anticholinergic
  - Scopolamine transdermal patch (Transderm Scop): Apply 4 hours prior to travel.
    - Contraindications: patients with angle-closure glaucoma or severe preeclampsia
    - Use with caution in patients with a history of psychosis or seizure disorder as use may exacerbate these conditions
    - Adverse effects: drowsiness, dizziness, blurred vision, dry mouth, urinary retention, slowed GI motility
    - Apply (1 mg) patch behind ear over the mastoid. Replace every 3 days.

ADDITIONAL THERAPIES

The most effective long-term management of motion sickness is habituation. It is superior to medications used to manage motion sickness and also without their potential side effects.

COMPLEMENTARY & ALTERNATIVE MEDICINE

- Acupressure on point PC6 (*Neiguan* on pericardium meridian) has been shown to reduce feelings of nausea and vomiting during pregnancy, after surgery, and in cancer chemotherapy. However, limited evidence of efficacy has been found for motion sickness; point PC6: 2 cm proximal of transverse crease of palmar side of wrist between tendons of the palmaris longus and the flexor carpi radialis (4)[B].
- Ginger: 1.0 to 1.5 g per 24 hours (250 mg PO 4 times a day); take 4 hours before travel; studies have shown ginger to be an effective treatment for nausea and vomiting (5)[B].

ONGOING CARE

DIET

- Eat before travel, avoid empty stomach; eat light, soft, bland, low-fat, and low-acid foods.
- Avoid alcohol.

PROGNOSIS

- Symptoms should resolve when motion exposure ends.
- Resistance to motion sickness seems to increase with age.

COMPLICATIONS

- Hypotension
- Dehydration
- Depression
- Panic
- Syncope

REFERENCES

1. Leung AK, Hon KL. Motion sickness: an overview. *Drugs Context*. 2019;8:2019-9-4.
2. Furman JM, Marcus DA, Balaban CD. Rizatriptan reduces vestibular-induced motion sickness in migraineurs. *J Headache Pain*. 2011;12(1):81–88.
3. Brainard A, Gresham C. Prevention and treatment of motion sickness. *Am Fam Physician*. 2014;90(1):41–46.
4. Lee EJ, Frazier SK. The efficacy of acupressure for symptom management: a systematic review. *J Pain Symptom Manage*. 2011;42(4):589–603.
5. Marx W, Kiss N, Isenring L. Is ginger beneficial for nausea and vomiting? An update of the literature. *Curr Opin Support Palliat Care*. 2015;9(2):189–195.

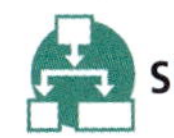

SEE ALSO

Algorithm: Dizziness

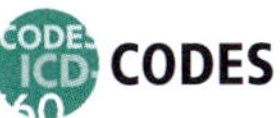

CODES

ICD10

T75.3XXA Motion sickness, initial encounter

CLINICAL PEARLS

- Prevention of motion sickness with behavioral interventions is more effective than pharmacologic treatment of symptoms.
- The scopolamine transdermal patch is a generally well tolerated first-line treatment for prevention of motion sickness. It should be applied at least 4 hours before travel.
- First-generation antihistamines are also effective, although sedating. They should be administered 30 to 60 minutes before travel.
- Although acupressure wristbands have been found to be effective by systematic reviews in postoperative and chemotherapy-induced nausea and vomiting, as well as hyperemesis gravidarum, conflicting data exist for use with motion sickness.

MULTIPLE MYELOMA

Poorva Bindal, MD

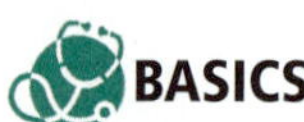

BASICS

DESCRIPTION

- Multiple myeloma (MM) is a malignant proliferation of a single clone of plasma cells. These malignant cells produce monoclonal protein (immunoglobulin [Ig]) that can be detected in the blood and/or urine as it is filtered in the kidneys.
- MM is characterized by bony lytic lesions, hypercalcemia, increased susceptibility to infections, and renal impairment.
- Monoclonal gammopathy of undetermined significance (MGUS) is a common disorder with limited monoclonal plasma cell proliferation that can progress to smoldering MM or symptomatic MM at rate of ~1% per year.

EPIDEMIOLOGY

- Median age: 65 to 74 years.
- ~2% of all cancers and 17% of hematologic malignancies in the United States
- African Americans about 2 to 3 times more commonly affected than Caucasians; less common in Asians

Incidence

7 cases per 100,000 in the United States annually

Prevalence

As of 2023, there are approximately 176,000 recognized cases of MM worldwide.

ETIOLOGY AND PATHOPHYSIOLOGY

- Arises from uncontrolled growth of a single clone of plasma cells in the bone marrow (BM), leading to an excessive production of abnormal monoclonal Ig, also called M proteins.
- Chromosomal translocations involving the Ig heavy chain loci, like t(11;14), t(4;14), or mutations in oncogenes or tumor suppressor genes, contribute to tumorigenesis and disease progression.
- The malignant plasma cells interact with the bone marrow stroma, inhibiting osteoblast function and stimulating osteoclast activity, which results in bone destruction, lytic lesions, and hypercalcemia that are commonly seen in patients with MM.

Genetics

Rarely occurs in familial clusters. A rare form of paratarg-7 protein might have pathogenic role.

RISK FACTORS

- Most cases have no known risks associated.
- Old age; immunosuppression; and exposure to chemicals, heavy metals, and ionizing radiation increase the risk of MM

COMMONLY ASSOCIATED CONDITIONS

Secondary amyloidosis with MM and polyneuropathy, organomegaly, endocrinopathy, monoclonal gammopathy, skin changes (POEMS).

DIAGNOSIS

HISTORY

- 34% of patients are asymptomatic at the time of presentation.
- Anemia (73%) is the most common presentation of MM.
- Hypercalcemia (28%): anorexia, abdominal pain, somnolence, polydipsia, polyuria, dehydration
- Elevated creatinine (48%), acute kidney injury
- Bony lesions (80%): lytic lesions causing bone pain (58%), osteoporosis, or pathologic fracture (26–34%)
- Other symptoms: fatigue (32%), peripheral neuropathy (PN), weight loss (24%), recurrent infections, hyperviscosity syndrome, and cord compression

PHYSICAL EXAM

- Dehydration, pallor, and bone tenderness
- Hyperviscosity syndrome in 7%: retinal hemorrhages, prolonged bleeding, neurologic changes
- Extramedullary plasmacytomas (large, purplish, subcutaneous masses)
- Skin: waxy papules, or plaques in the eyelids, retroauricular region, neck, or inguinal and anogenital regions

DIFFERENTIAL DIAGNOSIS

- Reactive plasmacytosis
- MGUS
- Smoldering MM (SMM): no end-organ damage (CRAB: hypercalcemia, renal insufficiency, anemia, bone lesions) features
- Metastatic carcinoma (kidney, breast, non–small cell lung cancer)
- Waldenström macroglobulinemia
- Reactive plasmacytosis
- AL amyloidosis
- Solitary plasmacytoma
- POEMS syndrome

DIAGNOSTIC TESTS & INTERPRETATION

The diagnosis of MM requires the following:

- BM involvement with ≥10% of plasma cells or the presence of a plasmacytoma and one or more of the following myeloma-defining events:
  - Evidence of end-organ damage:
    - Hypercalcemia: serum calcium >0.25 mmol/L (>1 mg/dL) higher than the upper limit of normal or >2.75 mmol/L (>11 mg/dL)
    - Renal insufficiency: creatinine clearance <40 mL/min or serum creatinine >177 μmol/L (>2 mg/dL)
    - Anemia: hemoglobin value of >2 g/dL below the lower limit of normal or a hemoglobin value <10 g/dL
    - Bone lesions: one or more osteolytic lesions on skeletal radiography, CT, or PET-CT
  - Any or more of the following findings is considered an MM-defining event (SLiM criteria):
    - Clonal BM plasma cell percentage ≥60% (S)
    - Involved: uninvolved serum free light chain (FLC) ratio ≥100 (Li) or <0.01%, with involved FLC ≥100 mg/L
    - >1 focal lesion (≥5 mm in size) on MRI studies, or PET-CT (M)

Initial Tests (lab, imaging)

- CBC with differential
- BUN, creatinine, serum electrolytes, albumin, and calcium
- Serum lactate dehydrogenase (LDH), β_2-microglobulin
- Serum protein electrophoresis (SPEP), serum immunofixation electrophoresis (SIFE): M protein level elevated
- Quantitative serum Ig levels: IgG, IgA, and IgM
- Quantitative serum FLC levels: κ and λ chains
- ESR, C-reactive protein: elevated
- Urinalysis: 24-hour urine for protein, urine protein electrophoresis (UPEP), urine immunofixation electrophoresis (UIFE); 20% positive urine protein:
  - Urinalysis dip is often negative for protein because this test identifies albumin, and the protein in MM is Bence Jones (BJ) monoclonal protein.
- Whole body low-dose CT is preferred for the detection of bone involvement.
- BM biopsy: plasma cell percentage, histology, immunohistochemistry, flow cytometry, cytogenetics, and fluorescence in situ hybridization (FISH)

Follow-Up Tests & Special Considerations

- For patients with suspected SMM, a whole body MRI or MRI of the spine and pelvis is recommended to evaluate for cord compression; PET/CT for those with extramedullary disease; baseline bone densitometry
- BM aspiration and biopsy to monitor response along with SPEP with SIFE: M protein helps to track progression of myeloma and response to treatment. Serum Igs and FLCs can be used to monitor response or relapse.

Diagnostic Procedures/Other

Multiple staging systems are used. The most common one is the Revised International Staging System (R-ISS). Durie-Salmon staging system is rarely used nowadays.

- International Staging System (ISS)
  - Stage I: albumin ≥3.5 g/dL and β_2-microglobulin <3.5 μg/mL
  - Stage II: neither stage I nor stage III
  - Stage III: β_2-microglobulin ≥5.5 μg/mL
- Mayo Stratification of Myeloma and Risk-Adapted Therapy (mSMART)
  - Standard risk: >t(11;14), t(6;14), and hyperdiploidy
  - Intermediate risk: t(4;14), del(13q) by cytogenetics, hypodiploidy
  - High risk: t(14;16), t(14;20), del(17 p)
- R-ISS combines ISS information with chromosomal abnormalities and LDH to provide better prognostic information for MM. High-risk patients often receive intensified therapy, including quadruplet induction (adding daratumumab), early transplant, and consideration for clinical trials.

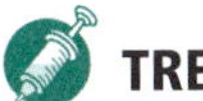

TREATMENT

Treatment is individualized based on disease characteristics, patient age, comorbidities, and risk stratification.

GENERAL MEASURES

Adequate hydration to prevent renal insufficiency; antimicrobial prophylaxis during treatment

MEDICATION

- A risk-adapted, multiphase approach; the three phases of treatment for newly diagnoses MM are induction phase, consolidation (often ASCT for whom are eligible), and maintenance phase.
- Agents include chemotherapy, proteasome inhibitors (PIs), immunomodulatory agents, steroids, bispecific antibodies, monoclonal antibodies and chimeric antigen receptor (CAR) T-cell therapy.
- Induction phase: The backbone of induction phase for transplant eligible patients is increasingly becoming a quadruplet regimen comprising a PIs, immunomodulatory drugs (IMiDs), corticosteroids, and anti-CD38 monoclonal antibody based on recent clinical trials and systematic reviews showing significant improvement in overall response rate, minimal residual disease negativity, progression free survival (PFS), and overall survival (OS).
- Consolidation therapy: Eligible patients undergo high-dose melphalan chemotherapy followed by ASCT as consolidation after induction. ASCT improves depth of response, PFS, and OS. Some centers use early transplant after initial induction, whereas others consider delayed transplant at relapse depending on patient preference and disease response.
- Induction chemotherapy for ASCT-ineligible patients is similar either with doublet or triplet (e.g., lenalidomide/low-dose dexamethasone or bortezomib/dexamethasone or daratumumab/lenalidomide/dexamethasone).
- Maintenance treatment: Lenalidomide is the most preferred agent for maintenance therapy after induction or transplant. For high-rise disease, maintenance may include PIs or combination approaches.

First Line

- PIs
  - Block ubiquitin-proteasome catalytic pathway in cells by binding to the 20S proteasome complex
  - Consider herpes simplex virus (HSV) prophylaxis with acyclovir.
  - Bortezomib: PI, IV or SC; SC has lower risk of PN; toxicity: PN, cytopenia, nausea, anorexia, leukopenia, thrombocytopenia, rash
  - Carfilzomib: IV, 2nd-generation PI; toxicity: cardiomyopathy and other cardiac adverse events, fever, diarrhea, thrombotic microangiopathy, fatigue; can have hypersensitivity reaction after infusion
  - Ixazomib—oral PI; toxicity: PN, diarrhea, thrombocytopenia, neutropenia, back pain, edema
- Cyclophosphamide
  - Nitrogen mustard–derivative alkylating agent
  - Toxicity: cytopenia, anaphylaxis, interstitial pulmonary fibrosis, hemorrhagic cystitis, impaired fertility
- Immunomodulators:
  - Thalidomide, lenalidomide, and pomalidomide
  - Antiangiogenesis inhibition, immunomodulation
  - Toxicity: birth defects (thalidomide), deep vein thrombosis (DVT), neuropathy, rash, nausea, bradycardia
- Dexamethasone: dose (40 mg/week)
- Daratumumab, isatuximab: IgGκ1 monoclonal antibodies against CD38; toxicity: fatigue, back pain, lymphocytopenia, neutropenia, anemia including Coombs positive hemolytic anemia, thrombocytopenia, cough, flu-like symptoms, and infusion-related reaction
- Bisphosphonates or RANK ligand inhibitors (zoledronic acid or denosumab)
  - No effect on mortality but decrease pain, pathologic fractures

Second Line

- Progression of MM is usually identified by a rise in monoclonal M protein in the serum or the urine or in the serum free light chain ratio with new or worsening end-organ damage.
- At relapse, review prior treatments, depth and duration of response, refractory status (primary refractory or refractory to specific agents), and patient fitness. If relapse occurs >6 months after completing therapy with an agent, the disease is still considered sensitive to that agent and can consider using previously effective drugs.
- Combination regimens, often triplets or quadruplets, are preferred for deeper responses in the second line. The combinations in the second-line involve PIs (carfilzomib, ixazomib), IMiDs (pomalidomide), monoclonal antibodies (daratumumab, isatuximab, elotuzumab) based on prior therapy and duration of response.
- CAR T-cell therapy with ciltacabtagene autoleucel has also been approved for second-line therapy for relapsed/refractory MM and should be considered for patients with early relapse and high-risk disease.
- Several other agents have been in development for second and subsequent relapses. Options include selinexor, antibody-drug conjugates, bispecific antibodies, and CAR T-cell therapy. Clinical trial enrollment is also strongly encouraged.
- Bispecific antibodies are monoclonal antibodies and a bispecific B-cell maturation antigen (BCMA)-directed T-cell engager. These agents can be used for 4th and higher disease recurrence.
- BCMA can also be targeted through the two recently FDA-approved CAR T-cell therapy agents; idecabtagene vicleucel, and ciltacabtagene autoleucel

ISSUES FOR REFERRAL

- For spinal or other bone pathology, refer to orthopedics.
- Referral to a large center is recommended after three lines of treatment for trial evaluation.

ADDITIONAL THERAPIES

- Local radiation therapy for uncontrolled bone pain or plasmacytoma
- Avoid NSAIDs due to nephrotoxicity.
- Aspirin 81 to 325 mg for patients on immunomodulators for DVT prophylaxis.
- Erythropoietin for selected patients with anemia
- IVIg infusion for patients with recurrent life-threatening infections
- Patients should receive vaccines for pneumococcus, influenza, and SARS-CoV2.
- Do not administer live-virus vaccines.

ADMISSION, INPATIENT, AND NURSING CONSIDERATIONS

Indications: pain, infections, cytopenia, renal failure, bone complications, spinal cord compression, dehydration

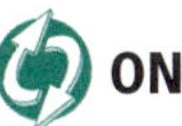

ONGOING CARE

PATIENT EDUCATION

International Myeloma Foundation: http://myeloma.org/Main.action

PROGNOSIS

- The survival depends heavily on the cytogenetic risk and stage of the disease.
- Median survival by R-ISS stage:
  - Stage I: has not been reached
  - Stage II: 83 months
  - Stage III: 43 months

COMPLICATIONS

Infections, pain, fractures, hypercalcemia, hyperuricemia, spinal cord compression, hyperviscosity syndrome, amyloidosis and dialysis

ADDITIONAL READING

- Ebraheem MS, Chakraborty R, Rochwerg B, et al. Quadruplet regimens for patients with newly diagnosed multiple myeloma: a systematic review and meta-analysis. *Blood Adv*. 2024;8(23):5993–6002.
- Sonneveld P, Dimopoulos MA, Boccadoro M, et al. Daratumumab, bortezomib, lenalidomide, and dexamethasone for multiple myeloma. *N Engl J Med*. 2024;390(4):301–313.

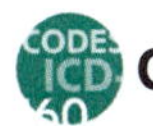

CODES

ICD10

- C90.0 Multiple myeloma
- C90.00 Multiple myeloma not having achieved remission
- C90.01 Multiple myeloma in remission

CLINICAL PEARLS

- MM is a plasma cell malignancy that causes end-organ damage.
- Look for presence of "CRAB."
- Avoid nephrotoxins (radiographic contrast material, NSAIDs, dehydration).
- Patients with MM are immunocompromised.

MULTIPLE SCLEROSIS

Adedamola Ayo Omole, MD

BASICS

Multiple sclerosis (MS) is an autoimmune disease that targets the neural myelin sheath causing demyelination and resulting in progressive axonal loss and CNS atrophy. While it primarily affects white matter, it can also impact grey matter and meninges, leading to a range of sensory, motor, behavioral, and cognitive symptoms.

DESCRIPTION

Subtypes of MS (1):

- Clinically isolated syndrome (CIS): Patient's initial symptoms are characteristic of CNS demyelination that may be due to MS but does not fulfill the criteria of dissemination in time; ~80% of patients with CIS will later relapse and be diagnosed with MS.
- Radiologically isolated syndrome (RIS): incidental brain or spinal cord MRI findings highly suggestive of MS, in an asymptomatic patient; no evidence of clinical attacks suggestive of MS; ~30–40% of patients with RIS later meet criteria for CIS or MS.
- Relapsing-remitting MS (RRMS): most common type at disease-onset; defined by relapse (attacks or exacerbations) followed by partial or complete improvement; recovery of residual deficits may ensue following each episode.
- Secondary progressive MS (SPMS): progressive worsening of neurologic function following initial RRMS; may be associated with acute exacerbations; often diagnosed retrospectively
- Primary progressive multiple sclerosis (PPMS): progressive decline in disease status and accumulation of disability from onset of disease without initial relapsing-remitting disease course (~10% of patients) (2)

Pregnancy Considerations

- If treatment is clinically necessary during pregnancy, preferred treatments include interferon-β and glatiramer acetate (3).
- Majority of patients experience reduced disease exacerbations during pregnancy, but relapse in the postpartum period.
- All drugs licensed for MS treatment are contraindicated during breastfeeding.

EPIDEMIOLOGY

Most often affects Caucasian women in their 2nd and 3rd generations of life.

Incidence

2.1 per 100,000 persons/year (1)

Prevalence

- Differs by latitude, higher rates among those living further from the equator (1)
- Americas: 117.49 per 100,000 people
- Worldwide: 43.95 per 100,000 people

ETIOLOGY AND PATHOPHYSIOLOGY

- Predominately an autoimmune process driven by T cells and B cells against the myelin sheath. Dysregulation and mistaken antigen identity lead CD4 T cells to cross the blood–brain barrier and recognize proteins on the surface of the myelin sheath. Cytokines, interferon-γ, and tumor necrosis factor-α are subsequently released, and activation of macrophages and B-cells leads to oligodendrocyte and myelin destruction, resulting in slower saltatory nerve conduction velocities.
- Oligodendrocytes, which have survived or formed from precursor cells, are able to partially remyelinate stripped axons, producing scars which overtime can lead to irreversible axonal loss and brain atrophy.
- The majority of axons are typically lost from the lateral corticospinal (motor) tracts of the spinal cord (2).

Genetics

Over 100 genetic loci have been associated with MS suggesting that it is ultimately an antigen-specific autoimmune process. Most commonly, these are mapped to the class II region of the HLA gene clusters. The most common being the HLA-DRB1 locus on chromosome 6, which produces major histocompatibility complexes with high-binding affinity for myelin basic proteins.

RISK FACTORS

- Age: peak incidence ages 20 to 40 years, but can present at any age (slightly earlier in women than men)
- Sex: female > male
- Race: Caucasian > Afro-Caribbean > East Asian
- Prior infections: Epstein-Barr virus; mononucleosis
- Substance: tobacco smoking
- Historically, proximity to the equator and its correlation with increased vitamin D exposure were inversely proportional to MS incidence. However, this association has been less noted and may be due to lifestyle changes leading to decreased sun exposure in these areas (2).
- Anti-TNF-α inhibitors like etanercept and infliximab have been associated with developing MS.

COMMONLY ASSOCIATED CONDITIONS

Internuclear ophthalmoplegia; optic neuritis; transverse myelitis; association with other autoimmune processes

DIAGNOSIS

A person with MS may present with a number of neurologic signs and symptoms depending on the locations of the lesion. The essential means of diagnoses is to demonstrate evidence of CNS lesions congruent with an objective history or a current clinical isolated attack that are separated by time and lesion location, that are not due to a separate disease process.

HISTORY

Common symptoms may include but not limited to: cognitive dysfunction, fatigue, dizziness, visual disturbances, facial palsy, dysphagia, muscle weakness or spasms, hyperesthesia or paresthesia, pain, bowel or bladder incontinence, urinary frequency or retention, or sexual dysfunction (2).

PHYSICAL EXAM

- Weakness, internuclear ophthalmoplegia, gait disturbance, hyperesthesia or paresthesia, cerebellar dysarthria, and spasticity (especially in lower extremities)
- Uhthoff phenomenon: Symptoms are worse with exposure to higher than usual temperature.
- Lhermitte phenomenon (barber chair phenomenon): Electric-like shocks extending down the spine caused by neck movement, especially flexion

DIFFERENTIAL DIAGNOSIS

- Infectious: Lyme disease, syphilis, acute disseminated encephalomyelitis, progressive multifocal leukoencephalopathy (PML), Guillain-Barré syndrome, primary cerebral angiitis, amyotrophic lateral sclerosis, Huntington disease, and HIV
- Autoimmune: systemic lupus erythematosus, antiphospholipid syndrome, neurosarcoidosis, Behçet disease, vasculitis, and Bell palsy
- CNS: neuromyelitis optica spectrum disorder, neoplasms, stroke, migraine, and normal pressure hydrocephalus
- Medications and substances: alcohol, anticholinergic drugs, cocaine, etanercept, infliximab, isoniazid, methanol
- Other: cobalamin (vitamin B12) deficiency, manganese toxicity, paraneoplastic syndrome, hypothyroidism, psychiatric disease (anxiety disorder, conversion disorder), Charcot-Marie-Tooth disease

DIAGNOSTIC TESTS & INTERPRETATION

- Blood tests to rule out alternative diagnosis: antinuclear antibody, antineutrophil cytoplasmic antibody, anti–double-stranded DNA antibody, antiphospholipid antibody, erythrocyte sedimentation rate, immunoglobulin G, immunoglobulin M, rheumatoid factor, HIV screening, rapid plasma reagin, thyroid-stimulating hormone (TSH), vitamin B_{12} level, complete blood count (CBC), comprehensive metabolic panel (CMP), Lyme disease antibody, anti-aquaporin-4 (AQP4) IgG autoantibody, MOG-IgG antibody (2)[B]
- MRI of head/spine with gadolinium: Periventricular and juxtacortical regions, and callosal and infratentorial lesions, and the cervical segment of the spinal cord are relatively specific for MS.
- Lumbar puncture: cerebrospinal fluid with elevated or normal protein levels; oligoclonal immunoglobulin G bands are seen in approximately 90% of MS but may be absent in early disease process.
- McDonald criteria for diagnosing MS (4): apply primarily when clinical suspicion for MS; not used for ruling out other neurologic conditions; dependent upon number of attacks and number of CNS lesions:
  - Two or more clinical attacks and two or more lesions with objective clinical evidence; MS is confirmed; may start treatment *or*
  - Two or more attacks and one lesion, with dissemination in space on MRI or an additional relapse causing new symptoms that effect another CNS region *or*
  - One attack and two lesions, with dissemination in time on MRI or another disease relapse or a positive test for oligoclonal bands in the CNS (3) *or*
  - One attack and one lesion, with dissemination in space and time
  - Formal diagnosis of PPMS can be made if symptoms gradually progress for at least 1 year and two of the following criteria are met:
    - At least one lesion in the brain is detected on MRI.
    - At least two spinal cord lesions are detected on MRI.
    - Oligoclonal bands in CSF

Initial Tests (lab, imaging)

MRI brain/spine

Follow-Up Tests & Special Considerations

Lumbar puncture, EMG

Diagnostic Procedures/Other

Evoked potentials: Assess function of visual, auditory, and somatosensory motor CNS pathways; measure CNS electric potentials evoked by neural stimulation. Visual evoked potentials are delayed in 80–90% of MS patients (1).

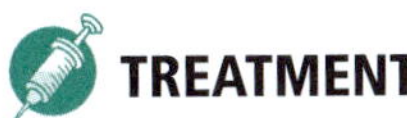

TREATMENT

GENERAL MEASURES

- Multidisciplinary team approach is paramount, including PT, OT and speech therapy, mental health specialist, pharmacists, urologist, neurologist, and dietitian.
- Three main categories currently exist for treatment: treatment for acute relapses, reducing MS-related activity using disease-modifying agents, and symptomatic therapy.
- Steroids: treatment for initial presentation and acute episodes of MS (1)
- Disease-modifying treatments (DMTs) early in the disease process is likely to slow overall disease progression; should be managed by MS specialist (2)[C]
- Smoking cessation is encouraged (1).

MEDICATION

- Acute relapse treatment—high-dose short-term glucocorticoid therapy (2)[A]
  - Methylprednisolone 1 g PO/IV daily for 3 to 5 days; without subsequent tapering; a second course may be given.
    - Side effects (S/E): infection risk, adrenal insufficiency, Cushing syndrome, fluid retention, hypokalemia, GI disturbances, headache, emotional lability, delirium, osteoporosis, hyperglycemia
  - Alternative therapy for those who cannot tolerate high-dose glucocorticoids: ACTH gel 80 to 120 units IM/SC daily for one week followed or not followed by taper
  - Plasmapheresis
- DMT: to decrease clinical attacks and delay disability progression (1),(2)[B]
  - Platform injection therapies
    - IFN-β_{1a} (Avonex) 30 μg IM weekly or IFN-β_{1a} (Rebif) 22 or 44 μg SC 3 times per week; IFN-β_{1b} (Betaseron/Betaferon/Extavia) 250 μg SC every other day
      - Monitor CBC, LFTs, TSH
      - S/E: flu-like symptoms, depression, skin site reactions, thyroid dysfunction, liver enzyme abnormalities
    - Glatiramer acetate (Copaxone) 20 mg SC daily
      - S/E: skin site reactions, postinjection reaction, lipoatrophy
  - Monoclonal antibodies (monitor CBC, LFTs, TSH)
    - Rituximab (Rituxan) 1 g IV once every 2 weeks ×2 doses; repeat 1 g once every 6 to 12 months. Rule out hepatitis B prior to use; S/E: hypogammaglobulinemia, infection, and PML
    - Natalizumab (Tysabri) 300 mg IV every 4 weeks
      - S/E: dizziness, nausea, increased risk of infection, PML
      - Alemtuzumab (Lemtrada) 12 mg/day × 5 days; 12 months later, 12 mg/day × 3 days
        - S/E: infusion reaction, increased risk of infection, thyroid problems, blood clots, immune thrombocytopenia
  - Oral therapies—for those who prefer self-administered oral medication
    - Dimethyl fumarate (Tecfidera) 120 to 240 mg PO BID × 7 days and then 240 mg BID
      - Monitor CBC, LFTs; S/E: diarrhea, cramps, nausea, flushing
    - Teriflunomide (Aubagio) 7 to 14 mg PO daily
      - Monitor CBC, LFTs, UA; S/E: headache, diarrhea, fatigue, arthralgia, hair thinning nausea
      - Fingolimod (Gilenya) 0.5 mg PO daily
        - Monitor ECG, CBC, LFTs, eye exam; S/E: 1st degree AV block, arrhythmia, infection risk
- Symptomatic therapies (1),(2)[B]
  - Spasticity: baclofen, dantrolene, tizanidine, cannabis extract (nabiximols), botulinum toxin, benzodiazepines, physiotherapy
  - Pain: amitriptyline, pregabalin, gabapentin, nabiximols, capsaicin
  - Trigeminal neuralgia: carbamazepine, oxcarbazepine, baclofen, gabapentin
  - Bladder dysfunction: imipramine, muscarinics, catheterization, intravesical botulinum toxin; avoid spicy, acidic foods, caffeine and alcohol for detrusor spasm.
  - Fatigue: amantadine, modafinil, SSRI
  - Tremors: diazepam, β-blockers
  - Depression: SSRI, SNRI, TCA
  - Movement disorder: ataxia (baclofen, dantrolene, tizanidine, deep brain stimulation); impaired walking (behavioral change therapy, physiotherapy)

ISSUES FOR REFERRAL

- Neurology: diagnosis and treatment
- Physical therapy and rehabilitation: physical therapy

ADDITIONAL THERAPIES

Hematopoietic stem cell transplants are being tested in clinical trials and may alter treatment and prevention of MS in the future (2).

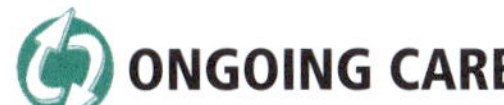

ONGOING CARE

FOLLOW-UP RECOMMENDATIONS

Patient Monitoring

- Assessing the severity of neurologic impairment from MS can be done using the Kurtzke Expanded Disability Status Scale (EDSS), which quantifies disability across eight functional systems: pyramidal, cerebellar, brainstem, sensory, bowel and bladder, visual, and cerebral. The EDSS scoring system is as follows:
  - 1.0: No disability, minimal signs in 1 functional system (FS); 2.0: minimal disability in 1 FS; 3.0: moderate disability in 1 FS; mild disability in 3 to 4 FS; fully ambulatory; 4.0: ambulatory without aid or rest for ~500m m; 5.0: ambulatory without aid or rest for ~200 m; 6.0: requires unilateral aid (cane, crutch), can walk 100 m; 7.0: unable to walk beyond 5 m even with aid, restricted wheelchair use for ~12 hour/day, self-propels and transfers alone; 8.0: essentially restricted to bed, chair, or wheelchair; out of bed most of the day; retains self-care functions, generally effective use of arms; 9.0: helpless, bedbound; can communicate and eat; 10: death due to MS
- This scale helps track disease progression and guide treatment.

PROGNOSIS

Average life expectancy is 5 to 10 years less than the unaffected population (2).

COMPLICATIONS

Mortality secondary to MS relapse is unusual; death is more commonly associated with a complication of MS such as infection.

REFERENCES

1. Saguil A, Farnell Iv EA, Jordan TS. Multiple sclerosis: a primary care perspective. *Am Fam Physician*. 2022;106(2):173–183.
2. Raffel J, Wakerley B, Nicholas R. Multiple sclerosis. *Medicine*. 2016;44(9):537–541.
3. Varytė G, Arlauskienė A, Ramašauskaitė D. Pregnancy and multiple sclerosis: an update. *Curr Opin Obstet Gynecol*. 2021;33(5):378–383.
4. Thompson AJ, Banwell BL, Barkhof F, et al. Diagnosis of multiple sclerosis: 2017 revisions of the McDonald criteria. *Lancet Neurol*. 2018;17(2):162–173. doi:10.1016/S1474-4422(17)30470-2.

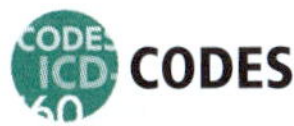

CODES

ICD10

G35 Multiple sclerosis

CLINICAL PEARLS

- MS is an immune-mediated inflammatory disease-causing demyelination, neuronal loss, and scarring within the CNS.
- Most common cause of nontraumatic neurologic disability in young adults
- Diagnosis is made with the McDonald criteria.
- Treatment is complex and rapidly changing; MS specialist and multiprofessional therapy is necessary.

M

MUMPS

Donna Marie Kaminski, DO, MPH, FAAFP • Brandis Belt, MD, MPH

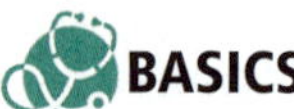

BASICS

An acute, self-limiting paramyxovirus infection, typically presenting with parotitis

DESCRIPTION

- Incubation period is 12 to 25 days, followed by 2 to 3 days symptomatic phase
- Asymptomatic in up to 30% of nonimmune and 60% of previously vaccinated individuals
- Painful parotitis in 95% of symptomatic cases
- Epidemics in late winter and in the spring
- Transmission by respiratory droplets, direct contact, or any surface (dish, doorknob, article of clothing)

EPIDEMIOLOGY

- 85% of mumps cases occur prior to 15 years of age, usually in children >2 years of age.
- Adult cases are typically more severe; predominant sex: male = female; geriatric population: Most U.S. adults are immune.
- Acute epidemic mumps: highly contagious in susceptible populations
  - Greatest number of cases occur in unvaccinated children 5 to 15 years of age.
- Mumps is unusual in children <2 years of age.
- Period of maximal communicability is 24 hours before to 72 hours after onset of parotitis.

Incidence

- Worldwide, 387,327 cases of mumps were reported in 2023. In the United States, there were a total of 357 cases reported in 2024.
- Since 1967 (start of U.S. national vaccination program), cases decreased by >99% due to the mumps vaccination program.
- Occasional regional epidemic outbreaks occur among individuals who have been fully vaccinated, primarily in settings with intense or frequent close contact, such as universities and correctional facilities.
- Incidence of mumps highest among those aged 1 to 4 years during 2021 to 2023 with a maximum 0.67 per 100,000 persons in 2023.

ETIOLOGY AND PATHOPHYSIOLOGY

Mumps is an RNA virus (*Rubulavirus*) of the *Paramyxovirus* genus. Mumps virus replicates in glandular epithelium of parotid gland, pancreas, and testes, and rarely kidneys, leading to interstitial edema and inflammation.

- Interstitial glandular hemorrhage may occur.
- Pressure caused by testicular edema against the tunica albuginea can lead to necrosis and loss of function.

RISK FACTORS

- Global travel: 1/3 of countries in Africa and Asia do *not* mandate mumps vaccination and continue to have pediatric epidemics (roughly every 4 years). Many areas of South and Central America do not have high mumps vaccine coverage. Travel from an area of recent epidemic should be noted.
- Crowded environments such as dormitories, barracks, or detention facilities show an increase risk of transmission.
- It is considered a human-only virus, but infectious viral particles have been found in bats.
- Immunity wanes rapidly after single-dose vaccination. With a 2-dose schedule, immunity drops from 95% to 86% after 9 years.

GENERAL PREVENTION

- Vaccination is effective and essential, especially for pediatric travelers (1) and should be considered 3 months post-cancer chemotherapy if antibody titers are low.
  - 2 doses of live attenuated mumps vaccine or mumps, measles, rubella (MMR) (or MMR with varicella [MMR-V]) vaccine recommended, first at age 12 to 15 months and second at 4 to 6 years; may start early at 6 months of age if travel is planned, but this dose does not count toward the 2-dose schedule.
  - Prevention may require 95% first dose and >80% second-dose adherence. Vaccine failure may increase 10–27% each year after vaccination.
  - Adverse effects of Jeryl-Lynn vaccine: seizure 25/100,000; fever 8/100,000; thrombocytopenic purpura 3/100,000
  - No relationship between MMR vaccine and autism, celiac disease, or multiple sclerosis; recent data show a reduced autism risk in girls after MMR vaccination (aHR 0.79, overall for both genders aHR 0.93) (2).
- Immunoglobulin (Ig) postexposure does not prevent mumps. Postexposure vaccination does not protect from recent exposure.
- Institute respiratory droplet isolation for hospitalized patients for 5 days after onset of parotitis.
- Isolate nonimmune individuals for 26 days after last case onset (social quarantine) due to incubation period as long as 25 days.
- In an epidemic situation, a third dose of MMR is indicated to decrease the attack rate (3)[A]. The boosted immunity from a third dose has been observed to last up to 3 years (4).
- The neutralizing antibodies from vaccination are still effective against variant strains of mumps virus.
- Although there are no reports of disseminated mumps from MMR vaccine in HIV patients, live vaccines (MMR) are contraindicated in immunocompromised patients (e.g., HIV with CD4 <200).

Pregnancy Considerations

Live viral vaccines are typically contraindicated in pregnancy; however, vaccination of children should not be delayed if a family member is pregnant. MMR and MMR-V given to breastfeeding mothers has not shown adverse effects in their infants.

DIAGNOSIS

HISTORY

- Up to 50% of cases are mild. Parotid swelling peaks in 1 to 3 days; lasts 3 days usually, rarely up to 7 days; if complications occur, they occur after the parotitis.
- Clinical diagnosis: swelling of one or both parotid glands 12 to 25 days after possible exposure
  - Parotid pain lasting ≥2 days
  - Meningitis without parotitis (rare; 1–10%)
- Rare prodrome of fever, neck ache, myalgias, malaise, and anorexia
- Sour foods cause pain in parotid gland region.
- Moderate fever, usually not >104°F (40°C):
  - High fever is often associated with complications.

PHYSICAL EXAM

- Painful parotid swelling (95% bilateral) obscures angle of mandible and elevates earlobe.
- Often redness at Stensen (buccal surface opposite the upper second molar) duct without pus
- Meningeal signs (15%); rare altered consciousness or seizures from encephalitis (<1%), rare bilateral optic neuritis
- Rare maculopapular, erythematous rash
- Rare sternal swelling (pathognomonic for mumps)

DIFFERENTIAL DIAGNOSIS

- If not epidemic, consider testing for influenza, parainfluenza parotitis, Epstein-Barr virus, coxsackievirus, adenovirus, parvovirus B19, influenza parotitis.
- Suppurative parotitis: often associated with *Staphylococcus aureus* (Presence of pus within Wharton duct with parotid massage essentially excludes diagnosis of mumps.)
- Recurrent allergic parotitis
- Salivary calculus with intermittent swelling (usually unilateral)
- Lymphadenitis from any cause, including HIV infection
- Cytomegalovirus parotitis (immunocompromised)
- Mikulicz syndrome: chronic, painless parotid, and lacrimal gland swelling of unknown cause that occurs in tuberculosis, sarcoidosis, lupus, leukemia, lymphosarcoma, and salivary gland tumors
- Sjögren syndrome, diabetes mellitus, uremia, malnutrition
- Drug-related parotid enlargement (iodides, guanethidine, phenothiazine)
- Mumps orchitis must be differentiated from testicular torsion and from chlamydial or bacterial orchitis.

DIAGNOSTIC TESTS & INTERPRETATION

Buccal swab and serum tests recommended: https://www.cdc.gov/mumps/lab/specimen-collect.html

- Swab of fluid from parotid duct or other affected salivary ducts after gland massage for (rRT-PCR plus viral culture)—send to state lab or CDC; most sensitive day 1 to day 3 of parotitis, especially important for vaccinated persons
- IgM titer (positive by day 5 in 100% of nonimmunized patients), rapid EIA for IgM, low sensitivity in previously immunized persons
- Rise in IgG titer samples; if not previously immunized: first, sample within 5 days of onset and second, 2 weeks later
- Urine for PCR (not as sensitive as oral specimens); may not be positive until ≥4 days after symptom onset; 50 mL in sterile container; send to state lab (or recognized public health lab).
- Other potential findings: elevated serum amylase; CSF leukocytosis, or leukopenia
- Testicular ultrasound may help differentiate mumps orchitis from testicular torsion.

Initial Tests (lab, imaging)

Buccal or oral swab PCR for mumps is recommended, especially in an epidemic setting as is an acute-phase serum specimen (mumps IgM, IgG, or RT-PCR). If not epidemic, consider testing for influenza in addition to mumps virus.

Follow-Up Tests & Special Considerations

Mumps is a reportable disease. Contact local health department.

Diagnostic Procedures/Other

If meningitis signs and symptoms present, lumbar puncture to exclude bacterial process; CSF pleocytosis, usually lymphocytic, in 65% of patients with parotitis

Test Interpretation

Periductal edema and lymphocytic infiltration of affected glands would be expected for mumps on biopsy.

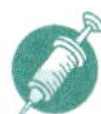

TREATMENT

- No specific antiviral therapy; supportive care (3)[A]
- Immediately place mask on patients with any suspected mumps exposures who present for evaluation, to decrease transmission.
- Analgesics to relieve pain
- Avoid corticosteroids for mumps orchitis because they can reduce testosterone and increase testicular atrophy.
- IVIG can reduce certain autoimmune-based sequelae, such as:
  - Postinfectious encephalitis; Guillain-Barré syndrome; ITP
- Interferon-α2b improves bilateral orchitis but not testicular atrophy.

GENERAL MEASURES

- Hospitalize patients with high fever, pancreatitis, or CNS signs and symptoms for supportive care, IVIG, or interferon. Mask the patient and use respiratory droplet isolation precautions.
- Orchitis
  - Ice packs to scrotum can help to relieve pain.
  - Scrotal support with adhesive bridge while recumbent and/or athletic supporter while ambulatory

MEDICATION

First Line

- Analgesics and anti-inflammatory medications (acetaminophen, nonsteroidal anti-inflammatory drugs [NSAIDs]) may diminish pain and swelling in acute orchitis and arthritis of mumps.
- May use acetaminophen for fever and/or pain
- Precautions: Avoid aspirin for pain in children (previously associated with Reye syndrome).

Second Line

Interferon-α2b for severe orchitis

COMPLEMENTARY & ALTERNATIVE MEDICINE

Medicinal herbs or acupuncture have not shown benefit in randomized controlled trials.

ADMISSION, INPATIENT, AND NURSING CONSIDERATIONS

- Hospitalize only if CNS signs and symptoms or severe complications occur.
- Use respiratory droplet precautions.
- Provide outpatient supportive care if no complications.
- Give IV fluids if severe nausea or vomiting accompanies pancreatitis.

ONGOING CARE

FOLLOW-UP RECOMMENDATIONS

Mumps orchitis:

- Bed rest and local supportive clothing (e.g., two pairs of briefs) or adhesive-tape bridge
- Withhold from school until no longer contagious (5 days after onset of parotid pain).
- Any unvaccinated school contacts should be excluded for 26 days.

Patient Monitoring

Most cases will be mild. Monitor hydration status.

DIET

Liquid diet if unable to chew

PATIENT EDUCATION

Orchitis is common in older children but rarely results in sterility, even if bilateral.

PROGNOSIS

- Complete recovery is typical; immunity is lifelong.
- Transient sensorineural hearing loss in 4% of adults; some degree of permanent unilateral hearing loss 1/1,000 children; mumps is the most common cause of pediatric hearing loss in some countries.
- Recurrence after 2 weeks may be nonmumps viral parotitis, but mumps RNA has been found in some recurrent parotitis swabs.

COMPLICATIONS

- Orchitis more common (20–30%) in postpubertal boys: Starts within 8 days of onset of parotitis; impaired fertility in 13%; absolute sterility is rare.
- Meningitis may present 5 to 10 days after first symptoms. Aseptic meningitis is typically mild, but meningoencephalitis may lead to seizures, paralysis, hydrocephalus, or death (in 2% of encephalitis cases).
- Acute cerebellar ataxia has been reported after mumps infections; self-resolving in 2 to 3 weeks
- Oophoritis in 7% of postpubertal females; no decreased fertility; mastitis has been reported in females. Pancreatitis, (usually mild), nephritis, thyroiditis, and arthralgias are rare.
- Myocarditis: usually mild but may depress ST segment; may be linked to endocardial fibroelastosis
- Deafness: 1/15,000 unilateral nerve deafness unrelated to encephalitis; may be permanent

Pediatric Considerations

- Orchitis is more common in adolescents. Young children are less likely to develop complications.
- Most complications occur in postpubertal group. Avoid aspirin use in children with viral symptoms.

Pregnancy Considerations

May increase risk of spontaneous pregnancy loss in first trimester; perinatal mumps often has a benign course.

REFERENCES

1. Bangs AC, Gastañaduy P, Neilan AM, et al. Clinical and economic impact of measles-mumps-rubella vaccinations to prevent measles importation from US pediatric travelers returning from abroad. *J Pediatric Infect Dis Soc*. 2022;11(6):257–266.
2. Hviid A, Hansen JV, Frisch M, et al. Measles, mumps, rubella vaccination and autism. *Ann Intern Med*. 2019;171(5):388.
3. Lam E, Rosen JB, Zucker JR. Mumps: an update on outbreaks, vaccine efficacy, and genomic diversity. *Clin Microbiol Rev*. 2020;33(2):e00151–e00119.
4. Kaaijk P, Wijmenga-Monsuur AJ, Ten Hulscher HI, et al. Antibody levels at 3-year follow-up of a third dose of measles-mumps-rubella vaccine in young adults. *Vaccines (Basel)*. 2022;10(1):132.

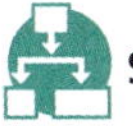

SEE ALSO

CDC Manual for the Surveillance of Vaccine-Preventable Diseases. https://www.cdc.gov/vaccines/pubs/surv manual/index.html. Accessed October 26, 2025.

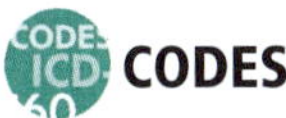

CODES

ICD10

- B26.3 Mumps pancreatitis
- B26.2 Mumps encephalitis
- B26.81 Mumps hepatitis

CLINICAL PEARLS

- Mumps is a clinical diagnosis based on swelling of ≥1 parotid glands for ≥2 days without other obvious cause. Confirm with buccal swab PCR, viral culture, and IgM and IgG serology to identify early in epidemic setting. Work with local health authorities to ensure appropriate specimen collection and report positive results to public health authorities.
- Ultrasound helps distinguish testicular torsion from testicular pain in the setting of mumps orchitis.
- A history of vaccination with MMR does not exclude mumps, especially if vaccination >9 years prior.
- The MMR vaccine is 68–95% effective after two immunizations. Immunity wanes over time.

MYALGIC ENCEPHALOMYELITIS/CHRONIC FATIGUE SYNDROME (CFS)

Allison H. Ferris, MD • Raphael Khella, DO

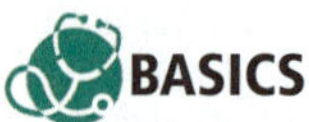

BASICS

DESCRIPTION

- A chronic and complex physical illness characterized by a new or definitive onset of debilitating fatigue that persists for >6 months with moderate to severe intensity at least half of the time, which significantly reduces a person's ability to perform activities, and can't be fully explained by an underlying medical condition.
- Key features include impaired memory or concentration, joint/muscle pain, nonrestorative sleep, postexertional malaise (PEM), and orthostatic intolerance.
- Synonyms: myalgic encephalomyelitis (ME)/chronic fatigue syndrome (CFS), chronic Epstein-Barr virus syndrome, postviral fatigue syndrome, chronic fatigue immune dysfunction, systemic exertion intolerance disease

EPIDEMIOLOGY

- Can affect all ages; incidence peaks at 10 to 19 years and 30 to 39 years.
- Females are twice as likely to be affected.

Prevalence

- Affects all racial and ethnic groups; more prevalent in minority and low socioeconomic
- Estimated at 519 to 1,038 diagnosed per 100,000; 1.7 to 3.4 million patients may have ME/CFS.
- Up to 90% of cases may stay undiagnosed (1).

ETIOLOGY AND PATHOPHYSIOLOGY

The cause is unknown and likely multifactorial.

- Suspected initiating stressors:
  - Viral, bacterial, or parasitic infection: Epstein-Barr virus, retroviruses, Lyme disease, Q fever, human herpesvirus type 6 (HHV6), enteroviruses, Ross River virus, Borna disease virus.
  - Recent vaccination; overexertion, chronic sleep deprivation; toxin exposure (e.g., organophosphate pesticides) or an atypical adverse reaction to a medication; significant physical or emotional trauma
- Hypothesized contributing factors:
  - Cellular metabolism (e.g., reduced oxidative phosphorylation and mitochondrial function in T cells); neuroendocrine system (e.g., diminished cortisol response to increased corticotropin; low catecholamines in CSF); immune system (e.g., increased proinflammatory cytokines, C-reactive protein, and β_2-microglobulin; higher ratio of naive B cells to memory B cells); muscular system (e.g., reduced oxygen uptake); autonomic system (e.g., orthostatic hypotension); serotonergic system (e.g., upregulation of serotonin receptors); gastrointestinal system (e.g., increased wall permeability, altered gut microbiota, irritable bowel syndrome [IBS] comorbidity)

Genetics

- Higher concordance in monozygotic twins
- Genetic polymorphisms in several neuroimmunoendocrine-related genes may contribute to developing disease.

RISK FACTORS

- Family history of ME or CFS
- Personality characteristics (neuroticism and introversion); comorbid depression or anxiety
- Long-standing medical and/or mental health conditions in childhood; childhood inactivity or overactivity; childhood trauma (emotional, physical, or sexual abuse)
- Prolonged idiopathic chronic fatigue

COMMONLY ASSOCIATED CONDITIONS

- Fibromyalgia
- IBS
- Gynecologic conditions (pelvic pain, endometriosis) and surgeries (hysterectomy, oophorectomy)
- Anxiety disorders and/or major depressive disorders; posttraumatic stress disorder (PTSD), including physical and/or past sexual abuse; domestic violence; attention deficit hyperactivity disorder (ADHD)
- Postural orthostatic tachycardia syndrome (POTS); sleep disorders, including obstructive sleep apnea (OSA)
- Reduced left ventricular size and mass; prolapsed mitral valve; temporomandibular joint syndrome
- Multiple chemical sensitivities; migraines, myofascial pain syndrome
- Hashimoto thyroiditis, Raynaud phenomenon; interstitial cystitis, sicca syndrome, allergies

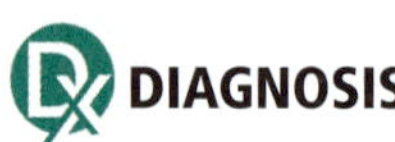

DIAGNOSIS

HISTORY

A thorough medical history and psychosocial history is required for an accurate diagnosis. Current diagnostic criteria require three symptoms and at least one of two additional manifestations:

- A substantial reduction or impairment in the ability to engage in preillness levels of activity (occupational, educational, social, or personal life) that:
  - Lasts for 6 months and is accompanied by fatigue that is often profound, of new onset (not lifelong), not the result of ongoing or unusual excessive exertion, and not substantially alleviated by rest
- PEM—worsening of symptoms after physical, mental, or emotional exertion that would not have caused a problem before the illness; often causes relapse lasting days, weeks, or longer
- Nonrestorative sleep—may not feel better even after full night of sleep despite absence of objective sleep alterations
- At least one of the following:
  - Cognitive impairment—problems with thinking, memory, executive function, and information processing, attention deficit, impaired psychomotor functions
  - Orthostatic intolerance—worsening of symptoms upon assuming and maintaining upright posture as measured by objective heart rate and blood pressure abnormalities during standing, bedside orthostatic vital signs, or head-up tilt testing

PHYSICAL EXAM

Complete physical exam (including mental status) to rule out other medical causes for symptoms. A complete mental status examination should be performed as well.

DIFFERENTIAL DIAGNOSIS

- Idiopathic chronic fatigue (i.e., fatigue of unknown cause for >6 months without meeting criteria for CFS)
- Psychiatric disorders: depression, anxiety, somatization disorder, substance abuse
- Physiologic: poor sleep hygiene, menopause, pregnancy until 3 months postpartum
- Sleep disorders: insomnia, OSA, narcolepsy
- Endocrine disorders: hypothyroidism or hyperthyroidism, primary adrenal insufficiency, hypercortisolism, diabetes mellitus, hypercalcemia
- Chronic infections: Lyme disease, chronic hepatitis B or C, fungal disease (e.g., histoplasmosis, coccidioidomycosis), parasitic disease (e.g., amebiasis, giardiasis, helminth infestation), HIV, tu.berculosis, chronic or subacute bacterial diseases (e.g., endocarditis, occult abscess), long COVID-19
- Acute infections: Epstein-Barr virus, parvovirus B19, Q fever, West Nile virus
- Iatrogenic (e.g., medication side effects), toxic agent exposure, substance abuse
- Rheumatologic diseases: systemic lupus erythematosus, rheumatoid arthritis, polymyositis, polymyalgia rheumatica
- Chronic inflammatory diseases: sarcoidosis, granulomatosis with polyangiitis, celiac disease, inflammatory bowel disease
- Neurologic disorders: multiple sclerosis, myasthenia gravis, Parkinson disease, traumatic brain injury
- Cardiovascular diseases: cardiomyopathy, pulmonary hypertension, valvular heart disease, arrhythmias
- Other: small intestinal bacterial overgrowth, obesity, malignancy

DIAGNOSTIC TESTS & INTERPRETATION

There is no validated diagnostic test. An abnormal result does not always indicate the cause of fatigue. Renew the search if the suspected problem is treated and patient remains fatigued.

Initial Tests (lab, imaging)

Standard laboratory tests are recommended to rule out other causes for symptoms:

- CBC; CMP; urinalysis; TSH and free T_4
- ESR or CRP; magnesium and phosphorus; vitamin B_{12}; serum folate; creatine kinase
- 25-hydroxy-cholecalciferol (vitamin D); serum iron, iron-binding capacity, ferritin

Follow-Up Tests & Special Considerations

- Additional laboratory studies, based on clinical features:
  - Antinuclear antibodies and rheumatoid factor, tuberculin skin test, salivary cortisol, HIV, RPR, Lyme serology, IgA tissue transglutaminase, urine drug screen

- Age/gender-appropriate cancer screening
- Electroencephalogram and/or magnetic resonance imaging if CNS symptoms
- Polysomnography and/or multiple sleep latency test if features of sleep disorder
- Assess for personality and psychosocial factors and maladaptive coping styles.

Diagnostic Procedures/Other

Potential biomarkers (e.g., HHV6 infection markers and antibodies against adrenergic and muscarinic receptors) are emerging.

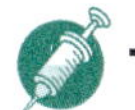

TREATMENT

- While large numbers of randomized clinical trials have not been performed, those that have suggest more positive results with nonpharmacologic treatments than pharmacologic treatments (2)[A]; most recommendations are based on expert opinion and standard symptom management (e.g., sleep disturbances, depression, and pain).
- Patients commonly use earplugs, earphones, sunglasses, and eye glasses to relieve sensitivity to light and sound (1).
- Focus on changes in lifestyle and insight with a goal to avoid complicating treatments (e.g., addictive medications, invasive testing) or interventions that support secondary gain. A multidisciplinary approach is recommended.
- Evidence surrounding cognitive-behavior therapy (CBT) and graded exercise therapy (GET) has been mixed, with some studies showing benefit and others not (1)[A],(2)[A]. Pacing has been suggested as an individualized approach to combat PEM (2)[A].

GENERAL MEASURES

Treatment involves symptom control and guided self-management. The aim is to reduce symptoms and improve quality of life. Identify the most troublesome symptoms (typically pain and insomnia) and address those first.

- Individual CBT: not curative; may improve coping strategies and/or assist in rehabilitation (e.g., social, occupational)
- GET: Track amount of exercise patient can do without exacerbating symptoms and gradually increase intensity and duration. Strike a balance between activity and rest. GET should only be performed in the presence of a trained professional to prevent illness exacerbation.
- Pacing: to mitigate the frequency, duration, and severity of PEM; individualized plans to conserve energy and manage activities

MEDICATION

- There are no established pharmacologic treatments. Medications are used primarily for specific symptoms.
- Use lowest effective dose; increase cautiously.
- Attempt to use medications that treat more than one symptom to limit polypharmacy (1)[C].
  - Studies have been conducted with antivirals, antidepressants, immunoglobulins, steroids (hydrocortisone or fludrocortisone), modafinil, staphylococcus toxoid, methylphenidate, melatonin, gabapentin and galantamine. None show clear benefit.
  - Agomelatine, an antidepressant with agonist activity at melatonin receptors, has been promising in early studies.
  - Rintatolimod, a synthetic drug with antiretroviral and immunomodulatory properties has shown promise in phase III trials.
- If insomnia is present, use of nonaddicting sleep aids (hydroxyzine, trazodone, doxepin, etc.) may improve outcomes.

ISSUES FOR REFERRAL

Psychiatrist for comorbid behavioral disorders; rehabilitative medicine; sleep or pain management specialist

COMPLEMENTARY & ALTERNATIVE MEDICINE

- Acupuncture, massage, and chiropractic have been shown to benefit some patients.
- Other helpful nonpharmacologic interventions may include physical therapy, stretches, hydrotherapy, yoga, tai chi, qigong, meditation, hot or cold packs, warm baths, electrical massagers, transcutaneous electrical nerve stimulations.
- Equivocal evidence for homeopathy and biofeedback

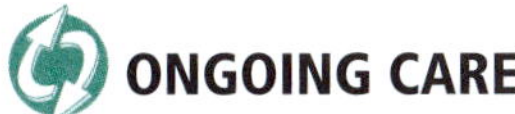

ONGOING CARE

FOLLOW-UP RECOMMENDATIONS

Patient Monitoring

No consensus exists; periodic reevaluation is appropriate for support, reevaluation, and assessment for other causes of symptoms.

DIET

No particular diet program has been shown to be effective for treatment of CFS. Unknown if weight loss is of benefit.

PATIENT EDUCATION

- Gradually increase exercise tolerance. Explain PEM and aerobic metabolism impairment for patients to not exceed their "energy envelope" (1). "Paced" activity management can help patients not exceed their energy limits (1).
- Avoid extended periods of rest, but ensure adequate rest between sessions. Relaxation techniques may also be helpful.
- Promote the benefits of cognitive therapies, lifestyle changes, and pharmacologic therapy. Educate patient's family on the condition and assist with applications for disability (1).
- The Solve ME/CFS Initiative: http://solvecfs.org/; Centers for Disease Control and Prevention, Myalgic Encephalomyelitis/Chronic Fatigue Syndrome: http://www.cdc.gov/cfs/

PROGNOSIS

- Disease severity can be classified as mild, moderate, severe, or very severe.
- A fluctuating course with relapse is common. Improvement is generally slow over months to years.
- Up to 75% of patients are unable to return to work, and 25% remain bedridden or housebound.

COMPLICATIONS

- Reduced physical activity out of fear it may worsen symptoms
- Depression
- Polypharmacy
- Unemployment: <1/3 of patients in trials return to work even if improved symptoms. The Social Security Administration considers CFS to be a disability. Receipt of third-party disability pay (secondary gain) has been associated with treatment nonresponse.
- Chronic immune activation or associated infection may increase risk for non-Hodgkin lymphoma in elderly (aged >80 years).

REFERENCES

1. Barry PW, Kelley K, Tan T, et al. NICE guideline on ME/CFS: robust advice based on athorough review of the evidence. *J Neurol Neurosurg Psychiatry*. 2024;95(7):671–674. doi:10.1136/jnnp-2023-332731.
2. Seton KA, Espejo-Oltra JA, Giménez-Orenga K, et al. Advancing research and treatment: an overview of clinical trials in myalgic encephalomyelitis/chronic fatigue syndrome (ME/CFS) and future perspectives. *J Clin Med*. 2024;13(2):325. doi:10.3390/jcm13020325.

ADDITIONAL READING

Gravelsina S, Vilmane A, Svirskis S, et al. Biomarkers in the diagnostic algorithm of myalgic encephalomyelitis/chronic fatigue syndrome. *Front Immunol*. 2022;13:928945. doi:10.3389/fimmu.2022.928945.

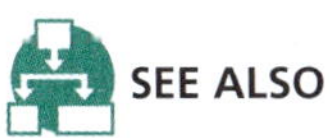

SEE ALSO

Algorithm: Fatigue

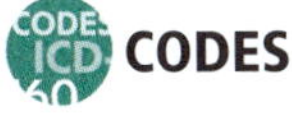

CODES

ICD10

R53.82 Chronic fatigue, unspecified

CLINICAL PEARLS

- Use established criteria for diagnosis.
- There are many more patients with idiopathic chronic fatigue than true CFS.
- No pharmacologic agents (e.g., antidepressants, immune modulators) are consistently effective for treating CFS.
- Management focuses on reducing the burden of disease and improving quality of life by managing symptoms, assessing patient needs, and providing support.

MYASTHENIA GRAVIS

Melody A. Jordahl-Iafrato, MD, MPH, FAAFP

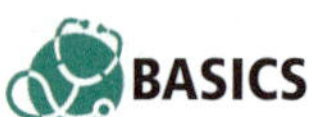

BASICS

DESCRIPTION

A disorder of neuromuscular transmission characterized by fluctuating muscle weakness:

- Ocular myasthenia gravis (MG) (15%): weakness limited to eyelids and extraocular muscles
- Generalized MG (85%): commonly affects ocular as well as a variable combination of bulbar, proximal limb, and respiratory muscles
- 50% of patients who present with ocular symptoms develop generalized MG within 2 years.
- Onset may be sudden and severe, but it is typically mild and intermittent over many years, maximum severity reached within 3 years for 85%.
- System(s) affected: neurologic, hematologic, lymphatic, immunologic, musculoskeletal

EPIDEMIOLOGY

Occurs at any age but a bimodal distribution to the age of onset:

- Female: 20 to 40 years
- Male: 60 to 80 years

Prevalence

In the United States, 70 to 320/1 million; increasing over the past 5 decades

Pediatric Considerations

A transient form of neonatal MG seen in 10–20% of infants born to mothers with MG. It occurs as a result of the transplacental passage of maternal antibodies that interfere with function of the neuromuscular junction; resolves in weeks to months; autoimmune juvenile MG makes up 10–15% of cases of MG in North America.

ETIOLOGY AND PATHOPHYSIOLOGY

An autoimmune disorder resulting in the reduction in the function of acetylcholine receptors (AChRs) at muscle end plates, resulting in insufficient neuromuscular transmission

- Seropositive/antiacetylcholine receptor (anti-AChR): a humoral, antibody-mediated, T-cell–dependent attack of the AChRs or receptor-associated proteins at the postsynaptic membrane of the neuromuscular junction; found in 85% of generalized MG and 50% of ocular MG; thymic abnormalities common (1)
- Muscle-specific kinase (MuSKs): 5% of generalized MG patients; typically females; is a severe form, respiratory and bulbar muscles involved; thymic abnormalities are rare (1).
- In remainder of seronegative, 12–50% with anti-LRP4, a molecule that forms a complex with MuSK, mild generalized weakness most common (1)
- Seronegative MG (SNMG): 5%; may have anti-AChR detectable by cell-based assay; clinically similar to anti-AChR; thymic hyperplasia may be present (1).
- Also documented immediately after viral infections (measles, Epstein-Barr virus [EBV], HIV, and human T-lymphotropic virus [HTLV])

Genetics

Familial predisposition is seen in 5% of cases.

RISK FACTORS

- Familial MG
- D-penicillamine (drug-induced MG)
- Other autoimmune diseases

COMMONLY ASSOCIATED CONDITIONS

- Thymic hyperplasia (60–70%)
- Thymoma (10–15%)
- Autoimmune thyroid disease (3–8%)

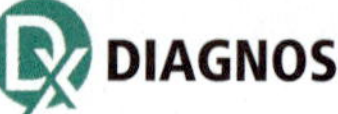

DIAGNOSIS

Myasthenia Gravis Foundation of America Clinical Classification:

- Class I: any eye muscle weakness, possible ptosis, no other evidence of muscle weakness elsewhere
- Class II: eye muscle weakness of any severity; mild weakness of other muscles:
  - Class IIa: predominantly limb or axial muscles
  - Class IIb: predominantly bulbar and/or respiratory muscles
- Class III: eye muscle weakness of any severity; moderate weakness of other muscles:
  - Class IIIa: predominantly limb or axial muscles
  - Class IIIb: predominantly bulbar and/or respiratory muscles
- Class IV: eye muscle weakness of any severity; severe weakness of other muscles:
  - Class IVa: predominantly limb or axial muscles
  - Class IVb: predominantly bulbar and/or respiratory muscles (can also include feeding tube without intubation)
- Class V: intubation needed to maintain airway

HISTORY

The hallmark of MG is fatigability.

- Fluctuating weakness, often subtle, that worsens during the day and after prolonged use of affected muscles; may improve with rest
- Early symptoms are transient with asymptomatic periods lasting days or weeks.
- With progression, asymptomatic periods shorten, and symptoms fluctuate from mild to severe.
- >50% of patients present with ocular symptoms (ptosis and/or diplopia). Eventually, 90% of patients with MG develop ocular symptoms.
- Ptosis might be unilateral, bilateral, or shifting from eye to eye.
- 15% present with bulbar symptoms.
- <5% present with proximal limb weakness alone.

ALERT

Myasthenic crisis: respiratory muscle weakness producing respiratory insufficiency and pending respiratory failure

PHYSICAL EXAM

- Ptosis may worsen with propping of opposite eyelid (curtain sign) or sustained upward gaze.
- "Myasthenic sneer," in which the midlip rises but corners of mouth do not move
- Muscle weakness is usually proximal and symmetric.
- Test for muscle fatigability by repetitive or prolonged use of individual muscles.
- Important to test and monitor respiratory function

DIFFERENTIAL DIAGNOSIS

- Thyroid ophthalmopathy
- Oculopharyngeal muscular dystrophy
- Myotonic dystrophy
- Brainstem and motor cranial nerve lesions
- Botulism
- Motor neuron disease (e.g., amyotrophic lateral sclerosis [ALS])
- Dermatomyositis/polymyositis

DIAGNOSTIC TESTS & INTERPRETATION

Initial Tests (lab, imaging)

- Anti-AChR antibody (74–85% are seropositive):
  - Generalized myasthenia: 75–85%
  - Ocular myasthenia: 50%
  - MG and thymoma: 98–100%
  - Poor correlation between antibody titer and disease severity (1)[C]
  - False-positive results in thymoma without MG, Lambert-Eaton myasthenic syndrome, small cell lung cancer, and rheumatoid arthritis treated with penicillamine
- Anti-MuSK antibody:
  - Used if MG is suspected and patient seronegative for AChR antibodies
  - Strong correlation between titer and disease severity (1)[C]
- LRP4 and clustered anti-AChR:
  - Used if MG suspected and the patient is seronegative for AChR antibodies
- Thyroid and other autoimmune testing anti-striated muscle (anti-SM) antibody:
  - Present in 84% of patients with thymoma who are <40 years of age
  - Can be present without thymoma in patients >40 years of age
- Chest radiographs or CT scans may identify a thymoma.
- MRI of brain and orbits to rule out other causes of cranial nerve deficit

Diagnostic Procedures/Other

- Tensilon (edrophonium) test:
  - Rarely done as edrophonium is no longer available in the United States and many other countries
  - A positive test shows improvement of strength within 30 seconds of administration.
  - Sensitivity 80–90% (2)[C]
  - Cardiac disease and bronchial asthma are relative contraindications, especially in elderly.
  - Atropine: 0.4 to 0.6 mg IV may rarely be required as antidote; must be available
- Ice pack test:
  - Ice pack applied to closed eyelid for 60 seconds, then removed; extent of ptosis immediately assessed
  - Ice will decrease the ptosis induced by MG.
  - Sensitivity 80% in patients with prominent ptosis
- Electrophysiology testing:
  - Repetitive nerve stimulation (RNS):
    - Widely available, most frequently used
    - Sensitivity generalized MG 76%; ocular MG 50% (2)[C]
  - Single-fiber electromyogram (SFEMG):
    - Assesses temporal variability between two muscle fibers within same motor unit (jitter)
    - Sensitivity 99%
    - Technically difficult to perform; limited availability, use if suspected and negative RNS (2)[C]

Test Interpretation
- Lymphofollicular hyperplasia of thymic medulla occurs in 65% of patients with MG, thymoma in 15%.
- Immunofluorescence: IgG antibodies and complement on receptor membranes in seropositive patients

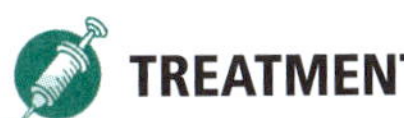

TREATMENT

GENERAL MEASURES
Three basic approaches: symptomatic, immunosuppressive, and supportive. Most should receive symptomatic treatment along with immunosuppressive and/or supportive modalities.

MEDICATION
First Line
Symptomatic treatments (anticholinesterase agents)
- Pyridostigmine bromide (Mestinon):
  - *Most commonly prescribed because available in oral tablet*
  - Starting dose of 60 mg PO TID with food
  - Maximum dose: 120 mg q3–4h
  - Long acting is available, but effect is not consistent.
  - Side effects are common, which can result in dose reduction or slower titration of dose: gastrointestinal disturbances, hypotension, syncope, urinary frequency (3).
- Neostigmine methylsulfate (Prostigmin):
  - Starting dose of 0.5 mg SC or IM q3h
  - Titrate dosage to clinical need.
  - Useful for patients who cannot absorb medications orally
  - May cause excessive salivary secretions, which may exacerbate swallowing difficulties (3)
- Patients with anti-MuSK may not respond well to these medications.

Second Line
- Immunosuppressants: Oral corticosteroids are the first choice of drugs when immunosuppression is necessary.
  - Prednisone:
    - May exacerbate symptoms short-term in up to 50% of patients
    - If inpatient and on other acute treatment, start with 60 mg/day PO.
    - If outpatient, start at lower dose (10 to 20 mg/day PO).
    - Titrate dose by 5 mg every 3 to 7 days to attain lowest effective dose (4)[B].
    - Use caution regarding long-term side effects from corticosteroids, including but not limited to weight gain, fluid retention, gastritis, ulcer formation, hyperglycemia, risk of infection, and osteoporosis.
- Azathioprine: 100 to 200 mg/day PO (4)[B]
  - *Most frequently used for long-term immunomodulation*, similar efficacy to steroids and IVIG
  - Consider screening for thiopurine S-methyltransferase (TPMT) levels prior to initiation of azathioprine.
  - Benefit may not be apparent for up to 18 months after initiation of therapy.
  - Prednisolone + azathioprine may be effective when used as a corticosteroid-sparing agent.
- Mycophenolate: 1 g PO or IV BID
- Cyclosporine: dosing varies; may give IV or PO (Use caution due to nephrotoxicity and drug interactions.)
- Acute immunomodulating treatments:
  - Plasmapheresis: bulk removal of 2 to 3 L of plasma 3 times per week, repeated until rate of improvement plateaus
    - Improves weakness in nearly all patients and can last up to 3 months
  - Immunoglobulin: 2 g/kg IV over 2 to 5 days (4)[B]
  - *Plasmapheresis and immunoglobulin have comparable efficacy in treating moderate to severe MG.*
  - Rapid onset of effect but short duration of action
  - Used for acute worsening of MG to improve strength prior to surgery, prevent acute exacerbations induced by corticosteroids, and as a chronic intermittent treatment to provide relief in refractory MG
- Other immunosuppressant therapies, typically used in refractory cases:
  - Eculizumab
  - Efgartigimod alfa: only for use in AChR antibody positive MG
  - Ravulizumab
  - Rituximab:
    - Seronegative MuSK-antibody positive MG patients may have better response to rituximab than conventional therapies.
  - Tacrolimus
  - Cyclophosphamide

ALERT
Use caution with drugs that can precipitate weakness: aminoglycosides, fluoroquinolones, β-blockers, calcium channel blockers, neuromuscular blockers, statins, diuretics, oral contraceptives, gabapentin, phenytoin, lithium, among others.

SURGERY/OTHER PROCEDURES
Pediatric Considerations
- Infants with severe weakness from transient neonatal myasthenia may be treated with oral pyridostigmine; general support is necessary until the condition clears.
- Corticosteroids limited only to severe disease

ADMISSION, INPATIENT, AND NURSING CONSIDERATIONS
- Management of pulmonary infections
- Myasthenic/cholinergic crises
- Plasmapheresis
- IV γ-globulin

ONGOING CARE

PATIENT EDUCATION
Myasthenia Gravis Foundation of America (MGFA): https://myasthenia.org/

PROGNOSIS
- Overall good but highly variable
- Myasthenic crisis associated with substantial morbidity and 4% mortality
- Seronegative patients are more likely to have purely ocular disease, and those with generalized SNMG have a better outcome after treatment.

COMPLICATIONS
Acute respiratory arrest; chronic respiratory insufficiency

REFERENCES

1. Berrih-Aknin S, Frenkian-Cuvelier M, Eymard B. Diagnostic and clinical classification of autoimmune myasthenia gravis. *J Autoimmun*. 2014;48–49:143–148.
2. Pasnoor M, Dimachkie MM, Farmakidis C, et al. Diagnosis of myasthenia gravis. *Neurol Clin*. 2018;36(2):261–274.
3. Farrugia ME, Goodfellow JA. A practice approach to managing patients with myasthenia gravis—opinions and a review of the literature. *Front Neurol*. 2020;11:604.
4. Gotterer L, Li Y. Maintenance immunosuppression in myasthenia gravis. *J Neurol Sci*. 2016;369:294–302.

ADDITIONAL READING

Menon D, Barnett C, Bril V. Novel treatments in myasthenia gravis. *Front Neurol*. 2020;11:538.

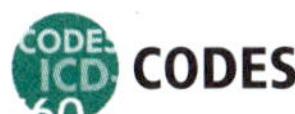

CODES

ICD10
- G70.01 Myasthenia gravis with (acute) exacerbation
- G70.00 Myasthenia gravis without (acute) exacerbation
- G70.0 Myasthenia gravis

CLINICAL PEARLS
- An autoimmune disease, marked by abnormal fatigability and weakness of selected muscles, which is relieved by rest
- >50% of patients present with ocular symptoms (ptosis and/or diplopia).
- Anticholinesterase medication and a thymectomy lessen symptom severity.
- Steroid therapy, plasma exchange, or immunoglobulin can be used in severely affected patients.

MYELODYSPLASTIC SYNDROMES (MDS)

Tara Baney, MS, CRNP • Allison Holmes, DO

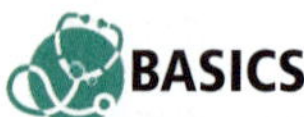

BASICS

DESCRIPTION

- Myelodysplastic syndromes (MDS) are a heterogeneous group of clonal stem cell disorders characterized by dysplastic cells and peripheral blood cytopenias: anemia, thrombocytopenia, and/or neutropenia.
- Dysplasia refers to an abnormality of development or differentiation in specific cell lines within the bone marrow. MDS has similar pathologic/cellular characteristics with acute myelogenous leukemia. MDS has a lower percentage of blast (<20%) in the peripheral blood and bone marrow. MDS has the ability to transform into AML as a premalignant condition.

EPIDEMIOLOGY

Incidence

- The incidence in the United States is approximately 4.5 cases per 100,000 population and increases with age (majority >80 years).
- The incidence rate between 70 and 79 years of age increases to 26.9 per 100,000 people.
- The incidence rate for those >80 years of age is 55.4 per 100,000 people.
- Median age is 77 years old which complicates the treatment/management.

ETIOLOGY AND PATHOPHYSIOLOGY

- MDS arises from mutations in hematopoietic stem cell lines due to various genetic/chromosomal abnormalities. Mutations are due to genetic abnormalities/damage to hematopoietic cells. Bone marrow is replaced with mutated cells which crowd out the normal cells and cause cytopenias of one or more cell lines.
- 80% of cases have no know cause or exposure.
- Environmental exposures: benzenes
- Chemotherapy and/or radiation therapy have been known to cause MDS which is classified as iatrogenic/secondary MDS. MDS can occur up to 10 years after treatment.
- De novo MDS or primary MDS may occur due to somatic mutations.
- Two classification systems of MDS exist.
  - World Health Organization (WHO) 2022
  - International Consensus Classification (ICC) 2022 includes cytogenetics/karyotype abnormalities, degree of dysplasia and percentage of blast; recent changes: MDS/AML 10–19% blast, MDS with multiple hit PT53 mutations and MDS due to cytotoxic agents (1)

Genetics

- Cytogenetic anomalies are observed in >90% of MDS patients which include translocations or aneuploidy (loss or gain of a chromosome).
- Deletion of the long arm of chromosome 5 (5q) is the most common abnormal karyotype due to either treatment-related MDS with 5q deletion, associated with chemotherapeutic agents versus de novo isolated 5q deletion. Patients with 5q deletion due to exposure to chemotherapeutic agents usually have other cytogenetic abnormalities and/or TP53 mutations. These tend to have a poorer prognosis. Isolated 5q deletion without other cytogenetic anomalies generally have better prognosis. Other cytogenetic anomalies commonly studied include normal karyotype, deletion 7q (-7), trisomy 8, and -Y (1).

RISK FACTORS

- Age: increased risk in patients >60 years old
- Tobacco use
- Chronic exposure to chemicals: benzene, pesticides, insecticides, and petroleum
- Prior chemotherapy or radiation therapy
- Inherited disorders: Fanconi anemia, Shwachman-Diamond syndromes, severe congenital neutropenia, and familial platelet disorder
- Autoimmune disorders such as vasculitis, connective tissue disease, and inflammatory arthritis
- End-stage renal disease on dialysis

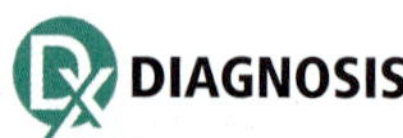

DIAGNOSIS

HISTORY

- The clinical course of MDS patients is driven by the type and degree of cytopenias.
- Recurrent infections, bleeding issues, fatigue, weight loss, and exertional dyspnea
- Fatigue is the most common symptom and tends to be out of proportion to anemia.
- Fevers, night sweats, and weight loss are not common.
- Evaluate for toxin exposure, including alcohol or previous chemotherapy.

PHYSICAL EXAM

- Generalized pallor, fatigue, petechiae, and ecchymosis as result of the anemia and thrombocytopenia
- Hepatosplenomegaly, although rare, as consequence of extramedullary hemopoiesis is present, especially in MDS/MPN overlapping syndromes.
- Lymphadenopathies are not common.

DIFFERENTIAL DIAGNOSIS

- Acute leukemia: AML or AMML
- Vitamin B_{12} and folate deficiencies
- HIV
- Chronic liver disease
- Excessive alcohol use
- Infections of the bone marrow human immunodeficiency virus, tuberculosis, atypical mycobacterium, and Epstein-Barr virus
- Other hematopoietic disorders that do not fulfill diagnostic criteria for MDS such as idiopathic cytopenia of unknown significance, idiopathic dysplasia of unknown significance, clonal hematopoiesis of indeterminate potential (CHIP), and clonal cytopenia of unknown significance

DIAGNOSTIC TESTS & INTERPRETATION

Initial Tests (lab, imaging)

A complete blood count with peripheral smear, peripheral flow cytometry, chemistry, viral studies (HIV and hepatitis panel), erythropoietin levels, and vitamin levels (B_{12} and folate) should be evaluated.

Diagnostic Procedures/Other

- *Histopathology*. A bone marrow evaluation MDS versus AML and to perform karyotype studies, fluorescent in situ hybridization (FISH), and mutational studies.
  - Blast %: <20% is consistent with MDS; ≥20% is diagnostic of AML.
- *Cytogenetics*. Clonal chromosome abnormalities are observed in 30–80% of MDS patients. In the rest of the patients (20–70%), submicroscopic alterations (microdeletions, point mutations) provide diagnostic evidence.

Test Interpretation

- Hematologic findings in the blood smear include macrocytic anemia with possible basophilic stippling, hyposegmented neutrophils (pseudo Pelger-Huet), and thrombocytopenia.
- A low reticulocyte index reflects the hypoproliferative nature of the disease.

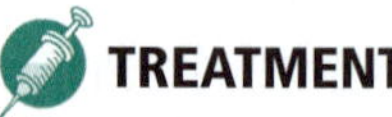

TREATMENT

GENERAL MEASURES

- Treatment is based on severity of symptoms and cytopenias, MDS classification, patient factors, and prognostic category (2).
- Patient factors that contribute to the patient's ability to tolerate treatments and selection of overall management
  - Patient age
  - Performance status
  - Comorbidities

- IPSS-M or IPSS-R scoring system should be used to guide treatment.
  - Lower risk MDS—Treatment is based on severity of cytopenias and symptoms.
  - Asymptomatic—monitoring rather than immediate treatment
  - Symptomatic patients
- Anemia—symptoms related to anemia (e.g., dyspnea, fatigue, weakness) and hemoglobin (Hb) <10 g/dL
- Thrombocytopenia—platelets <20,000/μL or excessive bleeding or bruising with platelets <50,000/μL
- Neutropenia—recurrent and/or severe infections with absolute neutrophil count (ANC) <500 neutrophils/μL or ANC <1,000 neutrophils/μL with recurrent infections

MEDICATION

First Line

- IPSS-R low, intermediate-risk disease
  - MDS-related anemia (5q del)
    - Blood transfusions and erythropoiesis-stimulating agents (ESA) (2)
    - ESA have a 30–60% response rate in LR-MDS; indications: Hb <10 g/dL and erythropoietin level <500; uncommon complications: worsening hypertension and thromboembolism
    - Need to be mindful of transfusions of packed red blood cells (PRBCs) as can cause iron overload.
    - Epoetin alfa or darbepoetin serum epo level <500 mU/ml
    - Lenalidomide; used in anemia in MDS with isolated del (5q); decreased need for transfusions (2)
    - If no response to ESA or luspatercept, can use Imetelstat
    - If mIDH1 mutation can use ivosidenib or olutasidenib if no response with other options.
- MDS-related anemia SF3B1 no 5q del
- Luspatercept or imetelstat (ineligible for ESA)
- MDS-related thrombocytopenia and neutropenia IPSS-R low, intermediate risk disease (2)
  - Thrombopoietin receptor agonists (romiplostim, eltrombopag) (close monitoring for leukemic transformation)
  - Neutropenia may be managed with G-CSF/antibiotics.
    - Azacitidine, decitabine, or oral decitabine + cedazuridine (2)

Second Line

- MDS-related anemia IPSS-R, low, intermediate-risk disease
- If no response to hypomethylating agent (HMA) or disease progression can consider ivosidenib or olutasidenib (if mIDH1 mutation).
- Thrombocytopenia or neutropenia IPSS-R, low, intermediate risk disease
  - Lack of response to supportive therapy, can use HMAs if have not been used
  - If no response to HMA or disease progression, can consider ivosidenib or olutasidenib (if mIDH1 mutation)
- High-intensity chemotherapy with stem cell transplant IPSS-R intermediate-, high-, very high-risk disease
  - Allogenic SCT only curative treatment option but reserved for high-risk disease or disease nonresponsive to other treatments in medically appropriate; rarely used (2)
    - Combination therapy
      - Azacitidine + ivosidenib or olutasidenib (if mIDH1) followed by allo-HCT
      - Azacitidine + venetoclax
      - Decitabine + venetoclax
      - Oral decitabine + cedazuridine + venetoclax

ADDITIONAL THERAPIES

- *Management of iron overload*. Iron chelation is often considered in patient with transfusion dependency.
- Iron levels, ferritin, and organ damage (heart, liver and pancreas) should be monitored.
- Iron chelators such as deferoxamine and deferasirox can be used; should be avoided in patients with EGFR <40 mL/min

ADMISSION, INPATIENT, AND NURSING CONSIDERATIONS

Complications such as bleeding, neutropenic fever, and undergoing SCT warrant a hospital admission.

ONGOING CARE

FOLLOW-UP RECOMMENDATIONS

Patient Monitoring

- Complete blood count to monitor cytopenias
- Repeat bone marrow examination for worsening cytopenias or evaluate response to therapy.
- Temperature and other vital signs to assess for signs of infection, bleeding, and anemia.
- Quality of life assessment

DIET

Alcohol consumption, meat, vegetable, and fruit intake do not appear to have significant influence in the risk of developing disease.

PATIENT EDUCATION

- Regular follow-up and compliance with medications; smoking cessation
- Instruct about symptoms that should prompt the patient to seek out medical care for treatment of infection, bleeding, and/or anemia.

PROGNOSIS

Overall, the outcome of MDS patients is variable, with medial survival ranging from 6 months to >5 years depending on classification and or management.

COMPLICATIONS

- Infection and bleeding are the leading causes of death, rather than AML conversion.
- Increased risk of cardiovascular disease either secondary to iron overload or chronic anemia
- Possibility of hepatic dysfunction from iron overload

REFERENCES

1. Arber DA, Orazi A, Hasserjian RP, et al. International Consensus Classification of Myeloid Neoplasms and Acute Leukemias: integrating morphologic, clinical, and genomic data. *Blood*. 2022;140(11):1200–1228.
2. Garcia-Manero G, Chien KS, Montalban-Bravo G. Myelodysplastic syndromes: 2021 update on diagnosis, risk stratification and management. *Am J Hematol*. 2020;95(11):1399–1420.

ADDITIONAL READING

Norman M, Yamartino K, Gerstein R, et al. A review of the isocitrate dehydrogenase inhibitors in management of adult patients with AML and MDS. *Expert Rev Hematol*. 2024;17(11):755–767. doi:10.1080/17474086.2024.2422554.

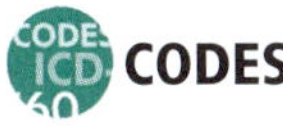

CODES

ICD10

- D46.9 Myelodysplastic syndrome, unspecified
- D46.4 Refractory anemia, unspecified
- D46.B Refract cytopenia w multilin dysplasia and ring sideroblasts

CLINICAL PEARLS

- MDS are a heterogeneous group of clonal stem cell disorders characterized by blood cytopenias and tendency for leukemic transformation.
- Different molecular and genetic mechanisms of pathogenesis translate into the same phenotypic manifestation of the disease.
- Infection and bleeding are the leading causes of death.
- Allogeneic stem cell transplant is ultimately the only curative treatment.

MYELOPROLIFERATIVE NEOPLASMS

Ronak S. Patel, DO • Daniel Michniuk, MS, DO

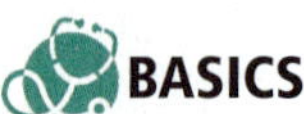

BASICS

DESCRIPTION

Myeloproliferative neoplasms (MPNs) are a group of clonal disorders that all originate in the pluripotent hematopoietic stem cell. This topic focuses on chronic myelogenous leukemia (CML), polycythemia vera (PV), essential thrombocythemia (ET), and primary myelofibrosis (PMF).

- The 2016 World Health Organization (WHO) MPN classification also includes chronic neutrophilic leukemia (CNL), chronic eosinophilic leukemia-not otherwise specified (CEL-NOS), and MPN-unclassifiable, all rarer.
- CML is characterized by uninhibited proliferation of myeloid precursor cells.
- PV is characterized by erythrocytosis.
- ET is characterized by thrombocytosis.
- PMF is characterized by bone marrow fibrosis and extramedullary hematopoiesis.
  - As MPNs share common origins, they often share common features, and they can transform into one another.

EPIDEMIOLOGY

The median age of diagnosis is >60 years.

Incidence

- CML: 1.4 to 2.4/100,000/year
- PV: 0.4 to 2.8/100,000/year
- ET: 1.0 to 2.5/100,000/year
- PMF: 0.8 to 2.1/100,000/year

ETIOLOGY AND PATHOPHYSIOLOGY

Genetic mutations activating hematopoiesis result in proliferation of cells of myeloid, erythroid, and/or megakaryocyte lineages.

Genetics

- CML is characterized by a 9:22 translocation (the Philadelphia chromosome) resulting in the oncogenic BCR-ABL1 fusion gene producing the constitutively active tyrosine kinase leading to cell proliferation, particularly of granulocytes.
- PV, ET, and PMF share "driver" mutations, most often of Janus kinase 2 (JAK2), myeloproliferative leukemia protein (MPL), and calreticulin (CALR) genes, that activate hematopoiesis. Mutation in one of these three genes is found in >90% of BCR-ABL negative MPNs.
  - JAK2 mutations: JAK2 specifically regulates hematopoiesis via erythropoietin (EPO), GM-CSF, thrombopoietin, growth hormone, leptin, IL-3 and IL-5 signaling (1). Mutations constitutively activating the JAK2 protein lead to cell proliferation and prolonged survival.
    - JAK2 V617F mutations: 95% of PV, 55% of ET, and 65% of PMF cases (1)
    - JAK2 exon 12 mutations: 4% of PV cases (1)
  - MPL gene mutations: The MPL gene encodes the thrombopoietin receptor, which regulates hematopoietic stem cells, especially megakaryocytes; mutations can cause cell overproduction.
    - MPL mutations: 3% of ET, 5% of PMF (1)
  - CALR gene mutations: specific frameshift mutations of CALR, which encodes calreticulin protein, lead to activated hematopoiesis, particularly of the megakaryocyte lineage. The mechanism may be via constitutive activation of the thrombopoietin receptor (1).
    - CALR mutations: 25% of ET, PMF cases (1)

RISK FACTORS

- Age ≥50 years
- Exposure to high levels of radiation from radiation therapy, as well as to chemicals like benzene or toluene, or cytotoxic agents such as chemotherapy
- Family history of MPNs
- History of blood clots

COMMONLY ASSOCIATED CONDITIONS

- Thrombotic events (e.g., CVA, TIA, DVT, portal vein thrombosis)
- Major and minor hemorrhagic events (e.g., acquired von Willebrand disease)
- Anemia
- Bone marrow fibrosis
- Osteosclerosis
- Extramedullary hematopoiesis
- Blast transformation into acute leukemia

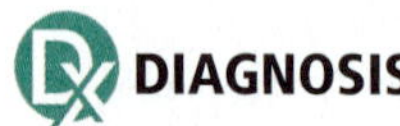

DIAGNOSIS

HISTORY

Constitutional symptoms are common, although a significant minority are asymptomatic.

- Any MPN may have these symptoms:
  - Constitutional: fatigue, weakness, night sweats, fevers, weight loss
  - Gastrointestinal: abdominal fullness, discomfort, or pain; early satiety
  - Musculoskeletal: bone pain
  - Neurologic: headaches, dizziness, trouble concentrating, transient visual disturbances
  - Psychiatric: depression, sexual dysfunction, insomnia
- Symptoms more common with certain MPNs:
  - CML: excess sweating, gout
  - PV: aquagenic pruritus, erythromelalgia, facial plethora, gout, tinnitus
  - PMF: abdominal fullness or pain, early satiety, gastrointestinal bleeding, weight loss, arthralgias, bone pain
  - ET: light-headedness, transient visual disturbance, atypical chest pain, erythromelalgia, livedo reticularis, pregnancy loss

PHYSICAL EXAM

- Any MPN may present with pallor, splenomegaly, hepatomegaly.
- Signs more common with certain MPNs:
  - CML: gouty tophi
  - PV: gouty tophi, increased blood pressure, conjunctival injection, facial plethora
  - ET: petechiae, livedo reticularis
  - PMF: petechiae, lymphadenopathy, marked splenomegaly

DIFFERENTIAL DIAGNOSIS

Generally, when one MPN is suspected, every MPN may be considered a possibility.

- CML: leukemoid reaction, other leukemias
- PV: secondary polycythemia, EPO receptor activating mutations
- ET: reactive thrombocytosis, myelodysplastic syndrome, thrombopoietin gene mutations
- PMF: secondary myelofibrosis, multiple myeloma, lymphoma, autoimmune disorders

DIAGNOSTIC TESTS & INTERPRETATION

Initial Tests (lab, imaging)

- Complete blood count
- Peripheral smear
- Renal and liver function, electrolytes
- Lactate dehydrogenase (LDH), uric acid

Follow-Up Tests & Special Considerations

- Testing for BCR-ABL (Philadelphia chromosome)
  - Karyotype to detect the 9;22 translocation
  - Detecting the BCR-ABL1 fusion gene via peripheral blood fluorescence in situ hybridization (FISH) or reverse transcription polymerase chain reaction (RT-PCR)
- Testing for JAK2, MPL, CALR gene mutants
- Bone marrow biopsy (BMBx) and aspiration
- Depending on the clinical scenario, consider:
  - EPO level, for detecting secondary causes of polycythemia
  - Iron studies (ferritin, transferrin, iron level)
  - von Willebrand factor, for detecting acquired von Willebrand disease, and assessing for increased bleeding risk

Test Interpretation

- CML
  - Leukocytosis, granulocytosis (neutrophil predominant), and mature and immature forms in peripheral smear
  - The Philadelphia chromosome/BCR-ABL1 fusion gene establishes the diagnosis.
  - Chronic CML can progress to an accelerated phase or a blast crisis phase.
    - CML accelerated phase—there are eight hematologic/cytogenetic criteria in the WHO guidelines.
    - CML blast phase—WHO criteria
      - 20% or more blasts in PB or BM, *or*
      - Infiltrative proliferation of blasts at an extramedullary site
- PV—WHO criteria
  - Either all three major criteria or the first two major criteria and the minor criterion
    - Major criteria
- Hemoglobin >16.5 g/dL in men >16 g/dL in woman; or hematocrit >49%/48%; or increased red cell mass (RCM)
- BMBx showing hypercellularity for age with trilineage growth including prominent erythroid, granulocytic, and megakaryocytic proliferation with pleomorphic, mature megakaryocytes
- Presence of JAK2V617F or JAK2 SH2
- Minor criterion: subnormal serum EPO level
- ET—WHO criteria
  - Either all four major criteria or the first three major criteria and the minor criterion
    - Major criteria

- Platelet count ≥450 × 10^9/L
- BMBx showing proliferation mainly of the megakaryocyte lineage with increased numbers of enlarged, mature megakaryocytes with hyperlobulated nuclei; no significant increase or left shift in neutrophil granulopoiesis or erythropoiesis and very rarely minor (grade 1) increase in reticulin fibers
- Not meeting WHO criteria for BCR-ABL1+ CML, PV, PMF, myelodysplastic syndromes, or other myeloid neoplasms
- Presence of JAK2, CALR, or MPL mutation
- Minor criterion: presence of a clonal marker or absence of evidence for reactive thrombocytosis
- PMF
  - PMF has been subdivided into prefibrotic/early stage and overt fibrotic stage
  - Overt PMF—WHO criteria
    - Diagnosis requires all three major criteria and at least one minor criterion.
    - Major criteria
    - Presence of megakaryocytic proliferation and atypia, accompanied by either reticulin and/or collagen fibrosis grades 2 and 3
    - Not meeting WHO criteria for ET, PV, BCR-ABL1+ CML, MPNs, or other myeloid neoplasms
    - Presence of JAK2, CALR, or MPL mutation or in the absence of these mutations, presence of another clonal marker, or absence of reactive myelofibrosis
  - Minor criteria: presence of at least one of the following, confirmed in two consecutive determinations
    - Leukoerythroblastosis
    - LDH above upper limit of normal
    - Palpable splenomegaly
    - Leukocytosis ≥11 × 10^9/L
    - Anemia not attributed to other condition

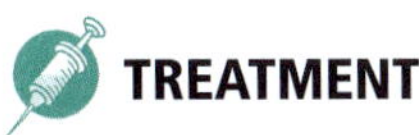

TREATMENT

GENERAL MEASURES

- PV: Phlebotomy is first line; goal hematocrit <45% in men and <42% in women (1)[A]. Achieving goal hematocrit decreases mortality from cardiovascular or thrombotic events 4-fold (1).
- PMF: transfusions for symptomatic anemia or thrombocytopenia
- Address hypertension, hyperlipidemia, diabetes, smoking, etc.

MEDICATION

- CML
  - First-line medications
    - Tyrosine kinase inhibitors (TKIs) for all patients with CML, regardless of which phase
    - The first-generation TKI (1GTKI) is imatinib; second-generation TKIs (2GTKI) include nilotinib, dasatinib, bosutinib; third-generation TKI (3GTKI) is ponatinib.
      - Low-risk chronic phase: 1GTKI or 2GTKI recommended
      - High-risk chronic phase: 2GTKI preferred
      - Accelerated phase: 2GTKI or 3GTKI are preferred; stem cell transplant (SCT) or chemotherapy may be considered.
      - Blast phase: TKIs often in combination with chemotherapy while awaiting SCT
- PV
  - First-line medications
    - Aspirin (81 to 100 mg); prevention of thrombotic complications (e.g., ocular migraine, transient ischemic attacks, and erythromelalgia) (1)[A]
    - High-risk PV patients (older age or history of thrombosis) or who don't tolerate phlebotomy: cytoreduction with hydroxyurea or interferon-α (1)[C]
  - Second-line medications
    - For high-risk patients with inadequate response to cytoreductive medication, consider JAK2 inhibitor ruxolitinib (1)[C].
- ET
  - First-line medications
    - Aspirin (81 to 100 mg) with prior history of thrombosis, JAK2 mutation, microvascular complications, or vasomotor symptoms (1)[C].
    - Cytoreduction in hydroxyurea is indicated for high-risk ET patients (thrombosis, or age >60 + JAK2 mutation), or patients with progressive thrombocytosis, acquired von Willebrand syndrome, significant bleeding, or splenomegaly (1)[C]
  - Second-line medications
    - Interferon-α or anagrelide (1)[C].
    - For symptoms not controlled with aspirin alone, cytoreduction with hydroxyurea can be considered.
- PMF
  - First-line medications
    - If SCT is not planned, and platelets ≥50 × 10^9/L, consider the JAK2 inhibitor ruxolitinib (1)[A].
  - Second-line medication therapy
    - Low-risk patients with bothersome symptoms may consider ruxolitinib, hydroxyurea, or interferon-α (1)[C].
    - Patients with disease progression on ruxolitinib may be considered for a newer JAK2 inhibitor (1)[C].
    - Patients with anemia who are not adequately responsive to nutrient repletion and/or transfusion: (1)[C]
      - EPO <500 mUmL: erythropoiesis-stimulating agents
      - EPO >500 mUmL: Consider danazol, prednisone, lenalidomide, thalidomide.

SURGERY/OTHER PROCEDURES

- Allogeneic SCT may be considered in CML accelerated phase and blast crisis, as well as in high-risk PMF (1)[A].
- Splenectomy may be considered in severe cases, most often in PMF (1)[C].
- Palliative radiation can be considered for foci of extramedullary hematopoiesis.

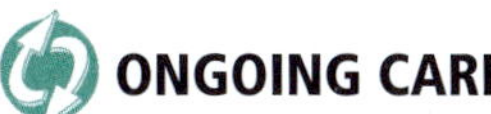

ONGOING CARE

PROGNOSIS

- CML prognosis is strongly tied to disease phase (chronic, accelerated, blast) and therapy response.
  - Patients in chronic phase responding well to therapy have a near-normal lifespan.
  - Patients in blast phase have a median survival of 1 year.
- Although PV, ET, and PMF share driver mutations, prognosis varies considerably:
  - PV: median survival 14 years (24 years if age <60) (1)
  - ET: median survival 20 years (33 years if age <60) (1)
  - PMF: median survival 6 years (15 years if age <60) (1)
    - Driver mutation affects prognosis: CALR generally confers a better prognosis, whereas JAK2 or "triple-negative" (no JAK2, MPL, or CALR mutation) status confers worse prognoses (1)
  - Transformation from PV or ET into overt PMF confers a worse prognosis.
  - Transformation into acute leukemia confers a poor prognosis; occurs most often in PMF (20%) and less often in PV and ET (8%) (1)

REFERENCES

1. Patel AB, Vellore NA, Deininger MW. New strategies in myeloproliferative neoplasms: the evolving genetic and therapeutic landscape. *Clin Cancer Res*. 2016;22(5):1037–1047.

ADDITIONAL READING

Grinfeld J, Nangalia J, Baxter EJ, et al. Classification and personalized prognosis in myeloproliferative neoplasms. *N Engl J Med*. 2018;379(15):1416–1430.

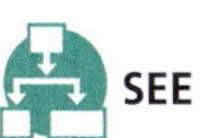

SEE ALSO

Leukemia, Chronic Myelogenous; Polycythemia Vera

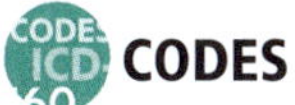

CODES

ICD10

- D47.1 Chronic myeloproliferative disease
- C92.10 Chronic myeloid leukemia, BCR/ABL-positive, not having achieved remission
- D45 Polycythemia vera

CLINICAL PEARLS

- MPNs result from mutations that activate hematopoiesis, resulting in proliferation of cells of myeloid, erythroid, and/or megakaryocyte lineages.
- CML is characterized by granulocytosis, PV is characterized by erythrocytosis, ET is characterized by thrombocytosis, and PMF is characterized by bone marrow fibrosis and extramedullary hematopoiesis, often also with thrombocytosis.
- As MPNs share common mutational origins, multiple cell lines may be increased, they often share common symptoms (such as constitutional symptoms) and clinical features, and they can transform into one another.
- Often the natural history lasts decades, but each MPN carries the risk of complications, such as thrombotic events, as well as transformation into acute leukemia or bone marrow fibrosis.

NARCOLEPSY

Waiz Wasey, MD, FAAFP

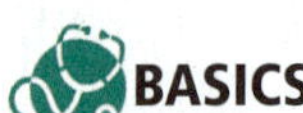

BASICS

DESCRIPTION

- A sleep disorder characterized by excessive daytime sleepiness (EDS) and may be associated with cataplexy (sudden loss of muscle control), hypnagogic hallucinations (vivid perceptual experiences while falling asleep), hypnopompic (vivid perceptual experiences while waking up from sleep), or sleep paralysis (temporary inability to move or speak that happens during transition from sleeping to awake state).
- Two types identified by American Academy of Sleep Medicine: type 1 (60–70%) (formerly narcolepsy with cataplexy) and type 2 (formerly narcolepsy without cataplexy)
- No cure, symptomatic management

EPIDEMIOLOGY

Incidence

- Bimodal distribution, age of onset peak at 15 years and again at 35 years with male predominance
- African Americans are more likely to present without cataplexy and at a younger age.

Prevalence

- Narcolepsy type 1: 25 to 50/100,000 people
- Narcolepsy type 2: 20 to 34/100,000 people

ETIOLOGY AND PATHOPHYSIOLOGY

- Primarily caused by degeneration of hypothalamic neurons that produce orexin (hypocretin); neurodegeneration may be caused by autoimmune process, stimulated by infections (influenza A or group A *Streptococcus*) or environmental factors.
- Orexin is crucial to promote wakefulness; it stimulates the reticular activating system (RAS) and inhibits rapid eye movement (REM). Loss of orexin leads to disorganization of sleep wake cycle, leading to sleepiness.
- Rarely, secondary narcolepsy can be caused by structural lesions (tumor, ischemia).
- *International Classification of Sleep Disorders* 3rd edition (*ICSD-3*) classification:
  - Narcolepsy
  - Narcolepsy type 1
  - Narcolepsy type 2
  - Narcolepsy due to medical conditions
- Cataplexy is a result of hypocretin cell deficiency.

Genetics

- 98% of patients with narcolepsy type 1 have human leukocyte antigen (HLA) DQB1*0602; 40–50% of patients with narcolepsy type 2 express this antigen. HLA DQB1*0602 is present in 12–30% of the general population.
- Autosomal recessive inheritance pattern
- Affects 12% of Asian people and 25% of White people; 38% of African American people are gene carriers.

RISK FACTORS

Age (peaks at 15 and 35 years), usually underdiagnosed before age of 18 years, head trauma, CNS infections, positive family history, recent influenza A, streptococcal infection or H1N1 vaccine; no evidence of COVID-19 leading to narcolepsy yet (1).

COMMONLY ASSOCIATED CONDITIONS

Obstructive sleep apnea (OSA) (up to 25%), obesity, anxiety

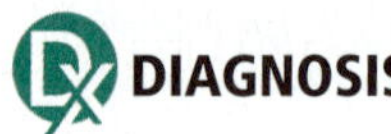

DIAGNOSIS

HISTORY

- Classic pentad of EDS, cataplexy, sleep paralysis, and hypnagogic/hypnopompic hallucinations, and disrupted/fragmented nocturnal sleep (five most common symptoms): Only 10–20% have all five.
- EDS and sleep attacks:
  - EDS is present in 100% of patients, usually the first initial symptom.
  - *ICSD-3* classification for both type 1 and 2 requires EDS occurring almost daily for at least 3 months.
  - Patients may report refreshing daytime naps, with a possible return of EDS in 1 to 2 hours.
  - Sudden sleep attacks (seconds) during stimulating situations such as driving and walking
- Cataplexy (65–75% patients); cardinal symptom:
  - Mainly associated with type 1 narcolepsy; type 2 may develop in the long run.
  - Sudden transient (seconds to minutes) episodes of total or partial loss of motor tone (buckling of knees, head dropping, sagging of jaw or weakness in arms, slurred speech, facial droop or grimace, etc.), usually triggered by strong positive emotions (such as laughing)
  - Symptoms can be subtle as much as slurred speech to loss of muscle strength leading to collapse.
  - Consciousness and memory are not impaired.
- Sleep paralysis
  - Transient (several minutes) inability to move, speak, or open the eyes either while falling asleep or upon awakening
  - During the event, breathing may be difficult because intercostal muscles are paralyzed and chest feels heavier.
  - Patients are aware of their surroundings and are able to recall the event.
  - Seen in 67% of patients who have narcolepsy with cataplexy and 49% narcolepsy without cataplexy
- Hypnagogic or hypnopompic hallucinations:
  - Vivid dreamlike experience in 30–60% patients with type 1 narcolepsy occurs during awakening (hypnopompic hallucinations) or at sleep onset (hypnagogic). Hypnopompic hallucinations are more indicative of narcolepsy than hypnagogic.
  - Hallucination commonly visual, tactile, or auditory.
  - Characteristic hallucinations include being attacked by animals
  - 15% of type 2 patients experience these as well.
- Other reported history
  - Nocturnal insomnia and sleep fragmentation; dreaming is common during naps.
  - Retrograde amnesia
  - Increased periodic limb movements
  - Dream enactment behaviors
  - Weight gain seen with progression

PHYSICAL EXAM

- Unremarkable, but complete exam may help rule out other causes.
- Deep tendon reflexes are either diminished or absent during an episode of cataplexy.

DIFFERENTIAL DIAGNOSIS

EDS is present in 4–28% of the general population, although most individuals are not narcoleptic:

- Sleep apnea syndromes
- Epileptic seizures and syncope
- Idiopathic hypersomnia (5–10% with EDS)
- Psychiatric (depression, bipolar 2, and substance abuse/withdrawal)
- Sleep-related movement disorders (restless leg syndrome, periodic limb movements of sleep)
- Iatrogenic/secondary to medication (benzodiazepines; barbiturates; opioids; antihistamines; β-blockers; and some antipsychotics, antidepressants, and anticonvulsants)
- Poor sleep hygiene and habits leading to sleep deficit and chronic sleep deprivation
- Circadian rhythm disorders (jet lag, shift work, delayed or advanced sleep phase disorders)
- Cataplexy disorders (Niemann-Pick type C, Prader-Willi syndrome, Norrie disease)
- Hypersomnia in Parkinson disease
- Stroke (slurred speech and facial sagging seen in partial cataplexy)

Pediatric Considerations

Narcolepsy is rare before the age of 5 years. EDS is more often attributable to OSA, poor sleep hygiene, and the increased sleep requirements early in life. The recommended amount of sleep decreases with age: newborns 16 to 18 hours/day; preschool-aged children 11 to 12 hours/day; school-aged children and teens 10 hours/day; adults 7 to 8 hours/day. Children can gain excessive weight, from 20 to 40 lb (2). Symptoms of EDS, sleep paralysis, and cataplexy might last longer than compared to adult population.

DIAGNOSTIC TESTS & INTERPRETATION

- Sleep log/actigraphy: First, ensure patient is getting adequate duration of sleep at night for at least 7 to 14 days.
- Prerequisites for valid multiple sleep latency test (MSLT) → normal polysomnography (PSG) with at least 360 minutes of sleep, free of drugs that may alter REM sleep (SSRIs, SNRIs and tricyclic antidepressants), and drugs that alter sleep architecture (stimulants, wake promoting agents, sedatives) for at least 2 weeks, standardized sleep schedule for 7 days
- Primary diagnostic tool
  - An overnight PSG to rule out other causes of EDS
  - MSLT: performed the day after PSG if at least 6 hours of sleep and no sleep disorder explained by PSG
    - Four to five 20-minute naps at 2-hour intervals
    - Positive if rapid onset of REM (<15 minutes) in at least 2 of 5 sleeps (including baseline PSG) and shortened mean sleep latency (<8 minutes)
    - If MSLT negative, but strong clinical suspicion, repeat the test.
    - Antidepressants and stimulants should be discontinued for at least 2 weeks prior to the test.

- Scoring tools
  - Epworth Sleepiness Scale (ESS): scored 0 to 24: >10 is suggestive of a sleep disorder rather than generalized fatigue; helpful for detecting response to medications
- Narcolepsy Severity Scale: a 15-item scale to assess the frequency, severity, and consequences of symptoms of narcolepsy type 1

Initial Tests (lab, imaging)

Urine drug screen to rule out use of recreational drugs or stimulants

Follow-Up Tests & Special Considerations

- Lumbar puncture for orexin level; ≤110 pg/mL in the cerebrospinal fluid (CSF) is indicative of narcolepsy; rarely performed
- HLA typing (HLA-DQB1*–06:02): particularly in children; it is supportive of diagnosis, lacks specificity; generally not recommended because 30% of healthy patient population has the gene (1).

Diagnostic Procedures/Other

- Narcolepsy type 1
  - EDS daily for ≥3 months
  - One of the following:
    - Cataplexy with positive MSLT
    - Low CSF orexin level <110 pg/mL or <1/3 of mean values in normal subjects; can lead to REM intrusion
- Narcolepsy type 2
  - All the above (with or without cataplexy) and normal CSF orexin level

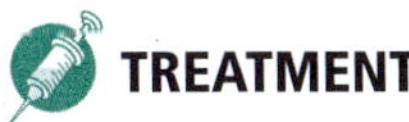

TREATMENT

GENERAL MEASURES

- Medications do not cure, but the goal is to minimize EDS and cataplectic episodes.
- Drug therapy, if used, should be supplemented by various behavioral strategies.
- Proper sleep hygiene and a regular sleep schedule.
- Well-timed 20-minute naps may be helpful.
- Avoid stimulants (alcohol, heavy meals, caffeine, nicotine).
- Use safety precautions, particularly when driving.

MEDICATION

First Line

- EDS
  - Modafinil (Provigil):
    - Works on dopaminergic, adrenergic, and histaminergic receptors of hypothalamus
    - Adult dose: 200 mg/day; start with 100 mg; max dose 400 mg/day in divided dosing
    - Adverse effects: headache, GI upset, tachycardia, and does not affect blood pressure (BP); tolerance limited, risk of Stevens-Johnson syndrome
    - Caution with oral contraceptive use as it decreases the efficacy
  - Armodafinil (Nuvigil):
    - Enantiomeric form of modafinil with the same half-life but lower adverse effect profile
    - Adult dose: 150 to 250 mg every morning
    - Headache, xerostomia, Stevens-Johnson syndrome, and toxic epidermal necrolysis
  - Pitolisant (Wakix): FDA approved for narcolepsy and cataplexy; doses up to 35.6 mg demonstrated effectiveness (2)
  - Solriamfetol (Sunosi):
    - Start with 75 mg QD; increase dose based on response every 3 days to a max dose of 150 mg/day.
    - Contraindicated with concomitant or recent MAOI use
    - Abuse potential: Use caution in patients with a history of drug use.
  - Clarithromycin: acts on GABA-A receptor; can be used for hypersomnia if alternative primary medication fails; dose 500 mg BID (start with a 2-week trial period); adverse effect: GI distress
- Cataplexy:
  - Sodium oxybate (Xyrem):
    - FDA approved for both EDS and cataplexy; now approved for ages ≥7 years.
    - For moderate to severe cases and best option for improving nighttime sleep
    - Dose: 6 to 9 g/day twice nightly; start with 2.25 g/day and increase by 1.5 g/day qwk; max dose: 9 g/day
    - May take 8 to 12 weeks for a full response
    - Is a date rape drug; abuse potential
    - May worsen sleep-disordered breathing in patients with OSA
  - Sodium oxybate, calcium, magnesium, potassium (Xywav) (3):
    - Approved by FDA for cataplexy and EDS in children aged ≥7 years
    - Once a night dosing options available
  - Sodium oxybate (Lumryz)
    - Once a night dosing
  - Pitolisant (Wakix): FDA approved for narcolepsy and cataplexy; doses up to 35.6 mg demonstrated effectiveness
  - Tricyclic antidepressants
    - Clomipramine: dose: 25 to 75 mg/day
    - Anticholinergic side effect profile: dry mouth, sedation, urinary retention, impotence
  - Serotonin-norepinephrine reuptake inhibitors
    - Venlafaxine: dose: 75 to 300 mg/day; start at 37.5 mg, max dose 375 mg/day. Taper dose to discontinue.
    - Fluoxetine: dose: 20 to 80 mg/day

Second Line

EDS

- Amphetamines: used if first line fail or patient unable to tolerate
  - Methylphenidate (Ritalin): dose: initial dose 5 to 10 mg/day divided BID or TID; max dose 60 mg/day, short-acting, most potent amphetamine available; can be used in combination with modafinil and armodafinil
  - Dextroamphetamine/amphetamine: dose: initial dose 10 mg/day; can increase by 10 mg qwk to a max dose 60 mg/day divided BID or TID; once a day dosing if extended-release formulary is used
  - Adverse reactions: headaches, irritability, HTN, psychosis, anorexia, habituation, rebound hypersomnia
- Frequent nocturnal awakenings
  - Temazepam: Dose 15 to 30 mg at bedtime
  - Zolpidem: Dose 5 to 10 mg at bedtime

ISSUES FOR REFERRAL

Unresponsive to primary medication and severe cataplexy may benefit from neurology referral.

ADDITIONAL THERAPIES

Cognitive-behavioral therapy for hypersomnia (limited availability)

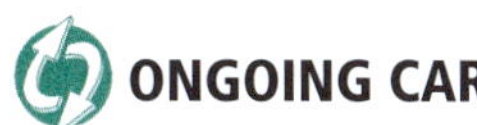

ONGOING CARE

FOLLOW-UP RECOMMENDATIONS

Patient Monitoring

Monitoring using scoring tools to gauge treatment effectiveness

PATIENT EDUCATION

Narcolepsy Network: https://www.narcolepsynetwork.org

PROGNOSIS

Improvements seen in 60–80%; symptoms can worsen with aging.

REFERENCES

1. Anderson D. Narcolepsy: a clinical review. *JAAPA*. 2021;34(6):20–25.
2. Meskill G, Davis C, Zarycranski D, et al. Assessment of the clinical benefits of pitolisant on excessive daytime sleepiness and cataplexy in adults with narcolepsy. *Sleep*. 2021;44(2):A189–99.
3. Bogan RK, Thorpy MJ, Dauvilliers Y, et al. Efficacy and safety of calcium, magnesium, potassium, and sodium oxybates (lower-sodium oxybate [LXB]; JZP-258) in a placebo-controlled, double-blind, randomized withdrawal study in adults with narcolepsy with cataplexy. *Sleep*. 2021;44(3):zsaa206.

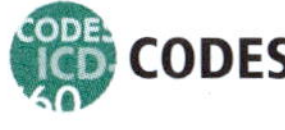

CODES

ICD10

- G47.429 Narcolepsy in conditions classified elsewhere w/o cataplexy
- G47.411 Narcolepsy with cataplexy
- G47.419 Narcolepsy without cataplexy

CLINICAL PEARLS

- Narcolepsy is an incurable, REM disorder.
- The classic tetrad includes EDS, cataplexy, sleep paralysis, and hypnagogic hallucinations, only cataplexy is pathognomonic for the disorder.

NASAL POLYPS

Daniel Perez, MD • Sagar Saoji, MD

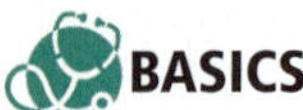

BASICS

- Painless, benign inflammatory, and hyperplastic lesions of sinonasal mucosa (1)
- Arise from near the ethmoid sinus but can infrequently arise from maxillary sinus mucosa
- Usually associated with chronic rhinosinusitis (CRS)

DESCRIPTION

- Appearance of edematous pedunculated mass in the nasal cavity or within the paranasal sinus
- Often causes symptoms of blockage, discharge, or loss of smell
- Most commonly bilateral; if unilateral, malignancy should be on the differential.

EPIDEMIOLOGY

Incidence

- Typical age at diagnosis ranges from 40 to 60 years.
- Increases with age to a peak in the sixth decade
- Men are more commonly affected, though women are more likely to have severe disease.

Prevalence

- ~1–4% in general population (2)
- Much rarer in children: ~0.1% and associated with cystic fibrosis
- Asthma is present in up to 65% of patients.

ETIOLOGY AND PATHOPHYSIOLOGY

- Separate T helper 1–driven and T helper 2–driven pathways
- In the Western Hemisphere, nasal polyps are due to the T helper 2–driven eosinophilia, IgE causing inflammation, and elevated levels of interleukin-5, which is often associated with environmental and/or seasonal allergic triggers.

Genetics

Patients with nasal polyps are more likely than controls to report having a first-degree relative with nasal polyps (3)[B].

RISK FACTORS

- An increased prevalence of nasal polyps has been described among textile workers who have been exposed to occupational dust, particularly among those with longer-duration exposure (3)[B].
- Nasal irritants such as smoke and other common allergens.

GENERAL PREVENTION

- The use of intranasal corticosteroids after polyp removal surgery has shown effectiveness against recurrence.
- Using a humidifier will help keep your nasal passages moist. This can help improve the flow of mucus in your sinuses and prevent blockage or inflammation, thus preventing nasal polyps from occurring or recurring.

COMMONLY ASSOCIATED CONDITIONS

- Asthma
- Bronchiectasis
- Aspirin hypersensitivity
- Allergic rhinitis
- Chronic sinusitis
- Allergic fungal sinusitis
- Cystic fibrosis (pediatric patients)
- Primary ciliary dyskinesia (Kartagener syndrome)
- Laryngopharyngeal reflux

DIAGNOSIS

- Made on the basis of the presence of sinonasal symptoms for >3 months and the visualization of polyps in the nasal cavity, usually initially via nasal endoscopy
- CT or MRI scans of the sinuses can also be used.
- A biopsy of the mass may be done to help differentiate a benign versus malignant growth.

HISTORY

Symptoms

- Rhinorrhea
- Nasal congestion
- Postnasal drainage
- Hyposmia/anosmia
- Inability to breathe through the nose
- Dull headaches
- Facial pain/pressure over the middle third of the face
- Sleep disturbance
- In some cases, there may be no symptoms.

PHYSICAL EXAM

Besides rhinorrhea, sinus tenderness to palpation and/or visualization of polyp, there are no other definitive physical exam findings.

DIFFERENTIAL DIAGNOSIS

- CRS without nasal polyps, rhinitis, structural abnormalities of the nose, and neurologic causes of hyposmia
- Other benign or malignant tumors (e.g., fibroma, hemangioma, osteoma, chondroma, encephalocele)
- Squamous cell carcinoma
- Malignant melanoma
- Meningocele
- Nasal foreign body

DIAGNOSTIC TESTS & INTERPRETATION

Initial Tests (lab, imaging)

Anterior rhinoscopy shows a pale, translucent mass

- Most commonly on the lateral wall of the middle meatus

Follow-Up Tests & Special Considerations

- If large posterior nasal polyps, examine the tympanic membrane for eustachian tube dysfunction.
- If unilateral polyp, a biopsy should be done to exclude malignancy.
- Test for cystic fibrosis in children with polyps.
- Sinus CT scan:
  - It may be helpful to corroborate history and endoscopic findings
  - Unable to differentiate polyp from other soft tissue masses
  - Reveals the extent of the disease and is necessary to formulate a plan for surgical intervention if indicated
- MRI:
  - May aid in diagnosis if concern for neoplasia, mycetoma, or encephalocele

Diagnostic Procedures/Other

Flexible/rigid endoscopy is required to assess the nasal cavity fully (3).

- The gold standard for diagnosis

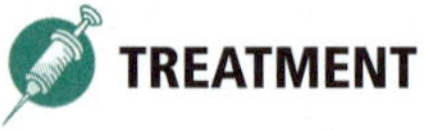

TREATMENT

GENERAL MEASURES

- Goal is to reduce the size or eliminate nasal polyps because they can obstruct the nasal cavity and impair the sense of smell, restrict breathing ability through the nose, and obstruct drainage of sinuses.
- Assess symptom severity with a 22-item Sinonasal Outcome Test (SNOT-22) or the Visual Analog Scale in primary care settings.

MEDICATION

First Line

Daily intranasal corticosteroid use with saline irrigation is the first-line therapy (4)[A].

- In patients who do not have significant nasal blockage by polyps, intranasal saline, and intranasal glucocorticoids can be administered for 1 to 3 months.
- Intranasal corticosteroids are shown to decrease nasal polyp size, lessen sinonasal symptoms, and improve quality of life
  - Budesonide 256 μg/day (one 64 μg spray in each nostril BID)
  - Beclomethasone dipropionate 168 to 320 μg/day (1 to 2 sprays per nostril BID)
  - Fluticasone propionate 400 to 744 μg/day (1 to 2 sprays per nostril twice daily)
  - Mometasone furoate 400 μg/day (2 sprays per nostril BID)
  - For children, mometasone furoate is preferred.

Second Line

- In patients with severe symptoms or those who cannot tolerate intranasal steroids, consider a short course of oral corticosteroids (14 to 21 days) and/or doxycycline (21 days) (4)[B].
  - Prednisone 30 to 50 mg daily (taper when indicated)
  - Prednisolone 20 to 60 mg daily (taper when indicated)
  - Doxycycline 200 mg once, followed by 100 mg daily (contraindicated in pregnancy or if breastfeeding)
- There are more risks associated with the use of oral steroids; can lead to serious side effects such as elevated blood sugar, cataracts, glaucoma, osteoporosis, bone fractures, and heart problems

ISSUES FOR REFERRAL

- If unilateral polyp, send for a biopsy.
- Consider referral to an otorhinolaryngologist for endoscopic sinus surgery if severe obstruction symptoms or conservative management is ineffective.

ADDITIONAL THERAPIES

Patients with persistent symptoms and have concurrent allergic rhinitis, consider:

- Injectable steroids—steroid medication can be injected directly into the nasal polyp. It is generally as effective as oral steroids but has less associated side effects (5).
  - One major side effect that can occur though is short-term vision loss.
- Systemic antihistamine—does not treat nasal polyps directly but can help reduce associated symptoms.
- Leukotriene pathway antagonist
- Allergy immunotherapy
- Aspirin desensitization
- Intralesional bleomycin A5 (BLE) injection may treat eosinophilic-type nasal polyps.
- Biologics:
  - Based on two multicentered randomized double-blinded studies, adding dupilumab to daily mometasone furoate nasal spray reduced polyp size, sinus opacification, and symptom severity; it was well-tolerated and decreased systemic corticosteroid treatment and surgery (6)[B].
  - Dupilumab works by blocking interleukin-4 and interleukin-13.
  - Other biologics that have efficacy and/or relief of symptoms: omalizumab, mepolizumab (7)

SURGERY/OTHER PROCEDURES

- Most surgeries are approached endonasally.
  - The external (Caldwell-Luc) approach is used for more difficult cases but carries a higher risk of complications.
- Functional endonasal sinus surgery has a slightly lower revision rate than intranasal polypectomy. Both modalities provide effective symptom relief.
- Postoperative use of nasal corticosteroids delay the recurrence of nasal polyps and hence the timing of revision surgery.
- Postoperative use of steroid-releasing stents to prevent polyp recurrence by decreasing mucosal inflammation

ONGOING CARE

- Recurrence up to ~40% (3)
- The use of intranasal corticosteroids after polyp removal surgery has shown effectiveness against recurrence.
- Recurrence is twice as likely in those with asthma

PROGNOSIS

Persons who undergo surgery have great improvements in symptoms, but the recurrence rate is high (8),(9)[B].

COMPLICATIONS

- Acute/chronic sinus infections
- Heterotrophic bone formation within the sinus cavity may occur.

REFERENCES

1. del Toro E, Portela J. *Nasal Polyps*. Treasure Island, (FL): StatPearls Publishing; 2023. https://pubmed.ncbi.nlm.nih.gov/32809581/. Accessed October 3, 2023.
2. Raciborski F, Arcimowicz M, Samoliñski B, et al. Recorded prevalence of nasal polyps increases with age. *Postepy Dermatol Alergol*. 2021;38(4):682–688. doi:10.5114/ada.2020.99365.
3. Hopkins C. Chronic rhinosinusitis with nasal polyps. *N Engl J Med*. 2019;381(1):55–63.
4. Rudmik L, Soler ZM. Medical therapies for adult chronic sinusitis: a systematic review. *JAMA*. 2015;314(9):926–939.
5. Zamzam SM, Elshazly M, Salah M, et al. Comparative study between intrapolyp steroid injection and oral steroid for treatment of sinonasal polyposis in Egyptian patients. *Egyptian J Otolaryngol*. 2020;36(59). doi:10.1186/s43163-020-00062-w.
6. Bachert C, Han JK, Desrosiers M, et al. Efficacy and safety of dupilumab in patients with severe chronic rhinosinusitis with nasal polyps (LIBERTY NP SINUS-24 and LIBERTY NP SINUS-52): results from two multicentre, randomised, double-blind, placebo-controlled, parallel-group phase 3 trials. *Lancet*. 2019;394(10209):1638–1650.
7. Han JK, Bachert C, Fokkens W, et al. Mepolizumab for chronic rhinosinusitis with nasal polyps (SYNAPSE): a randomised, double-blind, placebo-controlled, phase 3 trial. *Lancet Respir Med*. 2021;9(10):1141–1153.
8. Sharma R, Lakhani R, Rimmer J, et al. Surgical interventions for chronic rhinosinusitis with nasal polyps. *Cochrane Database Syst Rev*. 2014;2014(11):CD006990.
9. Rimmer J, Fokkens W, Chong LY, et al. Surgical versus medical interventions for chronic rhinosinusitis with nasal polyps. *Cochrane Database Syst Rev*. 2014;2014(12):CD006991.

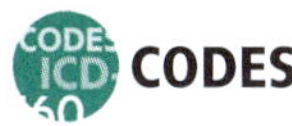

CODES

ICD10

- J33.9 Nasal polyp, unspecified
- J33.0 Polyp of nasal cavity
- J33.8 Other polyp of sinus

CLINICAL PEARLS

- Intranasal corticosteroid use has been demonstrated to reduce polyp size and recurrence as well as to improve nasal congestion.
- Short-course oral corticosteroids may be considered in those with persistent symptoms.
- Asthma is a common concomitant diagnosis and is often previously undiagnosed.
- Aggressive medical and surgical treatment improves asthma outcomes.
- Allergy testing can be helpful.
- If unilateral nasal polyp, refer for biopsy.

NEPHROTIC SYNDROME

Nahid N. Molaie, MD • John Cheng, MD

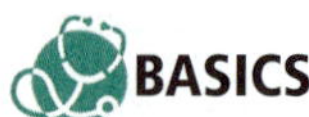

BASICS

DESCRIPTION

- A constellation of clinical and laboratory features defined by the presence of massive proteinuria (>3.5 g/1.73 m^2/24 hr), hypoalbuminemia (<2.5 g/dL), and peripheral edema, with hypercoagulability and susceptibility to infection
- In children nephrotic proteinuria is defined as >40 mg/m^2/hr
- It can be due to intrinsic renal disease or caused by congenital infections, diabetes mellitus, systemic lupus erythematosus, neoplasia or certain drug use (1),(2).

EPIDEMIOLOGY

- Diabetic nephropathy
- Minimal change disease (MCD)
  - Most common cause of nephrotic syndrome in children aged <10 years (90%)
  - Idiopathic condition in adults associated with NSAID use or Hodgkin lymphoma
- Amyloidosis: 4–17% of idiopathic nephrotic syndrome—two renal types primary (AL) and secondary (AA)
- Lupus nephropathy (LN): Adult women are affected about 10 times more often than men.
- Focal segmental glomerulosclerosis (FSGS)
  - 35% of nephrotic syndrome in adults, most common primary nephrotic syndrome in African Americans
  - Has both primary (idiopathic) and secondary forms (associated with HIV, morbid obesity, reflux nephropathy, previous glomerular injury)
- Membranous nephropathy
  - Most common cause of primary nephrotic syndrome in adults (40%)
  - Most often primary (idiopathic) but can be secondary associated with malignancy, hepatitis B, autoimmune diseases, thyroiditis, and certain drugs including NSAIDs, penicillamine, gold and captopril
- Membranoproliferative glomerulonephritis (MGN)
  - May present in the setting of a systemic viral or rheumatic illness

Incidence

- Worldwide, children have an incidence of 1.15 to 16.9 per 100,000 children, with lower incidence in Europe and North America, and higher in Southeast Asia and East Asia (1).
- Approximately 3 cases per 100,000 per year in adults. There is increased incidence and development of severe disease in African American and Hispanic population.

ETIOLOGY AND PATHOPHYSIOLOGY

- Primary renal disease (e.g., MCD, FSGS, MGN, IgA nephropathy)
- Secondary renal disease (e.g., diabetic nephropathy, amyloidosis, and paraproteinemias)
- Increased glomerular permeability to protein macromolecules, especially albumin
- Edema results primarily from renal salt retention, with arterial underfilling from decreased plasma oncotic pressure playing an additional role.
- The hypercoagulable state is likely due to loss of antithrombin III in urine.

Genetics

Mutations in genes regulating podocyte proteins identified in families with inherited nephrotic syndrome.

RISK FACTORS

- Children
  - Often idiopathic, with kidney biopsy showing MCD
  - Family history of nephrotic syndrome may be associated with genetic mutations.
  - Viral infections, including HIV, hepatitis B, cytomegalovirus, and parvovirus B19
  - Sickle cell disease (2)
- Adults
  - Drug addiction (e.g., heroin [FSGS])
  - Hepatitis B and C, HIV, CMV, Parvovirus B1, toxoplasmosis, other infections
  - Immunosuppression
  - Nephrotoxic drugs (lithium, bisphosphonates, interferon therapy, gold, bucillamine, and penicillamine)
  - Vesicoureteral reflux (FSGS)
  - Cancer (usually MGN, may be MCD)
  - Chronic analgesic use/abuse (NSAIDs)
  - Preeclampsia
  - Diabetes mellitus

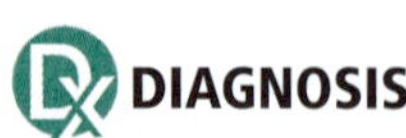

DIAGNOSIS

HISTORY

- Inquire about signs or symptoms of systemic disease: joint complaints, rash, edema, infectious symptoms, fever, anorexia, oliguria, foamy frothy urine, acute flank pain, and hematuria.
- Medication history, especially NSAIDs
- Inquire about any prior history of venous thromboembolism as it could be the first indication of nephrotic syndrome.

PHYSICAL EXAM

- Fluid retention: abdominal distention, abdominal fluid shift, extremity edema, puffy eyelids, scrotal swelling, weight gain, shortness of breath; pericardial rub and decreased breath sounds with pleural effusions may develop.
- Arterial hypertension is found in 25% of the cases.
- Orthostatic hypotension

> **ALERT**
> Pulmonary embolism is one of the most life-threatening aspects of a patient with active nephrotic syndrome.

DIFFERENTIAL DIAGNOSIS

- Edema and proteinuria: See "Etiology and Pathophysiology."
- Edema alone: congestive heart failure, cirrhosis, hypothyroidism, nutritional hypoalbuminemia, protein-losing enteropathy

DIAGNOSTIC TESTS & INTERPRETATION

Initial Tests (lab, imaging)

- Confirm proteinuria if present: by urine dipstick initially (3+ or 4+ readings) and then quantitate by 24-hour or spot urine protein-to-creatinine ratio. Spot urine protein-to-creatinine ratio is easier to perform, and follows 24-hour values in a linear fashion.
- Urine culture
- CBC and PT/INR and PTT
- Chemistry panel including electrolytes, urea, eGFR, liver function tests
- HbA1c and lipid panel
- Serum albumin that is often <2.5 g/dL
- Antinuclear antibody and/or anti–double-stranded DNA (lupus); rheumatoid factor; antinuclear cytoplasmic antibody
- Antistreptococcal antibodies, particularly in children
- Complement levels (C3/C4 and total hemolytic complement): A low C3 may suggest a postinfectious or membranoproliferative process, whereas both low C3 and C4 point to lupus.
- Phospholipase A receptor antibody (PLA2R), positive in 70% of cases of idiopathic membranous nephropathy
- Serum protein electrophoresis/urine immune electrophoresis to rule in a paraproteinemia
- Hepatitis B, C, HIV and syphilis serology
- Renal US to evaluate for renal abnormalities
- Chest x-ray to detect presence of pleural effusion or infection
- Doppler US of the lower extremities if deep vein thrombosis is suspected

Follow-Up Tests & Special Considerations

Consider genetic testing for the NPHS1 and NPHS2 mutations for infants and testing for NPHS2 in children who are resistant to steroid therapy.

Diagnostic Procedures/Other

- Adults often require kidney biopsy to determine the underlying cause of nephrotic syndrome.
- Biopsy is rarely done in children with first episode of nephrotic syndrome.
  - Biopsy is indicated if not responsive to steroids, or if hematuria (microscopic or macroscopic) is present, or persistent hypertension, or presence of rash or arthritis (2).

Test Interpretation

- Light microscopy: may show nothing in MCD; sclerosis may be seen in FSGS or diabetic nephropathy; diffuse mesangial hypercellularity suggests a proliferative disease such as IgA nephropathy, LN, or postinfectious GN.
- Immunofluorescence: Detect immunoreactants IgG, IgA, IgM, C3, C4, C1q, light chains; detect target antigens such as PLA2R, THDS7A, DNAJB9, or specific amyloid species.
- Electron microscopy: Define extent and characteristics of immune or monoclonal deposits.

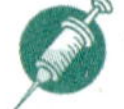

TREATMENT

Depends on the type of renal pathology and varies between children and adults; KDIGO issued guidelines in 2021 on the treatment for nephrotic syndrome in adults and children; a revised guideline is pending review in 2024 (1).

GENERAL MEASURES

- Weight, height, and blood pressure should be monitored closely along with urine output.
- Lifestyle modifications: sodium restriction, moderate protein restriction, heart healthy diet, target ideal body weight, increased physical activity, smoking cessation, reduce alcohol consumption

- Immunizations, preferably before starting immunosuppressive therapy
  - Pneumococcal vaccination and *Haemophilus influenza* immunization
  - Annual flu and COVID vaccination
  - Patient receiving complement antagonist should be vaccinated with both meningococcal conjugate vaccine and serogroup B meningococcal vaccine.
  - Herpes zoster vaccine
- Management of other cardiovascular risk factors, including hypertension and hyperlipidemia
- Screen for tuberculosis prior to immunosuppressive therapy.
- Prophylactic trimethoprim-sulfamethoxazole (TMP-SMZ) should be considered in patients with high dose prednisone or other immunosuppressive therapy (2).

MEDICATION

First Line

- Decreasing proteinuria:
  - Reduction in proteinuria is important as it reflects control of the primary disease, reduction of glomerular hypertension, and also reduction of podocyte damage.
  - ACE inhibitors or angiotensin II receptor blockers reduce proteinuria, hyperlipidemia, thrombotic tendencies, progression of renal failure, and control hypertension.
  - If ACE/ARB is not tolerated, control of BP with nondihydropyridine calcium channel blocker or β-blocker can also decrease proteinuria.
  - Protein restriction can slow the progression of the disease, but evidence is unclear.
  - Glucocorticoids: for steroid responsive disease (MCD and FSGS), steroids dosed in consultation with nephrologist; relapse is common and may require prolonged course of corticosteroids.
- Treatment of edema:
  - Loop diuretics are first-line treatment for edema and twice daily administration is preferred, as patients are often diuretic resistant, even with normal GFR.
    - Dosing a thiazide-like diuretic (hydrochlorothiazide, metolazone, or chlorthalidone) 2 to 5 hours prior to a loop diuretic can overcome diuretic resistance.
    - IV diuresis may be necessary as gastrointestinal absorption of diuretics may be limited due to intestinal wall edema.
    - Continuous infusion of a loop diuretic may mitigate the toxic effect and provide a sustained diuresis.
  - IV salt-poor albumin can be added to IV diuretic therapy to improve intravascular volume, diuresis, and natriuresis.
  - Salt restriction to <2 g sodium per day
    - Water restriction is usually not necessary, as patients are often intravascularly volume depleted. However, water restriction may be necessary in patients who develop hyponatremia.
  - Target weight loss of 0.5 to 1.0 kg/day (1 to 2 lb/day); edema should be corrected slowly to avoid acute hypovolemia, electrolyte disturbances, acute renal failure, and thromboembolism as a result of hemoconcentration.
- Treatment of hyperlipidemia
  - Statins have been shown to improve endothelial function and may decrease proteinuria with the exception of rosuvastatin which can worsen proteinuria, but effect on GFR and preservation of renal function is small. The major role for statin use is in cardiovascular risk reduction.
- Anticoagulation
  - Patients who have had thromboembolic event or who are at high risk (e.g., lower albumin levels) require anticoagulation. Prophylactic anticoagulation should not be given to patients at increased risk of bleeding.
  - Anticoagulation can be given as low-molecular-weight heparin followed by warfarin, or DOACs, or direct thrombin inhibitors.

Second Line

- Many of the nephrotic diseases will require escalation in therapy above steroids. These include rapidly relapsing forms as well as MGN, LN, and IgA nephropathy. Bolus steroids and other immunosuppressives are required in this circumstance (cyclophosphamide and levamisole for steroid-responsive nephrotic syndrome; for steroid-resistant, mycophenolate mofetil, chlorambucil, cyclosporine, or tacrolimus).
- Rituximab (anti-CD20 agent) and abatacept (anti–B7-1), combined with steroids or other immunosuppressive agents, has demonstrated early promise in the treatment of refractory nephrotic syndrome

ISSUES FOR REFERRAL

Nephrology for renal biopsy to confirm diagnosis and to assist with management

ADMISSION, INPATIENT, AND NURSING CONSIDERATIONS

Patients may require admission due to acute decompensation (2).

ONGOING CARE

FOLLOW-UP RECOMMENDATIONS

Patient Monitoring

- Frequent monitoring is required for relapse, disease progression, and for detecting signs of toxicity of medical management. Minimize length and dose of corticosteroid therapy.
- If on prolonged corticosteroid therapy, dual-energy x-ray absorptiometry (DEXA) should be checked every 12 to 18 months along with ophthalmologic exam annually, to evaluate for glaucoma and cataracts.

DIET

Muscle wasting and malnutrition are major problems in severe nephrotic syndrome. Optimal diet includes:

- Adequate protein (1 g/kg/day), low fat (cholesterol), reduced sodium (<2 g/day)
- Supplemental multivitamins and minerals, especially vitamin D, calcium, and iron
- Supplemental dietary proteins are of no value.

PROGNOSIS

Nephrotic syndrome in children (MCD) is typically self-limited and carries a good prognosis. Complete remission is expected if the basic disease is treatable (infection, malignancy, drug induced); otherwise, a relapsing and remitting course is possible, with progression to dialysis seen in more aggressive forms (diabetic glomerulosclerosis and FSGS).

COMPLICATIONS

- Deep vein, renal vein, or central venous thrombosis may occur.
- Increased risk of infections
- Pleural effusion, ascites
- Hyperlipidemia, cardiovascular disease
- Acute renal failure, progressive renal failure
- Protein malnutrition/muscle wasting

REFERENCES

1. Kidney Disease: Improving Global Outcomes (KDIGO) Glomerular Diseases Work Group. KDIGO 2021 clinical practice guideline for the management of glomerular diseases. *Kidney Int*. 2021;100(4S):S1–S276. doi:10.1016/j.kint.2021.05.021.
2. Noone DG, Iijima K, Parekh R. Idiopathic nephrotic syndrome in children [published correction appears in *Lancet*. 2018;392(10144):282. doi:10.1016/S0140-6736(18)31608-8]. *Lancet*. 2018;392(10141):61–74. doi:10.1016/S0140-6736(18)30536-1.

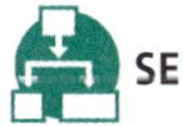

SEE ALSO

Acute Kidney Injury; Amyloidosis; Diabetes Mellitus, Type 1; Diabetes Mellitus, Type 2; Glomerulonephritis, Acute; HIV/AIDS; Lupus Erythematosus, Discoid; Multiple Myeloma

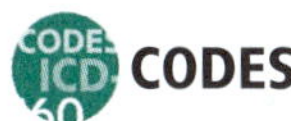

CODES

ICD10

- N04.0 Nephrotic syndrome with minor glomerular abnormality
- N04 Nephrotic syndrome
- N04.3 Nephrotic syndrome with diffuse mesangial proliferative glomerulonephritis

CLINICAL PEARLS

- Nephrotic syndrome is a clinical syndrome of >3.5 g/1.73 m^2/day proteinuria, hypoalbuminemia, hyperlipidemia, and edema often associated with diabetes and NSAIDs use.
- Pediatric nephrotic syndrome typically carries a good prognosis and is more easily treated with steroids, although recurrences are common.
- Nondiabetic adults with nephrotic syndrome will often require a renal biopsy to determine cause.
- Have a high index of suspicion for symptoms that may represent an embolic event in patients with nephrotic syndrome.

NEUROPATHIC PAIN

Raye Reeder, MD, MPH

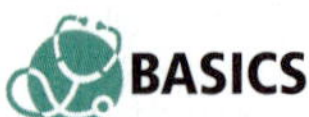

BASICS

DESCRIPTION

- The term neuropathic pain represents a broad spectrum of pain syndromes and encompasses a wide variety of peripheral and central disorders.
- Defined as injury of the nociceptive pathway in the central or peripheral nervous system (CNS and PNS) that result in either impairment, absence, or paradoxically augmentation of pain
- Symptoms are usually burning, tingling, sharp, stabbing, shooting, and electric shock-like quality.
- Often severe and resistant to standard treatments for pain

EPIDEMIOLOGY

Incidence

There is insufficient evidence on the general incidence rate of neuropathic pain as most studies target a single type of neuropathic pain. In a Dutch study targeted between 1996 and 2003, 9,135 new cases of neuropathic pain out of 362,693 persons contributing to the study were identified, yielding 8.2 new cases per 1,000 person-years (PY). The study approximates an annual incidence of almost 1% of the general population, affecting more women and middle-aged population.

Prevalence

Includes chronic conditions that affect up to 10% of the population, accounting for 20–25% of individuals with chronic pain

- Malignancy: Up to 20% have neuropathic pain from either cancer or treatment.
- Poststroke patients: up to 8%
- Spinal cord injury: 60–69%, a large majority of whom present with a syringomyelia
- Herpes zoster: lifetime incidence ~25%; up to 10% develop chronic postherpetic neuralgia.
- HIV: up to 50%
- Diabetes: ~50% will eventually develop neuropathy; 34% will develop neuropathic pain.

ETIOLOGY AND PATHOPHYSIOLOGY

- A variety of mechanisms contribute to neuropathic pain and many are poorly understood.
- One proposed mechanism suggests that damaged primary afferents, including nociceptors, become highly sensitive to mechanical stimuli and may generate impulses in the absence of stimulation. This increase in sensitivity and spontaneous activation without apparent stimulation is thought to be caused by an increase in the density of sodium channels in the damaged nerve fibers, leading to increased excitability and signal transduction.

Genetics

Studies have demonstrated that $Na_v1.7$ and $Na_v1.8$, two types of voltage-gated sodium channels encoded by the *SCN9A* and *SCN10A* genes, respectively, are expressed at high levels on the peripheral nociceptive neurons in the dorsal root ganglion.

RISK FACTORS

- General risk factors include older age, female, physical inactivity, and manual occupation.
- Diabetes mellitus (DM) types I & II, multiple sclerosis, Guillain-Barré syndrome, herpes zoster, trigeminal neuralgia, HIV, Lyme disease, malignancy/chemotherapy, nutrition (vitamins B_6 and B_{12} deficiencies), medications (isoniazid, ethambutol, chloroquine, paclitaxel, cisplatin, amiodarone, vincristine).

GENERAL PREVENTION

- Use of herpes zoster vaccines, which reduces both herpes zoster infections in patients >50 years of age and postherpetic neuralgia
- Use of antiviral or analgesic treatment in patients with herpes zoster infection
- Perioperative treatment of surgical patients to prevent chronic postsurgical pain; use of multimodal analgesia with gabapentin and local anesthetics to prevent acute and chronic pain after breast surgery for cancer
- Proper management of associated health conditions, such as DM

COMMONLY ASSOCIATED CONDITIONS

Depression and anxiety, sleep disturbances, substance abuse, impaired cognition, polypharmacy, and suicidal ideation

DIAGNOSIS

Diagnosis is based primarily on clinical history and the findings on physical examination.

HISTORY

- Onset and duration of symptoms, location, intensity (0 to 10), exacerbating factors
- Pain often described as burning, shooting, tingling, or electric shock-like
- Temporal profile: Symptoms become worse towards the end of the day.
- Sensory descriptors: numbness; weakness; reduced sensation to touch, pinprick, temperature, or vibration; decreased proprioception
- Effect on function: effect on sleep, ambulation, self-care, and sexual function
- Past medical, surgical, and psychosocial history, substance use (especially alcohol)
- Previous treatments: Neuropathic pain is generally resistant to acetaminophen or NSAIDs.
- Different screening tools in the form of questionnaires have emerged: Leeds Assessment of Neuropathic Symptoms and Signs, Douleur Neuropathique 4 questions, Neuropathic Pain Questionnaire, Pain-DETECT, Neuropathic Pain Symptom Inventory.

PHYSICAL EXAM

- Positive symptoms:
  - Hyperalgesia (abnormally increased pain response to stimulus) evoked by sharp or blunt pressure, heat or cold
  - Allodynia (pain from nonpainful stimulus) evoked by light touch, clothing, or bedsheets
- Negative symptoms: Hypoesthesia (abnormally reduced sensation of a tactile stimulus) to touch or temperature
- Gross motor examination
  - Weakness, fatigue, decreased range of motion, stiffness, and muscle spasm
  - Hypotonia, tremor, dystonia, ataxia, hyporeflexia/hyperreflexia, motor neglect
- Sensory examination
  - Light touch, pinprick, vibration sense, and proprioception may be either diminished or amplified.
  - Sensory disturbance may extend beyond a discrete nerve territory.
- Skin examination
  - Alterations in temperature, color, sweating, and hair growth suggestive of sympathetic nervous system involvement, such as in complex regional pain syndrome (CRPS)
  - Residual dermatomal scars can indicate previous herpes zoster infection.
  - Acanthosis nigricans can indicate diabetes.

DIFFERENTIAL DIAGNOSIS

- Nociceptive pain due to tissue damage
- Somatic symptom disorder
- Conversion disorder

DIAGNOSTIC TESTS & INTERPRETATION

Neurologic testing establishes distribution but does not yet provide benefit in determining treatment (1)[C].

- Confirmatory tests include the following (in order of increasing invasiveness):
  - Sensory assessment: touch, pinprick, pressure, cold, heat, vibration, temporal summation
  - Quantitative sensory testing: uses standardized mechanical and thermal stimuli to test the afferent nociceptive and non-nociceptive systems
  - Blink reflex testing: assesses trigeminal afferent system
  - Nerve conduction study/electromyography: assesses non-nociceptive large fiber function of the peripheral nerves
  - Somatosensory-evoked potentials and laser-evoked potentials (LEP): assesses afferent fiber function
  - Skin biopsy: assesses quantification of the intraepidermal nerve fiber
  - Corneal confocal microscopy: assesses corneal innervation and small nerve fibers
- CT/MRI: facilitate specific diagnosis such as herniated disk, nerve compression by tumor

Initial Tests (lab, imaging)

None specifically for neuropathic pain but can rule in or out a possible cause: serum vitamin B_{12}, TSH, syphilis screening, fasting glucose/HbA1C, CBC, CMP, Lyme serology, HIV testing

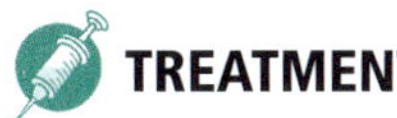

TREATMENT

GENERAL MEASURES

- Due to multiple neuropathic pain pathways, all medications have limited efficacy and minority of patients have significant benefit at tolerable doses.
- Physical and occupational therapy can help with functional goals.

MEDICATION

- The efficacy of systemic drug treatments is generally not dependent on the etiology of the underlying disorder.
- Combined therapy likely more effective than increasing dose of single medicine
- Thought to be resistant to acetaminophen and NSAIDs but often used with some benefit in treatment of acute pain (2)[C]

First Line

- Calcium channel $\alpha 2\delta$ ligands
  - Gabapentin: number needed to treat (NNT) = 7 for significant pain improvement (3)[A]
    - Dosing: up to 3,600 mg in 3 divided doses
    - Precautions: requires renal dosing
    - Common side effects: sedation, dizziness, peripheral edema, weight gain
    - Also in the form of extended release or enacarbil
  - Pregabalin NNT = 8 (3)[A]
    - Dosing: up to 600 mg in 2 doses
    - Precautions: requires renal dosing
    - Common side effects: sedation, dizziness, peripheral edema, weight gain
- Tricyclic antidepressants: NNT = 4 (3)[A]
  - Nortriptyline, desipramine, amitriptyline clomipramine, imipramine
    - Dosing: Start 10 to 25 mg at bedtime and then increase by 10 to 25 mg every 4 to 7 days up to 150 mg/day as tolerated.
    - Precautions: cardiac disease, glaucoma, prostatic adenoma, seizure, tramadol use
    - Geriatric: falls; limit dose to <75 mg.
    - Common side effects: somnolence, weight gain, anticholinergic effects, cardiac conduction block
    - Increased suicidality warning in children, adolescents, and young adults
- Serotonin norepinephrine reuptake inhibitors (SNRIs): NNT = 6 (3)[A]
  - Duloxetine
    - Dosing: 20 mg once daily to 60 mg twice daily; effective doses 60 to 120 mg daily
    - Precautions: hepatic disorder, tramadol use, hypertension
    - Common side effect: nausea, constipation; relatively the safest medication for neuropathic pain
  - Venlafaxine
    - Dosing: 37.5 mg to 225.0 mg daily
    - Effective doses: 150 to 225 mg daily
    - Precautions: cardiac disease, tramadol use, hypertension
    - Common side effects: nausea, hypertension at higher doses

Second Line

- Lidocaine, 5% patches (3)[B]
  - As effective as pregabalin for localized neuropathic pain from diabetes or herpes
  - Dosage: 1 to 3 patches for 12 hours daily to cover the painful area
  - Common side effects: local erythema, itch, rash
- Capsaicin high-concentration patches (8%): NNT = 11 (3)[A]
  - Dosing: 1 to 4 patches to cover the painful area; 30 minutes application to feet, 60 minutes application to remainder of body; avoid use on face; benefits for up to 3 months
  - Common side effects: pain (initial increase), erythema, itching, rare cases of hypertension, progressive neuropathy
  - No benefit from low concentration capsaicin cream

Third Line

- Botulinum toxin type A (3)[B]
  - Limited evidence based on small studies, no quality of life improvement
    - Dosage: 50 to 200 units subcutaneously to the painful area; repeat every 3 months.
    - Common side effects: pain and infection at injection site, weakness
- Cannabinoids (dronabinol and nabilone): low quality evidence
  - NNT = 20 for 50% improvement in pain
  - Number needed to harm (NNH) = 3 for adverse events
    - NNH = 25 for withdrawal due to adverse events
- Opioids (including tramadol): no proven long-term benefit; utility for neuropathic pain questioned (4)[A]
  - Chronic opioids decrease number and sensitivity of μ-opioid receptors, increasing hyperalgesia.

ISSUES FOR REFERRAL

Refer to pain clinic if refractory to initial treatment for trial of additional therapies.

ADDITIONAL THERAPIES

- Interventional pain management (epidural or peripheral nerve injections) will provide partial, lasting relief in 40–60% of patients (1)[B].
- Spinal cord stimulation (SCS): Pain that is continuous and unchanging responds best; best evidence for failed back surgery syndrome with leg pain (1)[B]
- Intrathecal drug delivery: reserved for refractory pain; ziconotide has demonstrated efficacy (1)[B].
- Transcutaneous electrical nerve stimulation is widely used; evidence shows slight benefit (1)[B],(3)[B].
- Cognitive behavioral and mindfulness therapies have some benefit as an adjunct to other therapies, especially in postherpetic neuropathy (1)[B],(3)[B].

SURGERY/OTHER PROCEDURES

Nerve destructive procedures haven't shown effectiveness and may cause insult/injury (an exception is treatment of terminal cancer) (1)[B].

- Sympathectomy dorsal root entry zone lesion (dorsal rhizotomy)
- Lateral cordotomy
- Trigeminal nerve ganglion ablation

COMPLEMENTARY & ALTERNATIVE MEDICINE

Acupuncture: limited evidence for improvement in pain

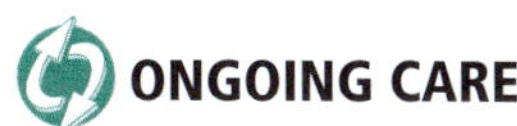

ONGOING CARE

PROGNOSIS

Chronic course of pain symptoms often requires management with numerous medications and adjunctive therapies. Pain management requires ongoing evaluation, patient education, and reassurance. Complete pain relief is rare.

COMPLICATIONS

Long-term disability and drug addiction are possible.

REFERENCES

1. Jones RCW III, Lawson E, Backonja M. Managing neuropathic pain. *Med Clin North Am*. 2016;100(1):151–167.
2. Gilron I, Baron R, Jensen T. Neuropathic pain: principles of diagnosis and treatment. *Mayo Clin Proc*. 2015;90(4):532–545.
3. Moisset X, Bouhassira D, Avez Couturier J, et al. Pharmacological and non-pharmacological treatments for neuropathic pain: systematic review and French recommendations. *Rev Neurol (Paris)*. 2020;176(5):325–352.
4. Zhang Y, Ahmed S, Vo T, et al. Increased pain sensitivity in chronic pain subjects on opioid therapy: a cross-sectional study using quantitative sensory testing. *Pain Med*. 2015;16(5):911–922.

ADDITIONAL READING

- Colloca L, Ludman T, Bouhassira D, et al. Neuropathic pain. *Nat Rev Dis Primers*. 2017;3:17002.
- Fornasari D. Pharmacotherapy for neuropathic pain: a review. *Pain Ther*. 2017;6(Suppl 1):25–33.

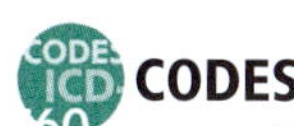

CODES

ICD10

- M79.2 Neuralgia and neuritis, unspecified
- E10.40 Type 1 diabetes mellitus with diabetic neuropathy, unsp
- E11.40 Type 2 diabetes mellitus with diabetic neuropathy, unsp

CLINICAL PEARLS

- Neuropathic pain is a common syndrome, affecting up to 10% of the population with major impacts on quality of life.
- Due to numerous mechanisms in neuropathy, potential benefit from any single treatment is limited.
- Narcotics likely have more harm than benefit; chronic use will likely increase pain.
- Functional goals and realistic pain targets are essential.

NEUROPATHY, PERIPHERAL

Christine S. Persaud, MD, MBA • Brianna K. Sarowa, MD • Anter Suarez Gonzales, MD

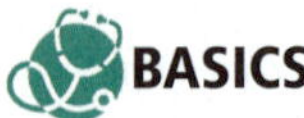

BASICS

A disease of the peripheral nervous system (PNS) that has multiple etiologies including diabetes, neurotoxic agents, alcohol use, nutrition deficiencies, immune-mediated causes, nerve compression, nerve injury, genetic mutations, and idiopathic (1).

DESCRIPTION

- A functional or structural disorder of the PNS, affecting any combination of motor, sensory, or autonomic nerves
- Peripheral motor involvement causes muscle atrophy, weakness, cramps, and fasciculations.
- Disorders of sensory nerves produce negative phenomena (loss of sensibility, lack of balance) or heightened phenomena (tingling or pain). Large sensory fiber dysfunction impairs touch and vibration sensation, whereas small fiber sensory neuropathy (SFSN) affects pin and thermal sensation and causes neuropathic pain.
- The autonomic nervous system (ANS) dysfunction causes cardiovascular, gastrointestinal, and sudomotor symptoms.
- Peripheral neuropathy (PN) can be subdivided as mononeuropathies, multifocal neuropathies, and polyneuropathies.

EPIDEMIOLOGY

- Diabetic PN is the most common cause of neuropathy globally (2).
- Approximately 50% of diabetics will develop PN (3).
- Chemotherapy-induced PN (CIPN) is a frequent side effect of chemotherapeutic agents with an estimated 30% of patients experiencing CIPN at 6 months after chemotherapy (1).

Prevalence

- Prevalence rises significantly with age, affecting up to 7–8% of people aged >55 years.
- The prevalence of diabetic PN is approximately 10–34% in type 1 diabetes and 8–25% in type 2 diabetes, prevalence increases with longer disease duration and poorer glycemic control.

ETIOLOGY AND PATHOPHYSIOLOGY

- The most common cause of acquired PN is diabetes mellitus, which manifests most commonly at approximately 75% in the pattern of a distal sensory polyneuropathy (DSP).
- Other causes include:
  - Vascular: ischemia, vasculitis
  - Infectious: HIV, hepatitis C, cryoglobulinemia, Lyme disease, varicella zoster
  - Traumatic: compression, crush, stretch, or transection (e.g., due to broken or dislocated bones, slipped disks between vertebrae, or arthritis)
  - Autoimmune: rheumatoid arthritis, Sjögren syndrome, lupus
  - Metabolic: renal failure, hypothyroidism, vitamin B_{12} deficiency, celiac disease, porphyria
  - Iatrogenic/toxic: chemotherapy, platinum, taxanes, metronidazole, colchicine, infliximab, lead, alcoholism
  - Neoplastic/paraneoplastic: paraproteinemia, Waldenström macroglobulinemia, multiple myeloma, amyloidosis, neurofibromatosis

Genetics

Approximately 50% of undiagnosed PN is hereditary.

RISK FACTORS

Diabetes and alcoholism

GENERAL PREVENTION

Management of underlying preventable causes of PN such as glycemic control, nutritional deficiencies, and avoiding neurotoxic agents.

DIAGNOSIS

Diagnosis is made by a detailed patient history, clinical symptoms, laboratory tests, and diagnostic testing of nerve conductions studies/electromyography (NCS/EMG) and possibly nerve biopsy (4).

HISTORY

- A detailed inquiry for symptoms of sensory, motor, or autonomic dysfunction:
  - Numbness, tingling, prickling, burning pain, a "tightly wrapped" sensation, and an "unsteady gait"
  - Distal weakness manifests as foot drop (tripping, foot slapping) or difficulty with grip; proximal weakness (e.g., difficulty arising from a chair) is less common.
  - Orthostatic dizziness, abnormal sweating, constipation, erectile dysfunction, or voiding difficulties
- Symptom onset:
  - Acute: Consider infection (e.g., Lyme disease), postinfectious dysimmune process (e.g., GBS), ischemia (e.g., vasculitis), toxin, or trauma.
  - Subacute: Consider metabolic, neoplastic, paraneoplastic, or dysimmune processes.
  - Chronic: Consider dysimmune process (CIDP), idiopathic, or hereditary.
- Progression: stable or indolent; slowly or rapidly progressive; monophasic or relapsing or remitting
- Anatomic pattern: focal, multifocal, diffuse
- Inquire about family history and comorbidities to help determine if condition is inherited.

PHYSICAL EXAM

- Based on exam, a functional (*sensory*: small fiber vs. large fiber vs. mixed, *sensorimotor*, *motor*, *autonomic*) and anatomic pattern of PN (*distal symmetric*, *multifocal*, or *focal*) should be established.
- Cognition is preserved in isolated PN.
- Cranial nerves may be involved with focal or multifocal PN (e.g., bifacial weakness may occur with GBS, Lyme disease, sarcoidosis, among other causes).
- Stocking/glove sensory loss is typical of distal symmetric sensory PN (e.g., diabetes).
- Isolated reduced pin or thermal sensation or allodynia suggests a pure SFSN.
- Reduced vibration and proprioception suggests large-fiber sensory neuropathy; when severe, a Romberg sign is present, and gait is wide based or ataxic.
- Distal muscle atrophy and weaknesses of toe extension and finger abduction are often present with distal symmetric axonal PN.
- In acquired demyelinating PN (e.g., GBS or CIDP), weakness is commonly both proximally and distally.
- Deep tendon reflexes may be reduced or absent, distally at the ankles in large-fiber axonal PN, or diffusely in demyelinating PN.
- High arched or flat feet or hammer toes suggest hereditary PN.

ALERT

Hyperreflexia and spasticity are upper motor neuron signs not seen with isolated PN.

DIFFERENTIAL DIAGNOSIS

- Mononeuropathy most likely due to compression, entrapment, or trauma
- Mononeuropathy multiplex (plexopathy, polyradiculopathy)

DIAGNOSTIC TESTS & INTERPRETATION

Initial Tests (lab, imaging)

- CBC, Cr, HbA1C, vitamin B_{12} with methylmalonic acid, LFTs, serum protein immunofixation electrophoresis, TSH
- NCS (the gold standard for the diagnosis of diabetic painful neuropathy [DPN]) (5) and EMG delineate axonal versus demyelinating, anatomic pattern, chronicity, and severity of PN.
- Autonomic reflex screen, testing of sweat function, quantitative sensory testing, and epidermal skin biopsy to evaluate small nerve fiber function (6)
- Specialized epidermal skin biopsy if suspected SFN and NCS/EMG is normal.
- Neuroimaging generally not indicated in evaluation of PN but useful in evaluation of brachial plexopathies, radiculopathies, or where findings are attributable to the CNS.

Follow-Up Tests & Special Considerations

- Based on the medical history, the PN type, and NCS/EMG findings; such as vitamins A, D, and E; zinc, copper, ESR, CRP, ANA, hepatitis B/C; antitissue transglutaminase
- Screen for alcohol use with distal symmetric PN.

Diagnostic Procedures/Other

Nerve biopsy (sural or superficial peroneal nerve): useful if vasculitis, amyloidosis, granulomatous disorders, or neoplastic infiltration is suspected; rarely helpful in late-onset chronic, slowly progressive distal symmetric PN

Test Interpretation

- Demyelinating PN: disproportionate slowing of conduction velocities, conduction block, increased temporal dispersion, or prolonged distal latencies on NCS; EMG findings including decreased recruitment and myokymia
- Axonal PN: reduced amplitude in sensory or motor responses, with relatively preserved conduction velocities and distal latency on NCS; EMG findings include abnormal spontaneous activity, decreased recruitment, increased duration and amplitude, and polyphasicity.
- Reduced ENFD on distal leg skin biopsies is supportive of SFN.

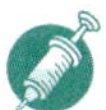

TREATMENT

GENERAL MEASURES

- Counsel on foot care and monitoring for signs of skin breakdown.
- Targeted treatment for underlying systemic conditions
- For diabetic PN, improved glucose control reduces risk of developing and reducing PN, especially in type 1 diabetes mellitus
- Lifestyle interventions, including exercise and weight loss, improves nerve function, nerve regeneration, and quality of life (7)

MEDICATION

First Line

Treatment of neuropathic pain: evidence of efficacy derived from clinical trials in diabetic painful neuropathy (DPN), postherpetic neuralgia (PHN), or trigeminal neuralgia:

- Anticonvulsants: gabapentin, for PHN; pregabalin, for DPN and PHN, gabapentin (off-label), for DPN; oxcarbazepine for DPN; carbamazepine, for trigeminal neuralgia
- SNRI: duloxetine or venlafaxine for DPN
- Tricyclic antidepressants (TCA): amitriptyline or nortriptyline
- Patches: lidocaine 5%, capsaicin 8%
- Supplements: α-lipoic acid, acetyl-L-carnitine

Second Line

Mexiletine

Third Line

Tapentadol: for DPN

ISSUES FOR REFERRAL

- Neurology for rapidly progressive symptoms
- Rheumatology for vasculitic PN
- Hematology/skeletal survey for paraproteinemia
- Physical therapy for gait and balance training

ADDITIONAL THERAPIES

- Combination therapy (e.g., gabapentin with TCA or venlafaxine or tramadol) can be more effective than monotherapy for neuropathic pain.
- Botulinum toxin subcutaneous, intradermal, or direct nerve injections can be considered for trigeminal neuralgia, DPN, or complex regional pain syndrome (CRPS) (8)[A].
- Additional immunosuppressant agents (e.g., cyclophosphamide) may be used in refractory chronic dysimmune PN.
- Treatment of autonomic symptoms
  - Compression stockings, abdominal binder, hydration, midodrine, and fludrocortisone for orthostatic hypotension
  - Pyridostigmine for immune-mediated dysautonomia (off-label)

SURGERY/OTHER PROCEDURES

Decompressive surgery for entrapment neuropathy (e.g., carpal tunnel syndrome) syndrome

COMPLEMENTARY & ALTERNATIVE MEDICINE

Low-intensity transcutaneous electrical nerve stimulation (TENS), acupuncture, meditation, supplements (G-agmatine, methylcobalamin, inositol) may be helpful.

ALERT

Vitamin B_6 supplementation may cause peripheral neurotoxicity and should be avoided except for a deficiency state.

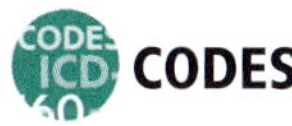

ONGOING CARE

For diabetic patients, PN is a sign of poor glycemic control and increased risk of diabetic complications; patients should follow up more frequently.

FOLLOW-UP RECOMMENDATIONS

- Exercises to improve muscle strength
- Avoid flu vaccination the first year following GBS.

DIET

Assess for vitamin B_{12} deficiency, ingestion of heavy metal toxins, thiamine deficiency in those with alcohol use disorder, and high carbohydrate intake for those with diabetes.

PATIENT EDUCATION

Seek care for any foot injury, maintain foot care, follow up with podiatrist regularly.

PROGNOSIS

- Late-onset idiopathic distal symmetric axonal PNs are indolent.
- 80% of GBS have a near complete or good recovery. 80% of CIDP have moderate or good response with treatment but can be relapsing.
- In diabetes, PN is a marker of systemic microvascular disease, increases cardiovascular risk and mortality.

COMPLICATIONS

PN can lead to foot ulcers, infections, increased fall risk, chronic pain, autonomic dysfunction, and increased cardiovascular and mortality risk.

REFERENCES

1. Zajączkowska R, Kocot-Kępska M, Leppert W, et al. Mechanisms of chemotherapy-induced peripheral neuropathy. *Int J Mol Sci*. 2019;20(6):1451. doi:10.3390/ijms20061451.
2. Iqbal Z, Azmi S, Yadav R, et al. Diabetic peripheral neuropathy: epidemiology, diagnosis, and pharmacotherapy. *Clin Ther*. 2018;40(6):828–849. doi:10.1016/j.clinthera.2018.04.001.
3. Hicks CW, Selvin E. Epidemiology of peripheral neuropathy and lower extremity disease in diabetes. *Curr Diab Rep*. 2019;19(10):86. doi:10.1007/s11892-019-1212-8.
4. Castelli G, Desai KM, Cantone RE. Peripheral neuropathy: evaluation and differential diagnosis. *Am Fam Physician*. 2020;102(12):732–739.
5. Selvarajah D, Kar D, Khunti K, et al. Diabetic peripheral neuropathy: advances in diagnosis and strategies for screening and early intervention. *Lancet Diabetes Endocrinol*. 2019;7(12):938–948.
6. Barrell K, Smith AG. Peripheral neuropathy. *Med Clin North Am*. 2019;103(2):383–397.
7. Look AHEAD Research Group. Effects of a long-term lifestyle modification programme on peripheral neuropathy in overweight or obese adults with type 2 diabetes: the Look AHEAD study. *Diabetologia*. 2017;60(6):980–988.
8. Park J, Park HJ. Botulinum toxin for the treatment of neuropathic pain. *Toxins (Basel)*. 2017;9(9):260.

CODES

ICD10

- G62.9 Polyneuropathy, unspecified
- G60.9 Hereditary and idiopathic neuropathy, unspecified
- G60.8 Other hereditary and idiopathic neuropathies

CLINICAL PEARLS

- Diagnosis is made by history and physical exam, targeted laboratory testing, NCS/EMG, skin biopsy, or ANS testing.
- Consider hereditary neuropathy if patient has an early age of PN symptom onset, family history of PN, or foot deformity.
- GBS is monophasic and progresses for up to 4 weeks; CIDP progresses beyond 8 weeks, and if untreated, usually has a progressive course.
- Distal symmetric polyneuropathy ("stocking-glove pattern") is the most common form of PN in diabetes.
- PN in diabetes is an independent marker of increased cardiovascular disease and significantly higher mortality risk.

NICOTINE ADDICTION

Jason I. Dailey, MD • Erik K. Hunsaker, MD

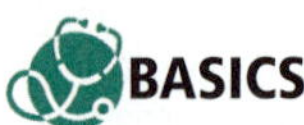

BASICS

DESCRIPTION

Nicotine addiction is characterized by the compulsive use of nicotine products coupled with a lack of control over using, withdrawal symptoms, and/or continued use despite knowledge of or experiencing adverse consequences.

EPIDEMIOLOGY

Prevalence

- Among people aged 12 or older in 2020, 8.5% (or about 23.6 million people) had nicotine dependence in the past 30 days. 22% (or about 61.6 million people) reported using tobacco products or vaping nicotine in the past 30 days.
- 15.6% (or about 43.6 million people) reported smoking cigarettes in the past 30 days. An estimated 8.7% of 8th graders, 15.1% of 10th graders, and 24.8% of 12th graders. 4.7% (or about 13.2 million people) reported vaping nicotine in the past 30 days.

ETIOLOGY AND PATHOPHYSIOLOGY

- Similar to other addictive drugs, nicotine affects neural pathways that control reward and pleasure.
- Nicotine exerts its biologic effects through nicotinic acetylcholine receptors (nAChRs), which modulate neurotransmission with acetylcholine and other chemical messengers including glutamate, GABA, dopamine, serotonin, acetylcholine, and norepinephrine. In this way, it induces euphoria, assists in information processing, reduces anxiety, and mitigates fatigue.
- Upregulation of these receptors occurs over time, leading to tolerance and dependence.
- Polymorphisms in neuronal nAChR genes are associated with increased susceptibility to dependence.
- Nicotine is metabolized by cytochrome P450 2A6 (CYP2A6). Individuals who are fast metabolizers tend to smoke more cigarettes, are more likely to suffer intense withdrawal symptoms, and have a lower probability of quitting than slow metabolizers.
- Nicotine withdrawal involves the release of corticotropin-releasing factor in the amygdala, which induces the perception of anxiety and stress.

Pregnancy Considerations

- Smoking is a risk factor associated with placenta previa, abruptio placentae, decreased maternal thyroid function, preterm premature rupture of membranes, and ectopic pregnancy.
- Carbon monoxide and nicotine interfere with fetal oxygen supply, resulting in decreased birth weights and intrauterine growth restriction.
- Maternal smoking adversely affects fetal lung development, with lifelong decreases in pulmonary function and increased risk of asthma.
- Maternal smoking is associated with increased risk for sudden infant death syndrome, learning and behavioral problems, and obesity.

RISK FACTORS

- Mental illness (depression, posttraumatic stress disorder, bipolar disorder, and schizophrenia)
- Low socioeconomic status, low educational status
- Early firsthand nicotine experience, home and peer influence
- Concurrent substance abuse

GENERAL PREVENTION

- The U.S. Preventive Services Task Force (USPSTF) recommends the following:
  - Screening all adults for tobacco use, providing cessation interventions for those who screen positive
  - Screening all pregnant women for tobacco use and providing pregnancy-tailored counseling to those who screen positive
- The USPSTF recommends that clinicians provide interventions, including education or brief counseling to prevent initiation of tobacco use among school-age children and adolescents.

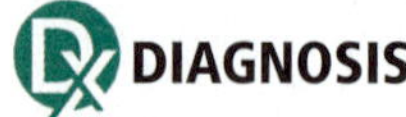

DIAGNOSIS

HISTORY

- Identify types, amount, and duration of nicotine products used.
- Review previous attempts to quit (methods used and duration of cessation).

PHYSICAL EXAM

- Pulmonary exam: wheezing, decreased breath sounds, prolonged expiration
- Cardiovascular exam: tachycardia, hypertension
- HEENT exam: epithelial dysplasia, squamous cell carcinoma, leukoplakia, stained teeth, hoarseness
- Skin exam: In combustible tobacco users, yellow-brown staining of the digits, "Harlequin nail" (bicolor nail seen after acute illness cause cessation of tobacco consumption, as unstained nail bed grows in), and clubbing may be seen.

DIAGNOSTIC TESTS & INTERPRETATION

- Lung cancer screening with low-dose CT is recommended annually by USPSTF for patients between 50 and 80 years old with a history of >20 pack-years of tobacco use who are currently smoking or have quit within the past 15 years (except those with life-limiting comorbidities).
- Neither spirometry nor regular chest x-rays are recommended for routine screening.

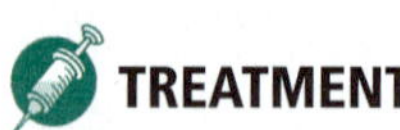

TREATMENT

GENERAL MEASURES

- American Society of Addiction Medicine (ASAM) recommends the following (1)[C]:
  - Screen all patients for nicotine/tobacco use disorder.
  - Offer evidence-based treatment to all patients.
  - Use motivational and harm reduction strategies for patients ambivalent about quitting.
- Brief strategies to help the patient willing to quit tobacco—use the "5 As":
  - Ask patient if he/she/they use nicotine.
  - Advise to quit.
  - Assess willingness to make a quit attempt.
  - Assist those willing to make a quit attempt.
  - Arrange follow-up contact to prevent relapse.
- Patients should be given a choice of methods to quit as this is shown to improve treatment compliance.

MEDICATION

- There are currently seven FDA-approved medications: nicotine replacement therapy (NRT), both long-acting (i.e., patch) and short-acting (i.e., gum, inhaler, lozenge, nasal spray) types, and non-NRT meds, bupropion SR and varenicline.
- The choice of a first-line medication depends on patient preference, though varenicline (NNT 11) may be more efficacious than bupropion (NNT 13) or NRT alone (NNT 15).
- Duration of nicotine pharmacotherapy is strongly recommended to be >12 weeks.
- Varenicline is a nicotinic acetylcholine partial agonist. It is probably the single most effective pharmacologic intervention for smoking cessation.
  - Neuropsychiatric symptoms: varenicline and bupropion previously had a black box warning for neuropsychiatric side effects; however, this warning was removed in December 2016 after further research demonstrated no elevated risk of neuropsychiatric side effects over placebo (2).
  - Initiation: Start 1 week before target quit date due to time needed to reach steady state.
    - Starter pack: 0.5 mg/day for 3 days, 0.5 mg BID for 4 days, 1 mg/day starting day 7
    - Maintenance pack of 1 mg BID for 12 weeks; if successful, may continue for another 12 weeks
  - Varenicline + bupropion is not more effective than either alone and confers increased side effects.
- Bupropion SR is an atypical antidepressant and norepinephrine-dopamine reuptake inhibitor. Contraindications: history of seizure, stroke, brain injury, brain tumors, anorexia/bulimia, recent use of MAOI (within 14 days).
  - Use 150 mg/day for 3 days and then 150 mg BID for 7 to 12 weeks.
  - Start 1 week before target quit date due to time needed to reach steady state.
- NRT:
  - Patch: For <10 cigarettes per day or <2 cans per pouches of smokeless tobacco, start with 14 mg/day for 6 weeks; for 10 to 29 cigarettes per day or 2 to 3 cans per pouches of tobacco, start 21 mg/day for 6 weeks; for 30 to 39 cigarettes per day or >3 pouches per cans of tobacco, start 35 mg (21 mg/day + 14 mg/day patch) for 4 weeks; for >40 cigarettes per day, start 42 mg (21 mg/day patch for 2 weeks) for 4 weeks. Titrate to patient symptoms; extending use of the patch beyond 12 weeks may improve abstinence rates.

- Gum: For >25 cigarettes per day, start 4 mg gum q1–2h for 6 weeks; for <25 cigarettes per day, start 2 mg gum q1–2h; then double dosing interval every 3 weeks (i.e., q2–4h and then q4–8h). Chew then tuck between cheek and gingiva once nicotine flavor is released, repeat for up to 30 minutes and then discard. Avoid using with acidic foods (i.e., coffee, soda), which decrease nicotine absorption.
- Lozenges: For patients who smoke their first cigarette within 30 minutes of waking, start 4 mg lozenge PO q1–2h for 6 weeks; if first cigarette >30 minutes after waking, start 2 mg lozenge PO q1–2h for 6 weeks; then double dosing interval every 3 weeks (i.e., q2–4h and then q4–8h).
- Nasal spray: Start 1 to 2 sprays (0.5 mg per spray) each nostril q1h for 8 weeks and then taper; max 10 sprays per hour and 80 sprays per day
- Inhaler: 6 to 16 cartridges inhaled (4 mg per cartridge) per day for 6 to 12 weeks and then taper; incorporates the behavioral and sensory aspects of smoking

- Combination NRT:
  - Using a combination of nicotine replacement + varenicline or bupropion may improve outcomes over monotherapy.
  - All forms of NRT increase quit rate 50–70%. Combining long-acting maintenance with short-acting breakthrough NRTs is more effective than using any single method alone. If combining patch with lozenge or gum, limit to one to three 2 mg. Avoid combined NRT use for patients with serious arrhythmias, unstable angina, MI within the prior 2 weeks, or those aged <18 years.
- E-cigarette is an electronic device that delivers aerosolized liquid with or without nicotine and includes various flavorings and other chemicals. Insufficient evidence exists regarding this product's safety and efficacy. Low-quality evidence suggests that e-cigarettes can help patients cut down on the number of cigarettes smoked but not nicotine consumption. Other research demonstrates poor efficacy of abstinence with long-term follow-up. Long-term safety has not been established.

Pregnancy Considerations

- Tobacco cessation prior to 15 weeks' gestation provides the greatest benefit for both the woman and fetus, but quitting any time is beneficial.
- Pregnant and breastfeeding women should be considered for NRT when the fetal risk of continued smoking is greater than the risk of NRT. Medications should be reserved for patients needing additional assistance due to limited safety data.
- NRT is metabolized faster in pregnant women, which may lead to higher dose requirements.
- Pregnant women may perceive e-cigarettes to be safer than conventional cigarettes; however, given limited evidence regarding this NRT and concerns regarding fetal nicotine exposure, e-cigarettes are not recommended in pregnancy.

Pediatric Considerations

- Behavioral therapy (including CBT) is recommended as first-line treatment. There is evidence that group counseling is superior to individual counseling and group messaging for tobacco cessation in youth. There are currently no FDA-approved pharmacologic treatments for youth. AAP recommends using NRT only for youth with moderate to severe substance use disorder.
- Risk of long-term addiction is much higher when smoking is initiated in adolescence than later in life, likely reflecting changes induced by nicotine in the developing brain. The biology of addiction, including withdrawal, occurs with fewer daily cigarettes in teens than in adults. Explanation of these biologic factors may help adolescents to stop or defer smoking.
- E-cigarette use in adolescents is reliably associated with subsequent smoking. An intervention to reduce smoking initiation was found to reduce the likelihood of ever smoking, suggesting there is a role for interventions to reduce smoking initiation even in adolescents who use e-cigarettes.

COMPLEMENTARY & ALTERNATIVE MEDICINE

No consistent evidence of efficacy for either Acupuncture or hypnotherapy

ADMISSION, INPATIENT, AND NURSING CONSIDERATIONS

- Consider NRT for inpatients who use nicotine to decrease withdrawal symptoms (use with caution in patients with unstable angina, serious arrhythmias, or MI within the previous 2 weeks).
- Bupropion may not adequately control acute withdrawal symptoms.

ONGOING CARE

FOLLOW-UP RECOMMENDATIONS

- Patients who have initiated therapy should follow up after 1 to 2 weeks to monitor response and side effects.
- Monitor for signs of nicotine withdrawal syndrome and start medication-assisted treatment or adjust dosage:
  - Increased appetite/weight gain (4 to 5 kg over 10 weeks)
  - Dysphoric, depressed mood, or anhedonia; insomnia, irritability, frustration, or anger, anxiety
  - Difficulty concentrating, restlessness
- Follow-up should continue periodically in person or via telephone, especially during the first 3 months.
- Pharmacotherapy is generally recommended for 3 months duration.

PATIENT EDUCATION

- Smokefree: https://smokefree.gov/; 1-800-QUIT-NOW (1-800-784-8669)
- BecomeAnEx: https://www.becomeanex.org/
- Text Messaging Support—National Texting Portal; text "QUITNOW" to 333888
- Tobacco Education Resource Library (resources include smoking cessation education posters and interactive games): https://digitalmedia.hhs.gov/tobacco/
- Freedom From Smoking Program (sponsored by the American Lung Association) (one of the most effective cessation programs in the country, available in various options to help individuals quit smoking): https://www.lung.org/quit-smoking/
- quitSTART (application and other phone apps): https://smokefree.gov/tools-tips/quitstart

PROGNOSIS

- Roughly 50% of all smokers will die from a tobacco-related illness.
- Former smokers have a 50% reduction in risk of CAD 1 year after quitting, a 50% reduction in head and neck cancers by 2 to 5 years, and a 50% reduction in lung cancer mortality by 10 years. The risk of stroke is reduced to that of nonsmokers 2 to 5 years after quitting.
- 22% of smokers relapse within 3 months of quitting. Multiple attempts are usually required.
- Individuals receiving support from significant others are more likely to quit.

COMPLICATIONS

- Chronic obstructive pulmonary disease (COPD) (emphysema and chronic bronchitis)
- Cancers (i.e., lung, oral/pharyngeal, kidney, bladder, cervical, anal, squamous cell)
- Atherosclerotic disease, peptic ulcer disease, periodontal disease
- Osteoporosis and hip fracture (in women), delayed wound healing

REFERENCES

1. ASAM Quality Improvement Council. Integrating tobacco use disorder interventions in addiction treatment: a guide for addiction treatment and clinicians program. American Society of Addiction Medicine. https://www.asam.org/quality-care/clinical-recommendations/tobacco. Accessed October 18, 2024.
2. Anthenelli RM, Benowitz NL, West R, et al. Neuropsychiatric safety and efficacy of varenicline, bupropion, and nicotine patch in smokers with and without psychiatric disorders (EAGLES): a double-blind, randomised, placebo-controlled clinical trial. *Lancet*. 2016;387(10037):2507–2520. doi:10.1016/S0140-6736(16)30272-0.

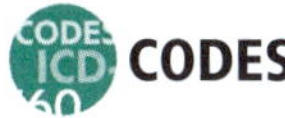

CODES

ICD10

- F17.200 Nicotine dependence, unspecified, uncomplicated
- F17.201 Nicotine dependence, unspecified, in remission
- F17.203 Nicotine dependence unspecified, with withdrawal

CLINICAL PEARLS

- Nicotine dependence is a chronic disease and will often require repeated interventions and multiple cessation attempts.
- Varenicline may be more efficacious than bupropion or NRT alone, though the choice should be based on patient preference and risk factors for side effects.

NONFATAL DROWNING

Nergess T. Taheri, DO, MSBI

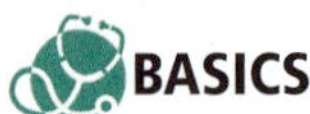

BASICS

DESCRIPTION

Respiratory impairment resulting from submersion or immersion in liquid; a drowning event in which the process of respiratory impairment is stopped before death and the victim survives

EPIDEMIOLOGY

Incidence

- From 2011 to 2020, an average of 4,012 fatal unintentional drownings and an average of 8,061 emergency room (ER) visits due to nonfatal drowning occurred each year in the United States (1)
- Three age-related peaks: toddlers and young children (1 to 5 years old), adolescents and young adults (15 to 25 years old), and the elderly
- Nearly 80% of people who die from drowning are male (1).
- In swimming pools, black children aged 10 to 14 years drown at rates 7.6 times higher than white children, whereas in natural water, American Indian or Alaska Native children drown at rates 2.7 times higher than white children (1).

Prevalence

- Most common injury-related cause of death for children aged 1 to 4 years in the United States (2)
- Second most common injury-related cause of death for children aged 5 to 14 years in the United States after motor vehicle crashes (1)
- For every child aged $<$18 years who dies from drowning, seven more children are seen in the ER for nonfatal submersion injuries (1).

ALERT

Proper water supervision and safety techniques are critical in avoiding morbidity and mortality from drowning.

ETIOLOGY AND PATHOPHYSIOLOGY

Hypoxemia via aspiration and/or reflex laryngospasm causing cerebral hypoxia and multisystem organ dysfunction

- 10–20% of victims drown without aspiration, likely due to prolonged laryngospasm; bathtub and bucket drowning in children aged $<$1 year; swimming pool drowning in children and young adults; motor vehicle accidents (vehicle submerged in water); head trauma while swimming or diving
- Pulmonary: morbidity primarily caused by hypoxia; aspiration of 1 to 3 mL/kg of liquid causes dilution of surfactant with decreased gas transfer across alveoli, atelectasis, development of intrapulmonary right-to-left shunting; acute respiratory distress syndrome (ARDS); obstruction due to laryngospasm and bronchospasm (2)
- Cardiac: hypoxic-ischemic injury and arrhythmia (primary or secondary); renal: acute tubular necrosis from hypoxemia, shock, hemoglobinuria, myoglobinuria
- Neurologic: hypoxic-ischemic brain injury with damage especially to the hippocampus, insular cortex, and basal ganglia; cerebral edema and increased intracranial pressure
- Coagulation: hemolysis and coagulopathy

RISK FACTORS

- Inadequate physical barriers surrounding pools, alcohol ingestion, male sex, low socioeconomic status
- Use of illicit drugs, seizure disorder, inability to swim or overestimation of swimming capabilities, hyperventilation prior to underwater swimming
- Boating mishaps and trauma during water sports, particularly when not wearing a life jacket; scuba diving
- Inadequate adult supervision of children, lack of appropriate instruction on how to swim, concomitant stroke or myocardial infarction (MI), hypothermia
- Cardiac arrhythmias: familial long QT and polymorphic ventricular tachycardia (VT)

GENERAL PREVENTION

- Periodic education regarding proper supervision and drowning prevention for caretakers of young children; proper adult supervision of children, particularly around water; pool alarms, buddy system; knowledge of water safety guidelines
- Mandatory physical barriers surrounding pools; four-sided fencing; self-closing gate at least 48 inches above the ground (1)
- Avoid alcohol or recreational drugs around water; swimming instruction at an early age; cardiopulmonary resuscitation (CPR) instruction for pool owners and parents; boating safety knowledge; personal flotation device and rescue equipment (e.g., preserver, if necessary)

Pediatric Considerations

Children should never be left alone near water. Young children can drown in very small amounts of water (bathtubs, buckets of water, and toilets).

COMMONLY ASSOCIATED CONDITIONS

- Trauma, seizure disorder, alcohol or illicit drug use
- Hypothermia, concomitant stroke or MI, cardiac arrhythmias: familial long QT and familial polymorphic VT, hyperventilation
- Pneumonia, hypotension

DIAGNOSIS

HISTORY

The Revised Utstein-style approach provides a standardized template for evaluating drowning incidents and provides guidance for the history, physical exam, and appropriate management by categorizing information into core (considered important and feasible to be reported in most systems worldwide) and supplemental data:

- Victim information core data: (i) victim identifier—unique number or code; (ii) sex; (iii) age; (iv) incident date and time of day; (v) precipitating event; (vi) Was the face submerged at any time before or at the time of rescue? (vii) preexisting illness; supplemental: (viii) race/ethnicity
- Scene information core data: (i) water temperature; (ii) Who witnessed the drowning? (iii) Was bystander (non-EMS) CPR performed? (iv) Was bystander ventilation given? (v) Did a trained first responder perform CPR or ventilation only? (vi) vital status at first trained responder assessment: Was the victim responsive? Breathing normally? Pulse palpable? (vii) initial cardiac rhythm; supplementary data: (viii) vital signs at first EMS assessment; (ix) pulmonary status at first EMS assessment; (x) type of water/liquid; (xi) body of water
- Time points and intervals from EMS core data: (i) time face was first seen to be underwater; (ii) time victim was removed from water; (iii) duration underwater (submersion duration); (iv) time of first trained responder treatment; (v) time trained responder started CPR on scene; (vi) time return of spontaneous circulation achieved; (vii) time first conscious/awake; (viii) interval from face first submerged to first treatment/CPR

PHYSICAL EXAM

- Airway status and degree of respiratory distress
- Pulse: absent, weak, or normal; vital signs, including pulse oximetry
- Pulmonary: rales, wheezing; cardiac: rate, rhythm; neurologic examination

DIFFERENTIAL DIAGNOSIS

Syncopal event, head trauma, arrhythmia, seizure, MI, stroke, alcohol or other substance overdose, nonaccidental trauma

DIAGNOSTIC TESTS & INTERPRETATION

Initial Tests (lab, imaging)

- Primary focus starts with the respiratory system, get pulse oximetry and arterial blood gas (ABG). Further testing will be unnecessary if GCS and pulse oximetry are normal (and remain so for 6 to 8 hours).
- Otherwise consider:
  - CBC with differential. ABG: hypoxia, hypercarbia, acidosis
  - Electrolytes: hypokalemia, hyponatremia, hypernatremia; blood glucose: increased levels may impair neurologic recovery after ischemic brain injury; BUN, creatinine: acute tubular necrosis
  - ECG, cardiac monitoring, and serial troponin: MI; creatine kinase (CK) and urine myoglobin: rhabdomyolysis; coagulation studies: coagulopathy
  - Toxicology screen; blood alcohol level
  - Chest x-ray (CXR) unnecessary if:
    - Normal initial GCS and pulse oximetry; no evidence of respiratory distress; no change after 4 to 6 hours of observation
  - CXR may show evidence of aspiration, atelectasis, pneumothorax, or ARDS in more severe cases.
  - Head CT and/or C-spine imaging for trauma

Follow-Up Tests & Special Considerations

- Observe patients with an initial GCS of 15 and pulse oximetry $>$95% for 4 to 6 hours in the emergency department (ED). Four factors predicted safe discharge: normal mentation, normal respiratory rate, absence of dyspnea, and hypotension (3).
- CXR findings may be minimal or absent early on.

Diagnostic Procedures/Other

Continuous cardiac monitoring and pulse oximetry; continuous core temperature monitoring if hypothermic; 12-lead ECG; central venous pressure (CVP) monitoring for critically ill with hypotension refractory to IV fluids; electroencephalogram (EEG) if seizure suspected

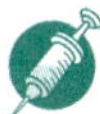

TREATMENT

Early resuscitation and reversal of hypoxemia/acidosis are key.

GENERAL MEASURES

- Prehospital
  - Never approach a struggling victim alone. Initiate basic life support (BLS) and advanced cardiovascular life support (ACLS) evaluation. Rescue breathing may be helpful if the victim is in the water and cannot be removed; chest compressions not as effective while in the water and may harm the rescuer and the victim
  - Remove the victim from the water and begin effective resuscitation as quickly as possible. Immediate CPR (airway, breathing, and circulation [ABC] sequence)
  - Start CPR if pulse is not definitely felt within 10 seconds, even in the hypothermic victim whose heart rate may be severely bradycardic. Routine cervical collar use and spinal precautions are not needed unless trauma is suspected; supplemental oxygen and early intubation with mechanical ventilation, if needed
  - Rapid crystalloid infusion if there is hypotension that is not corrected by oxygenation
  - Ventricular fibrillation is rare in drowning, but if an AED is available, use during the initial resuscitation phase; AED use is not contraindicated in a wet environment (3). If patient is breathing on his or her own and does not need spinal precautions, consider placing in the right lateral decubitus position to prevent aspiration of vomit or gastric contents. Evacuate patients with abnormal lung sounds, severe cough, frothy sputum, foamy material in the airway, depressed mentation, or hypotension to advanced medical care (3).
  - An asymptomatic patient with normal lung exam can be considered for release from the scene if another person can be with them for the next 4 to 6 hours for symptom monitoring (3).
- ED
  - Oxygen, as needed, to maintain saturation between 92% and 96%
  - Continuous positive airway pressure (CPAP), bilevel positive airway pressure (BiPAP), or intubation if supplemental oxygen alone is inadequate
  - If intubation is indicated, employ lung-protective ventilator settings (lower end-inspiratory airway pressures, lower tidal volumes of 6 mL/kg, higher positive end-expiratory pressures of 6 to 12 cm H_2O) to avoid barotrauma.
  - Indications for intubation
    - Neurologic deterioration; inability to protect the airway; inability to maintain oxygen saturation >90% or PaO_2 >60 mm Hg on high-flow supplemental oxygen; $PaCO_2$ >50 mm Hg
  - Remove wet clothing and initiate rewarming.
  - Obtain core temperature to rule out hypothermia.
  - If hypothermic, rewarm with minimally invasive core techniques such as warm IV fluids, warm/humidified oxygen, and external blanketing.
  - Active core rewarming only for refractory cases

MEDICATION

First Line

- High-flow oxygen, as needed
- For bronchospasm: aerosolized bronchodilator (2)[C]: albuterol (Proventil, Ventolin), 3 mL of 0.083% solution or 0.5 mL of 0.5% solution diluted in 3 mL of saline
- Vasopressors, as needed, for hypotension refractory to IV fluid resuscitation
- Prophylactic antibiotics are not recommended.

Second Line

For pneumonia: antibiotics based on sputum or endotracheal lavage culture

ADMISSION, INPATIENT, AND NURSING CONSIDERATIONS

- Admit all symptomatic patients or patients with abnormal vital signs, mental status, oxygenation, CXR, or laboratory analysis.
- Monitor vital signs and reassess neurologic status, continuous cardiac, and pulse oximetry monitoring.
- After initial resuscitation, induce hypothermia with core temperature maintained between 32°C and 34°C for 24 hours; may be neuroprotective for patients that remain comatose or have neurologic deterioration
- Patients can be discharged from the ED after 4 to 6 hours if they have a normal mental status and respiratory function with no further deterioration (3).

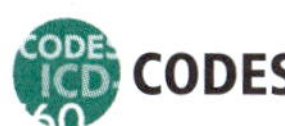

ONGOING CARE

FOLLOW-UP RECOMMENDATIONS

Appropriate follow-up with primary care provider, orthopedic, neurologic, cardiac, pulmonary, and additional specialists as indicated

Patient Monitoring

- ABG monitoring, as indicated
- A pulmonary artery catheter may be needed for hemodynamic monitoring in unstable patients (2)[C].
- Intracranial pressure monitoring in selected patients (2)[C]
- Serum electrolyte determinations

DIET

NPO until mental status normalizes

PATIENT EDUCATION

Reemphasize preventive measures on discharge from hospital and educate parents regarding supervision and preventive practices.

PROGNOSIS

- 75% of drowning victims survive; 6% will have residual neurologic deficits.
- Patients with an initial GCS ≥13 and an oxygen saturation ≥95% have a low risk of complications and an excellent chance for a full recovery.
- Patients who are comatose or receiving CPR at the time of presentation and those who have dilated and fixed pupils and no spontaneous respiratory activity have a poor prognosis.
- Neurogenic pulmonary edema may occur within 48 hours of initial presentation.

COMPLICATIONS

- Early
  - Bronchospasm, vomiting, aspiration
  - Hypoglycemia, hypothermia, seizures
  - Hypovolemia, electrolyte abnormalities
  - Arrhythmia from hypoxia or hypothermia (rarely from electrolyte imbalance)
  - Hypotension
- Late
  - ARDS, pneumonia, lung abscess, empyema
  - Anoxic encephalopathy, barotrauma, seizure
  - Renal failure, coagulopathy, sepsis

REFERENCES

1. Girasek DC, Hargarten S. Prevention of and emergency response to drowning. *N Engl J Med*. 2022;387(14):1303–1308.
2. Mott TF, Latimer KM. Prevention and treatment of drowning. *Am Fam Physician*. 2016;93(7):576–582.
3. Schmidt AC, Sempsrott JR, Hawkins SC, et al. Wilderness Medical Society clinical practice guidelines for the treatment and prevention of drowning: 2019 update. *Wilderness Environ Med*. 2019;30(4S):S70–S86.

ADDITIONAL READING

Peri F, De Nardi L, Canuto A, et al. Drowning in children and predictive parameters: a 15-year multicenter retrospective analysis. *Pediatr Emerg Care*. 2023;39(7):516–523.

CODES

ICD10

- T75.1XXA Unsp effects of drowning and nonfatal submersion, init
- T75.1XXD Unsp effects of drowning and nonfatal submersion, subs
- T75.1XXS Unsp effects of drowning and nonfatal submersion, sequel

CLINICAL PEARLS

- The most important treatment for near-drowning victims is prompt reversal of hypoxia.
- Water safety education (physical and behavioral modifications) helps prevent drowning.
- Encourage pool owners and parents with young children to become CPR certified.
- Patients remain at risk for ARDS for hours after submersion. All resuscitated patients require careful monitoring.
- Use lung-protective ventilator settings for intubated patients to prevent barotrauma.
- Patients with an initial GCS ≥13 and an oxygen saturation ≥95% have a low risk of complications and an excellent chance for a full recovery.

OBESITY

Vicente T. San Martin, MD • Nicole Baldera-Rodriguez, MD

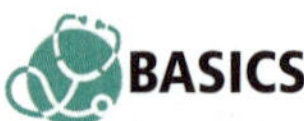

BASICS

DESCRIPTION

- A complex, multifactorial, chronic disease characterized by excess or dysfunctional adipose tissue that impairs health
- Obesity is categorized as (1):
  - Preclinical: excess adiposity with preserved organ function, associated with increased risk of clinical obesity and related diseases (e.g., type 2 diabetes, cardiovascular disease [CVD])
  - Clinical: excess adiposity with organ dysfunction (e.g., hypertension [HTN], sleep apnea) or significant limitations in daily living
- Traditionally quantified using body mass index (BMI) (BMI ≥30 kg/m^2), although BMI should not be used as a sole criterion for diagnosis:
  - Overweight: 25.0 to 29.9 kg/m^2
  - Class 1 obesity: 30.0 to 34.9 kg/m^2
  - Class 2 obesity: 35.0 to 39.9 kg/m^2
  - Class 3 obesity (severe obesity): ≥40 kg/m^2

EPIDEMIOLOGY

Incidence

Obesity rises in the early 20s and peaks at 40 to 59 years old.

Prevalence

- Obesity affects 40.3% of the U.S. population (National Health and Nutrition Examination Survey [NHANES]), with similar rates in men (39.2%) and women (41.3%).
- Severe obesity (BMI ≥40) affects 9.4%, more common in women across all age groups.
- In children and adolescents (ages 2 to 19 years), prevalence is 19.7%, increasing with age and peaking in adolescence.

Pediatric Considerations

- The United States Preventive Services Task Force (USPSTF) recommends obesity screening in children ≥6 years old, with referral to intensive behavioral interventions for positive cases (grade B).
- CDC age- and sex-specific BMI percentiles:
  - Overweight: BMI ≥85th to <95th percentile
  - Class I obesity: BMI ≥95th to 119th percentile
  - Severe obesity: class II: BMI ≥120th to 139th percentile of the 95th percentile; class III: BMI ≥140th percentile of the 95th percentile
- Obesity during adolescence is strongly associated with obesity in adulthood, and increases risk of musculoskeletal injuries, mental illness, low self-esteem, and reduced quality of life.

ETIOLOGY AND PATHOPHYSIOLOGY

- Multifactorial process involving genetic, environmental, behavioral, and psychosocial factors causing energy imbalance
- Adipocytes produce adiponectin and leptin: adiponectin improves insulin sensitivity; leptin deficiency is linked to severe obesity.
- Adipocyte hypertrophy drives local and systemic inflammation.
- Obesity alters neuronal signaling, reducing satiety.

Genetics

- Syndromes like Prader-Willi and Bardet-Biedl are rare causes.
- Multiple genes influence obesity and weight loss response to diet.

RISK FACTORS

Parental obesity, sedentary lifestyle, poor nutrition (especially high-calorie foods), limited access to fresh produce/foods, stress and mental illness

GENERAL PREVENTION

- Encourage ≥150 minutes/week of moderate activity (e.g., 30 minutes of exercise, 5 days per week), and a balanced diet with controlled portions.
- Avoid or eliminate calorie-dense and nutrient-poor foods such as sugary drinks and processed items.
- Early preventive counseling, especially in youth through motivational interviewing and using preferred weight-related terminology

COMMONLY ASSOCIATED CONDITIONS

- Type 2 diabetes, HTN, hyperlipidemia
- Coronary artery disease (CAD), congestive heart failure
- Obstructive sleep apnea
- Osteoarthritis, sports-related injuries
- Nonalcoholic fatty liver disease
- Chronic kidney disease
- Mood disorders: anxiety, depression
- Cognitive impairment and dementia
- Polycystic ovarian syndrome

Geriatric Considerations

Aging leads to changes in body composition including sarcopenia, reduced bone mineral density, and increase visceral fat, leading to frailty, impaired mobility, and higher cardiometabolic risk despite possible normal BMI.

Pregnancy Considerations

- >50% of women enter pregnancy with overweight or obesity, increasing the risk of gestational diabetes, preeclampsia, cesarean delivery, stillbirth, and prolonged neonatal hospitalizations.
- Prepregnancy BMI ≥30 warrants counseling and weight optimization.
- Pregnant women with obesity should receive screening for gestational diabetes and sleep apnea at the first prenatal visit.
- Recommended gestational weight gain is 11 to 20 pounds for singleton pregnancies

DIAGNOSIS

HISTORY

- Assess diet, physical activity, prior weight loss attempts, and readiness to change lifestyle.
- Evaluate life stressors, social support, and access to resources.
- Screen for eating disorders and medications associated with weight gain (e.g., antipsychotics).
- Identify functional limitations in daily activities.

PHYSICAL EXAM

- Common findings: large neck habitus, acanthosis nigricans, striae
- Measure waist circumference at the level of the umbilicus; elevated: men: >40 inches (102 cm); women: >35 inches (88 cm)

DIFFERENTIAL DIAGNOSIS

Cushing syndrome, hypothyroidism, binge eating disorder, depression

DIAGNOSTIC TESTS & INTERPRETATION

- Screen for physiologic causes and comorbid conditions.
- BMI is a useful screening tool but does not assess fat distribution or functional impact. Visceral fat better predicts cardiometabolic risk, especially in the elderly. Muscular individuals may have high BMI without excessive adiposity.
- Assess degree and significance of adiposity using (1):
  - Anthropometric tools (waist circumference, waist-to-height ratio, waist-to-hip ratio)
  - Body composition analysis (dual-energy x-ray absorptiometry (DEXA), bioelectrical impedance)
  - In patients with BMI ≥40 kg/m^2, excess adiposity can be pragmatically assumed.
  - Obesity-related complications such as insulin resistance/diabetes, fatty liver, HTN, obstructive sleep apnea

Initial Tests (lab, imaging)

Initial evaluation includes screening for metabolic complications with glucose, HbA1c, lipid profile, liver enzymes, and renal function tests. Additional studies such as TSH, endocrine tests, ECG, or sleep study are obtained based on clinical suspicion.

Follow-Up Tests & Special Considerations

Fatigue may suggest obstructive sleep apnea; consider sleep study.

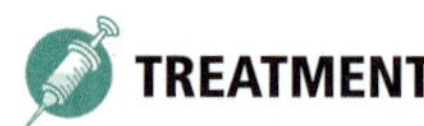

TREATMENT

GENERAL MEASURES

- Assess motivation to lose weight, patient goals of therapy, and interest in medication or surgery.
- Review nutritional intake and physical activity.
- Goal: ≥5% weight loss
- USPSTF advises clinicians to prioritize behavioral interventions.
- Treat obesity-related comorbidities.

MEDICATION

- Begin pharmacologic therapy after ≥3 to 6 months of lifestyle intervention if weight loss is <5% or not sustained; consider it for:
  - BMI ≥30
  - BMI ≥27 + comorbidities (e.g., CAD, diabetes, sleep apnea, HTN, hyperlipidemia)
  - Patients with clinical obesity based on excess adiposity or related complications, even if BMI is below these thresholds.
- USPSTF found that pharmacotherapy combined with behavioral interventions improves weight loss and maintenance more than behavioral therapy alone. Long-term use is often needed.
- Medication cost, insurance coverage, and availability may determine choice of medication.

First Line

- For long-term treatment, incretin-based therapies are generally preferred. Medication choice may also be influenced by diabetes and cardiovascular risk
- The most common side effects are GI related (nausea, vomiting, diarrhea, abdominal pain).
- Glucagon-like peptide-1 (GLP-1) receptor agonists are effective in lowering HbA1c and reducing body weight without increased incidence of hypoglycemic reactions (2).
- Tirzepatide (Mounjaro, Zepbound): dual GLP-1 agonist and glucose-dependent insulinotropic polypeptide (GIP) receptor agonist; dose 2.5 mg SC per week × 4 weeks then increasing slowly by 2.5 mg/week every 4 weeks to max tolerated or 15 mg/week
- Semaglutide (Ozempic, Rybelsus, Wegovy): GLP-1 agonist; dose: 0.25 mg SC once weekly × 4 weeks, and then increase dose at 4-week intervals to a target dose of 2.4 mg once weekly
- Liraglutide (Saxenda, Victoza): GLP-1 agonist; dose: 0.6 mg SC daily for 1 week, and then increase at weekly intervals to target dose of 3 mg daily

Second Line

- Phentermine/topiramate (Qsymia): likely most effective oral option; combines appetite suppression via increasing norepinephrine in the hypothalamus (phentermine), and GABA modulation (topiramate); schedule IV medication (3).
  - Dose: phentermine 3.75 mg/topiramate 23 mg once daily for 14 days, then titrate up to 15 mg/92 mg once daily
  - Adverse effects: misuse potential, tachycardia, mood changes, dry mouth, teratogenicity (oral clefts)
- Orlistat: inhibitor of pancreatic lipase that reduces intestinal absorption of fat and increases excretion
  - Dose: 120 mg 3 times daily with fat-containing meals
  - Adverse effects: GI side effects (cramps, flatus, fecal incontinence, oily spotting); should be taken with vitamin supplements because of slight decrease in fat-soluble vitamins (A, D, E, and K); generally poorly-tolerated
- Naltrexone/bupropion (Contrave): appetite suppression via β-endorphins blockade (naltrexone) and by acting on adrenergic and dopaminergic receptors in the hypothalamus (bupropion)
  - Dose: naltrexone 8 mg/bupropion 90 mg once daily for the first week, and up titrate to a goal of 16 mg/180 mg twice daily by week 4
  - Adverse effects: increased blood pressure, dry mouth, headache, insomnia, skin tingling, or numbness
- Plenity: hydrogel of cellulose and citric acid creates feeling of fullness; taken twice daily, 30 minutes before lunch and dinner with at least 16 oz of water; listed as an FDA-approved medical device and not a medication
- Short-term medications (<12 weeks) are older, sympathomimetic drugs that suppress appetite via early satiety; adverse effects: tachycardia, HTN, insomnia, dry mouth; contraindicated in uncontrolled HTN, CVD, hyperthyroidism, glaucoma, or exposure to monoamine oxidase inhibitors during or within 14 days of administration; used with caution in pulmonary HTN
  - Phentermine: (Schedule IV medication.): Dose: 15.0 to 37.5 mg daily or divided twice daily
  - Diethylpropion: (Schedule IV medication.): Dose: 25 mg 3 to 4 times daily before meals

ADDITIONAL THERAPIES

- Physical activity
  - Results in modest weight loss (1 to 3 kg/year) when added to dietary intervention
  - The type of exercise (aerobic vs. resistance) or intensity (high vs. low) does not seem to affect overall weight loss; dose-response relationship between duration of physical activity and weight loss, although still some interindividual variability
  - Should be individualized to patient's goals, exercise history, motivation, and overall health status; exercise is beneficial regardless of effect on weight.
- Comprehensive behavioral therapy (CBT): most effective in-person with high intensity (≥14 sessions in 6 months) by a trained interventionist; components: (i) reduced-calorie diet (ii) increased physical activity (iii) behavioral strategies to support adherence

SURGERY/OTHER PROCEDURES

- Consider bariatric surgery for:
  - BMI ≥40
  - BMI ≥35 with at least one serious obesity-related comorbidity
  - BMI 30.0 to 34.9 with inadequately controlled type 2 diabetes or metabolic disease despite optimal medical therapy
- Candidate should be evaluated for surgical risk, psychological readiness, and ability to commit to long-term follow-up and lifestyle changes.
- Surgical procedures include biliopancreatic diversion, Roux-en-Y gastric bypass, sleeve gastrectomy, laparoscopic adjustable gastric banding, vagal blocking therapy, and gastric aspiration (AspireAssist).

ONGOING CARE

FOLLOW-UP RECOMMENDATIONS

Continue to discuss weight, lifestyle modifications, and address both current and new goals. Long-term treatment is needed to maintain weight loss. A new treatment plan should be implemented if no clinical meaningful weight loss after 3 to 4 months.

DIET

- Net calorie reduction (~500 kcal/day) with a sustainable diet is most effective; targets: 1,200 to 1,500 kcal/day (women), 1,500 to 1,800 kcal/day (men); a reduction of 500 kcal/day can result in ~1 lb (0.45 kg) weight loss per week, but long-term significant weight loss maintenance is difficult.
- Very low calorie diet (200 to 800 kcal/day) leads to greater short-term weight loss, but similar long-term results compared to low-calorie diets; requires medical supervision
- Mediterranean: primarily plant-based foods, olive oil, nuts, legumes, whole grain, fruits, vegetables, fish and poultry; shown to reduce weight, BMI, HbA1c, fasting glucose, and CVD risk
- Balanced-nutrient, moderate calorie: 1,200 to 1,800 kcal/day; e.g., DASH diet: emphasizes fruits, vegetables, fiber, and low saturated fat (based on MyPlate food guide)

PATIENT EDUCATION

Build a healthy eating routine: https://odphp.health.gov/sites/default/files/2021-08/DGA-FactSheet-2021-03-26-compressed.pdf

PROGNOSIS

Patients who have obesity compared to those with a normal weight are at an increased risk for many serious health conditions.

COMPLICATIONS

CVD, osteoarthritis, higher death rates from cancer: colon, breast, prostate, endometrial, gallbladder, liver, kidney

REFERENCES

1. Rubino F, Cummings DE, Eckel RH, et al. Definition and diagnostic criteria of clinical obesity. *Lancet Diabetes Endocrinol*. 2025;13(3):221–262. doi:10.1016/S2213-8587(24)00316-4.
2. Xie Z, Hu J, Gu H, et al. Comparison of the efficacy and safety of 10 glucagon-like peptide-1 receptor agonists as add-on to metformin in patients with type 2 diabetes: a systematic review. *Front Endocrinol (Lausanne)*. 2023;14:1244432.
3. Siebenhofer A, Winterholer S, Jeitler K, et al. Long-term effects of weight-reducing drugs in people with hypertension. *Cochrane Database Syst Rev*. 2021;1(1):CD007654.

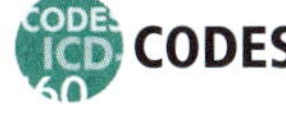

CODES

ICD10

- E66.9 Obesity, unspecified
- E66.3 Overweight
- R63.5 Abnormal weight gain

CLINICAL PEARLS

- Most U.S. adults are overweight or have obesity and the prevalence is increasing.
- Lifestyle modification is the cornerstone of therapy.
- Long-term medication may be indicated when nonpharmacologic treatment for 3 to 6 months has been ineffective.
- Consider bariatric surgery in patients who have failed conservative treatment, particularly if there are associated risk factors

OBSESSIVE-COMPULSIVE DISORDER (OCD)

Matthew J. Filippo, DO • Rebecca Feltman-Frank El Zoghbi, MD

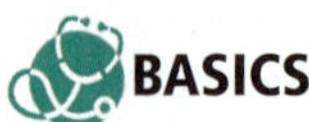

BASICS

DESCRIPTION

- A disorder characterized by pathologic obsessions (recurrent intrusive thoughts, ideas, or images) and/or compulsions (repetitive, ritualistic behaviors or mental acts) that are time-consuming and cause significant distress
- Not to be confused with obsessive-compulsive (anankastic) personality disorder

EPIDEMIOLOGY

Incidence

- Three subtypes: child/adolescent-onset (age <18 years), adult-onset (age 18 to 39 years) and late-onset (age ≥40 years).
- Child/adolescent-onset in 50% of cases (usually by age 18 years) (1).
- Consider pediatric acute-onset neuropsychiatric syndrome (PANS)/pediatric autoimmune neuropsychiatric disorders associated with streptococcal infections (PANDAS) in acute presentation of obsessive-compulsive disorder (OCD) and tics in children (2).
- Consider neurologic or neurodegenerative disorders in new-onset OCD.

Prevalence

~2% lifetime prevalence; slight female predominance when including postpartum OCD

ETIOLOGY AND PATHOPHYSIOLOGY

- Although the exact etiology of OCD is unknown, genetic, anatomical, neurochemical, autoimmune, and environmental factors are believed to contribute to the disorder.
- Dysregulation of serotonergic, catecholaminergic, and glutamatergic pathways
- Dysfunction of cortico-striatal-thalamo-cortical (CSTC) circuit, involving the orbitofrontal cortex (OFC) and anterior cingulate cortex (ACC)
- Stressors, trauma, and learned behaviors may be contributing factors to development of OCD symptoms.

Genetics

- First-degree relatives of individuals with child/adolescent-onset OCD have a 7–15% prevalence rate of the disorder.
- ~45–65% of the variance of OCD is explained by genetics. To date, no specific gene has been found.

RISK FACTORS

- Family history of OCD
- Advanced paternal and maternal age
- Coexisting psychiatric disorders, most commonly anxiety disorders and schizophrenia
- Antipsychotics such as clozapine and olanzapine with greater serotonergic blockade may cause symptoms of OCD.
- Brain insult (i.e., encephalitis, pediatric streptococcal infection, or head injury)
- History of childhood traumatic events, including social isolation and physical abuse
- Stressful life events can exacerbate OCD symptoms.

GENERAL PREVENTION

Although primary prevention strategies are limited, secondary prevention via early diagnosis and treatment decreases distress and impairment.

COMMONLY ASSOCIATED CONDITIONS

- Major depressive disorder
- Anxiety disorders including panic disorder/phobia/social phobia/generalized anxiety disorder
- Tourette syndrome/tic syndromes
- Autism spectrum disorder
- Substance abuse/eating disorder/body dysmorphic disorder
- Other obsessive-compulsive spectrum disorders including body-focused repetitive behaviors (trichotillomania, excoriation disorder), body dysmorphia, and hoarding disorder

DIAGNOSIS

HISTORY

- Obsessions, compulsions or both, which cause marked distress, are time-consuming (>1 hour/day), and cause significant occupational/social impairment.
- Two criteria support the diagnosis of obsessions:
  - Presence of recurrent, persistent, intrusive and inappropriate thoughts, causing significant anxiety and distress
  - The individual makes attempts to suppress or neutralize such thoughts with some other thought or activity (i.e., by performing a compulsion).
- Two criteria support the diagnosis of compulsions:
  - Repetitive, rigid behaviors (e.g., handwashing) or mental acts (e.g., counting silently), performed in response to an obsession
  - Although aimed at reducing stress, the response is either not realistically connected with the obsession or is excessive.

PHYSICAL EXAM

OCD is highly comorbid with body focused repetitive behaviors including trichotillomania and excoriation disorder. These may be thought of as part of an obsessive-compulsive spectrum.

- Chapped hands caused by excessive handwashing
- Scars and/or sores from skin picking and/or biting
- Patchy hair loss caused by compulsive pulling/picking/twisting of hair
- Weight loss from food restriction due to contamination fears

DIFFERENTIAL DIAGNOSIS

- Impulse-control disorders, involving compulsive gambling, sex, or substance use
- Tic disorder and stereotypic movement disorder (tics are often preceded by premonitory sensations and not aimed at neutralizing the obsession)
- Generalized anxiety disorder, phobic disorders, separation anxiety (excessive worry/anxious rumination, but without compulsion)
- Obsessive-compulsive personality disorder (characterized by perfectionism and control; usually ego-syntonic)

DIAGNOSTIC TESTS & INTERPRETATION

OCD is a clinical diagnosis based on *DSM-5* criteria as listed under history portion of this section.

Initial Tests (lab, imaging)

Consider obtaining basic labs to rule out OCD symptoms as result of a medical condition, substance, or medication. Consider strep testing in pediatric populations with sudden onset of symptoms.

Diagnostic Procedures/Other

- Free-form interviews are the most common method for determining an OCD diagnosis.
- Yale-Brown Obsessive-Compulsive Scale (Y-BOCS) or obsessive-compulsive inventory to assess severity of OCD and monitor progress

Test Interpretation

- Common obsessive themes and associated rituals/compulsions
  - Contamination, dirt, or disease; handwashing or cleaning
  - Symmetry or orderliness; ordering, rearranging, counting
  - Harm (i.e., being responsible for an accident) or doubt (windows locked, stove off); checking, repeating
  - Unacceptable thoughts (sexual, thoughts, taboo thoughts)
- 80–90% of patients with OCD have obsessions and compulsions.
- 10–19% of patients with OCD are pure obsessional.

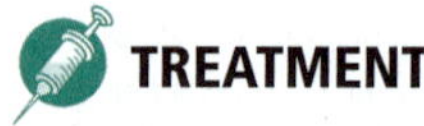

TREATMENT

GENERAL MEASURES

- Exposure and response prevention (ERP), a specialized form of cognitive-behavioral therapy (CBT), is first-line treatment. Combining ERP with medication is typically the most effective treatments for OCD.
- Electroconvulsive therapy (ECT), deep transcranial magnetic stimulation (TMS), and/or deep brain stimulation for severe illness

MEDICATION

First Line

- Adequate trial of antidepressants for at least 10 to 12 weeks (3)
- Doses may exceed typical doses for depression.
- Varying degrees of efficacy between agents; no one SSRI is superior to the other.
- SSRIs are recommended first-line agents.
  - Fluoxetine (Prozac)
    - Adults: 20 mg/day; increase by 10 to 20 mg q4–6wk until response (20 to 80 mg/day)
    - Children (7 to 17 years of age): 10 mg/day; increase gradually q4–6wk until response (20 to 60 mg/day).
  - Sertraline (Zoloft)
    - Adults: 50 mg/day; increase by 50 mg q4–7d until response; range: 50 to 200 mg/day; may divide if >100 mg/day
    - Children (6 to 17 years of age): 25 mg/day; increase by 25 mg every 7 days until response (50 to 200 mg/day).

– Fluvoxamine (Luvox)
  ◦ Adults: 50 mg QHS initially; may increase by 50 mg/day q4–7d up to 100 to 300 mg/day
  ◦ Doses >100 mg/day should be divided q12h.
- Precautions: Watch for suicidal behavior/worsening depression during first few months of therapy/after dosage changes with antidepressants, particularly in children, adolescents, and young adults.

Second Line

- Try switching to another SSRI:
  – 40–70% of patients show an adequate response to a trial of SSRI, with a remission rate of 10–40%
  – Citalopram/escitalopram do not have FDA approvals for OCD but can be effective.
  – Paroxetine is FDA approved for OCD. Given a higher side effect burden this is best reserved as a second-line option.
- If no response, switch to the tricyclic antidepressant (TCA), clomipramine (Anafranil)
  – Adults: 25 mg/day; increase gradually over 2 weeks to 100 mg/day and then to 250 mg/day (max dose) over next several weeks, as tolerated.
  – Children (10 to 17 years of age): 25 mg/day; titrate as needed and tolerated up to 3 mg/kg/day or 200 mg/day (whichever is less).
  – Clomipramine is associated with a higher side effect burden than alternative available treatments for OCD. Please be aware of variety of side effects along with contraindications before prescribing (including but not limited to myocardial infarction [MI], concomitant use within 14 days of MAOI, AV block, angle closure glaucoma)

Pregnancy Considerations

Although SSRIs are generally considered okay to use during pregnancy, they come with potential risks including preterm birth, neonatal adaption syndrome, among others. Paroxetine has higher risks than other SSRIs in pregnancy including potential cardiac defects. There is very limited data available about safety with clomipramine during pregnancy with humans; however, data available with animals demonstrate some concern for adverse effects on fetus.

ISSUES FOR REFERRAL

- Referral for ERP.
- Psychiatric evaluation if significantly interfering with patient's functioning

ADDITIONAL THERAPIES

- Antipsychotic agents alone are not effective in treating OCD. They can augment serotonergic agent(s) for treatment-resistant OCD; clozapine is known to worsen OCD symptoms.
  – Risperidone (Risperdal): initial dose: 0.5 mg/day; target dose: 0.5 to 2.0 mg/day for at least 8 weeks.
  – Aripiprazole (Abilify): initial dose: 5 mg/day; target dose: 10 mg/day for at least 8 weeks.
- Research is undergoing for benefit of augmentation from novel glutaminergic agents including N-acetylcysteine or memantine, and serotonergic agents such as ondansetron.
- Serotonin-norepinephrine reuptake inhibitor (SNRI) including venlafaxine and duloxetine and atypical antidepressants such as mirtazapine show efficacy as well.
- Deep transcranial magnetic stimulation (dTMS) is FDA approved for OCD.

SURGERY/OTHER PROCEDURES

For severe treatment resistant cases, consider neurosurgical procedure(s) including anterior cingulotomy or capsulotomy. These can be done via neurosurgery or via stereotactic radiotherapy (SRT). Also consider deep brain stimulation.

COMPLEMENTARY & ALTERNATIVE MEDICINE

Although evidence is limited, some explore practices like mindfulness (which can complement ERP by increasing awareness of thoughts without judgment), yoga, and/or supplements (e.g., inositol has been studied with mixed results, St. John's Wort is generally not recommended due to risk of serotonin syndrome). For highly treatment-resistant OCD, investigational approaches include psychedelic-assisted therapy (e.g., with psilocin), although these require further research in controlled settings.

ADMISSION, INPATIENT, AND NURSING CONSIDERATIONS

Average time from symptom onset to treatment is 11 years. Individuals may have significant embarrassment over intrusive thoughts and be reluctant to admit them. It is important to build rapport and maintain a safe, nonjudgmental space with open dialogue.

ONGOING CARE

FOLLOW-UP RECOMMENDATIONS

- Y-BOCS survey to track progress
- Continue medication 1 to 2 years at full dose.
- Discontinuation of medication is associated with high relapse rate. Some individuals may require long-term medication treatment.

Patient Monitoring

Monitor for decrease in obsessions and time spent performing compulsions.

DIET

A healthy diet with focus on fiber, protein, natural whole foods while eliminating excessive sugar, salt, caffeine, and alcohol can support therapeutic and pharmacologic interventions for OCD.

PATIENT EDUCATION

- International OCD Foundation: https://iocdf.org/
- Obsessive Compulsive Anonymous: http://obsessivecompulsiveanonymous.org

PROGNOSIS

- Chronic waxing and waning course in most patients
- 50% have suicidal thoughts.
- Early age of onset is associated with poorer prognosis and a more chronic course.

COMPLICATIONS

- Depression, anxiety, and panic attacks
- Avoidant behavior (Children may drop out of school; adults may become homebound.)

REFERENCES

1. Goodman WK, Grice DE, Lapidus KA, et al. Obsessive-compulsive disorder. *Psychiatr Clin North Am*. 2014;37(3):257–267.
2. American Psychiatric Association. Practice guideline for the treatment of patients with obsessive-compulsive disorder. Arlington, VA: American Psychiatric Association; 2007.
3. Roh D, Jang KW, Kim CH. Clinical advances in treatment strategies for obsessive-compulsive disorder in adults. *Clin Psychopharmacol Neurosci*. 2023;21(4):676–685. doi: 10.9758/cpn.23.1075.

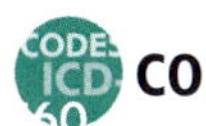

CODES

ICD10

- F42 Obsessive-compulsive disorder
- F42.2 Mixed obsessional thoughts and acts
- F42.3 Hoarding disorder

CLINICAL PEARLS

- Exposure with response (ritual) prevention (ERP) is first-line treatment.
- ERP plus an SSRI is first-line treatment for moderate to severe OCD.
- The majority of patients with OCD respond to treatment with an SSRI and ERP but do not fully remit.

OCULAR CHEMICAL BURNS

Jonathan C. Tsui, MD

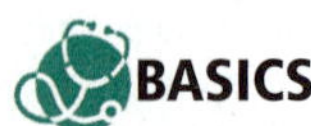

BASICS

DESCRIPTION

- Chemical exposure to the eye can result in rapid, devastating, and permanent damage and is one of the true emergencies in ophthalmology.
  - Alkali burns: more severe; alkaline compounds are lipophilic and penetrate rapidly into eye tissue; saponification of cell membranes leads to necrosis and may cause injury to lids, conjunctiva, cornea, sclera, iris, and lens.
  - Acid burns: less severe; associated anions from acidic compounds cause protein denaturation, creating a barrier to further acid penetration (hydrofluoric acid is an exception to this rule; see below). Injury is often limited to lids, conjunctiva, and cornea.
- System(s) affected: skin/exocrine, nervous
- Synonym(s): chemical ocular injuries

EPIDEMIOLOGY

Incidence

- Estimated 5 to 6 cases/100,000 persons per year (accounting for 11–22% of all ocular injuries)
- Median age is 32 years, but children between ages 1 and 2 years represent the highest-risk group.
- Male > female
- Most common in workplace and residential settings

ETIOLOGY AND PATHOPHYSIOLOGY

- Alkaline compounds (pH >7)
  - Alkali burns are twice as common as acid burns.
  - Typical sources include ammonia (most common), calcium hydroxide (lime), sodium/potassium hydroxide (lye), and ammonium hydroxide.
  - Lipophilic compounds that penetrate into deep structures dissociate into cations and hydroxide. Hydroxide causes saponification of fatty acids in cell membranes, leading to cell death. Cations cause hydration of glycosaminoglycans, leading to hydration of collagen, rapid shortening and thickening of collagen fibrils, and resultant corneal opacification and acute elevation in intraocular pressure (IOP).
  - Long-term elevation in IOP may occur from accumulation of inflammatory debris within the trabecular meshwork.
  - Penetration into deep structures may affect perfusing vessels, leading to ischemia.
- Acidic compounds (pH <7)
  - Typical sources include sulfuric acid (most common), sulfurous acid, hydrochloric acid, acetic acid, hydrofluoric acid.
  - Anion leads to protein denaturing and protective barrier formation by coagulation necrosis forming an eschar. This more superficial mechanism of injury reduces further tissue penetration but may lead to more prominent scarring.
  - Hydrofluoric acid is an exception. In its nonionized form, it behaves like an alkaline substance that can penetrate the corneal stroma and lead to extensive anterior segment lesions. When ionized, it may combine with intracellular calcium and magnesium to form insoluble complexes, leading to potassium ion movements and cell death. Once systemically absorbed, severe hypocalcemia can occur.

RISK FACTORS

- Industrial work, including chemical labs
- Construction work (plaster, cement, whitewash)
- Use of cleaning agents (drain cleaners, ammonia)
- Automobile battery explosions (sulfuric acid)
- Assault

GENERAL PREVENTION

- Safety glasses/goggles
- Safe handling training for occupational exposures

COMMONLY ASSOCIATED CONDITIONS

Facial (including eyelids) cutaneous chemical or thermal burns

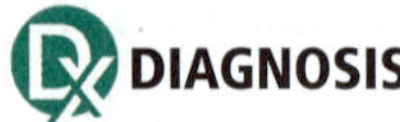

DIAGNOSIS

HISTORY

- Patient presents with pain, photophobia, blurred vision, and foreign body sensation.
- Ask about chemical involved, temperature, volume, timing and duration of exposure, velocity of impact, and involved area.
- In alkali burns, can have initial pain that later diminishes

PHYSICAL EXAM

- Alkaline compounds may present with corneal opacification secondary to glycosaminoglycan hydration; however, severe acid burns may also present with this finding.
- Acidic compound may present with a ground-glass appearance secondary to superficial scar formation.

DIFFERENTIAL DIAGNOSIS

- Thermal burns
- Ruptured globe
- Traumatic corneal abrasion or epithelial defects
- Infectious keratoconjunctivitis
- Intraocular/superficial ocular foreign body
- Ocular cicatricial pemphigoid

DIAGNOSTIC TESTS & INTERPRETATION

Initial Tests (lab, imaging)

- Examine the eye before initiating irrigation to rule out open globe (may require emergent surgical exploration if high index of suspicion for open globe that would be exacerbated by irrigation).
- Measure pH of tear film on both eyes and immediately initiate irrigation (if nonneutral) prior to additional tests.
- Imaging is not necessary unless suspicion of intraocular or orbital foreign body is present. In this case, CT should be used—MRI is contraindicated.

Follow-Up Tests & Special Considerations

- Complete ophthalmic exam include measuring visual acuity, IOP, and examining both anterior and posterior segments
- Grade degree of injury based on corneal, conjunctival, and limbal involvement using the Roper-Hall or Dua classification schemes to guide prognosis and treatment. It is important to establish baseline at time of injury and document changes over time as the patient is followed.
- Stem cell survival is the rate-limiting mechanism of recovery after corneal injury; limbal ischemia is a surrogate measure to estimate the degree of stem cell loss.

Diagnostic Procedures/Other

- Measure pH of tear film with litmus paper or electronic probe: Irrigating fluid with nonneutral pH (e.g., normal saline has pH of 4.5) may alter results; wipe away all excess topical anesthetics before measuring.
- Careful slit-lamp exam, fundus ophthalmoscopy, tonometry, and measurement of visual acuity
- Using fluorescein to evaluate the state of the corneal epithelium is essential.
- Examination of posterior segment may be challenging but should be attempted carefully using nonvasoconstrictive mydriatics to avoid potential worsening of ischemia.
- Full extent of damage from alkali burns may not be apparent until 48 to 72 hours after exposure.

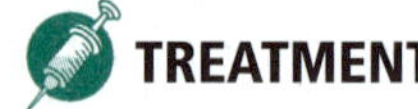

TREATMENT

Immediate copious irrigation and removal of corneal or conjunctival foreign bodies are always the initial treatment and paramount to minimizing long-term sequelae (1),(2),(3)[A]:

- Passively open patient's eyelid and have patient look in all directions while irrigating.
- Remove all chemical reservoirs from the eyes via lid eversion while flushing.
- Continue irrigation until the tear film and superior/inferior cul-de-sac is of neutral pH (7.2 ± 0.1) and stable, testing every 30 minutes (1)[A]:
  - Severe burns should be irrigated for at least 15 to 30 minutes and up to 2 to 4 hours; this irrigation should not be interrupted during transportation to hospital (1)[B].
  - Irrigation via Morgan lens (polymethylmethacrylate scleral lens) is a good way to achieve continuous irrigation over a prolonged period of time.

- Perform initial pH testing on both eyes even if the patient claims to only have unilateral ocular pain/irritation so that a contralateral injury is not overlooked.
- Use any available nontoxic fluid for irrigation on scene including bottled or tap water. In the clinic/hospital, sterile water, normal saline, normal saline with bicarbonate, balanced salt solution (BSS), or lactated Ringer solution may be used.
- A topical anesthetic can be used to provide patient comfort (e.g., proparacaine, tetracaine).
- Sweep the conjunctival fornices every 12 to 24 hours to prevent symblepharon formation and adhesions.

MEDICATION

First Line

- After initial irrigation, further treatment aims to decrease inflammation and collagen degradation and aid in collagen synthesis and recovery of corneal epithelium. Selection of medications depends on severity and associated conditions.
  - Topical prophylactic antibiotics: any broad-spectrum agent (e.g., bacitracin–polymyxin B ointment q2–4h, ciprofloxacin drops q2–4h)
    - Some experts suggest adding systemic tetracycline such as doxycycline 100 mg PO BID to encourage healing and prevent corneal ulceration (1),(2)[C].
  - Preservative-free artificial tears: carboxymethylcellulose (Refresh Plus) drops q1h for first 24 hours
    - Promotes reepithelialization, reduces recurrent erosion risk, and increases visual rehab (1),(2)[A]
  - Cycloplegics for photophobia and/or uveitis: cyclopentolate 1% TID (3)[C]
  - Topical corticosteroids for intraocular inflammation: prednisolone 1% or equivalent q1–2h for 7 to 10 days; and if severe, prednisone 20 to 60 mg PO daily for 5 to 7 days; taper rapidly if epithelium is intact, by day 10 to 14 (1)[C].
  - Vitamin C (ascorbic acid) 500 mg PO QID and topical 10% q2h ascorbate solution in artificial tears
    - Using vitamin C in conjunction with steroids reduces incidence of corneal thinning, ulceration, and perforation (1),(2)[A].
  - Acetylcysteine (Mucomyst) 10–20% topically q4h may promote wound healing (1)[B].
  - Ocular antihypertensives if IOP >30 to reduce risk of optic nerve damage: latanoprost 0.005% QHS, timolol 0.5% BID *or* levobunolol 0.5% BID, *and/or* acetazolamide 125 to 250 mg PO q6h *or* methazolamide 25 to 50 mg PO BID (2)[B]
  - Bandage contact lens: After initial injury, lenses with high oxygen permeability and hydrophilic properties may aid in epithelial migration/adhesion and basement membrane regeneration (3)[B].
- Precautions
  - Timolol and levobunolol: history of cardiac/pulmonary disease including bradycardia and asthma/COPD
  - Acetazolamide and methazolamide: history of nephrolithiasis or metabolic acidosis
  - Mannitol: history of heart failure, renal failure, or sickle cell
  - Scopolamine: history of urinary retention
  - Ascorbic acid: history of renal impairment
  - Tetracycline/doxycycline: Avoid systemic use in children <8 years old and pregnant patients.
  - Topical corticosteroids: Use with caution in the presence of damaged corneal epithelium because iatrogenic infection can occur. Use of corticosteroids >6 days may inhibit repair and cause corneoscleral melt (1)[B]. Daily follow-up with an ophthalmologist is recommended.

SURGERY/OTHER PROCEDURES

- The goals of subacute treatment are restoration of the normal ocular surface anatomy and corneal clarity and control of glaucoma.
- Surgical options include the following:
  - Débridement of necrotic tissue and inflammatory debris (1),(3)[A]
  - Conjunctival/tenon advancement (tenoplasty) to restore vascularity in severe burns
  - Tissue adhesive (e.g., cyanoacrylate) for impending or actual corneal perforation
    - Tectonic keratoplasty for acute perforation >1 mm
  - Limbal autograft transplantation for epithelial stem cell restoration
  - Amniotic membrane transplantation or umbilical cord serum drops to promote faster epithelial regeneration and improvement in visual acuity (1)[B]
  - Conjunctival or mucosal membrane transplant to restore ocular surface in severe injury
  - Corneal transplant (penetrating keratoplasty, anterior lamellar keratoplasty) for extensive scarring
  - Enucleation for blind, painful eyes

ONGOING CARE

FOLLOW-UP RECOMMENDATIONS

Patient Monitoring

- Ranges from daily to weekly visits initially depending on severity of ocular injury
- May need to be admitted if noncompliant or pediatric patient
- If on mannitol or prednisone, consider frequently checking serum electrolytes.

PATIENT EDUCATION

- Need for immediate ocular irrigation with water following ocular chemical exposure
- Shield at all times during acute care
- Safety glasses for future protection

PROGNOSIS

- Depends on severity of initial injury: increased limbal involvement in clock hours and greater percentage of conjunctival involvement correlate with poorer prognosis (Dua classification system)
- For mildly injured eyes, complete recovery is common.
- For severely injured eyes, permanent loss of vision is not uncommon.

COMPLICATIONS

- Orbital compartment syndrome
- Keratoconjunctivitis sicca (dry eye)
- Corneal ulcer/perforation/scarring
- Cicatricial ectropion/entropion
- Symblepharon
- Glaucoma
- Cataract
- Astigmatism
- Phthisis bulbi
- Blindness

REFERENCES

1. Sharma N, Kaur M, Agarwal T, et al. Treatment of acute ocular chemical burns. *Surv Ophthalmol*. 2018;63(2):214–235.
2. Baradaran-Rafii A, Eslani M, Haq Z, et al. Current and upcoming therapies for ocular surface chemical injuries. *Ocul Surf*. 2017;15(1):48–64.
3. Eslani M, Baradaran-Rafii A, Movahedan A, et al. The ocular surface chemical burns. *J Ophthalmol*. 2014;2014:196827.

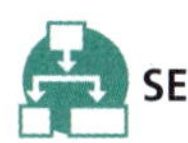

SEE ALSO

Burns

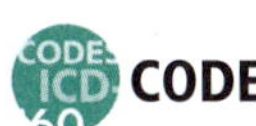

CODES

ICD10

- T26.50XA Corrosion of unsp eyelid and periocular area, init encntr
- T26.60XA Corrosion of cornea and conjunctival sac, unsp eye, init
- S05.00XA Inj conjunctiva and corneal abrasion w/o fb, unsp eye, init

CLINICAL PEARLS

- Prompt irrigation of all chemical burns, with any available nontoxic fluid such as water, as soon as possible (prior to arrival in the emergency department), is essential to ensure the best outcomes.
- All patients with ocular chemical injuries should have urgent ophthalmology evaluation.
- Prognosis is guarded depending on type of chemical injury.

ONYCHOMYCOSIS

Karl T. Clebak, MD, MHA, FAAFP • Maria Fowler, MD

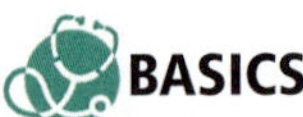

BASICS

DESCRIPTION

- Fungal infection of fingernails/toenails, caused mostly by dermatophytes, less commonly yeasts and nondermatophyte molds
- Toenails are more commonly affected than fingernails.
- Synonym: tinea unguium

EPIDEMIOLOGY

Prevalence

- Worldwide prevalence is approximately 5.5%.
- More common in adults than children, prevalence increases with age; 35% of adults aged >65 years
- Rare before puberty
- Estimated 50% of all nail disorders in the outpatient setting

ETIOLOGY AND PATHOPHYSIOLOGY

- Inoculation of nail with dermatophytes, non-nondermatophyte molds or yeasts
- Dermatophytes (60–70%): *Trichophyton* (*Trichophyton rubrum* most common), *Epidermophyton*, *Microsporum*
- Yeasts (30–40%): *Candida albicans* (most common), *Candida parapsilosis*, *Candida tropicalis*, *Candida krusei*
- Molds: *Scopulariopsis brevicaulis*, *Hendersonula toruloidea*, *Aspergillus* spp., *Alternaria tenuis*, *Cephalosporium*, *Scytalidium hyalinum*
- Dermatophytes, notably *Trichophyton*, cause 90% of toenail and 75% of fingernail onychomycoses.
- Yeasts, especially *Candida*, may involve fingernails (not uncommonly) or toenails.

Genetics

Possible autosomal dominant inheritance pattern

RISK FACTORS

- Older age, occlusive footwear, tinea pedis (particularly interdigital)
- Cancer, diabetes, psoriasis, peripheral vascular disease
- Nail injury
- Living with others with onychomycosis, communal swimming pools
- Smoking
- Immunodeficiency

GENERAL PREVENTION

- Keeping feet cool and dry
- Avoiding occlusive footwear
- Using sandals in public locker rooms and swimming pools
- Discarding or treating infected footwear and socks (1)

COMMONLY ASSOCIATED CONDITIONS

- Immunodeficiency (acquired immune deficiency syndrome and transplant patients), and chronic metabolic disease (e.g., diabetes)
- Tinea pedis/manuum

DIAGNOSIS

HISTORY

Discoloration of nail plate with thickening and onycholysis; slowly progressive onset with involvement of a single or multiple nails with varying degrees of involvement

PHYSICAL EXAM

- Dermatophytes: commonly preceded by dermatophyte infection at another site; 80% involve toenails, especially hallux; simultaneous infection of fingernails and toenails is rare. Five clinical forms occur:
  - Distal/lateral subungual onychomycosis (most common): mainly due to *T. rubrum*. Spreads from distal/lateral margins to nail bed to nail plate, causing linear channels or "spikes"; subungual hyperkeratosis; onycholysis; nail dystrophy; discoloration—yellow-white or brown-black, *bois vermoulu* ("worm-eaten wood"); onychomadesis
  - Proximal subungual onychomycosis (rare <1% of cases): typically caused by *T. rubrum* and *Fusarium* spp; can affect hands/feet; leukonychia—begins at proximal part of nail plate near cuticle and distally, appearing to occur from the proximal underside of the nail (or direct invasion of the nail plate from above); spreads to nail plate and lunula; seen with immunosuppressive conditions
  - Superficial onychomycosis (~10% of cases): infection of surface of nail plate; merging opaque white spots on nail plate eventually can involve entire surface of the nail; most commonly due to *Trichophyton mentagrophytes*
  - Endonyx onychomycosis involves interior of nail plate, sparing nail bed. Nail develops milky appearance with indentations and lamellar splitting. Subungual hyperkeratosis is absent.
  - Totally dystrophic onychomycosis causes complete destruction of nail plate by fungus, resulting in thickened and ridged nail bed covered with keratotic debris; considered end stage that may follow any subtype
- Candidal
  - Hands commonly involved (70%), especially the 3rd digit
  - Pain is mild, unless secondarily infected; increases on prolonged contact with water
  - Primarily affects tissue surrounding nail
  - Begins with cuticle detachment and produces white or white-yellow nail discoloration
  - Secondary ungual changes: convex, irregular, striated nail plate with dull, rough surface
  - Onycholysis, especially on hands; distal subungual onychomycosis may occur.
  - Primary involvement of the nail plate is uncommon.
  - Periungual edema/erythema may occur (club-shaped, bulbous fingertips).
- Molds (nondermatophyte)
  - Most common in those >60 years of age, more common in nails of hallux
  - Resembles distal and lateral onychomycosis

Pediatric Considerations

- Candidal infection presents more commonly as superficial onychomycosis.
- Topical treatments may be more effective in children due to thinner nails and faster nail growth rate.
- The U.S. Food and Drug Administration (FDA) has not approved any systemic antifungal agents for treatment of onychomycosis in children although sometimes used off label.

DIFFERENTIAL DIAGNOSIS

- Psoriasis (most common alternate diagnosis)
- Traumatic dystrophy
- Lichen planus
- Onychogryphosis ("ram's horn nails")
- Eczematous conditions
- Hypothyroidism
- Drugs and chemicals
- Yellow nail syndrome
- Neoplasms (0.7–3.5%) of all melanoma cases are subungual. In a brownish yellow nail, if dark pigment extends into periungual skin fold, consider subungual melanoma.
- Alopecia areata
- Chronic paronychia
- Pemphigus vulgaris
- Paronychia congenita
- Scabies

DIAGNOSTIC TESTS & INTERPRETATION

- Accurate diagnosis includes both laboratory and clinical evidence. Diagnostic accuracy ranges from 66% to 75%.
- About 50% of nail dystrophy seen on visual inspection is not fungal in origin.
- A nail plate biopsy or partial/full removal of nail with culture is needed to diagnose proximal subungual onychomycosis.

Initial Tests (lab, imaging)

- Direct microscopy with potassium hydroxide (KOH) preparation from nail sample (sensitivity 48–60%, specificity 38–78%)
- Fungal cultures: Low sensitivity of 60–65%, but high specificity of 83–100% results may take 3 to 6 weeks.
- In-office dermatophyte test, medium culture indicates dermatophyte growth; results in 3 to 7 days; limited studies
- Histologic examination of nail clippings/nail plate punch biopsy: proximal lesions; stain both with periodic acid–Schiff (PAS) stain (sensitivity 82–88%).
- Fluorescence microscopy can be used as a rapid screening tool for identification of fungi in nail specimens.
- Discontinue all topical medication for at least 1 week before obtaining a sample.

Follow-Up Tests & Special Considerations

Laboratory confirmation prior to treatment is cost-effective and should be considered to avoid misdiagnosis and unnecessary treatment.

Diagnostic Procedures/Other

A nail plate biopsy or partial/full removal of nail with culture is needed to diagnose proximal subungual onychomycosis.

Test Interpretation

Pathogens within the nail keratin indicate a positive result.

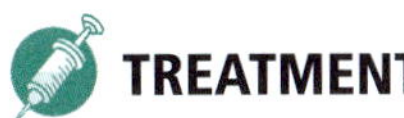

TREATMENT

GENERAL MEASURES

Avoid factors that promote fungal growth (i.e., heat, moisture, occlusion, tight-fitting shoes). Treat underlying disease risk factors. Treat secondary infections.

MEDICATION

Pregnancy Considerations

Oral antifungals and ciclopirox are pregnancy Category B (terbinafine, ciclopirox) or C (itraconazole, fluconazole, and griseofulvin). Griseofulvin is not advised in pregnancy due to risks of teratogenicity. Ideally, postpone treatment of onychomycosis until after pregnancy.

First Line

- Medication therapy is indicated for immunocompromised patients, complications including cellulitis or discomfort, or for cosmetic concerns.
- Oral antifungals are preferred due to higher rates of cure and shorter courses of treatment but have systemic adverse effects and many drug–drug interactions; recommended when >50% of nail is affected, multiple nails, involvement of nail matrix, or presence of dermatophytoma; recurrence following treatment is common—25–50% within 5 years.
- Terbinafine: 250 mg/day PO for 6 weeks for fingernails and 12 weeks for toenails; terbinafine offers the most effective clinical and mycologic cure rates compared to other treatments (2)[A]. Continuous terbinafine treatment has similar efficacy as pulse treatment.
- Alternative therapies for terbinafine resistant infections includes posaconazole, voriconazole, and itraconazole.
- Itraconazole pulse: 200 mg PO BID for 1 week and then 3 weeks off, repeat for two cycles for fingernails and three to four cycles for toenails; does not need to monitor liver function tests (LFTs) with pulse dosing
- Itraconazole continuous: 200 mg/day PO for 6 weeks for fingernails and 12 weeks for toenails (less effective than itraconazole pulse for dermatophytes, more effective than terbinafine for *Candida* and molds)

Second Line

- Fluconazole pulse: 150 to 300 mg PO weekly for 6 months; not FDA approved for onychomycosis
- Griseofulvin: 500 to 1,000 mg/day PO for up to 18 months; less effective with significant adverse events
- Posaconazole: 100, 200, or 400 mg once daily for 24 weeks; 400 mg once daily for 12 weeks; higher cost
- Topical agents: Use limited to disease not involving the lunula (proximal nail plate) or when <3 nails are affected. Topical therapy does not cause systemic toxicity but is much less effective than oral therapy.
- Efinaconazole solution 10%, apply directly to affected nails once daily for 48 weeks; complete or almost-complete cure after 48 weeks in range of 15–18%
- Ciclopirox: 8% nail lacquer: Apply once daily to affected nails for up to 48 weeks; remove lacquer with alcohol every 7 days, and then file loose nail material and trim nails. Application after PO treatment may reduce recurrences; systematic review >60% failure rate after 48 weeks of use (3)[A]
- Tavaborole 5% solution, indicated for onychomycosis of the toenails due to *T. rubrum* or *T. mentagrophytes*; complete or almost-complete cure 15–18% after 48 weeks; reserve topical treatment for those with less extensive disease and no proximal involvement who wish to avoid oral medication
- Contraindications for oral antifungals: hepatic disease, pregnancy, current/history of congestive heart failure (CHF) or ventricular dysfunction (itraconazole), porphyria (griseofulvin)
- Precautions/adverse effects:
  - Oral antifungals: rhinitis (itraconazole); CHF, peripheral edema, pulmonary edema (itraconazole), chronic kidney disease (avoid terbinafine for patients with creatinine clearance [CrCl] <50 mL/min; decrease fluconazole dose), photosensitivity, lupus-like symptoms, proteinuria (griseofulvin), hypersensitivity; hepatotoxicity/neutropenia

SURGERY/OTHER PROCEDURES

- Trimming, avulsion, débridement, or nail abrasion to reduce fungal load and enhance penetration of antifungal agents
  - Mechanical: File with abrasive stone or curette.
  - Chemical: Protect peripheral tissue with adhesive strips; apply ointment of 30% salicylic acid, 40% urea, or 50% potassium iodide under occlusive dressing.
  - Débridement may be combined with topical antifungal therapy.
  - Surgical avulsion if few nails are involved for pain control
- Laser treatment has shown some positive results but poor statistical power and limited efficacy or safety data.
- Limited data with using photodynamic therapy using topical photosensitizing agents and irradiation

COMPLEMENTARY & ALTERNATIVE MEDICINE

Melaleuca alternifolia (tea tree oil): Cochrane review found no evidence of benefit (3)[A]. Vicks VapoRub application to nails daily for 48 weeks has been found safe, but efficacy is uncertain.

ONGOING CARE

FOLLOW-UP RECOMMENDATIONS

Formation of a new fingernail takes 4 to 6 months, and a new toenail takes 12 to 18 months.

Patient Monitoring

- Topical agents: Slow response is expected; visits every 6 to 12 weeks
- Terbinafine, griseofulvin: baseline, and as needed, LFTs and CBC
- Itraconazole continuous: baseline, and as needed, LFTs

PATIENT EDUCATION

Advise patient to: Keep affected area clean and dry, avoid occlusive footwear, wear absorbent socks, discard old sneakers, and avoid sharing nail implements and using on both infected and uninfected nails. Cure may not be attainable.

PROGNOSIS

- Complete clinical cure in 25–50% (higher mycologic cure rates) with oral therapy
- Recurrence rate due to relapse or reinfection 10–50%
- Poor prognostic factors
  - Areas of nail involvement >50%
  - Significant proximal/lateral disease
  - Subungual hyperkeratosis >2 mm
  - White/yellow or orange/brown streaks in the nail (includes dermatophytoma)
  - Total dystrophic onychomycosis (with matrix involvement)
  - Nonresponsive organisms (e.g., *Scytalidium* mold)
  - Patients with immunosuppression
  - Diminished peripheral circulation

COMPLICATIONS

- Secondary infections with progression to soft tissue infection/osteomyelitis particularly in immunocompromised
- Toenail discomfort/pain that can limit physical mobility or activity
- Anxiety, negative self-image

REFERENCES

1. Lipner SR, Scher RK. Onychomycosis: treatment and prevention of recurrence. *J Am Acad Dermatol*. 2019;80(4):853–867.
2. Kreijkamp-Kaspers S, Hawke K, Guo L, et al. Oral antifungal medication for toenail onychomycosis. *Cochrane Database Syst Rev*. 2017;7(7):CD010031.
3. Crawford F, Hollis S. Topical treatments for fungal infections of the skin and nails of the foot. *Cochrane Database Syst Rev*. 2007;(3):CD001434.

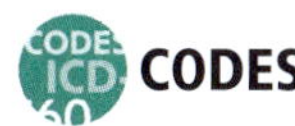

CODES

ICD10

- B35.1 Tinea unguium
- B37.2 Candidiasis of skin and nail

CLINICAL PEARLS

- Psoriasis and chronic nail trauma are commonly mistaken for fungal infection.
- Diagnosis should be based on both clinical and mycologic laboratory evidence.
- Oral medication is much more effective than topical, but recurrence following treatment is common.

OPIOID USE DISORDER

Daniel Albrecht, MD

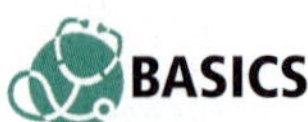

BASICS

DESCRIPTION

Opioid use disorder (OUD) describes the persistent use of opioids in the setting of clinical dysfunction with or without the manifestations of tolerance and withdrawal to opioids. Diagnosis is made by a checklist of symptoms defined by the *Diagnostic and Statistical Manual of Mental Disorders, 5th edition* (*DSM-5*). The criteria are not considered to be met for individuals taking opioids solely under appropriate medical supervision.

EPIDEMIOLOGY

Prevalence

In 2018, an estimated 10,250,000 people reported opioid misuse (3.7% of population ≥12 years old)

- 2,028,000 of those met *DSM-5* criteria for a diagnosis of OUD (0.7% of population ≥12 years old) (1).

RISK FACTORS

- Prior history of substance use disorder
- More severe reported pain
- Co-occurring mental disorders (2)

GENERAL PREVENTION

- Opioid prescriptions have been reduced by 29% between 2006 and 2018, which reduces access to prescription opioids.
- Harm reduction practices can prevent complications from OUD such as clean needle exchanges and safe injection sites.
- Access to intranasal naloxone can prevent opioid-related deaths.

COMMONLY ASSOCIATED CONDITIONS

- Mood disorders
- Personality disorders
- Posttraumatic stress disorder (PTSD)
- Other substance use disorders
- Sexually transmitted infections
- Hepatitis A, B, C
- HIV

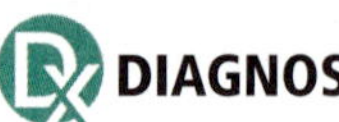

DIAGNOSIS

- The *DSM-5* describes 11 criteria to support the diagnosis of OUD, with severity defined as mild with 2 to 3 symptoms present, moderate with 4 to 5 symptoms present and severe with ≥6 symptoms present. The following criteria are generally referenced when assessing severity:
  - Opioids taken in larger amounts or for longer periods of time than required to treat pain, with a great deal of time is spent in activities obtaining and using the opioid, or to recover from adverse effects.
  - There are cravings to use opioids and the ongoing use resulting in a failure to fulfill expected social obligations.
  - Despite use, there is a persistent desire, often unsuccessful, to decrease opioid use.
  - Continued opioid use results in failures to fulfill major role obligations at work, school, or home, and use continues despite persistent social or interpersonal problems.
  - Recurrent opioid use in situations in which it is physically hazardous
- Tolerance, as defined by either a need for markedly increased amounts of opioids or markedly diminished effect with continued use of the same amount of an opioid.

PHYSICAL EXAM

- Patients in withdrawal from opioids may exhibit symptoms of sweating, restlessness, severe body aches, pupillary dilation, tremor, anxiety, and diarrhea.
- Patient under the effects of opioids may be more confused, lethargic, and have a decreased level of awareness. Opioids reduce respiratory drive and in severe cases can lead to apnea and death. Pupillary constriction can be used to differentiate opioid intoxication from other illicit substances, but the high prevalence of contamination in the illicit opioid supply makes this finding less reliable.

DIFFERENTIAL DIAGNOSIS

- Physical dependence on an opioid
- Disorders causing psychosis
- Mood disorders
- Effects of trauma including PTSD
- Another substance use disorder
- Polysubstance use disorder

DIAGNOSTIC TESTS & INTERPRETATION

One could make the diagnosis of OUD without additional testing; however, a medical professional may choose to obtain data from a prescription drug monitoring program or by urine or saliva drug testing.

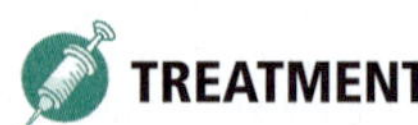

TREATMENT

GENERAL MEASURES

- Treatment mainstays include both medications for OUD (MOUD) and a variety of therapy interventions performed by trained professionals.
- Intranasal naloxone (Narcan) should be prescribed to all patients.
  - Family, friends, and bystanders can administer in the setting of an overdose with a brief training.
  - Narcan reverses the effects of opioids causing respiratory and CNS depression almost immediately.
  - Narcan given to a person without experiencing an opioid overdose has minimal side effects.

MEDICATION

First Line

- Opioid agonists act by binding the opioid receptors stronger than prescription or illicit opioids. These medications include:
  - Methadone: a long-acting, full opioid agonist whose half-life allows for once daily dosing; available in an oral solution or tablet, methadone for maintenance medication-assisted treatment (MAT) is only available at designated distribution sites, but can also be used as a chronic pain agent
  - Buprenorphine: a partial mu-opioid agonist; buprenorphine is available in transmucosal films or tablets as well as newer products including implants and injectable solutions; it is often paired with naloxone (Suboxone), to discourage abuse of buprenorphine
    - Injectable buprenorphine is now available and widely used as a MOUD.
- Opioid antagonists are also a potential therapy and include naltrexone, which comes in both injectable and oral forms. As full antagonists, these medications have the potential to send patients into withdrawal if they have not been off of opioids for roughly 1 week.

ISSUES FOR REFERRAL

Pregnancy Considerations

- Will face challenges with pain management and potential for neonatal abstinence syndrome (NAS) in newborns
- The American College of Obstetricians and Gynecologists recognizes usual prenatal guidelines may need adjustment for women with co-occurring OUD and therefore may benefit from a provider with more experience caring for pregnant women with OUD.
- Newborns born to mothers with OUD even on MAT should be monitored by a provider trained in evaluating for NAS.

ADDITIONAL THERAPIES

Patients are also recommended engaging with psychosocial interventions. These psychosocial interventions should be individualized and patient autonomy to decline these interventions should be respected (3).

ADMISSION, INPATIENT, AND NURSING CONSIDERATIONS

Pain management is challenging with patients diagnosed with OUD or who have a history of opioid misuse and may require higher doses of opioid analgesia or alternative medications.

ONGOING CARE

PATIENT EDUCATION

- All patients with OUD should discuss harm reduction practices to reduce chronic illnesses, including using needle exchanges or pharmacies to obtain clean needles for injecting and intranasal or oral opioid use as opposed to IV administration.
- Intranasal naloxone (Narcan) prescriptions should be sent to all patients with OUD and close acquaintances.

PROGNOSIS

Mortality is high due to death by unintentional overdose and significant medical complications.

- In the United States in 2023, of 105,007 overdose-related deaths, 72,776 were related to the use of synthetic opioids other than methadone, primarily illicitly manufactured fentanyl (4).

REFERENCES

1. National Center for Injury Prevention and Control. Annual Surveillance Report of Drug-Related Risks and Outcomes. Centers for Disease Control and Prevention. 2019. https://www.cdc.gov/overdose-prevention/media/pdfs/pubs/2019-cdc-drug-surveillance-report.pdf. Accessed December 16, 2025.
2. Kaye AD, Jones MR, Kaye AM, et al. Prescription opioid abuse in chronic pain: an updated review of opioid abuse predictors and strategies to curb opioid abuse: part 1. *Pain Physician*. 2017;20(2S):S93–S109.
3. Cunningham C, Edlund MJ, Fishman M, et al. The ASAM national practice guideline for the treatment of opioid use disorder: 2020 focused update. *J Addict Med*. 2020:14(2S Suppl 1):1–91.
4. National Institute on Drug Abuse. Drug Overdose Deaths: Facts and Figures. Retrieved from https://nida.nih.gov/research-topics/trends-statistics/overdose-death-rates on 2025, July 9. Accessed December 12, 2025.

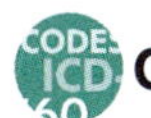

CODES

ICD10

- F11.10 Opioid abuse, uncomplicated
- F11.90 Opioid use, unspecified, uncomplicated
- F11.1 Opioid abuse

CLINICAL PEARLS

- Treatment includes both MAT and therapy interventions performed by trained professionals.
- Intranasal naloxone (Narcan) should be prescribed to all patients and close acquaintances.

OPTIC NEURITIS

Teri T. Kleinberg, MD, MSc

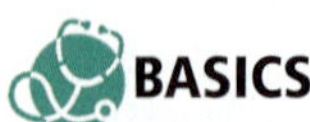

BASICS

DESCRIPTION

- Inflammation of the optic nerve (cranial nerve II) causing an optic neuropathy
- Commonly presents as acute demyelinating optic neuritis associated with multiple sclerosis (MS) (presenting complaint in 25% of MS patients), but other causes include infectious disease and systemic autoimmune disorders.
- Optic disc often normal in appearance at onset (retrobulbar ON, 67%) or swollen (papillitis, 33%).
- Key features:
  - Abrupt central visual loss (typically monocular)
  - Periorbital pain with eye movement (90%)
  - Dyschromatopsia: color vision deficits
  - Relative afferent pupillary defect (RAPD)
- Usually unilateral in adults; bilateral disease more common in children
- In children, headaches are common.
- System(s) affected: nervous
- Synonym(s): papillitis, demyelinating optic neuropathy; retrobulbar ON

EPIDEMIOLOGY

Incidence

- 5/100,000 cases per year
- More common in whites than in other races
- Predominant age: 18 to 45 years; mean age 30 years
- Predominant sex: female > male (3:1)

ETIOLOGY AND PATHOPHYSIOLOGY

- Cause is presumed to be a demyelinating autoimmune reaction.
- Neuromyelitis optica (NMO) IgG autoantibody, which targets the water channel aquaporin-4 (AQP4) in neuromyelitis optica spectrum disorder (NMOSD)
- Myelin oligodendrocyte glycoprotein (MOG) autoantibody in myelin oligodendrocyte glycoprotein antibody-associated disease (MOGAD)
- Viral infections: measles, mumps, varicella-zoster, coxsackievirus, adenovirus, hepatitis A and B, HIV, herpes simplex virus, cytomegalovirus, SARS-CoV-2 (MOGAD can be seen with COVID-19) (1)
- Nonviral infections: syphilis, tuberculosis, meningococcus, cryptococcosis, cysticercosis, bacterial sinusitis, *Streptococcus B*, *Bartonella*, typhoid fever, Lyme disease
- Systemic inflammatory disease: sarcoidosis, systemic lupus erythematosus, vasculitis
- Local inflammatory disease: intraocular or contiguous with the orbit, sinus, or meninges

Genetics

Genetics: Some people have genetic mutations that increase their chance of optic neuritis (i.e., MS) and several immune-mediated inflammatory diseases (IMIDs).

COMMONLY ASSOCIATED CONDITIONS

- MS (common): ON is associated with an increased risk of MS (30% risk in Optic Neuritis Treatment Trial [2])
- Other demyelinating diseases: NMO (Devic disease), multifocal demyelinating neuropathy, acute disseminated encephalomyelitis (ADEM)

DIAGNOSIS

- Clinical criteria
  - A: Monocular, subacute loss of vision associated with orbital pain worsening on eye movements, reduced contrast and color vision, and relative afferent pupillary deficit
  - B: Painless with all other features of (A).
  - C: Binocular loss of vision with all features of (A) or (B).
- Paraclinical criteria
  - Optical coherence tomography (OCT): Corresponding optic disc swelling acutely or an inter-eye difference in the mGCIPL of >4% or >4 μm or in the pRNFL of >5% or >5 μm within 3 months after onset.
  - MRI: contrast enhancement of the symptomatic optic nerve and sheaths acutely or an intrinsic signal (looking brighter) increase within 3 months
  - Biomarker: AQP4, MOG, or CRMP5 antibody seropositive, or intrathecal CSF IgG (oligoclonal bands).
- Application of the clinical and paraclinical criteria
  - Definite optic neuritis
    - (A) and one paraclinical test
    - (B) and two paraclinical tests of different modality
    - (C) and two different paraclinical tests of which one is MRI
- Possible optic neuritis
  - (A), (B), or (C) if seen acutely but in absence of paraclinical tests, with fundus examination typical for optic neuritis and consistent with the natural history during follow-up
  - Positive paraclinical test or tests, with a medical history suggestive of optic neuritis (3)

HISTORY

- *Decreased visual acuity*, deteriorating in hours to days, usually reaching lowest level after 1 week
- Usually unilateral but can also be bilateral
- Brow ache, globe tenderness, deep orbital *pain* exacerbated by *eye movement* (92%)
- Periorbital pain may precede visual loss.
- Desaturation of color vision (dull or faded colors), especially red tones
- Apparent dimness of light intensities
- Impairment of depth perception (80%); worse with moving objects (*Pulfrich phenomenon*)
- Transient increase in visual symptoms with increased body temperature and exercise (*Uhthoff phenomenon*)
- *Phosphenes*: fleeting colors and flashes of light (30%)
- May present with a recent flulike viral syndrome
- Detailed history and review of systems, looking for a history of demyelinating, infectious, or systemic inflammatory disease

PHYSICAL EXAM

Complete general exam, full neurologic exam, and ophthalmologic exam (with visual field) looking for the following:

- Decreased visual acuity and color perception
- Central, cecocentral, arcuate, or altitudinal visual field deficits
- Optic disc edema: (1/3) swollen disc or often (2/3) normal disc exam
- RAPD: The pupil of the affected eye dilates with a swinging light test unless disease is bilateral.

DIFFERENTIAL DIAGNOSIS

- Demyelinating diseases including MS, NMO, MOG
- Infectious/systemic inflammatory disease including sarcoidosis
- Acute papilledema (bilateral disc edema)
- Compression from a tumor/abscess compressing the optic nerve
- Temporal arteritis or other vasculitides
- Nonarteritic ischemic optic neuropathy (NAION)
- Diabetic papillopathy

DIAGNOSTIC TESTS & INTERPRETATION

Initial Tests (lab, imaging)

- Gadolinium-enhanced brain MRI and orbits to evaluate optic nerve and evaluate for white matter lesions to assess MS risk and differentiate between possible etiologies
- Serum NMO (AQP4-IgG) and MOG antibody testing is suggested for individuals without clear diagnosis of MS or atypical presentation as prompt initiation of immunotherapy required (4).
- For atypical presentations, including absence of pain, a very swollen optic nerve, >30 days without recovery, or retinal exudates:
  - Labs: ESR, CBC, CRP, ACE, FTA-ABS, SARS-CoV-2 PCR, QuantiFERON-TB gold, tick-bourne diseases, as directed by clinical history
  - Chest x-ray (CXR) or CT scan if high clinical suspicion of sarcoidosis
  - Lumbar puncture (LP) for CSF composition and oligoclonal bands

Follow-Up Tests & Special Considerations

- OCT of the retinal nerve fiber layer (RNFL); a noninvasive imaging technique of the optic nerve; may serve as a diagnostic tool to quantify thickness of the nerve fiber layer objectively and monitor structural change (axonal loss) of the optic nerve over time
- Visual field test (Humphrey 30–2) to evaluate for visual field loss: diffuse and central visual loss more predominant in the affected eye at baseline
- Low-contrast visual acuity

Diagnostic Procedures/Other

In atypical cases, including bilateral deficits, young age, or suspicion of infectious etiology, LP with neurology consultation indicated

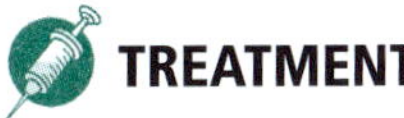

TREATMENT

Most recover spontaneously.

MEDICATION

First Line

- IV methylprednisolone (IVMP) hastens recovery of idiopathic and MS-associated disease by approximately 15 days but does not affect final visual outcome per the Optic Neuritis Treatment Trial (4); consider for patients who require fast recovery (i.e., monocular patients or those whose occupation requires high-level visual acuity) or more severe presenting vision loss.
  - Observation without treatment acceptable with typical presentation and mild vision loss (4)
  - High-dose IV MP (250 mg q6h for 3 days) followed by oral corticosteroids (1 mg/kg/day PO for 11 days, taper over 1 to 2 weeks) (5)
  - Longer steroid taper (1 to 3 months) if high suspicion of NMOSD or MOGAD (4)
- Discuss benefits and potential side effects of corticosteroids with patient (i.e., weight gain, osteoporosis, mood changes, gastrointestinal disturbances, hyperglycemia, insomnia)

ALERT

Avoid oral prednisone alone at intermediate doses (1 mg/kg/day), as the primary treatment because this may increase the risk for recurrent ON as compared to IV MP or no treatment.

Second Line

- Plasmapheresis (PLEX) considered in patients failing to respond to IVMP to temporarily remove pathologic antibodies especially in suspected NMOSD or atypical optic neuritis (2),(4)
- Disease-modifying agents, such as interferon-β1a (IFN-β1a; Avonex, Rebif) and IFN-β1b (Betaseron), are used to prevent or delay the development of MS in people with ON with $\geq$2 brain lesions evident on MRI (6).
- Long-term immunosuppressive therapy should be initiated promptly, especially after diagnosis of NMOSD (eculizumab, inebilizumab, satralizumab all recently FDA-approved) or MOGAD (monthly intravenous immunoglobulin infusions) (4).

Pediatric Considerations

- Optic disc swelling and bilateral disease are more common in children as is severe loss of visual acuity (20/200 or worse).
- Obtain serologic marker for antibodies to myelin oligodendrocyte glycoprotein antibody (MOG-Ab) (7).
- No systematic study defining high-dose corticosteroids in children with pediatric optic neuritis has been conducted.
  - Consensus recommends: 3 to 5 days of IV MP (4 to 30 mg/kg/day), followed by a 2- to 4-week taper of oral steroids
- Consider infectious and postinfectious causes of optic nerve impairment.

ADMISSION, INPATIENT, AND NURSING CONSIDERATIONS

In acute severe visual loss, admission to expedite diagnosis workup and treatment

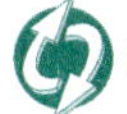

ONGOING CARE

FOLLOW-UP RECOMMENDATIONS

Patient Monitoring

Monthly to monitor visual changes and steroid side effects

PATIENT EDUCATION

North American Neuro-Ophthalmology Society (NANOS): https://www.nanosweb.org/files/Patient%20Brochures/English/2021/Optic_Neuritis.pdf (available in other languages)

PROGNOSIS

- Orbital pain usually resolves within 1 week.
- Improvement of visual acuity begins over 2 to 4 weeks and steadily continues over 6 to 12 weeks. Visual acuity often returns to normal (20/40 or better) within 1 year (90–95%), even after severe presenting visual deficit
- Other visual disturbances (e.g., contrast sensitivity) often persist after acuity returns to normal.
- Recurrence risk of 35% within 10 years: 14% affected eye, 12% contralateral, 9% bilateral; recurrence is higher in MS patients (48%).
- ON is associated with an increased risk of developing MS: 35% risk at 7 years, and 58% at 15 years.
- Poor prognostic factors include absence of pain, severe initial vision loss, and involvement of intracanalicular optic nerve.
- Children with bilateral visual loss have a better prognosis than adults.

COMPLICATIONS

Permanent loss of vision

REFERENCES

1. Benito-Pascual B, Gegúndez JA, Díaz-Valle D, et al. Panuveitis and optic neuritis as a possible initial presentation of the novel coronavirus disease 2019 (COVID-19). *Ocul Immunol Inflamm*. 2020;28(6):922–925.
2. Gostimir M, Sergott RC. Biomarker defined acute optic neuritis: a review and perspective. *Curr Treat Options Neurol*. 2023;25(9):307–322.
3. Petzold A, Fraser CL, Abegg M, et al. Diagnosis and classification of optic neuritis. *Lancet Neurol*. 2022;21(12):1120–1134. doi:10.1016/S1474-4422(22)00200-9.
4. Bergeron E, Bouffard MA. Evidence-based management of optic neuritis. *Curr Opin Ophthalmol*. 2024;35(1):73–82.
5. Vedula SS, Brodney-Folse S, Gal RL, et al. Corticosteroids for treating optic neuritis. *Cochrane Database Syst Rev*. 2007;(1):CD001430.
6. Balk LJ, Cruz-Herranz A, Albrecht P, et al. Timing of retinal neuronal and axonal loss in MS: a longitudinal OCT study. *J Neurol*. 2016;263(7):1323–1331.
7. Zhou S, Jones-Lopez EC, Soneji DJ, et al. Myelin oligodendrocyte glycoprotein antibody-associated optic neuritis and myelitis in COVID-19. *J Neuroophthalmol*. 2020;40(3):398–402.

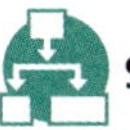

SEE ALSO

Multiple Sclerosis

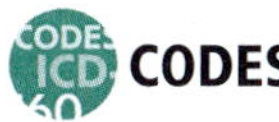

CODES

ICD10

- H46.9 Unspecified optic neuritis
- H46.00 Optic papillitis, unspecified eye
- H46.10 Retrobulbar neuritis, unspecified eye

CLINICAL PEARLS

- Key features include an abrupt visual loss (typically monocular), with periorbital pain with eye movement
- Brain MRI and orbits with contrast is the diagnostic procedure of choice for determining etiology and MS treatment recommendations
- High-dose IV MP followed by oral prednisone speeds visual recovery but does not improve 1-year visual outcome, whereas treatment with oral prednisone alone did not improve the outcome and was associated with an increased rate of recurrence of ON.

OSGOOD-SCHLATTER DISEASE (TIBIAL APOPHYSITIS)

Jacob Ringenberg, MD, CAQSM, MUSC, AHEC • Daniel D. Divilbiss, MD

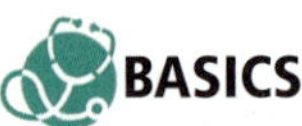

BASICS

DESCRIPTION

- Osgood-Schlatter disease (OSD) is a syndrome associated with traction apophysitis and patellar tendinosis that is most common in adolescent boys and girls.
- Patients classically present with pain and swelling of the anterior tibial tubercle.
- System(s) affected: musculoskeletal
- Synonym(s): tibial tubercle apophysitis

EPIDEMIOLOGY

Incidence

The incidence in girls is rising with increased participation in organized youth sports; almost equal to boys in the United States

Prevalence

- A common apophysitis in childhood and adolescence affecting athletes more than twice as frequently as nonathletes
- Estimated point prevalence of 10% in the general population aged 12 to 15 years

ETIOLOGY AND PATHOPHYSIOLOGY

Traction apophysitis of the tibial tubercle due to repetitive strain on the secondary ossification center of the tibial tuberosity; concurrent patellar tendinosis, disruption of the proximal tibial apophysis, and avulsion microfractures at the tibial tuberosity are contributing factors.

- Jumping and pivoting sports place the highest strain on the tibial tubercle. Repetitive trauma and deceleration with an eccentric load are the most likely inciting factors.
- Likely biomechanical association with tight iliopsoas, quadriceps, and hamstring muscles; increased quadriceps strength relative to hamstring strength in adolescence contributes

RISK FACTORS

- Affects children and adolescents most commonly from the ages of 8 to 18 years
  - Girls 8 to 13 years old
  - Boys 10 to 15 years old
- OSD is slightly more common in boys than girls but likely equally common with similar sports participation.
- Early sport specialization increases the risk of OSD 4-fold.
- Rapid skeletal growth
- Weak core stabilizing muscles
- Increased weight/BMI/height
- Patellofemoral malalignment
- Overload training volume
- Quadriceps tightness and/or shortening
- Hamstring tightness or relative weakness in ratio to the quadriceps
- Participation in repetitive-jumping sports and sports with heavy quadriceps activity (football, volleyball, basketball, hockey, soccer, skating, gymnastics)
- Ballet (2-fold risk compared with nonathletes)

GENERAL PREVENTION

- Avoid sports with heavy quadriceps loading (especially deceleration activities and eccentric loading).
- Increase hamstring and quadriceps flexibility.
- Reduce sports specialization.
- Increase cross-training.

COMMONLY ASSOCIATED CONDITIONS

- Shortened (tight) rectus femoris found in 75% with OSD
- Hamstring tightness
- Possible association with ADD/ADHD; adolescents with ADD/ADHD are at risk for other musculoskeletal injuries.
- Sinding-Larsen-Johansson apophysitis
- Calcaneal apophysitis (Sever disease)

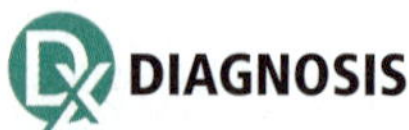

DIAGNOSIS

HISTORY

- Unilateral or bilateral (30%) pain of the tibial tuberosity
- Pain exacerbated by exercise; particularly jumping, landing, and squatting
- Pain upon kneeling on the affected side(s)
- Antalgic or straight-legged gait
- Heavy or increasing intensity of jumping/cutting sports

PHYSICAL EXAM

- Knee pain with squatting or crouching
- Absence of effusion or condyle tenderness
- Tibial tuberosity swelling and tenderness
- Pain increased with resisted knee extension or kneeling
- Erythema over tibial tuberosity
- Hamstring/quadriceps tightness
- Core muscle weakness
- Functional testing: Single-leg squat (SLS) and standing broad jump reproduce pain.

DIFFERENTIAL DIAGNOSIS

- Stress fracture of the proximal tibia
- Pes anserinus bursitis
- Quadriceps tendon avulsion
- Patellofemoral stress syndrome
- Chondromalacia patellae (retropatellar pain)
- Proximal tibial neoplasm
- Osteomyelitis of the proximal tibia
- Tibial plateau fracture
- Sinding-Larsen-Johansson syndrome (patellar apophysitis)—pain over inferior patellar tendon
- Patellar fracture or stress fracture
- Infrapatellar bursitis
- Patellar tendinitis—pain over inferior patellar tendon and inferior pole of patella
- Plica syndrome
- Osteochondroma of the tibial tubercle
- Tibial tuberosity fracture
- Patellar tendon lipoma
- Bacterial apophysitis
- Osteosynchondroses
- Osteochondritis dissecans
- Iliotibial band syndrome
- Hoffa disease (infrapatellar fat pad syndrome)
- Saphenous neuritis

DIAGNOSTIC TESTS & INTERPRETATION

Initial Tests (lab, imaging)

- Generally a clinical diagnosis; no tests are indicated unless other diagnoses are under consideration.
- Radiographic imaging of the proximal tibia and knee may show heterotopic calcification in the patellar tendon on the lateral view and primarily serves to rule out other pathology:
  - X-rays are rarely diagnostic, but appearance of a separate fragment at the tibial tuberosity identifies candidates for potential surgical intervention.
  - Calcified thickening of the tibial tuberosity with irregular ossification at tendon insertion on the tibial tubercle, fragmentation of the apophysis (1)[B]

Diagnostic Procedures/Other

- Bone scan may show increased uptake in the area of the tibial tuberosity:
  - Increased uptake in apophysitis is normal in children, but with OSD, there may be more uptake on the affected side.
- Ultrasound is a useful imaging modality, showing thickening of the distal patellar tendon, occasional infrapatellar bursa effusion, irregular ossification, and neovascularity of the patellar tendon insertion (1)[B].
- MRI shows fragmentation of the tibial tubercle and hyperintense T2 signal of the apophysis and patellar tendon insertion in more advanced cases.

Test Interpretation

Biopsy is not necessary but would show osteolysis and fragmentation of the tibial tubercle.

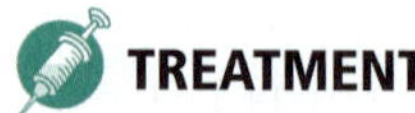

TREATMENT

GENERAL MEASURES

- No randomized controlled studies have been published to demonstrate clear benefit of any treatment over another.
- Frequent ice applications 2 to 3 times per day for 15 to 20 minutes
- Rest and activity modification—avoid activities that increase pain and/or swelling.
- Physical therapy helps with hamstring and quadriceps strengthening and stretching.
- Open- and closed-chain eccentric quadriceps strengthening

- Avoid aggressive dynamic stretching if pain is significant to avoid risk of tibial tubercle avulsion.
- Consult orthopedic surgery for tibial tuberosity fracture or complete avulsion.
- Electrical stimulation and iontophoresis have been reported (1)[B].
- Patients with marked midfoot pronation may benefit from orthotics.
- Various bracing options can be used including infrapatellar straps.
- With more severe disease, longer-term removal from sports may be indicated.

MEDICATION

First Line

- Common OTC analgesics may be considered.
- NSAIDs may be beneficial for pain relief.
- Opioids are not recommended as first line.

Second Line

- More potent analgesics, such as opioids, may *only* be considered for short-term use in extreme situations.
- Corticosteroid injections are not recommended.
- Hyperosmolar dextrose injections (prolotherapy) have shown benefit in randomized controlled trials (2)[B].
- Autologous conditioned plasma (ACP) has shown benefit in limited case studies (3)[C].
- Leukocyte-rich (LR) platelet-rich plasma has shown benefit in limited case studies.

ISSUES FOR REFERRAL

When conservative therapy is unsuccessful and symptoms persist into adulthood, consider surgical referral.

SURGERY/OTHER PROCEDURES

- Radial extracorporeal shockwave therapy (ESWT) has been used safely and effectively in retrospective observational studies.
- Débridement of a thickened, cosmetically unsatisfactory tibial tubercle (rare) or removal of mobile heterotopic bone
- Surgical excision of a painful tibial tubercle is rarely needed (<5%) and may be successfully done with bursoscopy instead of an open procedure.
- Recent report of successful pain elimination in OSD with percutaneous screw fixation of the tibial tuberosity (1)[C]
- Reduction wedge osteotomy has been recently reported as 100% successful in a small case series.

COMPLEMENTARY & ALTERNATIVE MEDICINE

Acupuncture has been used successfully as a treatment modality.

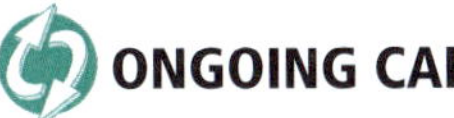

ONGOING CARE

FOLLOW-UP RECOMMENDATIONS

- Athletes may return to play if pain is controlled.
- Presence of pain does not preclude competition.

Patient Monitoring

With worsening of symptoms only

PATIENT EDUCATION

- Avoid jumping sports or reduce activities that increase pain and swelling.
- Assure patients and their family that symptoms and physical findings will diminish with time and rest.
- Patients can safely play sports with mild pain.
- Quadriceps and hamstring stretching and strengthening are important.
- Surgical options are rarely needed, but good results can be expected.

PROGNOSIS

- Usually, this is a self-limited condition that resolves within 2 years of full skeletal maturation. However, recent data suggest that many are affected into adulthood and must reduce sports and physical activity.
- Most patients with OSD will have residual prominence of the tibial tubercle that may never completely resolve.

COMPLICATIONS

- Rarely, a heavily fragmented and inflamed tibial ossicle will avulse and require surgery.
- Although 90% are reported to resolve, recent studies suggest that chronic pain and reduction of activity may continue into adulthood.
- Rare complications in adulthood include pseudarthrosis of the tibial tubercle, genu recurvatum, patella alta, and ossicle fragmentation possibly leading to osteoarthritis of the knee.

REFERENCES

1. Ladenhauf HN, Seitlinger G, Green DW. Osgood-Schlatter disease: a 2020 update of a common knee condition in children. *Curr Opin Pediatr*. 2020;32(1):107–112.
2. Wu Z, Tu X, Tu Z. Hyperosmolar dextrose injection for Osgood-Schlatter disease: a double-blind, randomized controlled trial. *Arch Orthop Trauma Surg*. 2022;142(9):2279–2285.
3. Danneberg DJ. Successful treatment of Osgood-Schlatter disease with autologous-conditioned plasma in two patients. *Joints*. 2017;5(3):191–194.

ADDITIONAL READING

Guldhammer C, Rathleff MS, Jensen HP, et al. Long-term prognosis and impact of Osgood-Schlatter disease 4 years after diagnosis: a retrospective study. *Orthop J Sports Med*. 2019;7(10):2325967119878136.

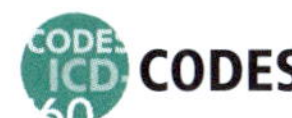

CODES

ICD10

- M92.50 Juvenile osteochondrosis of tibia and fibula, unsp leg
- M92.51 Juvenile osteochondrosis of tibia and fibula, right leg
- M92.52 Juvenile osteochondrosis of tibia and fibula, left leg

CLINICAL PEARLS

- Infrapatellar pain in an adolescent athlete is most commonly OSD, patellar tendinosis, or Sinding-Larsen-Johansson syndrome.
- OSD is generally self-limited. Athletes should modify activity based on pain. Mild pain is not a contraindication to athletic participation.
- Treatment focuses on strengthening and stretching of the hamstrings and quadriceps.
- ≥10% of adolescents with OSD will be symptomatic as adults.
- Persistent, employment hampering symptoms in adults may require surgical intervention.

OSTEOARTHRITIS

Patrick Wakefield Joyner, MD, MS

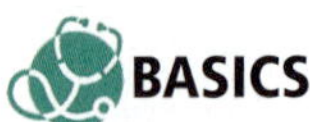

BASICS

DESCRIPTION

- Progressive loss of articular cartilage with reactive changes at joint margins and in subchondral bone
- Primary osteoarthritis (OA)
  - Idiopathic: categorized by clinical features (localized, generalized, erosive)
- Secondary OA
  - Posttraumatic (e.g., ACL rupture, distal radius fracture, shoulder dislocation)
  - Childhood anatomic abnormalities (e.g., congenital hip dysplasia, slipped capital femoral epiphysis [SCFE])
  - Inheritable metabolic disorders (e.g., Wilson disease, alkaptonuria, hemochromatosis)
  - Neuropathic arthropathy (Charcot joints)
  - Endocrinopathies: acromegalic arthropathy, hyperparathyroidism, hypothyroidism
  - Noninfectious inflammatory arthritis (e.g., rheumatoid arthritis [RA], spondyloarthropathies)
  - Gout, calcium pyrophosphate deposition disease (pseudogout)
- Synonym(s): osteoarthrosis; degenerative joint disease (DJD)

EPIDEMIOLOGY

- Most common joint disease globally and in the United States
- The knee is the most commonly involved joint, followed by hips and hands.
- Symptomatic OA most common in patients >40 years
- Leading cause of disability and activity limitation, particularly in patients >65 years of age
- Predominant sex: Diagnosis in women is increasing.
- Predominantly impacts weight-bearing joints

Incidence

- Hip (symptomatic)—88/100,000 per year
- Knee (symptomatic)—240/100,000 per year

Prevalence

- >30 million patients affected in United States
- Increases with age; radiographic evidence of OA is present in many patients >65 years old.
- 16–20% of patients >65 years old have radiographic evidence of glenohumeral OA.
- 113% increase from 1990 to 2019
- Knee OA contributes to the most overall burden of any joint with OA.

ETIOLOGY AND PATHOPHYSIOLOGY

Failure of chondrocytes to maintain the balance between degradation and synthesis of extracellular collagen matrix; collagen loss results in alteration of proteoglycan matrix and increased susceptibility to degenerative change.

Genetics

- Up to 65% of OA cases may have a genetic component.
- The heritability of end-stage hip OA is up to 27%.
- >100 polymorphic DNA variants have been associated with OA; these variants account for >20% OA heritability.

RISK FACTORS

- Increasing age: >50 years
- Emerging evidence for an association with atopy
- Age as a risk factor is greatest for hip, knee, and shoulder OA.
- Obesity (weight-bearing joints); BMI >35 kg/m^2
- Trauma, infection, or inflammatory arthritis
- Female gender (knee and hand)

GENERAL PREVENTION

Weight management; regular physical activity, perijoint muscle strengthening ("prehabbing")

COMMONLY ASSOCIATED CONDITIONS

- Obesity
- History of trauma
- Shoulder arthritis can be associated with a rotator cuff tear.

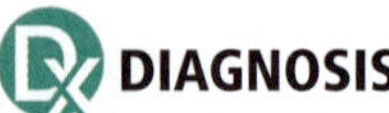

DIAGNOSIS

HISTORY

- Distinguish OA from other types of arthritis by:
  - Absence of systemic findings
  - Minimal articular inflammation
  - Distribution of involved joints (e.g., distal interphalangeal [DIP] and proximal interphalangeal [PIP] joints)
- OA characterized by slowly developing joint pain. Pain often described as aching or burning in nature. Anecdotally, many patients describe pain changes with alterations in weather conditions.
- Transient stiffness (especially after awakening in morning and after sitting) that tends to lessen 10 to 15 minutes after joint movement
- Most common joints in hand are as follows:
  - DIP > thumb carpometacarpal (CMC) > PIP > MCP

PHYSICAL EXAM

- Joint bony enlargement
- Decreased range of motion of affected joints
- Mechanical symptoms (clicking, locking) may be present, especially in knees with degenerative meniscal injury.
- Meniscus tear in the setting of severe/end-stage knee OA is an OA problem and should be treated as an OA ailment.
- OA is the most common cause of joint effusions.
- Local pain and stiffness with OA of spine; radicular pain (if compression of nerve roots)
- Changes in joint alignment (genu varum [bowlegs] and genu valgum [knock-knees])

DIFFERENTIAL DIAGNOSIS

- Crystalline arthropathies (gout; pseudogout): inflammatory arthritides (RA), spondyloarthropathies (reactive arthritis; psoriatic arthritis), septic arthritis
- Fibromyalgia; avascular necrosis; Lyme disease

DIAGNOSTIC TESTS & INTERPRETATION

Initial Tests (lab, imaging)

- Routine chemistries are not helpful in diagnosis.
- X-rays are usually normal early in disease process.
- As OA progresses, plain films show: Narrowed, asymmetric joint space, osteophyte formation, subchondral bony sclerosis, subchondral cyst formation
- MRI may particularly demonstrate chondral degeneration and associated meniscal tears. 5–10% weight loss is associated with slowing of arthritic changes and decreased chondral loss on follow-up studies, subchondral bone edema.

Follow-Up Tests & Special Considerations

- Monitor treatment with NSAIDs (renal insufficiency and GI bleeding).
- In secondary OA, abnormal lab results associated with underlying disorder (e.g., hemochromatosis [abnormal iron studies])

Diagnostic Procedures/Other

Joint aspiration (not usually necessary for diagnosis)

- OA: cell count usually <500 cells/mm^3, predominantly mononuclear
- Inflammatory: cell count usually >2,000 cells/mm^3, predominantly neutrophils
- Birefringent crystals in gout (−) and pseudogout (+)

Test Interpretation

- Patchy cartilage damage and bony hypertrophy
- Histologic phases:
  - Extracellular matrix edema and cartilage microfissures, subchondral fissuring and pitting, erosion and formation of osteocartilaginous loose bodies
- Subchondral bone trabecular microfractures and sclerosis with osteophyte formation

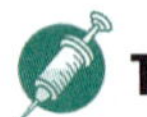

TREATMENT

GENERAL MEASURES

- Weight management combined with exercise/physical therapy to maintain or regain joint motion and muscle strength
  - Quadriceps-strengthening for knee OA—closed chain exercises
  - Periscapular strengthening and range of motion for shoulder OA
  - Abductor and core strengthening as well as gait mechanics for hip OA
- Transition to non–weight-bearing exercises (i.e., elliptical, stationary bike, swimming)
- All forms of exercise therapy improved outcome measures in knee arthritis (1).
- Bracing, joint supports, or insoles in patients with biomechanical instability:
  - Bracing is more beneficial in patients with unicompartmental disease of the knee.
- For knee OA in particular, several nonpharmacologic modalities are strongly recommended: aerobic, aquatic, and/or resistance exercise and weight loss.

MEDICATION

First Line

- Weight management: 1 lb of weight loss reduces pressure on lower extremities by ~4 lb
- Manage pain and inflammation:
  - Acetaminophen up to 1,000 mg TID: effective for pain relief in OA of knee and hip
  - Topical NSAID gels, creams have short-term (<4 weeks) benefits. Topical NSAIDs are a core treatment for hand and joints with minimal soft tissue–coverage (i.e., elbow, ankle, AC joint) OA.

 – If acetaminophen or topical NSAIDs are insufficient, consider an oral NSAID/COX-2 inhibitor. Use the lowest effective dose for the shortest time possible.
 – May use nonacetylated salicylates (e.g., salsalate, choline-magnesium salicylate) or low-dose ibuprofen ≤1,600 mg/day; consider a once-daily NSAID, if necessary, to help maintain compliance.

ALERT
- NSAIDs are associated with an increased risk of adverse cardiovascular events. The absolute risk is dependent on patient age, comorbidities, particular NSAID used, dose, and duration of use.

- All PO NSAIDs/COX-2 inhibitors have analgesic effects of a similar magnitude but vary in their potential GI and cardiorenal toxicity. Avoid NSAIDs in patients with renal disease, CHF, HTN, active peptic ulcer disease, and previous hypersensitivity to an NSAID or aspirin (ASA). Combination of NSAIDs and full-strength ASA (325 mg) is contraindicated. In patients at high cardiovascular risk: Combination of a nonselective NSAIDs and low-dose ASA (81 mg) is recommended. Oral or parenteral corticosteroids are contraindicated.
- Precautions:
  - If PO NSAIDs/COX-2 inhibitor use is necessary for a patient aged >65 years or a patient <65 years with increased GI bleeding risk factors, proton pump inhibitors are recommended.
  - Significant possible interactions:
    - NSAIDs reduce effectiveness of ACE inhibitors and diuretics. ASA and NSAIDs (except COX-2 inhibitors) may increase effects of anticoagulants. Salicylates reduce effectiveness of spironolactone (Aldactone) and uricosurics. Corticosteroids and some antacids increase salicylate excretion, whereas ascorbic acid and ammonium chloride reduce salicylate excretion and may cause toxicity.

Pregnancy Considerations
- ASA and NSAIDs have reported fetal risk during 1st and 3rd trimesters of pregnancy.
- Compatible with breastfeeding

Second Line
- Topical NSAIDs, CBD, and capsaicin can lower gastric and renal risks associated with oral NSAIDs.
- Bracing; medial and lateral unloader braces are effective; long leg alignment x-rays can help determine the appropriate brace.
- TENS modalities for pain may be more beneficial than hyaluronic acid (HA) injection.

Third Line
- Intra-auricular corticosteroid injections can be used for acute flares and for patients failing first- and second-line treatments. Minimize injections (≤3 per joint per year).
- Platelet-rich plasma (PRP) for patients with mild to moderate OA and patellofemoral OA
- In selected patients, PRP and bone marrow aspirate concentrate (BMAC) are equivalent in providing better and longer outcomes than HA injections alone (2).
- Combining HA with corticosteroids has longer relief than either alone (3).

ISSUES FOR REFERRAL
Disease that fails conservative management; concern for a septic joint or gout; musculoskeletal injury as a result of OA

ADDITIONAL THERAPIES
- Emerging therapies such as liposome-based dexamethasone and microspore-based triamcinolone show emerging promise.
- Address psychosocial factors (i.e., self-efficacy, coping skills). Screen for and appropriately treat anxiety and depression. Improve social support.

SURGERY/OTHER PROCEDURES
- Total knee arthroplasty (TKA), total hip arthroplasty (THA), total shoulder arthroplasty (TSA), reverse total shoulder arthroplasty (RTSA), and total ankle arthroplasty (TAA) all remain options for patients that fail conservative management for these respective joints. Total elbow arthroplasty (TEA) carries the highest complication and failure rate. TEA also results in lifelong weightbearing limitation of 5 lb.
- Ligament reconstruction and tendon interposition (LRTI) is an option for patients failing conservative treatment of the CMC joints.
- Arthroscopic débridement for patients >60 years of age with OA and meniscal pathology can experience long-term benefit (4).
- Patients possible too young for TKA can consider an osteotomy or unicompartmental knee arthroplasty (UKA).

COMPLEMENTARY & ALTERNATIVE MEDICINE
- Nutritional supplements (glucosamine and chondroitin sulfate) may benefit some patients and have low toxicity. There is lack of standardized outcome assessments. Trial results using glucosamine and chondroitin have been mixed. If no response is apparent within 6 months, discontinue use.
- TENS, yoga, and acupuncture have shown benefit.

ONGOING CARE

FOLLOW-UP RECOMMENDATIONS
- Follow-up at 3-month intervals for assessment of conservative management treatment and future options
- Recommend plain films of effected joint annually.

Patient Monitoring
Regularly assess range of motion and functional status. Monitor for GI blood loss and cardiac, renal, and mental status in older patients on NSAIDs or ASA; periodic CBC, renal function tests, stool for occult blood in patients on chronic NSAID therapy

DIET
Continue to ensure patients have adequate vitamin D intake and levels to maximize bone health.

PATIENT EDUCATION
- American College of Rheumatology: https://www.rheumatology.org/I-Am-A/Patient-Caregiver/Diseases-Conditions/Osteoarthritis
- Arthritis Foundation: https://www.arthritis.org

PROGNOSIS
- Progressive and chronic disease: early in course, pain relieved by rest; later, pain may persist at rest and at night.
- Joint effusions and enlargement may occur (especially in knees) as disease progresses.
- Osteophyte (spur) formation, especially at joint margins

COMPLICATIONS
Leading cause of musculoskeletal pain and disability

REFERENCES

1. Mo L, Jiang B, Mei T, et al. Exercise therapy for knee osteoarthritis: a systematic review and network meta-analysis. *Orthop J Sports Med*. 2023;11(5):23259671231172773.
2. Courties A, Kouki I, Soliman N, et al. Osteoarthritis year in review 2024: epidemiology and therapy. *Osteoarthritis Cartilage*. 2024;32(11):1397–1404. doi:10.1016/j.joca.2024.07.014.
3. Siddiq MAB, Oo WM, Hunter DJ. New therapeutic strategies in osteoarthritis. *Joint Bone Spine*. 2024;91(6):105739. doi:10.1016/j.jbspin.2024.105739.
4. Fuchs L, Givon A, Shweiki F, et al. Arthroscopic knee débridement in osteoarthritis in older age can be satisfactory. *J Clin Orthop Trauma*. 2023;38:102130.

ADDITIONAL READING

Baker MC, Robinson WH, Ostrom Q. Genetic association between atopic disease and osteoarthritis. *Osteoarthritis Cartilage*. 2024;32(2):220–225. doi:10.1016/j.joca.2023.11.003.

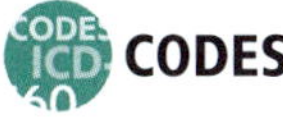

CODES

ICD10
- M19.239 Secondary osteoarthritis, unspecified wrist
- M19.9 Osteoarthritis, unspecified site
- M19.212 Secondary osteoarthritis, left shoulder

CLINICAL PEARLS
- Patients with OA typically have morning stiffness lasting for <15 minutes.
- OA most commonly affects the hips, knees, and hands (PIP and DIP joints).
- NSAID use is associated with increased risk of cardiovascular events.
- If used, intra-articular steroid injections should be limited to no more than 3 per joint per year.
- Emerging therapies (liposome-based dexamethasone and microspore-based triamcinolone) show promise.

OSTEOMYELITIS

Muneeza Khan, MD, FAAFP

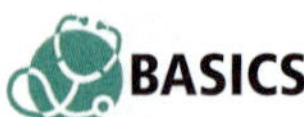

BASICS

DESCRIPTION

- An acute or chronic bone infection with associated inflammation; can occur as a result of hematogenous seeding, contiguous spread of infection, or direct inoculation into intact bone (trauma or surgery)
- Two major classification systems:
  - Lew and Waldvogel: classified according to duration (acute or chronic) and source of infection (hematogenous or contiguous)
  - Cierny-Mader classification: based on the portion of bone affected, physiologic status of the host, and risk factors
- Special situations
  - Vertebral osteomyelitis
    - Results from hematogenous seeding (most common), direct inoculation, or contiguous spread; back pain is most common initial symptom. Lumbar spine is most commonly involved, followed by thoracic spine.
  - Prosthetic joint infections
    - X-ray and three-phase bone scan; MRI/CT is of limited use with prostheses.
  - Posttraumatic infections
    - Risk factors include type and severity of fracture, as well as contamination. Tibia is the most common location.

EPIDEMIOLOGY

- More common in older adults; predominant sex: male > female
- Hematogenous osteomyelitis
  - Adults (most >50 years of age): vertebral
  - Children: long bones
- Contiguous osteomyelitis: related to diabetic foot infections (DFIs), decubitus ulcers, and infected total joint arthroplasties in older adults; trauma and surgery in younger adults
- *Mycobacterium tuberculosis* (MTB) is the most common cause of vertebral osteomyelitis worldwide. It is more likely to involve multiple vertebral bodies—especially of the thoracic spine—and is associated with paraspinal abscess formation.

Incidence

Generally low; normal bone is resistant to infection. The incidence of vertebral osteomyelitis has been estimated at 2.4 cases per 100,000 population, with an increasing incidence with advancing age.

Prevalence

Up to 66% of diabetics with foot ulcerations

ETIOLOGY AND PATHOPHYSIOLOGY

- Acute: suppurative infection of bone with edema and vascular compromise leading to sequestrum (segments of necrotic bone, may contain pus)
- Chronic: presence of necrotic bone or sequestrum or recurrence of previous infection
- Hematogenous osteomyelitis (typically monomicrobial)
  - *Staphylococcus aureus* (most common); coagulase-negative staphylococci and aerobic gram-negative bacteria; *Pseudomonas aeruginosa* (intravenous [IV] drug user); *Salmonella* sp. (sickle cell disease); MTB and fungal (rare; in endemic areas or in immunocompromised hosts)
- Contiguous focus osteomyelitis (polymicrobial)
  - Diabetes or vascular insufficiency
    - Coagulase-positive and coagulase-negative staphylococci; streptococci, gram-negative bacilli, anaerobes (*Peptostreptococcus* sp.)
  - Sacral decubitus ulcer
    - Pressure-related skin ulceration and necrosis
  - Puncture wound through shoe
    - *P. aeruginosa*
- Prosthetic device
  - Coagulase-negative staph and *S. aureus*

RISK FACTORS

- Diabetes mellitus (particularly, diabetic foot ulcer); recent trauma/surgery; foreign body (e.g., prosthetic implant)
- Neuropathy and vascular insufficiency; immunosuppression (including dialysis); sickle cell disease; injection drug use; previous osteomyelitis; bacteremia

GENERAL PREVENTION

- Comprehensive annual foot exam for diabetic patients; screen for peripheral artery disease; optimize glycemic control in diabetes.
- Antibiotic prophylaxis for posttraumatic infection
  - Clean bone surgery
    - Administer IV antibiotics within an hour of skin incision, keep at therapeutic level throughout surgery, and continue ≤24 hours postprocedure.
  - Closed fractures
    - Cefazolin, cefuroxime, clindamycin (β-lactam allergy), or vancomycin (β-lactam allergy or MRSA infection)
  - Open fractures
    - In patients who can receive antibiotics within 3 hours of injury with prompt operative treatment, 1st-generation cephalosporins are preferred (clindamycin or vancomycin if allergic); ceftriaxone for type III fractures; add metronidazole if associated with soil or fecal matter contamination.

COMMONLY ASSOCIATED CONDITIONS

Diabetes, kidney failure, HIV, sickle cell disease, immunosuppression, cancer, peripheral arterial disease, prosthetic joints, IV drug use, chronic skin infections

DIAGNOSIS

HISTORY

- Fever, chills, pain, swelling, and erythema, particularly in acute osteomyelitis. These features may be absent in chronic osteomyelitis.
- Hematogenous osteomyelitis
  - Elicit a history of conditions predisposing to bacteremia (diabetes, hemodialysis, invasive procedures, IV drug use, immunosuppression).
- Contiguous osteomyelitis and vascular insufficiency
  - Recent trauma/surgery within 1 to 2 months; presence of prosthetic device; history of diabetes/DFI
- Chronic osteomyelitis
  - History of acute osteomyelitis; draining sinus tract

PHYSICAL EXAM

- Fever, restricted range of motion, tenderness, signs of localized inflammation; motor and sensory deficits can be seen with vertebral infection in 1/3 of patients. Exposed bone in the setting of DFI is highly suspicious.
- Classic signs and symptoms of infection may be masked in diabetics due to vascular disease and neuropathy.

DIFFERENTIAL DIAGNOSIS

Systemic infection from other source, aseptic bone infarction, localized inflammation, or infection of overlying skin and soft tissues (e.g., gout), Brodie abscess (subacute osteomyelitis), neuropathic joint disease (Charcot foot), fractures/trauma, tumor

DIAGNOSTIC TESTS & INTERPRETATION

Initial Tests (lab, imaging)

Labs

- WBC is not reliable (can be normal or elevated) (1).
- A normocytic normochromic anemia may be present in chronic cases (1).
- CRP is usually elevated (nonspecific). ESR is high in most cases:
  - ESR >70 mm/hr increases likelihood >10-fold.
- Procalcitonin may also be elevated.
- For vertebral/hematogenous osteomyelitis, definitive diagnosis is made by vertebral disc aspiration or blood culture.
- Patients with positive blood cultures (with a pathogen likely to cause vertebral/hematogenous osteomyelitis) and with radiographic evidence of osteomyelitis do not need bone biopsy. Antibiotics given prior to culture may alter results.
- Immunosuppression (including diabetes), chronic inflammatory disease, and other sites of infection may alter lab results.
- Routine radiography is first-line imaging: Classic triad for osteomyelitis is demineralization, periosteal reaction, and bone destruction:
  - Bone destruction is not apparent on plain films until after 10 to 21 days of infection.
  - Bone scan is first test after plain x-ray for evaluation of prosthesis-related infection.
- Radionuclide scanning (e.g., technetium, indium, or gallium) helps if diagnosis is ambiguous or unsure of extent of disease; limited by low sensitivity/specificity
- MRI
  - Best for visualization of septic arthritis, spinal infection, and DFI
  - T1-weighted image: low signal intensity; T2-weighted image: high signal intensity; MRI: sensitivity 90% and specificity 80% for osteomyelitis in diabetic foot ulcers
  - Not as accurate for diagnosis of osteomyelitis with presence of Charcot neuroarthropathy joint disease or after recent surgery
  - MRI does not help assess the response to therapy due to persistence of bony edema.
- CT
  - Better than standard radiography to evaluate bony fragments and sequestration; inferior to MRI for soft tissue and bone marrow assessment

Follow-Up Tests & Special Considerations

- A persistently elevated CRP (4 to 6 weeks) can be associated with osteomyelitis but is nonspecific. CRP decreases faster than ESR, but a decrease in ESR after treatment is a good prognostic sign.
- Bone biopsy and culture remain gold standard for definitive diagnosis and isolation of causative organism.

Diagnostic Procedures/Other

- Probe-to-bone in DFI has high pooled sensitivity and specificity for osteomyelitis of 0.87 (95% CI 0.75 to 0.93) and 0.83 (95% CI 0.65 to 0.93), respectively.

- A probe-to-bone test can be used to help diagnose osteomyelitis; a sterile blunt metal instrument deep into the wound—positive if a hard gritty sensation is felt.
- Ulcer >2-cm wide and >2-cm deep increases likelihood for osteomyelitis in DFI.
- Positive probe-to-bone test and ulcer area >2 cm^2 are physical exam findings that best support osteomyelitis in the setting of DFI.
- Bone biopsy
  - For contiguous osteomyelitis, definitive diagnosis is made by bone biopsy for culture and histology.
  - Avoid wound swabs or needle aspiration in DFI and decubitus ulcers because these do not correlate well with bone biopsy culture (1).
  - Can obtain bone biopsy at same time as surgical débridement

Test Interpretation

Pathology of bone revealing inflammatory process with pyogenic bacteria and necrosis is diagnostic.

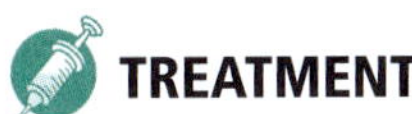

TREATMENT

GENERAL MEASURES

Adequate nutrition, smoking cessation, glycemic control, foot care, IV drug use cessation; check status of tetanus prophylaxis in patients with foot osteomyelitis caused by puncture wound.

MEDICATION

- In clinically stable patients, delay initiation of empiric antibiotics until biopsy and/or blood cultures have been obtained.
- Direct empiric therapy toward probable organism and tailor according to culture results. Optimal antimicrobial concentration at infected site is essential (consider vascular perfusion). Adjust antibiotic dosing according to renal function.
- 4 to 6 weeks of therapy is appropriate for most cases of acute osteomyelitis. In the setting of amputation or complete removal of infected bone, a 2-week course of pathogen-directed antibiotics may be adequate (1).
- Uncomplicated acute hematogenous vertebral osteomyelitis can be treated with 6 weeks of antibiotics.
- If a prosthetic joint or other orthopedic hardware cannot be removed or completely débrided, a prolonged 6-week course of parenteral antibiotics is indicated.
- Consider longer treatment courses for chronic osteomyelitis or MRSA infection (minimum of 8 weeks).
- Empiric therapy:
  - For vertebral/hematogenous osteomyelitis, include coverage for MRSA and gram-negative organisms.
  - IV vancomycin plus 3rd- or 4th-generation IV cephalosporin +/− metronidazole for DFI/contiguous osteomyelitis

First Line

- *S. aureus* or coagulase-negative staphylococci
  - MSSA: β-lactam at high dose (nafcillin or oxacillin 2 g IV q4h) *or* cefazolin 1 to 2 g IV q8h (use 2 g for patients >80 kg)
  - MRSA: vancomycin 15 to 20 mg/kg IV q8–12h (use q8h interval if CrCl >70 mL/min) with target trough of 15 to 20 μg/mL, not to exceed 2 g/dose
- *Streptococcus* sp.
  - Ceftriaxone 2 g IV q24h or cefazolin 2 g IV q8h
- *Enterobacter* sp.
  - Ciprofloxacin 750 mg PO q12h (or 400 mg IV q12h) or cefepime 2 g IV q12h
- *P. aeruginosa*
  - Cefepime 2 g IV q8h or ciprofloxacin 750 mg PO q12h (or 400 mg IV q8h)

Second Line

- *S. aureus*
  - MSSA: ceftriaxone 2 g IV q24h
  - MRSA: linezolid 600 mg PO/IV q12h *or* daptomycin 6 mg/kg IV q24h
- *Streptococcus* sp.
  - Penicillin G 4 million U q4–6h
- *P. aeruginosa*
  - Piperacillin-tazobactam 3.375 q IV q6h

ALERT

The combination of vancomycin plus piperacillin-tazobactam can increase risk of acute renal failure (number needed to harm = 11).

ADDITIONAL THERAPIES

Recent studies have demonstrated that there may be benefit of hyperbaric oxygen therapy in the management of chronic osteomyelitis.

SURGERY/OTHER PROCEDURES

- Surgical drainage, minimizing dead space, adequate soft tissue coverage, restoration of blood supply, and removal of necrotic tissues improve cure rates. Surgery indicated with presence of neurologic symptoms or infection of spinal implant; surgical débridement to healthy bone and/or soft tissue coverage/surgical flap (1)
- Evidence suggests antibiotics alone may be sufficient for DFI.
- Use of antibiotic-loaded cement or antibiotic coated polymethyl methacrylate cement beads for patients with vascular insufficiency to manage dead space and help control the infection.

ADMISSION, INPATIENT, AND NURSING CONSIDERATIONS

- Evaluate for peripheral vascular disease.
- Off-load pressure.
- Discharge criteria: clinical and laboratory evidence of resolving infection and appropriate outpatient therapy

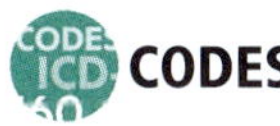

ONGOING CARE

FOLLOW-UP RECOMMENDATIONS

Patient Monitoring

Antimicrobial levels, ESR, CRP, and repeat plain radiography as clinical course dictates; CRP correlates better with clinical response than ESR. Monitor vancomycin dosing and renal function.

DIET

Glycemic control for diabetics; proper nutrition for malnourished patients

PATIENT EDUCATION

Diabetic glycemic control and foot care; IV drug use cessation

PROGNOSIS

- Superficial and medullary osteomyelitis treated with antimicrobial and surgical therapy have a response rate of 90–100%.
- Up to 36% recurrence rate in diabetics; increased mortality after amputation

COMPLICATIONS

- Abscess formation; bacteremia; fracture/nonunion; loosening of prosthetic implant; postoperative infection
- Sinus tract formation can be associated with neoplasms (e.g., Marjolin ulcer), especially in presence of long-standing infection.

REFERENCES

1. Masters EA, Ricciardi BF, Bentley KLM, et al. Skeletal infections: microbial pathogenesis, immunity and clinical management. *Nat Rev Microbiol*. 2022;20(7):385–400. doi:10.1038/s41579-022-00686-0.

ADDITIONAL READING

- Bury DC, Rogers TS, Dickman MM. Osteomyelitis: diagnosis and treatment. *Am Fam Physician*. 2021;104(4):395–402.
- Senneville É, Albalawi Z, van Asten SA, et al. IWGDF/IDSA guidelines on the diagnosis and treatment of diabetes-related foot infections (IWGDF/IDSA 2023). *Diabetes Metab Res Rev*. 2024;40(3):e3687. doi:10.1002/dmrr.3687.

CODES

ICD10

- M86.03 Acute hematogenous osteomyelitis, radius and ulna
- M86.032 Acute hematogenous osteomyelitis, left radius and ulna
- M86.01 Acute hematogenous osteomyelitis, shoulder

CLINICAL PEARLS

- Hematogenous osteomyelitis is usually monomicrobial. Osteomyelitis due to contiguous spread or direct inoculation is usually polymicrobial.
- Pain associated with acute osteomyelitis is typically gradual in onset.
- Treatment of chronic osteomyelitis often requires both surgical débridement and ≥6 weeks of antimicrobial therapy.
- Unlike diabetic foot ulcers, a positive probe-to-bone test (or frankly exposed bone) and abnormal MRI findings are not diagnostic of osteomyelitis in stage IV sacral pressure ulcers. Definitive treatment of osteomyelitis in stage IV sacral pressure ulcers often requires surgical débridement to healthy bone.
- Follow-up MRI is not needed for patients who are clinically improving with appropriate treatment.
- In diabetic foot wounds with no signs or symptoms of soft tissue or bone infection, antibiotic therapy is unnecessary.

OSTEOPOROSIS AND OSTEOPENIA

Candace Ripperda, MD • Jennifer Cherry Bohannan, MD

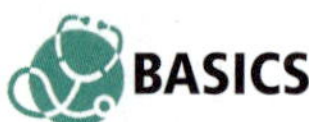

BASICS

DESCRIPTION

- Metabolic bone disease (MBD) is characterized by low bone mass and deteriorated bone microarchitecture.
- Leads to compromised bone strength and increased risk of fragility fracture
- Includes osteopenia (low bone mass) and osteoporosis (pathologic loss)
- Combined MBD affects >53 million Americans as over 2023, with 2 million new cases in 2022

ETIOLOGY AND PATHOPHYSIOLOGY

- Imbalance between bone resorption and formation resulting in a net loss of bone mass and density over time
- Age-related decrease in osteoblast activity and estrogen decline

Genetics

- Familial predisposition
- More common in Caucasians and Asians than in African Americans and Hispanics
- More common in females

COMMONLY ASSOCIATED CONDITIONS

- Lifestyle factors: alcohol abuse, excessive thinness, smoking, obesity, immobilization
- Malabsorption: inflammatory bowel disease, celiac disease
- Hypoestrogenism: premature menopause, hypogonadism, eating disorders
- Endocrinopathies: hyperparathyroidism, hyperthyroidism, diabetes mellitus
- Hematologic disorders: sickle cell disease, multiple myeloma
- Medications: glucocorticoids, anticonvulsants, aromatase inhibitors, GnRH agonists, anticoagulants, chemotherapy

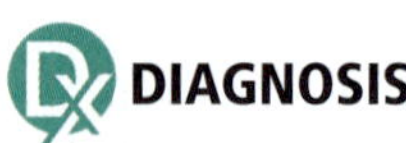

DIAGNOSIS

HISTORY

- Review modifiable (smoking, excessive alcohol, physical inactivity, and poor nutrition) and non-modifiable (age, gender, race, and family history) risk factors.
- History of fragility fracture
- Assess for commonly associated conditions and causes of secondary osteoporosis.

PHYSICAL EXAM

- Thoracic kyphosis (stooped posture) and rounded shoulders known as "dowager's hump"
- Poor balance, deconditioning
- Historical height loss >1.5 inches (difference between current height and peak height at age 20 years)
- Prospective height loss >0.8 inches (difference between current height and previously documented height)

DIFFERENTIAL DIAGNOSIS

- Primary hyperparathyroidism
- Multiple myeloma/other neoplasms
- Paget disease of bone

DIAGNOSTIC TESTS & INTERPRETATION

Initial Tests (lab, imaging)

- Dual energy x-ray absorptiometry (DEXA) is considered the gold standard for diagnosis.
  - T-score: The T-score compares an individual's bone mineral density (BMD) to that of healthy young adult of the same sex.
    - T-score between +1 and −1: normal bone density
    - T-score between −1 and −2.5: osteopenia (low bone density)
    - T-score ≤−2.5: osteoporosis
  - Z-score: The Z-score compares BMD to an age-matched group of individuals of the same sex.
    - Z-score <−2 SD: may indicate a secondary cause of bone loss
- Additionally, calculate the online country-specific fracture risk assessment tool (FRAX) for diagnosis of osteoporosis: https://www.shef.ac.uk/FRAX/
- A fragility fracture at any age and regardless of BMD is diagnostic of osteoporosis.
- Trabecular bone score (TBS) can help stratify those with osteopenic range BMD.
- Initial laboratory tests: Measure calcium, vitamin D (25-OH), parathyroid hormone (PTH), thyroid function tests, albumin, chemistry levels, renal function. Consider CBC, LFTs, and markers of bone turnover (bALP, urinary NTX).
- Plain radiographs lack sensitivity to diagnose osteoporosis, but an abnormality (e.g., widened intervertebral spaces, rib fractures) should prompt evaluation.

Follow-Up Tests & Special Considerations

Consider further lab work based on: Z-score ≤−2.5, to investigate secondary cause, or diagnosis at a young age (1)[C].

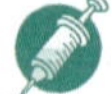

TREATMENT

Criteria for patients who benefit from treatment for their osteoporosis includes the following (1)[C]:

- Patients with a T-score ≤−2.5 with or without risk factors
- Patients with a history of a fragility fracture
- Postmenopausal women and men >50 years old with a history of fractures in vertebrae, hip, wrist, pelvis, or humerus
- Postmenopausal women and men >50 years old with osteopenia and a 10-year hip fracture risk ≥3% or any major fracture risk ≥20%, based on FRAX scoring

GENERAL MEASURES

- Initiate 1,200 mg of calcium per day (total of diet and supplement).
- Initiate 800 to 2,000 international units of vitamin D daily or amount needed to keep vitamin D (25-OH) ideally >30 ng/mL.
- Exercise prescription for regular weight-bearing and strength-building exercise
- Fall risk modification with balance training to reduce fall risk (RR 0.76, 95% CI 0.7 to 0.8) (1)[C]
- Smoking and alcohol cessation

MEDICATION

First Line

Bisphosphonates:

- Inhibit bone resorption by osteoclasts in skeletal tissue
  - Alendronate 10 mg PO daily or 70 mg PO weekly
  - Risedronate 5 mg PO daily, 35 mg PO weekly, or 150 mg PO monthly
  - Ibandronate 150 mg PO monthly or 3 mg IV every 3 months
  - Zoledronic acid 5 mg IV yearly
- Bisphosphonates reduced hip (RR 0.65, 95% CI 0.43 to 0.97), vertebral (RR 0.46, 95% CI 0.24 to 0.89), and any clinical fractures (RR 0.68, 95% CI 0.51 to 0.92) (2)[B].
- For secondary prevention of mild to moderate osteoporosis, oral bisphosphonates are preferred (3)[C].
- Side effects include esophagitis and gastritis.
- Osteonecrosis of the jaw (ONJ) is a rare risk that increases in incidence after 2 to 3 years on therapy (3)[C].
- ONJ is primarily seen in patients with cancer who receive high doses and those who receive IV treatment.
- There is a possible risk of atypical femur fractures in patients receiving bisphosphonates for >5 years (1)[C].
- Reassess therapy after 5 years; consider continuing up to 10 years if high risk or taking a drug holiday (1)[C],(3)[C].
- Bisphosphonates remain the least cost-prohibited of the treatment options.
- Avoid oral bisphosphonates in patients with:
  - Delayed esophageal emptying
  - Inability to stay upright for at least 30 to 60 minutes after taking the bisphosphonates
  - Hypocalcemia (Correct prior to initiating therapy.)
  - Severe renal impairment (creatinine clearance [CrCl] ≤30 mL/min for risedronate and ≤35 mL/min for alendronate and zoledronic acid)

Second Line

- Monoclonal antibody therapy:
  - Denosumab 60 mg SC every 6 months
    - Human monoclonal antibody receptor activator of nuclear factor κ-B ligand (RANKL) receptor, blocking, inhibiting osteoclast formation, and decreasing bone resorption
    - Reduced vertebral (RR 0.32, 95% CI 0.21 to 0.48), clinical (RR 0.81, 95% CI 0.69 to 0.96), and hip fractures risk (RR 0.61, 95% CI 0.37 to 0.98) (2)[B]

- Agent of choice in patients with renal insufficiency
- Side effects can include dermatologic reactions, hypocalcemia, and less commonly ONJ, atypical femur fracture, and serious infections.
- Increased risk of rebound bone turnover and fracture following discontinuation; therefore, subsequent bisphosphonate or alternative therapy is recommended (1)[C].

– Romosozumab 210 mg (split in two separate injections) once monthly for 1 year
- Monoclonal antibody that inhibits sclerostin, leading to increased bone formation
- Reduces vertebral fractures by 73–82% at 12 months ($p < .001$) (1)[C],(2)[B]
- Romosozumab therapy (12 months) followed by alendronate for women with severe osteoporosis or at high risk for fractures
- May increase risk of adverse cardiovascular events (pairing with a bisphosphonate may reduce this risk); should be avoided in patient with recent MI or stroke (1)[C]

- Recombinant formulations of PTH:
  - Anabolic agents that stimulate bone through osteoblastic activation
  - Used in severe osteoporosis patients due to their capability of reducing fracture risk more quickly (1)[C]
    - Teriparatide 20 mg SC daily
      - Use is limited to high risk for fractures (or previous therapy unsuccessful) as only approved for use up to 2 years in duration.
      - Reduced any clinical fracture (RR 0.50, 95% CI 0.32 to 0.74) (2)[B]
      - Bone loss may rapidly occur after discontinuation; therefore, sequential therapy with antiresorptive agent (bisphosphonate) is recommended.
      - Must have GFR >30
    - Abaloparatide 80 μg SC daily
      - Similar safety profile to teriparatide
      - Can be used in CKD and ESRD
      - Higher number of adverse events reported (2)[B]

ISSUES FOR REFERRAL
- Endocrinology referral for severe disease, young age of onset, rapid bone loss, poor response to treatment
- Dental referral for oral examinations prior to starting medication and for monitoring during treatment

ADDITIONAL THERAPIES
- Calcitonin: although not commonly used can help reduce bone breakdown and pain in some cases (1)[C]
- Hormone replacement therapy (HRT): Consider for select cases in postmenopausal women (1)[C].
- Selective estrogen receptor modulators (SERMs) and tissue selective estrogen complex: Consider for select cases in postmenopausal women.

SURGERY/OTHER PROCEDURES
Surgical options are focused on the sequelae of MBD and intractable pain, such as:
- Vertebroplasty: Orthopedic cement is injected into the compressed vertebral body.
- Kyphoplasty: Balloon is expanded within compressed vertebral body; cement is injected.

COMPLEMENTARY & ALTERNATIVE MEDICINE
- Acupuncture: may help manage pain
- Yoga and tai chi: can improve balance, strength, and flexibility

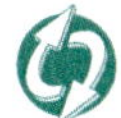

ONGOING CARE
Regular bone density monitoring, medication management, lifestyle modifications, fall prevention strategies, nutritional support, and patient education to optimize bone health and reduce fracture risk

FOLLOW-UP RECOMMENDATIONS
The duration of medication therapy is determined based on treatment guidelines and involves shared decision-making with the patient, considering the balance between treatment benefits and potential risks.

Patient Monitoring
- Yearly height measurement
- Most recommendations suggest repeating a DEXA scan to assess BMD 2 years after starting bisphosphonate therapy.
- Perform a risk assessment after 3 to 5 years of treatment. If BMD T-score at the hip is ≥2.5 and there has not been a hip or vertebral fracture, consider stopping treatment. If BMD remains low or high risk for fractures, the patient may benefit by continuing treatment beyond 5 years.
- Patients on bisphosphonates for 5 years (3 years of IV of zoledronic acid) and if a stable BMD, no prior fracture, and a low risk for fracture can be considered for a drug holiday
- Patients on bisphosphonates for 5 years at high fracture risk (prior fragility fracture, older age, frailty, and high fall risk) should be continued on therapy and a drug holiday can be reconsidered after 6 to 10 years.
- Continue to regularly monitor both serum calcium and vitamin D (25-OH).

DIET
- Calcium-rich foods: dairy products, fortified plant milks, leafy greens
- Vitamin D sources: fatty fish, egg yolks, and fortified cereals
- Limit sodium and caffeine.
- Limit alcohol consumption.

PROGNOSIS
- With treatment, there is an increase in bone mass and mobility, and reduced pain.
- Vertebral and hip fractures may lead to the need for chronic care and/or premature death.

COMPLICATIONS
- Recurrent fractures (spine, hips, wrists, ribs)
- Chronic back pain and loss of height
- Reduced mobility and muscle weakness
- Decreased quality of life and independence

REFERENCES

1. Subarajan P, Arceo-Mendoza RM, Camacho PM. Postmenopausal osteoporosis: a review of latest guidelines. *Endocrinol Metab Clin North Am*. 2024;53(4):497–512. doi:10.1016/j.ecl.2024.08.008.
2. Ayers C, Kansagara D, Lazur B, et al. Effectiveness and safety of treatments to prevent fractures in people with low bone mass or primary osteoporosis: a living systematic review and network meta-analysis for the American College of Physicians. *Ann Intern Med*. 2023;176(2):182–195. doi:10.7326/M22-0684.
3. Qaseem A, Hicks LA, Etxeandia-Ikobaltzeta I, et al; for Clinical Guidelines Committee of the American College of Physicians. Pharmacologic treatment of primary osteoporosis or low bone mass to prevent fractures in adults: a living clinical guideline from the American College of Physicians. *Ann Intern Med*. 2023;176(2):224–238. doi:10.7326/M22-1034.

ADDITIONAL READING

- Camacho PM, Petak SM, Binkley N, et al. American Association of Clinical Endocrinologists/American College of Endocrinology clinical practice guidelines for the diagnosis and treatment of postmenopausal osteoporosis—2020 update. *Endocr Pract*. 2020;26(Suppl 1):1–46.
- Nicholson WK, Silverstein M, Wong JB, et al; for US Preventative Services Task Force. Screening for osteoporosis to prevent fractures: US Preventative Services Task Force recommendation statement. *JAMA*. 2025;333(6):498–508. doi:10.1001/jama.2024.27154.

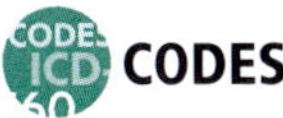

CODES

ICD10
- M85.80 Other specified disorders of bone density and structure, unspecified site
- M81.0 Age-related osteoporosis w/o current pathological fracture
- M80.00XA Age-rel osteopor w current path fracture, unsp site, init

CLINICAL PEARLS
- The cornerstone of prevention and treatment is to modify risk factors, including maximizing calcium, vitamin D (25-OH), and physical activity
- The diagnosis of BMD is based on DEXA and FRAX scoring.
- Any fragility fracture is diagnostic of osteoporosis and need evaluation with treatment.
- First-line pharmacotherapy continues to be bisphosphonates with consideration for patient preference, individual risks, and level of MBD.
- There is promising research into the benefits of sequential therapy and the utilization of bone density markers in evaluating treatment.

OTITIS EXTERNA

Laura Critchfield, PA-C • Karl T. Clebak, MD, MHA, FAAFP

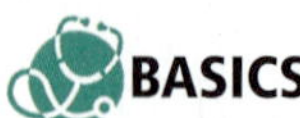

BASICS

DESCRIPTION

Inflammation of the external auditory canal:

- Acute otitis externa (AOE) (<3 weeks): most common form; infectious etiology most commonly bacterial (*Pseudomonas aeruginosa* and *Staphylococcus aureus*); less commonly fungal (*Aspergillus* and *Candida*)
- Chronic otitis externa (≥3 months): commonly due to inadequately treated AOE, persistent allergies, or chronic skin conditions
- Eczematous otitis externa: may accompany atopic eczema or other primary skin conditions
- Malignant (necrotizing) otitis externa: an infection that extends into the deeper tissues adjacent to the canal; may include osteomyelitis of the mastoid or temporal bone; a medical emergency requiring urgent referral; can be life-threatening; rare, especially in children
- Synonym: swimmer's ear

EPIDEMIOLOGY

Incidence

- Annual incidence of ~1% (1)
- Higher in the summer months and in warm, wet climates
- Can affect all age groups but has a peak incidence in 7- to 12-year-olds (2)

Prevalence

Lifetime prevalence of 10% (1)

ETIOLOGY AND PATHOPHYSIOLOGY

- Factors associated with pathogenesis:
  - Skin, cerumen, and surrounding structures provide protection for the integrity of external auditory canal.
  - Cerumen, being a hydrophobic and sticky substance, provides a physical barrier against many foreign particles. Normal cerumen production also creates an environment that is slightly acidic and not favorable for most pathogens.
  - Disruption of the protective skin-cerumen barrier, followed by the subsequent inflammation, swelling, and obstruction of the canal, and impaired cerumen production, are all factors in the development of AOE.
- AOE, infectious etiology (2):
  - Bacterial infection (>90%): *P. aeruginosa* (22–62%), *S. aureus* aureus (11–34%), polymicrobial infection is common.
  - Fungal infection (<10%, more commonly associated with chronic otitis externa): *Aspergillus* (60–90%), *Candida* spp. (10–40%).
- Chronic otitis externa etiology: often occurs due to inadequately treated AOE, persistent allergies, or chronic skin conditions (1)
- Eczematous otitis externa (associated with primary skin disorder) etiology:
  - Eczema, seborrhea, psoriasis
  - Contact dermatitis
  - Purulent otitis media
  - Sensitivity to topical medications
- Malignant (necrotizing) otitis externa etiology (3):
  - Invasive bacterial infection: *Pseudomonas*, increasing incidence of methicillin-resistant *S. aureus* (MRSA)
  - Associated with patients with diabetes or immunosuppression
  - More common in older adults

RISK FACTORS

- Acute and chronic otitis externa
  - Water exposure—typically swimming in fresh water
  - Hot, humid weather; sweating
  - Trauma to the external canal—cleaning, scratching, use of instruments
  - Foreign body
  - Use of external devices—hearing aids, ear plugs
  - Anatomic abnormalities—narrow canal, exostoses
  - Dermatologic conditions—eczema, seborrhea, psoriasis
  - Cerumen buildup
  - Excessive hair in canal
  - Previous ear surgery
  - Previous local radiotherapy
- Eczematous: primary skin disorder
- Necrotizing otitis externa in adults
  - Advanced age
  - Diabetes mellitus (DM)
  - Immunosuppression (e.g., AIDS, malignancy)

GENERAL PREVENTION

- Avoid prolonged exposure to moisture.
- Use a hair dryer on a low setting to dry the canal.
- Use a head-tilt maneuver to remove excess water.
- Treat predisposing skin conditions.
- Eliminate self-inflicted trauma to canal with cotton swabs and other foreign objects.
- Treat underlying systemic conditions.
- Ear plugs when swimming.
- Use acidifying ear drops before or after swimming.

DIAGNOSIS

HISTORY

- Associated symptoms: ear pain (70%), itching (60%), aural fullness (22%), +/− conductive hearing loss (32%), +/− jaw pain (3)
- Onset: rapid (within 48 hours), within the past 3 weeks
- Duration of symptoms: acute lasting <3 weeks, chronic lasting ≥3 months
- Assess: risk factors, predisposing conditions, history of prior ear infections or known tympanic membrane perforation, prior surgeries, local radiation therapy (3)
- Consider malignant otitis externa in older patients with a history or diabetes or an immunocompromised state that present with refractory purulent discharge and severe pain (1).

PHYSICAL EXAM

- Inspect the ear for erythema, swelling, discharge, signs of trauma, condition of the skin in and around the canal.
- Pain on manipulation of the pinnae (when pulled) and/or tragus (when pushed) is a classic finding—pain is often disproportionate to visual findings.
- Palpate mastoid area and surrounding lymph nodes
- Otoscopy—assess for signs of otitis media (pneumatic otoscopy or tympanometry can differentiate between otitis media and otitis externa); determine if the tympanic membrane is intact, an important factor for treatment options as the treatment options are more limited if the tympanic membrane is perforated (1),(3),(4).
- Assess for cranial nerve (VII, IX to XII) involvement (rare).
- High fever and granulation tissue in the external canal, particularly at the bone-cartilage junction is a clinical finding of malignant otitis externa (1),(3).

DIFFERENTIAL DIAGNOSIS

- Otitis media +/− perforation
- Foreign body
- Seborrheic dermatitis
- Psoriasis
- Eczema
- Contact dermatitis
- Furunculosis (infected hair follicle)
- Viral infections (varicella, measles, or herpes virus)
- Herpes zoster oticus (Ramsay-Hunt syndrome)
- Myringitis
- Otomycosis
- Cholesteatoma
- Temporomandibular joint (TMJ) syndrome
- Dental pathologies (caries, impacted molars) or other sources of referred pain
- Malignant otitis externa (osteomyelitis)
- Basal cell or squamous cell carcinoma

DIAGNOSTIC TESTS & INTERPRETATION

Initial Tests (lab, imaging)

AOE is a clinical diagnosis based on the patient's history and physical exam findings (1).

Follow-Up Tests & Special Considerations

- Culture otorrhea if (1): No improvement after initial treatment, the patient has predisposing risk factors, or there is concern for extension beyond the external canal.
- Radiologic evaluation of deep tissues with high-resolution CT scan, MRI, gallium scan, and bone scan if concerns for necrotizing otitis externa (3).

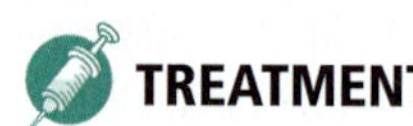

TREATMENT

GENERAL MEASURES

- Clean the external canal (aural toilet)—helps to facilitate the delivery of otic drops and healing process
- Analgesics as appropriate for pain—acetaminophen, nonsteroidal anti-inflammatory drugs, or in rare cases, a short-term opioid (4)

MEDICATION

- For diffuse, uncomplicated AOE, topical antibiotic preparations with or without topical corticosteroids are recommended for initial therapy (3).
  - Limited evidence to show that one preparation is more effective than another.
  - If there is a known or suspected perforation of the tympanic membrane, recommend a non-ototoxic topical preparation (ofloxacin or ciprofloxacin).
  - Advise patient on proper administration of topical preparations:
    - Patient lies down with affected side facing up. Topical preparation is administered into the canal (patient can gently move the pinna around to facilitate delivery). Patient is to remain in this position for 3 to 5 minutes.
- If the canal is obstructed, perform an aural toilet and/or place a wick using either compressed cellulose or ribbon gauze.
- Use systemic antibiotics only if the infection extends outside the external canal, if the patient has specific predisposing risk factors (diabetes, immunocompromised states, prior local radiotherapy, etc.), if unable to deliver topical preparation effectively, or if the patient fails initial therapeutic option (1),(3).
- Reassess diagnosis and treatment adherence within 48 to 72 hours if the patient does not respond to the initial therapeutic option (1),(3).

First Line

- Acute bacterial otitis externa, uncomplicated
  - Ciprofloxacin/dexamethasone 0.3%/0.1% suspension: children >6 months of age and adults: 4 drops instilled in affected ear twice daily for 7 days
  - Ofloxacin 0.3% solution (generic): children aged 6 months to 13 years: 5 drops instilled in affected ear once a day for 7 days; for patients aged ≥13 years: 10 drops instilled in affected ear once a day for 7 days
  - Neomycin/polymyxin B/hydrocortisone otic (Cortisporin): children: 3 drops in affected ear(s) 3 to 4 times daily for 7 days; adults: 4 drops in affected ear(s) 3 to 4 times daily for 7 days; do not continue for longer than 10 days.
  - Acetic acid 2%: children aged ≥3 years and adults: 3 to 5 drops every 4 to 6 hours with ear wick for 24 hours, wick may be removed after 24 hours then instill 5 drops 3 to 4 times a day for a total of 7 days. Recommend lower end of dosage range for children due to smaller capacity of the ear canal.
- Acute bacterial otitis externa, complicated—for severe or refractory cases, infection spreading beyond the ear canal, or patient with predisposing conditions (diabetes, immunocompromised states, etc.)
  - Topical and systemic treatment
  - Systemic options: Consider ciprofloxacin.
- Chronic otitis externa
  - Treat the underlying cause; remove any offending agents.
  - Consider the use of a corticosteroid (topical vs. systemic) for inflammation.
- Fungal otitis externa
  - Clean external canal.
  - If the tympanic membrane is intact:
    - Can use acidifying agents (acetic acid topical preparations)
    - If the patient fails acidifying agents, consider topical antifungal (clotrimazole 1% or tolnaftate 1% if TM perforation).
- Malignant otitis externa
  - Seek emergent otolaryngology consultation and hospitalization
  - Oral +/− IV antibiotics
  - Débridement

ISSUES FOR REFERRAL

Severe and/or resistant cases, concerns for malignant otitis externa (medical emergency), or those requiring surgical intervention

SURGERY/OTHER PROCEDURES

For malignant (necrotizing) otitis externa or furuncle

ADMISSION, INPATIENT, AND NURSING CONSIDERATIONS

Malignant (necrotizing) otitis media requiring parenteral antipseudomonal antibiotics, hospitalization, and emergent otolaryngology referral.

ONGOING CARE

FOLLOW-UP RECOMMENDATIONS

Patient Monitoring

For AOE, reassess diagnosis and treatment adherence within 48 to 72 hours if the patient does not respond to the initial therapeutic option or if symptoms do not completely resolve in 2 weeks (3). For chronic otitis externa, return every 2 to 3 weeks for repeated cleansing of canal.

PROGNOSIS

- With repeated cleansing and antibiotic therapy, most cases of chronic otitis externa will resolve. Occasionally, surgical intervention is required for resistant cases.
- Malignant (necrotizing otitis externa) managed inpatient with débridement and antipseudomonal antibiotics. Surgical intervention may be necessary in resistant cases or if there is cranial nerve involvement (3).

COMPLICATIONS

- Malignant (necrotizing) otitis externa may spread to infect contiguous bone causing osteomyelitis and infect other CNS structures, including causing cranial nerve palsies.
- AOE may spread to pinna, causing chondritis.

REFERENCES

1. Schaefer P, Baugh RF. Acute otitis externa: an update. *Am Fam Physician*. 2012;86(11):1055–1061.
2. Wiegand S, Berner R, Schneider A, et al. Otitis externa. *Dtsch Arztebl Int*. 2019;116(13):224–234. doi:10.3238/arztebl.2019.0224.
3. Rosenfeld RM, Schwartz SR, Cannon CR, et al. Clinical practice guideline: acute otitis externa. *Otolaryngol Head Neck Surg*. 2014;150(Suppl 1):S1–S24.
4. Jackson EA, Geer K. Acute otitis externa: rapid evidence review. *Am Fam Physician*. 2023;107(2):145–151.

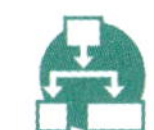

SEE ALSO

Algorithm: Ear Pain/Otalgia

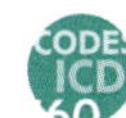

CODES

ICD10

- H60.523 Acute chemical otitis externa, bilateral
- H60.593 Other noninfective acute otitis externa, bilateral
- B37.84 Candidal otitis externa

CLINICAL PEARLS

- For diffuse, uncomplicated AOE, topical preparations with or without topical corticosteroids are recommended for initial therapy
- If there is a known or suspected perforation of the tympanic membrane, recommend a non-ototoxic topical preparation (ofloxacin or ciprofloxacin).
- If the canal is obstructed, perform an aural toilet and/or place a wick (use either compressed cellulose or ribbon gauze).
- Use systemic antibiotics only if the infection extends outside the external canal, if the patient has specific predisposing risk factors (diabetes, immunocompromised states, prior local radiotherapy, etc.), if unable to deliver topical preparation effectively, or if the patient fails initial therapeutic option.
- Reassess diagnosis and treatment adherence within 48 to 72 hours if the patient does not respond to the initial therapeutic option or if symptoms do not completely resolve within 2 weeks.
- Consider malignant otitis externa in older patients with a history or diabetes or an immunocompromised state that present with refractory purulent discharge and severe pain. Malignant otitis externa is a medical emergency that requires urgent referral and treatment.

OTITIS MEDIA

Sahil Mullick, MD, FAAFP • Aneeta Wadhawan, MD

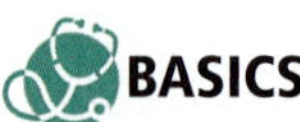

BASICS

DESCRIPTION

- Inflammation of the middle ear; usually accompanied by fluid collection
- Acute otitis media (AOM): inflammation of the middle ear; rapid onset; cause may be infectious (either viral [AOM-v] or bacterial [AOM-b] also known as suppurative otitis media) or sterile etiology (AOM-s)
- Recurrent AOM: ≥3 episodes in 6 months or ≥4 episodes in 1 year with ≥1 in the past 6 months
- Otitis media with effusion (OME): fluid in the middle ear without signs or symptoms of infection; this is also referred to as serous, secretory, or nonsuppurative otitis media.
- Chronic suppurative otitis media (CSOM) also known as chronic otitis media (COM): recurrent or chronic infection of the middle ear and mastoid cavity without an intact tympanic membrane; may present with or without cholesteatoma
- System(s) affected: nervous

EPIDEMIOLOGY

Incidence

- AOM
  - Predominant age: 6 to 24 months; declines >7 years; rare in adults
  - 50–85% of children have had at least 1 episode of AOM by age 3 years; 24% have had ≥3 episodes.
- OME: 90% of children have had at least 1 episode by age 4 years

Prevalence

Multiple factors (children): immature anatomy (shorter ET tube, > bone to cartilage ratio), genetic, physiologic

ETIOLOGY AND PATHOPHYSIOLOGY

- AOM-b: Usually, a preceding viral upper respiratory infection (URI) can produce eustachian tube dysfunction, leading to reduced clearance.
  - *Streptococcus pneumoniae*, *Haemophilus influenzae*, and *Moraxella catarrhalis* are the most frequent pathogens and account for 80% of AOM-b infections. *Streptococcus pyogenes*, *Mycoplasma spp.*, *Chlamydia*, anaerobes and other organisms are less frequent.
- AOM-v: 15–44% of AOM infections are caused by viruses (e.g., rhinovirus, respiratory syncytial virus, parainfluenza, influenza, enteroviruses, adenovirus, human metapneumovirus, and bocavirus). But only RSV, human metapneumovirus, and influenza were associated with office visits.
- AOM-s: 25–30%
- OME: middle ear inflammation and eustachian tube dysfunction

Genetics

Immunologic defects and genetic disorders (e.g., Down syndrome) can predispose changes in physical anatomy (e.g., more horizontal ear canals) that increase the likelihood of developing otitis media.

RISK FACTORS

- Developing AOM prior to 1 year of age is a risk for recurrent AOM.
- Bottle feeding while supine; pacifier use
- Routine daycare attendance
- Family history of AOM, particularly in children with siblings (1)
- Environmental smoke exposure
- Absence of breastfeeding during the first 6 months of life
- Low socioeconomic status
- Atopy (such as eczema, asthma)
- Underlying ENT abnormalities (e.g., cleft palate)

GENERAL PREVENTION

- PCV-7, PCV-13, and influenzae vaccines (2)[B]
- Breastfeeding for ≥6 months is protective (2)[B].
- Avoiding supine bottle-feeding, passive smoke, and pacifiers >6 months may be helpful.
- Secondary prevention: Adenoidectomy and adenotonsillectomy for recurrent AOM have limited short-term efficacy and are associated with their own adverse risks.

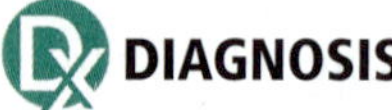

DIAGNOSIS

Clinical diagnosis: done by otoscope

- The most specific finding is a bulging tympanic membrane.
- Perforation of the tympanic membrane with discharge from the ear

HISTORY

- AOM:
  - Otalgia
  - Preceding or accompanying URI symptoms
  - Decreased hearing
- AOM in adults can present with only otalgia without fever, or unilateral hearing loss.

ALERT

- AOM in infants and toddlers may present with only irritability in early months of life.
- OME: usually asymptomatic and may only present with decreased hearing and, less frequently, complaints of tinnitus and ear-fullness (3)

PHYSICAL EXAM

- AOM:
  - Fever (not required for diagnosis)
  - Decreased eardrum mobility (with pneumatic otoscopy)
  - Moderate to severe bulging of tympanic membrane
  - Red, yellow, or cloudy tympanic membrane
  - Otorrhea
- OME:
  - Eardrum often dull but not bulging
  - Decreased eardrum mobility (pneumatic otoscopy)
  - Presence of air-fluid level
  - Weber test lateralizes to affected ear for an ear with effusion
  - Tympanometry if pneumatic otoscopy has no findings

DIFFERENTIAL DIAGNOSIS

Otitis externa or otitis media with effusion

DIAGNOSTIC TESTS & INTERPRETATION

Initial Tests (lab, imaging)

AOM is a clinical diagnosis requiring middle ear effusion and signs of middle ear inflammation on exam.

Diagnostic Procedures/Other

- Otoscopy—to document the presence of middle ear fluid
- Pneumatic otoscopy—to detect middle ear fluid (supplement with tympanometry and acoustic reflex measurement); pneumatic otoscopy is contraindicated with known tympanic perforation.
- Hearing testing if hearing loss persists for ≥3 months or if suspecting language delay.
- Tympanocentesis for microbiologic diagnosis helpful if child is immunocompromised, or has failed previous courses of antibiotic therapy; may be followed by myringotomy

Test Interpretation

Pneumatic otoscopy—tympanic mobility will be impaired if middle ear fluid is present.

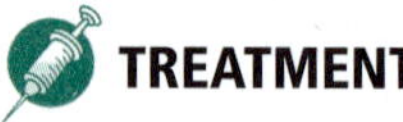

TREATMENT

GENERAL MEASURES

- Assess pain and treat with ibuprofen and/or acetaminophen.
- Majority will recover without antibiotic treatment.
- AOM: Observation with watchful waiting for those age >6 months with mild AOM. Prescribe antibiotics if no improvement or clinical worsening within 24 to 48 hours.
- OME watchful waiting for 3 months, and if no improvement, then refer to ENT for possible surgery. Antibiotics, decongestants, antihistamines, and steroids are not recommended.

MEDICATION

First Line

- Controversy exists about the usefulness of antibiotic treatment for this often self-resolving condition. Overdiagnosis of AOM is widespread, which can lead to the injudicious use of antibiotics and contributes to antibiotic resistance. Studies suggest number needed to treat for an additional beneficial outcome (NNTB) is 20 when looking at relief of pain at 2 to 3 days after start of antibiotics; the number needed to harm (primarily diarrhea and vomiting) is 9.
- AAP/AAFP recommends:
  - Treatment for <6 months of age: Treat with amoxicillin if >2 weeks old.
  - >6 months: Antibacterial therapy is recommended with severe otitis media (i.e., moderate to severe otalgia, otalgia >48 hours or fever ≥39°C) or otorrhea or bilateral otitis media between 6 months and 2 years of age.
- Observation is an option with nonsevere otitis media at >6 months to 2 years (otalgia <48 hours, temperature <39°C). However, there is a high risk of treatment failure and recommended antibiotics.
- Immunocompetent children >2 years of age can be observed. Parents/guardians must understand risks/benefits of observation.

- AOM: AAP/AAFP consensus guideline recommends treating with antibiotics if:
  - Between 2 weeks and 6 months, *or*
  - If >6 months with severe otitis media (e.g., moderate to severe otalgia, otalgia >48 hours, or fevers >39°C) *or*
  - Otorrhea *or*
  - Bilateral otitis media in infants between 6 months and 23 months of age without severe signs/symptoms
- Treat with amoxicillin, 90 mg/kg/day in 2 divided doses (maximum of 3 g/day) in those without risk of antibiotic resistance. Use a 10-day course for children aged <2 years; 5- to 7-day course for children aged ≥2 years.
- If penicillin allergic:
  - Cefdinir, 14 mg/kg/day in 1 to 2 doses (maximum 600 mg/day) for 10 days *or*
  - Cefpodoxime, 10 mg/kg/day in 2 divided doses (maximum 400 mg/day) for 10 days *or*
  - Cefuroxime 30 mg/kg/day in 2 divided doses (maximum 1 g/day) for 10 days *or*
  - Ceftriaxone 50 mg/kg IM/IV per day for 1 to 3 days depending on symptomatic improvement
  - Azithromycin 10 mg/kg on day 1 and 5 mg/kg days 2 to 5
- OME: No apparent benefit to medications which promote transitory resolution in 10–15%, but the effect is short-lived.

Second Line

- Alternative antibiotics are indicated for the following:
  - Persistent symptoms after 48 to 72 hours of amoxicillin
  - AOM within 1 month of amoxicillin therapy
  - Severe earache
  - Age <6 months with high fever
  - Immunocompromised
    - Amoxicillin-clavulanate; 90 mg/kg/day of amoxicillin, with 6.4 mg/kg/day of clavulanate in 2 divided doses; recommended in children who have taken amoxicillin in the previous 30 days and those with concurrent purulent conjunctivitis or history of AOM unresponsive to amoxicillin
    - Ceftriaxone, 50 mg/kg IM or IV q24h for 2 to 3 consecutive days can be reserved for those who are too sick to take oral medications or who unsuccessfully took amoxicillin-clavulanate.
- Neither erythromycin nor trimethoprim-sulfamethoxazole should be used as a second-line agent in treatment failures.
- Recurrent AOM: Antibiotic prophylaxis for recurrent AOM (>3 distinct, well-documented episodes in 6 months) is not recommended (2)[B].

ISSUES FOR REFERRAL

- If hearing loss occurs for >2 weeks after AOM resolution, follow up with audiogram.
- If >2 episodes in a 6-month period, consider ENT referral for fiberoptic nasopharyngoscopy to rule out malignancy.
- Refer to ENT for recurrent COM for consideration of tympanostomy tubes.

ADDITIONAL THERAPIES

Pain control: acetaminophen, ibuprofen

SURGERY/OTHER PROCEDURES

- Recurrent AOM: No definitive guidelines agreed upon as indications for surgery.
- Tympanostomy tubes may be effective in children aged <2 years with recurrent AOM.
- Adenotonsillectomy reduced the rate of AOM by 0.7 episode per child only in the 1st year after surgery and had a 15% complication rate.
- COM: Referral for surgery for tympanostomy should be individualized. It can be considered if >4 to 6 months of bilateral OME and/or >6 months of unilateral OME and/or hearing loss >25 dB or for high-risk individuals at any time.
- Tympanostomy tubes may reduce recurrence of AOM minimally, but it does not lower the risk of hearing loss.

ONGOING CARE

FOLLOW-UP RECOMMENDATIONS

Patients with otitis media who do not respond within 48 to 72 hours should be reevaluated. Consider changing the antibiotic.

Patient Monitoring

- AOM: Up to 40% may have persistent middle ear effusion at 1 month, with 10–25% at 3 months.
- OME/COM: Repeat otoscopic or tympanometric exams at 3 months, as indicated, as long as OME persists or sooner if there are red flags (see earlier discussion).

PROGNOSIS

Most cases of uncomplicated, non-severe AOM resolve without antibiotics.

COMPLICATIONS

- AOM: Tympanic membrane perforation/otorrhea, acute mastoiditis, facial nerve paralysis, otitic hydrocephalus, meningitis, labyrinthitis and hearing impairment, myringosclerosis, petrositis, brain abscess, epidural or subdural abscess, lateral or cavernous sinus thrombosis, or cholesteatoma
- COM: Speech and language disabilities may occur. Hearing loss is not caused by OME, but in children who are at risk for speech, language, or learning problems (e.g., autism spectrum, syndromes, craniofacial disorders, developmental delay, and children already with speech/language delay), it could lead to further problems because they are less tolerant of a hearing impairment.
- Recurrent AOM and COM: atrophy and scarring of eardrum, chronic perforation and otorrhea, cholesteatoma, permanent hearing loss, chronic mastoiditis, other intracranial suppurative complications

REFERENCES

1. Kaur R, Morris M, Pichichero ME. Epidemiology of acute otitis media in the postpneumococcal conjugate vaccine era. *Pediatrics*. 2017;140(3):e20170181. doi:10.1542/peds.2017-0181.
2. Lieberthal AS, Carroll AE, Chonmaitree T, et al. The diagnosis and management of acute otitis media. *Pediatrics*. 2013;131(3):e964–e999.
3. Lee DH, Yeo SW. Clinical diagnostic accuracy of otitis media with effusion in children, and significance of myringotomy: diagnostic or therapeutic? *J Korean Med Sci*. 2004;19(5):739–743. doi:10.3346/jkms.2004.19.5.739.

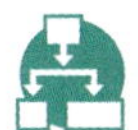

SEE ALSO

Algorithm: Ear Pain/Otalgia

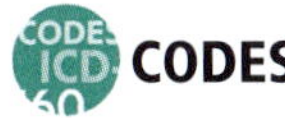

CODES

ICD10

- H65 Nonsuppurative otitis media
- H65.0 Acute serous otitis media
- H65.00 Acute serous otitis media, unspecified ear

CLINICAL PEARLS

- Pneumatic otoscopy is the single most specific and clinically useful test for diagnosis.
- Consider a delay of antibiotics for 24 to 48 hours in uncomplicated presentations (>6 months of age) who do not have severe illness or otorrhea.
- First-line treatment is amoxicillin, 80 to 90 mg/kg/day for 10 days for children aged <2 years; consider a 5- to 7-day course in >2 years of age.
- Erythema and effusion can persist for weeks.
- Antibiotics, antihistamines, and steroids are not indicated for COM.
- OME rarely develops in adults. Persistent unilateral effusion should be investigated to rule out neoplasm, particularly if there is a cranial nerve palsy.

OTITIS MEDIA WITH EFFUSION

Hobart Lee, MD, FAAFP

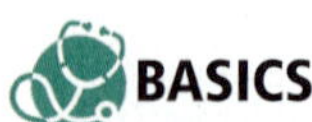

BASICS

DESCRIPTION

- Also called serous otitis media, secretory otitis media, nonsuppurative otitis media, "ear fluid," or "glue ear"
- Otitis media with effusion (OME) is defined as the presence of fluid in the middle ear in the absence of acute signs or symptoms of infection.
- More commonly, a pediatric disease
- May occur spontaneously from poor eustachian tube function or as an inflammatory response after acute otitis media (AOM)

EPIDEMIOLOGY

Approximately 90% of children have OME before school age, mostly between the ages of 6 months and 4 years.

Incidence

Approximately 2.2 million new cases annually in the United States

Prevalence

Less prevalent in adults and is usually associated with an underlying disorder

ETIOLOGY AND PATHOPHYSIOLOGY

- Chronic inflammatory condition where an underlying stimulus causes an inflammatory reaction with increased mucin production creating a functional blockage of the eustachian tube and thick accumulation of mucin-rich middle ear effusion
- Young children are more prone to OME due to shorter and more horizontal eustachian tubes, which become more vertical around 7 years of age.
- Biofilms, anatomic variations, and AOM caused by viruses or bacteria have been implicated as stimuli causing OME. The common pathogens causing AOM include nontypeable *Haemophilus influenzae*, *Streptococcus pneumoniae*, and *Moraxella catarrhalis*.
- In adults, OME is often associated with paranasal sinus disease (66%), smoking-induced nasopharyngeal lymphoid hyperplasia and adult onset adenoidal hypertrophy (19%), or head and neck tumors (4.8%).

RISK FACTORS

- Risk factors include a family history of OME, early daycare, exposure to cigarette smoke, bottle-feeding, and low socioeconomic status (1).
- Eustachian tube dysfunction may be a predisposing factor, although the evidence is unclear (2).
- Gastroesophageal reflux is associated with OME (2).

GENERAL PREVENTION

OME is generally not preventable, although lowering smoke exposure, breastfeeding, and avoiding daycare centers at an early age may decrease the risk.

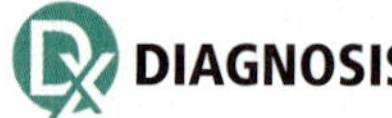

DIAGNOSIS

HISTORY

- OME is transient and asymptomatic in many pediatric patients.
- Most common reported symptom is hearing loss (2). There may be mild discomfort present in the ear, fullness, or "popping."
- Infants may have ear rubbing, excessive irritability, sleep problems, or failure to respond appropriately to voices or sounds.
- Clinical features may include "a history of hearing difficulties, poor attention, behavioral problems, delayed speech and language development, clumsiness, and poor balance" (2).
- There may be a history of recent or recurrent episodes of AOM or a recent upper respiratory tract infection (2).

PHYSICAL EXAM

- Cloudy tympanic membrane (TM) with distinctly impaired mobility; air-fluid level or bubble may be visible in the middle ear (1),(2).
- Color may be abnormal (yellow, amber, or blue), and the TM may be retracted or concave (2).
- Distinct redness of the TM may be present in approximately 5% of OME cases (1).
- Clinical signs and symptoms of acute illness should be absent in patients with OME (1).

DIFFERENTIAL DIAGNOSIS

- AOM
- Bullous myringitis
- Tympanosclerosis (may cause decreased/absent motion of the TM)
- Sensorineural hearing loss

DIAGNOSTIC TESTS & INTERPRETATION

Initial Tests (lab, imaging)

The primary standard to make the diagnosis is pneumatic otoscopy, which demonstrates reduced/absent mobility of the TM secondary to fluid in the middle ear. Pneumatic otoscopy has 94% sensitivity and 80% specificity for diagnosing OME. Accuracy of diagnosis with an experienced examiner is between 70% and 79% (1)[C].

Follow-Up Tests & Special Considerations

- Tympanometry may also be used to support or exclude the diagnosis in infants >4 months old, especially when the presence of middle ear effusion is difficult to determine (1)[C].
- Acoustic reflectometry (64% specificity and 80% sensitivity) may be considered instead of tympanometry (3)[B].
- Audiogram may show mild conductive hearing loss (2)[C].
- Hearing tests are recommended for OME lasting >3 months (1)[C].
- Language testing is recommended for children with abnormal hearing tests (1)[C].

Diagnostic Procedures/Other

Myringotomy is the gold standard but is not practical for clinical use (2)[C].

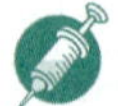

TREATMENT

- OME improves or resolves without medical intervention in most patients within 3 months, especially if secondary to AOM (1)[C].
- Current guidelines support a 3-month period of observation with optional serial exams, tympanometry, and language assessment during that wait time (1),(2)[C].
- Adults found to have OME should be screened for an underlying disorder and treated accordingly (2)[C].

MEDICATION

- The 2016 AAOHNS guideline recommends against routine use of antibiotics in treatment of OME. A 2016 Cochrane review, however, found that children treated with oral antibiotics were more likely to have tympanogram confirmed OME resolution in 2 to 3 months (number needed to treat = 5). Adverse events included diarrhea, vomiting, skin rash, and allergic reactions (number needed to harm = 20). Importantly, there were no reported patient-oriented outcomes (e.g., cognitive development, language, quality of life, or speech). Outcomes regarding short-term hearing, reduction of AOM infections, or need for ventilation tubes are unknown (1)[C],(4)[A].
- The 2016 AAOHNS and a 2006 Cochrane review found that antihistamines and decongestants have no benefit over placebo in OME treatment with possible adverse side effects such as insomnia, hyperactivity, and drowsiness (5)[A].

- The 2016 AAOHNS guideline recommends against administering oral or intranasal corticosteroids. No long-term benefit was shown, and adverse side effects such as weight gain and behavioral changes are possible (1)[C].
- In adults, eustachian tube dysfunction secondary to allergic rhinitis or recent upper respiratory infection can be the cause of OME. It is unknown whether decongestants, antihistamines, or nasal steroids improve outcomes in adults.

ISSUES FOR REFERRAL

The following are indications for referral to a surgeon for evaluation of tympanostomy tube placement:

- Chronic bilateral OME (≥3 months) with hearing difficulty
- Chronic OME with symptoms (e.g., vestibular problems, poor school performance, behavioral issues, ear discomfort, or reduced quality of life)
- At-risk children (speech, language, or learning problems due to baseline sensory, physical, cognitive, or behavioral factors) with chronic OME or type B (flat) tympanogram

ADDITIONAL THERAPIES

Hearing aids may be an acceptable alternative to surgery (2)[C].

SURGERY/OTHER PROCEDURES

- Tympanostomy tubes are recommended as initial surgery. Risks include purulent otorrhea, myringosclerosis, retraction pockets, and persistent TM perforations (1)[C].
- Adenoidectomy with myringotomy has similar efficacy to tympanostomy tubes in children >4 years of age but with added surgical and anesthetic risks (1)[C],(6).
- Adenoidectomy should not be performed in children with persistent OME alone unless there is a distinct indication for the procedure for another problem (e.g., adenoiditis/chronic sinusitis/nasal obstruction) (1)[C].
- Adenoidectomy (and concurrent tube placement) may be considered when repeat surgery for OME is necessary (e.g., when effusion recurs after tubes have fallen out or are removed). In these cases, adenoidectomy has been shown to decrease the need for future procedures for OME (1),(2)[C].
- Tonsillectomy or myringotomy alone is not recommended for treatment (1)[C].

COMPLEMENTARY & ALTERNATIVE MEDICINE

Autoinflation, which refers to the process of opening the eustachian tube by raising intranasal pressure (e.g., by forced exhalation with closed mouth and nose), may be beneficial in improving patients' tympanogram or audiometry and quality of life scores and may reduce overall persistence.

ONGOING CARE

FOLLOW-UP RECOMMENDATIONS

Patient Monitoring

- Children who are at risk for developmental difficulties should be evaluated for OME at the time of diagnosis and at 12 to 18 months (if initial diagnosis occurred <12 months). At-risk conditions include permanent hearing loss independent of OME, suspected or confirmed speech and language delay, autism spectrum disorder or other pervasive developmental disorder, Down syndrome or other craniofacial disorder, blindness or other uncorrectable visual impairment, cleft palate, and unspecified developmental delay (1)[C].
- For patients diagnosed with OME, reevaluation and repeat hearing tests should be performed every 3 to 6 months until the effusion has resolved or until the child develops an indication for surgical referral (1)[C].

PROGNOSIS

Approximately 50% of children >3 years of age have OME resolution within 3 months.

COMPLICATIONS

- The most significant complication of OME is permanent hearing loss, leading to possible language, speech, and developmental delays.
- Underventilation of the middle ear can cause a cholesteatoma (1)[C].

REFERENCES

1. Rosenfeld RM, Shin JJ, Schwartz SR, et al. Clinical practice guideline: otitis media with effusion executive summary (update). *Otolaryngol Head Neck Surg*. 2016;154(2):201–214.
2. Qureishi A, Lee Y, Belfield K, et al. Update on otitis media—prevention and treatment. *Infect Drug Resist*. 2014;7:15–24.
3. Shekelle P, Takata G, Chan LS, et al. Diagnosis, natural history, and late effects of otitis media with effusion. *Evid Rep Technol Assess (Summ)*. 2002;(55):1–5.
4. Venekamp RP, Burton MJ, van Dongen TMA, et al. Antibiotics for otitis media with effusion in children. *Cochrane Database Syst Rev*. 2016;2016(6):CD009163.
5. Griffin G, Flynn CA. Antihistamines and/or decongestants for otitis media with effusion (OME) in children. *Cochrane Database Syst Rev*. 2011;2011(9):CD003423.
6. Casselbrant ML, Mandel EM, Rockette HE, et al. Adenoidectomy for otitis media with effusion in 2–3-year-old children. *Int J Pediatr Otorhinolaryngol*. 2009;73(12):1718–1724.

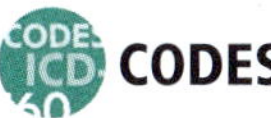

CODES

ICD10

- H65.90 Unspecified nonsuppurative otitis media, unspecified ear
- H65.00 Acute serous otitis media, unspecified ear
- H65.20 Chronic serous otitis media, unspecified ear

CLINICAL PEARLS

- OME is defined as the presence of a middle ear effusion in the absence of acute signs of infection.
- In children, OME most often arises following an AOM. In adults, it often occurs in association with eustachian tube dysfunction.
- The primary standard for diagnosis is pneumatic otoscopy.
- There is no benefit in antihistamines, decongestants, or corticosteroids for the treatment of OME in children.
- Management usually includes watchful waiting and surgery (when indicated); which strategy is chosen depends on many factors, including the risk/presence of any associated speech, language, or learning delays, and on the severity of any associated hearing loss.

OVARIAN CYST, RUPTURED

Kristina Gracey, MD, MPH

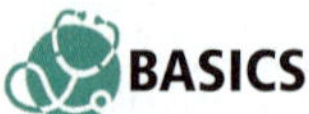

BASICS

- Ovarian cysts are frequent in reproductive-aged women.
- Patients with a symptomatic ruptured cyst usually complain of acute onset unilateral lower abdominal pain.
- Rupture can be caused by sexual intercourse, luteal phase, exercise, trauma, or pregnancy, or it can be idiopathic.
- Evaluation of the patient should include exclusion of other emergent causes: ectopic pregnancy, ovarian torsion, and nongynecologic sources of acute unilateral lower abdominal pain.
- Once the diagnosis of a ruptured cyst is confirmed, most patients can be managed conservatively as outpatients with adequate pain control. Surgical intervention is rarely indicated.

DESCRIPTION

Most ovarian cysts are benign physiologic follicles created by the ovary at the time of ovulation. Ovarian cysts can cause symptoms when they become enlarged and exert a mass effect on surrounding structures, or when they rupture and the cyst contents irritate the peritoneum or nearby pelvic organs.

EPIDEMIOLOGY

- The actual incidence of ovarian cysts is difficult to calculate as many ruptured cysts are asymptomatic or found incidentally.
- Ovarian cysts can be seen on transvaginal ultrasounds in nearly all premenopausal women and in up to 18% of postmenopausal women. The vast majority of these cysts are benign or functional.
- About 13% of ovarian masses in reproductive-aged women are malignant, as opposed to 45% in postmenopausal women. About 70% of ovarian malignancies are diagnosed at a late stage.
- Ruptured ovarian cysts most commonly affect the right ovary, 63%.

Incidence

About 7% of women worldwide experience a symptomatic cyst during their lifetime.

Prevalence

During pregnancy, prevalence varies from 1 to 5.3%; of those, just 0.63% are symptomatic and 1% are malignant.

ETIOLOGY AND PATHOPHYSIOLOGY

Normal ovulation occurs when a follicle matures and ruptures, releasing an oocyte, leaving a corpus luteum, which subsequently involutes. If the follicle fails to rupture and continues to grow, a follicular cyst is formed. If a corpus luteum fails to involute and continues to grow, then a corpus luteum cyst occurs. These are the most common cysts. Both types are physiologic (termed "functional") without malignant potential. Other cyst types include endometriomas (filled with menstrual blood), dermoid cysts that contains mature tissue of ectodermal, mesodermal, and/or endodermal origin, and ovarian malignancy originating from any of the structures of the ovary.

RISK FACTORS

Medications or conditions associated with increased ovulation and/or increased risk of cyst rupture.

- Ovulation induction agents (i.e., clomiphene [Clomid], aromatase inhibitors, GnRH agonists)
- Tamoxifen increases the risk of ovarian cysts in reproductive-aged women.
- Polycystic ovarian syndrome (PCOS) (common), fibrous dysplasia/McCune-Albright syndrome (rare)
- Ovarian endometriosis

GENERAL PREVENTION

Ovulation suppression with combined hormonal contraceptives is the mainstay therapy for prevention of recurrent ovarian cyst.

COMMONLY ASSOCIATED CONDITIONS

- Endometriomas located on or adjacent to the ovaries are found in 20–55% of women with endometriosis.
- PCOS

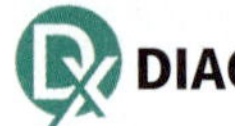

DIAGNOSIS

The characteristic symptoms of ruptured cyst may resemble ectopic pregnancy. Ectopic pregnancy should be ruled out when a ruptured cyst is suspected (1)[C].

HISTORY

- Questions that should be addressed if a ruptured ovarian cyst is suspected include:
  - Onset and characteristics of pain
  - Pain associated with timing of sexual intercourse, strenuous activity, or trauma
  - Date of last menstrual period
  - Presence or absence of vaginal bleeding
  - Nausea or vomiting
  - Shoulder or upper abdominal pain due to subphrenic extravasation
- Symptoms of hypotension/hypovolemia, including palpitations, shortness of breath, sensation of being hot or clammy, dizziness
- Additional information that will guide diagnosis should include patient age, known or previous ovarian cysts, and reproductive history.

ALERT

Patients with bleeding diathesis or undergoing anticoagulation therapy may experience significant bleeding from hemorrhagic cysts.

PHYSICAL EXAM

- Vital signs are usually normal unless significant blood loss has occurred.
- Rupture characterized by significant blood loss may be present in the form of pallor, pale mucosal membranes, and tachycardia.
- Patients will have significant tenderness to palpation or an acute abdomen if the peritoneum is irritated or inflamed.
- On some occasions, a palpable adnexal mass can be felt on bimanual exam. Care should be taken not to cause further injury with a forceful exam.

DIFFERENTIAL DIAGNOSIS

Includes all causes of acute abdominal pain, both gynecologic and nongynecologic

- Ectopic pregnancy should always be excluded with a negative pregnancy test (1)[C].
- Common gynecologic etiologies include:
  - Functional ovarian cysts
  - Ovarian torsion
  - Tubo-ovarian abscess
  - Teratomas
  - Degenerating fibroids
  - Endometrioma
  - Cystadenoma (mucinous or serous)
  - Hydrosalpinx
- Malignant gynecologic etiologies can usually be attributed to the various gynecologic cancers of the reproductive tract.
- Benign nongynecologic causes of acute lower abdominal pain include:
  - Appendicitis
  - Diverticulitis
  - Infections of the urinary tract
  - Renal colic
- Malignant nongynecologic causes of acute lower abdominal pain can be attributed to neoplastic processes of the lower GI tract.

DIAGNOSTIC TESTS & INTERPRETATION

- In all premenopausal women, pregnancy must be ruled out by a urine test.
- Complete blood count may reveal a significant drop in hematocrit if there is ongoing hemorrhage (2)[B]. Leukocytosis should raise the suspicion of an infectious process (1)[C].
- Urinalysis and STD testing should be obtained to evaluate for infectious causes, PID, or symptomatic renal stones (1)[C].
- A type and screen is indicated if surgical intervention is planned or blood products are being considered.

Initial Tests (lab, imaging)

- Ultrasonography
- Serial quantitative β-hCG if pregnancy of unknown location
- Complete blood count
- Urinalysis and STD Testing

Follow-Up Tests & Special Considerations

Computed tomography (CT) or magnetic resonance imaging (MRI) may narrow the differential diagnosis when ultrasonography is indeterminate.

- Sonographic imaging along with CT and MRI can aid in diagnosis of gynecologic emergencies (3)[C].
- CT is useful to confirm a hemoperitoneum, and MRI can assist when the diagnosis remains unclear after CT and ultrasound (3)[C].
- Ultrasound and CT imaging for diagnosis has decreased the need for diagnostic surgical intervention (2)[B].
- Additionally, ultrasound is useful in confirming normal Doppler flow to the affected ovary and adnexa (1)[C].

Diagnostic Procedures/Other

Laparoscopy may be diagnostic and therapeutic in emergent cases.

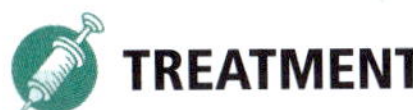

TREATMENT

GENERAL MEASURES

- For many patients, pain associated with a ruptured cyst will be transient and self-limiting.
- Cyst rupture in a stable healthy patient can be managed conservatively in 80% of cases (2)[B].
- Patient with anticoagulation can also be managed conservatively with cyst rupture using a multidisciplinary team (4)[C].

MEDICATION

Scheduled NSAIDs or oral narcotics can be prescribed depending on pain severity.

First Line

For patients with multiple episodes or a single severe occurrence, OCPs can be considered for ovulation suppression and prevention. They are not effective for treatment of ovarian cysts which are already present.

ISSUES FOR REFERRAL

- Obstetrician (OB)/GYN
  - Consider referral to an obstetrician if an adnexal mass is diagnosed during pregnancy. Such masses have a low risk of malignancy or acute complication for the pregnancy.
  - Most cysts resolve without intervention within 2 to 3 weeks; those that do not resolve in 12 weeks require referral for surgical assessment (5)[A].
  - Unstable patients with hemodynamic compromise or patients with significant hemoperitoneum should be resuscitated, and laparoscopy or a laparotomy should be considered. Surgical exploration should also be considered if there is a concern for malignancy.
- Gynecologic oncology: Referral to a gynecologic oncologist should be considered for complex adnexal masses with an elevated CA-125 and associated symptoms concerning for malignancy such as ascites, thick septation noted on ultrasound, early satiety, pleural effusion, enlarging abdominal mass, or bowel obstruction.
- General surgery: Acute lower abdominal pain that is nongynecologic and suspicious for bowel involvement should be referred to general surgery or a gastroenterologist.

ADDITIONAL THERAPIES

Guided cyst aspiration is not recommended for either diagnosis or treatment but could be considered in patients at high risk who are not good surgical candidates.

SURGERY/OTHER PROCEDURES

- Although the need for surgical intervention is rare, it is usually of an emergent nature.
- Patients with a low diastolic blood pressure and a large amount of hemoperitoneum often need surgery (2)[B].
- In most cases, laparoscopy is diagnostic and therapeutic. The decision to proceed with cystectomy or oophorectomy should be made intraoperatively after a thorough evaluation of the intra-abdominal environment has been completed.
- The advantages of a laparoscopic approach include a shorter length of stay, faster recovery, small scar, and few adhesions. Postoperative recovery time as well as patient satisfaction is significantly improved with a minimally invasive approach.
- Laparotomy should be performed in cases of critical hemodynamic instability or lack of laparoscopically trained surgeons. If there is a concern for malignancy or metastases, laparotomy may be the preferred method of surgery.

ADMISSION, INPATIENT, AND NURSING CONSIDERATIONS

Patients who require inpatient management should be managed with serial abdominal exams, analgesia, and intravenous resuscitation as indicated by their initial presentation.

ONGOING CARE

FOLLOW-UP RECOMMENDATIONS

- Follow-up for patients managed conservatively should be scheduled in 72 hours from the initial onset of symptoms. Patients should present sooner for new or worsening symptoms.
- Patients with complete resolution of symptoms within a few days can follow up as needed. However, these patients should be counseled on risk of reoccurrence and options for prevention.
- In patients who had surgery, postop follow-up should be scheduled 2 weeks from the date of surgery.
- Patients in whom an ovarian cyst was diagnosed incidentally should follow-up based on the size of their cyst.

Pregnancy Considerations

- The management of adnexal masses during pregnancy is controversial.
- Most adnexal masses in pregnancy can be managed expectantly because the risk of malignancy is low (1)[C]. If there is a risk for ruptured endometriotic cyst, early surgical intervention can reduce the risk of cyst fluid leakage, thus preventing adhesions and preserving fertility. MRI can help further characterize a mass safely in pregnancy (1)[C]. However, the possible risk of torsion or rupture should not be considered as an indication for surgery.

PATIENT EDUCATION

Reassurance of the benign nature of most ovarian cysts is an important cornerstone of patient education.

COMPLICATIONS

- Surgical procedure complications related to any laparoscopic surgery
- Ovarian reserve reduction may occur following any ovarian surgery. Desire for future fertility should be factored into surgical decisions. Cysts with a diameter of ≥5 cm can themselves cause compromise in ovarian reserve. It is unclear if the effect is temporary or permanent.

REFERENCES

1. Biggs WS, Marks ST. Diagnosis and management of adnexal masses. *Am Fam Physician*. 2016;93(8):676–681.
2. Kim JH, Lee SM, Lee JH, et al. Successful conservative management of ruptured ovarian cysts with hemoperitoneum in healthy women. *PLoS One*. 2014;9(3):e91171.
3. Iraha Y, Okada M, Iraha R, et al. CT and MR imaging of gynecologic emergencies. *Radiographics*. 2017;37(5):1569–1586.
4. Gupta A, Gupta S, Manaktala U, et al. Conservative management of corpus luteum haemorrhage in patients on anticoagulation: a report of three cases and review of the literature. *Arch Gynecol Obstet*. 2015;291(2):427–431.
5. Seehusen DA, Earwood JS. Oral contraceptives are not an effective treatment for ovarian cysts. *Am Fam Physician*. 2014;90(9):623.

ADDITIONAL READING

American College of Obstetricians and Gynecologists, Committee on Practice Bulletins—Gynecology. Practice Bulletin No. 174: evaluation and management of adnexal masses. *Obstet Gynecol*. 2016;128(5):e210–e226.

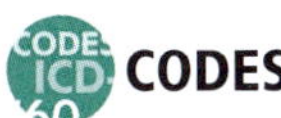

CODES

ICD10

- N83.20 Unspecified ovarian cysts
- N83.0 Follicular cyst of ovary
- N83.1 Corpus luteum cyst

CLINICAL PEARLS

- Functional ovarian cysts are very common in reproductive-aged women and are usually self-limiting.
- Always exclude ectopic pregnancy.
- Management of symptomatic ruptured cysts is usually accomplished with outpatient pain control and follow-up.
- Combined hormonal contraception is the mainstay of preventive treatment.

PALLIATIVE CARE

Erika Zimmons, DO, MS

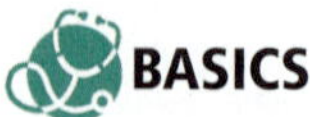

BASICS

DESCRIPTION

- The principal goal of palliative care is to prevent and alleviate suffering—whether physical (pain, breathlessness, nausea, etc.), emotional, social, or spiritual regardless of the underlying etiology.
- Palliative care is an interdisciplinary approach to caring for patients and families that aims to improve or maintain quality of life despite serious illness.
- The palliative care team helps to identify goals of care based on patient preferences and values.
- Hospice: In the United Sates, hospice is available for patients whose average life expectancy is ≤6 months and whose principal goal is to stay at home (including long-term care or assisted living facility), avoid hospitalizations, and forego disease-directed care with a curative intent. Unlike regular home nursing services, hospice does not require a patient to be homebound. Hospice offers backup support for patients 24 hours a day and 7 days per week. Hospice will also provide bereavement support for family and friends for 1 year after the patient's death.

RISK FACTORS

- Cancer
- Early-onset dementia
- Advanced heart failure

COMMONLY ASSOCIATED CONDITIONS

Common symptoms/syndromes encountered in palliative care:

- Pain: chronic pain, neuropathic pain, pain from bone metastases
- GI symptoms: ascites, anorexia/cachexia, bowel obstruction, constipation and stool impaction, diarrhea, dysphagia, mucositis/stomatitis, sialorrhea, xerostomia, nausea, and vomiting
  - For nausea and vomiting consider underlying etiology and treat accordingly.
    - GI causes: constipation, bowel (full or partial) obstruction, ileus, reflux, inflammation
    - Intrathoracic causes: cardiac, effusions (cardiac, pulmonary), mediastinal causes, esophageal disease
    - Autonomic dysfunction
    - Centrally mediated: intracranial pressure change, inflammation, cerebellar, vestibular, medication or metabolic cause stimulating vomiting center, and/or chemoreceptor trigger zone
    - Medication side effects
- General medical symptoms: delirium and fatigue
- Pulmonary symptoms: cough, breathlessness, dyspnea
- Psychological symptoms: anxiety, depression, insomnia
- Skin: decubitus ulcer, pruritus, complex wounds

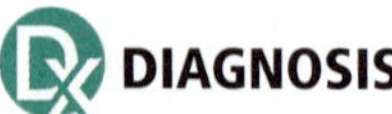

DIAGNOSIS

HISTORY

A comprehensive assessment includes:

- Underlying medical conditions and associated physical symptoms
- Communication with empathic inquiry and open-ended questions
  - Framework for breaking bad news—Set up interview, assess Perception, obtain Invitation, impart Knowledge, address Emotions with empathic responses, Strategy and Summary (SPIKES) (1)
  - The serious illness conversation provides a structure for discussion of prognosis and key topics such as feelings and goals related to health conditions (2).
- Comprehensive pain assessment and review of systems (e.g., Edmonton Symptom Assessment Scale)
  - The revised Edmonton Symptom Assessment Scale includes evaluation of symptoms of tiredness, drowsiness, nausea, lack of appetite, shortness of breath, depression, anxiety, well-being and other problems.
- Psychological symptom assessment
- Cultural, social, financial, and practical concerns
- Spiritual and existential issues
  - **F**aith, **I**mportance and influence, **C**ommunity, **A**ddress assessment (FICA—how does the patient wish these items to be addressed?)
- Presence and sources of suffering
- Goals of care: posthospital care, practical needs, hopes, and fears
- Prognosis: functional status and interest in knowing prognosis
  - The ability to complete functional tasks can be evaluated by tools such as the Karnofsy Performance Status Scale, the Eastern Cooperative Oncology Group (ECOG) performance status, or the Palliative Performance Scale

PHYSICAL EXAM

The physical examination is directed by underlying diagnosis, symptoms, and functional decline in the context of meeting the goals of the patient and family to maximize function, comfort, and support.

DIAGNOSTIC TESTS & INTERPRETATION

Initial Tests (lab, imaging)

Laboratory and radiology testing depends upon the underlying diagnosis and any associated symptoms. Avoid unnecessary testing.

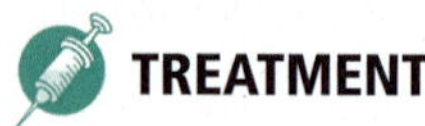

TREATMENT

GENERAL MEASURES

- Targeted interventions to maximize quality of life and minimize symptom burden considering patient's values, goals, fears, and social setting
- Treatment should involve an interdisciplinary team to address potential and realized suffering (physical, emotional, social, and/or spiritual).

MEDICATION

- Minimize polypharmacy; discontinue medications that offer little improvement in the quality of life.
- Focus the use of medications for symptom management. Continue use of disease-modifying medications especially if they lessen symptom burden and enhance immediate quality of life.
- In patients with cognitive impairment consider that they may not be able to verbalize symptoms.

- Consider medications to address symptoms:
  - *Pain*
    - Use immediate-release opioids—titrate to adequate control.
    - Once pain is controlled, convert to long-acting opioids with short-acting agents made available because tolerance develops and/or patient develops breakthrough pain.
  - Bone pain: NSAIDs added to narcotics are more effective than narcotics alone.
  - Neuropathic pain: may use adjuvant treatment, such as gabapentin or other anticonvulsants

ALERT
Avoid morphine in patients with renal failure; can induce delirium, hyperalgesia, agitation, and seizures

- *Vomiting* associated with a particular opioid may be relieved by substitution with an equianalgesic dose of another opioid or a sustained-release formulation.
  - Dopamine receptor antagonists (metoclopramide, prochlorperazine) may improve nausea symptoms.
  - Droperidol: insufficient evidence on the use for the management of nausea and vomiting
- *Constipation*: Consider prophylactic stimulants (bisacodyl or senna), or osmotic laxatives. Avoid nonessential medications that may cause constipation.

ALERT
Consider laxatives with opioid treatment to avoid constipation.

- Subcutaneous methylnaltrexone may be used for inducing bowel movements without inducing withdrawal in opioid-induced constipation.
- Dyspnea: Consider oxygen. Consider benzodiazepines if increased anxiety.
  - Treat the underlying cause of breathlessness. In addition, as the disease advances, low-dose opioids may be beneficial to patients. Immediate-release opioids PO/IV treat dyspnea effectively and typically at doses lower than necessary for the relief of moderate pain.
- *Delirium*: Consider review of medications or other causes that may be contributing to delirium. Consider the lowest doses of antipsychotics (haloperidol or risperidone, etc.) or in some cases benzodiazepines (only when necessary).
  - Monitor patient safety and use nonpharmacologic strategies to assist orientation (clocks, calendars, environment, and redirection).
- Pruritus: no optimal therapy; general measures include moisturizing skin and avoiding irritants.
- Anxiety: insufficient data for recommendations of specific medication
- Megestrol acetate improves appetite and slight weight gain in patients with anorexia-cachexia syndrome. However, consider possible side effects.

ISSUES FOR REFERRAL

- Referral to palliative care
  - Any patient with a serious, life-limiting illness who could use help with burdensome symptoms or suffering and/or complex goals of care discussion
  - Early referral to palliative care may improve quality of life and longevity for patients with advanced cancer.
- Referral to hospice care
  - Any patient with an average life expectancy of ≤6 months
  - Consider patients who have multiple hospitalizations and/or emergency department visits in the prior 6 months.
  - Refer to local hospice guidelines for additional disease-specific criteria.

ONGOING CARE

PATIENT EDUCATION

- Hospice Foundation of America: https://hospicefoundation.org/
- National Institute on Aging, "What Are Palliative Care and Hospice Care?": https://www.nia.nih.gov/health/what-are-palliative-care-and-hospice-care

REFERENCES

1. Baile W, Buckman R, Lenzi R, et al. SPIKES—a six-step protocol for delivering bad news: application to the patient with cancer. *Oncologist*. 2000;5(4):302–311.
2. Bernacki R, Hutchings M, Vick J, et al. Development of the serious illness care program: a randomised controlled trial of a palliative care communication intervention. *BMJ Open*. 2015;5(10):e009032.

ADDITIONAL READING

- Borneman T, Ferrell B, Puchalski CM. Evaluation of the FICA tool for spiritual assessment. *J Pain Symptom Manage*. 2010;40(2):163–173.
- Radbruch L, De Lima L, Knaul F, et al. Redefining palliative care—a new consensus-based definition. *J Pain Symptom Manage*. 2020;60(4):754–764.

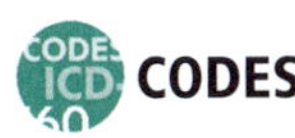

CODES

ICD10

Z51.5 Encounter for palliative care

CLINICAL PEARLS

- Palliative care is undergoing a shift toward earlier, integrated care for patients with serious illness. This includes active, holistic care for patients of all ages who are enduring serious health-related suffering (not just end-of-life scenarios) aiming to improve quality of life for all involved (patients, families, caregivers)
- The addition of adjuvant treatments may be more effective than narcotics alone for managing pain.
- Use laxatives with opioid treatment to avoid constipation.

PANCREATITIS, ACUTE

Joseph Daniel Hogue, MD, MBA • Farukh Ali Mirza, MD • Vicenda Augustin, MD

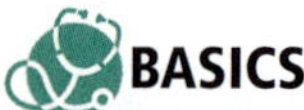

BASICS

DESCRIPTION

Acute inflammation of the pancreas with variable involvement of regional tissue or remote organ systems

- Symptoms relate to intrapancreatic activation of enzymes with pain, nausea and vomiting, and associated intestinal ileus
- Complete structural and functional recovery if there is no necrosis or pancreatic ductal disruption

EPIDEMIOLOGY

Incidence

13 to 49/100,000 per year; no predominant sex but increases with age; higher incidence in African American population

Prevalence

- 19/10,000
- Most common gastrointestinal diagnosis for inpatient hospitalizations with >300,000 admissions per year in the United States

ETIOLOGY AND PATHOPHYSIOLOGY

- Together, gallstones (including microlithiasis) and chronic alcohol use account for >80% of cases.
- Postendoscopic retrograde cholangiopancreatography (post-ERCP)
- Medications (most common)
  - ACE inhibitors; angiotensin receptor blockers (ARBs); thiazide diuretics and furosemide
  - Antimetabolites (mercaptopurine and azathioprine) and checkpoint inhibitors
  - Corticosteroids; glyburide; exenatide
  - Mesalamine; sulfamethoxazole/trimethoprim, pentamidine; valproic acid; statins
  - NSAIDs, opiates
- Metabolic causes
  - Hypertriglyceridemia (classically >1,000 mg/dL); even nonfasting levels as low as ~≥177 mg/dL (third overall most common cause, ~10% of cases)
  - Hypercalcemia; acute renal failure
  - Diet with high glycemic load
  - Systemic lupus erythematosus/polyarteritis/other vascular disease
  - Autoimmune; type I with elevated IgG4 and type II with normal IgG4
  - Infections: mumps, coxsackie, CMV, EBV, cryptosporidiosis, ascaris, Clonorchis; SARS CoV-2
- Penetrating peptic ulcer (rare)
- AIDS
- Cystic fibrosis, CFTR gene mutations, and other mutations
- Tumors (e.g., pancreatic, ampullary)
- Trauma/surgery
- Miscellaneous obstruction: celiac disease; Crohn disease; pancreas divisum; sphincter of Oddi dysfunction; choledochocele
- Scorpion venom
- Acute fatty liver of pregnancy
- Pancreatic fat deposition
- Associated coexisting risk factors: obesity; type II diabetes; smoking
- Pathophysiology—enzymatic autodigestion of the pancreas with interstitial edema and third spacing of fluid.
- Cellular injury alters membrane trafficking, which alters lysosomal function leading to trypsin formation and zymogen activation. A robust inflammatory response ensues resulting in increased vascular permeability, hemorrhage, edema, and necrosis.
- The severity of the first episode of acute pancreatitis, alcohol abuse, and smoking all increase the risk of acute recurrent pancreatitis, which, in turn, increases the risk of progression to chronic pancreatitis.
- Clinical features associated with an increasing severity of acute pancreatitis: age ≥60 years; obesity; long-term, heavy alcohol use; altered mental status

Genetics

Hereditary pancreatitis is rare; autosomal dominant

GENERAL PREVENTION

- Avoid excess alcohol consumption.
- Tobacco cessation
- Correct underlying metabolic processes (hypertriglyceridemia or hypercalcemia).
- Discontinue offending medications.
- Cholecystectomy (symptomatic cholelithiasis)
- Diet: There is an increased risk of gallstone pancreatitis with diets high in saturated fats, cholesterol, red meat, and eggs.

COMMONLY ASSOCIATED CONDITIONS

- Alcohol withdrawal, alcoholic hepatitis, diabetic ketoacidosis, and ascending cholangitis
- Morbid obesity, a pro-inflammatory state, increases severity and adverse outcomes (organ failure, mortality).

DIAGNOSIS

Symptoms do not always correlate with objective findings. Diagnosis requires two of three of the following:

- Typical symptoms
- Elevation of amylase or lipase (preferred) >3× ULN
- Characteristic imaging findings on CT/MRI or ultrasound; ultrasound preferred for evaluation of gallstones; CT/MRI typically reserved for diagnostic uncertainty or failure to improve clinically in 48 to 72 hours

HISTORY

- Acute onset of epigastric pain, which may radiate posteriorly
- Nausea/vomiting
- Alcohol use
- Personal or family history of gallstones
- Medication use—look for inciting medications
- Abdominal trauma
- Recent significant rapid weight loss

PHYSICAL EXAM

- Vital signs—Assess hemodynamic stability; fever; tachycardia; hypotension.
- Abdominal findings: epigastric tenderness, loss of bowel sounds, peritoneal signs
- Other findings: jaundice, rales/percussive dullness
- Rare (with hemorrhagic pancreatitis): flank discoloration (Grey Turner sign) or umbilical discoloration (Cullen sign)

DIFFERENTIAL DIAGNOSIS

- Penetrating peptic ulcer
- Acute cholecystitis or cholangitis
- Macroamylasemia, macrolipasemia
- Mesenteric vascular occlusion and/or infarction
- Intestinal obstruction; perforated viscus
- Aortic aneurysm (dissecting or rupturing)
- Inferior wall myocardial infarction
- Lymphoma

DIAGNOSTIC TESTS & INTERPRETATION

- Interpret laboratory and radiographic findings in the context of the clinical history.
- Diagnosis typically requires two of the following three criteria:
  - Upper abdominal pain
  - Serum lipase or amylase >3× ULN
  - Characteristic findings on CT
- There are several scoring systems to assess severity (BISAP, Ranson criteria, HAPS, etc.); however, none have been shown to be superior.
- Presence of SIRS is more easily adaptable and its presence for ≥48 hours indicates poor prognosis.
- Lipase is more specific to the pancreas than amylase. In addition, lipase has a longer half-life, and is preferred in patients who present later after pain onset.
- Elevated total bilirubin. If >3 mg/dL, consider common bile duct obstruction.
- A 3-fold elevation in the alanine aminotransferase (ALT) in the setting of acute pancreatitis has a 95% positive predictive value for gallstone pancreatitis. Triglyceride levels >1,000 mg/dL suggest hypertriglyceridemia as the cause.
- Glucose and calcium increased in severe disease.
- WBC elevation to 10,000 to 25,000/μL possible and not indicative of active infection
- Elevated baseline hematocrit >44 or rising hematocrit is poor prognostic sign (severe third spacing with associated hemoconcentration).

Initial Tests (lab, imaging)

- Use follow-up labs to assess renal function, hydration, sepsis, biliary obstruction, and tissue oxygenation.
- Chest x-ray (CXR) to evaluate for early acute respiratory distress syndrome (ARDS), pleural effusion, and perforation
- Ultrasound to look for gallbladder/biliary stones
- CT scan
  - Confirms the diagnosis, assesses severity, establishes a baseline, provides prognostic information, and rules out most other pathologies (excluding noncalcified cholelithiasis)
  - IV contrast is not essential for the initial CT scan; avoid contrast in volume-depleted patients.
  - The presence of gas in the peripancreatic collection is strong evidence for infection, but its absence does not rule it out.

Follow-Up Tests & Special Considerations

If patients fail to improve, and renal function is stable, a contrast-enhanced CT scan at day 3 to assess for necrosis; CT-guidance assists aspiration and drainage of abscess—mainly recommended if a fungal or drug-resistant infection is suspected.

P

Diagnostic Procedures/Other

- Magnetic resonance cholangiopancreatography (MRCP) helps assess choledocholithiasis, pancreas divisum, dilated pancreatic duct, and ductal changes.
- Esophagogastroduodenoscopy (EGD) is useful to rule out a penetrating duodenal ulcer or an obstructing ampullary neoplasm.
- ERCP may be necessary to decompress common bile duct due to an impacted stone.
- Endoscopic ultrasonography (EUS) is useful if patients present with "idiopathic pancreatitis."
- EUS-guided fine needle aspiration if autoimmune pancreatitis is suspected.

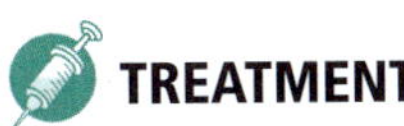

TREATMENT

GENERAL MEASURES

Many cases of acute pancreatitis require hospitalization; ICU if multiorgan dysfunction or hypotension/respiratory failure; 15–20% of cases of acute pancreatitis progress from mild to severe (including persistent organ failure).

- Fluid resuscitation
  - Patients may have significant volume deficit due to third spacing
  - Infuse bolus of 10 mL/kg, followed by 1.5 mL/kg/hr. Larger volumes may be required for patients presenting with severe pancreatitis, preferably with CVP monitoring (1)[A].
  - Lactated Ringer solution preferred over normal saline for initial fluid resuscitation, in patients without hypercalcemia, to decrease risk of systemic inflammation/SIRS and due to its less acidic pH
  - Target urine output should be 0.5 to 1.0 mL/kg/hr. 4 L should be the maximum total fluid on day 1.
  - Fluid resuscitation is of limited value after 24 hours, and fluid overload results in significant complications.
    - Eliminate unnecessary medications, especially those implicated as causes of pancreatitis.
    - Nasogastric (NG) tube for intractable emesis
    - Follow renal function, volume status, calcium, and oxygenation. Organ failure is more important prognostic indicator than pancreatic necrosis.
    - Nutritional support: Begin oral alimentation after pain, tenderness, and ileus have resolved; small amounts of high-carbohydrate, low-fat, and low-protein foods; advance as tolerated. In cases of mild pancreatitis, a soft low-fat diet may be started as soon as tolerated even before enzymes elevation and pain have completely resolved. Enteral nutrition can be considered for severe pancreatitis at 72 hours (or earlier if tolerated); nasogastric, nasoduodenal, and nasojejunal are all safe routes that can be used. However, nasojejunal tube route is preferred if there is digestive intolerance from gastric outlet obstruction or delayed gastric emptying. Discontinue with increases in pain, increases in amylase/lipase levels, or fluid retention; TPN (without lipids if triglycerides are elevated) if oral or nasoenteric feedings are not tolerated

MEDICATION

First Line

- Analgesia: no consensus; *avoid* meperidine (Demerol) due to the potential of accumulation of a toxic metabolite.
- Antibiotics
  - In the clear absence of infection, the use of prophylactic antibiotics is not recommended.
  - In patients with ascending cholangitis or necrotizing pancreatitis, if there is a strong suspicion of active infection, consider empiric imipenem class or β-lactam/β-lactamase inhibitor (e.g., piperacillin/tazobactam 4.5 g IV q8h) for initial treatment before cultures (especially aspirates) return.
  - Levofloxacin 500 mg QD IV if cholangitis and there is an allergy to penicillin
  - Watch for fungal superinfections when giving prophylactic antibiotics.

ISSUES FOR REFERRAL

Refer to a tertiary center if pancreatitis is severe or actively evolving and when advanced imaging or endoscopic therapy is being considered.

SURGERY/OTHER PROCEDURES

- Consider cholecystectomy before discharge in patients with uncomplicated acute biliary (nonnecrotizing) pancreatitis to reduce risk of recurrence.
- Necrosectomy should be performed nonsurgically for either infected or noninfected necrosis. Walled-off necrosis should be observed for 4 weeks and treated with antibiotics if infected.
- ERCP early if evidence of acute cholangitis or at 72 hours if evidence of ongoing biliary obstruction; ERCP with pancreatic ductal stent placement, if ductal disruption persists longer than 1 to 2 weeks.
- Plasma exchange with insulin within 24 hours of presentation if severe necrotizing pancreatitis secondary to hypertriglyceridemia

ADMISSION, INPATIENT, AND NURSING CONSIDERATIONS

Discharge criteria

- Pain controlled
- Tolerating oral diet
- Alcohol rehabilitation and tobacco cessation
- Low-grade fever and mild leukocytosis do not necessarily indicate infection and may take weeks to resolve. Infections may occur even after 10 days (33% of patients with necrotizing pancreatitis) due to secondary infection of necrotic material, requiring surgical débridement.

ONGOING CARE

FOLLOW-UP RECOMMENDATIONS

- Follow-up imaging in several weeks if the original CT scan showed a fluid collection or necrosis or if the amylase/lipase continue to be elevated. Follow-up findings may include:
  - Pseudocyst (occurs in 10%) or abscess (sudden onset of fever)
  - Splenic vein thrombosis in 16–18% with necrotizing pancreatitis
  - Pseudoaneurysm (splenic, gastroduodenal, intrapancreatic) hemorrhage can be life-threatening.
- Mild exocrine and endocrine dysfunction is usually subclinical. Patients with necrotizing pancreatitis, steatorrhea, or ductal obstruction should receive enzyme supplementation.
- After the first episode of acute pancreatitis, the risk of lifetime diabetes doubles, the risk of developing acute recurrent pancreatitis is ~17%, and the risk for developing chronic pancreatitis is ~8%.

DIET

Advance diet as tolerated; reduce fat, alcohol, and added sugars.

PROGNOSIS

85–90% of cases of acute pancreatitis resolve spontaneously; 3–5% mortality (17% in necrotizing pancreatitis)

COMPLICATIONS

AKI, ARDS, ascites, chronic pancreatitis/pancreatic insufficiency, DIC, multiorgan failure, necrotizing pancreatitis, pancreatic abscess, intestinal or bowel obstruction, pseudocyst, pseudoaneurysm, venous thrombosis

REFERENCES

1. Tenner S, Vege SS, Sheth SG, et al. American College of Gastroenterology Guidelines: management of acute pancreatitis. *Am J Gastroenterol*. 2024;119(3):419–437.

ADDITIONAL READING

- Beij A, Verdonk RC, van Santvoort HC, et al. Acute pancreatitis: an update of evidence-based management and recent trends in treatment strategies. *United European Gastroenterol J*. 2025;13(1):97–106.
- Trikudanathan G, Yazici C, Evans Phillips A, et al. Diagnosis and management of acute pancreatitis. *Gastroenterology*. 2024;167(4):673–688.

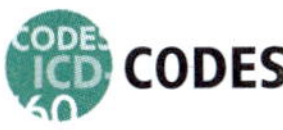

CODES

ICD10

- K85.9 Acute pancreatitis, unspecified
- K85.8 Other acute pancreatitis
- K85.2 Alcohol induced acute pancreatitis

CLINICAL PEARLS

- Gallstones and alcohol misuse are the leading causes of pancreatitis.
- Review all medications and discontinue any that may cause (or contribute to) pancreatitis.
- Start oral feeding as soon as possible in the absence of severe pain, vomiting, or ileus.
- Refer to tertiary center if acute pancreatitis is severe or evolving/worsening.

PANIC DISORDER

Christine Ramos Camacho, MD, MS

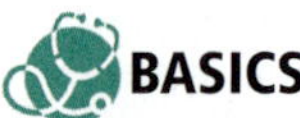

BASICS

DESCRIPTION
- A classic panic attack is characterized by rapid onset of a brief period of sympathetic nervous system hyperarousal accompanied by intense fear.
- In panic disorder, multiple panic attacks occur (including at least two without a recognizable trigger). Patients experience at least 1 month of worried anticipation of additional attacks and/or maladaptive (e.g., avoidance) behaviors.

EPIDEMIOLOGY
Prevalence
5% lifetime prevalence; median age of onset 24 years

ETIOLOGY AND PATHOPHYSIOLOGY
A combination of vulnerability factors (genetics, childhood hardships, and personality characteristics), with life stressors

Genetics
Higher incidence of panic disorder among family members

RISK FACTORS
- Life stressors of any kind can precipitate attacks, including history of sexual or physical abuse.
- Substance abuse, smoking, bipolar disorder, major depression, obsessive-compulsive disorder (OCD), and simple phobia

GENERAL PREVENTION
- Healthy lifestyle, including healthy diet, regular exercise and stress reduction techniques (such as mindfulness) are useful.
- The USPSTF recommends screening children and teens for anxiety and made a draft recommendation to screen adults aged ≤64 years.

COMMONLY ASSOCIATED CONDITIONS
- Other psychiatric diagnoses: PTSD, social phobia, simple phobia, major depression, bipolar disorder, substance abuse, OCD, separation anxiety disorder
- More common in patients with asthma, migraine, headaches, hypertension, mitral valve prolapse, reflux esophagitis, interstitial cystitis, irritable bowel syndrome, fibromyalgia, nicotine dependence
- Panic disorder increases the risk of suicide attempts and ideation.

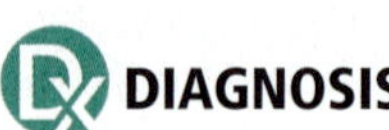

DIAGNOSIS
- Panic attack: an abrupt surge of intense fear, reaching a peak within minutes in which ≥4 of the following symptoms develop abruptly: (i) palpitations, pounding heart, or accelerated heart rate; (ii) sweating; (iii) trembling or shaking; (iv) sensation of shortness of breath or smothering; (v) a choking sensation; (vi) chest pain or discomfort; (vii) nausea or abdominal distress; (viii) feeling dizzy, unsteady, light-headed, or faint; (ix) derealization (feelings of unreality) or depersonalization (feeling detached from oneself); (x) fear of losing control or going crazy; (xi) fear of dying; (xii) paresthesias; (xiii) chills or hot flashes (1)[C]
- Panic disorder: recurrent panic attacks, at least two without known trigger, not better accounted for by another psychiatric condition (eg., PTSD, OCD, separation anxiety disorder, social anxiety disorder, or specific phobia) *and* not induced by drugs of abuse, medical conditions, or prescribed drugs *and* with >1 month of at least one of the following: (i) worry about additional attacks or worry about the implications of the attack (eg., losing control, having a heart attack, "going crazy"), (ii) a significant maladaptive change in behavior related to the attacks (1)[C]

HISTORY
- Obtain a good history through tactful, nonjudgmental questioning. Information should be elicited about physical and emotional symptoms, current life stress, separations, recent deaths, patient's concerns and fears, interpersonal problems.
- A medication and substance abuse history
- Review *DSM-5* diagnostic criteria. Ask for avoidance patterns that have developed since the onset of panic attacks.

PHYSICAL EXAM
- During an attack, there can be tachycardia, hyperventilation, and diaphoresis.
- Thyroid exam for fullness or nodules; look for exophthalmos or lid lag.
- Cardiac exam for murmur or arrhythmias
- Lung exam to rule out asthma (limited airflow, wheezing)

DIFFERENTIAL DIAGNOSIS
- Medication use may mimic panic disorder and create anxiety: Paradoxically, antidepressants used to treat panic may, initially, worsen panic; antidepressants in bipolar patients can cause anxiety/mania/panic; short-acting benzodiazepines (alprazolam), β-blockers (propranolol), and short-acting opioids can cause interdose rebound anxiety; benzodiazepine treatment causes panic when patients take too much and run out of these medicines early; bupropion, levodopa, amphetamines, steroids, albuterol, sympathomimetics, fluoroquinolones, and interferon can cause panic; rare medication side effect syndromes such as serotonin syndrome or malignant hyperthermia
- Substance withdrawal or abuse
- Medical conditions: cardiovascular, pulmonary, endocrine (hypothyroidism/hyperthyroidism, premenstrual dysphoric disorder, menopause, pregnancy, hypoglycemia [in diabetes], carcinoid syndrome, pheochromocytoma, Cushing syndrome, hyperaldosteronism, hyperparathyroidism), neurologic (transient ischemic attacks [TIAs], preictal and postictal states), others; note: It is unusual to have a first panic attack after the age of 40 years, making it more important to consider other medical conditions for those patients.
- Psychiatric conditions that have overlapping symptomatology include mood, anxiety, and personality disorders such as major depression, bipolar disorder, PTSD, borderline personality disorder, social phobia, OCD, and generalized anxiety disorder. In PTSD, there is always a recollection or visual image that precedes the panic attack. In social phobia, fear of scrutiny precedes the panic attack. In bipolar disorder, major depression, borderline personality disorder, and particularly substance abuse, the patient often complains first of panic symptoms and anxiety and minimizes other potentially relevant symptoms and behaviors.

DIAGNOSTIC TESTS & INTERPRETATION
No specific lab tests are indicated except to rule out conditions in the differential diagnosis.
- If chest discomfort, do appropriate workup; electrocardiogram (ECG) and pulse oximetry; consider Holter monitoring, stress testing, and/or chest CT scan in select patients.
- Fingerstick blood sugar in acute setting in a diabetic patient
- Thyroid-stimulating hormone (TSH), complete metabolic panel, CBC
- If nocturnal panic attacks, consider sleep study to evaluate for possible sleep apnea.
- Other testing as indicated, for instance if typical signs and symptoms of rare conditions like pheochromocytoma or carcinoid

Diagnostic Procedures/Other
- If a medical cause of anxiety is strongly suspected, do the workup appropriate for that condition.
- Panic Disorder Severity Scale (PDSS) can be used for monitoring changes in severity of symptoms and response to treatment. Also, the PhQ-PD can be used if screening is desired.

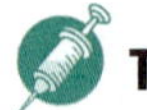

TREATMENT
Combined antidepressant therapy and psychotherapy is superior to either alone during initial treatment for panic disorder (2)[A],(3). Most effective therapy includes cognitive-behavioral therapy (CBT), mindfulness-based therapy, and exposure therapy. Psychotherapy provides long-lasting treatment, often without subsequent need for medications.

GENERAL MEASURES
Patient education is a vital part of treatment. A useful mnemonic is HR BET (think of Babe Ruth as the person you would have betted on to get a home run or your "HR BET").
- Harmless: Explain to patients why they are having their symptoms. For instance, hyperventilation may change the acid/base balance of the blood causing dizziness, extremity tingling, and odd out-of-body sensations.
- Resistance: Explain how resistance can prolong the panic and make it worse. People get anxious about being anxious.

- Breathing: Teach mindful diaphragmatic breathing (paying attention to the sensation of one breath at a time, with the abdomen expanding with each inhalation).
- Energy: Discuss that adrenaline can be felt as anxiety or excitement. Instead of calling it a panic attack, reframe it as an energy burst and see if patients can feel the energy flowing through their veins.
- Thoughts: Develop the skill of noticing thoughts without believing them all. People can also be taught to dispute irrational thoughts and beliefs (e.g., disputing "I'm dying now," with "I've had many of these attacks before; they have been thoroughly evaluated by my doctor, and they are not harmful; if I don't resist them and just do my diaphragmatic breathing, they resolve more quickly.").

MEDICATION

- Medication management is indicated if psychotherapy is not successful and/or symptoms are severe and may be combined with psychotherapy.
- Selective serotonin reuptake inhibitor (SSRI), serotonin-norepinephrine reuptake inhibitor (SNRI), tricyclic antidepressant (TCA), monoamine oxidase inhibitor (MAOI), and benzodiazepines have shown efficacy in treating panic disorder.
- It is recommended that medications be maintained for at least 1 year after symptom control to reduce risk of relapse.

First Line

- SSRIs and SNRIs are first line given efficacy, relatively benign side effect profile, and lack of abuse potential.
- Start a low-dose SSRI or SNRI, for example, fluoxetine 5 to 10 mg, paroxetine 10 mg, sertraline 25 mg, citalopram 10 mg, escitalopram 5 mg, or venlafaxine extended release (ER) 37.5 mg once daily in the morning (If sedation occurs, this can be changed to nightly dosing). Titrate up slowly every 1 to 2 weeks to therapeutic doses. If indicated, further dose increases usually happen no more frequently than monthly. Side effects include irritability, diarrhea, and sexual dysfunction, with less frequent side effects such as hyponatremia, GI bleeding, manic episodes (if patient is bipolar), elevated LFT's, QT prolongation (more often with citalopram), and serotonin syndrome. Warn people starting escitalopram that nausea is very frequent but usually resolves after 1 week of treatment. Suicidality can be seen in young patients. When stopping SSRI, taper over several weeks or months because of risk of discontinuation syndrome. This is more important for medications with a shorter half-life like paroxetine and venlafaxine compared with medications such as fluoxetine.
- Among SNRIs, venlafaxine (ER), if not effective after a month of 75 mg daily, can be slowly titrated up to a maximum dose of 225 mg/day with risk of hypertension at higher doses. Other side effects are similar to SSRIs. SNRIs such as desvenlafaxine or duloxetine can also be tried.

Second Line

- Mirtazapine can be used started at 15 mg QHS and potentially increasing to 30 mg QHS. Side effects of sedation and weight gain may limit use, but for people suffering from weight loss and insomnia, this medication could be helpful.
- TCAs, particularly imipramine, may be an option, but are seldom used (because of difficulty in dosing, more side effects, and greater risk associated with overdose compared with SSRIs). Screen for cardiac conduction system in patients >40 years of age with an ECG.
- MAOIs like phenelzine and tranylcypromine are also efficacious compared to placebo. Avoid with serotonergic agents given risk for serotonin syndrome. Dietary restrictions and drug interactions limit use of these medications.
- Benzodiazepines should be either avoided or used only for crisis and short-term relief of severe symptoms. Alprazolam (start 0.25 mg TID PRN) and clonazepam (start at 0.5 mg BID PRN) are FDA-approved for panic disorder. Clonazepam has a longer half-life, less interdose anxiety, and lower abuse potential than alprazolam. Benzodiazepines are associated with sedation, dependence, increased falls, increased car accidents, and increased mortality. Prescribing benzodiazepines to patients on opiates increases risk of overdose.

ISSUES FOR REFERRAL

- Refer to a counselor who treats anxiety with CBT, mindfulness-based therapy, and/or exposure therapy.
- Consider psychiatrist referral for comorbid bipolar disorder, borderline personality disorder, schizophrenia, suicidality, alcohol, substance abuse, or for patients unresponsive to initial treatment.

ADDITIONAL THERAPIES

Mindfulness meditation, aerobic exercise, yoga, or tai chi helps reduce symptoms.

COMPLEMENTARY & ALTERNATIVE MEDICINE

Kava kava should be avoided because of the risks of liver failure. Omega-3 fatty acids 2 g daily with EPA <60% may reduce symptoms (4)[C].

ADMISSION, INPATIENT, AND NURSING CONSIDERATIONS

Consider admission for concrete suicidal ideation.

ONGOING CARE

FOLLOW-UP RECOMMENDATIONS

Full therapeutic effect of antidepressants often does not occur until 4 to 6 weeks. Monitor (usually within 1 to 2 weeks) for suicidal ideation when starting antidepressants in patients ≤24 years of age.

DIET

Limiting caffeine may be helpful.

PATIENT EDUCATION

National Institute of Mental Health: http://www.nimh.nih.gov/health/publications/panic-disorder-when-fear-overwhelms/index.shtml

PROGNOSIS

Remission occurs in 64.5% in 6 months, but recurrence occurs in 21%. Predictors of remission are female gender, absence of ongoing stressors, and a low initial frequency of attacks.

COMPLICATIONS

Iatrogenic benzodiazepine dependence

REFERENCES

1. American Psychiatric Association. *Diagnostic and Statistical Manual of Mental Disorders*. 5th ed. Arlington, VA: American Psychiatric Association; 2013.
2. Furukawa TA, Watanabe N, Churchill R. Combined psychotherapy plus antidepressants for panic disorder with or without agoraphobia. *Cochrane Database Syst Rev*. 2007;2007(1):CD004364.
3. DeGeorge KC, Grover M, Streeter GS. Generalized anxiety disorder and panic disorder in adults. *Am Fam Physician*. 2022;106(2):157–164.
4. Su KP, Tseng PT, Lin PY, et al. Association of use of omega-3 polyunsaturated fatty acids with changes in severity of anxiety symptoms: a systematic review and meta-analysis. *JAMA Netw Open*. 2018;1(5):e182327.

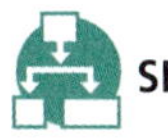

SEE ALSO

Algorithm: Anxiety

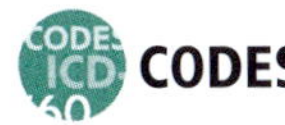

CODES

ICD10

F41.0 Panic disorder [episodic paroxysmal anxiety]

CLINICAL PEARLS

First-line pharmacologic treatment is usually an SSRI or SNRI; patient education is also important and counseling, particularly CBT, is often helpful. Consider assessing suicidality because patients with panic disorder are at increased risk for suicide, particularly if depressed.

PARKINSON DISEASE

Robert A. Baldor, MD, FAAFP

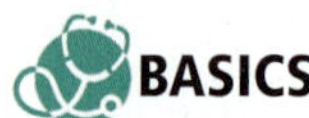

BASICS

DESCRIPTION

- An adult onset, progressive, neurodegenerative disorder caused by loss of dopaminergic neurons in the substantia nigra and other dopaminergic regions of the brain
- Cardinal symptoms include resting tremor, rigidity, bradykinesia, and postural instability.

EPIDEMIOLOGY

Prevalence

- Second most common neurodegenerative disease after Alzheimer disease.
- Average age of onset: ~60 years; slightly more common in men than women
- 1 to 2/1,000 persons; 0.3% of general population and 1–2% of those ≥60 years of age and up to 4% of those ≥80 years of age; affects 1+ million people in the United States and 6+ million worldwide

ETIOLOGY AND PATHOPHYSIOLOGY

Dopamine depletion in the substantia nigra and the nigrostriatal pathways results in the classic motor signs of Parkinson disease (PD) such as tremor, bradykinesia and rigidity.

- Loss of neurons accompanied by presence of Lewy bodies (hyaline inclusion bodies) and Lewy neuritis

Genetics

Mutations in multiple autosomal dominant and autosomal recessive genes are linked to PD/parkinsonian syndrome particularly when the age at symptom onset is <50 years.

RISK FACTORS

Age and family history of PD or tremor; lifelong pesticide use (rotenone, carbamate) is associated with risk of developing PD; repeated head trauma and living in rural areas, drinking well water; high dietary iron intake, low vitamin D level and women with low bone density/osteoporosis (1)

GENERAL PREVENTION

Caffeine consumption, cigarette smoking, and physical activity have been linked to decreased risk of development of PD include weight training, running, dancing, yoga, and traditional Chinese martial arts (2).

COMMONLY ASSOCIATED CONDITIONS

Cognitive abnormalities, autonomic dysfunction (e.g., constipation, urinary urgency), sleep disturbances, mental status changes (depression, psychosis, hallucinations, dementia), orthostatic hypotension, and pain

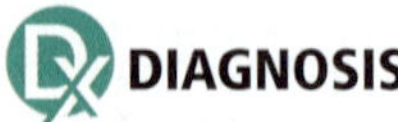

DIAGNOSIS

- Diagnosis is based on clinical features (rest tremor, rigidity, bradykinesia, postural instability) and response to dopaminergic therapy.
- PD is clinical diagnosis and gold standard for diagnosis are history and neuropathologic exam.
- Generally, bradykinesia plus either tremor or rigidity must be present.
- Idiopathic rapid eye movement sleep behavior disorder is a possible prodrome for PD.

HISTORY

Symptoms often subtle or attributed to aging

- Decreased emotion displayed in facial features
- General motor slowing and stiffness (One or both arms do not swing with walk.)
- Resting tremor (often initially one hand)
- Speech soft/mumbling
- Falls/difficulty with balance; seen with disease progression
- Psychiatric symptoms including depression, anxiety, hallucinations, and dementia
- Urinary symptoms including increased frequency and urgency, constipation

PHYSICAL EXAM

- Tremor
  - Resting tremor (4 to 6 Hz) that is often asymmetric; disappears with voluntary movement; frequently emerges in a hand while walking and may present as pill rolling; may also present in jaw, chin, lips, tongue
- Bradykinesia—generalized slowness of movements
- Rigidity: cogwheel (catching and releasing) or lead pipe (continuously rigid), tested by passively manipulating the limbs
- Postural instability—decreased ability to prevent falling

DIFFERENTIAL DIAGNOSIS

- Essential tremor: Bradykinesia is not present; often symmetric and occurs mostly during action or when holding hands outstretched, nonresponsive to levodopa (L-dopa).
- Depression can cause psychomotor slowing that may appear similar to bradykinesia in PD.
- Dementia with Lewy bodies: characterized clinically by visual hallucinations, fluctuating cognition, and parkinsonism; dementia occurs concomitantly with or before the development of parkinsonism.
- Multiple system atrophy: presets with parkinsonism and varying degrees of dysautonomia, cerebellar involvement, and pyramidal signs; poor response to L-dopa.
- Progressive supranuclear palsy: impairment in vertical eye movements (particularly down gaze), hyperextension of neck, and early falling; pseudobulbar palsy
- Associated neurodegenerative disorders: late stages of Alzheimer disease, Huntington disease, frontotemporal dementia, spinocerebellar ataxias
- Secondary parkinsonism (drug induced: reversible; may take weeks/months after offending medication is stopped; often bilateral symptoms): neuroleptics (most common); antiemetics (e.g., prochlorperazine and promethazine), metoclopramide; SSRIs; calcium channel blockers; amiodarone; lithium/valproic acid; amphotericin B; estrogens

DIAGNOSTIC TESTS & INTERPRETATION

Initial Tests (lab, imaging)

- Diagnosis is mainly clinical, and there are no confirmatory physiologic or blood tests.
- Reduction in α-synuclein and DJ-1 protein can act as a qualitative feature in PD diagnosis.
- MRI of brain is nondiagnostic but can be used to rule out structural abnormalities.

Follow-Up Tests & Special Considerations

Single-photon emission computerized tomography (SPECT) might be helpful to differentiate PD from secondary parkinsonism.

Diagnostic Procedures/Other

PET and MR spectroscopy are not recommended.

Test Interpretation

Diagnosis is clinical and no tests are recommended to confirm diagnosis of PD.

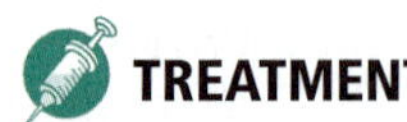

TREATMENT

GENERAL MEASURES

Multidisciplinary rehabilitation with standard physical and occupational therapy components to improve functional outcomes

MEDICATION

- PD treatment goal: Improve motor and nonmotor symptoms. Start treatment when symptoms impair functioning or quality of life.
- Agents are chosen based on patient age and symptoms present.
- "Off" periods describe the development of symptoms (often dyskinesias) while patient is on PD medication. This especially occurs among elderly patients taking L-dopa medications.

First Line

- First-line agents in early PD: L-dopa, dopamine agonists, monoamine oxidase B (MAO-B) inhibitors (3)[A],(4)[A].
  - L-dopa combined with carbidopa is still the most effective treatment for symptoms of PD, particularly bradykinesia. L-dopa by itself requires frequent dosing because of peripheral conversion.
  - L-dopa versus dopamine agonist is controversial:
    - Most patients eventually will develop involuntary motor fluctuations or dyskinesias with L-dopa
    - Older patients are often less able to tolerate the adverse events of dopamine agonists.
    - All patients eventually will require L-dopa.
  - For patients who experience dyskinesias while on L-dopa, can consider MAO-B inhibitors (rasagiline) or catechol-O-methyltransferase (COMT) inhibitors (entacapone) as adjuvants
- Carbidopa + L-dopa (Carbidopa inhibits peripheral conversion of L-dopa.)
  - Immediate release (Sinemet)
  - Orally disintegrating (Parcopa)
- Carbidopa + L-dopa + entacapone (Stalevo)
  - Addition of entacapone as a single agent should be initiated prior to use of this combination: once daily dose of carbidopa/L-dopa has been identified; may convert to Stalevo
  - Side effects are the same, plus diarrhea and brownish orange urine.

- Dopamine-receptor agonists (nonergot): use when mild symptoms, preference for once-daily medication and in younger patients; side effects: nausea, vomiting, hypotension, sedation, vivid dreaming, compulsive behavior, confusion, light-headedness, and hallucinations:
  - Pramipexole (Mirapex)
  - Ropinirole (Requip)
  - Rotigotine (transdermal patch)
- Selective MAO-B inhibitors: side effects: insomnia, jitteriness, hallucinations; mostly found with selegiline; rasagiline similar adverse events as placebo in clinical trials; rasagiline is metabolized via *CYP1A2*; caution with other medications using this enzyme system (e.g., ciprofloxacin):
  - Selegiline (Eldepryl)
  - Rasagiline (Azilect)

Second Line

- Second-line agents in early PD: β-adrenergic antagonists (postural tremor), amantadine, anticholinergics (young patients with tremor); lack of good evidence for symptom control
- Dopamine agonists (ergot): Increased adverse event profile makes these agents nonpreferred to nonergot dopamine agonists; bromocriptine (Parlodel)
- Treatment of L-dopa-induced motor complications
  - End of dose wearing off (i.e., decreased responsiveness to PD medication resulting in return of PD symptoms)
  - Entacapone (with each L-dopa dose) or rasagiline preferred
  - Dyskinesias: typically occur at peak dopamine level
  - Amantadine may be considered; however, efficacy is questionable.
  - The FDA has approved istradefylline (Nourianz) as the first adenosine A2A receptor antagonist to be approved in the United States as an oral agent for use as an adjunct to carbidopa/L-dopa in adults with PD who experience "off" episodes.
- Anticholinergic agents: avoided due to lack of efficacy (only useful for tremor) and increased adverse event profile: trihexyphenidyl; benztropine (Cogentin)
- *N*-methyl-D-aspartic acid antagonist: exact mechanism unknown, efficacy is questionable; may be useful for dyskinesias; side effects: confusion, dizziness, dry mouth, livedo reticularis, and hallucinations: amantadine (Symmetrel)
- COMT inhibitors: entacapone preferred due to hepatotoxicity associated with tolcapone; adverse events include nausea and orthostatic hypotension:
  - Entacapone (Comtan); tolcapone (Tasmar)
    - Requires LFT monitoring
- Apomorphine (Apokyn): nonergot-derived dopamine agonist given SC for off episodes in advanced disease; adverse events: nausea, vomiting, dizziness, hallucinations, orthostatic hypotension, somnolence
  - Only for "off" episodes with L-dopa therapy

ISSUES FOR REFERRAL

Neurology for suspected PD

ADDITIONAL THERAPIES

- Emotional and psychological support of patient and family; refer patients to community resources to promote social engagement.
- Physical therapy and endurance exercise to improve balance, muscle strength, walking speed
- Speech therapy: may be helpful in improving speech volume and maintaining voice quality
- Treatment of nonmotor symptoms:
  - Psychosis
    - In 2016, the FDA-approved pimavanserin (Nuplazid) as the first drug specifically designed to treat PD psychosis (PDP).
    - Quetiapine (Seroquel) had been widely used for people with PDP before pimavanserin.
    - Insomnia: rotigotine; FDA approved in transdermal form to treat insomnia in PD
    - Orthostatic hypotension: in addition to increasing salt and fluid intake can also use FDA-approved droxidopa
      - Can also consider midodrine, fludrocortisone, use of compression stockings
    - Dementia: Rivastigmine can be considered for cognitive impairment (i.e., mild to moderate dementia in PD).
    - Depression in PD: can consider pramipexole, nortriptyline, desipramine, venlafaxine, and CBT

SURGERY/OTHER PROCEDURES

- Deep brain stimulation (DBS) is an effective therapeutic option for patients with motor complications refractory to the best medical treatment who are healthy, have no significant comorbidities, are responsive to L-dopa, and do not have depression or dementia.
- Patients, who are not candidates for DBS, might benefit from MRI-guided focused ultrasound lesioning (unilateral pallidotomy) for relief from disabling motor symptoms.

COMPLEMENTARY & ALTERNATIVE MEDICINE

Music therapy may help to improve quality of life and motor symptoms in PD patients.

ADMISSION, INPATIENT, AND NURSING CONSIDERATIONS

- Fall risk precaution when admitted
- Note that small variation in medication dosage can impact PD symptoms. Make sure patient has home PD medications and takes them at the correct time.
- Avoid dopamine-blocking agents such as antipsychotics and antiemetics (prochlorperazine, metoclopramide).

ONGOING CARE

FOLLOW-UP RECOMMENDATIONS

- Avoid drug holidays is patient is having "off" time on L-dopa.
- Consider switching to dopamine agonist (non-ergot preferred), MAO-B inhibitors, or COMT inhibitors if patient develops dyskinesias on L-dopa/carbidopa therapy.
- Severe motor symptoms; at this point patient should not be allowed to drive self. This should be noted and reported to licensing agency.

Patient Monitoring

If on dopamine agonists—monitor for development of impulse control behaviors

DIET

- For dysphagia, consider soft food, swallowing evaluation, and increased time for meals.
- Avoid large, high-fat meals that slow digestion and interfere with medication absorption.

PATIENT EDUCATION

- Parkinson's Foundation: https://www.parkinson.org
- For caregivers: https://www.caregiver.org/resource/parkinsons-disease-caregiving/

PROGNOSIS

- PD is a chronic progressive disease; prognosis varies based on patient-specific symptoms.
- Increased mortality in PD; on average, survival is reduced by 5% every year of follow-up.

REFERENCES

1. Park KY, Jung JH, Hwang HS, et al. Bone mineral density and the risk of Parkinson's disease in postmenopausal women. *Mov Disord*. 2023;38(9):1606–1614. doi:10.1002/mds.29579.
2. Fan B, Jabeen R, Bo B, et al. What and how can physical activity prevention function on Parkinson's disease? *Oxid Med Cell Longev*. 2020;2020:4293071.
3. Halli-Tierney AD, Luker J, Carroll DG. Parkinson disease. *Am Fam Physician*. 2020;102(11):679–691.
4. Drugs for Parkinson's disease. *Med Lett Drugs Ther*. 2021;63(1618):25–32.

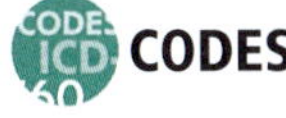

CODES

ICD10

- G21.11 Neuroleptic induced parkinsonism
- G21.8 Other secondary parkinsonism
- G21.4 Vascular parkinsonism

CLINICAL PEARLS

- The classic description for PD is shaky (pill-rolling tremor at rest), stiff (cogwheel rigidity), slow (bradykinesia), and stumbling (shuffling gait).
- No cure—goals are to delay disease progression and relieve symptoms.
- Emphasize the importance of exercise and movement to help preserve function.
- Pharmacotherapeutic regimens need to be individualized based on age/specific symptoms.

PARONYCHIA

Nancy V. Nguyen, DO

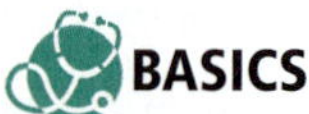

BASICS

DESCRIPTION

- Superficial inflammation of the lateral and posterior nail folds surrounding the fingernail or toenail. Develops after breakdown of barrier between nail plate and the adjacent nail fold
- Acute: characterized by pain, erythema, and swelling (1) lasting <6 weeks; usually a bacterial infection appearing after nail biting, trauma, manicures, ingrown nails, and hangnail manipulation. It also occurs as an adverse effect from several drugs. It can progress to abscess formation.
- Chronic: characterized by swelling, tenderness, cuticle elevation, and nail dystrophy and separation lasting at least 6 weeks, or recurrent episodes of acute eponychial inflammation and drainage
- Chemotherapy-associated paronychia (CAP) starts 4 to 8 weeks after chemotherapy initiation (2).
- May be considered work-related among bartenders, restaurant servers, dishwashers, nurses, and others who often wash their hands
- Usually involves one finger but drug-induced paronychia may involve multiple fingers
- Relevant anatomy: nail bed, nail plate, and perionychium
- Synonym(s): eponychia, perionychia, retronychia

Pediatric Considerations

Less common in pediatric age groups; commonly caused by trauma to periungual skin, such as thumb/finger-sucking or other injuries (*Staphylococcus aureus* and group A *Streptococcus* may be present). Paronychia is also a frequent adverse effect of BRAF and MEK inhibitor anticancer drugs.

EPIDEMIOLOGY

Incidence

- One of the most common hand infections in the United States
- Predominant age: all ages
- Predominant sex: female > male

ETIOLOGY AND PATHOPHYSIOLOGY

- Acute: mixed aerobic and anaerobic bacterial flora in 50% of cases. *Staphylococcus aureus* most common and *Streptococcus pyogenes*; less frequently, *Pseudomonas aeruginosa* and other gram-negative bacteria (with chronic paronychia)
- Chronic: eczematous reaction with secondary *Candida albicans* (~95%)
- Pediatric age groups: mixed anaerobic (*Fusobacterium*, *Peptostreptococcus*) and aerobic infections (*Eikenella corrodens*, *S. aureus*, streptococci) from oral flora
- A paronychial infection commonly starts in the lateral nail fold.
- Acute paronychia of the fingers is often due to trauma; acute paronychia of the toes is often due to ingrown nails (3).
- Recurrent inflammation, persistent edema, and fibrosis of nail folds cause nail folds to round up and retract, exposing nail grooves to irritants, allergens, and pathogens.
- Inflammation compromises ability of proximal nail fold to regenerate cuticle leading to decreased vascular supply. This can cause decrease efficacy of topical medications.
- Early in the course, cellulitis alone may be present.
- An abscess can form if the infection does not resolve quickly.

RISK FACTORS

- Acute: direct or indirect trauma to cuticle or nail fold, manicured/sculptured nails, nail biting, thumb sucking, manipulating a hangnail, ingrown toenail
- Chronic: frequent immersion of hands in water with excoriation of the lateral nail fold (e.g., chefs, bartenders, housekeepers, swimmers, dishwashers, nurses)
- Predisposing conditions such as diabetes mellitus (DM) and immunosuppression
- Medications such as EGFR inhibitors, systemic retinoids, chemotherapy, and antiretroviral agents

GENERAL PREVENTION

- Acute: Avoid trauma such as nail biting or manipulating a hangnail. Prevent ingrown toenails.
- Chronic: Avoid exposure to allergens and contact irritants; keep fingers/hands dry; wear rubber gloves with a cotton liner. Prevent excoriation of the skin.
- Keep nails short; avoid manicures.
- Apply moisturizer after washing hands.

COMMONLY ASSOCIATED CONDITIONS

DM, eczema or atopic dermatitis, immunosuppression

DIAGNOSIS

HISTORY

- Localized pain or tenderness, swelling, and erythema of posterior or lateral nail folds
  - Acute: fairly rapid onset (2 to 5 days after trauma)
  - Chronic: at least 6 weeks' duration
- Previous trauma (i.e., bitten nails, ingrown nails, manicured nails)
- Contact with herpes infections
- Contact with allergens or irritants (frequent water immersion, latex)
- Immunosuppressive therapy

PHYSICAL EXAM

- Acute: red, warm, tender, tense posterior or lateral nail fold ± abscess
- Chronic:
  - Initially appears as swollen, tender, boggy nail fold ± abscess
  - Later appears as retraction of nail fold and absence of adjacent healthy cuticle, thickening of nail plate with prominent transverse ridges known as Beau lines and discoloration; multiple digits typically involved
- Occasional elevation of nail bed or separation of nail fold from nail plate
- Fluctuance, purulence at the nail margin, or purulent drainage
- An untreated infection of the toe may lead to the formation of granulation tissue around the nail fold (3).
- Secondary changes of nail platelike discoloration
- Suspect *Pseudomonas* if with green changes in nail (chloronychia).

DIFFERENTIAL DIAGNOSIS

- Felon (abscess of fingertip pulp; urgent diagnosis required)
- Cellulitis
- Eczema
- Herpetic whitlow (similar in appearance, very painful, often associated with vesicles)
- Allergic contact dermatitis (latex, acrylic)
- Psoriasis (especially acute flare)
- Proximal/lateral onychomycosis (nail folds not predominantly involved)
- Retronychia
- Pemphigus vulgaris
- Acute osteomyelitis of the distal phalanx
- Reiter disease
- Pustular psoriasis
- Dermatomyositis
- Malignancy: squamous cell carcinoma of the nail, malignant melanoma, metastatic disease

DIAGNOSTIC TESTS & INTERPRETATION

None required unless condition is severe; resistant to treatment or if recurrence or methicillin-resistant *S. aureus* (MRSA) is suspected, then

- Gram stain
- Culture and sensitivity
- Potassium hydroxide wet mount plus fungal culture especially in chronic paronychia
- Drugs that may alter lab results: use of over-the-counter antimicrobials or antifungals

Initial Tests (lab, imaging)

Consider ultrasonography if uncertain about presence of an abscess.

Diagnostic Procedures/Other

- Incision and drainage recommended for suppurative cases or cases not responding to conservative management or empiric antibiotics
- Tzanck testing or viral culture in suspected viral cases
- Biopsy in cases not responding to conservative management or when malignancy suspected

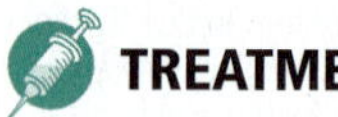

TREATMENT

GENERAL MEASURES

- Acute inflammation without abscess: warm water soaks or antiseptic soaks, and topical antibiotics (2). Consider oral antibiotics for more severe cases that do not respond to topical treatment alone.
- Abscesses should be drained.
- Antibiotics may not be necessary for successful I&D of uncomplicated infections.
- Chronic: Keep fingers dry; apply moisturizing lotion after hand washing; avoid exposure to irritants; improved diabetic control
- Pediatric cases should be treated with systemic antibiotics.

MEDICATION

First Line

- Acute paronychia (mild cases, no abscess formation):
  - Warm water soaks or antiseptic soaks (chlorhexidine, povidone-iodine) multiple times a day for 10 to 15 minutes each time, and topical antibiotics with *S. aureus* coverage (triple antibiotic ointment, mupirocin, bacitracin)
  - Antibiotic cream applied TID–QID after warm soak for 5 to 10 days
  - If eczematous: high-potency topical steroid applied BID (e.g., betamethasone 0.05% cream) for 7 to 14 days
- Acute paronychia (no abscess formation, not responding to topical treatment). Treat for 5 to 7 days.
  - Dicloxacillin 250 mg QID
  - Cephalexin 500 mg TID–QID
- Acute paronychia (exposure to oral flora, no abscess formation). Treat for 7 days. Cover for Eikenella.
  - Amoxicillin-clavulanate: 875 mg/125 mg BID; pediatric, 45 mg/kg q12h (for <40 kg) *or*
  - One of the following for Eikenella coverage:
    - Doxycycline 100 mg BID
    - Trimethoprim/sulfamethoxazole BID
    - Penicillin VK 500 mg QID
    - Ciprofloxacin 500 to 750 mg BID (Reserve fluoroquinolones for severe infection due to risks from this class of antibiotic.)
  - *PLUS* one of the following for anaerobic coverage:
    - Clindamycin 450 mg TID (pediatric, 10 mg/kg q8h)
    - Metronidazole 500 mg TID
- Acute paronychia (with risk factors for MRSA including but not limited to: recent hospitalization, recent surgery, ESRD on hemodialysis, HIV/AIDS, IVDU, resident of long term care facility). Treat for 7 days.
  - Trimethoprim/sulfamethoxazole 160 mg/800 mg BID
  - Doxycycline 100 mg BID
  - Clindamycin 300 to 450 mg TID–QID
- Acute paronychia with abscess formation:
  - Incision and drainage
    - Consider digital block anesthesia. Then, insert nail elevator, #11 scalpel blade, or hypodermic needle along nail plate at junction of the affected nail fold and nail to facilitate drainage. If no drainage occurs, use a needle or scalpel to open skin directly above abscess.
  - If ingrown nail involved or abscess extends to nail bed, consider partial nail removal.
  - Consider oral antibiotics for extension of cellulitis. Otherwise, usually no antibiotics indicated after I&D

Pediatric Considerations

- Without abscess formation: use systemic antibiotics as first-line treatment. Empiric treatment with beta-lactamase-resistant antibiotics (e.g., dicloxacillin, cloxacillin).
- With abscess formation: incision and drainage
- Chronic paronychia: Stop source of irritation, control inflammation, and restore natural protective barrier.
  - Topical high-potency steroids: betamethasone 0.05%; applied BID for 7 to 14 days
  - Topical antifungal: clotrimazole or nystatin; applied topically TID for up to 30 days
  - Topical calcineurin inhibitor: Tacrolimus 0.1% ointment BID for up to 21 days has been shown to be more effective than betamethasone but is more expensive.
- For paronychia caused by EGFR inhibitors, treat with topical antibiotics and potent topical corticosteroids without discontinuing the EGFR inhibitor for mild cases. For more severe cases, discontinue EGFR inhibitor temporarily.
- For paronychia caused by oncology pharmacotherapy, treat with corticosteroid ointment and phenol chemical matricectomy. Prompt treatment enables patients to continue anticancer drug treatment without impairing their quality of life.

Second Line

- Systemic antifungals (rarely needed, use if topical fails)
  - Itraconazole 200 mg for 90 days (may have longer action because it is incorporated into nail plate); pulse therapy may be useful (i.e., 200 mg BID for 7 days, repeated monthly for 2 months).
  - Terbinafine 250 mg/day for 6 weeks (fingernails) or 12 weeks (toenails)
  - Fluconazole 100 mg daily for 7 to 14 days
  - Ciclopirox 0.77% topical suspension BID for 2 to 4 weeks along with strict irritant avoidance
- Antipseudomonal drugs (e.g., ceftazidime, aminoglycosides) when pseudomonas is suspected

ISSUES FOR REFERRAL

- Acute: Severe infection may spread to underlying tendons, requiring evaluation and treatment by a hand surgeon as it often involves débridement, washout, or amputation, based on the severity of the infection.
- Chronic: In treatment failure, consider biopsy and/or, in cases of chronic paronychia, referral for possible partial excision of the nail fold or eponychial marsupialization with or without complete nail removal or Swiss roll technique.
- Failure to respond to therapy or chronic redness, tenderness and swelling of nail folds without abscess can be concerning for malignancy. Consider biopsy (3).

ADDITIONAL THERAPIES

Topical betaxolol 0.25% eye drops once daily on paronychia and pyogenic granuloma-like lesions covered with bandage

SURGERY/OTHER PROCEDURES

- Incision and drainage of abscess, if present. A subungual abscess or ingrown nail requires partial or complete removal of nail with phenolization of germinal matrix.
- Swiss roll technique for chronic and severe acute paronychia with runaround abscess involving both nail folds
- Recalcitrant cases may also need nail removal.

COMPLEMENTARY & ALTERNATIVE MEDICINE

Nail braces as a noninvasive alternative to nail extraction for patients with severe paronychia induced by EGFR inhibitors

ONGOING CARE

FOLLOW-UP RECOMMENDATIONS

- Acute: Postdrainage care consists of warm soaks or antiseptic soaks. Follow up in 24 to 48 hours after I&D to monitor for worsening infection.
- Chronic: Avoid frequent immersion, triggers, allergens, nail biting, or finger sucking.

DIET

Maintain good glucose control.

PATIENT EDUCATION

- Avoid trimming cuticles; avoid nail trauma; and stress importance of good diabetic control and diabetic education.
- Avoid contact irritants; use rubber gloves with cotton liners to avoid exposure to excess moisture.
- Use moisturizing lotion after washing hands; do not bite nails/suck on fingers.

PROGNOSIS

- With adequate treatment and prevention, healing can be expected in 1 to 2 weeks.
- Chronic paronychia may respond slowly to treatment, taking weeks to months.
- If no response in chronic lesions, rarely benign or malignant neoplasm may be present and referral to dermatology should be considered.

COMPLICATIONS

- Acute: subungual abscess
- Chronic: nail thickening, discoloration of nail, and nail loss

REFERENCES

1. Leggit JC. Acute and chronic paronychia. *Am Fam Physician*. 2017;96(1):44–51.
2. Relhan V, Bansal A. Acute and chronic paronychia revisited: a narrative review. *J Cutan Aesthet Surg*. 2022;15(1):1–16.
3. Lomax A, Thornton J, Singh D. Toenail paronychia. *Foot Ankle Surg*. 2016;22(4):219–223.

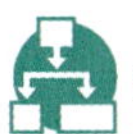

SEE ALSO

Onychomycosis, Retronychia

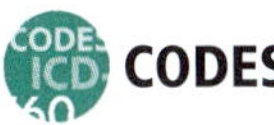

CODES

ICD10

- L03.019 Cellulitis of unspecified finger
- L03.039 Cellulitis of unspecified toe
- L03.011 Cellulitis of right finger

CLINICAL PEARLS

- Consider incision and drainage when appropriate.
- For chronic paronychia, topical steroid is the first-line treatment. Consider other differentials in nonresponders (e.g., rare causes: Raynaud, metastatic cancer, psoriasis, drug toxicity).
- Consider presence of more than one nail disease at the same time (e.g., paronychia and onychomycosis).

PAROTITIS, ACUTE AND CHRONIC

Erin W. DeLaney, MD

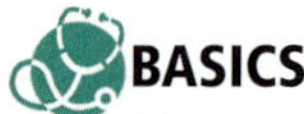

BASICS

DESCRIPTION

- Parotitis is caused by inflammation of the parotid gland due to infection, systemic illnesses, mechanical obstruction, or medications.
- The parotid gland is the largest salivary gland, located lateral and anterior to the masseter muscle, and extends posteriorly over the sternocleidomastoid muscle behind the angle of the mandible. It produces serous secretions, which lack bacteriostatic properties, making it more susceptible to infection than other salivary glands.
- The parotid duct, also called the Stensen duct, pierces the buccinator muscle and enters the buccal mucosa opposite the second maxillary molar.
- The branches of the facial nerve bisect the gland into lobes.

EPIDEMIOLOGY

- Viral parotitis is the most common cause of parotitis in children.
- Acute bacterial parotitis is less common but occurs more frequently in elderly patients, neonates, and postoperative patients.
- Juvenile recurrent parotitis (JRP): second most common inflammatory cause of parotitis in children in the United States; first episode usually occurs between ages 3 and 6 years.
- Chronic parotitis primarily affects adults; typically presents between ages 40 and 60 years
- Chronic bilateral parotid enlargement is a common manifestation of HIV infection.

Incidence

Elderly patients account for the majority of parotitis cases.

ETIOLOGY AND PATHOPHYSIOLOGY

- Acute viral parotitis begins as a systemic infection that localizes to the parotid gland, resulting in inflammation and swelling.
  - Mumps, or paramyxovirus, has a predilection for the parotid gland and classically has been linked to parotitis 16 to 18 days after infection. Mumps is a nationally reportable disease.
  - Other viral pathogens: parainfluenza, enterovirus, echovirus, influenza A, coxsackievirus, Epstein-Barr virus (EBV), human herpes virus (HHV6)
  - Also more common in pediatric patients with SARS-CoV-2 infection in the setting of multisystem inflammatory system
- Acute bacterial parotitis results from stasis of salivary flow that allows retrograde introduction of bacterial pathogens into the gland, resulting in localized infection.
  - *Staphylococcus aureus* is most common, followed by *Streptococcus pneumoniae* and anaerobes. Less common are *Streptococci viridans*, *Escherichia coli*, and *Haemophilus influenzae*.
  - *Klebsiella*, *Enterobacter*, and *Pseudomonas* can be seen in chronically ill or hospitalized patients.
  - Consider *Bartonella henselae* with cat exposure.
  - May be a manifestation of late onset group B *Streptococcus* (rare)
  - *Mycobacterium tuberculosis* has been seen in immunocompromised patients.
- Fungal
  - *Candida* has been isolated in chronically ill or hospitalized patients.
  - *Actinomyces* in patients with a history of trauma or dental caries
- Acute, recurrent parotitis
  - Mechanical: Repeated sialolith formation leads to ductal wall damage, fibrosis, and stricture formation.
  - Pneumoparotitis occurs when air is trapped in the parotid gland ducts; seen in wind instrument players, glassblowers, scuba divers, and rarely with dental cleaning
- "Anesthesia mumps": may be due to transient mechanical compression of the Stensen duct by airway devices, loss of muscle tone around the Stensen orifice after neuromuscular relaxants, increased salivary secretion, and increased flexion or rotation of the head during general anesthesia
- Chronic parotitis in patients with HIV can be due to presence of benign lymphoepithelial cysts, follicular hyperplasia of parotid lymph nodes, or diffuse infiltrative lymphocytosis syndrome, causing infiltration of the parotid gland by CD8 cells. Parotitis may be secondary to immune reconstitution after initiation of antiretroviral therapy.
- There are case reports of acute parotitis as a symptom of Kawasaki disease.

RISK FACTORS

- Immunosuppression, HIV, chemotherapy, radiation, malnutrition, alcoholism
- Acute viral parotitis: lack of mumps, measles, rubella (MMR) vaccination
- Acute bacterial parotitis: dehydration, debilitation, poor oral hygiene, cystic fibrosis, bulimia/anorexia, sialolithiasis (stones), ductal stenosis, trauma
- Neonatal parotitis: prematurity, dehydration, low birth weight, ductal obstruction, oral trauma, structural abnormalities
- JRP: dental malocclusion, congenital duct malformation, immunologic anomalies, disrupted enzyme activity
- Drug-induced parotitis: anticholinergics, ACE inhibitors (captopril), antihistamines, tricyclic antidepressants, antipsychotics (phenylbutazone, thioridazine, clozapine), iodine (contrast media), and L-asparaginase
- Chronic parotitis: ductal stenosis, HIV, tuberculosis, sarcoidosis, uremia, diabetes, gout, and atopy

GENERAL PREVENTION

- Complete MMR vaccine series. Pregnant women should not receive the mumps vaccine. Pregnancy should be avoided for 4 weeks after vaccination.
- Maintain adequate hydration, good dental hygiene, smoking cessation, alcohol abstinence, and avoidance of chronic purging.

COMMONLY ASSOCIATED CONDITIONS

Mumps, HIV, Sjögren syndrome, sarcoidosis, sialolithiasis

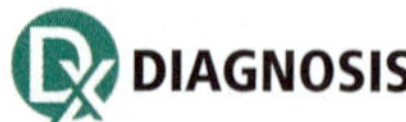

DIAGNOSIS

HISTORY

- Acute parotitis presents with sudden-onset pain and swelling of the cheek.
  - Viral parotitis is usually bilateral and accompanied by malaise, anorexia, headaches, myalgias, arthralgias, and fever.
  - Bacterial parotitis is associated with fever.
- JRP is usually unilateral, with pain and swelling resolving within 2 weeks.
- Other symptoms: trismus, pain exacerbated by chewing or worsened by foods that stimulate production of saliva, dry mouth with abnormal taste, difficulty with drinking/eating, anorexia, or dehydration
- Sialolithiasis is characterized by recurrent acute swelling and pain, exacerbated by eating. It may be associated with swelling around the Stensen duct.
- Chronic parotitis presents with recurrent or chronic nontender swelling of one or both parotid glands.

PHYSICAL EXAM

- Swelling or enlargement of the parotid gland(s); it may obscure the angle of the mandible or cause the ear to protrude upward and outward.
- Palpate with one hand starting at the attachment of the earlobe and proceed anteriorly and inferiorly along the mandibular ramus while the other hand simultaneously palpates the Stensen duct inside the oral cavity.
  - Bilateral tenderness suggests viral etiology, whereas unilateral tenderness, erythema, and warmth suggests a bacterial etiology.
  - Chronic parotitis is typically nontender.
- Trismus, halitosis, and dental decay may be noted.
- Drainage from the Stensen duct suggests bacterial parotitis or superinfection.
- In JRP, the Stensen duct is often enlarged, dilated, erythematous, and swollen.
- Facial nerve palsy can be seen in severe cases.

DIFFERENTIAL DIAGNOSIS

Lymphoma, neoplasm, lymphangitis, cervical adenitis, otitis externa, odontogenic infections, Ludwig angina, and cellulitis

DIAGNOSTIC TESTS & INTERPRETATION

- History and physical exam are sufficient for diagnosis.
- In cases where there is some diagnostic uncertainty, a CT scan of the head with IV contrast can help confirm the diagnosis and can also help rule out other types of orofacial infections.
- Aerobic culture of purulent drainage from Stensen duct, or aerobic and anaerobic culture from needle aspiration of gland or abscess can be obtained.
  - Anaerobic culture from the Stensen duct will likely contain oropharyngeal contamination, thus perform anaerobic cultures only from needle aspirate fluid.
  - It is reasonable to treat for common pathogens based on local antibiograms if needle aspirate fluid cannot be obtained.

- Acute bacterial parotitis can be associated with leukocytosis and elevated amylase; yet, these tests are generally nonspecific and are not necessary to make the diagnosis.
- For suspected mumps, the CDC recommends collecting a buccal swab for mumps RT-PCR if ≤3 days of symptom onset. If >3 days since onset of symptoms, obtain both buccal swab and a serum specimen for IgM.
  - Mumps RT-PCR is best obtained from a buccal swab performed after massaging the parotid gland for 30 seconds. In areas of high vaccination rates, IgM may be falsely negative necessitating correlation with clinical symptoms.
  - If initial IgM and RT-PCR obtained ≤3 days of symptom onset are negative, and there is strong clinical suspicion for mumps, consider repeating serum testing, as IgM response may not be detectable for 5 days after symptom onset.
- Send CMV titers in immunocompromised patients.
- For chronic, recurrent, or nontender parotitis, obtain HIV testing, PPD, SS-A/SS-B antibodies, rheumatoid factor, and antinuclear antibodies to evaluate for underlying etiology.

Initial Tests (lab, imaging)
- Imaging should be used primarily to rule out other pathology including abscess, masses, ductal stenosis, or sialolithiasis.
- Ultrasound (US) is the first-line diagnostic modality for detecting sialadenitis and has high sensitivity for identifying abscess and ductal lithiasis (1)[B].
- CT scan or MRI are both specific and sensitive for parotitis and outperform US in terms of their ability to rule out other similar appearing pathology.

Follow-Up Tests & Special Considerations
Consider sialography in chronic parotitis to assess the anatomy and functional integrity of the gland (diagnostic and therapeutic) (1)[C].

Diagnostic Procedures/Other
- Consider biopsy or fine-needle aspiration if there is suspicion for tuberculosis, Sjögren syndrome, or sarcoidosis.
- Noncaseating granulomas may be seen in sarcoidosis. Caseating granulomas may be seen in tuberculosis and *B. henselae* infections.

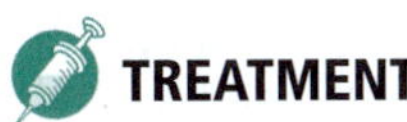

TREATMENT

GENERAL MEASURES
- Usually a self-limited course; treat with supportive care: rest, hydration, analgesia, and antipyretics.
  - Stimulate saliva production by eating hard candies. Sour candies may be more effective sialogogues.
  - Local heat application and gentle massage
  - Chronic parotitis: Encourage good dental hygiene and treat the underlying etiology.
- Patients with mumps should be isolated with standard and droplet precautions for 5 days after onset of parotid swelling.
- During a mumps outbreak, the CDC recommends administration of MMR vaccine even in fully vaccinated individuals, as a 3rd vaccine dose can decrease risk, especially in those whose second MMR was >13 years ago (2)[A].

MEDICATION
- Viral parotitis: no evidence for the use of immunoglobulin for postexposure prophylaxis or treatment; may initiate antibiotics if patient is toxic appearing
- Acute bacterial parotitis
  - Outpatient: amoxicillin/clavulanate or ciprofloxacin and clindamycin
  - Chronically ill or hospitalized: ampicillin/sulbactam or cefuroxime and metronidazole; if MRSA is probable, consider vancomycin or linezolid.
- Sjögren syndrome recurrent parotitis: Pilocarpine and cevimeline can stimulate saliva production and inhibit ascending infection and provide symptomatic relief. Alternatively, botulism toxin injection may be a consideration in these patients because it limits production of saliva and sialectasis (3)[B].

ISSUES FOR REFERRAL
Refer to otolaryngology for sialolithiasis, ductal stenosis, malignancy is suspected, no improvement with antibiotics, chronic obstruction due to Sjögren syndrome, or >1 recurrence per year (4)[B].

SURGERY/OTHER PROCEDURES
- Consider needle aspiration for bacterial parotitis with abscess, or clinical deterioration with increasing pain, erythema, and swelling not responding to medication.
- Consider superficial parotidectomy for severe recurrent parotitis in patients with underlying predisposing etiology.
- JRP: sialography; sialendoscopy with steroid irrigation is effective and safe for the treatment; performing US is recommended first to differentiate JRP from ductal stones (4)[A].
- Sclerotherapy with methyl violet or tetracycline is effective in the treatment of cysts in HIV parotitis and is also considered definitive treatment for chronic parotitis (5)[C].

ADMISSION, INPATIENT, AND NURSING CONSIDERATIONS
Admit those with comorbidities, systemic involvement, inability to tolerate PO, or neonates.

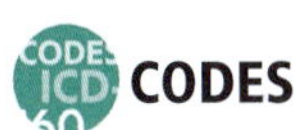

ONGOING CARE

FOLLOW-UP RECOMMENDATIONS
Antibiotic therapy for bacterial parotitis combined with adequate hydration should result in improvement within 48 hours; if not, patient should be reevaluated.

DIET
Ensure adequate fluid intake and promote salivary flow with hard or sour candy.

PROGNOSIS
- Viral infection in immunocompetent individuals often resolves with excellent prognosis.
- Parotid cysts in patients with HIV are usually benign lymphoepithelial lesions with infrequent malignant transformation.

COMPLICATIONS
- Complications of mumps may include orchitis, oophoritis, mastitis, aseptic meningitis, encephalitis, pancreatitis, myocarditis, sensorineural hearing loss, and nephritis.
- Untreated bacterial parotitis can lead to abscess formation and facial paralysis.
- Neoplasm can result from chronic autoimmune parotitis.
- Facial nerve paralysis can result from chronic inflammatory parotitis.

REFERENCES

1. Nation J, Panuganti B, Manteghi A, et al. Pediatric sialendoscopy for recurrent salivary gland swelling: workup, findings, and outcomes. *Ann Otol Rhinol Laryngol*. 2019;128(4):338–344.
2. Cardemil CV, Dahl RM, James L, et al. Effectiveness of a third dose of MMR vaccine for mumps outbreak control. *N Engl J Med*. 2017;377(10):947–956.
3. O'Neil LM, Palme CE, Riffat F, et al. Botulinum toxin for the management of Sjögren syndrome—associated recurrent parotitis. *J Oral Maxillofac Surg*. 2016;74(12):2428–2430.
4. Wood J, Toll EC, Hall F, et al. Juvenile recurrent parotitis: review and proposed management algorithm. *Int J Pediatr Otorhinolaryngol*. 2021;142:110617.
5. Berg EE, Moore CE. Office-based sclerotherapy for benign parotid lymphoepithelial cysts in the HIV-positive patient. *Laryngoscope*. 2009;119(5):868–870.

ADDITIONAL READING

Hernandez S, Busso C, Walvekar RR. Parotitis and sialendoscopy of the parotid gland. *Otolaryngol Clin North Am*. 2016;49(2):381–393.

CODES

ICD10
- K11.20 Sialoadenitis, unspecified
- K11.21 Acute sialoadenitis
- K11.23 Chronic sialoadenitis

CLINICAL PEARLS
- History and physical exam are sufficient for diagnosis (parotid swelling, tenderness, with or without purulent drainage from the Stensen duct).
- *S. aureus*, *S. pneumoniae*, and anaerobes are the most common organisms isolated in acute bacterial parotitis.
- In recurrent or chronic cases, consider other underlying etiologies, such as HIV.
- Usually self-limited with supportive care (local heat and gentle massage of gland, adequate hydration, analgesia, and antipyretics)
- Encouraging good oral hygiene and hydration in chronically ill, debilitated, and hospitalized patients can reduce risk of occurrence.

PARVOVIRUS B19 INFECTION

Christina Conrad, DO

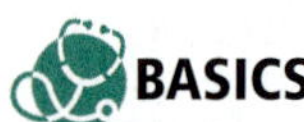

BASICS

DESCRIPTION

- Human parvovirus B19 is the cause of erythema infectiosum (fifth disease, morbus quintus).
- Individuals with increased red blood cell (RBC) turnover (sickle-cell anemia, spherocytosis, thalassemia) are more susceptible to transient aplastic crisis (TAC). In immunocompromised individuals, pure red cell aplasia (PRCA) may lead to transfusion-dependent anemia. In immunocompetent individuals, arthritis and arthralgias are common complications of parvovirus B19 infection.
- Systems affected: hematologic/lymphatic/immunologic, musculoskeletal, skin/exocrine, central nervous system, cardiac, renal, hepatobiliary

Pregnancy Considerations

Documented acute infection during pregnancy should prompt referral to maternal–fetal medicine specialist (concern for fetal anemia, hydrops). There is 30% chance of fetal transmission with acute maternal infection—this may be higher during epidemic outbreaks.

EPIDEMIOLOGY

- Global resurgence noted in aftermath of COVID-19 pandemic
- Common in childhood; may be asymptomatic
- Erythema infectiosum has an extremely low mortality rate.
- Peak age for erythema infectiosum is 4 to 12 years.
- Males and females are equally affected.
- Women are more likely to develop postinfectious arthritis.
- No known racial predilection
- In temperate climates, infections often occur from late winter to early summer.
- Local outbreaks may occur every 2 to 5 years.

Prevalence

In 2024, positivity rates rose to 10–32%—highest in children (0 to 10 years old), adults 41 to 50 years old, and pregnant women.

ETIOLOGY AND PATHOPHYSIOLOGY

- First described in 1974, parvovirus B19 is a small (20 to 25 nm) nonenveloped, single-stranded DNA virus in the *Erythrovirus* genus of the *Parvoviridae* family.
- Parvovirus B19 spreads primarily through respiratory droplets; has predilection for erythroid progenitor cells (temporary impact on erythropoiesis)
- The incubation period is typically 4 to 14 days.
- Prodromal symptoms are usually mild and include low-grade fever, headache, malaise, and myalgia.
- Rash and joint symptoms usually occur 2 to 3 weeks after initial infection. These are thought to be due to immune complex formation, and are associated with viral clearance (and decreased risk of transmission).
- Patients infected with parvovirus B19 are most contagious 5 to 10 days after exposure, well before the rash typically manifests.
- Cytotoxic infection of erythroid progenitor cells decreases RBC production, which can lead to TAC in patients with increased RBC turnover.

Genetics

Erythrocyte P antigen–negative individuals (approximately 1 in 200,000 people) are resistant to infection.

RISK FACTORS

- School-related epidemic and nonimmune household contacts have a secondary attack rate of 20–50%.
- Highest secondary attack rates are for daycare providers and school personnel in contact with affected children.
- Conditions with increased RBC turnover (spherocytosis, sickle-cell anemia, thalassemia) increase the risk of TAC.
- Immunodeficiency (congenital, due to HIV or malignancy) increases risk of PRCA and chronic anemia.
- As many as 40% of pregnant women are not immune; 1.5% seroconversion rate per year

GENERAL PREVENTION

- Respiratory spread; handwashing, cough/sneeze hygiene, and barrier precautions
- Droplet precautions are recommended around patients with TAC and in immunocompromised patients.
- Difficult to eliminate exposure because the period of maximal contagion occurs prior to the onset of the typical rash.
- No significant risk of infection based on occupational exposure if proper isolation precautions are followed; exclusion from the workplace is neither necessary nor recommended.
- No preventive vaccine is currently available.

COMMONLY ASSOCIATED CONDITIONS

- Nondegenerative arthritis
  - In children, joint symptoms are uncommon, and typically involve the knees and ankles (symmetric or asymmetric joint involvement).
  - In adults, joint symptoms are much more common, usually symmetric, involving the hands, with less frequent involvement of larger joints. Women are affected with joint symptoms more often than men.
  - Joint symptoms generally resolve within 3 weeks, but may persist for months or years. Longer-duration symptoms are more common in women. Routine radiography is not necessary.
- TAC
  - Involves patients with increased RBC turnover (sickle-cell disease, spherocytosis, thalassemia) or decreased RBC production (iron deficiency anemia)
  - Presents with fatigue, weakness, lethargy, and pallor (symptoms of anemia); may have dyspnea/shortness of breath
  - Aplastic event may be life-threatening but is typically self-limited. Reticulocytes typically reappear in 7 to 10 days with full recovery in 2 to 3 weeks.
  - In children with sickle-cell hemoglobinopathies and hereditary spherocytosis, fever is the most common symptom (73%); rash uncommon in these patients.
- Chronic anemia
  - Seen in immunocompromised individuals (HIV, cancer, transplant) with poor antibody response
  - Usually no clinical manifestations (fever, rash, or joint symptoms).
  - Patients may be transfusion-dependent.
- Fetal/neonatal infection (1)
  - Risk of transplacental spread of virus is ~30% in infected mothers.
  - Up to 50% of infected pregnant women may be asymptomatic, but vertical transmission can still occur.
  - Check IgM and IgG levels in pregnant women with symptoms consistent with parvovirus B19 infection.
  - Test pregnant women with known exposure to individuals with acute parvovirus B19.
    - If IgG positive and IgM negative, consider immune, and no further intervention is needed.
    - If IgM and IgG negative, repeat serologic testing in several weeks to look for seroconversion.
    - If IgM positive, test further to determine if acute infection is present (false-positive result).
  - Overall fetal death may occur in 5–10% of fetal infections and can occur with or without fetal hydrops.
  - Fetal bone marrow is primarily impacted. RBC survival is shortened resulting in anemia and (potentially) high-output cardiac failure. Other complications can result from fetal hypoalbuminemia, myocarditis, hepatitis, and placentitis.
  - Risk of fetal loss is highest in 1st trimester (19%).
  - Intrauterine fetal RBC transfusion can decrease fetal loss rate if fetal hydrops is present.
  - Infants who have undergone intrauterine transfusions are at risk for delays in psychomotor development.
- Parvovirus has also been associated with a gloves and socks syndrome (2).
  - Typically in younger adults, there is symmetric painful erythema and edema of feet and hands.
  - Gradually progresses to petechiae/purpura/vesicles/bullae and then skin sloughing
  - May have no other symptoms but can have fevers or arthralgias
  - Generally resolves in 1 to 3 weeks without scarring

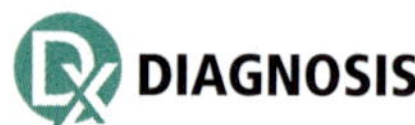

DIAGNOSIS

HISTORY

- Biphasic—may have a prodrome of fever, coryza, pharyngitis, headache, rhinorrhea, nausea
- Followed by rash and arthralgias
- Arthralgias may last for weeks or longer.

P

PHYSICAL EXAM

- The characteristic rash usually presents in several stages. The first stage is the characteristic "slapped cheek" appearance which spares the nasolabial folds. During the second stage, the rash spreads to the trunk and extremities in a diffuse, macular, erythematous pattern sparing the palms and soles. Central clearing leads to a commonly seen lacy/reticulated appearance. Within 3 weeks, the rash typically resolves.
- B19 may manifest as painful pruritic papules and purpura on the hands and feet (glove and sock distribution).

DIFFERENTIAL DIAGNOSIS

- Rubella, measles, enteroviral disease
- Systemic lupus erythematosus, drug reaction, rheumatoid arthritis

DIAGNOSTIC TESTS & INTERPRETATION

Initial Tests (lab, imaging)

- No need for routine lab studies in typical cases. Diagnosis is clinical and the illness is mild and self-limiting.
- IgG and IgM serology in immunocompetent patients; IgM detectable 10 to 12 days post infection.
- Nucleic acid amplification testing (NAAT) for fetal infection (via cord blood or amniotic fluid) as well as for patients with chronic infection or those who are immunocompromised.
- For patients with TAC, anemia and reticulocytopenia are present. IgM antibodies are noted by day 3, and IgG antibodies are detectable at time of clinical recovery. PCR shows high levels of viremia.
- Pregnant women exposed to B19 require NAAT and serologic testing to assess fetal risk.

Follow-Up Tests & Special Considerations

Fetal/neonatal infection

- To exclude congenital B19 in infants with negative B19 IgM, follow IgG serology over the 1st year of life.
- Serial fetal ultrasound (US) to assess for hydrops in cases of documented acute maternal infection in the 1st trimester.
- Weekly peak systolic velocity measurements of the middle cerebral artery by Doppler US is recommended to evaluate for heart failure, fetal anemia, and the potential need for intrauterine transfusion (>1.5 MoM).

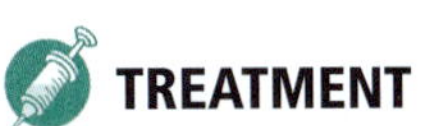

TREATMENT

GENERAL MEASURES

- No therapy is usually needed.
- Cessation of immunosuppressive therapy allows some patients to clear chronic infections.
- B19-associated anemia in HIV-positive patients may resolve with antiretroviral therapy and immune reconstitution.

MEDICATION

First Line

- Anti-inflammatory agents for arthritic symptoms
- Antipyretics for fever

Second Line

- May require RBC transfusions for TAC
- Intravenous immunoglobulin (IVIG) for B19-related refractory anemia or PRCA, especially in immunodeficient states
- Consider reduction of immunosuppressive therapy while on IVIG therapy.
- Intrauterine RBC transfusions reduce mortality in cases of fetal hydrops.

ISSUES FOR REFERRAL

- Acute infection during pregnancy should prompt referral to a maternal–fetal medicine specialist.
- Patients with chronic or abnormal B19 infections may benefit from consultation with immunology or infectious disease specialists.

ADMISSION, INPATIENT, AND NURSING CONSIDERATIONS

- Outpatient management is typical for erythema infectiosum.
- Inpatient management for aplastic crisis, which may require RBC transfusions
- In the inpatient setting, droplet isolation is appropriate for acute infections, TAC, and chronic infections in the immunocompromised.

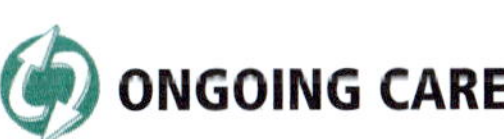

ONGOING CARE

FOLLOW-UP RECOMMENDATIONS

Patient Monitoring

Periodic blood counts for anemic patients until they have reticulocyte recovery

PATIENT EDUCATION

- Parvovirus B19 (fifth disease): http://www.cdc.gov/parvovirusB19/fifth-disease.html
- Parvovirus B19 infection and pregnancy: http://www.cdc.gov/parvovirusB19/pregnancy.html
- Healthy Children.org Parvovirus: https://www.healthychildren.org/English/health-issues/conditions/skin/Pages/fifth-disease-parvovirus-b19.aspx
- Children with typical rash are no longer infectious and may attend childcare or school.

PROGNOSIS

- Usually self-limited
- Joint symptoms usually subside within 3 weeks but may last months to years.
- ~20% of infections result in delayed virus elimination and viremia persisting for several months to years.
- Full recovery from aplastic crisis in 2 to 3 weeks

COMPLICATIONS

Conditions associated with B19 but where causality is unconfirmed

- Hepatitis—may predispose to acute fulminant hepatic failure
- Neurologic manifestations
- Myocarditis, pericarditis
- Membranoproliferative glomerulonephritis, focal segmental glomerulosclerosis, nephrotic syndrome
- Henoch-Schönlein purpura, idiopathic thrombocytopenic purpura, vasculitis, lymphocytic histiocytosis/hemophagocytic syndrome

REFERENCES

1. Ranno S, Russo C, Colagrossi L, et al. Parvovirus B19 rebound. *J Med Virol*. 2025;97(5):e70380. doi:10.1002/jmv.70380.
2. Leung AKC, Lam JM, Barankin B, et al. Erythema infectiosum: a narrative review. *Curr Pediatr Rev*. 2024;20(4):462–471 doi:10.2174/1573396320666230428104619.

ADDITIONAL READING

Venturoli S, Bertoldi A, Manaresi E, et al. Epidemiology of parvovirus B19 infection in an Italian metropolitan area, 2012–2024: COVID-19 pre-pandemic, pandemic and post-pandemic trends. *J Med Virol*. 2025;97(3):e70296. doi:10.1002/jmv.70296.

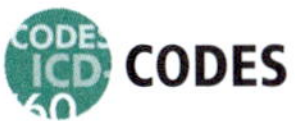

CODES

ICD10

- B34.3 Parvovirus infection, unspecified
- B08.3 Erythema infectiosum [fifth disease]

CLINICAL PEARLS

- Parvovirus B19 infection is usually a benign, self-limited illness with no long-term effects.
- Patients are no longer infectious by the time the "slapped cheek" rash of erythema infectiosum appears.
- Patients with increased RBC turnover (sickle-cell disease, thalassemia, spherocytosis) are at risk for TAC.
- Immunocompromised patients are at risk for chronic anemia, which may be transfusion-dependent.
- Documentation of acute infection in pregnant women merits maternal–fetal consultation.

PATELLOFEMORAL PAIN SYNDROME (PFPS)

Joshua A. Go, DO • Sean T. Matsuwaka, MD • Jaret Nishikawa, MD

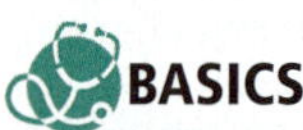

BASICS

DESCRIPTION

- Pain in or around the patella that is aggravated with increased patellar loading (e.g., prolonged sitting, squatting, kneeling, or ascending/descending stairs); not attributable to other causes
- Synonyms: anterior knee or retropatellar pain syndrome, chondromalacia patellae, runner's knee
- System(s) affected: musculoskeletal

EPIDEMIOLOGY

Incidence

- Incidence rates in military recruits ranged from 9.7 to 571.4/1,000 person-years.
- Incidence in amateur runners in the general population was 1,080.5/1,000 person-years.

Prevalence

- Annual prevalence for patellofemoral pain in the general population was reported as 22.7% and adolescents as 28.9%.
- More commonly occurs in females > males.

ETIOLOGY AND PATHOPHYSIOLOGY

Increased patellofemoral joint loading, which is often multifactorial:

- Patellar malalignment or maltracking
- Abnormal anatomy (e.g., patella alta, trochlear dysplasia)
- Quadriceps asymmetry, weakness and/or tightness
- Hamstring tightness
- Laxity of the patellofemoral joint or a tight lateral retinaculum
- Increased hip joint internal rotation
- Altered tibiofemoral joint mechanics

RISK FACTORS

- Activities such as running, squatting, and climbing up and down stairs
- Sudden increase in activities
- Female gender
- Dynamic valgus
- Patellar instability
- Quadriceps weakness
- Foot abnormalities (e.g., pes pronatus, rearfoot eversion) (1)
- In adolescents: increased hip adduction strength, although this may represent increased activity level
- Factors of uncertain significance: age, height, weight, body mass index, body fat, Q angle, and hip weakness

GENERAL PREVENTION

Strengthening and stretching exercises, particularly hip abductors and terminal extension of the quadriceps

COMMONLY ASSOCIATED CONDITIONS

- Overuse
- Knee ligament injury/surgery
- Patellar tendinopathy
- Prolonged synovitis
- Iliotibial (IT) band friction syndrome

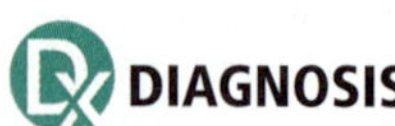

DIAGNOSIS

HISTORY

- An accurate history to differentiate between pain and instability (pain quality, location, swelling, giving way, locking, grinding, inciting events, overuse, changes in activity/training, and history of trauma)
- Most common symptom: diffuse anterior knee pain exacerbated during or after physical activity
- Pain with squatting, descending or ascending stairs, ambulating over uneven surfaces, or running

PHYSICAL EXAM

- Observation: Look for vastus medialis atrophy, localized erythema, effusion, knee (valgus/varus) and foot (pronation, supination) alignment abnormalities.
- Palpation: pain on palpation of the patellar edges (medial or lateral)
- Evaluate knee range of motion.
- Compression/patellar grind test: With patient supine, place one hand superior to the patella and push the patella inferiorly. Ask the patient to contract the quadriceps; pain upon contraction is consistent with PFPS; grinding may indicate chondromalacia of the patellofemoral joint.
- Single leg squat: 80% of patients with PFPS will demonstrate pain with this maneuver (2)[A]; also helpful in assessing for dynamic valgus
- Patellar apprehension test: With the patient supine with the knee flexed to 30 degrees, medial pressure is applied to the patella (to displace it laterally); pain or apprehension with passive patellar displacement is a positive test; not sensitive for PFPS (7–32%), but specific (86–92%)
- Passive patellar tilt test: With the patient supine with the knee extended, the patella is grasped, and the examiner lifts the lateral edge of the patella from the lateral femoral condyle, assessing for a tight lateral retinacular restraint; not sensitive for PFPS (42%), but specific (92%)
- Gait and posture may indicate any imbalances (e.g., femoral internal rotation, hip height, scoliosis, quadriceps atrophy) that may contribute to PFPS.
- Footwear evaluation may detect pes pronatus or rearfoot eversion which could contribute to PFPS (1)[A].

DIFFERENTIAL DIAGNOSIS

- Prepatellar bursitis
- Patellofemoral osteoarthritis
- Patellar and quadriceps tendinopathy
- Chondromalacia patellae
- Patellofemoral arthrosis
- Patellar subluxation and dislocation
- Knee ligamentous and meniscal pathology
- IT band syndrome
- Plica syndrome
- Osteochondral defect
- Osteochondritis dissecans
- Sinding-Larsen-Johansson syndrome
- Osgood-Schlatter disease
- Knee infection
- Neuroma or nerve entrapment
- Benign or malignant tumors
- Referred pain from hip or spine

DIAGNOSTIC TESTS & INTERPRETATION

- None indicated; typically a clinical diagnosis; in general, imaging is not necessary for the diagnosis of PFPS. If imaging is indicated because of severity, atypical symptoms, or persistence of symptoms despite treatment, plain films with four views of the knee are recommended to view patellar tilt and to rule out other etiologies of anterior knee pain:
  - Lateral, merchant or sunrise, standing anteroposterior (AP), posteroanterior (PA) tunnel views
- CT can be used to grade patellar malalignment.
- MRI can be used to evaluate for cartilage wear, osteochondral defects.
- Radiographic findings may not correlate with symptoms.

Follow-Up Tests & Special Considerations

Radiographic images may be normal until late stages, when the posterior patellar surface becomes irregular and cartilage erosion is radiographically detectable.

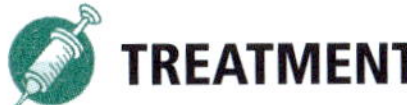

TREATMENT

GENERAL MEASURES

- Conservative therapy of activity modification, physical therapy, and rehabilitation is the gold standard (1)[A].
- Initial goal of therapy is to increase strength, flexibility, and ROM to enable practice of correct motion.
- Evidence supports both hip and knee exercises to help with recovery and short-term regain of function (3)[A].
- Hip abductors/external rotators, IT band, knee extensors, knee flexors, feet (excessive or insufficient pronation), and core muscle strengthening should be the main focus (1)[A].
- Stretching of the muscles surrounding the hip and knee, particularly proprioceptive neuromuscular facilitation stretches (1)[A]
- Education remains a pillar in the overall management of this syndrome (3)[A].

MEDICATION

- Acetaminophen or NSAIDs for pain management can help in the short term (2 to 3 weeks), but there is no evidence to support long-term use.
- The evidence for oral glucosamine and chondroitin sulfate is lacking and is not routinely recommended for treatment of patellofemoral pain.
- Injection of steroids, hyaluronic acid, and platelet-rich plasma (PRP) are lacking data for effectiveness in treating PFPS.

ISSUES FOR REFERRAL

- Referral for surgery after all conservative measures fail; surgery is rarely needed and may not be beneficial.
- Recalcitrant cases can be associated with psychosocial issues including depression, catastrophization, and central sensitization. Multimodal care, including referral to a mental health care professional, may be necessary.

ADDITIONAL THERAPIES

- Combination therapy in addition to an exercise program with other modalities, such as patellar taping or manual therapy may be beneficial (3)[A]
- Ankle and foot orthoses may offer some relief in the short term, but there is lack of evidence to support its use, particularly in the long term (3)[A].
- Dry needling may improve pain, but only a small improvement in function when combined with exercise therapy.

SURGERY/OTHER PROCEDURES

- For patients with a tight lateral retinaculum and lateral patellar tilt: operative realignment of the patella
- For patients with a defect in the cartilage of the patellofemoral joint: cartilage resurfacing/restoration

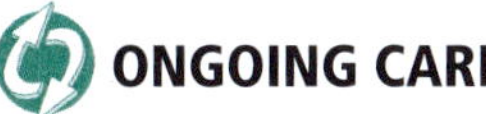

ONGOING CARE

PATIENT EDUCATION

- Patient education materials, including home exercise programs, may be provided, but this should not be considered a replacement for formal physical therapy.
- Educate the patient on the importance of participation and compliance in a specialized exercise program with a physical therapist for a specified duration (at least 6 weeks).
- The presence of significant quadriceps atrophy or an effusion precludes a return to full activity and sports
- Patients should have no complaints of nocturnal pain or pain with ADLs prior to restarting sports.
- Patients should be educated that if the condition becomes chronic, long-term pain does not typically correlate with damage to the knee.

PROGNOSIS

- PFPS may not be self-limiting and can become chronic.
- Patellofemoral pain for >12 months duration is associated with long-term pain and lack of full resolution of symptoms.
- 50% of people report persistent pain at 5 years postdiagnosis despite treatment.
- Long-term PFPS has not clearly been linked to structural patellofemoral joint OA.

REFERENCES

1. Gaitonde DY, Ericksen A, Robbins RC. Patellofemoral pain syndrome. *Am Fam Physician*. 2019;99(2):88–94.
2. Crossley KM, Stefanik JJ, Selfe J, et al. 2016 Patellofemoral pain consensus statement from the 4th International Patellofemoral Pain Research Retreat, Manchester. Part 1: terminology, definitions, clinical examination, natural history, patellofemoral osteoarthritis and patient-reported outcome measures. *Br J Sports Med*. 2016;50(14):839–843.
3. Neal BS, Lack SD, Bartholomew C, et al. Best practice guide for patellofemoral pain based on synthesis of a systematic review, the patient voice and expert clinical reasoning. *Br J Sports Med*. 2024;58(24):1486–1495. doi:10.1136/bjsports-2024-108110.

ADDITIONAL READING

- Halabi MH, Alturkistani BA, Abuhadi RH, et al. The efficacy of hip and knee muscles strengthening versus knee muscle strengthening alone in managing patellofemoral pain syndrome: a systematic review and meta-analysis. *Musculoskeletal Care*. 2025;23(1):e70059. doi:10.1002/msc.70059.
- Lankhorst NE, van Middelkoop M, Crossley KM, et al. Factors that predict a poor outcome 5–8 years after the diagnosis of patellofemoral pain: a multicentre observational analysis. *Br J Sports Med*. 2016;50(14):881–886.
- Smith BE, Selfe J, Thacker D, et al. Incidence and prevalence of patellofemoral pain: a systematic review and meta-analysis. *PLoS One*. 2018;13(1):e0190892. doi:10.1371/journal.pone.0190892.
- van der Heijden RA, Lankhorst NE, van Linschoten R, et al. Exercise for treating patellofemoral pain syndrome. *Cochrane Database Syst Rev*. 2015;(1):CD010387.

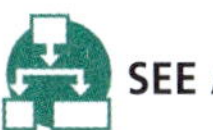

SEE ALSO

Algorithm: Knee Pain

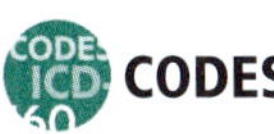

CODES

ICD10

- M25.569 Pain in unspecified knee
- M25.561 Pain in right knee
- M25.562 Pain in left knee

CLINICAL PEARLS

- PFPS is the most common cause of anterior knee pain in active adults.
- The clinical diagnosis is made by an accurate history and physical exam.
- Well-designed exercises geared at core, hip, and lower extremity flexibility and strength are the most effective evidence-based treatments.

PEDICULOSIS (LICE)

Sangili Chandran, MD • Batoul C. Zalkout, DO • Mohammed Mirza, MD

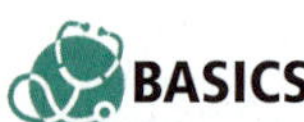

BASICS

DESCRIPTION

- A contagious parasitic infection caused by ectoparasitic blood-feeding insects (lice)
- Two species of lice infest humans:
  - *Pediculus humanus* has two subspecies: the head louse (var. *capitis*) and the body louse (var. *corporis*). Both species are 1 to 3 mm long, flat, and wingless and have three pairs of legs that attach closely behind the head.
  - *Pthirus pubis* (pubic or crab louse): resembles a sea crab and has widespread claws on the 2nd and 3rd legs

EPIDEMIOLOGY

Incidence

- In the United States: 6 to 12 million new cases per year
- Head lice are most common in children 3 to 11 years of age; more common in girls than boys. Pubic lice are more common in adults

Prevalence

Head lice: 1–3% in industrialized countries

ETIOLOGY AND PATHOPHYSIOLOGY

- Characteristics of lice:
  - An adult louse is dark grayish and moves quickly by crawling (does not jump or fly). It has claws that allow it to cling to individual strands of hair. Eggs (nits) camouflage with the individuals' hair color and are cemented to the base of the hair shaft (within 4 mm of the scalp). Nits (empty egg casings) appear white (opalescent) and remain cemented to the hair shaft.
  - Lice feed solely on human blood by piercing the skin, injecting saliva (anticoagulant properties to allow for blood meal), and then ingesting blood.
  - Itching is a delayed hypersensitivity reaction to the saliva of the feeding louse, which may take four to six weeks to develop after the first exposure. Subsequent exposures may take 1 to 2 days for symptoms to develop (1).
- Transmission: direct human-to-human contact
  - Head lice: direct head-to-head contact or contact with infested fomite (less likely)
  - Body lice: contact with contaminated clothing or bedding
  - Pubic lice: typically transmitted sexually (fomite transmission much less likely)

RISK FACTORS

- General: overcrowding and close personal contact
- Head lice
  - School-aged children, gender (girls; longer hair). Sharing combs, hats (including helmets), clothing, and bed linens
- Body lice: poor hygiene, homelessness
- Pubic lice: promiscuity (very high transmission rate)

GENERAL PREVENTION

- Environmental measures: Wash, dry-clean, or vacuum items that may have contacted infected individuals.
- Screen and treat affected household contacts.
- Head lice: Follow-up by school nurses may help to prevent recurrence and spread. Pubic lice: Limit the number of sexual partners (condoms do not prevent transmission nor does shaving pubic hair). Body lice: proper body hygiene

COMMONLY ASSOCIATED CONDITIONS

Up to 30% of patients with pubic lice have at least one concomitant STI.

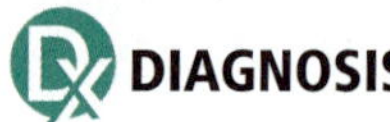

DIAGNOSIS

HISTORY

- Pruritus is common, often worse at night.
- Often associated with "outbreak" in school settings
- Investigate contacts of infected individuals.

PHYSICAL EXAM

- Diagnosis is confirmed by visualization of live lice.
- *P. humanus capitis* (head lice)
  - Found most often on the back of the head and neck and behind the ears (warmer areas)
  - Eyelashes may be involved.
  - Eggs, found cemented on the base of a hair shaft, are difficult to remove.
  - Pruritus may be accompanied by local erythema and small papules.
  - May see excoriations around hairline
  - Scratching can cause inflammation and secondary bacterial infection.
  - Pyoderma and lymphadenopathy may occur in severe infestation.
- *P. humanus corporis* (body lice)
  - Poor general hygiene
  - Adult lice and nits in the seams of clothing
  - Intense pruritus involving area covered by clothing (trunk, axillae, and groin)
  - Uninfected bites present as erythematous macules, papules, and wheals. Pyoderma and excoriation may be seen.
  - Transmit *Bartonella quintana* (trench fever) and *Borrelia recurrentis* (louse-borne relapsing fever) and *Rickettsia prowazekii* (epidemic typhus)
- *P. pubis* (pubic lice)
  - Pubic hair is the most common site, but lice may spread to hair around anus, abdomen, axillae, chest, beard, eyebrows, and eyelashes.
  - Eggs are present at the base of hair shafts. Anogenital pruritus; blue macules may be seen in surrounding skin.
  - Delay in treatment may lead to development of groin infection and regional adenopathy.

DIFFERENTIAL DIAGNOSIS

- Scabies and other mite species that can cause cutaneous reactions in humans
- Dandruff and other hair debris sometimes look like head lice eggs and nits but are less adherent.

DIAGNOSTIC TESTS & INTERPRETATION

- Diagnosis is based on visualization of live louse.
- Head lice: Comb hair thoroughly with a fine-toothed louse comb (0.2 to 0.3 mm between teeth) to identify live lice (2)[C]. Wet the hair to limit static electricity, which repels lice. Simple visual inspection has same sensitivity as wet combing but is only ~25% as effective as dry combing with a metal comb (3).
- Body lice: Examine the seams of clothing to locate lice and eggs.
- Lice and eggs are more easily visualized with a microscope.
- In contrast to dandruff, eggs and nits cannot be removed easily from a hair shaft.

Follow-Up Tests & Special Considerations

- Empty nits remain on hair shafts for months after eradication of the live infestation. Wood lamp exam: Live nits fluoresce white and empty nits fluoresce gray.
- Pubic lice: Evaluate for concurrent STIs.

TREATMENT

GENERAL MEASURES

- Head lice: Clean items that have been in contact with the head of the infected individual within 48 hours.
- Wash all bedding, towels, clothes, headgear, combs, brushes, and hair accessories in hot water (>60°C).
- Vacuum furniture and carpets. Seal any personal articles that cannot be washed in hot water, dry-cleaned, or vacuumed in a plastic bag and store for at least 2 weeks. Examine and treat household members and close contacts concurrently.
- Insecticide sprays are not necessary. Pubic lice: Avoid sexual activity until all partners are successfully treated.
- Nit and egg removal:
  - Remove eggs within 1 cm of the scalp to prevent reinfestation. After treatment with shampoo or lotion, eggs and nits remain in the scalp or pubic hair until mechanically removed. Hair conditioner facilitates nit removal. Eggs and nits best removed with a fine nit comb

MEDICATION

Permethrin (over the counter [OTC]), synergized pyrethrin (OTC), spinosad (Rx), benzyl alcohol (Rx), malathion (Rx), and topical ivermectin (Rx) are all effective for head lice (2)[A],(3)[C]. Permethrin, synergized pyrethrin, and malathion are effective for pubic lice (3)[C]

- Permethrin generally preferred because it may have residual activity for up to 3 weeks. However, use of newer shampoos and conditioners may reduce the residual effect (2)[C].
- Malathion and spinosad are considered second line for head lice but may not require a second application due to ovicidal activity (2)[B],(3)[C].
- Ivermectin 0.5% lotion and benzyl alcohol 5% lotion are also effective for head lice (2),(3)[C].

First Line

- Head and pubic lice:
  - Pyrethrum insecticides: Permethrin 1% (Nix Crème Rinse) or pyrethrins 0.33% with piperonyl butoxide 4% (synergized pyrethrin, Rid, Pronto) are first line unless there is proven resistance in the community.
    - Apply for 10 minutes and then wash. Reapply synergized pyrethrin in 7 to 10 days (day 9 is optimal); also be necessary with permethrin, if live lice are observed
    - Side effects: application-site erythema, ocular erythema, and application-site irritation

- Body lice: best treated with synergized pyrethrin lotion applied once and left on for several hours
- Eyelash infestation: Apply petroleum jelly BID for 10 days.
- Precautions:
  - Pyrethrin: Avoid in patients with ragweed allergy (may cause respiratory symptoms).
  - Pediculicides should never be used to treat eyelash infections.

Second Line

- Head lice and pubic lice
  - Malathion 0.5% lotion (Ovide)
    - Apply for 8 to 12 hours and then wash off.
      - Flammable and has a bad odor. Despite ovicidal activity, a second application may be necessary after 7 to 10 days (day 9 is optimal) if live lice are observed
  - Abametapir 0.74%, lotion
    - Apply once in age group ≥6 months. Mechanism of action: inhibits metalloproteinases in adult lice and eggs; side effects: erythema, rash, and skin burning sensation
- Head lice
  - Spinosad 0.9% lotion (Natroba)
    - Apply to dry hair and scalp for 10 minutes and then rinse with warm water. Repeat in 7 days if live lice are observed.
    - Side effects: application-site erythema, ocular erythema, and application-site irritation
  - Benzyl alcohol 5% lotion (Ulesfia)
    - Apply to dry hair using enough to saturate scalp and hair (amount depends on hair length), rinse after 10 minutes; repeat in 1 week.
    - Side effects: pruritus, erythema, pyoderma, ocular irritation, application-site irritation
  - Ivermectin 0.5% lotion (Sklice)
    - Apply to dry hair by using enough to saturate the scalp and hair (max. 4 oz) and then rinse after 10 minutes.
    - Side effects: burning sensation at application site, dandruff, dry skin, eye irritation
- Mechanical removal of lice and nits by wetting hair and then systematically combing with a fine-toothed comb every 3 to 4 days for 2 weeks to remove all lice as they hatch

Pediatric Considerations

- Ivermectin lotion 0.5% and abametapir lotion 0.74% recently approved by FDA for children aged ≥6 months. Benzyl alcohol also approved for children >6 months.
- Avoid synergized pyrethrin and permethrin in infants <2 months of age. Avoid topical ivermectin, and spinosad in children <6 months of age and avoid malathion in children <2 years of age.
- Lindane: not recommended

Pregnancy Considerations

Permethrin, synergized pyrethrin, malathion, spinosad, and benzyl alcohol are pregnancy Category B. Lindane and topical ivermectin are pregnancy Category C.

ADDITIONAL THERAPIES

- For "difficult to treat" cases of head lice, oral ivermectin 400 μg/kg (not approved by the FDA for lice), given twice at a 7-day interval, is superior to topical 0.5% malathion lotion (4).
- Ivermectin: 200 μg/kg PO repeated after 10 days or 300 μg/kg PO repeated after 7 days; should not be used in children <15 kg; pregnancy Category C; not approved by the FDA for lice
- Dual therapy with permethrin 1% and oral trimethoprim/sulfamethoxazole (TMP/SMX) only for cases of multiple treatment failures or suspected cases of lice-related resistance to therapy (TMP/SMX is not approved by the FDA for lice.)
- Permethrin 5% cream (Rx) is not FDA approved for lice and is unlikely to be effective for lice that are resistant to 1% cream rinse (2)[B].

COMPLEMENTARY & ALTERNATIVE MEDICINE

- Cetaphil lotion: dry-on, suffocation-based pediculicide (not approved by the FDA for lice)
  - Apply thoroughly to hair, comb, and then dry with hair dryer; shampoo after 8 hours. Repeat once a week until cured, up to a maximum of three applications.
- Dimethicone 4% lotion: Apply to hair for 8 hours; repeat in 1 week (not approved by the FDA for lice).
- No home remedies (e.g., vinegar, isopropyl alcohol, olive oil, ylang ylang oil, mayonnaise, melted butter, and petroleum jelly) are proven effective.
- Herbal shampoos and pomades have not been evaluated in clinical trials. Lavender oil and tea tree oil have been implicated in triggering prepubertal gynecomastia in boys and should not be used to treat lice.
- Electronic louse combs have not proven effective and are not approved by the FDA.
- Repellents: A placebo-controlled clinical trial demonstrated that rosemary, citronella, and piperonal essential oils were clinically effective as repellents when applied topically to the head of children.

ONGOING CARE

FOLLOW-UP RECOMMENDATIONS

Children may return to school after completing topical treatment, even if nits remain in place. No-nit policies are unnecessary.

Patient Monitoring

Drug resistance should be suspected if no dead lice are observed 8 to 12 hours after treatment.

PATIENT EDUCATION

- National Pediculosis Association: https://www.headlice.org/comb/
- CDC: https://www.cdc.gov/lice/index.html
- National Guideline Clearinghouse: http://www.guideline.gov/content.aspx?id=46429&search=lice

PROGNOSIS

- With appropriate treatment, >90% cure rate
- Recurrence is common, mainly from reinfection or treatment nonadherence. Resistance to synthetic pyrethroids is increasing.

COMPLICATIONS

- Poor sleep due to pruritus. Persistent itching may be caused by too frequent use of the pediculicide.
- Missed school; social stigma
- Secondary bacterial infections. Body lice can transmit typhus and trench fever.

REFERENCES

1. Gunning K, Kiraly B, Pippit K, et al. Lice and scabies: treatment update. *Am Fam Physician*. 2019;99(10):635–642.
2. Devore CD, Schutze GE; for Council on School Health and Committee on Infectious Diseases, American Academy of Pediatrics. Head lice. *Pediatrics*. 2015;135(5):e1355–e1365.
3. Coates SJ, Thomas C, Chosidow O, et al. Ectoparasites: pediculosis and tungiasis. *J Am Acad Dermatol*. 2020;82(3):551–569.
4. Patel PU, Tan A, Levell NJ. A Clinical review and history of pubic lice. *Clin Experimental Dermatol*. 2021;46(7):1181–1188. doi:10.1111/ced.14666.

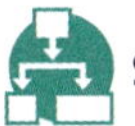

SEE ALSO

Arthropod Bites and Stings; Scabies

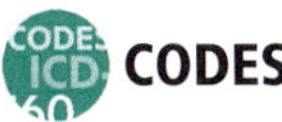

CODES

ICD10

- B85.0 Pediculosis due to Pediculus humanus capitis
- B85.1 Pediculosis due to Pediculus humanus corporis
- B85.3 Phthiriasis

CLINICAL PEARLS

- School-based no-nit policies are not necessary because empty nits may remain on hair shafts for months after successful eradication.
- Improper product application is a common cause of treatment failure.
- Prevalence of resistant infestations is increasing; if no dead lice are observed 8 to 12 hours after treatment, suspect resistance and use an alternative agent.
- Routine retreatment on day 9 is recommended for nonovicidal products (permethrin and synergized pyrethrin).
- With all treatment options, reinspect hair after 7 to 9 days, and if live lice are detected, repeat treatment on day 9.

PELVIC INFLAMMATORY DISEASE

Chirag N. Shah, MD • Daniel Scott Morrison, MD • Aarsh Shah, DO

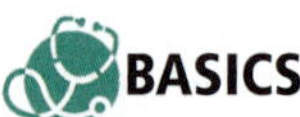

BASICS

DESCRIPTION

- Pelvic inflammatory disease (PID) is an infection of the upper female genital tract, including the uterus, fallopian tubes, and ovaries. PID is commonly an ascending polymicrobial infection acquired through retrograde movement of microorganisms from the lower genital tract.
- PID is concerning due to its potential impact on fertility.
- Mild to moderate PID is defined by the absence of a tubo-ovarian abscess (TOA). Severe PID involves systemic symptoms *or* presence of a TOA.
- Diagnosis is challenging due to nonstandardized definitions, lack of definitive tests, and varying symptoms (1)[C].

EPIDEMIOLOGY

Most commonly affects sexually active patients aged 15 to 24 years (1)[C].

Incidence

More than 1 million patients are diagnosed with PID annually.

Prevalence

Estimated lifetime PID prevalence is 4.4% in sexually active cisgender women aged 18 to 44 years. ~2.5 million U.S. women of reproductive age have had a PID diagnosis.

- Without a history of prior sexually transmitted infection (STI), lifetime prevalence is higher in Black than White women (6% vs. 2.7%).
- With a history of STI, lifetime prevalence was similar across races (10% vs. 10.3%).

ETIOLOGY AND PATHOPHYSIOLOGY

Multiple organisms cause PID, and polymicrobial infections are common.

- *Chlamydia trachomatis* and *Neisseria gonorrhoeae*, once considered the primary pathogens, are now identified in only 22–50% of cases.
- *Mycoplasma genitalium* infection is seen in ~4–22% of females diagnosed with PID, with some studies reporting upward of 60%. The latest study showed a 67% increase in odds of developing PID with an *Mycoplasma genitalium* infection (2)[A].
- Common flora and causes of bacterial vaginosis including aerobic and anaerobic species (e.g., *Gardnerella vaginalis* and *Escherichia coli*) are increasingly implicated (2)[A].
- Possible mechanisms for ascent from the lower genital tract include (i) travel from cervix to endometrium to salpinx to peritoneal cavity; (ii) lymphatic spread via infection of the parametrium; and (iii) hematogenous route, which is rare.

RISK FACTORS

- Sexually active and age <25 years
- New sexual partner or sexual partner with symptoms or known STI
- Two or more sexual partners in the last year (1)[C]
- Inconsistent condom use
- Gynecologic procedures that break the cervical barrier including endometrial biopsy, curettage, hysterosalpingography (HSG), hysteroscopy, in vitro fertilization, and insertion of IUD in the last 3 weeks.
- Other factors associated with PID:
  - Previous history of PID (10–25% recurrence)
  - Cervical ectopy
  - History of *C. trachomatis*; 10–40% develop PID.
  - History of gonococcal cervicitis; 10–20% develop PID (3)[A].

GENERAL PREVENTION

- Educational programs about safe sex practices such as condom use
- The U.S. Preventive Services Task Force recommends annual chlamydia screening for all sexually active women <25 years and for those ≥25 years at increased risk (e.g., new or multiple sex partners), with moderate evidence that it reduces cases of PID (1)[C].
- Routine STI screening in pregnancy
- STI screenings for those with new genital lesions or abnormal discharge

COMMONLY ASSOCIATED CONDITIONS

- In a patient with an IUD and a pelvic abscess, suspect *Actinomyces* infection and treat with penicillin.
- Rupture of an adnexal abscess is rare but life-threatening, requiring early surgical exploration (1)[C].
- Chlamydial or gonococcal perihepatitis, called Fitz-Hugh-Curtis syndrome, can accompany PID, causing severe pleuritic right upper quadrant pain, in 4–6% of PID cases (2)[A].
- Women presenting with acute pyelonephritis should also be evaluated for PID and STIs.

DIAGNOSIS

- Clinical diagnosis has a positive predictive value of 65–90% compared to laparoscopy.
- The CDC advises empiric PID treatment for females at risk with pelvic/lower abdominal pain of unknown etiology and one or more of the following: uterine, adnexal, or cervical motion tenderness.
- Fever >101°F, new/abnormal cervical mucopurulent discharge or friability, presence of abundant WBCs on wet prep, elevated C-reactive protein (CRP) or erythrocyte sedimentation rate (ESR), and laboratory documentation of genitourinary infection with *N. gonorrhoeae* or *C. trachomatis* help confirm PID diagnosis.
- Tubal thickening on ultrasound or MRI is highly specific (>90%) (2)[A].

HISTORY

- Lower abdominal/pelvic pain: dull, aching/crampy, bilateral, constant; worsened by motion, exercise, or coitus
- New/abnormal vaginal discharge (~75% of cases) or unanticipated/postcoital bleeding (~40% of cases)
- Fever, chills, dyspareunia
- Low back pain
- Dysuria
- Recent HSG or other procedure breaking the uterine barrier
- IUD insertion in the past 21 days

PHYSICAL EXAM

Fever; lower abdominal pain; cervical motion, uterine, or adnexal tenderness; evidence of cervicitis with/without vaginal discharge

DIFFERENTIAL DIAGNOSIS

Appendicitis, constipation, gastroenteritis, ectopic pregnancy, ovarian tumor/torsion, hemorrhagic/ruptured ovarian cyst, endometriosis/dysmenorrhea, functional pelvic pain, inflammatory bowel disease, diverticulitis, UTI/pyelonephritis, nephrolithiasis

DIAGNOSTIC TESTS & INTERPRETATION

Initial Tests (lab, imaging)

- Pregnancy test
- Chlamydia and gonorrhea testing with urine or cervical swab nucleic acid amplification test (NAAT); a negative result does not exclude PID
- Urinalysis
- Saline microscopy of vaginal fluid
- HIV and syphilis screening
- Transvaginal ultrasound

Pediatric Considerations

Consider sexual abuse in children presenting with PID.

Follow-Up Tests & Special Considerations

Follow-up ultrasound as an outpatient for resolution of TOA

Diagnostic Procedures/Other

- Consider laparoscopy in ill patients with a competing diagnosis, failed outpatient therapy, or no improvement after 72 hours of inpatient treatment.
- Endometrial biopsy (indicated only if laparoscopy shows no evidence of salpingitis) reveals endometritis.

Test Interpretation

If suspicion is high, treat empirically since NAAT take 1 to 3 days to result (1)[C].

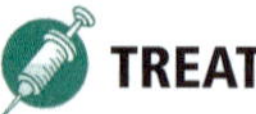

TREATMENT

- Patient education: Avoid intercourse until patient and partner(s) have been adequately treated. Counsel both parties on possible long-term implications.
- Outpatient treatment is advised, if appropriate.

GENERAL MEASURES

- An IUD does not need to be removed. Reassess the patient in 48–72 hours; if no clinical improvement, consider removal.
- Treatment should cover key pathogens (CT, NG, and polymicrobial infections with anaerobic coverage), regardless of test results (3)[A].

MEDICATION

First Line

Outpatient treatment regimen: long-acting cephalosporin, macrolide or tetracycline, and metronidazole.

- Ceftriaxone 500 mg IM single dose *plus* doxycycline 100 mg PO BID for 14 days plus metronidazole 500 mg PO BID for 14 days; patients weighing >150 kg need 1 g of ceftriaxone.
- As of 2021, the CDC recommends adding PO metronidazole to the standard outpatient regimen.

- Moxifloxacin 400 mg, PO, QID monotherapy for 14 days, can be considered for mild to moderate PID, especially in patients with a cephalosporin allergy (3)[A]. A regimen of doxycycline 100 mg PO BID for 7 days followed by moxifloxacin 400 mg PO daily for 7 days offers the best coverage against *M. genitalium* but is not recommended where fluoroquinolone-resistant gonorrhea is prevalent (2)[A].

Second Line

- Because of emerging resistance, culture for sensitivity testing and cure is advised 2 weeks after completion of treatment.
- Outpatient treatment regimen
  - Cefoxitin 2 g IM single dose and probenecid 1 g PO single dose, or cefotaxime (1 g IM), or ceftizoxime (1 g IM) *plus* doxycycline 100 mg PO BID for 14 days plus metronidazole 500 mg PO BID for 14 days
- In persons with documented severe allergic reactions to penicillin:
  - Skin testing is important to confirm penicillin allergy
  - Cross-reactivity between penicillin and third-generation cephalosporins is low (<1%) (1)[C].
  - Levofloxacin 500 mg PO BID for 14 days can be substituted for cephalosporins.
- Special consideration
  - Treat sex partners from the past 60 days. If last sexual encounter was >60 days prior, treat the most recent partner. Provide expedited partner therapy when possible (1)[C].
  - Treat HIV-infected patients with acute PID like non–HIV-infected patients but monitor closely for TOA, especially in patients with CD4 counts <200/mm^3.

SURGERY/OTHER PROCEDURES

Reserved for failures of medical treatment and suspected ruptured adnexal abscess causing acute surgical abdomen

ADMISSION, INPATIENT, AND NURSING CONSIDERATIONS

- Criteria for hospitalization if any of the following:
  - Surgical emergencies (e.g., appendicitis) can't be excluded.
  - Pregnancy
  - TOA
  - Severe illness, nausea or vomiting, unable to follow or tolerate outpatient regimen, or fever >101°F
  - Failure to respond to 72 hours of oral antibiotics (1)[C]
- For inpatient treatment of PID, the CDC recommends the following:
  - Parenteral regimen A
    - Ceftriaxone 1 g IV every 24 hours plus doxycycline 100 mg PO or IV every 12 hours plus metronidazole 500 mg PO or IV every 12 hours.
    - Alternatively, cefotetan 2 g IV BID or cefoxitin 2 g IV q6h plus doxycycline 100 mg PO or IV BID; this regimen does not require additional anaerobic coverage with metronidazole.
    - Parenteral therapy for 24 to 48 hours after clinical improvement; oral doxycycline is preferred due to its similar bioavailability to IV. Continue doxycycline and metronidazole for a total of 14 days.
  - Parenteral regimen B
    - Clindamycin 900 mg IV q8h plus gentamicin loading dose IV or IM (2 mg/kg) followed by a maintenance dose (1.5 mg/kg) q8h or single daily dosing at 3 to 5 mg/kg can be substituted.
    - Parenteral therapy may be discontinued 24 hours after clinical improvement. Oral therapy with doxycycline (as above) or clindamycin 450 mg PO QID should be continued to complete 14 days.
  - Parenteral regimen C: ampicillin/sulbactam 3 g IV every q6h doxycycline 100 mg PO or IV BID
- PID in pregnancy requires hospitalization, infectious disease consultation, and parenteral antibiotics due to high risk of maternal morbidity, perinatal mortality, and preterm delivery (1)[C].

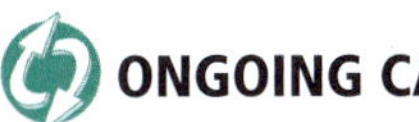

ONGOING CARE

FOLLOW-UP RECOMMENDATIONS

Arranging follow-up within 48 to 72 hours and providing clear patient education are key to ensuring good patient outcomes.

Patient Monitoring

- Follow up 72 hours after starting treatment, especially in patients with moderate or severe symptoms.
- Observe for worsening fever, abdominal pain, and cervical motion tenderness.
- Retest for gonorrhea and chlamydia 3 months post-treatment (1)[C].
- Track adnexal abscess size and position with serial ultrasounds.

PATIENT EDUCATION

- Abstain from sexual contact until complete treatment of patient and partner.
- Consistent and correct condom use
- Offer hepatitis B and human papillomavirus (HPV) vaccines to eligible patients.
- Advise comprehensive STI screening.
- Offer HIV preexposure prophylaxis (PrEP) to patients with new STI or PID.
- IUD insertion poses a low risk of PID, even with prior/current STI diagnosis.

PROGNOSIS

- PID has a high morbidity: ~18% become infertile, 29% develop chronic pelvic pain, and 0.6% have an ectopic pregnancy.
- Prognosis is good with early effective therapy but poor if delayed.
- Nongonococcal, nonchlamydial PID is linked to more severe PID and worse fertility outcomes.

COMPLICATIONS

- TOA occurs in 7–16% of patients before presentation; 1/3 of those hospitalized with PID
- Recurrent infection occurs in 20–25% of patients.
- Risk of ectopic pregnancy increases 7- to 10-fold with prior PID.
- Tubal infertility in 8%, 19.5%, and 40% of patients after 1, 2, and 3 episodes of PID, respectively.
- Chronic pelvic pain in 20–30% of cases is related to adhesions, chronic salpingitis, or recurrent infection.
- Hydrosalpinx: After PID resolves, fallopian tube fills with sterile fluid and becomes blocked, associated with pain and infertility.

REFERENCES

1. Shroff S. Infectious Vaginitis, cervicitis, and pelvic inflammatory disease. *Med Clin North Am*. 2023;107(2):299–315. doi:10.1016/j.mcna.2022.10.009.
2. Htaik K, Vodstrcil LA, Plummer EL, et al. Systematic review and meta-analysis of the association between *Mycoplasma genitalium* and pelvic inflammatory disease (PID). *Clin Infect Dis*. 2024:ciae295. doi:10.1093/cid/ciae295.
3. Chen F, Dong Q, Hong W, et al. Moxifloxacin monotherapy for treatment of uncomplicated pelvic inflammatory disease: a systematic review and meta-analysis with trial sequential analysis of randomized controlled trials. *Pharmacoepidemiol Drug Saf*. 2023;32(11):1189–1199. doi:10.1002/pds.5677.

ADDITIONAL READING

https://www.cdc.gov/std/treatment-guidelines/pid.htm

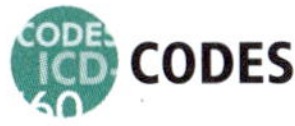

CODES

ICD10

- N70.0 Acute salpingitis and oophoritis
- N70 Salpingitis and oophoritis
- N71.0 Acute inflammatory disease of uterus

CLINICAL PEARLS

- PID often starts with gonorrhea or chlamydia but can be polymicrobial.
- Treat based on clinical suspicion (pelvic pain, cervical motion, or adnexal/uterine tenderness) without waiting for confirmatory testing.
- PID is a common cause of infertility.
- Complications include hydrosalpinx, adhesions, pelvic pain, and an increased risk of ectopic pregnancy.

PEPTIC ULCER DISEASE

Nergess T. Taheri, DO, MSBI • Sabari Nair, DO

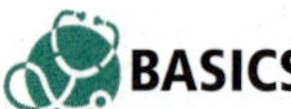

BASICS

Defects in the stomach and/or duodenal mucosa lead to inflammation and erosion of the underlying tissue by gastric acid and pepsin.

DESCRIPTION

- Mucosal breaks extending into the submucosa or muscularis propria located in the stomach or duodenum
- Peptic ulcer disease (PUD) is an endoscopic diagnosis versus dyspepsia which is a clinical diagnosis.
- *Helicobacter pylori* and aspirin/NSAIDs use are the leading causes of PUD.
- NSAIDs use plus *H. pylori* infection increases the risk of PUD by 60-fold.
- Multiple ulcers/ulcers distal to the second portion of duodenum and/or jejunum raise the possibility of gastrinoma (Zollinger-Ellison syndrome [ZES]).
- Idiopathic ulcers account for 20% of PUD (1).

EPIDEMIOLOGY

Incidence

United States: incidence approximately 500,000 cases/year (2)

Prevalence

- Highest prevalence in South Asia
- Low-/middle-income countries have higher prevalence of *H. pylori* infections and PUD (1).

RISK FACTORS

- *H. pylori* infection
- Long-term NSAIDs use
- Other medications: corticosteroids, bisphosphonates, potassium chloride, clopidogrel, sirolimus, chemotherapeutic agents, SSRIs
- Hypersecretion syndromes: gastrinoma (ZES), systemic mastocytosis, cystic fibrosis, hyperparathyroidism, carcinoid syndrome, antral G-cell hyperplasia
- Tobacco, alcohol, stress, radiation therapy, obesity

GENERAL PREVENTION

- Limit NSAIDs, aspirin, alcohol, tobacco, caffeine.
- If NSAIDs are necessary, use the lowest possible dose with a proton pump inhibitor (PPI) or misoprostol. Test for and eradicate *H. pylori*.
- Treat with PPIs or H_2 blockers for patients at risk for complications and recurrence.
- Strong association between obesity and PUD; counsel patients on weight loss.

COMMONLY ASSOCIATED CONDITIONS

Gastrinoma (ZES); multiple endocrine neoplasia type 1 (MEN 1); carcinoid syndrome

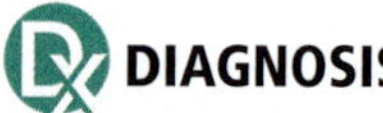

DIAGNOSIS

HISTORY

- NSAID-induced ulcers can present with bleeding/perforation.
- Epigastric pain: gnawing/burning, nonradiating, recurring and episodic
  - Duodenal ulcer: relieved by food or antacids
  - Gastric ulcer: aggravated by food, relieved by antacids
- Indigestion, nausea, vomiting, loss of appetite, belching, heartburn, epigastric fullness, early satiety
- Specific symptoms that increase the likelihood of PUD: pain relieved by food (LR+ = 3.3; LR− = 0.7), nighttime awakening due to pain that is relieved by food (LR+ = 2.8; LR− = 0.6), and episodic pain (LR+ = 2.3; LR− = 0.3) (3)
- Red flag symptoms: onset age ≥55 years, progressive dysphagia, GI bleeding (melena or hematochezia), iron deficiency anemia, persistent vomiting, severe abdominal pain, unintentional weight loss, anorexia, family history of gastric malignancy
- Tobacco, alcohol, and drug use

PHYSICAL EXAM

Monitor weight; signs of anemia; epigastric tenderness (absent in ~30% of older patients); heme-positive stool

DIFFERENTIAL DIAGNOSIS

- Functional dyspepsia, gastritis, drug-induced dyspepsia, GERD, biliary disease, gastroenteritis, pancreatitis, cholecystitis, Crohn disease, GI malignancy
- Life-threatening conditions: myocardial infarction, mesenteric ischemia, mesenteric vasculitis

DIAGNOSTIC TESTS & INTERPRETATION

Initial Tests (lab, imaging)

- CBC, liver function tests, amylase and lipase
- *H. pylori* testing: urea breath test, stool antigen test; false-negative results if patient was recently treated with antibiotics, bismuth, or PPIs, or in patients with active bleeding
  - Stop antibiotics and bismuth for at least 4 weeks and PPIs for at least 2 weeks prior to testing.
  - 25–55% of patients with *H. pylori* infection have false-negative results in the setting of acute upper GI bleed (1).
- Urea breath test: identifies active infection; screening and posttreatment testing; high positive predicted (PPV) and negative predicted value (NPV)
- Stool antigen: identifies active infection; screening and posttreatment testing; sensitivity 87%; specificity 70%; patients may not want to collect full stool sample.
- Serology: low utility as it does not distinguish past from active infection

Follow-Up Tests & Special Considerations

If multiple/refractory ulcers: Consider fasting serum gastrin to rule out ZES.

Diagnostic Procedures/Other

- Esophagogastroduodenoscopy (EGD): most accurate test for diagnosing PUD and *H. pylori* infection; patients of age >55 years with new dyspepsia and any patient with red flag symptoms should have an EGD. EGD is costly and invasive (4)[B].
- Can obtain barium swallow if EGD contraindicated or not possible

TREATMENT

Identify and mitigate risk factors: tobacco, alcohol, NSAIDs, obesity; gastroprotective medications: PPIs, H_2 blockers, and prostaglandin analogues

MEDICATION

First Line

- Gastroprotective agents
  - PPIs: most ulcers heal within 4 weeks, length of treatment 4 to 8 weeks
    - Omeprazole 20 to 40 mg/day; lansoprazole 30 mg/day; rabeprazole 20 mg/day; esomeprazole 20 to 40 mg/day; pantoprazole 40 mg/day; dexlansoprazole 30 to 60 mg/day
    - Precautions
      - May decrease bone density—monitor interval bone densitometry with long-term use
      - Associated with community-acquired pneumonia and *Clostridium difficile* infection
      - May cause hypomagnesemia
  - H_2 blockers: length of treatment: 4 to 8 weeks
    - Ranitidine or nizatidine 150 mg twice daily (BID) or 300 mg bedtime; cimetidine 400 mg BID or 800 mg bedtime; famotidine 20 mg BID or 40 mg bedtime; decrease dose by 50% if CrCl <50 mL/min
- NSAID-induced or aspirin-induced ulcers
  - PPIs, H_2 blockers, sucralfate or misoprostol; PPIs are most effective (2).
  - Discontinue NSAIDs.
  - Length of treatment: 6 to 8 weeks
  - *H. pylori*–induced ulcers

- Bismuth-based quadruple therapy and concomitant therapies are first line. Treatment duration is 10 to 14 days (4).
- Bismuth-based quadruple therapy: PPI BID plus metronidazole or tinidazole 500 mg four times daily (QID) plus tetracycline 500 mg QID plus bismuth subsalicylate 535 mg or bismuth subcitrate 300 mg QID (3)
- Concomitant therapy: PPI BID plus clarithromycin 500 mg BID plus amoxicillin 1 g BID plus metronidazole or tinidazole 500 mg BID (3)
- Clarithromycin-based triple therapy can be considered—duration 14 days: PPI BID plus clarithromycin 500 mg BID plus amoxicillin 1 g BID or metronidazole 500 mg TID (1)

- Refractory and idiopathic ulcers
  - Double-strength PPI for refractory ulcers, which are ulcers that have not healed after 8 to 12 weeks of therapy (~5–10% ulcers) (1)
  - Endoscopy after an additional 12 weeks of PPI therapy to demonstrate ulcer healing
  - Idiopathic ulcers warrant further workup to exclude rare causes.

Second Line

- *H. pylori* eradication: Use one of the following if first-line regimen fails:
  - Levofloxacin triple therapy: PPI high dose BID, amoxicillin 1 g BID, levofloxacin 500 mg daily; treatment duration 14 days (3)
  - High-dose dual therapy: PPI high dose BID, amoxicillin 1 g TID or 750 mg QID; treatment duration 14 days (3)
  - Rifabutin triple therapy: PPI high dose BID, amoxicillin 1 g TID, rifabutin 300 mg daily or rifabutin 150 mg BID; treatment duration 10 days (3)
- Significant possible interactions:
  - Cimetidine: Avoid with theophylline, warfarin, phenytoin, and lidocaine.
  - Omeprazole may prolong elimination of diazepam, warfarin, and phenytoin.
  - Sucralfate reduces absorption of tetracycline, norfloxacin, ciprofloxacin, and theophylline, leading to subtherapeutic levels.

Pregnancy Considerations

- Mild symptoms: Postpone treatment until after delivery; more severe symptoms(hyperemesis gravidarum); consider 7 days of treatment with a PPI, amoxicillin, and metronidazole in the first trimester (3).
- PPIs are *not* associated with increased risk of major birth defects, spontaneous abortions, or preterm delivery.
- Breastfeeding: H_2 blockers and PPIs are safe.

ISSUES FOR REFERRAL

Red flag symptoms: onset age ≥55 years, progressive dysphagia, overt GI bleeding, iron deficiency anemia, persistent/recurrent vomiting, severe abdominal pain, unintentional weight loss, anorexia, and/or family history of gastric malignancy

ADDITIONAL THERAPIES

Vonoprazan: potassium-competitive acid blocker; antisecretory agent; achieves ulcer healing in >90% patients (1)

SURGERY/OTHER PROCEDURES

- Endoscopy: ≥55 years of age with new-onset symptoms, treatment failure, red flag symptoms
  - Biopsy for *H. pylori*; biopsy ulcer margin for malignancy
  - Stop active bleeding or prevent rebleeding: Inject with epinephrine, heater probe treatment, or placement of endoscopic clips.
- Surgery indications: refractory ulcers; patients at high risk for complications (e.g., transplant recipients, on chronic steroids/NSAIDs); bleeding not responding to endoscopic therapy
  - Duodenal ulcers: truncal vagotomy and drainage (pyloroplasty/gastrojejunostomy), selective vagotomy (preserving the hepatic and/or celiac branches of the vagus) and drainage, or highly selective vagotomy (4)
  - Gastric ulcers: partial gastrectomy, Billroth I or II

ADMISSION, INPATIENT, AND NURSING CONSIDERATIONS

Bleeding peptic ulcers

- If hemodynamically stable: PPI therapy oral PPIs equivalent to IV PPIs
- If not hemodynamically stable, surgery (4)

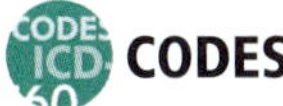

ONGOING CARE

FOLLOW-UP RECOMMENDATIONS

Patient Monitoring

- *H. pylori* eradication is expected in >90% (with double antibiotic regimen).
- Confirm eradication 4 weeks after completing therapy with urea breath test or fecal antigen test.
- Acute gastric ulcer: Confirm healing via EGD in 6 to 8 weeks; if not healed, obtain biopsy to rule out gastric cancer (2).

PATIENT EDUCATION

Lifestyle modifications: smoking cessation, decreased alcohol and caffeine, weight loss, limited NSAIDs use

PROGNOSIS

- NSAID-induced ulcer: Healing occurs >85% of the time with full PPI course and discontinuing offending medication (2).
- Once *H. pylori* is successfully eradicated, low risk of recurrence.
- Recurrence of PUD is common (up to >60%).

COMPLICATIONS

- Hemorrhage (≤25% of patients), perforation (<5%), gastric outlet obstruction (<5%), refractory PUD (5–10%)
- Risk of gastric adenocarcinoma increased in *H. pylori*–infected patients.

REFERENCES

1. Almadi MA, Lu Y, Alali AA, et al. Peptic ulcer disease. *Lancet*. 2024;404(10447):68–81. doi:10.1016/S0140-6736(24)00155-7.
2. Narayanan M, Reddy KM, Marsicano E. Peptic ulcer disease and *Helicobacter pylori* infection. *Mo Med*. 2018;115(3):219–224.
3. McConaghy JR, Decker A, Nair S. Peptic ulcer disease and *H. pylori* infection: common questions and answers. *Am Fam Physician*. 2023;107(2):165–172.
4. Lanas A, Chan FKL. Peptic ulcer disease. *Lancet*. 2017;390(10094):613–624.

CODES

ICD10

- K27.9 Peptic ulc, site unsp, unsp as ac or chr, w/o hemor or perf
- K26.9 Duodenal ulcer, unspecified as acute or chronic, without hemorrhage or perforation
- K25.9 Gastric ulcer, unspecified as acute or chronic, without hemorrhage or perforation

CLINICAL PEARLS

- PPIs: higher efficacy than H_2 blockers; almost twice ulcer-healing rate
- Eradicate *H. pylori* to assist healing and reduce risk of recurrence.
- EGD indications: patients with suspected peptic ulcers, red flag symptoms, treatment failure

PERICARDITIS

Munima Nasir, MD, FAAFP • Zakary S. Newberry, MD

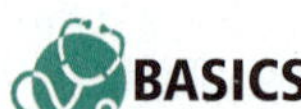

BASICS

DESCRIPTION

Inflammation of the pericardium; this may be associated with other pericardial syndromes including effusion, tamponade, or constrictive pericarditis, and may also involve the myocardium as in myopericarditis or perimyocarditis.

EPIDEMIOLOGY

Incidence

- Incidence is approximately 27.7 cases per 100,000 per year (1).
- After first episode of acute pericarditis, about 30% of patients experience recurrence within 18 months.

ETIOLOGY AND PATHOPHYSIOLOGY

- Inflammation of the pericardial sac can be acute, subacute, chronic, or recurrent (2).
- Can lead to production of serous/purulent fluid/dense fibrinous material, which may lead to hemodynamic compromise
- Idiopathic: 85–90% of cases; likely related to viral infection, which may trigger immune-related process
- Infectious
  - Viral (80–85% of cases): coxsackievirus, echovirus, adenovirus, Epstein-Barr virus, cytomegalovirus, hepatitis viruses, influenza virus, HIV, measles, mumps, varicella, SARS-CoV-2, parvovirus B19
  - Bacterial: *Mycobacterium tuberculosis* (in endemic countries)
  - Fungal (in immunocompromised populations): *Blastomyces dermatitidis, Candida* spp., *Histoplasma capsulatum*
  - Parasites: *Echinococcus*, *Toxoplasma*
- Noninfectious causes (15–20% of cases)
  - Acute MI (2 to 4 days after MI), Dressler syndrome (weeks to months after MI); aortic dissection; renal failure, uremia, dialysis-associated; malignancy-associated; radiation therapy; trauma; after cardiac procedures (e.g., catheterization, pacemaker placement, ablation, pericardiotomy)
  - Autoimmune disorders: connective tissue disorders, systemic lupus erythematosus (SLE), rheumatoid arthritis, scleroderma, hypothyroidism, inflammatory bowel disease, Wegener granulomatosis, spondyloarthropathies, sarcoidosis, IgG4-related
  - Suspected vaccination associations: smallpox, influenza, SARS-CoV-2 mRNA vaccine (incidence of ~4.8 per 1 million)
- Medication-induced: dantrolene, doxorubicin, hydralazine, isoniazid, mesalamine, methysergide, penicillin, phenytoin, procainamide, rifampin

Genetics

Familial Mediterranean fever and tumor necrosis factor receptor-associated periodic syndrome (TRAPS) are related to recurrent pericarditis (3).

RISK FACTORS

Thoracic surgery, chronic kidney disease, pneumonia, autoimmune diseases, lung or breast cancer especially if treated with radiation therapy

DIAGNOSIS

- Acute pericarditis (<4 to 6 weeks) must meet at least two of four criteria:
  - New/worsening pericardial effusion (60–80% of cases) on imaging
  - ECG changes with widespread ST elevations or PR depressions (up to 60% of cases)
  - Pericardial friction rub (<33% of cases)
  - Typical (pleuritic) chest pain
- Subacute pericarditis: symptoms above persist for >4 to 6 weeks but <3 months; recurrent pericarditis: return of symptoms after a 4- to 6-week symptom-free interval; chronic pericarditis: symptoms >3 months
- Myopericarditis: definite pericarditis *plus*
  - Symptoms (dyspnea, chest pain, or palpitations) *and* ECG changes not previously documented *or* focal/diffuse depressed left ventricular (LV) function documented on imaging
  - Absence of evidence of other cause
  - One of the following: elevated cardiac enzymes (creatine kinase [CK]-MB, troponin I or T) *or* new focal/diffuse depressed LV function *or* abnormal imaging consistent with myocarditis

HISTORY

- Prodrome of fever, malaise, myalgias, recent viral upper respiratory infection
- Acute, sharp/stabbing chest pain, pathognomonic if pain radiates to trapezius
- Pleuritic pain reduced by leaning forward, worsened by lying supine
- Shortness of breath

PHYSICAL EXAM

Pericardial friction rub (35–85% of cases): coarse, high-pitched sound heard during end expiration at left lower sternal border with patient leaning forward

- Highly specific but not sensitive for diagnosis
- May be transient and monophasic, biphasic, or triphasic
- New S_3 may suggest myopericarditis.

DIFFERENTIAL DIAGNOSIS

Myocardial ischemia/acute coronary syndrome, pulmonary embolism, aortic dissection, gastroesophageal reflux disease, pneumonia, costochondritis

DIAGNOSTIC TESTS & INTERPRETATION

Initial Tests (lab, imaging)

- CBC: typically shows leukocytosis
- Inflammatory markers: elevated erythrocyte sedimentation rate (ESR), C-reactive protein (CRP), and lactate dehydrogenase (LDH)
- Cardiac biomarkers: typically elevated CK, troponin
  - Elevated troponin associated with younger age, male sex, pericardial effusion at presentation, and ST segment elevation on ECG
  - Adverse outcomes are not predicted by elevated troponin.
- Classic ECG findings include widespread upward concave ST segment elevation (in all or most leads, a diffuse, nonregional process) and PR segment depression
  - ECG may be normal/show nonspecific abnormalities.
  - May demonstrate low voltage and electrical alternans with large effusions and tamponade
- Transthoracic echocardiogram is recommended to evaluate for pericardial effusion, tamponade, or myocardial disease.
- Chest x-ray to rule out pulmonary/mediastinal pathology
  - Enlarged cardiac silhouette suggests large pericardial effusion (at least 300 mL)
- CT scan and MRI to assess for pericardial inflammation and complications
  - Can assist in planning of pericardiectomy if necessary
- Additional testing may include thyroid stimulating hormone (TSH), tuberculin skin test, sputum cultures, rheumatoid factor, antinuclear antibody, and HIV serology.

Diagnostic Procedures/Other

Pericardiocentesis indicated for:

- Cardiac tamponade
- Suspected purulent, tuberculous, or neoplastic pericarditis
- Effusions >20 mm on echocardiography

Test Interpretation

- Microscopic examination may reveal hyperemia, leukocyte accumulation, or fibrin deposition.
- Purulent fluid with neutrophilic predominance if bacterial etiology; lymphocytic predominance in viral, tuberculous, and neoplastic pericarditis
- Do not use Light criteria (set of three criteria to determine if pleural fluid is exudative) for evaluation of pericardial fluid (3).

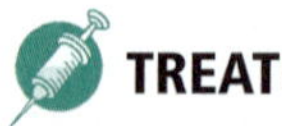

TREATMENT

GENERAL MEASURES

Specific therapy directed toward underlying disorder for patients with identified cause; restrictions of physical activity are an important part of treatment for recurrences.

MEDICATION

First Line

- NSAIDs are the mainstay of therapy for acute pericarditis:
  - Ibuprofen 600 mg TID for 7 to 10 days (2 to 4 weeks for recurrence) then taper (1)[C]
  - Aspirin 1,000 mg TID for 7 to 10 days (2 to 4 weeks for recurrence) then taper; preferred in patients with recent MI as other NSAIDs impair scar formation in animal studies (1)[C]

P

- Indomethacin 50 mg TID for 7 to 10 days (2 to 4 weeks for recurrence) then taper; avoid in elderly and coronary artery disease (1)[C].
- GI protection should be provided (proton pump inhibitor) (1)[C].
- Tapering should be done only if the patient is asymptomatic and CRP/ESR are normal. Repeat CRP/ESR every 1 to 2 weeks (1)[C].
- Monitoring: NSAIDs: CBC and CRP at baseline and weekly until CRP normalizes
- Contraindications: hypersensitivity to aspirin or NSAIDs, active peptic ulcer/GI bleeding
- Precautions: Use with caution in patients with asthma, 3rd-trimester pregnancy, coagulopathy, elderly, and renal/hepatic dysfunction.

- Colchicine:
  - Use in combination with NSAIDs to decrease incidence of recurrence, treatment failure, and for faster symptomatic response; not recommended for monotherapy (2)[A]
  - 0.5 to 0.6 mg BID for up to 3 months (6 months for recurrence); taper is not required. Adjust for weight, renal, and hepatic function (1)[C],(3)[C]
  - Only agent proven to prevent recurrences in RCTs; adjunctive therapy can reduce recurrence rate by 50% (2)[A].
  - Monitoring: Consider CBC, transaminases, CK, and creatinine at baseline and after 1 month at a minimum; follow CRP weekly until normal (1)[C]
  - Adverse reactions: diarrhea, abdominal pain, nausea
- Pregnancy: <20 weeks' gestation: Aspirin is first-line, but NSAIDs and prednisone are also allowed; >20 weeks' gestation: Prednisone is allowed with avoidance of NSAIDs, aspirin, and colchicine (3)[C].

Second Line

- Corticosteroid treatment is indicated in connective tissue disease, tuberculous pericarditis, contraindications to NSAIDs or colchicine, or severe recurrent symptoms unresponsive to NSAIDs or colchicine. Steroids should be avoided in uncomplicated acute pericarditis or if infectious etiology is suspected. Corticosteroid use alone has been found to be an independent risk factor for recurrence
- Use low dose (0.2 to 0.5 mg/kg/day) until resolution of symptoms and normalization of CRP and then perform slow tapering (1)[C].
- Consider prophylactic treatment with calcium/vitamin D, and conditionally use bisphosphonates in men or postmenopausal women for osteoporosis prevention for those continuing on corticosteroid (1)[C].
- If recurrence while tapering, do not increase dose or restart corticosteroids.
- Intrapericardial administration of steroids may be effective and limits systemic side effects.
- Anakinra (interleukin-1 [IL-1] antagonist)—for recurrent pericarditis
  - 2 mg/kg (up to 100 mg) subcutaneously daily for 2 to 6 months; adjust for renal function
- Decreased incidence of recurrence in one RCT (2)[A]
  - Adverse reactions—injection site reactions, elevated liver enzymes, herpes zoster reactivation
- Rilonacept (IL-1 antagonist)—for recurrent pericarditis
  - 320 mg subcutaneously once followed by 160 mg dose weekly for 12 weeks
  - Decreased recurrence rate compared to placebo (3)[C]
  - Adverse effects—injection site reactions, increased risk for upper respiratory tract infections

ISSUES FOR REFERRAL

Hospitalization recommended for patients with major medical comorbidities, refractory cases, uremic/dialysis-related cases, suspected/threatened tamponade, poor prognostic factors, or presentation that suggests an underlying systemic inflammatory disease (1)[C].

SURGERY/OTHER PROCEDURES

- Pericardiocentesis indicated in cardiac tamponade, tuberculous/purulent/neoplastic pericarditis, and moderate-to-large symptomatic effusions refractory to medical therapy
- Pericardial biopsy may be considered for diagnosis of persistent worsening pericarditis without a definite cause.
- Pericardial window may be performed in cases of recurrent cardiac tamponade with large pericardial effusion despite medical therapy.
- Pericardiectomy is standard of care for chronic constrictive pericarditis with persistent symptoms, such as NYHA class III or IV. Mortality is high at 6–12% so is reserved only after careful evaluation by experienced surgeons at hospitals with specific interest in pericardial disease.

ADMISSION, INPATIENT, AND NURSING CONSIDERATIONS

- Inpatient therapy is recommended for pericarditis associated with clinical predictors of poor prognosis:
  - Fever >38°C, subacute onset, large pericardial effusion, cardiac tamponade, lack of response to NSAIDs/aspirin therapy after 1 week, immunosuppression, trauma, anticoagulation therapy, myopericarditis
- IV fluids considered for hypotension or in pericardial tamponade

ONGOING CARE

FOLLOW-UP RECOMMENDATIONS

- 1 week to check treatment response, CBC, CRP
- Those with predictors of poor prognosis may require closer follow-up based on lab data and echocardiogram findings.

Patient Monitoring

Myopericarditis

- Use lower doses of anti-inflammatory drugs to treat symptoms for 1 to 2 weeks while minimizing deleterious effects
- Exercise restrictions for 4 to 6 weeks or until symptoms resolve and biomarkers normalize. For athletes, restriction should be a minimum of 3 months after symptom onset.
- Echocardiographic monitoring at 1, 6, and 12 months, especially in those with LV dysfunction

PROGNOSIS

- Overall good prognosis but depends on etiology; disease usually benign and self-limiting; purulent and tuberculosis pericarditis with high mortality
- Major markers of poor prognosis include, fever, subacute/recurrent presentation, large pericardial effusion, and signs of tamponade on echocardiogram

COMPLICATIONS

- Recurrent pericarditis: occurs in 15–30% of patients, with most resulting from idiopathic, viral, or autoimmune pericarditis; inadequate treatment of the initial attack; and, less commonly, neoplastic etiologies; recurrence usually within 1 week following initial episode but may occur months to years later
- Cardiac tamponade: rare complication with increased incidence in neoplastic, purulent, and tuberculous pericarditis
- Effusive-constrictive pericarditis: reported in 24% of patients undergoing surgery for constrictive pericarditis and in 8% of patients undergoing pericardiocentesis and cardiac catheterization for cardiac tamponade; failure of right atrial pressure to fall by 50% or to a level below 10 mm Hg after pericardiocentesis is diagnostic.
- Constrictive pericarditis: rare complication in which rigid pericardium produces abnormal diastolic filling with elevated filling pressures; pericardiectomy is definitive therapy; found to be associated with subacute pericarditis; mortality without diagnosis is up to 90%.
- Atrial fibrillation/flutter

REFERENCES

1. Lazarou E, Tsioufis P, Vlachopoulos C, et al. Acute pericarditis: update. *Curr Cardiol Rep*. 2022;24(8):905–913. doi:10.1007/s11886-022-01710-8.
2. Melendo-Viu M, Marchán-Lopez Á, Guarch CJ, et al. A systematic review and meta-analysis of randomized controlled trials evaluating pharmacologic therapies for acute and recurrent pericarditis. *Trends Cardiovasc Med*. 2023;33(5):319–326.
3. Bizzi E, Picchi C, Mastrangelo G, et al. Recent advances in pericarditis. *Eur J Intern Med*. 2022;95:24–31. doi:10.1016/j.ejim.2021.09.002.

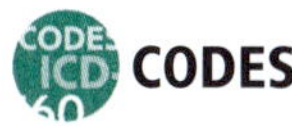

CODES

ICD10

- I31.9 Disease of pericardium, unspecified
- I30.9 Acute pericarditis, unspecified
- I30.1 Infective pericarditis

CLINICAL PEARLS

Therapy aimed at symptomatic relief and NSAIDs with colchicine are first-line treatment. Colchicine has been shown to decrease risk of recurrence by 50%.

PERIODIC LIMB MOVEMENT DISORDER (PLMD)

Joanna Drowos, DO, MPH, MBA

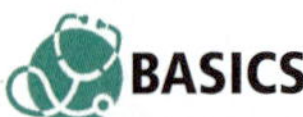

BASICS

DESCRIPTION

- Periodic limb movement disorder (PLMD) is a sleep-related movement disorder characterized by periodic limb movements of sleep (PLMS) with significant sleep disturbance and/or daytime functional impairment (1).
- PLMS are repetitive contractions of tibialis anterior muscles occurring mainly in the first hour of non–rapid eye movement (NREM) sleep (1).
- Movements can be unilateral or bilateral, simultaneous or not, and involve rhythmic extension of the big toe and ankle dorsiflexion (1).
- Generalized movements or arm movements occur less commonly (2).
- Movements may be associated with cortical arousals from sleep (PLMA) (2).
- PLMD is a diagnosis of exclusion when PLMS are not explained by other sleep disorders like obstructive sleep apnea (OSA), restless leg syndrome (RLS), or narcolepsy (1).
- Requires significant sleep disturbance and/or daytime functional impairment (2)
- Complaints include insomnia, nonrestorative sleep, daytime fatigue, somnolence (3).
- No associated restlessness or dysesthesia while awake (2)
- System(s) affected: musculoskeletal, nervous
- Synonym(s) for PLMS: nocturnal myoclonus; sleep myoclonus

EPIDEMIOLOGY

Incidence

PLMD is estimated to affect 4–11% of the general adult population and 5–8% of the pediatric population (3).

Prevalence

- PLMS increase with age: occur in 45% of patients aged >65 years and are more common in women (1)
- PLMS occurs in >15% of patients with insomnia and 85% of patients with RLS (1).

ETIOLOGY AND PATHOPHYSIOLOGY

- Etiology is uncertain.
- Suprasegmental disinhibition of the descending inhibitory pathways may be a factor.
- Evidence supports neuronal hyperexcitability with involvement of the central pattern generator for gait resulting in decreased dopamine transition.
- Triggering and exacerbating factors:
  - Peripheral neuropathy
  - Arthritis
  - Renal failure
  - Spinal cord injury
  - Pregnancy
  - Medication side effects: antidepressants, lithium, antipsychotics, antidementia, antiemetics (antidopaminergic) and sedating antihistamines

Genetics

Possible underlying genetic component mediated via single nucleotide polymorphisms in BTBD9, TOX3/BC034767, and MEIS1 (4)

RISK FACTORS

- Family history of RLS
- Iron deficiency anemia and associated conditions
- History of prematurity
- Older age
- Female gender
- Shift work
- Stress
- Caffeine intake

GENERAL PREVENTION

- Promote adequate sleep.
- Avoid PLMS triggers.
- Treat iron deficiency, frequently observed in children.

COMMONLY ASSOCIATED CONDITIONS

- Narcolepsy
- RLS (includes sensation of movement)
- End-stage renal disease
- Cardiovascular disease, stroke
- Gastric surgery
- Pregnancy
- Arthritis
- Lumbar spine disease, spinal cord injury
- Peripheral neuropathy
- Insomnia, insufficient sleep, parasomnias
- ADHD, anxiety, oppositional behaviors

Pediatric Considerations

- Association with RLS more common; may precede overt RLS by years
- Associated with and differential includes restless sleep disorder, ADHD, oppositional behaviors, mood disorders, growing pains (4)

Pregnancy Considerations

- May be secondary to iron or folate deficiency
- Most severe in the 3rd trimester
- Usually resolves after delivery

Geriatric Considerations

- May cause or exacerbate circadian disruption and "sundowning"
- PLMS may increase risk of atrial fibrillation in elderly.

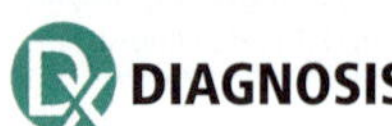

DIAGNOSIS

HISTORY

- Sleep disturbance is key.
- Insomnia: difficulty maintaining sleep, nonrestorative sleep
- Daytime fatigue, tiredness, somnolence
- Oppositional behaviors, ADHD, memory impairment, depression

PHYSICAL EXAM

No specific physical findings

DIFFERENTIAL DIAGNOSIS

- PLMS occurring with RLS, REM-sleep behavior disorder, narcolepsy, or associated with respiratory events from OSA, are considered secondary to the sleep disorder, not PLMD.
- Sleep-related leg cramps (isolated, painful, muscle knots)
- Fragmentary myoclonus (75 to 150 ms of electromyographic [EMG] activity, minimal movement, no periodicity)
- Nocturnal seizures (epileptiform EEG, motor pattern incongruent with PLMS)
- Fasciculations/tremor (no sleep association)
- Sleep-related rhythmic movement disorder (voluntary movement during wake–sleep transition; higher frequency than PLMS)
- Restless sleep disorder(large body movements, no periodicity)

DIAGNOSTIC TESTS & INTERPRETATION

- Polysomnography (PSG) demonstrating PLMS
- Tibialis anterior EMG activation lasting 0.5 to 10.0 seconds; amplitude increase >8μV from baseline (1).
- Movements occur in sequence at ≥4 at intervals of 5 to 90 seconds.
- Associated with heart rate variability from autonomic-level arousals; night-to-night PLMS variability is common.

Initial Tests (lab, imaging)

Iron studies: serum iron, ferritin, transferrin, iron-binding capacity

Follow-Up Tests & Special Considerations

Repeat ferritin if suspected change, or nonresponsive to treatment.

Diagnostic Procedures/Other

Rule out neuropathy: EMG or nerve conduction studies if indicated.

Test Interpretation

PSG results: PLMSI >5/hr in children, and >15/hr in adults (1)

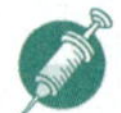

TREATMENT

Treatment paradigm similar to that for RLS, except that all medications are off-label for PLMD

GENERAL MEASURES

- Assess for and correct iron insufficiency.
- Adequate nightly sleep
- Regular exercise, low impact in the evening
- Weighted blanket, warm the legs (long socks, leg warmers, electric blanket, etc.)
- Hot/leg baths/warm soaks before bedtime
- Avoid caffeine, alcohol, and other triggers.

MEDICATION
- Use minimum effective dose to improve subjective sleep quality, reduce daytime somnolence, and control PLMS.
- Consider risks, side effects, interactions in different populations (e.g., benzodiazepines in elderly).
- Treatment should decrease daytime somnolence.

First Line
- Benzodiazepines and agonists most commonly used because of their effect on sleep; caution in the elderly (4)
  - Clonazepam (Klonopin): 0.5 to 2.0 mg QHS
  - Zaleplon, zolpidem, temazepam, triazolam, alprazolam, diazepam
- Anticonvulsants (gabapentinoids): useful for associated neuropathy; decrease PLMS and improve sleep architecture; caution with renal impairment (4)
  - Gabapentin enacarbil (Horizant): 600 mg early evening
  - Gabapentin (Neurontin) 300 to 600 mg HS
  - Pregabalin (Lyrica): 75 to 300 mg HS
- Dopamine agonists reduce PLMS, increase sleep efficiency; start low, titrate slowly (4)
  - Caveat: no data on long-term effects of dopamine agonists on PLMD
    - Pramipexole (Mirapex): 0.125 to 0.500 mg; titrate by 0.125 mg; take 2 hours HS
    - Ropinirole (Requip): 0.25 to 4.00 mg; titrate by 0.25 mg; take 1/2 to 1 hour HS; preferred in renal impairment
    - Transdermal rotigotine (Neupro): 1 to 3 mg/24 hr patch; initiate with 1 mg/24 hr; titrate up by 1 mg slowly to effectiveness.
- Avoid dopamine agonists in psychotic patients, especially if taking dopamine antagonists (4).
- Dopamine agonists may exert a stimulant effect, further disturbing sleep (4).

ISSUES FOR REFERRAL
To sleep medicine clinic, neurology and movement disorders clinic:
- Requiring high-dose medications
- Symptoms worsening while on medications
- Intractable iron deficiency
- Uncontrolled symptoms in adults or special populations

Pediatric Considerations
- First-line treatment: nonpharmacologic (3)
- Assess/correct iron deficiency (3).
- Consider low-dose clonidine with sleep-onset insomnia 0.1 to 0.3 mg HS; caution: orthostatic hypotension (3)

Pregnancy Considerations
- Initial approach: iron supplementation, nonpharmacologic therapies
- In 2nd and 3rd trimester, can use clonazepam 0.25 to 1.00 mg QHS (4)
- Carbidopa/levodopa 25/100 to 50/200 ER (4)
- Refractory PLMD—may use oxycodone in 2nd and 3rd trimester: discontinue 2 weeks prior to delivery (4)

Geriatric Considerations
- In weak or frail patients, avoid medications that may cause dizziness or unsteadiness.
- Avoid medications that may exacerbate PLMS, such as antidepressants and antihistamines (4).

ADDITIONAL THERAPIES
If iron deficient, iron supplementation (4):
- 325 mg ferrous sulfate with 200 mg vitamin C between meals QD
- Repletion may require months of treatment.

SURGERY/OTHER PROCEDURES
Correction of orthopedic, neuropathic, or peripheral vascular problems if indicated

COMPLEMENTARY & ALTERNATIVE MEDICINE
Vitamin/mineral supplements, including calcium, magnesium, vitamin D, vitamin B_{12}, folate maybe helpful.

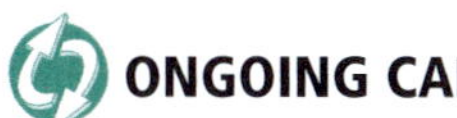

ONGOING CARE

FOLLOW-UP RECOMMENDATIONS

Patient Monitoring
- At monthly intervals until stable
- Assess symptom severity, medication side effects, augmentation.
- Annual and PRN follow-up thereafter
- Repeat iron blood work if previously low.

DIET
Avoid caffeine and alcohol, particularly later in the day.

PATIENT EDUCATION
- National Sleep Foundation: https://www.thensf.org
- American Academy of Sleep Medicine: http://www.sleepeducation.org/

PROGNOSIS
- Primary PLMD: lifelong, no current cure
- Secondary PLMD: may subside with resolution of cause or underlying disease
- Current therapies usually control symptoms.
- PLMD often precedes the emergence of RLS.

COMPLICATIONS
- Tolerance to medication requiring increased dose
- Augmentation (increased PLMs and sleep disturbance, emergence of RLS) from dopamine agonists:
  - Higher doses increase risk
  - Iron deficiency increases augmentation risk.
  - Add alternative medication and then gradually discontinue dopaminergic agent.
- Iatrogenic PLMD (from antidepressants, other medications)

REFERENCES

1. Hornyak M, Feige B, Riemann D, et al. Periodic leg movements in sleep and periodic limb movement disorder: prevalence, clinical significance and treatment. *Sleep Med Rev*. 2006;10(3):169–177.
2. Stiasny K, Oertel WH, Trenkwalder C. Clinical symptomatology and treatment of restless legs syndrome and periodic limb movement disorder. *Sleep Med Rev*. 2002;6(4):253–265.
3. DelRosso LM, Picchietti DL, Sharon D, et al; for International Restless Legs Syndrome Study Group (IRLSSG). Periodic limb movement disorder in children: a systematic review. *Sleep Med Rev*. 2024;76:101935.
4. Winkelman JW, Berkowski JA, DelRosso LM, et al. Treatment of restless legs syndrome and periodic limb movement disorder: an American Academy of Sleep Medicine systematic review, meta-analysis, and GRADE assessment. *J Clin Sleep Med*. 2025;21(1):153–199.

ADDITIONAL READING

American Academy of Sleep Medicine. Periodic limb movement disorder. In: *International Classification of Sleep Disorders*. 3rd ed. Darien, IL: American Academy of Sleep Medicine; 2014:292–299.

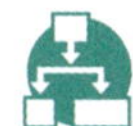

SEE ALSO

Restless Legs Syndrome

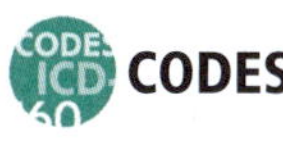

CODES

ICD10
G47.61 Periodic limb movement disorder

CLINICAL PEARLS
- Diagnosing PLMD requires significant sleep disturbance and/or daytime functional impairment in addition to PLMS when other diseases are excluded.
- Polysomnography demonstrating PLMS >5/hr in children and >15/hr in adults is diagnostic.
- Initial treatment involves correcting iron deficiency, keeping limbs warm and avoiding triggers.
- Pharmacologic treatment options are similar to those for RLS and are off-label for PLMD, including benzodiazepines, anticonvulsants, and dopamine agonists.

PERIPHERAL ARTERIAL DISEASE

D. Melessa Phillips, MD, MPH • Eric L. Wilkerson II, MD

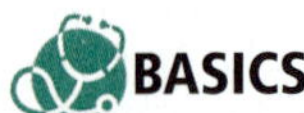

BASICS

DESCRIPTION

Peripheral arterial disease (PAD) represents an atherosclerotic occlusive disease of the peripheral arteries, most commonly in the lower extremities.

- It is an underdiagnosed form of cardiovascular disease strongly associated with health care disparities, an increased risk of amputation, myocardial infarction (MI), stroke, death, and significantly impaired functionality and quality of life.
- Definition: (generally) lower extremity atherosclerotic arterial obstruction that occurs from the aortoiliac segments to the pedal arteries (1).
- 4 clinical presentations:
  - Asymptomatic PAD
  - Chronic symptomatic PAD (Intermittent claudication [IC])
  - Chronic (critical) limb-threatening ischemia (CLTI)
  - Acute limb ischemia (ALI)

EPIDEMIOLOGY

- Affects >1:20 Americans aged >50 years, >230 million people globally
- Prevalence is equivalent between sexes or slightly higher in women (3.5%) than in men (2.5%) (1).

Prevalence

- Uncommon in those <40 years old (4.3%), prevalence rises rapidly with ages >70 years (14.3%) and >80 years (20%)
- Black Americans: disproportionally affected (1):
  - PAD rates are twice as high as other ethnicities at any given age
  - More advanced and severe disease (gangrene, foot sepsis) at presentation
  - 77% higher risk of major amputations
  - Less likely to be prescribed statin or antiplatelet therapy
- Black, Hispanic, and Native Americans with PAD are less likely to undergo revascularization procedures; have 10–30% higher complication rates than white PAD patients.

ETIOLOGY AND PATHOPHYSIOLOGY

PAD begins as a complex inflammatory cascade within the intimal layer of a large lower extremity artery wall, leading to progressive lipoprotein accumulation, atherosclerosis, and eventual arterial diameter narrowing.

- Compromised blood flow distal to arterial occlusion is unable to match muscle oxygen demand with exercise despite collateral vessel formation; producing symptoms of ischemia (see below)
- On average, Black Americans with PAD have increased markers of vascular aging (increased arterial stiffness, oxidative stress, lower skeletal mitochondrial function) compared to white Americans with PAD.

Genetics

Several of the risk factors for PAD (as noted below) are heritable, and genome-wide association studies to isolate PAD-specific single nucleotide polymorphisms are being explored.

- A positive family history of PAD may double the odds of PAD in family members.
- Factor V Leiden gene mutation (most common inherited cause of venous system blood clots) may be associated with development of PAD.

RISK FACTORS

- Conventional: smoking, diabetes, hypertension (HTN), sedentary lifestyle, increased levels of total cholesterol, LDL, lipoprotein(a) (Lp[a]) and apolipoprotein B (apoB), dyslipidemia, hypertriglyceridemia, chronic kidney disease (CKD), obesity (1)
- Nonconventional: lead and cadmium exposure, air pollution, depression (1)
- Risk amplifiers: race, ethnicity, geography, structural racism, implicit bias, and age (1)

GENERAL PREVENTION

Smoking abstinence or cessation, regular physical activity, heart-healthy nutrition, healthy weight, evidence-based control of blood pressure, blood sugar and lipids, preventive foot hygiene, regular foot inspections (self and professional)

COMMONLY ASSOCIATED CONDITIONS

Coronary artery disease, stroke, MI, carotid artery disease, transient ischemic attack (TIA), atrial fibrillation, congestive heart failure, HTN, diabetes, vascular dementia, cognitive decline, sleep apnea

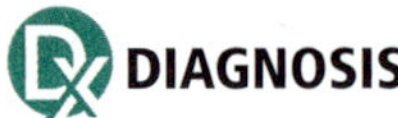

DIAGNOSIS

Made by history, physical examination, and ankle-brachial index (ABI) results

HISTORY

- Asymptomatic: 20–59%
  - Significant proportion of patients who report no exertional leg pain will develop symptoms during a 6-minute walk test
- Chronic symptomatic PAD: 10–35%
  - Aching, burning; cramping pain or discomfort or fatigue in buttock, thigh, calf, ankle or foot
  - Symptoms consistently induced by walking; consistently relieved (usually within 10 minutes) by rest
  - Leg weakness, numbness, or fatigue during walking; without pain
  - Progressively lower physical activity levels, worsening walking endurance and velocity, poorer balance
  - Without treatment, progresses over time to more advanced stages of CLTI and ALI
- CLTI: 2%
  - Claudication symptoms + ischemic rest pain, especially of forefoot
  - Pain worse with elevation of the limb; relieved by dependent position
  - Nonhealing wounds or ulcers
  - Dry or wet gangrene, tissue loss, and necrosis
  - Responsible for most major and minor limb amputations in PAD
- ALI: (1%)
  - Severest form of PAD; a surgical/endovascular emergency
  - Acute (<2 weeks) history of increasing lower limb severe pain, pallor, coolness, pulselessness, paresthesias
  - Hypoperfusion due to acute thrombosis/embolism; viability of limb threatened
  - Risk increased with history of previous revascularization, atrial fibrillation, and progressively lower ABI scores
  - Rutherford classification limb status (viable, salvageable/marginally threatened, salvageable/immediately threatened, irreversible) used to guide clinical decision-making regarding urgency of intervention.
- Symptoms often misdiagnosed as common orthopedic and neurologic comorbidities of aging (hip or knee arthritis, spinal stenosis, peripheral neuropathy)
- A history of erectile dysfunction in men may be an indication of undiagnosed PAD (1).

PHYSICAL EXAM

- Diminished femoral, popliteal, dorsalis pedis, or posterior tibial artery palpable pulses
- Dry, shiny, smooth, hairless skin, thickened toenails
- Nonhealing leg/foot ulcers
- Dry or wet gangrene
- Pain, pallor, coolness, pulselessness, paresthesias
- Tissue loss
- Calf atrophy
- Vascular bruit (epigastric, periumbilical, groin)

Geriatric Considerations

Older patients (aged >75 years) with PAD should be assessed for frailty, sarcopenia, malnutrition, and functional decline. These concurrent geriatric syndromes may obscure symptoms until PAD reaches an advanced state.

DIFFERENTIAL DIAGNOSIS

- Arterial aneurysm or dissection
- Deep vein thrombosis (DVT)
- Thromboangiitis obliterans (Buerger disease) or other vasculopathies
- Acute/chronic lymphedema or cellulitis
- Restless leg syndrome
- Spinal stenosis or nerve root compression (pseudoclaudication)

DIAGNOSTIC TESTS & INTERPRETATION

- Routine screening in asymptomatic patients not recommended due to insufficient evidence (USPSTF)
- High-risk patients: screening recommended by AHA (1); no interval specified
  - Aged >65 years
  - Ages 50 to 64 years with diabetes, history of smoking, dyslipidemia, HTN, CKD, family history of PAD
  - Aged >50 years with diabetes and one additional ASCVD risk factor
  - Known ASCVD in another vascular bed
- Screening is by ABI:
  - Normal = 0.9 to 1.4
  - Borderline = 0.9 to 1.0 (cannot rule out PAD)
  - Mild PAD = 0.81 to 0.90
  - Moderate PAD = 0.5 to 0.8
  - Severe PAD = 0 to 0.49
  - Sensitivity of 69–79%, specificity of 83–93% in symptomatic patients

Initial Tests (lab, imaging)

- Fasting lipid profile, Lp(a), apoB, basic metabolic profile, coagulation studies; Consider c-reactive protein, interleukin-6, D-dimer, homocysteine levels
- Exercise treadmill ABI is useful in patients who are symptomatic but have normal resting ABI.

Follow-Up Tests & Special Considerations

Most patients with PAD should be screened for abdominal aortic aneurysm (AAA) due to the high prevalence in such patients.

Diagnostic Procedures/Other

For ABI results other than 0.9 to 1.4 (2)[C]:

- Duplex ultrasound: noninvasive, cost-effective; complements history, physical, and ABI screening diagnosis; used for surveillance after endovascular/surgical procedures.
- Magnetic resonance angiography (MRA) and computed tomography angiography (CTA): determination of sites of occlusion and assess candidates for revascularization procedures
- Catheter-based angiography: limited to those receiving Percutaneous/endovascular (EVR) (see below) (1)
- Contraindications to MRA and CTA: CKD, implantable electronic devices (pacemakers), cochlear implants, metallic clips, or foreign bodies

Test Interpretation

See Surgery (below)

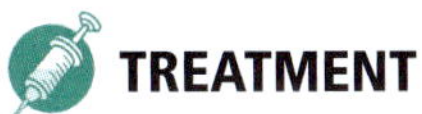

TREATMENT

GENERAL MEASURES

- Treatment goals:
  - Improve function, walking ability, and quality of life
  - Lower morbidity and mortality from PAD and associated CVD
- Smoking cessation, structured (supervised/community-based) exercise therapy, lipid-lowering agents, glycemic control, and antihypertensives can delay disease progression and provide symptomatic relief (1)[C]:
  - Exercise therapy: clinician-prescribed walking sessions: 30 to 45 minutes, 2 to 4 times/wk, minimum of 12 weeks
  - HTN: goal BP <130/80, selective use of ACE inhibitors or ARB to reduce major adverse cardiovascular events (MACE)
  - DM: use of GLP-1 agonists and SGLT-2 inhibitors to reduce MACE
  - High-intensity statin therapy to achieve >50% reduction in LDL-C
  - If LDL-C is ≥70 on maximally tolerated statin, reasonable to add PCSK9 inhibitor or ezetimibe.

MEDICATION

First Line

- Statins are recommended by AHA/ACC and AAFP guidelines for all individuals with symptomatic and asymptomatic PAD to LDL goal of at least <100 mg/dL; individualized depending on comorbid conditions.
- Recommendations
  - Patients with symptomatic PAD:
    - Single antiplatelet therapy (aspirin 75 to 325 mg or clopidogrel 75 mg daily) is indicated to reduce the risk of MACE (3)[A].
    - Rivaroxaban (2.5 mg daily) combined with low-dose aspirin is recommended to reduce the risk of MACE or major adverse limb events (MALE). Risk of bleeding is increased, so individualize decision-making (3)[A].
  - Patients who have undergone endovascular or surgical revascularization:
    - Rivaroxaban (2.5 mg daily) combined with low dose aspirin is recommended to reduce the risk of MACE or MALE (3).
  - Full-intensity oral anticoagulations should not be used in patients with PAD who do not have another indication (e.g., atrial fibrillation) to reduce the risk of MACE or MALE.
  - Cilostazol (100 mg orally BID) is recommended to improve leg symptoms and increase walking distance; should not be given to patients with CHF of any severity.
  - It is reasonable to prescribe antiplatelet monotherapy in asymptomatic patients who have an ABI diagnostic of PAD.

ISSUES FOR REFERRAL

See Surgery below

ADDITIONAL THERAPIES

Routine vaccines for age and comorbid conditions, including influenza and COVID-19, preventive foot care education

SURGERY/OTHER PROCEDURES

- Percutaneous/endovascular (EVR) or open surgical (OSR) revascularization should be considered in patients with functionally limiting claudication and an inadequate response to guideline-directed medical therapy; who have a favorable risk-benefit ratio
- Revascularization should not be performed solely to prevent progression of disease (2)[B].
  - EVR: percutaneous luminal balloon angioplasty, atherectomy, stenting (maybe drug-eluting) primarily suitable for aortoiliac and femoropopliteal disease
  - OSR: surgical bypass, endarterectomy—technique suitable for lesions at bifurcations and distal sites
  - Choice of EVR or OSR is highly individualized and based on the historical course of the disease, subspecialist availability, previous failed interventions, site(s) of artery obstruction, anesthetic risk, extent of tissue loss, severity of comorbid conditions, life expectancy, and durability of the intervention

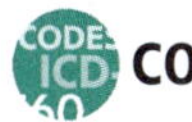

ONGOING CARE

FOLLOW-UP RECOMMENDATIONS

- Best outcomes: multispecialty PAD care team (primary care physician, podiatrist, vascular and wound care specialists, structured exercise therapists) focused on comprehensively addressing risk factor management, pharmacologic reconciliation and compliance, foot care, and early diagnosis of disease progression (2)
- All PAD patient should be seen at least twice a year for evaluation with history, exam, ABI, and determination of disease progression or emergence of new PAD risk factors
- Revascularization patients should be seen within 30 days of procedure and quarterly for assessment of symptoms with ABI and ultrasound surveillance.

DIET

Heart-healthy DASH or Mediterranean diet

PATIENT EDUCATION

Symptoms of progressive disease, preventive foot care, control of glucose, lipids, blood pressure

PROGNOSIS

- Limb ischemia and IC: 15–20% will have worsening claudication, 5–10% will require endovascular or surgical intervention, and 2–5% will undergo amputation (most commonly smokers and diabetics).
- At 5 years, 20% of patients with PAD will experience a nonfatal cardiovascular event, and 15–20% will die, most commonly of cardiovascular disease.

COMPLICATIONS

Amputations, diminished physical activity, increased functional impairment, poor quality of life

REFERENCES

1. Criqui MH, Matsushita K, Aboyans V, et al; for American Heart Association Council on Epidemiology and Prevention, Council on Arteriosclerosis, Thrombosis and Vascular Biology, Council on Cardiovascular Radiology and Intervention, Council on Lifestyle and Cardiometabolic Health, Council on Peripheral Vascular Disease, and Stroke Council. Lower extremity peripheral artery disease: contemporary epidemiology, management gaps, and future directions: a scientific statement from the American Heart Association. *Circulation*. 2021;144(9):e171–e191.
2. Parwani D, Ahmed MA, Mahawar A, et al. Peripheral arterial disease: a narrative review. *Cureus*. 2023;15(6):e40267.
3. Willems LH, Maas DPMSM, Kramers K, et al. Antithrombotic therapy for symptomatic peripheral arterial disease: a systematic review and network meta-analysis. *Drugs*. 2022;82(12):1287–1302.

CODES

ICD10

- I73.9 Peripheral vascular disease, unspecified
- I70.209 Unsp athscl native arteries of extremities, unsp extremity
- I70.219 Athscl native arteries of extrm w intrmt claud, unsp extrm

CLINICAL PEARLS

- PAD is significantly underdiagnosed; ABI testing should be available and is a best practice in all primary care offices for those with symptoms and those at high risk
- 70% of nontraumatic lower extremity amputations in the United States occur in diabetics (2).

PERITONITIS, ACUTE

Marie L. Borum, MD, EdD, MPH • Susie J. Park, MD

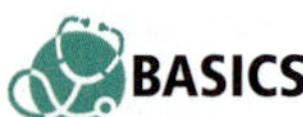

BASICS

DESCRIPTION

- Definition: inflammation of the peritoneum
- Classification:
  - Aseptic: chemical irritation or systemic inflammation of peritoneum
  - Bacterial: infection of peritoneal fluid
- Bacterial peritonitis types:
  - Primary/spontaneous bacterial peritonitis (SBP): infection of ascitic fluid without an identifiable intra-abdominal source
  - Secondary bacterial peritonitis: infection of ascitic fluid from a detectable intra-abdominal source
    - Secondary bacterial peritonitis can be further classified as either perforation peritonitis or nonperforation peritonitis.
  - Tertiary bacterial peritonitis: >48 hours of infection despite source control
  - Peritoneal dialysis–associated (PD) peritonitis

EPIDEMIOLOGY

Incidence

Annual incidence of SBP is around 1/3 in hospitalized patients with cirrhosis (1).

Prevalence

- In asymptomatic patients with cirrhosis and ascites, the outpatient prevalence of SBP is low.
- In patients with cirrhosis and ascites, 5% of peritonitis is secondary.
- Secondary peritonitis is the most common cause of sepsis in surgical ICU.

ETIOLOGY AND PATHOPHYSIOLOGY

- Mechanism
  - SBP:
    - Bacterial translocation via lymphatic spread through mesenteric lymph nodes
    - Often develops in the setting of large-volume ascites with advanced cirrhosis
    - Cirrhotic patients have:
      - Alterations to gut microbiota with higher prevalence of pathogenic organisms
      - Small intestinal bacterial overgrowth and increased intestinal mucosal permeability to bacteria
      - Decreased cellular and humoral immunity limiting peritoneal bacterial clearance
  - Secondary:
    - Introduction of bacteria from inflamed or perforated intraperitoneal (IP) organs or through instrumentation
  - Tertiary: evolves from secondary peritonitis
  - PD peritonitis:
    - Contamination with skin flora during exchanges or exit-site infection
- Microbiology
  - Most cases of SBP are monomicrobial.
    - Most common gram-negative pathogens are *Escherichia coli* and *Klebsiella* spp.
    - Most common gram-positive pathogens are *Streptococcus* and *Staphylococcus* spp.
  - Secondary: Organism depends on cause of peritonitis; gram-positive organisms more common with upper GI pathology, whereas gram-negative organisms more common with lower GI pathology. Common species include *E. coli*, *Klebsiella*, *Proteus*, *Streptococcus*, *Enterococcus*, *Bacteroides*, and *Clostridium* (1).
  - PD peritonitis is most commonly due to *Staphylococcus epidermidis* and *S. aureus* (2).

RISK FACTORS

- SBP: advanced cirrhosis with ascites, malnutrition, variceal hemorrhage, acid-suppressive therapy, and prior SBP (1)
  - Acid suppression (most commonly with PPIs) promotes gut bacterial growth and translocation.
  - 70% of SBP cases are in patients with Child-Pugh class C cirrhosis.
  - Low ascites protein (<1 g/dL) increases risk.
- Secondary: perforated peptic ulcers, mesenteric ischemia causing bowel necrosis, severe pancreatitis, trauma, or IBD causing bowel perforation
- PD peritonitis:
  - Nonsterile technique
  - Recent instrumentation

GENERAL PREVENTION

- SBP prophylaxis decreases mortality in patients at high risk (e.g., ascitic fluid protein concentration <1 g/dL, esophageal varices, or history of previous SBP).
  - Primary prophylaxis: antibiotics including norfloxacin, ciprofloxacin, trimethoprim-sulfamethoxazole
  - Patients with cirrhotic ascites who have low ascitic fluid protein (<1.5 g/dL), renal impairment (creatinine ≥1.2 mg/dL, BUN ≥25 mg/dL, serum sodium [Na] ≤130 mEq/L), or liver failure (Child-Pugh score ≥9 and serum bilirubin ≥3 mg/dL) should receive SBP prophylaxis (1).
- Limit use of PPI therapy.
- PD peritonitis:
  - Adherence to sterile technique
  - Antibiotic prophylaxis prior to procedures

COMMONLY ASSOCIATED CONDITIONS

SBP often occurs in the setting of decompensated cirrhosis (3).

DIAGNOSIS

HISTORY

- SBP: history of cirrhosis and/or ascites, fever, chills, mental status changes, abdominal pain (diffuse, continuous; may be subtle due to presence of ascites), nausea/vomiting, diarrhea, GI bleeding
- Secondary: may be clinically indistinguishable from SBP unless history of perforation, abscess, other intra-abdominal pathology, or recent surgical intervention is present
- Tertiary: persistent signs and symptoms despite initial treatment or history of recurrent peritonitis
- PD peritonitis: presumptive diagnosis in PD patients with cloudy effluent (2)

ALERT
Up to 1/3 of patients are asymptomatic (3).

PHYSICAL EXAM

- Tachycardia, tachypnea, altered mental status (can be subtle), hypotension, hyperthermia, or hypothermia
- Abdominal pain and distention, ascites, abdominal wall guarding, rebound tenderness, hypoactive/absent bowel sounds, diarrhea
  - There is no rigidity because ascites separates parietal layer of peritoneum from visceral layer.

DIFFERENTIAL DIAGNOSIS

- Liver disease: hepatitis, decompensated cirrhosis
- Luminal disease: abscess formation, ileus, volvulus, intussusception, mesenteric adenitis, pancreatitis, cholecystitis, malignancy, peritoneal carcinomatosis, IBD
- Extraluminal disease: ruptured ectopic pregnancy, tubo-ovarian abscess, PID, UTI, pyelonephritis
- Systemic disease: tuberculosis, pneumonia, MI, porphyria, SLE

DIAGNOSTIC TESTS & INTERPRETATION

ALERT
Early diagnosis and treatment reduce mortality.

Initial Tests (lab, imaging)

- CBC: leukocytosis, anemia
  - Thrombocytopenia <100,000/mL predicts SBP
- BMP: metabolic acidosis, azotemia
- LFTs, coagulation panel often abnormal at baseline in patients with cirrhosis
- CRP >60 mg/L + cirrhotic ascites is highly specific for SBP (96.5%).
- Secondary: Abdominal x-rays or CT may show free air or source of infection (abscess, perforation, etc.).

Follow-Up Tests & Special Considerations

- Obtain ascites, blood, and urine cultures before antibiotics are given.
- If culture is monomicrobial but PMN <250 cells/mm^3, colonization generally resolves if patient is asymptomatic but generally progresses to SBP if patient is symptomatic (1).
- If culture is polymicrobial but PMN <250 cells/mm^3, cause is likely traumatic paracentesis (1).
- If culture is negative but PMN >250 cells/mm^3, still likely to be SBP and requires broad-spectrum antibiotics (1)
- Alcoholic hepatitis and SBP can occur concurrently.

Diagnostic Procedures/Other

- Most important is diagnostic paracentesis with ascites fluid analysis: culture, Gram stain, cell count with differential, albumin; for secondary peritonitis, include LDH, total protein, glucose, alkaline phosphatase (ALP), and CEA.
- SBP:
  - PMN >250 cells/mm^3 (3)
  - Serum-ascites albumin gradient <1.1 g/dL rules out portal hypertension, making SBP unlikely.
- Secondary peritonitis: PMN >250 cells/mm^3 on ascitic fluid analysis with polymicrobial culture and/or two of the following (Runyon criteria): ascitic fluid total protein >1 g/dL, glucose <50 mg/dL, and LDH > upper limit of normal for serum
  - Effluent amylase level may suggest intra-abdominal pathology (2).

- PD peritonitis:
  - Two of positive effluent culture, consistent clinical features, and peritoneal fluid WBC >100 mm^3 with PMN >50% (2).

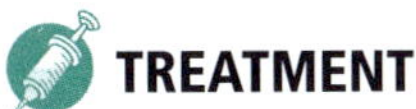

TREATMENT

GENERAL MEASURES

- Control ascites with salt restriction, spironolactone ±, furosemide, albumin infusion after large-volume paracentesis, and/or lactulose for encephalopathy.
- Discontinue β-blockers in SBP in patients who are hypotensive and/or have acute kidney injury (AKI).
- Avoid nephrotoxic medications.

MEDICATION

- SBP
  - First line: If low prevalence of multidrug-resistant organisms (MDRO): 3rd-generation cephalosporins, preferably IV cefotaxime (2 g IV q8h); course typically 5 to 7 days depending on clinical response
  - In absence of previous quinolone use, vomiting, shock, hepatic encephalopathy, or serum creatinine >3 mg/dL: can substitute oral fluoroquinolones (must be renally dosed) for cefotaxime (1)
  - Consider broader coverage if high prevalence of MDRO and/or for critically ill patients (3).
- SBP with renal or hepatic impairment (serum creatinine >1 mg/dL, BUN >30 mg/dL, or total bilirubin >5 mg/dL): Add albumin 1.5 g/kg within 6 hours and 1 g/kg on day 3 to prevent progression of AKI (3).
- If hypotension (MAP <65 mm Hg) or AKI, clinicians should hold nonselective β-blockers
- Reassess patient after 2 days of antibiotic therapy with repeat paracentesis.
  - If <25% decrease in PMN from baseline, indicates lack of response; consider broadening antibiotic coverage and evaluate for secondary bacterial peritonitis.
- Secondary:
  - Empiric broad-spectrum antibiotic coverage for polymicrobial infection; IV cefotaxime (2 g IV q8h) or other 3rd- to 4th-generation cephalosporin plus metronidazole
- Tertiary:
  - If no unrepaired perforations or leaks, continue with medical management: broad-spectrum antibiotics (guided by susceptibilities), early enteral nutrition
  - Consider adding antifungal coverage.
  - Consider removing catheter if recurrent or persistent PD–associated infection (2).
- PD peritonitis:
  - IP route for antibiotics preferred over IV route unless patient is septic.
  - Gram-positive coverage: vancomycin or a 1st-generation cephalosporin (e.g., cefazolin)
  - Gram-negative coverage: 3rd-generation cephalosporin (e.g., ceftazidime, cefepime), an aminoglycoside, or a carbapenem
  - Most patients usually improve within 48 hours of initiation of antibiotic therapy.
    - Clinical improvement, less cloudy efferent, and/or lower cell count in peritoneal fluid all demonstrate infection is resolving.
  - PD does not have to be discontinued (2).
  - Remove catheter if:
    - Fungal or mycobacterial peritonitis
    - Culture-negative peritonitis with persistent symptoms and elevated WBC in peritoneal fluid
    - PD effluent is not clear after a 5-day course of antibiotics (refractory peritonitis).
    - Peritonitis recurrence within 4 weeks of completion of antibiotic course
    - Laparotomy required
- If catheter removed, can be replaced after 2 weeks if symptoms have resolved (2)

SURGERY/OTHER PROCEDURES

- SBP: medical management only (high mortality if patient with SBP receives exploratory laparotomy)
- Secondary: emergent surgical management, including source control with open laparotomy to repair any perforated viscus and remove infected material
- Tertiary: If there are no unrepaired perforations or leaks, additional surgery for severe abdominal infection correlates with deterioration and mortality.

ADMISSION, INPATIENT, AND NURSING CONSIDERATIONS

- Acute peritonitis typically warrants hospitalization.
- In patients with cardiogenic or septic shock, use invasive monitoring with goal-directed fluid therapy.
- Patients who present with peritonitis can be severely hypovolemic, and volume resuscitation is critical.
- Patients with cirrhosis are often on β-blockers. During an episode of SBP, β-blockers can increase mortality, hepatorenal syndrome, and hospital stay.

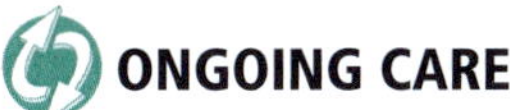

ONGOING CARE

FOLLOW-UP RECOMMENDATIONS

Patient Monitoring

Normalization of vital signs with resolution of leukocytosis is a sign of improvement.

- PMN decrease >25% is expected if repeat paracentesis is performed after 48 hours.

DIET

- NPO, total parental nutrition (TPN) as necessary, especially in secondary peritonitis
- Resume enteral feeding after return of bowel function.
- Sodium restriction can reduce future development of ascites.

PROGNOSIS

- SBP:
  - Mortality is low with prompt diagnosis and treatment.
  - Prognosis improves if antibiotics are started early and prior to onset of shock or renal failure.
  - Renal insufficiency is the strongest negative prognostic indicator.
- Secondary:
  - In-hospital mortality is generally higher with secondary peritonitis than those with SBP.
  - Prognosis is worse in perforation peritonitis (vs. nonperforation peritonitis) and mortality of perforation is high if not treated surgically.
- PD peritonitis
  - 2–6% mortality (highest in fungal, gram-negative, and *S. aureus* infections) (2)

COMPLICATIONS

- Renal and hepatic failure, encephalopathy, coagulopathy, secondary infection, iatrogenic infection, abscess, fistula formation, abdominal compartment syndrome
- Sepsis/septic shock, cardiovascular collapse, adrenal insufficiency, respiratory failure, ARDS
- Complications related to diagnostic paracentesis (e.g., bleeding, infection)

REFERENCES

1. Long B, Gottlieb M. Emergency medicine updates: spontaneous bacterial peritonitis. *Am J Emerg Med*. 2023;70:84–89. doi:10.1016/j.ajem.2023.05.015.
2. Li PK, Chow KM, Cho Y, et al. ISPD peritonitis guideline recommendations: 2022 update on prevention and treatment. *Perit Dial Int*. 2022;42(2):110–153.
3. Biggins SW, Angeli P, Garcia-Tsao G, et al. Diagnosis, evaluation, and management of ascites, spontaneous bacterial peritonitis and hepatorenal syndrome: 2021 practice guidance by the American Association for the study of liver diseases. *Hepatology*. 2021;74(2):1014–1048.

SEE ALSO

Appendicitis, Acute; Cirrhosis of the Liver; Diverticular Disease; Peptic Ulcer Disease

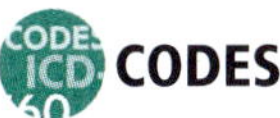

CODES

ICD10

- K65.0 Generalized (acute) peritonitis
- K65.2 Spontaneous bacterial peritonitis
- K65.8 Other peritonitis

CLINICAL PEARLS

- Maintain a high index of suspicion for SBP in cirrhotic patients with ascites and start treatment early.
- SBP is usually monomicrobial. Paracentesis is the gold standard for diagnosis.
- *E. coli* is the most common bacterial isolate from cases of SBP. 3rd-generation cephalosporins are first-line treatment.
- Ascitic fluid analysis stratifies patients at risk for secondary peritonitis who require additional imaging.
- Renal function is an important prognostic indicator for SBP.

PERTUSSIS

Susan McDiarmid, EdD, MS, PA-C • Michelle E. Duffelmeyer, MD

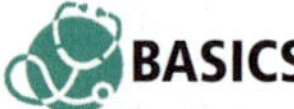

BASICS

- Highly contagious respiratory illness among close contacts
- Synonyms: "whooping cough," "the cough of 100 days"

DESCRIPTION

- Host: humans
- Most common reservoir: adults
- Ages: all
- Distribution: worldwide
- Pattern: endemic or epidemic with outbreaks every 3 to 5 years
- Seasonality: peaks late summer–autumn; can occur year-round
- Transmission: person to person via aerosolized droplets
- Effective vaccine: available
- Immunity: neither 100% nor lifelong immunity with either infection or vaccine
- System(s) affected: respiratory
- Classic clinical manifestations include paroxysmal cough, inspiratory whoop, and posttussive emesis.

EPIDEMIOLOGY

- Caused by *Bordetella pertussis*
- Typical incubation period: 7 to 10 days

Incidence

- United States: per CDC, >10,000 cases (higher than prepandemic levels)
- Incidence decreased during COVID-19 pandemic and now is rising in the United States and worldwide.

ETIOLOGY AND PATHOPHYSIOLOGY

- Toxin mediated
- Infectious process with predilection for ciliated respiratory epithelium
- Common organisms:
  - *B. pertussis*
  - *Bordetella parapertussis*

Genetics

No known genetic predisposition

RISK FACTORS

- Exposure to a confirmed case
- Non- or under-immunized infants and children
- Premature birth
- Chronic lung disease
- Immunodeficiency (e.g., AIDS)
- Obesity and preexisting asthma
- Age <6 months (accounts for ~90% pediatric pertussis hospitalizations)

GENERAL PREVENTION

- Public health measures
  - Surveillance
  - Outbreak management
  - Care of exposed individuals
- Prevention programs
- Immunizations
  - Primary childhood immunization series against pertussis followed by boosters
  - Maternal immunization during each pregnancy
  - Adults, including health care providers in close contact with infants <1 year of age, should be immunized.

Pediatric Considerations

Strategies to reduce neonatal pertussis:

- Tdap with each pregnancy, ideally between 27 and 36 weeks' gestation
- Cocooning
- Tdap recommended for all persons in close contact with infants <1 year of age

Geriatric Considerations

Older adults are at increased risk for pertussis complications due to:

- Age-related changes in immunity
- Comorbid medical conditions

COMMONLY ASSOCIATED CONDITIONS

- Apnea in infants
- Secondary bacterial pneumonia
- Sinusitis
- Seizures
- Encephalopathy
- Urinary incontinence
- Death

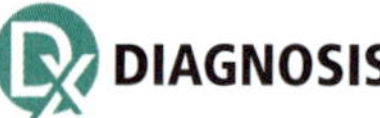

DIAGNOSIS

HISTORY

- Exposure to pertussis
- Insidious onset
- Classic clinical manifestations include paroxysmal cough, inspiratory whoop, and posttussive emesis.
- Incubation period 7 to 10 days (range: 5 to 21 days)

PHYSICAL EXAM

- Classic pertussis has three phases, which occur over 6 to 10 weeks:
  - Catarrhal phase: rhinorrhea, mild cough, and low-grade fever
  - Paroxysmal phase: Cough occurs in bursts, with increased frequency and intensity, often followed by an inspiratory whoop and/or posttussive vomiting.
  - Convalescent phase: Coughing paroxysms decrease in frequency and intensity.
- Classic presentation is more common in adults and unvaccinated children.

ALERT

- In the absence of paroxysms or complications, the physical exam may be normal.
- Infants <6 months of age may have atypical presentations.

DIFFERENTIAL DIAGNOSIS

Sporadic, prolonged cough can also be caused by:

- *B. parapertussis*
- *Mycoplasma pneumoniae*
- *Chlamydia trachomatis*
- *Chlamydophila pneumoniae*
- *Bordetella bronchiseptica*
- *Bordetella holmesii*
- Respiratory syncytial virus
- Adenovirus

DIAGNOSTIC TESTS & INTERPRETATION

Initial Tests (lab, imaging)

- Nasopharyngeal culture (gold standard): best results within 2 weeks of cough onset
- False results can occur in:
  - Previously immunized individuals
  - After initiation of appropriate antibiotic
  - After 2 weeks from cough onset
  - With incorrect collection or handling
- Polymerase chain reaction (PCR) assays: rapid turn-around time; good within first 3 weeks
- Serology:
  - Commercially available assay
  - Not FDA-approved for diagnosis

Follow-Up Tests & Special Considerations

- Evaluation and follow-up for associated conditions and complications
- Chest radiograph (two views) to evaluate for the presence of pneumonia
- EEG/neuroimaging may be considered in infant with seizure or apparent life-threatening events (ALTEs).
- Infants <1 month of age who are treated with macrolides should be monitored for the possible development of hypertrophic pyloric stenosis.

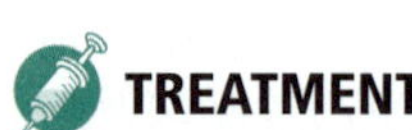

TREATMENT

GENERAL MEASURES

- Hospitalization with continuous cardiopulmonary monitoring is recommended for neonates with pertussis.
- Supplemental oxygen and/or mechanical ventilatory support may be needed.

MEDICATION

- Start empiric antibiotic therapy once diagnostic testing is performed in cases with strong clinical suspicion or in those at high risk for complications.
- Antibiotic therapy after cough is established may help to limit spread but is not expected to change clinical symptoms.
- Preferred antibiotics:
  - For patients >6 months:
    - Azithromycin, clarithromycin, or erythromycin
    - Alternative agent is trimethoprim/sulfamethoxazole (TMP/SMX) (Bactrim).
  - For infants <1 month of age, azithromycin is preferred but with caution.

First Line

Azithromycin is the first line for treatment and for postexposure prophylaxis (5-day course).

ALERT

- Infantile hypertrophic pyloric stenosis has been associated with the use of macrolides in infants <1 month of age.
- Consultation and monitoring are recommended.

ALERT

- *Fatal cardiac dysrhythmias* have been reported with azithromycin.
- Caution is recommended in individuals with prolonged QT and proarrhythmic conditions.

Second Line

TMP/SMX (for persons >2 months of age) if:

- Macrolide intolerance
- Macrolide resistance

ALERT

- TMP/SMX is *contraindicated* in infants <2 months of age.
- Clarithromycin is not recommended in infants <1 month of age.

ISSUES FOR REFERRAL

Evaluation and treatment of infants <6 months of age, especially those born prematurely, who are unimmunized and those who require hospitalization

ADDITIONAL THERAPIES

Symptomatic treatment of the cough in pertussis (e.g., corticosteroids, β_2-adrenergic agonists) has not shown benefit.

ADMISSION, INPATIENT, AND NURSING CONSIDERATIONS

- In infants, considerations for hospitalization include respiratory distress, evidence of pneumonia, inability to feed, cyanosis, apnea, seizures, and age <4 months.
- Small, frequent meals may be necessary to ensure adequate nutrition.
- IV fluids indicated for dehydration and when oral fluids are either contraindicated or poorly tolerated
- In addition to standard precautions, hospitalized patients should be isolated with respiratory precautions for 5 days after the initiation of effective antibiotic treatment and for 3 weeks after the onset of paroxysms in older patients if antibiotics are not used.
- Gentle suctioning of nasal secretions
- Avoid stimuli that trigger paroxysms.
- Respiratory monitoring, including pulse oximetry
- Educate each family about the importance of immunization.
- Discuss chemoprophylaxis with each family.

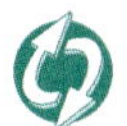

ONGOING CARE

FOLLOW-UP RECOMMENDATIONS

- Monitor infants who received erythromycin ethylsuccinate or azithromycin for hypotrophic pyloric stenosis.
- Neurologic and/or pulmonary follow-up as necessary

Patient Monitoring

ICU care may be necessary for severely ill or compromised patients.

DIET

IV fluids/nutrition may be required to treat dehydration or supplement poor oral intake.

PATIENT EDUCATION

- American Academy of Pediatrics: https://www.aap.org
- Centers for Disease Control and Prevention: https://www.cdc.gov/pertussis/index.html

PROGNOSIS

- Complete recovery in most cases
- Most severe morbidity and highest mortality in infants <6 months of age
- Worldwide overall mortality estimated at 160,799 deaths/year

COMPLICATIONS

- Highest and most severe in infants; may include apnea, cyanosis, and sudden death
- In children: may include conjunctival hemorrhage, inguinal hernia, pneumonia, and seizures
- More frequent in adults than adolescents: may include sinusitis, otitis media, pneumonia, weight loss, fainting, rib fracture, urinary incontinence, seizures, and encephalopathy

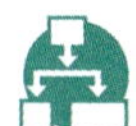

SEE ALSO

Centers for Disease Control and Prevention. Pertussis Surveillance and Trends. https://www.cdc.gov/pertussis/php/surveillance/index.html

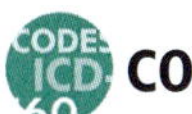

CODES

ICD10

- A37.10 Whooping cough due to Bordetella parapertussis without pneumonia
- A37 Whooping cough
- A37.91 Whooping cough, unspecified species with pneumonia

CLINICAL PEARLS

- Classic clinical manifestations include paroxysmal cough, inspiratory whoop, and posttussive emesis.
- Hospitalizations for pertussis is highest in infants <4 months of age.
  - Maternal Tdap is effective in protecting young infants against pertussis, especially during first 2 months of life.
- Neither immunization nor active infection confers lifelong immunity.

PHARYNGITIS

Munima Nasir, MD, FAAFP • Makayla B. Lagerman, MD

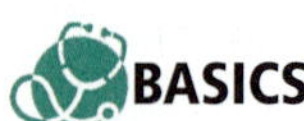

BASICS

DESCRIPTION

- Acute or chronic inflammation of the pharyngeal mucosa
- Group A *Streptococcus* (GAS) pharyngitis is notable for preventable suppurative (e.g., retropharyngeal or peritonsillar abscess) and nonsuppurative (e.g., rheumatic sequelae) complications
- Synonyms: sore throat; tonsillitis; "strep throat"

EPIDEMIOLOGY

- 1–2% of all outpatient and 6% of all pediatric visits to primary care physicians
- ~50% of cases of acute pharyngitis occur <18 years of age, and incidence declines in adults after 40 years of age
  - Low likelihood at <3-years-old
- Most commonly viral (50–80% of cases)
- GAS is the most common bacterial cause of acute pharyngitis, accounting for 15–30% of pediatric cases (with peak incidence in 7 to 8 year olds) and 5–15% of adult cases
- Less common causes of pharyngitis include *Fusobacterium necrophorum*, non-GAS, and *Neisseria gonorrhoeae* if sexually active.
- Rheumatic fever is a serious sequela but is rare in the United States (<1 case per 100,000). Early antibiotic use has reduced occurrence.
- 3,000 to 4,000 patients with GAS must be treated to prevent one case of acute rheumatic fever.

Pediatric Considerations

The highest incidence of rheumatic fever is in children 5 to 18 years old as a rare sequela of streptococcal pharyngitis.

ETIOLOGY AND PATHOPHYSIOLOGY

- Acute, viral
  - Most common pathogens: rhinovirus; adenovirus; coronavirus; enterovirus; influenza; parainfluenza virus; coxsackievirus; respiratory syncytial virus
  - Less common pathogens: herpes simplex virus; Epstein-Barr virus (EBV); cytomegalovirus (CMV); HIV
- Acute, bacterial (associated with higher fevers)
  - Group A, C, or G Streptococcus
  - *N. gonorrhoeae*; *Corynebacterium diphtheriae* (diphtheria); *Haemophilus influenzae*
  - *Moraxella catarrhalis*; *Chlamydia pneumoniae*
  - *Fusobacterium necrophorum* (20% young adult cases)
  - *Arcanobacterium haemolyticum*; *Mycoplasma pneumoniae*; *Francisella tularensis* (tularemia)
- Acute, noninfectious
  - May be caustic, mechanical, or trauma-related
- Chronic, more likely noninfectious
  - Allergic rhinitis
  - Gastroesophageal reflux disease (GERD)
  - Smoking or smoke exposure
  - Dry air exposure
  - Vocal strain
  - Medication side effects
  - Neoplasms
  - Vasculitis
  - Radiation

Genetics

Patients with family history of rheumatic fever have a higher risk of rheumatic sequelae following an untreated GAS infection.

RISK FACTORS

- Epidemics of GAS
- Cold season (late fall through early spring)
- Age (rheumatic fever possible, especially in children/adolescents 5 to 15 years)
- Close contact with infected people
- Immunosuppression
- Smoking or smoke exposure
- Allergic rhinitis
- GERD
- Oral sex
- Recent illness
- Chronic colonization of bacteria in tonsils/adenoids

GENERAL PREVENTION

- Avoid close contact with infectious people.
- Wash hands frequently.
- Vaccinations
- Avoid smoking or secondhand smoke.
- Manage preventable causes (e.g., GERD, allergic rhinitis).

DIAGNOSIS

Diagnosis is clinical, but suspicion for bacterial cause may warrant testing based on prediction rules.

HISTORY

- Sore throat
- Cough, coryza, and hoarseness (associated with viral infections)
- Dysphagia/odynophagia
- Rhinorrhea
- Fever
- Anorexia
- Chills
- Malaise; fatigue
- Headache
- Dysuria and arthralgias (suggesting gonococcal etiology)
- Sick contacts with similar symptoms or confirmed diagnosis

PHYSICAL EXAM

- Enlarged tonsils with or without exudate
- Pharyngeal erythema; palatal petechiae
- Cervical adenopathy (anterior suggestive of GAS, posterior associated with infectious mononucleosis)
- Fever (higher in bacterial infections)
- More concerning findings
  - Unilateral tonsillar swelling or uvular deviation (concern for peritonsillar abscess)
  - Trismus; stridor; drooling (concern for peritonsillar/retropharyngeal abscess or epiglottitis)
  - Neck stiffness or pain with neck extension (concerning for retropharyngeal abscess)
- Associations with specific infections
  - Pharyngeal ulcers (CMV, HIV, Crohn, other autoimmune vasculitides)
  - Punctate erythematous macules with reddened flexor creases and circumoral pallor (Scarlet fever—GAS)
  - Gray oral pseudomembrane suggests diphtheria or infectious mononucleosis (EBV/CMV).
  - Characteristic erythematous-based clear vesicles (HSV or coxsackie A virus)
  - Conjunctivitis (adenovirus)
  - Hepatomegaly (EBV/CMV)

DIFFERENTIAL DIAGNOSIS

- Viral infection, including acute HIV, EBV, and CMV
- Streptococcal infection
- Allergic rhinitis
- GERD
- Malignancy (lymphoma, squamous cell carcinoma)
- Irritants/chemicals (detergent/caustic ingestion)
- Atypical bacterial (e.g., gonococcal, chlamydial, syphilis, pertussis, diphtheria)
- Oral candidiasis (patients typically complain of dysphagia)
- Thyroiditis (can be painful or painless, possibly associated with hyperthyroid syndrome)
- Epiglottitis (associated with stridor, drooling, and respiratory distress)
- Referral from extrapharyngeal source (e.g., otitis media, dental abscess)
- Foreign body

DIAGNOSTIC TESTS & INTERPRETATION

- Prediction rules determine need for further testing (see below).
- Testing is generally not needed with overt viral clinical features (e.g., cough, rhinorrhea, hoarseness, oral ulcers)
- Avoid testing for GAS pharyngitis in children <3 years old as acute rheumatic flare is rare, unless there is a close sick contact who is GAS-positive.
- Modified Centor (McIsaac) clinical prediction rule for GAS infection:
  - +1 point: tonsillar exudates or swelling
  - +1 point: tender anterior chain cervical adenopathy
  - +1 point: absence of cough
  - +1 point: fever by history
  - +1 point: age <15 years
  - 0 point: age 15 to 44 years
  - −1 point: age >44 years
- Scoring:
  - 4 points: positive predictive value ~80%; treat empirically
  - 2 to 3 points: positive predictive value ~50%, rapid strep antigen; treat if GAS-positive
  - 0 or 1 point: positive predictive value <20%; do not test; treat symptomatically with follow-up as needed.

Initial Tests (lab, imaging)

- Testing is usually for GAS, as clinical features do not reliably discriminate between GAS and viral etiologies. Options include:
  - Rapid antigen detection test (RADT); quick adjunct to throat culture with 96% specificity and 86% sensitivity (1)[A]
    - Not needed for individuals scoring as low-risk with validated clinical decision-making tool

– Blood agar throat culture; gold standard (90–95% sensitivity) (1)[A]
  - Not needed for adults with negative RADT but recommended for children with negative RADT due to the higher likelihood of complications
– Antistreptolysin O is not recommended for diagnosis.
- Other tests if history suggests a different diagnosis:
  – NAAT (*N. gonorrhoeae*)
  – Viral cultures (HSV)
  – Monospot (EBV)
  – IgM serology (CMV)
  – HIV viral load
- Imaging may be indicated if sequelae of pharyngitis such as retropharyngeal abscess are suspected.

Follow-Up Tests & Special Considerations
- Assess for signs of severe infection, such as muffled voice, stridor, or respiratory distress as this may indicate impending airway compromise requiring immediate stabilization or transfer to higher level of care.
- Recurrent GAS infection may indicate β-lactamase production by host and may require anti-β-lactamase therapy.

Test Interpretation
Bacitracin disk sensitivity of hemolytic colonies suggests GAS

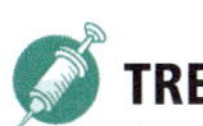

TREATMENT

Treatment is aimed at symptomatic relief, unless bacterial infection is suspected or confirmed.

GENERAL MEASURES
Conservative therapy recommended for viral cases:
- Salt water gargles
- Acetaminophen 10 to 15 mg/kg/dose q4h PRN (pediatric); in adults, do not exceed >4 g/day
- Nonsteroidal anti-inflammatory drugs (NSAIDs) are more effective than acetaminophen for GAS pharyngitis.
- Although not generally recommended, a single dose of steroids may hasten pain relief for patients aged >5 years.
- Anesthetic lozenges
- Cool-mist humidifier
- Hydration (PO or IV if PO is not tolerated)
- Viscous lidocaine (2%) 5 to 10 mL PO q4h swish/spit (severe pain)

Pediatric Considerations
Lower threshold to start antibiotics given higher risk of rheumatic fever

MEDICATION
- Antibiotics are used primarily to prevent complications of GAS.
  – 60–70% primary care visits by children with pharyngitis result in antibiotic prescriptions, contributing to antibiotic overuse (2)
  – Antibiotics minimally reduce risk of poststreptococcal glomerulonephritis
  – Antibiotics shorten symptom duration by ~16 hours.
  – Antibiotics may prevent pharyngitis/fever by day 3 (NNT 4 if GAS-positive, 6.5 if GAS-negative, 14.4 if untested).
- Corticosteroids, when used with antibiotics, may provide a small reduction in the duration of symptoms (24 hours); routine use is not currently recommended (1)[B]

First Line
Recommended first-line antibiotic therapies for GAS include:
- Penicillin V: children (<27 kg): 250 mg PO TID (BID dosing sufficient if compliant); adolescents and adults (>27 kg): 250 mg PO QID or 500 mg PO BID for 10 days
- Penicillin G benzathine: children <60 lb (27 kg): 600,000 units IM 1 dose; children ≥60 lb and adults: 1.2 million units IM 1 dose
- Amoxicillin: 50 mg/kg PO once daily (max 1,000 mg/dose) or 25 mg/kg PO BID (max = 500 mg/dose) for 10 days
  – Use with caution if unclear diagnosis as using amoxicillin with EBV infection may induce rash.
- In patients who need oral liquids, oral amoxicillin is usually preferred over penicillin.

Second Line
- If type IV hypersensitivity without anaphylactic penicillin allergy:
  – Cephalexin 20 mg/kg PO BID or (children) 25 to 50 mg/kg/day divided BID or (adults) 1,000 mg PO QID (max = 4 g/day) for 10 days
  – Cefadroxil 30 mg/kg PO once daily (max = 1 g/day) for 10 days
- If history of anaphylactic penicillin allergy (type I hypersensitivity):
  – Azithromycin 12 mg/kg PO once daily (max = 500 mg/dose), then 6 mg/kg (max = 250 mg/dose) once daily for 4 days after
  – Clarithromycin 7.5 mg/kg PO BID (max = 250 mg/dose) or (adults) 250 to 500 mg PO BID for 10 days
  – Clindamycin 7 mg/kg PO TID (max = 300 mg/dose) or (children) 10 to 30 mg/kg/day PO divided TID–QID or (adults) 150 to 450 mg PO TID–QID for 10 days
- Penicillin is most commonly used to prevent rheumatic sequelae; cephalosporins have a lower rate of failure for streptococcal pharyngitis.
- For children with lab-confirmed recurrence of GAS pharyngitis, treatment can include a previously used agent.

ISSUES FOR REFERRAL
- Document GAS-confirmed episodes to support need for future tonsillectomy/adenoidectomy.
- Tonsillectomy is recommended for those who have had ≥7 throat infections in 1 year, ≥5 infections/year for the past 2 years, or ≥3 infections/year for the past 3 years
  – Tonsillectomy is also recommended in patients who are difficult to treat medically, such as those with allergies to many antibiotics or history of peritonsillar abscess.

ONGOING CARE

FOLLOW-UP RECOMMENDATIONS
- Follow-up culture is not recommended.
- If symptoms worsen or persist >5 days, consider peritonsillar abscess.

DIET
As tolerated; ice, tea, soups, and honey may be used for symptom relief with adequate fluid intake.

PROGNOSIS
- Acute viral and bacterial infections are typically self-limited to 5 to 7 days.
  – GAS symptoms resolve without treatment, but rheumatic complications are still possible.
- Treatment failures (symptoms >10 days) may be due to antibiotic resistance, poor compliance, or untreated contacts.
  – Without confounding factors, prolonged symptoms should prompt workup for alternative cause.

COMPLICATIONS
- Rheumatic fever (e.g., carditis, valve disease, arthritis)
- Poststreptococcal glomerulonephritis
- Peritonsillar abscess: considered a clinical diagnosis and does not warrant imaging
  – Generally requires percutaneous/transoral drainage
  – Treatment may involve tonsillectomy, but most sources recommend resolution of infection before surgery.
- Acute airway compromise can often be bypassed with nasal trumpets; consult anesthesiologist/otolaryngologist.
- Repeated positive GAS tests may represent a chronic carrier of GAS. Antibiotics to treat GAS carriage is not recommended as risk of complications and transmission is low.

REFERENCES

1. Sauve L, Forrester AM, Top KA. Group A streptococcal pharyngitis: a practical guide to diagnosis and treatment. *Paediatr Child Health*. 2021;26(5):319–320.
2. Hamilton JL, Mccrea L. Streptococcal pharyngitis: rapid evidence review. *Am Fam Physician*. 2024;109(4):343–349.

ADDITIONAL READING

Miller JM, Binnicker MJ, Campbell S, et al. Guide to utilization of the microbiology laboratory for diagnosis of infectious diseases: 2024 update by the Infectious Diseases Society of America (IDSA) and the American Society for Microbiology (ASM). *Clin Infect Dis*. 2024:ciae104. doi:10.1093/cid/ciae104.

SEE ALSO

- Herpes Simplex; Infectious Mononucleosis, Epstein-Barr Virus Infections; Rheumatic Fever
- Algorithm: Pharyngitis

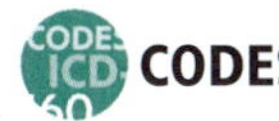

CODES

ICD10
- J31.1 Chronic nasopharyngitis
- A54.5 Gonococcal pharyngitis
- B08.5 Enteroviral vesicular pharyngitis

CLINICAL PEARLS

- Most cases of pharyngitis are viral and do not require antibiotics.
- The risk associated with undiagnosed and untreated GAS is rheumatic sequelae.
- The Modified Centor score helps guide testing and treatment.
- Penicillin is the preferred first-line therapy for GAS infection, children may prefer amoxicillin for adherence.

PILONIDAL DISEASE

Tam T. Nguyen, MD

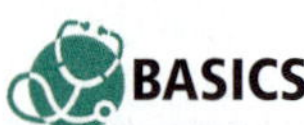

BASICS

DESCRIPTION

- Pilonidal disease results from an abscess, or sinus tract, in the upper part of the natal (gluteal) cleft.
- Synonym(s): jeep disease

EPIDEMIOLOGY

Incidence

- 16 to 26/100,000 per year
- Predominant sex: male > female (3 to 4:1)
- Predominant age: 2nd to 3rd decade, rare in age >45 years
- Ethnic/racial consideration: White > Black > Asian

Prevalence

Surgical procedures show male:female ratio of 4:1, yet incidence data are 10:1.

ETIOLOGY AND PATHOPHYSIOLOGY

Pilonidal means "nest of hair"; hair in the natal cleft allows hair to be drawn into the deeper tissues via negative pressure caused by movement of the buttocks (50%); follicular occlusion from stretching and blocking of pores with debris (50%) creating a pilonidal cyst

- Inflammation of SC gluteal tissues with secondary infection and sinus tract formation
- Polymicrobial, likely from enteric pathogens given proximity to anorectal contamination

Genetics

- Congenital dimple in the natal cleft/spina bifida occulta
- Follicular-occluding tetrad: acne conglobata, dissecting cellulitis, hidradenitis suppurativa, pilonidal

RISK FACTORS

- Sedentary/prolonged sitting
- Excessive body hair
- Obesity/increased sacrococcygeal fold thickness
- Congenital natal dimple
- Trauma to coccyx

GENERAL PREVENTION

- Weight loss
- Trim hair in/around gluteal cleft weekly.
- Hygiene
- Ingrown hair prevention/follicle unblocking

COMMONLY ASSOCIATED CONDITIONS

Obesity, hirsutism, and sedentary lifestyle

DIAGNOSIS

HISTORY

Three distinct clinical presentations

- Asymptomatic: painless cyst or sinus at the top of the gluteal cleft, fever is rare
- Acute abscess: severe pain, swelling, discharge from the top of the gluteal cleft that may or may not have drained spontaneously
- Chronic abscess: persistent drainage from a sinus tract at the top of the gluteal cleft

PHYSICAL EXAM

- Common: inflamed cystic mass at the top of the gluteal cleft with limited surrounding erythema ± drainage or a sinus tract
- Inflamed sinus accompanied by ≥1 pits with or without hair debris
- Less common: significant cellulitis of the surrounding tissues near the gluteal cleft

DIFFERENTIAL DIAGNOSIS

- Furunculosis or folliculitis
- Hidradenitis suppurativa
- Anal fistula
- Perirectal abscess
- Crohn disease

DIAGNOSTIC TESTS & INTERPRETATION

Generally, no tests are needed because it can be diagnosed clinically.

Initial Tests (lab, imaging)

- Consider CBC and wound culture but generally not necessary for less severe infections.
- Ultrasound or MRI might be considered to differentiate between perirectal abscess and pilonidal disease.

Diagnostic Procedures/Other

Wound culture if infection is suspected

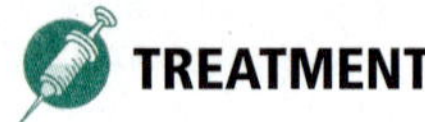

TREATMENT

GENERAL MEASURES

- Shave hair area; remove hair from crypts weekly (1).
- Asymptomatic disease does not need surgical treatment.
- Lifestyle modification with regular exercise and weight loss (1),(2),(3)

MEDICATION

- Antibiotics are not indicated unless there is significant cellulitis.
- If antibiotics are needed, a culture to guide therapy might be useful.
- Cefazolin plus metronidazole or amoxicillin-clavulanate are often used empirically if cellulitis is suspected.
- For penicillin allergy, may consider clindamycin plus a fluoroquinolone.

P

ISSUES FOR REFERRAL
- Patients who cannot comply with frequent dressing changes required after incision and drainage (I&D)
- Patients who have recurrence after I&D
- Patients who have complex disease with multiple sinus tracts

ADDITIONAL THERAPIES
- I&D with only enough packing to allow the cyst to drain; overpacking not indicated
- Antibiotics only if significant cellulitis and abscess; temporizing, not curative
- Negative pressure wound therapy
- Laser epilation of hair in the gluteal fold
- Phenol infusion treatment can be used especially for recurring disease.

SURGERY/OTHER PROCEDURES
- Several surgical techniques have proposed with limited data on superiority of one over another.
- Six levels of care based on severity or recurrence of disease; recent innovations in technique are aimed at expediting healing and minimizing recurrence.
  - I&D, remove hair, curette granulation tissue (3)[C]
  - Excision of midline "pits" allows drainage of lateral sinus tracts (pit picking) (1),(2),(4)[A].
  - Pilonidal cystotomy: Insert probe into sinus tract, excise overlying skin, and close wound.
  - Marsupialization: Excise overlying skin and roof of cyst, and suture skin edges to cyst floor (3).
  - Excision: use of flap closure; no clear benefit for open healing over surgical closure
  - Off-midline surgical excision (cleft lift or modified Karydakis procedure): A systematic review showed a clear benefit in favor of off-midline rather than midline wound closure. When closure of pilonidal sinuses is the desired surgical option, off-midline closure should be the standard management (2),(3),(4)[A].
  - Endoscopic pilonidal sinus treatment (EPSiT): minimally invasive procedure
- Endoscopic treatment such as EPSiT
- Fibrin glue in conjunction with some type of minimally excision

ADMISSION, INPATIENT, AND NURSING CONSIDERATIONS
- Severe cellulitis
- Large area excision

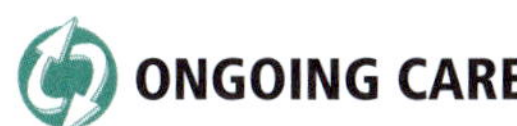

ONGOING CARE

FOLLOW-UP RECOMMENDATIONS
- Frequent dressing changes required after I&D
- Follow-up wound checks to assess for recurrence

Patient Monitoring
Monitor for fever; more extensive cellulitis

PATIENT EDUCATION
- Wash area briskly with washcloth daily.
- Shave the area weekly.
- Remove any embedded hair from the crypt.
- Avoid prolonged sitting.

PROGNOSIS
- Simple I&D has a 55% failure rate; median time to healing is 5 weeks.
- More extensive surgical excisions involve hospital stays and longer time to heal.

COMPLICATIONS
Malignant degeneration is a rare complication of untreated chronic pilonidal disease.

REFERENCES

1. Gil LA, Deans KJ, Minneci PC. Management of pilonidal disease: a review. *JAMA Surg*. 2023;158(8):875–883.
2. Johnson EK, Vogel JD, Cowan ML, et al. The American Society of Colon and Rectal Surgeons' clinical practice guidelines for the management of pilonidal disease. *Dis Colon Rectum*. 2019;62(2):146–157.
3. Humphries AE, Duncan JE. Evaluation and management of pilonidal disease. *Surg Clin North Am*. 2010;90(1):113–124.
4. Bi S, Sun K, Chen S, et al. Surgical procedures in the pilonidal sinus disease: a systematic review and network meta-analysis. *Sci Rep*. 2020;10(1):13720.

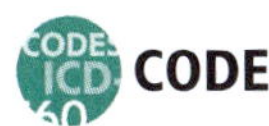

CODES

ICD10
- L05.91 Pilonidal cyst without abscess
- L05.92 Pilonidal sinus without abscess
- L05.01 Pilonidal cyst with abscess

CLINICAL PEARLS
- Avoid prolonged sitting.
- Lose weight.
- Trim hair in gluteal cleft weekly.
- Refer recurring infections for more definitive surgical management.

PINWORMS

Jonathan Edward MacClements, MD, FAAFP

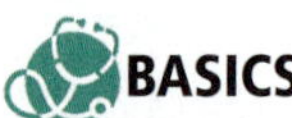

BASICS

DESCRIPTION

- Intestinal infection with *Enterobius vermicularis*
  - Characterized by perineal and perianal itching
  - Usually worse at night
- System(s) affected: gastrointestinal; skin/exocrine
- Synonym(s): enterobiasis

EPIDEMIOLOGY

Predominant age: 5 to 14 years

Prevalence

- Most common helminthic infection in the United States
  - 20 to 42 million people harbor the parasite.
- ~30% of children are infected worldwide.

Pediatric Considerations

More common in children, who are more likely to become reinfected

ETIOLOGY AND PATHOPHYSIOLOGY

- Small white worms (2 to 13 mm) inhabit the cecum, appendix, and adjacent portions of the ascending colon following ingestion; associated with multiple case reports of appendicitis
- Female worms migrate to the perineal areas at night to deposit eggs; this causes local irritation and itching.
- Scratching leads to autoingestion of the eggs and continuation of pinworm's life cycle within the host. Eggs incubate 1 to 2 months in the host small intestine. When mature, female pinworms migrate to the colon where they lay eggs around the anus at night, and the lifecycle continues.
- Infestation by the intestinal nematode *E. vermicularis*

RISK FACTORS

- Institutionalization (prevalence over 50%)
- Crowded living conditions
- Poor hygiene
- Warm climate
- Handling of infected children's clothing or bedding

GENERAL PREVENTION

- Hand hygiene, especially after bowel movements
- Clip and maintain short fingernails.
- Wash anus and genitals at least once a day, preferably during shower.
- Avoid scratching anus and putting fingers near nose (pinworm eggs can also be inhaled) or mouth.

COMMONLY ASSOCIATED CONDITIONS

- Pruritus ani
- Appendicitis

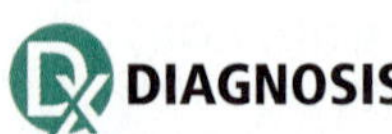

DIAGNOSIS

HISTORY

Many patients are asymptomatic. Common symptoms include the following:

- Perianal or perineal itching
- Vulvovaginitis
- Dysuria
- Abdominal pain (rare)
- Insomnia (typically due to pruritus)

PHYSICAL EXAM

Perineal and perianal exam; particularly in early morning to look for evidence of migrating worms

DIFFERENTIAL DIAGNOSIS

- Idiopathic pruritus ani
- Atopic dermatitis, contact dermatitis
- Psoriasis; lichen planus
- Human papillomavirus (HPV)
- Herpes simplex virus (HSV)
- Fungal infections; erythrasma
- Scabies
- Vaginitis; hemorrhoids
- Chron disease; ulcerative colitis

DIAGNOSTIC TESTS & INTERPRETATION

- Adhesive tape test
  - Place cellophane tape on the perianal skin in the early morning before bathing and affix to a microscope slide to look for pinworm eggs.
  - 90% sensitivity if performed on three consecutive mornings
  - Alternatively, use anal swabs or a pinworm paddle coated with adhesive material.
  - Scrapings from under fingernails of affected individuals can reveal pinworm eggs.
- Digital rectal exam with saline slide preparation of stool on gloved finger
- Stool samples are not helpful.
- *Routine stool examination for ova and parasites is positive in only 10–15% of infected patients.*

Initial Tests (lab, imaging)

Serologic tests are currently not available for diagnosing pinworm infections.

Test Interpretation

Identification of ova on low-power microscopy or direct visualization of the female worm (10-mm long); ova are asymmetric, flat on one side, and measure 56 × 27 μm.

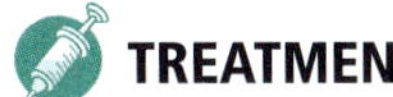

TREATMENT

MEDICATION

First Line

- Treatment options include:
  - Albendazole (Albenza): 400 mg PO as a single dose in adults and children >20 kg; may repeat in 2 weeks; 200 mg PO as a single dose repeated in 2 weeks in children ≤ 20 kg
  - Mebendazole (Emverm, Vermox): chewable 100-mg tablet as a single dose in adults and children >2 years of age; may repeat in 2 to 3 weeks; use with caution in children <2 years of age.
  - Pyrantel pamoate (OTC—Pin-X, Reese Pinworm Medicine): oral liquid or tablet 11 mg/kg as a single dose in adults and children >2 years of age; maximum dose 1 g. Use with caution in children <2 years of age.
- Repeat treatment after 2 weeks is often recommended due to the high frequency of reinfection. Refractory cases may (rarely) require retreatment every 2 weeks for 4 to 6 cycles.
- All symptomatic family members should be treated.

Pregnancy Considerations

Avoid drug therapy in pregnancy as all three drugs are FDA Pregnancy Category C. Treat after delivery but may consider treating in 3rd trimester if infection is compromising the pregnancy. Breastfeeding is allowed during mebendazole therapy.

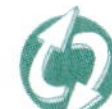

ONGOING CARE

FOLLOW-UP RECOMMENDATIONS

Unnecessary unless symptoms recur after initial therapy

PATIENT EDUCATION

- Take medicine with food.
- Practice good hygiene: handwashing and perianal hygiene; particularly after bowel movements
- Encourage frequent and careful handwashing.
- Clip fingernails.
- Wash clothing and bedding after diagnosis to prevent reinfection. Do not shake linen and clothing before laundering because this may spread the eggs.
- Do not share washcloths.
- Do not allow children to cobathe during treatment and for 2 weeks after treatment; showering is preferred.

PROGNOSIS

- Asymptomatic carriers are common.
- Drug therapy is 90% curative.
- Reinfection is common, especially among children.

COMPLICATIONS

- Perianal scratching may lead to bacterial superinfection.
- Females: vulvovaginitis, urethritis, endometritis, and salpingitis (1)
- UTIs
- Appendicitis
- Rarely: ectopic disease with granulomas of the pelvis, genitourinary tract, and appendix; colonic intussusception (2)

REFERENCES

1. Kang WH, Jee SC. *Enterobius vermicularis* (pinworm) infection. *N Engl J Med*. 2019;381(1):e1. doi:10.1056/NEJMicm1811156.
2. Sousa J, Hawkins R, Shenoy A, et al. Enterobius vermicularis-associated appendicitis: a 22-year case series and comprehensive review of the literature. *J Pediatr Surg*. 2022;57(8):1494–1498. doi: 10.1016/j.jpedsurg.2021.09.038.

ADDITIONAL READING

- Clinical Overview of Pinworm Infections. Centers for Disease Control and Prevention. Updated February 20, 2024. https://www.cdc.gov/pinworm/hcp-clinical/index.html. Accessed June 12, 2025.
- Julien C, Omouri A. Parasite in the appendix. *N Engl J Med*. 2020;383(11):e72.

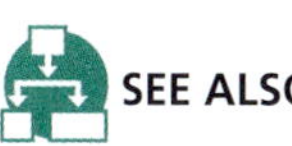

SEE ALSO

Pruritus Ani

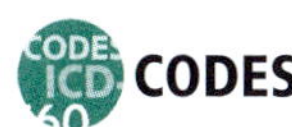

CODES

ICD10

B80 Enterobiasis

CLINICAL PEARLS

- Nocturnal or early morning perianal itch with restless sleep or insomnia (particularly in children) is the hallmark of symptomatic pinworm infection.
- Treatment includes mebendazole, albendazole, or pyrantel pamoate.
- Treat close contacts.
- Retreatment after 2 weeks is generally recommended.

PITUITARY ADENOMA

Anup Sabharwal, MD, MBA, FACC, FACE, FASPC, FNLA, FEAA

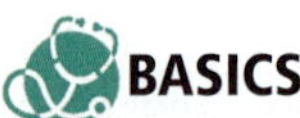

BASICS

DESCRIPTION

Typically benign, slow-growing (noncancerous) tumors that arise from cells in the pituitary gland

- Presenting symptoms include neurologic deficits, visual changes including diplopia, and headaches.
- Subtypes (hormonal): prolactinoma (PRL) 25–40%, nonfunctioning pituitary adenomas 30%, somatotroph adenoma (growth hormone [GH]) 15–20%, corticotroph adenoma (adrenocorticotropic hormone [ACTH]) 5–10%, thyrotroph adenoma (thyroid-stimulating hormone [TSH]) <1%, gonadotropinoma (luteinizing hormone/follicle-stimulating hormone [LH/FSH]), mixed (1)[A]
- Defined as microadenoma <10 mm and macroadenoma ≥10 mm
- May secrete hormones and/or cause mass effects, or visual changes
- Functioning (secreting) adenomas: adenomas that release excess pituitary hormones which can cause certain symptoms and/or conditions depending on the hormone it releases.
- Nonfunctioning (non-secreting) adenomas: adenomas that may not release hormones, but they can impinge or compress adjacent structures if they continue to grow.

EPIDEMIOLOGY

Incidence

- Autopsy studies have found microadenomas in 3–27% and macroadenomas in <0.5% of people without any pituitary disorders.
- Clinically apparent pituitary tumors are seen in 18/100,000 persons.

ETIOLOGY AND PATHOPHYSIOLOGY

- Monoclonal adenohypophysial cell growth
- Hormonal effects of functional microadenomas often prompt diagnosis before mass effect.
- PRL increased by functional PRLs or inhibited dopaminergic suppression by stalk effect

Genetics

Familial isolated pituitary adenomas: ~15% have mutations in the aryl hydrocarbon receptor–interacting protein gene (*AIP*); present at a younger age and are larger in size (2)

RISK FACTORS

Multiple endocrine neoplasias

COMMONLY ASSOCIATED CONDITIONS

- McCune-Albright syndrome
- Multiple endocrine neoplasia type 1 (MEN1)

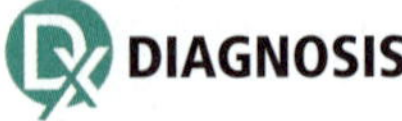

DIAGNOSIS

HISTORY

- Common
  - Hyperprolactinemia: infertility, amenorrhea, galactorrhea, gynecomastia, impotence
  - Headache (sellar expansion)
  - Visual disturbances: bitemporal hemianopsia
- Less common
  - Hypersomatotropinemia: acromegaly (coarse facial features, hand/foot swelling, carpal tunnel syndrome, hyperhidrosis, left ventricular hypertrophy)
  - Hyposomatotropinemia: failure to thrive (FTT) (children), asymptomatic (adults)
  - Intracranial pressure (ICP) elevation: headache, nausea, seizures
  - Hypercorticotropinemia: Cushing disease (supraclavicular/dorsocervical fat pad thickening, moon face, hirsutism, acne, plethora, abdominal striae, centripetal obesity with thin limbs, easy bruising and bleeding, hyperglycemia)
- Rare
  - Apoplexy: headache, sudden collapse
  - Secondary hyperthyroidism: palpitations, diaphoresis, heat intolerance, diarrhea
  - Secondary adrenal insufficiency: weakness, irritability, anorexia, nausea/vomiting
- Hypothalamic compression: temperature, thirst/appetite disorders

PHYSICAL EXAM

- Common
  - Visual disturbances: bitemporal hemianopsia
  - Hyperprolactinemia: hypogonadism, galactorrhea, gynecomastia
  - Hypersomatotropinemia: acromegaly (coarse features, hand/foot swelling, diaphoresis)
  - Hyposomatotropinemia: FTT (children)
- Less common
  - ICP elevation: papilledema, dementia
  - Cushing disease: centripetal obesity, supraclavicular fat pad thickening, moon face, hirsutism, acne
- Rare
  - Apoplexy: hypotension, hypoglycemia, tachycardia, oliguria
  - Secondary hyperthyroidism: tachycardia, tachypnea, diaphoresis, warm/moist skin, tremor
  - Adrenal crisis: orthostatic hypotension
- Hypothalamic compression: temperature dysregulation, obesity, increased urination

DIFFERENTIAL DIAGNOSIS

Pituitary hyperplasia (e.g., pregnancy, primary hypothyroidism, menopause), Rathke cleft cyst, granulomatous disease (e.g., tuberculosis), lymphocytic hypophysitis, metastatic tumor, germinoma, craniopharyngioma

DIAGNOSTIC TESTS & INTERPRETATION

- Somatotrophic (GH secreting: 40 to 130/million)
  - Acromegaly/hypersomatotropinemia: serum IGF-1 elevated; oral glucose tolerance test with GH given at 0, 30, and 60 minutes (normally suppresses GH to <1 g/L)
  - Hyposomatotropinemia: low GH-releasing hormone response
  - Macimorelin is a noninvasive oral test to evaluate for adult GH deficiency (3)[A].
- Corticotropic
  - Cushing disease/hypercorticotropinemia
  - 24-hour urinary-free cortisol >50 μg
  - Overnight low-dose dexamethasone suppression test (DMST): normal free plasma cortisol (FPC) >1.8 μg/dL at 8 AM (after 1 mg given at 11 PM on night prior)
  - ACTH level assay (if DMST results abnormal): <20 pg/mL = adrenal tumor; ≥20 pg/mL = ectopic/pituitary source
  - Hypocorticotropinemia/secondary glucocorticoid deficiency: high-dose corticotropin stimulation test: FPC <10 g/dL at baseline, with an increase of <25% 1 hour after 250 μg; metyrapone test: 11-deoxycortisol <150 ng/L after 2 g given (Prepare to give steroids because test may worsen insufficiency.)
- Gonadotrophic/hypogonadotropism: gonadotropin-releasing hormone stimulation of LH/FSH blunted in pituitary hypergonadism but increased in primary hypogonadism
- Lactotrophic (PRL secreting): hyperprolactinemia: serum PRL >20 ng/mL
- Thyrotrophic (TSH secreting): hyper-/hypothyroidism: TSH and free T_4 both increased for pituitary hyperthyroidism and both decreased for pituitary hypothyroidism.

Initial Tests (lab, imaging)

- A typical panel for asymptomatic tumors: PRL, GH, IGF-1, ACTH, 24-hour urinary-free cortisol or overnight DMST, β-HCG, FSH, LH, TSH, free T_4
- MRI preferred (>90% sensitivity and specificity) after biochemically confirmed
- Octreotide scintigraphy is useful in identifying tumors with somatostatin receptors (4)[B].

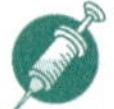

TREATMENT

Medical therapy is primary therapy for prolactinomas and adjunct for other tumors.

MEDICATION

First Line

- Hyperprolactinemia: Dopamine agonists increase dopaminergic suppression of PRL.
  - Cabergoline (Dostinex): D_2 receptor–specific
    - Initial dose: 0.25 mg PO once or twice weekly
    - Maintenance dose: Increase q4wk by 0.25 mg 2 times per week per PRL (max 2 mg/week).
    - Contraindications: hypersensitivity (ergots), uncontrolled hypertension (HTN), pregnancy
    - Precautions: caution with liver impairment
    - Interactions: may be inhibited by tricyclic antidepressants, phenothiazines, opiates
    - Adverse reactions: orthostatic hypotension, vertigo, dyspepsia, hot flashes
  - Bromocriptine (Parlodel): D_2 receptor–specific
    - Initial dose: 1.25 to 2.50 mg PO daily (give with food)
    - Maintenance dose: Increase by 2.5 mg/day q2–7d (max 15 mg/day).
    - Contraindications: hypersensitivity (ergots), uncontrolled HTN, pregnancy; preferred over cabergoline if required
    - Precautions: caution with liver impairment
    - Interactions: may be inhibited by tricyclic antidepressants, phenothiazines, opiates
    - Adverse reactions: orthostatic hypotension, seizures, hallucinations, stroke, myocardial infarction

- Somatotropinoma
  - Long-acting analogues of somatostatin (Sandostatin LAR and lanreotide Autogel)
    - Sandostatin LAR: 20 mg q28d (4)[A]; lanreotide autogel 90 mg q28d; titrate per package insert.
    - Contraindication: hypersensitivity
    - Precautions: caution with biliary, thyroid, cardiac, liver, or kidney disease
    - Interactions: Pimozide increases risk of QT prolongation; variable effects with β-blockers, diuretics, oral glycemic agents
    - Adverse reactions: ascending cholangitis, arrhythmias, congestive heart failure, glycemic instability
    - More effective as adjuvant than as primary treatment for somatotropinomas
    - Consider use of somatostatin analogue or pegvisomant in patients with severe residual disease (4)[A].
    - Consider use of cabergoline in patients with mild residual disease (5)[B].
  - Pegvisomant (Somavert): GH receptor antagonist
    - Initial dose: 40 mg SC × 1, then 10 mg daily and titrate by 5 mg q4–6wks based on IGF-1 levels (max 30 mg/day maintenance dose)
    - Contraindication: hypersensitivity
    - Precautions: caution if GH-secreting tumors, diabetes mellitus, impaired liver function
    - Interactions: NSAIDs, opiates, insulins, oral glycemic agents
    - Adverse reactions: hepatitis, tumor growth, GH secretion
- Corticotropinemia: peripheral inhibitors
  - Mitotane (Lysodren)
    - Initial dose: 2 to 6 g/day divided PO TID (max 19 g/day)
    - Maintenance dose: 2 to 16 g TID
    - Contraindication: hypersensitivity
    - Precautions: caution with liver dysfunction and brain damage
    - Interactions: contraindicated with rotavirus vaccine; caution with other vaccines
    - Adverse reactions: HTN, orthostatic hypotension, hemorrhagic cystitis, rash
  - Ketoconazole
    - Dosing: 200 mg PO TID (max 1,200 mg/day)
    - Contraindications: hypersensitivity, achlorhydria, fungal meningitis, impaired liver function
    - Precautions: caution with liver dysfunction
    - Interactions: contraindicated with dronedarone, methadone, statins, pimozide, sirolimus; caution with other antifungals
    - Adverse reactions: adrenal insufficiency, thrombocytopenia, hepatic failure, hepatotoxicity, anaphylaxis, leukopenia, hemolytic anemia
  - Pasireotide (Signifor)
    - Dosing: initially, 0.6 to 0.9 mg BID and then 0.3 to 0.9 mg BID
    - Contraindication: none
    - Precautions: hypocortisolism, hyperglycemia, bradycardia or QT prolongation, liver test elevations, cholelithiasis, and other pituitary hormone deficiencies
  - Mifepristone (Korlym)
    - Dosing: Administer PO once daily with a meal. The recommended starting dose is 300 mg once daily; not to exceed 600 mg daily in renal impairment
  - Contraindication: pregnancy, use of simvastatin or lovastatin and CYP3A substrates with narrow therapeutic range, concurrent long-term corticosteroid use, women with history of unexplained vaginal bleeding, women with endometrial hyperplasia with atypia or endometrial carcinoma
  - Precautions: adrenal insufficiency, hypokalemia, vaginal bleeding and endometrial changes, QT interval prolongation, use of strong CYP3A inhibitors
  - Interactions: potential interactions with drugs metabolized by CYP3A, CYP2C8/9, CYP2B6, and hormonal contraceptives. Nursing mothers should discontinue drug or discontinue nursing.
- Gonadotropinemia
  - Bromocriptine: See earlier discussion.
- Thyrotropinemia
  - Somatostatin analogues: See earlier discussion.

Second Line

- Corticotropinemia: peripheral inhibitors
  - Metyrapone
    - Dose: 250 mg PO QID
    - Contraindication: porphyria
    - Precautions: caution in liver/thyroid disease
    - Interactions: Dilantin increases metabolism.
    - Adverse reactions: nausea, hypotension
- Gonadotropinemia
  - Octreotide: See earlier discussion.

ISSUES FOR REFERRAL

Neurosurgery consultation for symptomatic tumors (except for PRL)

ADDITIONAL THERAPIES

- Fractionated radiotherapy: often effective as adjunctive when surgery is inadequate (5)[B]
- Stereotactic radiosurgery: alternative to surgery in high-risk patients or as adjunct (5)[B]

SURGERY/OTHER PROCEDURES

Most are now done endoscopically via translabial/transsphenoidal approach (6)[A].

ONGOING CARE

FOLLOW-UP RECOMMENDATIONS

Patient Monitoring

- Follow-up MRIs at 6 and 12 months after surgery
- Involved hormone(s) are followed postoperatively, especially after radiation because hypopituitarism may develop 10 to 15 years after treatment.

PROGNOSIS

Depends on type, size, symptoms, therapy

COMPLICATIONS

- Postoperative diabetes insipidus and/or hypogonadism (usually transient/common)
- Pituitary apoplexy (acute/uncommon): acute hemorrhagic pituitary infarction; adrenal crisis with severe headache; surgical decompression required to prevent shock, coma, and death
- Nelson syndrome (subacute/uncommon): rapid adenoma growth postadrenalectomy
- Pituitary hormone insufficiency (chronic/uncommon): often years after treatment
- Optic nerve neuropathy and brain necrosis after >60 Gy radiotherapy (chronic/rare)

REFERENCES

1. Dworakowska D, Grossman AB. The pathophysiology of pituitary adenomas. *Best Pract Res Clin Endocrinol Metab*. 2009;23(5):525–541.
2. Georgitsi M, Raitila A, Karhu A, et al. Molecular diagnosis of pituitary adenoma predisposition caused by aryl hydrocarbon receptor-interacting protein gene mutations. *Proc Natl Acad Sci U S A*. 2007;104(10):4101–4105.
3. Agrawal V, Garcia JM. The macimorelin-stimulated growth hormone test for adult growth hormone deficiency diagnosis. *Expert Rev Mol Diagn*. 2014;14(6):647–654.
4. Tichomirowa MA, Daly AF, Beckers A. Treatment of pituitary tumors: somatostatin. *Endocrine*. 2005;28(1):93–100.
5. Mondok A, Szeifert GT, Mayer A, et al. Treatment of pituitary tumors: radiation. *Endocrine*. 2005;28(1):77–85.
6. Buchfelder M. Treatment of pituitary tumors: surgery. *Endocrine*. 2005;28(1):67–75.

SEE ALSO

Cushing Disease and Cushing Syndrome; Galactorrhea

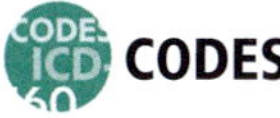

CODES

ICD10

D35.2 Benign neoplasm of pituitary gland

CLINICAL PEARLS

- An incidentaloma is an asymptomatic microadenoma found on imaging. General labs include PRL, GH, IGF-1, ACTH, 24-hour urinary-free cortisol/overnight DMST, β-subunit FSH, LH, TSH, and free T_4. Obtain follow-up MRIs at 6 and 12 months if normal, but consult endocrinology if not.
- Initial treatment selected for symptomatic pituitary adenoma includes a dopamine agonist for PRLs and surgical resection for all others.
- Pituitary apoplexy is a rapid hemorrhagic pituitary infarction due to compression of the blood supply. It is fatal within hours unless surgically decompressed.

PLANTAR FASCIITIS

Krystyna G. Golden, MD • Michael R. McNeely, MD • Blake R. Shaffer, MD

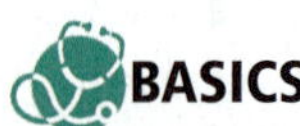

BASICS

DESCRIPTION

- Degenerative change of plantar fascia at origin on medial tuberosity of calcaneus
- Classically presents as pain on plantar surface of foot, usually at calcaneal insertion of plantar fascia, with weight-bearing especially in morning or on initiation of walking after prolonged rest
- Also referred to as: plantar fasciopathy, plantar heel pain syndrome, plantar fasciosis, painful heel syndrome

EPIDEMIOLOGY

Incidence

Estimated 1 million patient visits yearly in the United States

Prevalence

- Most common cause of plantar heel pain
- Lifetime: 10–15% of population; peak incidence between age 40 and 60 years, earlier in runners

ETIOLOGY AND PATHOPHYSIOLOGY

- Plantar fascia is composed of fibrous and dense connective tissue.
  - Three bands: medial, lateral, and central
  - Supports longitudinal plantar arch, assists intrinsic foot musculature, may assist in energy storage
- Repetitive microtrauma and collagen degeneration of plantar fascia
- Chronic degenerative change (-osis/-opathy rather than -itis) of plantar fascia generally at insertion on medial tuberosity of calcaneus

RISK FACTORS

- Intrinsic
  - Age (40 to 60 years)
  - Female, pregnancy
  - Obesity (BMI >30 kg/m^2)
  - Pes planus (flat feet), pes cavus (high arch), overpronation, leg length discrepancy
  - Hamstring, calf, and Achilles tightness
  - Calf and intrinsic foot muscle weakness
  - Decreased ankle range of motion with dorsiflexion (equinus or tight heel cord; <15 degrees of dorsiflexion)
  - Systemic connective tissue disorders
- Extrinsic
  - Dancers, runners, court sport athletes (e.g., tennis, volleyball)
  - Occupations with prolonged standing, especially on hard surfaces (nurses, letter carriers, warehouse/factory workers)
  - Overuse and rapid increase in activities involving repetitive loading

GENERAL PREVENTION

- Maintain normal body weight.
- Avoid training errors (increasing intensity, distance, duration, and frequency of high-impact activities too rapidly); avoid overtraining.
- Proper footwear (appropriate cushion/arch support)
- Runners should replace footwear every 250 to 500 miles.

COMMONLY ASSOCIATED CONDITIONS

- Heel spurs commonly seen but are not a marker of severity nor pathognomonic; surgical removal of unclear benefit
- Posterior tibial neuropathy

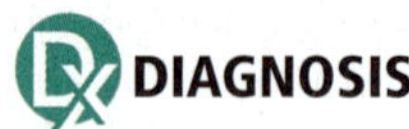

DIAGNOSIS

HISTORY

- Pain on plantar surface of foot, usually at fascial insertion at calcaneus (medial calcaneal tubercle) but can have pain anywhere along length of plantar fascia
- Pain is typically worse with first few steps in the morning or after prolonged rest or standing (poststatic dyskinesia).
- Pain typically improves after first few steps only to recur toward the end of the day or after prolonged ambulation.
- Pain commonly unilateral but can be bilateral in 1/3 of cases
- Pain can be dull and constant in chronic cases.
- Limp with excessive toe walking
- Numbness and burning of medial hindfoot is more suggestive of posterior tibial nerve compression.

PHYSICAL EXAM

- Point tenderness on medial tuberosity of calcaneus at insertion of plantar fascia
- Pain along plantar fascia with dorsiflexion of foot
- Windlass test: Extend MTP while allowing passive flexion of IP joint of hallux—pain indicates a positive test; high specificity, low sensitivity; sensitivity improves (13.5→31.8%) if performed while standing.
- Dorsiflexion-eversion test: pain with dorsiflexion plus eversion of the subtalar joint
- Decreased passive range of motion with dorsiflexion
- Loss of heel fat pad suggests heel fat pad syndrome.
- Point tenderness on posterosuperior aspect of heel suggests Achilles tendinopathy.
- Inability to abduct 5th toe, atrophy to abductor digiti minimi, or positive Phalen maneuver may suggest Baxter nerve entrapment.

DIFFERENTIAL DIAGNOSIS

- Calcaneal stress fracture
- Heel fat pad syndrome (painful or atrophic heel pad)
- Longitudinal arch strain
- Nerve entrapment (posterior tibial nerve—tarsal tunnel syndrome, medial calcaneal branch of posterior tibial nerve, abductor digiti quinti, first branch of the lateral plantar nerve [Baxter nerve])
- Tarsal coalition
- Achilles tendinopathy
- Calcaneal contusion
- Plantar calcaneal bursitis
- Tendonitis of posterior tibialis
- Plantar fascia tear
- S1 radiculopathy
- Adolescents: calcaneal apophysitis (Sever disease)

DIAGNOSTIC TESTS & INTERPRETATION

- Usually not necessary; typically a clinical diagnosis
- Consider applying a navicular sling; improvement confirms pronation induced plantar fasciitis.
- Consider imaging only to rule out other causes or persistent heel pain after 4 to 6 months of conservative therapy.
- Radiographs: two views of foot to evaluate for fracture, tumor, cyst, periostitis, bony erosions; weight-bearing films preferred; calcaneal spurs common but not diagnostic
- Ultrasound: hypoechoic at insertion, thickened plantar fascia ($\geq$4 mm), may additionally see partial thickness tears (1)
- MRI typically only used in recalcitrant cases to evaluate for other soft tissue etiologies.
- CT or technetium-99m bone scan can rule out calcaneal stress fracture and evaluate for infection.
- Nerve conduction studies can rule out nerve entrapment.
- Inflammatory markers: can consider if bilateral heel pain or young patients

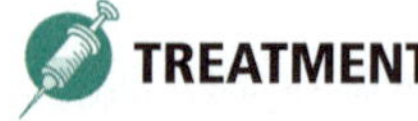

TREATMENT

GENERAL MEASURES

- Weight reduction if BMI >25 kg/m^2
- Intrinsic foot muscle strengthening to stabilize the arch
- Strengthen calf and intrinsic foot muscles, using the towel drag/pickup exercise and barefoot single leg balance.
- Relative rest/activity modification with avoidance of high-impact causative activities

- Stretching: Plantar fascia stretches more effective than Achilles tendon/gastrocnemius-soleus stretches, non–weight-bearing stretches preferable.
- Plantar fascia mobilization done in office and taught to patients.
  - Massage of tibialis anterior (tennis ball) followed by mobilization
  - Foot to inversion; compress tender point while moving foot to eversion; repeat along plantar fascia.
- Ice (frozen water bottle roll) and Massage
- Supportive footwear with stable midfoot or orthoses may be helpful.
  - For relief of acute pain (2 to 3 weeks); continued use may contribute to continued intrinsic muscle weakness.
  - Options include: heel cup, soft heel pad, navicular pad, medial heel wedge, Thomas heel, and night splint (2)
  - Custom orthoses show no benefit over prefabricated orthoses and are more costly.
  - Improved effectiveness of night splints when used in association with orthoses
- Surgical treatment of "heel spurs" is not indicated.

MEDICATION

First Line

- NSAIDs scheduled for 2 to 3 weeks: naproxen 500 mg PO BID *or* ibuprofen 600 to 800 mg PO TID PRN for pain
- Acetaminophen 1,000 mg PO TID PRN for pain

ISSUES FOR REFERRAL

- Physical therapy for patient instruction on proper stretching and strengthening techniques, manipulative treatments (joint and soft tissue mobilization), and massage. For chronic cases, consider analysis of gait and biomechanical factors.
- Podiatry: Consider if conservative measures fail after 3 to 6 months.
- Surgery: Consider if conservative measures fail after 6 to 12 months.

ADDITIONAL THERAPIES

- Corticosteroid injections (CSI)
  - Can provide short-term pain relief
  - Risk for plantar fascia rupture and calcaneal fat pad atrophy with resultant permanent heel pain
- Extracorporeal shock wave therapy (ESWT) (1)
  - Is an effective alternative to CSI in relieving pain and improving function
  - Optimal regimen for ESWT is still undetermined.
- Platelet-rich plasma (PRP) injections (3)
  - More effective than CSI and ESWT in reducing visual analogue scale (VAS) pain
  - Lower risk of complications than CSI but more pain associated with the procedure; consider tibial nerve block prior to PRP and walking boot for comfort after.
- Dextrose prolotherapy (1)
  - Inferior in short term pain relief when compared to corticosteroid injection but may be more effective long term and associated with lower risk of complication
  - Optimal regimen is still undetermined; typically use 2 to 10 mL 15–20% dextrose injectate per procedure.
  - Consider tibial nerve block prior to procedure.
- Botulinum toxin A injections
  - May be a safe and effective treatment option, limited studies comparing efficacy to other injection options
- Radiofrequency thermal lesioning (RTL)
- Low-dye and calcaneal taping
- Short walking cast

SURGERY/OTHER PROCEDURES

- Necessary in <10% of patients; more likely beneficial in severely obese
- Recommended if conservative treatment fails after 6 to 12 months and pain is unrelenting
- Open/endoscopic plantar fasciotomy (less risk and complications with endoscopic technique but requires specialized equipment and skills; not widely used)

COMPLEMENTARY & ALTERNATIVE MEDICINE

Acupuncture may reduce pain in short term but insufficient evidence for the long-term treatment of plantar fascitis.

ONGOING CARE

FOLLOW-UP RECOMMENDATIONS

- Ensure patient adherence to proper stretching technique.
- Following 3 to 6 months of unsuccessful conservative treatment, consider additional therapies or referrals.

PATIENT EDUCATION

- Weight reduction if BMI >25 kg/m^2
- Home plantar fascia mobilization exercises
- Strengthen foot muscles: place a towel on the floor, pull toward yourself with ball of foot and toes without lifting the heel; progressive one-leg standing
- Proper footwear (adequate cushion and arch support)
- Stretch plantar fascia: Pull toes into dorsiflexion prior to walking after prolonged sitting or sleep.
- Ice the foot using a frozen water bottle: Roll foot over bottle for 10 minutes in the morning and after work.
- Decrease repetitive stress.

PROGNOSIS

Self-limited (resolves within 12 months) in up to 80–90% of patients

COMPLICATIONS

- Rupture of plantar fascia (more common with repeated CSI)
- Chronic pain, gait abnormality

REFERENCES

1. Tseng WC, Chen YC, Lee TM, et al. Plantar fasciitis: an updated review. *J Med Ultrasound*. 2023;31(4):268–274. doi:10.4103/jmu.jmu_2_23.
2. Choo YJ, Park CH, Chang MC. Rearfoot disorders and conservative treatment: a narrative review. *Ann Palliat Med*. 2020;9(5):3546–3552.
3. Herber A, Covarrubias O, Daher M, et al. Platelet rich plasma therapy versus other modalities for treatment of plantar fasciitis: a systematic review and meta-analysis. *Foot Ankle Surg*. 2024;30(4):285–293. doi:10.1016/j.fas.2024.02.004.

ADDITIONAL READING

Li Z, Yu A, Qi B, et al. Corticosteroid versus placebo injection for plantar fasciitis: a meta-analysis of randomized controlled trials. *Exp Ther Med*. 2015;9(6):2263–2268.

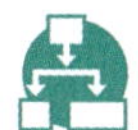

SEE ALSO

Algorithm: Heel Pain

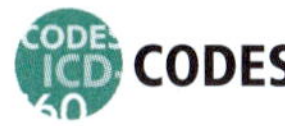

CODES

ICD10

M72.2 Plantar fascial fibromatosis

CLINICAL PEARLS

- Plantar fasciitis occurs due to degeneration of plantar fascia at origin (medial calcaneal tuberosity).
- Plantar medial heel pain with weight-bearing (most noticeable with initial steps in the morning or after period of inactivity) is hallmark presentation.
- Generally self-limited (resolution within 12 months)
- Strengthen intrinsic foot muscles, modify activity, stretch plantar fascia, ice (water bottle roll), massage (golf ball roll), and over-the-counter orthoses.
- Weight loss for BMI ≥25 kg/m^2
- Various nonsurgical treatment options exist for persistent symptoms.

PLEURAL EFFUSION

Erik Colegrove, MD

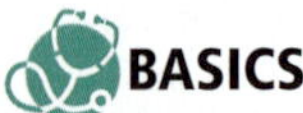

BASICS

Abnormal accumulation of fluid in the pleural space

DESCRIPTION

Types: transudate (low protein/low specific gravity) and exudate (high protein and cellular debris); transudate: commonly caused by congestive heart failure (CHF): 40%; exudates: pneumonia 25%, malignancy 15%, and pulmonary embolism (PE) 10%

EPIDEMIOLOGY

Incidence

Estimated 1.5 million cases per year in the United States; CHF: 500,000; pneumonia: 300,000; malignancy: 150,000; PE: 150,000; cirrhosis: 150,000; tuberculosis (TB): 2,500; pancreatitis: 20,000; collagen vascular disease: 6,000

Prevalence

Estimated 320 cases per 100,000 people in industrialized countries; in hospitalized patients with AIDS, prevalence is 7–27%; no gender predilection: ~2/3 of malignant pleural effusions occur in women.

ETIOLOGY AND PATHOPHYSIOLOGY

- Imbalance between pleural fluid formation and pleural fluid absorption due to and imbalance between oncotic and hydrostatic pressures between the vascular and pleural space
  - Favors pleural effusion: hydrostatic pressure in vessel greater than pleural space, oncotic pressure vessel less than pleural space, elevated capillary permeability from baseline
  - Favors fluid retention in the vessel: hydrostatic pressure in vessel less than pleural space, oncotic pressure vessel greater than pleural space, decreased capillary permeability from baseline
- Transudates: pleural fluid migration that results from imbalances in hydrostatic/oncotic forces, increase in capillary permeability, lymphatic obstruction/impaired drainage, translocation of fluid from another compartment (e.g., peritoneal or retroperitoneal)
- Transudates: CHF: 40% of transudative effusions; 80% bilateral; constrictive pericarditis, atelectasis; superior vena cava syndrome.; cirrhosis (hepatic hydrothorax), nephrotic syndrome, hypoalbuminemia; myxedema; urinothorax, central line misplacement; peritoneal dialysis; Dressler syndrome (postmyocardial infarction syndrome); yellow nail syndrome: yellow nails, lymphedema, and pleural effusion; SARS-CoV-2
- Exudates: lung parenchyma infection: bacterial (parapneumonic, tuberculous pleurisy), fungal, viral, parasitic (amebiasis, *Echinococcus granulosus*); cancer: lung cancer, metastases (breast, lymphoma, ovaries), mesothelioma; PE: 25% of PEs are transudate; collagen vascular disease: rheumatoid arthritis, systemic lupus erythematosus (SLE), Wegener granulomatosis, sarcoidosis, Churg-Strauss syndrome, Sjogren syndrome, granulomatosis with polyangitis; GI: pancreatitis, esophageal rupture, abdominal abscess, after liver transplant; chylothorax: thoracic duct tear, malignancy; hemothorax: trauma, PE, malignancy, coagulopathy, aortic aneurysm; others: after coronary artery bypass graft, uremia, asbestos exposure, radiation, drugs; drugs: nitrofurantoin, bromocriptine, amiodarone, procarbazine, hydralazine, procainamide, quinidine, methotrexate, methysergide, interleukin-2, mitomycin, practolol, minoxidil, bleomycin, cyclophosphamide, procarbazine, imatinib, all-trans retinoic acid, gemcitabine, dantrolene, valproic acid, sulfasalazine, minocycline, acebutolol, phenytoin, practolol, minoxidil, methysergide, L-tryptophan, dasatinib, docetaxel, filgrastim, ergot alkaloids
  - Meigs syndrome; yellow nail syndrome; ovarian stimulation syndrome; lymphangiomatosis; acute respiratory distress syndrome (ARDS); chylothorax: thoracic duct tear, malignancy, associated with lymphoma
  - Pleural effusions of extravascular origin (PEEVO)
  - Transudative PEEVO: hepatic hydrothorax, peritoneal dialysis, urinothorax, extravascular migration of central venous catheter, duropleural fistula, ventriculoperitoneal and ventriculopleural shunts, glycinothorax
  - Exudative PEEVO: esophageal or gastric perforation, misplaced enteral feeding tube, pancreaticopleural fistula and pancreatic pseudocyst, bilothorax

RISK FACTORS

Occupational exposures/drugs; PE, TB, bacterial pneumonias; opportunistic infections (in HIV patients when CD4 count is <150 cells/μL)

COMMONLY ASSOCIATED CONDITIONS

Hypoproteinemia, heart failure, cirrhosis, kidney disease

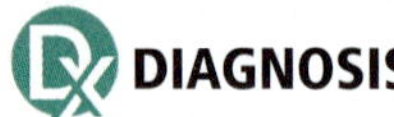

DIAGNOSIS

Presumptive diagnosis in 50% of cases; small pleural effusions; radiographic area <2 intercostal spaces (<300 mL) are asymptomatic

HISTORY

Dyspnea, fever, malaise, and weight loss; chest pain, cough, hemoptysis, and dull pain

PHYSICAL EXAM

- Pleural effusion >300 mL: tachypnea, asymmetric expansion of the thoracic cage; decrease/absent tactile fremitus; dullness to percussion; decreased/inaudible breath sounds, egophony, pleural friction rub
- Ascites suggest hepatic hydrothorax, ovarian cancer, and Meigs syndrome. If associated with unilateral swelling in lower extremity, consider DVT with PE. Lymphadenopathy may suggest malignancy.

DIFFERENTIAL DIAGNOSIS

Pseudochylothorax: accumulation of cholesterol or lecithin-globulin complexes in pleural space

DIAGNOSTIC TESTS & INTERPRETATION

Initial Tests (lab, imaging)

- Thoracocentesis: Use of thoracic ultrasound lowers rate of pneumothorax (4% vs. 9.5%); ultrasonography (US): detects as little as 5 to 50 mL of pleural fluid; identifies loculated effusions; site for thoracentesis, pleural biopsy, or pleural drainage; chest CT scan with contrast for patients with undiagnosed pleural effusion; CT pulmonary angiography if PE is suspected; CT scan of the chest with contrast is recommended if the pleural fluid has complex ultrasonographic features such as septations and loculations.
- Pleural fluid: appearance, pH, WBC differential, total protein, lactate dehydrogenase (LDH), glucose, Gram stain and culture, and acid-fast bacilli staining; consider polymerase chain reaction (PCR) for *Mycobacterium tuberculosis* and *Streptococcus pneumoniae*. If comorbidities implying risk, consider amylase, triglycerides, cholesterol, LE cells, cytology, antinuclear antibodies (ANAs), adenosine deaminase, tumor markers, rheumatoid factor, cytology, creatinine
  - PH ≤7.2, high risk of infection, insert intercostal drain
  - PH >7.2 <7.4, intermediate risk of infection, measure LDH, consider drain if LDH >900 IU/L
  - PH ≥7.4, low risk of pleural infection, ICD (drain) not needed
- Light criteria, transudate versus exudate (98% sensitivity; 80% specificity); fluid is considered an exudate if any of the following: ratio of pleural fluid-to-serum protein levels >0.5; ratio of pleural fluid-to-serum LDH levels >0.6; pleural fluid LDH level >2/3 the upper limit for serum LDH level; 99.5% sensitive for detecting exudative effusion; Light criteria may misdiagnose as high as 20% of transudates as exudative, thus clinical correlation remains important.
- Other exudate criteria: serum-effusion albumin gradient ≤1.2 (sensitivity 87%; specificity 92%); cholesterol effusion >45 mg/dL and LDH effusion >200 mg/dL (sensitivity 90%; specificity 98%); empyema: pus, putrid odor; culture; a putrid odor suggests an anaerobic empyema: LDH levels >1,000 IU/L (normal serum = 200 IU/L); glucose, <60 mg/dL; low pH; malignancy: cytology, red, bloody; glucose, normal to low, depending on the tumor burden; RBCs, >100,000/mm^3
- Lupus pleuritis: LE cells present; pleural fluid-to-serum ANAs ratio >1; glucose <60 mg/dL; pleural fluid-to-serum glucose ratio <0.5; fungal: positive KOH, culture; peritoneal dialysis: protein, <1 g/dL; glucose, 300 to 400 mg/dL; urinothorax: creatinine: pleural/blood >0.5; high LDH pleural fluid, with low protein levels
- Hemothorax: hematocrit: pleural/blood >0.5; benign asbestos effusion: unilateral, exudative; have elevated eosinophil count

- TB pleuritis: lymphocytes >80% predominance effusion; elevated levels of adenosine deaminase (ADA) >50 U/L and interferon-γ >140 pg/mL; positive acid-fast bacillus (AFB) stain, culture; total protein >4 g/dL; nuclear acid amplification (NAA), LDH levels elevated in about 75% of patients (often >500 units/L)
  - High prevalence populations: use ADA +/− IFN gamma
- Low prevalence populations use ADA (i.e., lower risk of a false positive).
- Chylothorax: milky; triglycerides >110 mg/dL; lipoprotein electrophoresis (chylomicrons); pseudochylothorax: cholesterol level >200 mg/dL or presence of cholesterol crystals; amebic liver abscess: anchovy paste effusion; Waldenström macroglobulinemia and multiple myeloma: protein >7 g/dL
- Esophageal rupture: high salivary amylase; pleural fluid acidosis, pH <6; amylase rich: acute pancreatitis, chronic pancreatic pleural effusion, malignancy, esophageal rupture; rheumatoid pleurisy: glucose <60 mg/dL; pleural fluid/serum glucose <0.5
- Lymphocytosis: tuberculous pleurisy, lymphoma, sarcoidosis, chronic rheumatoid pleurisy, yellow nail syndrome, or chylothorax (80–95% of the nucleated cells); carcinomatosis in half of cases (50–70% are lymphocytes.)
- Neutrophils >50% suggest parapneumonic effusion, empyema, PE, abdominal disease, malignant pleural effusion, and acute TB pleurisy. COVID-19 5.88% of pleural effusion
- Eosinophilia (>10% of total nucleated cells): pneumothorax, hemothorax, malignancy, drugs, pulmonary infarction, parasitic infection (lung fluke, amoebiasis, and echinococcus/ruptured hydatid cyst), fungal (coccidioidomycosis, cryptococcosis, histoplasmosis), benign asbestos pleural effusion
- Low glucose (<60 mg/dL): TB, malignancy, rheumatoid pleurisy, parapneumonic, empyema, hemothorax, paragonimiasis, Churg-Strauss syndrome. RBC count >100,000/mm^3: trauma, malignancy, PE, injury after cardiac surgery, asbestos pleurisy, pancreatitis, TB
- Pleural fluid LDH >1,000 IU/L: suggests empyema, malignant effusion, rheumatoid effusion, or pleural paragonimiasis; pH >7.3: rheumatoid pleurisy, empyema, malignant effusion, TB, esophageal rupture, or lupus nephritis pH <7.2 necessitates fluid drainage in patient with parapneumonic effusion.
- Mesothelial cells in exudates: TB is unlikely if there are >5% of mesothelial cells. ADA >35 units/L suggest TB pleurisy, empyema, complicated parapneumonic effusion, and malignancy. ADA >250 units/L consider empyema or lymphoma over TB. *S. pneumoniae* accounts for 50% of cases of parapneumonic effusions in AIDS patients, followed by *Staphylococcus aureus*, *Haemophilus influenzae*, *Mycoplasma pneumoniae*, *Legionella*, *Nocardia*, and *Bordetella bronchiseptica*; exudate with low count of nucleated cells. *Pneumocystis jiroveci* is an uncommon cause in HIV. Usually, it is a small effusion, unilateral or bilateral, and serous to bloody in appearance. Demonstration of the trophozoite or cyst is mandatory; cancer-related HIV pleural effusion: Kaposi sarcoma, Castleman disease, and primary effusion lymphoma; Kaposi sarcoma: mononuclear predominance, exudate, pH >7.4; LDH, 111 to 330 IU/L; glucose >60 mg/dL
- Comparison of specific imaging modalities
- Chest x-ray (CXR): posteroanterior–anteroposterior views: upright x-rays show a concave meniscus in the costophrenic angle that suggests >250 mL of pleural fluid; homogeneous opacity, with visibility of pulmonary vessels through diffuse haziness and absence of air bronchogram; 75 mL of fluid will obliterate the posterior costophrenic sulcus. Lateral x-rays show blunting of the posterior costophrenic angle and the posterior gutter; decubitus x-rays to exclude a loculated effusion and underlying pulmonary lesion or pulmonary thickening; supine x-rays show costophrenic blunting, haziness, obliteration of the diaphragmatic silhouette, decreased visibility of the lower lobe vasculature, and widened minor fissure.
- Chest US: uses artifacts in the lung fields to determine underlying level of free-flowing fluid, consolidation; increasing levels of consolidation results in more echogenic (whiter) tissue.
- Chest CT: better location of loculations and pleural thickening compared to x-ray, resulting in the "split pleural sign" enhancement of visceral and parietal layers at the margin of the effusion
- Chest MRI: Distinguish between transudates and exudates and evaluate for extent of tissue extension.

Diagnostic Procedures/Other

Diagnostic thoracentesis indicated for the following: clinically significant pleural effusion (>10-mm thick on US or lateral decubitus x-ray with no known cause)

TREATMENT

MEDICATION

First Line

CHF: diuretics (75% clearing in 48 hours); parapneumonic effusion: antibiotics; rheumatologic conditions/inflammation: steroids and NSAID

Second Line

Intrapleural treatments for fibrinopurulent stage

- Fibrinolytic/enzymatic therapy
- Streptokinse (250,000 IU per day)
- Patients with pleural infection: no benefit on mortality, rate of surgery, length of hospital stay
- Urokinase (100,000 to 200,000 IU per day)
  - More expensive than tPA/DNAase but lower hemothorax rate
- tPA (5 to 10 mg BID, 10 mg QD)
- DNAase
- Saline washes
- Intrapleural irrigation with saline in the pleural space, then manual aspiration until clear, reduces intrapleural enzyme administration and shortens chest tube removal time (1).

ISSUES FOR REFERRAL

Uncertain etiology; malignant effusion; high-risk diagnostic thoracentesis; decortication

ADDITIONAL THERAPIES

Pleurodesis for symptomatic patients whose pleural effusion reaccumulates too quickly for repeat therapeutic thoracentesis

SURGERY/OTHER PROCEDURES

- Percutaneous pleural biopsy if a cause is not clear after thoracentesis
- Contraindications for thoracentesis: anticoagulation, bleeding diathesis, thrombocytopenia <20,000/mm^3, mechanical ventilation
- Bronchoscopy: when malignancy is suspected (pulmonary infiltrate or mass on CXR or CT scan, hemoptysis, massive pleural effusion, or shift of the mediastinum toward the side of effusion)
- Video-assisted thoracoscopic surgery may reduce length of hospital stay and have better overall surgical outcomes compared to thoracostomy.

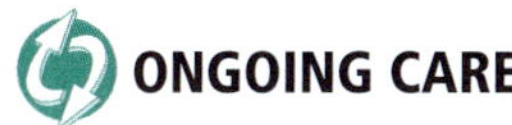

ONGOING CARE

COMPLICATIONS

Pleural effusion: constrictive fibrosis, pleurocutaneous fistula; 40% of pneumonia patients will developed up to 40% parapneumonic effusion, and close to 10% will progress to empyema. Mortality approaches 20% and up to 30% in patients with comorbidities; thoracentesis: pneumothorax (5–10%); hemothorax (~1%); empyema; spleen/liver laceration; reexpansion pulmonary edema (REPE) (if >1.5 L is removed); complications related to large-volume thoracentesis include REPE and pneumothorax ex vacuo.

REFERENCES

1. Sorino C, Mondoni M, Lococo F, et al. Optimizing the management of complicated pleural effusion: from intrapleural agents to surgery. *Respir Med*. 2022;191:106706.

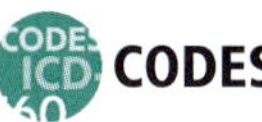

CODES

ICD10

- J86.9 Pyothorax without fistula
- J86.0 Pyothorax with fistula
- J91.0 Malignant pleural effusion

CLINICAL PEARLS

Rare causes of pleural exudates include constrictive pericarditis, urinothorax, and Meigs syndrome. Most common pleural exudates include malignancy, parapneumonic effusions, TB, and empyema.

PNEUMONIA, BACTERIAL

Jocelyn C. Young, DO, MSc

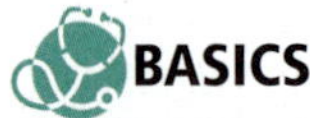

BASICS

Bacterial pneumonia is an acute infection of the pulmonary parenchyma by a bacterial organism.

DESCRIPTION

Bacterial pneumonia can be classified as follows:

- Community-acquired pneumonia (CAP); further classified by severity:
  - CAP in an outpatient setting
  - Nonsevere CAP in an inpatient setting
  - CAP in an ICU *or* severe CAP is based on illness severity criteria and defined as the presence of one major criterion *or* at least three minor criteria.
    - Major criteria: septic shock requiring vasopressors, respiratory failure requiring mechanical ventilation
    - Minor criteria: respiratory rate (RR) ≥30, PaO_2/FiO_2 ratio ≤250, multilobar infiltrates, confusion, BUN ≥20, WBC ≤4, platelets <100,000/μL, hypothermia, and hypotension
- Nosocomial pneumonia: acquired in health care settings
  - Hospital-acquired pneumonia (HAP): occurs ≥48 hours after admission and did not appear to be incubating at the time of admission
  - Ventilator-associated pneumonia (VAP): develops ≥48 hours after endotracheal intubation

EPIDEMIOLOGY

- In the United States, the annual incidence of CAP is 24.8 cases per 10,000 adults with higher rates as age increases. Pneumonia is the eighth leading cause of death and first among infectious causes of death.
- Worldwide, pneumonia kills more children than any other infectious disease. Respiratory viruses are the most commonly detected causes of pneumonia.

Incidence

- CAP: 5 to 6 cases per 1,000 persons with increased incidence occurring in the winter months
- HAP: 5 to 20 cases per 1,000 admissions; incidence increases 6- to 20-fold in ventilated patients

ETIOLOGY AND PATHOPHYSIOLOGY

- Adults, outpatient CAP
  - Typical (85%): *Streptococcus pneumoniae*, *Haemophilus influenzae*, *Staphylococcus aureus*, group A *Streptococcus*, *Moraxella catarrhalis*
  - Atypical (15%): *Legionella* spp., *Mycoplasma pneumoniae*, *Chlamydophila pneumoniae*
- Adults, inpatient nonsevere or severe CAP, HAP, VAP
  - Aerobic gram-negative bacilli: *Pseudomonas aeruginosa*, *Escherichia coli*, *Klebsiella pneumoniae*, and *Acinetobacter* spp.
  - Gram-positive cocci: *Streptococcus* spp. and *S. aureus* (including MRSA)
- Pediatric
  - Birth to 3 weeks: *E. coli*, group B *Streptococci*, *Listeria monocytogenes*
  - <3 months: *Chlamydia trachomatis*, *S. pneumoniae*, *H. influenzae*
  - 3 months to 18 years: Typical: *S. pneumoniae;* Atypical: *C. pneumoniae*, *M. pneumoniae*

RISK FACTORS

- Immunosuppression:
  - Chronic steroid use (>20 mg/day or >2 mg/kg/day of prednisone for >14 days)
  - HIV/immunoglobulin deficiencies/solid organ transplant/TNF-α inhibitor therapy
- Chronic health conditions: asthma, COPD, type 2 diabetes mellitus (DM), chronic renal failure, CHF, liver disease, tobacco use
- Age >65 years, antibiotic therapy in the past 6 months/resistance to antibiotics
- Hospitalization for ≥2 days during past 90 days
- Poor functional status

GENERAL PREVENTION

Vaccination recommendations:

- All children should be vaccinated with PCV15 or 20 at 2, 4, 6, and 12 to 15 months of age.
- Pneumococcal vaccination is recommended for all adults aged ≥65 years.
- Adults aged 19 to 64 years with chronic diseases, defined by the CDC, should receive 1 dose of PCV20 or 21. For those who have only received PPSV23, give PCV20 or PCV21 1 year after their most recent PPSV23.
- Annual influenza and COVID-19 vaccine

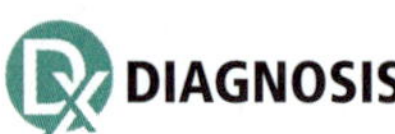

DIAGNOSIS

HISTORY

- Fever, chills, rigors, malaise, fatigue, dyspnea, cough (with/without sputum), pleuritic chest pain, myalgias
- Pediatric patients: lethargy, hypotonia, poor feeding, dry mucus membranes, vomiting

ALERT

History of advanced neurodegenerative disease who develop sudden high fever and cough should raise suspicion for aspiration pneumonia.

Geriatric Considerations

Older adults with pneumonia present with weakness, mental status change, agitation, or history of falls.

PHYSICAL EXAM

- Vitals: fever >100.4°F (38°C), tachypnea, tachycardia, hypoxemia
  - Severe cases may also present with hypothermia, bradycardia, or hypotension.
- Pulmonary exam: decreased breath sounds unilaterally with rales, rhonchi, egophony, increased fremitus, bronchial breath sounds, dullness to percussion, asymmetric breath sounds, abdominal tenderness
- Pediatric exam findings: grunting, retractions

DIFFERENTIAL DIAGNOSIS

Viral pneumonia, bronchitis, asthma or COPD exacerbation, pulmonary edema, lung cancer, pulmonary tuberculosis, pneumonitis, rheumatologic etiologies (i.e., sarcoidosis)

DIAGNOSTIC TESTS & INTERPRETATION

Initial Tests (lab, imaging)

- Outpatient setting:
  - No routine laboratory testing or imaging in outpatients is indicated
  - Clinical diagnosis with fever, tachypnea, and physical exam findings
- Inpatient and noncritical care setting:
  - CBC, CRP, chest x-ray
  - Procalcitonin is not recommended.
  - Urine *Legionella* antigen testing if there is travel to an endemic area *or* exposure to an outbreak
- Inpatient and critical care setting or severe CAP:
  - CBC, CRP, chest x-ray
  - Blood culture and sputum culture are recommended for severe CAP, history of or active MRSA or *P. aeruginosa* infections, or treated with parental antibiotics within the previous 90 days
  - Urine pneumococcal and *Legionella* antigen testing should be performed.
  - Procalcitonin is not recommended.
  - If MRSA is suspected, nasal testing for rapid MRSA is preferred, and if negative, coverage for MRSA is not indicated.
  - Evidence of necrotizing/cavitary pneumonia should raise suspicion for MRSA pneumonia.

Follow-Up Tests & Special Considerations

- Viral testing including influenzae and respiratory syncytial virus (RSV) as up to 80% of children <2 years old will have a viral cause.
- Obtain blood cultures only if no improvement on antibiotics or with severe CAP.
- Follow-up imaging is not indicated for patients with CAP symptoms improved in 5 to 7 days.

Diagnostic Procedures/Other

For HAP and VAP: By bronchoscopic or nonbronchoscopic means, obtain a lower respiratory tract sample for culture prior to initiation/change of therapy.

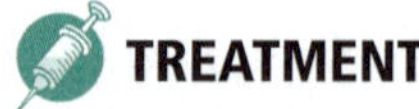

TREATMENT

GENERAL MEASURES

ALERT

Use a risk calculator to determine need for hospitalization and efficacy of treatment:

- Pneumonia Severity Index: https://www.thecalculator.co/health/Pneumonia-Severity-Index-(PSI)-Calculator-977.html
- CURB-65: https://www.mdcalc.com/curb-65-score-pneumonia-severity

MEDICATION

First Line

- Adults (1)
  - CAP, outpatient empiric treatment: no risk factors for MRSA *or P. aeruginosa* and no comorbidities
    - Amoxicillin 1 g 3 times daily
    - Doxycycline 100 mg twice daily
    - If local resistance <25%, azithromycin 500 mg on day 1 and then 250 mg daily

- CAP, outpatient empiric treatment: with comorbidities but without risk factors for MRSA or *P. aeruginosa*
  - Combination therapy:
    - Doxycycline 100 mg BID *plus*
    - Amoxicillin/clavulanate 875 mg/125 BID, cefpodoxime 200 mg BID, or cefuroxime 500 mg BID
  - Monotherapy with a respiratory fluoroquinolone
- Minimum duration of therapy is 5 days.

- CAP, inpatient: nonsevere pneumonia without risk factors for MRSA or *P. aeruginosa*
  - IV antibiotics initially, transition to PO with improvement
  - Minimum duration of therapy is 5 days.
  - Combination of:
    - β-Lactam (ampicillin/sulbactam, 1.5 to 3.0 g IV q6h *or* cefotaxime, 1 to 2 g IV q8h *or* ceftaroline, 600 mg IV q12h *or* ceftriaxone, 1 to 2 g IV daily) *plus*
    - Macrolide (azithromycin 500 mg PO/IV daily *or* clarithromycin 500 mg PO q12h) *or*
  - Monotherapy with a respiratory fluoroquinolone
  - If contraindications to macrolides and fluoroquinolones, use doxycycline 100 mg BID with β-lactam
- CAP, inpatient: severe pneumonia without risk factors for MRSA or *P. aeruginosa*
  - β-Lactam *plus* macrolide
  - β-Lactam *plus* respiratory fluoroquinolone
- CAP, inpatient: severe pneumonia with locally validated risk factors for MRSA or *P. aeruginosa*
  - Add approprite coverage as follows:
    - For MRSA risk factors: linezolid *or* vancomycin
    - For *P. aeruginosa* risk factors: aztreonam *or* cefepime *or* meropenem *or* piperacillin/tazobactam *or* ceftazidime
- Corticosteroids only in cases with refractory shock
- Routine administration of anaerobic coverage for suspected aspiration pneumonia is not recommended.
- When there is clinical and radiographic evidence of CAP in patients who tested positive for influenza, antibacterial, and anti-influenza treatments are recommended.
- HAP, inpatient (2)
  - Patients without MRSA risk factors and not at high risk of mortality, choose one of the following:
    - Piperacillin-tazobactam 4.5 mg IV q6h *or* cefepime 2 g IV q8h *or* levofloxacin 750 mg IV q24h *or* imipenem 500 mg IV q6h *or* meropenem 1 g IV q8h
  - Patients with MRSA risk factors add either vancomycin 15 mg/kg IV q8–12h based on trough *or* linezolid 600 mg IV q12h
- VAP, inpatient (2)
  - Empirically cover *S. aureus*, *P. aeruginosa*, and other gram-negative bacilli.
  - Cover MRSA if at risk for antimicrobial resistance or if prevalence of MRSA is not known.
  - Include double pseudomonas coverage from two different classes if at risk for antimicrobial resistance or in an ICU where susceptibility rates are not known.
- Pediatric, outpatient (≥3 months)
  - Antibiotic treatment in children 4 months to 4 years old is not routinely required because viral pathogens are more common.
  - 5 days of antibiotic therapy is recommended, and 7 days duration for those aged <6 months.
  - Presumed typical bacterial pneumonia
    - Amoxicillin 90 mg/kg/day PO BID (max 4 g/day)
    - For patients with penicillin allergy, clindamycin 13 mg/kg/dose PO TID
    - For children who are not up-to-date with vaccination and have penicillin allergy, use levofloxacin.
  - Presumed atypical bacterial pneumonia
    - Doxycycline 1 to 2 mg/kg/dose PO BID if >7 years old
    - Azithromycin 10 mg/kg PO on day 1 (max 500 mg) and then 5 mg/kg/day (max 250 mg) on days 2 to 5
    - Clarithromycin 15 mg/kg/day PO BID (max 1 g/day); or erythromycin 40 mg/kg/day PO daily
- Pediatric, inpatient (≥3 months)
  - Uncomplicated CAP
    - First-line empirical treatment is ampicillin 50 mg/kg/dose IV q6h.
    - For low- or medium-risk penicillin allergy/not fully immunized, ceftriaxone 50 to 100 mg/kg/day IV q12–24h (max 2,000 mg)
    - For high-risk allergy, levofloxacin 10 mg/kg/dose
  - Complicated CAP
    - First-line empirical treatment is ceftriaxone 100 mg/kg once followed by 50/mg/kg/dose IV q12h.
    - Add vancomycin or clindamycin if suspecting community-acquired MRSA.
    - Due to inferior in vitro-activity of oral cephalosporins, transition from empiric ceftriaxone should be to amoxicillin-clavulanate.
    - For high-risk allergy, substitute levofloxacin, 10 mg/kg/dose and vancomycin
    - Presumed atypical bacterial pneumonia
      - Azithromycin 10 mg/kg IV daily on days 1 and 2 (max 500 mg) and then 5 mg/kg/day PO (max 250 mg) on days 3 to 5
      - Alternatives: clarithromycin, erythromycin, doxycycline (if >8 years old), levofloxacin (if reached growth maturity)

ADMISSION, INPATIENT, AND NURSING CONSIDERATIONS

- Pulse oximetry and oxygen supplementation
- Positioning minimize aspiration risk

Pediatric Considerations

- Approximately 15% of all deaths worldwide in children <5 years of age can be traced back to CAP.
- Tachypnea along with high temperature lasting >3 days with cyanosis and respiratory distress is highly indicative of pneumonia.
- Inpatient treatment is recommended for infants ≤3 to 6 months or presence of respiratory distress.
- Discharge criteria: clinical stability for 12 to 24 hours including temperature ≤100°F (37.8°C); HR ≤100 bpm; RR ≤24; O_2 sat ≥90% on room air; maintain PO intake; normal mental status

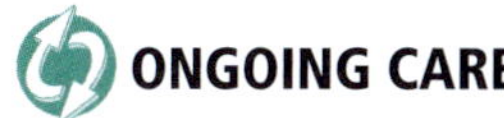

ONGOING CARE

PATIENT EDUCATION

Smoking cessation, vaccinations

COMPLICATIONS

Necrotizing pneumonia, respiratory failure, empyema, abscesses, cavitation, bronchopleural fistula, sepsis

REFERENCES

1. Metlay JP, Waterer GW, Long AC, et al. Diagnosis and treatment of adults with community-acquired pneumonia. An official clinical practice guideline of the American Thoracic Society and Infectious Diseases Society of America. *Am J Respir Crit Care Med*. 2019;200(7):e45–e67.
2. Kalil AC, Metersky ML, Klompas M, et al. Management of adults with hospital-acquired and ventilator-associated pneumonia: 2016 clinical practice guidelines by the Infectious Diseases Society of America and the American Thoracic Society. *Clin Infect Dis*. 2016;63(5):e61–e111.

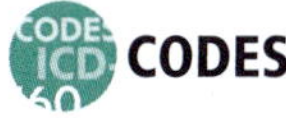

CODES

ICD10

- J15.9 Unspecified bacterial pneumonia
- J15.4 Pneumonia due to other streptococci
- J14 Pneumonia due to Hemophilus influenzae

CLINICAL PEARLS

Severity of illness calculators are helpful in determining need for hospitalization but does not replace clinical judgment.

PNEUMONIA, MYCOPLASMA

Kenneth A. Ballou, MD

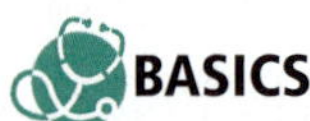

BASICS

DESCRIPTION

- Bronchopulmonary infection caused by one of several *Mycoplasma spp.*, *Mycoplasma pneumoniae* being the most common pathogen of the class
- Smallest, free-living organism; fastidious and slow-growing; first isolated in cattle in 1898
- Most frequently affects children/young adults but can also occur in the elderly; often causes epidemics in close communities (i.e., skilled nursing facilities, dormitories, military barracks)
- Infection may be asymptomatic, most often confined to the upper respiratory tract; however, may progress to pneumonia (5–10%)
- Course is usually acute with an incubation period of 1 to 4 weeks.
- Synonym(s): primary atypical pneumonia (PAP); Eaton agent pneumonia; cold agglutinin–positive pneumonia; walking pneumonia

Pediatric Considerations

- Increased incidence of asthma exacerbation in older children
- Infants 3 to 6 months of age with suspected bacterial pneumonia should be hospitalized.

EPIDEMIOLOGY

Incidence

- ~1 million cases/year in the United States; annual infection rate of 1% in the United States
- 20% of community-acquired pneumonia (CAP) requiring hospitalizations annually
- Most frequently in autumn/winter seasons

Prevalence

- Predominant sex: male = female
- Predominant age group affected: 5 to 20 years
  - May occur at any age
  - Rare in children <5 years of age
- Responsible for up to 15–20% of all cases of CAP yearly
  - Most common cause of pneumonia in school children and young adults who do not have a chronic underlying condition

ETIOLOGY AND PATHOPHYSIOLOGY

- *M. pneumoniae* is a short-rod mucosal pathogen, which lacks a cell wall and thus not visible on Gram stain.
- Can grow under both aerobic and anaerobic conditions
- Highly contagious, transmitted by aerosol droplets
- Pathogenicity linked to its filamentous tips, which adhere selectively to respiratory epithelial cell membrane proteins with production of H_2O_2 and superoxide radicals, damaging cilia
- Decreased ciliary movement produces prolonged paroxysmal, hacking cough.
- Incubation period is 2 to 3 weeks.

ALERT

- *M. pneumoniae* infection may worsen asthma symptoms as well as cause wheezing in children without asthma.
- *M. pneumoniae* infection may worsen chronic obstructive pulmonary disease (COPD) or other chronic pulmonary condition symptoms in adults.

RISK FACTORS

- Immunocompromised state (e.g., HIV, transplant recipients, chemotherapy)
- Smoking
- Close communal living (e.g., military barracks, prisons, hospitals, dormitories, schools, household contacts, skilled nursing facilities)
- Patients with functional asplenia (e.g., sickle cell anemia) tend to have a more severe course.

COMMONLY ASSOCIATED CONDITIONS

- Asthma exacerbations as a result of proinflammatory cytokine release
- COPD

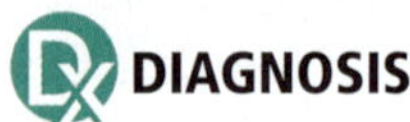

DIAGNOSIS

HISTORY

- Infection may be asymptomatic.
- Gradual onset of headache, malaise, low-grade fevers, chills
- Symptoms of upper respiratory infection, including incessant, nonproductive cough, worsening cough (which may become mildly productive late in the disease) and pleurisy; rhinorrhea, pharyngitis, and otalgia; sinusitis may subsequently occur.
- Pneumonia may occur with associated pleural effusion.
- The presence of pleuritic chest pain warrants a higher suspicion of *M. pneumoniae*.
- Extrapulmonary findings may develop in 5–10% of patients, including arthralgias, skin rashes, pharyngitis, bullous myringitis, cervical adenopathy (uncommon), hemolysis, hepatitis, congestive heart failure (CHF), and cardiac conduction abnormalities (1)[A].
- Neurologic symptoms develop more commonly in children and may include encephalitis, aseptic meningitis, cranial nerve palsies, cerebellar ataxia, ascending paralysis, and coma.
- Persistent cough is common during convalescence; other sequelae are rare.

PHYSICAL EXAM

- Hacking/pertussis-like cough may be present along with fever and lassitude.
- Normal lung findings with early infection, but rhonchi, rales, and/or wheezes may develop several days later.
- Mild pharyngeal injection without exudates
- Minimal/no cervical adenopathy
- Some patients may develop an audible pleural friction rub.
- Various exanthems, including erythema multiforme and Stevens-Johnson syndrome

DIFFERENTIAL DIAGNOSIS

- Viral/bacterial/fungal pneumonia
- Tuberculosis
- Other atypical pneumonias, including *Chlamydia pneumoniae*, *Chlamydophila psittaci*, *Coxiella burnetii* (Q fever), *Francisella tularensis* (tularemia), *Pneumocystis jiroveci*, *Legionella pneumophila*, and other CAPs
- Must differentiate from COVID-19 related pulmonary infection; COVID-19 testing recommended

DIAGNOSTIC TESTS & INTERPRETATION

- *M. pneumoniae* is typically a clinical diagnosis and treated empirically; however, when specific pathogen testing is indicated, polymerase chain reaction (PCR) is the test of choice.
- No clinical or radiographic findings can differentiate between *M. pneumoniae* and other atypical pneumonia pathogens (*Chlamydia*/*Legionella*).

Initial Tests (lab, imaging)

- WBC count may be normal or elevated.
- Hemolytic anemia is rare.
- Elevated inflammatory markers (erythrocyte sedimentation rate [ESR] or C-reactive protein [CRP]) may be present but is nonspecific.
- Procalcitonin (PCT) levels may be helpful.
- When indicated, PCR for *M. pneumoniae* DNA in nasopharyngeal and throat swabs as well as bronchoalveolar lavage respiratory secretions, CSF, and tissue samples may be the most sensitive and specific. PCR of a throat-swab is the gold-standard test (1),(2)[A].
- Radiography of the chest shows reticulonodular pattern with patchy areas of lower lobe consolidation. Small pleural effusion may be present in 10–15% cases.

Follow-Up Tests & Special Considerations

- Sputum Gram stains are not helpful because *M. pneumoniae* lacks a cell wall and cannot be stained.
- *M. pneumoniae* is difficult to culture and requires 7 to 21 days to grow; does not provide information to guide treatment.
- Complement fixation serologic assay shows 4-fold rise in IgM antibody titer at 2 to 4 weeks after symptom onset; this is an older technique.
- Positive cold agglutinins (titer of ≥1:128 or rising 4-fold) in 50% of infections but can take 1 to 2 weeks to develop; not sensitive/specific; not routinely recommended
- CT scan of chest may show a combination of patchy tree-in-bud opacities with segmental ground glass opacities.

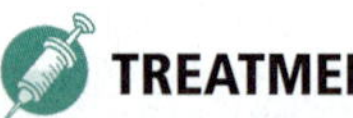

TREATMENT

GENERAL MEASURES

- Supportive care indicated, especially for very ill patients who may require inpatient treatment
- Treatment is initially empiric and must be comprehensive to cover all likely pathogens in the context of the clinical setting.
- Calculation of pneumonia severity score (CAP score: http://www.mdcalc.com/psi-port-score-pneumonia-severity-index-adult-cap) may be helpful in determining inpatient versus outpatient treatment.

ALERT

There is insufficient evidence regarding the efficacy of antibiotics in pediatric patients <24 months of age infected with *M. pneumoniae*. However, some studies show benefit to treating with a macrolide and amoxicillin to cover *M. pneumoniae* in addition to other likely agents causing CAP.

P

Pregnancy Considerations

- Azithromycin: pregnancy Category B (preferred treatment)
- Clarithromycin, levofloxacin, and moxifloxacin: pregnancy Category C

MEDICATION

First Line

- Doxycycline (drug of choice for CAP)
  - Children <8 years of age: not recommended due to tooth discoloration
  - Children >8 years of age (≤45 kg): 2 to 4 mg/kg/day up to 200 mg/day PO divided BID for 10 to 14 days
  - Children >8 years of age (≥45 kg): Refer to adult dosing.
  - Adults: 100 mg PO BID × 14 days
  - Useful in macrolide-resistant strains of *M. pneumoniae*
- Clarithromycin
  - Children <6 months of age: not established
  - Patients >6 months of age: 15 mg/kg/day PO divided q12h for 10 to 14 days
  - Adults: 500 mg PO BID for 14 to 21 days
- Azithromycin
  - <3 months of age: not established (2)
  - >3 months of age: day 1: 10 mg/kg PO × 1 (not to exceed 500 mg); days 2 to 5: 5 mg/kg PO daily (not to exceed 250 mg/day)
  - Adults: 500 mg PO on the first day, followed by 250 mg PO daily × 4 days
- Erythromycin
  - Children: 20 to 50 mg/kg/day (base) PO divided q6–8h for 10 to 14 days
  - Adults: 500 mg (base) PO q6h × 14 to 21 days

Second Line

- Levofloxacin
  - Children <18 years of age: not recommended
  - Adults: 750 mg PO/IV daily × 5 days
- Moxifloxacin
  - Children <18 years of age: not recommended
  - Adults: 400 mg PO/IV daily for 7 to 14 days
- Gemifloxacin
  - Children <18 years of age: not recommended
  - Adults: 320 mg PO daily for 5 to 7 days
- Levofloxacin and moxifloxacin show good activity against *M. pneumoniae*. Consider use with comorbid conditions and other pneumonia pathogens; also useful if macrolide resistance is suspected

ADDITIONAL THERAPIES

- Albuterol inhaler: 2 puffs q4–6h as needed for wheezing
- Dexamethasone may downregulate cytokine release, particularly if symptoms outside the respiratory tract are present.
- Supplemental oxygen as needed; up to 10.9% of hospitalized patients may require mechanical ventilation.
- Plasmapheresis in cases of severe hemolytic anemia

ADMISSION, INPATIENT, AND NURSING CONSIDERATIONS

- CAP score risk class IV/V
- Advanced age with comorbidities
- Complicating neoplastic disease
- Significant cerebrovascular, cardiac, renal, liver, or GI symptoms
- Altered mental status
- Inability to maintain oxygen saturation
- Tachycardia/tachypnea
- Hypotension
- Neurologic symptoms
- Signs of Stevens-Johnson syndrome
- Significant hemolysis (autoimmune hemolytic anemia, cold agglutinin disease)
- Change from IV to PO antibiotic may be made when:
  - Respiratory distress and hypoxia have resolved.
  - Patients are tolerating PO hydration.
  - No significant complications are present.
  - Utilization of PCT may aid in this decision.
- Generally, no need for 24-hour observation on PO antibiotics prior to discharge.

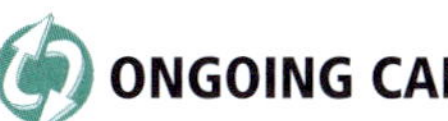

ONGOING CARE

FOLLOW-UP RECOMMENDATIONS

- Clearing of condition on CXR should be documented in patients >50 years of age.
- In smokers, document a clear CXR in 6 to 8 weeks.
- Worsening symptoms/development of rash or meningeal/neurologic signs should prompt immediate presentation to medical attention.
- Antibiotic prophylaxis for exposed contacts is not routinely recommended.
- For household contacts who may be predisposed to severe mycoplasmal infection, macrolide or doxycycline prophylaxis should be used.

DIET

Ensure adequate hydration.

PATIENT EDUCATION

- Smoking cessation
- Contact and droplet precautions
- Adequate handwashing techniques

PROGNOSIS

- Symptoms usually resolve in 2 weeks.
- Some constitutional symptoms may persist for several weeks.
- With correct therapy, even most severe cases can expect complete recovery.

COMPLICATIONS

- All complications are rare, except reactive airway disease, hemolytic anemia, and erythema multiforme.
- Reactive airway disease may persist indefinitely and can cause acute chest syndrome in patients with sickle cell anemia.
- Meningoencephalitis, aseptic meningitis
- Peripheral neuropathy
- Transverse myelitis/acute transverse myelitis
- Cerebellar ataxia
- Acute disseminated encephalomyelitis
- Guillain-Barré syndrome
- Encephalitis (especially in children)
- Polyneuritis/polyarthritis
- Stevens-Johnson syndrome
- Pericarditis/myocarditis
- Respiratory distress syndrome
- Cerebral ataxia
- Thromboembolic phenomena
- Pleural effusion
- Nephritis
- Occasional deaths occur primarily among the elderly and persons with sickle cell disease.

REFERENCES

1. Tahmasebi H, Babaeizad A, Mohammadlou M, et al. Reemergence of *Mycoplasma pneumoniae* disease: pathogenesis and new approaches. *Microb Pathog*. 2024;196:106944. doi:10.1016/j.micpath.2024.106944.
2. Rowlands RS, Meyer Sauteur PM, Beeton ML, et al. *Mycoplasma pneumoniae*: not a typical respiratory pathogen. *J Med Microbiol*. 2024;73(10):001910. doi:10.1099/jmm.0.001910.

ADDITIONAL READING

Garin N, Marti C, Skali Lami A, et al. Atypical pathogens in adult community-acquired pneumonia and implications for empiric antibiotic treatment: a narrative review. *Microorganisms*. 2022;10(12):2326. doi:10.3390/microorganisms10122326.

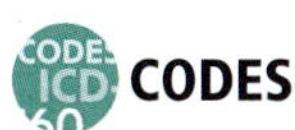

CODES

ICD10

J15.7 Pneumonia due to Mycoplasma pneumoniae

CLINICAL PEARLS

- Mycoplasma (*M. pneumoniae*) is one of the most common atypical respiratory pathogens seen in CAP.
- Atypical pneumonia is usually a clinical diagnosis.
- Atypical pneumonia with *M. pneumoniae* usually responds to empiric treatment (doxycycline).
- Outbreaks of *M. pneumoniae* can be seen in close communities (i.e., dormitories).

PNEUMONIA, *PNEUMOCYSTIS JIROVECI*

Thomas J. Hansen, MD

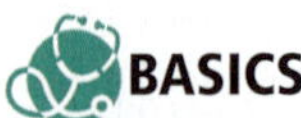

BASICS

DESCRIPTION

- *Pneumocystis jiroveci* is a potentially life-threatening infection that occurs primarily in immunocompromised patients.
- The fungus that causes this pneumonia in humans was previously called *Pneumocystis carinii*.
- The name was formally changed to *P. jiroveci* in 2001, following the discovery that the fungus that infects humans is unique and distinctive from the fungus that infects animals.
- *P. jiroveci* is extremely resistant to traditional antifungal agents, including both amphotericin and azole agents.
- To prevent confusion, the term PCP, which used to represent *P. carinii* pneumonia, now represents *Pneumocystis* pneumonia.

ALERT

No combination of symptoms, signs, blood chemistries, or radiographic findings is diagnostic of *P. jiroveci* pneumonia (1).

EPIDEMIOLOGY

- *P. jiroveci* has a worldwide distribution, and most children have been exposed to the fungus by age 2 to 4 years (2).
- The reservoir and mode of transmission for *P. jiroveci* is still unclear.
  - Human studies favor an airborne transmission model, with person-to-person spread being the most likely mode of infection acquisition (1).

Incidence

The incidence of PCP has decreased with the use of PCP prophylaxis. In the United States, one study shows a decrease in PCP incidence from 3 per 100 person-years between 1994 and 1997 to 0.39 per 100 person-years between 2008 and 2010 (3).

Prevalence

- The prevalence of *P. jiroveci* colonization among healthy adults is 0–20%.
- Recent studies have demonstrated the transient nature of *P. jiroveci* colonization in asymptomatic, immunocompetent patients (1).
- 50% of patients with PCP are coinfected with ≥2 strains of *P. jiroveci* (2).
- There is evidence that distinct strains are responsible for each episode in patients who develop multiple episodes of PCP (2).

ETIOLOGY AND PATHOPHYSIOLOGY

Mode of transmission is unknown; likely respiratory from infected host

RISK FACTORS

Individuals at risk (1)

- Patients with HIV infection and a low CD4 count, especially if not receiving prophylactic treatment for PCP
- Patients who are receiving high doses of glucocorticoids
- Patients who have an altered immune system not due to HIV
- Patients who are receiving chronic immunosuppressive medications
- Patients who have hematologic or solid malignancies resulting in malignancy-related immune depression

GENERAL PREVENTION

- Indications for prophylaxis
  - HIV-infected adults (4)
    - When CD4 count is 100 to 200 cells/μL and HIV viral load is above detection limits
    - When CD4 count is <100 cells/μL
  - HIV-infected children (2)
    - Prophylaxis should be provided for children aged ≥6 years based on adult guidelines.
    - For children aged 1 to 5 years, start when CD4 count is <500 cells/μL.
    - For infants 4 to 6 weeks to 12 months, prophylax for 1st year of life.
  - Non–HIV-infected adults receiving immunosuppressive medications or with underlying immune system deficits should receive PCP prophylaxis, but currently, there are no specific guidelines on when to start this.
- Medication
  - Trimethoprim-sulfamethoxazole (TMP-SMX)
    - Adults: 1 double-strength tablet daily or 1 single-strength tablet daily (preferred regimen) or 1 double-strength tablet 3 times/week
    - Children aged ≥4 weeks: TMP 5 to 10 mg/kg/day; and SMX, 25 to 50 mg/kg/day PO; the total daily dose should not exceed 320 mg TMP and 16,000 mg SMX; acceptable dosing intervals and schedules: in divided doses twice daily, 3 days/week on consecutive or alternate days; in divided doses twice daily, 2 days/week on consecutive or alternate days; total dose once daily, given 7 days/week.
  - Atovaquone suspension (alternate regimen)
    - Adults: 1,500 mg PO once daily with food
    - Children: not to exceed 1,500 mg/day
      - 1 to 3 months: 30 mg/kg/day PO once daily
      - 4 to 24 months: 45 mg/kg/day PO once daily
      - >24 months: 30 mg/kg/day PO once daily
      - Adolescents aged ≥13 years: Refer to adult dosing.
  - Dapsone (alternate regimen)
    - Adults only: 50 mg twice daily or 100 mg once daily
    - Children aged ≥1 month: 2 mg/kg (maximum 100 mg), PO, once a day or 4 mg/kg (maximum 200 mg), PO every week.
  - Pentamidine (alternate regimen)
    - Adults only: 300 mg aerosolized q4wk
- Discontinuation of prophylaxis
  - Discontinue if combined antiretroviral therapy has been administered for ≥6 months and the CD4+ T-lymphocyte cell count is ≥200 cells/μL and have been sustained for >3 consecutive months patients aged ≥6 years.
  - In children aged 1 to 5 years, discontinue if combined antiretroviral therapy has been administered for ≥6 months and the CD4+ T-lymphocyte cell count is ≥500 cells/μL and have been sustained for >3 consecutive months.

COMMONLY ASSOCIATED CONDITIONS

- HIV infection
- Chronic obstructive pulmonary disease (COPD)
- Interstitial lung disease
- Connective tissue diseases treated with corticosteroids
- Cancer and organ transplant patients on immunosuppressive medication

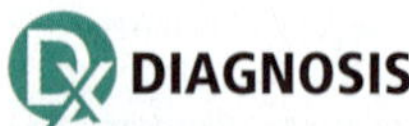

DIAGNOSIS

HISTORY

- HIV-infected patients
  - Subacute onset over several weeks
    - Progressively worsening dyspnea
    - Tachypnea
    - Cough: nonproductive or productive of clear sputum
    - Low-grade fever, chills
    - Weakness, fatigue, malaise
- Non–HIV-infected immunocompromised patients
  - More acute onset with fulminant respiratory failure
    - Abrupt tachypnea, dyspnea
    - Fever
    - Dry cough

PHYSICAL EXAM

- Fever
- Tachypnea
- Tachycardia
- Lung exam is often normal; if abnormal, reveals inspiratory crackles

DIFFERENTIAL DIAGNOSIS

- Tuberculosis
- Bacterial pneumonia
- Fungal pneumonia
- Viral pneumonia

DIAGNOSTIC TESTS & INTERPRETATION

P. jiroveci cannot be cultured. Therefore, a diagnosis relies on detection of the organism by colorimetric or immunofluorescent stains or by polymerase chain reaction (PCR) (2)[C].

- ABG: reveals hypoxemia and increased alveolar–arterial gradient that varies with severity of disease
- Lactate dehydrogenase (LDH): Serum LDH is frequently increased (nonspecific; likely due to underlying lung inflammation and injury).
- CD4 cell count is generally <200 cells/μL in HIV-infected patients with PCP.
- S-adenosylmethionine levels are significantly lower in a patient with PCP. The levels increase with successful treatment.
- Comprehensive metabolic profile
- Chest x-ray (CXR) (1)[C]
  - Bilateral, symmetric, fine, reticular interstitial infiltrates involving perihilar areas; becomes more homogeneous and diffuse as severity of infection progresses
  - Less common patterns include upper lobe involvement in patients receiving aerosolized pentamidine, solitary or multiple nodular opacities, lobar infiltrates, pneumatoceles, and pneumothoraces.
  - May be normal in up to 30% of patients with PCP
- High-resolution CT scan is more sensitive than CXR.

Diagnostic Procedures/Other

- Fiberoptic bronchoscopy with bronchoalveolar lavage (BAL) is the preferred diagnostic procedure to obtain samples for direct fluorescent antibody staining.
  - Sensitivities range from 89% to >98%.

- *Pneumocystis* trophic forms or cysts obtained from induced sputum, BAL fluid, or lung tissue, which can be visualized using conventional stains
- PCR can detect *Pneumocystis* from respiratory sources, but the potential remains for false positives (1)[C].

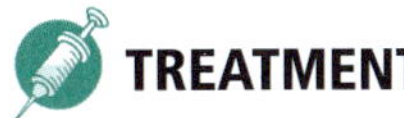

TREATMENT

The recommended duration of therapy differs in patients who are with/without AIDS:

- In patients with PCP who do not have AIDS, the typical duration of therapy is 14 days.
- Treatment of PCP in patients who have AIDS was increased to 21 days due to the risk for relapse after only 14 days of treatment (1)[C].

MEDICATION

First Line

- TMP-SMX (1)[C]
- Adult dosing
  - TMP-SMX: 15 to 20 mg/kg/day, PO or IV, divided into 3 or 4 divided doses
- Pediatric dosing (>2 months) (1)[C]
  - TMP: 15 to 20 mg/kg/day in divided doses q6–8h
- Reduce doses of TMP-SMX in patients with renal failure.
- Patients should receive 21 days of therapy.
- Treatment response to *Pneumocystis* therapy often requires at least 7 to 10 days before clinical improvement is documented.
- Pregnancy risk factor: category C (1)[C]
- Precautions
  - History of sulfa allergy
  - There is an emergence of drug-resistant PCP, especially against TMP-SMX.

Second Line

- Pentamidine (for moderate to severe cases)
  - Adults and children: 4 mg/kg IV once daily
- Dapsone + TMP (adults only)
  - Dapsone 100 mg PO once daily, *plus*
  - TMP 5 mg/kg PO TID
    - Check the glucose-6-phosphate dehydrogenase level before beginning dapsone because hemolysis may result.
- Clindamycin + primaquine (adults only)
  - Clindamycin 900 mg IV q8h or 600 mg IV q6h or 600 mg PO TID or 450 mg PO QID, *plus*
  - Primaquine 30 mg PO once daily
- Atovaquone
  - Adults: 750 mg PO BID (>13 years of age)
  - Children: 40 mg/kg/day PO divided BID (max 1,500 mg)
- Note: Pentamidine has greater toxicity than TMP-SMX: hypotension, hypoglycemia, pancreatitis (1)[C].

ADDITIONAL THERAPIES

Adjunctive corticosteroid (prednisone or methylprednisolone) (1)[C]

- Adjunctive corticosteroids are shown to provide benefits in patients who have HIV and symptoms of moderate to severe PCP.
- Corticosteroids provide the greatest benefit to HIV patients who have hypoxemia manifested as a partial pressure of arterial oxygen <70 mm Hg or an alveolar–arterial gradient >35 mm Hg on room air.
- Adults and children >13 years of age: prednisone, 40 mg PO BID on days 1 to 5; 40 mg daily on days 6 to 11; 20 mg daily on days 12 to 21

ADMISSION, INPATIENT, AND NURSING CONSIDERATIONS

- No set criteria for hospital admission
- Five predictors of mortality in HIV-associated *Pneumocystis* pneumonia
  - Increased age of the patient
  - Recent IV drug use
  - Total bilirubin >0.6 mg/dL
  - Serum albumin <3 g/dL
  - Alveolar–arterial oxygen gradient ≥50 mm Hg

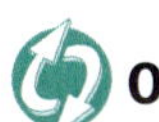

ONGOING CARE

FOLLOW-UP RECOMMENDATIONS

In patients with HIV/AIDS: Patients with previous episodes of PCP should receive lifelong secondary prophylaxis unless they respond well to highly active antiretroviral therapy (HAART) and have a CD4 count >200 cells/μL for at least 3 months.

Patient Monitoring

Serum LDH levels, pulmonary function test results, and ABG measurements generally normalize with treatment.

DIET

No special diet needed

PATIENT EDUCATION

- Centers for Disease Control and Prevention: https://www.cdc.gov/dpdx/pneumocystis/index.html
- FamilyDoctor.org: http://familydoctor.org/familydoctor/en/diseases-conditions/hiv-and-aids/complications/pneumocystis-pneumonia-pcp-and-hiv.html

REFERENCES

1. Krajicek BJ, Thomas CF Jr, Limper AH. *Pneumocystis* pneumonia: current concepts in pathogenesis, diagnosis, and treatment. *Clin Chest Med*. 2009;30(2):265–278.
2. Kovacs JA, Masur H. Evolving health effects of *Pneumocystis*: one hundred years of progress in diagnosis and treatment. *JAMA*. 2009;301(24):2578–2585.
3. Buchacz K, Lau B, Jing Y, et al; North American AIDS Cohort Collaboration on Research and Design (NA-ACCORD) of IeDEA. Incidence of AIDS-defining opportunistic infections in a multicohort analysis of HIV-infected persons in the United States and Canada, 2000–2010. *J Infect Dis*. 2016;214(6):862–872. doi:10.1093/infdis/jiw085.
4. Panel on Guidelines for the Prevention and Treatment of Opportunistic Infections in Adults and Adolescents with HIV. Guidelines for the Prevention and Treatment of Opportunistic Infections in Adults and Adolescents with HIV. https://clinicalinfo.hiv.gov/en/guidelines/hiv-clinical-guidelines-adult-and-adolescent-opportunistic-infections/whats-new. Accessed June 9, 2025.

ADDITIONAL READING

Green H, Paul M, Vidal L, et al. Prophylaxis for *Pneumocystis* pneumonia (PCP) in non-HIV immunocompromised patients. *Cochrane Database Syst Rev*. 2007;(3):CD005590.

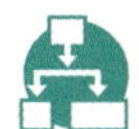

SEE ALSO

HIV/AIDS

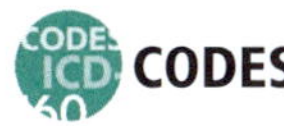

CODES

ICD10

B59 Pneumocystosis

CLINICAL PEARLS

- Colonization with *P. jiroveci* is common in the pediatric population.
- PCP only occurs in immunocompromised patients.
- Patients with HIV are at risk once their CD4 count is <200 cells/μL. At that time, TMP-SMX should be initiated as prophylaxis. Prophylaxis may end after HAART has been initiated and the CD4 count is >200 cells/μL for 3 months.
- Patients who are immunocompromised are also at risk. Currently, no clear clinical guidelines are available as to when to initiate or end prophylaxis.
- The first-line treatment is TMP-SMX. The typical duration of therapy is 14 days in non–HIV-infected patients and 21 days in HIV-infected patients.

POLYARTERITIS NODOSA

Ratnesh Chopra, MD • Yevgeniy Popov, DO, MPH

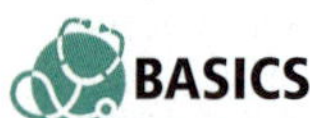

BASICS

DESCRIPTION

- Polyarteritis nodosa (PAN) is an antineutrophil cytoplasmic antibody (ANCA)-negative necrotizing arteritis of medium-sized muscular arteries and (occasionally) small arteries. Arterioles, capillaries, and venules are spared (1).
- Involved systems include gastrointestinal (GI) tract, peripheral nervous system (sensory and motor), CNS, genitourinary, skin, and cardiovascular. Glomerulonephritis and pulmonary capillaritis are rare (1).
- Features depend on location of vasculitis: for example, mesenteric ischemia–related symptoms, new onset or worsening hypertension (HTN), mononeuritis multiplex, purpuric or nodular skin lesions, or livedo reticularis.
- Renal disease in PAN usually manifests as HTN and mild proteinuria with/without azotemia.
- PAN formerly encompassed several distinct entities (classic PAN, microscopic PAN, and cutaneous PAN). With ANCA testing, microscopic PAN appears pathophysiologically unrelated to the other two.
  - Idiopathic generalized PAN (classic PAN) is clinically variable, ranging from single organ involvement to polyvisceral failure (1).
  - HBV-associated PAN patients are positive for active hepatitis B infection and can present in similar fashion to idiopathic generalized PAN (1).
  - Microscopic PAN has ANCAs directed against myeloperoxidase (MPO) and involvement of small arterioles (microscopic polyangiitis [MPA]). This is now classified as ANCA-associated vasculitis.
  - Cutaneous (or limited) PAN is generally limited to the deep dermal and subcutaneous (SC) levels of the skin with characteristic histopathologic features of PAN. There are few systemic manifestations, although myalgias and peripheral motor neuropathy (mononeuritis multiplex) or sensory neuropathy may be present.

EPIDEMIOLOGY

Incidence

Incidence of 0 to 1.6 cases per million; predominant age: peaks in 5th to 6th decade; incidence rises with age. Mean age at diagnosis is 50 years; male predominance.

Prevalence

Rare: up to 31 cases per 1 million adults (1)

ETIOLOGY AND PATHOPHYSIOLOGY

- Segmental, transmural, necrotizing inflammation of medium and small muscular arteries, with intimal proliferation, thrombosis, and ischemia of the end-organ/tissue supplied by the affected vessels; aneurysm formation at vessel bifurcations.
- Hepatitis B–related PAN results in direct vessel injury due to viral replication or deposition of immune complexes, with complement activation and subsequent inflammatory response.
- Most cases are idiopathic; 20% are related to hepatitis B or C infection.
- In patients with PAN and hepatitis B, HBsAg has been recovered from involved vessel walls.

Genetics

Mutations of adenosine deaminase 2 (ADA 2) have been identified in families with PAN (1).

RISK FACTORS

Hepatitis B > hepatitis C infection (cutaneous PAN)

COMMONLY ASSOCIATED CONDITIONS

- Hepatitis B (strong association with classic PAN); hepatitis C (less strongly linked to cutaneous PAN)
- Hairy cell leukemia; rare following hepatitis B vaccination
- Minocycline (symptoms resolve on stopping drug, reoccur if rechallenged.); case-based associations with CMV infection, amphetamines, and interferon

DIAGNOSIS

- There are no formal diagnostic criteria for PAN.
- Suspect PAN with:
  - Acute, sometimes fulminant multisystem disease with a relatively short prodrome (i.e., weeks to months); vasculitic skin rash with sensorimotor symptoms/findings; recent-onset HTN with systemic symptoms; unexplained sensory and/or motor neuropathy with systemic symptoms; hepatitis B infection with multisystem disease

HISTORY

Symptoms reflect specific organ involvement.

- Constitutional symptoms (fever, weight loss, malaise)
- Organ-specific symptoms
  - Focal muscular weakness/extremity numbness; myalgia and arthralgia
  - Rash (nodules, purpura, livedo)
  - Recurrent postprandial abdominal pain, intestinal angina, nausea, vomiting, and bleeding
  - Altered mental status, headaches, mononeuritis multiplex
  - Testicular/epididymal pain, neurogenic bladder (rare)

PHYSICAL EXAM

Findings/course reflect specific organ involvement.

- Peripheral nervous system: peripheral neuropathy, mononeuritis multiplex
- Renal: HTN
- Skin: purpura, urticaria, polymorphic rashes, SC nodules (uncommon but characteristic), livedo reticularis; deep skin ulcers, especially in lower extremities; Raynaud phenomenon (rare); single digit gangrene (rare)
- GI: acute abdomen; rebound, guarding, tenderness
- CNS: seizures, altered mental status, papillitis
- Lung: signs of pleural effusion—dullness to percussion; decreased breath sounds
- Cardiac: signs of congestive heart failure and/or myocardial infarction—S_3 gallop; pericarditis (Friction rub is rare.)
- Genitourinary: testicular/epididymal tenderness (can mimic testicular torsion)
- Musculoskeletal: arthritis (usually large joint in lower extremities)

DIFFERENTIAL DIAGNOSIS

- Other forms of vasculitis (ANCA-associated, such as granulomatosis with polyangiitis [GPA—formerly Wegener granulomatosis], Churg-Strauss syndrome, and MPA; Henoch-Schönlein purpura, drug-induced vasculitis, cryoglobulinemia, Goodpasture syndrome)
- Buerger disease; systemic lupus erythematosus (SLE); embolic disease (atrial myxoma, cholesterol emboli); thrombotic disease (antiphospholipid antibody syndrome); dissecting aneurysm; Ehlers-Danlos syndrome; multiple sclerosis, systemic amyloidosis; infection (subacute endocarditis, HIV infection, trichinosis, rickettsial diseases); fibromuscular dysplasia; ergotamine use; segmental arterial mediolysis

DIAGNOSTIC TESTS & INTERPRETATION

- ANCA typically negative; no specific laboratory abnormalities; confirm diagnosis with biopsy if possible.
- Angiography (conventional, CT angiography, or MR angiography) may reveal microaneurysms and/or beading of bifurcating blood vessels.
- Avoid contrast in renal disease.
- Nonspecific laboratory abnormalities:
  - Elevated ESR and CRP; mild proteinuria, elevated creatinine
  - Hepatitis B surface antigen positive in 10–50%; hepatitis C antibody/hepatitis C virus RNA
  - ANCA, anti-proteinase 3 (PR3), and anti-MPO are negative. Positive ANCA argues against PAN. Rheumatoid factor may be positive.
  - Anemia of chronic disease

Initial Tests (lab, imaging)

Look for evidence of systemic disease and rule out other causes

- CBC (thrombocytosis), ESR, and CRP (elevated)
- Chemistries: elevated creatinine/BUN
- Hepatitis B serology: often positive; hepatitis C is less commonly positive
- LFTs: abnormal if associated hepatitis B, C, or involvement of hepatobiliary tract
- Urinalysis: proteinuria/hematuria, generally no cellular casts or active urinary sediment
- ANA, cryoglobulins
- ANCA, anti-MPO, and anti-PR3
- Complement levels (C3, C4)
- Angiographic demonstration of aneurysmal changes/beading of small and medium-sized arteries

Diagnostic Procedures/Other

- Electromyography and nerve conduction studies in patients with suspected mononeuritis multiplex; if abnormal, consider sural nerve biopsy.
- Arterial/tissue biopsy (least invasive approach preferable)
- Skin biopsy from edges of ulcers; include deep dermis and SC fat to assess small muscular artery involvement (excisional *not* punch biopsy).

Test Interpretation

- Necrotizing inflammation with fibrinoid necrosis of small- and medium-sized muscular arteries; segmental, often at bifurcations and branchings; venules are not involved in classic PAN.
- Capillaritis/other lung parenchymal involvement by vasculitis *strongly suggests* another process (microscopic PAN, GPA, Churg-Strauss syndrome, or antiglomerular basement membrane disease).
- Acute lesions with infiltration of polymorphonuclear cells through vessel walls into perivascular area; necrosis, thrombosis, and infarction of involved tissue
- Aneurysmal dilatations, including aortic dissection.
- Peripheral nerves: 50–70% (vasa nervorum with necrotizing vasculitis)
- Testicular vessels involved in symptomatic males
- *The key differences from other necrotizing vasculitides are lack of granuloma formation and sparing of veins and pulmonary arteries.*

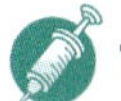

TREATMENT

GENERAL MEASURES

Treat HTN aggressively to prevent complications (stroke, myocardial infarction, heart failure).

MEDICATION

First Line

- Severe (life-threatening) disease: corticosteroids (CS) (high-dose oral prednisone [1 mg/kg/day] or intravenous [IV] methylprednisolone [0.5 to 1.0 g/day] for 3 days, then transition to prednisone 1 mg/kg/day, and taper according to response) (1)[A].
  - Only 50% of patients achieve and maintain remission with CS. Other patients require additional immunosuppressive therapy, and CS monotherapy is not recommended (1).
  - IV cyclophosphamide (0.6 g/m^2 every 2 weeks for 3 doses and then monthly for 4 to 12 months) in combination with CS: improves survival and spares use of chronic steroids in moderate/severe PAN (1)[A].
    - Cyclophosphamide has risk of infertility and malignancy.
  - Plasma exchange for severe refractory disease, such as progressive renal disease or catastrophic disease; the benefit of plasma exchange is unknown (1)[A].
- Less severe disease: CS alone ± other immunosuppressive agents (azathioprine 2 mg/kg/day, methotrexate 20 to 25 mg/week, mycophenolate mofetil 2,000 to 3,000 mg daily); hydroxychloroquine (5 mg/kg/day) use has been reported.
- Cutaneous PAN: Nonsteroidal anti-inflammatory drugs, dapsone, and colchicine are used.
- HBV-associated PAN: antiviral agents, short-term CS, plasma exchange
- Tocilizumab has been reported in treatment refractory, hepatitis B–negative PAN.
- Tumor necrosis inhibitors should be used in patients with clinical manifestations of deficiency of the enzyme Adenosine Deaminase 2 (DADA2) (1).

Second Line

- There is no well-defined second-line therapy in PAN.
- Infliximab (3 to 5 mg/kg IV at 0, 2, and 6 weeks, and every 4 to 8 weeks thereafter) and rituximab (1,000 mg IV on days 0 and 14 and then every 6 months *OR* 375 mg/m^2 IV weekly for 4 weeks) anecdotally reported to be of benefit in refractory PAN.

ADDITIONAL THERAPIES

- For patients receiving IV cyclophosphamide, mercaptoethanesulfonate reduces bladder exposure to carcinogenic metabolites.
- Prophylactically treat patients on cyclophosphamide for *Pneumocystis jiroveci (carinii)* pneumonia with trimethoprim-sulfamethoxazole (use dapsone 100 mg/day or atovaquone 1,500 mg/day in intolerant/allergic patients).

COMPLEMENTARY & ALTERNATIVE MEDICINE

Physical therapy is recommended for patients with muscular or nerve disease (1).

ADMISSION, INPATIENT, AND NURSING CONSIDERATIONS

Depends on extent and involvement of specific organs

ONGOING CARE

FOLLOW-UP RECOMMENDATIONS

- For patients with severe abdominal disease who become asymptomatic, follow-up vascular imaging is recommended (1).
- For patients with peripheral motor neuropathy symptoms, serial neurologic exams over periodic EMGs are recommended (1).

Patient Monitoring

- CBC, urinalysis, renal and hepatic function tests; acute-phase reactants (e.g., ESR, CRP) may help monitor disease activity.
- The Five Factor Score (FFS) can predict mortality and guide treatment strategies. Factors used in the evaluation of patients with PAN, include age, renal insufficiency, cardiac involvement, and GI manifestations. The fifth factor, ENT manifestations, is only applied to patients with ANCA-associated vasculitis.
- Be alert for side effects of immunosuppressant medications; delayed appearance of neoplasms, especially bladder malignancy in patients treated with cyclophosphamide (check annual U/A, urinary cytology with urologic evaluation if microscopic hematuria.); steroid-induced osteoporosis

DIET

- Low-salt diet (HTN); Mediterranean diet for cardiovascular health
- Calcium and vitamin D–rich diets for patients on CS therapy

PATIENT EDUCATION

American College of Rheumatology: https://rheumatology.org/

PROGNOSIS

- Expected outcome of untreated PAN is poor. Patients presenting with proteinuria, renal insufficiency, GI tract involvement, cardiomyopathy, CNS involvement, or aged >65 years have a worse prognosis.
- Steroid and cytotoxic treatment increases 5-year survival rate to 75–80%.
- Survival is greater for hepatitis B–related PAN as a result of the introduction of antiviral treatments.

COMPLICATIONS

- End-organ damage from ischemia
- Complications from immunosuppressive agents

REFERENCES

1. Chung SA, Gorelik M, Langford CA, et al. 2021 American College of Rheumatology/Vasculitis Foundation guideline for the management of polyarteritis nodosa. *Arthritis Rheumatol*. 2021;73(8):1384–1393. doi:10.1002/art.41776.

SEE ALSO

Hepatitis B; Hepatitis C

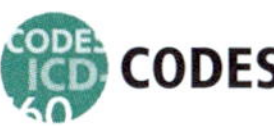

CODES

ICD10

- M30.0 Polyarteritis nodosa
- M30.1 Polyarteritis with lung involvement [Churg-Strauss]
- M30.8 Other conditions related to polyarteritis nodosa

CLINICAL PEARLS

- PAN is a necrotizing vasculitis of small- to medium-sized muscular arteries with lack of granuloma formation that spares veins and pulmonary arteries.
- Clinical features of PAN depend on target organ involvement
- Skin biopsies at ulcer edges (include deep dermis and SC fat) improve diagnostic yield.
- Check hepatitis B and C serologies.
- ANCA is negative in classic PAN.
- At diagnosis, the revised FFS can determine prognosis and guide therapy.
- Treatment involves use of immunosuppressive drugs; choice depends on the extent and severity of disease.

POLYCYSTIC KIDNEY DISEASE

Anila Khaliq, MD, FAAFP

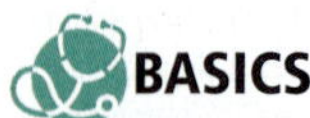

BASICS

DESCRIPTION

- A group of monogenic disorders that results in renal cyst development
- Autosomal dominant polycystic kidney disease (ADPKD) and autosomal recessive polycystic kidney disease (ARPKD)
- ADPKD is one of the most common human genetic disorders.

EPIDEMIOLOGY

- ADPKD is generally late onset with end-stage kidney disease (ESKD) developing in older adults.
- ARPKD usually present in infants.

Prevalence

As ESKD, ADPKD: 8.7/1 million in the United States; 7/1 million in Europe

ETIOLOGY AND PATHOPHYSIOLOGY

- ADPKD results from *PKD1* and *PKD2* mutations, which encode for polycystin 1 (PC1) and polycystin 2 (PC2). The disrupted polycystin function results in fluid-filled cysts that progressively increase in size, leading to gross enlargement of the kidney, and distortion of the renal architecture.
- ARPKD secondary to *PKHD1* mutations

Genetics

- ADPKD autosomal dominant inheritance
  - *PKD1* on chromosome 16p13.3 (85% of patients) encodes PC1.
  - *PKD2* on chromosome 4q21 (15% of patients) encodes PC2.
- ARPKD: autosomal recessive inheritance
  - Gene *PKHD1* on chromosome 6p21.1–p12 encodes fibrocystin.

RISK FACTORS

Family history

GENERAL PREVENTION

Genetic counseling

COMMONLY ASSOCIATED CONDITIONS

ADPKD

- Cysts in other organs
  - Polycystic liver disease in 58% of young age group to 94% of 45-year-olds
  - Pancreatic (5%); seminal (40%); arachnoid (8%)
- Vascular manifestations
  - Intracerebral aneurysms in 6% of patients without family history and in 16% with family history
  - Aortic root dilation, dissections
- Cardiac manifestations: mitral valve prolapse (25%); left ventricular hypertrophy
- Diverticular disease
- ARPKD: liver involvement: affected in inverse proportion to renal disease; congenital hepatic fibrosis with portal HTN

DIAGNOSIS

HISTORY

- ADPKD
  - Positive family history (15% are de novo mutations.)
  - Flank pain: 60%
  - Hematuria
  - UTI
  - HTN: 50% aged 20 to 34 years; 100% with ESKD
  - Renal failure
  - Presymptomatic screening of ADPKD is not currently recommended for at-risk children (1).
- ARPKD
  - 30% of affected neonates die:
    - Enlarged echogenic kidneys and oligohydramnios are diagnosed in utero.
    - Later in childhood: HTN
  - Adolescents and adults present with complications of portal HTN: esophageal varices
  - Hypersplenism

PHYSICAL EXAM

- HTN
- Flank masses

DIFFERENTIAL DIAGNOSIS

- ADPKD and ARPKD
- Tuberous sclerosis: prevalence 1/6,000
- Von Hippel-Lindau syndrome: prevalence 1/36,000
- Nephronophthisis: accounts for 10–20% of cases of renal failure in children; medullary cystic kidney disease
- Renal cystic dysplasias: multicystic dysplastic kidneys: grossly deformed kidneys; most common type of bilateral cystic diseases in newborns (prevalence: 1/4,000)
- Simple cysts: most common cystic abnormality
  - Localized or unilateral renal cystic disease
  - Medullary sponge kidney
  - Acquired renal cystic disease
- Renal cystic neoplasms: benign multilocular cyst (cystic nephroma)

DIAGNOSTIC TESTS & INTERPRETATION

Electrolytes, BUN/creatinine, urinalysis plus urinary citrate

Initial Tests (lab, imaging)

- ADPKD
  - Renal dysfunction
    - Impaired renal concentration (2), hypocitraturia aciduria
    - Hyperfiltration
    - Elevated creatinine
  - Urinalysis: hematuria and mild proteinuria
- ARPKD
  - Electrolyte abnormalities and renal insufficiency
  - Anemia, thrombocytopenia, leukopenia
- ADPKD
  - US: It is the easiest diagnostic method; however, it is suboptimal for disease exclusion at age <40 years (1)[C].
    - Renal enlargement is universal.
    - In at-risk patients: By age 30 years, two renal cysts (bilateral or unilateral) are 100% diagnostic. In children, it sometimes appears similar to ARPKD; may be diagnosed in utero
    - Presence of hepatic cysts in young adults is pathognomonic for ADPKD.
    - In the absence of family history, bilateral renal enlargement and cysts make the diagnosis.
    - In subjects between ages 16 and 40 years and without an established family history, the presence of >10 cysts is considered diagnostic.
  - CT scan/MRI ideally should be part of the initial evaluation (1)[C].
    - Kidney volume assessed by CT scan or MRI is a main predictor of progression.
    - Helpful in identifying cysts in other organs
    - In subjects aged <40 years, <5 cysts by MRI excludes the diagnosis (1)[B].
    - In at-risk subjects aged <40 years, ≥10 cysts by MRI is considered sufficient for diagnosis with a sensitivity and specificity of 100%.
- ARPKD
  - US: Kidneys are enlarged, homogeneously hyperechogenic (cortex and medulla).
  - CT scan is more sensitive if diagnosis is in doubt.
  - Presence of hepatic fibrosis helps the diagnosis.

Follow-Up Tests & Special Considerations

- Diagnosis and prevention of secondary problems because of renal and liver abnormalities
- Beyond age 2 years, renal size decreases in ARPKD but continues to grow in ADPKD at an average rate of 5.27% per year. Total kidney volume identifies patients with progressive disease (1).
- Consensus recommendations advise HTN screening in children with a family history of ADPKD from the age of 5 years onward with an interval of 3 years in cases where the child is normotensive.

Diagnostic Procedures/Other

- Genetic testing is available for *PKD1* and *PKD2* in ADPKD when imaging results are equivocal and for potential living related donors (3)[C].
- For *PKHD1* in ARPKD, a prenatal diagnosis is feasible in about 72% of patients.

Test Interpretation

- ADPKD
  - Kidneys are diffusely cystic and, although enlarged, retain their general shape.
  - Cysts range from a few millimeters to several centimeters and are distributed evenly throughout the cortex and medulla.

- They arise in all segments of the nephron, although they arise initially from the collecting ducts.
- One kidney may be larger than the other.
- In patients without established family history, the detection of >10 cysts per kidney by ultrasonography is usually considered diagnostic.
- ARPKD
  - Disease is a spectrum, ranging from severe renal disease with mild liver damage to mild renal disease with severe liver damage.
  - Renal enlargement is due to fusiform dilatation of the collecting ducts in the cortex and medulla in the newborn period.
  - Liver lesion is diffuse but limited to fibrotic portal areas.
  - Diagnosis is likely based on clinical imaging in severe neonatal or infantile cases on the basis of enlarged echogenic kidneys, a negative family history, and lack of additional features.
  - Molecular diagnostic analysis is the gold standard for diagnosing this disorder.
  - Kidneys decrease in size over time as the amount of fibrosis increases.

TREATMENT

GENERAL MEASURES

- Liberal water intake; vasopressin stimulate cystogenesis, increasing water intake throughout the day suppresses pituitary vasopressin release.
- Salt restriction; high salt intake is associated with higher increase in kidney volume and faster drop in kidney function.
- Maintain healthy weight. Overweight and obesity are linked to rapid decline in kidney function and higher increase in kidney volume.
- Smoking cessation; smoking is associated with an increase in cardiovascular risk, increase in proteinuria, and intracranial aneurysm development and rupture.
- Exercise; contact sports should be avoided.
- No caffeine restriction; caffeine intake does not affect kidney volume or kidney function.

MEDICATION

- Treatments that directly target cytogenic mechanisms such as decreasing cAMP levels in cystic tissues are now available. Tolvaptan slowed the rate of kidney growth and estimated GFR decline in patients with early ADPKD.
- Monitoring hepatic safety should be considered when prescribing tolvaptan.
- HTN: should be very well controlled to prevent complications; ACE inhibitors are preferred if no contraindications are present.
- The use of antihypertensive medications has been found to decrease mortality (4)[B].
- Hyperlipidemia: statins preferred

ISSUES FOR REFERRAL

- Nephrologist primary management
- Urologic consultation for management of symptomatic/infected cysts
- Genetic counseling is critical.

SURGERY/OTHER PROCEDURES

- Indications for surgical intervention
  - Uncontrollable HTN
  - Severe back and loin pain, abdominal fullness
  - Renal deterioration due to enlarging cysts
  - Hematuria/hemorrhage or recurrent UTI
- Open and laparoscopic cyst unroofing: may decrease pain and narcotics requirements; has not been proven to prevent renal failure or to prolong current renal function
- Percutaneous cyst aspiration ± injection of sclerosing agent; not usually performed secondary to recurrent fluid accumulation
- Renal transplant for ESKD

ADMISSION, INPATIENT, AND NURSING CONSIDERATIONS

Severe pain, gross hematuria with clots

ONGOING CARE

FOLLOW-UP RECOMMENDATIONS

None in early stages of the disease; avoid vigorous activity if disease advances. Recurrent gross hematuria is secondary to trauma, associated with faster decline of renal function.

Patient Monitoring

- Monitor blood pressure (BP) and renal function. Encourage hydration. Treat UTI and stone disease aggressively.
- Avoid nephrotoxic drugs.
- Creatinine and BP monitoring at least twice a year; more often as needed
- Screening for intracranial aneurysms (5)
- No matter the severity of disease GFR remains within normal limits for decades reducing its practicality as a marker for prognosis and progression of the disease state.

DIET

- Low-protein diet may retard renal insufficiency.
- Limit caffeine because this might increase cyst growth.
- High water intake to decrease ADH >3 L/day (6)[C]
- Limiting salt intake to ≤5 g/day

PROGNOSIS

- Renal failure in 2% by age 40 years; 23% by age 50 years; 48% by age 73 years
- ADPKD accounts for 10–15% of dialysis patients.
- No increased incidence of renal cell cancer
- Prognosis is variable and progression to ESRD is not predestined. Certain patients with PKD2 genotype or atypical PCKD may never progress to ESRD.

COMPLICATIONS

- Cyst rupture, infection, or hemorrhage
- Progression to renal failure
- Renal calculi
- Cholangitis

REFERENCES

1. Chapman AB, Devuyst O, Eckardt KU, et al. Autosomal-dominant polycystic kidney disease (ADPKD): executive summary from a Kidney Disease: Improving Global Outcomes (KDIGO) controversies conference. *Kidney Int*. 2015;88(1):17–27. doi:10.1038/ki.2015.59.
2. Zittema D, Boertien WE, van Beek AP, et al. Vasopressin, copeptin, and renal concentrating capacity in patients with autosomal dominant polycystic kidney disease without renal impairment. *Clin J Am Soc Nephrol*. 2012;7(6):906–913.
3. Harris PC, Rossetti S. Molecular diagnostics for autosomal dominant polycystic kidney disease. *Nat Rev Nephrol*. 2010;6(4):197–206.
4. Patch C, Charlton J, Roderick PJ, et al. Use of antihypertensive medications and mortality of patients with autosomal dominant polycystic kidney disease: a population-based study. *Am J Kidney Dis*. 2011;57(6):856–862.
5. Rozenfeld MN, Ansari SA, Shaibani A, et al. Should patients with autosomal dominant polycystic kidney disease be screened for cerebral aneurysms? *AJNR Am J Neuroradiol*. 2014;35(1):3–9.
6. Mahnensmith RL. Novel treatments of autosomal dominant polycystic kidney disease. *Clin J Am Soc Nephrol*. 2014;9(5):831–836.

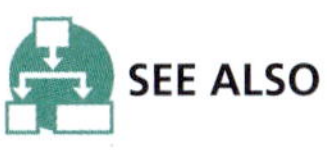

SEE ALSO

Chronic Kidney Disease

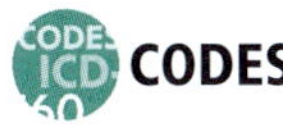

CODES

ICD10

- Q61.3 Polycystic kidney, unspecified
- Q61.2 Polycystic kidney, adult type
- Q61.1 Polycystic kidney, infantile type

CLINICAL PEARLS

- Most PKD patients eventually develop ESKD. No specific treatment has been proven to prevent ESKD, but hydration and control of BP are reasonable goals.
- Patients may benefit from a nephrology consultation after the initial diagnosis to counsel regarding disease progression prevention. Then, they can be followed by primary care if the disease was an incidental finding or no significant kidney dysfunction is present.

POLYCYSTIC OVARIAN SYNDROME (PCOS)

Jeremy Golding, MD, FAAFP

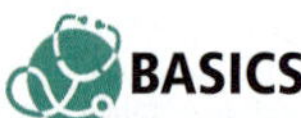

BASICS

DESCRIPTION

- Polycystic ovarian syndrome (PCOS) is a common endocrine disorder with heterogeneous manifestations. It is characterized by hyperandrogenism, insulin resistance, and anovulation, typically presenting as amenorrhea or oligomenorrhea.
- Clinical characteristics include menstrual dysfunction, infertility, hirsutism, acne, obesity, and metabolic syndrome. The ovaries are often polycystic on imaging, but are not required for diagnosis.
- The Rotterdam diagnostic criteria include two of the following three: (i) oligo- and/or anovulation; (ii) clinical and/or biochemical signs of hyperandrogenism; (iii) polycystic ovaries on ultrasound.
- The etiology of PCOS is unknown but presentation and course can be modified by lifestyle factors.
- System(s) affected: reproductive, endocrine/metabolic, skin/exocrine
- Synonym(s): Stein-Leventhal syndrome; polycystic ovary disease

ALERT

- Obesity may amplify PCOS, but it is not diagnostic. 20% of women with PCOS are not obese.
- Predisposes to and is associated with obesity, hypertension, diabetes, metabolic syndrome, hyperlipidemia, infertility, insulin-resistance syndrome, endometrial hyperplasia, and uterine cancer

EPIDEMIOLOGY

Incidence

Incidence and prevalence are still highly debated due to a wide spectrum of diagnostic features; the National Institutes of Health (NIH) criteria require chronic anovulation and hyperandrogenism.

Prevalence

The prevalence based on NIH criteria is around 5–18% of reproductive age women (1).

ETIOLOGY AND PATHOPHYSIOLOGY

- Cause(s) are complex, and include genetic and epigenetic susceptibility, hypothalamic and ovarian dysfunction, excess androgen exposure, insulin resistance, and adiposity-related mechanisms (1).
- Increased GnRH pulsations in the hypothalamus lead to increased production of LH with limited production of FSH.
- Hyperandrogenism: Ovaries are the main source of excess androgens (75% of circulating testosterone originates in the ovary). Polycystic ovaries have thickened thecal layers and overexpressed LH receptors, which cause excess androgen secretion.
- Obesity results in compensatory hyperinsulinemia: Women with PCOS have insulin resistance similar to that in type 2 diabetes. Elevated levels of insulin decrease sex hormone–binding globulin (SHBG), increasing bioavailability of testosterone. Insulin may also act directly on adrenal glands, ovaries, and hypothalamus to enhance androgen production.
- Insulin resistance causes elevated insulin levels and the frequently associated metabolic syndrome or frank diabetes mellitus.

Genetics

Likely a combination of polygenic and environmental factors. Implicated genes include *DENND1A* and *THADA*.

RISK FACTORS

See "Commonly Associated Conditions"; cause and effect are difficult to extricate in this disorder.

GENERAL PREVENTION

None known; focus on early diagnosis and treatment to prevent long-term complications.

COMMONLY ASSOCIATED CONDITIONS

Infertility, obesity, obstructive sleep apnea, hypertension, diabetes mellitus, endometrial hyperplasia/carcinoma, fatty liver disease, mood disturbances and depression, hirsutism

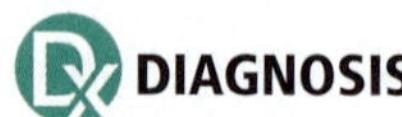

DIAGNOSIS

HISTORY

A comprehensive history, including a family history of diabetes and premature onset of cardiovascular disease, is important in the differential diagnosis. Focus on the onset and duration of the various signs of androgen excess, menstrual history, and concomitant medications, including the use of exogenous androgens; unpredictable, heavy, or absent menstrual cycles

PHYSICAL EXAM

- Vital signs: elevated body mass index (BMI), hypertension
- General appearance: central obesity (40–85% of women), hirsutism, acne
- Skin: male hair pattern, balding, acne, seborrhea, acanthosis nigricans
- Pelvic: ovarian enlargement, clitoromegaly

ALERT

Look specifically for signs of virilization, such as hair pattern, deepened voice, and clitoromegaly because they indicate significant testosterone levels beyond that of PCOS.

DIFFERENTIAL DIAGNOSIS

- Cushing syndrome, androgen-secreting ovarian or adrenal tumor
- HAIR-AN syndrome
- Thyroid disease, acromegaly, prolactin-producing pituitary adenoma
- Adult-onset adrenal hyperplasia, partial congenital adrenal hyperplasia (21-hydroxylase deficiency)
- 11β-hydroxylase deficiency or 17β-hydroxysteroid dehydrogenase deficiency
- Drug-induced hirsutism, oligo-ovulation (e.g., danazol, steroids, valproic acid)
- Idiopathic hirsutism

DIAGNOSTIC TESTS & INTERPRETATION

- Most commonly used diagnostic criteria is the Rotterdam criteria (need any 2 of 3): oligomenorrhea or amenorrhea, clinical and/or biochemical signs of hyperandrogenism, transvaginal ultrasonographic evidence of polycystic ovaries
- Ultrasonographic polycystic ovaries are not necessary for the diagnosis of PCOS.
- More recent criteria also focus on similar criteria while acknowledging that there may be forms of PCOS without overt evidence of hyperandrogenism.

Initial Tests (lab, imaging)

- Screening workup should rule out pregnancy, thyroid disease, hyperprolactinemia, congenital adrenal hyperplasia, and premature ovarian failure. Serum testing includes human chorionic gonadotropin (hCG), TSH, prolactin, 17-OH progesterone, and FSH.
- Hirsute women should have a free testosterone determination (total testosterone minus SHBG) and a DHEA-S.
- Workup to rule out hypothalamic amenorrhea (LH and FSH), androgen-secreting tumors (FSH, estradiol, testosterone, DHEA-S), Cushing syndrome (24-hour urinary free cortisol), and acromegaly (IGF-1) should be considered based on clinical characteristics (2).
- Typical findings in PCOS include testosterone increased but $<$200 ng/dL (6.94 nmol/L), mild elevation in DHEA-S but $<$800 μg/dL (20.8 μmol/L), mild increase in 17-OH progesterone level, increased estrogen level, and decreased SHBG.
- Anovulation can be determined by a midluteal phase progesterone level ($>$3 ng/mL if the woman has ovulated).
- LH/FSH level $\geq$2.5 to 3 in ~50% of women with PCOS, but such testing is not generally necessary.
- Drugs that may alter lab results: oral contraceptive pills (OCPs), steroids, antidepressants
- Transvaginal ultrasound findings: one or both ovaries with $\geq$12 follicles measuring 2 to 9 mm or increased ovarian volume to 10 cm^3

Follow-Up Tests & Special Considerations

- Consider fasting serum glucose, insulin level, and plasminogen activator inhibitor-1 determinations to establish presence of insulin resistance and glucose intolerance, especially if diagnosis is in doubt.
- Endometrial biopsy to rule out hyperplasia and/or carcinoma, if indicated
- If the syndrome is diagnosed, determination of fasting glucose and fasting lipid levels should be performed and formal glucose tolerance test is considered.

ALERT

Prolonged or heavy bleeding should prompt an endometrial biopsy for evaluation of endometrial hyperplasia and possible cancer generally in women over age 30 to 35 years.

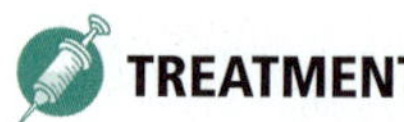

TREATMENT

GENERAL MEASURES

Lifestyle changes including appropriate nutrition and exercise to decrease body weight by as little as 5% can restore ovulation and increase insulin sensitivity (2)[A]. Treatment plans should be individualized based on patient needs and desires.

P

MEDICATION

- The goal of treatment in PCOS depends on symptoms and patient's goals for fertility.
- Treatment can be divided into four main categories: (i) restore menses, (ii) decrease insulin resistance, (iii) ameliorate androgen excess, and (iv) assist in fertility.

First Line

- Restore menses when pregnancy is not desired:
  - OCPs and progestins provide improvement in menstrual irregularity and provide endometrial protection.
  - Low-dose OCPs (30 to 35 μg); newer formulations containing progestins with lower androgenicity (e.g., norethindrone, desogestrel, norgestimate, drospirenone) may be particularly beneficial, but all OCPs increase SHBG and decrease excess androgens. Discuss benefits and balance against slightly increased thrombotic potential of third- and fourth-generation progestins as compared with older progestins.
  - Levonorgestrel IUD offers endometrial protection and pregnancy prevention but will not counteract hyperandrogenism.
  - If unable to tolerate OCPs, then intermittent medroxyprogesterone (Provera) 10 mg PO, or *micronized* progesterone (Crinone and Prometrium) 200 mg PO, for 10 to 14 days can be given every 1 to 3 months. These offer endometrial protection. However, these will not counteract hyperandrogenism or protect against pregnancy.
- Decrease insulin resistance:
  - Metformin may help to correct metabolic abnormalities in women who are insulin resistant. Initial dose is 500 mg daily for 1 week, increasing by 500 mg/week to a total of 1,500 to 2,000 mg/day divided BID; take with food. Overall, data support the usefulness of metformin on both cardiometabolic risk, weight loss, and reproduction assistance in women with PCOS. Thiazolidinediones may increase likelihood of ovulation and treat insulin resistance, but do not increase live birth rate.
  - GLP-1 agonists and other weight loss drugs may be of significant benefit in obese patients.
- If pregnancy is desired:
  - Letrozole (an aromatase inhibitor) has increased ovulation rates, clinical pregnancy rates, and live birth rates compared to clomiphene (Clomid) (3)[A]. Dosing starts on day 3, 4, or 5 with 2.5 mg daily for 5 days; can increase to 5 mg daily with max dose 7.5 mg daily for 5 days
  - Counsel patients that letrozole is not approved by the FDA for ovulation induction.
  - Metformin: 500 to 2,000 mg PO divided BID has been shown to improve hyperandrogenism and restore ovulation. Some providers will choose to continue metformin throughout the 1st trimester or the entire pregnancy if there is a history of spontaneous abortion or glucose intolerance. It does improve ovulation rates and insulin resistance but does not improve live birth rates alone or in combination with clomiphene when used for ovulation induction.
  - Metformin reduces the incidence of gestational diabetes.
  - All ovulation induction drugs increase the risk of multiple births and obstetric complications, such as preterm birth and hypertensive disorders.

Second Line

- Acne:
  - OCPs with low-androgenicity progestins for example, norethindrone, desogestrel, norgestimate, drospirenone
  - Spironolactone: 50 to 200 mg daily in 1 to 2 divided doses for acne and hirsutism not addressed by OCP therapy. This medication is unsafe in pregnancy, and potassium levels must be followed when used.
- Hirsutism:
  - Eflornithine hydrochloride 13.9% cream BID
  - Finasteride 2.5 to 5.0 mg daily; must be on very reliable contraception as this medication is teratogenic

ISSUES FOR REFERRAL

To reproductive endocrinologist for all women who cannot achieve pregnancy with clomiphene (Clomid) or letrozole

ADDITIONAL THERAPIES

If excess hair is uncomfortable, mechanical means of hair removal, including laser, electrolysis, waxing, and depilatory, may improve cosmesis.

SURGERY/OTHER PROCEDURES

Ovarian wedge resection and laparoscopic laser drilling are considered second line therapies, but can be considered controversial and are rarely used today; bariatric surgery for weight loss

ONGOING CARE

FOLLOW-UP RECOMMENDATIONS

6-month intervals to evaluate response to therapy and to monitor weight and medication side effects

Patient Monitoring

- Counsel patient about the risk of endometrial and breast carcinoma, insulin resistance, and diabetes as well as obesity and its role in infertility.
- See patient frequently throughout the menstrual cycle, depending on which drug combination is used to induce ovulation.
- All patients with PCOS who have not received medication or IUD for endometrial protection and have been amenorrheic for 1 year should undergo endometrial biopsy.

DIET

In overweight patients, weight loss is the most successful therapy because it improves cardiovascular risk, insulin sensitivity, menstrual patterns, and infertility: counsel on lifestyle dietary changes; consider referral to nutritionist and weight center. No specific diet plan is proven to be better than another.

PATIENT EDUCATION

- Provide patient with information about PCOS, such as from http://www.acog.org/.
- Review the importance of exercise and weight loss, if applicable. Modest weight loss of 5–10% of initial body weight has been demonstrated to improve many of the features of PCOS.

PROGNOSIS

- Fertility prognosis is good but may need assisted reproductive technologies.
- Proper follow-up and screening can prevent endometrial carcinoma.
- Early detection of diabetes may decrease morbidity and mortality associated with cardiovascular risk factor.

COMPLICATIONS

- Predisposes to endometrial hyperplasia and as high as 9% lifetime risk of endometrial cancer
- Women with PCOS appear to be at increased risk of complications of pregnancy including gestational diabetes and hypertensive disorders.

REFERENCES

1. Joham AE, Norman RJ, Stener-Victorin E, et al. Polycystic ovary syndrome. *Lancet Diabetes Endocrinol*. 2022;10(9):668–680.
2. Tang T, Lord JM, Norman RJ, et al. Insulin-sensitising drugs (metformin, rosiglitazone, pioglitazone, D-chiro-inositol) for women with polycystic ovary syndrome, oligo amenorrhoea and subfertility. *Cochrane Database Syst Rev*. 2010;(1):CD003053.
3. Franik S, Le QK, Kremer JA, et al. Aromatase inhibitors (letrozole) for ovulation induction in infertile women with polycystic ovary syndrome. *Cochrane Database Syst Rev*. 2022;9(9):CD010287.

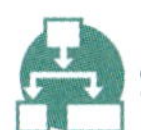

SEE ALSO

Algorithm: Amenorrhea, Secondary

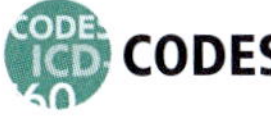

CODES

ICD10

- E28.2 Polycystic ovarian syndrome
- L68.0 Hirsutism

CLINICAL PEARLS

- PCOS is diagnosed based on 2 of 3 of (i) oligo-ovulation, (ii) signs of hyperandrogenism, and (iii) polycystic ovaries.
- Treat chronic anovulation to reduce risk of endometrial hyperplasia.
- In overweight people, weight loss may improve or eliminate many biochemical and clinical abnormalities.

POLYCYTHEMIA VERA

Jill W. Marsh, MD

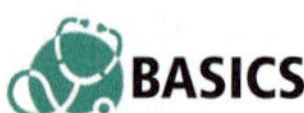

BASICS

DESCRIPTION

- Polycythemia vera (PV) is a chronic myeloproliferative neoplastic disorder marked by overproduction of red blood cells (erythrocytosis) which most often is diagnosed after 60 years of age. It is caused by a *JAK2* mutation and is typically discovered incidentally on CBC (increased H/H; often increased WBC and platelets too). The most frequent initial symptoms are pruritus, splenomegaly, or vasomotor abnormalities.
- Morbidity and mortality are primarily related to complications from blood hyperviscosity leading to venous or arterial thrombosis and/or from leukemic transformation or myelofibrosis (MF).
- The average survival after diagnosis of untreated PV is 6 to 18 months, but with adequate treatment, median survival is 13 years.
- Synonyms: primary polycythemia; PV rubra; Osler-Vaquez disease

EPIDEMIOLOGY

Incidence

- Median age at diagnosis: 61 years, one-quarter of cases present prior to age 50, and 10% prior to age 40
- Incidence in the United States in 2012: 2.8/100,000 population of men and 1.3/100,000 population of women; highest for men aged 70 to 79 years at 23.5/100,000 persons per year

Prevalence

In the United States in 2010, estimates ranged from 45 to 57 cases per 100,000 patient.

ETIOLOGY AND PATHOPHYSIOLOGY

Caused by a *JAK2* (tyrosine kinase) mutation which causes abnormal stem cells to suppress normal stem cells and turns on uncontrolled activation of hematopoietic signaling, particularly of the erythroid line and, to a lesser extent, the myeloid and megakaryocytic lines

Genetics

Most cases are not inherited. They are caused by either a *JAK2 V617F* mutation (95%) or a *JAK2* exon 12 mutation (4%). Compared with heterozygous mutations, homozygous mutations are associated with worse disease outcomes, including more severe symptoms and higher likelihood of disease progression (1).

RISK FACTORS

- Almost none
- Rare familial disposition but most cases are not inherited.
- Possible association with exposure to ionizing radiation or other toxins but most cases have no exposure risk.

GENERAL PREVENTION

None

COMMONLY ASSOCIATED CONDITIONS

- Arterial emboli (including ischemic digits, myocardial infarction, transient ischemic attack [TIA], stroke)
- Venous emboli (including DVT, pulmonary embolism, splanchnic thrombosis leading to complications like Budd-Chiari and splenomegaly)
- Major or microhemorrhage (including acquired von Willebrand disease)
- Gout
- Acute myeloid leukemia (AML) or myelodysplastic syndrome (MDS)
- Secondary MF

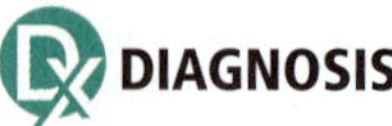

DIAGNOSIS

HISTORY

- Most cases are found incidentally but may present with non-specific, disease-related symptoms or complications.
- Disease-related vasomotor symptoms include headaches, dizziness, vision changes, pruritus, early satiety, fatigue, malaise, insomnia, excessive sweating, low mood, and gout.
- Erythromelalgia and aquagenic pruritus (AP) are classic, common PV complaints (~30% of patient):
  - Erythromelalgia: burning pain of feet/hands, occasionally with erythema, pallor, cyanosis, or paresthesias
  - AP: intense itching or stinging after warm bath or shower

PHYSICAL EXAM

- Hypertension (46%)
- Splenomegaly (75%), palpable spleen (36%)
- Hepatomegaly (30%)
- Facial plethora (ruddy cyanosis)
- Bone tenderness (especially ribs and sternum)
- Skin excoriations from significant pruritus
- Gouty tophi or arthritis
- Injection of the conjunctival small vessels and/or engorgement of the veins of the optic fundus

DIFFERENTIAL DIAGNOSIS

- Chronic myeloproliferative neoplasms (including chronic myeloid leukemia, primary MF, essential thrombocytopenia)
- Hemoglobinopathy
- Secondary erythrocytosis/polycythemia (common; secondary: primary PV cases are 10:1):
  - Pulmonary/chronic hypoxia: sleep apnea; tobacco use; emphysema; alveolar hypoventilation; high-altitude acclimatization
  - Cardiovascular: Eisenmenger syndrome from congenital heart defect
  - Endocrine disorders: pheochromocytoma, Bartter, aldosterone-secreting tumor
  - Renal artery stenosis
  - Carbon monoxide poisoning
  - Drugs: SGLT-2 inhibitors, diuretics, testosterone replacement, erythropoietin (EPO)
- Relative polycythemia (diuretics, severe dehydration, spurious/Gaisbock)
- Erythropoietin (EPO) receptor mutations (rare)
- Ectopic EPO production (rare)

DIAGNOSTIC TESTS & INTERPRETATION

Initial Tests (lab, imaging)

- Simplest algorithm:
  - Check CBC. If Hgb/hematocrit (Hct) >16/48 *and* any high clinical suspicion (common symptoms), obtain EPO level and gene testing for *JAK2 V617F*.
    - If *JAK2 V617F* positive = PV
    - If *JAK2 V617F* negative and EPO subnormal, check for *JAK2* exon 12 mutation; if positive = PV
- 2016 World Health Organization diagnostic criteria requires all three major criteria or the first 2 major criteria and the minor criterion* (*criterion number 2 [BM biopsy] may not be required in cases with substantive absolute erythrocytosis: Hgb >18.5 g/dL in men [Hct, 55.5%] or >16.5 g/dL in women [Hct, 49.5%] if major criterion 3 and minor criterion are present.)
  - Major criteria:
    - Hgb >16.5 g/dL (men); Hgb >16 g/dL (women) *or* Hct >49% (men); Hct >48% (women) *or* increased cell mass (>25% above mean normal predictive value)
    - Bone marrow biopsy showing hypercellularity for age with trilineage growth (panmyelosis) including prominent erythroid, granulocytic, and megakaryocytic proliferation with pleomorphic, mature megakaryocytes (difference in sizes)
    - Presence of *JAK2 V617F* or similar mutation such as *JAK2* exon 12 mutation
  - Minor criteria:
    - Subnormal serum EPO level
- Other lab findings that are common but not specific:
  - Hyperuricemia, hypercholesterolemia, elevated serum vitamin B_{12} levels, prolonged PT, aPTT due to low plasma volume
- Optional imaging: CT or US to assess for hepato- and/or splenomegaly

Follow-Up Tests & Special Considerations

- Prognostic considerations
- High risk: age >60 years and/or history of thrombosis
- Low risk: age ≤60 years and/or no history of thrombosis

Diagnostic Procedures/Other

- Bone marrow aspiration (if performed) shows hypercellularity of erythroid, granulocytic and megakaryocytic lines, or MF.
  - Initial MF (present in up to 20% of patients) can only be detected by performing a bone marrow biopsy; this finding may predict a more rapid progression to overt MF (post-PV MF).
- Cytogenetic testing (*JAK2 V617F*, exon 14 and 12)

Test Interpretation

- If *JAK2 V617F* mutation testing is negative and the EPO level is normal or high, then PV is excluded; investigate causes of secondary erythrocytosis.
- *JAK2 V617F* mutation in exon 14 is a distinguishing feature versus secondary polycythemia but not specific to PV as it can also be present in essential thrombocytopenia and primary MF.
- Other causes of erythrocytosis such as ectopic EPO production from a renal tumor, hypoxia from chronic lung, or cyanotic heart disease can be excluded with low or undetectable serum EPO level and normal oxygen saturation.

TREATMENT

GENERAL MEASURES

- Goals are to (i) decrease red blood cell mass, (ii) treat symptoms, and (iii) prevent complications like thrombosis (2).
  - Low dose aspirin is recommended for all patients.
  - For low risk patients, treatment is often as simple as daily aspirin and serial phlebotomy to reduce Hct.
  - For high risk patients, aspirin, phlebotomy, and/or other cytoreductive treatments are likely needed.
- Although not curative, current therapy for PV can relieve symptoms and prolong survival.
- If secondary PV, address etiology: aggressive treatment of causes like obstructive sleep apnea, COPD (especially smoking cessation), renal disease; consider lowering dose of testosterone replacement.
- Phlebotomy reduces the blood hyperviscosity, improves platelet function, restores systemic pressures, and decreases risk of thrombosis.
  - Reduce Hct to <45%; will significantly lower rate of cardiovascular death and major thrombosis
  - Performed initially as often as every 2 to 3 days until normal Hct reached; phlebotomies of 250 to 500 mL (1 unit—500 mL—phlebotomy should reduce Hct by 3 percentage points). Reduce to 250 to 350 mL in elderly patients or patients with cerebrovascular disease.
  - Frail patients should have volume replaced with saline solution to avoid postural hypotension.
  - High risk for thrombosis or presence of elevated platelet count is indication for cytoreductive therapy.
  - Complications of phlebotomy: chronic iron deficiency (symptomatology: pica, angular stomatitis, and glossitis), possible muscle weakness, and dysphagia that is the result of esophageal webs (very rare)

MEDICATION

First Line

- Primary therapies:
  - All patients should be given aspirin (50 to 100 mg) in daily or BID dosing to decrease microvascular symptoms and reduce death from CV or thromboembolic events. Aspirin should be used with caution in those with acquired von Willebrand disease or those with other contraindications.
  - Pegylated interferon α-2a (IFNa) can lessen symptoms and decrease erythrocytosis and can be use in both low and high risk patients.
  - Hydroxyurea is recommended for patients at high risk for thrombosis (age >60 years or history of thrombotic event) and with splenomegaly and hepatomegaly; common starting dose 500 to 1,500 mg PO daily, titrating to control Hct and platelet count; hydroxyurea can lead to skin ulcer, myelosuppression, and higher risk of leukemic transformation.
  - Ruxolitinib is approved for refractory PV or for patients who are intolerant to hydroxyurea.
  - Radioactive phosphorus (^{32}P) may control Hgb level and platelet count by destroying overactive marrow cells; may take up to 3 months before affecting cells; consider for patients intolerant or nonadherent to hydroxyurea or short expected survival due to mutagenic potential.
  - Refer to hematologist/oncologist for further dosing and instructions.
- Symptomatic/adjunctive:
  - Pruritus: cyproheptadine; cimetidine; SSRIs (paroxetine or fluoxetine); UV light therapy; oatmeal baths
  - Uric acid reduction: allopurinol
  - Erythromelalgia: aspirin should help this too

Second Line

Myelosuppression: chlorambucil or busulfan; busulfan at 2 to 4 mg daily may be effective option for elderly patients with advanced PV refractory or intolerant to other agents such as hydroxyurea and interferon, but significant rate of transformation was observed.

ISSUES FOR REFERRAL

Referral to a hematologist to assist in treatment and management particularly high-risk cases or intolerant to first-line therapy.

COMPLEMENTARY & ALTERNATIVE MEDICINE

Osteopathic manipulative medicine to promote circulation

ADMISSION, INPATIENT, AND NURSING CONSIDERATIONS

DVT prophylaxis should be given.

ONGOING CARE

FOLLOW-UP RECOMMENDATIONS

Monitor for secondary malignancies such as myeloproliferative neoplasms.

Patient Monitoring

Monitor Hct often and phlebotomize as needed to maintain target goal.

DIET

- Avoid high-sodium diet; can cause fluid retention
- Avoid iron supplement; a permissive chronic state of iron deficiency can help decrease blood production.

PATIENT EDUCATION

- Perform leg and ankle exercises to prevent clots.
- Continuous education regarding possible complications and seeking treatment early for any change or increase in symptoms

PROGNOSIS

- PV cannot be cured but can be controlled with treatment.
- Survival is >15 years with treatment.
- Patients are at risk for developing post polycythemic MF (PPMF) and an increased risk of malignant transformation.

COMPLICATIONS

- Splenomegaly or hepatomegaly
- Vascular thrombosis (major cause of death) including Budd-Chiari, DVT, arterial thrombosis (20%)
- Transformation to acute leukemia (5%)
- Transformation to MF (10%)
- Hemorrhage
- Peptic ulcer
- Uric acid stones or gout
- Increased risk for complications and mortality from surgical procedures; assess risk/benefits and ensure optimal control of disorder before any elective surgery.

REFERENCES

1. Cuthbert D, Stein BL. Polycythemia vera-associated complications: pathogenesis, clinical manifestations, and effects on outcomes. *J Blood Med*. 2019;10:359–371.
2. Tefferi A, Barbui T. Polycythemia vera: 2024 update on diagnosis, risk-stratification, and management. *Am J Hematol*. 2023;98(9):1465–1487.

ADDITIONAL READING

Kim TY, Kwag D, Lee JH, et al. Clinical features, gene alterations, and outcomes in prefibrotic and overt primary and secondary myelofibrotic patients. *Cancers (Basel)*. 2022;14(18):4485. doi:10.3390/cancers14184485.

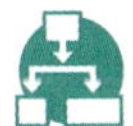

SEE ALSO

Myeloproliferative Neoplasms

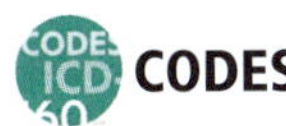

CODES

ICD10

D45 Polycythemia vera

CLINICAL PEARLS

- Erythrocytosis: Hgb >16.5 g/dL in men, >16 g/dL in women
- *JAK2* mutations are an important component of myeloproliferative disorders.
- *Bone marrow biopsy can help in diagnosis showing hypercellularity and trilineage growth.*
- Common complications include thrombosis, cardiovascular events, malignant transformation, and MF.
- All patients should take low-dose aspirin unless there is major bleeding risk or GI intolerance.
- Phlebotomy is first-line treatment and consultation with an experienced hematologist is recommended.

POLYMYALGIA RHEUMATICA

Tharani Ravi, MD • Edith Torres, DO

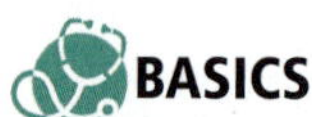

BASICS

DESCRIPTION

- An inflammatory clinical syndrome characterized by pain and morning stiffness of the shoulder, hip girdles, and neck; primarily impacts patients aged >50 years; associated with morning stiffness and elevated markers of inflammation
- Can be associated with giant cell arteritis (GCA)
- System(s) affected: musculoskeletal; hematologic/lymphatic/immunologic
- Synonym(s): senile rheumatic disease; polymyalgia rheumatica (PMR) syndrome; pseudo-polyarthrite rhizomélique

Geriatric Considerations

Incidence increases with age (age >50 years).

Pediatric Considerations

Rare in patients <50 years of age (1)

EPIDEMIOLOGY

Incidence

- Incidence increases after age 50 years. Incidence of PMR and GCA in the United States is 50 and 18 per 100,000 people, respectively.
- Predominant sex: female > male (2 to 3:1)
- Most common in Caucasians, especially those of northern European ancestry and in Scandinavian countries
- Peak incidence occurs between ages 70 and 80.

Prevalence

Prevalence in those >50 years old: 700/100,000

ETIOLOGY AND PATHOPHYSIOLOGY

- Unknown; symptoms relate to enhanced immune system and periarticular inflammatory activity.
- Pathogenesis
  - Polygenic; involves multiple environmental and genetic factors
  - Significant association between histologic evidence of GCA and parvovirus B19 DNA in temporal artery specimen

Genetics

Associated with human leukocyte antigen determinants (HLA-DRB1*04 and DRB1*01 alleles)

RISK FACTORS

- Aged >50 years
- Presence of GCA

COMMONLY ASSOCIATED CONDITIONS

Concurrent GCA (temporal arteritis) in ~15–30% of patients; more commonly in females than males

DIAGNOSIS

HISTORY

- Suspect PMR in elderly patients with new onset of proximal limb pain and stiffness (neck, shoulder, hip). Patients may use the term "stiffness" and "pain" interchangeably (2). Shoulder pain is most typically present.
- Symptoms often have a rapid onset.
- Difficulty rising from chair or combing hair (proximal muscle involvement) or putting on clothes like shirt or coat
- Nighttime pain
- Can be unilateral; however, soon it becomes symmetrical
- Severe morning stiffness
- Nonspecific systemic symptoms in ~25% (fatigue, weight loss, low-grade fever, depression, anorexia and low grade fever)
- Carpal tunnel syndrome can be seen in 10–15% of patients.
- Duration usually >2 weeks

PHYSICAL EXAM

- Decreased range of motion (ROM) of shoulders, neck, and hips
- Muscle strength is usually normal—may be limited by pain and/or stiffness.
- Muscle tenderness
- Disuse atrophy
- Synovitis of the small joints and tenosynovitis; feet and ankles never affected
- Coexisting carpal tunnel syndrome

DIFFERENTIAL DIAGNOSIS

- Rheumatoid arthritis (RA)
- Palindromic rheumatism
- Late-onset seronegative spondyloarthropathies (e.g., psoriatic arthritis, ankylosing spondylitis)
- Systemic lupus erythematosus; Sjögren syndrome; fibromyalgia
- Polymyositis-dermatomyositis (Check creatine phosphokinase, aldolase.)
- Thyroid disease; hyperparathyroidism, hypoparathyroidism
- Hypovitaminosis D
- Osteoarthritis
- Rotator cuff syndrome; adhesive capsulitis
- Remitting seronegative symmetrical synovitis with pitting edema (RS3PE) syndrome
- Occult infection or malignancy (e.g., lymphoma, leukemia, myeloma, solid tumor)
- Myopathy (e.g., steroid, alcohol, electrolyte depletion)
- Depression; fibromyalgia

DIAGNOSTIC TESTS & INTERPRETATION

ACR/EULAR classification criteria (3):

- Patients aged ≥50 years with bilateral shoulder aching and abnormal C-reactive protein concentrations or ESR, plus at least 4 points (without ultrasonography) or 5 points or more (with ultrasonography) from:
  - Morning stiffness for >45 minutes (2 points)
  - Hip pain or restricted range of motion (1 point)
  - Absence of rheumatoid factor (RF) or anti-citrullinated protein antibodies (2 points)
  - Absence of other joint involvement (1 point)
  - If ultrasonography is available, at least one shoulder with subdeltoid bursitis, biceps tenosynovitis or glenohumeral synovitis (either posterior or axillary); and at least one hip with synovitis or trochanteric bursitis (1 point)
  - If ultrasonography is available, both shoulders with subdeltoid bursitis, biceps tenosynovitis, or glenohumeral synovitis (1 point)
- Temporal artery biopsy if symptoms of GCA is present
- ESR (Westergren) elevation >40 mm/hr
  - ESR generally elevated, sometimes >100 mm/hr
  - ESR normal (<40 mm/hr) in 7–22% of patients
- Elevated C-reactive protein
- Normochromic/normocytic anemia
- Anti–cyclic citrullinated peptide (anti-CCP) antibodies usually negative (in contrast to elderly-onset RA).
- RF: negative (5–10% of patients aged >60 years have positive RF without RA.)
- Mild elevations in liver function tests, especially alkaline phosphatase
- Antibodies to ferritin peptide may be a useful diagnostic marker.
- Prednisone may alter lab results.
- Other disorders may cause elevation of ESR (e.g., infection, neoplasm, renal failure).
- Normal EMG
- Normal muscle histology
- CK is always normal.

Initial Tests (lab, imaging)

- ESR (usually >40 mm/hr); C-reactive protein; CBC (normocytic anemia)
- MRI is not necessary for diagnosis but may show periarticular inflammation, tenosynovitis, and bursitis.
- US may show bursitis, tendinitis, and synovitis.
- MRI, PET, and temporal artery US may help in diagnosis of PMR.
- ACR/EULAR classification criteria help confirm the clinical diagnosis.
- ^{18}F-fluorodeoxyglucose PET scan prior to therapy improves diagnostic accuracy.
- A scoring algorithm was devised consisting of the following: morning stiffness >45 minutes (2 points), hip pain/limited ROM (1 point), absence of RF and ACPA (2 points), and absence of peripheral joint pain (1 point).
- A score of >4 has 68% sensitivity and 78% specificity for PMR.

Diagnostic Procedures/Other

Temporal artery biopsy in patients with symptoms suggestive of GCA; treat empirically pending results.

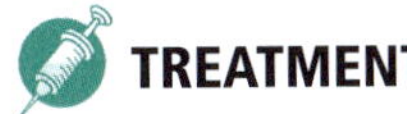

TREATMENT

GENERAL MEASURES

- Address risk of steroid-induced osteoporosis.
  - Obtain dual energy x-ray absorptiometry and check 25-OH vitamin D levels if necessary.
  - Consider antiresorptive therapies (bisphosphonates) for treatment of corticosteroid-induced osteoporosis.
- Encourage adequate calcium (1,500 mg/day) and vitamin D (800 to 1,000 U/day) supplementation.
- Physical therapy for ROM exercises, if needed

MEDICATION

First Line

- Prednisone: 12.5 to 25.0 mg/day PO initially; expect a dramatic (diagnostic) response within days; 15 mg/day is effective in almost all patients.
  - May increase to 25 mg/day if no immediate response
  - If no response within a week, reconsider diagnosis.
- Divided-dose steroids (BID or TID) may be useful initially (especially if symptoms recur in the afternoon).
- Consider using delayed-release prednisone taken at bedtime, which may help treat morning stiffness compared to immediate-release prednisone.
- Begin slow taper by 2.5 mg decrements every 2 to 4 weeks to a dose of 7.5 to 10.0 mg/day. Below this dose, taper by 1 mg/month to prevent relapse.
- Increase prednisone for symptom relapse (common).
- Corticosteroid treatment often lasts several years.
- May stop after 6 to 12 months if symptom free and ESR is normal
- Contraindications
  - Use steroids with caution in patients with chronic heart failure, diabetes mellitus (or other immunocompromised state), and systemic fungal or bacterial infection.
  - Treat any concurrent infections.
- Precautions
  - Long-term steroid use (>2 years) is associated with sodium and water retention, exacerbation of chronic heart failure, hypokalemia, increased susceptibility to infection, osteoporosis, fractures, hypertension, cataracts, glaucoma, avascular necrosis, depression, and weight gain.
  - Patients may develop temporal arteritis while on low-dose corticosteroid treatment for PMR. This requires an increase in prednisone dosing (up to 40 to 60 mg).
  - Alternate-day steroids are not effective.

Second Line

- Routine use of adjunctive therapy not recommended
- NSAIDs usually are not adequate for pain relief.
- Methotrexate modestly reduces relapse rate and lowers the cumulative dose of steroid therapy but has not been formally studied in PMR.
- Tocilizumab (IL-6 inhibitor) has been reported in case reports and small studies.
- There is conflicting evidence for anti-tumor necrosis factor (anti-TNF) agents (infliximab, etanercept).
- Rituxan may have a role in treatment based on small proof of concept trial (4)
- Corticosteroid injections (primarily for the shoulder) may help reduce pain and duration of morning stiffness, allowing for increased levels of activity.

ONGOING CARE

FOLLOW-UP RECOMMENDATIONS

Patient Monitoring

- Monthly evaluations initially and during medication taper; every 3 months otherwise
- Follow ESR as steroids are tapered; ESR and C-reactive protein should decline as symptoms improve.
- Follow up immediately for symptoms of GCA (e.g., headache, visual loss, and diplopia).
- Monitor side effects of corticosteroid therapy (osteoporosis, hypertension, and hyperglycemia).
- If patient is asymptomatic, do not treat elevated ESR (do not increase steroid dose to normalize ESR).

DIET

- Regular diet
- Adequate calcium and vitamin D

PATIENT EDUCATION

- Review adverse effects of corticosteroids.
- Discuss the symptoms of GCA (headache, visual loss, diplopia) and present immediately if any occur.
- Follow up if symptoms recur during steroid taper.
- Do not abruptly stop steroids.
- Ensure adequate calcium and vitamin D intake.
- Patient resources:
  - Arthritis Foundation: https://www.arthritis.org/
  - American College of Rheumatology: https://rheumatology.org/patients/polymyalgia-rheumatica

PROGNOSIS

- Most patients require at least 2 years of corticosteroid treatment.
- Exacerbation or relapse is common if steroids are tapered too quickly.
- Prognosis is very good with proper treatment.
- Relapse is common (in 25–50% of patients).
- Higher age at diagnosis, female sex, high baseline ESR, increased levels of soluble IL-6 receptor, and high initial steroid dose have been associated with a prolonged disease course and more disease flares.

COMPLICATIONS

- Complications related to chronic steroid use
- Exacerbation of disease with taper of steroids; development of GCA (may occur when PMR is being treated adequately)

REFERENCES

1. El Chami S, Springer JM. Update on the treatment of giant cell arteritis and polymyalgia rheumatica. *Med Clin North Am*. 2021 Mar;105(2):311–324.
2. García-Porrúa C, Heras-Recuero E, Blázquez-Sánchez T, et al. Traditional and emerging strategies for managing polymyalgia rheumatica: insights into new treatments. *J Clin Med*. 2024;13(21):6492. doi:10.3390/jcm13216492.
3. Dasgupta B, Cimmino MA, Maradit-Kremers H, et al. 2012 Provisional classification criteria for polymyalgia rheumatica: a European League Against Rheumatism/American College of Rheumatology collaborative initiative. *Ann Rheum Dis*. 2012;71(4):484–492.
4. Espígol-Frigolé G, Dejaco C, Mackie SL, et al. Polymyalgia rheumatica. *Lancet*. 2023;402(10411):1459–1472. doi:10.1016/S0140-6736(23)01310-7.

ADDITIONAL READING

Sun MM, Pope JE. Polymyalgia rheumatica and giant cell arteritis: diagnosis and management. *Curr Opin Rheumatol*. 2025;37(1):32–38.

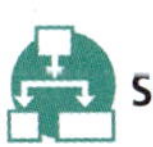

SEE ALSO

Arteritis, Temporal; Arthritis, Rheumatoid (RA); Depression; Fibromyalgia; Osteoarthritis; Polymyositis/Dermatomyositis

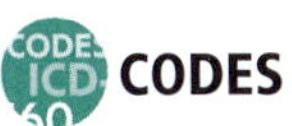

CODES

ICD10

- M35.3 Polymyalgia rheumatica
- M31.5 Giant cell arteritis with polymyalgia rheumatica

CLINICAL PEARLS

- Consider PMR in patients aged >50 years who present with hip, neck, and/or shoulder pain and stiffness.
- A normal ESR does not exclude PMR.
- Corticosteroids are the treatment of choice. If there is not a dramatic and rapid response, reconsider the diagnosis.
- Adjust steroids according to symptoms, not ESR.

POLYMYOSITIS/DERMATOMYOSITIS

Christopher M. Wise, MD • Nehal R. Shah, MD

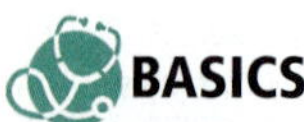

BASICS

DESCRIPTION

- Systemic connective tissue disease characterized by inflammatory and degenerative changes in proximal muscles, sometimes accompanied by characteristic skin rash
  - If skin manifestations (Gottron sign [symmetric, scaly, violaceous, erythematous eruption over the extensor surfaces of the metacarpophalangeal and interphalangeal joints of the fingers]; heliotrope [reddish violaceous eruption on the upper eyelids]) are present, it is designated as dermatomyositis.
  - Different types of myositis include the following (1):
    - Idiopathic polymyositis
    - Idiopathic dermatomyositis
    - Polymyositis/dermatomyositis as an overlap (usually with lupus or systemic sclerosis or as part of mixed connective tissue disease)
    - Myositis associated with malignancy
    - Necrotizing autoimmune myositis (often statin associated)
    - Inclusion body myositis (IBM), a variant with atypical patterns of weakness and biopsy findings
- System(s) affected: cardiovascular, musculoskeletal, pulmonary, skin/exocrine
- Synonym(s): myositis; inflammatory myopathy; antisynthetase syndrome (subset with certain antibodies)

EPIDEMIOLOGY

Incidence

- Estimated at 1.2 to 2 per 100,000 population per year
- Predominant age: 5 to 15 years, 40 to 60 years, peak incidence in mid-40s
- Predominant sex: female > male (2:1)

Prevalence

2.4 to 33.8 patients per 100,000 population

Geriatric Considerations

Elderly patients with myositis or dermatomyositis are at increased risk of neoplasm.

Pediatric Considerations

Childhood dermatomyositis is likely a separate entity associated with cutaneous vasculitis and muscle calcifications.

ETIOLOGY AND PATHOPHYSIOLOGY

- Inflammatory process, mediated by T cells and cytokine release, leading to damage to muscle cells (predominantly skeletal muscles)
- In patients with IBM, degenerative mechanisms may be important.
- Unknown; potential viral, genetic factors

Genetics

Mild association with human leukocyte antigen (HLA)-DR3, HLA-DRw52

RISK FACTORS

Family history of autoimmune disease (e.g., systemic lupus erythematosus [SLE], myositis) or vasculitis

COMMONLY ASSOCIATED CONDITIONS

- Malignancy more common in dermatomyositis subtype, older patients
- Progressive systemic sclerosis
- Vasculitis
- SLE
- Mixed connective tissue disease

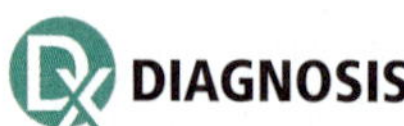

DIAGNOSIS

HISTORY

- Symmetric proximal muscle weakness causing difficulty when
  - Arising from sitting or lying positions
  - Climbing stairs
  - Raising arms
- Joint pain/swelling
- Dysphagia
- Dyspnea
- Rash on face, eyelids, hands, arms

PHYSICAL EXAM

Proximal muscle weakness

- Shoulder muscles
- Hip girdle muscles (trouble standing from seated or squatting position, weak hip flexors in supine position)
- Muscle swelling, stiffness, induration
- Distal muscle weakness is seen only in patients with IBM.
- Rash over face (eyelids, nasolabial folds), upper chest, dorsal hands (especially knuckle pads), fingers ("mechanic's hands")
- Periorbital edema
- Calcinosis cutis (childhood cases)
- Mesenteric arterial insufficiency/infarction (childhood cases)
- Cardiac impairment; arrhythmia, heart failure

DIFFERENTIAL DIAGNOSIS

- Vasculitis
- Progressive systemic sclerosis
- SLE
- Rheumatoid arthritis
- Muscular dystrophy
- Lambert-Eaton syndrome
- Sarcoidosis
- Amyotrophic lateral sclerosis
- Endocrine disorders
  - Thyroid disease
  - Cushing syndrome
- Infectious myositis (viral, bacterial, parasitic)
- Drug-induced myopathies:
  - Cholesterol-lowering agents (statins)
  - Colchicine
  - Corticosteroids
  - Ethanol
  - Chloroquine
  - Zidovudine
- Electrolyte disorders (magnesium, calcium, potassium)
- Heritable metabolic myopathies
- Sleep apnea syndrome

DIAGNOSTIC TESTS & INTERPRETATION

- Diagnosis of muscle component (myositis) usually relies on four findings:
  - Weakness
  - Creatine kinase (CK) and/or aldolase elevation
  - Abnormal electromyogram (EMG)
  - Findings on muscle biopsy
- Presence of compatible skin rash of dermatomyositis
- There is an emerging role for myositis-specific antibody (MSA) profiles. MSAs can be used to guide the appropriate workup for malignancy and interstitial lung disease (ILD) (2).

Initial Tests (lab, imaging)

- Increased CK, aldolase
- Increased serum aspartate aminotransferase (AST)
- Increased lactate dehydrogenase (LDH)
- Myoglobinuria
- Increased ESR
- Positive rheumatoid factor (<50% of patients)
- Positive antinuclear antibody (ANA) (>50% of patients)
- Leukocytosis (<50% of patients)
- Anemia (<50% of patients)
- Hyperglobulinemia (<50% of patients)
- Anti-3-hydroxy-3-methylglutaryl-coenzyme A reductase (HMGCR) and anti-SRP antibodies seen in patient with necrotizing autoimmune myositis
- Antisynthetase antibodies (anti–Jo-1 and non–Jo-1 synthetases) present in antisynthetase syndrome
  - Associated with an increased incidence of ILD
- Anti–MDA-5 antibody seen in overlap myositis with atypical rashes and severe ILD
- Anti–U1 RNP, anti–PM/Scl, and anti-Ku antibodies seen in overlap myositis
- Chest radiograph as part of initial evaluation to assess for associated pulmonary involvement or malignancy

Follow-Up Tests & Special Considerations

- Changes in muscle enzymes (CK or aldolase) correlate with improvement and worsening.
- MRI to assess muscle edema and inflammation may be used in some patients to determine best biopsy site or response to therapy.

Diagnostic Procedures/Other

- EMG: muscle irritability, low-amplitude potentials, polyphasic action potentials, fibrillations
- Muscle biopsy (deltoid or quadriceps femoris)

Test Interpretation

- Microscopic findings:
  - Muscle fiber degeneration
  - Phagocytosis of muscle debris
  - Perifascicular muscle fiber atrophy
  - Inflammatory cell infiltrates in adult form
  - Via electron microscopy: inclusion bodies (IBM only)
  - Sarcoplasmic basophilia
- Muscle fiber increased in size
- Vasculopathy (childhood polymyositis/dermatomyositis)

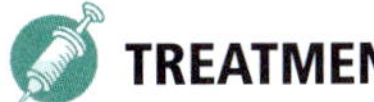

TREATMENT

GENERAL MEASURES

Approach to treatment has varied by specialty involved (dermatology, rheumatology, neurology). Treatment approach should be informed by lesion type, degree of muscle involvement, presence of systemic symptoms, presence of MSAs, and patient's age (2)[C]

MEDICATION

First Line

- Prednisone
  - 0.5 to 1.0 mg/kg/day PO in divided doses
  - IV pulse dose methylprednisolone 1,000 mg daily for 3 to 5 days in acute and severe cases
  - Consolidate doses and reduce prednisone slowly when enzyme levels are normal.
  - Probably need to continue 5 to 10 mg/day for maintenance in most patients
- Immunosuppressive maintenance therapy in parallel to steroids—recommended in most patients:
  - Azathioprine 1 to 2 mg/kg PO (arthritis dose) once daily or BID, or
  - Methotrexate 10 to 25 mg PO weekly, or
  - Mycophenolate mofetil 2 to 3 mg daily
- Rash of dermatomyositis may require topical steroids or oral hydroxychloroquine.
- Patients with IBM have very poor response to steroids and other first- and second-line drugs in general.

Second Line

- Other immunosuppressant drugs (e.g., cyclophosphamide, chlorambucil, cyclosporin, tacrolimus) can be added to steroids in refractory cases. Adrenocorticotropic gel (ACTH gel) may have a role in refractory cases.
- Combination methotrexate and azathioprine also may be useful in refractory cases.
- IVIG and rituximab have been reported to be helpful in patients with refractory disease. Rituxan may be more effective in patients with autoantibodies positive myositis (especially anti–Jo-1 and anti–Mi-2). IVIG can be a reasonable alternative in patients whom steroids or other immunosuppressive drugs are contraindicated such as infection and neoplasm.
- Cyclophosphamide is usually reserved for severe cases with lung or heart involvement.
- Contraindications: Methotrexate is contraindicated with previous liver disease, alcohol use, pregnancy, and underlying renal disease (use with extreme caution in patients with serum creatinine >1.5 mg/dL in general).
- Precautions
  - Prednisone: Adverse effects associated with long-term steroid use include adrenal suppression, sodium and water retention, hypokalemia, osteoporosis, cataracts, and increased susceptibility to infection.
  - Azathioprine: Adverse effects include bone marrow suppression, increased liver function tests, and increased risk of infection.
  - Methotrexate: Adverse effects include stomatitis, bone marrow suppression, pneumonitis, and risk of liver fibrosis and cirrhosis with prolonged use.

ISSUES FOR REFERRAL

- Diagnostic uncertainty, usually related to elevated muscle enzymes without typical symptoms of findings of muscle weakness
- Poor response to initial steroid therapy
- Excessive steroid requirement (unable to taper prednisone to <20 mg/day after 4 to 6 months)

SURGERY/OTHER PROCEDURES

None indicated, other than initial biopsy

COMPLEMENTARY & ALTERNATIVE MEDICINE

Benefits and harms of physical therapy are not well established, especially in active muscle disease (3)[A], although there is some suggestion of benefit in quiescent disease (4)[A]. Research is of low quality in this area.

ADMISSION, INPATIENT, AND NURSING CONSIDERATIONS

- Inability to stand, ambulate, respiratory difficulty, fever or other signs of infection
- Inpatient evaluation seldom needed

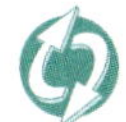

ONGOING CARE

FOLLOW-UP RECOMMENDATIONS

Patient Monitoring

- Follow muscle enzymes along with muscle strength and functional capacity.
- Monitor for steroid-induced complications (e.g., hypokalemia, hypertension, and hyperglycemia).
- Bone densitometry and consideration of calcium, vitamin D, and bisphosphonate therapy
- If azathioprine, methotrexate, or other immunosuppressant is used, appropriate laboratory monitoring should be done periodically (e.g., hematology, liver enzymes, and creatinine).
- Attempt to decrease and/or discontinue steroid dose as patient responds to therapy.
- Maintain immunosuppression until patient's muscle strength stabilizes for prolonged period depending on individual patient parameters, risks of medication, risk of relapse; time period undefined but most patients (80%) require prolonged maintenance immunosuppressive therapy.

DIET

Moderation of caloric and sodium intake to avoid weight gain from corticosteroid therapy

PATIENT EDUCATION

Curtail excess physical activity in early phases when muscle enzymes are markedly elevated. Emphasize range of motion exercises. Gradually introduce muscle strengthening when muscle enzymes are normal or improved and stable.

PROGNOSIS

- Residual weakness: 30%, persistent active disease: 20%
- 5 to 10 year survival is 80% and 75%, but mortality is 3- to 5-fold higher than general population. Most of the increase in mortality occurs in the 1st year after diagnosis. Survival is worse for women and African Americans and those with dermatomyositis, IBM, or cancer.
- Most patients improve with therapy.
- Patient with ILD have poor prognosis.
- Patients with IBM respond poorly to most therapies.
- 20–50% have full recovery
- Most patients require prolonged maintenance immunosuppresive therapy, with only 20% able to discontinue therapy over a 7-year period of time

COMPLICATIONS

Pneumonia, infection, myocardial infarction, carcinoma (especially breast, lung), severe dysphagia, respiratory impairment due to muscle weakness, ILD, aspiration pneumonitis, steroid myopathy, steroid-induced diabetes, hypertension, hypokalemia, osteoporosis

REFERENCES

1. Senécal JL, Raynauld JP, Troyanov Y. Editorial: a new classification of adult autoimmune myositis. *Arthritis Rheumatol*. 2017;69(5):878–884.
2. Waldman R, DeWane ME, Lu J. Dermatomyositis: diagnosis and treatment. *J Am Acad Dermatol*. 2020;82(2):283–296.
3. Voet NB, va der Kooi EL, van Engelen BG, et al. Strength training and aerobic exercise training for muscle disease. *Cochrane Database Syst Rev*. 2019;12(12):CD003907.
4. Van Thillo A, Vulsteke JB, Van Assche D, et al. Physical therapy in adult inflammatory myopathy patients: a systematic review. *Clin Rheumatol*. 2019;38(8):2039–2051.

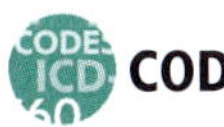

CODES

ICD10

- M33.20 Polymyositis, organ involvement unspecified
- M33.90 Dermatopolymyositis, unspecified, organ involvement unspecified
- M33.92 Dermatopolymyositis, unspecified with myopathy

CLINICAL PEARLS

- Corticosteroids alone may be sufficient in patients who have rapid improvement in weakness and muscle enzymes. However, most patients require azathioprine, methotrexate, or other immunosuppressive medications.
- Elevated muscle enzymes (e.g., CK and aldolase) are seen frequently as transient phenomena in patients with febrile illness and injuries; may return to normal on repeat
- In patients with persistently elevated muscle enzymes and symptoms and findings of muscle weakness, EMG followed by muscle biopsy should be the initial studies considered.
- Suspect IBM in older patients with very slow onset and progression of symptoms, poor response to steroids and immunosuppressive therapy, and atypical patterns (asymmetric, sometimes distal) of muscle weakness.

POPLITEAL (BAKER) CYST

Shane L. Larson, MD • Christopher Morrow, PA-C

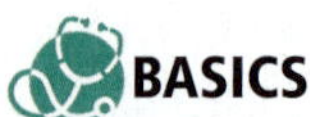

BASICS

DESCRIPTION

- A fluid-filled synovial sac arising in the popliteal fossa as a distention of (typically) the gastrocnemial-semimembranous bursa; not a true cyst
- Can be unilateral or bilateral
- Most frequent cystic mass around the knee
- Primary cysts are a distention of the bursa (arise independently without an intra-articular disorder).
- Secondary cysts occur if there is a communication between the bursa and knee joint, allowing articular fluid to fill the cyst.
- Associated with synovial inflammation

EPIDEMIOLOGY

Incidence

- Bimodal distribution
  - Children ages 4 to 7 years
  - Adults increasing with age
- Primary cysts usually seen in children <15 years
- Secondary cysts seen in adults

Prevalence

- Variable adult prevalence of 19–47% in symptomatic knees and 2–5% in asymptomatic knees
- In children: 6.3% in symptomatic knees; 2.4% in asymptomatic knees

ETIOLOGY AND PATHOPHYSIOLOGY

Associated intra-articular pathology includes

- Meniscal tears, mostly of the posterior horn
- Anterior cruciate ligament (ACL) insufficiency
- Degenerative articular cartilage lesions
- Rheumatoid arthritis (20%)
- Osteoarthritis (50%)
- Osteochondritis
- Gout (14%)
- Other potential factors
  - Infectious arthritis
  - Polyarthritis
  - Villonodular synovitis
  - Lymphoma
  - Sarcoidosis
  - Connective tissue diseases
- Extension or herniation of synovial membrane of the knee joint capsule or connection of normal bursa with the joint capsule
- May result from increased intra-articular pressure
- Commonly seen with knee effusions
- Direct trauma to the bursa is likely the primary cause in children because of no communication between the bursa and the joint.
- A valve-like mechanism allowing one-way passage of fluid from the joint to the bursal connection has been described.

RISK FACTORS

- Osteoarthritis of knee (most common)
- Rheumatoid arthritis
- Meniscal degeneration or tear
- Advancing age
- Ligamentous trauma
- Ligamentous insufficiency

COMMONLY ASSOCIATED CONDITIONS

Any condition causing knee joint effusion

DIAGNOSIS

HISTORY

- Painless mass arising in the popliteal fossa
- Most cysts are asymptomatic.
- Dull ache if cyst is large enough to impede joint motion—typically a restriction of flexion
- Painful if cyst ruptures
- Large cysts may cause entrapment neuropathy of the tibial nerve.
- Vascular compression, most commonly of the popliteal vein, may produce claudication or thrombophlebitis.
- Activity alters the cyst size.

PHYSICAL EXAM

- Examine in full extension and 90 degrees of flexion.
- Foucher sign: Mass increases with extension and disappears with flexion.
- Most commonly found in medial aspect of popliteal fossa lateral to the head of the gastrocnemius and medial to the neurovascular bundle
- Cyst is easiest to palpate when knee is slightly flexed and may occasionally be fluctuant or tender.
- Transillumination helps distinguish cyst from solid mass.
- Ruptured cysts are typically painful with associated swelling and bruising over the ipsilateral calf and ankle at the medial malleolus (crescent sign).
- Ruptured cysts also are associated with pseudothrombophlebitis, and rarely, compartment syndrome (1).

DIFFERENTIAL DIAGNOSIS

- Deep venous thrombosis
- Infection/abscess
- Ganglion cyst
- Hematoma
- Thrombophlebitis
- Lipoma, liposarcoma
- Fibroma, fibrosarcoma
- Vascular tumor
- Popliteal vein varices
- Xanthoma
- Aneurysm (rare)
- Muscular herniation (rare, related to trauma)

DIAGNOSTIC TESTS & INTERPRETATION

Initial Tests (lab, imaging)

- CBC, ESR (if septic arthritis suspected)
- Ensure not a popliteal aneurysm prior to aspiration. Send aspirate for cell count and culture to determine if fluid is infectious, inflammatory, or mechanical.
- Ultrasound confirms presence and size; Doppler can differentiate Baker cysts from popliteal vessel aneurysms, DVT, or soft tissue tumors (2).
- MRI helps assess derangements of internal joint structures and to identify cyst leakage.

Follow-Up Tests & Special Considerations

- Consider observation over invasive testing in children.
- Radiographs may show soft tissue density posteriorly.
- Arthrography may demonstrate communication with joint capsule or rupture.
- CT arthrography is superior for visualizing cystic details and can help distinguish lipomas, aneurysms, and malignancies from cysts.

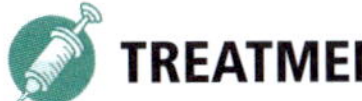

TREATMENT

GENERAL MEASURES

- No treatment if asymptomatic
- Treat any associated underlying conditions.
- Compressive wrap or sleeve for comfort

MEDICATION

If etiology is identified from cellular fluid examination, treat the underlying condition.

First Line

Analgesics and NSAIDs for symptomatic relief

ADDITIONAL THERAPIES

- Physical therapy improves knee ROM and strength, particularly with coexisting pathology.
- Temporary relief with needle aspiration; recurrence common
- Improvement in joint ROM, knee pain, swelling, accompanied reduction in bursa size after aspiration, and intra-articular/intracystic corticosteroid injection (3)[B]
- A combination of physical therapy and corticosteroid injection with or without aspiration leads to best improvements in pain, function, and reduction in cyst size (4)[A].
- Sclerotherapy injections of ethanol or dextrose/sodium morrhuate shown to have good results in small studies (5)[B].

SURGERY/OTHER PROCEDURES

- Consider excision when symptoms persist despite treatment or no etiology is found.
- Surgery usually not required in children
- Recurrence after standard surgery is common and is highest if chondral lesions are present.
- Arthroscopic surgery is highly successful if a valvular mechanism is identified and intra-articular pathology is treated (6)[B].
- Excision via arthroscopy or open procedure often requires concomitant treatment of underlying pathology.

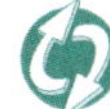

ONGOING CARE

PROGNOSIS

- Variable; many cysts remain asymptomatic.
- Some cysts resolve with treatment of underlying etiology (e.g., gout, rheumatoid arthritis).
- In children, most cysts resolve without treatment.

COMPLICATIONS

- Compartment syndrome in ruptured cyst
- Thrombophlebitis from compression of the popliteal vein
- Infection of popliteal cyst
- Hemorrhage into cyst if on anticoagulants

REFERENCES

1. Chatzopoulos D, Moralidis E, Markou P, et al. Baker's cysts in knees with chronic osteoarthritic pain: a clinical, ultrasonographic, radiographic and scintigraphic evaluation. *Rheumatol Int*. 2008;29(2):141–146.
2. Sanchez JE, Conkling N, Labropoulos N. Compression syndromes of the popliteal neurovascular bundle due to Baker cyst. *J Vasc Surg*. 2011;54(6):1821–1829.
3. Acebes JC, Sánchez-Pernaute O, Díaz-Oca A, et al. Ultrasonographic assessment of Baker's cysts after intra-articular corticosteroid injection in knee osteoarthritis. *J Clin Ultrasound*. 2006;34(3):113–117.
4. Di Sante L, Paoloni M, Dimaggio M, et al. Ultrasound-guided aspiration and corticosteroid injection compared to horizontal therapy for treatment of knee osteoarthritis complicated with Baker's cyst: a randomized, controlled trial. *Eur J Phys Rehabil Med*. 2012;48(4):561–567.
5. Centeno CJ, Schultz J, Freeman M. Sclerotherapy of Baker's cyst with imaging confirmation of resolution. *Pain Physician*. 2008;11(2):257–261.
6. Lie CW, Ng TP. Arthroscopic treatment of popliteal cyst. *Hong Kong Med J*. 2011;17(3):180–183.

ADDITIONAL READING

- Akagi R, Saisu T, Segawa Y, et al. Natural history of popliteal cysts in the pediatric population. *J Pediatr Orthop*. 2013;33(3):262–268.
- Akgul O, Guldeste Z, Ozgocmen S. The reliability of the clinical examination for detecting Baker's cyst in asymptomatic fossa. *Int J Rheum Dis*. 2014;17(2):204–209.
- Han JH, Bae JH, Nha KW, et al. Arthroscopic treatment of popliteal cysts with and without cystectomy: a systematic review and meta-analysis. *Knee Surg Relat Res*. 2019;31(2):103–112.
- Su C, Kuang S-D, Zhao X, et al. Clinical outcome of arthroscopic internal drainage of popliteal cysts with or without cyst wall resection. *BMC Musculoskelet Disord*. 2020;21(1):440.
- Van Nest DS, Tjoumakaris FP, Smith BJ, et al. Popliteal cysts: a systematic review of nonoperative and operative treatment. *JBJS Rev*. 2020;8(3):e0139.

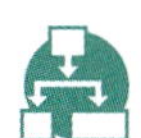

SEE ALSO

Algorithm: Knee Pain

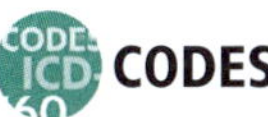

CODES

ICD10

- M71.20 Synovial cyst of popliteal space [Baker], unspecified knee
- M71.21 Synovial cyst of popliteal space [Baker], right knee
- M71.22 Synovial cyst of popliteal space [Baker], left knee

CLINICAL PEARLS

- Baker cyst: a fluid-filled synovial sac arising in the popliteal fossa as a distention of (typically) the gastrocnemial-semimembranous bursa; not a true cyst; often secondary to meniscal tear, osteoarthritis, etc.
- Conservative treatment of Baker cysts is preferred in children, as most will spontaneously resolve.
- In adults, treatment of underlying cause may resolve Baker cysts.
- Pain, bruising, and swelling over the medial malleolus (crescent sign) suggest cyst rupture.

PORTAL HYPERTENSION

Walter M. Kim, MD, PhD

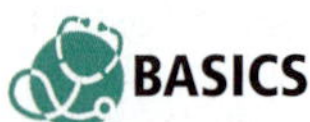

BASICS

DESCRIPTION

- Increased portal venous pressure that occurs in association with splanchnic vasodilatation, portosystemic collateral formation, and hyperdynamic circulation
- Most commonly secondary to an elevated hepatic venous pressure gradient (HVPG) (the gradient between portal and central venous pressures) >5 mm Hg
- Course is progressive, with risk of development of acute variceal bleeding, ascites, hepatic encephalopathy, portopulmonary syndrome, and hepatorenal syndrome.

EPIDEMIOLOGY

Prevalence

- Prevalence of clinically significant portal hypertension (HVPG >10 mm Hg): 0.98% in the United States
- Predominant sex: male > female adults

ETIOLOGY AND PATHOPHYSIOLOGY

- Develops as a consequence of resistance to blood flow in the portal venous system
- Cirrhosis is the most common cause of portal hypertension.
- Schistosomiasis is the most common cause of non-cirrhotic portal hypertension.
- Causes generally classified as follows:
  - Prehepatic (portal vein thrombosis or obstruction)
  - Intrahepatic (most commonly cirrhosis or schistosomiasis)
  - Posthepatic (hepatic vein thrombosis, Budd-Chiari syndrome, right-sided heart failure)
- 90% of intrahepatic cases are due to cirrhosis secondary to the following:
  - Virus (hepatitis B, hepatitis C, hepatitis D)
  - Alcoholism
  - Metabolic dysfunction-associated steatotic liver disease (MASLD)
  - Wilson disease
  - Hemochromatosis
  - Primary biliary cholangitis (PBC)
  - Sarcoidosis
- Increased HVPG (>10 mm Hg) results in venous collateral formation in the distal esophagus, proximal stomach, rectum, and umbilicus.
- Progression of portal hypertension results in splanchnic vasodilation and angiogenesis.
- Gastroesophageal variceal formation is found in 40% of patients with portal hypertension.

RISK FACTORS

Pediatric Considerations

Portal vein thrombosis is the most common extrahepatic cause; intrahepatic causes are more likely to be biliary atresia, viral hepatitis, and metabolic liver disease.

COMMONLY ASSOCIATED CONDITIONS

- Alcoholism
- Cirrhosis
- MASLD
- Schistosomiasis
- Extrahepatic portal vein thrombosis

DIAGNOSIS

HISTORY

- History of chronic liver disease
- Alcoholic hepatitis
- Jaundice
- Ascites; symptoms of heart failure including chest pain, shortness of breath, and/or edema
- Clinical features of upper gastrointestinal bleeding (hematemesis, melena)
- Weakness/fatigue
- Alcohol abuse
- Oliguria

PHYSICAL EXAM

- Exam findings may be general or related to specific complications.
- General
  - Pallor
  - Icterus
  - Digital clubbing
  - Palmar erythema
  - Splenomegaly
  - Caput medusa
  - Spider angiomata
  - Umbilical bruit
  - Hemorrhoids
  - Gynecomastia
  - Testicular atrophy
- Gastroesophageal varices
  - Hypotension
  - Tachycardia
- Ascites
  - Distended abdomen
  - Fluid wave
  - Shifting dullness with percussion
- Hepatic encephalopathy
  - Confusion/coma
  - Asterixis
  - Hyperreflexia

DIFFERENTIAL DIAGNOSIS

- Gastroesophageal varices with hemorrhage
  - Portal hypertensive gastropathy
  - Hemorrhagic gastritis
  - Peptic ulcer disease
  - Mallory-Weiss tear
- Ascites
  - Spontaneous bacterial peritonitis (SBP)
  - Pancreatic ascites
  - Peritoneal carcinomatosis
  - Tuberculous peritonitis
  - Hepatic malignancy
  - Fluid overload from heart failure
  - Nephrotic syndrome
- Hepatic encephalopathy
  - Delirium tremens
  - Intracranial hemorrhage
  - Sedative abuse
  - Uremia
- Hepatorenal syndrome
  - Drug nephrotoxicity
  - Renal tubular necrosis

DIAGNOSTIC TESTS & INTERPRETATION

Initial Tests (lab, imaging)

Direct calculation of HVPG (approximation of the gradient in pressure between portal vein and inferior vena cava [IVC]) is the gold standard in diagnosing portal hypertension:

- HVPG = wedged hepatic venous pressure (WHVP)—free hepatic venous pressure (FHVP)
- WHVP is estimated by occlusion of the hepatic vein by a balloon catheter and measurement of the proximal static column of blood.
- FHVP is estimated by direct measurement of the patent hepatic vein, intra-abdominal IVC, or right atrium.
- Esophageal varices generally develop when HVPG >10 mm Hg in compensated cirrhosis and HVPG >16 mm Hg in decompensated cirrhosis.
- Nonspecific changes associated with underlying disease:
  - Hypersplenism: anemia (also may be due to malnutrition or bleeding), leukopenia, thrombocytopenia
  - Hepatic dysfunction
    - Hypoalbuminemia
    - Hyperbilirubinemia
    - Elevated alkaline phosphatase
    - Elevated liver enzymes (AST, ALT)
    - Abnormal clotting (prothrombin time, international normalized ratio, partial thromboplastin time)
  - GI bleeding
    - Iron deficiency anemia
    - Elevated serum ammonia
    - Fecal occult blood
    - Thrombocytopenia
  - Hepatorenal syndrome
    - Elevated serum creatinine (Cr), blood urea nitrogen (BUN)
    - Urine sodium <5 mEq/L (<20 mmol/L)
  - US and CT scan/MRI may detect cirrhosis, splenomegaly, ascites, and varices.
  - US/duplex Doppler
    - Can determine presence and direction of flow in portal and hepatic veins
    - Useful in diagnosing portal vein thrombosis, shunt thrombosis, or the presence of ascites
  - CT scan/MRI: angiographic measurement of hepatic venous wedge pressure via jugular or femoral vein
    - Correlates with portal pressure
    - Risk of variceal bleeding is increased if HVPG >10 mm Hg.
  - Transient elastography and MRI elastography are noninvasive methods to determine hepatic fibrosis/cirrhosis and to predict portal hypertension.

Follow-Up Tests & Special Considerations

- If portal hypertension is diagnosed in a patient with no risk factors, the patient should first be evaluated for the presence of cirrhosis.
- HVPG response to nonselective β-blockers is associated with a significant reduction in risk of variceal bleeding and decompensation.

Diagnostic Procedures/Other

- Diagnostic paracentesis and calculation of the serum-ascites albumin gradient (SAAG) can differentiate between portal hypertensive (SAAG >1.1 g/dL) and nonportal hypertensive (SAAG <1.1 g/dL) causes of ascites.
- Upper endoscopy should be performed in patients with cirrhosis for variceal screening and can diagnose the presence of esophageal and gastric varices and portal hypertensive gastropathy.

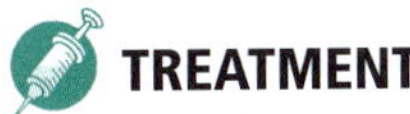

TREATMENT

GENERAL MEASURES

- Avoid sedatives that may precipitate encephalopathy.
- Limit sodium intake because cirrhotic patients avidly retain sodium (<2 g sodium/day)

MEDICATION

First Line

- Prophylaxis against variceal bleeding with nonselective β-blockers (NSBB) (1)
  - Compensated cirrhosis
    - Carvedilol: 6.25 mg PO daily (maximum dose of 12.5 mg daily)
  - Decompensated cirrhosis
    - Nadolol: 20 to 40 mg PO daily (maximum dose of 80 mg daily with ascites and 160 mg daily without ascites)
    - Propranolol: 20 to 40 mg PO 2 to 3 times daily (maximum dose of 160 mg daily with ascites and 320 mg daily without ascites)
  - Doses may be titrated up as tolerated to maximum recommended doses; goal resting heart rate of 55 to 60 beats/min
- Therapy for acute variceal hemorrhage:
  - Octreotide: 50 μg IV bolus followed by 25 to 50 μg/hour continuous infusion; pediatric dose: 1 μg/kg bolus followed by 1 μg/kg/hour is used traditionally; treat for up to 5 days.
  - Somatostatin: 250 μg IV bolus followed by 250 to 500 μg/hour continuous infusion
- β-Blockers should be used with caution in setting of severe refractory ascites and previous history of SBP.
- Initial treatment for ascites (along with salt and fluid restriction):
  - Furosemide: 20 to 40 mg/day PO; pediatric dose: 1 to 2 mg/kg/dose PO
  - Spironolactone: 50 to 100 mg/day PO; pediatric dose: 1 to 3 mg/kg/day PO

Second Line

- Terlipressin (2 mg IV q4h; titrate down to 1 mg IV q4h once hemorrhage is controlled; may be used for up to 48 hours) is a more selective splanchnic vasoconstrictor and may be associated with fewer complications. It is currently used when standard therapy with somatostatin or octreotide fails.
- Addition of nitrates, such as nitroglycerin or isosorbide mononitrate, reduces portal pressures and bleeding rates and has been shown to reduce mortality. Because the risk–benefit ratio is not clear, nitrates are not considered first-line treatment.

SURGERY/OTHER PROCEDURES

- Treatments available for specific complications of portal hypertension (in addition to or if refractory to medications):
  - Gastroesophageal varices without hemorrhage
    - Endoscopic variceal ligation (EVL) is the preferred therapy for prevention of bleeding of large (grade II or grade III) varices and requires serial interventions every 2 to 4 weeks until the varices are eradicated.
  - Gastroesophageal varices with hemorrhage
    - EVL or sclerosis (the first-line treatment in many cases for acute hemorrhage) within 12 hours of presentation (2)[A]
    - Balloon tamponade (not used commonly when endoscopic treatment is available)
    - Transjugular intrahepatic portosystemic shunt (TIPS)
    - Portacaval shunting
  - Ascites refractory to medical management
    - Large-volume paracentesis
    - Peritoneovenous shunt
    - TIPS (relatively contraindicated in patients with acute or recurrent hepatic encephalopathy)
- Liver transplantation should be considered for patients with advanced liver disease.

ADMISSION, INPATIENT, AND NURSING CONSIDERATIONS

- Acute bleeding from the intestinal tract, either vomiting or per rectum
- Acute confusional state/mental status changes suggestive of hepatic encephalopathy
- If acute variceal bleeding is present:
  - Type and cross patient's blood.
  - Initial resuscitation with isotonic fluid until packed RBCs are available
  - Correct coagulopathy with vitamin K and fresh frozen plasma (FFP)
  - Upper endoscopy as soon as the patient is stabilized (for diagnosis and treatment)
  - Avoid sedatives that may precipitate encephalopathy.
  - Limit sodium administration because cirrhotic patients avidly retain sodium.
  - Restrict protein only if encephalopathic.

ALERT

If the patient is an active alcohol drinker, assess for alcoholic hepatitis by laboratory testing and watch for signs and symptoms of withdrawal. Follow inpatient protocols for alcohol withdrawal management.

- Use isotonic fluid for hydration.
- Discharge criteria
  - For GI bleeding:
    - No active bleeding in 24 hours
    - Stable hemoglobin and hematocrit
    - Hemodynamically stable (especially heart rate)
  - For encephalopathy: improvement in or resolution of mental status changes to baseline

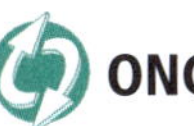

ONGOING CARE

DIET

- In cirrhosis, patients retain sodium, so restrict sodium intake to <2 g daily.
- Alcohol abstinence

PROGNOSIS

- Hepatic reserve defined by Child-Pugh classification: rating based on encephalopathy, ascites, bilirubin, albumin, prothrombin
- Variceal bleeding
  - 1/3 of patients with known varices will bleed eventually.
  - 50% rebleed, usually within 2 years, unless portal pressure is reduced by surgical or TIPS procedure.
  - 15–20% mortality rate
- Ascites and encephalopathy often recur.
- Prognosis of patients with ascites is poor: 50% 1-year survival without liver transplant (compared with 90% for patients with cirrhosis and no ascites).

COMPLICATIONS

- Acute gastroesophageal variceal bleed
- Ascites
- Hepatic encephalopathy
- Hepatic hydrothorax
- Hepatorenal syndrome
- Portal hypertensive gastropathy
- Portopulmonary hypertension
- Splenomegaly
- SBP

REFERENCES

1. Kaplan DE, Ripoll C, Thiele Maja, et al. AASLD practice guidance on risk stratification and management of portal hypertension and varices in cirrhosis. *Hepatology*. 2024;79(5):1180–1211.
2. de Franchis R; for Baveno VI Faculty. Expanding consensus in portal hypertension: report of the Baveno VI Consensus Workshop: stratifying risk and individualizing care for portal hypertension. *J Hepatol*. 2015;63(3):743–752.

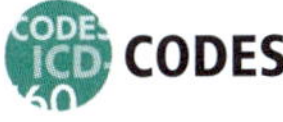

CODES

ICD10

K76.6 Portal hypertension

CLINICAL PEARLS

- Portal hypertension can be diagnosed based on physical examination in the setting of known risk factors, specifically cirrhosis.
- Endoscopic treatment is successful for acute variceal hemorrhage 85% of the time.
- Prognosis of patients with ascites is poor: 50% 1-year survival without liver transplant (compared with 90% for patients with cirrhosis and no ascites)

POSTCONCUSSION SYNDROME (MILD TRAUMATIC BRAIN INJURY)

Vicki R. Nelson, MD, PhD

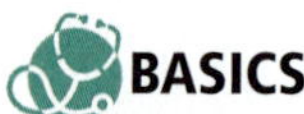

BASICS

DESCRIPTION

- Postconcussion syndrome (PCS) is defined by the persistence of symptoms following a concussion (mild traumatic brain injury [mTBI]) beyond 4 weeks from the time of injury; language changing to "persistent symptoms following concussion"
- Persistent symptoms include:
  - Cognitive (attention, memory, delayed processing speed)
  - Somatic (headache, neck pain)
  - Vestibular/ocular (visual change, light/noise sensitivity)
  - Emotional (depression, irritability)
  - Autonomic (sleep changes, exercise intolerance)

EPIDEMIOLOGY

Incidence

The reported frequency of patients persistent symptoms varies widely, around 18–31%. Variability in incidence is largely due to differing diagnostic criteria regarding symptom burden and duration.

- 80–90% of individuals with concussion recover *symptomatically* within 7 to 10 days, longer in children/adolescents.

Prevalence

Female sex, youth and adolescents, as well as older age are risk factors for prolonged concussion symptoms.

ETIOLOGY AND PATHOPHYSIOLOGY

- Controversial; exact mechanism(s) is unknown. It is likely that PCS results as a combination of multiple neurobiologic and psychogenic factors.
- Only some individuals with mTBI develop persistent symptoms; it is unclear what causes postconcussion symptoms to persist leading to PCS.
- Behavioral factors are commonly associated with (and may play a role in) the development of persistent symptoms. It can be challenging to differentiate exacerbation of preexisting neuropsychological disorders from persistent postconcussive symptoms.

RISK FACTORS

- Strongest predictor is severity of initial concussion symptoms.
- Initial symptoms including retrograde amnesia, difficulty concentrating, disorientation, insomnia, loss of balance, sensitivity to noise, or visual disturbance
- Preexisting psychiatric disorders including depression, anxiety, personality disorder, and posttraumatic stress disorder (PTSD)
- Preexisting expectation of poor outcomes following mTBI
- Nonsport concussion/mTBI
- Low socioeconomic status
- Loss of consciousness is *not* predictive of persistent symptoms.

GENERAL PREVENTION

- Prevention of concussion (see mTBI) including education, public health, and policy is key.
- Early clinical evaluation and treatment following concussion prevents persistent symptoms.
- Identified symptom constellations should be treated early.
- Treatment of preexisting comorbidities such as anxiety, depression, attention disorders, migraines, or insomnia early in concussion treatment may reduce the likelihood of developing persistent symptoms following concussion.

COMMONLY ASSOCIATED CONDITIONS

- PTSD
- Anxiety
- Depression
- Fibromyalgia
- ADHD

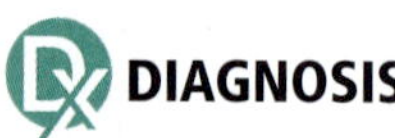

DIAGNOSIS

HISTORY

- Confirmation of appropriate concussion diagnosis including history of recent impact and closed head injury, including the following:
  - Mechanism of injury
  - Thorough characterization of associated symptom intensity, duration and timing of onset following injury
  - Previous head injuries, including concussion, and timing of those injuries
  - Previous medical history with special attention to potential diagnoses with overlapping symptoms (e.g., headache disorders, visual deficits, behavioral and psychological disorders)
  - Evaluation of psychosocial stressors, particularly those associated with injury or temporal association (e.g., traumatic stress following a concussive injury during a motor vehicle accident)
- Screening for psychological symptoms (depression, anxiety)
- Many screening and diagnostic tools are available (e.g., Sport Concussion Assessment Tool [SCAT], Sport Concussion Office Assessment Tool [SCOAT], NFL Sideline Concussion Assessment Tool) and may be used for diagnosis of concussion (1).

PHYSICAL EXAM

- Complete neurologic exam with special considerations to
  - Ocular tracking, nystagmus, and convergence
  - Cervical spine and paracervical musculature
  - Occipital nerve entrapment/neuralgia
  - Vestibular and ocular assessments
- Review of vital signs and comparison to prior may aid in identification of autonomic disruption.

DIFFERENTIAL DIAGNOSIS

- Concussion/mTBI
- Acute stress disorder/PTSD
- Anxiety, depression
- Migraine, headache disorders
- Chronic fatigue syndrome, fibromyalgia
- Whiplash injury
- Insomnia, sleep disorder
- ADHD

DIAGNOSTIC TESTS & INTERPRETATION

Diagnosis is made on the presence of persistent symptoms in the setting of appropriate history and trauma. There is no single diagnostic test.

Initial Tests (lab, imaging)

- Brain imaging at initial evaluation of mTBI is not routinely indicated.
- Consider advanced imaging if there is concern for cervical spine injury or central neurologic processes (e.g., if an appropriate history of trauma is not present to support the diagnosis of concussion, or symptom history [timing, constellation, etc.] is not consistent).
- There is insufficient evidence to support the use of other advanced neuroimaging such as functional MRI, magnetic resonance spectroscopy, and diffusion tensor imaging (DTI)

Diagnostic Procedures/Other

- Several computerized neuropsychiatric (CNP) tests are available to help guide treatment, particularly if objective data is needed to support workplace and academic accommodations.
  - Immediate Post-Concussion Assessment and Cognitive Testing (ImPACT)
  - CNS Vital Signs
  - Axon Sports Computerized Cognitive Assessment Tool (CCAT)
  - Automated Neuropsychological Assessment Metrics (ANAM)
- Formal neuropsychiatric consultation is superior to CNP testing when available and there is concern for diagnostic uncertainty, preexisting history, overlapping neuropsychiatric concern, or need for therapeutic intervention.

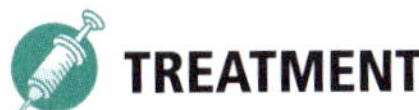

TREATMENT

GENERAL MEASURES

- Treatment consists primarily of symptomatic management and targeted treatment of symptom groups.
- Progressive return to usual demands, rather than avoidance of symptoms, can be helpful for resolution of PCS.
- Return to full activity should be guided by existing evidence-based recommendations for return to activity (work, school, sport) after concussion in the early months after injury (1).
- Noncontact, aerobic activity that does not exacerbate symptoms can be beneficial to recovery.
- After a period of initial avoidance of higher risk (contact) activities and symptom stabilization, the return to higher risk activities such as sport or driving can be approached as a shared decision with the patient given consideration of risks and benefits.
- Physical therapy for coexisting cervical, vestibular, and/or autonomic symptoms is beneficial.
- Psychologist or psychiatrist involvement may help with persistent mood, anxiety, or trauma as well as coping and adaptation strategies for persistent pain and symptoms.

MEDICATION

First Line

- Pharmacotherapy is targeted based on patient symptoms.
- Chronic headache
  - Avoid prolonged NSAID use to avoid overuse headaches.
  - Prophylactic medications should be considered if addressing underlying causes of headache are not effective or to provide relief which pursuing treatment (e.g., amitriptyline, topiramate, gabapentin)
- Emotional dysregulation (irritability, sadness, anxiety, depression)
  - SSRI (e.g., sertraline 25 mg daily titrated to effective dose with maximum 200 mg daily) for persistent depressive symptoms or anxiety
- Sleep dysregulation
  - Melatonin (up to 5 mg in adults)
  - Trazodone (25 to 50 mg at night)
- Cognitive disorders
  - Continue preexisting medications (e.g., amphetamines or methylphenidate for ADHD) and consider temporary increases in dose if needed to manage symptom.

ISSUES FOR REFERRAL

- If symptoms persist, consider referral to a concussion expert or multidisciplinary clinic.
- Physical therapy for vestibular/ocular rehabilitation, neck pain/whiplash, autonomic dysregulation, and activity intolerance
- Neuropsychiatric referral including comprehensive cognitive evaluation for potential TBI rehabilitation
- Cognitive-behavioral therapy for emotional, behavioral, or psychological symptoms
- Occupational therapy for vocational rehabilitation
- Neurology referral if interventions are unsuccessful or additional neurologic concerns present

COMPLEMENTARY & ALTERNATIVE MEDICINE

- Massage therapy, osteopathic manipulative treatment, acupuncture for headaches and neck pain
- Potential benefits shown with hyperbaric oxygen therapy in military veterans with concurrent PCS and PTSD

ONGOING CARE

FOLLOW-UP RECOMMENDATIONS

Regular follow-up to evaluate for persistent symptoms, treatment efficacy, need for neuropsychologic evaluation, and the efficacy of and/or need for pharmacologic therapy; predominant symptoms may evolve with treatment success and improvement of previously targeted symptoms

PATIENT EDUCATION

- Centers for Disease Control and Prevention: http://www.cdc.gov/headsup/
- Brain Injury Association of America: http://www.biausa.org/; (800) 444-6443

PROGNOSIS

- Symptoms and disability after concussion are greatest within the first 1 to 2 weeks. Most patients recover within 3 months.
- Patients with persistent symptoms following concussion typically require multidisciplinary treatment; about 90% will experience resolution of symptoms within a year following injury.
- Adolescents may recover more slowly than adults.

COMPLICATIONS

Repeat head injury before resolution of PCS can worsen or prolong symptoms.

REFERENCES

1. Patricios JS, Schneider KJ, Dvorak J, et al. Consensus statement on concussion in sport: the 6th International Conference on Concussion in sport-Amsterdam, October 2022. *Br J Sports Med*. 2023;57(11):695–711. doi:10.1136/bjsports-2023-106898.

ADDITIONAL READING

- McIntosh SJ, Vergeer MH, Galarneau JM, et al. Factors associated with Persisting symptoms after concussion in adults with mild TBI: a systematic review and meta-analysis. *JAMA Network Open*. 2025;8(6):e2516619. doi:10.1001/jamanetworkopen.2025.16619.
- Renga V. Clinical evaluation and treatment of patients with postconcussion syndrome. *Neurol Res Int*. 2021;5567695. doi:10.1155/2021/5567695.

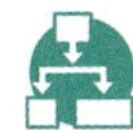

SEE ALSO

Concussion (Mild Traumatic Brain Injury)

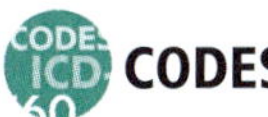

CODES

ICD10

- F07.81 Postconcussional syndrome
- S06.9X0A Unsp intracranial injury w/o loss of consciousness, init
- S06.9X9A Unsp intracranial injury w LOC of unsp duration, init

CLINICAL PEARLS

- Imaging is rarely useful for patients experiencing persistent symptoms following a concussion.
- Customize multidisciplinary treatment plans for patients based on their unique symptoms.
- Graduated return to daily activities, driving, work, and academics should be advanced as symptoms permit and may require accommodations. Efforts to completely avoid symptom exacerbation are not necessary beyond the acute period following concussion.

POSTTRAUMATIC STRESS DISORDER (PTSD)

Ulunma Natalie Umesi, MD, MBA

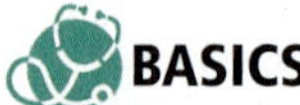

BASICS

A psychiatric disorder that may occur in people who have experienced, witnessed, perceived, or been threatened by a traumatic event such as with death, sexual violence, or serious injury.

DESCRIPTION

- The disorder can appear at any age. In children >6 years of age, young adults, and adults; it presents with four trauma-associated symptom groups:
  - Intrusion symptoms like flashbacks, nightmares, distressing recollections
  - Avoidance of anything related to the traumatic event and/or numbing of general responsiveness
  - Increased arousal and reactivity
  - Negative alterations in mood and cognition
- Symptoms of PTSD usually develop within 3 months after a trauma
- Expression of symptoms can be delayed 6 months to years after trauma exposure.
- For diagnosis of PTSD, symptoms should be present for >1 month.

EPIDEMIOLOGY

- Probability of PTSD was assessed in about 29 types of traumatic experiences, divided into groups: sexual relationship violence, interpersonal violence, exposure to organized violence, participation in organized violence, and other life-threatening traumatic experiences.
- Unexpected death of loved one, rape, other sexual assault were associated with the highest rate of PTSD.
- 5–8% of children and adolescents exposed to trauma develop PTSD depending on trauma exposure and other risk factors.

Prevalence

The lifetime prevalence of PTSD is 6–10%, with higher rates in combat veterans and victims of interpersonal violence.

ETIOLOGY AND PATHOPHYSIOLOGY

- Biologic dimensions: hypersensitivity of catecholamine pathways and overactivity of the central opioid pathways is seen; the amygdala and hippocampus dysfunction, with possible atrophy from overexposure to catecholamines, serotonergic dysregulation, glutamatergic dysregulation, and increased thyroid activity
- Learning theory: Life-threatening fear is classically conditioned by event exposure; any internal or external cue reminiscent of the event produces an intense "fight-or-flight" fear response.
- Cognitive theories: These models suggest that severe trauma becomes represented in complex memory structures. The activation of these memories triggers intense thoughts and emotions that cause discomfort/dysfunction.
- Psychodynamic theory: Traumatic memories overwhelm defense mechanisms. Repeated recall of the traumatic event with associated fear is an effort to understand the event in a less threatening way.

RISK FACTORS

- Preexisting factors:
  - Female sex
  - Younger age
  - Psychiatric history
  - Low socioeconomic status
  - Ethnicity
- Peritrauma factors:
  - Severity of the trauma
  - Peritrauma emotionality
  - Perception of threat to life
  - Perpetration of the trauma
- Posttrauma environment:
  - Perceived injury severity
  - Medical complications
  - Perceived social support
  - Persistent dissociation from traumatic event

GENERAL PREVENTION

Trauma-focused cognitive-behavioral therapy (TF-CBT) and prolonged exposure delivered within weeks of a potentially traumatic event for people showing signs of distress have the most evidence in the prevention of PTSD.

COMMONLY ASSOCIATED CONDITIONS

- Major depressive disorder
- Alcohol/substance abuse
- Panic disorder/agoraphobia/social phobia/obsessive-compulsive disorder
- Smoking (especially with assaultive trauma)
- Major neurocognitive disorders, dementia, or amnesia
- Traumatic brain injury/postconcussion syndrome

Pediatric Considerations

Oppositional defiant disorder and separation anxiety are common comorbid conditions.

DIAGNOSIS

Diagnosis is based on *DSM-5* criteria (1):

- Criterion A: exposure to trauma (≥1 of the following):
  - Direct experience of a traumatic event
  - In-person witnessing of a traumatic event
  - Learning of a traumatic event involving a close friend or family member
  - Repeated exposure to details of a traumatic event
- Criterion B: intrusive symptoms associated with the traumatic event (≥1 of the following):
  - Recurrent, involuntary, and intrusive distressing memories of the event
  - Recurrent distressing dreams related to the event
  - Dissociative reactions that simulate a recurrence of the event
  - Intense or prolonged distress to stimuli that resemble an aspect of the event
- Criterion C: avoidance of stimuli associated with the trauma (≥1 of the following):
  - Avoidance of memories, thoughts, or feelings about the event
  - Avoidance of external reminders that trigger memories, thoughts, or feelings about the event
- Criterion D: negative cognitive and mood changes associated with the trauma (≥2 of the following):
  - Inability to remember aspects of event
  - Persistent and exaggerated negative opinion of self, others, or the world
  - Distorted beliefs about the cause or consequences of the event
  - Negative emotional state
  - Diminished interest in significant activities
  - Feeling detached from others
  - Inability to experience positive emotions
- Criterion E: hyperarousal (≥2 of the following):
  - Difficulty sleeping/falling asleep
  - Decreased concentration
  - Hypervigilance
  - Outbursts of anger/irritable mood
  - Exaggerated startle response
  - Self-destructive behavior
- Criterion F: Duration of the relevant criteria symptoms should be >1 month.
- Criterion G: clinically significant distress/impairment in functioning
- Criterion H: relevant criteria not attributed to substance effects or other medical conditions

Pediatric Considerations

- Reactions can include a fear of being separated from a parent, or regressive behavior.
- Older children may show extreme withdrawal, disruptive behavior, and/or an inability to pay attention. Regressive behaviors, nightmares, sleep problems, irrational fears, irritability, refusal to attend school, outbursts of anger, fighting, somatic complaints with no medical basis, and decline in schoolwork performance.
- Parental posttraumatic stress has been shown to be a robust predictor of pediatric PTSD (2)[A].

HISTORY

Symptoms of intrusion, avoidance, alternations of mood and cognition, and hyperarousal must have lasted >1 month. Of note, PTSD may be diagnosed in children; avoidance is not a requirement.

PHYSICAL EXAM

- Patients may present with physical injuries from the traumatic event.
- Mental status examination:
  - Thoughts and perceptions (e.g., hallucinations, delusions, suicidal ideation, phobias)
  - General appearance: disheveled, poor hygiene
  - Behavior: agitation; startle reaction extreme
  - Psychological numbness
  - Orientation may be affected.
  - Memory: forgetfulness, especially concerning the details of the traumatic event
  - Poor concentration
  - Poor impulse control
  - Altered speech rate and flow
  - Mood and affect may be changed: depression, anxiety, guilt, and/or fear.

Pediatric Considerations

Elevated heart rate immediately following trauma is associated with development of PTSD (2)[A].

DIFFERENTIAL DIAGNOSIS

- Generalized anxiety disorder/adjustment disorder
- Obsessive-compulsive disorder
- Schizophrenia
- Major depressive disorder/mood disorder with psychotic features
- Substance abuse
- Personality/dissociative/conversion disorders
- Factitious disorder or malingering

DIAGNOSTIC TESTS & INTERPRETATION

- Diagnosis is based on *DSM-5* criteria (1).
- Screening tools are often used to assess for criteria and the extent of symptoms.
  - Primary Care PTSD Screen for *DSM-5* (PC-PTSD-5) (3)
  - PTSD Checklist for DSM-5 (PCL-5)
  - Trauma Screening Questionnaire (TSQ)

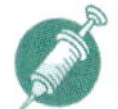

TREATMENT

Combination psychotherapy and pharmacotherapy, initiated soon after the trauma, results in better prognosis (4).

MEDICATION

Both paroxetine and sertraline are FDA-approved drugs for the treatment of PTSD, but other SSRIs may also be effective.

First Line

- Depression, panic attacks, startle response, sleep disruption: may improve with SSRIs (5)[A]:
  - Sertraline: 50 to 200 mg every day (FDA-approved)
  - Paroxetine: starting dose: 10 mg every day; maybe increased in 10 mg increments at intervals ≥1 week (FDA-approved)
  - Fluoxetine: 20 mg every day/BID not to exceed 80 mg/day (demonstrates some efficacy for all three symptom clusters)
- Sleep disruption: Sleep disruption due to hyperarousal is ubiquitous in PTSD; standard sedatives, such as trazodone 50 to 300 mg at bedtime, mirtazapine 7.5 to 30 mg QHS, or amitriptyline 25 to 100 mg QHS
- Nightmares/nighttime hyperarousal: prazosin 2 to 15 mg QHS (6)[A], clonidine 0.1 to 0.2 mg QHS, amitriptyline 25 to 100 mg QHS

Second Line

Refractory/residual symptoms: Consider augmentation with:

- Depression: mirtazapine 15 to 45 mg/day; consider switch to a serotonin-norepinephrine reuptake inhibitor (SNRI), such as venlafaxine XR 37.5 to 300 mg/day, duloxetine 60 to 120 mg/day, or desvenlafaxine 50 to 100 mg/day. Nefazodone 300 to 600 mg/day in divided doses can be very effective but requires quarterly LFTs.
- Reexperiencing/intrusive thoughts: 1st-/2nd-generation antipsychotic medications: aripiprazole 5 to 15 mg/day, risperidone 0.5 to 2.0 mg/day, olanzapine 2.5 to 10.0 mg/day, quetiapine 50 to 400 mg/day (7)[A]. 2nd-generation Rx less prone to extrapyramidal symptoms (EPS): cognitive dulling
- Hyperarousal: clonidine, start 0.05 mg BID/TID; slowly titrate to as much as 0.45 mg/day divided doses; guanfacine 1 to 3 mg/day in divided doses (long-acting forms of both clonidine and guanfacine now available). Also consider 2nd-generation antipsychotics quetiapine, risperidone, and olanzapine as above; divided doses often more helpful
- Impulsivity/explosiveness: anticonvulsants: valproic acid 500 to 2,000 mg/day, carbamazepine 200 to 600 mg/day, topiramate 50 to 200 mg/day
- Anxiety: Benzodiazepines (especially short-acting) should be avoided given the risk of substance abuse and questionable benefit in PTSD (8)[A]. Consider hydroxyzine 25 to 50 mg TID/QID PRN or risperidone 0.25 to 0.5 mg TID PRN.

ADDITIONAL THERAPIES

- Exposure therapies, particularly prolonged exposure therapy and TF-CBT, have shown the highest effectiveness for treatment of PTSD (9)[A]:
- Eye movement desensitization and reprocessing (EMDR) has been shown to benefit patients with PTSD.
- Telemedicine-based collaborative care (nurse, case manager, pharmacy, psychology, psychiatry)

Pediatric Considerations

Little evidence to support use of pharmacologic interventions for pediatric PTSD

ONGOING CARE

- The initial stabilization phase can be prolonged.
- Ongoing exposure to trauma can undermine the improvement.
- Patients with a history of childhood sexual abuse (complex PTSD) are often challenging to treat; they have significant difficulties with affect regulation and trust.

PATIENT EDUCATION

National Center for PTSD: https://www.ptsd.va.gov

PROGNOSIS

- In 50% of cases, the symptoms spontaneously remit after 3 months; however, symptoms may persist and cause long-term impairment in life functioning.
- Factors associated with a good prognosis include rapid engagement of treatment with early and ongoing social support, avoidance of retraumatization, and the absence of other psychiatric disorders/substance abuse.

COMPLICATIONS

- Increased risk for panic disorder, agoraphobia, obsessive-compulsive disorder, social phobia, specific phobia, major depressive disorder, somatization disorder; impulsive behavior, suicide, and homicide
- Victims of sexual assault are at especially high risk for developing mental health problems and committing suicide.

REFERENCES

1. American Psychiatric Association. *Diagnostic and Statistical Manual of Mental Disorders*. 5th ed. Arlington, VA: American Psychiatric Association; 2013.
2. Brosbe MS, Hoefling K, Faust J. Predicting posttraumatic stress following pediatric injury: a systematic review. *J Pediatr Psychol*. 2011;36(6):718–729.
3. Prins A, Ouimette P, Kimerling R, et al. The primary care PTSD screen (PC-PTSD): development and operating characteristics. *Primary Care Psychiatry*. 2003;9(1):9–14.
4. Weber M, Schumacher S, Hannig W, et al. Long-term outcomes of psychological treatment for posttraumatic stress disorder: a systematic review and meta-analysis. *Psychol Med*. 2021;51(9):1420–1430. doi:10.1017/S003329172100163X.
5. Stein DJ, Ipser JC, Seedat S. Pharmacotherapy for post traumatic stress disorder (PTSD). *Cochrane Database Syst Rev*. 2006;2006(1):CD002795.
6. Writer BW, Meyer EG, Schillerstrom JE. Prazosin for military combat-related PTSD nightmares: a critical review. *J Neuropsychiatry Clin Neurosci*. 2014;26(1):24–33.
7. Han C, Pae CU, Wang SM, et al. The potential role of atypical antipsychotics for the treatment of posttraumatic stress disorder. *J Psychiatr Res*. 2014;56:72–81.
8. Jeffreys M, Capehart B, Friedman MJ. Pharmacotherapy for posttraumatic stress disorder: review with clinical applications. *J Rehabil Res Dev*. 2012;49(5):703–715.
9. Kornør H, Winje D, Ekeberg Ø, et al. Early trauma-focused cognitive-behavioural therapy to prevent chronic post-traumatic stress disorder and related symptoms: a systematic review and meta-analysis. *BMC Psychiatry*. 2008;8:81.

ADDITIONAL READING

- National Institute of Mental Health. Post-traumatic stress disorder. https://www.nimh.nih.gov/health/topics/post-traumatic-stress-disorder-ptsd#part_2237
- U.S. Department of Veterans Affairs. PTSD treatment basics. National Center for PTSD. https://www.ptsd.va.gov/understand_tx/tx_basics.asp

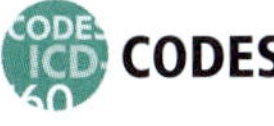

CODES

ICD10

- F43.10 Post-traumatic stress disorder, unspecified
- F43.11 Post-traumatic stress disorder, acute
- F43.12 Post-traumatic stress disorder, chronic

CLINICAL PEARLS

Treatment is often best accomplished with a combination of psychotherapy and pharmacotherapy.

PREECLAMPSIA AND ECLAMPSIA (TOXEMIA OF PREGNANCY)

Ann M. Aring, MD, FAAFP, FASAM

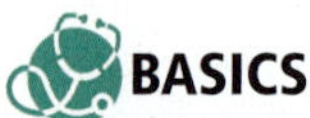

BASICS

DESCRIPTION

- Preeclampsia: A disorder of pregnancy occurring after 20 weeks' gestation characterized by new-onset hypertension (HTN), new-onset proteinuria, ± impaired organ function
- Eclampsia: New-onset grand mal seizure activity with no history of underlying neurologic disease
- Most postpartum cases of preeclampsia and eclampsia occur within 48 hours of delivery but can occur up to 6 weeks postpartum.

EPIDEMIOLOGY

Incidence

Preeclampsia occurs in 5–8% of all pregnancies.

Prevalence

- Predominant age
  - Most in younger women, primiparous women
  - Older (age >40 years) patients with preeclampsia have 4 times the incidence of seizures compared with patients in their 20s.
- 40% of eclamptic seizures occur before delivery; 16% occur >48 hours after delivery.
- Eclampsia is a main cause of perinatal mortality and morbidity (2–8% of all pregnancies).

ETIOLOGY AND PATHOPHYSIOLOGY

- Cause of preeclampsia is becoming clearer.
  - Genetic predisposition and abnormal placental implantation
  - Angiogenic factors
  - Vascular endothelial damage and oxidative stress
- Systemic disorders in eclampsia include the following:
  - Cardiovascular: generalized vasospasm
  - Hematologic: decreased plasma volume, increased blood viscosity, hemoconcentration, coagulopathy
  - Renal: decreased glomerular filtration rate
  - Hepatic: periportal necrosis, hepatocellular damage, subcapsular hematoma
  - CNS: cerebral vasospasm and ischemia, cerebral edema, cerebral hemorrhage

Genetics

2 to 4 times increased risk in pregnant women with family history of preeclampsia

RISK FACTORS

- Nulliparity
- Age >40 years
- Family history of preeclampsia
- Maternal medical problems: diabetes, chronic HTN, chronic renal disease, obesity, systemic lupus erythematosus
- Multiple gestation
- Prior pregnancy with preeclampsia
- In vitro fertilization

GENERAL PREVENTION

- Adequate prenatal care
- Good control of preexisting HTN
- Low-dose aspirin (ASA) (60 to 80 mg): ASA started early after 12 weeks' gestational age (GA) may lower the risk of developing preeclampsia and the rate of preterm delivery and neonatal death in moderate- to high-risk patients (see "Risk Factors" as mentioned earlier).
- Low-dose calcium supplementation has been shown to reduce the risk and severity of preeclampsia in calcium-deficient populations.

COMMONLY ASSOCIATED CONDITIONS

Abruptio placentae, placental insufficiency, fetal growth restriction, preterm delivery, fetal demise, maternal seizures (eclampsia), maternal pulmonary edema, maternal liver/kidney failure, or maternal death

DIAGNOSIS

Preeclampsia diagnosis:

- Blood pressure:
  - New-onset elevated blood pressure (BP): systolic BP (SBP) ≥140 mm Hg or diastolic BP (DBP) ≥90 mm Hg (on two occasions at least 4 hours apart) after 20 weeks' gestation *and new onset of one or more of the following:*
    - Proteinuria:
      - Proteinuria >300 mg/24 hours
      - Spot protein: creatinine ≥0.3 mg protein/mg Cr
      - Urine dipstick ≥2+ if quantitative measurement is not available
    - Or, without proteinuria and new onset of ANY of these features:
      - Platelets <100,000/μL
      - Liver transaminase levels >2 times normal and right upper quadrant (RUQ) pain
      - Creatinine >1.1 mg/dL or doubling of serum creatinine levels
      - Pulmonary edema
      - Headache or visual symptoms
  - Preeclampsia with severe features occurs with new-onset BP ≥160/110 mm Hg after 20 weeks of gestation OR lesser BP elevation and new onset of one or more of the following:
    - Platelets <100,000/μL
    - Severe persistent RUQ, epigastric pain, or both
    - Creatinine >1.1 mg/dL or doubling of serum creatinine levels
    - Visual symptoms
    - New-onset severe headache
    - Pulmonary edema
- Eclampsia diagnosis:
  - New-onset tonic-clonic, focal, or multifocal seizures
  - No history of neurologic disease

HISTORY

- May be asymptomatic. In some cases, rapid excessive weight gain (>5 lb/week; >2.3 kg/week); more severe cases are associated with epigastric/RUQ pain, headache, altered mental status, and visual disturbance. Note: Headache, visual symptoms, and epigastric or RUQ pain often precede seizure.
- Seizures may occur once/repeatedly.

PHYSICAL EXAM

BP criteria:

- Preeclampsia *without* severe features: elevated BP ≥140/90 mm Hg
- Preeclampsia *with* severe features: elevated BP ≥160 systolic mm Hg or 110 mm Hg diastolic
- Normal BP, even in response to treatment; does not rule out potential for seizures

DIFFERENTIAL DIAGNOSIS

- Chronic HTN: HTN before pregnancy; high BP before the 20th week
- Chronic HTN with superimposed preeclampsia
- Gestational HTN: Increased BP first discovered after 20 weeks, often close to term, with no proteinuria and without evidence of organ dysfunction. BP becomes normal by 12 weeks postpartum, or it is reclassified as chronic HTN.
- Seizures in pregnancy: epilepsy, cerebral tumors, meningitis/encephalitis, and ruptured cerebral aneurysm. Until other causes are proven; however, all pregnant women with convulsions should be considered to have eclampsia.

DIAGNOSTIC TESTS & INTERPRETATION

Initial Tests (lab, imaging)

- Urinalysis for protein should be done at each prenatal visit
- Complete blood count (CBC) with platelets, serum creatinine, serum transaminase levels, lactate dehydrogenase (LDH), and uric acid
- Coagulation studies including prothrombin time (PT), partial thromboplastin time (PTT), and fibrinogen: Abnormalities suggest severe disease.
- 24-hour urine or spot protein/creatinine ratio if urine protein dips 1+ on more than one occasion or if preeclampsia is being considered
- Daily fetal movement monitoring by mother ("kick counts")
- US imaging is used to monitor growth and cord blood flow; perform, as indicated, based on clinical stability and laboratory findings.
- Nonstress test (NST) at diagnosis and then twice weekly until delivery
- Biophysical profile (BPP) if NST is nonreactive
- US imaging for growth progress every 3 weeks, and amniotic fluid volume at least once weekly
- With seizures, CT scan and MRI should be considered if focal findings persist or uncharacteristic signs/symptoms are present.

Follow-Up Tests & Special Considerations

Disseminated intravascular coagulation, thrombocytopenia, liver dysfunction, and renal failure can complicate preeclampsia associated with HELLP (hemolysis, elevated liver enzymes, low platelet) syndrome.

Test Interpretation

CNS: cerebral edema, hyperemia, focal anemia, thrombosis, and hemorrhage; cerebral lesions account for 40% of eclamptic deaths.

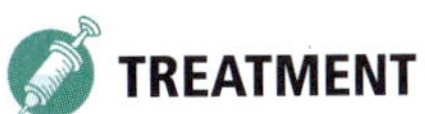

TREATMENT

GENERAL MEASURES

- Health care providers must balance timing of delivery with maternal and fetal risks.
- Delivery recommended for pre-eclampsia of any severity at ≥37 weeks' gestation.
- Preeclampsia without severe features:
  - Consider outpatient care
  - Maternal: daily BP monitoring; daily weights; weekly labs (CBC, creatinine, liver function test [LFT])
  - Fetal:
    - Patient-measured: daily "kick counts"
    - NST/BPP/US (see "Initial Test (lab, imaging)" section above)
    - Induction of labor at 37 0/7 weeks' gestation
    - Steroids for gestation <37 weeks
- Preeclampsia with severe features:
  - Inpatient care
  - Maternal:
    - Daily labs (CBC, serum creatinine, LFTs)
    - Use magnesium sulfate ($MgSO_4$) IV as seizure prophylaxis and continue 24 hours after delivery
    - Antihypertensive therapy titrated to keep SBP <160 mm Hg and DBP <110 mm Hg (some recommend <150/100 mm Hg postpartum)
  - Fetal:
    - Continuous heart monitoring
    - Daily US with BPP
    - Check amniotic fluid levels and fetal growth.
  - Definitive management (delivery) depends on GA
  - At 23 to 34 weeks:
    - Antihypertensives
    - Evaluate maternal–fetal condition.
    - Use steroids such as betamethasone 12 mg IM daily × 2 doses or dexamethasone 6 mg every 12 hours × 4 doses to enhance fetal lung maturity
    - Plan delivery at 34 weeks with $MgSO_4$ prophylaxis.
    - If HELLP syndrome (full or partial), severe oligohydramnios, significant renal dysfunction, persistent symptoms, fetal growth restriction, onset of labor, or premature rupture of membranes (PROM), proceed to delivery.
  - At ≥34 weeks: delivery is recommended. Start $MgSO_4$ IV. Do not delay delivery to give steroids in the late preterm period.

ALERT

- A severe BP reading ≥160/110 mm Hg requires pharmacologic treatment within 30 to 60 minutes of confirming the diagnosis.
- Regardless of GA, emergent delivery is recommended if there are signs of maternal hypertensive crisis, abruptio placentae, uterine rupture, or fetal distress. Delivery is the definitive treatment.
- Seizures: control of convulsions, correction of hypoxia and acidosis, lowering of BP, steps to delivery baby as soon as convulsions are controlled.

MEDICATION

First Line

- Seizure prophylaxis for women with severe preeclampsia:
  - $MgSO_4$: loading dose 4 g IV in 200 mL normal saline over 20 to 30 minutes; maintenance dose 1 to 2 g/hr IV continuous infusion (Although recent guidelines suggest it not be universally administered for seizure prophylaxis to prevent eclampsia, the quality of the evidence is low, and the strength of the recommendation is qualified.)
- BP control:
  - Antihypertensives are not advised for mildly elevated BP without severe features.
  - Start antihypertensive treatment for severe HTN ≥160/110 mm Hg within 30 minutes of meeting diagnostic criteria.
    - Labetalol (IV): 20 mg over 2 minutes followed at 20 to 30 minutes intervals with doses of 20 to 80 mg titrated to keep BP <160/110 mm Hg; max of 300 mg/24 hr (contraindicated in asthma, heart disease, congestive heart failure)
    - Hydralazine (IV): 5 to 10 mg over 2 minutes, followed at 20-minute intervals with 5- to 10-mg IV boluses; titrated to keep BP <160/110 mm Hg; max of 25 mg/24 hr
    - Nifedipine immediate release 10 mg oral followed by 20 mg in 20 minutes if needed for severe range. Sustained release (PO) (used in the postpartum): 30 to 120 mg/day (caution with combination of nifedipine and $MgSO_4$ resulting in hypotension and neuromuscular blockade)
- Eclampsia/seizures:
  - $MgSO_4$ for seizures
    - 4 to 6 g IV over 15 to 20 minutes followed by 1 to 2 g/hr infusion
    - Further boluses of magnesium may be given for recurrent convulsions with the amount given based on the neurologic examination and patellar reflexes.
    - Contraindications: myasthenia gravis, renal failure, pulmonary edema
  - Levels of 6 to 8 mEq/mL are considered therapeutic, but monitor clinical status of:
    - Patellar reflexes are present.
    - Respirations are not depressed.
    - Urine output is ≥25 mL/hr.
  - May be given safely, even in the presence of renal insufficiency
- Fluid therapy
  - Ringer lactated solution with 5% dextrose at 60 to 120 mL/hr, with careful attention to fluid volume status
- Calcium gluconate or chloride (1 g, administered slowly IV) may reverse magnesium-induced respiratory depression.

Second Line

For refractory seizures unresponsive to $MgSO_4$, consider using:

- Diazepam 2 mg/min until resolution or 20 mg given *or*
- Lorazepam 1 to 2 mg/min up to total of 10 mg *or*
- Phenytoin 15 to 20 mg/kg at a maximum rate of 50 mg/min *or*
- Phenobarbital 20 mg/kg infused at 50 mg/min; may repeat with additional 5 to 10 mg/kg after 15 minutes

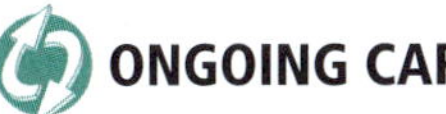

ONGOING CARE

FOLLOW-UP RECOMMENDATIONS

Women with a history of preeclampsia should report this to physicians caring for them in later life. It is an important cardiovascular disease risk factor.

DIET

Do not recommend salt restriction because the patient often experiences intravascular hypovolemia.

PATIENT EDUCATION

American College of Obstetricians and Gynecologists: http://www.acog.org/

PROGNOSIS

- For nulliparous women with preeclampsia before 30 weeks of gestation, the recurrence rate for the disorder may be as high as 40% in future pregnancies.
- 25% of eclamptic women will have HTN during subsequent pregnancies
- Preeclamptic, multiparous women may be at higher risk for subsequent essential HTN; they also have higher mortality during subsequent pregnancies than primiparous women do.

COMPLICATIONS

- Most women do not have long-term sequelae from eclampsia, although many may have transient neurologic deficits.
- Maternal and/or fetal death

ADDITIONAL READING

Bryant A, Cahill A, Kuller J, et al; American College of Obstetricians and Gynecologists; Society for Maternal-Fetal Medicine. Low-dose aspirin use for the prevention of preeclampsia and related morbidity and mortality. 2021. https://www.acog.org/clinical/clinical-guidance/practice-advisory/articles/2021/12/low-dose-aspirin-use-for-the-prevention-of-preeclampsia-and-related-morbidity-and-mortality.

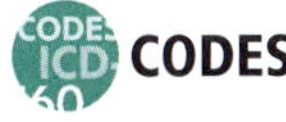

CODES

ICD10

- O14.90 Unspecified pre-eclampsia, unspecified trimester
- O15.00 Eclampsia in pregnancy, unspecified trimester
- O14.00 Mild to moderate pre-eclampsia, unspecified trimester

CLINICAL PEARLS

- Management of preeclampsia depends on both the severity of the condition and the GA of the fetus.
- $MgSO_4$ is the drug of choice for preeclampsia with severe features.
- Start daily low-dose ASA in the late 1st trimester in high-risk patients to prevent preeclampsia.
- Continue to monitor maternal BP postpartum. The patient is still at risk for developing preeclampsia.

PREMENSTRUAL SYNDROME (PMS) AND PREMENSTRUAL DYSPHORIC DISORDER (PMDD)

Ulunma Natalie Umesi, MD, MBA

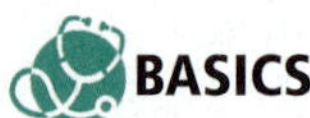

BASICS

DESCRIPTION

- Premenstrual syndrome (PMS), a complex of physical and emotional symptoms sufficiently severe to interfere with everyday life, occurs cyclically during the luteal phase of menses.
- Premenstrual dysphoric disorder (PMDD) is a severe form of PMS characterized by severe recurrent depressive and anxiety symptoms, with premenstrual (luteal phase) onset, that typically begins within 10 to 14 days and that remits within a few days after the start of menses (1), as defined in the 5th edition of the *Diagnostic and Statistical Manual of Mental Disorders* (*DSM-5-TR*).
- System(s) affected: endocrine/metabolic, nervous, reproductive

EPIDEMIOLOGY

Prevalence

- Many women have some physical and psychological symptoms before menses that can encompass a spectrum from mild molimina to severe and disabling symptoms.
- The prevalence of PMS is reported anywhere between 20% and 30% of menstruating women. 1.2% to 6.4% of women have PMDD based on *DSM-5-TR* criteria with upwards of 18% of menstruating women meeting partial *DSM* criteria (2).

ETIOLOGY AND PATHOPHYSIOLOGY

Two main ideas on the pathophysiology are postulated and widely accepted:

- Changing levels of the progesterone metabolite allopregnanolone interacts with serotonin and γ-aminobutyric acid (GABA) receptors, provoking downstream effects of decreased GABA-mediated inhibition and decreased serotonin levels.
- Decreased function of the serotonin system (in particular the serotonin transporter) serves as the primary abnormality and thus when modulated by sex hormones leads to decreased serotonin levels in patients with PMS/PMDD.

Genetics

- The role of genetic predisposition is controversial; however, twin studies do suggest a genetic component.
- Involvement of gene coding for the serotonergic *5HT1A* receptor and allelic variants of the estrogen receptor-α gene (*ESR1*) is suggested.

RISK FACTORS

- Age: typically presents in the late 20s to mid-30s; there is evidence to demonstrate that initial onset of PMDD may be later.
- History of mood disorder (major depression, bipolar disorder), anxiety disorder, personality disorder, or substance abuse
- Family history
- Low parity
- Cigarette smoking and other nicotine-containing products
- Psychosocial stressors/history of trauma
- High BMI (>27.5 kg/m^2)

COMMONLY ASSOCIATED CONDITIONS

There is a high prevalence of cooccurring mood disorders and/or anxiety disorders in patients with PMS/PMDD.

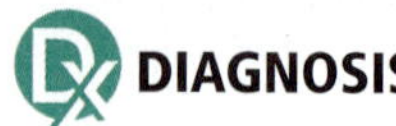

DIAGNOSIS

HISTORY

- Criteria for the diagnosis of PMS has been established by the International Society for Premenstrual Disorders (ISPMD) and include the following:
  - Physical or emotional symptoms
  - Symptoms are present during the luteal phase and abate as menstruation begins.
  - A symptom-free week
  - Symptoms are associated with significant impairment during the luteal phase.
- Criteria for the diagnosis of PMDD was established by the American Psychiatric Association in 2013 and included in the *DSM-5*.
- Symptoms occur 1 week before menses, improve in the first few days after menses begin, and are minimal/absent in the week following menses (over most menstrual cycles during the past year).
- ≥5 of the following (1 must be among the first 4):
  - Marked depressed mood, feelings of hopelessness, or self-deprecating thoughts
  - Marked anxiety, tension, and/or feelings of being keyed up or on edge
  - Marked affective lability (mood swings)
  - Marked irritability or anger or increased interpersonal conflicts
  - Decreased interest in usual activities and social withdrawal
  - Lethargy, easy fatigability, or lack of energy
  - Appetite change, overeating, food cravings
  - Hypersomnia or insomnia
  - Feeling out of control or overwhelmed
  - Subjective difficulty concentrating
  - Physical symptoms, such as abdominal bloating, breast tenderness, headaches, weight gain, and joint/muscle pain
- Emotional symptoms must be sufficiently severe to interfere with work, school, usual social activities, or relationships with others.
- Symptoms may be superimposed on an underlying psychiatric disorder but may not be an exacerbation of another condition, such as panic disorder/major depression.
- Criteria should be confirmed by prospective patient record of symptoms for a minimum of two consecutive menstrual cycles (without confirmation, "provisional" should be noted with diagnosis) (2).
- Symptoms should not be attributable to drug abuse, medications, or other medical conditions.
- Diagnosis can be established through the use of a validated tool such as the Daily Record of Severity of Problems or similar inventory.

PHYSICAL EXAM

No specific physical exam is required; may consider thyroid and pelvic exams if indicated by additional patient symptoms

DIFFERENTIAL DIAGNOSIS

- Premenstrual exacerbation of underlying psychiatric disorder
- Psychiatric disorders (especially bipolar disorder, major depression, anxiety)
- Thyroid disorders
- Perimenopause
- Premenstrual migraine
- Chronic fatigue syndrome
- Irritable bowel syndrome (painful symptoms)
- Seizures
- Anemia
- Endometriosis (painful symptoms)
- Drug/alcohol abuse

DIAGNOSTIC TESTS & INTERPRETATION

- The repetitive nature of symptoms precludes the need for labs if a classic history is present.
- Consider hemoglobin to rule out anemia and serum thyroid-stimulating hormone (TSH) to rule out hypothyroidism.
- Imaging with pelvic ultrasound to diagnose causes of pelvic pain and dysmenorrhea may be needed.

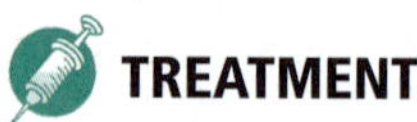

TREATMENT

GENERAL MEASURES

Exercise increases β-endorphins in the brain, but the role of physical activity in the treatment of premenstrual disorders remains unclear.

MEDICATION

First Line

- SSRIs are recommended as the first-line therapy in the treatment of physical, functional, and behavioral symptoms of PMS and PMDD compared to placebo (3)[A]:
  - Continuous SSRI (daily) dosing may be somewhat more effective than intermittent luteal phase dosing (3)[A], but both appear significantly better than placebo (1).
  - All SSRIs tested appeared effective.
  - SSRIs are effective at low doses but may require titration of the dose for the desired response in certain patients. Higher doses have increased effect but are accompanied by increased side effects.
- Fluoxetine (Prozac, Sarafem) 20 mg/day every day or 20 mg/day only during the luteal phase, or 90 mg once a week for 2 weeks in the luteal phase
- Sertraline (Zoloft) 50 to 150 mg/day every day or 50 to 150 mg/day only during the luteal phase
- Citalopram (Celexa) 10 to 30 mg/day every day or 10 to 30 mg/day only during the luteal phase
- Adverse effects (number needed to harm [NNH] with moderate-dose SSRI): nausea (NNH = 7), asthenia (NNH = 9), somnolence (NNH = 13), fatigue (NNH = 14), decreased libido (NNH = 14), and sweating (NNH = 14)

- Contraindications: patients taking monoamine oxidase inhibitors (MAOIs)
- Precautions
  - Increased risk of suicidal thinking and behavior in children and adolescents with depressive disorders; uncertain if this risk applies to those taking SSRIs for PMDD
  - Bipolar disorder
  - Seizure disorder
  - QTc prolongation (with citalopram)
  - Hepatic dysfunction
  - Renal dysfunction

Second Line

Alternative therapies should be considered if no response to SSRIs:

- Spironolactone (Aldactone) 50 to 100 mg/day for 7 to 10 days during the luteal phase; helpful for fluid retention
  - Adverse reactions: lethargy, headache, irregular menses, hyperkalemia
  - Regular monitoring of electrolytes is recommended due to the risk of hyperkalemia.
- Oral contraceptive pills (OCPs): decrease overall symptoms but may not alter affective symptoms (4)[A]
  - OCPs can cause adverse effects similar to PMDD symptoms.
  - Extended-cycle use of OCPs (e.g., 12 weeks on and 1 week off) or a shorter placebo interval (e.g., 24 active pills with 4 placebo days [24/4] compared with 21/7 preparations) may be beneficial.
  - OCPs containing the progestin drospirenone (structurally similar to spironolactone) may improve physical symptoms and mood changes associated with PMDD. Caution: Side effects (5)[A] and the risk of venous thromboembolism may be modestly higher than with other OCPs.
  - Continuous administration of levonorgestrel/ethinyl estradiol may improve patient symptoms in PMDD.
    - Suggested OCP formulations:
      - Ethinyl estradiol 0.02 to 0.03 mg/drospirenone 3 mg (Gianvi/Loryna/Nikki/Ocella/Syeda/Vestura/Yasmin/Yaz Zarah): 1 tablet/day
      - Ethinyl estradiol 0.02 to 0.03 mg/drospirenone 3 mg/levomefolate 0.451 mg (Beyaz/Safyral): 1 tablet/day
      - Levonorgestrel 90 μg/ethinyl estradiol 20 μg (Amethyst/Lybrel): 1 tablet/day
- Anxiolytics
  - Alprazolam (Xanax) 0.25 mg TID–QID only during luteal phase; taper at the onset of menses (other benzodiazepines not studied for PMDD); caution: addictive potential
  - Buspirone (BuSpar) 10 to 30 mg/day divided BID–TID in the luteal phase
- Ovulation inhibitors
  - Gonadotropin-releasing hormone (GnRH) agonists: leuprolide (Lupron) depot 3.75 mg/month IM; precautions: Menopause-like side effects (e.g., osteoporosis, hot flashes, headaches, muscle aches, vaginal dryness, irritability) limit treatment to 6 months; may be the first step if considering bilateral oophorectomy for severe, refractory PMDD
  - Danazol (Danocrine) 300 to 400 mg BID; adverse reactions: androgenic and antiestrogenic effects (e.g., amenorrhea, weight gain, acne, fluid retention, hirsutism, hot flashes, vaginal dryness, emotional lability)
  - Estrogen, transdermal preferred, 100 to 200 μg:
    - Precautions: increased risk of blood clots, stroke, heart attack, and breast cancer
    - Requires concomitant progesterone add-back therapy to protect against uterine hyperplasia and endometrial cancer
- Progesterone: insufficient evidence to support use

ISSUES FOR REFERRAL

Short-term follow-up (within 1 to 3 months) can assess if the patient has an adequate response to treatment. If not, referral to a psychiatrist may be indicated for further evaluation. Safety and risk assessments should be included during evaluation of PMDD symptoms.

ADDITIONAL THERAPIES

Cognitive-behavioral therapy (CBT) is theoretically helpful for PMS/PMDD given its application for symptom reduction in other mood disorders, but direct evidence is lacking.

SURGERY/OTHER PROCEDURES

Bilateral oophorectomy, usually with concomitant hysterectomy, is an option for rare, refractory cases with severe, disabling symptoms.

COMPLEMENTARY & ALTERNATIVE MEDICINE

Acupuncture demonstrated superiority to progestins, anxiolytics, and sham acupuncture with no evidence of harm (6)[A].

- Some data support the use of the following:
  - Calcium: 600 mg BID
  - Vitamin B_6: 50 to 100 mg/day
  - Chasteberry (*Vitex agnus-castus*): 4 mg/day of extract containing 6% of agnuside (or 20 to 40 mg/day of fruit extract)
  - Omega-3 fatty acids 2 g/day
- Data insufficient regarding the following: magnesium: 200 to 400 mg/day; vitamin D: 2,000 IU/day; vitamin E: 400 IU/day; manganese: 1.8 mg/day; St. John's wort: 900 mg/day; soy: 68 mg/day isoflavones; ginkgo: 160 to 320 mg/day; saffron: 30 mg/day
- Evidence supporting efficacy and/or safety of herbal products is lacking; the following products/interventions have not been found useful for PMS/PMDD, although not all studies are of high quality and able to eliminate the possibility of benefit completely: evening primrose oil, black currant oil, black cohosh, wild yam root, dong quai, kava kava, light-based therapy.

ONGOING CARE

FOLLOW-UP RECOMMENDATIONS

Patient Monitoring

Increased risk of suicidal thinking and behavior in children and adolescents with depressive disorders on initiation of SSRIs; uncertain if this risk applies to those taking SSRIs for PMDD

DIET

- Reduce consumption of salt, sugar, caffeine, dairy products, and alcohol (anecdotal reports).
- Eat small, frequent portions of food high in complex carbohydrates (limited data).

PATIENT EDUCATION

- Counsel patients to eat a balanced diet rich in calcium, vitamin D, and omega-3 fatty acids and low in saturated fat and caffeine.
- Counsel patients to quit tobacco and other nicotine use (more research is needed on the benefit of smoking cessation in PMS and PMDD).
- Counsel women that they are not "crazy." PMDD is a real disorder with a physiologic basis.
- Although incompletely understood, successful treatment is often possible.

PROGNOSIS

- Many patients can have their symptoms adequately controlled. PMS disappears at menopause.
- PMS can continue after hysterectomy if ovaries are left in place.

REFERENCES

1. Biggs WS, Romeu JM, Gaudard T, et al. Premenstrual syndrome and premenstrual dysphoric disorder: common questions and answers. *Am Fam Physician*. 2025;111(4):345–350.
2. Carlini SV, Deligiannidis KM. Evidence-based treatment of premenstrual dysphoric disorder: a concise review. *J Clin Psychiatry*. 2020;81(2):19ac13071.
3. Jespersen C, Lauritsen MP, Frokjaer VG, et al. Selective serotonin reuptake inhibitors for premenstrual syndrome and premenstrual dysphoric disorder. *Cochrane Database Syst Rev*. 2024;8(8):CD001396.
4. de Wit AE, de Vries YA, de Boer MK, et al. Efficacy of combined oral contraceptives for depressive symptoms and overall symptomatology in premenstrual syndrome: pairwise and network meta-analysis of randomized trials. *Am J Obstet Gynecol*. 2021;225(6):624–633.
5. Ma S, Song SJ. Oral contraceptives containing drospirenone for premenstrual syndrome. *Cochrane Database Syst Rev*. 2023;6(6):CD006586.
6. Kim SY, Park HJ, Lee H, et al. Acupuncture for premenstrual syndrome: a systematic review and meta-analysis of randomized controlled trials. *BJOG*. 2011;118(8):899–915.

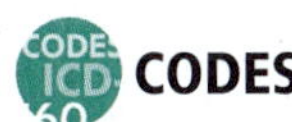

CODES

ICD10

N94.3 Premenstrual tension syndrome

CLINICAL PEARLS

- Have the patient keep a daily log of their symptoms and menses. Symptoms beginning in the week before menses and abating before the end of menses, occurring over at least 2 months, and sufficiently severe to interfere with daily functioning are diagnostic of PMS/PMDD, with PMDD typically more severe.
- Daily SSRIs may be slightly more effective than luteal phase treatment but has more side effects. Onset of noticeable clinical improvement with SSRIs is typically faster than with treatment of PMDD.

PRENATAL CARE AND TESTING

Henry Del Rosario, MD

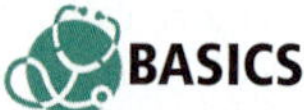

BASICS

The goal of prenatal care is to ensure the well-being of mother and baby using the best available evidence and a patient-centered approach. General concepts include estimating the gestational age (GA) accurately; identifying risk for complications; encouraging and empowering the patient for motherhood, newborn care, and breastfeeding; and intervening when fetal abnormalities are present to prevent morbidity and mortality.

GENERAL PREVENTION

In the United States, the typical prenatal visit schedule consists of monthly visits for weeks 4 to 28 of pregnancy, visits twice monthly from 28 to 36 weeks, weekly after week 36 (until delivery, typically at weeks 38 to 41).

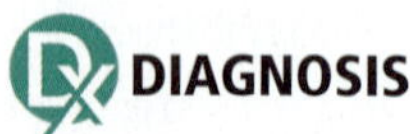

DIAGNOSIS

HISTORY

Collect the following histories in the initial prenatal visit and continually update throughout the pregnancy (1),(2):

- Medical history, with an emphasis on the following but not limited to prediabetes/DM, obesity/overweight, thyroid disorders, pregestational hypertension (HTN) or history of hypertensive disease in pregnancy (e.g., chronic HTN, gestational HTN, pre-eclampsia with or without severe features, HELLP syndrome), maternal age at delivery, previous DVT/PE, known uterine anomaly, autoimmune disease (e.g., systemic lupus erythematosus, rheumatoid arthritis, Sjögren), strong family history of diseases in pregnancy or congenital/inheritable conditions
- Obstetrical history, including but not limited to:
  - History of preterm delivery or PTL
  - History of hypertensive disease in pregnancy
  - History of gestational diabetes (GDM) or early onset GDM
  - Other medical conditions raising maternal risk: HIV/AIDS or other STIs in the past, sickle cell disease, intrahepatic cholestasis of pregnancy
  - Personal history of delivering a newborn with birth defects/trisomies or congenital/inheritable condition
- Psychosocial history, including but not limited to:
  - Depression screening (use EPDS or PHQ-9), intimate partner violence (ACOG guidelines: Screen *all* pregnant patients at the first prenatal visit, 1x/trimester, and at postpartum checkup.)
  - Tobacco, alcohol, and drug use
  - Lifestyle, nutrition, toxin exposures, travel to areas with endemic diseases, stressors/supports; potential barriers to care (preferred language, housing, transportation, child care issues, economic constraints, work schedule)

PHYSICAL EXAM

- A full physical exam on intake (1),(2)
- At each subsequent prenatal visit, the following should be recorded (1),(2):
  - Weight gain recommendations (2009 IOM)
    - BMI $<$18.5 kg/m^2 (underweight): 28 to 40 lb (12.5 to 18 kg)
    - BMI 18.5 to 24.9 kg/m^2 (normal weight): 25 to 35 lb (11.5 to 16 kg)
    - BMI 25 to 29.9 kg/m^2 (overweight): 15 to 25 lb (7 to 11.5 kg)
    - BMI $\geq$30 kg/m^2 (obese): 11 to 20 lb (5 to 9 kg)
  - BP (mm Hg): Assess for mild ($\geq$140 to $<$160/$\geq$90 to $<$110) or severe range ($\geq$160/$\geq$110) BP if not normal
  - Fundal height: Start after weeks 20 to 24.
  - Fetal heart rate: usually audible by 8 to 12 weeks' GA with a Doppler device
  - Pelvic/cervical exam if indicated
  - Fetal position by Leopold maneuver at weeks 32 to 36; confirm by ultrasound (US) if available.

DIAGNOSTIC TESTS & INTERPRETATION

- First prenatal visit (1):
  - Lab tests
    - Hematocrit or hemoglobin, blood type, Rhesus type, and antibody screen
    - Hemoglobin electrophoresis: Screen for sickle cell disease, SCT, or thalassemia.
    - Urine culture
    - Ab titers for Rubella and Varicella
    - STI screen: RPR/VDRL, GC/C, hepatitis B, HIV
    - Not recommended: routine screening for bacterial vaginosis, toxoplasmosis, CMV, and parvovirus; thyroid and vitamin D deficiency
  - Carrier screening (including, but not limited to):
    - Cystic fibrosis screening: Counseling is needed first, and screening should be offered when one partner is of Caucasian, European, or Ashkenazi Jewish descent.
    - Spinal muscular atrophy
    - Hemoglobinopathies (i.e., risk for sickle cell disease, thalassemia)
  - Screening for fetal aneuploidy:
    - Counseling should be provided before any shared decision-making on testing.
    - All women should be offered screening or diagnostic testing, regardless of maternal age.
    - US nuchal translucency (NT): measures thickness at the back of the neck of the fetus
    - Blood screens: human chorionic gonadotropin (hCG), pregnancy-associated plasma protein A (PAPP-A), quadruple test: α-fetoprotein (AFP), unconjugated estriol (UE3), hCG, dimeric inhibin-A (DIA)
    - Cell-free DNA testing: should not be used as a substitute for diagnostic testing due to potential for false-positive or false-negative results; all women with positive screening test should have a diagnostic procedure before any irreversible action is taken.
    - 1st-trimester "combined test" between 11 and 13 weeks' GA using both NT and hCG/PAPP-A blood testing is an effective protocol; may be performed either as a single combined stand-alone test (US NT 1 blood [HCG and PAPP-A]) or as part of a sequential "step-by-step" 1st- and 2nd-trimester screening process (See the following discussion.)
    - Women who undergo 1st-trimester screening should be offered 2nd-trimester assessment for open fetal defects and US screening for other fetal structural defects.
    - 2nd-trimester screening: Obtain quadruple test ideally at weeks 15 to 18 but can be done as late as week 22.
    - If risk is found, all pregnant women should be offered invasive prenatal diagnostic testing regardless of maternal age or other risk factors (3); diagnostic tests for genetic disorders:
      - CVS: 1st trimester: usually done weeks 10 to 12; small sample of the placenta; chorionic tissue sample obtained either transcervical (TC) or transabdominal (TA)
      - Amniocentesis: usually done weeks 15 to 18; small sample of amniotic fluid from the amniotic sac surrounding the developing fetus is obtained by a US-guided TA approach.
      - The rate of procedure-related pregnancy loss that is attributable to a prenatal diagnostic procedure is 0.1–0.3% when performed by experienced health care providers (3).
      - Chromosomal microarray analysis: can detect a pathogenic copy number variant in about 1.7% of patients with normal US and normal karyotype; make available to any patient choosing to undergo invasive diagnostic testing; primary test for patients undergoing diagnostic testing for indication of a fetal structural abnormality detected by US examination (3)
  - Cervical cancer screening:
    - A Pap smear or approved high-risk HPV screen should be obtained when indicated by standard Pap screening guidelines, regardless of gestation, to start at age 21 years.
    - Squamous intraepithelial lesions can progress during pregnancy but often regress postpartum.
    - LSIL/CIN1 in pregnancy: Colposcopy is preferred, but it is acceptable to defer colposcopy to 6 weeks postpartum.
    - CIN 2 or CIN 3 in pregnancy: In the absence of invasive disease or advanced pregnancy, additional colposcopic and cytologic examinations are acceptable; repeat biopsy is recommended only if appearance of lesion worsens or if cytology suggests invasive cancer; it is acceptable to defer reevaluation until 6 weeks postpartum.
    - Endocervical sampling is contraindicated in pregnancy.
- Subsequent prenatal visits (1),(2):
  - Urinalysis for glucose and protein: limited evidence for benefit or harm; the baseline during initial intake may be useful for high-risk patients (e.g., chronic HTN).
- 24- to 28-week prenatal visits (1),(2):
  - Obtain diabetes screen.
  - Repeat hematocrit or hemoglobin, and repeat antibody screen in Rh-negative mother prior to receiving prophylactic Rh immunoglobulin. Repeat syphilis testing in the 3rd trimester around 28 weeks in all cases (2018 CDC, ACOG and AAP guidelines due to rising cases of congenital syphilis). Retest for HIV at 28 weeks in high-risk cases. Retest for syphilis and HIV at delivery in high-risk cases.

P

- GDM screening (2)
  - The ADA and ACOG define increased risk of diabetes in pregnancy who need earlier screening based on BMI ≥25 kg/m^2 (≥23 kg/m^2 in Asian Americans) plus one or more of the following:
    - Previous pregnancy history of GDM, fetal macrosomia (≥4,000 g BW prior delivery), or stillbirth
    - HTN (140/90 mm Hg or being treated for HTN)
    - HDL cholesterol ≤35 mg/dL (0.90 mmol/L)
    - Fasting triglyceride ≥250 mg/dL (2.82 mmol/L)
    - Hemoglobin A1C ≥5.7%, impaired glucose tolerance or impaired fasting glucose
    - PCOS, acanthosis nigricans, nonalcoholic steatohepatitis, morbid obesity prepregnancy BMI ≥40 kg/m^2, and other conditions associated with insulin resistance
    - Current or past history of cardiovascular disease
    - Family history of diabetes—first-degree relative (parent or sibling)
    - High-risk ethnicity or communities
  - Early onset diagnosis is made via 2-step testing (see below) ideally between weeks 12 to 16 of pregnancy for at risk cases.
  - For typical low-risk cases, employ 2-step testing starting week 24 to 28: Screen using a 1-hour glucola test and, if needed and appropriate (see below*), a 3-hour diagnostic test.
  - The risk of developing type 2 diabetes with the personal history of GDM is up to 50% in the next 20 years after delivery. Therefore, a fasting 75-g 2-hour oral glucose tolerance test (OGTT), because it is only 1 step, may be helpful in diagnosing postpartum diabetes or glucose intolerance. It is unclear if the 75-g 2-hour GTT is comparable to the 2-step approach in diagnosing GDM*.
  - Assess for readiness for change in diet +/− exercise. Provide counseling, nutrition, and other support on diagnosis of GDM. Continue to support during the postpartum period and beyond.
  - Diagnosing GDM (ACOG and AAFP guidelines):
    - Setting cutoff for "elevated 1-hour GCT": Setting the cutoff at 130 or 135 may be prudent for a practice with higher local prevalence of GDM. Setting the cutoff at 140 may be prudent for a practice with low local prevalence of GDM.
    - Routine screening for GDM (~week 24 to 28): 50 g PO nonfasting glucose load with blood glucose testing 1 hour later; if elevated, then proceed to 3-hour testing for diagnosis.
      - *Each practice or institution may have internal guidelines for 1-hour results if ≥180 to 185 and proceed with fasting BG monitoring instead of proceeding with 3-hour GTT.
    - Diagnostic test: 3-hour GTT is achieved, on a separate day from 1-hour GCT, by 100 g PO glucose load after fasting for ≥8 hours with blood drawn: fasting, 1, 2, and 3 hours after ingestion of glucose. A positive diagnosis of GDM requires that ≥2 positive thresholds by either of the criteria listed below.
      - NDDG standard: ≥105 (fasting), ≥190 (1-hour), ≥165 (2-hour), ≥145 (3-hour)
      - Carpenter and Coustan standard: ≥95 (fasting), ≥180 (1-hour), ≥155 (2-hour), ≥140 (3-hour)
    - ACOG states, due to known adverse events, one elevated value from the 3-hour GTT may be sufficient to demonstrate evidence of glucose intolerance.
    - 1-step approach (75-g OGTT) on all women will increase the diagnosis of GDM, but sufficient prospective studies demonstrating improved outcomes are still lacking and need further research. ACOG does acknowledge that some centers may opt for "1 step" if warranted based on their population.
- 35 to 37 week prenatal visits (1):
  - Group B *Streptococcus* (GBS) culture: Screen all low-risk cases at 35 to 37 weeks' GA to identify women colonized with GBS. For cases requiring induction at 37 weeks or earlier, screen as soon as possible.
  - High-risk patients: High-risk patients should be screened again for gonorrhea, chlamydia, syphilis, and HIV.
- Postterm pregnancy:
  - The rate of stillbirth increases with GA by 1/3,000 per week at 41 weeks, 3/3,000 per week at 42 weeks, and 6/3,000 at 43 weeks. In one meta-analysis, routine induction of labor at 41 weeks' GA reduced rates of perinatal death without increased rates of cesarean delivery.
  - For prenatal care >41 to 42 weeks, fetal well-being should be assessed with nonstress testing and US assessment of amniotic fluid volume.

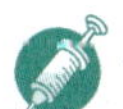

TREATMENT

ISSUES FOR REFERRAL

Abnormal screening labs or imaging may prompt referral to maternal–fetal medicine specialist or other medical specialists as indicated.

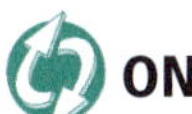

ONGOING CARE

PATIENT EDUCATION

- Immunizations during pregnancy per CDC:
  - Tdap during each pregnancy (should be given between 27 and 36 weeks' GA); hepatitis B and influenza; likely safe include meningococcal, rabies; contraindicated or safety not established: live vaccines including BCG, MMR, and varicella
  - Vaccination against COVID-19 is recommended in pregnancy. COVID-19 increases the risk for patient and fetus.
- Recommendations for use of dietary supplements in pregnancy (1),(2)
  - Folic acid 0.4 mg/day beginning at least 1 month prior to attempting conception and continuing throughout pregnancy; 1 to 4 mg for women at higher risk of having child with neural tube defect beginning 1 to 3 months before conception, continued through first 12 weeks of gestation, and then reduced to 0.4 mg/day
  - Calcium: 1,000 to 1,300 mg/day; supplement may be beneficial for women with high risk for gestational HTN or communities with low dietary calcium intake.
  - Caffeine: Limit to <200 mg/day; more research needed
  - Iron: Screen for anemia (hemoglobin/hematocrit) and order extra iron supplementation if necessary.
  - Vitamin A: Pregnant women in industrialized countries should limit to <5,000 IU/day.
  - Vitamin D: 200 to 1,200 IU (dose in standard prenatal vitamin) is recommended until more evidence is available to support different dose.
- Other important counseling topics during pregnancy (2):
  - Airline travel: generally safe until up to week 35; >2 hours without ambulation increases the risk of thrombosis.
  - Exercise: Healthy women with uncomplicated pregnancies should continue to exercise.
  - Seat belts/airbags: Wear lap and shoulder seat-belts; working airbags (ACOG and AAFP)
  - Sexual activity: Intercourse while pregnant is not associated with adverse outcomes. Avoiding sex may be necessary in cases of low-lying placenta, placenta previa, or vasa previa.
  - Alcohol, cigarettes, and illicit drugs are injurious to fetal and maternal health.
  - Pregnancy-safe medications (teratogenicity)
  - Avoid large fish such as shark, tuna, swordfish, and mackerel (high levels of mercury).
  - Preconception counseling offers the opportunity to discuss individualized risks.

REFERENCES

1. Zolotor AJ, Carlough MC. Update on prenatal care. *Am Fam Physician*. 2014;89(3):199–208.
2. Kilpatrick SJ, Papile L, Macones GA, et al, eds. *Guidelines for Perinatal Care*. 8th ed. Elk Grove Village, IL: American Academy of Pediatrics, 2017.
3. American College of Obstetricians and Gynecologists' Committee on Practice Bulletins—Obstetrics, Committee on Genetics, Society for Maternal-Fetal Medicine. Practice Bulletin No. 162: prenatal diagnostic testing for genetic disorders. *Obstet Gynecol*. 2016;127(5):e108–e122.

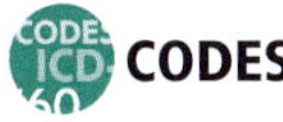

CODES

ICD10

- Z34.90 Encntr for suprvsn of normal pregnancy, unsp, unsp trimester
- Z36 Encounter for antenatal screening of mother
- Z34.00 Encntr for suprvsn of normal first pregnancy, unsp trimester

CLINICAL PEARLS

Given the complexity of screening and counseling, checklists and team-based care help ensure consistent application of recommended interventions.

PREOPERATIVE EVALUATION OF THE NONCARDIAC SURGICAL PATIENT

Anush Pillai, DO, FAAFP

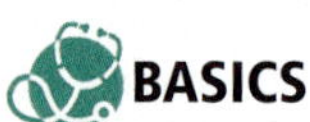

BASICS

DESCRIPTION

- Preoperative medical evaluation involves assessing risks specific to the patient, assessment of the risk of the surgery itself, assessing functional status of the patient, consideration regarding medication management, and evaluation for any preoperative testing.
- Following the above assessment, the examiner formulates recommendations for the surgeon and anesthesiologist. Additional recommendations may be given to the patient as well.

EPIDEMIOLOGY

45% of patients age ≥45 years undergoing surgery have several comorbidities and 25% have atherosclerotic cardiovascular disease (ASCVD). There is an approximate 3% risk of death, myocardial infarction (MI), or stroke for noncardiac surgery. Preoperative patient evaluation and subsequent optimization of perioperative care reduce both postoperative morbidity and mortality.

RISK FACTORS

Factors influencing risk of adverse surgical outcomes may be divided as follows:

- Patient's functional capacity (1): Exercise tolerance is one of the most important determinants of cardiac risk:
  - Self-reported exercise tolerance may be a useful predictive tool when assessing risk. Patients with poor functional status (unable to achieve >4 metabolic equivalents (METs) or Duke Activity Status Index (DASI) score >34 have an almost 2-fold greater risk of inpatient cardiovascular (CV) events. The BASEL-PMI study showed 1.63× higher rate of death, MI, acute heart failure (HF), or life-threatening arrhythmias at 30 days in patients with poor functional capacity.
  - Patients who report good exercise tolerance require minimal, if any, additional testing.
- Risk of the surgery: High-risk surgeries (>5% risk) include intrathoracic, intra-abdominal, suprainguinal vascular procedures, and emergency surgeries. Low risk surgeries (<1% risk) are superficial procedures, breast surgery, endoscopic procedures, and most ambulatory surgeries. All others would fall under intermediate risk (1–5%). Urgent and emergent surgeries have higher risk.
- Risks associated with patient medical conditions (2)
  - History of ischemic heart disease, significant valvular heart disease, the presence of decompensated HF or a history of HF, poorly controlled HTN, CVA, diabetes mellitus (especially) requiring insulin, and renal insufficiency (creatinine >2 mg/dL)
  - Bleeding risk/history of bleeding, prior anesthesia complications, uncontrolled asthma/COPD/obstructive sleep apnea (OSA), and immunosuppression may also increase risk.
  - Patients >70 years of age are at higher risk for complications, longer length of stay, and mortality. Assess frailty risk using available calculators for geriatric patients.

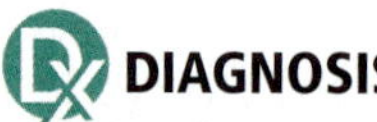

DIAGNOSIS

HISTORY

- Obtain complete H&P, past medical history, OB-GYN history, medication history, allergy history, PSH, and anesthesia history. Review substance use (tobacco, alcohol, drug use, and cessation). Obtain patients current activity and exercise level/tolerance. Ask about any systemic steroid use in last 6 months.
- Review of systems
  - General: recent illness, infections, stress, unexplained weight loss/gain
  - Cardiovascular: exercise capacity, angina, dyspnea on exertion, palpitations, edema, presyncope, syncope
    - 1 MET: can take care of self, eat, dress, and use toilet; walk around house indoors; walk a block or two on level ground at 2 to 3 mph.
    - 4 METs: can climb 2 flights of stairs or walk uphill, walk on level ground at 4 mph, run a short distance, do heavy work around house, participate in moderate recreational activities
    - 10 METs: can participate in strenuous sports such as swimming, singles tennis, football, basketball, or skiing
    - Note presence of HF, cardiomyopathy, ischemic heart disease (stable vs. unstable), valvular disease, HTN (status of control) arrhythmias, new or worsening murmurs, pericarditis, history of pacemaker or implantable cardioverter defibrillator (ICD)
  - Pulmonary: smoking status, poorly controlled asthma, COPD, HF, pulmonary hypertension, nutritional status, sleep apnea
  - GI: hepatic disease, reflux, ulcers, inflammatory bowel disease, hernias (especially hiatal), nausea, vomiting, NSAID use
  - Hematologic: anemia, serious bleeding, clotting problems, blood transfusions, hereditary disorders, unexplained bruising
  - Renal: kidney failure, dialysis, infections, stones, changes in urinary function
  - Endocrine: hypothyroid or hyperthyroid symptoms, parathyroid, pituitary, adrenal disease, glycemic control in diabetics
  - Neuropsychiatric: seizures, stroke, paralysis, tremor, weakness, paresthesias, depression, anxiety, mania, psychosis, neuromuscular disorders affecting respiration or cardiac function
  - Musculoskeletal: functional limitations, fall risk, inflammatory/autoimmune conditions, and steroids or immunosuppressant use, NSAID use; assess for frailty in geriatric patients using screening tools.
  - Reproductive: menstrual history, contraception
- Mouth/upper airway: dentures, crowns, partials, bridges, teeth (loose, chipped, cracked, capped)

PHYSICAL EXAM

- Assess vital signs.
- Oropharynx: Assess Mallampati class.
- Neck: Check for carotid pulses, bruits, thyroid tenderness/masses.
- Pulmonary: Assess for dyspnea, tachypnea, abnormal breathing patterns, air movement, any issues for chest expansion, and if any abnormal sounds.
- Cardiovascular system: heart rate, rhythm, murmurs, extra beats, pulses
- Neuromuscular exam: gait, fall risk, ROM, strength, cranial nerves
- Skin: rash, bruising, petechiae, purpura, open wounds, skin infections
- Psychiatric: mental status, psychosis

DIAGNOSTIC TESTS & INTERPRETATION

Initial Tests (lab, imaging)

Laboratory testing should never be "routine" prior to surgery. Tests should be obtained only when indicated by specific conditions or risk factors. "Routine" testing results in unnecessary delays and disruptions to planned surgery. Specific tests should be requested if the evaluator suspects findings from the clinical evaluation that may influence perioperative patient management. Recent labs (<3 months) are reliable, unless there are any clinical changes or medication changes.

- CBC: if symptoms of anemia, procedure with major blood loss, liver disease, kidney disease, medication use that may affect bleeding/clotting function, concerns for infection/inflammation/myeloproliferative disorder, or immunosuppression
- CMP: Check if diabetic, CKD, history abnormal LFTs or liver disease, CHF or if patient is on medications that may affect electrolytes, liver, or kidney function.
- PT/PTT: if history of a bleeding disorder, chronic liver disease, or malnutrition, or those on medications that may affect these levels
- Urinalysis: indicated in certain urogynecologic procedures or if patient may have foreign body implants to ensure no obvious underlying infection
- Pregnancy test: all female patients of childbearing age
- Chest X-ray (CXR): if significant heart or lung disease or if recent change of symptoms
- BNP or NT-proBNP: Consider in patients with known CVD, or age ≥65 years, or age ≥45 years with symptoms suggestive of CVD undergoing elevated risk noncardiac surgery (NCS)
- Cardiac troponin (cTn): Consider in patients with known CVD, or age ≥65 years, or age ≥45 years with symptoms suggestive of CVD undergoing elevated risk NCS (1).

Diagnostic Procedures/Other

- ECG
  - Not indicated for asymptomatic patients undergoing low-risk procedures (1)
  - Reasonable for patients with known CAD, peripheral vascular disease, cerebrovascular disease, significant arrhythmia, or known significant structural heart disease; recommended in patients undergoing vascular surgery and in patients undergoing intermediate risk or other high-risk surgery with at least one clinical risk factor (1)
- Echocardiogram (ECHO): not routinely recommended (2); consider for dyspnea, worsening HF, moderate to severe valvular disease with change in clinical status or valvular disease with no prior ECHO evaluation in over 1 year (1)

- Stress testing or cardiac catheterization:
  - No need for low-risk patients or patients with good functional capacity with stable symptoms undergoing low risk procedures (1)
  - Use Revised Cardiac Risk Index or the ACS NSQIP online risk calculators to estimate risk of MACE in the perioperative period.
    - If low risk (<1%), then proceed with surgery.
    - If the risk is >1%, assess functional capacity.
      - For patients with functional capacity >4 METs, proceed with surgery.
      - If functional capacity <4 METs or unknown, consider exercise or pharmacologic stress testing with nuclear imaging if it will change management.
        - If abnormal stress testing, may need cardiac catheterization and revascularization depending on findings, patient status, and patient's symptoms
  - Stress testing is appropriate in patients undergoing high-risk surgery with poor or unknown functional capacity and high risk for perioperative CV events.
- PFTs: no evidence except for thoracic surgery
- Coronary CT angiography: Avoid in low-risk patients with adequate functional capacity, stable symptoms, and undergoing low-risk procedures (1).

Test Interpretation

- Low-risk patient, low-risk surgery—proceed to surgery.
- Low-risk patient, asymptomatic, intermediate-/high-risk surgery, good functional capacity—proceed to surgery.
- Intermediate-risk patient, intermediate-risk surgery, good functional capacity—proceed to surgery
- Intermediate-/high-risk patient, intermediate-/high-risk surgery, low functional capacity, or unable to determine functional capacity—further evaluation needed with labs, EKG, ECHO, or stress testing; if initial testing abnormal, will need to optimize condition prior to surgery

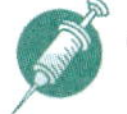

TREATMENT

DVT prophylaxis should be addressed as per guidelines.

GENERAL MEASURES

Delaying surgery:

- Delay or cancel elective surgery if patient has unstable coronary syndromes, recent MI (<30 days), decompensated CHF, significant arrhythmias, or severe valvular disease.
- Wait at least 60 days after MI if patient did not require a coronary intervention. Waiting at least 6 to 9 months after a CVA for elective/nonurgent surgery.
- If recent percutaneous coronary intervention (PCI) without stent placement, delay NCS for 14 days to reduce perioperative major adverse cardiovascular events (MACE).
- Delay surgery >1 year if PCI with drug-eluting stent (DES) done for ACS if antiplatelets need to be held for surgery to minimize MACE. Delay for 6 months if PCI with DES done for chronic coronary disease (CCD) to minimize MACE

MEDICATION

Reducing cardiac risk (3)

- β-blockers:
  - When indicated, perioperative β-blockade is most beneficial when initiated minimum of 1 to 4 weeks preoperatively and continued for one month postoperatively.
  - If no immediate need for β-blockade, do *not* initiate on date of surgery in β-blocker–naive patients (1).
  - Patients chronically on β-blockers should have the medication continued in the perioperative period (1).
- Reducing pulmonary risk: Smoking cessation at least 8 weeks prior to elective surgery. Optimize asthma and COPD control.
- Antihypertensives:
  - Hold diuretics and clonidine on date of surgery.
  - Okay to continue ACE-I/ARBs on date of surgery if normal/stable renal function, normal electrolytes, and hemodynamically stable in those with indications other than hypertension for these medications. For patients on ACE-I/ARB for HTN only, could hold 24 hours preoperative to limit intraoperative hypotension.
  - Okay to continue other BP medications on date of surgery (1).
- Hypoglycemics:
  - Hold regular insulin on morning of surgery, take 1/3 or 1/2 dose of basal insulin if NPO. Hold oral hypoglycemics and use insulin. Hold metformin 48 hours preoperative and prior to contrast studies (1).
  - SGLT2i: Hold 3 to 4 days prior to surgery when feasible to reduce risk of perioperative metabolic acidosis (1).
- Stress dose steroids: Consider perioperative steroids if patient had >2 weeks of systemic corticosteroids in prior 3 to 6 months to reduce risk of adrenal crisis.
- Antiplatelet agents:
  - Dual antiplatelet therapy (DAPT) for minimum 30 days for patients with bare metal stents and 1 year for DESs.
  - Postpone elective surgery if DAPT needs to be stopped for surgery. Clinical correlation for emergency surgery based on type of surgery, bleeding risk, cardiovascular risk.
  - Discontinue aspirin 7 to 10 days prior to surgery if used for primary prevention or if no indications.
  - Continue perioperatively if used for secondary prevention unless high bleeding risk.
- Oral anticoagulation (OAC): For patients with CVD with high thrombotic risk, preoperative bridging is appropriate with parenteral heparin (2).
- Statins:
  - Continue perioperative statins.
  - Initiate statin several weeks preoperative in patients undergoing vascular surgery or those with clinical indications undergoing high-risk noncardiac surgeries (2).

SURGERY/OTHER PROCEDURES

Cataract surgery under topical/regional anesthesia does *not* require preoperative exams or testing.

COMPLEMENTARY & ALTERNATIVE MEDICINE

Stop all supplements, vitamins, herbs 7 to 10 days preoperative.

ADMISSION, INPATIENT, AND NURSING CONSIDERATIONS

Discharge planning, medication reconciliation, family support, follow-up care

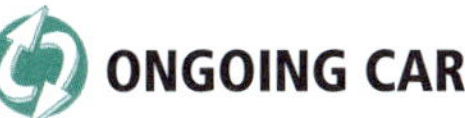

ONGOING CARE

FOLLOW-UP RECOMMENDATIONS

Follow up with PCP in 1 to 2 weeks and surgeon as directed.

REFERENCES

1. Thompson A, et al. 2024 AHA/ACC/ACS/ASNC/HRS/SCA/SCCT/SCMR/SVM guideline for perioperative cardiovascular management for noncardiac surgery: a report of the American College of Cardiology/American Heart Association Joint Committee on Clinical Practice Guidelines. *Circulation*. 2024;150(10):e351–e442.
2. Smilowitz NR, Berger JS. Perioperative cardiovascular risk assessment and management of noncardiac surgery: a review. *JAMA*. 2020;32(3):279–290.
3. Mikhail MA, Mohabbat AB, Ghosh AK. Perioperative cardiovascular medication management in noncardiac surgery: common questions. *Am Fam Physician*. 2017;95(10):645–650.

ADDITIONAL READING

- Cohn S. Update in perioperative cardiac medicine 2021. *Clev Clin J Med*. 2021;88(4):216–220.
- Kumar C, Salzman B, Colburn JL. Preoperative assessment in older adults: a comprehensive approach. *Am Fam Physician*. 2018;98(4):214–220.
- Mierle DM, Raslau D, Regan DW, et al. Preoperative evaluation before noncardiac surgery. *Mayo Clinic Proceedings*. 2020;95(4):807–822.

SEE ALSO

Algorithm: Preoperative Evaluation of Noncardiac Surgical Patient

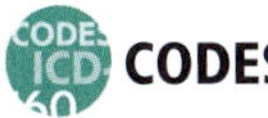

CODES

ICD10

- Z01.818 Encounter for other preprocedural examination
- Z01.811 Encounter for preprocedural respiratory examination
- Z01.812 Encounter for preprocedural laboratory examination

CLINICAL PEARLS

- Preoperative good functional capacity (as evaluated by a combination of self-reporting using >4 METs and DASI score >34) is a strong predictor of good outcome in the perioperative period.
- Provide guidance on management of chronic medications for preoperative/perioperative/postoperative care.
- No preoperative tests are or should be routine.
- Active cardiac conditions should lead to delay or cancellation of nonemergent surgery.

PRESBYCUSIS

Darnel Viray Dabu, MD, MPH, FAAFP, DipABLM • Sabari Nair, DO

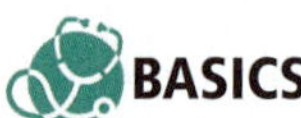

BASICS

DESCRIPTION

- Age-related hearing loss (HL).
- Represents a lifetime of insults to the auditory system from toxic noise exposure and natural decline resulting in gradual, progressive, bilateral HL
- Usually presents as high-frequency HL with tinnitus (ringing)
- Impacts the "clarity" of sounds (i.e., ability to detect, identify, and localize sounds) making it difficult to hear in noisy conditions and reduced ability to understand speech.
- Central and peripheral causes:
  - Central presbycusis: age-related change in the auditory portions of the central nervous system negatively impacting auditory perception, speech-communication performance, or both
  - Peripheral presbycusis: age-related, bilateral sensorineural HL (SNHL) typically symmetric
- No cure for presbycusis exists to date; management consists of mitigating risk factors and auditory amplification.
- Hearing aids (HA) are the mainstay of treatment and are now sold over the counter for mild-to-moderate HL.
- Can lead to adverse effects on physical, cognitive, emotional, behavioral, and social function in the elderly (e.g., depression, social isolation) and is a contributor to all-cause dementia

EPIDEMIOLOGY

Prevalence

- Increases with age—ages 60 to 69 years, 27%; ages 70 to 79 years, 55%; ages >80 years, 81%
- Predominant sex: male > female

ETIOLOGY AND PATHOPHYSIOLOGY

- The external ear transmits sound energy to the tympanic membrane. The middle ear ossicles amplify and conduct the sound waves into the inner ear (cochlea) via the oval window. The organ of Corti, located in the cochlea, contains hair cells that detect these vibrations and depolarize, producing electrical signals that travel through the auditory nerve to the brain. These hair cells are susceptible to damage from a variety of insults and cannot be regenerated leading to cell death and permanent HL.
- Presbycusis is caused by the accumulated effects of noise exposure, systemic disease, oxidative damage, ototoxic drugs, and genetic susceptibility.

Genetics

Presbycusis has a clear familial aggregation:

- Genetic polymorphisms in genes encoding detoxification enzymes have been linked to age-related HL including GSTM1, GSTT1, and NAT2*6A (1).
- Other genes linked to age-related HL include GRM7, GRHL2, DFNA5, and KCNQ4 (1)
- Mitochondrial DNA mutations/deletions have also been implicated in age-related HL.

RISK FACTORS

- Advancing age
- Noise exposure (military, industrial, leisure etc.)
- Ototoxic substances (organic solvents, heavy metals, carbon monoxide)
- Drugs (aminoglycosides, cisplatin [dose dependent], salicylates, NSAIDs, diuretics, antimalarials)
- Cigarette smoking
- Alcohol abuse
- Lower socioeconomic status
- Family history of presbycusis
- Head trauma (temporal bone fractures)
- Cardiovascular disease (hypertension, atherosclerosis, hyperlipidemia)
- Diabetes mellitus
- Autoimmune disease (auto cochleitis/labyrinthitis)
- Metabolic bone disease
- Endocrine medical conditions: levels of aldosterone
- Otologic conditions (e.g., Ménière disease or otosclerosis)

GENERAL PREVENTION

- Avoid hazardous noise exposure. 70 dBA or lower is considered safe.
- Use hearing protection (earmuffs, earplugs).
- Screening
  - Based on a 2021 review, according to the USPSTF, there is insufficient evidence to assess the relative benefits and harms of HL screening in adults aged ≥50 years.
  - Hearing Handicap Inventory for the Elderly Screening (2)
  - RCT published in 2010 on screening for HL, HA use was significantly higher in three screened groups (4.1% in those using a questionnaire, 6.3% using handheld audiometry, and 7.4% using both modalities) versus unscreened control participants (3.3%) at 1-year follow-up (3)[B].

COMMONLY ASSOCIATED CONDITIONS

- Accelerated multidomain cognitive decline, cognitive impairment, and dementia (4)[A]
- A variety of cognitive, behavioral, and psychosocial disorders (5)
- Smoking, central adiposity, poorly controlled diabetes (6)

DIAGNOSIS

HISTORY

- Reduced hearing sensitivity and speech understanding in noisy/public environments
- Impaired localization of sound sources
- Increased difficulty understanding conversations, especially with women, due to higher frequency of spoken voice
- Presents bilaterally and symmetrically
- If unilateral HL, alternative diagnosis should be pursued.
- Cardiac risk factors
- Exposure to ototoxic medications
- Family history of age-related HL
- Additional history if HL is suspected or detected:
  - Time course of HL
  - Symptoms of tinnitus, otalgia, otorrhea, or vertigo
  - History of noise exposure, ear trauma, or head trauma
  - Presence of any neurologic deficit
- Reports from patient/family/caregiver
  - Confusion in social situations
  - Excessive volume of television/radio/computer
  - Social withdrawal
  - Anxiety in group settings

PHYSICAL EXAM

- Whispered voice test
- Otoscopic examination to rule out other etiologies like infection, tumors, cerumen impaction, or tympanic membrane perforation
- Pneumatic otoscopy to evaluate for simple middle ear effusion as cause of conductive HL
- Rinne and Weber tests are helpful for determining conductive versus SNHL but not recommended for general screening.

DIFFERENTIAL DIAGNOSIS

- Complete canal occlusion (cerumen, foreign body)
- Large external or middle ear tumors
- Chronic otitis media or effusion
- Cholesteatoma
- Otosclerosis
- Osteogenesis imperfecta
- Perilymph fistula (trauma/iatrogenic)
- Ménière disease
- Acoustic neuroma (usually unilateral)
- Vascular anomaly
- Acute noise-induced traumatic loss (explosion)
- Autoimmune HL

DIAGNOSTIC TESTS & INTERPRETATION

- Central: synthetic sentence identification test with ipsilateral competing message and the dichotic sentence identification test (2)[C]
- Peripheral: handheld audiometry; insert probe in ear (sealing canal) and have patient indicate if tones can be heard.
  - Positive likelihood ratio (LR) range, 3.1 to 5.8; negative LR range, 0.03 to 0.4
- Screening audiometry
  - Symmetric high-frequency HL in descending slope pattern
  - SNHL frequencies >2 KHz initially
  - Essential to determine global clinical hearing status and if etiology is conductive HL versus SNHL or pseudohypacusis (conversion)

Initial Tests (lab, imaging)

Imaging studies are not indicated for the diagnosis of presbycusis.

Follow-Up Tests & Special Considerations

Asymmetric HL should have evaluation via MRI for acoustic neuroma.

TREATMENT

- Treatment consists of HAs, cochlear implants (CIs), active middle ear implants (AMEIs), electrical acoustic stimulation, hearing-assistive technologies (HATs), and aural rehabilitation.
- Analog HA: picks up sound waves through a microphone; converts them into electrical signals; amplifies and sends them through the ear canal to the tympanic membrane
- Digital HA: programmable; may reduce acoustic feedback, reduce background noise, detect and automatically accommodate different listening environments, control multiple microphones
  - HAs have an average decibel gain of 16.3 dB.
  - Associated with hypersensitivity to loud sounds ("loudness recruitment")
- HATs (2)
  - Can be used alone or in combination with HAs (for difficult listening conditions)
  - Addresses face-to-face communication, broadcast or other electronic media (radio, TV), telephone conversation, sensitivity to alerting signals, and environment stimuli (doorbell, baby's cry, alarm clock, etc.)
  - Includes personal FM systems, infrared systems, induction loop systems, hardwired systems, telephone amplifier, telecoil, telecommunication device for the deaf (TDD), situation-specific devices (e.g., television), alerting devices
- Aural rehabilitation (also known as audiologic orientation or auditory training)
  - Adjunct to HA or HATs
  - Involves education regarding proper use of amplification devices, coaching on how to manage the auditory environment, training in speech perception and communication, and counseling for coping strategies to deal with the difficulties of HAs or HATs

ISSUES FOR REFERRAL

- Sudden SNHL is atypical and an otologic emergency warranting urgent otolaryngologic evaluation/audiometry.
- Refer to audiologist for formal evaluation and optimal fitting of HAs and/or HATs

ADDITIONAL THERAPIES

- Gene therapy: Ongoing research targets include investigation of various transcription factors, cell cycle modulators, and cyclin-dependent kinase inhibitors associated with formation and regeneration of hair cells, and maintenance of supporting cells.
- Pharmacotherapy: Ongoing research includes cellular signaling pathways and molecules as the most investigated targets for pharmacotherapy. Wnt and Notch signaling cascades are implicated in proliferation of supporting cells and associated with limited hair cell growth.
- Stem cell therapy: Mesenchymal stem cells have also shown success in regenerating cochlear spiral ganglion neurons. Endogenous stem cells show the most promising results (2).
- Antioxidants paired with anti-inflammatory drugs or neurotrophic factors being explored

SURGERY/OTHER PROCEDURES

- CIs
  - Bypasses the ear canal, middle ear, and hair cells in the cochlea to provide electric stimulation directly to the auditory nerve
  - Indications include hearing no better than identifying ≤50% of keywords in test sentences in the best aided condition in the worst ear and 60% in the better ear.
  - Incoming sounds are received through the microphone in the audio processor component (resembles a small HA), which converts them into electrical impulses and sends them to the magnetic coil (located on the skin). The impulses transmit these across intact skin via radio waves to the implanted component (directly subjacent to the coil). The pulses travel to the electrodes in the cochlea and stimulate the cochlea at high rates.
  - Receiving a unilateral CI is most common; some may receive bilateral CIs (either sequentially or in the same surgery). Others may wear a CI in one ear and an HA in the contralateral ear (bimodal fit).
  - Younger age at CI placement derives the greatest benefit.
- AMEIs
  - Suitable for elderly adults who cannot wear conventional HAs for medical or personal (cosmetic) reasons and whose HL is not severe enough for a CI
  - Different models available and may include components that are implantable under the skin
- Electric acoustic stimulation: use of CI and HA together in one ear
  - Addresses the specific needs of patients presenting with good low-frequency hearing (a mild-to-moderate SNHL in frequencies up to 1,000 Hz) but poorer hearing in the high frequencies (sloping to 60 dB or worse HL >1,000 Hz)
    - Contraindications: progressive HL, autoimmune disease; HL related to meningitis, otosclerosis, or ossification; malformation of the cochlea; a gap in air conduction and bone conduction thresholds of >15 dB; external ear contraindications, active infection, or unwillingness to use amplification device (2)

ONGOING CARE

FOLLOW-UP RECOMMENDATIONS

Patient Monitoring

- Check for proper fit of HA and assess and address any patient concerns to improve compliance, as 25–40% of adults will either stop wearing them or use them only occasionally.
- Annual audiograms

PATIENT EDUCATION

- Communication should be face-to-face; spoken clearly and unhurriedly, without competing background noise (e.g., radio, TV); and include a confirmation that the message is received.
- Formal speech reading classes may be beneficial.

REFERENCES

1. Wang J, Puel JL. Presbycusis: an update on cochlear mechanisms and therapies. *J Clin Med*. 2020;9(1):218. doi:10.3390/jcm9010218.
2. Vaisbuch Y, Santa Maria PL. Age-related hearing loss: innovations in hearing augmentation. *Otolaryngol Clin North Am*. 2018;51(4):705–723.
3. Yueh B, Collins MP, Souza PE, et al. Long-term effectiveness of screening for hearing loss: the screening for auditory impairment—which hearing assessment test (SAI-WHAT) randomized trial. *J Am Geriatr Soc*. 2010;58(3):427–434.
4. Loughrey DG, Kelly ME, Kelley GA, et al. Association of age-related hearing loss with cognitive function, cognitive impairment, and dementia: a systematic review and meta-analysis. *JAMA Otolaryngol Head Neck Surg*. 2018;144(2):115–126.
5. Fishman J, Fisher E. Impact of coronavirus disease 2019 on otolaryngological practice, effect of presbylarynx and presbycusis in the elderly, and suicidal ideation in patients with tinnitus. *J Laryngol Otol*. 2021;135(12):1035–1036. doi:10.1017/S0022215121003431.
6. Cunningham LL, Tucci DL. Hearing loss in adults. *N Engl J Med*. 2017 Dec 21;377(25):2465–2473. doi:10.1056/NEJMra1616601.

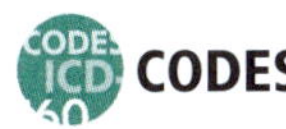

CODES

ICD10

- H91.10 Presbycusis, unspecified ear
- H91.13 Presbycusis, bilateral
- H91.11 Presbycusis, right ear

CLINICAL PEARLS

- Presbycusis is age-related HL, showing increased prevalence with age. It is often bilateral and initially begins as high-frequency HL. It presents as difficulty communicating in noisy conditions.
- HL is significantly associated with social isolation, depression, and progressive cognitive impairment leading to dementia.
- Early audiology referral for individuals with suspected HL may improve treatment efficacy.
- Use of auditory assistive devices such as HAs, CIs, and AMEIs are associated with improvement in cognitive function, social isolation, and depression.

PRESSURE ULCER

Ramanpreet Grewal, MD

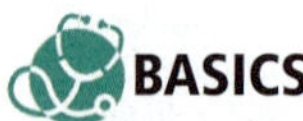

BASICS

DESCRIPTION
- Breakdown in a localized area of skin or underlying tissue, primarily caused by prolonged pressure and/or shear
- Usually over a bony prominence where the skin is in proximity with the underlying bone (e.g., sacrum, calcaneus, ischium)
- Classified in stages according to the National Pressure Injury Advisory Panel (NPIAP):
  - Stage I: nonblanchable erythema—intact skin with nonblanchable redness; darkly pigmented skin may not have visible blanching.
  - Stage II: partial-thickness skin loss—shallow open ulcer with a viable red-pink, moist wound bed, without slough; or intact or open/ruptured serum-filled blister
  - Stage III: full-thickness skin loss—subcutaneous fat may be visible, but bone, tendon, or muscle is not exposed; slough, if present, does not obscure depth of tissue loss.
  - Stage IV: full-thickness tissue loss—exposed bone, tendon, or joint; slough or eschar may be present but does not completely obscure wound base.
  - Unstageable: depth unknown—base of the ulcer is covered by slough and/or eschar in the wound bed.
  - Suspected deep tissue injury: depth unknown—purple or maroon area of intact skin or blood-filled blister. Pain and temperature change precede skin color changes.
- Synonyms: bedsores, decubitus ulcers, pressure sores, pressure injuries, pressure wounds, pressure points, pressure damage, pressure-related skin injuries, skin breakdown, ischemic ulcers

EPIDEMIOLOGY

Incidence
Ranges widely depending on setting and population: 0–53.4% (1)

Prevalence
Ranges widely depending on setting and population: 0–72.5% (1)

ETIOLOGY AND PATHOPHYSIOLOGY
Complex process of risk factors interacting with external forces (pressure and/or shear, friction, and moisture)

RISK FACTORS
- Mobility impairment
- Malnutrition
- Reduced skin perfusion
- Sensory impairment
- Medical devices

GENERAL PREVENTION
- Structured risk assessment
- Skin and tissue assessment
- Preventive skin care
- Nutrition screening
- Repositioning
- Early mobilization
- Support surfaces
- Microclimate control
- Prophylactic dressings
- Electrical stimulation of the muscles

COMMONLY ASSOCIATED CONDITIONS
- Advanced age
- Immobility
- Trauma
- Hip fractures
- Diabetes
- Cerebrovascular and cardiovascular disease
- Incontinence

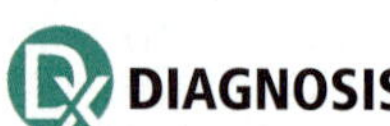

DIAGNOSIS

HISTORY
- Risk factors
- Nutritional assessment
- Pain assessment
- Date of ulcer diagnosis
- Treatment course

PHYSICAL EXAM
- Full skin examination on initial contact and repeatedly throughout visits
- Assess location, stage, size (length, width, depth), identify the presence of sinus tracts, undermining, tunneling, exudate, necrosis, odor, and signs of healing (e.g., granulation tissue) (1).
- Identify factors that may affect healing (impaired perfusion, sensation, presence of infection).

DIFFERENTIAL DIAGNOSIS
- Venous ulcers
- Arterial ulcers
- Diabetic foot ulcer
- Cellulitis and erysipelas
- Incontinence associated dermatitis
- Skin tears
- Intertrigo
- Neuropathic ulcers
- Cutaneous squamous cell carcinomas
- Hypertensive ulcers
- Pyoderma gangrenosum, cancers, vasculitides, and other dermatologic conditions

DIAGNOSTIC TESTS & INTERPRETATION

Initial Tests (lab, imaging)
- Laboratory tests:
  - Complete blood count (CBC) and consider C-reactive protein (CRP) to check for infection/inflammation or anemia
  - Albumin and prealbumin to assess nutritional status
  - Electrolytes to assess overall metabolic status
  - Blood urea nitrogen (BUN) and creatinine to assess kidney function
  - Hemoglobin A1c (HbA1c) to assess long-term blood sugar control
  - Wound culture: Do not culture surface drainage. If culture is necessary, do deep tissue culture/bone biopsy.
- Imaging studies:
  - X-rays, MRI, or ultrasound may be used to assess the depth of the ulcer and determine if there is underlying bone involvement.
  - Ankle-brachial index and Doppler ultrasound (for lower extremity wounds)

Follow-Up Tests & Special Considerations
- Nutrition management: Ensure adequate nutrition, especially in at-risk patients.
- Pressure redistribution: Use support surfaces to reduce pressure on vulnerable areas.
- Diabetes management: Monitor and manage blood sugar in diabetic patients.
- Mobility and positioning: Encourage regular position changes to prevent ulcers.
- Patient education: Educate patients and caregivers on wound care and prevention.
- Addressing underlying causes: Manage medical conditions contributing to ulcers.
- Physical therapy: Involve physical therapists to improve mobility and healing.
- Pain management: Address pain to improve patient comfort.
- Patient compliance: Encourage adherence to the treatment plan and follow-up appointments.

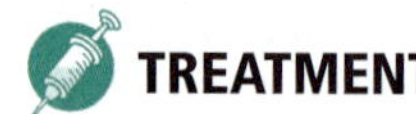

TREATMENT

GENERAL MEASURES
- Comprehensive initial assessment of the patient
- Pressure reduction/redistribution (2)[A]
- Nutritional support (e.g., protein-containing supplements) (3)[B]
- Wound assessment and treatment
  - Wound bed preparation (tissue management, infection and inflammation control, moisture balance, epithelial edge advancement) (1)
  - Wound cleansing (1)[C]
  - Debridement (1)[C]
- Address immobility.
- Manage incontinence.
- Address pain.
- Assess goals of care and advance directives.

MEDICATION

First Line
- Wound dressings as appropriate for the category of ulcer (transparent film, hydrocolloid, hydrogel, alginate, foam, silver-impregnated, honey-impregnated, cadexomer iodine, gauze, silicone, collagen matrix, composite) (1)[C].
- Individual studies comparing dressings are generally of low quality. Systematic reviews comparing dressings have been unable to find superiority of one dressing over another (4)[A].
- Enzymatic débriding agents

Second Line
- Activated charcoal
- Topical antiseptics (hydrogen peroxide, Dakin solution, povidone-iodine)

ISSUES FOR REFERRAL
- Consider referral to a wound care specialist (if available) for complex or nonhealing wounds.
- Consider vascular surgery for improvement of blood flow to wound via vascular bypass if appropriate.
- Consider a surgical consultation for possible urgent drainage and/or débridement if advancing cellulitis; suspected source of sepsis; undermining, tunneling, sinus tracts, and/or extensive necrotic tissue that cannot otherwise be removed by nonsurgical debridement methods; or for stage III or IV that are not closing with conservative management (1)[C].
- Consider plastic surgery for skin graft/flap if appropriate.
- Consider dermatology referral if suspected pyoderma gangrenosum, cancer, vasculitis, or other dermatologic conditions.

ADDITIONAL THERAPIES
- Direct contact electrical stimulation for recalcitrant stage II and any category/stage III and IV (1)[C]
- Electromagnetic field for recalcitrant category/stage II and any stage III and IV (1)[C]
- Pulsed radio frequency energy for recalcitrant stage II and any stage III and IV (1)[C]

SURGERY/OTHER PROCEDURES
- Débridement: removal of dead or infected tissue from the ulcer
- Flap surgery: transplanting healthy tissue from nearby areas to cover the ulcer
- Skin grafting: using healthy skin from another part of the body to cover the ulcer
- Negative pressure wound therapy (NPWT): applying vacuum to the wound to promote healing
- Muscle flap rotation: rotating a muscle with its blood supply to cover the wound
- Implants and bioengineered tissues: Using surgical implants or bioengineered tissues to aid healing

COMPLEMENTARY & ALTERNATIVE MEDICINE
- Low-frequency ultrasound for débridement of necrotic soft tissue (not eschar) (1)[C]
- High-frequency ultrasound as adjunct for infected pressure ulcers (1)[C]
- NPWT as an early adjuvant treatment for deep, stage III and IV (1)[C]
- Consider course of hydrotherapy with pulsed lavage with suction for wound cleansing and débridement (1)[C].
- Phototherapy: short-term UVC light if traditional therapies fail (1)[C]; laser not recommended; infrared is not recommended (1)[C].
- Hyperbaric and topical oxygen therapy not recommended for routine use (1)[C]
- Hydrotherapy with whirlpool should not be considered for routine use (1)[C].
- Vibration therapy not recommended (1)[C]
- Consider sterile maggot débridement therapy.

ADMISSION, INPATIENT, AND NURSING CONSIDERATIONS
- Admission criteria/initial stabilization: refractory cellulitis, osteomyelitis, systemic infection, advanced nutritional decline, suspected patient mistreatment, inability to care for self
- Dressing changes 1 to 3 times daily based on wound assessment and plan of care
- Assess risk factors according to scales.
- Assess for changing or new wounds.
- Discharge criteria: clinical improvement in wound and systemic illness; when applicable, safe and appropriate location for discharge

ONGOING CARE

FOLLOW-UP RECOMMENDATIONS
- Wound assessment: Regularly assess the pressure ulcer for progress and changes.
- Wound measurement: Periodically measure the ulcer's dimensions to track healing and treatment effectiveness.

Patient Monitoring
- Home health nursing
- Change plan of care if no improvement in 2 to 3 weeks.

DIET
- Approximately 1.0 to 1.5 kg/day of protein
- Strict glycemic control
- Include micronutrients in diet or as supplements (vitamin C and zinc).

PATIENT EDUCATION
- Check skin regularly.
- Signs and symptoms of infection
- Report new or increased pain.
- Prevention of new wound where old wound healed
- Skin care, moisture prevention
- Smoking cessation

PROGNOSIS
Variable, depending on the following:
- Removal of pressure
- Nutrition
- Wound care

COMPLICATIONS
- Infection
- Amputation
- Increased mortality

REFERENCES

1. Haesler E, ed. *Prevention and Treatment of Pressure Ulcers: Clinical Practice Guideline*. Osborne Park, Western Australia: Cambridge Media; 2014.
2. Bergstrom N, Horn SD, Rapp MP, et al. Turning for Ulcer Reduction: a multisite randomized clinical trial in nursing homes. *J Am Geriatr Soc*. 2013;61(10):1705–1713.
3. Smith ME, Totten A, Hickam DH, et al. Pressure ulcer treatment strategies: a systematic comparative effectiveness review. *Ann Intern Med*. 2013;159(1):39–50.
4. Westby MJ, Dumville JC, Soares MO, et al. Dressings and topical agents for treating pressure ulcers. *Cochrane Database Syst Rev*. 2017;6(6):CD011947.

ADDITIONAL READING

- Pieper B, ed. *Pressure Ulcers: Prevalence, Incidence, and Implications for the Future*. Washington, DC: NPUAP; 2012.
- Qaseem A, Humphrey LL, Forciea MA, et al; for Clinical Guidelines Committee of the American College of Physicians. Treatment of pressure ulcers: a clinical practice guideline from the American College of Physicians. *Ann Intern Med*. 2015;162(5):370–379.
- Reddy M, Gill SS, Rochon PA. Preventing pressure ulcers: a systematic review. *JAMA*. 2006;296(8):974–984.
- Stansby G, Avital L, Jones K, et al. Prevention and management of pressure ulcers in primary and secondary care: summary of NICE guidance. *BMJ*. 2014;348:g2592.

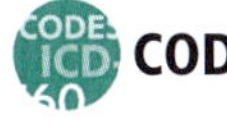

CODES

ICD10
- L89.95 Pressure ulcer of unspecified site, unstageable
- L89.91 Pressure ulcer of unspecified site, stage 1
- L89.92 Pressure ulcer of unspecified site, stage 2

CLINICAL PEARLS
- Create assessment and prevention protocols for all patients.
- Identify risk factors, reduce/redistribute pressure, maximize nutrition, regular skin checks, and assess and treat wounds appropriately.
- All care needs to be done in a time-sensitive, patient-centered fashion.

PRETERM LABOR

Bindusri Paruchuri, MD

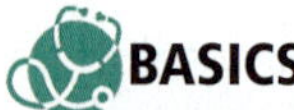

BASICS

Preterm birth is defined as birth between 20 + 0 weeks' and 36 + 6 weeks' gestation.

DESCRIPTION

Regular contractions occurring between 20 weeks to 36 weeks and 6 days with either a change in effacement and cervical dilation or cervical dilation of ≥2 cm on presentation

EPIDEMIOLOGY

Preterm birth is the leading cause of perinatal morbidity and mortality in the United States.

Incidence

- 10–15% of pregnancies experienced at least one episode of preterm labor.
- Causes of preterm births in the United States: Spontaneous preterm labor makes up 40–45% of preterm births, preterm premature rupture of membranes makes up 30–35% of preterm births, medically indicated delivery due to maternal or neonatal etiology associated with 30–35% of preterm births, and multiple gestation.

Prevalence

- Non-Hispanic Black patients are 50% more likely to have a preterm birth than Hispanic or White patients.
- 10% of all births in the United States in 2019 were preterm: 50% of preterm deliveries are due to spontaneous preterm labor, 25% following preterm prelabor rupture of membranes, and 25% due to maternal or fetal medical indications due to complications (1).

ETIOLOGY AND PATHOPHYSIOLOGY

- Premature formation and activation of myometrial gap junctions
- Abnormal placental implantation/placental abruption/placental ischemic disease (preeclampsia and fetal growth restriction)
- Systemic inflammation/infections (e.g., UTI, autoimmune conditions)/immunopathology (e.g., antiphospholipid antibodies)
- Local inflammation/infections (e.g., intraamniotic infections, GBS) → colonization with infectious organism noted in 25–40% of all preterm births
- Uterine abnormalities/overdistension (multiple gestation, polyhydramnios)/cervical insufficiency/premature dilation
- Preterm premature rupture of membranes
- Trauma
- Fetal abnormalities
- Hypertensive disorders of pregnancy

Genetics

Familial predisposition; numerous gene candidates mediating various pathways have been identified, but causality and gene–environment interactions are not well defined.

RISK FACTORS

- Prior preterm delivery (most significant risk factor): 3-fold greater if previous preterm birth
- Demographic factors, including social and economic disadvantages and Black race with concern for chronic stress from structural racism
- Short interpregnancy interval (<18 months)
- Prepregnancy weight <45 kg (100 lb), body mass index <18.5 kg/m^2
- Substance abuse (e.g., cocaine, tobacco)
- Unintended pregnancy
- Cervical insufficiency/short cervical length of less <25 mm
- Abdominal surgery/trauma during pregnancy/history of dilation and curettage
- Uterine structural abnormalities, such as large fibroids or müllerian abnormalities
- Serious maternal infections/diseases/bacterial vaginosis and genital tract infections/bacteriuria
- Multiple gestation, intrauterine growth restriction, polyhydramnios
- Placenta previa, vaginal bleeding, premature placental separation (abruption)

GENERAL PREVENTION

- Patient education at each visit in 2nd and 3rd trimesters for those at risk and periodically in the last two trimesters for the general population
- For women with a singleton pregnancy and no history of spontaneous preterm births, visualization of the cervix on routine fetal anatomical scan between 18 0/7 and 22 6/7 should be performed. If found to be shortened, a transvaginal ultrasound should be done for further evaluation (1)[C]. This recommendation is the same for multiple gestation and women with a history of medically induced preterm birth. Twin pregnancies are more likely to have a shortened cervix during the second trimester, and women with a history of medically induced preterm birth are more likely to have a subsequent preterm birth (1).
- For women with history of spontaneous preterm birth and singleton pregnancy, a screening transvaginal ultrasound to evaluate cervix length should be done at 16 0/7 weeks and repeated every 1 to 4 weeks (protocols vary) until 24 0/7 weeks (1).
- Primary prevention involves counseling on interval contraception to optimize pregnancy spacing and smoking cessation. If previous preterm birth, evaluate if etiology is likely to recur and target intervention to specific condition. Women with history of spontaneous preterm birth and singleton pregnancy should be offered vaginal or intramuscular progesterone to prevent preterm birth with a shared decision model (1).
- Secondary prevention:
  - For patients with a cervix of <25 mm in length with or without a history of previous spontaneous preterm delivery and singleton pregnancy, it is recommended to give vaginal progesterone if not already on progesterone. Most protocols give 200 mg daily at diagnosis at 18 0/7 to 25 6/7 to continue until 36 to 37 weeks (1). An FDA advisory committee voted in late 2022 to withdraw approval of 17-hydroxy progesterone and its generic equivalents based on results from postmarket confirmatory trial data in the PROLONG study, released in October 2019, showing lack of efficacy. Data is insufficient to recommend vaginal progesterone for multiple gestation (1).
  - Women with a singleton pregnancy and history of spontaneous preterm birth with shortened cervix should be considered for a cerclage (1). Cerclage can be considered for any patient who is noted to have cervical insufficiency on physical exam (1).
- Tocolysis

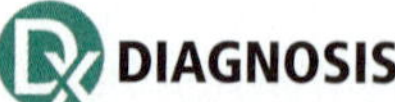

DIAGNOSIS

- Diagnosis is generally based on a combination of significant cervical changes (such as dilation, effacement) with regular contractions. However, there is no single test that will reliably diagnose or predict true preterm labor.
- ACOG defines preterm labor as regular contractions noted with change in cervical dilation, effacement, or both, or regular contractions and cervical dilation of at least 2 cm at presentation.

HISTORY

- Address risk factors
- Regular uterine contractions or cramping/dull, low backache or pain/intermittent lower abdominal pain/increased low pelvic pressure
- Change in vaginal discharge/vaginal bleeding
- Fluid leakage

PHYSICAL EXAM

- Sterile speculum exam for membrane rupture evaluation, cultures, and cervical inspection
- Bimanual cervical exam if intact membranes

ALERT

Avoid bimanual examination when possible if rupture of the membranes is suspected.

DIFFERENTIAL DIAGNOSIS

- Braxton-Hicks contractions/false labor
- Round ligament pain
- Lumbosacral muscular back pain
- UTI or vaginal infections
- Adnexal torsion
- Appendicitis
- Nephrolithiasis

DIAGNOSTIC TESTS & INTERPRETATION

Initial Tests (lab, imaging)

- There are no specific tests that completely accurately predict preterm birth, although they help with risk stratification.
- In symptomatic women from 22 to 34 weeks' gestation with intact membranes and no intercourse or bleeding in past 24 hours, obtain a fetal fibronectin (FFN) swab from the posterior vaginal fornix.
  - If results are positive (≥50 ng/mL), patient is at a modest increased risk for preterm birth (positive predictive value [PPV] 13–30% for delivery within 2 weeks). However, if results are negative, >97% of patients will not deliver in 14 days, so can consider avoiding complicated or high-risk interventions.
  - FFN and shortened cervix alone has low predictive value, so other data should be used as well in acute management of patient (2).
- Urinalysis and urine culture; cultures for gonorrhea, chlamydia, and wet prep
- Vaginal introitus and rectal culture for group B *Streptococcus* if indicated
- pH and ferning test of vaginal fluid to evaluate for rupture of membranes
- CBC with differential and Kleihauer-Betke test if abruption suspected

- US to identify number of fetuses and fetal position, confirm gestational age, estimate fetal weight, quantify amniotic fluid, and look for conditions that contraindicate tocolysis
- Transvaginal US to evaluate cervix length, funneling, and dynamic changes after obtaining FFN (if clinical assessment of the cervix is uncertain or if the cervix is closed on digital exam). ACOG and Society for Maternal-Fetal Medicine (SMFM) recommend transvaginal cervical length screening in patients with history of previous spontaneous preterm birth.

Diagnostic Procedures/Other

Monitor contractions with external tocodynamometer.

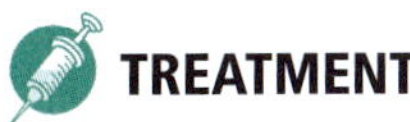

TREATMENT

GENERAL MEASURES

Treat underlying risk factors. Hospitalization is necessary if the patient needs IV tocolysis.

MEDICATION

Tocolysis may allow time for interventions such as transfer to tertiary care facility and administration of corticosteroids but may not prolong pregnancy significantly (2).

First Line

- Corticosteroids (2):
  - Corticosteroids decrease neonatal respiratory distress, intraventricular hemorrhage, necrotizing enterocolitis, and overall perinatal mortality.
  - Give if the mother is at 24 to 34 weeks' gestation and is at risk for delivery in the next 7 days (2); can consider if mother is 23 weeks to 23 weeks and 6 days and at risk for delivery in the next 7 days
  - Rescue course considered if <34 weeks' gestation, at risk for delivery in next 7 days, and previous course of corticosteroids was administered 14 days prior (2)
  - Betamethasone 12 mg IM × 2 doses 24 hours apart *or* dexamethasone 6 mg IM q12h for 4 doses (2).
  - Steroids may reduce the risk of respiratory morbidities in singleton infants born to nondiabetic mothers in the late preterm period (34 + 0 to 36 + 6 weeks' gestation). If delivery is likely during this time period, administration of steroids may be considered as above. Tocolysis is not recommended.
- Tocolysis: reserved for women who benefit from a 48-hour delay to receive corticosteroids as there is no evidence showing tocolysis causes improvement in neonatal outcomes up to 34 weeks' gestation (2).
  - Nifedipine is a calcium channel blocker (CCB) that can be used for tocolysis: 20 mg PO loading dose, and then 10 to 20 mg q4–6h for 48 hours (do not use sublingual route); check BP often and avoid hypotension. Concurrent use with magnesium sulfate is discouraged due to the theoretical risk of neuromuscular blockade (3); contraindications: hypotension, preload dependent cardiac abnormalities such as aortic insufficiency (2)
  - Indomethacin is a nonsteroidal anti-inflammatory drug used for tocolysis: 50 to 100 mg PO initial dose and then 25 to 50 mg q6–8h; best to use in combination with magnesium if it is being used for neuroprotection (2),(3). Consider for use up to 32 weeks (2); contraindications: platelet dysfunction, bleeding disorder, gastrointestinal ulcerative disease, and asthma (if hypersensitive to aspirin) (2)
  - Terbutaline is a β-adrenergic receptor agonist given for tocolysis. Given via SC administration. If contractions persist or pulse >120 beats/min, change to another tocolytic agent (3). Due to reports of serious cardiovascular events and maternal deaths, PO or long-term SC administration of terbutaline should not be given (3); contraindications: tachycardia-sensitive maternal cardiac disease and poorly controlled diabetes mellitus (2)
  - Contraindications to tocolysis: severe preeclampsia, eclampsia, hemorrhage with hemodynamic instability, preterm premature rupture of membranes, chorioamnionitis, advanced labor, intrauterine growth restriction, fetal distress, or lethal fetal abnormalities
- Magnesium sulfate: recommended for imminent delivery prior to 32 weeks for neuroprotection as it reduces the risk and severity of cerebral palsy
- Antibiotics for group B *Streptococcus* prophylaxis if culture is indicated

Second Line

- Magnesium sulfate by IV infusion has not been shown to be superior to placebo in prolonging pregnancy beyond 48 hours. The side effects are generally greater than those with calcium channel blockers or NSAIDs. Therefore, this agent should be used cautiously; contraindication: myasthenia gravis
- Antibiotics should not be used as tocolysis or to improve neonatal outcomes for preterm labor with intact membranes and may be associated with harm.

ISSUES FOR REFERRAL

- If delivery is inevitable but not immediate, consider transport to a tertiary care center or hospital equipped with a neonatal ICU.
- Consider consultation with maternal–fetal medicine specialist.

ADDITIONAL THERAPIES

- Data to prove efficacy of pelvic rest (e.g., no douching or intercourse) is lacking. Bed rest and hydration have not been shown to be effective in the prevention of preterm delivery and are not recommended (2).
- If there is preterm prelabor rupture of membranes, latency antibiotics are indicated.

SURGERY/OTHER PROCEDURES

Consider cerclage with history of recurrent 2nd trimester losses and diagnosis of cervical insufficiency, ultrasound finding of shortened cervix (<25 mm) and history of preterm birth, and rescue cerclage can be done emergently when cervical insufficiency is noted in patient with threatened preterm labor.

ADMISSION, INPATIENT, AND NURSING CONSIDERATIONS

Suspected/threatened preterm labor management: IV access with IV hydration, continuous fetal and contraction monitoring, assessing cervical dilatation and effacement, and monitoring for fluid overload

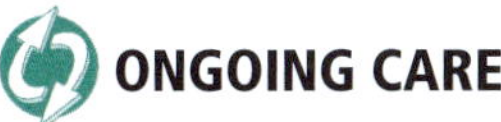

ONGOING CARE

FOLLOW-UP RECOMMENDATIONS

Patient Monitoring

- Weekly office visits with contraction monitoring, cervical checks or cervical US if at high risk for recurrence
- Routine use of maintenance tocolysis is ineffective in preventing recurrent preterm labor or preterm birth.

PATIENT EDUCATION

Call physician or proceed to hospital whenever regular contractions last >1 hour, bleeding, increased vaginal discharge or fluid, decreased fetal movement.

PROGNOSIS

If membranes are ruptured and no infection is confirmed, delivery often occurs within 3 to 7 days. If membranes are intact, 20–50% deliver preterm.

COMPLICATIONS

Labor resistant to tocolysis, pulmonary edema, intraamniotic infection

REFERENCES

1. American College of Obstetricians and Gynecologists. Prediction and prevention of spontaneous preterm birth: ACOG practice bulletin, number 234. *Obstet Gynecol*. 2021;138(2):e65–e90.
2. American College of Obstetricians and Gynecologists. Practice bulletin no. 171 summary: management of preterm labor. *Obstet Gynecol*. 2016;128(4):931–933.
3. Rundell K, Panchal B. Preterm labor: prevention and management. *Am Fam Physician*. 2017;95(6):366–372.

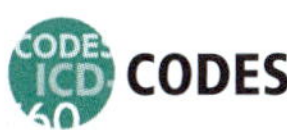

CODES

ICD10

- O60.03 Preterm labor without delivery, third trimester
- O60.0 Preterm labor without delivery
- O60.02 Preterm labor without delivery, second trimester

CLINICAL PEARLS

- Treatment of preterm labor/tocolysis may delay delivery to facilitate short-term interventions such as administration of corticosteroids, which improve neonatal outcomes.
- Magnesium sulfate is recommended for neuroprotection for imminent deliveries prior to 32 weeks.

PRIAPISM

Dongsheng Jiang, MD, MSc • Joseph P. Wiedemer, MD

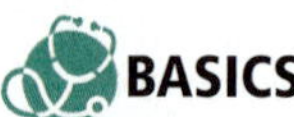

BASICS

DESCRIPTION

- Penile (or less common clitoral) erection lasting for >4 hours and unrelated to sexual stimulation or arousal
- Classification:
  - Ischemic (low-flow, veno-occlusive): accounts for 95% of priapism cases. It is associated with ischaemia of the corpora cavernosa.
  - Nonischemic (high-flow, arterial): less common and often painless and does not require urgent treatment
  - Recurrent ischemic ("stuttering") priapism: episodic, short-lived, and may not require intervention
- Malignant priapism: rare, resulting most commonly from penile metastases related to primary bladder, prostatic, rectosigmoid, and renal tumors
- System(s) affected: reproductive and vascular
- Functional impairment: neurophysiologic, sexual, psychosocial

Pediatric Considerations

In children, the most common etiology is sickle cell disease (SCD) (63% of cases). Less common etiologies, occurring more typically in the adolescent years, are leukemia, idiopathic, penile trauma (e.g., post circumcision), or illicit drugs (up to 35% of cases).

EPIDEMIOLOGY

Incidence

- About 5.3 per 100,000 men per year
- Age: There has been an age shift since 2008 toward men in their 40s. The incidence doubles in men aged >40 years (2.9 vs. 1.5/100,000 person-years).
- Race: 61.1% African American (correlated with incidence of SCD), 30% Caucasian, 6.3% Hispanic

ETIOLOGY AND PATHOPHYSIOLOGY

- Anatomy and physiology:
  - The penis consists of three longitudinally oriented corpora: two dorsolaterally paired corpora cavernosa that are responsible for penile erection and a single ventral corpus spongiosum that surrounds the glans penis and extends distally to form the glans penis.
  - In general, the penile artery supplies the penis. It divides into three branches: dorsal artery, bulbar artery (supplies the corpus spongiosum), and cavernosal artery (the main blood supply to the erectile tissue).
  - In ischemic priapism, decreased venous outflow results in increased intracavernosal pressure. This leads to erection, decreased arterial inflow, blood stasis, local hypoxia, and acidosis (a compartment syndrome). Penile tissue necrosis and fibrosis may occur if priapism persists >24 hours. Pathophysiology mechanisms thought to contribute to impaired smooth muscle relaxation and decreased venous outflow include dysregulation of the NO/cGMP, RhoA/Rho kinase, and opiorphin signaling pathways as well as excessive adenosine signaling (1).
- In nonischemic priapism, increased arterial flow without decreased venous outflow results in a sustained, nonpainful, partially rigid erection.
- Causes:
  - Ischemic priapism:
    - Idiopathic: about 50% cases
    - Hematologic dyscrasias: SCD, thalassemia, leukemia, multiple myeloma, fat emboli during hyperalimentation, hemodialysis, glucose-6-phosphate dehydrogenase (G6PD) deficiency, factor V Leiden mutation
    - Infections (toxin mediated): urinary tract infections, scorpion sting, spider bite, rabies, malaria
    - Metabolic disorders: nephrolithiasis, amyloidosis, Fabry disease, gout
    - Neurogenic disorders: syphilis, spinal cord injury, cauda equina syndrome, autonomic neuropathy, lumbar disc herniation, spinal stenosis, cerebrovascular accident, brain tumor, spinal anesthesia
    - Neoplasms: penis, urethra, bladder, prostate, kidney and rectum
    - Medications:
      - Vasoactive erectile agents (i.e., papaverine, phentolamine, prostaglandin E1/alprostadil)
      - α-Adrenergic receptor antagonists (i.e., prazosin, terazosin, doxazosin, tamsulosin)
      - Antidepressants and antipsychotics (i.e., trazodone, bupropion, fluoxetine, sertraline, lithium, clozapine, risperidone, olanzapine, chlorpromazine, thioridazine, phenothiazines)
      - Antihypertensives (i.e., hydralazine, guanethidine, propranolol)
      - Hormones (i.e., gonadotropin-releasing hormone, testosterone)
      - Anxiolytics (hydroxyzine)
      - Anticoagulants (heparin, warfarin)
      - Recreational drugs (i.e., alcohol, marijuana, cocaine)
  - Nonischemic priapism (2):
    - Almost universally associated with penile or perineal trauma resulting in a fistula between the cavernous artery and the corpus cavernosum
    - Acute spinal cord injury
    - Treatment of ischemic priapism

RISK FACTORS

- SCD has a lifetime risk of ischemic priapism 29–42%.
- Dehydration correlated with SCD or trait
- Prior history of priapismic episodes

GENERAL PREVENTION

- Avoid dehydration (SCD cases).
- Avoid excessive sexual stimulation.
- Avoid or limit causative drugs.
- Avoid trauma to the genital area

COMMONLY ASSOCIATED CONDITIONS

- SCD (42.9%) or sickle cell trait (2.5%)
- Drug abuse (7.9%)
- G6PD deficiency
- Leukemia
- Neoplasm

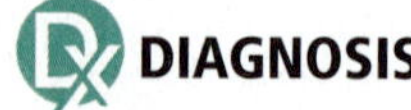

DIAGNOSIS

HISTORY

- Prior priapism episodes or prolonged erections after waking and degree of pain
- Duration of erection
- Perineal or penile trauma (blunt force or needle injury)
- Urination difficult during erection
- History of any hematologic abnormalities (e.g., SCD or trait)
- Cardiovascular disease
- Medications
- Recreational drug use

PHYSICAL EXAM

- In general, physical examination should include the following:
  - A complete penile, scrotal, and perineal exam to identify the presence of trauma, gangrene (rare), or prosthesis
  - An abdominal and lymph noted exam to rule out underlying conditions
- Common findings:
  - Ischemic (or stuttering): Penis is fully erect, painful, or tender; corpora cavernosa are rigid; and corpora spongiosum and glans are flaccid.
  - Nonischemic: Penis is partially erect (not tender or painful), and the corpora cavernosa are semirigid and nontender, with the glans and corpora spongiosum flaccid.

DIAGNOSTIC TESTS & INTERPRETATION

- CBC with reticulocyte count
- Sickling hemoglobin (Hgb) solubility test and Hgb electrophoresis
- Coagulation profile
- Urinalysis/urine toxicology

- Corporal blood gas (CBG): Nonischemic blood gas analysis is identical to normal arterial blood, whereas the following is concerning for ischemic priapism: pH <7.25, pO_2 <30 mm Hg, and pCO_2 >60 mm Hg.
- A color Doppler ultrasound:
  - Ischemic—low arterial flow
  - Nonischemic—high arterial flow
- Penile arteriography can be used to identify the presence and arterial cavernous fistula or pseudoaneurysms (nonischemic).
- Penile MRI can be used for cases >48- to 72-hour duration to evaluate for corporal smooth muscle necrosis and candidacy for immediate penile prosthesis implantation.

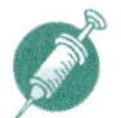

TREATMENT

- Based on the type:
  - Ischemic priapism: requires immediate treatment and urology consultation
    - Initial conservative management with encouraging ejaculation, vigorous physical exercise, cold bath, icing
    - Cold enemas are *not* recommended especially if those measures lead to delay in starting more evidence based treatment (2).
    - Cavernosal aspiration with a large-bore needle
    - Cavernosal injection of phenylephrine 200 μg repeated to a maximum of 1,500 μg (with BP monitoring)
    - If this fails, shunt procedures are considered.
  - Nonischemic priapism: not an emergency
    - Observation, icing, site specific compression; causative fistula may close spontaneously.
    - If persists, may consider selective arteriography and embolization (2)
  - Stuttering priapism
    - The initial goal is to prevent recurrence. But, if the episode is prolonged, there is a risk of conversion to ischemic priapism.
    - Initial conservative treatment including ejaculation, physical exercise, icing, and/or cold shower.
    - Manage acute episodes as ischemic cases—aspiration then intracavernous injections of:
      - Phenylephrine: 200 μg every 3 to 5 minutes to a maximum of 1 mg within 1 hour
      - Etilefrine: 2.5 mg diluted in 1 to 2 mL saline
      - Adrenaline: 2 mL of 1/100,000 solution given up to 5 times in a 20-minute period
      - Methylene blue: 50 to 100 mg
- In all cases, particularly SCD cases, treat the underlying condition (e.g., SCD does not delay intracavernous treatment).
- Although blood transfusion is an option, particularly in SCD cases, other interventions should be explored and exhausted first.

GENERAL MEASURES

- Treat any underlying cause or disease process.
- In SCD cases: IV hydration; supplemental oxygen; partial exchange or repeated transfusions to reduce percentage of sickle cells to <50%

MEDICATION

- Analgesics (e.g., opioids) for pain, if needed
- May try oral pseudoephedrine or terbutaline while waiting for intracavernous injection

Second Line

- Ischemic priapism:
  - Etilefrine (intracavernous) is the second most used sympathomimetic.
  - Methylene blue (intracavernous) can be used for pharmacologically induced priapism (cGMP inhibitor).
  - Epinephrine (intracavernous) has a higher success rate than phenylephrine but greater cardiovascular side effects.
- Stuttering priapism:
  - Prevention of recurrence with daily oral medications:
    - Adrenergic agonists: pseudoephedrine and etilefrine
    - Androgen suppression: antiandrogens, 5α-reductase inhibitors (finasteride), and ketoconazole
    - PDE5 inhibitors: sildenafil
    - Smooth muscle regulation: digoxin or terbutaline
    - Others: gabapentin, baclofen, hydroxyurea

ISSUES FOR REFERRAL

A urologist should be consulted in all cases of suspected priapism.

SURGERY/OTHER PROCEDURES

- For ischemic priapism, surgical options after medical therapy include the following:
  - Distal cavernoglandular shunts
    - Percutaneous: Ebbehoj, Winter, or T shunt
    - Open: Al-Ghorab or Burnett
  - Proximal cavernoglandular shunts
    - Open: Quackles or Sacher
  - Venous shunts
    - Grayhack (saphenous vein shunt)
    - Barry (deep dorsal vein shunt)
  - Immediate penile prothesis placement: Relative indications include failure of intracavernous therapies or corporal smooth muscle necrosis or MRI/biopsy; early surgery avoids cavernosus fibrosis, which offers the opportunity to maintain penile size, and prevent penile curvature due to cavernosal fibrosis.
- For nonischemic priapism, surgical options include the following:
  - Selective embolization with autologous blood clot, absorbable (gel foam or sponge) or nonabsorbable materials (coils or acrylic glue), or surgical ligation as a last resort

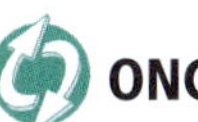

ONGOING CARE

PROGNOSIS

- Even with excellent treatment for a prolonged priapism, complete detumescence may require several weeks secondary to edema.
- Impotence due to irreversible corporal fibrosis is likely in ischemic priapism and is up to 90% if the priapism lasts >24 hours.

COMPLICATIONS

- Patient can have mental illnesses such as suicidality, depression, and anxiety. When treating those condition, drugs such as fluoxetine, citalopram, and trazodone should be avoided due to potential in precipitating priapism (3).
- Erectile dysfunction

REFERENCES

1. Anele UA, Morrison BF, Burnett AL. Molecular pathophysiology of priapism: emerging targets. *Curr Drug Targets*. 2015;16(5):474–483.
2. Ericson C, Baird B, Broderick GA. Management of priapism: 2021 update. *Urol Clin North Am*. 2021;48(4):565–576.
3. Idris IM, Burnett AL, DeBaun MR. Epidemiology and treatment of priapism in sickle cell disease. *Hematology Am Soc Hematol Educ Program*. 2022;2022(1):450–458.

SEE ALSO

Anemia, Sickle Cell; Erectile Dysfunction

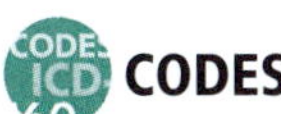

CODES

ICD10

- N48.30 Priapism, unspecified
- N48.39 Other priapism
- N48.31 Priapism due to trauma

CLINICAL PEARLS

- If priapism lasts >24 hours, it likely results in permanent sexual impairment.
- Priapism can occur in children, particularly in SCD. Treatment should address both the underlying disease as well as developmental needs.
- In evaluating priapism, the clinician must distinguish ischemic from nonischemic priapism by history and physical exam as well as cavernosal blood gas and possibly ultrasound or MRI, if indicated.
- Ischemic priapism is an emergent condition that requires immediate urologic evaluation and treatment.

PROSTATE CANCER

Daniel R. Matta, MD, DFPHM, FAAFP • Brittney Bennett, MBBS

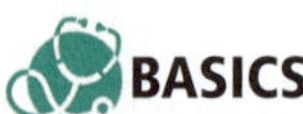

BASICS

DESCRIPTION

- The prostate is a male reproductive gland that contributes seminal fluid to the ejaculate.
- In an adult male, the prostate gland is approximately the size of a walnut, weighing 20 to 25 g and commonly enlarges after age 50 years.
- Three distinct zones delineate the functional anatomy of the prostate: peripheral zone (largest, adjacent to the rectal wall, palpable on digital rectal exam [DRE] and the most common location for prostate cancer), central zone (contains the ejaculatory ducts), and transition zone (located centrally, adjacent to the urethra).
- Prostatic epithelial cells produce prostate-specific antigen (PSA), which is used as a tumor marker and in screening.

EPIDEMIOLOGY

Incidence

Approximately 300,000 men in the United States will be newly diagnosed with carcinoma of the prostate (CaP) in 2025, representing approximately 15% of all new cancer diagnoses.

Prevalence

- Approximately 35,000 men in the United States will die of CaP in 2025, representing 5.8% of all cancer deaths.
- Median age at diagnosis is 67 years.
- Autopsy studies find foci of latent CaP in 50% of men in their 8th decade of life.

ETIOLOGY AND PATHOPHYSIOLOGY

- Adenocarcinoma: >95%; nonadenocarcinoma: <5% (most common transitional cell carcinoma)
- Location of CaP: 70% peripheral zone, 20% transitional zone, 5–10% central zone

Genetics

The most strongly implicated genes are BRCA2, and BRCA1. HOXB13 mutations and DNA mismatch repair genes are associated with hereditary prostate cancer.

RISK FACTORS

Age >50 years, African American race, positive family history

GENERAL PREVENTION

Finasteride use associated with moderate risk reduction in low-grade CaP but associated with an increased risk of high-grade disease.

ALERT

- Screening for prostate cancer is controversial:
  - U.S. Preventive Services Task Force (USPSTF): "for men aged 55 to 69 years, the decision to undergo periodic PSA-based screening for prostate cancer should be an individual one and should include discussion of the potential benefits and harms of screening with their clinician. Screening offers a small potential benefit of reducing the chance of death from prostate cancer in some men. However, many men will experience potential harms of screening" (1)[A]. USPSTF recommends against PSA screening for men ≥70 years old (1).
  - The American Urological Association (AUA) panel recommends for men 55 to 69 years old shared decision-making between physician and patient regarding PSA screening.
  - PSA screening is not recommended in men age <40 years or any man with <10 years of estimated life expectancy.
  - When providing informed consent, data shows if you screen 1,000 men between 55 and 69 years old:
    - 240 will have a positive result; only ~100 will truly have CaP; of the 100 with cancer, 80 will agree to treatment.
    - Treatment will result in one less person dying but 50 will develop erectile dysfunction (ED); 15 permanent incontinence

COMMONLY ASSOCIATED CONDITIONS

Obesity, hyperlipidemia, diabetes, hypertension

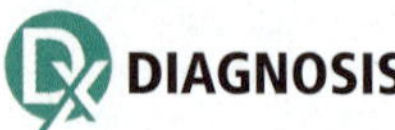

DIAGNOSIS

HISTORY

Early prostate cancer can be asymptomatic, but patients may experience lower urinary tract symptoms, hematuria, hematospermia, ED, bone pain (metastatic disease).

PHYSICAL EXAM

DRE to assess for prostatic masses, firmness, or asymmetry.

DIFFERENTIAL DIAGNOSIS

Benign prostatic hyperplasia, prostatitis, prostatic intraepithelial neoplasia (PIN), prostate stones, atypical small acinar proliferation (ASAP)

DIAGNOSTIC TESTS & INTERPRETATION

Initial Tests (lab, imaging)

- In general, total PSA ≥4 ng/mL is concerning for CaP (sensitivity 21%, specificity 91%).
  - Rectal manipulation will not significantly elevate PSA.
  - 5-α-reductase inhibitors decrease PSA by ~50%.
  - Consider MRI to guide decision to biopsy and then location.
- Other PSA metrics used to aid in CaP diagnosis:
  - Total PSA velocity: ≥0.75 ng/mL/year or >20% baseline for higher values increases CaP risk.
  - Free PSA and age-/race-adjusted PSA are helpful in evaluating risk. With PSA 4 to 10 ng/mL, a low percent free PSA is associated with higher risk of CaP.
  - PSAD ≥0.15 associated with higher prevalence of CaP

Follow-Up Tests & Special Considerations

- PSMA-PET has increased sensitivity and specificity over conventional imaging (CT, bone scan).
- Germline and/or somatic testing can be undertaken based on factors related to personal/family history or pathologic features.

Diagnostic Procedures/Other

Prostate biopsy

- Decision to biopsy involves PSA, DRE, MRI, and consideration of comorbidities and life expectancy.
- Standard biopsy: systematic random cores from peripheral zone base, mid-gland, and apex, 8 to 12 cores
- Prebiopsy MRI used to identify suspicious prostate lesions
  - The Gleason grade ranks specimens from 1 (most differentiated) to 5 (least differentiated).
  - Primary and secondary patterns are identified and reported, and the sum is the Gleason score (e.g., 3 + 4 = 7).
  - Most prostate cancer are scored 6 to 10, with 10 having the worst prognosis.
  - Grade group 1 = Gleason 6; group 2 = Gleason 3 + 4 = 7; group 3 = Gleason 4 + 3 = 7; group 4 = Gleason 8; group 5 = Gleason 9 and 10.
- Biopsies can be performed by either a transrectal or transperineal approach; both approaches used transrectal ultrasound guidance.

Test Interpretation

Staging

- Tumor, node, and metastasis (TNM) staging used to generate a clinical and pathologic stage, which directs treatment. Clinical staging is as follows:
  - T1: cancer found incidentally on TURP or found on biopsy for elevated PSA
  - T2: cancer found on DRE but confined to the prostate
  - T3: cancer found to be extended locally outside the prostate and/or the seminal vesicle
  - T4: cancer invading adjacent organs
  - N1: denotes local lymph node spread
  - M1: distant metastasis

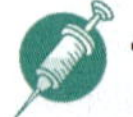

TREATMENT

- Use Prostate Predict Calculator to help patient consider treatment options: https://prostate.predict.nhs.uk
- Treatment options include:
  - Watchful waiting: monitoring with expectation to provide palliation with symptoms
  - Active surveillance: close monitoring of PSA, DRE, and repeat biopsy at regular intervals
    - ProtecT trial (2023) found watchful waiting had equal cancer-specific and all-cause mortality compared to surgery or radiotherapy. In the treatment arms, there was less disease progression (including metastatic disease) but resulted in significantly more morbidity (urinary and bowel dysfunction, ED) (2).
  - Radical prostatectomy: ± pelvic lymph node dissection (PLND)
  - Radiation therapy: external beam (EBRT)
  - Brachytherapy: radioactive implants placed in prostate; option for early clinical stage localized to the prostate
  - Antiandrogen therapy
    - Bilateral orchiectomy (surgical castration)
    - Gonadotropin-releasing hormone (GnRH) agonist, antagonist, or antiandrogen (medical castration)
    - Abiraterone: 17α-hydroxylase inhibitor (CYP17A adrenal androgen production)
    - Bicalutamide/nilutamide/flutamide/enzalutamide/apalutamide: androgen receptor antagonists

- Chemotherapy: includes multiple chemotherapeutic agents used to treat castrate-resistant prostate cancer (CRPC)
- Risk factors
  - Treatment options based on risk: very low-, low-, favorable intermediate-, unfavorable intermediate-, high-, and very high-risk categories; this is based on risk of recurrence after definitive treatment.
  - Must meet all three criteria to be low risk; any one criterion moves patient to a higher risk group: risk category clinical stage/serum PSA (ng/mL)/grade group: low T1–T2a/<10/1; intermediate T2b–T2c/10–20/2–3; high T3a/>20/4–5
  - Very low and very high-risk categories, as well as differentiating favorable versus unfavorable intermediate risk, are based on additional clinical/pathologic criteria.
  - Updated risk stratification algorithms include additional groups of very low risk, favorable and unfavorable intermediate risk, and very high risk.
  - Localized CaP
    - Very low and low risk:
      - Mainstay of therapy is active surveillance.
      - Radical prostatectomy and radiation therapy may be offered.
    - Intermediate risk:
      - Mainstay of therapy is radical prostatectomy or radiation therapy.
      - Radical prostatectomy has shown a possible survival benefit in intermediate prostate cancer.
      - Active surveillance may be offered to patients in the favorable intermediate risk group.
    - High and very high risk:
      - Mainstay of therapy is radical prostatectomy or radiation therapy.
      - Adjuvant radiation may be considered based on adverse pathologic findings after prostatectomy.
  - Patients with unfavorable intermediate disease or worse are recommended to undergo additional staging evaluation with soft tissue and bone imaging.

ALERT
Life expectancy determination and risks and benefits of surveillance and treatment options is critical.

- Locally advanced CaP:
  - Mainstay of therapy is androgen deprivation therapy (ADT) and radiation; surgery and adjuvant radiation also used
  - Adding abiraterone + prednisone in patients commencing long-term ADT for high risk (T3–T4, Gleason 8 to 10, PSA >40), locally advanced prostate cancer has been shown to significantly increase overall survival.
- Metastatic CaP:
  - Mainstay of therapy is RT and ADT.
  - Early chemotherapy (docetaxel) with ADT may be considered for high-volume disease; ADT with abiraterone + prednisone for lower volume disease
  - ADT specifics:
    - GnRH agonists include leuprolide, goserelin, histrelin, or triptorelin.
    - GnRH antagonists include degarelix: an alternative to GnRH agonists; suppresses testosterone production and avoids flare phenomenon observed with GnRH agonists
    - Side effects of ADT: osteoporosis, gynecomastia, ED, decreased libido, obesity, lipid alterations, diabetes, and cardiovascular disease
    - Flare phenomenon (disease flare: hot flashes, fatigue) can occur owing to transient increase in testosterone levels on initiation of GnRH agonist therapy.
    - If spinal cord metastases are present, the concern for cord compression with a testosterone flare can be avoided by starting antiandrogen therapy prior to initiation of a GnRH agonist.
    - Combined androgen blockade with GnRH agonist and antiandrogen (e.g., bicalutamide, nilutamide, or flutamide) may be used to prevent flare.
- CRPC—CRPC is defined as progression of disease following ADT. Treatment includes the following:
  - Treatment (prior docetaxel, prior novel hormone therapy):
    - Preferred: cabazitaxel or docetaxel rechallenge
  - Treatment (prior docetaxel, no prior novel hormone therapy):
    - Preferred: abiraterone, cabazitaxel, or enzalutamide
  - Treatment (no prior docetaxel, prior novel hormone therapy):
    - Preferred: docetaxel
    - Preferred if BRCA mutation: olaparib or rucaparib
  - Treatment (no prior docetaxel, no prior novel hormone therapy):
    - Preferred: abiraterone, docetaxel, enzalutamide
  - Metastatic: tumor and germline testing recommended
  - Nonmetastatic
    - Continue ADT; add antiandrogen (apalutamide, darolutamide, or enzalutamide) if PSA doubling time ≤10 months.
- Bone health: Men with prostate cancer, especially on ADT, are at elevated risk of pathologic fractures; consider bone density.
  - Denosumab (RANK-ligand inhibitor—prevents osteoclast activation) and zoledronic acid (bisphosphonate) can be offered for prevention.

ONGOING CARE

FOLLOW-UP RECOMMENDATIONS

- Prostatectomy: PSA and DRE; some combination of CT/MRI/PET/bone scan is obtained at recurrence. If the PSA recurrence is due to local disease, salvage radiation +/− ADT is considered. For metastatic disease, androgen deprivation is considered.
- XRT: PSA and DRE are recommended at regular intervals. Biochemical recurrence is defined as PSA increase ≥2 ng/mL above nadir; some combination of CT/MRI/PET/bone scan is usually obtained. If the PSA recurrence is thought to be from local disease, salvage prostatectomy, cryosurgery, brachytherapy, or high-intensity focused ultrasound (HIFU) are considered. For metastatic disease, androgen deprivation is considered.

PROGNOSIS

- Localized disease is frequently curable; advanced disease has a favorable prognosis if lesions are hormone sensitive.
- 5-year CaP survival by stage: local 100%, regional 100%, distant 30.2%
- Recurrence risk increased if: extraprostatic extension, seminal vesicle invasion, positive surgical margins

COMPLICATIONS

- Prostatectomy: Urinary incontinence and ED are the most common long-term issues.
- Radiation therapy: urinary incontinence, ED, radiation cystitis, and radiation proctitis
- Treatment options for ED: PDE5 inhibitors, intracavernosal injections, intraurethral suppositories, vacuum pump, penile prosthesis
- Treatment options for incontinence: oral medications, urethral sling, artificial sphincter

REFERENCES

1. Grossman DC, Curry SJ, Owens DK, et al; and US Preventive Services Task Force. Screening for prostate cancer: US Preventive Services Task Force recommendation statement. *JAMA*. 2018;319(18):1901–1913.
2. Hamdy FC, Donovan JL, Lane JA, et al; ProtecT Study Group. Fifteen-year outcomes after monitoring, surgery, or radiotherapy for prostate cancer. *N Engl J Med*. 2023;388(17):1547–1558. doi:10.1056/NEJMoa2214122.

ADDITIONAL READING

Xu J, McPharlin S, Mulhem E. Prostate cancer screening: common questions and answers. *Am Fam Physician*. 2024;110(5):493–499.

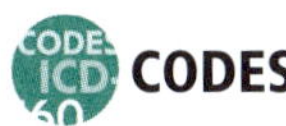

CODES

ICD10

- C61 Malignant neoplasm of prostate
- Z80.42 Family history of malignant neoplasm of prostate
- D07.5 Carcinoma in situ of prostate

CLINICAL PEARLS

- Use of PSA for CaP screening is controversial; shared decision-making is recommended.
- Care must be taken when interpreting PSA levels in patients taking 5-α-reductase inhibitors.
- Decision to treat localized CaP is based on risk group and patient factors. Survival outcomes are excellent for patients with localized CaP, but treatment can carry significant morbidity impacting quality of life.

PROSTATIC HYPERPLASIA, BENIGN (BPH)

Bliss Puthenpurayil, MD

BASICS

- Benign prostatic hyperplasia (BPH) is due to proliferation of both smooth muscle and epithelial cell lines of the periurethral prostate which causes increased prostate volume and may lead to compression of the urethra and obstructive symptoms.
- BPH presents clinically with storage and/or voiding symptoms known collectively as lower urinary tract symptoms (LUTS). These include difficulty initiating a variable urinary stream, incomplete bladder emptying, frequency, urgency, and nocturia.
- Symptoms do not directly correlate to prostate volume. It is estimated that only half of all men with histologic evidence of BPH experience moderate to severe LUTS.
- Progression may result in upper and lower urinary tract infections and may progress to direct bladder outlet obstruction and acute renal failure (ARF).

EPIDEMIOLOGY

Age related with nearly universal development in men

Incidence

Incidence increases with age with an estimated prevalence varying from 70% to 90% by the age of 80 years (estimated at 8–20% by age 40 years).

ETIOLOGY AND PATHOPHYSIOLOGY

- Unknown etiology
- Develops in prostatic periurethral or transition zone
- Hyperplastic nodules of stromal and epithelial components increase glandular components.

RISK FACTORS

- Increasing age
- Higher free prostate-specific antigen (PSA) levels, heart disease, and use of β-blockers
- Low androgen levels from cirrhosis/chronic alcoholism reduces the risk of BPH
- Obesity and sedentary lifestyle can worsen LUTS.
- No evidence of increased or decreased risk with smoking, alcohol, or any dietary factors

GENERAL PREVENTION

Symptoms can be managed through weight loss, regulation of fluid intake (especially in the evening), decreased intake of bladder irritants including artificial sweeteners, tea, carbonated drinks, alcohol, caffeine, and increased physical activity.

COMMONLY ASSOCIATED CONDITIONS

- LUTS can be divided into two groups:
  - Irritative symptoms: frequency, nocturia, urgency, and urge incontinence
  - Obstructive symptoms: difficulty initiating urinary stream, incomplete voiding, or weak stream
- LUTS can also be secondary to cardiovascular, respiratory, or renal disease (1).

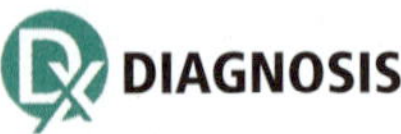

DIAGNOSIS

HISTORY

- Screen for other causes such as infection, procedural history, or neurogenic causes.
- Evaluate symptom severity with the American Urological Association Society Symptom Index (AUA-SI) or the International Prostate Symptom Score (IPSS).
- Evaluate for comorbid conditions such as diabetes, congestive heart failure (CHF), or Parkinson disease.
- Review medication list and family history of BPH/prostate cancer.
- Screen for gross hematuria.
- Nocturia >2 times per night warrants a frequency/volume chart for 2 to 3 days to detect urinary patterns

PHYSICAL EXAM

- Digital rectal exam (DRE): symmetrically enlarged prostate (*size does not always correlate with symptoms*)
- Signs of renal failure due to obstructive uropathy (edema, pallor, pruritus, ecchymosis, nutritional deficiencies)

DIFFERENTIAL DIAGNOSIS

- Obstructive:
  - Prostate cancer
  - Urethral strictures
  - Bladder neck contracture (usually secondary to prostate surgery)
  - Inability of bladder neck or external sphincter to relax appropriately during voiding
- Neurogenic:
  - Spinal cord injury or stroke
  - Parkinsonism
  - Multiple sclerosis
- Medical:
  - Poorly controlled diabetes mellitus
  - CHF
- Pharmacologic:
  - Diuretics (increased urine production)
  - Decongestants (increased sphincter tone)
  - Opioids (impaired autonomic function)
  - Tricyclic antidepressants (anticholinergic)
- Other:
  - Bladder carcinoma
  - Overactive bladder
  - Nocturnal polyuria
  - Bladder calculi
  - UTI and prostatitis
  - Urethritis/sexually transmitted infections
  - Obstructive sleep apnea (OSA) (nocturia)
  - Bladder irritants

DIAGNOSTIC TESTS & INTERPRETATION

Initial Tests (lab, imaging)

- Complete urinalysis including microscopic exam and urine culture in all patients presenting with LUTS to evaluate other etiologies such as bladder/kidney stones, cancer, UTI, or urethral strictures.
- PSA (especially for men with a life expectancy of 10 years or more who would be surgical candidates if prostate cancer was identified)
- PSA levels correlate with prostate volume which can help guide treatment choice.
- With bladder cancer risk factors (smoking history, exposure to radiation/chemicals or microscopic or gross hematuria), obtain urine cytology, CT urogram/renal US, and cystoscopy based on the current AUA guidelines.
- If nocturia is the main concern, consider using a frequency volume chart for urine output.
- Uroflow: volume voided per unit time (Peak flow <10 mL/sec is abnormal.)
- Postvoid residual (PVR): either with catheterization or bladder ultrasound (>100 mL = incomplete emptying)
- Sleep study if OSA or primary nocturnal polyuria is suspected

Follow-Up Tests & Special Considerations

- No additional testing is recommended in uncomplicated LUTS.
- Further testing if symptoms do not respond to medical management or if initial evaluation suggests underlying disease
- Transrectal ultrasound or cross-sectional imaging (MRI/CT): assessment of prostate gland size; not necessary in the routine evaluation
- Abdominal ultrasound: can demonstrate increased PVR or hydronephrosis; not necessary in the routine evaluation

Diagnostic Procedures/Other

- Pressure-flow studies (urine flow vs. voiding pressures) to determine etiology of symptoms
  - Obstructive pattern shows high voiding pressures with low flow rate.
- Urodynamic study to assess bladder function
- Cystoscopy
  - Demonstrates presence, configuration, cause (stricture, stone), and site of obstructive tissue
  - Not recommended in routine evaluation unless other factors, such as hematuria, persistent dysuria, recurrent UTI, are present

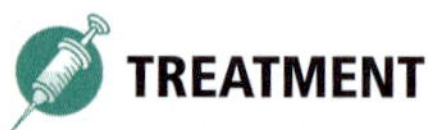

TREATMENT

GENERAL MEASURES

- Treatment ranges from watchful waiting to lifestyle modifications, medications, or surgical management.
- Mild symptoms (score of <7) or moderate symptoms (score 8 to 15) on the IPSS that are non-bothersome require no treatment with repeat evaluation performed annually.
- For moderate to severe symptoms, attempt lifestyle interventions including fluid restriction (especially in the evening) avoidance of alcohol and caffeine, timed voiding, pelvic floor therapy exercises, diet, and eliminating or reducing contributing medications.

MEDICATION

- α-Adrenergic antagonists:
  - First-line option for moderate/severe and bothersome LUTS (2)
  - Affects contraction of smooth muscle in the prostatic urethra and bladder neck
  - Clinical improvement typically takes 2 to 4 weeks with an average 5- to 8-point improvement in the IPSS
  - Side effects may include orthostatic hypotension, retrograde ejaculation.
  - AUA recommends alfuzosin (Uroxatral), doxazosin (Cardura), silodosin (Rapaflo), and tamsulosin (Flomax) because they are thought to be more selective and have less effect on blood pressure. Prazosin (Minipress) and phenoxybenzamine (Dibenzyline) have insufficient evidence and are not recommended.
    - Tamsulosin (Flomax): 0.4 to 0.8 mg/day PO
    - Alfuzosin (Uroxatral): 10 mg/day PO
    - Terazosin (Hytrin): Start at 1 mg PO daily at bedtime, max 20 mg daily
    - Doxazosin (Cardura): 1 to 8 mg/day PO
    - Silodosin (Rapaflo): 8 mg/day PO
  - Terazosin and doxazosin are nonuroselective and require dose titration to avoid vascular-related events.

- Contraindications:
  - Use caution in patients who have low blood pressure, using phosphodiesterase type 5 inhibitors for erectile dysfunction.
  - Do not use in men pursuing cataract surgery until they are postoperative due to the risk for perioperative floppy iris syndrome.
  - Do not use concomitantly with other α-adrenergic antagonists.
  - Due to the similar efficacy, AUA does not recommend switching between alpha blockers if patients fail to have sufficient improvement with the first drug; can consider switching based on side effects
- 5-α-Reductase inhibitors
  - Blocks conversion of testosterone to dihydrotestosterone to gradually reduce prostatic volume
  - Greatest clinical benefit when prostate volume exceeds 30 g on imaging, a PSA >1.5 ng/mL, or palpable prostate enlargement on DRE
  - Generally requires 6 months to show clinical benefits
    - Finasteride (Proscar): 5 mg/day PO
    - Dutasteride (Avodart): 0.5 mg/day PO
  - Shows reduced risk of acute urinary retention and less need for surgical intervention
  - Used in patients with refractory hematuria after other causes have been ruled out
  - Side effects include decreased libido, depressive symptoms, and erectile dysfunction.
  - When used alone or in combination with α-blockers, can reduce the risks of urinary retention and need for future prostate-related surgery

ALERT

A PSA value in a patient taking a 5-α-reductase inhibitors will be artificially reduced by up to 50%. Test before and after initiating treatment.

- Combination therapy of α-blocker plus 5-α-reductase inhibitor is superior to monotherapy with an α-blocker only in men with evidence of enlarged prostates (≥30 mL).
- Anticholinergic agents are appropriate for moderate to severe predominant storage LUTS without an elevated PVR. Options include solifenacin (VESIcare), tolterodine, or oxybutynin (Ditropan XL), darifenacin (Enablex), trospium (Sanctura); should be avoided in patients with PVR >250 mL
- β3-agonists (Mirabegron, Vibegron) combined with an α-blocker is a treatment option for patients with moderate to severe storage LUTS.
- Phosphodiesterase-5 inhibitors lead to mild improvement of LUTS; can use tadalafil (Cialis): 5 mg/day PO but avoid use in combination with α-blockers or in those with CrCl <30 mL/min irrespective of comorbid erectile dysfunction

Geriatric Considerations

Use caution with anticholinergics, antihistamines, sympathomimetics, tricyclic antidepressants, and opioids.

ISSUES FOR REFERRAL

- Moderate or severe LUTS that do not respond to medical management
- BPH-related complications such as recurrent UTIs or hematuria, renal insufficiency, and urinary retention
- Abnormal PSA or prostate exam
- Any history of urethral trauma or stricture, or neurologic disease of the bladder/urinary system

SURGERY/OTHER PROCEDURES

- Indications for surgery:
  - Recurrent urinary retention due to prostatic obstruction refractory to medical therapy
  - Intractable symptoms secondary to prostatic obstruction with AUA score >8
  - Obstructive uropathy (renal insufficiency)
  - Recurrent or persistent UTIs due to prostatic obstruction
  - Recurrent gross hematuria due to enlarged prostate
  - Bladder calculi
- Surgical procedures: TURP remains the gold standard surgical procedure; however, for selected patient populations, there are other options available.
- Common complications of TURP:
  - Bleeding, retrograde ejaculation, urinary incontinence
  - TURP syndrome: hyponatremia secondary to absorption of hypotonic irrigation fluid
- Other options include transurethral vaporization of the prostate (TUVP), transurethral microwave thermotherapy (TUMT), transurethral incision of the prostate (TUIP), photoselective vaporization of the prostate (PVP), prostatic urethral lift (PUL), water vapor thermal therapy (WVTT), laser enucleation, and robotic waterjet treatment (RWT).
- Holmium laser enucleation (HoLEP), thulium laser enucleation of the prostate (ThuLEP), and PVP are options for patients on anticoagulation.
- PUL and WVTT can be offered as a treatment option for patients who prefer conservation of erectile and ejaculatory function.
- Transurethral needle ablation and prostate artery embolization are not supported by current data.

COMPLEMENTARY & ALTERNATIVE MEDICINE

- There are no recommended complementary or alternative treatments for BPH (2).
- Saw palmetto (*Serenoa repens*) has been thoroughly studied in a Cochrane review and did not improve LUTS.

ONGOING CARE

FOLLOW-UP RECOMMENDATIONS

Recommend 4 to 12 weeks after initiating treatment (if adverse events do not require earlier consultation) to assess response to therapy.

Patient Monitoring

- DRE and PSA yearly in patients who choose watchful waiting; PSA should not be checked while patient is in retention, recently catheterized, or within a week of any prostate-related surgery.
- Consider monitoring PVR, if elevated.

DIET

Large boluses of oral/IV fluids, alcohol, or caffeine may exacerbate LUTS.

PATIENT EDUCATION

National Kidney and Urologic Diseases Information Clearinghouse: https://www.niddk.nih.gov/health-information/community-health-outreach/information-clearinghouses

PROGNOSIS

- Symptoms improve or stabilize in 70–80% of patients.
- 25% of men with LUTS will have persistent storage symptoms after prostatectomy.
- Of men with BPH, 11–33% have occult prostate cancer.

COMPLICATIONS

- Urinary retention (acute or chronic)
- Bladder stones, prostatitis, hematuria

REFERENCES

1. McVary KT, Roehrborn CG, Avins AL, et al. Update on AUA guideline on the management of benign prostatic hyperplasia. *J Urol*. 2011;185(5):1793–1803.
2. Pearson R, Williams PM. Common questions about the diagnosis and management of benign prostatic hyperplasia. *Am Fam Physician*. 2014;90(11):769–774.

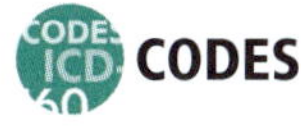

CODES

ICD10

- N40.0 Enlarged prostate without lower urinary tract symptoms
- N40.1 Enlarged prostate with lower urinary tract symptoms

CLINICAL PEARLS

- Although medical therapy has changed the management of BPH, it has only delayed the need for TURP by 10 to 15 years, not eliminated it.
- Urinary retention, obstructive uropathy, recurrent UTIs, elevated PSA, bladder calculi, hematuria, and failure of medical therapy are indications for surgical management of BPH.

PROSTATITIS

Julie A. Creech, DO • Ogechukwu Nwanegwo, MD

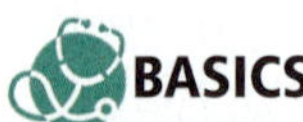

BASICS

DESCRIPTION

- Painful or inflammatory condition affecting the prostate gland with or without bacterial etiology, often characterized by urogenital pain, voiding symptoms, and/or sexual dysfunction
- National Institutes of Health's (NIH) classification
  - *Class I*: *acute bacterial prostatitis*: symptomatic with fever, chills, sudden onset pelvic/perineal pain, dysuria, and obstructive symptoms; polymorphonuclear leukocytes (PMNL) and bacteria in urine
  - *Class II*: *chronic bacterial prostatitis*: symptomatic chronic or recurrent bacterial infection with pain and voiding disturbances; PMNL and bacteria in expressed prostatic secretions (EPS), or urine after prostate massage, or in semen
  - *Class III*: *chronic prostatitis/chronic pelvic pain syndrome* (CP/CPPS)
    - Inflammatory (subtype IIIA): chronic symptoms with PMNL in EPS/urine after prostate massage or in semen
    - Noninflammatory (subtype IIIB): chronic symptoms without presence of PMNL in EPS/urine after prostate massage or in semen
  - *Class IV*: asymptomatic *inflammatory prostatitis*: incidental finding during prostate biopsy; presence of PMNL and/or bacteria in EPS/urine after prostatic massage or in semen
- System(s) affected: genitourinary, renal, reproductive

EPIDEMIOLOGY

Incidence

- 2 million cases annually in the United States, with bimodal: 20 to 40 and >60 years old
- CP is more common after 50 years.
- Bacterial prostatitis is more frequent in HIV.

Prevalence

- Affects approximately 16% of men, up to 10% of cases are acute with confirmed bacterial origin
- Accounts for 8% of visits to urologists and 1% of visits to primary care physicians

ETIOLOGY AND PATHOPHYSIOLOGY

- Acute bacterial prostatitis (NIH class I)
  - Etiology is likely from ascending urethral infection with intraprostatic reflux of infected urine into prostatic ducts, often associated with cystitis
  - Can occur after instrumentation of prostate
  - Usually, gram-negative bacteria (*Escherichia coli* [most common]; *Proteus*, *Klebsiella*, *Serratia*, and *Enterobacter* species; *Pseudomonas aeruginosa*)
  - Rarely, gram-positive bacteria (*Staphylococcus aureus*, *Streptococcus*, and *Enterococcus* spp.)
  - Staphylococcal prostatitis warrants evaluation for hematogenous spread (endovascular).
  - Atypical bacteria include *Chlamydia trachomatis*, *Trichomonas vaginalis*, *Ureaplasma urealyticum*, Mycobacterium tuberculosis and fungal etiologies in immunocompromised hosts.
  - Consider *Neisseria gonorrhoeae* or *C. trachomatis* in sexually active men <35 years.
- Chronic bacterial prostatitis (NIH class II)
  - Similar pathogens as class I
  - Often as recurrent episodes of same organism
  - Progression from acute to CP is poorly understood
- CP/CPPS (NIH class III): most common
  - Unclear etiology
  - Inciting agent may cause inflammation or neurologic damage around the prostate and leads to pelvic floor neuromuscular and/or neuropathic pain.
  - No correlation between histologic inflammation of prostate and presence or absence of symptoms
  - Patients with chronic inflammation on histology have shorter time to symptomatic progression.

RISK FACTORS

- Urinary tract infections (including STIs)
- HIV infection
- Prostatic calculi
- Urethral stricture
- Urinary catheterization: indwelling and intermittent
- Genitourinary instrumentation: prostate biopsy (especially with prior quinolone intake), transurethral resection of the prostate (TURP), cystoscopy
- Urinary retention
- Benign prostatic hypertrophy
- Unprotected sexual intercourse
- Prostate cancer

GENERAL PREVENTION

- Antibiotic prophylaxis for genitourinary instrumentation and prostatic biopsy
- Increased physical activity associated with reduced risk for CP/CPPS

COMMONLY ASSOCIATED CONDITIONS

- Benign prostatic hyperplasia, cystitis, urethritis
- Sexual dysfunction (erectile dysfunction, premature ejaculation)

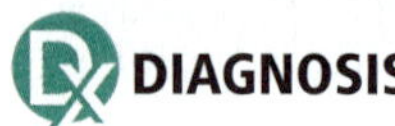

DIAGNOSIS

HISTORY

- Acute prostatitis (NIH class I):
  - Acutely ill with fever, chills, malaise
  - Low back pain, myalgias
  - Nausea, vomiting
  - Frequency, urgency, dysuria, nocturia
  - Prostatodynia, pelvic pain, perineal pain
  - Cloudy urine
  - Obstructive voiding symptoms: poor stream, hesitancy, retention, urge incontinence
  - Recent prostate instrumentation
- CP (NIH classes II and III) (symptoms vary from patient to patient and may include the following):
  - More insidious presentation than class I
  - Symptoms for 3 of 6 previous months
  - Low-grade fever (class II only)
  - Prostatodynia, perineal pain
  - Dysuria, frequency, urgency
  - Lower abdominal pain
  - Low back, testicular, and/or penile pain
  - Hematospermia
  - Sexual dysfunction/painful ejaculation
  - Associated with high caffeine and alcohol intake

PHYSICAL EXAM

- Vital signs (Unstable vitals suggest sepsis.)
- Back exam (CVA tenderness)
- Abdominal exam (bladder distension)
- Prostate exam
  - NIH class I (acute bacterial prostatitis): Prostate is very tender, warm, firm, and edematous.
  - NIH class II (chronic bacterial prostatitis): Prostate is often nontender and normal in size, but enlarged, tender, edematous, and nodular prostate may also be encountered.
  - NIH class III (CP/CPPS): often normal prostate on exam

ALERT
Avoid vigorous massage of the prostate in acute bacterial prostatitis; may induce iatrogenic bacteremia.

DIFFERENTIAL DIAGNOSIS

- Lower urinary tract infection
- Pyelonephritis
- Cystitis (bacterial, interstitial) and urethritis
- Epididymitis
- Proctitis
- Prostatic abscess
- Acute/chronic urinary retention
- Benign prostatic hypertrophy or malignancy (prostate, bladder)
- Obstructive calculi
- Prostate Cancer (1)[B]

DIAGNOSTIC TESTS & INTERPRETATION

Initial Tests (lab, imaging)

- Suspected acute prostatitis (NIH class I)
  - Urinalysis, urine culture and sensitivity
  - Complete blood count with differential, blood culture if immunocompromised or signs of SIRS/sepsis are present
  - Prostate-specific antigen (PSA) is not recommended unless specific indications
  - Imaging is optional and used as indicated to rule out complications, for example, transrectal prostatic ultrasound (TRUS) or CT scan of abdomen to rule out abscess, pelvic ultrasound (US)/bladder scan if symptoms of urinary retention. Initial imaging of prostate is not recommended.
  - STI testing (higher risk in men age <35 years old or >35 years old with risky risk sexual behavior)
- Suspected chronic bacterial prostatitis (NIH class II)
  - Microbiologic localization cultures of lower urinary tract 4- or 2-glass test (pre-massage and post-massage urine culture)
  - Semen cultures are not recommended
  - TRUS is not recommended
  - Urodynamics studies are optional and could help to document obstruction/bladder problems.
- Suspected CP/CPPS (NIH class III)
  - Diagnosis of exclusion (especially to rule out urinary tract infection/STI with history/physical exam and appropriate laboratory investigation if indicated)
  - Administration of NIH Chronic Prostatitis Symptom Index (NIH-CPSI): Nine-question symptom survey (http://www.prostatitis.org/symptomindex.html) is useful for symptom evaluation (not diagnosis) at diagnosis and with ongoing treatment.
  - 4- or 2-glass test pre-massage and post-massage test with urine microscopy considered optional (prostatic massage rarely and anecdotally associated with sepsis; proceed with caution)
  - Urodynamic studies are optional and could be helpful to investigate obstructive symptoms.
  - Semen cultures are not recommended.

- Cystoscopy may be indicated for select patients (i.e., with hematuria or obstructive symptoms refractory to treatment).
- TRUS is not recommended.
- Serum PSA levels are not recommended unless specific indications (e.g., abnormal DRE age >45 years, family history of prostate cancer or risk factors)
- Psychological assessment
- If the following additional symptoms are present, consider the following additional work-up:
  - Hematuria: urine cytology, cystoscopy, CT urography with or without contrast
  - Urethral symptoms (dysuria, discharge, penile pain): urethral swab
  - Concomitant abdominal pain: CT scan
  - Testicular pain: scrotal US
  - Lumbar radiculopathy: MRI of spine

Follow-Up Tests & Special Considerations

If not improving: US, CT scan, TRUS or MRI, or referral to urology

Diagnostic Procedures/Other

- Urodynamic testing if obstructive symptoms present
- Cystoscopy

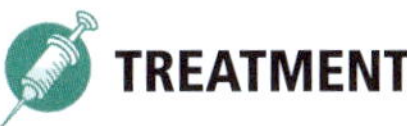

TREATMENT

GENERAL MEASURES

- NSAIDs for analgesia
- α_1-Blockers for lower urinary tract symptoms (obstructive/voiding symptoms)
- Antipyretics/stool softeners
- Hydration
- Sitz baths to relieve pain and spasm
- Urinary drainage for urine retention

MEDICATION

First Line

- Acute bacterial NIH class I (outpatient)
  - Fluoroquinolones are preferred first-line agents.
    - Trimethoprim-sulfamethoxazole 160/800 mg PO q12h (consider local *E. coli* resistance rates)
    - Ciprofloxacin 500 mg PO q12h or levofloxacin 500 to 750 mg PO once daily
  - Duration of therapy is 2 to 4 weeks (some support for 4 to 6 weeks).
  - If at risk for STI: ceftriaxone 250 mg IM for 1 dose (or cefixime 400 mg PO 1 dose) plus doxycycline 100 mg PO q12h for 10 days
  - α_1-Blockers for symptomatic relief of lower urinary tract symptoms and NSAIDs for analgesia
- Acute bacterial NIH class I (inpatient)
  - Urinary drainage (indwelling, intermittent, or suprapubic catheterization)
  - Obtain both blood and urine cultures
  - Initial broad-spectrum IV antibiotic therapy in acutely ill patients:
    - Not severely ill (2)[B]:
      - Ceftriaxone 1 to 2 g IV q24h + levofloxacin 500 to 750 mg IV q24h *or*
      - Zosyn 3.375 g IV q6h
    - Severely ill (2)[B]:
      - Zosyn q6h + aminoglycoside *or*
      - Cefotaxime 2 g q4h + aminoglycoside *or*
      - Ceftazidime 2 g q8h + aminoglycoside
  - De-escalate to oral regimen pending blood/urine culture results and with clinical improvement for additional 2 to 4 weeks of therapy.
- Chronic bacterial NIH class II
  - Ciprofloxacin 500 mg PO q12h or levofloxacin 500 to 750 mg PO daily for 4 to 6 weeks or trimethoprim-sulfamethoxazole (160/800 mg PO q12h for 8 to 12 weeks)
  - If gram-positive bacteria (*Enterococcus faecalis*) and failed ciprofloxacin or levofloxacin consider moxifloxacin 400 mg PO once daily or linezolid 600 mg PO q12h
  - Refractory cases: can consider intermittent antimicrobial treatment of acute symptomatic episodes (cystitis), low-dose antimicrobial suppression, radical TURP or open prostatectomy if all options failed
  - α-Blockers combined with antimicrobial therapy reduce the high recurrence rate and optimal for patients with obstructive symptoms.
- CP/CPPS NIH class III
  - Unclear source of disease, limited evidence on effective treatment
  - Treatment choice is patient-centered, focusing on symptom relief in four domains: pain, lower urinary tract symptoms, psychological stress, and sexual dysfunction.
  - Empiric trial of eliminating caffeine and alcohol
  - α_1-Blockers (tamsulosin 0.4 mg PO daily) can be beneficial, especially in men with lower urinary tract symptoms; however, studies do not show statistically significant differences.
  - Fluoroquinolones (ciprofloxacin 500 mg PO BID) may help for symptoms in patients, but studies do not show it is statistically significant.
  - NSAIDs can help with symptoms.

Second Line

Chronic bacterial prostatitis

- Fosfomycin is another antimicrobial option that can be used for the treatment of multi-drug resistant gram-negative organisms (i.e., *E. coli*) in CP as it has been known to have adequate penetration of prostatic tissues
  - Low toxicity profile
  - Consider in cases of intolerance to first-line treatment
  - Fosfomycin 3 g q48hr for 6 weeks

ISSUES FOR REFERRAL

Urology referral if antibiotic treatment fails, symptoms persist (especially obstructive voiding symptoms), hematuria, elevated PSA; or for surgical drainage if an abscess persists after ≥1 week of therapy

ADDITIONAL THERAPIES

- Cognitive-behavioral therapy (CBT) for psychosocial stressors or sexual dysfunction
- Pudendal nerve block or neurolysis if due to pudendal nerve entrapment.

SURGERY/OTHER PROCEDURES

Surgical resection may be considered for refractory cases of recurrent bacterial prostatitis or to drain an abscess.

ADMISSION, INPATIENT, AND NURSING CONSIDERATIONS

- Sepsis
- PO intolerance
- Urinary retention
- Proven or suspected abscess
- Risk factors for resistance (recent prostatic instrumentation or recent fluoroquinolone use)
- Immunocompromised

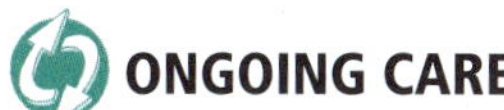

ONGOING CARE

FOLLOW-UP RECOMMENDATIONS

Negative urine culture at 7 days predictive of cure after completion of treatment course

PROGNOSIS

- Fever and dysuria usually resolve in 2 to 6 days.
- Acute infection usually improves in 3 to 4 weeks.
- Course of CP is often prolonged; 55–97% cure rate depending on population and drug used
- 20% have reinfection or persistent infection.
- 10% with acute bacterial prostatitis may progress to CP.

COMPLICATIONS

- Prostatic abscess (common in patients who are HIV infected)
- Pyelonephritis
- Urinary retention
- Epididymitis
- Infertility
- Chronic bacterial prostatitis (following acute prostatitis)
- Metastatic infection (spinal, sacroiliac)
- Erectile dysfunction

REFERENCES

1. Sharp VJ, Takacs EB, Powell CR. Prostatitis: diagnosis and treatment. *Am Fam Physician*. 2010;82(4):397–406.
2. Coker TJ, Dierfeldy DM. Acute bacterial prostatitis: diagnosis and management. *Am Fam Physician*. 2016;93(2):114–120.

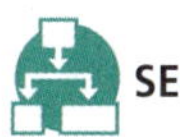

SEE ALSO

- Prostate Cancer; Prostatic Hyperplasia, Benign (BPH); Urinary Tract Infection (UTI) in Males
- Algorithm: Hematuria

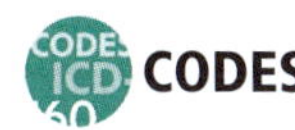

CODES

ICD10

- N41.8 Other inflammatory diseases of prostate
- N41 Inflammatory diseases of prostate
- N41.4 Granulomatous prostatitis

CLINICAL PEARLS

- Prostatic massage is contraindicated in acute prostatitis.
- Fluoroquinolones are recommended first-line antibiotic for bacterial prostatitis.
- At least 14 to 30 days of antibiotic therapy is required for acute prostatitis; longer for chronic bacterial prostatitis

PROTEIN C DEFICIENCY

Kyle J. Fletke, MD

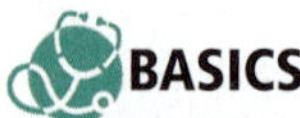

BASICS

Protein C deficiency (PCD) is a rare heritable disorder or acquired risk factor resulting in a prothrombotic state. Symptoms range from an asymptomatic presentation to recurrent venous thromboembolism (VTE), life-threatening neonatal purpura fulminans, or severe disseminated intravascular coagulation (DIC).

DESCRIPTION

- Protein C is a vitamin K–dependent anticoagulant protein synthesized in an inactive form by the liver.
- Activated protein C (APC) inhibits generation of thrombin by inactivating factors Va and VIIIa, using protein S as a cofactor.
- Deficiency in protein C activity therefore leads to a prothrombotic state.
- System(s) affected: cardiovascular, pulmonary, integumentary, hematologic, and immunologic

EPIDEMIOLOGY

Incidence

The estimated incidence is between 1 in 200 and 1 in 500 (1). Clinically substantial PCD is estimated to be 1 in 20,000. Severe PCD is rare, predicted in 1 in 4 million infants.

Prevalence

- 0.3% of the general population
- 3–5% of persons with VTE
- Mean age of first thrombosis is 45 years.
- There is no known gender predominance.

ETIOLOGY AND PATHOPHYSIOLOGY

- PCD can be inherited or acquired.
- Genetic mutations can lead to two types of PCD; however, the distinction between the two is clinically irrelevant.
  - Type I (most common) results in the reduction of protein C levels.
  - Type II results in a decreased functionality, despite having normal levels of protein C.
- Acquired PCD is more common and can occur in many disease states such as:
  - Liver disease
  - DIC
  - Severe infections (especially meningococcemia)
  - Autoantibody inhibitors directed toward protein C
  - Cancer and chemotherapy (i.e., L-asparaginase, 5-FU, methotrexate, and cyclophosphamide)
  - Initial use of vitamin K antagonists (warfarin)
  - Vitamin K deficiency (secondary to malnutrition or malabsorption of fat-soluble vitamins)
- Heterozygous PCD and mild deficiency can cause a wide range of symptom severity from asymptomatic to recurrent thromboses.
  - There is an increased risk of DVT, PE, and sequelae such as ischemic arterial stroke and pregnancy-associated thrombosis.

Genetics

- Autosomal dominant inheritance pattern with incomplete penetrance
- At least 270 genetic mutations have been described in the protein C (PROC) gene that can lead to a functional deficiency.
- Heterozygous patients often have mild or asymptomatic disease.
- Homozygous patients, or those with another coexisting genetic thrombophilia, often have more severe disease.
- Additionally, mutations in other genes (GCKR, EDEM2, BAZ1B, etc.) are associated with variability in the levels of protein C expression in the general population, although their clinical significance is currently unknown.
- Patients with PCD who start warfarin without concomitant heparin are at increased risk of developing warfarin-induced skin necrosis (WISN). This is thought to be due to the shorter half-life of protein C (5 to 8 hours) compared to other vitamin K–dependent clotting factors. However, not all patients who develop WISN have PCD.

ALERT

The prevention of warfarin necrosis has been achieved by avoiding loading doses of warfarin and the use of heparin bridging. Screening all patients for inherited or acquired forms of PCD prior to initiating warfarin is neither cost-effective nor prognostic because many patients with documented deficiency do not progress to WISN.

RISK FACTORS

Acquired conditions such as heart failure, severe liver disease, DIC, vitamin K antagonists

GENERAL PREVENTION

Because PCD is usually a congenital disease, there are no preventive measures.

COMMONLY ASSOCIATED CONDITIONS

- VTE at any site, often spontaneous
- Arterial thrombosis is rare, and a causative relationship has not been clearly demonstrated.
- Homozygosity can be associated with catastrophic thrombotic complications at birth (e.g., purpura fulminans).
- Recurrent pregnancy losses

DIAGNOSIS

HISTORY

- Recurrent VTE
- VTE at <40 years of age
- Thrombosis in unusual locations (e.g., mesentery, sagittal sinus, portal vein)
- Thrombosis at a young age (<50 years)
- Family history of thrombosis, spontaneous abortion, or WISN

PHYSICAL EXAM

Normal unless patient is presenting with active thrombosis and/or has physical stigmata of illness associated with PCD

DIFFERENTIAL DIAGNOSIS

- Factor V Leiden
- Protein S deficiency
- Antithrombin deficiency
- Dysfibrinogenemia
- Dysplasminogenemia
- Hyperhomocysteinemia
- Prothrombin G20210A mutation
- Elevated factor VIII, IX, or XI levels
- Antiphospholipid antibody syndrome
- DIC
- Heparin-induced thrombocytopenia (HIT)

DIAGNOSTIC TESTS & INTERPRETATION

PCD can be diagnosed using clotting assays, ELISA, and chromogenic tests to assess protein C levels. PROC gene mutational analysis is also available.

Initial Tests (lab, imaging)

- CBC with peripheral smear, INR, aPTT, hepatic and renal function tests, appropriate imaging
- Testing for heritable causes of thrombophilia in unselected patients presenting with a first-time VTE (provoked or unprovoked) is not indicated (2).
- Consider screening for antiphospholipid syndrome rather than other thrombophilia (PCD) for women with recurrent early pregnancy loss (three loses prior to 10 weeks' gestation) (3)[B].

Follow-Up Tests & Special Considerations

- Testing for heritable or acquired thrombophilia is suggested in the following circumstances:
  - First episode of VTE and patient age <40 years
  - Recurrent VTE regardless of the presence of risk factors
  - Patients with VTE at unusual sites
- Testing for PCD should be considered in patients with history of WISN.
- Testing for protein C and S deficiencies should be done urgently in neonates and children suspected to have purpura fulminans (2).
- Testing for hereditary thrombophilia should only be considered in asymptomatic first-degree relatives of those with proven hereditary thrombophilia if they are female, of childbearing age, and have no history of prior pregnancy complications (3)[C].
- When ordering additional testing for hereditary or acquired thrombophilia, the following conditions should be considered:
  - Antiphospholipid antibody syndrome
  - Antithrombin III deficiency
  - Factor V Leiden
  - PCD
  - Protein S deficiency
  - Prothrombin G20210A mutation

Diagnostic Procedures/Other

Testing for PCD is done using two separate lab tests:

- An immunoassay for a quantitative assessment of protein C levels
- A functional activity assay using a snake venom protease to activate protein C

Test Interpretation

- Drugs that may alter lab results:
  - Oral contraceptives can raise protein C levels.
  - Warfarin reduces protein C levels and should be discontinued 2 to 3 weeks before reliable testing.
- Liver disease reduces protein C levels.

ALERT

Acute thrombosis can lower protein C levels. Repeat confirmatory test of low protein C level at a separate time is advisable. If a normal level of protein C is obtained at presentation, then deficiency can be excluded.

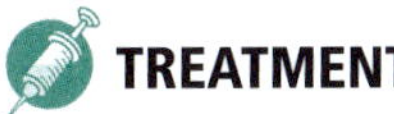

TREATMENT

GENERAL MEASURES

- Individuals with PCD should be educated regarding signs and symptoms of VTE.
- Women with any of the following history should avoid estradiol-containing contraceptives and hormone replacement therapy during menopause:
  - Diagnoses of PCD
  - First-degree relative with PCD
  - First-degree relative with VTE at age <50 years
- Women may use progestin-only hormonal contraception options.
- Routine anticoagulation for asymptomatic patients with PCD is not recommended (3)[C].
- Anticoagulation is recommended for at least 3 months in patients with inherited thrombophilia following their first VTE (2). Shared decision-making should be used to discuss duration of therapy >3 months.
- Treat VTE as an outpatient when possible if clinically stable (3)[B].
- Severe congenital PCD may be treated with protein C concentrates.

Pregnancy Considerations

- The VTE risk per pregnancy in patients with no prior history of VTE is 0.1–1.7%. The VTE risk per pregnancy in patients with prior VTE is 4–17%.
- Heparin-based products should be used during pregnancy when therapeutic or prophylactic treatment of VTE is needed.
- For pregnant women with known PCD but no personal history of VTE or additional thrombotic risk factors (i.e., family history of VTE in first-degree relative <50 years of age, obesity, prolonged immobility), antepartum and postpartum clinical monitoring is recommended over prophylactic therapy.
- For pregnant women with known PCD, no personal history of VTE but with an additional thrombotic risk factor, antepartum surveillance is recommended with postpartum prophylactic therapy for 6 weeks of either prophylactic or intermediate dose. Individuals with a high risk of thrombosis may be treated with protein C concentrate at the time of surgery or delivery.
- For pregnant women with known PCD and previous VTE, it is recommended to treat antepartum and postpartum patients with either prophylactic or intermediate-dose LMWH/UFH.

MEDICATION

First Line

- LMWH (3)[A]: initially started with warfarin for a minimum of 5 days and two consecutive INRs between 2 and 3 to bridge; additionally, LMWH may be started 5 to 10 days prior to starting dabigatran or edoxaban.
  - Enoxaparin (Lovenox) 1 mg/kg SC BID or 1.5 mg/kg/day SC
  - Tinzaparin (Innohep): 175 anti-Xa IU/kg/day SC
  - Dalteparin (Fragmin) 200 U/kg/day
- Novel oral anticoagulants (NOACs):
  - Rivaroxaban (Xarelto) 15 mg PO BID with food for 21 days and then 20 mg PO QD with food
  - Apixaban (Eliquis) 10 mg PO BID for 7 days and then 5 mg PO BID
  - Dabigatran (Pradaxa) 150 mg PO BID (after 5 to 10 days of parenteral anticoagulation)
  - Edoxaban (Savaysa) 60 mg PO QD (after 5 to 10 days of parenteral anticoagulation)
- Oral vitamin K antagonist:
  - Warfarin (Coumadin) titrated to an INR of 2.0 to 3.0 (3)[A]
- Factor Xa inhibitors:
  - Fondaparinux (Arixtra) <50 kg: 5 mg/day SC; 50 to 100 kg: 7.5 mg/day SC; >100 kg: 10 mg/day SC; contraindicated if CrCl <30 mL/min
- Contraindications
  - Active bleeding
  - Risk of bleeding is a relative contraindication to long-term anticoagulation.
- Precautions
  - Observe patient for signs of embolization, further thrombosis, or bleeding.
  - Monitor kidney function, drug–drug interactions, and CBC (including platelets to monitor for HIT).

Second Line

- Heparin 80 U/kg IV bolus followed by 18 U/kg/hr; adjust dose depending on PPT.
- In patients requiring large daily doses of heparin, measure an anti-Xa level for dose guidance.
- Alternatively, and for outpatients, unfractionated heparin can be given at 333 U/kg and then 250 U/kg SC, without monitoring (3)[C].
- May be treatable with replacement protein C concentrate; neonatal purpura fulminans can be controlled with protein C replacement from fresh frozen plasma (FFP).

SURGERY/OTHER PROCEDURES

- Anticoagulation may be held for surgical interventions.
- In patients with acute proximal DVT of the lower extremity *and* an absolute contraindication to anticoagulation, inferior vena cava (IVC) filters are recommended; otherwise, the use of an IVC filter in addition to anticoagulants is not recommended (3)[B].

ADMISSION, INPATIENT, AND NURSING CONSIDERATIONS

- Life-threatening VTE
- Significant bleeding while on anticoagulant therapy

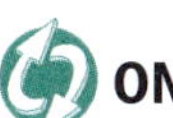

ONGOING CARE

FOLLOW-UP RECOMMENDATIONS

Patient Monitoring

- Warfarin requires periodic monitoring of the INR to maintain a range of 2.0 to 3.0 (monthly, after initial stabilization).
- LMWH is the treatment of choice in pregnancy. Periodic monitoring with anti-Xa levels is recommended in these patients.

DIET

Unrestricted (except if on warfarin—avoid varying diet with foods that have significant amounts of vitamin K)

PATIENT EDUCATION

- Patients should be educated about signs and symptoms of VTE as well as the use of oral anticoagulant therapy if taking such.
- Avoid NSAIDs while on warfarin.
- Avoid estrogen containing OCPs because of increased risk of thrombosis.

PROGNOSIS

When compared with normal individuals, persons with PCD have normal life spans.

COMPLICATIONS

Primary or recurrent VTE

REFERENCES

1. Tait RC, Walker ID, Reitsma PH, et al. Prevalence of protein C deficiency in the healthy population. *Thromb Haemost*. 1995;73(1):87–93.
2. Baglin T, Gray E, Greaves M, et al; for British Committee for Standards in Haematology. Clinical guidelines for testing for heritable thrombophilia. *Br J Haematol*. 2010;149(2):209–220.
3. Guyatt GH, Akl EA, Crowther M, et al; for American College of Chest Physicians Antithrombotic Therapy and Prevention of Thrombosis Panel. Executive summary: antithrombotic therapy and prevention of thrombosis, 9th ed: American College of Chest Physicians evidence-based clinical practice guidelines. *Chest*. 2012;141(Suppl 2):7S–47S.

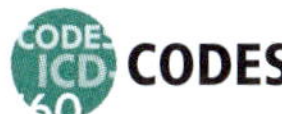

CODES

ICD10

D68.59 Other primary thrombophilia

CLINICAL PEARLS

- Screening of asymptomatic family members is not justified with the possible exception of females of childbearing age with no previous history of pregnancy complications.
- Asymptomatic patients with PCD do not need prophylactic anticoagulation because the risk of thrombosis is low.
- Patients with PCD presenting with first-time VTE should be anticoagulated for at least 3 months. Other risk factors and shared decision-making should be used to determine if anticoagulation should be used for a longer duration.
- Recurrent VTE is an indication for indefinite anticoagulation.

PROTEIN S DEFICIENCY

Opeoluwa Olukorede, MD, MS

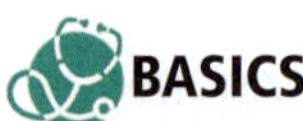

BASICS

DESCRIPTION

- Protein S is a vitamin K–dependent glycoprotein, produced mainly in the liver that acts as a cofactor for protein C. It is also produced by megakaryocytes and endothelial cells.
- Protein C becomes activated when thrombin binds to the endothelial receptor, thrombomodulin.
- Activated protein C, with protein S (a cofactor), inactivates clotting factors Va and VIIIa enhancing fibrinolysis.
- Protein S is also able to directly inhibit factors Va, VIIa, and Xa independently of activated protein C.
- Protein S deficiency is a congenital thrombophilia, which increases the risk of thromboembolism.
- It primarily affects the venous system.
- System(s) affected: cardiovascular, hematologic/immunologic, pulmonary

EPIDEMIOLOGY

Incidence

- Mean age of first thrombosis: 2nd decade
- Predominant sex: male = female

Prevalence

- ~0.2% of general population
- Found in ~1% of persons with venous thrombosis embolism (VTE)

ETIOLOGY AND PATHOPHYSIOLOGY

- It is an autosomal dominant disease.
- Only the free form of protein S (30–40%) acts as a cofactor for activated protein C. Protein S reversibly binds to the C4b protein, which leads to conditions in which free protein S is low, but total protein S is normal. These individuals are prone to thrombosis.
- Conditions with reduced protein S: pregnancy, disseminated intravascular coagulation (DIC), liver disease, nephrotic syndrome, HIV, acute thrombosis, and acute varicella-zoster virus infection
- Drugs: oral contraceptives, warfarin, and L-asparaginase chemotherapy

Genetics

- Due to mutations in the PROS1 gene on chromosome 3; most individuals are heterozygous.
- Heterozygotes have an odds ratio (OR) of VTE of 1.6 to 11.5.
- Homozygosity or compound heterozygosity, if untreated, is usually incompatible with adult life.
- Homozygotes can have a fulminant thrombotic event in infancy, termed *neonatal purpura fulminans*.

RISK FACTORS

- Oral contraceptives, pregnancy, and the use of hormone replacement therapy (HRT) increase the risk of VTE in patients with protein S deficiency.
- Patients with protein S deficiency and other prothrombotic states have further increased rate of thrombosis.
- Arterial thrombosis is more frequent in patients with protein S deficiency who smoke.
- Patients heterozygous for protein S deficiency who are initiated on warfarin without concomitant heparin can develop warfarin-induced skin necrosis because the half-life of other vitamin K–dependent clotting factors (e.g., prothrombin, factor IX, and factor X) is much longer than the anticoagulant protein S (4 to 8 hours), leading to a transient hypercoagulable state when protein S becomes depleted. These patients develop extremely low levels of protein S and develop necrosis of the skin over central areas of the body such as the breast, abdomen, buttocks, and genitalia.

Pregnancy Considerations

Increased thrombotic risk and pregnancy losses

GENERAL PREVENTION

There are no preventive measures.

COMMONLY ASSOCIATED CONDITIONS

- Deep and superficial VTE, often unprovoked
- Up to 50% of homozygotes will have thrombosis.
- Homozygosity is associated with catastrophic thrombotic complications at birth: *neonatal purpura fulminans*.
- Sites of thrombosis can be unusual, including the mesentery, cerebral veins, and axillary veins.
- Arterial thrombosis is rare but reported in several case reports.
- Skin necrosis in patients treated with warfarin
- Recurrent pregnancy losses

DIAGNOSIS

HISTORY

Inherited thrombophilias should be suspected in:

- Unprovoked VTE at age <50 years
- VTE with a strong family history of VTE or known familial protein S deficiency
- VTE in unusual sites as mesenteric or cerebral vein
- Recurrent VTE

PHYSICAL EXAM

Normal

DIFFERENTIAL DIAGNOSIS

Other inherited thrombophilias:

- Factor V Leiden (most common; usually in Caucasians)
- Protein C deficiency (in Caucasians)
- Antithrombin deficiency
- Dysfibrinogenemia
- Dysplasminogenemia
- Homocystinemia
- Prothrombin G20210A mutation
- Elevated factor VIII levels
- Acquired VTE risk factors: surgery, immobility, cancer, myeloproliferative neoplasms, trauma, antiphospholipid syndrome, paroxysmal nocturnal hemoglobinuria, pregnancy, HRT, postpartum, DIC

DIAGNOSTIC TESTS & INTERPRETATION

Initial Tests (lab, imaging)

- For evaluation of new clot in a patient at risk: CBC with peripheral smear, PT/INR, aPTT, thrombin time, lupus anticoagulant, antiphospholipid antibodies, anticardiolipin antibody, anti-β_2-glycoprotein I antibody, activated protein C resistance, protein S antigen and resistance, antithrombin III assay, fibrinogen, factor V Leiden, prothrombin G20210A
- Immunoassay for quantitative assessment of total and free protein S levels
- Protein S activity assay (mainly after obtaining activated protein C resistance)
- Disorders that may alter lab results: acute thrombosis, vitamin K antagonists (VKA), any acute illness response, liver disease, and pregnancy-reduced protein S levels; direct oral anticoagulants affect protein S activity assay.
- Heparin and low-weight heparin do not alter lab results.
- Total protein S levels are markedly decreased in newborns and young infants; use age-adjusted norms.

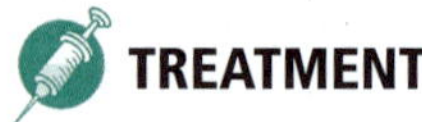

TREATMENT

GENERAL MEASURES

- Routine anticoagulation for asymptomatic patients with protein S deficiency is not recommended.
- Antithrombotic therapy recommendations for patients with protein S deficiency can be guided by antithrombotic therapy for VTE disease guidelines.
- Patients with unprovoked VTE and who have a low or moderate bleeding risk are suggested to receive extended anticoagulant therapy (no scheduled stop date) >3 months of therapy (1), and those who have a high bleeding risk are recommended to receive 3 months of anticoagulant therapy (1),(2)[B].
- Patients with a second unprovoked VTE and who have a low-to-moderate bleeding risk are recommended to receive extended anticoagulant therapy >3 months (1),(2)[B]; those who have high bleeding risk are suggested to receive 3 months of anticoagulant therapy (1).

- Patients with VTE and no history of cancer are suggested to receive dabigatran, rivaroxaban, apixaban, or edoxaban over VKA therapy as long-term (first 3 months) anticoagulant therapy; VKA therapy over low-molecular-weight heparin (LMWH) (1)
- Patients with VTE and active cancer are suggested to receive LMWH, rivaroxaban, or edoxaban for long-term anticoagulation (3). It is recommended that these patients receive extended anticoagulant therapy (1).
- Treatment of thrombosis with LMWH is recommended over unfractionated heparin, unless the patient has severe renal failure.
- Treat as outpatient, if possible.
- Prophylaxis should be considered in risk situations such as surgery, immobility, or postpartum, especially in patients with family history.
- The role of family screening for protein S deficiency is unclear because most patients with this mutation do not have thrombosis. Screening should be considered for women considering oral contraceptives or pregnancy and who have a family history of protein S deficiency (4)[B].

MEDICATION

- LMWH
  - Enoxaparin (Lovenox) 1 mg/kg SC BID
    - Alternatively, 1.5 mg/kg/day SC
  - Tinzaparin (Innohep) 175 anti-Xa U/kg/day SC
  - Dalteparin (Fragmin) 200 U/kg/day SC divided QD–BID
- Factor Xa inhibitor
  - Fondaparinux (Arixtra) <50 kg: 5 mg/day SC; 50 to 100 kg: 7.5 mg/day SC; >100 kg: 10 mg/day SC; contraindicated if CrCl <30 mL/min
- Dual oral anticoagulants (DOACs):
  - Dabigatran 150 mg PO BID (after 5 to 10 days of parenteral anticoagulation)
  - Rivaroxaban 15 mg PO BID for 21 days and then 20 mg PO QD
  - Apixaban 10 mg PO BID for 7 days and then 5 mg PO BID
  - Edoxaban: person weighs ≤60 kg: 30 mg PO QD; >60 kg: 60 mg PO QD (after 5 to 10 days of parenteral anticoagulation)
- Oral anticoagulant: warfarin (Coumadin): 2 to 5 mg PO QD then adjusted to an INR of 2 to 3; LMWH initially for a minimum of 5 days and two consecutive INRs between 2 and 3, at which time it can be stopped; contraindications
  - Active bleeding precludes anticoagulation; risk of bleeding is a relative contraindication to long-term anticoagulation.
  - Warfarin is contraindicated in patients with a prior history of warfarin-induced skin necrosis.
- Precautions
  - Observe patient for signs of embolization, further thrombosis, or bleeding.
  - Avoid IM injections.
  - Periodically, check stool and urine for occult blood; monitor CBC, including platelets.
  - Heparin: thrombocytopenia and/or paradoxical thrombosis with thrombocytopenia
  - Warfarin: necrotic skin lesions (typically breasts, thighs, and buttocks)
  - LMWH: Adjust dose in renal insufficiency.
- Significant possible interactions
  - Agents that intensify the response to oral anticoagulants: ethanol, allopurinol, amiodarone, anabolic steroids, androgens, many antimicrobials, cimetidine, chloral hydrate, disulfiram, NSAIDs, sulfinpyrazone, tamoxifen, levothyroxine, vitamin E, ranitidine, salicylates, and acetaminophen
  - Agents that diminish the response to oral anticoagulants: aminoglutethimide, antacids, barbiturates, carbamazepine, cholestyramine, diuretics, griseofulvin, rifampin, and oral contraceptives

ISSUES FOR REFERRAL

- Patients with suspected protein S deficiency should be seen by a hematologist.
- Screening and prophylactic treatment of asymptomatic family members is not justified (5).

SURGERY/OTHER PROCEDURES

- Anticoagulation must be held for surgical interventions.
- For most patients with DVT, recommendations are against routine use of vena cava filter in addition to anticoagulation. IVC filter is only recommended in case of contraindication to anticoagulation (1)[A].

COMPLEMENTARY & ALTERNATIVE MEDICINE

Diet modifications if taking VKA

ADMISSION, INPATIENT, AND NURSING CONSIDERATIONS

- Life-threatening VTE
- Significant bleeding while on anticoagulant therapy
- Look for signs of bleeding while on anticoagulation therapy.

ONGOING CARE

FOLLOW-UP RECOMMENDATIONS

Patient Monitoring

- Warfarin requires periodic (monthly after initial stabilization) monitoring of the INR.
- Periodic measurement of INR to maintain a range of 2 to 3
- LMWH is the treatment of choice in pregnancy. Periodic monitoring with anti-Xa levels is recommended in some cases, such as overweight and borderline renal failure.

DIET

Unrestricted, unless taking VKA

PATIENT EDUCATION

- Patients should be educated about the use of oral anticoagulant therapy if taking such.
- Patients undergoing warfarin therapy should avoid drinking alcohol on a daily basis.
- Avoid NSAIDs while on warfarin.

PROGNOSIS

- Persons with protein S deficiency have normal lifespan.
- By the age of 45 years, 50% of the people heterozygous for protein S deficiency will have VT; half will be spontaneous.

COMPLICATIONS

Recurrent thrombosis (requires indefinite anticoagulation)

REFERENCES

1. Kearon C, Akl EA, Ornelas J, et al. Antithrombotic therapy for VTE disease: CHEST Guideline and Expert Panel Report. *Chest*. 2016;149(2):315–352.
2. Moll S. Thrombophilias—practical implications and testing caveats. *J Thromb Thrombolysis*. 2006;21(1):7–15.
3. Key NS, Khorana AA, Kuderer NM, et al. Venous thromboembolism prophylaxis and treatment in patients with cancer: ASCO clinical practice guideline update. *J Clin Oncol*. 2020;38(5):496–520.
4. Langlois NJ, Wells PS. Risk of venous thromboembolism in relatives of symptomatic probands with thrombophilia: a systematic review. *Thromb Haemost*. 2003;90(1):17–26.
5. Hornsby LB, Armstrong EM, Bellone JM, et al. Thrombophilia screening. *J Pharm Pract*. 2014;27(3):253–259.

ADDITIONAL READING

Ameku K, Higa M. Rivaroxaban treatment for warfarin-refractory thrombosis in a patient with hereditary protein S deficiency. *Case Rep Hematol*. 2018;2018:5217301.

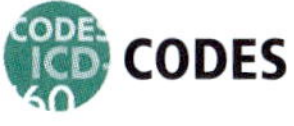

CODES

ICD10

D68.59 Other primary thrombophilia

CLINICAL PEARLS

- Asymptomatic patients with protein S deficiency do not require prophylactic anticoagulation because the risk of thrombosis is low; asymptomatic patients do not require anticoagulation.
- Patients with protein S deficiency and DVT should be anticoagulated for at least 6 months, especially if first episode.

PROTEINURIA

Maham Haq, MD

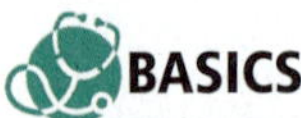

BASICS

DESCRIPTION

- Proteinuria: urinary protein excretion of >150 mg/day
- Nephrotic-range proteinuria: urinary protein excretion of ≥3.5 g/day; also called heavy proteinuria

Pediatric Considerations

- Proteinuria: Normal is daily excretion of up to 100 mg/m^2 (body surface area) for children. For neonates, daily excretion may be up to 300 mg/m^2 due to decreased reabsorption of filtered proteins.
- Nephrotic-range proteinuria: daily excretion of >1,000 mg/m^2 (body surface area)

Pregnancy Considerations

- Proteinuria in pregnancy beyond 20 weeks' gestation is a hallmark of preeclampsia/eclampsia and demands further workup.
- Proteinuria in pregnancy before 20 weeks' gestation is suggestive of underlying renal disease.

EPIDEMIOLOGY

Prevalence

The prevalence of proteinuria varies based on the definition used; maybe as high as 10% in school-aged children

ETIOLOGY AND PATHOPHYSIOLOGY

Normal protein filtration up to 150 mg/day, of which approximately 20 mg is albumin

- Glomerular proteinuria: increased glomerular capillary wall permeability due to both the increased size of glomerular basement membrane pores and loss of negatively charged barrier from glycosaminoglycans
  - Primary glomerulonephropathy
    - Minimal-change disease
    - Idiopathic/primary membranous glomerulonephritis
    - Focal segmental glomerulosclerosis/ glomerulonephritis
    - Membranoproliferative glomerulonephritis
    - IgA nephropathy (Berger disease)
  - Secondary glomerulonephropathy
    - Chronic disease (diabetes, hypertension, chronic kidney disease [CKD])
    - Autoimmune/collagen vascular disorders (e.g., lupus nephritis, Henoch-Schönlein purpura, Goodpasture syndrome)
    - Genetic disorders (Alport syndrome, Fabry disease)
    - Amyloidosis, sarcoidosis
    - Preeclampsia
    - Infection (HIV, CMV, hepatitis B and C, post-streptococcal, endocarditis, syphilis, malaria)
    - Malignancy (GI, lung, lymphoma)
    - Renal transplant rejection
    - Structural (reflux nephropathy, polycystic kidney disease)
    - Drug-induced (NSAIDs, penicillamine, lithium, heavy metals, gold, heroin)
    - Sickle cell disease
- Tubulointerstitial proteinuria: Tubulointerstitial disease prevents proximal tubular reabsorption of smaller proteins (β_2-microglobulin, immunoglobulin [Ig] light chains, retinol-binding protein, amino acids).
  - Medications (NSAIDs, aminoglycosides, penicillins, cephalosporins, quinolones, sulfonamides, amphotericin B, cisplatin, radiocontrast media)
  - Toxins (lead, copper, mercury)
  - Uric acid nephropathy
  - Interstitial nephritis
  - Fanconi syndrome
  - Acute tubular necrosis
- Overflow proteinuria: Plasma concentration of low-molecular-weight proteins exceed capacity of the tubules to reabsorb filtered protein.
  - Multiple myeloma (light chains; also tubulotoxic)
  - Hemoglobinuria
  - Myoglobinuria (in rhabdomyolysis)
  - Lysozyme (in acute monocytic leukemia)
- Benign proteinuria
  - Functional (fever, exercise, cold exposure, stress, dehydration, seizures, CHF)
  - Idiopathic transient
  - Orthostasis (postural)—usually found in older children and adolescents

GENERAL PREVENTION

Control of weight, BP, and blood glucose reduces the risk of chronic disease that leads to proteinuria.

COMMONLY ASSOCIATED CONDITIONS

Nephrotic syndrome, glomerulonephritis, CKD

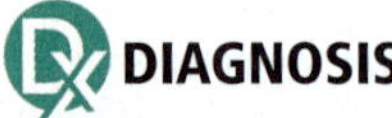

DIAGNOSIS

HISTORY

- Fever
- Frothy/foamy urine
- Change in urine output
- Blood- or cola-colored urine
- Recent weight change
- History of UTIs
- Dysuria, flank pain
- Swelling
- Rule out systemic illness: diabetes, heart failure, autoimmune, recent streptococcal infection.
- If pregnant: swelling of hands or face, headaches, blurry vision, abdominal pain

PHYSICAL EXAM

- Vitals (temperature, BP)
- Weight
- Peripheral edema
- Periorbital/facial edema
- Abdominal or CVA tenderness
- Ascites
- Palpation of kidneys
- Check lungs and heart for signs of CHF.

DIFFERENTIAL DIAGNOSIS

Includes all causes listed under "Etiology and Pathophysiology"

DIAGNOSTIC TESTS & INTERPRETATION

All patients with CKD risk factors should be screened via serum creatine determination for GFR estimation and analysis of random urine sample for proteinuria.

Initial Tests (lab, imaging)

- Urinalysis (UA) quantitatively estimates proteinuria:
  - Only sensitive to albumin; will not detect low-molecular proteins of overflow/tubular etiologies
  - False-positive: if urine pH >7, highly concentrated (specific gravity [SG] >1.015), gross hematuria, mucus, semen, leukocytes, iodinated contrast agents, penicillin analogues, sulfonamide metabolites
  - False-negative: If urine is dilute (SG 1.005), albumin excretion <20 to 30 mg/dL, urinary protein is low-molecular weight.
  - Sensitivity, 32–46%; specificity, 97–100%
  - Negative urine dipstick with positive sulfosalicylic acid test may indicate Bence-Jones protein.
- Protein results interpretation on dipstick urinalysis
  - 1+ = 30 mg/dL
  - 2+ = 100 mg/dL
  - 3+ = 300 mg/dL
  - 4+ = 1000 mg/dL
- If UA shows trace to 2+ protein, rule out transient proteinuria with repeat UA at another visit:
  - More common than persistent proteinuria
  - Reassure patient that transient proteinuria is benign and requires no further workup.
- If initial UA shows 3+ to 4+ protein or repeat UA is positive, measure creatinine clearance and quantify proteinuria with first morning spot urine to calculate urine protein-to-creatinine (P/C) ratio, which is preferred over 24-hour urine test due to inconsistent collection and inconvenience to patients (1),(2),(3)[A]. 24-hour urine test remains the gold standard.
  - Numerical P/C ratios correlate with total protein excreted in grams per day (i.e., ratio of 0.2 correlates with 0.2 g during a 24-hour collection).
  - Consider orthostatic proteinuria if P/C ratio <0.3 after recumbent position and P/C ratio >0.3 after prolonged standing activity.

Follow-Up Tests & Special Considerations

If urine P/C ratio >0.3, consider further evaluation, which can include the following:

- CBC, ferritin, ESR, serum iron
- Electrolytes, LFTs
- Lipid profile (ideally, fasting)
- Prothrombin time/international normalized ratio to assess for concurrent coagulopathy
- Anti-phospholipase A2 receptor antibody: positive in ~70% of primary membranous nephropathy
- Antinuclear antibodies: elevated in lupus
- Antistreptolysin O titer: elevated after streptococcal infection
- Complement C3/C4: low in most glomerulonephritis
- HIV, syphilis, and hepatitis serologies: all associated with glomerular proteinuria
- Serum and urine protein electrophoresis: abnormal in multiple myeloma

- Patients with persistent proteinuria not explained by orthostatic changes should undergo renal ultrasound to rule out structural abnormalities. (e.g., reflux nephropathy, polycystic kidney).
- Patients with nephrotic-range proteinuria are at increased risk for hypercholesterolemia and thromboembolic events (~25% of adult patients) with the highest risk in membranous nephropathy. Optimal duration of prophylactic anticoagulation is unknown but may extend for the duration of the nephrotic state (4).
- Proteinuric pregnant patients beyond 20 weeks' gestation should be examined for other signs/symptoms of preeclampsia (e.g., hypertension, thrombocytopenia, elevated liver transaminases).

TREATMENT

- Treat any identified underlying etiology.
- BP goal for both diabetic and nondiabetic is ≤140/90 mm Hg (5)[C].
- Proteinuria goal is <0.5 g/day (6)[A].
- BP goal of 130/80 mm Hg for patients with normal urinary albumin concentration
- BP goal of 125/75 mm Hg for patients with ≥1 g/24 hours proteinuria.

GENERAL MEASURES

- Limit protein intake to 0.8 g/kg/day with DM or without DM and glomerular filtration rate (GFR) <30 mL/min/1.73 m^2. Soy protein may be renoprotective. Monitor protein intake with 24-hour urine urea excretion (6)[A].
- Limit sodium chloride intake to <2 g/day to optimize antiproteinuric medications (5)[B].
- Effect on BP is further protective (6)[A].
- Limit fluid intake for urine output goal of <2 L/day. Larger urine volumes are associated with increased proteinuria and later GFR decline (6)[B],(7).
- Smoking cessation: Smoking is associated with increased proteinuria and faster kidney disease progression (6)[B].
- Encourage supine posture (up to 50% reduction vs. upright) (6)[B].
- Discourage severe exertion (6)[B].
- Encourage weight loss (6)[B].

MEDICATION

First Line

Loop diuretics, ACE inhibitors (ACEis), or angiotensin II receptor blockers (ARBs) use is a conservative management approach with nephrotic syndrome.

- ACEi: first-line therapy; if persistent proteinuria >0.5 g/day; use maximally tolerated doses; use even if normotensive (6),(8)[A].
- ARBs: proven antiproteinuric and renoprotective; ARBs are first choice if ACEis are not tolerated (6)[A].
  - Combination ACEi and ARB should not be used. Although shown to reduce proteinuria, combination does not reduce poor CV outcomes and does increase risk of adverse drug reactions (7),(9)[A].
  - May continue therapy with ACEi or ARB up to 30% increase in serum creatinine (8).
- Loop diuretics: first-line therapy if edema is present; may be used as additional therapy for BP control and proteinuria reduction

Second Line

- β-Blockers: antiproteinuric and cardioprotective (6)[A]
- Dihydropyridine calcium channel blockers (non-DHCCB): antiproteinuric, may be renoprotective (6)[B]
- Aldosterone antagonists: antiproteinuric independent of BP control (6)[B]
- NSAIDs: antiproteinuric but also nephrotoxic; generally should be avoided (6)

ISSUES FOR REFERRAL

Consider nephrology referral for possible renal biopsy if impaired creatinine clearance, nephrotic-range proteinuria, or unclear.

ADDITIONAL THERAPIES

Corticosteroids: No proven benefit in mortality or need for renal replacement in adults with nephrotic syndrome, although steroids are recommended in some patients who do not respond to conservative treatment. Classically, children with nephrotic syndrome respond better than adults, especially those with minimal-change disease (7)[A].

COMPLEMENTARY & ALTERNATIVE MEDICINE

- Regular exercise and smoking cessation
- Antioxidant therapy: may be antiproteinuric in diabetic nephropathy (6)[C]
- Avoid excessive caffeine consumption: antiproteinuric in diabetic rat models (6)[C]
- Avoid iron overload (6)[C].

ONGOING CARE

FOLLOW-UP RECOMMENDATIONS

Patient Monitoring

All patients with persistent proteinuria should be followed with serial BP checks, UA, and renal function tests.

DIET

- Restrict dietary sodium to <2 g/day
- Restrict caloric intake to achieve normal BMI with target 35 kcal/kg/day
- Restrict dietary fat to <30% of total calories

PROGNOSIS

- Transient and orthostatic proteinuria are benign conditions.
- Clinical significance of persistent proteinuria varies greatly and depends on underlying etiology.
- Degree of proteinuria is associated with disease progression in CKD.
- Independent of GFR, higher levels of proteinuria likely convey an increased risk of mortality, myocardial infarction, and progression to kidney failure.

COMPLICATIONS

- Progression to chronic renal failure
- Hypercholesterolemia
- Hypercoagulable state
- Increased risk for infection for patient with nephrotic syndrome

REFERENCES

1. Mazaheri M, Assadi F. Simplified algorithm for evaluation of proteinuria in clinical practice: how should a clinician approach? *Int J Prev Med*. 2019;10:35. doi:10.4103/ijpvm.IJPVM_557_18.
2. Hull RP, Goldsmith DJ. Nephrotic syndrome in adults. *BMJ*. 2008;336(7654):1185–1189.
3. National Kidney Foundation. K/DOQI clinical practice guidelines for chronic kidney disease: evaluation classification and stratification: guideline 5. Assessment of proteinuria. http://www2.kidney.org/professionals/KDOQI/guidelines_ckd/toc.htm. Accessed November 16, 2017.
4. Kerlin BA, Ayoob R, Smoyer WE. Epidemiology and pathophysiology of nephrotic syndrome—associated thromboembolic disease. *Clin J Am Soc Nephrol*. 2012;7(3):513–520.
5. James PA, Oparil S, Carter BL, et al. 2014 Evidence-based guideline for the management of high blood pressure in adults: report from the panel members appointed to the Eighth Joint National Committee (JNC 8). *JAMA*. 2014;311(5):507–520.
6. Wilmer WA, Rovin BH, Hebert CJ, et al. Management of glomerular proteinuria: a commentary. *J Am Soc Nephrol*. 2003;14(12):3217–3232.
7. Kodner C. Diagnosis and management of nephrotic syndrome in adults. *Am Fam Physician*. 2016;93(6):479–485.
8. Rovin BH, Adler SG, Barratt J, et al. KDIGO 2021 clinical practice guideline for the management of glomerular diseases. *Kidney Int*. 2021;100(4S):S1–S276. doi:10.1016/j.kint.2021.05.021.
9. Fried LF, Emanuele N, Zhang JH, et al; for VA NEPHRON-D Investigators. Combined angiotensin inhibition for the treatment of diabetic nephropathy. *N Engl J Med*. 2013;369(20):1892–1903.

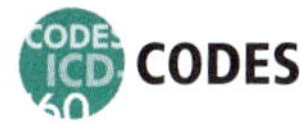

CODES

ICD10

- R80.9 Proteinuria, unspecified
- R80.2 Orthostatic proteinuria, unspecified
- R80.1 Persistent proteinuria, unspecified

CLINICAL PEARLS

- Transient and orthostatic proteinuria are benign conditions that do not convey a poor prognosis.
- Proteinuria >2 g/day likely represents glomerular malfunction and warrants a nephrology consultation.
- Clinical course varies greatly but, in general, the degree of proteinuria correlates with kidney disease progression.
- First-line therapy for persistent proteinuric patients is a high-dose ACEi.

PROTHROMBIN 20210 (MUTATION)

Touqir Zahra, MD, FACP • Raksha Sharma, MD

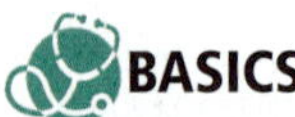

BASICS

DESCRIPTION

- The G20210A is a gain of function mutation where adenine is substituted for a guanine at the 20210 noncoding position of the prothrombin (a.k.a. factor II) gene.
- Prothrombin 20210 mutation is the second most common venous thrombophilia after the factor V Leiden mutation.
- The mechanism of increasing the risk of thrombosis is incompletely understood but has been attributed to increased prothrombin or factor II levels in circulation by increased prothrombin protein translation without changing the levels of prothrombin mRNA transcription.
- Autosomal dominant condition, where heterozygotes have a 30% higher prothrombin level and a 3- to 4-fold increased risk of venous thromboembolism (VTE)
- System(s) affected: cardiovascular, hematologic/lymphatic/immunologic, nervous, pulmonary, reproductive, and hepatic
- Synonym(s): prothrombin G20210A mutation; prothrombin G20210A gene polymorphism; prothrombin gene mutation; and factor II A^{20210} mutation

EPIDEMIOLOGY

- Mean age of first thrombosis is in the 2nd decade of life.
- Inheritance is similar between both genders (autosomal).

Incidence

In patients with the prothrombin 20210 mutation, the cumulative incidence of VTE complications after 10 years was 61.3% (1).

Prevalence

- Found largely in Caucasian population with a prevalence ranging between 1% and 6%, but overall, it is about 2%.
- In patients presenting with a VTE, prothrombin 20210 mutation has a prevalence that ranges from 4.6% to 18% with increased prevalence attributed to highly thrombophilic families.

ETIOLOGY AND PATHOPHYSIOLOGY

- Noncoding substitution of adenine for guanine at the 20210 position at the terminal nucleotide of the 3′ resulting in a gain of function of prothrombin gene, leading to increased levels of prothrombin (factor II), by increased translation of prothrombin mRNA but not transcription
- The base change location is in the 3′ terminal nucleotide of the untranslated region associated with the mRNA sequence for polyadenylation. The gain of function is possible due to increased rate of processing, alteration of the site of cleavage, or increased mRNA stability.
- In the coagulation cascade, prothrombin (factor II) is the precursor of thrombin, which cleaves fibrinogen to fibrin. Elevated prothrombin activity leads to elevated thrombin levels and subsequent clot formation.
- The majority of thrombus formation occurs in the venous circulation: deep venous thrombosis (DVT)/PE, mesenteric, and cerebral. Recent studies have shown that prothrombin 20210 mutation did not correlate with Budd-Chiari syndrome or a portal or hepatic vein thrombosis.
- G20210A mutation is not known to be a risk factor for some arterial thrombotic events (myocardial infarction or acute ischemic stroke); however, studies have shown an increased prevalence of the mutation in patients with critical limb ischemia.

Genetics

- Caused by the G20210A mutation of the *F2* gene (prothrombin gene) located in the short (p) arm of chromosome 11 that causes a gain of function
- Heterozygotes have a 30% increased levels of prothrombin levels, with a 3- to 4-fold increase of VTE events. Homozygotes are at an even greater risk.
- There are three other prothrombin mutations not related to the G20210A area:
  - Yukuhashi: missense mutation G1787T, arginine for leucine at amino acid 596, leading to prolonged procoagulant activity
  - C20209T: adjacent to G20210A mutation, primarily found in African individuals; newer studies have suggested a possible relationship between this mutation and recurrent pregnancy loss, although it is not fully understood.
  - A19911G: located in the intron of the prothrombin gene; may affect the G20210A mutation by increasing the odds ratio of the venous thromboembolic event. Mechanism is still unknown.

RISK FACTORS

- Being a hereditary condition, the presence of such mutation in the parents poses risk of transmission to offspring.
- Regarding the risk of developing VTE:
  - Patients with both the prothrombin 20210 mutation and factor V Leiden mutation increases the odds ratio of VTE by 20-fold.
  - Virchow triad of thrombogenesis consists of stasis, endothelial injury, and thrombophilia. Any condition that promotes stasis and endothelial injury will consequently increase the risk of VTE, for example, oral contraceptive, pregnancy, malignancy, orthopedic surgery, congestive heart failure, cerebrovascular accident in the past 3 months, air travel, obesity, and smoking.

Pregnancy Considerations

- Increased thrombotic risk in patients with prothrombin 20210 mutation during pregnancy and in the postpartum state is attributed to relative stasis.
- Anticoagulation should begin in the 1st trimester because the risk of VTE increases early in pregnancy and should be discontinued at onset of labor or before scheduled induction/cesarean delivery. Postpartum risk of VTE is usually greater, and anticoagulation can resume 4 to 6 hours after a vaginal delivery or 6 to 12 hours after surgery. Warfarin may begin immediately due to slow onset of action.
- C20209T mutation may have some relation with recurrent pregnancy loss; however, it is not well studied.

GENERAL PREVENTION

Asymptomatic individuals with the mutation do not require any prophylactic anticoagulation. Exceptions are generally made for pregnant women with very high-risk thrombophilic mutations (usually factor V Leiden) with a strong family history. After the first VTE, lifelong prophylaxis may be warranted if some features are present: unprovoked or in a nontraditional area like hepatic, portal, mesenteric, or cerebral.

COMMONLY ASSOCIATED CONDITIONS

- VTE
- Factor V Leiden

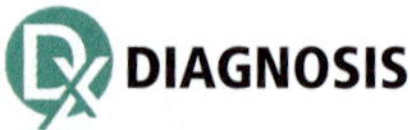

DIAGNOSIS

HISTORY

- Previous VTE
- Family history of VTE
- Family history of prothrombin 20210 mutation

PHYSICAL EXAM

- Unilateral swollen, erythematous, and tender calf is significant for a possible DVT.
- Positive Homans sign, sensitivity of 10–54%, specificity of 39–89% for DVT
- Tachycardia is the most common sign of a pulmonary embolism; however, patients may have chest pain and hypotension depending on the severity of the pulmonary embolus.
- A tender abdomen may be indicative of mesenteric veins thrombosis; however, other causes of an acute abdomen should be worked up as appropriate.

DIFFERENTIAL DIAGNOSIS

- Factor V Leiden mutation
- Protein C deficiency
- Protein S deficiency
- Antithrombin deficiency
- Other causes of activated protein C resistance (e.g., antiphospholipid antibodies)
- Dysfibrinogenemia
- Dysplasminogenemia
- Homocystinemia
- Elevated factor VIII levels

DIAGNOSTIC TESTS & INTERPRETATION

Screening for prothrombin G20210A mutation in asymptomatic individuals is not recommended, except for those with very strong family history. Testing can take place in patients with thrombosis at a very early age, recurrent unprovoked VTE, or those with thrombosis in unusual locations.

Initial Tests (lab, imaging)

- This mutation can be diagnosed using PCR with electrophoresis or immunoassays.
- Imaging should be obtained as appropriate for the suspected site of thrombosis: ultrasound with Doppler, computed tomography scan with contrast to evaluate venous phase, and V/Q scan.
- Testing for an inherited thrombophilic condition is reliable during an acute embolic event or with anticoagulation use.

Follow-Up Tests & Special Considerations

Although prothrombin levels are elevated, this is not a sensitive test to make the diagnosis.

Diagnostic Procedures/Other

MR angiography (MRA), venography, or arteriography to detect thrombosis

Test Interpretation

Imaging is likely to show presence of arterial or venous thrombus.

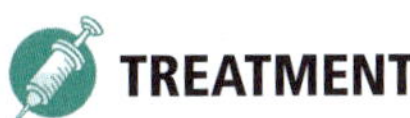

TREATMENT

GENERAL MEASURES

Management of patients with a first-time VTE with or without an acquired thrombophilic condition remains overall very similar.

MEDICATION

Is directed to treat those patients with VTE (prophylactic doses may vary). We recommend the reader to check the most updated doses, dose adjustments, and contraindications for the medications listed below. The doses listed apply to most adults.

First Line

In adult patients without cancer, the following oral anticoagulants are preferred over warfarin and low-molecular-weight heparin (LMWH): dabigatran, rivaroxaban, apixaban, or edoxaban is preferred over warfarin.

- Apixaban (Eliquis): Initial dose is 10 mg BID for 7 days, followed by 5 mg BID.
- Dabigatran (Pradaxa): requires initial parenteral anticoagulation for 5 to 10 days, followed by 150 mg BID
- Edoxaban (Savaysa): requires initial parenteral anticoagulation for 5 to 10 days, followed by 60 mg daily
- Rivaroxaban (Xarelto): Initial dose is 15 mg BID with food for 21 days, followed by a daily dose of 20 mg with food.

Second Line

For patients without cancer that cannot be treated with DOAC, warfarin is preferred over LMWH.

- Warfarin (Coumadin): Initial dose may range from 2 to 10 mg PO daily and then adjusted to an INR of 2 to 3.
- Enoxaparin (Lovenox): 1 mg/kg SC injection every 12 hours

ISSUES FOR REFERRAL

- Recurrent thrombosis on anticoagulation
- Difficulty anticoagulating
- Genetic counseling

SURGERY/OTHER PROCEDURES

- Anticoagulation must be held for surgical interventions.
- For most patients with DVT, recommendations are against routine use of vena cava filter in addition to anticoagulation, except in case with contraindication to anticoagulation.
- Thrombectomy may be necessary in some cases.

ADMISSION, INPATIENT, AND NURSING CONSIDERATIONS

- Admission criteria/initial stabilization: complicated thrombosis, such as pulmonary embolus; required heparin drip
- Patient can be safely discharged if patient is stable on anticoagulation.

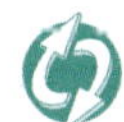

ONGOING CARE

- Compression stockings for prevention
- DVT prophylaxis as appropriate if patient admitted to hospital

FOLLOW-UP RECOMMENDATIONS

Patient Monitoring

- Warfarin use requires periodic (weekly and then monthly after initial stabilization) INR measurements, with a goal of 2 to 3.
- Heterozygosity for the prothrombin 20210 mutation increases the risk for recurrent VTE only slightly; thus, its presence does not alter the length of anticoagulation treatment decision.

DIET

- No restrictions; unless taking warfarin
- Food rich in vitamin K may interfere with warfarin anticoagulation.
- Grapefruit and St. John's wort interfere with the cytochrome P450 and can alter the levels and clearance of anticoagulant therapy.

PATIENT EDUCATION

Patients should be educated about:

- Use of oral anticoagulant therapy
- Signs and symptoms of acute blood loss
- Avoidance of NSAIDs while on warfarin

PROGNOSIS

When compared with normal individuals, persons with prothrombin 20210 have normal lifespans.

COMPLICATIONS

- Recurrent thrombosis on anticoagulation
- Bleeding on anticoagulation
- Complications are usually location dependent and can lead to death, possibly from a massive pulmonary embolism.
- Venous stasis ulcers

REFERENCES

1. Simioni P, Prandoni P, Lensing AW, et al. Risk for subsequent venous thromboembolic complications in carriers of the prothrombin or the factor V gene mutation with a first episode of deep-vein thrombosis. *Blood*. 2000;96(10):3329–3333.

ADDITIONAL READING

- Kearon C, Akl EA. Duration of anticoagulant therapy for deep vein thrombosis and pulmonary embolism. *Blood*. 2014;123(12):1794–1801.
- Moll S. Thrombophilias—practical implications and testing caveats. *J Thromb Thrombolysis*. 2006;21(1):7–15.
- Wells PS, Forgie MA, Rodger MA. Treatment of venous thromboembolism. *JAMA*. 2014;311(7):717–728.

SEE ALSO

Antithrombin Deficiency, Deep Vein Thrombophlebitis; Factor V Leiden; Protein C Deficiency; Protein S Deficiency

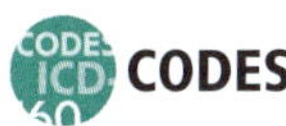

CODES

ICD10

D68.52 Prothrombin gene mutation

CLINICAL PEARLS

- Prothrombin 20210 mutation is the second most common inherited risk factor for VTE after factor V Leiden mutation.
- Asymptomatic patients with prothrombin 20210 mutation do not need anticoagulation or screening.
- Management of VTE is no different with or without the prothrombin G20210A mutation. However, indefinite anticoagulation may be considered in people with an unprovoked VTE or thrombus in a nontraditional area (mesenteric or cerebral).

PRURITUS ANI

Marie L. Borum, MD, EdD, MPH • Justin Paul Canakis, DO • Jacob Thomas Newman, DO

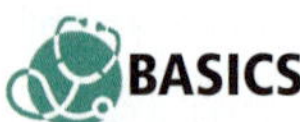

BASICS

DESCRIPTION

- Intense anal/perianal itching and/or burning
- Usually acute (defined as <6 weeks of symptoms)
- Classified as primary (idiopathic) or secondary (25–75% of cases) to anorectal pathology

EPIDEMIOLOGY

Incidence

- 1–5% of the general population
- Predominant age: 30 to 50 years; although seen in all age groups
- Predominant sex: male > female (4:1)

Prevalence

Difficult to estimate because many patients do not report symptoms; affects 1–5% of the population

ETIOLOGY AND PATHOPHYSIOLOGY

- Multiple etiologies categorized by inflammatory, infectious, systemic, neoplastic, anorectal disorders, neuropathic, neurogenic, and psychogenic causes (1),(2)
- Most cases are idiopathic (25–90%), which are likely due to trauma from wiping or scratching and perianal fecal contamination.
  - Soilage can be due to an abnormality of rectoanal inhibitory reflex and a lower threshold or transient internal anal sphincter relaxation.
- Depending on underlying etiology, itch pathway may be histamine mediated or nonhistamine mediated (1).
- Pruritus ani is typically intensely perceived by the patient due to dense innervation.
- Etiologies of secondary pruritus ani:
  - Inflammatory dermatologic diseases:
    - Allergic contact dermatitis (soaps, perfumes, or dyes in toilet paper, topical anesthetics, oral antibiotics)
    - Atopic dermatitis ± lichen simplex chronicus (Patients may also have asthma and/or eczema.)
    - Psoriasis (Lesions tend to be poorly demarcated, pale, and nonscaling.)
    - Seborrheic dermatitis
    - Scleroderma
    - Lichen planus (may be seen in patients with ulcerative colitis and myasthenia gravis)
    - Hidradenitis suppurativa
    - Radiation dermatitis (2)
  - Colorectal/anorectal diseases: rectal prolapse, hemorrhoids, fissures or fistulas, proctitis, chronic diarrhea/constipation, polyps
  - Infectious etiologies may be sexually transmitted: bacteria (gonorrhea, chlamydia, syphilis), viruses (herpes simplex virus [HSV], condyloma acuminata from human papillomavirus [HPV], molluscum), parasites (pinworms, lice, scabies, or bed bugs), fungi (*Candida* or dermatophytes like tinea); other bacteria (*Staphylococcus aureus*, β-hemolytic *Streptococcus*, *Corynebacterium minutissimum* [erythrasma]) (2)
  - Malignancies: melanoma, basal cell/squamous cell carcinoma, colorectal cancer, leukemia, lymphoma, or (uncommon) the presenting symptom of Bowen or Paget disease
  - Mechanical factors: vigorous cleaning and scrubbing, tight-fitting clothes, synthetic undergarments
  - Systemic diseases (often presents as generalized pruritus): diabetes mellitus (most common), cholestasis, chronic liver disease, renal failure, hyperthyroidism, anemia, HIV, vitamin or iron deficiencies, lumbosacral radiculopathy (particularly in the elderly)
  - Chemical irritants: local anesthetics, chemotherapy, diarrhea (often from antibiotic use)
  - Dietary elements (citrus, milk products, coffee, tea, cola, chocolate, beer, wine, tomatoes, nuts)
  - Psychogenic factors: anxiety–itch–anxiety cycle

RISK FACTORS

- Obesity
- Excess perianal hair growth and/or perspiration
- Underlying anorectal pathology
- Atopic disease
- Underlying anxiety disorder
- Caffeine intake has been correlated with symptoms.

GENERAL PREVENTION

- Good perianal hygiene; avoid overzealous cleaning.
- Avoid mechanical irritation of skin (vigorous cleaning or rubbing with dry toilet paper or baby wipes, harsh soaps or perfumed products, excessive scratching with fingernails, or tight/synthetic undergarments).
- Minimize moisture in perianal area (absorbent cotton in anal cleft may help keep area dry).
- Avoid laxative use (loose stool is an irritant).

COMMONLY ASSOCIATED CONDITIONS

- Psoriasis is seen in 5–55% of patients with pruritus ani.
- Coexisting anorectal disease, such as hemorrhoids, can be seen in up to 52% of patients with pruritus ani.

DIAGNOSIS

HISTORY

- Patients present with complaints of anal and/or perianal itching, burning, or excoriation.
- Inquire about:
  - Timing (when it started, when it is worse)
  - Perianal hygiene (frequency of cleansing and products used)
  - Change in bowel habits
  - Bleeding (spotting of toilet paper, melena, hematochezia)
  - Recent antibiotic use
  - Skin disorders (psoriasis, eczema)
  - Rectal or vaginal discharge, menstrual cycle
  - Dietary history: Focus on the "C's": caffeine, coffee, cola, chocolate, citrus, calcium (dairy) (2).
  - Medical history (hepatitis, iron deficiency anemia, and diabetes in particular)
  - Family history of colorectal cancer
  - Anal receptive intercourse
  - Change in toiletry products
  - Household members (particularly children) with itching (possible pinworms)
  - Pets
  - Clothing preference (tight, synthetic) (3)

PHYSICAL EXAM

- Perianal visual inspection for erythema, hemorrhoids, anal fissures, maceration, lichenification, warts, polyps, excoriations, neoplasia, stool seepage
- Classification based on gross appearance
  - Stage 1: erythema, inflamed appearance
  - Stage 2: lichenification
  - Stage 3: lichenification, coarse skin, potential fissures or ulcerations (3)
- Digital rectal exam to evaluate for masses, internal sphincter tone, pain
- Valsalva to evaluate for prolapse
- Anoscopy to evaluate for hemorrhoids, fissures, other internal lesions

DIFFERENTIAL DIAGNOSIS

"ITCHeS" acronym (4)

- **I**nfection: *Candida*, parasites (scabies, pinworms), HPV, HSV, bacterial (gram-positive bacteria, gonorrhea, chlamydia, syphilis)
- **T**opical irritants: soaps/detergents, garments, deodorants, perfumes, stool leakage
- **C**utaneous/**C**ancer/**C**olorectal: eczema, psoriasis, lichen planus, lichen sclerosus, seborrhea, skin cancer, extramammary Paget disease, Bowen disease, fistula, fissure, prolapse, hemorrhoids, colorectal cancer
- **H**ypersensitivity: foods, medications (colchicine, quinidine, mineral oil)
- e**S**ystemic: diabetes, iron deficiency anemia, uremia, cholestasis, hematologic malignancy

DIAGNOSTIC TESTS & INTERPRETATION

Initial Tests (lab, imaging)

Use history and exam to suggest a specific etiology, and guide testing:

- Pinworm tape test; stool for ova and parasites
- CBC, comprehensive metabolic panel, A1c, thyroid studies to identify underlying systemic disease
- Wood lamp examination will show coral-red fluorescence in erythrasma (2).
- Skin scraping with potassium hydroxide (KOH) prep for dermatophytes or candidiasis (as etiology or as superinfection) and mineral oil prep for scabies
- Perianal skin culture (bacterial superinfection)
- Hemoccult testing of stool

Pediatric Considerations

Pinworms are common in children. Consider perianal Crohn disease.

Follow-Up Tests & Special Considerations

Anal DNA polymerase chain reaction (PCR) probe for gonorrhea and chlamydia; may perform anal speculum exam and test for anal HPV if receptive anal intercourse; HIV testing in patients with HIV risk factors

Diagnostic Procedures/Other

- Biopsy suspicious lesions (e.g., lichenification, ulcerated epithelium, refractory cases) to exclude neoplasia; evaluate etiology.
- Consider colonoscopy if history, exam, or testing suggests colorectal pathology (family history of colorectal disease, especially if age >40 years, weight loss, rectal bleeding, change in bowel habits).

Geriatric Considerations

- Stool incontinence may be a predisposing factor.
- Consider systemic disease.
- Higher likelihood of colorectal pathology

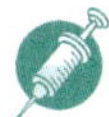

TREATMENT

GENERAL MEASURES

- Proper anal/perianal hygiene; avoid vigorous rubbing while cleansing after bowel movement. Use cotton swabs moistened with warm water instead of tissue paper. Avoid chemical and mechanical irritants and wear proper undergarments.
- High-fiber diet and/or bowel regimen to maintain regular bowel movements
- Avoid tight-fitting clothing. Use cotton undergarments.
- Avoiding moisture; absorbent cotton, talcum powder, or cornstarch if there is an excess moisture; can use hair dryer on cool setting to dry anal area (3)[C]
- Cotton gloves at night to control nocturnal scratching

MEDICATION

First Line

- Treat underlying infections: fungal or dermatophyte infection with topical imidazoles, bacterial infection with topical antibacterials.
- Treat underlying anorectal anatomic pathology: banding of prolapsing internal hemorrhoids, treat fistulas, or fissures.
- Break itch–scratch cycle with low-potency steroid cream such as hydrocortisone 1% ointment applied sparingly up to 4 times daily (3)[C]. Discontinue when itching subsides. Avoid use >2 weeks due to risk of skin atrophy.
- If no response with low-potency steroid, consider high-potency steroid cream.
- Antihistamines, particularly sedating antihistamines, may be useful in reducing nighttime itching until local measures take effect. Avoid in elderly patients due to anticholinergic properties.
- Tricyclic antidepressants may reduce nighttime scratching. SSRIs or gabapentin may be used in resistant cases (1)[C].
- Zinc oxide can be used after steroid course for barrier protection (2); petroleum jelly is another barrier. Avoid mineral oil as it can worsen pruritus.
- Albendazole for pinworm

Second Line

- Low-dose topical capsaicin cream in combination with steroid cream if refractory symptoms (3)[C]
- 0.03% tacrolimus ointment can be considered in cases not responsive to high potency steroids (3)[C].
- Intradermal methylene blue injections, sometimes known as anal tattooing, may be used to destroy nerve endings and create permanent anesthesia in cases not responsive to medical management (3)[C].
- Biologics, such as the IL-4 inhibitor dupilumab, show promise for recalcitrant cases, although there is limited data currently.

ISSUES FOR REFERRAL

- Intractable pruritus: Consider referral to gastroenterology (for colonoscopy) or dermatology (for additional treatment, possibly injections, or biopsies). Refractory or persistent symptoms should signal the possibility of underlying neoplasia because pruritus ani of long duration is associated with a greater likelihood of colorectal pathology.
- Refer for colonoscopy if at risk for colon cancer.

SURGERY/OTHER PROCEDURES

As above, especially if concern for malignancy is identified

ONGOING CARE

FOLLOW-UP RECOMMENDATIONS

- See patient every 2 weeks if not improving.
- Ensure proper hygiene and avoidance of irritants.
- Work up for systemic disease, and check for persistent lichenification. If refractory pruritus or lichenification does not resolve, consider underlying malignancy.

DIET

- Eliminate foods and beverages known or suspected to exacerbate symptoms: coffee, tea, chocolate, beer, cola, vitamin C tablets in excessive doses, citrus fruits, tomatoes, or spices.
- Eliminate foods or drugs contributing to loose bowel movements or dermatitis.
- Add fiber supplementation to bulk stools and prevent fecal leakage in patients who have fecal incontinence or partially formed stools.

PATIENT EDUCATION

- Review proper anal hygiene:
  - Resist overuse of soap and rubbing.
  - Avoid products with irritating perfumes and dyes.
  - Avoid use of ointments and mineral oil.
  - Wear loose, light cotton clothing.
  - If moisture is a problem, use cotton, unmedicated talcum powder, or cornstarch to keep the area dry.
  - Cleanse perianal area after bowel movements with water-moistened cotton.
  - Dry the area after bathing by patting with a soft towel or by using a hair dryer on cool setting (3)[C].
- Avoid medications that cause diarrhea or constipation.
- Avoid caffeine, cola, chocolate, citrus, tomatoes, tea, alcohol, nuts, and milk products (2).
- Use barrier protection if engaging in anal intercourse.
- If unable to completely empty rectum with defecation, use small plain-water enema (infant bulb syringe) after each bowel movement to prevent soiling and irritation.
- If persists, consider underlying medical disease.

PROGNOSIS

- Conservative treatment successful in ~90% of cases
- Idiopathic pruritus ani is often chronic—waxes and wanes.

COMPLICATIONS

- Bacterial superinfection at site of excoriations and potential abscess formation or penetrating infection via self-inoculation with colonic pathogens
- Lichenification
- Significant effect on quality of life

REFERENCES

1. Jakubauskas M, Dulskas A. Evaluation, management and future perspectives of anal pruritus: a narrative review. *Eur J Med Res*. 2023;28(1):57.
2. Sacks OA, Beresneva O. Causes and management of pruritus ani. *Dis Colon Rectum*. 2023;66(1):10–13.
3. Ortega AE, Delgadillo X. Idiopathic pruritus ani and acute perianal dermatitis. *Clin Colon Rectal Surg*. 2019;32(5):327–332.
4. Andrade A, Kuah CY, Martin-Lopez JE, et al. Interventions for chronic pruritus of unknown origin. *Cochrane Database Syst Rev*. 2020;1(1):CD013128.

ADDITIONAL READING

- Davies D, Bailey J. Diagnosis and management of anorectal disorders in the primary care setting. *Prim Care*. 2017;44(4):709–720.
- Felemovicius I, Ganz RA, Saremi M, et al. SOOTHER TRIAL: observational study of an over-the-counter ointment to heal anal itch. *Front Med (Lausanne)*. 2022;9:890883.

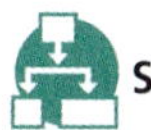

SEE ALSO

Pinworms; Pruritus Vulvae

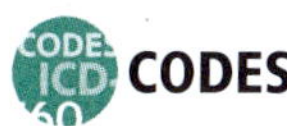

CODES

ICD10

L29.0 Pruritus ani

CLINICAL PEARLS

- Pruritus ani is characterized by anal/perianal itching and/or burning. It is a skin irritation with itch–scratch–itch cycle.
- Conservative treatment with perianal hygiene and reassurance is successful in 90% of patients.
- Consider trial of dietary elimination of "C's"—citrus, vitamin C supplements, calcium products, caffeine, coffee, cola, chocolate.
- Rule out infection (viral, bacterial, parasitic) in immunosuppressed patients.
- Consider underlying malignancy if refractory.

PRURITUS VULVAE

Livia Yumi Maruoka Nishi, MD • Trinity Simone Rosa Belgrave, BS, MS, MBBS

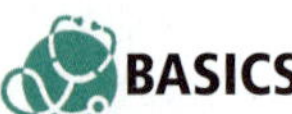

BASICS

DESCRIPTION

- Pruritus vulvae may be a symptom of any of several disorders or can itself be a primary diagnosis.
- Underlying conditions may cause vulvar pruritus, or it may be a primary diagnosis.
- It can be acute (<6 weeks) duration or chronic.
- Pruritus vulvae as a primary diagnosis may also be more appropriately documented as vulvodynia (see "Vulvodynia" topic) or burning vulva syndrome.

EPIDEMIOLOGY

Symptoms may occur at any age during a woman's lifetime.

- Young girls most commonly have infectious or hygiene etiology.
- The primary diagnosis is more common in postmenopausal women.

Incidence

The exact incidence is unknown, although most women complain of vulvar pruritus at some point in their lifetime.

Prevalence

- Prevalence not known
- Small US study found 6.6% women aged 20 to 59 experienced persistent genital itching or burning (1).

ETIOLOGY AND PATHOPHYSIOLOGY

- Etiology of condition can be due to inflammatory, infectious, and neoplastic processes that affect female genitalia. Nonlocal causes include systemic, genetic, psychogenic and neurogenic conditions (2).
- Age-related hormonal changes result in different risk factors in various age groups (2).
  - Early childhood (age 2 to 7 years) physiologic and skin and vaginal flora changes
  - Prepubertal atopic and irritant dermatitis, dermatoses, and infections
  - Postmenopausal atrophy increases risk of infection, irritation.

RISK FACTORS

Vary depending on etiology

- High-risk sexual behavior
- Immunosuppression
- Autoimmune disease
- Medication

GENERAL PREVENTION

- Hygiene
- Avoid irritants.
- Tight-fitting clothing should be avoided.
- Only cotton underwear should be worn.
- Management of associated systemic conditions

COMMONLY ASSOCIATED CONDITIONS

- Infectious etiology
  - Vaginal or vulvar candida
  - *Gardnerella vaginalis*
  - *Trichomonas*
  - Human papillomavirus
  - Herpes simplex virus
  - Dermatophytosis
  - Parasites: scabies, *Pthirus pubis*
- Vulvar vestibulitis
- Dermatoses
  - Lichen sclerosus (LS)
  - Lichen planus (LP)
  - Lichen simplex chronicus (LSC)
- Malignant or premalignant conditions
- Immune mediated
  - Autoimmune progesterone dermatitis: perimenstrual eruptions
  - Irritant or allergic contact dermatitis
  - Atopic dermatitis
  - Psoriasis
- Fecal or urinary incontinence
- Neurogenic
  - Small fiber polyneuropathy (SFPN)—amyloidosis, vitamin B_{12} deficiency, sarcoidosis (3)
- Extramammary Paget disease
- Dietary: methylxanthines (e.g., coffee, cola), tomatoes, peanuts

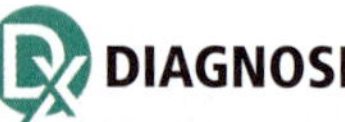

DIAGNOSIS

Diagnosis depends on etiology. Delayed diagnosis can have profound negative effect on women's sexual comfort and quality of life (4).

HISTORY

- Duration of symptoms
- Timing of symptoms (scabies often worse at night)
- Other medical diagnosis (eczema, psoriasis, renal failure)
- Medications SGLT-2, repeated courses of steroids, antibiotics: increased risk of candida infections
- Associated change in vaginal discharge
- Dyspareunia/postcoital bleeding

PHYSICAL EXAM

- Visual inspection of the vulva, vagina, perineum, and anus
- Superior surfaces of the labia majora—extending from mons to the anal orifice—are most involved
- Vulvar skin is leathery or lichenified in appearance.
- Papillomatosis may be a sign of chronic inflammation.
- Cotton swab–applied pressure to area of pain and to vestibular glands
- Musculoskeletal evaluation to confirm not contributing if persistent vulvar pain
- Oral cavity: several conditions have oral manifestations (LP)

DIFFERENTIAL DIAGNOSIS

- Acute pruritus
  - Infection: vaginal candidiasis, bacterial vaginosis
- Acute/chronic
  - Inflammatory: atopic dermatitis, dermatoses, contact dermatitis, psoriasis
  - Postmenopausal/estrogen suppression atrophic vaginitis/Zoon vulvitis
- Neoplastic

DIAGNOSTIC TESTS & INTERPRETATION

Diagnostic testing determined by specific considerations based on history and exam

Initial Tests (lab, imaging)

- Infectious cause
- Microscopy
  - Sodium chloride: *Gardnerella* or *Trichomonas*
  - 10% potassium hydroxide: *Candida*
- Culture
  - Viral culture or polymerase chain reaction: herpes simplex virus
  - Repeated yeast infections consider culture for resistant *Candida* species
- Systemic cause: HbA1c, HIV, vitamin B_{12}
- Neurogenic: imaging (L4–S2)
- Colposcopy with acetic acid or Lugol solution of vagina and vulva

Follow-Up Tests & Special Considerations

- A patch test may be performed by a dermatologist to assist in identifying a causative agent if contact dermatitis is suspected or if topical products are suspected as source of dermatitis.
- Exam-directed tissue biopsies are essential in the postmenopausal population to rule out malignancy.

Diagnostic Procedures/Other

- Vulvar biopsy is recommended by ACOG for
  - Immunocompromised patients (HIV)
  - Concern for malignancy
  - Lesions which fail to respond or, worsen in response to standard treatment
  - Atypical lesion
  - Uncertain diagnosis
- Biopsies should be collected from any ulceration, discoloration, raised areas, macerated areas, and the area of most intense pruritus.

Test Interpretation

- Only in the absence of pathologic findings can the primary diagnosis of pruritus vulvae be made.
- Biopsies of visible lesions most commonly show LSC (25%), LS (20%), or chronic inflammation (15%).

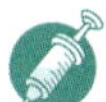

TREATMENT

Treatment guided by primary underlying etiology; considerations for possible exacerbating factors particularly in cases of chronic symptoms

GENERAL MEASURES

- Stop all potential irritants.
- Eliminate bacterial and fungal infection.
- Treat systemic disease
- Cool the affected area: Use cool gel packs (not ice packs, which may cause further injury).
- Sitz baths and bland emollients to soothe fissured or eroded skin

MEDICATION

First Line

- Inflammatory: topical steroids (2)
  - Ointments more effective
  - Short-term use (2 to 4 weeks)
- Eczema/psoriasis/allergic or irritant dermatitis, LS, LSC: mid- to high-potency steroids (triamcinolone, clobetasol)
- LP: low-potency steroids (hydrocortisone); patients with vulvovaginal LP typically do not achieve complete symptom control (5).
- Infections
  - Candidiasis: oral antifungals: fluconazole, topical antifungals: clotrimazole
  - Scabies: permethrin cream
  - Genital herpes: oral antivirals: valacyclovir, acyclovir
- Neuropathic:
  - Burns, scars, postradiation SFPN: topical anesthetics, oral SSRI, TCA (amitriptyline), gabapentin
- 1st-Generation antihistamines
  - Hydroxyzine: Initiate with 10 mg before bedtime (slowly increase up to 100 mg).
  - Doxepin: Initiate with 10 mg before bedtime.
- 2nd-Generation antihistamines are of little benefit.

Second Line

Inflammatory long term

- Calcineurin inhibitors such as 1% pimecrolimus (6)[A]

ISSUES FOR REFERRAL

- Persistent symptoms should prompt additional investigation and referral to a dermatologist, gynecologist, or gynecologic oncologist.
- Dermatology referral for patch testing to evaluate for contact dermatitis

ADDITIONAL THERAPIES

- Sacral neuromodulation device
- Laser therapy
- GnRH analogues
- Naltrexone

ONGOING CARE

- Frequent evaluation, repeat cultures, and biopsies are necessary for cases resistant to treatment.
- Refractory cases may require referral to gynecologist or gynecologic oncology for further management.

FOLLOW-UP RECOMMENDATIONS

Follow-up is typically recommended within 1 to 3 months of the initial evaluation, with subsequent visits tailored to the patient's condition, treatment response, and individual needs.

DIET

Dietary alterations include avoidance of the following:

- Coffee and other caffeine-containing beverages
- Tomatoes
- Peanuts

PATIENT EDUCATION

- American College of Obstetricians and Gynecologists: https://www.acog.org
- National Vulvodynia Association: https://www.nva.org

PROGNOSIS

Conservative measures and short-term topical steroids control most patients' symptoms.

COMPLICATIONS

- Contact dermatitis
  - Postinflammatory hypopigmentation or hyperpigmentation to skin
  - Secondary infections bacterial, dermatophytes, candida, viruses
  - Untreated contact dermatitis may with excessive itching progress to LSC.
- LS
  - Even with treatment may impact patient's quality of life, self-esteem, diminished sexual activity, and sexual disfunction
  - Progression to mental health conditions particularly anxiety-depressive disorder; risk for progression related to severity of symptoms
  - Progression to vestibulodynia, vulvodynia
  - Scaring may lead to architectural changes which may result in dyspareunia, urinary dysfunction and psychosexual distress
  - Not considered precancerous but vulvar cancer reported in 2–5% of patients
- LP
  - Vulvar SCC reported in 3–6% of patients with erosive LP

REFERENCES

1. Harlow BL, Wise LA, Stewart EG. Prevalence and predictors of chronic lower genital tract discomfort. *Am J Obstet Gynecol*. 2001;185(3):545–550.
2. Mashoudy KD, Tomlinson AF, Kim S, et al. Scratching the surface: a comprehensive guide to understanding and managing vulvovaginal itching. *Am J Clin Dermatol*. 2025;26(3):361–378.
3. Raef HS, Elmariah SB. Vulvar pruritus: a review of clinical associations, pathophysiology and therapeutic management. *Frontiers Med (Lausanne)*. 2021;8:649402.
4. Kellogg Spadt S, Kusturiss E. Vulvar dermatoses: a primer for the sexual medicine clinician. *Sex Med Rev*. 2015;3(3):126–136.
5. Tziotzios C, Brier T, Lee JYW, et al. Lichen planus and lichenoid dermatoses: Conventional and emerging therapeutic strategies. *J Am Acad Dermatol*. 2018;79(5):807–818.
6. Chi CC, Kirtschig G, Baldo M, et al. Systematic review and meta-analysis of randomized controlled trials on topical interventions for genital lichen sclerosus. *J Am Acad Dermatol*. 2012;67(2):305–312.

ADDITIONAL READING

- American College of Obstetricians and Gynecologists' Committee on Practice Bulletins—Gynecology. Diagnosis and management of vulvar skin disorders: ACOG practice bulletin, number 224. *Obstet Gynecol*. 2020;136(1):e1–e14. doi:10.1097/AOG.0000000000003944.
- Pichardo-Geisinger R. Atopic and contact dermatitis of the vulva. *Obstet Gynecol Clin North Am*. 2017;44(3):371–378.
- Savas JA, Pichardo RO. Female Genital Itch. *Dermatol Clin*. 2018;36(3):225–243. doi:10.1016/j.det.2018.02.006.

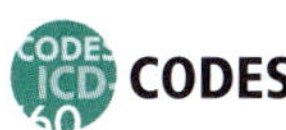

CODES

ICD10

- L29.2 Pruritus vulvae
- N94.819 Vulvodynia, unspecified

CLINICAL PEARLS

- Pruritus vulvae is a common complaint with many etiologies.
- Pruritus vulvae is a diagnosis of exclusion once other causes of itching have been ruled out.
- Initial treatment is conservative.
- Exam-directed biopsies from any ulceration, discoloration, raised areas, macerated areas, and the area of most intense pruritus are essential to rule out malignancy.
- Even with appropriate treatment, patients can suffer from significant impairment to quality of life and sexual function as a result of these conditions.

PSEUDOFOLLICULITIS BARBAE

George C. Umeh, MD

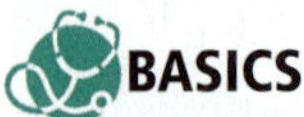

BASICS

DESCRIPTION

- Foreign body inflammatory reaction from an ingrown hair resulting in the appearance of papules and pustules. This is found mainly in the bearded area (barbae) but may occur in other hairy locations such as the scalp, axilla, or pubic areas where shaving is done.
- A mechanical problem: extrafollicular and transfollicular hair penetration
- System(s) affected: skin/exocrine
- Synonym(s): chronic sycosis barbae; pili incarnati; folliculitis barbae traumatica; razor bumps; shaving bumps; tinea barbae

EPIDEMIOLOGY

- Predominant age: postpubertal, middle age (14 to 25 years)
- Predominant sex: male > female (can be seen in females of all races who wax/shave)

Incidence

- Adult male African Americans: unknown
- Adult male whites: unknown

Prevalence

- Widespread in Fitzpatrick skin types IV to VI (darker complexions) who shave
- 45–83% of African American soldiers who shave

ETIOLOGY AND PATHOPHYSIOLOGY

- Transfollicular escape of the low-cut hair shaft as it tries to exit the skin is accompanied by inflammation and often an intraepidermal abscess.
- As the hair enters the dermis, more severe inflammation occurs, with downgrowth of the epidermis in an attempt to sheath the hair.
- A foreign body reaction forms at the tip of the invading hair, followed by abscess formation.
- Shaving too close
- Plucking/tweezing or wax depilation of hair may cause abnormal hair growth in injured follicles.

Genetics

- People with curly hair have an asymmetric accumulation of acidic keratin hHa8 on hair shaft.
- Single-nucleotide polymorphism (disruption Ala12Thr substitution) affects keratin of hair follicle.

RISK FACTORS

- Curly hair
- Shaving too close or shaving with multiple razor strokes
- Plucking/tweezing hairs
- South Mediterranean/American, Middle Eastern, Asian, or African descent (skin types IV to VI)

GENERAL PREVENTION

- Prior to shaving, rinse face with warm water to hydrate and soften hairs.
- Use adjustable hair clippers that leave very low hair length above skin.
- Shave with either a manual adjustable razor at coarsest setting (avoids close shaves), a single-edge blade razor (e.g., Bump Fighter), a foil-guarded razor (e.g., PFB razor), or electric triple "O-head" razor.
- Empty razor of hair frequently.
- Shave in the direction of hair growth. Do not overstretch skin when shaving.
- Use a generous amount of the correct shaving cream/gel (e.g., Ef-Kay shaving gel, Edge shaving gel, Aveeno therapeutic shave gel, Easy Shave medicated shaving cream).
- Daily shaving reduces papules/pruritus.
- Regular use of depilatories

COMMONLY ASSOCIATED CONDITIONS

- Keloidal folliculitis
- Pseudofolliculitis nuchae

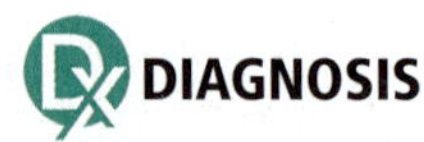

DIAGNOSIS

HISTORY

Pain on shaving; pruritus of shaved areas, irritated "razor bumps"?

PHYSICAL EXAM

- Tender, exudative, erythematous follicular papules or pustules in beard area (less commonly in scalp, axilla, and pubic areas); range from 2 to 4 mm
- Hyperpigmented "razor or shave bumps"?
- Alopecia
- Lusterless, brittle hair

DIFFERENTIAL DIAGNOSIS

- Bacterial folliculitis
- Impetigo
- Acne vulgaris
- Tinea barbae
- Sarcoidal papules

DIAGNOSTIC TESTS & INTERPRETATION

Initial Tests (lab, imaging)

- Clinical diagnosis
- Culture of pustules: usually sterile; may show coagulase-negative *Staphylococcus epidermidis* (normal skin flora)
- Additional hormonal testing may be indicated in females with hirsutism and/or polycystic ovary syndrome: dehydroepiandrosterone sulfate, luteinizing hormone (LH)/follicle-stimulating hormone (FSH), and free and total testosterone (1)[C].

Test Interpretation

Follicular papules and pustules

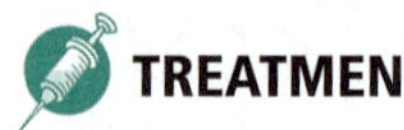

TREATMENT

GENERAL MEASURES

- Effective treatment for PFB requires a multifaceted approach that targets various aspects of the pathogenesis (2).
- Mild cases: Stop shaving or avoid close shaving for 30 days while keeping beard groomed and clean (3). Consider 5% benzoyl peroxide after shaving and application of 1% hydrocortisone cream at bedtime (or LactiCare-HC lotion after shaving); tretinoin 0.025% cream; apply daily.
- Acute treatment
  - Dislodge embedded hair with sterile needle/tweezers.
  - Discontinue shaving until red papules have resolved (minimum 3 to 4 weeks; longer if moderate or severe); can trim to length >0.5 cm during this time
  - Massage beard area with washcloth, coarse sponge, or a soft brush several times daily.
  - Hydrocortisone 1–2.5% cream to relieve inflammation
  - Selenium sulfide if seborrhea is present and to help reduce pruritus
  - Systemic antibiotics if secondary infection is present

Pregnancy Considerations

Do not use tretinoin (Retin-A) or tetracycline.

MEDICATION

First Line

- Topical or systemic antibiotic for secondary infection
  - Application of clindamycin (Cleocin T) solution BID or topical erythromycin
  - Low-dose erythromycin or tetracycline 250 to 500 mg PO BID for more severe inflammation
  - Benzoyl peroxide 5% and clindamycin 1% gel BID: Administer until papule/pustule resolves.
- Mild cases: tretinoin 0.025% cream at bedtime; combination of the above therapies
- Moderate disease/chemical depilatories
  - Disrupt cross-linking of disulfide bonds of hair to produce blunt (less sharp) hair tip.
  - Apply no more frequently than every third day: 2% barium sulfide (Magic shaving cream) or calcium thioglycolate (Surgex); calcium hydroxide (Nair)
- Contraindications
  - Clindamycin: hypersensitivity history; history of regional enteritis or ulcerative colitis; history of antibiotic-associated colitis
  - Erythromycin, tetracycline, tretinoin: hypersensitivity history
- Chemical depilatories: Use cautiously; frequent use and prolonged application may lead to irritant contact dermatitis and chemical burns.
- Tetracycline: Avoid in pregnancy
- Tretinoin: Avoid in pregnancy; severe skin irritation
- Benzoyl peroxide: skin irritation and dryness, allergic contact dermatitis
- Hydrocortisone cream: local skin irritation, skin atrophy with prolonged use, lightening of skin color

Second Line

- Chemical peels with either glycolic acid or salicylic acid
- Consider eflornithine HCl cream (Vaniqa) to reduce hair growth and stiffness in combination with other therapies.

ISSUES FOR REFERRAL

- Worsening or poor response to the above therapies after 4 to 6 weeks should prompt dermatology consultation.
- Occupational demands may also prompt earlier referral to dermatology for more aggressive therapy.

SURGERY/OTHER PROCEDURES

Laser treatment with long-pulsed Nd:YAG is helpful for severe cases.

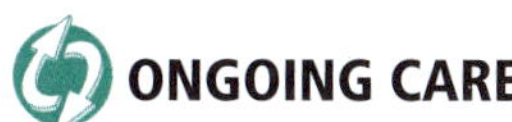

ONGOING CARE

FOLLOW-UP RECOMMENDATIONS

Patient Monitoring

Educate patient on curative and preventive treatment, including the possibility of growing out beard rather than shaving.

DIET

- No restrictions
- No dietary studies available

PATIENT EDUCATION

https://skinofcolorsociety.org/patient-dermatology-education/1408-2/

PROGNOSIS

- Good, with preventive methods
- Prognosis is poor in the presence of progressive scarring and foreign body granuloma formation.

COMPLICATIONS

- Scarring (occasionally keloidal)
- Foreign body granuloma formation
- Disfiguring postinflammatory hyperpigmentation (use sunscreens; can treat with hydroquinone 4% cream, Retin-A, clinical peels)
- Impetiginization of inflamed skin
- Epidermal (erythema, crusting, burns with scarring) and pigmentary changes with laser

REFERENCES

1. Quarles FN, Brody H, Johnson BA, et al. Pseudofolliculitis barbae. *Dermatol Ther*. 2007;20(3):133–136.
2. Dalia Y, Khatib J, Odens H, et al. Review of treatments for pseudofolliculitis barbae. *Clin Exp Dermatol*. 2023;48(6):591–598.
3. Nussbaum D, Friedman A. Pseudofolliculitis barbae: a review of current treatment options. *J Drugs Dermatol*. 2019;18(3):246–250.

ADDITIONAL READING

- Kundu RV, Patterson S. Dermatologic conditions in skin of color: part II. disorders occurring predominately in skin of color. *Am Fam Physician*. 2013;87(12):859–865.
- Taylor SC, Barbosa V, Burgess C, et al. Hair and scalp disorders in adult and pediatric patients with skin of color. *Cutis*. 2017;100(1):31–35.

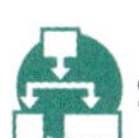

SEE ALSO

Folliculitis; Impetigo

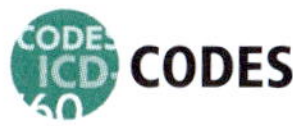

CODES

ICD10

- L73.1 Pseudofolliculitis barbae
- B35.0 Tinea barbae and tinea capitis
- L73.8 Other specified follicular disorders

CLINICAL PEARLS

- Electrolysis is not recommended as a treatment. It is expensive, painful, and often unsuccessful.
- Combination of laser therapy with eflornithine is more effective than laser alone.
- The unpleasant smell of sulfur could be a problem with some depilatory products.
- Have patient test for skin sensitivity with a small (coin sized) amount of the depilatory on the bearded area or forearm.

PSEUDOGOUT (CALCIUM PYROPHOSPHATE DIHYDRATE)

Sarah A. Pierotti, DO, FAAP, CAQSM • Oswald Ramos Tuarez, MD

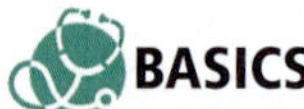

BASICS

- Terminology "pseudogout" falling out of favor
- Recommended nomenclature includes calcium pyrophosphate dihydrate (CPPD) deposition as it encompasses all conditions: CPPD deposition/disease, chondrocalcinosis, pseudogout, and pyrophosphate arthropathy

DESCRIPTION

- Acute or chronic, autoinflammatory arthropathy triggered by CPPD crystal deposition within cartilage or synovium of joints
- Should be differentiated from other crystal-induced arthropathies:
  - CPPD crystals: chondrocalcinosis, pseudogout, and pyrophosphate arthropathy
  - Monosodium urate crystals: gout
  - Hydroxyapatite: ankylosing spondylitis, osteoarthritis, or vascular calcification
- Clinical phenotypes:
  - Asymptomatic CPPD: incidental finding of chondrocalcinosis on XR
  - Acute CPPD arthritis (acute, self-limiting, synovitis) approximately 25% of CPPD (1)
    - Rule out septic arthritis promptly!
    - Can be brought on by joint trauma, medical illness, or surgery (hip replacement, post parathyroidectomy)
  - Chronic CPPD crystal inflammatory arthritis: often refer as "pseudorheumatoid arthritis," approximately 50% of CPPD disease (1); recurring inflammatory episodes result in more severe articular damage than OA
  - CPPD can occur in spinal tissues, intervertebral discs, spinal ligaments, and at C2 vertebra ("crowned dens syndrome").
  - Pseudoneuropathic arthropathy: similar to Charcot arthropathy with severe joint degeneration from CPPD but normal neurologic function; rare
  - Tumoral deposits of CPP crystals in soft tissues leading to damage can be confused for cancer; rare

Incidence

Poorly understood given difficulty in identifying asymptomatic cases

Prevalence

- Thought to affect 4–7% of adults in Europe and United States
- No gender predominance
- Chondrocalcinosis noted on appendicular XR demonstrates prevalence of 7–13% at 60 years of age, 50% in those >80 years of age (2)

ETIOLOGY AND PATHOPHYSIOLOGY

- Incompletely understood
- Two-part: crystal formation/deposition and inflammatory response:
  - Formation: complexation of anionic pyrophosphate (PPi) in articular cartilage; PPi binds to calcium to form CPP crystals; clearance dependent upon pyrophosphate driven by stimulation of anaplastic lymphoma kinase (ALK) by magnesium (2)
  - Deposition: Cartilage matrix is a complimentary environment for crystal formation, commonly within fibrocartilage (meniscus), hyaline cartilage, or those undergoing chondroid metaplasia (2).
  - Inflammatory response: triggered by monoclinic needle shape > triclinic rod shaped crystals; resulting IL-1β production and neutrophil recruitment into the joint leading to inflammation and damage

Genetics

- Most cases are sporadic; rare familial pattern with autosomal dominant inheritance (<1% of patients)
- Associated gene mutations: ANKH and TNFRSF11B

RISK FACTORS

Advanced age; joint trauma; osteoarthritis, medications (loop diuretics, pamidronate, GM-CSF)

GENERAL PREVENTION

- Colchicine 0.6 mg BID may be used prophylactically in recurrent CPPD.
- Treatment of underlying associated conditions may be beneficial

COMMONLY ASSOCIATED CONDITIONS

- Hypomagnesemia: Magnesium assists in clearance of CPP crystals, cofactor of pyrophosphatase.
- Hypophosphatasia: low functional alkaline phosphatase
- Hyperparathyroidism: altered calcium metabolism
- Hemochromatosis: Iron has an inhibitory action on pyrophosphatases
- Gout
- Amyloidosis
- Hypothyroidism
- Wilson disease
- Familial hypocalciuric hypercalcemia
- X-linked hypophosphatemic rickets
- Acromegaly

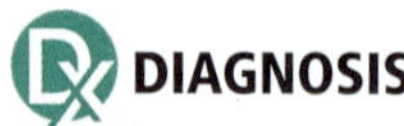

DIAGNOSIS

HISTORY

- Presentation may mimic gout or septic arthritis.
- Acute onset most common; may be chronic or recurrent
- Monoarticular or oligoarticular arthritis with associated redness, warmth, swelling, most commonly affecting knees (50% of cases), wrists, MCP, ankles, shoulders or elbows
- Possible low-grade fever during acute flares
- Symptoms last weeks to months (vs. gout: days)
- Can mimic RA with multiple symmetric joints involved, although rare (<5%)
- History: possible joint trauma, surgery, underlying metabolic disease; some concern for recent intra-articular hyaluronan
- Chronic CPPD: progressive degenerative arthritis with superimposed acute inflammatory attacks

PHYSICAL EXAM

- Signs of inflammation: erythema, edema, warm, and tender, may mimic osteo/rheumatoid or septic arthritis with joint deformity, swelling
- Decreased ROM

DIFFERENTIAL DIAGNOSIS

- Septic arthritis: *Rule out first.*
- Gout
- Osteoarthritis
- Rheumatoid arthritis
- Crystal arthropathies (e.g., hydroxyapatite deposition disease)
- Infection: Lyme disease, postinfectious/reactive arthritis
- Trauma/hemarthrosis

DIAGNOSTIC TESTS & INTERPRETATION

Validated classification criteria established in 2023 by ACR/EULAR (3)[B]

Initial Tests (lab, imaging)

- Labs: CBC, blood culture (if ruling out sepsis/septic joint)
- Joint aspiration with fluid analysis (cell count, gram stain, crystal search, culture)
  - Cell count 2,000 to 100,000 WBCs/mL with neutrophil predominance (80–90%)
    - >50,000 WBC count increases likelihood of septic arthritis
    - Majority of CPPD crystals are non-birefringent which can lead to high rates of false-negative fluid analysis.
- Imaging: XR affected joint
  - Effective in identifying calcification in cartilage, synovium, capsule or tendons
    - Punctate/linear calcifications in fibrocartilage (especially knee, hip, pubic symphysis and wrists)
      - Chronic CPPD: subchondral cysts and loose bodies found in joints not typically affected by degenerative disease
  - Neither sensitive nor specific

Follow-Up Tests & Special Considerations

- Labs: serum CMP, ALK, calcium, phosphorus, magnesium, iron, TIBC, ferritin, TSH, PTH
  - May rule out underlying conditions; but no utility in identifying CPPD
- Imaging: US or CT if XR is of low yield
  - Recent international guidelines provide criteria for identifying CPPD-related calcifications using US or CT
  - US: joint effusion, synovial thickening, hyperechoic deposits: May be more useful than plain radiography for diagnosis in peripheral joints (positive predictive value 92% and negative predictive value 93%) (4)[C]
  - CT more useful for challenging locations, can detect crowned dens syndrome which is diagnostic (5)

P

Diagnostic Procedures/Other

ALERT
Rule out septic joint with fluid aspiration.

Test Interpretation

- Synovial fluid analysis with demonstration of CPPD crystals is required for diagnosis.
- Crystal search: weakly positive birefringent, mostly rhomboid or rod-shaped CPPD crystals with polarizing light microscopy (*gold standard*) (3),(5)

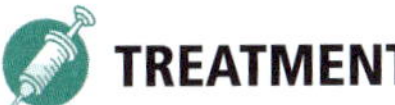

TREATMENT

GENERAL MEASURES

Conservative measures:

- Symptom relief: ice, rest, compresses
- Off-load: splinting, gait assistance with crutches/walker

MEDICATION

First Line

Intra-articular steroid (1 to 2 joints)

- Aspiration with glucocorticoid preferred (5)[C]
- If multiple joints/injection not feasible: systemic NSAIDs, colchicine, or oral/parenteral glucocorticoids
- Triamcinolone acetonide: 40 to 80 mg with 1 to 2 mL lidocaine (large joints)
- Prednisolone–sodium phosphate 4 to 20 mg

ALERT
Steroid should not be used until septic arthritis has been ruled out.

- NSAIDs (take with food) (5)[C]
- Ibuprofen 600 to 800 mg PO q6–8 h; max 3.2 g/day
- Naproxen 500 mg PO BID
  - Taper after symptoms improve; typical duration 1 to 2 weeks
- Other NSAIDs effective; indomethacin higher complication rates (relative risk [RR] = 2.2) versus ibuprofen (RR = 1.2)
- Colchicine (5)[C]
  - Acute flare: 1.2 to 1.8 mg on day 1 (e.g., 1 mg followed by 0.5 to 0.6 mg 1 hour later), then 0.5 to 0.6 mg twice daily until resolution
  - Chronic or prophylaxis: 0.5 to 0.6 mg twice daily to reduce frequency of attacks (5)
  - Side effects primarily gastrointestinal

Second Line

Oral prednisone or equivalent: 30 to 50 mg/day for 10 to 14 days with a taper to avoid rebound symptoms

- For patient unable to take oral route or contraindicated intra-articular injection, parenteral route has demonstrated efficacy; triamcinolone acetonide 40 mg IM once

ALERT
Recent randomized trial: no significant effect of methotrexate in chronic-recurrent CPPD

ISSUES FOR REFERRAL

For atypical, chronic, or failing first-line therapy, refer to rheumatology, orthopedics.

ADDITIONAL THERAPIES

- Conservative measures: ice, compression, heat
- Physical therapy: isometrics initially, progress to ROM and loading exercises as tolerated
- Magnesium supplementation: A small trial showed symptom improvement; placebo effects noted; further studies needed
- Additional therapies for chronic CPPD
  - ACTH, anakinra, hydroxychloroquine, infliximab, probenecid, magnesium, ethylenediaminetetraacetic acid (EDTA) suggested; large scale studies needed to evaluate effectiveness (6)[C]

SURGERY/OTHER PROCEDURES

- Hyaluronic acid: controversial as it may trigger flares in some cases
- Surgical intervention: severe joint damage/instability; lack of RCT; procedural recommendation based on clinical practice and patient needs based on arthritis management
  - Arthroplasty, synovectomy, joint débridement, lavage, arthroplasty
  - Consider removal of large/space-occupying tophaceous lesions.

ADMISSION, INPATIENT, AND NURSING CONSIDERATIONS

- No established admission criteria.
- Septic arthritis (synovial WBC >50,000/mL) admit promptly. Admission is prudent to expedite work up, antibiotic administration, and orthopedic consultation.
- Nonseptic joint: based on clinical judgment; focus on pain management and treatment; pain management: IV with transition to oral.

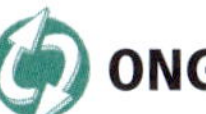

ONGOING CARE

FOLLOW-UP RECOMMENDATIONS

Multidisciplinary team approach: appropriate follow-up with primary care, specialists, and/or PT

Patient Monitoring

- Reevaluate response 48 to 72 hours after beginning treatment; reexamine in 1 week.
- Consider follow-up every 3 to 6 months for flares, symptom monitoring, and evaluation of joint damage.

PATIENT EDUCATION

- Educate on triggers: trauma, symptomps, metabolic imbalances.
- Promote joint health with activity/exercise.

PROGNOSIS

- Acute CPP crystal arthritis is self-limited. Inflammation typically resolves within days to weeks with appropriate treatment.
- Long-term outcomes depend on timely management of flares, control of inflammation, and treatment of associated metabolic disorders to limit joint damage. Patients may experience progressive joint damage and functional limitation with recurrent attacks.

COMPLICATIONS

CPPD may lead to:

- Chronic joint damage and cartilage breakdown, especially in patients with underlying joint comorbidities such as osteoarthritis and may require arthroplasty
- Tenosynovitis, carpal/cubital tunnel syndrome, or nodules ("tophi") due to periarticular crystal deposits
- Recurrent acute inflammatory attacks

Geriatric Considerations

- Higher risk for GI bleeding and acute renal insufficiency in elderly warranting close monitoring/education when taking NSAIDs
- Colchicine associated with high rates of renal insufficiency in elderly patients; avoid loading dose.

REFERENCES

1. Rosenthal AK, Ryan LM. Calcium pyrophosphate deposition disease. *N Engl J Med*. 2016;374(26):2575–2584.
2. Pascart T, Filippou G, Lioté F, et al. Calcium pyrophosphate deposition disease. *Lancet Rheumatol*. 2024;6(11):e791–e804.
3. Abhishek A, Tedeschi SK, Pascart T, et al. The 2023 ACR/EULAR classification criteria for calcium pyrophosphate deposition disease. *Ann Rheum Dis*. 2023;82(10):1248–1257.
4. Zhang W, Doherty M, Pascual E, et al. EULAR recommendations for calcium pyrophosphate deposition. Part II: management. *Ann Rheum Dis*. 2011;70(4):571–575.
5. Voulgari PV, Venetsanopoulou AI, Drosos AA. Recent advances in the therapeutic management of calcium pyrophosphate deposition disease. *Front Med (Lausanne)*. 2024;11:1327715.
6. Pascart T, Richette P, Flipo RM. Treatment of nongout joint deposition diseases: an update. *Arthritis*. 2014;2014:375202.

ADDITIONAL READING

Macmullan P, McCarthy G. Treatment and management of pseudogout: insights for the clinician. *Ther Adv Musculoskelet Dis*. 2012;4(2):121–131.

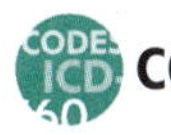

CODES

ICD10

- M11.20 Other chondrocalcinosis, unspecified site
- M11.269 Other chondrocalcinosis, unspecified knee
- M11.29 Other chondrocalcinosis, multiple sites

CLINICAL PEARLS

- Perform arthrocentesis to confirm diagnosis.
- Rule out septic arthritis before initiating treatment especially intraarticular steroids.
- NSAIDs are preferred pharmacologic treatment for acute flare (intraarticular or oral steroids are acceptable if appropriate).
- Suspect CPPD in arthritis cases that do not follow a pattern typical of degenerative joint disease.

PSORIASIS

Karl T. Clebak, MD, MHA, FAAFP • Roland W. Newman II, DO • Madeline E. Lee, MD

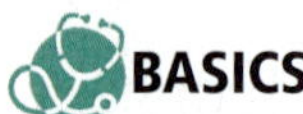

BASICS

DESCRIPTION

- A chronic, inflammatory disorder commonly characterized by cutaneous erythematous plaques with silvery scale, and varying phenotypes and severity
- Clinical phenotypes:
  - Plaque (vulgaris): ~80% of cases; well-demarcated, red plaques with silvery scale on the scalp, extensor surfaces, and trunk
  - Guttate: <2% of psoriasis patients, usually in patients <30 years of age; abrupt onset of 1- to 10-mm droplet-shaped papules with fine scale on the trunk/extremities, often after strep infection 2 to 3 weeks prior; typically, self-limiting and may resolve spontaneously
  - Inverse: affects intertriginous areas and flexural surfaces; pink-red plaques with minimal scale, without satellite pustules (vs. candidiasis)
  - Erythrodermic: affects ≥90% of body surface area (BSA) with generalized erythema and scaling; associated with desquamation; hair loss; nail dystrophy; and systemic symptoms (chills, malaise, lymphadenopathy, and/or high-output cardiac failure)
  - Pustular: Sterile pustules can present in localized or generalized forms. Generalized pustular psoriasis may lead to severe systemic illness, including superinfection.
  - Nail disease: pitting, oil spots, and onycholysis; nails involved in 50% with psoriasis at diagnosis with lifetime incidence of 80–90% with cutaneous psoriasis; increased association with psoriatic arthritis

EPIDEMIOLOGY

Incidence

Predominant age: two peaks of incidence between the ages of 20 to 30 years and 50 to 60 years

Prevalence

- 3.2% prevalence in the United States
- In the United States, the most commonly affected demographic group is non-Hispanic Caucasian.

ETIOLOGY AND PATHOPHYSIOLOGY

Psoriasis involves immune dysregulation of dendritic cells, T lymphocytes, and keratinocytes, triggered by infections, stress, and trauma. IL-23 and IL-17 signaling is one of the central signaling pathways in the propagation of psoriasis.

Genetics

- Genetic predisposition (polygenic)
- 40% have psoriasis in a first-degree relative.
- Multiple susceptibility loci contain genes involved in immune system regulation.
- HLA-C*06:02 is most strongly correlated with early onset psoriasis.

RISK FACTORS

- Family history
- Obesity
- Local trauma; local irritation (Koebner phenomenon)
- HIV
- Streptococcal infection
- Stress (may contribute to exacerbation)
- Medications: lithium, antimalarials, β-blockers, interferon, TNF-α inhibitors, steroid withdrawal
- Smoking
- Alcohol abuse
- Dysbiosis of gut microbiota

GENERAL PREVENTION

Avoid triggers like trauma, sunburn, smoking, certain medications, alcohol, and stress.

COMMONLY ASSOCIATED CONDITIONS

- Psoriatic arthritis
- Seborrheic dermatitis
- Obesity, metabolic syndrome, diabetes, chronic kidney disease
- Cardiovascular disease, atherosclerotic disease
- Nonalcoholic fatty liver disease (NAFLD)
- Other autoimmune conditions: Crohn disease, ulcerative colitis, ankylosing spondylitis
- Psychiatric/psychological conditions: depression, anxiety, suicidal ideation, low self-esteem, alcohol abuse, sexual dysfunction
- Myopathy

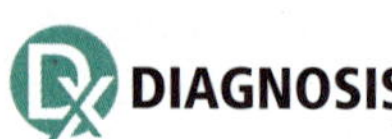

DIAGNOSIS

HISTORY

- May include: sudden onset of clearly demarcated, erythematous plaques with overlying silvery scales or exacerbation of chronic plaques, especially on extensor surfaces and scalp; typically, non or mild pruritus; triggers may include recent streptococcal infection or trauma.
- Family history of similar condition

PHYSICAL EXAM

- Well-demarcated salmon-pink plaques with silvery scale on scalp, ears, extensor surfaces (especially knees/elbows), umbilicus, lower back, and nails
- Nail findings: pitting, oil spots, onycholysis
- Auspitz sign: pinpoint bleeding with removal of scale
- Koebner phenomenon: new psoriatic lesions arising at sites of skin injury/trauma
- Woronoff ring is a pale blanching ring that may be seen around a psoriatic lesion.
- Sebopsoriasis: Psoriasis can overlap with seborrheic dermatitis as greasy scales on the scalp, eyebrows, nasolabial folds, postauricular, and presternal areas.

DIFFERENTIAL DIAGNOSIS

- Plaque: seborrheic dermatitis (may coexist), nummular eczema, atopic dermatitis, contact dermatitis, lichen simplex chronicus (may coexist), tinea, pityriasis rubra pilaris, dermatomyositis, squamous cell carcinoma in situ, reactive arthritis, pityriasis rosea, lichen planus, lichen sclerosis et atrophicus
- Guttate: secondary syphilis, pityriasis rosea, pityriasis lichenoides chronica, small plaque parapsoriasis
- Inverse: cutaneous candidiasis, tinea, seborrheic dermatitis, contact dermatitis
- Pustular: subcorneal pustulosis, acute generalized exanthematous pustulosis, folliculitis
- Erythrodermic: cutaneous T-cell lymphoma, drug-induced erythroderma, pityriasis rubra pilaris

DIAGNOSTIC TESTS & INTERPRETATION

Initial Tests (lab, imaging)

- Clinical diagnosis from history and physical exam; KOH is helpful for ruling out tinea in inverse psoriasis.
- Biopsy is rarely needed unless diagnosis unclear.
- Consider x-rays if complaints of joint pain to evaluate for psoriatic arthritis.

Diagnostic Procedures/Other

- Psoriasis Area and Severity Index (PASI) evaluates overall severity and BSA involvement.
- Dermatology Life Quality Index (DLQI)

Test Interpretation

Biopsy findings: thickening of the stratum corneum (hyperkeratosis) with retention of nuclei (parakeratosis); elongation, thickening, and clubbing of rete ridges; dilated tortuous capillary loops in the dermal papillae; perivascular lymphocytic infiltrate, Munro microabscesses: neutrophils in stratum corneum

TREATMENT

GENERAL MEASURES

Adequate topical hydration (emollients); avoidance of triggers; weight loss

MEDICATION

Management is based on severity of psoriasis and presence of inflammatory arthritis. First, assess for concurrent psoriatic arthritis, and if present start with therapies with dual approval for psoriasis and psoriatic arthritis, even if skin manifestations are mild due to risk of joint destruction secondary to psoriatic arthritis (1)[C]. In general, topical corticosteroids, vitamin D analogues, and tazarotene are used to treat mild to moderate disease. Systemic treatment with nonbiologic and biologic agents and ultraviolet B phototherapy are used for moderate to severe disease (2).

First Line

- Mild to moderate disease
  - Emollients: petrolatum/ointments to maintain skin hydration and minimize pruritus and risk of koebnerization
  - Topical corticosteroids
    - Anti-inflammatory, antiproliferative, immunosuppressive, and vasoconstrictive effects
    - Local side effects: skin atrophy, hypopigmentation, striae, acne, folliculitis, and purpura; systemic side effects: Risk is higher, with higher potency formulations used over a large surface for a prolonged period; pregnancy Category C
    - Apply BID daily until lesions resolve, then taper to PRN.
    - Scalp: high potency in solution/foam vehicle; shampoos and sprays also available
    - Face, intertriginous areas, infants: low-potency corticosteroids: 1% hydrocortisone
    - Adult initial therapy: medium-potency corticosteroids daily: 0.1% mometasone or triamcinolone; high-potency corticosteroids: 0.05% betamethasone or fluocinonide daily; superpotent corticosteroids: clobetasol, halobetasol; caution with use over 2 to 4 weeks; avoid occlusive dressings; reserved for recalcitrant plaques

P

- Vitamin D analogues: calcipotriene 0.005% cream daily to BID; may be used in combination with a superpotent corticosteroid; should not be used with products that can alter pH (e.g., topical lactic acid) local side effects: burning, pruritus, edema, peeling, dryness, and erythema; pregnancy Category C
- Topical retinoids: tazarotene 0.05% or 0.10% (Tazorac) daily; may be combined with corticosteroids; side effects: local irritation, photosensitivity; pregnancy Category X
- Topical calcineurin inhibitors: tacrolimus 0.1% or pimecrolimus 1.0% may be used as steroid-sparing agents, especially in facial and intertriginous areas.
- Topical phosphodiesterase-4 (PDE4) inhibitors: roflumilast topical (Zoryve) cream 0.15% or foam 0.30% applied daily; can be applied to face, intertriginous zones, and external genitalia
- Topical aryl hydrocarbon receptors (AHR) agonist: tapinarof 1% cream applied once daily for plaque psoriasis; usually well tolerated with most-common side effects being mild folliculitis and contact dermatitis
- Comparison of topical therapies: Vitamin D analogues have slower onset of action than topical corticosteroids but longer disease-free periods for body plaques; for scalp, potent and superpotent steroids are more effective.
- Combination of superpotent steroids and vitamin D analogues has better efficacy than either as monotherapy.

• Moderate to severe disease: may need combination therapy
  - Light therapy: UVB (broad/narrowband [BB/NB]) or PUVA: Treatment protocols are skin type dependent. PUVA with GI SE, photosensitivity, and increased risk of nonmelanoma skin cancer; can be used as adjunct therapy
  - Oral systemic therapies
    - Methotrexate: Start with 5-mg test dose, then increase to 7.5 to 15.0 mg/week IV, PO, IM, or SC, and then increase 2.5 mg every 2 to 3 weeks, up to 25 mg; contraindicated in pregnancy and use caution in women of childbearing age; supplement with folic acid 1 mg/day baseline chest x-ray, monitor LFTs, renal function, CBC, testing for latent tuberculosis (TB); consider liver biopsy when cumulative dose reaches 3.5 to 4.0 g; avoid alcohol and medications that interfere with folic acid metabolism including trimethoprim—sulfamethoxazole (Bactrim), NSAIDs, sulfamethoxazole, or hepatotoxic agents (e.g., retinoids).
    - Cyclosporine: Start 2.5 mg/kg/day; if insufficient response after 4 weeks, increase by 0.5 mg/kg/day; additional dosage increases every 2 weeks (max dose: 5 mg/kg/day); pregnancy Category C; side effects: renal toxicity and hypertension, limit use to 6 months to 1 year; monitor renal function and electrolytes with Mg^{2+}, CBC, lipids, and blood pressure.
    - Acitretin (Soriatane): Start at 10 to 25 mg/day; effective for pustular psoriasis and as a maintenance therapy after stabilization with other agents; pregnancy Category X: pregnancy test before starting; two forms of contraception 1 month before, during, and for at least 3 years after treatment; avoid alcohol; side effects: alopecia, dry skin, cheilitis, hepatotoxicity, hyperlipidemia; monitor labs and eye exams.
    - PDE4 enzyme inhibitor: apremilast (Otezla): Start at 10 mg PO, titrate to 30 mg BID by day 6; no routine labs needed; GI symptoms and depression are common; pregnancy Category C
  - Biologics—biologics are indicated for patients with moderate to severe psoriasis who do not respond to topical or other systemic therapies or have significant psoriatic arthritis involvement. They are very expensive and long-term outcomes and safety data are not available (3)[A], but they are also the most effective drugs for psoriasis (4). The clinical effectiveness of these drugs is generally similar.
    - General guidelines: baseline and yearly latent TB screening, baseline hepatitis panel, avoid live vaccines; monitor CBC with differential, and for signs/symptoms of infections, heart failure, malignancy, drug-induced lupus, demyelinating disorder. All should be considered effective first-line treatments; pregnancy Category B
      - TNF-α inhibitors: also approved for treatment of psoriatic arthritis; options include etanercept (Enbrel), adalimumab (Humira), infliximab (Remicade), and certolizumab (Cimzia).
      - IL-12/IL-23 antagonist: ustekinumab (Stelara); also approved for treatment of psoriatic arthritis
      - IL-17 antagonists: secukinumab (Cosentyx), brodalumab (Siliq), ixekizumab (Taltz); also approved for the treatment of psoriatic arthritis; avoid in patients with inflammatory bowel disease.

Second Line
• Immunosuppressives: azathioprine, hydroxyurea, 6-thioguanine, fumaric acid esters
• Topicals: salicylic acid, anthralin, coal tar

ISSUES FOR REFERRAL
Refer patients with psoriasis >20% of BSA, psoriatic arthritis, pustular psoriasis, severe extremity involvement, or disease not responding to topical therapy.

SURGERY/OTHER PROCEDURES
Psoriasis and psoriatic medications can affect wound healing postoperatively.

COMPLEMENTARY & ALTERNATIVE MEDICINE
Balneotherapy, climatotherapy, and stress management interventions

ADMISSION, INPATIENT, AND NURSING CONSIDERATIONS
Rule out sepsis; restoration of barrier function of skin with cleaning and bandaging; intensive topical corticosteroid therapy, initiate systemic therapy; management of electrolytes; erythrodermic psoriasis is at high risk for bacterial superinfection that can lead to sepsis and death and may require close inpatient monitoring.

ONGOING CARE

FOLLOW-UP RECOMMENDATIONS
Assess BSA; adjust therapy if no improvement.

DIET
Although evidence is inconsistent, a heart-healthy diet and regular exercise may reduce cardiovascular risk and improve overall quality of life in psoriasis patients.

PATIENT EDUCATION
National Psoriasis Foundation: https://www.psoriasis.org; (800) 723-9166.

PROGNOSIS
Plaque psoriasis is chronic with flares. Guttate psoriasis may resolve spontaneously in months.

COMPLICATIONS
Patients with psoriasis are at increased risk for cardiovascular disease due to chronic systemic inflammation. Early management of cardiovascular risk factors is recommended.

REFERENCES

1. Armstrong AW, Read C. Pathophysiology, clinical presentation, and treatment of psoriasis: a review. *JAMA*. 2020;323(19):1945–1960.
2. Garner KK, Hoy KDS, Carpenter AM. Psoriasis: recognition and management strategies. *Am Fam Physician*. 2023;108(6):562–573.
3. Sbidian E, Chaimani A, Afach S, et al. Systemic pharmacological treatments for chronic plaque psoriasis: a network meta-analysis. *Cochrane Database Syst Rev*. 2020;1(1):CD011535. doi:10.1002/14651858.CD011535.pub3.
4. Blauvelt A, Noe MH. The best psoriasis medications emerge. *JAMA Dermatol*. 2024;160(1):99–100.

ADDITIONAL READING

Mason AR, Mason J, Cork M, et al. Topical treatments for chronic plaque psoriasis. *Cochrane Database Syst Rev*. 2013;(3):CD005028.

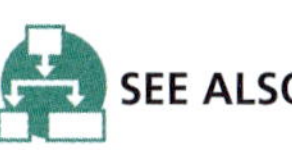
SEE ALSO

Arthritis, Psoriatic

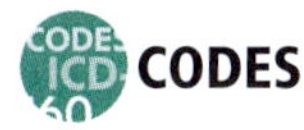

CODES

ICD10
• L40.2 Acrodermatitis continua
• L40.5 Arthropathic psoriasis
• L40.59 Other psoriatic arthropathy

CLINICAL PEARLS
Lifelong condition with remissions and exacerbations; set realistic expectations with patient. Disease burden is not limited to skin. Control cardiovascular risk factors.

PSYCHOSIS

Elizabeth M. Payment, MD

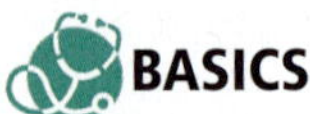

BASICS

DESCRIPTION

A disorder where thoughts and emotions are disrupted; seen in schizophrenia, mood disorders, substance use, medical problems, delirium, and dementia

- Positive symptoms: hallucinations and delusions (fixed false beliefs not typical of cultural background)
- Negative symptoms: anhedonia, poverty of speech, lack of motivation, social withdrawal, affective blunting, predictor of poor long-term functioning
- Cognitive symptoms: poor working memory, information processing, inattention, disorganized speech and/or behavior

EPIDEMIOLOGY

Prevalence

- Schizophrenia: peak onset: men ages 18 to 25 years and women ages 25 to 35 years
- 1% of the general population (50% of bipolar and 20% of unipolar depression cases)

ETIOLOGY AND PATHOPHYSIOLOGY

- Many causes including psychiatric, medical, substance use
- Positive symptoms: excessive dopaminergic activity in the mesolimbic pathway
- Negative symptoms: diminished dopaminergic activity in mesocortical pathway
- Cognitive symptoms: neurodevelopmental factors including childhood trauma, neurodegenerative factors such as smoking, obesity, and cortical disinhibition

Genetics

Schizophrenia: 50% concordance in monozygotic twins; many genes involved

RISK FACTORS

Family history, substance use (e.g., stimulants, THC), lower socioeconomic status

GENERAL PREVENTION

Community interventions for early detection and treatment of prodromal symptoms; patients with first episode should receive early intervention services

COMMONLY ASSOCIATED CONDITIONS

- Associated with metabolic syndrome, autonomic dysfunction, sudden cardiac death, and breast and lung cancer
- Substance use, including nicotine

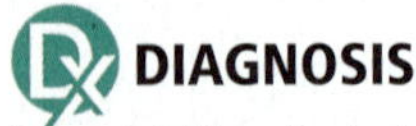

DIAGNOSIS

Rule out delirium: Psychotic disorders should not have fluctuating mentation.

HISTORY

- Delusions: persecutory, bizarre, somatic, referential, or grandiose
- Hallucinations: auditory, visual, tactile, gustatory, or olfactory
- Bipolar, unipolar depression, and dementia are associated with psychosis.
- Screen for drugs of abuse and history of epileptiform activity or TBI.
- Suicidality: higher risk with comorbid depression/mania, previous attempts, drug use, agitation/akathisia, poor adherence to medications

PHYSICAL EXAM

- Mental status exam: disorganized speech, behavior, and/or thought process; thought blocking; response latency; blunted affect; social withdrawal; lack of initiative; poverty of thought/speech; hallucinations
- Pay attention to focal neurologic signs, parkinsonism, tardive dyskinesia, and akathisia.
- May present with catatonia: lack of movement or extreme excitement, posturing, mutism, grimacing, waxy flexibility

DIFFERENTIAL DIAGNOSIS

- Schizophrenia: positive symptoms and negative symptoms, prodrome of social withdrawal, cognitive impairment
- Mood disorder with psychotic features: occur in mania and depression; mood congruent; psychosis remits as mood improves.
- Substance-induced: alcohol and benzodiazepine withdrawal, intoxication with cocaine, bath salts, PCP, THC, amphetamines, hallucinogens, and alcohol; may persist beyond acute intoxication
- Posttraumatic stress disorder: psychosis associated with traumatic recollections; often visual hallucinations
- Postpartum psychosis
- Psychosis due to general medical condition
- Medication-induced psychosis: steroids especially >40 mg prednisone equivalent, L-dopa, anticholinergics, antidepressants in bipolar patients, interferon, digoxin, stimulants

DIAGNOSTIC TESTS & INTERPRETATION

Labs: CBC, CMP, thyroid-stimulating hormone (TSH), lipid panel, EKG, pregnancy test, urine drug screen; consider rapid plasma reagin (RPR), HIV, ANA, ESR, vitamin B_{12}, vitamin D, urinalysis

Initial Tests (lab, imaging)

- Imaging: not necessary for diagnosis; consider CT or MRI if focal neurologic signs, first break or new onset in elderly or adolescents; sudden onset of symptoms, especially with comorbid fever or headache
- Consider EKG to assess QTc interval.

Follow-Up Tests & Special Considerations

- Consider Wilson disease, porphyria, metachromatic leukodystrophy, and inflammatory conditions.
- Consider lumbar puncture if unable to distinguish from delirium and/or rapid-onset psychosis.
- Consider electroencephalogram (EEG) for seizures and psychosis associated with ictal events.
- Consider anti-NMDA receptor antibodies in suspected autoimmune encephalitis.

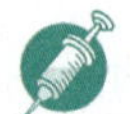

TREATMENT

GENERAL MEASURES

Ensure safety of person and environment and rule out medical causes particularly delirium.

MEDICATION

- Antipsychotics are mainstay of treatment (1),(2),(3)[B].
- For mania with psychotic features, a mood stabilizer may be used with an antipsychotic.
- For depression with psychotic features, antidepressant and antipsychotic combination improves response more than either alone
- In delirium, treat underlying cause; may not require antipsychotic therapy
- Side effects
  - Acute dystonia: benztropine 1 to 3 mg IM/IV then 0.5 to 2.0 mg BID–TID or diphenhydramine 50 to 100 mg IM/IV BID–TID max 400 mg/day
  - Parkinsonism: lower antipsychotic dose; switch to atypical (particularly, quetiapine or clozapine) and/or add benztropine 0.5 to 2.0 mg PO BID–TID
  - Akathisia (intense restlessness): lower antipsychotic dose; treat with β-blocker or benzodiazepine; may switch to antipsychotic with lower akathisia risk such as quetiapine or clozapine
  - Tardive dyskinesia: seen in ~1/3 of those treated long term with typicals, ~1/8 with atypicals switch to clozapine or quetiapine. Otherwise, minimize dose. Symptomatic treatment has been tried with low-dose benzodiazepines, botulinum toxin, and VMAT-2 inhibitors such as valbenazine and deutetrabenazine.
  - Neuroleptic malignant syndrome: potentially fatal; rigidity, tremor, fever, autonomic instability, mental status changes; discontinue neuroleptic; ICU; volume resuscitation; cooling blankets; no anticholinergics/antihistamines; consider dantrolene, amantadine, bromocriptine, and electroconvulsive therapy (ECT).
  - Metabolic syndrome, sudden cardiac death, stroke, heart failure, PNA (elderly), pulmonary embolus; can minimize metabolic risk by using anorexigenics and behavioral counselling

First Line

- Atypical antipsychotics: lower risk of extrapyramidal symptoms and dyskinesias (clozapine, quetiapine)
- Greater risk of weight gain, diabetes, and hyperlipidemia especially with olanzapine and clozapine
- Acute psychotic agitation:
  - Olanzapine 5 to 10 mg IM NTE 30 mg/day; do not administer with IM/IV benzodiazepine.
  - Ziprasidone 10 mg IM q2h or 20 mg q4h, NTE 40 mg/day
  - Haloperidol 2 to 5 mg +/− lorazepam 2 mg IM, can be given with 1 mg IM benztropine, NTE 20 mg haloperidol and 8 mg lorazepam per day
  - Droperidol, 2.5 to 5.0 mg IV or IM; high risk of QT prolongation
  - Dexmetomidine (sublingual) 120 to 180 μg q2h, NTE 360 μg/day
  - Risperidone (ODT), 1 to 2 mg PO
  - Loxapine: inhaled powder, 10 mg via oral inhaler; single dose in 24-hour period; can cause bronchospasm, especially in patients with preexisting lung disease

- Psychosis in schizophrenia
  - Risperidone: Start 1 to 2 mg QD; target dose of 2 to 8 mg/day reached over 1 to 2 weeks; >6 mg rarely more effective and higher risk of parkinsonism; higher risk of prolactinemia/parkinsonism due to D_2 blockade
  - Ziprasidone: Start 20 to 40 mg PO BID with at least 500 calories. Target dose 100 to 160 mg/day in divided doses over 2 weeks; prolongs QTc; less likely to cause weight gain than other atypicals; higher risk of akathisia/parkinsonism
  - Aripiprazole: Start 10 to 15 mg QD, may increase to 30 mg/day over 1 to 2 weeks; less weight gain but high rates of akathisia; lowers QTc
  - Lurasidone: Start 20 to 40 mg QD with at least 350 calories, increase up to 160 mg QHS over 2 to 4 weeks; less weight gain but high rates of akathisia/parkinsonism

Second Line

- Olanzapine: Start 5 to 10 mg QHS; target dose 5 to 20 mg/day within 2 days; more likely weight gain, hyperlipidemia, and hyperglycemia than other atypicals except clozapine; sedating; drug metabolism increased 50% by tobacco use
- Quetiapine: Start 25 mg BID, increase 25 to 50 mg q8–12h days 2 and 3, up to 300 to 400 mg by day 4; can then increase 50 to 100 mg/day, NTE 800 mg/day divided BID–TID; less risk of parkinsonism but more weight gain; sedation, restless legs syndrome; gradual titration better tolerated; prolongs QTc
- Paliperidone: Start 3 to 6 mg QD; target dose 6 to 12 mg QD; titrate over 1 to 2 weeks; higher risk of prolactinemia/parkinsonism than others; minimal hepatic metabolism, ideal for hepatic impairment
- Asenapine: Start 5 mg QHS or BID sublingually, increase to 10 mg BID if needed over 1 to 2 weeks; less weight gain than some, high rates of akathisia/parkinsonism; sedation, orthostatic hypotension; transdermal patch available, start on 3.8 mg/24 hours, may increase to 5.7 or 7.6/24 hours if needed after 1 week.
- Iloperidone: Start 1 mg BID, may increase by 2 mg daily, but slower can be better due to significant orthostasis (max 12 mg BID); little akathisia/parkinsonism, less weight gain but long titration, orthostasis, sedation; prolongs QTc
- Brexpiprazole: Start 1 mg QD for first 4 days, 2 mg QD days 5 to 7, can increase dose up to 4 mg/day based on response; lower rates of akathisia than aripiprazole but higher rates than others; less weight gain than others
- Cariprazine: Start at 1.5 mg QD, can be increased to 3 mg QD on day 2, dosed up to 6 mg QD based on response; in 6-week study, fasting glucose, cholesterol, triglycerides and weight were similar to placebo.
- Lumateperone: 42 mg daily; no titration required; mild average weight loss; moderate sedation and dry mouth
- First generation antipsychotics such as haloperidol which can be started at 0.5 to 2.0 mg q8–12h; target dose of 10 mg QD or less divided doses; high rates of tardive dyskinesia; decreased rates of metabolic syndrome
- Olanzapine/samidorphan: Start at 5 mg/10 mg QD. Increase olanzapine at weekly intervals of 5 mg pending response, up to 20 mg/10 mg QD; less weight gain risk attributed to samidorphan—a novel opioid-system modulator, similar to naltrexone
- Long-acting injectable antipsychotics
  - Haloperidol: decanoate—50 mg, 50 to 200 mg, q3–4 wk
  - Fluphenazine: decanoate—12.5 mg, 12.5 to 50.0 mg, q2–3 wk
  - Aripiprazole
    - Maintena: 400 mg qmo (2-week PO overlap), 300 to 400 mg qmo
    - Lauroxil: 441 to 1064 mg, 3-week PO overlap, 15 mg/day PO: 662 mg IM qmo
      - *Or* 30 mg PO and initio + lauroxil or 882 mg IM q6wk or 1064 mg IM q2mo
    - Asimtufii: 960 mg q2mo (2-week PO overlap)
  - Paliperidone
    - Sustenna: 234 mg then 156 mg in 1 week, 39 to 234 mg qmo
    - Trinza: 273 to 819 mg q3mo, needs 4 months of Sustenna
    - Hafyera: 1092 to 1560 mg q6mo; needs 4 months of Sustenna or one Trinza cycle
  - Olanzapine: Pamoate—210 to 405 mg
  - Risperidone
    - Consta: 12.5 to 50.0 mg q2wk (PO overlap), 12.5 to 50.0 mg q2wk
    - Perseris: 90 or 120 mg SubQ qmo (no PO overlap), 90 mg = 3 mg QD, 120 = 4 mg QD
    - Rykindo: 25 to 50 mg q2wk (PO overlap)
    - Uzedy: 50 to 250 mg SubQ monthly to q2mo
    - Risvan: 75 to 100 mg monthly

Geriatric Considerations

Antipsychotics increase risk of death in the elderly with dementia. Pimavanserin is approved for Parkinson disease psychosis.

ADDITIONAL THERAPIES

Psychotherapy, exercise, vocational, art, and group are effective adjuvants to antipsychotics (2)[B].

COMPLEMENTARY & ALTERNATIVE MEDICINE

- Vitamin treatments if there is a deficiency (common with folic acid, B_6, B_{12}, D), omega 3 supplements, glycine
- THC can precipitate psychosis.

ADMISSION, INPATIENT, AND NURSING CONSIDERATIONS

Admission if at risk for harm to self or others; extreme functional impairment; new-onset psychosis

ONGOING CARE

Medication management, psychotherapy

FOLLOW-UP RECOMMENDATIONS

Close follow-up for inpatient discharge (high risk for suicide); use therapy, exercise, smoking cessation, AIMS testing.

Patient Monitoring

- For patients treated with anti-psychotics, screen initially for metabolic syndrome (lipid panel, glucose, HbA1c, CBC, CMP, LFTs, weight, waist circumference) and AIMS testing. Continue monitoring with long-term use.
- EPS: Evaluate every week until dose is stable for 2 weeks. Once stabilized, assess EPS and TD at least every 6 to 12 months.

DIET

Avoid alcohol and sugar-sweetened beverages.

PATIENT EDUCATION

National Alliance on Mental Illness: https://www.nami.org/

PROGNOSIS

- Schizophrenia: fluctuating course; 70% first-episode psychosis patients improve in 3 to 4 months; 20–40% attempt suicide; 7% die of suicide.
- Medications are a mainstay of treatment but are only one component; others include community care models, psychosocial interventions, cognitive-behavioral therapy, self-help-based interventions, and motivational enhancement techniques.

COMPLICATIONS

- Metabolic disturbances secondary to antipsychotic medications, sedentary lifestyle, and smoking
- Life expectancy reduced over a decade compared to general population (largely mediated by heart disease)

REFERENCES

1. American Psychiatric Association. Clinical Practice Guidelines. https://www.psychiatry.org/psychiatrists/practice/clinical-practice-guidelines. Accessed November 19, 2025.
2. National Institute for Health and Care Excellence. Psychosis and schizophrenia in adults: prevention and management. http://www.nice.org.uk/guidance/cg178. Accessed November 19, 2025.
3. VA/DOD Clinical Practice Guidelines. Management of First-Episode Psychosis and Schizophrenia. http://www.healthquality.va.gov/guidelines/MH/scz/index.asp. Accessed October 12, 2025.

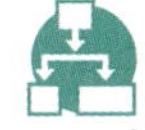

SEE ALSO

Delirium; Schizophrenia

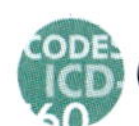

CODES

ICD10

- F29 Unsp psychosis not due to a substance or known physiol cond
- F20.9 Schizophrenia, unspecified
- F39 Unspecified mood [affective] disorder

CLINICAL PEARLS

- Antipsychotics are the mainstay of treatment; decrease all-cause mortality and increase quality of life
- Aripiprazole shortens QTc.
- Long-acting injectables may increase adherence.

PULMONARY ARTERIAL HYPERTENSION

Nasheena Jiwa, MD

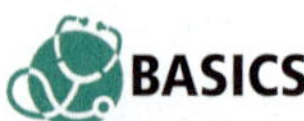

BASICS

DESCRIPTION

Pulmonary arterial hypertension (PAH) is characterized by abnormalities in the small pulmonary arteries (precapillary pulmonary hypertension [PH]) that produce increased pulmonary arterial pressure (PAP) and vascular resistance, eventually resulting in right-sided heart failure.

- Previously, PH was classified as primary PH (without cause, now idiopathic PAH [IPAH]) or secondary PH (with cause or associated condition); now, it is clear that some types of secondary PH closely match primary PH (IPAH) in their histology, natural history, and response to treatment. Therefore, WHO classifies PH into five groups based on mechanism, with PAH as group 1 in this classification.
- PAH is diagnosed by right-heart catheterization and defined by a mean PAP ≥20 mm Hg at rest and a pulmonary vascular resistance (PVR) of ≥3 Wood units when other groups of PH are ruled out; pulmonary capillary wedge pressure ≤15 mm Hg (excludes PH owing to left heart disease; i.e., group 2 PH) without:
  - Mild or absent chronic lung disease or other causes of hypoxemia (excludes PH owing to lung disease or hypoxemia; i.e., group 3 PH)
  - Venous thromboembolic disease (excludes chronic thromboembolic PH [CTEPH]; i.e., group 4 PH)
  - Systemic disorder (like sarcoidosis), hematologic disorders (like myeloproliferative disease), and metabolic disorders (like glycogen storage disease) (excludes group 5 PH)
- PAH is divided into following main categories:
  - Idiopathic: sporadic, with no family history or risk factors
  - Heritable: IPAH with mutations or familial cases with or without mutations
  - Drug or toxin induced: mostly associated with anorectics (e.g., fenfluramine), rapeseed oil, L-tryptophan, dasatinib (Bcr-Abl tyrosine kinase inhibitor), and illicit drugs such as methamphetamine, cocaine
  - Associated: connective tissue diseases (e.g., systemic lupus erythematosus, rheumatoid arthritis, scleroderma), HIV infection, portal hypertension, congenital heart disease, schistosomiasis (chronic hemolytic anemia added to group 5 PH—unclear/multifactorial mechanisms)
  - Pulmonary veno-occlusive disease (PVOD) and/or pulmonary capillary hemangiomatosis (PCH) and persistent PH of the newborn (PPHN) are classified as separate categories due to more differences than similarities with PAH.
    - PVOD and/or PCH: rare cause of PH characterized by extensive diffuse occlusion of the pulmonary veins (unlike PAH which involves the small muscular pulmonary arterioles)

EPIDEMIOLOGY

- Age: can occur at any age; mean age 37 years
- Sex (IPAH): female > male (female:male ratio ranges from 1.7 to 4.8:1)

Incidence

- Overall PAH: 5 to 52 cases per million
- IPAH: low, ~2 to 6 per million
- Drug-induced PAH: 1/25,000 with >3 months of anorectic use
- HIV associated: 0.5/100
- Portal hypertension associated: 1 to 6/100
- Scleroderma associated: 6–60%

Prevalence

PAH: ~15 to 50 cases per million; IPAH: ~6 cases per million

ETIOLOGY AND PATHOPHYSIOLOGY

- Pulmonary: inflammation, vasoconstriction, endothelial dysfunction, and intimal proliferation causing remodeling of pulmonary arteries produced by increased cell proliferation and reduced rates of apoptosis lead to obstruction
- Cardiovascular: Right ventricular hypertrophy (RVH), eventually leading to right-sided heart failure and right ventricular (RV) ischemia due to reduced right coronary artery flow causes RV remodeling associated with PAH.
- IPAH: by definition, unknown. True IPAH is mostly sporadic or sometimes familial in nature.
- Pulmonary arteriolar hyperactivity and vasoconstriction, occult thromboembolism, or autoimmune (high frequency of antinuclear antibodies)

Genetics

75% of heritable PAH (HPAH) cases and 25% of IPAH cases have mutations in *BMPR2* (autosomal dominant).

RISK FACTORS

Female sex, previous illicit anorectic drug use, recent pulmonary embolism, first-degree relatives of patient with familial PAH

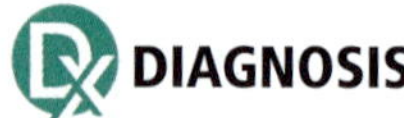

DIAGNOSIS

HISTORY

Dyspnea, weakness, syncope, dizziness, chest pain, palpitations, lower extremity edema

PHYSICAL EXAM

- Pulmonary component of S_2 (at apex in >90% of patients)
- Early systolic click of pulmonary valve
- Pansystolic murmur of tricuspid regurgitation
- Diastolic murmur of pulmonic insufficiency (Graham Steell murmur)
- Edema as jugular vein distention, ascites, hepatomegaly, or peripheral edema

DIFFERENTIAL DIAGNOSIS

Other causes of dyspnea:

- Pulmonary parenchymal disease such as chronic obstructive pulmonary disease, interstitial lung disease, or restrictive lung disease
- Pulmonary vascular disease such as pulmonary thromboembolism
- Cardiac disease such as cardiomyopathy

DIAGNOSTIC TESTS & INTERPRETATION

- Echocardiography (ECG): RVH and right axis deviation, or RV strain (increased P wave amplitude, incomplete right bundle branch block pattern, an R-to-S ratio >1 in lead V_1)
- Pulmonary function testing: reduced diffusion capacity
- Arterial blood gas: arterial hypoxemia, hypocapnia
- Ventilation/perfusion (V/Q) scan: Look for proximal pulmonary artery emboli and CTEPH; rule out group 4 PH.
- Exercise test: reduced maximal O_2 consumption, high-minute ventilation, low anaerobic threshold, increased PO_2 alveolar–arterial gradient; correlation to severity of disease with 6-minute walk distance (6MWD) test
- Antinuclear antibody test: positive (up to 40% of patients)
- LFTs: Evaluate for portopulmonary hypertension as a complication of chronic liver disease.
- HIV test, thyroid function tests, sickle cell disease screening
- Elevated brain natriuretic peptide (BNP) and N-terminal-proBNP may be useful for early detection of PAH in young, otherwise healthy patients with mild symptoms. It can also be used to assess disease severity and prognosis.
- Chest radiograph
  - Prominent central pulmonary arteries with peripheral hypovascularity of pulmonary arterial branches
  - RV enlargement is a late finding.
- Echo Doppler: should be performed with suspicion of PAH; echo suggests, but does not diagnose, PAH; most commonly used screening tool
  - Important to rule out underlying cardiac disease such as atrial septal defect with secondary PH or mitral stenosis
  - Right atrial and RV enlargement; tricuspid regurgitation
  - Estimates mean PAP and assesses cardiac structure and function, excludes congenital anomalies
- In patients at risk for HPAH, screen for gene mutations *BMPR2*.
- Polysomnography: for suspected symptoms of obstructive sleep apnea

Diagnostic Procedures/Other

- Pulmonary angiography
  - Should be done if V/Q scan suggests CTEPH
  - Use caution; can lead to hemodynamic collapse; use low-osmolar agents, subselective angiograms
- Right-sided cardiac catheterization (gold standard for diagnosis of PAH)
- Essential to confirm diagnosis and determine severity and prognosis by measuring PAPs and hemodynamics: Rule out underlying cardiac disease (e.g., left-sided heart disease) and assess response to vasodilator therapy.
- 6MWD: classifies severity of PAH and estimates prognosis

TREATMENT

- Treat underlying diseases/conditions that may cause PAH to relieve symptoms and improve quality of life and survival.
- Reasonable goals of therapy include:
  - Modified NYHA functional class (FC) I or II
  - ECG/CMR of normal/near-normal RV size and function
  - Hemodynamic parameters showing normalization of the RV function (right arterial pressure [RAP] <8 mm Hg and cardiac index [CI] >2.5 to 3 L/min/m^2)
  - 6MWD of >380 to 440 m
  - Cardiopulmonary exercise testing, including peak oxygen consumption of >15 mL/min/kg and $EqCO_2$ <45 L/min
  - Normal BNP levels (1)[C]

GENERAL MEASURES

- Supervised exercise training; avoid strenuous physical activity; psychosocial support (2)[C]
- Avoid pregnancy (2)[C].
- Influenza and pneumococcal immunization (2)[C]
- Oxygen—maintain arterial blood O_2 pressure >60 mm Hg (2)[C]

MEDICATION

- Acute vasodilator test during heart catheterization for all patients who are potential candidates for long-term oral calcium channel blocker (CCB) therapy (2)[C]
  - Screens for pulmonary vasoreactivity/responsiveness using inhaled nitrous oxide; epoprostenol (IV) or adenosine (IV): Positive response may be a prognostic indicator.
  - Contraindicated in right-sided heart failure or hemodynamic instability
- Chronic vasodilator therapy
  - If IPAH with positive response to acute vasodilator test (a fall in mean PAP of ≥10 mm Hg and to a value <40 mm Hg, with unchanged/increased cardiac output), use CCBs.
    - Adequate response confirmed after 3 to 4 months of treatment
    - ~13% will initially respond. Long-term clinical response to CCB therapy is small (~7%) (2)[C].
    - CCBs include nifedipine (long-acting), diltiazem, and amlodipine.
    - Avoid verapamil due to its significant negative inotropic effect.
  - CCBs are contraindicated in patients with a cardiac index of <2 L/min/m^2 or a right atrial pressure >15 mm Hg if PAH with negative response to acute vasodilator test or worsening on therapy; specific vasodilator choice based on risk stratification (2)[C]
    - Nonresponders to acute vasoreactivity who are in WHO-FC II should be treated with an oral compound (2)[B].
    - Nonresponders who remain or progress to WHO-FC III should be considered for treatment with any approved PAH drugs (2)[B].
    - Continuous IV epoprostenol is recommended as first-line therapy for WHO-FC IV PAH due to survival benefit (NNT = 5) (2)[A].
    - In case of inadequate clinical response, sequential combination therapy should be considered. Therapy includes ERA plus a phosphodiesterase type 5 (PDE5) inhibitor or a prostanoid plus ERA or a prostanoid plus a PDE5 inhibitor (2)[A].
    - WHO-FC II PAH-approved drugs: ambrisentan, bosentan, macitentan, riociguat, sildenafil, tadalafil (2)[B]
    - WHO-FC III PAH-approved drugs: ambrisentan, bosentan, epoprostenol (IV), macitentan, riociguat, sildenafil, tadalafil, treprostinil (SC, inhaled) (2)[B]
    - WHO-FC IV PAH-approved drugs: epoprostenol (IV) (2)[A]
  - Drug classes:
    - Prostacyclins: improve exercise capacity, cardiopulmonary hemodynamics: epoprostenol (IV), treprostinil (IV, SC, or inhaled), iloprost, beraprost
    - Prostacyclin IP: receptor agonist—selexipag
    - Endothelin receptor antagonists: improve exercise capacity; reducing mortality has been noted: bosentan (PO), ambrisentan (PO), macitentan. Pregnancy Category X; monitor LFTs monthly.
    - PDE5 inhibitor: suggested improvement in exercise capacity, cardiopulmonary hemodynamics, and symptoms (2)[C]: sildenafil (PO), tadalafil (PO), vardenafil
    - Guanylate cyclase stimulant: stimulators of the nitric oxide receptor, improves exercise capacity: riociguat (PO)
- Anticoagulation
  - Improved survival originally suggested in patients with IPAH only. Newer studies show some evidence for favorable effects of anticoagulation on survival in IPAH, HPAH, or PAH associated with anorexigens (2)[C].
  - Warfarin with international normalized ratio of 1.5 to 2.5 shows survival advantage in patients in multiple observational studies.
    - Contraindications: Avoid in patients with syncope or significant hemoptysis; consider drug interactions.
- Diuretics indicated in patients with RV volume overload (e.g., peripheral edema or ascites) (2)[B]
- Digoxin has little long-term data in PAH: used in RV failure and/or atrial dysrhythmias, increases cardiac output, and preserves RV contractility

ISSUES FOR REFERRAL

Refer to a pulmonologist and/or a cardiologist for further evaluation/treatment if PAH is suspected.

SURGERY/OTHER PROCEDURES

- Balloon atrial septostomy for severe PAH with right-sided heart failure despite optimized medical therapy to relieve symptoms prior to lung transplant or as a treatment on its own
- Heart–lung or lung transplantation

ADMISSION, INPATIENT, AND NURSING CONSIDERATIONS

Medical therapy is primarily palliative.

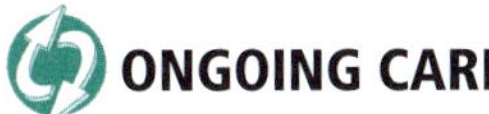

ONGOING CARE

FOLLOW-UP RECOMMENDATIONS

Exercise: walking or low-level aerobic activity, as tolerated, once stable; respiratory training

DIET

Fluid and salt restrictions, especially with RV failure

PATIENT EDUCATION

Discuss prognosis, lifestyle changes, and all therapeutic options (including transplant).

PROGNOSIS

- Median survival is 2 to 3 years from diagnosis; 5-year survival rate is 34% (NIH registry); newer data show 5-year survival ~70% with new treatment.
- Mode of death: right-sided heart failure (most common), pneumonia, sudden death, cardiac death
- Poor prognostic factors
  - Rapid symptom progression
  - Clinical evidence of RV failure
  - WHO functional PAH class IV (or NYHA functional class III or IV)
  - 6MWD <300 m
  - Peak VO_2 during cardiopulmonary exercise testing <10.4 mL/kg/min
  - ECG with pericardial effusion, significant RV enlargement/dysfunction, right atrial enlargement
  - Mean right atrial pressure >20 mm Hg
  - Cardiac index <2 L/min/m^2
  - Elevated mean PAP
  - Significantly elevated BNP and NT-proBNP; other markers also show promise in predicting survival: RDW, GDF-15, interleukin-6, creatinine.
  - Scleroderma spectrum of diseases

COMPLICATIONS

- Thromboembolism, heart failure, pleural effusion, and sudden death
- Pregnancy should be avoided due to high maternal mortality (30–50%) and fetal wastage.

REFERENCES

1. McLaughlin VV, Gaine SP, Howard LS, et al. Treatment goals of pulmonary hypertension. *J Am Coll Cardiol*. 2013;62(Suppl 25):D73–D81.
2. Galiè N, Corris PA, Frost A, et al. Updated treatment algorithm of pulmonary arterial hypertension. *J Am Coll Cardiol*. 2013;62(Suppl 25):D60–D72.

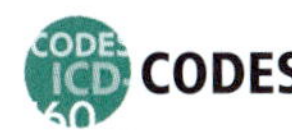

CODES

ICD10

- I27.0 Primary pulmonary hypertension
- I27.2 Other secondary pulmonary hypertension

CLINICAL PEARLS

- PAH involves abnormalities in the small pulmonary arteries (precapillary PH) which increase PAP and vascular resistance leading to right heart failure. Diagnosis is made by right heart catheterization.
- For positive vasodilator test, CCBs are the first-line agents to manage IPAH.

PULMONARY EMBOLISM

Srinath Ramakrishnan, MD • Scott Kopec, MD

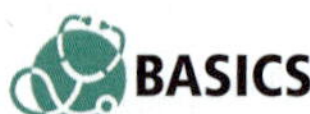

BASICS

Pulmonary embolism (PE) is an acute cardiovascular disorder that causes pulmonary vascular bed obstruction, which may result in acute right ventricular failure.

DESCRIPTION

- PE is the most serious presentation of venous thromboembolism (VTE).
- Classified based on severity:
  – Low-risk PE: no evidence of end organ damage or hemodynamic instability
  – Submassive PE: no systemic hypotension, but there is either myocardial necrosis (elevated troponin) or right ventricle (RV) dysfunction (RV dilation or systolic dysfunction on echocardiography [echo], RV/LV ratio >1 on computed tomography [CT], elevation of B-type natriuretic peptide [BNP] or N-terminal pro-BNP, or consistent electrocardiogram [ECG] changes)
  – Massive PE: hemodynamic instability with sustained hypotension; pulselessness; or persistent bradycardia, cardiogenic shock, acute manifesting RV failure

EPIDEMIOLOGY

Third leading cause of vascular death (after MI and stroke); case fatality rates vary (1–60%); ~11% at 2 weeks

Incidence

- Approximately 30 to 80/100,000, with higher incidence in African Americans and lower in Asians; >100,000 cases annually in the United States
- Incidence increases with age, most occurring at 60 to 70 years of age.
- 250,000 hospitalizations per year in the United States, 10–60% in hospitalized patients (highest risk for orthopedic and cancer patient; 1:1,000 pregnancies)

Prevalence

Within hospitalized patients: 17.3% prevalence of PE in hospitalized adults who were admitted for first episode of syncope (between 2012 and 2014) (1)

ETIOLOGY AND PATHOPHYSIOLOGY

- Venous stasis, endothelial damage, and changes in coagulation properties generate thrombus formation.
- Thrombus causes increased pulmonary vascular resistance, impaired gas exchange, and decreased pulmonary compliance. RV failure due to pressure overload is usually the primary cause of death.
- The most common source (85%) of PE is proximal lower extremity deep vein thrombosis (DVT).

Genetics

- Factor V Leiden: most common thrombophilia; +5.5% in White people; 2.2% in Hispanic people; 1.2% in African American; 0.5% in Asian; associated with 20% of VTE
- Prothrombin G20210A: 3% of White people; rare in African American, Asian, and Native American; 6% in patients with VTE
- Rarely deficiencies in protein C, S, and antithrombin

RISK FACTORS

- Older age, obesity, prolonged immobilization, surgery (total hip and knee, hip fracture cancer), major trauma, joint replacement, spinal cord injury, active cancer, hormonal replacement therapy, pregnancy/puerperium, previous thrombosis, antiphospholipid syndrome, genetics
- Oral contraceptive most frequent risk factor in women

GENERAL PREVENTION

- Low VTE risk: early ambulation after surgery, compression stockings, and intermittent pneumatic compression
- Use of thromboprophylaxis in COVID-19 infection is not commonly done but may be considered in those at high risk (prior VTE, recent surgery, limb immobilization, recent trauma, etc.).
- Hip or knee arthroplasty (high VTE risk): ≥10 days prophylaxis with low-molecular-weight heparin (LMWH), fondaparinux, apixaban, dabigatran, rivaroxaban, or low-dose unfractionated heparin (UFH)
- Spinal cord injury, hip fracture surgery, and trauma surgery (high VTE risk): 28 to 35 days with LMWH, fondaparinux, UFH, or vitamin K antagonists (VKA)
- Long-distance travel (>8 hours): hydration, walking, avoidance of constrictive clothing and frequent calf exercises, compression stockings below knee
- Patients with factor V Leiden, prothrombin G20210A with no previous thrombosis do not need prophylaxis.

COMMONLY ASSOCIATED CONDITIONS

COVID-19 infection, cancer, sepsis, illnesses leading to hospitalizations, surgery

DIAGNOSIS

Establish a pretest probability using a validated clinical prediction tool based on clinical criteria.

- Wells score (each predictor is +1; PE unlikely if 0 to 1, PE likely if >2)
- Geneva scores (Each predictor is +1 except for heart rate (HR) >95 beats/minute, which is +2; PE unlikely if 0 to 2 and PE likely if >3).
- If unlikely score: D-dimer: fibrin degradation product; levels are adjusted for age or adjusted to the YEARS algorithm for ruling out PE or the Wells score
- PE rule out criteria (PERC rule): Physicians can use this to rule out a need for imaging for PE where the clinical gestalt is low risk. All of these points should be negative to rule out a PE (age, HR >100, SaO_2 <95% on RA, unilateral leg swelling hemoptysis, recent surgery or trauma, prior PE or DVT, oral hormone therapy)

HISTORY

- Determine if the presentation is provoked or idiopathic. Approximately 30% of cases develop without identifiable risk factor.
- Bleeding risk (previous anticoagulation, history of bleeding, recent interventions/surgeries, liver disease, kidney disease)
- Sudden onset dyspnea (>85%), chest pain (>50%), cough (20%), syncope (14%), hemoptysis (7%)

PHYSICAL EXAM

- Dyspnea, syncope, hemoptysis, tachycardia, tachypnea, accentuated S_2; pleuritic chest pain, pleural friction rub, rales
- Signs of DVT: leg swelling, tenderness, visible collateral veins
- Signs of RV failure: jugular vein distention, S_3 or S_4, systolic murmur at left sternal edge, hepatomegaly

DIFFERENTIAL DIAGNOSIS

- Pulmonary: pneumonia, bronchitis, pneumothorax, pneumonitis, chronic obstructive pulmonary disease exacerbation, pulmonary edema
- Cardiac/vascular: myocardial infarction, pericarditis, congestive heart failure, aortic dissection
- Musculoskeletal: rib fracture(s), chest wall pain

DIAGNOSTIC TESTS & INTERPRETATION

- D-dimer ELISA: In patients with low pretest probability, it can rule out PE if it is negative (high negative predictive value [NPV]). It is not diagnostic if positive (low positive predictive value [PPV]), and it is not helpful if pretest probability is intermediate or high.
- CBC, creatinine, aPTT and PT, ABG: In young patients with idiopathic, recurrent, or significant family history of VTE, consider hypercoagulable test.
- Do not test for protein C, S, Factor VIII or antithrombin in the acute setting.
- Patients with intermediate or high pretest probability *or* low probability with elevated D-dimer need further diagnostic testing.
- Chest x-ray (CXR): Westermark sign (lack of vessels in an area distal to the embolus), Hampton hump (wedge-shaped opacity with base in pleura), Fleischner sign (enlarged pulmonary arteries), pleural effusion, hemidiaphragm elevation
- ECG: right heart strain, S1Q3T3
- CT pulmonary angiography: sensitivity 96–100%, specificity 86–89%; NPV 99.8%; if normal, it excludes PE if low or intermediate clinical probability.
- Ventilation/perfusion scintigraphy (V/Q scan): use if CT angiography is not available or contraindicated; a high-probability V/Q scan makes the diagnosis of PE; normal V/Q scan excludes PE.
- Pulmonary angiography: gold standard invasive and technically difficult: 2% morbidity and <0.01 mortality risk
- Echo: assesses RV function and thrombus in transit
- MR angiography: lower sensitivity and specificity than CT angiography
- Compression venous ultrasound (CUS): noninvasive; sensitivity >90%, specificity ~95%; it confirms the diagnosis of PE in patients with clinical suspicion.
- CT venography: can be done at the same time as CT angiography; increases diagnostic yield

ALERT

If preclinical probability is intermediate or high and patient has a low bleeding risk, start treatment while waiting for results.

Initial Tests (lab, imaging)

CBC, CMP, aPTT and PT, and D-dimers; EKG, and CXR

P

Follow-Up Tests & Special Considerations
CT pulmonary angiography or ventilation/perfusion scintigraphy

Diagnostic Procedures/Other
Pulmonary angiography—definitive test

Test Interpretation
- D-dimer (performed if Wells criteria for PE ≤4): normal: PE is ruled-out; high: Move on to imaging (spiral CTA).
- Spiral CTA (performed if Wells is >4 or D-dimer is high): diagnostic/positive: Treat for PE; nondiagnostic/contraindicated: Perform V/Q scan, CUS.
- V/Q scan, CUS negative: TEE or MR or pulmonary angiography; positive: Treat for PE.

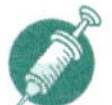

TREATMENT
- Patients with acute PE should be treated with anticoagulation for a minimum of 3 months. The duration may be extended based on individual risk assessments, whether the PE was unprovoked, ongoing risk factors (e.g., an underlying cancer), and bleeding risk.
- Treatment is based on risk stratification (2).
  - Low risk PE → Outpatient management is now recommended for selected low-risk PE patients. Patients with low complications risk, as determined by PE severity index (PESI) or simplified PESI (sPESI), and with adequate home support, may be safely treated at home. Hospitalization should be reserved for those with submassive/massive PE.
  - Intermediate-risk PE → anticoagulation (LMWH is recommended.)
  - High-risk PE → anticoagulation + definite INR consult for thrombolysis/embolectomy catheter/surgery

GENERAL MEASURES
Goal to maintain SaO_2 at >92%

MEDICATION
First Line
- Rivaroxaban (first line): 15 mg BID × 3 weeks and then 20 mg once daily to complete treatment; compared to warfarin, it has less major bleeding side effects while having same efficacy; ok to use in heparin-induced thrombocytopenia (HIT)
- Apixaban (first line): 10 mg BID for 7 days, then 5 mg once daily; less major bleeding episodes; ok to use in HIT
- Warfarin (second line) on day 1, if possible; 5 mg/day for 3 days in hospitalized or older patients and at a dose of 10 mg in <60 years of aged patients; adjust dose to maintain an INR of 2 to 3; needs to overlap with UFH, LMWH, or fondaparinux: 5 to 7 days, until 2 consecutive days of therapeutic INR
- LMWH (third line): preferred due to lower risk of major bleeding and HIT
  - Enoxaparin (Lovenox) 1 mg/kg/dose SC q12h or 1.5 mg/kg/dose SC QD
  - Dalteparin (Fragmin) 200 U/kg SC q24h
  - Fondaparinux (Arixtra) 5 mg (body weight <50 kg), 7.5 mg (body weight 50 to 100 kg), or 10 mg (body weight >100 kg) SC q24h
- UFH: IV bolus of 80 U/kg or 5,000 U followed by continuous infusion (initially 18 U/kg/hour or 1,300 U/hour) with dose adjustments to maintain aPTT that corresponds to anti-Xa levels of 0.3 to 0.7
- DOACs are generally preferred over LMWH for cancer-associated PE, except in patients with gastrointestinal malignancies or high bleeding risk, where LMWH may be favored.
- Systemic thrombolysis is strongly recommended for patients with hemodynamic instability (massive PE). IV systemic thrombolysis with weight-based dose of tenecteplase, alteplase at a dose of 0.6 mg/kg of body weight *or* alteplase at a dose of 100 mg administered over 1 to 2 hours.

ALERT
- Contraindications: active bleeding; heparin: HIT; LMWH: HIT, renal failure; warfarin: pregnancy; rivaroxaban and fondaparinux: renal failure; edoxaban: severe kidney or liver failure; apixaban: renal impairment and nonvalvular atrial fibrillation; dabigatran: severe kidney problems
- Contraindications to systemic thrombolysis: recent ischemic stroke, history of hemorrhagic stroke, active bleed, recent major surgery

Pregnancy Considerations
- Warfarin: teratogenic; safe while breastfeeding
- LMWH: dalteparin, enoxaparin, and fondaparinux are Category B; heparin is Category C: Use if the benefit outweighs risks.
- UFH: requires aPTT monitoring; can cause osteoporosis if used for prolonged period
- Rivaroxaban is Category C.
- Edoxaban and apixaban: Category B; increase risk of hemorrhage
- Dabigatran: Category C; only if benefit > risk.

ISSUES FOR REFERRAL
Hematology referral for unprovoked DVT in younger adults

SURGERY/OTHER PROCEDURES
- IVC filter placement if absolute contraindication for anticoagulation or recurrent PE despite adequate anticoagulation treatment
- Emergency embolectomy can be considered in patients with massive PE with contraindications for thrombolysis.
- Consider US-assisted catheter-directed thrombolysis with intermediate risk of death or submassive PE.

ADMISSION, INPATIENT, AND NURSING CONSIDERATIONS
Low-risk PE patients, identified using tools like the sPESI or Hestia criteria, may be considered for outpatient management, provided there is adequate support and follow-up

ONGOING CARE
Duration of anticoagulation
- Provoked PE (trigger no longer present): 3 months
- Unprovoked PE: >3 months; consider long-term or prolonged secondary prophylaxis if bleeding risk is low. HERDOO2 score provides guidance to determine duration of therapy in women with first unprovoked VTE. Low risk (0 to 1 criteria) can safely stop treatment after 6 months.
- Cancer-related PE: LMWH first 3 to 6 months; consider secondary prophylaxis as long as the patient has active cancer.
- Recurrent unprovoked PE: long-term anticoagulation

FOLLOW-UP RECOMMENDATIONS
If concomitant DVT, consider 30 to 40 mm Hg knee-high compression stockings.

Patient Monitoring
- INR should be checked regularly; target is 2 to 3.
- aPTT needs to be monitored in SC UFH.
- Anti-Xa can be checked in special circumstances if treated with LMWH, including pregnancy, younger patients, renal disease.
- Regular monitoring of renal function for patients on DOACs

PATIENT EDUCATION
Emphasize the importance of adherence to anticoagulation therapy and monitor for bleeding signs

PROGNOSIS
- Mortality: submassive 6–14%; massive PE 15–60%; PESI score predicts 30-day mortality.
- High risk: age >80 years, cancer, chronic CVD; pulse >110 beats/min, systolic BP <100 mm Hg, O_2 saturation <90%

COMPLICATIONS
Post-PE syndrome: permanent pulmonary vasculature changes, chronic dyspnea, reduced exercise capacity

REFERENCES

1. Lee LH, Gallus A, Jindal R, et al. Incidence of venous thromboembolism in Asian populations: a systemic review. *Thromb Haemost*. 2017;117(12):2243–2260.
2. Kahn SR, de Wit K. Pulmonary embolism. *N Engl J Med*. 2022;387(1):45–57.

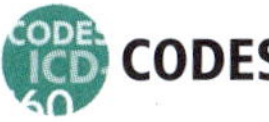

CODES
ICD10
- I26.02 Saddle embolus of pulmonary artery with acute cor pulmonale
- I26.92 Saddle embolus of pulmonary artery without acute cor pulmonale
- I26.01 Septic pulmonary embolism with acute cor pulmonale

CLINICAL PEARLS
- In low pretest probability patients, a negative D-dimer can rule out PE (high NPV).
- In moderate to high pretest probability, obtain CT pulmonary angiography.

PULMONARY FIBROSIS

Avignat S. Patel, MD

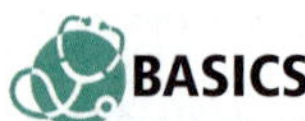

BASICS

DESCRIPTION

- Pulmonary fibrosis (PF) encompasses a group of interstitial lung diseases (ILDs), a family of >200 different lung diseases, characterized by inflammation, cellular proliferation, and fibrosis within lung interstitium and bronchial walls.
- ILD and PF can both be either idiopathic (without a known cause) or secondary.
- Idiopathic ILD is called idiopathic interstitial pneumonia. The most common idiopathic interstitial pneumonia is idiopathic PF (IPF).
- IPF is defined as a form of progressive fibrotic ILD associated with the histologic and/or radiologic appearance of usual interstitial pneumonia (UIP) when other causes have been excluded.

EPIDEMIOLOGY

- Most common ILD prevalent worldwide (25–30% of all ILD)
- Most common in men >60 years of age

Incidence

Higher in North America and Europe (3 to 9 cases per 100,000 person-years) than in South America and East Asia (fewer than 4 cases per 100,000 person-years)

Prevalence

In the United States, the prevalence has been reported to range from 10 to 60 cases per 100,000.

ETIOLOGY AND PATHOPHYSIOLOGY

- A favored model for the pathogenesis of IPF is that recurrent, alveolar epithelial damage with accelerated cell senescence leads to abnormal cellular repair and deposition of interstitial fibrosis by myofibroblasts.
- Causes of nonidiopathic PF include occupational and environmental exposures, drugs, and connective tissue diseases (CTDs).

Genetics

- The role of host genetic factors and their interactions with environmental factors is unknown.
- Mutations in genes involved in maintenance of telomere length are associated with increased risk of IPF.
- An SNP in the MUC5B promoter leads to gene over expression and is associated with increased risk of IPF. However, the mechanism linking MUC5B and IPF is not clear.

RISK FACTORS

- Family history of IPF
- Smoking—most significant association
- GERD, OSA
- Occupational and environmental exposures: wood (pine), metal dusts (lead, brass, steel), farming, birds, hairdressing, stone cutting, exposure to livestock, vegetable and animal dust, mold

GENERAL PREVENTION

Avoidance of above risk factors

COMMONLY ASSOCIATED CONDITIONS

- Pulmonary hypertension: 30–80% of patients with IPF
- GERD
- Nonidiopathic PF may be related to CTDs (RA and systemic sclerosis).

DIAGNOSIS

HISTORY

- Gradual onset
- Exertional breathlessness and nonproductive cough
- Constitutional symptoms (weight loss, fever, fatigue, myalgias, arthralgias) are uncommon.
- History of exposure (see "Risk Factors" section)

PHYSICAL EXAM

- Lung auscultation: bibasilar fine, late inspiratory crackles: "Velcro" crackles
- Clubbing in late stages, cyanosis (rare)
- Findings of pulmonary hypertension and right ventricular (RV) failure (elevated JVP, RV parasternal heave, loud P_2, LE edema)
- Signs of connective tissue disorders (skin/nailfold changes, arthritis)

DIFFERENTIAL DIAGNOSIS

- Other ILDs such as fibrotic hypersensitivity pneumonitis, nonspecific interstitial pneumonia, occupational lung disease, CTD-ILD, cryptogenic organizing pneumonia, post-COVID-19 ILD
- See below for histologic differential diagnosis of UIP.

DIAGNOSTIC TESTS & INTERPRETATION

Initial Tests (lab, imaging)

- Blood tests: Most routine labs are normal.
- Chest radiograph:
  - Reduced lung volumes and reticular opacities mostly at lung bases
  - Coarse reticular pattern and honeycombed cysts in advanced stages
- Pleural abnormalities (such as pleural plaques, effusions) are uncommon.

Follow-Up Tests & Special Considerations

- Chest CT scan:
  - Once diagnosis of IPF is suspected, obtain high-resolution CT (HRCT) chest, including prone and inspiratory/expiratory images with thin <1.25 mm slices.
  - In diagnosing IPF, HRCT is categorized into one of four patterns: UIP, probable UIP, indeterminate UIP, and alternative diagnosis (1)[C].
  - UIP pattern requires bilateral, primary peripheral, basilar reticulation, *and* honeycombing with or without traction bronchiectasis. UIP pattern on HRCT is diagnostic of IPF without need for surgical lung biopsy.
  - Probable UIP pattern has changes described previously with traction bronchiectasis but without honeycombing.
  - Atypical features on HRCT include upper- or mid-lung predominance, predominant consolidation, ground-glass opacities, and diffuse nodules or cysts; these increase the likelihood of an ILD other than IPF.
  - A diagnosis of ILD/IPF can be suspected based upon findings on a CT performed for other indications. Findings of possible ILD in patients without a known diagnosis are called interstitial lung abnormalities (ILAs). In some cases, ILAs may represent early ILD/IPF and patients should be evaluated (2).
- Serologic testing for CTDs to exclude nonidiopathic causes: ANA; RF; anti–CCP antibodies; myositis specific antibodies
- Echocardiogram to assess cardiac function, RV function, and pulmonary hypertension

Diagnostic Procedures/Other

- Pulmonary function testing (PFT):
  - PFTs in all patients undergoing evaluation and treatment of IPF/ILD
  - Findings include:
    - Decreased diffusion capacity for carbon monoxide (DLCO)
    - Decreased lung volumes (TLC, RV, FRC)
    - Decreased spirometric values: FVC and FEV_1 due to reduced lung volumes, with preserved FEV_1/FVC ratio
- ABG may show hypoxemia and respiratory alkalosis.
- 6-minute walk distance (6MWD): reduced distance and exertional hypoxemia
- Bronchoscopy:
  - Bronchoalveolar lavage (BAL):
    - Can be helpful in excluding other diagnoses like infection, malignancy, etc.
    - ATS/ERS does not recommend routine use of BAL for diagnosis of IPF.
  - Bronchoscopic transbronchial biopsy:
    - Not recommended for diagnosis of IPF as sensitivity and specificity is poor
    - May help exclude other ILDs
    - A genomic classifier run on transbronchial biopsy specimens can assist in diagnosing patients whose CT scan is not definite for UIP.
  - Transbronchial lung cryobiopsy is potential alternative to thoracoscopic biopsy (1)[B].
- Surgical lung biopsy:
  - Gold standard for diagnosis of ILD
  - When the combination of clinical and imaging data is not diagnostic, a thoracoscopic lung biopsy can be considered.
  - Biopsy samples should be taken from multiple lobes avoiding the most severely affected areas as they will show nondiagnostic fibrosis.
  - Procedure should not be performed in high-risk patients, including:
    - High oxygen requirements (>2 L/min)
    - Significant pulmonary hypertension
    - Rapid disease progression
    - Severely reduced FVC or DLCO

Test Interpretation

- Histopathology
  - Gross pathology distinctive nodular pleural surface
  - Histopathologic pattern in IPF is UIP.
    - UIP pattern requires dense fibrosis with architectural distortion, subpleural, and basal distribution, spatial and temporal heterogeneity, fibroblastic foci, and honeycomb changes plus absence of features suggestive of alternate diagnosis.
    - Differential diagnosis of UIP histologic pattern includes IPF, CTD-ILD, fibrotic hypersensitivity pneumonitis, asbestosis, chronic radiation pneumonitis, Hermansky-Pudlak syndrome and neurofibromatosis.

- Diagnostic strategies:
  - As per ATS/ERS statements of IPF in 2018 and 2022, diagnosis of IPF requires (1),(3)[C]:
    - Exclusion of other known causes of ILD and either of the following:
      - UIP or probable UIP pattern on HRCT
      - Specific combinations of HRCT patterns and histopathology patterns
  - UIP pattern on HRCT would be diagnostic with all histology patterns except alternate diagnosis findings.
  - UIP pattern on histology would be diagnostic with all HRCT patterns except alternate diagnosis findings.
  - Per ATS/ERS, for patients suspected of having IPF, a multidisciplinary discussion (pulmonologists, radiologists, pathologists, rheumatologists) is recommended for diagnostic decision-making.

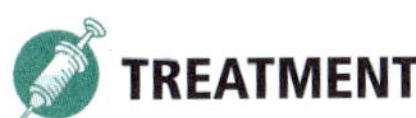

TREATMENT

GENERAL MEASURES

- Smoking cessation
- Vaccinations: pneumococcus, influenza, SARS-CoV2
- Pulmonary rehabilitation
- Referral to a transplant center
- Supplemental oxygen: Clinical practice guidelines strongly recommend supplemental oxygen if SpO_2 <88%.

MEDICATION

- Two medications, nintedanib and pirfenidone, have been shown to be safe, effective, and are recommended in the treatment of IPF.
  - In placebo-controlled, randomized trials, each drug slowed the rate of FVC decline by approximately 50% over the course of 1 year.
  - Both have shown some efficacy in reducing severe respiratory events, such as acute exacerbations and hospitalization.
  - Pooled data and meta-analyses also suggest reduced mortality.
  - The cost of each medication is estimated to exceed $100,000 annually.

First Line

- Nintedanib:
  - Mechanism of action: tyrosine kinase inhibitor that targets growth factor pathways including VEGF, FGF, and PDGF receptors.
  - Most common side effect is diarrhea (>2/3 of patients). It is also associated with a small risk of bleeding and should be used cautiously, if at all, in patients on therapeutic anticoagulation.
  - Liver function should be monitored as liver toxicity has been reported.
  - Also approved for progressive fibrotic ILDs other than IPF and systemic sclerosis-ILD
- Pirfenidone:
  - Mechanism of action: anti-inflammatory and antifibrotic effects, including inhibition of collagen synthesis, down regulation of TGF-β and TNF-α, and reduction in fibroblast proliferation
  - Common side effects: anorexia, nausea, vomiting, photosensitive rash, abnormal liver function
- Cannot recommend one agent over the other because there have been no head-to-head comparisons and efficacy is similar

Second Line

- No second-line agents available
- Treatment guidelines for IPF by ATS/ERS include:
  - Strong recommendations against use of:
    - Anticoagulation (warfarin)
    - Combination prednisone + azathioprine + *N*-acetylcysteine (NAC)
    - Selective endothelin receptor antagonist (ambrisentan)
    - Imatinib, a tyrosine kinase inhibitor with one target
  - Conditional recommendations against:
    - Dual endothelin receptor antagonists (macitentan, bosentan)
    - Phosphodiesterase-5 inhibitor (sildenafil)
    - NAC monotherapy

ISSUES FOR REFERRAL

- Referral to pulmonologist for diagnosis and management
- Thoracic surgeon referral is indicated if patient cannot be diagnosed by ATS clinical and radiographic criteria.
- Referral to lung transplant center is indicated early on for patients showing progressive worsening of the disease.

ADDITIONAL THERAPIES

Several investigational therapies are being studied in randomized controlled trials. A new antifibrotic, nerandomilast, recently completed a Phase 3 trial meeting primary endpoint and is awaiting U.S. Food and Drug Administration (FDA) approval.

SURGERY/OTHER PROCEDURES

Lung transplant:

- Can prolong survival and improve quality of life for highly selected candidates
- Only a minority of patients with IPF receive lung transplants
- Only 66% of lung transplant recipients survive for >3 years after transplant and only 53% survive for >5 years.
- Common complications include primary graft dysfunction, acute and chronic allograft rejection, opportunistic infections, and cancer.

COMPLEMENTARY & ALTERNATIVE MEDICINE

No proven benefit of any complementary and alternative medications

ADMISSION, INPATIENT, AND NURSING CONSIDERATIONS

- Patient with acute exacerbation of IPF should be admitted to the hospital for management.
- Need for mechanical ventilation portends a poor prognosis and should be avoided if possible.
- Palliative care consult is appropriate for all patients diagnosed with IPF.

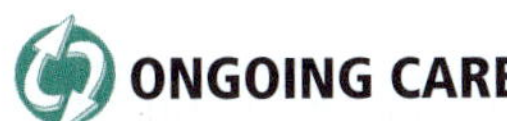

ONGOING CARE

FOLLOW-UP RECOMMENDATIONS

- Pulmonary clinic and, if possible, at an ILD clinic
- Monitoring with serial HRCT (at least yearly), PFT (at least every 6 months)
- If on antifibrotic medications, monitor LFTs.

PROGNOSIS

IPF carries a poor prognosis with a median survival of 3.8 years among adults ≥65 years of age in the United States.

COMPLICATIONS

- Acute exacerbation of IPF
  - 10–20% per patient per year
  - It is characterized by worsening hypoxemia, new bilateral ground-glass opacities, consolidation, or both on HRCT imaging that are not fully explained by volume overload or infection.
  - Triggers: infection, aspiration, drug toxicity or idiopathic
  - Treatment: Available guidelines make weak recommendations for the use of glucocorticoids (no definitive benefit based on available data) and do not recommend the use of mechanical ventilation. Consider palliative care referral.
- Increased risk for VTE, lung cancer, and pulmonary hypertension
  - Management of pulmonary hypertension-ILD should be in consultation with a pulmonary hypertension specialist. Inhaled treprostinil is the only treatment currently approved in pulmonary hypertension-ILD, including IPF, and can be considered.

REFERENCES

1. Raghu G, Remy-Jardin M, Richeldi L, et al. Idiopathic pulmonary fibrosis (an update) and progressive pulmonary fibrosis in adults: an official ATS/ERS/JRS/ALAT clinical practice guideline. *Am J Respir Crit Care Med*. 2022;205(9):e18–e47.
2. Podolanczuk AJ, Hunninghake GM, Wilson KC, et al. Approach to the evaluation and management of interstitial lung abnormalities: an official American Thoracic Society clinical statement. *Am J Respir Crit Care Med*. 2025;211(7):1132–1155.
3. Raghu G, Remy-Jardin M, Myers JL, et al; for American Thoracic Society, European Respiratory Society, Japanese Respiratory Society, Latin American Thoracic Society. Diagnosis of idiopathic pulmonary fibrosis. An official ATS/ERS/JRS/ALAT clinical practice guideline. *Am J Respir Crit Care Med*. 2018;198(5):e44–e68.

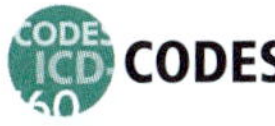

CODES

ICD10

- J84.10 Pulmonary fibrosis, unspecified
- J84.112 Idiopathic pulmonary fibrosis

CLINICAL PEARLS

- IPF is the most common idiopathic ILD and frequently misdiagnosed or has delayed diagnosis.
- HRCT scan is the cornerstone for diagnosis.
- Two antifibrotic drugs are the only approved therapy for IPF.
- Oxygen supplementation, pulmonary rehab, anti-reflux treatment, vaccinations against pneumococcus, influenza, and SARS-CoV2 should be considered in all patients.
- Referral to pulmonary clinic, ILD clinic, and lung transplant center should be considered early.

PYELONEPHRITIS

Dana G. Carroll, PharmD, BCPS, CDCES, BCGP • Randi Cheree Melton, DO • Jacquelynn Parks Luker, MD

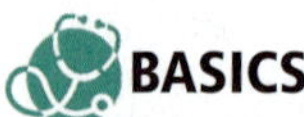

BASICS

DESCRIPTION

- Infection of the renal parenchyma and/or renal pelvis, often producing localized flank/back pain combined with systemic symptoms, such as fever, chills, nausea, and vomiting. There is a wide spectrum of illness ranging from mild symptoms to septic shock.
- Chronic pyelonephritis is the result of progressive inflammation of the renal interstitium and tubules due to recurrent infection, vesicoureteral reflux, or both.
- Considered uncomplicated if the infection is caused by a typical pathogen in an immunocompetent patient with normal urinary tract anatomy and renal function

Geriatric Considerations

May present as altered mental status; absence of fever is common in older adults. Older patients with diabetes and pyelonephritis are at higher risk of bacteremia, prolonged hospitalization, and mortality. The high prevalence of asymptomatic bacteriuria (ABU) in older adults makes the use of urine dipstick less reliable for diagnosing UTI. Culture and sensitivity (C&S) data are useful in guiding therapy for pyelonephritis in older adults and should be obtained.

Pregnancy Considerations

Pyelonephritis affects 1–2% of pregnancies and is the most common medical complication requiring hospitalization in pregnancy. Pregnant patients with untreated ABU have a 20–30% risk of developing acute pyelonephritis. Patients with pyelonephritis are at increased risk for developing acute respiratory distress syndrome and spontaneous preterm labor. Pregnant women with acute pyelonephritis should be considered for hospitalization and treated initially with a 2nd or 3rd generation IV cephalosporin.

Pediatric Considerations

UTI is present in ~5% of patients age 2 months to 2 years with fever and no apparent source on history and physical exam. A urine specimen, preferably by catheterization or suprapubic aspiration, should be obtained and sent for urinalysis prior to starting antibiotics. Treatment should be based on the clinical situation.

EPIDEMIOLOGY

Incidence

Community-acquired acute pyelonephritis: 3 to 4 cases per 10,000 males; 15 to 17 cases per 10,000 females; 28 cases per 10,000 women ages 18 to 49 years

Prevalence

Adult cases: 250,000/year, with 200,000 hospitalizations

ETIOLOGY AND PATHOPHYSIOLOGY

Escherichia coli (>80%); *Klebsiella* spp. second most common followed by:

- Other gram-negative pathogens: *Proteus*, *Serratia*, *Clostridium*, *Pseudomonas*, and *Enterobacter* spp.; *Enterococcus* spp.
- *Staphylococcus epidermidis*, *Staphylococcus saprophyticus* (second leading cause in young women), and *Staphylococcus aureus*
- *Candida* spp.

RISK FACTORS

Underlying urinary tract abnormalities, indwelling catheter/recent urinary tract instrumentation, nephrolithiasis, immunocompromised (diabetes), elderly, institutionalized patients (particularly women), prostatic enlargement, stress incontinence

COMMONLY ASSOCIATED CONDITIONS

Indwelling catheters, renal calculi; benign prostatic hyperplasia

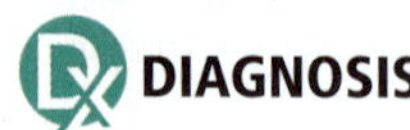

DIAGNOSIS

HISTORY

- Adults: fever, flank pain, nausea ± vomiting, malaise, anorexia, myalgia, dysuria, urinary frequency, urgency, suprapubic discomfort, mental status changes
- Infants and children: fever, irritability, poor feeding, GI symptoms

PHYSICAL EXAM

- Adults
  - Presentation ranges from no physical findings to septic shock.
  - Fever: ≥38°C (100.4°F)
  - Costovertebral angle tenderness
  - Mental status changes common in older adults.
- Infants and children: lethargy, fever, poor skin perfusion, inadequate weight gain/weight loss, jaundice, pallor

DIFFERENTIAL DIAGNOSIS

Obstructive uropathy, acute bacterial pneumonia (lower lobe), cholecystitis, acute pancreatitis, appendicitis, perforated viscus, aortic dissection, pelvic inflammatory disease, ectopic pregnancy, kidney stone, diverticulitis

DIAGNOSTIC TESTS & INTERPRETATION

Initial Tests (lab, imaging)

- Urinalysis: pyuria (>5 WBC/HPF) ± leukocyte casts, hematuria, nitrites (sensitivity 35–85%; specificity 92–100%), and mild proteinuria; urine leukocyte esterase positive (sensitivity 74–96%; specificity 94–98%); urine Gram stain, urine C and S (>100,000 colony forming units/mL or >100 colony forming units/mL + symptoms)
- CBC, BUN, serum creatinine, glomerular filtration rate (GFR), and pregnancy test (if indicated)
- C-reactive protein levels correlate with prolonged hospitalization and recurrence; serum albumin <3.3 g/dL also associated with increased risk for hospital admission
- Imaging not necessary in routine cases; ultrasound (US) if obstruction is suspected, stones suspected or no improvement in first 2 to 3 days of therapy
- Pediatrics: Guidelines recommend renal/bladder US (not voiding cystourethrogram) after first febrile UTI between ages 2 and 24 months.

Follow-Up Tests & Special Considerations

- Catheterization/suprapubic aspirate to obtain samples from non–toilet-trained children
- Blood culture(s): if hospitalized, diagnosis uncertain, suspected hematogenous source or immunosuppression; recent antibiotic use may alter results.
- If patient's condition does not improve within 72 hours, if obstruction/anatomic abnormality is suspected, in patients with immunosuppression or multiple comorbidities, and/or if certain lab abnormalities are present (urine pH >7, GFR <40, 50% decline in renal function), consider computed tomography (CT) scan of abdomen and pelvis ± contrast. Contrast-enhanced CT is typically the image of choice for children and adults with acute pyelonephritis; US of kidneys, ureter, bladder is not as sensitive as CT scan but is cheaper and more readily available; cystoscopy with ureteral catheterization

Test Interpretation

- Acute: abscess formation with neutrophil response
- Chronic: fibrosis with reduction in renal tissue

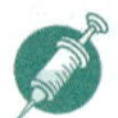

TREATMENT

- ≤7 days of treatment is equivalent to longer regimens in adults (including those with bacteremia) without urogenital abnormalities (1)[A].
- IV antibiotics for inpatients with severe illness or unable to tolerate oral

GENERAL MEASURES

- Broad-spectrum antibiotics initially based on severity of illness, health status, and risk factors for resistant pathogens; tailor to C&S results.
  - Risk factors for a multidrug-resistant (MDR) pathogens/infections if present within last 3 months: history of urinary MDR pathogen; inpatient stay at a health care facility (hospital, nursing home, etc.); use of fluoroquinolone, trimethoprim-sulfamethoxazole (TMP-SMX), or broad-spectrum β-lactam; travel to geographic regions with significant incidence of MDR pathogens (e.g., Asia, Middle East, Africa); obstructive uropathy (2)[A]
- Consider urinary analgesics (e.g., phenazopyridine 200 mg q8h) for dysuria.

MEDICATION

- For empiric oral therapy, a fluoroquinolone is recommended. Should fluoroquinolone resistance exceed 10% or if the patient has nausea/vomiting, ceftriaxone 1 gram IV daily for 10 days or until oral agents can be used.
- For IV therapy, fluoroquinolone, an aminoglycoside ± ampicillin, an extended-spectrum cephalosporin ±a β-lactamase inhibitor, an extended-spectrum penicillin ± an aminoglycoside, or a carbapenem are recommended.
- Contraindications: known drug allergy; fluoroquinolones are not recommended in children, adolescents, and pregnant women unless other alternatives are not available. Nitrofurantoin does not achieve reliable tissue levels to treat pyelonephritis.
- Precautions
  - Adjust antibiotic dosages in patients with renal insufficiency. Monitor aminoglycoside levels and renal function.
  - If *Enterococcus* is suspected based on Gram stain, ampicillin ± gentamicin or piperacillin-tazobactam are good empiric choices; if patient is penicillin allergic, vancomycin may be used. If outpatient, add amoxicillin to fluoroquinolone, pending C&S results. 3rd-generation cephalosporin should be avoided for suspected/proven enterococcal infections.
  - >20% *E. coli* strains are resistant to ampicillin and TMP-SMX in community-acquired infections.
  - Extended-spectrum β-lactamase (ESBL)-producing strains should be treated with a carbapenem ± β-lactamase inhibitor or ceftolozane-tazobactam.

First Line

- Adults
  - Oral (initial outpatient treatment)
    - Ciprofloxacin: 500 mg q12h for 5 to 7 days; Ciprofloxacin XR: 1,000 mg/day for 5 to 7 days
    - Levofloxacin: 750 mg/day for 5 to 7 days
    - TMP-SMX (160/800 mg): 1 tab q12h for 14 days provided uropathogen known to be susceptible ± ceftriaxone 1 g initial IM/IV dose
  - IV (initial inpatient treatment for patients with no risk factors for MDR organisms)
    - Ciprofloxacin: 400 mg q12h; levofloxacin: 750 mg/day
    - Ceftriaxone: 1 g/day
    - Gentamicin: 5 to 7 mg/kg body weight q24h
    - Ampicillin: 2 g q4–6h ± gentamicin for *Enterococcus*
  - IV (initial inpatient treatment for patients with at least one risk factor for MDR organisms)
    - Ertapenem 1 g q24h
    - Antipseudomonal carbapenem: meropenem: 1 g q8h; imipenem: 500 mg q6h
    - Add vancomycin for methicillin-resistant *S. aureus* (MRSA)
    - Use daptomycin or linezolid vancomycin-resistant *Enterococcus* (VRE).
  - Severe illness: IV therapy until afebrile for 48 hours and tolerating PO intake; switch to PO agents to complete a 7- to 14-day course.
- Pediatric
  - Oral: cefdinir: 14 mg/kg/day for 10 to 14 days; ceftibuten 9 mg/kg/day for 10 to 14 days; cefixime 8 mg/kg/day; amoxicillin-clavulanate weight-based divided q8–12h for 10 to 14 days
  - IV: ceftriaxone: 50 mg/kg/day (IM use acceptable in outpatient setting); cefotaxime: 150 mg/kg/day divided in 3 to 4 doses; ampicillin: 100 mg/kg/day divided in 4 doses + gentamicin

Second Line

Adults

- Oral
  - Use oral β-lactams with caution; if used, longer courses of therapy (10 to 14 days) recommended
  - Cefixime 400 mg q24h
  - Amoxicillin-clavulanate: 875/125 mg q12h
- IV
  - Piperacillin-tazobactam 3.375 mg q6h
  - Targeted therapy for MDR organisms
    - Ceftazidime-avibactam: 2.5 g q8h; ceftolozane-tazobactam: 1.5 g q8h; meropenem-vaborbactam: 4 g q8h

Pediatric Considerations

- Initial empiric antibiotic choice should cover *E. coli*. Add ampicillin if *Enterococcus* is suspected.
  - Oral antibiotics (ceftibuten, cefixime, cefdinir, and amoxicillin/clavulanate) may be used alone *or*
  - IV antibiotics (single daily dosing if an aminoglycoside is chosen) for 2 to 4 days, followed by PO antibiotics for a total of 10 to 14 days
- Complete outpatient antibiotic course.

Pregnancy Considerations

- Acute pyelonephritis should be aggressively treated. Hospital admission should be considered and IV therapy may be required.
- May consider low-dose suppressive antibiotics (nitrofurantoin or cephalexin) for the remainder of pregnancy following treatment of pyelonephritis (3)[A]

ISSUES FOR REFERRAL

Acute pyelonephritis unresponsive to therapy, chronic pyelonephritis, abnormal urogenital anatomy

SURGERY/OTHER PROCEDURES

Perinephric abscess may require surgical drainage.

ADMISSION, INPATIENT, AND NURSING CONSIDERATIONS

- Inpatient therapy for severe illness, risk factors for complicated pyelonephritis, pregnancy, or extremes of age
- Consider transitioning from IV to PO therapies after the patient is afebrile for 24 hours; outpatient therapy if mild to moderate illness, uncomplicated course, and tolerating PO intake; IV fluids for dehydration; blood cultures for patients admitted with pyelonephritis; discharge on PO agent after patient is afebrile 24 to 48 hours to complete up to 2 weeks of therapy

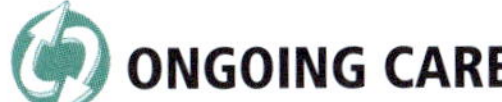

ONGOING CARE

FOLLOW-UP RECOMMENDATIONS

Adults and children: Patients treated in the outpatient setting should have follow-up at 48 to 72 hours to evaluate for improvement and consideration of further evaluations and/or broadening coverage if not improving. Repeat urine culture only needed for complicated cases.

Patient Monitoring

If no response within 48 to 72 hours (5% of patients): Reevaluate and review cultures, CT scan, or US to review anatomy; adjust therapy as needed; urologic or infectious disease consult; the two most common causes of failure to respond are a resistant organism and nephrolithiasis.

DIET

Encourage fluid intake.

PROGNOSIS

95% of treated patients respond within 48 hours.

COMPLICATIONS

Renal abscess, perinephric abscess, metastatic infection: skeletal system, endocardium, eye, meningitis with subsequent seizures, septic shock and death, acute/chronic renal failure

REFERENCES

1. Jones DE. Renal and urinary conditions: urinary tract infections. *FP Essent*. 2024;543:24–34.
2. Pianucci K, Cipriano F, Chung E. Review of urinary tract infections and pyelonephritis. *Pediatr Ann*. 2024;53(6):e217–e222. doi:10.3928/19382359-20240407-05.
3. American College of Obstetricians and Gynecologists. Urinary tract infections in pregnant individuals. *Obstet Gynecol*. 2023;142(2):435–445. doi:10.1097/AOG.0000000000005269.

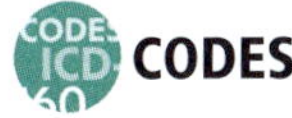

CODES

ICD10

- N12 Tubulo-interstitial nephritis, not spcf as acute or chronic
- N10 Acute tubulo-interstitial nephritis
- N11.9 Chronic tubulo-interstitial nephritis, unspecified

CLINICAL PEARLS

- Urine C&S is helpful for targeting antibiotic therapy and should be obtained when possible.
- The most common causes of poor response to treatment are antibiotic resistance and coexisting nephrolithiasis.
- Fluoroquinolones are generally the initial antibiotic of choice for pyelonephritis. Oral β-lactams are less effective. IV β-lactams may be used in cases of complicated UTIs.

PYLORIC STENOSIS

Shani H. Cunningham, DO, MEd, FAAP

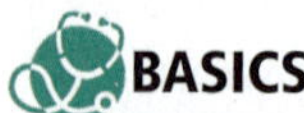

BASICS

DESCRIPTION

Acquired narrowing of the pyloric canal due to progressive hypertrophy of pyloric muscle leading to obstruction

EPIDEMIOLOGY

- Presentation is most common between 2 and 8 weeks of age, with a median presentation of 6 weeks.
- The most common condition requiring surgical intervention in the 1st year of life

Incidence

- Highest incidence found in first-born males
- Overall 1.56 per 1,000 live births
- Higher in Caucasian and Hispanic children

ETIOLOGY AND PATHOPHYSIOLOGY

- Impaired physiologic relaxation of the pyloric muscle leads to hypertrophy.
- Gastric outflow is obstructed, leading to gastric distension and forceful projectile postprandial vomiting.

Genetics

Five genetic loci linked to infantile hypertrophic pyloric stenosis (IHPS) have been identified. IHPS2 and IHPS5 have been associated with autosomal dominant inheritance of pyloric stenosis (1).

RISK FACTORS

- Maternal smoking during pregnancy
- C-section delivery
- Prematurity
- Formula feeding which may cause higher serum levels associated with pylorospasm
- Postnatal macrolide antibiotics, especially if administered in the first 2 weeks of life
- Multiple gestations:
  - 200-fold increased risk if monozygotic twin affected
  - 20-fold increased risk if dizygotic twin affected

GENERAL PREVENTION

Breast milk contains increased vasoactive intestinal peptides which are agents of smooth muscle relaxation.

COMMONLY ASSOCIATED CONDITIONS

Hiatal and inguinal hernias

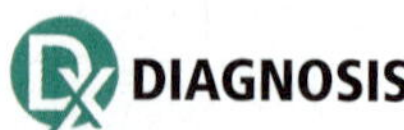

DIAGNOSIS

HISTORY

- Nonbilious projectile vomiting immediately after feeding with increasing in frequency and severity
- Hunger and irritability due to inadequate nutrition
- Weight loss
- Median duration of symptoms is 10 days.

PHYSICAL EXAM

- Firm "olive-like" mass palpable in the right upper quadrant
- Visible peristalsis after feeding
- Late signs include dry mucous membranes, poor skin turgor, tachycardia, and irritability.
- Rarely, jaundice when starvation leads to an elevated indirect hyperbilirubinemia

DIFFERENTIAL DIAGNOSIS

- Inappropriate feeding
- GERD
- Gastritis
- Adrenal crisis
- Antral or gastric web

DIAGNOSTIC TESTS & INTERPRETATION

Initial Tests (lab, imaging)

- Labs: hypokalemic, hypochloremic, metabolic alkalosis
- Pyloric ultrasound is the study of choice: Pathologic limits are 3-mm pyloric muscle thickness, 15-mm pyloric length, 11-mm pyloric diameter, and 12-mL pyloric volume with muscle thickness being the key factor. Although these measurements remain diagnostic, they may exclude younger (<3 weeks old), smaller infants who can be clinically diagnosed (2)[B].
- Upper GI series: rarely indicated: strong gastric contractions; pyloric canal outlined by string of contrast material (string sign) and parallel lines of barium in the narrow channel separated by mucosa (double-tract sign or railroad track sign).

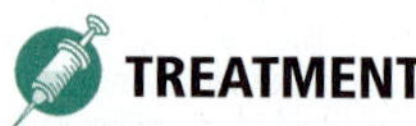

TREATMENT

GENERAL MEASURES

- Pyloric stenosis is a medical emergency but not a surgical emergency.
- Ensure proper nutrition and hydration; treat alkalosis or electrolyte deranges preoperatively if present.
- Definitive treatment is surgical pyloromyotomy.

ADDITIONAL THERAPIES

Medical treatment with oral or IV atropine is an alternative to surgical treatment (3)[A].

- Oral atropine: initial dose of 0.05 mg/kg/day and increased to max of 0.1 mg/kg/day
- IV atropine: initial dose of 0.1 mg/kg/day and increased by 0.01 mg/kg/day until vomiting ceases and then change to oral atropine at twice the effective IV dose

- Recommended for use in patients when anesthesia or surgery is not possible
- Takes 5 to 15 months for pyloric muscle to normalize on medical therapy, although vomiting will usually cease within 7 days
- Associated with lower success rates and longer stays as compared to surgery

SURGERY/OTHER PROCEDURES

- Pyloromyotomy (Ramstedt procedure) is curative.
  - The entire length of hypertrophied muscle is divided, with preservation of the underlying mucosa.
- Laparoscopic approach results in less postoperative pain, shorter hospital stays, shorter postoperative recovery, lower complication rates, improved cosmesis, and can be performed with no increase in operative time or complications (3),(4)[A],(5)[B].

ADMISSION, INPATIENT, AND NURSING CONSIDERATIONS

- Fluid resuscitation:
  - Initially, ≥1 20 mL/kg boluses needed
  - For optimal resuscitation in infants, use D5 1/2 NS with 20 mEq of KCl
  - Usually then placed on 1.5 to 2 times maintenance fluids
- Correct electrolyte abnormalities prior to anesthesia due to metabolic alkalosis reducing inspiratory drive and potentially causing postoperative apnea.

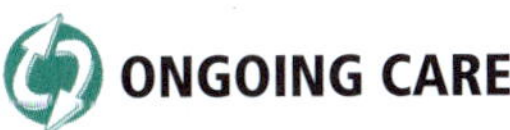

ONGOING CARE

FOLLOW-UP RECOMMENDATIONS

Discharge following surgery when tolerating 2 to 3 full feeds (6)[C].

Patient Monitoring

- Postoperative monitoring including monitoring for pain, emesis, apnea
- If significant emesis present after 1 to 2 weeks, then upper GI studies needed to rule out incomplete pyloromyotomy or duodenal leak (6)[C]

DIET

- Ad-lib feedings are recommended after pyloromyotomy as they decrease length of stay.
- Timing of first feed is not significant, but early feeding is associated with increased potential for emesis without impacting length of stay (7)[A].

PATIENT EDUCATION

Counsel caregivers on postoperative emesis, signs and symptoms of infection, and assessment of hydration status.

PROGNOSIS

Surgery is curative.

COMPLICATIONS

- Dehydration
- Failure to thrive
- Jaundice
- Chronic abdominal pain and pain-associated functional GI disorders following surgery
- Incomplete pyloromyotomy
- Mucosal perforation

REFERENCES

1. Zaghal A, El-Majzoub N, Jaafar R, et al. Brief overview and updates on infantile hypertrophic pyloric stenosis: focus on perioperative management. *Pediatr Ann*. 2021;50(3):e136–e141.
2. Said M, Shaul DB, Fujimoto M, et al. Ultrasound measurements in hypertrophic pyloric stenosis: don't let the numbers fool you. *Perm J*. 2012;16(3):25–27.
3. Wu SF, Lin HY, Huang FK, et al. Efficacy of medical treatment for infantile hypertrophic pyloric stenosis: a meta-analysis. *Pediatr Neonatol*. 2016;57(6):515–521.
4. Oomen MWN, Hoekstra LT, Bakx R, et al. Open versus laparoscopic pyloromyotomy for hypertrophic pyloric stenosis: a systematic review and meta-analysis focusing on major complications. *Surg Endosc*. 2012;26(8):2104–2110.
5. Mahida JB, Asti L, Deans KJ, et al. Laparoscopic pyloromyotomy decreases postoperative length of stay in children with hypertrophic pyloric stenosis. *J Pediatr Surg*. 2016;51(9):1436–1439.
6. Peters B, Oomen MWN, Bakx R, et al. Advances in infantile hypertrophic pyloric stenosis. *Expert Rev Gastroenterol Hepatol*. 2014;8(5):533–541.
7. Sullivan KJ, Chan E, Vincent J, et al; for the Canadian Association of Paediatric Surgeons Evidence-Based Resource. Feeding post-pyloromyotomy: a meta-analysis. *Pediatrics*. 2016;137(1).

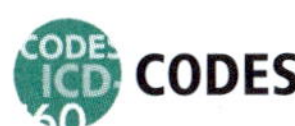

CODES

ICD10

Q40.0 Congenital hypertrophic pyloric stenosis

CLINICAL PEARLS

- Pyloric stenosis is the most common condition requiring surgical intervention in the 1st year of life.
- The condition classically presents between 1 and 5 months of life, with projectile vomiting after feeds and a firm, mobile mass in the right upper quadrant.
- Abdominal US is the study of choice.
- Surgery (laparoscopic Ramstedt pyloromyotomy is the preferred method) is curative, but conservative medical management with atropine can be safe and effective as well.

RAPE CRISIS SYNDROME

Ulunma Natalie Umesi, MD, MBA • Frantz Aubry, MD • Ambreka Benons, MD

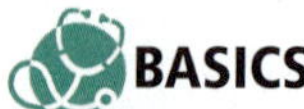

BASICS

- Known also as rape trauma syndrome
- Refers to trauma following sexual assault
- May be experienced by all sexual and gender identities

DESCRIPTION

- Definitions (vary by jurisdiction on local, state, and national levels):
  - Rape (a legal term), sexual assault (a medical term), or sexual violence (a general term): any form of sexual activity that occurs without consent between a victim and perpetrator(s)/suspect(s)
  - Rape/sexual assault/sexual violence: may be associated with the use of force and/or threats, alcohol, and/or illicit and/or prescription drugs
  - Rape crisis syndrome is a historical term that has previously been used to define what is now known as the following, differentiated by time lapsed since the inciting event:
  - Acute stress reaction (ASR)—up to 3 days following event (no longer recognized in *DSM*)
  - Acute stress disorder (ASD)—3 days to 1 month following event (*DSM*-5)
  - Posttraumatic stress disorder (PTSD)—>1 month following event (*DSM*-5)
- Psychological responses to sexual violence range from transient to chronic and debilitating.

EPIDEMIOLOGY

- In the United States, 33% of women and 25% of men have reported experiencing sexual violence during their lifetime.
- The following populations are especially vulnerable:
  - Adolescents and young children
  - Persons with disabilities
  - Elderly adults
  - Those with a low socioeconomic status and/or that are homeless
  - Sex workers and persons being trafficked
  - People living in institutions/areas of conflict/training environments
- 33% of female victims first experienced sexual violence before the age of 18 years; 13% first experienced it before the age of 10 years
- 25% of male victims first experienced sexual violence before the age of 18 years; 25% first experienced it before the age of 10 years
- Only 16–38% of victims report to law enforcement, and only 17–43% of victims obtain a medical evaluation.

RISK FACTORS

- History of sexual violence, psychological aggression, physical violence, trafficking, and/or stalking
- Early initiation of sexual activity
- Engagement in high-risk sexual behavior
- Exposure to familial and/or environmental violence
- Consumption of alcohol/use of illicit drugs
- Belief in traditional gender roles

GENERAL PREVENTION

- Primary prevention: Promoting gender equality, teaching skills to prevent sexual violence, empowering and supporting females, and creating protective environments decrease the occurrence of sexual violence perpetration.
- Secondary prevention:
  - HARK screening tool, which includes questions that assess if a patient has felt humiliated (H) and/or afraid (A), and been raped (R) and/or kicked (K) within the past year, is 81% sensitive and 95% specific for intimate partner violence as well as clinically useful (1).

DIAGNOSIS

History and/or objective physical exam findings concerning for sexual violence

HISTORY

- Medical and forensic histories and exams should ideally be performed by providers with specialized training in providing medical and forensic care (e.g., Sexual Assault Nurse Examiners [SANEs]) who should be willing to testify in court on behalf of the patient, if indicated.
- States usually require the completion of specific forms for documenting the history of a victim and/or suspect/perpetrator of sexual violence.
- Use a trauma-informed approach to patient care in order to help prevent retraumatization by incorporating the "four Rs" (1): (i) realizing the widespread impact of trauma; (ii) recognizing signs and symptoms of trauma; (iii) responding by integrating knowledge about trauma into practices, procedures, and policies; and (iv) resisting retraumatization (2)
- Avoid questioning that may imply that a patient is at fault and/or be interpreted as investigative.
- Inquire about patient safety.
- Record answers in the patient's own words, and request clarification on unclear terminology.
- Describe all types of physical trauma and sexual contact and whether it was actual/attempted and with/without use of force.
- Inquire about any alcohol and/or illicit drug use before and/or after the episode of sexual violence.
- Document the time of occurrence of activities that could potentially alter biologic specimens (e.g., taking a bath or shower, using a douche or mouthwash, brushing teeth, eating/drinking, and/or changing clothes).
- Obtain a thorough gynecologic history, including the LMP, last consenting sexual contact, last use of contraception, and prior surgeries.
- Inquire about a recent history of strangulation.
  - If positive, advise obtaining angiographic neck imaging (e.g., a CT angiogram [CTA]) to assess for a potential carotid artery dissection, embolus, hematoma, and/or edema around the larynx and/or trachea.

PHYSICAL EXAM

- Request for exams to be performed by SANEs, if available.
- Document all atypical physical findings and/or signs concerning for sexual and/or physical trauma.
- Document the patient's mental status and emotional state during the exam.
- In patients with a recent history of strangulation, examine the patient's scalp, eyes, eyelids, ears, face, oropharynx, neck, and chest; and assess for any neurologic, respiratory, voice, and throat-related changes.
- Obtain the patient's consent prior to each step of the examination, as it is both mandatory and empowering to patients.
- Pending the patient's preferences, may obtain confidential medical photographs (i.e., on a secure digital camera that is reserved solely for use on this unique patient population) prior to swabbing and physically examining the patient
- May use a UV light (Wood lamp) and orange-tinted forensic goggles to detect biologic specimens on clothing and/or skin prior to swabbing and physically examining the patient

ALERT

- A medical and forensic SAFE Kit (previously referred to as a "rape kit") contains sterile cotton swabs that can be used to collect biologic specimens from the oropharyngeal cavity, anogenital regions, and other bodily sites as clinically indicated.
- Perform a complete oropharyngeal, genital, and rectal exam and assess for physical signs concerning for physical and sexual trauma, blood and/or other biologic fluids, and/or foreign objects.
  - Use a nonlubricated, water-moistened speculum for patients with a vagina.
  - Perform testing and/or collect biologic specimens as indicated based on the patient's history and physical exam.

DIAGNOSTIC TESTS & INTERPRETATION

- Pregnancy test
- Drug and/or alcohol testing as indicated
- Testing for sexually transmitted infections (STIs) is medically indicated but not required prior to prescribing treatment.

Follow-Up Tests & Special Considerations

- Screen for safety following treatment, including suicidality.
- Counsel regarding pregnancy or transmission of STI following sexual assault.

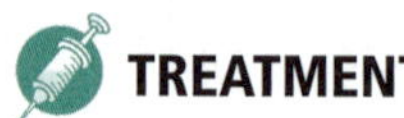

TREATMENT

GENERAL MEASURES

- Employ enhanced sensitivity and privacy measures as well as a trauma-informed care approach.
- All cases of sexual violence must be reported immediately to the appropriate law enforcement agency.
- With a victim's permission, enlist the help of personnel from local support agencies (e.g., sexual violence/"rape crisis" support centers) and in-house social services (e.g., SANEs, victim advocates, sexual assault response and care coordinators, sexual assault care providers, behavioral health specialists, and chaplains).
- Sensitivity of treatment may be best executed with use of a designated Sexual Assault Response Team (SART)
  - National Sexual Violence Resource Center offers both free and certificate courses (3).
- Discuss risks of STI exposure and test/treat as indicated.
- Evaluate for psychological sequelae, and refer for a further evaluation and treatment by behavioral health specialists.

MEDICATION

First Line

- Empirically and prophylactically, treat STIs (especially gonorrhea, chlamydia, trichomoniasis, bacterial vaginosis, hepatitis B, and human papillomavirus [HPV]), as well as considering treatment for human immunodeficiency virus (HIV) and syphilis, depending on a patient's level of risk (4). Cultures are not required before treatment.
- Gonorrhea: (adult dosing) (i) weight <150 kg: ceftriaxone 500 mg IM single dose, (ii) weight ≥150 kg: ceftriaxone 1 g IM single dose; (pediatric dosing) (i) weight ≤45 kg: ceftriaxone 25 to 50 mg/kg IV or IM single dose (not to exceed 250 mg), (ii) weight >45 kg: refer to adult dosing.
- Chlamydia: (adult dosing) azithromycin 1 g PO single dose, or doxycycline 100 mg PO BID for 7 days, or levofloxacin 500 mg PO daily for 7 days; (pediatric dosing) (i) age ≥8 years: azithromycin 1 g PO single dose, or doxycycline 100 mg PO BID for 7 days, (ii) age <8 years with weight ≥45 kg: azithromycin 1 g PO single dose, (iii) age <8 years with weight <45 kg: erythromycin base or ethylsuccinate 50 mg/kg/day PO divided into 4 doses daily for 14 days
- Trichomoniasis: (adult and pediatric dosing) (i) men: metronidazole or tinidazole 2 g PO single dose, (ii) women: metronidazole 500 mg BID for 7 days, or tinidazole 2 g PO single dose
- Bacterial vaginosis: (adult and pediatric dosing) metronidazole 500 mg PO BID for 7 days, or metronidazole gel 0.75% 5 g (one full applicator) intravaginally daily for 5 days, or clindamycin cream 2% 5 g (one full applicator) intravaginally nightly for 7 days
- HIV: nPEP (nonoccupational post exposure prophylaxis) for victims with a high-risk of HIV exposure (e.g., the suspect/perpetrator's HIV status is positive and/or history is positive for IV drug use)
  - nPEP options: (5)
    - Tenofovir disoproxil fumarate (Viread) 300 mg PO daily with emtricitabine (Truvada) 200 mg PO daily for 28 days plus
    - Raltegravir (Isentress) 400 mg PO BID or dolutegravir (Tivicay) 50 mg PO daily for 28 days
    - Pregnant: Dolutegravir should be cautiously prescribed, especially during the first 28 days, given the potential risk of congenital neural tube defects; recommend consulting an infectious disease (ID) provider.
    - Nonpregnant women: nPEP should be cautiously prescribed in nonpregnant women of childbearing age who are effectively using birth control.
    - Children (age ≤12 years): Consult ID provider.
  - Treatment is most effective if started within 4 hours of an episode of sexual assault and can reduce HIV transmission by ~80%; unlikely to be beneficial, if started after 72 hours.
- Hepatitis B: hepatitis B immunoglobulin 0.06 mL/kg IM single dose and initiate a 3 dose-total hepatitis B virus immunization series
  - No treatment if the victim has received a complete hepatitis B vaccine series and has documented levels of immunity.
- HPV: HPV vaccination is recommended for all victims between 9 and 26 years of age and may be considered after shared clinical decision-making in victims between 27 and 45 years of age. Administer 1st dose at initial exam.
- Syphilis: Patients with a high-risk of contracting syphilis may be treated with benzathine penicillin G 2.4 million units IM single dose.

Pregnancy Considerations

Discuss termination-related options listed in order of increasing effectiveness (6).

- Levonorgestrel 0.75 mg PO q12h × 2 doses (Plan B), or 1.5 mg PO single dose (Plan B One-Step); effective up to 72 hours
- Ulipristal acetate (Ella) 30 mg PO single dose; lacks a hormonal component; effective up to 120 hours; preferred for use in overweight and obese
- Copper IUD (Paragard) 313.4 mg IU single device; lacks a hormonal component; effective up to 120 hours

ADMISSION, INPATIENT, AND NURSING CONSIDERATIONS

Patients expressing suicidal or homicidal ideation meet criteria for inpatient psychiatric admission

ONGOING CARE

FOLLOW-UP RECOMMENDATIONS

Patient Monitoring

Follow-up medical care:

- 1 to 2 weeks: counseling; pregnancy and gonorrhea and chlamydia retesting, and vaginitis assessment
- 6, 12, and 24 weeks: syphilis and HIV retesting
- 4 to 8 weeks: HPV anogenital wart assessment

DIET

Higher prevalence in disordered eating following sexual assault in female victims of younger age

PATIENT EDUCATION

Provide community resources for support.

COMPLICATIONS

- PTSD
- MDD

REFERENCES

1. Nelson HD, Bougatsos C, Blazina I. *Screening Women for Intimate Partner Violence and Elderly and Vulnerable Adults for Abuse: Systematic Review to Update the 2004 U.S. Preventive Services Task Force Recommendation*. Rockville, MD: Agency for Healthcare Research and Quality; 2012. Evidence synthesis no. 92. AHRQ publication no. 12-05167-EF-1.
2. Ravi A, Little V. Providing trauma-informed care. *Am Fam Physician*. 2017;95(10):655–657.
3. National Sexual Violence Resource Center (NSVRC). National Sexual Violence Resource Center Web site. https://www.nsvrc.org/homepage. Accessed November 29, 2024.
4. Meehan PJ, Rosenstein NE, Gillen M, et al. Responding to detection of aerosolized Bacillus anthracis by autonomous detection systems in the workplace. *MMWR Recomm Rep*. 2004;53(RR-7):1–12.
5. Centers for Disease Control and Prevention, U.S. Department of Health and Human Services. *Updated Guidelines for Antiretroviral Postexposure Prophylaxis After Sexual, Injection Drug Use, or Other Nonoccupational Exposure to HIV—United States, 2016*. Atlanta, GA: U.S. Department of Health and Human Services, 2016; 2016.
6. Cheng L, Che Y, Gülmezoglu AM. Interventions for emergency contraception. *Cochrane Database Syst Rev*. 2012;(8):CD001324.

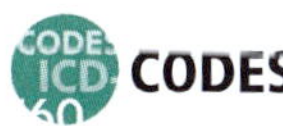

CODES

ICD10

- T74.21XA Adult sexual abuse, confirmed, initial encounter
- T74.22XA Child sexual abuse, confirmed, initial encounter
- Z04.41 Encounter for exam and obs following alleged adult rape

CLINICAL PEARLS

- Employ enhanced sensitivity and privacy measures, as well as a trauma-informed care approach, when providing care.
- All cases of sexual violence must be reported immediately to the appropriate law enforcement agency.

RAYNAUD PHENOMENON

Kelsey E. Phelps, MD

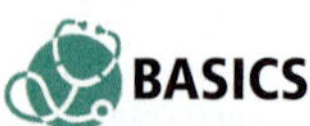

BASICS

DESCRIPTION

- Idiopathic intermittent episodes of vasoconstriction of digital arteries, precapillary arterioles, and cutaneous arteriovenous shunts in response to cold, emotional stress, or blunt trauma
  - A triphasic color change of the fingers (occasionally the toes, rarely nipples) is the principal physical manifestation.
    - The initial color is *white* from extreme pallor, then *blue* from cyanosis, and finally with warming/vasodilatation, the skin appears *red*.
    - Thumbs are rarely involved.
  - Swelling, throbbing, and paresthesias are associated symptoms.
  - Primary
    - 80% of patients have primary disease.
    - Episodes are bilateral and nonprogressive.
    - Diagnosis confirmed if after 2 years of symptoms, no underlying connective tissue disease develops
  - Secondary
    - Progressive and asymmetric
    - Vascular spasm is more frequent and more severe over time. Ulceration is rare; gangrene does not develop; 13% progress to digital fat pad atrophy and ischemic fingertip changes.
    - Typically associated with an underlying connective tissue disorder
- System(s) affected: hematologic, lymphatic, immunologic, musculoskeletal, dermatologic, exocrine

Pregnancy Considerations

- Raynaud phenomenon can appear as breast pain in lactating women.
- Positive breast milk bacterial culture distinguishes mastitis from Raynaud phenomenon.

Geriatric Considerations

Initial appearance of Raynaud phenomenon after age 40 years suggests underlying connective tissue disease.

Pediatric Considerations

Associated with systemic lupus erythematosus (SLE) and scleroderma

EPIDEMIOLOGY

Incidence

- Primary
  - Predominant age: 14 years; ~1/4 begin >40 years
  - Predominant sex: female > male (4:1)
- Secondary
  - Predominant age: >40 years
  - Predominant sex: no gender predilection

Prevalence

- Primary: 3–12% of men; 6–20% of women (based on clinical history)
- Secondary: ~1% of population

ETIOLOGY AND PATHOPHYSIOLOGY

Unknown. Dysregulation of vascular control mechanisms leads to imbalance between vasodilation and vasoconstriction. There is a reduced endothelin-dependent vasodilation activity and an increased vasoconstriction in peripheral vessels by overproduction of endothelin-1. 5-HT_2 serotonin receptors may be involved in secondary Raynaud phenomenon. Platelet and blood viscosity abnormalities in secondary disease contribute to ischemic pathology.

Genetics

Some studies suggest dominant inheritance pattern. ~1/4 of patients with primary condition also have a first-degree relative with Raynaud phenomenon.

RISK FACTORS

- Existing autoimmune or connective tissue disorder
- End-stage renal disease with hemodialysis may increase risk if a steal phenomenon develops in association with the arteriovenous shunt.
- Primary and secondary disease associated with elevated homocysteine levels
- Smoking is not associated with increased risk of Raynaud phenomenon but may worsen symptoms.

GENERAL PREVENTION

- Avoid cold exposure.
- Tobacco cessation
- No relationship has been established between Raynaud phenomenon and vibratory tool use.
- Stress and anxiety can trigger attacks.

COMMONLY ASSOCIATED CONDITIONS

Secondary Raynaud

- Scleroderma; SLE; polymyositis
- Sjögren syndrome; occlusive vascular disease
- Cryoglobulinemia

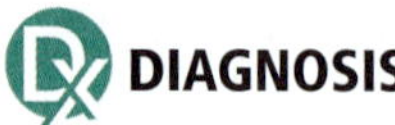

DIAGNOSIS

HISTORY

- Primary
  - Symmetric attacks involving fingers
  - Family history of connective tissue disorder
  - Absence of tissue necrosis, ulceration, or gangrene
  - If after ≥2 years of symptoms, no abnormal clinical or laboratory signs have developed, secondary disease is unlikely.
- Secondary
  - Onset typically after 40 years of age
  - Asymmetric episodes more intense and painful
  - Arthritis, myalgias, fever, dry eyes and/or mouth, rash, or cardiopulmonary symptoms
  - History of medication and/or recreational drug use
  - Exposure to toxic agents
  - Repetitive trauma

PHYSICAL EXAM

Pallor (whiteness) of fingertips with cold exposure, then cyanosis (blue), and then redness and pain with warming

- Ischemic attacks evidenced by demarcated or cyanotic skin limited to digits; usually starts on one digit and spreads symmetrically to remaining fingers of both hands. The thumb is typically spared.
- Rarely involves other tissues (e.g., tongue) (1),(2)
- Beau lines: transverse linear depressions in nail plate on most or all fingernails that occurs after exposure to cold or any insult that disrupts normal nail growth
- Livedo reticularis: mottling of the skin of the arms and legs; benign and reverses with warming
- Primary
  - Normal physical exam
  - Nail bed capillaries have normal appearance: Place 1 drop of type B immersion oil on skin at base of fingernail and view capillaries with handheld ophthalmoscope at 10 to 40 diopters.
- Secondary
  - Skin changes, arthritis, and abnormal lung findings suggest connective tissue disease.
  - Ischemic skin lesions: ulceration of finger pads (autoamputation in severe, prolonged cases)
  - Nail bed capillary distortion including giant loops, avascular areas, and increased tortuosity
  - Abnormal Allen test (Have patient open and close hand several times and then tightly into a fist. Sequentially occlude the ulnar and radial arteries while the patient opens hand to reveal the return of color as a measure of circulation.)

DIFFERENTIAL DIAGNOSIS

- Thromboangiitis obliterans (Buerger disease): primarily affects men; smoking related
- Rheumatoid arthritis (RA)
- Progressive systemic sclerosis (scleroderma): Raynaud phenomenon precedes other symptoms.
- SLE
- Carpal tunnel syndrome; thoracic outlet syndrome
- Hypothyroidism
- CREST syndrome (calcinosis cutis, Raynaud phenomenon, esophageal dysmotility, sclerodactyly, and telangiectasias)
- Cryoglobulinemia; Waldenström macroglobulinemia
- Acrocyanosis
- Polycythemia
- Occupational (e.g., especially from vibrating tools, masonry work, exposure to polyvinyl chloride)
- Drug induced (e.g., clonidine, ergotamine, methysergide, amphetamines, bromocriptine, bleomycin, vinblastine, cisplatin, cyclosporine)

DIAGNOSTIC TESTS & INTERPRETATION

Provocative test (e.g., ice water immersion) unnecessary

- Primary
  - Antinuclear antibody: negative
  - ESR: normal
- Secondary
  - Tests for secondary causes (e.g., CBC, ESR)
  - Positive autoantibody has low positive predictive value for connective tissue disease (30%).
  - Antibodies to specific autoantigens (e.g., scleroderma with anticentromere or antitopoisomerase antibodies)
  - Nailfold videocapillaroscopy is gold standard (200 times magnification).

Follow-Up Tests & Special Considerations

Periodic assessments for a connective tissue disorder

Diagnostic Procedures/Other

Diagnosis is determined by history and physical exam.

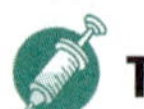

TREATMENT

Assess using a Raynaud Condition Score.

GENERAL MEASURES

- Dress warmly, wear gloves, avoid cold temperatures.
- During attacks, rotate the arms in a windmill pattern or place the hands under warm water or in a warm body fold to alleviate symptoms.
- Tobacco cessation

- Avoid β-blockers, amphetamines, ergot alkaloids, OTC medications containing pseudoephedrine, and sumatriptan.
- Temperature-related biofeedback may help patients increase hand temperature. 1-year follow-up is no better than control.
- Finger guards to protect ulcerated fingertips
- Recognition and avoidance of stressful situations

MEDICATION

First Line

- Calcium channel blockers (CCBs); nifedipine is the best studied and most frequently used. 30 to 180 mg/day (sustained-release form); seasonal (winter) use is effective with up to 75% of patients experiencing improvement.
- Compatible with breastfeeding
- Contraindications: allergy to drug, pregnancy, CHF
- Precautions: may cause headache, dizziness, light-headedness, edema, or hypotension
- Significant possible interactions
  - Increases serum level of digoxin

Second Line

- Amlodipine (5 to 10 mg/day) and nicardipine are effective and may have fewer adverse effects.
- No data exist to support switching CCB if initial drug is ineffective.
- Small studies support benefit from losartan and fluoxetine.
- Phosphodiesterase type 5 inhibitors (sildenafil, vardenafil) may reduce symptoms without increasing blood flow.
- Parenteral iloprost, a prostacyclin, in low doses (0.5 ng/kg/min over 6 hours), has improved ulcerations with severe Raynaud phenomenon when CCBs failed. Oral prostacyclin has not proven useful.
- Nitroglycerin patches may be helpful, but use is limited by the incidence of severe headache. Nitroglycerin gel has shown promise as a topical therapy.
- Topical sildenafil cream may also improve digital arterial blood flow in patients with secondary Raynaud phenomenon (3).
- Prazosin (1 to 2 mg TID) is the only well-studied α_1-adrenergic receptor blocker with modest effect; adverse effects may outweigh any benefit.
- ACE inhibitors are no longer recommended.

ISSUES FOR REFERRAL

If an underlying disease is suspected, consider rheumatology consultation for evaluation and treatment.

ADDITIONAL THERAPIES

- Botulinum toxin has shown promising evidence in the treatment of primary Raynaud phenomenon as well as systemic sclerosis-associated Raynaud phenomenon, including treatment of ischemic ulcers (4).
- Aspirin
- Digital or wrist block with lidocaine or bupivacaine (without epinephrine) for pain control
- Short-term anticoagulation with heparin if persistent critical ischemia, evidence of large-artery occlusive disease, or both

SURGERY/OTHER PROCEDURES

Surgical intervention is rare in Raynaud phenomenon. Effect of cervical sympathectomy is transient; symptoms return in 1 to 2 years. Digital fat grafting is a novel modality that has shown improved symptomatology.

COMPLEMENTARY & ALTERNATIVE MEDICINE

- *Ginkgo biloba* with unclear benefit
- Fish oil supplements may increase digital systolic pressure and time to onset of symptoms after exposure to cold; not proven in controlled trials
- Vitamin D supplementation led to improvement in self-reported symptoms in vitamin D–deficient patients with Raynaud phenomenon (5)[B].
- Evening primrose oil reduced severity of attacks in one study.
- Oral arginine is no better than placebo.
- Acupuncture and acupressure found to be helpful in symptom reduction, but studies have been small and evidence is not statistically significant (6).
- Traditional Chinese medicine (TCM) may have a positive effect on primary Raynaud phenomenon, but evidence is inconclusive due to weak methodology (7).
- Biofeedback is not likely helpful.

ONGOING CARE

FOLLOW-UP RECOMMENDATIONS

Avoid exposure to cold; reassess for secondary causes.

Patient Monitoring

Manage fingertip ulcers and rapidly treat infection.

DIET

No special diet

PATIENT EDUCATION

- Tobacco cessation
- Avoid triggers (e.g., trauma, vibration, cold).
- Dress warmly; wear gloves.
- Warm hands when experiencing vasospasm.

PROGNOSIS

- Attacks may last from several minutes to a few hours.
- 2/3 of attacks resolve spontaneously.
- ~13% of Raynaud phenomenon patients develop a secondary disorder, typically connective tissue diseases.

COMPLICATIONS

- Primary: very rare
- Secondary: gangrene, autoamputation of fingertips

REFERENCES

1. Wigley FM, Flavahan NA. Raynaud's phenomenon. *N Engl J Med*. 2016;375(6):556–565.
2. Devgire V, Hughes M. Raynaud's phenomenon. *Br J Hosp Med (Lond)*. 2019;80(11):658–664.
3. Wortsman X, Del Barrio-Díaz P, Meza-Romero R, et al. Nifedipine cream versus sildenafil cream for patients with secondary Raynaud phenomenon: a randomized, double-blind, controlled pilot study. *J Am Acad Dermatol*. 2018;78(1):189–190.
4. Ennis D, Ahmad Z, Anderson MA, et al. Botulinum toxin in the management of primary and secondary Raynaud's phenomenon. *Best Pract Res Clin Rheumatol*. 2021;35(3):101684.
5. Hélou J, Moutran R, Maatouk I, et al. Raynaud's phenomenon and vitamin D. *Rheumatol Int*. 2013;33(3):751–755.
6. Gladue H, Berrocal V, Harris R, et al. A randomized controlled trial of acupressure for the treatment of Raynaud's phenomenon: the difficulty of conducting a trial in Raynaud's phenomenon. *J Scleroderma Relat Disord*. 2016;1(2):226–233.
7. Zhang J, Hu J, He X, et al. Effectiveness of Chinese herbal medicine for primary Raynaud's phenomenon: a systematic review and meta-analysis of randomized controlled trials. *J Tradit Chin Med*. 2020;40(4):509–517.

ADDITIONAL READING

Herrick AL. Evidence-based management of Raynaud's phenomenon. *Ther Adv Musculoskelet Dis*. 2017,9(12):317–329.

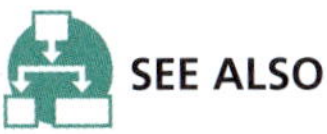

SEE ALSO

Algorithm: Raynaud Phenomenon

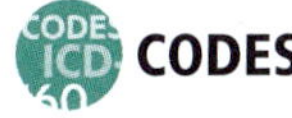

CODES

ICD10

- I73.00 Raynaud's syndrome without gangrene
- I73.01 Raynaud's syndrome with gangrene

CLINICAL PEARLS

- Raynaud phenomenon is a clinical diagnosis.
- Provocative testing is not recommended.
- Initial presentation of Raynaud phenomenon after age 40 years suggests underlying (secondary) disease.
- Cold avoidance and stress reduction are foundational in treating Raynaud phenomenon.
- Digital ulcers are not normal and always merit a workup for secondary disease.
- Acute digital ischemia is a medical emergency.

REACTIVE ARTHRITIS (REITER SYNDROME)

Laura Marsh, MD, CAQSM

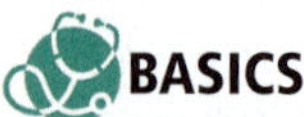

BASICS

Reiter syndrome is a seronegative, multisystem, inflammatory disorder classically involving joints, the eyes, the lower genitourinary (GU) tract, and the skin. It is a sterile, inflammatory arthritis that is triggered by an infection, usually in the gastrointestinal or GU tract. Lower limb joint, axial joint (e.g., spine, sacroiliac joints), and dermatologic manifestations are common (1)[C].

DESCRIPTION

The classic triad includes arthritis, conjunctivitis/iritis, and either urethritis or cervicitis ("can't see; can't pee; can't bend my knee"). The diagnosis is primarily clinical, and there are no formal diagnostic criteria.

- The epidemiology is similar to other reactive arthritides, typically characterized by sterile joint inflammation associated with infections originating at nonarticular sites. Active *Chlamydia* spp. have been detected in the joint fluid of some affected patients, although this is not the norm. A fourth feature (dermatologic involvement) may include buccal ulceration, balanitis, or a psoriasiform skin eruption. (Having only two features does not rule out the diagnosis.)
- Two forms of Reiter syndrome:
  - Sexually transmitted: Symptoms emerge 7 to 14 days after exposure to *Chlamydia trachomatis* and other sexually acquired pathogens.
  - Postenteric infection (including traveler's diarrhea), most typically *Salmonella*, *Shigella*, *Yersinia*, and *Clostridium difficile*.
- In individuals with new or frequent sexual partners, the triggering infection is likely sexually transmitted (rather than enteric). The infection has often been cleared by the time rheumatic symptoms appear, and genital chlamydia is often asymptomatic.
- In individuals with a history of recent enteric illness, the triggering event is more likely to be a bacterial enteric infection rather than sexual transmission.
- Has been associated with COVID-19 infection
- System(s) affected: musculoskeletal, renal/urologic, dermatologic/exocrine
- Synonym(s): idiopathic blennorrheal arthritis; arthritis urethritica; urethro-oculo-synovial syndrome; Fiessinger-Leroy-Reiter disease; reactive arthritis

Pediatric Considerations

Juvenile rheumatoid arthritis (RA) has many of the same clinical features as Reiter syndrome.

EPIDEMIOLOGY

- Predominant age: 20 to 40 years
- Predominant sex: male > female

Incidence

- 0.2–1% incidence after bacterial dysentery outbreaks
- Complicates 1–2% of nongonococcal urethritis cases

Prevalence

~1 to 5 cases per 100,000 individuals per year

ETIOLOGY AND PATHOPHYSIOLOGY

- The pathophysiology of all the seronegative reactive arthritis syndromes and the immunologic role of infectious diseases as precipitants for clinical illness are incompletely understood.
- Pro-inflammatory cytokines lead to synovitis. Toll-like receptors (TLR) have been implicated in the recognition of gram-negative lipopolysaccharide as part of the disease cascade.
- The role of HLA-B27 is incompletely understood, but there is an increased risk of developing reactive arthritis if patients are HLA-B27 positive. In these patients, the disease is more likely to be severe and longer lasting.
- Avoiding precipitant infections and early management of multiorgan inflammation is important.
- *C. trachomatis* is the most common sexually transmitted infection associated with Reiter syndrome.
- Dysentery-associated Reiter syndrome follows infection with *Shigella*, *Salmonella*, *Yersinia*, and *Campylobacter* spp. Enteric-associated Reiter syndrome is more common in women, children, and the elderly than the postvenereal form.

Genetics

HLA-B27 tissue antigen is present in 60–80% of patients, suggesting a genetic predisposition.

RISK FACTORS

- New or high-risk sexual contacts 1 to 4 weeks before the onset of clinical presentation; the primary infection may be subclinical and undiagnosed.
- Food poisoning or bacterial dysentery due to travel or incorrectly prepped/stored food.

GENERAL PREVENTION

- Avoidance of infectious precipitants is the most important general precaution (and potentially the most difficult to achieve).
- Safe sexual practices; proper food and water hygiene

DIAGNOSIS

- Clinical presentation with joint, eye, and GU inflammation and negative serologic testing
- Classic symptoms are not always present.
- HLA-B27 testing is not required for diagnosis.

HISTORY

The presence of the clinical syndrome plus

- Diarrhea, dysentery, urethritis, or genital discharge and appropriate exposure history
- Exposure risks, including travel or migration history and potential infectious exposure
- Arthritis associated with urethritis for >1 month (84% sensitive; 98% specific for diagnosis)
- Urethritis occurs 1 to 15 days after sexual exposure.
- Reiter syndrome onset within 10 to 30 days of either enteric infection or STI
- Mean duration of symptoms is 19 weeks.

PHYSICAL EXAM

- Musculoskeletal
  - Asymmetric arthritis (especially knees, ankles, and metatarsophalangeal joints)
  - Enthesopathy (inflammation at tendinous insertion into bone, such as plantar fasciitis, digital periostitis, polydactylitis and Achilles tendinitis)
  - Spondyloarthropathy (spine and sacroiliac joint involvement)
- Urogenital tract
  - Urethritis; prostatitis; cystitis (rare)
  - Balanitis
  - Cervicitis: usually asymptomatic
- Eye
  - Conjunctivitis of one or both eyes
  - Occasionally, scleritis, keratitis, and corneal ulceration
  - Rarely, uveitis and iritis
- Skin
  - Mucocutaneous lesions (small, painless superficial ulcers on oral mucosa, tongue, or glans penis)
  - Keratoderma blennorrhagica (hyperkeratotic skin lesions of palms and soles and around nails—can be mistaken for psoriasis)
- Cardiovascular: occasionally, pericarditis, murmur, conduction defects, and aortic incompetence
- Nervous system: rarely, peripheral neuropathy, cranial neuropathy, meningoencephalitis, and neuropsychiatric changes
- Constitutional
  - Fever, malaise, anorexia, and weight loss
  - Patient can appear seriously ill (e.g., fever, rigors, tachycardia, and exquisitely tender joints).

DIFFERENTIAL DIAGNOSIS

- Seropositive arthritides: RA and others
- Ankylosing spondylitis
- Arthritis associated with inflammatory bowel disease
- Psoriatic arthritis
- Juvenile RA
- Bacterial arthritis, including gonococcal
- Rheumatic fever

DIAGNOSTIC TESTS & INTERPRETATION

- Blood
  - Negative rheumatoid factor
  - Leukocyte count: 10,000 to 20,000 cells/mm^3
  - Neutrophil predominance
  - Elevated ESR and/or CRP
  - Moderate normochromic, normocytic anemia
  - Hypergammaglobulinemia
- Synovial fluid
  - Leukocyte count: 1,000 to 8,000 cells/mm^3
  - Bacterial culture negative
  - Crystals negative
- Supportive tests
  - Cultures, antigens, or PCR positive for *C. trachomatis* or stool test positive for *Salmonella*, *Shigella*, *Yersinia*, or *Campylobacter* spp.
  - HIV serology (acute retroviral syndrome)
  - HLA-B27 histocompatibility antigen is positive in 60–80% of cases in non–HIV-related Reiter syndrome; HLA testing is not required or recommended for diagnosis.
  - Rheumatoid factor is negative.
  - Screening for STI, COVID-19
- X-ray
  - Periosteal proliferation, thickening
  - Articular bony spurs
  - Erosions at articular margins
  - Joint space narrowing
  - Soft tissue swelling
  - Syndesmophytes (spine); sacroiliitis
  - Enthesitis is a hallmark finding but not always seen (2).

Test Interpretation

- Villous formation within joints; hyperemia, and inflammation
- Prostatitis and seminal vesiculitis
- Skin biopsy similar to psoriasis

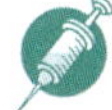

TREATMENT

GENERAL MEASURES

Treatment is determined by symptoms.

- Conjunctivitis does not require specific treatment.
- Iritis requires treatment.
- Mucocutaneous lesions do not require treatment.
- Physical therapy (PT) aids recovery.
- Arthritis may become prominent and disabling during the acute phase.

MEDICATION

First Line

- Symptomatic management:
  - NSAIDs, including indomethacin, naproxen, and others
    - Contraindications
      - GI bleeding
      - Peptic ulcer, gastritis, or ulcerative colitis
      - Renal insufficiency
  - Intra-articular or systemic corticosteroids for refractory arthritis and enteritis
  - Specific treatment of isolated microorganism:
    - *C. trachomatis*: doxycycline 100 mg PO BID for 7 to 14 days (*Note*: All STIs should be treated whether associated with Reiter syndrome or not.)
    - *Salmonella, Shigella, Yersinia,* and *Campylobacter* infections: ciprofloxacin 500 mg PO BID for 5 to 10 days (*Note*: Emerging antimicrobial resistance will limit the utility of ciprofloxacin. Antibiotic treatment does not reduce GI symptoms or duration of infection or prevent carrier state (*Salmonella* only).
    - Antibiotic treatment following onset of syndrome does not appear to benefit inflammatory joint, eye, or urinary tract symptoms, but it may be needed for the triggering infection.
- GI upset: antacids
- Iritis: intraocular steroids
- Keratitis: topical steroids

Second Line

- Sulfasalazine is promising but not FDA approved.
- Methotrexate or azathioprine in severe cases (experimental, not approved or known to be effective); immunosuppressive therapy is relatively contraindicated in HIV-related Reiter syndrome.
- Specialty consultation is recommended, particularly if considering immunomodulatory agents such as sulfasalazine, methotrexate, or azathioprine or for treatment with anti-TNF medications (etanercept and infliximab), which have shown benefit in isolated case reports.
- No published evidence supports the beneficial effect of antibiotics on the long-term outcome in patients with Reiter syndrome.

ISSUES FOR REFERRAL

Joint and eye complications; complex cases—consider consultation with rheumatology; ophthalmology

ADMISSION, INPATIENT, AND NURSING CONSIDERATIONS

- Based on severity of disease and associated complications
- Inpatient care may be needed during acute phase.

ONGOING CARE

FOLLOW-UP RECOMMENDATIONS

Activity modification until joint inflammation subsides

Patient Monitoring

Monitor clinical response to anti-inflammatory medications. Observe for complications, particularly with sulfasalazine and immunosuppressive drugs.

PATIENT EDUCATION

- Educate on risk factors for exposure and recurrence.
- Home PT program
- National Institute of Arthritis and Musculoskeletal and Skin Diseases: https://www.niams.nih.gov/

PROGNOSIS

Acute reactive arthritis typically lasts from 3 to 5 months. Approximately 25% of patients develop chronic reactive arthritis (longer than 6 months). Patients may develop secondary arthritis in the peripheral joints. Prognosis is poor in cases involving the heel, eye, or heart.

COMPLICATIONS

- Chronic or recurrent disease in 5–50% of patients
- Ankylosing spondylitis develops in 30–50% of patients who test positive for HLA-B27 antigen.
- Urethral strictures
- Cataracts and blindness
- Aortic root necrosis

REFERENCES

1. Schmitt SK. Reactive arthritis. *Infect Dis Clin North Am*. 2017;31(2):265–277.
2. Giraudo C, Astorri D, Reijnierse M. Reactive arthritis: a comprehensive journey through diagnostic findings. *Skeletal Radiol*. 2025;54(11):2443–2455. doi:10.1007/s00256-025-04965-8.

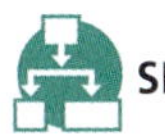

SEE ALSO

Ankylosing Spondylitis; Arthritis, Psoriatic; Behçet Syndrome

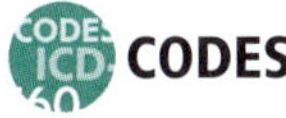

CODES

ICD10

- M02.30 Reiter's disease, unspecified site
- M02.39 Reiter's disease, multiple sites

CLINICAL PEARLS

- Diagnosis of reactive arthritis is based on the clinical presentation of the classic triad of joint, eye, and GU inflammation and negative serologic testing for rheumatoid factor (signs and symptoms may not all be present at the same time).
- Screen for STI (including HIV) if sexually acquired. Enteric studies are rarely clinically indicated.
- Refer patients with a chronic or recurrent course and those who have clinical complications.
- Treatment focuses on symptom relief and treating any underlying infection.

R

RELATIVE ENERGY DEFICIENCY IN SPORT (RED-S)

Rahul Kapur, MD • Kristofer Lee Setterstrom, MD, BSc

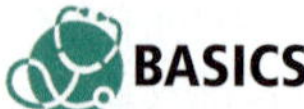

BASICS

Syndrome of three interrelated clinical entities: low energy availability (LEA) (with or without disordered eating [DE]), menstrual dysfunction (MD), and low bone mineral density (LBMD).

DESCRIPTION

- Relative energy deficiency in sport (RED-S) (female athlete triad) first described in 1992 to include DE, amenorrhea, and osteoporosis
- In 2007, American College of Sports Medicine (ACSM) updated definition to: components including LEA (with or without DE), MD, and LBMD with each component representing an interrelated spectrum ranging from health to dysfunction.
- LEA is fundamental to RED-S and full recovery is not possible without correction of it.
- 2014 International Olympic Committee's (IOC) position statement from 2014 deviated to consider "RED-S."
  - Focus on energy deficiency and its broader physiologic effects beyond bone and menstrual health, ranging from growth to cardiovascular.
  - Emphasized similar syndrome in males
- Male athlete triad; LEA, functional hypothalamic hypogonadism, and LBMD
- Concept of energy deficiency in men involving reproductive and bone abnormalities

EPIDEMIOLOGY

Prevalence

- Prevalence: 3/3 criteria (energy availability (EA), MD, LBMD): 0–16%; 2/3 criteria: 3–27%; 1/3 criteria: 16–60%
- DE higher than general population
- MD: prevalence of secondary amenorrhea ~60% in female athletes versus 2–5% in the general population
- LBMD: Using the WHO criteria for LBMD, prevalence of osteopenia (T-score between −1 and −2) ranges from 0% to 40% in female athletes versus ~12% in the general population
- Full triad is more prevalent in lean and weight-bearing sports (1.5–6.7%), including swimming and cross-country, versus non-lean sports (0–2%), including volleyball and softball.

ETIOLOGY AND PATHOPHYSIOLOGY

- EA is defined by energy intake minus exercise energy expenditure.
  - LEA can occur either intentionally or inadvertently (e.g., increasing training or DE).
  - Results in energy shunted from reproduction to more critical functions, (thermoregulation cellular maintenance)
  - Leads to suppression of luteinizing hormone (LH) pulse frequency and thus MD
    - This suppresses ovulation and estrogen concentrations, causing decreased bone formation and increased bone resorption, leading to LBMD.
- RED-S elements exist along a bidirectional continuum of severity, ranging from "healthy" to "unhealthy."
- Additionally, LEA effects endothelial dysfunction and lipids.

RISK FACTOR

- History of menstrual irregularities and amenorrhea; stress fractures and recurrent or nonhealing injuries; critical comments about eating or weight from parent or coach; depression; dieting; personality factors (perfectionism and/or obsessiveness), overtraining, and inappropriate coaching behaviors
- Lean physique sports with an aesthetic component (ballet, figure skating, gymnastics), or sports with weight classifications (wrestling); frequent weigh-ins, consequences for weight gain, and win-at-all-cost attitude all increase risk.
- A lack of family or social support; intense training hours; social isolation, or entering a new environment (boarding school or college); an athlete with comorbid psychological conditions (anxiety, depression, and/or obsessive-compulsive disorder)

GENERAL PREVENTION

- Education of athletes, coaches, trainers, parents, and physicians. Young athletes are extremely impressionable and may turn negative comments and unhealthy advice into maladaptive eating and exercising habits.
- General screening during preparticipation exam (PPE) and annual physicals
- Female Athlete Triad Coalition has 11-question screening to use during PPE.
- Screen athletes presenting with "red flag" conditions such as fractures, weight changes, fatigue, amenorrhea, bradycardia, orthostatic hypotension, syncope, arrhythmias, electrolyte abnormalities, or depression.
- Screen for other conditions that may accelerate bone loss, including steroid use, tobacco use, alcohol use, and hyperthyroidism.
- IOC consensus statement (2023) recommends only testing body composition in athletes <18 years of age for medical purposes due to risk of detrimental medical and psychological outcomes with unnecessary testing (1).

COMMONLY ASSOCIATED CONDITIONS

- Anorexia nervosa, bulimia nervosa, avoidant or restrictive food intake disorder, and other psychological disorders, including low self-esteem, depression, and anxiety
- LBMD predisposes athletes to stress fractures and may not be fully reversible. This may lead to a higher rate of fractures after menopause.

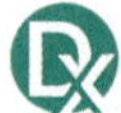

DIAGNOSIS

- RED-S is a clinical diagnosis based primarily on patient history; screening for RED-S at annual sports physicals or during routine exams and acute visits if there are concerns
- In 2015, the IOC RED-S clinical assessment tool (CAT) was developed to help screen for LEA and guide management.
- More recently, validated questionnaires include the Low Energy Availability in Females (LEAF-Q) to screen for LEA, as well as the Female Athlete Screening Tool (FAST) and Brief EDs in Athletes Questionnaire (BEDA-Q) to screen for eating disorders (2).
- LEA can be diagnosed with EA <30 kcal/kg of fat-free muscle mass per day (2).

HISTORY

- Assess menstrual history (including hormonal contraceptive use), fracture history, and symptoms of depression. Assess dietary practices, eating behaviors, and history of weight changes.
- Dietary intake logs (at least 3 days of intake, including one weekday, for comprehensive assessment [2]) and a nutritional assessment by a sports dietitian can help. Assess body image, fear of weight gain, fluctuations in weight, history of DE, and use of laxatives, diet pills, or enemas.

PHYSICAL EXAM

- Height, weight, body mass index (BMI) <17.5% kg/m^2, <85% of expected body weight in adolescents, or ≥10% weight loss in 1 month
- Bradycardia, orthostatic hypotension, hypothermia, cold or cyanotic extremities, lanugo, parotid gland enlargement or tenderness, epigastric tenderness, eroded tooth enamel, and knuckle or hand calluses (Russell sign)
- Patients with amenorrhea should undergo a pelvic exam to verify the presence of a uterus and evaluate for outflow tract abnormalities. Vaginal atrophy may be present if the patient is in a low estrogen state.

DIFFERENTIAL DIAGNOSIS

Screen for anorexia nervosa, bulimia nervosa, avoidant/restrictive food intake disorder, and rumination disorder using the *DSM-5* criteria. Rule out the following in amenorrheic patients: pregnancy, thyroid dysfunction, Cushing syndrome.

- Hypothalamic dysfunction: psychological stress-induced amenorrhea, medication-induced amenorrhea, Kallmann syndrome
- Pituitary dysfunction: prolactinoma, Sheehan syndrome, sarcoidosis, empty sella syndrome
- Ovarian dysfunction: polycystic ovarian syndrome, premature ovarian failure, menopause, gonadal dysgenesis, Turner syndrome, ovarian neoplasm, autoimmune disease
- Uterine dysfunction: Asherman syndrome, absence of uterus

DIAGNOSTIC TESTS & INTERPRETATION

Initial Tests (lab, imaging)

- Basic metabolic panel (BMP), magnesium (Mg), phosphorus, albumin, CBC with differential, ESR, thyroid stimulating hormone (TSH), calcium, 25-OH vitamin D, FSH, LH, prolactin, alkaline phosphatase (fractures) and urinalysis, urine hCG have been well established as initial tests. Consider testing for leptin, IGF-1, and carboxy-terminal propeptide of type 1 procollagen to evaluate for bone formation and resorption (2).
- Pelvic ultrasound in patients with hyperandrogenism to exclude polycystic ovaries or virilizing ovarian tumors
- ECG to rule out prolonged QT interval

Follow-Up Tests & Special Considerations

- BMD testing by DEXA; risk factors: DE, eating disorders >6 months, hypoestrogenism, amenorrhea, oligomenorrhea, and/or in patients with a history of stress fractures or fractures from minimal impact
- If components of RED-S persist, reevaluation by the same DEXA machine every 1 to 2 years.

TREATMENT

- A multidisciplinary team including a physician, registered dietitian, and behavioral health provider build open lines of communication with coaches, trainers, and family.
- Cognitive behavioral therapy (CBT) is necessary given the strong psychological components that can precipitate the condition (3).
- Physically active females should strive for an EA of >45 kcal/kg of fat-free muscle mass per day. If unable to accurately determine fat-free muscle mass, then an increase of caloric intake by 330 +/− 65 kcal/day has been demonstrated to help facilitate return of menstruation (2).
- Nonpharmacologic measures should be taken first and followed for at least 1 year.
- First step is optimizing nutritional status to increase energy intake.
- Goal is body weight associated with normal menses (proving return of acceptable estrogen levels). This often correlates with BMI >18.5 or >90% predicted weight.
- Encourage real food with proper balance of macronutrients/micronutrients over supplements if possible. Aim for 1.2 to 2.0 g/kg of body weight per day of protein intake (2).
- Calcium intake with goal of 1,000 to 1,300 mg/day; encourage calcium-rich foods; supplementation to reach goal if dietary intake is insufficient.
- A minimum of 600 IU of vitamin D should be consumed/supplemented; may require 1,500 to 2,000 IU to keep serum levels between 32 and 50 ng/mL.
- There may be a role for iron, at least in athletes with iron-deficiency anemia if not others.
- Mg (oxygen uptake and electrolyte balance) and zinc (lost in sweat, muscle breakdown) are also crucial; however, specific intake requirements in LEA have not been identified (2).
- Treat maladaptive behavioral disorders.

MEDICATION

Pharmacotherapy should only be considered if the patient has not achieved eumenorrhea after 1 year of recommended therapy.

First Line

For failed nutrition intervention and/or worsening symptoms (particularly fractures): 17-β-oestradiol transdermal patch continuously with cyclic oral micronized progesterone was found to be superior to combined oral contraceptive pills and placebo for improvement of bone density.

Second Line

- Other postmenopausal medications (bisphosphonates, denosumab) should not be recommended in reproductive-aged women, due to potential teratogenic effect.
- Experimental medications: recombinant insulin-like growth factor (rhIGF-1) and metreleptin (synthetic leptin analog)

ADMISSION, INPATIENT, AND NURSING CONSIDERATIONS

Potentially life-threatening conditions (bradycardia, severe orthostatic hypotension, significant electrolyte imbalances, hypothermia, arrhythmias, or prolonged QT interval.) require hospital admission (2).

ONGOING CARE

- Patients should have regular follow-up with a multidisciplinary treatment team.
- The Female Athlete TC consensus statement provided the first evidence-based clearance and return-to-play guidance, which considers the following factors: LEA (with emphasis on DE), BMI, delayed menarche, oligomenorrhea/amenorrhea, LBMD, stress fracture.
- RED-S released a CAT in 2014 (updated in 2015), which considers similar criteria as compared to the TC clearance guide, although classifies them into "green, yellow, red" categories.

PATIENT EDUCATION

All young female patients should be counseled on the importance of proper nutrition, calcium and vitamin D, and the benefits of regular weight-bearing exercise. Patients presenting with ≥1 components of RED-S should be educated about the short-term and long-term effects of LBMD.

PROGNOSIS

- The short-term and long-term prognosis for patients with RED-S depends on time to diagnosis and response to treatment.
- It is estimated that amenorrheic women will lose 2–3% of bone mass per year without intervention.
- With early diagnosis and treatment using a multidisciplinary team, the prognosis for patients with RED-S is good. Patients regain normal menstrual cycling and increase BMD.
- Because RED-S often occurs within the age window of optimal bone strengthening, patients with a prolonged disease course may suffer from complications of decreased BMD throughout their adolescent and adult life.
- Patients with DE behaviors often require long-term therapy to manage their disease.

REFERENCES

1. Mountjoy M, Ackerman KE, Bailey DM, et al. 2023 International Olympic Committee's (IOC) consensus statement on relative energy deficiency in sport (RED-S). *Br J Sports Med*. 2023;57(17):1073–1097.
2. Grabia M, Perkowski J, Socha K, et al. Female athlete triad and relative energy deficiency insport (RED-S): nutritional management. *Nutrients*. 2024;16(3):359.
3. Patel B, Schneider N, Vanguri P, et al. Effects of education, nutrition and psychology on preventing the female athlete triad. *Cureus*. 2024;16(3):e55380.

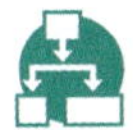

SEE ALSO

Algorithms: Amenorrhea, Primary (Absence of Menarche by Age 16 Years); Amenorrhea, Secondary; Weight Loss, Unintentional

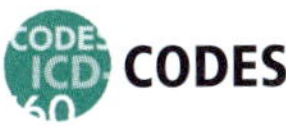

CODES

ICD10

- F50.9 Eating disorder, unspecified
- N91.2 Amenorrhea, unspecified
- R53.83 Other fatigue

CLINICAL PEARLS

- RED-S consists of LEA (with or without DE), MD, and LBMD.
- Early intervention by a multidisciplinary team, including physicians, registered dietitians, mental health professionals, coaches, trainers, and parents, is the most successful strategy to minimize further bone loss, recover BMD, and regain normal menstrual function.

R

RENAL TUBULAR ACIDOSIS

Anastasia Sokhan, MD • Merly Cubelo, DO • Bradley R. Brodie, MD

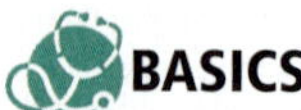

BASICS

DESCRIPTION

- Renal tubular acidosis (RTA) is a group of disorders characterized by an inability of the kidney to excrete fixed acids or resorb filtered bicarbonate (HCO_3), resulting in chronic normal anion gap hyperchloremic metabolic acidosis. Renal function must be normal or near normal.
- Several types have been identified:
  - Type I (distal) RTA: inability of the distal tubule to acidify the urine due to impaired hydrogen ion (H^+) excretion, increased back leak of secreted H^+, or impaired sodium (NA^+) reabsorption; urine pH >5.5
  - Type II (proximal) RTA: inability to reabsorb HCO_3 in proximal tubule with compensatory distal HCO_3 reabsorption accompanied by hypokalemia; urine pH <5.5
  - Type III (mixed) RTA: extremely rare autosomal recessive syndrome with associated osteopetrosis, cerebral calcification, intellectual disability.
  - Type IV (hyperkalemic) RTA: heterogenous group of disorders accompanied by hyperkalemia. Urine pH is usually <5.5 (1).

EPIDEMIOLOGY

The most prevalent subtype worldwide and in the United States is type IV, primarily caused by diabetic nephropathy and urinary tract obstruction. RTA incidence exceeds 20% postrenal transplant, particularly with rejection or immunosuppressive drugs. Type III mainly affecting children of Arabic, North African, and Middle Eastern descent.

Incidence

Incidence of distal RTA (DRTA) is 1 in 10,000 people; proximal RTA (PRTA) is less common

ETIOLOGY AND PATHOPHYSIOLOGY

- Type I—caused by conditions and medications that impair adequate urine acidification at the distal tubule (inability to generate bicarb); often associated with hypokalemia
  - Autoimmune diseases, obstructive uropathy, genetic inheritance and familial disorders, hematologic diseases; medications: NSAIDs, lithium, amphotericin b, aminoglycosides, topiramate, valproic acid, etc.; toxins: toluene, glue, etc.
  - Incomplete distal RTA—a form in which patients are unable to appropriately acidify their urine, however are able to excrete sufficient acid to maintain normal serum HCO_3 and pH.
  - Voltage-dependent RTA—a form of distal RTA in which the impairment in urine acidification is due to poor delivery of Na^+ to the distal tube, leading to disruption of favorable transepithelial voltage gradient, and retention of K^+ and H^+. This form will lead to hyperkalemia, as opposed to hypokalemia in classic distal RTA (2).
- Type II—caused by conditions and medications that impair adequate HCO_3 reabsorption in the proximal convoluted tubule causing bicarbonate leak. Often associated with hypokalemia:
  - Primary Fanconi syndrome or systemic diseases causing Fanconi syndrome (multiple myeloma and other dysproteinemic states, amyloidosis, paroxysmal nocturnal hemoglobinuria, tubulointerstitial nephritis).
  - Medications (carbonic anhydrase inhibitors, chemotherapy agents, antiretrovirals, anticonvulsant medications; other: deferasirox, apremilast, heavy metals, aminoglycosides)
  - Familial (cystinosis, tyrosinemia, hereditary fructose intolerance, galactosemia, glycogen storage disease type I, Wilson disease, Lowe syndrome, inherited carbonic anhydrase deficiency)
  - Defects in calcium metabolism (secondary hyperparathyroidism, vitamin D deficiency)
- Type IV—caused by aldosterone resistance or deficiency that results in hyperkalemia, which lead to impaired ammonia genesis in proximal tubule and decreased acidification of urine:
  - Medications: NSAIDs, ACE inhibitors, ARBs, heparin products, potassium-sparing diuretics, beta blockers, TMP/SMX, calcineurin inhibitors, renin inhibitors
  - Diabetic nephropathy; tubulointerstitial nephropathies; primary adrenal insufficiency; pseudohypoaldosteronism (PHA) (end-organ resistance to aldosterone) (3)

Genetics

- Type I RTA: hereditary forms due to mutations affecting intercalated cells in collecting tubules; loss of function mutations of a chloride-bicarbonate exchanger (AE1) is inherited in autosomal dominant and recessive manners and may be associated with hemolytic anemia, spherocytosis, or ovalocytosis.
- Type II RTA: Autosomal dominant form is extremely rare. Autosomal recessive form is associated with mutation in a basolateral electrogenic sodium-bicarbonate cotransporter (NBCe1) and can be seen with severe growth retardation, ophthalmologic abnormalities, and intellectual disability.
- Type III RTA: Mutations of chromosome 8q22 resulting in carbonic anhydrase II (CA II) deficiency.
- Type IV RTA: Some cases are familial, such as PHA type I (autosomal dominant).

GENERAL PREVENTION

Careful use/avoidance of causative agents

COMMONLY ASSOCIATED CONDITIONS

- Type I RTA in children: hypercalciuria leading to rickets, nephrocalcinosis
- Type I RTA in adults: autoimmune diseases (Sjögren syndrome, RA, SLE), obstructive uropathy, hypercalciuria
- Type II RTA: Fanconi syndrome (generalized proximal tubular dysfunction resulting in glycosuria, aminoaciduria, hyperuricosuria, phosphaturia, bicarbonaturia)
- Type II RTA in adults: multiple myeloma, carbonic anhydrase inhibitors, aminoglycosides
- Type IV RTA: diabetic nephropathy, solid-organ transplant (due to calcineurin inhibitors)

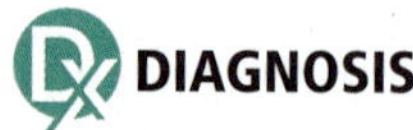

DIAGNOSIS

HISTORY

- Often asymptomatic (particularly type IV)
- In children: failure to thrive, rickets
- Osteomalacia in adults
- Anorexia, nausea/vomiting, constipation
- Polyuria and polydipsia
- Generalized weakness
- Heart palpitations/arrhythmia

DIFFERENTIAL DIAGNOSIS

- RTA should be considered in any patient with normal plasma anion gap metabolic acidosis. If not, evaluate for causes of anion-gap metabolic acidosis: ketoacidosis, ingestions (ASA, methanol, ethylene glycol, propylene glycol), lactic acidosis, D-lactic acidosis, uremia, pyroglutamic acid.
- Extrarenal HCO_3 losses: chronic diarrhea; small bowel obstruction, pancreatic or biliary fistulas; urinary diversion, etc.
- Acidosis of chronic renal failure (develops when GFR ≤20 to 30 mL/min)
- Excessive administration of acid load via chloride salts, including dilutional acidosis via normal saline (NaCl, HCl, NH_4Cl, lysine HCl, $CaCl_2$, $MgCl_2$)

DIAGNOSTIC TESTS & INTERPRETATION

Initial Tests (lab, imaging)

- Serum chemistries and electrolytes
  - Hyperchloremic metabolic acidosis with a normal anion gap (anion gap = $Na^+ - [Cl^- + HCO_3]$)
  - Plasma $HCO_3 > 10$ mEq/L
  - Plasma potassium:
    - Low: in type I RTA (due to impaired distal H^+ secretion/increased H^+ back leak) and type II RTA
    - High: in type IV RTA, and type I (if due to voltage-dependent RTA)
  - BUN and Cr should be normal/near baseline to rule out renal failure as a cause of acidosis.
  - Electrolyte abnormalities of Fanconi syndrome (hypophosphatemia, hyponatremia, hypoglycemia, hypoproteinemia) may be seen in type II RTA.
- Urine studies
  - Urine pH >5.5 in the presence of hyperchloremic metabolic acidosis is strongly suggestive of type I RTA, and type II RTA if serum HCO_3^- is above resorptive threshold of distal tubules (12 to 18 mEq/L). Urine pH is typically <5.5 in type IV RTA.

- Urine culture to rule out infection with urea-splitting organisms.
- Urine calcium is typically high in type I RTA. Increased fractional excretion of phosphate, uric acid, glucose, amino acids, low molecular weight proteins, and presence of urinary retinol-binding protein 4 (not readily available in most places) are sensitive for type II RTA.
- Urine anion gap (UAD; $U_{Na} + U_{K} - U_{Cl}$) is inversely related to urine NH_4^+ excretion (NH_4^+ cannot be directly measured in urine). Positive UAG in acidemic patient indicates impaired urine acid excretion, and is a sign of types I and IV RTA.
  - Accurate UAG requires U_{Na} >25 mEq/L. UAG will also be positive in renal failure, in which acid excretion is impaired. There is a limited utility of UAG in type II RTA, as patients may not have maximal ammonium excretion during acidosis, and UAG may not be appropriately negative.

Pregnancy Considerations

Studies have identified severe acid–base disturbances in pregnant women with inherited type I RTA, who presented with severe hypokalemia and metabolic acidosis.

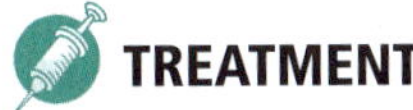

TREATMENT

MEDICATION

First Line

- Provide oral alkali to raise serum HCO_3 to normal.
- Type I RTA: typical doses 1 to 2 mEq/kg/day (in adults), 3 to 4 mEq/kg/day (in children) HCO_3 equivalent divided 3 to 4 times per day (require much higher doses if HCO_3 wasting is present); may require K^+ supplementation.
- Type II RTA: typical doses 10 to 15 mEq/kg/day HCO_3 equivalent, divided 4 to 6 times per day; very difficult to restore plasma HCO_3 to normal, as renal HCO_3 losses increase once plasma HCO_3 is corrected above resorptive threshold; exogenous HCO_3 increases K^+ losses, requiring supplemental K^+; often need supplemental PO_4 and vitamin D due to proximal PO_4 losses (3)
- Type IV RTA: Lowering K^+ concentration often leads to correction of acidosis. Stop nonessential potassium affecting medications. Facilitate K^+ excretion with loop diuretic, sodium zirconium cyclosilicate (Lokelma), or polystyrene sulfonate (Kayexalate) (4).
- Consider vitamin D and phosphate supplementation to avoid bone resorption due to decreased proximal phosphate resorption and decreased activation of vitamin D.
- Sodium-containing compounds will increase urinary calcium excretion, potentially increasing the risk of nephrolithiasis.

Second Line

- Thiazide diuretics may be used as adjunctive therapy in type II RTA (after maximal alkali replacement) to induce mild hypovolemia, which increases proximal Na^+/HCO_3^- reabsorption and reduces amount of alkali replacement needed but are likely to further increase urinary K^+ losses. They can also be considered in type I RTA to reduce calcium excretion.
- Indomethacin can also be considered to reduce severity of polyuria and hypokalemia in type I RTA.
- Fludrocortisone 0.1 mg daily help manage hyperkalemia due to aldosterone deficiency.

SURGERY/OTHER PROCEDURES

If distal RTA is due to obstructive uropathy—lithotripsy should be considered.

ADMISSION, INPATIENT, AND NURSING CONSIDERATIONS

Admit if severe acidosis, hyperkalemia, patient unreliable, emesis persistent, or infant with severe failure to thrive.

ONGOING CARE

FOLLOW-UP RECOMMENDATIONS

Patient Monitoring

Electrolytes 1 to 2 weeks following initiation of therapy, monthly until serum HCO_3 corrected to desired range, and then as clinically indicated; poor compliance common due to 3 to 6 times per day alkali dosing schedule.

DIET

Plant-based diet has lower acid load and less bioavailable phosphate. Increased intake of alkali-producing fruits and vegetables and limiting intake of acid-producing foods may correct acidosis (5)

PATIENT EDUCATION

- National Kidney Foundation: https://www.kidney.org/
- National Foundation for Rare Disorders (NORD): https://rarediseases.org/

PROGNOSIS

Depends on associated disease

- Type I RTA: Amount of alkali supplementation decreases with age due to increased release of H^+ from bone during skeletal growth. Primary disease is permanent and will require lifelong alkali replacement.
- Type II RTA: Long-term compliance to therapy is poor due to large amounts of supplementation required. Prognosis depends on cause; sporadic cases can improve over time and therapy stopped.
- Type IV RTA: Treatment and prognosis depends on underlying cause.

COMPLICATIONS

Nephrocalcinosis, nephrolithiasis (type I); hypercalciuria (type I); hypokalemia (type I, type II if given HCO_3); hyperkalemia (type IV, some causes of type I); osteomalacia (type II due to phosphate wasting), osteopenia (due to buffering of acid in bone)

REFERENCES

1. Corey HE, Eckstein D. Renal tubular acidosis. *Crit Care Nephrol*. 2019;405–408.e1. doi:10.1016/b978-0-323-44942-7.00068-6.
2. Giglio S, Montini G, Trepiccione F, et al. Distal renal tubular acidosis: a systematic approach from diagnosis to treatment. *J Nephrol*. 2021;34(6):2073–2083. doi:10.1007/s40620-021-01032-y
3. Soleimani M, Rastegar A. Pathophysiology of renal tubular acidosis: core curriculum 2016. *Am J Kidney Dis*. 2016;68(3):488–498.
4. Palmer BF, Kelepouris E, Clegg DJ. Renal tubular acidosis and management strategies: a narrative review. *Adv Ther*. 2021;38(2):949–968. doi:10.1007/s12325-020-01587-5.
5. Goraya N, Wesson DE. Management of the metabolic acidosis of chronic kidney disease. *Adv Chronic Kidney Dis*. 2017;24(5):298–304. doi:10.1053/j.ackd.2017.06.006.

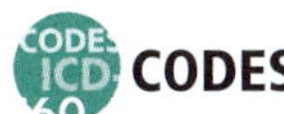

CODES

ICD10

N25.89 Oth disorders resulting from impaired renal tubular function

CLINICAL PEARLS

- Consider RTA in cases of normal anion gap metabolic acidosis with normal renal function.
- Type I RTA: urine pH >5.5 in setting of acidemia; positive UAG; acidemia can be severe.
- Type II RTA: urine pH <5.5 unless HCO_3 raised above the resorption threshold (12 to 18 mEq/L)
- Type IV RTA: most common subtype; hyperkalemia; urine pH <5.5; acidemia usually mild
- Treatment includes avoidance of inciting causes, provision of oral alkali (HCO_3 or citrate), and measures to supplement (type II, many type I) or restrict (type IV) potassium.
- Exclude urinary tract infection (UTI) before diagnosing RTA.
- Consider evaluating for monoclonal gammopathy in patient with Type II RTA.
- Incomplete distal RTA should be considered in any calcium stone formers with a urine pH persistently ≥5.5 in the absence of UTI and normal or near normal serum HCO_3 concentration.

R

RESPIRATORY DISTRESS SYNDROME, ACUTE (ARDS)

Srinath Ramakrishnan, MD • Scott Kopec, MD

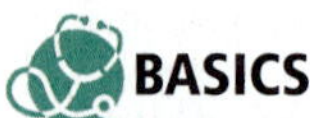

BASICS

DESCRIPTION

- Acute respiratory distress syndrome (ARDS) is a clinical syndrome of acute hypoxemic respiratory failure characterized by bilateral pulmonary infiltrates not fully explained by cardiac failure or fluid overload, developing within 7 days of a known clinical insult or new/worsening respiratory symptoms. This is not a primary diagnosis; rather, it is triggered by other primary diagnoses such as sepsis, trauma, pancreatitis, etc. ARDS presents as new or worsening respiratory symptoms with bilateral alveolar infiltrates on imaging.
- The severity of ARDS is defined by the extent of hypoxia present, measured by the PF ratio, which is the ratio of partial pressure of arterial oxygen (PaO_2) to the fraction of inspired oxygen (FiO_2).
  - Mild distress corresponds with a ratio of 200 mm Hg < PaO_2/FiO_2 ≤300 mm Hg.
  - Moderate distress corresponds with a ratio of 100 mm Hg < PaO_2/FiO_2 ≤200 mm Hg.
  - Severe distress corresponds with a ratio of PaO_2/FiO_2 ≤100 mm Hg.
- Synonym(s): acute lung injury; increased-permeability pulmonary edema; noncardiac pulmonary edema
- Systems affected: pulmonary, cardiovascular

EPIDEMIOLOGY

Incidence

- The incidence of ARDS in the United States is estimated to be 38.9 cases/100,000 person-years.
- An estimated 10–15% of all ICU patients and approximately 23% of ventilator-dependent patients meet the criteria for the diagnosis of ARDS.
- 30% of ARDS cases are classified as mild at the time of diagnosis, whereas the majority of cases (47%) are classified as moderate, and the least amount of cases (23%) are considered severe.

ETIOLOGY AND PATHOPHYSIOLOGY

- ARDS is a response to direct or indirect alveolar injury leading to diffuse alveolar damage.
  - Direct
    - Pneumonia (bacterial, viral, fungal, or opportunistic)
    - Aspiration of gastric contents
    - Near drowning
    - Pulmonary contusion
    - Inhalation injury
  - Indirect
    - Sepsis (nonpulmonary)
    - Shock
    - Transfusion-related acute lung injury (TRALI)
    - Major burn injury
    - Nonthoracic trauma
    - Drug overdose
    - Cardiopulmonary bypass
    - Reperfusion edema after lung transplant or embolectomy
- The progression of the diffuse alveolar damage in ARDS is divided into three phases.
  - Exudative phase—The initial highly inflammatory phase when alveolar macrophages are activated due to lung injury, leading to complement activation, release of pro-inflammatory mediators, and activation of neutrophils. This causes epithelial–endothelial barrier disruption, leading to intra-alveolar and extra-alveolar flooding with fluid. This is followed by hyaline membrane formation leading to alveolar collapse.
  - Proliferative phase—The second phase is characterized by fibroblasts, myofibroblasts, and alveolar epithelial cell (ACE) II mediated repair. Formation of new matrix, differentiation into ACE I, and formation of cellular junctions begins which leads to expression of aquaporin and ion channels, aiding in the reabsorption of fluid.
  - Fibrotic phase—The final phase, not experienced by every patient, is characterized by prolonged mechanical ventilation and associated with increased mortality.

Genetics

No single gene has been identified for clinical use.

RISK FACTORS

- Patients who are low risk may be identified by a lung injury prevention score; however, this score is less accurate in high-risk patients.
- There are several risk factors that predispose patients to developing ARDS. These include advanced age, female sex, smoking, alcohol use, aortic or cardiovascular surgeries, and traumatic brain injury.
- Increased levels of markers of systemic inflammation have been associated with adverse outcomes.

GENERAL PREVENTION

To date, there has been no effective strategy proven to prevent developing ARDS; however, measures can be taken to mitigate risk factors. Early lung protective ventilation and sepsis management have both been shown to improve clinical outcomes in ARDS.

COMMONLY ASSOCIATED CONDITIONS

- Pneumonia, sepsis, and aspiration of gastric contents cause 85% of ARDS cases in the medical ICU setting.
- Other causes can include:
  - Trauma
  - Burns
  - Cardiothoracic surgery
  - Pancreatitis
  - Inhalational injuries and near drownings
  - TRALI
  - Shock
  - Medication toxicity

DIAGNOSIS

HISTORY

Precipitating event (see "Etiology and Pathophysiology") followed by abrupt onset of respiratory distress and hypoxemia

PHYSICAL EXAM

- Progressive symptoms of dyspnea such as tachypnea and tachycardia
- Increased oxygen requirements
- Decreased breath sounds with or without rales

DIFFERENTIAL DIAGNOSIS

- Bilateral pneumonia (including COVID-19)
- Congestive heart failure
- Interstitial and airway diseases
- Hypersensitivity pneumonitis
- Endobronchial tuberculosis
- Diffuse alveolar hemorrhage
- Veno-occlusive disease
- Mitral stenosis: intravascular volume overload
- Drug-induced lung disease especially vascular leak syndrome with immunotherapy

DIAGNOSTIC TESTS & INTERPRETATION

Initial Tests (lab, imaging)

- Initial labs should include a CBC, CMP, and ABG with evidence of hypoxemia.
- ECG: can show sinus tachycardia; nonspecific ST-T wave changes
- Chest x-ray (CXR): bilateral opacities; air bronchograms can be common.
- Chest CT scan: bilateral opacities not fully explained by effusions, lobar/lung collapse, or nodules

Follow-Up Tests & Special Considerations

- Blood cultures, sputum cultures, COVID-19 PCR
- Consider transthoracic echocardiography (TTE) in patients when the diagnosis of cardiac failure cannot be excluded.
- Consider bronchoscopy when the cause of ARDS cannot be clearly identified.

Diagnostic Procedures/Other

- Old approach: Invasive monitoring of pulmonary artery wedge pressure (PAWP) has fallen out of favor after clinical trials have shown no increased benefit and an increase in catheter-related complications.
- New approach: Measuring esophageal pressure with a manometer to estimate pleural pressure allows for adjustment of PEEP to achieve a positive end-expiratory transpulmonary pressure gradient, an approach that is increasingly used in clinical care and especially useful in the morbidly obese (1)[C].

Test Interpretation

- With introduction of the Berlin criteria, a diagnosis of ARDS can be made with a calculated PaO_2/FiO_2 of ≤300 mm Hg along with radiologic evidence of new bilateral infiltrates. If an ABG is not available, ARDS can be diagnosed in nonintubated patients on high-flow nasal oxygen therapy who meet the Berlin criteria using the pulse oximeter saturation/% inhaled oxygen ratio (SpO_2/FiO_2) as a surrogate. A SpO_2/FiO_2 ratio of ≤315 would meet the criteria for ARDS.
- Severity of ARDS is based on the Berlin criteria:
  - Mild—200 mm Hg < PaO_2/FiO_2 ≤300 mm Hg
  - Moderate—100 mm Hg < PaO_2/FiO_2 ≤200 mm Hg
  - Severe—PaO_2/FiO_2 ≤100 mm Hg

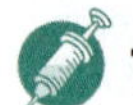

TREATMENT

As ARDS is not the primary diagnosis in patients, it is managed by first stabilizing the patient with appropriate pulmonary support and then ultimately managing the inciting illness or injury.

GENERAL MEASURES

- Identify and treat the cause of ARDS.
- Lung protective ventilation and conservative fluid therapy
- Using tidal volume ventilation (6 mL/kg of predicted body weight) and limiting plateau airway pressure goal to ≤30 cm H_2O has shown a decrease in mortality in comparison to higher volumes.
- Tidal volumes can be reduced to 4 mL/kg if plateau pressures exceed 30 cm H_2O (1)[A].
- Maintaining driving pressure (plateau pressure minus PEEP) should be maintained at ≤15 cm H_2O.

- Respiratory rate can be set to maintain adequate minute ventilation. Permissive hypercapnia is allowed as long as pH >7.3. Recent data supports lower respiratory rates (1)[C].
- Use a PEEP-FiO_2 table (e.g., ARDSNet low PEEP Table) to titrate oxygenation and avoid derecruitment. Routine use of high levels of PEEP in all patients is not recommended (1).
- Routine use of early continuous neuromuscular blockade is not recommended. It may be considered in patients with severe ventilator dyssynchrony or elevated plateau pressures not responsive to other strategies.
- Prone positioning has shown a decrease in mortality and has led to early extubation in patients with moderate to severe ARDS (PaO_2/FiO_2 <150 mm Hg and PEEP >5 cm H_2O) who have been intubated for <36 hours. Prone positioning should be used in adults with severe ARDS (PaO_2/FiO_2 <150) for at least 12 to 16 hours per day for up to 28 days or until a PaO_2/FiO_2 ratio is ≥150 mm Hg. While in the supine position, patients need a PEEP of ≤10 cm H_2O and an FiO_2 of ≤0.6 for >4 hours. The benefit of prone positioning is reduction in deleterious effects of positive pressure ventilation on nondependent and less injured airspaces.
- Extracorporeal membrane oxygenation (ECMO) is reserved for severe ARDS after standard supportive measures have failed. For certain patients with very severe ARDS (PaO_2/FiO_2 <80) refractory to optimal conventional strategies who have a reversible condition, referral to an ECMO center is recommended (1)[C].

MEDICATION

First Line

Dexamethasone should be considered in moderate to severe ARDS of early onset.

ADDITIONAL THERAPIES

- A conservative fluid strategy is recommended in ARDS without shock. For fluid management, central venous pressure (CVP) can be used to estimate fluid status. Fluid strategy of targeting CVP of 4 cm H_2O has led to increased ventilator-free days and a decreased stay in the ICU with no change in mortality.
- Airway pressure release ventilation may improve oxygenation, but studies have shown no mortality benefit (1)[C].
- Noninvasive ventilation should be avoided in patients with moderate to severe ARDS, but high-flow nasal cannula is preferred in mild ARDS (1)[C].
- Early corticosteroids use (dexamethasone 20 mg for 5 days and then 10 mg for 5 days) may be considered in moderate to severe ARDS. Initiating corticosteroids after 14 days of onset of ARDS should be avoided (1)[C].
- No benefit has been shown for using inhaled nitric oxide, β-agonist, surfactant, statins, nonsteroidal anti-inflammatory agents, antioxidants, or neutrophil elastase inhibitor in non-COVID ARDS.

Pregnancy Considerations

Supportive care while identifying the underlying cause of ARDS continues to be important in the management of pregnant women with ARDS. However, fetal well-being, possible need for delivery, and physiologic changes associated with pregnancy must be considered. All pregnant patient should be followed by an obstetrician.

ADMISSION, INPATIENT, AND NURSING CONSIDERATIONS

All patients with ARDS should be managed in an ICU setting.

- Use lung protective ventilation while providing adequate PEEP.
- Consider prone positioning and paralysis if PaO_2/FiO_2 is <120 to 150 mm Hg.
- If failing initial supportive measures, consider early referral to an ECMO center.
- If perfusion is inadequate after restoration of intravascular volume (e.g., septic shock), vasopressor therapy is indicated.
- Early physical therapy
- Nursing care may include any or all of the following:
  - Skin, eye, and mouth care
  - Deep vein thrombosis (DVT) prophylaxis
  - Stress ulcer prophylaxis
  - Suctioning of endotracheal tube
  - Adequate care while changing position of patient from supine to prone and vice versa
  - Ensure adequate level of sedation and/or paralysis while on mechanical ventilation.
  - Tracheostomy care
- Discharge criteria
  - Resolution or improvement of underlying cause, improving respiratory status, and return to baseline oxygen status

ONGOING CARE

FOLLOW-UP RECOMMENDATIONS

Patient Monitoring

- Monitoring driving pressure, lung compliance, and ventilator synchrony regularly to guide optimal ventilation
- Daily labs are needed until the patient is no longer critical.
- Daily CXRs are not needed but should be ordered when evaluating for endotracheal tube placement, the presence of progressing infiltrates, catheter placement, worsening hypoxia, or complications of mechanical ventilation (e.g., air leaks).

DIET

Trophic and full-calorie enteral nutrition have shown no difference in mortality, whereas early parenteral nutrition might be harmful (1)[C].

PATIENT EDUCATION

American Thoracic Society. What is acute respiratory distress syndrome? https://www.thoracic.org/patients/patient-resources/resources/acute-respiratory-distress-syndrome.pdf. Accessed October 9, 2025.

PROGNOSIS

Mortality rates range from 26% to 60% with a significant increase across the severity categories.

COMPLICATIONS

- Short-term complications include:
  - Barotrauma
  - Nosocomial infection
  - Delirium
  - Catheter-related infection
  - DVT
  - Gastrointestinal bleeding due to stress ulcer
  - Poor nutrition
  - Multiple-organ dysfunction syndrome
  - Death
- Long-term complications are related to the age and comorbidities of the patient.
  - Pulmonary dysfunction
  - Reduced health-related quality of life
  - Persistent reticular pattern/ground glass opacities on radiographic imaging
  - Neuropsychological disability, such as depression and PTSD

REFERENCES

1. Thompson BT, Chambers RC, Liu KD. Acute respiratory distress syndrome. *N Engl J Med*. 2017;377(6):562–572. doi:10.1056/NEJMra1608077.

ADDITIONAL READING

Matthay MA, McAuley DF, Ware LB. Clinical trials in acute respiratory distress syndrome: challenges and opportunities. *Lancet Respir Med*. 2017;5(6):524–534.

SEE ALSO

NHLBI ARDS Network. https://www.ardsnet.org/

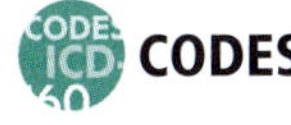

CODES

ICD10

J80 Acute respiratory distress syndrome

CLINICAL PEARLS

- ARDS is the acute onset of hypoxemia secondary to alveolar injury with a PaO_2/FiO_2 ≤300 mm Hg and bilateral infiltrates on CXR.
- Treatment includes identifying and treating the underlying cause, as ARDS is not a primary diagnosis.
- Lung protective mechanical ventilation can improve morbidity and mortality.
- Prone positioning and paralytics can be considered in PaO_2/FiO_2 <150 mm Hg.

RESPIRATORY DISTRESS SYNDROME, NEONATAL

Elizabeth T. Nguyen, MD, CAQSM, FAAP • Tanner J. Jennings, DO

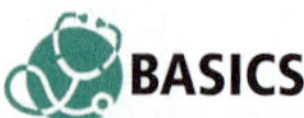

BASICS

DESCRIPTION

- Neonatal respiratory distress syndrome (NRDS) is a disorder primarily of prematurity manifested by respiratory distress. However, it can occur in early term neonates as well.
- System(s) affected: respiratory
- Synonym(s): hyaline membrane disease; surfactant deficiency

ALERT

A disorder of the neonatal period

EPIDEMIOLOGY

Incidence

- >80% incidence in infants born ≤28 weeks' gestation
- 1% all newborns, 10% of preterm infants
- Inversely proportional to gestational age
- Gender: male predominance
- Eighth leading cause of infant death in the United States in 2023: 12.5 infant deaths per 100,000 live births

ETIOLOGY AND PATHOPHYSIOLOGY

- Impaired surfactant synthesis and secretion
  - Usually secondary to deficient surfactant (dipalmitoyl lecithin) production in immature lungs
  - Leads to low lung compliance, low lung volume, and increased lung resistance
- High oxygen exposure and barotrauma during treatment can cause further damage to alveolar epithelium.

Genetics

NRDS is thought to be multifactorial with both genetic and environmental factors contributing to surfactant deficiency in both preterm and term infants, but no current conclusive data is known.

RISK FACTORS

- Premature birth
- Low birth weight
- Infants of diabetic/hypertensive mothers
- Absence of antenatal corticosteroid exposure
- Perinatal asphyxia
- History of RDS in a sibling
- Male sex
- White race
- Cesarean delivery or operative vaginal delivery
- Assisted reproductive technology/multiple gestation
- Lack of prenatal care

GENERAL PREVENTION

- Prevention of premature birth:
  - Education
  - Regular prenatal care
  - Management of maternal medical conditions
- Promote healthy behaviors during pregnancy focusing on:
  - Diet
  - Exercise
  - Avoidance of exposure to tobacco smoke, alcohol, and illegal drugs
- Antenatal corticosteroids:
  - For babies born between 24 weeks and 31 6/7 weeks' gestational age, antenatal corticosteroid use when administered 2 to 7 days prior decreased the risk of NRDS, surfactant use, death.
  - For women at risk for preterm delivery within 24 0/7 and 33 6/7 weeks' gestation, including those with ruptured membranes and multiple gestations

COMMONLY ASSOCIATED CONDITIONS

- Patent ductus arteriosus (PDA)
- Bronchopulmonary dysplasia (BPD)
- Pneumothorax
- Recurrent wheezing, asthma, respiratory infections, and PFT abnormalities
- Neurodevelopmental delay, cerebral palsy

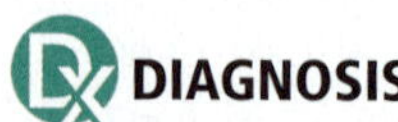

DIAGNOSIS

HISTORY

- Preterm neonates with worsening respiratory distress beginning at or shortly after birth and progressing over first few hours of life
- Early interventions can modify classic course.

PHYSICAL EXAM

- Tachypnea
- Tachycardia
- Expiratory grunting
- Low oxygen saturation
- Nasal flaring
- Subcostal and intercostal retractions
- Cyanosis
- Decreased breath sounds
- Pallor
- Diminished pulses
- Peripheral edema
- Decreased urine output

DIFFERENTIAL DIAGNOSIS

- Bacterial pneumonia
- Transient tachypnea of newborn
- Interstitial lung disease
- Persistent pulmonary hypertension
- Cyanotic congenital heart disease
- Meconium aspiration syndrome

DIAGNOSTIC TESTS & INTERPRETATION

Initial Tests (lab, imaging)

- Arterial blood gases (ABGs)
  - Evaluate for evidence of acid–base abnormalities (respiratory acidosis, metabolic acidosis), hypoxemia, and hypercarbia.
- Chest x-ray (CXR):
  - Microatelectasis
  - Diffuse reticulogranular pattern (ground-glass appearance)
  - Air bronchograms
  - Low lung volumes
- Lung ultrasound
  - Presence of subpleural consolidations
  - Significant correlation with CXR
  - Can also be used to monitor treatment response

Follow-Up Tests & Special Considerations

- Complete blood count with differential
- Blood culture
- Blood glucose
- Lumbar puncture/cerebrospinal fluid

Diagnostic Procedures/Other

- Echocardiogram: Consider if murmur is present to evaluate for PDA and contribution to lung disease due to L → R shunting.
- Lung pathology (autopsy findings)
  - Macroscopically: uniformly ruddy, airless appearance of lungs
  - Microscopically: diffuse atelectasis and hyaline membranes (eosinophilic and fibrinous membrane lining air spaces)

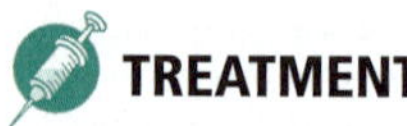

TREATMENT

GENERAL MEASURES

- Delivery room
  - Delayed cord clamping if possible to allow time for placental transfusion and improvement in hemodynamic transition
  - Optimal thermoregulation of delivery room
- Respiratory support
  - If no respiratory failure: early initiation of continuous positive airway pressure (CPAP) (1)
  - If respiratory failure: Intubate, ventilate as needed, and administer pulmonary surfactant.
    - The fraction of inspired oxygen (FiO_2) requirements exceeding 0.3 to 0.4 is still main indication for administration.
    - New research is being performed using lung ultrasound scores to help guide surfactant decisions (2).
- Respiratory monitoring options
  - Noninvasive
    - Transcutaneous monitor or end-tidal CO_2 monitor
    - Pulse oximetry: target >90% to <94% O_2 saturation
  - Invasive
    - Umbilical artery catheter placement
      - Direct sampling of ABGs
- Empiric antibiotic therapy with ampicillin and gentamicin pending evaluation of blood cultures
- Supportive care:
  - Thermoneutral environment
  - Maintain adequate perfusion.
  - Optimize fluid and electrolyte balance (avoid overhydration).
  - Routine use of diuretics is not indicated.
  - Provide for nutritional needs.

MEDICATION

- Pulmonary surfactant
  - Poractant alfa (Curosurf)—porcine lung minced extract
  - Calfactant (Infasurf)—bovine lung lavage extract
  - Beractant (Survanta)—bovine lung minced extract
  - Each surfactant has specific protocols for delivery; consult local standards.
    - Trials show similar efficacy among surfactants. Possible survival advantage of poractant alfa at a higher dose.
    - Possible benefit of surfactant with added budesonide to reduce BPD but further studies needed
  - Administer within first 30 to 60 minutes of life; should be balanced with less invasive forms of respiratory support
  - Strong evidence for use with gestational age <30 weeks, especially if requiring intubation for stabilization
  - Less invasive surfactant administration (LISA) preferred method of surfactant administration for spontaneously breathing babies on CPAP
  - Administration of prophylactic surfactant showed no decrease in intubation rates in first 120 hours of life (3)
  - Side effects
    - Bradycardia
    - Hypotension
    - Airway obstruction/endotracheal tube blockage with administration
    - Rapid changes in tidal volume (due to increased compliance) can cause a pneumothorax and small risk of pulmonary hemorrhage.
    - Transient adverse effects indicates surfactant administration should be temporarily stopped until neonate is stable and dosing can be continued.
  - Contraindications: presence of congenital anomalies incompatible with life beyond neonatal period; infant with laboratory evidence of lung maturity
- Caffeine: Early therapy may improve respiratory effort and improve neurodevelopmental outcomes in low birthweight infants requiring mechanical ventilation.
- Inhaled nitrous oxide (INO) is limited to those with documented pulmonary hypertension with severe respiratory distress and should be stopped if no response given adverse effects.
- No current data to support routine diuretic use

ISSUES FOR REFERRAL

Comorbid conditions associated with prematurity

- PDA (cardiology consult)
- Necrotizing enterocolitis (NEC) (gastroenterology)
- Retinopathy of prematurity (ROP) (ophthalmology)

ADDITIONAL THERAPIES

Treat associated problems of prematurity.

SURGERY/OTHER PROCEDURES

Surgical intervention typically not recommended unless structural or anatomical defect/etiology exists.

COMPLEMENTARY & ALTERNATIVE MEDICINE

No sufficient evidence regarding specific supplementation as effective for treating NRDS

ADMISSION, INPATIENT, AND NURSING CONSIDERATIONS

- All neonates with respiratory distress require immediate evaluation, monitoring, and treatment in the delivery room with transfer to a NICU.
- Supportive care
  - Thermoneutral environment
  - Respiratory monitoring
  - Establish relationship with family to provide education and emotional support.
- Discharge criteria
  - Should have stable vital signs and pulse oximetry before discharge
  - Medical home and support services should be in place.

ONGOING CARE

FOLLOW-UP RECOMMENDATIONS

Following discharge, infants should be followed closely by their physicians to monitor growth and respiratory symptomatology.

PATIENT EDUCATION

- Educate parents regarding the risks in subsequent pregnancies.
- Advise parents regarding potential issues with chronic lung disease.

PROGNOSIS

- Progressive worsening of clinical picture during first 2 days of life
- Prognosis and outcome are highly dependent on gestational age; significant neurodevelopmental delays in almost half infants ≤25 weeks' gestation

COMPLICATIONS

- Complications specific to NRDS
  - Pneumothorax
  - Chronic lung disease, BPD
  - Pulmonary interstitial edema (PIE)
- Additional complications may occur related to therapeutic interventions and comorbid conditions.

REFERENCES

1. Sweet DG, Carnielli VP, Greisen G, et al. European consensus guidelines on the management of respiratory distress syndrome: 2022 update. *Neonatology*. 2023;120(1):3–23.
2. De Luca D, Bonadies L, Alonso-Ojembarrena A, et al. Quantitative lung ultrasonography to guide surfactant therapy in neonates born late preterm and later. *JAMA Netw Open*. 2024;7(5):e2413446.
3. Murphy MC, Miletin J, Klingenberg C, et al. Prophylactic oropharyngeal surfactant for preterm newborns at birth: a randomized clinical trial. *JAMA Pediatr*. 2024;178(2):117–124.

ADDITIONAL READING

- Lemyre B, Laughon M, Bose C, et al. Early nasal intermittent positive pressure ventilation (NIPPV) versus early nasal continuous positive airway pressure (NCPAP) for preterm infants. *Cochrane Database Syst Rev*. 2016;12(12):CD005384.
- Murphy SL, Kockanek KD, Xu J, et al. Mortality in the United States, 2023. National Center for Health Statistics Data Brief No. 521. https://www.cdc.gov/nchs/products/databriefs/db521.htm. Accessed October 24, 2025.
- Roberts D, Brown J, Medley N, et al. Antenatal corticosteroids for accelerating fetal lung maturation for women at risk of preterm birth. *Cochrane Database Syst Rev*. 2017;3(3):CD004454.
- Selfic Pasic I, Riera Soler L, Vazquez Mendez E, et al. Comparison between lung ultrasonography and chest X-ray in the evaluation of neonatal respiratory distress syndrome. *J Ultrasound*. 2023;26(2):435–448.

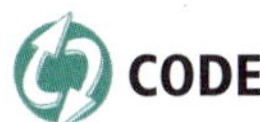

CODES

ICD10

P22.0 Respiratory distress syndrome of newborn

CLINICAL PEARLS

- NRDS is a disorder primarily of prematurity manifested by respiratory distress.
- Early treatment with CPAP or pulmonary surfactant can modify clinical course.
- Prognosis and outcome are highly dependent on gestational age.

RESPIRATORY SYNCYTIAL VIRUS (RSV) INFECTION

Sahil Mullick, MD, FAAFP • Maydolis Mosquera Garcia, MD

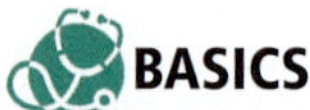

BASICS

Respiratory syncytial virus (RSV) is the primary etiologic pathogen of bronchiolitis and a common agent for pneumonia in infant and the elderly. Despite its global impact, treatment remains primarily supportive.

DESCRIPTION

- RSV remains one of the most common causes of childhood illness and the most common cause of hospitalization in infants, with 90–95% of children infected by 24 months of age.
- RSV-associated lower respiratory tract infections (LRTIs) are characterized as bronchiolitis or pneumonia, may end with respiratory failure, and death.
- In adults, RSV typically causes upper respiratory tract infection (URTI), but life-threatening LRTI/acute cardiac events and worsening of asthma/chronic obstructive pulmonary disease (COPD)/congestive heart failure (CHF) can occur in high-risk populations.
- Infections occur in seasons lasting between 3 and 5 months during autumn and winter. In tropical regions, the infection circulates all year long.

Incidence

- Worldwide, RSV is responsible for approximately 33 million LRTI per year and up to 199,000 childhood deaths.
- Annually, RSV causes an estimated 33.1 million acute LRTIs worldwide, and 3.2 million hospitalizations in children aged <5 years.
- Morbidity and mortality in the United States per year: 2.1 million outpatient visits and 80,000 hospitalizations for RSV in children aged <5 years; 160,000 hospitalizations and 10,000 deaths for RSV in adults aged ≥65 years.
- RSV cases are particularly increasing in the wake of the COVID-19 pandemic.

Prevalence

Difficult to conclude accurately

ETIOLOGY AND PATHOPHYSIOLOGY

- RSV is single-stranded negative-sense RNA virus, belonging to the Paramyxoviridae family. Two subtypes, A and B, are simultaneously present in most outbreaks, with A subtypes causing more severe disease.
- RSV is spread via direct contact or droplet aerosols. Incubation period ranges from 2 to 8 days, mean is 4 to 6 days.
  - Natural RSV infections result in incomplete immunity; recurrent infections are common.
  - RSV causes neutrophil-intensive airway inflammation. It develops in the cytoplasm of infected cells and matures by budding from the membrane.

Genetics

- Severe RSV infections may be associated with polymorphisms in cytokine-related genes, including *CCR5*; *IL4*; *IL8*, *IL10*, and *IL13*.
- RSV replicates in apical ciliated bronchial epithelial cells. The airway epithelium produces chemokines, which recruit neutrophils.

RISK FACTORS

- Significant association with RSV-associated acute LRTI
  - Infants born prematurely; low birth weight, male gender; underlying cardiopulmonary disease; HIV; Down syndrome
  - Any age group with persistent asthma; children <5 years with socioeconomic vulnerability; immunodeficiency; siblings with asymptomatic RSV infection; second-hand smoke; history of atopy, no breastfeeding; adult patients with COPD or functional disability
  - Other risk factors: daycare center attendance; exposure to indoor and environmental air pollutants; multiple births, malnutrition, higher altitude
- For severe or life-threatening RSV infection
  - Preterm infants born ≤28 weeks, 6 days of gestation, or who are <12 months at the start of RSV season; infants with bronchopulmonary dysplasia who are <1 year or <23 months and requiring treatment; infants ≤12 months of age who are being medically treated for acyanotic heart disease or have moderate to severe pulmonary hypertension
- Children <2 years with congenital heart disease, chronic lung disease, weakened immune systems, or who have neuromuscular disorders.
- Adults aged ≥75 years living in nursing homes or long-term care facilities or adults with chronic lung or heart disease (asthma, congestive heart failure, chronic obstructive pulmonary disease, diabetes mellitus, cerebrovascular disease, chronic kidney disease, severe obesity, weakened immune systems, organ transplant recipients, receiving chemotherapy)

GENERAL PREVENTION

- Good hygiene by covering coughs and sneezes, washing or sanitizing hands often, and cleaning frequently touched surfaces; avoid passive smoke exposure. Isolate patients with proven or suspected RSV.
- Immunizations:
  - Adult: single-dose RSV vaccine for everyone aged ≥75 years, and adults aged 60 to 74 years at increased risk for severe RSV disease. Adults who have received the RSV vaccine should not receive another dose.
  - Pregnancy: maternal vaccination with the RSVpreF vaccine between 32 0/7 and 36 6/7 weeks' gestation
  - Infants: administration of the long-acting monoclonal antibody (mAb) nirsevimab to infants aged <8 months entering their first RSV season if the mother is unimmunized, or for children between the ages of 8 and 19 months who are at increased risk for severe RSV disease before their second RSV season.
- Probiotics protect against RSV infection in neonatal mice through a microbiota-AM axis, suggesting that the probiotics may be a promising candidate to prevent and treat RSV infection, and deserve more research and development in the future.
- Breastfeeding can significantly reduce hospitalizations due to respiratory infections.

COMMONLY ASSOCIATED CONDITIONS

In hospitalized infants:

- Pulmonary infiltrates/atelectasis (42.8%); otitis media (25.3%); hyperinflation (20.8%); respiratory failure (14%)
- Hyperkalemia (10.1%, defined as K+ >6); apnea (8.8%); bacterial pneumonia (7.6%)

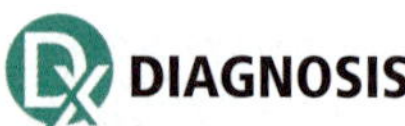

DIAGNOSIS

HISTORY

- History of prematurity, secondhand tobacco smoke exposure, daycare, number, and age of siblings
- Immunization history
- Family history of respiratory disease
- Children: nasal congestion, cough, and coryza. Low-grade fever, wheezing; nasal flaring, chest wall retraction
- Adults: young adults present with URI symptoms; mild fever, cough in 90%, wheeze in 40%

PHYSICAL EXAM

- Vital signs: fever, signs of increased work of breathing (tachypnea, grunting, flaring, retracting), apnea, pulse rate; pulse oximetry
- Dry mucous membranes; skin turgor (dehydration); serous otitis or acute otitis
- Upper respiratory findings: rhinorrhea, nasal congestion, cough, sneezing, and sometimes fever and myalgia
- Lower respiratory tract involvement: rhonchus breath sounds, tachypnea; accessory muscle use, wheezes and crackles; prolonged expiration

Pediatric Considerations

- Young infants with bronchiolitis may develop apnea.
- Hospital admission based on apnea, hypoxia, respiratory failure, reduced oral intake, and hydration status

DIFFERENTIAL DIAGNOSIS

- Mild illness/URTI: other respiratory viral infections: parainfluenza, metapneumovirus, influenza, rhinovirus, coronavirus, human bocavirus, and adenovirus; coinfection with other viruses (e.g., adenovirus, influenza), mycoplasma, or bacteria, including *Bordetella pertussis*, should be considered; allergic rhinitis, sinusitis; asthma exacerbation, croup
- Severe illness/LRTI: bronchiolitis, asthma, pneumonia, foreign body aspiration

DIAGNOSTIC TESTS & INTERPRETATION

Initial Tests (lab, imaging)

- The diagnosis of RSV is clinical. However, it is recommended in hospitalized patients being treated prophylactically with mAb.
- If obtained:
  - WBC count is normal or elevated. Virologic tests for RSV rarely change management decisions or outcomes. Septic workups are not necessary, unless the child is toxic appearing.
  - CXR findings include hyperinflation, peribronchiolar thickening, atelectasis, interstitial infiltrates, segmental, or lobar consolidation.

Follow-Up Tests & Special Considerations

Real-time NAAT (PCR) from nasopharyngeal swabs have superior sensitivity and specificity and are preferred to rapid antigen assays. Serology is not recommended.

Diagnostic Procedures/Other

Evidence of inadequate feeding or fluid intake, history of apnea, lethargy, or moderate to severe respiratory distress (nasal flaring, tachypnea, grunting, retractions or cyanosis), and/or an $SpO_2 \leq 92\%$ in room air (cutoffs for acceptable SpO_2 vary per country), warrant hospitalization, ideally in a secondary care level hospital

Test Interpretation

Antigen test for RSV: Sensitivity ranges from 72% to 94% and specificity 95–100%, in children up to 32 months of age, but sensitivity is 0–25% in older children and adults.

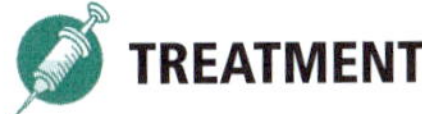

TREATMENT

GENERAL MEASURES

- Treatment for patients with RSV is supportive.
- Nasal suction and lubrication

MEDICATION

First Line

Oxygen as needed, control of fever and pain with acetaminophen and ibuprofen; encourage fluid intake to prevent dehydration

Second Line

- Nasogastric or intravenous fluids who cannot maintain hydration orally.
- While suctioning is often used to reduce secretions in nasopharynx, it prolongs duration of hospitalization particularly in infant aged 2 to 12 months.
- Nonspecific therapies to consider:
  - In severe cases with atelectasis, when conventional therapy is unsuccessful: deoxyribonuclease as nebulized or mucolytic
  - Albuterol (or salbutamol) or epinephrine in infants and children may reduce the risk of hospitalization.
  - Systemic corticosteroids, could be considered where reactive airway disease is strongly suspected (asthma, etc.)
  - In the emergency department, 3% hypertonic saline may reduce the risk of hospitalization, not recommended for inpatient management; may modestly reduce the duration of admission for infants admitted >72 hours—further studies needed
  - Chest physiotherapy for infants and children with a diagnosis of bronchiolitis when relevant comorbidities are present
  - Antibiotics, unless there is a concomitant bacterial infection or a strong suspicion
  - Routine use of ribavirin is discouraged but can be considered on case-by-case basis. It should be considered for treatment of RSV-LRTI in hematologic subjects. Oral formulation appears to be an easier, safe, and cost-effective alternative to aerosolized ribavirin.

ADDITIONAL THERAPIES

Bulb suctioning of the nares

Pediatric Considerations

Over-the-counter (OTC) cough and cold medications should not be used in children aged <6 years.

COMPLEMENTARY & ALTERNATIVE MEDICINE

No complementary, alternative, or integrative therapies are of proven benefit.

ADMISSION, INPATIENT, AND NURSING CONSIDERATIONS

- The main goal is to achieve an adequate fluid balance and normal oxygen saturation levels. Patients with worsening despite oxygen supplementation may benefit from CPAP.
- Mechanical ventilation is required in about 5% of infants hospitalized with RSV.
- Nursing considerations/education: Educate the family on handwashing and universal precautions.
- No set criteria for discharge; stable respiratory status with no oxygen requirement; ability to maintain oral intake and hydration status; adequate follow-up and patient education

ONGOING CARE

- Ad26.RSV.preF demonstrated protection from RSV infection through immunization in a human challenge model and therefore could potentially protect against natural RSV infection and disease.
- RSVpreF vaccine was effective against symptomatic RSV infection and viral shedding. No evident safety concerns were identified. Recently, FDA has approved bivalent RSVpreF vaccine in individuals aged ≥60 years. Clesrovimab is in clinical trials.

FOLLOW-UP RECOMMENDATIONS

Most infants and children can be monitored at home, with follow-up as needed.

Patient Monitoring

- Adequate fluid intake
- Maintaining oxygen saturation

PATIENT EDUCATION

- Bronchiolitis and Your Child: https://familydoctor.org/condition/rsv-respiratory-syncytial-virus/
- Parent education—emphasize use of alcohol-based hand gels/wash and/or to wash hands with soap and water. Clean surfaces with gloves and avoid daycare/kindergarten during recovery.

PROGNOSIS

Most patients recover fully within 7 to 10 days. Reinfection is common.

COMPLICATIONS

- The overall mortality for RSV is <1% with <400 deaths attributed to RSV each year.
- Infants hospitalized for RSV may be at increased risk for recurrent wheezing, allergic sensitization, and reduced pulmonary function, particularly during the 1st decade of life.
- Studies have shown early RSV infection is linked with development of childhood asthma.

ADDITIONAL READING

- Asseri AA. Respiratory syncytial virus: a narrative review of updates and recent advances in epidemiology, pathogenesis, diagnosis, management and prevention. *J Clin Med*. 2025;14(11):3880. doi:10.3390/jcm14113880.
- Centers for Disease Control and Prevention. Respiratory syncytial virus (RSV). https://www.cdc.gov/rsv/index.html. Accessed June 5, 2025.
- Jones JM, Fleming-Dutra KE, Prill MM, et al. Use of nirsevimab for the prevention of respiratory syncytial virus disease among infants and young children: recommendations of the advisory committee on immunization practices - United States, 2023. *MMWR Morb Mortal Wkly Rep*. 2023;72(34):920–925. doi:10.15585/mmwr.mm7234a4.
- Mazur NI, Caballero MT, Nunes MC. Severe respiratory syncytial virus infection in children: burden, management, and emerging therapies. *Lancet*. 2024;404(10458):1143–1156. doi:10.1016/S0140-6736(24)01716-1.

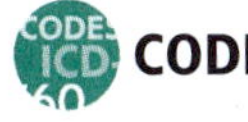

CODES

ICD10

- B97.4 Respiratory syncytial virus causing diseases classd elswhr
- J06.9 Acute upper respiratory infection, unspecified
- J21.0 Acute bronchiolitis due to respiratory syncytial virus

CLINICAL PEARLS

- RSV causes 50–90% of pediatric bronchiolitis.
- Hand sanitation is the key to RSV prevention.
- Diagnosis of RSV is typically clinical.
- Treatment of RSV is usually supportive.
- Consider RSV vaccination for individuals aged ≥60 years.

R

RESTLESS LEGS SYNDROME

Terrence Tsui, DO • Mable Tsui, DO

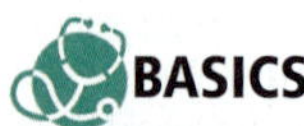

BASICS

DESCRIPTION

- Sensorimotor disorder consisting of a strong urge to move the limbs; legs commonly affected initially but may involve arms/other body parts
- Symptoms begin/worsen during rest or inactivity; relief of symptoms with movement
- Often occurs in the evening
- Involuntary leg jerks reported during wake/sleep
- Early-onset phenotype: 40–60% familial, stable, slow progression of symptoms
- Late-onset phenotype: more aggravating factors and rapid progression
- Synonym(s): Willis-Ekbom disease

EPIDEMIOLOGY

Prevalence

Estimated 5–15% of the population. Women are affected more than men (1).

Pregnancy Considerations

- 10–30% prevalence; triggers/exacerbates RLS
- Predictors: past history (Hx), family Hx, iron deficiency (ID), Hgb ≤11 g/dL (2)[C]
- Peaks in 3rd trimester
- Most symptoms are relieved by 1-month postpartum.

ETIOLOGY AND PATHOPHYSIOLOGY

- Brain iron deficiency (BID), from low serum iron or impaired transport of iron into the brain, leading to CNS dopamine dysregulation:
  - Higher than normal dopamine agonists (DA) levels in the morning leading to DA D_2 receptors downregulation
  - Lower than normal DA at night
  - Increased glutamate and decreased adenosine leading to hyperarousal and insomnia
- Sensorimotor pathways abnormalities and increased motor excitability
- Triggered by prolonged immobility, such as hospitalizations
- Medication induced:
  - Most antidepressants: mirtazapine, TCAs, SSRIs, SNRIs
  - DA-blocking antiemetics (e.g., metoclopramide, prochlorperazine).
  - Phenothiazine antipsychotics (risperidone, clozapine, olanzapine, quetiapine, etc.); possible exception: aripiprazole (partial D_2 agonist)
  - PPIs, H_2 blockers (increase risk)
  - Theophylline and other xanthines
  - Sedating antihistamines
  - Melatonin may exacerbate symptoms (3).

Genetics

- Susceptibility loci: 2p14, 2q, 6p21.2, 9p, 12q, 14q, 15q23, and 20p
- Genes: *MEIS1*, *BTBD9*, *PTPRD*, *TOX3*, *MAP2K5/LBXCOR1*

RISK FACTORS

- ID, vitamin D deficiency
- Family Hx
- End-stage renal disease
- Temperature (cold weather, other environmental factors may increase incidence/trigger symptoms) (4)
- Pregnancy

GENERAL PREVENTION

- Regular physical activity during the day, low-impact activity at night such as stretches, walks
- Adequate sleep quality/quantity; delay wake time if possible.
- Avoid caffeine, alcohol, nicotine mainly in the evening.
- Avoid meds that may trigger RLS (5)[C].

COMMONLY ASSOCIATED CONDITIONS

- Insomnia, delayed sleep phase
- ID, renal disease/uremia/dialysis, gastric surgery, IBS
- Parkinson disease, multiple sclerosis, peripheral neuropathy, Machado-Joseph disease, migraines
- Anxiety, depression, ADHD
- Cardiovascular disease, diabetes mellitus, pulmonary hypertension, COPD

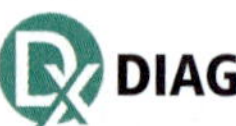

DIAGNOSIS

Clinical, based on Hx, "difficult to describe"; all criteria must be met for RLS diagnosis:

- An urge to move the legs, usually accompanied by or thought to be caused by uncomfortable and unpleasant sensations in the legs. The urge must:
  - Begin or worsen during periods of rest/inactivity such as lying down or sitting
  - Be partially or totally relieved by movement such as walking or stretching at least as long as the activity continues
  - Occur exclusively or predominantly in the evening rather than during the day
- The above features are not solely accounted for by "mimics" or another sleep, medical, or behavioral condition. (Mimics include leg cramps, positional discomfort, habitual foot tapping, arthralgias/arthritis, myalgias, leg edema, peripheral neuropathy, radiculopathy; even though some may coexist.)
- The symptoms of RLS cause concern/distress; sleep disturbance; or impairment in mental, physical, social, occupational, educational, behavioral, or other area of functioning.

HISTORY

- Signs/symptoms (see also "Description")
  - Painful in ~35% of patients
  - Example descriptions: antsy, burning, achy, itching, crawling sensation, "can't get comfortable"
  - Urge to move may be the only "discomfort."
  - Some patients must get up and walk.
  - Periodic limb movements of sleep (PLMS) in ~80% of patients
  - Insomnia, fatigue, anxiety, depression
- Severity range: from rare, minor problem to daily, mild to moderate, to severe impact on quality of life

Pediatric Considerations

Additional supportive findings:

- Insomnia or sleep disturbance
- RLS in immediate biologic relative
- PLMS

PHYSICAL EXAM

Usually normal

DIFFERENTIAL DIAGNOSIS

- Vascular compression: Single position change eliminates discomfort without requiring repetitive movements.
- Claudication: Movement does not relieve pain.
- Motor neuron disease: fasciculation/tremor, no discomfort or circadian pattern
- Peripheral neuropathy: prominent daytime component unresponsive to DAs
- Dermatitis/pruritus: movement only to scratch; no circadian pattern
- Sleep-related leg cramps: muscle knot
- PLMD, RSD: no wake time urge to move
- Growing pains: no urge to move or relief by movement

DIAGNOSTIC TESTS & INTERPRETATION

Initial Tests (lab, imaging)

Assessment of serum iron stores: ferritin, transferrin saturation (TSAT), iron-binding capacity, serum iron (see also "General Measures").

Follow-Up Tests & Special Considerations

If secondary causes suspected, other labs should be evaluated: BUN, serum glucose, creatinine, magnesium, vitamin B_{12}, folate, TSH.

Diagnostic Procedures/Other

- Sleep study (PSG) helpful but not required
  - Frequent, PLM during wake, prior to sleep
- Suggested immobilization test (SIT) or multiple SIT (m-SIT)
  - Patient attempts to sit still in bed for 1 hour (SIT) or four 1-hour periods, every 2 hours (m-SIT) while completing every 10 minutes a visual analogue scale (VAS) or m-SIT disturbance scale.
  - SIT >40 movements per hour suggest RLS.

TREATMENT

GENERAL MEASURES

- If iron insufficient, supplement (5)[C]:
  - 325 mg $FeSO_4$ with 100 mg vitamin C QHS
  - Repletion requires months until serum ferritin >75 ng/mL and TSAT >16%.
- Daily exercise; avoid activities that exacerbate RLS.
- Avoid exacerbating factors; maintain regular sleep.
- Treat obstructive sleep apnea (OSA) if present.
- Hot baths, warm soaks, leg massage
- In bed: long socks, electric blanket, weighted blanket
- Intense mental activity (games, puzzles, etc.)

MEDICATION

- Consider not initiating medications in mild to moderate cases until general measures have failed. Use minimum dose necessary (6).
- Assess symptom severity every encounter using a scale: for example, sIRLS, IRLS, or JHRLSS.
- Opt for longer acting/extended-release options (5)
- Refractory RLS may require combination therapy.

First Line

$\alpha 2\delta$ ligands—less risk for augmentation and more effective in DA-naive patients (5):

- Gabapentin enacarbil (Horizant): 300 to 1,200 mg QD ~5:00 PM (FDA-approved) (5)
- Pregabalin (Lyrica): 50 to 450 mg/day (off-label)
- Gabapentin (Neurontin): 100 to 1800 mg/day (off-label)

Second Line

- Off-label: opiates (5)
  - Buprenorphine/naloxone 2.0/0.5 mg, 1/4 to 2 strips QD
  - Methadone 2.5 to 20.0 mg, oxycodone (IR or ER) 5 to 30 mg
- DAs (FDA approved)—increased risk for augmentation (Rx-induced worsening of symptoms, symptoms occur earlier and spread to other body parts); at every encounter: assess for augmentation, impulse-control disorders (ICD) (5)[C].
  - Pramipexole IR 0.125 to 0.500 mg 1 to 2 hour before symptoms; titrate by 0.125 mg every 4 days.
  - Ropinirole IR (Requip) 0.25 to 4.00 mg 0.5 to 1 hour before symptoms; titrate by 0.25 mg every 4 days.
  - Transdermal rotigotine (Neupro): 1 to 3 mg/24 hr patch; start at 1 mg/day; titrate by 1 mg/week.
- Short-acting DAs for occasional symptoms:
  - Carbidopa/levodopa (Sinemet or Sinemet CR): initial: carbidopa 25 mg/levodopa 100 mg PRN before bedtime
- Avoid DAs in psychotic patients, particularly if taking dopamine antagonists.
- Avoid exceeding DA-recommended dose.
- Benzodiazepines and benzodiazepine receptor agonists if insomnia/anxiety present:
  - Clonazepam (Klonopin): 0.5 to 3.0 mg/day
  - Temazepam, triazolam, alprazolam, zaleplon, zolpidem, and diazepam

Pregnancy Considerations

- Nonpharmacologic therapies, assess/correct ID, vitamin D, folate
- If severe and failed above, 2/3 trimesters, consider low-dose clonazepam, clonidine, carbidopa/levodopa, or opioids (2)[B]

Pediatric Considerations

- First-line treatment: nonpharmacologic therapies, healthy sleep habits, assess/correct ID
- Consider low-dose, age-adjusted gabapentin, clonidine, melatonin for sleep.

Geriatric Considerations

- Avoid medications causing dizziness/unsteadiness.
- Many medications trigger/worsen RLS in the elderly. Consider reducing polypharmacy.

ISSUES FOR REFERRAL

Severe, intractable symptoms

ADDITIONAL THERAPIES

- Noninvasive peroneal nerve stimulator
- Vitamin/supplementation: Mg, vitamin D, folate

SURGERY/OTHER PROCEDURES

For orthopedic, neuropathic, or lower extremities vein disease (laser ablation, sclerotherapy)

COMPLEMENTARY & ALTERNATIVE MEDICINE

Compression stockings, pneumatic compression devices for the legs

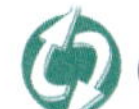

ONGOING CARE

FOLLOW-UP RECOMMENDATIONS

Patient Monitoring

- At 1- to 4-week intervals until stable and then annually
- If taking iron, reassess iron stores, at least ferritin.

DIET

Avoid caffeine and alcohol, mainly in the evening.

PATIENT EDUCATION

- RLS Foundation: https://www.rls.org
- National Sleep Foundation: https://www.sleepfoundation.org/

PROGNOSIS

- Early onset: lifelong condition with no current cure
- Late onset/secondary: may subside with resolution of precipitating factors; otherwise, chronic, progressive
- Current therapies usually control symptoms.

COMPLICATIONS

Augmentation of symptoms following DA therapy

- Higher doses increase risk, and increasing the dose makes symptoms worse.
- Greater risk with meds with shorter half-lives
- ID increases risk.
- Down-titrate and discontinue DAs for at least 10 days, may add alternative medication then or to continue treatment.

REFERENCES

1. Schormair B, Zhao C, Bell S, et al. Genome-wide meta-analyses of restless legs syndrome yield insights into genetic architecture, disease biology and risk prediction. *Nat Genet*. 2024;56(6):1090–1099.
2. Picchietti DL, Hensley JG, Bainbridge JL, et al; for International Restless Legs Syndrome Study Group. Consensus clinical practice guidelines for the diagnosis and treatment of restless legs syndrome/Willis-Ekbom disease during pregnancy and lactation. *Sleep Med Rev*. 2015;22:64–77.
3. Buntak V, Shukla A, Tobias L. Intriguing correlation between melatonin and restless legs syndrome. *Sleep*. 2024;47(Suppl 1):A508. doi:10.1093/sleep/zsae067.01189.
4. Castillo-Álvarez F, Marzo-Sola ME. Restless legs syndrome. Pathophysiology, diagnosis and treatment. *Med Clin (Barc)*. 2025;164(2):84–90. doi:10.1016/j.medcli.2024.05.026.
5. Garcia-Borreguero D, Silber MH, Winkelman JW, et al. Guidelines for the first-line treatment of restless legs syndrome/Willis-Ekbom disease, prevention and treatment of dopaminergic augmentation: a combined task force of the IRLSSG, EURLSSG, and the RLS-foundation. *Sleep Med*. 2016;21:1–11.
6. Silber MH, Buchfuhrer MJ, Earley CJ, et al; for Scientific and Medical Advisory Board of the Restless Legs Syndrome Foundation. The management of Restless Legs Syndrome: an updated algorithm. *Mayo Clin Proc*. 2021;96(7):1921–1937.

SEE ALSO

- Periodic Limb Movement Disorder (PLMD)
- International Restless Legs Syndrome Study Group: https://www.irlssg.org

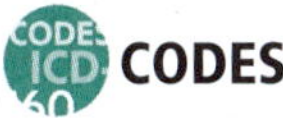

CODES

ICD10

G25.81 Restless legs syndrome

CLINICAL PEARLS

- Iron supplement is an often well-tolerated, easily available treatment for RLS.
- $\alpha 2\delta$ (gabapentinoids) should be considered as initial therapy.
- To avoid augmentation, titrate DAs only up to the minimum dose necessary to control symptoms.
- Antidepressants, antipsychotics, antiemetics, and sedating antihistamines can trigger or worsen RLS.
- Severity and change in symptoms can be monitored using a severity scale such as sIRLS, IRLS, or JHRLSS.
- Insomnia is often a symptom of RLS.

RETINAL DETACHMENT

Angela Rodgers, MD, FAAFP • Gena Damento, MD • Cheyenne Chinea, OD, FAAO

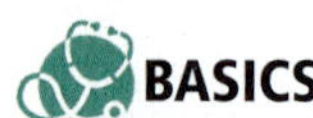

BASICS

DESCRIPTION

- A vision threatening condition where the retina is separated (lifts away) from the underlying retinal pigment epithelium (RPE).
- Three types: rhegmatogenous retinal detachment (RRD), exudative (a.k.a. serous), and traction retinal detachment (TRD)
- Each type has a different mechanism where fluid accumulates under the retina, allowing separation from back of the eye.
- System(s) affected: nervous

EPIDEMIOLOGY

Incidence

- Increases with age
- Male > female (3:2)
- Per year: 1/10,000 (1)

ETIOLOGY AND PATHOPHYSIOLOGY

- RRD: most common type; full-thickness retinal break allows fluid to enter the subretinal space, separating retina from RPE; tension from posterior vitreous detachment (PVD) causes most retinal tears; with aging, vitreous gel liquefies, separating vitreous from retina.
- Exudative (serous) detachment: when fluid accumulates under retina due to breakdown in blood-retinal-barrier; can occur in any disorder that affects retinal or choroidal vasculature, like uveitis, malignant hypertension or preeclampsia, tumors, or medications (2)
- TRD: separation of retina from underlying RPE due to vitreoretinal membranes that occur most frequently with neovascularization of retina, as occurs in proliferative diabetic retinopathy, retinopathy of prematurity, sickle-cell retinopathy; penetrating trauma is another cause that can put traction on retina through same mechanism (3).

Genetics

There is increased risk of RRD if parent or sibling has this condition. Risk increases with family history of myopia.

RISK FACTORS

- RRD:
  - Increasing age: average onset 55 years old but can occur in 20s in significant nearsightedness due to early liquefaction of the vitreous gel
  - Personal/family history of retinal detachment
  - Myopia (>6 diopters is considered high myopia)
  - Aphakia (not having a lens in the eye) or pseudophakia (having an intraocular lens implant)
- PVD
  - Lattice degeneration: areas of retinal thinning found in 7–8% of the general population (1); associated with atrophic retinal holes; <1% of lattice will convert to retinal detachment.
  - History ocular trauma (most often blunt trauma)
- TRD and exudative retinal detachment
  - Presence/history underlying conditions (see above) which could lead to retinal detachment

GENERAL PREVENTION

Pediatric Considerations

Retinopathy of prematurity can lead to TRDs—such patients requires frequent exams and prompt treatment to prevent permanent vision loss.

COMMONLY ASSOCIATED CONDITIONS

- Lattice degeneration
- High myopia
- Hypertension; diabetes

Pregnancy Considerations

Preeclampsia/eclampsia may be associated with exudative retinal detachment. No intervention is indicated, provided hypertension is controlled. Prognosis is usually good.

DIAGNOSIS

HISTORY

- Sudden flashes of light (photopsia)
- Shower of floaters
- Visual field loss is sometimes described as "a curtain coming across the vision."
- Central vision will be preserved if macula is not detached.
- Poor visual acuity (20/200 or worse)
- Vision distortion (most common with exudative retinal detachment)

PHYSICAL EXAM

- Vitals, blood pressure may be elevated.
- Visual acuity and field testing
- Pupillary reflex (relative afferent pupillary defect with larger retinal detachments or if macula involved)
- Fluorescein dye evaluation (Seidel test: rules out penetrating injury/ruptured globe in trauma)
- Anterior chamber evaluation for pigment ("Shafer's sign") with slit lamp
- Tono-Pen pressure assessment
- Dilated eye exam to rule out other differential diagnoses

DIFFERENTIAL DIAGNOSIS

Painless acute vision loss: vitreous hemorrhage, vitreous detachment, central retinal artery occlusion, central retinal vein occlusion, stroke; retinoschisis (splitting of the retina) and vasculitis such as giant cell arteritis (usually involves pain) may be considered.

DIAGNOSTIC TESTS & INTERPRETATION

Initial Tests (lab, imaging)

- A dilated fundus exam to determine presence of retinal detachment; fundus photography (using widefield cameras) may be used as an adjunct.
- Ultrasound can help differentiate retinal detachment from vitreous hemorrhage or vitreous detachment.
  - Point-of-care ultrasound (POCUS): Place linear probe onto closed eyelid viewing orbit in transverse and longitudinal views. Ask patient to look side to side with eyes closed. Detached retina will present as thin, bright (hyperechoic) structure attached to optic disc posteriorly and to ora serrata anteriorly (but separated from choroid) creating "V-shape." This is distinguished from vitreous hemorrhage (hyperechoic dots partially separated from retina) and vitreous detachment (thin hyperechoic structure "swaying seaweed" separated from retina) (4).

Diagnostic Procedures/Other

CRP, ESR, and CBC (looking for platelet elevation) are indicated if there is concern for possible vasculitis such as giant cell arteritis.

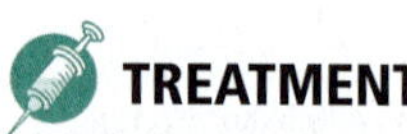

TREATMENT

GENERAL MEASURES

- A prompt referral to ophthalmology is required in cases of suspected retinal detachment.
- Retinal tears often precede RRD, therefore any patient with symptoms of PVD requires dilated exam (patients with new floaters, flashes, or "shadow" in their visual field). Tears are treated with laser procedure (usually performed by retinal specialist) to prevent fluid accumulation underneath retina, which would lead to retinal detachment. Round holes in retina and lattice degeneration are treated based on concern or chance of progression to retinal detachment.
- Exudative detachments are usually managed by treating the underlying disorder.
- Traction detachments can be observed if not vision threatening (not involving macula). If fovea is involved or threatened, surgical treatment, such as vitrectomy, is needed.

MEDICATION

First Line

- Treatment of RRD or TRD is surgical only, with goal of attaching retina back in anatomical position. Medications for exudative detachments are based on underlying cause of fluid buildup.
- This can include systemic steroids in case of inflammatory processes, medications to treat underlying infectious processes, and anti-hypertensive agents in case of hypertensive retinopathy. Rarely, intraocular injections of either a steroid or anti-VEGF agent can be used (2)[A].
- Central serous retinopathy is a choroidal disease known to be associated with corticosteroid use. In these cases, a discussion between ophthalmologist and patient's prescribing doctor is recommended to see if cessation of medication is appropriate.

SURGERY/OTHER PROCEDURES

- Pneumatic retinopexy (PR): when air/gas is injected intraocularly in the office followed by cryopexy in area of the break
- Pars plana vitrectomy (PPV): intraocular surgical procedure performed in the operating room which removes the vitreous, releasing any tension on the retina, which allows it to fall back into anatomical position; vitreous substitutes, such as gas, air, or silicone oil, may be placed into eye to tamponade retina into place. Laser is also used intraoperatively to scar off any tears or openings that could allow fluid to pass underneath the retina in the future. Head positioning is required when gas or air is left in the eye as described in PR above.
- Scleral buckle (SB): when a band is sewn around the outside of the eye which presses the eye inward, mechanically helping the retina to fall back into place; this is more commonly performed in younger patients as is considered less invasive than a PPV.
- Timing of repairs:
  - Macula attached: within 24 hours if possible; if the detachment is peripheral and does not have features suggestive of rapid progression (e.g., large and/or superior tears), repair can be performed within a few days.
  - Macula recently detached: within 7 days of development of a macula-off retinal detachment (1)[A]
  - Chronic macular detachment (>2 weeks duration): elective repair within 2 weeks

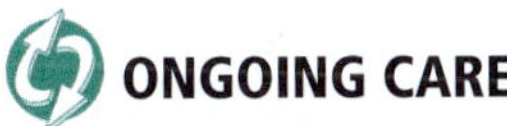

ONGOING CARE

FOLLOW-UP RECOMMENDATIONS

Patient Monitoring

- Patients with acute symptomatic PVD should be reexamined by the ophthalmologist in 4 to 6 weeks. Delayed retinal tears and RRDs can occur for several months after an acute PVD, so the patient should be monitored and be given the warning signs of an RRD.
- If acute symptomatic PVD is associated with gross vitreous hemorrhage that interferes with complete visualization of the retinal periphery by indirect ophthalmoscopy, the patient should be reexamined at shorter intervals with indirect ophthalmoscopy until the entire retinal periphery can be observed. Early PPV can be considered.
- Postoperative considerations
  - If intraocular gas has been used, the patient may need specific head positioning and should not travel to high altitudes to avoid expanding the intraocular gas bubble.
  - Patients should be monitored for development of postoperative infections and use topical antibiotics in the immediate postoperative period.

PATIENT EDUCATION

- It is important for patients to be educated on the symptoms of a retinal detachment in order to seek care from their provider.
- Ophthalmologists should be alerted if there is new onset of floaters or flashes, increase in floaters or flashes, sudden shower of floaters, curtain or shadow in the peripheral visual field, or reduced vision.
- Patients who have gas placed into the eye should be educated not to go into higher elevations unless cleared by their ophthalmologist.

PROGNOSIS

- RRD
  - Postoperative visual acuity depends primarily on the status of the macula preoperatively. Also important is the length of time between the detachment and the repair (75% of eyes with macular detachments of <1 week will obtain a final visual acuity of 20/70 or better).
  - 87% of eyes with a retinal detachment not involving the macula attain a visual acuity of 20/50 or better postoperatively. 37% of eyes with a detached macula preoperatively attain 20/50 or better vision postoperatively.
  - In 10–15% of successfully repaired retinal detachments not involving the macula preoperatively, visual acuity does not return to the preoperative level. This decrease is secondary to complications such as macular edema and macular pucker.
- Tractional retinal detachment
  - Vision may be preserved if not involving the fovea. In cases of proliferative diabetic retinopathy, vision may be limited due to poor overall retinal health even when the retinal detachment does not involve the retina.
- Exudative retinal detachment
  - Prognosis is dependent on control of the underlying disorder. If the underlying condition is treated, the prognosis generally is good.

COMPLICATIONS

- Redetachment of the retina or development of additional retinal tears in the same or other eye
  - PVR is the most common cause of failed retinal detachment repair, where presence of PVR decreases the success rate of the primary procedure to 68% (1)[A].
- Scleral buckles may erode the overlying conjunctiva and lead to an infection.
- Cataract formation is common following intraocular procedures (such as PPV), patients should therefore be monitored for cataract development.
- Rarely, intraocular pressure can be elevated following silicone oil placement due to oil migrating into the angle of the eye or if the eye is overfilled. Elevated intraocular pressure can also be seen in the postoperative period due to a side effect of topical steroid use.

REFERENCES

1. Sultan ZN, Agorogiannis EI, Iannetta D, et al. Rhegmatogenous retinal detachment: a review of current practice in diagnosis and management. *BMJ Open Ophthalmol*. 2020;5(1):e000474.
2. Amer R, Nalcı H, Yalçındağ N. Exudative retinal detachment. *Surv Ophthalmol*. 2017;62(6):723–769.
3. Ghazi NG, Green WR. Pathology and pathogenesis of retinal detachment. *Eye (Lond)*. 2002;16(4):411–421.
4. Lahham S, Ali Q, Palileo BM, et al. Role of point of care ultrasound in the diagnosis of retinal detachment in the emergency department. *Open Access Emerg Med*. 2019;11:265–270. doi:10.2147/OAEM.S219333.

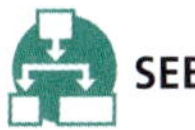

SEE ALSO

Retinopathy, Diabetic

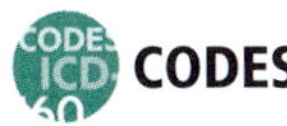

CODES

ICD10

- H33.059 Total retinal detachment, unspecified eye
- H33.20 Serous retinal detachment, unspecified eye
- H33.0 Retinal detachment with retinal break

CLINICAL PEARLS

- If a patient complains of new onset of floaters or flashes of light or loss of vision, the patient should undergo a dilated eye exam to rule out a retinal tear or retinal detachment.
- There is an increased risk of retinal detachment after cataract surgery.
- POCUS is a fast, highly sensitive and specific way to diagnose retinal detachment.

RETINOPATHY, DIABETIC

Haley Severin, DO, MS

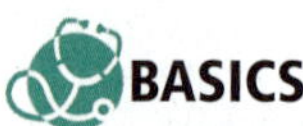

BASICS

DESCRIPTION

- Most patients with diabetes mellitus (DM) will develop diabetic retinopathy (DR). It is the leading cause of new cases of legal blindness among residents in the United States between the ages of 20 and 64 years.
- DR can be divided into three stages:
  - Nonproliferative DR (NPDR) (background)
  - Severe NPDR (preproliferative)
  - Proliferative DR (PDR)

Pregnancy Considerations

Pregnancy can exacerbate condition.

EPIDEMIOLOGY

Incidence

- Peak incidence of type 1, juvenile-onset DM is between the ages of 12 and 15 years.
- Peak incidence of type 2, adult-onset DM is between the ages of 50 and 70 years.

Prevalence

- Worldwide, DR affects 1 out of 3 persons with DM.
- 2/3 of type 1 DM (T1DM) patients who have had DM for at least 35 years will develop PDR, and 1/3 will develop diabetic macular edema (DME). Proportions are reversed for type 2 DM (T2DM).

ETIOLOGY AND PATHOPHYSIOLOGY

- Related to development of diabetic microaneurysms and microvascular abnormalities
- Vascular endothelial growth factor (VEGF) is elevated in patients with hypoxic retina. Intraocular levels of VEGF are elevated in patients with retinal or iris NV. Retinal hypoxia also contributes to DME, and VEGF is a major contributor to DME.

RISK FACTORS

- Renal disease
- Systemic hypertension (HTN)
- Smoking
- Elevated lipid levels

GENERAL PREVENTION

- Monitor and control of blood glucose.
- Schedule yearly ophthalmologic eye exams.

COMMONLY ASSOCIATED CONDITIONS

- Glaucoma; cataracts
- Retinal detachment; vitreous hemorrhage (VH)
- Disc edema (diabetic papillopathy)

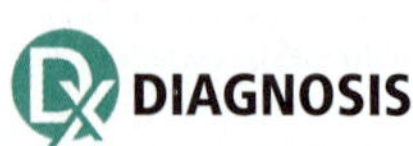

DIAGNOSIS

PHYSICAL EXAM

- Eye exam: measurement of visual acuity (VA) and documentation of the status of the iris, lens, vitreous, and fundus
- NPDR (background)
  - Microaneurysms
  - Intraretinal hemorrhage
  - Lipid deposits
- Severe NPDR (preproliferative)
  - Nerve fiber layer infarctions ("cotton wool spots")
  - Venous beading
  - Venous dilatation
  - Intraretinal microvascular abnormalities (IRMA)
  - Extensive retinal hemorrhage
  - The Early Treatment Diabetic Retinopathy Study (ETDRS) developed the 4:2:1 rule for severe NPDR. Severe NPDR was defined as having any one of the following features:
    - Severe intraretinal hemorrhages and microaneurysms in four quadrants
    - Venous beading in two or more quadrants
    - IRMAs in one or more quadrants
- PDR
  - New blood vessel proliferation: NV can be found on the retinal surface, optic nerve, and iris.
  - Visual loss caused by VH, traction retinal detachment; contraction of fibrovascular tissue on a vitreous scaffold can lead to VH and traction retinal detachment.

DIFFERENTIAL DIAGNOSIS

Other causes of retinopathy (e.g., radiation, retinal venous obstruction, HTN)

DIAGNOSTIC TESTS & INTERPRETATION

Diagnostic Procedures/Other

- Fluorescein angiography demonstrates retinal nonperfusion, retinal leakage, and PDR.
- Optical coherence tomography (OCT) can be used to help detect DME by measuring retinal thickness. Swept-source OCT angiography (SS-OCTA) can detect diabetic NV. OCT angiography (OCTA) can visualize the retinal vasculature.

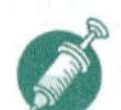

TREATMENT

GENERAL MEASURES

- The Diabetes Control and Complications Trial (DCCT) recommended that for most patients with T1DM with insulin-dependent DM, blood glucose levels should be as close to the nondiabetic range as is safe to reduce the risk and rate of progression of DR.
- The United Kingdom Prospective Diabetes Study (UKPDS) demonstrated patients with T2DM had slower progression of DR with intensive blood glucose control. It also showed that intensive control of blood pressure slowed progression of DR.
- Microvascular complications, including PDR, are increased when blood sugar levels are ≥200 mg/dL.
- Cataract surgery can cause retinopathy to worsen and increase the risk for development of DME.
- HTN has a detrimental effect on DR and must be controlled.
- Severe obstructive sleep apnea (OSA) is a risk factor for DME in patients with T2DM. Refractory continuous positive airway pressure (CPAP) may help prevent refractory DME in patients with OSA (1)[B].

MEDICATION

- Treatment of HTN with the angiotensin-receptor blocker candesartan has been shown to result in regression of DR in some patients.
- Statin therapy in patients with T2DM is associated with a decreased risk of DR. T2DM patients on lipid-lowering medications are less likely to develop NPDR, PDR, or DME.
- Treatment with fenofibrate are effective agents reducing progression of DR in patients with overt retinopathy (2).

SURGERY/OTHER PROCEDURES

- Preventive treatment of moderate to severe NPDR without centered-involved DME (CI-DME) with intravitreal aflibercept injection (IAI) reduced the development of PDR or vision-reducing CI-DME. After 2 years of follow-up, preventive treatment with IAI did not confer VA benefit compared with observation plus IAI only after development of PDR or vision-reducing CI-DME (3)[A].
- Treatment for DME
  - Intravitreal anti-VEGF is first-line treatment for DME:
    - Ranibizumab, an antibody fragment that binds VEGF, can be used to treat DME when injected intravitreally. Ranibizumab 0.3 mg (0.05 mL) injected intravitreally monthly resulted in improved vision and reduced central foveal thickness.
      - Anti-VEGF treatment by intravitreal injection (IVI) results in superior clinical outcomes compared to laser photocoagulation for DME.
      - Intravitreal ranibizumab injections (IRIs) are beneficial for patients with DME and concurrent macular nonperfusion.
      - IRI for DME may also improve DR severity and reduce the risk of DR progression.
      - Treat and extend dosing for IRI decreased the number of injections while giving similar visual and anatomic outcomes compared with monthly dosing at 1 year.
      - As-needed treatment after a loading dose of 3 monthly injections has been shown to result in comparable results to more frequent treatments.
      - Topical povidone-iodine prophylaxis is important to help prevent endophthalmitis from IVIs from anti-VEGF treatment.
    - Bevacizumab, a full-length antibody that binds VEGF, can be used to treat DME when injected intravitreally. Intravitreal bevacizumab injection (IBI) is an off-label use.
    - Aflibercept, a decoy receptor for VEGF that inhibits all isoforms of VEGF-A, B, and placental growth factor isoforms (4); aflibercept 2 mg (0.05 mL) injected intravitreally every 4 weeks for the first 5 injections followed by 2 mg (0.05 mL) intravitreally once every 8 weeks; it is indicated for patients with DME and for DR in patients without DME.
      - IAI has demonstrated significant superiority in functional and anatomic end points over macular laser photocoagulation.

- At worse levels of initial VA (20/50 or worse) in patients with DME, IAI was more effective in improving vision than ranibizumab or bevacizumab with 1-year follow-up. When the initial vision loss was mild (20/32 to 20/40) in patients with DME, there was no significant difference between aflibercept, ranibizumab, and bevacizumab.
  - Aflibercept had superior 2-year VA outcomes compared with bevacizumab. The superiority of aflibercept over ranibizumab, noted at 1 year, was no longer seen at 2 years of follow-up.
- Among eyes with CI-DME and good VA (20/25 or better), there was no significant difference in vision loss whether eyes were initially managed with observation plus IAI only if VA decreased, or with initial focal laser treatment plus IAI only if VA decreased, or prompt IAI. Observation without treatment unless VA worsens may be a reasonable plan of action for CI-DME (5)[A].
- As-needed IAI has been shown to maintain vision and reduce treatment frequency.

◦ Brolucizumab, a humanized single-chain antibody fragment that inhibits all isoforms of VEGF-A. It is injected intravitreally, at a dose of 6 mg every 6 weeks for the first 5 doses, followed by 1 injection every 8 to 12 weeks. There are reports of retinal vasculitis and/or retinal vascular occlusion after IVI of brolucizumab.

◦ Faricimab, inhibits both angiopoietin 2 and VEGF-A. It is injected intravitreally, at a dose of 6 mg monthly for the first 4 doses. Treatment is extended or reduced based on outcomes, with a range of 1 to 4 months between doses (6)[A].

– Focal laser treatment.

– Vitrectomy may benefit some with diffuse macular edema. This may apply especially to eyes with vitreomacular traction found on OCT and with persistent DME.

– Intravitreal triamcinolone may be used for DM-related macular edema that fails laser treatment; no long-term benefit of intravitreal triamcinolone relative to focal/grid photocoagulation in patients with DME. When anti-VEGF treatment is inappropriate or ineffective for DME, intravitreal corticosteroid treatment and/or macular focal/grid laser photocoagulation may be used.

– Intraocular steroid implants for DME; either a dexamethasone implant or a fluocinolone acetonide implant; complications of these implants include cataract and glaucoma.

- Treatment for PDR:
  - Thermal laser photocoagulation in a panretinal pattern is a common form of treatment for PDR. The goal of panretinal photocoagulation (PRP) is regression or involution of NV. PRP destroys ischemic retina and decreases the neovascular stimulus.
    - The DR study demonstrated that when PRP was used to treat PDR or severe NPDR, eyes treated with PRP had a reduction of ≥50% in the rates of severe vision loss compared with untreated control eyes. In certain subgroups, the incidence of severe visual loss in untreated eyes was as high as 36.9% at 2 years.
    - Patients with DME and high-risk proliferative disease can have simultaneous focal and PRP without adversely affecting the visual outcome.
  - Both IRI and IAI are alternative therapies to PRP for PDR. They can be used in conjunction with PRP to treat PDR.
  - Initial IAI or pars plana vitrectomy (PPV) with PRP can be used to treat PDR-related VH (7)[A].
  - IVI of anti-VEGF therapy for PDR does not increase the risk for TRD.
  - PPV recommended for patients with severe PDR, traction retinal detachment involving the macula, and nonclearing VH:
    - The Diabetic Retinopathy Vitrectomy Study (DRVS) demonstrated the benefits of early PPV (1 to 6 months after onset of VH) in T1DM and for eyes with very severe PDR.
    - Immediate PPV with endolaser may be considered for PDR-associated VH (<30 days).
    - Preoperative IBI can be used as an adjuvant to vitrectomy for complications of PDR. This is an off-label use.

ONGOING CARE

FOLLOW-UP RECOMMENDATIONS

Patient Monitoring

Scheduled ophthalmologic eye exams

- Yearly follow-up if no retinopathy
- Every 6 months with background DR
- At least every 3 to 4 months with pre PDR
- Every 2 to 3 months with active PDR
- Patients with DME should be followed every 4 to 6 weeks.

DIET

In middle-aged and older individuals with T2DM, intake of at least 500 mg/day of dietary long-chain omega-3 polyunsaturated fatty acids, achievable with 2 weekly servings of oily fish, is associated with a decreased risk of DR.

PATIENT EDUCATION

- Advise regular ophthalmic exams.
- Stress importance of glucose control.

PROGNOSIS

If the condition is diagnosed and treated early in development, outlook is good. If treatment is delayed, blindness may result.

COMPLICATIONS

- Repeated IVI of anti-VEGF therapy may increase the risk of sustained intraocular pressure elevation and the possible need for ocular hypotensive treatment.
- Blindness

REFERENCES

1. Chiang JF, Sun MH, Chen KJ, et al. Association between obstructive sleep apnea and diabetic macular edema in patients with type 2 diabetes. *Am J Ophthalmol*. 2021;226:217–225.
2. Kataoka SY, Lois N, Kawano S, et al. Fenofibrate for diabetic retinopathy. *Cochrane Database Syst Rev*. 2023;6(6):CD013318. doi:10.1002/14651858.CD013318.pub2.
3. Maturi RK, Glassman AR, Josic K, et al. Effect of intravitreous anti-vascular endothelial growth factor vs sham treatment for prevention of vision-threatening complications of diabetic retinopathy: the Protocol W randomized clinical trial. *JAMA Ophthalmol*. 2021;139(7):701–712.
4. Reddy SK, Devi V, Seetharaman ATM, et al. Cell and molecular targeted therapies for diabetic retinopathy. *Front Endocrinol (Lausanne)*. 2024;15:1416668. doi:10.3389/fendo.2024.1416668.
5. Glassman AR, Baker CW, Beaulieu WT, et al. Assessment of the DRCR Retina Network approach to management with initial observation for eyes with center-involved diabetic macular edema and good visual acuity: a secondary analysis of a randomized clinical trial. *JAMA Ophthalmol*. 2020;138(4):341–349.
6. Wykoff CC, Abreu F, Adamis AP, et al. Efficacy, durability, and safety of intravitreal faricimab with extended dosing up to every 16 weeks in patients with diabetic macular oedema (YOSEMITE and RHINE); two randomised, double-masked, phase 3 trials. *Lancet*. 2022;399(10326):741–755. doi:10.1016/S0140-6736(22)00018-6.
7. Glassman AR, Beaulieu WT, Maguire MG, et al. Visual acuity, vitreous hemorrhage, and other ocular outcomes after vitrectomy vs aflibercept for vitreous hemorrhage due to diabetic retinopathy: a secondary analysis of a randomized clinical trial. *JAMA Ophthalmol*. 2021;139(7):725–733.

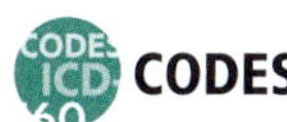

CODES

ICD10

- E11.319 Type 2 diabetes mellitus with unspecified diabetic retinopathy without macular edema
- E10.319 Type 1 diabetes mellitus with unspecified diabetic retinopathy without macular edema
- E10.329 Type 1 diab w mild nonprlf diabetic rtnop w/o macular edema

CLINICAL PEARLS

- Schedule yearly ophthalmologic eye exams.
- Options for the treatment of DME include focal laser treatment, intravitreal triamcinolone, intravitreal ranibizumab, intravitreal bevacizumab (off-label), intravitreal aflibercept, intraocular steroid implants, and vitrectomy.

RHABDOMYOLYSIS

Chirag N. Shah, MD • Daniel Scott Morrison, MD • Jaydip Desai, DO

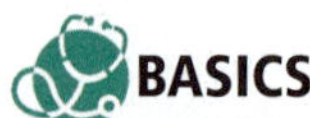

BASICS

DESCRIPTION

- Breakdown of muscle and release of intracellular contents into the bloodstream
- Most commonly caused by traumatic muscle injury
- Typically presents with muscle pain, weakness, and reddish-brown (tea-colored) urine
- Up to 50% of patients are asymptomatic.

EPIDEMIOLOGY

Most common among

- Males; <10 years old; >60 years old; BMI >40 kg/m^2
- Most commonly cited causes in adults are trauma and drugs. In pediatric cases, up to 1/3 can be due to infection (1)[A].

Incidence

- 25,000 reported cases annually in the United States (1)[A]
- Although muscle-related side effects of statins are the most common reason for discontinuation of statins, rhabdomyolysis is rare (0.5% of patients)

Prevalence

- The prevalence of acute kidney injury (AKI) is 5 to 30% with rhabdomyolysis, which contributes significantly to morbidity and mortality (1)[A]
- Without AKI, mortality is 20%; with AKI, mortality increases up to 50%

ETIOLOGY AND PATHOPHYSIOLOGY

- Direct muscle trauma (most common cause)
  - Crush injuries; fractures; extended periods of muscle pressure (during surgery, unconscious from alcohol ingestion, coma); burns, electrocution, lightning strike
- Muscle exertion
  - New strenuous and/or prolonged physical exercise (marathon runners, athletes, contact sports); seizures; delirium tremens; malignant hyperthermia; neuroleptic malignant syndrome (NMS)
- Drugs and toxins
  - Alcohol; cocaine (most common recreational drug), phencyclidine, heroin, bath salts, and synthetic marijuana has been associated with severe rhabdomyolysis.
  - Antipsychotics (due to NMS, malignant hyperthermia, and dystonia)
  - Antimalarials
  - HMG-CoA reductase inhibitors (statins)—develops about 2 to 3 weeks after initiating therapy (risk <0.01%, elevated with higher doses and in combination with fibrates) (1)[A]
  - Corticosteroids
  - Toxins: carbon monoxide, snake envenomation, scorpion bites
- Muscle ischemia
  - Thrombosis, embolism, sickle cell disease, compartment syndrome, tourniquets
- Infections
  - Viral: influenza A and B, coxsackievirus, HIV, varicella
  - Bacterial: *Streptococcus* or *Staphylococcus* sepsis, *Salmonella*, *Legionella*
  - Parasite: malaria
- Hypothermia; hyperthermia.
- Autoimmune disorders
  - Polymyositis, dermatomyositis
- Metabolic and endocrinologic:
  - Hypothyroidism or thyrotoxicosis; electrolyte imbalances (e.g., hyponatremia, hypernatremia, hypokalemia, hypocalcemia, hypophosphatemia); hyperosmolar state

Genetics

Hereditary causes of rhabdomyolysis are rare but should be suspected in children, patients with recurrent attacks, or patients who have attacks after minimal exertion, mild illness, or starvation.

- Genetic disorders
  - Muscular dystrophies; disorders of lipid metabolism (e.g., carnitine palmitoyltransferase deficiency)
  - Disorders of carbohydrate metabolism (i.e., phosphofructokinase deficiency); glycogen storage diseases (e.g., phosphorylase B kinase deficiency) and others (e.g., lactate dehydrogenase A deficiency)
  - Mitochondrial disorders

RISK FACTORS

- Bodyweight more than 30% above ideal body weight
- Immobilization/compression for 6 hours or more
- Extracellular volume loss
- Pre-existing azotemia
- Diabetes
- Hypertension

GENERAL PREVENTION

- Avoid excessive exertion; ensure adequate hydration.
- Avoid precipitating drugs, metabolic and electrolyte abnormalities.

COMMONLY ASSOCIATED CONDITIONS

- AKI
- Disseminated intravascular coagulation (DIC)
- Compartment syndrome

DIAGNOSIS

HISTORY

- Crush injuries
  - Direct trauma and/or prolonged compression/immobility
    - Motor vehicle accidents (MVA) and entrapment in collapsed buildings; the elderly are more susceptible to crush injury due to immobility and falls; prolonged immobilization "found down" syndrome
- Overexertion and/or use of drug/toxin (e.g., cocaine, amphetamine, statins), particularly in warm environments; agitation while patients are in restraints; prolonged periods of lying on a hard surface (e.g., intoxicated or obtunded individuals)
- Common symptoms
  - Malaise, muscle aches, weakness, cramps, fatigue, nausea, vomiting, diarrhea, fever, decreased urinary output, or tea-colored urine
  - Encephalopathy and confusion in severe cases

PHYSICAL EXAM

- Vital sign abnormalities
- Obvious crush injury
  - Discoloration or blisters seen in cases of prolonged pressure necrosis
  - Neurovascular compromise in severe cases with compartment syndrome
- May have muscle tenderness usually in the proximal muscles such as thighs, calves, and lower back with weakness and/or swelling on exam
- Tea-colored urine is indicative of myoglobinuria.

DIFFERENTIAL DIAGNOSIS

- Traumatic injuries
- Other diseases with dark urine:
  - Kidney stones; nephritic syndromes; hemoglobinuria; porphyria.
- Inflammatory myopathies; infection (bacterial or viral); phosphorylase, phosphofructokinase, carnitine palmityl transferase, phosphoglycerate mutase deficiency; Guillain-Barré syndrome; myocardial infarction

DIAGNOSTIC TESTS & INTERPRETATION

Initial Tests (lab, imaging)

- 12-lead ECG (hyperkalemia/peaked T-waves, may induce fatal arrhythmias)
- Creatine kinase (total CK) is the diagnostic test of choice: elevated >5 times the upper limit of normal or >1,000 U/L to diagnose rhabdomyolysis (2)[A]
  - CK levels >5,000 U/L are causally related to acute renal failure (ARF) and should prompt aggressive fluid resuscitation.
  - CK levels rise within 12 hours, peak within 24 to 72 hours, and return to normal in 3 to 5 days.
    - As a result, CK is a more sensitive marker than myoglobin, although it is responsible for renal damage.
    - Normal myoglobin levels do not rule out rhabdomyolysis (due to rapid clearance)
- Urinalysis: Dipstick test positive for blood without erythrocytes (RBCs) in sediment suggests injury from either hemoglobin or myoglobin.
  - Absence of myoglobinuria does not rule out rhabdomyolysis as the myoglobin can be cleared within 1 to 6 hours.
  - Urine pH is usually acidic; often positive for protein
- Other lab/electrolyte abnormalities:
  - Hyperkalemia: elevations of serum potassium from muscle injury can be compounded by ARF.
  - Calcium:
    - Initial hypocalcemia: Calcium enters the injured muscle cells and precipitates as calcium phosphate, leading to calcification of ischemic muscle cells.
      - Only correct initial hypocalcemia if patient is symptomatic or has ECG changes; resolves during the renal recovery phase (2)[A]
    - Hypercalcemia during renal recovery phase: unique to rhabdomyolysis-induced ARF for 20–30% of patients; as renal function improves, there is mobilization of the precipitated calcium (3)[B].

- Extreme hyperuricemia may or may not be present and can cause acute uric acid nephropathy.
- Elevations in blood urea nitrogen (BUN) and creatinine suggest ARF
- Transaminitis: reversible hepatic dysfunction
  - Elevations in alanine aminotransferase (ALT), aspartate aminotransferase (AST), and lactic dehydrogenase likely due to muscle injury rather than hepatic injury
- Hyperphosphatemia
- Increased PT/PTT, fibrin degradation products, and D-dimer with decreases in platelets and fibrinogen indicate DIC

Follow-Up Tests & Special Considerations

Ongoing muscle injury is manifested by rising creatine phosphokinase (CPK).

Diagnostic Procedures/Other

- Compartment pressures if compartment syndrome is suspected
- Ultrasound imaging can show muscle thickening, ground glass opacity, traits of edema, and anechoic areas.
- If the patient requires intubation, rocuronium is the paralytic of choice as patients can have severe hyperkalemia from rhabdomyolysis.

Test Interpretation

Muscle necrosis; myoglobin-related renal injury may resemble acute tubular necrosis from other causes.

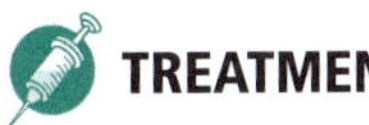

TREATMENT

GENERAL MEASURES

- Address underlying causes (e.g., medication cessation, temperature control, trauma, infection).
- Aggressive hydration with large volumes of IV fluids is often necessary.
  - In severe muscle trauma (crush injuries), up to 12 L of fluid may be sequestered in the muscles.
- Monitor CK levels, renal function, and electrolytes.
  - Follow potassium levels due to the potential for arrhythmias. Treat hyperphosphatemia and hypocalcemia cautiously as treatment may worsen calcium precipitation in the muscle tissue (3)[B].
    - Both should be transient and resolve over a few days.
- Recognize and treat compartment syndrome promptly.

MEDICATION

First Line

Aggressive fluid resuscitation is the most important intervention: normal saline (NS) and 5% glucose solution

- Target urine output of 200 to 300 mL/hr; alternating NS and 5% glucose is recommended to prevent volume overload. Infusion rate should be 500 mL/hr.

Second Line

- Alkalinization of the urine may decrease myoglobin-induced nephrotoxicity in the tubules (sodium bicarbonate to increase urine pH >6.5).
  - Use is controversial. Side effects include worsening hypocalcemia. May help patients with very high CK levels, acidosis, or coexisting hyperkalemia (2)[A]
  - 150 mEq (3 ampules) $NaHCO_3$ in 1 L of D5W and infuse at 200 mL/hr
- IV mannitol as a bolus if urine output remains low, 1 to 2 g/kg, but not to exceed 200 g in 24 hours with a cumulative dose of 800 g; it is used to prevent ARF only if diuresis is not adequate (<200 mL/hr) despite fluid therapy.
  - An osmotic agent, filtered but not reabsorbed by the tubules; this may remove necrotic cell debris and prevent the rise in compartment pressures. Use is controversial.
  - Consider adding furosemide to force diuresis if necessary (40 to 120 mg/day). Do not diurese in anuric renal failure; caution also in the elderly and patients with heart disease
- Hyperkalemia can result from massive release of intracellular potassium stores or ARF. Severe hyperkalemia may be life-threatening; treatment when ECG changes are present (tall, thin T waves; PR prolongation; QRS widening; P wave flattening)
  - Calcium gluconate: IV 1 to 2 grams (0.5 mL 10% calcium gluconate = 4 mg elemental calcium; give 4 mg/kg/hr for 4 hours.)
  - If acidosis is present: 1 to 2 ampules sodium bicarbonate (2 to 3 mL/kg) IV; sodium bicarbonate can worsen hypocalcemia. If tolerated: Oral sodium polystyrene sulfonate (Kayexalate) as much as 20 g (1 g/kg) can be given via enema and transiently drive potassium into the cells. Administration of glucose can prevent the hypoglycemic effects. Precautions: continuous monitoring of potassium levels to prevent overcorrecting with potential hypokalemia and arrhythmias
  - Indications for dialysis include resistant and symptomatic hyperkalemia (ECG), oliguria (<0.5 mL/kg over a 12-hour period), anuria, volume overload, or persistent acidosis (pH <7.1).

ISSUES FOR REFERRAL

Usually managed as an inpatient; diagnosis of compartment syndrome merits surgical consultation for consideration of fasciotomy. Renal dialysis may be indicated in ARF.

ADDITIONAL THERAPIES

- During the oliguric phase, symptomatic hypocalcemia (rare) may benefit from IV medication.
- Correction of hypocalcemia, if not symptomatic, should be avoided as in the recovery phase, hypercalcemia may develop (2)[A].

SURGERY/OTHER PROCEDURES

- Fasciotomy—for muscle entrapment/compartment syndrome
- Survivors of rhabdomyolysis with compartment syndrome may need further surgeries.

COMPLEMENTARY & ALTERNATIVE MEDICINE

Education on heat-related injuries.

ADMISSION, INPATIENT, AND NURSING CONSIDERATIONS

- Patients with significant elevations of CK or any signs of renal injury should be admitted for IV hydration and clinical monitoring; volume expansion with NS to increase urine output to at least 150 mL/hr
- CK usually peaks 24 to 36 hours after muscle injury; so, monitoring should confirm that the CK is trending down. Renal function should be stable/improving. Electrolytes should be normal.
- Patients with mild CK elevation, normal renal function, a clear etiology, and adequate follow-up may be discharged after the observation phase and hydration if CK is trending down

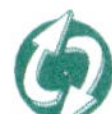

ONGOING CARE

FOLLOW-UP RECOMMENDATIONS

Follow up within a few days to recheck CK, electrolytes, urine studies, and renal function.

Patient Monitoring

Contingent on disease: essential for metabolic myopathies; myotoxic drugs should be discontinued/monitored closely.

DIET

With renal failure, restrict protein intake to lower BUN levels. With anuria, it is essential to restrict volume intake.

PROGNOSIS

Contingent on primary cause of rhabdomyolysis and recovery from ARF without complications

COMPLICATIONS

- Death, especially from hyperkalemia/renal failure
- Prognosis is very good with prompt initiation of fluids for IV rehydration, dialysis, and supportive care.

REFERENCES

1. Stanley M, Chippa V, Aeddula NR, et al. Rhabdomyolysis. In: *StatPearls* [Internet]. Treasure Island, FL: StatPearls Publishing; 2023. https://www.ncbi.nlm.nih.gov/books/NBK448168/.
2. Cabral BMI, Edding SN, Portocarrero JP, et al. Rhabdomyolysis. *Dis Mon*. 2020;66(8):101015.
3. Safari S, Aghili SH, Shahlaee MA, et al. Incidence of electrolyte imbalances following traumatic rhabdomyolysis: a systematic review and meta-analysis. *Cureus*. 2024;16(4):e59333. doi:10.7759/cureus.59333.

ADDITIONAL READING

Danaei B, Sharifi A, Mazloom H, et al. Prevalence of compartment syndrome and disseminated intravascular coagulation following rhabdomyolysis; a systematic review and meta-analysis. *Arch Acad Emerg Med*. 2023;11(1):e55. doi:10.22037/aaem.v11i1.2083.

SEE ALSO

Algorithm: Acute Kidney Injury (Acute Renal Failure)

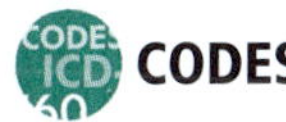

CODES

ICD10

- M62.82 Rhabdomyolysis
- T79.6 Traumatic ischemia of muscle
- T79.6xxS Traumatic ischemia of muscle, sequela

CLINICAL PEARLS

- Elevation of CK is the diagnostic hallmark of rhabdomyolysis.
- The cornerstone of treatment of rhabdomyolysis is aggressive fluid administration.
- Initial serum creatinine predicts mortality.
- Electrolyte abnormalities, acute kidney injury, hepatic injury, compartment syndrome, and (rarely) DIC are the most worrisome complications of rhabdomyolysis.

RHABDOMYOSARCOMA

Vincent Shaw, MD

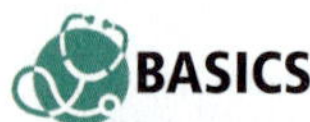

BASICS

DESCRIPTION

- Rhabdomyosarcoma (RMS) is a malignant soft tissue tumor presumed to originate from a mesenchymal cell line shared with striated skeletal muscle.
- Occurs mainly as primary malignancy but can also be a component of heterogeneous neoplasms
  - WHO classification of soft tissue tumors describes four main RMS subtypes:
    - Embryonal RMS (ERMS): 60% of RMS cases
      - Early onset and the most common subtype in children
      - Commonly presents in the head, neck, and genitourinary areas
    - Subdivided into:
      - Classic
      - Botryoid (6% overall embryonal): seen in infants, although can happen in <4-year-old patients
      - Spindle cell: 3% of cases and affects young children
      - Both botryoid and spindle cell variants have better prognosis than the classic variant
    - Alveolar RMS (ARMS): 20% of pediatric cases
      - Aggressive subtype
      - More common in the trunk, perineum/perianal area, and extremities
    - Spindle/Sclerosing: approximately 10% of cases
      - Mostly found in the paratesticular region
    - Anaplastic (children)/pleomorphic (adults): <10% of cases
      - Typically seen in patients aged 30 to 50 years (rarely in pediatric population)
      - Associated with Li-Fraumeni symptoms
      - Demonstrates hyperchromatic enlarged nuclei
  - Pathologic and molecular studies have now delineated up to five or six distinct subfamilies of RMS.
  - Common primary sites:
    - Head and neck (25%) presentation (common in young children, usually embryonal type)
    - Genitourinary (31%, mostly embryonal type)
    - Musculoskeletal (13%, most common in extremities primary sites in adolescents and adults, alveolar subtype)

EPIDEMIOLOGY

- RMS is most common soft tissue sarcoma in pediatric population.
- Common metastatic sites: bone marrow, lung, lymph nodes

Incidence

- 4.5 cases of RMS per 1 million children per year
- Accounts for 50% of all soft tissue sarcomas in children and adolescents
  - 50% of pediatric cases occur before the age of 10 years (often before age 6 years).

Prevalence

- Represents 3% of all pediatric tumors and 1% of all adult tumors
- Slight predilection for males (1.3:1 male-to-female ratio)
- More common in the African-American population

ETIOLOGY AND PATHOPHYSIOLOGY

- Originates from rhabdomyoblast cell
- Tumor is often >5 cm in size with poorly circumscribed border, white coloration, and infiltrative features.

Genetics

Genetic characteristics vary according to the RMS subtype:

- Alveolar:
  - Linked to recurrent Forkhead box O1 (FOXO1) fusions (identified in 90% of cases)
  - t(1;13)(p36;q14), causing PAX3-FOXO1 fusion
  - t(2;13)(q35;q14), causing *PAX7-FOXO1* fusion
- Embryonal:
  - Multiple complex genetic aberrations, including *MYOD1* mutations
  - Loss or uniparental disomy of 11p15.5 +2, +8, +11, +12, +13, +20 affecting genes *IGF-2*, *H19*, *CDKN1C*, and/or *HOTS*
- Spindle cell/sclerosing:
  - 8q13 rearrangements involving *SRF-NCOA2* and *TEAD1-NCOA2*

RISK FACTORS

Largely unknown; however, appears to be increased risk of RMS in setting of:

- Rapid growth in utero
- Radiation exposure in utero
- Lower socioeconomic status
- Recreational drug use during pregnancy

COMMONLY ASSOCIATED CONDITIONS

- Beckwith-Wiedemann syndrome (11p15 mutations)
- Costello syndrome (germline *HRAS* mutations)
- Li-Fraumeni syndrome (germline *TP53*; known as *p53* mutations)
- Neurofibromatosis type I (*NF1* mutations)
- Noonan syndrome (*PTPN11* mutations)

DIAGNOSIS

Thorough history and physical examination necessary but typically requires molecular genetic, immunohistochemical, and/or structural techniques to confirm diagnosis of RMS

HISTORY

Initial presenting symptoms variable based on location of mass, age of patient, etc.

- Manifests as a progressive, palpable mass
- When in the head/neck region, patients may report diplopia, recurrent sinusitis, or persistent nasal discharge.
- RMS of genitourinary tissue may present as urinary obstruction, hematuria, polyuria, or potentially vaginal bleeding in females.
- Other symptoms may be noted due to the mass effect of the primary/metastatic lesions.
- Personal or family history of genetic syndromes (e.g., Li-Fraumeni, Noonan, etc.)

PHYSICAL EXAM

- Painless, enlarging mass when in head/neck region, but may be painful when present in the extremities (with overlying erythema of skin)
- Polypoid mass protruding from the vagina (suggests botryoid subtype)
- Exophthalmos and chemosis (seen with orbital involvement)
- Abdominal pain and mass effect symptoms include seizures, visual field defects, nerve palsy, headaches, etc.

DIFFERENTIAL DIAGNOSIS

- Osteosarcoma
- Ewing sarcoma
- Liposarcoma
- Lipoma
- Wilms tumor
- Lymphoproliferative disorder
- Lymphadenopathy
- Neurofibromatosis type 1

DIAGNOSTIC TESTS & INTERPRETATION

Initial Tests (lab, imaging)

- Laboratory studies: Complete blood count, serum chemistries, liver function test, and coagulation profile should be obtained for clinical optimization prior to initiating treatment.
- Imaging studies should include:
  - MRI with/without contrast (or CT) of the primary tumor (to define anatomy)
  - CT chest and abdomen/pelvis
  - Bone scan
- Additional staging workup:
  - Lymph node biopsy
  - Bone marrow aspirate and biopsy

Follow-Up Tests & Special Considerations

Biopsy of the suspected RMS tumor is necessary for diagnosis.

Diagnostic Procedures/Other

- For pathological diagnosis:
  - Core needle biopsy, incisional biopsy, or excisional biopsy (based on size of the mass)
  - RMS tumors typically demonstrate eccentric eosinophilic cytoplasm with abundant thick/thin filaments
- Histologic classification:
  - Alveolar: rhabdomyoblasts grossly mimicking pulmonary alveoli arranged in interseptal nests within a network of intersecting fibrous septae
  - Embryonal: typically displays a myxoid matrix
    - Classic: rhabdomyoblasts configured in sheets, large nest, eosinophilic cytoplasm

Table 1. TNM Staging System for RMS

Stage	Site(s)	T	Tumor Diameter	N	M
1	Orbit; head and neck (excluding parameningeal), genitourinary—non-bladder and non-prostate, biliary tract	T1 or T2	a or b	Any N	M0
2	Bladder or prostate, extremity, cranial parameningeal, other	T1 or T2	a	N0 or NX	M0
3a	Bladder or prostate, extremity, cranial parameningeal, other	T1 or T2	a	N1	M0
3b	Bladder or prostate, extremity, cranial parameningeal, other	T1 or T2	b	Any N	M0
4	All sites (metastatic)	T1 or T2	a or b	N0 or N1	M1

T1, confined to organ of origin; T2, extends outside the organ of origin; a, ≤5 cm in diameter; b, >5 cm in diameter; M0, no distant metastasis; N0, regional nodes not clinically involved; NX, clinical status of regional nodes unknown; N1, regional nodes clinically involved by neoplasm; M1, distant metastasis.

    ◦ Botryoid: "grape-like" appearance with notable clustering in subepithelium forming the cambium layer
    ◦ Spindle cell: rhabdomyoblasts with spindle-like appearance
  – Anaplastic/pleomorphic: rhabdomyoblast with large hyperchromatic nuclei and multipolar mitotic morphologies
- Immunohistochemical (ICH) markers:
  – Positive for desmin, sarcomeric actin, myogenin, myoglobin
  – Usually negative for CD99, CK, S100, NKX2.2, NSE
- Molecular testing for PAX/FOXO1 fusion (tested by PCR and fluorescence in situ hybridization) (1)[A]
- Genetic profiling likely to become gold standard for diagnosis and prognosis
- Staging is based on the site, size, regional nodal involvement, and degree of spread (Table 1).

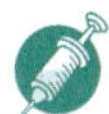

TREATMENT

- Spans surgical resection, radiation, and chemotherapy
- Treatment should be performed by interdisciplinary team that includes oncologist, surgeon, and radiologist

GENERAL MEASURES

The development of multimodal therapy protocols has led to improved outcomes

SURGERY/OTHER PROCEDURES

- Surgery:
  – Local resection of tumor along with metastases and nodal resection (2)[C]
  – Lymph node sampling is intended to identify unknown metastasis and guide decision for post-operative radiation.
- Radiation therapy: recommended to enhance local control, except in patients with embryonal type
  – Emergent therapy only considered in patients with compression symptoms
  – Ionizing radiation shown to decrease recurrence rates, especially in higher stage classifications
- Chemotherapy:
  – Selected based on prognosis/risk stratification (e.g., low, intermediate, or high)
    ◦ "VAC" regimen consists of vincristine, actinomycin D (dactinomycin), and cyclophosphamide
    ◦ "IVA" regimen includes ifosfamide, vincristine, and actinomycin D
  – Most common adverse reactions are the following:
    ◦ Vincristine: peripheral neuropathy
    ◦ Dactinomycin: myelosuppression and hepatotoxicity
    ◦ Cyclophosphamide: hemorrhagic cystitis (mesna is used for prophylaxis), transitional cell carcinoma, myelosuppression with leukopenia, and infertility
- In addition, ifosfamide, topotecan, doxorubicin, etoposide, and irinotecan may be used in alternative regimens.
- Administration protocol depends on risk stratification but, generally, ranges from 12 to 24 months given in separate cycles (up to 15 cycles).

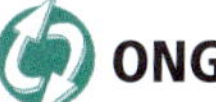

ONGOING CARE

FOLLOW-UP RECOMMENDATIONS

- Physical examination and imaging surveillance for the first 5 years (CT/MRI/x-ray) to assess for recurrence, metastatic disease, or development of secondary malignancies
  – Imaging should be done every 3 months for the 1st year, every 4 months for the following 2 years, and finally every 6 months for the subsequent 2 years
- After first 5 years, no more imaging surveillance is typically required.

DIET

There are no specific dietary limitations.

PATIENT EDUCATION

National Cancer Institute: https://www.cancer.gov/types/soft-tissue-sarcoma/patient/rhabdomyosarcoma-treatment-pdq

PROGNOSIS

- RMS (overall) 5-year survival: 61% (children) and 27% (adults)
- Metastatic RMS overall survival <25%
- RM of extremities and parameningeal RMS have worse prognosis.

COMPLICATIONS

- Recurrence
- Secondary neoplasm
- Growth abnormalities

REFERENCES

1. Gallagher KPD, van Heerden W, Said-Al-Naief N, et al. Molecular profile of head and neck rhabdomyosarcomas: a systematic review and meta-analysis. *Oral Surg Oral Med Oral Pathol Oral Radiol*. 2022;134(3):354–366.
2. Skapek SX, Ferrari A, Gupta AA, et al. Rhabdomyosarcoma. *Nat Rev Dis Primers*. 2019;5(1):1.

ADDITIONAL READING

Leiner J, Le Loarer F. The current landscape of rhabdomyosarcomas: an update. *Virchows Arch*. 2020;476(1):97–108.

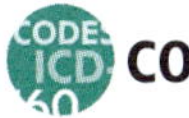

CODES

ICD10

- C49.9 Malignant neoplasm of connective and soft tissue, unsp
- C49.0 Malignant neoplasm of connective and soft tissue of head, face and neck
- C49.5 Malignant neoplasm of connective and soft tissue of pelvis

CLINICAL PEARLS

- RMS more common in children but can develop in adults, the latter having higher mortality.
- Genetic disorders and congenital syndromes increase risk of RMS.
- If a localized tumor is identified with concurrent lymph node involvement, implement more aggressive therapy.
- The most common site of metastasis is the lung, followed by bone marrow/bone and peritoneum.

R

RHEUMATIC FEVER

Lukus A. Berber, MD

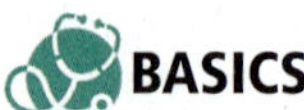

BASICS

DESCRIPTION

- Acute rheumatic fever (ARF) is an autoimmune, inflammatory response to infection with group A *Streptococcus* (GAS) that affects multiple organ systems.
- Untreated acute disease can lead to chronic rheumatic heart disease (RHD).
- Recurrence is common without adequate antibiotic treatment.

Pediatric Considerations

Most cases occur in children aged 5 to 15 years; rare in children <5 years

EPIDEMIOLOGY

- ARF and RHD are largely restricted to low-income countries and marginalized sections of wealthy countries.
- Male = female; females are more likely to develop chorea and RHD.
- Endemic regions include South Pacific, indigenous populations of Australia and New Zealand, Africa, and Asia (1).

Incidence

- Worldwide, incidence has been declining for 25 years. The large majority of new cases are in developing countries (1).
- Mean worldwide incidence ranges from 8 to 51/100,000 school-aged children; in endemic regions, prevalence can be >1,000 cases per 100,000 people (1).
- Incidence of ARF in the United States is currently <3.4 to 2/100,000 school-aged children (1).

Prevalence

- In developing areas, RHD affects >33 million people and is the leading cause of cardiovascular death during the first 5 decades of life.
- Prevalence has been rising due to improved medical care and longer survival.

ETIOLOGY AND PATHOPHYSIOLOGY

- ARF most commonly occurs 2 to 3 weeks after GAS pharyngitis infection, but GAS impetigo may also be a proceeding infection.
- Although pathogenicity is not completely understood, expert consensus implicates genetic and molecular mimicry leading to an inflammatory cascade as key to disease development.
- Immune cross-reactive response contributes to joint involvement due to accumulation of immune complexes.

Genetics

- Susceptibility is associated with certain indigenous populations.
- ARF is heritable, polygenic, and displays variable and incomplete penetrance.

RISK FACTORS

Poverty, household crowding, genetic susceptibility, ethnic predisposition, and social disadvantage are the strongest risk factors.

GENERAL PREVENTION

- Primary prevention: Appropriate treatment of streptococcal infection prevents ARF in most cases.
- Secondary prevention: long-term antibiotic prophylaxis (up to 5 to 10 years) to prevent recurrence (1)

DIAGNOSIS

- 2015 revised Jones criteria and lab evidence of preceding GAS infection are used for diagnosis.
- Initial ARF: 2 major *or* 1 major + 2 minor
- Recurrent ARF: 2 major *or* 1 major + 2 minor *or* 3 minor
- Sydenham chorea is independently sufficient to diagnosis ARF, even without lab evidence of preceding infection.

Low-Risk Population	Moderate- and High-Risk Population
Major criteria:	Major criteria:
• Carditis: clinical or subclinical (echocardiogram)	• Carditis: clinical or subclinical (echocardiogram)
• Polyarthritis *only*	• Polyarthritis *or* monoarthritis
• Chorea	• Chorea
• Erythema marginatum	• Erythema marginatum
• Subcutaneous nodules	• Subcutaneous nodules
Minor criteria:	Minor criteria:
• Polyarthralgia	• Monoarthralgia
• Fever ≥38.5°C	• Fever ≥38°C
• ESR ≥60 mm/hr	• ESR ≥30 mm/hr
• CRP ≥3 mg/dL	• CRP ≥3 mg/dL
• ↑PR interval	• ↑PR interval

- The revised criteria distinguish between low-risk and moderate-risk to high-risk patient populations. Patients can be considered low risk if they are from and among a low-incidence group.
- Subclinical carditis can be diagnosed with echocardiographic evidence of mitral or aortic valve regurgitation and can be supported by chest x-ray demonstrating cardiomegaly or left atrial enlargement.

HISTORY

- ARF typically presents 2 to 3 weeks following GAS pharyngitis or impetigo.
- Polyarthritis (knees, ankles, elbows, wrists) (35–66%) is self-limited and often the first symptom; each resolves in days, thus seems to "migrate." Rapid improvement occurs with anti-inflammatories, which may mask initial symptoms. Moderate and high-risk patients may only have monoarthritis.
- Fever
- Erythema marginatum rash
- Pancarditis or valvulitis (50–70%) can be subclinical (asymptomatic without auscultatory findings) or clinically apparent.
- Sydenham chorea (late manifestation [1 to 6 months after infection] in 10–30%): purposeless, involuntary, nonstereotypical movements, most commonly involving the face and hands
  - More common in 5 to 15 years old, females
  - Improves or ceases during sleep
  - Can have associated muscular weakness, may manifest as deteriorating handwriting
  - Psychiatric symptoms may have onset prior to chorea, with emotional lability and obsessive-compulsive symptoms.
  - Self-resolves over several months and can relapse

PHYSICAL EXAM

- Neuro: Sydenham chorea: Involuntary movements may be general or unilateral and involve the face. "Milkmaid grip" is intermittent hypotonia on test of grip strength.
- Cardiac: pericardial friction rub, holosystolic murmur of mitral/aortic regurgitation, rarely diastolic; rarely evidence of heart failure
- Skin
  - Subcutaneous nodules (<10%): firm, painless protuberances on extensor surfaces involving knees, elbows, wrists, occiput, and spinous process of thoracic and lumbar vertebrae; more common in severe ARF, persists several weeks
  - Erythema marginatum (5–13%): evanescent, pink rash with pale centers and rounded/serpiginous margins found on trunk and proximal extremities; rare to be found on face; typically nonpruritic; blanches with pressure and can be induced with heat

DIFFERENTIAL DIAGNOSIS

- Systemic lupus erythematosus
- Poststreptococcal reactive arthritis
- Juvenile rheumatoid arthritis
- Infectious arthritis
- Myocarditis (viral or idiopathic)
- Innocent cardiac murmur
- Cardiomyopathy
- Tourette syndrome
- Kawasaki syndrome
- Pediatric autoimmune neuropsychiatric disorders associated with streptococcal infections (PANDAS)
- Lyme disease
- Henoch-Schönlein purpura
- Wilson disease
- Substance abuse
- Tic disorder
- Encephalitis
- Huntington chorea
- Drug reaction

DIAGNOSTIC TESTS & INTERPRETATION

Initial Tests (lab, imaging)

- Serologic evidence of GAS infection is needed whenever possible, and diagnosis is in question when it cannot be obtained (chorea and chronic indolent rheumatic carditis being the exception due to delayed onset).
  - Rapid streptococcal antigen test with high pretest probability
  - Positive GAS throat culture
  - Elevated or rising antistreptococcal antibody titer (ASO or ADB); ASO peaks 3 to 5 weeks postinfection, ADB 6 to 8 weeks. A rise in titer is better than a single titer result.
- ESR and CRP are acute-phase reactants; almost always increased in ARF
- CBC with differential: leukocytosis, normocytic anemia
- ECG: PR prolongation, AV block, signs of pericarditis
- Joint aspiration and synovial fluid evaluation is indicated if significant effusion or septic arthritis is suspected.
- Echocardiogram: chamber size and function, pericardial effusion, and valve disease
- All cases of confirmed *or* suspected ARF should have an echocardiogram within 12 weeks due to 18% prevalence of subclinical carditis.

Follow-Up Tests & Special Considerations

- CRP is useful to monitor the acute disease process and can initially be trended twice weekly, followed by every 1 to 2 weeks until normalized.
- Due to morbidity associate with untreated cardiac disease, all confirmed cases of ARF should have serial echocardiograms, even if the initial screen was negative for carditis (1)[C].
- All household contacts should be screened with GAS throat cultures. Positive results should be treated with antibiotics, even if asymptomatic.

Test Interpretation

Prior treatment with aspirin or steroids may lead to falsely negative lab results.

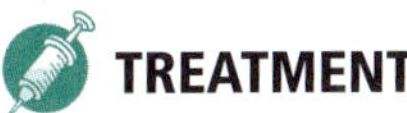

TREATMENT

GENERAL MEASURES

- Antibiotic
- Anti-inflammatory agent (naproxen)
- Manage other manifestations as indicated (e.g., chorea, dysrhythmia, carditis, or heart failure).

MEDICATION

First Line

- Eradication: GAS infection treatment should begin within 9 days of illness to prevent ARF. If ARF diagnosis is confirmed, begin secondary prophylaxis.
- If no penicillin allergy:
  - Penicillin VK 250 mg PO BID for 10 days, benzathine penicillin G IM for 1 day, or amoxicillin 50 mg/kg PO for 10 days (preferred in children)
- If penicillin allergy:
  - 1st-generation cephalosporin PO for 10 days, azithromycin 12 mg/kg PO for 5 days, clindamycin 7 mg/kg/dose PO for 10 days, or clarithromycin 7.5 mg/kg/dose PO for 10 days
- Arthritis: Naproxen 10 to 20 mg/kg/day divided BID is now recommended over aspirin, given superior side-effect profile and less risk of Reye syndrome.
- Carditis: If heart failure, 3rd-degree AV block, or other severe manifestations, appropriate traditional management should be initiated as indicated.
- NSAIDs, glucocorticoids, and IVIG are not recommended for carditis, although glucocorticoids can be considered in severe carditis with acute cardiac failure.
- Chorea: generally self-limited, not requiring treatment. Valproic acid or carbamazepine may be used for severe cases. IVIG and glucocorticoids are restricted to failure of initial management. Antipsychotics are not routinely used due to extrapyramidal side effects.

Second Line

- Penicillin allergy and severity should be confirmed prior to starting a second-line agent.
- If severe penicillin allergy is present, erythromycin is preferred by the New Zealand Guidelines Group but not by the Infectious Diseases Society of America.

ISSUES FOR REFERRAL

- A cardiologist should be involved in management of ARF.
- Pediatric neurologist or movement specialist can help guide therapy with severe chorea.

SURGERY/OTHER PROCEDURES

Valve stenosis is a late sequela resulting from fibrosis and calcification; mainstay of therapy is surgical correction (1).

ADMISSION, INPATIENT, AND NURSING CONSIDERATIONS

- Initial hospitalization may be helpful for diagnosis and to ensure stability.
- Heart failure requires prompt hospitalization.
- IV fluids
  - Only if signs of dehydration or hypotension; use caution in heart failure.
- Nursing
  - Activity as tolerated

ONGOING CARE

FOLLOW-UP RECOMMENDATIONS

- Secondary prophylaxis: antibiotic therapy from time of diagnosis until at least age 21 years, or 5 years after diagnosis (whichever comes later)
- In patients with ARF with carditis, antibiotic therapy from time of diagnosis until at least age 21 years, or 10 years after diagnosis (whichever comes later)
- Indefinite prophylactic antibiotics can be indicated if valvular disease is present, as recurrence of disease can worsen severity of carditis.
  - First-line prophylaxis is long-acting benzathine penicillin G monthly IM injections.
  - Penicillin V PO 250 mg BID is an alternative.
  - If penicillin allergy, sulfadiazine 0.5 to 1.0 g daily
  - If penicillin and sulfa drug allergy, azithromycin
  - Patients on penicillin prophylaxis who develop GAS pharyngitis while on penicillin should be treated with clindamycin.
- If ARF is possible, but uncertain, treat with 1 year of secondary antibiotic prophylaxis until repeat echocardiogram (1)[C].
- Routine antibiotic prophylaxis for dental procedures is no longer recommended for patients with RHD.

Patient Monitoring

Weekly monitoring after the initial diagnosis; every 6 months thereafter, based on clinical stability

Pediatric Considerations

Use aspirin with caution in children given the risk of Reye syndrome.

Pregnancy Considerations

May exacerbate valve disease, particularly mitral stenosis in RHD; refer pregnant patients to a cardiologist.

DIET

No dietary restrictions; low-sodium if heart failure present

PATIENT EDUCATION

- American Heart Association: http://www.heart.org
- Centers for Disease Control and Prevention: Clinical Guideline for Rheumatic Fever (https://www.cdc.gov/group-a-strep/hcp/clinical-guidance/acute-rheumatic-fever.html)

PROGNOSIS

Long-term sequelae are generally limited to the heart and depend on the severity of carditis during an acute attack. Recurrence is most common in the first year after diagnosis (1).

COMPLICATIONS

- Recurrence of ARF due to GAS reinfection
- RHD can occur 10 to 20 years after ARF, with mitral more common than aortic regurgitation, can lead to mitral stenosis. Heart failure is the worst complication.
- Jaccoud arthropathy is chronic and involves painless deformities of hands/feet.
- Patients with a history of ARF have a higher incidence of infective endocarditis in the future.

REFERENCES

1. Kumar RK, Antunes MJ, Beaton A, et al; and American Heart Association Council on Lifelong Congenital Heart Disease and Heart Health in the Young, Council on Cardiovascular and Stroke Nursing, and Council on Clinical Cardiology. Contemporary diagnosis and management of rheumatic heart disease: implications for closing the gap: a scientific statement from the American Heart Association. *Circulation*. 2020;142(20):e337–357.

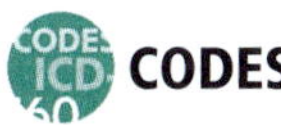

CODES

ICD10

- I00 Rheumatic fever without heart involvement
- I01.9 Acute rheumatic heart disease, unspecified
- I01.0 Acute rheumatic pericarditis

CLINICAL PEARLS

- ARF is an autoimmune, inflammatory disease that follows a GAS pharyngeal infection and affects multiple organ systems, most notably, the heart.
- Modified Jones criteria now delineates between low-risk and moderate-/high-risk patients. Diagnosis requires two major or one major plus two minor manifestations in the context of a preceding documented GAS infection.
- Early echocardiogram evaluation for subclinical carditis can expedite initial diagnosis and improve clinical outcomes.
- Treatment involves acute antibiotic eradication, ideally within 9 days of illness, followed immediately by long-term antibiotic prophylaxis to prevent CRHD. Supportive care includes NSAIDs such as naproxen or aspirin.

RHINITIS, ALLERGIC

Madhavi Singh, MD

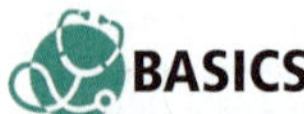

BASICS

Allergic rhinitis is the collection of symptoms involving mucous membranes of nose, eyes, ears, and throat after an exposure to allergens such as pollen, dust, or dander.

DESCRIPTION

- IgE-mediated inflammation of the nasal mucosa following exposure to an extrinsic protein; an immediate symptomatic response is characterized by sneezing, congestion, and rhinorrhea followed by a persistent late phase dominated by congestion and mucosal hyperreactivity.
- Allergic rhinitis can be classified into seasonal or perennial and can be intermittent or persistent.
- Seasonal responses are usually due to outdoor allergens such as tree pollen, flowering shrubs in spring, grasses and flowering plants in summer, and ragweed and mold in fall.
- Perennial responses, or year-round symptoms, are usually associated with indoor allergens like dust mites, mold, and animal dander.
- Occupational allergic rhinitis is caused by allergens at the workplace and can be sporadic or year-round.
- Nonallergic rhinitis (e.g., vasomotor, rhinitis of pregnancy, and rhinitis medicamentosa [RM]) can occur.

Pediatric Considerations

Chronic nasal obstruction can result in facial deformities, dental malocclusions, and sleep disorders.

Pregnancy Considerations

Physiologic changes during pregnancy may aggravate all types of rhinitis, frequently in the 2nd trimester.

EPIDEMIOLOGY

- Onset usually in first 2 decades, rarely before 6 months of age, with tendency declining with advancing age
- The mean age of onset is 8 to 11 years, and about 80% of cases have established allergic rhinitis by age 20 years.

Prevalence

- ~10–25% of the U.S. adult population and 9–42% of the U.S. pediatric population are affected.
- 44–87% of patients with allergic rhinitis have mixed allergic and nonallergic rhinitis, which is more common than either pure form (1).

ETIOLOGY AND PATHOPHYSIOLOGY

- Aeroallergen-driven mucosal inflammation due to resident and infiltrating inflammatory cells as well as vasoactive and proinflammatory mediators (e.g., cytokines)
- Inhalant allergens:
  - Perennial: house dust mites, indoor molds, animal dander, cockroach/insect detritus
  - Seasonal: tree, grass, and weed pollens; outdoor molds
  - Occupational: latex, plant products (e.g., baking flour), sensitizing chemicals, and certain animals for people working in farms and vet clinics

RISK FACTORS

- Family history of atopy, with a greater risk if both parents have atopy
- Higher socioeconomic status
- Tobacco smoke can exacerbate symptoms and increase risk of developing asthma.
- Unclear evidence regarding risk due to early, repeated exposure to offending allergen and early introduction of solid food
- Pets in house and houses infested with cockroaches can cause perennial allergic rhinitis.
- Male sex
- Exposure to pollutants increase the risk of Ige-mediated allergic disease

GENERAL PREVENTION

- Primary prevention of atopic disease has not been proven effective by maternal diet or maternal allergen avoidance.
- Exclusive breastfeeding to 6 months of age lowers risk of some atopic disorders.
- Symptomatic control by environmental avoidance is the "first-line treatment."
- No evidence to support use of acaricides with mite-proof mattress and pillow covers, carpet and drape removal, removal of plants in the home, and pet control
- Air conditioning and limited outside exposure during allergy season (1)[B]
- HEPA air cleaners and vacuum bags of unclear efficacy
- Close doors and windows during allergy season.
- Use a dehumidifier to reduce indoor humidity.

COMMONLY ASSOCIATED CONDITIONS

Other IgE-mediated conditions: asthma, atopic dermatitis, allergic conjunctivitis, food allergy

DIAGNOSIS

Diagnosis is made primarily by history and physical exam.

HISTORY

- History of atopic dermatitis and/or food allergies
- History of nasal congestion; rhinorrhea; pruritus of nose, eyes, ears, and/or palate; sneezing; itching; and watering eyes
- Family history of allergic diseases
- History of environmental and occupational exposure and various nasal stimuli can help differentiate between allergic and vasomotor rhinitis.

PHYSICAL EXAM

Many findings are suggestive of but not specific for allergic rhinitis:

- Dark circles under eyes, "allergic shiners" (infraorbital venous congestion)
- Transverse nasal crease from rubbing nose upward; typically seen in children
- Rhinorrhea, usually with clear discharge
- Pale, boggy, blue-gray nasal mucosa
- Postnasal mucus discharge
- Oropharyngeal lymphoid tissue hypertrophy

DIFFERENTIAL DIAGNOSIS

- Infectious rhinitis: usually viral, commonly with secondary bacterial infection
  - Usually associated with sinusitis and is known as rhinosinusitis
  - Viral rhinitis averages six episodes per year from ages 2 to 6 years.
  - IgA deficiency with recurrent sinusitis
- RM:
  - Rebound effect associated with continued use of certain medications; topical decongestant drops and sprays are the most common.
  - Other medications that may indue RM include ACE inhibitors, reserpine, β-blockers, oral contraceptive pills (OCPs), guanethidine, methyldopa, aspirin, and NSAIDs.
- Vasomotor (idiopathic) rhinitis caused by numerous nasal stimuli such as warm or cold air, scents and odors, light or particulate matter
  - Hormonal: pregnancy, thyroid, OCPs
  - Nonallergic rhinitis with eosinophilia syndrome (NARES)
  - Gustatory: watery rhinorrhea in response to alcohol or food
  - "Skier's nose": watery rhinorrhea in response to cold air
- Conditions associated with rhinitis:
  - Nasal polyps, tumor
  - Septal/anatomic obstruction
    - Adenoidal hypertrophy, particularly in children
    - Septal abnormality or deflected nasal septum (DNS) in adults

DIAGNOSTIC TESTS & INTERPRETATION

- Lab tests rarely needed
- Skin testing is done to identify the allergen for immunotherapy.

Initial Tests (lab, imaging)

- Testing is rarely indicated.
- If diagnosis implies other causes, consider the following:
  - CBC with differential may show elevated eosinophils.
  - Increased total serum IgE level
  - Nasal probe smear may show elevated eosinophils.
- Medications that may alter lab results:
  - Corticosteroids may decrease eosinophilia.
  - Antihistamines suppress reactivity to skin tests; stop antihistamines 7 days before testing.

Diagnostic Procedures/Other

- Consider testing in only those cases where allergic symptoms do not respond to 1st- and 2nd-line treatments and/or considering immunotherapy.
- Specific allergen sensitivity with allergen skin testing or radioallergosorbent test (RAST); clinical correlation based on history is essential in interpreting results.
- Diagnostic allergen prick tests are used to select agent to determine appropriate environmental control measures as well as to direct immunotherapy:
  - Prick or puncture: superficial injury to epidermis with application of test antigen
  - Intradermal

- RAST: more expensive and less sensitive than skin testing; typically used in patients to whom skin testing is not practical or a severe reaction is possible
- Rhinoscopy: useful to visualize intranasal and posterior pharyngeal structures, including adenoids, polyps, and larynx
- CT scan of sinuses is not routinely done but can be used to check for complete opacity, fluid level, and mucosal thickening.

Test Interpretation

- Nasal washing/scraping: eosinophils predominate but may see basophils, mast cells
- Nasal mucosa: submucosal edema but without destruction; eosinophilic infiltration; congested mucous glands and goblet cells

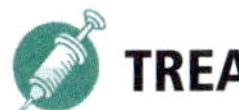

TREATMENT

There are three mainstays of treatment of allergic rhinitis:

- Allergen avoidance
- Medication
- Allergy immunotherapy

GENERAL MEASURES

Limit exposure to offending allergen.

MEDICATION

First Line

- Mild symptoms. 2nd-generation nonsedating antihistamines are the first-line therapy for mild to moderate allergic rhinitis (1).
  - Adverse effects: mild sedation, mild anticholinergic effects
  - Generic (cetirizine, fexofenadine, loratadine, levocetirizine)
- Intranasal antihistamine spray and intranasal steroid spray can also be used.
- Moderate to severe symptoms: Intranasal corticosteroids are first-line therapy for moderate to severe allergic rhinitis (1):
  - Beclomethasone dipropionate, budesonide, flunisolide, fluticasone propionate, mometasone furoate, and triamcinolone acetonide
  - Most effective drug class for symptoms of allergic rhinitis
  - Use nasal sprays after showering and direct the spray away from septum to improve deposition on mucosal surface.
  - May be used as needed; however, more effective with daily use (1)
  - Adverse effects: nosebleed, nasal septal perforation, and systemic corticosteroid effects
- Ciclesonide is a new-generation corticosteroid with previously demonstrated efficacy in the treatment of asthma when delivered through a metered-dose inhaler. Ciclesonide is also currently in clinical development as an intranasal formulation for use in the treatment of allergic rhinitis.
- Systemic steroids should be considered only in urgent cases and only for short-term use.
- Patients with comorbid moderate-to-severe asthma treated with omalizumab and dupilumab show improvement in symptoms.

Second Line

- Nasal antihistamines effective but may be systemically absorbed and may cause sedation: azelastine, olopatadine
- Intranasal anticholinergics such as ipratropium nasal spray: 2 sprays per nostril BID–TID
- Intranasal anticholinergics can increase efficacy in combination with steroid use.
- Leukotriene antagonists such as montelukast 10 mg/day PO
  - Should generally be used as an adjunct, not monotherapy
  - May be first line in those with concomitant asthma
- Mast-cell stabilizers such as cromolyn nasal spray: 1 spray per nostril TID–QID
  - May take 2 to 4 weeks of therapy for optimal efficacy
  - May be ineffective in patients with nonallergic rhinitis and nasal polyps
- 3rd-generation antihistamines, such as the following:
  - Brompheniramine: 12 to 24 mg PO BID
  - Chlorpheniramine: 4 mg PO q4–6h PRN
  - Clemastine: 1 to 2 mg PO BID PRN
  - Diphenhydramine: 25 to 50 mg PO q4–6h PRN:
    - May precipitate urinary retention in men with prostatism and/or hypertrophy
    - Adverse effects: sedation, prolonged QT interval, performance impairment, and anticholinergic effect
  - Decongestants
    - Phenylephrine: 10 mg PO q4h PRN
    - Pseudoephedrine: 60 mg PO q4–6h PRN
    - Oxymetazoline nasal spray (Afrin): 2 to 3 sprays per nostril q10–12h PRN (max of 3 days); intranasal agents should not be used for >3 days due to rebound rhinitis. Discourage use in patients with hypertension (HTN) or cardiac arrhythmia.
- Nasal saline sprays or irrigation used as needed, daily or twice a day for increased symptoms

ISSUES FOR REFERRAL

Refer to allergist for consideration of immunotherapy.

ADDITIONAL THERAPIES

- Nasal saline use has evidence of efficacy as sole agent or as adjunctive treatment (1).
- Other treatment strategies
  - When initiating intranasal steroids, consider starting with a "burst," using 2 sprays in each nostril daily for 2 weeks and then decreasing to 1 spray in each nostril daily thereafter.
  - To mitigate long-term side effects of intranasal steroids, consider a "5 days on, 2 days off" strategy, with the days off being the days of lowest exposure to allergens.
  - Allergen immunotherapy (desensitization)
    - Reserved when symptoms are uncontrollable with medical therapy or have a comorbidity (e.g., asthma)
    - Specific allergen extract is injected SC in increasing doses to induce patient tolerance.

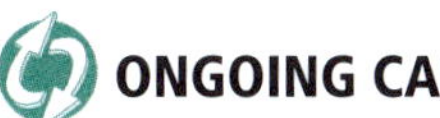

ONGOING CARE

DIET

Some patients with severe sensitivity to seasonal pollens may have oral allergy syndrome, which is associated with itching in the mouth with the ingestion of fresh fruits that may cross-react with the allergens.

PATIENT EDUCATION

- Asthma and Allergy Foundation of America: https://www.aafa.org/
- Other helpful information available at ACAAI: http://www.acaai.org/ and AAAAI: http://www.aaaai.org/home.aspx

PROGNOSIS

- Acceptable control of symptoms is the goal.
- Treatment is helpful to reduce the risk of comorbidities, such as sinusitis and asthma.

COMPLICATIONS

- Secondary infection such as otitis media or sinusitis
- Epistaxis
- Nasopharyngeal lymphoid hyperplasia
- Airway hyperreactivity with allergen exposure
- Asthma
- Facial changes, especially in children who are mouth breathers
- Sleep disturbance

REFERENCES

1. Wallace DV, Dykewicz MS, Bernstein DI, et al; for Joint Task Force on Practice Parameters for Allergy and Immunology. The diagnosis and management of rhinitis: an updated practice parameter. *J Allergy Clin Immunol*. 2008;122(Suppl 2):S1–S84.

SEE ALSO

Conjunctivitis, Acute

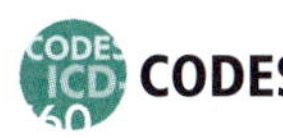

CODES

ICD10

- J30.89 Other allergic rhinitis
- J30.81 Allergic rhinitis due to animal (cat) (dog) hair and dander
- J30.2 Other seasonal allergic rhinitis

CLINICAL PEARLS

- Nasal saline irrigation (flushing 6 to 8 oz) may be very helpful in clearing upper airway of secretions and may precede the use of nasal corticosteroids.
- 2nd-generation antihistamines and intranasal corticosteroids are first-line therapies for allergic rhinitis.

ROCKY MOUNTAIN SPOTTED FEVER

Alicia Leandra Olowu, DO • Alexandria Quinere, MBS, DO

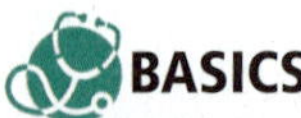

BASICS

Tick-borne rickettsial diseases include spotted fever rickettsiosis (SFR), ehrlichiosis, and anaplasmosis. In the United States, Rocky Mountain spotted fever (RMSF) is the SFR associated with the most severe and fatal outcomes (1).

DESCRIPTION

- RMSF is a tick-borne illness caused by the bacterium *Rickettsia rickettsii* (2)[C].
- Symptoms include fever, headache, and a petechial or maculopapular rash that typically begins at wrists and ankles, spreading toward palms, soles, and the trunk.
- System(s) affected: cardiovascular, musculoskeletal, skin, CNS, renal, hepatic, and pulmonary

EPIDEMIOLOGY

In the United States, ticks are both vectors and reservoirs. Important species in the United States include the American dog tick, *Dermacentor variabilis*, (the most common vector) found in eastern, central, and pacific coastal areas; the Rocky Mountain wood tick, *Dermacentor andersoni*, found in the western United States; and the brown dog tick, *Rhipicephalus sanguineus* is distributed throughout all states. Although it can be seen throughout the United States, RMSF is most common in the southeastern and south-central United States.

Incidence

- In the United States, the annual incidence of SFR increased from 1.7 cases per million persons in 2000 to 13 to 14 cases per million by 2012 to 2016. Cases have been reported in all states except Hawaii and Alaska. RMSF is also seen in Canada, Mexico, and throughout Central and South America (3)[B].
- Arkansas, Missouri, North Carolina, Tennessee, and Oklahoma account for 50–63% of SFR cases. There has also been increasing prevalence in Arizona, particularly among American Indian communities, likely due to the brown dog tick.
- Cases occur year round. Most cases are reported from April through September during the peak of outdoor activity.
- Highest incidence occurs in those aged 60 to 69 years. Highest number of reported deaths is in children aged <10 years (1).

Prevalence

In the United States, 5,207 cases were reported in 2019, although the highest peak was in 2017 with 5,248.

ETIOLOGY AND PATHOPHYSIOLOGY

- An adult tick releases *R. rickettsii*, from its salivary glands after 6 to 10 hours of feeding. Moreover, infection can occur by contact with tick tissues or fluids during the tick removal process.
- Pathogens infect vascular endothelial cells, causing small and medium vessel injury throughout the body leading to disseminated inflammation. Subsequent vascular permeability can cause pulmonary edema, cerebral edema, and hyponatremia. Local consumption of platelets and the small vessel injury results in the characteristic petechial rash.
- Subsequent end-organ injury may also result in meningoencephalitis, acute renal failure, ARDS, shock, arrhythmia, and seizure.
- It is unknown whether *R. rickettsii* crosses the placenta and causes in utero infection.
- RMSF can rarely be caused by direct inoculation of tick blood or fluid into open wounds or conjunctivae, or through inhalation of contaminated aerosols.

RISK FACTORS

- Known tick bite, engorged tick, or presence of tick for >20 hours
- Tick crushed during removal
- Accumulated outdoor exposure or residence in wooded areas; contact with outdoor pets, particularly dogs, or wild animals

GENERAL PREVENTION

- Limit tick exposure: Highest tick exposure is in tall grasses, open areas of low bushy vegetation or wooded areas.
- Wear light-colored clothing, long sleeves, pants, socks, and closed-toed shoes. Use 20–30% DEET-containing insect repellents.
- Permethrin spray-on clothing
- Regular tick checks, prompt, and proper tick removal; do not use bare hands to remove ticks.
- Wash hands and site of bite with soap and water after tick removal to avoid potential mucosal inoculation.
- Protect pets through ectoparasite control.

DIAGNOSIS

- Maintain high incidence of suspicion for rickettsial infections when patients present with "influenza-like" symptoms during summer months regardless of a known history of tick exposure (2)[C].
- Delay of empirical therapy increases risk of long-term sequelae and mortality.

HISTORY

Consider RMSF in acute febrile illness and rash, particularly with a history of potential tick exposure within previous 14 days, outdoor activities or travels to an endemic area, during late spring or summer months. *The tick bite goes unnoticed 30–50% of the time, and the lack of a clear history of a tick bite should not exclude the diagnosis*.

- Typically presents like a viral illness in the first 1 to 4 days with sudden onset of fever, severe frontal headache, malaise, myalgia, anorexia, nausea, vomiting, abdominal pain, and photophobia.
- Rash typically appears 3 to 5 days after onset of fever; starts as small blanching, pink macules on wrist and ankles before spreading to the trunk where rash may become maculopapular in appearance
- Involvement of palms and soles usually present by 5th to 6th day, along with generalized petechial rash, a sign of advanced disease. Rash generally spares the face and is not pruritic.
- Although children more frequently (>90%) have a rash, the classic triad of fever, rash, and tick bite occurs in <60% of children with RMSF. 10% of patients never develop a rash and decision to treat should not be based solely on presence of rash.
- Other symptoms include conjunctival injection, mental status impairments, restlessness, arthralgia, peripheral or periorbital edema, calf pain, and hearing loss.

PHYSICAL EXAM

- Fever is typically >102°F.
- The rash typically starts as an erythematous, macular, or maculopapular exanthema (1 to 4 mm in diameter); 50% become petechial or purpuric. In some cases, a petechial rash can occur without prior maculopapular eruption. Rash can be difficult to visualize on dark skin.
  - In severe cases, the rash can involve the entire body (including mucous membranes) and may progress to necrotic or gangrenous lesions, appearing similar to meningococcemia.
- AMS, focal neurologic deficits, lymphadenopathy, hepatosplenomegaly, and edema of dorsum of hands or feet can occur

DIFFERENTIAL DIAGNOSIS

- Viral exanthema (e.g., hand-foot-mouth disease, measles, rubella, roseola, parvovirus)
- Viral gastroenteritis, appendicitis, mononucleosis, upper respiratory infection
- TTP/ITP, toxic shock syndrome
- Meningoencephalitis, meningococcemia
- Other tick-borne infections: typhus, ehrlichiosis, Lyme disease, babesiosis, anaplasmosis, boutonneuse fever, leptospirosis
- Drug reaction or serum sickness
- Kawasaki disease, idiopathic vasculitides, infective endocarditis

DIAGNOSTIC TESTS & INTERPRETATION

Most cases of RMSF are diagnosed based on IgM and IgG serologic response to *R. rickettsii*, in conjunction with a high degree of clinical suspicion. Do not delay therapy awaiting results, as confirmation can take weeks (2)[C],(3)[A].

Initial Tests (lab, imaging)

- Specific laboratory diagnosis
  - Indirect fluorescent antibody (IFA) testing is gold-standard. Requires one sample in the first week, and a repeat in 2 to 4 weeks later to see a 4-fold change in antibody titers (3).
  - Sensitivity of IFA in the first 10 to 12 days of illness is low. 2 weeks after onset of illness the sensitivity is 95% but cannot distinguish between *R. rickettsii* and other spotted fever-group *Rickettsia* (3)[A].
  - Immunoglobulins (IgM, IgG) appear 7 to 10 days upon start of disease; the best time to obtain convalescent antibody titer is at the 14 to 21-day mark of onset of symptoms.
  - Due to seroprevalence, it is impossible to differentiate a single elevated IgG titer associated with acute illness from previous infections (3)[B].
  - Polymerase chain reaction (PCR) of blood samples can confirm diagnosis of RMSF if positive, but shows limited sensitivity, particularly in early stages. A negative result does not rule it out.
  - Skin biopsy using direct immunofluorescence or immunoperoxidase staining can help diagnose RMSF with high specificity and moderate sensitivity, but its value decreases after treatment initiation.

- Nonspecific laboratory tests:
  - WBC count: variable, frequently normal
  - Thrombocytopenia (<150,000 cells/μL) in 60% of children
  - Hyponatremia <135 mEq/dL
  - Elevated hepatic transaminases
  - Anemia, increase in BUN/creatinine, PT/PTT, hyperbilirubinemia, and hypoalbuminemia may also be present.
  - CSF may have lymphocytic pleocytosis, elevated protein, and normal glucose.
- Imaging procedures are rarely helpful.

Diagnostic Procedures/Other

Skin biopsy can offer definitive diagnosis; a 3-mm punch biopsy to perform a rapid direct fluorescent antibody (DFA) test (sensitivity 70%, specificity 100%). However, results are often delayed, and should not preclude initiation of treatment

Test Interpretation

- Test acute and convalescent phase sera in tandem
- Early treatment may limit antibody formation.
- Seropositivity increases with age in endemic states. In such situations, positive spotted fever group *Rickettsia* serologies do not necessarily signify an acute infection (this is why the 4-fold change is necessary for definitive diagnosis).

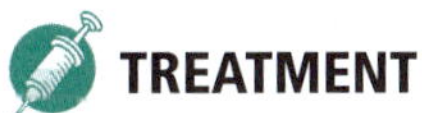

TREATMENT

MEDICATION

First Line

Doxycycline is the treatment of choice in both adults and children (2)[C].

- Untreated rickettsial infections have a high rate of morbidity and mortality (20–30% without prompt antibiotic treatment). Antibiotics should not be delayed while awaiting confirmatory testing. Other antibiotics are considerably less effective (2)[C].
- Dosing:
  - Adults and children who are >100 lbs (>45 kg): doxycycline 100 mg PO or IV q12h until 3 days after the fever subsides and there is clinical improvement
  - Children <100 lbs (<45 kg), including those <8 years old: doxycycline 2.2 mg/kg PO or IV q12h until 3 days after fever subsides and there is clinical improvement.
- Typical course of treatment is 5 to 7 days, at a minimum, possibly longer if severe or complicated disease.
- RMSF resistance to doxycycline has not been documented.
- Adverse effects may include:
  - Dyspepsia; take medication with food and water. Avoid dairy, iron, or antacids, as they may inhibit drug absorption.
  - Photosensitivity may occur. Minimize sun exposure and use sunscreen.
  - No risk of dental staining in children <8 years old (2)[C]
- Severe allergy is a contraindication to doxycycline; rapid desensitization may be considered for life-threatening disease in severe illness.

Second Line

In patients with allergies to tetracyclines/doxycycline, a thorough history to determine extent of allergy should be obtained since doxycycline is the best treatment. In setting of anaphylaxis or other contraindication to tetracyclines, chloramphenicol 50 to 75 mg/kg IV divided into 4 doses daily for 7 days is second-line therapy; chloramphenicol is the alternative to treat RMSF; associated with adverse hematologic effects (e.g., aplastic anemia) and increased case mortality

Pregnancy Considerations

- Doxycycline is appropriate for this life-threatening infection in pregnancy if suspicion is high. No current data have found evidence of teratogenicity, although studies are limited. There are some data on fatty liver of pregnancy with high dose doxycycline, but these doses exceeded what is used for RMSF.
- Short-term doxycycline is compatible with breastfeeding.
- Chloramphenicol may be considered but should be avoided in the 3rd trimester due to risk for gray baby syndrome.

ISSUES FOR REFERRAL

- Consider infectious disease consult along with immunology/allergist if patient is severely allergic to doxycycline.
- Report cases of RMSF to public health authorities.

ADDITIONAL THERAPIES

Patients with neurologic injury may require prolonged physical and cognitive therapy.

ADMISSION, INPATIENT, AND NURSING CONSIDERATIONS

- Admission criteria/initial stabilization
  - CNS dysfunction
  - Nausea/vomiting preventing oral antibiotic therapy
  - Immunocompromised patients
  - Specific acute organ failure
  - Failure of oral pain management
  - ICU for patients with shock
  - Severe allergy to tetracycline/doxycycline
- Discharge criteria
  - Resolution of fever
  - Ability to take oral therapy and nutrition

ONGOING CARE

FOLLOW-UP RECOMMENDATIONS

- Patients with mild disease may be treated as outpatients if close follow-up is available.
- Hospitalize patients with moderate to severe disease.
- Infection does not confer lifelong immunity.

Patient Monitoring

- Follow up patients treated as outpatients every 2 to 3 days until symptoms resolve.
- Follow-up CBC, electrolytes, LFTs, if clinically indicated

DIET

Consider nutritional supplementation if intake is poor.

PATIENT EDUCATION

General prevention and caution regarding tick avoidance during outside activities in endemic areas

PROGNOSIS

- Prognosis is closely related to timely administration of appropriate antibiotics.
- Delay in treatment may increase mortality by 3-fold if delayed to 5th day of illness.
- When treated promptly, prognosis is excellent with resolution of symptoms and no sequelae.
- Children aged <10 years and elderly aged >70 years are at higher risk of morbidity and/or mortality.
- Patients with G6PD deficiency are at high risk for fulminant RMSF, in which death can occur ≤5 days.

R

COMPLICATIONS

- Encephalopathy, most commonly transient impaired level of consciousness or meningismus
- Seizures, focal neurologic deficit
- Renal injury leading to acute renal failure
- Hepatitis, congestive heart failure (CHF), respiratory failure
- Proximal muscle weakness, changes in personality, paresthesias, deafness, secondary thromboses, and tissue necrosis may also be seen.

REFERENCES

1. Ho BM, Davis HE, Forrester JD, et al. Wilderness Medical Society clinical practice guidelines for the prevention and management of tick-borne illness in the United States. *Wilderness Environ Med*. 2021;32(4):474–494. doi:10.1016/j.wem.2021.09.001.
2. Pace EJ, O'Reilly M. Tickborne diseases: diagnosis and management. *Am Fam Physician*. 2020;101(9):530–540.
3. Binder AM, Nichols Heitman K, Drexler NA. Diagnostic methods used to classify confirmed and probable cases of spotted fever rickettsioses—United States, 2010–2015. *MMWR Morb Mortal Wkly Rep*. 2019;68(10):243–246.

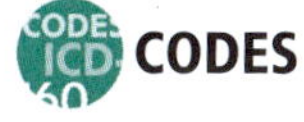

CODES

ICD10

A77.0 Spotted fever due to Rickettsia rickettsii

CLINICAL PEARLS

- Diagnosis of RMSF requires a high index of clinical suspicion.
- Tick bites are often unnoticed, and some patients (up to 15%) may never develop a rash. Treat empirically if index of suspicion is high.
- Begin treatment immediately without waiting for confirmatory testing in suspected cases. Doxycycline is drug of choice for RMSF in both adults, including pregnant women, and children. The only absolute contraindication is severe allergy to the drug.
- There is no evidence to support prophylaxis against RMSF in patients with known tick bite.

ROSEOLA

Jeffrey D. Quinlan, MD, FAAFP

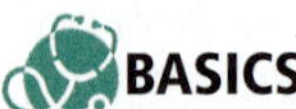

BASICS

Omnipresent infection occurring in infancy and childhood; majority of cases are caused by human herpesvirus 6 (HHV-6); may be associated with other diseases including encephalitis

DESCRIPTION

- Acute infection of infants or very young children
- Causes a high fever; once fever resolves, skin eruption begins
- Rash is a sudden, pink, maculopapular eruption on starting on the trunk and limbs and spreads distally (1).
- Transmission via contact with salivary secretions or respiratory droplet
- Incubation period of 9 to 10 days
- System(s) affected: skin/exocrine, metabolic, gastrointestinal, respiratory, neurologic
- Synonym(s): roseola infantum, exanthem subitum; pseudorubella; sixth disease; 3-day fever

Pediatric Considerations

A disease of infants and very young children

EPIDEMIOLOGY

- Predominant age
  - HHV-6
    - Infants and very young children (<2 years old)
    - Peak age infection 6 to 9 months, rarely congenital or perinatal infection
    - 95% of children have been infected with HHV-6 by 2 years of life.
  - HHV-7
    - Later childhood
    - Mean age of infection 26 months
    - >90% population with HHV-7 by 10 years
- Predominant sex: male = female
- No seasonal variance

Incidence

Common: accounts for 20% ED visits for febrile illness among children 6 to 8 months

Prevalence

- Peak prevalence is between 9 and 21 months.
- Nearly 100% population carrying HHV-6 by 3 years.
- Approximately 20% patients with primary HHV-6 have roseola.

ETIOLOGY AND PATHOPHYSIOLOGY

- HHV-6 and HHV-7
- Majority of cases (60–74%) due to HHV-6
  - HHV-6B > HHV-6A
  - HHV-6A seen in children in Africa
  - HHV-6 binds to CD46 receptors on all nucleated cells.
- Primary infection typically through respiratory droplets or saliva
- Congenital infection/vertical transmission occurs in 1% of cases.
  - Transplacental transmission
  - Chromosomal integration (clinical significance unknown)
- Lifelong latent or persistent asymptomatic infection occurs after primary infection.
  - 80–90% of population intermittently sheds HHV-6/HHV-7 in saliva.
  - Patients are viremic from 2 days prior to fever until defervescence and onset of rash.
  - HHV-6 latency is also implicated in CSF.

Genetics

HHV-6 is integrated into the chromosomes of 0.2–3% of the population. This leads to vertical transmission of the virus. Clinical significance of this is unknown.

RISK FACTORS

- Female gender
- Having older siblings
- At-risk adults: immunocompromised
  - Renal, liver, other solid organ, and bone marrow transplant (BMT)
  - HHV-6 reactivation can occur in first week post-transplant. HHV-6 viremia occurs in 30–45% of BMT within the first several weeks after transplantation.
    - Usually asymptomatic
    - Up to 82% of HHV-6 reactivation/reinfection in solid organ transplant
- Non-risk factors
  - Child care attendance
  - Method of delivery
  - Breastfeeding (HHV does not appear to pass through breast milk.)
  - Maternal age
  - Season

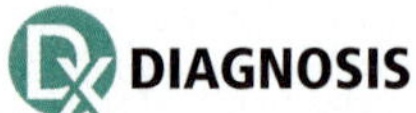

DIAGNOSIS

HISTORY

- 3 to 5 days abrupt fever 102.2 to 104.0°F (39 to 40°C) not associated with a rash
- The child may be fussy during this prodrome.
- Sudden drop of fever associated with appearance of rash: rash on trunk then spreads centrifugally mainly to neck, possibly also to peripheral extremities, and face
- Diarrhea
- Mild upper respiratory symptoms
- Rhinorrhea
- Febrile seizure occurs in 13% of cases.

PHYSICAL EXAM

- Rash (exanthem subitum)
  - Rose-pink macules and/or papules that blanch
  - First appears on the trunk then peripherally
  - May occur up to 3 days after fever resolves
  - Fades within 2 days
  - Occurs in approximately 20% of patients in the United States
- Mild inflammation of tympanic membrane, pharynx, and/or conjunctiva
- Ulcers on soft palate and uvula (Nagayama spots)
- Cervical lymphadenopathy
- Periorbital edema

DIFFERENTIAL DIAGNOSIS

- Enterovirus infection
- Adenovirus infection
- Epstein-Barr virus
- Fifth disease—parvovirus B_{19}
- Rubella
- Scarlet fever
- Drug eruption
- Measles

DIAGNOSTIC TESTS & INTERPRETATION

- Primarily a clinical diagnosis not requiring laboratory or radiologic testing
- Tests often cannot differentiate latent or active disease.
- Specific diagnosis only necessary in severe cases, unclear diagnosis where more serious disease needs to be ruled out, or if considering antiviral therapy

Initial Tests (lab, imaging)
- If necessary, HHV-6 and HHV-7 by PCR
  - Serum, whole blood, CSF, or saliva
  - Becoming more widely available
  - Not required in non-immunocompromised individuals
- HHV-6 IgM immunofluorescence
- Diagnostic for acute infection
  - Spike seen in first week of illness
- HHV-6 IgG immunofluorescence
  - Check at diagnosis and then 2 weeks later.
  - Use with IgM to show primary infection.
  - Negative initial test and rise on follow-up suggest primary infection.
- Viral culture
  - Rarely done
  - No clinical use (very time-consuming)
- Other laboratory findings
  - Decreased total leukocytes, lymphocytes, and neutrophils
  - Elevated transaminases
  - Thrombocytopenia

Diagnostic Procedures/Other
- Urine culture: to rule out UTI as source of fever
- Chest x-ray (CXR): if a child has respiratory symptoms

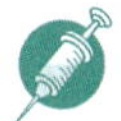

TREATMENT

No treatment necessary, resolves without sequelae

GENERAL MEASURES
- Symptomatic relief including antipyretics
- Hydration

MEDICATION
First Line
- No specific first-line treatment in immunocompetent hosts beyond supportive measures
  - Antivirals are not recommended in immunocompetent.
- No approved antiviral treatment in immunocompromised
- Second-line IV tested in vitro studies in stem cell transplant patients
  - HHV-6B susceptible: Ganciclovir or foscarnet
  - HHV-6A and HHV-7 are more resistant to ganciclovir.
- Antivirals suggested in individual cases of encephalitis (associated with reactivation of HHV-6)
- In bone marrow and stem cell transplant recipients receiving immunosuppression, prophylaxis is effective in preventing reactivation of HHV-6.

ONGOING CARE

FOLLOW-UP RECOMMENDATIONS
Patient Monitoring
- During febrile prodrome, monitor for dehydration.
- None after typical rash appears and fever resolves
- Mean duration of illness is 6 days.
- If febrile seizures occur, they will cease after fever subsides and will not likely recur.
- Symptomatic reactivation in immunocompromised

DIET
Encourage fluids.

PATIENT EDUCATION
- Parental reassurance that this is usually a benign, self-limited disease
- There is no specific, recommended period of exclusion from out-of-home care for affected children.
- Patient is viremic a few days prior to fever until time of defervescence and rash onset.

PROGNOSIS
- Course: acute, complete recovery without sequelae
- Reactivation in immunocompromised patients are common.

COMPLICATIONS
- Febrile seizures
  - 13% patients with roseola
  - Accounts for 1/3 of primary seizures in children $<$2 years old
- Medication hypersensitivity syndromes (drug reaction with eosinophilia and systemic symptoms)
- Reactivation can occur in transplant patients, HIV-1 infection, and other immunocompromised individuals.
- Meningoencephalitis occurs in immunocompetent and in immunosuppressed patients; poor association with multiple sclerosis
- Pityriasis rosea
- Possible association with progressive multifocal leukoencephalopathy

REFERENCES

1. Allmon A, Deane K, Martin KL. Common skin rashes in children. *Am Fam Physician*. 2015;92(3):211–216.

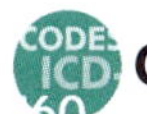

CODES

ICD10
- B08.20 Exanthema subitum [sixth disease], unspecified
- B08.21 Exanthema subitum [sixth disease] due to human herpesvirus 6
- B08.22 Exanthema subitum [sixth disease] due to human herpesvirus 7

R

CLINICAL PEARLS
- Roseola infection should be suspected if an infant or young child presents with a high temperature without other clinical findings.
- As the fever abates, a macular rash will be seen on the trunk, with eventual spread to the face and extremities in 20% of patients.
- Roseola is a clinical diagnosis, and laboratory testing is not necessary for most children with classic presentation.
- For atypical presentations, complications, and immunocompromised hosts, several laboratory tools are available, including serologic testing for antibody, viral PCR testing, and viral culture.
- Infection is typically self-limiting and without sequelae.
- Usually, only symptomatic treatment is needed.
- Consider prophylaxis in patients undergoing bone marrow or stem cell transplant and receiving immunosuppressive therapy.

ROTATOR CUFF IMPINGEMENT SYNDROME

Faren H. Williams, MD, MS • Minjin Fromm, MD

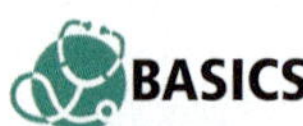

BASICS

DESCRIPTION

- Compression of rotator cuff tendons and subacromial bursa between the humeral head and the structures comprising the coracoacromial arch and proximal humerus
- Most common cause of atraumatic shoulder pain in patients >25 years of age
- Primary symptom is pain that is most severe when the arm is abducted between 60 and 120 degrees (the "painful arc").
- Classically divided into three stages:
  - Stage I: acute inflammation, edema, or hemorrhage of the underlying tendons due to overuse (typically in those aged <25 years)
  - Stage II: progressive tendinosis that leads to partial rotator cuff tear along with underlying thickening or fibrosis of surrounding structures (commonly, ages 25 to 40 years)
  - Stage III: full-thickness tear (typically in patients aged >40 years)

EPIDEMIOLOGY

Incidence

- Shoulder pain accounts for 1% of all primary care visits.
- Peak incidence of 25/1,000 patients per year occurs in patients aged 42 to 46 years.
- Impingement is responsible for 18–74% of shoulder pain diagnoses.

Prevalence

Prevalence of shoulder pain in general population ranges from ~7% to 30%.

RISK FACTORS

- Repetitive overhead motions (throwing, swimming)
- Glenohumeral joint instability or muscle imbalance
- Acromioclavicular arthritis or osteophytes
- Thickened coracoacromial ligament
- Shoulder trauma
- Increasing age
- Smoking

GENERAL PREVENTION

- Proper throwing and lifting techniques
- Proper strengthening to balance rotator cuff and scapula stabilizer muscles

DIAGNOSIS

HISTORY

- Gradual increase in shoulder pain with overhead activities (Sudden onset of sharp pain suggests a tear.)
- Night pain is common, exacerbated by lying on the affected shoulder or sleeping with the affected arm above the head.
- Anterolateral shoulder pain with overhead activities
- May progress to weakness and decreased range of motion if shoulder is not used through full range of motion

PHYSICAL EXAM

- Examine patient for atrophy/asymmetry. Observe how the patient takes off his or her shirt during exam.
- Neer impingement test: Examiner stabilizes the scapula and moves the affected upper extremity through a flexion arc. Positive result is pain with flexion of the shoulder; sensitivity: 78%; specificity: 58%
- Hawkins-Kennedy impingement test: Examiner places the arm in 90 degrees of forward flexion and then gently internally rotates the arm. End point for internal rotation is when the patient feels pain or when the rotation of the scapula is felt or observed by the examiner. Test is positive when patient experiences pain during the maneuver; sensitivity: 74%; specificity: 57%
- Empty can test (supraspinatus): Examiner asks the patient to elevate and internally rotate the arm with thumbs pointing downward in the scapular plane. Elbow should be fully extended. Examiner applies downward pressure on upper surface of the arm. Test is positive when patient complains of pain with resistance; sensitivity: 69%; specificity: 62%
- Lift-off test (subscapularis): Patient internally rotates the shoulder, placing the back of the hand on ipsilateral buttock, and then lifts hand off buttock against resistance. A tear in the subscapularis muscle produces weakness of this action; sensitivity: 42%; specificity: 97%
- Drop-arm test: Patient fully elevates arm and then slowly reverses the motion. If the arm is dropped suddenly or the patient has extreme pain, the test is positive for a possible rotator cuff tear; sensitivity: 21%; specificity: 92%
- Resisted external rotation: weakness suggestive of infraspinatus and/or teres minor tendon involvement
- Apprehension-relocation test for anterior glenohumeral joint instability: Have the patient supine or sitting; abduct the arm to 90 degrees and flex the patient's elbow to 90 degrees; examiner slowly rotates the humerus (pushes hand posteriorly while patient resists and then anteriorly while the patient resists). If the patient becomes anxious or has apprehension from this maneuver, test is positive implying instability and risk for dislocation. If pain is present, rather than instability, consider labral tear and/or impingement syndrome.
- Examine cervical spine to rule out cervical pathology as source of shoulder pain.
- Neurovascular exam of the upper extremity

DIFFERENTIAL DIAGNOSIS

- Labral injury
- Acromioclavicular arthritis (more common in older patients; positive cross-arm test—pain when affected arm is fully adducted across the chest in the horizontal plane)
- Adhesive capsulitis (rotator cuff tendonitis leads to decreased use and atrophy of rotator cuff muscles, followed by contracture; linked to diabetes and potentially prior trauma)
- Anterior shoulder instability (prior trauma; more common in patients <25 years old)
- Multidirectional instability
- Biceps tendonitis or rupture (Perform Speed and Yergason tests and look for visible or palpable defect of biceps—"Popeye sign.")
- Calcific tendonitis
- Cervical radiculopathy (spinal or foraminal stenosis, can test with Spurling maneuver)
- Glenohumeral arthritis (Evaluate with plain films.)
- Suprascapular nerve entrapment (Look for focal muscle atrophy of supraspinatus or infraspinatus.)
- Traumatic rotator cuff tear

DIAGNOSTIC TESTS & INTERPRETATION

Initial Tests (lab, imaging)

- Plain-film radiographs of the shoulder (three views): anteroposterior, axillary, scapular Y views
- Plain films may reveal:
  - Osteoarthritis of the acromioclavicular and glenohumeral joints
  - Superior migration of the humeral head (indicative of a large rotator cuff tear)
  - Cystic change of the humeral head and sclerosis of the inferior acromion (indicative of chronic rotator cuff disease)
  - Calcific tendonitis

- MRI is used to definitively assess rotator cuff tendinopathy, partial tears, and complete tears.
- MR arthrogram is preferred for labral pathology.
- Ultrasound is sensitive and specific for rotator cuff tears but is highly operator dependent.
- CT scan is preferred for bony pathology or for those unable to undergo MRI.

Diagnostic Procedures/Other

- Lidocaine injection test
  - Inject lidocaine into the subacromial space:
    - Repeat impingement tests; if pain is completely relieved and range of motion is improved, likely impingement syndrome (rather than cuff tear)
  - Allows for more accurate strength testing on physical examination:
    - If strength is intact, rule out rotator cuff tear.
    - If range of motion does not improve in any plane, more likely adhesive capsulitis
  - Some pain relief and improved range of motion occur after lidocaine injection with
    - Glenoid labral tear
    - Capsular strain
    - Glenohumeral osteoarthritis
    - Glenohumeral instability
- A lack of any pain relief suggests other sources (i.e., cervical radiculopathy) or inappropriate placement of injection.

Test Interpretation

May have tendinosis, tendonitis, or muscle/tendon tear

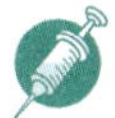

TREATMENT

Pain control in combination with aggressive rehabilitation improves and fully resolves rotator cuff tendonitis in most patients.

GENERAL MEASURES

- Rest initial and then mandatory supervised physical therapy for 6 to 8 weeks
- Ice or heat for symptom relief
- Activity modification, with avoidance of aggravating activities, particularly overhead motions
- Range-of-motion exercises
- Rotator cuff and adjacent muscle strengthening to enhance stability and prevent further injuries

MEDICATION

First Line

NSAIDs or other analgesic, often for 6 to 12 weeks

ISSUES FOR REFERRAL

Failure of conservative treatment, persistent pain, weakness, or complete tear of rotator cuff

ADDITIONAL THERAPIES

- Supervised- or home-exercise regimens provide significant pain reduction and improve function.
- Physical therapy is effective for short-term and long-term recovery of function (1)[A]:
  - Initial goal is to restore range of motion.
  - After pain resolves, gradually strengthen rotator cuff muscles in internal rotation, external rotation, and abduction

SURGERY/OTHER PROCEDURES

- Steroid injections may have a significant benefit on pain and function in the short term but do not appear to have a significant long-term effect (2)[A].
- No evidence that surgery is superior to conservative management or that one surgical technique is superior to another for impingement syndrome (3)[A]
- Platelet-rich therapies for musculoskeletal soft tissue injuries are increasingly common.
  - No apparent effect of platelet-rich plasma injection during arthroscopic rotator cuff repair on overall retear rates or shoulder-specific outcomes
- Extracorporeal shock wave therapy is currently under study as an emerging treatment for calcific tendonitis.

COMPLEMENTARY & ALTERNATIVE MEDICINE

Acupuncture is potentially beneficial for reducing pain and improving function, particularly when used with physical therapy.

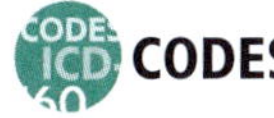

ONGOING CARE

PATIENT EDUCATION

- Physical rehabilitation is necessary, both in conservative course of treatment (i.e., NSAIDs, physical therapy, home exercises) and in surgical intervention.
- An aggressive trial of rehabilitation should be encouraged prior to extensive testing or surgical intervention. Providing pain relief prior to beginning a program of physical therapy improves adherence and outcomes.
- Symptoms often recur if not fully addressed.

PROGNOSIS

- Variable, depends on underlying pathology
- Most patients improve with conservative management. Recovery can be slow.
- Patients with more severe symptoms—those with symptoms for >1 year—are less likely to respond well with conservative therapies.

COMPLICATIONS

- Progression of injury
- Tendon retraction in complete rotator cuff tear

REFERENCES

1. Green S, Buchbinder R, Hetrick S. Physiotherapy interventions for shoulder pain. *Cochrane Database Syst Rev*. 2003;(2):CD004258.
2. Gaujoux-Viala C, Dougados M, Gossec L. Efficacy and safety of steroid injections for shoulder and elbow tendonitis: a meta-analysis of randomised controlled trials. *Ann Rheum Dis*. 2009;68(12):1843–1849.
3. Gebremariam L, Hay EM, Koes BW, et al. Effectiveness of surgical and postsurgical interventions for the subacromial impingement syndrome: a systematic review. *Arch Phys Med Rehabil*. 2011;92(11):1900–1913.

ADDITIONAL READING

- Burbank KM, Stevenson JH, Czarnecki GR, et al. Chronic shoulder pain: part I. Evaluation and diagnosis. *Am Fam Physician*. 2008;77(4):453–460.
- Burbank KM, Stevenson JH, Czarnecki GR, et al. Chronic shoulder pain: part II. Treatment. *Am Fam Physician*. 2008;77(4):493–497.
- Hanchard NCA, Lenza M, Handoll HHG, et al. Physical tests for shoulder impingements and local lesions of bursa, tendon or labrum that may accompany impingement. *Cochrane Database Syst Rev*. 2013;(4):CD007427.

CODES

ICD10

- M75.40 Impingement syndrome of unspecified shoulder
- M75.110 Incmpl rotatr-cuff tear/ruptr of unsp shoulder, not trauma
- M75.120 Complete rotatr-cuff tear/ruptr of unsp shoulder, not trauma

CLINICAL PEARLS

- Consider impingement syndrome in patients who engage in activities with repetitive overhead motions (e.g., swimming, throwing) who present with shoulder pain.
- Atraumatic shoulder pain in middle age often represents rotator cuff tendonitis.
- The supraspinatus tendon is most commonly affected in impingement syndrome.
- Neer and Hawkins tests specifically check for shoulder impingement.
- The empty can maneuver tests for weakness of supraspinatus muscle
- The drop-arm test is specific for rotator cuff tear.
- Physical therapy over 6 to 12 weeks promotes return to function.
- Most patients with shoulder impingement respond well to conservative management.

SALIVARY GLAND CALCULI/SIALADENITIS

Sahil Mullick, MD, FAAFP • Mateusz Ogledzinski, MD

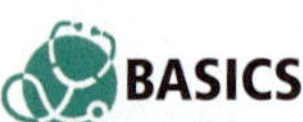

BASICS

DESCRIPTION

- Inflammation of one or more salivary glands
- Infectious, obstructive, or autoimmune
- "Sialolithiasis" is characterized by a painful swelling of the affected gland when eating due to an obstructing stones within the salivary glands or ducts.
- "Sialadenitis" is inflammation of the salivary gland classified as acute or chronic sialadenitis.
  - Acute can be caused by a primary infection (viral/bacterial) or secondary infection.
  - Chronic sialadenitis is due to repeated episodes of inflammation resulting in progressive loss of salivary gland function.
- Parotid gland and submandibular glands are commonly affected by sialadenitis. However, parotid gland is affected mostly by acute suppurative sialadenitis. The submandibular gland is more commonly affected (80–90% of cases) by stones than the parotid gland due to higher mucinous content of saliva, longer course of Wharton duct, and slow salivary flow against gravity.

EPIDEMIOLOGY

Incidence

- Peak incidence is 30 to 60 years of age; rarely in children
- Most common in debilitated and dehydrated patients
- 70% of the stones are single; 30% bilateral
- 7 to 14 per 100,000 person-years

ETIOLOGY AND PATHOPHYSIOLOGY

- Stagnation of salivary flow and elevated calcium concentrations are thought to be important.
- Decreased salivary outflow from anticholinergics, dehydration, or radiation
- Abnormal lipid levels induce impaired salivary flow and potential hyposalivation, contributing to salivary stasis and supersaturation, creating an environment conductive to calcium salt precipitation and sialolith formation.
- Salivary calculi are composed of calcium phosphate and hydroxyapatite with smaller amounts of magnesium, potassium, and ammonium.
- Predisposing factors include inflammation of the salivary gland or duct, salivary stasis, retrograde bacterial contamination from the oral cavity, increased alkalinity of saliva, and physical trauma to salivary duct or gland.
- Gout is associated with salivary stone development. In gout, sialoliths are composed of uric acid.
- Bacterial sialadenitis tends to be unifocal caused by *Staphylococcus aureus*, *Streptococcus viridans*, *Streptococcus pyogenes*, *Haemophilus influenzae*, *Escherichia coli*, *Pseudomonas aeruginosa*, and group B streptococci (neonates and children).
- Viral sialadenitis tends to be multifocal caused by mumps, cytomegalovirus, Epstein-Barr virus, HIV, and enteroviruses.
- Other common causes include radioiodine use, positive pressure ventilation use with anesthesia, Sjögren syndrome, and sarcoidosis (1).

Pediatric Considerations

Common causes of sialadenitis in children are mumps and idiopathic juvenile recurrent parotitis.

RISK FACTORS

- Hypovolemia
- Diuretic use
- Anticholinergic use
- Trauma
- Gout
- History of nephrolithiasis
- Poor oral hygiene, malnutrition, smoking, dehydration
- Head/neck radiation
- Dyslipidemia

GENERAL PREVENTION

- Maintain proper oral care and hygiene.
- Avoid anticholinergics and other causes of xerostomia.

COMMONLY ASSOCIATED CONDITIONS

- Radiation or drug-induced xerostomia
- Sjögren syndrome, Mikulicz syndrome
- Hypercalcemia

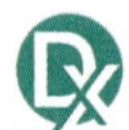

DIAGNOSIS

Diagnosis is most often clinical based on physical exam and characteristic history, which is often described as sudden onset swelling and pain in the affected gland. Pain is often worse with eating. Most (75–80%) salivary gland stones occur in the submandibular glands, 6–20% occur in the parotid gland and 1–2% occur in the sublingual or minor salivary glands. Submandibular stones are more often located in the duct. Parotid stones tend to be smaller than mandibular stones, are more often multiple, and located within the gland itself (1).

HISTORY

- Review history for
  - Alcoholism, bulimia, malnutrition; radiation therapy, past malignancy; TB or HIV exposure
- Acute onset of pain and swelling over the affected salivary gland, especially postprandial or following the anticipation of eating
- Dental pain, discharge, foul breath (halitosis) hypersalivation, and pain with chewing
- Xerostomia
- 33% of the patients with submandibular sialolithiasis present with painless swelling and 10% with pain but not swelling.
- Worsening pain, erythema and/or fever may indicate secondary infection.
- Pus drainage through the gland duct into the mouth

PHYSICAL EXAM

- Visual inspection of the glands and ducts; for submandibular gland, a stone may be felt within the Wharton duct or seen near the frenulum of the tongue. For parotid glands, a stone may be felt within Stensen duct or seen at the orifice.
- Bimanual exam of oral cavity palpating all salivary glands, floor of mouth, tongue, and neck to assess symmetry, tenderness, induration, edema, presence of stones, lymphadenopathy and the number of glands involved; a functioning gland is usually spongy and elastic.
- Examine duct openings for purulent discharge and presence of saliva. Purulent discharge at the orifice raises concern for acute bacterial sialadenitis.
- Gently palpate gland to express normal, thin absent or reduced amounts of saliva; assess for bubbling appearance or purulent drainage.
- Examine eyes for interstitial keratitis.
- Evaluation of facial nerve (CN VII) function, which is at risk for compromise if parotid gland is involved

Pediatric Considerations

Stones in children are often within the distal duct. Ultrasound with sialendoscopy is diagnostic and therapeutic.

DIFFERENTIAL DIAGNOSIS

- Bacterial parotitis
- Idiopathic juvenile recurrent parotitis; cystic fibrosis
- Mumps; tularemia
- Collagen vascular disease
- Metal poisoning
- Salivary gland tumors; lymphoma

DIAGNOSTIC TESTS & INTERPRETATION

Sialolithiasis is a clinical diagnosis based on a characteristic history and physical examination. There is typically sudden onset of swelling and pain in the affected gland associated with eating or anticipation of eating. A stone may be seen at the opening of the affected salivary duct or palpated along the course of the duct. Imaging is helpful when physical exam is equivocal or there is concern for tumor formation.

Initial Tests (lab, imaging)

- Consider CBC.
- Culture and sensitivity of any expressed pus
- Ultrasound is able to detect up to 90% of stones 2 mm or larger (2)[C].
- CT scan with IV contrast is more sensitive but has radiation exposure (3)[C].
- MR sialography for patients with an inconclusive ultrasound and persistent symptoms without the use of intraductal contrast
- Sonopalpation (concurrent ultrasound with transoral palpation) proved to have a sensitivity and specificity of 96.6% and 90% in finding a calculus (3)[B].

Follow-Up Tests & Special Considerations

- If autoimmune process is suspected, order rheumatoid factor (RF) and antinuclear antibodies (ANAs) (4)[C].
- Salivary gland biopsy

Diagnostic Procedures/Other

- Sialography to evaluate sialolithiasis and other obstructive lesions
- Sialendoscopy to find and remove sialoliths; in one study, sialendoscopy confirmed 221 (79%) parotid and 812 (93%) submandibular stones (5)[A].
- One study revealed that sonography, cone beam CT, and sialendoscopy all had excellent specificity and positive predictive value in diagnosing stones (3)[B].
- When sialendoscopy fails, a novel ultrasound-guided needle localization approach has been proposed.
- Technetium-99m pertechnetate scintigraphy showed decreased gland excretion and decreased uptake in patients with sialolithiasis.

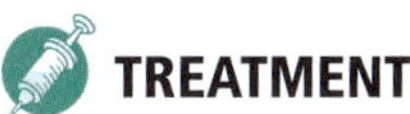

TREATMENT

GENERAL MEASURES

- Maintain hydration.
- Apply warm compresses.
- Massage the gland and milk the duct.
- Sialagogues (agents that promote salivary flow) like tart, lemon juice, and hard candies (lemon drops) may be helpful. Use throughout the day as tolerated.
- Maintain good oral hygiene.
- Chlorhexidine 0.12% mouth rinses 3 times a day will help to reduce the bacterial burden in oral cavity and will promote oral hygiene.
- Discontinue medications with anticholinergic effects that reduce salivary flow.
- Cholesterol level control

MEDICATION

- Pain management with NSAIDs
- Antibiotics for suspected secondary infection (fever, purulent discharge)

First Line

- Antistaphylococcal antibiotics such as dicloxacillin 500 mg or cephalexin 500 mg QID for 7 to 10 days
- If no improvement within 5 to 7 days, a culture of the duct discharge should be obtained and the antibiotic coverage broadened by substituting amoxicillin/clavulanate or clindamycin.
- Penicillin allergic: Use clindamycin 300 mg PO q8h.
- Gram negative: 3rd-generation cephalosporin or fluoroquinolone
- Anaerobic: metronidazole or clindamycin

Second Line

- 1st-generation cephalosporin (cephalexin or cefazolin) or clindamycin is also indicated for empiric coverage.
- If MRSA, then vancomycin

ISSUES FOR REFERRAL

- Dentist if poor dentition/dental abscess
- ENT if failure to improve with conservative management, recurrent symptoms (6)

ADDITIONAL THERAPIES

In the case of chronic sialadenitis with strictures, consider sialostent placement.

SURGERY/OTHER PROCEDURES

- Submandibular stones found in the anterior floor of the mouth can be excised intraorally (sialodochoplasty), whereas those in the hilum require gland excision. Parotid stones usually require parotidectomy (4)[A].
- Good results in patient symptom relief, quality of life, and safety have been reported in sialadenitis and sialolithiasis using sialendoscopy (4),(5). Complications include strictures, ranulas, and lingual nerve injury. However, sialendoscopy is contraindicated in acute sialadenitis.
- A combined approach using limited intraoral incision with sialendoscopy has shown an 86% success rate.
- Incision and drainage of parotid abscess is indicated after failing 3 to 5 days of medical management (7).
- Sialoliths >4 mm and stenoses can be successfully treated by radiologically or fluoroscopically controlled or sialendoscopically based methods in ~80% of cases. Extracorporeal shock wave lithotripsy (ESWL) is successful in up to 50% of cases.
- Transoral duct slitting for extraparenchymal submandibular stones; 90% success rate

COMPLEMENTARY & ALTERNATIVE MEDICINE

Consider lemon drops or other sialogogues to promote salivation. In one study, postoperative use of sialogogues nearly halved rates of sialadenitis (4)[C].

ADMISSION, INPATIENT, AND NURSING CONSIDERATIONS

- Parotid abscess
- Inability to tolerate PO intake

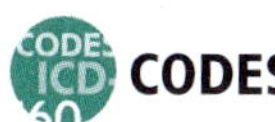

ONGOING CARE

FOLLOW-UP RECOMMENDATIONS

Avoid prescribing medications that cause xerostomia.

Patient Monitoring

Monitor patients with chronic sialadenitis because decreased salivary gland function due to fibrosis and loss of acini can lead to acute exacerbations.

DIET

- Avoid sialogogues during acute attacks.
- Maintain adequate hydration.

PATIENT EDUCATION

Maintaining excellent oral hygiene/hydration

PROGNOSIS

- Acute symptoms usually resolving in about a week with appropriate treatment. Complete resolution is expected after conservative outpatient treatment.
- Patients with autoimmune etiology may have prolonged course due to systemic involvement.
- In patients who undergo transoral surgical stone removal, recurrence has been reported in 18%.

COMPLICATIONS

- Local spreading of infection, causing cellulitis or Ludwig angina
- Facial nerve impingement, hypoglossal and lingual nerve injuries (e.g., transient marginal mandibular nerve palsy)
- Dental decay: Hypofunction of salivary gland causes decrease protection from acid erosion, promoting dental decay.
- Chronic obstruction may result in persistent inflammation, fibrosis, and eventual atrophy of the affected gland, with loss of function.
- Large or impacted stones may cause pressure necrosis, squamous metaplasia of the ductal epithelium.

REFERENCES

1. Kao WK, Chole RA, Ogden MA. Evidence of a microbial etiology for sialoliths. *Laryngoscope*. 2020;130(1):69–74.
2. Goncalves M, Mantsopoulos K, Schapher M, et al. Ultrasound supplemented by sialendoscopy: diagnostic value in sialolithiasis. *Otolaryngol Head Neck Surg*. 2018;159(3):449–455.
3. Schwarz D, Kabbasch C, Scheer M, et al. Comparative analysis of sialendoscopy, sonography, and CBCT in the detection of sialolithiasis. *Laryngoscope*. 2015;125(5):1098–1101.
4. Wilson KF, Meier JD, Ward PD. Salivary gland disorders. *Am Fam Physician*. 2014;89(11):882–888.
5. Atienza G, López-Cedrún JL. Management of obstructive salivary disorders by sialendoscopy: a systematic review. *Br J Oral Maxillofac Surg*. 2015;53(6):507–519.
6. Wallace E, Tauzin M, Hagan J, et al. Management of giant sialoliths: review of the literature and preliminary experience with interventional sialendoscopy. *Laryngoscope*. 2010;120(10):1974–1978.
7. Capaccio P, Torretta S, Pignataro L, et al. Salivary lithotripsy in the era of sialendoscopy. *Acta Otorhinolaryngol Ital*. 2017;37(2):113–121.

CODES

ICD10

- K11.5 Sialolithiasis
- K11.20 Sialoadenitis, unspecified
- K11.21 Acute sialoadenitis

CLINICAL PEARLS

- Mainstay of treatment is hydration, good oral hygiene, sialogogues, and possible surgical excision.
- Nonpharmacologic agents that promote salivary flow like tart and hard candies such as lemon drops may be helpful and should be used throughout the day.

S

SALMONELLA INFECTION

Marie L. Borum, MD, EdD, MPH • Robert S. Gordon III, DO, MS

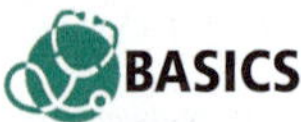

BASICS

DESCRIPTION

- Infection caused by any serotype of the bacterial genus *Salmonella*, a gram-negative facultatively anaerobic bacillus
- Nontyphoidal *Salmonella* (NTS) typically causes gastroenteritis via foodborne infection and sporadic outbreaks; less commonly causes infection outside the gastrointestinal (GI) tract
- Clinical syndromes
  - Enteric fever (see "Typhoid Fever")
  - Nontyphoidal gastroenteritis
    - Chronic carrier state (>1 year)
  - Nontyphoidal invasive disease
    - Bacteremia
      - Endovascular complications; localized infection outside GI tract (i.e., osteomyelitis, abscess)

Geriatric Considerations

Patients >65 years old have increased risk of invasive disease with bacteremia and endovascular complications due to comorbidities (atherosclerotic endovascular lesions, prostheses, etc.) that increase risk of bacterial seeding.

Pediatric Considerations

Neonates (<3 months) are more susceptible to invasive disease and complications.

EPIDEMIOLOGY

Incidence

- Global incidence of nontyphoidal *Salmonella enteritidis* estimated to be ~94 million per year (mostly foodborne).
  - Wide variation by region from 40 to 3,980 estimated cases per 100,000
- Global incidence of invasive nontyphoidal *Salmonella* infection was estimated to be 535,000 cases in 2017.
- Most commonly identified foodborne bacterial illness in the United States and a common cause of traveler's diarrhea.
  - Estimated 1.4 million cases per year in the United States, with annual incidence of 15 illnesses per 100,000
  - Estimated 25,000 hospitalizations and 420 deaths per year
- Second most common bacteria isolated from stool cultures in diarrheal illness (following *Campylobacter*) in the United States; highest incidence of bacteremia in children <5 years old; hospitalization rates higher in patients >50 years old; peak frequency: July to November
- Foodborne *Salmonella* outbreaks can be widespread—associated with fruit and raw poultry products; also spread by contact with reptiles/amphibians (turtles, snakes, lizards)

ETIOLOGY AND PATHOPHYSIOLOGY

- *Salmonella enterica*
  - Most pathogenic species in humans; 2,500 different serotypes
- Etiology
  - ~95% of cases are foodborne.
- Pathophysiology
  - Typical infectious dose in immunocompetent patients is ingestion of 1 million bacteria but can be lower in patients taking antibiotics or in the setting of gastric acid reduction. Bacteria ingested invade the distal ileal and proximal colonic mucosa to produce an inflammatory and cytotoxic response. Bacteria can enter the mesenteric lymphatic system and then the systemic circulation to cause disseminated/invasive disease.

RISK FACTORS

Recent travel to underdeveloped nations; consumption of undercooked meat, egg, or unpasteurized dairy products; nonanimal products have also been implicated in outbreaks; contact with live reptiles or poultry; contact with human carrier (*Salmonella* fecal shedding); impaired gastric acidity: H_2 receptor blockers, antacids, proton pump inhibitors (PPIs), gastrectomy, achlorhydria, pernicious anemia, infants; recent antibiotic use; reticuloendothelial blockade: sickle cell disease, malaria, bartonellosis; immunosuppression: HIV, diabetes, corticosteroid or other immunosuppressant use, chemotherapy; impaired phagocytic function: chronic granulomatous disease, hemoglobinopathies, malaria (1),(2)

GENERAL PREVENTION

Proper hygiene in production, transport, and storage of food (e.g., refrigeration during food storage and thoroughly cooking food prior to consumption). Control of animal reservoirs: Avoid contact with high-risk animals, feces, and polluted waters; hand hygiene. CDC tracks outbreaks (1),(2).

COMMONLY ASSOCIATED CONDITIONS

Gastroenteritis; bacteremia: immunocompromised or patients with underlying disease (e.g., cholelithiasis, prostheses); osteomyelitis: higher incidence in sickle cell disease; abscesses: higher incidence with malignant tumors; reactive arthritis.

DIAGNOSIS

HISTORY

- *Salmonella* infections are typically asymptomatic or result in mild, self-limited gastroenteritis (1).
- Exposure history: travel; contact with infected human, reptile, or poultry; improper food preparation; local outbreaks; host factors: age, immune status, other risk factors; symptoms typically begin 8 to 72 hours after ingestion and resolve within 4 to 10 days (1).
- Acute uncomplicated illness
  - Sudden onset of diarrhea
    - Not typically grossly bloody, but can be bloody especially among pediatric patients
  - Vomiting is infrequent. Abdominal cramping; headache; myalgias; fever.

PHYSICAL EXAM

- Fever
- Evidence of hypovolemia.
- Abdominal tenderness. Heme-positive stool in some patients.
- Hepatosplenomegaly in some patients

DIFFERENTIAL DIAGNOSIS

Viral gastroenteritis; bacterial enteritis due to other organisms; pseudomembranous colitis; inflammatory bowel disease

DIAGNOSTIC TESTS & INTERPRETATION

Initial Tests (lab, imaging)

- Gastroenteritis
  - Stool culture for *Salmonella*, *Escherichia coli*, *Shigella*, and *Campylobacter* (Optimal specimen is a diarrheal stool sample.)
  - Indications for stool culture include the following:
    - Severe diarrhea (≥6 loose stools daily); diarrhea >1 week in duration; diarrhea containing blood or mucous
    - Fever
    - Multiple cases suggesting an outbreak
  - Fecal leukocytes: positive
  - Blood cultures are warranted in:
    - Infants <3 months; people of any age with signs of septicemia or other systemic manifestations of infection; cases where enteric fever is suspected; immunocompromised patients
- Bacteremia
  - Blood cultures if febrile
  - Stool cultures: may also be positive
  - Culture CSF if patient is <3 months of age with positive blood culture.
- Endovascular infection
  - Consider angiography in bacteremic patients >50 years of age if aortic or vascular source is suspected.
- Local infections
  - Wound culture; consider CT or MRI for soft tissue or bone infections.
- Chronic carrier state
  - Stool culture positive for >1 year
  - Urine culture may be positive in chronic carriers.

Follow-Up Tests & Special Considerations

- Look for other causes in diarrhea lasting >14 days. Asymptomatic excretion of *Salmonella* may occur for weeks after infection; follow-up fecal cultures are routinely not indicated for patients with uncomplicated gastroenteritis (1).
- Follow-up blood cultures suggested for patients with bacteremia

Test Interpretation

Intestinal biopsies (if taken) may show mucosal ulceration, hemorrhage, and necrosis seen on along with reticuloendothelial hypertrophy/hyperplasia.

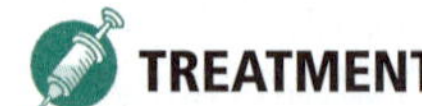

TREATMENT

- Treatment is supportive for nonsevere nontyphoidal *Salmonella* gastroenteritis in immunocompetent patients between 12 months and 50 years of age. The illness is typically self-limited. There is no proven benefit for treatment of mild disease. Treatment can suppress the host immunologic response. Higher rates of relapse have also been reported and there is the potential to extend asymptomatic carriage (1),(2).
- Consider antibiotics in immunocompetent hosts with severe diarrhea, high fever, or those requiring hospitalization (1),(2)

- Patients at increased risk of bacteremia benefit from antibiotics:
  - Infants <3 months of age
  - Patients >50 years old (risk particularly increases after age 65 years)
  - HIV-infected patients; cancer patients, especially those with hematologic, GI, or genitourinary malignancies
  - Patients with hemoglobinopathies, atherosclerotic lesions, and prosthetic valves, grafts, or joints or any immunosuppressed state
- Chronic carriage of nontyphoidal *Salmonella*
  - 4 to 6 weeks of antimicrobial therapy; prophylactic therapy in immunocompromised patients

GENERAL MEASURES

- Hydration and electrolyte replacement; handwashing and barrier precautions for inpatients (1),(2)
- Avoid antimotility drugs in patients with fever or dysentery. Antimotility drugs may increase contact time of the enteropathogen in the gut mucosa (1),(2)

MEDICATION

First Line

- Gastroenteritis, uncomplicated: No specific medications are necessary; supportive care (1),(2)
- Gastroenteritis, complicated (due to illness severity or host risk factors such as immunocompromised) (1),(2)
  - Adults (Treat for 14 days if immunocompromised.)
    - Ciprofloxacin: 750 mg/day PO for 1 day or 500 mg/day PO for 3 days, *or* (2)
    - Levofloxacin: 500 mg/day PO for 1 to 3 days, *or* (2)
    - Azithromycin: 500 mg/day PO for 3 days or 1 g PO single dose (2)
      - Preferred agent for febrile diarrhea or dysentery
  - Children
    - Ceftriaxone: 100 mg/kg/day IV or IM in 2 equally divided doses for 3 to 7 days, (3) *or*
    - Azithromycin: 10 mg/kg PO for first dose and then 5 mg/kg/day for subsequent doses daily for 5 days (3)
  - HIV patients
    - Increased duration (range of 2 to 6 weeks) of antimicrobial therapy and/or zidovudine may decrease relapse.
- Bacteremia: Due to resistance trends, treat life-threatening infections in adults with a fluoroquinolone *or* a 3rd-generation cephalosporin until susceptibilities are determined.
  - Adults
    - Ciprofloxacin (or other fluoroquinolone): 400 mg IV BID for 10 to 14 days, *or*
    - Ceftriaxone: 1 to 2 g/day IV for 10 to 14 days
  - Children
    - Cefotaxime: 50 mg/kg IV q6h for 7 to 10 days, *or* (3)
    - Ceftriaxone: 100 mg/kg IV daily (max 2 g) or 50 mg/kg IV BID 7 to 10 days, *or* (3)
    - Amoxicillin: 30 mg/kg/dose TID for 7 to 10 days, *or* (3)
    - Trimethoprim-sulfamethoxazole: 4 mg/kg PO BID for 7 to 10 days, *or* (3)
    - Azithromycin: 20 mg/kg PO for first dose and then 10 mg/kg/day for subsequent doses daily for 7 to 10 days (3)
- Localized infection (e.g., septic arthritis, osteomyelitis, cholangitis, and pneumonia); surgical drainage or débridement in addition to a minimum of 3 weeks of antimicrobial therapy
  - In sustained bacteremia, prolonged local infection, or immunocompromised patients, give antibiotics PO for 4 to 6 weeks.
- Chronic carrier state (shedding >1 year duration)
  - Amoxicillin: 1 g PO TID for 6 weeks, or
  - Trimethoprim-sulfamethoxazole 160 mg/800 mg PO BID for 12 weeks, *or*
  - Ciprofloxacin: 500 mg PO BID for 4 to 6 weeks

ALERT

- Strains resistant to ampicillin, amoxicillin, tetracyclines, and trimethoprim-sulfamethoxazole have been reported (1).
- Fluoroquinolone resistance is increasing, perhaps due to increasing use in livestock.
- Pet reptiles identified as having a 48% carrier-rate, 72% of which were multi-drug resistant organisms.

Second Line

- Azithromycin is an alternative agent that may be useful in patients with multiple allergies or if the organism demonstrates an unusual resistance pattern.
- Fluoroquinolones are now routinely given to children for 5 to 7 days in areas of the world where multidrug-resistant *Salmonella typhi* is common.

SURGERY/OTHER PROCEDURES

- Surgical excision and drainage for infected tissue sites, followed by a minimum of 3 weeks of antibiotic therapy
- If biliary tract disease is present, a preoperative 10- to 14-day course of parenteral antibiotics is recommended prior to cholecystectomy.

ONGOING CARE

FOLLOW-UP RECOMMENDATIONS

Patient Monitoring

- Asymptomatic shedding of *Salmonella* may occur for weeks after infection. Follow-up fecal cultures are generally not indicated for patients with uncomplicated gastroenteritis. Requirements may differ during a *Salmonella* outbreak.
- Criteria may vary by state and local regulations. Some public health departments require negative stool cultures for health workers and food handlers prior to returning to work. Shedding may last from 4 to 8 weeks.
- Serotyping of isolates can be performed at public health laboratories. Genomic techniques are available to identify and monitor outbreaks.

DIET

Easily digestible foods

PATIENT EDUCATION

Meticulous hand hygiene; caution handling raw meat, poultry, and eggs; fruits and vegetables should be thoroughly washed prior to consumption. Thoroughly cooking meats eliminates *Salmonella*; caution when handling animals with high fecal carriage rates.

PROGNOSIS

Most cases of *Salmonella* gastroenteritis are self-limited and have an excellent prognosis. Increased mortality is seen in the young (<3 months), elderly (>65 years), and immunocompromised. Increased mortality is seen with bacteremia and other invasive infections. Mortality is increased in multidrug-resistant strains.

COMPLICATIONS

Toxic megacolon, hypovolemic shock, metastatic abscess formation, endocarditis, infectious endarteritis, meningitis, septic arthritis, reactive arthritis, osteomyelitis, pneumonia, appendicitis, cholecystitis

REFERENCES

1. Shane AL, Mody RK, Crump JA, et al. 2017 Infectious Diseases Society of America clinical practice guidelines for the diagnosis and management of infectious diarrhea. *Clin Infect Dis*. 2017;65(12):e45–e80. doi:10.1093/cid/cix669.
2. Riddle MS, DuPont HL, Connor BA. ACG clinical guideline: diagnosis, treatment, and prevention of acute diarrheal infections in adults. *Am J Gastroenterol*. 2016;111(5):602–622. doi:10.1038/ajg.2016.126.
3. Wen SC, Best E, Nourse C. Non-typhoidal Salmonella infections in children: review of literature and recommendations for management. *J Paediatr Child Health*. 2017;53(10):936–941. doi:10.1111/jpc.13585.

ADDITIONAL READING

Kim S, Kang H, Excler JL, et al. The economic burden of non-typhoidal Salmonella and invasive non-typhoidal *Salmonella* infection: a systematic literature review. *Vaccines (Basel)*. 2024;12(7):758. doi:10.3390/vaccines12070758.

SEE ALSO

Gastroenteritis; Typhoid Fever

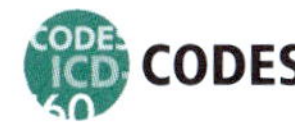

CODES

ICD10

- A02.25 Salmonella pyelonephritis
- A01.02 Typhoid fever with heart involvement
- A01.3 Paratyphoid fever C

CLINICAL PEARLS

- Nontyphoidal *Salmonella* infection is typically a foodborne infection associated with a self-limited gastroenteritis.
- Clinical syndromes include gastroenteritis, bacteremia, endovascular infection, localized infection outside the GI tract, and a chronic carrier state.
- Those at greatest risk of complications from *Salmonella* infection include the young, elderly, and the immunocompromised patients.
- Uncomplicated gastroenteritis in healthy patients can be treated with supportive care.
- Antibiotics should be used in infants, the elderly, immunocompromised patients, and for invasive infections such as bacteremia outside the GI tract.

SARCOIDOSIS

Donnah Mathews, MD, FACP

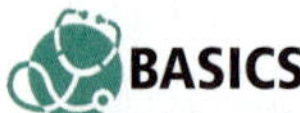

BASICS

Sarcoidosis is an inflammatory, multisystemic granulomatous disease of unknown cause

DESCRIPTION

- Sarcoidosis is characterized by noncaseating granulomas, affecting young and middle-aged adults.
  - Frequently presents with bilateral hilar adenopathy, pulmonary infiltrates, ocular or skin lesions
  - In ~50% of cases, it is diagnosed in asymptomatic patients with abnormal chest x-rays (CXRs).
  - Almost any organ may be involved.
- System(s) affected: primarily pulmonary but virtually any, including cardiovascular, gastrointestinal, hematologic, endocrine, renal, neurologic, dermatologic, ophthalmologic, musculoskeletal
- Synonym(s): Löfgren syndrome (erythema nodosum [EN], hilar adenopathy, fever, arthralgias); Heerfordt syndrome (uveitis, parotid enlargement, facial palsy, fever); lupus pernio; Besnier-Boeck-Schaumann disease; Boeck sarcoid; Scheuermann disease

EPIDEMIOLOGY

Incidence

Peaks at 30 to 50 years of age in men and 50 to 60 years in women. Rare in children

Prevalence

True prevalence unknown due to lack of diagnostic sensitivity and other factors.

ETIOLOGY AND PATHOPHYSIOLOGY

- Development requires both genetic predisposition and environmental exposure. Thought to be due to exaggerated cell-mediated immune response to unknown antigen(s)
- In the lungs, the initial lesion is CD4^{+} T-cell alveolitis, causing noncaseating granulomata, which may resolve or may undergo fibrosis. "Immune paradox" with affected organs showing an intense immune response and yet anergy exists elsewhere.

Genetics

- Although worldwide in distribution, increased prevalence in Scandinavians, Japanese, Black Americans, and women
- Link to the loci in the HLA Class II region and butyrophilin-like 2 genes (BTNL2)

RISK FACTORS

Multiple occupations and environmental exposures are associated with sarcoidosis including insecticides, agricultural employment, metal working, fire fighting exposure to inorganic dust, and the handling of building supplies (i.e., rescue workers in the World Trade Center)

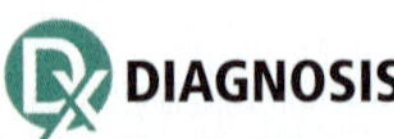

DIAGNOSIS

- Diagnosis is based on three criteria: clinical presentation, nonnecrotizing granulomatous inflammation in tissue samples (although not always required), and exclusion of other diagnoses.
- Löfgren syndrome: acute clinical presentation with erythema nodosum, bilateral hilar adenopathy, and polyarthralgia, often with a fever.

HISTORY

- Patients may be asymptomatic.
- Patients may have nonspecific complaints, such as the following:
  - Nonproductive cough or shortness of breath
  - Fever or night sweats
  - Weight loss
  - General fatigue
  - Eye pain
  - Chest pain/palpitations/arrhythmias
  - Skin lesions
  - Polyarthritis
  - Encephalopathy, seizures, hydrocephalus (rare)
  - Patients >70 years old more likely to have systemic symptoms

PHYSICAL EXAM

- Many patients have a normal physical exam.
- Lungs may reveal wheezing/fine interstitial crackles.
- ~30% of patients have extrapulmonary manifestations, including the following:
  - Uveitis, retinitis, or other eye findings: conjunctival nodules, lacrimal gland enlargement, cataracts, glaucoma, papilledema
  - Cranial nerve palsies, especially 7th nerve
  - Salivary gland swelling or lymphadenopathy
  - Arrhythmias
  - Hepatosplenomegaly
  - Polyarthritis
  - Rashes
    - Maculopapular of nares, eyelids, forehead, base of neck at hairline, and previous trauma sites
    - Waxy nodular of face, trunk, and extensor surfaces of extremities
    - Plaques (lupus pernio) of nose, cheeks, chin, and ears
    - EN (component of Löfgren syndrome)

DIFFERENTIAL DIAGNOSIS

- Infectious granulomatous disease, such as tuberculosis, nontuberculous mycobacteria, and fungal infections
  - Bacterial pneumonia, such as *Brucella*, *Tropheryma whipplei*, *Francisella tularensis*, *Bartonella henselae*, *Coxiella burnetii*
  - Viral, such as herpes zoster
  - Parasitic, such as *Toxoplasma gondii*, schistosomiasis, leishmaniasis
- Lymphoma
- Autoimmune such as vasculitides, Langerhans cell histiocytosis, inflammatory bowel disease
- Hypersensitivity pneumonitis

DIAGNOSTIC TESTS & INTERPRETATION

No definitive test for diagnosis, but diagnosis is suggested by the following:

- Clinical and radiographic manifestations
- Exclusion of other diagnoses
- Histopathologic detection of noncaseating granulomas (not always required)

Initial Tests (lab, imaging)

- Screening for extrapulmonary disease:
  - Complete blood cell count, HIV
  - Creatinine (renal sarcoidosis)
  - Alkaline phosphatase (hepatic sarcoidosis) +/− transaminase testing
  - Calcium
  - 25- and 1,25-OH vitamin D levels to determine if replacement needed
- Baseline eye exam
- Baseline ECG
  - If high risk symptoms or ECG changes (such as heart block) concerning for cardiac sarcoidosis, cardiac MRI or cardiac FDG PET-CT
- Biomarkers show evidence of inflammation and are not pathognomonic tests:
  - Serum ACE elevated in 50–60% of patients but lacks diagnostic specificity
  - CRP, serum amyloid A, chitotriosidase, interleukin-2 receptor also show inflammation and disease activity
- FDG PET-CT most effective for tissue-specific inflammatory activity if assessing for biopsy site
- CXR or CT scan may reveal granulomas/hilar adenopathy. CXRs are staged using Scadding classification.
  - Stage 0 = normal
  - Stage 1 = bilateral hilar adenopathy alone
  - Stage 2 = bilateral hilar adenopathy + parenchymal infiltrates (primarily upper lobes)
  - Stage 3 = parenchymal infiltrates with shrinking hilar adenopathy
  - Stage 4 = parenchymal infiltrates with volume loss, bronchiectasis, calcification, or cyst formation
- For patients with suspected pulmonary hypertension, transthoracic echocardiogram is suggested and may lead to right heart catheterization if indicated.

Follow-Up Tests & Special Considerations

Patients with asymptomatic bilateral hilar lymphadenopathy

- If high clinical suspicion for sarcoidosis (i.e., Löfgren syndrome, lupus pernio, Heerford syndrome), biopsy not needed
- If tissue sampling determined to be necessary, endobronchial ultrasound (EBUS)-guided lymph node sampling preferred over mediastinoscopy

Diagnostic Procedures/Other

- Pulmonary function tests (PFTs) may reveal restrictive pattern with decreased carbon monoxide diffusing capacity (DLCO).
- Ophthalmologic examination may reveal uveitis, retinal vasculitis, or conjunctivitis.
- ECG
- Tuberculin skin test
- Biopsy of lesions should reveal noncaseating granulomas.
- If lungs are affected, bronchoscopy with biopsy of central and peripheral airways is helpful. EBUS-guided transbronchial needle aspiration may have a better diagnostic yield.

ALERT
If signs indicate Löfgren syndrome (acute sarcoid with bilateral hilar lymphadenopathy, EN, and diffuse arthritis/arthralgias), it is not necessary to perform a biopsy as prognosis is good with observation alone, and biopsy would not change management.

Test Interpretation

Noncaseating epithelioid granulomas without evidence of fungal/mycobacterial infection

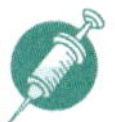

TREATMENT

- Many patients undergo spontaneous remission.
- Treatment depends on risk of organ failure and morbidity and the extent to which the patient's quality of life is impacted with symptoms.
- No treatment may be necessary in asymptomatic individuals, but treatment may be required for cardiac, CNS, renal, or ocular involvement.
- No treatment is indicated for asymptomatic patients with stage I to III radiographic changes with normal/mildly abnormal lung function, although close follow-up is recommended.
- Treatment of pulmonary manifestations is done on the basis of impairment.
  - Worsening pulmonary symptoms and deteriorating lung function and/or worsening radiographic findings

MEDICATION

Systemic therapy is indicated for hypercalcemia or cardiac, neurologic, or eye disease.

First Line

- No FDA-approved treatment for sarcoidosis
- Systemic corticosteroids in the symptomatic individual or with worsening lung function or radiographic findings
  - Optimal dose of glucocorticoids is not known. Prior to initiating glucocorticoids, must exclude tuberculosis
  - 0.3 to 0.6 mg/kg ideal body weight (20 to 40 mg/day) for 4 to 6 weeks
  - If stable, taper by 5 mg/week to 10 to 20 mg/day over the next 6 weeks.
  - If no relapse, 10 to 20 mg/day for 8 to 12 months; relapse is common.
  - Higher doses (80 to 100 mg/day) may be warranted in patients with acute respiratory failure and cardiac, neurologic, or ocular disease.
- In patients with skin disease, topical steroids may be effective.
- Inhaled steroids (800 to 1,600 μg BID) may be of some clinical benefit in early disease with mild pulmonary symptoms.
  - Contraindications and significant possible interactions: Refer to the manufacturer's profile of each drug.

Second Line

- All alternative agents to glucocorticoids carry substantial risk for toxicity, including myelosuppression, hepatotoxicity, and opportunistic infection. Prior to utilizing these medications, assess for adherence to steroid therapy, comorbid disease, or other complicating factors contributing to steroid failure. Referral to specialist is recommended.
- Glucocorticoid-sparing agents should be initiated early if patients require long-term suppression of inflammation. Could also be used as first line
  - Methotrexate
  - Other immunosuppressants include azathioprine, leflunomide, or mycophenolate.
  - Antimalarial agent hydroxychloroquine is particularly useful with cutaneous disease, hypercalcemia, and some cases of neurosarcoidosis
  - Use of immunosuppressants require regular monitoring of CBC and LFTs. Vaccinations should be up to date.
- Tumor necrosis factor antagonists, such as infliximab and adalimumab, have been useful in refractory cases.

ISSUES FOR REFERRAL

May be followed by a pulmonologist, with referrals to other specialists as dictated by involvement of other organ systems; if requiring a second-line therapy

SURGERY/OTHER PROCEDURES

Rarely, lung transplantation in severe, refractory cases with a 70% post-transplant survival rate at 5 years.

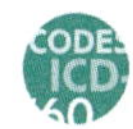

ONGOING CARE

FOLLOW-UP RECOMMENDATIONS

Patient Monitoring

- Approximately 30% of patients with sarcoidosis will develop a new disease manifestation within 3 years of baseline evaluation.
- Monitor serum calcium, creatinine, alkaline phosphatase annually
- Patients on prednisone for symptoms should be seen every 1 to 2 months while on therapy.
- Patients not requiring therapy should be seen every 3 months for at least the first 2 years after diagnosis, obtaining a history and physical exam, laboratory testing tailored to sites of disease activity, PFTs, and ambulatory pulse oximetry.
- If on hydroxychloroquine, obtain ophthalmologic exam every 6 to 12 months.
- Other testing per individual patient's symptoms, including HRCT, echocardiogram, Holter monitoring, urinalysis (UA), thyroid-stimulating hormone (TSH), bone density, MRI of brain, ophthalmologic exam

PATIENT EDUCATION

- The American Lung Association
- Sarcoidosis by MedlinePlus

PROGNOSIS

- 50% of patients will have spontaneous resolution within 2 years.
- 25% of patients will have significant fibrosis, but no further worsening of the disease after 2 years.
- 25% of patients (higher in some populations, including Black Americans) will have chronic disease.
- Patients on corticosteroids for >6 months have a greater chance of having chronic disease.
- Overall death rate: <10%; most fatal cases due to lung disease, followed by cardiac sarcoidosis.
- Poor prognostic factors include age of onset >40 years, black race, lower income (1), scadding sage III or IV, severe dyspnea or hypoxemia with minimal exertion on presentation; pulmonary hypertension, extrapulmonary involvement of lupus pernio; vitiligo, uveitis, hepatomegaly, splenomegaly, neurologic involvement, osseous involvement, hypercalcemia, nephrolithiasis, small fiver neuropathy

COMPLICATIONS

- Patients may develop significant respiratory involvement, including cor pulmonale. Pulmonary hemorrhage from infection with aspergillosis in the damaged lung is possible.
- Other organs, especially the heart (congestive heart failure, arrhythmias), eyes (rarely blindness), and CNS, can be involved with serious consequences.

REFERENCES

1. Belperio JA, Shaikh F, Abtin FG, et al. Diagnosis and treatment of pulmonary sarcoidosis: a review. *JAMA*. 2022;327(9):856–867. doi:10.1001/jama.2022.1570.

CODES

ICD10

- D86.89 Sarcoidosis of other sites
- D86.81 Sarcoid meningitis
- D86.2 Sarcoidosis of lung with sarcoidosis of lymph nodes

CLINICAL PEARLS

- Sarcoidosis is a noninfectious, multisystem, granulomatous disease of unknown cause, typically affecting young and middle-aged adults.
- Diagnosis is based on clinical findings, exclusion of other disorders, and pathologic detection of noncaseating granulomas.

SCABIES

Roland W. Newman II, DO

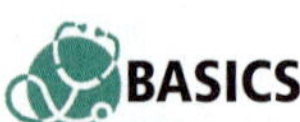

BASICS

DESCRIPTION

- A contagious parasitic infection of the skin caused by the mite *Sarcoptes scabiei*, var. *hominis*
- Typically, a clinical diagnosis based on history and physical exam
- System(s) affected: skin/exocrine

EPIDEMIOLOGY

- Global disease whose burden is highest in tropical areas, overcrowded regions, and in economically disadvantaged populations (1)
- Most commonly affected: children, adolescents, and elderly.
- In North America, case occurrence is more evenly distributed among all age groups.

Incidence

- Predominant age: children, sexually active young adults, and the elderly
- Male children from lower income quartiles were more likely to visit the ED in a retrospective analysis of nationally representative National Emergency Department Sample for 2013 to 2015, whereas older male patients, insured by Medicare, from the highest income quartile in the Midwest/West were most likely to be admitted to the hospital.

Prevalence

Prevalence varies substantially worldwide but is more common in resource-poor settings.

- More prevalent in areas of overcrowding and in developing countries, particularly tropical climates
- Added to World Health Organization list of neglected tropical diseases in 2017

ETIOLOGY AND PATHOPHYSIOLOGY

- *S. scabiei*, var. *hominis*
  - An obligate human parasite
  - Primarily transmitted by prolonged human-to-human direct skin contact
  - Infrequently transmitted via fomites (e.g., bedding, clothing, or furnishings)
- Female mite lays eggs in burrows in the stratum corneum and epidermis.
- Itching is caused by a delayed type IV hypersensitivity reaction to the mite saliva, eggs, or excrement.

RISK FACTORS

- Prolonged skin-to-skin contact (e.g., sexual, overcrowding, nosocomial infection)
- Poor nutritional status, poverty, and homelessness
- Hot, tropical climates
- Seasonal variation: Incidence may be higher in the winter than in the summer (due to overcrowding).
- Immunocompromised patients (drug-induced), those with leukemia, lymphoma, or those with congenital immune deficiencies, including those with HIV/AIDS, are at increased risk of developing severe (crusted/Norwegian) scabies.

GENERAL PREVENTION

Prevent outbreaks by prompt treatment and cleansing of fomites (see "General Measures").

DIAGNOSIS

HISTORY

- Generalized itching is often severe and worse at night.
- Identify potential contact with infected individuals.
- Initial/primary infection usually asymptomatic for the first 3 to 4 weeks (until sensitivity occurs)
- Subsequent reinfection typically develops symptoms after only 1 to 3 days.

PHYSICAL EXAM

- Lesions (inflammatory, erythematous, pruritic papules) most commonly located in the finger webs, flexor surfaces of the wrists, elbows, axillae, buttocks, genitalia, feet, and ankles; often spares the head/neck in adults
- Burrows (thin, curvy lines in the upper epidermis that measure 1 to 10 mm in length)—a pathognomonic sign of scabies most common in hands and wrists
- Secondary erosions and excoriations from scratching
- Pustules (if secondarily infected)
- Pruritic papular or nodular lesions in covered areas (buttocks, groin, axillae) resulting from an exaggerated scratching due to hypersensitivity reaction
- Crusted scabies (or Norwegian scabies) is a psoriasiform dermatosis occurring with hyperinfestation with thousands/millions of mites (more common in immunosuppressed patients).

Geriatric Considerations

The elderly often itch more severely despite fewer cutaneous lesions and are at risk for extensive infestations, perhaps related to a decline in cell-mediated immunity. There may be back involvement in those who are bedridden.

Pediatric Considerations

Infants and very young children often present with vesicles, papules, and pustules and have more widespread involvement, including the hands, palms, feet, soles, body folds, and head (rare for adults).

DIFFERENTIAL DIAGNOSIS

- Atopic dermatitis
- Contact dermatitis
- Dermatitis herpetiformis
- Eczema
- Folliculitis/impetigo
- Insect bites
- Papular urticaria
- Pediculosis corporis
- Psoriasis (crusted scabies)
- Pyoderma
- Seborrheic dermatitis
- Syphilis
- Tinea corporis

DIAGNOSTIC TESTS & INTERPRETATION

- Based on 2018 International Alliance Control for Scabies (IACS) criteria for the diagnosis of scabies:
  - Confirmed scabies diagnosis: based on microscopic identification of mites, eggs, or fecal pellets (scybala) *or* visualization of mite with dermoscopy
  - Clinical scabies diagnosis: detection of burrows, *or* typical lesions on male genitalia, *or* typical lesions in a typical distribution with two history features of itch and known infectious contact
  - Suspected scabies diagnosis: typical lesions in a typical distribution with one history feature of itch or known infectious contact, *or* atypical lesions or atypical distribution with two history features of itch and known infectious contact
- A failure to find mites does not rule out scabies.

Initial Tests (lab, imaging)

CBC is rarely needed but may show eosinophilia.

Diagnostic Procedures/Other

- Examination of skin with dermoscopy
  - Simplest and fastest method to identify the pathogen
  - Look for typical burrows in finger webs, on flexor aspect of the wrists, and on the penis.
  - Look for a dark point at the end of the burrow (the mite, also known as "delta wing sign").
- Skin scraping
  - Place a drop of mineral oil over a non-excoriated lesion or burrow.
  - Scrape the lesion with a surgical blade (no. 15).
  - Scraping under fingernails may be positive.
  - When mite is not found with scraping, biopsy may reveal mite, eggs, or feces.
- Potassium hydroxide (KOH) wet mount is *not* recommended because it can dissolve mite pellets.
- Burrow ink test
  - If burrows are not obvious, apply gentian violet or India ink to an area of rash. Wash off the ink with alcohol. A burrow should remain stained and become more evident. Then apply mineral oil, scrape, and observe microscopically, as noted previously.

Test Interpretation

Skin biopsy of a nodule (although rarely performed) will reveal portions of the mite in the corneal layer.

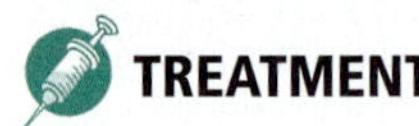

TREATMENT

GENERAL MEASURES

- Treat all intimate contacts (including close household and family members).
- Treat items in contact with skin. Wash all clothing, bed linens, and towels in hot (60°C) water and dry in hot dryer. Personal items that cannot be washed should be sealed in a plastic bag for at least 7 days.
- Itching and dermatitis can persist for up to 4 weeks despite appropriate treatment and can be treated with oral antihistamines and/or topical/oral corticosteroids. It is important to educate patients this is likely not a sign of treatment failure. However, persistent symptoms greater than 4 weeks posttreatment may need further workup for an alternative diagnosis, failure of initial treatment, or irritation secondary to treatment.

MEDICATION

First Line

- Permethrin 5% cream (Elimite) is generally accepted as first-line therapy.
  - After bathing or showering, apply cream from the neck to the soles of the feet, paying particular attention to areas that are most involved and then wash off after 8 to 14 hours.
  - It is recommended to repeat treatment 1 to 2 weeks later.
  - The adult dose is usually 30 g per treatment.
  - Side effects include itching, stinging, erythema, and burning. (minimal absorption).
- Ivermectin (Stromectol)
  - Not FDA approved for scabies; (i.e., off-label use)
  - 200 μg/kg PO as a single dose; repeated in 2 weeks due to limited ovicidal activity. Failure of a second dose of ivermectin has been shown to be a predictor of unsuccessful treatment.
  - Take with food to improve bioavailability and enhance penetration into the epidermis.
  - May need higher doses or may need to use in combination with topical scabicide for HIV-positive patients
  - Side effects may include headache and nausea.
- Both permethrin and ivermectin are associated with high clearance rates in the treatment of scabies without highly significant differences between the two.
- Choice between either permethrin or ivermectin can be based on availability, practicality, and associated cost depending on the individual situation.
- Crusted scabies often require more frequent applications of permethrin (q2–3d for 1 to 2 weeks) in combination with repeated doses of oral ivermectin on days 1, 2, 8, 9, and 15. Severe cases may need further dosing of on days 22 and 29.

Pediatric Considerations

- Permethrin may be used on infants >2 months of age. In children <5 years of age, the cream should be applied to the head and neck as well as to the entire body.
- PO ivermectin should be avoided in children aged <5 years and in those weighing <15 kg.

Second Line

- Crotamiton (Eurax) 10% cream may be used on infants >2 months of age.
  - Apply from the neck down for 24 hours, rinse off, reapply for an additional 24 to 48 hours, and then thoroughly wash off.
  - Nodular scabies: Apply to nodules for 24 hours, rinse off, reapply for an additional 24 hours, and then thoroughly wash off.
- Precipitated sulfur 2–10% in petrolatum
  - Not FDA-approved for scabies and must be compounded in the United States.
  - Apply to the entire body from the neck down for 24 hours, rinse by bathing and then repeat for 2 more days (3 days total).
  - It is malodorous and messy.
- Lindane (Kwell) 1% lotion
  - Lindane use is no longer recommended due to high potential for systemic absorption and subsequent CNS neurologic toxicity (2).
- Spinosad (Natroba) topical 0.9% suspension
  - Ovicidal
  - Previously used to treat head lice, spinosad was approved in 2021 by the U.S. FDA as a topical treatment for scabies (3).
  - Low risk of toxicity, highly effective, and requiring only single treatment.
  - Limitations of treatment include high-cost and need for a prescription (4).

Pediatric Considerations

Infants aged <2 months can be treated with sulfur ointment preparation.

Pregnancy Considerations

- Permethrin is pregnancy Category B, and ivermectin and crotamiton are pregnancy Category C.
- Permethrin is considered compatible with lactation (5).

ISSUES FOR REFERRAL

Consider referral to dermatology if unable to confirm diagnosis and/or resistant to repeated treatments.

ADDITIONAL THERAPIES

- Crusted scabies may require use of keratolytics to improve penetration of permethrin.
- Nodular scabies may require intralesional steroids for complete resolution, if they persist for several weeks after treatment.
- Benzyl benzoate lotion (not available in the United States but used widely in developing countries)
  - Not FDA-approved for scabies
  - Dose for adults is 25%; dilute to 12.5% for children.
  - After bathing, apply lotion from the neck to soles of feet for 24 hours.

COMPLEMENTARY & ALTERNATIVE MEDICINE

Tea tree oil (TTO) derived from the plant *Melaleuca alternifolia* is a safe, effective, and generally well tolerated alternative option as a treatment for scabies. 5% TTO has proven efficacy as a scabicidal agent in vitro. Topical application of TTO is generally associated with a low incidence of adverse effects (irritant or localized reactions to the oil). Most irritant skin reactions can be avoided by use of TTO concentrations of less than 20%.

ONGOING CARE

FOLLOW-UP RECOMMENDATIONS

Patient Monitoring

Recheck patient at weekly intervals only if rash or itching persists. Scrape new lesions and retreat if mites or products are found.

PATIENT EDUCATION

Patients should be instructed on proper application and cautioned not to overuse the medication when applying it to the skin. A patient fact sheet is available from the CDC.

PROGNOSIS

Lesions begin to regress in 1 to 2 days, but eczema and itching may persist for up to 4 weeks after treatment.

COMPLICATIONS

- Nodules (nodular scabies) may persist for weeks to months after treatment.
- Postscabetic pruritus; poor sleep due to pruritus
- Pyoderma; secondary bacterial infection (more common in developing countries); impetigo due to group A streptococci and *Staphylococcus aureus* may lead to sepsis, poststreptococcal glomerulonephritis, and rheumatic heart disease.
- Social stigma

REFERENCES

1. Richards RN. Scabies: diagnostic and therapeutic update. *J Cutan Med Surg*. 2021;25(1):95–101. doi:10.1177/1203475420960446.
2. Al-Dabbagh J, Younis R, Ismail N. The current available diagnostic tools and treatments of scabies and scabies variants: an updated narrative review. *Medicine (Baltimore)*. 2023;102(21):e33805. doi:10.1097/MD.0000000000033805.
3. Fernando DD, Fischer K. Spinosad topical suspension (0.9%): a new topical treatment for scabies. *Expert Rev Anti Infect Ther*. 2022;20(9):1149–1154. doi:10.1080/14787210.2022.2099376.
4. Wright TA. Spinosad: a low-risk, effective treatment for lice. *Am Fam Physician*. 2019;100(10):601.
5. Workowski KA, Bachmann LH, Chan PA, et al. Sexually transmitted infections treatment guidelines, 2021. *MMWR Recomm Rep*. 2021;70(4):1–187. doi:10.15585/mmwr.rr7004a1.

SEE ALSO

Arthropod Bites and Stings; Pediculosis (Lice)

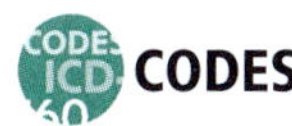

CODES

ICD10

B86 Scabies

CLINICAL PEARLS

- Prior to diagnosis, use of a topical steroid to treat pruritic symptoms may mask symptoms and is termed *scabies incognito*.
- Eczema and itching may persist for up to 4 weeks after treatment, causing many patients to falsely believe that they have failed treatment or are being reinfected.
- In patients with actual reinfection, it is possible the patient has not applied the medication properly or, more likely, the index patient has not been identified and treated.

SCARLET FEVER

Alicia Leandra Olowu, DO • Tyler Gopee, DO

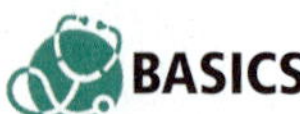

BASICS

DESCRIPTION

- A disease (typically in childhood) characterized by fever, pharyngitis, and rash caused by group A β-hemolytic *Streptococcus pyogenes* (GAS) that produces erythrogenic toxin
- Incubation period: 1 to 7 days; duration of illness: 4 to 10 days
- Rash (erythematous, blanchable 1 to 2 mm papules; "sand paper") usually appears within 24 to 48 hours after symptom onset
- Rash first appears in the groin, trunk, and axillae accompanied by strawberry tongue and circumoral pallor and then rapidly spreads outward all over the body, sparing palms and soles.
- Rash clears at the end of the 1st week and is followed by several weeks of desquamation.
- Rash is not dangerous but is a marker for GAS infection with suppurative and nonsuppurative complications.
- System(s) affected: head, eyes, ears, nose, throat, skin/exocrine
- Synonym(s): scarlatina

EPIDEMIOLOGY

Incidence

- In high-income countries, 15% of school age children and 4–10% of adults have an episode of GAS pharyngitis each year.
- Scarlet fever is rare in infancy because of maternal antitoxin antibodies.
- Predominant age: 4 to 15 years; peak age: 4 to 8 years
- Recent shift to older school-aged children; thought to reflect reduced early-life GAS exposure during COVID-19, changes in strain antigenicity, and enhanced detection of atypical cases
- Predominant sex: male = female
- Rare in the United States in persons aged >12 years because of high rates (>80%) of lifelong protective antibodies to erythrogenic toxins

Prevalence

- 15–30% of cases of pharyngitis in children are due to GAS; 5–15% in adults
- <10% of children with streptococcal pharyngitis develop scarlet fever.

ETIOLOGY AND PATHOPHYSIOLOGY

- Erythrogenic toxin (streptococcal pyrogenic exotoxin) production is necessary for scarlet fever to develop clinically.
- Multiple streptococcal superantigens (SpeA, SpeC, and SSA) are implicated, with GAS strains often carrying a repertoire of >10 superantigens encoded on prophages that can transfer between strains.
- The characteristic rash reflects a delayed, host-acquired hypersensitivity that occurs primarily in individuals with prior exposure to *Streptococcus pyogenes*.
- Antitoxin antibodies can reduce susceptibility to the rash (historically the basis of the Dick test) but do not protect against underlying GAS infection.
- The primary site of streptococcal infection is usually within the tonsils, but scarlet fever may also occur with infection of the skin, surgical wounds, or uterus (puerperal scarlet fever).

RISK FACTORS

- Winter/early spring seasonal increase; more common in school-aged children
- Contact with infected individual(s); crowded living conditions (e.g., barracks, child care, schools)
- Skin lesions due to trauma, surgery, or skin disorders, heart ailments, diabetes, and cancer are other risk factors. Injection drug users have shown a higher risk of invasive GAS infection owing to their immunocompromised status

GENERAL PREVENTION

- Spread by contact with airborne respiratory droplets, saliva, and nasal secretions
- Foodborne outbreaks have been reported, but are rare.
- Asymptomatic contacts do not require cultures/prophylaxis.
- Symptomatic contacts of a child with documented GAS infection who have recent or current clinical evidence of a GAS infection should undergo appropriate laboratory tests and should be treated if test results are positive.
- Children should not return to school/daycare until they are afebrile and have received 12 to 24 hours of antibiotic therapy.

COMMONLY ASSOCIATED CONDITIONS

Pharyngitis, impetigo, rheumatic fever, glomerulonephritis

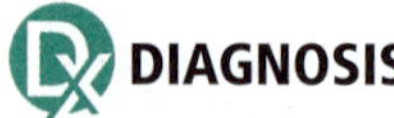

DIAGNOSIS

HISTORY

Prodrome 1 to 2 days

- Sore throat, headache, myalgias, malaise
- Fever (>38°C [100.4°F]), vomiting
- Abdominal pain (may mimic acute abdomen)
- Rash—scarlatiniform erythematous punctate eruption
- Cough, conjunctivitis, hoarseness, diarrhea, coryza, oral ulceration and rhinorrhea are more commonly associated with viral infections.

PHYSICAL EXAM

- Oral exam
  - Beefy red tonsils and pharynx with/without exudate
  - Petechiae on palate
  - Circumoral pallor
  - White coating on tongue: White strawberry tongue appears on days 1 to 2. This sheds by days 4 to 5, leaving a red strawberry tongue, which is shiny and erythematous with prominent papillae.
- Exanthem (appears within 1 to 5 days)
  - Scarlet, nonconfluent, 1 to 2 mm papules with generalized erythema; blanches when pressed
  - Orange-red punctate skin eruption with sandpaper-like texture, "sunburn with goose pimples"
  - Coarse "sandpaper" rash, initially appearing in groin, upper trunk, and axillae, and then spreading outward to extremities; prominent in skin folds, flexural surfaces (e.g., axillae, groin, buttocks), with sparing of palms and soles
  - Flushed face with circumoral pallor, red lips
  - Pastia lines: transverse red streaks in skin folds of abdomen, antecubital space, and axillae
  - Desquamation begins on face after 7 to 10 days and proceeds over trunk to hands and feet; may persist for 6 weeks
  - In severe cases, small vesicular lesions (miliary sudamina) may appear on abdomen, hands, and feet.

DIFFERENTIAL DIAGNOSIS

- Viral exanthem: measles; rubella; roseola; erythema infectiosum (Fifth disease)
- Infectious mononucleosis, mycoplasma pneumonia
- Secondary syphilis, toxic shock syndrome, staphylococcal scalded-skin syndrome
- Kawasaki disease
- Acute systemic lupus erythematosus

DIAGNOSTIC TESTS & INTERPRETATION

- The signs and symptoms of streptococcal and nonstreptococcal pharyngitis overlap too broadly for diagnosis to be made with precision on clinical grounds alone. Even patients with all clinical features are confirmed to have streptococcal pharyngitis only about 35–50% of the time, particularly in children.
- Use results from rapid antigen detection testing (RADT) or polymerase chain reaction (PCR) based rapid testing.
- Modified Centor clinical decision rule
  - Absence of cough 1 point
  - Swollen, tender anterior cervical nodes 1 point
  - Temperature 38°C (100.4°F) 1 point
  - Tonsillar exudate or swelling 1 point
  - Age:
    - 3 to 14 years: 1 point
    - 15 to 44 years: 0 point
    - ≥45 years: −1 point
- Cumulative score:
  - 0: risk of GAS pharyngitis 1–2.5%—no further testing or antibiotics indicated
  - 1: risk of GAS pharyngitis 5–10%—no further testing or antibiotics indicated—option to perform throat culture or RADT—treat if positive.
  - 2: risk of GAS pharyngitis 11–17%—perform throat culture or RADT—treat if positive.
  - 3: risk of GAS pharyngitis 28–35%—perform throat culture or RADT—treat if positive.
  - 4+: risk of GAS pharyngitis 51–53%—consider empiric treatment with antibiotics.
- Testing for GAS pharyngitis is *not recommended* for patients with symptoms suggesting a viral etiology (e.g., cough, coryza, diarrhea, conjunctivitis, rhinorrhea, hoarseness, oral ulcers).

Initial Tests (lab, imaging)

- RADT: diagnostic if positive, sensitivity approaches that of culture, 95% specific; in children, negative RADT should be confirmed by throat culture (not necessary in adults). Positive RADT does not require confirmatory culture.
- PCR: diagnostic if positive, 100% sensitive, 94.1% specific, 84.1% positive predictive value, 100% negative predictive value; positive PCR does not require confirmatory culture.
- Throat culture is the gold standard to confirm streptococcal infection (99% specific; 90–97% sensitive; 5–10% of healthy individuals are carriers).
- Serologic tests (antistreptolysin O titer and streptozyme tests, antihyaluronidase): Confirm recent GAS infection; not helpful or recommended for diagnosis of acute disease
- Gram stain: gram-positive cocci in chains
- CBC may show elevated WBC count (12,000 to 16,000/mm^3); eosinophilia later (second week)
- Follow-up (posttreatment) throat cultures or RADT/PCR not routinely recommended
- Diagnostic testing and empiric treatment of asymptomatic household contacts of patients with acute streptococcal pharyngitis is not routinely recommended (1)[B].

Follow-Up Tests & Special Considerations

- Recent antibiotic therapy may impact culture results.
- Within 5 days of symptoms, antibiotics can delay/abolish antistreptolysin O response.

Test Interpretation

Skin lesions reveal characteristic inflammatory reaction, specifically hyperemia, edema, and polymorphonuclear cell infiltration.

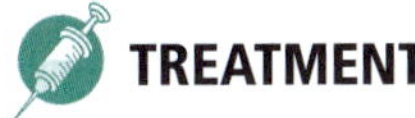

TREATMENT

GENERAL MEASURES

Supportive care; analgesic/antipyretic such as acetaminophen or NSAIDs, for moderate to severe symptoms or to control fever; symptomatic treatment can include medicated throat lozenges (2) and topical anesthetics.

MEDICATION

First Line

The primary reason for treating GAS is to decrease the risk of acute rheumatic fever. Early treatment decreases duration of symptoms by 1 to 2 days and decreases the period of contagiousness. Penicillin is the drug of choice for GAS pharyngitis given its proven efficacy, safety, narrow spectrum, and low cost.

- Penicillin (PO; penicillin V and others) for 10 days
  - 250 mg PO BID or TID for <27 kg (60 lb); 250 mg QID or 500 mg BID for >27 kg (60 lb) adolescents and adults (3)
  - If compliance is questionable, use penicillin G benzathine: single IM dose 600,000 U for <27 kg (60 lb); 1.2 mU for those >27 kg (60 lb)
- Amoxicillin (PO) 50 mg/kg (max dose 1,000 mg) once daily or 25 mg/kg (max dose 500 mg) twice daily for 10 days (use only for definitive GAS because it can induce rash with some viral infections)
  - Contraindications: penicillin allergy
  - Amoxicillin has similar efficacy to penicillin and is more palatable for children.
- Precautions: Avoid in patients with penicillin allergy (anaphylaxis).

Second Line

For patients allergic to penicillin

- Type IV hypersensitivity to penicillin:
  - Oral cephalosporins: Many are effective, but 1st-generation cephalosporins are less expensive:
    - Cephalexin 20 mg/kg dose twice daily for 10 days; max 500 mg every 12 hours
    - Cefadroxil 30 mg/kg once daily; max 1,000 mg for 10 days
- Type I hypersensitivity to penicillin:
  - Azithromycin: 12 mg/kg/day (max 500 mg) for 5 days
  - Clarithromycin: children >6 months: 7.5 mg/kg BID for 10 days; adults: 250 mg BID for 10 days
  - Clindamycin 7 mg/kg (max 300 mg/dose) TID for 10 days
- Antimicrobial resistance considerations:
  - Increasing macrolide (erythromycin, azithromycin), clindamycin, and tetracycline resistance
  - Tetracyclines and sulfonamides should not be used.

ALERT
Avoid aspirin in children due to risk of Reye syndrome.

ISSUES FOR REFERRAL

Peritonsillar abscess/retropharyngeal abscess; shock symptoms: hypotension, disseminated intravascular coagulation (DIC), cardiac, liver, renal dysfunction

SURGERY/OTHER PROCEDURES

- Tonsillectomy is recommended with recurrent bouts of pharyngitis (≥6 positive strep cultures in 1 year).
- Although children still may get streptococcal pharyngitis ("strep throat") after a tonsillectomy, the procedure reduces the frequency and severity of infections.

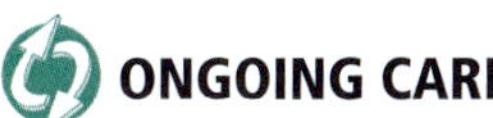

ONGOING CARE

FOLLOW-UP RECOMMENDATIONS

Follow-up throat culture not needed unless symptomatic

Patient Monitoring

GAS is uniformly susceptible to penicillin, treatment failures are typically due to poor adherence to recommended antibiotic therapy

PATIENT EDUCATION

- Delay in treatment awaiting culture results does not increase the risk of rheumatic fever.
- Complete the entire course of antibiotics.
- Children should not return to school/daycare until they have received >24 hours of antibiotic therapy.
- Can spread person to person. Personal hygiene is important (wash hands, do not share utensils).
- "Recurring strep throat: When is tonsillectomy useful?" (http://www.mayoclinic.org/diseasesconditions/strep-throat/expert-answers/recurringstrep-throat/faq-20058360)

PROGNOSIS

- Treatment shortens symptoms by 12 to 24 hours.
- Recurrent attacks are possible (different erythrogenic toxins).

COMPLICATIONS

- Suppurative
  - Sinusitis
  - Otitis media/mastoiditis
  - Cervical lymphadenitis
- Nonsuppurative
  - Rheumatic fever; glomerulonephritis; streptococcal toxic shock syndrome
  - Pediatric autoimmune neuropsychiatric disorder associated with GAS (PANDAS)

S

REFERENCES

1. Shulman ST, Bisno AL, Clegg HW, et al. Clinical practice guideline for the diagnosis and management of group A streptococcal pharyngitis: 2012 update by the Infectious Diseases Society of America. *Clin Infect Dis*. 2012;55(10):1279–1282.
2. Mohapatra RK, Kutikuppala LVS, Mishra S, et al. Rising global incidence of invasive group A streptococcus infection and scarlet fever in the COVID-19 era—our knowledge thus far. *Int J Surg*. 2023;109(3):639–640.
3. van Driel ML, De Sutter AI, Thorning S, et al. Different antibiotic treatments for group A streptococcal pharyngitis. *Cochrane Database of Syst Rev*. 2021;(3):CD004406.

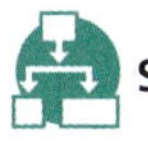

SEE ALSO

- Pharyngitis
- Algorithm: Pharyngitis

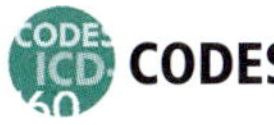

CODES

ICD10

- A38.9 Scarlet fever, uncomplicated
- J02.0 Streptococcal pharyngitis
- A38.0 Scarlet fever with otitis media

CLINICAL PEARLS

- Consider scarlet fever in the differential diagnosis of children with fever and an exanthematous rash.
- Key clinical findings include strawberry tongue, circumoral pallor, and a coarse sandpaper rash.
- Desquamation (7 to 10 days after symptom onset) may last for several weeks following scarlet fever.
- Diagnose GAS pharyngitis using a validated clinical decision rule (modified Centor score) and selective use of RADT.
- Penicillin remains the drug of choice; amoxicillin is as effective and is more palatable for children.
- Consider scarlet fever in older school-aged children, even if previously considered low-risk. Age-based clinical suspicion thresholds should be broadened in post-pandemic settings.

SCHIZOPHRENIA

Darnel Viray Dabu, MD, MPH, FAAFP, DipABLM • Michael F. Cascio, MD, MHA

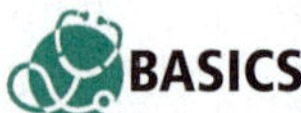

BASICS

A severe and persistent mental illness characterized by delusions, hallucinations, disorganization of thought and behavior, and cognitive dysfunction

DESCRIPTION

Major psychiatric disorder with a variable course, typically involving prodromal, active, and residual psychotic symptoms with disturbances in thought, speech, affect, behavior, and perception

EPIDEMIOLOGY

Prevalence

- Worldwide prevalence 7.2 per 1,000 people
- Age of onset: typically <30 years, earlier in males (late teens to mid-20s) than females (early 20s to early 30s)

ETIOLOGY AND PATHOPHYSIOLOGY

- Overstimulation of mesolimbic dopamine D_2 receptors, deficient prefrontal dopamine, and aberrant prefrontal glutamate (NMDA) activity results in perceptual disturbances, disordered thought process, and cognitive impairments
- Two genes, SRRM2 and AKAP11, associated with increased risk of schizophrenia; gene PLCO demonstrates a shared increased risk of both schizophrenia and autism.

Genetics

If first-degree relative has schizophrenia, risk is 8–10%.

RISK FACTORS

- Antenatal risk factors include prenatal infection or malnutrition, obstetric complications leading to hypoxia, winter births, postnatal infections requiring hospitalization, urban birth, and advanced paternal age.
- Additional risk factors: adolescent cannabis use, childhood trauma, urban residence, autoimmune disorders, severe and repeated stress, lower socioeconomic status, minority status, being an immigrant, inadequate social support

GENERAL PREVENTION

Educate all patients on the risks of marijuana use.

COMMONLY ASSOCIATED CONDITIONS

- Nicotine dependence (>50%) and substance use disorders
- Metabolic syndrome, diabetes mellitus

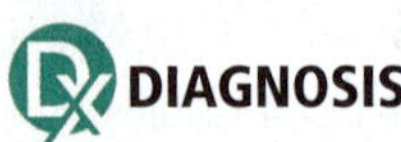

DIAGNOSIS

Focus on identifying an insidious social and functional decline over a ≥6-month period (differentiates schizophrenia from brief psychotic and schizophreniform disorders).

HISTORY

At least two of the following symptoms must be present for ≥1 month and at least one of these symptoms must be delusions, hallucinations, or disorganized speech (positive symptoms) (1)

- Delusions (fixed, false beliefs)
- Hallucinations (auditory is more common than visual disturbances.)
- Disorganized speech (derailed or incoherent speech)
- Grossly disorganized/catatonic behavior (hyperactive or hypoactive movements that are often repetitive)
- Negative symptoms (diminished emotional expression, poverty of speech and thought, amotivation, lack of social interest)

PHYSICAL EXAM

No physical findings; however, chronic treatment with neuroleptics may result in extrapyramidal symptoms, including dystonia (sustained muscle contractions), akathisia (restlessness), parkinsonism (tremor, shuffling gait), or tardive dyskinesia (repetitive, involuntary movements, especially of the face and mouth).

DIFFERENTIAL DIAGNOSIS

- Substance-induced psychosis, although 25% of patients with substance-induced psychosis will transition to schizophrenia, with highest in cannabis (2)[A].
- Personality disorders: paranoid, schizotypal, schizoid, borderline personality disorders
- Mood disorders: bipolar disorder, major depressive disorders with psychotic features or catatonia
- Autism spectrum disorder or neurodevelopmental disorders

DIAGNOSTIC TESTS & INTERPRETATION

Imaging (MRI), EEG, LP, and laboratory tests may be indicated to rule out other causes.

Initial Tests (lab, imaging)

- The following labs are often used to rule out a medical etiology of psychotic symptoms (3):
  - Thyroid-stimulating hormone (TSH), complete blood count (CBC), blood chemistries
  - Vitamin levels (thiamine/vitamin B_1, vitamin D, methylmalonic acid/vitamin B_{12}, folate/vitamin B_9)
  - Drug/alcohol screen of blood and urine, urinalysis
  - Syphilis, HIV, hepatitis B, hepatitis C
  - Heavy-metal blood test: lead, mercury
  - Ceruloplasmin, urine porphobilinogen
  - Erythrocyte sedimentation rate (ESR), antinuclear antibody (ANA)
- The following labs are used to assess for comorbidities and baseline values prior to antipsychotic initiation:
  - Electrocardiogram (ECG) for baseline QTc
  - CBC, blood chemistries, TSH, hemoglobin A1C, lipid panel
  - Pregnancy test, if indicated

Follow-Up Tests & Special Considerations

Clinical and laboratory tests for routine monitoring, at least yearly, if using antipsychotic medications:

- Weight, waist circumference, and blood pressure
- CBC, hemoglobin A1C, lipid panel
- Pregnancy test and prolactin level, if indicated
- ECG, monitoring for QTc prolongation
- Clinical assessment of extrapyramidal symptoms

Diagnostic Procedures/Other

Neuropsychological testing: can help assess cognitive level to predict functioning and need for assistance

Test Interpretation

Ventriculomegaly is frequently seen on MRI with whole brain gray matter loss and white matter loss in medial temporal lobe structures preferentially.

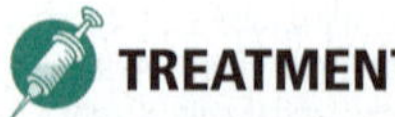

TREATMENT

GENERAL MEASURES

- Pharmacologic treatments are the mainstay of the treatment.
- If accessible, psychosocial intervention and rehabilitative therapies can help with successful community functioning.

MEDICATION

First Line

- Antipsychotic medications: atypical antipsychotics have a lower potential for extrapyramidal side effects.
  - Atypical (2nd generation)
    - Risperidone, olanzapine, ziprasidone, aripiprazole, quetiapine, paliperidone, iloperidone, asenapine, lurasidone, clozapine, brexpiprazole, lumateperone, cariprazine, pimavanserin (Parkinson disease–related psychosis)
  - Typical (1st generation)
    - Haloperidol, chlorpromazine, fluphenazine, trifluoperazine, perphenazine, thioridazine, thiothixene, loxapine
- Medication choice is based on clinical and subjective response and side-effect profile (4)
  - Sensitivity to extrapyramidal adverse effects: atypical
  - For least risk of tardive dyskinesia: quetiapine, clozapine
  - For least risk of metabolic syndrome: aripiprazole, ziprasidone, lurasidone, perphenazine, brexpiprazole
  - For least risk of QTc prolongation: aripiprazole
    - Avoid use of thioridazine and ziprasidone in patients with a prolonged QT interval.
- For poor compliance/high risk of relapse: Injectable form of long-acting antipsychotic may be used.
  - Haloperidol, fluphenazine, risperidone, olanzapine, aripiprazole, and paliperidone
- Usual maintenance daily range (initiation is commonly at a lower dose)
  - Chlorpromazine: 200 to 800 mg/day divided TID–QID
  - Aripiprazole: 10 to 30 mg/day
  - Asenapine: 5 to 10 mg BID (sublingual), 3.8 to 7.6 mg transdermal once daily patch
  - Fluphenazine: 1 to 5 mg/day
  - Haloperidol: 2 to 20 mg/day
  - Lurasidone: 40 to 160 mg/day (with meal)
  - Olanzapine: 10 to 30 mg/day
  - Paliperidone: 6 to 12 mg/day
  - Perphenazine: 8 to 64 mg/day divided BID–QID
  - Quetiapine: 400 to 800 mg/day up 3 times a day
  - Risperidone: 2 to 8 mg divided QD–BID
  - Ziprasidone: 20 to 80 mg BID (with meal)
  - Cariprazine: 1.5 to 6.0 mg/day PO
  - Brexpiprazole: 2 to 4 mg/day PO
  - Lumateperone: 42 mg/day PO
  - Clozapine: (for refractory schizophrenia)
    - Typical dosage range is 300 to 450 mg QD–BID dosing.
    - Effective if suicidal
    - Serious risk of agranulocytosis mandates registration with the Clozapine Risk Evaluation and Mitigation Strategy (CREMS) and weekly to monthly monitoring of CBC with differential.

- Significant risk of seizure at higher doses
- Side effects can include myocarditis, DVT, sialorrhea, tachycardia, QT prolongation, orthostasis, severe constipation, and weight gain (5)[A].

ALERT
All antipsychotics are associated with weight gain and carry the risk of tardive dyskinesia.

- Managing adverse effects of antipsychotics
  - Dystonic reaction (especially of head and neck): diphenhydramine 25 to 50 mg PO/IM/IV q6–q8h PRN or benztropine 1 to 2 mg IM/IV
  - Akathisia (restlessness): propranolol 20 to 30 mg BID or lorazepam 0.5 to 1.0 mg BID
  - Parkinsonism: trihexyphenidyl 2 mg BID (up to 15 mg daily) or benztropine 0.5 BID (1 to 4 mg/day); amantadine 100 mg daily (up to 300 mg daily)
  - Tardive dyskinesia: Consider switching to clozapine; otherwise, deutetrabenazine (6 to 24 mg BID), valbenazine (80 mg daily), or tetrabenazine (25 to 50 mg TID)
  - Neuroleptic malignant syndrome: hyperthermia, autonomic dysfunction, and extrapyramidal symptoms; requires hospitalization and supportive management (IVF and cessation of offending neuroleptic)
  - Weight gain/metabolic syndrome: Metformin up to 2,000 mg daily may attenuate weight gain (6).
  - Geriatric considerations: All antipsychotics have increased mortality risk in elderly patients with dementia.
- Adjunctive treatments
  - Benzodiazepines
    - May be effective adjuncts to antipsychotics during acute phase of illness
    - First-line short-term treatment of catatonia
    - Withdrawal reactions with psychosis or seizures; risk for dependence and cognitive impairment
    - Best when used only in the short-term; high total exposure to benzodiazepines may be associated with increased risk of death in patients with schizophrenia.
  - Mood stabilizers
    - Valproic acid may be effective adjunct for those with agitated/violent behavior (4).
    - Lithium may be effective adjunct for patients with affective symptoms or suicidal ideation (4).
  - Antidepressants:
    - Useful if comorbid depression and/or anxiety are present
    - Associated with a lower risk of psychiatric hospitalization when added to antipsychotic monotherapy compared to adding a second antipsychotic (7)[B]

ISSUES FOR REFERRAL

- Suicidality, coexistence of a substance use disorder, difficulty in engagement, or poor self-care
- Family members benefit from advocacy organizations such as National Alliance on Mental Illness (NAMI)

ADDITIONAL THERAPIES

- Psychoeducation and psychotherapy for patient and family; cognitive behavioral therapy and vocational support programs have been shown to be effective.
- Vocational support programs
- Negative symptoms typically respond better to these nonpharmacologic interventions than with medications.

SURGERY/OTHER PROCEDURES

Electroconvulsive therapy (ECT) should be considered for catatonic features, severe depression, or aggression and suicidality.

ADMISSION, INPATIENT, AND NURSING CONSIDERATIONS

The decision to admit is based on the risk of self-harm or harm to others and the inability to care for self.

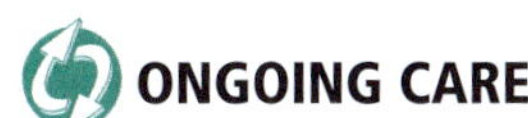

ONGOING CARE

FOLLOW-UP RECOMMENDATIONS

Continue to evaluate symptoms with regard to safety and psychosis. Treat emerging comorbidities and medication side effects and prevent complications.

DIET

Poor diet choices higher in cholesterol, saturated fat, and sodium. Results from dysregulation of reward pathways due to increased dopamine activity in the mesolimbic pathway and brain regions controlling cognition. Obesity, food cravings, and additive behavior are all linked to this pathway (8).

PATIENT EDUCATION

National Alliance on Mental Illness: https://www.nami.org

PROGNOSIS

- Typical course is one of remissions and exacerbations.
- Suicide risk is 4.5 times higher for those with schizophrenia compared to those patients without (9).

COMPLICATIONS

Medication side effects (tardive dyskinesia, orthostatic hypotension, QTc prolongation, metabolic syndrome)

REFERENCES

1. American Psychiatric Association. *Diagnostic and Statistical Manual of Mental Disorders*. 5th ed, text rev. Washington, DC: American Psychiatric Association Publishing; 2022.
2. Murrie B, Lappin J, Large M. Transition of substance-induced, brief, and atypical psychoses to schizophrenia: a systematic review and meta-analysis. *Schizophr Bull*. 2020;46(3):505–516.
3. Skikic M, Arriola JA. First episode psychosis medical workup: evidence-informed recommendations and introduction to a clinically guided approach. *Child Adolesc Psychiatr Clin N Am*. 2020;29(1):15–28.
4. Hasan A, Falkai P, Wobrock T, et al; WFSBP Task Force on Treatment and Guidelines for Schizophrenia. World Federation of Societies of Biological Psychiatry (WFSBP) guidelines for biological treatment of schizophrenia—a short version for primary care. *Int J Psychiatry Clin Pract*. 2017;21(2):82–90.
5. Dragoi AM, Radulescu I, Năsui BA, et al. Clozapine: an updated overview of pharmacogenetic biomarkers, risks, and safety—particularities in the context of COVID-19. *Brain Sci*. 2020;10(11):840. doi:10.3390/brainsci10110840.
6. Agarwal SM, Stogios N, Ahsan ZA, et al. Pharmacologic interventions for prevention of weight gain in people with schizophrenia. *Cochrane Database Syst Rev*. 2022;10(10):CD013337.
7. Stroup TS, Gerhard T, Crystal S, et al. Comparative effectiveness of adjunctive psychotropic medications in patients with schizophrenia. *JAMA Psychiatry*. 2019;76(5):508–515.
8. Onaolapo OJ, Onaolapo AY. Nutrition, nutritional deficiencies, and schizophrenia: an association worthy of constant reassessment. *World J Clin Cases*. 2021;9(28):8295–8311. doi:10.12998/wjcc.v9.i28.8295.
9. Olfson M, Stroup TS, Huang C, et al. Suicide risk in medicare patients with schizophrenia across the life span. *JAMA Psychiatry*. 2021;78(8):876–885. doi:10.1001/jamapsychiatry.2021.0841.

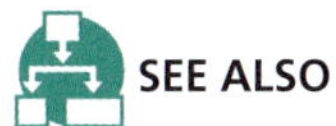

SEE ALSO

Algorithm: Delirium

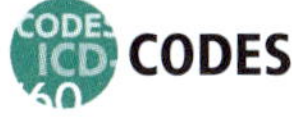

CODES

ICD10

- F20.3 Undifferentiated schizophrenia
- F20.5 Residual schizophrenia
- F20.2 Catatonic schizophrenia

CLINICAL PEARLS

- Schizophrenia is a severe and persistent mental illness that impacts cognition and functioning and requires a multidisciplinary team approach to assist with coping and treatment and to promote recovery.
- Presence of positive symptoms, including hallucinations and delusions and negative symptoms, including flattened affect, anhedonia, amotivation, and social withdrawal
- Higher rates of tobacco use and metabolic syndrome in schizophrenia with associated reduced life expectancy

SCLERITIS

Amethyst Wilder, MD

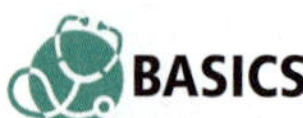

BASICS

DESCRIPTION

- Scleritis is a painful, inflammatory process of the sclera, below the conjunctiva and episclera.
  - Categorized by location (anterior or posterior) and subtype (diffuse, nodular, or necrotizing)
  - Commonly associated with systemic disorders
  - Potentially vision threatening
- In contrast, episcleritis is a self-limited inflammation of the superficial episclera with only mild discomfort.
- System(s) affected: ocular

EPIDEMIOLOGY

- Mean age is 54 years (ranges from 12 to 96 years).
- Predominant sex: female > male (1.6:1)

Incidence

Estimated to be 6 cases per 100,000 people in the general population (1)[C]

Prevalence

- Anterior scleritis, about 94% of cases (2)[B]
  - Diffuse anterior scleritis, about 75% (most common)
- Remaining 6% have posterior scleritis.

ETIOLOGY AND PATHOPHYSIOLOGY

- Frequently associated with a systemic illness (2)[B]
  - Most commonly rheumatoid arthritis
  - In about 38% of cases, scleritis is the presenting manifestation of an underlying systemic disorder.
- Other etiologies
  - Drug-induced scleritis has been reported in patients on bisphosphonate therapy.
  - Surgically induced necrotizing scleritis is exceedingly rare and occurs after multiple surgeries.
  - Infectious scleritis may be viral (HSV, HIV) but occurs most commonly after surgical trauma, and *Pseudomonas aeruginosa* in poorly controlled diabetic patients is the most common causative organism.

RISK FACTORS

Individuals with autoimmune disorders are most at risk.

COMMONLY ASSOCIATED CONDITIONS

- Autoimmune disorders
  - Rheumatoid arthritis (most common)
  - Sjögren syndrome
  - Systemic lupus erythematosus
  - Sarcoidosis
- Vasculitides
  - Granulomatosis with polyangiitis
  - Polyarteritis nodosa
  - Behçet disease
- Inflammatory bowel disease
- Herpes zoster, herpes simplex
- HIV, syphilis, Lyme disease, tuberculosis

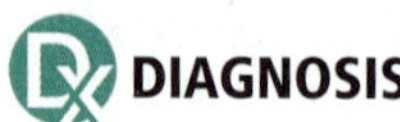

DIAGNOSIS

HISTORY

- Erythema and inflammation of the sclera
  - Can be bilateral in about 40% of cases (2)[B]
- Photophobia and tearing
- Pain ranging from mild discomfort to extreme localized tenderness
  - May be described as constant, deep, boring, or pulsating
  - Pain may be referred to the eyebrow, temple, or jaw.
  - Pain may awaken patient from sleep in early hours of morning.
  - Severe pain is most commonly associated with necrotizing scleritis (2)[B].

PHYSICAL EXAM

- Examine sclera in all directions of gaze by gross inspection.
  - A bluish hue may suggest thinning of sclera.
  - Inspect for degree of injection and extent of thinning.
- Different subtypes of scleritis are associated with varying presentations and distinct findings
  - Diffuse anterior scleritis: widespread inflammation
  - Nodular anterior scleritis: immovable, inflamed nodule
  - Necrotizing anterior scleritis with inflammation: sclera becomes transparent
  - Scleromalacia perforans without inflammation: painless and often associated with rheumatoid arthritis
- Check visual acuity.
  - Decrease in visual acuity of two or more Snellen lines occurs in about 16% of patients (2)[B].
- Slit-lamp exam
  - Episcleritis: conjunctival and superficial vascular plexuses displaced anteriorly; blanches with phenylephrine
  - Scleritis: Deep episcleral plexus is the maximum site of vascular congestion, displaced anteriorly due to edema of underlying sclera; characteristic blue or violet color, absent in patients with episcleritis
- Dilated fundus exam to rule out posterior involvement
  - Posterior scleritis: associated with retinal and choroidal complications; adjacent swelling of orbital tissues may occur.
- A complete physical exam, particularly of the skin, joints, heart, and lungs, should be done to evaluate for associated conditions.

DIFFERENTIAL DIAGNOSIS

- Conjunctivitis
- Episcleritis
- Iritis (anterior uveitis)
- Posterior uveitis
- Blepharitis
- Ocular rosacea

DIAGNOSTIC TESTS & INTERPRETATION

- Routine tests to exclude systemic disease: CBC, serum chemistry, urinalysis, ESR, and/or C-reactive protein
- Specific tests for underlying systemic illness: for example, rheumatoid factor, anti-cyclic citrullinated peptide antibodies
- B-scan US to detect posterior scleritis; look at thickness of sclera and for T-sign (fluid in Tenon space at interface between the optic nerve and sclera) (1)[C].

TREATMENT

GENERAL MEASURES

If scleral thinning, glasses/eye shield should be worn to prevent perforation; should be managed by an appropriate eye care physician.

MEDICATION

- First-line therapies for noninfectious scleritis (1)[C]
  - Oral NSAID therapy, choice based on availability, example is ibuprofen 600 to 800 mg PO TID–QID or indomethacin 50 mg PO TID provided no contraindications exists
    - About 37% successful (3)[B]
  - Systemic steroids, prednisone 40 to 60 mg PO QD or 1 mg/kg/day, taper over 4 to 6 weeks.
    - Use caution if suspect infectious etiology.
  - Antimetabolites including methotrexate, azathioprine, mycophenolate mofetil, cyclophosphamide, and cyclosporine may be used as steroid-sparing agents.
    - They are generally recommended if steroids cannot be tapered below 10 mg PO QD (3)[B]
- Second-line therapies (3)[B]
  - Immunomodulatory agents, infliximab, rituximab, and adalimumab can be used if patient has failed or is not a candidate for antimetabolites or calcineurin inhibitors.
    - Preferred over etanercept due to higher treatment success and its potential paradoxic effect on ocular inflammation.
- Adjunct therapy considerations
  - Topical steroids: prednisolone acetate 1% under ophthalmologist care
  - Subconjunctival triamcinolone acetonide injection only for nonnecrotizing, 40 mg/mL
    - 97% improvement after one injection
    - Increased risk of ocular HTN, cataract, and globe perforation
- Special consideration: necrotizing anterior scleritis and posterior scleritis
  - Preferentially IV steroid therapy if vision threatening; otherwise, use if failure of NSAIDs.
  - May require immunosuppressive therapy in addition to systemic steroids
  - Treat aggressively due to possible complications if left untreated; may need patch grafting to maintain globe integrity
- Infectious
  - Appropriate antiviral therapy if needed
  - Antibiotic therapy resolves about 18% of cases, whereas the remaining often requires surgical intervention such as débridement.

ISSUES FOR REFERRAL

- All patients with scleritis should be managed by an ophthalmologist familiar with this condition.
- Rheumatology referral for coexistent systemic disease is helpful for long-term success.

ADDITIONAL THERAPIES

Immunosuppressants used for autoimmune and collagen vascular disorders may be of help in active scleritis.

SURGERY/OTHER PROCEDURES

- In rare cases, scleral biopsy may be indicated to confirm infection or other etiology.
- Ocular perforation requires scleral grafting.

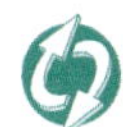

ONGOING CARE

FOLLOW-UP RECOMMENDATIONS

Avoid contact lenses.

Patient Monitoring

- Patient in the active stage of inflammation should be followed very closely by an ophthalmologist to assess the effectiveness of therapy.
- Medication use mandates close surveillance for adverse effects.

PATIENT EDUCATION

The Ocular Immunology and Uveitis Foundation: https://uveitis.org/patient_articles/scleritis/

PROGNOSIS

Scleritis is indolent, chronic, and often progressive.

- Diffuse anterior scleritis has the best prognosis
- Necrotizing anterior scleritis has the worst prognosis
- Recurrent bouts of inflammation may occur.
- Scleromalacia perforans has the highest risk of perforation of the globe.

COMPLICATIONS

- Decrease in vision, anterior uveitis, ocular HTN, and peripheral keratitis
- Cataract and glaucoma can result from disease or treatment with steroids.
- Ocular perforation can occur in severe stages.

REFERENCES

1. Beardsley RM, Suhler EB, Rosenbaum JT, et al. Pharmacotherapy of scleritis: current paradigms and future directions. *Expert Opin Pharmacother*. 2013;14(4):411–424.
2. Sainz de la Maza M, Molina N, Gonzalez-Gonzalez LA, et al. Clinical characteristics of a large cohort of patients with scleritis and episcleritis. *Ophthalmology*. 2012;119(1):43–50.
3. Sainz de la Maza M, Molina N, Gonzalez-Gonzalez LA, et al. Scleritis therapy. *Ophthalmology*. 2012;119(1):51–58.

ADDITIONAL READING

- Cao JH, Oray M, Cocho L, et al. Rituximab in the treatment of refractory noninfectious scleritis. *Am J Ophthalmol*. 2016;164:22–28.
- Diogo MC, Jager MJ, Ferreira TA. CT and MR imaging in the diagnosis of scleritis. *AJNR Am J Neuroradiol*. 2016;37(12):2334–2339.
- Levy-Clarke G, Jabs DA, Read RW, et al. Expert panel recommendations for the use of anti-tumor necrosis factor biologic agents in patients with ocular inflammatory disorders. *Ophthalmology*. 2014;121(3):785–796.e3.
- Hodson KL, Galor A, Karp CL, et al. Epidemiology and visual outcomes in patients with infectious scleritis. *Cornea*. 2013;32(4):466–472.

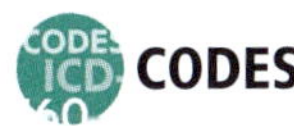

CODES

ICD10

- H15.009 Unspecified scleritis, unspecified eye
- H15.019 Anterior scleritis, unspecified eye
- H15.039 Posterior scleritis, unspecified eye

CLINICAL PEARLS

- Episcleritis is a self-limited inflammation of the eye with mild discomfort.
- Scleritis is a painful, severe, and potentially vision-threatening condition.
- It is key to differentiate between episcleritis and scleritis to guide treatment modalities (topical versus systemic).
- Investigation for underlying inflammatory diseases is prudent.

SCLERODERMA

Ann M. Lynch, BSP, PharmD

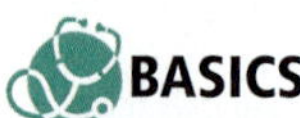

BASICS

DESCRIPTION

- Scleroderma (systemic sclerosis [SSc]) is a chronic disease of unknown cause involving connective tissue, characterized by diffuse fibrosis of skin and visceral organs and vascular abnormalities.
- Most manifestations have vascular features (e.g., Raynaud phenomenon), but frank vasculitis is rarely seen.
- Can range from a mild disease, affecting the skin, to a systemic disease that can cause death in a few months
- The disease is categorized into two major clinical variants.
  - Diffuse: distal and proximal extremity and truncal skin thickening
  - Limited
    - Restricted to the fingers, hands, and face
    - CREST syndrome (calcinosis, Raynaud phenomenon, esophageal dysmotility, sclerodactyly, telangiectasia)
- System(s) affected: include, but not limited to skin, renal, cardiovascular, pulmonary, musculoskeletal, gastrointestinal (GI)

Geriatric Considerations

Uncommon >75 years of age

Pediatric Considerations

Rare in this age group

Pregnancy Considerations

- Safe and healthy pregnancies are common and possible despite higher frequency of premature births.
- High-risk management must be standard care to avoid complications, specifically renal crisis.
- Diffuse scleroderma causes greater risk for developing serious cardiopulmonary and renal problems. Pregnancy should be delayed until disease stabilizes.

EPIDEMIOLOGY

Incidence

- In the United States: 1 to 5/100,000 per year
- Predominant age
  - Young adult (16 to 40 years); middle-aged (40 to 75 years); peak onset 30 to 50 years
  - Symptoms usually appear in the 3rd to 5th decades.
- Predominant sex: female > male (4:1)

Prevalence

In the United States: 1 to 25/100,000

ETIOLOGY AND PATHOPHYSIOLOGY

Pathophysiology involves both a vascular component and a fibrotic component. Both occur simultaneously. The inciting event is unknown, but there is an increase in certain cytokines after endothelial cell activation that are profibrotic (TGF-β and PDGF).

- Unknown
- Possible alterations in immune response
- Possibly some association with exposure to quartz mining, quarrying, vinyl chloride, hydrocarbons, toxin exposure
- Treatment with bleomycin has caused a scleroderma-like syndrome, as has exposure to rapeseed oil.

Genetics

Familial clustering is rare but has been seen.

RISK FACTORS

Unknown

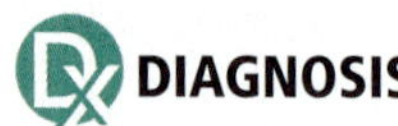

DIAGNOSIS

HISTORY

- Raynaud phenomenon is generally the presenting complaint (differentiated from Raynaud disease, generally affecting younger individuals and without digital ulcers).
- Skin thickening, "puffy hands," pruritus, and gastroesophageal reflux disease (GERD) are often noted early in the disease process.

PHYSICAL EXAM

- Skin
  - Digital ulcerations
  - Digital pitting
  - Tightness, swelling, thickening of digits
  - Hyperpigmentation/hypopigmentation
  - Narrowed oral aperture
  - SC calcinosis
- Peripheral vascular system
  - Telangiectasia
- Joints, tendons, and bones
  - Flexion contractures
  - Friction rub on tendon movement
  - Hand swelling
  - Joint stiffness
  - Polyarthralgia
  - Sclerodactyly
- Muscle
  - Proximal muscle weakness
- GI tract
  - Dysphagia
  - Esophageal reflux due to dysmotility (most common systemic sign in diffuse disease)
  - Malabsorptive diarrhea
  - Nausea and vomiting
  - Weight loss
  - Xerostomia
- Kidney
  - Hypertension
  - May develop scleroderma renal crisis: acute renal failure (ARF)
- Pulmonary
  - Dry crackles at lung bases
  - Dyspnea
- Nervous system
  - Peripheral neuropathy
  - Trigeminal neuropathy
- Cardiac (progressive disease)
  - Conduction abnormalities
  - Cardiomyopathy
  - Pericarditis
  - Secondary cor pulmonale

DIFFERENTIAL DIAGNOSIS

- Mixed connective tissue disease/overlap syndromes
- Scleredema
- Nephrogenic systemic fibrosis
- Toxic oil syndrome (Madrid, 1981, affecting 20,000 people)
- Eosinophilia–myalgia syndrome
- Diffuse fasciitis with eosinophilia
- Scleredema of Buschke

DIAGNOSTIC TESTS & INTERPRETATION

Initial Tests (lab, imaging)

- Nail fold capillary microscopy—drop out is most significant finding.
- CBC
- Creatinine
- Urinalysis (albuminuria, microscopic hematuria)
- Antinuclear antibodies (ANA): positive in >90% of patients
- Anti–Scl-70 (anti-topoisomerase [ATA]) antibody is highly specific for systemic disease and confers a higher risk of interstitial lung disease (ILD).
- Anticentromere antibody usually associated with CREST variant.
- Chest radiograph
  - Diffuse reticular pattern
  - Bilateral basilar pulmonary fibrosis
- Hand radiograph
  - Soft tissue atrophy and acroosteolysis
  - Can see overlap syndromes such as rheumatoid arthritis
  - SC calcinosis

Follow-Up Tests & Special Considerations

- Pulmonary function tests (PFTs)
  - Decreased maximum breathing capacity
  - Increased residual volume
  - Diffusion defect
- Antibodies to U3-RNP—higher risk for scleroderma-associated pulmonary hypertension
- Anti–PM-Scl antibodies (for myositis)
- Anti-RNA polymerase III—higher risk for diffuse cutaneous involvement and renal crisis
- ECG (low voltage): possible nonspecific abnormalities, arrhythmia, and conduction defects
- Echocardiography: pulmonary hypertension or cardiomyopathy
- Nail fold capillary loop abnormalities
- Upper GI
  - Distal esophageal dilatation
  - Atonic esophagus
  - Esophageal dysmotility
  - Duodenal diverticula
- Barium enema
  - Colonic diverticula
  - Megacolon
- High-resolution CT scan for detecting alveolitis, which has a ground-glass appearance or fibrosis predominant in bilateral lower lobes

Diagnostic Procedures/Other

- Skin biopsy
  - Compact collagen fibers in the reticular dermis and hyalinization and fibrosis of arterioles
  - Thinning of epidermis, with loss of rete pegs, and atrophy of dermal appendages
  - Accumulation of mononuclear cells is also seen.
- Right-sided heart catheterization: Pulmonary hypertension is an ominous prognostic feature.

Test Interpretation

- Skin
  - Edema, fibrosis, or atrophy (late stage)
  - Lymphocytic infiltrate around sweat glands
  - Loss of capillaries
  - Endothelial proliferation
  - Hair follicle atrophy
- Synovium
  - Pannus formation
  - Fibrin deposits in tendons
- Kidney
  - Small kidneys
  - Intimal proliferation in interlobular arteries
- Heart
  - Endocardial thickening
  - Myocardial interstitial fibrosis
  - Ischemic band necrosis
  - Enlarged heart
  - Cardiac hypertrophy
  - Pulmonary hypertension
- Lung
  - Interstitial pneumonitis
  - Cyst formation
  - Interstitial fibrosis
  - Bronchiectasis
- Esophagus
  - Esophageal atrophy
  - Fibrosis

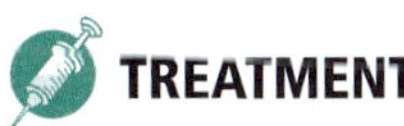

TREATMENT

GENERAL MEASURES

- Treatment is symptomatic and supportive.
- Esophageal dilation may be used for strictures.
- Avoid cold; dress appropriately in layers for the weather; be wary of air conditioning.
- Avoid smoking (crucial).
- Avoid fingersticks (e.g., blood tests).
- Elevate the head of the bed during sleep to help relieve GI symptoms.
- Use softening lotions, ointments, and bath oils to help prevent dryness and cracking of skin.
- Dialysis may be necessary in renal crisis.

MEDICATION

First Line

- ACE inhibitors (ACEIs): for preservation of renal blood flow and for treatment of hypertensive renal crisis
- Dihydropyridine calcium channel blockers (e.g., nifedipine, amlodipine) for Raynaud phenomenon
- Corticosteroids: for disabling myositis, pulmonary alveolitis, or mixed connective tissue disease, doses up to 15 mg daily (not recommended in high doses due to increased incidence of renal failure)
- NSAIDs: for joint or tendon symptoms; caution with long-term concurrent use with ACEIs (potential renal complications)
- Antibiotics: for secondary infections in bowel and active skin infections
- Antacids, proton pump inhibitors: for gastric reflux
- Metoclopramide: for intestinal dysfunction
- Hydrophilic skin ointments: for skin therapy
- Consider immunosuppressives for treatment of life-threatening or potentially crippling scleroderma or interstitial pneumonitis such as cyclophosphamide for ILD.
- Nitrates, dihydropyridine calcium-channel blockers, PDE5 antagonists, and fluoxetine for Raynaud phenomenon
- Avoidance of caffeine, nicotine, and sympathomimetics may ease Raynaud symptoms.
- PDE5 antagonists, prostanoids, and endothelin-1 antagonists are changing the management of pulmonary hypertension.
- Alveolitis: immunosuppressants and alkylating agents

ADDITIONAL THERAPIES

- Anti–TNF-α therapy: Preliminary suggestion is that this may reduce joint symptoms and disability in inflammatory arthritis, but small sample sizes and observational biases lend to the need for further well-designed, adequately powered, longitudinal clinical trials.
- Physical therapy to maintain function and promote strength
- Heat therapy to relieve joint stiffness

SURGERY/OTHER PROCEDURES

- Some success with gastroplasty for correction of GERD
- Limited role for sympathectomy for Raynaud phenomenon
- Lung transplantation for pulmonary hypertension and ILD
- Hematopoietic stem cell transplantation for selected patients with severe, refractory, or rapidly progressive SSc (1)

ONGOING CARE

FOLLOW-UP RECOMMENDATIONS

Patient Monitoring

- Monitor every 3 to 6 months for end organ and skin involvement and medications. Provide encouragement.
- Echocardiology and PFTs yearly

DIET

- Drink plenty of fluids with meals.
- Adjust eating habits if GI symptoms are present.

PATIENT EDUCATION

- Stay as active as possible, but avoid fatigue.
- Printed patient information available from the Scleroderma Federation: https://scleroderma.org/
- Advise the patient to report any abnormal bruising or nonhealing abrasions.
- Assist the patient about smoking cessation, if needed.

PROGNOSIS

- Possible improvement but incurable
- Prognosis is poor if cardiac, pulmonary, or renal manifestations present early.

COMPLICATIONS

- Renal failure
- Respiratory failure
- Flexion contractures
- Disability
- Esophageal dysmotility
- Reflux esophagitis
- Arrhythmia
- Megacolon
- Pneumatosis intestinalis
- Obstructive bowel
- Cardiomyopathy
- Pulmonary hypertension
- Possible association with lung and other cancers
- Death

REFERENCES

1. Zhao M, Wu J, Wu H, et al. Clinical treatment options in scleroderma: recommendations and comprehensive review. *Clin Rev Allergy Immunol*. 2022;62(2):273–291.

ADDITIONAL READING

Fernández-Codina A, Walker KM, Pope JE, et al; for Scleroderma Algorithm Group. Treatment algorithms for systemic sclerosis according to experts. *Arthritis Rheumatol*. 2018;70(11):1820–1828.

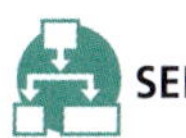

SEE ALSO

Morphea

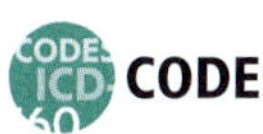

CODES

ICD10

- M34.2 Systemic sclerosis induced by drug and chemical
- M34.9 Systemic sclerosis, unspecified
- M34.0 Progressive systemic sclerosis

CLINICAL PEARLS

- Raynaud phenomenon is frequently the initial complaint.
- Skin thickening, "puffy hands," and GERD are often noted early in disease.
- Patients must be followed proactively for development of pulmonary hypertension or ILD.

S

SEASONAL AFFECTIVE DISORDER

Matthew J. Filippo, DO • Erica Minor, DO

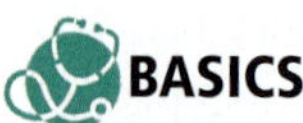

BASICS

DESCRIPTION

- Patients experience depressive episodes or, less commonly, hypomanic or manic episodes.
- Depressive episodes typically occur during winter months (fall-winter onset), with full remission in the spring and summer. Conversely, patients may experience a spring-summer onset with remission in fall-winter months, although this is less common.
- Ranges from a seriously disabling illness to milder subclinical symptoms colloquially termed "winter blues"

EPIDEMIOLOGY

Prevalence

- Affects up to 500,000 Americans every winter
- Up to 30% of patients visiting a primary care physician (PCP) during winter may report winter depressive symptoms.
- Predominant age: Although it may occur at any age, there is a peak in individuals in their 20s to 30s.
- Predominant sex: female > male (3:1)

ETIOLOGY AND PATHOPHYSIOLOGY

- Photoperiod and phase shift hypotheses: During the winter months, the period of natural daylight is shorter. When there is less sunlight, the pineal gland increases melatonin secretion (photoperiod hypothesis). This can lead to a phase shift, causing a misalignment of the circadian rhythm from the sleep-wake cycle. Light therapy in the morning or evening can suppress melatonin secretion to correct the phase shift and improve symptoms of depression. Reduced sunlight may also decrease vitamin D levels, which may contribute to symptoms of depression, although vitamin D's role appears more correlation than causation.
- Serotonin dysregulation hypothesis: This hypothesis poses there is increased serotonin transporter activity leading to enhanced clearance from the synaptic cleft. This altered secretion is thought to contribute to seasonal affective disorder (SAD) pathophysiology. Centrally acting serotonergic agents, such as SSRIs, have been shown to alleviate SAD symptoms.

Genetics

- Twin studies suggest a genetic component.
- There is an association with melanopsin gene (OPN4) and GPR50 melatonin receptor variants.

RISK FACTORS

- Most common during months of January and February
- Spending a prolonged period of time in an environment without windows or significant sunlight exposure
- Living at a higher latitude

GENERAL PREVENTION

- Increase time outside during daylight hours, or move to, or plan to vacation at, a more southern location. Bright light therapy may be effective as treatment but has not been shown beneficial as preventative treatment.
- Bupropion (Wellbutrin) is the only FDA-approved antidepressant for the prevention of SAD.
- The role of low-dose evening melatonin as prevention is not definitively established, with studies showing mixed results. It may have a role in symptom management (see "Treatment").

COMMONLY ASSOCIATED CONDITIONS

Comorbid psychiatric disorders such as alcohol use disorder, ADHD, and binge eating

DIAGNOSIS

Under *DSM-5*, SAD is not a standalone diagnosis, rather, it is a specifier, "with seasonal pattern," applied to major depressive disorder, bipolar I disorder, or bipolar II disorder.

- Remission of symptoms occurs during a characteristic time of year (usually spring or summer).
- Symptoms have occurred for the past 2 years.
- Seasonal episodes substantially outnumber any nonseasonal depressive episodes in the patient's lifetime.
- Carefully document the presence or absence of prior manic episodes.
- Screen for the existence of any suicidal ideation and safety risk factors.

HISTORY

- Symptoms of depression meeting the criteria for major depressive disorder are the following:
  - Sleep disturbance: either too much or too little
  - Lack of interest in life and absence of pleasure from hobbies/activities
  - Guilt: feelings of guilt or worthlessness
  - Energy: fatigue or constantly feeling tired
  - Concentration: difficulty with concentration and memory
  - Appetite: changes in appetite and weight
  - Psychomotor retardation: patients feeling slowed down with decreased activity
  - Suicidal thoughts: Patients report thoughts of suicide.
- In SAD episodes with fall-winter onset, hypersomnia, hyperphagia (craving for carbohydrates and sweets), and weight gain usually predominate. Despite sleeping more, patients report daytime sleepiness and fatigue. Cravings may lead to binge eating and weight gain >20 lbs.
- In SAD episodes with spring-summer onset, depression symptoms of insomnia and loss of appetite are more common.
- Obtain collateral history if patient is unable to provide insight into the seasonal component.

PHYSICAL EXAM

Use exam to exclude other organic causes for symptoms. Neurologic deficits, signs of endocrine dysfunction, or stigmata of substance abuse should prompt further testing.

DIFFERENTIAL DIAGNOSIS

- Organic causes of low energy and fatigue, such as hypothyroidism, anemia, autoimmune disorders, mononucleosis (or other viral syndromes)
- Substance use disorders

DIAGNOSTIC TESTS & INTERPRETATION

- Thyroid-stimulating hormone to rule out hypothyroidism, which can mimic depressive symptoms, CBC, electrolytes, glucose, and 25-OH vitamin D level
- Pregnancy test for women of childbearing potential
- Urine toxicology screen if substance use is a concern
- Imaging is not useful unless there are focal neurologic findings or when looking to exclude an organic cause.

Follow-Up Tests & Special Considerations

Polysomnography shows rapid eye movement sleep is increased in patients with SAD.

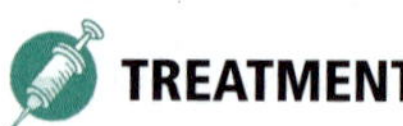

TREATMENT

MEDICATION

Both medication and bright light therapy are strong first-line contenders. The use of either is often guided by patient preference, severity, and contraindications. Combination therapy should be used for more severe cases (1),(2).

First Line

- SSRIs can be effective as first-line treatments for SAD. It may be reasonable to decrease a patient's dose during nonseasonal months when patients do not experience symptoms of depression (3)[C].
- SSRIs such as sertraline (Zoloft), paroxetine (Paxil), fluoxetine (Prozac), citalopram (Celexa), and escitalopram (Lexapro) can be used at typical antidepressant doses.
- Bupropion (Wellbutrin) is the only antidepressant currently approved by the FDA for the prevention of SAD.
- Studies using low-dose melatonin show mixed results. It appears most effective when given in the early evening paired with early morning light therapy.

Second Line

Short-acting β-blockers given before sunrise suppress melatonin release and may help in reducing SAD symptoms especially when paired with early morning bright light therapy.

ISSUES FOR REFERRAL

- Patients with ocular disease should be referred for an ophthalmologic exam before phototherapy and for serial monitoring.
- Patients who fail to respond or who develop manic symptoms or suicidal ideation once treatment is initiated should be considered for psychiatric referral.

ADDITIONAL THERAPIES

- Phototherapy using special light sources has been shown to be effective in 60–90% of patients and can be considered a first-line treatment, often providing relief with a few sessions.
- Variables that can regulate effect of bright light therapy are the following:
  - Light intensity: At least 2,500 lux is suggested (domestic lights emit, on average, 200 to 500 lux). There is stronger evidence using 7,000 to 10,000 lux.
  - Treatment duration is dependent on the intensity of light source. Typical effective regimens include 10,000 lux for 30 minutes daily, or 2,500 lux for 1 to 2 hours daily.
  - Time of treatment: Most patients respond better by using the light therapy early in the morning.
  - Color of light source: Research into blue-enriched light suggests potential for efficacy with shorter exposure durations.
- A light box is placed on table several feet away, and the light is allowed to shine onto the patient's retinas (sunglasses should be avoided).
- The most common side effects are eye strain and headache. Insomnia can result if the light box is used too late in the evening. Light boxes can rarely precipitate mania in some patients but can still be used in patients with bipolar disorder.
- Dawn simulators gradually increase illumination, simulating sunrise while using a less intense light source. They have been shown to be more effective than placebo and may be comparable to bright light therapy with better tolerability.

COMPLEMENTARY & ALTERNATIVE MEDICINE

- Work to reduce stress levels through meditation, progressive relaxation exercises, and/or lifestyle modification.
- Although correcting vitamin D deficiency is important for overall health and may support mood, current evidence is insufficient to recommend vitamin D as a standalone treatment for SAD. Its role is more relevant in individuals with coexisting deficiency.
- Getting regular physical activity ideally with sunlight exposure

ADMISSION, INPATIENT, AND NURSING CONSIDERATIONS

Consider for suicidal ideation or loss of the ability to function secondary to depression or mania.

ONGOING CARE

FOLLOW-UP RECOMMENDATIONS

Regular monitoring for response to treatment; rarely, patients may become manic when treated with SSRIs or light therapy.

Patient Monitoring

Patients should be monitored weekly after initiating light or pharmacotherapy to monitor treatment results, side effects, and any increased suicidal ideation if treating with SSRIs.

DIET

Although patients often report carbohydrate cravings, a balanced diet is encouraged. Counsel on choosing complex carbohydrates over simple sugars to help stabilize energy levels and mood. Managing binge eating, if present, is also crucial.

PATIENT EDUCATION

- Increase time outdoors during daylight.
- Rearrange home or work environment to get more direct sunlight through windows.

PROGNOSIS

Symptoms, if untreated, generally remit within 5 months with exposure to spring light and often return in subsequent winters. If treated, patients usually respond within 3 to 6 weeks.

COMPLICATIONS

Development of suicidal ideation and mania are two outcomes the clinician needs to monitor.

REFERENCES

1. Lam RW, Levitt AJ, Levitan RD, et al. The Can-SAD study: a randomized controlled trial of the effectiveness of light therapy and fluoxetine in patients with winter seasonal affective disorder. *Am J Psychiatry*. 2006;163(5):805–812.
2. Galima SV, Vogel SR, Kowalski AW. Seasonal affective disorder: common questions and answers. *Am Fam Physician*. 2020;102(11):668–672.
3. Nussbaumer-Streit B, Thaler K, Chapman A, et al. Second-generation antidepressants for treatment of seasonal affective disorder. *Cochrane Database Syst Rev*. 2021;3(3):CD008591. doi:10.1002/14651858.CD008591.pub3.

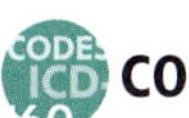

SEE ALSO

- Bipolar I Disorder; Bipolar II Disorder; Depression
- Algorithm: Depressive Episode, Major

CODES

ICD10

- F33.9 Major depressive disorder, recurrent, unspecified
- F33.0 Major depressive disorder, recurrent, mild
- F33.1 Major depressive disorder, recurrent, moderate

CLINICAL PEARLS

- SAD is diagnosed by applying the "with seasonal pattern" specifier to major depressive disorder or bipolar disorder. For patients with a mood disorder, specifically inquire whether depressive episodes demonstrate a regular temporal relationship with particular times of the year.
- Ensure that symptoms are not due to an organic process or better explained by substance use.
- Guidelines suggest using SSRIs first if the patient is more acute or has contraindications to light therapy.
- Light therapy boxes are available from numerous suppliers but are not extensively regulated; practitioners should take care to ensure patients use devices from reputable suppliers. Dawn simulators can be used as an alternative if bright light therapy is less tolerable.
- Some patients may experience increased suicidal thoughts after starting treatment with SSRIs. These patients should be closely monitored as outpatients.

SEIZURE DISORDER, ABSENCE

Zaiba Jetpuri, DO, MBA, FAAFP • Humza Feroz Siddiqi, MD

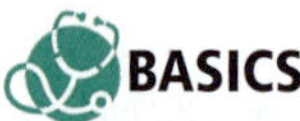

BASICS

DESCRIPTION

A type of generalized nonmotor seizure characterized by a brief lapse of awareness. Classified by the International League Against Epilepsy (ILAE):

- Definition: Childhood absence epilepsy (CAE) is characterized by recurrent brief episodes of impaired consciousness ("staring spells") with abrupt onset and termination and EEG showing 3 Hz spike-wave discharges.
  - Typical have an abrupt onset, last 5 to 30 seconds and offset of behavioral arrest, loss of awareness, and blank staring, sometimes with eyelid movements, eye-opening, or oral automatisms (e.g., lip smacking).
  - Atypical have a less abrupt onset, last 10 to 45 seconds and offset and often associated with loss of muscle tone or subtle myoclonic jerks. Brief postictal confusion can sometimes occur.
  - Myoclonic have an abrupt onset, last 10 to 60 seconds and offset of staring and loss of awareness with continuous rhythmic jerks of shoulders, arms, legs, head, or perioral muscles. They can have impairment of consciousness varying from complete loss of awareness to retained awareness.
  - Eyelid myoclonia have an abrupt onset, last <6 seconds and offset of repetitive, rhythmic jerks of the eyelids with simultaneous upward deviation of the eyeballs and extension of the head. They can also have incomplete impairment of consciousness, often with awareness mostly retained.

EPIDEMIOLOGY

- Accounts for 10–17% of childhood-onset epilepsy; most common pediatric epilepsy syndrome
- Predominant age of onset: between 4 and 10 years, with peak onset between 5 and 7 years
- Predominant gender: female > male (2:1) with male predominance in myoclonic absence seizure

ETIOLOGY AND PATHOPHYSIOLOGY

- Mainly genetic with complex, multifactorial inheritance; however, may be secondary to a variety of congenital or acquired brain disorders such as hypoxia–ischemia, trauma, CNS infection, cortical malformations, or inborn errors of metabolism
- Absences are triggered in the corticothalamic system when γ-aminobutyric acid (GABA)-mediated activity induces prolonged hyperpolarization and activates T-type ("low-threshold") calcium channels, resulting in sustained-burst firing of these neurons, causing absence seizures.

Genetics

- 75% concordance occurs in monozygotic twins; 84% share EEG features.
- 15–44% of patients with CAE have a family history of epilepsy.
- Mutations of GABA-A/B receptors—involved in spike wave discharges
- Mutations in calcium channels (CACNA1 A, CACNA1 H, CACNA1 I, CACNG3)—thalamocortical dysrhythmia
- Mutations of SLC21A, which encodes GLUT1—associated with a worse prognosis

RISK FACTORS

- Lack of medication compliance
- Lack of sleep
- Alcohol use
- Medications that lower seizure threshold
- Hyperventilation
- Febrile seizures in ~20%; family history in ~50%

GENERAL PREVENTION

- Primary prevention can't be studied and likely is not achievable because the causes are mostly, if not all, genetic.
- Secondary prevention is achievable by avoiding triggers including:
  - Adequate sleep per age-based recommendations
  - Adherence to an individualized medication regimen
  - There is a growing body of evidence that suggests exercise may help reduce episode frequency in some forms of epilepsy, but the effect with regard to CAE/juvenile absence epilepsy (JAE) is still undetermined.

COMMONLY ASSOCIATED CONDITIONS

Difficulties in visual attention and visuospatial skills, verbal learning and memory, fine motor skills, executive functions, reduced language abilities, ADHD, anxiety, depression, social isolation, and low esteem

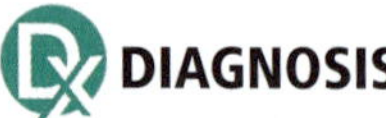

DIAGNOSIS

- Frequent (multiple/day), last ~9 to 10 seconds (range 4 to 20 seconds), abrupt pause/stare (80–95%); motor automatisms (40–60%); eyelid involvement (55%).
- Loss of awareness, no recall
- Easily provoked by hyperventilation (90% trigger efficacy)
- Variants: myoclonic absence, eyelid myoclonia, atypical absence (<2.5 Hz)
- Comorbidities: ADHD, anxiety, mood/learning disorders; often precede epilepsy onset and impact academics

HISTORY

- Detailed description of episode, including activity at onset, any automatisms, duration of episode, frequency of episodes, aura or postictal state, age of onset, and birth and developmental history
- Teachers report that child seems to daydream or zone out frequently and during episodes become unresponsive and unaware with a blank stare.
- Pallor is frequently reported.
- Child will forget portions of conversations.
- Child with normal IQ underperforms in school.

ALERT

Seizures are often so brief that untrained observers are not aware of the occurrence.

PHYSICAL EXAM

- Unless a child has another genetic or acquired abnormality, a neurologic exam usually is normal. Abnormal physical exam indicates the need for further diagnostic workup (e.g., MRI, metabolic, or genetic testing).
- Seizures may be induced by hyperventilation:
  - Have the child blow on a pinwheel or similar exercise for 3 to 5 minutes to provoke seizure.
  - Alternatively, ask the patient to perform hyperventilation with eyes closed and count. Patient will open eyes at onset of seizure and stop counting.
  - Hyperventilation: Provokes seizures in ~90% untreated.

ALERT

- Absence seizures are not associated with sensitivity to light or other photic stimuli (e.g., strobe lights).
- Voluntary hyperventilating (tantrums) may induce absences.

DIFFERENTIAL DIAGNOSIS

- JAE
- Juvenile myoclonic epilepsy (JME)
- Focal seizures with or without awareness
- Psychogenic nonepileptic seizures
- Confusional states and acute memory disorders
- Migraine variants
- Panic/anxiety attacks
- Breath-holding spells
- Nonepileptic staring spells/behavioral
- Status epilepticus

DIAGNOSTIC TESTS & INTERPRETATION

Initial Tests (lab, imaging)

- Video-EEG monitoring, including sleep and awake with hyperventilation resulting in spike-wave complexes from <2.5 to 6.0 Hz, depending on type of absence seizure, is standard for diagnosis.
- Ictal EEG = 2.5 to 5.5 Hz generalized spike-wave, classically 3 Hz, abrupt onset/termination; pre/postictal slowing may occur.
- Imaging is not routinely indicated in children with typical absence and normal neurologic exam and cognition. If imaging is performed, MRI is preferable to CT scan due to higher sensitivity for anatomic abnormalities.
- Presently, no laboratory values can definitively prove or rule out the diagnosis of an absence seizure. However, labs such as electrolytes, creatinine, liver and renal function tests, TSH, CBC, and toxicology screen can rule out endocrine, metabolic, toxic, or infectious etiologies (1)[C].

Follow-Up Tests & Special Considerations

- Drug levels are useful in evaluating symptoms of toxicity or for breakthrough seizures.
- Follow blood chemistry, hepatic function, blood counts, etc., specific to drug regimen.

Diagnostic Procedures/Other

Uncommonly, there may be a need for a lumbar puncture to rule out causes of treatment-resistant absences.

Test Interpretation

- CSF glucose levels
- Variations in GLUT-1 expression or SLC2A1 gene, etc.

TREATMENT

GENERAL MEASURES

ALERT

Patients should refrain from activities that would put them at risk if a seizure occurred (e.g., climbing heights, swimming unsupervised, cycling on busy roads, driving, operating heavy machinery, cooking with stoves unsupervised). Providers should be familiar with state laws concerning driving with epilepsy.

MEDICATION

ALERT

- Certain common anticonvulsants may exacerbate absence including carbamazepine, oxcarbazepine, phenytoin, phenobarbital, tiagabine, vigabatrin, pregabalin, and gabapentin.
- 20–25% of children with CAE (and probably also with JAE) are pharmacoresistant.

First Line

- Ethosuximide blocks T-type calcium channels:
  - High efficacy and fewer adverse attentional effects compared to valproic acid; however, is only effective against absence seizures (2)[A]
  - Possible disease-modifying, remission is achieved more frequently when ETX is introduced as a first drug.
  - Side effects: vomiting, diarrhea, abdominal discomfort, hiccups, headache, sedation
  - Adverse effects: aplastic anemia, skin reactions, and renal/hepatic impairment. Monitor CBC and CMP (1)[C].
  - Ethosuximide and valproate > lamotrigine; ethosuximide causes fewer attention problems.
- Valproic acid (alternative first line)
  - Attention deficits persist more frequently with valproic acid monotherapy compared to ethosuximide or lamotrigine.
  - Adverse effects: teratogenicity, behavior/cognitive abnormalities, hepatotoxicity, pancreatitis. Monitor CMP, amylase, and lipase; reduced bone mineral density and increased risk of osteoporosis and fractures
  - Side effects: tremor, drowsiness, dizziness, weight gain, alopecia, sedation, vomiting

Second Line

Lamotrigine affects sodium channels:

- Controls seizures but may be less efficacious than ethosuximide or valproic acid (3)[A]
- Side effects: rash, diplopia, headache, insomnia, dizziness, nausea, vomiting, diarrhea
- Adverse effects: rare Stevens-Johnson rash, more often when co-administered with valproic acid

ISSUES FOR REFERRAL

Failure to gain seizure control for at least 1 year with two AEDs should prompt referral to neurologist for confirmation of the diagnosis for seizure, search for a pathogenic genetic variant (i.e., GLUT-1 deficiency) and/or syndrome classification and, if appropriate, for consideration of epilepsy surgery.

Pediatric Considerations

- Neuropsychological testing, such as the Wechsler Intelligence Scale for Children (WISC) and the NEPSY-II, along with assessing developmental milestones, behavior, and teacher and parent reports, can help diagnose comorbid conditions caused by or associated with CAE.
- Prescribe vitamin D supplementation (usual dose 400 to 1,000 IU/day for children without deficiency and 1,000 to 2,000 IU or more daily for children with deficiency) in children taking valproic acid due to AE of reduced bone mineral density.
- Fatal hepatotoxicity with valproic acid risk is greatest in <2-year-olds (1)[C].

Pregnancy Considerations

Anticonvulsants, especially valproic acid, are associated with an increase in fetal malformations. Use of valproic acid in women of childbearing age, who are not using adequate birth control, is contraindicated.

SURGERY/OTHER PROCEDURES

- Epilepsy surgery including ablation and resection for medically refractive absence epilepsy
- Vagal nerve stimulator (VNS) may be considered as an option for medically refractory absence epilepsy.

COMPLEMENTARY & ALTERNATIVE MEDICINE

A ketogenic diet may reduce seizure frequency in children with drug-resistant epilepsy.

ADMISSION, INPATIENT, AND NURSING CONSIDERATIONS

Status epilepticus requires inpatient care.

ONGOING CARE

PATIENT EDUCATION

- Caregivers should be informed that tonic-clonic seizures are rare in absence seizures but should be taught how to manage a generalized tonic-clonic seizure.
- *Sarah Jayne Has Staring Moments*: a fictional children's book for child absence seizure epilepsy by Kate Lambert

PROGNOSIS

- Prognosis for CAE is excellent with 56–84% remission rate.
- Remission is less common in JAE, JME, and those who progress to generalized tonic-clonic seizures or myoclonic seizures.
- Patients whose shortest pretreatment EEG seizures are >20 seconds in duration are more likely to achieve seizure freedom, regardless of treatment.
- Typical absence seizures generally cease spontaneously by age 12 years or sooner. However, a subset may develop other forms of epilepsy or experience cognitive and behavioral difficulties.
- Cognitive outcomes: attentional deficits = most consistent long-term problem, correlate with reduced academic performance

COMPLICATIONS

- Reported frequencies of typical absence status epilepticus range from 5.8% to 9.4%.
- <10% develop generalized tonic-clonic seizures.

REFERENCES

1. Fisher RS, Cross JH, D'Souza C, et al. Instruction manual for the ILAE 2017 operational classification of seizure types. *Epilepsia*. 2017;58(4):531–542.
2. Min L, Chunyan W, Biaoxue R. Effects of valproic acid on skeletal metabolism in children with epilepsy: a systematic evaluation and meta-analysis based on 14 studies. *BMC Pediatr*. 2020;20(1):97.
3. Glauser TA, Cnaan A, Shinnar S, et al; for Childhood Absence Epilepsy Study Team. Ethosuximide, valproic acid and lamotrigine in childhood absence epilepsy: initial monotherapy outcomes at 12 months. *Epilepsia*. 2013;54(1):141–155.

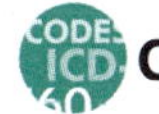

CODES

ICD10

- G40.409 Other generalized epilepsy and epileptic syndromes, not intractable, without status epilepticus
- G40.419 Oth generalized epilepsy, intractable, w/o stat epi
- G40.401 Oth generalized epilepsy, not intractable, w stat epi

CLINICAL PEARLS

- Children with CAE can exhibit cognitive, behavioral, and psychosocial comorbidities. For these children, attentional deficits are the most important marker of cognitive dysfunction and often associated with reduced academic performance, anxiety, depression, and behavioral disorders.
- If parents are unable to determine the cause of a staring spell, try suggesting that parents mention something exciting or unexpected like "ice cream" during a spell to get the child's attention rather than calling his or her name.
- Ethosuximide and valproic acid are first-line agents in treatment of absence seizures.
- Maintain a seizure diary to help identify type and cause of seizures.
- Review seizure precautions and create a seizure response plan.

S

SEIZURE DISORDER, FOCAL

Robert A. Baldor, MD, FAAFP

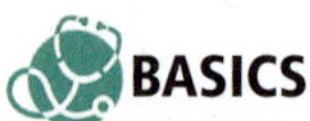

BASICS

DESCRIPTION

- Seizures occur when abnormal synchronous neuronal discharges in the brain cause transient cortical dysfunction.
- Focal or localization-related seizures have previously been referred to as partial seizures and originate from a discrete focus limited to one cerebral hemisphere.
- Focal seizures are further divided into aware versus unaware and motor versus nonmotor:
  - Focal seizures with impairment of awareness (formerly "complex partial seizures")
  - Focal seizures without impairment of awareness (formerly "simple partial seizures")

EPIDEMIOLOGY

Prevalence

Focal seizures occur in 20/100,000 persons in the United States.

ETIOLOGY AND PATHOPHYSIOLOGY

- Focal seizures begin when a localized seizure focus produces an abnormal, synchronized depolarization within a neuronal network limited to one cerebral hemisphere; it may stay discretely localized or be widely distributed throughout that hemisphere.
- The area of cortex involved in the seizure determines the symptoms; for example, an epileptogenic focus in motor cortex produces contralateral motor symptoms.
- Most common etiologies vary by life stage:
  - Early childhood: developmental/congenital malformation, trauma
  - Young adults: developmental, infection, trauma
  - Adults 40 to 60 years of age: cerebrovascular insult, infection, trauma
  - Adults >60 years of age: cerebrovascular insult, trauma, neoplasm

Genetics

Benign rolandic epilepsy has an autosomal dominant inheritance pattern.

RISK FACTORS

- History of traumatic brain injury (TBI)
- Thiamine-deficient formula

COMMONLY ASSOCIATED CONDITIONS

Depression

DIAGNOSIS

Duration: seconds to minutes, unless status epilepticus develops; status epilepticus may present as focal/generalized convulsions/altered mental status without convulsions.

- Focal seizures without impairment of awareness (simple partial seizures)
  - Motor onset: Seizure activity in motor strip causes contraction (tonic) or rhythmic jerking (clonic) movements that may involve one entire side of body or may be more localized (i.e., hands, feet, or face).
    - Jacksonian march: As discharge spreads through motor cortex, tonic–clonic activity spreads in predictable fashion (i.e., beginning in hand and progressing up arm and to the face).
  - Nonmotor onset:
    - Todd paralysis: after motor seizure, residual, temporary weakness in the affected area
    - Parietal lobe: sensory loss/paresthesias, dizziness
    - Temporal lobe: déjà vu, rising sensation in epigastrium, auditory hallucinations/forced memories, unpleasant smell/taste
    - Occipital: visual hallucinations
- Focal seizures with impairment of awareness (complex partial seizures):
  - May have aura; indicates the onset of the seizure
  - Amnesia for the event, postictal confusion
  - Most often, focus is temporal/frontal.
  - Motor manifestations may include dystonic posturing/automatisms (i.e., simple, repetitive movements of face and hands or more complex actions such as purposeless walking).
  - Frontal lobe seizure is characterized by brief, bilateral complex movements, vocalizations.

HISTORY

- A detailed description of the seizure should be obtained from an observer.
- Review medication list for drugs that lower seizure threshold (e.g., tramadol, bupropion, theophylline).
- Obtain history of drugs of abuse (e.g., cocaine) that may lower seizure threshold.
- Review history of prior TBI.

PHYSICAL EXAM

Include neurologic exam, with attention to lateralizing signs suggestive of structural lesion.

DIFFERENTIAL DIAGNOSIS

- Syncope/postanoxic myoclonus
- Hypoglycemia
- Psychogenic nonepileptic seizure
- TIA
- Migraine and headache disorder

DIAGNOSTIC TESTS & INTERPRETATION

- CBC; complete metabolic panel; urinalysis; urine drug screen; levels of antiepileptic drugs; chest x-ray
- Elevated prolactin, if measured within 10 to 20 minutes of suspected seizure, lactate, or elevated creatine phosphokinase; if measured within 6 to 24 hours, may help to differentiate generalized/focal seizure from psychogenic nonepileptic seizure
- Emergency evaluation of new seizure: CT scan to screen for hemorrhage and stroke
- CSF exam if infection is suspected (1)[B],(2)[B]
- EEG should be considered in patients with first time unprovoked seizure (2)[B].
- Yield of EEG is increased by being obtained in the first 24 hours following seizure and by sleep deprivation.
- If difficulty with diagnosis, continuous video–EEG monitoring may be appropriate.
- In patients without recent neuroimaging, consider CT or MRI (2)[B].

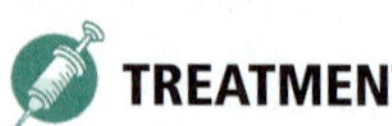

TREATMENT

GENERAL MEASURES

Maintain a seizure diary, noting potential triggers, such as stress, sleep deprivation, drug use, discontinuation of alcohol/benzodiazepines, menses.

MEDICATION

- Current guidelines do not recommend for or against starting an AED after a single unprovoked seizure. Patients should be counseled that AEDs will reduce risk of repeat seizure over 2 years but have no effect on long-term remission (3)[C].
- Initiating an AED after a single unprovoked seizure lowers the probability of recurrence within 5 years, but does not have an effect on remission or mortality. Additionally, there is increased risk of adverse effects with immediate treatment (4)[B].
- AEDs act on voltage-gated ion channels, affect neuronal inhibition via enhancement of γ-aminobutyric acid (GABA, an inhibitory neurotransmitter), or decrease neuronal excitation. End result is to decrease the abnormal synchronized firing and to prevent seizure propagation.
- 50% of those with newly diagnosed focal seizures respond to, and tolerate, first AED trial. Up to 50% of those who fail the first AED trial will also fail a second AED trial (5)[B].
- Choose AED based on seizure type, side effect profile, and patient characteristics. Increase dose until seizure control is obtained/side effects become unacceptable.
- Attempt monotherapy, but many patients will require adjunctive agents. Multiple effective add-on agents are available, but there is no clear evidence for one AED over another.
- AEDs may prevent seizures after a TBI in the short term, although they provide no efficacy in long-term prevention (6)[B].
- Several AEDs induce/inhibit cytochrome P450 enzymes (watch for drug interactions).

First Line

- Carbamazepine: affects sodium channels
  - Side effects include GI distress, hyponatremia, diplopia, dizziness, rare pancytopenia/marrow suppression, and exfoliative rash.
  - Patients of Asian ancestry should be screened for HLA-B*1502 prior to initiation to reduce risk of Stevens-Johnson syndrome or toxic epidermal necrolysis.
- Oxcarbazepine: affects sodium channels; side effects include dizziness, diplopia, hyponatremia, and headache.
- Lamotrigine: affects sodium channels
  - Side effects include insomnia, dizziness, and ataxia.
  - Risk of Stevens-Johnson syndrome reaction (potentially fatal exfoliative rash), especially when given with valproate, requires slow titration
- Levetiracetam: multiple mechanisms; side effects include sedation, ataxia, and irritability.

Second Line

- Phenytoin: affects sodium channels; side effects include ataxia, dizziness, diplopia, tremor, GI upset, gingival hyperplasia, and fever.
- Phenobarbital: multiple mechanisms; side effects include sedation and withdrawal seizures.
- Valproate: multiple mechanisms; side effects include GI upset, weight gain, alopecia, and tremor; less common, thrombocytopenia, hepatitis, pancreatitis
- Topiramate: multiple mechanisms; side effects include anorexia, cognitive slowing, sedation, nephrolithiasis, and anhidrosis.
- Gabapentin: multiple mechanisms; side effects include sedation, dizziness, and ataxia.
- Pregabalin: affects calcium channels; side effects include sedation, dizziness, and weight gain.
- Zonisamide: affects sodium channels:
  - Side effects include sedation, anorexia, nausea, dizziness, ataxia, anhidrosis, and nephrolithiasis.
  - Cross-reaction with sulfa allergy

Pregnancy Considerations

- Folate should be prescribed for all women of childbearing age who are taking AEDs. AED therapy during the 1st trimester is associated with doubled risk for major fetal malformations (6% vs. 3%).
- Phenytoin in pregnancy may result in fetal hydantoin syndrome.
- Valproate is associated with neural tube defects and should be avoided in pregnancy when possible.
- Fetal insult from seizures following withdrawal of therapy also may be severe. Risk-to-benefit balance should be evaluated with high-risk pregnancy and neurology consultations. Most patients remain on anticonvulsants.
- AED levels should be monitored at least every trimester.

ISSUES FOR REFERRAL

Epilepsy specialist for refractory seizures

ADDITIONAL THERAPIES

- Vagal nerve stimulator provides periodic stimulation to vagus nerve. High-frequency stimulation provides greater reduction in seizure frequency than low-frequency but has greater rates of side effects (6)[B].
- Deep brain stimulation may decrease seizure frequency in medically refractive epilepsy.
- Repetitive magnetic transcranial stimulation may reduce seizures with refractory focal seizures.

SURGERY/OTHER PROCEDURES

- For refractory focal seizures with identifiable focus
- Preoperative testing, such as Wada test, should be done to decrease likelihood of inducing aphasia and memory loss.
- 34–74% will be seizure free after temporal lobe surgery. Prognosis varies for surgical resection of extratemporal foci.
- Goal of surgical intervention is to reduce reliance on medications; most patients remain on anticonvulsants postoperatively.

ADMISSION, INPATIENT, AND NURSING CONSIDERATIONS

Admit for unremitting seizure (status epilepticus).

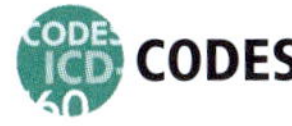

ONGOING CARE

FOLLOW-UP RECOMMENDATIONS

- Most states restrict driving for those with seizure disorders.
- May also recommend against activities such as swimming, climbing to heights, or operating heavy machinery

Patient Monitoring

AED levels if concern over toxicity, noncompliance, or for breakthrough seizures

DIET

Ketogenic or low-glycemic index diet may improve seizure control in some patients.

PATIENT EDUCATION

Avoid potential triggers such as alcohol or drug use and sleep deprivation.

PROGNOSIS

- Risk of seizure recurrence: ~30% after first seizure; of these, 50% will occur in the first 6 months, 90% in the first 2 years.
- ~25–30% of all seizures are refractory to current medications.
- AEDs initiated after an initial seizure can decrease the risk of seizure over the first 5 years but may not reduce long-term risk of recurrence or mortality.
- The risk of developing seizure after mild TBI remains high for a long period (>10 years).

COMPLICATIONS

- Risk of accidental injury
- Depression, anxiety, memory impairment

REFERENCES

1. Gavvala JR, Schuele SU. New-onset seizure in adults and adolescents: a review. *JAMA*. 2016;316(24):2657–2668.
2. Krumholz A, Wiebe S, Gronseth GS, et al. Evidence-based guideline: management of an unprovoked first seizure in adults: report of the Guideline Development Subcommittee of the American Academy of Neurology and the American Epilepsy Society. *Neurology*. 2015;84(16):1705–1713.
3. Leone MA, Giussani G, Nevitt SJ, et al. Immediate antiepileptic drug treatment, versus placebo, deferred, or no treatment for first unprovoked seizure. *Cochrane Database Syst Rev*. 2021;5(5):CD007144.
4. Bonnett LJ, Tudur Smith C, Donegan S, et al. Treatment outcome after failure of a first antiepileptic drug. *Neurology*. 2014;83(6):552–560.
5. Thompson K, Pohlmann-Eden B, Campbell LA, et al. Pharmacological treatments for preventing epilepsy following traumatic head injury. *Cochrane Database Syst Rev*. 2015;2015(8):CD009900.
6. Panebianco M, Rigby A, Marson AG. Vagus nerve stimulation for focal seizures. *Cochrane Database Syst Rev*. 2022;7(7):CD002896.

S

CODES

ICD10

- G40.109 Local-rel symptc epi w simp prt seiz,not ntrct, w/o stat epi
- G40.209 Local-rel symptc epi w cmplx prt seiz,not ntrct,w/o stat epi
- G40.119 Local-rel symptc epi w simple part seiz, ntrct, w/o stat epi

CLINICAL PEARLS

- Focal seizures originate from a discrete focus limited to one hemisphere in the cerebral cortex and are further divided into aware versus unaware and motor versus nonmotor, depending on patient presentation.
- It is controversial whether AED treatment is indicated after a first seizure. Treatment should be considered when a structural cause is identified or risk of injury from seizure is high.
- An EEG and neuroimaging (CT or MRI) should be considered in evaluating a first unprovoked seizure.

SEIZURE DISORDERS

Sahil Mullick, MD, FAAFP • Mohammad Sameer Ahmed Zidan, MBBS

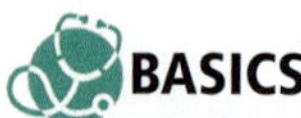

BASICS

DESCRIPTION

- Seizure disorders refer to a group of conditions characterized by recurrent, unprovoked seizures due to abnormal neuronal activity in the brain. Epilepsy, the most recognized seizure disorder, is diagnosed when an individual experiences two or more unprovoked seizures separated by at least 24 hours, or one unprovoked seizure with a high risk of recurrence.
- Status epilepticus is defined as a seizure lasting >5 minutes or recurrent seizures without recovery between them; prompt management is critical due to the risk of morbidity and mortality (1).

EPIDEMIOLOGY

Epilepsy affects approximately 50 million people globally, making it one of the most common neurologic conditions (2).

Prevalence

Prevalence of up to 1.2% in the U.S. population as of 2023

ETIOLOGY AND PATHOPHYSIOLOGY

Seizures arise due to imbalances between excitatory and inhibitory neuronal signaling. Etiologies include structural lesions (stroke, trauma), genetic mutations, infections (e.g., neurocysticercosis), metabolic derangements, or unknown causes (3)

Genetics

Family history increases the risk 5-fold, particularly in generalized epilepsies. Mutations in genes affecting ion channels (e.g., SCN1A, KCNQ2) are implicated in various syndromes.

RISK FACTORS

Risk factors include febrile seizures, traumatic brain injury, CNS infections, perinatal complications, and genetic predisposition (3).

GENERAL PREVENTION

Primary prevention includes managing CNS infections and head trauma. Secondary prevention targets early diagnosis and adherence to therapy to reduce recurrence (2).

COMMONLY ASSOCIATED CONDITIONS

Common comorbidities include depression, anxiety, cognitive impairment, and migraines. Neurodevelopmental disorders often coexist in pediatric populations (3).

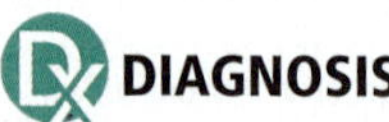

DIAGNOSIS

Diagnosis is clinical, supported by EEG and neuroimaging. Seizures are classified as focal, generalized, or unknown onset. EEG confirms epileptic activity; video-EEG is valuable for distinguishing from psychogenic nonepileptic seizures (PNES). Febrile seizures, common in children, are benign but may increase later epilepsy risk (2).

HISTORY

History should explore aura, seizure type, triggers, duration, postictal symptoms, and family history.

PHYSICAL EXAM

Physical exam may reveal focal neurologic signs or stigmata of genetic syndromes.

DIFFERENTIAL DIAGNOSIS

Includes syncope, PNES, transient ischemic attacks, migraines, and metabolic encephalopathy (3)

DIAGNOSTIC TESTS & INTERPRETATION

Initial tests: blood glucose, electrolytes, calcium, renal/liver function, toxicology; neuroimaging (MRI preferred) identifies structural causes. EEG within 24 to 48 hours improves yield. Lumbar puncture is indicated if infection is suspected (2).

Initial Tests (lab, imaging)

- Glucose, sodium, potassium, calcium, phosphorus, magnesium, BUN, ammonia; drug and toxin screens
- AED levels
- CBC, UA, ECG, lumbar puncture if needed
- Serum prolactin has limited utility; may be useful in differentiating generalized tonic-clonic and focal seizure from PNES
- Imaging is recommended for new-onset seizures. MRI is preferred than CT scan.
  - CT scan of the brain: indicated routinely as an initial evaluation, especially in the ER
  - Brain MRI: superior in evaluation of the temporal lobes, strokes, and other structural abnormalities

Follow-Up Tests & Special Considerations

Serial EEGs or ambulatory EEGs may be needed. Consider genetic testing in pediatric or syndromic cases.

Diagnostic Procedures/Other

Lumbar puncture is recommended if there is suspicion of intracranial infection.

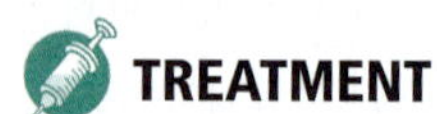

TREATMENT

GENERAL MEASURES

Ensure airway, breathing, and circulation in acute seizures. Educate patients and caregivers about triggers and safety.

MEDICATION

- AED: Select based on the type of seizure, potential adverse effects/drug interactions, and comorbid medical conditions.
- Treatment should begin with a single agent and the dose titrated until seizures are controlled or side effects become problematic. Consider switching to a different agent versus adding a second agent.

First Line

- The AAN and AES guidelines emphasize the use of lamotrigine and levetiracetam for focal-onset seizures and sodium valproate for generalized-onset seizures, with levetiracetam as an alternative for women of childbearing potential (4).
- First-line options include levetiracetam, lamotrigine, valproate, depending on seizure type (2).

Second Line

Second-line options include topiramate, carbamazepine, and others. Medication choice depends on age, sex, comorbidities, and side effect profiles (2).

Pregnancy Considerations

Use lowest effective dose of monotherapy. Avoid valproate if possible due to teratogenicity. Folic acid supplementation is essential (3).

ISSUES FOR REFERRAL

Refer patients with refractory seizures, diagnostic uncertainty, or need for advanced interventions.

SURGERY/OTHER PROCEDURES

Indicated for drug-resistant focal epilepsy; options include temporal lobectomy or laser ablation; neurostimulation devices (e.g., vagus nerve stimulation) may benefit selected patients (3).

COMPLEMENTARY & ALTERNATIVE MEDICINE

Some patients explore CBD or acupuncture; evidence remains limited; should be discussed with care team (3)

ADMISSION, INPATIENT, AND NURSING CONSIDERATIONS

Admit if status epilepticus, uncontrolled seizures, or new neurologic findings. Nursing care includes monitoring airway, seizure precautions, and medication adherence (1).

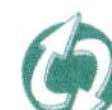

ONGOING CARE

FOLLOW-UP RECOMMENDATIONS

Regular follow-up ensures seizure control, medication adherence, and psychosocial support. Routine labs and EEGs may be repeated as needed (2).

Patient Monitoring

- Monitor drug levels and seizure frequency.
- CBC and lab values (e.g., calcium, vitamin D) as indicated
- Monitor for side effects and adverse reactions.
- All patients taking any AED should be monitored closely for notable changes in behavior that could indicate the emergence/worsening of suicidal thoughts/behavior/depression.

DIET

The ketogenic diet is effective in pediatric drug-resistant epilepsy. Modified Atkins or low–glycemic index diets may help some adults (3).

PATIENT EDUCATION

Educate about adherence, lifestyle modifications, seizure first aid, and driving restrictions (2).

PROGNOSIS

70% of patients achieve seizure freedom with appropriate treatment; poor prognostic factors include early onset, comorbid intellectual disability, and drug resistance.

COMPLICATIONS

Injury, status epilepticus, sudden unexpected death in epilepsy (SUDEP), and psychosocial impairment are key complications (1).

REFERENCES

1. Glauser T, Shinnar S, Gloss D, et al. Evidence-based guideline: treatment of convulsive status epilepticus in children and adults: report of the Guideline Committee of the American Epilepsy Society. *Epilepsy Curr*. 2016;16(1):48–61. doi:10.5698/1535-7597-16.1.48.
2. Centers for Disease Control and Prevention. Epilepsy facts and stats. https://www.cdc.gov/epilepsy/data-research/facts-stats/index.html. Accessed October 24, 2025.
3. World Health Organization (WHO). Epilepsy: a public health imperative. https://www.who.int/publications/i/item/epilepsy-a-public-health-imperative. Accessed October 24, 2025.
4. Kanner AM, Ashman E, Gloss D, et al. Practice guideline update summary: efficacy and tolerability of the new antiepileptic drugs I: treatment of new-onset epilepsy: report of the Guideline Development, Dissemination, and Implementation Subcommittee of the American Academy of Neurology and the American Epilepsy Society. *Neurology*. 2018;91(2):74–81.

SEE ALSO

Seizure, Febrile

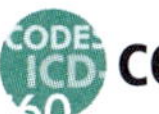

CODES

ICD10

- G40.B1 Juvenile myoclonic epilepsy, intractable
- G40.804 Other epilepsy, intractable, without status epilepticus
- G40.A0 Absence epileptic syndrome, not intractable

CLINICAL PEARLS

- Always rule out reversible causes in new-onset seizures.
- Status epilepticus is a medical emergency treat within 5 minutes.
- Tailor medication to seizure type and patient profile. Monitor drug levels and interactions in long-term care.
- Safety education is critical: driving, water safety, and work hazards.

S

SEIZURES, FEBRILE

Christina Conrad, DO • Priya Prasher, MBBS

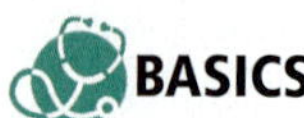

BASICS

DESCRIPTION

Febrile seizures (FS) occur in children aged 6 months to 6 years with fever ≥100.4°F (38°C) in the absence of an underlying neurologic abnormality, metabolic condition, or intracranial infection. There are three distinct categories (1),(2),(3):

- Simple febrile seizure (SFS) (70–75%; must meet all criteria):
  - Generalized clonic or tonic–clonic seizure activity without focal features
  - Duration <15 minutes
  - Does not recur within 24 hours
  - Resolves spontaneously
  - No history of previous afebrile seizure, seizure disorder, or other neurologic problem
- Complex febrile seizure (CFS) (20–25%; only one criterion must be met):
  - Partial seizure, focal activity
  - Duration >15 minutes but <30 minutes
  - Recurrence within 24 hours
  - Postictal focal neurologic abnormalities (e.g., Todd paralysis)
- Febrile status epilepticus (FSE) (5%): lasts >30 minutes

EPIDEMIOLOGY

Incidence

- About 500,000 FS in the United States annually
- Occurs in 3–5% of children 6 months to 6 years of age. Peak incidence is 18 months of age with 90% of children having their first FS before age 3 years. Only 6% of FS occur before age 6 months (3).
- Seasonal pattern that mirrors peaks of febrile respiratory (November to January) and gastrointestinal infections (June to August)

ETIOLOGY AND PATHOPHYSIOLOGY

The pathophysiology of FS remains unclear, but current research suggests the following mechanisms that lower seizure threshold:

- Age-dependent vulnerability of developing nervous system (2).
- Increased neuronal activity (i.e., seizures) secondary to temperature-sensitive ion channels and secretion of cytokines from inflammatory processes such as fever-promoting pyrogen interleukin-1β.
- Hyperthermia-induced hyperventilation and alkalosis, which provokes neuronal excitability.

Genetics

- More common in children with first-degree relatives who have had febrile seizures. Monozygotic twins have a higher concordance rate than dizygotic twins (1).
- Certain genes that have been identified as risk factors for family epilepsy syndromes may also increase the risk of FS (1).

RISK FACTORS

- Most common risk factors for developing first FS (1),(4):
  - Height of fever, more so than rate of rise.
  - Viral infection (80% of FS caused by virus)
  - Recently immunized, particularly with MMR and DTwP
  - Family history of FS
    - As many as 25–40% of cases have a positive family history of FS. Risk increases with number of affected first-degree (OR = 4.5%) and second-degree relatives (OR = 3.6%); greater concordance rate in monozygotic than dizygotic twins (1)
- Other general risk factors for FS: nicotine exposure in utero, NICU stay >28 days, developmental delay, or day care attendance
- Risk is slightly increased for males (2).
- Recent vaccination
  - Certain vaccines (e.g., MMR, DTwP, PCV13), method of preparation, vaccine coadministration, and associated age of administration have shown to increase risk of FS (3).
  - No evidence of increased risk with isolated influenza vaccination
- Perhaps increased risk with iron deficiency anemia and low zinc levels (1)

GENERAL PREVENTION

Choose vaccines with lower risk of developing FS and ask if the child has ever had a history of FS after vaccine administration (3),(4).

- Increased risk of FS if vaccine administrations are delayed.
- Separate MMR and varicella vaccine and administer between 12 and 15 months of age.
- Administer DTaP (acellular) rather than DTwP (whole cell) vaccine.

COMMONLY ASSOCIATED CONDITIONS

- Viral infections are the cause of fever in nearly 80% of FS cases, particularly human herpesvirus 6 (HHV-6), influenza, parainfluenza, adenovirus, and respiratory syncytial virus (RSV) (3).
- Bacterial infections: otitis media, pharyngitis, urinary tract infection (UTI), pneumonia, and gastroenteritis (specifically with *Shigella*).
- Vaccinations (3)
  - MMRV vaccination had 2-fold increase in risk of FS compared to separation of MMR and varicella vaccine.
  - DTwP vaccine had roughly 15% greater chance of causing FS compared to DTaP (1 per 2,835 vaccines and 1 per 19,496 vaccines, respectively).
  - There is a small increased risk for FS when activated influenza vaccine (flu shot) is given at the same time as either the PCV13 (pneumococcal) vaccine or the DTaP vaccine.
    - Also, small increased risk with PCV13 given alone
    - No increased risk if influenza or DTaP given alone

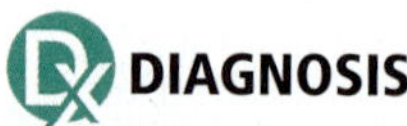

DIAGNOSIS

HISTORY

- Symptoms of underlying infection or neurologic deficits
- Onset, duration, type, and number of seizure
  - An SFS is generalized and associated with tonic–clonic movements of the limb and rolling back of the eyes. It may last a few seconds to 15 minutes, although generally <5 minutes, and does not recur within 24 hours.
- Presence of postictal state (such as weakness or paralysis)
  - Postictal drowsiness should resolve within 5 to 10 minutes. Encephalopathy beyond this range raises suspicion of CNS or systemic infection.
- Any interventions made to stop seizure
- Past medical history:
  - Immunization status, recent vaccines
  - Preexisting conditions: developmental delay, cerebral palsy, metabolic disorders, injury
  - Recent antibiotic course
- Family history: FS, afebrile seizures, epilepsy, metabolic disorders, and other neurologic conditions
- Factors concerning for child abuse or trauma

PHYSICAL EXAM

- Monitoring vital signs and close observation of neurologic status/change are essential in all children (1).
  - Unstable vital signs or toxic appearance warrants further evaluation.
  - Look for tachypnea, hypoxemia, lesions in oropharynx, or viral exanthem.
    - Observe for presence of closed eyes and a deep breath to indicate cessation of seizure. Children with persistently open and deviated eyes may still be seizing in absence of convulsive motor activities.
    - Average duration of FSE is 67 minutes.
  - Assess mental status and signs of meningitis—obtunded or comatose mental state, nuchal rigidity, prolonged focal seizure or petechial rash, and multiple seizures.
  - Duration of seizures >30 minutes, presence of postictal drowsiness, and neurologic deficits were predictive factors for meningitis.
- A thorough physical exam should not be deferred until postictal state has resolved. Although exam may be limited, prompt evaluation may reveal focal neurologic deficits or Todd paresis (2)[A].
- Assess for nonaccidental trauma with skin inspection, palpation for occult trauma, and retinal exam.

DIFFERENTIAL DIAGNOSIS

- Seizures due to other etiology: meningitis, encephalitis, primary epilepsy, intracranial mass, trauma, electrolyte abnormality, hypoglycemia, metabolic disorder
- Seizure mimics: rigors, crying, breath-holding spell, choking episode, tic disorder, parasomnia, dystonic reaction, shaking chills (shivering)

DIAGNOSTIC TESTS & INTERPRETATION

Initial Tests (lab, imaging)

- Routine laboratory tests not routinely recommended if the child is well appearing (4)
  - Blood workup if other symptoms such as vomiting, diarrhea, and poor fluid intake that points toward another etiology for seizure
  - Urinalysis only if indicated by current UTI rates in children with SFS are comparable to febrile children without seizure.
- Lumbar puncture (LP) not necessary in well-appearing children who quickly return to baseline
  - Following situations may warrant LP:
    - Meningeal signs and symptoms (4); infant 6 to 12 months of age without known *Haemophilus influenzae* type b (Hib) or *Streptococcus pneumoniae* immunization (4)
    - Child was treated with antibiotics as it can mask the signs and symptoms of meningitis (4).
- Neuroimaging is not routinely recommended to identify the cause of an FS (2)[A],(4).
  - Studies demonstrate limited utility of emergent imaging in most patients with FS; no advantage of MRI versus CT for management of FS in ED
  - Warranted if strong indication of acute/subacute bleeding or structural lesion
  - Nonurgent, outpatient MRI brain is recommended for patients with focal CFS especially with postictal neurologic deficits.
    - No evidence to support routine use of neuroimaging in absence of interictal or postictal focality.
- Check for anemia if iron deficiency is suspected.

Follow-Up Tests & Special Considerations

If there is a need to perform both EEG and MRI for a child presenting with FS, do EEG first. MRI in children will most often require complete sedation, which may alter the results of an EEG.

TREATMENT

Most FS are self-limited; however, if health care professionals are able to witness the FS, acute abortive treatment should be no different than any other seizure treatment. FSE rarely stops spontaneously and often requires more than one medication to control. Early intervention with AEDs is important for duration of FSE and outcome (2)[A].

GENERAL MEASURES

During an acute seizure management, continue to monitor patient's ABCs (1):

- Airway: Position the patient laterally, suction secretions, and place a nasopharyngeal airway.
- Breathing: Administer oxygen for cyanosis; consider bag-mask ventilation or intubation for inadequate ventilation.
- Circulation: Establish IV access for any medication and fluid bolus.

MEDICATION

First Line

- Treat seizures of $\geq$5 minutes duration with anticonvulsants. If seizures continue 5 minutes after administration of medication, can repeat dose (2):
  - Out of hospital (e.g., home or paramedics on route): rectal diazepam 0.5 mg/kg, buccal midazolam (0.2 to 0.4 mg/kg), or nasal midazolam (0.2 mg/kg)
  - In hospital: IV or IM lorazepam 0.05 to 0.1 mg/kg or IV diazepam 0.1 to 0.2 mg/kg; "out of hospital" options can also be used if IV option is not available.
- If seizures are prolonged or recurrent, administer IV fosphenytoin (20 mg phenytoin equivalent per kilogram); if seizures persist after 10 minutes of loading dose, can give additional dose (5 to 10 mg phenytoin equivalent per kilogram) (2)
  - There is some evidence that fosphenytoin should be avoided due to risk of worsening seizures in patients with SCN1A mutations (2).
- Antipyretics should be used to reduce fever as it often helps with overall comfort level of patients (1).
  - In one study, rectal acetaminophen (10 mg/kg, every 6 hours for 24 hours) showed potential to prevent FS recurrence during same fever episode (1).
  - Prophylactic antipyretics before vaccination is not recommended as not effective and could decrease immune response to certain vaccines.

Second Line

IV phenobarbital (15 to 20 mg/kg), valproic acid (20 to 40 mg/kg), or levetiracetam (20 to 60 mg/kg)

ISSUES FOR REFERRAL

Neurology consultation if persistent neurologic deficits, recurrent FS, or abnormal exam on evaluation (2)

ADMISSION, INPATIENT, AND NURSING CONSIDERATIONS

Abnormal or concerning findings on history or physical exam or prolonged/delayed recovery

ONGOING CARE

FOLLOW-UP RECOMMENDATIONS

Anticonvulsant prophylaxis during subsequent febrile episodes is not recommended, as adverse effects of anticonvulsants outweigh benefits (4).

PATIENT EDUCATION

Guidance for parents should focus on reassurance, emphasizing the benign nature of FS, overall excellent prognosis of the disease, and basic guidelines on interventions of FS were to reoccur (1).

- FS often do not cause brain damage, have a low risk for sequelae, and do not have a negative impact on intellect, behavior, or risk of death.
- The benefits of vaccinations greatly outweigh the side effects. The vaccine-induced FS risk is more affected by personal and family history rather than the sole act of receiving the vaccination (3).

PROGNOSIS

Favorable for children with normal neurodevelopmental status.

- A second FS occurs in about 1/3 of the patients; a third FS in 15% of patients.
- Risk factors for recurrent FS (2):
  - Age of onset: younger the age, higher the risk
  - Relatively low temp ($<$104°F) at time of first FS
  - Shorter interval ($<$1 hour) between onset of fever and seizure
  - First-degree relative with history of FS or epilepsy
  - First FS has complex FS features, particularly focal or prolonged CFS (continued topic of debate)
- Risk of FS developing into epilepsy:
  - Age $>$3 years at time of first FS
  - Developmental delay or abnormal neurologic exam prior to onset of first FS
  - CFS
  - Family history of epilepsy
  - Fever duration of 1 hour before seizure onset
- An unprovoked, afebrile seizure (epilepsy) after FS is estimated to be 1% for simple FS and 4–6% for CFS.

REFERENCES

1. Smith DK, Sadler KP, Benedum M. Febrile seizures: risks, evaluation, and prognosis. *Am Fam Physician*. 2019;99(7):445–450.
2. Whelan H, Harmelink M, Chou E, et al. Complex febrile seizures—a systematic review. *Dis Mon*. 2017;63(1):5–23.
3. Deng L, Gidding H, Macartney K, et al. Postvaccination febrile seizure severity and outcome. *Pediatrics*. 2019;143(5):e20182120.
4. Subcommittee on Febrile Seizures; American Academy of Pediatrics. Neurodiagnostic evaluation of the child with a simple febrile seizure. *Pediatrics*. 2011;127(2):389–394.

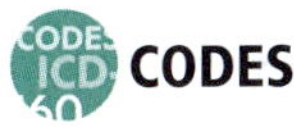

CODES

ICD10

- R56.00 Simple febrile convulsions
- R56.01 Complex febrile convulsions
- G40.901 Epilepsy, unsp, not intractable, with status epilepticus

CLINICAL PEARLS

- FS are generally benign and without sequelae if the underlying causes are ruled out.
- Labs, LP, neuroimaging, and EEG not routinely recommended in an acute setting in the absence of suspicion for underlying pathology.
- Prophylaxis with anticonvulsants or antipyretics during subsequent febrile episodes is not recommended.

SEROTONIN SYNDROME

Michael T. Partin, MD • Karl T. Clebak, MD, MHA, FAAFP • Munima Nasir, MD, FAAFP

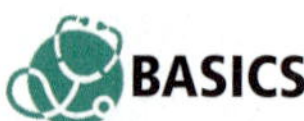

BASICS

DESCRIPTION

- A potentially life-threatening drug-induced syndrome that results from synaptic increase in serotonin (5-hydroxytryptamine [5-HT]) concentrations and stimulation of peripheral and CNS serotonergic receptors (1)
- Classic triad of symptoms that include mental status changes, neuromuscular hyperactivity, and autonomic instability
- Onset is usually within 24 hours with the majority occurring within 6 hours of exposure to, or change in, dosing of a serotonergic agent. Rarely, reported weeks after discontinuation of serotonergic agents
- It is a concentration-dependent toxicity that can develop in any individual who has ingested drug combinations that synergistically increase synaptic 5-HT.
- Serotonin toxicity occurs in three main settings: (i) therapeutic drug use, which often results in mild to moderate symptoms; (ii) intentional overdose of a single serotonergic agent, which typically leads to moderate symptoms; and (iii) as the result of a drug interaction between numerous serotonergic agents (most commonly, selective serotonin reuptake inhibitors [SSRIs], serotonin noradrenergic reuptake inhibitors [SNRIs], and monoamine oxidase inhibitors [MAOIs]), most often associated with severe serotonin toxicity.

Geriatric Considerations

Increased risk through polypharmacy given frequent use of serotonergic analgesics, antibiotics, and antidepressants

Pediatric Considerations

- Similar manifestations and management in children and adults
- Consider toxic ingestion of serotonergic agents prescribed to caregivers.
- Symptoms in neonates may include tremors, increased muscle tone, jitteriness, shivering, feeding/digestive disturbances, irritability, agitation, sleep disturbances, increased reflexes, excessive crying, and respiratory disturbances.

Pregnancy Considerations

Serotonin levels are increased from baseline during an uncomplicated pregnancy with preeclamptic patients demonstrating a 10-fold increase in serotonin levels.

EPIDEMIOLOGY

Seen in approximately 14–16% of SSRI overdose patients

Incidence

The exact incidence of serotonin syndrome is unknown. The number of cases is likely higher than reported due to its ability to mimic other clinical syndromes and potential for mild cases to go undiagnosed (1).

ETIOLOGY AND PATHOPHYSIOLOGY

- Increased synaptic 5-HT or agonist concentration as a result of one or more of the following mechanisms: (i) decreased 5-HT breakdown (e.g., MAOI), (ii) decreased 5-HT reuptake (e.g., SSRI), (iii) increased 5-HT agonists (e.g., tryptophan), (iv) increased 5-HT release (e.g., amphetamines), and (v) CYP2D6 and CYP3A4 inhibitors (e.g., erythromycin)
- Risk is mediated in a dose-related manner to the action of 5-HT/5-HT agonists on 5-HT_{1A} and/or 5-HT_{2A} receptors.
- A number of drugs are associated with serotonin syndrome, which usually involves combination with an SSRI. These include SSRIs (e.g., citalopram, escitalopram, fluoxetine, fluvoxamine, paroxetine, sertraline); MAOIs; SNRIs (duloxetine, venlafaxine, desvenlafaxine); tricyclic antidepressants (e.g., amitriptyline, clomipramine); other antidepressants (nefazodone, trazodone, mirtazapine); anxiolytic (buspirone); lithium; triptans; anticonvulsants (Depakote); analgesics (fentanyl, meperidine, pentazocine, tramadol); antibiotics/antivirals (linezolid, tedizolid [weak MAOI], ritonavir); over-the-counter (OTC) cough medications (dextromethorphan); some antipsychotics (risperidone, olanzapine); antiemetics (ondansetron, granisetron); other medications, such as metoclopramide, cyclobenzaprine, L-dopa; dietary supplements (tryptophan); herbal supplements (St. John's wort, nutmeg); methylene blue; and drugs of abuse (e.g., methylenedioxymethamphetamine [MDMA], cocaine, D-lysergic acid diethylamide [LSD], and amphetamine) (2)[A]

RISK FACTORS

- Recent dose adjustments or overdose of drugs associated with serotonin syndrome
- The greatest number of adverse events are associated with SSRIs in combination with other substances, and the combination of SSRIs and MAOIs carries the greatest risk of developing serotonin toxicity.

GENERAL PREVENTION

- Consider drug–drug interactions when a multidrug regimen is required and avoid if possible.
- Caution patients about taking SSRIs with OTC medications (e.g., dextromethorphan) or herbal supplements (e.g., St. John's wort) prior to consulting a physician.
- Avoid serotonergic agents for nonpsychiatric disorders (e.g., tramadol for pain relief).

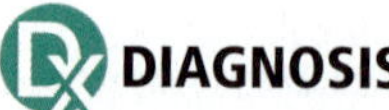

DIAGNOSIS

- Serotonin syndrome is a clinical diagnosis.
- *Hunter Toxicity Criteria Decision Rules* (3) aid in the diagnosis of clinically significant serotonin toxicity (sensitivity, 84%; specificity, 97%). A patient who took a serotonergic agent must have one of the following:
  - Spontaneous clonus
  - Inducible clonus with agitation or diaphoresis
  - Ocular clonus with agitation or diaphoresis
  - Hypertonia and hyperthermia (temperature >38°C) with inducible clonus or ocular clonus (3)[A]
  - Tremor and hyperreflexia

HISTORY

- Obtain a thorough drug history including OTC remedies, dietary and herbal supplements, and illicit drugs. Ask about dose, formulation, and recent changes.
- Review comorbidities (e.g., depression and chronic pain).
- Address possibility of drug overdose and obtain collateral information if intentional overdose is suspected.
- Elicit description of symptoms, including onset and progression.

PHYSICAL EXAM

Initially, patients can develop a peripheral tremor, confusion, and ataxia; systemic signs follow (e.g., agitation, diaphoresis, hyperreflexia, and shivering). Severe signs include fever, jerking, and diarrhea.

- Neuromuscular abnormalities:
  - Mild: hyperreflexia, myoclonus, and tremor all greater in lower extremities; bilateral Babinski sign
  - Moderate: opsoclonus, spontaneous or inducible clonus (involuntary muscle contractions, most commonly tested by rapid dorsiflexion of foot)
  - Severe: rigidity, respiratory failure, tonic–clonic seizure
- Autonomic dysfunction:
  - Mild: diaphoresis, mydriasis, tachycardia
  - Moderate: hyperactive bowel sounds, diarrhea, nausea, vomiting, hyperthermia (<40°C)
  - Severe: hyperthermia (≥40°C), labile blood pressure (BP)
- Mental status changes:
  - Mild: anxiety, akathisia (restlessness), insomnia
  - Moderate: agitation
  - Severe: coma, delirium, confusion
- Severe cases have led to altered level of consciousness, rhabdomyolysis, metabolic acidosis, disseminated intravascular coagulation (DIC), and acute respiratory distress syndrome (ARDS) (3)[A].

DIFFERENTIAL DIAGNOSIS

- Neuroleptic malignant syndrome (NMS): lead pipe rigidity and extrapyramidal features without clonus or hyperreflexia
- Anticholinergic fever (e.g., benztropine, diphenhydramine, oxybutynin, nifedipine, famotidine, atropine, scopolamine; plant poisoning from belladonna/"deadly nightshade"): urinary retention, decreased bowel sounds, normal reflexes
- Malignant hyperthermia: generally following administration of anesthetics or depolarizing muscle relaxants
- CNS infection (e.g., meningitis, encephalitis) and heat stroke
- Sympathomimetic toxicity (e.g., cocaine, methamphetamine, PCP)
- Hyperthyroidism (thyroid storm)
- Tetanus and rabies

DIAGNOSTIC TESTS & INTERPRETATION

- Serum serotonin levels do not correlate with clinical findings.
- Nonspecific lab findings may include:
  - Elevated WBC, creatine phosphokinase, hepatic transaminases
  - Decreased serum bicarbonate
- Consider urine toxicology screening for illicit drugs.

TREATMENT

Supportive care is the mainstay of therapy: administrating oxygen and aggressive IV fluids, continuous cardiac monitoring, monitoring urine output, and stabilizing vital signs.

- Benzodiazepines may be effective for the management of agitation.
- Administration of serotonin antagonists: Cyproheptadine may be useful if supportive measures and sedation (benzodiazepines) are unable to control agitation and correct vital signs. This agent does not reduce the duration of serotonin syndrome.
- Mild cases (afebrile, tachycardia, shivering, diaphoresis, mydriasis, hyperreflexia, intermittent tremor or myoclonus)
  - Discontinue precipitating agent(s).
  - Supportive care and sedation
  - Observe for 12 to 24 hours.
- Moderate cases (temperature >38°C, autonomic instability, hyperactive bowel sounds, diarrhea, diaphoresis, ocular clonus, hyperreflexia, tremor, mild agitation, or hypervigilance)
  - Interventions as listed above for mild cases
  - Aggressive treatment of autonomic instability
  - Treatment with cyproheptadine should be initiated if agitation and vital sign abnormalities are unimproved with benzodiazepines and supportive care.
  - Hypotension from MAOI interactions should be treated with low doses of direct-acting sympathomimetics (e.g., norepinephrine, phenylephrine, epinephrine); indirect serotonin agonists, such as dopamine, should be avoided.
  - Severe hypertension and tachycardia should be treated with short-acting agents, such as nitroprusside or esmolol.
- Severe cases (temperature >41.1°C, autonomic instability, delirium, muscular rigidity, and hypertonicity)
  - Discontinue precipitating agent(s).
  - Immediate sedation and endotracheal intubation as indicated
  - Paralysis as clinically indicated (maintained with nondepolarizing continuous paralytic agents such as vecuronium, cisatracurium, rocuronium)

MEDICATION

- Benzodiazepines: may be used to manage agitation in serotonin syndrome and also may correct mild increases in BP and heart rate. Use with caution in patients with delirium, given the known paradoxical effect of exacerbating delirium.
- Cyproheptadine (Periactin):
  - Adult: initial dose 12 mg PO (can also be crushed and given via nasogastric [NG] tube) followed by 2 mg q2h until clinical response observed; 12 to 32 mg of drug may be required in a 24-hour period.
  - Pediatric:
    - <2 years old: 0.06 mg/kg q6h
    - 2 to 6 years old: 2 mg q6h
    - 7 to 14 years old: 4 mg q6h

ISSUES FOR REFERRAL

- Psychiatry: for assistance with medication management and follow-up care (inpatient psychiatric care vs. outpatient psychiatric follow-up)
- Toxicology/clinical pharmacology service
- Poison control center

ADMISSION, INPATIENT, AND NURSING CONSIDERATIONS

- ICU admission is often indicated in severe cases.
- Discharge when mental status has returned to baseline, with stable vital and neurologic (e.g., clonus) signs. Ensure close follow-up.

ONGOING CARE

FOLLOW-UP RECOMMENDATIONS

- In mild cases, address risks and benefits of restarting offending agents. Serotonergic medications need to be titrated slowly, and patients must have close outpatient follow-up.
- In severe cases the offending agent should likely not be resumed unless precipitant for serotonin syndrome is found (e.g., combination with another serotonin agonist); the patient can be carefully monitored, or there is a clear benefit versus risk of restarting the medication.

PROGNOSIS

Most cases resolve within 24 hours of discontinuation of serotonergic agents; this can be longer depending on the drug's half-life:

- MAOIs can result in toxicity for several days.
- SSRIs can result in toxicity for up to several weeks after discontinuation.

COMPLICATIONS

Adverse outcomes, including death, are usually the consequence of poorly treated hyperthermia and may include acute renal failure, ARDS, arrhythmia, coma, DIC, seizure, metabolic acidosis, multiorgan failure, myoglobinuria, respiratory arrest, and rhabdomyolysis.

REFERENCES

1. Mikkelsen N, Damkier P, Pedersen SA. Serotonin syndrome—a focused review. *Basic Clin Pharmacol Toxicol*. 2023;133(2):124–129. doi:10.1111/bcpt.13912.
2. Moss MJ, Hendrickson RG; Toxicology Investigators Consortium (ToxIC). Serotonin toxicity: associated agents and clinical characteristics. *J Clin Psychopharmacol*. 2019;39(6):628–633.
3. Dunkley EJC, Isbister GK, Sibbritt D, et al. The hunter serotonin toxicity criteria: simple and accurate diagnostic decision rules for serotonin toxicity. *QJM*. 2003;96(9):635–642.

ADDITIONAL READING

Mas Serrano M, Pérez-Sánchez JR, Portela Sánchez S, et al. Serotonin syndrome in two COVID-19 patients treated with lopinavir/ritonavir. *J Neurol Sci*. 2020;415:116944.

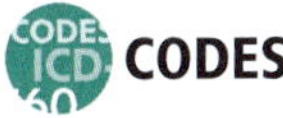

CODES

ICD10

G25.79 Other drug induced movement disorders

CLINICAL PEARLS

Consider serotonin syndrome in patients with recent use of a serotonergic agent (particularly if multiple proserotonergic agents are involved) presenting with unexplained tachycardia, hypertension, hyperthermia, clonus, hyperreflexia, and change in mental status.

SEXUAL DYSFUNCTION IN WOMEN

Shelby Takeshita, MD • Rachel KM McCool, MD

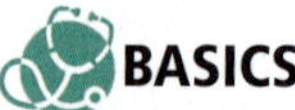

BASICS

- Female sexual dysfunction (FSD) is a common multifactorial concern faced by ~43% of women in the United States, impacting individuals of multiple ages and reproductive statuses.
- Evaluation should include exploration across biomedical, sexual, and psychosocial etiologies and may involve elements from multiple of these areas.
- Management includes a comprehensive laboratory assessment and treatment tailored to individual patient goals.

DESCRIPTION

- According to the *DSM-5*, FSD is defined as sexual concerns arising from desire, arousal, orgasm, or sexual pain leading to personal distress for >6 months and present >75% of the time (1).
- FSD often arises from four domains: female sexual interest and arousal, female orgasmic, genito-pelvic pain/penetration, or substance/medication-induced (2).
- FSD can be lifelong, acquired, generalized, or situational depending on the underlying cause.
- Note: For purposes of this article, discussion will focus on individuals assigned female at birth who identify as female, with the understanding that sexual dysfunction can occur across all genders with similar and unique challenges as those described below.

EPIDEMIOLOGY

According to data from the American College of Obstetricians and Gynecologists, 43% of women disclose sexual function concerns, of whom 12% endorse it causing personal distress (2).

Incidence

- Sexual dysfunction can occur at any age, with underlying etiology varying across the lifespan and rates increasing with age.
- In women treated for gynecologic (GYN) cancers, 74% endorse FSD and 40% experience dyspareunia.
- 83% of women experience FSD in first 3 months after childbirth and may never return to incidence in nulliparous peers (1).

Prevalence

- Sexual dysfunction prevalence varies by age, with the highest prevalence being 15% in women aged 45 to 65 years.
- Prevalence in women aged 18 to 44 years is 10%, whereas prevalence in women aged 65 to 85 years is 9% (2).
- Prevalence increases in women with pelvic organ prolapse, urinary incontinence, and subfertility (1).

ETIOLOGY AND PATHOPHYSIOLOGY

The female sexual response follows a nonlinear model requiring motivation, arousal (physical and subjective), willingness, and neural inputs (2). Thus, pathophysiology of sexual dysfunction is complex and multifactorial, with underlying cause varying between patients. These may include:

- Changes in sex hormones: Sex hormones are important in creating a neurochemical sexual response in the central nervous system and urogenital level, leading to changes in lubrication, clitoral engorgement, pelvic neurovasculature, and pelvic floor function.
- Central nervous system: Neuroendocrine circuits impact the emotional and behavioral aspects of sexual function including arousal, orgasm, and desire (3).
- Comorbid illness: Comorbidities such as diabetes, cardiovascular disease, malignancy, or neurologic disease can impact the above processes as well as psychological view of themselves and their sexuality.
- Psychological: Mood disorders, stress, alcohol/substance use impact the above model of the female sexual response.
- Iatrogenic: Multiple medications impact sexual functioning (2).
- Individual factors: Sleep, relationship concerns, body image, trauma, societal attitudes toward sexuality, and more all impact the above model of female sexual response (3).

RISK FACTORS

Sexual dysfunction in women is a multifactorial issue, often including a combination of biologic and psychosocial causes.

- Menopause: changing body image, genitourinary syndrome of menopause
- Education: lack of knowledge about sexual stimulation and response
- Psychological: mood disorders, personality disorders, substance abuse, or psychopathies
- Chronic medical problems: cardiovascular, endocrine, dermatologic, neurologic, malignancy, medication effects
- GYN issues: childbirth, pelvic floor or bladder dysfunction, endometriosis, uterine fibroids, chronic vulvovaginal candidiasis/vaginal infections, female genital mutilation, breastfeeding
- Relationship factors: safety, intimate partner violence, discrepancies in partners' expectations, cultural attitudes towards sexuality, sexual trauma (2)

GENERAL PREVENTION

Ways to help evaluate for, support, and assist in prevention include:

- Practice trauma-informed care in clinic.
- Perform sexual dysfunction screening at routine visits.
- Normalize FSD in discussion.
- Assess patient safety at every visit (2).

COMMONLY ASSOCIATED CONDITIONS

History of sexual trauma, marital/relationship discord, psychiatric disorders, malignancy, menopause, pregnancy/childbirth, abnormal uterine bleeding, pelvic pain, incontinence, pelvic organ prolapse

DIAGNOSIS

- Take a thorough sexual history and perform trauma-informed genitourinary exam if indicated based on areas of concern from history.
- Diagnosis will require assessment of the above multifactorial etiologies for FSD to determine cause/management.
- Helpful screening tools: Female Sexual Function Index, Female Sexual Distress Scale (2)

HISTORY

- Obtain current medical, obstetric, and psychiatric history.
- Obtain thorough sexual history including questions on safety, pain, sexuality, sexual partners, lubrication, arousal, libido, and orgasm.
- Evaluate current medication list for potential side effects.
- Discuss current life stressors and social circumstances.

PHYSICAL EXAM

- Follow trauma-informed principles during physical exam, allowing patient to guide speed and content of exam.
- Examine vulva visually for rashes/lesions and evaluate for pain with cotton swab on vestibule.
- Perform speculum exam to evaluate for lesions, prolapse, or cervical abnormalities.
- Perform bimanual exam, with focus on tense or painful pelvic floor muscles, cervical motion tenderness, or pelvic masses.
- During exam, pay attention to vascular and neurologic findings.

DIFFERENTIAL DIAGNOSIS

- Pelvic floor and uterine disorders: fibroids, endometriosis, sexually transmitted infection (STI), cancer, pregnancy, urinary incontinence, vaginismus, female orgasmic disorder, genito-pelvic pain disorder
- Vulvar disorders: genitourinary syndrome of menopause, lichen sclerosis, genital mutilation
- Hormonal concerns: menopause, pregnancy, breastfeeding
- Psychosocial concerns: stressors, mental health disorders, prior abuse, body image, societal stereotypes
- Cardiovascular history: hypertension, heart failure, vascular disease
- Neurologic disorders: stroke, multiple sclerosis, spinal cord injury
- Gastrointestinal disorders: irritable bowel disease, liver failure
- Endocrine disorders: diabetes, adrenal insufficiency, thyroid disease
- Iatrogenic: selective serotonin reuptake inhibitors (SSRIs), chemotherapy, surgical menopause, steroids

DIAGNOSTIC TESTS & INTERPRETATION

Labs and imaging can assist in identifying causes for FSD.

Initial Tests (lab, imaging)

- Lab testing is generally not indicated unless there is concern for underlying medical conditions (2)[C].
- Labs to consider based on unique patient history: FSH, estradiol, free androgen index and sex hormone binding globulin, thyroid function, prolactin, ferritin, lipid panel, HbA1c, STI screening (2)[C]
- Can consider pelvic or abdominal imaging if concern for structural issue

Follow-Up Tests & Special Considerations

Because there is no standard workup for FSD, testing must be individualized to the patient, the symptoms described, and patient history. During workup, it is important to validate and normalize FSD.

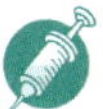

TREATMENT

Treatment should be multifactorial in nature and tailored to the patient. It is important to address underlying medical/psychiatric conditions and use a mixture of the medical and lifestyle therapies discussed below.

GENERAL MEASURES

- Identify if patient has underlying medical conditions influencing sexual function, or if the patient is taking medications which may impact function.
- Provide education on vulvovaginal care. Counsel on use of lubricants that are similar to vaginal pH and osmolarity (2)[C].
- Educate patient on relationship safety and communication.
- Lifestyle education surrounding sleep, nutrition, decreased alcohol/substance use, and smoking cessation

MEDICATION

- Lubricants improve dyspareunia due to vaginal dryness.
- Hormonal medications:
  - Low-dose vaginal estrogen: assists in postmenopausal dryness and pain by improving lubrication and vaginal pH; preferred hormonal treatment for FSD due to genitourinary syndrome of menopause (2),(3)[C]
  - Transdermal testosterone: can assist with libido and short-term use can be considered for postmenopausal women with sexual interest or arousal disorders; obtain baseline testosterone and repeat in 3 to 6 weeks to keep within normal range. Stop if patient has no response after 6-month trial (2)[C]; insufficient evidence for use in premenopausal women (3)[C]
  - Ospemifene: selective estrogen receptor modulator (SERM) approved for postmenopausal dryness and pain; can be considered in individuals not responsive to vaginal estrogen (2),(3)[C]
  - Estrogen or SERM therapy is only recommended for treatment of FSD due to hypoestrogenic state (2)[C].
- Central nervous system medications:
  - Bupropion: adjunct for SSRI-induced sexual dysfunction; may be used daily or prior to planned sexual activity
  - Flibanserin: serotonin agonist approved for hypoactive desire disorder in premenopausal women without depression (2),(3)[C]; patients should be counseled they cannot drink alcohol while on this therapy.
  - Bremelanotide: melanocortin agonist administered as an on-demand injection before sexual activity (3)[C]
- Tibolone: synthetic steroid used for menopausal symptoms; however, can have increased risk of stroke and is not approved in the United States (3)[C]

First Line

- First-line therapy should include lifestyle counseling and nonpharmacologic interventions.
- For postmenopausal dysfunction, vaginal estrogen is included in first-line therapies unless contraindicated.

Second Line

Second-line therapy will vary based on the underlying cause of FSD.

ISSUES FOR REFERRAL

Referrals are warranted for underlying muscular, structural, social, or psychological basis of pain.

ADDITIONAL THERAPIES

Nonpharmacologic therapies play a large role in managing FSD, including:

- Pelvic floor physical therapy (PT): helps patients with self-awareness, strength, control, and confidence while decreasing vaginismus and improving libido (2)[C]
- Vaginal dilators: helpful with vaginismus or vaginal stenosis; initiating treatment with a small dilator under supervision of a specialist, or in combination with other therapies is most beneficial.
- Psychotherapy: cognitive behavioral therapy, psychosexual counseling, sexual skills training, couples therapy, mindfulness-based therapy (2)[C]

SURGERY/OTHER PROCEDURES

Surgical interventions such as laser therapy and trigger point injections are under investigation, currently not recommended outside clinical trials (2)[C].

COMPLEMENTARY & ALTERNATIVE MEDICINE

- Self-stimulation devices
- Yoga
- Relaxation techniques or mindfulness based practices
- Hypnotherapy (1)

ADMISSION, INPATIENT, AND NURSING CONSIDERATIONS

Indications depend on individual underlying cause of dysfunction.

ONGOING CARE

Multiple visits may be necessary due to issues identified which require further exploration and to help destigmatize discussion of sexual function (2)[C].

FOLLOW-UP RECOMMENDATIONS

As needed for continued lifestyle and medication-based interventions

Patient Monitoring

Follow up with patients as needed for symptom level, and for underlying comorbid conditions

DIET

Encourage patient to consume healthy diet and maintain ideal body weight.

PATIENT EDUCATION

- American Association of Sexuality Educators, Counselors, and Therapists: https://www.aasect.org
- National Women's Health Resource Center: https://www.healthywomen.org
- Meet Rosy: https://meetrosy.com/ (online platform and app for sexual wellness)
- International Society for the Study of Women's Sexual Health: https://www.isswsh.org
- Come As You Are Workbook by Emily Nagoski

PROGNOSIS

Prognosis depends on the underlying cause for FSD. Certain therapies such as pelvic floor PT have been proven to improve function in 39% of women after 6 months of therapy.

COMPLICATIONS

If untreated, FSD can lead to decreased quality of life, relationship conflict, and mood-based symptoms.

S

REFERENCES

1. Kershaw V, Jha S. Female sexual dysfunction. *Obstet Gynecol*. 2022;24(1):12–23. doi:10.1111/tog.12778.
2. American College of Obstetricians and Gynecologists. Female sexual dysfunction: ACOG practice bulletin clinical management guidelines for obstetrician-gynecologists, number 213. *Obstet Gynecol*. 2019;134(1):e1–e18. doi:10.1097/AOG.0000000000003324.
3. Nappi RE, Tiranini L, Martini E, et al. Medical treatment of female sexual dysfunction. *Urol Clin North Am*. 2022;49(2):299–307. doi:10.1016/j.ucl.2022.02.001.

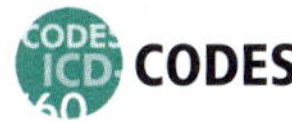

CODES

ICD10

- R37 Sexual dysfunction, unspecified
- F52.0 Hypoactive sexual desire disorder
- N94.1 Dyspareunia

CLINICAL PEARLS

- FSD is a common, complex, multifactorial problem.
- Causes of FSD can be identified with thorough history and physical exam.
- Symptoms of sexual dysfunction peak in women aged 45 to 64 years.
- Combination of behavioral, physical, and medical therapy leads to greater treatment success.

SHOULDER PAIN

Michael J. Maddaleni, MD, CAQSM

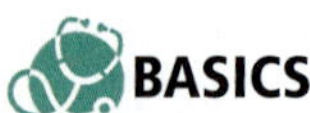

BASICS

DESCRIPTION

- Shoulder pain commonly affects patients of all ages.
- Causes include acute trauma, overuse during sports, infection, and activities of everyday living.
- Age plays an important role in determining the etiology of shoulder pain.
- Onset and characteristics of pain, mechanism of injury, and limitation in activity or sport narrow the differential diagnosis.

EPIDEMIOLOGY

- Shoulder pain accounts for 16% of all musculoskeletal (MSK) complaints.
- The lifetime prevalence of shoulder pain is ~70%.
- Predominant etiology varies with age:
  - <30 years: shoulder instability, overuse injuries, impingement syndrome
  - 30 to 60 years: rotator cuff (RTC) disorder, impingement syndrome, partial tears
  - >60 years: full-thickness tear, glenohumeral OA

Incidence

The incidence of shoulder pain is 7 to 25 cases per 1,000 patients, with a peak incidence in the 4th to 6th decades of life.

ETIOLOGY AND PATHOPHYSIOLOGY

Pathology varies with cause:

- Trauma—fracture, dislocation, ligament/tendon tear, acromioclavicular (AC) separation
- Overuse—RTC pathology, biceps tenosynovitis, bursitis, muscle strain, apophyseal injuries, labral injuries
- RTC disorders most commonly result from repetitive overhead activity, leading to RTC impingement with a three-stage progression:
  - Stage I: tendinopathy
  - Stage II: partial RTC tear
  - Stage III: full-thickness RTC tear
- Subacromial bursitis can occur with RTC disorders but is rarely an isolated diagnosis.
- Age related: In pediatric athletes, instability and physeal injuries are more common. With increasing age, the incidence of AC and glenohumeral joint OA, adhesive capsulitis, and RTC tear rises.
- Rheumatologic: rheumatoid arthritis, polymyalgia rheumatica, fibromyalgia
- Infectious: septic arthritis
- Referred pain: neck, gallbladder, diaphragm

RISK FACTORS

- Repetitive overhead activity
- Overhead and upper extremity weight-bearing sports (baseball, softball, swimming, tennis, volleyball, football)
- Weight lifting: AC joint disorders
- Rapid increases in training frequency or load (often associated with improper technique)
- Muscle weakness or imbalance
- Trauma or fall onto the shoulder
- Diabetes, thyroid disorders and other autoimmune diseases, female gender, and age 40 to 60 years are risk factors for adhesive capsulitis.

GENERAL PREVENTION

- Maintain strength and range of motion (ROM).
- Avoid repetitive overhead activities such as pitch counts in younger baseball athletes.
- Proper technique (pitching, weight lifting)

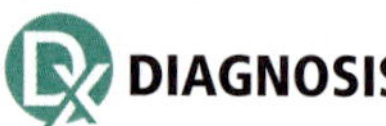

DIAGNOSIS

HISTORY

- Pain characteristics location:
  - Superior: AC pathology, trapezius strain
  - Lateral: RTC pathology, deltoid pathology
  - Anterior: proximal biceps tendinosis, labrum pathology, glenohumeral OA
  - Diffuse pain: RTC pathology, adhesive capsulitis, glenohumeral OA
- Descriptors:
  - Night pain, worse lying on affected side: RTC pathology, adhesive capsulitis, glenohumeral OA
  - Stiff shoulder, limited ROM: adhesive capsulitis, glenohumeral OA
- Aggravating movements:
  - Cross-body adduction, "scarf test": AC pathology
  - Abduction/external rotation (reaching behind): instability, RTC pathology, glenohumeral OA
  - Overhead activity: RTC pathology, AC pathology, labrum pathology, glenohumeral OA
  - Turning neck, pain past elbow: cervical pathology
- Mechanism of injury
  - Forceful abduction and external rotation: traumatic shoulder instability/dislocation
  - Fall directly onto lateral shoulder: AC joint sprain or separation, clavicular fracture
  - Repetitive overhead activity: RTC pathology
  - Fall on outstretched hand (FOOSH): shoulder separation; forearm/wrist fracture
- Age
  - Shoulder instability (subluxation, dislocation, multidirectional instability) is the most common cause of shoulder pain in young athletes (<30 years old).
  - RTC disorders are the most common cause of shoulder pain in patients >30 years old. Severity of RTC disorder increases with age.
  - Older patients (>60 years old) commonly have OA.
  - Trauma in a young person <40 years old is more commonly associated with dislocation/subluxation. In patients >40 years old, trauma is more commonly associated with RTC tear.

PHYSICAL EXAM

- Three main joints combine to create the shoulder: glenohumeral, AC, and sternoclavicular (SC).
- Four RTC muscles/tendons (SITS): supraspinatus (abduction), infraspinatus (external rotation), teres minor (external rotation, adduction), and subscapularis (adduction, internal rotation)
- Observe face and shoulder movements as patient disrobes, moves arm, and shakes hand.
- Inspect for malalignment, muscle atrophy, asymmetry, erythema, ecchymosis, and swelling. Scapular winging suggests long thoracic nerve or muscular (trapezius, serratus anterior) dysfunction. Prominent scapular spine with scalloped infraspinatus fossa suggests infraspinatus atrophy.
- Palpate SC joint, AC joint, acromion, biceps tendon for tenderness, warmth, or bony step-offs.
- Evaluate active *and* passive ROM and flexibility.
- Decreased active *and* passive ROM is more common with adhesive capsulitis. Normal abduction is to 180 degrees.
- Pain from 60 to 180 degrees suggests subacromial impingement; 120 to 180 degrees suggests AC joint pathology.
- Mildly decreased active and/or passive ROM may also indicate glenohumeral OA.
- Decreased active ROM with full passive ROM: RTC pathology
- Evaluate for muscle strength, including grip, biceps, triceps, and deltoid.
- Test RTC strength: supraspinatus (empty can test), infraspinatus/teres minor (resisted external rotation, external lag test), subscapularis (lift-off test, belly press, resisted internal rotation).
- Pain with RTC strength testing indicates RTC pathology. Weakness could suggest tear.
- Special diagnostic tests
  - Neer RTC impingement test: Examiner stabilizes the scapula and internally rotates the patient's arm and flexes the shoulder through the full ROM or until the patient reports pain.
  - Hawkins RTC impingement test: Examiner internally rotates the shoulder with the elbow, and shoulder flexed to 90 degrees to the end of ROM or until the patient reports pain.
  - Drop-arm test for RTC tear: positive if patient is unable to smoothly control the lowering of their arm or to hold the arm in 90 degrees of abduction
  - Cross-arm adduction (Scarf test) is painful in AC joint arthritis or sprain.
  - Speed test for biceps tendinopathy: With arm 30 degrees of flexion and palm supinated, patient attempts to flex the elbow against resistance. Pain over biceps is positive.
  - Yergason test for biceps tendinopathy: With the elbow stabilized to the patient's side and flexed to 90 degrees, place the patient's forearm in pronation and resist against supination.
  - Apprehension, relocation test for anterior glenohumeral joint instability: Examiner supports the elbow of the patient and with the other hand holding the wrist, slowly externally rotates the humerus with the shoulder at 90 degrees abduction, patient apprehensive with maneuver.
  - Sulcus sign for inferior glenohumeral joint instability: Examiner pulls down with the hand grasping the subject's elbow, positive if significant inferior movement of the arm, relative to shoulder.
  - O'Brien, clunk test for labral pathology: Move arm at 90 degrees of flexion, 10 degrees of adduction, thumb pointed down (arm in internal rotation), examiner resists flexion distally. Maintain same position, and have the patient turn thumb up. Pain with thumb down and no pain with thumb up is positive.
  - Spurling test for cervical pathology: rotation of head toward side of symptoms along with neck extension with applied downward force to reproduce radicular symptoms

DIFFERENTIAL DIAGNOSIS
- Fracture (clavicle, humerus, scapula), contusion
- RTC disorder: impingement, tear, calcific tendonitis
- Subacromial bursitis
- Scapulothoracic dyskinesis
- AC joint pathology (AC separation/OA, osteolysis)
- Biceps tenosynovitis or tear
- Acromial apophysitis or os acromiale
- Glenohumeral joint OA
- Glenohumeral joint instability (acute dislocation or chronic multidirectional instability)
- Adhesive capsulitis
- Labral tear or associated bony pathology
- Muscle strain (trapezius, deltoid, biceps)
- Cervical radiculopathy
- Other: autoimmune, rheumatologic, referred pain, septic joint (biliary/splenic, cardiac, pneumonia/lung mass)

DIAGNOSTIC TESTS & INTERPRETATION
Initial Tests (lab, imaging)
- A history of significant trauma, prolonged symptoms, or red flags (older age, fever, rest pain) suggests a need for imaging.
- Adults with nontraumatic shoulder pain of <4 weeks duration may not require initial imaging.
- Plain radiographs anteroposterior, scapular Y, axillary views
- EMG study of the upper extremity may help differentiate referred cervical pain and brachial plexopathy from a primary shoulder disorder.
- Obtain ECG if any suspicion for cardiac etiology.
- Serologic tests if autoimmune etiology is suspected

Follow-Up Tests & Special Considerations
- MRI is gold standard for noninvasive soft tissue imaging, including RTC, biceps tendon.
- MR arthrogram may be necessary to assess for labral tears and instability.
- Ultrasound (US) can assess for RTC tears, biceps tendinopathy, and AC joint pathology.
- US can be equivalent to MRI in detecting full-thickness tears (sensitivity 92%, specificity 94%) and partial-thickness tears (sensitivity 67%, specificity 94%).

Test Interpretation
- Tendinosis rather than tendonitis is common with stage I impingement.
- Capsular scarring is the hallmark of adhesive capsulitis.
- RTC enthesophytes visualized with calcific tendonitis
- Tear enlargement and pain development in asymptomatic tears are more common with involvement of the dominant shoulder.

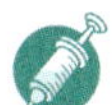

TREATMENT
- In general, conservative therapy includes activity modification, analgesics, and/or anti-inflammatory medicines in association with appropriate rehabilitative programs.
- Physical therapy almost always required for full resolution

MEDICATION
First Line
- Analgesics and anti-inflammatory medications for symptomatic relief
- Corticosteroid injections (subacromial, glenohumeral, AC, subscapular bursa) can be used to acutely relieve pain due to RTC pathology, adhesive capsulitis, OA, or scapulothoracic dyskinesis.
- Steroid injections can improve ability to engage in rehabilitative activities.
- Platelet-rich plasma (PRP) and prolotherapy techniques can also be used; evidence of their benefit is unclear.
- US guidance improves accuracy of anatomic placement of corticosteroid injections; long-term outcomes have thus far been shown to be similar between US-guided versus nonguided injections

ISSUES FOR REFERRAL
- If etiology remains unclear, patient is not responsive to conservative care, for complicated or displaced fractures.
- Full-thickness RTC tears >1 cm (acute or chronic) in patients <65 years old or any tear with significant changes in functional status require surgical referral. These tears have a high rate of progression, fatty infiltration, or retraction with nonoperative care.

ADDITIONAL THERAPIES
- Physical therapy can benefit persistent RTC disorders, adhesive capsulitis, and shoulder instability.
- Manual therapy and exercises may improve pain and increase function in RTC disease.
- Manual manipulative therapy (MMT) by osteopathic physicians or physical therapists improves pain with adhesive capsulitis, RTC, and soft tissue disorders. In adhesive capsulitis, MMT is generally less effective than glucocorticoid injections at 6-week mark, but both have similar long-term outcomes. Acupuncture may improve short-term pain and function in RTC impingement.
- Adhesive capsulitis: Treatment typically begins with a corticosteroid injection or a hydrodilatation of the capsule.

SURGERY/OTHER PROCEDURES
- Surgery is recommended for shoulder pain caused by acute displaced fractures, large RTC tears (criteria as above). It may also be recommended for multiple shoulder dislocation in patients <20 years of age.
- Surgery can be considered for shoulder pain unresponsive to conservative measures >3 to 6 months. Surgery is not more effective than active nonsurgical treatment in impingement syndrome.
- Orthobiologic techniques including PRP injections are more frequently being used in MSK medicine.

COMPLEMENTARY & ALTERNATIVE MEDICINE
Acupuncture may help with acute shoulder pain.

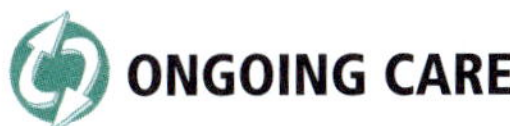

ONGOING CARE

PROGNOSIS
Shoulder pain generally has a favorable outcome with conservative care, but recovery can be slow, with 40–50% of patients complaining of persistent pain or recurrence at 12 months.

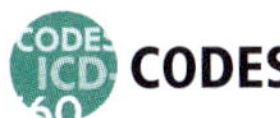

CODES

ICD10
M25.519 Pain in unspecified shoulder

CLINICAL PEARLS
- RTC disorders (tendinopathy, tears) are the most common cause of shoulder pain in individuals >30 years of age.
- Shoulder instability (acute dislocation/subluxation or chronic instability) is the most common source of shoulder pain in individuals <30 years of age.
- Patients with diabetes are at increased risk for adhesive capsulitis.
- Most patients do well with a structured program of pain control and rehabilitation.

SINUSITIS

Chirag N. Shah, MD • Grant Wei, MD, FACEP • James Mack, DO

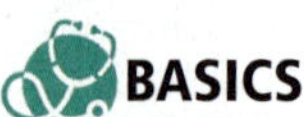

BASICS

DESCRIPTION

- Acute sinusitis is a symptomatic inflammation of ≥1 paranasal sinuses of <4 weeks duration resulting from impaired drainage and retained secretions accompanied by obstruction, facial pain/pressure/fullness. Rhinitis and sinusitis typically coexist; "rhinosinusitis" is the preferred term.
- Disease is subacute when symptomatic for 4 to 12 weeks, recurrent acute when ≥4 annual episodes without persistent symptoms in between, and chronic when symptomatic >12 weeks.
- Uncomplicated rhinosinusitis has no extension of inflammation beyond the paranasal sinuses and nasal cavity.

EPIDEMIOLOGY

- Affects 1 in 8 adults (>30 million people in the U.S. yearly diagnosed with rhinosinusitis)
- Acute bacterial rhinosinusitis remains the fifth leading reason for prescribing antibiotics.
- Viral cause in 90–98% of cases with 0.5–2.0% having a bacterial superinfection.

Incidence

Incidence is highest in early fall through early spring (related to the incidence of viral upper respiratory infection [URI]). Adults have two to three viral URIs yearly; 90% of colds are accompanied by viral rhinosinusitis. It is the fifth most common diagnosis during family physician visits.

ETIOLOGY AND PATHOPHYSIOLOGY

- Important features
  - Inflammation and edema of the sinus mucosa lead to obstruction of the sinus ostia causing impaired mucociliary clearance and stagnation of secretions that become hospitable to bacterial growth.
- Neutrophil influx and release of cytokines damage mucosal surfaces.
- Viral: majority cases (rhinovirus; influenza A and B; parainfluenza; respiratory syncytial, adenovirus, coronavirus, and enterovirus)
- Bacterial (complicates 0.5–2.0% of viral cases)
  - More likely if symptoms worsen within 5 to 6 days after initial improvement
  - No improvement within 10 days of symptom onset
  - 3 to 4 days of fever >102°F and facial pain and purulent nasal discharge
  - *Streptococcus pneumoniae*, *Haemophilus influenzae*, and *Moraxella catarrhalis* are most common bacterial pathogens.
  - Overdiagnosis may lead to overuse of and increasing resistance to antibiotics.
  - Methicillin-resistant *Staphylococcus aureus* present in 0–15.9% of patients
- Fungal: seen in immunocompromised hosts (uncontrolled diabetes, neutropenia, use of corticosteroids) or as a nosocomial infection; most common etiology is Aspergillus.

RISK FACTORS

- Viral URI
- Allergic rhinitis
- Asthma
- Cigarette smoking
- Dental infections and procedures
- Anatomic variations
  - Tonsillar and adenoid hypertrophy
  - Turbinate hypertrophy, nasal polyps
  - Cleft palate
  - Septal deviations
- Immunodeficiency (e.g., HIV)
- Cystic fibrosis (CF)
- Prolonged supine positioning (i.e., ICU patients)

GENERAL PREVENTION

Handwashing, vaccinations, avoiding symptomatic individuals, avoiding smoking, and exposure to secondhand smoke

DIAGNOSIS

- History and physical exam suggest and establish diagnosis but rarely helpful in distinguishing bacterial from viral causes.
- Use a constellation of symptoms rather than a particular sign or symptom in diagnosis.

HISTORY

- Symptoms somewhat predictive of bacterial sinusitis
  - Worsening of symptoms >5 to 6 days after initial improvement
  - Persistent symptoms for ≥10 days
  - Persistent purulent nasal discharge
  - Unilateral upper tooth or facial pain
  - Unilateral maxillary sinus tenderness
  - Fever
- Associated symptoms
  - Headache
  - Nasal congestion/discharge
  - Retro-orbital pain
  - Otalgia
  - Hyposmia
  - Halitosis
  - Chronic cough
- Symptoms requiring urgent attention
  - Visual disturbances, especially diplopia
  - Periorbital swelling or erythema
  - Altered mental status

PHYSICAL EXAM

- Fever
- Edema and erythema of nasal mucosa
- Purulent discharge
- Tenderness to palpation over sinus(es)
- Pain localized to sinuses bending forward
- Transillumination of the sinuses may confirm fluid in sinuses (helpful if asymmetric; not helpful if symmetric exam).

Pediatric Considerations

- Sinuses are not fully developed until 20 years of age. Maxillary and ethmoid sinuses are present at birth. Frontal sinuses are last to develop.
- Children are at risk for developing sinusitis because they average six to eight colds per year.

DIFFERENTIAL DIAGNOSIS

- Dental disease
- CF
- Wegener granulomatosis
- HIV infection
- Neoplasm
- Nasal foreign body
- Allergic rhinitis
- Headache: tension, cluster, or migraine

DIAGNOSTIC TESTS & INTERPRETATION

Diagnostic tests not routinely recommended; a diagnosis of sinusitis is best made through a history and physical examination.

- Diagnostic testing is often not needed after a clinical diagnosis of sinusitis is made.
- Imaging does not distinguish bacterial from viral etiology.
- CT of maxillofacial without intravenous contrast is recommended for acute recurrent sinusitis, chronic sinusitis, or with contrast if a complication is suspected (1)[C].
- Routine use of sinus radiography is also discouraged as three or more clinical findings have similar diagnostic accuracy as imaging.
- Culture and biopsy are indicated for chronic bacterial sinusitis and fungal sinusitis.

Test Interpretation

- Inflammation, edema, thickened mucosa
- Polyps

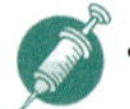

TREATMENT

Most cases resolve with supportive care (treating pain and nasal symptoms). Antibiotics should be reserved for symptoms that persist >10 days, onset with severe symptoms (high fever, purulent nasal discharge, facial pain) for at least 3 to 4 consecutive days, or worsening signs/symptoms that were initially improving (2)[A].

GENERAL MEASURES

- Hydration
- Steam inhalation 20 to 30 minutes TID
- Saline irrigation (Neti pot) or nasal drops
- Sleep with the head of the bed elevated.
- Avoid caffeine, alcohol, exposure to cigarette smoke or fumes.
- Acute viral sinusitis is self-limited; antibiotics only when findings suggest bacterial infection
- Analgesics, nonsteroidal anti-inflammatory drugs (NSAIDs)

MEDICATION

First Line

- Decongestants
  - Pseudoephedrine HCl
  - Phenylephrine nasal spray (limited use)
  - Oxymetazoline (Afrin) nasal spray (not to be used >3 days)
- Analgesics
  - Acetaminophen
  - NSAIDs
- Intranasal steroids
- Meta-analysis shows some small benefits with the addition of intranasal steroids, which may be greater with high doses and with longer course duration.
  - Budesonide (Rhinocort)
  - Mometasone furoate (Nasonex)
  - Fluticasone (Flonase)

- Antibiotics
  - Current professional society guidelines, supported by meta-analysis, suggest antibiotic treatment be restricted to patients that meet specific criteria:
    - Persistent symptoms (≥10 days)
    - Severe symptoms (3 to 4 days)
    - Worsening of symptoms after initial improvement of typical viral upper respiratory tract infection (3 to 4 days)
  - If antibiotics are prescribed, meta-analysis has shown that an antibiotic course of 5 days is noninferior to long courses (3)[A].
  - Reserve antibiotic use for patients with moderate to severe disease.
  - Antibiotics have not been shown to prevent recurrences or complications.
  - Choice should be based on antibiotic resistance in the community.
    - Amoxicillin-clavulanate 875/125 mg q12h; 2 g PO BID in regions with high rates of resistant *Streptococcus pneumoniae*
    - Doxycycline: 100 mg PO BID, an alternative to amoxicillin-clavulanate for initial therapy (adults only)
    - Trimethoprim-sulfamethoxazole (TMP/SMX) and 3rd-generation cephalosporins not recommended due to a high rate of resistance
  - Pediatrics
    - Amoxicillin: 45 to 90 mg/kg/day in 2 divided doses if uncomplicated acute bacterial sinusitis in children
    - Amoxicillin-clavulanate: 80 to 90 mg/6.4 mg/kg/day in 2 divided doses for children with severe illness, recent antibiotics, or attending daycare
    - Levofloxacin: 10 to 20 mg/kg/day max 750 mg/day for severe penicillin (PCN) allergy
    - Clindamycin (30 to 40 mg/kg/day) + cefixime (8 mg/kg/day in 2 divided doses) or cefpodoxime (10 mg/kg/day in 2 divided doses) for non-type 1 PCN allergy
    - Ceftriaxone: 50 mg/kg IM single dose if not able to tolerate oral meds
- Treat children 10 to 14 days if uncomplicated bacterial rhinosinusitis.
  - Inflammation, especially in the case of allergies, may be a predisposing factor, and patients may benefit from the use of the following agents for symptomatic relief.
    - Oral antihistamines
      - Loratadine (Claritin), fexofenadine (Allegra), cetirizine (Zyrtec), desloratadine (Clarinex), or levocetirizine (Xyzal)
      - Chlorpheniramine (Chlor-Trimeton)
      - Diphenhydramine (Benadryl)
    - Intranasal antihistamines
      - Azelastine (Astepro)
    - Ophthalmic antihistamines
      - Ketotifen (Zaditor)
    - Leukotriene inhibitors, especially in patients with asthma
      - Montelukast (Singulair)

Second Line

- Levofloxacin (Levaquin): 750 mg/day for 5 days or moxifloxacin 400 mg/day for 5 to 7 days (adults only)
- No response to first-line therapy >72 hours
  - Broaden antibiotic coverage or switch to a different class; evaluate for resistant pathogens or other causes.
- *Note*: Bacteriologic failure rates of up to 20–25% are possible with use of azithromycin and clarithromycin.
- If lack of response to 3 weeks of antibiotics, consider CT scan of sinuses and ENT referral.

ISSUES FOR REFERRAL

Complications such as periorbital edema, cranial nerve palsies, vision changes, and meningeal signs or failure of treatment

ALERT

- Meta-analyses have demonstrated no benefit of newer antibiotics over amoxicillin or doxycycline (2)[A].
- Higher antibiotic doses and antibiotic therapy taken longer than a standard 7- to 10-day course do not curtail symptom degree or duration.
- Antibiotic recommendations vary with different guidelines. Patients seen by specialists are different from those in a primary care setting. Patients usually do not have complicated sinusitis in a primary care or outpatient setting.
- Consider watchful waiting without antibiotics in patients with uncomplicated mild illness (mild pain and temperature <101°F) with assurance of follow-up within 7 days.
- Consider antihistamines and/or decongestants for symptomatic improvement
- PCV-13 pneumococcal vaccine can help reduce chronic sinusitis in children.
- Use of intranasal steroids shows small but significant improvement in symptoms when used alone or with antibiotics.
- The use of systemic steroids is not indicated.
- Precautions
  - Decongestants can exacerbate hypertension.
  - Intranasal decongestants are limited to 3 days to avoid rebound nasal congestion.

Pregnancy Considerations

- Nasal irrigation with saline, pseudoephedrine, antihistamines, and nasal steroids are safe during pregnancy and lactation.
- Antibiotics safe in pregnancy and lactation: amoxicillin, amoxicillin-clavulanate, cephalosporins
- Antibiotic contraindicated: doxycycline, fluoroquinolones
- Antibiotic safe in lactation but not pregnancy: levofloxacin

SURGERY/OTHER PROCEDURES

- If medical therapy fails, consider sinus irrigation.
- Functional endoscopic sinus surgery is the preferred treatment for medically recalcitrant cases.
- Absolute surgical indications include massive nasal polyposis, subperiosteal or orbital abscess, frontal soft tissue spread of infection, mucocele or mucopyocele, invasive or allergic fungal sinusitis, suspected obstructing tumor, or CSF rhinorrhea.

ADMISSION, INPATIENT, AND NURSING CONSIDERATIONS

Hospitalization for complications (e.g., meningitis, orbital cellulitis or abscess, brain abscess)

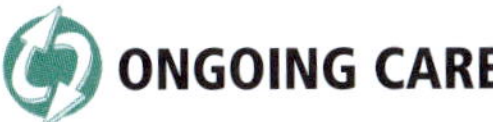

ONGOING CARE

FOLLOW-UP RECOMMENDATIONS

Return if no improvement after 72 hours or no resolution of symptoms after 10 days of antibiotics.

PROGNOSIS

Alleviation of symptoms within 72 hours with complete resolution within 10 to 14 days

COMPLICATIONS

Serious complications (meningitis, orbital cellulitis, brain abscess, cavernous sinus thrombosis, osteomyelitis, subdural empyema) are rare.

S

REFERENCES

1. Wilcox J, Lobo D, Anderson S. Sinusitis. *Prim Care*. 2025;52(1):87–97. doi:10.1016/j.pop.2024.09.010.
2. Shaikh N, Hoberman A, Shope TR, et al. Identifying children likely to benefit from antibiotics for acute sinusitis: a randomized clinical trial. *JAMA*. 2023;330(4):349–358.
3. Kuijpers SME, Buis DTP, Ziesemer KA, et al. The evidence base for the optimal antibiotic treatment duration of upper and lower respiratory tract infections: an umbrella review. *Lancet Infect Dis*. 2025;25(1):94–113. doi:10.1016/S1473-3099(24)00456-0.

ADDITIONAL READING

Conway, SJ, Mueller GD, Shaikh N. Antibiotics for acute sinusitis in children: a meta-analysis. *Pediatrics*. 2024;153(5):e2023064244.

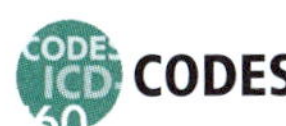

CODES

ICD10

- J01.41 Acute recurrent pansinusitis
- J01.0 Acute maxillary sinusitis
- J01.80 Other acute sinusitis

CLINICAL PEARLS

- Most cases resolve with supportive care (treating pain and nasal symptoms).
- Reserve antibiotics for symptoms >7 to 10 days of mild to moderate symptoms, or if >3 to 4 consecutive days of severe symptoms (high fever, purulent nasal discharge, facial pain).
- Intranasal corticosteroids offer a small therapeutic benefit in acute sinusitis.
- Significant patient symptom relief with antihistamines and saline nasal spray/irrigation

SJÖGREN SYNDROME

Julie A. Creech, DO • Devin Patrick Kearns, DO

BASICS

- First described by Swedish ophthalmologist Henrik Sjögren; chronic autoimmune disorder characterized by inflammation from lymphocytic infiltration of exocrine organs (especially lacrimal and salivary glands) resulting in decreased gland function; typically, presents with sicca symptoms such as dry eyes (xerophthalmia), dry mouth (xerostomia), and parotid enlargement
- Extraglandular manifestations: arthralgia, myalgia, Raynaud phenomenon, pulmonary disease, GI disease, leukopenia, anemia, lymphadenopathy, vasculitis, renal tubular acidosis, lymphoma, CNS involvement with longitudinal transverse myelitis (>4 vertebral segments), and optic neuritis associated with anti–aquaporin-4 antibodies, PNS involvement with small fiber neuropathy
- Primary Sjögren: not associated with other diseases; *HLA-DRB1*0301* and *HLA-DRB1*1501* are the most common
- Secondary Sjögren: occurs in conjunction with other autoimmune rheumatic disorders, such as rheumatoid arthritis (most common); associated with HLA-DR4, systemic lupus erythematous (SLE), or systemic sclerosis

EPIDEMIOLOGY

Incidence

Annual incidence: ~4/100,000

- No racial or geographic predilection
- Predominant sex: female > male (9:1)
- Predominant age at onset: 4th to 5th decades of life

Prevalence

Sjögren syndrome (SS) affects 1 to 4 million people in the United States.

ETIOLOGY AND PATHOPHYSIOLOGY

- Etiology is unknown; theorized to be a viral trigger (EBV, HCV, HTLV-1) in genetically predisposed people
- Pathophysiology involves multifactorial systemic autoimmune process characterized by infiltration of glandular tissue predominately by CD4 T lymphocytes.
  - Theorized that glandular epithelial cells present antigen to the T cells inducing cytokine production, ultimately leading to B-cell dysregulation, autoantibody production, chronic inflammation, and increased incidence of B-cell malignancies.

Genetics

A familial tendency suggests a genetic predisposition.

GENERAL PREVENTION

No known mode of prevention; complications can be prevented by early diagnosis and treatment. Oral health providers play a key role in early detection and management of salivary dysfunction.

COMMONLY ASSOCIATED CONDITIONS

Secondary SS is associated with rheumatoid arthritis, scleroderma, SLE, polymyositis, HIV, hepatitis C, MCTD, PBC, hypergammaglobulinemic purpura, necrotizing vasculitis, autoimmune thyroiditis, chronic active hepatitis, and mixed cryoglobulinemia

Pregnancy Considerations

Pregnant SS patients with high anti-SSA Abs have increased risk of delivering a fetus with congenital heart block. Currently, there are no established evidence-based protocols for screening, prophylaxis, or treatment.

DIAGNOSIS

- 2020 ACR/EULAR classification criteria (1):
  - Inclusion criteria applicable when patient is positive for one ocular/oral dryness symptom (see "History") or at least one positive domain from the EULAR SS disease activity index questionnaire, and a total score of ≥4 from the following:
    - Positive serum anti-SSA/Ro antibody—3 points
    - Focal lymphocytic sialadenitis with a focus score ≥1 foci/4 mm^2 from labial salivary gland biopsy—3 points
    - Abnormal ocular staining score of ≥5 or van Bijsterveld score of ≥4—1 point
    - Schirmer test result of ≤5 mm/5 min—1 point
    - Unstimulated salivary flow rate of ≤0.1 mL/min—1 point
- Ocular signs and symptoms
  - Troublesome dry eyes daily for ≥3 months
  - Recurrent sandy/gritty ocular sensation
  - Use of tear substitute ≥3 times per day
- Oral signs and symptoms
  - Daily dry mouth for ≥3 months
  - Recurrent feeling of swollen salivary glands
  - Need to drink liquid to help swallow dry foods
- Exclusion criteria: prior diagnosis to exclude diagnosis history of head and neck radiation; active hepatitis C (positive PCR) AIDS; sarcoidosis/amyloidosis; graft-versus-host disease
- Other manifestations: chronic arthritis, type 1 RTA, tubular interstitial nephritis, rheumatoid arthritis, vasculitis, vaginal dryness, pleuritis, pancreatitis

HISTORY

- Decreased tear production; burning, scratchy sensation in eyes
- Difficulty speaking or swallowing, dental caries, xerotrachea
- Enlarged or intermittent swelling of parotid glands (bilateral)
- Dyspareunia or vaginal dryness
- Questions for patients from consensus criteria and EULAR questionnaire:
  - Have you had daily, persistent, troublesome dry eyes for >3 months?
  - Do you have a recurrent sensation of sand or gravel in the eyes?
  - Do you use tear substitutes >3 times a day?
  - Have you had a daily feeling of dry mouth for >3 months?
  - Do you frequently drink liquids to aid in swallowing dry food?

PHYSICAL EXAM

- Eye exam: dry eyes (keratoconjunctivitis sicca), decreased tear pool in the lower conjunctiva, dilated conjunctival vessels, mucinous threads, filamentary keratosis (slit-lamp examination)
- Oral exam: dry mouth (xerostomia); decreased sublingual salivary pool (tongue sticks to tongue depressor); frequent oral caries (sometimes in unusual locations such as the incisor surface and along the gum line [cervical portion of the teeth]); dark red tongue from prolonged xerostomia
- Ear, nose, and throat exam: parotid enlargement, submandibular enlargement
- Skin exam: vasculitic purpura (typically 2 to 3 mm in diameter and on the lower extremities)

DIFFERENTIAL DIAGNOSIS

- Causes of ocular dryness: hypovitaminosis A, decreased tear production unrelated to autoimmune process (i.e., age related), chronic blepharitis or conjunctivitis, impaired blinking (i.e., due to Parkinson disease or Bell palsy), infiltration of lacrimal glands (i.e., amyloidosis, lymphoma, sarcoidosis), low estrogen levels
- Causes of oral dryness: medications (anticholinergics, antihistamines, antidepressants), dehydration, anxiety, sialadenitis due to chronic obstruction, chronic viral infections (e.g., hepatitis C or HIV), radiation of head/neck, candidiasis, burning mouth syndrome
- Causes of salivary gland swelling: unilateral: obstruction, chronic sialadenitis, bacterial infection, neoplasm; bilateral (asymmetric): IgG4-related disease, HIV; bilateral (symmetric) hepatic cirrhosis, DM, anorexia/bulimia, acromegaly, alcoholism, hypolipoproteinemia, chronic pancreatitis, acute or chronic viral infection (i.e., mumps, EBV, coxsackievirus, echovirus, granulomatous diseases (i.e., tuberculosis, sarcoidosis)

DIAGNOSTIC TESTS & INTERPRETATION

- Schirmer test (<5-mm wetness after 5 minutes)
- Rose Bengal test (slit lamp) to obtain ocular surface staining and tear break-up time (TBUT)
- Minor salivary gland biopsy (gold standard)
- Autoantibodies: +antinuclear antibodies (ANAs) (95%), +RF (75%)
- Primary SS: +anti-Ro (anti-SSA, 56%) and +anti-La (anti-SSB, 30%)

Initial Tests (lab, imaging)

- Preliminary lab workup
  - Basic labs: CBC w/ differential, chemistry panel, erythrocyte sedimentation rate (ESR), C-reactive protein (CRP), urinalysis
  - Special labs: ANA, rheumatoid factor (RF), anti-Ro/SSA, anti-La/SSB
    - Anti-SSA and anti-SSB antibodies present in 33–74% and 23–52% of SS patients, respectively.
- Imaging:
  - Salivary gland scintigraphy (insensitive, highly specific)
  - Parotid gland sialography (should not be used in acute parotitis)
  - MRI (correlates well with salivary gland biopsy)
  - Salivary gland US (SGUS), highly specific for salivary gland involvement in SS

Diagnostic Procedures/Other

- Salivary gland biopsy: to confirm suspected diagnosis or exclude other causes of xerostomia and bilateral glandular enlargement
- Parotid biopsy is indicated if malignancy is suspected; lymph node biopsy to rule out pseudolymphoma or lymphoma

Test Interpretation

- Salivary gland histology shows focal collections of lymphocytes; immunocytology shows CD4+ T-cell lymphocyte predominance
- SGUS parameters include:
  - Parenchymal nonhomogeneity—most useful diagnostic marker
  - US inflammatory findings include hypoechoic and hyperechoic bands; real-time sonoelastography to quantify tissue rigidity and assess glandular damage

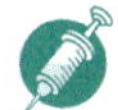

TREATMENT

- Goals of treatment: symptom palliation, improved quality of life, monitor and treat systemic manifestations
- Prior to treatment of oral dryness, assess baseline salivary gland function. Avoid medications that worsen oral dryness. Promote good oral hygiene and routine dental care. Address fatigue and pain.

MEDICATION

- Therapy for dry mouth:
  - Non-pharmacologic: gustatory stimulants (sugar-free candies, lozenges, xylitol), mechanical stimulants (xylitol containing sugar-free gum), fluoride-containing mouth wash/gel/spray or artificial saliva preparations such as Salivart, Saliment, Xero-Lube, MouthKote.
  - Pharmacologic therapy: Evoxac or Salagen; work via stimulation of salivary flow
  - Not recommended: immunosuppressive therapies, hydroxychloroquine (HCQ), oral glucocorticoids, or rituximab (1)
- Therapy for dry eyes:
  - Nonpharmacologic: artificial tears with hydroxyethylcellulose or dextran are more viscous and can last longer; (opt for preservative free) topical gel/ointment (assist in controlling nighttime symptoms take prior to going to bed)
  - If unresponsive to non-pharmacologic, consider ophthalmology evaluation to guide pharmacologic options such as topical NSAIDs/corticosteroids and topical Cyclosporin A (CyA). The evidence of serum teardrop benefits are inconsistent.
- Therapy for MSK-related pain
  - Inflammatory MSK pain: HCQ is first line (1).
  - In acute MSK pain: short course of acetaminophen or NSAIDs for <7 to 10 days
- Tumor necrosis factor inhibitors are strongly discouraged in sicca treatment and in most other primary Sjögren clinical contexts (1).

First Line

- Xerostomia: sugar-free lozenges, especially malic acid, artificial saliva; pilocarpine 5 mg PO starting at QD with titration to QID or cevimeline 30 mg PO TID
- Keratoconjunctivitis sicca: artificial tears and ocular lubricants for symptomatic relief
- Chronic MSK pain: regular aerobic exercise and physical activity

Second Line

- Xerostomia: Bromhexine and N-acetylcysteine; saliva substitutes can be used for those with no glandular function or whose glands cannot be stimulated (1)
- Keratoconjunctivitis sicca: topical glucocorticoids or topical NSAIDs (Use with caution—avoid long-term use—consider ophthalmic supervision.) Topical cyclosporine and autologous serum tear drops are used if symptoms are refractory to glucocorticoids or NSAIDs (1).
- Inflammatory MSK pain: if unresponsive to HCQ, consider short term (<1 month) of corticosteroids. Antidepressants and anticonvulsants are also effective (1).
- For life-threatening extraglandular manifestations, immunosuppressive agents (leflunomide, MTX, etc.) are used (1).

ISSUES FOR REFERRAL

Rheumatology to help manage systemic manifestations; oral health: At a minimum, patients should undergo annual dental examination with twice yearly dental cleanings; ophthalmology for grading of severity and management of xerophthalmia

ADDITIONAL THERAPIES

- Gynecologic Conditions:
  - Vaginal dryness: moisturizers (e.g., Replens, Vagisil) and lubricants (e.g., Sylk, Silken Secret); if unresponsive to above measures, vaginal estrogen creams/rings/tablets are options.
  - Be vigilant for and treat vaginal yeast infections.
- Keratoconjunctivitis sicca: Conserve tears with side shields or ski/swim goggles, humidifiers, and warm moist compresses.
- Fatigue
  - Dehydroepiandrosterone (DHEA) does not offer improvement in fatigue and well-being above placebo.
  - Counsel on exercise and role of reducing fatigue.

SURGERY/OTHER PROCEDURES

Punctal plug/occlusion: if keratoconjunctivitis is refractory to artificial tears, consider punctal plug.

COMPLEMENTARY & ALTERNATIVE MEDICINE

Acupuncture may benefit saliva production and symptoms of xerostomia.

ADMISSION, INPATIENT, AND NURSING CONSIDERATIONS

More likely from extraglandular manifestations such as cardiopulmonary disease, renal involvement, and CNS manifestations

ONGOING CARE

FOLLOW-UP RECOMMENDATIONS

Frequency of follow-up depends on severity.

Patient Monitoring

Monitor for complications, systemic manifestations, and relief of symptoms. Medicolegal pitfalls: Monitor for parotid tumor or lymphoma.

DIET

No specific diet identified to contribute to formation of SS. It is recommended to reduce sugar intake and avoid nonwater drinks between meals and 1 hour prior to bedtime.

PATIENT EDUCATION

In most cases, nonpharmacologic measures are adequate: humidifiers, adequate water intake, chewing gum, artificial tears, smoking cessation.

PROGNOSIS

No therapy has been shown to reverse glandular dysfunction, though, except in the early stages of the disease, dysfunction can remain stable for up to 12 years (1). Hypocomplementemia is an independent risk factor for premature death. Extraglandular involvement is associated with decreased quality of life and increased mortality. Primary SS is associated with increased risks of malignancy, non-Hodgkin lymphoma, and thyroid cancer.

COMPLICATIONS

Complications include dental caries, gum disease, dysphagia, salivary gland calculi, keratitis, conjunctivitis, and ocular scarring

REFERENCES

1. Ramos-Casals M, Brito-Zerón P, Bombardieri S, et al. EULAR recommendations for the management of Sjögren's syndrome with topical and systemic therapies. *Ann Rheum Dis*. 2020;79(1):3–18. doi:10.1136/annrheumdis-2019-216114.

ADDITIONAL READING

- Maleki-Fischbach M, Kastsianok L, Koslow M, et al. Manifestations and management of Sjögren's disease. *Arthritis Res Ther*. 2024;26(1):43. doi:10.1186/s13075-024-03262-4.
- Rathore T, Dattatri M. Exploring Sjögren's syndrome through interdisciplinary perspectives: a concise review. *J Immunoassay Immunochem*. 2024;45(3):153–177. doi:10.1080/15321819.2024.2353766.

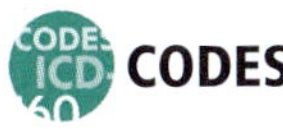

CODES

ICD10

- M35.01 Sjögren syndrome with keratoconjunctivitis
- M35.03 Sjögren syndrome with myopathy
- M35.00 Sjögren syndrome, unspecified

CLINICAL PEARLS

- Many symptoms of SS can be treated with nonpharmacologic interventions such as artificial tears and sugar-free candy/lozenges.
- Coordinate care management with rheumatology, ophthalmology and oral health.
- Consider SS in patients with unexplained lung disease and +ANA.
- Patients with primary SS may have an increased risk of lymphoma and incidence of celiac disease.

SLEEP APNEA, OBSTRUCTIVE

Thomas J. Hansen, MD

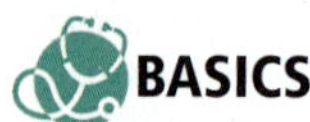

BASICS

DESCRIPTION

- Obstructive sleep apnea (OSA) is defined as repetitive episodes of cessation of airflow (apnea) through the nose and mouth during sleep due to obstruction at the level of the pharynx.
  - Repetitive apneas produce sleep disruption, leading to excessive daytime sleepiness (EDS).
  - Associated with oxygen desaturation and nocturnal hypoxemia
- System(s) affected: cardiovascular; nervous; pulmonary
- Synonym(s): sleep apnea syndrome; nocturnal upper airway occlusion

EPIDEMIOLOGY

Prevalence

The estimated prevalence rated of moderate to severe sleep-disordered breathing has substantially increased over the last two decades. The current prevalence is 10% among 30- to 49-year-old men and 17% among 50- to 70-year-old men. In women, the prevalence is 3% among those 30 to 49 years old and 9% among those 50 to 70 years old.

ETIOLOGY AND PATHOPHYSIOLOGY

OSA occurs when the nasopharynx or oropharynx collapses passively during inspiration. Anatomic and neuromuscular factors contribute to pharyngeal collapse, which leads to hypoxic arousal.

- Anatomic abnormalities, such as increased soft tissue in the palate, tonsillar hypertrophy, macroglossia, and craniofacial abnormalities, predispose the airway to collapse by decreasing the area of the upper airway or increasing the pressure surrounding the airway.
- During sleep, decreased muscle tone in the nasopharynx or oropharynx contributes to airway obstruction and collapse.
- Upper airway narrowing may be due to the following:
  - Obesity, redundant tissue in the soft palate
  - Enlarged tonsils/uvula or a low soft palate; large/posteriorly located tongue
  - Craniofacial abnormalities or neuromuscular disorders
  - Alcohol/sedative use before bedtime

RISK FACTORS

- Obesity (strongest risk factor)
- Age >40 years
- Alcohol/sedative intake before bedtime
- Smoking
- Nasal obstruction (due to polyps, rhinitis, or deviated septum)
- Anatomic narrowing of nasopharynx
- Hypothyroidism
- Neurologic syndromes (e.g., muscular dystrophy, cerebral palsy)

GENERAL PREVENTION

Weight control and avoidance of alcohol and sedatives at night can help.

COMMONLY ASSOCIATED CONDITIONS

- Hypertension
- Obesity
- Daytime sleepiness
- Metabolic syndrome
- Rare:
  - Cardiac arrhythmias
  - Cardiovascular disease
  - Congestive heart failure
  - Pulmonary hypertension
  - Nasal obstructive problems

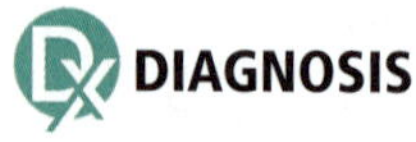

DIAGNOSIS

HISTORY

- Elicit a complete history of daytime and nighttime symptoms. Symptoms can be insidious and may have been present for years.
- Daytime symptoms
  - EDS or fatigue (cardinal symptom)
    - Mild symptoms are those that occur during quiet activities (e.g., reading, watching television).
    - More severe symptoms are those that occur during dynamic activities (e.g., work, driving).
  - Tired on morning awakening "nonrestorative sleep"
  - Sore/dry throat
  - Poor concentration, memory problems, irritability, mood changes, behavior problems (in children)
  - Morning headaches
  - Decreased libido
  - Depression
- Nighttime symptoms
  - Loud snoring (present in 60% of people with OSA)
  - Snort/gasp that arouses patient from sleep but not usually to full consciousness
  - Disrupted sleep
  - Witnessed apneic episodes at night

PHYSICAL EXAM

- OSA is commonly associated with obesity.
- Focused head and neck exam
  - Short neck with large circumference
  - Oropharynx
    - Narrowing of the lateral airway wall
    - Tonsillar hypertrophy; macroglossia
    - Micrognathia/retrognathia
    - Soft palate edema; high, arched hard palate
    - Long/thick uvula
  - Nasopharynx
    - Deviated nasal septum; poor nasal airflow

DIFFERENTIAL DIAGNOSIS

- Other causes of EDS such as the following:
  - Narcolepsy
  - Idiopathic daytime hypersomnolence
  - Inadequate sleep time
  - Depressive episodes with EDS
  - Periodic limb movements disorder
- Respiratory disorders with nocturnal awakenings such as the following:
  - Asthma
  - Chronic obstructive pulmonary disease
  - Congestive heart failure
- Central sleep apnea (Respiratory effort is absent as compared to OSA where effort is present.)
- Sleep-related choking/laryngospasm
- Gastroesophageal reflux
- Sleep-associated seizures (temporal lobe epilepsy)

DIAGNOSTIC TESTS & INTERPRETATION

Initial Tests (lab, imaging)

When clinically indicated

- Thyroid-stimulating hormone; CBC to evaluate anemia and polycythemia, which can indicate nocturnal hypoxemia; fasting glucose in obese
- Rare: arterial blood gases to evaluate daytime hypercapnia

Diagnostic Procedures/Other

- The gold standard for OSA is a full-night, in-laboratory polysomnography (PSG), a nighttime sleep study (1)[B].
  - Demonstrates severity of hypoxemia, sleep disruption, and cardiac arrhythmias associated with OSA and elevated end-tidal CO_2
  - Shows repetitive episodes of cessation/marked reduction in airflow despite continued respiratory efforts
  - Apneic episodes must last at least 10 seconds and occur 10 to 15 times per hour and cause decreased oxygen saturation to be considered clinically significant.
  - Complete PSG is expensive, and health insurance may not cover the cost.

- Multiple sleep latency testing is a diagnostic tool used to measure the time it takes from the start of a daytime nap period to the first signs of sleep (sleep latency). It provides an objective measurement of daytime sleepiness.
- The apnea-hypopnea index (AHI) is defined as the total number of apneas and hypopneas divided by the total sleep time in hours.
  - Mild OSA: AHI = 5 to 15
  - Moderate OSA: AHI = 15 to 30
  - Severe OSA: AHI >30
- Split-night PSG (as compared to a full-night PSG) occurs when patients are diagnosed with OSA within the first part of the night, and then positive pressure device titration is initiated during the second half of the night.
- Drugs that may alter the test results include benzodiazepines and other sedatives that can amplify the severity of apnea seen during the sleep study.
- In patients with a high pretest probability of moderate to severe uncomplicated OSA, home sleep apnea testing with a technically adequate device is an appropriate alternative to laboratory-based PSG provided there is no suspicion of nonrespiratory sleep disorders, the patient is not a mission-critical worker (defined as a job where falling asleep has a major negative impact), and a sleep expert is available to interpret it.

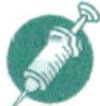

TREATMENT

- Lifestyle modification: weight loss, exercise, and avoidance of alcohol, smoking, and sedatives, especially before bedtime
- Weight loss decreases the severity of symptoms in obese. Lifestyle modifications should be seen as adjunctive rather than curative therapy (2)[A], and a lack of improvement of symptoms with lifestyle modification should not preclude patients from receiving other therapy such as continuous positive airway pressure (CPAP).
- Position changes—if OSA is present only when supine, keep the patient off his or her back when sleeping (e.g., tennis ball worn on back of nightshirt or using a sleep position trainer).
- Positive airway pressure—the most effective therapy for mild, moderate, or severe OSA is CPAP (3)[A]. Treatment with CPAP uses a mask interface and a flow generator to prevent airway collapse, thus helping to prevent apnea, hypoxia, and sleep disturbance.
- Several types of mask interfaces, including nasal masks, oral masks, and nasal pillows exist for CPAP therapy. Short-term data suggest that nasal pillows are the preferred interface in almost all patients. In patients with compliance difficulty, a different choice of interface may be appropriate.
- Hypoglossal nerve stimulation is an option for patients who fail or are intolerant of CPAP therapy. Indications include a diagnosis of moderate to severe OSA with an AHI between 15 and 65 events per hour, a body mass index <35 kg/m^2, and absence of complete concentric collapse at the level of velopharynx or soft palate on drug-induced sleep endoscopy.
- Oral appliances to treat OSA are available and often subjectively preferred by patients (mandibular advancement devices vs. tongue retaining devices). Although oral appliances have been shown to improve symptoms compared with inactive controls, they are not as effective for reduction of respiratory disturbances as CPAP over short-term data. Treatment with oral appliances may be considered in patients who fail to comply with or decline CPAP therapy.

MEDICATION

Medications are yet to be proven effective in treating OSA.

ISSUES FOR REFERRAL

If sleep apnea is suspected, patient should be referred for a sleep study evaluation.

ONGOING CARE

Lifelong compliance with weight loss or CPAP is necessary.

DIET

Overweight patients should be encouraged to lose weight.

PATIENT EDUCATION

- Weight loss and avoidance of alcohol and sedatives
- Significantly sleepy patients should not drive a motor vehicle/operate dangerous equipment.

PROGNOSIS

- Lifelong compliance with weight loss or CPAP is necessary for effective treatment of OSA, but long-term adherence is poor.
- Morbidity usually due to motor vehicle accidents or secondary to cardiac complications, including arrhythmias, cardiac ischemia, and hypertension; data insufficient on whether treatment changes outcomes.

COMPLICATIONS

Untreated OSA may increase the risk for development of hypertension, stroke, myocardial infarction, diabetes, cardiovascular disease, and work-related and driving accidents, but it is unclear that treatment reduces or prevents any of these problems.

Pediatric Considerations

- The most common cause is tonsillar hypertrophy. Additional causes are obesity and craniofacial abnormalities along with neuromuscular diseases, such as cerebral palsy and spinal muscular atrophy.
- Signs and symptoms
  - Nighttime: loud snoring, restlessness, and sweating
  - Daytime: hyperactivity and decreased school performance
- Diagnosis is with PSG. Abnormal AHI is different in children: >1 per hour is abnormal.
- Surgery is the first-line treatment in cases due to adenotonsillar hypertrophy. For cases due to obesity/craniofacial abnormalities, patients can use CPAP treatment.

Geriatric Considerations

The presence of sleep apnea in the geriatric population may be associated with earlier onset of mild cognitive impairment as well as Alzheimer dementia at an earlier age.

REFERENCES

1. Kapur VK, Auckley DH, Chowdhuri S, et al. Clinical practice guideline for diagnostic testing for adult obstructive sleep apnea: an American Academy of Sleep Medicine clinical practice guideline. *J Clin Sleep Med*. 2017;13(3):479–504.
2. Anandam A, Akinnusi M, Kufel T, et al. Effects of dietary weight loss on obstructive sleep apnea: a meta-analysis. *Sleep Breath*. 2013;17(1):227–234.
3. Giles TL, Lasserson TJ, Smith BJ, et al. Continuous positive airways pressure for obstructive sleep apnoea in adults. *Cochrane Database Syst Rev*. 2006;(3):CD001106.

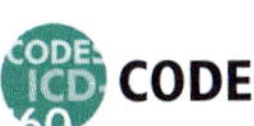

CODES

ICD10

- G47.33 Obstructive sleep apnea (adult) (pediatric)
- G47.30 Sleep apnea, unspecified

CLINICAL PEARLS

- OSA is characterized by repetitive episodes of apnea often terminating in a snort/gasp.
- Laboratory PSG is the key to diagnosis.
- CPAP is the most effective form of treatment for both mild to moderate and moderate to severe OSA.
- Central sleep apnea may mimic OSA.

SLEEP DISORDER, SHIFT WORK

Jennifer W. Caceres, MD

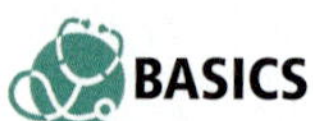

BASICS

DESCRIPTION

Shift work disorder (SWD), classified as a circadian rhythm sleep-wake disorder, is characterized by symptoms of insomnia and/or excessive sleepiness when required to work during usual sleep times. SWD is caused by a misalignment between the internal circadian rhythm and the required sleep-wake schedule defined by nontraditional work shifts including night shifts, afternoon or evening shifts, early morning shifts, irregular shifts, and rotating shifts (1).

EPIDEMIOLOGY

Prevalence

- In the United States, ~20% of employed adults are shift workers, particularly in service-related occupations such as health care, protective services, transportation, and food services (1).
- 1 in 3 shift workers is affected by insomnia or some form of sleep disturbance. ~90% of shift workers note daytime sleepiness or fatigue. SWD has an estimated prevalence of approximately 2–5% in the general population of the United States (1).
- Prevalence of SWD rises with age, particularly for adults age >50 years.

ETIOLOGY AND PATHOPHYSIOLOGY

In shift workers, there is a misalignment between one's endogenous circadian rhythm of sleep and wakefulness and a sleep-wake schedule based on nontraditional shift work. Dyssynchrony results in excessive sleepiness during the work shift and/or insomnia during desired sleep time (1),(2).

Genetics

One possibly genetically linked trait is a person's preference for the morning versus evening. This is partially linked to the polymorphism of the clock gene PERIOD3 (PER3) involved in sleep-wake regulation (1).

RISK FACTORS

- Age >50 years (1)
- Strong competing social and domestic needs

GENERAL PREVENTION

- Reduce or eliminate shift work. Try to rotate shifts forward if shifts must be rotated. Use bright light during shifts.
- Improve sleep hygiene. Schedule regular sleep including naps (<1 hour) just before a shift or, if possible, during a shift.

COMMONLY ASSOCIATED CONDITIONS

- SWD has been associated with functional consequences including impaired immediate free recall, decreased processing speed, and selective attention impairments.
- SWD has been associated with higher risk of vehicular accidents, job-related injuries.
- SWD has been associated with poor physical health (including increased incidence of gastrointestinal [GI] disorders, cardiovascular disease [CVD], diabetes, and possible increase risk of cancers) as well as poor mental health (including increased incidence of substance use disorders and mood disorders).

DIAGNOSIS

- This is a clinical diagnosis. Criteria for circadian rhythm disorder per *Diagnostic and Statistical Manual of Mental Disorders*, 5th edition (*DSM-5*) include all three of the following:
  - A persistent or recurrent pattern of sleep disruption that is primarily due to an alteration of the circadian system or to a misalignment between the endogenous circadian rhythm and sleep-wake schedule required by an individual's physical environment or social or professional schedule.
  - The sleep disruption leads to excessive sleepiness or insomnia, or both.
  - The sleep disturbance causes clinically significant distress or impairment in social, occupational, and other important areas of functioning.
- Additional specification per *DSM-5* for SWD includes:
  - Insomnia during the major sleep period and/or excessive sleepiness (including inadvertent sleep) during the major awake period associated with a shift work schedule (i.e., requiring unconventional work hours).
  - The disorder is classified as to whether it is episodic (symptoms at least 1 month but <3 months), persistent (symptoms at least 3 months or longer) or recurrent (two or more episodes occurring within 1 year).

HISTORY

- A careful history is critical. Assess work history, detailed sleep history, level of sleepiness, safety risk, and performance impairments during work shifts.
- Note the following in particular (2)[C]:
  - Sleep/wake habits, sleep environment; degree of alertness or sleepiness; light exposure before, during, and after the shift; job-related factors: occupation, work schedule, years of shift work, length of shift, number of consecutive shifts, and commute after shift; sedating or stimulating medications or substance use; impact on social and domestic responsibilities (including drowsy driving)
- Evaluate for symptoms of other sleep disorders, which often coexist and can exacerbate SWD such as the following (2):
  - Loud snoring and pauses in breathing during sleep (obstructive sleep apnea [OSA]); sudden sleep attacks and leg symptoms (restless legs syndrome [RLS]); falling asleep at inappropriate times, drop attacks, and daytime fatigue (narcolepsy)

PHYSICAL EXAM

Evaluate for findings suggestive of mood disorders, GI disease, diabetes, CVD, cancer signs of OSA such as obesity, and large neck (2)[C].

DIFFERENTIAL DIAGNOSIS

- Other primary sleep disorders: insomnia, sleep-related breathing disorders, central disorders of hypersomnolence, parasomnias, sleep-related movement disorders (2)
- Other circadian rhythm sleep disorders such as delayed sleep phase type or irregular sleep-wake type. Distinguishing among these can be challenging.

DIAGNOSTIC TESTS & INTERPRETATION

No diagnostic testing is required for the diagnosis. If concern for another sleep disorder, consider polysomnography or multiple sleep latency testing (testing for narcolepsy). Given possible increased risk, consider screen for potential medical comorbidities as discussed above including mood disorders and metabolic disorders among shift workers (1),(2).

Diagnostic Procedures/Other

- Sleep diaries can help identify sleep-wake disturbances related to shift work and should be recorded for 2 weeks.
- Standardized measures of sleepiness can be obtained using several tools including the Insomnia Severity Index (ISI) and Epworth Sleepiness Scale (ESS).

Test Interpretation

Sleep diaries often reveal:

- Increased sleep latency; decreased total sleep time; frequent awakenings
- Most people revert to nocturnal sleeping on their days off. Every work week, they must "start over" to shift circadian rhythms to align with work schedules.

TREATMENT

- The only standard recommendation by the American Academy of Sleep Medicine (AASM) is planned (prescribed) sleep schedules.
- Other commonly used strategies include promoting wakefulness while at work with bright light exposure, caffeine or rarely other stimulants, and/or promoting sleep with sleep hygiene optimization, melatonin, and hypnotics.

GENERAL MEASURES

- Sleep hygiene: an important first step in approaching the treatment of sleep disorders. This includes minimizing exposure to bright light before and during scheduled sleep periods (maintain a dark sleeping space, wear dark sunglasses following work shift, wear an eye mask to sleep), maintaining a quiet sleep environment (wear ear plugs to sleep, disconnect phone/doorbell, use a white noise generator), maintaining cool sleeping quarters to help retrain core body temperature to align with modified sleep-wake cycle, and avoiding use of stimulants during second half of work shift.
- Sleep time: protected time for sleep prior to and following work shifts with strategic naps where possible. Shift workers, particularly night shift workers, should be aware of postnap sleep inertia and avoid driving when drowsy (1).
- Anchor sleep: Schedule sleep periods so that at least 1 to 2 hours of designated sleep time overlap on work days and nonwork days. Anchor sleep can help increase sleep duration as well as allow workers to maintain time for socialization and recreation.
- Work/social/domestic factors: Treat psychosocial stress, depression; encourage healthy eating habits; limit substance use; increase exercise to at least 30 minutes, 5 times per week (not within 2 to 4 hours of bedtime). Seek family member and social support for protected sleep time (1).
- Work-related interventions: If possible, reduce number of consecutive shifts (<4) or reduce shift duration (<12 hours), allow adequate time between shifts (>11 hours), move heavy workload outside circadian nadir (04:00 PM to 07:00 PM).
- Light exposure: Timed bright light exposure can delay the physiologic nadir of alertness and thus, promote alertness during the night/early shift and possibly reduce circadian misalignment. Light avoidance during the day may also help with circadian adaption and improve sleep (1),(2).

MEDICATION

- Sleep-promoting medications:
  - Melatonin may help shift circadian rhythms and can increase the quality and duration of sleep as well as increase alertness during the work shift. AASM recommends 3 mg of melatonin for daytime sleep for shift workers (1); clinical effectiveness of melatonin is unclear.
  - Ramelteon (Rozerem), a melatonin receptor agonist, is FDA approved to treat insomnia, and may also provide benefit in SWD.
  - Doxepin (tricyclic antidepressant) given at low doses may improve sleep without residual daytime impairment. Trazodone is a non–first-line agent for treatment of insomnia; it may also provide some benefit in SWD.
  - Intermediate-acting hypnotics such as zolpidem (Ambien) or eszopiclone (Lunesta) can cause post-sleep sedation. Long-term use is discouraged due to potential dependence. Additionally, side effects such as anxiety or irritability may affect sleep (1).
- Wakefulness-promoting medications:
  - Modafinil (Provigil) and armodafinil (Nuvigil) are FDA approved for excessive sleepiness in patients with SWD and can reduce daytime sleepiness and improve cognitive performance. Notably, modafinil has been tied to rare instances of Stevens-Johnson syndrome (2).
  - Prophylactic caffeine use immediately prior to and during work shift. Limiting caffeine to the first half of the night shift is recommended to limit disruption of daytime sleep (2).

First Line

Circadian shift/sleep promoting: melatonin 3 mg PO or sublingual, 30 minutes before daytime sleep period. Take only when the patient is home and able to go to bed.

Second Line

- Wakefulness promoting:
  - Modafinil initially 200 mg PO 1 hour prior to work shift; armodafinil 150 mg PO 1 hour prior to work shift; long-acting (12 to 16 hours, depending on food intake) use judiciously in SWD to impede the patient's ability to sleep after the shift
- Sleep promoting:
  - Nonbenzodiazepine hypnotics:
    - Zolpidem 5 to 10 mg or eszopiclone 1 to 3 mg immediately prior to bed; suvorexant 10 to 20 mg PO 30 minutes prior to bed
  - Antidepressants
    - Doxepin (3 to 6 mg) and trazodone (25 to 150 mg), 1 to 2 hours prior to bed
  - Benzodiazepines: Estazolam, flurazepam, quazepam, temazepam, and triazolam are FDA approved for the treatment of insomnia. Due to high risk of tolerance/withdrawal, use cautiously for short-term treatment of insomnia.
  - In general, hypnotics may improve daytime sleep but does not appear to improve sleep maintenance or nighttime alertness. They may also cause residual sedation during work hours. This may worsen SWD symptoms.

ISSUES FOR REFERRAL

Refer to a sleep specialist for suspicion of other primary sleep disorders or dependence on hypnotics, alcohol, or stimulants.

ADDITIONAL THERAPIES

- Bright light therapy: Blue wavelengths are more effective and higher intensities (>2,000 lux) are recommended (1),(2).
- Cognitive-behavioral therapy for insomnia (CBT-I): It has been shown to have positive effects on sleep latency and total sleep time in small studies, but has not been evaluated in large, high-powered randomized control trials as of yet (2).
- Notably, there have been no high-powered, long-term studies to evaluate what effect these therapies have on comorbidities associated with SWD.

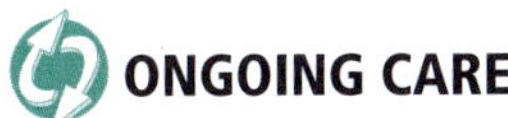

ONGOING CARE

PATIENT EDUCATION

Discuss sleep hygiene and optimizing the sleep environment. Shift workers who sleep in the daytime should ensure a cool, dark, quiet sleep environment. Reserve bedroom for sleeping and intimacy only. Remove televisions, cell phones, tablets, and laptop computers from the bedroom. When going to sleep, turn clock away from bed and discourage prolonged reading in bed. Blackout shades help achieve the proper darkness. Symptoms are associated with shift work and should resolve if shift work is eliminated, this may not be feasible for patients. Fatigue risk management programs to educate shift workers, especially night shift workers, about sleep and the hazards associated with sleep deficiency.

REFERENCES

1. Wickwire EM, Geiger-Brown J, Scharf SM, et al. Shift work and shift work sleep disorder: clinical and organizational perspectives. *Chest*. 2017;151(5):1156–1172.
2. Cheng P, Drake C. Shift work disorder. *Neurol Clin*. 2019;37(3):563–577.

ADDITIONAL READING

HelpGuide. Weekly sleep diary. https://www.helpguide.org/wp-content/uploads/2018/12/sleep-diary.pdf. Accessed November 6, 2022.

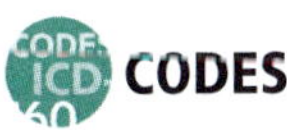

CODES

ICD10

G47.26 Circadian rhythm sleep disorder, shift work type

CLINICAL PEARLS

- SWD has been associated with increased risk for metabolic disorders and mood disorders.
- The first diagnostic step in SWD is to obtain a comprehensive sleep history and work history. Sleep diaries are helpful tools to assess sleep-wake patterns.
- Shift workers are at greater risk for accidents during night and early morning shifts.

S

SMELL AND TASTE DISORDERS

Beth K. Mazyck, MD • Daniel B. Kurtz, PhD, BS

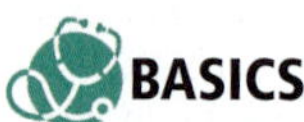

BASICS

DESCRIPTION

- Physiologically, the senses of smell and taste aid in normal digestion by triggering GI secretions.
- Loss of smell occurs more frequently than loss of taste, and patients frequently confuse the concepts of flavor loss (as a result of smell impairment) with taste loss (an impaired ability to sense sweet, sour, salty, or bitter).
- Smell depends on the functioning of olfactory nerve (CN I) and trigeminal nerve (CN V).
- Taste depends on the functioning of CNs VII, IX, and X. Because of these multiple pathways, total loss of taste (ageusia) is rare.
- Systems affected: nervous, upper respiratory

EPIDEMIOLOGY

Incidence

There are ~200,000 patient visits a year for smell and taste disturbances.

Prevalence

- Predominant sex: male > female. Men begin to lose their ability to smell earlier in life than women.
- Predominant age:
  - Age >80 years: 80% have major olfactory impairment; nearly 50% are anosmic.
  - Ages 65 to 80 years: 60% have major olfactory impairment; nearly 25% are anosmic.
  - Age <65 years: 1–2% have smell impairment.
- Prior to the COVID-19 pandemic, an estimated >2 million affected in the United States
- Commonly occurs with SARS-CoV-2, the virus responsible for COVID-19

ETIOLOGY AND PATHOPHYSIOLOGY

- Smell and/or taste disturbances:
  - COVID-19: Common in mildly symptomatic patients (~65%) but even more common in patients needing hospitalization (85%) (1),(2),(3). Unexplained chemosensory loss is a good predictor of COVID-19 (4),(5)[B].
  - Nutritional factors (e.g., malnutrition, vitamin deficiencies, liver disease, pernicious anemia)
  - Endocrine disorders (e.g., thyroid disease, diabetes mellitus, renal disease)
  - Migraine headache (e.g., gustatory aura, olfactory aura)
  - Sjögren syndrome
  - Toxic exposures
  - Neurodegenerative diseases (e.g., multiple sclerosis, Alzheimer disease, cerebrovascular accident, Parkinson disease)
  - Infections
- Smell specific disturbance:
  - Nasal and sinus disease (e.g., allergies, rhinitis, rhinorrhea, URI)
  - Cigarette smoking
  - Cocaine abuse (intranasal)
  - Hemodialysis
  - Neoplasm (e.g., brain tumor, nasal polyps, intranasal tumor)
  - Systemic lupus erythematosus (SLE)
  - Bell palsy
- Taste specific loss:
  - Oral appliances, procedures
  - Intraoral abscess, gingivitis
  - Damage to CNs VI, IX, or X
  - Stroke (especially frontal lobe)
- Selected medications:
  - Antibiotics: amikacin, ampicillin, azithromycin, ciprofloxacin, clarithromycin, doxycycline, griseofulvin, metronidazole, ofloxacin, tetracycline, terbinafine, β-lactamase inhibitors
  - Anticonvulsants: carbamazepine, phenytoin
  - Antidepressants: amitriptyline, doxepin, imipramine, nortriptyline
  - Antihistamines and decongestants: zinc-based cold remedies (Zicam)
  - Antihypertensives and cardiac medications: acetazolamide, amiloride, captopril, diltiazem, hydrochlorothiazide, nifedipine, propranolol, spironolactone
  - Anti-inflammatory agents: auranofin, gold, penicillamine
  - Antimanic drugs: lithium
  - Antineoplastics: cisplatin, doxorubicin, methotrexate, vincristine
  - Antiparkinsonian agents: levodopa, carbidopa
  - Antiseptic: chlorhexidine
  - Antithyroid agents: methimazole, propylthiouracil
  - Lipid-lowering agents: statins

Genetics

Unknown

RISK FACTORS

- Poor nutritional status
- Smoking

GENERAL PREVENTION

- Well-balanced diet
- Maintain good oral and nasal health.
- Avoid tobacco products, chemical exposures.

Geriatric Considerations

Anosmia also may be an early sign of degenerative disorders and has been shown to predict increased 5-year mortality (6)[B].

Pediatric Considerations

- In developing countries with poor nutrition (particularly zinc depletion), smell and taste disorders may occur.
- Delayed puberty in association with anosmia (± midline craniofacial abnormalities, deafness, or renal abnormalities) suggests the possibility of Kallmann syndrome (hypogonadotropic hypogonadism).

Pregnancy Considerations

Many women report increased sensitivity to odors during pregnancy as well as an increased dislike for bitterness and a preference for salty substances.

COMMONLY ASSOCIATED CONDITIONS

URI, allergic rhinitis, dental abscesses

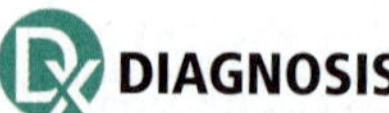

DIAGNOSIS

Smell and taste disturbances are symptoms; it is essential to look for possible underlying causes.

HISTORY

- Symptoms of URI, environmental allergies
- Fever, cough, sore throat suggestive of COVID-19 infection
- Oral pain, other dental problems
- Cognitive/memory difficulties
- Current medications
- Nutritional status, ovolactovegetarian
- Weight loss or gain
- Frequent infections (impaired immunity)
- Worsening of underlying medical illness
- Increased use of salt and/or sugar to increase taste of food
- Neurodegenerative disease

PHYSICAL EXAM

Thorough HEENT exam

DIFFERENTIAL DIAGNOSIS

- Epilepsy (gustatory or olfactory aura)
- Memory impairment
- Psychiatric conditions

DIAGNOSTIC TESTS & INTERPRETATION

Initial Tests (lab, imaging)

Consider (Not all patients require all tests.)

- SARS-CoV-2
- CBC, chemistry panel
- Vitamin B_{12} level
- Thyroid-stimulating hormone (TSH)
- Serum IgE
- CT scanning is the most useful and cost-effective technique for assessing sinonasal disorders and is superior to an MRI in evaluating bony structures and airway patency. Coronal CT scans are particularly valuable in assessing paranasal anatomy (7)[B].

Follow-Up Tests & Special Considerations

Diagnosis of smell and taste disturbances is usually possible through history; however, the following tests can be used to confirm:

- Olfactory tests
  - Smell identification test: evaluates the ability to identify 40 microencapsulated scratch-and-sniff odorants (8)[B]
  - Brief smell identification test (9)[B]
  - Taste tests (more difficult because no convenient standardized tests are presently available): Solutions containing sucrose (sweet), sodium chloride (salty), quinine (bitter), and citric acid (sour) are helpful.
  - An MRI is useful in defining soft tissue disease; therefore, a coronal MRI is the technique of choice to image the olfactory bulbs, tracts, and cortical parenchyma; possible placement of an accessory coil (TMJ) over the nose to assist in imaging

TREATMENT

GENERAL MEASURES

- Appropriate treatment for underlying cause
- Quit smoking.
- Treatment of underlying nasal congestion with nasal decongestants and/or nasal/oral steroids (10)[B]
- Surgical correction of nasal blockage/nasal polyps
- Drug-related smell or taste loss can be reversed with cessation of the offending medication, but it may take many months.
- Proper nutritional and dietary assessment (7)[C]
- Formal dental evaluation

MEDICATION

- Treat underlying causes as appropriate. Idiopathic cases will often resolve spontaneously.
- Consider trial of corticosteroids topically (e.g., fluticasone nasal spray daily to BID) and/or systemically (e.g., oral prednisone 60 mg daily for 5 to 7 days) (10)[B].
- Zinc and vitamins (A, B complex) when deficiency is suspected

ISSUES FOR REFERRAL

Consider referral to an otolaryngologist or neurologist for persistent cases.

ONGOING CARE

DIET

- Weight gain/loss is possible because the patient may reject food or may switch to calorie-rich foods that are still palatable.
- Ensure a nutritionally balanced diet with appropriate levels of nutrients, vitamins, and essential minerals.

PATIENT EDUCATION

- Caution patients not to overindulge as compensation for the bland taste of food. For example, patients with diabetes may need help in avoiding excessive sugar intake as an inappropriate way of improving food taste.
- Patients with chemosensory impairments should use measuring devices when cooking and should not cook by taste.
- Optimizing food texture, aroma, temperature, and color may improve the overall food experience when taste is limited.
- Patients with permanent smell dysfunction must develop adaptive strategies for dealing with hygiene, appetite, safety, and health.
- Natural gas and smoke detectors are essential; check for proper function frequently.
- Check food expiration dates frequently; discard old food.

PROGNOSIS

- COVID-19 infection associated smell loss:
  - Recovery of smell by 30, 60, 90, or 120 days was reported by 74%, 86%, 90%, and 96% respectively (11). A small number will experience long-term loss, although recovery can still occur beyond 6 months.
- A small number of those who lost smell due to COVID-19 experience phantosmia or parosmia (phantom smells, or previously pleasant smells become foul).
- In general, the olfactory system regenerates poorly after a head injury. Most patients who recover smell function following head trauma do so within 12 weeks of injury.
- Patients who quit smoking typically recover improved olfactory function and flavor sensation.
- Many taste disorders (dysgeusia) resolve spontaneously within a few years of onset.
- Phantosmias that are flow dependent may respond to surgical ablation of olfactory mucosa.
- Conditions such as radiation-induced xerostomia and Bell palsy generally improve over time.

COMPLICATIONS

- Permanent loss of ability to smell/taste
- Psychiatric issues with dysgeusia and phantosmia

REFERENCES

1. Spinato G, Fabbris C, Polesel J, et al. Alterations in smell or taste in mildly symptomatic outpatients with SARS-CoV-2 infection. *JAMA*. 2020;323(20):2089–2090.
2. Menni C, Valdes AM, Freidin MB, et al. Real-time tracking of self-reported symptoms to predict potential COVID-19. *Nat Med*. 2020;26(7):1037–1040.
3. Vaira LA, Hopkins C, Petrocelli M, et al. Smell and taste recovery in coronavirus disease 2019 patients: a 60-day objective and prospective study. *J Laryngol Otol*. 2020;134(8):703–709.
4. Parma V, Ohla K, Veldhuizen MG, et al. More than smell-COVID-19 is associated with severe impairment of smell, taste, and chemesthesis. *Chem Senses*. 2020;45(7):609–622.
5. Gerkin RC, Ohla K, Veldhuizen MG, et al. The best COVID-19 predictor is recent smell loss: a cross-sectional study. *medRxiv* [Preprint]. 2020;2020.07.22.20157263.
6. Pinto JM, Wroblewski KE, Kern DW, et al. Olfactory dysfunction predicts 5-year mortality in older adults. *PLoS One*. 2014;9(10):e107541.
7. Malaty J, Malaty IAC. Smell and taste disorders in primary care. *Am Fam Physician*. 2013;88(12):852–859.
8. Doty RL, Shaman P, Dann M. Development of the University of Pennsylvania Smell Identification Test: a standardized microencapsulated test of olfactory function. *Physiol Behav*. 1984;32(3):489–502.
9. Jackman AH, Doty RL. Utility of a three-item smell identification test in detecting olfactory dysfunction. *Laryngoscope*. 2005;115(12):2209–2212.
10. Seiden AM, Duncan HJ. The diagnosis of a conductive olfactory loss. *Laryngoscope*. 2001;111(1):9–14.
11. Tan BKJ, Han R, Zhao JJ, et al. Prognosis and persistence of smell and taste dysfunction in patients with covid-19: meta-analysis with parametric cure modelling of recovery curves. *BMJ*. 2022;378:e069503. doi:10.1136/bmj-2021-069503.

S

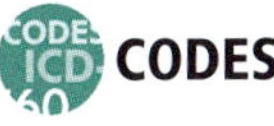

CODES

ICD10

- R43.9 Unspecified disturbances of smell and taste
- R43.1 Parosmia
- R43.2 Parageusia

CLINICAL PEARLS

- Smell loss is often the first and only symptom of mild cases of COVID-19.
- Smell disorders are often mistaken as decreased taste by patients.
- Most temporary smell loss is due to nasal passage obstruction.
- Actual taste disorders are often related to dental problems or medication side effects.
- Gradual smell loss is very common in the elderly; extensive workup in this population may not be indicated if no associated signs/symptoms are present but may be predictive of 5- to 13-year mortality.
- Sudden unexplained smell loss may be a predictor of COVID-19.

SOMATIC SYMPTOM (SOMATIZATION) DISORDER

Elizabeth M. Payment, MD

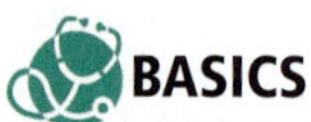

BASICS

DESCRIPTION

- Somatic symptom disorders (SSD) are a pattern of one or more somatic symptoms causing excessive thoughts, feelings or behaviors related to the somatic symptom or associated health concern recurring or persisting for >6 months that are distressing or result in significant disruption of daily life.
- Diagnosis is made based on having symptoms and abnormal thoughts, feelings and behaviors in response to symptoms as that are medically unexplained.
- Conceptualization and diagnostic criteria for somatic symptom presentations were significantly modified with the advent of *DSM-5*. SSD is similar in many aspects to the former somatization disorder, which required presentation with multiple physical complaints. No longer based on symptoms counts; current diagnosis is based on the way the patient presents and perceives his or her symptoms.
- SSD now includes most presentations that would formerly be considered hypochondriasis. Hypochondriasis has been replaced by illness anxiety disorder, which is diagnosed when the patient presents with significant preoccupation with having a serious illness in the absence or presence of mild illness-related somatic complaints.
- SSD also includes functional neurologic symptom disorders, formerly known as conversion disorder, and involves one or more symptoms of altered voluntary or sensory functions with clinical findings that are incompatible with current neurologic or medical.
- Somatization increases disability independent of comorbidity, and individuals with SSD have health-related functioning that is 2 standard deviations below the mean.
- Symptoms may be specific (e.g., localized pain) or relatively nonspecific (e.g., fatigue).
- Symptoms sometimes may represent normal bodily sensations or discomfort that does not signify serious disease.
- Suffering is authentic. Symptoms are not intentionally produced or feigned.
- SSDs are sometimes referred to as "functional disorders" to denote their nonphysical basis and with the assumption that the illness behavior is a function of the environment.

EPIDEMIOLOGY

Incidence

- Usually, first symptoms appear in adolescence.
- Predominant sex: female > male (10:1)
- Type and frequency of somatic complaints may differ among cultures, so symptom reviews should be adjusted based on culture; more frequent in cultures without Western/empirical explanatory models

Prevalence

- Expected 2% among women and <0.2% among men
- Somatization seen in up to 29% of patients presenting to primary care offices
- Somatic concerns may increase, but other features of the presentation decrease such that prevalence declines after age 65 years.

ETIOLOGY AND PATHOPHYSIOLOGY

Patients with SSD demonstrate different patterns of heart rate variability. Although this cannot be used to clinically differentiate, it does point to the differences in psychophysiology of SSD. Also, not to be used clinically, patients with SSD display differences in brain functional connectivity, with the possibility that deficits in attention distort perception of external stimuli, affecting regulation of externally responsive body functioning (1)[C]. Reduced density in the form of decreased cell counts and radiologic signaling have also been detected in brain areas related to somatic sensation and emotional experience.

Genetics

Consanguinity studies and single nucleotide polymorphism genotyping indicate that both genetic and environmental factors contribute to the risk of SSD.

RISK FACTORS

- Child abuse, particularly sexual abuse, has been shown to be a risk factor for somatization.
- Symptoms begin or worsen after losses (e.g., job, close relative, or friend).
- Greater intensity of symptoms often occurs with stress.

COMMONLY ASSOCIATED CONDITIONS

Comorbid with other psychiatric conditions is yet to be determined but is likely to be 20–50% with anxiety, depression, or personality disorders.

DIAGNOSIS

- Determining that a somatic symptom is medically unexplained is unreliable, and it is inappropriate to diagnose a mental disorder solely because a medical diagnosis is not demonstrated. Rely on symptoms and presentation rather than ruling out medical causes in making the SSD diagnosis.
- Up to 10% of patients meeting criteria for SSD will be false positives for these diagnoses (2)[B].
- Illness anxiety and somatic distress are independent but often co-occur.

HISTORY

- One or more somatic complaints that are distressing and cause significant disruption to everyday life
- SSD involves patient excessive thoughts, feelings, or behaviors associated with symptoms or associated health concerns manifested by at least one of the following:
  - Disproportionate and persistent thoughts about the seriousness of the symptoms
  - Persistent high level of anxiety about health or symptoms
  - Excessive time or energy devoted to symptoms or health concerns
- Specify if
  - With predominant pain
  - Persistent
- Specify current severity
  - Mild: 1 or more symptoms
  - Moderate: 2 or more symptoms
  - Severe: 2 or more symptoms with multiple somatic complaints or one very severe somatic symptom
- Diagnoses no longer rely on symptom counts, but common symptoms include:
  - Pain symptoms related to different sites such as head, abdomen, back, joints, extremities, chest, or rectum, or related to body functions such as menstruation, sexual intercourse, or urination
  - Gastrointestinal (GI) symptoms such as nausea, bloating, vomiting (not during pregnancy), diarrhea, intolerance of several foods
  - Sexual symptoms such as indifference to sex, difficulties with erection or ejaculation, irregular menses, excessive menstrual bleeding, or vomiting throughout all 9 months of pregnancy
  - Pseudoneurologic symptoms such as impaired balance or coordination, weak or paralyzed muscles, lump in throat or trouble swallowing, loss of voice, retention of urine, hallucinations, numbness (to touch or pain), double vision, blindness, deafness, seizures, amnesia or other dissociative symptoms, loss of consciousness (other than with fainting); none of these is limited to pain.
- Patients with SSD frequently use alternative treatments, which should be explored for their effects on health and physical functioning.

PHYSICAL EXAM

Physical exam remarkable for absence of objective findings to explain the many subjective complaints

DIFFERENTIAL DIAGNOSIS

- Other psychiatric illnesses must be ruled out:
  - Depressive disorders
  - Anxiety disorders
  - Schizophrenia
  - Other somatic disorders: illness anxiety disorder, conversion disorder
  - Factitious disorder
  - Body dysmorphic disorder
- Malingering

- General medical conditions, with vague, multiple, confusing symptoms, must be ruled out.
  - Systemic lupus erythematosus
  - Hyperparathyroidism
  - Hyper- or hypothyroidism
  - Lyme disease
  - Porphyria
  - Multiple system atrophy

DIAGNOSTIC TESTS & INTERPRETATION

Several screening tools are available that help to identify symptoms as somatic:

- Patient Health Questionnaire (PHQ)-15 (screens and monitors symptoms)
- Somatic Symptom Scale-8
- Somatic Symptom Disorder B-Criteria Scale (SSD-12)

Initial Tests (lab, imaging)

- Laboratory test results do not support the subjective complaints.
- Imaging studies do not support the subjective complaints.

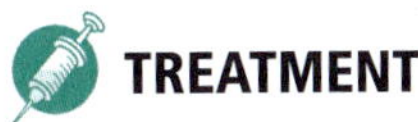

TREATMENT

GENERAL MEASURES

- The goal of treatment is to help the person learn to control the symptoms.
- Do not tell patients that the problems is in their head and that their symptoms are imaginary. Enhanced or structured care as follows can be as effective as psychological interventions in adults.
- The involvement of a single provider is important because a history of seeking medical attention and "doctor shopping" is common.
- Patients usually receive the most benefit from primary care providers who accept the limitations of treatment, listen to their patient's concerns, and provide reassurance.
- A supportive relationship with a sympathetic health care provider is the most important aspect of treatment:
  - Regular scheduled appointments should be maintained to review symptoms and the person's coping mechanisms (at least 15 minutes once a month).
  - Acknowledge and explain test results.
- Antidepressant or antianxiety medication and referral to a support group or mental health provider can help patients who are willing to participate in their treatment.

MEDICATION

Antidepressants (e.g., SSRIs) help to treat comorbid depression and anxiety. Fluoxetine has been shown to have efficacy with illness anxiety disorder (formerly hypochondriasis), although >50% of those patients did not respond to the medication

ISSUES FOR REFERRAL

- Discourage referrals to specialists for further investigation of somatic complaints.
- Referrals to support groups or to a mental health provider may be helpful.

ADDITIONAL THERAPIES

- There are multiple reviews in the literature which speak to the validity for this recently reformulated disorder. These add to the numerous studies with positive outcomes for child and adult patients with various forms of somatization or medically unexplained symptoms.
- Treatment typically includes long-term therapy, which has been shown to decrease the severity of symptoms.
- Individual or group cognitive-behavioral therapy addressing health anxiety, health beliefs, and health behaviors has been shown to be the most efficacious treatment for SSD. Cognitive processes modified in therapy include patient tendencies to ruminate and catastrophize.
- Emotional awareness and expression therapy is a promising new treatment. It targets emotional processing associated with trauma and conflict as a mechanism of symptom change.
- For children, SSD can result in missing school. School avoidance (malingering) and school anxiety should be your first considerations. Psychological interventions reduce symptom numbers and severity, disability, and school absence.
- Consideration should be given to providing integrated multidisciplinary care. For example, for patients with a functional gastrointestinal disorder, inclusion of dietitians, gut-focused hypnotherapists, psychiatrists, and behavioral (biofeedback) physiotherapists, has been shown to improved symptoms, specific functional disorders, psychological state, quality of life, and cost of care for the treatment of functional gastrointestinal disorders.

ONGOING CARE

FOLLOW-UP RECOMMENDATIONS

Patients should have regularly scheduled follow-up with a primary care doctor, psychiatrist, and/or therapist.

PATIENT EDUCATION

Encourage interventions that decrease stressful elements of the patient's life:

- Psychoeducational advice
- Increase in exercise
- Pleasurable private time

PROGNOSIS

- Chronic course, fluctuating in severity
- Full remission is rare.
- Individuals with this disorder have been found to have 4 times the risk for suicide and increased mortality for respiratory and GI disorder.
- Patients with this diagnosis do experience substantially greater functional disability and role impairment than nonsomatizing patients.

COMPLICATIONS

- May result from invasive testing and from multiple evaluations that are performed while looking for the cause of the symptoms
- A dependency on pain relievers or sedatives may develop.

REFERENCES

1. Kim SM, Hong JS, Min KJ, et al. Brain functional connectivity in patients with somatic symptom disorder. *Psychosom Med*. 2019;81(3):313–318.
2. Henningsen P. Management of somatic symptom disorder. *Dialogues Clin Neurosci*. 2018;20(1):23–31. doi:10.31887/DCNS.2018.20.1/phenningsen.

ADDITIONAL READING

Kurlansik SL, Maffei MS. Somatic symptom disorder. *Am Fam Physician*. 2016;93(1):49–54.

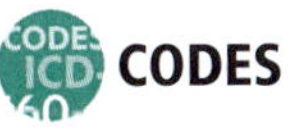

CODES

ICD10

- F45.9 Somatoform disorder, unspecified
- F45.20 Hypochondriacal disorder, unspecified
- F45.22 Body dysmorphic disorder

CLINICAL PEARLS

- Diagnosis is based on a pattern of symptoms rather than an absence of medical explanation.
- A clue is accumulation of several diagnoses with >13 letters (e.g., chronic fatigue syndrome, fibromyalgia syndrome, reflex sympathetic dystrophy, temporomandibular joint syndrome, carpal tunnel syndrome, mitral valve prolapse).
- Inability of more than three physicians to make a meaningful diagnosis suggests somatization.
- Acknowledge the patient's pain, suffering, and disability.
- Do not tell patients the symptoms are "all in their head."
- Emphasize that this is not a rare disorder.
- Discuss the limitations of treatment while providing reassurance that there are interventions that will lessen suffering and reduce symptoms.

SPINAL STENOSIS

Stephen W. Line, DO, CAQSM • Victoria Allon Nutting, DO, MS • Laura Marsh, MD, CAQSM

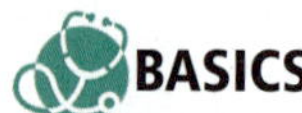

BASICS

DESCRIPTION

- A condition characterized by narrowing of either the central spinal canal, lateral recess, and/or neural foramen
- Symptoms may include pain, numbness, tingling, and muscle weakness.

EPIDEMIOLOGY

Prevalence

The prevalence of acquired spinal stenosis increases with age.

- Approximately 11–38% of adults will have some degree of lumbar stenosis on imaging (aged 19 to 93 years; mean age 62 years) (1).
- Lumbar spinal stenosis affects more than 200,000 people in the United States and is one of the most common reasons for spinal surgery in patients >65 years old (2).

ETIOLOGY AND PATHOPHYSIOLOGY

- Spinal stenosis can result from congenital or acquired causes (1).
  - Congenital spinal stenosis:
    - Developmentally short pedicles, achondroplasia, spinal dysraphism, spina bifida, and spondyloepiphyseal dysplasias.
  - Acquired spinal stenosis
    - Spondylosis, spondylolisthesis (degenerative or due to pars interarticular fracture), trauma, postoperative changes, inflammatory arthropathy (e.g., ankylosing spondylitis, rheumatoid arthritis), and space-occupying lesions (tumors, cysts)
- The most common cause of acquired spinal stenosis is degenerative spondylosis.
  - May involve the lumbar, cervical, thoracic spine (in order of prevalence)
    - Within the lumbar spine, the L4–L5 and L5–S1 levels are the most frequently involved.
  - Degenerative changes leading to spinal cord and nerve root compression include disc degeneration, facet arthropathy, osteophyte formation, and ligamentum flavum hypertrophy (3).
    - Disc dehydration leads to loss of height with bulging of the disc annulus and ligamentum flavum into the spinal canal.
    - Increased facet loading causes reactive sclerosis and osteophyte formation which compresses neural structures.
  - Not all patients with radiographic spinal stenosis are symptomatic, and the degree of radiographic stenosis does not always correlate with the patients symptoms.
  - Symptomatic spinal stenosis is likely caused by mechanical compression and ischemia of spinal nerve roots. Increased intrathecal pressure may also lead to development of symptoms (3).

RISK FACTORS

Spinal trauma, spinal surgery, spine inflammatory arthropathy, vitamin B_{12} deficiency, osteoporosis, renal osteodystrophy, Cushing disease, acromegaly, and Paget disease

COMMONLY ASSOCIATED CONDITIONS

- Cervical or lumbosacral radiculopathy
- Degenerative spondylolisthesis
- Pars interarticular fracture
- Scoliosis
- Cauda equina syndrome

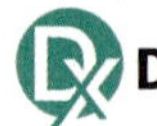

DIAGNOSIS

The diagnosis of spinal stenosis can be made clinically based on typical features and symptoms but is more commonly diagnosed radiographically. Anatomical narrowing can be seen in the absence of clinical symptoms.

HISTORY

- Insidious onset and slow progression are typical; discomfort with standing, paresthesias, and weakness (often bilateral) (3)
- Symptoms *worsen with extension* (prolonged standing, walking downhill or downstairs).
- Symptoms *improve with flexion* (sitting, leaning forward while walking, walking uphill or upstairs, lying in a flexed position, pushing a shopping cart, biking).
- Neurogenic claudication (i.e., pain, tightness, numbness, aching, and cramping of lower extremities) may mimic vascular claudication (2).
- The Zurich Claudication Questionnaire (ZCQ) is a self-administered measure to evaluate symptom severity, physical function, and satisfaction after treatment (2).

PHYSICAL EXAM

Neurologic exam may be normal. Key exam areas include the following:

- Inspection of spinal alignment:
  - Positive finding: loss of lordosis or scoliosis
- Palpation of the spinal region:
  - Positive finding: midline tenderness or paraspinal muscle tenderness
  - Most patients will not exhibit significant pain to palpation.
- Assessment of active or passive range of motion:
  - Positive finding: limitation in flexion, extension, sidebending, or rotation
  - Pain with extension of lumbar spine is typical.
- Muscle strength testing:
  - L4–L5 nerve root impingement may lead to weakness in hip abduction and great toe flexion.
  - S1 nerve root impingement may lead to hip extension weakness.
- Neurovascular evaluation:
  - Sensory changes (C5–T1 or L3–S1) may be detectable on light touch.
  - Deep tendon reflexes may be decreased.
  - About 50% of patients with LSS will have decreased Achilles reflex testing.
- Specialty testing:
  - Straight leg raise and Trendelenburg may be positive in nerve root impingement.
  - Positive Romberg test in the setting of low back pain (3)
  - FABER, FADIR, Ober, and log roll testing can help to rule out hip pathology
- Gait assessment:
  - A forward flexed gait, wide-based gate, or antalgic gait pattern is common.

DIFFERENTIAL DIAGNOSIS

- Vascular claudication
- Disc herniation or bulge
- Degenerative joint disease of the upper extremity (shoulder, elbow, or wrist)
- Degenerative joint disease of the lower extremity (hip, knee, or ankle)
- Peripheral neuropathy
- Cervical myelopathy

DIAGNOSTIC TESTS & INTERPRETATION

Generally, diagnosis is clinical. Diagnostic imaging is used to stage severity and formulate treatment plan.

Initial Tests (lab, imaging)

- CBC, ESR, C-reactive protein (if considering infection or malignancy)
- Plain radiographs (AP, lateral, oblique views)
  - Assists in excluding other causes of new back pain (e.g., malignant lytic lesions, vertebral compression fractures, degenerative spondylolisthesis, and scoliosis).
- MRI without contrast is the modality of choice (2),(3).

Follow-Up Tests & Special Considerations

- New back pain lasting >2 weeks or back pain accompanied by neurologic findings in patients >50 years generally warrants further evaluation, including evaluation for potential metastatic disease.
- CT myelography is an alternative to MRI but is invasive and has higher risk of complications.

Diagnostic Procedures/Other

- Electromyelography and nerve conduction studies are not required for diagnosis but may assist in ruling out other diagnosis such as peripheral neuropathy or cervical myelopathy.
- Ankle brachial index (ABI) testing can help diagnose or rule out peripheral arterial disease.

Test Interpretation

- Common radiograph findings include decreased disc height, facet hypertrophy, osteophyte formation, and spinal canal and/or foraminal narrowing.
- MRI will detail the extent and location of central canal stenosis, neuroforaminal stenosis, lateral recess stenosis, disc herniation/bulge, and other features of degenerative disc and spine disease.
- Radiologic abnormalities in general do not correlate with the clinical severity.

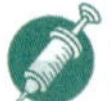

TREATMENT

- In general, nonoperative interventions are first line in the absence of progressive or debilitating neurologic symptoms:
  - Multimodal rehabilitation interventions, such as physical therapy, home exercise program, weight management (1)
  - Targeted injections (e.g., epidural steroid injections, facet joint injections) and radiofrequency ablation procedures (e.g., medial branch ablations) can help reduce symptoms (2),(3).
  - Expert consensus does not recommend the use of long-term NSAIDs, opioids, and adjunctive analgesics such as acetaminophen, methylcobalamin, and calcitonin in patients with LSS and neurogenic claudication (1).

- When conservative measures fail, neurosurgical or orthopedic spine consultation is warranted to prevent further neuropathy or myelopathy.
  - Patients should understand that the benefits of surgery may diminish over time.

MEDICATION

When pharmacotherapy is used, it is important to consider duration of treatment and the etiology of the symptoms as treatment of acute and low back pain can have varying recommendations.

First Line

- Nonsteroidal anti-inflammatory drugs (NSAIDs)
  - NSAIDs have been shown to provide modest relief in acute low back pain.
  - Consider potential for GI side effects, fluid retention, and renal failure. Use with caution in elderly.
  - COX-2 selective NSAIDs are associated with increased risk of serious cardiovascular events.
  - Typical treatment duration is 2 to 4 weeks and dose should be reduced once tolerated. Use with chronic low back pain is not recommended (1).
- Acetaminophen
  - Historically, acetaminophen has been considered a first-line medication for acute and chronic low back pain but recent evidence has shown mixed efficacy. Consider risk for hepatotoxicity (1).

Second Line

- Nonbenzodiazepine muscle relaxants
  - Have been shown to provide short-term effect symptomatic relief in acute low back pain
  - Provide mild analgesia in muscle spasm and modest skeletal muscle relaxation.
  - Side effect of sedation and dizziness is common.
    - Use with caution in geriatric population and those operating heavy machinery.
    - Consider dosing at bedtime to reduce sedation side effect.
- Management of chronic pain
  - Several medications may play a role in chronic pain management after assessment of risk profile. The following medications may be a reasonable option in select patients when contraindications exist to other pharmacotherapy options.
    - Gabapentin
    - Pregabalin
    - Duloxetine
    - Opiates (Tramadol often selected as first choice in this class)
      - Side effects of opioids include constipation, confusion, urinary retention, drowsiness, nausea, vomiting, and the potential for dependence and abuse. Use with caution in elderly.
  - Oral steroids, benzodiazepines, and antidepressants have inconsistent evidence for chronic pain and are typically not recommended as second-line agents.

ISSUES FOR REFERRAL

Nonsurgical patients with unremitting pain would benefit from pain management consultation. Consultation with neurosurgery or orthopedic spine specialist should be considered in patients with ongoing pain, progressive myelopathy, or worsening radicular symptoms that are refractory to conservative treatment.

ADDITIONAL THERAPIES

- Physical activity, core exercises, and gentle back mobility exercises are encouraged to prevent deconditioning.
- Modified exercise regimen (e.g., aquatic therapy, recumbent biking, walking, yoga, or Pilates)
- Lumbar spine bracing is controversial due to lack of evidence and due to concern for paraspinal muscle weakening with prolonged use.

SURGERY/OTHER PROCEDURES

- Surgery may be required for pain relief to increase mobility and improve quality of life.
- Surgical decompression is definitive for patients who are symptomatic after nonoperative treatment.
- Cognitive impairment, multiple comorbidities, and osteoporosis may increase the risk of perioperative complications.
- Surgical options include minimally invasive lumbar decompression (MILD), decompression with interspinous process spacers (IPS), and decompressive laminectomy (with or without fusion) (2),(3).

COMPLEMENTARY & ALTERNATIVE MEDICINE

Osteopathic manipulation, chiropractic techniques, acupuncture, massage, heat therapy, and cryotherapy can be considered.

- Severe spinal stenosis is a contraindication to high-velocity manipulation techniques.
- More clinical research is needed on these complementary modalities.

ADMISSION, INPATIENT, AND NURSING CONSIDERATIONS

- Admission criteria/initial stabilization: acute or progressive neurologic deficit.
- Discharge criteria: improved pain or after neurologic deficit has been addressed.

ONGOING CARE

FOLLOW-UP RECOMMENDATIONS

- Follow-up is based on stability or progression of symptoms.
- No specific limitations to activity; patients may be as active as tolerated.

DIET

Optimize nutrition for weight management as obesity can significantly contribute to progression of symptoms (3).

PATIENT EDUCATION

Educate on common symptoms, treatments, and diagnostic options. Maintaining and active lifestyle should be encouraged. Discuss monitoring for red flags of low back pain, including bowel/bladder dysfunction, saddle anesthesia, progressive extremity numbness, or weakness.

PROGNOSIS

- Spinal stenosis can usually be managed conservatively, but the pain can lead to limitation in ADLs and progressive disability.
- Surgery usually improves pain and symptoms in patients who fail nonoperative treatment.
- Surgical outcomes are similar in terms of pain relief and functional improvement for patients of all ages.

COMPLICATIONS

- Severe spinal stenosis can lead to bowel and/or bladder dysfunction and disabling weakness.
- Surgical complications include infection, neurologic injury, chronic pain, and disability.

REFERENCES

1. Bussières A, Cancelliere C, Ammendolia C, et al. Non-surgical interventions for lumbar spinal stenosis leading to neurogenic claudication: a clinical practice guideline. *J Pain*. 2021;22(9):1015–1039.
2. Diwan S, Sayed D, Deer TR, et al. An algorithmic approach to treating lumbar spinal stenosis: an evidence-based approach. *Pain Med*. 2019;20(Suppl 2):S23–S31.
3. Deer T, Sayed D, Michels J, et al. A Review of Lumbar Spinal Stenosis with Intermittent Neurogenic Claudication: Disease and Diagnosis. *Pain Med*. 2019;20(Suppl 2):S32–S44.

ADDITIONAL READING

Comer C, Ammendolia C, Battié MC, et al. Consensus on a standardised treatment pathway algorithm for lumbar spinal stenosis: an international Delphi study. *BMC Musculoskelet Disord*. 2022;23(1):550.

SEE ALSO

Algorithm: Low Back Pain, Acute

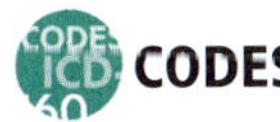

CODES

ICD10

- M48.00 Spinal stenosis, site unspecified
- M48.06 Spinal stenosis, lumbar region
- M48.04 Spinal stenosis, thoracic region

CLINICAL PEARLS

- Spinal stenosis most commonly affects the lumbar spine.
- Typical symptoms present as neurogenic claudication (pain, tightness, numbness, and subjective weakness of lower extremities). Flexion of the spine generally relieves symptoms associated with spinal stenosis, whereas extension of the spine tends to worsen symptoms.
- MRI is the diagnostic modality of choice.
- All patients with spinal stenosis should pursue lifestyle modifications.
- Additional conservative measures include physical therapy, home exercise programs, oral medications, and targeted epidural steroid injections. Consider surgical referral for decompression when spinal stenosis fails conservative management.

SPRAIN, ANKLE

Shane L. Larson, MD • Briana Lindberg, MD, CAQSM • Brock A. Benedict, DO

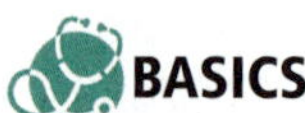

BASICS

DESCRIPTION

The most common cause of ankle injury comprising a significant proportion of injuries in the athletic and general populations:

- There are three types of ankle sprains: lateral, medial, and syndesmotic ("high ankle sprain"):
  - Lateral ankle sprains (LAS) are the most common. The anterior talofibular ligament (ATFL) is the most likely to be injured, followed by the calcaneofibular ligament (CFL) and then posterior talofibular ligament (PTFL) (1).
  - Medial ankle sprains (MAS) are the second most common and result from an injury to the deltoid ligament.
  - Syndesmotic injuries are the least common ankle sprains. These injuries result from injury to the syndesmosis between the distal tibia and distal fibula bones, consisting of the anterior, posterior, and transverse tibiofibular ligaments; the interosseous ligament; and interosseous membrane.
- Ankle sprains are classified according to the degree of ligamentous disruption:
  - Grade I: mild stretching of a ligament with possible microscopic tears
  - Grade II: incomplete tear of a ligament
  - Grade III: complete ligament tear

Geriatric Considerations

Increased risk of fracture in patients with preexisting bone weakness (osteoporosis/osteopenia)

Pediatric Considerations

- Increased risk of physeal injuries instead of ligament sprain because ligaments have greater tensile strength than physes
- Inversion ankle injuries in children may have a concomitant fibular physeal injury (Salter-Harris type I or higher fracture).
- Consider tarsal coalition with recurrent ankle sprains.

EPIDEMIOLOGY

Incidence

- Ankle sprains are very common in the general population and are some of the most commonly reported sport-related injuries. Nearly half of all ankle sprains occur during sports participation (1).
- The highest incidence of LAS occur in indoor/court sports (basketball, volleyball, tennis), followed by field sports such as football and soccer (1),(2).
- High ankle sprains are reported most frequently in men's football, wrestling, and soccer (1).

Prevalence

- 11–17% of high school and collegiate sports-related injuries in the United States (2)
- Although common in the general population, ankles sprains occur more frequently with athletic participation.

ETIOLOGY AND PATHOPHYSIOLOGY

- LAS result from an inversion force with the ankle in plantar flexion.
- MAS are due to forced eversion while the foot is in dorsiflexion.
- Syndesmotic sprains result from eversion stress/extreme dorsiflexion along with internal rotation of tibia.

RISK FACTORS

- Intrinsic risk factors
  - Limited ankle dorsiflexion range of motion
  - Reduced ankle proprioception
  - Decreased postural core strength/balance
  - Female gender
  - Low body mass index (BMI)
  - Poor strength, cardiorespiratory endurance, and/or coordination
  - Anatomical abnormalities of the knee, ankle, and/or foot
- Extrinsic risk factors
  - Type of sport played:
    - LAS: basketball, indoor volleyball, field sports and climbing
    - MAS: collegiate men's/women's soccer, men's football, women's gymnastics
    - Syndesmotic injury: football, wrestling, ice hockey
  - Higher heel height on footwear
- Prior history of ankle sprain may contribute to chronic ankle instability and increased risk for repeated ankle sprain (2).

GENERAL PREVENTION

- Address modifiable risk factors and improve overall physical conditioning:
  - Training in agility and flexibility
  - Single-leg balancing
  - Proprioceptive training
- Taping and/or bracing may help reduce the risk of both primary injury in selected sports (i.e., volleyball, basketball, football) or reinjury (1),(2). Taping and bracing do not reduce sprain severity.

COMMONLY ASSOCIATED CONDITIONS

- Contusions
- Fractures
  - Fibular head fracture/dislocation (Maisonneuve)
  - Fracture of the base of the 5th metatarsal
  - Distal fibula physeal fracture (includes Salter-Harris fractures in pediatric patients; most common type of pediatric ankle fracture)

DIAGNOSIS

HISTORY

- Elicit specific mechanism of injury (inversion vs. eversion).
- Popping/snapping sensation during the injury
- Previous history of ankle injuries
- Ability to ambulate immediately after the injury
- Rapid onset of pain, swelling, or ecchymosis
- Location of pain (lateral/medial)
- Difficulty bearing weight
- Past medical history of systemic disorders

PHYSICAL EXAM

- Timing: Initial assessment for laxity may be difficult due to pain, swelling, and muscle spasm. Repeating the exam ~5 days after injury often improves sensitivity.
- Compare to uninjured ankle for swelling, ecchymosis, weakness, and laxity.
- Assess the ability to bear weight, gait, and inspect for evidence of swelling, bruising, deformity, or other visible injuries.
- Palpate ATFL, CFL, PTFL, and deltoid ligament for tenderness.
- Palpate lateral and medial malleolus, base of 5th metatarsal, navicular, and entire fibula (concern for fibular head fracture with syndesmotic injury).
- Assess active and passive ankle range of motion with dorsiflexion, plantarflexion, inversion, and eversion.
- Determine strength in all ranges of motion.
- Evaluate neurovascular status.
- Special tests:
  - Anterior drawer test to check for ATFL laxity
  - Talar tilt test to check laxity in CFL (with inversion) or deltoid ligament (eversion)
  - Squeeze test: compress tibia and fibula midcalf to check for syndesmotic injury; sensitivity, 30%; specificity, 93.5%
  - Dorsiflexion/external rotation test: positive test is pain at syndesmosis with rotation; sensitivity, 20%; specificity, 85%
- Grade the injury.
  - Grade I sprain: mild swelling and pain; no laxity; able to bear weight/ambulate without pain
  - Grade II sprain: moderate swelling and pain; mild laxity with firm end point is noted; weight-bearing/ambulation is painful.
  - Grade III sprain: severe swelling, pain, and bruising; laxity with no end point; significant instability and loss of function/motion; unable to bear weight/ambulate

DIFFERENTIAL DIAGNOSIS

- Tendinopathy/tendon tear
- Fracture and/or dislocation of the ankle/foot
- Hindfoot/midfoot injuries
- Nerve injury
- Contusion

DIAGNOSTIC TESTS & INTERPRETATION

Initial Tests (lab, imaging)

- Ottawa ankle rules (sensitivity, 86–99%; specificity, 25–46%) may help determine need for radiographs to rule out ankle fractures (patient must be aged 18 to 55 years; certain patients, e.g., diabetics with diminished sensation, may still need radiographs):
  - Pain in malleolar zone
  - Inability to bear weight (walk ≥4 steps) immediately and in the exam room
  - Bony tenderness at distal 6 cm of the posterior edge of the lateral and/or medial malleolus
  - Bony tenderness with palpation of navicular
  - Tenderness on palpation at the base of 5th metatarsal
  - Although Ottawa ankle rules are highly sensitive, they should not overrule clinical judgment.
- If radiographs are indicated, obtain anteroposterior, lateral, and mortise views of the ankle.
  - Small avulsion fractures are associated with grade III sprains.
  - Stress views may assist in establishing the diagnosis of syndesmotic or deltoid ligament injuries (1).
- Ultrasound (US) is comparable to MRI in identifying major ligamentous injury, although it is operator-dependent. US also allows for dynamic assessment for stability and/or functional deficits (1).

- Consider CT if radiographs are negative but suspicion for occult fracture is high.
- MRI is the gold standard for soft tissue imaging but is expensive and rarely necessary.

Follow-Up Tests & Special Considerations

If the patient's condition does not improve in 6 to 8 weeks, consider CT, MRI, or US. Failure to resolve could indicate an injury such as a missed fracture, osteochondral defect, or syndesmotic injury.

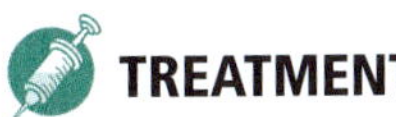

TREATMENT

GENERAL MEASURES

- Most grades I, II, and III lateral ankle sprains can be managed conservatively.
- Relative rest, ice, compression, and elevation (RICE) is a reasonable intervention in the acute phase (1)[A]. However, there is no evidence that RICE alone, cryotherapy alone, or compression alone impacts pain, swelling, or function for LAS but may improve pain, swelling, and function when used along with exercise (2)[A].
- Functional bracing (i.e., lace-up bracing) combined with exercise improves has better functional outcomes over immobilization (2)[A]. For significant pain/swelling, a short period of immobilization (<10 days) may improve pain and function prior to mobilization. For medial and syndesmosis sprains, a period of immobilization and protected weight-bearing for up to 2 weeks may prevent secondary injury (1)[B].
- Manual therapies (i.e., talocrural glides, talocrural distraction) following acute injury can improve ankle dorsiflexion, pain, and function (1)[A].
- Neuromuscular/proprioceptive training implemented within the first week following injury improves pain, swelling, return to activity, and it reduces the rate of reinjury when compared to RICE therapy (1)[A].

MEDICATION

- NSAIDs may be used judiciously in the acute phase to help with pain and swelling; however, there are some concerns that NSAID use may impair the normal inflammatory process necessary for healing (1),(2)[A].
  - Topical forms (e.g., 1% diclofenac gel) may be used to minimize gastrointestinal, renal, and cardiac side effects. PRN NSAID dosing has similar outcomes to scheduled dosing with improved safety profile.
  - Example: naproxen 500 mg BID PRN
- Acetaminophen 650 mg q4–6h (max outpatient therapy dose: 3,250 mg/day) is a reasonable alternative to NSAIDs to assist with reducing the pain in the first two weeks. Acetaminophen may be combined with NSAIDs without the risk of adverse drug interaction.
- Opioids (<5 days) if severe pain (rarely needed)
- Platelet-rich plasma (PRP) injections into the ATFL following LAS may improve short-term pain and function over bracing alone but are nonsuperior in the longer term. There is a limited evidence that PRP injection for syndesmosis injuries may lead to faster return to play over standard rehabilitation protocols (1)[A].

ISSUES FOR REFERRAL

- Malleolar/talar dome fracture
- Syndesmotic sprain
- Dislocation/subluxation
- Tendon rupture
- Ongoing instability
- Uncertain diagnosis

ADDITIONAL THERAPIES

Physical therapy:

- After the acute phase of the injury, early initiation of physical therapy can increase range of motion, strength, and flexibility, and it can improve proprioceptive balance (wobble board/ankle disk).
- Functional rehabilitation through physical therapy may prevent chronic instability and speeds healing.
- Athletes should undergo sport-specific rehabilitation before returning to play.

SURGERY/OTHER PROCEDURES

- Surgery is typically reserved for treatment of complicated recurrent sprains and certain syndesmotic sprains.
- Patients with chronic ankle instability who fail functional rehabilitation or with poor tissue quality may need anatomic repair/reconstructive surgery.

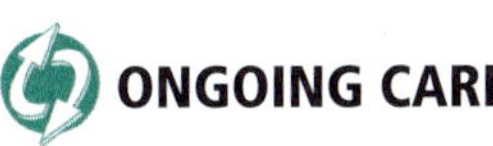

ONGOING CARE

FOLLOW-UP RECOMMENDATIONS

- After an ankle sprain, consider ankle-stabilizing orthoses (air-stirrup braces, lace-up supports, athletic taping, etc.) for athletes participating in high-risk sports to prevent future ankle sprains.
- Moderate and severe sprains require ankle orthoses for ≥6 months during sports participation.
- Gradual return to play for athletes with a grade I lateral ankle sprain can generally be accomplished in 1 to 2 weeks; grade II sprain return to play time is 2 to 3 weeks; grade III sprain is approximately 4 weeks.
- Syndesmotic sprains take longer (~8 to 9 weeks) to heal than lateral ankle sprains.

Patient Monitoring

If athletes continue to have symptoms when they return to play or if a patient has pain for 6 to 8 weeks after injury, repeat examination and imaging.

PATIENT EDUCATION

- Crutch training
- Provide training on proper use of elastic bandages, brace, and/or orthoses.
- Demonstrate mobilization exercises (alphabet trace and towel grab).

PROGNOSIS

- Earlier physical therapy and mobilization with bracing allow for faster return to daily living and/or sports.
- Higher grade sprains, older patient age, and initial non–weight-bearing status have poorer prognosis and longer recovery.
- Ligamentous strength does not return for months after the injury.

COMPLICATIONS

- Joint instability
- Intermittent swelling/pain if not properly treated
- 5–33% continue to have pain 1 year postinjury.
- Accumulation of cartilage damage, leading to degenerative changes

REFERENCES

1. Chen ET, Borg-Stein J, McInnis KC. Ankle sprains: evaluation, rehabilitation, and prevention. *Curr Sports Med Rep*. 2019;18(6):217–223.
2. Vuurberg G, Hoorntje A, Wink LM, et al. Diagnosis, treatment and prevention of ankle sprains: update of an evidence-based clinical guideline. *Br J Sports Med*. 2018;52(15):956.

ADDITIONAL READING

- Caldemeyer LE, Brown SM, Mulcahey MK. Neuromuscular training for the prevention of ankle sprains in female athletes: a systematic review. *Phys Sportsmed*. 2020;48(4):363–369.
- D'Hooghe P, Cruz F, Alkhelaifi K. Return to play after a lateral ligament ankle sprain. *Curr Rev Musculoskelet Med*. 2020;13(3):281–288.
- Ortega-Avila AB, Cervera-Garvi P, Marchena-Rodriguez A, et al. Conservative treatment for acute ankle sprain: a systematic review. *J Clin Med*. 2020;9(10):3128.

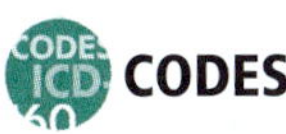

CODES

ICD10

- S96.919A Strain of unsp msl/tnd at ank/ft level, unsp foot, init
- S93.499A Sprain of other ligament of unspecified ankle, init encntr
- S93.419A Sprain of calcaneofibular ligament of unsp ankle, init

CLINICAL PEARLS

- Children are at an increased risk of physeal injuries because ligaments are stronger than physes.
- Conditioning, including proprioceptive training, before participating in sports and throughout the season helps to prevent ankle sprains.
- Functional rehabilitation, rather than total immobilization, is recommended for quicker return to sport and work.
- Patients who do not adequately rehabilitate an ankle sprain are at increased risk for recurrence and chronic ankle instability.
- If patient's condition is not improving in 6 to 8 weeks, consider advanced imaging with CT, MRI, or US.

SPRAINS AND STRAINS

Lee A. Mancini, MD, CAQSM, CSCS*D, CSN • Alec L. Tributino, DO • Grant Pierre, MD, CAQSM

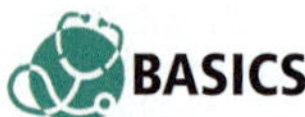

BASICS

DESCRIPTION

- *Sprains* are complete or partial ligamentous injuries either within the body of the ligament or at the site of attachment to bone.
  - Classified as grade 1, 2, or 3 (AMA Ligament Injury Classification)
    - Grade 1: stretch injury without ligamentous laxity
    - Grade 2: partial tear with increased ligamentous laxity but firm end point on exam
    - Grade 3: complete tear with increased ligamentous laxity and no firm end point on exam
  - Usually secondary to trauma (e.g., falls, twisting injuries, motor vehicle accidents)
  - Physical exam is the key to accurate diagnosis.
- *Strains* are partial or complete disruptions of the muscle, muscle–tendon junction, or tendon.
  - Classified as
    - First degree: minimal damage to muscle, tendon, or musculotendinous unit
    - Second degree: partial tear to the muscle, tendon, or musculotendinous unit
    - Third degree: complete disruption of the muscle, tendon, or musculotendinous unit
  - Often associated with overuse injuries

Geriatric Considerations

More likely to see associated bony injuries due to decreased joint flexibility and increased prevalence of osteoporosis and osteopenia

Pediatric Considerations

- Sprains and strains account for 24% of pediatric injuries.
- 3 million pediatric sports injuries occur annually.
- Consider physeal/apophyseal injuries in the skeletally immature patient.

EPIDEMIOLOGY

Incidence

~80% of all U.S. athletes experience a sprain or strain at some point.

Prevalence

- Ankle sprains are among the most common injuries in primary care, accounting for ~30% of sports medicine clinic visits. Most ankle sprains are due to inversion injuries (lateral sprains) involving the anterior talofibular ligament; account for 650,000 annual ER visits in the United States
- Predominant age
  - Sprains: any age in physically active patient
  - Strains: usually 15 to 40 years of age
- Predominant sex: male > female for most; female > male for sprain of anterior cruciate ligament (ACL)

ETIOLOGY AND PATHOPHYSIOLOGY

- Trauma, falls, motor vehicle accidents
- Excessive exercise; poor conditioning
- Improper footwear
- Inadequate warm-up and stretching before activity
- Prior sprain or strain

RISK FACTORS

- Prior history of sprain or strain is the greatest risk factor for future sprain/strain.
- Change in or improper footwear, protective gear, or environment (e.g., surface)
- Sudden increase in training schedule or volume
- Tobacco use, medication adverse effects

GENERAL PREVENTION

- Appropriate warm-up and cool-down exercises
- Use proper equipment and footwear.
- Balance training programs improve proprioception and reduce the risk of ankle sprains.
- Semirigid orthoses may prevent ankle sprains during high-risk sports, especially in athletes with history of sprain.
- Proprioception and strength training decrease injury risk; stretching does not

COMMONLY ASSOCIATED CONDITIONS

- Effusions, ecchymosis, hemarthrosis
- Stress, avulsion, and/or other fractures
- Syndesmotic injuries
- Contusions
- Dislocations/subluxations

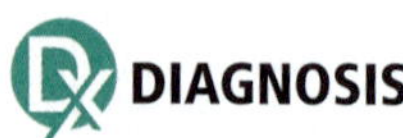

DIAGNOSIS

HISTORY

- Obtain a thorough description of mechanism of injury including activity, trauma, baseline conditioning, and prior musculoskeletal injuries.
- May describe feeling or hearing pop or snap

PHYSICAL EXAM

- Inspect for swelling, asymmetry, ecchymosis, and gait disturbance.
- Evaluate for neurovascular compromise.
- Palpate for tenderness.
- Evaluate for decreased range of motion (ROM) of joint and joint instability/laxity.
- Evaluate for strength.
- Sprains
  - Grade 1: tenderness without laxity; minimal pain, swelling; little ecchymosis; can bear weight
  - Grade 2: tenderness with increased laxity on exam but firm end point; more pain, swelling; often ecchymosis; some difficulty bearing weight
  - Grade 3: tenderness with increased laxity on exam and no firm end point; severe pain, swelling; obvious ecchymosis; difficulty bearing weight

DIFFERENTIAL DIAGNOSIS

- Tendonitis
- Bursitis
- Contusion
- Hematoma
- Fracture
- Osteochondral lesion
- Rheumatologic process

DIAGNOSTIC TESTS & INTERPRETATION

- Ankle
  - Anterior drawer test assesses integrity of anterior talofibular ligament.
  - Talar tilt test assesses integrity of calcaneofibular ligament.
  - Squeeze test assesses for syndesmotic injury.
  - Palpate lateral and medial malleoli.
- Knee
  - Lachman and anterior drawer tests assess integrity of ACL. Posterior drawer and sag tests assess integrity of posterior cruciate ligament.
  - Valgus/varus stress tests assess integrity of medial and lateral collateral ligaments, respectively.
- Shoulder
  - Load and shift test; sulcus sign; and the apprehension, relocation, surprise test assess for instability of the glenohumeral joint.
- Radiographs help rule out bony injury; stress views may be necessary. Obtain bilateral radiographs in children to rule out growth plate injuries.
- Use Ottawa Foot and Ankle Rules (ages 18 to 55 years) to determine if radiographs are necessary.
- Ottawa Ankle Rules: x-ray required if pain in the malleolar zone *and*
  - Bone tenderness in posterior aspect distal 6 cm of tibia or fibula *or*
  - Unable to bear weight immediately or in emergency department
- Ottawa Foot Rules: x-ray required if midfoot zone pain is present *and*
  - Bone tenderness at base of 5th metatarsal *or*
  - Bone tenderness at navicular *or*
  - Inability to bear weight immediately or in emergency department

Follow-Up Tests & Special Considerations

- Can consider repeat x-rays in 1 to 2 weeks if symptoms not improved to rule out occult fracture
- CT scan can be considered if occult fracture is suspected.
- MRI is the gold standard for imaging soft tissue structures, including muscle, ligaments, and intra-articular structures. If tibiofibular syndesmotic disruption is suspected, MRI is highly accurate for diagnosis. Contrast is usually not necessary for diagnosis of most ligamentous and labral injuries.
- Ultrasound evaluation of a variety of muscles, tendons, and ligaments by a skilled operator allows for dynamic evaluation of potential sprain/strain that can add to traditional diagnostic imaging.

Diagnostic Procedures/Other

Surgery may be required for some partial and complete sprains depending on location, mechanism, and chronicity.

TREATMENT

GENERAL MEASURES

- Acute: *p*rotection, relative *r*est (activity modification), *i*ce, *c*ompression, *e*levation, *m*edications, *m*odalities (PRICEMM) therapy
- Ankle sprains: should consist of functional support, possibly augmented by nonsteroidal anti-inflammatory drugs in the early phases after injury
- Grades 1 and 2 ankle sprain: functional treatment with brace, orthosis, taping, elastic bandage wrap
  - Ankle braces (lace-up, stirrup-type, air cast) are a more effective functional treatment than elastic bandages or taping (1)[A].
- Grade 3 ankle sprain: Short period of immobilization may be needed. Consider short walking boot and/or crutches.
- Refer for early physical therapy.
- For high-level athletes with more extensive damage (e.g., biceps or pectoralis disruption), consider surgical referral.

MEDICATION

First Line

- Acetaminophen: not to exceed 3 g/day
- NSAIDs
  - Ibuprofen: 200 to 800 mg TID
  - Naproxen: 250 to 500 mg BID
  - Diclofenac: 50 to 75 mg BID
- Acetaminophen and NSAIDs have similar efficacy in reducing pain after soft tissue injuries with less GI side effects; NSAIDs are better than narcotics.
- Topical diclofenac, ibuprofen, and ketoprofen are effective for pain related to strains and sprains, especially in gel form or patch (2)[A].

Second Line

- Platelet-rich plasma injections may aid recovery in treatment of muscle strains, but more studies are needed.
- Opioids should rarely be considered acutely for severe pain, but discretion is advised.

ISSUES FOR REFERRAL

- ACL sprain in athletes/physically active
- Salter-Harris physeal fractures
- Joint instability especially if chronic
- Tendon disruption (i.e., Achilles, biceps, ACL)
- Lack of improvement with conservative measures

ADDITIONAL THERAPIES

- Physical therapy is a useful adjunct after a sprain, particularly if early mobilization is crucial.
  - Proprioception retraining
  - Core strengthening
  - Eccentric exercises
  - Thera-Band exercises
- After hamstring strain, frequent daily stretching and progressive agility and trunk stabilization exercises may speed recovery and reduce risk of reinjury (3)[A]. Rehab protocols emphasizing eccentric/lengthening exercises are more effective than conventional exercises (4)[B].

SURGERY/OTHER PROCEDURES

- Casting and surgery are reserved for select partial and complete sprains. Need for surgery depends on the neurovascular supply to the injured area as well as the ability to attain full ROM and stability of the affected joint. The need for surgery also depends on activity level and patient preference.
- For primary management of acute lateral ankle sprains, there is no difference between surgical versus conservative therapy. Risks are increased with surgical intervention.
- Chronic ankle instability affects 10–20% of people who sustain an acute sprain. If conservative management fails and laxity is present, surgery is considered (5)[A].
- Percutaneous needle tenotomy versus surgical tenotomy are available as options for chronic tendinosis (chronic, recurrent strains).

ONGOING CARE

FOLLOW-UP RECOMMENDATIONS

If the affected joint has full strength and ROM, the patient can advance activity as tolerated using pain as a guide for return to activity.

Patient Monitoring

After initial treatment, consider early rehabilitation. Limit swelling and work on increasing ROM.

DIET

Weight loss if overweight

PATIENT EDUCATION

- Injury prevention through proprioceptive training and physical therapy
- ROM and strengthening exercises to restore functional capacity

PROGNOSIS

Favorable with appropriate treatment and rest. Duration of recovery depends on the severity and location of injury.

COMPLICATIONS

- Chronic joint instability
- Arthritis
- Muscle contracture
- Chronic tendinopathy

REFERENCES

1. Petersen W, Rembitzki IV, Koppenburg AG, et al. Treatment of acute ankle ligament injuries: a systematic review. *Arch Orthop Trauma Surg*. 2013;133(8):1129–1141.
2. Derry S, Moore RA, Gaskell H, et al. Topical NSAIDs for acute musculoskeletal pain in adults. *Cochrane Database Syst Rev*. 2015;2015(6):CD007402.
3. Pas HIMFL, Reurink G, Tol JL, et al. Efficacy of rehabilitation (lengthening) exercises, platelet-rich plasma injections, and other conservative interventions in acute hamstring injuries: an updated systematic review and meta-analysis. *Br J Sports Med*. 2015;49(18):1197–1205.
4. Askling CM, Tengvar M, Tarassova O, et al. Acute hamstring injuries in Swedish elite sprinters and jumpers: a prospective randomised controlled clinical trial comparing two rehabilitation protocols. *Br J Sports Med*. 2014;48(7):532–539.
5. McCriskin BJ, Cameron KL, Orr JD, et al. Management and prevention of acute and chronic lateral ankle instability in athletic patient populations. *World J Orthop*. 2015;6(2):161–171.

ADDITIONAL READING

- Hamilton BH, Best TM. Platelet-enriched plasma and muscle strain injuries: challenges imposed by the burden of proof. *Clin J Sport Med*. 2011;21(1):31–36.
- Kim TH, Lee MS, Kim KH, et al. Acupuncture for treating acute ankle sprains in adults. *Cochrane Database Syst Rev*. 2014;(6):CD009065.
- Monk AP, Davies LJ, Hopewell S, et al. Surgical versus conservative interventions for treating anterior cruciate ligament injuries. *Cochrane Database Syst Rev*. 2016;4(4):CD011166.
- Seah R, Mani-Babu S. Managing ankle sprains in primary care: what is best practice? A systematic review of the last 10 years of evidence. *Br Med Bull*. 2011;97:105–135.

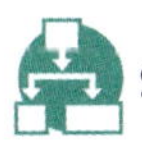

SEE ALSO

Tendinopathy

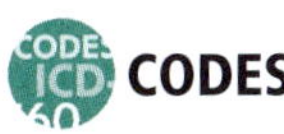

CODES

ICD10

- S93.6 Sprain of foot
- S93.4 Sprain of ankle
- S93.5 Sprain of toe

CLINICAL PEARLS

For acute injury, remember PRICEMM:

- Protection of the joint
- Relative rest (activity modification)
- Apply ice.
- Apply compression.
- Elevate joint.
- Medications/ice for pain
- Other modalities as needed
- Wean out of brace as tolerated to limit atrophy of stabilizing muscles.

SQUAMOUS CELL CARCINOMA, CUTANEOUS

Nathan J. Macedo, MD, MPH

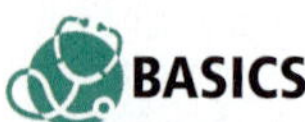

BASICS

DESCRIPTION

- Cutaneous squamous cell carcinoma (cSCC) is the second most common skin cancer after basal cell carcinoma (BCC), with >1 million cases diagnosed annually in the United States.
- Arises from epidermal keratinocytes and accounts for the majority of nonmelanoma skin cancer–related deaths

EPIDEMIOLOGY

Historically, cSCC has been thought to account for 20% of nonmelanoma skin cancers, thus is considered to be the second most common malignancy after BCC. However, recent data indicate that the ratio of BCC to SCC is 1 in the U.S. Medicare population.

Incidence

- The average age for incidence is around 60 years, more common in men.
- Incidence increases the closer the person gets to the equator or higher altitude.

Prevalence

>1 million cases of cSCC are diagnosed annually in the United States.

ETIOLOGY AND PATHOPHYSIOLOGY

- cSCC arises from malignant transformation of keratinocytes in the epidermis, primarily due to cumulative ultraviolet (UV) radiation exposure.
- UV radiation induces DNA damage and results in mutations in tumor suppressor genes (e.g., TP53) and proto-oncogenes.
- In immunosuppressed individuals, mutated keratinocytes escape detection and proliferate.

Genetics

Some hereditary disorders have genes that are associated with cSCC. They include:

- Xeroderma pigmentosum
- Oculocutaneous albinism
- Epidermodysplasia verruciformis
- Genes mutated include: CDKN2A, NOTCH1, Ras, and TP53

RISK FACTORS

- Cumulative UV exposure
- Fair skin types (Fitzpatrick I to III)
- Gender (more common in men)
- Increasing age (average age of onset is the mid-60s)
- Preexisting lesions of actinic keratosis (AK)
- Immunosuppression
  - Solid organ transplantation
  - HIV/AIDS, non-Hodgkin lymphoma, and chronic lymphocytic leukemia
- Chronic skin conditions
  - Burn scars, hidradenitis suppurativa, chronic osteomyelitis, discoid lupus erythematosus, lichen planus, lichen sclerosis et atrophicus, and xeroderma pigmentosum
- Inherited genetic conditions
  - Albinism, epidermolysis bullosa, xeroderma pigmentosum
- Prior history of ionizing radiation exposure
- Arsenic exposure
- Ulcers
- Bowen disease (squamous cell carcinoma [SCC] in situ)
- Erythroplasia of Queyrat (SCC in situ of the penis)
- HPV infection (6, 11, 16, 18)
- Treatment with BRAF inhibitors (vemurafenib and dabrafenib)

GENERAL PREVENTION

- Protect skin from sun exposure.
- Wear sunscreen, hats, and UV-protective clothing.
- The U.S. Preventive Services Task Force (USPSTF) recommends counseling about minimizing exposure to UV radiation for people aged 6 months to 24 years with fair skin types to decrease their risk of skin cancer (1).

COMMONLY ASSOCIATED CONDITIONS

AK is the precursor of cSCC, Bowen disease, and erythroplasia of Querat.

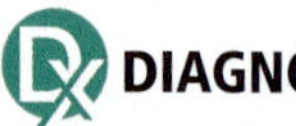

DIAGNOSIS

- Histopathology remains the gold standard for the diagnosis of cSCC. A punch or shave biopsy can be used to obtain a sample (2).
- Dermoscopy is a noninvasive technique that can help improve diagnostic accuracy (2).

HISTORY

Patients typically with known risk factors such as older age and fair skin type often present with a nonhealing lesion that bleeds with minimal trauma on a sun-exposed area of skin.

PHYSICAL EXAM

- Lesions occur mainly in chronically exposed areas: Face (especially lips, ear, nose, cheek, and eyelid)
- Lesions occur chiefly in chronically sun-exposed areas:
  - Face and backs of the forearms and hands
  - Bald areas of the scalp and top of ears in men
  - The sun-exposed "V" of the neck as well as the posterior neck below the occipital hairline
  - In elderly women, lesions tend to occur on the legs and other sun-exposed locations.
  - In African Americans, equal frequency in sun-exposed and unexposed areas
- Clinical appearance
  - Generally slow-growing, firm, hyperkeratotic papules, nodules, or plaques
  - Lesions may have a smooth, verrucous, or papillomatous surface.
  - Varying degrees of ulceration, erosion, crust, or scale
  - Color is often red to brown, tan, or pearly (indistinguishable from BCC).
- Clinical variants
  - Bowen disease (SCC in situ): a solitary lesion that resembles a scaly psoriatic plaque
  - Invasive SCC: often a raised, firm papule, nodule, or plaque; lesions may be smooth, verrucous, or papillomatous, with varying degrees of ulceration, erosion, crust, or scale.
  - Cutaneous horn: SCC with an overlying cutaneous horn. A cutaneous horn represents a thick, hard, fingernail-like keratinization produced by the SCC. Bowen disease may also have a cutaneous horn on its surface.
  - Erythroplasia of Queyrat refers to Bowen disease of the glans or prepuce penis, which manifests as one or more velvety red plaques.
  - Subungual SCC appears as hyperkeratotic lesions under the nail plate or surrounding periungual skin, often mimicking warts.
  - Marjolin ulcer: an SCC evolving from a new area of ulceration or elevation at the site of a scar or ulcer
  - HPV-associated SCC: virally induced; present as new or enlarging warty growth on the penis, vulva, perianal area, or periungual region
  - Verrucous carcinoma: a subtype of SCC that is extremely well-differentiated, can be locally destructive, but rarely metastasizes. Lesions are "cauliflower-like" verrucous nodules or plaques.
  - Basaloid SCC: less common than typical SCC; seen more often in men aged 40 to 70 years

DIFFERENTIAL DIAGNOSIS

- AK
- BCC

DIAGNOSTIC TESTS & INTERPRETATION

- Biopsy of the lesion will demonstrate characteristic histologic findings. Shave biopsy, punch biopsy, or excisional biopsy can be utilized (2).
- Histopathologic findings are as follows (2):
  - Pleomorphic, hyperchromatic squamous cells with nuclear pleomorphism (2)
  - Aggregates of glassy, eosinophilic keratinocytes (2)
  - Full-thickness atypia of the epidermis (2)
  - Keratinocyte mitoses (2)
  - Squamous pearls (2)
  - Inflammatory infiltrate of lymphocytes and plasma cells may be seen (2).

- Factors associated with local recurrence and metastases (3)
  - Tumor depth >2 mm or beyond subcutaneous fat
  - Poorly differentiated tumor
  - Perineural involvement of nerves >0.1 mm is associated with an increased risk of nodal metastases and increased mortality
  - Temple, ear, lip location
  - Diameter >2 cm
  - Arising from a scar
  - Immunosuppression
- Current staging systems (3)
  - Formal staging:
    - *AJCC Cancer Staging Manual* 8th edition (2017) applies only to tumors of the head and neck.
      - Tumor size, depth of invasion, perineural invasion, and bone involvement define T stage
- Alternative risk stratification: Brigham and Women's Hospital (BWH)
- Classification is more predictive of outcomes.
- Factors: tumor diameter ≥2 cm, poor differentiation, perineural invasion ≥0.1 mm, and invasion beyond subcutaneous fat.

Follow-Up Tests & Special Considerations

- For high-risk cSCC:
  - Complete skin exam and lymph node exam required every 2 to 6 months
    Every 6 to 12 months for the next 3 years
  - Annually after 5 years
- For high-risk cSCC with regional disease: These are the follow-up recommendations:
  - Complete skin exam and lymph node exam every 1 to 3 months
  - Every 2 to 4 months for the next year
  - Every 4 to 6 months until the 5th year
  - Every 6 to 12 months for the patient's lifetime

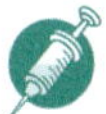

TREATMENT

Selecting the most appropriate treatment options should involve consideration of the following:

- Tumor location and characteristics
- High-risk areas
- Recurrence rate
- Patient expectations
- Patient's functional status and life expectancy

MEDICATION

First Line

- First-line treatment for cSCC is complete surgical excision with histopathologic control of excision margins.
- cSCC with a low risk of metastasis can be treated with wide local excision, electrodesiccation, curettage, or cryosurgery.
- Mohs micrographic surgery (MMS) is the gold-standard treatment for high-risk tumors instead of surgical excision.
- Cryotherapy, radiation, and topical medication can be used to treat patients who have bleeding disorders or contraindications to surgery (1).
  - Topical medications (chemotherapy drugs)—5-fluorouracil (5-FU), imiquimod

Second Line

Systemic therapies

- Monoclonal antibodies (cetuximab, panitumumab); FDA-approved for locally advanced or metastatic cSCC not amenable to surgery or radiation
- Tyrosine kinase inhibitors (erlotinib)
- Chemotherapy—used in locally advanced or metastatic skin SCC
  - Chemotherapeutic drugs used are methotrexate, bleomycin, doxorubicin, and cisplatin.
- Oral retinoids decrease the incidence of AK and cSCC.
- Radiation
  - Radiation can be primary or adjuvant therapy and is especially useful for patients who are poor surgical candidates or have positive margins, perineural invasion, or nodal disease (3).

SURGERY/OTHER PROCEDURES

Radiation-induced malignancy

ADMISSION, INPATIENT, AND NURSING CONSIDERATIONS

Examine sentinel lymph nodes for early detection of metastasis. This can decrease disease-related morbidity and mortality.

ONGOING CARE

PROGNOSIS

- cSCC is associated with a positive 5-year survival rate of about 98%.
- 30–50% of high-risk cSCC patients will develop second skin cancer within five years.
- Patients with high-risk cSCC have an increased risk of recurrence, lymph node, or distant metastases.
- Staging is essential for treating high-risk cutaneous SCC.
- After recurrence, the prognosis is inferior. There is a risk of distant metastasis and metastasis to regional lymph nodes.
- After resection of cancer, recurrent cancers have twice the risk of recurrence.
- For patients with metastatic disease, the long-term prognosis is poor.
  - For patients having distant metastasis, 10-year survival rates are <10%.
  - For patients having regional lymph node involvement, 10-year survival rates are <20%.
- Distant metastasis occurs in 15% of cases and involves these sites:
  - Brain
  - Lungs
  - Liver
  - Skin
  - Bone

COMPLICATIONS

- Local recurrence
- Metastasis

REFERENCES

1. Firnhaber JM. Basal cell and cutaneous squamous cell carcinomas: diagnosis and treatment. *Am Fam Physician*. 2020;102(6):339–346.
2. Combalia A, Carrera C. Squamous cell carcinoma: an update on diagnosis and treatment. *Dermatol Pract Concept*. 2020;10(3):e2020066.
3. Wysong A. Squamous-cell carcinoma of the skin. *N Engl J Med*. 2023;388(24):2262–2273.

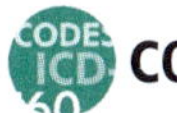

CODES

ICD10

- C44.92 Squamous cell carcinoma of skin, unspecified
- C44.320 Squamous cell carcinoma of skin of unspecified parts of face
- C44.42 Squamous cell carcinoma of skin of scalp and neck

CLINICAL PEARLS

- cSCC is the second most common form of skin cancer and is associated with UV light exposure and immunosuppression.
- Counsel patients about the importance of using and reapplying a broad spectrum (UVA/UVB) sunscreen of at least SPF 15 every day to prevent all types of skin cancer.
- The head and neck are the most common regions for invasive cSCC.
- MMS provides cure rates of 97% for primary cSCC.

S

STRESS FRACTURE

Dongsheng Jiang, MD, MSc • Joanna Jiang, MD

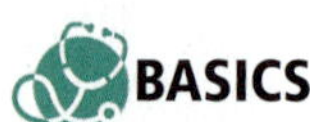

BASICS

DESCRIPTION

- Stress fractures are overuse injuries caused by cumulative microdamage from repetitive bone loading.
- Stress fractures occur in different situations:
  - Fatigue fracture: abnormal repetitive stress applied to normal bone (e.g., young college athletes or new military recruits with increased physical activity demands and inadequate conditioning); common sites include tibia, fibula, metatarsals, femoral neck, and navicular.
  - Insufficiency fracture: normal stress applied to structurally abnormal bone (e.g., femoral neck fracture in osteopenic bone, metabolic bone disease); common sites include spine, sacrum, femoral neck, and medial femoral condyle.
  - Combination fracture: abnormal stress applied to abnormal bone (e.g., female long-distance runners with premature osteoporosis from athletic triad)
- Weight-bearing bones of the lower extremity are most commonly affected at the following sites:
  - Tibia/fibula (most common)
  - Metatarsals (second most)
  - Navicular
  - Femoral neck
  - Pars interarticularis
- High-risk stress fractures occur in zones of tension or areas with poor blood supply and are more likely to result in fracture displacement and/or nonunion. High-risk sites include the following:
  - Femoral neck
  - Anterior tibial diaphysis
  - Sesamoids
  - Pars interarticularis of lumbar spine (L4, L5)
  - 5th metatarsal at metaphyseal–diaphyseal junction
  - Proximal 2nd metatarsal
  - Medial malleolus
  - Tarsal navicular
  - Patella
  - Talar neck
- Synonym(s): march fracture; fatigue fracture

EPIDEMIOLOGY

Incidence

- Greatest incidence in 15- to 27-year-olds
- Females > males
- Accounts for up to 20% of visits to sports medicine and orthopedic clinics

Prevalence

- Lifetime athletic stress fracture is 10% (1).
- Affects up to 6.9% of male and 21.0% of female military members

ETIOLOGY AND PATHOPHYSIOLOGY

- Bone is dynamic and constantly remodeling in response to applied physiologic stress.
- Repetitive loading or overuse causes microfractures that fail to heal due to imbalance between bone resorption and bone formation.
- If microdamage accumulates in excess of reparation, bony fatigue leads to stress fracture.

RISK FACTORS

- Intrinsic
  - Females are at 2.3 times higher risk than males.
  - Female athlete triad
  - Small tibial width
  - Later menarche, amenorrhea, or irregular menses
  - History of stress fracture
  - History of osteoporosis, osteomalacia, rheumatoid arthritis, prolonged corticosteroid therapy
  - BMI <19 kg/m^2
  - Skeletal malalignment: pes cavus/planus, leg length discrepancies, excessive forefoot varus, tarsal coalitions, prominent posterior calcaneal process, tight heel cords
  - Biomechanical factors such as increased vertical loading rate (e.g., heel-to-toe running instead of forefoot striking)
- Extrinsic
  - High-risk exercises—track and field, cross country
  - Training regimen—running >20 miles/week or training >5 hr/day
  - Nutritional—inadequate caloric intake or history of eating disorder
  - Chronic low vitamin D
  - Rapid increase in mileage, running pace, or training volume
  - Inappropriate footwear
  - Hard training/running surface
  - Inadequate recovery or rest and training with fatigued muscle
  - Lifestyle: high alcohol intake or smoking
  - Meds: glucocorticoids, anticonvulsants, antidepressants, depot-medroxyprogesterone acetate (DMPA), methotrexate, antiretrovirals, chronic cannabis use, >5 years of bisphosphonate use

GENERAL PREVENTION

- Prevention is the key especially in adolescent athletes (1).
- Graduated increments in training load intensity: no >10% per week
- Optimize energy balance.
- Diversify sports participation (minimizing sports specialization).
- Reduce intensity and duration of activity if new-onset pain.
- Proper footwear (Athletes should have a gait analysis prior to training.)
- Increasing dynamic physical activity (jumping; plyometric training) increases bone density and resistance to mechanical stress.
- Decrease vertical loading rate either by switching to forefoot strike running or (if continuing with heel-to-toe strike) by using a heel pad insert.
- Vitamin D supplementation (800 IU/day) in combination with calcium (2,000 mg/day)

COMMONLY ASSOCIATED CONDITIONS

- Osteoporosis/osteopenia
- Female athlete triad
- Metabolic bone disorders

DIAGNOSIS

HISTORY

- Insidious onset of vague bony pain over a period of weeks; pain is typically worse with physical activity.
- Initially relieved by rest and then pain persists with rest or slight activity
- If untreated, pain progresses and may occur earlier during training sessions. With time and repetitive loading, the pain also becomes more localized.
- History of recent change in training intensity, alteration in training terrain, and/or footwear
- Assess dietary practices: energy availability, disordered eating, weight fluctuations, and calcium and vitamin D intake.
- In female athletes, assess menstrual history: menarche, oligomenorrhea, or amenorrhea.

PHYSICAL EXAM

- Height, weight, BMI, and any stigmata of disordered eating (cold extremities, hypercarotenemia, lanugo hair, calluses on back of fingers, poor oral hygiene, parotid gland hypertrophy, or orthostatic hypotension)
- Antalgic gait (limp; limiting weight on affected leg)
- Point or percussion tenderness over injury site: A vibrating tuning fork over the fracture site may intensify pain.
- Swelling may be present.
- Specific tests:
  - Hop test for tibial stress fracture: With a stress fracture, the patient cannot hop on one leg 10 times; if able to perform test, consider shin splints (medial tibial stress syndrome).
  - Fulcrum test for femoral stress fracture: With patient seated, provoke pain by applying downward force on the distal femur while the other hand is under the midthigh on femoral shaft (if clinical suspicion is high, defer or use only with extreme caution to avoid completing a femoral neck stress fracture).
  - Single-leg hyperextension (Stork) test for pars interarticularis fracture of lumbar spine: Stand on one leg and extend lumbar spine; positive if painful on symptomatic side
- Anatomic malalignment may be present (leg length discrepancy, scoliosis, pes planus/cavus).

DIFFERENTIAL DIAGNOSIS

- Shin splints (medial tibial stress syndrome—pain resolves with rest; stress fracture pain does not)
- Infection (osteomyelitis)
- Soft tissue injury (sprain, tendonitis, and periostitis)
- Exertional compartment syndrome
- Bony fracture, pathologic fracture, insufficiency fracture
- Neoplasm (osteoid osteoma)
- Nerve entrapment syndromes
- Intermittent claudication

DIAGNOSTIC TESTS & INTERPRETATION

Initial Tests (lab, imaging)

- Laboratory tests are not required unless clinically indicated for suspected disease (e.g., female athlete triad, hyperparathyroidism, vitamin D deficiency).
- May consider CBC, CMP, TSH, 25-hydroxyvitamin D(25[OH]D), FSH, LH plus 24-hour urine calcium and PTH

- Plain films (x-ray):
  - First line in suspected stress fracture
  - Findings typically seen 2 to 8 weeks after pain onset
  - High false negative rate during early stages (1 to 2 weeks)
  - May see periosteal callus, "gray cortex sign" (region of decreased cortical intensity), osteopenia, endosteal reaction, or ill-defined cortical margin
  - Severe cases may show discrete fracture.

Follow-Up Tests & Special Considerations

- MRI:
  - Gold standard for imaging stress fractures
  - Early signs (edema of bone and surrounding soft tissue) can be identified as early as 1 to 2 days after the onset of symptoms.
  - Sensitivity is up to 88%; specificity up to 100%, accuracy 90% (1)
- Bone scan:
  - Sensitive but has potential for false positives
  - Can show signs of stress fracture as early as 3 to 5 days after onset of symptoms
  - Useful for suspected rib or spine stress fractures
  - Should not be used to assess healing
- CT scan:
  - Less sensitive than MRI or bone scan for early stress fractures but has an important role in evaluating longitudinal fracture lines and occult fractures of foot, tibia, carpal scaphoid, and pars interarticularis
  - Can distinguish conditions (osteoid osteoma, malignancy, and osteomyelitis) that mimic stress fracture on bone scan; useful when fractures are chronic and are associated with low bone turnover
  - Bony detail provided by CT scan allows differentiation of complete versus incomplete fracture, especially if MRI is equivocal.
- US: not routinely used but beneficial for superficial stress fracture
- Classification by radiographic findings (CT, MRI, bone scan, or x-ray)
  - Grade I: asymptomatic stress reaction; no pain, periosteal edema only, no fracture line
  - Grade II: symptomatic stress reaction; pain on exam, bone marrow edema, no fracture line seen on imaging
  - Grade III: nondisplaced fracture; pain on exam, nondisplaced fracture line seen on imaging
  - Grade IV: displaced fracture; pain on exam, displaced fracture >2 mm seen on imaging
  - Grade V: nonunion; pain on exam, nonunion characteristics on imaging, long-standing symptoms

TREATMENT

- Low-risk stress fractures are generally treated nonoperatively with a 2-phase protocol (2):
  - Cessation of sport activity for 6 to 8 weeks
  - After a period of pain-free rest of 10 to 14 days, gradually return to activity over the subsequent weeks, including continued physical therapy.
    - Protection, rest, ice, compression, and elevation (PRICE) for acute pain and edema
    - Activity modification: Decrease activity to the level of pain-free functioning.
    - Start alternative lower load exercises, such as hydrotherapy or swimming, antigravity treadmill cycling, and elliptical workouts, to maintain fitness.
    - Consider temporarily immobilizing patients who have pain at rest or with gentle range of motion.
    - If patients have pain with ambulation, use crutches with periodic walking trial to monitor readiness for nonaided (pain free) ambulation.
    - Pneumatic leg brace is effective in decreasing the return-to-play time for tibial shaft stress fracture.
    - Adequate recovery time is important to ensure proper healing of all stress fractures. The patient should be pain free before starting rehabilitation.
- High-risk fractures: typically require immediate immobilization and a period of non–weight-bearing; may require early surgical intervention to avoid nonunion and facilitate earlier return to sport
- Criteria for allowing an athlete to return:
  - A low-grade stress fracture at a high-risk location must heal fully prior to returning to full activity.
  - Complete resolution of symptoms with activities of daily living
  - 10 to 14 days after the patient is pain free
  - Radiographic evidence of healing
  - No tenderness to palpation at the injury site
  - Optimization of the athlete's nutritional, biomechanical, hormonal, and psychological status

MEDICATION

First Line

- Calcium (up to 2 g/day through diet sources)
- Vitamin D (800 to 4,000 IU/day) to maintain 25(OH)D levels between 32 ng/mL and 50 ng/mL (2)[C]
- Acetaminophen is useful for pain.
- NSAIDs are beneficial for pain and inflammation but may adversely affect fracture healing.

Second Line

- Bisphosphonates such as IV pamidronate or ibandronate may be useful (2)[C].
- Parathyroid hormone analog teriparatide is effective (2)[C].
- Oral contraceptives do not restore bone density in athletes (1).

ISSUES FOR REFERRAL

- Multidisciplinary team approach should always be considered to include parents, coaches, athletic trainers, PT, school nurse, nutritionist, rehab, team physician, PCP, gynecology, endocrinology, and orthopedics.
- Orthopedic consultation for high-risk fractures, failure to improve with standard treatment, evidence of nonunion within 3 to 4 weeks, or inability to tolerate rehabilitation

ADDITIONAL THERAPIES

- Electrical stimulation may be an adjunct for delayed union and nonunion.
- Extracorporeal shock wave therapy (ESWT) and pulsed US require additional study.
- Physical therapy

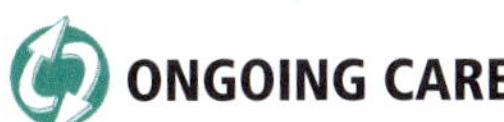

ONGOING CARE

FOLLOW-UP RECOMMENDATIONS

Once the patient is pain free, low-impact training can be started and be advanced gently as tolerated.

Patient Monitoring

Imaging every 4 to 6 weeks to assess healing

DIET

- Adequate caloric intake
- Adequate calcium and vitamin D

PATIENT EDUCATION

Correct training errors with gait retraining.

COMPLICATIONS

- Delayed union
- Nonunion

S

REFERENCES

1. Beck B, Drysdale L. Risk factors, diagnosis and management of bone stress injuries in adolescent athletes: a narrative review. *Sports (Basel)*. 2021;9(4):52.
2. da Rocha Lemos Costa TM, Borba VZC, Correa RGP, et al. Stress fractures. *Arch Endocrinol Metab*. 2022;66(5):765–773.

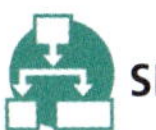

SEE ALSO

Algorithm: Foot Pain

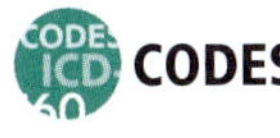

CODES

ICD10

- M84.38XA Stress fracture, other site, initial encounter for fracture
- M84.369A Stress fracture, unsp tibia and fibula, init for fx
- M84.376A Stress fracture, unspecified foot, init encntr for fracture

CLINICAL PEARLS

- The diagnosis of stress fractures requires a high index of suspicion. X-rays are often negative initially.
- Identify and treat female athletic triad or underlying metabolic conditions.
- To help prevent stress fractures, gradually increase training volume and avoid sudden increases in high-impact activity or running mileage. Ensure adequate nutrition intake including calcium, vitamin D.
- High-risk fractures require immediate immobilization and non–weight-bearing.
- Ensure gradual return to training with proper rehabilitation protocol for all stress fractures. Treat any underlying metabolic causes and mitigate risk factors.

STROKE, ACUTE (CEREBROVASCULAR ACCIDENT [CVA])

Austin Peppers, MD • Peter Koppenheffer, MD

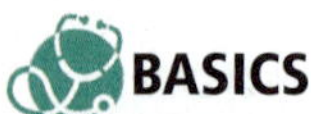

BASICS

DESCRIPTION

- An acute neurologic injury caused by a vascular event affecting the brain, spinal cord, or retina, most commonly resulting from arterial occlusion (ischemia) or intracranial bleeding (hemorrhage); transient ischemic attacks (TIA) are nonpersistent episodes of neurologic dysfunction caused by focal ischemia without evidence of acute infarction on neuroimaging.
- Stroke categories:
  - Ischemic stroke (≈80–87%): thrombotic, embolic, or hypoperfusion mechanisms
  - Hemorrhagic stroke: intracerebral hemorrhage (ICH), subarachnoid hemorrhage (SAH), and less commonly subdural/epidural hemorrhage

Pediatric Considerations

- Stroke is rare in children and adolescents:
  - Neonatal stroke: ~1 per 1,600 to 4,000 live births (often presenting with seizures)
  - Childhood arterial ischemic stroke: ~1–6 per 100,000 children per year
- Pediatric risk factors differ from adults: arteriopathies (e.g., moyamoya, cervical artery dissection); congenital heart disease (right-to-left shunts); sickle cell disease; infection/inflammation (e.g., varicella), trauma, and prothrombotic disorders.

EPIDEMIOLOGY

Incidence

~795,000 people in the United States experience a stroke each year (~610,000 are first-episode strokes and ~185,000 are recurrent). A stroke occurs about every 40 seconds, and someone in the United States dies from stroke-related approximately every 3 minutes (1).

Prevalence

Prevalence in the United States: 550/100,000; predominant age: risk increases >45 years of age; highest during the 7th and 8th decades; predominant sex: male > female at younger age but higher incidence in women with age ≥75 years (1)

ETIOLOGY AND PATHOPHYSIOLOGY

- Ischemic stroke: Arterial occlusion impedes cerebral blood flow. A segment of irreversibly injured tissue develops, surrounded by a penumbra that is often salvageable with timely reperfusion. Common ischemic stroke mechanisms include the following:
  - Large-artery atherosclerosis (extracranial or intracranial) with thromboembolism
  - Cardioembolic disease (e.g., atrial fibrillation (AFib), recent myocardial infarction (MI), valvular disease, cardiomyopathy)
  - Small-vessel disease (lacunar stroke) most commonly associated with chronic hypertension (HTN)
  - Other causes (e.g., cervical artery dissection, vasculitis, hypercoagulable states, drug-associated vasospasm)
- Hemorrhagic stroke types:
  - ICH: most often due to chronic HTN-related small-vessel arteriopathy or cerebral amyloid disease
  - SAH: typically due to rupture of an intracranial aneurysm

Genetics

Stroke risk is generally polygenic and mediated through multiple vascular risk factors. Consider heritable causes if stroke occurs at young age or is recurrent.

RISK FACTORS

- Nonmodifiable: age, gender, race, family history/genetics, prior stroke or TIA
- Modifiable: metabolic: diabetes, dyslipidemia; lifestyle: smoking, alcohol, cocaine/amphetamine use, physical inactivity
- Cardiovascular disease: HTN, AFib, valvular heart disease, endocarditis, recent MI, severe carotid artery stenosis, hypercoagulable states, patent foramen ovale (2)

GENERAL PREVENTION

Smoking cessation, regular exercise, avoid prolonged physical inactivity, weight control to maintain BMI<30 kg/m^2 and maximize glucose control, low salt diet, moderate alcohol use; control blood pressure (BP); manage hyperlipidemia; antiplatelet therapy (e.g., aspirin) in high-risk persons; treat anticoagulation therapy for nonvalvular AFib (3).

COMMONLY ASSOCIATED CONDITIONS

Coronary artery disease, heart failure, AFib, valvular disease; carotid and peripheral arterial disease; diabetes mellitus, metabolic syndrome, chronic kidney disease; obstructive sleep apnea; depression, cognitive impairment, and poststroke fatigue

DIAGNOSIS

HISTORY

- Determining time course is critical: Attempt to determine the time that patient was last known to be well.
- Typical symptoms: abrupt onset of focal deficits such as weakness, speech/language disturbance, vision loss/visual field cut, hemisensory loss, ataxia, vertigo
- Balance, eyes, face, arm, speech, time (BE-FAST)
- Assess risk factors.
- Vomiting, seizures, severe headache ("thunderclap") favor hemorrhagic stroke

PHYSICAL EXAM

- Assess airway, breathing, and circulation (ABC).
- Vital signs—pulse (character and rate) and BP
- Cardiovascular exam: bruits, rhythm (AFib); murmurs; gallops; peripheral stigmata of endocarditis, signs of heart failure
- Pulmonary exam: signs of fluid overload or bronchospasm
- Neurologic exam (stroke syndromes):
  - Anterior cerebral artery: motor/sensory deficit: (contralateral leg > face/arm), gait apraxia; abulia (inability to act willfully)
  - Middle cerebral artery:
    - Dominant: aphasia (inability to speak); motor/sensory deficit (face > arm > leg > foot); homonymous hemianopia
    - Nondominant: neglect, motor/sensory deficit (face/arm > leg > foot), homonymous hemianopia
  - Posterior cerebral artery: homonymous hemianopia; visual hallucinations; visual palsies; motor/sensory deficits; alexia (inability to read—"word blindness") without agraphia (inability to write)
  - Posterior (vertebrobasilar) circulation: diplopia, vertigo, gait and limb ataxia, facial paresis, Horner syndrome, dysphagia, dysarthria, alternating sensory loss
- The three most predictive findings for stroke on physical examination are (i) facial paresis, (ii) arm weakness or drift, and (iii) abnormal speech.
- National Institutes of Health (NIH) Stroke Scale (NIHSS): https://www.ninds.nih.gov/health-information/stroke

DIFFERENTIAL DIAGNOSIS

- Migraine (complicated); postictal state (Todd paralysis); systemic infection, including meningitis or encephalitis (infection may uncover or enhance previous deficits); toxic or metabolic disturbance (hypoglycemia, acute renal failure, liver failure, drug intoxication); brain tumor, primary or metastases; head trauma, encephalopathy, septic emboli (2)
- Other types of intracranial hemorrhage (epidural, subdural, subarachnoid)

DIAGNOSTIC TESTS & INTERPRETATION

Immediate priorities are to confirm stroke type, identify large vessel occlusion (LVO) and assess eligibility for reperfusion therapy (2).

Initial Tests (lab, imaging)

- Emergent noncontrast head CT (or MRI if immediately available) to exclude intracranial hemorrhage and assess early ischemic changes.
- CT angiography (CTA) head/neck (or MRA) to detect LVO and guide endovascular thrombectomy decisions; CT perfusion or MRI perfusion/diffusion-weighted imaging (DWI) (selected patients) to estimate infarct core versus salvageable tissue, especially for extended time windows, wake-up/unknown onset strokes, and large-core selection
- Point-of-care glucose
- Electrocardiogram (ECG); CBC; electrolyte panel; baseline troponin; coagulation studies: PT, PTT, INR

Follow-Up Tests & Special Considerations

- MRI brain with DWI (most sensitive for acute infarct; helpful for posterior circulation strokes and small infarcts)
- Vascular imaging for etiology and secondary prevention planning (carotid duplex, CTA/MRA, intracranial vessel imaging)
- Echocardiography (TTE/TEE) when cardioembolic source is suspected; consider bubble study for right-to-left shunt.
- Prolonged rhythm monitoring for cryptogenic stroke if initial telemetry is unrevealing.
- Secondary prevention labs: fasting lipid panel and HbA1c (often after the acute phase)
- Consider lumbar puncture for suspected SAH if CT is negative and clinical suspicion remains high (often after CTA, depending on local protocols).
- Consider liver tests, toxicology screen, blood alcohol, ABG; EEG if suspect seizures, blood type and cross
- Diffusion weighted (DW)-MRI is more sensitive than CT for acute ischemic stroke (AIS). MRI is better than CT for posterior fossa lesions.

Test Interpretation

- Noncontrast CT: identifies hemorrhage; may show early ischemic signs (loss of gray-white differentiation, sulcal effacement, insular ribbon sign, hyperdense artery sign)
- CTA: localizes arterial occlusion/stenosis and provides information on collateral circulation

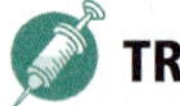

TREATMENT

Initial management includes rapid stroke team activation, stabilization, and emergent neuroimaging to distinguish ischemic from hemorrhagic stroke. Time-to-treatment metrics (door-to-imaging and door-to-needle/door-to-groin puncture) strongly influence outcomes (3).

GENERAL MEASURES

- Airway/oxygenation: provide supplemental oxygen to maintain SpO_2 >94%; intubate if unable to protect airway; glucose: treat hypoglycemia immediately; avoid severe hyperglycemia—commonly target 140 to 180 mg/dL in hospitalized patients. BP: AIS

without reperfusion therapy: permissive HTN is often allowed; treat only if markedly elevated (e.g., >220/120 mm Hg) or if other indication (aortic dissection, acute heart failure, etc.). If IV thrombolysis is planned, reduce BP to <185/110 mm Hg before treatment and maintain <180/105 mm Hg for at least 24 hours; spontaneous ICH: avoid overly aggressive BP lowering.
- Keep NPO until dysphagia screening is completed; aspiration precautions and early speech-language evaluation; continuous cardiac monitoring, frequent neurologic reassessment, and early stroke unit care when available.

MEDICATION

First Line

- AIS: reperfusion and antithrombotic therapy (2)
  - IV alteplase (tPA): 0.9 mg/kg (max 90 mg), with 10% as IV bolus over 1 minute and remainder infused over 60 minutes; most beneficial when started as early as possible and used in eligible patients within 4.5 hours of last known well (and in selected imaging-defined populations with unknown onset)
  - IV tenecteplase (TNK): single IV bolus thrombolytic; FDA-approved for AIS (current U.S. labeling specifies treatment initiation within 3 hours of symptom onset using a weight-based single-bolus regimen); many stroke systems use 0.25 mg/kg (max 25 mg) as an alteplase alternative (including some use up to 4.5 hours or imaging-selected scenarios per evidence and institutional protocols); dosing and eligibility should follow institutional protocol and current guidance.
  - Antiplatelet therapy: Start aspirin (commonly 160 to 325 mg) within 24 to 48 hours after ischemic stroke if no contraindication. If IV thrombolysis was given, delay antiplatelets and anticoagulants until 24-hour follow-up imaging excludes hemorrhage.
  - Short-term dual antiplatelet therapy (DAPT): For minor noncardioembolic ischemic stroke (often NIHSS ≤3) or high-risk TIA, initiate aspirin + clopidogrel as soon as safe (ideally within 24 hours) and continue for a short course (commonly 21 days; up to 90 days in select scenarios) before transitioning to single antiplatelet therapy. Long-term DAPT is generally not recommended for secondary prevention.
- BP management options include the following:
  - Labetalol 10 to 20 mg IV over 1 to 2 minutes, may be repeated once
  - Nicardipine infusion 5 mg/hr, titrate 2.5 mg/hr at 5- to 15-minute intervals to maximum of 15 mg/hr; reduce to 3 mg/hr when target BP is reached.
- Hemorrhagic stroke (4)
  - Rapid reversal of anticoagulation when present (e.g., four-factor PCC + vitamin K for warfarin; idarucizumab for dabigatran; andexanet alfa or PCC for factor Xa inhibitors—guided by institutional protocols)
  - BP lowering as above; manage pain, agitation, and nausea to avoid BP surges.
  - Aneurysmal SAH: Nimodipine is standard to reduce risk of delayed cerebral ischemia (unless contraindicated); definitive aneurysm treatment (coiling/clipping) is urgent.

Second Line

Carotid endarterectomy (CEA) is indicated for >70% ipsilateral stenosis; may be indicated for 50–69% stenosis in carefully selected patients, depending on risk factors, and the skill and experience of the surgeon

ISSUES FOR REFERRAL

Follow-up with neurologist 1 week after discharge

ADDITIONAL THERAPIES

If no contraindications, consider a trial of fluoxetine to improve motor outcomes. Deep vein thrombosis (DVT) prophylaxis; corticosteroids are *not* recommended for cerebral brain edema. Continue statin medication following acute stroke. Refer to PT, OT, and speech therapy as necessary.

SURGERY/OTHER PROCEDURES

- Endovascular thrombectomy (ischemic stroke): strongly recommended for eligible patients with anterior circulation LVO (e.g., ICA/proximal MCA) within 6 hours; and for selected patients in extended windows (up to 24 hours) using clinical/imaging criteria; thrombectomy for basilar artery occlusion in appropriately selected patients (including some presenting 6 to 24 hours after onset); some thrombectomy benefit in selected patients with large ischemic cores, expanding eligibility beyond traditional small-core criteria in some centers
- Surgical management of malignant infarction/ICH: Decompressive hemicraniectomy may reduce mortality in malignant MCA infarction (typically within 48 hours of onset in selected patients). Cerebellar infarction or cerebellar ICH with brainstem compression/hydrocephalus may require urgent decompression and/or ventricular drainage. Selected ICH patients may benefit from minimally invasive hematoma.
- Aneurysmal SAH: Secure aneurysm early (endovascular coiling or surgical clipping) to prevent rebleeding; manage in a specialized neurocritical care setting when possible.

COMPLEMENTARY & ALTERNATIVE MEDICINE

Acupuncture within 30 days of stroke onset may improve neurologic functioning.

ADMISSION, INPATIENT, AND NURSING CONSIDERATIONS

- Observe closely with frequent neurologic exams in first 24 hours for neurologic decline, particularly due to cerebral edema.
- Elevate head of bed to at least 30 degrees if elevated ICP is suspected. Patients with ischemic stroke may benefit from a horizontal bed position during the acute phase. Monitor cardiac rhythm for at least 24 hours to identify arrhythmias. Airway support and ventilatory assistance may be necessary due to diminished consciousness or bulbar involvement; reserve supplemental oxygen for hypoxic patients. Consider elective intubation for patients with malignant edema. Maintain oxygen saturation >94%. Correct hypovolemia with normal saline. Keep patients NPO until swallow evaluation has been performed; to reduce risk of aspiration pneumonia, elevate head of bed to 30 degrees.
- IV hydration with normal saline until swallowing status is assessed; correct hypoglycemia (especially <60 mg/dL). Avoid hyperglycemia within first 24 hours of stroke, insulin to maintain glucose levels 140 to 180 mg/dL.
- DVT prophylaxis; early PT and discharge planning for rehabilitation and placement; fall precautions; frequent repositioning to prevent skin breakdown

ONGOING CARE

FOLLOW-UP RECOMMENDATIONS

- Secondary prevention of stroke with aggressive management of risk factors; platelet inhibition using aspirin, clopidogrel, or aspirin plus extended-release dipyridamole based on physician and patient preference
- Stroke-like symptoms within 2 weeks of the initial event have a high chance of being recurrent stroke and should be followed up within 24 hours.

Patient Monitoring

Follow-up every 3 months for first year and then annually

DIET

Patients with impaired swallowing should receive nasogastric or percutaneous endoscopic gastrostomy feedings to maintain nutrition and hydration.

PATIENT EDUCATION

National Stroke Association: https://www.stroke.org

PROGNOSIS

Variable depends on subtype and severity of stroke; NIH SS may be used for prognosis.

COMPLICATIONS

- Acute: brain herniation, hemorrhagic transformation, MI, CHF, dysphagia, aspiration pneumonia, UTI, DVT, pulmonary embolism, malnutrition, pressure sores
- Chronic: falls, depression, dementia, orthopedic complications, contractures, OSA

REFERENCES

1. Martin SS, Aday AW, Allen NB, et al. 2025 heart disease and stroke statistics: a report of US and global data from the American Heart Association. *Circulation*. 2025;151(8):e41–e660. doi:10.1161/CIR.0000000000001303.
2. Powers WJ, Rabinstein AA, Ackerson T, et al. Guidelines for the early management of patients with acute ischemic stroke: 2019 update to the 2018 guidelines for the early management of acute ischemic stroke: a guideline for healthcare professionals from the American Heart Association/American Stroke Association. *Stroke*. 2019;50(12):e344–e418. doi:10.1161/STR.0000000000000211.
3. Kleindorfer DO, Towfighi A, Chaturvedi S, et al. 2021 Guideline for the prevention of stroke in patients with stroke and transient ischemic attack. *Stroke*. 2021;52(7):e364–e467. doi:10.1161/STR.0000000000000375.
4. Greenberg SM, Ziai WC, Cordonnier C, et al. 2022 guideline for the management of patients with spontaneous intracerebral hemorrhage. *Stroke*. 2022;53(7):e282–e361. doi:10.1161/STR.0000000000000407.

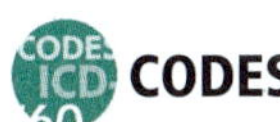

CODES

ICD10

- I63.9 Cerebral infarction, unspecified
- I61.9 Nontraumatic intracerebral hemorrhage, unspecified
- I63.50 Cereb infrc due to unsp occls or stenos of unsp cereb artery

CLINICAL PEARLS

- Suspected stroke is a medical emergency: Activate stroke protocol, obtain rapid glucose, and perform emergent brain imaging. Door-to-needle times correlate with outcomes.
- Distinguish ischemic versus hemorrhagic stroke before initiating antithrombotics or reperfusion therapy.
- Consider LVO in severe deficits—CTA head/neck early can expedite thrombectomy.

SUBCONJUNCTIVAL HEMORRHAGE

Nisarg Joshi, MD, BS

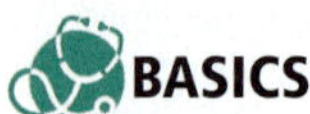

BASICS

DESCRIPTION

- Subconjunctival hemorrhage (SCH) is bleeding from small blood vessels underneath the conjunctiva, the thin clear skin covering the sclera (white outer layer) of the eye.
- SCH is diagnosed clinically:
  - Well-demarcated areas of extravasated blood can be seen just under the surface of the conjunctiva of the eye.
  - Lesions can be flat, elevated, or bullous.
- Typically, SCH self-resolves in a few days to weeks depending on the severity.

EPIDEMIOLOGY

Common; 3% rate of diagnosis in ophthalmology clinics (1)

Incidence

Incidence increases

- With increasing age
- In contact lenses wearers (5% of cases) (2)
- With systemic diseases such as diabetes, hypertension (HTN), and coagulation disorders
- With trauma
- During summer months, possibly due to trauma (1)

ETIOLOGY AND PATHOPHYSIOLOGY

- SCH results from damage to conjunctival and episcleral vessels from direct or indirect injury.
- Antithrombogenic and anticoagulated states (blood dyscrasias, thrombocytopenia, anemia, anti-platelet use, anticoagulant use) increase the risk and severity of SCH.
- Causes include
  - Idiopathic
  - Direct trauma from
    - Blunt or penetrating injury to the eye
      - If there is a large SCH from a trauma, the patient may have underlying globe rupture and should be evaluated for this.
    - Contact lenses placement or removal; improper contact lenses wear
    - Rubbing eyes
      - Commonly when sleeping which leads to patient waking up with eye redness
      - In patient on anticoagulation, even mild eye rubbing can induce SCH.
    - Foreign body in eye
    - Ocular surgery, injection, or other procedure
    - Related to ocular surface infection (i.e., viral conjunctivitis) or ocular surface lesion
  - Valsalva maneuvers causing sudden severe venous congestion such as coughing, sneezing, vomiting, straining, severe asthma or COPD exacerbation, weightlifting, or childbirth/labor
  - Damaged vessels from atherosclerotic disease or diabetes (which is a cause of recurrent SCH without trauma)
- In patients aged >60 years, HTN is the most common etiology.
- In patients aged <40 years, trauma, Valsalva, and contact lenses use are the most common etiologies.
- In patients aged >40 years, conjunctivochalasis (redundant conjunctival folds) and presence of pinguecula are strongly associated (2).

RISK FACTORS

- Trauma
- Age
- Contact lenses wearer
- Systemic diseases (HTN, diabetes)
- Bleeding disorders (1) or anticoagulant use
- Recent ocular procedure (cataract, laser-assisted in situ keratomileusis [LASIK], etc.)

GENERAL PREVENTION

- Avoid rubbing eyes.
- Proper cleaning and maintenance of contact lenses
- Protective eyewear during sports and hobbies
- Optimizing control of systemic diseases such as HTN, diabetes, and atherosclerotic disease, thrombocytopenia
- Control of PT/INR in patients on warfarin therapy (3)

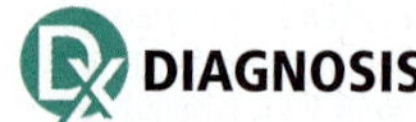

DIAGNOSIS

HISTORY

- Usually, the patient notices redness in the mirror or another person mentions it to the patient.
- Generally, patients do not have ocular symptoms like pain, light sensitivity, or decrease in vision.
- Patients may complain of mild irritation or foreign body sensation.
- Obtain history of trauma, recent ocular surgery, rubbing eyes, contact lenses use, eye infections, heavy Valsalva maneuvers (coughing, straining going to the bathroom, lifting heavy objects, etc.) (1). SCH can occur 12 to 24 hours after orbital fracture (4).
- Evaluate medical history of systemic disease like diabetes mellitus, HTN, and coagulopathy.
- Ask about medications that may increase risk: aspirin, clopidogrel, other anti-platelets, anticoagulants.
- Obtain history of other systemic symptomatology.

PHYSICAL EXAM

- Visual acuity, intra-ocular pressure, and pupils should be unaffected (3).
- Slit lamp exam shows bright red well-demarcated spots or patches. They are more often inferior due to gravity (2).
- Lesions can be flat, elevated, or bullous.
- The color of the conjunctiva changes over time. When the blood newly accumulates, the color is bright red. Older blood has a darker red color. The conjunctiva may have a yellow hue from blood-breakdown products as the hemorrhage dissipates.
- Fluorescein can be applied to assess for conjunctival and cornea abrasions/lacerations. Under cobalt blue light, there should be no stain uptake with a simple SCH.
- If the conjunctiva was lacerated, drops of blood can extrude from the conjunctiva onto the eyelid and periorbital skin.
- If a foreign body was involved, it could be hidden by the SCH.

- If there is concern for penetrating or perforating ocular trauma, a shield should be placed over the eye and the patient should be evaluated emergently by an ophthalmologist and/or trauma team.
- Measure blood pressure to evaluate for uncontrolled HTN (1).

Geriatric Considerations

In older adults, the area of SCH will be more widespread across the sclera (2). Elastic and connective tissues are more fragile with age, and underlying conditions such as HTN and diabetes may contribute.

DIFFERENTIAL DIAGNOSIS

- Viral, bacterial, allergic, or chemical conjunctivitis (enterovirus and coxsackievirus most common) (4)[B]
- Foreign body in/on the conjunctiva
- Penetrating or perforating trauma
- Recent ocular surgery/injection
- Contact lenses induced
- Child abuse (particularly if bilateral in an infant or toddler) (4)
- Occasionally found in newborns following vaginal delivery

DIAGNOSTIC TESTS & INTERPRETATION

- Typically, no testing is indicated; SCH is a clinical diagnosis. If a foreign body is suspected, perform a fluorescein exam.
- Fluorescein exam of a patient with a SCH should show no uptake of fluorescein (3)[C].
- If an orbital fracture is suspected, an orbital/maxillofacial CT scan may be obtained (5)[C].

Follow-Up Tests & Special Considerations

If history and physical exam suggest a bleeding disorder (3)[C], consider evaluating for a blood dyscrasia.

ALERT

- If a penetrating injury is suspected, may obtain a CT scan of the orbits
- Do not perform MRI because the foreign object may be metallic (5)[C].

TREATMENT

- Reassurance is important.
- SCH self-resolves with time.
- Artificial tears can be used 4 times a day as needed for eye irritation (3)[C].

GENERAL MEASURES

- Control BP.
- Control blood glucose.
- Control INR.
- Wear protective eyewear.

ISSUES FOR REFERRAL

- If there is a history of any significant trauma, even blunt trauma, seek emergent ophthalmology consultation.
- If the patient complains of any decreased visual acuity or visual disturbances (i.e., new floaters), refer to an ophthalmologist as soon as possible.
- If there is no resolution of SCH within 2 weeks or if SCH are recurrent, patient may need referral to an ophthalmologist.

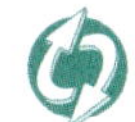

ONGOING CARE

FOLLOW-UP RECOMMENDATIONS

- Follow up only if the SCH does not self-resolve.
- If SCH recurs, then work up patient for systemic associations such as bleeding disorders (3)[C] or diabetes.

PATIENT EDUCATION

- Reassurance of the self-limited nature of the problem and typical time frame for resolution
- Education to return to clinic if the area does not heal or recurs.
- Correct cleaning and maintenance of contact lenses
- Eye lubricants for ocular irritation

PROGNOSIS

Excellent

COMPLICATIONS

Rare

REFERENCES

1. Mimura T, Usui T, Yamagami S, et al. Recent causes of subconjunctival hemorrhage. *Ophthalmologica*. 2010;224(3):133–137.
2. Mimura T, Yamagami S, Mori M, et al. Contact lens-induced subconjunctival hemorrhage. *Am J Ophthalmol*. 2010;150(5):656–665.e1.
3. Cronau H, Kankanala RR, Mauger T. Diagnosis and management of red eye in primary care. *Am Fam Physician*. 2010;81(2):137–144.
4. Tarlan B, Kiratli H. Subconjunctival hemorrhage: risk factors and potential indicators. *Clin Ophthalmol*. 2013;7:1163–1170.
5. Wirbelauer C. Management of the red eye for the primary care physician. *Am J Med*. 2006;119(4):302–306.

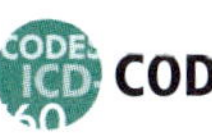

CODES

ICD10

- H11.30 Conjunctival hemorrhage, unspecified eye
- H11.31 Conjunctival hemorrhage, right eye
- H11.32 Conjunctival hemorrhage, left eye

CLINICAL PEARLS

- SCH is a clinical diagnosis. The condition is typically asymptomatic and most will self-resolve within 2 weeks.
- Risk factors include trauma, Valsalva, HTN, and diabetes.
- Indications for immediate referral to an ophthalmologist include eye pain, changes in vision, lack of pupil reactivity, and/or suspected penetrating eye injury.
- Reassurance and comfort measures (i.e., ocular lubrication) are mainstays of treatment.

SUBSTANCE USE DISORDERS

S. Lindsey Clarke, MD, FAAFP • Benjamin J. Velky, MD

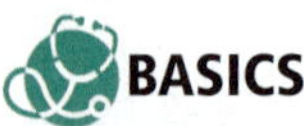

BASICS

DESCRIPTION

Any pattern of substance use causing significant physical, mental, or social dysfunction

- Substances of abuse include:
  - Alcohol
  - Cannabis (marijuana, hashish, cannabis oil, extracts); also sold as highly concentrated extracts for use in vaporizers
  - "Club drugs" (MDMA [ecstasy, Molly], PMMA [Superman], flunitrazepam, gamma-hydroxybutyrate [GHB])
  - Dissociative drugs (ketamine, phencyclidine [PCP], tenocyclidine [TCP])
  - Hallucinogens (lysergic acid diethylamide [LSD], salvia, ayahuasca, *N*,*N*-dimethyltryptamine [DMT])
  - Inhalants (glue, paint thinners, nitrous oxide "Whippets")
  - Opioids (carfentanil and other synthetic analogs of fentanyl, heroin, kratom, desomorphine [Krokodil], U-47700 [Pink])
  - Prescription medications
    - CNS depressants (barbiturates, benzodiazepines, hypnotics)
    - Dextromethorphan ("Robotripping")
    - Opioids and morphine derivatives (fentanyl, hydrocodone, oxycodone, others)
    - Stimulants (amphetamines, methylphenidate)
  - Stimulants (cocaine, amphetamines, methamphetamines, Khat)
  - Synthetic cannabinoids (Spice, K2, fake weed); often much more potent than marijuana; may be smoked or vaporized
  - Synthetic cathinones (bath salts, alpha-PVP [Flakka])
  - Tobacco

EPIDEMIOLOGY

Prevalence

- 70.5 million Americans (24.9%) reported illicit drug use in the past year in 2023.
- 14.7% of 12- to 17-year-olds; 39% of 18- to 25-year-olds
- >1 in 3 (36.5%) young adults used marijuana in past year.

ALERT

- Opioid overdose is the leading cause of death for persons 26 to 38 years of age years in the United States. >82% of these are due to synthetic opioids. There have been increasing cases of overdose and death related to synthetic opioids mixed with xylazine, which does not respond to naloxone administration.
- Many states require naloxone to be prescribed or offered when issuing a prescription of opioids to patients at increased risk of overdose, such as those receiving ≥50 morphine milligram equivalents per day of an opioid, those taking both opioids and benzodiazepines, and those with a history of substance abuse.

ETIOLOGY AND PATHOPHYSIOLOGY

Genetics

Substances of abuse affect dopamine and other neurotransmitter receptors. Variant alleles may account for differences in susceptibility to misuse of different substances.

RISK FACTORS

- Academic problems, school dropout
- Criminal involvement
- Depression, anxiety
- Family dysfunction or trauma
- Family history
- Peer or family use or approval
- Unemployment, low socioeconomic status

GENERAL PREVENTION

- Prescribe nonopioid therapies to treat pain and when necessary, use limited amounts to treat acute severe pain.
- Avoid prescribing narcotics for chronic conditions.
- Early identification and aggressive early intervention improve outcomes.
- Universal school-based interventions are modestly effective for prevention.

DIAGNOSIS

Substance use disorder (*DSM-5-TR* criteria): ≥2 of the following in past year; severity graded by number of criteria present:

- Using more than intended
- Failed attempts to quit
- Increased time spent obtaining, using, or recovering from the substance
- Craving
- Failed obligations at work, school, or home
- Continued use despite social or interpersonal problems
- Interference with important activities
- Use in hazardous situations
- Continued use despite health problems
- Tolerance
- Withdrawal

HISTORY

- Anxiety, depression, psychosis
- Frequent visits to emergency department
- History of blackouts, insomnia, mood swings, chronic pain, repetitive trauma
- History of infections (e.g., endocarditis, hepatitis B or C, HIV, TB, STI, or recurrent pneumonia)
- Incarceration
- Social or behavioral problems, including chaotic relationships and/or employment difficulties

PHYSICAL EXAM

- Abnormal vital signs
- Abnormally dilated or constricted pupils
- Cardiac dysrhythmias, pathologic murmurs
- Cutaneous needle marks
- Malnutrition
- Mental status changes

DIFFERENTIAL DIAGNOSIS

- Metabolic delirium: hypoxia, hypoglycemia, infection, thiamine deficiency, hypothyroidism, thyrotoxicosis, medication toxicity
- Mood, anxiety, and personality disorders

DIAGNOSTIC TESTS & INTERPRETATION

USPSTF recommends screening adults ≥18 years for unhealthy drug use when appropriate diagnosis and treatment services can be provided. USPSTF found insufficient evidence for or against such screening in adolescents.

- Substance Use Brief Screen and single-question screening tools (e.g., "How many times in the past year have you used an illegal drug or used a prescription medication for nonmedical reasons?") are sensitive (71–100%) and specific (61–96%) for identifying problem use in hospital and primary care settings (1)[A].
- Recommended screening tools for adults:
  - Tobacco, alcohol, prescription medication, and other substance use (TAPS): score ≥1 identifies problem use of illicit and prescription drugs (sensitivity 63–83%, specificity 93%)
  - Revised opioid risk tool (ORT-OUD): predicts risk of opioid use disorder in primary care patients with chronic pain (sensitivity 95%, specificity 85%)
- Recommended screening tools for teens:
  - Screening to Brief Intervention (S2B1)
  - Brief Screener for Tobacco, Alcohol, and Other Drugs (BSTAD)

Pregnancy Considerations

- Substance abuse may cause fetal abnormalities, morbidity, and fetal or maternal death.
- Screen for substance use at the first prenatal visit with a brief intervention, and refer for treatment to improve maternal and neonatal outcomes

Initial Tests (lab, imaging)

- Blood alcohol concentration
- Urine drug screen
- Standard screening immunoassays may miss synthetic cannabinoids and opioids.
- Approximate detection limits
  - Alcohol: 6 to 10 hours
  - Amphetamines and variants: 2 to 3 days
  - Barbiturates: 2 to 10 days
  - Benzodiazepines: 1 to 6 weeks
  - Cocaine: 2 to 3 days
  - Heroin: 1 to 1.5 days
  - LSD, psilocybin: 8 hours
  - Marijuana: 1 to 7 days; up to 1 month with chronic/heavy use
  - Methadone: 1 day to 1 week
  - Opioids: 1 to 3 days
  - PCP: 7 to 14 days
  - Anabolic steroids: oral, 3 weeks; injectable, 3 months; nandrolone, 9 months
- Liver transaminases
- HIV, hepatitis B and C

Follow-Up Tests & Special Considerations

- Blood cultures, echocardiogram for endocarditis
- Head CT scan for seizure, delirium, trauma
- Right upper quadrant abdominal ultrasound for cirrhosis

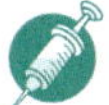

TREATMENT

Determine substances abused early (may influence disposition).

GENERAL MEASURES

- Treatment should combine pharmacotherapy and cognitive behavioral therapy or another evidence-based modality when applicable (2)[A].
- Nonjudgmental, medically oriented attitude
- Motivational interviewing and brief interventions can promote change.
- Community reinforcement and contingency management are effective psychosocial interventions.
- Self-help groups to aid recovery (Alcoholics Anonymous, other 12-step programs)
- Support groups for family (Al-Anon/Alateen)

MEDICATION

- Benzodiazepine or barbiturate withdrawal
  - Gradual taper preferable to abrupt discontinuation
  - Substitution of long-acting benzodiazepine (e.g., clonazepam) or phenobarbital
- Opioid dependence
  - Buprenorphine: 8 to 24 mg SL daily, 100 to 300 mg SC monthly or as 6-month subdermal implant; may precipitate a more severe withdrawal if initiated too soon (3)[A]
  - Buprenorphine/naloxone: 2/0.5 mg to 16/4 mg SL daily; available as SL tabs and films and buccal films; combination limits abuse potential compared with buprenorphine alone.
  - Methadone: 10 to 40 mg/day PO; use restricted to inpatient settings and licensed clinics (3)[A]
  - Naltrexone: 50 mg PO daily, 100 mg PO every 2 days, 150 mg PO every 3 days, or 380 mg IM every 4 weeks; must be opioid-free for 7 to 10 days prior to treatment to avoid precipitating withdrawal
  - Naloxone: For opioid overdose 0.4 to 2 mg IV/IM/SUBQ, repeat every 2 to 3 minutes as needed; intranasal 4 to 8 mg, repeat every 2 to 3 minutes as needed. Refer to state mandates for co-prescribing with opioid medications.
- Opioid withdrawal
  - Clonidine: 0.1 to 0.2 mg PO BID or TID for autonomic hyperactivity (3)[A]
  - Tramadol ER: 100 to 300 mg PO daily, then taper (off label) (3)[B]
- Adjuncts to therapy
  - Use all medications in conjunction with psychosocial behavioral interventions.
  - Antiemetics, nonaddictive analgesics for opioid withdrawal
  - Antidepressants, mood stabilizers, nonhabituating anxiolytics and hypnotics for symptoms that persist after detoxification
- Contraindications
  - Buprenorphine in breastfeeding, hepatic impairment
  - Methadone in hepatic impairment
  - Naltrexone in pregnancy, breastfeeding, hepatic impairment
- Precaution: Clonidine can cause hypotension.
- Significant possible interactions
  - Buprenorphine and opioids, CNS depressants, or HIV protease inhibitors
  - Methadone and opioids, CNS depressants, or strong inhibitors of CYP3A4 (clarithromycin, ketoconazole, HIV protease inhibitors)
  - Naltrexone and opioid medications (may induce or exacerbate withdrawal)

ISSUES FOR REFERRAL

- Consider addiction specialist, especially for opioid and polysubstance abuse.
- Medication-assisted treatment for opioid dependence (e.g., methadone).
- Psychiatrist for comorbid psychiatric disorders
- Social services

ADMISSION, INPATIENT, AND NURSING CONSIDERATIONS

- Indications for inpatient detoxification
  - History of severe withdrawal (e.g., seizures)
  - Mental status changes; hallucinations or psychotic features
  - Threat of harm to self or others
  - Obstacles to close monitoring/follow-up
  - Comorbid medical illness
  - Pregnancy
- Look for signs of infection (e.g., bacterial endocarditis).
- Monitor for signs of drug use in the hospital.
- Discharge when detoxification complete and a rehabilitation plan is in place

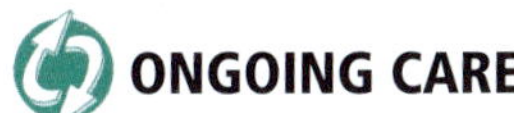

ONGOING CARE

FOLLOW-UP RECOMMENDATIONS

Initially frequent visits to monitor for medical stability and adherence and then progressive follow-up intervals

Patient Monitoring

Verify patient's adherence with the substance abuse treatment program.

PATIENT EDUCATION

- Substance Abuse and Mental Health Services Administration: https://www.samhsa.gov
- Alcoholics Anonymous: http://www.aa.org
- Narcotics Anonymous: http://www.na.org

PROGNOSIS

- Behavioral therapy and pharmacotherapy are most successful when used in combination.
- Patients in treatment for longer periods have higher success rates.

COMPLICATIONS

- Bacterial endocarditis
- Cirrhosis, hepatic malignancy, hepatitis, HIV, tuberculosis, syphilis
- Depression, psychosis
- Harm to self and others: accidents, violence
- Malnutrition
- Overdoses resulting in seizures, arrhythmias, cardiac and respiratory arrest, coma, death
- Sexual assault (alcohol, flunitrazepam, GHB)
- Social problems, including arrest, marital discord, and violence

REFERENCES

1. Han BH, Sherman SE, Link AR, et al. Comparison of the Substance Use Brief Screen (SUBS) to the AUDIT-C and ASSIST for detecting unhealthy alcohol and drug use in a population of hospitalized smokers. *J Subst Abuse Treat*. 2017;79:67–74.
2. Ray LA, Meredith LR, Kiluk BD, et al. Combined pharmacotherapy and cognitive behavioral therapy for adults with alcohol or substance use disorders: a systematic review and meta-analysis. *JAMA Netw Open*. 2020;3(6):e208279.
3. Srivastava AB, Mariani JJ, Levin FR. New directions in the treatment of opioid withdrawal. *Lancet*. 2020;395(10241):1938–1948.

ADDITIONAL READING

- Centers for Disease Control and Prevention. E-cigarette, or vaping, products visual dictionary. https://www.cdc.gov/tobacco/basic_information/e-cigarettes/pdfs/ecigarette-or-vaping-products-visual-dictionary-508.pdf.
- National Institute on Drug Abuse. Commonly used drugs charts. https://nida.nih.gov/research-topics/commonly-used-drugs-charts.

SEE ALSO

Alcohol Use Disorder (AUD); Alcohol Withdrawal; Tobacco Use and Smoking Cessation

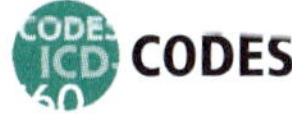

CODES

ICD10

- F18.951 Inhalant use, unspecified with inhalant-induced psychotic disorder with hallucinations
- F11.120 Opioid abuse with intoxication, uncomplicated
- F17.201 Nicotine dependence, unspecified, in remission

CLINICAL PEARLS

- Substance use disorders are prevalent, serious, and often unrecognized in clinical practice. Comorbid psychiatric disorders are common.
- Substance abuse is distinguished by family, social, occupational, legal, or physical dysfunction that is caused by persistent use of the substance.
- Dependence is characterized by tolerance, withdrawal, compulsive use, and repeated overindulgence.
- Treatment should combine pharmacotherapy and cognitive behavioral therapy or another evidence-based modality when applicable.
- Consider referring patients with opioid dependence to an addiction specialist or to a certified outpatient treatment program.

SUICIDE

Irene Coletsos, MD, MS • Harold J. Bursztajn, MD

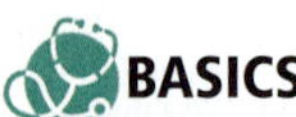

BASICS

DESCRIPTION

Suicide and attempted suicide are significant causes of morbidity and mortality.

EPIDEMIOLOGY

- Women *attempt* suicide 1.5 times more often than men. Men *complete* suicide 4 times more often than women.
- In the United States: predominant age: 10 to 14 years; 25 to 34 years (2nd leading cause of death), 11th leading cause of death overall, per final review of 2023 Centers for Disease Control and Prevention (CDC) data.
- In the United States, >49,300 died of suicide in 2024. Young adults who are gender nonconforming were 4 times more likely to attempt suicide than their gender conforming peers.
- The highest risk professions are: construction 65 per 100,000 for men, 25 per 100,000 for women; next highest risk: farming/fishing/forestry 49 per 100,000 for men; 26 per 100,000 for women in maintenance and repair.
- Suicide risk for women physicians in the United States was 53% higher than nonphysician women, in general (method most often used was poisoning or cutting); while the suicide risk for male physicians was 16 percent lower than male nonphysicians.
- Veterans have a 57.3% higher rate than nonveterans (with increased risk at time of discharge from service).
- Incarcerated persons are at increased risk (49 per 100,000 in jails—which house unsentenced persons and those with shorter sentences); state jails (27 per 100,000); federal prisons (14.47 per 100,000) (with highest risk the first day of incarceration and at release).
- Worldwide, suicide is the 14th cause of death leading cause of death, overall, and the 3rd cause of death among youths (ages 15 to 29 years), per World Health Organization reports from 2021.

RISK FACTORS

- 80% who complete suicide had a previous attempt.
- 90% who complete suicide meet *Diagnostic and Statistical Manual, Fifth Edition Text Revision* criteria for major depression, bipolar disorder, anorexia, panic, and personality disorders; schizophrenia or acute onset of psychosis are also risk factors due to command hallucinations and hopelessness that can accompany these states; delusional disorders—specifically persecutory and somatic delusions—associated with increased depression accompanying those symptoms (1)
- In addition to mental illness, other factors that could increase risk for suicide attempts include genetics, life history, and environmental factors. Retrospective studies have identified additional factors, which correlate to increased risk for suicide:
- Childhood trauma (adverse childhood experiences [ACEs])
- Substance use and withdrawal
- Family history of suicide
- Physical illness, including head injury (associated with 20% increased risk of death by suicide)
- For teenagers: not feeling "connected" to their peers or family; being bullied; perceiving lack of understanding about possible gender identity issues; poor grades
- Among veterans: childhood abuse; major depression; multiple psychiatric hospitalizations are the best predictors of suicide risk (2).
- For the general public: access to lethal means: firearms, poisons; including prescription and nonprescription drugs; pesticides

GENERAL PREVENTION

- Screen for risk: Screening instruments include the Patient Health Questionnaire-2 (PHQ-2), the PHQ-9, the Columbia Suicide Severity Rating Scale, Beck Scale for Suicide Ideation, Linehan Reasons for Living Inventory, and Risk Estimator for Suicide.
- Treat underlying mental and medical illnesses and substance abuse. Continuity of care has been identified as a key protective factor.
- Screen for possession of means of harm, including prescribed/unprescribed drugs, poisons, and firearms.
- Create a safety plan for patients at risk patients and their families, including how to access 24/7 emergency care.
- For additional resources, for needs ranging from quick support to educational:
  - Military: https://www.realwarriors.net/; suggested treatments include cognitive restructuring techniques (that their experience with adversity can be a source of strength) and help with problem-solving (so the service member does not feel like a "burden"), therapeutic martial arts training, and focus on vets' helping others: "Power of 1" initiative (any "one" helpful contact could save a life).
  - Within the United States for anyone in need: https://988lifeline.org/; text: Enter 988 to get a prompt allowing for communication via phone/text message/chat.
  - For teens, their families, and their educators: https://www.cdc.gov/healthy-youth/index.html/; https://www.stopbullying.gov/; https://988lifeline.org/help-yourself/youth/; Text: https://988/lifeline.org/chat/.
  - Members of "minority" populations (ethnic or gender) who are concerned that their cultures/life experiences might not be understood by the medical establishment: resources with counselors with specific knowledge/training include: https://988lifeline.org/help-yourself/black-mental-health/; https://988lifeline.org/help-yourself/native/.
  - For healthcare providers: multiple links available via the links above; additional resources at the national Suicide Prevention Resource Center (https://SPRC.org).

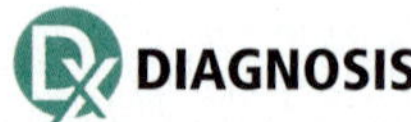

DIAGNOSIS

HISTORY

- Depressed patients should be asked about suicidal ideation and a potential plan:
  - "Have you ever felt that life isn't worth living? Do you ever wish you could go to sleep and not wake up? Are you having thoughts about killing yourself?"
- Use psychodynamic formulation: mental-state exam (including judgment, if the patient is able to make decisions, or affected by prescribed or nonprescribed drugs/drug withdrawal), history; if the patient is experiencing a loss, or is under stress, and does not have access to a previously sustaining resource (e.g., a significant other, a pet, sports ability, a job), that patient is under increased risk for suicide.
- Prior attempts: precipitants, lethality, intent to die, precautions taken to avoid being rescued, reaction to survival (a patient who is upset that the suicide was not completed is at increased risk for a subsequent attempt)
- History of psychiatric symptoms, substance abuse
- Also note strengths, such as reasons to live, hopes for future, social supports. A patient without these strengths is at increased risk.
- Gather collateral history (from friends, family, physicians). Break confidentiality if patient is at imminent risk.

PHYSICAL EXAM

- Medical conditions: chronic illnesses (which can increase risk for hopelessness) or acute illnesses, such as delirium, intoxication, withdrawal, medication side effects, all which can impair judgment
- Psychosis
- In adults: See "Risk Factors."
- In teens: may not appear to be depressed; therefore, screen for chronic risk factors:
  - ACEs
  - Identification as a gender minority (LGBTQIA: Lesbian, Gay, Bisexual, Transgender, Queer/Questioning, Intersex, Asexual)
  - Identification as an ethnic minority: American Indian/Alaska Native; Black
  - Screen for acute risk factors: substance abuse, social isolation and bullying (commonly through electronic media), poor grades.
  - Protective factors identified for young adults: identifying a parent/parental figure who is supportive and understanding.

DIFFERENTIAL DIAGNOSIS

Suicidal threats and gestures need to be immediately triaged to assess patient safety, although in some cases the threat could be an attempt to manipulate others, such as in the case of personality disorders.

DIAGNOSTIC TESTS & INTERPRETATION

Diagnostic Procedures/Other

- Columbia Suicide Severity Rating Scale, clinical instructions accessed at https://cssrs.columbia.edu/wp-content/uploads/C-SSRS_Pediatric-SLC_11.14.16.pdf
- Suicide Trigger Scale version 3 (STS-3), which measures a patient's "ruminative flooding" (self-critical, repetitive thoughts) and "frantic hopelessness" (feeling suicide is the only choice): https://www.ncbi.nlm.nih.gov/pmc/articles/PMC3443232/

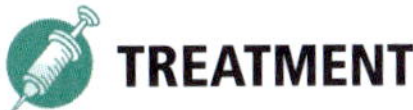

TREATMENT

GENERAL MEASURES

- Patients expressing active suicidal thoughts or who made an attempt require immediate evaluation for risk factors and a formal psychiatric consultation.
- Cognitive therapy decrease reattempt rate in prior suicide attempters by half (3),(4).
- Psychotherapy with suicidal patients is a challenge even for experienced clinicians. The countertransference, a clinician's feelings toward a patient, can evolve into wanting to be rid of the patient. If the patient detects this, the risk of suicide increases. Clinicians should be on the lookout for countertransference and get counseling if needed.
- Among military personnel: ACE campaign: Ask about suicidal thoughts; Care for the person, including removing access to lethal weapons; "Escort" the soldier/vet to help: an emergency room, a 911 call; call to a support hotline such as (800) 273-TALK (8255); text: 838255

MEDICATION

- Psychopharmacology "is not a substitute for getting to know the patient."
- Patients are at increased risk of suicide at the outset of antidepressant treatment and when it is discontinued. Consider tapering/switching medicines rather than sudden discontinuation. Monitor carefully.
- Anxiety, agitation, and delusions increasing in intensity should be treated aggressively.
- In the inpatient/emergency room setting, agitated or combative patients may require sedation with IV or IM benzodiazepines and/or antipsychotics.

Pediatric Considerations

FDA posted black box warning for antidepressant use in the pediatric population after increased suicidality was noted. Weigh risks versus benefits of starting an antidepressant and closely monitor.

ISSUES FOR REFERRAL

Consider a psychiatric consult.

ADMISSION, INPATIENT, AND NURSING CONSIDERATIONS

- Inpatient hospitalization if patient is suicidal with a plan, or otherwise at high risk; involuntary if at immediate risk
- Immediately after a suicide attempt, treat the medical problems resulting from the self-harm before initiating psychiatric care.
- Order lab work (e.g., solvent screen, blood and urine toxicology screen, aspirin, and acetaminophen levels). Patients may not disclose ingestions.
- Risk for self-harm continues while inpatient: Upon arrival, patients should be searched for potentially dangerous items; be on one-to-one observation; offered medication to ease symptoms; use restraints only if necessary for patient safety.
- The period after transfer (involuntary to voluntary hospitalization; postdischarge) are times of high risk.
- Discharge when no longer considered a danger to self/others. Look for signs that the patient is truly at reduced risk, such as improved appetite, sleep, engagement with staff and group therapy.

ONGOING CARE

FOLLOW-UP RECOMMENDATIONS

Patient Monitoring

- Increase monitoring at the beginning of treatment, when changing medications, and after hospital discharge.
- Educate family and other close contact to the warning signs of suicidality.
- Make sure that the patient is willing to accept recommended follow-up.
- Curtail access to firearms.
- Limit the number of pills to impulsive patients, but it might not prevent further attempts.

PATIENT EDUCATION

Patients who feel they are in acute danger of hurting themselves should consider one or several of these options:

- Call 911 or go directly to an emergency room.
- Contact treating therapist immediately.
- Call the National Suicide Prevention Hotline at (800) 273-TALK (8255)
- Service members and their families: call (800) 796-9699 or (800) 273-TALK (8255); text 838255.

PROGNOSIS

The key to a favorable prognosis is early recognition of risks, early treatment of disorders that had led to distress.

REFERENCES

1. González-Rodríguez A, Molina-Andreu O, Navarro Odriozola V, et al. Suicidal ideation and suicidal behaviour in delusional disorder: a clinical overview. *Psychiatry J*. 2014;2014:834901. doi:10.1155/2014/834901.
2. Koola MM, Ahmed AO, Sebastian J, et al. Childhood physical and sexual abuse predicts suicide risk in a large cohort of veterans. *Prim Care Companion CNS Disord*. 2018;20(4):18m02317.
3. Brown GK, Ten Have T, Henriques GR, et al. Cognitive therapy for the prevention of suicide attempts: a randomized controlled trial. *JAMA*. 2005;294(5):563–570.
4. Ghahramanlou-Holloway M, Neely L, Tucker J. A cognitive-behavioral strategy for preventing suicide. *Current Psychiatry*. 2014;13(8):18–28.

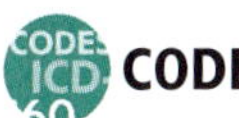

CODES

ICD10

- R45.851 Suicidal ideations
- T14.91 Suicide attempt
- Z91.5 Personal history of self-harm

CLINICAL PEARLS

- Key preventative measure is to listen to patients and take steps to keep them safe. This could include immediate hospitalization.
- Family and contacts of people who have attempted or committed suicide suffer from reactions ranging from rage to despair. Encourage counseling.
- Resources for clinicians: https://www.suicidology.org/; https://www.suicideassessment.com/
- Resources as noted in "General Prevention" section.

SUPERFICIAL THROMBOPHLEBITIS

Tomas P.J. Reilly, MD

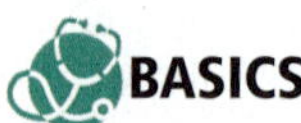

BASICS

DESCRIPTION

- Superficial thrombophlebitis refers to a thrombosis-related inflammatory process of superficial veins.
- Most common in the lower extremities with 60–80% of total cases involving the greater saphenous vein but can occur in any location
- Classically, it was considered a benign and self-limiting process, but recent evidence associates it with ≥10% risk of thromboembolic complications including progression to deep venous thrombosis (DVT) and pulmonary embolism (1).
- Traumatic thrombophlebitis types:
  - Injury
  - IV catheter related
  - Intentional/iatrogenic (i.e., sclerotherapy)
- Aseptic thrombophlebitis types:
  - Primary hypercoagulable states: disorders with measurable defects in the proteins of the coagulation and/or fibrinolytic systems
  - Secondary hypercoagulable states: clinical conditions with a risk of thrombosis (venous stasis, pregnancy, malignancy)
- Septic (suppurative) thrombophlebitis types:
  - Iatrogenic, long-term IV catheter use
  - Infectious, mainly syphilis and psittacosis
- Mondor disease—rare presentation of groin, penis, or anterior chest/breast veins
- System(s) affected: cardiovascular
- Synonym(s): phlebitis; phlebothrombosis, superficial vein thrombosis (SVT)

Geriatric Considerations

Septic thrombophlebitis is more common; prognosis is poorer.

Pediatric Considerations

Subperiosteal abscesses of adjacent long bone may complicate the disorder.

Pregnancy Considerations

- Associated with increased risk of aseptic superficial thrombophlebitis, especially during postpartum
- As NSAIDs are contraindicated during pregnancy, alternative therapeutic approaches are advised.

EPIDEMIOLOGY

- Mean age is 60 years old.
- 50–70% in women
- More common in those with varicose veins
- Epidemiology by thrombophlebitis types:
  - Traumatic/IV related has no predominant age/sex.
  - Suppurative more common in extremes of ages (neonates, elderly)
  - Aseptic primary hypercoagulable state
    - Childhood to young adult
  - Aseptic secondary hypercoagulable state
    - Mondor disease: women, ages 21 to 55 years
    - Thromboangiitis obliterans onset: ages 20 to 50 years

Incidence

- Current estimates put the incidence around 0.64 to 1.31 per 1,000 person-years (1), with increasing age associated with higher rates.
- Current incidence of catheter-associated septic thrombophlebitis is 0.5 per 1,000 days of peripherally inserted catheters.
- In pregnancy, incidence varies by trimester and postpartum. Per 1,000 person-years, incidence rates were 0.1, 0.2, 0.5, and 1.6 during the 1st, 2nd, and 3rd trimesters, and postpartum, respectively.
- Aseptic primary hypercoagulable state: Antithrombin III and heparin cofactor II deficiency incidence is 50/100,000 persons.
- Superficial migratory thrombophlebitis in 27% of patients with thromboangiitis obliterans

Prevalence

- Superficial thrombophlebitis is common with prevalence estimated between 3% and 11% of the general population.
- 1/3 of patients in a medical ICU develop thrombophlebitis that eventually progresses to the deep veins.

ETIOLOGY AND PATHOPHYSIOLOGY

- The process for thrombosis and phlebitis in superficial thrombophlebitis is variable but follows similar processes underlying thrombus formation in other vessels. These include venous stasis, vascular wall injury, microthrombi with subsequent platelet aggregation, and hypercoagulable states.
- Varicose veins play a primary role in etiology of lower extremity thrombophlebitis.
- Mondor disease pathophysiology not completely understood but thought to be related to local trauma/direct injury
- Less commonly due to infection (i.e., septic)
  - *Staphylococcus aureus, Pseudomonas, Klebsiella, Peptostreptococcus* spp.
  - *Candida* spp.
- Aseptic primary hypercoagulable state due to inherited disorders of hypercoagulability
- Aseptic secondary hypercoagulable states
  - Malignancy (Trousseau syndrome: recurrent migratory thrombophlebitis): most commonly seen in metastatic mucin or adenocarcinomas of the GI tract (pancreas, stomach, colon, and gallbladder), lung, prostate, and ovary
  - Pregnancy
  - Estrogen-based oral contraceptives
  - Behçet or Buerger disease

Genetics

Not applicable other than hypercoagulable states

RISK FACTORS

- Varicose veins
- Immobilization
- Obesity
- Advanced age
- Postoperative states
- Pregnancy or postpartum
- Hypercoagulable status
- Estrogen-based oral contraceptives
- History of previous superficial thromboembolism or venous thromboembolic event (VTE)
- Trauma (IV placement/IV drug use, burns, surgery)
- Tobacco use (thromboangiitis obliterans)

GENERAL PREVENTION

- Avoid catheterization when possible, especially of the lower extremity.
- Insert catheters under aseptic conditions, secure cannulas, and replace every 3 days.
- Early mobilization and use usual DVT prophylaxis in high-risk patients (i.e., ICU, immobilized)
- Minimize risk factors as able.

COMMONLY ASSOCIATED CONDITIONS

- Increasing evidence of association between superficial thrombophlebitis and VTE
- Estimated lifetime risk of VTE is 4 to 6 times higher in those with history of superficial thrombophlebitis.
- Frequently seen with concurrent DVT (6–53%)
- Symptomatic pulmonary embolism can also be seen concurrently (0–10%).
- Both DVT/PE can occur up to 3 months after onset of superficial thrombophlebitis.

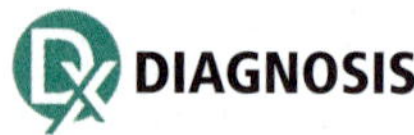

DIAGNOSIS

HISTORY

Patients classically complain of a section of firm, warm, and painful skin in a cord-like segment. This segment overlies the affected superficial vein. Patients may have risk factors as mentioned above.

PHYSICAL EXAM

- Swelling, tenderness, redness along the course of a vein or veins
- Examination often reveals a firm and tender palpable cord along the course of the vein with overlying cutaneous erythema.
- Fever in 70% of patients in septic phlebitis
- Sign of systemic sepsis in 84% of suppurative cases

DIFFERENTIAL DIAGNOSIS

- Cellulitis
- DVT
- Erythema nodosum
- Cutaneous polyarteritis nodosa
- Lymphangitis
- Contact dermatitis
- Other inflammatory vasculitides

DIAGNOSTIC TESTS & INTERPRETATION

Initial Tests (lab, imaging)

- H&P is usually adequate for diagnosis of superficial thrombophlebitis. If there is any uncertainty, venous ultrasonography can be completed.
- However, physical exam alone underestimates the extent of disease burden due to the association with DVT. Consequently, there is increasing recommendation for a comprehensive duplex ultrasound to evaluate for the presence of DVT.

Follow-Up Tests & Special Considerations

- Patients with recurrent SVT or found with concurrent unprovoked VTE may benefit from additional testing for thrombophilia.
- If suspicious for sepsis
  - Blood cultures (bacteremia in 80–90%)
  - Consider culture of the IV fluids being infused.
  - CBC demonstrates leukocytosis.
- In migratory thrombophlebitis, have a high index of suspicion for malignancy.
- Consider repeat venous ultrasound to assess effectiveness of therapy.
  - If thrombosis is extending, more aggressive therapy required

Diagnostic Procedures/Other

Typically, additional labs and imaging are not needed.

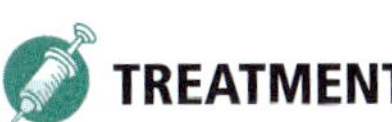

TREATMENT

GENERAL MEASURES

- Patients with concomitant VTE should be treated per VTE standard of care.
- Suppurative thrombophlebitis treatment depends on source of infection, with typical treatment requiring source control (i.e., catheter removal), broad-spectrum antibiotics, and consultation for urgent surgical venous excision.
- Treatment of aseptic low-risk superficial thrombophlebitis is generally conservative, including NSAIDs and compression.
  - Conservative management, antibiotics not useful
  - For varicosities, compression stockings; maintain activities.
  - Catheter/trauma associated
    - Immediately remove IV and culture tip.
    - Elevate with application of warm compresses.
    - If slow to resolve, consider LMWH.
- Large, severe, or septic thrombophlebitis
  - Inpatient care or bed rest with elevation and local warm compress
  - When the patient is ambulating, then start compression stockings or ACE bandages.

MEDICATION

First Line

- High-risk superficial thrombophlebitis
  - High-risk criteria: extensive SVT, involvement above the knee, particularly if close to the saphenofemoral junction; severe symptoms; involvement of the greater saphenous vein; history of VTE or SVT; active cancer; recent surgery (2)
  - Treat for 45 days with rivaroxaban 10 mg PO once daily or fondaparinux 2.5 mg SC once daily (2),(3)[A]
  - SVT within 3 cm of the deep venous system should be treated with full-dose anticoagulation, such as direct oral anticoagulants (DOACs) (1).
- Otherwise, best medication(s) and duration of treatment are not well defined, as 2018 Cochrane review found that most trials comparing NSAIDs, compression, elevation, other anticoagulation, surgical interventions were small and of poor quality (3)[A].
- Localized, mild thrombophlebitis (usually self-limited)
  - NSAIDs and ASA for inflammation/pain to reduce symptoms and local progression
  - Use of compression stockings can also provide symptomatic relief.

Second Line

- Septic/suppurative
  - May present or be complicated by sepsis
  - Requires IV antibiotics (broad spectrum initially) and anticoagulation
- Anticoagulation with fondaparinux or rivaroxaban treatment can prevent extension of SVT in addition to VTE prevention. As above, consider if thrombus is large, close to the junction with deep veins, or involves the long saphenous vein; may also consider 4 weeks of LMWH, such as enoxaparin
- Superficial thrombophlebitis related to inherited or acquired hypercoagulable states is addressed by treating the related disease.

ISSUES FOR REFERRAL

- Severely inflamed or very large superficial thrombophlebitis should be evaluated for excision.
- Septic superficial thrombophlebitis should be urgently referred in the inpatient setting.
- Refer to vascular surgeon when patients require anticoagulation but have contraindications.

SURGERY/OTHER PROCEDURES

- Septic
  - Surgical consultation for excision of the involved vein segment and involved tributaries
  - Drain contiguous abscesses.
  - Remove all associated cannula and culture tips.
- Aseptic: Manage underlying conditions.
  - Evaluate for saphenous vein ligation to prevent deep vein extension after acute phase resolved.
  - Consider referral for varicosity excision.

ADMISSION, INPATIENT, AND NURSING CONSIDERATIONS

- Septic: inpatient
- Aseptic: outpatient

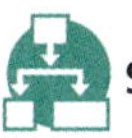

ONGOING CARE

FOLLOW-UP RECOMMENDATIONS

Patient Monitoring

- Septic: routine WBC count and differential; target treatment based on culture result.
- Aseptic: Some experts recommend follow-up D-dimer to ensure decreasing thrombotic burden.
- Local, mild thrombophlebitis typically resolves with conservative therapy and does not require specific monitoring unless there is a failure to resolve.

DIET

No restrictions

PATIENT EDUCATION

- Review local care, elevation, and use of compression hose for acute treatment and prevention of recurrence.
- Counsel on risk of recurrence or progression.
- Counsel on signs of progression or failure of therapy.
- Counsel on need for follow-up or referral when additional workup may be required (concern for thrombophilia, migratory thrombophlebitis).

PROGNOSIS

- Septic/suppurative: high mortality (50%) if untreated; depends on treatment delay, need for surgery, source of infection
- Aseptic
  - Usually benign course; recovery in 2 to 3 weeks
  - Depends on development of DVT and early detection of complications
  - Aseptic thrombophlebitis can be isolated, recurrent, or migratory.
  - Recurrence is likely if related to varicosity or if severely affected vein is not removed, or if related to a persistent hypercoagulable state.

COMPLICATIONS

- Septic: systemic sepsis, bacteremia (84%), septic pulmonary emboli (44%), metastatic abscess formation, pneumonia (44%), subperiosteal abscess of adjacent long bones in children
- Aseptic: DVT (6–53%), VTE (up to 10%), thromboembolic phenomena

REFERENCES

1. Piazza G, Krishnathasan D, Hamade N, et al. Superficial vein thrombosis: a review. *JAMA*. 2025;334(22):2020–2030. doi:10.1001/jama.2025.15222.
2. Stevens SM, Woller SC, Kreuziger LB, et al. Antithrombotic therapy for VTE disease: second update of the CHEST guideline and expert panel report. *Chest*. 2021;160(6):e545–e608.
3. Di Nisio M, Wichers IM, Middeldorp S. Treatment for superficial thrombophlebitis of the leg. *Cochrane Database Syst Rev*. 2018;2(2):CD004982.

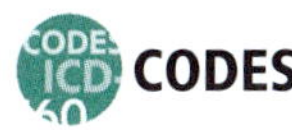

SEE ALSO

Deep Vein Thrombophlebitis

CODES

ICD10

- I80.9 Phlebitis and thrombophlebitis of unspecified site
- I80.00 Phlbts and thombophlb of superfic vessels of unsp low extrm
- I80.8 Phlebitis and thrombophlebitis of other sites

CLINICAL PEARLS

- Mild superficial thrombophlebitis is typically self-limiting and responds well to conservative care.
- High-risk superficial thrombophlebitis should be treated with anticoagulation due to risk of extension. Lower extremity disease involving large veins or proximal saphenous vein likely benefits from anticoagulation to prevent DVT.
- Septic thrombophlebitis requires admission for antibiotics and anticoagulation. If severe, consider surgical consultation for venous excision.

S

SYNCOPE

Santiago O. Valdes, MD, FAAP • Sarah Tucker, MD

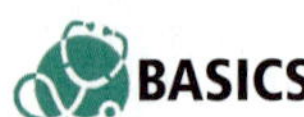

BASICS

DESCRIPTION

- Abrupt, transient loss of consciousness caused by cerebral hypoperfusion, characterized by unresponsiveness and loss of postural tone with spontaneous recovery
- System(s) affected: cardiovascular, nervous

EPIDEMIOLOGY

Prevalence

- Approximately 20–35% of adults and up to 25% of children <18 years of age report ≥1 episode during their lifetime.
- The prevalence in institutionalized elderly (>75 years of age) is 23%.

ETIOLOGY AND PATHOPHYSIOLOGY

- Systemic hypotension secondary to decreased cardiac output and/or systemic vasodilation leads to a drop in cerebral perfusion and resultant loss of consciousness. Syncope can be divided into cardiac and noncardiac etiologies:
  - Cardiac
    - Arrhythmogenic: bradyarrhythmias (e.g., sinus node dysfunction, heart block), tachyarrhythmias (e.g., ventricular tachycardia [VT], ventricular fibrillation, supraventricular tachycardia), and channelopathies (e.g., Brugada syndrome, long QT syndrome)
    - Structural: aortic stenosis, pulmonary embolism, hypertrophic cardiomyopathy, myocardial infarction, coronary anomalies, tamponade, vascular dissection
  - Noncardiac
    - Reflex (neurally mediated) syncope (NMS): vasovagal (inappropriate vasodilation leading to neurally mediated systemic hypotension and decreased cerebral blood flow); carotid sinus hypersensitivity; situational (micturition, defecation, cough, pain, emotions, hair combing)—most common cause in adult cases
    - Orthostatic hypotension (OHT): volume depletion, pregnancy, anemia, medications
    - Drug/alcohol induced
    - Primary autonomic failure: pure autonomic failure, Parkinson disease
    - Secondary autonomic failure: diabetes, amyloidosis
- The vast majority of pediatric cases represent benign alterations in vasomotor tone.

RISK FACTORS

- Heart disease (acquired or structural)
- Dehydration
- Medications (e.g., antihypertensives, antiarrhythmics, diuretics)
- Presence of a primary autonomic degenerative disorder

GENERAL PREVENTION

Preventative measures are aimed at addressing underlying etiology. Common measures include maintaining adequate hydration and salt intake, moving slowly from sitting to standing position, and lying down flat when experiencing light-headedness.

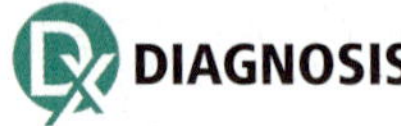

DIAGNOSIS

HISTORY

- Careful history, physical exam, and an ECG are more important than other investigations in determining the diagnosis (1).
- Make sure that the patient or witness (if present) is not referring to vertigo (i.e., sense of rotary motion, spinning, and whirling), seizure, or causes of fall without loss of consciousness. Onset of syncope is usually rapid, and recovery is spontaneous, rapid, and complete. Duration of syncopal episodes are typically brief (<60 seconds).
- Circumstances: Prolonged standing, urination, coughing, defecation, postprandial, and intense emotions are more likely to be associated with NMS. Consider carotid sinus hypersensitivity with abrupt neck movements. Consider cardiac cause with exertional syncope.
- Number of previous episodes (benign causes of syncope tend to be associated with a single episode)
- Presence of prodromal symptoms: Consider NMS.
  - Elderly patients are less likely to experience a prodrome.
- Palpitations, chest pain, dyspnea, or no prodrome: Consider cardiac.
- Position (supine: arrhythmia; erect: NMS; supine → erect: OHT)
- Prolonged syncope: Consider psychiatric or neurologic.
- Delayed recovery: Consider neurologic (postictal).
- Ask for family history of long QT syndrome, catecholaminergic polymorphic VT, Brugada syndrome, implantable cardioverter-defibrillator (ICD), hypertrophic cardiomyopathy, or unexplained sudden cardiac death in young family members (<50 years).
- High-risk findings: new-onset chest discomfort, breathlessness, abdominal pain, headache, syncope during exertion or when supine, or sudden palpitations immediately followed by syncope
- Even after careful evaluation, including diagnostic procedures and special tests, the cause will be found in only 50–60% of patients.

PHYSICAL EXAM

Check for orthostasis:

- Measure the BP and pulse after the patient is supine for 5 minutes and then have the patient stand and repeat BP and pulse immediately, after standing 1 and 3 minutes.
  - A drop in systolic blood pressure (SBP) of ≥20 mm Hg or diastolic blood pressure (DBP) of ≥10 mm Hg is consistent with OHT. Induction of prodromal symptoms with postural changes even without vital sign changes is indicative of orthostatic intolerance.
- Check for cardiac murmur/rubs/gallops or focal neurologic abnormality.
- High-risk findings: unexplained SBP <90 mm Hg, suggestion of GI bleed on rectal exam, persistent bradycardia (<40 bpm) in absence of physical training, or undiagnosed systolic murmur

DIFFERENTIAL DIAGNOSIS

Consider nonsyncope causes of transient loss of consciousness:

- Drop attacks
- Vertigo
- Seizure disorder
- Stroke/transient ischemic attack (TIA)
- Psychiatric (conversion, somatization): lack hemodynamic and/or autonomic changes

DIAGNOSTIC TESTS & INTERPRETATION

- Relevant testing should be performed to identify life-threatening conditions or those associated with significant risk of injury (2)[C].
- There are several risk stratification scores that can be considered for use in adult populations, including the Evaluation of Guidelines in Syncope Study (EGSYS) score which can be used to identify patients with a high risk of mortality (3)[C].

Initial Tests (lab, imaging)

- ECG: Consider cardiac cause if there are ischemic changes, bifascicular block, AV block, sinus bradycardia <40 bpm or sinus pause lasting >3 seconds, prolonged QTc, preexcitation, Brugada pattern, or alternating BBB.
- Other testing should be guided by history and physical:
  - CBC, electrolytes, BUN, creatinine
  - Glucose (rarely helpful if asymptomatic or presenting hours later)
  - BNP
  - Cardiac enzymes (only if history suggestive of MI or myocarditis)
  - D-dimer (for pulmonary embolism workup)
  - Urine pregnancy and urine drug screen
  - Initial cardiac or neuroimaging only if indicated
  - Lung scan or helical CT scan of chest if concern for PE

Follow-Up Tests & Special Considerations

- If history and physical suggest ischemic, valvular, or congenital heart disease (1),(2)[B]
  - Echocardiogram (1),(2)[B]
  - Exercise stress test (if syncope with exertion) (1),(2)[C]
  - Cross sectional imaging in select patients (CT scan or MRI) (1)[B]
- Ambulatory ECG monitoring, (e.g. Holter, external loop recorder, implantable loop recorder)
- Head imaging, carotid US, and EEG are not recommended in routine evaluation of syncope but may be useful if history and physical is concerning for neurologic issues (1)[C].
- Tilt-table testing (1),(2)[B]
  - Provocative test for vasovagal syncope
  - High false-positive rate
  - Often, results are not reproducible.
- Psychiatric evaluation (2)[C]: indicated when syncope is thought to be psychogenic

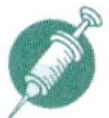

TREATMENT

- Initial therapy consists of maintaining good hydration status and normal salt intake. Educate patients of the premonitory signs of syncope (1).
- Majority of pediatric patients improve with nonpharmacologic measures.

GENERAL MEASURES

- NMS: reassurance, education, behavior modification (increased water and salt intake, lying down when experiencing prodromal symptoms)
- Elderly patients without previously recognized heart disease should be admitted if cardiac etiology of syncope is suspected.
- Patients without heart disease, especially young patients (age <60 years), can be worked up safely as outpatients.
- Prescribe antiarrhythmics for documented arrhythmias occurring simultaneously with syncope or symptoms of presyncope. Asymptomatic arrhythmias do not necessarily require treatment.
- Consider reduction or removal of medications that may be contributing to syncopal episodes.

MEDICATION

First Line

- Geared toward specific underlying etiology
- In cases of recurrent NMS and OHT (1)[B]
  - Mineralocorticoids (fludrocortisone)
  - α-Adrenergic agonists (midodrine)
  - Norepinephrine precursor (droxidopa)

Second Line

- SSRIs (1)[C] (paroxetine, sertraline, fluoxetine)
- Vagolytics (disopyramide)
- Acetylcholinesterase inhibitor (pyridostigmine)

ISSUES FOR REFERRAL

When cardiac or neurologic etiologies are suspected, obtain appropriate consultation, as indicated.

ADDITIONAL THERAPIES

For vasovagal/neurocardiogenic/NMS

- Counterpressure maneuvers and exercise improve vasovagal symptoms and recurrence (1).
- Head-up tilt sleeping (2)[C]
- Abdominal binders and/or support stockings (1),(2)[C]
- Increased fluid and salt intake to maintain intravascular volume in cases of recurrent NMS

SURGERY/OTHER PROCEDURES

- ICD placement for patients with cardiac conditions with high risk of sudden death and/or recurrent syncope on medications (e.g., long QT syndrome, Brugada syndrome, catecholaminergic polymorphic VT, hypertrophic cardiomyopathy) (1),(2)[B]
- Electrophysiology study (EPS) and ablation can be performed in arrhythmias (1)[B].
- Many recommend pacemaker implantation in patients with the following:
  - 2nd- (Mobitz type II) and 3rd-degree heart block
  - High risk of developing 3rd-degree heart block (bifascicular block, HV interval >100 ms by EPS)
  - Pacing-induced infranodal block
  - Sinus node recovery time ≥3 seconds

ADMISSION, INPATIENT, AND NURSING CONSIDERATIONS

A number of validated risk predictor tools have been published (i.e., ROSE rule, Syncope Risk Score, STePS) and may be useful in the determination of need for hospital admission. In the presence of ≥1 serious medical condition, inpatient evaluation should strongly be considered (3).

ONGOING CARE

FOLLOW-UP RECOMMENDATIONS

Patient Monitoring

- Frequent follow-up visits for patients with cardiac causes of syncope, especially if on antiarrhythmics
- Patients with an unknown cause of syncope rarely (5%) are diagnosed during the follow-up.
- Home video recording with smartphone technology is recommended for recurrent episodes.

DIET

No specific diet unless the patient has heart disease or NMS (see "Additional Therapies").

PATIENT EDUCATION

- Reassurance that most cardiac causes can be treated, and those with noncardiac causes do well, even if the cause is never discovered.
- Teaching of preventative and counter measures including avoidance of prolonged standing, awareness of position changes (particularly after lying or sitting), abdominal and or leg pumping movements/contractions while standing or crossing legs upon standing.
- Carefully consider whether the patient should drive while syncope is being evaluated. Physicians should be aware of pertinent local legislation.

PROGNOSIS

- The majority of patients (80%) have no recurrence of syncope.
- The identification of a cardiac etiology of syncope and/or the presence of other chronic medical conditions may alter prognosis.

COMPLICATIONS

Secondary traumatic injury from falling

REFERENCES

1. Shen WK, Sheldon RS, Benditt DG, et al. 2017 ACC/AHA/HRS guideline for the evaluation and management of patients with syncope: a report of the American College of Cardiology/American Heart Association Task Force on clinical practice guidelines and the Heart Rhythm Society. *Circulation*. 2017;136(5):e60–e122.
2. Brignole M, Moya A, de Lange FJ, et al; for ESC Scientific Document Group. 2018 ESC guidelines for the diagnosis and management of syncope. *Eur Heart J*. 2018;39(21):1883–1948.
3. Liang Y, Li X, Tse G, et al. Syncope prediction scores in the emergency department. *Curr Cardiol Rev*. 2022;18(5):1–7.

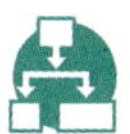

SEE ALSO

- Aortic Valvular Stenosis; Atrial Septal Defect; Carotid Sinus Hypersensitivity; Patent Ductus Arteriosus; Pulmonary Arterial Hypertension; Pulmonary Embolism; Seizure Disorders; Stokes-Adams Attacks
- Algorithms: Syncope; Transient Ischemic Attack and Transient Neurologic Defects

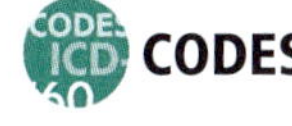

CODES

ICD10

R55 Syncope and collapse

CLINICAL PEARLS

- Careful history and physical exam are keys to a diagnosis.
- Use the ECG/event-recorder to evaluate for arrhythmias.
- Reflex-mediated vasovagal (NMS/neurocardiogenic) is the most common cause in children and adults.
- True neurologic causes of syncope are rare.

SYNCOPE, REFLEX (VASOVAGAL SYNCOPE)

Melinda Kwan, DO, MPH • Norton Winer, MD

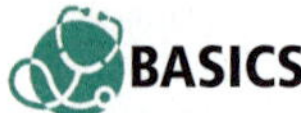

BASICS

A reversible loss of consciousness and postural tone secondary to systemic hypotension and cerebral hypoperfusion due to vasodilation and/or bradycardia (rarely, tachycardia) with spontaneous recovery and no neurologic sequelae; the term *syncope* excludes seizures, coma, shock, or other states of altered consciousness.

DESCRIPTION

- Derived from the Greek *syncopa*, "to cut short"
- Sudden, transient loss of consciousness characterized by unresponsiveness, falling, and spontaneous recovery
- Common cause of syncope in all age groups, especially in patients with no evidence of neurologic or cardiac disease
- Five main types of syncope: vasovagal or neurocardiogenic syncope, situational syncope, orthostatic hypotension, carotid sinus hypersensitivity, and glossopharyngeal/trigeminal neuralgia syncope (uncommon) (1)

EPIDEMIOLOGY

- Mortality: cardiac-related syncope 20–30% and 5% in idiopathic syncope
- Age: any age

Incidence

- Ranges from 7% in children aged <18 years and 15% in adults aged >70 years
- 36–62% of all syncopal episodes
- 30% recurrence rate

Prevalence

22% in the general population

ETIOLOGY AND PATHOPHYSIOLOGY

Cause: An abnormal response of the normal mechanisms that maintain blood pressure in an upright posture. Vasovagal syncope typically occurs when an individual is an upright position for a comparatively long duration (up to ≥10 minutes), compared with orthostatic hypotension which generally develops in a short period (such as a quick positional change).

- In normal individuals, upright posture results in venous pooling and transient decrease in BP.
- Neurally induced syncope may result from a cardioinhibitory response, a vasodepressor response, or a combination of the two.
- Increased cardiovagal tone leads to bradycardia or asystole, and decreased peripheral sympathetic activity leads to venodilation and hypotension (2).
- Vasovagal syncope usually has a precipitating event, often related to fright, pain, panic, exercise, noxious stimuli, or heat exposure (2).
- Carotid sinus syncope is precipitated by position change, turning head, or wearing a tight collar (possible neck tumors or surgical scarring).
- Situational syncope is related to micturition, defecation, postexercise, cough, or swallow.
- Glossopharyngeal syncope is related to throat or facial pain.

Genetics

Vasovagal syncope is associated with certain genetic markers, particularly involving serotonin and dopamine signaling (3).

RISK FACTORS

- Low-resting BP
- Age: older age
- Prolonged supine position with resulting deconditioning of autonomic control

GENERAL PREVENTION

Avoid precipitating events or situations. Optimize diabetes control, use of elastic stockings, adequate hydration.

COMMONLY ASSOCIATED CONDITIONS

- Cardiopulmonary disorders: CHF, MI, arrhythmias, hypertrophic obstructive cardiomyopathy, HTN, pulmonary embolism (PE)
- Neurologic disorders: autonomic dysfunction, Shy-Drager syndrome, Parkinson disease, multiple system atrophy, transient ischemic attack, vertebrobasilar insufficiency, peripheral neuropathy
- Psychiatric disorders:
  - Generalized anxiety disorder
  - Panic disorder
  - Major depression
  - Alcohol dependence

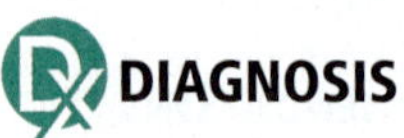

DIAGNOSIS

HISTORY

- History of syncope during or immediately after exertion is concerning for cardiac syncope.
- Neurally mediated syncope is preceded by blurred vision, palpitations, nausea, warmth, diaphoresis, or light-headedness, or there may be history of nausea, warmth, diaphoresis, or fatigue *after* syncope.
- Vasovagal syncope
  - Three phases: prodrome, loss of consciousness, and postsyncope
  - Precipitating event or stimulus is usually identified, such as panic, fright, pain, or exercise.
  - May be postexertional in athletes (diagnosis of exclusion)
  - Position: *can be preceded by prolonged standing but can occur from any position; generally resolves when the patient becomes supine*
    - Preceding events: as discussed above
    - Prodrome: as listed above for neurally mediated syncope
  - Duration: generally brief (seconds to minutes)
  - Recovery: may be prolonged with persistent nausea, pallor, and diaphoresis but without neurologic change or confusion
- Carotid sinus syncope is precipitated by position change, after turning head, or wearing a tight collar.
- Situational syncope is related to micturition, defecation, or coughing.
- Glossopharyngeal syncope (less common) is related to throat or facial pain.
  - Precipitating events or situations may include panic, pain, exercise, micturition, defecation, coughing, or swallowing.
- Pregnant women can have reflex syncope when moving from supine to lateral decubitus or upright positions.

PHYSICAL EXAM

- Vital signs, including orthostatics and bilateral BP
- Cardiac exam: volume status, murmurs, rhythm, carotid bruits
- Neurologic exam: signs of focal deficit
- Assess for occult blood loss.
- Dix-Hallpike if benign paroxysmal vertigo is suspected

DIFFERENTIAL DIAGNOSIS

- Seizure
- Arrhythmia
- Hypoglycemia
- Cardiac syncope
- Cerebrovascular syncope
- Orthostatic hypotension
- Drop attacks
- Psychiatric illness

DIAGNOSTIC TESTS & INTERPRETATION

Guided by history and physical, includes basic tests to rule out three primary causes of syncope: hypoglycemia, arrhythmia, and anemia

Initial Tests (lab, imaging)

- Blood glucose (hypoglycemia)
- ECG should be ordered for all patients. Abnormal ECG findings are common in patients with cardiac syncope (arrhythmia).
- CBC (rule out anemia)
- Head CT, MRI/MRA, carotid ultrasound only if history or physical exam suggests a neurologic cause
  - Radiology studies are not indicated for insignificant trauma in the presence of a normal neurologic exam.

Follow-Up Tests & Special Considerations

- 24-hour Holter monitoring only if a high probability of cardiac cause and/or abnormal ECG findings is present
- A low hemoglobin without obvious cause of bleed warrants stool guaiac, head CT (rule out subarachnoid hemorrhage), abdominal CT (rule out retroperitoneal bleed)
- Negative imaging prompts workup for alternative causes.

- Stroke, bleed, or carotid stenosis require appropriate disease-oriented management.
- EEG only if history or physical exam suggests seizure
- Implantable loop recorder

Diagnostic Procedures/Other

- Head-up tilt table testing:
  - Contraindicated in patients with known cardiac or neurovascular disease or in pregnancy
  - Indicated for recurrent syncope or single episode accompanied by injury or risk to others (e.g., pilots, surgeons)
  - Uses positional changes to reproduce symptoms
  - Positive test diagnostic for vasovagal syncope
- Carotid sinus massage, only in a monitored setting (i.e., BP and HR monitoring, IV access):
  - Contraindicated in patients with carotid disease (careful auscultation prior to massage is essential)
  - Pressure at the angle of the jaw for 5 seconds with simultaneous ECG monitoring
  - Positive tests (causing syncope or cardiac pause >3 seconds) are diagnostic of carotid sinus syncope.
- Psychiatric evaluation: to rule out anxiety, depression, and alcohol abuse

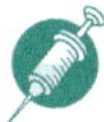

TREATMENT

Therapy is primarily for recurrent syncope. Situational syncope does not warrant specific treatment.

GENERAL MEASURES

Identify and avoid precipitating events or situations.

MEDICATION

First Line

Nonpharmacologic treatment

- Patient counseling
  - Increased salt and fluid intake
- Moderate exercise training
  - Isometric muscle contractions
    - These maneuvers increase cardiac output and arterial blood pressure.
  - Yoga
- Tilt-table training
  - Progressively prolonged periods of enforced upright posture

Second Line

- α-Agonists mainly used for orthostatic hypotension
  - Midodrine is commonly used, particularly in younger, healthy patients with a high "syncope burden" (4). It increases peripheral vascular resistance and venous return. Side effects include HTN, paresthesia, urinary retention, "goose bumps," hyperactivity, dizziness, tremor, and nervousness.
- SSRIs: Paroxetine and fluoxetine are useful in treating neurocardiogenic/vasovagal syncope.
  - Serotonin affects BP and HR via the central nervous system. Serotonin decreases a sympathetic withdrawal response to rapid increases in serotonin levels.
  - Side effects include weight gain, nausea, anxiety, sexual dysfunction, and insomnia.
- Mineralocorticoids: Fludrocortisone has been found helpful mainly in orthostatic hypotension.
  - Helpful in renal sodium absorption and increasing the vasoconstrictive peripheral vascular response
  - Adverse reactions include fluid retention, HTN, CHF, peripheral edema, and hypokalemia.
- β-Blockers: metoprolol, atenolol, or pindolol mainly for postural orthostatic tachycardia syndrome (POTS)
  - Block peripheral vasodilators and ventricular mechanoreceptor stimulation
  - Stabilization of HR and BP
  - Side effects: hypotension and bradycardia (with worsening of syncope), fatigue, depression, and sexual dysfunction
  - Contraindicated in asthma

ISSUES FOR REFERRAL

Neurology or cardiology, as needed

ADDITIONAL THERAPIES

Use of support/pressure stockings

SURGERY/OTHER PROCEDURES

Pacemaker placement may be of use in patients with frequent neurocardiogenic/vasovagal syncope that is refractory to other therapies.

- Prevents prolonged bradycardia or asystole during syncopal episodes
- Long-term effect
- Invasive placement procedure

COMPLEMENTARY & ALTERNATIVE MEDICINE

Treatments for underlying heart disease or precipitating factors (e.g., anxiety); none are proven therapies.

- Nutrition and supplements: omega-3 fatty acids, multivitamin, CoQ10, acetyl-L-carnitine, α-lipoic acid, and L-arginine
- Herbs: green tea (*Camellia sinensis*), bilberry (*Vaccinium myrtillus*), ginkgo (*Ginkgo biloba*)
- Homeopathy: carbo vegetabilis, opium, sepia
- Acupuncture: It may precipitate fainting.

ADMISSION, INPATIENT, AND NURSING CONSIDERATIONS

Hospital admission or intense evaluation for:

- Severe coronary artery disease or structural heart disease (severe CHF, low ejection fraction or previous myocardial infarction, aortic stenosis)
- Arrhythmic syncope:
  - ECG may show bifascicular block, sinus bradycardia <40 without SA block or β-blockers, Brugada syndrome, abnormal QT interval, etc.
- Severe anemia or electrolyte abnormalities
- Family history of sudden death
- Isotonic crystalloids, as needed
- Vital sign monitoring
- Discharge when hemodynamically stable and workup satisfactory

ONGOING CARE

DIET

- Increased salt intake may help if not otherwise contraindicated (2)[C].
- Maintain fluid intake.

PATIENT EDUCATION

- Identify and avoid precipitating events or situations.
- Avoid dehydration, alcohol consumption, warm environments, tight clothing, and long periods of standing motionless.
- Recognize presyncopal symptoms.
- Use behaviors, such as lying down, to avoid syncope.

PROGNOSIS

May be recurrent but not life-threatening

COMPLICATIONS

May result in injury from falls

S

REFERENCES

1. Zou R, Wang S, Lin P, et al. The clinical characteristics of situational syncope in children and adults undergoing head-up tilt testing. *Am J Emerg Med*. 2020;38(7):1419–1423.
2. Rocha BML, Gomes RV, Cunha GJL, et al. Diagnostic and therapeutic approach to cardioinhibitory reflex syncope: a complex and controversial issue. *Rev Port Cardiol (Engl Ed)*. 2019;38(9):661–673.
3. Behnoush AH, Yazdani K, Khalaji A, et al. Pharmacologic prevention of recurrent vasovagal syncope: a systematic review and network meta-analysis of randomized controlled trials. *Heart Rhythm*. 2023;20(3):448–460. doi:10.1016/j.hrthm.2022.12.010.
4. Sheldon R, Faris P, Tang A, et al. Midodrine for the prevention of vasovagal syncope: a randomized clinical trial. *Ann Intern Med*. 2021;174(10):1349–1356. doi:10.7326/M20-5415.

SEE ALSO

Algorithms: Syncope; Transient Ischemic Attack and Transient Neurologic Defects

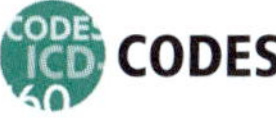

CODES

ICD10

R55 Syncope and collapse

CLINICAL PEARLS

- A careful history of the events preceding the syncopal episode helps guide evaluation and management.
- Rule out cardiac or neurogenic syncope.
- Prodrome is common with reflex syncope.
- Recovery may be prolonged, with persistent symptoms but there is no residual neurologic deficit or confusion.
- Patients should avoid precipitating situations or events.

SYNDROME OF INAPPROPRIATE ANTIDIURETIC HORMONE SECRETION (SIADH)

Ashraf Elamin, MD • Matthew A. Niemi, MD

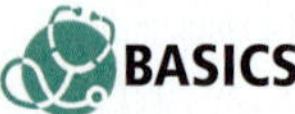

BASICS

The syndrome of inappropriate antidiuretic hormone secretion (SIADH) is a disorder with impaired water excretion (concentrated urine), caused by abnormal production of antidiuretic hormone (ADH) despite low serum osmolality.

DESCRIPTION

- Decreased urinary electrolyte-free water excretion leads to dilutional hyponatremia (total body sodium [Na] levels may be normal or near-normal, but the patient's total body water is increased).
- Often secondary to medications but may be associated with an underlying pulmonary disorder or central nervous system (CNS) disease
- Common cause of hyponatremia in hospitalized patients
- Synonym(s): SIADH; syndrome of inappropriate antidiuresis

EPIDEMIOLOGY

Incidence

- Often found in the hospital setting, especially perioperative patients in response to stress, intravenous fluids, and drugs; the incidence can be as high as 35%.
- Predominant age: elderly
- Predominate sex: females > males

ETIOLOGY AND PATHOPHYSIOLOGY

- Drugs:
  - Antidepressants (e.g., SSRIs, tricyclics, monoamine oxidase inhibitors [MAOIs])
  - Antineoplastic drugs (e.g., vincristine, vinblastine, cisplatin, cyclophosphamide)
  - Antipsychotic agents (e.g., risperidone, quetiapine, phenothiazines, haloperidol)
  - Analgesics (e.g., duloxetine, pregabalin, tramadol, NSAIDs)
  - Anticonvulsants (e.g., carbamazepine, oxcarbazepine, valproic acid, phenytoin)
  - Others (e.g., vasopressin, desmopressin [DDAVP], oxytocin, ciprofloxacin, α-interferon, ecstasy)
- Malignancies (ectopic ADH production):
  - Bronchogenic or small cell carcinoma of the lung
  - Lymphoma
  - Mesothelioma
  - Pancreatic adenocarcinoma
  - Thymoma
- Pulmonary conditions:
  - Asthma/COPD
  - Atelectasis/pneumothorax
  - Cystic fibrosis
  - Positive pressure mechanical ventilation
  - Pneumonia (viral, bacterial)
  - Pulmonary tuberculosis (TB)
  - Sarcoidosis
- Neurologic causes:
  - Brain tumor
  - CNS injury (i.e., subarachnoid hemorrhage, trauma, stroke, surgery)
  - CNS lupus
  - Encephalitis, meningitis
  - Epilepsy
  - Guillain-Barré syndrome
  - Multiple sclerosis
- Acute intermittent porphyria
- Delirium tremens
- HIV infection/AIDS
- Rocky Mountain spotted fever

Genetics

- 10% of patients have an X-linked mutation for vasopressin 2 receptors (V2R).
- Polymorphisms in TRPV4 gene

RISK FACTORS

- Advanced age
- Postoperative status
- Institutionalization
- Use of predisposing drugs

GENERAL PREVENTION

Avoid high-risk medications, if drug-induced.

COMMONLY ASSOCIATED CONDITIONS

See "Etiology and Pathophysiology."

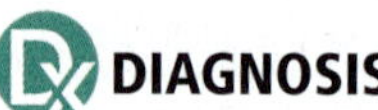

DIAGNOSIS

- Bartter and Schwartz criteria for SIADH:
  - Decreased osmolality (<275 mOsm/kg) with inappropriately concentrated urine (>100 mOsm/kg) and euvolemia
- Signs and symptoms depend upon the acuity and severity of hyponatremia and the degree of cerebral edema.

HISTORY

Symptoms:

- Fatigue, lethargy
- Anorexia, nausea, vomiting
- Increased thirst
- Headaches
- Dizziness, changes in vision
- Unsteady gait, falls
- Myalgias/weakness
- Confusion
- Seizures, coma

PHYSICAL EXAM

- Euvolemic state
- Mild hyponatremia (serum Na 125 to 135 mEq/L)
  - Slow cognition and reaction times
  - Hyporeflexia
  - Ataxia
- Moderate to severe hyponatremia (serum Na <125 mEq/L)
  - Altered mental status, coma
  - Lethargy
  - Seizures
  - Psychosis

DIFFERENTIAL DIAGNOSIS

- Intravascular volume depletion and thiazide-diuretic induced
- Appropriate ADH secretion secondary to decreased effective arterial blood volume (e.g., congestive heart failure [CHF], nephrotic syndrome, liver cirrhosis)
- Low solute intake hyponatremia ("tea and toast" diet; beer potomania)
- Reset osmostat (can be differentiated from SIADH by checking fractional excretion of urate (high in SIADH) (1)
- Psychogenic polydipsia (water intake >10 L/day—self-correction when intake is stopped)
- Endocrinopathies (adrenal insufficiency, hypothyroidism)
- Translocational hyponatremia: caused by hyperglycemia, mannitol, sucrose, glycine
- Pseudohyponatremia (lab artifact caused by hyperlipidemia, paraproteinemias, administration of IVIG)
- Postoperative complications (nonosmotic release of ADH, stimulated by pain, nausea, vomiting, hypotension)
- Cerebral salt-wasting syndrome (hyponatremia, extracellular fluid depletion, CNS insult)

DIAGNOSTIC TESTS & INTERPRETATION

- Serum Na level: low
- Serum urea level: normal to low
- Serum osmolality: low
- Urine osmolality: high; urine osmolality >100 mOsm/kg H_2O (2)
- Urine Na concentration: high; urine Na >30 mEq/L (2)
- Fractional excretion of Na >0.5% (2)
- Serum ADH level: high (not clinically useful)
- Not usually required for diagnosis but to assist in the diagnosis and assess for other causes:
  - Serum uric acid, glucose, creatinine (Cr)
  - Thyroid function
  - Morning cortisol

Initial Tests (lab, imaging)

- Serum osmolality
- Urine electrolytes (urine Na and urine potassium [K]) and urine osmolality

Follow-Up Tests & Special Considerations

- Consider chest X-ray as part of SIADH workup to evaluate for pulmonary disease.
- Patients with nausea, vomiting, headache, vision changes, and confusion should have a head CT scan to look for signs of trauma or space-occupying lesions.

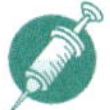

TREATMENT

Depends on clinical picture and acute versus chronic (3).

GENERAL MEASURES

- Treat underlying cause; remove the offending agent.
- Fluid restriction (usually <1,000 mL/day) is recommended.
- Avoid isotonic saline because this can worsen the hyponatremia.
- Correct hypokalemia.
- Mild asymptomatic hyponatremia (serum Na >125 mEq/L [>125 mmol/L]): Restrict fluid and treat the underlying cause.
- Moderate hyponatremia (serum Na 120 to 125 mEq/L):
  - Restrict free water intake; increase oral solute intake.
  - Calculate urine/plasma electrolyte ratio ([urine Na + K]/[serum Na + serum K]) to determine efficacy of fluid restriction; ineffective if ratio >1 (4) and may need pharmacologic therapy.
- Severe or with neurologic manifestations
  - Hypertonic saline (3% sodium chloride [NaCl] IV bolus)
  - Can increase serum Na more rapidly with hypertonic saline by 4 to 6 mEq/L over 4 to 6 hours in the initial treatment period, but not to exceed 8 mEq/L total in 24 hours (2),(5)[C].
- Chronic (≥48 hours duration)
  - Goal correction is 6 to 8 mEq/L per 24-hour period
- Acute (<48 hours duration)
  - Can initially correct rapidly, but the 24-hour goal is the same as in chronic hyponatremia (5)[C]

MEDICATION

- If severe or neurologic symptoms: IV 3% NaCl to increase serum Na cautiously (6)[B]:
  - If serum Na <120 mEq/L or severe neurologic symptoms, consider bolus of hypertonic saline to increase serum Na by 4 to 6 mEq/L over the first 4 to 6 hours.
- NaCl oral tablets
- Oral urea is an option but limited due to bitter taste.
- Loop diuretics: furosemide + K replacement
- V2R antagonist (the vaptans: tolvaptan, conivaptan) (6)[B]
  - Good efficacy and safety profiles in the treatment of moderate hyponatremia due to SIADH
  - Liberal fluid intake is encouraged.
  - Must be initiated in the hospital setting
  - Conivaptan only available IV and limited to 4 days maximum
  - Avoid tolvaptan in patients with liver disease.
- Demeclocycline (limited use)
  - Blocks ADH at renal tubule; produces nephrogenic diabetes insipidus
  - Dosage for long-term management: 300 to 600 mg PO BID
  - Onset of action within 1 week; therefore, not best for acute management
  - Adverse effects of GI intolerance and nephrotoxicity limit its use.
  - Paucity of evidence for efficacy
- Contraindications: Avoid tolvaptan in patients with cirrhosis due to possible liver injury. Avoid conivaptan in patients with Cr clearance <30 mL/minute.
- Precautions: Overly rapid correction (>10 mEq/L/day) can increase the risk for osmotic demyelination syndrome (ODS):
  - Permanent CNS damage in pons leading to quadriplegia and pseudobulbar palsy
  - Increased risk in women, alcoholics, malnutrition, hypoxia, chronic hyponatremia of <110 mEq/L, and hypokalemia

ALERT

Increase Na levels slowly, not >8 mEq/L/24 hours to prevent ODS (2)[C].

ISSUES FOR REFERRAL

Nephrology consultation recommended for severe hyponatremia.

ADDITIONAL THERAPIES

In chronic SIADH, SGLT-2 inhibitors (empagliflozin 25 mg daily) may increase serum Na by 4 mmol/L after 4 weeks due to its osmotic diuretic effect (7). Renal function and volume status should be monitored if SGLT-2 inhibitors used.

ADMISSION, INPATIENT, AND NURSING CONSIDERATIONS

Neurologic exam with vital signs if symptomatic or moderate/severe hyponatremia.

ONGOING CARE

FOLLOW-UP RECOMMENDATIONS

Patient Monitoring

- Careful continuous clinical and laboratory monitoring of hyponatremic state during the acute phase:
  - Hourly urine output
  - Urine Na, urine K, urine osmolality
  - Goal Na increase is <8 mEq/L/24 hours until Na reaches 130 mEq/L (2),(5)[C].
  - If moderate/severe, check serial serum chemistry every 4 to 8 hours to ensure an appropriate rate of correction.
- Chronic management: Treat underlying cause; continue fluid restriction and NaCl tablets as needed; referral to nephrologist

DIET

Increase protein/solute intake and decrease water/fluid intake.

PATIENT EDUCATION

Diet and fluid restrictions

PROGNOSIS

- Higher risk of ICU admission and increased risk of 30-day hospital readmission in hyponatremic patients (8)
- If symptomatic (seizure, coma): high mortality due to cerebral edema if serum Na <120 mEq/L

COMPLICATIONS

- Falls and hip fractures
- Cerebral edema (see "Prognosis")
- Osmotic demyelination with overcorrection (see "Treatment" precautions): central pontine and extrapontine irreversible myelinolysis (5)
- Chronic hyponatremia is associated with osteoporosis (8)[C].

REFERENCES

1. Imbriano LJ, Ilamathi E, Ali NM, et al. Normal fractional urate excretion identifies hyponatremic patients with reset osmostat. *J Nephrol*. 2012;25(5):833–838. doi:10.5301/jn.5000074.
2. Decaux G, Musch W. Clinical laboratory evaluation of the syndrome of inappropriate secretion of antidiuretic hormone. *Clin J Am Soc Nephrol*. 2008;3(4):1175–1184.
3. Miller NE, Rushlow D, Stacey SK. Diagnosis and management of sodium disorders: hyponatremia and hypernatremia. *Am Fam Physician*. 2023;108(5):476–486.
4. Furst H, Hallows KR, Post J, et al. The urine/plasma electrolyte ratio: a predictive guide to water restriction. *Am J Med Sci*. 2000;319(4):240–244.
5. Adrogué HJ, Madias NE. The challenge of hyponatremia. *J Am Soc Nephrol*. 2012;23(7):1140–1148.
6. Esposito P, Piotti G, Bianzina S, et al. The syndrome of inappropriate antidiuresis: pathophysiology, clinical management and new therapeutic options. *Nephron Clin Pract*. 2011;119(1):c62–c73.
7. Refardt J, Imber C, Sailer CO, et al. A randomized trial of empagliflozin to increase plasma sodium levels in patients with the syndrome of inappropriate antidiuresis. *J Am Soc Nephrol*. 2020;31(3):615–624. doi:10.1681/ASN.2019090944.
8. Usala RL, Fernandez SJ, Mete M, et al. Hyponatremia is associated with increased osteoporosis and bone fractures in a large US health system population. *J Clin Endocrinol Metab*. 2015;100(8):3021–3031.

SEE ALSO

Hyponatremia

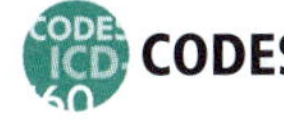

CODES

ICD10

E22.2 Syndrome of inappropriate secretion of antidiuretic hormone

CLINICAL PEARLS

- Treatment of the underlying cause is key. Review all medications for potential culprits.
- ODS is a cerebral demyelination syndrome that causes quadriplegia, pseudobulbar palsy, seizures, coma, and death. It is caused by an overly rapid rate of Na correction. Increase Na levels slowly, not >8 mEq/L/24 hours, to prevent ODS.
- Safe correction of hyponatremia is important. Online calculators are available: http://www.medcalc.com/sodium.html.

SYPHILIS

Melissa E. Badowski, PharmD, MPH • Mahesh C. Patel, MD

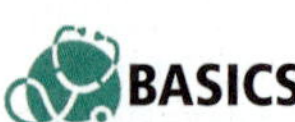

BASICS

DESCRIPTION

- A chronic, systemic infectious disease caused by the spirochete *Treponema pallidum*
- Transmitted sexually by direct contact with an active lesion; also transmitted vertically (maternal–fetal) and via blood transfusions
- Untreated disease includes four overlapping stages.
  - Primary: single (usually) painless chancre at point of entry (genital, oral, anal); appears in 10 to 90 days; chancre heals without treatment in 3 to 6 weeks.
  - Secondary: appears 2 to 8 weeks after primary chancre; nonpruritic rash on palms or soles of feet, mucous membrane lesions, headache, fever, lymphadenopathy, and alopecia
  - Latent: seroreactive without evidence of disease
    - Early latent: acquired within the last year
    - Late latent: exposure >12 months prior to diagnosis
  - Tertiary (late): Serology may be negative (fluorescent treponemal antibody absorption [FTA-ABS] test typically positive).
    - Gumma, cardiovascular, and late neurosyphilis; may be fatal
  - Neurosyphilis: any type of CNS involvement; can occur at any stage
    - Psychosis, delirium, dementia

Pediatric Considerations

In noncongenital cases, consider child abuse.

Pregnancy Considerations

- Screen all patients who are pregnant with venereal disease research laboratory (VDRL) test or rapid plasma reagin (RPR) test early in pregnancy, (i.e., first prenatal visit). If ongoing risk, repeat at 28 weeks and at delivery (1)[A].
- Use the same nontreponemal test for initial screening and for follow-up (1)[A].

EPIDEMIOLOGY

Incidence

- Syphilis case rates increased 60% globally and in the United States from 2019 through 2023.
- Case rates of congenital syphilis have increased as well.
- Highest rates remain in men who have sex with men (MSM).

ETIOLOGY AND PATHOPHYSIOLOGY

T. pallidum enters through intact mucous membranes or breaks in skin. The organism quickly enters the lymphatics to cause systemic disease; highly infectious; exposure to as few as 60 spirochetes is associated with ~50% chance of infection.

RISK FACTORS

MSM, multiple sexual partners, exposure to infected body fluids, injection drug use, transplacental transmission, adult individuals in custody, high-risk sexual behavior, people with HIV (PWH)

GENERAL PREVENTION

Education regarding safe sex; condoms reduce but do not eliminate transmission (1)[A].

COMMONLY ASSOCIATED CONDITIONS

HIV infection, hepatitis B, and other sexually transmitted infections (STIs)

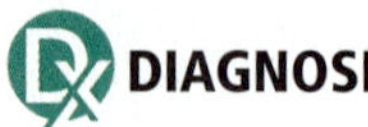

DIAGNOSIS

HISTORY

- As a "great imitator," a high index of suspicion is often required for accurate diagnosis.
- Previous sexual contact with partner with known infection or high-risk sexual behavior
- Genital lesions (chancre—primary syphilis)
- Rash, alopecia, malaise, headache, anorexia, nausea, fatigue (secondary syphilis)
- Mental status changes (tertiary syphilis)

PHYSICAL EXAM

Signs/symptoms depend on stage

- Primary: single (occasionally multiple), usually painless ulcer (chancre) in groin or at other point of entry; regional adenopathy
- Chancres begin as solitary firm, raised painless papules that erode and ulcerate. Spontaneous healing occurs in 4 to 8 weeks regardless of treatment.
- Secondary
  - Rash: skin/mucous membranes
    - Rough, red-brown macules, usually on palms and soles
    - May appear with chancre or after it has healed
    - Condylomata lata
    - Alopecia
  - Nonspecific symptoms: fever, adenopathy, malaise, headache, hair loss
- Tertiary (late) syphilis
  - Focal neurologic findings (hearing loss, vision loss; meningeal findings; loss of pain, temperature; proprioception)
  - Gummas (skin, mucous membranes, other organ systems)

DIFFERENTIAL DIAGNOSIS

- Primary: chancroid, lymphogranuloma venereum, granuloma inguinale, condylomata acuminata, herpes simplex, Behçet syndrome, trauma, carcinoma, mycotic infection, lichen planus, psoriasis, fungal infection
- Secondary: pityriasis rosea, drug eruption, psoriasis, lichen planus, viral exanthema, Stevens-Johnson syndrome
- Positive serology, asymptomatic: previously treated syphilis/other spirochetal disease (yaws, pinta)

DIAGNOSTIC TESTS & INTERPRETATION

Initial Tests (lab, imaging)

- Dark-field microscopy demonstrating *T. pallidum* spirochetes in lesion exudate/tissue biopsy; molecular PCR-based assays increasingly used in ulcerative lesions to detect *T. pallidum*
- Nontreponemal tests (VDRL/RPR) (1)
  - Primary screening test: positive within 7 days of exposure
  - Nonspecific false-positive results are common; must confirm diagnosis with treponemal tests
  - Positive test should be quantified and titers followed regularly after treatment.
    - Titers usually correlate with disease activity; 4-fold change is clinically significant. Titers decrease with time/treatment; following adequate treatment for primary/secondary disease, a 4-fold decline is typical in 6 to 12 months. Absence of a 4-fold decline suggests potential treatment failure.
    - With appropriate treatment, titers should become negative (see Serofast reaction).
    - Titers of patients treated in latent stages decline more gradually.
  - Prozone phenomenon: negative results from high titers of antibody; test with diluted serum.
  - Serofast reaction: persistently positive results years after treatment; new infection diagnosed by 4-fold rise in titer
  - Conditions that may alter treponemal testing (All stages of syphilis can have a false-negative RPR result, especially in primary syphilis.)
    - Pregnancy, autoimmune disease, mononucleosis, malaria, leprosy, viral pneumonia, cardiolipin antigens, injection drug use, acute febrile illness, HIV infection; elderly can have false-positive results.
- *T. pallidum* particle agglutination (TP-PA) increasingly used for primary testing as high sensitivity overcomes challenges of nontreponemal tests
- Treponemal tests (confirmatory test after positive nontreponemal screening test): for example, FTA-ABS, TP-PA, others (1)[A]:
  - Confirmatory test; usually positive for life after treatment; titers of no benefit; 15–25% of patients treated during primary stage revert to serologic nonreactivity after 2 to 3 years.
- Lumbar puncture (LP) indicated for (1)[A]:
  - Neurologic, ocular, or auditory manifestations; some advise LP in all secondary and early latent cases—even without neurologic symptoms; patients with late latent/latent disease of unknown duration if nonpenicillin therapy planned; treatment failures; evidence of active tertiary syphilis (e.g., aortitis, gumma, iritis); children to rule out neurosyphilis; VDRL, not RPR, used on CSF; send CSF for protein, glucose, and cell count.
  - Negative FTA-ABS or microhemagglutination (MHA)-TP on CSF excludes neurosyphilis (highly sensitive).

TREATMENT

GENERAL MEASURES

- Advise patients to notify partner(s) and to avoid intercourse until treatment is complete (1)[A].
- Test for HIV infection.
- 200 mg of doxycycline within 72 hours of unprotected exposure reduces transmission, particularly for MSM.
- Management of sexual contacts (2)[A]
  - Presumptively treat partners exposed within 90 days of diagnosis. Presumptively treat partners exposed >90 days before diagnosis if serologic results are not available immediately and follow-up is uncertain.
  - Long-term sex partners of patients with latent infection should be evaluated clinically (including serologies) and treated accordingly.

MEDICATION

ALERT

Use Bicillin L-A instead of Bicillin C-R (combination benzathine–procaine penicillin).

First Line

- Benzathine penicillin G remains the initial drug of choice. The formulation is determined by the disease stage and clinical presentation.
- Primary, secondary, and early latent <1 year (2)[A]
  - Penicillin G benzathine 2.4 million U IM × 1 dose
  - Penicillin-allergic patients: doxycycline 100 mg PO BID for 2 weeks, or ceftriaxone 1 to 2 g IM or IV daily for 10 to 14 days
    - Azithromycin 2 g PO for 1 dose (early syphilis only; should not be used in HIV, MSM, or pregnancy); resistance and treatment failures have been noted in several U.S. regions.
- Late latent/latent of unknown duration and tertiary without evidence of neurosyphilis (2)[A]
  - Penicillin G benzathine 2.4 million U IM weekly × 3 doses
  - Penicillin-allergic patients: Attempt desensitization and treatment with penicillin or doxycycline 100 mg PO BID for 28 days; adherence may be an issue.
- Ocular or neurosyphilis (2)[A]
  - Aqueous crystalline penicillin G 3 to 4 million U IV q4h as a continuous infusion for 10 to 14 days
  - Alternative: penicillin G procaine 2.4 million U IM daily in conjunction with probenecid 500 mg PO QID for 10 to 14 days (if compliance can be ensured)
  - Penicillin-allergic patients: Attempt desensitization and treat with penicillin; if unable to desensitize, administer ceftriaxone 2 g IV daily for 10 to 14 days
  - If late latent, latent of unknown duration, or tertiary in addition to neurosyphilis, consider treating as late latent after completion of neurosyphilis treatment regimen.
- Congenital (2)[A]
  - Aqueous crystalline penicillin G 50,000 U/kg/dose IV q12h for the first 7 days of life and q8h thereafter for a total of 10 days, or penicillin G procaine 50,000 U/kg/dose IM daily for 10 days
  - If negative CSF serologies, normal physical exam, and maternal titer then give 50,000 U/kg penicillin G benzathine IM in single dose; if >1 day of drug is missed, restart course.
  - Children (after newborn period): aqueous crystalline penicillin G 50,000 U/kg/dose IV q4–6h for 10 days; late latent, 50,000 U/kg IM as 3 doses at 1-week intervals; for contacts without symptoms: Treat as primary disease after serologies are obtained.
  - Do not give benzathine or procaine penicillins IV.
- Children (after newborn period) (2)[A]: aqueous crystalline penicillin G 50,000 U/kg/dose IV q4–6h for 10 days; late latent, 50,000 U/kg IM as 3 doses at 1-week intervals
- Pregnancy (2)[A]
  - Treatment is same as for nonpregnant patients. Some recommend second dose of penicillin G benzathine 2.4 million U IM 1 week after initial dose in 3rd trimester or with primary, secondary, or early latent syphilis.
  - Penicillin sensitivity: no proven alternatives to penicillin available for treatment during pregnancy; penicillin-allergic patients: Desensitize and treat with penicillin.
- Treat contacts without symptoms as primary disease after obtaining serologies.
- History of penicillin allergy:
  - Confirmed IgE-mediated reaction: desensitization; questionable history of IgE-mediated hypersensitivity: penicillin skin testing if major and minor penicillin determinants available; doxycycline (100 mg PO BID for 14 days) or tetracycline (500 mg PO QID for 14 days) are alternatives for primary and secondary syphilis.
- Precautions (2)[A]
  - PWH and pregnant patients may show poor response to recommended IM doses. Use IV therapy for all treatment failures in these patients.

ONGOING CARE

FOLLOW-UP RECOMMENDATIONS

- Clinical and serologic evaluation 6 to 12 months after treatment; if >1 year duration, check at 24 months (2)[A].
- In PWH, clinical and serologic evaluation at 3, 6, 9, 12, and 24 months after therapy (2)[A]

Patient Monitoring

- Use VDRL or RPR test to monitor therapy: 4-fold rise (two dilutions) in titer indicates new infection, whereas failure to decrease 4-fold (two dilutions) in 6 to 12 months may indicate treatment failure (although definitive criteria for cure not established); always use same test (preferably same lab) (2)[A].
- Retreatment for persistent clinical signs or recurrence, 4-fold rise in titers, or failure of initially high titer to decrease 4-fold by 6 to 12 months
- Neurosyphilis: Repeat LP every 6 months to check for normalization of CSF cell count (± CSF-VDRL and protein evaluation) (2)[A].

PATIENT EDUCATION

No intimate contacts until 4-fold titer drop

PROGNOSIS

- Excellent in all cases except patients with late syphilis complications and with HIV infection
- Syphilis in PWH
  - Treatment same as for HIV-negative patients; more often false-negative treponemal and nontreponemal tests or unusually high titers; response to therapy less predictable; early syphilis: increased risk of neurosyphilis and higher rates of treatment failure; late neurosyphilis: harder to treat; can occur up to ≥20 years after infection

COMPLICATIONS

- Membranous glomerulonephritis; paroxysmal cold hemoglobinuria; meningitis and tabes dorsalis; cardiovascular aneurysms; valvular damage; irreversible organ damage
- Jarisch-Herxheimer reaction
  - Fever, chills, headache, myalgias, new rash; common when starting treatment (of primary/secondary disease; less common with tertiary) owing to treponemal lysis; should not be confused with drug reaction; managed with analgesics and antipyretics

REFERENCES

1. Chevalier FJ, Bacon O, Johnson KA, et al. Syphilis: a review. *JAMA*. 2025;334(21):1927–1940. doi:10.1001/jama.2025.17362.
2. Workowski KA, Bachmann LH, Chan PA, et al. Sexually transmitted infections treatment guidelines, 2021. *MMWR Recomm Rep*. 2021;70(4):1–187.

ADDITIONAL READING

Hamill MM, Ghanem KG, Tuddenham S. State-of-the-art review: neurosyphilis. *Clin Infect Dis*. 2024;78(5):e57–e68. doi:10.1093/cid/ciad437.

SEE ALSO

Chlamydia Infection (Sexually Transmitted); Gonococcal Infections

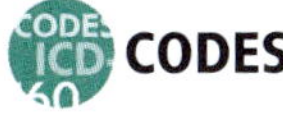

CODES

ICD10

- A52.71 Late syphilitic oculopathy
- A51.0 Primary genital syphilis
- A52.74 Syphilis of liver and other viscera

CLINICAL PEARLS

- Screen all PWH and all individuals with high-risk sexual behaviors for syphilis.
- Penicillin remains the treatment of choice for syphilis.
- Syphilis rates are rising, particularly congenital cases and among women—prevalence remains highest among MSM.

TARSAL TUNNEL SYNDROME

Terrence Tsui, DO

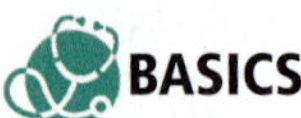

BASICS

DESCRIPTION

Tarsal tunnel syndrome is an entrapment neuropathy of the posterior tibial nerve as it travels within the tarsal tunnel beneath the flexor retinaculum at the medial ankle.

EPIDEMIOLOGY

Unknown incidence and prevalence

ETIOLOGY AND PATHOPHYSIOLOGY

- Contents within the tarsal tunnel: the posterior tibial tendon, the flexor digitorum longus tendon, the posterior tibial artery and veins, the posterior tibial nerve, and the flexor hallucis tendon
- The posterior tibial nerve passes through the tarsal tunnel, which is formed by three osseus structures—sustentaculum tali, medial calcaneus, and medial malleolus—covered by the flexor retinaculum (aka laciniate ligament).
- There are three terminal branches of the posterior tibial nerve:
  - The medial calcaneal nerve provides sensation to the medial heel.
  - The medial and lateral plantar nerves supply sensation to their respective sides of the sole of the foot and motor innervation to the deep muscles of the plantar aspect of the foot.
- Patient presentation can vary because the posterior tibial nerve can branch proximal, within, or distal to the tarsal tunnel.
- Chronic compression of the posterior tibial nerve within the tarsal tunnel can damage the endoneurial microvasculature, leading to edema and demyelination.
- Increased pressure in the tarsal tunnel is caused by a variety of mechanical and biochemical mechanisms. The specific cause for compression is identifiable in only 60–80% of cases.
- Three general categories: trauma, space-occupying lesions, deformity
  - Trauma including displaced fractures, deltoid ligament sprains, or tenosynovitis
  - Varicosities
  - Hindfoot varus or valgus
  - Fibrosis of the perineurium
- Other causes:
  - Osseous prominences; osteophytes
  - Ganglia; lipoma; neurilemmoma
  - Inflammatory synovitis
  - Pigmented villonodular synovitis
  - Tarsal coalition
  - Accessory musculature
- In patients with systemic disease (e.g., diabetes), the "double crush" syndrome refers to the development of a second compression along the same nerve at a site of anatomic narrowing in patients with previous proximal nerve damage.

RISK FACTORS

- Tarsal tunnel syndrome is associated with certain occupations and activities involving repetitive and prolonged weight-bearing on the foot and ankle (walking, running, dancing).
- Other possible risk factors include
  - Varicosities
  - Heel varus or valgus
  - Bifurcation of the posterior tibial nerve into medial and lateral plantar nerves proximal to the tarsal tunnel

COMMONLY ASSOCIATED CONDITIONS

Diabetes, systemic inflammatory arthritis, connective tissue disorders, obesity

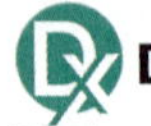

DIAGNOSIS

Tarsal tunnel syndrome is a clinical diagnosis, characterized by pain and paresthesias in a predictable distribution along the medial aspect of the ankle and plantar surface of the foot. There is no single confirmatory test.

HISTORY

- May have history of trauma to the foot prior to the onset of symptoms
- Pain, burning, and numbness/tingling in the medial retro-malleolar region radiating to the medial heel and/or the plantar aspect of foot
- Pain usually worsens during standing or weight-bearing activities.
- Pain radiates proximally up the medial leg (Valleix phenomenon) in 33% of patients with severe compression.
- Some patients have substantial night pain (may be related to venostasis).
- Symptoms improve with rest, wearing loose footwear, and elevation.
- In advanced nerve compression, motor involvement may cause weakness, atrophy, and digital contractures of the intrinsic foot muscles.

PHYSICAL EXAM

- Inspect: foot alignment
  - Examine for excessive foot pronation during standing or walking.
  - Examine for hindfoot varus or valgus deformity while standing.
- Palpate the tarsal tunnel and the course of the tibial nerve for tenderness and swelling.
- Tinel sign: Percussion over the tibial nerve may reproduce paresthesias that radiate distally.
- Valleix sign: Percussion over the tibial nerve may produce paresthesias that radiate proximally.
- Compression test: Applying pressure to the tarsal tunnel for 60 seconds may reproduce symptoms.
- Triple compression test aka dorsiflexion/eversion test: reproduction of symptoms with stretching of the nerve with exaggerated dorsiflexion and eversion of the foot/ankle
- Sensory examination
  - The medial calcaneal nerve usually is spared, but numbness and altered sensation may be present in the distribution of the medial or lateral plantar nerves.
  - Vibratory sensation and two-point discrimination are decreased early in the disease process.
- Motor examination
  - Intrinsic foot muscle weakness (difficult to assess)
  - Weakness of toe plantar flexion may be present (rare).
  - Toe contractures in flexion and atrophy of the abductor hallucis or abductor digiti minimi may be seen late in the disease process.

DIFFERENTIAL DIAGNOSIS

- Peripheral neuropathies (diabetes, alcoholism, HIV, or drug related)
- Inflammatory arthritis (rheumatoid arthritis)
- Morton neuroma
- Metatarsalgia
- Subtalar joint arthritis
- Tibialis posterior tendinopathy
- Plantar fasciitis
- Plantar callosities
- Peripheral vascular disease
- Lumbar radiculopathy
- Proximal injury or compression of the tibial branch of the sciatic nerve

DIAGNOSTIC TESTS & INTERPRETATION

Initial Tests (lab, imaging)

- Routine lab tests help evaluate for other conditions that may mimic tarsal tunnel syndrome, including diabetic neuropathy, rheumatoid arthritis, thyroid dysfunction, or other systemic illnesses.
- Weight-bearing radiographs, followed by CT scan (if necessary) to assess for fracture or structural abnormality
- Consider evaluation of lumbar spine x-ray if double crush (injury to lumbar nerve results in compensatory injury to posterior tibial nerve) is suspected.
- MRI: helps assess the tarsal tunnel for soft tissue masses or other sources of nerve compression before surgery
- Ultrasound (US): gaining importance and with several advantages over MRI; dynamic testing in positions where the nerve may be stretched or compressed; can assess for space-occupying lesions (ganglia, varicose veins, lipomas, etc.) and tenosynovitis

Pregnancy Considerations

- Tarsal tunnel syndrome can occur during pregnancy, typically secondary to local compression caused by fluid retention and volume changes.
- Treatment is supportive care as most cases resolve after pregnancy.

Pediatric Considerations

MRI is recommended for evaluating pediatric tarsal tunnel syndrome to exclude a neoplastic mass.

Diagnostic Procedures/Other

- Electrodiagnostic studies
  - Electromyography (EMG) of the intrinsic muscles of the foot can confirm the diagnosis of tarsal tunnel syndrome. A normal EMG does not exclude the diagnosis (false-negative rate is ~10%).
  - Nerve conduction studies (NCS) may reveal slowed conduction of the tibial nerve.
  - EMG/NCS findings are often normal, but it does not exclude the diagnosis.
  - EMG/NCS may expose a more proximal nerve compression such as a lumbar radiculopathy.
- Diagnostic injection
  - A diagnostic/therapeutic injection with lidocaine +/− corticosteroid into the tarsal tunnel may help confirm the diagnosis if symptoms temporarily improve. This may also help determine if surgical intervention may be beneficial.

TREATMENT

- Conservative management is initially recommended, except for acute onset tarsal tunnel syndrome or in the setting of a known space-occupying lesion.
- The goal of conservative treatment is to decrease compressive forces of the posterior tibial nerve in the tarsal tunnel reducing patient symptoms.

GENERAL MEASURES

- If possible, identify and treat the causative factor of the nerve compression.
- Conservative management starts with activity modification or immobilization, rest, physical therapy, and anti-inflammatory medications.
- Rest and immobilization (ankle brace of cam walker boot) reduces mechanical compression from activity.
- Physical therapy to strengthen the intrinsic and extrinsic muscles of the foot, nerve mobilization exercises, and to restore the medial longitudinal arch of the foot.
- Orthotics, taping, and/or bracing may help alter weight-bearing mechanics decreasing pressure in the tarsal tunnel.

MEDICATION

First Line

- Analgesics and anti-inflammatory medications: acetaminophen, NSAIDs
- Medications that alter neurogenic pain: gabapentin, pregabalin, tricyclic antidepressants

Second Line

Image-guided corticosteroid injection into the tarsal tunnel

ISSUES FOR REFERRAL

Surgery is indicated:

- If nonoperative measures fail following a 6-month trial
- In the setting of acute tarsal tunnel syndrome
- If there are signs of motor involvement/weakness or muscle atrophy
- If a space-occupying lesion is identified

ADDITIONAL THERAPIES

Weight loss in obese patients

SURGERY/OTHER PROCEDURES

- The procedure involves releasing the flexor retinaculum and decompression of the posterior tibial nerve.
- Tarsal tunnel release surgery has mixed results with reports varying between 50% and 91% improvement in symptoms postoperatively.
- The main adverse outcome is an unsuccessful surgical intervention characterized by lack of improvement or recurrence of symptoms.
- Causes for a failed tarsal tunnel release include:
  - Incorrect diagnosis
  - Incomplete release
  - Adhesive neuritis (external scar formation)
  - Intraneural damage (systemic disease, direct nerve injury)
  - Failure to treat all sources of nerve compression in a double crush phenomenon
- Electrodiagnostic studies are rarely helpful in determining the cause of a failed tarsal tunnel release.
- Results with surgical revision are poorer than those for the primary surgical release.

ADDITIONAL READING

- Bojovic M, Dimitrijevic S, Olory BCR, et al. Overview of nerve entrapment syndromes in the foot and ankle. *Int Orthop*. 2025;49(4):853–862.
- Bowley MP, Doughty CT. Entrapment neuropathies of the lower extremity. *Med Clin North Am*. 2019;103(2):371–382.
- Ferkel E, Davis WH, Ellington JK. Entrapment neuropathies of the foot and ankle. *Clin Sports Med*. 2015;34(4):791–801.
- Fortier LM, Leethy KN, Smith M, et al. An update on posterior tarsal tunnel syndrome. *Orthop Rev (Pavia)*. 2022;14(4):35444.
- Madani S, Doughty C. Lower extremity entrapment neuropathies. *Best Pract Res Clin Rheumatol*. 2020;34(3):101565.
- McSweeney SC, Cichero M. Tarsal tunnel syndrome—a narrative literature review. *Foot (Edinb)*. 2015;25(4):244–250.
- Nelson SC. Tarsal tunnel syndrome. *Clin Podiatr Med Surg*. 2021;38(2):131–141.
- Sha I I. Tarsal tunnel syndrome—a comprehensive review. *Iowa Orthop J*. 2024;44(2):32–36.

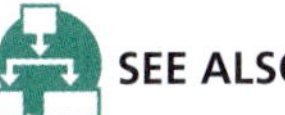

SEE ALSO

Algorithm: Foot Pain

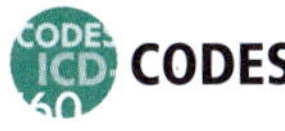

CODES

ICD10

- G57.50 Tarsal tunnel syndrome, unspecified lower limb
- G57.51 Tarsal tunnel syndrome, right lower limb
- G57.52 Tarsal tunnel syndrome, left lower limb

CLINICAL PEARLS

- Tarsal tunnel syndrome typically presents with pain and numbness/tingling/burning/paresthesias of the medial ankle and plantar foot.
- Tarsal tunnel syndrome is a clinical diagnosis which can be supported with imaging and electrodiagnostic studies.
- Conservative management is recommended, except for patients with an acute onset tarsal tunnel syndrome or known space-occupying lesion.

T

TELOGEN EFFLUVIUM

Sahil Mullick, MD, FAAFP • Sreelakshmi Surendran Pillai, MD

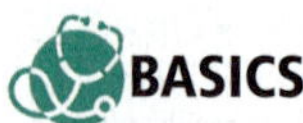

BASICS

Acute, self-limited diffuse hair loss or hair thinning

DESCRIPTION

Telogen effluvium (TE) is a transient condition in which there is a premature conversion of a significant proportion of anagen (growth phase) hairs into telogen (resting phase) hairs resulting in subsequent increased shedding of these resting hair follicles when the follicles re-enter anagen, and the clinical appearance of moderate to severe hair thinning. Normally, each hair follicle cycles independently of others through anagen, catagen (end-of-growth transformation), and telogen, with the large majority of hair follicles in anagen at any given time.

- Five proposed types of TE:
  - Immediate anagen release: a highly common form, lasting 3 to 4 weeks, in which follicles meant to remain in anagen phase enter telogen prematurely due to a signal, including high fever, drug induced, or stress
  - Delayed anagen release: large group of hair follicles that have remained in the anagen phase for an extended period all together enter the telogen phase, resulting in hair loss; common in postpartum
  - Short anagen: a speculative type in which at least 50% of the hair follicles have an idiopathic shortening of the anagen phase; results in a doubling of the follicles in the telogen phase
  - Immediate telogen release: Normal resting club hairs remain within the hair follicle until an unknown signal causes their release, initiating the anagen stage to begin. In this type, the resting club hairs are prematurely released, ending the telogen phase abruptly and causing diffuse shedding.
  - Delayed telogen release: The presence of increased visible light, whether it be a seasonal or environmental change, is thought to end a prolonged telogen phase and initiate the anagen phase; results in diffuse shedding of hair follicles

EPIDEMIOLOGY

Most of the cases of TE are subclinical; therefore, true incidence is not clearly known. No racial predilection of the disease has been recognized, and it affects both males and females with a higher incidence rate in females. However, it should be taken into account that women take hair shedding problem more seriously than men and are likely overrepresented in seeking medical treatment. The association of TE with age is unclear; however, elderly women are known to be more susceptible to acute TE following fever, trauma, hemorrhage, or psychological stress. Studies have reported the incidence of TE in children to be around 2.7%.

Incidence

Second most common cause of alopecia

Prevalence

Unknown

ETIOLOGY AND PATHOPHYSIOLOGY

- The hair cycle consists of two predominant phases: the anagen (growth phase) and the telogen (resting phase), which last ~3 years and 3 months, respectively. In a normal scalp, ~10–15% of hairs are in the telogen phase. Due to the presence of some types of external/internal stress, there may be an increase in the percentage of telogen hairs. As new anagen hairs emerge, these telogen hair follicles are forced out. The preceding event usually occurs 2 to 3 months prior to the appearance of hair loss.
- It is hypothesized that substance P plays a key role in the pathogenesis of TE through various mechanisms. Studies have been conducted on human hair follicles in vitro and mice hair follicles in vivo, which support this theory.
- The role of substance P includes the following:
  - Upregulation of substance P receptor, NK1, at the gene and protein level, leading to premature catagen development and hair growth inhibition
  - Upregulation of nerve growth factor (NGF) and subsequently its hair apoptosis–producing receptor, p75NTR
  - Downregulation of hair growth–promoting receptor, TrkA
  - Upregulation of major histocompatibility class (MHC) I and β_2-microglobulin resulting in loss of hair follicle immune-privilege
  - Increase in tumor necrosis factor-α release by mast cells resulting in hair keratinocyte apoptosis
- Decreased cortisol levels in chronic stress states may also enhance the effects of substance P.

RISK FACTORS

- Infection
- Trauma
- Major surgery
- Thyroid disorder
- Febrile illness
- Malignancy
- Allergic contact dermatitis
- Iron deficiency anemia
- Excess vitamin A
- Protein-calorie restriction
- End-stage liver or renal disease
- Hormonal changes (including pregnancy, delivery, and estrogen-containing medications)
- Chronic stress
- Drug induced (β-blockers, anticonvulsants, antidepressants, anticoagulants, retinoids, ACE-inhibitors, etc.)
- Immunizations

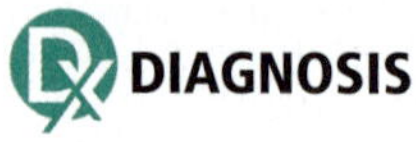

DIAGNOSIS

HISTORY

- Commonly, an inciting event 2 to 6 months previous to noted hair loss
- Fear of becoming bald
- Patients often present with evidence of hair loss with collections of hair or photographs

PHYSICAL EXAM

- Decreased density of hair on the scalp, most commonly involving the crown and temples
- In rare cases of chronic TE, there is a hair loss at the eyebrows and pubic region.
- May have diffuse shedding of hair when fingers are run through the scalp
- Shed hairs are telogen hairs, which have a small bulb of unpigmented or pigmented keratin on the root end (so-called "club" hairs).
- May affect nail growth, resulting in the appearance of Beau lines, which are transverse grooves on the nails of the hands and feet

DIFFERENTIAL DIAGNOSIS

- Hypothyroidism
- Hyperthyroidism
- Alopecia areata (diffuse pattern)
- Androgenetic alopecia
- Drug-induced alopecia
- Systemic lupus erythematosus
- Secondary syphilis
- Trichotillomania

DIAGNOSTIC TESTS & INTERPRETATION

Most often, TE is a clinical diagnosis based on typical history and exclusion of other scalp pathology and medical conditions. Blood work may be collected primarily to rule out other possible causes of hair loss. Nutritional deficiencies in iron and zinc have been associated with TE.

Initial Tests (lab, imaging)

If indicated:

- CBC, ferritin
- TSH
- Creatinine
- Consider iron profile and zinc.
- Consider hepatic enzymes.
- Consider RPR/VDRL.

Diagnostic Procedures/Other

- Hair pull test: unreliable; performed by gently pulling 25 to 30 hairs from various sites on a patient's scalp; each pull should elicit <5 normal club hairs; increased quantity may indicate possibility of TE.
- Hair clip test: performed by cutting 25 to 30 hairs from the patient's scalp and examining them under a microscope; a negative test (not indicative of TE) will demonstrate <10% of hair shafts of small diameter. A positive test will demonstrate >10% of hair shafts of small diameter.
- Trichogram: ~50 hairs are plucked using a hemostat from the patient's scalp, and the number of telogen and anagen hairs present are counted. In TE, there will be >10% of hairs in the telogen phase.
- Scalp biopsy: rarely needed; it is recommended that several 4-mm punch biopsies be obtained, all horizontally embedded to determine an accurate anagen-to-telogen ratio. Histologically, catagen-to-telogen hairs have numerous apoptotic cells in the outer sheath epithelium. >12–15% of hair follicles in telogen phase is consistent with TE.

TREATMENT

TE is a benign, self-limited process. Identify and correct the underlying cause. The patient should be reassured that hair growth will resume in 3 to 6 months, with full growth to return in 12 to 18 months (1). No treatment is required; however, when a nutritional deficiency is identified, there may be some benefit in taking a specific supplement.

MEDICATION

- Minoxidil stimulates hair regrowth via arteriolar smooth muscle vasodilation; not effective in TE
- Oral zinc therapy: new medication that may have benefits for patients with TE through various mechanisms all essential to hair growth, including the following (2)[C]:
  - Cofactor for enzymes needed in nucleic acid and protein synthesis and cell division
  - Inhibition of the catagen phase by blocking certain enzymes involved in hair apoptosis
  - Involved in hair growth regulation via hedgehog signaling

COMPLEMENTARY & ALTERNATIVE MEDICINE

- Combination oral vitamin therapy: A formulation of zinc; biotin; iron; vitamins A, C, E, and B complex; folic acid; magnesium; and amino acids of keratin and collagen was associated with statistically significant improvement compared to a formulation of calcium pantothenate, cystine, thiamine nitrate, medicinal yeast, keratin, and aminobenzoic acid in the following measures after 180 days of use: hair loss, hair volume, scalp hair density, hair shine, and hair strength (3)[C].
- An extract from millet mixed with polar lipids has been found to enhance the cell proliferation in the hair bulb, reduce hair density in the telogen phase, improve scalp dryness, and improve hair brightness.

ONGOING CARE

DIET

If a measurable deficiency has been found, it should be corrected. A balanced diet and stable body weight are important. Although the use of polyphenolic compounds such as those in green tea has been reported to improve hair loss in mice, no such controlled studies are available for humans.

REFERENCES

1. Malkud S. Telogen effluvium: a review. *J Clin Diagn Res*. 2015;9(9):WE01–WE03.
2. Karashima T, Tsuruta D, Hamada T, et al. Oral zinc therapy for zinc deficiency-related telogen effluvium. *Dermatol Ther*. 2012;25(2):210–213.
3. Sant'Anna Addor FA, Donato LC, Melo CSA. Comparative evaluation between two nutritional supplements in the improvement of telogen effluvium. *Clin Cosmet Investig Dermatol*. 2018;11:431–436.

ADDITIONAL READING

Mounsey AL, Reed SW. Diagnosing and treating hair loss. *Am Fam Physician*. 2009;80(4):356–362.

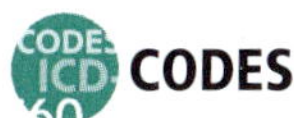

CODES

ICD10

L65.0 Telogen effluvium

CLINICAL PEARLS

- TE is a self-limited form of nonscarring alopecia, most often acute.
- TE is due to a premature conversion of a significant proportion of anagen (growth phase) hairs into telogen (resting phase) hairs, resulting in increased shedding of these resting hair follicles and the clinical appearance of moderate to severe hair thinning and loss when growth resumes.
- There are many potential causes of TE, both emotional and physiologic. Often, it is hard to determine the etiology, but eliminating the stressor is the key to resolving TE and stimulating new hair growth.
- No treatment is needed. Patient should be reassured that complete hair regrowth will occur in 12 to 18 months.

TEMPOROMANDIBULAR JOINT DISORDER (TMD)

Zakary S. Newberry, MD • Roland W. Newman II, DO • Caitlyn Haines, MD

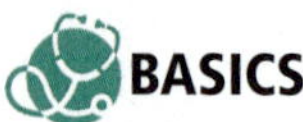

BASICS

DESCRIPTION

- Syndrome characterized by:
  - Pain and tenderness involving the muscles of mastication and surrounding tissues
  - Sound, pain, stiffness, or grating in the temporomandibular joint (TMJ) with movement
  - Limitation of mandibular movement with possible locking or dislocation
  - Recent research suggests that TMD is a complex disorder with multiple causes consistent with a biopsychosocial model of illness.
- System(s) affected: musculoskeletal
- Synonym(s): TMJ syndrome; TMJ dysfunction; myofascial pain–dysfunction syndrome; bruxism; orofacial pain

EPIDEMIOLOGY

Incidence

- Annual first-onset incidence is 3.9%.
- Age of onset most commonly between 18 and 44 years

Prevalence

- May be as high as 31% in adults and 11% in children
- 1.5 times higher prevalence in females compared with males
- Up to 70% of people may show signs of TMD, but only 5–12% of people report symptoms and seek treatment.

ETIOLOGY AND PATHOPHYSIOLOGY

- Pathophysiology is multifactorial and includes anatomic, behavioral, emotional, and cognitive origins, akin to other chronic pain disorders.
- The American Academy of Orofacial Pain categorizes TMD according to three anatomic origins of pain, including the following:
  - Muscular disorders involving the muscles of mastication
    - Bruxism
    - Masticatory muscle spasm
    - Myositis
    - Myofibrosis
    - Poorly fitting oral devices (dentures, splints)
    - Contracture
    - Neoplasia
  - Articular disorders of the joint
    - Congenital disorders
    - Inflammatory disorders (synovitis, arthritides, capsulitis, ankyloses)
    - Avascular necrosis
    - TMJ disk derangement, osteoarthritis
    - Hyper- or hypomobile TMJ
    - TMJ trauma (condylar fractures, dislocation)
  - Cranial bone disorders including the mandible
    - Congenital and developmental disorders
    - Acquired disorders (fracture, neoplasm)

Genetics

Gene polymorphisms, such as catechol O-methyltransferase (COMT), are thought to be associated with predisposition to developing TMD, largely due to changes in pain responsiveness.

RISK FACTORS

- Trauma to the face, jaw, and neck
- Rheumatologic and degenerative conditions involving the TMJ
- Psychosocial stress and poor adaptive capabilities
- Repetitive microtrauma from dental malocclusion, including inappropriate dental treatment
- Inconsistent association with bruxism and jaw/teeth clenching
- Hormonal contraceptive use
- Repetitive jaw motions and positions may be associated

GENERAL PREVENTION

- Elimination of tension-causing oral habits
- Stress reduction
- Reduction in overall muscle tension

COMMONLY ASSOCIATED CONDITIONS

Craniomandibular disorders, somatization disorder, somatoform pain disorder, fibromyalgia, juvenile idiopathic arthritis, tension headache, irritable bowel syndrome, sleep disturbance, tobacco use, other chronic pain syndromes

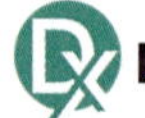

DIAGNOSIS

TMD is a clinical diagnosis, and localized pain is the unifying feature.

HISTORY

- Most common presenting symptoms include:
  - Facial pain (96%)
  - Ear discomfort (82%)
  - Headache (79%)
  - Jaw discomfort or dysfunction (75%)
- Clicking, grinding, popping of TMJ may be present, although this is present in up to 50% of asymptomatic patients.

PHYSICAL EXAM

- Physical examination may reveal:
  - Abnormal mandibular movement (jaw deviation, teeth misalignment)
  - Decreased TMJ range of motion (ROM) (interincisal distance <25 mm; normal 35 to 55 mm)
  - Tenderness over the TMJ or muscles of mastication
  - Crepitus to palpation of TMJ
  - Pain with dynamic loading of TMJ
  - Tooth wear on intraoral examination
  - Postural asymmetry
- Evaluation of oral cavity, inner ear, and neck can exclude other causes of facial pain

DIFFERENTIAL DIAGNOSIS

- Condylar fracture/dislocation
- Trigeminal, glossopharyngeal, or post-herpetic neuralgia
- Dental or periodontal conditions
- Neoplasm of the jaw, orofacial muscles, or salivary glands
- Acute, nondental infection: parotitis, sialadenitis, otitis, mastoiditis
- Jaw claudication: giant cell arteritis
- Migraine, cluster, or tension-type headache
- Ramsay Hunt syndrome (zoster auricular syndrome)

DIAGNOSTIC TESTS & INTERPRETATION

Blood work only useful to rule out other conditions and is often not required for diagnosis

Initial Tests (lab, imaging)

- There is poor correlation between pain severity and pathologic changes seen in joint or muscle tissues.
- Consider the following for traumatic, infectious, severe, or treatment-resistant cases, with MR or CT more useful as part of surgical workup:
  - Panoramic dental radiographs
  - CT scan allows fine detail of bony structures, preferred for trauma
  - US: Effusion and findings correlate with MRI and subjective pain.
  - MRI: noninvasive study for disc position; more sensitive than US; can help determine need for surgical management

Diagnostic Procedures/Other

- Local anesthetic nerve block can differentiate orofacial pain of articular versus muscular origin.
- Arthroscopy can be diagnostic for cartilage and bony pathology.

Test Interpretation

Positive findings include:

- Condylar head displacement
- Anterior disc displacement
- Posterior capsulitis
- Loosening of disc and capsular attachments
- Chondroid metaplasia of disc leading to disc perforation and degeneration

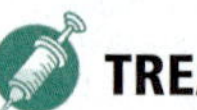

TREATMENT

Signs and symptoms will abate without intervention in most patients, with 50% reporting improvement at 1 year and 85% by 3 years. With conservative therapy, symptoms resolve in 75% of cases within 3 months.

- Conservative therapy includes:
  - Patient education and setting expectations, as most patients will improve with limited intervention

- Psychosocial interventions, including cognitive-behavioral therapy with or without biofeedback (1)[A]
- Behavior modification to eliminate oral habits including heavy chewing of food and nonfood items as well as potential strain from playing musical instruments that stress or strain the jaw (wind, brass, or string) (1)[A]
- Therapeutic exercises and formal physical therapy, especially if displacement is present.

- The American Dental Association recommends a "less is often best" stepwise approach and offers the following stepwise progression for therapy:
  - Eating softer foods
  - Avoiding chewing gum and nail-biting
  - Modifying pain with heat or ice
  - Relaxation techniques including meditation and biofeedback
  - Exercises to strengthen jaw muscles
  - Medications
  - Night guards and orthotics
- Occlusal adjustment cannot be recommended for the management or prevention of TMD because there is an absence of evidence from RCTs that occlusal adjustment treats or prevents TMD [A](2).
- Insufficient evidence exists either for or against the use of stabilization splint therapy for the treatment of TMD

MEDICATION

First Line

- NSAIDs:
  - Naproxen: 500 mg BID has stronger evidence than other NSAIDs
  - Ibuprofen, if osteoarthritis is suspected
  - Topical diclofenac (avoid contact with eyes or mucous membranes) if oral medication is contraindicated
- Gabapentin: Titrate up to 1,800 mg/day divided.
- Acetaminophen

Second Line

- Cyclobenzaprine 10 mg QHS is more effective than placebo for pain reduction (3)[B].
- Tricyclic antidepressants: nortriptyline or amitriptyline, at low (10 to 35 mg) doses
- Acupuncture and dry needling can reduce pain (2)
- Opiates should be reserved for perioperative or severe cases (4)[B].
- DMARDs may benefit inflammatory arthropathies such as rheumatoid or psoriatic arthritis.
- Ineffective medications (4)[B]
  - The following medications when compared with placebo in RCTs were shown to be ineffective in improving pain and should not be used for the treatment of TMD:
    - Benzodiazepines
    - Topical capsaicin
    - Celecoxib

ISSUES FOR REFERRAL

Referral to maxillofacial surgery should be considered in cases of severe pain, ineffective conservative therapy, or history of trauma.

ADDITIONAL THERAPIES

Joint and muscle injections:

- A systematic review of arthrocentesis with injection of hyaluronic acid and platelet rich plasma showed no clinical improvement (5).
- Steroids given >3 times annually may accelerate degenerative changes.
- Injections into inferior space or double spaces have better effect than superior space injections alone.
- A systematic review evaluating botulinum toxin type A injections revealed mixed results (2)
- For advanced structural abnormalities, referral for discectomy, arthroplasty, or joint replacement can be considered; however, strong evidence is lacking for lavage or surgical treatments over conservative management (2).

COMPLEMENTARY & ALTERNATIVE MEDICINE

- Glucosamine may be effective if pain is secondary to osteoarthritis of the TMJ (4)[B].
- Multiple electronic diagnostic and treatment modalities are currently marketed to patients; however, the scientific literature does not support the use of electronic diagnostic and treatment devices for TMD at this time.

ONGOING CARE

FOLLOW-UP RECOMMENDATIONS

- Relax jaw by disengaging teeth
- Avoid wide, uncontrolled opening, such as yawning
- Trial soft diets
- Stress management and behavior modification counseling may be helpful.
- Be aware of any teeth-clenching or grinding habits

Patient Monitoring

- Ongoing assessment of clinical response to conservative therapies is necessary.
- Surgical intervention may be considered after 3 to 6 months of treatment in patients with persistent functional limitations and structural or intraarticular disorders.

DIET

Soft diet to reduce chewing

PROGNOSIS

- With conservative therapy, symptoms resolve in 75% of cases within 3 months
- 90% of patients respond to noninvasive therapy.
- Patients benefit most from a comprehensive treatment approach including (3):
  - Restoration of normal muscle function
  - Pain control
  - Stress management
  - Behavior modification

COMPLICATIONS

- Secondary degenerative joint disease
- Chronic TMJ dislocation
- Loss of joint ROM
- Depression and significant reduction in quality of life
- Chronic pain syndromes
- Secondary headache disorder

REFERENCES

1. Aggarwal VR, Lovell K, Peters S, et al. Psychosocial interventions for the management of chronic orofacial pain. *Cochrane Database Syst Rev*. 2011;(11):CD008456.
2. Gil-Martínez A, Paris-Alemany A, López-de-Uralde-Villanueva I, et al. Management of pain in patients with temporomandibular disorder (TMD): challenges and solutions. *J Pain Res*. 2018;11:571–587.
3. Gauer RL, Semidey MJ. Diagnosis and treatment of temporomandibular disorders. *Am Fam Physician*. 2015;91(6):378–386.
4. Mujakperuo HR, Watson M, Morrison R, et al. Pharmacological interventions for pain in patients with temporomandibular disorders. *Cochrane Database Syst Rev*. 2010;(10):CD004715.
5. Derwich M, Mitus-Kenig M, Pawlowska E. Mechanisms of action and efficacy of hyaluronic acid, corticosteroids and platelet-rich plasma in the treatment of temporomandibular joint osteoarthritis—a systematic review. *Int J Mol Sci*. 2021;22(14):7405.

SEE ALSO

Headache, Tension

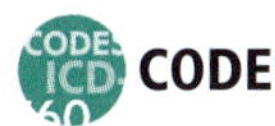

CODES

ICD10

- M26.60 Temporomandibular joint disorder, unspecified
- M26.62 Arthralgia of temporomandibular joint
- M26.63 Articular disc disorder of temporomandibular joint

CLINICAL PEARLS

- TMD refers to a number of potential underlying joint and muscle conditions involving the jaw. Characteristics of all conditions are pain and functional limitation.
- TMD is a clinical diagnosis; imaging and labs are often of limited utility.
- Cognitive-behavioral therapy reduces pain, depression, and limitation of function.
- Exercises may improve function and pain.
- Evidence is lacking to support occlusion correction or splinting.
- Naproxen, gabapentin, topical methyl salicylate, glucosamine, amitriptyline, acupuncture, and botulinum toxin injections have some evidence of efficacy.

TESTICULAR TORSION

Scott Geiger, MD

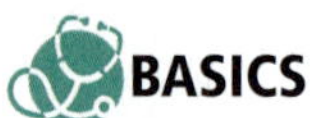

BASICS

DESCRIPTION

- Twisting of testis and spermatic cord, resulting in acute ischemia and loss of testis if unrecognized:
  - Intravaginal torsion: occurs within tunica vaginalis, only involves testis and spermatic cord; most commonly seen in practice
  - Extravaginal torsion: involves twisting of testis, cord, and processus vaginalis as a unit; typically seen in neonates
- System(s) affected: reproductive

Geriatric Considerations

Rare in this age group

Pediatric Considerations

Peak incidence at age 14 years

EPIDEMIOLOGY

Incidence

- ~1/4,000 males before age 25 years
- Predominant age:
  - Occurs from newborn period to 7th decade
  - 65% of cases occur in 2nd decade, with peak at age 14 years; rare beyond the age of 30 years.
  - Second peak in neonates (in utero torsion usually occurs around week 32 of gestation)

ETIOLOGY AND PATHOPHYSIOLOGY

- Initial incomplete twisting of spermatic cord causes venous obstruction, edema of testis, leading to congestion and then ischemia.
- Complete twisting of the spermatic cord causes arterial occlusion, in addition to the above, leading to rapid ischemia.
- Congenital bell clapper deformity, which is bilateral in at least 2/5th of cases: A high mesorchium (the posterior-lateral attachment of the testis to the tunica vaginalis) allows more room for the testis to twist within the tunica vaginalis and is associated intravaginal testicular torsion (TT).
- No clear anatomic defect is associated with extravaginal TT:
  - In neonates, the tunica vaginalis is not yet well attached to scrotal wall, allowing torsion of entire testis including tunica vaginalis.
- Usually spontaneous and idiopathic
- 20% of patients have a history of trauma.
- 1/3 have had prior episodic testicular pain.
- Contraction of cremaster muscle or dartos may play a role and is stimulated by trauma, exercise, cold, and sexual stimulation.
- Increased incidence may be due to increasing weight and size of testis during pubertal development.
- Possible alterations in testosterone levels during nocturnal sex response cycle; possible elevated testosterone levels in neonates
- Testis must have inadequate, incomplete, or absent fixation within scrotum.
- Torsion may occur in either clockwise or counterclockwise direction.

Genetics

- Unknown
- Familial TT, although previously rarely reported, may involve as many as 10% of patients.

RISK FACTORS

- May be more common in colder months
- Paraplegia
- Previous contralateral TT

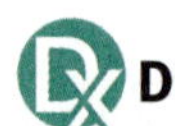

DIAGNOSIS

TT is a clinical diagnosis. A good history and physicals are the most important and helpful tools in evaluating and managing TT. If history and physical are highly suggestive of TT, imaging studies may be skipped and immediate urologic consult should be done, as time is of the utmost essence (1).

HISTORY

- Acute onset of unrelenting pain, often during period of inactivity
- Onset of pain usually sudden but may start gradually with subsequent increase in severity
- Nausea and vomiting are common:
  - Presence may increase the likelihood of TT versus other differential diagnoses.
- Prior history of multiple episodes of testicular pain with spontaneous resolution in an episodic crescendo pattern may indicate intermittent TT.

PHYSICAL EXAM

- Scrotum is enlarged, red, edematous, and painful unilaterally.
- Testicle is swollen and exquisitely tender.
- "Bell clapper" deformity: an asymmetrically high-riding testis oriented transversely instead of longitudinally occurring due to shortening spermatic cord from the torsion
- Testis may be high in scrotum with a transverse lie; this is called Brunzel sign.
- Prehn sign: when elevation of the testis does not decrease pain in the affected testicle
- Absent cremasteric reflex. Elicit cremasteric reflex by lightly stroking the inner thigh of the suspected side.

DIFFERENTIAL DIAGNOSIS

- Torsion appendix testis (this may account for 35–67% of acute scrotal pain cases in children)
- Epididymitis (8–18% of acute scrotal pain cases)
- Orchitis
- Incarcerated or strangulated inguinal hernia
- Acute hydrocele
- Traumatic hematoma
- Testicle rupture
- Idiopathic scrotal edema
- Acute varicocele
- Epididymal hypertension (venous congestion of testicle or prostate due to sexual arousal that does not end in orgasm)
- Testis tumor
- Henoch-Schönlein purpura
- Scrotal abscess
- Leukemic infiltrate

DIAGNOSTIC TESTS & INTERPRETATION

- Doppler ultrasound (US) may confirm testicular swelling but is diagnostic by demonstrating a lack of blood flow to the testicle; PPV of 89.4%; a normal testicular US does not rule out TT.
- In boys with intermittent, recurrent TT, both Doppler US and radionuclide scintigraphy findings will be normal.
- The Testicular Workup for Ischemia and Suspected Torsion (TWIST) was developed in 2013, which consists of a 7-point risk assessment tool based on:
  - Testicular swelling (2 points)
  - Hard testis (2 points)
  - High-riding testis (1 point)
  - Absence of cremasteric reflex (1 point)
  - Nausea/vomiting (1 point)
- Multiple scoring systems exist; however, a commonly used system created by Barbosa et al. stratifies 0 to 2 as low risk (rule out torsion), 3 to 4 as intermediate risk (proceed with US), and 5 to 7 as high risk (proceed with surgical intervention). This is a beneficial diagnostic tool as it is simple, fast, and proves useful in clinical settings where US access is limited (2).

Initial Tests (lab, imaging)

Urinalysis to rule out any infection such as epididymitis, orchitis, UTI

Diagnostic Procedures/Other

- Doppler US flow detection demonstrates absent or reduced blood flow with torsion and increased flow with inflammatory process (reliable only in first 12 hours).
- Radionuclide testicular scintigraphy with technetium-99m pertechnetate demonstrates absent/decreased vascularity in torsion and increased vascularity with inflammatory processes (including torsion of appendix testes).

Test Interpretation

- Venous thrombosis
- Tissue edema and necrosis
- Arterial thrombosis
- Decreased Doppler flow also seen in hydrocele, abscess, hematoma, or scrotal hernia
- Sensitivity of radionuclide testicular scintigraphy is decreased relative to ultrasonography because hyperemia in the torsed testicle can mimic flow.

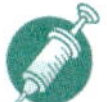

TREATMENT

- Manual reduction/detorsion: best performed by an experienced physician, especially if a surgeon is not available; may be successful, facilitated by lidocaine 1% (plain) injection at level of external ring:
  - Performed by rotating the affected testicle in a medial-to-lateral direction described as the "open book"; 1/3 of torsion, however, is medial to lateral on presentation.
  - If successful will usually provide immediate relief; may need to rotate anywhere from 180 to 360 degrees, resulting in possible partial untwisting (3)
  - Difficult to determine success of manual reduction, especially after giving local anesthesia
  - Manual reduction might require sedation, and the entire process may delay definitive treatment.
  - Even if successful, must always be followed by surgical exploration, urgently but not emergently
- Surgical exploration via scrotal approach with detorsion, evaluation of testicular viability, orchidopexy of viable testicle, orchiectomy of nonviable testicle
- In boys with a history of intermittent episodes of testicular pain, scrotal exploration is warranted with testicular fixation if abnormal testicular attachments are confirmed.

GENERAL MEASURES

Early exam is crucial because necrosis of the testicle can occur after 6 to 8 hours.

MEDICATION

Studies are ongoing on medications used to prevent reperfusion injury and increase blood flow.

ISSUES FOR REFERRAL

All patients diagnosed with TT should receive urgent/emergent referral to urology.

SURGERY/OTHER PROCEDURES

Operative testicular fixation of the torsed testicle after detorsion and confirmation of viability:

- At least 3- or 4-point fixation with nonabsorbable sutures between the tunica albuginea and the tunica vaginalis
- Excision of window of tunica albuginea with suture to dartos fascia
- Any testis that is not clearly viable should be removed.
- Testes of questionable viability that are preserved and fixated invariably atrophy.
- Bilateral testicular fixation is recommended by many surgeons.
- Contralateral testicle frequently has similar abnormal fixation and should be explored.

COMPLEMENTARY & ALTERNATIVE MEDICINE

No complementary or alternative medicine recommended. Patients should be educated on the acuity of illness, and the need for immediate intervention.

ADMISSION, INPATIENT, AND NURSING CONSIDERATIONS

Patients can usually be discharged from recovery.

ONGOING CARE

FOLLOW-UP RECOMMENDATIONS

Patient Monitoring

- Postoperative visit at 1 to 2 weeks
- Yearly visits until puberty may be needed to evaluate for atrophy.
- Counsel high-risk patients during primary care visits on emergency room return precautions.

DIET

Regular diet

PATIENT EDUCATION

Possibility of testicular atrophy in salvaged testis with depressed sperm counts; importantly, fertility rates in patients with one testicle remain excellent.

PROGNOSIS

- Testicular salvage:
  - Salvage is related directly to duration of torsion (85–97% if within 6 hours, 20% after 12 hours <10% if >24 hours).
  - The degree of torsion is related to testicular salvage:
    - The median degree of torsion is <360 in patients who are explored and orchidopexy performed.
- 80–94% may have depressed spermatogenesis related to duration of ischemic injury (possibly related to autoimmune-mediated injury).
- Up to 45% of patients undergoing orchidopexy for TT will develop atrophy of testicle.
- Preoperative manual detorsion is associated with improved surgical salvage in patients with TT.

COMPLICATIONS

- Possible testicular atrophy
- Abnormal spermatogenesis
- Infertility:
  - Fertility rates with one testicle remain excellent.
  - Nearly 36% of patients who experience torsion have sperm counts <20 million/mL.

REFERENCES

1. Sharp VJ, Kieran K, Arlen AM. Testicular torsion: diagnosis, evaluation, and management. *Am Fam Physician*. 2013;88(12):835–840.
2. Qin KR, Qu LG. Diagnosing with a TWIST: systematic review and meta-analysis of a testicular torsion risk score. *J Urol*. 2022;208(1):62–70.
3. Bowlin PR, Gatti JM, Murphy JP. Pediatric testicular torsion. *Surg Clin North Am*. 2017;97(1):161–172.

ADDITIONAL READING

Jacobsen FM, Rudlang TM, Fode M, et al. The impact of testicular torsion on testicular function. *World J Mens Health*. 2020;38(3):298–307.

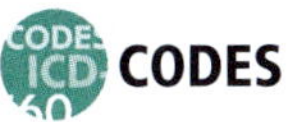

CODES

ICD10

- N44.03 Torsion of appendix testis
- N44.0 Torsion of testis
- N44.02 Intravaginal torsion of spermatic cord

CLINICAL PEARLS

- The diagnosis of TT is usually made by physical exam. Patients with suspected torsion should be taken to the OR without delay. If the diagnosis is in question, a testicular Doppler US may be done to evaluate blood flow. If US is unavailable, the TWIST score can be utilized to help with clinical decision-making in a timely fashion.
- Although testicular necrosis may be present within 6 to 8 hours of torsion, this is highly variable.
- Preoperative manual detorsion is warranted and is associated with improved surgical salvage in patients with TT
- Infertility can be a problem even if the testicle is viable. Autoimmune anti-sperm antibodies may be produced, and they may affect subsequent fertility.

TESTOSTERONE DEFICIENCY

Jennifer M. Corliss, MD, FAAFP • Rachel S. Rodriguez, MD, FAAFP

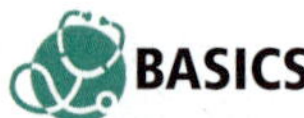

BASICS

DESCRIPTION

- Testosterone (T) is the principle circulating androgen in males. Testosterone deficiency (TD) is characterized by low levels of T in addition to signs and symptoms.
- No universally accepted threshold of T concentration to distinguish eugonadal from hypogonadal men, but the U.S. Food and Drug Administration (FDA) definition is T <300 ng/dL.
- T levels correlate with overall health and may be associated with sexual dysfunction.
- Synonym(s): hypogonadism; hypoandrogenism; androgen deficiency; low T

EPIDEMIOLOGY

Prevalence

- Estimates of TD vary; typically 20% of men >60 years, 30% >70 years, and 50% >80 years of age
- Symptomatic TD in United States ages 40 to 69 years is 6–12.3%
- Affects 2.4 million men in United States ages 40 to 69 years

ETIOLOGY AND PATHOPHYSIOLOGY

Hypothalamus produces gonadotropin-releasing hormone (GnRH), which stimulates pituitary to produce follicle-stimulating hormone (FSH) and luteinizing hormone (LH). LH stimulates Leydig cells to produce T. Leydig cells are responsible for 90% of the body's T.

- Primary hypogonadism: Testes produce insufficient amount of T; FSH/LH levels are elevated.
- Secondary hypogonadism: low T from inadequate production of LH
- Congenital syndromes: cryptorchidism, Klinefelter, hypogonadotropic hypogonadism (Kallmann)
- Acquired: cancer, trauma, orchiectomy, steroids
- Infectious: mumps (orchitis), HIV, tuberculosis
- Systemic: Cushing, hemochromatosis, autoimmune, severe illness (e.g., renal and liver disease), metabolic syndrome, obesity, obstructive sleep apnea
- Medications and drugs: LHRH agonists, corticosteroids, ethanol, marijuana, opioids, SSRIs
- Elevated prolactin: prolactinoma, dopamine antagonists (neuroleptics and metoclopramide)

Genetics

- Klinefelter syndrome: XXY karyotype
- Kallmann syndrome: abnormal GnRH secretion

RISK FACTORS

- Obesity, diabetes, COPD, depression, thyroid disorders, malnutrition, alcohol, stress
- Chronic infections, inflammatory states, chronic steroid use, narcotic use
- Undescended testicles, varicocele
- Testicular trauma, cancer, testicular radiation, chemotherapy, disorders of the pituitary and/or hypothalamus

GENERAL PREVENTION

General health maintenance and treatment of obesity

COMMONLY ASSOCIATED CONDITIONS

- Infertility, erectile dysfunction, low libido
- Osteopenia/osteoporosis
- Diabetes, insulin resistance, metabolic syndrome
- Depressed mood, poor concentration, irritability

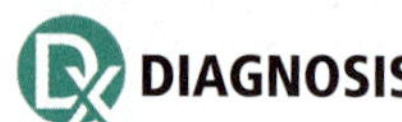

DIAGNOSIS

HISTORY

- Congenital and developmental abnormalities
- Infertility, loss of libido, erectile dysfunction
- Depression, fatigue, difficulty with concentration
- Decreased muscle strength, energy level
- Increase in body fat, development of diabetes
- Bone fractures from relatively minor trauma
- Testicular trauma, infection, radio- or chemotherapy
- Decrease in testicle size or consistency
- Headaches or vision changes
- Medications, narcotic use

PHYSICAL EXAM

- Infancy: ambiguous genitalia
- Puberty
  - Impaired growth of penis, testicles
  - Lack of secondary male characteristics
  - Gynecomastia, eunuchoid habitus
- Adulthood
  - Decreased muscular development, visceral fat distribution
  - Presence of gynecomastia
  - Small and/or soft testicles
  - Digital rectal exam, and International Prostate Symptom Score (IPSS)

DIFFERENTIAL DIAGNOSIS

- Delayed puberty
- Obesity, depression, chronic illness, hypothyroidism
- Normal aging
- Prior anabolic steroid abuse

DIAGNOSTIC TESTS & INTERPRETATION

- T levels vary widely and are subject to diurnal, seasonal, and age-related variations.
- Measurement should be obtained between 6 and 10 AM. Confirmation with a second measurement is necessary. Free T with total T may be preferred in some cases. Measurements should not be obtained during acute illness. T circulates in blood primarily bound to SHBG or albumin. Only 2–3% of total T is found free. Free and albumin-bound T is considered bioavailable. Laboratory findings must be interpreted in the appropriate clinical setting.

Initial Tests (lab, imaging)

Morning T level is initial test. If initial morning T is low, and confirmed on repeat test, further evaluation is appropriate.

- Evaluation should include LH and FSH to differentiate between primary versus secondary hypogonadism.
- Consider estradiol and prolactin, especially if LH is low, or if breast symptoms and gynecomastia.
- If primary hypogonadism of unknown origin and physical exam reveals severe testis atrophy, consider obtaining karyotype (Klinefelter 1:500 to 1,000 risk).
- If secondary hypogonadism, consider prolactin, iron saturation, pituitary function testing, and/or MRI.

Follow-Up Tests & Special Considerations

- Prior to initiating therapy:
  - Hemoglobin and hematocrit (to determine risk of polycythemia)
  - Prostate-specific antigen (PSA) in men >40 years of age (to exclude prostate cancer diagnosis)
  - Estradiol in men with breast symptoms or gynecomastia
- Dual energy x-ray absorptiometry (DEXA) in men with severe TD or fracture from minimal trauma
- Pituitary MRI: if there is elevation of prolactin more than twice the upper limit of normal or LH/FSH below normal range

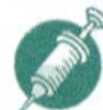

TREATMENT

Testosterone therapy (TT) recommended for symptomatic men (e.g., low libido and/or erectile dysfunction, low energy level, constitutional symptoms) with low T levels ≤300 ng/dL obtained in the morning; not recommended for older men with low T levels in absence of signs or symptoms (1)[C]

- Recent data suggests T replacement can significantly increase hemoglobin levels in men with low T and unexplained anemia.
- Recent data suggests men with low bone mineral density and low T can increase bone density and bone strength with T replacement.
- In older men with low T and age-associated memory impairment, T replacement was not found to be beneficial.

GENERAL MEASURES

- Future fertility: Impact of exogenous T should be discussed regarding its association with infertility.
- Prostate cancer: Safety of TT is uncertain and a contraindication (2)[B].
  - 2018 American Urological Association (AUA) guidelines: Patients with TD and history of prostate cancer should be informed that there is inadequate evidence to quantify the risk–benefit ratio of TT (1)[B].
  - 2018 endocrine guidelines: Patients with organ-confined prostate cancer who have undergone radical prostatectomy and disease free for ≥2 years with undetectable PSA may be considered for TT on an individualized basis.
  - TT should be avoided in men with PSA >4 or PSA >3 and increased risk of prostate cancer (African Americans, men with first-degree relative with prostate cancer).

- TT should not be used in men with metastatic prostate cancer, breast cancer, hematocrit >54%, untreated obstructive sleep apnea, uncontrolled congestive heart failure (CHF), severe lower urinary tract symptoms with an IPSS >19 (1).
- TT is not recommended for mood or strength improvement in otherwise healthy men or asymptomatic men with low T (1).
- Cardiovascular disease (CVD) risk
  - TD is also a risk factor for CVD (1).
  - Even in men with CVD or a high risk of developing CVD, TT was not found to cause an increased risk of cardiac events (3).
- Consider short-term TT as an adjunctive in men with HIV and low T to promote weight maintenance and gains in lean body mass and strength.

MEDICATION

ALERT

Avoid TT gel contact with women (especially pregnant women) or children

- Oral therapy with methyltestosterone is not recommended due to association with significant hepatotoxicity.
  - Oral testosterone undecanoate (Jatenzo) was FDA approved in March 2019.
- FDA cautions that TT is approved for men with confirmed low T by blood work with signs and symptoms, not solely due to aging.
- FDA warning for blood pressure elevation with TT.
- TT should NOT be started for a period of 3 to 6 months in patients with acute cardiovascular event.
- Topical gels/solutions: most common
  - Mimics normal daily circadian rhythm
  - Good absorption, 15–20% are nonresponders
- Transdermal patch (Androderm)
  - Achieves less robust levels
  - High incidence of skin irritation
- Testosterone enanthate (Xyosted) SC weekly injection
  - Boxed warning for increased blood pressure
- Testosterone cypionate (IM every 1 to 3 weeks)
  - Starting dose: 100 mg/week or 200 mg/2 weeks
- Testosterone undecanoate (IM every 8 to 12 weeks)
  - Small risk of oil embolism, needs observation in office for 30 minutes postinjection
- Testosterone pellets (Testopel)
  - Minor office procedure
  - Long-acting formulation, 3 to 4 months
  - 1–2% risk of infection or pellet extrusion
- Buccal application (Methyltestosterone) BID dosing
  - Adheres to gum line, can cause irritation
- Nasal gel (Natesto) TID dosing
  - Nasal irritation
  - May be protective of fertility
- Oral testosterone undecanoate (Jatenzo or Tlando) BID dosing
  - FDA warning for blood pressure elevation
  - Titration required to determine appropriate dose
  - 2-year data demonstrates good efficacy, with safety profile similar to other testosterone formulations

ISSUES FOR REFERRAL

PSA elevation, abnormal prostate exam, worsening BPH (IPSS >19), refractory to replacement therapy should be referred to urology.

ONGOING CARE

FOLLOW-UP RECOMMENDATIONS

Patient Monitoring

- Monitor T 3 to 6 months after treatment initiation, then every 6 to 12 months
  - Adjust dosing to achieve a total T in the middle tertile of the normal reference range.
- Measure hematocrit at baseline, at 3 to 6 months, and then annually.
- Stop treatment 3 to 6 months after starting in patients who experience normalization of T but fail to achieve symptom improvement.
- Bone mineral density after 1 to 2 years of therapy in men with osteoporosis
- PSA and prostate exam every 6 to 12 months

DIET

Lifestyle changes and weight loss may raise testosterone levels without the need for T replacement.

PATIENT EDUCATION

- TD can be chronic and may need lifelong therapy.
- T replacement comes with risks, and it is very important to regularly monitor outcomes.
- Women and children must not be allowed to come in contact with TT gel products.

PROGNOSIS

There is evolving evidence that TT may improve metabolic functions such as glycosylated hemoglobin, blood sugar, total cholesterol, and visceral fat in diabetics; bone mineral density, and also unexplained anemia.

COMPLICATIONS

Complications of T replacement

- Decreased testicular volume, azoospermia in 40% of patients on TT, infertility
- Fluctuations in mood or libido
- Gynecomastia and growth of breast cancer
- Acne and oily skin
- Erythrocytosis
- Exacerbation of sleep apnea
- Hepatotoxicity with prolonged oral use
- Possible prostate enlargement, worsening BPH symptoms

REFERENCES

1. Mulhall JP, Trost LW, Brannigan RE, et al. Evaluation and management of testosterone deficiency: AUA guideline. *J Urol*. 2018;200(2):423–432.
2. Debruyne FMJ, Behre HM, Roehrborn CG, et al; for RHYME Investigators. Testosterone treatment is not associated with increased risk of prostate cancer or worsening of lower urinary tract symptoms: prostate health outcomes in the Registry of Hypogonadism in Men. *BJU Int*. 2017;119(2):216–224.
3. Lincoff AM, Bhasin S, Flevaris P, et al; TRAVERSE Study Investigators. Cardiovascular safety of testosterone-replacement therapy. *N Engl J Med*. 2023;389(2):107–117. doi:10.1056/NEJMoa2215025.

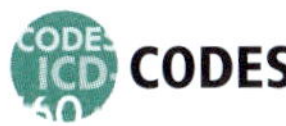

CODES

ICD10

- E29.1 Testicular hypofunction
- E89.5 Postprocedural testicular hypofunction

CLINICAL PEARLS

- TD is common, and prevalence increases with age.
- Men with sexual dysfunction, obesity, unexplained anemia, bone density loss, chronic steroid or narcotic use, and metabolic diseases should be tested for TD.
- Initial test of choice is a morning total and free T. If low, repeat measurements.
- TT in the appropriately selected population can increase lean mass, reduce fat mass, increase bone mineral density, improve libido, improve unexplained anemia, and improve erections. However, it has not been shown to improve cognition or memory impairment in the elderly.
- Lifestyle changes such as diet and exercise may restore testosterone levels.

T

THALASSEMIA

Rafia Ali, MD

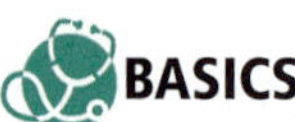

BASICS

DESCRIPTION

- A group of inherited hematologic disorders that affect the synthesis of adult hemoglobin tetramer (HbA)
- α-Thalassemia is due to a deficient synthesis of α-globin chain, whereas β-thalassemia is due to a deficient synthesis of β-globin chain:
  - The synthesis of the unaffected globin chain proceeds normally.
  - This unbalanced globin chain production causes unstable hemoglobin tetramers, which leads to hypochromic, microcytic red blood cells (RBCs), and hemolytic anemia.
- α-Thalassemia is more common in persons of Mediterranean, African, and Southeast Asian descent, whereas β-thalassemia is more common in patients of African and Southeast Asian descent.
- Types
  - Thalassemia (minor) trait (α or β): absent or mild anemia with microcytosis and hypochromia
  - α-Thalassemia major with hemoglobin Barts: usually results in fatal hydrops fetalis (fluid in ≥2 fetal compartments secondary to anemia and fetal heart failure).
  - α-Thalassemia intermedia with hemoglobin H (hemoglobin H disease): results in moderate hemolytic anemia and splenomegaly
  - β-Thalassemia, transfusion-dependent: results in severe anemia, growth retardation, hepatosplenomegaly, bone marrow expansion, and bone deformities; transfusion therapy is necessary to sustain life.
  - β-Thalassemia, non–transfusion-dependent: milder disease; transfusion therapy may not be needed or may be needed later in life, or during periods of erythropoietic stress (e.g., infection, pregnancy).
  - β-Thalassemia minor: asymptomatic carrier state with mild anemia
- Other variants include hemoglobin E/β-thalassemia in Southeast Asians, which often mimics the severity of α-thalassemia major; δ-thalassemia; hemoglobin H constant spring
- System(s) affected: hematologic/lymphatic/immunologic, cardiac, hepatic
- Synonym(s): Mediterranean anemia; hereditary leptocytosis; Cooley anemia

Pediatric Considerations

- β-Thalassemia major causes symptoms during early childhood, usually starting at 6 months of age, and requires periodic transfusions to sustain life.
- Newborn's cord blood or heel stick should be screened for hemoglobinopathies with hemoglobin electrophoresis or comparably accurate test, although this primarily detects sickle cell disease.

Pregnancy Considerations

- Preconception genetic counseling is advised for individuals with thalassemia and their first-degree relatives. Testing is also appropriate for those with reasonable likelihood of thalassemia based on ethnicity, country of origin, or other patient concerns.
- Once pregnant, a chorionic villus sample at 10 to 11 weeks' gestation or an amniocentesis at 15 weeks' gestation can be done to detect point mutations or deletions with polymerase chain reaction (PCR) technology.

EPIDEMIOLOGY

Incidence

- Occurs in ~4.4/10,000 live births
- Predominant age: Symptoms start to appear 6 months after birth with β-thalassemia major.
- Predominant sex: male = female

Prevalence

- Worldwide, ~200,000 people are alive with β-thalassemia major and <1,000 patients are in the United States.
- In the worldwide population, an estimated 1.5% are β-thalassemia carriers and 5% α-thalassemia carriers.

ETIOLOGY AND PATHOPHYSIOLOGY

Disruption in the balance of globin chain synthesis leads to imbalance in α- and α-globin chains and subsequent abnormalities in RBC formation and function. Unmatched globin chains cause hemolysis and ineffective erythropoiesis.

Genetics

- Inherited in an autosomal recessive pattern
- α-Thalassemia results from a deletion of ≥1 of the 4 genes, 2 on each chromosome 16, responsible for α-globin synthesis. 1-gene deletion is a silent carrier state, 2-gene deletion is the trait, 3-gene deletion results in hemoglobin H, and 4-gene deletion results in hemoglobin Bart, causing fatal hydrops fetalis.
- Non-deletional forms do occur rarely. Hemoglobin H constant spring is the most common non-deletional form.
- β-Thalassemia is caused by mutations or deletions in the β-globin gene (HBB) on chromosome 11; 20 alleles account for >80% of the mutations.
- Significantly disparate phenotype with the same genotype occurs because β-globin chain production can range from near-normal to absent.

RISK FACTORS

Family history of thalassemia

GENERAL PREVENTION

- Prenatal information: genetic counseling regarding partner selection and information on the availability of diagnostic tests during the pregnancy
- Complication prevention
  - For offspring of adult thalassemia patients, an evaluation for thalassemia by 1 year of age
  - Severe forms
    - Avoid exposure to sick contacts.
    - Keep immunizations up-to-date.
  - Promptly treat bacterial infections. (After splenectomy, patients should maintain a supply of an appropriate antibiotic to take at the onset of symptoms of a bacterial infection.)
  - Dental checkups every 6 months
  - Avoid activities that could increase the risk of bone fractures.

DIAGNOSIS

Thalassemia does not always find anemia but presents with microcytosis (low mean corpuscular volume [MCV]) and normal or elevated RBC count, normal or high ferritin, and a relatively normal red cell distribution width (RDW). Iron deficiency anemia presents with anemia and low hemoglobin, low MCV, low mean corpuscular hemoglobin (MCH), low ferritin, and increased RDW.

HISTORY

Poor growth, excessive fatigue, cholelithiasis, pathologic fractures, shortness of breath

PHYSICAL EXAM

Pallor, splenomegaly, jaundice, maxillary hyperplasia/frontal bossing due to massive bone marrow expansion, dental malocclusion

DIFFERENTIAL DIAGNOSIS

- Iron deficiency anemia
- Anemia of chronic disease/anemia of inflammation
- Lead toxicity, sideroblastic anemia
- Other hemolytic anemias
- Other hemoglobinopathies

DIAGNOSTIC TESTS & INTERPRETATION

Special tests

- Bone marrow aspiration to evaluate for causes of microcytic anemia is rarely needed.
- Multiple indices have been evaluated to discriminate β-thalassemia trait from iron deficiency anemia, yet none is sensitive enough to exclude β-thalassemia.
- Hemoglobin: usual range 10 to 12 g/dL with thalassemia trait and 3 to 8 g/dL with β-thalassemia major before transfusions
- Hematocrit
  - 28–40% in thalassemia trait
  - May fall to <10% in β-thalassemia major
- Peripheral blood
  - Microcytosis (MCV <70 fL)
  - Hypochromia (MCH <20 pg)
  - High percentage of target cells
  - Reticulocyte count is elevated.
  - Variation in size and shape (anisocytosis and poikilocytosis)
  - Target cells, Heinz bodies
- RDW
  - A normal RDW with a microcytic hypochromic anemia is almost always thalassemia trait.
  - The RDW can be elevated in ~50% of thalassemia trait patients. This is in contrast to iron deficiency anemia, where the RDW is almost always elevated (90%).
- Hemoglobin electrophoresis
  - In α-thalassemia trait, no recognizable electrophoretic pattern occurs in adults.
  - However, in the neonatal period, 3–10% of trait patients will have hemoglobin H or hemoglobin Bart at birth, which would confirm α-thalassemia.
  - If HbA_2 is below normal (<2.5%) with a normal HbF level, the diagnosis is α-thalassemia intermedia (HbH disease).
  - In the neonatal period with β-thalassemia trait, the electrophoresis is normal. However, in adults, elevated HbA_2 levels (>4%) may be present but are usually normal.
  - β-Thalassemia major or intermedia has elevated HbA_2, elevated HbF, and reduced or absent HbA.
- DNA analysis
  - α-Thalassemia can definitively be diagnosed with genetic testing of hemoglobin A1 and A2 (for deletions and point mutations), but this is not routinely done due to the high cost.
  - High-performance liquid chromatography
  - Cost-effective primary screening tool for children and adolescents
  - Equivocal results should be confirmed with DNA analysis.

Pediatric Considerations

For children, calculate Mentzer index (MCV/RBC count).

- <13: suggests thalassemia
- >13: suggests iron deficiency anemia
- Liver iron concentrations can be assessed with MRI (FerriScan).

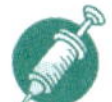

TREATMENT

- Outpatient for mild cases
- Inpatient for transfusion therapy

GENERAL MEASURES

- Mild cases (trait or minor) require no therapy.
- Thalassemia intermedia: No therapy is necessary unless hemoglobin falls to a level that causes symptoms; then, transfusion therapy is needed. Decision is based on patient's quality of life.
- Iron supplements should not be given unless iron deficiency occurs and is confirmed with low ferritin. Supplements increase the risk of iron overload.
- Thalassemia major
  - A regular transfusion schedule to increase post-transfusion hemoglobin to 13 to 14 g/L and maintain a mean hemoglobin level of at least 9.3 g/dL (1.4 mmol/L)
  - Patients require >8 transfusion events per year. An event may be multiple transfused units.
  - Iron overload
    - Patients receiving transfusion therapy increase total body iron 4 times the normal amount.
    - Therapy is iron chelation. (See "Medication.")

MEDICATION

Thalassemia intermedia and major: folic acid supplements (1 mg/day)

First Line

β-Thalassemia major

- Iron chelation with deferoxamine (Desferal)
  - Usually continuous SC or IV infusion
  - Acute toxicity: initial—1,000 mg IV, may be followed by 500 mg every 4 hours for 2 doses; subsequent doses of 500 mg every 4 to 12 hours based on response (max 6,000 mg/day)
  - Chronic: 20 to 40 mg/kg over 8 to 12 hours daily
  - Usually started by 5 to 8 years of age
  - Treatment lasts 3 to 5 years to reach serum ferritin <1,000 ng/mL.
- Deferasirox (Exjade): 20 to 30 mg/kg/day PO acceptable alternative; approved for transfusion and non–transfusion-dependent patients with hepatic iron concentrations ≥5 mg/g of dry weight and serum ferritin >300 μg/L; renal and hepatic monitoring is recommended.

Second Line

Chelation with deferiprone (Ferriprox) 25 mg/kg TID PO initially is an acceptable alternative for patients who have not responded to may provide more cardioprotection. A drawback is weekly CBC because ~1% of patients develop agranulocytosis.

ADDITIONAL THERAPIES

β-Thalassemia intermedia

- Hydroxyurea may improve hemoglobin 1 to 2 g/dL.
- Psychological support seems appropriate for this chronic disease. However, no conclusions can be made regarding specific psychological therapies.

SURGERY/OTHER PROCEDURES

- Splenectomy
  - May be needed if hypersplenism causes an increase in the transfusion requirements (>180 to 200 mL/kg/year)
  - Defer surgery until patient is at least 4 years of age (due to increased infection risk).
  - Administer pneumococcal polyvalent-23 vaccine 1 month before splenectomy. Children should complete their pneumococcal conjugate vaccine series before surgery.
  - Daily penicillin prophylaxis, 250 mg BID, after splenectomy for 2 years for all patients and for children until age 16 years
- Bone marrow transplantation with HLA-identical related donor stem cells in children before developing hepatitis or iron overload has high likelihood of remission but may impair fertility.
- Mitapivat
  - Small molecule that activates RBC pyruvate kinase
  - Can increase hemoglobin levels for both α- and β-Thalassemia patients

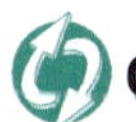

ONGOING CARE

FOLLOW-UP RECOMMENDATIONS

- Thalassemia trait requires no restrictions.
- β-Thalassemia major
  - Avoid strenuous activities (e.g., football, soccer).
  - Acceptable activity levels will be determined on an individual basis depending on the severity of the disorder.

Patient Monitoring

- Thalassemia-trait patients require no special follow-up.
- For β-thalassemia major, lifelong monitoring is necessary because the therapy and disease progression have numerous potential complications.

DIET

- Thalassemia trait requires no restrictions.
- β-Thalassemia major
  - Limit intake of iron-rich foods (e.g., red meats such as liver and some cereals)

PATIENT EDUCATION

Printed patient information available from Cooley's Anemia Foundation

PROGNOSIS

- Thalassemia-trait patients live a normal lifespan.
- β-Thalassemia major patients live an average of 17 years and usually die by age 30 years.
- Iron overload causes most of the morbidity and mortality:
  - Cardiac events are the primary cause of death.
  - Myocardial iron deposition is best assessed with MRI T2.
  - Effective iron chelation improves longevity.

COMPLICATIONS

- Chronic hemolysis
- Susceptibility to infections after splenectomy
- Infections from blood transfusion
- Jaundice
- Leg ulcers
- Cholelithiasis
- Osteoporosis and low-trauma fractures
- Impaired growth rate
- Delayed or absent puberty
- Hypogonadism
- Hepatic siderosis
- Splenomegaly
- Cardiac disease from iron overload
- Thromboembolic phenomenon
- Aplastic and megaloblastic crises
- Increased risk of hematologic and abdominal cancer
- Increased risk of dementia

ADDITIONAL READING

Baird DC, Batten SH, Sparks SK. Alpha- and beta-thalassemia: rapid evidence review. *Am Fam Physician*. 2022;105(3):272–280.

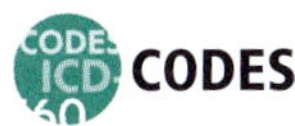

CODES

ICD10

- D56.5 Hemoglobin E-beta thalassemia
- D56.3 Thalassemia minor
- D56.0 Alpha thalassemia

CLINICAL PEARLS

- Thalassemia (group of inherited hematologic disorders that affect the synthesis of adult hemoglobin tetramer) is a genetic condition; hemoglobin will not improve over time.
- α-Thalassemia is due to a deficient synthesis of the α-globin chain, whereas β-thalassemia is due to a deficient synthesis of the β-globin chain.
- Hemoglobin electrophoresis is needed for genetic counseling but not to make the diagnosis of thalassemia minor when evaluating a patient with mild hypochromic, microcytic anemia, and normal serum ferritin.
- Anemia from thalassemia minor is not due to inadequate iron availability or iron storage. Therefore, iron supplements will not improve the anemia and could be harmful due to GI distress and iron overload. If coexisting iron deficiency is proven, then iron therapy is appropriate.

THORACIC OUTLET SYNDROME

Robert A. Baldor, MD, FAAFP

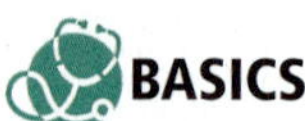

BASICS

DESCRIPTION

- This syndrome consists of a constellation of symptoms that affect the head, neck, shoulders, and upper extremities caused by compression of the neurovascular structures (brachial plexus and subclavian vessels) at the thoracic outlet.
- Three forms of thoracic outlet syndrome (TOS) have been described:
  - Neurogenic (nTOS)
  - Venous (vTOS)
  - Arterial (aTOS)
- Synonym(s): scalenus anticus syndrome; cervical rib syndrome; costoclavicular syndrome; 1st rib syndrome

EPIDEMIOLOGY

- There are no universal diagnostic criteria to accurately determine epidemiology.
- nTOS
  - Approximately 90–95% of all TOS cases (1)
  - Predominant in 20- to 50-year-old females
- vTOS
  - Approximately 5–10% of all TOS cases (1)
  - Predominant in 20- to 35-year-old physically active males
- aTOS
  - Approximately 1% of all TOS cases (1)
  - No gender preference

ETIOLOGY AND PATHOPHYSIOLOGY

- TOS primarily impacts three anatomic spaces within the thoracic outlet (1):
  - Scalene triangle
    - Bordered by the anterior scalene, middle scalene and 1st rib
    - Contains trunks of the brachial plexus and subclavian artery
  - Costoclavicular space
    - Bordered by the clavicle, 1st rib and upper portion of the scapula
    - Contains divisions of the brachial plexus, subclavian artery, and subclavian vein
  - Subcoracoid space
    - Bordered by the pectoralis muscle, 2nd to 4th ribs and coracoid process
    - Contains cords of the brachial plexus
- Proposed etiologies include (1):
  - Congenital—cervical rib, 1st rib
  - Traumatic—motor vehicle accidents
  - Functional—overuse activity of the upper extremity, particularly shoulder abduction/extension

RISK FACTORS

- Trauma to the shoulder girdle
- Presence of a cervical rib (1% of population)
- Exostosis of clavicle or 1st rib
- Postural abnormalities (e.g., drooping of shoulders, scoliosis)
- Occupational exposure via repetitive activity (e.g., computer users; musicians; overhead athletes; repetitive upper body work)

GENERAL PREVENTION

Consider workplace evaluation for proper occupational ergonomics, including proper posture.

COMMONLY ASSOCIATED CONDITIONS

- Paget–von Schrötter syndrome: effort thrombosis of subclavian vein
- Gilliatt-Sumner hand: neurogenic atrophy of abductor pollicis brevis
- Pancoast tumor

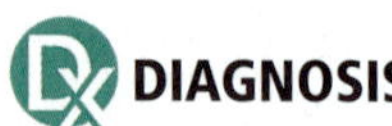

DIAGNOSIS

HISTORY

Sports play can be an initial presentation of symptom provocation, particularly for pediatric patients (2).

- nTOS
  - High index of suspicion if there is a history of neck trauma or repetitive overhead activity
  - Upper extremity pain and paresthesias are considered common presenting symptoms (1).
  - Additional symptoms:
    - Occipital and orbital headache
    - Muscle atrophy of the upper extremity
    - Raynaud phenomenon secondary to sympathetic nerve irritation (1)
- vTOS
  - High index of suspicion if symptoms worsen with shoulder abduction particularly in overhead lifting athletes
  - Common symptoms: unilateral arm claudication, cyanosis, swelling, pain, venous enlargement
- aTOS
  - 85% of cases estimated to be related to cervical rib
  - Highest morbidity of all types due to risk for limb ischemia
  - Common symptoms: unilateral arm weakness, pallor, paresthesia, pain, weak or absent pulse, blood pressure asymmetry

PHYSICAL EXAM

- Initial considerations
  - Posture
  - Cervical alignment
  - Scapular stability
  - Inspection and palpation of thoracic outlet anatomy
  - Upper extremity and cranial nerve neurologic examination
- Specialized testing
  - Adson maneuver (aTOS): head rotation to the affected side with cervical extension and then deep inhalation
    - Positive if paresthesias occur or if radial pulse is not palpable during maneuver
  - Morley test (vTOS): manual compression of brachial plexus for 30 seconds in the supraclavicular area of the scalene triangle
    - Positive with reproduction of an aching sensation and typical localized paresthesia
  - Hyperabduction test (aTOS): elevation of arm above the head
    - Positive if diminished of radial pulse
  - Military maneuver (i.e., costoclavicular bracing): patient elevates chin and pushes shoulders posteriorly in an extreme "at-attention" position
    - Positive test reproduces symptoms
  - 1-minute Roos test: Shoulders and arms are braced in a 90-degree abducted and externally rotated position; patient is required to clench and relax fists repetitively for 1 minute.
    - Positive test reproduces symptoms.

DIFFERENTIAL DIAGNOSIS

- Cervical disc or carpal tunnel syndrome
- Orthopedic shoulder problems (shoulder strain, rotator cuff injury, tendonitis)
- Cervical spondylitis
- Ulnar nerve compression at elbow and hand
- Multiple sclerosis
- Spinal cord tumor/disease
- Angina pectoris
- Migraine
- Complex regional pain syndromes
- C3–C5 and C8 radiculopathies
- Pancoast tumor

DIAGNOSTIC TESTS & INTERPRETATION

Initial Tests (lab, imaging)

- History and physical are the strongest clinical indicators for TOS. However, additional imaging helps to confirm subtype to guide proper treatment.
- Chest x-ray is often an appropriate initial imaging modality for all subtypes (3).
- EMG may be a beneficial initial test to narrow differential between neurogenic and vascular types.

Follow-Up Tests & Special Considerations

American College of Radiology recommends a variety of imaging modalities. MRI and CT assist with definitive subtype diagnosis after initial workup (3).

- nTOS: Chest MRI can consider use of contrast although not required if contraindicated for a patient.
- aTOS: chest CTA, chest MRA, duplex US over the subclavian vessels
- vTOS: chest CT with contrast; catheter venography of the upper extremity; duplex US of the subclavian vessels

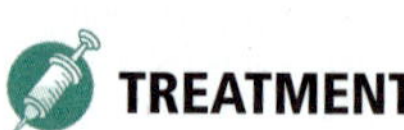

TREATMENT

GENERAL MEASURES

Conservative management usually involves approaches to reduce and redistribute pressure and traction on the thoracic outlet.

- Physical therapy is first-line treatment along with activity modification, rest, and NSAIDs if no vascular alarm symptoms exist (4)[B].
- Adjunctive therapies including taping, adhesive elastic bandages, moist heat, TENS, or US may be used, but should not substitute active exercise and correction of posture and muscle imbalance (4)[B].

MEDICATION

No firm evidence exists for any specific pharmacologic approach to the three types of TOS.

- Anti-inflammatory (ibuprofen)
  - Adult dose: 400 to 800 mg PO q8h; not to exceed 3,200 mg/day
  - Pediatric dose: <12 years: 10 mg/kg/dose q6–8h
  - Contraindications: documented hypersensitivity, active PUD, renal or hepatic impairment, recent use of anticoagulants, hemorrhagic conditions
- Neuropathic pain: Tricyclic antidepressants, carbamazepine, gabapentin, phenytoin, pregabalin; muscle relaxants such as baclofen, metaxalone, or tizanidine may be helpful.
- Severe pain: Consider procedural alternatives as listed below.

ISSUES FOR REFERRAL

- If vascular type TOS is suspected, immediate referral to vascular surgery should be made due to risk for limb ischemia.
- Sports medicine or PM&R providers can be considered for diagnostic and therapeutic injections.
- Vascular surgery (aTOS and vTOS), orthopedic surgery (nTOS), or neurosurgery (nTOS) can be considered for surgical evaluation.

SURGERY/OTHER PROCEDURES

- Botulinum toxin—type A injection therapy
  - Benefit from decreased muscular tension and pain
  - 64–69% of patients have relief for up to 3 months although with a risk of prolonged duration of symptoms (5). Alternative injection therapies show the best efficacy when combined with physical therapy modalities (5).
    - Trigger point
    - Corticosteroid
    - Local anesthetic
- Surgical options can provide greater relief to symptoms than conservative management alone (6).
- Complete 1st rib resection and anterior scalenectomy are common combined surgical interventions to provide pressure relief to the thoracic outlet structures in all subtypes.
- Thrombolytic may be necessary for acute vTOS with consideration of venoplasty thereafter.

ADMISSION, INPATIENT, AND NURSING CONSIDERATIONS

Conservative, outpatient treatment is reasonable first-line therapy except in cases of thromboembolic phenomena and acute ischemia, symptoms of chronic vascular occlusion, stenosis, arterial dilatation, or progressive neurologic deficit

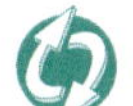

ONGOING CARE

FOLLOW-UP RECOMMENDATIONS

Patient Monitoring

Office follow-up visits every 3 to 4 weeks

PATIENT EDUCATION

Physical therapy, postural exercises, ergonomic workstation

PROGNOSIS

Durable long-term functional outcomes can be achieved predicated on a highly selective approach to the surgical management of patients with TOS. A majority of operated patients will not require adjunctive procedures or chronic narcotic use (7)[C].

COMPLICATIONS

- Postoperative shoulder, arm, hand pain, and paresthesias: 10%
- Patients who will have symptomatic recurrences at 1 month to 7 years postoperatively (usually within 3 months): 1.5–2.0%
- Patients who will have brachial plexus injury, probably due to intraoperative traction: 0.5–1.0%
- Reoperation is indicated for symptomatic recurrence with long posterior remnant of 1st rib (posterior approach) or with disrupted fibrous adhesions (transaxillary approach).
- Venous obstruction or arterial emboli; usually responds to thrombolytics

REFERENCES

1. Cavanna AC, Giovanis A, Daley A, et al. Thoracic outlet syndrome: a review for the primary care provider. *J Osteopath Med*. 2022;122(11):587–599. doi:10.1515/jom-2021-0276.
2. Garraud T, Pomares G, Daley P, et al. Thoracic outlet syndrome in sport: a systematic review. *Front Physiol*. 2022;13:838014. doi:10.3389/fphys.2022.838014.
3. Zurkiya O, Ganguli S, Kalva SP, et al; for Expert Panels on Vascular Imaging, Thoracic Imaging, and Neurological Imaging. ACR appropriateness criteria® thoracic outlet syndrome. *J Am Coll Radiol*. 2020;17(5S):S323–S334.
4. Vanti C, Natalini L, Romeo A, et al. Conservative treatment of thoracic outlet syndrome. A review of the literature. *Eura Medicophys*. 2007;43(1):55–70.
5. Li N, Dierks G, Vervaeke HE, et al. Thoracic outlet syndrome: a narrative review. *J Clin Med*. 2021;10(5):962.
6. Balderman J, Abuirqeba AA, Eichaker L, et al. Physical therapy management, surgical treatment, and patient-reported outcomes measures in a prospective observational cohort of patients with neurogenic thoracic outlet syndrome. *J Vasc Surg*. 2019;70(3):832–841.
7. Scali S, Stone D, Bjerke A, et al. Long-term functional results for the surgical management of neurogenic thoracic outlet syndrome. *Vasc Endovascular Surg*. 2010;44(7):550–555.

ADDITIONAL READING

- Dengler NF, Ferraresi S, Rochkind S, et al. Thoracic outlet syndrome part I: systematic review of the literature and consensus on anatomy, diagnosis, and classification of thoracic outlet syndrome by the European Association of Neurosurgical Societies' Section of Peripheral Nerve Surgery. *Neurosurgery*. 2022;90(6):653–667. doi:10.1227/neu.0000000000001908.
- Hock G, Johnson A, Barber P, et al. Current clinical concepts: rehabilitation of thoracic outlet syndrome. *J Athl Train*. 2024;59(7):683–695. doi:10.4085/1062-6050-138.22.

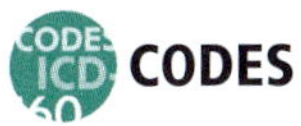

CODES

ICD10

G54.0 Brachial plexus disorders

CLINICAL PEARLS

- This syndrome is caused by compression of the neurovascular structures (brachial plexus and subclavian vessels) at the thoracic outlet, specifically in the area superior to the 1st rib and posterior to the clavicle.
- Three subtypes exist: neurogenic, arterial, venous.
- Physical therapy, activity modification, rest and NSAIDs are the first-line treatment if no alarm symptoms exist.
- If vascular type TOS (venous or arterial) is suspected, immediate referral to vascular surgery should be made due to risk for limb ischemia.

T

THROMBOPHILIA AND HYPERCOAGULABLE STATES

Allen Zhou, MD • Halle Elizabeth Field, MD

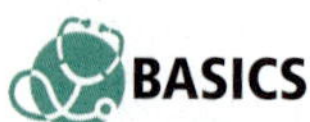

BASICS

DESCRIPTION

- A coagulation disorder that predisposes an individual to inappropriate clot formation of the venous, and less commonly, the arterial vasculature
- May be inherited or acquired
- Common examples of venous thromboembolism (VTE): deep venous thrombosis (DVT), pulmonary embolism (PE)
- Common examples of arterial thromboembolism: myocardial infarction, ischemic stroke
- Synonym(s): hypercoagulable disorder; prothrombotic state

EPIDEMIOLOGY

- VTE incidence is higher in women than men during ages 16 to 44 years; then, higher in men when age >45 years
- VTE incidence is higher in African American populations.
- Hereditary thrombophilias
  - An inherited thrombophilic defect or risk can be detected in 40–50% of patients with first idiopathic VTE.
  - Factor V Leiden (FVL) is the most common inherited thrombophilia (half of all currently characterizable inherited thrombophilia cases involve the FVL mutation).

Thrombophilia	Prevalence
Factor V Leiden	3–7%
Prothrombin G20210A	2%
Protein C deficiency	0.02–0.05%
Protein S deficiency	0.01–1.00%
Antithrombin III (ATIII) deficiency	0.04%

- Acquired thrombophilias:
  - Cancer: 20% of all VTEs occur in patients with cancer.
  - Pregnancy: VTE affects 0.1–0.2% of pregnancies.
  - Antiphospholipid antibodies (APLA): 20% of patients with VTE have moderate to high levels of APLA before a thrombotic event.
  - See "Risk Factors."

Prevalence

In patients with symptomatic VTE, the prevalence of any thrombophilia is 38%.

ETIOLOGY AND PATHOPHYSIOLOGY

- Underlying mechanism depends on whether thrombophilia is inherited or acquired.
- Associated with Virchow triad which includes blood flow stasis, hypercoagulable state, and vascular endothelial injury
- An imbalance between the hemostatic and fibrinolytic pathways leads to thrombus formation.

Genetics

- The most common hereditary thrombophilias (FVL, prothrombin G20210A, proteins C and S defects, and ATIII deficiency) are inherited in an autosomal dominant pattern.
- Homozygous mutations have a higher risk of VTE.
- FVL: mutated form of factor V that is resistant to proteolysis by activated protein C (aPC)
- Prothrombin G20210A: increases gene expression of prothrombin
- Protein C and S deficiencies: result in overactivity of factors Va and VIIIa
- ATIII deficiency: decreases inhibition of thrombin and factor Xa as well as other coagulation factors

RISK FACTORS

- Acquired risk factors (common)
  - Ages ≥65 years
  - Previous thromboembolism
  - Immobilization or prolonged travel (e.g., flight time >8 hours)
  - Trauma
  - Surgery
  - Malignancy (especially pancreatic, ovarian, brain, and lymphoma)
  - Pregnancy and postpartum state
  - Medications including oral contraceptives (OCPs), hormonal therapy (e.g., tamoxifen), thalidomide, lenalidomide, bevacizumab, L-asparaginase, erythropoiesis-stimulating agents, pomalidomide, tranexamic acid
  - Presence of central venous catheter
  - COVID-19/COVID-19 vaccine
  - Cardiovascular disease including heart failure
  - Kidney disease including end-stage kidney disease and nephrotic syndrome
  - Gastrointestinal disease including inflammatory bowel disease and chronic liver disease
  - Hematologic disease including heparin-induced thrombocytopenia (HIT) and hyperviscosity syndromes (e.g., sickle cell disease, myeloproliferative syndromes)
  - Antiphospholipid syndrome (APS)
  - Hyperhomocysteinemia secondary to vitamin deficiencies (B_6, B_{12}, folic acid)
  - Rare genetic factors: dysfibrinogenemia, methylene tetrahydrofolate reductase mutation
  - Indeterminate factors: elevated factor VIII
- Inherited risk factors
  - FVL; prothrombin G20210A; protein C deficiency; protein S deficiency; ATIII deficiency

GENERAL PREVENTION

- Consider medication prophylaxis in any hospitalized patient with VTE risk factors.
- Consider mechanical prophylaxis in patients at increased risk for VTE when anticoagulation is contraindicated.
- Consider prophylaxis with low-molecular-weight heparin (LMWH) plus aspirin in pregnant patients with APS.
- Consider prophylaxis with anticoagulation in patients with solid tumors who have additional risk factors for VTE per Khorana score.
- Consider prophylaxis with unfractionated heparin (UFH) or LMWH in patients with genetic or acquired risks of thrombosis and an anticipated additional risk such as immobilization associated with surgery.
- Use caution with procoagulant medicines (e.g., OCP) in asymptomatic individuals with known hereditary predisposition.

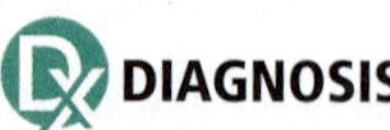

DIAGNOSIS

HISTORY

Consider hypercoagulable assessment for the following:

- Recurrent thrombosis
- VTE event in patient aged <45 years
- First-degree relative with VTE before age 45 years
- VTE in unusual vascular beds (e.g., hepatic, portal, mesenteric, cerebral veins)
- Thrombosis in multiple venous sites
- Arterial thrombosis
- Warfarin-induced skin necrosis
- Recurrent fetal loss

PHYSICAL EXAM

- DVT: unilateral extremity swelling, erythema, warmth, tenderness
- PE: tachypnea, tachycardia, fever, pleural friction rub, hypoxia

DIAGNOSTIC TESTS & INTERPRETATION

- Rationale for screening (1)[C],(2)[C]
  - Helps to inform future risk assessment
  - Helps to guide evaluation and management of first-degree relatives, particularly female relatives considering hormonal therapy or pregnancy
- Appropriate tests for patients with a family history of VTE
  - FVL, prothrombin G20210A, protein S, protein C, and ATIII assays
- Appropriate tests for unprovoked VTE, recurrent VTE, unusual sites of VTE, or VTE secondary to pregnancy, OCPs or hormonal therapy
  - FVL, prothrombin G20210A, protein S, protein C, and ATIII assays
  - APLA assays
- Appropriate tests for arterial thrombosis
  - APLA assays
- When testing patients for hereditary thrombophilia, all tests should be performed a minimum of 2 weeks after completing anticoagulation course.
  - In particular, protein C, protein S, and ATIII levels are affected by acute thrombosis and anticoagulation.
  - This approach avoids repeated testing and recurrent office visits.

Initial Tests (lab, imaging)

- Complete blood count
- FVL: performed by genetic testing or functional aPC resistance assay. Genetic testing directly analyzes DNA. Therefore, it is not affected by anticoagulation. However, it cannot detect acquired or other hereditary causes of aPC resistance (1)[C].
- Prothrombin G20210A genetic assay
- ATIII functional assay: may be low with acute thrombosis and heparin therapy; may be falsely high with direct oral anticoagulants (DOACs)
- Protein C functional assay: may be low with acute thrombosis; will be lower on warfarin and DOACs
- Protein S functional assay and free protein S: may be low with acute thrombosis; will be lower on warfarin and DOACs
- APLA: anti-β2-glycoprotein, anticardiolipin, lupus anticoagulant; lupus anticoagulant may be unreliable on heparin and DOACs.
- Consider evaluation for malignancy in an unprovoked thrombosis in those aged >40 years or at greater risk.
- Consider HIT antibody immunoassay or functional assay if high clinical suspicion.
- Pregnancy test if of reproductive age

Follow-Up Tests & Special Considerations

Special situations (1)[C]

- APS
  - APS can present as arterial and/or venous thrombosis.
  - Other clinical manifestations may include pregnancy complications such as fetal demise, premature birth due to eclampsia or severe preeclampsia, or recurrent unexplained spontaneous abortions.
  - Testing for APLA on two separate occasions at least 12 weeks apart is needed for diagnosis.
- Malignancy
  - There is an increased risk of VTE in cancer, especially with mucin-producing adenocarcinoma.
  - Thrombophilia testing is not suggested in patients with active cancer and VTE.
- Thrombosis at unusual sites
  - Sites include the splanchnic veins (e.g., hepatic, portal, mesenteric) and cerebral veins
  - Consider cirrhosis, extrinsic tumor compression, and local inflammation (e.g., pancreatitis) in patients with portal vein thrombosis.
  - Consider paroxysmal nocturnal hemoglobinuria and myeloproliferative neoplasms in patients with unexplained splanchnic vein thrombosis.
- Combination OCPs
  - Smoking and obesity in women taking combined OCPs are associated with increased risk of VTE.

Pediatric Considerations

- Warfarin is teratogenic and should be avoided in pregnancy.
- LMWH or UFH are preferred for all prophylactic and treatment options.
- There is lack of safety data on DOACs on fetus.

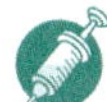

TREATMENT

- Assess VTE context: provoked or unprovoked.
- Assess VTE risk.
  - Low-risk inherited thrombophilias: heterozygous FVL, heterozygous prothrombin 20210 mutation
  - High-risk inherited thrombophilias: protein C deficiency, protein S deficiency, ATIII deficiency
- Duration of treatment (2)[C]
  - Duration is individualized and may be indefinite if the VTE is unprovoked, recurrent, life-threatening, or at an unusual site.
- Consider extended thromboprophylaxis postdischarge with major prothrombotic risk factors such as history of VTE or major surgery as long as bleeding risk is not high (e.g., post-hip arthroplasty).

MEDICATION

First Line

- DOACs: Apixaban, dabigatran, edoxaban, and rivaroxaban are recommended over vitamin K antagonists for initial and long-term oral anticoagulation (3)[C].
- Parenteral anticoagulation: LMWH has largely replaced UFH as first-line therapy for all inherited thrombophilia.
- Pregnancy: low-dose aspirin and/or LMWH or UFH; warfarin is contraindicated.
- APS: Warfarin and LMWH remain first-line agents for anticoagulation.

Second Line

Usually indicated when contraindication to heparin or LMWH, such as heparin-associated thrombocytopenia and thrombosis

- Factor Xa inhibitors (fondaparinux)
- Direct thrombin inhibitors (argatroban)

SURGERY/OTHER PROCEDURES

- Thrombolysis (3)[C]
  - Consider for patients with PE and hemodynamic instability
  - Should be followed by anticoagulation
- Thrombectomy
  - Consider for patients either with PE or extensive DVT who are also suitable candidates for thrombolysis
- Inferior vena cava filter
  - Consider for patients with contraindications to anticoagulation
  - Reduces short-term risk of PE but may increase long-term risk of recurrent VTE

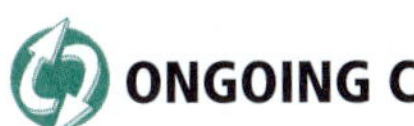

ONGOING CARE

FOLLOW-UP RECOMMENDATIONS

Patient Monitoring

Monitor warfarin with INR goal of 2 to 3 (most indications).

DIET

- Vitamin K–stable diet if patient is taking warfarin
- Rivaroxaban should be taken with food to aid absorption.

PATIENT EDUCATION

- Signs and symptoms of VTE
- Modifiable risk factors (e.g., long periods of immobilization)
- Seek evaluation for any trauma.
- Medical alert bracelets

PROGNOSIS

- Recommend 3 to 6 months of treatment for provoked VTE with consideration for long-term anticoagulation in those with unprovoked VTE.
- HERDOO2 and DASH score may be considered in females with first unprovoked episode of VTE to consider discontinuation of long-term anticoagulation.
- Risk of recurrence among those with provoked VTE not currently on anticoagulation is 3.3% in the first year and lower thereafter.
- Patients with an unprovoked VTE not receiving chronic anticoagulation have risks of recurrence of 10% (year 1), 25% (year 5), and 36% (year 10).

REFERENCES

1. Middeldorp S, Nieuwlaat R, Baumann Kreuziger L, et al. American Society of Hematology 2023 guidelines for management of venous thromboembolism: thrombophilia testing. *Blood Adv*. 2023;7(22):7101–7138.
2. Connors JM. Thrombophilia testing and venous thrombosis. *N Engl J Med*. 2017;377(12):1177–1187.
3. Ortel TL, Neumann I, Ageno W, et al. American Society of Hematology 2020 guidelines for management of venous thromboembolism: treatment of deep vein thrombosis and pulmonary embolism. *Blood Adv*. 2020;4(19):4693–4738.

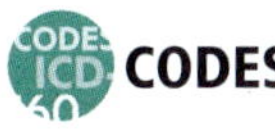

CODES

ICD10

- D68.59 Other primary thrombophilia
- D68.51 Activated protein C resistance
- D68.2 Hereditary deficiency of other clotting factors

CLINICAL PEARLS

- Assess for risk factors including malignancy, especially in those aged >50 years.
- The majority of patients with VTE should not be tested for thrombophilia.
- Use thrombophilia testing to guide future VTE prophylaxis, family screening, and evaluation of severe or fatal VTE. Do not use test results alone to determine anticoagulation duration.
- When assessing for hereditary thrombophilia, all tests should be performed a minimum of 2 weeks after completing anticoagulation course as protein C, protein S, and ATIII levels are affected by both acute thrombosis and anticoagulation.

THROMBOTIC THROMBOCYTOPENIC PURPURA

Chirag N. Shah, MD • Grant Wei, MD, FACEP • Jay Patel, DO

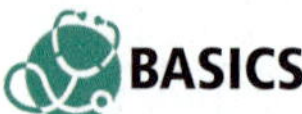

BASICS

DESCRIPTION

- An acute syndrome of microangiopathic hemolytic anemia (MAHA) and consumptive thrombocytopenia with deposition of hyaline thrombi in terminal arterioles and capillaries leads to ischemic multiorgan damage.
- Thrombotic thrombocytopenic purpura (TTP) is characterized by MAHA (schistocytes on peripheral smear) and thrombocytopenia (generally <30,000), with or without the following signs and symptoms:
  - Neurologic symptoms, renal dysfunction, fever
  - Most patients do not show the historic pentad of MAHA, thrombocytopenia, renal dysfunction, neurologic abnormalities, and fever because treatment is initiated before the pentad can develop.

EPIDEMIOLOGY

Incidence

- First episode mostly in adulthood (~90%) with a median age of 41 years and 10% in childhood to adolescence (1)[C]
- Predominant sex: female > male (2:1); higher relapse in females (1)[C]
- Incidence ratio of blacks to whites is 7:1.
- Other features with increased risk: high body mass index and pregnancy
- Annual incidence of ~3 new cases per million people

Prevalence

Annual prevalence of ~10 cases per million people

ETIOLOGY AND PATHOPHYSIOLOGY

- In TTP, the aggregating agent responsible for platelet thrombi is unusually large von Willebrand factor (UL vWF) multimers, which are far larger than those found in normal plasma.
- A metalloprotease, ADAMTS13, which normally enzymatically cleaves UL vWF multimers to prevent clumping within vessels, is deficient, defective, or absent, allowing UL vWF to react with platelets. This leads to endothelial cell damage and disseminated thrombi characteristic of TTP.
- Arterioles often affected: brain, kidney, pancreas, heart, adrenal glands; lungs and liver are relatively spared.
- In familial TTP, patients have an inherited deficiency of ADAMTS13.
- In acquired idiopathic TTP, autoantibodies are directed against the metalloprotease ADAMTS13 (1)[C].
- Endothelial injury, either directly from a drug/toxin or indirectly via platelet/neutrophil activation, has been proposed as a cause of secondary TTP especially in those without ADAMTS13 deficiency.

Genetics

- TTP is most often an acquired disorder. A congenital form of inherited TTP (Upshaw-Schulman syndrome) is due to a mutation at the ADAMTS13 gene locus on chromosome 9q34. This has an autosomal-recessive pattern of inheritance.
- USS typically presents in infancy and is rarely diagnosed after 10 years of age. It does not have the female predominance seen in idiopathic TTP, more often has notable renal impairment, and there is some heterogeneity among siblings.

RISK FACTORS

- Pregnancy, oral contraceptives, AIDS and early HIV infection, bacterial infection/sepsis, acute pancreatitis
- Autoimmune disease: antiphospholipid antibody syndrome, systemic lupus erythematosus, scleroderma
- Cancer, hematopoietic stem cell transplantation, and solid organ transplant
- Drugs of abuse: MDMA, cocaine, oxymorphone ER
- Drug toxicity
  - Antimicrobials: trimethoprim, ciprofloxacin, famciclovir
  - Chemotherapy: mitomycin C and gemcitabine, pentostatin and vincristine, bleomycin and cisplatin, oxaliplatin, bevacizumab and sunitinib, adalimumab, bortezomib, carfilzomib, and ixazomib
  - Calcineurin inhibitors: tacrolimus and cyclosporine
  - Immune mediated: quinine and quinidine, ticlopidine and clopidogrel

COMMONLY ASSOCIATED CONDITIONS

- TTP/hemolytic uremic syndrome (HUS)/atypical HUS have similar presentations with MAHA and thrombocytopenia and multiorgan involvement.
- TTP generally presents with minimal renal involvement and may have neurologic abnormalities, whereas the opposite is more characteristic of HUS/atypical HUS. Creatinine of >2 to 3 is not suggestive of TTP.
- However, patients with HUS and TTP may have both prominent renal and neurologic manifestations, often making the diagnosis unclear—hence the historical hybrid name "TTP-HUS."
- ADAMTS13 levels are diminished (generally <10%) in adults with familial or acquired idiopathic TTP but are normal in children diagnosed with HUS.

DIAGNOSIS

- Screening ADAMTS13 activity level
  - <10% defines severe deficiency and makes TTP more likely. Levels of 10–20% suggest possible TTP especially if drawn after plasma exchange (PEX) has been initiated. >20% makes TTP less likely.
  - Due to the high mortality associated with TTP, do not wait for the results of ADAMTS13 determination to initiate therapy.
- Most common symptoms are nonspecific: nausea, vomiting, weakness, abdominal pain, fatigue, and fever.
- Related to thrombocytopenia: easy bruising, purpura, petechiae, epistaxis, menorrhagia, bleeding gums, GI bleeding, intracranial hemorrhage—visual symptoms are due to retinal hemorrhages
- Related to hemolytic anemia (MAHA): jaundice, fatigue; end-organ ischemia
  - Neurologic: occurs in ~60% of the patients (1)[C]; headache, altered mental status, seizures, or stroke
  - Cardiac: arrhythmia, myocardial infarction, heart failure
  - Renal: hematuria, proteinuria, oliguria, or anuria
- A scoring system (PLASMIC) was devised to predict ADAMTS13 activity <10% in adults with unexplained thrombocytopenia and MAHA. It is used to support the diagnosis of TTP while the ADAMTS13 lab test is pending; 1 point each for:
  - Platelet count <30,000/μL
  - Hemolysis (reticulocyte count >2.5%, undetectable haptoglobin, or indirect bilirubin >2 mg/dL)
  - No active cancer
  - No solid organ or stem cell transplant history
  - MCV <90 fL
  - INR <1.5
  - Creatinine <2 mg/dL
  - Score of 6 to 7 predictive of ADAMTS13 activity of <10%; score of 0 to 4 predictive of ADAMTS13 activity was >10%.

HISTORY

- Generally, acute onset of symptoms but subacute in about 1/4 of patients
- In about 50% of cases, a trigger/risk factor of some kind is identified.

PHYSICAL EXAM

- Fever
- Mental status/neurologic: confusion, coma, stupor, weakness
- HEENT: retinal hemorrhage, scleral icterus, epistaxis
- Abdomen/GI: nonspecific tenderness
- Skin: jaundice, petechiae, purpura, ecchymoses

DIFFERENTIAL DIAGNOSIS

- HUS and atypical HUS
- Antiphospholipid antibody syndrome: prolonged partial thromboplastin time (PTT) and presence of lupus anticoagulant
- Systemic lupus erythematosus
- Malignant hypertension: diastolic blood pressure >130 mm Hg, papilledema, retinal hemorrhages
- Pregnancy-associated preeclampsia/eclampsia or hemolysis, elevated liver enzymes, and low platelets (HELLP) syndrome
- Disseminated intravascular coagulation
- Idiopathic thrombocytopenic purpura (ITP): no hemolysis, normal LDH, and bilirubin, presence of antiplatelet antibodies
- Malignancy-associated microangiopathy
- Evan syndrome (autoimmune hemolytic anemia and thrombocytopenia): positive direct Coombs test
- Sclerodermal kidney

DIAGNOSTIC TESTS & INTERPRETATION

Initial Tests (lab, imaging)

- CBC
  - Hemoglobin (decreased): Average is 8 to 10 g/dL; platelets decreased: in the 10 to 30,000/μL range
- High reticulocyte count (>120 × 10^9/L)
- Undetectable haptoglobin (hemolysis)
- Peripheral smear
  - Schistocytes (prominent, >1% of RBCs)
  - Helmet cells, RBC fragments, nucleated RBCs, polychromasia (reticulocytosis)
- Coagulation studies
  - Normal in most; mild elevation in 15%; fibrinogen is normal.
- Coombs test: negative direct Coombs test
- Electrolytes, BUN/creatinine: mild elevation of BUN and creatinine (creatinine <3 mg/dL)

- Liver function studies: increased indirect bilirubin (hemolysis)
- LDH: 5 to 10 times normal
- Urinalysis
  - Proteinuria, microscopic hematuria; positive dipstick for large blood but minimal RBCs on microscopic exam
- ECG changes (10%): sinus tachycardia, heart block
- Stool for Shiga toxin
- Increased troponin in 60% of cases (>0.1 μg/L)
- HIV, hepatitis A, B, and C testing: Exclude underlying viral precipitant.
- Pregnancy test (women with inherited TTP often have their first episode during their pregnancy)
- Head CT/MRI scan: in patients with mental status changes to rule out possible intracranial pathology

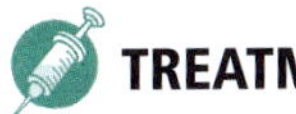

TREATMENT

ALERT

- Prompt treatment of presumptive or confirmed TTP is necessary due to the high mortality (90%).
- Complete response to treatment is defined by a platelet count $>150 \times 10^9$/L for 2 consecutive days, together with normal or normalizing LDH and clinical recovery (1)[C].
- In the absence of another apparent cause, the dyad of MAHA and thrombocytopenia is sufficient to begin treatment for TTP while the workup proceeds (1)[C].
  - PEX transfusion is the cornerstone of the treatment of TTP and should begin immediately.
  - The most effective therapy for TTP is PEX with fresh frozen plasma (FFP) (2)[A].
  - PEX replaces deficient or defective metalloprotease (ADAMTS13) and removes UL vWF and antimetalloprotease antibodies.
  - Optimal PEX duration is variable. Continue for 2 days after platelet count is ≥150,000 and then consider tapering.
  - FFP: temporary until PEX can be initiated; reserve for those with active bleeding.

MEDICATION

First Line

- Glucocorticoids have adjunctive benefit in some patients. The International Society on Thrombosis and Haemostasis guidelines recommend its use for all patients, due to the potential life-saving benefits compared to the adverse effects of short-term steroids (3)[C]. Steroids may work by suppressing the autoantibodies inhibiting ADAMTS13 activity.
  - May be used in patients with severe ADAMTS13 deficiency, in the setting of exacerbation when PEX is stopped or in relapse after remission; little benefit of steroids when used as monotherapy
  - Doses: prednisone 1 kg/day and taper once in remission or methylprednisolone 1 g/day IV for 3 days
- Rituximab, an anti-CD20 antibody that deletes B cells, may reduce relapse when given in conjunction with PEX and steroids; dose: 375 mg/m^2 IV once weekly for 4 weeks

Second Line

The following medications are used in refractory cases:

- Caplacizumab: a monoclonal antibody that inhibits vWF-glycoprotein 1b interaction; in patients with TTP, caplacizumab has been shown to reduce the time it takes for platelets to normalize, the length of the PEX, and the length of the hospital stay while not significantly raising the risk of adverse events.
- Intravenous immunoglobulin (IVIG)
- Splenectomy in the acute phase

ISSUES FOR REFERRAL

- Hematology or blood bank for PEX
- Nephrology for dialysis; cardiology for heart block or ischemia; neurosurgery for hemorrhage

ADDITIONAL THERAPIES

Recombinant ADAMTS13 is under investigation to be used as an alternative therapeutic agent.

SURGERY/OTHER PROCEDURES

Splenectomy is reserved for severe, refractory cases (1)[C].

ADMISSION, INPATIENT, AND NURSING CONSIDERATIONS

- ABCs, oxygen, IV access, telemetry
- Volume resuscitation if hypotensive/actively bleeding; packed RBCs can be transfused safely.
- Platelet transfusion may be used for the treatment of hemorrhage.
- Discharge on normalization and stabilization of neurologic symptoms, LDH, platelets, and renal function

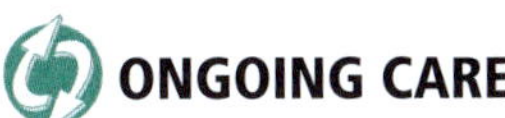

ONGOING CARE

FOLLOW-UP RECOMMENDATIONS

After PEX is discontinued, blood counts and ADAMTS13 activity should be monitored for months to evaluate for relapse.

PATIENT EDUCATION

- Self-monitor for signs of relapse (e.g., fever, headache, bruising) and prolonged periods of fatigue following the acute phase
- National Heart, Lung, and Blood Institute: https://www.nhlbi.nih.gov/health/thrombotic-thrombocytopenic-purpura

PROGNOSIS

- Most recover fully from idiopathic TTP when treated promptly:
  - 30-day mortality is 10% in those who receive PEX.
  - 70% respond within 14 days; 90% respond within 28 days; 80% survival in idiopathic TTP treated with PEX (1)
- Prior to widespread PEX treatment, TTP carried up to a 90% mortality rate.
- Initial LDH and platelet counts are not predictive of response to treatment.
- Final platelet count and LDH or the length or intensity of treatment do not predict relapse.
- Low levels of ADAMTS13 activity during remission are associated with higher risk of relapse (1)[C].
- Patients with severe ADAMTS13 deficiency had a risk of relapse which is estimated to be 41% at 7.5 years, with the greatest risk being in the 1st year.
- In patients with autoimmune TTP, there is a 40% relapse rate.

COMPLICATIONS

- Mild cognitive impairments in attention, concentration, and memory following ≥1 episode of TTP
- Complications of PEX: central line infections and hemorrhage, citrate toxicity, hypersensitivity reactions to frequent plasma exposure, electrolyte abnormalities

REFERENCES

1. Joly BS, Coppo P, Veyradier A. Thrombotic thrombocytopenic purpura. *Blood*. 2017;129(21):2836–2846.
2. Michael M, Elliott EJ, Ridley GF, et al. Interventions for haemolytic uraemic syndrome and thrombotic thrombocytopenic purpura. *Cochrane Database Syst Rev*. 2009;2009(1):CD003595.
3. Zheng XL, Vesely SK, Cataland SR, et al. ISTH guidelines for treatment of thrombotic thrombocytopenic purpura. *J Thromb Haemost*. 2020;18(10):2496–2502.

ADDITIONAL READING

Chen B, Li X, Xiao D, et al. Comparison of the efficacy and safety of caplacizumab versus placebo in thrombotic thrombocytopenic purpura: a meta-analysis and systematic review based on randomized controlled trials. *Ann Transl Med*. 2022;10(12):657.

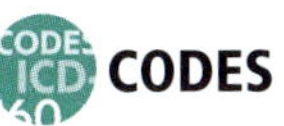

CODES

ICD10

- M31.1 Thrombotic microangiopathy
- D69.42 Congenital and hereditary thrombocytopenia purpura
- D69.3 Immune thrombocytopenic purpura

CLINICAL PEARLS

- The diagnosis of TTP is made clinically; symptoms are nonspecific: nausea; vomiting; weakness; abdominal pain; fatigue; fever; and easy bruising, purpura, or petechiae.
- The pentad of fever, neurologic symptoms, renal dysfunction, MAHA, and thrombocytopenia is not present in most patients.
- The dyad of MAHA (schistocytes on peripheral smear) and severe thrombocytopenia (<30,000) is sufficient to initiate treatment with PEX.
- Do not wait for the results of ADAMTS13 determination to initiate therapy.

THYROID MALIGNANT NEOPLASIA

Jennifer L. Gilley, DO • Jared Dendy, MD, FACP, ECNU

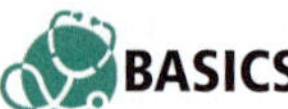

BASICS

Thyroid cancer accounts for 2.2% of all newly diagnosed cancers and 0.4% of cancer related deaths. Thyroid cancer has an overall five-year survival rate around 98.4% (2014–2020) in the United States. Thyroid cancers subclassified as papillary, follicular, medullary, or anaplastic. Thyroid nodules are very common—only 5% are malignant. Diagnosis involves imaging and tissue sampling with most treatments with surgical resection, some with radioactive iodine ablation, and very few with systemic chemotherapy.

DESCRIPTION

- Papillary thyroid carcinoma (PTC)
  - Most common type, 75–80% of thyroid cancers
  - Peak age of incidence: 40 to 60 years
  - Most common form of pediatric thyroid cancer
  - Associated with radiation exposure, especially if exposure occurred in childhood
  - Metastasizes by lymphatic route (15–30% have palpable cervical lymphadenopathy at time of diagnosis)
  - Many subtypes: conventional (classic), follicular variant, oxyphilic, cribriform-morular, and more aggressive forms such as tall cell or diffuse sclerosing
- Follicular carcinoma
  - Makes up around ~10% of thyroid cancers in iodine sufficient areas (up to 25–40% in areas that are iodine deficient)
  - Peak age of incidence: 60 years
  - Associated with radiation exposure and iodine deficiency
  - Metastasizes by the hematogenous route
  - Can be divided into invasive and minimally invasive forms based on morphology
    - Oncocytic carcinoma (formerly Hürthle cell carcinoma) which tends to be more aggressive was originally considered a variant of follicular thyroid carcinoma; it is now suggested that it is its own distinct entity variant
      - Overall poorer prognosis
- Medullary thyroid carcinoma (MTC)
  - 3–4% of all thyroid carcinoma
  - 25–35% are associated with multiple endocrine neoplasia (MEN) syndromes.
  - Peak age of incidence: 50 to 60 years
  - MTC associated with MEN2B occur in childhood, those with MEN2A occur in young adults, and those with familial non-MEN medullary thyroid cancer (FMTC) occur in middle age.
  - Calcitonin is a serologic marker and is used in diagnostic workup for this form of thyroid cancer only.
  - *RET* proto-oncogene mutation is used for germline mutation screening; family members who carry the *RET* gene may consider early prophylactic thyroidectomy.
- Anaplastic carcinoma
  - 1–3% of thyroid tumors
  - Most common in elderly patients
  - Most aggressive form of thyroid neoplasia
  - Almost uniformly fatal (median survival 2 to 6 months)
- Other: poorly differentiated thyroid carcinoma, lymphoma, sarcoma, or metastatic (renal, breast, or lung)

Geriatric Considerations

Risk of malignancy (ROM) increases, and prognosis is worse if >60 years old.

Pediatric Considerations

- Thyroid nodules are more frequently malignant (22–25% in children vs. 5–10% in adults).
- <2% of thyroid malignancies occur in children and adolescents.
- Increased tumor size (>4 cm), extrathyroidal extension, and multifocal disease are independent factors associated with nodal metastases in pediatric differentiated thyroid cancer and require further evaluation with fine needle aspiration (FNA) for suspicious nodes to consider neck dissection (1)[C].

EPIDEMIOLOGY

- Incidence: 13.5/100,000 per year for men and women in the United States from 2017 to 2021.
- Deaths: 0.5/100,000 per year for men and women in the United States from 2018 to 2022.
- Predominant age: usually >40 years old
- Predominant sex: female > male (3:1) prevalence

ETIOLOGY AND PATHOPHYSIOLOGY

- No established etiologic factors of pathogenesis; most cases arise spontaneously.
- Radiation exposure likely has a role in the development of thyroid malignancies.

Genetics

Gene mutations that activate the MAPK pathway (e.g., *BRAF*) and PI3K-AKT pathway (e.g., PTEN) have been implicated.

RISK FACTORS

- Family history (first-degree relative)
- Radiation exposure: papillary carcinoma
- Iodine deficiency: follicular carcinoma
- MEN2: medullary carcinoma

GENERAL PREVENTION

- Screening is only recommended for high-risk groups such as individuals with MEN2A or MEN2B
- Screening includes calcitonin stimulation screening, physical exam, and testing for the RET proto-oncogene

COMMONLY ASSOCIATED CONDITIONS

- Papillary carcinoma: Hashimoto thyroiditis
- Medullary carcinoma: pheochromocytoma, hyperparathyroidism, ganglioneuroma of the GI tract, neuroma of mucosal membranes

DIAGNOSIS

HISTORY

- If not found incidentally, can present with a firm immobile neck mass with or without cervical lymphadenopathy
- More concerning symptoms includes the following:
  - Change in voice (dysphonia)
  - Difficulty swallowing (dysphagia)
  - Difficulty breathing (dyspnea or orthopnea)
  - Stridor (in aggressive cancer)

PHYSICAL EXAM

Fixed immobile thyroid nodule with or without cervical lymphadenopathy (nodules will often move with swallowing)

DIFFERENTIAL DIAGNOSIS

- Multinodular goiter
- Thyroid adenoma
- Thyroglossal duct or dermoid cyst
- Thyroiditis
- Thyroid cyst
- Ectopic thyroid

DIAGNOSTIC TESTS & INTERPRETATION

Initial Tests (lab, imaging)

- When a thyroid nodule is found, first steps include obtaining a TSH and thyroid ultrasound including ultrasound of cervical lymph nodes (2),(3)[C].
  - Most thyroid cancers show up as "cold" (nonhormone producing) nodules. TSH therefore is typically normal.
- The appearance of the thyroid nodule is graded using TI-RADS diagnostic criteria as more or less suspicious for malignancy on a 5-point scale with 5 being highly suspicious. TI-RADS provides guidance regarding if more invasive investigation is needed and how often a nodule should be reevaluated for change.
  - Characteristics concerning for malignancy include hypoechoic pattern, shape that is taller than wide, microcalcifications, and irregular margins.
- When there is adequate suspicion for malignancy, an ultrasound guided FNA should be obtained (3)[C].
- FNA samples are graded as more or less suspicious for malignancy using the BETHESDA criteria (3)[C].
- Molecular studies (point mutations, translocations, etc.) can be considered if an indeterminate BETHESDA score (III or IV) is given to help further classify risk (3)[C]

Follow-Up Tests & Special Considerations

- CT or MRI neck: useful to evaluate large substernal masses, extent of invasion, if suspicion of MTC with neck disease or calcitonin >500 pg/mL, and to evaluate for recurrent disease (3)[C]
- Calcitonin levels: Measure in patients with FNA results suggestive of MTC or personal or family history of MEN2 (consider IV pentagastrin stimulation test to increase sensitivity; not available in United States or Canada).
- In patients with MTC, can consider genetic testing for *RET* proto-oncogene
- Thyroid scan: 12–15% of cold nodules are malignant; rate is higher in patients <40 years of age and those with microcalcifications on ultrasound. ^{18}F-FDG PET scan can help if the cytology is indeterminate; also helpful with recurrent disease when patient has a negative ^{131}I scan and an elevated thyroglobulin (TG) level (2)[C].
- Thyroglobulin (TG): not recommended in initial evaluation as it can be elevated in multiple diseases; used only as postoperative tumor marker for recurrence (2)[C].

Diagnostic Procedures/Other

Flexible fiberoptic laryngoscopy: if vocal cord paralysis is suspected and in high-risk disease

Test Interpretation

- FNA: The 2023 Bethesda System for Reporting Thyroid Cytopathology classification of cytology
  - Nondiagnostic (BETHESDA I): 5–20% ROM
  - Benign (BETHESDA II): 2–7% ROM
  - Atypia of undetermined significance (AUS) (BETHESDA III): 13–30% ROM
  - Follicular neoplasm (BETHESDA IV): 23–34% ROM
  - Suspicious for malignancy (BETHESDA V): 67–83% ROM
  - Malignant (BETHESDA VI): 97–100% ROM
  - *BETHESDA III and BETHESDA IV can be considered indeterminate and may warrant genetic markers testing
- Papillary: psammoma bodies, anaplastic epithelial papillae, nuclear grooves, and "Orphan Annie Eye" nuclei
- Follicular: anaplastic epithelial cords with colloid filled follicles similar in appearance to thyroid adenoma except that capsular or vascular invasion is evident
- Oncocytic (formerly Hürthle cell): large eosinophilic cells with granular cytoplasm
- Medullary: large amounts of amyloid stroma; originates from C-Cells
- Anaplastic: Numerous mitotic figures and atypical mitoses are present with extensive necrosis.

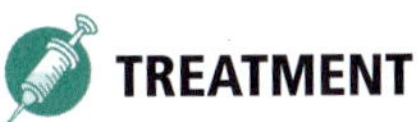

TREATMENT

GENERAL MEASURES

- Most cases of thyroid cancer are managed surgically (either a total thyroidectomy or lobectomy) and medically with a good prognosis (2)[C].
- Palliative support has a role in case of advanced thyroid malignancy.
- Papillary and follicular: ^{131}I thyroid remnant ablation or adjuvant therapy
- In cases of multiple comorbidities (high surgical risk) or limited life expectancy observation without surgical intervention can be considered (2)[C].

MEDICATION

After total thyroidectomy, hormone replacement therapy with levothyroxine (T4) will be required.

- TSH suppression therapy may reduce recurrence with goal to keep TSH <0.1 mU/L for patients with a high recurrence risk, 0.1 to 0.5 mU/L for patients with a moderate recurrence risk, and 0.5 to 2.0 mU/L for patients at low risk for recurrence (2)[C].

ADDITIONAL THERAPIES

- External beam radiation or chemotherapy may be considered for radioactive iodine insensitive tumors, inoperable recurrence, and for palliative care.
- ^{131}I is used in high-risk patients with papillary and follicular tumors. The role is to ablate any remnant thyroid tissue to improve specificity of future TG assays to monitor for recurrence, and to eliminate any microscopic residual cancer not removed at the time of surgery. ^{131}I is also used to treat metastatic papillary or follicular tumors.

SURGERY/OTHER PROCEDURES

- Papillary: total thyroidectomy with elective neck dissection for suspicious lymph nodes in central or lateral neck compartments or for large tumors (>4 cm in size); lobectomy with isthmectomy can be considered if lesion <1 cm in low-risk patient (controversial).
- Follicular and Hürthle cell: similar management as papillary carcinoma
- Medullary: total thyroidectomy with central node dissection; unilateral or bilateral modified radical neck dissection if lateral nodes are suspicious
- Anaplastic: palliative care; no adequate treatment available and surgery is controversial; consider tracheostomy (to protect airway) and clinical trials using chemotherapy/radiation.

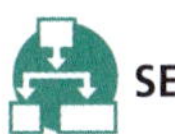

ONGOING CARE

FOLLOW-UP RECOMMENDATIONS

Patient Monitoring

- 10–30% of initially disease-free patients will develop recurrence and/or metastases. 80% recur in neck and 20% with distant metastases (lung).
- TSH, TG, and anti-TG antibodies at 6 months, 12 months, then annually; can screen more frequently if results are concerning.
- Periodic ultrasound to monitor for recurrence is recommended in intermediate- to high-risk patients; may also consider TSH-stimulated radioiodine whole body imaging in high-risk patients.
- Medullary thyroid cancer: Calcitonin level should be done yearly (3)[C].

DIET

Low-iodine diet recommended in patients undergoing radioactive iodine therapy following surgery

PATIENT EDUCATION

- National Cancer Institute: https://www.cancer.gov/types/thyroid/patient/thyroid-treatment-pdq
- American Thyroid Association: https://www.thyroid.org/thyroid-information/

PROGNOSIS

- 5-year survival of thyroid cancer is 98.4%.
- Papillary carcinoma: Overall 5-year survival rate taking into account all stages: 99.6%. Survival rate with distant metastasis is 67.8%.
- Follicular carcinoma: Overall 5-year survival rate taking into account all stages: 98.5%. Survival rate with distant metastasis is 67.8%.
- Oncocytic carcinoma (formerly Hürthle cell carcinoma): 93% 5-year survival rate and 83% survival rate overall; grossly invasive tumor survival <25%
- Medullary carcinoma: Overall 5-year survival taking into account all stages: 91%. Survival rate with distant metastasis is 43%.
- Anaplastic carcinoma: Overall five year survival taking into account all stages: <10%. Survival rate with distant metastasis is <5%.

COMPLICATIONS

- Hoarseness either from tumor invasion or iatrogenic injury to recurrent laryngeal nerve
- Hypocalcemia/hypoparathyroidism from devascularization of parathyroid glands during surgery (usually transient)

REFERENCES

1. Francis GL, Waguespack SG, Bauer AJ, et al; for American Thyroid Association Guidelines Task Force. Management guidelines for children with thyroid nodules and differentiated thyroid cancer. *Thyroid*. 2015;25(7):716–759.
2. Haugen BR, Alexander EK, Bible KC, et al. 2015 American Thyroid Association management guidelines for adult patients with thyroid nodules and differentiated thyroid cancer: the American Thyroid Association Guidelines Task Force on thyroid nodules and differentiated thyroid cancer. *Thyroid*. 2016;26(1):1–133.
3. Wells SA Jr, Asa SL, Dralle H, et al; for American Thyroid Association Guidelines Task Force on Medullary Thyroid Carcinoma. Revised American Thyroid Association guidelines for the management of medullary thyroid carcinoma. *Thyroid*. 2015;25(6):567–610.

ADDITIONAL READING

- Ali SZ, Baloch ZW, Cochand-Priollet B, et al. The 2023 Bethesda System for reporting thyroid cytopathology. *J Am Soc Cytopathol*. 2023;12(5):319–325.
- Boucai L, Zafereo M, Cabanillas ME. Thyroid cancer: a review. *JAMA*. 2024;331(5):425–435.

SEE ALSO

Multiple Endocrine Neoplasia (MEN) Syndromes

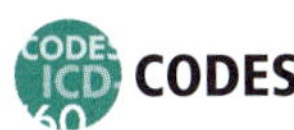

CODES

ICD10

C73 Malignant neoplasm of thyroid gland

CLINICAL PEARLS

- Workup for all patients with a thyroid nodule includes TSH and thyroid and neck ultrasound then, and based on TI-RADS score of any found nodules, either observation or FNA
- FNA results will be graded using BETHESDA criteria and result in surgical intervention or observation.
- In those with confirmed thyroid cancer, serial monitoring with TG, TG-antibody, and thyroid/neck ultrasound is recommended along with TSH suppression.

THYROIDITIS

Munima Nasir, MD, FAAFP • Sonali Bhat, MD

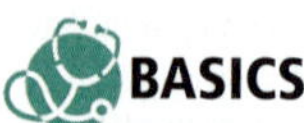

BASICS

DESCRIPTION

- Inflammatory dysfunction of the thyroid gland
- Painful thyroiditis:
  - Subacute granulomatous thyroiditis—nonsuppurative thyroiditis, de Quervain thyroiditis, giant cell thyroiditis
  - Infectious/suppurative thyroiditis is most commonly associated with *Streptococcus* and *Staphylococcus* spp. but can be due to fungal, mycobacterial, or parasitic thyroid infections. Radiation-induced thyroiditis: from radioactive iodine therapy (1%) or external irradiation
- Painless thyroiditis
  - Hashimoto (autoimmune) thyroiditis: most common etiology of chronic hypothyroidism; 90% of patients with high-serum antithyroid peroxidase (TPO) antibodies
  - Postpartum thyroiditis (PPT): thyrotoxicosis followed by hypothyroidism in the 1st year postpartum or after spontaneous/induced abortion
  - Painless (silent) thyroiditis: mild hyperthyroidism
  - Riedel (fibrous) thyroiditis: rare inflammatory process involving the thyroid and surrounding cervical tissues
  - Drug-induced: interferon-α, interleukin-2, amiodarone, kinase inhibitors, or lithium
  - Radiation-induced: from radioactive iodine therapy (1%) or external irradiation

EPIDEMIOLOGY

- Subacute granulomatous thyroiditis: most common cause of thyroid pain; peaks during summer; incidence: 3/100,000/year; female > male (4:1); peak age: 40 to 50 years
- Hashimoto thyroiditis (HT): peak onset 30 to 50 years of age; can occur in children; female > male (7:1)
- PPT: occurs within 12 months of pregnancy in 1–18% of pregnancies
- Painless (silent) thyroiditis: accounts for 1–5% of cases; female > male (4:1) with peak age 30 to 40 years; common in areas of iodine sufficiency
- Riedel thyroiditis: female > male (4:1); highest prevalence age 30 to 60 years; rare with estimated incidence of 1.06 cases per 100,000 patients

ETIOLOGY AND PATHOPHYSIOLOGY

- Subacute granulomatous thyroiditis: probably viral; can be associated with COVID-19 infection; the mechanism of thyroid injury can be due to direct destruction of thyroid tissue, as well as indirect immune-mediated responses, medicines used to treat COVID-19, and less frequently COVID-19 vaccinations (1).
- Hashimoto disease: Antithyroid antibodies may be produced in response to an environmental antigen and cross-react with thyroid proteins (molecular mimicry). Precipitating factors include infection, stress, sex steroids, pregnancy, iodine intake, and radiation exposure.
- PPT: autoimmunity-induced discharge of preformed hormone from the thyroid
- Painless (silent) thyroiditis: autoimmune
- Riedel (fibrous) thyroiditis: rare inflammatory process involving the thyroid and surrounding cervical tissues; associated with various forms of systemic fibrosis

Genetics

Autoimmune thyroiditis is associated with the CT60 polymorphism of cytotoxic T-cell lymphocyte–associated antigen 4; also associated with HLA-DR4, HLA-DR5, and HLA-DR6 in whites

RISK FACTORS

- Subacute granulomatous thyroiditis: recent viral respiratory infection, such as COVID-19 infection, or HLA-B35
- Hashimoto disease: family/personal history of thyroid/autoimmune disease, high iodine intake, cigarette smoking, selenium deficiency

GENERAL PREVENTION

Emerging evidence may support vitamin D or selenium supplementation, but more research is needed (2).

DIAGNOSIS

HISTORY

- Hypothyroid symptoms (e.g., constipation, heavy menstrual bleeding, fatigue, weakness, dry skin, hair loss, cold intolerance)
- Hyperthyroid symptoms (e.g., irritability, heat intolerance, increased sweating, palpitations, loose stools, disturbed sleep, and lid retraction)
- Subacute granulomatous thyroiditis: sudden/gradual onset, with preceding upper respiratory infection/viral illness (fever, fatigue, malaise, anorexia, and myalgia are common); pain may be limited to thyroid region or radiate to upper neck, jaw, throat, or ears. Patients with COVID-19 infection may be more likely to have a painless presentation (1). Post-COVID-19 fatigue may be associated with hypothyroid phase of subacute thyroiditis.
- Classic triphasic course (thyrotoxic, hypothyroid, recovery) but variable in the following: subacute, silent, and PPT

PHYSICAL EXAM

- Hashimoto disease: 90% have a symmetric, diffusely enlarged, painless thyroid gland, with a firm, pebbly texture; 10% have atrophy.
- PPT: painless, small, nontender, firm goiter (2 to 6 months after delivery)
- Riedel thyroiditis: rock-hard, wood-like, fixed, painless goiter, often accompanied by symptoms of esophageal/tracheal compression (stridor, dyspnea, a suffocating feeling, dysphagia, and hoarseness); should be considered when restrictive and infiltrative symptoms are out of proportion of the size of the mass on exam.
- Signs of hypothyroid: delayed relaxation phase of deep tendon reflexes, nonpitting edema, dry skin, alopecia, bradycardia
- Signs of hyperthyroid: moist palms, hyperreflexia, tachycardia/atrial fibrillation

DIFFERENTIAL DIAGNOSIS

Simple goiter; iodine-deficient/lithium-induced goiter; Graves' disease (GD); lymphoma; oropharynx and trachea infections; thyroid cancer; amiodarone; contrast dye; amyloid

DIAGNOSTIC TESTS & INTERPRETATION

- Subacute granulomatous (de Quervain) thyroiditis
  - In the thyrotoxic phase, decreased TSH; elevated T4, ESR, CRP, WBC count; mild anemia
  - 25% of patients have low concentrations of antithyroid antibodies.
  - ESR normalizes during hypothyroid phase.
  - Consider ultrasound (US) to rule out thyroid cancer.
- Suppurative (acute) thyroiditis (thyroid abscess)
  - Generally, patients are euthyroid; occasionally presents with destructive thyrotoxicosis
  - US or CT scan is usually diagnostic. Fine needle aspiration (FNA) can confirm diagnosis (3)[C].
- HT
  - Anti-TPO antibodies present in 95% of cases.
  - Antithyroglobulin antibodies present in 60–80%.
  - Ultrasonography may demonstrate decreased echogenicity and hypoechoic nodules with an echogenic rim (4)[C].
- PPT
  - Thyroid antibodies (TPOAb, TgAb) present
    - If Ab positive in the first trimester, higher risk of developing PPT
    - Higher Ab titers, higher risk of PPT
  - Must distinguish from thyrotoxicosis caused by GD (which has a positive TSH receptor antibody, high radioiodine uptake, and specific physical findings [e.g., goiter, ophthalmopathy])
  - After the thyrotoxic phase, obtain a TSH level in 4 to 8 weeks (or if the patient develops new symptoms) to screen for the hypothyroid phase.
  - If the patient has a history of PPT, screen for permanent hypothyroidism with an annual TSH level.
- Painless (silent) thyroiditis
  - 5–20% of patients undergo a thyrotoxic phase that lasts 3 to 4 months.
  - Thyroid function normalizes within 12 months.
  - ~50% of patients have anti-TPO antibodies.
  - Absence of TSH receptor antibodies distinguishes from GD (3)[C].
- Riedel thyroiditis
  - Thyroglobulin and TPO antibody titers are elevated (likely due to simultaneous Hashimoto disease).
  - 72% of individuals have elevated CRP and 97% have elevated ESR.
  - Parathyroid involvement can cause hypocalcemia.
  - Histology confirms diagnosis and reveals a fibroinflammatory process.
- Drug-induced thyroiditis
  - Thyroid function test results vary and depend on the offending medication. Thyrotoxicosis is common. Lithium is associated with hypothyroidism (3)[C].

Initial Tests (lab, imaging)

TSH, free T4, T3; antithyroid antibodies

Follow-Up Tests & Special Considerations

- US: shows variable heterogeneous texture, hypoechogenic in subacute, painless (silent), and PPT
- Thyroid RAIU scan: decreased in all forms of thyroiditis but not helpful in establishing diagnosis of Hashimoto disease; high RAIU in hashitoxicosis, GD
- Random urine iodine measurement may be helpful to distinguish from other causes of low RAIU.
  - Urine iodine <500 μg/L (subacute granulomatous thyroiditis)
  - Urine iodine >1,000 μg/L (in patients with exposure to excess exogenous iodine/radiocontrast material)

Diagnostic Procedures/Other

- Hashimoto with a dominant nodule should have FNA to rule out thyroid carcinoma.
- Open biopsy is necessary for a definitive diagnosis of Reidel thyroiditis.

Test Interpretation

- Subacute granulomatous thyroiditis: giant cells, mononuclear cell infiltrate
- Hashimoto: lymphocytic infiltration with Hürthle cells, fibrosis, thyroid atrophy
- Postpartum and painless (silent) thyroiditis: lymphocytic infiltration

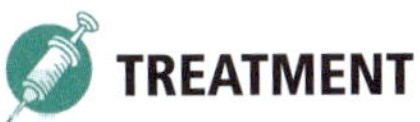

TREATMENT

GENERAL MEASURES

- If thyrotoxic and symptomatic: propylthiouracil and propranolol, except not used in PPT or painless thyroiditis
- An elevated TSH level in a woman who is pregnant or attempting to become pregnant is an indication for thyroid replacement.

MEDICATION

- Subacute granulomatous thyroiditis
  - β-Blockers and NSAIDs may be used to treat mild symptomatic cases.
  - Prednisone 40 mg QD × 1 to 2 weeks, followed by 2- to 4-week taper in severe cases
  - Levothyroxine may be used in the hypothyroid phase. Discontinue after 3 to 6 months with normalization of thyroid function (3)[C].
- Suppurative (acute) thyroiditis (thyroid abscess)
  - Systemic antibiotics
  - Abscess drainage or removal
  - Excision or occlusion of the pyriform sinus (3)[C]
- HT
  - Levothyroxine 1.6 to 1.8 μg/kg
- PPT
  - Treatment is guided by stage.
  - Metoprolol and propranolol for lactating women in the thyrotoxic state; antithyroid medications are not recommended.
  - If lactating or trying to conceive, treat symptomatic hypothyroidism.
  - Levothyroxine may be tapered starting at 12 months postpartum. Monitor TSH every 6 to 8 weeks. Avoid tapering if a woman is trying to conceive or is pregnant (5)[C].
- Painless (silent) thyroiditis
  - If symptomatic during hyperthyroid state, treat with β-blocker.
  - Antithyroid medications are unnecessary.
  - For severe cases, corticosteroids may reduce the severity and length of the hyperthyroid state (3)[C].
- Reidel thyroiditis (no management consensus)
  - Medical therapy is first line in absence of obstructive symptoms. Medical therapies have not been validated by RCTs due to the rarity of the condition. However, glucocorticoids are recommended as first line, and tamoxifen is second-line treatment.
  - Treat hypothyroidism with levothyroxine and hypoparathyroidism with calcium and calcitriol.
  - Debulking surgery if obstruction present
- Drug-induced thyroiditis
  - Discontinue offending drug.

COMPLEMENTARY & ALTERNATIVE MEDICINE

- Emerging evidence that vitamin D and selenium have positive impacts on the treatment of HT (6),(7).
- Studies show a combination of myoinositol + selenium may reduce the presence of thyroid antibodies and proinflammatory chemokines. However, more research is needed (2).

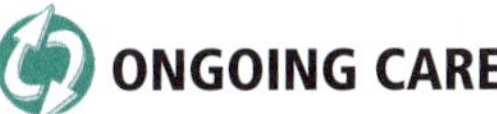

ONGOING CARE

FOLLOW-UP RECOMMENDATIONS

Patient Monitoring

- Subacute granulomatous thyroiditis: Repeat thyroid function tests every 3 to 6 weeks until euthyroid and then every 6 to 12 months.
- Hashimoto disease: Repeat thyroid function tests every 3 to 12 months.
- PPT: Check TSH annually.
- Reidel thyroiditis: Consider CT scan if extrathyroidal disease is suspected.
- Check thyroid function before and after 3 months of starting amiodarone. Then monitor every 3 to 6 months.

Pregnancy Considerations

^{131}I is contraindicated in breastfeeding women.

PROGNOSIS

- Subacute granulomatous thyroiditis: Most patients are euthyroid at 12 months. 5–15% have persistent hypothyroidism.
- Hashimoto disease: persistent goiter; eventual thyroid failure
- PPT: Thyroid function normalizes in 12 months. 10–20% of patients have persistent hypothyroidism.
- Painless (silent) thyroiditis: 5–20% of patients undergo a thyrotoxic phase that lasts 3 to 4 months.
- Riedel Thyroiditis: 90% have improvement or resolution of symptoms within 12 months. It is unclear at this time what factors contribute to poor prognosis due to the rarity of the condition.

REFERENCES

1. Meftah E, Rahmati R, Zari Meidani F, et al. Subacute thyroiditis following COVID-19: a systematic review. *Front Endocrinol (Lausanne)*. 2023;14:1126637.
2. Tywanek E, Michalak A, Świrska J, et al. Autoimmunity, new potential biomarkers and the thyroid gland—the perspective of Hashimoto's thyroiditis and its treatment. *Int J Mol Sci*. 2024;25(9):4703.
3. Ross DS, Burch HB, Cooper DS, et al. 2016 American Thyroid Association guidelines for diagnosis and management of hyperthyroidism and other causes of thyrotoxicosis. *Thyroid*. 2016;26(10):1343–1421.
4. Ralli M, Angeletti D, Fiore M, et al. Hashimoto's thyroiditis: an update on pathogenic mechanisms, diagnostic protocols, therapeutic strategies, and potential malignant transformation. *Autoimmun Rev*. 2020;19(10):102649.
5. Alexander EK, Pearce EN, Brent GA, et al. 2017 Guidelines of the American Thyroid Association for the diagnosis and management of thyroid disease during pregnancy and the postpartum. *Thyroid*. 2017;27(3):315–389.
6. Lebiedziński F, Lisowska KA. Impact of vitamin D on immunopathology of Hashimoto's thyroiditis: from theory to practice. *Nutrients*. 2023;15(14):3174.
7. Huwiler VV, Maissen-Abgottspon S, Stanga Z, et al. Selenium supplementation in patients with Hashimoto thyroiditis: a systematic review and meta-analysis of randomized clinical trials. *Thyroid*. 2024;34(3):295–313.

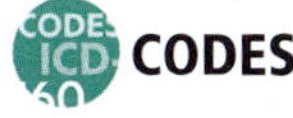

CODES

ICD10

- E06.5 Other chronic thyroiditis
- E06.0 Acute thyroiditis
- E06 Thyroiditis

CLINICAL PEARLS

HT is the most common etiology of chronic hypothyroidism.

TINEA (CAPITIS, CORPORIS, CRURIS)

Daniel Scott Morrison, MD • Chirag N. Shah, MD • Shivam Kaushik, DO

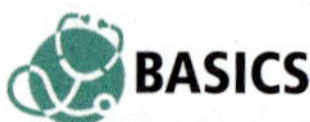

BASICS

DESCRIPTION

- Superficial fungal infections of the skin/scalp; various forms of dermatophytosis; the names relate to the particular area affected.
  - Tinea cruris: infection of crural fold and gluteal cleft
  - Tinea corporis: infection involving the face, trunk, and/or extremities; often presents with ring-shaped lesions, hence the misnomer *ringworm*
  - Tinea capitis: infection of the scalp and hair; affected areas of the scalp can show characteristic black dots resulting from broken hairs.
- Dermatophytes have the ability to subsist on protein, namely keratin.
- They cause disease in keratin-rich structures such as skin, nails, and hair.
- Infections result from contact with infected persons/animals.
  - Zoophilic infections are acquired from animals.
  - Anthropophilic infections are acquired from personal contact (e.g., wrestling) or fomites.
  - Geophile infections are acquired from the soil
- System(s) affected: skin, exocrine
- Synonym(s): jock itch; ringworm

EPIDEMIOLOGY

Incidence

- Tinea cruris
  - Predominant age: any age; rare in children
  - Predominant sex: male > female
- Tinea corporis
  - Predominant age: postpubertal children and young adults
  - Predominant sex: male = female
- Tinea capitis
  - Predominant age: 3 to 9 years; almost always occurs in young children
  - Predominant sex: male = female

Prevalence

Common worldwide with dramatic increase over the past two decades due to more frequent international travel, socioeconomic problems, and contact with animals, specifically pets

Pediatric Considerations

- Tinea cruris is rare prior to puberty.
- Tinea capitis is common in young children.

Geriatric Considerations

Tinea cruris is more common in the geriatric population due to an increase in risk factors.

Pregnancy Considerations

Tinea cruris and capitis are rare in pregnancy.

ETIOLOGY AND PATHOPHYSIOLOGY

Superficial fungal infection of skin/scalp

- Tinea cruris: Source of infection is usually the patient's own tinea pedis, with agent being transferred from the foot to the groin via the underwear when dressing; most common causative dermatophyte is *Trichophyton interdigitale*; rare cases caused by *Epidermophyton floccosum* and *Trichophyton mentagrophytes* (1).
- Tinea corporis: most commonly caused by *Trichophyton rubrum*; other notable causes include *Trichophyton tonsurans*, *Microsporum canis*, *Trichophyton interdigitale*, *Microsporum gypseum*, *Trichophyton violaceum*, and *Microsporum audouinii*. It can also be caused by Epidermophyton (1).
- Tinea capitis: *T. tonsurans* found in 90% and *Microsporum* sp. in 10% of patients. There may be a geographic predilection for certain organisms (2)[A],(3)[B].

Genetics

Evidence suggests a genetic susceptibility in certain individuals.

RISK FACTORS

- Warm climates; summer months and/or copious sweating; wearing wet clothing/multiple layers (tinea cruris)
- Daycare centers/schools/confined quarters (tinea corporis and capitis)
- Depression of cell-mediated immune response (e.g., individuals with atopy or AIDS)
- Obesity (tinea cruris and corporis)
- Direct contact with an active lesion on a human, an animal, or rarely, from soil; working with animals (tinea corporis)
- Cushing syndrome (tinea corporis)

GENERAL PREVENTION

- Avoidance of risk factors, such as contact with suspicious lesions
- Fluconazole or itraconazole may be useful in wrestlers to prevent outbreaks during competitive season.

COMMONLY ASSOCIATED CONDITIONS

Tinea pedis, tinea barbae, tinea manus

DIAGNOSIS

HISTORY

- Lesions range from asymptomatic to pruritic.
- In tinea cruris, acute inflammation may result from wearing occlusive clothing; chronic scratching may result in an eczematous appearance.
- Previous application of topical steroids, especially in tinea cruris and corporis, may alter the overall appearance causing a more extensive eruption with irregular borders and erythematous papules. This modified form is called *tinea incognito*.

PHYSICAL EXAM

- Tinea cruris: well-marginated, erythematous, half-moon–shaped plaques in crural folds that spread to medial thighs; advancing border is well-defined, often with fine scaling and sometimes vesicular eruptions. Lesions are usually bilateral and do not include the scrotum/penis (unlike *Candida* infections) but may migrate to the perineum, perianal area, and gluteal cleft and onto the buttocks in chronic/progressive cases. The area may be hyperpigmented on resolution.
- Tinea corporis: scaling, round or oval pruritic plaques characterized by a sharply defined annular pattern with peripheral activity and central clearing (ring-shaped lesions) involving the face, trunk, and/or extremities; papules and occasionally pustules/vesicles present at border and, less commonly, in center
- Tinea capitis: commonly begins with round patches of scale involving scalp (alopecia less common). In its later stages, the infection frequently takes on patterns of chronic scaling with either little/marked inflammation or alopecia. Less often, patients will present with multiple patches of alopecia and the characteristic black-dot appearance of broken hairs. Extreme inflammation results in kerion formation (exudative, pustular nodulation). Severity of kerion is from one (few pustules with erythema) to four (pustules and erythema with alopecia and scarring).

DIFFERENTIAL DIAGNOSIS

- Tinea cruris
  - Intertrigo: inflammatory process of moist-opposed skin folds, often including infection with bacteria, yeast, and fungi; painful longitudinal fissures may occur in skin folds.
  - Erythrasma: diffuse brown, scaly, noninflammatory plaque with irregular borders, often involving groin; caused by bacterial infection with *Corynebacterium minutissimum*; fluoresces coral red with Wood lamp
  - Seborrheic dermatitis of groin
  - Psoriasis of groin ("inverse psoriasis")
  - Candidiasis of groin (typically involves the scrotum)
  - Acanthosis nigricans
- Tinea capitis
  - Psoriasis
  - Seborrheic dermatitis
  - Pyoderma
  - Alopecia areata and trichotillomania
  - Aplasia cutis congenital
  - Acne
  - Cellulitis
- Tinea corporis
  - Pityriasis rosea
  - Eczema (nummular)
  - Contact dermatitis
  - Secondary syphilis
  - Psoriasis
  - Seborrheic dermatitis
  - Subacute systemic lupus erythematosus (SLE)
  - Erythema annulare centrifugum
  - Erythema multiforme; erythema migrans
  - Impetigo circinatum
  - Granuloma annulare

DIAGNOSTIC TESTS & INTERPRETATION

Initial Tests (lab, imaging)

- Wood lamp exam reveals no fluorescence in most cases (*Trichophyton* sp.); 10% of infections, those caused by *T. rubrum*, will fluoresce with a green light.
- Potassium hydroxide (KOH) preparation of skin scrapings from dermatophyte leading border shows characteristic translucent, branching, rod-shaped hyphae.
- Fungal culture with Mycosel agar containing cycloheximide and chloramphenicol is the best method for diagnosis of tinea capitis (3).
- PCR is another method gaining popularity for the diagnosis of tinea capitis (3).

Follow-Up Tests & Special Considerations

- Reevaluate to assess response, especially in resistant/extensive cases.
- Fungal culture using Sabouraud dextrose agar/dermatophyte test medium

Test Interpretation

- Skin scrapings show fungal hyphae in epidermis; the best yield from scrapings from active border
- Arthrospores found in hair shafts; spores and/or hyphae seen on KOH exam (1)
- Fungal growth on Mycosel medium is confirmatory for tinea capitis (3)

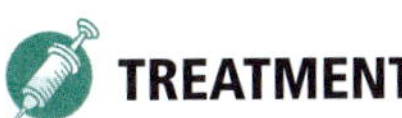

TREATMENT

GENERAL MEASURES

- Careful handwashing and personal hygiene; laundering of towels/clothing of affected individual; no sharing of towels/clothes/headgear/pillows
- Avoid predisposing conditions such as hot baths and tight-fitting clothing (boxer shorts are better than briefs).
- Avoid contact sports (e.g., wrestling) temporarily while starting treatment.
- Evaluate other family members, close contacts, or household pets (especially kittens and puppies).
- Use of prophylactic antifungal shampoo by all household members for 2 to 4 weeks in cases of tinea capitis (3)[A]
- Itching can be alleviated by over-the-counter (OTC) preparations such as Sarna or Prax.
- Topical steroid preparations should be avoided, unless absolutely needed to control itching and only after definitive diagnosis and initiation of antifungal treatment.
- Nystatin should be avoided in tinea infections but is indicated for cutaneous candidal infections.
- Keep area as dry as possible (talcum/powders may be beneficial).

MEDICATION

First Line

- Tinea cruris/corporis
  - Topical terbinafine 1% (Lamisil): OTC inexpensive and effective compound; can be applied once or BID for 1 to 3 weeks
  - Topical econazole 1% (Spectazole), ketoconazole (Nizoral): usually applied BID for 2 to 3 weeks
  - Topical butenafine 1% (Mentax): applied once daily for 2 weeks; also very effective. To prevent relapse, use for 1 week after resolution.
  - Topical naftifine 1% cream applied once daily
- Tinea capitis; PO terbinafine for 4 weeks, PO griseofulvin for 8 weeks, and PO itraconazole are about equally effective in children, although terbinafine might have a slight advantage in *Trichophyton* whereas griseofulvin may be preferable with *Microsporum* sp. Griseofulvin is the best choice when the causative species is unknown (2)[A].
  - PO griseofulvin for *Trichophyton* and *Microsporum* sp.; microsized preparation available; dosage of 10 to 20 mg/kg/day (max 1,000 mg); taken BID or as a single dose daily for 6 to 12 weeks
  - PO terbinafine can be used for *Trichophyton* sp. at 62.5 mg/day in patients weighing 10 to 20 kg; 125 mg/day if weight 20 to 40 kg; 250 mg/day if weight >40 kg; use for 4 to 6 weeks. There is little evidence for use in children <4 years of age.
  - PO itraconazole can be used for *Microsporum* sp. and matches griseofulvin efficacy while being better tolerated; dosage of 3 to 5 mg/kg/day (maximum 400 mg daily), but most studies have used 100 mg/day for 6 weeks in children >2 years of age

Second Line

Tinea cruris/corporis

- Oral antifungal agents are effective but not indicated in uncomplicated tinea cruris/corporis cases. They can be used for resistant and extensive infections or if the patient is immunocompromised. If topical therapy fails, consider possible oral therapy.
- The following oral regimens have been reported in medical literature as being effective but currently are not specifically approved by FDA for tinea cruris:
  - PO terbinafine (Lamisil): 250 mg/day for 1 to 2 weeks
  - PO itraconazole (Sporanox): children 3 to 5 mg/kg/day with maximum dose of 200 mg/day; adults 100 mg BID once and repeated 1 week later
  - PO fluconazole (Diflucan): children 6 mg/kg once weekly with maximum dose of 200 mg weekly; adults 200 mg once per week for 4 weeks
- Topical terbinafine 1% solution has been studied recently and appears effective as a once-daily application for 1 week.
- Oral antifungals have many interactions including warfarin, oral contractive pills (OCPs), and alcohol; advise checking for drug interactions prior to use; contraindicated in pregnancy. Monitor for liver toxicity when using oral antifungals.

ISSUES FOR REFERRAL

Refer if disease is nonresponsive/resistant, especially in immunocompromised host.

ADDITIONAL THERAPIES

Treatment of secondary bacterial infections

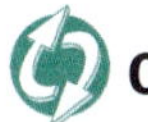

ONGOING CARE

FOLLOW-UP RECOMMENDATIONS

Reevaluate response to treatment.

Patient Monitoring

Liver function testing before therapy and at regular intervals during the course of therapy for patients requiring oral terbinafine, fluconazole, itraconazole, and griseofulvin (3)[B]

PATIENT EDUCATION

Explain the causative agents, predisposing factors, and prevention measures.

PROGNOSIS

- Excellent prognosis for cure with therapy in tinea cruris and corporis
- In tinea capitis, lesions will heal spontaneously in 6 months without treatment, but scarring is more likely.
- Areas of hair loss in tinea capitis will regrow with adequate treatment.

COMPLICATIONS

- Secondary bacterial infection
- Generalized, invasive dermatophyte infection
- Secondary eruptions called dermatophytid reactions (associated with primary/inflammatory skin disorders) may occur at distant sites.
- Majocchi granuloma is a rare complication in tinea corporis when the fungus invades the follicle and advances into the dermis (3)[B].

REFERENCES

1. Kinoshita-Ise M, Sachdeva M. Update on trichoscopy: Integration of the terminology by systematic approach and a proposal of a diagnostic flowchart. *J Dermatol*. 2022;49(1):4–18. doi:10.1111/1346-8138.16233.
2. Gupta AK, Bamimore MA, Renaud HJ, et al. A network meta-analysis on the efficacy and safety of monotherapies for tinea capitis, and an assessment of evidence quality. *Pediatr Dermatol*. 2020;37(6):1014–1022. doi:10.1111/pde.14353.
3. Ion A, Popa LG, Porumb-Andrese E, et al. A current diagnostic and therapeutic challenge: tinea capitis. *J Clin Med*. 2024;13(2):376. doi:10.3390/jcm13020376.

ADDITIONAL READING

Chen X, Jiang X, Yang M, et al. Systemic antifungal therapy for tinea capitis in children. *Cochrane Database Syst Rev*. 2016;2016(5):CD004685. doi:10.1002/14651858.CD004685.pub3.

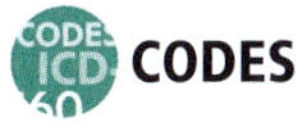

CODES

ICD10

- B35.0 Tinea barbae and tinea capitis
- B35.4 Tinea corporis
- B35.6 Tinea cruris

CLINICAL PEARLS

- Tinea corporis is characterized by scaly plaque, with peripheral activity and central clearing.
- Tinea cruris is characterized by erythematous plaque in crural folds usually sparing the scrotum. Treatment of concomitant tinea pedis is advised.
- Tinea capitis is a fungal infection of the scalp affecting hair growth. Topical therapy is ineffective for this infection.

T

TINEA PEDIS

William Andrew Pleasant, MD • Chirag N. Shah, MD • Daniel Scott Morrison, MD

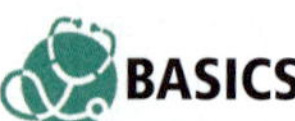

BASICS

DESCRIPTION

- Superficial fungal infection of the skin of the feet caused by dermatophytes
- Most common dermatophyte infection encountered in clinical practice; contagious
- Often accompanied by tinea manuum, tinea unguium, and tinea cruris
- Clinical forms: interdigital (most common), hyperkeratotic (moccasin type), vesiculobullous (inflammatory), and rarely ulcerative
- System(s) affected: skin/exocrine
- Synonym(s): athlete's foot, foot ringworm

EPIDEMIOLOGY

- Predominant age: 20 to 50 years, although can occur at any age
- Predominant gender: males infected about 3 times as frequently as females

Prevalence

- 4–10% of the population
- >70% of population will experience during a lifetime.

Pediatric Considerations

Rare in younger children; common in adolescents

Geriatric Considerations

Elderly are more susceptible to outbreaks because of immunocompromised and impaired perfusion of distal extremities.

ETIOLOGY AND PATHOPHYSIOLOGY

Superficial infection caused by dermatophytes that release enzymes called keratinases to invade and thrive only in nonviable keratinized tissue

- *Trichophyton interdigitale* (acute)
- *Trichophyton rubrum* (chronic): most common
- *Trichophyton tonsurans*
- *Epidermophyton floccosum*

Genetics

No known genetic pattern

RISK FACTORS

- Hot, humid weather
- Sweating
- Occlusive/tight-fitting footwear
- Immunosuppression
- Prolonged application of topical steroids

GENERAL PREVENTION

- Good personal hygiene
- Wearing rubber or wooden sandals in community showers, bathing places, locker rooms
- Careful drying between toes after showering or bathing; blow-drying feet with hair dryer may be more effective than drying with a towel
- Changing socks and shoes frequently
- Applying drying or dusting powder
- Applying topical antiperspirants

COMMONLY ASSOCIATED CONDITIONS

- Hyperhidrosis
- Onychomycosis
- Tinea manuum/unguium/cruris/corporis

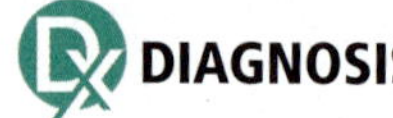

DIAGNOSIS

HISTORY

- Itchy, scaly rash on foot, usually between toes; may progress to fissuring/maceration in toe web spaces
- May be associated with onychomycosis and other tinea infections
- May be complicated by secondary bacterial infections

PHYSICAL EXAM

- Acute form: self-limited, intermittent, recurrent; scaling, thickening, and fissuring of sole and heel; silvery white scaling or fissuring of toe webs; or pruritic vesicular/bullous lesions between toes or on soles
- Chronic form: most common; slowly progressive, pruritic erythematous erosion/scales between toes, in digital interspaces; extension onto soles, sides/dorsum of feet (moccasin distribution); if untreated, may persist indefinitely
- Other features: strong odor, hyperkeratosis, maceration, ulceration
- Tinea pedis may occur unilaterally or bilaterally.
- Secondary presumably immune-mediated eruptions called dermatophytid reactions may occur at distant sites

DIFFERENTIAL DIAGNOSIS

- Interdigital type: erythrasma, impetigo, pitted keratolysis, candidal intertrigo
- Moccasin type: psoriasis vulgaris, chronic contact dermatitis, eczematous dermatitis, pitted keratolysis
- Inflammatory/bullous type: impetigo, allergic contact dermatitis, dyshidrotic eczema (negative potassium hydroxide [KOH] examination of scrapings), bullous disease

DIAGNOSTIC TESTS & INTERPRETATION

Wood's lamp exam will not fluoresce unless complicated by another fungus, which is uncommon: *Malassezia furfur* (yellow to white), *Corynebacterium* (red), or *Microsporum* (blue-green)

Initial Tests (lab, imaging)

Testing is not needed in typical presentation.

- Microscopic exam using KOH applied to scrapings of the affected area
- Culture (Sabouraud medium)

Follow-Up Tests & Special Considerations

Real-time PCR is increasingly being used; helpful in cases of recurrence as it identifies species.

Test Interpretation

- KOH preparation: confirmed with detection of segmented hyphae
- Culture: dermatophyte

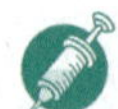

TREATMENT

Treatment is generally with topical antifungal medications for up to 4 weeks and is more effective than placebo (1)[C]

- Acute treatment
  - Aluminum acetate soak (Burow solution; Domeboro, 1 pack to 1 quart warm water) to decrease itching and acute eczematous reaction
  - Antifungal cream of choice BID after soaks: allylamines (naftifine, terbinafine) which are slightly more effective than azoles (imidazoles including clotrimazole, econazole, ketoconazole, miconazole, oxiconazole, sertaconazole, and tioconazole), and triazoles (which include: fluconazole, itraconazole, posaconazole, voriconazole, efinaconazole, terconazole, butoconazole)
- Chronic treatment:
  - Antifungal creams BID, continuing for 3 days after the rash is resolved: terbinafine 1%, clotrimazole 1%, econazole 1%, ketoconazole 2%, tolnaftate 1%, etc. (2)[A]
  - May try systemic antifungal therapy (see below); consider if concomitant onychomycosis or after failed topical treatment

GENERAL MEASURES

- Soak with aluminum chloride 30% or aluminum acetate for 20 minutes BID.
- Perform careful removal of dead/thickened skin after soaking or bathing.
- Treat shoes with antifungal powders.
- Avoid occlusive footwear.
- Chronic, extensive disease, or nail involvement requires oral antifungal medication for systemic therapy.

MEDICATION

Oral therapy is indicated for extensive infections, disease refractory to topical treatment, and immunocompromised patients. Topical treatments as noted above are generally first-line.

First Line

- Systemic antifungals (3)[A]:
  - Itraconazole: 200 mg PO BID for 7 days (cure rate >90%)
  - Terbinafine: 250 mg PO daily for 14 days (more efficacious than itraconazole)
- If concomitant onychomycosis:
  - Itraconazole: 200 mg PO BID for 1st week of the month for 3 months (Liver function testing is recommended.)
  - Terbinafine: 250 mg PO daily for 12 weeks, or pulse dosing: 500 mg PO daily for 1st week of the month for 3 months (not recommended if creatinine clearance <50 mL/min)

- Pediatric dosing options: weight based with treatment duration similar to adults
  - Griseofulvin: 10 to 15 mg/kg/day or divided
  - Terbinafine:
    - 10 to 20 kg: 62.5 mg/day
    - 20 to 40 kg: 125 mg/day
    - >40 kg: 250 mg/day
  - Itraconazole: 3 to 5 mg/kg/day
  - Fluconazole: 6 mg/kg/week
- Contraindications: itraconazole, pregnancy Category C
- Precautions: All systemic antifungal drugs may have potential hepatotoxicity.
- Dose reduction is required for patients with moderate to severe chronic kidney disease.
- Significant possible interactions: Itraconazole requires gastric acid for absorption; effectiveness is reduced with antacids, H_2 blockers, proton pump inhibitors, etc. Take with acidic beverages, such as soda, if on antacids.
- Side effects: Itraconazole and terbinafine may cause gastrointestinal distress, including diarrhea; itraconazole may also cause peripheral edema, especially if used in conjunction with calcium channel blockers.

Second Line

- Systemic antifungals: griseofulvin microsize (Grifulvin V) 250 to 500 mg daily for 21 days
- Contraindications (griseofulvin):
  - Patients with porphyria, hepatocellular failure Patients with history of hypersensitivity to griseofulvin
- Precautions (griseofulvin):
  - Should be used only in severe cases
  - Periodic monitoring of organ system functioning, including renal, hepatic, and hematopoietic
  - Possible photosensitivity reactions
  - Lupus erythematosus, lupus-like syndromes, or exacerbation of existing lupus erythematosus has been reported.
- Significant possible interactions (griseofulvin):
  - Decreases activity of warfarin-type anticoagulants
  - Barbiturates usually depress griseofulvin activity.
  - May potentiate the effect of alcohol, producing tachycardia and flush

ISSUES FOR REFERRAL

Consider dermatology referral if extensive or resistant disease, especially in immunocompromised host.

ADDITIONAL THERAPIES

- Treatment of secondary bacterial infections
- Treatment of eczematoid changes

COMPLEMENTARY & ALTERNATIVE MEDICINE

- Baking soda soak (1/2 cup in 1 quart warm water) has been shown to provide antifungal activity.
- White vinegar soak (1:1 white vinegar to warm water) may be used to aid in gram-negative bacterial coinfection.

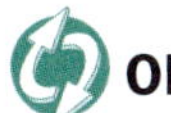

ONGOING CARE

FOLLOW-UP RECOMMENDATIONS

Avoid sweat buildup along feet.

Patient Monitoring

Evaluate for response, recognizing that infections may be chronic/recurrent.

DIET

No restrictions

PATIENT EDUCATION

See "General Prevention"

PROGNOSIS

- Although control is usually attainable, long-term cure is not always possible. Relapse is common.
- Infections tend to be chronic with exacerbations (e.g., in hot, humid weather)
- Personal hygiene and preventive measures, such as open-toed sandals, careful drying, and frequent sock changes are essential.

COMPLICATIONS

- Tinea pedis is commonly the cause of tinea cruris. Patients presenting with tinea in the groin area should be examined for presence of infection of the foot which is transferred to the groin on undergarments.
- Secondary bacterial infections (common portal of entry for streptococcal infections, producing lymphangitis/cellulitis of lower extremity)
- Eczematoid changes/dermatophytid reactions

REFERENCES

1. Thomas B, Falk J, Allan GM. Topical management of tinea pedis. *Can Fam Physician*. 2021;67(1):30.
2. Ward H, Parkes N, Smith C, et al. Consensus for the treatment of tinea pedis: a systematic review of randomised controlled trials. *J Fungi (Basel)*. 2022;8(4):351.
3. Bell-Syer SE, Khan SM, Torgerson DJ. Oral treatments for fungal infections of the skin of the foot. *Cochrane Database SystRev*. 2012;10:CD003584.

ADDITIONAL READING

- Crawford F, Hollis S. Topical treatments for fungal infections of the skin and nails of the foot. *Cochrane Database Syst Rev*. 2007;3:CD001434.
- Hawkins DM, Smidt AC. Superficial fungal infections in children. *Pediatr Clin North Am*. 2014;61(2):443–455.
- Leung AKC, Barankin B, Lam JM, et al. Tinea pedis: an updated review [published online ahead of print June 29, 2023]. *Drugs Context*. doi:10.7573/dic.2023-5-1.
- Rotta I, Sanchez A, Goncalves PR, et al. Efficacy and safety of topical antifungals in the treatment of dermatomycosis: a systematic review. *Br J Dermatol*. 2012;166(5):927–933.

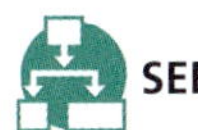

SEE ALSO

Dermatitis, Contact; Dyshidrosis

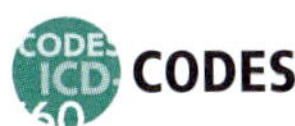

CODES

ICD10

B35.3 Tinea pedis

CLINICAL PEARLS

- Tinea pedis is often recurrent or chronic in nature.
- Careful drying between toes after showering or bathing helps prevent recurrences; blow-drying feet with a hair dryer may be more effective than drying with a towel.
- Treatment with topical antifungal medications for up to 4 weeks is usually sufficient.
- Oral therapy should be reserved for severe disease, topical therapy failure, or immunocompromised patients.
- Dusting and desiccating powders (containing antifungal agents) may help prevent recurrences.

TINEA VERSICOLOR

Dori Goldberg, MD • Yuying Zhang, BS

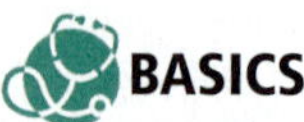

BASICS

DESCRIPTION

- A benign superficial skin infection commonly caused by *Malassezia* yeast species that leads to well-demarcated scaly hypopigmented or hyperpigmented macules/patches, primarily located on the upper trunk, neck, and upper arms.
- System(s) affected: skin/exocrine
- Synonym(s): pityriasis versicolor

EPIDEMIOLOGY

Incidence

- Common, occurs worldwide, especially in tropical climates
- Predominant age: adolescents and young adults between 21 and 30 years of age
- Predominant sex: male = female

Pediatric Considerations

Skin eruptions usually occur after puberty, when sebaceous glands are more active. However, tinea versicolor can also be seen in children, especially in tropical climates; facial lesions are more common in children.

Geriatric Considerations

Not common in the geriatric population

Prevalence

Prevalence can reach up to 50%, especially in warm climates.

ETIOLOGY AND PATHOPHYSIOLOGY

- Hypopigmented lesions (more commonly noted in darker skin tones) is likely due *Malassezia* species producing azelaic acid that damages melanocytes by inhibiting tyrosinase. The small melanosomes and lipid-like material accumulates in the stratum corneus blocking ultraviolet light.
- Hyperpigmented lesion is due to inflammatory response to pathogen leading to thicker stratum corneum and abnormally large melanosome.
  - Tinea versicolor is caused by saprophytic yeast: *Pityrosporum orbiculare* (also known as *Plasmodium ovale*, *Malassezia furfur*, or *Malassezia ovalis*), which is a known colonizer of all humans.
  - Development of clinical disease is associated with transformation of *Malassezia* from yeast cells to pathogenic mycelial form. Several endogenous (host) and exogenous/external factors may play a role in the transformation to active disease.
  - Tinea versicolor is generally not contagious.

Genetics

Genetic predisposition may exist.

RISK FACTORS

- Hot, humid weather
- Application of oily lotion or cream to the skin
- Wearing masks
- Hyperhidrosis
- HIV infection/immunosuppression
- High cortisol levels (Cushing syndrome/disease, prolonged steroid administration)
- Pregnancy
- Malnutrition and poor general health
- Oral contraceptives

GENERAL PREVENTION

- Prophylactic use of antifungal products including ketoconazole 2% shampoo or selenium sulfide 2.5% lotion once weekly for 6 to 12 months after initial cure in patients with ≥2 episodes/year
- Wear loose clothes
- Avoid tanning bed or sun lamp
- Avoiding oily skin products
- Avoid excessive sun exposure

COMMONLY ASSOCIATED CONDITIONS

- Seborrheic dermatitis and *Malassezia* folliculitis share similar yeast
- Atopic dermatitis, HIV or other immunodeficiency, Cushing disease and biologic induced dermatomycoses increase risk of tinea versicolor

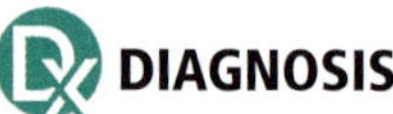

DIAGNOSIS

- The diagnosis is usually based on clinical presentation.
- If needed, a Wood's lamp and microscopic examination of scales soaked in potassium hydroxide can help confirm with finding includes hyphae and spores often liken to "spaghetti and meatball" (1).

HISTORY

- Onset: usually when weather turns hot/humid, after travel to tropical areas, and summer sports
- Daily activities: use of heavy moisturizer, tight synthetic athletic wear, use of tanning bed, use of topical steroids
- Hormonal changes: pregnancy, use of oral contraceptives
- Skin presentation: failure to obtain an even tan, pruritus worst with heat or exercise
- Prior history: family or personal history of recurrence
- Comorbidities: immunocompromised or abnormal endocrine states (Cushing disease, biological therapy, etc.)

PHYSICAL EXAM

- Rash appears round or oval macules 1 to 3 cm, symmetrically appearing in the upper trunk commonly. In children, facial involvement more likely.
- Lesion often coalesce into well-demarcated irregular patches.
- Color of lesions may vary depending on presentation and individual skin tone (hypopigmented, hyperpigmented, erythematous)
- Lesion changes color with season: lighter than surrounding skin during summer, darker than surrounding skin in the winter
- Hypopigmentation more common in individual with darker skin
- Mild to moderate pruritus
- Fine scales are present over the lesions and become more visible with scraping.

DIFFERENTIAL DIAGNOSIS

Other skin diseases with discolored macules and plaques or patches include the following:

- Pityriasis alba/rosea ("Christmas tree-like" distribution visible in *P. rosea*)
- Vitiligo (presents without scaling)
- Seborrheic dermatitis (more erythematous; thicker scales)
- Nummular eczema
- Secondary syphilis
- Erythrasma
- Mycosis fungoides

DIAGNOSTIC TESTS & INTERPRETATION

Wood lamp examination: affected area may appear fluorescent yellow to yellow-green (1).

Initial Tests (lab, imaging)

- Direct microscopy of scales with 10% potassium hydroxide (KOH) preparation shows hyphae and spores ("spaghetti and meatballs" pattern).
- Dermatoscopy: "contrast-halo" pigment ring, perifollicular scale and follicular plug
- Routine lab tests are usually not necessary.
- Fungal culture is not useful.

Follow-Up Tests & Special Considerations

- Extensive recurrent or treatment resistance: consider liver-function test (LFT) for planning of oral azole therapy
- Test for other comorbidity: HbA1C or fasting glucose, HIV test, review of system to evaluate for metabolic/immune screen

Diagnostic Procedures/Other

- Gold Standard microscopy: KOH and fluorescence stain
- Wood Lamp or dermoscopy

Test Interpretation

- KOH (positive) hyphae and spores → confirms active *Malassezia* overgrowth
- KOH (negative) but Wood lamp (positive) → likely washed off chromophores; repeat scraping from active border

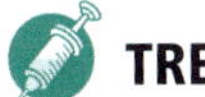

TREATMENT

GENERAL MEASURES

- Keep skin cool, dry, and nonocclusive: shower and change clothes after exercise; avoid heavily oils and tanning bed.
- Sun behavior: sunscreen prevents posttreatment hyperpigmented "contrast" tanning
- Patients who fail topical treatment can be treated with an oral/systemic medication.

MEDICATION

Topical antifungal therapy is the treatment of choice in limited disease and is safe and usually effective. Evidence is generally of poor quality, but data suggest that longer durations of treatment and higher concentrations of active agents produce greater cure rates.

First Line

- Ketoconazole 2% shampoo applied to damp skin for 1 to 3 days and left on for 5 minutes (Ketoconazole is contraindicated in pregnancy.) before rinsing (2)
- Selenium sulfide shampoo 2.5% (Selsun):
  - Applied daily for 1 week to the affected areas and allowed to dry and remain on skin for 10 minutes prior to showering
- Terbinafine (Lamisil) 1% solution twice daily for 1 to 4 weeks (2)
- Topical ciclopirox Olamine 1% cream twice daily for 2 weeks
- Newer preparations include 2.25% selenium sulfide foam and ketoconazole 2% gel
- Cure rates of topical anti-yeast preparations typically 70–80%; healing continues after active treatment. Even pigmentation may take months to return.

Second Line

- Can be used for extensive and recalcitrant disease (nonresponders)
- Oral fluconazole 300 mg once weekly for 2 weeks (2)
- Itraconazole 200 mg/day PO for 1 week (7 days); cure rate >90% (2)
- Oral ketoconazole is no longer recommended by the FDA due to risks of hepatotoxicity, adrenal insufficiency, and drug–drug interactions.
- Oral terbinafine or griseofulvin is not effective.

ISSUES FOR REFERRAL

- If resistant to treatment
- If extensive disease occurs in immunocompromised host

ADDITIONAL THERAPIES

Tacrolimus 0.03% ointment nightly for 8 weeks showed shortened repigmentation lag

SURGERY/OTHER PROCEDURES

Photodynamic therapy and narrow-band ultraviolet B (NB-UVB) light have both been shown to be effective alternative treatments in tinea versicolor (3).

ADMISSION, INPATIENT, AND NURSING CONSIDERATIONS

Hospital admission is rare and not required unless it is presented as secondary presentation for immunocompromised patients.

ONGOING CARE

- Ketoconazole 2% or selenium sulfide 2.5% shampoo can be used weekly for maintenance or monthly for prophylaxis.
- Follow up: repeat LFTs if on >2 weeks of systemic azole. Reassess relapse frequency and discontinue prophylaxis after one clear year or continue only through humid season.

FOLLOW-UP RECOMMENDATIONS

Inform patients that pigment changes/variations may remain for several months after treatment.

Patient Monitoring

- Topicals: watch for irritant dermatitis
- Failure to respond should prompt reassessment or dermatology referral.
- Resistance to treatment, frequent recurrences, or widespread disease may point to immunodeficiency.

DIET

There is no proven diet to treat and prevent recurrence of tinea versicolor.

PATIENT EDUCATION

- Condition is not contagious.
- Color change lags behind fungal cure; expect 1 to 3 months for repigmentation
- Symptoms can relapse in one year without maintenance, weekly shampoo reduces prevents recurrence to <25%.
- Seek care if patches spread despite treatment or become painful

PROGNOSIS

- Lesions may last for months to years.
- Lesions may recur periodically because *Malassezia* yeast organisms are known human colonizers and natural inhabitants of the skin.
- Pigment changes/variations may take months to resolve.
- First-line topical therapy has 90% clear rate

COMPLICATIONS

- Post-inflammatory dyschromia, will fade over months
- Azole induced hepatotoxicity, ensures baseline LFT check
- Uncommon, but can selenium, propylene glycol can cause irritant dermatitis

REFERENCES

1. Leung AK, Barankin B, Lam JM, et al. Tinea versicolor: an updated review. *Drugs Context*. 2022;11:2022-9-2. doi:10.7573/dic.2022-9-2.
2. Tirado-Sánchez A, Ungson-Garcia MG, Isa-Pigmentel M, et al. Recurrent pityriasis versicolor: a short review of clinical features and antifungal and non-antifungal treatment options. *Our Dermatol Online*. 2023;14(4):436–447.
3. Alberdi E, Gómez C. Successful treatment of pityriasis versicolor by photodynamic therapy mediated by methylene blue. *Photodermatol Photoimmunol Photomed*. 2020;36(4):308–312.

ADDITIONAL READING

- Committee on Infectious Disease, American Academy of Pediatrics. Red Book: 2024–2027 Report of the Committee on Infectious Diseases, 33rd Edition. American Academy of Pediatrics; 2024.
- Kallini JR, Riaz F, Khachemoune A. Tinea versicolor in dark-skinned individuals. *Int J Dermatol*. 2014;53(2):137–141. doi:10.1111/ijd.12345.
- Singla P, Sharma NR, Mane P, et al. Epidemiological, clinical and mycological characteristics of pityriasis versicolor: results of a study from a teaching hospital in rural part of Northern India. *J Family Med Prim Care*. 2022;11(9):5236–5240. doi:10.4103/jfmpc.jfmpc_2317_21.
- Vishwanath T, Kapadia FM, Mahajan SA, et al. Dermoscopic perspective of pityriasis versicolor in a cross-sectional study. *Indian Dermatol Online J*. 2024;15(2):218–225. doi:10.4103/idoj.idoj_319_23.

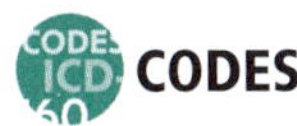

CODES

ICD10

B36.0 Pityriasis versicolor

CLINICAL PEARLS

- Tinea versicolor, also called pityriasis versicolor, is characterized by noncontagious, finely scaling macules of varying colors.
- Recurrence is common in summer months.
- Lesions tend to become more apparent after tanning because they typically do not tan; hypopigmented patches become more visible.
- Inform patients that discoloration/pigment variations may remain for several months after treatment.

T

TINNITUS

Donna I. Meltzer, MD

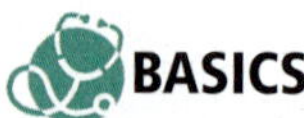

BASICS

DESCRIPTION

- Tinnitus is a perceived sensation of sound in the absence of an external acoustic stimulus; often described as a ringing, hissing, buzzing, clicking, or whooshing
- Derived from the Latin word *tinnire*, meaning "to ring"
- May be heard in one or both ears or centrally within the head
- Two types: subjective (most common) and objective tinnitus
  - Subjective tinnitus: perceived only by the patient; can be continuous, intermittent, or pulsatile
  - Objective tinnitus: audible to the examiner; rare
- Primary tinnitus: idiopathic with or without sensorineural hearing loss (SNHL) (1)
- Secondary tinnitus: associated with a specific cause (other than SNHL)

EPIDEMIOLOGY

Incidence

- Incidence increasing in association with excessive noise exposure
- Higher rates of tinnitus in smokers, hypertensives, diabetics, and obese patients

Prevalence

- Tinnitus reported by 35 to 50 million adults in the United States; although underreported, 12 million seek medical care.
- Affects 10–15% of adults (2)
- Prevalence increases with age and peaks in 6th decade; estimated 8% prevalence reported post COVID-19 infection
- Prevalence of 13–53% in general pediatric population
- Ethnicity/race: White > Black and Hispanic
- Gender: men > women

ETIOLOGY AND PATHOPHYSIOLOGY

- Precise pathophysiology is unknown; numerous theories have been proposed. Ototoxic agents or noise exposure damage hair cells so that there is abnormal neural activity in the auditory cortex. Inflammation may play a role.
- Causes of secondary tinnitus (2)
  - Otologic: cholesteatoma, cerumen impaction, foreign body, middle ear effusion, otosclerosis, Ménière disease, vestibular schwannoma, patulous eustachian tube
  - Medications: anti-inflammatory agents (aspirin, NSAIDs); antimalarial agents, antimicrobial drugs (aminoglycosides, macrolides); antineoplastic agents, loop diuretics, miscellaneous drugs (antiarrhythmics, antiulcer, anticonvulsants, antihypertensives); anesthetics
  - Somatic: temporomandibular joint (TMJ) dysfunction, head or neck injury
  - Neurologic: multiple sclerosis, spontaneous intracranial hypertension, vestibular migraine, type I Chiari malformation, palatal myoclonus, idiopathic stapedial muscle spasm
  - Infectious: viral (impact of COVID-19 on tinnitus is not clear) bacterial, fungal
  - Metabolic: diabetes mellitus, dyslipidemia, vitamin B_{12} deficiency
  - Vascular: aortic or carotid stenosis, venous hum, arteriovenous fistula or malformation, vascular tumors, high cardiac output state (anemia)

Genetics

Limited evidence to support a genetic component

RISK FACTORS

- Hearing loss (but can have tinnitus with normal hearing)
- High-level noise exposure
- Advanced age
- Use of ototoxic medications (some are irreversible)
- Otologic disease (otosclerosis, Ménière disease, cerumen impaction)
- Depression and anxiety associated with increased odds of tinnitus

GENERAL PREVENTION

- Avoid loud noise exposure and wear appropriate ear protection to prevent hearing loss.
- Monitor ototoxic medications and avoid prescribing >1 ototoxic agent concurrently.
- Consuming fruit, fiber, caffeine, and dairy may be associated with a reduced incidence of tinnitus (3).

COMMONLY ASSOCIATED CONDITIONS

- SNHL caused by presbycusis (age-associated hearing loss) or prolonged loud noise exposure
- Conductive hearing loss due to cerumen, otosclerosis, cholesteatoma
- Psychological disorders: depression, anxiety, insomnia, suicidal ideation
- Despair, frustration, interference with concentration and social interactions, work hindrance

DIAGNOSIS

HISTORY

- Onset gradual (presbycusis) or abrupt (following loud noise exposure)
- Duration: acute versus chronic (>6 months)
- Timing: can be continuous (hearing loss) or intermittent (Ménière disease)
- Pattern: nonpulsatile > pulsatile (often vascular cause)
- Location: bilateral > unilateral (vestibular schwannoma, cerumen, Ménière disease)
- Pitch: high pitch (with SNHL) > low pitch (Ménière disease)
- Associated symptoms: hearing loss, headache, noise intolerance, vertigo, TMJ dysfunction, neck pain
- Exacerbating factors: loud noise; jaw, head, or neck movements
- Alleviating factors: hearing aid, position change, medications
- Medication use (prescription, OTC, supplements)
- Hearing and past noise exposure (occupational, military, recreational)
- Psychosocial history (depression, anxiety, sleep habits)
- Impact of tinnitus: bothersome or nonbothersome; Tinnitus Handicap Inventory, Tinnitus Functional Index

PHYSICAL EXAM

- HEENT, neck, neurologic, and vascular examinations to help with etiology or guide next steps
- Ear: cerumen impaction, effusion, cholesteatoma
- Check hearing; air and bone conduction testing with 512- or 1,024-Hz tuning fork (Weber and Rinne tests)
- Eye: funduscopic exam for papilledema (intracranial hypertension) or visual field change (mass)
- TMJ: Palpate for tenderness and crepitus with movement.
- Cranial nerve, Romberg test (equilibrium), finger to nose, gait; assess for nystagmus.
- Auscultate for bruits or murmurs; compress jugular vein (suspect venous etiology if maneuver reduces tinnitus)

DIFFERENTIAL DIAGNOSIS

- Pulsatile tinnitus: carotid stenosis, aortic valve disease, AV malformation, high cardiac output state (anemia, hyperthyroidism), paraganglioma (glomus tumor)
- Nonpulsatile tinnitus: auditory hallucinations

DIAGNOSTIC TESTS & INTERPRETATION

- Tinnitus is a symptom; no objective test to confirm diagnosis
- Complete audiologic examination
  - Pure tone audiometry (air and bone conduction)
  - Tympanometry
  - Weber test, Rinne test
- Carotid Doppler ultrasonography (neck bruit)

Initial Tests (lab, imaging)

- Little evidence to support lab testing other than targeted lab studies based on history and physical exam. Use clinical judgment and consider the following:
  - CBC, BUN/creatinine, fasting glucose, lipid panel
- Guidelines advise against imaging studies unless have unilateral, pulsatile tinnitus; focal neurologic abnormality; or asymmetric hearing loss (1)[C]

- The American College of Radiology (ACR) updated the evidence-based recommendations for patients presenting with tinnitus; history, physical, and associated symptoms guide initial imaging (4)[C].
  - Pulsatile tinnitus (unilateral or bilateral) with normal otoscopy: initial imaging includes MRA head with IV contrast, MRI head and internal auditory canal (IAC) without and with contrast, or CTA head alone or head and neck with IV contrast; carotid artery duplex scan is no longer recommended.
  - Pulsatile tinnitus (unilateral or bilateral) with suspected retrotympanic lesion on otoscopy: CT temporal bone without IV contrast; might consider CTA head and neck with IV contrast.
  - Unilateral nonpulsatile tinnitus if no hearing loss and no neurologic deficit: MRI head and IAC without and with IV contrast; might consider MRI study without contrast.
  - Bilateral nonpulsatile tinnitus: imaging not indicated if no hearing loss, neurologic deficit, or trauma

Follow-Up Tests & Special Considerations

Consider TSH, HIV, RPR, autoimmune panel, Lyme test, vitamin B_{12} and vitamin D levels; low-quality evidence for some of these studies (2)

Diagnostic Procedures/Other

Electronystagmography (vestibular testing for Ménière disease)

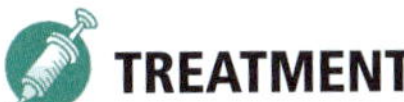

TREATMENT

GENERAL MEASURES

- Individualize treatment based on the severity of tinnitus and impact on function.
- Cognitive behavioral therapy (CBT), education, relaxation therapy
- Reassure patient.
- Manage treatable pathology.
- Hearing aids (corrects hearing and might mask tinnitus) can be tried if there is hearing loss and bothersome tinnitus (1)[C].
- Protect hearing against future loud noise.
- Discontinue ototoxic medications (some medications have reversible ototoxic effects).

MEDICATION

No pharmacologic agent has been shown to consistently alleviate tinnitus.

First Line

- Antidepressants (SSRIs or TCAs): probably help with psychological distress; insufficient evidence that antidepressant drug therapy improves tinnitus (2).
- Anxiolytics (benzodiazepines) do not provide consistent benefit and risk side effect of dependency (2).

Second Line

Anticonvulsants: potentially suppress central auditory hyperactivity but not recommended (1)[C]

ISSUES FOR REFERRAL

- Audiologist for comprehensive hearing evaluation and management
- Otolaryngologist, neurologist, or neurosurgeon depending on pathology
- Dental referral for TMJ treatment and dental orthotics (splint, night guard)
- Therapists for CBT, biofeedback, education, and relaxation techniques

ADDITIONAL THERAPIES

- CBT employs relaxation exercises, coping strategies, and deconditioning techniques to reduce arousal levels and reverse negative thoughts about tinnitus; might reduce negative impact of tinnitus on quality of life; recommended as beneficial based on randomized controlled trials (1)[C]
- Sound therapy (masking): Patients wear low-level noise generators to mask the tinnitus noise; optional therapy (1)[C]
- Tinnitus retraining therapy (TRT) combines counseling, education, and acoustic therapy (soft music, sound machine) to minimize bothersome nature of tinnitus. TRT might reduce tinnitus, but probably no benefit over standard counseling with enriched sound.
- Internet-based technology or smartphone apps to mask tinnitus may hold promise, but high-quality studies are lacking.
- Transcranial magnetic stimulation (TMS): a noninvasive method to stimulate neurons in the brain by rapidly changing magnetic fields; not recommended as randomized trials were inconclusive (1)[C]
- Botulism toxin (for palatal myoclonus)
- Intratympanic steroid injections not recommended (1)[C]

SURGERY/OTHER PROCEDURES

- Cochlear implants (for severe SNHL) might improve severity of tinnitus.
- Ablation of cochlear nerve (destroys hearing)
- Otosclerosis: stapedectomy surgery with implantation of ossicular prosthesis
- Severe Ménière disease not alleviated by medications: installation of endolymphatic shunt, labyrinthectomy, or vestibular neurectomy
- Auditory neoplasms: surgical resection/radiation
- Pulsatile tinnitus due to atherosclerotic carotid artery disease: carotid endarterectomy

COMPLEMENTARY & ALTERNATIVE MEDICINE

Acupuncture, *Gingko biloba*, melatonin, zinc, cannabis, or antioxidants might alleviate tinnitus in some patients; however, many conflicting studies report no benefit with these methods.

ONGOING CARE

FOLLOW-UP RECOMMENDATIONS

- Audiologist: for hearing evaluation and therapy
- Counseling: as needed for psychological distress
- Family physician: as needed for support and guidance

PATIENT EDUCATION

- American Tinnitus Association: https://www.ata.org/
- National Institute on Deafness and Other Communication Disorders: https://www.nidcd.nih.gov/health/tinnitus

PROGNOSIS

- Tinnitus persisted in 80% of older patients and increased in severity in 50%.
- Focus on managing tinnitus and reducing severity, not curing.

REFERENCES

1. Tunkel DE, Bauer CA, Sun GH, et al. Clinical practice guideline: tinnitus executive summary. *Otolaryngol Head Neck Surg*. 2014;151(4):533–541.
2. Dalrymple SN, Lewis SH, Philman S. Tinnitus: diagnosis and management. *Am Fam Physician*. 2021;103(11):663–671.
3. Zhang M, Wang X, Zhang S, et al. Association of 15 common dietary factors with tinnitus: a systematic review and meta-analysis of observational studies. *BMJ Open*. 2025;15(3):e091507.
4. Jain V, Policeni B, Juliano AF, et al; for Expert Panel on Neurological Imaging. ACR appropriateness criteria® tinnitus: 2023 update. *J Am Coll Radiol*. 2023;20(Suppl 11):S574–S591.

ADDITIONAL READING

- Grundfast KM, Jamil TL. Evaluation and management of tinnitus: are there opportunities for improvement? *Otolaryngol Head Neck Surg*. 2023;168(1):45–58.
- Lee HY, Jung DJ. Recent updates on tinnitus management. *J Audiol Otol*. 2023;27(4):181–192.
- Meijers S, Stegeman I, van der Leun JA, et al. Analysis and comparison of clinical practice guidelines regarding treatment recommendations for chronic tinnitus in adults: a systematic review. *BMJ Open*. 2023;13(9):e072754.

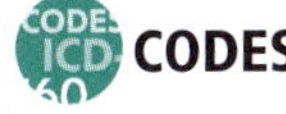

CODES

ICD10

- H93.19 Tinnitus, unspecified ear
- H93.11 Tinnitus, right ear
- H93.12 Tinnitus, left ear

CLINICAL PEARLS

- People have different levels of tolerance to tinnitus. It may affect sleep, concentration, and emotional state. Many patients with chronic tinnitus have depression.
- To prevent tinnitus from worsening, avoid loud noises and minimize stress.
- Optimal management may involve multiple strategies.

TOBACCO USE AND SMOKING CESSATION

Christine Ramos Camacho, MD, MS

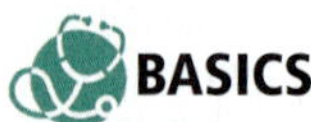

BASICS

DESCRIPTION

- Nicotine sources: cigars, pipes, water pipes, hookahs, cigarettes, and electronic cigarettes (e-cigarettes; vapes; e-hookahs, vape pens), smokeless tobacco such as dip, snuff and chewing tobacco.
- Electronic nicotine delivery system (ENDS) use is common

EPIDEMIOLOGY

Smoking causes more deaths each year than alcohol use, motor vehicle accidents, illegal drug use, firearm-related injuries combined.

Incidence

- >2 million new smokers annually in the U.S.
- Over half of new smokers are <18 years of age (6% initiation rate for teens).
- Over half of individuals who have ever smoked cigarettes have successfully quit.

Prevalence

- Age: highest among those ages 45 to 64 years (16%). Gender: male > female (15% vs. 12%)
- Cigarette smoking among adults has declined significantly since the 1960s. Cigarette smoking is responsible for >480,000 deaths per year in the United States, including >41,000 deaths from secondhand smoke exposure. This is about 1 in 5 deaths annually or 1,300 deaths every day.
- Each day, about 2,000 people <18 years smoke their first cigarette.
- In 2020, ~31 million U.S. adults were current cigarette smokers, this represents 14% of men and 11% of women. In 2019, 14% of all adults (34.1 million people) currently smoked cigarettes: 15.3% in men, 12.7% of women.

ETIOLOGY AND PATHOPHYSIOLOGY

- Addiction due to nicotine's rapid stimulation of the brain's dopamine system (teenage brain especially susceptible)
- Atherosclerotic risk due to adrenergic stimulation, endothelial damage, carbon monoxide, and adverse effects on lipids
- Direct airway damage from cigarette tar, and carcinogens in all tobacco products
- E-cigarettes produce an aerosol by heating liquid nicotine, flavoring, and chemicals. Potential adverse effects of e-cigarettes are related to exposure to nicotine as well as to other vapor components produced by the devices.

RISK FACTORS

- Presence of a smoker in the household.
- Easy access to cigarettes.
- Comorbid stress and psychiatric disorders
- Low self-esteem/self-worth.
- Poor academic performance
- Boys: high levels of aggression and rebelliousness Girls: preoccupation with weight and body image

GENERAL PREVENTION

- Most first-time tobacco use occurs before high school graduation. Restricting minors' access to tobacco by limiting tobacco advertisements and encouraging tobacco-free sports initiatives.
- Smoking bans in public areas and workplaces
- Health warnings on tobacco products

COMMONLY ASSOCIATED CONDITIONS

- Coronary artery disease, cerebrovascular disease, peripheral vascular disease, and abdominal aortic aneurysm (AAA)
- Chronic obstructive pulmonary disease (COPD); cancer of the lip, oral cavity, pharynx, larynx, lung, esophagus, stomach, pancreas, kidney, urinary bladder, cervix, and blood' pneumonia, osteoporosis; periodontitis; alcohol use; depression, anxiety, reduced fertility
- E-cigarette use associated with several cases of idiopathic acute eosinophilic pneumonia

Pregnancy Considerations

Smoking during pregnancy can increase the risk of miscarriage, congenital anomalies, stillbirth, fetal growth restriction, preterm birth, placental abruption. Patients are encouraged to quit smoking completely as the evidence on pharmacotherapy interventions for tobacco smoking cessation in pregnancy is insufficient.

Pediatric Considerations

Secondhand smoke increases the risk for sudden infant death syndrome, acute upper and lower respiratory tract infections, exacerbations of asthma, otitis media. Nicotine passes through breast milk and decreases the production of milk by suppressing the prolactin levels.

DIAGNOSIS

HISTORY

- Ask about (and document) tobacco use, secondhand smoke exposure at every encounter
- Type and quantity of tobacco used: "Heavy smoking" is ≥20 cigarettes per day or ≥20 pack-years.
  - Pack-years = packs/day × years
  - Assess for awareness of health risks and interest in quitting.
- Identify triggers: stress, habit, pleasure
- Prior attempts to quit: method, duration of success, reason for relapse

PHYSICAL EXAM

- General: tobacco odor, staining of nails, hair
- Skin: premature wrinkling, especially the face
- Mouth: nicotine-stained teeth, poor oral dentition; inspect for mucosal changes, hypertrophy, fungating lesions
- Lungs: crackles, wheezing, increased or decreased volume, chronic cough
- Vessels: carotid or abdominal bruits, abdominal aortic enlargement or aneurysm, weak peripheral pulses, stigmata of peripheral vascular disease

DIAGNOSTIC TESTS & INTERPRETATION

- The U.S. Preventive Services Task Force (USPSTF) recommends that clinicians ask all adults about tobacco use, advise them to stop using tobacco, and assist with behavioral interventions and FDA-approved pharmacotherapy for cessation to nonpregnant adults who use tobacco.
- The USPSTF recommends one-time screening abdominal ultrasound (US) for AAA in men ≥65 years of age who ever smoked (number needed to screen to prevent one AAA = 500).
- USPSTF recommends yearly screening for lung cancer with low-dose CT for individuals aged 55 to 80 years with a 30 pack-years history of smoking, current smokers, or those who have quit within past 15 years.

Initial Tests (lab, imaging)

- Nicotine can be measured in the blood and urine by checking cotinine levels.
- Fagerström Test to assess for nicotine dependence

Diagnostic Procedures/Other

Pulmonary function tests (PFTs) for smokers with chronic pulmonary symptoms, such as wheezing, cough, or dyspnea.

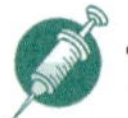

TREATMENT

ALERT

Report cases of lung injury of unclear etiology and a history of e-cigarette or vaping product use within the past 90 days to state or local health department.

GENERAL MEASURES

- Behavioral counseling (5 As):
  - Ask about tobacco use at every office visit.
  - Advise all smokers to quit.
  - Assess the patient's willingness to quit.
  - Assist the patient in his or her attempt to quit and provide quit line number (1-800-QUIT-NOW).
  - Arrange follow-up and support.
- 50% of adult smokers try to quit every year. Fewer than 1 in 10 succeed. Less than 50% of adult smokers receive professional advice to quit. Even very brief advice promotes successful attempts at quitting.
- Patients ready to quit smoking should set a quit date within the next 2 weeks; no difference in success rates between patients who taper prior to their quit date and those who stop abruptly
- Behavioral interventions and use of FDA-approved pharmacotherapy for tobacco smoking cessation are effective in helping people to quit.
- Current evidence is insufficient to recommend the use of electronic cigarettes for tobacco cessation in adults.
- Text messaging, contingency planning and financial incentives boost quit rates

MEDICATION

Varenicline and nicotine gum therapy may each reduce relapse in patients who had stopped smoking.

First Line

- Varenicline (Chantix): 0.5 mg/day PO for 3 days, then 0.5 mg BID for 4 days, and then 1 mg BID for 11 weeks:
  - Start 1 to 4 weeks prior to smoking cessation and continue for 12 to 24 weeks.
  - Superior versus placebo and bupropion; number needed to treat = 6 and 15, respectively
  - May be combined with nicotine replacement therapy (NRT) for those with cravings
  - Side effects: nausea, insomnia, headache, depression, suicidal ideation; safety not established in adolescents or patients with psychiatric or cardiovascular disease; pregnancy Category C
- NRT (e.g., patch, gum, lozenge, inhaler, nasal spray) (1)[A]:
  - Improves quit rates by 50–70% versus placebo. Combination (patch, plus fast acting) is most effective with quit rates similar to varenicline
  - Available over the counter
  - Patch (NicoDerm CQ 21, 14, and 7 mg):
    - 1 patch q24h; start with 21 mg if smoking ≥10 cigarettes/day; otherwise, start with 14 mg.
    - 6 weeks on initial dose and then taper
    - 2 weeks each on subsequent doses
    - No proven benefit beyond 8 weeks
  - Electronic nicotine delivery systems (ENDS)
    - Contain less nicotine than cigarette
    - Controversial if less "dangerous" than tobacco
    - Conflicting data on whether teen use increases or decreases risk to cigarette progression.
    - Insufficient evidence to recommend as adjunct for tobacco cessation
  - Gum (Nicorette, 2 and 4 mg):
    - Use 4 mg if smoking ≥25 cigarettes per day.
    - Chew 1 piece q1–2h for 6 weeks, then 1 piece q2–4h for 3 weeks, and then 1 piece q4–8h for 3 weeks.
    - May use in combination with bupropion; monitor for hypertension.
    - Side effects: headache, pharyngitis, cough, rhinitis, dyspepsia; all mainly with inhaler and spray forms
    - Pregnancy Category D
  - NRT is reasonable in hospitalized smokers because NRT products immediately treat nicotine withdrawal symptoms, whereas varenicline and bupropion take time to reach steady state.
- Cytisine (available in Europe and Canada). A plant-based alkaloid that, similar to varenicline, is a partial agonist of nicotinic acetylcholine receptors. More effective than NRT and similar to varenicline in quit rates.

Second Line

- Bupropion SR: 150 mg PO for 3 days and then 150 mg BID (2)[A]:
  - Start 1 week prior to smoking cessation and continue for 7 to 12 weeks.
  - Twice as effective as placebo
  - Drug of choice for patients with depression or schizophrenia; additional benefit of weight loss
  - May be combined with varenicline and NRT in men who smoke >1 PPD
  - Side effects: tachycardia, headache, nausea, insomnia, dry mouth; contraindicated in patients who have seizure disorders or anorexia/bulimia; pregnancy Category C
- Nortriptyline: 25 to 75 mg/day PO or in divided doses:
  - Start 10 to 14 days prior to smoking cessation and continue for at least 12 weeks.
  - Efficacy similar to bupropion, but side effects are more common; pregnancy Category D
  - The antidepressants bupropion and nortriptyline aid long-term smoking cessation.
- Clonidine: 0.1 mg PO BID or 0.1 mg/day transdermal patch weekly: Side effects: hypotension, bradycardia, depression, fatigue; pregnancy Category C

ADDITIONAL THERAPIES

- Pharmacotherapy and behavior health support increase success compared with minimal intervention or usual care.
- Naltrexone: can be used in addition to other pharmacotherapy as it shows decreased nicotine use and craving without significant weight gain (3).

COMPLEMENTARY & ALTERNATIVE MEDICINE

- Acupuncture and hypnotherapy may help smoking cessation in short-term.
- Avoid situations and activities that are associated with smoking.

ADMISSION, INPATIENT, AND NURSING CONSIDERATIONS

Intense counseling interventions in hospitalized patients combined with follow-up for >1 month after discharge showed significant improvement in smoking cessation rates at 6 months or more postdischarge.

ONGOING CARE

35–40% of patients relapse between years 1 and 5 after quitting. 2/3 of smokers who relapse report wanting to quit again within 30 days.

FOLLOW-UP RECOMMENDATIONS

Follow up 3 to 7 days after scheduled quit date and at least monthly for 3 months thereafter. Refraining from tobacco products for first 2 weeks is critical to long-term abstinence. Inpatient counseling plus four postdischarge telephone calls effective for relapse prevention in hospitalized smokers

Patient Monitoring

- Short-term withdrawal symptoms include dysphoria, depressed mood, irritability, anxiety, insomnia, increased appetite, and poor concentration.
- Nicotine withdrawal syndrome: dysphoric or depressed mood, insomnia, irritability, frustration, or anger; anxiety, difficulty concentrating, restlessness, and increased appetite or weight gain. Within 2 to 5 years after quitting, risk for stroke approximate to that of a nonsmoker
- Risk for cancer of the mouth, throat, esophagus, and bladder drops by half within 5 years of quitting. Ten years after quitting, the risk of dying from lung cancer drops by 50%.

DIET

Limit unhealthy foods, and avoid alcohol use which is often linked to smoking.

PATIENT EDUCATION

1-800-QUIT-NOW

PROGNOSIS

- Smoking increases the risk for coronary heart disease (2-fold to 4-fold), stroke (2-fold to 4-fold), and lung cancer (25-fold). Smokers are more likely to die from COPD than nonsmokers (12-fold increased risk). Tobacco cessation reduces the risk of coronary heart disease sharply in the first 2 years after quitting (more slowly after that).
- Tobacco cessation slows the progression of COPD and reduces the loss of lung function over time. Tobacco cessation also reduces the risk of acute myeloid leukemia, cancer of the lung, cervix, colon, rectum, bladder esophagus, kidney, liver, mouth and throat. The risk of developing diabetes is 30–40% higher for active smokers than nonsmokers.
- People who quit smoking after a heart attack or cardiac surgery reduce their risk of death by 1/3. Relapse rates initially >60% but decrease to 2–4% after 2 years of abstinence. The incidence of myocardial infarction (MI) is increased 6-fold in women and 3-fold in men who smoke at least 20 cigarettes per day, when compared with nonsmokers.
- Tobacco cessation reduces the risk of premature death and can add as much as 10 years of life expectancy.

COMPLICATIONS

- Disability and premature death due to heart attack, stroke, cancer, COPD
- Causation proven cancers associated with smoking: colorectal, head and neck, esophagus, kidney, liver, lower urinary tract, renal pelvis, ureter, and bladder, lung, mesothelioma, nasal cavity, paranasal sinuses, pancreas, penis, stomach, uterine, cervix; evidence equivocal: breast, skin
- Smoking doubles the risk of coronary artery disease and stroke.

REFERENCES

1. Lindson N, Chepkin SC, Ye W, et al. Different doses, durations and modes of delivery of nicotine replacement therapy for smoking cessation. *Cochrane Database Syst Rev*. 2019;4(4):CD013308.
2. Livingstone-Banks J, Lindson N, Hartmann-Boyce J. Effects of interventions to combat tobacco addiction: Cochrane update of 2021 to 2023 reviews. *Addiction*. 2024;119(12):2101–2115. doi:10.1111/add.16624.
3. Gaddey HL, Dakkak M, Jackson NM. Smoking cessation interventions. *Am Fam Physician*. 2022;106(5):513–522.

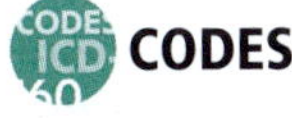

CODES

ICD10

- F17.210 Nicotine dependence, cigarettes, uncomplicated
- F17.213 Nicotine dependence, cigarettes, with withdrawal
- F17.211 Nicotine dependence, cigarettes, in remission

CLINICAL PEARLS

- Most adult cigarette smokers want to quit.
- Nicotine replacement improves cessation rates.
- Establish a quit date and provide resources to promote success.

TOURETTE SYNDROME

Alicia Leandra Olowu, DO

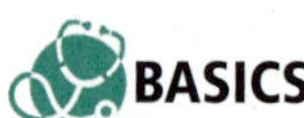

BASICS

DESCRIPTION

Tourette syndrome (TS) is a childhood-onset neurobehavioral disorder characterized by the presence of multiple motor and at least one phonic tic.

- Tics are sudden, brief, repetitive, stereotyped motor movements (motor tics), or sounds (phonic tics) produced by moving air through the nose, mouth, or throat.
- Patients can suppress their tics, but this often causes inner tension that eventually results in more forceful tics.
- System(s) affected: nervous

EPIDEMIOLOGY

Incidence

- Average age of onset 7 years (1)
- Male > female (3:1); heterogeneous disorder, but non-Hispanic White (2:1) compared with Hispanic and/or Black

ETIOLOGY AND PATHOPHYSIOLOGY

Recent neuroimaging and electrophysiology research have pointed to possible abnormalities in frontal cortical volume and its connectivity. This supports circuit dysfunction contributing to excess dopamine/glutamate signaling, which is thought to be significant contributor to tic generation, involving decreased inhibitory output from the basal ganglia, which results in an imbalance of inhibition and excitation in the motor cortex (2).

- Thought to result from a complex interaction between social, environmental, and multiple genetic abnormalities
- Controversial pediatric autoimmune neuropsychiatric disorder associated with streptococcal infection (PANDAS); TS/OCD cases linked to immunologic response to previous group A β-hemolytic *Streptococcus* (GABHS)

Genetics

- Predisposition: frequent familial history of tic disorders and OCD
- Recent studies suggest polygenic inheritance with evidence for a locus on chromosome 17q; sequence variants in *SLITRK1* gene on chromosome 13q also are associated with TS.

RISK FACTORS

- Risk of TS among relatives: 9.8–15%
- Low birth weight, maternal stress, nausea/vomiting in 1st trimester, maternal smoking (3)

COMMONLY ASSOCIATED CONDITIONS

- OCD (28–67%), ADHD (50–60%), conduct disorder, learning disabilities (23%)
- Depression/anxiety including phobias, panic attacks, and stuttering; increased risk of contemplating suicide (1)
- Impairments of visual perception, sleep disorders, restless leg syndrome, and migraine headaches
- Cardiometabolic disorders, especially obesity, circulatory system diseases, type 2 diabetes (50%) (4)

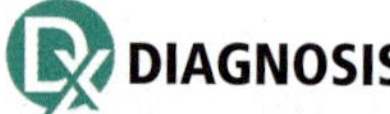

DIAGNOSIS

HISTORY

Diagnosis of TS is based on history and clinical presentation (i.e., observation of tics with/without presence of coexisting disorders). Identify comorbid conditions.

PHYSICAL EXAM

- Typically, the physical exam is normal.
- Motor and vocal tics are the clinical hallmarks.
  - Tics fluctuate in type, frequency, and anatomic distribution over time.
  - Multiple motor tics include facial grimacing, blinking, head/neck jerking, tongue protruding, sniffing, touching, and burping.
  - Vocal tics include grunts, snorts, throat clearing, barking, yelling, hiccupping, sucking, and coughing.
  - Tics are exacerbated by anticipation, emotional upset, anxiety, or fatigue.
  - Tics subside when patient is concentrating/absorbed in activities but may persist during sleep.
- *Diagnostic and Statistical Manual of Mental Disorders* (5th ed.; *DSM-5*) criteria:
  - Both multiple motor and one or more vocal tics have been present at some time, although not necessarily concurrently.
  - Tics may wax and wane in frequency but have persisted for >1 year since onset.
  - Onset before age 18 years
  - Not attributable to the physiologic effects of a substance (e.g., cocaine) or another medical condition (e.g., Huntington disease, postviral encephalitis)

DIFFERENTIAL DIAGNOSIS

- Chorea/Huntington disease
- Myoclonus
- Essential tremor
- Headache
- Dementia
- Wilson disease
- Sydenham chorea
- Multiple sclerosis
- Postviral encephalitis
- Toxin exposure (e.g., carbon monoxide, cocaine)
- Drug effects (e.g., dopamine agonists, fluoroquinolones)

DIAGNOSTIC TESTS & INTERPRETATION

Initial Tests (lab, imaging)

- No definitive lab tests diagnose TS; based on clinical features
- Measure thyroid-stimulating hormone (TSH) due to association of tics with hyperthyroidism.
- EEG shows nonspecific abnormalities; useful only to differentiate tics from epilepsy

Test Interpretation

Smaller caudate volumes and increased striatal dopaminergic terminals

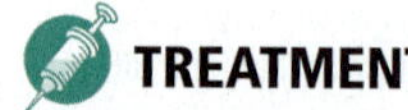

TREATMENT

GENERAL MEASURES

- Goal of treatment should be to improve social functioning, self-esteem, and quality of life. Patients should play an active role in treatment decisions and be educated that tics are not voluntary or psychiatric.
- Watchful waiting is an acceptable approach to treatment in patients without functional impairments (1)[A].
- Valid, reliable, responsive Tic severity scales for treatment assessment (5): Yale Global Tic Severity Scale (most extensively used and validated (1); Shapiro Tourette Syndrome Severity Scale; Tourette's Disorder Scale
- Educate patient, family, teachers, and friends to identify and address psychosocial stressors and environmental triggers.
- No cure for tics: Treatment is purely symptomatic, and multimodal treatment usually is indicated.
- TS clusters with several comorbid conditions; each disorder must be evaluated for associated functional impairment because patients often are more disabled by their psychiatric conditions than by the tics; choice of initial treatment depends largely on worst symptoms (tics, obsessions, or impulsivity).
- Comprehensive behavioral intervention for tics (CBIT) should be offered as an initial treatment before medications (1)[B].
  - Includes habit reversal training, relaxation training, and function intervention
  - Reduced tic severity with CBIT compared to psychoeducation and supportive therapy
- When pharmacotherapy is employed, monotherapy is preferred to polytherapy. Additionally, physicians should routinely reevaluate the necessity of pharmacotherapy (1)[A].

MEDICATION

First Line

- Recommendations should be individualized based on shared decision-making after considering benefits and harms along with treating comorbid conditions (1).
- Most of the data points to antipsychotics being most effective, but use is limited by side effects and other medications (i.e., α_2-agonists) are generally used first (6).
- Antipsychotics (6)
  - Haloperidol, risperidone, aripiprazole, tiapride are probably more likely than placebo to reduce tic severity (1).
  - Pimozide and ziprasidone are possibly more likely than placebo to reduce tic severity (1).
  - Prescribe the lowest effective dose to decrease risk of side effects (1)[A].

- Atypical (risk of weight gain and other metabolic disturbances, EPS)
  - Risperidone: Initiate 0.25 mg BID; titrate up to 4 mg/day.
  - Olanzapine: Initiate 2.5 to 5 mg/day; titrate up to 20 mg/day.
  - Quetiapine: Initiate 12.5 to 25 mg/day; titrate to 300 to 400 mg/day.
  - Ziprasidone: Initiate 5 to 10 mg/day; titrate up to 10 to 40 mg/day.
    - Must be given under ECG monitoring (1)[A]
  - Aripiprazole: Initiate 2 mg/day; titrate up to 10 to 20 mg/day.
- Typical (high risk for EPS)
  - Haloperidol: Initiate 0.5 mg/day; titrate up to 2 to 10 mg at bedtime.
    - FDA-approved for treating tics but considered last option of typical antipsychotics due to lower efficacy and increased side effects
  - Pimozide: Initiate 0.05 mg/kg per dose; titrate up to 0.2 mg/kg/day QHS with a max of 10 mg/day
    - FDA-approved for treating tics; good for long-term control of tics, not exacerbations
    - Risk of cardiac toxicity (prolonged QTc) so give under ECG monitoring
  - Fluphenazine: Initiate 0.5 to 1 mg/day; titrate up to 3 mg/day in kids and 10 mg/day in adults.

- α_2-Adrenergic receptor agonists (7)[B]
  - Historically first line due to favorable side effects, but suboptimal efficacy in limited clinical trials
  - Good choice in patients with comorbid ADHD due to efficacy in treating both conditions (1)
  - Side effects: bradycardia, sedation, and hypotension. Monitor heart rate and blood pressure (1)[A].
  - Clonidine 0.1 to 0.3 mg/day given BID to TID; maximum dose 0.5 mg/day
  - Guanfacine 1 to 3 mg/day given daily or BID
    - Less sedating and longer duration of action compared with clonidine
    - Monitor QTc interval in patients with a history of cardiac conditions, patients taking QT-prolonging drugs, or patients with family history of long QT syndrome (1)[A].
- Alternative treatments
  - Topiramate: 25 to 200 mg/day (7)[A]
  - Tetrabenazine
  - Baclofen: Initiate 10 mg/day; titrate up to 10 to 80 mg/day (6).
  - Preliminary data for deutetrabenazine and valbenazine (vesicular monoamine transporter-2 [VMAT2] inhibitors) and ecopipam (novel D1 receptor antagonist) (6)
- Comorbid ADHD:
  - Stimulants: methylphenidate: 2.5 to 30 mg/day; dextroamphetamine: 5 to 30 mg/day
  - α_2-Adrenergic agonists: guanfacine, clonidine
  - Other medications: atomoxetine, desipramine
- Comorbid OCD (8)[B]:
  - SSRIs: fluoxetine: 10 to 80 mg/day, fluvoxamine: 50 to 300 mg/day, or sertraline: 50 to 200 mg/day
    - First-line treatment of OCD; can be used in TS as well
    - Side effects: nausea, insomnia, sexual dysfunction, headache, agitation, suicidality
    - SSRIs are not as effective in treating OCD symptoms in children with tics compared to those without tics; however, cognitive-behavioral therapy was effective in both populations making this intervention first line for OCD in patients with tic disorders (1).
  - Tricyclic antidepressants: clomipramine: 25 to 200 mg/day
    - Can be used in patients refractory to SSRIs or to augment SSRIs in partial responders
    - Side effects: weight gain, dry mouth, lowered seizure threshold, and constipation; ECG changes, including QT prolongation and tachycardia

ADDITIONAL THERAPIES

- Botulinum toxin injections for localized simple motor ticks and disabling vocal tics (1)
- Habit-reversal training for tic suppression treatment: works equally for motor and vocal tics

SURGERY/OTHER PROCEDURES

Thalamic ablation and deep brain stimulation have been used experimentally and can be considered for severe, self-injurious tics (1)[C]. Patients must have failed multiple classes of medications and behavioral therapy (1)[A].

COMPLEMENTARY & ALTERNATIVE MEDICINE

- Reassurance and environmental modification
- Identification and treatment of triggers
- CBIT, hypnotherapy, biofeedback, acupuncture
- Cannabinoids: insufficient evidence to recommend; small trials show small positive effects (9).
- Physical exercise (10)

ONGOING CARE

FOLLOW-UP RECOMMENDATIONS

Patient Monitoring

Observe for associated psychiatric disorders and inquire about suicidal thoughts (1).

PATIENT EDUCATION

- Reassurance that many patients with tics do not need medication, simply education, and/or therapy
- National Tourette Syndrome Association: http://www.tsa-usa.org

PROGNOSIS

- Symptoms will fluctuate throughout illness.
- Tic severity typically stabilizes by age 25 years.
- 60–75% of young adults show some improvement in symptoms; 10–40% of patients will exhibit full remission.

REFERENCES

1. Pringsheim T, Okun MS, Müller-Vahl K, et al. Practice guideline recommendations summary: treatment of tics in people with Tourette syndrome and chronic tic disorders. *Neurology*. 2019;92(19):896–906.
2. Choi CY, Agin-Liebes J, Kuo SH. Emerging therapies and recent advances for Tourette syndrome. *Heliyon*. 2023;9(1):e12874. doi:10.1016/j.heliyon.2023.e12874.
3. Ayubi E, Mansori K, Doosti-Irani A. Effect of maternal smoking during pregnancy on Tourette syndrome and chronic tic disorders among offspring: a systematic review and meta-analysis. *Obstet Gynecol Sci*. 2021;64(1):1–12.
4. Brander G, Isomura K, Chang Z, et al. Association of Tourette syndrome and chronic tic disorder with metabolic and cardiovascular disorders. *JAMA Neurol*. 2019;76(4):454–461.
5. Martino D, Pringsheim TM, Cavanna AE, et al. Systematic review of severity scales and screening instruments for tics: critique and recommendations. *Mov Disord*. 2017;32(3):467–473.
6. Quezada J, Coffman KA. Current approaches and new developments in the pharmacological management of Tourette syndrome. *CNS Drugs*. 2018;32(1):33–45.
7. Huys D, Hardenacke K, Poppe P, et al. Update on the role of antipsychotics in the treatment of Tourette syndrome. *Neuropsychiatr Dis Treat*. 2012;8:95–104.
8. Pringsheim T, Steeves T. Pharmacological treatment for attention deficit hyperactivity disorder (ADHD) in children with comorbid tic disorders. *Cochrane Database Syst Rev*. 2011;(4):CD007990.
9. Curtis A, Clarke CE, Rickards HE. Cannabinoids for Tourette's syndrome. *Cochrane Database Syst Rev*. 2009;2009(4):CD006565.
10. Reilly C, Grant M, Bennett S, et al. Review: physical exercise in Tourette syndrome—a systematic review. *Child Adolesc Ment Health*. 2019;24(1):3–11.

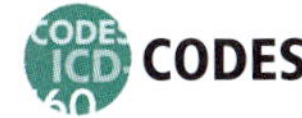

CODES

ICD10

F95.2 Tourette's disorder

CLINICAL PEARLS

- TS is diagnosed by history and witnessing tics; have parent video patient's tics if not present on exam.
- Many patients require no treatment; patient should play an active role in treatment decisions.
- Nearly 50% of children with tics also have ADHD. Stimulants may be used as first-line treatment for ADHD (tics are not a contraindication, as previously believed).

TOXOPLASMOSIS

Jonathan Edward MacClements, MD, FAAFP

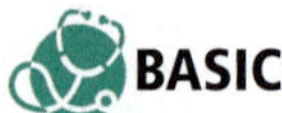

BASICS

- *Toxoplasma gondii* is an obligate intracellular protozoan parasite.
- Clinically significant disease typically manifests only in pregnancy or in an immunocompromised patient.

DESCRIPTION

- Acute self-limited infection in immunocompetent individuals
- Acute symptomatic or reactivated latent infection in immunocompromised patients
- Congenital toxoplasmosis (acute primary infection during pregnancy)
- Ocular toxoplasmosis

Pediatric Considerations

- The earlier a fetal infection occurs, the more severe the resulting disease.
- Risk of perinatal death is 5% if infected in 1st trimester.

Pregnancy Considerations

- Pregnant immunocompromised and HIV-infected women should undergo serologic testing.
- Counsel pregnant women regarding risks of toxoplasmosis.
- Serologic testing during pregnancy is controversial.

EPIDEMIOLOGY

Incidence

- Prevalence of congenital toxoplasmosis in the United States: 10 to 100/100,000 live births
- Predominant sex: male > female

Prevalence

- Present in every country with prevalence differing worldwide (1)[A].
- In the United States, 11% of individuals aged 6 to 49 years are seropositive.
- Age-adjusted prevalence in the United States is 10%.
- Toxoplasmosis is considered a neglected parasitic infection in the United States and has been targeted by CDC for public health action.

ETIOLOGY AND PATHOPHYSIOLOGY

- *T. gondii* has two life cycles. The sexual portion of the life cycle is exclusive to felines. The asexual cycle occurs in humans. Cats become infected by eating contaminated meat (birds, mice). Oocysts form within the tract of the cat and are shed in the stool.
- Transmission to humans
  - Ingestion of raw or undercooked meat, food, or water containing tissue cysts or oocytes that is usually from soil contaminated with feline feces
  - Transplacental passage from infected mother to fetus; risk of transmission is 30% on average.
  - Blood product transfusion or solid-organ transplantation
  - Ingested *T. gondii* oocysts enter host's gastrointestinal (GI) tract where bradyzoites/tachyzoites are released, penetrate contiguous cells, replicate, and are transported to susceptible tissues causing clinical disease.

Genetics

Human leukocyte antigen (HLA) DQ3 is a genetic marker for susceptibility in HIV/AIDS patients.

RISK FACTORS

- Immunocompromised states, including HIV infection with CD4 cell count <100/μL
- Primary infection during pregnancy; risk of fetal transmission increases with gestational age at seroconversion. Transmission in the 1st trimester is associated with more severe consequences.
- Chronically infected immunocompromised pregnant women are at increased risk for transmitting congenital toxoplasmosis.

GENERAL PREVENTION

- Avoid eating undercooked meat: Cook at 152°F (66°C) or freeze for 24 hours at ≤−12°C.
- Avoid drinking unfiltered water.
- Wash produce thoroughly.
- Wear gloves and wash hands after gardening and handling soil
- Wear gloves and wash hands after handling raw meat or cat litter.
- Avoid shellfish (*Toxoplasma* cysts).

COMMONLY ASSOCIATED CONDITIONS

- Chorioretinitis; self-limiting, febrile lymphadenopathy; mononucleosis-like illness
- Potential association with schizophrenia

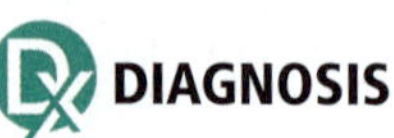

DIAGNOSIS

HISTORY

- Congenital toxoplasmosis
  - Clinical presentation varies widely; 80% of patients are asymptomatic at birth.
  - Classic triad (*uncommon*): chorioretinitis, hydrocephalus, cerebral calcifications
  - Manifestations may include prematurity, intrauterine growth retardation (IUGR).
  - Jaundice, rash with a mononucleosis-like illness
  - Mental retardation, seizures, visual defects, spasticity, sensorineural hearing loss
- Ocular toxoplasmosis
  - Chorioretinitis: focal necrotizing retinitis
  - Yellowish-white elevated cotton patch
  - Congenital disease usually bilateral; acquired is more often unilateral.
  - Symptoms include blurred vision, scotoma, pain, and photophobia.
- Acute toxoplasmosis (immunocompetent host)
  - ~90% of patients are asymptomatic.
  - Most common manifestation is bilateral, symmetric, nontender cervical lymphadenopathy.
  - Constitutional symptoms such as fever, chills, and sweats are usually mild.
  - Headaches, myalgias, pharyngitis, hepatosplenomegaly, and diffuse nonpruritic maculopapular rash may occur.
  - Pregnant women are often asymptomatic.
  - CNS: encephalitis
  - Headache; focal neurologic deficits and seizures
  - Fever usually present
  - Extracerebral toxoplasmosis: pneumonitis, chorioretinitis; rarely: GI system, liver, musculoskeletal system, heart, bone marrow, bladder, and orchitis

PHYSICAL EXAM

- In adults: fever, lymphadenopathy, nonpruritic maculopapular rash (spares palms and soles); hepatosplenomegaly; visual changes; funduscopic changes
- In newborns: hydrocephalus, neurologic abnormalities, hepatosplenomegaly, chorioretinitis, microcephaly, mental retardation

DIFFERENTIAL DIAGNOSIS

Syphilis, lymphoma, progressive multifocal leukoencephalopathy, cryptococcal meningitis, congenital TORCH infections, HIV; *Listeria* infection, tuberculosis (TB), tularemia; CMV infection; leukemia; erythroblastosis fetalis

DIAGNOSTIC TESTS & INTERPRETATION

- CBC: atypical lymphocytosis, anemia, thrombocytopenia
- Serology interpretation
  - IgM antibodies appear in the 1st week if acute infection
  - Initial test demonstrates positive IgM and negative IgG, with both tests being positive 2 weeks later.
  - If follow-up IgG is negative 2 to 4 weeks later and IgM is positive, this is likely a false positive.
  - Negative IgG rules out prior infection (IgG persists for life).
- Types of serologic tests
  - ELISA: most commonly used
  - Sabin-Feldman dye test: Gold standard against which all other serologic assays are compared.
  - IFA test: more available in commercial labs
  - ISAGA: widely available commercially; more sensitive and specific than IFA for detecting IgM
  - Avidity testing: confirmatory test to establish if positive IgM/IgG reflects recent or chronic infection
- PCR: *T. gondii* DNA amplification in blood or amniotic fluid; used for diagnosis of fetal infection
- Culture (rarely necessary): Organism can be isolated either by cell culture or by mouse inoculation.

Initial Tests (lab, imaging)

- Diagnosis of primary infection is typically based on history and confirmed by serology.
- Serum *Toxoplasma*-specific IgG and IgM are first step.
- According to IgM result, determine IgG avidity.
- Diagnosis of maternal infection and congenital toxoplasmosis
  - Test pregnant women who have mononucleosis-like illness but negative heterophile test for toxoplasmosis.
  - Diagnose maternal infection based on two blood samples at least 2 weeks to show seroconversion.
  - High avidity of IgG during 1st trimester argues against maternal primary infection.
  - Real-time PCR analysis of amniotic fluid predicts fetal infection and guides treatment.
  - Fetal ultrasound is useful for prognosis.
  - Routine screening for toxoplasmosis is not recommended in pregnancy.
- Neonatal diagnosis of congenital toxoplasmosis
  - Serology requires repeat testing for IgM and IgA.
  - Sample cord or peripheral blood within 2 weeks
  - Ophthalmologic, auditory, and neurologic examinations; lumbar puncture and head CT scan

- Diagnosis of toxoplasmic encephalitis
  - Serology for IgG
  - Imaging: MRI is more sensitive than CT scan to identify characteristic ring-enhancing lesions.
- SPECT and PET scans can help distinguish toxoplasmosis from CNS lymphoma.

Diagnostic Procedures/Other
- Lymph node biopsy
- Brain biopsy in CNS disease
- Amniocentesis with PCR (risk of false negatives and false positives)
- Placental isolation of *Toxoplasma* is diagnostic.

Test Interpretation
- Confirmatory, meningocerebritis ± abscesses with necrosis, Giemsa
- Lymph node histology with reactive follicular hyperplasia, irregular clusters of epithelioid histiocytes blurring margins of germinal centers, and distension of sinuses with monocytoid cells

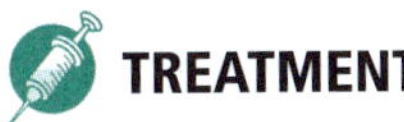

TREATMENT

GENERAL MEASURES
Immunocompetent patients usually require no treatment.

MEDICATION
Recommended treatment drugs for toxoplasmosis target the tachyzoite stage of the parasite and do not eradicate encysted parasites in the tissues

First Line

ALERT
Important: All pyrimethamine-containing regimens should include leucovorin (folinic acid 10 to 25 mg/day PO) during and 1 week after completion of pyrimethamine to prevent drug-induced hematologic toxicity (2)[A].

- Treatment in immunocompromised hosts
  - Initial regimen of choice is pyrimethamine 200 mg loading dose PO, followed by 50 mg/day *plus* sulfadiazine 4 to 6 g/day PO in 4 divided doses; for those intolerant or allergic to sulfadiazine, clindamycin 600 to 1,200 mg IV or 450 mg PO QID can be used instead.
  - Alternative regimens for patients intolerant to sulfadiazine and clindamycin include the following:
    - Pyrimethamine: 200 mg loading dose PO, followed by 50 mg/day *plus* azithromycin 900 to 1,200 mg PO once daily
    - Pyrimethamine: 200 mg loading dose PO and then 50 mg/day *plus* atovaquone 1,500 mg PO BID
    - Sulfadiazine: 1,000 to 1,500 mg QID *plus* atovaquone 1,500 mg BID
    - Trimethoprim-sulfamethoxazole: 10/50 mg/kg/day PO or IV divided BID (for 30 days) may be a cost-effective alternative.
  - Duration of therapy: typically 6 weeks, lower doses for secondary prophylaxis (2)[A]
  - Use adjunctive steroids in patients with signs of increased intracranial pressure.
  - Anticonvulsants, if there is a history of seizures
- Prophylaxis in immunocompromised patients
  - Primary prophylaxis: indicated for patients with HIV infection and CD4 count <100 cells/μL who are *T. gondii* IgG–positive
    - Trimethoprim-sulfamethoxazole-DS: 1 tablet PO daily; alternative for sulfa allergy is dapsone 50 mg/day PO *plus* pyrimethamine 50 mg PO weekly *plus* leucovorin 25 mg PO weekly *or* atovaquone 1,500 mg PO daily.
  - Secondary prophylaxis: Following 6 weeks of therapy, administer lower doses of drugs:
    - Sulfadiazine 2 to 4 g/day in 2 to 4 divided doses *plus* pyrimethamine 25 to 50 mg/day is the first choice.
    - Alternative regimens include clindamycin 600 mg PO q8h *plus* pyrimethamine 25 to 50 mg/day PO *or* atovaquone 750 mg PO BID to QID ± pyrimethamine 25 mg PO daily.
- Pregnant women
  - Although typically offered, it is unsure if antenatal treatment reduces congenital transmission.
  - <18 weeks' gestation: spiramycin 1 g PO q8h without food until delivery if amniotic fluid PCR is negative; does not treat infection in the fetus
  - >18 weeks' gestation: Pyrimethamine and sulfadiazine should be considered only if fetal infection is documented by positive amniotic fluid PCR (pyrimethamine is teratogenic):
    - Pyrimethamine: 50 mg PO q12h for 2 days, then 50 mg/day *plus* sulfadiazine 75 mg/kg PO × 1 dose and then 50 mg/kg q12h (max 4 g/day)
- Treat infected newborns regardless of clinical manifestations:
  - Pyrimethamine 2 mg/kg/day (max 50 mg) for 2 days; then 1 mg/kg/day (max 25 mg) for 2 to 6 month and then 1 mg/kg (max 25 mg) on Monday, Wednesday, and Friday; sulfadiazine 100 mg/kg/day divided BID; and leucovorin 10 mg 3 times per week during pyrimethamine and 1 week after discontinuation
- Immunocompetent nonpregnant patients generally do not require treatment unless symptoms are severe or prolonged; one of two regimens can be used:
  - Pyrimethamine: 100 mg loading dose PO, followed by 25 to 50 mg/day *plus* sulfadiazine 2 to 4 g/day in 4 divided doses
  - Pyrimethamine: 100 mg loading dose PO, followed by 25 to 50 mg/day *plus* clindamycin 300 mg PO QID

Second Line
- Clindamycin: 900 to 1,200 mg TID IV used for ocular and CNS toxoplasmosis alone and in combination with pyrimethamine; as effective as the sulfadiazine-pyrimethamine with fewer adverse effects
- Corticosteroids (prednisone 1 to 2 mg/kg/day) are added for macular chorioretinitis or CNS infection.
- Alternatives: atovaquone (Mepron), azithromycin (Zithromax), clarithromycin (Biaxin), or dapsone *plus* pyrimethamine and leucovorin
- Trimethoprim-sulfamethoxazole appears to be equivalent to pyrimethamine-sulfadiazine in AIDS patients with CNS disease.

ADDITIONAL THERAPIES
For prevention of recurrent episode of chorioretinitis, trimethoprim-sulfamethoxazole-DS q12h for 45 days

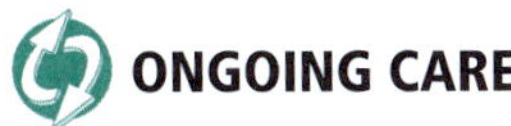

ONGOING CARE

FOLLOW-UP RECOMMENDATIONS

Patient Monitoring
Precautions
- Monitor for bone marrow, renal, or liver toxicity.
- Good hydration: Sulfadiazine is poorly soluble and may crystallize in the urine.
- Watch for antibiotic-associated diarrhea.
- Sulfonamides may alter phenytoin and warfarin levels or interfere with oral hypoglycemic agents.

PROGNOSIS
- Immunodeficient patients often relapse if treatment or suppression therapy is stopped.
- Treatment may prevent the development of untoward sequelae in infants with congenital toxoplasmosis.

REFERENCES

1. Dubey JP. Outbreaks of clinical toxoplasmosis in humans: five decades of personal experience, perspectives and lessons learned. *Parasit Vectors*. 2021;14(1):263. doi:10.1186/s13071-021-04769-4.
2. Dunay IR, Gajurel K, Dhakal R, et al. Treatment of toxoplasmosis: historical perspective, animal models, and current clinical practice. *Clin Microbiol Rev* 2018;31(4):e00057–17.

ADDITIONAL READING

- Centers for Disease Control and Prevention. Clinical Overview of Toxoplasmosis. https://cdc.gov/toxoplasmosis/hcp/clinical-overview/index.html. Accessed June 12, 2025
- Maldonado YA, Read JS; for Committee on Infectious Disease. Diagnosis, treatment, and prevention of congenital toxoplasmosis in the United States. *Pediatrics*. 2017;139(2):e20163860.

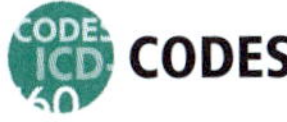

CODES

ICD10
- B58.9 Toxoplasmosis, unspecified
- P37.1 Congenital toxoplasmosis
- B58.2 Toxoplasma meningoencephalitis

CLINICAL PEARLS
- Toxoplasmosis is typically asymptomatic in immunocompetent patients.
- Primary prevention is important, particularly for pregnant women and immunodeficient patients.
- The most common manifestation of acute toxoplasmosis in immunocompetent host is bilateral, symmetric, nontender cervical lymphadenopathy.
- Universal screening for congenital toxoplasmosis is not currently recommended.

TRACHEITIS, BACTERIAL

Cliff C. Moeckelmann, MD

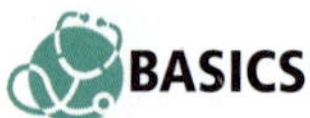

BASICS

DESCRIPTION

- Acute, life-threatening upper airway obstruction due to infraglottic bacterial infection following a primary viral infection (typically parainfluenza or influenza)
- Historically high mortality rates of up to 20% in children; more recent evidence suggests lower mortality rates, as low as 2.7% in the Casazza et al. case series (1). Improving prompt recognition and airway management has lowered mortality; however, it can still result in severe, acute, upper airway obstruction and death.
- Affects two major groups of patients in the pediatric age range
  - Those with a native intact airway
  - Those with an artificial airway
- Often preceded by viral infection, such as influenza, parainfluenza, or respiratory syncytial virus
- Staphylococcus is the most common bacteria identified in those with an intact native airway.
- Diagnostic hallmarks on endoscopy: ulceration, pseudomembranes in the trachea with thick mucopurulent exudates, and mucosal sloughing that can cause airway obstruction
- System(s) affected: pulmonary
- Synonym(s): laryngotracheobronchitis; bacterial croup; pseudomembranous croup

EPIDEMIOLOGY

Incidence

- Incidence: <1 per 100,000 children per year
- Peak incidence in children: fall and winter
- Mean age: 5 years
- Infections in adolescents and adults have been reported.

Prevalence

- Most data on prevalence are limited due to the rarity of the condition.
- Methicillin-resistant *Staphylococcus aureus* (MRSA) may contribute to changing epidemiology and virulence.

ETIOLOGY AND PATHOPHYSIOLOGY

- Methicillin-sensitive *S. aureus* (MSSA) accounted for 33% of cases and *Haemophilus influenzae* 12.1% in Barengo et al. cohort study (2)
- Mixed respiratory flora
- *Streptococcus pneumoniae*
- In children with artificial airway, most common organisms in order of frequency are *Pseudomonas aeruginosa*, *S. aureus*, *H. influenzae*, *S. pneumoniae*, and other gram-negative organisms.
- Viral-induced injury to the respiratory epithelium in conjunction with localized immune impairment can predispose individuals to bacterial superinfection.

Genetics

No known genetic predisposition

RISK FACTORS

- Periods of increased seasonal activity of respiratory viruses
- Reports following tonsillectomy, adenoidectomy, with chronic tracheal aspiration, and with evidence of other concurrent infections, including sinusitis, otitis, pneumonia, or pharyngitis
- Presence of an artificial airway

GENERAL PREVENTION

- Standard precautions, with scrupulous attention to handwashing
- Age-appropriate Centers for Disease Control and Prevention (CDC) scheduled pediatric immunization against *H. influenzae* and viruses that may predispose to bacterial tracheitis

COMMONLY ASSOCIATED CONDITIONS

- Consider anatomic abnormalities, foreign bodies, as well as recent pharyngeal or laryngeal surgery.
- Predisposing: Down syndrome, immunodeficiency, subglottic hemangioma, tracheoesophageal fistula repair, tracheobronchomalacia
- More common in children with tracheostomy
- Viral coinfection may occur.

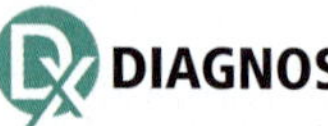

DIAGNOSIS

- Careful history and physical exam are the best methods to help distinguish bacterial tracheitis from croup and other rare causes of upper airway obstruction.
- X-ray imaging of anterior/posterior and lateral neck can show characteristic signs of intratracheal opacities and subglottic airway narrowing.
- The diagnosis of bacterial tracheitis is confirmed by flexible laryngoscopy, operative bronchoscopy, and/or autopsy. Findings include mucopurulent exudates, ulcerations, and pseudomembranes within the subglottis and/or trachea.

HISTORY

- Presentation can be variable from mild to severe with high fever and systemic toxicity.
- Classic presentation:
  - The most common presenting symptoms in children are difficulty breathing, sore throat, and painful cough.
  - Gradual progression of mild upper airway symptoms over 1 hour to 6 days to acute, febrile phase of rapid respiratory decompensation
  - Drooling usually absent
  - No response to aerosolized and/or systemic corticosteroids (Differentiation from croup)
- Individuals with artificial airways may have a more indolent case and are also more likely to experience recurrence.

PHYSICAL EXAM

- Acute onset
- High fever
- Inspiratory stridor
- Respiratory distress
- Toxic appearance
- Voice hoarseness
- Drooling uncommon
- Atypical presentations can also occur and some may present with URI symptoms.
- Children with artificial airways can have more indolent onset.

DIFFERENTIAL DIAGNOSIS

- Severe croup (viral)
- Foreign body aspiration
- Spasmodic croup
- Angioneurotic edema
- Bronchiolitis
- Epiglottitis
- Bacterial pneumonia
- Diphtheria in unimmunized individuals
- Retropharyngeal abscess

DIAGNOSTIC TESTS & INTERPRETATION

- Tracheal endoscopy (rigid bronchoscopy in children with intact airway or tracheoscopy in those with artificial airway) provides a definitive diagnosis.
- Diffuse inflammation of larynx, trachea, and bronchi
- Mucopurulent exudate; microabscesses may be present.
- Semi-adherent membranes (containing numerous neutrophils and cellular debris) may be identified within the trachea.

Initial Tests (lab, imaging)

Obtain Gram stain and aerobic, anaerobic, and viral cultures of tracheal secretions during the tracheal endoscopy. Bacterial cultures of tracheal secretions are required for culture isolates and sensitivities.

- Tracheal biopsy is rarely indicated but may be considered in immunodeficient child or child with ulcerative colitis.
- Routine laboratory studies are not required to make the diagnosis and are rarely helpful.
- Rapid antigen or polymerase chain reaction (PCR) based testing for respiratory viruses may be helpful.
- CBC results may vary.
  - WBC count may show marked leukocytosis or may be normal.
  - Increased band cell count
- Chest radiographs are neither definitive nor diagnostic of bacterial tracheitis but may be helpful in identifying associated pneumonia.
- Anteroposterior (AP) and lateral neck x-rays show subglottic and tracheal narrowing (i.e., steeple sign on AP film).

Follow-Up Tests & Special Considerations

- In patients with pneumonia, follow-up chest films may be required.
- Repeat bronchoscopies may be needed to remove pseudomembranes.
- Children with or at risk for acute airway obstruction should be carefully monitored in a setting and with personnel capable of securing a pediatric airway.

Diagnostic Procedures/Other
Bronchoscopy

Test Interpretation
Findings include mucopurulent exudates, ulcerations, and pseudomembranes within the subglottis and/or trachea.

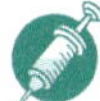

TREATMENT

- Consider as a potentially life-threatening airway emergency.
- Children with suspected or actual bacterial tracheitis should be cared for in a pediatric ICU.
- Assess and monitor respiratory status; supplemental oxygen may be necessary.
- Airway protection and support, as necessary (at least 50% require intubation; some studies report up to 100% [80% require intubation; 94% admitted to PICU]).
- Ventilatory support may be required.

GENERAL MEASURES
- Consider bacterial tracheitis as a potentially life-threatening airway emergency.
- Support care and monitoring in PICU care are often required.
- Supplemental oxygen, endotracheal intubation, and/or mechanical ventilation may be required.

MEDICATION
- Empiric therapy should cover the most common pathogens until sensitivities are available: antistaphylococcal agent (nafcillin or oxacillin IV) and a 3rd-generation cephalosporin (e.g., ceftriaxone or cefotaxime).
- Vancomycin if MRSA or highly resistant penicillin *S. pneumoniae* suspected.
- In the case of technology-dependent children with tracheostomy, make initial antibiotic choices based on previous tracheal culture.
- Narrow regimen when isolated pathogen's cultures and sensitivities are available
- Usual duration of antibiotics is 10 to 14 days, can transition to oral regimen when patient is afebrile >48 hours and can tolerate swallowing oral medication.
- Systemic or inhaled corticosteroids or racemic epinephrine has no proven efficacy in relieving airway obstruction in bacterial tracheitis (differentiation from viral croup).
- Contraindications: Refer to the manufacturer's literature for each drug.
- Precautions: Refer to the manufacturer's literature for each drug.
- Significant possible interactions: Refer to the manufacturer's literature for each medication.

ISSUES FOR REFERRAL
- All children with suspected or actual bacterial tracheitis should be cared for in a pediatric ICU.
- Critical care teams may include ID, ENT, and pulmonary consultants in addition to the pediatric intensivist.

SURGERY/OTHER PROCEDURES
- Therapeutic bronchoscopy may be needed to facilitate the removal of inspissated secretions and accumulated debris .
- Tracheostomy is usually not necessary.

COMPLEMENTARY & ALTERNATIVE MEDICINE
No evidence to support use

ADMISSION, INPATIENT, AND NURSING CONSIDERATIONS
- Diagnostic endoscopic evaluation of the upper airway
- Airway stabilization and support
- Pediatric intensive care admission

Pediatric Considerations
- Suctioning and pulmonary toilet
- Hydration
- Antibiotics as described above
- Nursing
  - Provide a calm, quiet environment for child once endoscopy and cultures are done.
  - Airway monitoring
  - Frequent suctioning
  - Monitor fluid balance.
  - Establish and maintain open lines of communication with child and parent.

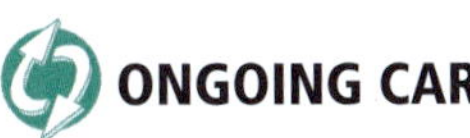

ONGOING CARE

FOLLOW-UP RECOMMENDATIONS

Patient Monitoring
Children with artificial airway will require ongoing follow-up.

DIET
Varies with clinical situations

PATIENT EDUCATION
Keep immunizations up to date.

PROGNOSIS
- Intubation generally requires hospitalization of 3 to 11 days.
- Usually requires 3 to 7 days of hospitalization
- With effective early recognition and management, complete recovery can be expected.
- Cardiopulmonary arrest and death have occurred.
- Higher recurrence rates in children with artificial airways

COMPLICATIONS
- Pneumonia
- Pneumothorax
- Tracheal stenosis, especially with prolonged intubation
- Toxic shock syndrome
- Septic shock
- Acute respiratory distress syndrome (ARDS)
- Disseminated intravascular coagulation
- Cardiopulmonary arrest

REFERENCES

1. Casazza G, Graham ME, Nelson D, et al. Pediatric bacterial tracheitis—a variable entity: case series with literature review. *Otolaryngol Head Neck Surg*. 2019;160(3):546–549. doi:10.1177/0194599818808774.
2. Barengo JH, Redmann AJ, Kennedy P, et al. Demographic characteristics of children diagnosed with bacterial tracheitis. *Ann Otol Rhinol Laryngol*. 2021;130(12):1378–1382. doi:10.1177/00034894211007250.

ADDITIONAL READING

- García-Boyano M, Alcalá FJC, Alonso AR, et al. Microbiological patterns of bacterial infections in tracheostomized children: reducing uncertainty in continuous care. *Pediatr Pulmonol*. 2023;58(12):3507–3515. doi:10.1002/ppul.26684.
- Russell CJ, Shiroishi MS, Siantz E, et al. The use of inhaled antibiotic therapy in the treatment of ventilator-associated pneumonia and tracheobronchitis: a systematic review. *BMC Pulm Med*. 2016;16:40.

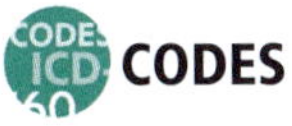

CODES

ICD10
- J04.10 Acute tracheitis without obstruction
- J04.11 Acute tracheitis with obstruction
- J05.0 Acute obstructive laryngitis [croup]

CLINICAL PEARLS

- Bacterial tracheitis is an acute, potentially life-threatening, infraglottic bacterial infection that generally follows a primary viral infection.
- Bacterial tracheitis should be suspected in croup-like cases who fail to respond to oral or inhaled corticosteroids and racemic epinephrine.
- Bronchoscopy (or tracheoscopy in the child with an artificial airway) provides a definitive diagnosis.
- Initial treatment priorities include broad-spectrum antibiotic coverage, aggressive airway protection, and supportive care.

T

TRANSGENDER HEALTH

Kiran A. Lorick, MD

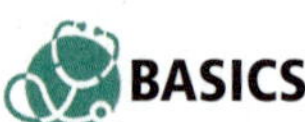

BASICS

DESCRIPTION

- Transgender and gender diverse (TGD) is a term meant to be inclusive of people of various global communities whose gender identity and/or expression is incongruent with societal attributes typically associated with their sex assigned at birth.
- There are a number of social and health disparities that exist amongst TGD people, including increased rates of harassment, homelessness, anxiety, depression, suicidality, cardiovascular disease, and substance abuse, in part due to discrimination faced or fear of discrimination within the community and when seeking health care.
- Better education of clinicians is imperative to bridge some of the gaps in care and improve the health of the TGD population; such education begins with creating a welcoming and safe environment for transgender individuals to speak openly with knowledgeable and culturally sensitive clinicians.

EPIDEMIOLOGY

- Approximately 1.3 million U.S. adults (4.6% of adults assigned male at birth and 3.2% of adults assigned female at birth) and up to 2.7% of children and adolescents identify as transgender. These populations have approximately doubled in the past decade and are expected to continue to grow (1).
- It is difficult to estimate the size of the TGD population worldwide due to the lack of standardized methodologies and systematically reviewed data from studies aiming to assess the number or proportion of TGD people (2).

DIAGNOSIS

- Gender dysphoria is an outdated term previously used to describe the TGD population and is classified as a mental health condition in the *Diagnostic and Statistical Manual of Mental Disorders* (*DSM-5*); this classification has contributed to the stigmas faced by TGD people; therefore, the World Health Organization (WHO) now uses "gender incongruence" and has moved it from the mental disorders to the sexual health chapter. This change is also reflected in the most recent version of the *International Classification of Diseases* (*ICD-11*) and is divided by stage of life:
  - Gender incongruence of childhood refers to a strong desire in a prepubertal child to be a gender different from their assigned sex for at least 2 years; this may include a dislike of the associated sexual characteristics or anatomy of their assigned sex, desire for those of their experienced gender. Gender variant behaviors and preferences may also be noted, but alone are not the basis for assigning the diagnosis as these can be part of gender identity exploration, typical of normal development.
    - Caregiver involvement is recommended as part of the assessment unless their involvement would be considered harmful to the patient or is not feasible (2).
    - Of note, any underlying mental health concerns that may impact ability to make the diagnosis should be addressed (2).
  - Gender incongruence of adolescence or adulthood refers to a disparity between an individual's assigned sex and their experienced gender; this may present as a desire to align one's body with the experienced gender via medical and/or surgical interventions; this diagnosis is NOT made prior the onset of puberty. Additionally, gender variant behaviors and preferences alone are not the basis for assigning the diagnosis.
- There is no single assessment to diagnose gender incongruence, but the information needed to make the diagnosis is gathered through history-taking.

HISTORY

- Inquiry about gender identity should be included in history-taking. This may include specifically asking about chosen name, chosen pronouns, and the terminology used to describe their gender identity and sexual organs/genitalia. Additional inquiry may be helpful such as duration of the patient's experience, social impact (which may be adjusted based on patient's age and can include a formal evaluation of social determinants of health), a sexual organ/anatomic inventory, asking about sexual health practices (e.g., tucking or chest binding, partners, etc.), any prior medical/surgical/health care interventions or desire for such interventions, menstrual history, etc.
- It is recommended that health care providers ask open-ended questions and make clear that the expectation is for the patient to share only as much as they feel comfortable and also emphasizing that the information would be important to identify the patient's individualized health needs.
- TGD persons may use terms that are specific to their own personal and cultural beliefs; and so, mirroring their language is important to providing effective care.
- Overall, an age-appropriate biopsychosocial assessment, which includes medical, surgical, family, and social histories, is recommended

PHYSICAL EXAM

Transgender patients may experience discomfort during the physical examination because of their desire to have the physical attributes of a gender other than their assigned sex or prior negative experiences. Examinations should be based on the patient's current anatomy and specific needs for the visit and should always be explained, chaperoned when necessary, and stopped as indicated by the patient's comfort level.

TREATMENT

GENERAL MEASURES

- Care of TGD people, including providing gender-affirming medical and/or surgical treatments (GAMSTs) is dependent upon health care providers' ability to create a safe, inclusive environment where TGD patients feel comfortable to seek care; this requires education of not just the healthcare providers but the entirety of the health care team—administrative staff who may be first to greet the patient and clinical staff who may be rooming the patient and aiding in the delivery of care—in terms of appropriate use of terminology in verbal and written communication, etc; this may also include the design of the clinic space—decor, accessibility to gender-neutral restrooms, etc.
- Care of the TGD population can be provided by primary care providers or specialists but should include multidisciplinary care and may incorporate multiple treatment modalities based on patient's age, preferences, medication, surgery, behavioral health care, voice therapy, aesthetic medicine, etc.)
- Treatment options may be affected by local legal guidelines and should be considered by the health care provider
- Treatment of any kind has proved to provide significant benefit for patients with regard to improved mental and physical health outcomes, as well as overall quality of life.
- Education is a key component of all treatments, including reviewing reversibility of therapies, effects of therapies on fertility, effects on body image, need for monitoring/aftercare, etc.

MEDICATION

First Line

- Puberty suppression: use of reversible "puberty blockers," often gonadotropin-releasing hormone (GnRH) agonists is recommended for TGD adolescents at Tanner stage 2. These may be considered at later stages of puberty or postpuberty (Tanner stage 4 or later) such as those who have not yet started gender-affirming hormone therapy (GAHT), do not desire GAHT, or may benefit from its use for suppression of menstrual bleeding or to treat breakthrough bleeding; of note, progestin may be used as an alternative when GnRH agonists are not available.
  - A typical prescription would be intramuscular leuprolide 11.25 mg every 3 months.
- GAHT: use of sex hormones to promote the development of secondary physical/sexual characteristics that align with gender identity/desired image.
  - For TGD patients with feminine embodiment goals, estrogen (ideally in the form of estradiol) AND an androgen-lowering medication such as spironolactone is recommended. These aid in redistribution of body fat, decrease in muscle mass and strength, softening of skin/decreased oiliness, decreased sexual desire, decreased spontaneous erections, male sexual dysfunction, breast growth, decreased testicular volume, decreased sperm production, and possible scalp hair; typical prescriptions include (2):
    - Oral 17β-estrogen: initiate at 5 μg/kg/day and titrate every 6 months by 5 μg/kg/day up to 20 μg/kg/day based on estradiol levels in prepubertal youth; for postpubertal patients, the dose is increased more rapidly such as 1 mg/day for 6 months, followed by 2 mg/day and up according to estradiol levels; typical adult dose: 2 to 6 mg/day
    - Transdermal 17β-estrogen: initial dose of 6.25 to 12.5 μg/24hr (which may require matrix patches that can be cut into 1/4 and 1/2) and then titrating by 12.5 μg/24hr every 6 months based on estradiol levels; typical adult dose: 50 to 200 μg/24hr. Patches are usually applied every 3 to 4 days.

  - Androgen-lowering medication: spironolactone 25 mg BID for prepubertal youth; titrate by 25 mg BID every 3 to 6 months for postpubertal patients; typical dose adult dose: 100 to 300 mg/day with a maximum dose of 400 mg/day.
- For TGD patients with masculine embodiment goals, testosterone is recommended. It aids with skin oiliness/acne, facial/body hair growth, scalp hair loss, increased muscle mass/strength, fat redistribution, cessation of menses, clitoral enlargement, vaginal atrophy, and deepening of voice. Typical prescription (2):
  - Injectable testosterone: 25 mg/m^2 every 2 weeks, increase by 25 mg/m^2 every 2 weeks every 6 months based on testosterone levels or until adult dose for prepubertal youth; for post-pubertal patients, the dose may be increased more rapidly such as 75 mg every 2 weeks for 6 months; typical adult dose: 100 to 200 mg every 2 weeks with a maximum adult dose of 200 mg every 2 weeks
- GAHT is appropriate for TGD youth who have already entered puberty or following a period of puberty suppression with adequate psychosocial support and who have demonstrated emotional and cognitive maturity to provide consent/assent. This is NOT recommended for children who have not begun endogenous puberty.
- GAHT may be increased more quickly in older patients as desired (e.g., every 3 months)
- GAHT is typically continued for lifetime as discontinuation may result in bone loss.

SURGERY/OTHER PROCEDURES

- Multiple gender-affirming surgeries (GAS) are available depending on patients' goals:
  - TGD patients assigned female at birth may consider "top/chest surgery" via subcutaneous mastectomy or "bottom surgery" such as metoidioplasty, phalloplasty, vaginectomy, hysterectomy with or without salpingo-oophorectomy, or uterine transplant.
  - TGD patients assigned male at birth may consider breast augmentation, orchiectomy, vaginoplasty and vulvoplasty, or penile transplant.
  - Cosmetic surgeries such as brow lifts/augmentation/reduction, hair removal/transplant, facelift, chin reshaping, pectoral/hip/gluteal/calf implants, hair removal, and liposuction/filling may be considered.
- Surgeons should ensure that a multidisciplinary team of health professionals is involved in the decision-making process before proceeding with GAS
- For TGD patients seeking GAS, adults should have been on GAHT for at least 6 months and adolescents for at least 12 months to achieve the desired surgical result, unless GAHT is not desired or contraindicated.
- Guidance on practices such as chest binding and genital tucking/packing should also be reviewed with patients.

ONGOING CARE

FOLLOW-UP RECOMMENDATIONS

Patient Monitoring

- Regular monitoring of sex hormone levels occurs to ensure endogenous sex hormones are lowered and the administered sex hormone levels are maintained at appropriate levels to meet the individualized patient's needs, maintain good bone health, and are not at supraphysiologic levels.
  - Monitor sex hormone levels every 3 months during the first year of hormone therapy or with dose changes until stable adult dosing is achieved; then 1 to 2 times per year.
    - For TGD patients on parenteral testosterone: serum total testosterone should be measured midway between injections and should be between 400 to 700 ng/dL; some also measure peak and trough peaks to ensure levels remain in the range of reference male.
    - Transdermal testosterone: testosterone should be measured no sooner than 1 week of daily application and at least 2 hours after application of the product
      - Patients should also have hematocrit or hemoglobin measures at baseline and approximately every 3 months or with dose changes for the first year and then 1 to 2 times per year.
    - For TGD patients on estrogen: Serum testosterone should be <50 ng/dL and serum estradiol should be 100 to 200 pg/mL.
    - For patients on spironolactone, serum electrolytes and renal function should be monitored.
- Routine preventive care should be continued and should incorporate information obtained from the organ/anatomy inventory and any pertinent medical/family/social histories, including:
  - Mental health screenings
  - Breast cancer screening for TGD patients on estrogen therapy and/or with any amount of breast tissue (may need to review operative reports) should receive the same breast cancer screening as cisgender women; taking into consideration the length of time of estrogen therapy
  - Cervical cancer screening for those with a cervix according to age-related guidelines
  - Prostate cancer screening for TGD patients should follow the recommendations for cisgender men.
  - Appropriate sexual health screenings, including for human immunodeficiency virus (HIV) and sexually transmitted infections, and education based on patient's behaviors and present anatomy, for example, pre- and post-exposure HIV prophylaxis for patients who meet criteria or anal cancer screening with anal pap smear for those at increased risk
  - Evaluation of cardiovascular risk factors
  - Evaluation of osteoporosis risk factors to determine the optimal age and necessity for screening
  - Age-appropriate and behavior-specific immunizations (e.g., human papillomavirus)
  - Screening for intimate partner violence
  - Screening for tobacco use, use of electronic cigarettes/vaping, alcohol use, and illicit drug use
  - Screening for social determinants of health (1)
- Fertility, pregnancy, contraception, and abortion considerations include:
  - Fertility and parenting desires should be discussed early in the process of transition, before the initiation of GAMSTs. Fertility preservation options should be addressed accordingly
  - For TGD patients with a uterus who would like to carry a pregnancy, health care providers should review preconception care, prenatal use and cessation of GAHTs, pregnancy care, labor and delivery, chest/breastfeeding supportive services, and postpartum support; along with any associated costs that may vary by state/insurance.
  - Contraception counseling should occur with all TGD patients who are able to become pregnant, and should include:
    - GAHT is not an effective contraception.
    - Lack of menses does not mean TGD patients are unable to conceive.
    - Testosterone use is not a specific contraindication to using any form of contraception.
  - All patients should be counseled on barrier use for prevention of sexually transmitted infections.
  - Pregnancy termination options/services should be discussed with patients desiring an abortion; and when possible, refer to providers that offer procedural options which are gender-affirming (2).

T

REFERENCES

1. Dakkak M, Kriegel DL II, Tauches K. Caring for transgender and gender-diverse people: guidelines from WPATH. *Am Fam Physician*. 2023;108(6):626–629.
2. Coleman E, Radix AE, Bouman WP, et al. Standards of care for the health of transgender and gender diverse people, version 8. *Int J Transgend Health*. 2022;23(Suppl 1):S1–S259. doi:10.1080/26895269.2022.2100644.

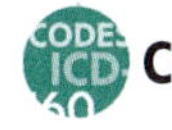

CODES

ICD10

- F64.1 Gender identity disorder in adolescence and adulthood
- Z11.4 Encounter for screening for human immunodeficiency virus
- Z72.52 High risk homosexual behavior

CLINICAL PEARLS

- The World Professional Association for Transgender Health (WPATH) publishes the Standards of Care for Health of Transgender and Gender Diverse People, currently on version 8 (SOC-8), which should be referenced for specific care guidelines when treating TGD patients.
- In general, primary care for TGD patients aligns with local guidelines for the cisgender population.

TRANSIENT ISCHEMIC ATTACK (TIA)

Veerauo Vera Konkankit, MD, MSc • George Edsel Reusser, MD

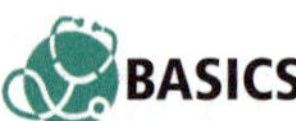

BASICS

DESCRIPTION

- Transient episode of neurologic dysfunction due to focal brain, retinal, or spinal cord ischemia without acute infarction
- 7.5–17.4% of patients with transient ischemic attack (TIA) experience a stroke within 3 months (1).
- Synonym: ministroke

EPIDEMIOLOGY

Prevalence

- Prevalence: ~2%
- Risk increases >60 years of age; highest in 7th and 8th decades of life
- Predominant sex: male > female
- Predominant race/ethnicity: African American > Hispanic > White

ETIOLOGY AND PATHOPHYSIOLOGY

Temporary reduction/cessation of cerebral blood flow adversely affecting neuronal function; common subtypes:

- Embolic from unknown source (36%)
- Cardioembolic events (29%):
  - Valvular pathology; mural hypokinesias with thrombosis
  - Atrial fibrillation (AFib): 5–20% incidence
- Large artery atherothrombosis (16%)
- Small vessel ischemic diseases (16%)
- Uncommon causes (3%): arterial dissection, hypercoagulable states, vasculitis, vasospasms, or sickle cell occlusive disease

RISK FACTORS

- Older age (i.e., >60 years)
- HTN, cardiac diseases (AFib, MI, valvular disease)
- Atherosclerotic disease (carotid/vertebral stenosis)
- Obesity, diabetes mellitus (DM), hyperlipidemia
- Cigarette smoking
- Thrombophilias

GENERAL PREVENTION

- Strict control of *DM*, *HTN*, *hyperlipidemia*
- Anticoagulation when high risk of cardioembolism (e.g., AFib, mechanical valves)
- Antiplatelet therapy for preventing recurrence, if previous TIA (2)

ALERT

1.5–3.5% risk of stroke in first 48 hours after TIA

Geriatric Considerations

- Older patients have a higher mortality rate—highest in 7th and 8th decades of life.
- AFib is a frequent cause.

Pediatric Considerations

- Congenital heart disease is a common cause.
- Genetic: Marfan syndrome, moyamoya, or sickle cell disease

Pregnancy Considerations

- Preeclampsia, eclampsia, and HELLP syndrome
- Thrombotic thrombocytopenic purpura (TTP) and hemolytic uremic syndrome
- Hypercoagulable states related to pregnancy

COMMONLY ASSOCIATED CONDITIONS

- AFib, uncontrolled HTN, carotid stenosis
- Some disease processes mimic TIA presentation (seizures, migraines, metabolic disturbances, syncope, multiple sclerosis); difference: gradual onset with nonspecific symptoms (headache, memory loss) versus acute onset with specific neurologic deficits (TIA)

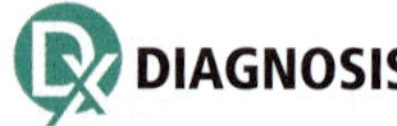

DIAGNOSIS

HISTORY

- Emphasis on symptom onset, progression, and recovery
- Carotid circulation (hemispheric): monocular visual loss, hemiplegia, hemianesthesia, neglect, aphasia, visual field defects (amaurosis fugax); less often, headaches, seizures, amnesia, confusion
- Vertebrobasilar (brain stem/cerebellar): bilateral visual obscuration, diplopia, vertigo, ataxia, facial paresis, Horner syndrome, dysphagia, dysarthria; also headache, nausea, and vomiting
- Past medical history, baseline functional status
- ABCD2 with imaging or ABCD3-I score: helps predict CVA risk after TIA (3)[B]
  - Score of 0 to 1: 0%; 2 to 3: 1.3%; 4 to 5: 4.1%; 6 to 7: 8.1%
  - **A**ge ≥60 years: 1 point
  - **B**lood pressure (BP) ≥ 140/90 mm Hg: 1 point
  - **C**linical presentation
    - U/L weakness: 2 points
    - Speech impaired without weakness: 1 point
  - **D**uration: 10 to 59 minutes: 1 point, ≥60 minutes: 2 points
  - **D**iabetes: 1 point
  - **Dual TIA** (within 7 days preceding): 2 points
  - **I**maging (new lesion or carotid stenosis): 2 points

PHYSICAL EXAM

- Vital signs, oxygen saturation
- Thorough neurologic and cardiac exams
- Ocular exam for examination of emboli

DIFFERENTIAL DIAGNOSIS

- Stroke, ischemic or hemorrhagic
- Carotid artery dissection
- Meningitis
- Labyrinthine disorder
- Migraine (hemiplegic)
- Focal seizure (Todd paralysis)
- Bell palsy
- Neoplasm of brain
- Subarachnoid hemorrhage
- Intoxication
- Glucose or other electrolyte abnormalities
- Multiple sclerosis

DIAGNOSTIC TESTS & INTERPRETATION

Initial Tests (lab, imaging)

- Neuroimaging within 24 hours of symptom onset
- Typically, noncontrast head computed tomography (CT) scan to rule out hemorrhage and guide thrombolysis (1)
- MRI, including diffusion-weighted imaging, is the preferred brain diagnostic modality to rule out stroke (1).
- Noninvasive imaging of the cervicocephalic vessels should be performed routinely in suspected TIA by carotid US/TCD, MRA, or CTA depending on availability and expertise and characteristics of the patient (4)[B].
- Routine blood tests (CBC, chemistry profile, UPT, coagulation screen, fasting lipid panel, ECG) are reasonable in evaluation of patient with TIA (4)[B].
- Screening for DM: fasting serum glucose or hemoglobin A1C (4)
- Consider hypercoagulability blood panel with risk factors and comorbidities (4).

Follow-Up Tests & Special Considerations

- Transesophageal echocardiogram (TEE) to identify patent foramen ovale (PFO), aortic arch atherosclerosis, and valvular disease (4)[B]
- Prolonged cardiac monitoring if unclear etiology after initial brain imaging and ECG (4)[B]
- EEG: if suspected seizure

Diagnostic Procedures/Other

- CT scan is typically the first neuroimaging test. Preferred variant is noncontrast, but probability of detecting acute tissue changes after ischemic symptoms resolve within 24 hours is 4% (1).
- Diffusion-weighted MRI can identify brain ischemia within minutes of onset and is highly sensitive (88% sensitivity within 24 hours) and specific (95% specificity) for acute infarction and will guide management (1).

Test Interpretation

Clinical suspicion increases if carotid bruits heard or emboli are noticed in the eyes.

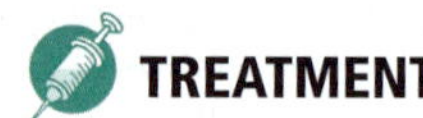

TREATMENT

GENERAL MEASURES

- Patients with high-risk TIAs require rapid referral and a 24-hour admission for observation and work-up.
- Outpatient investigations may be considered based on patient's stroke risk, follow-up arrangement, and social circumstances.
- Antiplatelet therapy to prevent recurrence or future CVA
- Treatment/control of underlying associated conditions

MEDICATION

The use of antiplatelet agents rather than oral anticoagulation is recommended to reduce risk of recurrent stroke and other cardiovascular events, except for cardioembolic etiologies (4)[A].

First Line

- Antiplatelets within first 24 hours, after intracranial hemorrhage has been ruled out
- Cardioembolic: anticoagulation (first two weeks)
  - Warfarin 2 to 5 mg/day initially, adjust according to target INR (5)
  - Direct thrombin inhibitor:
    - Dabigatran (Pradaxa) 150 mg BID
    - Idarucizumab (Praxbind) reversal agent

- Factor Xa inhibitors
  - Apixaban (Eliquis) 5 mg BID
  - Rivaroxaban (Xarelto) 20 mg/day
  - Edoxaban (Savaysa) 60 mg/day
- Large artery: antiplatelet therapy
  - Aspirin (ASA) 50 to 325 mg/day and clopidogrel 75 mg/day
    - Combined aspirin and clopidogrel therapy has shown to reduce incidence of subsequent stroke for high-risk TIA patients by 21% without increased risk of bleeding when used for a duration of ≤3 months immediately following TIA or CVA (2)[A]
    - Contraindications (CI): active PUD and hypersensitivity to aspirin or NSAIDs
    - Precautions: may aggravate preexisting PUD; or worsen symptoms of asthma
- Small-vessel
  - ASA 50 to 325 mg/day
    - CI: active PUD and hypersensitivity to aspirin or NSAIDs
    - Precautions: may aggravate preexisting PUD; or worsen symptoms of asthma.
  - Clopidogrel 75 mg/day
    - If allergy to aspirin (5)[B]
    - Precautions: TTP can occur and increases risk of bleeding when combined with aspirin.
    - May be very slightly more effective than aspirin alone (5)[B]
  - Dual antiplatelet therapy with ASA 50 to 325 mg/day and clopidogrel 300 to 600 mg as loading dose, followed by 75 mg/day (1)
  - ASA/dipyridamole 25 mg/200 mg BID (1)
    - Combined therapy with dipyridamole and ASA not proven to have greater efficacy (4)

Second Line

- Cardioembolic
  - ASA 325 mg/day or ASA 325 mg/day and clopidogrel 75 mg/day
    - Reserved for patients who cannot take anticoagulation for reasons other than bleeding risk
- Large artery
  - ASA 50 to 325 mg/day and ticagrelor 90 mg BID (6)
- Small vessel
  - ASA 50 to 325 mg/day and ticagrelor 180 mg as a loading dose, followed by 90 mg BID
- Ticlopidine (Ticlid): 250 mg BID:
  - If unable to tolerate other agents
  - CI: hypersensitivity, presence of hematopoietic/hemostatic disorders, conditions associated with bleeding, severe liver dysfunction
  - Precautions: neutropenia (0.8% severe), which is reversible with cessation of the drug; monitor blood counts every 2 weeks for first 3 months. TTP can occur.

ISSUES FOR REFERRAL

Interventional radiology or vascular surgery if carotid endarterectomy appropriate

ADDITIONAL THERAPIES

- High (≤75 years of age) or moderate statin (>75 years of age) (safe to start after first 48 hours), ezetimibe 10 mg/day (7)
- BP should be reduced after 24 hours. Thiazides, ACE inhibitors, and ARBs have shown to be of benefit. β-Blockers have not shown benefit in reducing TIA recurrence or stroke.
- Patients with DM or pre-DM should be advised to maintain glycemic control.

SURGERY/OTHER PROCEDURES

Consider carotid endarterectomy if carotid artery stenosis ≥70%, recommended within 2 weeks if there are no contraindications to early revascularization.

ADMISSION, INPATIENT, AND NURSING CONSIDERATIONS

Symptoms <72 hours and the following:

- ABCD2-I score of >3
- ABCD2-I score of 0 to 3 and uncertainty that diagnostic workup can be completed within 2 days as outpatient. Alternatively: If urgent imaging not available through ED or urgent neurology follow-up not available, admit ABCD2-I score ≥3 with evidence of focal ischemia.

ONGOING CARE

FOLLOW-UP RECOMMENDATIONS

Patient Monitoring

- Strict control of BP and smoking cessation
- Monitor lipids every 3 to 12 months determined by individual need (5).

DIET

- DASH diet or as appropriate for medical problems
- Any level of physical activity is beneficial, but at least 30 minutes of moderate-intensity physical activity daily is preferred (150 minutes/week).

PATIENT EDUCATION

- Keep a BP log; avoid tobacco; limit alcohol; keep a healthy weight.
- Call 911 with the following warning signs:
  - Weakness, tingling, or loss of feeling in one side of the body
  - Sudden double vision or loss of vision in one eye
  - Sudden severe headaches
  - Trouble speaking
  - Trouble understanding others

PROGNOSIS

High mortality risk associated with TIA, up to 25% of patients will die within 1 year of TIA.

COMPLICATIONS

Stroke and functional impairment

REFERENCES

1. Kleindorfer DO, Towfighi A, Chaturvedi S, et al. 2021 Guideline for the prevention of stroke in patients with stroke and transient ischemic attack: a guideline from the American Heart Association/American Stroke Association. *Stroke*. 2021;52(7):e364–e467.
2. Pan Y, Elm JJ, Li H, et al. Outcomes associated with clopidogrel-aspirin use in minor stroke or transient ischemic attack: a pooled analysis of clopidogrel in high-risk patients with acute non-disabling cerebrovascular events (CHANCE) and platelet-oriented inhibition in new TIA and minor ischemic stroke (POINT) trials. *JAMA Neurol*. 2019;76(12):1466–1473.
3. Zhao M, Wang S, Zhang D, et al. Comparison of stroke prediction accuracy of ABCD2 and ABCD3-I in patients with transient ischemic attack: a meta-analysis. *J Stroke Cerebrovasc Dis*. 2017;26(10):2387–2395.
4. Coutts SB. Diagnosis and management of transient ischemic attack. *Continuum (Minneap Minn)*. 2017;23(1):82–92.
5. Lansberg MG, O'Donnell MJ, Khatri P, et al. Antithrombotic and thrombolytic therapy for ischemic stroke: *Antithrombotic Therapy and Prevention of Thrombosis, 9th ed*: American College of Chest Physicians evidence-based clinical practice guidelines. *Chest*. 2012;141(Suppl 2):e601S–e636S.
6. Johnston SC, Amarenco P, Denison H, et al. Ticagrelor and aspirin or aspirin alone in acute ischemic stroke or TIA. *N Engl J Med*. 2020;383(3):207–217.
7. National Institute for Health and Care Excellence. *Stroke and Transient Ischaemic Attack in Over 16s: Diagnosis and Initial Management*. 2022.

SEE ALSO

Algorithms: Stroke; Transient Ischemic Attack

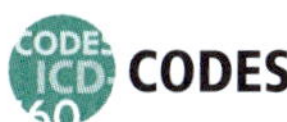

CODES

ICD10

- G45.9 Transient cerebral ischemic attack, unspecified
- G45.1 Carotid artery syndrome (hemispheric)
- G45.0 Vertebro-basilar artery syndrome

CLINICAL PEARLS

- Use the ABCD2-I or ABCD3-I scoring systems to help with risk stratification.
- Encourage smoking cessation, exercise, weight loss, limited ETOH intake, and control of HTN, hyperlipidemia, and DM.
- Antiplatelet therapy (e.g., aspirin, clopidogrel, or aspirin-clopidogrel) should be initiated.
- Anticoagulation therapy (e.g., warfarin, apixaban) should be initiated in patients with AFib or cardioembolic risk factors.

TRANSIENT STRESS CARDIOMYOPATHY

Saleha Ozair, MD • Adedapo Iluyomade, MD, MBA

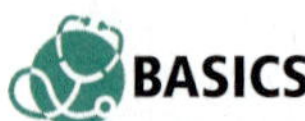

BASICS

DESCRIPTION

- Transient stress cardiomyopathy (TSC) is a unique cause of reversible left ventricle (LV) dysfunction with a presentation indistinguishable from the acute coronary syndromes (ACS), particularly ST-segment elevation myocardial infarction (STEMI).
- Typically, the patient is a postmenopausal woman who presents with acute chest pain, dyspnea, or syncope and an identifiable "trigger" (i.e., an acute emotional or physiologic stressor).
- First reported by authors from Japan as "takotsubo" (the Japanese word for octopus trap, due to the characteristic shape of the LV at the end of systole) cardiomyopathy (1)
- Presenting clinical features include:
  - Chest pain/pressure, dyspnea and/or syncope
  - ECG changes, including ST-segment elevations or diffuse T-wave inversions
  - Mild elevation in cardiac biomarkers (creatine kinase [CK], troponin)
  - Transient wall motion abnormalities that may involve the base, midportion, and/or lateral walls of the LV
  - The apex of the right ventricle (RV) may be affected in up to 25% of cases.
- Clinical features may vary on a case-by-case basis, and formal diagnostic criteria have not been established.
- Authors from the Mayo Clinic have proposed that three of the four following criteria establish the diagnosis (1):
  - Transient akinesis or dyskinesis of the LV apical and midventricular segments with regional wall motion abnormalities extending beyond a single epicardial vascular distribution
  - Absence of obstructive coronary artery disease (CAD) or angiographic evidence of acute plaque rupture
  - New ECG abnormalities, either ST-segment elevation or T-wave inversion
  - Absence of recent significant head trauma, intracranial bleeding, pheochromocytoma, obstructive epicardial CAD, myocarditis, hypertrophic cardiomyopathy
- Synonym(s): takotsubo cardiomyopathy; apical ballooning syndrome; stress cardiomyopathy; broken heart syndrome; ampulla cardiomyopathy

EPIDEMIOLOGY

Incidence

- Recent studies indicate that TSC accounts for approximately 1.8% of patients presenting with suspected acute coronary syndrome (ACS) (2). Among patients with STEMI, TSC represents 0.4–2.8% of cases.
- The incidence of TSC has been increasing over time, from 2.3 per 100,000 person-years in 2006 to 7.1 per 100,000 person-years in 2017 in the United States.
- Predominant sex: 82–100% of cases occur in women; predominant age: Mean age of patients is 62 to 75 years.

ETIOLOGY AND PATHOPHYSIOLOGY

- The precise pathophysiologic mechanisms of TSC are not well understood (3).
- There is considerable evidence that sympathetic stimulation is central to its pathogenesis. A clear emotional or physiologic triggering event precipitates the syndrome in most cases, and TSC has been associated with conditions of catecholamine excess (e.g., pheochromocytoma, central nervous system disorders) and activated specific cerebral regions.
- Occurs primarily in subjects with increased susceptibility of the coronary microcirculation and of cardiac myocytes to stress hormones leading to temporary left ventricular dysfunction with secondary myocardial inflammation
- A perturbation in the brain–heart axis, originating in the insular cortex, may be the inciting event.
- Subsequent overwhelming activation of the sympathetic nervous system initiates a cascade of events, including the following: catecholamine-induced LV dysfunction: "biased agonism" of for β_2-adrenergic receptors, located predominantly at the cardiac apex; endothelial dysfunction and vasospasm; cellular metabolic injury: myocardial norepinephrine release, calcium overload, contraction band necrosis

Genetics

No genetic associations have been described to date.

RISK FACTORS

Female sex, postmenopausal state; emotional stress (i.e., argument, death of family member); physiologic stress (i.e., acute medical illness); chronic neurologic or psychiatric disease

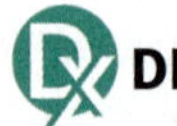

DIAGNOSIS

Because TSC is often indistinguishable from an ACS, it should be treated initially as such: Activate emergency medical services or report to emergency department; provide oxygen if needed, IV access, and ECG monitoring; and obtain urgent cardiology consultation.

HISTORY

- In 2/3 of patients, there is exposure to a "trigger event."
  - Emotional stress: argument, death of family member, divorce, public speaking, etc.
  - Physiologic stress: acute medical condition such as head trauma, asthma attack, seizure, etc.
- In 1/3 of patients, there is no identifiable trigger.
- Acute onset of dyspnea or chest pain; palpitations and/or syncope may occur

PHYSICAL EXAM

Exam may be unremarkable or may include any of the following: tachypnea, tachycardia, hypotension, jugular venous distension, bibasilar rales, S_3 gallop, systolic ejection murmur due to dynamic LV outflow tract gradient, holosystolic murmur of mitral regurgitation

DIFFERENTIAL DIAGNOSIS

Acute STEMI, pulmonary embolism, myopericarditis, pheochromocytoma, hypertrophic cardiomyopathy, subarachnoid hemorrhage or stroke

DIAGNOSTIC TESTS & INTERPRETATION

The InterTAK Diagnostic Score comprises seven parameters (female sex, emotional trigger, physical trigger, absence of ST-segment depression [except in lead aVR], psychiatric disorders, neurologic disorders, and QT prolongation) ranked by their diagnostic importance with a maximum attainable score of 100 points.

- In patients with non–ST-segment elevation, the InterTAK Diagnostic Score can be considered. Patients with a low probability (InterTAK score ≤70 points) should undergo coronary angiography with left ventriculography, whereas in patients with a high score (score ≥70), transthoracic echocardiography should be considered.
- The InterTAK Diagnostic Score has been validated for differentiating TSC from ACS.

Initial Tests (lab, imaging)

- ECG should be done urgently and may show the following: Q waves, diffuse ST-segment elevations; diffuse and often dramatic T-wave inversions; QTc interval prolongation
- Laboratory tests typically reveal a mild elevation in cardiac biomarkers such as
  - CK (rarely >500 U/mL); Troponin I, Troponin T or high-sensitivity cardiac troponin
  - B-type natriuretic peptide (BNP); markers of high filling pressures (e.g., BNP) tend to be higher than markers of necrosis (e.g., CK, troponin).
  - TSC can be distinguished from AMI with 95% specificity using a BNP/TnT ratio ≥1,272 (sensitivity 52%).
- Chest radiograph: cardiomegaly, pulmonary edema
- Echocardiogram:
  - Reduced LV systolic function
  - Abnormal diastolic function, including evidence of increased filling pressures
  - Regional wall motion abnormalities in one of the following patterns:
    - Classic or "takotsubo-type" ballooning of the apex with a hypercontractile base
    - "Reverse takotsubo": apical hypercontractility with basal akinesis
    - "Midventricular" akinesis with apical and basal hypercontractility
    - Focal or localized akinesis of an isolated segment
  - Dynamic intracavitary LV gradient
  - Mitral regurgitation
  - Variable involvement of the RV

Follow-Up Tests & Special Considerations

Cardiac MRI

- Reduced LV function
- Wall motion abnormalities as described for transthoracic echocardiography
- Absence of delayed hyperenhancement with gadolinium
- Allows for differentiation between reversible and irreversible changes

Diagnostic Procedures/Other

- The diagnosis of TSC is often challenging because its clinical phenotype may closely resemble STEMI regarding electrocardiographic abnormalities and biomarkers. Coronary angiography with left ventriculography is considered the "gold standard" diagnostic tool to exclude or confirm TSC.
- Coronary angiography reveals nonocclusive CAD; endothelial dysfunction as measured by fractional flow reserve or TIMI frame counts; and rarely, epicardial coronary spasm.
- Left-sided heart catheterization: increased LV end-diastolic pressure to a similar degree as AMI
- Ventriculography: wall motion abnormalities as described for transthoracic echocardiography
- Right-sided heart catheterization
  - Increased pulmonary capillary wedge pressure
  - Secondary pulmonary hypertension
  - Increased right ventricular filling pressures
  - Reduced cardiac output or cardiogenic shock (cardiac index <2 L/min/m^2 and mean arterial pressure [MAP] <60 mm Hg)

Test Interpretation

Characteristic pathologic findings of involved myocardium have not been described.

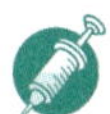

TREATMENT

- Due to the lack of randomized clinical trials, treatment strategies for TSC are based largely on expert consensus.
- Activation of emergency medical services and Advanced cardiac life support therapies as needed
- Oxygen, IV access, ECG monitoring

MEDICATION

After diagnostic cardiac catheterization, empirical treatment goals are as follows:

- Management of hypotension: differentiation between cardiogenic shock and dynamic LV cavity gradient
- Management of increased filling pressures and congestive states using standard practices for treatment of congestive heart failure
- Attenuation of sympathetic drive

First Line

- Although β-blockers are of theoretical benefit, their use has not been associated with improved outcomes in observational cohorts. Due to the potential risk of pause-dependent torsades de pointes, β-blockers should be used cautiously, especially in patients with bradycardia and QTc >500 ms.
- If there is evidence of left ventricular systolic dysfunction or pulmonary edema, consider the following:
  - Furosemide 20 to 40 mg IV/PO BID as needed to reduce LV filling pressures and dyspnea
  - The use of angiotensin-converting enzyme inhibitors or angiotensin receptor blockers was associated with improved survival at 1-year follow-up even after propensity matching: Lisinopril 10 to 40 mg/day PO (or equivalent) or valsartan 80 to 160 mg PO BID (or equivalent) has been associated with improved outcomes in observational cohorts.

Second Line

Short-term anticoagulation should be considered in patients with severely reduced LV function to prevent LV thrombus formation; unfractionated heparin 80 U/kg IV bolus followed by 18 U/kg/hr IV or enoxaparin sodium (Lovenox) 1 mg/kg SC BID

ISSUES FOR REFERRAL

All patients with TSC generally should be inpatient and referred to cardiology as an outpatient.

ADDITIONAL THERAPIES

- Urgent cardiology consultation and consideration of cardiac catheterization
- Hypotension may require the following:
  - Vasopressors (e.g., or dopamine or norepinephrine bitartrate [Levophed]) if there is no LV outflow tract gradient
  - IV fluids to increase afterload in the presence of an LV outflow tract gradient
  - Cardiogenic shock that is not due to an LV outflow tract gradient may require placement of an intra-aortic balloon pump.

COMPLEMENTARY & ALTERNATIVE MEDICINE

Psychiatric evaluation: Despite psychiatric disorders being recognized as a clear substrate and trigger for TSC, studies show that only 32% of patients are treated during their incident hospitalization.

ADMISSION, INPATIENT, AND NURSING CONSIDERATIONS

- Normal saline infusion to support BP, if necessary, and no evidence of heart failure
- Discharge criteria is generally considered after exclusion of ACS and resolution of congestive state, hypotension, and major impairment of systolic function.

ONGOING CARE

FOLLOW-UP RECOMMENDATIONS

- Impairments in systolic function typically resolve in 2 to 3 days but may last as long as 1 month.
- Patients should follow up with cardiology and serial echocardiography to document improved LV function.

Patient Monitoring

Inpatient monitoring for cardiac arrhythmias and hemodynamic compromise is warranted.

DIET

Eating a variety of fruits, vegetables, whole grains, lean meats, and fish can improve heart health, while managing sodium intake can reduce leg swelling from fluid retention.

PROGNOSIS

- Although TSC has generally been considered a benign disease, recent studies (4) suggest that TSC may have rates of cardiogenic shock and mortality comparable to ACS patients treated according to current guidelines.
- Recurrence is rare; it also has been reported in 0–8% of patients.

COMPLICATIONS

- Left-sided heart failure, pulmonary edema, cardiogenic shock and hemodynamic compromise
- Dynamic LV outflow tract gradient complicated by hypotension
- Mitral regurgitation
- Ventricular arrhythmias
- LV thrombus formation
- LV free wall rupture
- Death (rare, 0–8%)

REFERENCES

1. Ghadri JR, Wittstein IS, Prasad A, et al. International expert consensus document on takotsubo syndrome (part 1): clinical characteristics, diagnostic criteria, and pathophysiology. *Eur Heart J*. 2018;39(22):2032–2046.
2. Singh T, Khan H, Gamble DT, et al. Takotsubo syndrome: pathophysiology, emerging concepts, and clinical implications. *Circulation*. 2022;145(13):1002–1019.
3. Lyon AR, Bossone E, Schneider B, et al. Current state of knowledge on Takotsubo syndrome: a position statement from the taskforce on Takotsubo syndrome of the Heart Failure Association of the European Society of Cardiology. *Eur J Heart Fail*. 2016;18(1):8–27.

T

SEE ALSO

Algorithm: Chest Pain/Acute Coronary Syndrome

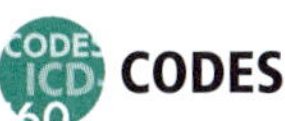

CODES

ICD10

I51.81 Takotsubo syndrome

CLINICAL PEARLS

- TSC is poorly recognized and often regarded as a benign condition. However, it may be associated with severe clinical complications including death, and its prevalence is likely underestimated.
- Echocardiography may strongly suggest the diagnosis.
- Treatment is supportive and should include diuretics and ACE inhibitors or ARB in patients with CHF.

TRICHOMONIASIS

Michael Arnold, MD • Christopher M. Beaumont, PA

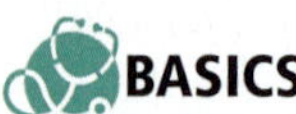

BASICS

DESCRIPTION

- Sexually transmitted urogenital infection caused by a pear-shaped, parasitic protozoan
- Causes vaginitis/urethritis in women, nongonococcal urethritis in men
- Association with infertility in epidemiologic studies
- In pregnancy, increases risk of preterm labor, preterm premature rupture of membranes, small for gestational age infant, and possibly stillbirth
- Synonym(s): trich; trichomonal urethritis

EPIDEMIOLOGY

Incidence

- The most common curable sexually transmitted infection (STI); in 2008, >275 million new cases worldwide, over half of curable STIs
- Estimated 1.1 million new cases annually in United States
  - 10–25% of vaginal infections
  - In males, up to 17% of nongonococcal urethritis; French study shows decreasing prevalence in men since 2007.
- Predominant age: middle-aged adults
  - Rare until onset of sexual activity
  - Common in postmenopausal women; age is not protective, and long-term carriage is common.

Pediatric Considerations

- Rare in prepubertal children; diagnosis should raise concern of sexual abuse.
- Neonatal infections occur most often in the lungs, also vaginal

Prevalence

- 2.1% in U.S. women aged 14 to 59 years
- 0.5% of U.S. men aged 14 to 59 years
- Racial disparity demonstrated
  - 9.6% of black women versus 0.8% of other women
  - 3.4% of black men versus 0.03% of other men

ETIOLOGY AND PATHOPHYSIOLOGY

- *Trichomonas vaginalis*: pear-shaped, flagellated, parasitic protozoan
- Grows best at 35–37°C in anaerobic conditions with pH 5.5 to 6.0
- Divides by binary fission; does not have a cyst form so does not survive externally
- STI, but nonsexual transmission possible because it can survive several hours in moist environment

Genetics

No known genetic considerations

RISK FACTORS

- Multiple sexual partners
- Unprotected intercourse
- Lower socioeconomic status
- Other STIs
- Untreated partner with previous infection
- Use of douching or feminine powders
- Hormonal contraception use does NOT increase risk.

GENERAL PREVENTION

- Use of male or female condoms
- Limiting sexual partners
- Male circumcision may be protective.

COMMONLY ASSOCIATED CONDITIONS

- Other STIs, including HIV, increases risk of STI
- Bacterial vaginosis, increases risk of bacterial vaginosis

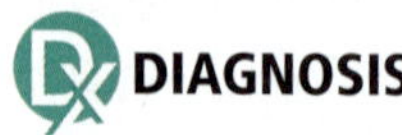

DIAGNOSIS

HISTORY

- Women—up to 85% may be asymptomatic.
  - Yellow-green, malodorous vaginal discharge
  - Vulvovaginal pruritus
  - Dysuria
  - Symptoms often worsen during menses.
- Men—77% are asymptomatic.
  - Dysuria
  - Urethral discharge, often scant
  - Pruritus or burning after intercourse

PHYSICAL EXAM

- Women
  - Vaginal erythema
  - Yellow-green, frothy, malodorous vaginal discharge
  - Cervical petechiae ("strawberry cervix"; seen in <5% of patients on pelvic exam, more with colposcopy)
  - Pelvic exams do not improve STI diagnosis.
- Men: penile discharge, spontaneous and with expression

DIFFERENTIAL DIAGNOSIS

- Women (other vaginitides)
  - Bacterial vaginosis
  - Vaginal candidiasis
  - Chlamydial infection
  - Gonorrheal infection
- Men (other urethritis)
  - Chlamydial infection
  - Gonorrheal infection

DIAGNOSTIC TESTS & INTERPRETATION

Initial Tests (lab, imaging)

- Wet mounts of vaginal or urethral discharge: direct visualization of motile trichomonads; most common because inexpensive and available
  - Sensitivity: as low as 26%; declines rapidly within 1 hour from collection
  - Specificity: 99.8%
- Culture: sensitivity >95%, specificity >99%; takes 4 to 7 days for growth
- Nucleic acid amplification test (NAAT)
  - Gold standard for diagnosis
  - Sensitivity and specificity 95–99%
  - Vaginal, endocervical, or urine specimens
  - British analysis shows that combined NAAT for *Trichomonas*, gonorrhea, *Chlamydia*, and *Mycoplasma genitalium* is the most cost-effective.
- Antigen detection
  - ELISA and direct fluorescent antibody tests: sensitivity of 80–90%
  - Limited clinical availability

Follow-Up Tests & Special Considerations

Detection on cervical Papanicolaou smear

- Treat because highly specific (97–99%)
- Not effective for *Trichomonas* screening—sensitivity as low as 60%

Diagnostic Procedures/Other

In males, urethral meatal swab increases *Trichomonas* detection rate by 4 times over urine.

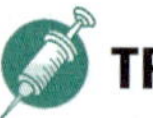

TREATMENT

- Symptomatic individuals require treatment.
- Sexual partners should be treated presumptively.
- Patients should abstain from sexual intercourse during treatment and until they are asymptomatic.

GENERAL MEASURES

The nitroimidazole class is only proven effective antimicrobial treatment. If metronidazole resistance is suspected, use tinidazole.

MEDICATION

It is essential to treat partners to prevent reinfection.

First Line

- Metronidazole: 500 mg PO BID for 7 days
  - FDA pregnancy risk Category B
  - Cure rate: 84–98%
  - Single 2-g dose is no longer recommended.
    - 7-day course increases cure rate with number needed to treat (NNT) of 13 compared to single 2-g dose
    - Single dose has double the rate of repeat infection.
  - Increasing resistance—study of PID treatment showed that metronidazole did not improve *T. vaginalis* rate compared to control.
- Tinidazole: 2 g PO, 1 dose
  - FDA pregnancy risk Category C
  - Abstain from breastfeeding during treatment and for 3 days after the dose.
  - More expensive
  - Reaches higher levels in genitourinary tract
  - Cure rate: 92–100%

Second Line

- Secnidazole, 2 g PO, 1 dose
  - Longer half-life than metronidazole and tinidazole, approved for treatment of both *T. vaginalis* and bacterial vaginosis with single dose
  - Approval is based on study of 147 women with 92% cure rate at 6 to 12 days after single 2-g dose.
- Can dose with metronidazole or tinidazole or 2 g daily for 7 days if infection persists
- Consider IV dosing of metronidazole based on case report demonstrating cure after multiple failed oral regimens.
- Recommendations for metronidazole resistance include tinidazole with intravaginal paromomycin, intravaginal boric acid, and intravaginal metronidazole with miconazole.

Pregnancy Considerations

Metronidazole is effective for trichomoniasis infection during pregnancy but may increase risk of preterm delivery and low-birth weight babies.

- Studies showed risk in patients receiving 4 times the standard dosing.
- Trichomoniasis is also associated with prematurity.

ISSUES FOR REFERRAL

- Multidrug-resistant organism
- Patient allergy to metronidazole: Desensitization to metronidazole is recommended.

ADDITIONAL THERAPIES

- Limited clinical trials assessing effectiveness of alternative therapies
- Intravaginal metronidazole gel is only effective if adding miconazole.

COMPLEMENTARY & ALTERNATIVE MEDICINE

See "Additional Therapies."

ONGOING CARE

FOLLOW-UP RECOMMENDATIONS

- If symptoms persist after initial treatment, repeat testing.
- Repeat infections occur in up to 37% of cases, treat with metronidazole at same or higher dosage
- Retest *T. vaginalis* recommended between 3 weeks and 3 months of treatment
- HIV-positive patients should be screened for *Trichomonas* at time of HIV diagnosis and at least annually.
- Patients with multiple partners should be screened annually.

DIET

Abstain from alcohol during treatment and for 24 hours following last dose of metronidazole or 48 to 72 hours following last dose of due to disulfiram-like reaction.

PATIENT EDUCATION

Educate about the sexually transmitted aspect.

- Advise patient to notify sexual partner to be treated.
- Discuss STI prevention—condom use can prevent recurrence.
- Abstain from intercourse while undergoing treatment; use condoms if abstention is not feasible.
- Avoid alcohol during treatment with metronidazole or tinidazole.

PROGNOSIS

- Excellent
- Usually eliminated after one course of antibiotics although resistance is increasing

COMPLICATIONS

Pregnancy Considerations

Linked to low birth weight, preterm premature rupture of membranes, and preterm birth; associations with infertility, but not proven

ADDITIONAL READING

- Akter T, Festin M, Dawson A. Hormonal contraceptive use and the risk of sexually transmitted infections: a systematic review and meta-analysis. *Sci Rep*. 2022;12(1):20325.
- Daugherty M, Glynn K, Byler T. Prevalence of Trichomonas vaginalis infection among US males, 2013–2016. *Clin Infect Dis*. 2019;68(3):460–465.

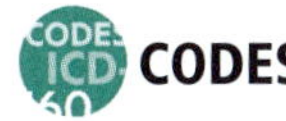

CODES

ICD10

- A59.02 Trichomonal prostatitis
- A59 Trichomoniasis
- A59.0 Urogenital trichomoniasis

CLINICAL PEARLS

- Both partners need to be treated for trichomoniasis.
- Retest patients between 3 weeks and 3 months of treatment.
- Avoid alcohol during treatment.
- Treatment in pregnancy does not reduce risk of adverse pregnancy outcomes.
- Annual screening is recommended for HIV-positive patients and patients with multiple partners.
- Not a nationally notifiable condition

TRIGEMINAL NEURALGIA

Haley Severin, DO, MS

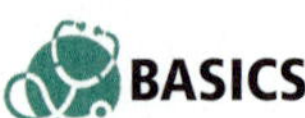

BASICS

DESCRIPTION

- Trigeminal neuralgia (TN) is a painful disorder of the sensory nucleus of the 5th cranial (trigeminal) nerve that commonly produces episodic, paroxysmal, severe, lancinating facial pain lasting seconds to minutes.
- Often precipitated by stimulation of well-defined, ipsilateral trigger zones: usually perioral, perinasal, and occasionally intraoral (e.g., by talking, washing your face, shaving, or exposure to cold air)
- Subtypes:
  - Classical: secondary to neurovascular compression, as evidenced by MRI
  - Idiopathic: when the criterion for TN is met, with evidence on MRI or electrophysiologic testing, suggestion no apparent or visible etiology
  - Secondary: diagnosed based on fulfillment of criteria for TN but attributed to a separate causative comorbid condition; the three subtypes of secondary TN are attributed to multiple sclerosis (MS), space-occupying lesions (cerebellopontine angle tumors, meningioma, etc.), or to other causes (1)[A].
- System(s) affected: nervous
- Synonym(s): tic douloureux; Fothergill neuralgia; trifacial neuralgia; prosopalgia

EPIDEMIOLOGY

Incidence

- 4 to 29/100,000 per year
- Mean onset of 55 years

Pregnancy Considerations

Teratogenicity of medication therapy limits their use during 1st and 2nd trimesters.

ETIOLOGY AND PATHOPHYSIOLOGY

- Compression of the trigeminal nerve root by an anomalous artery, vein, or tumor such as meningioma or acoustic neuroma
- Demyelination from compression, or other cause such as MS, leads to an ectopic impulse generation with erratic responses such as hyperexcitability of damaged nerves and transmission of action potentials along adjacent, undamaged, and unstimulated sensory fibers.

Genetics

- Prevalence of familial TN is about 1–2%.
- Autosomal dominant inheritance pattern suggested
- Other presentations may be attributed to gene mutations of calcium channels, sodium channels, MPZ gene, etc.

RISK FACTORS

MS associated with a 20-fold increased risk of developing TN

COMMONLY ASSOCIATED CONDITIONS

- Sjögren syndrome; rheumatoid arthritis
- Acute polyneuropathy
- Charcot-Marie-Tooth neuropathy

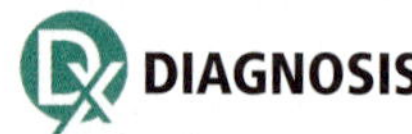

DIAGNOSIS

HISTORY

Paroxysms of pain in the distribution of the trigeminal nerve, which include the ophthalmologic (V1), maxillary (V2), and mandibular (V3) branches. Patients typically experience unilateral pain in the V2 and V3 dermatomes, although pain can be bilateral. Attacks are stereotyped in the individual often triggered by stimuli such as light touch, chewing, talking, brushing teeth, cold air, smiling, or grimacing. Autonomic symptoms such as lacrimation, conjunctival injection, or rhinorrhea can be associated with TN. Pain can be continuous and mild between attacks. MS-associated secondary TN differs significantly in regard to classic TN. In general, it often presents at a younger age and more commonly, occurs bilaterally.

PHYSICAL EXAM

Exam findings are typically benign due to the paroxysmal nature of the disorder. Light touch to affected trigger zone(s) may elicit pain attacks.

DIFFERENTIAL DIAGNOSIS

Other forms of neuralgia usually have sensory loss. Presence of sensory loss nearly excludes the diagnosis of TN.

- Neoplasia in cerebellopontine angle
- Vascular malformation of brainstem
- Demyelinating lesion (MS)
- Migraine, cluster headache
- Giant cell arteritis
- Postherpetic neuralgia
- Short-lasting unilateral neuralgiform headache attacks (SUNHA)

DIAGNOSTIC TESTS & INTERPRETATION

International Classification of Headache Disorders 3rd edition (*ICHD-3*) diagnostic criteria for TN:

- A. Recurrent paroxysms of unilateral facial pain in the distribution(s) of one of more divisions of the trigeminal nerve, with no radiation beyond, and fulfilling criteria B and C
- B. Pain has all of the following characteristics:
  - Lasting from a fraction of a second to 2 minutes
  - Severe intensity
  - Electric shock-like shooting, stabbing, or sharp in quality
- C. Precipitated by innocuous stimuli within the affected trigeminal distribution
- D. Not better accounted for by another *ICHD-3* diagnosis
  - Additional criteria for classical: demonstration on MRI or surgical findings of neurovascular compression with nerve root changes (not simply contact)
  - Subclassifications of TN with concomitant continuous pain: presence of background pain between episodes in the same distribution; typically burning, throbbing, or aching
  - Secondary TN is caused by underlying disease known to cause TN, including MS, space occupying lesions, AV malformations, and genetic malformations

Initial Tests (lab, imaging)

Imaging is indicated without an obvious cause to rule out secondary causes.

- MRI, with and without contrast with trigeminal sequences, offers more detailed imaging.

Follow-Up Tests & Special Considerations

- Labs (e.g., electrolytes, liver and kidney function) and ECG prior to initiating medications.
- Screen for HLA-B*1502 allele in patients of Han Chinese descent before initiating carbamazepine/oxcarbazepine.

Test Interpretation

Diagnosis of classical TN requires imaging or surgical confirmation of morphologic changes to the trigeminal nerve indicating neurovascular compression such as dislocation, distortion, atrophy, or compression of the nerve at its origin from the pons.

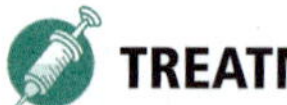

TREATMENT

GENERAL MEASURES

- Avoid stimulation (e.g., air, heat, cold) of trigger zones, including lips, cheeks, and gums.
- Medication treatment is first line.
- Invasive procedures are reserved for patients who fail to respond to drug treatment.

MEDICATION

First Line

- Carbamazepine (Tegretol)100 to 200 mg BID; increase gradually (100 mg every other day up to 1,600 mg) to avoid adverse reactions until pain relieved or side effects occur:
  - First-line therapy along with oxcarbazepine; offers meaningful and initial pain control in almost 90% of patients; limited by side effects that lead to withdrawal in up to 40% of patients (1)[A]
  - Common side effects: sedation, GI upset, hyponatremia, rash, dizziness, visual disturbance

- Contraindications: AV block, serious blood dyscrasias
- Precautions: decreased dose in impaired liver function; monitor for Steven-Johnson syndrome and toxic epidermal necrolysis; avoid in patients with the HLA-B*1502 allele.

- Oxcarbazepine (Trileptal): 150 to 300 mg BID; effective dose usually 375 mg BID; max 1,800 mg/day:
  - Faster, with less drowsiness and fewer drug interactions than carbamazepine
  - Common side effects: sedation, GI upset, and hyponatremia

Second Line

- Phenytoin (Dilantin): can be used in refractory cases or as rescue therapy (off label); 250 to 1,000 mg IV at a rate no faster than 50 mg/minute.
- Baclofen (Lioresal): 40 to 80 mg/day; start 5 mg TID and titrate up (as an adjunct to phenytoin or carbamazepine); maintenance dose 50 to 60 mg/day, use limited by side effects: drowsiness, weakness, nausea, vomiting
- Gabapentin (Neurontin): Start 300 mg daily; can increase dose up to 300 to 600 mg TID–QID; can be used as monotherapy or in combination with other medications
- Lamotrigine: Titrate up to 200 mg BID over weeks; use limited by medication interactions and side effects: aseptic meningitis, blood dyscrasias, hypersensitivity reactions, suicidal ideation
- Botulinum toxin injection may be beneficial; can provide significant relief up to 12 weeks, side effects: facial asymmetry and swelling form injections (2)[A]
- Pimozide: dopamine receptor agonist; can be used in refractory cases, limited by side effects: sedation, arrhythmias, anticholinergic effects, extrapyramidal symptoms, parkinsonism

ISSUES FOR REFERRAL

Initial treatment failure or positive findings on imaging studies; evaluation at pain clinic prior to surgical referral

ADDITIONAL THERAPIES

Stereotactic radiosurgery has been shown to be effective after drug failure. Due to its non-invasive nature, it is preferred when there is no evidence of neurovascular contact, or when there are significant comorbidities limiting surgical procedures (2).

- 24–71% of patients achieved continued pain relief 1 to 2 years after the procedure
- Most common side effect: sensory disturbance (facial numbness)

SURGERY/OTHER PROCEDURES

- Microvascular decompression (MVD) of cranial nerve (CN) V at its entrance to (or exit from) brainstem
  - >90% are pain free after MVD with 80% pain free at 1 year, 75% at three years, and 73% at 5 years (1)[A].
  - Most common side effect: transient facial numbness and diplopia, headache, nausea, vomiting
  - Pain relief after procedure strongly correlates with the type of TN pain: paroxysmal results in better outcomes than concomitant continuous (aching pain between paroxysms).
- Peripheral nerve ablation:
  - Radiofrequency thermocoagulation; neurectomy; partial sensory rhizotomy
  - Higher rates of failure and facial numbness than decompression surgery
- 4% tetracaine dissolved in 0.5% bupivacaine nerve block; also, ropivacaine or lidocaine can provide temporary relief.
- Alcohol block or glycerol injection into trigeminal cistern: unpredictable side effects (dysesthesia and anesthesia dolorosa) and temporary relief
- Peripheral block or section of CN V proximal to Gasserian ganglion
- Balloon compression of Gasserian ganglion

COMPLEMENTARY & ALTERNATIVE MEDICINE

Acupuncture noted to aid in pain; further studies are needed to support this modality (3)[A].

ADMISSION, INPATIENT, AND NURSING CONSIDERATIONS

Severe acute exacerbations leading to dehydration or anorexia due to trigger avoidance

ONGOING CARE

FOLLOW-UP RECOMMENDATIONS

Follow up, every 3 to 6 months in initial few years, to monitor symptoms and treatment efficacy.

Patient Monitoring

- Medication serum levels if indicated
- If carbamazepine is prescribed: CBC and platelets at baseline, then weekly for a month, then monthly for 4 months, and then every 6 to 12 months if dose is stable (Regimens for monitoring vary.)
- Reduce drugs after 4 to 6 weeks to determine whether condition is in remission; resume at previous dose if pain recurs. Withdraw drugs slowly after several months, again to check for remission or if lower dose of drugs can be tolerated.

PATIENT EDUCATION

- The Facial Pain Association: https://www.facepain.org/
- Living with Facial Pain: https://www.livingwithfacialpain.org/

PROGNOSIS

- 50–60% eventually fail pharmacologic treatment.
- Of those, relapse is seen in ~50% of stereotactic radiosurgeries and ~27% of surgical microvascular decompressions.

COMPLICATIONS

- Mental and physical sluggishness; dizziness with carbamazepine
- Paresthesias and corneal reflex loss with stereotactic radiosurgery
- Surgical mortality and morbidity associated with microvascular decompression

REFERENCES

1. Xu R, Xie ME, Jackson CM. Trigeminal neuralgia: current approaches and emerging interventions. *J Pain Res*. 2021;14:3437–3463. doi:10.2147/JPR.S331036.
2. Lambru G, Zakrzewska J, Matharu M. Trigeminal neuralgia: a practical guide. *Pract Neurol*. 2021;21(5):392–402. doi:10.1136/practneurol-2020-002782.
3. Chen Q, Yi DI, Perez JNJ, et al. The molecular basis and pathophysiology of trigeminal neuralgia. *Int J Mol Sci*. 2022;23(7):3604. doi:10.3390/ijms23073604.

ADDITIONAL READING

- Allam AK, Sharma H, Larkin MB, et al. Trigeminal neuralgia: diagnosis and treatment. *Neurol Clin*. 2023;41(1):107–121.
- Cruccu G, Di Stefano G, Truini A. Trigeminal neuralgia. *N Engl J Med*. 2020;383(8):754–762.

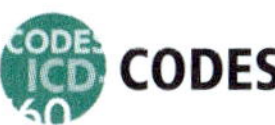

CODES

ICD10

- B02.22 Postherpetic trigeminal neuralgia
- G50.0 Trigeminal neuralgia

CLINICAL PEARLS

- Patients with TN typically have a normal physical exam.
- Imaging, ideally MRI, should be obtained to rule out secondary causes in newly presenting patients with clinical suspicion of TN.
- First-line treatment: carbamazepine or oxcarbazepine
- If pharmacotherapy fails, stereotactic radiosurgery or surgical microvascular decompression often is successful.

T

TRIGGER FINGER (DIGITAL STENOSING TENOSYNOVITIS)

Leigh Romero, MD, CAQSM • Jayshree S. Thomas, DO

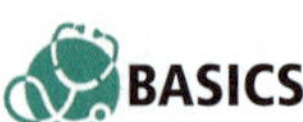

BASICS

DESCRIPTION

Trigger finger, also known as digital stenosing tenosynovitis, is a disruption of the smooth tendon gliding complex of an affected digit in flexion resulting in a transient catching and/or locking sensation, followed by a painful release or "trigger" as an inflamed tendon passes through a narrow pulley sheath on extension of the affected digit.

EPIDEMIOLOGY

Incidence

- Adult population: 2–3% of adults
  - Women > Men (6:1)
  - Typically, presents in the 5th and 6th decades of life
- Rare in children: affects <0.05%
  - Women = Men
  - 90% are trigger thumbs
  - Associated with mucopolysaccharidoses (MPS)
- 20% of patients with diabetes mellitus (1)

Prevalence

Lifetime prevalence in the general adult population is 2–3%.

ETIOLOGY AND PATHOPHYSIOLOGY

- The result of fibrocartilaginous metaplasia of the flexor digitorum superficialis tendon and/or pulley from prolonged inflammation causing narrowing around the pulley.
- This can occur at any of the five pulleys along the flexor tendon—A1 pulley is the most common.
- If flexor tendon becomes nodular, the triggering phenomenon is worse because the nodule has difficulty passing under the A1 pulley.
- Because intrinsic flexor muscles are stronger than extensors, the finger can get stuck in the flexed position.
- The ring finger and thumb of the dominant hand are most commonly affected.
- No clear association with repetitive movements (1).

Genetics

No specific Mendelian inheritance or high-penetrance familial syndrome has been identified in current literature.

RISK FACTORS

- Diabetes mellitus
- Rheumatoid arthritis
- Hypothyroidism
- Mucopolysaccharide disorders
- Amyloidosis

GENERAL PREVENTION

- Most cases are idiopathic.
- No clear association with occupational-related or repetitive activities (1)

COMMONLY ASSOCIATED CONDITIONS

- Orthopedic conditions:
  - Rheumatoid arthritis
  - Calcific peritendinitis
  - Septic tenosynovitis
  - Carpal tunnel syndrome
  - Congenital trigger thumb
- Medical conditions:
  - Diabetes
  - Amyloidosis
  - Hypothyroidism
  - Sarcoidosis
  - Gout
  - Pseudogout

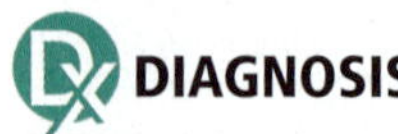

DIAGNOSIS

HISTORY

- Clicking, catching, snapping, or locking of a digit during flexion—usually painless initially, then progresses to painful episodes
- The finger may become locked in the flexed position requiring passive manipulation of the finger into extension in more severe cases.
- Functional limitations tend to include difficulty with grasping and holding objects, manipulating coins, or buttoning clothing
- Green classification for severity of trigger finger symptoms (1)
  - Grade 1: pre-triggering—tenderness and pain at A1 pulley
  - Grade 2: active—catching with active full extension
  - Grade 3A: passive—catching requiring passive extension
  - Grade 3B: passive—inability to actively flex
  - Grade 4: contracture—catching with fixed contracture of proximal interphalangeal joint (PIP) joint

PHYSICAL EXAM

- May visualize locking/catching or "triggering" of the affected digit, specifically while flexing the digit
- Can be painful or painless—pain may radiate proximally into the palm or distally into the finger
- If active triggering is not present, place a finger on the PIP as the finger is actively flexed and extended, noting the presence of loss of smooth motion or a clicking sensation.
- Palpable and tender nodule may be present at the affected pulley near the metacarpophalangeal (MCP) joint.
- Fixed flexion of the affected joint in more severe cases

DIFFERENTIAL DIAGNOSIS

- Dupuytren contracture
- Ganglion of flexor tendon sheath
- Osteoarthritis
- Diabetic cheiroarthropathy
- MCP joint sprain

DIAGNOSTIC TESTS & INTERPRETATION

Initial Tests (lab, imaging)

- Clinical diagnosis based on history and physical exam
- No labs or imaging necessary
- Ultrasound and MRI may be potentially useful to rule out other conditions.
- If concerned for an underlying metabolic disorder in pediatric patients, proceed with appropriate evaluation as indicated.

Diagnostic Procedures/Other

- Ultrasound can be used for diagnostic (static and dynamic evaluation) and therapeutic purposes.
- Ultrasound is more appropriate for pediatric patients as MRI commonly requires sedation for children.

Test Interpretation

MRI/ultrasound

- Thickening of the affected pulley (global or nodular) and hypervascularization
- Flexor tendons with focal or diffuse tendinosis, partial tear, longitudinal split, intratendinous cyst degeneration, and dynamic snapping
- Possible synovial sheath effusion, synovial hypertrophy, synovial hypervascularization, and synovial cyst around the tendon
- Increased blood flow (vascular hyperplasia) on doppler imaging.

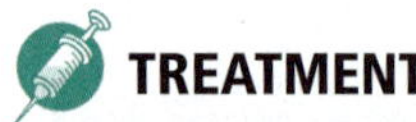

TREATMENT

GENERAL MEASURES

- Goals of treatment are to alleviate pain and to allow smoother movement of the digit.
- Start with conservative interventions such as: oral NSAIDs, activity modification, and splinting followed by corticosteroid injection.
- Activity modification can be helpful in early disease.
- Splinting may be more effective in preventing recurrence than initial treatment choice.
  - The splint can isolate and block at the MCP, PIP, or DIP joints.
- Splinting the MCP joint at 10 to 15 degrees of flexion for 6 to 10 weeks for 24 hours/day with the distal joints free to move:
  - Splinting is more effective for fingers than thumbs (70% vs. 50%).
  - Splinting is less effective with severe symptoms, symptoms >6 months, or if multiple digits are involved.
- Most recommend attempting steroid injection prior to surgery.
- Initial injection of long-acting corticosteroid may provide symptom relief. Subsequent injections are less likely to help.
- Surgery is often successful for patients unresponsive to splinting/corticosteroid injections or who suffered recurrence.

MEDICATION

First Line

- Oral NSAIDs may reduce pain and discomfort but have not been shown to alter underlying disease.
- NSAIDs do not reduce symptoms of snapping/locking/catching.
- Steroid injection of the tendon sheath/surrounding subcutaneous tissue has 57–90% success rate.
- Triamcinolone appears more effective than dexamethasone.
- Injection in surrounding tissues is as efficacious as injecting into the tendon sheath.
- Injection into the palmar surface at the mid-proximal phalanx is associated with less pain than injection of tendon sheath at MCP joint.
- Corticosteroid injection has higher success rate than splinting; however, a systematic review quotes the efficacy of orthotic use as 47–93% effective.

Second Line

- Injection with diclofenac may be an alternative to corticosteroid for patients with diabetes mellitus if increase in blood sugar is a concern.
- Corticosteroids are more effective than diclofenac during the first 3 weeks postinjection. Efficacy is similar to other modalities by 3 months postinjection.

ISSUES FOR REFERRAL

Refer to a hand surgeon if symptoms are refractory to conservative measures with oral NSAIDs, physical therapy, splinting, and/or corticosteroid injections.

ADDITIONAL THERAPIES

- Splinting—dependent on what provides the patient the most relief. Lower success rates in patients with severe or chronic symptoms
  - Can take 6 to 10 weeks
  - Can splint at DIP joint—resolution of 50% of symptoms
  - Can splint at MCP joint with 15 degrees of flexion—resolution of 92.9% of symptoms
  - Can night splint: better compliance versus continuous splinting—resolution in 55% of grade 1 and 2 trigger finger
- Exercises—can be useful particularly after surgical release
  - Digit blocking—blocking MCP joint while allowing PIP joint to bend; can perform at DIP joint
  - Tendon gliding
  - Active range of motion
- Heat/ice, ultrasound, electric stimulation, massage, stretching, and joint motion

SURGERY/OTHER PROCEDURES

- Suggested after failure to reduce symptoms despite conservative therapy and up to three corticosteroid injections in the same digit
- No apparent differences in success or rates of complications between surgical approaches
- Surgery has lower rate of recurrence than corticosteroid injection but has disadvantage of being more painful initially.
- Methods
  - Percutaneous release of A1 pulley
    - Can be performed using ultrasound guidance
    - Success rate >90%
    - Shorter recovery time
  - Open surgical débridement and release of the A1 pulley
    - Gold standard
    - Success rate >90%
    - Better visualization of the pulley
    - Less risk of damage to other structures

COMPLEMENTARY & ALTERNATIVE MEDICINE

Extracorporeal shock wave therapy (ESWT)

- Believed to suppress ongoing inflammation reducing thickening of the flexor tendon and its sheath

ADMISSION, INPATIENT, AND NURSING CONSIDERATIONS

- In-office trigger finger release
  - Minimally invasive procedure performed under local anesthesia
  - Can be performed using percutaneous approach versus small open incision
  - Not suitable for all cases, especially for trigger thumb
- Day surgery for trigger finger release

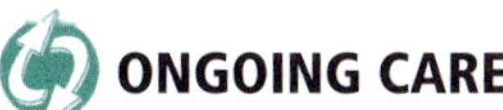

ONGOING CARE

FOLLOW-UP RECOMMENDATIONS

- Follow-up is needed only if symptoms persist or if complications develop after surgery
- Splinting of the affected digit to minimize flexion/extension of the MCP joint helps symptom resolution

Patient Monitoring

Pain level, post-procedure or postoperative guidelines, and adherence to treatment regimen

DIET

No specific diet is recommended for prevention, treatment, or after receiving corticosteroid injections unless diabetic

PROGNOSIS

Prognosis is excellent with conservative treatment or surgical intervention. Recurrence following corticosteroid injection is more likely for patients with type 1 diabetes mellitus, younger patients, involvement of multiple digits, and history of other upper extremity tendinopathies.

COMPLICATIONS

- Diabetic patients may have increased blood sugar levels for up to 5 days following steroid injection.
- Other minor steroid injection complications include skin hypopigmentation and subcutaneous fat atrophy; tendon attrition or rupture is rare.
- Complications from surgery include infection, bleeding, digital nerve injury, persistent pain, and loss of range of motion of the affected finger. The rate of major complications is low (3%). The rate of minor complications (including loss of range of motion) is higher (up to 28%).
- Another surgical complication, injury to the A2 pulley, may result in bowstringing (bulging of the flexor tendon in the palm with flexion) and pain.

REFERENCES

1. Johnson E, Stelzer J, Romero AB, et al. Recognizing and treating trigger finger. *J Fam Pract*. 2021;70(7):334–340.

ADDITIONAL READING

Amirfeyz R, McNinch R, Watts A, et al. Evidence-based management of adult trigger digits. *J Hand Surg Eur Vol*. 2017;42(5):473–480.

T

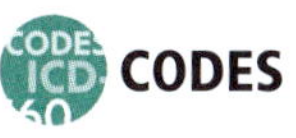

CODES

ICD10

- M65.30 Trigger finger, unspecified finger
- M65.319 Trigger thumb, unspecified thumb
- M65.329 Trigger finger, unspecified index finger

CLINICAL PEARLS

- Trigger finger is the inhibition of smooth tendon gliding due to narrowing around the flexor pulley that causes pain, clicking, catching, and locking.
- More common in females >50 years of age.
- Diagnosis is based on clinical presentation (history and physical exam).
- Initial conservative therapy consists of NSAIDs, splinting, physical therapy, or corticosteroid injection.
- Long-acting corticosteroid injections are effective for treatment of trigger finger but have a higher recurrence rate than surgery.
- Diabetic patients are at increased risk of developing trigger finger but are less likely to respond to steroid injections.
- Open and percutaneous surgical release have high success rates for patients not responsive to splinting or injections.

TROCHANTERIC BURSITIS (GREATER TROCHANTERIC PAIN SYNDROME)

Daniel L. Warden, MD • Nicholas Moore, MD, FAAFP, CAQSM • Kyle M. Samyn, DO, MS

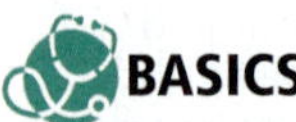

BASICS

Trochanteric bursitis is often used as a general term to describe lateral hip pain and tenderness over the greater trochanter. There may be inflammation at one of a number of bursa at the lateral hip, but more commonly, the pain is due to hip abductor tendon injury and external snapping hip. More recently, there has been a shift to describe this condition as greater trochanteric pain syndrome (GTPS) (1).

DESCRIPTION

- Bursae are fluid-filled sacs found primarily at tendon attachment sites with bony protuberances:
  - Multiple bursae are in the area of the greater trochanter of the femur.
  - These bursae are associated with the tendons of the gluteus muscles, iliotibial band (ITB), and tensor fasciae latae.
  - The subgluteus maximus bursa is implicated most commonly in lateral hip pain (1).
- Other structures of the lateral hip include the following:
  - ITB, tensor fasciae latae, gluteus maximus tendon, gluteus medius tendon, gluteus minimus tendon, quadratus femoris muscle, vastus lateralis tendon, piriformis tendon
- *Bursitis* refers to bursal inflammation.
- *Tendinopathy* refers to any abnormality of a tendon, inflammatory or degenerative.
- *Enthesopathy* refers to abnormalities of the zones of attachment of ligaments and tendons to bones.

EPIDEMIOLOGY

Incidence

- 1.8/1,000 persons/year
- Peak incidence in 4th to 6th decades

Prevalence

- Predominant sex: female > male
- More common in running and contact athletes
  - Football, rugby, soccer

ETIOLOGY AND PATHOPHYSIOLOGY

- Acute: Abnormal gait or poor muscle flexibility and strength imbalances lead to bursal friction and secondary inflammation.
  - Tendon overuse and inflammation
  - Direct trauma from contact or frequently lying with body weight on hip can cause an inflammatory response.
- Chronic
  - Fibrosis and thickening of bursal sac due to chronic inflammatory process
  - Tendinopathy due to chronic overuse and degeneration: gluteus medius and minimus most commonly involved (1)

Genetics

No known genetic factors

RISK FACTORS

Multiple factors have been implicated (1):

- Female gender
- Obesity
- Tight hip musculature (including ITB)
- Direct trauma
- Total hip arthroplasty
- Abnormal gait or pelvic architecture
  - Leg length discrepancy
  - Sacroiliac (SI) joint dysfunction
  - Knee or hip osteoarthritis
  - Abnormal foot mechanics (e.g., pes planus, overpronation)
  - Neuromuscular disorder: Trendelenburg gait

GENERAL PREVENTION

- Maintain ITB, hip, and lower back flexibility and strength.
- Avoid direct trauma (use of appropriate padding in contact sports).
- Avoid prolonged running on banked or crowned surfaces.
- Wear appropriate shoes.
- Appropriate bedding and sleeping surface
- Maintain appropriate body weight loss.

COMMONLY ASSOCIATED CONDITIONS

- Biomechanical factors (1)
  - Tight ITBs, leg length discrepancy, SI joint dysfunction, pes planus
  - Width of greater trochanters greater than width of iliac wings
- Other associated pathology (1):
  - Low back pain
  - Knee and hip osteoarthritis
  - Obesity

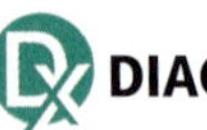

DIAGNOSIS

HISTORY

General history (1)

- Pain localized to the lateral hip or buttock
- Pain may radiate to groin or lateral thigh (pseudoradiculopathy).
- Pain exacerbated by:
  - Prolonged walking or standing
  - Rising after prolonged sitting
  - Sitting with legs crossed
  - Lying on affected side
- Other historical features:
  - Direct trauma to affected hip
  - Chronic low back pain
  - Chronic leg/knee/ankle/hip pain
  - Recent increase in running distance or intensity
  - Change in running surfaces

PHYSICAL EXAM

- Palpate for point tenderness with direct palpation over the lateral hip is characteristic of GTPS (1)[B].
- Other exam features have lower sensitivity (1)[B]:
  - Pain with extremes of passive rotation, abduction, or adduction
  - Pain with resisted hip abduction and external or internal rotation
  - Trendelenburg sign
- Other tests to rule out associated conditions:
  - Patrick-FABERE (flexion, abduction, external rotation, extension) test for SI joint dysfunction
  - Ober test for ITB pathology
  - Flexion and extension of hip for osteoarthritis
  - Leg length measurement
  - Foot inspection for pes planus or overpronation
  - Lower extremity neurologic assessment for lumbar radiculopathy or neuromuscular disorders
  - Hip lag sign

DIFFERENTIAL DIAGNOSIS

- ITB syndrome
- Piriformis syndrome
- Osteoarthritis or avascular necrosis of the hip
- Lumbosacral osteoarthritis/disc disease with nerve root compression
- Fracture or contusion of the hip or pelvis—particularly in setting of trauma
- Stress reaction/fracture of femoral neck—particularly in female runners
- Septic bursitis/arthritis

DIAGNOSTIC TESTS & INTERPRETATION

No routine lab testing is recommended.

Initial Tests (lab, imaging)

- Diagnosis can be made by history and exam (2).
- If imaging is ordered:
  - US can aid in diagnosis and guide aspiration and/or injection.
  - Anteroposterior and frog-leg views of affected hip to rule out specific bony pathology (OA, stress fracture, etc.)
  - Consider lumbar spine radiographs if back pain is thought to be a contributing factor.
  - MRI is image of choice in recalcitrant pain or to formally exclude stress fracture.

Follow-Up Tests & Special Considerations

- If there is a concern for a septic bursitis, then aspiration or incision and drainage may be necessary.
- Advanced imaging rarely necessary; detection of abnormalities on MRI is a poor predictor of GTPS.

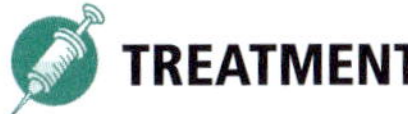

TREATMENT

GENERAL MEASURES

- Physical therapy to address underlying dysfunction and weakness
- Correct pelvic/hip instability.
- Correct lower limb biomechanics.
- Low-impact conditioning and aquatic therapy
- Gait training
- Weight loss (if applicable)
- Minimize aggravating activities such as prolonged walking or standing.
- Avoid lying on affected side.
- Runners
  - May need to decrease distance and/or intensity of runs during treatment. Some need to stop running. Amount of time is case specific but may range from 2 to 4 weeks.
  - Avoid banked tracks or roads with excessive tilt.

MEDICATION

First Line

- NSAIDs (1)[B]: Treat for 2 to 4 weeks.
  - Naproxen: 500 mg PO BID
  - Ibuprofen: 800 mg PO TID
- Corticosteroid injection is effective for pain relief (3)[C] and can be considered first-line therapy for selected cases:
  - Dexamethasone: 4 mg/mL or
  - Kenalog: 40 mg/mL; use 1 to 2 mL.
  - Consider adding a local anesthetic (short- and/or long-acting) for more immediate pain relief.
  - Can be repeated with similar effect if original treatment showed a strong response
  - Goal is pain relief.
  - Corticosteroid injections may not be effective for certain cases (4). A noninflammatory cause, such as a chronic tendinopathy or referred pain, should be considered and further explored in these cases.

ISSUES FOR REFERRAL

- Septic bursitis
- Recalcitrant bursitis
- Positive sag test concerning for gluteal tendon tear

ADDITIONAL THERAPIES

- Ice
- Low-energy shock wave therapy has been shown to be superior to other nonoperative modalities.
- Focus on achieving flexibility of hip musculature, particularly the ITB.
- Address contributing factors:
  - Low back flexibility
  - If leg length discrepancy, consider heel lift.
  - If pes planus or overpronation, consider arch supports or custom orthotics.

SURGERY/OTHER PROCEDURES

- Surgery rare but effective in refractory cases
- If surgery is indicated, potential options include:
  - Arthroscopic bursectomy
  - ITB release
  - Gluteus medius tendon repair
- Tenotomy

COMPLEMENTARY & ALTERNATIVE MEDICINE

- Acupuncture
- Prolotherapy
- Growth factor injection techniques
- Platelet-rich plasma injection

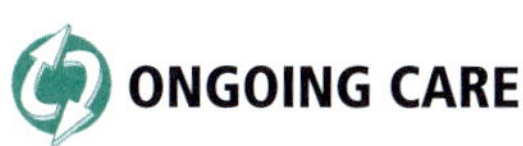

ONGOING CARE

FOLLOW-UP RECOMMENDATIONS

4 weeks posttreatment, sooner if significant worsening

PATIENT EDUCATION

- Maintain hip musculature flexibility, including ITB.
- Correct issues that may cause abnormal gait:
  - Low back pain
  - Knee pain
  - Leg length discrepancy (heel lift)
  - Foot mechanics (orthotics)
- Gradual return to physical activity

PROGNOSIS

Depends on chronicity and recurrence, with more acute cases having an excellent prognosis

COMPLICATIONS

Bursal thickening and fibrosis

REFERENCES

1. Williams BS, Cohen SP. Greater trochanteric pain syndrome: a review of anatomy, diagnosis and treatment. *Anesth Analg*. 2009;108(5):1662–1670.
2. Chowdhury R, Naaseri S, Lee J, et al. Imaging and management of greater trochanteric pain syndrome. *Postgrad Med J*. 2014;90(1068):576–581.
3. Stephens MB, Beutler AI, O'Connor FG. Musculoskeletal injections: a review of the evidence. *Am Fam Physician*. 2008;78(8):971–976.
4. Nissen MJ, Brulhart L, Faundez A, et al. Glucocorticoid injections for greater trochanteric pain syndrome: a randomised double-blind placebo-controlled (GLUTEAL) trial. *Clin Rheumatol*. 2019;38(3):647–655.

ADDITIONAL READING

- Barratt PA, Brookes N, Newson A. Conservative treatments for greater trochanteric pain syndrome: a systematic review. *Br J Sports Med*. 2017;51(2):97–104.
- Pretell J, Ortega J, García-Rayo R, et al. Distal fascia lata lengthening: an alternative surgical technique for recalcitrant trochanteric bursitis. *Int Orthop*. 2009;33(5):1223–1227.

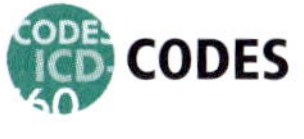

CODES

ICD10

- M70.60 Trochanteric bursitis, unspecified hip
- M70.62 Trochanteric bursitis, left hip
- M70.61 Trochanteric bursitis, right hip

CLINICAL PEARLS

- Patients with GTPS often present with an inability to lie on the affected side.
- Femoral neck stress fractures are a do-not-miss diagnosis, particularly in young female runners.
- Corticosteroid injection helps as an initial therapy, particularly for pain relief to allow for aggressive physical therapy.
- Physical therapy is treatment mainstay for correcting biomechanical imbalances and restoring proper function.

TUBERCULOSIS

Crystal L. Romero, MD, MPH

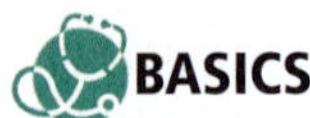

BASICS

DESCRIPTION

- Active tuberculosis (TB) infection caused by *Mycobacterium tuberculosis*
  - Primary infection or reactivation of latent infection; risk increases with immunosuppression: highest risk first 2 years after infection; reactivation risk increases with comorbid disease (e.g., HIV, diabetes).
  - Well-described forms: pulmonary (85%), miliary (disseminated), meningeal, abdominal, lymphadenitis (scrofula)
- Usually acquired by inhalation of airborne bacilli from an individual with active TB; bacilli multiply in alveoli and spread via macrophages, lymphatics, and blood. Outcomes include: eradication (tissue hypersensitivity stops infection; primary TB; latent TB [LTBI]).

EPIDEMIOLOGY

Incidence

- Worldwide (2023): estimated 10.8 million; 134/100,000
- ~7% of cases involve people living with HIV; mostly from Southeast Asia and Africa
- United States (2023): 9,633 (2.9/100,000); 76% of U.S. cases were in non-U.S. born. TB case rates rose in the United States from 2022 to 2023

Prevalence

- Worldwide (2023): World Health Organization estimates 10.8 million new cases of TB in 2023.
- Mortality
  - Worldwide (2023): 1.25 million deaths due to TB.

ETIOLOGY AND PATHOPHYSIOLOGY

- Causative organisms: *M. tuberculosis* (mostly); less likely *Mycobacterium bovis* or *Mycobacterium africanum*
- Spread by aerosol droplets and reach alveolar space; alveolar macrophages ingest and migrate.
- Cell-mediated response by activated T lymphocytes and macrophages forms a granuloma ("tubercle") that limits bacterial replication. If replication continues, the tubercle grows with spread to regional lymph nodes. An expanding tubercle within the lung parenchyma with regional lymph node enlargement is called a Ranke complex.
- As the infection is contained, destruction of the macrophages produces early "solid necrosis." In 2 to 3 weeks, "caseous necrosis" develops and LTBI ensues. In the immunocompetent, granuloma undergoes "fibrosis" and calcification. In the immunocompromised, primary progressive TB develops. Cavitary lesions may form.

RISK FACTORS

- For latent infection: homeless, correctional facility, close contact with infected, living in area with high incidence of active TB, health care worker; medically underserved, low income, substance use
- For development of disease once infected: renal failure; lymphoma; silicosis; diabetes; cancer of head, neck, or lung; children <5 years old; malnutrition; systemic corticosteroids; HIV; immunosuppressive drugs; IV drug use, alcohol misuse, cigarette smokers; <2 years since infection with *M. tuberculosis*; <90% ideal body weight

GENERAL PREVENTION

- Screen for and treat LTBI. Report active TB to health department; test and treat all close contacts. Without treatment LTBI will progress to active TB disease in 5–10%.
- Bacillus Calmette-Guérin (BCG) vaccine: Used primarily in endemic countries; high-risk children, negative PPD; ongoing exposure; not recommended in the United States.

COMMONLY ASSOCIATED CONDITIONS

Immunosuppression; HIV coinfection; malignancy

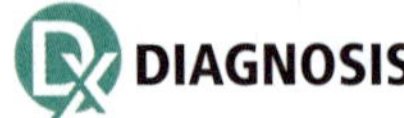

DIAGNOSIS

HISTORY

Signs and symptoms

- General: fever, night sweats, unintentional weight loss, malaise, painless lymph node swelling, arthralgias
- Pulmonary TB: unexplained cough >2 to 3 weeks, hemoptysis, pleuritic chest pain
- Abdominal TB: acutely as surgical abdomen; chronic abdominal TB varies (vague abdominal symptoms, abdominal mass, "doughy" abdomen)

PHYSICAL EXAM

- Can be normal; specific findings depend on organs involved: hepatosplenomegaly, adenopathy, rales; poor weight gain in children
- Late findings: renal, bone, or CNS disease

DIFFERENTIAL DIAGNOSIS

- Pulmonary TB: pneumonia, malignancy, actinomycosis, coccidiomycosis, sarcoidosis, tularemia, etc.
- Extrapulmonary TB: other mycobacterial infections, syphilis, cat-scratch disease, leishmaniasis, erythema nodosum, rheumatologic disease, erythema induratum

DIAGNOSTIC TESTS & INTERPRETATION

Diagnosis based on rapid nucleic acid amplification tests (NAATs) for detection of *M. tuberculosis* and identification of drug resistance. Sputum culture is the gold standard for confirmation of active TB and drug susceptibility testing. Molecular methods are used for initial management.

Initial Tests (lab, imaging)

Active TB

- Three sputum samples for acid-fast bacilli (AFB) stain and mycobacterial culture by aerosol induction, gastric aspirate (children), or bronchoalveolar lavage (1)[B]
- NAAT: (Xpert MTB/RIF and next-generation sequencing); faster than culture and more reliable than AFB smear (1)[C]. Positive result supports presumptive diagnosis of TB while culture pending. Negative NAAT does not rule out TB.
- Chest radiograph primary TB: infiltrate with or without atelectasis, effusion, or adenopathy.
- CT chest: good sensitivity, tree-in-bud (centrilobular nodules with branching linear opacities)

Follow-Up Tests & Special Considerations

- Baseline CBC, creatinine, liver function tests, visual acuity, and red-green color discrimination (regimens involving ethambutol [EMB])
- HIV: If positive, get baseline CD4 count, viral load, and genotype. Check hepatitis B and C if injection drug users, Africa or Asia born, HIV infected, or otherwise high risk.
- Extrapulmonary: urine, CSF, bone marrow, and liver biopsy for culture as indicated; interferon-gamma (IFN-γ) and adenosine deaminase levels
- Nonspecific findings: anemia, thrombocytosis, SIADH, hypergammaglobulinemia, monocytosis, sterile pyuria

Diagnostic Procedures/Other

- Culture: takes several weeks for definitive results
- Xpert MTB/RIF (rapid molecular test): FDA-approved molecular assay for pulmonary TB diagnosis and detection of drug resistance, particularly in areas with high prevalence of multi-drug resistant (MDR) TB

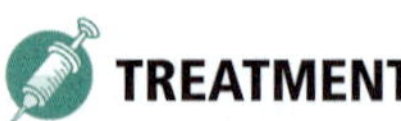

TREATMENT

GENERAL MEASURES

If clinical suspicion, treat immediately. Prescribing physician is responsible for treatment completion. Respiratory and droplet precautions, airborne isolation; not infectious if favorable clinical response after 2 to 3 weeks of therapy and each of three repeat AFB smears are negative

MEDICATION

Dose by ideal body weight; directly observed therapy (DOT) preferred

First Line

- LTBI—see "Tuberculosis, Latent (LTBI)."
- Active TB
  - Drug-susceptible TB
    - Rifapentine, moxifloxacin, isoniazid (INH), and pyrazinamide (PZA) daily for 4 months; this is an alternative to the traditional 6-month regimen of INH, rifampin (RIF), PZA, and EMB, as long fluoroquinolone resistance has been excluded. The 4-month regimen is not recommended for children, pregnant individuals, or those with extrapulmonary TB outside of clinical trials. DOT is preferred, but self-administered therapy may be used where DOT is not feasible.
  - RIF or MDR TB
  - BPaL—6 months of oral bedaquiline (400 mg daily for 2 weeks, then 200 mg 3 times weekly), pretomanid (200 mg daily), and linezolid (600 mg daily, with dose reduction to 300 mg daily if toxicity occurs)
  - BPaLM—also oral: bedaquiline (400 mg daily for 2 weeks, then 200 mg 3 times weekly), pretomanid (200 mg daily), linezolid (600 mg daily for 16 weeks, then 300 mg daily for 8 weeks), and moxifloxacin (400 mg daily for 24 weeks)
- Regimen 3

Pregnancy Considerations

- Treatment initiated whenever the probability of maternal disease is moderate to high.
- Treat TB in pregnancy with INH/RIF/EMB daily for 2 months; followed by INH/RIF daily or twice per week for 7 months
- Streptomycin is harmful and PZA not advised given unclear fetal effects.
- Breastfeeding: OK while taking TB drugs; supplement with pyridoxine 25 to 50 mg/day

Pediatric Considerations

- Children may attend school if they are taking the appropriate medications.
- Commonly have severe disease and faster rate of progression to disease.
- Pediatric TB treatment should be directly observed using four drugs.

ALERT

- Continue EMB until organism susceptibility to INH *plus* RIF is determined.
- Initiation of ART therapy in HIV-positive patients infected with TB carries an increased risk of immune reconstitution inflammatory syndrome (IRIS) with pulmonary TB (2)[A].

Second Line

- Fluoroquinolones and injectable aminoglycosides; use when MDR suspected or intolerance; pretomanid approved for use in XDR-TB (BPaL regimen: with bedaquiline and linezolid)
- >12 years old with drug susceptible TB: 2 months INH/RIF/PYR/moxifloxacin then 2 months INH/RIF/moxifloxacin (3)

ISSUES FOR REFERRAL

ALERT

Notify public health authorities for all cases of active TB. Consult infectious disease specialist for drug-resistant TB and HIV-positive patients on ART. Case management referral is recommended.

ADDITIONAL THERAPIES

- Pyridoxine: 50 mg for persons at risk for INH neuropathy; 100 mg daily to patients with preexisting neuropathy
- Steroids: recommended for TB meningitis; not for TB pericarditis

SURGERY/OTHER PROCEDURES

For extrapulmonary complications (spinal cord compression, bowel obstruction, constrictive pericarditis)

ADMISSION, INPATIENT, AND NURSING CONSIDERATIONS

- Negative pressure isolation room with personal respirators and droplet precaution
- Three consecutive negative sputum AFB smears are necessary for release from isolation.

ONGOING CARE

FOLLOW-UP RECOMMENDATIONS

Patient Monitoring

- Monthly sputum for AFB smear and culture until two consecutive cultures are negative; must confirm prior to starting continuation phase. Monthly visits to monitor medication adherence and adverse effects; CXR after 2 months of treatment
- Liver enzymes monthly for chronic liver disease, alcohol use, pregnant, or postpartum patients. Drug induced liver injury is most common side effect of treatment. Temporarily halt medications for enzyme increase ≥5 × ULN if asymptomatic or ≥3 × ULN if symptomatic.
- Visual acuity and red-green color monthly if on EMB >2 months or doses >20 mg/kg/day
- If culture positive after 2 months of therapy, reassess drug sensitivity, initiate DOT, coordinate with public health authorities, and consider infectious disease consultation.

PATIENT EDUCATION

- Emphasize medication adherence. Screen and treat close contacts.
- Alert patient that health authorities must be notified.

PROGNOSIS

Few complications and full resolution of infection if medications are taken for full course as prescribed.

COMPLICATIONS

- Cavitary lesions can become secondarily infected.
- Risk for drug resistance increases with HIV positive, treatment nonadherence, or residence in area with high incidence of resistance.

REFERENCES

1. Lewinsohn DM, Leonard MK, LoBue PA, et al. Official American Thoracic Society/Infectious Diseases Society of America/Centers for Disease Control and Prevention clinical practice guidelines: diagnosis of tuberculosis in adults and children. *Clin Infect Dis*. 2017;64(2):111–115.
2. Nahid P, Dorman SE, Alipanah N, et al. Official American Thoracic Society/Centers for Disease Control and Prevention/Infectious Diseases Society of America clinical practice guidelines: treatment of drug-susceptible tuberculosis. *Clin Infect Dis*. 2016;63(7):e147–e195.
3. Saukkonen JJ, Duarte R, Munsiff SS, et al. Updates on the treatment of drug-susceptible and drug-resistant tuberculosis: an official ATS/CDC/ERS/IDSA clinical practice guideline. *Am J Respir Crit Care Med*. 2025;211(1):15–33.

ADDITIONAL READING

- Kontsevaya I, Cabibbe AM, Cirillo DM, et al. Update on the diagnosis of tuberculosis. *Clin Microbiol Infect*. 2024;30(9):1115–1122.
- Motta I, Boeree M, Chesov D, et al. Recent advances in the treatment of tuberculosis. *Clin Microbiol Infect*. 2024;30(9):1107–1114.

SEE ALSO

- WHO tuberculosis program: https://www.who.int/teams/global-tuberculosis-programme/overview
- Tuberculosis, CNS; Tuberculosis, Latent (LTBI); Tuberculosis, Miliary

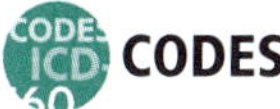

CODES

ICD10

- A15.9 Respiratory tuberculosis unspecified
- A15.0 Tuberculosis of lung
- A19.9 Miliary tuberculosis, unspecified

CLINICAL PEARLS

- TB is fully curable when treated appropriately.
- Children and elderly patients exhibit fewer classic features of TB.
- TST/IGRA cannot discern active TB from LTBI.
- Notify public health authorities about cases of active TB. Consult infectious disease for drug-resistant TB and HIV-positive patients on ART.

TUBERCULOSIS, LATENT (LTBI)

Jennifer M. Romeu, MD, FAAFP, MSM

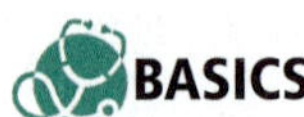

BASICS

DESCRIPTION

- Latent tuberculosis infection (LTBI) is an asymptomatic, noninfectious condition following exposure to an active case of tuberculosis. LTBI is usually detected by a screening skin/blood test. LTBI affects ~25% of the global population.
- Active tuberculosis (TB) occurs in 5–10% of untreated LTBI patients. Chance of active TB increases with immunosuppression and is highest for all individuals within 2 years of infection; 85% of the cases are pulmonary, which can be spread person-to-person via aerosol route.
- >80% of active TB cases in the United States result from untreated LTBI.
- LTBI treatment is a key component of the US TB elimination strategy.

ALERT

- Nitrosamine particles have been isolated in rifampin and rifapentine products in 2020–2022. They are potential or probable carcinogens- due to the life-threatening nature of TB, the FDA has approved ongoing production of these antimicrobials with close monitoring (1).
- The current pace of decline in TB incidence will not eliminate TB in the US in the 21st century. Extra effort is needed to identify patients with LTBI (2).

EPIDEMIOLOGY

- LTBI is not reportable in many states.
- In the United States, high-risk groups include immigrants from countries with a high TB rate (countries other than Canada, Australia, New Zealand, or a country in western/northern Europe); persons with a history of drug use or homelessness; HIV-infected or immunocompromised individuals; persons living or working in high-risk congregate settings such as nursing homes, carceral facilities, and health care workers (2).
- Newly exposed individuals (particularly children) are also at higher risk.
- On average, 5–10% of those infected with LTBI will go on to develop active TB during their lifetime, most typically within 5 years (1)
- In 2023, there were 9,615 TB cases reported in the United States (3).
- The highest TB incidence for US-born persons occurred among people of non-Hispanic White race/ethnicity and the most likely medical diagnostic risk factor was a diagnosis of diabetes.
- Some studies suggest reactivation of LTBI after use of certain immunotherapies, most notably in patients treated for psoriasis (4).

Prevalence

- Globally, ~2 billion people are estimated to be infected with TB. Globally, ~10 million people were diagnosed with active TB in 2020, ~1.1 million were children.
- The CDC estimates 13 million people with LTBI (5).

ETIOLOGY AND PATHOPHYSIOLOGY

Mycobacterium tuberculosis, *Mycobacterium bovis*, and *Mycobacterium africanum*

RISK FACTORS

Immigrants from TB-endemic countries, including most countries of Africa, Asia, and Eastern Europe; close contact with infected individual; living or working in a congregate setting; use of illicit drugs; lower socioeconomic status or experiencing homelessness; healthcare workers; laboratory personnel working with mycobacteria

GENERAL PREVENTION

- Screen for LTBI and treat individuals with positive tests.
- If a person has fibrotic lung changes on imaging and no evidence of TB treatment, these patients should be screened for LTBI.
- Special population: Organ donors should be screened. If donor is deceased, interferon-γ release assay (IGRA) testing is still possible.

COMMONLY ASSOCIATED CONDITIONS

- HIV infection (see "Initial Tests [lab, imaging]")
- Immunosuppression
- IV drug use and substance use disorders

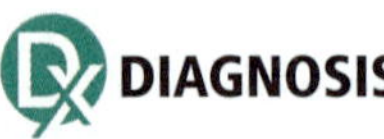

DIAGNOSIS

HISTORY

- Assess risk; history of immigration from high-risk area including those with temporary visas for school or work, history of IV drug use and/or drug treatment, HIV, recent incarceration or experience of homelessness, immunosuppression; known exposure to TB case; caring for an individual with TB.
  - If household contact has LTBI, test all household contacts.
- Assess for active TB cough for more than 2 to 3 weeks, fevers, night sweats, weight loss, hemoptysis.

PHYSICAL EXAM

- There are no active signs of infection on exam in patients with LTBI.
- Assess for signs active TB: vital signs, weight, pulmonary and lymph node exams.

DIFFERENTIAL DIAGNOSIS

- Fungal infections; atypical mycobacteria or *Nocardia*
- Immunosuppression from conditions such as HIV

DIAGNOSTIC TESTS & INTERPRETATION

Initial Tests (lab, imaging)

- Test for TB infection with tuberculin skin (PPD) or IGRA (2). IGRA preferred for individuals with history of BCG vaccine and/or those who would have difficulty returning for second test (to read tuberculin skin test [TST])
- Chest x-ray to rule out active TB
- If concern for active disease, perform acid fast bacilli sputum smear and culture (2).
- Screen at-risk patients for HIV (2).
- Baseline lab testing prior to treatment is recommended for patients at risk for liver disease.

Follow-Up Tests & Special Considerations

- Repeat liver transaminases recommended during LTBI treatment if symptoms develop concerning for hepatotoxicity.
- Discontinue treatment if ALT elevation is >5 times the upper limit of normal or >3 times the upper limit of normal with signs/symptoms consistent with hepatic damage.
- Without known exposure or evidence of TB transmission, health care workers in the United States do not need to serial TB screening at any interval after a baseline test.

Test Interpretation

- TST: PPD: 5 U (0.1 mL) intermediate-strength intradermal volar forearm; measure induration at 48 to 72 hours:
  - Positive if induration is (2)
    - >5 mm and patient has HIV infection (or suspected), is immunosuppressed (including patients on TNF-α inhibitor therapy), had recent close TB contact, or has clinical evidence of active or old disease on CXR
    - >10 mm and patient age <4 years or recent immigrant from high-prevalence country, injection drug user, resident or employee of high-risk congregate settings, or other high-risk medical conditions
    - >15 mm and patient age >4 years and has no risk factors
  - Negative if induration <5 mm on initial test and, if indicated, on second test
  - Use the two-step test (administer a second intradermal test 1 to 3 weeks after initial test; measure and interpret as usual) if patient has had no recent PPD and is age >55 years or is a nursing home resident, prison inmate, or health care worker.
  - Preferred for children <2 years
  - False positives can occur with patients who received BCG vaccine (6).
- IGRA (QuantiFERON-TB and QuantiFERON-TB GOLD; T-SPOT) measure release of interferon by sensitized lymphocytes when exposed to *M. tuberculosis* antigens
  - IGRA unaffected by prior BCG vaccination; requires only one visit for the lab draw; improved sensitivity and specificity; more costly
- Pulmonary immunity assays; measure cytokine response to *M. tuberculosis* antigens; IFN-γ; TNF-α; IL-2 have shown promise differentiating LTBI from active TB.
- Next-generation MTB skin tests (TBST) elicit response from *M. tuberculosis* specific antigens such as ESAT-6 and CFP-10; less impacted by prior BCG vaccination (improved specificity).
- Special considerations
  - Measles vaccine: may suppress tuberculin activity; simultaneous PPD and measles vaccine recommended; if not simultaneous, defer PPD for 4 to 6 weeks after measles vaccine.
  - False-negative skin test: Recent viral infection; new (<10 weeks) infection; severe malnutrition; HIV; anergy; age <6 months; active TB; steroid use.

TREATMENT

GENERAL MEASURES

- First exclude active TB by completing thorough history, physical exam, and lung imaging; obtain chest x-ray within 2 months of starting LTBI therapy.
- Treatment for LTBI is critical for the control and elimination of TB disease. LTBI treatment decreases the risk of active TB and decreases risk of potential spread to others. Treat all persons with LTBI.
- Directly observed therapy (DOT) is recommended if patient adherence is not assured. Video DOT is effective.
- Treat LTBI during pregnancy if patient has recent infection or is HIV positive (use isoniazid [INH] with pyridoxine, and monitor liver enzymes); otherwise, postpone treatment until after delivery.
- Consult public health or infectious disease specialist for suspected INH resistance in HIV patients.

MEDICATION

The CDC and National Tuberculosis Controllers Association (NTCA) recently convened in 2020 to complete a systemic review and update the treatment recommendations.

First Line

- Short-term rifamycin-based therapy. Rifamycins have many drug interactions (via CYP3A4 pathway); use a drug-interaction tool before prescribing.
  - Rifamycins can reduce the effectiveness of hormonal contraception; persons using hormonal contraception should consider the copper IUD, switch to, or add a barrier method for the full duration of latent TB treatment.
  - Rifamycins can interact with warfarin—patients require increased monitoring.
  - Monitor for hypersensitivity reaction and hepatotoxicity.
  - Monitor for hypotensive or flulike reaction to weekly INH/rifapentine and discontinue if this occurs.
  - Rifamycins cause temporary red-orange discoloration of body fluids (urine, sweat, tears, saliva); this reverses on discontinuation of medication.
- INH should be closely monitored for hepatotoxicity, especially in patients with a history of alcohol use disorder, HBV, HCV, fatty liver, NASH, or other signs of liver dysfunction or injury.
  - Peripheral neuritis and hypersensitivity are possible. Consider concurrent pyridoxine (vitamin B_6) 25 to 50 mg/day.

Regimens:

- Once-weekly INH + rifapentine (3HP)
  - 3 months duration, weekly administration with DOT
  - INH (15 mg/kg/day—max 900 mg) for weekly dosing
  - Rifapentine weekly dosing
    - 10 to 14 kg, 300 mg
    - 14.1 to 25.0 kg, 450 mg
    - 25.1 to 32.0 kg, 600 mg
    - 32.1 to 49.9 kg, 750 mg
    - >50 kg, 900 mg (max weekly dose)
- 4 months of daily rifampin (RIF)
  - 10 mg/kg/day (max daily dose of 600 mg)
- 3 months of daily RIF and INH
- Daily INH for 6 to 9 months if rifamycin-based therapy contraindicated
  - 5 mg/kg/day (max daily dose of 300 mg)

Second Line

Alternative options include INH daily for 6 or 9 months.

- Reduced adherence when compared to shorter-course regimens
- Longer duration could increase risk for hepatotoxicity.
- These two durations have not been directly compared.

ISSUES FOR REFERRAL

Consult public health or infectious disease specialist for suspected INH resistance in HIV patients. Consult public health or infectious disease specialist for complicated medication interactions, especially in the circumstance of nitrosamine products in RIF and rifapentine. Consult infectious disease specialists for concerns for multidrug resistant cases.

ADDITIONAL THERAPIES

Pediatric Considerations

- Follow public health recommendations for assessing and treating newborns.
- If mother has disease and is possibly contagious, evaluate infant for congenital TB and test for HIV as well; separating newborn from mother is an individualized risk-benefit discussion.
- Treat or refer for treatment if you suspect congenital TB.

ADMISSION, INPATIENT, AND NURSING CONSIDERATIONS

Geriatric Considerations

Before entering a long-term care setting, patients should have two-step PPD using facility protocols. INH side effects are more pronounced. No isolation required.

ONGOING CARE

FOLLOW-UP RECOMMENDATIONS

Patient Monitoring

- During treatment course for LTBI, monthly visits to assess adherence and monitor for signs and symptoms of active TB or signs of adverse treatment effects; consider partnering with local public health offices for DOT monitoring if appropriate.
- Check liver enzymes if patient is symptomatic, HIV positive, has chronic liver disease, uses alcohol, or is pregnant or postpartum. Modify drugs as needed.
- In a patient who has elected to defer LTBI treatment, there is no indication to repeat chest x-ray unless symptoms develop or the patient elects to initiate treatment.

DIET

Regular; in patients treated with INH, consider pyridoxine 10 to 50 mg/day.

PROGNOSIS

Generally, there are few complications, and treatment is effective if medications are taken as prescribed. If LTBI treatment is erroneously offered to a patient with active TB, it can result in monotherapy of active disease. Nonadherence during LTBI treatment does not lead to drug resistance but does result in untreated LTBI. Retreatment is not necessary.

COMPLICATIONS

Active TB

REFERENCES

1. Carnero Canales CS, Marquez Cazorla J, Furtado Torres AH, et al. Advances in diagnostics and drug discovery against resistant and latent tuberculosis infection. *Pharmaceutics*. 2023;15(10):2409.
2. Sterling TR, Njie G, Zenner D, et al. Guidelines for the treatment of latent tuberculosis infection: recommendations from the national tuberculosis controllers association and CDC, 2020. *MMWR Recomm Rep*. 2020;69(1):1–11.
3. Williams PM, Pratt RH, Walker WL, et al. Tuberculosis—United States, 2023. *MMWR Morb Mortal Wkly Rep*. 2024;73(12):265–270.
4. Seeburruth D, McGuinty J, Sood S, et al. Characteristics, management, and outcomes of latent tuberculosis reactivation following the use of biologics for psoriasis: a systematic review. *J Cutan Med Surg*. 2025:12034754251351851. doi:10.1177/12034754251351851.
5. Mangione CM, Barry MJ, Nicholson WK, et al. Screening for latent tuberculosis infection in adults: US Preventive Services Task Force recommendation statement. *JAMA*. 2023;329(17):1487–1494. doi:10.1001/jama.2023.4899.
6. Palanivel J, Sounderrajan V, Thangam T, et al. Latent tuberculosis: challenges in diagnosis and treatment, perspectives, and the crucial role of biomarkers. *Curr Microbiol*. 2023;80(12):392.

ADDITIONAL READING

Centers for Disease Control and Prevention. LTBI: a guide for primary health care providers. https://www.cdc.gov/tb/publications/ltbi/default.htm.

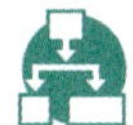

SEE ALSO

Tuberculosis; Tuberculosis, Miliary

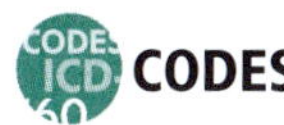

CODES

ICD10

R76.11 Nonspecific reaction to skin test w/o active tuberculosis

CLINICAL PEARLS

- Treatment of LTBI is crucial to the control and elimination of TB disease in the United States.
- Screen persons from TB-endemic countries, and treat those who are positive. Screen household contacts of patients who are LTBI positive. Screen individuals exposed to active cases of TB.
- The IGRA blood test is unaffected by prior BCG vaccination.

ULCER, APHTHOUS

Velyn Wu, MD, MACM

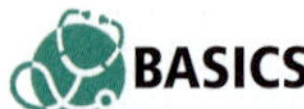

BASICS

Aphthous ulcers are the most common ulcerative disease of the oral mucosa.

DESCRIPTION

- Self-limited, painful ulcerations of the nonkeratinized oral mucosa, which are often recurrent
  - Affects chewing, eating, and speaking
- Synonyms: canker sores; aphthae; aphthous stomatitis
  - Comes from *aphthi* meaning "to set on fire" or "to inflame" in Greek; first used by Hippocrates to categorize oral disease
- Classification based on severity
  - Simple aphthosis
    - Common, episodic, infrequent (<7 episodes annually)
    - Prompt healing (resolution in 1 to 2 weeks), few ulcers
    - Minimal pain, little disability, limited to oral cavity
    - Self-limiting, responds well to local treatments
  - Complex aphthous ulcers
    - Uncommon, episodic or continuous, slow healing
    - Few to many ulcers, frequent or continuous ulceration
    - Short or nonexistent disease-free intervals
    - Marked pain, major disability
    - Often need systemic treatments
    - May have genital aphthae
- Classification based on ulcer morphology
  - Minor aphthous ulcers (Mikulicz aphthae)
    - Age of onset 5 to 19 years
    - Usually <10 mm in diameter
    - Number of ulcers: 1 to 5
    - Self-limited, healing within 4 to 14 days
    - Distribution: lips, cheeks, tongue, floor of mouth
    - Rarely affects the roof of the mouth
    - Nonscarring
    - Affects males and females equally
  - Major aphthous ulcers (Sutton disease), 10% of all aphthae
    - Age of onset 10 to 19 years
    - Usually >10 mm in diameter
    - Number of ulcers: 1 to 10
    - Distribution: lips, soft palate, pharynx
    - May take weeks to months to heal
    - Generally more painful than minor aphthous ulcers
    - May cause scarring and be accompanied by fever and malaise
    - Affects males and females equally
  - Herpetiform ulcers, 5% of all aphthae
    - Age of onset 20 to 29 years
    - Usually 1 to 2 mm in diameter, form larger lesions when coalesced
    - No association with herpes simplex virus
    - Occur in small clusters numbering 10s to 100s, lasting 1 to 4 weeks
    - Generally more painful than minor aphthous ulcers
    - Scarring unusual
    - May also affect the palate, gingiva, and pharynx
    - Affects more females than males

EPIDEMIOLOGY

- Recurrent aphthous stomatitis (RAS) is the most common ulcerative disease of the oral mucosa and accounts for 25% of recurrent ulcers in adults and 40% in children.
- More common in patients <40 years of age, Caucasians, nonsmokers, and those of higher socioeconomic status

Incidence

5% to 60% depending on ethnic and socioeconomic groups

Prevalence

Lifetime prevalence of 5–85%

ETIOLOGY AND PATHOPHYSIOLOGY

Associated with stress-induced rise in salivary cortisol, multiple HLA antigens, cell-mediated immunity and inflammation

Genetics

Associations with specific HLA subtypes

RISK FACTORS

- Local trauma: sharp teeth, dental treatments, or mucosal injury secondary to toothbrushing
- Sodium lauryl sulfate–containing toothpaste
- Increased stress and anxiety
- Nutritional deficiencies: iron, zinc, vitamin B complex, and folate
- Immunodeficiency: HIV
- Recent cessation of tobacco use
- Medications (numerous)
- Endocrine alterations (i.e., menstrual cycle)
- *Helicobacter pylori* infection
- Underlying medical disorders (e.g., celiac disease, inflammatory bowel disease [IBD], Behçet)

GENERAL PREVENTION

- Avoid sodium lauryl sulfate–containing toothpaste
- Vitamin supplementation: B_{12}, D, zinc

DIAGNOSIS

HISTORY

- Patients typically complain of oral ulcerations, which are painful and exacerbated by movement of the mouth. Exacerbation may also be reported with certain foods (hot, spicy, acidic, or carbonated foods or drinks).
- May experience prodrome of burning or pruritic sensation of the oral mucosa 2 to 48 hours prior to appearance of ulcers, progressing to pain which peaks before ulceration
- Aphthae typically begin between the ages of 5 and 29 and are recurrent.
- Ask about ulcerative lesions of other anatomic areas, family history, prior history of aphthous ulcers and new medications prior to onset of ulcers. Ask about the risk factors and take a comprehensive review of systems in order to prioritize the differential.

PHYSICAL EXAM

- Round or ovoid ulcerations generally <10 mm in size; covered with a grayish-white pseudomembrane surrounded by an erythematous halo
- Ulcers are typically found in the buccal or lip mucosa, ventral tongue, soft palate, or oral vestibule; rarely on the roof of the mouth or lips.
- Evaluate for signs of secondary infection: elevated temperature, lymphadenopathy, increased surrounding edema, or pus drainage.

DIFFERENTIAL DIAGNOSIS

- Oral trauma (biting, dentures)
- Infection
  - Herpes virus (HSV stomatitis): vesicular lesions on keratinized tissue (dorsal tongue, vermillion border); generally not present on mucosa, often with prodromal symptoms (fever, headache, malaise, etc.)
  - HIV: Ulcerations have lengthened healing time and tend to be more painful; may be seen in acute seroconversion syndrome or in advanced disease (low CD4 count)
  - Hand-foot-mouth disease: small vesicles within the oral cavity, along with lesions on the hands and feet
  - COVID-19
  - Association with *H. pylori* remains controversial
- Mucocutaneous syndromes (lichen planus, pemphigus); especially if chronic or nonhealing
- Medication induced
  - Fixed drug eruptions
  - Linear IgA bullous dermatosis: tense vesicles or bullae appearing 1 to 15 days after initiation of medication, most commonly caused by vancomycin
- Malignancy: nonhealing lesions, leukoplakia or ipsilateral cervical lymphadenopathy.
- Systemic disease should be considered, causing aphthous-like ulcerations, in adults with their first episode (late onset) or lesions elsewhere (atypical presentation)
  - Behçet syndrome: autoimmune systemic vasculitis usually involving mucous membranes
    - In 80% of Behçet syndrome, ulcers are the presenting sign.
    - Genital and oral ulceration, more likely major than minor aphthae
    - Signs and symptoms can include uveitis, arthritis, skin lesions, or central nervous system deficits.
  - Reiter syndrome: reactive arthritis, preceded by infection, usually of the genital tract, predominantly found in men
    - Uveitis; urethritis; HLA-B27–associated arthritis
  - Sweet syndrome
  - IBD: crohn disease, ulcerative colitis
  - PFAPA syndrome: periodic fevers, aphthous ulcers, pharyngitis, adenitis, abdominal pain, and joint pain
  - Systemic lupus erythematosus (SLE): autoimmune vascular collagen disease
  - Gluten-sensitive enteropathy (celiac disease)
  - Herpangina and hand-foot-and-mouth disease

DIAGNOSTIC TESTS & INTERPRETATION

Lab work may be useful for evaluation for other etiologies of aphthae.

Initial Tests (lab, imaging)

Consider complete blood count, zinc, folic acid, iron, ferritin and B vitamins to evaluate for systemic causes in severe or recurrent cases (1)[C]

Follow-Up Tests & Special Considerations

- Biopsy and viral testing for nonhealing ulcers or atypical presentations
- Rheumatologic serology if underlying systemic disease is suspected
- Gastroenterology evaluation if gastroenterologic disease is suspected

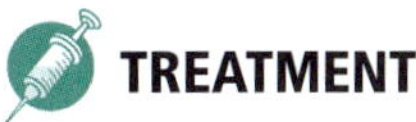

TREATMENT

GENERAL MEASURES

Management is symptomatic. Goal is to reduce inflammation, relieve pain, promote healing, and decrease frequency of recurrence.

MEDICATION

In general, treatment is supportive. Topicals can be helpful and effective for minor aphthae, but systemic treatment may be needed for major aphthae.

First Line

- Topical corticosteroids (to improve healing time and symptoms) (1)[C],(2)[C],(3)[C]
  - Adverse effects: may increase risk of oral candidiasis (more likely with higher potency formulations)
  - Topical steroid preparations
    - Triamcinolone acetonide 0.1% dental paste
      - Apply sparingly to ulcers 2 to 4 times daily for up to 2 weeks or until ulcer resolution.
    - Fluocinonide 0.05% gel or ointment
      - Apply sparingly to ulcer 4 times daily for up to 2 weeks or until ulcer resolution.
- Topical anesthetics (to reduce symptoms only) (1)[B],(3)[A]
  - Preparations
    - Lidocaine 5% ointment or 10% spray
      - Apply 4 times daily or prior to eating as needed for pain for up to 2 weeks or until ulcer resolution.
    - Hyaluronic acid 2.5% gel
      - Apply 2 times per day for 2 weeks until ulcer resolution.
    - Benzocaine topical (OTC)
  - Adverse effects: may cause initial stinging; benzocaine rarely causes methemoglobinemia, especially in children aged <2 years.
- Antimicrobial/antiseptic mouth rinses (improve healing time, decrease pain, and may prevent recurrence) (1)[A],(3)[A]
  - Preparations
    - Chlorhexidine aqueous mouthwash 0.12% or 0.2%
      - Use 3 times daily while lesions persist.
      - May cause superficial tooth staining
    - Doxycycline
      - 100 mg in 10 mL of water
      - Use rinses for 2 to 3 minutes 4 times per day for 3 days.
    - May consider rinses of hydrogen peroxide with menthol
- Topical immunomodulators (improves healing time, reduces symptoms, and prevents recurrence when used in prodromal phase) (1)[B],(3)[A]
  - Adverse effects: may cause stinging sensation
  - Preparation
    - Amlexanox 5% oral paste
      - Apply to ulcers 4 times daily for up to 2 weeks or until ulcer resolution.
      - Not available in the United States

Second Line

Oral Medications (may extend time between recurrence) (1)[B],(3)[A]

- Systemic corticosteroids—rescue therapy in acute, severe, recurrent outbreaks
  - Prednisone 0.75 mg/kg/day, tapered by 0.25 mg/kg/day every 2 weeks
- Montelukast 10 mg daily can have similar efficacy to steroids.
- Colchicine, pentoxifylline, thalidomide, and dapsone have been used with variable success but should be used with caution due to side effects.
- Levamisole—immune modulator, typically well tolerated, pregnancy Category C
- Antibiotics—penicillin G potassium, 50 mg 4 times daily for 4 days

ISSUES FOR REFERRAL

Otolaryngology or dental referral if lesions have not resolved as expected

ADDITIONAL THERAPIES

- Vitamin B_{12} 1,000 μg sublingual daily may be effective in decreasing the duration of outbreaks, number of ulcers, and level of pain (1)[B].
- Vitamin C 2,000 mg/day may also be an effective adjunctive therapy given its anti-inflammatory properties (3)[A].
- *H. pylori* eradication has been associated with lower number of aphthous lesions (3)[A].

SURGERY/OTHER PROCEDURES

Low-level laser therapy at wavelength of 658 nm can improve pain and promote healing (1)[A],(3)[A]

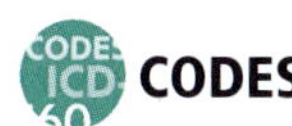

ONGOING CARE

FOLLOW-UP RECOMMENDATIONS

Evaluation for infection, mucocutaneous or systemic disease, or malignancy should be pursued for nonhealing lesions or lesions with lymphadenopathy or unusual presentation.

Patient Monitoring

Aphthous ulcers are often recurrent, so patients should be monitored for recurrence.

DIET

Deficiencies of iron, vitamin B_{12}, and folic acid are significantly associated with recurrent aphthous ulcers.

PATIENT EDUCATION

- Avoid
  - Acidic food or drink
  - Abrasive, hard foods
  - Sodium laurel sulfate–containing toothpaste
- Behavior modification to reduce dental trauma with toothbrush or bruxism
- Maintain proper nutrition.

PROGNOSIS

Varies from single or infrequent recurrences of few, mild, self-resolving lesions to chronic, large, or deep painful lesions; symptoms improve with age.

COMPLICATIONS

- Aphthous ulcers can provide a site for infection and can leave scars.
- Disability from ulcers can affect mental health.

REFERENCES

1. Lau CB, Smith GP. Recurrent aphthous stomatitis: a comprehensive review and recommendations on therapeutic options. *Dermatol Ther*. 2022;35(6):e15500.
2. Gasmi Benahmed A, Noor S, Menzel A, et al. Oral aphthous: pathophysiology, clinical aspects and medical treatment. *Arch Razi Inst*. 2021;76(5):1155–1163.
3. Edgar NR, Saleh D, Miller RA. Recurrent aphthous stomatitis: a review. *J Clin Aesthet Dermatol*. 2017;10(3):26–36.

ADDITIONAL READING

- Shinkre R, Mukherji I, Bharadwaj A, et al. Depression, anxiety, stress, and pain severity in patients with recurrent aphthous stomatitis: a cross-sectional study. *Cureus*. 2024;16(6):e62694.
- Wang Z, Cao H, Xiong J, et al. Recent advances in the aetiology of recurrent aphthous stomatitis (RAS). *Postgrad Med J*. 2022;98(1155):57–66.

CODES

ICD10

K12.0 Recurrent oral aphthae

CLINICAL PEARLS

- Aphthous ulcers are the most common chronic disease of the oral cavity.
- Most cases are mild, self-limited episodes.
- Appropriate treatment should be aimed at symptom control and promotion of healing.
- Nonhealing ulcers, extraoral involvement, and sudden onset in adulthood require additional workup.

U

ULCERATIVE COLITIS

Abbas Rupawala, MD

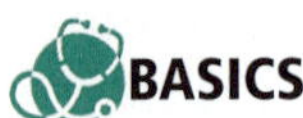

BASICS

DESCRIPTION

- Ulcerative colitis (UC) is a chronic inflammatory bowel disease (IBD) characterized by diffuse mucosal inflammatory changes limited to the colon.
- Most cases involve the rectum and may extend proximally in a continuous fashion involving part or the entire large intestine (1).
- Frequently manifested by recurrent episodes of bloody and mucoid diarrhea often associated with abdominal pain, rectal urgency, stool incontinence, fever, and weight loss
- Clinical course includes exacerbations and spontaneous or treatment induced remissions.
- Colonic involvement is universal and may be accompanied by other extraintestinal manifestations.

EPIDEMIOLOGY

Incidence

Although incidence of UC was highest in Western nations, incidence has been increasing worldwide:

- Asia/Middle East: 0.75 to 3.64/100,000 person-years
- North America: 10 to 15/100,000 person-years
- Europe: 10 to 40/100,000 person-years

Prevalence

Due to young age at diagnosis and relatively low mortality, prevalence continues to rise:

- North America: 305 to 400/100,000 persons
- Europe: 286 to 505/100,000 persons

ETIOLOGY AND PATHOPHYSIOLOGY

- Idiopathic inflammatory disorder hypothesized to result from immune dysfunction in a genetically predisposed individual in response to environmental triggers and gut microbiome alterations
- Inflammation starts in rectum (>95% of patients) and extends proximally (50% rectosigmoid), and 20% have pancolitis. Rectum may be spared in <5% adults and up to 1/3 of pediatric patients.

Genetics

- Polygenic disease with >200 genetic loci in genome-wide studies; increased risk with Turner syndrome
- Higher incidence in first-degree relative.

RISK FACTORS

- Peak incidence at age 20 to 40 years and second peak at age 50 to 80 years
- Higher incidence in White and Ashkenazi Jewish populations; rising in Black and Latinx populations
- Environmental risk factors include enteric infection, diet (Western diet, ultraprocessed foods), antibiotic use, lack of breastfeeding in infant, obesity, and NSAIDs use. Smoking may lower risk of UC.

GENERAL PREVENTION

Pregnancy Considerations

- Patient should be advised to conceive during remission if planning a pregnancy; 3 to 6 months of remission before conception decreases risk of exacerbation during pregnancy (2).
- There is increased risk of preterm delivery and small for gestational age in women with active disease.
- Ideally, pregnant women should be monitored by both gastroenterologist and maternal-fetal medicine specialist (2).

COMMONLY ASSOCIATED CONDITIONS

- Common: arthritis/arthralgias: small and large joints, sacroiliitis, aphthous ulcers, erythema nodosum, anemia, osteoporosis, fatty liver
- Rare: episcleritis, scleritis and uveitis, autoimmune hepatitis, liver cirrhosis, primary sclerosing cholangitis (PSC), bile duct carcinoma, ankylosing spondylitis, pyoderma gangrenosum, colon cancer

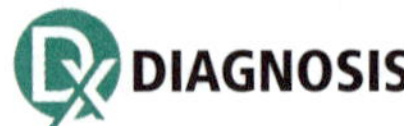

DIAGNOSIS

HISTORY

- Symptoms may include:
  - Small frequent bloody or mucoid diarrhea associated with tenesmus, rectal urgency, fecal incontinence and abdominal pain; onset is gradual and progressive over weeks.
  - Weight loss, anorexia, fatigue, fever
  - Extraintestinal manifestation including joint, skin, ocular, oral, hepatobiliary-related symptoms
- Potential precipitating factors: recent smoking cessation, NSAIDs use, enteric infection
- Assess for a family history of IBD.

PHYSICAL EXAM

- Exam may often be normal.
- Weight loss, signs of fluid depletion (tachycardia, hypotension), signs of anemia (pallor)
- Severe disease: fever, hypotension, tachycardia, pallor, loss of subcutaneous fat, muscle wasting, peripheral edema, clubbing
- Abdominal tenderness, blood on rectal exam

DIFFERENTIAL DIAGNOSIS

- Crohn disease
- Infectious colitis: bacterial, parasitic, or viral (cytomegalovirus [CMV]), *Clostridium difficile* infection
- Ischemic colitis
- Irritable bowel syndrome
- Diverticular associated colitis
- Diversion colitis in patients with diverting ostomy
- Medication-induced colitis (NSAIDs, mycophenolate, checkpoint inhibitors)
- Radiation colitis
- Graft versus host disease
- Celiac disease

DIAGNOSTIC TESTS & INTERPRETATION

Initial Tests (lab, imaging)

- CBC: leukocytosis and anemia
- BMP: abnormal urea and electrolytes, especially hypokalemia
- LFTs: can be abnormal; low albumin indicates severe disease.
- CRP may be elevated, especially in more severe disease.
- Fecal calprotectin (FC): elevated; FC may also use to differentiate IBD from irritable bowel syndrome with varying cutoffs 50 to 150 μg/g. FC can also be used to monitor treatment response (1).
- Stool studies to rule out infectious cause: *C. difficile (CDI in newly diagnosed or relapsing IBD ranges from 5% to 47%)*, stool cultures, Shiga toxin, ova and parasite microscopy, *Giardia* antigen (1)
- Perinuclear antineutrophil cytoplasmic antibody (pANCA) commonly present in patients with UC, but testing for them is not currently recommended for diagnosis (1).
- Abdominal x-ray to exclude dangerous colonic dilation and assess disease severity
- Limited value to cross-sectional imaging

Diagnostic Procedures/Other

Diagnosis of UC requires colonoscopy with at least two biopsies from each of five sites along the entire colon (unaffected and affected areas). In severe cases, complete colonoscopy may be contraindicated due to risk of perforation and sigmoidoscopy with biopsy may suffice (1).

Test Interpretation

- Endoscopic findings: mucosal engorgement with altered vascular markings, erythema, friability, granularity, and erosions; in severe UC, deep ulcerations and active bleeding may be found (1).
- Histologic findings: mucosal separation, crypt architecture distortion, and atrophy of the crypts; chronic inflammatory cells in lamina propria; lymphocytes and plasma cells in crypt bases, Paneth cell metaplasia
- Mild ileal inflammation ("backwash ileitis") may be present in UC.
- Assess disease extent as per Montreal classification and severity (mild, moderate, or severe) to help prognosticate and select appropriate management. Multiple criteria can be used to assess severity, including the Mayo Score and the proposed American College of Gastroenterology Ulcerative Colitis Activity Index (1).

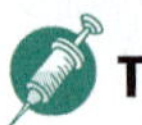

TREATMENT

- Disease severity and extent dictate treatment approach: step up versus top down therapy
- Goals of treatment are to restore normal bowel function, reverse inflammatory changes of the intestinal mucosa, and to maintain a steroid-free remission without extraintestinal manifestations and minimal side effects (1).
  - Drugs initiated for induction of remission may be continued for maintenance if they are effective.
  - Steroids are not recommended for maintenance. Chronic steroid use can cause adrenal suppression, gastrointestinal bleeding, heart disease, osteoporosis, thinning of skin, and compromised vascular wall integrity.
  - Advanced therapies and side effects should be reviewed: infections, infusion/injection reactions, cancer risk, cardiovascular risks, paradoxical side effects, etc. should be reviewed.
  - Shared decision-making including risks versus benefits of medications, goals of treatment should be practiced.

MEDICATION

First Line

- Induction of remission in mild to moderately active UC
  - Proctitis
    - Rectal 5-ASA 1 g/day
    - If 5-ASA fails, use topical steroid suppository, foam or enema and tacrolimus suppository.

- Left-sided/extensive colitis
  - Rectal 5-ASA enema/suppository and oral 5-ASA
  - If 5-ASA fails, use budesonide MMX 9 mg/day (1)[B] or oral systemic corticosteroid (1)[C].
- Reassess within 4 to 8 weeks to determine response.

- Maintenance of remission in mild to moderately active UC:
  - Proctitis: rectal 5-ASA
  - Left-sided/extensive colitis: oral 5-ASA
- Induction of remission in moderate to severe active UC:
  - Budesonide MMX or oral systemic corticosteroids (1)[B]
  - Advanced therapy naive: S1P modulator, IL-23, or IL-12/23 inhibitor, anti-integrin or anti-TNF
    - S1P modulator (ozanimod, etrasimod)
    - IL-23 inhibitor: guselkumab, mirikizumab, risankizumab
    - IL-12/23 inhibitor: ustekinumab or biosimilars
    - Anti-TNFs: infliximab and biosimilars, adalimumab and biosimilars, golimumab
  - Advanced therapy exposed patients: JAK inhibitors (tofacitinib, upadacitinib) or other advanced therapies
- Maintenance of remission in patient with previously moderate to severe active UC: continuation of advanced therapy

Second Line

Pediatric Considerations

- Pediatric growth and development can be affected due to malabsorption.
- Oral 5-ASA regimens are first line for both induction and maintenance therapy in mild to moderate pediatric UC. Combination of oral and topical rectal 5-ASA is more effective than oral 5-ASA alone even in extensive disease.
- Oral steroids can be used for induction of remission in moderate disease (with systemic symptoms) to severe disease.
- Consider biologics (infliximab, adalimumab) for children with UC that is persistently active, steroid-dependent, or uncontrolled by 5-ASA.

Pregnancy Considerations

- Risks and benefits of medications versus untreated disease are important for pregnancy/lactation consideration.
- Stop methotrexate at least 3 months prior to conceiving. It is contraindicated in pregnancy.
- In general, aminosalicylate, biologic, and immunomodulator therapies may be continued during pregnancy and lactation.
- Corticosteroids may be used for induction therapy but not maintenance therapy due to increased risks for preterm birth, low fetal weight, and gestational diabetes.

ISSUES FOR REFERRAL

- Referral to gastroenterologist recommended for management of moderate to severe disease, especially if immunomodulator drugs are used
- Referral to general or colorectal surgery recommended if surgical intervention is anticipated (indications as follows)

SURGERY/OTHER PROCEDURES

- Surgery is indicated for those who are refractory or intolerant to medical therapy (particularly with high-dose steroids).
- Emergent surgery (typically total or subtotal abdominal colectomy with end ileostomy) for massive hemorrhage, perforation, and toxic dilatation
- Total colectomy with ileostomy is curative.

COMPLEMENTARY & ALTERNATIVE MEDICINE

There is ongoing research into the role of probiotics, dietary changes, and fecal microbiota transplant as treatment for UC. The current evidence is insufficient to support the efficacy of any particular alternative therapy for achieving or maintaining remission.

ADMISSION, INPATIENT, AND NURSING CONSIDERATIONS

- Admission for UC or its complications warrants gastroenterology consultation.
- Severe UC may require emergent surgical intervention. Consultation with surgery is indicated.
- Imaging studies help assess disease activity and colon size.
- Initiate IV corticosteroids and rule out infectious etiologies (*C. difficile*, CMV, shigella/amoeba).

ONGOING CARE

Management of patient with acute severe ulcerative colitis (ASUC) (1):

- Hospitalization
- Sigmoidoscopy without bowel preparation within 24 to 36 hours of admission
- DVT prophylaxis
- Test for CDI.
- 60 mg methylprednisolone or hydrocortisone 100 mg 3 or 4 times per day to gain remission; if 3 to 5 days IV corticosteroids fail, use infliximab, cyclosporine, or JAK inhibitors and obtain a surgical consultation.
- Monitor stool frequency, rectal bleeding, serial CRP, abdominal x-ray for signs of toxic megacolon.
- Toxic megacolon, large intestine perforation, severe hemorrhage, lack of response to medical therapy are all indications for colectomy.
- Avoid anticholinergic, NSAIDs, and opioids.

FOLLOW-UP RECOMMENDATIONS

Patient Monitoring

Routine monitoring visits during maintenance phase should review:

- Vaccinations to reduce risk of vaccine preventable infections (flu, pneumonia, shingles)
- Bone health: vitamin D and calcium supplementation, DEXA scans
- Cancer screening: skin, cervical cancer
  - Colon cancer screening: starting at 8 years from diagnosis in left sided or extensive disease; at diagnosis in UC with PSC
- Mental health screening for anxiety and depression
- Lab monitoring of blood counts, renal and liver chemistries, nutritional deficiencies

DIET

- Low-residue diet during exacerbations
- There are otherwise no specific dietary recommendations.

PATIENT EDUCATION

Crohn and Colitis Foundation: https://www.ccfa.org/

PROGNOSIS

Poor prognostic factors as measured by the likelihood of colectomy

- <40 years old at prognosis
- Extensive UC
- Severe endoscopic disease
- Previous hospitalization for colitis
- Elevated CRP
- Low serum albumin

COMPLICATIONS

- Perforation
- Venous thromboembolism
- Anemia
- Fulminant colitis
- Toxic megacolon
- Liver disease
- Stricture formation
- Osteoporosis
- Colorectal cancer

REFERENCES

1. Rubin DT, Ananthakrishnan AN, Siegel CA, et al. ACG clinical guideline update: ulcerative colitis in adults. *Am J Gastroenterol*. 2025;120(6):1187–1224.
2. Mahadevan U, Seow CH, Barnes EL, et al; for Global Consensus Group for Pregnancy and IBD. Global consensus statement on the management of pregnancy in Inflammatory bowel disease. *Inflamm Bowel Dis*. 2025;31(10):2615–2664.

SEE ALSO

Algorithm: Hematemesis (Bleeding, Upper Gastrointestinal)

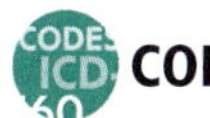

CODES

ICD10

- K51.90 Ulcerative colitis, unspecified, without complications
- K51.919 Ulcerative colitis, unspecified with unspecified complications
- K51.80 Other ulcerative colitis without complications

CLINICAL PEARLS

- Diffuse, uninterrupted colonic mucosal inflammation
- The hallmark symptom is bloody diarrhea.
- Common medical treatments include 5-ASA, steroids, and advanced therapies.
- Refractory disease or severe complications may require surgical intervention.
- Annual or biannual surveillance colonoscopy after 8 to 10 years of colitis due to increased risk of colorectal cancer (1)

URETHRITIS

Chirag N. Shah, MD • William Andrew Pleasant, MD • Matthew R. Carroll, DO

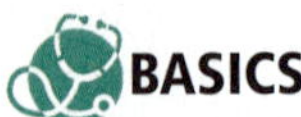

BASICS

DESCRIPTION
- Inflammation of the urethra
- Common manifestation of sexually transmitted infection (STI)
- Frequently associated with dysuria, pruritus, and/or urethral discharge; classified as gonococcal (caused by *Neisseria gonorrhoeae*) and nongonococcal (caused by other bacteria, or less common autoimmune disorders [Reiter syndrome], trauma, or chemical irritation)

EPIDEMIOLOGY

Incidence
- In 2022, 648,056 cases of gonorrhea were reported, a 9.2% decrease in the overall rate from the previous year. This was the first decrease in the rate of gonorrhea observed since 2009.
- Gonorrhea is the second most commonly reported STD.
- 40% of gonorrhea cases occurred in men who have sex with men (MSM).
- In 2022, there were 1,649,716 cases of chlamydia reported, making it the most common STD in the United States.
- The rate of chlamydia in 2022 (459.0 per 100,000) was similar to the rate in 2021 (459.5 per 100,000), but the rate in men increased by 1.8%, and the rate in women decreased by 1.2%.
- Highest incidences of gonorrhea and chlamydia among young men and women, ages 15 to 24 years (61% of all cases)
- Chlamydial infections are 5 times more likely in young adult women than gonococcal infections.
- In 2022, there were 207,255 reported cases of syphilis, the greatest number of cases reported since 1950; representing a 17.3% increase since 2021.
- The number of primary and secondary syphilis cases—the most infectious stages of syphilis—increased to 59,016 cases.

ETIOLOGY AND PATHOPHYSIOLOGY
- Most common cause is infection via sexual transmission of *N. gonorrhoeae*, a gram-negative diplococcus.
- *N. gonorrhoeae* is a gram-negative diplococcus that interacts with nonciliated epithelial cells → cellular invasion → inflammation, neutrophil production, and bacterial cell phagocytosis.
- Sexually transmitted *Chlamydia trachomatis* infection is the most common cause of nongonococcal urethritis.
- Other established pathogens:
  - *Mycoplasma genitalium*, *Trichomonas vaginalis*, *Ureaplasma urealyticum*, Herpes simplex virus (rare), Adenovirus (rare)
- Noninfectious causes (less common)
  - Chemical irritants (i.e., soaps, shampoos, douches, spermicides), foreign bodies, urethral instrumentation

RISK FACTORS
- Age 15 to 24 years
- New sex partner/one or more sex partner(s), history of or coexisting STI, sex partner with concurrent partner(s)
- Inconsistent condom use outside a mutually monogamous relationship; exchanging sex for money or drugs
- Members of the population with increased prevalence of infection, including incarcerated populations, military recruits, and economically disadvantaged populations

GENERAL PREVENTION
- Use of male condoms, female condoms, or cervical diaphragms
- Abstinence or reduction in the number of sex partners; behavioral counseling

COMMONLY ASSOCIATED CONDITIONS

ALERT
Annual chlamydia and gonorrhea screening is recommended for all sexually active women aged <24 years and women aged >25 years with risk factors (B recommendation). There is insufficient evidence to recommend screening in men (1)[A]

DIAGNOSIS

- Chief complaint
  - Urethral discharge (mucopurulent suggestive of *N. gonorrhoeae*), dysuria, erythema of the urethral meatus, symptom onset 2 to 8 days following exposure
- History
  - Sexual history, including condom use, number of partners, sexual behaviors
  - Previous STIs, substance abuse, recent travel
  - Symptoms indicative of complications or additional sites of infection (i.e., men: testicular pain and swelling, anal itching, rectal pain or bleeding; women: lower abdominal pain, dyspareunia, irregular vaginal bleeding)
- Male genitourinary (GU) exam (possible findings)
  - Urethral discharge, meatal erythema, testicular tenderness; palpate scrotum to check for epididymitis or orchitis; assess for ulcers and inguinal lymphadenopathy
- Female GU exam (possible findings)
  - Vaginal discharge, endocervical discharge, hyperemia, and/or friability

Pediatric Considerations
Pediatric infections with gonorrhea and chlamydia after the neonatal period strongly suggest sexual contact. If indicated, investigations should be initiated promptly.

DIFFERENTIAL DIAGNOSIS
- Other GU tract diseases: cystitis/urinary tract infection, epididymitis, prostatitis, pelvic inflammatory disease (PID), pyelonephritis, chronic pelvic pain syndrome
- Vaginal atrophy, especially in postmenopausal women
- Stevens-Johnson syndrome, Wegener granulomatosis, Reiter syndrome: uveitis, urethritis, arthritis
- Urethral syndrome (pain without infection or purulence), longstanding or intermittent symptoms
- Chemical irritation/trauma, mucositis

DIAGNOSTIC TESTS & INTERPRETATION

ALERT
Health care providers are required to report all gonorrhea and chlamydia infections following local and state requirements.

Initial Tests (lab, imaging)
- Diagnostic criteria for urethritis—any of the following in a patient with history, signs, or symptoms consistent with urethritis:
  - Gram stain of urethral secretion with >2 WBC per oil immersion field
  - Microscopic examination of first-void urine sediment shows >10 WBC per high-power field
  - Observation of mucopurulent or purulent discharge on examination
  - Positive leukocyte esterase test with first-void volume
- Gonorrhea
  - Nucleic acid amplification test (NAAT); sensitivity: 90–100%, specificity: 97–100%
  - Preferred specimen collection in first void (men) and vaginal swab (women) (2)[A]
  - Tissue culture was the traditional gold standard but is typically only used now in suspected chlamydial pneumonia or chlamydial ophthalmia.
- Chlamydia
  - NAAT—sensitivity: 85–95%, specificity: 93–99%
  - Preferred specimen collection is the same as for gonorrhea.
  - Tissue culture is currently NOT recommended.
- Gram stain diagnosis criteria
  - Urethral secretions with ≥2 WBC per oil immersion
  - Mucopurulent or purulent discharge
  - First-void urine sediment with ≥10 WBC per high-power field
  - Symptom onset 2 to 8 days following exposure
- Methylene blue/gentian violet (MB/GV)
  - Alternative to gram staining
  - Does not require heat fixation
  - Sensitivity: 97.3% (same as gram stain)
- If concern for *Trichomonas*: NAAT (urine, urethral, vaginal, or endocervical swab), wet mount, or culture
- There is no FDA-approved diagnostic test available for *M. genitalium*, an emerging pathogen with a greater prevalence than gonorrhea in many populations.

ALERT
Due to the similarity in clinical symptoms and high rates of coinfection, cotesting for gonorrhea and chlamydia infection is recommended. In addition, given that risk factors for gonorrhea and chlamydia indicate risks for other STIs, screening for HIV, syphilis (RPR), hepatitis C, and hepatitis B may also be indicated.

Follow-Up Tests & Special Considerations
- Test of cure (TOC) for chlamydia and gonorrhea is recommended in pregnant women or when treatment noncompliance is suspected.
- Repeat testing in 3 months is recommended due to rates of reinfection.
- HIV infection: Persons with HIV infection should receive the same treatment as patients without HIV infection.

Diagnostic Procedures/Other

Cystourethroscopy for cases with suspected foreign body, intraurethral warts, or urethral stricture

Test Interpretation

Urethral strictures (untreated gonorrhea), intraurethral lesions (venereal warts, congenital anomalies), PID, or tubo-ovarian abscesses are possible.

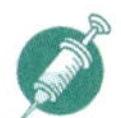

TREATMENT

- Most cases can be treated in the outpatient setting.
- Single-dose regimens with direct observation are preferred and have higher rates of adherence.
- Preferred agents for empiric treatment with unknown cause of urethritis—500 mg IM ceftriaxone for 1 dose PLUS 100 mg PO doxycycline BID for 7 days

MEDICATION

CDC recommendations

- *Chlamydia trachomatis*
  - First line—100 mg PO doxycycline for 7 days
    - Alternate regimens: 500 mg PO erythromycin QID for 7 days *or* 800 mg PO erythromycin ethylsuccinate QID for 7 days *or* 500 mg PO levofloxacin for 7 days *or* 300 mg PO ofloxacin BID for 7 days
      - Of note, 1 g PO 1 dose azithromycin for 7 days is no longer first line due to increasing resistance (3)[C]
- *Neisseria Gonorrhea*
  - First line—500 mg IM ceftriaxone for 1 dose for patients $<$150 kg *or* 1,000 mg IM ceftriaxone for 1 dose for patients $>$150 kg (safe in pregnancy)
    - Alternative regimens: 800 mg PO cefixime for 1 dose *or* 240 mg IM gentamicin for 1 dose *plus* 2 g PO azithromycin for 1 dose
- *Trichomonas vaginalis*
  - First Line—2 g PO metronidazole for 1 dose *or* 2 g PO tinidazole for 1 dose
    - Alternative regimen: 500 mg PO metronidazole BID for 7 days
- *Mycoplasma genitalium*
  - First Line—400 mg PO moxifloxacin for 7 to 14 days *or* 1 g PO azithromycin for 1 dose
    - Alternative regimen: 100 mg PO doxycycline BID for 7 days
- Recurrent and persistent urethritis
  - If it was initially used, consider repeating doxycycline, or a trial of moxifloxacin 400 mg PO QD × 7 days or 1 g PO × 1 dose, with TOC
- General considerations
  - Contraindications: sensitivity to any of the indicated medications
  - Precautions: Patients taking tetracyclines may have increased photosensitivity.
  - Significant possible interactions
    - Tetracyclines should not be taken with milk products or antacids.
    - Oral contraceptives may be rendered less effective by oral antibiotics. Patients and partners should use a backup method of birth control for the remainder of the cycle.

Pregnancy Considerations

- Chlamydia:
  - Screen all pregnant patients: All pregnant women at increased risk should be screened for chlamydia at their prenatal visit and again in the 3rd trimester.
  - TOC 3 weeks after therapy to check for chlamydial eradication and retest in 3 months
  - 1 g PO azithromycin for 1 dose
  - Alternative regimens:
    - 500 mg PO amoxicillin TID for 7 days
- Gonorrhea:
  - Screen all pregnant patients: All pregnant women at increased risk should be screened for gonorrhea at their prenatal visit and again in the 3rd trimester.
  - Standard first-line treatment is safe in pregnancy.
  - TOC 3 weeks after therapy to check for gonococcal eradication and retest in 3 months
  - Quinolones are contraindicated.
  - If there is a cephalosporin allergy and spectinomycin is not available, an infectious disease consult is recommended.

ONGOING CARE

FOLLOW-UP RECOMMENDATIONS

- Sexual activity should be avoided for 7 days following administration of single-dose therapy or until completion of a multiday regimen.
- All sexual partners who came in contact with the patient within 60 days should be referred for evaluation, testing, and presumptive treatment.
- Expedited partner therapy (EPT) is an acceptable alternative; EPT—the practice of treating the diagnosed patient's sex partner(s) for chlamydia or gonorrhea by providing medications to the partner(s) without clinical evaluation

Patient Monitoring

- Instruct patients to return if symptoms persist or recur after completing treatment.
- Screen for reinfection in all patients at 3 months.

PATIENT EDUCATION

- Behavioral counseling interventions are recommended. Evidence of benefit increases with the intensity of intervention.
- Successful approaches include basic information about STIs and transmission, assessing risk for transmission, and training skills (i.e., condom use, communication about safe sex, problem solving, goal setting).

PROGNOSIS

If the diagnosis is firmly established, appropriate medications are prescribed, and the patient is compliant with treatment, relief of symptoms occurs within days, and the problem will resolve without sequela.

COMPLICATIONS

Stricture formation, epididymitis, prostatitis, PID in women, disseminated gonococcal infection, gonococcal meningitis, gonococcal endocarditis, perinatal transmission (chlamydial conjunctivitis, chlamydial pneumonia, ophthalmia neonatorum), Reiter syndrome; chronic cervical chlamydial infection has been proposed to increase the risk of cervical cancer.

REFERENCES

1. Cantor A, Dana T, Griffin JC, et al. Screening for chlamydial and gonococcal infections: updated evidence report and systematic review for the US Preventive Services Task Force. *JAMA*. 2021;326(10):957–966. doi:10.1001/jama.2021.10577.
2. Aaron KJ, Griner S, Footman A, et al. Vaginal swab vs urine for detection of *Chlamydia trachomatis*, *Neisseria gonorrhoeae*, and *Trichomonas vaginalis*: a meta-analysis. *Ann Fam Med*. 2023;21(2):172–179. doi:10.1370/afm.2942.
3. Sell J, Nasir M, Courchesne C. Urethritis: rapid evidence review. *Am Fam Physician*. 2021;103(9):553–558.

ADDITIONAL READING

Centers for Disease Control and Prevention. National overview of STIs, 2022. https://www.cdc.gov/std/statistics/2022/overview.htm. Accessed October 4, 2024.

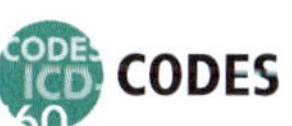

CODES

ICD10

- N34.2 Other urethritis
- A56.01 Chlamydial cystitis and urethritis
- A54.01 Gonococcal cystitis and urethritis, unspecified

CLINICAL PEARLS

- Inflammation of the urethra, frequently associated with dysuria, pruritus, and/or urethral discharge
- NAAT preferred method of diagnosis for men and women
- In cases of gonorrhea or chlamydia infection, in-person follow-up or EPT is recommended for all partners of patients within the last 60 days.
- Given that risk factors for gonorrhea and chlamydia indicate risk for other STIs, screening for HIV, syphilis (RPR), hepatitis C, and hepatitis B may also be indicated.
- Repeat testing for gonorrhea and chlamydia in 3 months is recommended due to rates of reinfection.
- Treatment in persons with HIV infection is the same as in patients without HIV infection.

URINARY TRACT INFECTION (UTI) IN WOMEN

Narmina Khanmammadova, MD • Akhil K. Das, MD, FACS

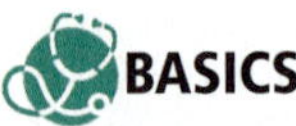

BASICS

DESCRIPTION

- Urinary tract infection (UTI) is the presence of pathogenic microorganisms in the urinary tract causing symptoms (see "History").
- Uncomplicated UTI: UTI in patients with an anatomically normal urinary tract with no obstruction, no predisposing risk factors and symptoms confined to the lower urinary tract
- Complicated UTI: UTI in the presence of anatomical or functional abnormality, immunocompromised host, or a multidrug resistant organism (see "Risk Factors")
- Recurrent UTI: symptomatic; occurs following complete treatment and resolution of documented infection; ≥2 culture-proven infections in 6 months, or ≥3 in 12 months.
- Asymptomatic bacteriuria (ASB): presence of bacteria in urine with no symptoms
- Synonym(s): cystitis

EPIDEMIOLOGY

UTIs are highly prevalent among women (1).

Incidence

Accounts for >8 million office visits with 21% of these being emergency room visits (84% women) and >100,000 hospital admissions with a cost of >$2 billion annually

Prevalence

- >50% of women will have at least one UTI in their lifetime.
- About 20–40% of women with a prior UTI episode will experience another UTI.

ETIOLOGY AND PATHOPHYSIOLOGY

- Ascension of bacteria into the bladder via the urethra is the most common etiology.
- Pathogenic organisms possess adherence factors (pili or fimbriae) and toxins that allow the initiation and propagation of UTIs.
- Most UTIs are caused by bacteria originating from bowel flora:
  - *Escherichia coli* is the causative organism in 75–95% of cases of uncomplicated UTIs.
  - Less common: *Staphylococcus saprophyticus*, *Klebsiella pneumoniae*, *Proteus* mirabilis

Genetics

Women with nonsecretor Lewis antigen have increased bacterial adherence.

RISK FACTORS

- Biologic:
  - Urinary stasis/obstruction: pelvic organ prolapse, bladder diverticula, neurogenic bladder, voiding dysfunction, urethral stricture, anatomic anomalies of the urinary tract
  - Urinary calculi
  - Immunosuppression: diabetes, HIV, malignancy, malnutrition
- Behavioral practices that promote colonization:
  - Sexual intercourse
  - Use of spermicides or antimicrobials
  - Poor hygiene

GENERAL PREVENTION

- Resolve urinary obstruction/stasis
- Adequate hydration
- Women with frequent/intercourse-related UTI should empty bladder immediately before and after intercourse.
- Avoid feminine hygiene sprays, diaphragms, spermicidal agents, and douches.
- Vaginal estrogen in postmenopausal women may help prevent recurrent UTI (2)[C].

COMMONLY ASSOCIATED CONDITIONS

See "Risk Factors."

Geriatric Considerations

- Elderly patients due to underlying urinary tract abnormality or voiding dysfunction, or other comorbidities:
  - Poor hygiene, urinary/fecal incontinence, pelvic organ prolapse
  - Low estrogen levels increase vaginal pH and alter microbial flora, leading to increased colonization with pathogenic organisms.
- May present with atypical symptoms such as altered mental status or urinary incontinence
- Treatment of ASB does not improve outcomes and should be avoided.

Pediatric Considerations

Bowel and bladder dysfunction or congenital urinary tract abnormalities such as vesicoureteral reflux (VUR) or duplicated collecting system are risk factors.

DIAGNOSIS

HISTORY

- Dysuria, urgency, frequency, sensation of incomplete bladder emptying, hematuria, suprapubic pain, malodorous urine, altered mental status, nocturia, sudden onset or worsening of urinary incontinence, dyspareunia
- Number of UTIs, recent sexual activity or new sexual partner(s)

PHYSICAL EXAM

- Suprapubic tenderness
- Urethral and/or vaginal tenderness; evaluate for diverticulum or other urethral masses.
- Fever or costovertebral angle tenderness indicates upper UTI.

DIFFERENTIAL DIAGNOSIS

Vaginitis, STDs causing urethritis/pyuria, neoplasm, calculi, interstitial cystitis

DIAGNOSTIC TESTS & INTERPRETATION

Initial Tests (lab, imaging)

- Clean catch midstream voided urine may be contaminated with vaginal or perineal organisms. Suspect contamination: growth of normal vaginal flora (lactobacillus) or mixed cultures with >1 organism.
- Urinalysis (microscopic):
  - Pyuria (≥10 WBC/HPF in a centrifuged specimen)
  - Bacteriuria: not reliable
  - Hematuria (≥3 RBCs/HPF)
  - >10 squamous cells/HPF indicate poor collection/quality/contamination
- Dipstick urinalysis:
  - Leukocyte esterase (indicates presence of 5 to 15 WBC/HPF; 80–92% sensitivity, 64–84% specificity, when ≥10^5 CFU/mL)
  - Nitrite tests are specific but not sensitive for UTI. A positive test indicates that nitrite-reducing organisms (e.g., *E. coli*, *Klebsiella*, *Proteus*) are present. A negative test does not exclude other pathogens.
- Urine culture: not indicated for uncomplicated UTI; necessary for unclear diagnosis, recurrent, or complicated UTI

Follow-Up Tests & Special Considerations

- Empiric antibiotics may be given without urine culture for uncomplicated UTI.
- Imaging:
  - Consider renal and bladder ultrasound (RBUS) and abdominal and pelvic CT scan for: recurrent UTIs, immunocompromised patients, signs of obstruction, or patients with persistent symptoms after treatment
  - Consider CT scan or MR urogram only for patients with recurrent UTIs or those with risk factors for anatomic abnormalities.

Pediatric Considerations

An RBUS, and/or voiding cystourethrogram (VCUG) can be used to evaluate for VUR and other abnormalities such as pelvocaliectasis or ureteral dilatation.

Diagnostic Procedures/Other

- If the urine specimen is suspected to be contaminated, a catheterized specimen may be necessary.
- Suprapubic bladder aspiration or urethral catheterization: to obtain specimens from infants
- Cystourethroscopy: to evaluate patients with recurrent UTIs, history of nephrolithiasis, previous anti-incontinence surgery, or hematuria in the absence of an active infection

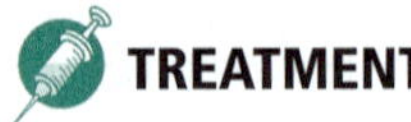

TREATMENT

GENERAL MEASURES

- ASB in a nonpregnant woman should not be treated.
- Maintain adequate hydration with ≥2 L water daily.
- Many women with uncomplicated UTIs have resolution without treatment and rarely progress to serious infections.

MEDICATION

First Line

- Symptomatic:
  - Phenazopyridine 100 to 200 mg TID is a urinary topical analgesic and should only be used for rapid symptom relief, not definitive treatment. Urinalysis interpretation on this medication may be inaccurate; doesn't affect urine culture results.
  - NSAIDs may offer some relief for symptoms; option for those with mild symptoms wishing to avoid antibiotics

- Uncomplicated UTI:
  - Trimethoprim/sulfamethoxazole (TMP/SMX; Bactrim): 160/800 mg PO BID for 3 days, best where resistance of *E. coli* strains <20%; rash may be higher than with other antibiotics; preferred first line
  - Nitrofurantoin (Macrobid): 100 mg PO BID for 5 days should be used in patients with allergy to TMP/SMX and in areas where *E. coli* resistance to TMP/SMX >20%; ineffective in treating upper UTI; also, should also be avoided if creatinine clearance is <30 mL/min
  - Fosfomycin (Monurol): 3 g PO single dose
- UTI in pregnancy:
  - Nitrofurantoin: 100 mg PO BID for 7 days. Discontinue at 35 weeks for risk of neonatal hemolytic anemia.
  - Cephalexin (Keflex): 250 to 500 mg PO TID for 7 days
  - TMP/SMX: 800/160 mg PO q12h for 5 to 7 days; avoided if possible during the 1st (possible risk of neural tube defects) and 3rd (risk of kernicterus) trimesters
  - Fosfomycin: 3 g PO once
  - Fluoroquinolones: contraindicated
- Postcoital UTI:
  - Single dose TMP/SMX or nitrofurantoin or cephalexin
- Complicated UTI:
  - Extend course to 7 to 10 days; may begin with fluoroquinolone, TMP/SMX, or cephalosporin (Avoid using nitrofurantoin for complicated UTI due to lack of tissue penetration.)

Second Line

- Uncomplicated UTI
  - β-Lactams (amoxicillin/clavulanate, cefdinir, cefpodoxime) for 3 to 7 days
  - Fluoroquinolones should not be used in uncomplicated UTI due to risk of adverse reactions, which may occur even with single doses (see FDA box warnings regarding hypoglycemia, tendon rupture risk, neuropathy).
- Recurrent UTIs
  - Aim for the shortest antibiotic course and symptom resolution. Urine culture is required. Consider 3 to 12 months of prophylactic antibiotics, followed by observation for reinfection. Continuous antimicrobial prophylaxis: daily TMP 100 mg, or TMP/SMX 40/200 mg, or nitrofurantoin 50 to 100 mg, or cephalexin 125 to 250 mg, or fosfomycin 3 g every 10 days
  - Other options are patient-initiated antibiotic treatment for early UTI symptoms (minimizes office visits, antibiotic use), postcoital prophylaxis, and intermittent-dosed prophylaxis (e.g., Monday-Wednesday-Friday).
  - For those wishing to avoid antibiotics, methenamine may be used for prophylaxis of recurrent UTI (3)[A],(4)[C].

Pediatric Considerations

Long-term antibiotics might lower recurrent UTI risk in susceptible children, but raise risk of resistance.

ISSUES FOR REFERRAL

Refer to a urologist if recurrent/complicated UTIs.

Pediatric Considerations

UTI in children, especially <1 year of age, might prompt referral to a pediatric urologist.

SURGERY/OTHER PROCEDURES

- Sepsis from urinary tract obstruction requires prompt drainage often in the setting of upper tract obstruction/dilation requiring ureteral stent or percutaneous nephrostomy tube.
- Children with febrile UTIs and VUR may need antireflux surgery such as ureteral reimplantation.

COMPLEMENTARY & ALTERNATIVE MEDICINE

- *Vaccinium macrocarpon* (cranberry, not cranberry juice cocktail) may help to prevent and treat UTIs by inhibiting bacterial adherence to the bladder epithelium.
- Vaginal estrogen can prevent recurrent UTIs in peri- and postmenopausal women.
- There is not enough evidence to support the use of probiotics for UTI prophylaxis. Evidence for D-mannose is weak.

ADMISSION, INPATIENT, AND NURSING CONSIDERATIONS

Inpatient evaluation is reserved for patients with complicated UTIs. Majority of uncomplicated UTIs are managed in an outpatient setting.

ONGOING CARE

FOLLOW-UP RECOMMENDATIONS

First UTI: Reproductive-age and middle-age, nonpregnant females require no follow-up if UTI is clinically cured after 3-day therapy (4)[C]. Obtain urine culture if symptoms persist after 2 to 3 days of treatment.

Pregnancy Considerations

- During pregnancy, UTI always requires culture and usually requires a 7- to 14-day treatment.
- Following the treatment of acute infection, consider a single follow-up urine culture 1 to 2 weeks posttherapy.
- In patients with recurrent UTIs, prophylactic antibiotics for the rest of pregnancy could be considered.

Patient Monitoring

- Repeat culture in asymptomatic patients after completing therapy for a UTI to document bacterial clearance is unnecessary, and may promote overtreatment of ASB.
- Obtain repeat urine cultures in patients with persistent symptoms after treatment. An empiric course of alternate antibiotics can be started preferably after a urine sample is obtained.

DIET

Reduce/prevent glycosuria.

PATIENT EDUCATION

Urology Care Foundation: https://www.urologyhealth.org/

PROGNOSIS

Symptoms resolve within 2 to 3 days of antibiotic treatment in almost all patients.

COMPLICATIONS

Pyelonephritis or sepsis, renal abscess, urinary outlet obstruction

Pregnancy Considerations

Pregnant females with UTI are at higher risk for pyelonephritis, low birth weight, or premature birth.

REFERENCES

1. He Y, Zhao J, Wang L, et al. Epidemiological trends and predictions of urinary tract infections in the global burden of disease study 2021. *Sci Rep*. 2025;15(1):4702. doi:10.1038/s41598-025-89240-5.
2. Schmiemann G, Kranz J, Mandraka F, et al. The diagnosis, treatment, and prevention of recurrent urinary tract infection. *Dtsch Arztebl Int*. 2024;121(11):373–382. doi:10.3238/arztebl.m2024.0068.
3. Harding C, Mossop H, Homer T, et al. Alternative to prophylactic antibiotics for the treatment of recurrent urinary tract infections in women: multicentre, open label, randomised, non-inferiority trial. *BMJ*. 2022;376:e068229. doi:10.1136/bmj-2021-0068229.
4. Anger JT, Bixler BR, Holmes RS, et al. Updates to recurrent uncomplicated urinary tract infections in women: AUA/CUA/SUFU guideline. *J Urol*. 2022;208(3):536–541. doi:10.1097/JU.0000000000002860.

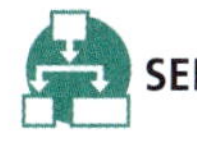

SEE ALSO

Algorithm: Dysuria

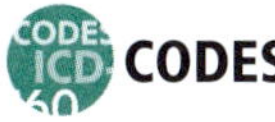

CODES

ICD10

- N39.0 Urinary tract infection, site not specified
- N30.90 Cystitis, unspecified without hematuria
- N30.91 Cystitis, unspecified with hematuria

CLINICAL PEARLS

- Urine culture is generally not indicated for women with uncomplicated UTIs.
- Uncomplicated UTIs should be treated for 3 days (TMP/SMX) or 5 days (nitrofurantoin).
- Pregnant women with bacteriuria should be treated due to the risk of poor outcomes.
- Nonpregnant women and elderly with ASB should not be treated.

U

URINARY TRACT INFECTION (UTI) IN MALES

Suzanne Florczyk, PharmD • Laura Ross, MD

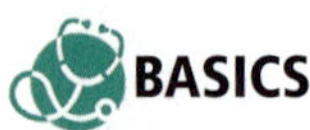

BASICS

DESCRIPTION

- Cystitis is an infection of the lower urinary tract usually resulting from a single gram-negative enteric bacteria (see also Prostatitis, Pyelonephritis, and Urethritis).
- System(s) affected: renal/urologic
- Synonym(s): urinary tract infection (UTI); cystitis
- In otherwise healthy males aged 15 to 50 years, UTI is uncommon and considered uncomplicated.
- In male newborns, infants, and elderly men, UTI is considered complicated, with associated functional/structural mechanisms.

EPIDEMIOLOGY

Incidence

- Predominant age: increases with age
- Uncommon in men <50 years of age; 6 to 8 infections per 10,000 men aged 21 to 50 years (1)

Prevalence

Lifetime prevalence approximately 14%

ETIOLOGY AND PATHOPHYSIOLOGY

- *Escherichia coli* (majority of infections)
- *Klebsiella* spp.
- *Enterobacter*
- *Enterococcus*
- *Proteus*
- *Citrobacter*
- *Providencia*
- *Streptococcus faecalis* and *Staphylococcus* sp.
- *Pseudomonas* and *Morganella* (more common in elderly and catheterized patients)
- Pathogenesis—bacterial entry into urinary tract via ascension or bladder instrumentation

Genetics

Not applicable

RISK FACTORS

- Age
- Obesity
- History of prior UTI
- Outlet obstruction
  - Benign prostatic hypertrophy (BPH)—incidence of 33% of men with UTIs (2)
  - Urethral stricture
  - Calculi
- Fecal incontinence
- Urinary incontinence
- Recent urologic surgery
- Urinary tract instrumentation/catheterization
- Infection of the prostate/kidney
- Immunocompromised
- Diabetes
- Bladder diverticula
- Neurogenic bladder
- Cognitive impairment
- Institutionalization
- Uncircumcised
- Anal intercourse
- Intercourse with an infected female partner (1)

GENERAL PREVENTION

- Prompt treatment of predisposing factors
- Use a catheter only when necessary; if needed, use aseptic technique and closed system and remove as soon as possible.
- Cranberry products are not recommended for preventing UTI.

COMMONLY ASSOCIATED CONDITIONS

- Acute bacterial pyelonephritis
- Chronic bacterial pyelonephritis
- Urethritis
- Prostatitis
- Prostatic hypertrophy
- Prostate cancer

Geriatric Considerations

Bacteriuria is more common among the elderly, usually is transient, and may be related to functional status. Of men >65 years of age, 5–10% have asymptomatic bacteriuria (ASB). If ASB is noted, no treatment is needed (1).

Pediatric Considerations

Can be associated with obstruction to normal flow of urine, such as vesicoureteral reflux. Unique diagnostic criteria and evaluation recommendations exist.

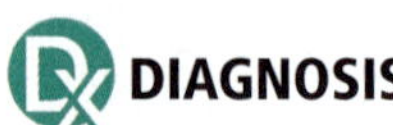

DIAGNOSIS

HISTORY

- Urinary frequency
- Urinary urgency
- Dysuria
- Hesitancy
- Slow urinary stream
- Dribbling of urine
- Nocturia
- Suprapubic discomfort or perineal pain
- Constipation
- Low back pain
- Hematuria
- Systemic symptoms (chills, fever) or flank pain, nausea, vomiting present with concomitant pyelonephritis or prostatitis

PHYSICAL EXAM

- Suprapubic tenderness
- Costovertebral angle (CVA) tenderness and/or fever may be present with concomitant pyelonephritis/prostatitis/epididymitis.
- Perform genital examination.
- Consider digital rectal exam, including palpation of the prostate gland, to rule out bacterial prostatitis.

DIFFERENTIAL DIAGNOSIS

- Anatomic/functional pathology of the urinary tract
- Urethritis/STIs
- Infections in other sites of the genitourinary tract (e.g., epididymis, prostatitis). >90% of men with febrile UTI have concomitant prostate infection (1)[A].

DIAGNOSTIC TESTS & INTERPRETATION

- Urine dipstick/manual microscopy of clean catch midstream void showing the following:
  - Pyuria (>10 WBCs)
  - Bacteriuria
  - Leukocyte esterase is more sensitive, and nitrite is more specific in detecting UTI.
  - Positive leukocyte esterase (in males: sensitivity, 78%; specificity, 59%; positive predictive value [PPV], 71%; negative predictive value [NPV], 67%)
  - Positive nitrite (in males: sensitivity, 47%; specificity, 98%; PPV, 96%; NPV, 59%)

ALERT

All patients presenting with dysuria should be tested for STIs, as gonorrhea, chlamydia, and syphilis are epidemic in the United States.

- Automated microscopy/flow cytometry that measures cell counts and bacterial counts can be used to improve screening characteristics (sensitivity, 92%; specificity, 55%; PPV, 47%; NPV, 97%). The high NPV of these screening tests allows for more judicious use of urine culture.
- Urine culture: >100,000 colony-forming units (CFU; >10^5 CFU) of bacteria per milliliter of urine confirm diagnosis.
- Lower counts, such as >10^3 CFU, also may be indicative of infection, especially in the presence of pyuria.
- Diagnosis in infants and children <24 months old made on the basis of both pyuria and 50,000 CFU on culture
- Renal and bladder ultrasound recommended in infants and young children after first confirmed UTI

Follow-Up Tests & Special Considerations

- Consider assessing for risk factors for STIs because chlamydial/gonococcal urethritis can mimic a UTI. If risk factors are present, use urine nucleic acid amplification tests to identify gonococcal and *Chlamydia* infections and treat as necessary.
- Further urologic evaluation is warranted to rule out other disorders in men with recurrent UTI, febrile UTI, or pyelonephritis. This may include the following:
  - Ultrasound
  - Cystoscopy
  - Urodynamics
  - IV pyelography
- Value of a urologic evaluation in a single uncomplicated UTI has not been determined.
- Antibiotics prior to culture or phenazopyridine prior to urine dipstick can alter results.
- Blood cultures are not routine; perform if concern for sepsis or bacteremia.

Test Interpretation

Depends on site of infection

TREATMENT

- Catheter management: In general, avoid unnecessary catheterization.
- Minimize the use of indwelling catheters. Those who require extended catheterization should be managed by intermittent catheterization, if possible. There is no benefit of using prophylactic antibiotics to reduce the risk of catheter-associated UTIs.
- Exchange the Foley for acute infections when initiating antibiotics.

GENERAL MEASURES

- Hydration
- Analgesia, if required
- Aggressive treatment to prevent constipation with both soluble (psyllium) and insoluble (wheat germ) fiber
- Patient with indwelling catheters
  - If asymptomatic bacterial colonization, no need to treat (Sterilization of urine is not possible, and resistant organisms may take up residence.)
  - If symptomatic of acute infection, institute treatment.

MEDICATION

First Line

- Acute, uncomplicated cystitis
  - Treat empirically; strongly consider if nitrite positive, using local resistance patterns or based on culture and sensitivity results for 5–7 days.
  - For empirical therapy, a fluoroquinolone or trimethoprim-sulfamethoxazole DS usually used to treat the most likely pathogens. Fosfomycin, nitrofurantoin, and beta-lactams do not achieve reliable tissue concentration in the prostate.
- Complicated, febrile, or recurrent infection
  - Prescribe a minimum of 2 weeks antibiotics based on antimicrobial sensitivities with repeat urine check after the treatment. In men with febrile UTI or pyelonephritis, prostatic involvement also must be considered. Total duration of antimicrobial therapy generally ranges from 10 to 14 days. Five- to 7-day regiments of fluoroquinolones are comparable to longer durations. Treatment of concomitant prostatitis requires antimicrobials with good prostatic tissue and fluid penetration (fluoroquinolones).

Second Line

According to culture and sensitivity results and patient's history

ISSUES FOR REFERRAL

Further urologic evaluation and referral are warranted to rule out other disorders in male infants and men with recurrent UTI, febrile UTI, or pyelonephritis.

ADDITIONAL THERAPIES

- Probiotics
- Polyethylene glycol 3350 for constipation
- Phenazopyridine—limit use to 48 hours when used concomitantly with an antibacterial agent.

ADMISSION, INPATIENT, AND NURSING CONSIDERATIONS

- Inability to tolerate oral medications
- Acute renal failure
- Suspected sepsis

ONGOING CARE

FOLLOW-UP RECOMMENDATIONS

Patient Monitoring

Any patients who have worsening symptoms following initiation of antimicrobials, persistent symptoms after 48 to 72 hours of appropriate therapy, or recurrent symptoms within a few weeks of treatment should have additional evaluation.

DIET

Encourage adequate fluid intake.

PATIENT EDUCATION

National Kidney Foundation: https://www.kidney.org

PROGNOSIS

Clearing of infections with appropriate antibiotic treatment

COMPLICATIONS

- Pyelonephritis
- Ascending infection
- Recurrent infection
- Prostatitis

REFERENCES

1. Wagenlehner FME, Weidner W, Pilatz A, et al. Urinary tract infections and bacterial prostatitis in men. *Curr Opin Infect Dis*. 2014;27(1):97–101.
2. Drekonja DM, Rector TS, Cutting A, et al. Urinary tract infection in male veterans: treatment patterns and outcomes. *JAMA Intern Med*. 2013;173(1):62–68.

ADDITIONAL READING

- Coupat C, Pradier C, Degand N, et al. Selective reporting of antibiotic susceptibility data improves the appropriateness of intended antibiotic prescriptions in urinary tract infections: a case-vignette randomised study. *Eur J Clin Microbiol Infect Dis*. 2013;32(5):627–636.
- Foxman B. Urinary tract infection syndromes: occurrence, recurrence, bacteriology, risk factors, and disease burden. *Infect Dis Clin North Am*. 2014;28(1):1–13.

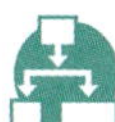

SEE ALSO

- Prostate Cancer; Prostatic Hyperplasia, Benign (BPH); Prostatitis; Pyelonephritis; Urethritis
- Algorithms: Dysuria; Urethral Discharge

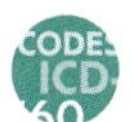

CODES

ICD10

- N39.0 Urinary tract infection, site not specified
- N30.90 Cystitis, unspecified without hematuria
- N30.91 Cystitis, unspecified with hematuria

CLINICAL PEARLS

- Cystitis is an infection of the lower urinary tract, usually resulting from a single gram-negative enteric bacteria.
- Risk factors/causes: age, obesity, history of UTI, BPH/outlet obstruction, incontinence, urinary tract instrumentation or catheterization, infection of the prostate/kidney, immunocompromised or diabetes, cognitive impairment, institutionalization, neurogenic bladder, uncircumcised, anal intercourse, intercourse with infected female partner
- Evaluation: urinalysis, urine culture, STI testing (e.g., gonorrhea, *Chlamydia* by culture/DNA probe)
- Treat empirically with fluoroquinolones or trimethoprim-sulfamethoxazole DS for 5 to 7 days.

UROLITHIASIS

Roland W. Newman II, DO

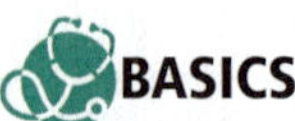

BASICS

DESCRIPTION

- Stone formation within the urinary tract: Urinary crystals bind to form a nidus, which grows to form a calculus (stone).
- Range of symptoms: asymptomatic to obstructive; febrile morbidity if result of infection

EPIDEMIOLOGY

- Vesical calculosis (bladder stones) due to malnutrition during early life is frequent in the Middle East and in Asian countries.
- Incidence in industrialized countries seems to be increasing, probably due to improved diagnostics and increasingly rich diets.
- Increased incidence in patients with surgically induced absorption issues (IBD, gastric bypass)

Incidence

- In industrialized countries: 100 to 200/100,000 per year
- Predominant age: Mean age is 40 to 60 years.
- Predominant sex: male > female (~3:1)

Prevalence

- 10–15% in the United States
- 15% globally (1)
- Lifetime risk of >14% in men, >6% in women
  - Incidence is increasing in female, pediatric, and adolescent populations.
  - Median age of presentation in pediatric cases—boys: 4.4 years of age; girls: 7.3 years of age

ETIOLOGY AND PATHOPHYSIOLOGY

- Supersaturation and dehydration lead to high salt content in urine which congregates.
- Stasis of urine
  - Renal malformation (e.g., horseshoe kidney, ureteropelvic junction obstruction).
  - Incomplete bladder emptying (e.g., neurogenic bladder, prostate enlargement, multiple sclerosis)
- Crystals may form in pure solutions (homogeneous) or on existing surfaces, such as other crystals or cellular debris (heterogeneous).
- Balance of promoters and inhibitors: organic (Tamm-Horsfall protein, glycosaminoglycan, uropontin, nephrocalcin) and inorganic (citrate, pyrophosphate)
- Calcium oxalate and/or phosphate stones (80%)
  - Hypercalciuria
    - Absorptive hypercalciuria: increased jejunal calcium absorption
    - Renal leak: increased calcium excretion from renal proximal tubule
    - Resorptive hypercalciuria: mild hyperparathyroidism
  - Hypercalcemia
    - Hyperparathyroidism
    - Sarcoidosis
    - Malignancy
    - Immobilization
    - Paget disease
- Hyperoxaluria
  - Enteric hyperoxaluria
    - Intestinal malabsorptive state associated with irritable bowel disease, celiac sprue, or intestinal resection
    - Bile salt malabsorption leads to formation of calcium soaps.
  - Primary hyperoxaluria: autosomal recessive, types I and II
  - Dietary hyperoxaluria: overindulgence in oxalate-rich food
- Hyperuricosuria
  - Seen in 10% of calcium stone formers
  - Caused by increased dietary purine intake, systemic acidosis, myeloproliferative diseases, gout, chemotherapy, Lesch-Nyhan syndrome
  - Thiazides, probenecid
- Hypocitraturia
  - Caused by acidosis: renal tubular acidosis, malabsorption, thiazides, enalapril, excessive dietary protein
- Uric acid stones (10–15%): hyperuricemia causes as discussed earlier
- Struvite stones (5–10%): infected urine with urease-producing organisms (most commonly *Proteus* sp.)
- Cystine stones (<1%): autosomal recessive disorder of renal tubular reabsorption of cystine
- Bladder stones: seen with chronic bladder catheterization and some medications (indinavir)
- In children: usually due to malnutrition

Genetics

- Up to 20% of patients have a family history. However, spouses of those who form stones have higher calcium excretion rates than controls, suggesting strong dietary–environmental factors.
- Autosomal dominant: idiopathic hypercalciuria
- Autosomal recessive
  - Cystinuria, Lesch-Nyhan syndrome, hyperoxaluria types I and II
  - Ehlers-Danlos syndrome, Marfan syndrome, Wilson disease, familial renal tubular acidosis

RISK FACTORS

- White > Asian > African American
- Male
- Family history (increases risk by up to 2.5 times)
- Diet rich in protein, refined carbohydrates, and sodium; carbonated drinks; low calcium diet, low fluid intake
- Occupations associated with a sedentary lifestyle or with a hot, dry workplace
- Incidence rates peak during summer secondary to dehydration, hot climates.
- Obesity
- Surgically/medically induced malabsorption (Crohn disease, gastric bypass, celiac, primary hyperparathyroidism)
- Horseshoe kidney (incidence of 21–60%)
- Medications that can increase risk of forming calcium, uric acid stones
- Recent literature suggesting possible association between microbiome (gut and urinary) and urolithiasis

GENERAL PREVENTION

- Hydration (2)
  - Aim for 2.5 to 3.0 L of fluid intake per day (3).
- Diet
  - Decrease salt and meat intake.
  - Avoid oxalate-rich foods.
  - Balanced diet with low animal protein, lower sodium, and normal calcium intake (3)

Pediatric Considerations

- Increasing in prevalence due to obesity, diabetes, hypertension
- Additional risk factor considerations include renal disease or immaturity, preterm birth, and low birth weight.
- Ultrasound should be considered in children before CT imaging to reduce radiation exposure.
- Consider additional work-up to evaluate for metabolic abnormality or hereditary etiology.
- Children with uncomplicated ureteral stones of ≤10 mm can be offered observation with or without medical expulsive therapy (MET) using α-blockers.

Pregnancy Considerations

- Pregnant women have the same incidence of renal colic as do nonpregnant women.
- Most symptomatic stones occur during the 2nd and 3rd trimesters, heralded by symptoms of flank pain/hematuria.
- Most common differential diagnosis is physiologic hydronephrosis of pregnancy. Use ultrasound to avoid irradiation. Noncontrast-enhanced CT scan also is diagnostic.
- 30% require intervention, such as stent placement.
- Pregnant women who have ureteral stones with symptoms that are generally well controlled should be offered observation as first-line therapy.

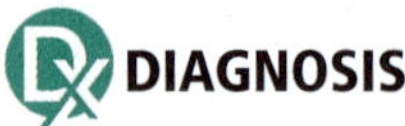

DIAGNOSIS

HISTORY

- Pain
  - Renal colic: acute onset of severe groin and/or flank pain
  - Distal stones may present with referred pain in labia, penile meatus, or testis.
- Microscopic/gross hematuria occurs in 95% of patients.
- Nausea, vomiting, tachycardia, diaphoresis, low-grade fever
- Frequency and dysuria occur with stones at the vesicoureteric junction (VUJ).

PHYSICAL EXAM

Tender costovertebral angle with palpation/percussion and/or iliac fossa

DIFFERENTIAL DIAGNOSIS

- Appendicitis
- Ruptured aortic aneurysm
- Musculoskeletal strain
- Pyelonephritis (upper UTI)
- Pyonephrosis (obstructed upper UTI; emergency)
- Perinephric abscess
- Pelvic or ovarian pathology: ectopic pregnancy, cyst, torsion
- Salpingitis
- Myocardial infarction
- Additional GI pathology: biliary colic, diverticulitis, obstruction, incarcerated hernia

DIAGNOSTIC TESTS & INTERPRETATION

- Urinalysis for RBCs, leukocytes, nitrates, pH (acidic urine <5.5 is associated with uric acid stones; alkaline >7 with struvite stones), send for culture and sensitivity
- Blood: urea, creatinine, electrolytes, calcium, and urate; consider CBC.
- Parathyroid hormone only if calcium is elevated
- Stone analysis if/when stone passed

Initial Tests (lab, imaging)

- Noncontrast-enhanced helical CT scan of the abdomen and pelvis has replaced IV pyelogram.
  - Stone is found most commonly at levels of ureteric luminal narrowing: pelviureteric junction, pelvic brim, and VUJ.
  - Acute obstruction: Proximal ureter and renal pelvis are dilated to the level of obstruction, and perinephric stranding is possible on imaging.
- Renal ultrasound may be as effective with lower radiation at diagnosis as well as identifying obstruction.
- X-ray of kidneys, ureter, and bladder to determine if stone is radiopaque or lucent
  - Calcium oxalate/phosphate stones are radiopaque.
  - Uric acid stones are radiolucent.
  - Staghorn calculi (that fill the shape of the renal calyces) are usually struvite and opaque.
  - Cystine stones are faintly opaque (ground-glass appearance).
- Ultrasound has low sensitivity and specificity but is often the first choice for pregnant women and children.

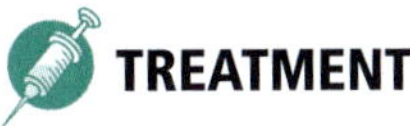

TREATMENT

GENERAL MEASURES

- 75% of patients are successfully treated conservatively and pass the stone spontaneously.
- Most stones <5 mm will pass spontaneously with conservative treatment.
- Stones between 5 to 10 mm may pass with MET.
- Stones >10 mm generally require surgical intervention.
- 30–50% of patients will have recurrent stones within 5 to 10 years.

MEDICATION

- MET: α_1-Antagonists (e.g., tamsulosin) may improve likelihood of spontaneous stone passage.
- Passage of larger stones (i.e., 5 to 10 mm) increased with tamsulosin
- Category C in pregnancy
- Pain control with NSAIDs (anti-inflammatory effect decreases smooth muscle stimulation and spasms)

ISSUES FOR REFERRAL

- Urgent referral of patients with UTI, sepsis, acute renal failure, anuria
- Early referral of pregnant patients, children, adults >60 years of age, large stones (>8 mm), bilateral obstruction, solitary kidney, chronic renal failure, transplanted kidney

ADDITIONAL THERAPIES

- Uric acid stone dissolution therapy
  - Alkalinize urine with potassium citrate; keep pH >6.5.
  - Allopurinol 100 to 300 mg/day PO (for those who continue to form stones despite alkalinization of urine)
- Cystine stone dissolution/prevention
  - Alkalinize urine with potassium citrate; keep pH >6.5.
  - Chelating agents: captopril, α-mercaptopropionylglycine, D-penicillamine
- Consider altering medications that increase risk of stone formation: probenecid, loop diuretics, salicylic acid, salbutamol, indinavir, triamterene, and acetazolamide.
- Vitamin D supplementation does *not* induce stone formation; with calcium supplementation ≤1,200 mg/day (or as antacid) with vitamin D supplementation does not increase the risk of stone formation and may lower risk.
- Treat hypercalciuria with thiazides on an acute basis only.
- Treat hypocitraturia with potassium citrate and high-citrate juices (e.g., orange, lemon).
- Treat enteric hyperoxaluria with oral calcium/magnesium, cholestyramine, and potassium citrate.

SURGERY/OTHER PROCEDURES

- Immediate relief of obstruction is required for patients with the following conditions:
  - Sepsis, renal failure (obstructed solitary kidney, bilateral obstruction), uncontrolled pain, despite adequate analgesia
- Emergency surgery for obstruction
  - Placement of a retrograde stent (i.e., endoscopic surgery, usually requires an anesthetic)
  - Radiologic placement of a percutaneous nephrostomy tube
- Elective surgery for stone treatment
  - Extracorporeal shock wave lithotripsy
  - Ureteroscopy with basket extraction/lithotripsy (laser/pneumatic)
  - Percutaneous nephrolithotomy
    - First choice for stones >2 cm
- Open surgery is uncommon.

ADMISSION, INPATIENT, AND NURSING CONSIDERATIONS

Analgesia

- Combination of NSAIDs (ketorolac 30 to 60 mg) and oral opiate
- Parenteral opioid if vomiting or if preceding fails to control pain (morphine 5 to 10 mg IV or IM q4h)
- Antiemetic if required or prophylactically with parenteral narcotics

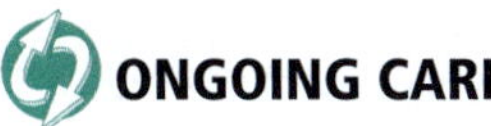

ONGOING CARE

FOLLOW-UP RECOMMENDATIONS

- Patients being treated conservatively should be followed until imaging is clear or stone is visibly passed.
  - Strain urine and send stone for composition.
  - Tamsulosin and nifedipine (MET) in selected patients to speed passage
  - If pain management is suboptimal or stone does not progress or pass within 4 to 6 weeks, patient should be referred to a urologist.
- Patients with recurrent stone formation should have metabolic workup: 24-hour urine for volume, pH, creatinine, calcium, cystine, phosphate, oxalate, uric acid, and magnesium.
  - PTH if serum calcium is found elevated
  - Ultrasonography to evaluate for renal anomaly if indicated

DIET

ALERT

- Increased fluid intake for life cannot be overemphasized for decreasing recurrence. Encourage intake of 2 to 3 L/day; advise patient to have clear urine rather than yellow.
- Decrease or eliminate carbonated drinks.
- Patients who form calcium stones should minimize high-oxalate foods such as green leafy vegetables, rhubarb, peanuts, chocolates, and beer.
- Decrease protein and salt intake.
- Lowering calcium intake is inadvisable and may even increase urine calcium excretion.
- Increase phytate-rich foods (natural dietary bran, legumes and beans, whole cereal)
- Avoid excessive vitamin C.

PATIENT EDUCATION

- Multiple dietary factors play a role in stone formation: hydration, carbohydrate, protein, and calcium, sodium chloride, and oxalate intake
- Reducing dietary intake of calcium oxalate is effective in correcting risk factors for stone formation (4).

PROGNOSIS

- Spontaneous stone passage depends on stone location (proximal vs. distal) and stone size (<5 mm, 90% pass; >8 mm, 10% pass).
- Stone recurrence: 50% of patients at 10 years

U

REFERENCES

1. Anan G, Kikuchi D, Hirose T, et al. Impact of sodium-glucose cotransporter-2 inhibitors on urolithiasis. *Kidney Int Rep*. 2023;8(4):925–928. doi:10.1016/j.ekir.2023.01.034.
2. Bao Y, Tu X, Wei Q. Water for preventing urinary stones. *Cochrane Database Syst Rev*. 2020;2(2):CD004292.
3. Kiremit MC, Boyuk A, Petkova K. Fluid intake recommendations in urolithiasis and general advice to patients without metabolic risk factors. *World J Urol*. 2023;41:1251–1259. doi:10.1007/s00345-023-04285-3.
4. Siener R. Nutrition and kidney stone disease. *Nutrients*. 2021;13(6):1917. doi:10.3390/nu13061917.

SEE ALSO

Algorithms: Dysuria; Renal Calculi; Urethral Discharge

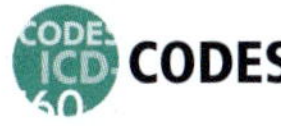

CODES

ICD10

- N20.9 Urinary calculus, unspecified
- N20.0 Calculus of kidney
- N20.1 Calculus of ureter

CLINICAL PEARLS

- MET may improve likelihood of spontaneous stone passage
- SGLT-2 inhibitors are less likely to contribute to urolithiasis compared to other antidiabetic agents (1).
- Patients with calcium stones should minimize high oxalate foods (rhubarb, peanuts, chocolate, beer). Lowering calcium intake may increase calcium excretion.

URTICARIA

Dori Goldberg, MD • Yuying Zhang, BS

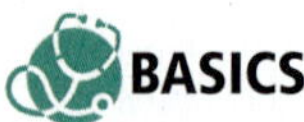

BASICS

DESCRIPTION

- Urticaria: an inflammatory skin disorder characterized by hives with or without angioedema
- Urticaria can be classified as acute or chronic.
  - Acute: recurring lesions that persist for <6 weeks
  - Chronic: recurring lesions that persist for >6 weeks
- The causes of urticaria vary; acute urticaria is often self-limited and trigger may not be identifiable. In chronic urticaria, further allergen testing may be warranted.
- Presentation: a cutaneous lesion or lesions involving edema of the epidermis and/or dermis presenting with rapid onset and pruritus; individual lesions will change over minutes to hours with no individual lesions persisting >24 hours without change
- Etiology of urticaria is either spontaneous or induced.
- System(s) affected: integumentary
- Synonym(s): hives; wheals

EPIDEMIOLOGY

Urticaria may be spontaneous or induced.

Incidence

- The peak onset happens around 20 to 40 years of age, and affects women more frequently than men. However, urticaria can also affect children, adult, and geriatric population to similar extent.
- Chronic urticaria is also associated with autoimmune disorders and prevalence increase with variety of chronic infections.
- In 20% of patients, chronic urticaria lasts >10 years.

Prevalence

- It is a common disorder that occurs in 15–25% of individuals some point in their lives.
- Up to 36% of patients with acute urticaria can progress to CSU.
- The prevalence of CSU is about 0.12–0.30% for adult and children

ETIOLOGY AND PATHOPHYSIOLOGY

- Core mechanism
  - Mast-cell activation (IgE-dependent, autoimmune IgG binding to IgE docking site, or non-IgE "pseudoallergic" triggers) → rapid degranulation of histamine, leukotrienes, cytokines, proteases
  - Mediator release in superficial dermis → transient wheals; in deep dermis/subcutis → angioedema
- Trigger categories
  - Acute spontaneous urticaria (ASU)
    - Viral and bacterial infections
    - IgE mediated food allergy (peanuts, seafood, eggs, etc.); pseudoallergenic foods such as strawberries, tomatoes, preservatives, and coloring agents contain histamine.
    - Drugs: IgE-mediated (e.g., penicillin and other antibiotics), direct mast cell stimulation (e.g., aspirin, NSAIDs, opiates)
    - Others: inhalant, contact, ingestion, or occupational exposure (e.g., latex, cosmetics)
    - Transfusion reaction
  - Chronic spontaneous urticaria (CSU)
    - Autoimmune thyroid disease, other auto-antibodies
    - Indolent infections (*Helicobacter pylori*, parasites)
    - Chronic meds (NSAIDs, ACE-I, hormones)
    - Hormonal shifts (pregnancy, progesterone)
    - Collagen-vascular disease, malignancy
  - Chronic inducible urticaria (CIU)
  - Physical stimuli
    - Dermographism (most common)
    - Cold, heat, solar/UV, delayed pressure, vibration
    - Cholinergic (exercise, emotion, hot bath)
    - Contact (latex, chemicals)
    - Aquagenic (water)

Genetics

No consistent pattern known: Chronic urticaria displays an autoimmune-like genetic signature with HLA-B44 and vitamin D receptor variants being susceptible markers.

RISK FACTORS

Chronic urticaria

- Female sex
- Obesity with BMI ≥30 kg/m^2
- Autoimmune thyroid disease
- NSAIDs sensitivity
- Psychological stress
- *H. pylori*

GENERAL PREVENTION

Avoidance of known triggers is the mainstay of prevention.

COMMONLY ASSOCIATED CONDITIONS

- Autoimmune thyroid disease
- Atopic dermatitis/allergic rhinitis
- Anxiety and depression
- Angioedema (common)
- Anaphylaxis (somewhat common)

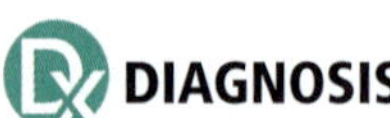

DIAGNOSIS

The diagnosis of urticaria is based primarily on a thorough clinical history and physical exam; however, diagnostic tests may be helpful in some instances (1).

HISTORY

- It is important to assess for the following:
  - Timeline—When did hives start? How often? Do individual spots clear within 24 hours and itch?
  - Lesion appearance/morphology—Note size, shape, body sites involved.
  - Triggers—Ask about heat/cold, pressure, exercise, foods, insect stings, new drugs (especially NSAIDs), recent infections.
  - Background—Family history of hives/allergy and what treatments the patient has tried
- Red flag: Painful welts that last > 48 hours and leave bruising suggest urticarial vasculitis, not ordinary urticaria

ALERT

Important to rule out underlying anaphylaxis in those patients presenting with acute onset of urticaria. Presentation for anaphylaxis include hypotension, respiratory distress, tachycardia, GI symptoms including nausea, vomiting, and diarrhea may occur.

PHYSICAL EXAM

- Typical hives: well-circumscribed, erythematous round, oval, or polymorphic indurated plaques, variable in size, with central pallor and surrounding erythema
- Blanchable with pressure
- Dermographism: linear wheal after stroking skin with tongue depressor; appear within 10 minutes
- Angioedema: painful, non-pitting swelling of lips, eyelids, extremities, may last 24 to 72 hours.
- Evaluate for underlying conditions including thyroid abnormalities (nodules), bacterial, viral, or fungal infection (e.g., fever).

DIFFERENTIAL DIAGNOSIS

- Urticarial vasculitis
- Anaphylaxis (may present with urticaria)
- Morbilliform or fixed drug eruptions
- Erythema multiforme
- Systemic lupus erythematosus (SLE), vasculitis, and polyarteritis
- Angioedema without urticaria
- Urticaria pigmentosa/systemic mastocytosis
- Bullous pemphigoid (urticarial stage)
- Arthropod bite
- Atopic/contact dermatitis
- Viral exanthem

DIAGNOSTIC TESTS & INTERPRETATION

- Diagnosis is usually clinical.
- Skin prick tests and serum-specific IgE tests can help confirm diagnosis of acute urticaria due to type 1 mediated reaction.
- Other laboratory studies that may help identify specific underlying disease include CBC, ESR, C-CRP, and thyroid studies. Skin biopsy may be warranted (1).

Initial Tests (lab, imaging)

- Acute: generally not indicated
- Chronic: directed by clinical suspicion of underlying cause
  - Allergy skin tests and radioallergosorbent test (RAST) for inhaled allergens, insects, drugs, or foods
  - Infection: Consider pharyngeal culture, LFTs, mononucleosis test, urinalysis in appropriate setting.

Follow-Up Tests & Special Considerations

Chronic urticaria (CIU/CSU): Extensive lab testing is not indicated and has not proven to improve outcome nor is it cost-effective. Limit lab testing according to clinical history and indication. Skin or IgE testing should be limited to specific history of provoking allergen (1).

- Baseline (every chronic case)—CBC, ESR/CRP
- Routine add-ons—TSH ± anti-TPO, LFTs, urinalysis

- Targeted tests (only if history suggests)
  - Allergy: skin-prick/specific-IgE
  - Autoimmune/vasculitis: ANA, RF, C3/C4/CH50, cryoglobulins
  - Infection: *H. pylori* screen, stool ova and parasite (O&P)
- Specialized
  - Autologous serum skin test (autoimmune CSU)
  - Serum protein electrophoresis (SPEP)/immunofixation electrophoresis (IFE) when malignancy is a concern

Diagnostic Procedures/Other

- Food and drug reactions: elimination of (or challenges with) suspected agents
- Physical-trigger challenge tests
  - Dermographism: light stroke → wheal within minutes
  - Cold urticaria: ice cube 5 minutes, watch 10 to 15 minutes for wheal
  - Cholinergic: exercise or 42°C bath 10 minutes → pinpoint wheals
  - Solar: controlled exposure to specific light wavelengths
  - Delayed pressure: 2 to 3 kg weight 20 minutes on skin, inspect ~6 hours later
  - Aquagenic: Apply water of differing temperatures to skin.
  - Vibratory: 4 to 5 minutes localized vibration, then observe
- Skin biopsy
  - Reserve for lesions persisting > 24 hours or when vasculitis is suspected (1).

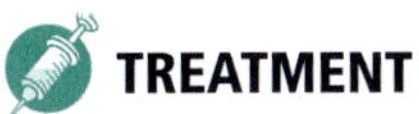

TREATMENT

GENERAL MEASURES

The mainstay of therapy for urticaria is to avoid identifiable triggers.

MEDICATION

First Line

- First-line management include avoidance of trigger and lifestyle management. Medication includes starting with 2nd-generation antihistamine (H_1) blockers for any urticaria in which avoidance of stimulus is impossible or not feasible. If needed, increase dose of 2nd-generation H_1 blockers up to 4-fold usual dose (2). Standard starting doses:
  - Fexofenadine (Allegra): 120 mg/day
  - Loratadine (Claritin): 10 mg/day 5 to 10 mL/day for pediatric formula
  - Desloratadine (Clarinex): 5 mg/day; children formula includes 2.5 to 5.0 mL
  - Cetirizine (Zyrtec): 10 to 20 mg/day; in pediatrics, 5 to 10 mL daily children formula
  - Rupatadine: novel H_1 antagonist with antiplatelet-activating factor activity; recommend 10 mg/day
- Acute urticaria with unknown triggers usually treated with antihistamines at standard or highest doses. The use of corticosteroids is commonly paired with antihistamine; however current published studies does not have strong support of the protective impact of steroids use in combination with antihistamine on the development of chronic urticaria (3).

Second Line

- If first-line treatment after doubling dosage is inadequate after 2 to 4 weeks, adding another 2nd-generation H_1 blocker can be considered. Also:
  - Omalizumab 300 mg SC q4wk, if needed increase to 600 mg SC q2wk (2)
  - H_2-specific antihistamines (beneficial as adjuvants): cimetidine, ranitidine, nizatidine, famotidine
  - 1st-generation antihistamines (H_1; for patients with sleep disturbed by itching):
    - Older children and adults: hydroxyzine or diphenhydramine 25 to 50 mg q6h
    - Children <6 years of age: diphenhydramine 12.5 mg q6–8h (5 mg/kg/day) or hydroxyzine (10 mg/5 mL) 2 mg/kg/day divided q6–8h
- If continue to show no improvement after 6 months, consider adding another 2nd-generation antihistamine, or cyclosporine 1.5 to 5.0 mg/kg/day (1).

Geriatric Considerations

1st-generation H_1 blockers may cause excessive drowsiness as well as dry mouth and eyes.

ISSUES FOR REFERRAL

Referral to an allergist, immunologist, or dermatologist for recalcitrant cases, especially if lesions fail to respond to first-line treatment and/or severe presentation of urticaria presents including angioedema and atypical features including fever, arthritis, anaphylaxis, etc.

ADDITIONAL THERAPIES

- Anti-IgE mAb-ligelizumab 72 mg q4wk showed to achieve complete hive control in 51% versus 26% with omalizumab at week 12
- Other off label drugs such as include dupilumab, remibrutinib, and benralizumab also showed potential for treatment of refractory and resistant chronic urticaria.

ADMISSION, INPATIENT, AND NURSING CONSIDERATIONS

Educating patient on use of EpiPen as pathophysiology is similar to anaphylaxis; if the airway is threatened, immediate consultation to evaluate for laryngeal edema and need for definitive airway management

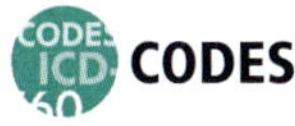

ONGOING CARE

FOLLOW-UP RECOMMENDATIONS

Follow-up is recommended within 6 weeks as nearly 1/3 of acute patient develop chronic urticaria.

Patient Monitoring

- Use the urticaria activity score (UAS7) for assessing CSU.
- Recently developed tool to assess disease control in patients with chronic urticaria (spontaneous and inducible) is the urticaria control test (UCT). If UCT score ≥12, disease is considered controlled.
- If patient is started on omalizumab or ligelizumab; monitor for anaphylaxis 2 hours post-first dose.

PROGNOSIS

- Resolution of acute symptoms: 70% <72 hours
- Chronic urticaria: 35% symptom-free in a year; another 30% will see symptom reduction.
- 50% of chronic urticaria remits within 5 years, but flares are unpredictable.
- Vaccination and infections can transiently worsen hives, preempt with antihistamines.

REFERENCES

1. Ben-Shoshan M, Kanani A, Kalicinsky C, et al. Urticaria. *Allergy Asthma Clin Immunol*. 2024;20(Suppl 3):64. doi:10.1186/s13223-024-00931-6.
2. McSweeney SM, Christou EAA, Maurer M, et al. Physical urticaria: clinical features, pathogenesis, diagnostic work-up, and management. *J Am Acad Dermatol*. 2023;89(2):324–337. doi:10.1016/j.jaad.2023.02.062.
3. Badloe FMS, Grosber M, Ring J, et al. Treatment of acute urticaria: a systematic review. *J Eur Acad Dermatol Venereol*. 2024;38(11):2082–2092. doi:10.1111/jdv.19904.

ADDITIONAL READING

- Dressler C, Werner RN, Eisert L, et al. Chronic inducible urticaria: a systematic review of treatment options. *J Allergy Clin Immunol*. 2018;141(5):1726–1734. doi:10.1016/j.jaci.2018.01.031.
- Konstantinou GN, Podder I, Dhabal A. Is there a role of genetics in acute and chronic urticaria—a systematic review and meta-analysis. *Clin Transl Allergy*. 2025;15(7):e70072. doi:10.1002/clt2.70072.
- Powell RJ, Leech SC, Till S, et al. BSACI guideline for the management of chronic urticaria and angioedema. *Clin Exp Allergy*. 2015;45(3):547–565.

CODES

ICD10

- L50.9 Urticaria, unspecified
- L50.1 Idiopathic urticaria
- L50.8 Other urticaria

CLINICAL PEARLS

- Rapid onset, individual lesions resolve within 24 hours, multiple crops of lesions can occur in stages.
- Mainstay of therapy is to avoid identified triggers.
- Antihistamines best studied and most efficacious therapy but may require higher-than-normal doses for efficacy.
- If individual lesions last >24 hours, patient should be evaluated for urticarial vasculitis and other more serious diagnoses.

UTERINE AND PELVIC ORGAN PROLAPSE

Electra Korn, MD • Deepali Maheshwari, DO, MPH

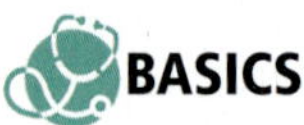

BASICS

DESCRIPTION

- Symptomatic descent of ≥1 of the following:
  - The anterior vaginal wall (known as a cystocele)
  - The posterior vaginal wall (known as a rectocele)
  - The vaginal apex (the uterus and cervix, or cuff scar after total hysterectomy)
- Prolapse above or to the level of the hymen are generally not symptomatic.
- Associated symptoms
  - Feeling of pelvic pressure or heaviness
  - Vaginal bulge
  - Difficulty with voiding or defecation
  - Discomfort with intercourse
- Cost associated with treatment is >$1 billion annually (~200,000 surgeries per year)

EPIDEMIOLOGY

Incidence

- The incidence of pelvic organ prolapse (POP) ranges from 1.5 to 1.8 per 1,000 woman-years.
  - Peaks in women aged 60 to 69 years
- In the United States, there are approximately 300,000 surgeries for POP each year.
- A woman's lifetime risk of undergoing surgery for pelvic floor prolapse ranges from 6% to 18%.

Prevalence

- The prevalence varies when defined by patient symptoms alone (2.9–8.0%) or by exam findings (41.1%).
- It is estimated that 50% of women will develop prolapse, but only 10–20% of those will seek care for their condition.

ETIOLOGY AND PATHOPHYSIOLOGY

- Pelvic organs are supported by attachments between pelvic floor muscles, connective tissue, and the bony pelvis. Defects in this support can lead to prolapse in one or multiple compartments.
- Symptomatic women frequently have defects in >1 compartment, as well as damage to the levator ani muscle complex (a critical component of utero-vaginal support) and its attachments to the pelvis.
- Gradual process that often begins long before symptoms develop

RISK FACTORS

- Vaginal childbirth: Each additional vaginal birth increases risk.
- Increasing age
- Family history
- Obesity (BMI >30 kg/m^2)
- Chronic straining (constipation, chronic cough from pulmonary disease, repeated heavy lifting)
- Connective tissue disorders (1)

GENERAL PREVENTION

- There is some evidence that pelvic floor muscle training ("Kegel exercises") may decrease the risk of symptomatic POP.
- Weight loss and proper management of conditions that cause increase in intra-abdominal pressure such as constipation may help prevent prolapse.

COMMONLY ASSOCIATED CONDITIONS

- Constipation
- Fecal incontinence
- Urinary incontinence or retention
- Other urinary symptoms, such as hesitancy, urgency, or frequency

DIAGNOSIS

Less than half of women discuss symptoms with PCP. Only 10–12% seek medical attention. Barriers include embarrassment, social stigma, ability to cope, belief that POP is part of the aging process, belief that treatment options are limited, and fear of surgery.

HISTORY

- Common symptoms include the following:
  - Feeling a bulge in vagina
  - Something "falling out" of vagina
  - Pelvic pressure with activity or prolonged standing
  - Difficulty with voiding or defecation
  - Splinting the bulge to evacuate
  - Urinary or fecal urgency
  - Urinary frequency
  - Urinary or fecal incontinence
  - Constipation
- Document the presence, duration, and severity of coexisting urinary or bowel symptom.
- Assess impact on sexual function and quality of life.
- Assess past medical and surgical history:
  - Gravidity and parity/obstetric history
  - Chronic constipation
  - Pulmonary disease
  - Prior pelvic procedures

PHYSICAL EXAM

- Abdominal examination to document any distention or masses
- Complete pelvic and rectal examination
  - Patient can be evaluated in supine position.
  - If prolapse is not well demonstrated, have patient cough or strain in an upright (standing) position to assess maximum descent.
- The standard to measure prolapse is the validated Pelvic Organ Prolapse Quantification (POP-Q) scale.
  - Describes prolapse of each compartment in relationship to the vaginal hymen
  - Patient is supine with the head of the bed at 45 degrees, performing Valsalva maneuver.
    - Stage 1: prolapse in which the distal point is ≥1 cm above hymen
    - Stage 2: prolapse in which the distal point is between 1 cm above and 1 cm below hymen
    - Stage 3: prolapse in which the distal point is >1 cm below the hymen, but <2 cm the total vaginal length
    - Stage 4: complete vaginal vault eversion ("procidentia"); entire vaginal mucosa everted
- A split speculum should be used to observe apical, anterior, and posterior compartments successively.

DIFFERENTIAL DIAGNOSIS

- Rectal prolapse
- Hemorrhoids
- Bartholin cyst
- Vaginal cyst
- Urethral diverticulum
- Cervical elongation

DIAGNOSTIC TESTS & INTERPRETATION

Initial Tests (lab, imaging)

Postvoid residual to evaluate bladder emptying

Follow-Up Tests & Special Considerations

- Consider urodynamic testing if results would alter treatment plan (e.g., if evaluating concurrent urinary retention or voiding dysfunction, or if evaluating for occult stress urinary incontinence).
- Selective use of upper urinary tract imaging if observation is planned or if evidence of obstruction (e.g., abnormal postvoid residual).
- If fecal incontinence or significant change in bowel habits, selective use of lower GI tract imaging or endoscopy
- Consider defecography for patients with bowel symptoms/defecatory dysfunction.

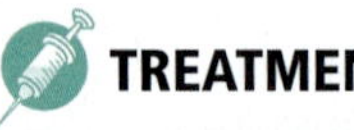

TREATMENT

GENERAL MEASURES

- Treatment is generally guided by degree of bother for the patient. It is important to document the patient's desire, goals, and expectations (2).
- Treatment should consider type and severity of symptoms, patient's age, other comorbid conditions, prior surgical history, sexual function, desire for future fertility, and risk of recurrence.

- Treatment for asymptomatic patients:
  - Stage 1 or 2: clinical observation
  - Stage 3 or 4: regular follow-up and evaluation (every 3 to 6 months)
- Expectant management is an acceptable option for patients without evidence of urinary or bowel obstruction.
- Treatment is indicated when there is urinary/bowel obstruction or hydronephrosis regardless of the degree of prolapse.
- A vaginal pessary should be considered in all women presenting with symptomatic prolapse.
  - There are >13 types of pessaries.
  - The most commonly used pessaries are the ring pessary and Gellhorn.
  - Most women can be successfully fitted with a pessary.
  - Satisfaction rate for patients using pessaries is very high.
  - Minor complications such as vaginal discharge and odor can often be treated with vaginal estrogen.
  - Vaginal erosion is rare and can be treated by removal of pessary and optional vaginal estrogen supplementation.
  - Complications such as erosions, abrasions, ulcerations, vaginal bleeding, and fistulas may be seen with neglected pessaries.

MEDICATION

- There are no data to support the use of vaginal estrogen or other medications for the prevention or treatment of POP.
- Constipation should be managed with an appropriate bowel regimen that includes daily fiber supplementation.

ISSUES FOR REFERRAL

Referral is indicated when pessary or surgery is necessary or desired by the patient.

ADDITIONAL THERAPIES

Pelvic floor muscle training may reduce the symptoms of POP but does not affect the degree of prolapse.

SURGERY/OTHER PROCEDURES

- Reconstructive procedures are performed with the goal of restoration of vaginal anatomy and resolution of symptoms.
- Surgical repair should focus on repairing all affected compartments in a single procedure.
- For anterior and posterior vaginal wall repairs, a native tissue only approach is most frequently offered, due to FDA warnings regarding vaginal mesh.
- For apical repairs:
  - Concomitant hysterectomy is generally performed with apical repair.
    - Uterine preservation via hysteropexy is also an option, with research ongoing regarding the risks and benefits of this approach.
  - Native tissue repairs, such as uterosacral ligament suspension and sacrospinous ligament fixation, offer a vaginal approach.
  - Sacral colpopexy, which can be performed via abdominal, laparoscopic, or robotic approaches, uses surgical mesh and has higher success rates and overall durability.
    - The risk of recurrent prolapse is considered lower with sacral colpopexy than vaginal approaches; there may be an elevated risk of complications.
- Reconstructive surgery using native tissue is associated with an increased rate of failure (one in three lifetime risk of repeat surgery) as compared to procedures using surgical mesh.
- Coexisting stress incontinence should be addressed at the same time as the prolapse repair.

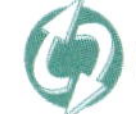

ONGOING CARE

FOLLOW-UP RECOMMENDATIONS

Patient Monitoring

- Patients who choose a pessary for management should be seen regularly.
- There is no standard of care established for follow-up but commonly:
  - Within 7 to 14 days of initial fitting and then at 3 to 12 month intervals depending on patient's independence with the pessary, proficiency with placement and removal and cognitive and motor abilities.
  - Pessary should be removed regularly and cleaned with soap and water, at least every 3 to 6 months.
- Patients who undergo prolapse surgery should be evaluated postoperatively and follow-up intervals vary by provider.

PATIENT EDUCATION

- Patients should have POP explained to them with diagrams and descriptions of their anatomy.
- It is important to emphasize that surgery is geared toward improving quality of life.
- Patients should be educated about potential pessary complications.
- Patients should be informed about possible symptoms of POP if they are still asymptomatic.
- Using fiber supplementation may help patients with bowel complaints such as constipation.

COMPLICATIONS

- Recurrence rates after surgery are variable and quoted between 3.4% and 29.2%.
- There is a risk of dyspareunia and pelvic pain after any surgical repair.
- Repairs using mesh may also be complicated by mesh erosion.
- Potential complications of pessary use include vaginal erosion and fistula in patients that are lost to follow-up.
- Severe prolapse can lead to urinary retention and defecatory dysfunction that may go unrecognized in the elderly.

REFERENCES

1. Schulten SFM, Claas-Quax MJ, Weemhoff M, et al. Risk factors for primary pelvic organ prolapse and prolapse recurrence: an updated systematic review and meta-analysis. *Am J Obstet Gynecol*. 2022;227(2):192–208.
2. Raju R, Linder BJ. Evaluation and management of pelvic organ prolapse. *Mayo Clin Proc*. 2021;96(12):3122–3129.

ADDITIONAL READING

- Baessler K, Christmann-Schmid C, Maher C, et al. Surgery for women with pelvic organ prolapse with or without stress urinary incontinence. *Cochrane Database Syst Rev*. 2018;8(8):CD013108.
- Larouche M, Belzile E, Geoffrion R. Surgical management of symptomatic apical pelvic organ prolapse: a systematic review and meta-analysis. *Obstet Gynecol*. 2021;137(6):1061–1073.

U

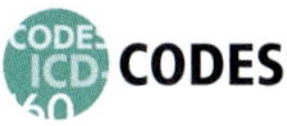

CODES

ICD10

- N81.9 Female genital prolapse, unspecified
- N81.10 Cystocele, unspecified
- N99.3 Prolapse of vaginal vault after hysterectomy

CLINICAL PEARLS

- Many women do not bring up POP with their doctor—providers should ask routinely.
- Vaginal pessary is a nonsurgical treatment option in any patients with symptomatic prolapse.
- Treatment should be guided by degree of bother and impact on patient's quality of life.

UTERINE MYOMAS

Rashmi Rode, MD, FAAFP • Sally Khoury, MD

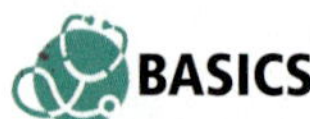

BASICS

DESCRIPTION

- Uterine fibroids are benign monoclonal, pseudoencapsulated, hormone-dependent neoplasms of the myometrium, representing the most common tumors in women worldwide.
- Depending on the location of tumor, four variants of uterine fibroids are identified:
  - Submucous uterine leiomyoma—~5% of all cases; internal, evoking abnormal uterine bleeding and infection; occasionally protruding from cervix
  - Intramural leiomyoma—common; within myometrium; may cause marked uterine enlargement
  - Subserous leiomyoma—common; external; may become pedunculated
  - Unspecified leiomyoma (code used for primary gynecological examination)
  - Rare locations: cervix, broad, round, and uterosacral ligaments
- System affected: reproductive
- Synonym(s): fibroids; myoma; fibromyoma; myofibroma; leiomyoma

EPIDEMIOLOGY

Uterine fibroids are extremely prevalent, particularly among women of reproductive age. The cumulative incidence by age 50 years approaches 70–80%, depending on racial and ethnic background (1).

Incidence

Ranged widely (217 to 3,745 cases per 100,000 women-years); highest among non-Hispanic Black women and women aged ≥40 years (1).

Prevalence

Ranging from 4.5% to 68.6% (1)

- African American women: 60% by age 35 years; up to 80% by age 50 years.
- White women: 40% by age 35 years; up to 70% by age 50 years.
- Fibroids are rarely seen before puberty and tend to regress after menopause unless influenced by exogenous hormone therapy.

ETIOLOGY AND PATHOPHYSIOLOGY

- Fibroids arise through a multistep, multifactorial process involving genetic, hormonal, and environmental influences. They represent monoclonal tumors, meaning each arises from a single transformed smooth muscle cell.
- Hormonal influences:
  - Estrogen and progesterone both play significant roles in fibroid growth (2).
  - Myomas express more estrogen and progesterone receptors than adjacent normal myometrium.
  - Estrogen promotes cellular proliferation and matrix production.
  - Progesterone promotes fibroid growth through upregulation of growth factors and inhibition of apoptosis.
- Growth factors:
  - Transforming growth factor beta (TGF-β), basic fibroblast growth factor (bFGF), platelet-derived growth factor (PDGF), epidermal growth factor (EGF), and insulin-like growth factor (IGF) contribute to proliferation and extracellular matrix accumulation (2).
  - Vascular endothelial growth factor (VEGF) promotes angiogenesis.

Genetics

- Somatic chromosomal rearrangements are seen in 40% of fibroids.
- MED12 gene mutations are present in ~70% of fibroids, particularly in women of African descent (2).
- Higher levels of aromatase in fibroid tissue contribute to increased local estrogen production.

RISK FACTORS

- Race: African American women are 3 times more likely to develop fibroids than Caucasian women; fibroids are more numerous, larger, and symptomatic (2).
- Early menarche (<10 years of age)
- Nulliparity: inverse relationship with fibroid risk
- Oral contraceptive use before 16 years old, protective if used past adolescence
- Obesity: risk increases by 21% for every 10 kg of excess weight
- Hypertension: associated with earlier onset and increased risk
- Family history: 2.5-fold increased risk with affected first-degree relatives
- Vitamin D deficiency
- Alcohol consumption

GENERAL PREVENTION

Protective factors

- Use of progesterone-only contraception
- Parity
- Diets rich in citrus fruits, green vegetables, fish, and low-fat dairy; limited intake of red meat

COMMONLY ASSOCIATED CONDITIONS

- Endometrial cancer: due to unopposed estrogen stimulation
- Breast cancer: similar hormonal milieu may contribute

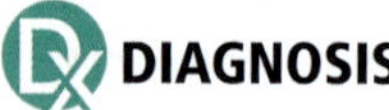

DIAGNOSIS

HISTORY

Most fibroids are asymptomatic and found incidentally. When symptomatic (~30%), presentations can include the following:

- Abnormal uterine bleeding: menorrhagia (heavy/prolonged menses), metrorrhagia
- Pelvic pressure: due to uterine enlargement compressing bladder (causing frequency, urgency) or rectum (constipation, back pain)
- Pelvic pain: typically due to degeneration or torsion of a pedunculated myoma
- Infertility: Submucosal fibroids can interfere with implantation or cause recurrent pregnancy loss.

ALERT

Rapid fibroid growth in perimenopausal or postmenopausal women raises suspicion for uterine sarcoma (very rare, 0.1–0.3% of fibroid cases)

PHYSICAL EXAM

- Often an incidental finding
- Bimanual exam may reveal an enlarged, irregular, mobile uterus with firm nodules.
- Generally nontender unless complications are present

DIFFERENTIAL DIAGNOSIS

- Intrauterine pregnancy
- Gynecologic malignancies: ovarian, uterine, leiomyosarcoma
- Gastrointestinal or urinary tract masses: diverticulitis, pelvic kidney, adnexal tumors

DIAGNOSTIC TESTS & INTERPRETATION

Initial Tests (lab, imaging)

- Urine or serum pregnancy test
- Complete blood count (CBC) to assess for anemia; consider vitamin D level.
- Pelvic ultrasound (transvaginal preferred): identifies hypoechoic, well-circumscribed masses

Follow-Up Tests & Special Considerations

- Saline infusion sonohysterography: for intracavitary fibroid detection
- MRI: superior for surgical planning, mapping fibroids, evaluating degeneration
- CT scan: generally not first line but may help in complex or atypical cases

Diagnostic Procedures/Other

- Hysteroscopy: direct visualization of endometrial cavity; useful for submucosal fibroids
- Hysterosalpingogram (HSG): evaluates cavity contour and tubal patency
- Diagnostic laparoscopy: helpful in complex cases or when malignancy or other pelvic pathology is suspected
- Endometrial sampling or dilation and curettage (D&C): if abnormal bleeding or malignancy suspected

Test Interpretation

- Pathology: Fibroids consist of whorled bundles of smooth muscle cells with varying degrees of connective tissue.
- Degeneration types:
  - Hyaline: most common
  - Calcific: common in older women
  - Cystic, red, or hemorrhagic
  - Necrosis: often in pedunculated fibroids, secondary to torsion
  - Suppuration/infection: especially in submucosal types

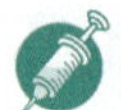

TREATMENT

Management should be individualized based on symptom severity, fibroid size and location, patient age, reproductive plans, and proximity to menopause.

GENERAL MEASURES

- Iron supplementation and NSAIDs may address heavy bleeding and dysmenorrhea.
- Conservative management
  - Observation is appropriate for asymptomatic fibroids, particularly in perimenopausal women, as fibroids often regress after menopause.
  - Monitor with pelvic exams and imaging (ultrasound) every 6 to 12 months if stable.

MEDICATION

Medical management can control symptoms and reduce fibroid size, often serving as a bridge to surgery or as definitive therapy in select patients.

- Hormonal therapies: first line
  - Combined oral contraceptives (COCs): useful for menorrhagia but do not reduce fibroid size
  - Progestins:
    - Norethindrone acetate 5 to 10 mg daily
    - Medroxyprogesterone acetate 10 mg daily or 150 mg IM every 3 months
    - Levonorgestrel-releasing intrauterine device (LNG-IUD): controls bleeding and may modestly reduce uterine volume
- Gonadotropin-Releasing Hormone (GnRH) agonists: GnRH agonists, either with or without add-back hormonal therapy, are recommended for the short-term treatment of abnormal uterine bleeding leiomyoma and uterine enlargement associated with uterine leiomyomas and as a bridge to other treatment strategies (3).
  - Leuprolide acetate (monthly IM or depot)
    - Induces hypoestrogenic state, reducing fibroid size by 30–50% within 3 months
    - Often used preoperatively to facilitate less invasive surgery
    - Side effects: menopausal symptoms, bone loss (limit use to ≤6 months or 12 months with add back hormones)
- GnRH antagonists:
  - Elagolix (oral): with or without hormonal "add-back" therapy for bleeding symptoms
  - Combination of elagolix (300 mg twice daily) with add-back therapy (1 mg estradiol and 0.5 mg norethindrone acetate once daily) is U.S. Food and Drug Administration (FDA)-approved for up to 24 months (3).
- Selective progesterone receptor modulators (SPRMs):
  - Ulipristal acetate:
    - Effective in reducing bleeding and fibroid volume
    - Contraindicated in patients with hepatic dysfunction
- Antifibrinolytics: tranexamic acid: nonhormonal treatment for menorrhagia
- Antiprogestins: mifepristone: reduces size and bleeding; investigational in the United States
- Consider vitamin D supplementation in patients with deficiency. Regimens vary. 50,000 IU weekly for 8 to 12 weeks has been used.

First Line

Hormonal therapy

Second Line

GnRH antagonists

ISSUES FOR REFERRAL

- Medical therapy may be initiated by a primary care physician after adequate pelvic examination.
- Gynecologic evaluation for persistent symptoms or surgical planning
- Interventional radiology consultation for Uterine artery embolization (UAE)

SURGERY/OTHER PROCEDURES

Surgery is indicated for fibroids causing significant symptoms, infertility, or suspicion of malignancy. Surgical options vary depending on fibroid location, size, and patient reproductive goals.

- Myomectomy:
  - Preferred for women desiring future fertility
  - Approaches: hysteroscopic (for submucosal), laparoscopic, robotic, or open (laparotomy)
  - Risks: bleeding, recurrence (~15–30%), adhesion formation
- Hysterectomy: The most minimally invasive route is recommended whenever possible, and the vaginal approach is preferred (3)[C].
  - Definitive treatment eliminates recurrence risk
  - Routes: vaginal, laparoscopic, robotic, abdominal
  - Consider for women with no future fertility desires and large/multiple fibroids.
  - FDA caution: avoid power morcellation due to risk of disseminating occult malignancy
- Endometrial Ablation:
  - For small submucosal fibroids and menorrhagia in women not desiring fertility
  - Less effective in larger fibroids or distorted cavities
- UAE
  - Recommended in patients who desire uterine preservation (3)[C]
  - Minimally invasive; performed by interventional radiology
  - Reduces fibroid size by ~50% and bleeding by ~85–90%
  - Potential complications: postembolization syndrome, ovarian dysfunction, infection
  - Not recommended for women planning pregnancy
- MRI-guided focused ultrasound surgery (MRgFUS):
  - Noninvasive; uses thermal ablation to induce necrosis
  - Symptom relief in appropriately selected patients
  - Limited availability and not suitable for all fibroid types

COMPLEMENTARY & ALTERNATIVE MEDICINE

- Limited evidence
- Some patients pursue acupuncture, herbal therapies, or dietary interventions.

ADMISSION, INPATIENT, AND NURSING CONSIDERATIONS

- Usually outpatient
- Inpatient for some surgical procedures

ONGOING CARE

FOLLOW-UP RECOMMENDATIONS

- After total hysterectomy, patients should refrain from sexual activity within 1 to 2 months.
- After organ-preserving myomectomy, women should use contraception for 6 to 12 months. Pregnancy is safe in 6 to 12 months following surgery.

Patient Monitoring

- Monitor symptoms, hemoglobin, and fibroid size every 6 to 12 months.
- Repeat imaging (ultrasound or MRI) as indicated by clinical course.

PATIENT EDUCATION

- Encourage informed decision-making; discuss all treatment risks and benefits.
- Reliable resources:
- Society of Interventional Radiology: https://www.sirweb.org
- Women's Health.gov: https://www.womenshealth.gov
- American College of Obstetricians and Gynecologists: http://www.acog.org

PROGNOSIS

- Symptom resolution is common with appropriate treatment.
- Myomectomy is associated with a ~10–30% recurrence rate; most do not require further intervention.
- Submucosal fibroid resection may improve fertility.

COMPLICATIONS

- Anemia due to heavy bleeding
- Infertility or pregnancy complications (malpresentation, preterm labor, cesarean delivery)
- Rarely, fibroid prolapse or degeneration with acute pain
- Masking of malignancies (e.g., uterine sarcoma)

Pregnancy Considerations

- Rapid fibroid growth may occur.
- Placental abnormalities and fetal growth restriction may result from fibroid interference
- Cesarean delivery is often indicated if uterine cavity has been surgically breached.

Geriatric Considerations

New or enlarging fibroids warrant evaluation for malignancy (e.g., leiomyosarcoma).

REFERENCES

1. Stewart EA, Cookson CL, Gandolfo RA, et al. Epidemiology of uterine fibroids: a systematic review. *BJOG*. 2017;124(10):1501–1512. doi:10.1111/1471-0528.146402.
2. Yang Q, Ciebiera M, Bariani MV, et al. Comprehensive review of uterine fibroids: developmental origin, pathogenesis, and treatment. *Endocr Rev*. 2022;43(4):678–719. doi:10.1210/endrev/bnab039.
3. Management of symptomatic uterine leiomyomas: ACOG practice bulletin, number 228. *Obstet Gynecol*. 2021;137(6):e100–e115.

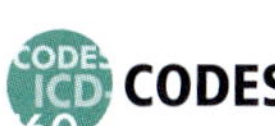

CODES

ICD10

- D25.9 Leiomyoma of uterus, unspecified
- D25.2 Subserosal leiomyoma of uterus
- D25.1 Intramural leiomyoma of uterus

CLINICAL PEARLS

- Uterine myomas are the most common hormone-dependent benign tumors in women.
- Usually asymptomatic and incidental finding on pelvic exam or ultrasound but may cause pelvic pain and pressure, abnormal uterine bleeding, and/or infertility
- Management ranges from observation to medical to surgical management.

U

UVEITIS

Mikayla L. Spangler, PharmD • Laura K. Klug, PharmD • Matthew A. Halfar, MD

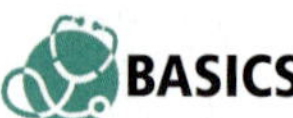

BASICS

DESCRIPTION

- A nonspecific term used to describe any intraocular inflammatory disorder
- The uvea is the middle layer of the eye between the sclera and retina. The anterior part of the uvea includes the iris and ciliary body. The posterior part of the uvea is the choroid.
  - Anterior uveitis: refers to ocular inflammation limited to the iris (iritis) alone or iris and ciliary body (iridocyclitis)
  - Intermediate uveitis: refers to inflammation of the structures just posterior to the lens (pars planitis or peripheral uveitis)
  - Posterior uveitis: refers to inflammation of the choroid (choroiditis), retina (retinitis), or vitreous near the optic nerve and macula
  - Panuveitis: refers to inflammation of all of the above areas of the uvea
- System(s) affected: nervous
- Synonym(s): iritis; iridocyclitis; choroiditis; retinochoroiditis; chorioretinitis; anterior uveitis; posterior uveitis; pars planitis; panuveitis; synonyms are anatomic descriptions of the focus of the uveal inflammation.

Pediatric Considerations

- Infection should be the primary consideration.
- Allergies and psychological factors (depression, stress) may serve as a trigger.
- Trauma is also a common cause in this population.

EPIDEMIOLOGY

Predominant sex: male = female, except for human leukocyte antigen B27 (HLA-B27) anterior uveitis: male > female, autoimmune etiology: female > male

Incidence

Overall incidence is 17 to 52 cases/100,000 per year in the developed world.

Prevalence

- Overall prevalence is 38 to 714 cases/100,000 population.
- Anterior uveitis is the most common (80% of cases) with iritis being 4 times more prevalent than posterior uveitis.

ETIOLOGY AND PATHOPHYSIOLOGY

- Infectious: may result from viral, bacterial, parasitic, or fungal etiologies
- Suspected immune mediated: possible autoimmune or immune complex–mediated mechanism postulated in association with systemic (especially rheumatologic) disorders
  - Autoimmune uveitis (AIU) patients should be referred to an ophthalmologist for local treatment.
- Isolated eye disease
- Undifferentiated (~25%)
- Some medications may cause uveitis. The most causative medications include rifabutin, bisphosphonates, sulfonamides, metipranolol, brimonidine, prostaglandin analogs, immune checkpoint inhibitors, TNF-α inhibitors, protein kinase inhibitors (BRAF and MEK), anti-vascular endothelial growth factor (VEGF) agents, Bacillus Calmette-Guérin (BCG) vaccination, and systemic and intraocular cidofovir (1)
- Masquerade syndromes: diseases such as malignancies that may be mistaken for primary inflammation of the eye

Genetics

- Iritis: 50–70% are HLA-B27 positive.
- Predisposing gene for posterior uveitis associated with Behçet disease may include HLA-B51.

RISK FACTORS

No specific risk factors

COMMONLY ASSOCIATED CONDITIONS

- Viral infections: herpes simplex, herpes zoster, HIV, cytomegalovirus, congenital Zika virus
- Bacterial infections: brucellosis, leprosy, leptospirosis, Lyme disease, *Propionibacterium* infection, syphilis, tuberculosis (TB), Whipple disease
- Parasitic infections: acanthamebiasis, cysticercosis, onchocerciasis, toxocariasis, toxoplasmosis
- Fungal infections: aspergillosis, blastomycosis, candidiasis, coccidioidomycosis, cryptococcosis, histoplasmosis, sporotrichosis
- Suspected immune mediated: ankylosing spondylitis, Behçet disease, Crohn disease, drug or hypersensitivity reaction, interstitial nephritis, juvenile rheumatoid arthritis, Kawasaki disease, multiple sclerosis, psoriatic arthritis, Reiter syndrome, relapsing polychondritis, sarcoidosis, Sjögren syndrome, systemic lupus erythematosus, ulcerative colitis, vasculitis, vitiligo, Vogt-Koyanagi (Harada) syndrome
- Isolated eye disease: acute multifocal placoid pigmentary epitheliopathy, acute retinal necrosis, birdshot choroidopathy, Fuchs heterochromic cyclitis, glaucomatocyclitic crisis, lens-induced uveitis, multifocal choroiditis, pars planitis, serpiginous choroiditis, sympathetic ophthalmia, trauma
- Masquerade syndromes: leukemia, lymphoma, retinitis pigmentosa, retinoblastoma

DIAGNOSIS

HISTORY

- Decreased visual acuity
- Pain, photophobia, blurring of vision (2)[C]
  - Usually acute
- Anterior uveitis
  - Generally acute in onset
  - Deep eye pain
  - Photophobia (consensual)
- Intermediate and posterior uveitis
  - Unresolving floaters
  - Generally insidious in onset
  - More commonly bilateral

PHYSICAL EXAM

Slit-lamp exam and indirect ophthalmoscopy are necessary for precise diagnosis (2)[C].

- Anterior uveitis
  - Conjunctival vessel dilation
  - Perilimbal (circumcorneal) dilation of episcleral and scleral vessels (ciliary flush)
  - Small pupillary size of affected eye
  - Hypopyon or hyphema (WBCs or RBCs pooled in the anterior chamber)
  - Frequently unilateral (95% of HLA-B27—associated cases); if first occurrence and otherwise asymptomatic, no further diagnostic testing is needed (2)[C].
  - Bilateral involvement and systemic symptoms (fever, fatigue, abdominal pain) may be associated with interstitial nephritis (2)[C].
  - Systemic disease is most likely to be associated with anterior uveitis (in one study, 53% of patients were found to have systemic disease) (2)[C].
- Intermediate and posterior uveitis
  - More commonly bilateral
  - Posterior inflammation will generally cause minimal pain or redness unless associated with an iritis.

DIFFERENTIAL DIAGNOSIS

- Acute angle-closure glaucoma
- Conjunctivitis; episcleritis; keratitis; scleritis

DIAGNOSTIC TESTS & INTERPRETATION

No specific test for the diagnosis of uveitis.; tests for etiologic factors or associated conditions should be based on history and physical exam (2)[C].

Initial Tests (lab, imaging)

- CBC, BUN, creatinine (interstitial nephritis) (2)[C]
- HLA-B27 typing (ankylosing spondylitis, Reiter syndrome) (2)[C],(3)
- Antinuclear antibody, ESR (systemic lupus erythematosus, Sjögren syndrome) (2)[C],(3)
- Venereal disease research laboratory (VDRL) test, fluorescent titer antibody (syphilis) (2)[C],(3)
- Fluorescent treponemal antibody absorption (FTA-ABS) or microhemagglutination assay for antibodies to *Treponema pallidum* (MHA-TP) (2)[C]
- Purified protein derivative (PPD) tuberculin skin test (TB) (2)[C]
- Lyme serology (Lyme disease) (2)[C],(3)
- Chest x-ray (sarcoidosis, histoplasmosis, TB, lymphoma) (2)[C],(3)
- Sacroiliac radiograph (ankylosing spondylitis) (2)[C]

Diagnostic Procedures/Other

Slit-lamp exam (2)[C],(3)

Test Interpretation

- Keratic precipitates
- Inflammatory cells in anterior chamber or vitreous
- Synechiae (fibrous tissue scarring between iris and lens)
- Macular edema
- Perivasculitis of retinal vessels

TREATMENT

GENERAL MEASURES

- Urgent ophthalmologic consultation
- Medical therapy is best initiated following full ophthalmologic evaluation.
- Treatment of underlying cause, if identified
- Anti-inflammatory therapy

MEDICATION

First Line

- The treatment depends on the etiology, location, and severity of the inflammation.
- Prednisolone acetate 1% ophthalmic suspension: 1 to 2 drops to the affected eye 2 to 4 times per day, during first 24 to 48 hours, dosing frequency may be increased *or* dexamethasone 0.1% ophthalmic suspension: 1 to 2 drops to affected eye 4 to 6 times per day, may use hourly in severe disease; other corticosteroid options include prednisolone sodium phosphate 1% solution, dexamethasone sodium phosphate 0.1% solution, and loteprednol etabonate 0.5% (Lotemax) suspension, difluprednate (Durezol) 0.05% emulsion (2),(3)[C].
  - Taper prior to discontinuation
  - Contraindications
    - Hypersensitivity to the medication or component of the preparation
    - Topical corticosteroid therapy is contraindicated in uveitis secondary to infectious etiologies, unless used in conjunction with appropriate anti-infectious agents.
  - Precautions
    - Topical corticosteroids may increase intraocular pressure, increase susceptibility to infections, impair corneal or scleral wound healing, or cause corneal epithelial toxicity or crystalline keratopathy. Prolonged use may cause cataract formation and exacerbate existing herpetic keratitis, which may masquerade as iritis.
    - Significant possible interactions
- Cycloplegic agents may be used to dilate the eye and relieve pain. Agents include atropine 1% 1 to 2 drops up to QID or homatropine hydrobromide (Isopto) 5% 1 to 2 drops q3–4h (2)[C].
  - Contraindications
    - Patients known to have, or be predisposed to glaucoma.
  - Precautions
    - Use extreme caution in infants, young children, and elderly because of increased susceptibility to systemic effects.

Second Line

- Systemic corticosteroids are useful for maintenance therapy for patients with noninfectious posterior uveitis or for severe ocular inflammation. These should always be used with other immunosuppressive medications for steroid-sparing effects; prednisone ≤7.5 mg daily (3)[B]
- Intravitreal corticosteroid deposits may also be used for long-term maintenance; fluocinolone acetonide ([Retisert 590 μg released over 30 months], [Yutiq 180 μg released over 36 months], and [Iluvien 190 μg released over 36 months]), dexamethasone (Ozurdex) 0.7 mg released slowly >3 to 6 months (3),(4)[C]
  - Retisert has caused nearly all patients to develop cataracts and significant increases in intraocular pressure in just over 75% of patients, whereas Ozurdex resulted in less occurrence of an increase in intraocular pressure and cataract development (3),(4)[C].
- Intravitreal triamcinolone acetonide injections can be given (3)[C].
- Immunosuppressive agents including antimetabolites (methotrexate, azathioprine, and mycophenolate mofetil), T-cell inhibitors (cyclosporine and tacrolimus), and alkylating agents (cyclophosphamide, chlorambucil) may be employed in cases resistant or intolerant to initial treatment, or used for their corticosteroid-sparing effect. Close monitoring is required (4)[C].
- Advancing research suggests benefit of the biologic agents in refractory uveitis. Adalimumab is the only biologic agent with FDA approval for this indication. Other biologic agents, including infliximab, golimumab, certolizumab-pegol, abatacept, and tocilizumab, have also been studied (3),(4)[C].
  - Benefits of biologic therapy include glucocorticoid sparing effects, but limitations may include high cost and adverse effect potential.
- Systemic and ophthalmic preparations of NSAIDs may provide some symptom relief (2)[C].

ISSUES FOR REFERRAL

Caution when using empiric treatment; referral to an ophthalmologist is recommended in most cases.

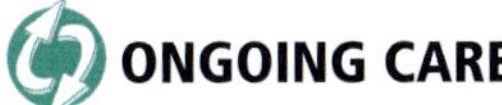

ONGOING CARE

FOLLOW-UP RECOMMENDATIONS

Patient Monitoring

- Complete history and physical exam to evaluate for associated systemic disease
- Ophthalmologic follow-up

PATIENT EDUCATION

- Instruct on proper method for instilling eye drops.
- Wear dark glasses if photophobia is a problem.

PROGNOSIS

- Depends on the presence of causal diseases or associated conditions
- Uveitis resulting from infections (systemic or local) tends to resolve with eradication of the underlying infection.
- Uveitis associated with seronegative arthropathies tends to be acute (lasting <3 months) but frequently recurrent.

COMPLICATIONS

- Cycloplegia: paralysis of the ciliary muscle of the eye, resulting in a loss of accommodation
- Loss of vision as a result of the following:
  - Keratic precipitate deposition on the corneal or lens surfaces
  - Increased intraocular pressure, acute angle-closure glaucoma
  - Formation of synechiae
  - Cataract formation
  - Vasculitis with vascular occlusion, retinal infarction
  - Macular edema
  - Optic nerve damage

REFERENCES

1. Abdalla Elsayed MEA, Kozak I. Pharmacologically induced uveitis. *Surv Ophthalmol*. 2021;66(5):781–801.
2. Harthan JS, Optiz DL, Fromstein SR, et al. Diagnosis and treatment of anterior uveitis: optometric management. *Clin Optom (Auckl)*. 2016;8:23–35.
3. Burkholder BM, Jabs DA.Uveitis for the non-ophthalmologist. *BMJ*. 2021;372:m4979.
4. Pleyer U, Neri P, Deuter C. New pharmacotherapy options for noninfectious posterior uveitis. *Int Ophthalmol*. 2021;41(6):2265–2281.

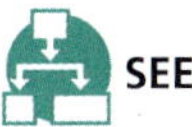

SEE ALSO

Conjunctivitis, Acute; Glaucoma, Primary Closed-Angle; Scleritis

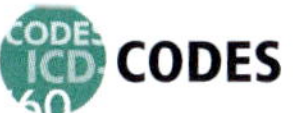

CODES

ICD10

- H20.9 Unspecified iridocyclitis
- H30.90 Unspecified chorioretinal inflammation, unspecified eye
- H20.019 Primary iridocyclitis, unspecified eye

CLINICAL PEARLS

- Symptoms vary depending on depth of involvement and associated conditions but should be suspected when eye pain is associated with visual changes.
- Severe or unresponsive uveitis may require therapy, including periocular injection of corticosteroids, sustained-release corticosteroid implants, systemic corticosteroids, cytotoxic agents, immunosuppressive agents, immunomodulatory agents, or tumor necrosis factor inhibitors.

U

VAGINAL ADENOSIS

Carolina Isabel Burgos-Burgos, MD

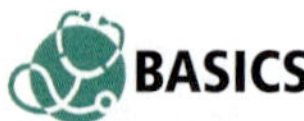

BASICS

DESCRIPTION

- The normal vagina is lined with squamous epithelium. Adenosis is characterized by the presence of columnar epithelium or glandular tissue in the wall of the vagina.
- Around week 15 of embryologic development, the müllerian system, which forms the upper 2/3 of the vagina, fuses with the invaginating cloaca or urogenital sinus to form the lower 1/3 of the vagina. Squamous metaplasia from the cloacal region then produces squamous epithelium within the vagina (1).
- *Adenosis* occurs when this squamous epithelium fails to epithelialize the vagina completely.
- Three main types of adenosis epithelium:
  - Endocervical
  - Endometrial
  - Tubal
- System(s) affected: reproductive

Geriatric Considerations

- Adenosis is a disorder of the young female. By menopause, the vagina and cervix should be completely epithelialized.
- In a postmenopausal patient, the presence of glandular epithelium is an indication for excision and evaluation, given the risk of well-differentiated adenocarcinoma.

Pregnancy Considerations

Pregnancy produces a wide eversion of the transformation zone of the cervix. This can become so widely everted that it will extend onto the vaginal fornices, leading to the impression of adenosis. This will resolve after pregnancy.

EPIDEMIOLOGY

- Spontaneous (non-diethylstilbestrol [DES]) adenosis is common in young women and usually resolves with age; prevalence decreases after puberty and is rare after age 30.
- DES-associated adenosis: Up to 90% of "DES daughters" develop adenosis, with a 40-fold increased risk of clear cell adenocarcinoma

Incidence

- Although the cumulative incidence of vaginal adenosis is unknown, the incidence of cloacal malformations is 1/20,000 to 1/25,000 live births.
- Although spontaneous vaginal adenosis appears to be fairly common (10% of adult women), it is mostly an insignificant coincidental finding. Widespread symptomatic involvement is rare (2).

Prevalence

- In the United States, adenosis is common in young women, affecting 10–20%. As maturation progresses with puberty, epithelialization occurs.
- Predominant age
  - Age <1 month: 15%
  - Prepubertal: typically absent
  - Age 13 to 25 years: 13%
  - Age >25 years: decreasing prevalence, uncommon beyond age 30 years (2)

ETIOLOGY AND PATHOPHYSIOLOGY

- In most young females, the etiology is incomplete squamous metaplasia or epithelialization. This occurs as a natural phenomenon and resolves with age.
- Described as congenital or acquired:
  - Congenital: proliferation of the remnant müllerian epithelium in the vagina due to exposure to DES in utero ("DES daughters"). DES is a synthetic, nonsteroidal estrogen used to prevent miscarriage or premature deliveries from 1938 to 1971. An estimated 5 million women were prescribed DES during this period (3).
  - Transformation-related protein 63 (TRP63/p63) marks the cell fate of müllerian duct epithelium to become squamous epithelium in the cervix and vagina. DES disrupts the TRP63 expression and induces adenosis lesions (3). It has also been suggested that DES induces vaginal adenosis by inhibiting the BMP4 and Activin A-regulated vaginal cell fate through a downregulation of RUNX1.
  - Acquired: trauma and inflammation causing spontaneous de novo changes or changes in an acquired lesion in the vaginal epithelium
  - Additional reports documented adenosis subsequent to sulfonamide-induced Stevens–Johnson syndrome and after treatment of vaginal condylomas with 5-fluorouracil (4).

Genetics

- Vaginal adenosis is not linked to inherited genetic mutations or familial syndromes.
- Primarily associated with disrupted embryologic signaling, particularly after in utero exposure to DES. DES interferes with pathways such as BMP4 and Activin A-SMAD/RUNX1, leading to persistence of glandular epithelium in the vagina.
- Genetic mutations such as TP53 and PTEN are implicated in vaginal adenocarcinoma, but not in benign adenosis.

RISK FACTORS

Adenosis of the vagina/cervix may arise in up to 90% of DES daughters and has a 40-fold increased risk of developing into clear cell adenocarcinoma.

GENERAL PREVENTION

None: Last DES exposure was in the 1970s.

COMMONLY ASSOCIATED CONDITIONS

DES exposure

- Adenosis from DES exposure should lead to an evaluation of other DES-related abnormalities.
- Müllerian tract anomalies associated with DES exposure include cervical hood, cervical ridge, shortened cervix, incompetent cervix, and T-shaped uterine cavity.
- Patients with known DES exposure should have their reproductive tract evaluated prior to conception.
- Most patients with adenosis have not been DES-exposed and do not require evaluation of the reproductive system.
- The FDA issued a drug bulletin in 1971 advising physicians to stop prescribing DES to pregnant women because of its link to vaginal clear cell adenocarcinoma in DES daughters.

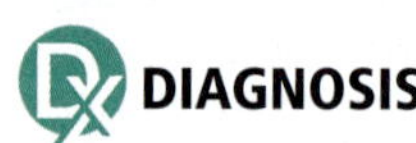

DIAGNOSIS

HISTORY

- Maternal DES exposure
- Complaints of
  - Profuse mucoid vaginal discharge from the glandular epithelium
  - Pruritus
  - Pain/soreness of the vaginal introitus
  - Postcoital bleeding
  - Dyspareunia

PHYSICAL EXAM
On pelvic exam, adenosis appearance is varied: patchy or diffuse red stippling, granularity or nodularity, single or multiple cysts, erosions, ulcers, or warty protuberances that may even extend to the vulva.

DIFFERENTIAL DIAGNOSIS
- Erosive lichen planus
- Fixed drug eruption
- Erythema multiforme
- Bullous skin disease
- Vaginal adenocarcinoma

DIAGNOSTIC TESTS & INTERPRETATION

Initial Tests (lab, imaging)
Four-quadrant Pap smear should be used liberally to isolate quadrants of the vagina that may contain abnormalities. No imaging is indicated, unless diagnosed with underlying malignancy.

Follow-Up Tests & Special Considerations
Pap smear can be followed by colposcopy and biopsy.

Diagnostic Procedures/Other
- Colposcopy should be used to outline areas of adenosis to ensure that no malignancy is present.
- A thorough evaluation for adenocarcinoma of the vagina arising in adenosis should be done.
- A biopsy may be necessary to ensure that the process represents only benign adenosis.

Test Interpretation
- Biopsy will show benign glandular epithelium.
- Biopsies may show areas of ongoing squamous metaplasia.

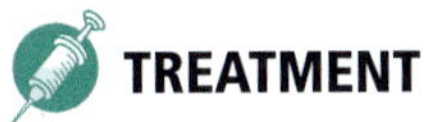

TREATMENT

GENERAL MEASURES
- Unless malignancy is present, treatment is conservative.
- In most young females with this condition, it will resolve with expectant management.
- Treatment is warranted in women with severe subjective symptoms that impair the quality of life.
- First-line treatment: If indicated in patients with focal lesions and no history of DES exposure, simple excision is an effective treatment (4).

ISSUES FOR REFERRAL
Malignancy found on biopsy warrants referral to gynecologic oncology specialist.

SURGERY/OTHER PROCEDURES
- Aggressive therapy, such as laser or surgical excision, is necessary if premalignant or malignant changes arise.
- Symptomatic treatment has been performed with carbon dioxide laser coagulation, unipolar coagulation, or vaginal resection.

ADMISSION, INPATIENT, AND NURSING CONSIDERATIONS
Outpatient management

ONGOING CARE

FOLLOW-UP RECOMMENDATIONS

Patient Monitoring
If the initial colposcopy is normal, a yearly four-quadrant Pap smear of the vagina and of the cervix should be performed.

DIET
No special diet is recommended.

PATIENT EDUCATION
- No limitations
- It is not necessary to avoid intercourse or placing objects in the vagina.
- The patient should be educated to keep normal guideline-recommended pelvic and Pap smear appointments. In most situations, this is benign, and expectant management is all that is necessary.
- https://www.acog.org/

PROGNOSIS
- Most patients will have squamous metaplasia and epithelialization with complete resolution of the adenosis.
- 1/1,000 to 1/10,000 may develop adenocarcinoma in the adenosis and will require definitive therapy as for vaginal cancer. Cumulative incidence of progression of adenosis to adenocarcinoma is 1.5/1,000 for DES daughters.

COMPLICATIONS
- Infertility with DES association
- Adverse pregnancy outcome with DES association
- Adenocarcinoma of vagina
- Clear cell adenocarcinoma with DES association

REFERENCES

1. Reich O, Fritsch H. The developmental origin of cervical and vaginal epithelium and their clinical consequences: a systematic review. *J Low Genit Tract Dis*. 2014;18(4):358–360.
2. Kranl C, Zelger B, Kofler H, et al. Vulval and vaginal adenosis. *Br J Dermatol*. 1998;139(1):128–131.
3. Laronda MM, Unno K, Butler LM, et al. The development of cervical and vaginal adenosis as a result of diethylstilbestrol exposure in utero. *Differentiation*. 2012;84(3):252–260.
4. Martin AA, Atkins KA, Lonergan CL, et al. Vaginal adenosis as a dermatologic complaint. *J Am Acad Dermatol*. 2013;69(2):e92–e93.

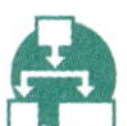

SEE ALSO

Vaginal Malignancy

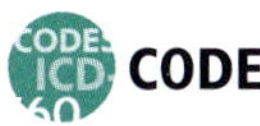

CODES

ICD10
- Q52.4 Other congenital malformations of vagina
- N89.8 Other specified noninflammatory disorders of vagina
- T38.5X5A Adverse effect of other estrogens and progestogens, initial encounter

CLINICAL PEARLS
- Adenosis is characterized by the presence of columnar epithelium or glandular tissue in the wall of the vagina.
- Adenosis is common among the daughters of women exposed to DES.
- Rarely, adenosis can be associated with an underlying vaginal malignancy.

VAGINAL BLEEDING DURING PREGNANCY

Kristina Gracey, MD, MPH • Vernon L. Wheeler, MD • Opeoluwa Olukorede, MD, MS • Anne M. Knierim, MD

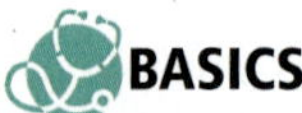

BASICS

DESCRIPTION

- Vaginal bleeding during pregnancy has many causes and ranges in severity from benign, with normal pregnancy outcome to life-threatening for both infant and mother.
- Origin of blood can be from the vagina, cervix, uterus, fetus, or placenta. The differential diagnosis is guided by the gestational age of the fetus.

EPIDEMIOLOGY

Prevalence

- In early pregnancy: 7–25% of patients
- In late pregnancy: 0.3–2% of patients

ETIOLOGY AND PATHOPHYSIOLOGY

- Many times, the cause is unknown.
- Anytime in pregnancy:
  - Cervicitis (infectious or noninfectious)
  - Vaginitis (infectious or noninfectious)
  - Vaginal or cervical trauma (including postcoital)
  - Cervical lesion (including polyps or warts) or neoplasia
  - Hyperemia of cervix (increased blood flow from pregnancy)
- Early pregnancy:
  - For up to 50% of early pregnancy bleeding, no cause is ever found; bleeding in the 1st trimester is a risk factor for multiple adverse pregnancy outcomes (1)[A]
  - Ectopic pregnancy: leading cause of 1st-trimester maternal death in the United States—must be excluded in every pregnant patient with bleeding.
  - Spontaneous abortion: occurs in 10–15% of clinically recognized early pregnancies.
  - Loss of one fetus from a multiple gestation ("vanishing twin")
  - Implantation bleeding: benign, about 6 days after fertilization
  - Uterine fibroids
  - Subchorionic bleeding (or hematoma): in late 1st trimester
  - Low-lying placenta
  - Gestational trophoblastic disease: hydatidiform mole (most common), choriocarcinoma, or placental-site trophoblastic tumors
- Late pregnancy:
  - Cervical change
  - Placenta previa: painless bleeding; prevalence of 2.9% in North America; however, prevalence varies by geographical region; occurs in 0.5% of pregnancies in the United States
  - Placental abruption: (typically) painful bleeding; occurs in 1–2% deliveries in the United States.
  - Vasa previa: minimal bleeding with fetal distress; rare (1:2,500 deliveries)
  - Placenta accreta, increta, percreta
  - Uterine rupture: typically presents with vaginal bleeding, abnormal fetal heart rate, and disordered or hypertonic uterine contractions with or without pain

Genetics

No genetic risk factors have been determined to increase the risk of bleeding during pregnancy

RISK FACTORS

See specific etiologies in earlier discussion.

GENERAL PREVENTION

- Address modifiable risk factors such as domestic violence and tobacco and drug use.
- If placenta or vasa previa, nothing per vagina

COMMONLY ASSOCIATED CONDITIONS

See specific risk factors in earlier discussion.

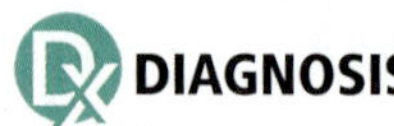

DIAGNOSIS

HISTORY

- Anytime in pregnancy: quality of pregnancy dating, context (e.g., following bowel movement, during voiding, after intercourse, drug use, or trauma including domestic violence), amount of bleeding, obstetrical history, personal or family history of inherited bleeding disorders
- Early pregnancy: severe nausea/vomiting (can be associated with molar pregnancy); amount of bleeding, pelvic pain, or suprapubic cramping (e.g., spontaneous abortion, ectopic) complications in previous pregnancies (e.g., spontaneous abortion, abruption, 1st-trimester vaginal bleeding)
- Late pregnancy: contractions (labor), abdominal pain especially between contractions (abruption, uterine rupture), presence or absence of fetal movement, rupture of membranes
- See "Etiology and Pathophysiology" for additional pertinent history.

PHYSICAL EXAM

- Vital signs: When present, signs of hemodynamic instability include tachycardia and tachypnea, hypotension and thready pulse.
- Abdomen: uterine tenderness, fundal height (increasing fundal height may be associated with placental abruption)
- Speculum: Visualize cervix and identify source of bleeding (from cervical os or from within vagina).
- Cervix: digital exam to assess for dilation; required to assess for labor but should not be performed until placenta previa ruled out via ultrasound and may be done visually on speculum exam
- Fetal monitoring: Doppler heart tones in early pregnancy; external fetal monitoring for gestational age of >26 weeks

DIFFERENTIAL DIAGNOSIS

- Hematuria (UTI, kidney stones)
- Rectal bleeding

DIAGNOSTIC TESTS & INTERPRETATION

Initial Tests (lab, imaging)

- CBC
- Blood type and screen if more than minimal bleeding; if significant hemorrhage, type and crossmatch. The World Health Organization does not recommend giving RhoGAM until 12 weeks' gestation and later (2) while the Society for Maternal-Fetal Medicine recommends screening for Rh-negative status and administering RhoGAM to all Rh-negative patients with vaginal bleeding under 12 weeks' gestation (3).
- Quantitative β-human chorionic gonadotropin (β-hCG):
  - Prior to 12 weeks, levels can be followed serially every 48 to 72 hours with characteristic trends:
    - Although many texts cite at least 66% rise in 48 hours in normal pregnancy, when initial β-hCG levels is <1,500 mIU/mL, between 1,500 to 3,000 mIU/mL, or >3,000 mIU/mL, subsequent level is expected to increase by at least 49%, 40%, and 33%, respectively over 48 hours.
    - Falls by ~50% every 48 to 72 hours in spontaneous abortion
    - Rises gradually (<50% in 48 hours) or plateaus in ectopic pregnancy
    - Extremely high in molar pregnancy
- Transabdominal or transvaginal ultrasound should be used to confirm an intrauterine pregnancy (IUP) when the quantitative β-hCG >2,000.
- Other lab tests based on clinical scenario:
  - Wet mount, gonorrhea/chlamydia/trichomoniasis, Pap smear
  - Progesterone level occasionally used to determine viability in threatened abortion (<5 indicates not viable, >25 indicates viability, 5 to 25 is equivocal)
  - Prothrombin time with international normalized ratio (INR), partial thromboplastin time, fibrinogen, and fibrin split products: if suspect coagulopathy or abruption
  - Kleihauer-Betke: assesses for fetal–maternal hemorrhage; low sensitivity and specificity for abruption; helpful for dosing RhoGAM
- Transvaginal ultrasound is the preferred imaging modality if evaluating for possible ectopic pregnancy.
  - Early pregnancy:
    - Gestational sac seen at 5 to 6 weeks; fetal heartbeat observed by ≥6 weeks
    - Diagnostic of ectopic with nearly 100% sensitivity when β-hCG level is 1,500 to 2,000 mIU/mL; if no IUP is present and ultrasound does not confirm ectopic pregnancy, serial quantitative β-hCG values should be followed.
  - Late pregnancy:
    - Proceed to rule out placenta previa with ultrasound, labor with serial cervical exams, and abruption with external fetal monitoring.

ALERT
Confirm fetal presentation and placental position prior to cervical exam (to avoid complications in placenta previa).

Diagnostic Procedures/Other

Ultrasound: Can be used to follow the size of a hematoma or to follow the progression of a pregnancy in early 1st trimester bleeding.

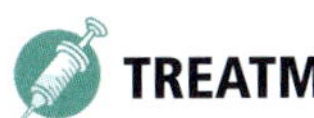

TREATMENT

GENERAL MEASURES

Treat the underlying cause of the bleeding if identified.

MEDICATION

First Line

- If the mother is Rh-negative, give RhoGAM to prevent autoimmunization. In late pregnancy, dose according to the amount of estimated fetal–maternal hemorrhage.
- If cause of bleeding is preterm labor, consider steroid administration for fetal lung maturity if <36 weeks' gestation. Tocolytics may be used to prolong pregnancy to allow for course of steroids.
- If threatened abortion and patient with shortened cervix on transvaginal ultrasound: Consider progesterone vaginally; shown to improve live birth outcomes in subgroups of women with history of three or more spontaneous abortions; no benefit is seen on patients without a history of spontaneous abortion.
- If mother has an inherited bleeding disorder or if bleeding is severe, consider recombinant or donor blood products.
- If early pregnancy loss is determined to be the cause, consider expectant managementor medication management by using the combination of mifepristone and misoprostol to accelerate return to prepregnant state.

ISSUES FOR REFERRAL

If bleeding ectopic pregnancy is found, immediate referral to OB-GYN for management.

SURGERY/OTHER PROCEDURES

- Cesarean section may be indicated for recurrent or uncontrolled bleeding with placenta previa or vasa previa.
- If ectopic is diagnosed, immediate surgical treatment may be needed. Some early ectopic pregnancies can be treated medically if certain criteria are met.
- Surgical uterine evacuation is necessary for molar pregnancy due to malignant potential.
- Incomplete or inevitable spontaneous abortion: Management is patient centered and should include psychological support. In the absence of infection, patient may elect expectant, medical, or surgical management.
- If history of cervical insufficiency resulting in preterm delivery, can consider cerclage placement in the 2nd trimester.

COMPLEMENTARY & ALTERNATIVE MEDICINE

Acupuncture: may increase blood flow to the uterine lining to help prevent threatened miscarriage.

ADMISSION, INPATIENT, AND NURSING CONSIDERATIONS

- In early pregnancy: based on quantity of bleeding, need for surgical treatment for ectopic pregnancy, or presence of infection in case of spontaneous abortion
- In late pregnancy, consider admission if significant bleeding and/or presence of maternal or fetal compromise; consider admission with trauma if ≥2 contractions per 10 minutes
- In late pregnancy, may discharge when bleeding has stopped; labor, previa, and abruption have been ruled out; and fetal heart tracing is normal.
- After trauma in late pregnancy, may discharge home if normal fetal heart tracing for ≥4 hours with <2 contractions per 10 minutes (Consider mechanism of injury when deciding on duration of observation.)

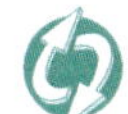

ONGOING CARE

FOLLOW-UP RECOMMENDATIONS

Patient Monitoring

- Patient should be instructed to report any increase in the amount or frequency of bleeding and to seek immediate care if experiencing fever, dizziness, abdominal pain, or sudden increased bleeding and to seek immediate care if experiencing fever, dizziness, abdominal pain, or sudden increase in bleeding. Patient should save any tissue passed vaginally for examination.
- Frequency of outpatient follow-up as indicated based on etiology of bleeding

PATIENT EDUCATION

- American Academy of Family Physicians (AAFP): https://www.aafp.org/pubs/afp/issues/2009/0601/p993.html
- American College of Obstetricians and Gynecologists (ACOG): https://www.acog.org/womens-health/faqs/bleeding-during-pregnancy

PROGNOSIS

- Prognosis depends on the etiology of vaginal bleeding, severity of bleeding, and rapidity of diagnosis; ectopic pregnancies result in 9–14% of maternal mortality in the 1st trimester and 5–10% of all pregnancy related deaths
- Approximately half of patients with early pregnancy bleeding will continue with a normal pregnancy; if fetal heart activity (ultrasound) present during the episode of 1st-trimester bleeding, there is a <10% chance of pregnancy loss.
- Heavy bleeding in early pregnancy, particularly when accompanied by pain, is associated with higher risk of spontaneous abortion.
- Subchorionic bleeding has about 2- to 3-fold increased risk of spontaneous abortion. Smaller hemorrhage and presence of viable fetal heart rate confer lower risk of loss; most resolve spontaneously.
- Bed rest has not been shown to affect the outcome of bleeding in early pregnancy but may be indicated for bleeding in late pregnancy with placenta or vasa previa or with maternal hypertension.

COMPLICATIONS

- Pregnancy loss
- Preterm labor
- Hemorrhage
- Increased rates of cesarean delivery when the cause of bleeding (i.e. placental) leads to fetal distress

REFERENCES

1. Karimi A, Sayehmiri K, Vaismoradi M, et al. Vaginal bleeding in pregnancy and adverse clinical outcomes: a systematic review and meta-analysis. *J Obstet Gynaecol*. 2024;44(1):2288224.
2. World Health Organization. Abortion care guideline. 2022. https://iris.who.int/bitstream/handle/10665/349316/9789240039483-eng.pdf
3. Society for Maternal-Fetal Medicine; Prabhu M, Louis JM, Kuller JA; SMFM Publications Committee. Society for Maternal–Fetal Medicine Statement: RhD immune globulin after spontaneous or induced at less than 12 weeks gestation. *Am J Obstet Gynecol*. 2024;230(5):B2–B5.

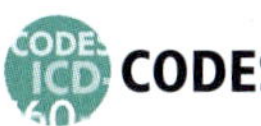

CODES

ICD10

- O20.9 Hemorrhage in early pregnancy, unspecified
- O46.90 Antepartum hemorrhage, unspecified, unspecified trimester
- O20.0 Threatened abortion

CLINICAL PEARLS

- For up to 50% of early pregnancy bleeding, no cause is ever found.
- Always consider ectopic pregnancy in 1st-trimester bleeding.
- Do not perform digital exam in late pregnancy bleeding until placenta has been located on ultrasound.

V

VAGINAL MALIGNANCY

Kristina Gracey, MD, MPH • Akanksha Srivastava, MD • Sharmilee Korets, MD

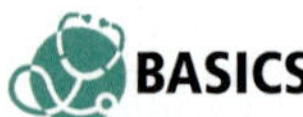

BASICS

DESCRIPTION

- Primary carcinomas of the vagina are rare: 2–3% of gynecologic malignancies and 1,372 new cases annually in the United States as of 2021 (1)
- Vaginal intraepithelial neoplasia (VAIN), the precursor lesion for vaginal cancer, is defined by squamous cell atypia and is classified by the depth of epithelial involvement (2)
  - VAIN 1: 1/3 thickness
  - VAIN 2: 2/3 thickness
  - VAIN 3: >2/3 thickness
  - Carcinoma in situ (CIS): designating full-thickness neoplastic changes without invasion through the basement membrane
- Invasive malignancies: Vaginal malignancies include squamous cell carcinoma (85–90%), adenocarcinoma (5–10%), sarcoma (2–3%), and melanoma (2–3%). Clear cell carcinoma is a subtype of adenocarcinoma. Invasive vaginal cancer can spread by direct extension to adjacent tissues, lymphatic dissemination to locoregional lymph nodes (pelvic and para-aortic, or inguinal), or via hematogenous squamous cell carcinoma; has the potential for hematogenous metastasis to other sites including the lungs and liver.
- To be classified as a primary vaginal malignancy, only the vagina can be involved. If the cervix or vulva is involved, then the tumor is classified as a primary cancer arising from the cervix or the vulva. Additionally, if the patient has had a diagnosis of invasive cervical or vulvar cancer in the preceding 5 years, it cannot be classified as a primary vaginal malignancy.
- If the patient has a cervix, then a primary cervical malignancy should be conclusively ruled out before vaginal cancer diagnosis can be made.
- Most vaginal malignancies are metastatic tumors from other primary sites (e.g., cervix, vulva, endometrium).

Pregnancy Considerations

This malignancy is not typically associated with pregnancy (3).

EPIDEMIOLOGY

Incidence

Predominant age is dependent on type:

- CIS: mid-40 to 60 years
- Invasive squamous cell malignancy: mid-60 to 70 years
- Adenocarcinoma: can occur at any age; 50 years is the mean age, with peak incidence between 17 and 21 years of age.
- Clear cell adenocarcinoma occurs most often in females aged <30 years with a history of exposure to diethylstilbestrol (DES) in utero.
- Mixed Müllerian sarcomas and leiomyosarcomas in the adult population: mean age is 60 years.

Pediatric Considerations

Vaginal tumors are extremely rare. Rhabdomyosarcoma (botryoid and embryonal subtype) is the most common malignant neoplasm of the vagina in children, and can be part of a cancer syndrome (NF-1, Li-Fraumeni, Beckwith-Wiedemann). Less common entities are germ cell tumor and clear cell adenocarcinoma.

Prevalence

In the United States, it is one of the rarest of all gynecologic malignancies

ETIOLOGY AND PATHOPHYSIOLOGY

- Women with a history of cervical malignancy have a higher probability of developing squamous cell malignancy in the vagina, even after hysterectomy.
- Human papillomavirus (HPV) is found in 80–93% of patients with vaginal CIS and 50–65% of the patients with invasive vaginal carcinoma.
- HPV-16 is the most common, found in 66% of CIS and 55% of invasive vaginal cancers.
- There is a higher risk of vaginal cancer in patients who smoke cigarettes.
- Clear cell adenocarcinoma of the vagina in young women has been associated with DES exposure in utero. The incidence, however, is exceedingly rare, estimated at 1/1,000 to 1/10,000 exposed females.
- Metastatic lesions can involve the vagina, spreading from the other gynecologic organs.
- Although rare, renal cell carcinoma, lung adenocarcinoma, GI cancer, pancreatic adenocarcinoma, ovarian germ cell cancer, trophoblastic neoplasm, and breast cancer can all metastasize to the vagina

Genetics

There is no known genetic pattern

RISK FACTORS

- Similar risk factors as cervical cancer, including smoking, HPV exposure, immunodeficiency
- Age
- African American
- Multiple sex partners, early age of first sexual intercourse
- History of squamous cell cancer of the cervix or vulva
- Vaginal adenosis, often associated with DES exposure
- Vaginal irritation
- DES exposure in utero
- Prior pelvic radiation

COMMONLY ASSOCIATED CONDITIONS

Due to field effect, patients with vaginal cancer are more likely to develop malignancy in the cervix or vulva and should be followed closely.

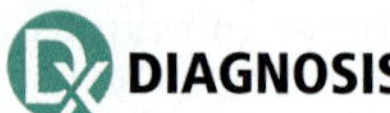

DIAGNOSIS

HISTORY

- Abnormal bleeding is the most common symptom.
- Postcoital bleeding can result from direct trauma to the tumor.
- Vaginal discharge
- Dyspareunia
- Urinary symptoms, including hematuria and increased frequency
- Constipation
- Pain along with symptoms and signs of hydroureter/nephrosis are late findings when the tumor has spread into the paravaginal tissues and extends to the pelvic sidewall.

Pediatric Considerations

In children, sarcomas can present either as a mass protruding from the vagina or as abnormal genital bleeding.

PHYSICAL EXAM

Pelvic examination

- The vagina, uterus, adnexa (fallopian tubes and ovaries), bladder, and rectum should be evaluated for unusual changes by direct visual inspection and by palpation.
- Vaginal malignancies are found most commonly on the posterior wall in the upper 1/3 of the vagina.

DIFFERENTIAL DIAGNOSIS

- Premalignant changes: VAIN 1, 2, 3, and CIS
- Adequate biopsies ensure that invasive lesions are not overlooked. Invasive lesions penetrate the basement membrane and cannot be treated conservatively.
- Other malignancies, such as endometrial, cervix, bladder, or colon cancer, can invade directly into the vagina or metastasize to the vagina.
- In the childbearing years, trophoblastic disease should be considered.
  - The vagina is a common site of metastases; however, biopsy in the office should be done with care because the implants are highly vascularized and may hemorrhage if sampled.
  - The clinical presentation is typically obvious so histopathologic confirmation before treatment is not always required.

DIAGNOSTIC TESTS & INTERPRETATION

Initial Tests (lab, imaging)

- Pap smear and gynecologic exams may incidentally detect asymptomatic lesions.
- Biopsy suspicious lesions.
- Vaginal colposcopy and directed biopsies should be undertaken in women with abnormal vaginal cytology.
- In the case of suspected dysplasia, wide excision under anesthesia may be necessary to ensure that invasive cancer is not present.
- In known or suspected invasive cancer, exam under anesthesia, cystoscopy to rule out bladder invasion, and proctosigmoidoscopy to rule out rectal invasion can be undertaken.
- Chest x-ray (CXR): to evaluate for metastatic disease
- MRI with vaginal gel can be used to evaluate for direct locoregional extension.
- CT scan: to evaluate the liver and retroperitoneum, especially the lymph nodes in the pelvic, para-aortic, and inguinal regions.
- PET scan detects primary and secondary metastatic lesions more often than CT scan.

Follow-Up Tests & Special Considerations

- Lymphoscintigraphy (sentinel lymph node mapping) as part of the pretreatment evaluation can result in a change in the radiation fields and improve comprehensive treatment planning in women with vaginal cancer.

- PET and CT can diagnose local and regional lymphatic involvement and result in a change of radiation fields, improving considerations for treatment.
- HPV vaccination: Implementation of prophylactic HPV vaccination could theoretically prevent ~2/3 of the intraepithelial lesions in the lower genital tract; however given the low incidence of vaginal dysplasia and cancer, this has not yet been directly studied.

Test Interpretation

The International Federation of Gynecology and Obstetrics (FIGO) system is used and the clinical stage of vaginal cancer which is not changed once treatment has started.

- Tumors are staged clinically:
  - Stage I: carcinoma limited to the vaginal wall (26%)
  - Stage II: involves the subvaginal tissues but has not extended to the pelvic wall (37%)
  - Stage III: extends to the pelvic sidewall (24%)
  - Stage IV: extends beyond the true pelvis (13%)
    - IVa: Tumor invades bladder and/or rectal mucosa and/or direct extension beyond the true pelvis.
    - IVb: spread to distant organs
- The pTNM classification of the American Joint Committee on Cancer (AJCC) is used for pathologic staging.

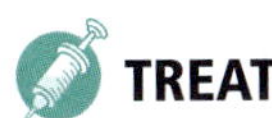

TREATMENT

GENERAL MEASURES

Patients with premalignant or invasive malignancies of the vagina should be referred to a gynecologist or gynecologic oncologist. Diagnoses and presence or absence of invasion must be established with certainty prior to treatment. Treatment methods for premalignant changes such as VAIN and CIS include the following:

- Wide local excision
- Partial or total vaginectomy
- Topical therapy with imiquimod or fluorouracil (5-FU) cream
- Laser therapy
- Intracavitary radiation therapy (very rarely used for premalignant diagnoses)

TREATMENT OF INVASIVE DISEASE

These patients are often elderly, and aggressive therapy may be limited by the patient's performance status and ability to tolerate radical surgery, chemotherapy, or radiation.

- Treatment with radiotherapy or surgery depends on the stage of disease; it is common to use radiotherapy and radiosensitizing cisplatin chemotherapy (chemoradiation) for better cancer control.
- Early-stage primary squamous cell carcinoma treated with radiation alone has shown good results.
- Neoadjuvant chemotherapy followed by radical surgery may benefit selected patients.
- Immunotherapies may offer benefit in specific types of metastatic vaginal cancers
- With one exception, no chemotherapeutic agents have shown a survival advantage. The exception is childhood sarcomas, which have been treated with combinations of the following: actinomycin-D, Cytoxan, VP-16

SURGERY/OTHER PROCEDURES

- Whenever there is a doubt as to the presence or absence of invasive disease, vaginectomy must be performed.
- Invasive lesions usually are treated by radiation therapy, but stage I lesions can be treated with radical hysterectomy or radical vaginectomy with pelvic lymph node dissection.
- If the lesion involves the lower vagina, inguinal node dissection also must be done because cancer involving the lower vagina can metastasize to the groin region (inguinal–femoral nodes).
- Premenopausal women who desire to retain ovarian function are better candidates for radical surgery for early-stage disease, with vaginal reconstruction possible afterward.
- Patients who have not completed their family can occasionally be treated with limited resection and localized radiation to the area.
- Sarcomas are treated by radiation therapy followed by pelvic exenteration if persistent disease is present.

Pediatric Considerations

The treatment of vaginal tumors today mainly consists of neoadjuvant chemotherapy followed by local control with surgery or radiotherapy.

Geriatric Considerations

Treatment of older patients, who often have more comorbidities and increased frailty, needs to be tailored properly based on anticipated tolerance of treatment and potential side effects as well as goals of care.

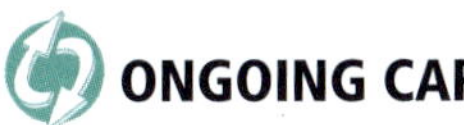

ONGOING CARE

FOLLOW-UP RECOMMENDATIONS

- Patients are usually ambulatory and able to resume full activity by 6 weeks after surgery, depending on the extent of the procedure undertaken.
- Many patients are fully active while receiving chemotherapy and radiation therapy.

Patient Monitoring

Is dependent on the initial stage and grade of the cancer and subsequent risk of recurrence; interval pelvic exam with direct inspection and palpation of the vaginal mucosa are paramount; cytology and imaging can be used dependent on prior therapies and probability of recurrence; in general, routine imaging is not recommended in the absence of clinical suspicion for disease.

PATIENT EDUCATION

- National Cancer Center: https://www.cancer.gov/types/vaginal
- Foundation For Women's Cancer: https://foundationforwomenscancer.org/gynecologic-cancers/gynecologic-cancer-types/vaginal-cancer/
- Centers for Disease Control and Prevention: https://www.cdc.gov/vaginal-vulvar-cancers/resources/index.html
- Medscape: https://emedicine.medscape.com/article/2156399-overview

PROGNOSIS

Stage is the most important determinant of survival; tumor size >2 cm, correlated with worse survival outcome; stage and 5-year survival:

- I: 77.6%
- II: 52.2%
- III: 42.5%
- IVA: 20.5%
- IVB: 12.9%

COMPLICATIONS

- Those typically associated with major abdominal surgery or radiation therapy
- Common complications of treatment include rectovaginal or vesicovaginal fistulas, rectal/vaginal strictures, radiation cystitis, and/or proctitis.
- Most recurrences occur within the first 2 years after initial diagnosis.

REFERENCES

1. U.S. Cancer Statistics Data Visualizations Tool. Centers for Disease Control and Prevention. https://www.cdc.gov/united-states-cancer-statistics/dataviz/index.html. Accessed December 24, 2024.
2. Jhingran A. Updates in the treatment of vaginal cancer. *Int J Gynecol Cancer*. 2022;32(3):344–351. doi:10.1136/ijgc-2021-002517.
3. Soo-Hoo S, Luesley D. Vulval and vaginal cancer in pregnancy. *Best Pract Res Clin Obstet Gynaecol*. 2016;33:73–78.

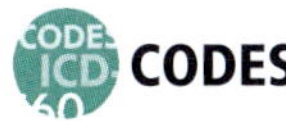

CODES

ICD10

- C52 Malignant neoplasm of vagina
- D07.2 Carcinoma in situ of vagina
- N89.3 Dysplasia of vagina, unspecified

CLINICAL PEARLS

- Vaginal cancer is rare; 85–90% of vaginal cancers are squamous cell.
- Vaginal malignancies are found most commonly on the posterior wall in the upper 1/3 of the vagina.
- Most vaginal malignancies are metastatic (from cervix, vulva, endometrium, breast, or ovary).

VAGINITIS AND VAGINOSIS

Tatiana Cordova, MD • Andrea Soto Abarca, MD • Prit M. Dhagat, DO, MPH

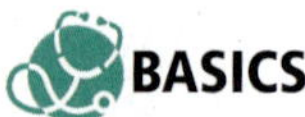

BASICS

DESCRIPTION

- "Vaginosis" and "vaginitis" are broad terms indicating any process of the vagina caused by or leading to infection, inflammation, or changes in the normal vaginal flora. The difference between vaginitis and vaginosis is the presence (vaginitis) or absence (vaginosis) of inflammation.
- The most common causes are bacterial vaginosis (BV), vulvovaginal candidiasis (VVC), trichomoniasis, and cytolytic vaginosis. Noninfectious causes (<10%) can include atrophic, irritant, allergic, and inflammatory vaginitis.
- Normal physiologic vaginal discharge is clear to white, not malodorous, not associated with pain or pruritus, and the quantity varies during menses.

EPIDEMIOLOGY

- Vaginal symptoms represent one of the most frequent reasons women seek medical care, accounting for approximately 10 million office visits each year (1).
- BV is the most common cause with an estimated 7.4 million cases per year, followed by VVC as the second most common cause of vaginitis in reproductive-aged women (2).

Prevalence

- Prevalence rates of BV are of 15% in pregnant women, 20–25% in young females at student health clinics, and up to 30–40% among women seen at sexually transmitted infection (STI) clinics (1).
- Non-White women have higher rates of BV (African American 51%, Mexican Americans 32%) than White women (23%).
- 29–40% of all females report at least one episode of VVC.
- Vaginal trichomoniasis is a common STI with 3 to 5 million cases diagnosed in the United States yearly (2).
- African-American women are 10 times more commonly affected by vaginal trichomoniasis when compared to White and Hispanic women (2).
- Desquamative inflammatory vaginitis (DIV) is found in 2–20% of women (1).

ETIOLOGY AND PATHOPHYSIOLOGY

- BV is caused by a change in the normal vaginal flora with an increase of facultative anaerobic organisms and the lack of hydrogen peroxide producing lactobacilli (2).
  - Increased pH, and a malodorous, clear, white, or gray discharge with fishy odor
  - Organisms associated include *Gardnerella vaginalis, Prevotella* spp., *Bacteroides* spp., *Peptostreptococcus* spp., *Mycoplasma hominis, Ureaplasma urealyticum*, *Fusobacterium* spp., or *Atopobium vaginae.*
  - Not directly caused by sexual transmission, although strongly associated with other STI's
- VVC is caused by *Candida* spp., particularly *Candida albicans* (80–92%) and *Candida glabrata* (<10%).
  - *Candida* can be identified in the lower genital tract in healthy women, and it is thought to gain access via rectal and perianal colonization and migration.
  - Symptoms occur when candidal organisms overwhelm the normal vaginal flora and invade the superficial vaginal epithelial cells.
  - Complicated VVC should be considered in immunocompromised patients (pregnancy, diabetes, etc.), those who experience ≥4 episodes of VVC in a year or those who have only budding yeast on wet mount.
- Trichomoniasis is caused by an infection via *Trichomonas vaginalis*. The organism infects the squamous epithelium of the vagina, urethra, and paraurethral glands; primarily transmitted during intercourse
- DIV is a chronic, purulent vaginitis with uncertain etiology or pathogenesis. Inflammation is cardinal feature. The vagina is colonized with facultative bacteria, not the obligate anaerobic bacteria that colonize the vagina in BV (1).
- Atrophic vaginitis symptoms result from a lack of estrogen while irritant/allergic vaginitis symptoms can result from mechanical, chemical, or allergic irritation.

RISK FACTORS

- BV
  - Although traditionally *not* considered an STI, there is mounting evidence that sexual transmission is a key driver of persistence and recurrence (3)[B].
  - Women who have sex with women, smoking, vaginal douching, low socioeconomic status, other STIs such as HSV-2, use of an IUD.
  - Male circumcision decreases risk.
- VVC—diabetes, recent antibiotics use, immunosuppression, higher estrogen levels, estrogen-containing contraceptives
- Trichomoniasis—inconsistent use of barrier contraception, multiple sexual partners, limited education and low socioeconomic status, illicit drug use, smoking, coexistent STIs, douching, incarceration (2)
- Other risk factors associated with vaginitis/vaginosis: decreased estrogen; smoking; use of creams, gels, or lubricants; tight-fitting clothing; poor hygienic practice; changes in diet; condoms, sex toys, tampons

GENERAL PREVENTION

- Vulvar hygiene with warm water and unscented cleanser; advise patients not to douche. Wear cotton underwear.
- Except in cases of trichomoniasis, treatment of sexual partners is not recommended but may be considered in recurrent cases.

COMMONLY ASSOCIATED CONDITIONS

- STIs (gonorrhea, chlamydia, HSV, or HIV)
- Vaginal intraepithelial neoplasia and cancer can present with symptoms of vaginitis.

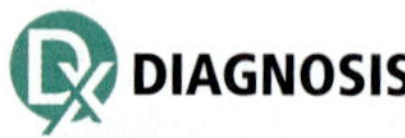

DIAGNOSIS

HISTORY

- General principles:
  - It is important to distinguish vulvar versus vaginal symptoms.
  - Onset, timing, severity, duration, and character of the vaginal symptoms are important to discern.
  - Symptomatic patients complain of itching, burning, irritation, dyspareunia, and abnormal discharge.
  - Other topics to discuss: age, menstrual status and relation to cycle, discharge characteristics (color, consistency, amount, odor), recurrence of symptoms, sexual history (including risk factors for STIs, number of partners, gender identification, specific sexual practices), vulvovaginal hygiene practices (shaving, douching), self-treatment (OTC medications), and other underlying medical conditions (DM, HIV, IBD) (2)
- BV: thin, homogenous discharge characterized by a "fishy" odor; pain and pruritus are uncommon.
- VVC: itching, burning, irritation, dyspareunia, dysuria, and a white thick discharge; odor is uncommon.
- Trichomoniasis: Majority will have minimal or no genitourinary symptoms (70–85%). Symptomatic patients will complain of abnormal discharge, itching, burning, or postcoital bleeding (2).
- DIV: Purulent discharge with burning, dyspareunia, and/or introital pain; homogenous yellowish discharge with no fishy smell (1)

PHYSICAL EXAM

- Physical exam should begin with a thorough evaluation of the vulva and the skin surrounding the anus (2).
- BV—thin, watery discharge (clear to gray or tan colored) with an amine or "fishy" smell; vaginal epithelium should appear normal and noninflamed; does not affect vulva
- VVC—erythema and swelling of the vulva and vaginal mucosa with cottage cheese-like discharge of variable thickness; vulvar excoriations and fissures may be present; lack of odor
- Trichomoniasis—yellow/green, frothy discharge with foul odor; discharge can appear purulent. Vulvar or vaginal erythema can be visualized. Punctate hemorrhages can be seen on the cervix ("strawberry cervix").
- DIV—purulent discharge and vaginal inflammation; submucosal cervicovaginal petechiae; no fishy smell

DIFFERENTIAL DIAGNOSIS

Physiologic discharge; leukorrhea of pregnancy; STIs; foreign body; contact dermatitis; cervicitis; urinary tract infection; atrophic vaginitis; dermatoses: lichen sclerosus, lichen planus, seborrheic dermatitis, psoriasis; genitourinary syndrome of menopause (2)

DIAGNOSTIC TESTS & INTERPRETATION

Initial Tests (lab, imaging)

- BV
  - Clinical diagnosis is established with Amsel criteria (2); positive diagnosis can be made if meeting 3 out of 4:
    - Thin, homogenous discharge that smoothly coats vaginal wall
    - Vaginal pH >4.5
    - A positive amine or "Whiff" test with use of KOH solution added to discharge
    - >20% of the epithelial cells identified as "clue cells"; most reliable indicator
  - Nucleic acid amplification tests (NAAT) for multiple bacterial species may be considered if Amsel criteria cannot be reliably collected in symptomatic patients suspected of having recurrent BV (4)
- VVC
  - Visualization of blastospores or pseudohyphae on saline or 10% KOH microscopy
  - Culture or NAAT may be useful if recurrent symptomatic infection.
- Trichomoniasis
  - Visualization of motile trichomonads on saline microscopy
  - NAAT is preferred as microscopy has limited sensitivity (50–60%) (2).
  - Several POC tests, including patient performed, are available with increased sensitivity compared to microscopy but are expensive.
- DIV
  - Wet mount with increase in inflammatory cells and parabasal (immature) squamous epithelial cells, pH >4.5
  - Wet mount is preferred diagnostic method.

Follow-Up Tests & Special Considerations

- BV/VVC/trichomoniasis—new testing modalities such as oligonucleotide probes and NAATs may be used for patient comfort, but outcomes are not clearly improved compared to more standard diagnostic methods, and the tests are expensive.
- It is important to consider other vaginitis/vaginosis causes such as cytolytic vaginosis and atrophic vaginitis when symptoms persist despite treatment or negative testing.
- Cytolytic vaginosis can have similar presentation as VVC by history and physical exam and can be associated with periods of high estrogen such as luteal phase of menses.

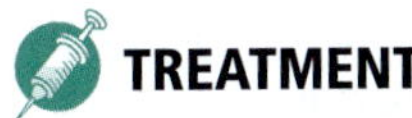

TREATMENT

GENERAL MEASURES

- Avoid douching and tight-fitting clothing.
- Regular use of condoms may help to prevent BV (2).
- Consider avoiding use of tampons during intravaginal treatment to ensure adequate dispersion of medication.
- BV and vulvovaginal candidal infections only require treatment if symptomatic, incidental findings on Pap smear or other tests need not be treated if patient is asymptomatic (2).

MEDICATION

Medication recommendations based on Centers for Disease Control and Prevention (CDC) treatment guidelines and American College of Obstetricians and Gynecologists (ACOG) practice bulletin

First Line

- BV
  - Metronidazole 500 mg orally BID for 7 days, or 0.75% gel 1 full applicator (5 g) vaginally daily for 5 days, or clindamycin 2% cream vaginally daily for 5 to 7 days
  - Recurrent infection may require repeated intravaginal treatment twice weekly for 4 to 6 months. In addition to standard therapy, oral metronidazole 400 mg BID and topical (clindamycin 2% cream BID) antimicrobial treatment of male partners, reduces the risk of BV recurrence (3)[B]. Advise patients to avoid alcohol during treatment with oral metronidazole and for 24 hours following.
- VVC
  - Uncomplicated infections can be treated with a one-time dose of fluconazole 150 mg tab or topical/vaginal suppository antifungal regimens such as clotrimazole, miconazole, or nystatin creams. Treatment can range from 3 to 7 days.
  - Severe infections may require multi dose treatment of oral fluconazole (2 to 3 doses every 3 days).
  - Recurrent infections (≥4 in 1 year) may require fluconazole 150 mg 3 times in 1st week, then weekly for up to 6 months. Evidence is insufficient to recommend one specific regimen over another.
  - Avoid oral azoles in pregnant women.
  - Advise patients that topical medications may weaken rubber or latex condoms.
- Trichomoniasis
  - Metronidazole 500 mg orally BID for 7 days
  - Partner should be treated as well and counseled to abstain from sex until both patients have completed treatment and are asymptomatic (2).
  - Test of cure is not necessary, although retesting 3 months after initial treatment is acceptable (2).
- DIV
  - Address estrogen deficiency.
  - Clindamycin 2% cream intravaginally at bedtime for 1 to 3 weeks
  - May need additional maintenance therapy

Second Line

- BV—secnidazole 2 g orally once or tinidazole/ clindamycin orally for 2 to 5 days; avoid alcohol during treatment with and 72 hours after tinidazole.
- VVC
  - Recurrent infections benefit from speciation to help determine treatment course.
  - Nonalbican candidiasis may require longer duration of treatment with topical or oral azoles, boric acid (vaginal suppository 600 mg daily for 7 days for acute VVC, 2 weeks for recurrent VVC).
- Trichomoniasis—one-time 2 g oral dose of either tinidazole or metronidazole
- DIV—topical glucocorticoid such as hydrocortisone cream 300 to 500 mg intravaginally nightly for 3 weeks or clobetasol intravaginally nightly for 1 week

ONGOING CARE

FOLLOW-UP RECOMMENDATIONS

- Delay sexual relations until symptoms clear/ discomfort resolves. Use of condoms may reduce recurrence of BV.
- Consider suppressive therapy for recurrent infection, and partner treatment when appropriate. Monthly treatment may help reduce colonization of bacteria associated with BV.

Patient Monitoring

No specific follow-up needed; if symptoms persist or recur within 2 months, repeat pelvic exam and culture.

PATIENT EDUCATION

ACOG: https://www.acog.org

PROGNOSIS

VVC: 80–90% of uncomplicated cases cured with appropriate treatment; 30–50% of recurrent infections return after discontinuation of maintenance therapy; high spontaneous remission rate of untreated symptoms as well

COMPLICATIONS

- BV has been associated with an increased risk of HIV and other STIs.
- BV has been associated with increased risk of preterm birth, chorioamnionitis, postpartum and postabortal endometritis, and pelvic inflammatory disease.
- VVC may occur following treatment of BV.

REFERENCES

1. Paavonen J, Brunham RC. Bacterial vaginosis and desquamative inflammatory vaginitis. *N Engl J Med*. 2018;379(23):2246–2254.
2. American College of Obstetricians and Gynecologists. Vaginitis in nonpregnant patients: ACOG practice bulletin, number 215. *Obstet Gynecol*. 2020;135(1):e1–e17.
3. Vodstrcil LA, Plummer EL, Fairley CK, et al. Male-partner treatment to prevent recurrence of bacterial vaginosis. *N Engl J Med*. 2025;392(10):947–957.
4. Yazdy GM, Mitchell C, Sobel JD, et al. Recurrent infectious vaginitis: a practical approach for the primary care clinician. *Med Clin North Am*. 2024;108(2):373–392.

ADDITIONAL READING

Paladine HL, Desai UA. Vaginitis: diagnosis and treatment. *Am Fam Physician*. 2018;97(5):321–329.

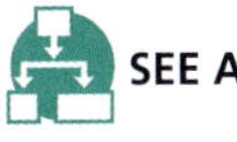

SEE ALSO

Algorithm: Vaginal Discharge

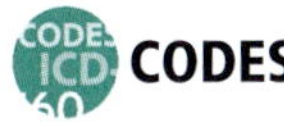

CODES

ICD10

- N76.0 Acute vaginitis
- B37.3 Candidiasis of vulva and vagina
- N95.2 Postmenopausal atrophic vaginitis

CLINICAL PEARLS

- Most women experience relief of symptoms with appropriate therapy chosen.
- Vaginal pH is underused as a diagnostic tool for evaluation of vaginitis.
- Asymptomatic BV and VVC infections do not require treatment.

V

VARICOSE VEINS

Christopher George Bentsen, MD • Daniel Michniuk, DO, MS

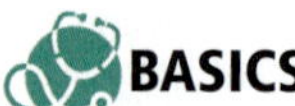

BASICS

Varicose veins (VV), or varicosities, are dilated, tortuous, subcutaneous veins of at least 4 mm in diameter, measured with the patient in the upright position. VV is part of a spectrum of chronic venous disorders ranging from telangiectasias to chronic venous insufficiency. Ovarian vein failure can also cause pelvic VV and subsequently pelvic congestion syndrome.

DESCRIPTION

- Lower extremity venous drainage is accomplished via a network of superficial veins > small perforator veins > deep veins; diseases in any of these systems may result in VV.
- VV usually form in the great and small saphenous veins and their branches.

Geriatric Considerations

- Surgeries have low morbidity and mortality in patients aged >60 years, with significant self-reported improvement despite more advanced disease on presentation.
- High-risk geriatric patients should avoid hybrid procedures and general anesthesia when possible.

Pregnancy Considerations

External compression is first-line treatment in pregnant females.

EPIDEMIOLOGY

Treatment of late complications of VV, such as chronic venous ulcerations, costs an estimated $3 billion per year in the United States.

Prevalence

Approximately 23% of US adults have VV, affecting an estimated 22 million women and 11 million men between 40 and 80 years old; 2 million will develop symptoms.

ETIOLOGY AND PATHOPHYSIOLOGY

Exact pathophysiology is debated, but involves: venous hypertension, valve dysfunction, structural changes in the vessel wall, inflammation, alteration of shear wall stress, and genetic disposition.

- Venous hypertension is caused by reflux from valvular incompetence, outflow obstruction, calf muscle failure, increased intra-abdominal pressure from pregnancy, obesity, chronic constipation, tumors, or other proximal obstruction.
- Valve dysfunction may be due to deformation, tearing, thinning, adhesion of the valve leaflets, vein wall stiffening with failed leaflet fit, trauma, deep thrombophlebitis, and congenital valvular incompetence.
- Structural changes in the vein wall (disruption of smooth muscle cells and elastic fibers, etc.) leads to vessel dilation and weakening.
- Turbulent flow, reflux, and increases in shear stress, promotes inflammatory and prothrombotic changes that further contribute to the loss of wall and leaflet integrity.
- Deep venous insufficiency can lead to secondary VV via enlarging collaterals.

Genetics

VV is highly polygenic; a cohort study of >500,000 individuals has linked genetic associations with 30 new loci, the strongest occurring in intron region CASZ1 (implicated in blood pressure) and 16q24 (genes encoding a vascular mechanosensory channel).

RISK FACTORS

- Inherited: gender, tall height (>180 cm), congenital syndromes
- Acquired: age, deep vein thrombosis (DVT), pregnancy, decreased leg impedance
- Lifestyle: prolonged standing and/or sitting, tobacco use, obesity
- Hormonal: female gender (high estrogen state)
- Socioeconomic: lower education level

GENERAL PREVENTION

Maintain a healthy body mass index, avoid sitting or standing for prolonged periods of time, and wear compression stockings.

COMMONLY ASSOCIATED CONDITIONS

- Stasis dermatitis
- Lipodermatosclerosis (chronic inflammation and fibrosis causing skin hyperpigmentation and underlying fat hardening)
- Venous ulceration (usually near medial malleolus/gaiter area)

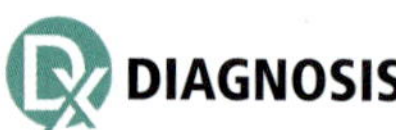

DIAGNOSIS

HISTORY

- Symptoms range from asymptomatic, cosmetic concerns, to debilitating complaints.
- Localized symptoms: pain/tingling, burning, itching
- Generalized symptoms: leg cramp, fatigue, swelling and heaviness
- Symptoms often worse at the end of the day and after prolonged standing
- Women are more prone to symptoms due to hormonal influences; usually worse during menses

PHYSICAL EXAM

- Inspection
  - Performed while the patient is standing; VV in proximal femoral ring and distal legs may not be visible when the patient is supine.
  - Telangiectasias (spider veins) are small, dilated blood vessels (arteriole, venule or capillary)
  - VV features:
    - Dilated, tortuous superficial veins, ≥4 mm in diameter
    - Dark purple/blue and raised above the surface of the skin
    - Often twisted, bulging, and cord-like
    - Most commonly found on the posterior/medial lower extremity
  - Skin changes may include erythema, eczema, hemosiderosis, atrophie blanche, lipodermatosclerosis, and ulcers (most often above the medial malleus).
  - Edema of the affected limb may be present.
  - Atrophy blanche, fan shaped VV in ankle (corona phlebectatica) and lipodermatosclerosis are signs of advanced venous disease.
  - Vulva, perineal, or groin VV may be a sign of pelvic vein incompetence or obstruction due to abdominal, pelvic or renal mass.
- Palpation
  - Palpate saphenofemoral junction (SFJ) ~4 cm inferolateral to pubic tubercle for any saphena varix.
- Bedside tests have limited value, as follows:
  - Tap test: Examiner place 1 finger on the SFJ and uses another hand to tap along the VV. A thrill will be felt on the SFJ if the examiner taps on a defective vein. A healthy valve will block the transmission of the thrill.
  - Cough test: Examiner palpates the SFJ for a thrill when the patient coughs.
- Duplex ultrasound has largely replaced the tourniquet tests.
  - Trendelenburg positioning locates the defective valves. Patient lies supine and elevates the leg. Once venous blood is drained, the examiner ties a tourniquet on the leg, and the patient stands. If the VV remains flat, the defect is above the tourniquet level. If the VV fills back up, the defect is below the tourniquet level. The examiner repeats the test until the site of the defect is found.
  - Perthes test assesses the deep system. Patient lies supine and the examiner ties a tourniquet around the upper thigh. Patient then walks for 5 minutes. Persistent VV indicates deep vein pathology. VV disappears if deep venous system is competent.

DIFFERENTIAL DIAGNOSIS

- For lower extremity pain: arthritis, peripheral neuritis, deep vein thrombosis, superficial thrombophlebitis, ischemia
- For lower extremity ulcers: arterial/venous insufficiency, neuropathic, infection, trauma, vasculitis, drugs (e.g., warfarin skin necrosis, heparin-induced thrombocytopenia), inflammatory disorders (e.g., pyoderma gangrenosum, panniculitis)

DIAGNOSTIC TESTS & INTERPRETATION

Initial Tests (lab, imaging)

Venous duplex ultrasonography is recommended for severe disease requiring intervention. It can determine saphenous junction competency, the junction diameter, the extent of the reflux, and the location and size of the affected vein. It can also assess for DVT and thrombophlebitis (1).

Follow-Up Tests & Special Considerations

- Lab tests are only needed to rule out other differentials.
- Magnetic resonance imaging, venography, and plethysmography are used if venous ultrasound is inconclusive or for complex surgical situations.

Test Interpretation
- The clinical, etiologic, anatomic, pathophysiologic (CEAP) is the gold standard of classification for chronic venous disorders.
- Uncomplicated:
  - C0: no visible or palpable signs of venous disease
  - C1: telangiectasias or reticular veins
- Local symptoms and complication:
  - C2: VV; CV2r: recurrent VV
  - C3: edema
- Complex varicose disease:
  - C4a: pigmentation or eczema; C4b: lipodermatosclerosis or atrophie blanch, C4c: corona phlebectatica
  - C5: healed venous ulcer
  - C6: active venous ulcer; C6r: recurrent active venous ulcer

TREATMENT
- VV is not curable due to irreversible damage to the veins and valves.
- Indications for treatment include pain, aching, heaviness, fatigue, burning, edema, stasis dermatitis, recurrent superficial phlebitis, or ulceration
- Management options (most treatment involves multiple modalities and repetition): lifestyle modifications, compression therapy, local ablative therapies, surgery, and endovenous ablative therapies
- Lifestyle modification
  - Elevation of feet to at least heart level for 30 minutes 4 times daily
  - Avoid prolonged standing (moving side to side when possible), sitting, and sitting with legs hanging down.
  - Weight loss, exercise (walking), and foot flexion exercises to improve calf muscle pump function
- Compression stockings while awake; indicated as first line in pregnant women, if interventional treatment is ineffective, and presence of active or healed venous ulcer. Trial of compression therapy may be required before approval of interventional therapies by insurance. Non-adherence rate ~60% due to difficulty with application.

MEDICATION
- Low-dose diuretics have minimal effect.
- Topical steroids are helpful with stasis dermatitis.
- Oral and topical therapies called phlebotonics may reduce symptoms of chronic venous insufficiency. Diosmiplex (Vasculera) is a prescription medical food not FDA-approved or regulated as a drug.

ISSUES FOR REFERRAL
National Institute for Health and Care Excellence (NICE) recommends referral of patients with:
- Symptomatic primary (or recurrent) VV
- Skin changes
- Superficial venous thrombosis
- Active and healed leg ulcers

SURGERY/OTHER PROCEDURES
- Sclerotherapy, surgery, and endovenous ablation: Indicated if noninvasive measures fail, cosmetic concerns, recurrent hemorrhage, and superficial thrombophlebitis; contraindicated in pregnancy, acute venous thromboembolism, and peripheral artery disease (PAD) (ankle brachial index <0.9); sclerotherapy is likely safe and at least somewhat effective for cosmesis and symptoms (2)[A].
- Local ablative therapy: for telangiectasias and reticular veins
  - Chemical (sclerotherapy) or heat-based (thermoregulation, cutaneous laser) endothelial injury resulting in sclerosis of the vein's endothelium, converting the vein into connective tissue over time
  - Liquid or foam sclerotherapy
    - Results in cosmetic improvement in 70% of patients and a patient satisfaction rate >70%
    - Gives best result when compression stocking are worn 7 to 10 days after the procedure.
    - Complications include allergic reactions to the sclerosant, hyperpigmentation, superficial thread-like capillaries causing a blue discoloration (matting), cellulitis, and rarely, ulceration or thromboembolism.
    - Ultrasound-guided foam sclerotherapy (UFGS) is useful in treating perforator vein reflux with improved outcomes from increased adhesion to the veins (3)[C].
    - Notably, sclerotherapy does not have the same long-term success compared to endovenous thermal ablation (EVTA) methods in thick-walled veins but is the preferred method for small-diameter of thin-walled veins (3)[C].
- Surgery: for large branch, residual postablation VV and saphenous VV
  - Surgical stripping
    - Less used with the development of less invasive procedures and up to 50% recurrence rate by 5 years
    - Complications include extensive ecchymosis, scarring, hematoma, lymphocele, infection, nerve damage, and DVT
  - CHIVA/stab phlebectomy:
    - French acronym for Conservatrice Hémodynamique de l'Insuffisance Veineuse en Ambulatoire (ambulatory conservative hemodynamic treatment of venous insufficiency); aims to alleviate signs and symptoms without destroying the vein
    - The surgeon maps the affected veins with ultrasound, makes a few small incisions, and ties off the veins.
    - Only requires local anesthesia and leaves minimal scars; thus reducing VV recurrence and fewer side effects than vein stripping
- EVTA: indicated for saphenous VV; radiofrequency ablation (RFA) uses thermal energy (85–120°C) to seal the incompetent veins via thermal damage. Endovenous laser ablation (EVLA) uses laser and fiber-optic catheters to generate thermal energy (up to 800°C) to induce venous fibrosis.
  - 3 years estimated pooled success rates of 84% for RFA, 92% for EVLA compared to 78% in surgical stripping
  - Recommended by NICE as first-line treatment of truncal vein incompetence
  - RFA has a much lower subsequence incidence of thromboembolism and PAD compared to other treatments.
  - Mechanochemical endovenous ablation (MOCA) is a hybrid system composed of a nonthermal rotating tip with simultaneous injection of liquid sclerosant. The least painful option and least risk of nerve damage.

COMPLEMENTARY & ALTERNATIVE MEDICINE
Phlebotonics, including horse chestnut seed extract, may ease pain, edema, and itching, but long-term safety and efficacy evidence is lacking (1)[C].

ADMISSION, INPATIENT, AND NURSING CONSIDERATIONS
Encourage compression stockings and frequent ambulation. Ensure both chemical and mechanical VTE prevention.

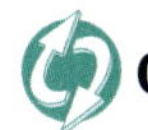

ONGOING CARE

DIET
A low-salt, high-fiber, high-omega3 fatty acid diet and weight-loss are beneficial.

PATIENT EDUCATION
- Avoid long periods of standing and crossing legs.
- Maintain a healthy weight and exercise regularly to improve leg strength and circulation.
- Wear elastic support stockings and avoid clothing that constricts the legs.

PROGNOSIS
- Approximately 10% will progress to advanced chronic venous diseases without treatment or correction of underlying cause, but progression is not linear and is individual to each patient
- Associated with a 5-fold increased risk of DVT and linked to PAD

COMPLICATIONS
- Venous stasis dermatitis, edema, eczema, pigmentation, lipodermatosclerosis
- Venous ulcers +/− superimposed infection, such as superficial thrombophlebitis, and petechial hemorrhages from varicosities
- Recurrence after surgical treatment

REFERENCES

1. Raetz J, Wilson M, Collins K. Varicose veins: diagnosis and treatment. *Am Fam Physician*. 2019;99(11):682–688.
2. de Ávila Oliveira R, Riera R, Vasconcelos V, et al. Injection sclerotherapy for varicose veins. *Cochrane Database Syst Rev*. 2021;12(12):CD001732.
3. Fayyaz F, Vaghani V, Ekhator C, et al. Advancements in varicose vein treatment: anatomy, pathophysiology, minimally invasive techniques, sclerotherapy, patient satisfaction, and future directions. *Cureus*. 2024;16(1):e51990. doi:10.7759/cureus.51990.

ADDITIONAL READING

Alsaigh T, Fukaya E. Varicose veins and chronic venous disease. *Cardiol Clin*. 2021;39(4):567–581.

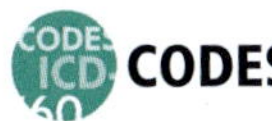

CODES

ICD10
- I83.2 Varicose veins of lower extremities with both ulcer and inflammation
- I83.011 Varicose veins of right lower extremity with ulcer of thigh
- I83.228 Varicose veins of left lower extremity with both ulcer of other part of lower extremity and inflammation

CLINICAL PEARLS
EVTA methods such as RFA and EVLA have been demonstrated to be superior to open surgical techniques for VV treatment with similar improvement in quality of life.

VASCULITIS

Irene J. Tan, MD, FACR

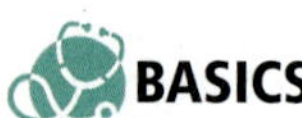

BASICS

DESCRIPTION

An inflammatory disorder of blood vessels

- Clinical features result from the destruction of blood vessel walls with subsequent thrombosis, ischemia, bleeding, and/or aneurysm formation.
- Vasculitis is a heterogeneous group of diseases classified by the size, type, and location of involved blood vessels.
  - Small-vessel vasculitis
    - Antineutrophil cytoplasmic antibodies (ANCA)-associated vasculitis (AAV)
      - Microscopic polyangiitis (MPA)
      - Granulomatosis with polyangiitis (GPA; formerly Wegener granulomatosis)
      - Eosinophilic granulomatosis with polyangiitis (EGPA; formerly Churg-Strauss syndrome)
    - Immune complex small vessel vasculitis
      - Antiglomerular basement membrane (anti-GBM) disease
      - Cryoglobulinemic vasculitis
      - IgA vasculitis (formerly Henoch-Schönlein purpura [HSP])
      - Hypocomplementemic urticarial vasculitis
  - Medium-vessel vasculitis
    - Polyarteritis nodosa (PAN)
    - Kawasaki disease (KD)
  - Large-vessel vasculitis
    - Takayasu arteritis (TAK)
    - Giant cell arteritis (GCA)
- Vasculitis occurs as a primary disorder or secondary to infection, a drug reaction, malignancy, or connective tissue disease.
  - Variable vessel vasculitis
    - Behçet disease
    - Cogan syndrome
  - Single-organ vasculitis
    - Cutaneous leukocytoclastic angiitis
    - Cutaneous arteritis
    - Primary CNS vasculitis
  - Vasculitis associated with systemic disease
    - Lupus vasculitis
    - Rheumatoid vasculitis
    - Sarcoid vasculitis
  - Vasculitis associated with other etiology
    - Hepatitis C–associated cryoglobulinemic vasculitis
    - Hepatitis B–AAV
    - Syphilis-associated aortitis
    - Drug-induced immune complex vasculitis
    - Drug-associated ANCA-AAV
    - Cancer-AAV
- Protean features often delay definitive diagnosis.

EPIDEMIOLOGY

Highly variable, depending on the particular syndrome

- Hypersensitivity vasculitis is most commonly encountered in clinical practice.
- KD, IgA vasculitis, and dermatomyositis are more common in children.
- TAK is most prevalent in young Asian women. GPA, MPA, and EGPA are more common in middle-aged males.
- GCA occurs exclusively in those >50 years of age and is rare in the African-American population.

Incidence

Annual incidence in adults (unless otherwise specified)

- IgA vasculitis: 200 to 700/1 million in children <17 years of age
- GCA: 100 to 170/1 million in white people aged >50 years
- KD: depends on race/age; ~200/1 million
- PAN: 2 to 33/1 million
- GPA: 4 to 15/1 million
- MPA: 1 to 24/1 million
- EGPA: 1 to 3/1 million
- TAK: 2/1 million
- Primary CNS vasculitis: 2/1 million in adults
- Hypersensitivity vasculitis: depends on drug exposure
- Viral-/retroviral-AAV unknown; >90% of cases of cryoglobulinemic vasculitis are associated with hepatitis C.
- Connective tissue disorder–AAV: variable

ETIOLOGY AND PATHOPHYSIOLOGY

- Three major immunopathogenic mechanisms
  - Immune-complex formation: systemic lupus erythematosus (SLE), IgA vasculitis (HSP), and cryoglobulinemic vasculitis
  - ANCA autoantibodies: GPA, MPA, and EGPA
  - Pathogenic T-lymphocyte response: GCA and TAK
- Pathophysiology best understood where known drug triggers have been identified (e.g., antibiotics, sulfonamides, and hydralazine)

Genetics

- Mutation in CECR1 encoding adenosine deaminase 2 is associated with PAN.
- Behçet's syndrome is associated with HLA-B*51.
- IgA vasculitis is associated with HLA-DQA1*01:01, HLA-DQB1*05:01 and HLA-DRB1*01:01.

RISK FACTORS

A combination of genetic susceptibility and environmental exposure likely triggers onset.

GENERAL PREVENTION

Early identification is the key to prevent irreversible organ damage in severe forms of systemic vasculitis.

COMMONLY ASSOCIATED CONDITIONS

Hepatitis C (cryoglobulinemic vasculitis), hepatitis B (PAN), cytomegalovirus (CMV), Epstein-Barr virus (EBV), HIV (viral-/retroviral-AAV), SLE, rheumatoid arthritis (RA), Sjögren syndrome, mixed connective tissue disease (MCTD), dermatomyositis, ankylosing spondylitis, Behçet disease, relapsing polychondritis (CTD-AAV), respiratory tract methicillin-resistant *Staphylococcus aureus* (MRSA) in GPA, levamisole-adulterated cocaine, medications: propylthiouracil, methimazole, hydralazine, minocycline; SARS-CoV-2 infection

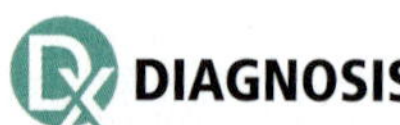

DIAGNOSIS

HISTORY

- Consider age, gender, and ethnicity.
- Comprehensive medication history
- Family history of vasculitis
- Constitutional symptoms: fever, weight loss, malaise, fatigue, diminished appetite, sweats
- CNS/PNS: mononeuritis multiplex, polyneuropathy, headaches, visual loss, tinnitus, stroke, seizure, encephalopathy
- Heart/lung: myocardial infarction, cardiomyopathy, pericarditis, cough, chest pain, hemoptysis, dyspnea
- Renal: hematuria, hypertension
- GI: abdominal pain, hematochezia, perforation
- Musculoskeletal: arthralgia, myalgia
- Miscellaneous: hemoptysis; unexplained ischemic or hemorrhagic events, chronic sinusitis, and recurrent epistaxis
- Note the organs affected and estimate the size of blood vessels involved.
- Demographics, clinical features, and the predominant vessel size/organ involvement help identify specific type of vasculitis.
- Vasculitis is a presenting condition in SARS-CoV-2/COVID-19 infection.

PHYSICAL EXAM

- Vital signs: blood pressure (hypertension) and pulse (regularity, rate, and palpability)
- Skin: palpable purpura, livedo reticularis, nodules, ulcers, gangrene, nail bed capillary changes
- Neurologic: cranial nerve exam, sensorimotor exam
- Ocular exam: visual fields, scleritis, episcleritis
- Cardiopulmonary exam: rubs, murmurs, arrhythmias
- Abdominal exam: tenderness, organomegaly

DIFFERENTIAL DIAGNOSIS

- Fibromuscular dysplasia
- Embolic disease (atheroma, cholesterol emboli, atrial myxoma, mycotic aneurysm with embolization)
- Drug-induced vasospasm (cocaine, amphetamines, ergots)
- Thrombotic thrombocytopenic disorders (disseminated intravascular coagulation [DIC], thrombotic thrombocytopenic purpura [TTP], antiphospholipid syndrome, heparin- or warfarin-induced thrombosis), thromboangiitis obliterans
- Systemic infection (infective endocarditis, fungal infections, disseminated gonococcal infection, Lyme disease, syphilis, Rocky Mountain spotted fever [RMSF], bacteremia, ehrlichiosis, babesiosis)
- Malignancy (lymphomatoid granulomatosis, angioimmunoblastic T-cell lymphoma, intravascular lymphoma)
- Miscellaneous (Goodpasture syndrome, sarcoidosis, amyloidosis, Whipple disease, congenital coarctation of aorta)

DIAGNOSTIC TESTS & INTERPRETATION

ALERT

- Diagnosis rests on a structured clinical evaluation (looking for end-organ involvement).
- Renal disease is often clinically silent. Routine serum creatinine and urinalysis with microscopy are needed to identify underlying glomerulonephritis.
- Tissue specific biopsy is diagnostic (e.g., temporal artery, sural nerve, renal biopsy).

- Initial tests exclude alternate diagnoses and guide therapy.
- Routine tests
  - CBC, serum creatinine, liver enzymes, urinalysis with microscopy, random urine for protein and creatinine
  - Specific serology when appropriate
    - Antinuclear antibodies (ANA); C3, C4
    - Rheumatoid factor (RF); cryoglobulin
    - Rapid plasma reagin/venereal disease reaction level (RPR/VDRL)
    - RMSF titers; Lyme titers
    - ANCA, antiproteinase 3 (anti-PR3), and antimyeloperoxidase (anti-MPO) antibodies
    - Hepatitis screen for B and C; HIV
    - Anti-GBM titer; SARS-CoV-2 RT-PCR and antigen test
    - Serum and urine protein electrophoresis
- Miscellaneous
  - ESR, C-reactive protein; drug screen; creatine kinase (CK); blood culture; ECG
  - Electromyography (EMG); LP
- CXR, high-resolution CT scan, MRI, and arteriography may be required to delineate extent of organs involved.

Diagnostic Procedures/Other

- EMG with nerve conduction can document neuropathy and target nerve for biopsy.
- If biopsy is not practical, angiography may be diagnostic for large- and medium-vessel vasculitides.
- Bronchoscopy may be required to differentiate pulmonary infection from potentially life-threatening hemorrhagic vasculitis in patients with hemoptysis.

Test Interpretation

Blood vessel biopsy shows immune cell infiltration into vessel wall layers with varying degrees of necrosis. Granuloma formation in some, depending on the type.

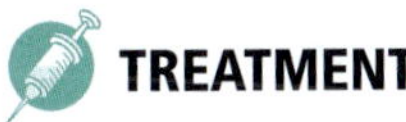

TREATMENT

GENERAL MEASURES

- Discontinue offending drug (hypersensitivity vasculitis).
- Simple observation for mild cases of pediatric IgA vasculitis
- ANCA-AAV has two-phase treatment: initial induction followed by maintenance (steady tapering of corticosteroids with immunosuppressants or immunomodulators).

MEDICATION

First Line

- Therapy moving towards targeted (less-toxic) regimens
- Rituximab often first line (for remission and maintenance), can be in association with (lower dose) glucocorticoids
- Oral 5Ca receptor antagonists emerging as steroid-sparing therapy (particularly if renal involvement)

Second Line

- Cyclophosphamide, methotrexate, and azathioprine in severe/refractory cases
- Plasma exchange is no longer generally recommended except in severe cases.
- Emerging therapies (targeted immunomodulation) include B-cell depleting agents, complement inhibitors, and cell-based therapies.

ISSUES FOR REFERRAL

- Rheumatology for comanagement with biologic agents
- Nephrology referral for persistent hematuria or proteinuria, rising creatinine, or a positive ANCA titer
- Pulmonary referral for persistent pulmonary infiltrate unresponsive to antibiotic therapy or if gross hemoptysis

ADDITIONAL THERAPIES

Plasma exchange does not improve mortality or progression to ESRD in severe ANCA-AAV.

SURGERY/OTHER PROCEDURES

Rarely, corrective surgery is required to repair tissue damage as a result of aggressive vasculitis.

ADMISSION, INPATIENT, AND NURSING CONSIDERATIONS

- Hemoptysis, acute renal failure, intestinal ischemia, any organ-threatening symptoms or signs, and/or need for biopsy
- Initial therapy is guided by the organ system involved.
  - If pulmonary hemorrhage is present, life-saving measures may include mechanical ventilation and immunosuppression.
  - If acute renal failure is present, attend to electrolyte and fluid balance and immunosuppression.
  - If signs of intestinal ischemia are present, make NPO and consider immunosuppression, and parenteral nutrition.
- Discharge criteria: stabilization or resolution of potential life-threatening symptoms

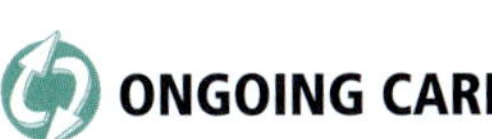

ONGOING CARE

FOLLOW-UP RECOMMENDATIONS

If significant coronary artery disease is involved in KD, moderate activity restriction may be of benefit.

Patient Monitoring

Frequent clinical follow-up supported by patient self-monitoring to identify disease relapse

DIET

Alter diets for patients with renal involvement or hyperglycemia/dyslipidemia.

PROGNOSIS

Prognosis is good for patients with limited organ involvement. Relapsing courses, renal, intestinal, or extensive lung involvement have a poorer prognosis.

COMPLICATIONS

Early morbidity/mortality is due to active vasculitic disease; delayed morbidity/mortality may also be secondary to complications of chronic therapy with cytotoxic medications or subsequent tissue scarring.

ADDITIONAL READING

- Free ME. Emerging cell therapies in the vasculitis field. *Rheumatology (Oxford)*. 2025;64(Suppl 1): i11–i14. doi:10.1093/rheumatology/keae518.
- Kronbichler A, Bajema IM, Bruchfeld A, et al. Diagnosis and management of ANCA-associated vasculitis. *Lancet*. 2024;403(10427):683–698. doi:10.1016/S0140-6736(23)01736-1.
- Robson JC, Grayson PC, Ponte C, et al; for DCVAS Investigators. 2022 American College of Rheumatology/European Alliance of Associations for rheumatology classification criteria for granulomatosis with polyangiitis. *Ann Rheum Dis*. 2022;81(3):315–320.

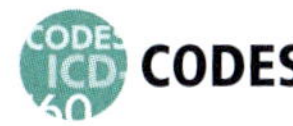

CODES

ICD10

- M31.7 Microscopic polyangiitis
- M31.30 Wegener's granulomatosis without renal involvement
- M31.9 Necrotizing vasculopathy, unspecified

CLINICAL PEARLS

- Suspect vasculitis in patients with a petechial rash, palpable purpura, glomerulonephritis, pulmonary-renal syndrome, intestinal ischemia, or mononeuritis multiplex.
- Exclude silent renal involvement by routinely obtaining serum creatinine, urinalysis with microscopy, and random urine and creatinine.
- Vasculitis has "skip" lesions, which may complicate diagnostic biopsy.
- In patients with vasculitis, look for an underlying inciting process such as medication, infection, thrombosis, or malignancy.

VENOUS INSUFFICIENCY ULCERS

Sahoko Hirano Little, MD, PhD

BASICS

- Venous stasis ulcers are the most common type of chronic leg ulcers, affecting 1–3% of the American population.
- Venous stasis ulcers are the most serious consequence of chronic venous insufficiency, which is a condition that occurs when the venous wall and/or valves in the leg veins are not working effectively, making it difficult for blood to return to the heart and causing stasis.
- Diagnosis is based on history and physical examination with characteristic appearances and location of the ulcers along with signs of chronic venous insufficiency.
- Important to rule out coexisting arterial insufficiency, wound infection, and other etiologies.
- Treatment consists of compression and absorbable dressing.

DESCRIPTION

- Irregular and shallow skin ulcers with well-defined borders, red granulation on the wound bed, and large amount of serous discharge
- Most common locations are lower legs below calves and malleolar regions.
- Surrounding tissue shows signs of venous insufficiency, such as edema, varicose veins, hyperpigmentation, scaly skin, fibrotic skin, atrophie blanche (scars from previous ulcers), and lipodermatosclerosis (champagne bottle appearance).
- Usually mild pain unless infected or complicated with arterial insufficiency.
- They can spontaneously develop, or after minor trauma failing to heal without proper treatment.

EPIDEMIOLOGY

Chronic leg ulcers are caused by venous insufficiency, arterial insufficiency, or mixed venous and arterial insufficiency (48%, 15%, and 18%, respectively).

Incidence

- The overall incidence of venous ulcers is 18/100,000 persons; more common in women than men (20.4 versus 14.6/100,000); incidence increases with age in both men and women.
- >20,000 patients are newly diagnosed with venous ulcers in the United States yearly.

Prevalence

- Prevalence of venous stasis ulcers is estimated to be 4% worldwide.
- Venous insufficiency is a chronic condition with a high recurrence rate of 66% within 5 years of closure.

ETIOLOGY AND PATHOPHYSIOLOGY

- Venous insufficiency is a chronic condition with a high recurrence rate of 66% within 5 years of closure.
- Venous hypertension comes from the following:
  - Venous obstruction (e.g., tumor compression, thrombus, obesity)
  - Incompetent venous valves (primary or secondary after thrombus)
  - Calf muscle pump dysfunction (e.g., debility, myopathies, neuropathies)

RISK FACTORS

- Obesity, older age, female, family history of venous disease
- History of deep venous thrombosis (DVT); history of venous insufficiency disease
- Failure of the calf muscle pump (e.g., ankle fusion, inactivity, debility, paralysis)
- Prolonged standing or sitting; history of multiple pregnancies

GENERAL PREVENTION

- Wear compression garments if any signs of venous insufficiency (e.g., edema, venous dermatitis, varicose veins) with or without history of DVT
- For patients who had venous stasis ulcers, lifelong compression therapy is recommended due to severity and chronic nature of venous insufficiency.

COMMONLY ASSOCIATED CONDITIONS

- Secondary lymphedema due to venous insufficiency, or obesity related lymphedema of the legs is common.
- Coexisting infection and arterial insufficiency are also common.

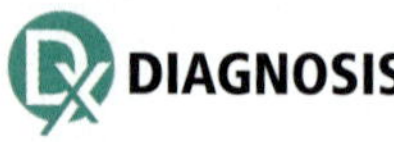

DIAGNOSIS

HISTORY

- Skin ulcer(s) formed between ankle and calf with or without trauma
- Copious weeping drainage from the ulcer
- Chronic edema of the leg preceding the ulcer formation with or without history of DVT
- No severe pain; pain can be up to moderate but usually mild.

PHYSICAL EXAM

- Basic examination for chronic skin ulcers:
  - Length, width, and depth in centimeters to document size; document the depth in relation to dermis, fat, muscle, or bone.
  - Evaluate amount and type of drainage.
  - Evaluate skin edge and periwound for maceration and undermining.
- Look for signs of venous stasis ulcers:
  - Irregular and shallow skin ulcers with well-defined borders
  - Large amount of seeping serous discharge
- Look for evidence of venous insufficiency:
  - Pitting or nonpitting edema
  - Hemosiderin staining
  - Stasis dermatitis (scaly skin)
  - Atrophie blanche, ivory colored stellate scars
  - Lipodermatosclerosis
  - Thickened skin (sign of lymphedema)
- Assess arterial circulation.
  - Palpate pulses at dorsalis pedis and posterior tibialis.
  - Obtain ankle-brachial index (ABI) if pulses are not strongly palpated (toe-brachial index [TBI] if diabetic as well).

DIFFERENTIAL DIAGNOSIS

- Arterial insufficiency ulcer (alone or with venous stasis)
- Neuropathic ulcer
- Cellulitis/wound infection
- Malignancy
- Autoimmune disease/vasculitis
- Calciphylaxis
- Pyoderma gangrenosum
- Factitious disorder/self-picking

DIAGNOSTIC TESTS & INTERPRETATION

Initial Tests (lab, imaging)

ABIs are recommended especially when foot pulses are not strongly palpated or the patient has risk factor for peripheral vascular disease (1)[C].

Follow-Up Tests & Special Considerations

Biopsy of leg ulcers that failed to respond to current treatment, or have atypical features.

Diagnostic Procedures/Other

Venography followed by vascular surgery consultation.

Test Interpretation

- ABI <0.5 is contraindication for compression.
- ABI 0.5 to 0.9: Mild compression can be used. ABI 0.9 to 1.3 is normal.
- ABI can be falsely elevated due to calcification of arteries and calcification of the skin and subcutaneous tissue.
- Patients with abnormal ABI and symptomatic peripheral artery disease should be referred to vascular surgery.

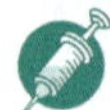

TREATMENT

Compression therapy with absorbable dressing is the standard care.

GENERAL MEASURES

- Compression therapy is the standard of care for venous ulcers and chronic venous insufficiency (2)[A]. Compression therapy reduces edema, improves venous reflux, enhances healing, and reduces pain.
  - Inelastic compression bandages: provides pressure during ambulation and muscle contraction but no resting pressure (e.g., Unna boot and short stretch bandages).
  - Elastic compression bandages: sustains compression during rest. It can become tighter after application and is not effective when the patients apply it looser than recommended (e.g., ACE wrap)

- Multilayer compression bandages: consist of inelastic and elastic bandages and more effective than either alone.
- Compression stockings: Pressure should be at least 20 to 30 mm Hg. If stockings can be worn over the dressings, it can be used instead of bandages.
- Other compression garments: tubular compression garments or Velcro compression wraps can be used effectively over dressings.

- Dressings are used under compression garment to promote healing and to prevent infection and injury from compression garment.
- Barrier cream or skin prep applied to the periulcer skin to prevent maceration of the surrounding skin.

MEDICATION

- Micronized purified flavonoid fraction and pentoxifylline have been proven to aid in healing venous limb ulcers and are recommended as effective adjuvant therapies to compression therapy (3)[A]. Sulodexide is shown to be effective, but it is not available in the United States (3)[A].
- Oral antibiotic therapy is indicated if infection is suspected.

First Line

Compression therapy (2)[A], local wound care such as interactive dressings and débridement, medical treatment (pentoxifylline) (3)[A], and lifestyle modification (elevation of legs, increasing exercise)

Second Line

- Surgical therapy (sclerotherapy, endovenous ablation, open vascular surgery, radiofrequency ablation) showed mixed results in healing venous stasis ulcers. They may reduce recurrence (1)[B].
- Treatment of lymphedema when lymphedema is present (e.g., manual drainage by lymphedema specialists and intermittent pneumatic compression device designed for lymphedema treatment)
- Graft of skin substitutes can be performed for large ulcers that shorten the time to heal the ulcers (1)[B].

ISSUES FOR REFERRAL

- With prominent toe or foot edema, fibrotic skin, or edema that persists after elevation, consider lymphedema. Refer to a certified lymphedema therapist (CLT).
- Refer to a wound clinic for complex, large, or ulcers that are not responding to the current therapy.
- Refer to a vascular specialist for abnormal ABI.
- Use home health nurses if the patient is unable to perform dressing change or compression treatment.

ADDITIONAL THERAPIES

- Exercise (e.g., activation of calf muscle pump with ankle flexion and extension).
- Infection control if likelihood is high (elevated WBC, unilateral, sudden onset, patient ill, etc.)
  - Mechanical and surgical débridement of necrotic tissue and biofilm to reduce bioburden.
  - Topical antimicrobials, such as dressing containing cadexomer iodine (Silver dressing and honey are widely used, but definitive data are lacking.) to treat suspected critical colonization.
  - Systemic antibiotics when wound infection is suspected (increased pain and worsening wound).
- Hyperbaric oxygen therapy is not indicated for venous stasis ulcers.

SURGERY/OTHER PROCEDURES

- Current evidence does not support the superiority of surgical interventions (open or endovascular) over compression alone for ulcer healing and recurrence (1)[B].
- If necrotic tissue, consider sharp, enzymatic, mechanical, larval or autolytic débridement (1)[C].
- Skin grafting generally is not effective if there is a persistent edema and the underlying venous disease is not addressed.

COMPLEMENTARY & ALTERNATIVE MEDICINE

Micronized purified flavonoid fraction is supplement that can be tried with good evidence (3)[B].

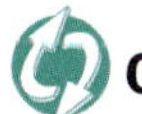

ONGOING CARE

The ulcers should be treated and examined regularly. Once ulcers are healed, patients should be reminded to continue to use compression stockings, and should be changed every 3 to 6 months.

FOLLOW-UP RECOMMENDATIONS

- Due to high recurrence rate and chronic and severe venous stasis disease in the patients with venous stasis ulcers, lifelong compression therapy is recommended even after the ulcers are healed.
- Consider ordering compression stocking when the ulcer is getting close to heal. Compression strength should be at least 20 mm Hg to be worn at all times outside the bed and should be changed every 3 to 6 months.

Patient Monitoring

The ulcers should be treated and examined ideally weekly, at least monthly to ensure the improvement, and document measurement of the size and order the wound care materials.

DIET

Low-sodium diet and weight loss for patients with a high BMI; high-protein diet, unless kidney disease, to promote wound healing.

PATIENT EDUCATION

Patient education on importance of compression therapy and how to do wound care.

PROGNOSIS

- Venous insufficiency is a lifelong medical problem.
- Poor prognostic factors
  - Ulcer duration >3 months
  - Ulcer >10 cm
  - Presence of arterial disease in the lower limbs
  - Advanced age
  - Elevated BMI

COMPLICATIONS

Wound infection, resulting in deep tissue infection, lymphedema, and chronic infection and chronic inflammation.

REFERENCES

1. Gould LJ, Dosi G, Couch K, et al. Modalities to treat venous ulcers: compression, surgery, and bioengineered tissue. *Plast Reconstr Surg*. 2016;138(Suppl 3):199S–208S.
2. Shi C, Dumville JC, Cullum N, et al. Compression bandages or stockings versus no compression for treating venous leg ulcers. *Cochrane Database Syst Rev*. 2021;7(7):CD013397.
3. Pompilio G, Nicolaides A, Kakkos SK, et al. Systematic literature review and network meta-analysis of sulodexide and other drugs in chronic venous disease. *Phlebology*. 2021;36(9):695–709.

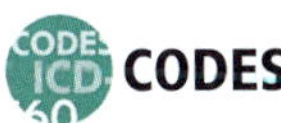

CODES

ICD10

- I87.2 Venous insufficiency (chronic) (peripheral)
- I83.009 Varicose veins of unsp lower extremity w ulcer of unsp site
- I89.0 Lymphedema, not elsewhere classified

CLINICAL PEARLS

- The diagnosis of venous ulcers is clinical; however, exams such as ABI and color duplex ultrasonography may be helpful if the diagnosis is unclear.
- Compression therapy is the standard of care for venous ulcers and chronic venous insufficiency, but arterial insufficiency needs to be ruled out.
- Treat critical colonization with topical antimicrobials cadexomer iodine (topical antibiotics are not effective due to resistance).
- Refer patients with venous ulcers failing to improve with current treatment to a wound specialist.
- Referral to vascular surgeon for concomitant arterial disease (abnormal ABI).

VENTRICULAR SEPTAL DEFECT

Jeremy Golding, MD, FAAFP • Luay Sarsam, MD

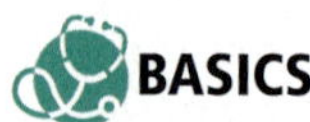

BASICS

DESCRIPTION

- Congenital (usually) or acquired defect in the interventricular septum that allows communication of blood between the left and the right ventricles
- Second most common congenital heart malformation reported in infants and children. It can also occur as a late complication of acute myocardial infarction (MI).
- Severity of the defect is correlated with its size, with large defects being the most severe.
- Blood flow across the defect typically is left to right, depending on defect size and pulmonary vascular resistance (PVR).
- Prolonged left-to-right shunting of blood can lead to pulmonary hypertension (HTN). This may eventually lead to a reversal of flow across the defect and cyanosis (Eisenmenger complex)

Geriatric Considerations

Almost entirely associated with late complication of MI

Pediatric Considerations

Congenital defect

ALERT

- Pregnancy may exacerbate symptoms and signs of a ventricular septal defect (VSD).
- Can be tolerated during pregnancy if VSD is small
- May be associated with an increased risk of preeclampsia in women with an unrepaired VSD

EPIDEMIOLOGY

Incidence

- Congenital defect: no gender predilection, occurs in ~2/1,000 live births and accounts for 30% of all congenital cardiac malformations
- Post-MI: Some studies suggest that gender may play a role.

Prevalence

In the United States:

- Occurs in ~50% of all children with congenital heart disease
- Low prevalence in adults (~0.3 per 1,000) due to spontaneous closure
- Post-MI complication in ~0.2–3% of cases

ETIOLOGY AND PATHOPHYSIOLOGY

- Congenital
- In adults, late complication of MI
- Some reports of iatrogenic causes

Genetics

Multifactorial etiology; autosomal dominant and recessive transmissions have been reported.

RISK FACTORS

- Congenital VSD:
  - Risk of sibling being affected: 4.2%
  - Risk of offspring being affected: 4%
  - Prematurity
- Post-MI VSD:
  - Advanced age
  - Arterial HTN
  - First MI
  - Most frequent within 1st week after MI
  - Most commonly after anterior wall acute MI

GENERAL PREVENTION

Avoid prenatal exposure to known risk factors (ibuprofen cyclooxygenase [COX] inhibitors, marijuana, organic solvents, febrile illness). For adults, avoid risk factors for MI and obtain evaluation before pregnancy.

COMMONLY ASSOCIATED CONDITIONS

- Congenital:
  - Tetralogy of Fallot
  - Aortic valvular deformities, especially aortic insufficiency and bicuspid aortic valve
  - Down syndrome (trisomy 21), endocardial cushion defect
  - Transposition of great arteries
  - Coarctation of aorta
  - Tricuspid atresia
  - Truncus arteriosus
  - Patent ductus arteriosus
  - Atrial septal defect
  - Pulmonic stenosis
  - Subaortic stenosis
- Adult: coronary artery disease

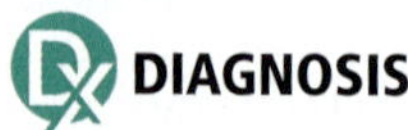

DIAGNOSIS

HISTORY

- Presentation depends on degree of shunting across the defect; may be completely asymptomatic with small defects
- Respiratory distress, tachypnea, tachycardia
- Diaphoresis with feeds, poor weight gain in infants

PHYSICAL EXAM

- Small defect:
  - Harsh holosystolic murmur loudest at left lower sternal border
  - Detected after PVR drops at 4 to 8 weeks of life
- Moderate defect:
  - Harsh holosystolic murmur at left lower sternal border associated with a thrill
  - Forceful apical impulse with lateral displacement
  - Increased intensity of P_2
  - Diastolic rumble at apex due to increased flow across the mitral valve
- Large defect:
  - Holosystolic murmur heard throughout the precordium with diastolic rumble at apex with precordial bulge and hyperactivity, although large defects may have little or no murmur initially
  - If congestive heart failure (CHF) exists: tachycardia, tachypnea, and hepatomegaly
  - If pulmonary HTN exists: cyanosis with exertion
  - If severe, irreversible pulmonary HTN (Eisenmenger complex) exists: cyanosis, clubbing, syncope, arrhythmias, and polycythemia

DIFFERENTIAL DIAGNOSIS

- Patent ductus arteriosus, atrial septal defect
- Children: tetralogy of Fallot
- Adults: mitral regurgitation

DIAGNOSTIC TESTS & INTERPRETATION

Initial Tests (lab, imaging)

- A 12-lead ECG may show left ventricular hypertrophy and left atrial enlargement initially. As pulmonary HTN develops, right ventricular hypertrophy and right atrial enlargement may be seen.
- A chest x-ray (CXR) may demonstrate increased pulmonary vascularity and/or cardiomegaly.
- A 2D echocardiogram using color Doppler and bubble study for visualization of location, size of defect, and shunt direction
- Color flow Doppler for direction and velocity of VSD jet; may be used to estimate right ventricular pressure
- Ventriculography in conjunction with above imaging modalities can aid in characterization of VSD but is invasive

Follow-Up Tests & Special Considerations

- Weight and hematocrit check
- Serial echocardiograms
- Cardiac catheterization performed occasionally for perioperative planning or to assess need for closure of defect

Diagnostic Procedures/Other

- Cardiac catheterization (left and right sides of heart) can confirm the diagnosis, document number of defects, quantify ratio of pulmonary blood flow to systemic blood flow (Qp/Qs), and determine PVR.
- Demonstration of an oxygen saturation step up from the right atrium to the distal pulmonary artery

Test Interpretation

- Congenital VSD (four major anatomic types)
  - Membranous (70%)
  - Muscular (20%)
  - Atrioventricular canal type (5%)
  - Supracristal (5%; higher in Asians)
- Post-MI VSD predominantly involves muscular septum.
- Right bundle branch block is common after surgical repair

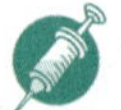

TREATMENT

- Small VSD tends to close spontaneously during childhood and has low risk for complications.
- Larger VSD tends to persist into adulthood and has more risk for complications.
- Start diuretic therapy if signs of fluid overload.
- Minimize IV fluids.
- Consider ACE inhibitor and/or digoxin.
- Nasogastric feeds for neonates
- Correct anemia via iron supplementation or a possible RBC transfusion.

GENERAL MEASURES

- Appropriate health care maintenance
- Outpatient, until surgical repair is indicated
- Inpatient management in setting of acute MI
- Inpatient for treatment of severe CHF

MEDICATION

First Line

- Per the 2007 American Heart Association guidelines, endocarditis antibiotic prophylaxis is not recommended for most VSDs. It is recommended for VSDs associated with complex cyanotic heart disease, during the first 6 months after surgical repair, or for residual VSDs located near the patch following surgery.
- Pediatric: Medications aim to control pulmonary edema, decrease work of breathing, and allow for growth:
  - Furosemide 1 to 2 mg/kg PO/IV once to twice a day
  - Spironolactone 1 to 2 mg/kg/day divided BID
  - Captopril
    - Infants: oral: 0.3 to 2.5 mg/kg/day divided every 8 to 12 hours; max 2 mg/kg/day
    - Children and adolescents: oral: 0.3 to 6.0 mg/kg/day divided every 8 to 12 hours; maximum daily dose: 150 mg/day
  - Digoxin: infants <2 years of age, 10 μg/kg/day PO divided BID; children, 2 to 10 years of age, 5 to 10 μg/kg/day PO divided BID; children >10 years of age, 2 to 5 μg/kg/day PO divided BID
- Adults: Digoxin and diuretics may be beneficial in some circumstances.
- Side effects:
  - Drugs that increase systemic vascular resistance may increase left-to-right shunting and cause signs and symptoms of pulmonary overcirculation.
  - HTN

Second Line

- Surgical closure is indicated if the pulmonic-to-systemic flow is >2:1 or with poorly controlled pulmonary overcirculation despite maximal medical and dietary interventions.
- If an infant with a VSD has persistent pulmonary HTN or failure to grow, surgical repair is recommended prior to 6 months of age even if patient is otherwise asymptomatic.
- For post-MI VSDs, afterload reduction, inotropic support, intra-aortic balloon pump, and left ventricular assist device may be used to stabilize the patient prior to surgery. Surgical repair includes septal débridement and patch placement.

ISSUES FOR REFERRAL

Close follow-up of a congenital VSD is necessary until primary intracardiac repair is performed to ensure that significant pulmonary HTN does not develop.

ADDITIONAL THERAPIES

- Infant caloric requirements up to 150 kcal/kg/day or more for adequate weight gain
- Treatment of iron deficiency anemia to increase oxygen-carrying capacity

SURGERY/OTHER PROCEDURES

- Surgical correction with either a VSD patch or repair is commonly used. Postsurgical outcomes for isolated VSD are excellent. Complications are rare and include reoperation for residual VSD, extended hospital stay, arrhythmias, valve injury, depressed ventricular function, and heart block (1).
- Percutaneous transcatheter device closure has become a safe and effective option for some children with small to moderate VSDs. Complications include valvular regurgitation, residual defects, and heart block. There is a greater risk of conduction abnormality with this technique compared to surgical closure. Recent studies have shown steroids may decrease this risk (2)[C].
- Perventricular device closure (hybrid technique) of some subtypes of isolated VSDs without cardiopulmonary bypass is feasible under transesophageal echocardiographic (TEE) guidance. Complications are similar to percutaneous closure (3)

ADMISSION, INPATIENT, AND NURSING CONSIDERATIONS

- Failure to thrive
- Pulmonary overcirculation/CHF
- Stabilize airway.
- Reduce temperature stress.
- Frequent vital sign monitoring; daily weight and calorie counts
- Discharge criteria: CHF stabilization, weight gain, or successful repair

ONGOING CARE

FOLLOW-UP RECOMMENDATIONS

- Small VSDs without evidence of CHF or pulmonary HTN generally can be followed every 1 to 5 years after the neonatal period.
- Moderate to large VSDs require more frequent follow-up.
- Potential complications of VSDs include right ventricular outflow obstruction and aortic valve prolapse.

Patient Monitoring

- Physical growth and development monitoring
- Influenza vaccine for children >6 months of age
- RSV prophylaxis with nirsevimab for children <24 months of age with hemodynamically significant lesions entering both 1st and 2nd RSV season. Children with small VSDs do not need RSV prophylaxis beyond that recommended for healthy infants.

DIET

- Low sodium in heart failure
- High calorie in failure to thrive

PATIENT EDUCATION

- No activity restriction in absence of pulmonary HTN
- Parents need support and instructions for prevention of complications until the child is ready for surgery.

PROGNOSIS

- Congenital:
  - Course is variable depending on the size of the VSD.
  - Small VSD: Many will close spontaneously by age 3 years. Muscular defects are more likely to close spontaneously.
  - Large VSD: CHF or failure to thrive in infancy necessitating surgical repair
  - 20-year cumulative survival rate after surgery for isolated VSD is 87%; 40 years is 78%.
  - Progressive pulmonary vascular disease and pulmonary HTN are the most feared complications of VSD caused by left-to-right shunting and may eventually lead to reversal of the shunt (Eisenmenger complex). Death usually occurs in the 4th decade of life if untreated.
- Post-MI:
  - With medical management alone, 80–90% mortality in the first 2 weeks
  - Prognosis worse with inferior MI compared with anterior MI

COMPLICATIONS

- CHF
- Aortic insufficiency
- Sudden death
- Hemoptysis
- Cerebral abscess
- Paradoxical emboli
- Cardiogenic shock
- Heart block rarely may accompany surgical closure.
- Pulmonary HTN, particularly Eisenmenger complex

REFERENCES

1. Scully BB, Morales DLS, Zafar F, et al. Current expectations for surgical repair of isolated ventricular septal defects. *Ann Thorac Surg*. 2010;89(2):544–549.
2. Yang L, Tai B-C, Khin LW, et al. A systematic review on the efficacy and safety of transcatheter device closure of ventricular septal defects (VSD). *J Interv Cardiol*. 2014;27(3):260–272.
3. Yin S, Zhu D, Lin K, et al. Perventricular device closure of congenital ventricular septal defects. *J Card Surg*. 2014;29(3):390–400.

ADDITIONAL READING

Penny DJ, Vick GW III. Ventricular septal defect. *Lancet*. 2011;377(9771):1103–1112.

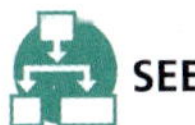

SEE ALSO

Acute Coronary Syndromes: NSTE-ACS (Unstable Angina and NSTEMI); Down Syndrome; Tetralogy of Fallot

CODES

ICD10

- Q21.0 Ventricular septal defect
- I23.2 Ventricular septal defect as current comp following AMI
- Q21.3 Tetralogy of Fallot

CLINICAL PEARLS

- A loud 2/6 to 3/6 low-pitched harsh holosystolic murmur at the left lower sternal border is typical.
- A diastolic rumble at the apex indicates moderate to large VSD or ratio of pulmonary to systemic blood flow (Qp/Qs) >2:1, which likely will require surgical or percutaneous closure.
- Disappearance of the murmur could be secondary to spontaneous closure of the defect or the development of pulmonary HTN.

VERTIGO

Molly Zhao, MD • Richard A. Sacra, MD

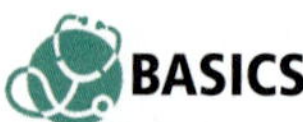

BASICS

DESCRIPTION

Vertigo is a symptom, a sensation of perceived motion ("room spinning") when no motion is happening, whereas dizziness is a disturbance of orientation without movement.

- One of 4 types of dizziness (vertigo, presyncope, lightheadedness, disequilibrium)

EPIDEMIOLOGY

Incidence

The 1-year incidence for new onset vertigo was 1.4%; incidence in women nearly twice that of men (1).

Geriatric Considerations

- High index of suspicion for cardiovascular disease, neurologic disorders, arrhythmias, and orthostatic hypotension (2)
- Benign paroxysmal positional vertigo (BPPV) is more common in ages 50 to 70 years, possibly due to the aging inner ear and otoconia degeneration (2).
- Medications implicated 1/4 of the time (3).

Prevalence

The lifetime prevalence of vertigo in adults aged 18 to 79 years was 7.4%, with a one-year prevalence of 4.9%. Prevalence was two to three times higher in women than men, and three times higher in the elderly (1).

ETIOLOGY AND PATHOPHYSIOLOGY

- Dysfunction of the rotational velocity sensors of the inner ear results in asymmetric central processing: a combination of sensory disturbance of motion and malfunction of the central vestibular apparatus (3).
- Peripheral causes: acute vestibular neuritis, BPPV caused by loose canaliths getting stuck in the posterior canal (85–95%) and lateral canal (5–15%), Ménière disease, otosclerosis, acute labyrinthitis, cholesteatoma, perilymphatic fistula, superior canal dehiscence syndrome, motion sickness.
- Central causes: cerebellar tumor, vestibular schwannoma, stroke, migraine, vertebrobasilar ischemia (3)
- Numerous drug causes such as aminoglycosides (3)

Genetics

Unclear

RISK FACTORS

- History of migraines
- History of CVD/risk factors for CVD
- Use of ototoxic medications
- Trauma/barotrauma/heavy weightlifting
- Psychosocial stress/depression
- Exposure to toxins

GENERAL PREVENTION

If due to motion sickness, consider pretreatment with anticholinergics, such as meclizine, scopolamine.

COMMONLY ASSOCIATED CONDITIONS

- Hypertension
- Hyperlipidemia
- Multiple sclerosis

DIAGNOSIS

HISTORY

- Review current medications, specifically recent additions or change in dosage as medication are a common cause of vertigo (3).
- Do not rely on symptom quality—often unreliable. Focus on timing and triggers.
  - TiTrATE is a clinically useful evaluation tool: **Ti**ming, **Tr**iggers, **A**nd a **T**argeted **E**valuation (3).
  - **Ti**ming: episodic or continuous. Episodic may last seconds to a few hours. Continuous lasts days to weeks (3).
    - If episodic and spontaneous, vestibular migraine, panic attacks, vasovagal syncope, and Ménière disease; dangerous causes include TIA, arrhythmia, MI, pulmonary embolism, CO poisoning, and hypoglycemia (4).
    - If continuous, assess for trauma or toxins (including prescribed and recreational).
    - If continuous and spontaneous, evaluate for vestibular neuritis, which is the most common cause. Perform HINTS exam (see "Physical Exam") in patient with nystagmus and full neurologic exam to evaluate for central lesions.
  - **Tr**iggers: present or absent
    - If triggers, perform Dix-Hallpike maneuver and orthostatic vitals (see "Physical Exam").
      - Positional changes are the most common trigger, precipitating BPPV or orthostatic hypotension. A central mimic, central paroxysmal positional vertigo does not respond to Epley and elicits persistent vertical nystagmus, which differentiates it from BPPV.
    - Do not confuse *worsening* of symptoms with motion with triggering. Many central vertigos are worse with movement.
  - **A**nd a **T**argeted **E**valuation: See "Physical Exam" for more details
- Specific history items that suggest a diagnosis:
  - Unilateral hearing loss and tinnitus suggest Ménière disease versus vestibular schwannoma (both chronic) versus acute labyrinthitis. Further assess to determine if sensorineural versus conductive; the latter suggests otosclerosis.
  - Recent viral infection suggests acute labyrinthitis or vestibular neuritis.
  - Symptoms triggered by sudden change in head position suggests BPPV.
  - Symptoms triggered when going from sitting to standing suggests orthostatic hypotension.
  - History of migraines suggests vestibular migraine. Differentiate from nonmigrainous headaches, which can also be present with CNS tumors.
  - Depressed mood/anxiety with episodic vertigo that has since become continuous suggests psychiatric causes.
  - History of unilateral sensory or motor symptoms indicates a central cause such as TIA or CVA until proven otherwise.
  - Onset after decompression (diving, flying) suggests decompression sickness or barotrauma and warrants emergency evaluation (3).

PHYSICAL EXAM

- Cardiovascular: orthostatic blood pressure assessment on patients with episodic symptoms (3)
- HEENT: Identify barotrauma, otosclerosis, cholesteatoma. Check Rinne and Weber tests, if hearing loss (3).
- Neurologic: Assess for nystagmus in all patients (3).
- Dix-Hallpike maneuver: for episodic, triggered vertigo: Rapidly move the patient from a seated to supine position with the head turned 45 degrees to the right and held just over (below)the edge of the exam table. Observe for nystagmus and patient report of vertigo. Nystagmus/vertigo may not appear immediately. Wait until symptoms resolve and then return the patient to the sitting position. Repeat on left (3).
  - The presence of extinguishing horizontal nystagmus (transient, upbeat) is a positive test for BPPV. If induced nystagmus does not subside however, consider central causes and perform HINTS (3).
  - Vertical nystagmus always indicates a central cause even if triggered by Dix-Hallpike.
  - If Dix-Hallpike is negative, check for lateral canal BPPV with a log roll test.
  - If duration and trigger of symptoms are not consistent with BPPV, do not perform Dix-Hallpike; a positive result could encourage you to overlook a central cause.
  - A negative Dix-Hallpike does not rule out BPPV, if symptoms are consistent and suspicion is low for other causes.
- HINTS exam: Perform for continuous, spontaneous vertigo with spontaneous nystagmus.
  - Horizontal **H**ead **I**mpulse: Rapidly and repeatedly rotate patient's head to midline from 20 degrees while maintaining their gaze on examiner's nose. Patients with peripheral vertigo will show rapid saccades to refocus on the target. Eyes staying on the target during rotation (normal function) suggests the possibility of central causes.
  - Direction changing **N**ystagmus: Having already assessed for presence and direction of nystagmus, now check for changing direction. Nystagmus that changes direction with eye motion indicates a central lesion.
  - **T**est of **S**kew: Vertical eye movement during cover-uncover test indicates a central lesion. A normal test has no movement.
  - A combination of these findings is 96.8% sensitive and 98.5% specific for CVA/other central cause (HINTS positive).
  - If a patient meets criteria for HINTS exam, do not perform Dix-Hallpike.
- Finger rub test to exclude unilateral hearing loss in patients with nystagmus as most stroke patients with vertigo have hearing loss as well (5)[A].
- Gait assessment in patients without nystagmus (5)[A].
- Perform a full neuro exam if diagnosis not already clear, paying attention to sensation, gait, and Romberg test (3).

DIFFERENTIAL DIAGNOSIS

Causes (3):

- Peripheral vertigo: BPPV, vestibular neuritis, Ménière disease
- Central vertigo: CVD, vestibular migraine, posterior fossa tumor
- Orthostatic hypotension (episodic, triggered, positive orthostatic blood pressure drop)
- Psychiatric (associated psych symptoms)
- Medication/toxin (continuous, medication/substance history, evaluation otherwise negative)
- Other cardiovascular such as arrhythmia (episodic, often no triggers or triggered by exertion)
- Hypoglycemia (episodic, associated medications or comorbidities)
- Degenerative neurologic disease (often progressive by history, associated neurologic findings)
- Peripheral neuropathy

DIAGNOSTIC TESTS & INTERPRETATION

Initial Tests (lab, imaging)

- Labs not routinely necessary unless abnormal neuro exam, and identify a cause in <1% of patients (3).
- Obtain ECG, Holter monitoring, 28-day event monitoring, and possibly carotid doppler ultrasonography for patients with symptoms suggestive of cardiovascular disease (3).
- Obtain STAT MRI if a central cause is suspected to rule out stroke. CT cannot reliably see the posterior fossa and will not show changes in an early stage of infarct. Vertigo may be the only symptom of acute stroke (3).
- Ear, nose, and throat (ENT)/audiology referral if Ménière disease is suspected (3).
- If vestibular schwannoma is suspected, either CT or MRI to evaluate internal auditory canal (3).

Diagnostic Procedures/Other

- Consider electronystagmography if Ménière disease is suspected (3).
- Audiometry is needed for evaluation of hearing loss.

TREATMENT

GENERAL MEASURES

Treatments depend on cause (3).

- If medication is likely cause: stop medication and reassess.
- BPPV: Epley maneuver and modified Epley maneuver (Epley maneuver–YouTube) (3)
- Vestibular neuritis and labyrinthitis (see "Labyrinthitis")
  - Vestibular-suppressant medications
  - Vestibular rehabilitation exercises
  - Corticosteroid course for sudden onset of hearing loss and emergent referral to ENT.
- Ménière disease (see "Ménière Disease"):
  - Low-salt diet (<1 to 2 g/day)
  - Diuretics such as hydrochlorothiazide
- Perilymphatic fistula, canal dehiscence—consult ENT.
- Vascular ischemia: prevention of future events through blood pressure reduction, lipid lowering, smoking cessation, antiplatelet therapy, and anticoagulation, if necessary; MRI or CT if suspected
- Vertiginous migraines: dietary and lifestyle modifications, vestibular rehab, prophylactic and abortive medications
- Psychological: SSRIs are better than benzodiazepines for anxiety-related vertigo.

MEDICATION

Avoid use of medication in mild cases. Use for a few days only because longer use may impair adaptation/compensation by the brain; medications not recommended for BPPV (3)

- Meclizine: 12.5 to 50.0 mg PO q4–8h
- Dimenhydrinate: 25 to 50 mg PO q6h
  - Precautions: prostatic hyperplasia, glaucoma
- Prochlorperazine: 5 to 10 mg PO or IM q6–8h; 25 mg rectally q12h; 5 to 10 mg by slow IV over 2 minutes
  - Contraindications: blood dyscrasias, age <2 years, hypotension
  - Precautions: acutely ill children, glaucoma, breast cancer history, impaired cardiac function, prostatic hyperplasia
- Psychiatric causes
  - SSRIs preferred for frequent vertigo related to depression/anxiety
  - Lorazepam 0.5 to 2.0 mg PO, IM, or IV q4–8h for short-term relief of more severe anxiety-related vertigo
  - Diazepam 2 to 10 mg PO or IV q4–8h for short-term relief of more severe symptoms

Geriatric Considerations

Use vestibular-suppressant medications with caution due to increased risk of falls and urinary retention.

Pregnancy Considerations

Meclizine and dimenhydrinate are pregnancy Category B.

ISSUES FOR REFERRAL

Consider referral to otolaryngologist, vestibular rehabilitation therapist, or neurologist if patient needs further care.

ONGOING CARE

FOLLOW-UP RECOMMENDATIONS

Adhere to balance exercises for symptom reduction and return to normal activities of daily living (ADLs).

Patient Monitoring

After 1 to 2 weeks, assess for recurrence or new symptoms.

DIET

- Restricted salt intake for Ménière disease
- Dietary modifications for vertiginous migraine

PATIENT EDUCATION

- Avoid triggers such as caffeine/alcohol (vertiginous migraine).
- Epley maneuver: MedlinePlus Medical Encyclopedia

PROGNOSIS

Depends on diagnosis and response to treatment

COMPLICATIONS

- Anxiety, depression
- Disability, injuries from falls

REFERENCES

1. Neuhauser HK. The epidemiology of dizziness and vertigo. *Handb Clin Neurol*. 2016;137:67–82.
2. Fancello V, Hatzopoulos S, Santopietro G, et al. Vertigo in the elderly: a systematic literature review. *J Clin Med*. 2023;12(6):2182.
3. Rogers TS, Noel MA, Garcia B. Dizziness: evaluation and management. *Am Fam Physician*. 2023;107(5):514–523.
4. Newman-Toker DE, Edlow JA. TiTrATE: a novel, evidence-based approach to diagnosing acute dizziness and vertigo. *Neurol Clin*. 2015;33(3):577–599, viii.
5. Edlow JA, Carpenter C, Akhter M, et al. Guidelines for reasonable and appropriate care in the emergency department 3 (GRACE-3): acute dizziness and vertigo in the emergency department. *Acad Emerg Med*. 2023;30(5):442–486.

SEE ALSO

- Ménière Disease; Motion Sickness; Vertigo, Benign Paroxysmal Positional (BPPV)
- Algorithm: Dizziness

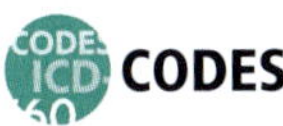

CODES

ICD10

- R42 Dizziness and giddiness
- H81.10 Benign paroxysmal vertigo, unspecified ear
- H81.49 Vertigo of central origin, unspecified ear

CLINICAL PEARLS

- Ensure no medications are cause of symptoms.
- TiTrATE your assessment.
- Acute, spontaneous, continuous vertigo with a normal horizontal head impulse, direction-changing nystagmus, and skew deviation (HINTS positive) is highly sensitive and specific for CVA.
- If patient warrants a HINTS exam, do not perform Dix-Hallpike because central cause can also produce a positive Dix-Hallpike.
- For patients with hearing loss, rule out central cause before assuming a peripheral cause.

VERTIGO, BENIGN PAROXYSMAL POSITIONAL (BPPV)

Chirag N. Shah, MD • Daniel Scott Morrison, MD • Jacqueline O. Nicholas, MD, BA

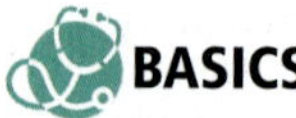

BASICS

DESCRIPTION

- Benign paroxysmal positional vertigo (BPPV) is a mechanical disorder of the inner ear. It is characterized by a brief period of an altered sensation of motion experienced when the position of the patient's head is changed relative to gravity.
- Vertigo results from the mismatch in the perception of movement by the visual, vestibular, and proprioceptive systems when no mismatch exists.
- The brief period of vertigo is caused by abnormal stimulation of 1 or more of the 3 semicircular canals of the inner ear, with the posterior canal most commonly affected (85–95% of cases).
- BPPV is the most common cause of vertigo.

EPIDEMIOLOGY

- Age of onset is most commonly between the 5th and 7th decades of life.
- Incidence increases with each decade of life.
- Prevalent sex: female > male
- BPPV affects the quality of life of elderly patients and is associated with reduced activities of daily living scores, falls, and depression (1)[A].

Incidence

1-year incidence 0.6%; lifetime cumulative 10%

Prevalence

1-year prevalence 1.6%; lifetime 2.4%

ETIOLOGY AND PATHOPHYSIOLOGY

- In BPPV, calcite particles (otoconia), which normally weigh the sensory membrane of the maculae, become dislodged and settle into the semicircular canal, changing the dynamics of the canal. Reorientation of the canal relative to gravity causes the otoconia to move to the lowest part of the canal, causing displacement of the endolymph, deflection of the cupula, and activation of the primary afferent. This results in the generation of nystagmus and the associated sensation of vertigo.
- BPPV may be idiopathic, posttraumatic, or associated with viral neurolabyrinthitis.

RISK FACTORS

Hypertension, diabetes mellitus, stroke, vitamin D deficiency, osteoporosis, migraine, and head trauma (1)[A]

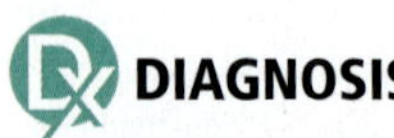

DIAGNOSIS

- The diagnosis is established based on history and findings on positional testing, clarified by Dix and Hallpike in 1952.
- Positional tests place the plane of the canal being tested into the plane parallel with gravity.
- A systematic approach prevents misdiagnosis or failure in recognizing a stroke, notably posterior stroke.

HISTORY

- Most common form of triggered episodic vestibular syndrome
- Brief in duration with head motion intolerance
- Patients present with a usual chief complaint of dizziness, "room spinning" sensation, and/or feeling "off balance."
- Brief episodes of vertigo are associated with:
  - Rolling over in bed
  - Getting into or out of bed
  - Looking up (referred to as "top-shelf syndrome")
  - Bending forward
  - Quick head movements
- Frequently, patients complain of nausea and, if severe enough, vomiting.

PHYSICAL EXAM

- The Dix-Hallpike test (DHT) is used to diagnose BPPV. The test provokes the characteristic nystagmus associated with the symptoms of vertigo, with an estimated sensitivity of 79% (95% CI 65–94) and specificity of 75% (95% CI 33–100).
  - To perform the DHT, rapidly move the patient from seated to the supine position with the head turned 45 degrees to the right and held extended just over the edge of the exam table. This position is maintained for 45 to 60 seconds. Observe for nystagmus and patient report of vertigo. Nystagmus/vertigo may not appear immediately. Wait until symptoms resolve and then return the patient to the sitting position. Repeat on the left.
- The direction of the fast phase of the nystagmus, any latency period before onset, and the duration of the nystagmus before it ceases are recorded.
- BPPV is consistent with a latency period of <30 seconds between lowering the head and the subsequent onset of nystagmus; the eye movements peak, then slowly resolve within 40 seconds. The direction of the nystagmus reverses when the patient's head is brought back upright and to the neutral position. Repeated testing results in diminished vertiginous symptoms and nystagmus fatigue.
- The following characteristics help to distinguish a peripheral etiology (BPPV, Meniere, labyrinthitis) of vertigo versus a central (stroke) cause:
  - Triggered nystagmus (vs. spontaneous or gaze)
  - Onset is sudden (vs. sudden or slow).
  - Severity of intense spinning (vs. less intense)
  - Pattern is paroxysmal (vs. constant).
  - Symptoms are aggravated by movement (vs. variable).
  - Nausea or diaphoresis is frequent (vs. variable).
  - Nystagmus has rotatory-vertical, horizontal eye movements (vs. vertical).
  - Symptoms fatigue (vs. ongoing)
  - Progressive hearing loss, tinnitus, no change (vs. acute ipsilateral hearing loss or no change)
  - An abnormal TM may be seen (vs. this is not an associated finding).
- Red flags in vertigo
  - Neurologic deficit, ipsilateral hearing loss, gait abnormality, direction-changing nystagmus (nystagmus that changes its direction with different body and head positions).
- Head Impulse, Nystagmus, Test of Skew (HINTS) + no hearing loss:
  - Head impulse test of vestibulo-ocular reflex function:
    - Normally, eye movement will correct with rapid head movement so that the center of the vision remains on a target. This reflex fails in peripheral causes of vertigo.
    - Have the patient fix their eyes on your nose, and move their head in the horizontal plane to the left and then to the right.
    - When the head is turned toward the normal side, the vestibulo-ocular reflex remains intact and eyes are fixated on the examiner's nose.
    - When the head is turned toward the affected side, the vestibulo-ocular reflex fails and the eyes make a corrective saccade to refixate on the examiner's nose.
    - It is reassuring if the reflex is *abnormal* (due to dysfunction of the peripheral nerve).
  - Unidirectional gaze-evoked nystagmus.
  - Test for skew deviation "vertical dysconjugate gaze":
    - Skew deviation is a fairly specific predictor of a central lesion in patients with acute vestibular syndrome.
    - The presence of skew may help identify stroke when a positive head impulse test falsely suggests a peripheral lesion.
    - Have the patient look at your nose with their eyes and start by covering one eye and then rapidly move to cover the other eye, do this rapidly back and forth.
    - When each eye is uncovered, quickly look to see if the eye has movement or refixation. Horizontal is normal, vertical is not.
  - In the setting of acute dizziness and vertigo, ABCD2 ≥4 in combination with HINTS was found to be the most sensitive (100%) and specific (100%) in detecting acute stroke, and outperforms MRI obtained within the first 2 days after symptom onset (2)[B].
  - Use of HINTS is limited in evaluation in the ED to specifically rule out a stroke in those presenting with acute vestibular syndromes.

DIFFERENTIAL DIAGNOSIS

- Orthostatic hypotension and other disorders that cause low BP; symptoms usually occur when the patient stands up.
- Damage to the brainstem or cerebellum can cause positional vertigo but is accompanied by other neurologic signs and usually has a different pattern of nystagmus.
- Low spinal fluid pressure may cause positional symptoms that are better when the patient lies down.

- Migraine-associated vertigo
- Traumatic brain injury
- Brain tumors, hemorrhage, or infarction
- Vestibular neuronitis

DIAGNOSTIC TESTS & INTERPRETATION

Systematic approach: triage, TiTrATE, then treatment

- TiTrATE approach: Timing, Triggers, and Targeted examinations:
  - Timing classifies the disease processes into episodic versus continuous.
  - Triggers further seek to find underlying causes by looking at exam findings (e.g., DHT).
  - Targeted examination and ancillary tests are based on findings.
- Combination of all this information allows the clinician to further evaluate with CT or MRI.

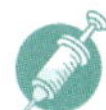

TREATMENT

- The canalith repositioning procedure (CRP) or Epley maneuver is effective in the treatment of posterior canal BPPV. Using a particle repositioning maneuver, the clinician moves the patient through a series of positions. Most studies evaluating the effectiveness of CRP have been performed in specialist clinics. However, in a randomized controlled trial out of primary care offices, a single CRP administered by a general practitioner demonstrated significant improvement in symptoms compared to a sham maneuver.
- The clinician moves the patient through a series of four provoking positions:
  - Placement of the right posterior canal (involved canal) in the right head-hanging position of the DHT.
  - The head is then rotated a total of 90 degrees toward the left (uninvolved side) into 45 degrees of left head rotation.
  - Maintaining 45 degrees of left head rotation, the patient is rolled onto the left side (uninvolved side) with the head slightly elevated from the supporting surface.
  - The patient then sits up and flexes the neck 36 degrees. Each position is maintained for a minimum of 45 seconds or as long as the nystagmus lasts.
- CRP is the best maneuver for posterior BPPV and should be offered to all age groups.
- Other maneuvers include Semont and Lempert Roll Maneuver.
- Contraindications are cervical spine disease, carotid vascular disease, and retinal detachment. If the CRP is ineffective, self-administered CRP is performed at home. The patient performs the CRP on the bed with the head extended over the edge of a pillow. Better outcomes are achieved with a combination of CRP with self-administered CRP.
- CRP and Semont are ineffective for horizontal BPPV; variations of the Lempert maneuver, barbecue roll, or Gufoni maneuver are widely used treatment methods for horizontal BPPV.
- Postmaneuver activity restrictions were previously advocated, but in controlled trials, they did not differ in clinical outcomes.

MEDICATION

- Vestibular suppressant medications are not recommended for the treatment of BPPV, other than for the short-term management of vegetative symptoms. Canal repositioning maneuvers are superior (3)[A].
- Antiemetics such as ondansetron may be considered for prophylaxis for patients who have had severe nausea or vomiting with the DHT.
- Vestibular suppressants such as benzodiazepines and antihistamine anticholinergics (e.g., meclizine) should be avoided as they may suppress nystagmus during the DHT and treatment.

ISSUES FOR REFERRAL

Several factors, most notably history of head trauma, idiopathic BPPV, vitamin D deficiency, are associated with failure of first CRP, requiring additional sessions (1)[A]. Consider a referral to a specialist if BPPV is unresponsive to treatment or if the patient is diagnosed with atypical BPPV involving the anterior or lateral canal. Consider referring to a physical therapist, neurologist, or otolaryngologist (1)[A].

ADDITIONAL THERAPIES

- Vestibular rehabilitation therapy (VRT) has been shown to have some efficacy in reducing symptom burden on quality of life in patients with BPPV. This therapy modality consists of exercises that focus on strengthening vestibular compensation to changes in positioning.
- Hypertension, diabetes mellitus, hyperlipidemia, osteoporosis, hypothyroidism, and vitamin D deficiency have been identified as potential risk factors for BPPV occurrence/recurrence; therefore, treatment of these comorbidities may be protective against BPPV occurrence, reduce relapse of attacks, and improve responsiveness to CRP (1)[A].
- Surgical intervention is rarely indicated, except for refractory BPPV, and includes posterior canal occlusion and singular neurectomy.

ONGOING CARE

FOLLOW-UP RECOMMENDATIONS

The patient should follow up within a week after treatment to ensure resolution.

PATIENT EDUCATION

A number of illustrative YouTube videos are available for education and self-CRP maneuvers.

PROGNOSIS

- 80% cure rate with CRP maneuvers, with a 30% recurrence rate at 1 year, and 44% redevelop BPPV within 2 years.
- High rates of reoccurrence are seen with comorbid hypertension, hyperlipidemia, diabetes mellitus.

COMPLICATIONS

During the maneuvers, a canal conversion may occur. The debris from the canal being treated may reflux into another canal.

REFERENCES

1. Alolayet H, Murdin L. Benign paroxysmal positional vertigo a systematic review of the effects of comorbidities. *Front Neurol*. 2025;16:1595693. doi:10.3389/fneur.2025.1595693.
2. Wang W, Zhang Y, Pan Q, et al. Central nystagmus plus ABCD^2 identifying stroke in acute dizziness presentations. *Acad Emerg Med*. 2021;28(10):1118–1123. doi:10.1111/acem.14295.
3. Sharif S, Khoujah D, Greer A, et al. Vestibular suppressants for benign paroxysmal positional vertigo: a systematic review and meta-analysis of randomized controlled trials. *Acad Emerg Med*. 2023;30(5):541–551. doi:10.1111/acem.14608.

ADDITIONAL READING

Edlow JA, Carpenter C, Akhter M, et al. Guidelines for reasonable and appropriate care in the emergency department 3 (Grace-3): acute dizziness and vertigo in the emergency department. *Acad Emerg Med*. 2023;30(5):442–486. doi:10.1111/acem.14728.

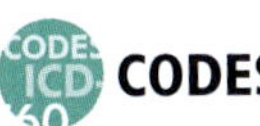

CODES

ICD10

- H81.10 Benign paroxysmal vertigo, unspecified ear
- H81.12 Benign paroxysmal vertigo, left ear
- H81.11 Benign paroxysmal vertigo, right ear

CLINICAL PEARLS

- The diagnosis of BPPV is based on history and findings on positional testing.
- The typical presentation is a report of transient episodes of vertigo (sensation that the room is spinning) associated with a change in position of the head relative to gravity.
- BPPV may be treated effectively with particle-repositioning maneuvers in the office and at home.
- Vestibular suppressant medications and antiemetics are not recommended for the treatment of BPPV, other than for the short-term management of symptoms.
- Patients should always be ambulated in order to verify normal gait prior to discharge.

VINCENT STOMATITIS

Daniel V. Girzadas Jr., MD • Anna Krzywiec, DO

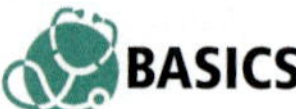

BASICS

An inflammatory infection of the gingiva, characterized by pain, ulcerations, and necrotizing damage to interdental papillae

DESCRIPTION

- Caused by an imbalance of oral flora, resulting in a predominance of anaerobic bacteria that invade the gingival mucosa and form a gray pseudomembranous exudate
- Clinical presentation includes oral pain, fetid breath, gingival ulcerations, necrosis, and bleeding
- Whereas other periodontal diseases develop over time, necrotizing periodontal disease is characterized by its rapid onset, pain, ulcerated gingival mucosa, and "punched out" crater-like lesions of interdental papillae (1).
- The most common bacteria include *Fusobacterium* spp., *Prevotella intermedia*, and spirochetes. Concomitant infection with Epstein-Barr virus, herpes simplex virus, and type 1 human cytomegalovirus is common.
- Synonym(s): Vincent angina; Vincent disease; Vincent stomatitis, trench mouth; fusospirochetal gingivitis; acute necrotizing ulcerative gingivitis (ANUG); necrotizing ulcerative gingivitis (NUG)
- Necrotizing gingivitis, necrotizing periodontitis, and necrotizing stomatitis are classified together under the umbrella term "necrotizing periodontal disease (NPD)."

EPIDEMIOLOGY

Colloquially called "trench mouth," necrotizing periodontal disease predominantly affects younger populations with poor oral hygiene and inadequate nutrition.

Incidence

- Predominant age: 18 to 30 years in developed countries, malnourished children ages 3 to 14 years
- Affects both genders with similar frequency
- Historically, incidence increased in military personnel due to poor battlefield conditions and psychological stress, hence the use of the informal phrase, "trench mouth" (1).

Prevalence

- The true prevalence is unknown, but likely <1% overall (1).
- Worldwide prevalence has declined since World War II (1).
- A rare disease in developed countries; however, recent data demonstrated a prevalence rate of 6.7% in Chilean students between 12 and 21 years and approaching 25% in children in sub-Saharan African countries (2),(3).

ETIOLOGY AND PATHOPHYSIOLOGY

- Immunocompromised state resulting in poor host response to invasive anaerobic bacteria
- Disruption of normal oral flora with a predominance of invasive anaerobic bacteria (*Treponema* spp., *Selenomonas* spp., *Fusobacterium* spp., and *Prevotella intermedia*) (2)
- Invasive anaerobic bacteria produce metabolites such as collagenase, endotoxins, and fibrinolysin that destroy tissue, leading to loss of integrity and necrosis of the gingival mucosa and interdental papillae (4).
- Stress increases adrenocortical hormones and reduces gingival microcirculation and salivary flow, which alters leukocyte and lymphocyte function. Stress may also result in behavioral changes that lead to poor oral hygiene and malnutrition (2).
- Increased bacterial attachment with active herpesvirus infection

RISK FACTORS

- Malnutrition
- Immunosuppression (diabetes, alcohol use, HIV, cancer, chemotherapy, steroid use)
- Low socioeconomic status
- Tobacco use
- Poor oral hygiene, infrequent or absent dental care
- Orthodontics
- Herpesvirus infection
- Psychological stress

GENERAL PREVENTION

- Appropriate nutrition
- Proper oral hygiene
- Regular dental care
- Prompt recognition and institution of therapy
- Management of medical problems such as cancer and HIV infection
- Smoking cessation
- Stress management

COMMONLY ASSOCIATED CONDITIONS

- Most commonly seen in malnourished patients, patients undergoing cancer treatment, or those from underdeveloped countries
- Bacteremia
- Tooth loss
- Chronic gingivitis
- Noma (cancrum oris), a gangrenous infection of the oral mucosa
- Aspiration pneumonia

DIAGNOSIS

A gray pseudomembranous exudate on exam, gingival ulcerations, damage to interdental papillae, rapid onset of symptoms, and risk factors ultimately make the diagnosis of Vincent stomatitis.

HISTORY

- Presentation typically includes the triad of rapid onset of gingival pain, bleeding, and ulcerations/necrosis of interdental papillae (4).
- Fetid odor of breath, metallic taste in the mouth
- Systemic symptoms: regional lymphadenopathy, fever, malaise
- Presence of risk factors including tobacco use, poor oral hygiene, malnourishment, and immunocompromise
- Active herpesvirus infection or HIV

PHYSICAL EXAM

- Fever
- Fetid odor of the breath
- Ulceration of gingival mucosa
- Inflamed, erythematous gingiva
- Necrosis of interdental papillae
- Gingival bleeding
- Formation of gray, pseudomembranous exudate
- Cervical and submandibular lymphadenopathy

DIFFERENTIAL DIAGNOSIS

- Herpes simplex virus
- Recurrent aphthous stomatitis
- Medication side effects
- Oral malignancy
- Diphtheria
- Lymphoma/leukemia
- Primary syphilis
- Ascorbic acid deficiency
- Behçet disease or granulomatosis with polyangiitis
- Oral histoplasmosis

DIAGNOSTIC TESTS & INTERPRETATION

Initial Tests (lab, imaging)

Diagnosis is primarily based on clinical presentation, but if systemic illness or invasive spread to deeper tissue or bone is suspected, the following studies should be considered:

- Aerobic and anaerobic cultures of inflamed or débrided tissue
- Group A strep rapid antigen detection assay or throat culture
- Blood cultures if systemic involvement
- Dental radiographs
- CT imaging of the face and neck if there is concern that the infection has spread to deeper tissue

Diagnostic Procedures/Other

Although biopsy could be performed for histopathology, the diagnosis is largely clinical in nature. Microbiology testing often does not add relevant diagnostic information given many of these bacterial pathogens are typical of healthy gingiva and other nonspecific cases of gingivitis and periodontitis (1).

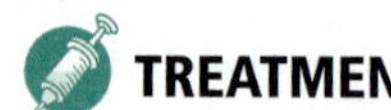

TREATMENT

Goals of care include sequential steps of alleviating the acute phase, management of preexisting conditions, and treating disease sequelae (2).

GENERAL MEASURES

- Manage the acute phase of disease with superficial débridement, oral hygiene (gentle brushing), antimicrobial mouthwash, and oral antibiotics. Some experts recommend treatment of all patients with oral antibiotics, others recommend treatment only for those with systemic symptoms such as fever, malaise, and vomiting.
  - Débridement can be accomplished by a cotton-topped swab soaked with hydrogen peroxide for gentle local débridement, rinse with hydrogen peroxide or chlorhexidine, ultrasonic débridement with a dental specialist, or surgical débridement under local anesthesia.
- Once the acute disease is controlled, the patient will require ongoing outpatient dental cleanings, specifically scaling and root planing.
- Elimination of tobacco, improved nutritional status, and better oral hygiene will increase the rate of healing and reduce the risk of future gingival disease.

MEDICATION

Most cases are treatable on an outpatient basis. Severe disease with systemic effects and/or neck involvement requires inpatient treatment. Other than chlorhexidine, there is no role for topical antibiotics given they cannot effectively penetrate the periodontal tissue (2).

First Line

- Chlorhexidine gluconate 0.12% 15 mL 30 seconds rinse/spit twice daily (1)[C]
- The following antibiotics can be considered
  - Metronidazole 250 to 500 mg PO or IV q8h for 7 to 10 days (1)[C],(2)[C],(4)[C]; pediatric dosing: 30 to 50 mg/kg/day divided q8h (3)[A] *or*
  - Amoxicillin-clavulanate 875 mg PO q12h for 7 to 10 days; pediatric dosing: 25 to 45 mg/kg/day divided q12h amoxicillin *or*
  - Amoxicillin 250 to 500 mg PO q8h PO for 7 days (4)[C]; pediatric dosing: 25 to 45 mg/kg/day divided q12h *or*
  - Penicillin V potassium 250 to 500 mg PO q6h PO for 5 to 7 days for adults and children >12 years of age *or*
  - Some historical data suggests combination therapy of metronidazole with either amoxicillin or penicillin V potassium
  - Ampicillin/sulbactam offers effective coverage for immunocompromised patients requiring hospitalization.

Second Line

- Doxycycline 100 mg PO BID 7 to 10 days (do not use for children <8 years of age); for children aged ≥8 years dosing is 2 mg/kg per dose up to 100 mg PO BID max.
- Clindamycin 450 mg PO or 600 mg IV q8h for 7 to 10 days; pediatric dosing: 8 to 25 mg/kg/day divided q6–8h—no longer recommended as a first-line agent due to resistance patterns
- Erythromycin 250 to 500 mg q6–12h PO for 10 days; pediatric dosing: 30 to 50 mg/kg/day divided q6–8h

Pediatric Considerations

- Chlorhexidine gel may be prescribed in place of mouth rinses due to concern for risk of ingestion.
- Alternatively, can consider 3% hydrogen peroxide diluted by half with water as a safer mouthwash in children to help remove the pseudomembranous coating and decrease bleeding (3)
- In addition to amoxicillin or amoxicillin-clavulanate, metronidazole may be considered as first-line oral therapy (refer to dosing above) (3)[A].

ISSUES FOR REFERRAL

Severe disease requires débridement by a consultant dentist, oral surgeon, or ENT specialist.

ADDITIONAL THERAPIES

- Warm saline rinses q2h
- Sodium bicarbonate toothpaste, brush q2h
- Viscous lidocaine 2% 1 tbsp rinse/spit q6–8h (with caution in pediatric patients)
- NSAID medications q4–12h
- Opioid analgesics q4–6h (severe pain)
- Treatment of underlying immunodeficiency (if present)

SURGERY/OTHER PROCEDURES

- Débridement of inflamed/necrotic gingival tissue
- Dental extraction
- Gingival restoration
- Adjuvant therapies
  - Low-level laser therapy (LLLT) has been shown in one case series to decrease pain and accelerate healing.
  - Photochemotherapy has been shown to reduce bleeding ulcers and bacterial counts compared to conventional therapy alone.

COMPLEMENTARY & ALTERNATIVE MEDICINE

3% hydrogen peroxide and warm sterile saline in a 1:1 ratio q2–3h as an oral rinse (1)[C]

ADMISSION, INPATIENT, AND NURSING CONSIDERATIONS

- Severe disease, failure of oral antibiotics, or ongoing comorbidities
- Parenteral antibiotics, analgesia requirement, or inability to tolerate PO

ONGOING CARE

FOLLOW-UP RECOMMENDATIONS

- Close dental follow-up
- Specialty follow-up (if underlying immunodeficiency)

DIET

- Soft diet until healed
- Balanced nutritional diet with multivitamin supplementation

PATIENT EDUCATION

- Oral hygiene with emphasis on twice daily brushing, flossing, and routine dental care
- Proper nutrition
- Tobacco cessation

PROGNOSIS

- Lack of treatment can lead to rapid tissue destruction, necrotizing ulcerative periodontitis, and cancrum oris, an often fatal gangrenous orofacial infection
- The maintenance of adequate oral hygiene is needed to prevent recurrence.

COMPLICATIONS

- Malnutrition/dehydration
- Gingival/tooth loss
- Deep infection of neck

REFERENCES

1. Dufty J, Gkranias N, Donos N. Necrotising ulcerative gingivitis: a literature review. *Oral Health Prev Dent*. 2017;15(4):321–327.
2. Malek R, Gharibi A, Khlil N, et al. Necrotizing ulcerative gingivitis. *Contemp Clin Dent*. 2017;8(3):496–500.
3. Marty M, Palmieri J, Noirrit-Esclassan E, et al. Necrotizing periodontal diseases in children: a literature review and adjustment of treatment. *J Trop Pediatr*. 2016;62(4):331–337.
4. Atout RN, Todescan S. Managing patients with necrotizing ulcerative gingivitis. *J Can Dent Assoc*. 2013;79:d46.

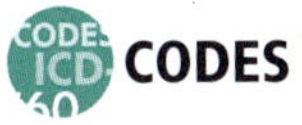

CODES

ICD10

A69.1 Other Vincent's infections

CLINICAL PEARLS

- Diagnosis is largely clinical based on symptoms of oral pain, fetid breath, gingival ulcerations, interdental papillary necrosis, and grayish exudate on the gingival surface.
- Immunosuppression, malnourishment, smoking, and poor oral hygiene are key risk factors for NUG.
- Most patients experience rapid improvement following appropriate treatment with gentle débridement, chlorhexidine rinses, oral antibiotics, and improved oral hygiene.
- Smoking cessation and treatment of malnutrition or underlying illness are additional important treatment considerations.
- Severe disease requires extensive débridement of necrotic gingival tissue and close follow-up with a periodontal specialist or oral surgeon to limit recurrence and prevent rapid destruction of the periodontium.

VITAMIN B_{12} DEFICIENCY

Sahil Mullick, MD, FAAFP • Aya Allam, MD

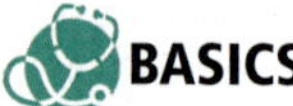

BASICS

- Vitamin B_{12} deficiency is related to inadequate intake or absorption of cobalamin.
- Cobalamin is critical for central nervous system myelination, red blood cell production, immune cell cytogenesis, and DNA synthesis (1).
- Deficiency can cause megaloblastic anemia, bone marrow dysfunction, cytopenia including lymphopenia, and diverse and potentially irreversible neuropsychiatric changes.
- Neuropsychiatric disorders are due to demyelination of cervical, thoracic dorsal, and lateral spinal cords; white matter; and cranial and peripheral nerves.
- Elevated MMA and homocysteine levels MMA are more sensitive and specific and persist for several days even after treatment.

DESCRIPTION

Normal vitamin B_{12} absorption and diet recommendations

- Vitamin B_{12} is a water-soluble vitamin present in animal-source foods and foods fortified with vitamin B_{12}.
- Dietary vitamin B_{12} (cobalamin) bound to food is cleaved by acids in stomach and bound to haptocorrin that are secreted in saliva (commonly known as R-factor).
- Pancreatic proteases cleave vitamin B_{12} from haptocorrin.
- In duodenum, vitamin B_{12} uptake depends on binding to intrinsic factor (IF) secreted by gastric parietal cells.
- Vitamin B_{12}-IF complex is absorbed by terminal ileum into portal circulation.
- Small amount of ingested vitamin B_{12} (<1 percent) can be absorbed by passive diffusion and is the basis for use of high dose oral vitamin B_{12} in pernicious anemia (PA).
- Total body stores of vitamin B_{12} are in 2 to 5 mg range. Most of it are stored in liver.
- Vitamin B_{12} excreted in bile is effectively reabsorbed through enterohepatic circulation.
- Typical Western diet: 5 to 30 mg/day; however, only 1 to 5 mg/day is effectively absorbed.
- Recommend 2.4 mg/day for adults and 2.6 mg/day during pregnancy and 2.8 mg/day during lactation (most prenatal vitamins contain vitamin B_{12}).

EPIDEMIOLOGY

Prevalence

- National Health and Nutrition Examination Survey documented 6.9% and 15% prevalence of B_{12} deficiency in U.S. adults aged 51 to 70 and >70 years, respectively (2).
- Morbidity increases vitamin B_{12} deficiency occurrence, ranging from 4% to 5% in community-living elderly to about 30–40% in institutionalized subjects with multiple comorbidities.
- Prevalence in those <60 years old is 6% versus 20% in those >60 years.
- Increasing recognition in breastfed-only infants with vitamin B_{12}–deficient mothers
- Among patients with clinical macrocytosis (defined as a mean corpuscular volume [MCV] >100), 18–20% were due to vitamin B_{12} deficiency (3).
- Vitamin B_{12} deficiency due to PA is more common in people of Northern European ancestry and lower in people of African descent.

ETIOLOGY AND PATHOPHYSIOLOGY

- Decreased oral intake
  - Vegetarians and vegans: Vitamin B_{12} is found in animal-source foods.
- Decreased IF
  - PA: can be associated with autoantibodies directed against gastric parietal cells and/or IF; 15–30% of all cases; most frequent cause of severe disease; neurologic disorders are common presenting complaints.
  - Chronic atrophic gastritis: autoimmune attack on gastric parietal cells causing autoimmune gastritis and leading to decreased IF production
  - Gastrectomy: removal of entire or part of stomach
- Decreased absorption
  - Crohn disease: Terminal ileal inflammation decreases body's ability to absorb vitamin B_{12}.
  - Chronic alcoholism: decreases body's ability to absorb vitamin B_{12}
  - Gluten hypersensitivity (celiac disease) intestinal villi atrophy and subsequent malabsorption
  - Ileal resection
  - Pancreatic insufficiency: Pancreatic proteases are required to cleave the vitamin B_{12}–haptocorrin bond to allow vitamin B_{12} to bind to IF.
  - *Helicobacter pylori* infection: impairs release of vitamin B_{12} from bound proteins
- Medications:
  - Proton pump inhibitors (PPIs), H_2 antagonists, and antacids decrease gastric acidity, inhibiting vitamin B_{12} release from dietary protein; metformin
  - Metformin usage can cause calcium-dependent membrane inhibition, interfering with vitamin B_{12}–IF absorption.
- Hereditary (rare): transcobalamin II deficiency

Genetics

Imerslund-Gräsbeck disease (juvenile megaloblastic anemia) caused by mutations in the amnionless (AMN) or cubilin (CUBN) genes with autosomal recessive pattern of inheritance; inadequate ileal uptake of vitamin B_{12}-IF complex and decreased vitamin B_{12} renal protein reabsorption.

COMMONLY ASSOCIATED CONDITIONS

- Gastric abnormalities: PA, gastritis, gastrectomy/bariatric surgery
- Small bowel disease: malabsorption syndrome, ileal resection, IBD, celiac disease
- Pancreatic insufficiency
- Diet: breastfed infant in vitamin B_{12} deficient mother, strict vegan diet
- Medications: neomycin, metformin, PPI, histamine 2 receptor antagonists, nitrous oxide (N_2O) abuse

DIAGNOSIS

- Asymptomatic; incidental finding of anemia or elevated MCV.
- Neuropsychiatric
  - Frequent: sensory polyneuritis, paresthesias, positive Babinski sign, weakness, gait unsteadiness, loss of proprioception (impaired vibratory sensation, positive Romberg, ataxia, hyperreflexia)
  - Classic but uncommon: subacute combined degeneration of spinal cord associated with PA; areflexia, ataxia, proprioception and vibration loss, bowel and bladder incontinence, orthostatic hypotension, decreased memory, mania, delirium, psychosis, depression
- Digestive
  - Classic: Hunter glossitis, jaundice, and high lactate dehydrogenase and bilirubin
  - Possible: abdominal pain, dyspepsia, nausea, vomiting, diarrhea
  - Rare: mucocutaneous ulcers
- Other
  - Frequent: fatigue with exertion, skin pallor, palpitations, edema, jaundice

HISTORY

- Underlying disease associated with vitamin B_{12} deficiency
- Fatigue, anorexia, depression
- Falls (due to diminished proprioception), loss of sensation in "stocking-glove" distribution
- Glossitis/loss of sense of taste

PHYSICAL EXAM

- Lymphadenopathy, hepatosplenomegaly, enlarged tongue (glossitis)
- Neurologic exam: impaired vibratory sense, altered proprioception possible ataxia, diminished sensations in light touch, and/or weakness

DIFFERENTIAL DIAGNOSIS

Folate deficiency, copper deficiency, hypothyroidism, syphilis, multiple sclerosis, HIV myelopathy

DIAGNOSTIC TESTS & INTERPRETATION

- Measurement of vitamin B_{12}, complete blood count (MCV)
- Measurement of vitamin B_{12} may be low or low normal depending on cutoff value.
  - 95–97% sensitive levels <200 pg/mL
  - May need additional tests such as MMA and homocysteine if vitamin B_{12} level is low normal (<350 pg/mL)
- MCV is often increased, although it is not necessarily present if the condition is associated with other kinds of anemia.
- Measurement of MMA
  - More sensitive and specific than homocysteine
  - Levels increased in renal failure and volume depletion
- Measurement of homocysteine
  - Levels increased in folate deficiency, renal failure, homocystinuria; vitamin B_6 deficiency and hypothyroidism
- MMA and homocysteine levels only reliable in an untreated patient because levels fall with supplementation
- Other tests: folate and other markers of anemia (iron studies)
- Holotranscobalamin (holo-TC) accounts for approximately 10% of the circulating vitamin B_{12} and is the earliest marker showing vitamin B_{12} depletion. It is also known as active vitamin B_{12}, the only form of vitamin B_{12} that is taken up and used by the cells in the body.

ALERT
- Low levels of vitamin B_{12} are seen in folate deficiency, HIV, and multiple myeloma.
- Elevated levels of vitamin B_{12} are seen in renal disease, occult malignancy, and alcoholic liver disease.
- Macrocytosis may be due to folate deficiency, reticulocytosis, medications, bone marrow dysplasia, and hypothyroidism or be masked by concomitant microcytic anemia.
- In asymptomatic individuals, vitamin B_{12} deficiency is associated with reductions in the binding protein haptocorrin. However, this condition may be difficult to discriminate from true vitamin B_{12} deficiency in the presence of symptoms.
- Check antibody to IF; positive test is confirmatory for PA, but sensitivity is only 50–70%.
- Antibodies to parietal cells, present in 90% of patients with PA, are less specific and can occur in simple atrophic gastritis and in autoimmune thyroid disease.
- For patients with negative anti-IF result and high suspicion for PA, check serum gastrin level (elevated in PA).

Pregnancy and Newborn Considerations
- Pregnant women with low vitamin B_{12} have higher risk of having children with neural tube defects, developmental delay, failure to thrive, hypotonia, ataxia, and anemia.
- Exclusively breastfed infants of mothers who are vitamin B_{12} deficient are at risk of developing vitamin B_{12} deficiency. Infants might not show signs or symptoms until 4 to 6 months of age, which may include developmental regression, feeding difficulties, lethargy, or hypotonia.
- Children born to mothers with normal to high folate levels and low serum vitamin B_{12} values have higher truncal adiposity and insulin resistance which may influence long-term risk of development of type 2 diabetes and cardiovascular disease.
- Low vitamin B_{12} has a negative influence on children's development and cognitive functioning, may cause growth and motor retardation.
- Untreated severe vitamin B_{12} deficiency during pregnancy can lead to severe anemia, peripheral neuropathy, cognitive decline, and a variety of neuropsychiatric manifestations.
- May also manifest with microangiopathic hemolytic anemia and thrombocytopenia, mimicking other thrombotic microangiopathy disorders such as atypical hemolytic uremic syndrome, HELLP syndrome, and thrombotic thrombocytopenic purpura

Initial Tests (lab, imaging)
Vitamin B_{12}, MMA, and homocysteine levels

Diagnostic Procedures/Other
Bone marrow exam is usually unnecessary.

Test Interpretation
- If vitamin B_{12} level is:
  - >400 pg/mL, no deficiency
  - Between 150 to 399 pg/mL, obtain MMA level and homocysteine level.
  - <150 pg/mL, deficiency is present
- If MMA and homocysteine level testing is warranted
  - If MMA levels and homocysteine levels are high, vitamin B_{12} deficiency is confirmed.
  - If MMA levels are normal but homocysteine levels are high, folate deficiency is confirmed.
  - If both are normal, vitamin B_{12} deficiency is unlikely.

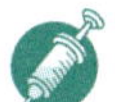

TREATMENT

All individuals with documented vitamin B_{12} deficiency should be treated, unless there's a strong reason not to such as patient refusal or palliative care setting.

GENERAL MEASURES
- Repleting deficiency can be done over weeks, must be done urgently in symptomatic patients, unless there is a strong reason not to do so (e.g., palliative care setting or patient refusal).
- If asymptomatic, repletion can be instituted over a period of weeks
- Urgent replacement with:
  - Symptomatic anemia or neurologic or neuropsychiatric findings, due to risk of adverse events and irreversibility of neurologic deficits
  - Pregnancy, as the developing fetus may be affected
  - Neonates and infants, whose development may be impacted

MEDICATION
- Parenteral cyanocobalamin replacement recommended in patients with severe neurologic symptoms or severe anemia: IM cyanocobalamin
  - 1,000 μg injected every other day for 1 to 2 weeks, then
  - 1,000 μg every week for 1 month, then
  - 1,000 μg once a month for life
- Can also use high-dose, daily oral cyanocobalamin at doses of 1,000 to 2,000 μg

ALERT
Folic acid without vitamin B_{12} in patients with PA is contraindicated; it will not correct neurologic abnormalities.

ONGOING CARE

FOLLOW-UP RECOMMENDATIONS

Patient Monitoring
- Hematologic
  - Reticulocytosis in 1 week
  - Hemoglobin will usually return to normal in 6 to 8 weeks.
  - Monitor potassium in profoundly anemic patients.
- Neurologic: improvement within 6 weeks to 3 months of treatment; however, maximum improvement noticed at 6 to 12 months; some symptoms may be irreversible.

DIET
Meat, animal protein, foods fortified with vitamin B_{12} unless contraindicated

PROGNOSIS
- Deficiency typically resolves by 4 to 8 weeks.
- It takes longer to resolve and might not completely resolve in severe or longstanding illness. If expected response is not achieved, then additional testing should be indicated.

COMPLICATIONS
- Vision problems
- Memory loss
- Pins and needles (paraesthesia)
- Loss of physical coordination (ataxia)
- Peripheral neuropathy, particularly in the legs

REFERENCES

1. Layden AJ, Täse K, Finkelstein JL. Neglected tropical diseases and vitamin B_{12}: a review of the current evidence. *Trans R Soc Trop Med Hyg*. 2018;112(10):423–435.
2. Vincenti A, Bertuzzo L, Limitone A, et al. Perspective: practical approach to preventing subclinical B_{12} deficiency in elderly population. *Nutrients*. 2021;13(6):1913.
3. Devi A, Rush E, Harper M, et al. Vitamin B_{12} status of various ethnic groups living in New Zealand: an analysis of the Adult Nutrition Survey 2008/2009. *Nutrients*. 2018;10(2):181.

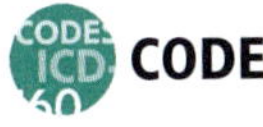

CODES

ICD10
- D51 Vitamin B_{12} deficiency anemia
- D51.3 Other dietary vitamin B_{12} deficiency anemia
- D51.8 Other vitamin B_{12} deficiency anemias

CLINICAL PEARLS
- Vitamin B_{12} deficiency can coexist with other anemia; thus, MCV can be normal, decreased, or increased.
- Common presenting symptoms include fatigue, depression, falls, glossitis/loss of taste, stocking/glove neuropathy.
- For PA, cyanocobalamin must be lifelong.

VITAMIN D DEFICIENCY

Ramanpreet Grewal, MD

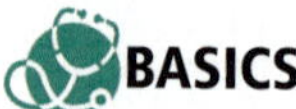

BASICS

This topic covers the commonly acquired vitamin D deficiency and not type II vitamin D–resistant rickets/type I pseudovitamin D–resistant rickets (both rare autosomal recessive disorders).

DESCRIPTION

- Vitamin D is a hormone and a vitamin.
- D_3 is synthesized in the skin by exposure to ultraviolet B (UV-B) radiation; D_2 and D_3 are present in foods.
- D_2 and D_3 are hydroxylated in the liver to 25 vitamin D (calcidiol), the major circulating form.
- Calcidiol is further hydroxylated in the kidney to the active metabolite 1,25 vitamin D.
- Hypocalcemia stimulates parathyroid hormone (PTH) secretion, which prompts increased conversion of 25 vitamin D to 1,25 vitamin D.
  - 1,25 vitamin D decreases renal calcium and phosphorus excretion, increases intestinal calcium and phosphorus absorption, and increases osteoclast activity. The net result is an increase in serum calcium.

EPIDEMIOLOGY

The overall prevalence rate of vitamin D deficiency has been reported to be around 40%. Rates are the highest rate in blacks (82%), followed by Hispanics (69%). Vitamin D deficiency was more common among individuals who were obese, had no college education, in poor overall health, had hypertension, low high-density lipoprotein (HDL), and did not consume milk regularly.

Pediatric Considerations

NHANES data suggest 70% of children do not have sufficient 25-OH vitamin D serum levels (9% deficient and 61% insufficient); deficiency has been associated with an increase in BP and decrease in HDL cholesterol.

ETIOLOGY AND PATHOPHYSIOLOGY

- Insufficient dietary intake of vitamin D and/or lack of UVB exposure (in sunlight) results in low levels of vitamin D.
  - This limits calcium absorption, causing excess PTH release.
- PTH stimulates osteoclast activity, which helps to normalize calcium and phosphorous but results in osteomalacia.
- Dietary deficiency
  - Inadequate vitamin D intake
- Inadequate sunlight exposure
  - Institutionalized/hospitalized patients
- Chronic illness: liver/kidney disease
- Malabsorptive states (including inflammatory bowel diseases [IBD])

RISK FACTORS

- Inadequate sun exposure; dark skin
- Female; elderly; obesity
- Low socioeconomic status; immigrant populations; rates higher in Blacks and Hispanics.
- Latitudes >38°
- Institutionalized; depression
- Medications, gastric bypass surgery/malabsorption syndromes

GENERAL PREVENTION

- Adequate exposure to sunlight and dietary sources of vitamin D (plants, fish); many foods are fortified with vitamin D_2 and D_3
- The recommended minimum daily requirement is 600 IU/day from age 1 to 70 years and 800 IU/day for those aged >70 years; up to 4,000 IU/day is safe in healthy adults without risk of toxicity
- For ages 51 to 70 years, minimally recommended supplementation is 800 IU/day to prevent nonvertebral fractures.

Pediatric Considerations

- The American Academy of Pediatrics (AAP) recommends all breastfed babies receive 400 IU/day of vitamin D beginning "within the first few days of life."
- 2016 Global Consensus Recommendations suggest all infants, regardless of feeding method, begin vitamin D 400 IU within a few days of birth.
- Midgestational vitamin D deficiency doubled the risk of autism spectrum disorder in European cohort.
- The AAP states percentage of U.S. infants who meet the AAP's guidelines for vitamin D intake has not increased; only 27% of infants overall and <40% of infants in nearly all demographic subgroups met intake recommendations.

Pregnancy Considerations

Insufficient data to recommend routine screening of all pregnancies; only "at risk" should be screened; it is safe to take 1,000 to 2,000 IU/day during pregnancy.

COMMONLY ASSOCIATED CONDITIONS

- Osteomalacia, osteoporosis
- Premenstrual syndrome
- Rickets
- Celiac disease; gastric bypass
- Chronic renal disease
- Bacterial vaginosis in pregnant women
- Hypertension
- Cohort study found that vitamin D deficiency is correlated with increased risk of all-cause mortality.

ALERT
Vitamin D deficiency is associated with risk of myocardial infarction (MI) and all-cause mortality.

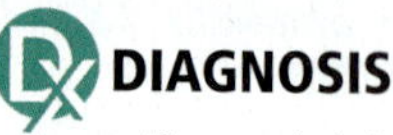

DIAGNOSIS

- Nonspecific musculoskeletal complaints
- Weak antigravity muscles
- Fracture with minimal trauma

HISTORY

- Senior citizens at risk of falling
- Renal disease
- GI (malabsorption) disorders; liver dysfunction
- Immigration from tropical to colder climates
- Dark-skinned/veiled individuals
- Housebound patients
- Women at perimenopause

PHYSICAL EXAM

- Vague neurologic signs: numbness, proximal myopathy, paresthesias, muscle cramps, laryngospasm
- Chvostek sign: contraction of the facial muscles by tapping along the facial nerve
- Trousseau phenomenon: carpal spasms and paresthesia produced by pressure on nerves and vessels of the upper arm, by inflation of a BP cuff
- Tetany, seizures
- Bowed legs

DIFFERENTIAL DIAGNOSIS

- Malabsorptive disease (e.g., IBD, gastric bypass, celiac disease)
- Malnutrition

DIAGNOSTIC TESTS & INTERPRETATION

Initial Tests (lab, imaging)

- Only test patients at increased risk of deficiency (poor dietary intake, limited sun exposure, etc.) or if suspected due to risk factors (malabsorption, symptoms, etc.)
- Measure 25-OH vitamin D (most sensitive measure of vitamin D status).
- Vitamin D deficiency
  - IOM: <20 ng/mL
  - Optimal serum levels: 40 to 80 ng/mL
- PTH elevation: not routinely obtained unless severe deficiency
- Low-normal/low calcium and phosphorous
- Elevated alkaline phosphatase (in later disease)
- Plain radiographs: If atypical fracture, radiographs may show osteomalacia (pseudofractures/looser zones) in pelvis, femur, and fibula.

- Osteoporosis screen
  - Women aged ≥65 years with no risk factors
  - Women aged ≥60 years at risk: body weight <70 kg (best predictor)
  - Less evidence: smoking, low body mass index, family history, decreased activity, alcohol or caffeine use
  - African American women have higher bone density than Caucasians.

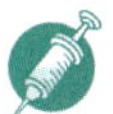

TREATMENT

- Treatment goals remain unclear, but current "normal" 25-OH vitamin D levels are based on suppression of PTH.
- Obesity: Treatment of VDD in obesity, especially those who are obese and depressed, improves depressive symptoms and may improve weight loss.

ALERT
All-cause mortality: A Cochrane Systematic Review found that vitamin D supplementation lowers all-cause mortality. Recent long-term data shows treatment to 25 vitamin D levels >30 ng/ml lowered both MI and all-cause mortality risk.

Geriatric Considerations

In senior citizens, serum 25-OH vitamin D of 20 ng/mL resulted in improved physical performance scores; recent data suggest supplementation may not improve fracture risk and remains unclear about a true benefit.

MEDICATION

- Vitamin D sufficient (25-OH vitamin D ≥20 ng/mL)
  - Vitamin D 800 to 2,000 (50 mcg) IU/day D_3
  - D_3 (animal derived) may be slightly more effective than D_2 (plant derived).
  - Calcium supplementation: unclear benefit and may increase some CHD risk in patients; no supplementation currently required (see below)
- Vitamin D deficiency (25-OH vitamin D <20 ng/mL)
  - D_3 50,000 IU/week for 8 weeks, followed by 1,000 to 2,000 IU/day of vitamin D_3
- Calcium: meta-analysis data support dietary intake of calcium rather than calcium supplementation
  - Dietary intake of ~700 mg/day leads to best outcomes; higher doses did NOT decrease the risk of osteoporotic fractures.
  - Dietary calcium may be more beneficial than calcium supplementation. Supplementary calcium associated with an increased risk of MI, especially in women, but this data remain controversial.
  - Supplementation of both vitamin D and calcium may increase risk of renal stone formation.

ISSUES FOR REFERRAL

Endocrinology if no response to treatment

ADDITIONAL THERAPIES

Aggressive calcium in ICU patients with ionized calcium <3.2 mg/dL or if symptomatic (tetany, seizures, QT prolongation, bradycardia, or hypotension or ventilated patient with decreased diaphragmatic function)

ADMISSION, INPATIENT, AND NURSING CONSIDERATIONS

- Symptoms of severe hypocalcemia
- Malabsorption syndromes

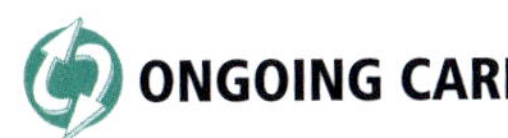

ONGOING CARE

FOLLOW-UP RECOMMENDATIONS

Follow-up of abnormal 25-OH vitamin D not required

DIET

- Cod liver oil is the most potent source of vitamin D and has ~1,300 IU vitamin D/tablet/tablespoon.
- Fatty fish (tuna, salmon)
- Fortified milk (100 IU/8 oz), cereal, and foods

PROGNOSIS

- Cancer:
  - Systematic review of 63 observational studies found adequate 25-OH vitamin D levels correlate with lower rates of colon, breast, and prostate cancer.
  - Observational data show inverse relationship between serum 25-OH vitamin D levels and breast cancer.
  - Serum level >30 ng/ml lowered risk of bladder cancer
  - Vitamin D supplementation lowers cancer mortality and all-cause mortality.
- Cardiovascular disease: A serum 25 vitamin D level >30 ng/ml may lower MI risk and CV mortality.
- Asthma:
  - A Cochrane Systematic Review found that vitamin D supplement reduced the risk of severe asthma attacks requiring hospital admission or emergency department from 6% to ~3% and vitamin D supplementation reduced the rate of asthma attacks needing treatment with steroids.
- Upper respiratory infections: Vitamin D supplementation lower risk of URI.
- Fractures: Vitamin D_3 supplementation in general population of midlife and older adults did not result in a significantly lower risk of fractures versus placebo who were not selected for vitamin D deficiency, low bone mass, or osteoporosis
- Other outcomes: Adequate vitamin D levels may lower pain scores in osteoarthritis of the knee, decrease PMS symptoms, lower risk of metabolic syndrome in women, lower dementia risk, and improve depression symptoms.

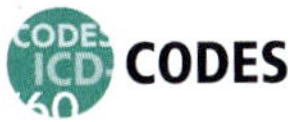

CODES

ICD10

- E55 Vitamin D deficiency
- E55.0 Rickets, active
- E55.9 Vitamin D deficiency, unspecified

CLINICAL PEARLS

- Common risk factors for vitamin D deficiency include inadequate sun exposure or dietary intake, obesity, Black or Hispanic ethnicity, and obesity.
- 25-OH vitamin D (most sensitive measure of vitamin D status) is the most sensitive laboratory test for diagnosis.
- Vitamin D deficiency is defined by serum levels <20 ng/mL.
- Up to 2,000 IU/day of supplemental vitamin D is safe in healthy adults without risk of toxicity.
- The AAP recommends all breastfed babies receive 400 IU/day of vitamin D beginning within a few days of birth.

VITAMIN DEFICIENCY

Christine Ramos Camacho, MD, MS

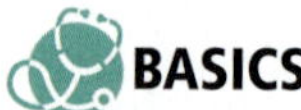

BASICS

DESCRIPTION

- Vitamins are essential micronutrients required for normal metabolism, growth, and development.
- Vitamin supplementation in food products, adequate food security, and availability of supplements make vitamin deficiencies less common in developed countries. Certain populations are at increased risk.
- Toxicity is rare for water-soluble vitamins. It is possible for fat-soluble vitamins (A, D, E, K).

EPIDEMIOLOGY

Incidence

- Higher incidence seen in geriatric patients, pregnant women, exclusively breastfed infants, individuals with highly restricted diets or certain chronic disease states.
- True incidence is unknown because most vitamin deficiencies are asymptomatic.

Prevalence

- Varies by age groups, comorbid conditions, geography, and setting (i.e., urban, rural)
- The prevalence of vitamin B_{12} deficiency is ~6% in patients <60 years old and increases to ~20% after age of 60 years (1).
- Vitamin D deficiency prevalence is increased in individuals with darker skin pigmentation, obesity, low dietary intake of vitamin D, or low sunlight exposure. This deficiency is seen in ~5% of the general population, with non-Hispanic Blacks having the highest prevalence.

ETIOLOGY AND PATHOPHYSIOLOGY

- Deficiency usually develops from one of five mechanisms: reduced intake, diminished absorption, increased use, increased demand, or increased excretion
- Chronic disease states: HIV, malabsorption (i.e., celiac sprue, short bowel syndrome), chronic liver and kidney disease, alcoholism, malignancies, pernicious anemia, inborn errors of metabolism
- Bariatric surgeries: gastric bypass, gastrectomy, small or large bowel resection
- Certain drugs predispose to vitamin deficiencies: prednisone, phenytoin, isoniazid, protease inhibitors, methotrexate, phenobarbital, alcohol, nitrous oxide, H_2 receptor antagonists, metformin, colchicine, cholestyramine, 5-fluorouracil, 6-mercaptopurine, azathioprine, chloramphenicol, proton pump inhibitors, chronically used antibiotics, penicillamine, hydralazine
- Malnutrition, imbalanced nutrition, obesity, fad diets, extreme vegetarianism, total parenteral nutrition, bulimia/anorexia, other eating disorders, parasitic infection

Genetics

- Cystic fibrosis
- Hartnup disease, A-β-lipoproteinemia
- Rare genetic predisposition
  - Autoimmune disease (i.e., pernicious anemia)
  - Congenital enzyme deficiencies (i.e., biotinidase or holocarboxylase synthetase deficiency)
  - Transcobalamin II deficiency
  - Ataxia with vitamin E deficiency (AVED)

RISK FACTORS

Poverty, malnutrition, chronic excessive alcohol intake, chronic disease states, advanced age, dietary restrictions, bariatric surgery, certain medications, and exclusively breastfed infants

GENERAL PREVENTION

- Ingesting large and varied amounts of vitamin supplements increases risk of toxicity and drug–drug interactions and is not recommended.
- Antioxidant supplements have not been shown to impact cancer incidence; *increased* mortality risk seen in some studies.
- Avoid restrictive diets.
- USPSTF recommends against low-dose supplementation with vitamin D (<400 IU) and calcium (<1,000 mg) to reduce fracture risk in community-dwelling postmenopausal women.
- USPSTF concludes current evidence is insufficient to assess benefits and harms of daily supplementation with doses >400 IU of vitamin D and >1,000 mg of calcium for primary prevention of fractures in
  - Community-dwelling, postmenopausal women
  - Men and premenopausal women.
  - Note: Above recommendations are not applicable if history of osteoporotic fractures, increased risk for falls or diagnosis of osteoporosis, or vitamin D deficiency.
- USPSTF recommends all women planning or capable of pregnancy take a daily supplement containing 0.4 to 0.8 mg of folic acid (2),(3)[A].
- USPSTF recommends against using β-carotene or vitamin E supplements for the prevention of cardiovascular disease or cancer.
- Adults without regular, effective sun exposure year round should consume 600 to 800 IU/day of vitamin D_3. Elderly confined indoors and other high-risk groups may require higher doses (800 to 1,000 IU/day)
- All infants should receive 400 IU/day of vitamin D soon after birth if exclusively or partially breastfed.

COMMONLY ASSOCIATED CONDITIONS

Anemia, neuropathies, dermatitis, visual disturbances

DIAGNOSIS

HISTORY

- Review dietary intake and supplement use.
- Decreased visual acuity, night blindness
- Poor wound healing, easy bruising
- Skin changes, new rash
- Neuropathy
- Abnormal food cravings (pica)
- Osteomalacia, history of pathologic fracture
- Birth of a child with spina bifida
- Previous GI or bariatric surgery
- Recurrent or persistent vomiting or diarrhea
- Prior or current medical conditions
  - Tuberculosis (TB), HIV infection, hepatitis, cancer
  - Hypermetabolic state: thyrotoxicosis, 2nd- or 3rd-degree burns, extensive or chronic wound, any systemic infection
- Chronic disease requiring steroids, disease-modifying antirheumatic drugs (DMARDs), or immunosuppressants
- Malabsorptive or chronic GI disorder: celiac disease, sprue, Crohn disease, ulcerative colitis, GERD
- Parenteral or enteral nutrition via tube feeding
- Pregnancy
- Amenorrhea or infertility issues
- Medications, supplements
- Food allergies or intolerances, fad or restrictive diet

PHYSICAL EXAM

- Neurologic exam: gait, memory/cognitive impairment, reflexes, sensory or motor impairment, peripheral neuropathy
- Oropharyngeal exam: glossitis, bleeding gums, hyperemic pharynx, stomatitis, cheilitis
- Skin exam: maculosquamous dermatitis, photosensitive pigmented dermatitis, ecchymosis, petechiae
- Visual assessment

DIFFERENTIAL DIAGNOSIS

Multiple conditions mimic signs and symptoms of vitamin deficiencies.

- Diabetes mellitus, thyroid disorders, hyperparathyroidism, heart failure, Alzheimer disease, multiple sclerosis, substance abuse, toxic ingestions, hematologic disorders/malignancies

DIAGNOSTIC TESTS & INTERPRETATION

Initial Tests (lab, imaging)

- No routine screening indicated
- Test if symptomatic, history indicates high risk, or clinical characteristics are present:
  - 25-OH vitamin D
    - Sufficient levels are >20 ng/mL (20 to 50 ng/mL is a level that is safe and sufficient for skeletal health).
    - Vitamin D insufficiency is 12 to 20 ng/mL.
    - Vitamin D deficiency is <12 ng/mL (increased risk of rickets and osteomalacia) (4).
  - Prothrombin time (PT)/partial thromboplastin time (PTT)
  - Vitamin B_{12} and folate levels
  - Serum homocysteine and methylmalonic acid (if high suspicion of vitamin B_{12} deficiency with normal B_{12} level)
  - Retinol serum level, retinol-binding protein
- Cyanocobalamin, thiamine, and vitamin A
- Ancillary tests:
  - BUN, calcium, phosphorus, magnesium
  - Albumin, liver function tests
  - CBC
  - Parathyroid hormone
- Bone densitometry for:
  - Women ≥65 years old without previous fractures or risk factors
  - Women <65 years old whose 10-year fracture risk is equal to a 65-year-old white woman without additional risk factors

- Disease states from vitamin deficiency
  - Vitamin A (retinol): night blindness, complete blindness, xerophthalmia
  - Vitamin B_1 (thiamine)
    - Wernicke encephalopathy: acute syndrome with memory disturbance, truncal ataxia, nystagmus, ophthalmoplegia
    - Korsakoff syndrome: anterograde and retrograde amnesia, confabulation
    - Dry beriberi: symmetric motor and sensory peripheral neuropathy, paresthesias, loss of reflexes
    - Wet beriberi: neuropathy with cardiovascular symptoms of peripheral vasodilation, high-output failure, dyspnea, and tachycardia
    - Infantile beriberi: loud piercing cry, cyanosis, tachycardia, cardiomegaly, dyspnea, vomiting, seizures
  - Vitamin B_2 (riboflavin): glossitis, stomatitis, cheilitis, hyperemia of the pharyngeal mucosal membranes, normocytic-normochromic anemia
  - Vitamin B_3 (niacin): pellagra = photosensitive pigmented dermatitis, dementia, and diarrhea
  - Vitamin B_5 (pantothenic acid): paresthesias and dysesthesias ("burning feet syndrome"), anemia
  - Vitamin B_6 (pyridoxine): dermatitis, cheilosis, atrophic glossitis, stomatitis, neuropathy
  - Vitamin B_9 (folate): megaloblastic anemia, rarely manifest neurologic symptoms
  - Vitamin B_{12} (cobalamin): pernicious anemia, leukopenia, pancytopenia, shuffling broad-based gait, atrophic glossitis, loss of vibration and position sense, cognitive impairment, areflexia, olfactory impairment, peripheral neuropathy, hyperpigmentation, jaundice, vitiligo
  - Vitamin C (ascorbic acid): scurvy = ecchymoses, bleeding gums and petechiae; hyperkeratosis, arthralgias, impaired wound healing
  - Vitamin D (calciferol): rickets, osteomalacia
  - Vitamin E: neuromuscular disorders and hemolysis
  - Vitamin K: easy bruising, mucosal bleeding, melena, hematuria
  - Biotin: changes in mental status, dysesthesias, nausea, maculosquamous dermatitis of the extremities

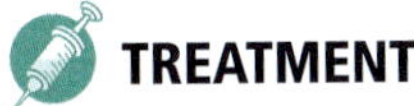

TREATMENT

MEDICATION

- Ask patients about supplement use; encourage patients to bring vitamin and supplement bottles for review.
- Assess for potential adverse drug effects/reactions. Patients with alcohol use disorders should receive thiamine, folic acid, and MVI.
- Give patients with suspected thiamine deficiency 100 mg thiamine prior to IV fluids containing glucose to prevent precipitating Korsakoff psychosis.
- Treat vitamin D deficiency with short-term, high-dose cholecalciferol (4,000 to 10,000 IU/day) is advised, followed by maintenance dose. To maintain serum 25-hydroxy vitamin D levels between 75 to 125 nmol/L (30 to 50 ng/mL), prophylactic supplementation ranges from 800 to 2,000 IU/day in healthy individuals to 3,000 to 5,000 IU/day in high-risk groups. Recommended daily supplementation for children, adolescents, and adults up to aged 70 years is 600 IU/day. Those aged >71 years old is 800 IU/day.
- If there is concomitant B_{12} and folate deficiency, start vitamin B_{12} first to avoid precipitating subacute combined degeneration of the spinal cord.
- Consider obtaining prealbumin/albumin levels and a dietary consult for malnourished patients.
- After bariatric surgery, patients should receive 3,000 IU of D_3 daily to maintain a 25(OH)D level of >30 ng/mL.

Geriatric Considerations

- Vitamin B_{12} deficiency exists in ~20% of patients aged >60 years. Treat symptomatic or severe deficiency with an IM injection of cyanocobalamin 1,000 μg/day 3 times a week for 2 weeks. For neurologic symptoms, give same dose every other day for 3 weeks or until symptom resolution. To prevent recurrence or treat mild deficiency, take daily oral vitamin B_{12} 1,000 μg or monthly IM vitamin B_{12} 1,000 μg every month. High-dose (1,000 to 2,000 μg/day) oral treatment is as effective as monthly IM injections, but use caution with malabsorption or compliance issues.
- Vitamin D deficiency target level of >30 ng/mL minimizes risk of falls and fractures in the elderly.

Pediatric Considerations

- Vitamin K deficiency increases bleeding risk.
  - More common in neonates because they lack intestinal flora that produces vitamin K during the 1st week of life.
  - Condition peaks 2 to 10 days after birth: bleeding from the umbilical stump and/or circumcision site, generalized bruising, and GI hemorrhage.
  - Infrequent in developed countries due to routine injection of newborns with vitamin K (1 mg)
- Vitamin D deficiency increases risk of rickets.
  - Vitamin D supplementation (400 IU/day) is recommended for all infants starting in the first few days of life.
  - 600 IU/day of vitamin D is recommended for children >12 months and adults either through diet or supplementation.
  - Morbidly obese and minority children are at increased risk for vitamin D deficiency.
- In children aged >6 months in developing countries, vitamin A supplementation has been shown to decrease mortality.

Pregnancy Considerations

All pregnant women and women of childbearing age considering pregnancy are strongly encouraged to take a multivitamin containing at least 0.4 mg folic acid daily to prevent neural tube defects (3)[A].

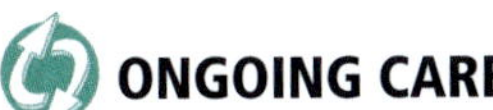

ONGOING CARE

DIET

Vitamins are best used by the body from food intake. Supplements should be used where it is not feasible to ingest the recommended amount of a particular vitamin.

PATIENT EDUCATION

- Drug–drug interactions may occur between vitamins and medications. Patients should report all supplements and medications to their health care provider.
- Risk of vitamin toxicity is most common with fat-soluble vitamins (A, D, E, K).
- Bariatric surgery patients must be monitored for vitamin deficiencies before and after surgery.

PROGNOSIS

Most vitamin deficiencies are fully reversible if treated without undue delay.

COMPLICATIONS

- Vitamin toxicities, liver failure (vitamins A, D, E, K), desquamation of skin (vitamin A), neuropathy (vitamin B_6)
- Kidney stones (vitamin C, vitamin D), hypercoagulability (vitamin K), pseudohyperparathyroidism (vitamin D)
- Masking of pernicious anemia (folic acid)

REFERENCES

1. Obeid R, Andrès E, Češka R, et al; for The Vitamin B Consensus Panelists Group. Diagnosis, treatment and long-term management of vitamin B_{12} deficiency in adults: a delphi expert on consensus. *J Clin Med*. 2024;13(8):2176.
2. Grygorieva N, Tronko M, Kovalenko V, et al. Ukrainian consensus on diagnosis and management of vitamin D deficiency in adults. *Nutrients*. 2024;16(2):270.
3. Bibbins-Domingo K, Grossman DC, Curry SJ, et al; for U.S. Preventive Services Task Force. Folic acid supplementation for the prevention of neural tube defects: US Preventive Services Task Force recommendation statement. *JAMA*. 2017;317(2):183–189.
4. Giustina A, Adler RA, Binkley N, et al. Controversies in vitamin D: summary from an international conference. *J Clin Endocrinol Metab*. 2019;104(2):234–240.

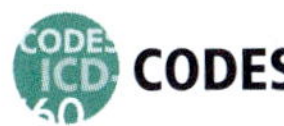

CODES

ICD10

- E56.9 Vitamin deficiency, unspecified
- E56.0 Deficiency of vitamin E
- E55.9 Vitamin D deficiency, unspecified

CLINICAL PEARLS

- In healthy adults, multivitamins have no value if dietary intake is adequate.
- Vitamin D supplementation (400 IU/day) is recommended for all infants.
- No routine screening for vitamin D deficiency is indicated.

V

VITILIGO

Matthew J. Kor, MD

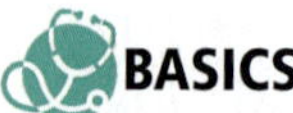

BASICS

DESCRIPTION

- An acquired depigmentation of the epidermis due to a loss of melanocytes. There are two major clinical variants.
- Nonsegmental vitiligo: Represents 80–90% of cases, is often bilateral, symmetrical and enlarges over time (1); subtypes include: the following
  - Acrofacial: on face and distal extremities ("lip-tip" pattern)
  - Generalized: progressive, with flares, commonly associated with autoimmunity; common locations are acral, periorificial, and in sites sensitive to pressure/friction (Koebner phenomenon).
  - Mixed: coexistence of nonsegmental and segmental
  - Mucosal (multifocal): only mucosal surfaces
  - Universal: involves >80% of the body surface area; most likely to have family history; comorbidities are common and associated with poorest quality-of-life (QOL).
- Segmental vitiligo: typically unilateral distribution and earlier onset than nonsegmental (face > trunk > extremities). Lesions may present within a dermatome (i.e., trigeminal), follow Blaschko lines, and involve melanocytes of hair follicles causing leukotrichia. These lesions are less responsive to treatment. Subtypes include:
  - Bisegmental: bilaterally distributed
  - Plurisegmental: multiple segments
  - Unisegmental: single segment
- Undetermined/unclassified:
  - Focal: few lesions, random distribution; may be able to later classify as on one of the forms above after 1 to 2 years
  - Mucosal (focal type): only mucosal surfaces

EPIDEMIOLOGY

- 50% begin before age 20 years; females in 1st decade; males in 5th decade; onset earlier with positive family history
- Predominance: male = female; however, females are more likely to seek treatment.

Prevalence

Approximately 0.5–2% the world; except in Africa and India where prevalence can be almost 10% in certain regions

ETIOLOGY AND PATHOPHYSIOLOGY

Likely a spectrum of disorders with a common phenotype and multiple mechanisms contribute to the pathology.

- Autoimmune: humoral autoantibodies and skin-homing T cells
- Neural: dysregulation of nerve endings leading to decreased melanin production/increased destruction
- Oxidative stress: Exogenous and endogenous stressors increase reactive oxygen species like hydrogen peroxide.

Genetics

- Polygenic/multifactorial inheritance
- 20% of patients report affected relative; however, monozygotic twins have only 23% concordance.

RISK FACTORS

- Family history: vitiligo/autoimmune disorders
- Personal history: associated conditions

COMMONLY ASSOCIATED CONDITIONS

Common comorbidities include (2):

- Autoimmune and connective tissue diseases: systemic sclerosis, alopecia areata, discoid lupus erythematous, Sjögren syndrome, myasthenia gravis, systemic lupus erythematous, rheumatoid arthritis, pernicious anemia
- Endocrine: thyroid disease (hypothyroidism/hyperthyroidism), hypoparathyroidism, Addison disease, insulin-dependent diabetes, metabolic syndrome
- Allergic and dermatologic: psoriasis, atopic dermatitis, lichen planus, chronic urticaria, allergic rhinitis, asthma
- Psychiatric: body dysmorphic disorder, adjustment disorder, impulse control disorder, developmental disorder, suicide and intentional self-inflicted injury, attention deficit hyperactive disorder
- Sensorineural hearing hypoacusis and ophthalmic abnormalities

Pediatric Considerations

Association with Hashimoto thyroiditis; screening at onset and possibly annually may be beneficial.

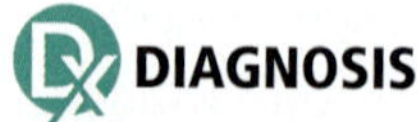

DIAGNOSIS

HISTORY

- Inquire about recent history of sunburns, pregnancy, skin trauma, or emotional stress.
- Discuss family history of premature graying, vitiligo, and autoimmune disorders.
- Complete a review of systems for related associated conditions.
- Ascertain psychological impact on QOL, Dermatology Life Quality Index.

PHYSICAL EXAM

- Complete a full-body skin exam with Wood lamp (depigmentation appears bright blue-white)
- Lesions are rounded well-demarcated, uniform, white macules and nonscaly patches.

DIFFERENTIAL DIAGNOSIS

- Infectious: tinea versicolor, leprosy, leishmaniasis, onchocerciasis, treponematoses
- Postinflammatory hypopigmentation: psoriasis, atopic dermatitis, pityriasis alba, systemic lupus erythematosus, scleroderma
- Inherited hypomelanosis: piebaldism, tuberous sclerosis, Waardenburg syndrome, hypomelanosis of Ito, Vogt-Koyanagi-Harada disease
- Malformations: nevus anemicus, nevus depigmentosus
- Paraneoplastic: hypopigmented mycosis fungoides, melanoma-associated leukoderma
- Occupational/chemical/drug induced leukoderma
- Melasma: Normal skin may be confused as vitiligo in the setting of surrounding hyperpigmentation.
- Halo nevi
- Lichen sclerosus
- Idiopathic guttate hypomelanosis
- Progressive macular hypomelanosis

DIAGNOSTIC TESTS & INTERPRETATION

Initial Tests (lab, imaging)

Obtain thyroid labs and consider other autoimmune labs based on history.

Diagnostic Procedures/Other

- Skin biopsy is rarely needed.
- Consider ophthalmologic and audiologic evaluations.

TREATMENT

- Lesions that respond best are on the face, of recent onset, in darker skin type, and in younger patients.
- Combination therapy is more effective than monotherapy with recurrence and failure of therapy being common.

GENERAL MEASURES

Sunscreen

MEDICATION

- Topical corticosteroids (TCS): Avoid use on face/axilla/groin.
  - Side effects: skin atrophy, telangiectasia, hypertrichosis, acneiform eruptions, and striae; regular steroid holidays for several weeks are recommended.
- Systemic corticosteroids: short term or pulsed; oral or intramuscular
  - Side effects: tachyphylaxis, Cushing syndrome, growth retardation
- Topical calcineurin inhibitors (TCI): slightly inferior to TCS as monotherapy but better side effect profile; significantly more expensive
  - Side effects: black box warning for a theoretical risk of lymphoma or skin cancer; local reactions include burning sensation, pruritus, erythema, and rare transient hyperpigmentation.
  - Pediatric: for children >2 years of age
- Phototherapy: Narrowband ultraviolet B (NBUVB) is superior to ultraviolet A (UVA).
  - Side effects: pruritus and erythema

First Line

- For stabilization of rapidly progressive disease (weeks to months), systemic corticosteroids are recommended with reassessment in 46 weeks.
  - When used in combination with phototherapy, stabilization is expected in <3 months.
  - If systemic corticosteroids are contraindicated, NBUVB is recommended.
    - Conventional immunosuppressants (i.e. methotrexate) have also been used.
- For stable limited disease, TCS of mid (e.g., mometasone furoate 0.1%) to high (e.g., clobetasol propionate 0.05%) potency or TCI are recommended with reassessment in 3 months.
  - TCS: can be used BID for mid potency or daily for high potency safely for 2 to 3 months
  - TCI: Tacrolimus (0.03% in children and 0.1% in adults) or pimecrolimus 1% are preferred at high risk for skin atrophy regions.
- For stable extensive disease, NBUVB is recommended 2 to 3 times a week with reassessment after 15 to 20 sessions.
  - Intermittent TCS or TCI may be added.

Second Line

- Janus kinase (JAK) inhibitors (i.e., ruxolitinib) may be applied BID for nonsegmental vitiligo when affected areas are <10% with plans to reassess in 24 weeks.
  - Use cautiously with known history of atherosclerotic cardiovascular disease, risk of malignancy, and venous thromboembolism.
- Psoralen plus UVA (PUVA) photochemotherapy: Avoid use in children and pregnant women.
  - Side effects: erythema, pruritus, chronic actinic damage, carcinogenesis
- Topical vitamin D_3 analogs: less effective than TCS alone
  - Side effects: burning sensation; avoid exposure to phototherapy due to cutaneous hyperpigmentation.

ISSUES FOR REFERRAL

Referrals depend on severity of symptoms and associated conditions

ADDITIONAL THERAPIES

Prostaglandins and analogues, afamelanotide, cell based therapies, Wnt/β-catenin signaling agonists (3)

SURGERY/OTHER PROCEDURES

- Skin grafting and micropigmentation are common treatments. However, a mini-graft test is recommended to monitor for a Koebner phenomenon at donor site.
- Tattoos or cosmetic camouflage (i.e., 6% dihydroxyacetone cream) provide permanent and temporary therapies, respectively.

COMPLEMENTARY & ALTERNATIVE MEDICINE

Limited evidence in vitamins, alpha-lipoic acid, *Ginkgo biloba*

ONGOING CARE

FOLLOW-UP RECOMMENDATIONS

- Monitor for symptoms of related conditions.
- With topical steroids, follow at regular intervals to avoid steroid atrophy, telangiectasia, and striae distensae.

DIET

No restrictions

PATIENT EDUCATION

- Disease course, progression, and cosmesis
- Trauma/friction and Koebner phenomenon

PROGNOSIS

- Spontaneous repigmentation is uncommon.
- Generalized vitiligo is often progressive with flares. Focal vitiligo often has rapid onset and then stabilizes.

COMPLICATIONS

Psychiatric morbidity associated with stigmatization and low self-esteem

REFERENCES

1. AL-smadi K, Imran M, Leite-Silva VR, et al. Vitiligo: a review of aetiology, pathogenesis, treatment, and psychosocial impact. *Cosmetics*. 2023;10(8):84.
2. Lee JH, Ju HJ, Seo JM, et al. Comorbidities in patients with vitiligo: a systematic review and meta-analysis. *J Invest Dermatol*. 2023;143(5):777–789.e6.
3. Iwanowski T, Kołkowski K, Nowicki RJ, et al. Etiopathogenesis and emerging methods for treatment of vitiligo. *Int J Mol Sci*. 2023;24(11):9749.

ADDITIONAL READING

- Bergqvist C, Ezzedine K. Vitiligo: a review. *Dermatology*. 2020;236(6):571–592. doi:10.1159/000506103.
- Kussainova A, Kassim L, Akhmetova A, et al. Vitiligo and anxiety: a systematic review and meta-analysis. *PLoS One*. 2020;15(11):e0241445.
- Salloum A, Bazzi N, Maalouf D, et al. Microneedling in vitiligo: a systematic review. *Dermatol Ther*. 2020;33(6):e14297. doi:10.1111/dth.14297.

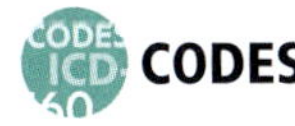

CODES

ICD10

- L80 Vitiligo
- H02.739 Vitiligo of unspecified eye, unspecified eyelid and periocular area
- H02.735 Vitiligo of left lower eyelid and periocular area

CLINICAL PEARLS

- Vitiligo can be a psychologically devastating skin disease.
- Screen for associated diseases, particularly if onset occurs later in life.
- Consult dermatology for extensive disease, facial involvement, and when advanced treatments are considered.

VON WILLEBRAND DISEASE

Ashten Duncan, MD, MPH, CPH • William McCormick Bowen, MD • Nora Elizabeth Kratz, MD

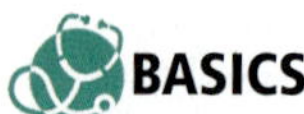

BASICS

DESCRIPTION

- von Willebrand disease (vWD) is a lifelong bleeding disorder resulting from either a quantitative or qualitative (e.g., structural or functional) defect in von Willebrand factor (vWF).
- vWF is a large glycoprotein that plays an essential role in primary hemostasis, which facilitates the adherence of platelets to the injured blood vessel. It also serves as a carrier for factor VIII (FVIII) circulating in the blood.
- The most common clinical consequences mucocutaneous bleeding, bleeding during childbirth, dental procedures, easy bruising, and menorrhagia.
- vWD is most commonly diagnosed as an autosomal-dominant condition but can also be autosomal recessive. In rare cases, this condition can also be acquired (AvWD).
- vWD can be broken down into three different types:
  - Type 1: mildest type—associated with a mild-to-moderate quantitative vWF deficiency
  - Type 2: qualitative defect in vWF (e.g., issues with the protein folding, binding, polypeptide chain structure)
  - Type 3: most severe type—associated with a complete deficiency in vWF

EPIDEMIOLOGY

Prevalence

- vWD is the most common inherited bleeding disorder.
- Prevalence of the inherited forms of vWD is about 109 to 2,200 per 100,000 of the general population with men and women acquiring the disorder at equal frequency.
- Women are diagnosed more often due to the increased bleeding that is seen during menstrual periods, during pregnancy, and after childbirth.
- Exact prevalence of the AvWD is unknown but is estimated to be up to 0.1% of the general population (1).

ETIOLOGY AND PATHOPHYSIOLOGY

- vWF is a large, multimeric glycoprotein that is *released* from endothelial cells and stored within the α-granules of platelets.
- vWF binds to subendothelial collagen at sites of vascular injury and facilitates platelet adhesion to these sites via its interaction with the platelet GP1b receptor. This process forms a platelet plug, allowing for the initial arrest of bleeding (i.e., primary hemostasis). The formation of a fibrin clot follows the creation of a platelet plug, which requires normal amounts of and function of coagulation factors (i.e., secondary hemostasis).
- vWF acts as a carrier for FVIII in the circulation, protecting it from degradation. A deficiency in vWF may result in decreased FVIII levels.
- When vWF is deficient or dysfunctional, primary hemostasis is compromised, resulting in the clinical symptoms described above.
- There are three distinct types of inherited vWD. Within this classification scheme, type 2 vWD has several subtypes, described below. Whereas types 1 and 3 are associated with quantitative deficiencies in vWF (decreased in type 1, absent in type 3), type 2 vWD results from functional defects in the glycoprotein.
  - Type 1, the most common and mildest form, represents 70–80% of cases.
  - Type 2, caused by qualitative defects in vWF, accounts for 10–15% of cases. The various subtypes are described below:
    - Type 2A results from the absence of high- and intermediate-molecular-weight vWF multimers.
    - Type 2B occurs due to a gain-of-function mutation in vWF, which increases its affinity for the platelet GP1b receptor. Complexes of platelets and vWF form as a result and are subsequently removed from circulation. Removal of these aggregates results in loss of the high-molecular-weight vWF multimers as well as thrombocytopenia.
    - Type 2M results from a defect in the platelet-binding domain of vWF; however, in contrast to types 2A and 2B, the entire vWF multimer remains intact.
    - Type 2N results from a mutation in the FVIII binding domain of vWF, resulting in low FVIII levels with an intact multimer.
  - Type 3 represents 1–5% of cases, the least common and most severe form.
    - Most severe form with markedly decreased to undetectable levels of vWF and FVIII
  - Platelet-type vWD (PLT-vWD), also known as pseudo-vWD, results from a hyperaffinity mutation in the platelet GP1b receptor gene, causing increased binding to vWF. Consequently, many platelet-vWF complexes form, which are then cleared from circulation. Similar to vWD type 2B, these patients demonstrate loss of high-molecular-weight vWF multimers in addition to thrombocytopenia.
  - AvWD may be due to cardiovascular, hematologic, or autoimmune conditions as well as tumors and medications. The pathophysiology of AvWD is related to underlying quantitative and/or qualitative changes in vWF and may result from shear-induced cleaving of vWF in cardiovascular conditions, increased adsorption of vWF by certain tumor cells or activated platelets, or presence of anti-vWF autoantibodies in hematologic disorders.

Genetics

- The 178-kb gene for vWF is located on the short arm of chromosome 12.
- Most cases of type 1 vWD follow an autosomal-dominant inheritance pattern, with variable expressivity. Rarer occurrences of type 1 are inherited in an autosomal-recessive manner.
- Types 2A, 2B, and 2M are inherited in an autosomal-dominant manner, whereas 2N is inherited in an autosomal-recessive manner.
- Type 3 follows an autosomal-recessive inheritance pattern.

RISK FACTORS

- Inherited vWD: personal and/or family history of bleeding disorders.
- AvWD: Risk factors include lymphoproliferative disorders, myeloproliferative disorders, autoimmune disorders, states of high vascular flow (e.g., aortic stenosis, presence of LVAD or ventricular septal defect).

COMMONLY ASSOCIATED CONDITIONS

Individuals with type O blood have accelerated clearance of vWF leading to vWF levels that are 25–30% lower than other those with blood type A, B, or AB. Therefore, type 1 disease is diagnosed more frequently in individuals with type O blood.

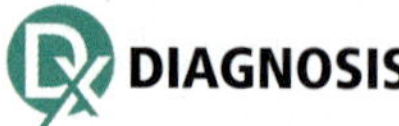

DIAGNOSIS

- For patients with low probability of vWD: Use a validated bleeding assessment tool (BAT) as first-line screening prior to ordering laboratory studies (https://www1.wfh.org/docs/en/Resources/Assessment_Tools_ISTHBAT.pdf).
- For patients with moderate to high probability of vWD (e.g., family history of bleeding disorders, personal history of unusual bleeding diathesis, abnormal initial laboratory tests): In addition to screening with a BAT, also order the following:
  - vWF antigen (vWF:Ag), platelet-dependent vWF activity (e.g., VWF:GPIbM), and FVIII:C lab studies
  - vWF is an acute-phase reactant that increases in response to a variety of stimuli (e.g., bleeding, trauma, pregnancy). vWD diagnostic testing should be performed when patients are at a baseline state of health.

HISTORY

- A positive family history of a bleeding disorder is the most common and suggestive finding.
- vWD should be in the differential diagnosis for heavy menstrual bleeding at any age.

PHYSICAL EXAM

Common locations of bleeding include oral mucosa, gingiva, endometrium, and gastrointestinal mucosa.

DIFFERENTIAL DIAGNOSIS

Congenital thrombocytopenia, qualitative platelet defects, coagulation factor deficiencies, hemophilia, dysfibrinogenemias, fibrinolytic disorders, liver disease, uremia, connective tissue disorders, coagulation factor inhibitors

DIAGNOSTIC TESTS & INTERPRETATION

- Initial evaluation of a suspected bleeding abnormality
  - Complete blood count (CBC)
  - Prothrombin time (PT/INR)
  - Partial thromboplastin time (PTT)
  - Fibrinogen level
  - Peripheral blood smear
- Initial evaluation of suspected inherited vWD
  - vWF:Ag: determines total amount of vWF present
  - vWF activity (vWF:RCo): functional assay tests vWF function by assessing its ability to agglutinate platelets in the presence of the antibiotic ristocetin
  - FVIII: C level
- Note: Multimeric analysis is not recommended in the initial evaluation of vWD.

Follow-Up Tests & Special Considerations

vWF is an acute-phase reactant, so elevations may be seen in proinflammatory conditions, liver disease, pregnancy (which may correct mild deficits), or with estrogen use. vWF levels also increase with age; however, it is unclear if this decreases bleeding risk.

Condition	Description	vWF:RCo (IU/dL)	vWF:Ag (IU/dL)	FVIII	vWF:RCo/ VWF:Ag
Type 1	Partial quantitative vWF deficiency (75% of symptomatic vWD patients)	<30*	<30*	↓ or Normal	>0.5–0.7
Type 2A	↓ vWF-dependent platelet adhesion with selective deficiency of high-molecular-weight multimers	<30*	<30–200*†	↓ or Normal	<0.5–0.7
Type 2B	↑ Affinity for platelet GPIb	<30*	<30–200*†	↓ or Normal	Usually <0.5–0.7
Type 2M	↓ vWF-dependent platelet adhesion without selective deficiency of high-molecular-weight multimers	<30*	<30–200*†	↓ or Normal	<0.5–0.7
Type 2N	Markedly decreased binding affinity for FVIII	30–200	30–200	↓↓	>0.5–0.7
Type 3	Virtually complete deficiency of vWF (Severe, rare)	<3	<3	↓↓↓ (<10 IU/dL)	Not applicable
"Low vWF"**		30–50	30–50	Normal	>0.5–0.7
Normal		50–200	50–200	Normal	>0.5–0.7

↓ refers to a decrease in the test result compared to the laboratory reference range. ↑ refers to an increase in the test result compared to the laboratory reference range.

*<30 IU/dL is designated as the level for a definitive diagnosis of vWD; some patients with type 1 or 2 vWD have levels of vWF:RCo and/or vWF:Ag of 30–50 IU/dL.

†The vWF:Ag in the majority of individuals with type 2A, 2B, or 2M vWD is <50 IU/dL.

**This does not preclude the diagnosis of vWD in patients with vWF:RCo of 30–50 IU/dL if there is supporting clinical and/or family evidence for vWD. This also does not preclude the use of agents to increase vWF levels in those who have vWF:RCo of 30–50 IU/dL and who may be at risk for bleeding.

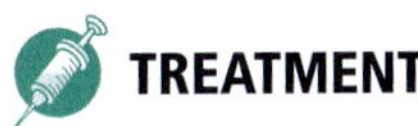

TREATMENT

GENERAL MEASURES

- Minor bleeding episodes generally do not require therapeutic intervention. Individuals receive treatment prior to undergoing surgeries, dental procedures, and following injury.
- In mild disease, trauma-related and spontaneous bleeding events may be managed with desmopressin acetate (DDAVP)
- Chronic menorrhagia can be managed with hormonal contraception (i.e., oral contraceptive pills [OCPs], progestin-containing intrauterine device [IUD]), endometrial ablation (for women no longer desiring future pregnancy), DDAVP, or antifibrinolytic agents.

MEDICATION

First Line

- Desmopressin (i.e., DDAVP)
  - Enhances release of vWF from endothelial cells
  - Effective for type 1 vWD; not indicated in type 2B or type 3
  - Trial of DDAVP should initially be measured in nonbleeding state to determine response.
- Factor-replacement therapy (i.e., vWF and/or FVIII concentrates)
  - Most effective treatment for patients with types 2 and 3 vWD
  - In cases of PT-vWD, administration of exogenous platelets is the treatment of choice
  - Dose of vWF concentrate may be adjusted for FVIII levels and ristocetin cofactor activity.
  - FVIII levels should be monitored to avoid supranormal levels and possible venous thromboembolism (VTE).
  - Contraindicated if patient develops alloantibodies to vWF
  - In patients with severe bleeding phenotype, prophylactic treatment is used.
- Antifibrinolytics (i.e., aminocaproic acid and tranexamic acid)
  - Contraindicated in patients with hematuria due to risk of retention of large blood clots in the renal collecting system
  - Given as adjunct to DDAVP
- Recombinant FVIIa (NovoSeven)
  - Used for patients who develop alloantibodies to vWF
  - Used effectively in the treatment of patients with type 3 vWD

Second Line

- OCPs and progestin-containing IUDs can raise vWF and FVIII levels in the blood and also have a role in the treatment of chronic menorrhagia.
- Platelets may be given as an adjunct to factor concentrates if hemostasis has not been achieved during an active bleeding event.
- Intravenous immunoglobulin has been useful in some patients with AvWD associated with monoclonal gammopathy.

ADMISSION, INPATIENT, AND NURSING CONSIDERATIONS

- If the patient is being admitted to observation for condition(s) with low thrombotic risk, mechanical VTE prophylaxis (i.e., sequential compression devices) or regular ambulation on the unit is preferred.
- If the patient is being admitted for a long hospitalization requiring immobilization and/or for a condition with high thrombotic risk, VTE chemoprophylaxis (e.g., low-molecular-weight heparin) can be considered if the patient has largely preserved qualitative and quantitative vWF levels with close monitoring for bleeding.

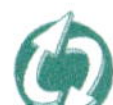

ONGOING CARE

FOLLOW-UP RECOMMENDATIONS

Patients should be seen by a hematologist prior to invasive procedures to reduce risk of excessive bleeding.

Patient Monitoring

- Repeat laboratory studies only for patients with moderate to severe vWD if frequency of their bleeding events changes.
- Aspirin and other NSAIDs should be avoided to prevent bleeding events.

DIET

No dietary restrictions are recommended.

PATIENT EDUCATION

- National Bleeding Disorders Foundation: https://www.hemophilia.org/NHFWeb/MainPgs/MainNHF.aspx?menuid=182&contentid=47&rptname=bleeding
- Centers for Disease Control and Prevention: https://www.cdc.gov/ncbddd/vwd/facts.html

PROGNOSIS

- Most patients with vWD have normal life expectancy. Shortened life expectancy is often a direct result of massive hemorrhage from a major injury (e.g., high-velocity motor vehicle collision, extremity crush injuries).
- In the United States, about 15% of individuals with vWD will experience one or more major bleeding events within a 4-year period. Of these events, almost 90% will be gastrointestinal bleeds with many resulting in hospitalizations.

COMPLICATIONS

Multiple transfusions may result in alloantibodies against vWF.

REFERENCES

1. Du P, Bergamasco A, Moride Y, et al. Von Willebrand disease epidemiology, burden of illness and management: a systematic review. *J Blood Med*. 2023;14:189–208.

SEE ALSO

Algorithms: Bleeding Gums; Ecchymosis

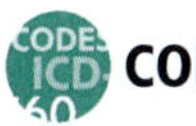

CODES

ICD10

D68.0 Von Willebrand's disease

CLINICAL PEARLS

- vWD is the most common inherited bleeding disorder in American adults
- Treatment should be administered for recurrent bleeding episodes in all types of vWD, but prophylaxis is not required for minor bleeding events.
- First-line therapies for vWD include DDAVP, factor-replacement therapy, antifibrinolytics, and recombinant FVIIa.

VULVAR MALIGNANCY

Jeremy Golding, MD, FAAFP

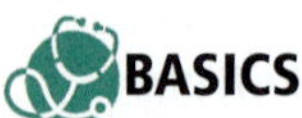

BASICS

DESCRIPTION

- Premalignant lesions of the vulva are collectively known as vulvar intraepithelial neoplasia (VIN).
- Exposure to human papillomavirus (HPV) has been linked to >70% of VIN.
- Invasive squamous cell carcinoma is the most common malignancy involving the vulva (90% of patients).
- Melanoma is the second most common type of vulvar malignancy (8%) and sarcoma is the third.
- Other invasive cell types include basal cell carcinoma, Paget disease, adenocarcinoma arising from Bartholin gland or apocrine sweat glands, adenoid cystic carcinoma, small cell carcinoma, verrucous carcinoma, and sarcomas.
- Sarcomas are usually leiomyosarcoma and probably arise at the insertion of the round ligament in the labium major; however, sarcoma can arise from any structure of the vulva, including blood vessels, skeletal muscle, and fat.
- Rarely, breast carcinoma has been reported in the vulva and is thought to arise from ectopic breast tissue.
- System(s) affected: reproductive

Geriatric Considerations

- The surgery is usually well tolerated.
- Patients who are not surgical candidates can be treated with combination chemotherapy and/or radiation.
- In the elderly, palliative vulvectomy provides relief of symptoms for ulcerating symptomatic advanced disease.

EPIDEMIOLOGY

Incidence

- Yearly incidence of high-grade VIN around 3.26/100,000 women-years and rising (1)
- 6,900 estimated new cases and 1,630 deaths in 2024 (2),(3)
- Mean age at diagnosis is 65 years; in situ disease: mean age is 40 years; invasive malignancy: mean age is 60 years

ETIOLOGY AND PATHOPHYSIOLOGY

- Patients with cervical cancer are more likely to develop vulvar cancer later in life, secondary to "field effect" phenomenon with a carcinogen involving the lower genital tract.
- HPV has been associated with squamous cell abnormalities of the cervix, vagina, and vulva; 55% of vulvar cancers are attributable to oncogenic HPV, predominantly HPV 16 and 33; vaginal intraepithelial neoplasia (VAIN) 2/3 and anal intraepithelial neoplasia (AIN) are attributable to HPV.
- Squamous cell carcinoma
  - There are two etiologic pathways for developing vulvar squamous cell carcinoma: lichen sclerosus and HPV.
  - The International Society for the Study of Vulvovaginal Disease (ISSVD) proposed a revised terminology in 2015: low-grade squamous intraepithelial lesion (LSIL), which includes flat condyloma and HPV effect, high-grade squamous intraepithelial lesion (HSIL), and differentiated VIN (dVIN) type. The ISSVD previously used a three level system grading VIN as 1, 2, 3, which has been abandoned.
  - Differentiated type occurs in older age groups, is associated with lichen sclerosus and chronic venereal diseases, and is not related to HPV. It carries a higher risk of progression to malignancy.
- The warty basaloid type, also known as bowenoid type, is related to HPV infection and occurs in younger women. Melanoma, second most common histology, is often identified in postmenopausal women; often pigmented but can be amelanotic, arising de novo; often found on clitoris or labia minora; prognosis is poor, 5-year survival <50%.
- Smoking is associated with squamous cell disease of the vulva, possibly from direct irritation of the vulva by the transfer of tars and nicotine on the patient's hands or from systemic absorption of carcinogen.

Genetics

No known genetic pattern

RISK FACTORS

- VIN or cervical intraepithelial neoplasia (CIN)
- Smoking
- Lichen sclerosus (vulvar dystrophy)
- HPV infection, condylomata, or sexually transmitted diseases (STD) in the past
- Low economic status
- Autoimmune processes
- Immunodeficiency syndromes or immunosuppression
- Northern European ancestry
- Risk factors for recurrence: age >50 years, positive excision margins, concurrent VAIN

GENERAL PREVENTION

- HPV vaccination has the potential to decrease vulvar cancer by 60%.
- Abstinence from smoking/smoking cessation counseling

COMMONLY ASSOCIATED CONDITIONS

- Patients with invasive vulvar cancer are often elderly and have associated medical conditions.
- High rate of other gynecologic malignancies

DIAGNOSIS

HISTORY

Complaints of pruritus or raised lesion in the vaginal area, vaginal bleeding, discharge

PHYSICAL EXAM

- In situ disease: a small raised area associated with pruritus, single vulvar plaque, ulcer, or mass on labia majora, perineum, clitoris; most commonly found on labia majora
- Vulvar bleeding, dysuria, enlarged lymph nodes less common symptomatology
- Invasive malignancy: an ulcerated, nonhealing area; as lesions become large, bleeding occurs with associated pain and foul-smelling discharge; enlarged inguinal lymph nodes indicative of advanced disease

DIFFERENTIAL DIAGNOSIS

- Infectious processes can present as ulcerative lesions and include syphilis, lymphogranuloma venereum, and granuloma inguinale.
- Disorder of Bartholin gland, seborrheic keratosis, hidradenomas, lichen sclerosus, epidermal inclusion cysts
- Crohn disease can present as an ulcerative area on the vulva.
- Rarely, lesions can metastasize to the vulva.

DIAGNOSTIC TESTS & INTERPRETATION

Initial Tests (lab, imaging)

- Hypercalcemia can occur when metastatic disease is present.
- Squamous cell antigen can be elevated with invasive disease.

Follow-Up Tests & Special Considerations

- Upon examination, any suspicious lesions should be biopsied.
- Diagnosis based on histologic findings following vulvar biopsy
- The vulva can be washed with 3% acetic acid to highlight areas and visualized with a colposcope, allows for visualization of acetowhite lesions and vascular lesions.
- For patients with new onset of pruritus, the area of pruritus should be biopsied.
- Liberal biopsies must be used to diagnose in situ disease prior to invasion and to diagnose early invasive disease.
- The patient should not be treated for presumed benign conditions of the vulva without full exam and biopsy, including Pap smear and colposcopy of cervix, vagina, and vulva.
- When symptoms persist, reexamine and rebiopsy.
- Treatment of benign condyloma of the vulva has not been shown to decrease the eventual incidence of in situ or invasive disease of the vulva.
- CT scan to evaluate pelvic and periaortic lymph node status if tumor >2 cm or if suspicion of metastatic disease

Diagnostic Procedures/Other

Office vulvar biopsy is done to establish the diagnosis.

Test Interpretation

A surgical staging system is used for vulvar cancer (International Federation of Gynecology and Obstetrics classification system).

- Stage I: tumor confined to the vulva
  - Stage IA: lesions ≤2 cm in size, confined to the vulva or perineum and with stromal invasion ≤1 mm, no node metastasis
  - Stage IB: lesions >2 cm in size or with stromal invasion >1 mm, confined to the vulva or perineum, with negative nodes
- Stage II: tumor of any size with extension to adjacent perineal structures (lower 1/3 urethra, lower 1/3 vagina, anus) with negative nodes
- Stage III: tumor of any size with or without extension to adjacent perineal structures (lower 1/3 urethra, lower 1/3 vagina, anus) with positive inguinofemoral lymph nodes

- Stage IIIA
  - With 1 lymph node metastasis (≥5 mm), or
  - 1 to 2 lymph node metastases (<5 mm)
- Stage IIIB
  - With ≥2 lymph node metastases (≥5 mm), or
  - ≥3 lymph node metastases (<5 mm)
- Stage IIIC: with positive nodes with extracapsular spread
- Stage IV: Tumor invades other regional (upper 2/3 urethra, upper 2/3 vagina) or distant structures.
- Stage IVA: Tumor invades any of the following:
  - Upper urethral and/or vaginal mucosa, bladder mucosa, rectal mucosa, or fixed to pelvic bone
  - Fixed or ulcerated inguinofemoral lymph nodes
- Stage IVB: any distant metastasis, including pelvic lymph nodes

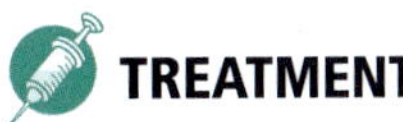

TREATMENT

GENERAL MEASURES

- Surgery in combination with radiation therapy is standard treatment (3).
- Wide excision can be performed for carcinoma in situ, and any suspicious lesion should be excised for definitive diagnosis.
- Cystoscopy and sigmoidoscopy should be performed if there is a question of invasion into the urethra, bladder, or rectum.

MEDICATION

- Neoadjuvant therapy is being investigated with bleomycin-cisplatin and paclitaxel-based regimens showing high-response rates and tolerable side effects.
- As an adjuvant therapy, fluorouracil (Efudex) cream for in situ disease can produce occasional results but is not well tolerated because of irritation of the vulva.
- Chemoradiotherapy with cisplatin and 5-fluorouracil (5-FU) has been successful in advanced or recurrent disease, although local morbidity is increased.
- Contraindications: elderly patients: If chemotherapeutic agents are used, pay close attention to the patient's performance status and ability to tolerate aggressive chemotherapy.

ADDITIONAL THERAPIES

- Preoperative radiation therapy can be used in those with advanced vulvar cancer.
- Adjuvant radiation should be considered with tumor size >4 cm, evidence of lymphovascular invasion, positive surgical margins, or lymph node involvement.
- Preoperative chemoradiation allows for a less radical surgical procedure in patients who are not surgical candidates.
- Postoperative radiation decreases recurrence frequency and may improve survival.
- Radiation is contraindicated with verrucous carcinoma because it induces anaplastic transformation and increases metastases.

SURGERY/OTHER PROCEDURES

- In situ disease can be treated with wide excision or laser vaporization of the affected area. Laser vaporization is preferable in the younger patient, whereas wide excision is preferable in the elderly patient, in whom the risk of invasive disease.
- If tumor extension within <1 cm from structures that will not be removed, preoperative radiation to prevent inadequate surgical margins prior to excision 1-cm tumor-free margin is required because smaller margin would increase risk of recurrence.
- Inguinofemoral lymphadenectomy: removal of superficial inguinal and deep femoral lymph nodes
- Targeted dissection of grossly involved nodes, termed "nodal debulking," is being investigated due to high rates of complication after full inguinofemoral lymphadenectomy.
- Stage IA: radical local excision without lymph node dissection
- Stage IB: radical local excision with either sentinel lymph node biopsy (SLNB) or ipsilateral inguinofemoral lymph node dissection because the risk of metastases is >8%
- Stage II: modified radical vulvectomy and/or chemoradiation and groin node dissection
- Stages III and IV: neoadjuvant chemoradiation and less radical surgery
- Pelvic exenteration after radiation provides effective therapy for advanced or recurrent malignancies involving the bladder or rectum.
- More limited surgery has been undertaken for early invasive lesions, especially in young patients, to preserve the clitoris and sexual function.
- SLNB also has been advocated for early invasive lesion (stage IB or higher). It has shown to accurately diagnose groin metastases in women with early vulval cancer and unknown groin node status. This will limit the surgical morbidity associated with inguinofemoral lymphadenectomy in those with early stage disease.
- Radical vulvectomy with bilateral groin node dissection through separate incisions provides better cosmetic results than en bloc technique.
- Unilateral lymphadenectomy should be considered when lesion <2 cm, lateral lesion >2 cm from vulvar midline, or no palpable groin nodes.

ADMISSION, INPATIENT, AND NURSING CONSIDERATIONS

- Concurrent chemotherapy with radiation is considered standard of care.
- In advanced malignancy involving the urethra and rectum, concomitant cisplatin/5-FU chemotherapy with radiation produces a significant decrease in size of the primary tumor, usually obviating the need for pelvic exenteration.

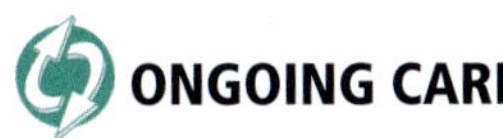

ONGOING CARE

FOLLOW-UP RECOMMENDATIONS

Patient Monitoring

- Early stage, treated with surgery alone: clinical exam of the groin nodes and vulvar area every 6 months for 2 years and then annually
- Following chemoradiation, assessment for further treatment within 6 to 12 weeks of therapy completion
- Advance stage, clinical exam of the groin nodes and vulvar area every 3 months for 2 years, then every 6 months for 3 years, and then annually
- Cervical and/or vaginal cytology annually
- Majority of relapses occur within 1st year.

PATIENT EDUCATION

American College of Obstetricians and Gynecologists: https://www.acog.org/

PROGNOSIS

The 5-year survival is based on stage: stage I: 78.5%; stage II: 58.8%; stage III: 43.2%; stage IV: 13%; inguinal and/or femoral node involvement is the most important determinant of survival.

COMPLICATIONS

- The major complications are wound breakdown, lymphedema, urinary stress incontinence, and psychosexual consequences.
- In the immediate postoperative period, ~50% of patients experience breakdown of the wound. This requires aggressive wound care by visiting nurses as often as twice a day. The wounds usually granulate and heal over a period of 6 to 10 weeks.
- ~15–20% of patients experience some form of mild to moderate lymphedema after the groin node dissection. These patients should be instructed in the use of leg elevation and support hose. <1% of patients experience severe, debilitating lymphedema.

REFERENCES

1. Thuijs NB, van Beurden M, Bruggink AH, et al. Vulvar intraepithelial neoplasia: incidence and long-term risk of vulvar squamous cell carcinoma. *Int J Cancer*. 2021;148(1):90–98.
2. Siegel RL, Giaquinto AN, Jemal A. Cancer statistics, 2024. *CA Cancer J Clin*. 2024;74(1):12–49.
3. Merlo S. Modern treatment of vulvar cancer. *Radiol Oncol*. 2020;54(4):371–376. doi:10.2478/raon-2020-0053.

ADDITIONAL READING

Dockery LE, Soper JT. Vulvar intraepithelial neoplasia: a review of the disease and current management. *Obstet Gynecol Surv*. 2021;76(1):55–62.

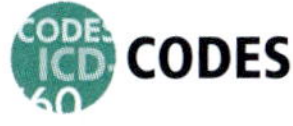

CODES

ICD10

- C51.9 Malignant neoplasm of vulva, unspecified
- D07.1 Carcinoma in situ of vulva
- C51.0 Malignant neoplasm of labium majus

CLINICAL PEARLS

- 55% of vulvar cancers are attributable to oncogenic HPV. VAIN 2/3 and AIN are attributable to HPV. Therefore, HPV vaccination has the potential to decrease vulvar cancer by 1/3.
- Biopsy all suspicious or nonhealing vulvar lesions.

V

VULVODYNIA

Andrea B. Dotson, MD, MSPH, IBCLC, NABBLM-C, FAAFP

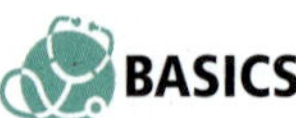

BASICS

DESCRIPTION

- Vulvar pain ≥3 months duration without visible findings, lab abnormalities, or an identifiable neurologic disorder (1),(2)
- Vulvodynia is differentiated from vulvar pain caused by a specific disorder (i.e., infectious, neoplastic, hormonal deficiencies) (2).
- Vulvodynia descriptors include provoked (caused by insertion or contact) versus unprovoked, localized (pain to vaginal vestibule) versus diffuse (generalized pain to entire vulvar area), and primary (pain present at first tampon use/intercourse) versus secondary (2),(3)

EPIDEMIOLOGY

- Can occur at any age, but most women diagnosed between age 20 and 40 years (3).
- Nearly half of women opt not to seek treatment (4).
- Women with and without vulvodynia have similar rates of marital satisfaction, but women with vulvodynia have poorer sexual satisfaction (4).

Incidence

- Annual rate of new onset vulvodynia 1.8%, although newer estimates may be close to 4.2 cases per 100 person-years (5),(6).
- Lifetime incidence approaches 15%, suggesting nearly 14 million U.S. women will experience vulvar discomfort at some point in their lives (5),(6).
- Provoked vulvodynia considered the most common cause of sexual pain in women <30 years old (3).

Prevalence

- Between 8.3% and 16% (4),(5),(6)
- More prevalent in Latina women when compared with White and Black women.

ETIOLOGY AND PATHOPHYSIOLOGY

- Multifactorial with unknown exact cause (4)
- Neuropathically mediation:
  - Neurogenic inflammation sensitizes afferent nerves, and transmits impulses to the CNS, where reinforcing signals sustain pain loop.
  - Vulvar biopsy specimens show increased neuronal proliferation and branching.
- Pelvic floor pathology:
  - Hypertonic pelvic floor at the superficial muscle layer, weaker vaginal muscle contraction, and decreased relaxation after contraction (5)
- Other contributing factors:
  - Recurrent vulvovaginal candidiasis or other infections
  - Immune-mediated chronic neuroinflammatory process within vulvar tissues
  - Chemical exposure (trichloroacetic acid) or physical trauma
  - Reduced estrogen receptor expression/changes in estrogen concentration
  - CNS etiology, similar to other regional pain syndromes
  - Trauma: episiotomy, forceps delivery, abuse, pelvic floor injury

RISK FACTORS

- Recurrent vulvovaginal infections, specifically candidiasis (4)
- Hormonal factors: Pain onset or increased severity may be associated with perimenopause/menopause.
- Pelvic floor dysfunction
- Interstitial cystitis/painful bladder syndrome
- Childhood physical or sexual abuse (5)
- Depression and anxiety (4)
- Other neuropathic and chronic pain disorders, including regional pain syndrome

GENERAL PREVENTION

- Wear 100% cotton underwear in the daytime and no underwear to sleep.
- Avoid douching and other vulvar irritants such as perfumes, dyes, and detergents.
- Avoid abrasive activities and tight, synthetic clothing.
- Avoid panty liners.
- Clean the vulva with water only and pat area dry after bathing.
- Avoid use of hair dryers in the vulvar area.

COMMONLY ASSOCIATED CONDITIONS

Chronic pain syndromes, chronic cystitis, irritable bowel syndrome, fibromyalgia, migraines, depression, anxiety, endometriosis, low back pain, pelvic floor dysfunction (4)

DIAGNOSIS

- Vulvodynia is a clinical diagnosis; there is no definitive test for diagnosis.
- Pain should be characterized using a standard measure such as the McGill Pain Questionnaire.
- Use physical exam to rule out other causes of vulvovaginal pain. Negative fungal culture, along with relevant history and positive cotton swab test, confirms diagnosis.

HISTORY

Adequate sexual, social, and pain history should be taken to assess degree of symptoms. Visual pain scales and pain diaries may be helpful (7)[B]:

- Pain may be described as generalized and unprovoked or feeling as though the vagina is blocked or too small during penetrative intercourse.
- Quality of pain is burning or stinging (4).
- Screen for bowel or bladder dysfunction.
- History of trauma or abuse
- History of infections, including herpes, candidiasis, other STIs
- Assess for precipitants of vulvar pain: tight garments, bicycle riding, tampon use, prolonged sitting, perfumed or deodorant soaps, douching (4).
- Assess for complaints of dyspareunia: vaginismus (involuntary vaginal muscle spasm), adequate lubrication, anorgasmia, partner problems, abuse.

PHYSICAL EXAM

- Ask patient to show where pain is localized or most painful.
- Examine for lesions suggestive of lichen planus or lichen sclerosus.
- Vaginal exam:
  - Vulva may be erythematous, especially at the vestibule; discomfort with separation of the labia minora
  - Spontaneous or elicited pain at the lower 1/2 of anterior vaginal wall suggests bladder etiology.
- Bulbocavernosus and anal wink reflexes to assess for peripheral neuropathy

DIFFERENTIAL DIAGNOSIS

- Infections: candidiasis, herpes, human papillomavirus (HPV), bacterial vaginosis, trichomoniasis, dermatophytes
- Inflammation: lichen planus, immunobullous disorder, allergic vulvitis, lichen sclerosus, atrophic vaginitis
- Neoplasia: Paget disease, vulvar or vaginal intraepithelial neoplasia, squamous cell carcinoma
- Neurologic/muscular: herpes neuralgia, spinal nerve compression, vaginismus

DIAGNOSTIC TESTS & INTERPRETATION

- Tampon test: reproduces pain in real-life settings
- Test for concurrent infections.
- Biopsy skin lesions

Initial Tests (lab, imaging)

- Vaginal pH, wet mount, and yeast culture are recommended to rule out vaginitis.
- Gonorrhea and chlamydia with risk factors present
- No need for advanced testing or other imaging unless symptoms dictate

TREATMENT

GENERAL MEASURES

- Multidisciplinary treatment has the best outcomes.
- Combination of medical treatments, and psychotherapy, physical therapy, and complementary treatments alleviate symptoms more than medication alone.
- Cognitive-behavioral therapy (CBT) superior to supportive therapy (7)[C]

MEDICATION

- Oral therapies
  - Tricyclic antidepressants (TCAs): first-line treatment for unprovoked vulvodynia (7)[B]; fatigue, constipation, sweating, palpitations, and weight gain are most common side effects.
    - Amitriptyline, nortriptyline: Start at 10 mg daily; dose titrated to pain control; average effective dose is 60 mg daily. In one study, a 47% complete response rate was recorded (8)[B].
  - Anticonvulsant therapies:
    - Gabapentin: 300 mg QHS, increase by 300 mg every 3 days. Maximum recommended dose is 3,600 mg daily divided into 3 doses.
    - Topiramate and lamotrigine have been recommended if other therapies are not effective.
  - Selective serotonin reuptake inhibitor (SSRI)/ serotonin norepinephrine reuptake inhibitors (SNRIs): not commonly used; but there is some benefit for generalized vulvodynia (9); consider use in patients who cannot tolerate TCAs.
  - Opioids/NSAIDs: not recommended
- Topical therapies
  - Preferred with provoked vulvodynia (9)
  - Lidocaine 5% ointment: for provoked vestibulodynia
    - Application 15 to 20 minutes before intercourse; penile numbness and possible toxicity with ingestion can occur.
    - Overnight (average of 8 hours) QHS for 6 to 8 weeks; resulted in nonpainful intercourse for 76% of women (5)[C]
  - Cromolyn 4% cream: decreases mast cell degranulation in vulvar tissue; recommended application TID (4)[C]
  - Capsaicin 0.025%: decreases discomfort and increases frequency of intercourse with 20-minute daily application (5)[B]
  - Topical amitriptyline 2% combined with baclofen 2% is helpful in patients with comorbid vaginismus.
  - Topical corticosteroids and testosterone creams have not been shown to alleviate symptoms of vulvodynia.
  - Topical estrogen
- Botulinum toxin A injectable may be helpful.

ISSUES FOR REFERRAL

A team approach is recommended for most effective management. Referral to psychosexual medicine, psychology, partner therapy, and pain management teams should be strongly considered (7)[B].

ADDITIONAL THERAPIES

- CBT: associated with a 30% decrease in vulvar discomfort with sexual intercourse (10)[B]
- Biofeedback/pelvic floor physical therapy: treats both generalized and localized vulvar pain; treatment duration of 12 to 16 weeks is recommended.
- Vaginal dilators

SURGERY/OTHER PROCEDURES

- Vestibulectomy surgery may be considered for patients with localized/provoked symptoms who have failed to respond to other measures; not recommended for generalized vulvodynia (7)[B]
- 60–80% of women who undergo surgery report a significant reduction in pain symptoms; however, when surveyed, patients prefer behavioral therapies than surgical intervention.
- Vestibulectomy is less successful in patients with vaginismus (9).
- Surgical approaches
  - Local excision: precise localization of painful areas; tissue closed in elliptical fashion
  - Total vestibulectomy: Tissue is removed from Skene ducts to perineum. The vagina is then brought down to cover defect.
  - Perineoplasty: vestibulectomy plus removal of perineal tissue; incision usually terminated above the anal orifice; reserved for severe cases (4)[B]

COMPLEMENTARY & ALTERNATIVE MEDICINE

Acupuncture significantly reduces pain for some women (7)[C].

ONGOING CARE

PATIENT EDUCATION

- Reassure patients that vulvodynia is not transmissible and does not predispose to cancer (7)[C].
- Goal of treatment is symptom control, not cure. Remission can be achieved, but can relapse.
- Encourage treatment with home remedies, including ice packs, sitz baths with baking soda, olive oil, and barrier cream to preserve moisture after bathing.

PROGNOSIS

- Traditionally viewed as a chronic pain disorder, but new evidence suggests remission is possible.
- 1 in 10 vulvodynia patients reported remission regardless of treatment.

REFERENCES

1. Bornstein J, Goldstein AT, Stockdale CK, et al; consensus vulvar pain terminology committee of the International Society for the Study of Vulvovaginal Disease (ISSVD); International Society for the Study of Women's Sexual Health (ISSWSH); International Pelvic Pain Society (IPPS). 2015 ISSVD, ISSWSH, and IPPS consensus terminology and classification of persistent vulvar pain and vulvodynia. *J Sex Med*. 2016;13(4):607–612.
2. Goldstein AT, Pukall CF, Brown C, et al. Vulvodynia: assessment and treatment. *J Sex Med*. 2016;13(4):572–590.
3. Sadownik LA. Etiology, diagnosis, and clinical management of vulvodynia. *Int J Womens Health*. 2014;6:437–449.
4. Shah M, Hoffstetter S. Vulvodynia. *Obstet Gynecol Clin North Am*. 2014;41(3):453–464.
5. Boardman LA, Stockdale CK. Sexual pain. *Clin Obstet Gynecol*. 2009;52(4):682–690.
6. Reed BD, Legocki LJ, Plegue MA, et al. Factors associated with vulvodynia incidence. *Obstet Gynecol*. 2014;123(2 Pt 1):225–231.
7. Nunns D, Mandal D, Byrne M, et al; for British Society for the Study of Vulval Disease (BSSVD) Guideline Group. Guidelines for the management of vulvodynia. *Br J Dermatol*. 2010;162(6):1180–1185.
8. Stockdale CK, Lawson HW. 2013 Vulvodynia guideline update. *J Low Genit Tract Dis*. 2014;18(2):93–100.
9. Stenson AL. Vulvodynia: diagnosis and management. *Obstet Gynecol Clin North Am*. 2017;44(3):493–508.
10. De Andres J, Sanchis-Lopez N, Asensio-Samper JM, et al. Vulvodynia—an evidence-based literature review and proposed treatment algorithm. *Pain Pract*. 2016;16(2):204–236.

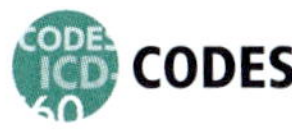

CODES

ICD10

- N94.819 Vulvodynia, unspecified
- N94.818 Other vulvodynia
- N94.810 Vulvar vestibulitis

CLINICAL PEARLS

- Vulvodynia is a clinical diagnosis; it should be suspected in any woman with chronic pain at the introitus and vulva.
- A decrease in pain may take weeks to months and may not be complete.
- No single treatment is proven in all women; improvement over time is common even without treatment.

VULVOVAGINITIS, ESTROGEN DEFICIENT

Mark T. Nadeau, MD • Elliana Kae V. Yap, MD, BS

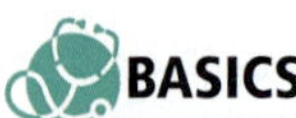

BASICS

DESCRIPTION

- Estrogen-deficient vulvovaginitis is a hypoestrogenic state with external genital, urologic, and sexual sequelae.
- Estrogen deficiency affects all tissues in the female body; however, the genital tissues are especially hormone responsive and are most affected.
- Decreased estrogen leads to decreased blood flow to vaginal tissues and thinning of vaginal tissues, dryness, and atrophy. Patients with estrogen-deficient vulvovaginitis may present with urinary incontinence, vaginal burning and itching, dyspareunia, increased urinary frequency, recurrent UTIs, or various other symptoms.
- This condition is also referred to as genitourinary syndrome of menopause when associated with the postmenopausal state, although this condition may occur in women of all ages.

EPIDEMIOLOGY

Incidence

Predominant age: postmenopausal females. The average age of menopause in the United States is 51.3 years but ranges from 45 to 55 years old.

Prevalence

- Approximately 40–54% of postmenopausal women are affected, and approximately 15% of premenopausal women are also affected.
- This condition is likely underdiagnosed because patients may be reluctant to report symptoms because of embarrassment or the misconception that symptoms should be accepted as a natural part of aging.

ETIOLOGY AND PATHOPHYSIOLOGY

- Estrogen is vasoactive, increasing blood flow to target tissues, lubrication, and elasticity. The duration of estrogen deficiency is a major factor in the development and severity of genitourinary syndrome of menopause.
- Decreased estrogen levels in the vagina and vulva result in decreased blood flow and decreased lubrication and elasticity of vaginal and vulvar tissues as well as thinning of these tissues.
- Decreased cellular maturation results in decreased glycogen stores, which affects the normal vaginal flora and consequently the pH.
- The resulting increased pH impairs the viability of the normal flora, permitting the proliferation of fecal and other flora, resulting in UTIs and vaginal infections.
- Estrogen deficiency may be caused by the following:
  - Menopause (surgical or natural)
  - Premature ovarian failure (chemotherapy, radiation, autoimmune, anorexia, genetic)
  - Postpartum estrogen deficiency in lactating women
  - Medications that alter hormonal concentration, such as gonadotropin-releasing hormone agonists or antagonists, oral contraceptives, selective estrogen receptor modulators (SERMs), and aromatase inhibitors
  - Elevated prolactin from hypothalamic–pituitary disorders with subsequent reduction in estrogen secretion
- Abstinence from sexual activity appears to exacerbate atrophic changes, whereas, regular sexual activity can help to preserve the vaginal epithelium.

Genetics

No known pattern

RISK FACTORS

- Estrogen-deficient states, including lactation and postpartum, natural menopause, oophorectomy
- Immunologic disorders and endocrine disorders
- Premature ovarian failure
- Antiestrogen medications
- Smoking; alcohol abuse
- Sexual abstinence or decreased frequency of coital activity
- No previous vaginal birth
- Chemotherapy, radiation therapy

COMMONLY ASSOCIATED CONDITIONS

- Urge and stress urinary incontinence, pelvic organ prolapse
- Frequent UTIs
- Bacterial or fungal vulvovaginitis
- Vaginal stenosis
- Loss of libido, dyspareunia

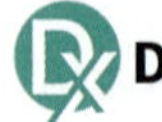

DIAGNOSIS

Clinical diagnosis through thorough history taking.

HISTORY

- All female patients should be asked about symptoms because many women are embarrassed to discuss these issues with their health care providers. Providers should ask about: vaginal dryness, dyspareunia, pruritus, vaginal burning, pressure, tender areas, vaginal discharge (leukorrhea or yellow/malodorous); urinary symptoms: dysuria, hematuria, frequency, infections, stress, and urge urinary incontinence
- Ask about menstrual history and thorough sexual history
- Ask about exposure to radiation therapy and medications.
- Ask about self-treatment and products used.
- Determine exposure to irritants (e.g., soaps, feminine sprays, lotions, lubricants, constant pad use).

PHYSICAL EXAM

Evidence for the diagnosis includes the following:

- Loss of pubic hair, decreased elasticity/friability of vaginal tissues, decreased vulvar and vaginal fullness/adipose tissue
- Prominence of urethral meatus, introital narrowing
- Fusion or resorption of labia minora
- Vulvar erythema or ecchymosis
- Pale-appearing, shiny, smooth vaginal and urethral epithelium
- Vaginal shortening, intolerance to speculum exams
- Loss of vaginal rugation
- Pelvic organ prolapse
- Cervical atrophy and stenosis of os

DIFFERENTIAL DIAGNOSIS

- Malignancy
- Sexual trauma
- Infection secondary to foreign bodies (e.g., piercings)
- Dermatologic conditions of vulva and vagina:
  - Dermatitis
  - Lichen sclerosis: hypopigmented, waxy appearing tissue
  - Lichen planus: painful, red plaques with white lacy edges
  - Lichen simplex chronicus: thick, lichenified, erythematous skin
- Bacterial or fungal vulvovaginitis

DIAGNOSTIC TESTS & INTERPRETATION

Because vulvovaginitis is a clinical diagnosis, labs are not always necessary, but if a dermatologic or oncologic condition is suspected, biopsy is recommended.

Initial Tests (lab, imaging)

Lab tests are generally unnecessary to make the diagnosis. However, the following labs and imaging may be obtained as corroborative of clinical impression:

- Follicle-stimulating hormone (FSH) and estrogen levels. FSH rises and estrogen drops with menopause.
- Evaluate for infections via wet preparation and vaginal pH (usually >5).
- Urinalysis if suspected concomitant UTI
- Cytology for maturation index: Higher proportion of parabasal cells and lower proportion of intermediate and superficial cells indicate decreased maturation index.
- Transvaginal ultrasound: Endometrial stripe <5 mm indicates loss of estrogen stimulation.

Follow-Up Tests & Special Considerations

Drugs that may alter lab results:

- Estrogen therapy will alter the maturation index but may improve symptoms.
- Progestins, SERMs, and gonadotropin-releasing hormone agonists may produce a reversible pseudomenopausal state.

Diagnostic Procedures/Other

- Clinical diagnosis; however, use caution on pelvic exam as high risk of pain and bleeding.
- Two tests may be used to support the diagnosis: vaginal pH and vaginal maturation index (VMI)

Test Interpretation

- A pH of 4.6 or greater indicates VVA, assuming the patient does not have bacterial vaginosis. Premenopausal women without VVA typically have a pH of 4.5 or less
- VMI (1) is the criterion standard for VVA confirmation but is generally not used or needed in clinical practice. This test assesses the relative proportion of parabasal, intermediate, and superficial vaginal epithelial cell types. In premenopausal women, $>15\%$ superficial cells would be considered normal; however, in postmenopausal women with VVA, the typical proportion would be $<5\%$.

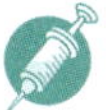

TREATMENT

Nonhormonal and/or hormonal approaches may be tried

GENERAL MEASURES

- Wear loose-fitting, undyed cotton underwear; avoid prolonged pad use, especially scented pads; avoid feminine deodorant sprays and douching.
- Symptomatic relief, if needed (e.g., cool baths or compresses); lactating postpartum women with high levels of prolactin are in a hypoestrogenic state; these women should be instructed to use lubrication for symptoms of dyspareunia and reassured that the symptoms will resolve when they are no longer breastfeeding.
- Increase coital activity
- Smoking cessation

MEDICATION

- Nonhormonal vaginal moisturizers and lubricants are generally regarded as first-line therapy for mildly symptomatic estrogen-deficient vulvovaginitis (2), although one recent study has shown that neither nonhormonal vaginal moisturizers nor lubricants and vaginal estrogen provided greater benefit than placebo gel or tablet. Importantly, nonhormonal vaginal moisturizers will not reverse most atrophic vaginal changes (3),(4).
- Estrogen therapy is preferred for moderate to severe symptoms: Local hormonal therapy (vaginal estrogen) is the first-line hormonal treatment and can reverse atrophic changes and alleviate symptoms.
  - Vaginal cream: Insert via applicator 2 to 4 g daily for 1 to 2 weeks, then 1 to 2 g daily for 1 to 2 weeks and then 1 g 1 to 3 times a week.
  - Vaginal 10-μg tablet: Insert via preloaded applicator each night for 14 days and then twice weekly.
  - Estradiol-containing vaginal ring 2 mg: Insert into vagina and replace every 3 months.
  - Adverse side effects are uncommon, but patients may complain of vaginal irritation, vaginal bleeding or breast tenderness.
  - Systemic hormonal therapy is typically reserved for patients wanting treatment for vasomotor symptoms associated with estrogen deficiency in addition to atrophic vulvovaginitis. Transdermal preparations may be safer from a cardiovascular standpoint than oral preparations. Systemic estrogen therapy should be used in the lowest possible dose for the shortest duration of time. Long-term therapy may be necessary due to the chronic nature of estrogen-deficient vulvovaginitis. Contraindications to systemic estrogens include:
    - Breast or estrogen-dependent cancers, endometrial hyperplasia or cancer
    - Undiagnosed vaginal bleeding
    - Thromboembolic disorders
    - Uncontrolled hypertension; severe dyslipidemia
    - Liver disease
    - History of stroke or coronary heart disease
    - Smoking in ages >35 years
    - Migraines with neurologic symptoms
    - Acute cholecystitis/cholangitis
- Precautions: Any abnormal vaginal bleeding must be evaluated. Monitor for DVT and stroke.

First Line

Local, vaginally administered estrogens such as cream, vaginal tablets, or a low-dose vaginal ring

ISSUES FOR REFERRAL

- Refer to urogynecologist for evaluation if symptomatic due to pelvic organ prolapse and/or refractory stress and urge urinary incontinence.
- Recurrent UTIs should be further evaluated and may require a referral to urogynecology and/or urology.

ADDITIONAL THERAPIES

- Laser therapy with fractional CO_2 has demonstrated promise in initial studies. Benefits thought to be due to modeling of vaginal tissue; however, randomized controlled trials with long-term follow-up are still needed. Not FDA approved.
- Lasofoxifene (Fablyn, Oporia) and oxytocin vaginal gel (Vagitocin) are under development but not yet approved.

SURGERY/OTHER PROCEDURES

Surgical intervention is not typically indicated; however, atrophic vulvovaginitis is commonly seen with pelvic organ prolapse which can have surgical indication depending on severity.

COMPLEMENTARY & ALTERNATIVE MEDICINE

- One study found that Vitamin E and phytoestrogen applied locally as gel improved symptoms.
- Another randomized controlled trial evaluating dietary supplementation of soy showed no improvement.

ADMISSION, INPATIENT, AND NURSING CONSIDERATIONS

Management of this condition occurs primarily in the outpatient setting.

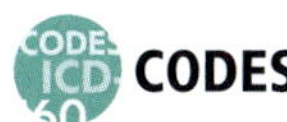

ONGOING CARE

FOLLOW-UP RECOMMENDATIONS

Follow up as needed to determine response to treatment and for adjustment of treatment regimen.

Patient Monitoring

Instruct the patient that symptoms should improve within 30 to 60 days. If they do not, reevaluate and reexamine for other causes.

DIET

Increased consumption of cranberry juice or extract to prevent recurrent UTIs has been recommended but not well supported by evidence.

PATIENT EDUCATION

American College of Obstetricians and Gynecologists (ACOG): https://www.acog.org/womens-health

PROGNOSIS

The prognosis is good. Most symptoms will be alleviated with vaginal estrogen replacement therapy. Of note, one limiting factor to treatment includes that patients regard their symptoms as natural processes of aging and do not seek help. This makes the diagnosis difficult in about 75% of cases due to patient's embarrassment to discuss with specialists.

COMPLICATIONS

- Recurrent UTIs may occur in women with vaginal atrophy.
- Vaginal atrophy predisposes patients to vaginal infections.

REFERENCES

1. Mac Bride MB, Rhodes DJ, Shuster LT. Vulvovaginal atrophy. *Mayo Clin Proc*. 2010;85(1):87–94. doi:10.4065/mcp.2009.0413.
2. Potter N, Panay N. Vaginal lubricants and moisturizers: a review into use, efficacy, and safety. *Climacteric*. 2021;24(1):19–24.
3. National Library of Medicine. Management of symptomatic vulvovaginal atrophy: 2013 position statement of The North American Menopause Society. *Menopause*. 2013;20(9):888–902.
4. Lynch C. Vaginal estrogen therapy for the treatment of atrophic vaginitis. *J Womens Health (Larchmt)*. 2009;18(10):1595–1606.

CODES

ICD10

- N95.2 Postmenopausal atrophic vaginitis
- E28.39 Other primary ovarian failure

CLINICAL PEARLS

- Estrogen-deficient vulvovaginitis affects virtually all postmenopausal women to some degree as well as some premenopausal women.
- This disorder is associated with genital, urologic, and sexual symptoms including vaginal itching, vaginal dryness, urinary incontinence, increased urinary frequency, recurrent UTIs, and dyspareunia.
- Estrogen-deficient vulvovaginitis is a clinical diagnosis; lab tests are generally unnecessary.
- Vaginal moisturizers and lubricants are first-line therapy for mild symptoms, and vaginal estrogen preparations, rather than systemic preparations, are the preferred hormonal therapy for women with moderate to severe symptoms of estrogen-deficient vulvovaginitis.

VULVOVAGINITIS, PREPUBESCENT

Simon B. Griesbach, MD • Laura Horowitz, DO

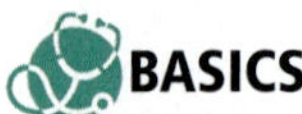

BASICS

DESCRIPTION

- Vulvitis is inflammation of the external genitalia.
- Vaginitis is inflammation involving the vaginal mucosa, and can be characterized with or without odor or bleeding.
- In premenarchal females, vulvitis is usually primary with secondary extension into the vagina.
- Vulvovaginitis can be classified as either nonspecific (not likely infectious, but rather hygienic/behavioral cause) or specific (likely infectious cause).
- Systems affected: reproductive, integumentary
- Clinical features: vaginal/vulvar itching, soreness, dysuria, redness, discharge, bleeding, odor, and pain

EPIDEMIOLOGY

Incidence

Unknown

Prevalence

Most common gynecologic problem in prepubertal females

ETIOLOGY AND PATHOPHYSIOLOGY

- In the prepubertal child, levels of estrogen are low, leading to thin, immature, and fragile vaginal epithelium.
- Anatomically, underdeveloped labia minora, absence of pubic hair, minimal adiposity of the labia majora, and close proximity of the introitus to the anus make contamination more likely (1).
- The prepubertal child also has an alkaline vaginal pH due to a relative deficiency of lactobacilli (which is lactic acid forming) as compared to adolescent and adult females (1).
- Infectious organisms causing vulvovaginitis are typically respiratory, enteric, or rarely sexually transmitted.
- Most cases (~75%) of pediatric vulvovaginitis are classified as nonspecific vulvovaginitis and do not have an infectious etiology.
- Nonspecific vulvovaginitis causes include:
  - Poor perineal hygiene (wiping back to front) (2)
  - Chemical irritants (bubble baths, scented soaps, wipes, laundry detergents)
  - Tight-fitting clothing or underwear made of synthetic materials
- Specific vulvovaginitis causes include:
  - Bacterial:
    - *Streptococcus pyogenes* is typically a respiratory pathogen and can cause vulvitis in the absence of respiratory symptoms.
    - *Escherichia coli* is the most common fecal pathogen.
    - *Shigella* vaginitis is associated with mucopurulent bloody discharge and is not always accompanied by a history of diarrhea.

ALERT

Presence of *Neisseria gonorrheae* or *Chlamydia trachomatis* strongly suggests sexual transmission and should prompt consideration of sexual abuse.

- *Enterobius vermicularis* (pinworms)
  - Most common symptom is nocturnal perineal itching.
  - Should be considered in children with vaginal itching and irritation
  - Very common in young children and certain populations
- Considerations for recurrent/chronic vulvovaginitis:
  - Anatomic abnormalities could include double vagina with fistula, ectopic ureter, and urethral prolapse.
  - Systemic inflammatory diseases
  - Other conditions, such as Crohn disease, lichen sclerosus, vitiligo, psoriasis, and atopic dermatitis are possible.
  - Foreign body
    - Presents with foul-smelling, bloody, or brown discharge from the vagina
    - Should be considered in patients with recurrent vulvovaginitis after other causes are ruled out
    - Most common objects: toilet paper, small toys, hair clips
    - If there is gray watery discharge, consider possibility of battery as foreign body (1).

RISK FACTORS

- Inadequate handwashing or perineal cleansing after urination and defecation (2)
- Wearing of tight-fitting or wet clothing
- Obesity
- Immunosuppression
  - Diabetes
  - Recent antibiotic use
- Anatomic abnormalities

GENERAL PREVENTION

- Good perineal hygiene (including wiping from front to back)
- Urination with legs spread apart and labia separated
- Avoidance of tight-fitting clothing and nonabsorbent underwear
- Avoidance of irritants such as harsh/perfumed soaps and bubble baths

COMMONLY ASSOCIATED CONDITIONS

- Urinary tract infections are common in children with vulvovaginitis.
- Constipation predisposes to vulvovaginitis and vice versa.

DIAGNOSIS

HISTORY

- In taking the history from pediatric patient, develop good rapport with the patient and family as both the history and physical exam are sensitive to discuss.
- Symptoms may include:
  - Vaginal discharge
  - Vaginal or anal itching, burning or discomfort
  - Vulvar redness
  - Dysuria or perineal pain during urination
  - Prepubertal vaginal bleeding
  - Enuresis or encopresis
- Obtain careful history addressing any recent respiratory or enteric infections in the patient or close contacts.
- Ask questions to determine character of any vaginal discharge, if present.
- Determine exposure to irritants that may predispose to vulvovaginitis.
- Question when symptoms most often occur/worsen.
- Inquire about patient's toileting habits:
  - Wiping technique
  - Position of legs while urinating
  - If rushing to the bathroom and inadequate voiding
  - If not voiding/stooling while away at school

PHYSICAL EXAM

- Inform patients and family that exam may be embarrassing and uncomfortable but not painful.
- Explain physical exam thoroughly to the patient and caregivers prior to beginning, giving opportunities to ask questions.
- If exam provokes significant anxiety, consider deferring exam or, for urgent/emergent concerns, performing exam under anesthesia.
- Examine pediatric patients in two positions for best visualization:
  - Supine in frog-leg position: provides view of external anatomy; Valsalva brings distal vagina into view
  - Prone in knee-chest position: Taking deep breath separates vaginal walls and provides view of internal vagina and cervix; foreign body can be seen in this position.
- Look for excoriation, erythema, swelling of the introitus, discharge, foreign body, lichenification of external skin and evaluate degree of estrogenized tissue.
- Perform rectovaginal exam if vaginal bleeding, abdominal pain or in cases concerning for tumor or foreign body.
- Perform culture collection if necessary.

DIFFERENTIAL DIAGNOSIS

- Lichen sclerosus
- Contact dermatitis
- Eczema
- Psoriasis

DIAGNOSTIC TESTS & INTERPRETATION

Diagnosis is often clinical with testing only necessary in patients with history or exam concerning for an infectious cause.

Initial Tests (lab, imaging)

- Definitive diagnosis of bacterial vulvovaginitis requires a culture of vulvar and vaginal secretions.
  - Collect this specimen with a moistened small-diameter collection swab.
- Perform PCR for STI or herpes virus if suspected.
- Potassium hydroxide and saline smears of vaginal discharge, if present, can aid in diagnoses of fungal or certain bacterial causes. They have limited sensitivity and specificity.
- Urinalysis and urine culture can be considered; evaluate for concurrent urinary infection.
- Tape test can be considered to evaluate for pinworm; some treat based on history and exam alone due to low sensitivity of testing.

Diagnostic Procedures/Other

- Exploration of the vagina for a foreign body may be necessary in cases of persistent, recurrent symptoms.
- If an anatomic abnormality is suspected, imaging may be necessary to confirm.
- If available, consider referral to a pediatric or adult gynecologist provider with specific training/experience to determine next steps.

Test Interpretation

Culture often reveals organisms identical to those cultured in asymptomatic individuals.

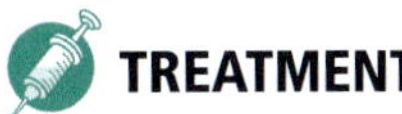

TREATMENT

- Treatment is appropriate in the outpatient health care setting, except where systemic illness requires hospital care.
- No specific infectious cause is identified in 75% of patients. In this case, treating clinicians should recommend general hygiene/behavioral changes as first-line treatment, with recommendations tailored to patient's history.
- A known concomitant respiratory illness or visualized purulent vaginal discharge suggests infection. Obtain a culture and use antibiotic directed against the species with the highest colony count.

GENERAL MEASURES

- Avoid irritants, including scented soaps, wipes, and bubble baths.
- Soak the vulva/perineum in a small amount of clear, warm water for 15 minutes 1 to 4 times per day.
- Recommend the patient avoid wearing underwear to bed or instead wear loose-fitting boxer-shorts bottoms with loose pajamas.

MEDICATION

- Non-antibiotic options
  - To break the itching–scratching–infection cycle, consider clobetasol propionate 0.05% as initial treatment and hydrocortisone cream 1% to follow for short-term maintenance.
  - For estrogen deficiency with labial adhesion/agglutination or urethral prolapse: estrogen cream 0.625 mg to fused area nightly for 2 weeks
  - Emollients or barrier creams (unscented) may offer symptomatic relief.
- Antibiotic options
  - Antibiotic use should be restricted to cases of bacterial infection only and based on culture and sensitivity analysis when available. Most durations will be 5 to 10 days (1).
  - Common bacterial organisms include *S. pyogenes, Streptococcus pneumoniae, Haemophilus influenzae, Staphylococcus aureus, Shigella* spp., and *E. coli*.
    - *C. trachomatis*:
      - ≤45 kg: erythromycin base, 50 mg/kg/day QID for 14 days
      - ≥45 kg and <8 years old: azithromycin, 1 g PO single dose
      - ≥45 kg and ≥8 years old: azithromycin, 1 g PO single dose or doxycycline 100 mg BID for 7 days
    - *N. gonorrhoeae*:
      - ≤45 kg: ceftriaxone, 25 to 50 mg/kg up to 250 mg IM or IV once
      - >45 kg: ceftriaxone, 500 mg IM or IV once
      - Consider treatment for chlamydia if not excluded.
    - *Trichomonas vaginalis*:
      - Metronidazole, 500 mg PO divided TID for 7 days
    - *Candida* spp:
      - Topical nystatin, miconazole, clotrimazole, or terconazole
    - Pinworms:
      - Mebendazole, 100 mg PO once, repeated in 2 weeks

ISSUES FOR REFERRAL

- Suspected sexual abuse
- Suspected anatomic abnormality (except minor labial agglutination)
- Persistent, severe, or recurrent infections
- Inability to tolerate physical exam with serious cause suspected

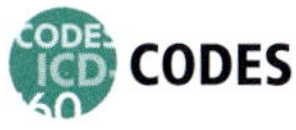

ONGOING CARE

Consider the need for further psychological support for both parent (most often mother) and child:

- Parents play a large role in trial and error process of hygiene changes for their child which adds stress. Normalize this is not something the parent did wrong.
- Often this can feel a "taboo" subject. Offer psychological support if there have been lifestyle changes that have affected socialization of the child (e.g., scared to go to sleep overs without parental support overnight).
- Delays in diagnosis may result in traumatic experiences and cause sequelae such as vaginismus.

FOLLOW-UP RECOMMENDATIONS

Patient Monitoring

Monitor for fever, pruritus, and vaginal discharge.

DIET

- Healthy balanced diet, high in fiber to prevent constipation
- Adequate fluid intake

PATIENT EDUCATION

Hygiene

- Urinate with legs apart, sitting forward to decrease likelihood urine will collect in the vagina.
  - Consider facing "backward" on toilet seat to facilitate this.
- Wipe front to back after elimination and avoid reuse of toilet paper.
- Avoid bubble baths and other irritating products, including all scented products.
- Clean daily with mild soap and water and dry gently with soft towel or cool hair dryer.
- Defer hair shampooing to the end of bath time; consider washing hair while standing up.
- Apply unscented ointments or barrier creams for skin protection.
- Avoid tight clothing, underwear made of synthetic materials, sitting in wet swimsuits, or wearing full body sleeper pajamas.

COMPLICATIONS

- If an STI is identified and not treated effectively, the patient is at risk for pelvic inflammatory disease (PID).
- Untreated vulvovaginitis can cause labial adhesions.
- Vaginismus

REFERENCES

1. Romano ME. Prepubertal vulvovaginitis. *Clin Obstet Gynecol*. 2020;63(3):479–485.
2. Cemek F, Odabaş D, Şenel Ü, et al. Personal hygiene and vulvovaginitis in prepubertal children. *J Pediatr Adolesc Gynecol*. 2016;29(3):223–227.

CODES

ICD10

- N76.0 Acute vaginitis
- N77.1 Vaginitis, vulvitis and vulvovaginitis in dis classd elswhr

CLINICAL PEARLS

- Vulvovaginitis is the most common gynecologic problem in prepubescent females.
- The hypoestrogenic state and prepubescent anatomy may increase susceptibility to vulvar and vaginal infection.
- Treatment is typically supportive (avoid scratching, warm soaks) but may require antibiotics if a bacterial infection is suspected.
- Isolating an infection with known sexual transmission should prompt further investigation.
- Recurrent or persistent vulvovaginitis, especially with foul-smelling discharge, should prompt a skilled exam of the vagina for a retained foreign body (most commonly toilet paper).
- Good perineal hygiene will limit this condition.

WARTS

Karl T. Clebak, MD, MHA, FAAFP • Makayla B. Lagerman, MD

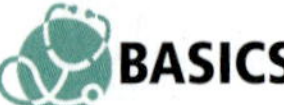

BASICS

- Warts (verrucae) are benign growths that are confined to the epidermis. All warts are caused by the human papillomavirus (HPV). Warts can appear on any area of the skin or mucous membranes. Common warts are predominantly seen in children and young adults.
- Clinically, warts are described as follows:
  - Common warts (verrucae vulgaris)
  - Plantar warts (verrucae plantaris)
  - Flat warts (verrucae plana)
  - Genital warts (condyloma acuminatum)
  - Epidermodysplasia verruciformis is a rare, lifelong hereditary disorder characterized by chronic infection with HPV

DESCRIPTION

Common warts are most often found at sites subject to frequent trauma, such as the hands and feet. Because warts often vary widely in shape, size, and appearance, the various descriptive names for them generally reflect their clinical appearance, location, or both. For example:

- Filiform (fingerlike) warts are threadlike, planar warts are flat, and plantar warts are located on the plantar surfaces (soles) of the feet.
- Genital warts, or condyloma acuminata, may be large and cauliflower-like, or they may consist of small papules.
- Warts on mucous membranes (mucosal papillomas), such as those in the mouth or vagina, tend to be white in color due to moisture retention.

EPIDEMIOLOGY

Incidence

- Predominant age: young adults and children
- No sex predominance: female = male

Prevalence

- ~7–10% of the U.S. population
- ~10% of all school children and young adults experience common warts
- Common warts appear 2 times as frequently in patients who are White compared to Black or Asian.

ETIOLOGY AND PATHOPHYSIOLOGY

- HPV is a nonenveloped, double-stranded circular DNA virus that infects epidermal keratinocytes, stimulating cell proliferation.
- Various strains of DNA HPV: To date, >200 different subtypes have been identified; there are high- and low-risk strains.
- The virus is passed primarily through skin-to-skin contact or from the recently shed virus kept intact in a moist, warm environment.

RISK FACTORS

- HIV/AIDS and other immunosuppressive diseases (e.g., lymphomas)
- Immunosuppressive drugs that decrease cell-mediated immunity (e.g., and chemotherapeutic agents)
- Pregnancy
- Handling raw meat, fish, or other types of animal matter in one's occupation (e.g., butchers)
- Previous wart infection
- Use of communal shower room
- Close contact recreational activities
- Close contact with affected person
- Trauma

GENERAL PREVENTION

- Avoid sharing shoes, socks, towels, tools (nail file, razors), underwear.
- Maintain personal hygiene, keep feet clean and dry, wear breathable footwear and wear footwear in communal shower room.
- Avoid scratching or manipulating warts.
- The HPV vaccine (Gardasil) can help prevent genital warts in both males and females.
- Precaution to avoid contact with HPV particles should be taken during surgical treatment of warts.

COMMONLY ASSOCIATED CONDITIONS

Warts, hypogammaglobulinemia, infections, myelokathexis (WHIM) syndrome; warts, immunodeficiency, lymphedema, dysplasia (WILD) syndrome; hyper-IgE recurrent infection syndrome

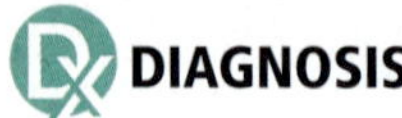

DIAGNOSIS

Most often made on clinical appearance

HISTORY

History of a growing skin lesion; usually asymptomatic; however, warts on soles of feet or around nails may cause discomfort.

PHYSICAL EXAM

- Distribution of warts is generally asymmetric, and lesions are often clustered or may appear in a linear configuration due to scratching (autoinoculation).
- Common wart: rough-surfaced, hyperkeratotic, papillomatous, raised, skin-colored papules, 5 to 10 mm in diameter; several may coalesce into a larger cluster (mosaic wart); most frequently seen on hands, knees, and elbows; usually asymptomatic but may cause cosmetic disfigurement or tenderness
- Filiform warts: These are long, slender, delicate, fingerlike growths, usually seen on the face around the lips, eyelids, or nares.
- Plantar warts often have a rough surface and appear on the plantar surface of the feet in children and young adults.
  - Can be tender and painful; extensive involvement on the sole of the foot may impair ambulation, particularly when present on a weight-bearing surface.
  - Most often seen on the metatarsal area, heels, and toes in an asymmetric distribution (pressure points)
  - Pathognomonic "black dots" (thrombosed dermal capillaries); punctate bleeding becomes more evident after paring with a no. 15 blade.
  - Both common and plantar warts generally demonstrate the following clinical findings:
    - A loss of normal skin markings (dermatoglyphics) such as finger, foot, and hand prints
    - Lesions may be solitary or multiple, or they may appear in clusters (mosaic warts).
- Flat warts: slightly elevated, smooth, numerous, flat-topped, skin-colored or tan papules, small (1 to 3 mm) in diameter
  - Commonly found on the face, arms, dorsa of hands, knees, and shins (women)
  - Sometimes exhibit a linear configuration caused by autoinoculation
  - In men, shaving spreads flat warts.
  - In women, they often occur on the shins where leg shaving spreads lesions.
- Epidermodysplasia verruciformis (rare): Widespread flat, reddish brown pigmented papules and plaques that present in childhood with lifelong persistence on the trunk, hands, upper and lower extremities, and face are characteristics.
- Focal epithelial hyperplasia (rare): multiple painless, 1- to 5-mm whitish painless, soft, sessile papules or plaques on the oral mucosa, gingiva, tongue or lips

DIFFERENTIAL DIAGNOSIS

- Molluscum contagiosum, seborrheic keratosis, epidermal nevus, acrochordon (skin tag), solar keratosis, cutaneous horn, acquired digital fibrokeratoma, squamous cell carcinoma (SCC), keratoacanthoma, lichen planus, lichen nitidus, talon noir (black heel)
- Corns/calluses
  - Corns (clavi) are sometimes difficult to distinguish from plantar warts. Like calluses, corns are thickened areas of the skin and most commonly develop at sites subjected to repeated friction and pressure, such as the tops and the tips of toes and along the sides of the feet.

ALERT

- A melanoma on the plantar surface of the foot can mimic a plantar wart.
- Verrucous carcinoma, a slow-growing, locally invasive, well-differentiated SCC, also may be easily mistaken for a common or plantar wart.

DIAGNOSTIC TESTS & INTERPRETATION

Initial Tests (lab, imaging)

- Warts are typically a clinical diagnosis by visual exam.
- In atypical skin lesions with concern for cancer, biopsy with pathology and HPV genotyping can be performed.
- For genital HPV, 3–5% acetowhite test is recommended.

Test Interpretation

In the granular layer, HPV-infected cells may have coarse keratohyalin granules and vacuoles surrounding wrinkled-appearing nuclei. These koilocytic (vacuolated) cells are pathognomonic for warts.

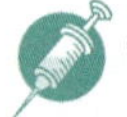

TREATMENT

The abundance of therapeutic modalities described below is reflects that none is uniformly or clearly effective in trials. Placebo treatment response rate is significant, and quality of evidence in general is poor. Whereas first-line treatments with salicylic acid and cryotherapy have low cure rates, other treatments such as CPA formulation, immunotherapy, and intralesional bleomycin have higher cure rates with need for further high-quality research.

GENERAL MEASURES

- There is no ideal treatment.
- Removing warts and addressing any related infections as early as possible may help prevent recurrence.
- In children and immunocompetent adults, most warts regress spontaneously.
- In many adults and immunocompromised patients, warts are often difficult to eradicate.
- Painful, aggressive therapy should be avoided unless there is a need to eliminate the wart(s).
- For surgical procedures, especially in anxious children, pretreat with anesthetic cream such as EMLA (emulsion of lidocaine and prilocaine).

MEDICATION

First Line

- Self-administered topical therapy
  - Keratolytic (peeling) agents: The affected area(s) should be hydrated first by soaking in warm water for 5 minutes before application. Apply daily for 12 weeks. Most over-the-counter agents contain and/or lactic acid: agents such as Duofilm, Occlusal-HP, Trans-Ver-Sal, and Mediplast. Salicylic acid had a mean cure of 13.6%. Avoid use on face due to hyper- and hypopigmentation. Many patients abandon therapy before sufficient time has been given for treatment to work.
- Office based:
  - Cryotherapy is effective and can be used as second-line treatment with mean cure rate of 45.6%.
  - Cantharidin 0.7% is an extract of the blister beetle that causes epidermal necrosis and blistering but may be difficult to obtain as a solution in the United States; it may be compounded in compounding pharmacies.
  - Plantar warts had high rates of clearance with combination cantharidin 1%, salicylic acid 20–30%, and podophyllin resin 5% in flexible collodion even after single treatment. Warts were thoroughly débrided, followed by an application of a thin topical coating, then occluded for several hours, and finally washed off.
  - Generally well-tolerated and effective
  - Potential adverse effects: pain, blistering, scarring, hyper-/hypopigmentation

Second Line

- Home based:
  - 5% (Aldara) cream, a local inducer of interferon, is applied at home by the patient. It is approved for external genital and perianal warts and is used off-label and may be applied to warts under duct tape occlusion. It is applied at bedtime and washed off after 6 to 10 hours; applied to flat warts without occlusion. Use 5 times a week up to 16 weeks.
  - Topical retinoids (e.g., 0.025–0.1% cream or gel) for flat warts
- Office based:
  - Bleomycin, 5-fluorouracil, and cidofovir local injections are suggested for common warts that are refractory or recurrent
  - Immunotherapy: induction of delayed-type hypersensitivity with the following:
    - Diphenylcyclopropenone (DPCP) or diphencyprone (DCP): cure rate 44–88%; mutagenic effects in vitro.
    - Dinitrochlorobenzene (DNCB): cure rate 66–95%; its mutagenicity limits its use.
    - Squaric acid dibutylester (SADBE): Cure rate 58–86%; there is possible mutagenicity; side effects: erythema, edema, itching, burning.
    - Efficacy compared to other treatment modalities requires further research. Contact immunotherapy requires sensitization before rechallenge.
  - Intralesional injections using mumps, *Candida* antigen, interferon, and MTB antigen used occasionally.
  - Oral therapy
    - Oral high-dose: possibly works better in children (40 mg/kg/day; max 1,600 mg) or isotretinoin (oral retinoids)
  - Other treatments (All have all been used with varying results.)
    - Dichloroacetic acid, trichloroacetic acid, podophyllin, formic acid, aminolevulinic acid in combination with blue light, 5-fluorouracil, formaldehyde, levamisole, topical or IV for recalcitrant warts in the setting of HIV, and glutaraldehyde
  - There are isolated case reports of resolution of recalcitrant, chronic oral, and cutaneous warts with the quadrivalent HPV vaccine, although this is off-label and investigational.

ISSUES FOR REFERRAL

Consider referral to dermatology immunocompromised patients who do not respond to initial treatments.

SURGERY/OTHER PROCEDURES

- Cryotherapy with liquid nitrogen (LN_2) may be applied with a cotton swab or with a cryotherapy gun (Cryogun). Aggressive cryotherapy may be more effective than, but it is associated with increased adverse effects (blistering and scarring).
- Light electrocautery with or without curettage
- Photodynamic therapy: Topical 5-aminolevulinic acid is applied to warts followed by photoactivation; better cosmetic outcome for recalcitrant facial flat warts
- CO_2 laser ablation: expensive; clearance rate 50–200%; adverse effects: postprocedure pain, delayed wound healing, scarring, pigment changes
- Pulse-dye laser: expensive; clearance rate 32–92%; adverse effects: mild pain, dyspigmentation, mild scaring; safe for children and adults
- For filiform warts: Dip hemostat into LN_2 for 10 seconds, then gently grasp the wart for 10 seconds and repeat. Wart sheds in 7 to 10 days.

COMPLEMENTARY & ALTERNATIVE MEDICINE

- Duct tape: Cover wart with waterproof tape (e.g., duct tape). Leave the tape on for 6 days and then soak, pare with emery board, and leave uncovered overnight; then reapply tape cyclically for eight cycles; unclear efficacy as single agent.
- Hyperthermia: safe and inexpensive approach; immerse affected area into 45°C water bath for 30 minutes 3 times per week.
- Oral daily zinc therapy at a maximum dose of 600 mg/day increased clearance rates compared to placebo

Pregnancy Considerations

The use of some topical chemical approaches may be contraindicated during pregnancy or in women who are likely to become pregnant during the treatment period.

ONGOING CARE

FOLLOW-UP RECOMMENDATIONS

Patient Monitoring

1/3 of the warts of epidermodysplasia may become malignant.

PATIENT EDUCATION

- The HPV types causing common, plantar, or flat warts are usually different from HPV causing genital warts.
- Vaccine is available to protect against those causing genital warts.

PROGNOSIS

- More often than not (especially in children), warts tend to "cure" themselves over time.
- In many adults and immunocompromised patients, warts often prove difficult to eradicate.

COMPLICATIONS

- Autoinoculation (pseudo-Koebner reaction)
- Scar formation
- Chronic pain after plantar wart removal or scar formation
- Nail deformity after injury to nail matrix

ADDITIONAL READING

Zhu P, Qi RQ, Yang Y, et al. Clinical guideline for the diagnosis and treatment of cutaneous warts (2022). *J Evid Based Med*. 2022;15(3):284–301. doi:10.1111/jebm.12494.

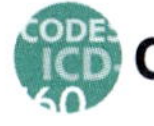

CODES

ICD10

- A63.0 Anogenital (venereal) warts
- B07 Viral warts
- B07.9 Viral wart, unspecified

CLINICAL PEARLS

- No single therapy for warts is uniformly effective or superior; thus, treatment involves a certain amount of trial and error.
- Because most warts in children tend to regress spontaneously within 2 years, benign neglect is often a prudent option.
- Conservative, nonscarring, least painful, least expensive treatments are preferred.

ZOLLINGER-ELLISON SYNDROME

Justin T. Ertle, MD

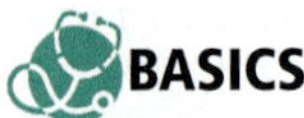

BASICS

DESCRIPTION

- Zollinger-Ellison syndrome (ZES) describes a chronic clinical syndrome of acid peptic disease due to gastric acid hypersecretion caused by a gastrinoma (a neuroendocrine tumor-secreting ectopic gastrin).
- It is often associated with severe and refractory peptic ulcers and gastroesophageal reflux disease (GERD); diarrhea, abdominal discomfort, or other symptoms may be present.
- Gastrinomas, which are typically found in the duodenum or pancreas, are most often sporadic but are associated with multiple endocrine neoplasia type 1 (MEN1) in a significant minority of patients.
- System(s) affected: endocrine/metabolic, gastrointestinal
- Synonym(s): Z-E syndrome; pancreatic ulcerogenic tumor syndrome; multiple endocrine neoplasia, partial; ulcerogenic islet cell tumor

EPIDEMIOLOGY

Incidence

- 2–5 per million people per year (1)
- Age: Mean age of onset is 40 years (2).
- ZES may tend to occur earlier in patients with MEN1.
- Diagnosis is made on average 5 to 6 years after onset (2).
- Sex: slight male predominance, male > female (1.3:1) (2)

Pediatric Considerations

ZES has been diagnosed in patients as young as 1 year old.

ETIOLOGY AND PATHOPHYSIOLOGY

- Gastrinomas (neuroendocrine tumors-secreting ectopic gastrin) prompt the gastric acid hypersecretion that causes ZES. Gastrinomas arise in the duodenum in 70–80% of cases, and the next most common site is the pancreas; other sites do occur rarely (1).
- Gastrinomas are neuroendocrine tumors that secrete ectopic gastrin.
- Hypergastrinemia leads to increased parietal cell mass/gastric mucosal hypertrophy and acid hypersecretion.

Genetics

Gastrinomas are sporadic in 70–80% of cases and are associated with MEN1 in 20–30% of cases (1).

RISK FACTORS

- MEN1
- Family history of ulcer disease

GENERAL PREVENTION

Screen first-degree relatives of patients with MEN1.

COMMONLY ASSOCIATED CONDITIONS

- Gastrinoma
- MEN1 (associated with tumors of the pancreas, pituitary, and parathyroid)
- Peptic ulcer disease (PUD)
- GERD

DIAGNOSIS

HISTORY

- Most common signs/symptoms:
  - Abdominal pain/discomfort (77%) (2)
  - Diarrhea (72%) (2)
  - Peptic ulcer history (67%) (2)
  - GERD (moderate/severe) (44%) (2)
  - GI bleeding (23%) (2)
- Other associated symptoms include:
  - Weight loss
  - Malabsorption
  - Nausea
- In an era when may patients in the general population take proton pump inhibitors (PPIs) and histamine (H_2) blockers, it is important to note that these may mask symptoms of ZES.
- Diagnosis is made on average 5–6 years after the onset of symptoms (2).
- ZES/Gastrinoma should be considered in patients with:
  - Ulcer disease that is recurrent or refractory
  - Ulcers and gastric hypertrophy
  - Duodenal and Jejunal ulcers
  - Ulcers associated with diarrhea, hypercalcemia, kidney stones, pituitary disease, or family history of MEN1

PHYSICAL EXAM

- Physical examination may be normal
- Associated examination findings may include the following:
  - Epigastric tenderness
  - Dental erosions
  - Complications of severe PUD, including hemorrhage, perforation, and obstruction
    - Melenic or Heme positive stool (from bleeding)
    - Conjunctival pallor (if anemic)
  - Hepatomegaly (with liver metastasis)
  - Jaundice (tumor compression of common bile duct)
  - Signs of MEN1 can include cushing syndrome, hypercalcemia, hyperparathyroidism.

DIFFERENTIAL DIAGNOSIS

- PUD or GERD
- Causes of elevated serum gastrin other than ZES:
  - Assay error (1)
  - Elevated serum gastrin with hypochlorhydria/achlorhydria (physiologic) (1)
    - Atrophic gastritis
    - Pernicious anemia
    - Drug induced (associated with PPIs or other antisecretory agents)
    - Gastric cancer
    - Chronic renal failure
    - *Helicobacter pylori* infection (pangastritis)
    - Postvagotomy
  - Elevated serum gastrin with normal or increased gastric acid (inappropriate) (1)
    - Antral G-cell hyperfunction
    - Chronic renal failure
    - *Helicobacter pylori* infection (antral predominant)
    - Gastric outlet obstruction
    - Short bowel syndrome
    - Retained gastric antrum
    - Juvenile polyposis of the stomach

DIAGNOSTIC TESTS & INTERPRETATION

The recommended diagnostic strategy for ZES involves initially confirming inappropriate hypergastrinemia, distinguishing ZES from other causes of inappropriate hypergastrinemia and localizing the tumor. (See "Differential Diagnosis.")

Initial Tests (lab, imaging)

Confirm inappropriate hypergastrinemia:

- Fasting serum gastrin (FSG), in the absence of antisecretory therapy, is the recommended initial test to assess for hypergastrinemia (>1,000 pg/mL) (1)[A].
  - Elevated FSG is sensitive for ZES (sensitivity 97–99%) but is not specific (1). (See "Differential Diagnosis.")
  - No level of hypergastrinemia alone is diagnostic of ZES.
- If hypergastrinemia is confirmed, gastric pH and/or acid output should be assessed to confirm that the hypergastrinemia is inappropriate, to support the diagnosis of ZES (1)[A]. This may require specialist consultation.
  - >99% of patients with ZES have a basal gastric pH ≤2 off antisecretory drugs (1).

ALERT

PPIs and H_2 blockers increase gastric pH and serum gastrin and must be held prior to serum gastrin and gastric pH testing. Holding PPIs at least 7 days and H_2 blockers 2 days prior to testing. However, not all patients may be able to tolerate holding these medications; gastroenterology consultation and alternate means of testing are necessary for some patients.

- FSG increased >10-fold (>1,000 pg/ml, with normal <100 pg/mL) and gastric pH is ≤2, is considered diagnostic for ZES.
- If FSG is increased, but <10-fold, and the gastric pH is ≤2, ZES is possible and additional testing is recommended.
  - For example, FSG >200 pg/mL (off PPI/H_2 blocks), with ulcers, is still suggestive of ZES.

Follow-Up Tests & Special Considerations

- If FSG is increased, but <10-fold, and the gastric pH is ≤2:
  - A secretin test (performed off PPIs) demonstrating an increase in serum gastrin of >120 pg/ml, with the FSH/pH changes above, has a sensitivity of 94% and specificity of 100% for ZES (1).
  - A basal acid output (BAO) of >15 mEq/hr (no previous gastric surgery; >5 mEq/hr after previous gastric acid reducing surgery), with the FSG/pH changes above, establishes the diagnosis of ZES (1).
- Chromogranin A is a marker for neuroendocrine tumors that may be commonly measured during diagnostic evaluation for ZES/gastrinoma; it is not specific for gastrinomas (or neuroendocrine tumors) and is less sensitive than gastrin level testing.
  - Endoscopic US: finds 24–38% of primary tumors in pancreas, much less effective in duodenum
  - Abdominal CT scan: most useful for pancreatic tumors and metastasis >3 cm
  - Abdominal US, MRI, and angiography are not typically useful except in large tumors.

- Newest modality is ^{68}Gallium labeled somatostatin PET/CT scanning which is showing excellent sensitivity and specificity
- Check serum calcium, phosphorus, cortisol, and prolactin to rule out MEN1 (3)

Diagnostic Procedures/Other

If ZES has been definitively diagnosed and tumor localization is the next step, or if ZES is suspected but some of the above tests are difficult to obtain, perform, or interpret, direct visualization and imaging tests are often appropriate.

- CT/PET imaging with gallium-68 or 68Ga-dotatate is imaging test of choice for tumor localization.

Test Interpretation

- Endoscopy may reveal tumors in the duodenal or stomach wall; multiple ulcers, including jejunal ulcers; and prominent gastric and duodenal folds.
- Biopsy shows hyperplasia of antral gastrin-producing cells; histology appears similar to carcinoid.
- 50% of gastrinomas stain positive for adrenocorticotropic hormone (ACTH), vasoactive intestinal polypeptide, insulin, or neurotensin.
- 90% of gastrinomas are found in the gastric triangle (bordered by the bile duct, the junction of second and third portions of the duodenum, and the junction of the head and body of pancreas).
- ~30% of gastrinomas are in the head of the pancreas (more likely >3 cm, metastasis to liver).
- ~70% of gastrinomas are in the wall of the first or second portion of duodenum (more likely small and solitary).
- 2/3 of gastrinomas are malignant.
- 1/3 of patients have metastasis on presentation: regional nodes > liver > bone > peritoneum, spleen, skin, and mediastinum.

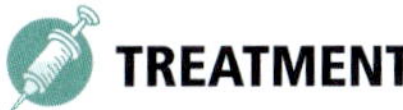

TREATMENT

GENERAL MEASURES

- Goals are to control acid hypersecretion and resect the tumor.
- Advanced imaging initially to evaluate for resection
- Surgical removal when primary tumor can be identified and as adjunct to control symptoms. Surgical resection of primary may enable stopping acid secretion and need for medical treatment.
- Medical treatment for symptom control when primary tumor is not found or metastasis on initial diagnosis.

MEDICATION

- PPIs are the first-line treatment; add H_2 blockers if PPI not tolerated or insufficient.
- Medications heal 80–85% of ulcers, most of which recur. Lifelong medication use should be anticipated.
- 4- to 8-fold higher H_2 dose often necessary; may need up to double dose of PPI
  - Start at a lower dose and titrate to symptoms (or maximum recommended dosage).
- If hyperparathyroidism is present (MEN1), correct hypercalcemia.

First Line

- PPIs
  - Omeprazole 60 to 120 mg/day
  - Lansoprazole 60 to 180 mg/day (doses >120 mg need to be divided BID)
  - Rabeprazole 60 to 100 mg/day up to 60 mg BID
  - Pantoprazole 40 to 240 mg/day PO; 80 to 120 mg q12h IV
- H_2 blockers
  - Cimetidine 300 mg q6h up to 2.4 g/day
  - Ranitidine 150 mg q12h up to 6 g/day
  - Famotidine 20 mg q6h; up to 640 mg/day
- Contraindications
  - Known hypersensitivity to the drug
  - H_2 blockers: antiandrogen effects, drug interactions due to cytochrome P450 inhibition
  - PPIs: none
- Precautions
  - Adjust doses for geriatric patients and patients with renal insufficiency.
  - Gynecomastia has been reported with high-dose cimetidine (>2.4 g/day).
  - PPIs may induce a profound and long-lasting effect on gastric acid secretion, thereby affecting the bioavailability of drugs depending on low gastric pH (e.g., ketoconazole, ampicillin, iron).
- Significant possible interactions: Consider drug–drug interactions and consult prescribing materials accordingly.

Second Line

- Octreotide may slow growth of liver metastases or (occasionally) promote regression. Octreotide LAR can be given every 28 days.
- Chemotherapy regimens using streptozocin, 5-fluorouracil, and doxorubicin shows limited response.
- Interferon shows a limited response but may be useful in combination with octreotide.

ISSUES FOR REFERRAL

Patients with known or suspected ZES should be referred to specialty consultation for coordination of diagnosis and management.

SURGERY/OTHER PROCEDURES

- Laparotomy to search for resectable tumors unless patient has liver metastasis on presentation or MEN1; surgery improves outcomes.
- Definitive therapy: removal of identifiable gastrinomas (95% of tumors are found at the time of surgery; 5-year cure is 40% when all are removed). Second surgeries are worth considering if there is radiologic evidence of new or growing tumors and resection may prolong life span.
- Total gastrectomy is rarely indicated.
- In MEN1, parathyroidectomy, by lowering calcium, may also decrease acid production and decrease antisecretory drug use. Gastrinomas in MEN1 are generally small, benign, and multiple, and surgery is not usually curative in this situation.

ADMISSION, INPATIENT, AND NURSING CONSIDERATIONS

- Titrate medication to symptom control.
- Appropriate surveillance postoperatively to look for metastasis

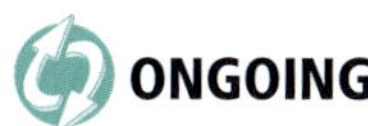

ONGOING CARE

FOLLOW-UP RECOMMENDATIONS

Patient Monitoring

- Longitudinal follow-up to evaluate for tumor recurrence or metastases. Reoperation may be considered.
- Titrate medical therapy to control symptoms.
- Advise patients of potential danger of stopping antisecretory treatment. Rare cases have been reported of severe adverse outcomes within 2 days of stopping PPIs. Gastric acid analysis can help guide medical therapy to maintain basal gastric acid output at <10 mEq/hr (<2 mEq/hr if patient has complications such as perforation or esophagitis).

DIET

Restrict foods that aggravate symptoms.

PATIENT EDUCATION

Inform patients as to the nature of disease and prognosis.

PROGNOSIS

- Overall survival rate: 5 to 10 years: 69–94%
- The prognosis improves with complete surgical removal of the tumor.
- If liver metastasis is present on initial surgery, 5-year survival is 30–40%; 10-year survival is 25%.
- Mortality is directly related to liver metastasis, tumor size, and presence of pancreatic tumors.

COMPLICATIONS

- Complications of peptic ulcer disease (bleeding, perforation, obstruction)
- 2/3 of gastrinomas are malignant with metastasis.
- Paraneoplastic phenomena (e.g., production of ACTH with resulting Cushing syndrome) is possible.
- Decrease in vitamin B_{12} levels is possible with long-term PPI use.

REFERENCES

1. Metz DC, Cadiot G, Poitras P, et al. Diagnosis of Zollinger-Ellison syndrome in the era of PPIs, faulty gastrin assays, sensitive imaging and limited access to acid secretory testing. *Int J Endocr Oncol*. 2017;4(4):167–185.
2. Ito T, Ramos-Alvarez I, Jensen RT. Successful lifetime/long-term medical treatment of acid hypersecretion in Zollinger-Ellison syndrome (ZES): myth or fact? Insights from an analysis of results of NIH long-term prospective studies of ZES. *Cancers (Basel)*. 2023;15(5):1377.
3. Sok C, Ajay PS, Tsagkalidis V, et al. Management of gastric neuroendocrine tumors: a review. *Ann Surg Oncol*. 2024;31(3):1509–1518.

ADDITIONAL READING

Zollinger RM, Ellison EH. Primary peptic ulcerations of the jejunum associated with islet cell tumors of the pancreas. *Ann Surg*. 1955;142(4):709–728.

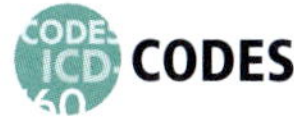

CODES

ICD10

E16.4 Increased secretion of gastrin

CLINICAL PEARLS

- Consider ZES if peptic ulcers recur or if unusually high doses of PPI are needed to control symptoms.
- Abdominal pain and diarrhea should be totally controllable with adequate medical treatment.
- ~25–30% of cases of ZES occur in association with MEN1.
- Once ZES is diagnosed, search for gastrinomas in the head of the pancreas and the first or second portion of the duodenum.
- PPI can mask symptoms and elevate gastrin levels, complicating diagnosis.

INDEX

NOTE: Page numbers preceded by A- indicate Algorithms.

J